Robbins

PATHOLOGIC BASIS *of* DISEASE

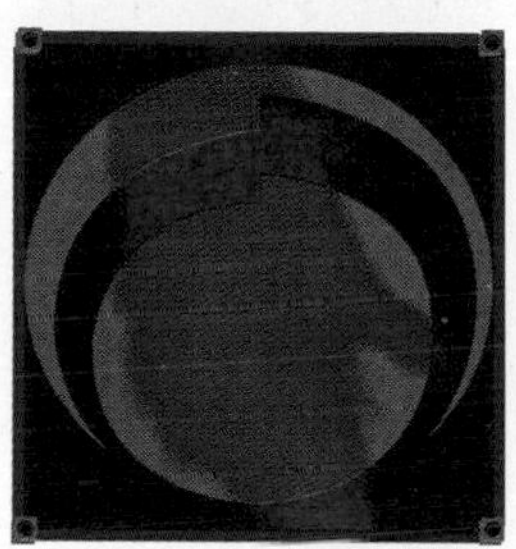

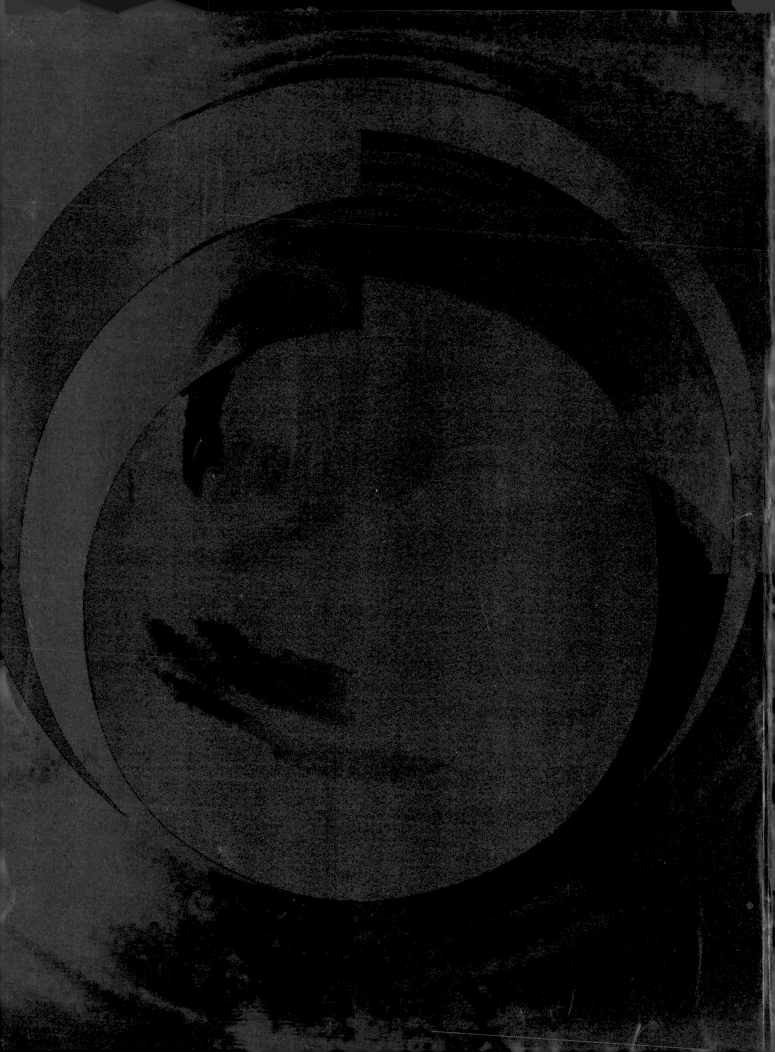

Robbins

PATHOLOGIC BASIS of DISEASE

Sixth Edition

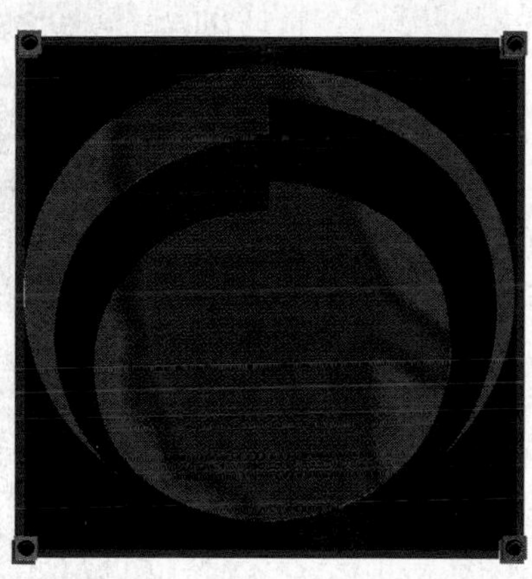

Ramzi S. Cotran, M.D.
Frank Burr Mallory Professor of Pathology
Harvard Medical School
Chairman, Department of Pathology
Brigham and Women's Hospital
The Children's Hospital
Boston, Massachusetts

Vinay Kumar, M.D., F.R.C.Path.
Vernie A. Stembridge Chair in Pathology
Department of Pathology
The University of Texas
Southwestern Medical School
Dallas, Texas

Tucker Collins, M.D., Ph.D.
Professor of Pathology
Harvard Medical School
Pathologist
Brigham and Women's Hospital
Boston, Massachusetts

W.B. Saunders Company
An Imprint of Elsevier Science
Philadelphia London New York St. Louis Sydney Toronto

W.B. SAUNDERS COMPANY
An Imprint of Elsevier Science

The Curtis Center
Independence Square West
Philadelphia, Pennsylvania 19106

Library of Congress Cataloging-in-Publication Data

Cotran, Ramzi S.

Robbins pathologic basis of disease.—6th ed./Ramzi S. Cotran, Vinay Kumar, Tucker Collins.

p. cm.

Includes bibliographical references and index.

ISBN 0-7216-7335-X

1. Pathology. I. Kumar, Vinay. II. Collins, Tucker. III. Robbins, Stanley L. (Stanley Leonard). IV. Title.
[DNLM: 1. Pathology. QZ 4C845r 1999]

RB 111.R62 1999 616.07—dc 21

DNLM/DLC 98-36022

ROBBINS PATHOLOGIC BASIS OF DISEASE ISBN 0-7216-7335-X

Printed in the United States of America.

Last digit is the print number: 9 8

To Kerstin

To Raminder

To Mary

With love.

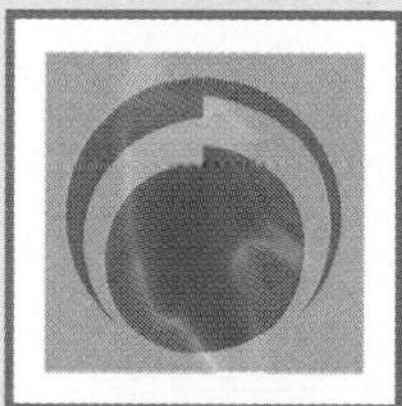

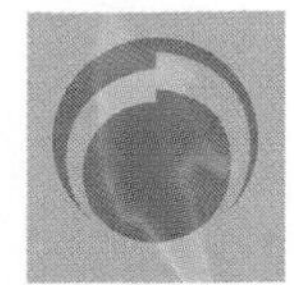

Contributors

Daniel M. Albert, M.D., M.S.
F.A. Davis Professor and Chair, Department of Ophthalmology and Visual Sciences, University of Wisconsin Medical School, Madison, WI
The Eye

Douglas C. Anthony, M.D., Ph.D.
Associate Professor of Pathology, Harvard Medical School; Director of Neuropathology, Children's Hospital, Boston, MA
Peripheral Nerve and Skeletal Muscle; The Central Nervous System

Jon Aster, M.D., Ph.D.
Assistant Professor of Pathology, Harvard Medical School; Pathologist, Brigham and Women's Hospital, Boston, MA
White Cells, Lymph Nodes, Spleen, and Thymus

James M. Crawford, M.D., Ph.D.
Associate Professor of Pathology, Director, Program in Gastrointestinal Pathology, Yale University School of Medicine, New Haven, CT
The Gastrointestinal Tract; The Liver and the Biliary Tract; The Pancreas

Christopher P. Crum, M.D.
Professor of Pathology, Harvard Medical School; Director, Women's and Perinatal Pathology, Brigham and Women's Hospital, Boston, MA
The Female Genital Tract

Umberto De Girolami, M.D.
Associate Professor of Pathology, Harvard Medical School; Director of Neuropathology, Brigham and Women's Hospital; Neuropathologist, Children's Hospital, Boston, MA
Peripheral Nerve and Skeletal Muscle; The Central Nervous System

Thaddeus P. Dryja, M.D.
David Glen Denning Cogan Professor, Department of Ophthalmology, Massachusetts Eye and Ear Infirmary, Harvard Medical School, Boston, MA
The Eye

Matthew P. Frosch, M.D., Ph.D.
Assistant Professor of Pathology, Harvard Medical School; Neuropathologist, Brigham and Women's Hospital, Boston, MA
Peripheral Nerve and Skeletal Muscle; The Central Nervous System

Agnes B. Kane, M.D., Ph.D.
Chair and Professor, Department of Pathology, Brown University School of Medicine, Providence, RI
Environmental and Nutritional Pathology

Lester Kobzik, M.D.
Associate Professor of Pathology, Harvard Medical School; Pathologist, Brigham and Women's Hospital, Boston, MA
The Lung

Susan C. Lester, M.D., Ph.D.
Assistant Professor of Pathology, Harvard Medical School; Pathologist, Brigham and Women's Hospital, Boston, MA
The Breast

Martin C. Mihm, Jr., M.D.
Clinical Professor of Pathology, Harvard Medical School; Senior Dermatopathologist, Massachusetts General Hospital, Boston, MA
The Skin

Richard N. Mitchell, M.D., Ph.D.
Assistant Professor of Pathology, Harvard Medical School; Pathologist, Brigham and Women's Hospital, Boston, MA
Hemodynamic Disorders, Thrombosis, and Shock

George F. Murphy, M.D.
Professor of Pathology, Jefferson Medical College; Director of Cutaneous Pathology and Medical Education, Department of Pathology, Thomas Jefferson University, Philadelphia, PA
The Skin

Andrew Rosenberg, M.D.
Associate Professor of Pathology, Harvard Medical School; Associate Pathologist, Massachusetts General Hospital, Boston, MA
Bones, Joints, and Soft Tissue Tumors

John Samuelson, M.D., Ph.D.
Associate Professor, Department of Immunology and Infectious Diseases, Harvard School of Public Health, Boston, MA
Infectious Diseases

Frederick J. Schoen, M.D., Ph.D.
Professor of Pathology, Harvard Medical School; Director, Cardiac Pathology, and Vice-Chairman, Department of Pathology, Brigham and Women's Hospital, Boston, MA
Blood Vessels; The Heart

Deborah Schofield, M.D., M.B.A.
Associate Professor of Pathology, University of Southern California; Attending Pathologist, Children's Hospital of Los Angeles, Los Angeles, CA
Diseases of Infancy and Childhood

Preface

We present this sixth edition of *Robbins Pathologic Basis of Disease* with considerable excitement, for these are heady times for pathology as a science and medical practice.

The rapid, sometimes frenetic pace of the discovery of genes and molecules has had a profound impact on the core of the science of pathology—the study of the *pathogenesis* of disease. While much still needs to be uncovered to link abnormal genes and the expression of disease, gone are the times when the mechanisms of most diseases were "unknown," or "obscure" or "mysterious." Those of us who toiled with these unknowns found it exhilarating, in completing this revision, to witness this extraordinary change in virtually every field of pathology.

We thus have attempted to weave the new discoveries of mechanisms throughout the text, blending them with the classic morphologic descriptions and clinical manifestations of diseases. It was difficult, but essential, to avoid information overload by making distinctions between new but unproven hypotheses and fundamental discoveries that will stand the test of time. However, while the latter received more attention, unsolved problems have not been eliminated because of our conviction that textbooks must not only provide explanations but also cajole open minds to pursue the path of discovery. Indeed, although the torrent of new knowledge appears daunting, in many cases it simplifies the task of both authors and readers, because long and wordy speculations are replaced by concise and rational molecular explanations.

The molecular advances are also changing pathology as a medical practice. While morphology remains at the heart of diagnostic pathology, immunologic, cytogenetic, and molecular analyses of tissues and cells are increasingly becoming guides to render diagnoses, to assess prognosis, and to suggest therapy. A golden era for genetic pathology is at hand, and we attempt in the chapters on organ systems to present critical molecular analyses relevant to specific diseases or tumors.

Although new knowledge has meant extensive revision, our goals remain essentially the same.

- To integrate into the discussion of pathologic processes and disorders the newest established information available—morphologic and molecular.
- To organize the presentations into logical and uniform approaches, thereby facilitating readability, comprehension, and learning.
- Not to permit the book to become larger and more cumbersome, and yet to provide adequate discussion of the significant lesions, processes, and disorders, allotting space in proportion to their clinical and biologic importance.
- To place great emphasis on clarity of writing and good usage of language in the recognition that struggling to comprehend is time-consuming and wearisome and gets in the way of the learning process.
- To make this first and foremost a student text—used by students throughout their four years of medical school and into their residencies—but, at the same time, to provide sufficient detail and depth to meet the needs of more advanced readers.

We hope that we have in some measure achieved these goals in a manner that will keep this text useful into the next millennium.

The basic organization of the book also remains largely unchanged. The chapters on general principles and processes, such as cell injury and inflammation, are confined to the first part of the text, while the remainder of the book is concerned with the disorders of various organs and systems. Every chapter has been carefully updated, and many have been largely rewritten. The previous Chapter 1, which included both cell injury and adaptations, has been divided into two chapters. The first includes a more thorough discussion of cell death and the expanded understanding of apoptosis and its role in disease. The second considers the important adaptations, the intracellular accumulations, and recent insights into the mechanisms of cell aging. In systemic pathology, emphasis has remained on the origins of functional and structural changes, but the essential morphology, highlighted by a shaded background, has been carefully preserved. Whenever appropriate, genetic techniques relevant to the identification of particular lesions or tumors have been incorporated. The clinical significance of these changes has been integrated throughout the text.

In addition to revisions in text, there have been extensive changes in the illustrative material. Virtually all black and white photographs have been replaced by those in color. A large number of new schematics and diagrams that provide a three-dimensional view of cells and tissues have also been incorporated, but only where they can illuminate the text. We hope that this new infusion not only reinforces the textual matter but also makes the reading more pleasurable.

A liberal but judicious number of references are incorporated into the writing to provide source material for those who wish to pursue subjects of their own interest. Great effort was made in selecting these references for their quality, authenticity, and completeness. Most are recent—indeed some appeared in 1998—but older classics have been retained precisely because they are "classic."

While welcoming a new coauthor, Dr. Tucker Collins, and two additional chapter contributors to this edition, the senior authors reviewed, edited, and critiqued all of the chapters to ensure uniformity of style and flow that have been the hallmarks of this text. The authors were greatly helped by the advice and reviews of many experts who were sought out to confirm the accuracy, completeness, and authenticity of areas of their expertise, as detailed in the Acknowledgments section.

We hope that we have succeeded in transmitting to the readers of this text the beauty of the expanding knowledge of the nature of many diseases and have stimulated them to learn more about the pathologic basis of disease.

RSC

VK

TC

Acknowledgments

No textbook of this size can be completed without the help of many, many individuals. Hence, thanks and gratitude are owed to all of them for help in various ways in the completion of this edition.

First and foremost, all three of us wish to offer a salute to Dr. Stanley Robbins, who conceived this book and nourished it for more than 40 years. His principles of emphasizing clear writing and his uncompromising standards of accuracy continue to guide us. His mark on this book remains indelible. Second, we thank our contributing authors, trusted colleagues who have added to the luster of this book by preparing chapters in their areas of expertise. Their names appear in the Table of Contents and in the chapters themselves, and so it suffices here to note our gratitude to them for their willingness to lend their names and writing to this edition.

We also wish to acknowledge, with enormous gratitude, consultant colleagues who are not named as authors but who have reviewed, criticized, and sometimes even rewritten sections of this book in their specialty areas. Such excellence as the book may have is owed in part to them; any errors are ours. Foremost among those were:

- Dr. Manjeri Venkatachalam (Chapter 1—Cell Injury)
- Dr. Louis Picker (Chapter 3—Inflammation)
- Dr. Patricia D'Amore (Chapter 4—Tissue Repair)
- Dr. Nancy Schneider (Chapter 6—Genetic Disorders)
- Dr. Brian Dawson (Chapter 6—Genetic Disorders)
- Dr. William Edwards (Chapter 13—The Heart)
- Dr. Jon Aster (Chapter 14—Red Cells)
- Dr. David Dorfman (Chapter 15—The Thymus)
- Dr. Steven Kroft (Chapter 15—White Cells)
- Dr. David Sacks (Chapter 20—Diabetes)
- Dr. Helmut Rennke (Chapter 21—The Kidney)
- Dr. Andrew Renshaw (Chapter 22—Lower Urinary Tract)
- Dr. William Murphy (Chapter 22—Lower Urinary Tract)
- Dr. Dennis Burns (Chapter 26—Endocrine System)
- Dr. Christopher Fletcher (Surgical Pathology, several chapters)

Many other colleagues made their contributions by providing oversight and critiques in their special areas of interest or personal insights that influenced our writing. We particularly thank Drs. Abul Abbas, Amin Arnaout, Alan Beggs, Steven Blacklow, Carsten Bönnemann, Jonathan Epstein, David Genest, Robert Handin, Donald Ingber, David Louis, Richard Mitchell, James Morris, George Mutter, William Schoene, Charles Serhan, Mark Tanter, F.S. Vogel, Xiaodong Wang, Gayle Winters, and Ms. Nancy L. Robinson.

We thank Mr. John Boucher, our principal editorial assistant, on whose shoulders lay the burden of orchestrating the flow of manuscripts, galleys, page proofs, and illustrations among W.B. Saunders Company, the authors, illustrators, and sundry contributors. His help has been indispensable in the completion of the book on schecule. Personal assistance also was afforded by Margarita Rosado, Julie Smith, Beverly Shackelford, Patricia Nuckolls, Elizabeth Thurston, and Marilyn Gibson. Their efforts maintained the progress of the work and ultimately put the book together.

We owe thanks to many, many members of the staffs of the Brigham and Women's Hospital, The Children's Hospital, and the University of Texas Southwestern Medical School in Dallas, as well as other colleagues and friends who have added to this book by providing us with prize photographic and graphic gems. We emphasize that it would hardly have been possible to put together the many excellent new color illustrations without the outstanding collaboration of our fellows, residents, and colleagues. All are acknowledged with their specific contributions in the legends to the illustrations, but in addition, we wish to single out a few for special gratitude: Drs. Scott Granter, James Gulizia, Saba Jamal, Susan Lester, Robert McKenna, Helmut Rennke, Andrew Renshaw, Mary Sunday, Arthur Weinberg, and Trace Worrell.

Most of the new graphic art was created by Mr. James Perkins, Assistant Professor of Medical Illustration at Rochester Institute of Technology. His efforts were supplemented by Ms. Emiko-Rose Koike and Mr. Quade Paul from the Observatory Group. To all, our deepest thanks.

We are also indebted to our publisher, W.B. Saunders Company, and the many in the company who participated in the production of the book. Outstanding among them is Mrs. Hazel Hacker, our Senior Developmental Editor. Without her care, concern, and uncompromising standards of excellence, this book would have been much poorer. Also deserving of our thanks are Mr. William R. Schmitt, our Editorial Manager, Ms. Carolyn Naylor, Assistant Director of Book Production, Ms. Linda R. Garber, Senior Production Manager, Ms. Arlene Friday Chappelle, Senior Copy Editor, and the late Mr. David Harvey, Copy Editing Supervisor. Undoubtedly there are many other "unsung heroes" who should be recognized for their contributions—to all of them we say thanks and ask forgiveness for their not being individually singled out.

And finally, once again we acknowledge our wives, Kerstin Cotran, Raminder Kumar, and Mary Whitley, for their tolerance of our absences and their unflinching support of this seemingly endless task.

RSC

VK

TC

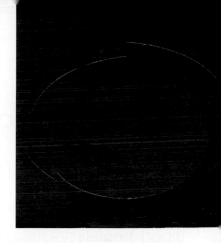

Contents

GENERAL PATHOLOGY

1
Cellular Pathology I: Cell Injury and Cell Death 1

2
Cellular Pathology II: Adaptations, Intracellular Accumulations, and Cell Aging 31

3
Acute and Chronic Inflammation 50

4
Tissue Repair: Cellular Growth, Fibrosis, and Wound Healing 89

5
Hemodynamic Disorders, Thrombosis, and Shock 113
RICHARD N. MITCHELL
RAMZI S. COTRAN

6
Genetic Disorders 139

7
Diseases of Immunity 188

8
Neoplasia 260

9
Infectious Diseases 329
JOHN SAMUELSON

10
Environmental and Nutritional Pathology 403
AGNES B. KANE
VINAY KUMAR

11
Diseases of Infancy and Childhood 459
DEBORAH SCHOFIELD
RAMZI S. COTRAN

DISEASES OF ORGAN SYSTEMS

12
Blood Vessels 493
FREDERICK J. SCHOEN
RAMZI S. COTRAN

13
The Heart 543
FREDERICK J. SCHOEN

14
Red Cells and Bleeding Disorders...... 601

15
White Cells, Lymph Nodes, Spleen, and Thymus 644
JON ASTER
VINAY KUMAR

16
The Lung 697
LESTER KOBZIK

17
Head and Neck 756

18
The Gastrointestinal Tract 775
JAMES M. CRAWFORD

19
The Liver and the Biliary Tract 845
JAMES M. CRAWFORD

20
The Pancreas................................ 902
JAMES M. CRAWFORD
RAMZI S. COTRAN

21
The Kidney 930

22
The Lower Urinary Tract 997

23
The Male Genital Tract.................... 1011

24
The Female Genital Tract................ 1035
CHRISTOPHER P. CRUM

25
The Breast 1093
SUSAN C. LESTER
RAMZI S. COTRAN

26
The Endocrine System 1121

27
The Skin...................................... 1170
GEORGE F. MURPHY
MARTIN C. MIHM, JR.

28
Bones, Joints, and Soft Tissue Tumors .. 1215
ANDREW ROSENBERG

29
Peripheral Nerve and Skeletal Muscle **1269**
UMBERTO DE GIROLAMI
DOUGLAS C. ANTHONY
MATTHEW P. FROSCH

30
The Central Nervous System **1293**
UMBERTO DE GIROLAMI
MATTHEW P. FROSCH
DOUGLAS C. ANTHONY

31
The Eye **1359**
DANIEL M. ALBERT
THADDEUS P. DRYJA

Index **1379**

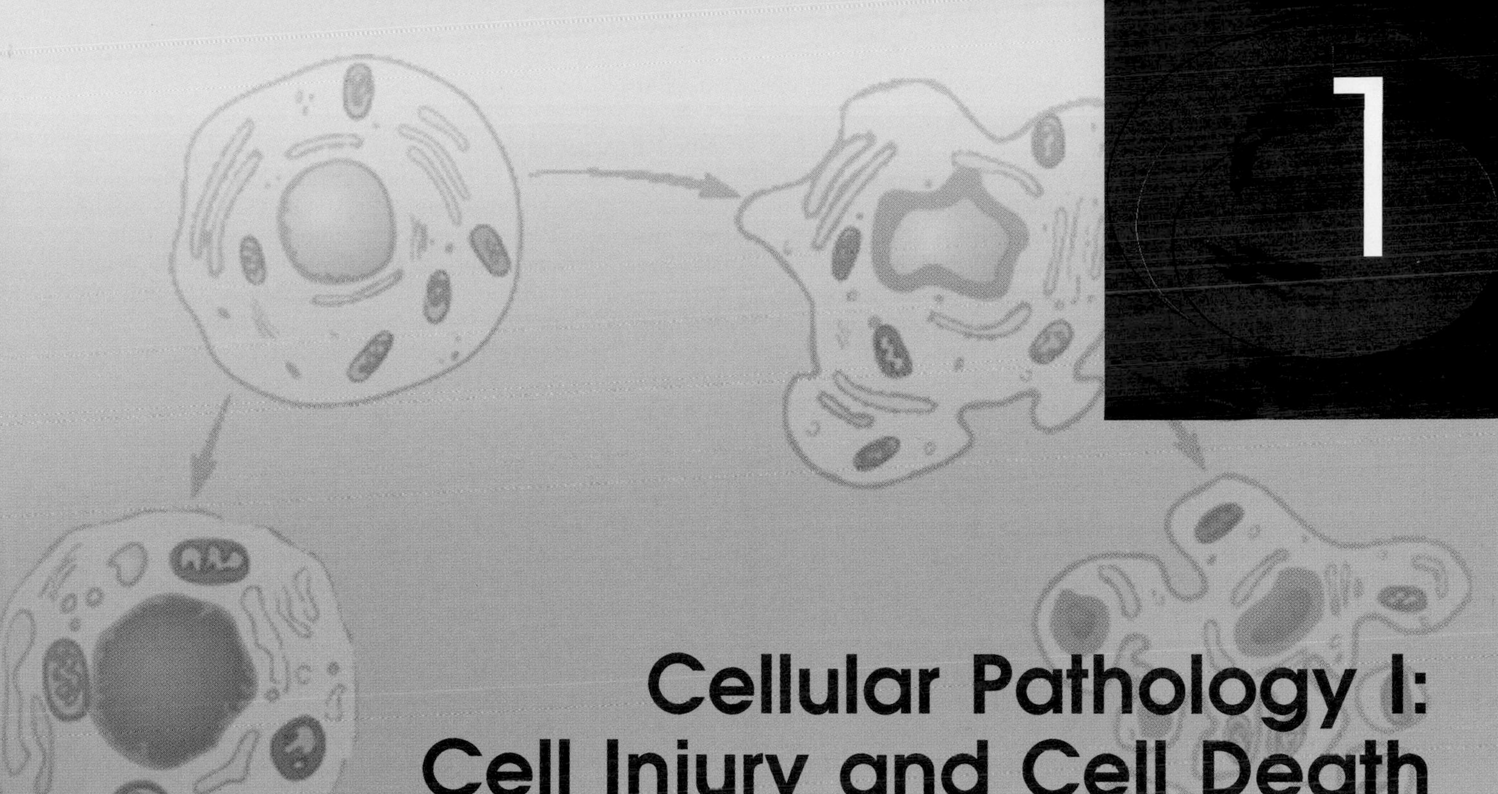

1

Cellular Pathology I: Cell Injury and Cell Death

INTRODUCTION TO PATHOLOGY

DEFINITIONS

CAUSES OF CELL INJURY

CELL INJURY AND NECROSIS

GENERAL BIOCHEMICAL MECHANISMS

ISCHEMIC AND HYPOXIC INJURY

Cell Injury During Ischemia/Hypoxia

Reversible Cell Injury

Irreversible Cell Injury

Ischemia/Reperfusion Injury

FREE RADICAL-INDUCED CELL INJURY

Chemical Injury

MORPHOLOGY OF REVERSIBLE CELL INJURY AND NECROSIS

Reversible Injury

Necrosis

APOPTOSIS

DEFINITION AND CAUSES

BIOCHEMICAL FEATURES

MECHANISMS

SPECIFIC EXAMPLES OF APOPTOSIS

SUBCELLULAR RESPONSES TO CELL INJURY

LYSOSOMAL CATABOLISM

INDUCTION (HYPERTROPHY) OF SMOOTH ENDOPLASMIC RETICULUM

MITOCHONDRIAL ALTERATIONS

CYTOSKELETAL ABNORMALITIES

INTRODUCTION TO PATHOLOGY

Pathology is literally the study *(logos)* of suffering *(pathos).* More specifically, it is a bridging discipline involving both basic science and clinical practice and is devoted to the study of the structural and functional changes in cells, tissues, and organs that underlie disease. By the use of molecular, microbiologic, immunologic, and morphologic techniques, pathology attempts to explain the whys and wherefores of the signs and symptoms manifested by patients while providing a sound foundation for rational clinical care and therapy.

Traditionally, the study of pathology is divided into general pathology and special or systemic pathology. The former is concerned with the basic reactions of cells and tissues to abnormal stimuli that underlie all diseases. The latter examines the specific responses of specialized organs and tissues to more or less well defined stimuli. In this book, we first cover the principles of general pathology and then proceed to specific disease processes as they affect particular organs or systems.

The four aspects of a disease process that form the core of pathology are its cause *(etiology),* the mechanisms of its development *(pathogenesis),* the structural alterations induced in the cells and organs of the body *(morphologic changes),* and the functional consequences of the morphologic changes *(clinical significance).*

Etiology or Cause. The concept that certain abnormal symptoms or diseases are "caused" is as ancient as recorded history. For the Arcadians (2500 B.C.), if someone became ill, it was the patient's own fault (for having sinned) or the makings of outside agents, such as bad smells, cold, evil spirits, or gods.[1] In modern terms, there are the two major classes of etiologic factors: intrinsic or genetic and acquired (e.g., infectious, nutritional, chemical, physical). Knowledge or discovery of the primary cause remains the backbone on which a diagnosis can be made, a disease understood, or a treatment developed. The concept, however, of one etiologic agent to one disease—developed from the study of infections or single-gene disorders—is no longer sufficient. Genetic factors are clearly involved in some of the common environmentally induced maladies, such as atherosclerosis and cancer, and the environment may also have profound influences on certain genetic diseases.

Pathogenesis. Pathogenesis refers to the sequence of events in the response of the cells or tissues to the etiologic agent, from the initial stimulus to the ultimate expression of the disease. The study of pathogenesis remains one of the main domains of pathology. Even when the initial infectious or molecular cause is known, it is many steps removed from the expression of the disease. For example, to understand cystic fibrosis is to know not only the defective gene and gene product but also the biochemical, immunologic, and morphologic events leading to the formation of cysts and fibrosis in the lung, pancreas, and other organs. Indeed, as we shall see throughout the book, the molecular revolution has already identified mutant genes underlying a great number of diseases and promises to map the entire human genome before too long. Nevertheless, the functions of the encoded proteins and how mutations induce disease are often still obscure. Thus, the study of pathogenesis has never been more exciting scientifically or more relevant to the development of new therapies.

Morphologic Changes. The morphologic changes refer to the structural alterations in cells or tissues that are either characteristic of the disease or diagnostic of the etiologic process.

Functional Derangements and Clinical Significance. The nature of the morphologic changes and their distribution in different organs or tissues influence normal function and determine the clinical features (symptoms and signs), course, and prognosis of the disease.

Virtually all forms of organ injury start with molecular or structural alterations in *cells*, a concept first put forth in the 19th century by Rudolf Virchow, known as the father of modern pathology. We therefore begin our consideration of pathology with the study of the origins, molecular mechanisms, and structural changes of cell injury. Yet different cells in tissues constantly interact with each other, and an elaborate system of *extracellular matrix* is necessary for the integrity of organs. Cell-cell and cell-matrix interactions contribute significantly to the response to injury, leading collectively to *tissue* and *organ injury*, which are as important as cell injury in defining the morphologic and clinical patterns of disease.[2]

DEFINITIONS

The normal cell is confined to a fairly narrow range of function and structure by its genetic programs of metabolism, differentiation, and specialization; by constraints of neighboring cells; and by the availability of metabolic substrates. It is nevertheless able to handle normal physiologic demands, so-called *normal homeostasis*. Somewhat more excessive physiologic stresses or some pathologic stimuli may bring about a number of physiologic and morphologic *cellular adaptations*, during which new but altered steady states are achieved, preserving the viability of the cell and modulating its function as a response to such stimuli. For example, the bulging muscles of the bodybuilders engaged in "pumping iron" result from cellular adaptations, the increase in muscle mass reflecting the increase in size of the individual muscle fibers. The workload is thus shared by a greater mass of cellular components, and each muscle fiber is spared excess work and so escapes injury. The enlarged muscle cell achieves a new equilibrium, permitting it to survive at a higher level of activity. This adaptive response is called *hypertrophy*. Conversely, *atrophy* is an adaptive response in which there is a decrease in the size and function of cells. These and other cell adaptations are considered in Chapter 2.

If the limits of adaptive response to a stimulus are exceeded, or in certain instances when adaptation is not possible, a sequence of events follows, loosely termed *cell injury*. Cell injury is *reversible* up to a certain point, but if the stimulus persists or is severe enough from the beginning, the cell reaches the "point of no return" and suffers *irreversible cell injury* and *cell death*. For example, if the blood supply to a segment of the heart is cut off for 10 to 15 minutes and is then restored, the myocardial cells experience injury but can recover and function normally. If blood flow is not restored until 1 hour later, however, irreversible injury ensues, and many myocardial fibers die. *Adaptation, reversible injury, irreversible injury*, and *cell death* can be considered states of progressive encroachment on the cell's normal function and structure (Fig. 1–1).

Cell death, the ultimate result of cell injury, is one of the most crucial events in pathology, affecting every cell type and being the major consequence of ischemia (lack of blood flow), infection, toxins, and immune reactions. In addition, it is critical during normal embryogenesis, lymphoid tissue development, and hormonally induced involution and is the aim of cancer radiotherapy and chemotherapy.

There are two principal patterns of cell death, *necrosis* and *apoptosis*.[2]

- *Necrosis* or *coagulation necrosis* is the more common type of cell death after exogenous stimuli, occurring after such stresses as ischemia and chemical injury. It is manifested by severe cell swelling or cell rupture, denaturation and coagulation of cytoplasmic proteins, and breakdown of cell organelles.
- *Apoptosis* occurs when a cell dies through activation of an internally controlled suicide program. It is a subtly orchestrated disassembly of cellular components designed to eliminate unwanted cells during embryogenesis and in various physiologic processes. Doomed cells are removed with minimum disruption to the surrounding tissue. It also occurs, however, under pathologic conditions, in which it is sometimes accompanied by necrosis. Its chief morphologic features are chromatin condensation and fragmentation. Although the mechanisms of necrosis and apoptosis differ, as we shall see, there is

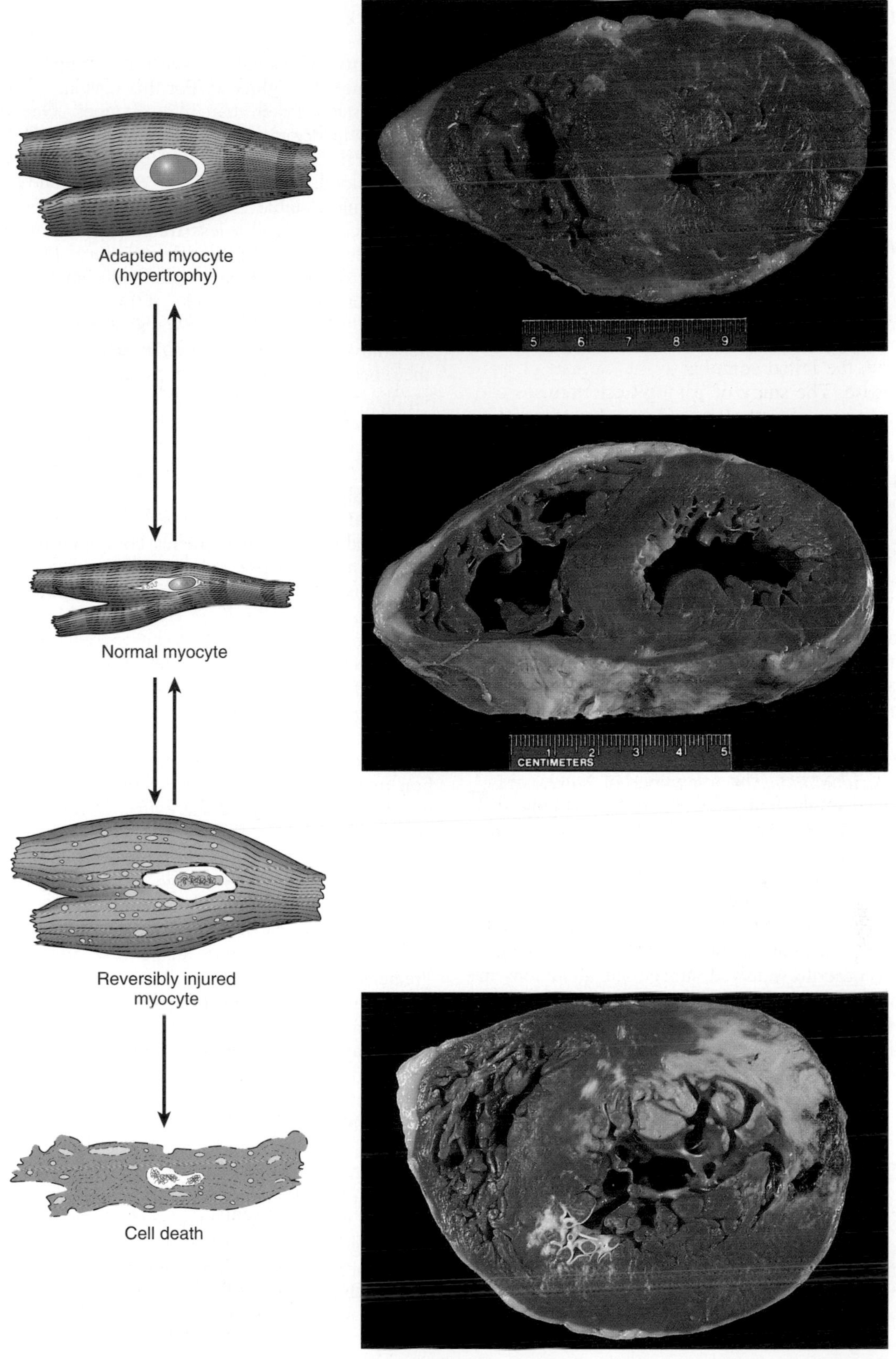

Figure 1–1

The relationships between normal, adapted, reversibly injured, and dead myocardial cells. The cellular adaptation depicted here is hypertrophy, and the type of cellular injury is ischemic necrosis. In reversibly injured myocardium, there are generally only functional effects, without any readily apparent gross or even microscopic changes. In the example of myocardial hypertrophy, the left ventricular wall is more than 2 cm in thickness (normal is 1 to 1.5 cm). In the specimen showing necrosis, the transmural light area in the posterolateral left ventricle represents an acute myocardial infarction. All three transverse sections have been stained with triphenyltetrazolium chloride, an enzyme substrate that colors viable myocardium magenta. Failure to stain is due to enzyme leakage after cell death.

Table 1–1. CELLULAR RESPONSES TO INJURY

- Acute cell injury (Chapter 1)
  - Reversible injury
  - Cell death
    - Necrosis
    - Apoptosis
- Subcellular alterations in sublethal and chronic injury (Chapter 1)
- Cellular adaptations (Chapter 2)
  - Atrophy, hypertrophy, hyperplasia, metaplasia
- Intracellular accumulations (Chapter 2)
- Pathologic calcification (Chapter 2)
- Cell aging (Chapter 2)

considerable overlap between these two processes. Recently, a new term has been introduced—*oncosis*—to define the prelethal changes preceding necrotic cell death.[2] These are characterized by cell swelling (*oncos*, Greek for swelling) and can be distinguished from the prelethal changes in apoptosis, associated largely with cell shrinkage.[3] Whether the term will achieve the status sought by its creators is still unclear.

The cellular changes described—reversible and irreversible cell injury leading to *necrosis* or *apoptosis*—are morphologic patterns of *acute cell injury* induced by various stimuli. Other groups of morphologic cellular alterations are listed in Table 1–1: *subcellular alterations*, which occur usually as a response to sublethal or chronic stimuli; *intracellular accumulations* of a number of substances—proteins, lipids, carbohydrates—which occur largely as a result of metabolic derangements in cells; *pathologic calcification*, a common consequence of cell and tissue injury; and *cell aging*.

In this chapter, we first consider the broad categories of stimuli that cause cell injury; then discuss the various forms of acute cell damage, including necrosis and apoptosis; and finally describe selected subcellular alterations induced by sublethal stimuli. Chapter 2 completes the discussion of cellular pathology with a consideration of cellular adaptations, intracellular accumulations, pathologic calcification, and cell aging.

CAUSES OF CELL INJURY

The causes of reversible cell injury and cell death range from the external gross physical violence of an automobile accident to internal endogenous causes, such as a subtle genetic lack of a vital enzyme that impairs normal metabolic function. Most adverse influences can be grouped into the following broad categories.

Oxygen Deprivation. Hypoxia, an extremely important and common cause of cell injury and cell death, impinges on aerobic oxidative respiration. Hypoxia should be distinguished from *ischemia*, which is a loss of blood supply from impeded arterial flow or reduced venous drainage in a tissue. In contrast to hypoxia, during which glycolytic energy production can continue, ischemia compromises the availability of metabolic substrates (supplied by flowing blood) including glucose. For this reason, ischemia tends to injure tissues faster than hypoxia does. One cause of hypoxia is inadequate oxygenation of the blood due to cardiorespiratory failure. Loss of the oxygen-carrying *capacity* of the blood, as in anemia or carbon monoxide poisoning (producing a stable carbon monoxyhemoglobin that blocks oxygen carriage), is a less frequent basis of oxygen deprivation that results in significant injury. Depending on the severity of the hypoxic state, cells may adapt, undergo injury, or die. For example, if the femoral artery is narrowed, the skeletal muscle cells of the leg may shrink in size (atrophy). This reduction in cell mass achieves a balance between metabolic needs and the available oxygen supply. More severe hypoxia induces injury and cell death.

Physical Agents. Physical agents include mechanical trauma, extremes of temperature (burns and deep cold), sudden changes in atmospheric pressure, radiation, and electric shock (Chapter 10).

Chemical Agents and Drugs. The list of chemicals that may produce cell injury defies compilation. Simple chemicals such as glucose or salt in hypertonic concentrations may cause cell injury directly or by deranging electrolyte homeostasis of cells. Even oxygen, in high concentrations, is severely toxic. Trace amounts of agents known as *poisons*, such as arsenic, cyanide, or mercuric salts, may destroy sufficient numbers of cells within minutes to hours to cause death. Other substances, however, are our daily companions: environmental and air pollutants, insecticides, and herbicides; industrial and occupational hazards, such as carbon monoxide and asbestos; social stimuli, such as alcohol and narcotic drugs; and the ever-increasing variety of therapeutic drugs.

Infectious Agents. These agents range from the submicroscopic viruses to the large tapeworms. In between are the rickettsiae, bacteria, fungi, and higher forms of parasites. The ways by which this heterogeneous group of biologic agents cause injury are diverse and are discussed in greater detail in Chapter 9.

Immunologic Reactions. Although the immune system serves in the defense against biologic agents, immune reactions may, in fact, cause cell injury. The anaphylactic reaction to a foreign protein or a drug is a prime example, and reactions to endogenous self-antigens are thought to be responsible for a number of autoimmune diseases (Chapter 7).

Genetic Derangements. Genetic defects as causes of cell injury are of major interest to biologists today (Chapter 6). The genetic injury may result in a defect as gross as the congenital malformations associated with Down syndrome or as subtle as the single amino acid substitutions in hemoglobin S in sickle cell anemia. The many inborn errors of metabolism arising from enzymatic abnormalities, usually an enzyme lack, are excellent examples of cell damage due to subtle alterations at the level of DNA.

Nutritional Imbalances. Even today, nutritional imbalances continue to be major causes of cell injury. Protein-calorie deficiencies cause an appalling number of deaths, chiefly among underprivileged populations. Deficiencies of specific vitamins are found throughout the world (Chapter 10). Nutritional problems can be self-imposed, as in anorexia nervosa, or self-induced starvation. Ironically, nutritional excesses have also become important causes of cell injury. Excesses of lipids predispose to atherosclerosis, and obesity is an extraordinary manifestation of the overloading of some cells in the body with fats. Atherosclerosis is virtually endemic in the United States, and obesity is rampant. In addition to the problems of undernutrition and overnutrition, the composition of the diet makes a significant contribution to a number of diseases.

CELL INJURY AND NECROSIS

In this section, we consider reversible cell injury and the pattern of cell death known as necrosis. Some of the mechanisms clearly overlap with those leading to apoptosis, which is discussed separately.

The biochemical mechanisms responsible for reversible cell injury and cell death are complex. As we have seen, injury to cells has many causes, and there are multiple pathways to cell death that interact with one another. There are, however, a number of principles that are relevant to most forms of cell injury.

- *The cellular response to injurious stimuli depends on the type of injury, its duration, and its severity.* Thus, small doses of a chemical toxin or brief periods of ischemia may induce reversible injury, whereas large doses of the same toxin or more prolonged ischemia might result either in instantaneous cell death or in slow, irreversible injury leading in time to cell death.
- *The consequences of cell injury depend on the type, state, and adaptability of the injured cell.* The cell's nutritional and hormonal status and its metabolic needs are important in its response to injury. How vulnerable is a cell, for example, to loss of blood supply and hypoxia? The striated muscle cell in the leg can be placed entirely at rest when it is deprived of its blood supply; not so the striated muscle of the heart. Exposure of two individuals to identical concentrations of a toxin, such as carbon tetrachloride, may be without effect in one and may produce cell death in the other. This may be due, as we shall see, to the genetic variations affecting amount and activity of hepatic enzymes that convert carbon tetrachloride to toxic byproducts (Chapter 10).
- Although the precise biochemical sites of action for many stimuli are difficult to pinpoint, four intracellular systems are particularly vulnerable: (1) *maintenance of the integrity of cell membranes,* on which the ionic and osmotic homeostasis of the cell and its organelles depends; (2) *aerobic respiration* involving mitochondrial oxidative phosphorylation and production of adenosine triphosphate (ATP); (3) *protein synthesis;* and (4) *preservation of the integrity of the genetic apparatus* of the cell.
- *The structural and biochemical elements of the cell are so closely interrelated that whatever the precise point of initial attack, injury at one locus leads to wide-ranging secondary effects.* For example, impairment of aerobic respiration disrupts the energy-dependent membrane sodium pump that maintains the ionic and fluid balance of the cell, resulting in alterations in the intracellular content of ions and water.
- *The morphologic changes of cell injury become apparent only after some critical biochemical system within the cell has been deranged.* As would be expected, the morphologic manifestations of lethal damage take more time to develop than those of reversible damage. For example, cell swelling is a reversible morphologic change, and this may occur in a matter of minutes. Unmistakable light microscopic changes of cell death, however, do not occur in the myocardium until 10 to 12 hours after total ischemia, yet we know that irreversible injury occurs within 20 to 60 minutes (see Fig. 1–1). Obviously, ultrastructural alterations are visible earlier than light microscopic changes.

General Biochemical Mechanisms

With certain injurious agents, the biochemical loci of attack are well defined. Many toxins cause cell injury by interfering with endogenous substrates or enzymes. Particularly vulnerable are *glycolysis,* the *citric acid cycle,* and *oxidative phosphorylation* in mitochondrial inner membranes. Cyanide, for example, inactivates cytochrome oxidase, and fluoroacetate interferes with the citric acid cycle, both resulting in ATP depletion. Certain anaerobic bacteria, such as *Clostridium perfringens,* elaborate phospholipases, which attack phospholipids in cell membranes. Yet with many injurious stimuli, the precise pathways that lead to cell death are not fully understood.

Nevertheless, there are several common biochemical themes that are important in the mediation of cell injury and cell death by necrosis, *whatever the inciting agent.* These include the following:

- *ATP depletion.* High-energy phosphate in the form of ATP is required for many synthetic and degradative processes within the cell. These include membrane transport, protein synthesis, lipogenesis, and the deacylation-reacylation reactions necessary for phospholipid turnover. ATP is produced in two ways. The major one in mammalian cells is *oxidative phosphorylation* of adenosine diphosphate (ADP), in a reaction that results in reduction of oxygen by the electron transfer system of mitochondria. The second is the *glycolytic pathway,* which can generate ATP in the absence of oxygen using glucose derived either from body fluids or from the hydrolysis of glycogen. Thus, tissues with greater glycolytic capacity (e.g., liver) have an advantage when ATP levels are falling because of inhibition of oxidative metabolism by injury. *ATP depletion and decreased ATP synthesis are common consequences of both ischemic and toxic injury.*
- *Oxygen and oxygen-derived free radicals* (Fig. 1–2). Cells generate energy by reducing molecular oxygen to water. During this process, small amounts of partially reduced reactive oxygen forms are produced as an unavoidable byproduct of mitochondrial respiration. Some of these forms are free radicals that can damage lipids,

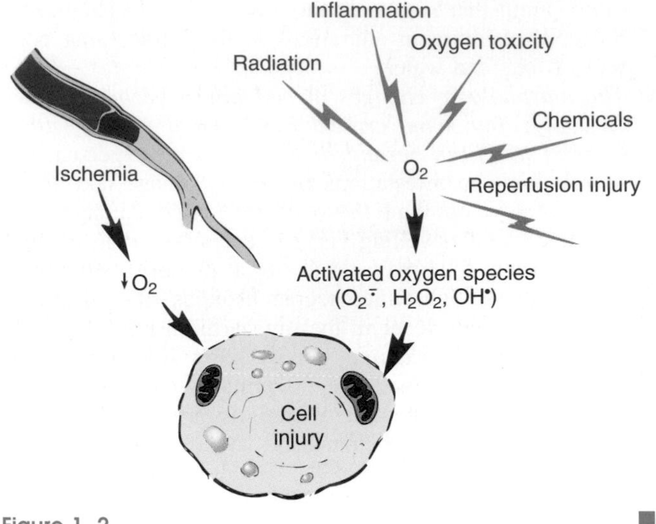

Figure 1–2

The critical role of oxygen in cell injury. Ischemia causes cell injury by reducing cellular oxygen supplies, whereas other stimuli, such as radiation, induce damage by toxic activated oxygen species.

proteins, and nucleic acids, as described later in the chapter. They are referred to as *reactive oxygen species*. Cells have defense systems to prevent injury caused by these products. An imbalance between free radical–generating and radical-scavenging systems results in *oxidative stress*, a condition that has been associated with the cell injury seen in many pathologic conditions, as we describe throughout the book.

- *Intracellular calcium and loss of calcium homeostasis.*[3] Cytosolic free calcium is maintained at extremely low concentrations (less than 0.1 μmol) compared with extracellular levels of 1.3 mmol, and most intracellular calcium is sequestered in mitochondria and endoplasmic reticulum. Such gradients are modulated by membrane-associated, energy-dependent Ca^{2+}, Mg^{2+}-ATPases. Ischemia and certain toxins cause an early increase in cytosolic calcium concentration, owing to the net influx of Ca^{2+} across the plasma membrane and the release of Ca^{2+} from mitochondria and endoplasmic reticulum. Sustained rises in cell Ca^{2+} subsequently result from nonspecific increases in membrane permeability. Increased Ca^{2+} in turn activates a number of enzymes, with potential deleterious cellular effects. The enzymes known to be activated by calcium include *phospholipases* (thus promoting membrane damage), *proteases* (which break down both membrane and cytoskeletal proteins), *ATPases* (thereby hastening ATP depletion), and *endonucleases* (which are associated with chromatin fragmentation) (Fig. 1–3). Although cell injury results in increased intracellular calcium and this in turn mediates a variety of deleterious effects, including cell death, loss of calcium homeostasis is not always a necessary proximal event in irreversible cell injury.
- *Defects in membrane permeability.* Early loss of selective membrane permeability leading ultimately to overt membrane damage is a consistent feature of all forms of cell injury. Such defects may be the result of a series of events involving ATP depletion and calcium-modulated activation of phospholipases, as discussed in detail later. This type of damage may affect the mitochondria, the plasma membrane, and other cellular membranes. The plasma membrane, however, can also be damaged directly by certain bacterial toxins, viral proteins, lytic complement components, products of cytolytic lymphocytes (perforins), and a number of physical and chemical agents.
- *Irreversible mitochondrial damage.* Mammalian cells are obligately dependent on oxidative metabolism for long-term survival, regardless of glycolytic ability. Thus, irreparable damage to mitochondria will ultimately kill cells. Directly or indirectly, mitochondria are important targets for virtually all types of injurious stimuli, including hypoxia and toxins. They can be damaged by increases of cytosolic Ca^{++}, by oxidative stress, by breakdown of phospholipids through the phospholipase A_2 and sphingomyelin pathways, and by lipid breakdown products derived therefrom, such as *free fatty acids and ceramide*. The damage is commonly expressed as the formation of a high-conductance channel, the so-called *mitochondrial permeability transition*, in the inner mitochondrial membrane[4] (Fig. 1–4). Although reversible in its early stages, this nonselective pore becomes permanent if the inciting stimuli persist, precluding maintenance of mitochondrial proton motive force, or potential. Because maintenance of potential is critical for mitochondrial oxidative phosphorylation, *it follows that irreversible mitochondrial permeability transition is a death blow to the cell.* Mitochondrial damage can also be associated with leakage of cytochrome *c* into the cytosol. Because cytochrome *c* is a soluble but integral component of the electron transport chain and can trigger

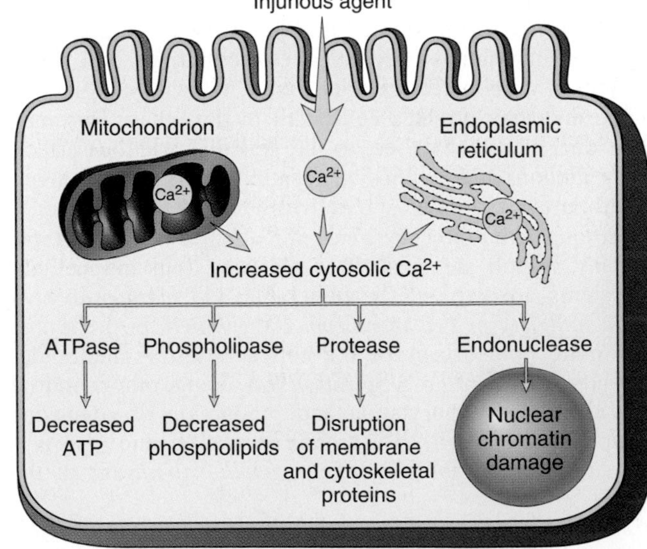

Figure 1–3

Sources and consequences of increased cytosolic calcium in cell injury. ATP, adenosine triphosphate.

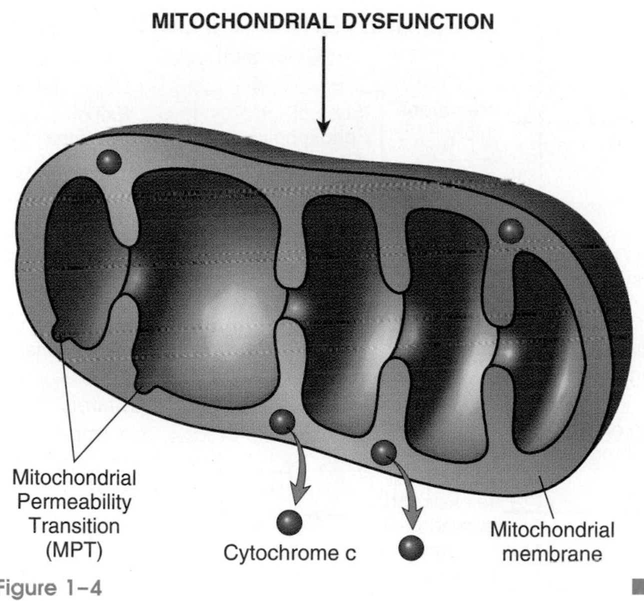

Figure 1–4

Mitochondrial dysfunction, induced by a variety of stimuli, causes mitochondrial permeability transition (MPT) and leakage of cytochrome *c* into the cytosol. The MPT is in the inner mitochondrial membrane.

apoptotic death pathways in the cytosol (see later), this pathologic event is also likely to be a key determinant of cell death.

Having briefly reviewed these general mechanisms, we now concentrate on three common forms of cell injury: (1) ischemic and hypoxic injury; (2) injury induced by free radicals, including activated oxygen species; and (3) some types of toxic injury.

Ischemic and Hypoxic Injury

This is the most common type of cell injury in clinical medicine and has been studied extensively in humans, in experimental animals, and in culture systems.[1, 5–7] Reasonable scenarios concerning the mechanisms underlying the morphologic changes have emerged. In contrast to hypoxia, during which glycolytic energy production can continue, ischemia compromises the delivery of substrates for glycolysis. Thus, in ischemic tissues, anaerobic energy generation will stop after glycolytic substrates are exhausted or glycolytic function becomes inhibited by the accumulation of metabolites that would have been removed otherwise by blood flow. For this reason, *ischemia tends to injure tissues faster than hypoxia.*

Types of Ischemic Injury. Ischemic injury is the most common clinical expression of cell injury by oxygen deprivation. The most useful models to study ischemic injury involve complete occlusion of one of the end-arteries to an organ (e.g., a coronary artery) and examination of the tissue (e.g., cardiac muscle) in areas supplied by the artery. Complex pathologic changes occur in diverse cellular systems during ischemia. With time, these alterations progress in severity, ultimately compromising vital structural and biochemical components and resulting in cell death. However, up to a certain point, for a duration that varies among different types of cells, the injury is amenable to repair, and the affected cells can recover if oxygen and metabolic substrates are again made available by restoration of blood flow. Pathologic changes characteristic of ischemic cells that can recover when they are given an opportunity to do so are described as *reversible ischemic injury.* With further extension of the ischemic duration, cell structure continues to deteriorate, owing to relentless progression of ongoing injury mechanisms. With time, the energetic machinery of the cell—the mitochondrial oxidative powerhouse and the glycolytic pathway—becomes irreparably damaged. In that all ischemic disease can ultimately be traced back to cellular depletion of ATP, inability to generate high-energy compounds when given an opportunity to do so can be considered to be a *point of no return,* at which time reperfusion cannot rescue the damaged cell. Even if the cellular energetic machinery were to remain intact, irreparable damage to the genome or to cellular membranes will ensure a lethal outcome regardless of reperfusion. This is *irreversible ischemic injury.*

Under certain circumstances, when blood flow is restored to cells that have been previously made ischemic but have not died, injury is often paradoxically exacerbated and proceeds at an accelerated pace. As a consequence, tissues sustain loss of cells in *addition to those that are irreversibly damaged at the end of ischemia.* This is a clinically important process that contributes to net tissue damage during myocardial and cerebral infarction, as described in Chapters 13 and 30. This so-called *ischemia/reperfusion injury* is particularly significant because appropriate medical treatment has the potential to decrease the fraction of cells that may otherwise be destined to die in the "area at risk."

CELL INJURY DURING ISCHEMIA/HYPOXIA

Reversible Cell Injury

The first point of attack of hypoxia is the cell's aerobic respiration, that is, oxidative phosphorylation by mitochondria.[5, 6] As the oxygen tension within the cell decreases, there is loss of oxidative phosphorylation and decreased generation of ATP. The resulting depletion of ATP has widespread effects on many systems within the cell (Fig. 1–5).

- The activity of the *plasma membrane energy-dependent sodium pump* (ouabain-sensitive Na^+, K^+-ATPase) is reduced. *Failure of this active transport system, due to diminished ATP concentration and enhanced ATPase activity, causes sodium to accumulate intracellularly with diffusion of potassium out of the cell.* The net gain of solute is accompanied by isosmotic gain of water, *cell swelling*, and dilation of the endoplasmic reticulum. A second mechanism for cell swelling in ischemia is the *increased intracellular osmotic load* engendered by the accumulation of catabolites, such as inorganic phosphates, lactate, and purine nucleosides.
- *Cellular energy metabolism is altered.* When oxygen

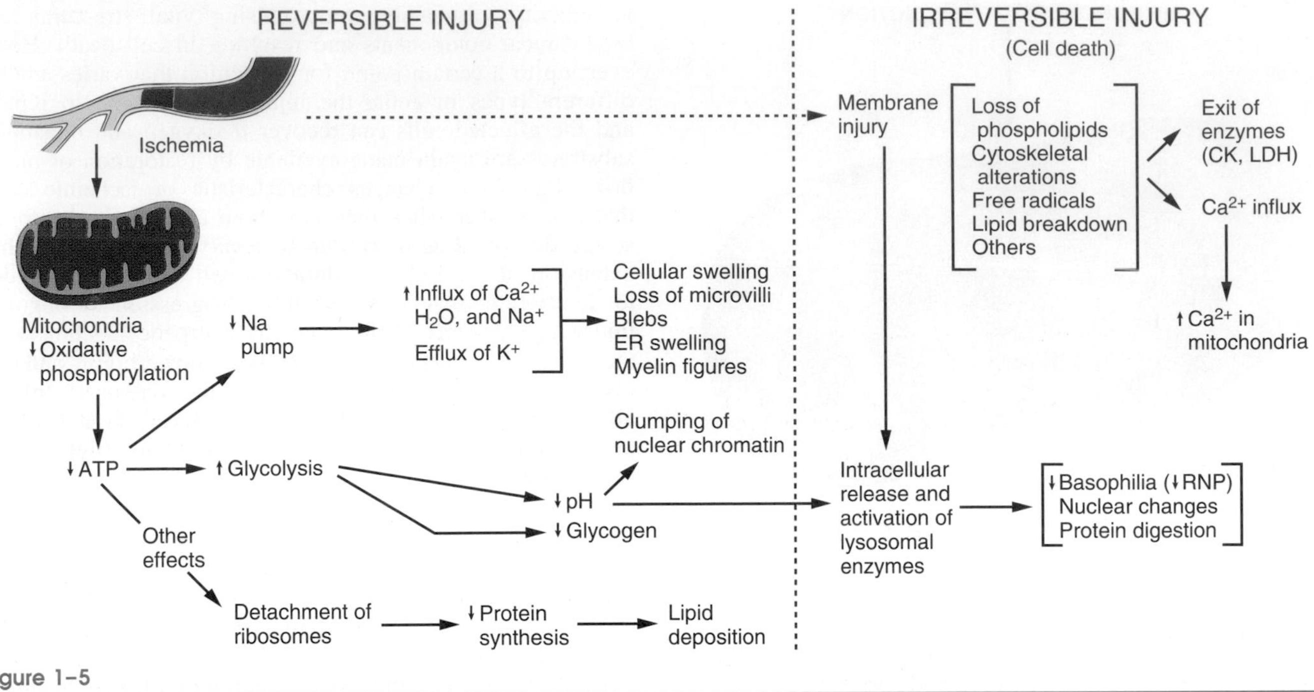

Figure 1–5

Postulated sequence of events in ischemic injury. Note that although reduced oxidative phosphorylation and ATP levels have a central role, ischemia can cause direct membrane damage. ER, endoplasmic reticulum; CK, creatine kinase; LDH, lactate dehydrogenase; RNP, ribonucleoprotein.

levels are low, oxidative phosphorylation ceases and cells rely on glycolysis for energy production. This switch to anaerobic metabolism is controlled by energy pathway metabolites acting on glycolytic enzymes. The decrease in cellular ATP and associated increase in adenosine monophosphate stimulate phosphofructokinase and phosphorylase activities. This results in an increased rate of *anaerobic glycolysis* designed to maintain the cell's energy sources by generating ATP through metabolism of glucose derived from glycogen. As a consequence, *glycogen stores are rapidly depleted.* Glycolysis results in the accumulation of lactic acid and inorganic phosphates from the hydrolysis of phosphate esters. *This reduces the intracellular pH.*

- The next phenomenon to occur is structural disruption of the protein synthetic apparatus manifested as *detachment of ribosomes from the granular endoplasmic reticulum* and *dissociation of polysomes into monosomes,* with a consequent *reduction in protein synthesis.*
- Functional consequences can occur in reversible cell injury. Heart muscle ceases to contract within 60 seconds of coronary occlusion. Note, however, that noncontractility does not mean cell death.

If hypoxia continues, worsening ATP depletion causes further morphologic deterioration. The cytoskeleton disperses, resulting in the loss of ultrastructural features such as microvilli and the formation of "blebs" at the cell surface (Fig. 1–6 and 1–7). "Myelin figures," derived from plasma as well as organellar membranes, may be seen within the cytoplasm or extracellularly. They are thought to result from dissociation of lipoproteins with unmasking of phosphatide groups, promoting the uptake and intercalation of water between the lamellar stacks of membranes. At this time, the mitochondria are usually swollen, owing to loss of volume control by these organelles; the endoplasmic reticulum remains dilated; and the entire cell is markedly swollen, with increased concentrations of water, sodium, and chloride and a decreased concentration of potassium. *If oxygen is restored, all of these disturbances are reversible.*

Irreversible Cell Injury

If ischemia persists, irreversible injury ensues. This process has morphologic hallmarks, but the biochemical explanation for the critical transition from reversible injury to cell death has remained elusive.

Irreversible injury is associated morphologically with severe swelling of mitochondria (see Figs. 1–5 and 1–6*C*), extensive damage to plasma membranes, and swelling of lysosomes. *Large, flocculent, amorphous densities develop in the mitochondrial matrix* (see Fig. 1–7*C*). In the myocardium, these are indications of irreversible injury and can be seen as early as 30 to 40 minutes after ischemia. Massive influx of calcium into the cell then occurs, particularly if the ischemic zone is reperfused. There is continued loss of proteins, enzymes, coenzymes, and ribonucleic acids from the hyperpermeable membranes. The cells may also leak metabolites, which are vital for the reconstitution of ATP, thus further depleting net intracellular high-energy phosphates.

At this stage, *injury to the lysosomal membranes occurs, followed by leakage of their enzymes into the cytoplasm and activation of their acid hydrolases.* Lysosomes contain

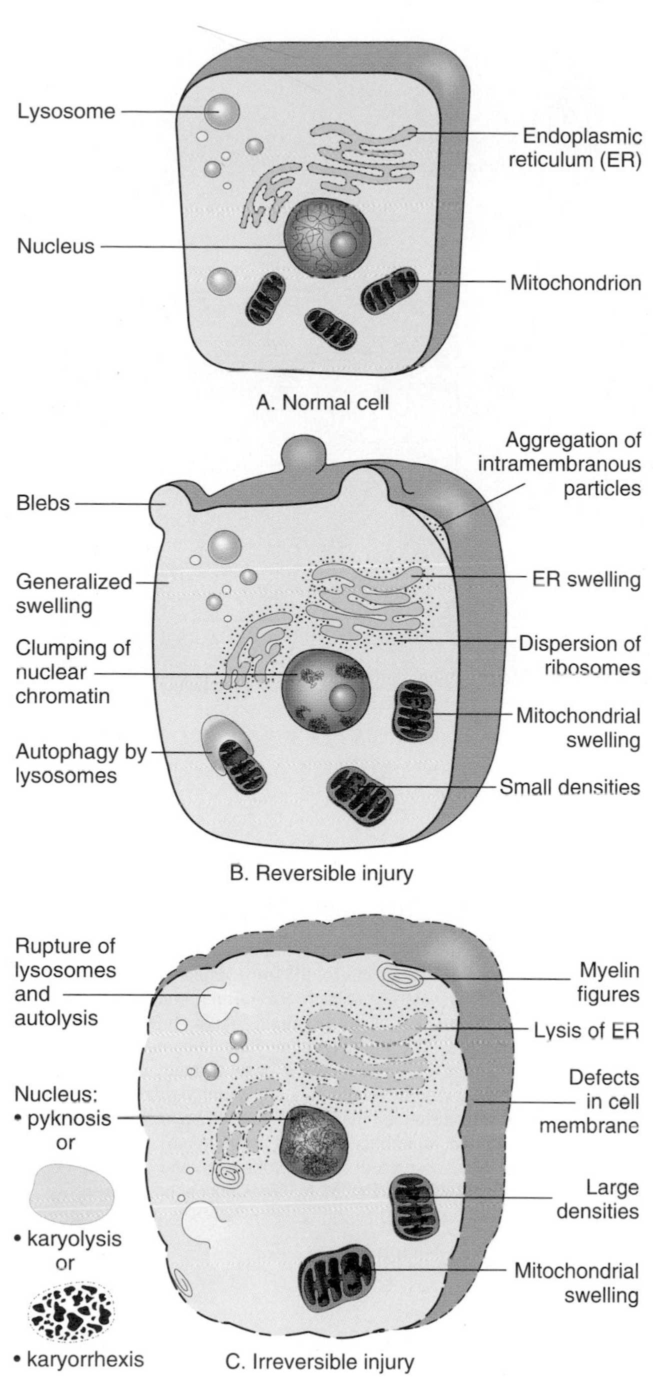

Figure 1–6

Schematic representation of a normal cell *(A)* and the ultrastructural changes in reversible *(B)* and irreversible *(C)* cell injury (see text).

RNases, DNases, proteases, phosphatases, glucosidases, and cathepsins. Activation of these enzymes leads to enzymatic digestion of cell components evidenced by loss of ribonucleoprotein, deoxyribonucleoprotein, and glycogen and the various *nuclear changes* described later. Although these changes have traditionally been ascribed to falling pH, more recent studies suggest that the early fall in pH is followed by a shift to neutral or even alkaline pH as irreversible injury proceeds. Indeed, acidosis protects against lethal injury in many models of ischemia and reperfusion, probably as a result of the inhibitory effect of low pH on enzymatic reactions such as phospholipase activity and processes such as mitochondrial permeability transition.[8] Early clumping of nuclear chromatin, also seen during ischemia, could also be caused by reduction in cell pH.

After death, cell components are progressively degraded, and there is widespread leakage of cellular enzymes into the extracellular space and, conversely, entry of extracellular macromolecules from the interstitial space into the dying cells. Finally, the dead cell may become replaced by large masses composed of phospholipids in the form of myelin figures. These are then either phagocytosed by other cells or degraded further into fatty acids. *Calcification* of such fatty acid residues may occur with the formation of calcium soaps.

At this point in the story, we should note that leakage of intracellular enzymes and other proteins across the abnormally permeable plasma membrane, and into the plasma, provides important clinical parameters of cell death. Cardiac muscle, for example, contains transaminases, lactate dehydrogenase, creatine kinase (CK), and cardiac-specific proteins (troponins). Elevated serum levels of such molecules (e.g., creatine kinase MB, troponin) are valuable clinical criteria of myocardial infarction, a locus of cell death in heart muscle (Chapter 13).

Mechanisms of Irreversible Injury. The sequence of events for hypoxia was described as a continuum from its initiation to the ultimate digestion of the lethally injured cell by lysosomal enzymes. But at what stage did the cell actually die? And what is the critical biochemical event (the "lethal hit") responsible for the point of no return? Two phenomena consistently characterize irreversibility. The first is the *inability to reverse mitochondrial dysfunction causing marked ATP depletion,* and the second is the development of *profound disturbances in membrane function. ATP depletion* clearly contributes to the functional and structural consequences of ischemia, as described earlier (see Fig. 1–3), and may also lead to membrane damage (see later).[13]

A great deal of evidence indicates that membrane damage is a central factor in the pathogenesis of irreversible cell injury. Loss of mitochondrial membrane function, increased permeability to extracellular molecules, and demonstrable plasma membrane ultrastructural defects occur in the earliest stages of irreversible injury.

Several biochemical mechanisms may contribute to such membrane damage (Fig. 1–8).

1. *Mitochondrial dysfunction.* Increase of cytosolic calcium associated with ATP depletion results in increased uptake of Ca^{2+} by mitochondria, activating mitochondrial phospholipases and resulting in accumulation of free fatty acids. Acting in concert, they cause changes in the permeability of the inner mitochondrial membrane, such as the mitochondrial permeability transition,[4,9] as well as of the outer mitochondrial membrane, as we have seen.
2. *Loss of membrane phospholipids.* In ischemic tissues, irreversible ischemic injury is associated with a decrease in the content of membrane phospholipids. This degra-

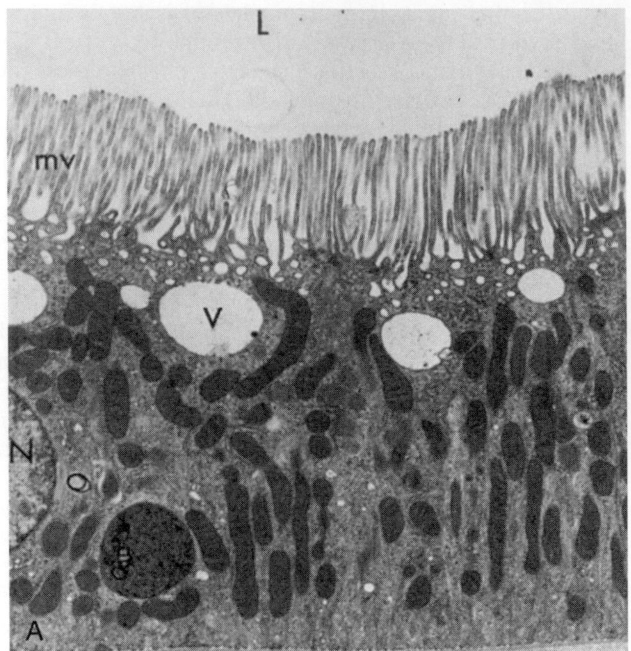

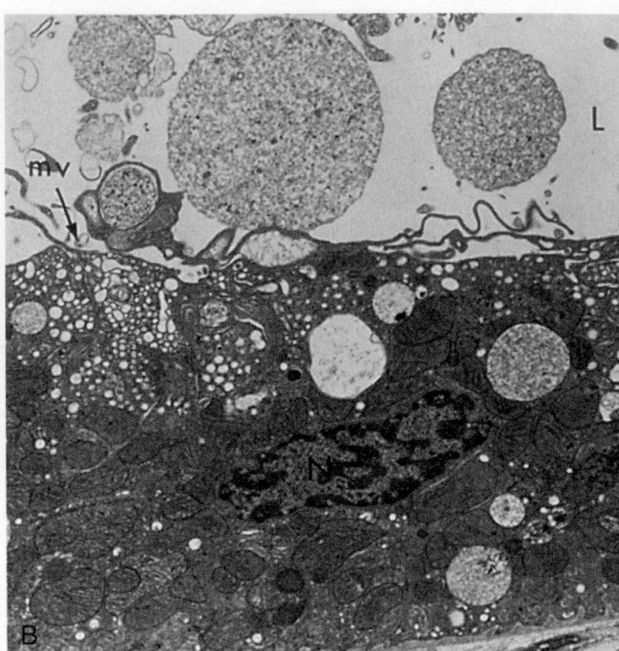

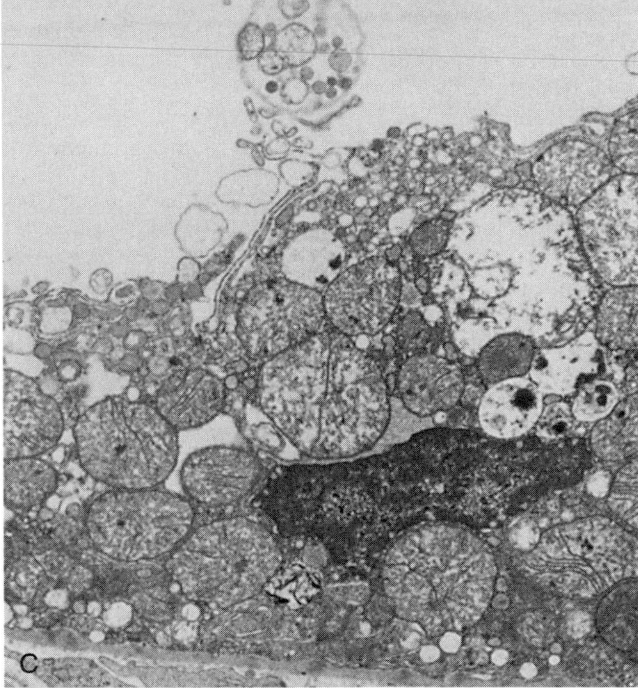

Figure 1–7 ■

A, Electron micrograph of a normal epithelial cell of the proximal kidney tubule. Note abundant microvilli (mv) lining the lumen (L). N, nucleus; V, apical vacuoles (which are normal structures in this cell type). *B*, Epithelial cell of the proximal tubule showing reversible ischemic changes. The microvilli (mv) are lost and have been incorporated in apical cytoplasm; blebs have formed and are extruded in the lumen (L). Mitochondria are slightly dilated. (Compare with *A*.) *C*, Proximal tubular cell showing irreversible ischemic injury. Note the markedly swollen mitochondria containing amorphous densities, disrupted cell membranes, and dense pyknotic nucleus. (Courtesy of Dr. M.A. Venkatachalam, University of Texas, San Antonio, TX.)

dation is likely to be due to activation of endogenous phospholipases by ischemia-induced increases of cytosolic calcium.[10, 11] Phospholipid loss can also occur secondary to decreased ATP-dependent reacylation or diminished de novo synthesis of phospholipids (Fig. 1–8).

3. *Cytoskeletal abnormalities*. Cytoskeletal filaments serve as anchors connecting the plasma membranes to the cell interior. Activation of proteases by increased cytosolic calcium may cause damage to elements of the cytoskeleton.[12] In the presence of cell swelling, this damage results, particularly in myocardial cells, in detachment of the cell membrane from the cytoskeleton, rendering it susceptible to stretching and rupture.
4. *Reactive oxygen species*. Partially reduced oxygen free radicals are highly toxic molecules that cause injury to cell membranes and other cell constituents.[13] Such free radicals are present at low levels in myocardium during ischemia, but there is an increase in free radical production *on restoration of blood flow* (see Ischemia/Reperfusion Injury).
5. *Lipid breakdown products*. These include unesterified

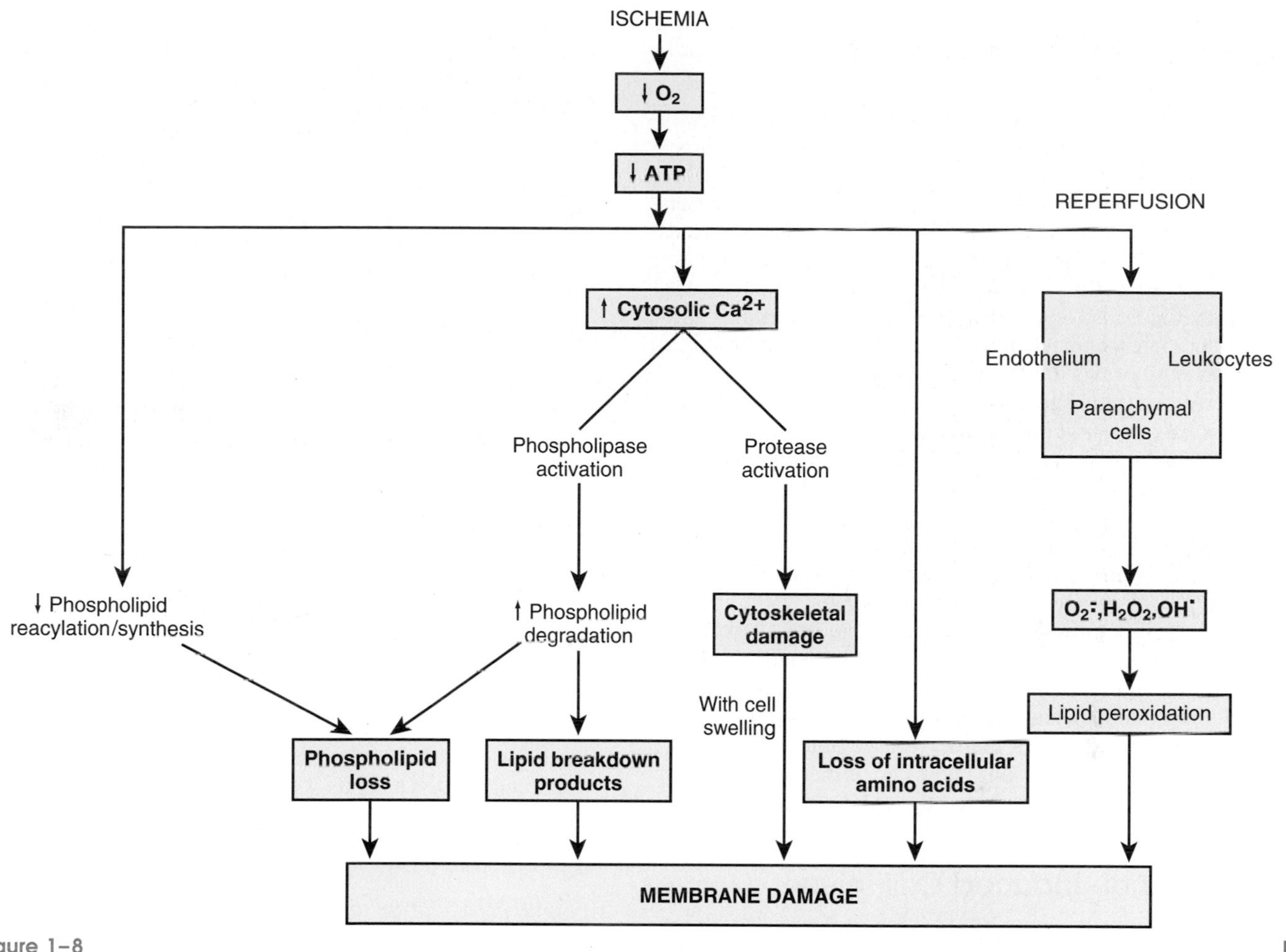

Figure 1–8 ■

Mechanisms of membrane damage in ischemia and reperfusion.

free fatty acids, acyl carnitine, and lysophospholipids, catabolic products that are known to accumulate in ischemic cells as a result of phospholipid degradation. They have a detergent effect on membranes. They also either insert into the lipid bilayer of the membrane or exchange with membrane phospholipids, potentially causing changes in permeability and electrophysiologic alterations.[7]

6. *Loss of intracellular amino acids.* Addition of certain amino acids, principally glycine, protects hypoxic cells from irreversible membrane damage in vitro, suggesting that loss of such amino acids—which occurs in hypoxia—predisposes to membrane structural injury.[14] Glycine also enables ATP-depleted cells to resist the lethal effects of high calcium and thus remain viable.[14a]

Whatever the mechanism of membrane injury, the resultant loss of membrane integrity causes further influx of calcium from the extracellular space. When, in addition, the ischemic tissue is reperfused to some extent, as may occur in vivo, the scene is set for massive influx of calcium. Calcium is taken up avidly by mitochondria after reoxygenation and permanently poisons them, inhibits cellular enzymes, denatures proteins, and causes the cytologic alterations characteristic of coagulative necrosis.[3, 11]

In summary, hypoxia affects oxidative phosphorylation and hence the synthesis of vital ATP supplies. Membrane damage is critical to the development of lethal cell injury, and calcium is an important mediator of the biochemical and morphologic alterations leading to cell death.

ISCHEMIA/REPERFUSION INJURY

Restoration of blood flow to ischemic tissues can result in recovery of cells if they are reversibly injured, or not affect the outcome if irreversible cell damage has occurred. However, depending on the intensity and duration of the ischemic insult, variable numbers of cells may proceed to die *after* blood flow resumes, by necrosis as well as by apoptosis.[15–17] The affected tissues often show neutrophilic infiltrates.[18, 19] As noted earlier, this ischemia/reperfusion injury is a clinically important process in such conditions as myocardial infarction and stroke and may be amenable to therapeutic interventions.

How does reperfusion injury occur? One possibility is that a number of ischemic cells are structurally intact, that is, not necrotic as yet, but are biochemically compromised nevertheless and lose integrity during reperfusion. Another is that *new damaging processes* are set in motion during reperfusion, causing the death of cells that might have recovered otherwise. Several mechanisms have been proposed.

- New damage may be initiated during reoxygenation by increased generation of *oxygen free radicals* by parenchymal and endothelial cells and infiltrating leukocytes.[18, 19] Superoxide anions can be produced in reperfused tissue as a result of incomplete and vicarious reduction of oxygen by damaged mitochondria or because of the action of oxidases derived from leukocytes, endothelial cells, or parenchymal cells.[2, 20] Cellular antioxidant defense mechanisms may also be compromised by ischemia, favoring the accumulation of radicals.
- Reactive oxygen species can further promote the *mitochondrial permeability transition,* referred to earlier, which, when it occurs, precludes mitochondrial energization and cellular ATP recovery and leads to cell death.[9, 21]
- Ischemic injury is associated with the production of *cytokines and increased expression of adhesion molecules* by hypoxic parenchymal and endothelial cells. These agents recruit circulating polymorphonuclear leukocytes to reperfused tissue; the ensuing inflammation causes additional injury (Chapter 3). The importance of neutrophil influx in reperfusion injury has been demonstrated by experimental studies that have used anti-inflammatory interventions, such as antibodies to either cytokines or adhesion molecules, to reduce the extent of the injury.[22]

Free Radical–Induced Cell Injury

One important mechanism of membrane damage, alluded to in the discussion of reperfusion injury, is injury induced by free radicals, particularly by activated oxygen species. It contributes to such varied processes as chemical and radiation injury, oxygen and other gaseous toxicity, cellular aging, microbial killing by phagocytic cells, inflammatory damage, tumor destruction by macrophages, and others[23, 24] (see Fig. 1–2).

Free radicals are chemical species that have a single unpaired electron in an outer orbit. Energy created by this unstable configuration is released through reactions with adjacent molecules, such as inorganic or organic chemicals—proteins, lipids, carbohydrates—particularly with key molecules in membranes and nucleic acids. Moreover, free radicals initiate autocatalytic reactions whereby molecules with which they react are themselves converted into free radicals to propagate the chain of damage.

Free radicals may be *initiated* within cells by

- *Absorption of radiant energy* (e.g., ultraviolet light, x-rays). For example, ionizing radiation can hydrolyze water into hydroxyl ($OH^{\bullet}$) and hydrogen ($H^{\bullet}$) free radicals.[25]
- *Enzymatic metabolism of exogenous chemicals or drugs* (e.g., carbon tetrachloride [CCl_4] can generate [$CCl_3^{\bullet}$], described later in this chapter).
- *The reduction-oxidation reactions that occur during normal metabolic processes.* For example, during normal respiration, molecular oxygen is sequentially reduced by the addition of four electrons to generate water. In this process, small amounts of toxic intermediates are produced; these include *superoxide anion radical ($O_2^{-}\cdot$), hydrogen peroxide (H_2O_2),* and *hydroxyl ions ($OH^{\bullet}$)* (Fig. 1–9). Rapid bursts of superoxide production occur in activated polymorphonuclear leukocytes during inflammation. This occurs by a precisely controlled reaction in a plasma membrane multiprotein complex that uses NADPH oxidase for the redox reaction (Chapter 3). In addition, some intracellular oxidases (such as xanthine oxidase) generate superoxide radicals as a consequence of their activity.
- *Transition metals* such as iron and copper donate or accept free electrons during intracellular reactions and catalyze free radical formation, as in the Fenton reaction ($H_2O_2 + Fe^{2+} \rightarrow Fe^{3+} + OH^{\bullet} + OH^{-}$) (Fig. 1–9). Because most of the intracellular free iron is in the ferric (Fe^{3+}) state, it must be first reduced to the ferrous (Fe^{2+}) form to participate in the Fenton reaction. This reduction can be enhanced by superoxide, and *thus sources of iron and superoxide are required for maximal oxidative cell damage.*
- *Nitric oxide* (NO), an important chemical mediator generated by endothelial cells, macrophages, neurons, and other cell types (Chapter 3), can act as a free radical and can also be converted to highly reactive peroxynitrite anion ($ONOO^{-}$) as well as $NO_2^{\bullet}$ and NO_3^{-}.

The effects of these reactive species are wide-ranging, but three reactions are particularly relevant to cell injury.

1. *Lipid peroxidation of membranes.* Free radicals in the presence of oxygen may cause peroxidation of lipids within plasma and organellar membranes. Oxidative damage is *initiated* when the double bonds in unsaturated fatty acids of membrane lipids are attacked by oxygen-derived free radicals, particularly by $OH^{\bullet}$.[26] The lipid-radical interactions yield peroxides, which are themselves unstable and reactive, and an autocatalytic chain reaction ensues (called *propagation*), which can result in extensive membrane, organellar, and cellular damage. Other more favorable *termination* options take place when the free radical is captured by a scavenger, such as vitamin E, embedded in the cell membrane.
2. *Oxidative modification of proteins.* Free radicals promote oxidation of amino acid residue side chains, formation of protein-protein cross-linkages (e.g., sulfhydryl mediated), and oxidation of the protein backbone resulting in protein fragmentation.[27] Oxidative modification enhances degradation of critical enzymes by the multicatalytic proteasome complex,[28] raising havoc throughout the cell.
3. *Lesions in DNA.* Reactions with thymine in nuclear and mitochondrial DNA produce single-stranded breaks in DNA. This DNA damage has been implicated in cell aging (Chapter 2) and in malignant transformation of cells (Chapter 8).

Cells have developed multiple mechanisms to remove free radicals and thereby minimize injury. Free radicals are

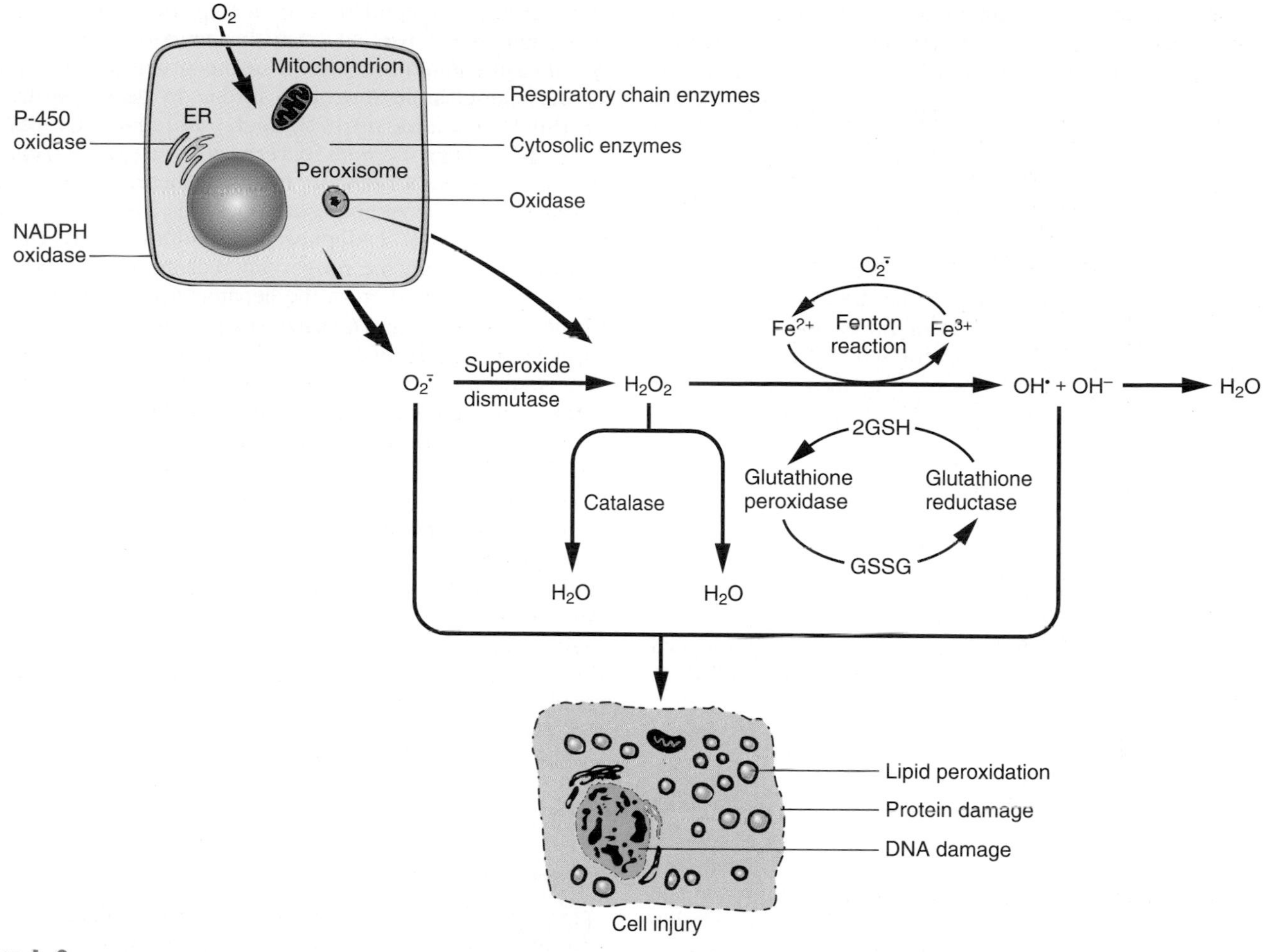

Figure 1–9

Formation of reactive oxygen species and antioxidant mechanisms in biologic systems. O_2 is converted to superoxide ($O_2^{\bar{\cdot}}$) by oxidative enzymes in the endoplasmic reticulum (ER), mitochondria, plasma membrane, peroxisomes, and cytosol. $O_2^{\bar{\cdot}}$ is converted to H_2O_2 by dismutation and thence to $OH^{\cdot}$ by the Cu^{2+}/Fe^{2+}–catalyzed Fenton reaction. H_2O_2 is also derived directly from oxidases in peroxisomes. Not shown is another potentially injurious radical, singlet oxygen. Resultant free radical damage to lipid (peroxidation), proteins, and DNA leads to various forms of cell injury. Note that superoxide catalyzes the reduction of Fe^{3+} to Fe^{2+}, thus enhancing $OH^{\cdot}$ generation by the Fenton reaction. The major antioxidant enzymes are superoxide dismutase, catalase, and glutathione peroxidase. GSH, reduced glutathione; GSSG, oxidized glutathione; NADPH, reduced form of nicotinamide adenine dinucleotide phosphate.

inherently unstable and generally decay spontaneously. Superoxide, for example, is unstable and decays (dismutes) spontaneously into oxygen and hydrogen peroxide in the presence of water. There are, however, several nonenzymatic and enzymatic systems that contribute to inactivation of free radical reactions. These include the following:

- *Antioxidants,* which either block the initiation of free radical formation or inactivate (e.g., scavenge) free radicals and terminate radical damage. Examples are the lipid-soluble vitamins E and A as well as ascorbic acid and glutathione in the cytosol.
- As we have seen, iron and copper can catalyze the formation of reactive oxygen species. The levels of these reactive forms are minimized by binding of the ions to storage and transport proteins (e.g., *transferrin, ferritin, lactoferrin,* and *ceruloplasmin*), thereby minimizing $OH^{\cdot}$ formation.
- A series of *enzymes* act as free radical–scavenging systems and break down hydrogen peroxide and superoxide anion. These enzymes are located near the sites of generation of these oxidants and include the following:
  - *Catalase,* present in peroxisomes, which decomposes H_2O_2 ($2\ H_2O_2 \rightarrow O_2 + 2\ H_2O$).
  - *Superoxide dismutases* are found in many cell types and convert superoxide to H_2O_2 ($2\ O_2^{\bar{\cdot}} + 2\ H \rightarrow H_2O_2 + O_2$). This group includes both manganese–superoxide dismutase, which is localized in mitochondria, and copper-zinc–superoxide dismutase, which is found in the cytosol.
  - *Glutathione peroxidase* also protects against injury by catalyzing free radical breakdown ($H_2O_2 + 2\ GSH \rightarrow$

GSSG [glutathione homodimer] + 2 H_2O, or 2 $OH^•$ + 2 GSH → GSSG + 2 H_2O). The intracellular ratio of oxidized glutathione (GSSG) to reduced glutathione (GSH) is a reflection of the oxidative state of the cell and is an important aspect of the cell's ability to detoxify reactive oxygen species.

In many pathologic processes, the final effects induced by free radicals depend on the net balance between free radical formation and termination. As stated earlier, free radicals are now thought to be involved in many pathologic and physiologic processes, to be reviewed throughout this book. We now discuss certain forms of chemical injury because the toxicity of several chemicals and drugs can be attributed either to conversion of these chemicals to free radicals or to the formation of oxygen-derived metabolites.

CHEMICAL INJURY

The mechanisms by which chemicals, certain drugs, and toxins produce injury are described in greater detail in Chapter 10 in the discussion of environmental disease. Here we will describe two forms of chemically induced injury as examples for the sequence of events leading to cell death.

Chemicals induce cell injury by one of two general mechanisms.[29]

- Some chemicals can act *directly* by combining with some critical molecular component or cellular organelle. For example, in *mercuric chloride poisoning*, mercury binds to the sulfhydryl groups of the cell membrane and other proteins, causing increased membrane permeability and inhibition of ATPase-dependent transport. In such instances, the greatest damage is usually to the cells that use, absorb, excrete, or concentrate the chemicals—in the case of mercuric chloride, the cells of the gastrointestinal tract and kidney. *Cyanide* poisons mitochondrial cytochrome oxidase and blocks oxidative phosphorylation. Many antineoplastic chemotherapeutic agents and antibiotic drugs also induce cell damage by direct cytotoxic effects.
- Most other chemicals are not biologically active but must be converted to reactive toxic metabolites, which then act on target cells. This modification is usually accomplished by the P-450 mixed function oxidases in the smooth endoplasmic reticulum of the liver and other organs.[30] Although these metabolites might cause membrane damage and cell injury by *direct covalent binding* to membrane protein and lipids, by far the most important mechanism of membrane injury involves the formation of *reactive free radicals* and subsequent lipid peroxidation.

Carbon tetrachloride (CCl_4) is used widely in the dry-cleaning industry. The toxic effect of CCl_4 is due to its conversion by P-450 to the *highly reactive toxic free radical* $CCl_3^•$ ($CCl_4 + e \rightarrow CCl_3^• + Cl^-$). The free radicals produced locally cause auto-oxidation of the polyenic fatty acids present within the membrane phospholipids. There, oxidative decomposition of the lipid is initiated, and organic peroxides are formed after reacting with oxygen (lipid peroxidation). This *reaction is autocatalytic* in that new radicals are formed from the peroxide radicals themselves. Thus, rapid breakdown of the structure and function of the endoplasmic reticulum is due to decomposition of the lipid. *It is no surprise, therefore, that CCl_4-induced liver cell injury is both severe and extremely rapid in onset.* Within less than 30 minutes, there is a decline in hepatic protein synthesis; and within 2 hours, there is swelling of smooth endoplasmic reticulum and dissociation of ribosomes from the rough endoplasmic reticulum[31] (Fig. 1–10). Lipid export from the hepatocytes is reduced owing to their inability to synthesize apoprotein to complex with triglycerides and thereby facilitate lipoprotein secretion. The result is the fatty liver of CCl_4 poisoning (Fig. 1–11). Mitochondrial injury then occurs, and this is followed by progressive swelling of the cells due to increased permeability of the plasma membrane. Plasma membrane damage is thought to be caused by relatively stable fatty aldehydes, which are produced by lipid peroxidation in the smooth endoplasmic reticulum but are able to act at distant sites. This is followed by massive influx of calcium and cell death (Fig. 1–11).

Acetaminophen (Tylenol), a commonly used analgesic drug, is detoxified in the liver through sulfation and glucuronidation, and small amounts are converted by cytochrome P-450–catalyzed oxidation to an electrophilic, highly toxic metabolite. This metabolite itself is detoxified by interac-

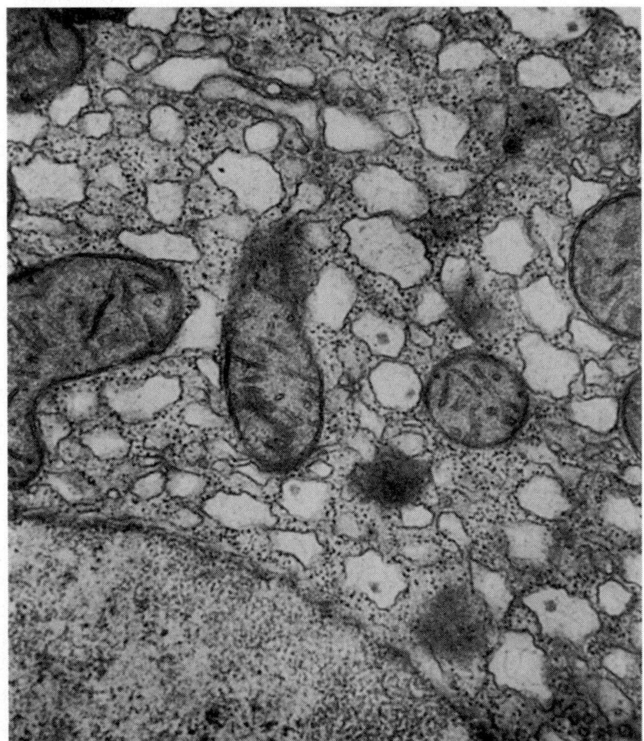

Figure 1–10

Rat liver cell 4 hours after carbon tetrachloride intoxication, with swelling of endoplasmic reticulum and shedding of ribosomes. At this stage, mitochondria are unaltered. (Courtesy of Dr. O. Iseri, University of Maryland, Baltimore, MD.)

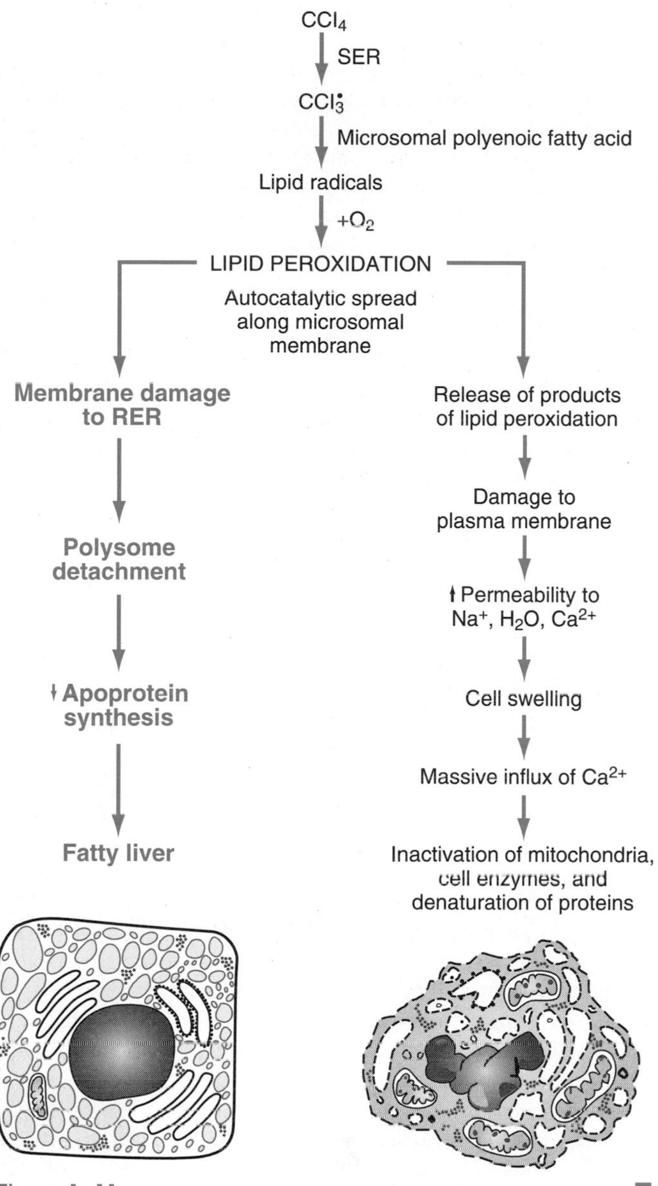

Figure 1–11

Sequence of events leading to fatty change and cell necrosis in carbon tetrachloride (CCl_4) toxicity. RER, rough endoplasmic reticulum; SER, smooth endoplasmic reticulum.

tion with GSH. When large doses of the drug are ingested, GSH is depleted, and thus the toxic metabolites accumulate in the cell, destroy nucleophilic macromolecules, and covalently bind proteins and nucleic acids. The decrease in GSH concentration, coupled with covalent binding of toxic metabolites, increases drug toxicity, resulting in massive liver cell necrosis, usually 3 to 5 days after the ingestion of toxic doses. This hepatotoxicity correlates with lipid peroxidation and can be reduced by administration of antioxidants, suggesting that the oxidative damage may be more important than covalent binding in the ultimate toxicity of the drug.[32]

Morphology of Reversible Cell Injury and Necrosis

All stresses and noxious influences exert their effects first at the molecular level. The time lag required to produce the morphologic changes of cell injury or death varies with the sensitivity of the methods used to detect these changes. With histochemical or ultrastructural techniques, changes may be seen in minutes to hours after ischemic injury; however, it may take considerably longer (hours to days) before changes can be seen by light microscopy or on gross examination.

REVERSIBLE INJURY

Two patterns of reversible cell injury can be recognized under the light microscope: *cellular swelling* and *fatty change*. Cellular swelling appears whenever cells are incapable of maintaining ionic and fluid homeostasis; its pathogenesis has been described earlier. Fatty change occurs in hypoxic injury and various forms of toxic or metabolic injury. It is manifested by the appearance of small or large lipid vacuoles in the cytoplasm and occurs in hypoxic and various forms of toxic injury. It is principally encountered in cells involved in and dependent on fat metabolism, such as the hepatocyte and myocardial cell (Chapter 2).

MORPHOLOGY. Cellular swelling is the first manifestation of almost all forms of injury to cells. It is a difficult morphologic change to appreciate with the light microscope; it may be more apparent at the level of the whole organ. When it affects all cells in an organ, it causes some pallor, increased turgor, and increase in weight of the organ. On microscopic examination, small clear vacuoles may be seen within the cytoplasm; these represent distended and pinched-off segments of the endoplasmic reticulum. This pattern of nonlethal injury is sometimes called **hydropic change** or **vacuolar degeneration.** Swelling of cells is reversible.

The ultrastructural changes of reversible cell injury previously described (see Figs. 1–6 and 1–7) include (1) **plasma membrane alterations**, such as blebbing, blunting, and distortion of microvilli; creation of myelin figures; and loosening of intercellular attachments; (2) **mitochondrial changes**, including swelling, rarefaction, and the appearance of small phospholipid-rich amorphous densities; (3) **dilation of the endoplasmic reticulum** with detachment and disaggregation of polysomes; and (4) **nuclear alterations**, with disaggregation of granular and fibrillar elements.

NECROSIS

Necrosis refers to a spectrum of morphologic changes that follow cell death in living tissue, largely resulting from the progressive degradative action of enzymes on the lethally injured cell (cells placed immediately in fixative are dead but not necrotic). As commonly used, necrosis is the gross and histologic correlate of cell death occurring in the setting of irreversible exogenous injury. Its most common manifestation is *coagulative necrosis,* characterized by denaturation of cytoplasmic proteins, breakdown of cell organelles, and cell swelling.

The morphologic appearance of necrosis is the result of two essentially concurrent processes: (1) enzymic digestion of the cell and (2) denaturation of proteins. The catalytic enzymes are derived either from the lysosomes of the dead cells themselves, in which case the enzymic digestion is referred to as *autolysis,* or from the lysosomes of immigrant leukocytes, termed *heterolysis.* These processes require hours to develop, and so there would be no detectable changes in cells if, for example, a myocardial infarct caused sudden death. The only telling evidence might be occlusion of a coronary artery. The earliest histologic evidence of myocardial necrosis does not become manifest until 4 to 12 hours later, but loss of cardiac-specific enzymes and proteins from necrotic muscle can be detected in the bloodstream as early as 2 hours after myocardial cell death (Fig. 1–12).

MORPHOLOGY. The necrotic cells show **increased eosinophilia** attributable in part to loss of the normal basophilia imparted by the RNA in the cytoplasm and in part to the increased binding of eosin to denatured intracytoplasmic proteins (Fig. 1–12*B*). The cell may have a more glassy homogeneous appearance than that of normal cells, mainly as a result of the loss of glycogen particles. When enzymes have digested the cytoplasmic organelles, the cytoplasm becomes vacuolated and appears moth-eaten. Finally, calcification of the dead cells may occur. By electron microscopy, necrotic cells are characterized by overt discontinuities in plasma and organelle membranes, marked dilation of mitochondria with the appearance of large amorphous densities, intracytoplasmic myelin figures, amorphous osmiophilic debris, and aggregates of fluffy material probably representing denatured protein (see Fig. 1–7*C*).

Nuclear changes appear in the form of one of three patterns, all due to nonspecific breakdown of DNA (see Fig. 1–6*C*). The basophilia of the chromatin may fade (**karyolysis**), a change that presumably reflects DNase activity. A second pattern (also seen in apoptotic cell death) is **pyknosis**, characterized by nuclear shrinkage and increased basophilia. Here the DNA apparently condenses into a solid, shrunken basophilic mass. In the third pattern, known as **karyorrhexis**, the pyknotic or partially pyknotic nucleus undergoes fragmentation. With the passage of time (a day or two), the nucleus in the necrotic cell totally disappears.

Once the necrotic cells have undergone the early alterations described, the mass of necrotic cells may have several morphologic patterns. Although the terms are somewhat outmoded, they are routinely used and their meanings are understood by both pathologists and clinicians. When denaturation is the primary pattern, **coagulative necrosis** develops. In the instance of dominant enzyme digestion, the result is **liquefactive necrosis;** in special circumstances, **caseous necrosis and fat necrosis** may occur.

Coagulative necrosis implies preservation of the basic outline of the coagulated cell for a span of at least some days (Fig. 1–13*A*). The affected tissues exhibit a firm texture. Presumably, the injury or the subsequent increasing intracellular acidosis denatures not only structural proteins but also enzymic proteins and so blocks the proteolysis of the cell. The myocardial infarct is an excellent exam-

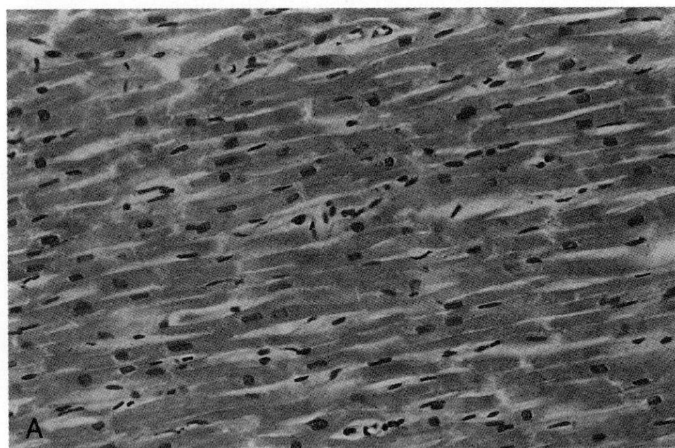

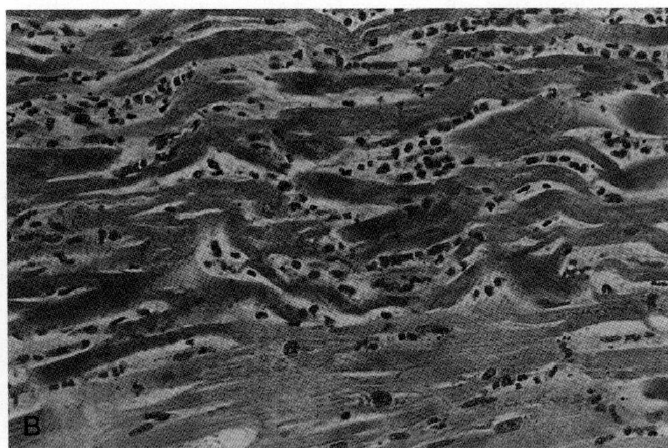

Figure 1–12

A, Normal myocardium. *B,* Myocardium with coagulation necrosis (upper two thirds of figure), showing strongly eosinophilic anucleate myocardial fibers. Leukocytes in the interstitium are an early reaction to necrotic muscle. Compare with *A* and with normal fibers in the lower part of the figure.

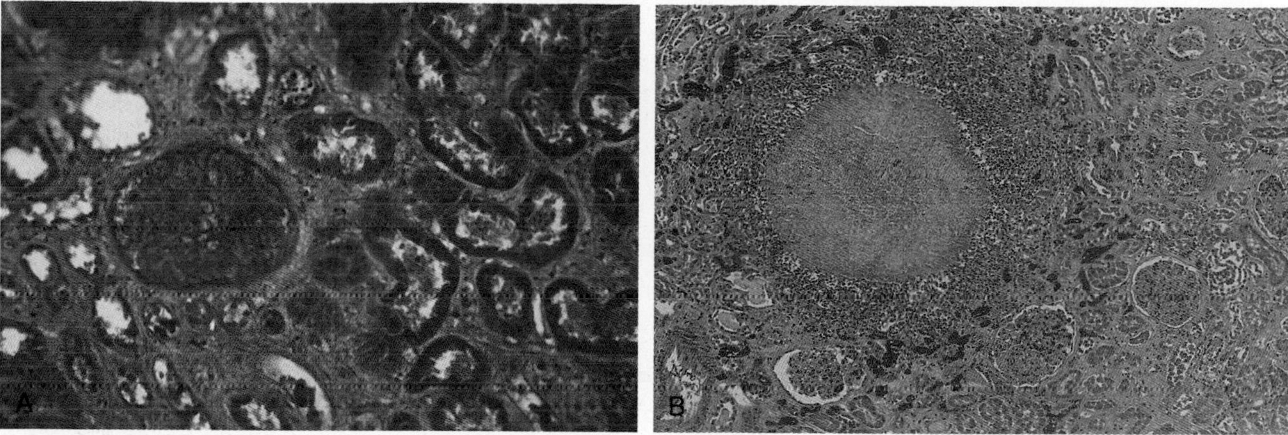

Figure 1–13

Coagulative and liquefactive necrosis. *A*, Kidney infarct exhibiting coagulative necrosis, with loss of nuclei and clumping of cytoplasm but with preservation of basic outlines of glomerular and tubular architecture. *B*, A focus of liquefactive necrosis in the kidney caused by fungal seeding. The focus is filled with white cells and cellular debris, creating a renal abscess that obliterates the normal architecture.

ple in which acidophilic, coagulated, anucleated cells may persist for weeks. Ultimately, the necrotic myocardial cells are removed by fragmentation and phagocytosis of the cellular debris by scavenger white cells and by the action of proteolytic lysosomal enzymes brought in by the immigrant white cells. The process of coagulative necrosis, with preservation of the general tissue architecture, is characteristic of hypoxic death of cells in all tissues except the brain.

Liquefactive necrosis is characteristic of focal bacterial or occasionally fungal infections, because these agents constitute powerful stimuli to the accumulation of inflammatory cells (Fig. 1–13*B*). For obscure reasons, hypoxic death of cells within the central nervous system often evokes liquefactive necrosis. Whatever the pathogenesis, liquefaction completely digests the dead cells. The end result is transformation of the tissue into a liquid viscous mass. If the process had been initiated by acute inflammation (Chapter 3), the material is frequently creamy yellow because of the presence of dead white cells and is called pus. Although **gangrenous necrosis** is not a distinctive pattern of cell death, the term is still commonly used in surgical clinical practice. It is usually applied to a limb, generally the lower leg, that has lost its blood supply and has undergone coagulation necrosis. When bacterial infection is superimposed, coagulative necrosis is modified by the liquefactive action of the bacteria and the attracted leukocytes (so-called wet gangrene).

Caseous necrosis, a distinctive form of coagulative necrosis, is encountered most often in foci of tuberculous infection (Chapter 9). The term caseous is derived from the gross appearance (white and cheesy) of the area of necrosis (Fig. 1–14). On microscopic examination, the necrotic focus appears as amorphous granular debris seemingly composed of fragmented, coagulated cells and amorphous granular debris enclosed within a distinctive inflammatory border known as a granulomatous reaction (Chapter 3). Unlike coagulative necrosis, the tissue architecture is completely obliterated.

Fat necrosis is a term that is well fixed in medical parlance but does not in reality denote a specific pattern of necrosis. Rather, it is descriptive of focal areas of fat destruction, typically occurring as a result of release of activated pancreatic lipases into the substance of the pancreas and the peritoneal cavity. This occurs in the calamitous abdominal emergency known as acute pan-

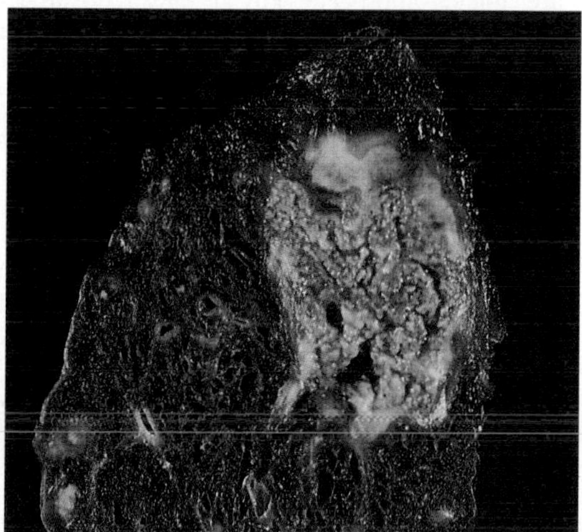

Figure 1–14

A tuberculous lung with a large area of caseous necrosis. The caseous debris is yellow-white and cheesy.

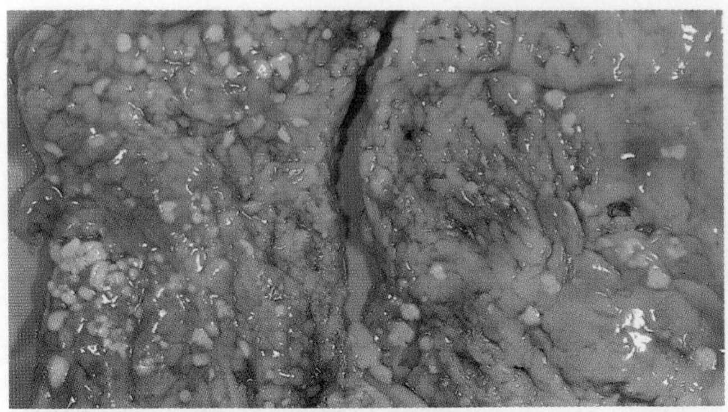

Figure 1–15

Foci of fat necrosis with saponification in the mesentery. The areas of white chalky deposits represent calcium soap formation at sites of lipid breakdown.

creatitis (Chapter 20). In this disorder, activated pancreatic enzymes escape from acinar cells and ducts; the activated enzymes liquefy fat cell membranes, and the activated lipases split the triglyceride esters contained within fat cells. The released fatty acids combine with calcium to produce grossly visible chalky white areas (fat saponification), which enable the surgeon and the pathologist to identify the lesions (Fig. 1–15). On histologic examination, the necrosis takes the form of foci of shadowy outlines of necrotic fat cells, with basophilic calcium deposits, surrounded by an inflammatory reaction.

Ultimately, in the living patient, most necrotic cells and their debris disappear by a combined process of enzymic digestion and fragmentation, with phagocytosis of the particulate debris by leukocytes. If necrotic cells and cellular debris are not promptly destroyed and reabsorbed, they tend to attract calcium salts and other minerals and to become calcified. This phenomenon, called *dystrophic calcification*, is considered in Chapter 2.

APOPTOSIS

This morphologic pattern of cell injury, long recognized by pathologists, is now accepted as a distinctive and important mode of cell death. Although several features distinguish apoptosis from coagulative necrosis (Fig. 1–16), it overlaps and shares certain common mechanisms with necrotic cell death. In addition, at least some types of cell death are expressed either as apoptosis or necrosis, depending on the intensity and duration of the stimulus, the rapidity of the death process, and the extent of ATP depletion suffered by the cell.

Definition and Causes

Apoptosis was initially recognized in 1972 by its distinctive morphology and named after the Greek designation for "falling off."[33, 33a] It is a form of cell death designed to eliminate unwanted host cells through activation of a coordinated, internally programmed series of events effected by a dedicated set of gene products. It occurs in the following general settings: (1) during development; (2) as a homeostatic mechanism to maintain cell populations in tissues; (3) as a defense mechanism such as in immune reactions; (4) when cells are damaged by disease or noxious agents; and (5) in aging.[34, 35] It is responsible for numerous physiologic, adaptive, and pathologic events, including the following:

- *The programmed destruction of cells during embryogenesis,* including implantation, organogenesis, developmental involution, and metamorphosis. Although apoptosis is a morphologic event, which may not always underlie the functionally defined "programmed cell death" of embryologists, the terms are currently used synonymously by most workers.
- *Hormone-dependent involution in the adult,* such as endometrial cell breakdown during the menstrual cycle, ovarian follicular atresia in the menopause, the regression of the lactating breast after weaning, and prostatic atrophy after castration.

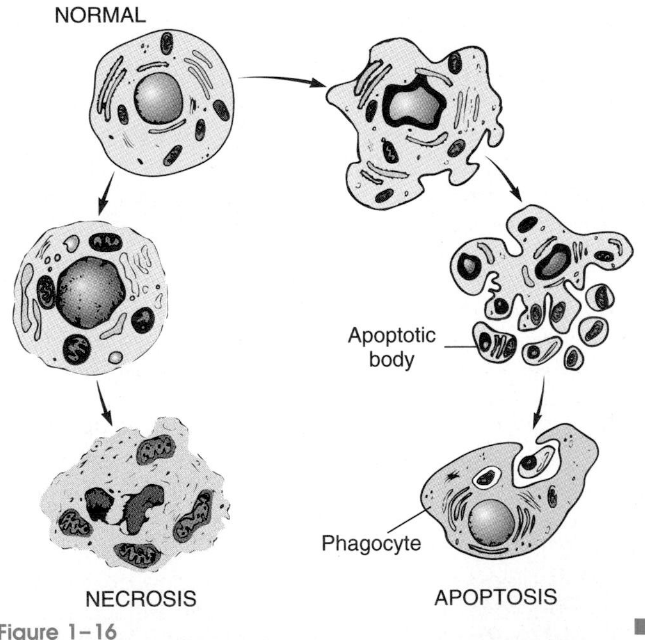

Figure 1–16

The sequential ultrastructural changes seen in coagulation necrosis *(left)* and apoptosis *(right)*. In apoptosis, the initial changes consist of nuclear chromatin condensation and fragmentation, followed by cytoplasmic budding and phagocytosis of the extruded apoptotic bodies. Signs of *coagulation necrosis* include chromatin clumping, organellar swelling, and eventual membrane damage. (Adapted from Walker NI, et al: Patterns of cell death. Methods Archiv Exp Pathol 13:18–32, 1988. Reproduced with permission of S. Karger AG, Basel.)

- *Cell deletion in proliferating cell populations,* such as intestinal crypt epithelia.
- *Cell death in tumors,* most frequently during regression but also in tumors with active cell growth.
- Death of neutrophils during an *acute inflammatory response.*
- *Death of immune cells,* both B and T lymphocytes after cytokine depletion, as well as deletion of autoreactive T cells in the developing thymus.
- *Cell death induced by cytotoxic T cells,* such as in cellular immune rejection and graft-versus-host disease.
- *Pathologic atrophy in parenchymal organs after duct obstruction,* such as occurs in the pancreas, parotid gland, and kidney.
- *Cell injury in certain viral diseases,* as for example in viral hepatitis, in which apoptotic cells in the liver are known as *Councilman bodies.*
- *Cell death produced by a variety of injurious stimuli* that are capable of producing necrosis, but when given in low doses. For example, heat, radiation, cytotoxic anticancer drugs, and hypoxia can induce apoptosis if the insult is mild, but large doses of the same stimuli result in necrotic cell death.

Before the mechanisms of apoptosis are discussed, we describe the morphologic and biochemical events characteristic of this process.

MORPHOLOGY. The following morphologic features, some best seen with the electron microscope, characterize cells undergoing apoptosis (Fig. 1–16).

- **Cell shrinkage.** The cell is smaller in size; the cytoplasm is dense; and the organelles, although relatively normal, are more tightly packed.
- **Chromatin condensation.** This is the most characteristic feature of apoptosis. The chromatin aggregates peripherally, under the nuclear membrane, into well-delimited dense masses of various shapes and sizes (Fig. 1–17). The nucleus itself may break up, producing two or more fragments.
- **Formation of cytoplasmic blebs and apoptotic bodies.** The apoptotic cell first shows extensive surface blebbing, then undergoes fragmentation into a number of membrane-bound apoptotic bodies composed of cytoplasm and tightly packed organelles, with or without a nuclear fragment.
- **Phagocytosis of apoptotic cells or bodies** by adjacent healthy cells, either parenchymal cells or macrophages. The apoptotic bodies are rapidly degraded within lysosomes, and the adjacent cells migrate or proliferate to replace the space occupied by the now deleted apoptotic cell.

Plasma membranes are thought to remain intact during apoptosis, until the last stages, when they become permeable to normally retained solutes. This classical description is accurate with respect to apoptosis during physiologic conditions such as embryogenesis and deletion of immune cells. However, indeterminate forms of cell death with features of necrosis as well as of apoptosis are not uncommon after injurious stimuli, described as **secondary necrosis** by Wyllie.[34] Under such conditions, the severity, rather than the specificity of stimulus, determines the form in which death is expressed. If necrotic features are predominant, early plasma membrane damage occurs, and cell swelling, rather than shrinkage, is seen.

On histologic examination, in tissues stained with hematoxylin and eosin, apoptosis involves single cells or small clusters of cells. The apoptotic cell appears as a round or oval mass of intensely eo-

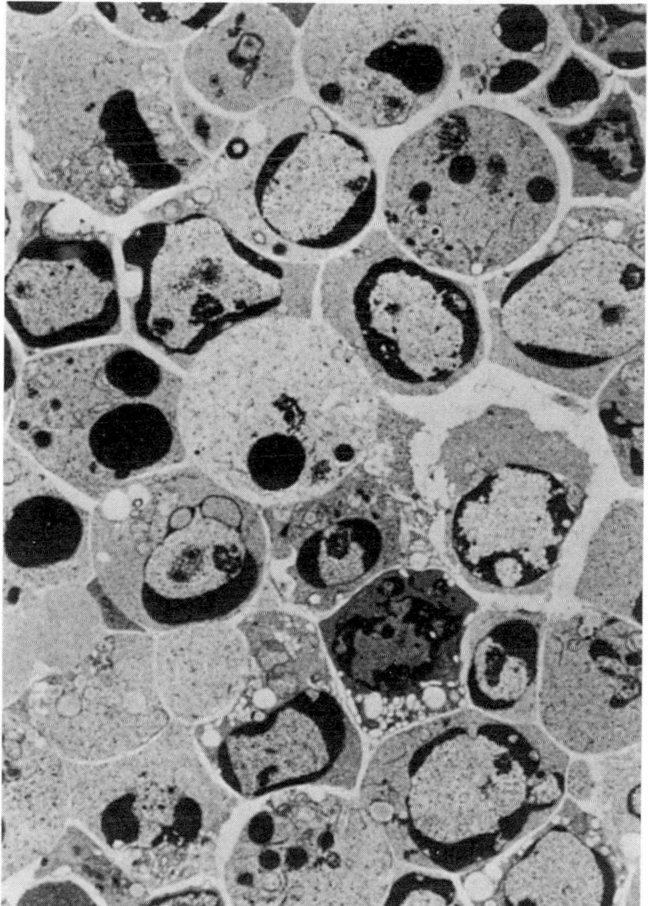

Figure 1–17

Ultrastructural features of apoptosis. Some nuclear fragments show peripheral crescents of compacted chromatin, whereas others are uniformly dense. (From Kerr JFR, Harmon BV: Definition and incidence of apoptosis: a historical perspective. In Tomei LD, Cope FO (eds): Apoptosis: The Molecular Basis of Cell Death. Cold Spring Harbor, NY, Cold Spring Harbor Laboratory Press, 1991, pp 5–29.)

sinophilic cytoplasm with dense nuclear chromatin fragments (Fig. 1–18). Because the cell shrinkage and formation of apoptotic bodies are rapid and the fragments are quickly phagocytosed, degraded, or extruded into the lumen, **considerable apoptosis may occur in tissues before it becomes apparent in histologic sections.** In addition, **apoptosis—in contrast to necrosis—does not elicit inflammation,** making it more difficult to detect histologically.

Biochemical Features

Apoptotic cells usually exhibit a distinctive constellation of biochemical modifications that underlie the structural pathology described before (Fig. 1–18). Some of these features may be seen in necrotic cells also, but other alterations are more specific.

Protein Cleavage. A specific feature of apoptosis is protein hydrolysis involving the activation of several members of a newly discovered family of cysteine proteases named *caspases*.[36] Caspase cleavage of the nuclear scaffold and cytoskeletal proteins (together with protein cross-linking) underlies the distinctive nuclear and cytoplasmic structural alterations seen in apoptotic cells. Caspase activity also triggers endonucleases (see later).

Protein Cross-Linking. Extensive protein cross-linking by transglutaminase activation[37] converts cytoplasmic proteins into covalently linked shrunken shells that may break into apoptotic bodies.

DNA Breakdown. Apoptotic cells exhibit a characteristic breakdown of DNA into large 50- to 300-kilobase pieces.[38] Subsequently, there is internucleosomal cleavage of DNA into oligonucleosomes in multiples of 180 to 200 base pairs by Ca^{2+} and Mg^{2+} dependent endonucleases. The fragments are visualized by agarose gel electrophoresis as DNA ladders (Fig. 1–19). Endonuclease activity also forms the basis for detecting cell death by cytochemical techniques that recognize double-stranded breaks of DNA.[39] However, internucleosomal DNA cleavage is not specific for apoptosis. Moreover, the "smear" pattern of DNA fragmentation thought to be indicative of necrosis may be only a late autolytic phenomenon, and typical DNA ladders may be seen in necrotic cells as well.[39, 40]

Phagocytic Recognition. Apoptotic cells express phosphatidylserine in the outer layers of their plasma membranes, the phospholipid having "flipped" out from the inner layers. In some types of apoptosis, thrombospondin, an adhesive glycoprotein, is also expressed on the surfaces of apoptotic bodies. These alterations permit the early recognition of dead cells by macrophages and adjacent cells for phagocytosis, without the release of proinflammatory cellular components.[41] In this way, the apoptotic response disposes of cells with minimal compromise to the surrounding tissue.

Mechanisms

From examining the conditions in which apoptosis occurs, listed earlier, it can be deduced that apoptosis can be

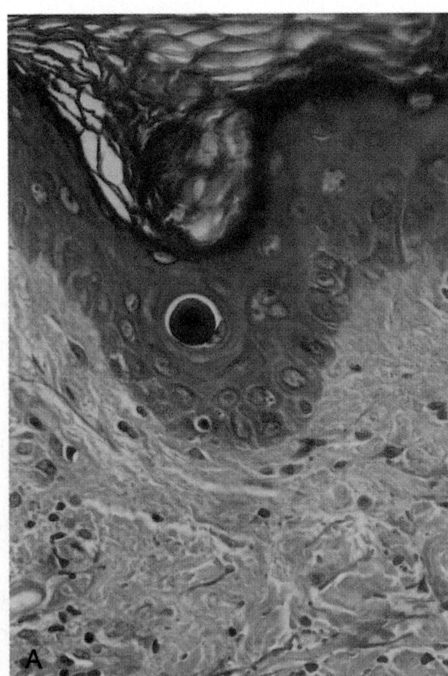

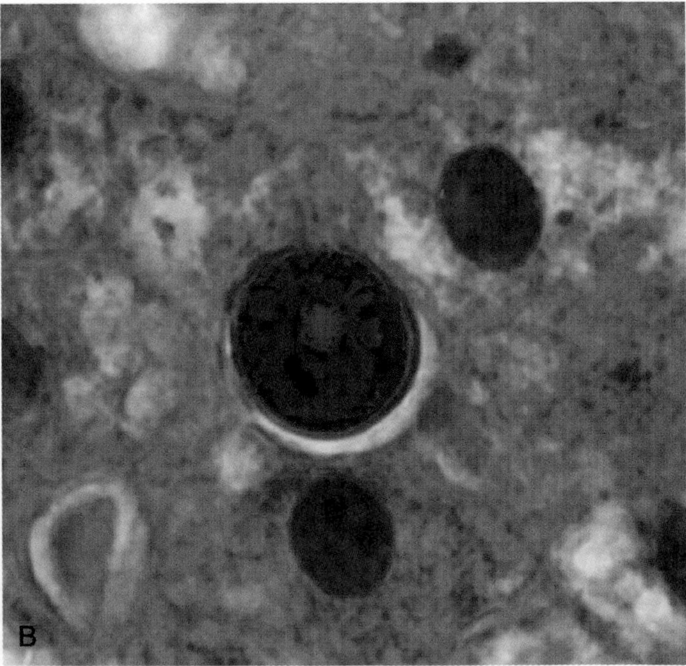

Figure 1–18

A, Apoptosis in the skin in an immune-mediated reaction. The apoptotic cells are visible in the epidermis with intensely eosinophilic cytoplasm and small, dense nuclei. H&E stain. (Courtesy of Dr. Scott Granter, Brigham and Women's Hospital, Boston, MA.) *B*, High power of apoptotic cell in liver in immune-mediated hepatic cell injury. (Courtesy of Dr. Dhanpat Jain, Yale University New Haven, CT.)

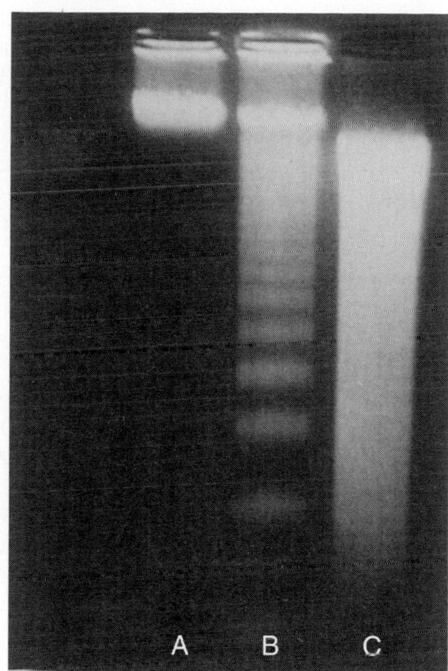

Figure 1–19

Agarose gel electrophoresis of DNA extracted from culture cells. Ethidium bromide stain; photographed under ultraviolet illumination. *Lane A*, Control culture. *Lane B*, Culture showing extensive apoptosis; note ladder pattern of DNA fragment induced by heat. *Lane C*, Culture showing massive necrosis; note diffuse smearing of DNA. *These patterns are characteristic of but not specific for apoptosis and necrosis, respectively.* (From Kerr JFR, Harmon BV: Definition and incidence of apoptosis: a historical perspective. In Tomei LD, Cope FO [eds]: Apoptosis: The Molecular Basis of Cell Death. Cold Spring Harbor, NY, Cold Spring Harbor Laboratory Press, 1991, p 13.)

activated by a variety of death-triggering signals, ranging from a *lack of growth factor or hormone*, to *a positive ligand-receptor interaction*, to *specific injurious agents*. In addition, there is a coordinated but often inverse relationship between cell growth and apoptosis. Indeed, as we shall see in the discussion of cell growth (Chapter 4) and neoplasia (Chapter 8), apoptosis is important in the regulation of normal cell population density, and suppression of cell death by apoptosis is a determinant of the growth of cancer. For these reasons, the mechanisms underlying apoptosis are the subject of intense investigation. Observations made in the nematode *Caenorhabditis elegans*, in which development of the worm pursues a highly reproducible, programmed pattern of cell growth followed by cell death, have greatly enhanced our understanding of the mechanisms; they have allowed the identification of specific genes (the so-called *ced* genes, for *C. elegans* death) and their mammalian counterparts that can either initiate or inhibit cell death.

Apoptosis is the endpoint of an energy-dependent cascade of molecular events, initiated by certain stimuli, and consisting of four separable but overlapping components[42–45] (Fig 1–20):

1. *Signaling pathways* that initiate apoptosis
2. *Control and integration*, in which intracellular positive and negative regulatory molecules inhibit, stimulate, or forestall apoptosis and thus determine the outcome
3. *A common-execution phase* consisting of the actual death program and accomplished largely by the caspase family of proteases
4. *Removal of dead cells* by phagocytosis (Fig. 1–20)

Signaling Pathways. Apoptotic stimuli generate signals that are either transmitted across the plasma membrane to intracellular regulatory molecules or addressed more directly at targets present within the cell.

Transmembrane signals may be negative or positive determinants of apoptosis. For example, certain hormones, growth factors, and cytokines generate signal transduction cascades that suppress preexisting death programs and are thus normal *survival* stimuli. Conversely, absence of some of such factors leads to failure of suppression of death programs and thus triggers apoptosis. Other transmembrane positive regulators of apoptosis are receptor-ligand interactions at the plasma membrane that generate signals to *activate* death programs. The most important examples in this group are death pathways initiated by ligand binding of plasma membrane receptors of the tumor necrosis factor receptor (TNFR) superfamily. Morphogens, growth factors, and differentiation factors involved in embryonic development may act as either positive or negative regulators.

Intracellular signaling may also cause apoptosis. Examples include the binding of glucocorticoids to nuclear receptors; physicochemical agents such as heat, radiation, xenobiotics, and hypoxia; and viral infections.

Control and Integration Stage (Fig. 1–20). This is performed by specific proteins that connect death signals to the execution program. These proteins are important because their actions may result in either "commitment" (i.e., determination of the inevitability of cell death) or abortion of potentially lethal signals. The proteins involved in this regulation have clinical significance: by determining the life or death of cell communities involved in important biologic processes (such as the immune response or cancer), they can affect the outcomes of disease.

There are commonly two broad schemes for this stage, which are not mutually exclusive. One involves the direct transmission of signals by specific *adapter proteins* to the execution mechanism, as described for the Fas–Fas ligand model and target cell killing by cytotoxic T lymphocytes (see later).[46–48] The second involves members of the Bcl-2 family of proteins[49] which play major and ubiquitous roles in apoptotic regulation largely by *regulating mitochondrial function*.[50] As previously described (see Fig. 1–4), death agonists can generate signals that affect mitochondria in two ways (Fig. 1–21):

- Apoptotic signals result in mitochondrial permeability transitions.[50a] Formation of pores within the inner mitochondrial membrane results in reduction of membrane potential and mitochondrial swelling.
- The signals also cause increased permeability of outer mitochondrial membranes, releasing an apoptotic trigger, cytochrome *c*, from mitochondria into the cytosol.[51, 52] Cytochrome *c* is located between the inner and outer

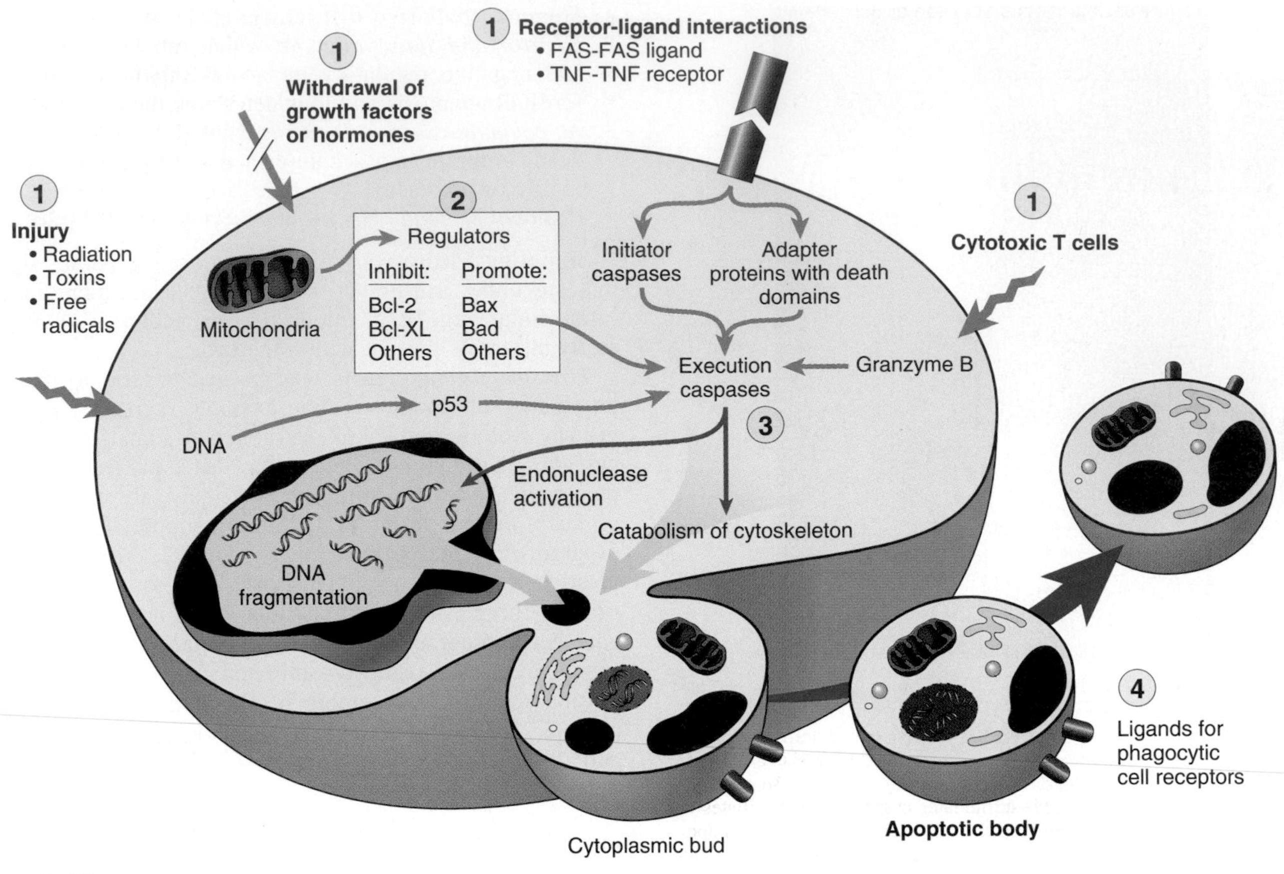

Figure 1–20

Schematic representation of apoptotic events. Labeled (1) are multiple stimuli of apoptosis. These include specific death ligands (tumor necrosis factor [TNF] and Fas ligand), withdrawal of growth factors or hormones, or injurious agents (e.g., radiation). Some stimuli (such as cytotoxic cells) directly activate execution caspases *(right).* Others act by way of adapter proteins and initiator caspases (see Fig. 1–22), or by mitochondrial events involving cytochrome *c.* (2) Control and regulation are influenced by members of the Bcl-2 family of proteins, which can either inhibit or promote the cell's death. (3) Execution caspases activate latent cytoplasmic endonuclease, and proteases that degrade cytoskeletal and nuclear proteins. This results in a cascade of intracellular degradation, including fragmentation of nuclear chromatin and breakdown of the cytoskeleton. Not shown is transglutaminase-induced cross-linking of proteins. (4) The end result is formation of apoptotic bodies containing various intracellular organelles and other cytosolic components; these bodies also express new ligands for binding and uptake by phagocytic cells.

mitochondrial membranes and is an integral but soluble component of the respiratory pathway. *Cytochrome c release precedes the morphologic changes of apoptosis, showing that it occurs early, consistent with a regulatory function.*

Several proteins regulate such mitochondrial permeability events, but the most important are members of the Bcl-2 family, detailed in Chapter 8 and involved in an important way in cancer formation. Bcl-2, the mammalian homolog of the anti-apoptotic *ced-9* gene in *C. elegans,* is situated in the outer mitochondrial membrane, endoplasmic reticulum, and nuclear envelope. Its function is regulated by other family members. By selectively binding to Bcl-2, these related proteins can alter Bcl-2's activities and either promote apoptosis (e.g., Bax, Bad) or inhibit the process (e.g., Bcl-XL). *Bcl-2 suppresses apoptosis in two ways: by direct action on mitochondria to prevent increased permeability, and by effects mediated by interactions with other proteins.* Indeed, it is thought that *mitochondrial permeability is determined by the ratio of pro-apoptotic and anti-apoptotic members of the Bcl-2 family in the membrane.*[49, 50]

In certain cells Bcl-2 can also suppress apoptosis by serving as a *docking protein,* binding proteins from the cytosol and sequestering them on the mitochondrial membrane (Fig. 1–21). Protein binding may modulate the function of Bcl-2 itself or target the docked protein for interaction with other proteins. Notable among these Bcl-2-binding proteins is the *pro-apoptotic protease activating factor (Apaf-1),* the mammalian homolog of the nematode gene ced-4.[53, 54] This protein also associates with inactive zymogen forms of certain *initiator* caspases (e.g., caspase 9), so called to distinguish them from the *execution* caspases described later. It is speculated that when cytochrome *c* is released from mitochondria by death signals, it binds Apaf-1 and activates it, triggering an initiator caspase and setting in motion the proteolytic events that kill the cell (Fig. 1–21). In this scenario, Bcl-2 binding protects because it sequesters Apaf-1 and inhibits its catalytic caspase-triggering function, even if cytochrome *c* has leaked out of mitochondria.

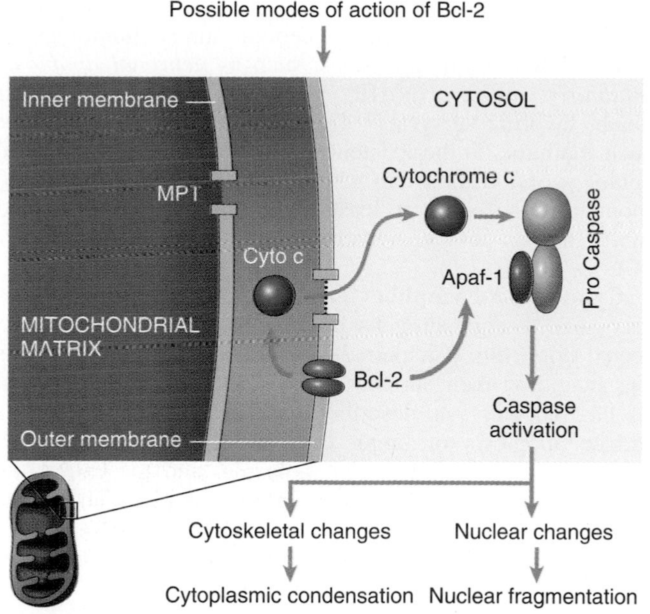

Figure 1–21

Mitochondrial events and the effects of Bcl-2 in apoptosis. Death agonists cause changes in the inner mitochondrial membrane, resulting in the mitochondrial permeability transition (MPT) and release of cytochrome *c* into the cytosol by currently unclear mechanisms. Released cytochrome *c* disrupts the binding between Bcl-2 and pro-apoptotic protease activating factor (Apaf). The latter activates an initiator caspase, which initiates the proteolytic events that eventually kill the cell. Bcl-2 thus suppresses apoptosis by inhibition of cytochrome *c* release and by binding and thus inactivating Apaf-1.

The two scenarios for the anti-apoptotic actions of Bcl-2, that is, to directly prevent cytochrome *c* release and to inhibit Apaf-1–induced caspase activation despite cytochrome *c* release, are not mutually exclusive.[52] Other important proteins are also involved in apoptotic regulation. These include the p53 protein and certain mammalian homolog of viral protease inhibitor proteins (see later).

The Execution Phase. This phase of apoptosis is the final pathway, a proteolytic cascade, toward which a plethora of heterogeneous signaling and regulatory mechanisms converge. Even accounting for variations, it exhibits common themes generally applicable to all forms of apoptosis. The proteases that trigger and mediate the execution phase are highly conserved across species and belong to the *caspase family,* as already described. They are mammalian homologs of the *ced-3* gene in *C. elegans*.[52,55] The term caspase is based on two catalytic properties of this family of enzymes: the "c" reflects a cysteine protease mechanism, and "aspase" refers to their unique ability to cleave after aspartic acid residues.[56] The caspase family, now including more than ten members, can be divided functionally into two basic groups—initiator and execution, depending on the order by which they are activated before final cell death.[36] Initiator caspases, as we have seen, include caspase 9, which binds to Apaf-1, and caspase 8, which is triggered by Fas–Fas ligand interactions (see later).

Like many proteases, caspases exist as zymogens and must undergo an activating cleavage for apoptosis to be initiated. Caspases have their own cleavage sites that can be hydrolyzed not only by other caspases but autocatalytically. After an initiator caspase is triggered, the enzymatic death program is set in motion by rapid and sequential activation. Execution caspases disrupt the cytoskeleton by cleavage of cytoskeletal and nuclear matrix proteins.[56] The targets of caspase activation in the nucleus include proteins involved in transcription, DNA replication, and DNA repair. In particular, caspase 3 activation converts a cytoplasmic DNase (CAD) into an active form by cleaving an inhibitor of the enzyme and resulting in the characteristic internucleosomal cleavage of DNA, described earlier.[57]

Removal of Dead Cells. As already alluded to, apoptotic cells and their fragments have marker molecules on their surfaces, which facilitates early recognition by adjacent cells or phagocytes for phagocytic uptake and disposal. The process is so efficient that dead cells disappear without leaving a trace, and inflammation is virtually absent.

Specific Examples of Apoptosis

Signaling by Tumor Necrosis Factor (TNF) Family of Receptors. The TNFR family includes members that bind not only the important cytokine TNF (Chapter 3) but other clinically significant ligands as well. Some initiate apoptosis, some initiate cell proliferation, and others initiate both. A subfamily of TNFR including Fas and TNFR1 (see later) exhibit homologous cytoplasmic 80–amino acid "death recognition domains."[58] Two important examples of cell death are mediated by this subfamily. Death signaling in both requires clustering of receptors by a trimeric ligand, and homotypic binding of such receptors with cytoplasmic "adapter proteins" that exhibit corresponding death domains (FADD, or Fas-associated protein with a death domain) (Fig. 1–22). These adapter proteins, through separate "death effector domains," in turn bind to homologous domains in initiator caspases (pro-caspase 8). This results in an autocatalytic activation to sequentially trigger the execution phase. We now consider the two examples of such cell death.

- **Fas–Fas ligand–mediated apoptosis**. This type of apoptosis is caused by a cell surface receptor designated Fas (CD95). A membrane-bound or soluble ligand, called Fas ligand (FasL or CD95L), produced by cells of the immune system, binds to Fas on T cells and activates a death program, as shown in Figure 1–22. This system is important in that it eliminates activated lymphocytes from an immune reaction, thereby limiting the host response (Chapter 7).
- **TNF-induced apoptosis**. Activation of one of the TNF receptors (TNFR1) by the cytokine TNF can lead to apoptosis by inducing the association of the receptor with the adapter protein TRADD (TNFR–adapter protein with a death domain). As with the Fas–Fas ligand system, TRADD in turn binds to FADD and leads to apoptosis through caspase activation, as discussed[59] (Fig. 1–23). In contrast to Fas, however, under certain condi-

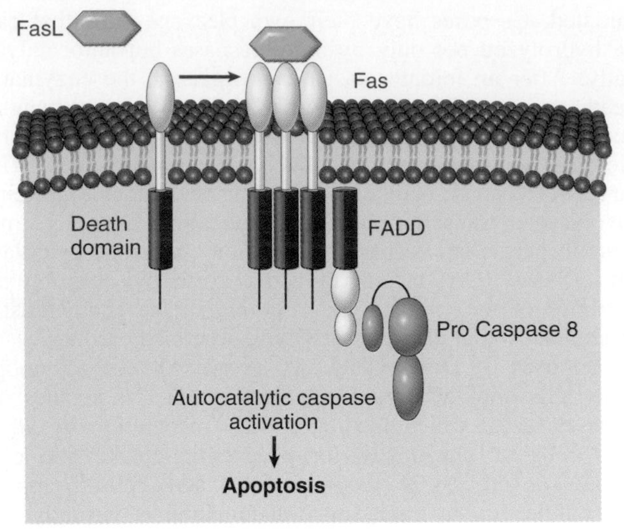

Figure 1–22

A model of Fas-mediated signaling, caspase activation, and the induction of a death signal (see text). FADD, Fas-associating protein with a death domain.

tions, TNFR1 binding to TRADD is followed by binding to other adapter proteins, leading to activation of the important transcription factor nuclear factor–κB (NF-κB) by stimulating degradation of its inhibitor (IκB)[60] (Fig. 1–23). The NF-κB/IκB transcriptional regulatory system is important for cell survival and, as we shall see (Chapter 3), for a number of inflammatory responses.

But what determines this yin and yang of TNF action? The answer is unclear, but the constitutive presence of activated NF-κB (such as occurs in tumors) is thought to favor survival.[61] In addition, certain human homologs of certain inhibitors of apoptosis, such as *neuronal apoptosis inhibitory protein* (NAIP), suppress TNF-induced cell death, favoring survival.[62] Testimony to the importance of such inhibitors is the existence of a genetic disorder, called *spinal muscle atrophy*, in which mutations of the NAIP are thought to account, at least in part, for the spinal cord motor neuron loss characteristic of the disease[63] (Chapter 30).

Cytotoxic T-Lymphocyte–Stimulated Apoptosis. CTLs recognize foreign antigens presented on the surface of infected host cells (Chapter 7). On recognition, they express Fas ligand on their surfaces and kill target cells by ligation of Fas receptors, as described earlier. Alternatively, CTLs induce apoptosis of target cells by secreting *perforin,* a transmembrane pore-forming molecule, and the exocytotic release of cytoplasmic granules into target cells. The serine protease *granzyme B* is the critical cytotoxic component in this process.[47] Granzyme B has the ability to cleave proteins at aspartate residues and is able to activate a variety of cellular caspases.[48] *In this way, the CTL kills target cells through bypassing the upstream signaling events and directly induces the effector phase of apoptosis.*

Apoptosis After Growth Factor Deprivation. Survival of many cells depends on a supply of cytokines or growth factors. In the absence of the factor, the cells undergo apoptosis. For example, neurons are dependent on nerve growth factor for their support, and withdrawal of such support during development can lead to apoptotic cell death.[64] On withdrawal of growth factor, pro-apoptotic members of the Bcl-2 family of proteins are thought to move from the cytosol to the outer mitochondrial membrane and change the ratio of pro-apoptotic and anti-apop-

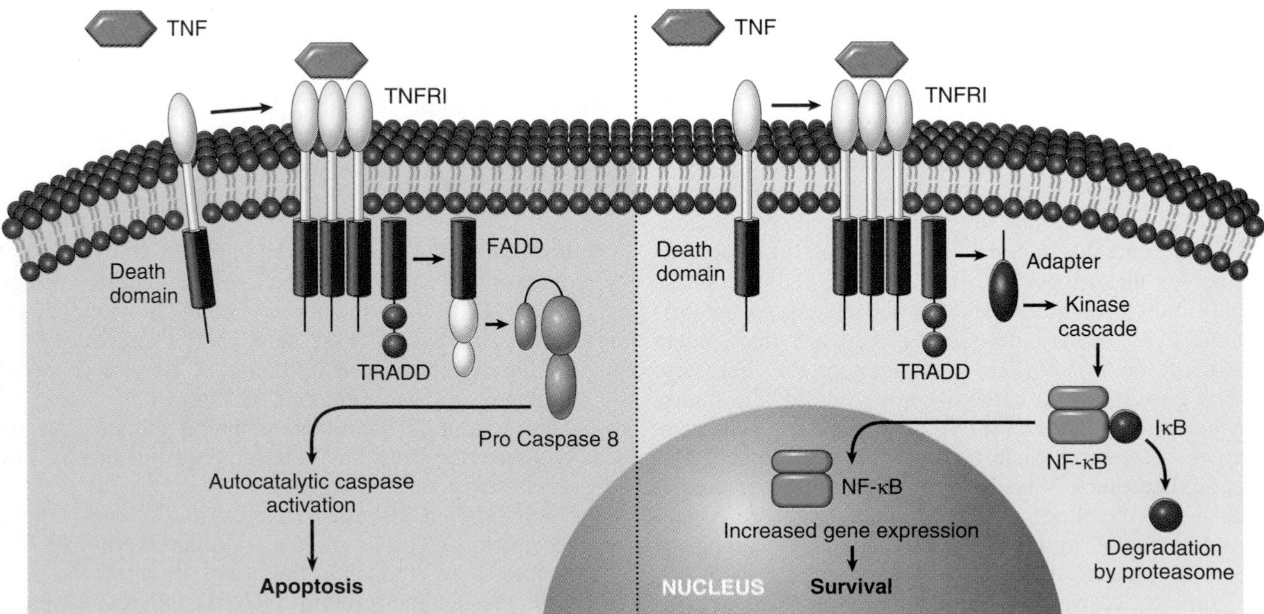

Figure 1–23

Apoptosis vs. survival induced by TNF. A model of TNF-receptor–mediated signaling and the induction of *apoptosis* (*left*), or NF-κB activation and cell *survival signals* (*right*).

totic members of the Bcl-2 family at this site. This change causes increased permeability of the membrane, leakage of cytochrome *c*, and activation of the proteolytic cascade as described previously.

DNA Damage–Mediated Apoptosis. Exposure of cells to radiation or chemotherapeutic agents induces apoptosis by a mechanism that is initiated by DNA damage (genotoxic stress) and that involves the tumor-suppressor gene *p53*. *p53* accumulates when DNA is damaged and arrests the cell cycle (at the G_1 phase) to allow additional time for repair (Chapters 4 and 8). However, if the repair process fails, *p53* triggers apoptosis. Thus, *p53* normally stimulates apoptosis, but when it is mutated or absent (as it is in certain cancers), it favors cell survival. Thus, *p53* seems to serve as a critical "life or death" switch in the case of genotoxic stress. The mechanism by which DNA damage engages the distal death effector machinery—the caspases—is complex but seems to involve its well-characterized function in transcriptional regulation.[58]

To end this discussion of apoptosis, one must note that a concept of *dysregulated apoptosis ("too little or too much")* has emerged to explain components of a wide range of diseases discussed throughout the book.[58, 65] In essence, two groups of disorders may result from such dysregulation:

- *Disorders associated with inhibited apoptosis and increased cell survival.* Here, an inappropriately low rate of apoptosis may prolong survival of abnormal cells. These accumulated cells can give rise to. (1) *cancers,* especially those carcinomas with *p53* mutations, or hormone-dependent tumors, such as breast, prostate, or ovarian cancers (Chapter 8); and (2) *autoimmune disorders,* which could arise if autoreactive lymphocytes are not removed after an immune response (Chapter 7).
- *Disorders associated with increased apoptosis and excessive cell death.* These diseases are characterized by a marked loss of normal or protective cells and include (1) *neurodegenerative diseases,* manifested by loss of specific sets of neurons, such as in the spinal muscular atrophies (Chapter 29); (2) *ischemic injury,* such as in myocardial infarction (Chapter 13) and stroke (Chapter 30); and (3) *virus-induced lymphocyte depletion,* such as occurs in acquired immune deficiency syndrome (AIDS) (see Chapter 7).

To summarize, apoptosis is a distinctive form of cell death manifested by characteristic chromatin condensation and DNA fragmentation, whose function is the deletion of cells in normal development, organogenesis, immune function, and tissue growth, but which can also be induced by pathologic stimuli. The mechanism of apoptosis has several key stages: first, there are multiple pathways of commitment to cell death; second, there is a control stage, in which the apoptotic threshold is established by the relative expression and activity of different positive and negative regulators, including the Bcl-2 family of proteins; and third, there is a conserved execution stage, involving the activation of caspases that perform the terminal proteolysis. Apoptotic bodies are then engulfed by macrophages by receptor-mediated phagocytosis. Dysregulation of this process may contribute to a variety of disease states.

SUBCELLULAR RESPONSES TO CELL INJURY

To this point in the chapter, the focus has been on the cell as a unit. Certain conditions, however, are associated with distinctive alterations in cell organelles or the cytoskeleton. Some of these alterations coexist with those described for acute lethal injury; others represent more chronic forms of cell injury, and still others are adaptive responses that involve specific homeostatic mechanisms or cellular organelles. Here we touch on only some of the more common or interesting of these reactions.

Lysosomal Catabolism

Primary lysosomes are membrane-bound intracellular organelles that contain a variety of hydrolytic enzymes, including acid phosphatase, glucuronidase, sulfatase, ribonuclease, and collagenase. These enzymes are synthesized in the rough endoplasmic reticulum and then packaged into vesicles in the Golgi apparatus (Fig. 1–24). Primary lysosomes fuse with membrane-bound vacuoles that contain material to be digested, forming *secondary lysosomes* or *phagolysosomes*. Lysosomes are involved in the breakdown of phagocytosed material in one of two ways: heterophagy and autophagy.

- **Heterophagy.** Materials from the external environment are taken up through the general process of *endocytosis*. Uptake of particulate matter is known as *phagocytosis;* uptake of soluble smaller macromolecules is called *pinocytosis*. Endocytosed vacuoles and their contents eventually fuse with a lysosome, resulting in degradation of the engulfed material. Heterophagy is most common in the "professional" phagocytes, such as neutrophils and macrophages, although it may also occur in other cell types. Examples of heterophagocytosis include the uptake and digestion of bacteria by neutrophilic leukocytes and the removal of apoptotic cells and bodies by macrophages.
- **Autophagy.** In this process, intracellular organelles and portions of cytosol are first sequestered from the cytoplasm in an *autophagic vacuole* formed from ribosome-free regions of the rough endoplasmic reticulum, which then fuses with preexisting primary lysosomes or Golgi elements to form an *autophagolysosome*.[66] Autophagy is a common phenomenon involved in the removal of damaged organelles during cell injury and the cellular remodeling of differentiation, and it is particularly pronounced in cells undergoing atrophy induced by nutrient deprivation or hormonal involution.

The enzymes in the lysosomes are capable of degrading most proteins and carbohydrates, but some lipids remain undigested. Lysosomes with undigested debris may persist

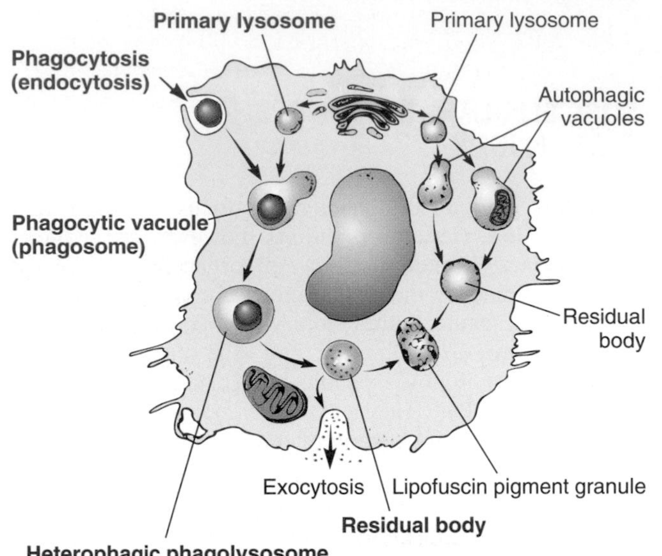

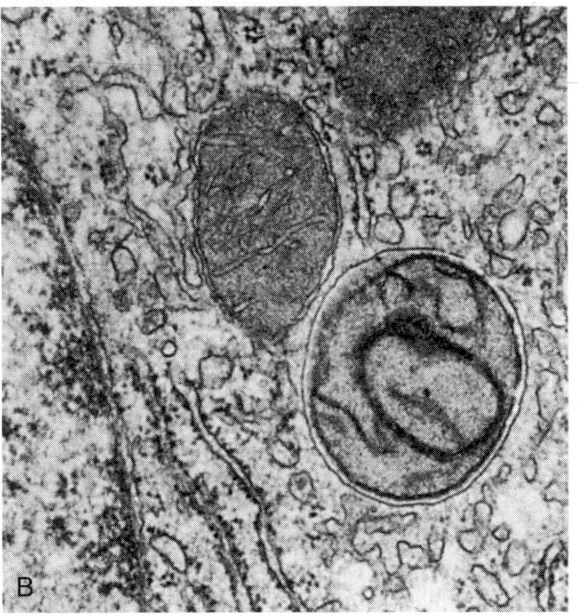

Figure 1–24

A, Schematic representation of autophagy *(right)* and heterophagy *(left)*. (Redrawn from Fawcett DW: A Textbook of Histology, 11th ed. Philadelphia, WB Saunders, 1986, p 17.) *B*, Electron micrograph of an autophagolysosome containing a degenerating mitochondrion and amorphous material.

within cells as *residual bodies* or may be extruded. *Lipofuscin pigment* granules represent undigested material that results from intracellular lipid peroxidation. Certain indigestible pigments, such as carbon particles inhaled from the atmosphere or inoculated pigment in tattoos, can persist in phagolysosomes of macrophages for decades.

Lysosomes are also repositories where cells sequester abnormal substances that cannot be completely metabolized. Hereditary *lysosomal storage disorders*, caused by deficiencies of enzymes that degrade various macromolecules, result in the accumulation of abnormal amounts of these compounds in the lysosomes of cells all over the body, particularly neurons, leading to severe abnormalities (Chapter 6). Certain drugs can disturb lysosomal function and *cause acquired or drug-induced (iatrogenic) lysosomal diseases*. Drugs in this group include cloroquine, an antimalarial agent that raises the internal pH of the lysosome, thus inactivating its enzymes, and the antiarrhythmic drug amiodarone, which binds to phospholipids within the lysosome, rendering them resistant to breakdown.

Induction (Hypertrophy) of Smooth Endoplasmic Reticulum

Protracted use of barbiturates leads to a state of increased tolerance, so repeated doses lead to progressively shorter periods of sleep. Patients are therefore said to have "adapted" to the medication. This adaptation is due to induction of an increased volume (hypertrophy) of the smooth endoplasmic reticulum of hepatocytes, which metabolizes the drug[67] (Fig. 1–25). Barbiturates are modified in the liver by oxidative demethylation, which involves the P-450 mixed function oxidase system found in the smooth endoplasmic reticulum. The role of these enzyme modifications is to increase the solubility of a variety of compounds (e.g., alcohol, steroids, eicosanoids, and carcinogens as well as insecticides and other environmental pollutants) and thereby facilitate their secretion.[30] Although this is often thought of as "detoxification," many compounds are rendered *more* injurious by P-450 modification. In addition, the products formed by this oxidative metabolism include reactive oxygen intermediates, which can cause oxidative injury within the cell. In any case, the barbiturates (and many other agents) stimulate the synthesis of more enzymes, as well as more smooth endoplasmic reticulum. In this manner, the cell is better able to modify the drugs and adapt to its altered environment. It is noteworthy that cells adapted to one drug have increased capacity to metabolize other drugs handled by the system or endogenous metabolic products, such as bilirubin and bile acids. Thus, patients taking phenobarbital for epilepsy who increase their alcohol intake may have subtherapeutic levels of the antiseizure medication.

Mitochondrial Alterations

We have seen that mitochondrial dysfunction plays an important role in acute cell injury and apoptosis. In addition, various alterations in the number, size, and shape of mitochondria occur in some pathologic conditions. For example, in cell hypertrophy and atrophy, there is an increase and a decrease, respectively, in the number of mitochondria in cells (Chapter 2). Mitochondria may assume extremely large and abnormal shapes (megamitochondria), as can be seen in the liver in alcoholic liver disease and in certain nutritional deficiencies (Fig. 1–26). In certain inherited metabolic diseases of skeletal muscle, the *mitochondrial myopathies*, defects in mitochondrial metabolism are asso-

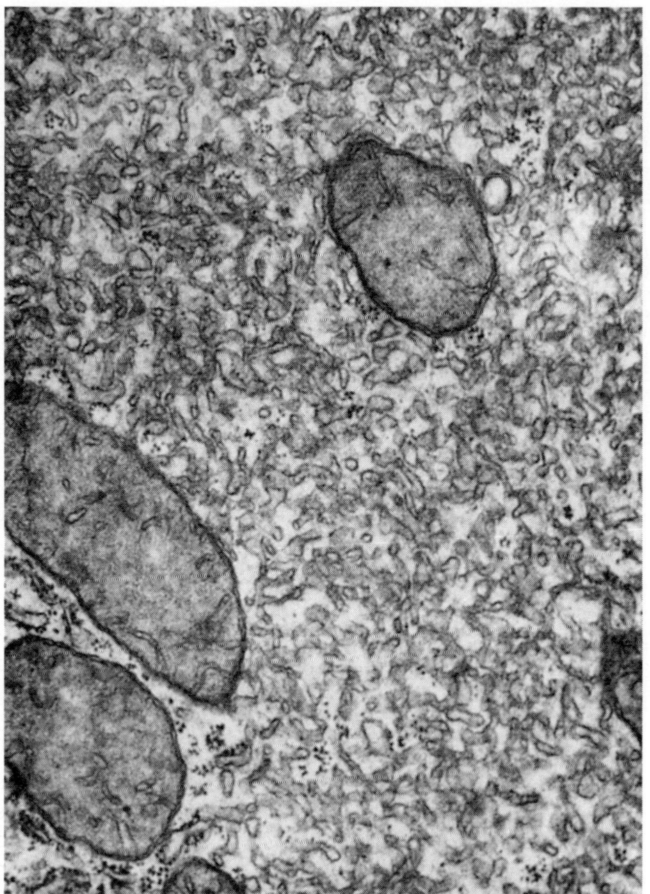

Figure 1–25

Electron micrograph of liver from phenobarbital-treated rat showing marked increase in smooth endoplasmic reticulum. (From Jones AL, Fawcett DW: Hypertrophy of the agranular endoplasmic reticulum in hamster liver induced by phenobarbital. J Histochem Cytochem 14:215, 1966. Courtesy of Dr. Fawcett.)

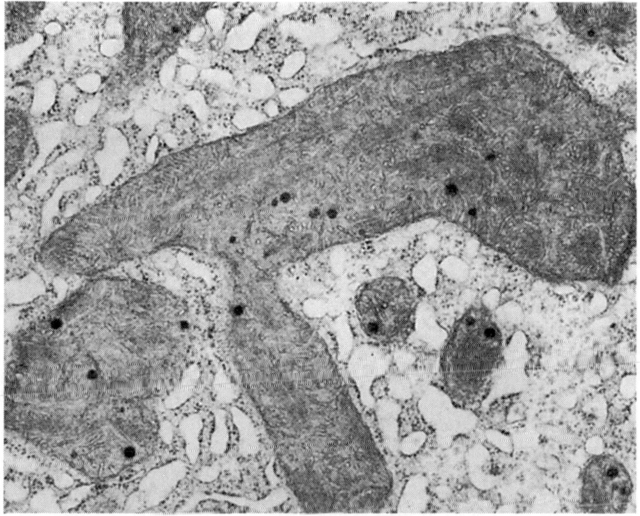

Figure 1–26

Enlarged, abnormally shaped mitochondria from the liver of a patient with alcoholic cirrhosis. Note also crystalline formations in the mitochondria.

ciated with increased numbers of mitochondria that are often unusually large, have abnormal cristae, and contain crystalloids (Chapter 29). In addition, certain benign tumors called *oncocytomas* (found in a salivary glands, thyroid, parathyroids, and kidneys) consist of cells with abundant enlarged mitochondria, giving the cell a distinctly eosinophilic appearance.

Cytoskeletal Abnormalities

Abnormalities of the cytoskeleton underlie a variety of pathologic states. The *cytoskeleton* consists of microtubules (20 to 25 nm in diameter), thin actin filaments (6 to 8 nm), thick myosin filaments (15 nm), and various classes of intermediate filaments (10 nm). Several other nonpolymerized and nonfilamentous forms of contractile proteins also exist. Cytoskeletal abnormalities may be reflected by (1) defects in cell function, such as cell locomotion and intracellular organelle movements, or (2) in some instances by intracellular accumulations of fibrillar material. Only a few examples are cited.

- *Thin filaments.* Thin filaments are composed of actin, myosin, and their associated regulatory proteins.[68] Functioning thin filaments are essential for various stages of leukocyte movement or the ability of such cells to perform phagocytosis adequately. Some drugs and toxins target actin filaments and thus affect these processes. For example, cytochalasin B prevents polymerization of actin filaments, and phalloidin, a toxin of the mushroom *Amanita phalloides*, also binds actin filaments.
- *Microtubules.* Defects in the organization of microtubules can inhibit sperm motility, causing male sterility, and at the same time can immobilize the cilia of respiratory epithelium, causing interference with the ability of this epithelium to clear inhaled bacteria, leading to bronchiectasis (Kartagener or the *immotile cilia syndrome*). Microtubules, like microfilaments, are essential for various stages of leukocyte migration and phagocytosis. Drugs such as colchicine bind to tubulin and prevent the assembly of microtubules. The drug is used in acute attacks of gout to prevent leukocyte migration and phagocytosis in response to deposition of urate crystals. Microtubules are an essential component of the mitotic spindle, which is required for cell division. Drugs that bind to microtubules (e.g., vinca alkaloids) can be antiproliferative and therefore act as antitumor agents.
- *Intermediate filaments.* These components provide a flexible intracellular scaffold that organizes the cytoplasm and resists forces applied to the cell.[69] The intermediate filaments are divided into five classes, including keratin filaments (characteristic of epithelial cells), neurofilaments (neurons), desmin filaments (muscle cells), vimentin filaments (connective tissue cells), and glial filaments (astrocytes). Accumulations of keratin filaments and neurofilaments are associated with certain types of cell injury. For example, the *Mallory body*, or "alcoholic hyalin," is an eosinophilic intracytoplasmic inclusion in liver cells that is characteristic of alcoholic liver disease,[70] although it can be present in other condi-

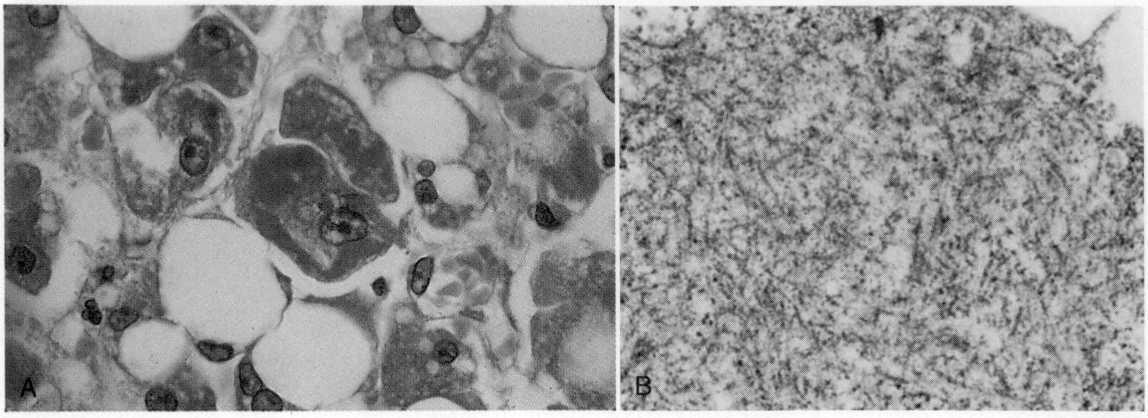

Figure 1–27

A, The liver of alcohol abuse (chronic alcoholism). Hyaline inclusions in the hepatic parenchymal cell in the center appear as eosinophilic networks disposed about the nuclei. *B*, Electron micrograph of alcoholic hyalin. The material is composed of intermediate (prekeratin) filaments and an amorphous matrix.

tions. Such inclusions are now known to be composed predominantly of *keratin* intermediate filaments (Fig. 1–27). In the nervous system, neurofilaments are present in the axon where they provide structural support. The *neurofibrillary tangle* found in the brain in Alzheimer disease contains microtubule-associated proteins and neurofilaments, a reflection of a disrupted neuronal cytoskeleton. Mutations in intermediate filament genes cause multiple human disorders.[71] For example, alterations in one of the keratin filament genes cause the skin disorder epidermolysis bullosa simplex.

This ends our general discussion of acute cellular injury and its principal manifestations: reversible injury, necrosis, and apoptosis. References are made to these cellular events throughout the book because all organ injury and ultimately all clinical disease arise from derangements in cell structure and function.

We wish to thank Dr. M. A. Venkatachalam, University of Texas, San Antonio, for invaluable help in preparation of this chapter.

REFERENCES

1. Majno G: The Healing Hand: Man and Wound in the Ancient World. Boston, Harvard University Press, 1975, p 43.
2. Majno G, Joris I: Apoptosis, oncosis, and necrosis. An overview of the cell death. Am J Pathol 146:3, 1995.
3. Trump BJ, Berezesky I: The reactions of cells to lethal injury: oncosis and necrosis—the role of calcium. In Lockshin RA, et al (eds): When Cells Die—A Comprehensive Evaluation of Apoptosis and Programmed Cell Death. New York, Wiley-Liss, 1998, pp 57–96.
4. Bernardi P: The permeability transition pore. Control points of a cyclosporine A–sensitive mitochondrial channel involved in cell death. Biochim Biophys Acta 1275:5, 1996.
5. Jennings RB, Reimer KA: The cell biology of acute myocardial ischemia. Annu Rev Med 42:225, 1991.
6. Weinberg JM: The cell biology of ischemic renal injury. Kidney Int 39:476, 1991.
7. Choi DW: Ischemia-induced neuronal apoptosis. Curr Opin Neurobiol 6:667, 1996.
8. Lemasters JJ, et al: Reperfusion injury to heart and liver cells: protection by acidosis during ischemia and a "pH paradox" after reperfusion. In Hochachka PW, et al (eds): Surviving Hypoxia: Mechanisms of Control and Adaptation. Boca Raton, FL, CRC Press, 1993, pp 495–507.
9. Lemasters JJ, et al: The mitochondrial permeability transition in toxic, hypoxic and reperfusion injury. Mol Cell Biochem 174:159, 1997.
10. Nakamura H, et al: Subcellular characteristics of phospholipase A_2 activity in the rat kidney. Enhanced cytosolic, mitochondrial, and microsomal phospholipase A_2 enzymatic activity after renal ischemia and reperfusion. J Clin Invest 87:1810, 1991.
11. Farber JL: Membrane injury and calcium homeostasis in the pathogenesis of coagulative necrosis. Lab Invest 47:114, 1982.
12. Nishimura Y, et al: Mitochondrial dysfunction and cytoskeletal disruption during chemical hypoxia to cultured rat hepatic sinusoidal endothelial cells: the pH paradox and cytoprotection by glucose, acidotic pH and glycine. Hepatology 27:1039, 1998.
13. Farber JL: Mechanisms of cell injury by activated oxygen species. Environ Health Perspect 102:17, 1994.
14. Dong Z, et al: Development of porous defects in plasma membranes of ATP depleted Madin-Darby canine kidney cells and its inhibition by glycine. Lab Invest 78:657, 1998.
14a. Dong Z, et al: Intracellular Ca^{2+} thresholds that determine survival or death of energy deprived cells. Am J Path 152:231, 1998.
15. Choi DW: Ischemia-induced neuronal apoptosis. Curr Opin Neurobiol 6:667, 1996.
16. Lieberthal W, Levine JS: Mechanisms of apoptosis and its potential role in renal tubular epithelial cell injury. Am J Physiol 271:F477, 1996.
17. MacLellan WR, Schneider MD: Death by design. Programmed cell death in cardiovascular biology and disease. Circ Res 81:137, 1997.
18. Lefer AM, Lefer DJ: Pharmacology of the endothelium in ischemia-reperfusion and circulatory shock. Annu Rev Pharmacol Toxicol 33:71, 1993.
19. Thiagarajan RR, et al: The role of leukocyte and endothelial adhesion molecules in ischemia-reperfusion injury. Thromb Haemost 78:310, 1997.
20. Kurose I, Granger DN: Evidence implicating xanthine oxidase and neutrophils in reperfusion-induced microvascular dysfunction. Ann NY Acad Sci 723:158, 1994.
21. Qian T, et al: Mitochondrial permeability transition in pH-dependent reperfusion injury to rat hepatocytes. Am J Physiol 273:C1783, 1997.
22. Grinyo JM: Reperfusion injury. Transplant Proc 29:59, 1997.
23. Knight JA: Diseases related to oxygen-derived free radicals. Ann Clin Lab Sci 25:111, 1995.

24. Lubec G: The hydroxyl radical: from chemistry to human disease. J Invest Med 44:324, 1996.
25. Riley PA: Free radicals in biology: oxidative stress and the effects of ionizing radiation. Int J Radiat Biol 65:27, 1994.
26. Farber JL, et al: The mechanisms of cell injury by activated oxygen species. Lab Invest 62:670, 1990.
27. Bertlett BS, Stadtman ER: Protein oxidation in aging, disease and oxidative stress. J Biol Chem 272:20313, 1997.
28. Mitch WE, Goldberg AL: Mechanisms of muscle wasting. The role of the ubiquitin-proteasome pathway. N Engl J Med 335:1897, 1996.
29. Snyder JW: Mechanisms of toxic cell injury. Clin Lab Med 10:311, 1990.
30. Coon MJ, et al: Cytochrome P450: peroxidative reactions of diversozymes. FASEB J 10:428, 1996.
31. Farber E, et al: Dissociation of effects on protein synthesis and ribosomes from membrane changes induced by carbon tetrachloride. Am J Pathol 64:601, 1971.
32. Cohen SD, Khairallah EA: Selective protein arylation and acetaminophen-induced hepatotoxicity. Drug Metab Rev 29:59, 1997.
33. Kerr JF, et al: Apoptosis: a basic biological phenomenon with wide-ranging implications in tissue kinetics. Br J Cancer 26:239, 1972.
33a. Cummings MC, et al: Apoptosis. Am J Surg Pathol 21:88, 1997.
34. Wyllie AH: Apoptosis: an overview. Br Med Bull 53:451, 1997.
35. Jacobson MD, et al: Programmed cell death in animal development. Cell 88:347, 1997.
36. Salvesen GS, Dixit VM: Caspases: intracellular signaling by proteolysis. Cell 91:443, 1997.
37. Nemes Z, et al: Expression and activation of tissue transglutaminase in apoptotic cells of involuting rodent mammary tissue. Eur J Cell Biol 70:125, 1996.
38. Bortner CD, et al: The role of DNA fragmentation in apoptosis. Trends Cell Biol 5:21, 1995.
39. McCarthy NJ, Evan GI: Methods for detecting and quantifying apoptosis. Curr Top Dev Biol 36:259, 1998.
40. Dong Z, et al: Internucleosomal DNA cleavage triggered by plasma membrane damage during necrotic cell death. Involvement of serine but not cysteine proteases. Am J Pathol 151:1205, 1997.
41. Savill J: Recognition and phagocytosis of cells undergoing apoptosis. Br Med Bull 53:491, 1997.
42. Nagata S: Apoptosis by death factor. Cell 88:355, 1997.
43. Golstein P: Controlling cell death. Science 275:1081, 1997.
44. Wyllie AH: The genetic regulation of apoptosis. Curr Opin Genet Dev 5:97, 1995.
45. Raff MC. Social controls on cell survival and cell death. Nature 356: 397, 1992.
46. Nagata S, Golstein P: The Fas death factor. Science 267:1449, 1995.
47. Heusel JW, et al: Cytotoxic lymphocytes require granzyme B for the rapid induction of DNA fragmentation and apoptosis in allogenic target cells. Cell 76:977, 1994.
48. Darmon AJ: Activation of the apoptotic protease CPP32 by cytotoxic T-cell–derived granzyme B. Nature 377:446, 1995.
49. Yang E, Korsmeyer SJ: Molecular thanatopsis: a discourse on the Bcl-2 family and cell death. Blood 88:386, 1996.
50. Reed JC: Double identity for proteins of the Bcl-2 family. Nature 387:773, 1997.
50a. Pastorino JG, et al: The overexpression of Bax produces cell death upon the induction of the mitochondrial permeability transition. J Biol Chem 273:7770, 1998.
51. Reed JC: Cytochrome *c*: can't live with it—can't live without it. Cell 91:559, 1997.
52. Hengartner MO: Death cycle and Swiss army knives. Nature 391:441, 1998.
53. Li P, et al: Cytochrome *c* and dATP-dependent formation of Apaf-1/caspase-9 complex initiates an apoptotic protease cascade. Cell 91: 479, 1997.
54. Vaux DL: CED-4—the third horseman of apoptosis. Cell 90:389, 1997.
55. Hengartner MO, Horvitz HR: Programmed cell death in *Caenorhabditis elegans*. Curr Opin Genet Dev 4:581, 1994.
56. Porter AG, et al: Death substrates come alive. Bioessays 19:501, 1997.
57. Enari M, et al: A caspase-activated DNase that degrades DNA during apoptosis, and its inhibitor ICAD. Nature 391:43, 1998.
58. Webb SJ, et al: Apoptosis. An overview of the process and its relevance in disease. Adv Pharmacol 41:1, 1997.
59. Hsu H, et al: TRADD-TRAF2 and TRADD-FADD interactions define two distinct TNF receptor 1 signal transduction pathways. Cell 84: 299, 1996.
60. Maniatis T: Catalysis by a multiprotein IκB kinase complex. Science 278:828, 1997.
61. Gilmore TD: Clinically *rel*evant findings. J Clin Invest 100:2935, 1997.
62. Liston P, et al: Suppression of apoptosis in mammalian cells by NAIP and a related family of IAP genes. Nature 379:349, 1996.
63. Roy N, et al: The gene for neuronal apoptosis inhibitory protein is partially deleted in individuals with spinal muscular atrophy. Cell 80: 167, 1995.
64. Park DS, et al: Ordering the multiple pathways of apoptosis. Trends Cardiovasc Med 7:294, 1997.
65. Thompson CB: Apoptosis in the pathogenesis and treatment of diseases. Science 267:1456, 1995.
66. Dunn WA: Studies on the mechanisms of autophagy. J Cell Biol 110: 1923, 1990.
67. Jones AL, Fawcett DW: Hypertrophy of the agranular endoplasmic reticulum in hamster liver induced by phenobarbital. J Histochem Cytochem 14:215, 1966.
68. Mermall V, et al: Unconventional myosins in cell movement, membrane traffic and signal transduction. Science 279:527, 1998.
69. Fuchs E, Cleveland DW: A structural scaffolding of intermediate filaments in health and disease. Science 279:514, 1998.
70. Kachi K, et al: Synthesis of Mallory body, intermediate filament, and microfilament proteins in liver cell primary cultures. Lab Invest 68: 71, 1993.
71. Bonifas JM, et al: Epidermolysis bullosa simplex: evidence in two families for keratin gene abnormalities. Science 254:1202, 1991.

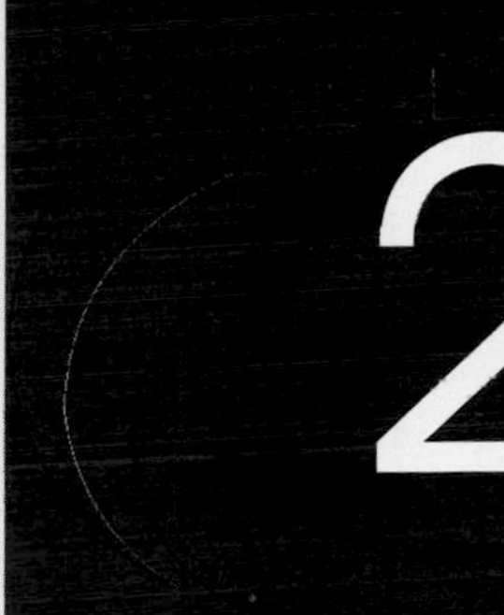

Cellular Pathology II: Adaptations, Intracellular Accumulations, and Cell Aging

CELLULAR ADAPTATIONS OF GROWTH AND DIFFERENTIATION
HYPERPLASIA
Physiologic Hyperplasia
Pathologic Hyperplasia
HYPERTROPHY
ATROPHY
METAPLASIA
INTRACELLULAR ACCUMULATIONS
LIPIDS
Steatosis (Fatty Change)
Cholesterol and Cholesterol Esters
PROTEINS
Defects in Protein Folding
GLYCOGEN
PIGMENTS
PATHOLOGIC CALCIFICATION
DYSTROPHIC CALCIFICATION
METASTATIC CALCIFICATION
HYALINE CHANGE
CELLULAR AGING
TIMING OF THE AGING PROCESS—THE CONCEPT OF A CLOCK
METABOLIC EVENTS, GENETIC DAMAGE, AND AGING
CONCLUSION

In Chapter 1, we discussed the morphologic expression and mechanisms of reversible cell injury and cell death. As noted, however, cells can respond to excessive physiologic stresses or pathologic stimuli by undergoing a number of physiologic and morphologic *cellular adaptations*, in which a new but altered steady state is achieved, preserving the viability of the cell and modulating its function as a response to such stimuli. Some of these adaptations involve changes in cellular growth, size, or differentiation and include *hyperplasia*, an increase in cell number; *hypertrophy*, an increase in cell size; *atrophy*, a decrease in the size and function of cells; and *metaplasia*, an alteration of cell differentiation. *Pathologic adaptations* may share the same underlying mechanisms as physiologic adaptations, but they provide the cells with the ability to survive in their environment and perhaps escape injury. Adaptive responses also can include the *intracellular accumulation* and storage of products in abnormal amounts. In special situations, storage becomes the primary mode of responding to substances that cannot be metabolized or excreted. These intracellular accumulations may consist of (1) *normal substances*, such as lipids, proteins, glycogen, iron, melanin, and bilirubin; (2) *abnormal endogenous products*, which include the proteins generated by genetically altered genes, such as α_1-antitrypsin in α_1-antitrypsin deficiency; or (3) *exogenous products*, which include environmental agents such as anthracotic pigment or soot. These accumulations can give rise to both structural changes and functional impairment.

There are numerous molecular mechanisms for cellular adaptations. Some are due to direct stimulation of cells by factors produced by other cells or to the cells themselves as is the case in cell growth (see discussion in Chapter 4). Others involve *up-regulation or down-regulation of specific cellular receptors* involved in metabolism of certain components—for example, in the regulation of cell surface receptors participating in the uptake and degradation of low-density lipoproteins (Chapter 6). Still others are associated with the *induction of new protein synthesis by the target cells*, as in the heat-shock response or the chronic response to hypoxia. Adaptations can also involve a switch by cells from producing one type of a family of proteins to another or markedly overproducing one protein; such is the case in cells producing various types of collagens and extracellular matrix proteins in chronic inflammation and fibrosis (Chapters 3 and 4). Adaptations then involve all steps in cellular metabolism of proteins—*receptor binding; signal transduction; transcription or translation; or regulation of protein synthesis, packaging, and release.*

This chapter discusses common adaptive changes in cell growth and differentiation that are particularly important in pathologic states—hyperplasia, hypertrophy, atrophy, and metaplasia and the intracellular accumulations of lipids, proteins, carbohydrates, and pigments. We also discuss the manifestations of cellular aging since they represent adaptations to environmental determinants of cell structure and function.

CELLULAR ADAPTATIONS OF GROWTH AND DIFFERENTIATION

Hyperplasia

Hyperplasia constitutes an increase in the number of cells in an organ or tissue, which may then have increased volume. Although hyperplasia and hypertrophy are two distinct processes, frequently both occur together, and they may well be triggered by the same mechanism. Estrogen-induced growth in the uterus involves both increased DNA synthesis and enlargement of smooth muscle and epithelium. In certain instances, however, even cells capable of dividing, such as renal epithelial cells, undergo hypertrophy but not hyperplasia. Growth inhibitors, such as transforming growth factor-β (TGF-β), may be involved in this phenomenon. In *nondividing cells* (e.g., myocardial fibers), only hypertrophy occurs. Nuclei in such cells have a much higher DNA content than that of normal myocardial cells, probably because the cells arrest in the cell cycle without undergoing mitosis. Hypertrophy does not involve cell division, but hyperplasia takes place if the cellular population is capable of synthesizing DNA, thus permitting mitotic division. Hyperplasia can be *physiologic or pathologic*.

PHYSIOLOGIC HYPERPLASIA

Physiologic hyperplasia can be divided into (1) *hormonal hyperplasia*, best exemplified by the proliferation of the glandular epithelium of the female breast at puberty and during pregnancy and the physiologic hyperplasia that occurs in the pregnant uterus, and (2) *compensatory hyperplasia*, for example, the hyperplasia that occurs when a portion of the liver is removed (partial hepatectomy).

Mechanisms of Hyperplasia: Lessons From Hepatic Regeneration. In the myth of Prometheus, the ancient Greeks recognized the capacity of the liver to regenerate. Having stolen the secret of fire from the Gods, Prometheus was chained to a mountain, and his liver was devoured daily by a vulture, only to regenerate anew every night.[1] The experimental model of partial hepatectomy has been especially useful in examining mechanisms of compensatory hyperplasia. In the normal mature liver, only 0.5 to 1.0% of cells are undergoing DNA replication. After partial hepatectomy, all the existing mature cellular populations composing the intact organ proliferate to rebuild the lost hepatic tissue. Hepatocytes are the first cell type to proliferate, and remarkably, these cells can maintain their normal metabolic functions while proliferating.[1] An increase in the number of DNA-synthesizing cells begins as early as 12 hours after hepatectomy and peaks between 1 and 2 days later, when about 10% of all cells may be involved in DNA synthesis (Fig. 2–1). Initiation of cell proliferation is associated with specific and sequential increases in proteins involved in an intracellular signaling cascade leading to DNA synthesis, as will be detailed in Chapter 4.[2] These include the induction of transcription factors (e.g., c-*fos*, c-*jun*, nuclear factor-κB [NF-κB], signal transducer and activator of transcription [STAT]) as well as proteins linked to the cell cycle (e.g., *myc*, *p53*, and cyclins) (Fig. 2–1).[3]

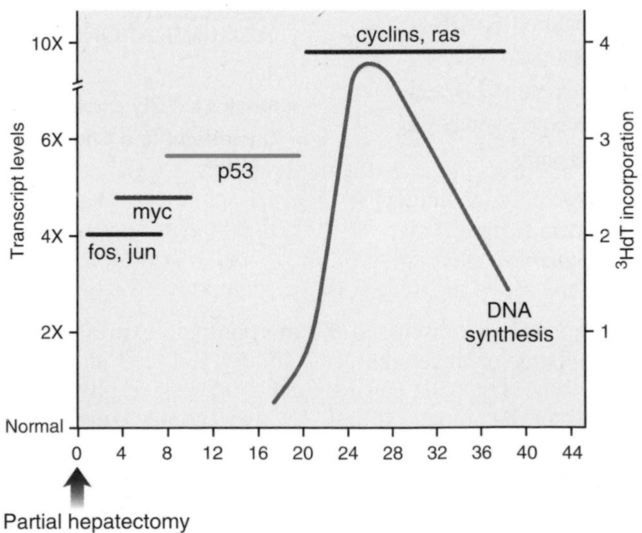

Figure 2–1

Expression of protooncogenes after partial hepatectomy and its relation to DNA synthesis by hepatocytes. (Courtesy of Nelson Fausto, University of Washington, Seattle, WA).

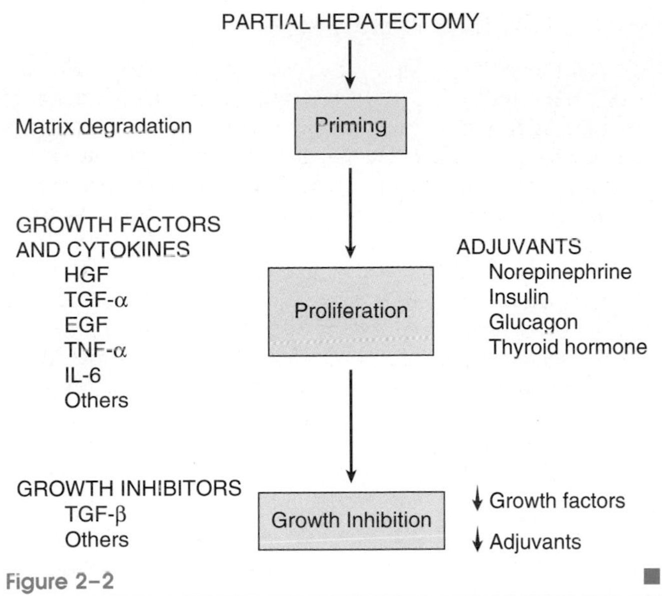

Figure 2–2

Postulated sequence of events in the compensatory hyperplasia after partial hepatectomy.

Subsequently, DNA synthesis declines, and by the time the liver mass is restored (at 1 to 2 weeks), the liver cells become quiescent again.

There is substantial evidence that cell proliferation in this setting is dependent on the action of polypeptide growth factors and cytokines (see Chapter 4 for a detailed discussion of cell growth). Factors implicated include the following:

- *Growth factors*: *Hepatocyte growth factor* (HGF) and its receptor c-Met are key factors for liver growth and function.[4] HGF (also called *scatter factor*) initially identified in the serum of hepatectomized rats as a potent mitogen for cultured hepatocytes, is produced in the liver by nonparenchymal cells and by mesenchymal cells in many organs. Plasma HGF levels rise rapidly after partial hepatectomy. Both *TGF-α* and *epidermal growth factor (EGF)* are also mitogenic for hepatocytes in culture, and experimental studies suggest that EGF may play a mitogenic role in the early stages after partial hepatectomy, while *TGF-α* acts at later times.
- *Cytokines*: *Interleukin-6 (IL-6)* and *tumor necrosis factor-α (TNF-α)* are important components of the early signaling pathways involved in regeneration. The functional relevance of IL-6 was demonstrated in transgenic mice lacking the cytokine. In these animals, defective hepatocyte regeneration results in massive hepatic necrosis after partial hepatectomy, which can be prevented by administration of IL-6.[5]

None of these growth factors or cytokines, however, are sufficient to induce proliferation in normal liver cells in vivo, and it has been proposed that an initial *priming* signal to the remnant hepatic cells is necessary for the full effect of these mitogens (Fig. 2–2). Such priming signals include degradation of the extracellular matrix, which would convert inactive matrix-associated HGF to its active, receptor binding form. Certain hormones, such as norepinephrine, whose blood level also increases after hepatectomy, and insulin, may function as adjuvants for cell proliferation. Cessation of cell growth, after the liver mass has been restored, appears to be caused by *growth inhibitors* produced in the liver itself. One of these inhibitors is TGF-*β*, which is produced by nonparenchymal cells of the liver.

In addition to proliferating differentiated hepatocytes, adult livers contain a small population of *stem cells* located in the junction between hepatocytes and the smallest segments of the biliary tree.[6] These stem cells have a variety of developmental options, including differentiating into hepatocytes and biliary duct epithelium. Stem cells do not play a major role in the hyperplasia after hepatectomy but may participate in the regeneration that occurs after certain forms of liver injury, such as hepatitis.

PATHOLOGIC HYPERPLASIA

Most forms of *pathologic hyperplasia are instances of excessive hormonal stimulation or are the effects of growth factors on target cells.* An example of hormonally induced hyperplasia is hyperplasia of the endometrium. After a normal menstrual period, there is a rapid burst of proliferative activity. As is well known, this proliferation is potentiated by pituitary hormones and ovarian estrogen. It is brought to a halt by the rising levels of progesterone, usually about 10 to 14 days before the anticipated menstrual period. In some instances, however, the balance between estrogen and progesterone is disturbed. This results in absolute or relative increases in the amount of estrogen, or both, with consequent hyperplasia of the endometrial glands. Although this form of hyperplasia is a common cause of abnormal menstrual bleeding, the hyperplastic process remains controlled nonetheless: If the estrogenic stimulation abates, the hyperplasia disappears. Thus, it responds to regular growth control of cells. As is discussed in Chapter 8, Neoplasia, it is this response to normal regulatory control mechanisms that differentiates benign pathologic hyperplasias from cancer. *Pathologic hyperplasia, however, constitutes a fertile soil in which cancerous proliferation may eventually arise.* Thus, patients with hyperplasia of the endometrium are at increased risk for developing endometrial cancer (Chapter 24).

Hyperplasia is also an important response of connective tissue cells in wound healing, in which proliferating fibroblasts and blood vessels aid in repair (Chapter 4). Under these circumstances, growth factors are responsible for the hyperplasia. Stimulation by growth factors is also involved in the hyperplasia that is associated with certain *viral infections*, such as papillomaviruses, causing skin warts and a number of mucosal lesions composed of masses of hyperplastic epithelium.

Hypertrophy

Hypertrophy refers to an increase in the size of cells and, with such change, an increase in the size of the

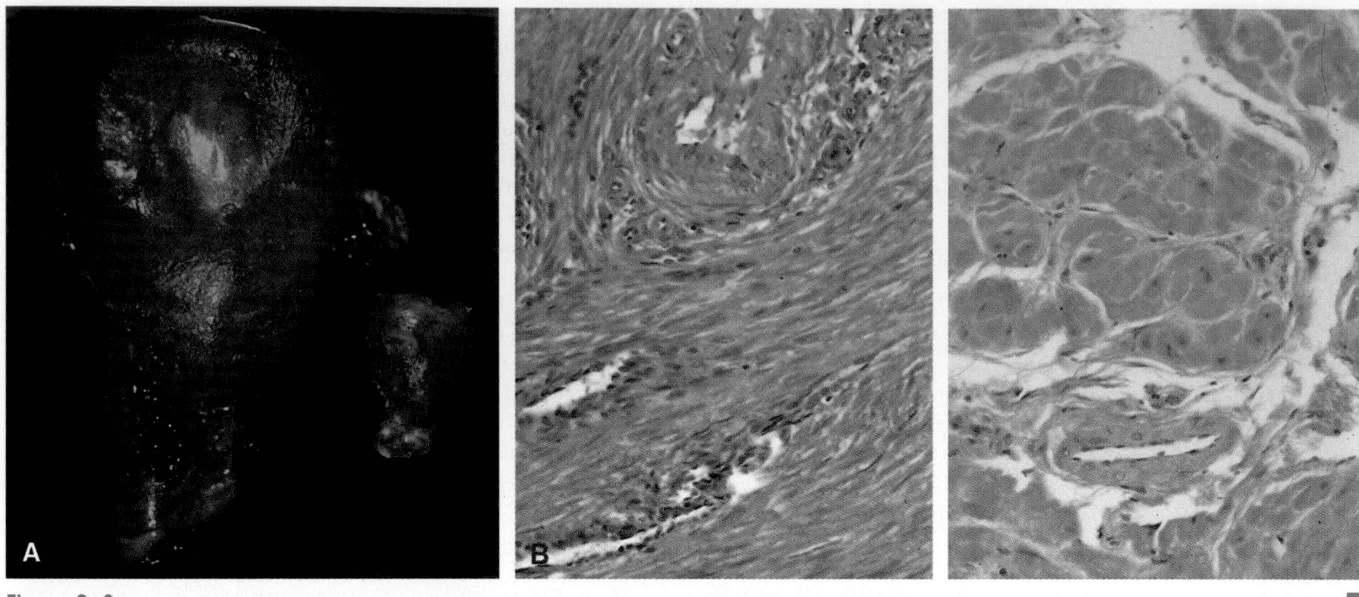

Figure 2–3

Physiologic hypertrophy of the uterus during pregnancy. *A*, Gross appearance of a normal uterus *(right)* and a gravid uterus (removed for postpartum bleeding) *(left)*. *B*, Small spindle-shaped uterine smooth muscle cells from a normal uterus *(left)* compared with large plump cells in gravid uterus *(right)*.

organ. Thus, the hypertrophied organ has no new cells, just larger cells. The increased size of the cells is due not to cellular swelling but to the synthesis of more structural components.

Hypertrophy can be *physiologic* or *pathologic* and is caused by increased functional demand or by specific hormonal stimulation. The massive physiologic growth of the uterus during pregnancy is a good example of hormone-induced hypertrophy involving both hypertrophy and hyperplasia (Fig. 2–3*A*). The cellular hypertrophy is stimulated by estrogenic hormones through smooth muscle estrogen receptors, which allow for interactions of the hormones with nuclear DNA, eventually resulting in increased synthesis of smooth muscle proteins and an increase in cell size (Fig. 2–3*B*). Similarly, prolactin and estrogen cause hypertrophy of the breasts during lactation. These are ex-

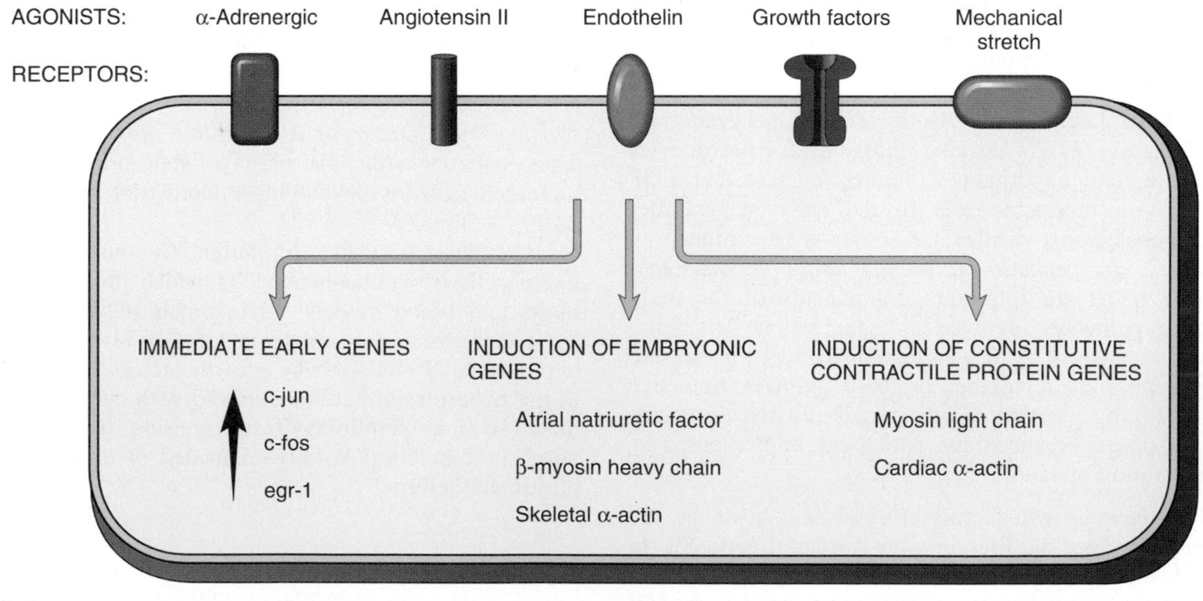

Figure 2–4

Phenotypic changes in hypertrophy, shown here in myocardial fibers subjected to hemodynamic overload (see text).

amples of physiologic hypertrophy effected by hormonal stimulation.

Hypertrophy as an adaptive response is exemplified by muscular enlargement seen in two settings. The striated muscle cells in both the heart and the skeletal muscles are most capable of hypertrophy, perhaps because they cannot adapt to increased metabolic demands by mitotic division and formation of more cells to share the work. The most common stimulus appears mainly to be increased workload. In the heart, it is usually *chronic hemodynamic overload*, owing either to hypertension or to faulty valves, and in skeletal muscles, heavy work. Synthesis of more proteins and filaments occurs, achieving a balance between the demand and the cell's functional capacity. The greater number of myofilaments permits an increased workload with a level of metabolic activity per unit volume of cell not different from that borne by the normal cell. Thus, the draft horse readily pulls the load that would break the back of a pony.

Not only the size, but also the phenotype of the individual myocytes is altered in hypertrophy (Fig. 2–4).[7] In volume overload in the myocardium, genes that are expressed only during early development are re-expressed. For example, in the embryonic heart, the gene for atrial natriuretic factor (ANF) is expressed in both the atrium and the ventricle. After birth, ventricular expression of the gene is selectively down-regulated.[8] Cardiac hypertrophy, however, results in the reinduction of ANF gene expression.[9] ANF is a peptide hormone that causes salt secretion by the kidney, decreases blood volume and pressure, and therefore serves to *reduce* hemodynamic load.

There is also a switch of contractile proteins from adult to fetal or neonatal forms. For example, the expression of the α-myosin heavy chain (α-MHC) is replaced by that of the β-MHC, which leads to decreased myosin adenosine triphosphatase (ATPase) activity and a slower, more energetically economical contraction. A number of other genes are likewise activated during hypertrophy, including those encoding some of the early regulatory factors (c-*fos*, c-*jun*, egr-1); growth factors (TGF-β, insulin-like growth factor-1 [IGF-1], fibroblast growth factor [FGF]); vasoactive agents (α-adrenergic agonists, endothelin-1, and angiotensin II); and components involved in receptor mediated signaling pathways, such as receptors (e.g., IGF-1 receptor) and kinases (e.g., protein kinase C).[10] These factors are discussed in detail in Chapter 4.

What are the triggers for hypertrophy and for these changes in gene expression? In the heart, there are at least two groups of signals: *mechanical triggers*, such as stretch, and *trophic triggers*, such as polypeptide growth factors and vasoactive agents (angiotensin II, α-adrenergic agonists). Current models suggest that growth factors or vasoactive agents produced by cardiac nonmuscle cells or by myocytes themselves in response to hemodynamic stress selectively regulate the expression of genes leading to myocyte hypertrophy.[11]

Whatever the exact mechanism of hypertrophy, it eventually reaches a limit beyond which enlargement of muscle mass is no longer able to compensate for the increased burden, and cardiac failure ensues. At this stage, a number of *degenerative* changes occur in the myocardial fibers, of which the most important are lysis and loss of myofibrillar contractile elements. Myocyte death can occur by either apoptosis or necrosis.[12] The limiting factors for continued hypertrophy and the causes of the cardiac dysfunction are poorly understood; they may be due to limitation of the vascular supply to the enlarged fibers, diminished oxidative capabilities of mitochondria, alterations in protein synthesis and degradation, or cytoskeletal alterations.

Atrophy

Shrinkage in the size of the cell by loss of cell substance is known as atrophy. It represents a form of adaptive response. When a sufficient number of cells are involved, the entire tissue or organ diminishes in size or becomes atrophic. Atrophy can be physiologic or pathologic. *Physiologic atrophy* is common during early development. Some embryonic structures, such as the notocord or thyroglossal duct, undergo atrophy during fetal development. The uterus decreases in size shortly after parturition, and this is a form of physiologic atrophy. *Pathologic atrophy* depends on the basic cause and can be local or generalized. The common causes of atrophy are the following:

- *Decreased workload (atrophy of disuse)*: When a broken limb is immobilized in a plaster cast or when a patient is restricted to complete bed rest, skeletal muscle atrophy rapidly ensues. The initial rapid decrease in cell size is reversible when activity is resumed. With more prolonged disuse, skeletal muscle fibers decrease in number as well as in size and can be accompanied by increased bone resorption, leading to osteoporosis of disuse.
- *Loss of innervation (denervation atrophy)*: Normal function of skeletal muscle is dependent on its nerve supply. Damage to the nerves leads to rapid atrophy of the muscle fibers supplied by those nerves (Chapter 29).
- *Diminished blood supply*: A decrease in blood supply (ischemia) to a tissue as a result of arterial occlusive disease results in atrophy of tissue owing to progressive cell loss. In late adult life, the brain undergoes progressive atrophy, presumably as atherosclerosis narrows its blood supply (Fig. 2–5).
- *Inadequate nutrition*: Profound protein-calorie malnutrition (marasmus) is associated with the use of skeletal muscle as a source of energy after other reserves such as adipose stores have been depleted. This results in marked muscle wasting.
- *Loss of endocrine stimulation*: Many endocrine glands, the breast, and the reproductive organs are dependent on endocrine stimulation for normal function. The loss of estrogen stimulation after the menopause results in physiologic atrophy of the endometrium, vaginal epithelium, and breast.
- *Aging (senile atrophy)*: The aging process is associated with cell loss. Morphologically, it is seen in tissues containing permanent cells, particularly in the brain and heart.

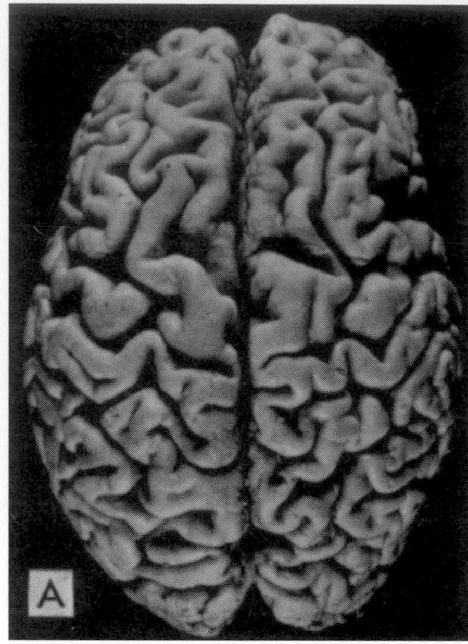

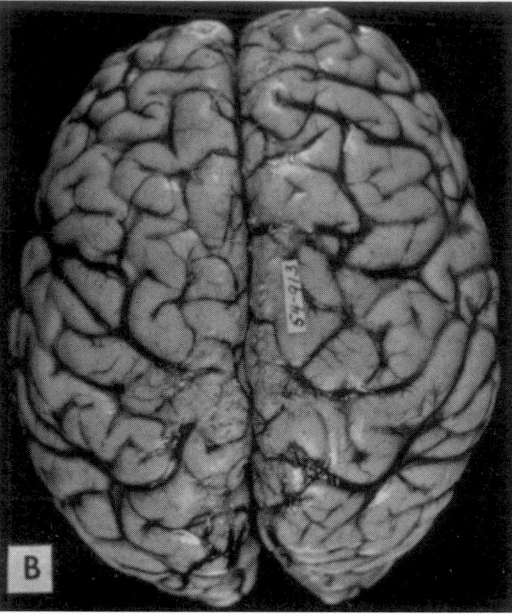

Figure 2–5

A, Physiologic atrophy of the brain in an 82 year-old male. The meninges have been stripped. *B*, Normal brain of a 36-year-old male.

- *Pressure*: Tissue compression for any length of time can cause atrophy. An enlarging benign tumor can cause atrophy in the surrounding compressed tissues. Atrophy in this setting is probably the result of ischemic changes caused by a blood supply that has been compromised by the expanding mass.

The fundamental cellular changes are identical in all of these settings, representing a retreat by the cell to a smaller size at which survival is still possible. Atrophy represents a reduction in the structural components of the cell. In muscle, the cells contain fewer mitochondria and myofilaments and a lesser amount of endoplasmic reticulum. By bringing into balance cell volume and lower levels of blood supply, nutrition, or trophic stimulation, a new equilibrium is achieved. Although *atrophic cells may have diminished function, they are not dead. Apoptosis* or programmed cell death (Chapter 1), however, may be induced by the same signals that cause atrophy and thus may contribute to loss of organ mass. For example, apoptosis contributes to the regression of endocrine organs after hormone withdrawal and the shrinkage of secretory glands after obstruction of their ducts.

The biochemical mechanisms responsible for atrophy are incompletely understood but are likely to affect the balance between protein synthesis and degradation. The regulation of protein degradation probably plays a key role in atrophy. Mammalian cells contain multiple proteolytic systems that serve distinct functions. *Lysosomes* contain acid hyrolases (e.g., cathepsins) and other enzymes that degrade endocytosed proteins from the extracellular environment and the cell surface as well as some cellular components. The *ubiquitin-proteasome pathway* is responsible for the degradation of many cytosolic and nuclear proteins.[13] Proteins degraded by this process are first conjugated to ubiquitin and then degraded within a large cytoplasmic proteolytic complex, or proteasome. This pathway is thought to be responsible for the accelerated proteolysis in a variety of catabolic conditions, including cancer cachexia. Hormones, particularly glucocorticoids and thyroid hormone, stimulate proteasome-mediated protein degradation; insulin opposes these actions. Additionally, cytokines, such as TNF-α and IL-1β, are capable of signaling accelerated muscle proteolysis by way of this mechanism.

In many situations, atrophy is also accompanied by marked increases in the number of *autophagic vacuoles*. As stated earlier, these are membrane-bound vacuoles within the cell that contain fragments of cell components (e.g., mitochondria, endoplasmic reticulum), which are destined for destruction and into which the lysosomes discharge their hydrolytic contents. The cellular components are then digested. Some of the cell debris within the autophagic vacuole may resist digestion and persist as membrane-bound residual bodies that may remain as a sarcophagus in the cytoplasm. An example of such *residual bodies* is the *lipofuscin granules*, discussed in Chapter 1. When present in sufficient amounts, they impart a *brown discoloration* to the tissue (brown atrophy).

Obviously, atrophy may progress to the point at which cells are injured and die. If the blood supply is inadequate even to maintain the life of shrunken cells, injury and cell death may supervene. The atrophic tissue may then be replaced by fatty ingrowth.

Metaplasia

Metaplasia is a reversible change in which one adult cell type (epithelial or mesenchymal) is replaced by another adult cell type.[14] It, too, may represent an adaptive substitution of cells that are sensitive to stress by cell types better able to withstand the adverse environment.

The most common epithelial metaplasia is *columnar* to *squamous* (Fig. 2–6*A*), as occurs in the respiratory tract in response to chronic irritation. In the habitual cigarette

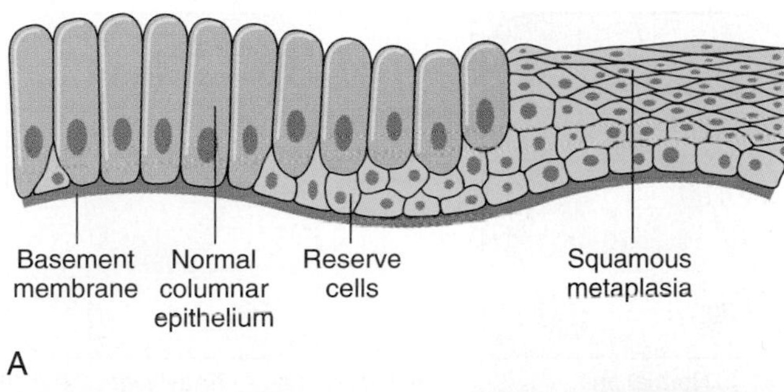

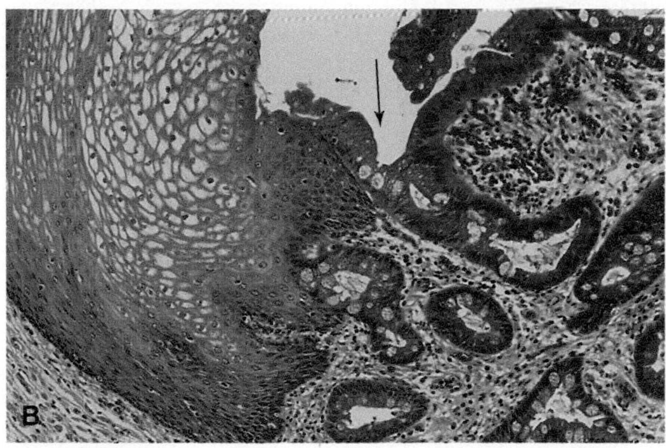

Figure 2–6

Metaplasia. *A*, Schematic diagram of columnar to squamous metaplasia. *B*, Metaplastic transformation of esophageal stratified squamous epithelium (left) to mature columnar epithelium (so-called Barrett metaplasia).

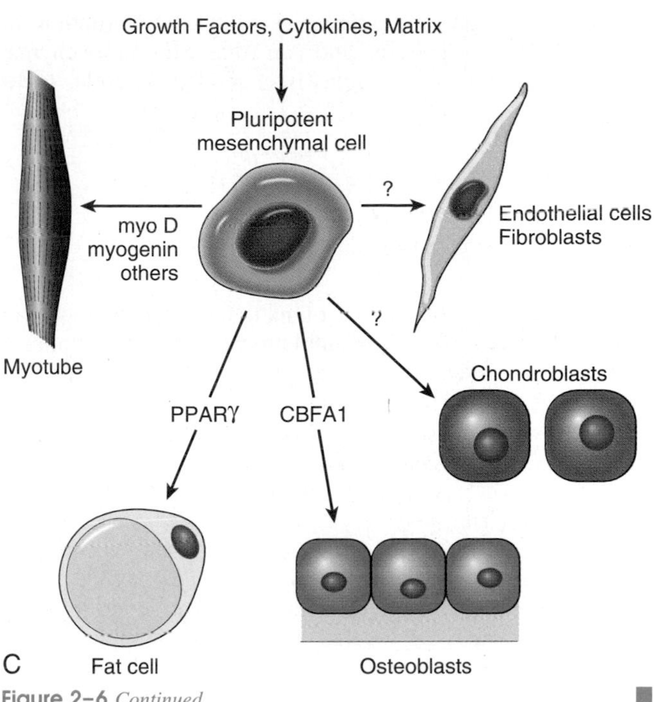

Figure 2–6 *Continued*

C, Differentiation pathways for stem cells. Activation of key regulatory proteins by growth factors, cytokines, or matrix components leads to commitment of stem cells to differentiate into specific cellular lineages. Differentiation of myotubes requires the combined action of several factors (e.g., myo D, myogenin); fat cells require PPARγ; the osteogenic lineage requires CBFA1, while factors for endothelial cells and fibroblasts are not yet known. (*C*, Adapted and redrawn from Rodan GA, Harada S: The missing bone. Cell 89:677, 1997.)

smoker, the normal columnar ciliated epithelial cells of the trachea and bronchi are often replaced focally or widely by stratified squamous epithelial cells. Stones in the excretory ducts of the salivary glands, pancreas, or bile ducts may cause replacement of the normal secretory columnar epithelium by nonfunctioning stratified squamous epithelium. A deficiency of vitamin A (retinoic acid) induces squamous metaplasia in the respiratory epithelium, and vitamin A excess *suppresses* keratinization (Chapter 10). In all these instances, the more rugged stratified squamous epithelium is able to survive under circumstances in which the more fragile specialized epithelium most likely would have succumbed. Although the squamous metaplastic cells in the respiratory tract, for example, are capable of surviving, an important protective mechanism—mucus secretion—is lost. Thus, epithelial metaplasia is a two-edged sword and, in most circumstances, represents an undesirable change. *Moreover, the influences that predispose to such metaplasia, if persistent, may induce cancer transformation in metaplastic epithelium.* Thus, the common form of cancer in the respiratory tract is composed of squamous cells.

Metaplasia from squamous to columnar type may also occur, as in *Barrett esophagitis,* in which the squamous esophageal epithelium is replaced by intestinal-like columnar cells (Chapter 18) (Fig. 2–6*B*). The resulting cancers that may arise are glandular (adeno) carcinomas.

Connective tissue metaplasia is the formation of cartilage, bone, or adipose tissue (mesenchymal tissues) in tissues that normally do not contain these elements. For example, bone formation in muscle, designated *myositis ossificans*, occasionally occurs after bone fracture. This type of metaplasia is less clearly seen as an adaptive response.

Metaplasia is thought to arise from a reprogramming of stem cells that are known to exist in most epithelia (called *reserve* cells) or of undifferentiated mesenchymal cells present in connective tissue. In a metaplastic change, these precursor cells differentiate along a new pathway. This is brought about by changes in signals generated by mixtures of cytokines, growth factors, and extracellular matrix components in the cell's environment. Tissue-specific and differentiation genes are involved in the process and an increasing number of these are being indentified. For example, bone morphogenetic proteins (BMPs), members of the TGF-β superfamily, induce chondrogenic or osteogenic expression in mesenchymal stem cells, while suppressing differentiation into muscle or fat.[15] These growth factors, acting as external triggers, then induce specific transcription factors that lead the cascade of phenotype-specific genes toward a fully differentiated cell (Fig. 2–6*C*). Such transcription factors include MyoD for muscle, PPARγ for adipose tissue, and CBFA-1 for osteoblastic differentiation.[16] How these normal pathways run amuck to cause metaplasia is unclear in most instances. In the case of vitamin A deficiency or excess, it is known that retinoic acid regulates cell growth, differentiation, and tissue patterning.[17] Certain *cytostatic* drugs cause a disruption of DNA methylation patterns and can transform mesenchymal cells from one type (fibroblast) to another (muscle, cartilage).

INTRACELLULAR ACCUMULATIONS

One of the manifestations of metabolic derangements in cells is the intracellular accumulation of abnormal amounts of various substances. The stockpiled substances fall into three categories: (1) a *normal cellular constituent* accumulated in excess, such as water, lipid, protein, and carbohydrates; (2) an *abnormal substance*, either exogenous, such as a mineral or products of infectious agents, or endogenous, such as a product of abnormal synthesis or metabolism; and (3) a *pigment*. These substances may accumulate either transiently or permanently, and they may be harmless to the cells, but on occasion they are severely toxic. The substance may be located in either the cytoplasm (frequently within lysosomes) or the nucleus. In some instances, the cell may be producing the abnormal substance, and in others it may be merely storing products of pathologic processes occurring elsewhere in the body.

Many processes result in abnormal intracellular accumulations in non-neoplastic cells, but most can be divided into three general types (Fig. 2–7).

1. *A normal endogenous substance is produced at a normal or increased rate, but the rate of metabolism is inadequate to remove it.* An example of this type of process is fatty change in the liver because of intracellular accumulation of triglycerides (see later). Another is the appearance of reabsorption protein droplets in renal tubules because of increased leakage of protein from the glomerulus.
2. *A normal or abnormal endogenous substance accumulates because of genetic or acquired defects in the metabolism, packaging, transport, or secretion of these substances.* One example is the group of conditions caused by genetic defects of specific enzymes involved in the metabolism of lipid and carbohydrates resulting in intracellular deposition of these substances, largely in lysosomes. These so-called storage diseases are discussed in Chapter 5. Another is *alpha$_1$-antitrypsin* deficiency, in which a single amino acid substitution in the enzyme results in defects in protein folding and accumulation of the enzyme in the endoplasmic reticulum of the liver in the form of globular eosinophilic inclusions (see later and Chapter 19).
3. *An abnormal exogenous substance is deposited* and accumulates because the cell has neither the enzymatic machinery to degrade the substance nor the ability to transport it to other sites. Accumulations of carbon particles and such nonmetabolizable chemicals as silica particles are examples of this type of alteration.

Whatever the nature and origin of the intracellular accumulation, it implies the storage of some product by individual cells. If the overload is due to a systemic derangement

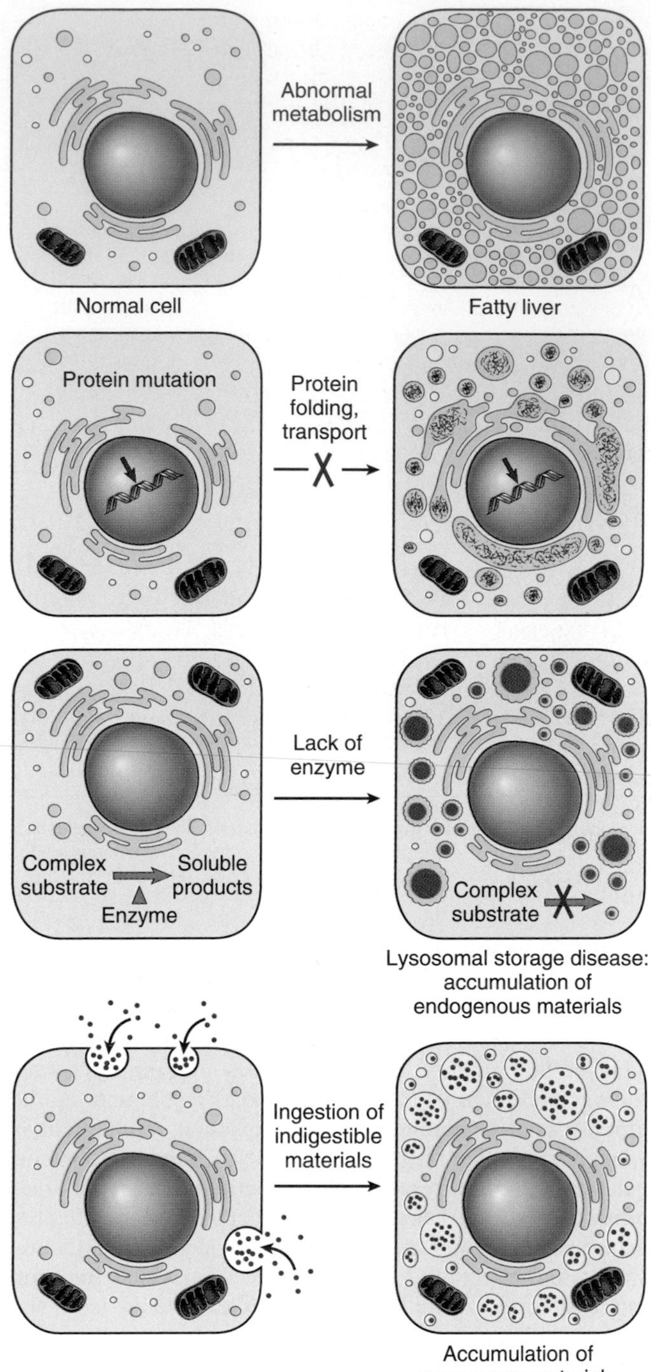

Figure 2–7

General mechanisms of intracellular accumulation: (1) abnormal metabolism, as in fatty change in the liver; (2) mutations causing alterations in protein folding and transport, as in alpha$_1$-antitrypsin deficiency; (3) deficiency of critical enzymes that prevent breakdown of substrates that accumulate in lysosomes, as in lysosomal storage diseases; and (4) inability to degrade phagocytosed particles, as in hemosiderosis and carbon pigment accumulation.

and can be brought under control, the accumulation is reversible. In genetic storage diseases, accumulation is progressive, and the cells may become so overloaded as to cause secondary injury, leading in some instances to death of the tissue and the patient.

Lipids

All major classes of lipids can accumulate in cells: triglycerides, cholesterol/cholesterol esters, and phospholipids. Phospholipids, as we have seen, are components of the myelin figures found in necrotic cells. In addition, abnormal complexes of lipids and carbohydrates accumulate in the lysosomal storage diseases (Chapter 6). Here we concentrate on triglyceride and cholesterol accumulations.

STEATOSIS (FATTY CHANGE)

The terms *steatosis* and *fatty change* describe abnormal accumulations of triglycerides within parenchymal cells. Fatty change is often seen in the liver because it is the major organ involved in fat metabolism, but it also occurs in heart, muscle, and kidney. The causes of steatosis include toxins, protein malnutrition, diabetes mellitus, obesity, and anoxia. *In industrialized nations, by far the most common cause of significant fatty change in the liver (fatty liver) is alcohol abuse*[18] (Chapter 19).

Different mechanisms account for triglyceride accumulation in the liver. Free fatty acids from adipose tissue or ingested food are normally transported into hepatocytes. In the liver, they are esterified to triglycerides, converted into cholesterol or phospholipids, or oxidized to ketone bodies. Some fatty acids are synthesized from acetate as well. Release of triglycerides from the hepatocytes requires association with apoproteins to form lipoproteins, which may then traverse the circulation (Chapter 5). *Excess accumulation of triglycerides within the liver may result from defects in any one of the events in the sequence from fatty acid entry to lipoprotein exit* (Fig. 2–8*A*). A number of such defects are induced by alcohol, a hepatotoxin that alters mitochondrial and microsomal functions. CCl_4 and protein malnutrition act by decreasing synthesis of apoproteins. Anoxia inhibits fatty acid oxidation. Starvation increases fatty acid mobilization from the peripheral stores.

The significance of fatty change depends on the cause and severity of the accumulation. When mild, it may have no effect on cellular function. More severe fatty change may impair cellular function, but unless some vital intracellular process is irreversibly impaired (e.g., in CCl_4 poisoning), fatty change per se is reversible. As a severe form of injury, fatty change may be a harbinger of cell death, *but cells may die without undergoing fatty change.*

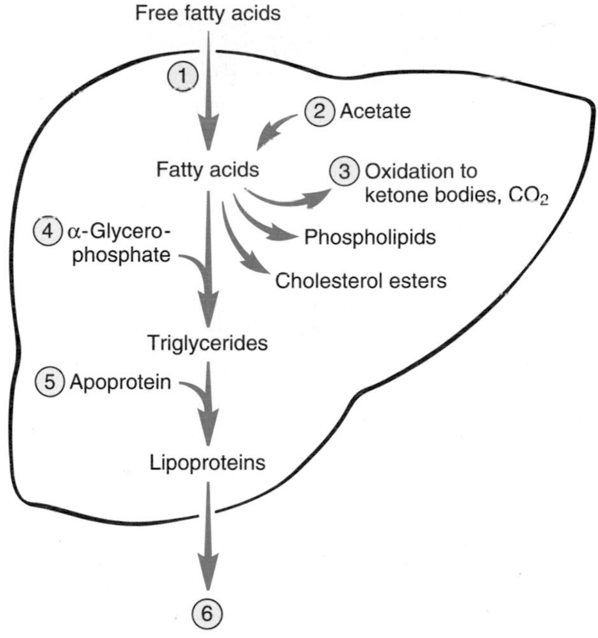

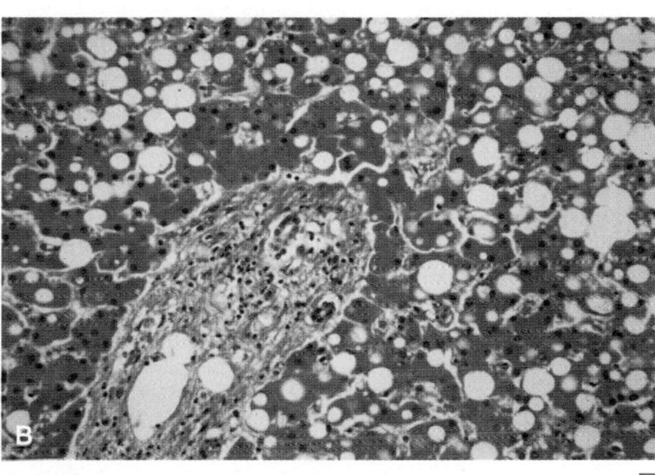

Figure 2–8

Fatty liver. *A*, Schematic diagram of the possible mechanisms leading to accumulation of triglycerides in fatty liver. Defects in any of the six numbered steps of uptake, catabolism, or secretion can result in lipid accumulation. *B*, High-power detail of fatty change of the liver. In most cells, the well-preserved nucleus is squeezed into the displaced rim of cytoplasm about the fat vacuole. (*B*, Courtesy of Dr. James Crawford, Department of Pathology, Yale University School of Medicine.)

MORPHOLOGY. Fatty change is most often seen in the liver and heart. In all organs, fatty change appears as clear vacuoles within parenchymal cells. Intracellular accumulations of water or polysaccharides (e.g., glycogen) may also produce clear vacuoles, and it becomes necessary to resort to special techniques to distinguish these three types of clear vacuoles. The identification of lipids requires the avoidance of fat solvents commonly used in paraffin embedding for routine hematoxylin and eosin stains. To identify the fat, it is necessary to prepare frozen tissue sections of either fresh or aqueous formalin-fixed tissues. The sections may then be stained with Sudan IV or Oil Red-O, both of which impart an orange-red color to the contained lipids. The periodic acid–Schiff (PAS) reaction is commonly employed to identify glycogen, although it is by no means specific. When neither fat nor polysaccharide can be demonstrated within a clear vacuole, it is presumed to contain water or fluid with a low protein content.

Liver. In the liver, mild fatty change may not affect the gross appearance. With progressive accumulation, the organ enlarges and becomes increasingly yellow until, in extreme instances, the liver may weigh 3 to 6 kg and be transformed into a bright yellow, soft, greasy organ.

Fatty change begins with the development of minute, membrane-bound inclusions (liposomes) closely applied to the endoplasmic reticulum. Fatty change is first seen by light microscopy as small vacuoles in the cytoplasm around the nucleus. As the process progresses, the vacuoles coalesce, creating cleared spaces that displace the nucleus to the periphery of the cell (Fig. 2–8*B*). Occasionally, contiguous cells rupture, and the enclosed fat globules coalesce, producing so-called fatty cysts.

Heart. Lipid is found in cardiac muscle in the form of small droplets, occurring in two patterns. In one, prolonged moderate hypoxia, such as that produced by profound anemia, causes intracellular deposits of fat, which create grossly apparent bands of yellowed myocardium alternating with bands of darker, red-brown, uninvolved myocardium **(tigered effect)**. The other pattern of hypoxia is produced by more profound hypoxia or by some forms of myocarditis (e.g., diphtheria) and shows more uniformly affected myocytes.

CHOLESTEROL AND CHOLESTEROL ESTERS

The cellular metabolism of cholesterol (discussed in detail in Chapter 6) is tightly regulated such that most cells use cholesterol for the synthesis of cell membranes without intracellular accumulation of cholesterol or cholesterol esters. Accumulations, however, manifested histologically by intracellular vacuoles, are seen in several pathologic processes.

- *Atherosclerosis*: In atherosclerotic plaques, smooth muscle cells and macrophages within the intimal layer of the aorta and large arteries are filled with lipid vacuoles, most of which are made up of cholesterol and cholesterol esters. Such cells have a foamy appearance (*foam cells*), and aggregates of them in the intima produce the yellow cholesterol-laden atheromas characteristic of this serious disorder. Some of these fat-laden cells rupture, releasing lipids into the extracellular space. The mechanisms of cholesterol accumulation in both cell types in atherosclerosis are discussed in detail in Chapter 12. The extracellular cholesterol esters may crystallize in the shape of long needles, producing quite distinctive clefts in tissue sections.
- *Xanthomas*: Intracellular accumulation of cholesterol within macrophages is also characteristic of acquired and hereditary hyperlipidemic states. Clusters of foamy cells are found in the subepithelial connective tissue of the skin and in tendons producing tumorous masses known as xanthomas.
- *Inflammation and necrosis*: Foamy macrophages are frequently found at sites of cell injury and inflammation, owing to phagocytosis of cholesterol from the membranes of injured cells, including parenchymal cells, leukocytes, and erythrocytes. Phospholipids and myelin figures are also found in inflammatory foci. When abundant, the cholesterol-laden macrophages impart a yellowish discoloration to such inflammatory foci.
- *Cholesterolosis*: This refers to the focal accumulations of cholesterol-laden macrophages in the lamina propria of the gallbladder. The mechanism of accumulation is unknown (Fig. 2–9).

Proteins

Excesses of proteins within the cells sufficient to cause morphologically visible accumulation have diverse causes. They usually appear as rounded, eosinophilic droplets, vacuoles, or aggregates in the cytoplasm. By electron microscopy, they can be amorphous, fibrillar, or crystalline in appearance. Accumulations of cytoskeletal proteins have already been alluded to in the discussion of cytoskeletal alterations. In some disorders, such as certain forms of amyloidosis, both intra- and extracellular accumulation of the same protein occurs (Chapter 7).

Some of the causes of intracellular accumulation of proteins are obvious. Excesses may be presented to the cell beyond its capacity to rapidly metabolize them, as is the case in the accumulation of

- *Reabsorption droplets in proximal renal tubules*. This is seen in renal diseases associated with protein loss in the urine (proteinuria). In the kidney, small amounts of protein filtered through the glomerulus are normally reabsorbed by pinocytosis in the proximal tubule. In disor-

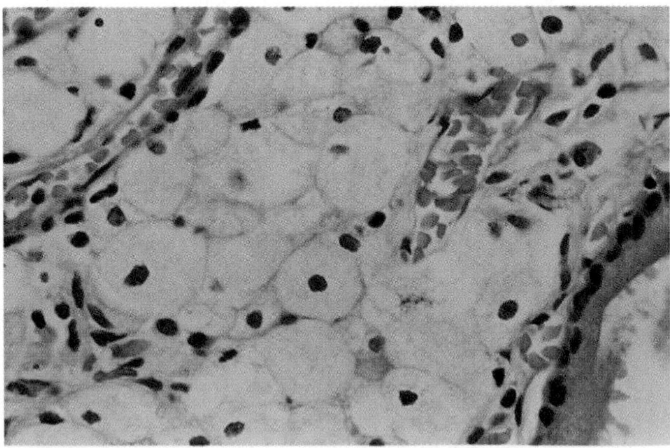

Figure 2–9

Cholesterolosis. Cholesterol-laden macrophages (foam cells) from a focus of gallbladder cholesterolosis. The gallbladder mucosa is in the upper left.

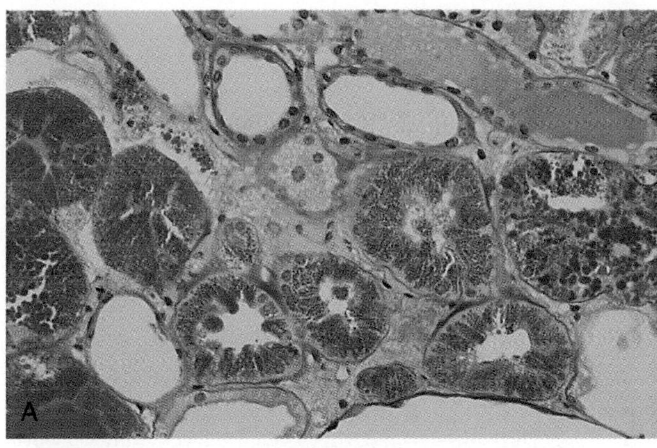

Figure 2–10

A, Protein reabsorption droplets in the renal tubular epithelium. (Courtesy of Dr. Helmut Rennke, Department of Pathology, Brigham and Women's Hospital.)

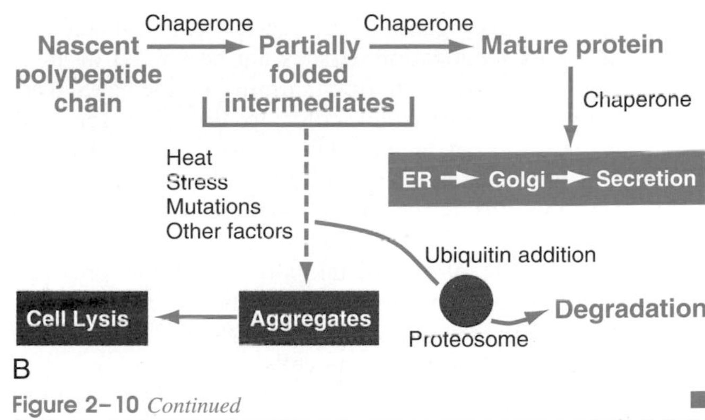

Figure 2–10 *Continued*

B, Simplified scheme of protein folding and how defects can lead to protein aggregation and abnormal cellular translocation (see text).

ders with heavy protein leakage across the glomerular filter, however, there is increased reabsorption of the protein. These pinocytotic vesicles fuse with lysosomes to produce phagolysosomes, which appear as pink hyaline droplets within the cytoplasm of the tubular cell (Fig. 2–10*A*). The process is reversible; if the proteinuria diminishes, the protein droplets are metabolized and disappear.

- A second cause is synthesis of excessive amounts of normal secretory protein, as occurs in certain plasma cells engaged in active synthesis of immunoglobulins. The ER becomes hugely distended, producing large, homogeneous eosinophilic inclusions called *Russell bodies*.

However, it has become clear that defects in *protein folding* may underlie some of these depositions in a variety of unrelated diseases, and we will briefly review the salient points in these events.

DEFECTS IN PROTEIN FOLDING

Nascent polypeptide chains of proteins, made on ribosomes, are ultimately arranged into either α helices or β sheets, and the proper configuration of these arrangements (protein folding) is critical to the individual protein's function and its transport across the cell organelles.[19] In the process of folding, partially folded intermediates arise, and these may be particularly vulnerable to form intracellular aggregates among themselves or by entangling other proteins. Under normal conditions, however, these intermediates are stabilized by a number of molecular *chaperones,* which interact with proteins directly (Fig. 2–10*B*). Chaperones aid in proper folding and in transport across the endoplasmic reticulum (ER), Golgi complex, and beyond. Some chaperones are synthesized constitutively and affect normal protein intracellular metabolism, whereas others are induced by stress, such as heat (heat-shock proteins, e.g., hsp70, hsp90), and "rescue" shock-stressed proteins from misfolding. If the folding process is not successful, the chaperones facilitate degradation of the damaged protein. This degradative process often involves ubiquitin (a heat-shock protein), which is added to the abnormal protein and marks it for degradation by the proteasome complex.[20] There are several mechanisms by which protein folding defects can cause intracellular accumulations or result in disease.

- *Defective intracellular transport and secretion of critical proteins.* As noted, in *α1-antitrypsin deficiency* mutations in the protein significantly slow folding, resulting in the build-up of partially folded intermediates, which aggregate in the ER of the liver and are not secreted. The resultant deficiency of the circulating enzyme causes emphysema (Chapter 16). In *cystic fibrosis,* frequent mutation delays dissociation of a chloride channel protein from one of its chaperones, resulting in abnormal folding and loss of function (Chapter 6).
- *Toxicity of aggregated, abnormally folded proteins.* Aggregation of abnormally folded proteins, caused by genetic mutations, aging, or unknown environmental factors, is now recognized as a feature of a number of neurodegenerative diseases, including Alzheimer, Huntington, and Parkinson diseases, as well as certain forms of amyloidosis.[21] The deposits can be intracellular, extracellular, or both, and there is accumulating evidence that the aggregates may either directly or indirectly cause the pathologic changes. These disorders, now euphemistically called the *proteinopathies* or *protein-aggregation diseases,* and the possible mechanisms leading to protein misfolding are described in Chapter 7 for amyloidosis and Chapter 30 for the neurodegenerative diseases.

Glycogen

Glycogen is a readily available energy store that is present in the cytoplasm. Excessive intracellular deposits of glycogen are seen in patients with an abnormality in either glucose or glycogen metabolism. Whatever the clinical setting, the glycogen masses appear as clear vacuoles within the cytoplasm. Glycogen is best preserved in nonaqueous fixatives; for its localization, tissues are best fixed in absolute alcohol. Staining with Best carmine or the PAS reaction imparts a rose-to-violet color to the glycogen, and diastase digestion of a parallel section before staining serves as a further control by hydrolyzing the glycogen.

Diabetes mellitus is the prime example of a disorder of glucose metabolism. In this disease, glycogen is found in the epithelial cells of the distal portions of the proximal convoluted tubules and sometimes in the descending loop of Henle as well as within liver cells, β cells of the islets of Langerhans, and heart muscle cells.

Glycogen also accumulates within the cells in a group of closely related disorders, all genetic, collectively referred to as the *glycogen storage diseases*, or *glycogenoses* (Chapter 6). In these diseases, enzymatic defects in the synthesis or breakdown of glycogen result in massive stockpiling, with secondary injury and cell death.

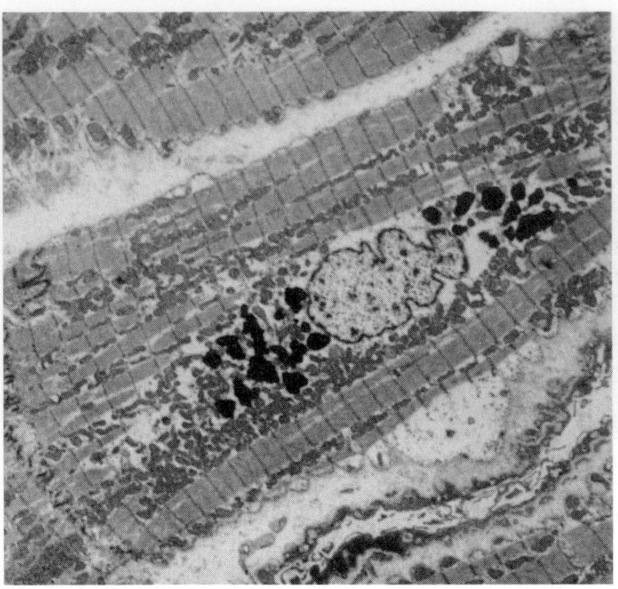

Figure 2–11

Lipofuscin granules in a cardiac myocyte as shown by electron microscopy. Low magnification. Note the perinuclear, intralysosomal location.

Pigments

Pigments are colored substances, some of which are normal constituents of cells (e.g., melanin), whereas others are abnormal and collect in cells only under special circumstances. Pigments can be either exogenous, coming from outside the body, or endogenous, synthesized within the body itself.

Exogenous. The most common *exogenous pigment* is *carbon* or coal dust, which is a virtually ubiquitous air pollutant of urban life. When inhaled, it is picked up by macrophages within the alveoli and is then transported through lymphatic channels to the regional lymph nodes in the tracheobronchial region. Accumulations of this pigment blacken the tissues of the lungs (*anthracosis*) and the involved lymph nodes. In coal miners and those living in heavily polluted environments, the aggregates of carbon dust may induce a fibroblastic reaction or even emphysema and thus cause a serious lung disease known as *coal worker's pneumoconiosis* (Chapter 16). *Tattooing* is a form of localized, exogenous pigmentation of the skin. The pigments inoculated are phagocytized by dermal macrophages, in which they reside for the remainder of the life of the embellished. The pigments do not usually evoke any inflammatory response.

Endogenous. *Lipofuscin* is an insoluble pigment, also known as lipochrome and *wear-and-tear* or aging pigment. Lipofuscin is composed of polymers of lipids and phospholipids complexed with protein, *suggesting that it is derived through lipid peroxidation of polyunsaturated lipids of subcellular membranes.* Lipofuscin is not injurious to the cell or its functions. Its importance lies in its being the telltale sign of free radical injury and lipid peroxidation. The term is derived from the Latin (*fuscus* = brown), thus brown lipid. In tissue sections, it appears as a yellow-brown, finely granular intracytoplasmic, often perinuclear pigment. It is seen in cells undergoing slow, regressive changes and is particularly prominent in the liver and heart of aging patients or patients with severe malnutrition and cancer cachexia. On electron microscopy, the granules are highly electron dense, often have membranous structures in their midst, and are usually in a perinuclear location (Fig. 2–11).

Melanin, derived from the Greek (*melas* = black), is an endogenous, non–hemoglobin-derived, brown-black pigment formed when the enzyme tyrosinase catalyzes the oxidation of tyrosine to dihydroxyphenylalanine in melanocytes. It is discussed further in Chapter 27. For all practical purposes, melanin is the *only endogenous brown-black pigment.* The only other that could be considered in this category is homogentisic acid, a black pigment that occurs in patients with *alkaptonuria*, a rare metabolic disease. Here the pigment is deposited in the skin, connective tissue, and cartilage, and the pigmentation is known as ochronosis.

Hemosiderin is a hemoglobin-derived, golden yellow–to–brown, granular or crystalline pigment in which form iron is stored in cells. Iron metabolism and the synthesis of ferritin and hemosiderin are considered in detail in Chapter 14. Iron is normally carried by specific transport proteins, transferrins. In cells, it is stored in association with a protein, apoferritin, to form ferritin micelles. Ferritin is a constituent of most cell types. *When there is a local or systemic excess of iron, ferritin forms hemosiderin granules*, which are easily seen with the light microscope (Fig. 2–12). Thus, hemosiderin pigment represents aggregates of ferritin micelles. Under normal conditions, small amounts of hemosiderin can be seen in the mononuclear phagocytes of the bone marrow, spleen, and liver, all actively engaged in red cell breakdown.

Excesses of iron cause hemosiderin to accumulate within cells, either as a localized process or as a systemic derangement. *Local excesses* of iron and hemosiderin result from gross hemorrhages or the myriad minute hemorrhages that accompany severe vascular congestion. The best example of localized hemosiderosis is the common bruise. After local hemorrhage, the area is at first red-blue. With lysis of

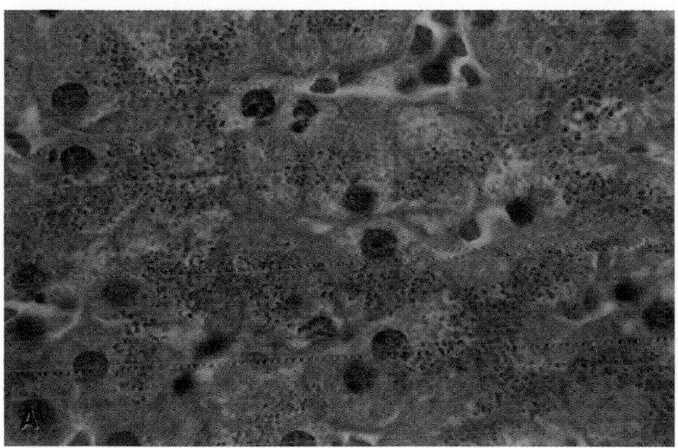

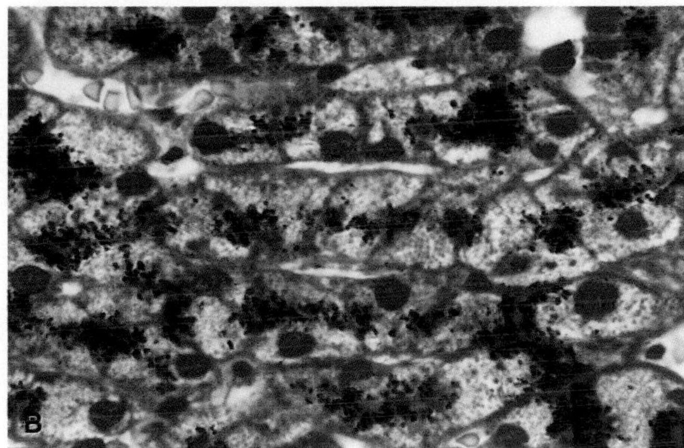

Figure 2–12

Hemosiderin granules in liver cells. *A*, H&E section showing golden-brown, finely granular pigment. *B*, Prussian blue reaction, specific for iron.

the erythrocytes, the hemoglobin eventually undergoes transformation to hemosiderin. Macrophages take part in this process by phagocytizing the red cell debris, and then lysosomal enzymes eventually convert the hemoglobin, through a sequence of pigments, into hemosiderin. The play of colors through which the bruise passes reflects these transformations. The original red-blue color of hemoglobin is transformed to varying shades of green-blue, comprising the local formation of biliverdin (green bile), then bilirubin (red bile), and thereafter the iron moiety of hemoglobin is deposited as golden yellow hemosiderin.

Whenever there are causes for *systemic overload of iron*, hemosiderin is deposited in many organs and tissues, a condition called *hemosiderosis*. It is seen with (1) increased absorption of dietary iron, (2) impaired use of iron, (3) hemolytic anemias, and (4) transfusions because the transfused red cells constitute an exogenous load of iron. These conditions are discussed in Chapter 18.

MORPHOLOGY. The pigment appears as a coarse, golden, granular pigment lying within the cell's cytoplasm. When the basic cause is the localized breakdown of red cells, the pigmentation is found at first in the reticuloendothelial cells in the area. In systemic hemosiderosis, it is found at first in the mononuclear phagocytes of the liver, bone marrow, spleen, and lymph nodes and in scattered macrophages throughout other organs such as the skin, pancreas, and kidneys. With progressive accumulation, parenchymal cells throughout the body (principally in the liver, pancreas, heart, and endocrine organs) become pigmented. Iron can be visualized in tissues by the Prussian blue histochemical reaction, in which colorless potassium ferrocyanide is converted by iron to blue-black ferric ferrocyanide (Fig. 2–12).

In most instances of systemic hemosiderosis, the pigment does not damage the parenchymal cells or impair organ function. The more extreme accumulation of iron, however, in a disease called **hemochromatosis** is associated with liver and pancreatic damage, resulting in liver fibrosis, heart failure, and diabetes mellitus (Chapter 18).

Bilirubin is the normal major pigment found in bile. It is derived from hemoglobin but contains no iron. Its normal formation and excretion are vital to health, and jaundice is a common clinical disorder caused by excesses of this pigment within cells and tissues. Bilirubin metabolism and jaundice are discussed in Chapter 19.

PATHOLOGIC CALCIFICATION

Pathologic calcification implies the abnormal deposition of calcium salts, together with smaller amounts of iron, magnesium, and other mineral salts. It is a common process occurring in a variety of pathologic conditions.[22] There are two forms of pathologic calcification. When the deposition occurs locally in nonviable or dying tissues, it is known as *dystrophic calcification*; it occurs despite normal serum levels of calcium and in the absence of derangements in calcium metabolism. In contrast, the deposition of calcium salts in vital tissues is known as *metastatic calcification*, and it almost always reflects some disturbance in calcium metabolism, leading to hypercalcemia.

Dystrophic Calcification

Dystrophic calcification is encountered in areas of necrosis, whether they are of coagulative, caseous, or liquefactive type, and in foci of enzymatic necrosis of fat. Calcification is almost inevitable in the atheromas of advanced atherosclerosis. It also commonly develops in aging or damaged heart valves, further hampering their function (Fig. 2–13). Whatever the site of deposition, the calcium salts appear macroscopically as fine, white granules or

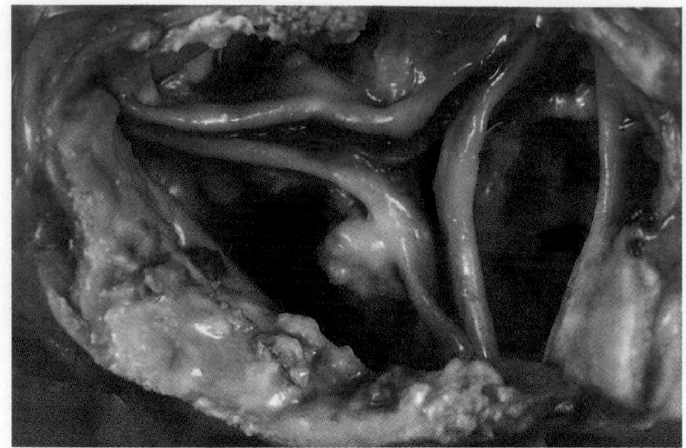

Figure 2–13

View looking down onto the unopened aortic valve in a heart with calcific aortic stenosis. The semilunar cusps are thickened and fibrotic. Behind each cusp are seen irregular masses of piled-up dystrophic calcification.

clumps, often felt as gritty deposits. Sometimes a tuberculous lymph node is virtually converted to stone.

MORPHOLOGY. Histologically, with the usual hematoxylin and eosin stain, the calcium salts have a basophilic, amorphous granular, sometimes clumped appearance. They can be intracellular, extracellular, or in both locations. In the course of time, **heterotopic** bone may be formed in the focus of calcification. On occasion, single necrotic cells may constitute seed crystals that become encrusted by the mineral deposits. The progressive acquisition of outer layers may create lamellated configurations, called **psammoma bodies** because of their resemblance to grains of sand. Some types of papillary cancers (e.g., thyroid) are apt to develop psammoma bodies. Strange concretions emerge when calcium iron salts gather about long slender spicules of asbestos in the lung, creating exotic, beaded dumbbell forms.

Pathogenesis. In the *pathogenesis* of dystrophic calcification, the final common pathway is the formation of crystalline calcium phosphate mineral in the form of an apatite similar to the hydroxyapatite of bone. The process has two major phases: *initiation* (or nucleation) and *propagation*; both can occur intracellularly and extracellularly.[23] Initiation of *intracellular calcification* occurs in the *mitochondria* of dead or dying cells that accumulate calcium, as described in Chapter 1. Initiators of *extracellular* dystrophic calcification include phospholipids found in membrane-bound *vesicles* about 200 nm in diameter; in cartilage and bone, they are known as *matrix vesicles,* and in pathologic calcification, they are derived from degenerating or aging cells. It is thought that calcium is concentrated in these vesicles by a process of membrane-facilitated calcification, which has several steps (Fig. 2–14): (1) Calcium ion binds to the phospholipids present in the vesicle membrane; (2) phosphatases associated with the membrane generate phosphate groups, which bind to the calcium; (3) the cycle of calcium and phosphate binding is repeated, raising the local concentrations and producing a deposit near the membrane; and (4) a structural change occurs in the arrangement of calcium and phosphate groups generating a microcrystal, which can then propagate and perforate the membrane. Propagation of crystal formation depends on the concentration of Ca^{2+} and PO_4 and the presence of inhibitors and other proteins in the extracellular space, such as the connective tissue matrix proteins.

In the process of normal bone calcification, several noncollagenous matrix proteins regulate the growth of apatite crystals. These are multifunctional proteins that facilitate interaction with mineral, other matrix molecules, and cells and may regulate dystrophic calcification. They include the

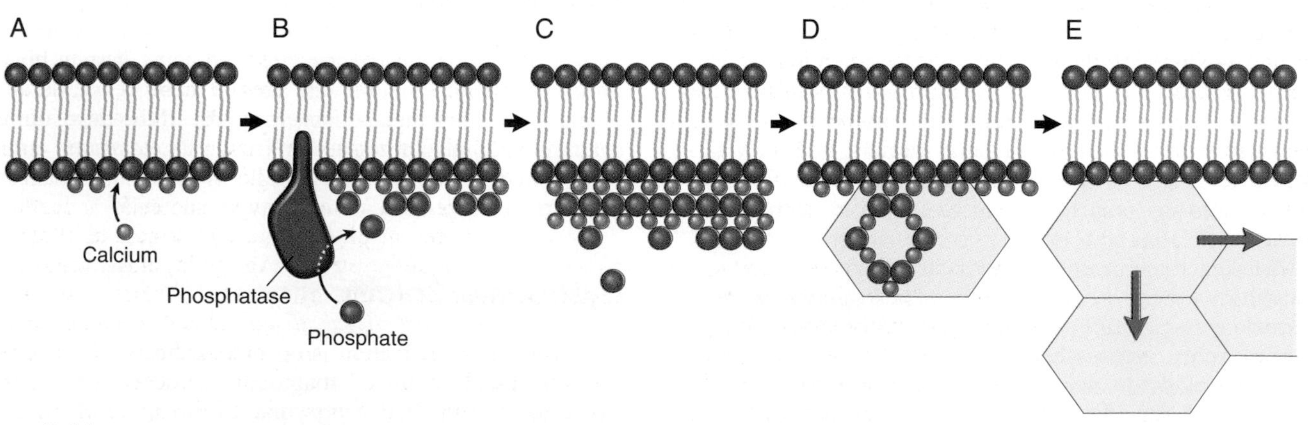

Figure 2–14

Model of membrane-facilitated calcification. Calcium ions bind the phospholipids present in a membrane. Membrane-associated phosphatases generate phosphate groups that bind to the bound calcium. The cycle of phosphate and calcium binding is repeated, increasing the size of the deposit. A microcrystal develops after a rearrangement in the phosphate and calcium ions. (Adapted and redrawn from Majno G, Joris I: Cells, Tissues and Disease: Principles of General Pathology. Cambridge, MA, Blackwell Scientific, 1996.)

following proteins: (1) *osteopontin,* an acidic calcium-binding phosphoprotein with high affinity to hydroxyapatite that is abundant in foci of dystrophic calcification[24]; (2) *osteonectin,* also known as secreted protein acidic rich in cysteine (SPARC), which binds minerals and inhibits cell spreading and migration during new blood vessel formation or angiogenesis (Chapter 4)[25]; (3) *osteocalcin*[26]; and (4) γ-carboxyglutamic acid (GLA)–containing proteins, such as *matrix GLA protein* (Mgp).[27] GLA is formed from glutamic acid by carboxylation in the presence of vitamin K, and Mgp binds tightly to mineral ions through these modified residues. Mice lacking Mgp exhibit inappropriate calcification of cartilage and die as a result of arterial calcification and blood vessel rupture.[28] This suggests that inhibition of calcification in arteries and cartilage requires Mgp and that this family of proteins may be negative regulators of calcification. They are under intense study as potential leads for therapy to prevent harmful dystrophic calcifications.

Although dystrophic calcification may be simply a telltale sign of previous cell injury, it is often a cause of organ dysfunction. Such is the case in calcific valvular disease and atherosclerosis, as becomes clear in further discussion of these diseases.

Metastatic Calcification

Metastatic calcification may occur in normal tissues whenever there is hypercalcemia. Hypercalcemia also accentuates dystrophic calcification. There are four principal causes in groups of patients who present with hypercalcemia[29]: (1) *increased secretion of parathyroid hormone* (PTH) with subsequent bone resorption, as in hyperparathyroidism due to parathyroid tumors and ectopic secretion of PTH by malignant tumors (Chapter 8); (2) *destruction of bone tissue,* occurring with primary tumors of bone marrow (e.g., multiple myeloma, leukemia) or diffuse skeletal metastasis (e.g., breast cancer), accelerated bone turnover (e.g., Paget disease), or immobilization; (3) *vitamin D–related disorders,* including vitamin D intoxication, sarcoidosis (in which macrophages activate a vitamin D precursor), and idiopathic hypercalcemia of infancy (Williams syndrome) characterized by abnormal sensitivity to vitamin D; and (4) *renal failure,* which causes retention of phosphate, leading to secondary hyperparathyroidism. Less common causes include aluminum intoxication, which occurs in patients on chronic renal dialysis, and milk-alkali syndrome, which is due to excessive ingestion of calcium and absorbable antacids such as milk or calcium carbonate.

Metastatic calcification may occur widely throughout the body but principally affects the interstitial tissues of the gastric mucosa, kidneys, lungs, systemic arteries, and pulmonary veins. Although quite different in location, all of these tissues *lose acid* and therefore have an internal alkaline compartment that predisposes them to metastatic calcification. In all these sites, the calcium salts morphologically resemble those described in dystrophic calcification. Thus, they may occur as noncrystalline amorphous deposits or, at other times, as hydroxyapatite crystals.

In general, the mineral salts cause no clinical dysfunction, but, on occasion, massive involvement of the lungs produces remarkable x-ray films and respiratory deficits. Massive deposits in the kidney (nephrocalcinosis) may in time cause renal damage (Chapter 21).

HYALINE CHANGE

The term *hyaline* is widely used as a descriptive histologic term rather than a specific marker for cell injury. *It usually refers to an alteration within cells or in the extracellular space, which gives a homogeneous, glassy, pink appearance in routine histologic sections stained with hematoxylin and eosin.* This tinctorial change is produced by a variety of alterations and does not represent a specific pattern of accumulation. Intracellular accumulations of protein, described earlier (reabsorption droplets, Russell bodies, Mallory alcoholic hyalin), are examples of intracellular hyaline deposits.

Extracellular hyalin has been somewhat more difficult to analyze. Collagenous fibrous tissue in old scars may appear hyalinized, but the physiochemical mechanism underlying this change is not clear. In long-standing hypertension and diabetes mellitus, the walls of arterioles, especially in the kidney, become hyalinized, owing to extravasated plasma protein and deposition of basement membrane material. With hematoxylin and eosin stains, the protein group of proteins referred to as *amyloid* (discussed in Chapter 7) also have a hyaline appearance. These, however, have a specific fibrillar structure with a characteristic biochemical composition. Amyloid can be identified by its special staining pattern with the Congo red stain, with which it appears red and shows bipolar refringence. Thus, although the term *hyaline* is convenient to use, it is important to recognize the multitude of mechanisms that produce this change and the implications of the alteration when it is seen in different pathologic conditions.

CELLULAR AGING

Shakespeare probably characterized aging best in his elegant description of the seven ages of man. It begins at the moment of conception, involves the differentiation and maturation of the organism and its cells, at some variable point in time leads to the progressive loss of functional capacity characteristic of senescence, and ends in death.

With age, there are physiologic and structural alterations in almost all organ systems. Aging in individuals is affected to a great extent by genetic factors, diet, social conditions, and occurrence of age-related diseases, such as atherosclerosis, diabetes, and osteoarthritis. In addition, there is good evidence that aging-induced alterations in *cells* are an important component of the aging of the organism. Here we discuss cellular aging because it could represent the progressive accumulation over the years of sublethal injury that may lead to cell death or at least to the diminished capacity of the cell to respond to injury.

A number of cell functions decline progressively with

age. Oxidative phosphorylation by mitochondria is reduced, as is synthesis of nucleic acids and structural and enzymatic proteins, cell receptors, and transcription factors. Senescent cells have a decreased capacity for uptake of nutrients and for repair of chromosomal damage. The morphologic alterations in aging cells include irregular and abnormally lobed nuclei, pleomorphic vacuolated mitochondria, decreased endoplasmic reticulum, and distorted Golgi apparatus. Concomitantly, there is a steady accumulation of the pigment lipofuscin, which, as we have seen, represents a product of lipid peroxidation and evidence of *oxidative damage; advanced glycation end products,* which result from nonenzymatic glycosylation and are capable of cross-linking adjacent proteins[30]; and *abnormally folded proteins.* The role of oxidative damage is discussed later. Advanced glycation end products are important in the pathogenesis of diabetes mellitus and are discussed in Chapter 20 but may also participate in aging. For example, age-related glycosylation of lens proteins may underlie senile cataracts. The nature of abnormally folded proteins was discussed earlier in the chapter.

Although several mechanisms have been proposed to account for cellular aging, recent concepts center on two interrelated processes: the existence of a genetically determined *clock* that times aging, and the effects of continuous exposure to exogenous influences that result in the progressive accumulation of cellular and molecular damage. Both of these processes are reviewed next.

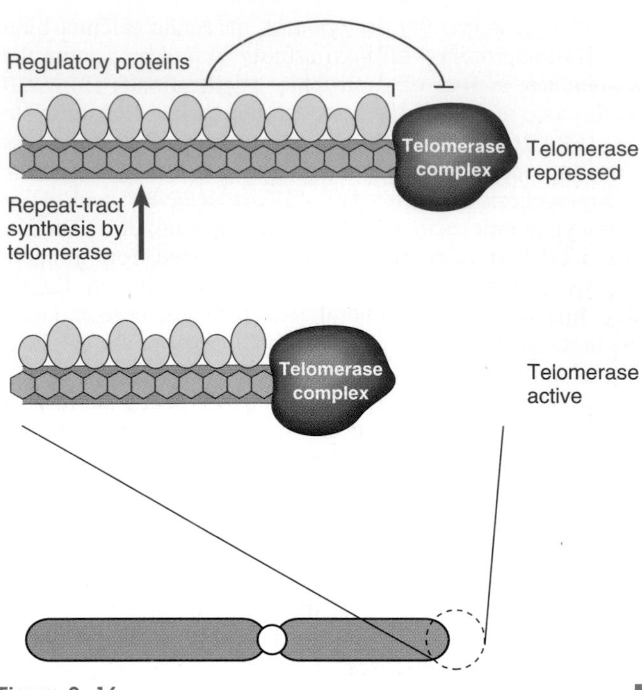

Figure 2–16 ■

Telomeres *(bottom)* and proposed mechanism of length determination by regulation of telomerase activity. Active telomerase *(middle)* adds repeated sequences and regulatory proteins *(top),* which in turn repress telomerase activity. (Modified and redrawn with permission from Shore D: Different means to common ends. Nature 385:676, 1997. Copyright 1997, Macmillan Magazines Limited.)

Timing of the Aging Process—the Concept of a Clock

The concept of a clock was developed from a simple experimental model for aging. Normal human fibroblasts when placed in tissue culture have limited division potential.[31] Cells from children undergo more rounds of replication than cells from older people (Fig. 2–15). In contrast, cells from patients with *Werner's syndrome*, a rare disease characterized by premature aging, have markedly reduced in vitro life span. After a fixed number of divisions, all cells become arrested in a terminally nondividing state, known as *cellular senescence.* Many changes in gene expression occur during cellular aging, but a key question is which of these are causes and which are effects of cellular senescence. For example, some of the proteins that inhibit progression of the cell growth cycle (as detailed in Chapter 4)—such as the products of the cyclin-dependent kinase inhibitor genes (e.g., *p21*)—are overexpressed in senescent cells.[32]

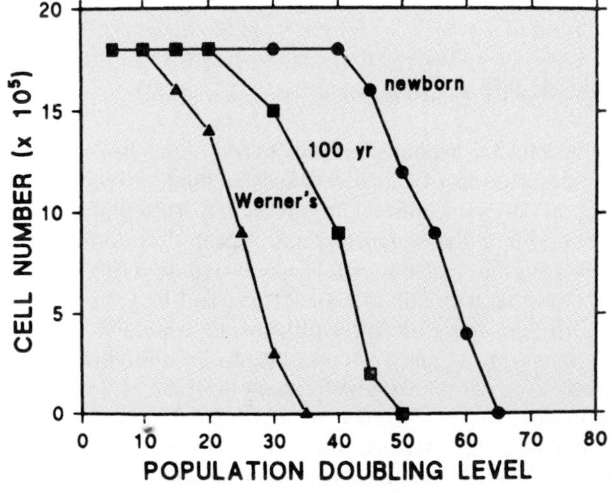

Figure 2–15 ■

Finite population doublings of primary human fibroblasts derived from a newborn, a 100-year-old person, and a 20-year-old patient with Werner syndrome. The ability of cells to grow to a confluent monolayer decreases with increasing population-doubling levels. (From Dice JF: Cellular and molecular mechanisms of aging. Physiol Rev 73:150, 1993.)

How dividing cells can *count* their divisions is under intensive investigation and several mechanisms are being explored.

- *Incomplete replication of chromosome ends (telomere shortening)*: *Telomeres* are short repeated sequences of DNA (TTAGGG) that compose the linear ends of chromosomes and are important in (1) ensuring the complete replication of chromosome ends and (2) protecting chromosomal termini from fusion and degradation.[33] The sequences are formed by a specialized ribonucleoprotein, *telomerase*, an enzyme that stabilizes telomere length by adding to the ends of chromosomes.[34] The activity of telomerase is repressed by regulatory proteins, which restrict telomere elongation, thus providing a length

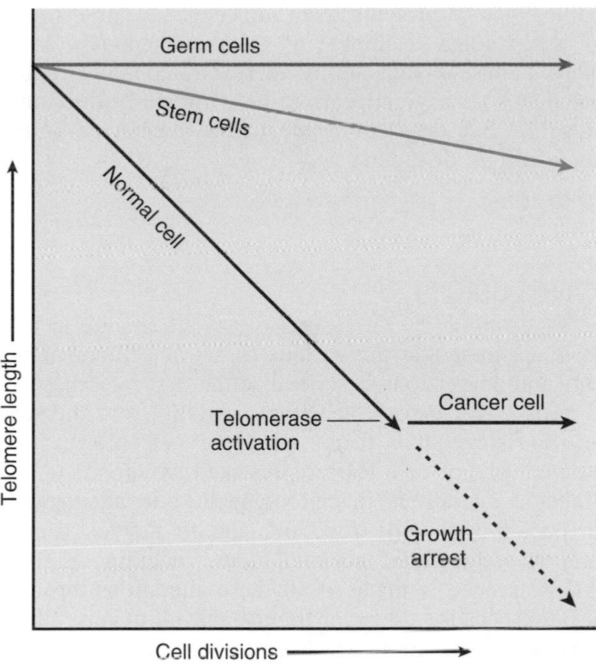

Figure 2–17

Telomere-telomerase hypothesis and proliferative capacity. Telomere length is plotted against the number of cell divisions. In normal somatic cells, there is no telomerase activity and telomeres progressively shorten with increasing cell divisions until growth arrest, or senescence, occurs. Germ cells and stem cells both contain telomerase activity, but only the germ cells have sufficient levels of the enzyme to stabilize telomere length completely. Telomerase activation in cancer cells inactivates the teleomeric clock that limits the proliferative capacity of normal somatic cells. (Modified and redrawn with permission from Holt SE, et al.: Refining the telomer-telomerase hypothesis of aging and cancer. Nature Biotech 14:836, 1996. Copyright 1996, Macmillan Magazines Limited.)

sensing mechanism (Fig. 2–16).[35] Telomerase activity is expressed in germ cells and is present at low levels in stem cells, but it is usually absent in most somatic tissues. When somatic cells replicate, a small section of the telomere is not duplicated, and telomeres become progressively shortened (Fig. 2–17). Shortened telomeres are proposed to signal a growth checkpoint allowing cells to become senescent. Conversely in immortal cancer cells, telomerase is reactivated, and telomeres are not shortened, suggesting that telomere elongation might be an important—possibly essential—step in tumor formation.[36] Despite such alluring observations, however, the relationship of telomerase activity and telomeric length to aging and cancer still needs to be more fully established.[37]

- *Clock genes*: The concept that genetically set clocks are involved in controlling the rate and timing of aging is being supported by the identification of clock genes, particularly in lower forms. For example, *clk-1*, a gene of the nematode *Caenorhabditis elegans*, appears to alter growth rate and timing of developmental processes.[38] Worms that have a mutant form of the gene have life spans that are 50% longer than those of normal worms and display a decreased rate of development as well as a slowing of some rhythmic behaviors seen as adults (e.g., swimming). Mammalian homologs of these genes are being vigorously pursued.[39]

Metabolic Events, Genetic Damage, and Aging

In addition to the importance of timing and a genetic clock, cellular life span may also be determined by the balance between cellular damage resulting from *metabolic events* occurring within the cell and counteracting molecular responses that can repair the damage. Smaller animals have generally shorter life spans and faster metabolic rates, suggesting that the life span of a species is limited by fixed total metabolic consumption over a lifetime.[40] One group of products of normal metabolism are reactive oxygen metabolites. As we have seen (Chapter 1), these byproducts of oxidative phosphorylation cause covalent modifications of proteins, lipids, and nucleic acids (Fig. 2–18).[41] The amount of oxidative damage, which increases as an organism ages, may be an important component of senescence, and the accumulation of lipofuscin in aging cells is seen as the telltale sign of such damage. Consistent with this proposal are the following observations: (1) Restriction of caloric intakes lowers steady-state levels of oxidative damage, slows age-related changes, and extends the maximal life span in mammals; (2) variation in the longevity among different species is inversely correlated with the rates of mitochondrial generation of superoxide anion radical; (3) overexpression of the antioxidative enzymes superoxide dismutase (SOD) and catalase extends life span in transgenic forms of *Drosophila*; and (4) a gene that helps control the life span of *C. elegans*, *daf-2*, encodes the worm version of the insulin receptor, thereby providing a possible link between aging and glucose metabolism.[42] Thus, part of the mechanism that times aging may be the cumulative damage that is generated by toxic byproducts of metabolism, such as oxygen radicals. Increased oxidative damage could result from repeated environmental exposure to such influences as ionizing radiation, or progressive reduction of antioxidant defense mechanisms (e.g., vitamin E, glutathione peroxidase), or both.

A number of protective responses counterbalance progressive damage in cells, and an important one is the recognition and repair of unrepaired damaged DNA.[43] Although most DNA damage is repaired by endogenous DNA repair enzymes, some persists and accumulates as cells age. Several lines of evidence point to the importance of DNA repair in the aging process. Patients with *Werner's syndrome* show premature aging, and the defective gene product is a DNA helicase—a protein involved in DNA replication and repair and other functions requiring DNA unwinding.[44] A defect in this enzyme causes rapid accumulation of chromosomal damage that mimics the injury that normally accumulates during cellular aging. Genetic instability in somatic cells is also characteristic of other disorders in which patients display some of the manifestations of aging at an increased rate, such as *Cockayne syndrome*[45] and *ataxia telangiectasia* (Chapter 8). Studies of mutants of budding yeast and *C. elegans* show that life span is

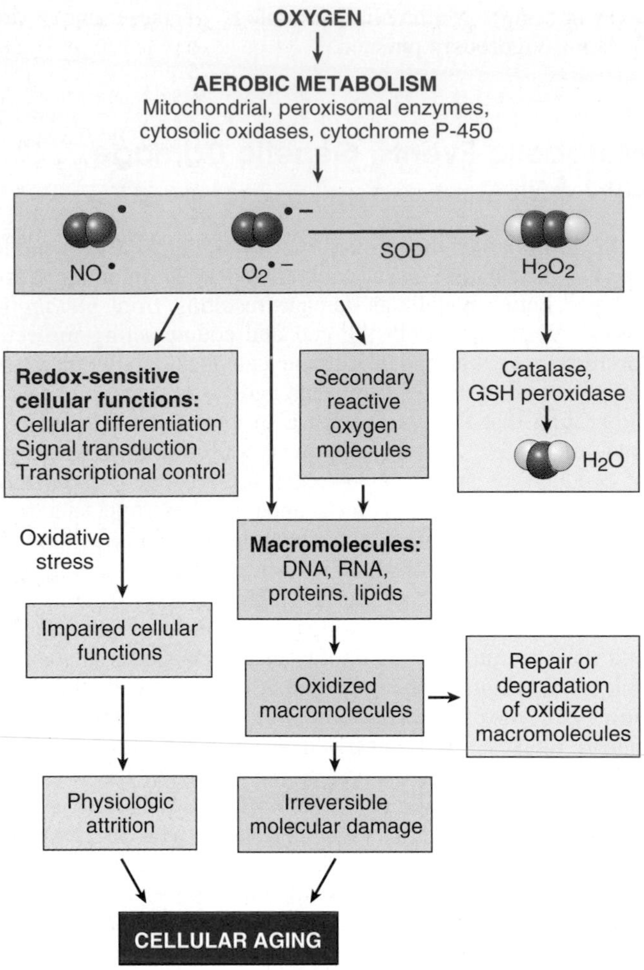

Figure 2–18

Oxidative stress and aging. Aerobic metabolism generates reactive oxygen metabolites such as hydrogen peroxide, superoxide anion, and nitric oxide. These reactive species can be inactivated by antioxidant defense mechanisms, or give rise to a variety of secondary reactive oxygen metabolites (e.g., peroxynitrite). Interactions between the reactive species and macromolecules may cause both reversible and irreversible oxidative modifications. The accumulation of irreversible oxidative damage may be a causal factor in aging and certain diseases. Antioxidant defense mechanisms include glutathione, vitamin E, vitamin C, and urate. SOD, superoxide dismutase. (Modified and redrawn from Weindruch R, Sohal RS: Caloric intake and aging. N Engl J Med 337:986, 1997.)

increased if responses to DNA damage are enhanced.[46] Thus, the balance between cumulative metabolic damage and the response to that damage could determine the rate at which we age.[47] In this scenario, aging can be delayed by decreasing the accumulation of damage or by increasing the response to that damage.

Much more might be said about the mechanisms of cellular aging, but it suffices here to say that these mechanisms involve both programmed events in cell proliferation and differentiation—such as telomere shortening and the activity of clock genes—and the consequences of progressive environmental injury overwhelming the cell's defense mechanisms (Fig. 2–18). Oxidative free radical damage to proteins, lipids, and DNA as well as post-translational modifications of proteins (e.g., nonenzymatic glycation) are two well-studied examples of such exogenously induced effects. Failure in the ability to repair oxidative injury or repair DNA damage appears to be particularly important in cell aging and may contribute to the premature aging of cells in certain disorders.

CONCLUSION

It is apparent that the various forms of cellular derangements and adaptations described in the first two chapters of this book cover a wide spectrum, ranging from the reversible and irreversible forms of acute cell injury; to the regulated type of cell death represented by apoptosis; to the pathologic alterations in cell organelles; to adaptations in cell size, growth, and function; and to the less ominous forms of intracellular accumulations, including pigmentations. Reference is made to all these alterations throughout this book because all organ injury and ultimately all clinical disease arise from derangements in cell structure and function.

REFERENCES

1. Michalopoulos GK, DeFrances MC: Liver regeneration. Science 276: 60, 1997.
2. Diehl AM, Rai RM: Regulation of signal transduction during liver regeneration. FASEB J 10:215, 1996.
3. Taub R: Transcriptional control of liver regeneration. FASEB J 10: 413, 1997.
4. Fausto N, et al: Role of growth factors and cytokines in hepatic regeneration. FASEB J 9:1527, 1995.
5. Cressman DE, et al: Liver failure and defective hepatocyte regeneration in interleukin-6-deficient mice. Science 274:1379, 1996.
6. Thorgeirsson SS: Hepatic stem cells in liver regeneration. FASEB J 10:1249, 1996.
7. Chien KR, Grace AA: Principles of cardiovascular molecular and cellular biology. In Braunwald E (ed): Heart Disease: A Textbook of Cardiovascular Medicine, 5th ed. Philadelphia, WB Saunders, 1996, pp 1626–1649.
8. Rosenzweig A, Seidman CE: Atrial natriuretic factor and related peptide hormones. Annu Rev Biochem 60:229, 1991.
9. Saito Y, et al: Augmented expression of atrial natriuretic polypeptide gene in ventricle of human failing heart. J Clin Invest 83:298, 1989.
10. Hudlicka O, Brown MD: Postnatal growth of the heart and its blood vessels. J Vasc Res 33:266, 1996.
11. Schwartz K, Mercadier JJ: Molecular and cellular biology of heart failure. Curr Opin Cardiol 11:227, 1996.
12. Anversa P, et al: Myocyte death in heart failure. Curr Opin Cardiol 11:245, 1996.
13. Mitch WE, Goldberg AE: Mechanisms of muscle wasting: the role of the ubiquitin-proteosome pathway. N Engl J Med 335:1897, 1996.
14. Lugo M, Putong PB: Metaplasia: an overview. Arch Pathol Lab Med 108:185, 1984.
15. Reddi HA: BMPs: actions in flesh and bone. Nat Med 3:837, 1997.
16. Rodan GA, Haroda S: The missing bone. Cell 89:677, 1997.
17. Means AL: The roles of retinoids in vertebrate development. Annu Rev Biochem 64:201, 1995.
18. Lee RJ: Fatty change and steatohepatitis. In Lee RJ (ed): Diagnostic Liver Pathology. St. Louis, Mosby–Year Book, 1994, pp 167–194.
19. Taubes G: Misfolding the way to disease. Science 271:1493, 1996.
20. Baumeister W, et al: The proteasome: paradigm of a self-compartmentalizing protease. Cell 92:367, 1998.
21. Welch WJ, Gambelt P: Chaperoning brain diseases. Nature 392:23, 1998.

22. Vyavahare NR, et al: Current progress in anticalcification for bioprosthetic and polymeric heart valves. Cardiovasc Pathol 6:219, 1997.
23. Majno G, Joris I: Cells, Tissues, and Disease: Principles of General Pathology. Cambridge, MA, Blackwell Science, 1996, pp 229–246.
24. Giachelli CM: Osteopontin is elevated during neointima formation in rat arteries and is a novel component of human atherosclerotic plaques. J Clin Invest 92:1696, 1993.
25. Motamed K, Sage HE: Regulation of vascular morphogenesis by the matricellular protein SPARC. Kidney Int 51:1383, 1997.
26. Ducy P, et al: Increased bone formation in osteocalcin-deficient mice. Nature 382:448, 1996.
27. Hauschka PV, et al: Ostocalcin and matrix Gla proteins: vitamin K-dependent proteins in bone. Physiol Rev 69:990, 1989.
28. Luo G, et al: Spontaneous calcification of arteries and cartilage in mice lacking matrix GLA protein. Nature 386:78, 1997.
29. Potts JT: Diseases of the parathyroid gland and other hyper- and hypocalcemic disorders. In Isselbacher KJ, et al (eds): Harrison's Principles of Internal Medicine, 13th ed. New York, McGraw-Hill, 1994, pp 2151–2165.
30. Bucala R, Cerami A: Advanced glycosylation: chemistry, biology, and implications for diabetes and aging. Adv Pharmacol 23:1, 1992.
31. Hayflick L, Moorhead PS: The serial cultivation of human diploid cell strains. Exp Cell Res 25:585, 1961.
32. Smith JR, Pereira-Smith OM: Replicative senescence: implications for in vivo aging and tumor suppression. Science 273:63, 1996.
33. Blackburn E, Greider C (eds): Telomeres. New York, Cold Spring Harbor Laboratory Press, 1995.
34. Morin GB: The human telomere terminal transferase enzyme is a ribonucleoprotein that synthesizes TTAGGG repeats. Cell 59:521, 1991.
35. van Steensel B, Lange T: Control of telomere length by the human telomeric protein TRF1. Nature 385:740, 1997.
36. Kim NW, et al: Specific association of human telomerase activity with immortal cells and cancer. Science 266:2011, 1994.
37. Holt SE, et al: Refining the telomere-telomerease hypothesis of aging and cancer. Nat Biotech 14:836, 1996.
38. Lakowski B, Hekimi S: Determination of life-span in *Caenorhabditis elegans* by four clock genes. Science 272:1010, 1996.
39. Pennisi E: Worm genes imply a master clock. Science 272:949, 1996.
40. Sohal RS, Weindruch R: Oxidative stress, caloric restriction and aging. Science 273:59, 1996.
41. Weindruch R, Sohal RS: Caloric intake and aging. N Engl J Med 337:986, 1997.
42. Kimura KD, et al: daf-2, an insulin receptor-like gene that regulates longevity and diapause in *Caenorhabditis elegans*. Science 277:942, 1997.
43. Gilchrest BA, Bohr VA: Aging processes, DNA damage, and repair. FASEB J 11:322, 1997.
44. Yu C-E, et al: Positional cloning of the Werner's syndrome gene. Science 272:258, 1996.
45. Nance MA, Berry SA: Cockayne syndrome: review of 140 cases. Am J Med Genet 42:68, 1994.
46. Jazwinski SM: Longevity, genes and aging. Science 273:54, 1996.
47. Guarente L: What makes us tick? Science 275:943, 1997.

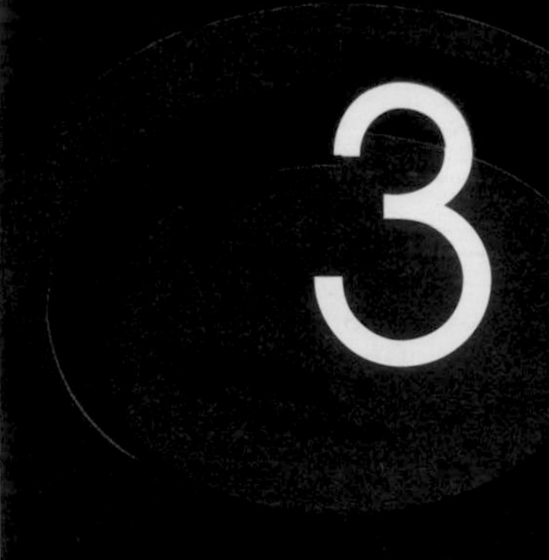

Acute and Chronic Inflammation

GENERAL FEATURES OF INFLAMMATION
HISTORICAL HIGHLIGHTS
ACUTE INFLAMMATION
VASCULAR CHANGES
Changes in Vascular Flow and Caliber
Increased Vascular Permeability (Vascular Leakage)
CELLULAR EVENTS: LEUKOCYTE EXTRAVASATION AND PHAGOCYTOSIS
Adhesion and Transmigration
Chemotaxis
Leukocyte Activation
Phagocytosis
Recognition and Attachment
Engulfment
Killing or Degradation
Release of Leukocyte Products and Leukocyte-Induced Tissue Injury
Defects in Leukocyte Function
SUMMARY OF THE ACUTE INFLAMMATORY RESPONSE
CHEMICAL MEDIATORS OF INFLAMMATION
VASOACTIVE AMINES
Histamine
Serotonin
PLASMA PROTEASES
Complement System
Kinin System
Clotting System
ARACHIDONIC ACID METABOLITES: PROSTAGLANDINS, LEUKOTRIENES, AND LIPOXINS
PLATELET-ACTIVATING FACTOR
CYTOKINES AND CHEMOKINES
Terms and Definitions
General Properties and Functional Classes
Interleukin-1 and Tumor Necrosis Factor
Chemokines
NITRIC OXIDE
LYSOSOMAL CONSTITUENTS OF LEUKOCYTES
OXYGEN-DERIVED FREE RADICALS
NEUROPEPTIDES
SUMMARY OF CHEMICAL MEDIATORS OF ACUTE INFLAMMATION
OUTCOMES OF ACUTE INFLAMMATION
CHRONIC INFLAMMATION
DEFINITION AND CAUSES
HISTOLOGIC FEATURES
MONONUCLEAR INFILTRATION: CELLS AND MECHANISMS
OTHER CELLS IN CHRONIC INFLAMMATION
GRANULOMATOUS INFLAMMATION
LYMPHATICS IN INFLAMMATION
MORPHOLOGIC PATTERNS IN ACUTE AND CHRONIC INFLAMMATION
SEROUS INFLAMMATION
FIBRINOUS INFLAMMATION
SUPPURATIVE OR PURULENT INFLAMMATION
ULCERS
SYSTEMIC EFFECTS OF INFLAMMATION

GENERAL FEATURES OF INFLAMMATION

In Chapter 1, we saw how various exogenous and endogenous stimuli can cause cell injury. These same stimuli also can provoke a *complex reaction in the vascularized connective tissue called inflammation.* Invertebrates with no vascular system, single-celled organisms, and multicellular parasites all have their own responses to local injury. These include phagocytosis of the injurious agent; entrap-

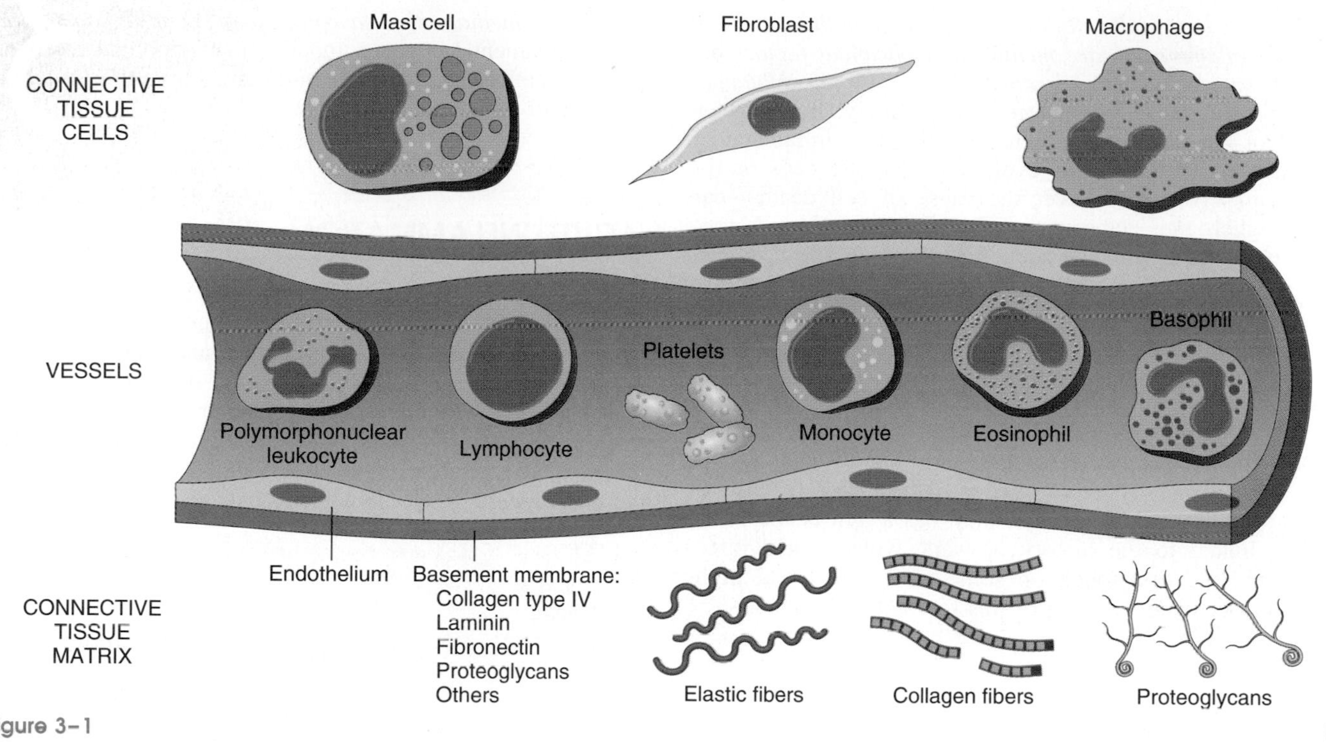

Figure 3–1

Intravascular cells and connective tissue matrix and cells involved in the inflammatory response.

ment of the irritant by specialized cells (hemocytes), which then ingest it; and neutralization of noxious stimuli by hypertrophy of the cell or one of its organelles. All these reactions have been retained in evolution, but what characterizes the inflammatory process in higher forms is the *reaction of blood vessels, leading to the accumulation of fluid and leukocytes in extravascular tissues.*

The inflammatory response is closely intertwined with the process of repair. Inflammation serves to destroy, dilute, or wall off the injurious agent, but it, in turn, sets into motion a series of events that, as far as possible, heal and reconstitute the damaged tissue. Repair begins during the early phases of inflammation but reaches completion usually after the injurious influence has been neutralized. During repair, the injured tissue is replaced by *regeneration* of native parenchymal cells, by filling of the defect with fibroblastic tissue *(scarring)*, or, most commonly, by a combination of these two processes.

Inflammation is fundamentally a protective response the ultimate goal of which is to rid the organism of both the initial cause of cell injury (e.g., microbes, toxins) and the consequences of such injury (e.g., necrotic cells and tissues). Without inflammation, infections would go unchecked, wounds would never heal, and injured organs might remain permanent festering sores. *Inflammation and repair may be potentially harmful, however.* Inflammatory reactions, for example, underlie life-threatening hypersensitivity reactions to insect bites, drugs, and toxins as well as some common chronic diseases, such as rheumatoid arthritis, atherosclerosis, and lung fibrosis. Repair by fibrosis may lead to disfiguring scars or fibrous bands that cause intestinal obstruction or limit the mobility of joints. For this reason, our pharmacies abound with anti-inflammatory drugs, which ideally would enhance the salutary effects of inflammation yet control its harmful sequelae.

The inflammatory response occurs in the vascularized connective tissue, including plasma, circulating cells, blood vessels, and cellular and extracellular constituents of connective tissue (Fig. 3–1). The circulating cells include *neutrophils, monocytes, eosinophils, lymphocytes, basophils,* and *platelets*. The connective tissue cells are the *mast cells,* which intimately surround *blood vessels*; the connective tissue *fibroblasts*; and occasional *resident macrophages* and *lymphocytes*. The extracellular matrix, as described in Chapter 4, consists of the structural fibrous proteins (*collagen, elastin*), adhesive glycoproteins (*fibronectin, laminin, nonfibrillar collagen, tenascin,* and others), and proteoglycans. The basement membrane is a specialized component of the extracellular matrix consisting of adhesive glycoproteins and proteoglycans.

Inflammation is divided into acute and chronic patterns. *Acute inflammation* is of relatively short duration, lasting for minutes, several hours, or a few days, and its main characteristics are the exudation of fluid and plasma proteins (edema) and the emigration of leukocytes, predominantly neutrophils. *Chronic inflammation* is of longer duration and is associated histologically with the presence of lymphocytes and macrophages, the proliferation of blood vessels, fibrosis, and tissue necrosis. Many factors modify the course and histologic appearance of both acute and chronic inflammation, and these become apparent later in this chapter.

The vascular and cellular responses of both acute and chronic inflammation are mediated by chemical factors derived from plasma or cells and triggered by the inflammatory stimulus. Such mediators, acting singly, in combinations, or in sequence, then amplify the inflammatory response and influence its evolution. Necrotic cells or tissues themselves—whatever the cause of cell death—can also trigger the elaboration of inflammatory mediators. Such is the case with the acute inflammation after myocardial infarction. Inflammation is *terminated* when the injurious stimulus is removed and the mediators are either dissipated or inhibited.

This chapter first describes the sequence of events in acute inflammation as well as the structural and molecular mechanisms underlying them, then reviews the various classes of specific mediators that contribute to these events. This is followed by a discussion of the major features of chronic inflammation. Inflammation has a rich history, intimately linked to the history of wars, wounds, and infections, and we first touch on some of the historical highlights in our understanding of this fascinating process.[1, 2]

HISTORICAL HIGHLIGHTS

Although signs of inflammation were described in an Egyptian papyrus (3000 BC), Celsus, a Roman writer of the first century AD, first listed the four cardinal signs of inflammation: *rubor, tumor, calor,* and *dolor* (redness, swelling, heat, and pain). A fifth clinical sign, loss of function (*functio laesa*), was later added by Virchow. In 1793, the Scottish surgeon *John Hunter* noted what is now considered an obvious fact: that inflammation is not a disease but a nonspecific response that has a *salutary* effect on its host.[3] *Julius Cohnheim* (1839–1884) first used the microscope to observe inflamed blood vessels in thin, transparent membranes, such as the mesentery and tongue of the frog. Noting the initial changes in blood flow, the subsequent edema caused by increased vascular permeability, and the characteristic leukocyte emigration, he wrote descriptions that can hardly be improved on.[4]

The Russian biologist *Elie Metchnikoff* discovered the process of *phagocytosis* by observing the ingestion of rose thorns by amebocytes of starfish larvae and of bacteria by mammalian leukocytes (1882).[5] He concluded that the purpose of inflammation was to bring phagocytic cells to the injured area to engulf invading bacteria. At that time, Metchnikoff contradicted the prevailing theory that the purpose of inflammation was to bring in factors from the serum to neutralize the infectious agents. It soon became clear that both cellular (phagocytes) and serum factors (antibodies) were critical to the defense against microorganisms, and in recognition of this, both Metchnikoff and Paul Ehrlich (who developed the humoral theory) shared the Nobel Prize in 1908.

To these names must be added that of *Sir Thomas Lewis*, who, on the basis of simple experiments involving the inflammatory response in skin, established the *concept that chemical substances, such as histamine locally induced by injury, mediate the vascular changes of inflammation.* This fundamental concept underlies the important discoveries of chemical mediators of inflammation and the potential to use anti-inflammatory agents.

ACUTE INFLAMMATION

Acute inflammation is the immediate and early response to an injurious agent. Since the two major defensive components against microbes—antibodies and leukocytes—are normally carried in the bloodstream, it is not surprising that vascular phenomena play a major role in acute inflammation. Therefore, acute inflammation has three major components: (1) *alterations in vascular caliber that lead to an increase in blood flow,* (2) *structural changes in the*

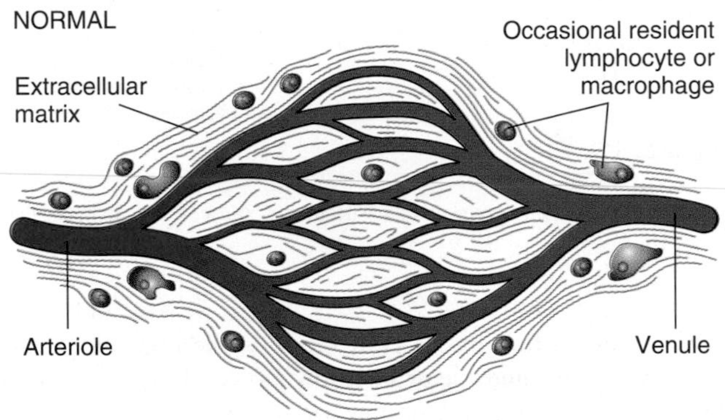

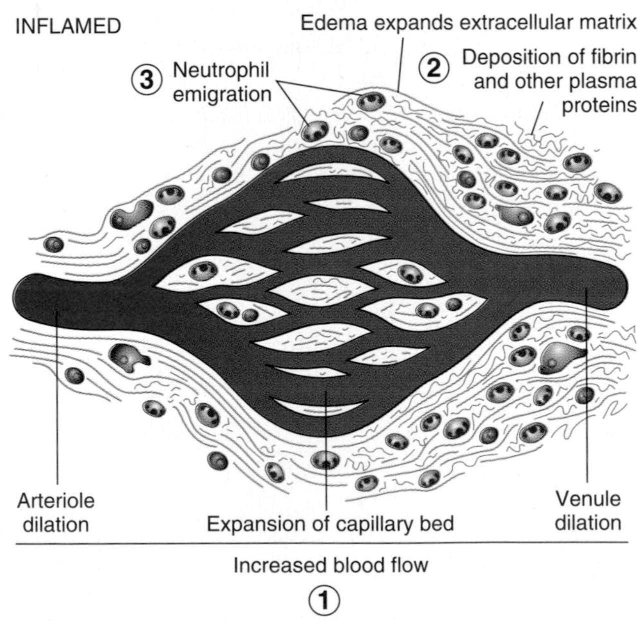

Figure 3–2

The major local manifestations of acute inflammation, compared to normal. (1) Vascular dilation (causing erythema and warmth), (2) extravasation of plasma fluid and proteins (edema), and (3) leukocyte emigration and accumulation in the site of injury.

microvasculature that permit the plasma proteins and leukocytes to leave the circulation, and (3) *emigration of the leukocytes from the microcirculation and their accumulation in the focus of injury* (Fig. 3–2).

Certain terms must be defined before specific features of inflammation are described. The escape of fluid, proteins, and blood cells from the vascular system into the interstitial tissue or body cavities is known as *exudation*. An *exudate* is an inflammatory extravascular fluid that has a high protein concentration, much cellular debris, and a specific gravity above 1.020. It implies significant alteration in the normal permeability of small blood vessels in the area of injury. In contrast, a *transudate* is a fluid with low protein content (most of which is albumin) and a specific gravity of less than 1.012. It is essentially an ultrafiltrate of blood plasma and results from hydrostatic imbalance across the vascular endothelium. In this situation, the permeability of the endothelium is normal. *Edema* denotes an excess of fluid in the interstitial or serous cavities; it can be either an exudate or a transudate. *Pus*, a *purulent* exudate, is an inflammatory exudate rich in leukocytes (mostly neutrophils) and parenchymal cell debris.

Vascular Changes

CHANGES IN VASCULAR FLOW AND CALIBER

Changes in vascular flow and caliber begin early after injury and develop at varying rates, depending on the severity of the injury. The changes occur in the following order:

- After an inconstant and transient vasoconstriction of arterioles, lasting a few seconds, *vasodilation* occurs. Vasodilation first involves the arterioles and then results in opening of new capillary beds in the area. Thus comes about *increased blood flow*, which is the cause of the heat and the redness (Fig. 3–2). How long vasodilation lasts depends on the stimulus, but it is eventually followed by the next event, slowing of the circulation.
- *Slowing of the circulation* is brought about by *increased permeability of the microvasculature*, with the outpouring of protein-rich fluid into the extravascular tissues, a process that is described in detail presently. The loss of fluid results in concentration of red cells in small vessels and increased viscosity of the blood, reflected by the presence of dilated small vessels packed with red cells—a condition termed *stasis*.
- As *stasis* develops, one begins to see peripheral orientation of leukocytes, principally neutrophils, along the vascular endothelium, a process called *leukocytic margination*. Leukocytes then stick to the endothelium, at first transiently (rolling), then more avidly, and soon afterward they migrate through the vascular wall into the interstitial tissue, in processes that are reviewed later.

The time scale of changes in vascular caliber is variable. With mild stimuli, stasis may not become apparent until 15 to 30 minutes have elapsed, whereas with severe injury, stasis may occur in a few minutes.

INCREASED VASCULAR PERMEABILITY (VASCULAR LEAKAGE)

Increased vascular permeability leading to the escape of a protein-rich fluid (exudate) into the interstitium *is the hallmark of acute inflammation*. The loss of protein from the plasma reduces the intravascular osmotic pressure and increases the osmotic pressure of the interstitial fluid. Together with the increased hydrostatic pressure owing to vasodilation, this leads to a marked *outflow* of fluid and its

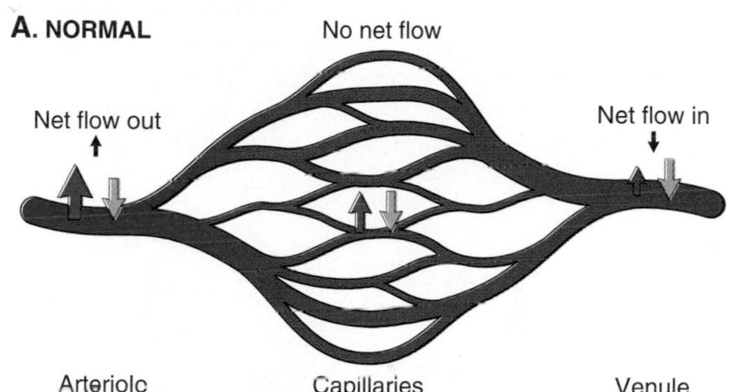

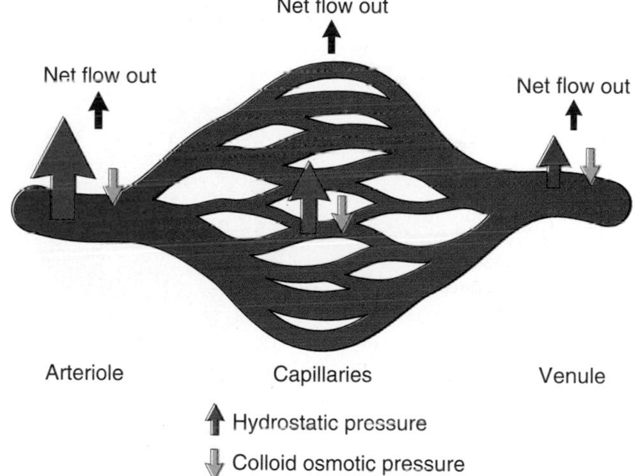

Figure 3–3

Blood pressure and plasma colloid osmotic forces in normal and inflamed microcirculation. *A*, Normal hydrostatic pressure *(red arrows)* is about 32 mm Hg at the arterial end of a capillary bed and 12 mm Hg at the venous end; the mean colloid osmotic pressure of tissues is approximately 25 mm Hg *(green arrows)*, which is equal to the mean capillary pressure. Although fluid tends to leave the precapillary arteriole, it is returned in equal amounts via the postcapillary venule, so that the net flow *(black arrows)* in or out is zero. *B*, Acute inflammation. Arteriole pressure is increased to 50 mm Hg, the mean capillary pressure is increased because of arteriolar dilation, and the venous pressure increases to approximately 30 mm Hg. At the same time, osmotic pressure is reduced (averaging 20 mm Hg) because of protein leakage across the venule. The net result is an excess of extravasated fluid.

MECHANISMS OF VASCULAR LEAKAGE IN ACUTE INFLAMMATION

Gaps: Endothelial contraction

- Venules
- Vasoactive mediators (histamine, leukotrienes, etc.)

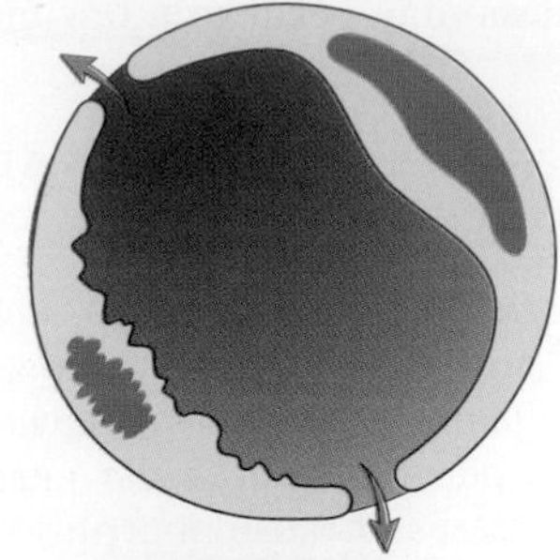

Gaps: Cytoskeletal reorganization

- Mostly venules; capillaries
- Cytokines (e.g., interleukin-1 and tumor necrosis factor)
- Hypoxia

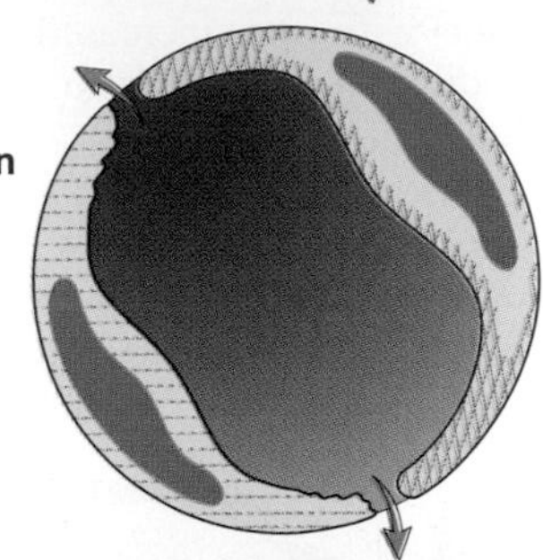

Direct injury

- Arterioles, capillaries, and venules
- Toxins, burns, chemicals

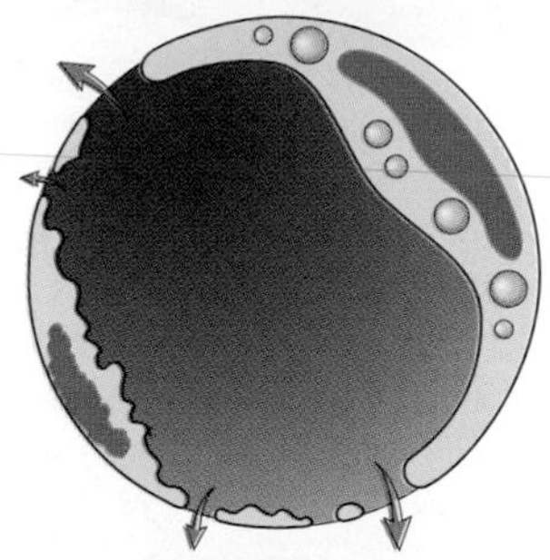

Leukocyte-dependent injury

- Mostly venules
- Pulmonary capillaries
- Late response

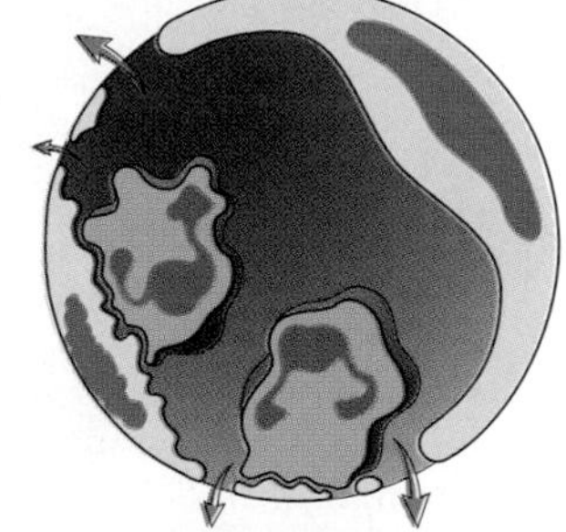

Increased transcytosis

- Venules
- VEGF; Other mediators?

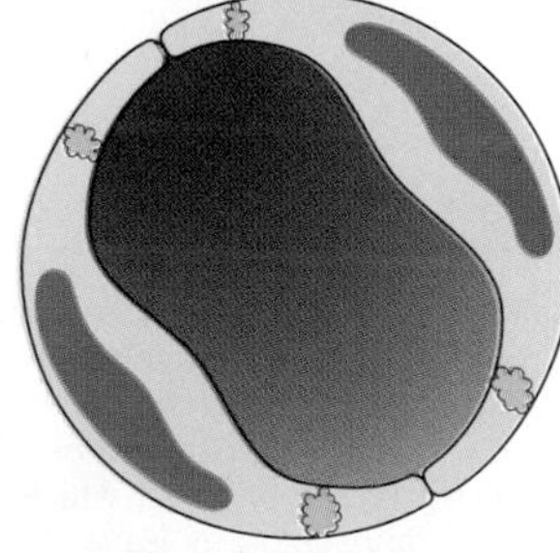

Figure 3–4

Diagrammatic representation of five mechanisms of increased vascular permeability in inflammation (see text).

accumulation in the interstitial tissue (Fig. 3–3). This net increase of extravascular fluid is called *edema*.

Normal fluid exchange and microvascular permeability are critically dependent on an intact endothelium. How then does the endothelium become leaky in inflammation? The following mechanisms have been proposed (Fig. 3–4):

- *Formation of endothelial gaps in venules:*[6] This is the most common mechanism of vascular leakage and is elicited by histamine, bradykinin, leukotrienes, substance P, and many other classes of chemical mediators. It occurs rapidly after exposure to the mediator and is usually reversible and short-lived (15 to 30 minutes); it is thus known as the *immediate transient response*.

  Classically, this type of leakage affects only venules 20 to 60 μm in diameter, leaving capillaries and arterioles unaffected[7] (Fig. 3–5). The precise reason for this restriction to venules is uncertain, but studies suggest that it is related to a greater density of receptors to the putative mediator (shown for histamine and substance P)[8] in venular endothelium. Parenthetically, many of the later leukocyte events in inflammation—adhesion and emigration—also occur predominantly in the venules in most organs. The gaps are largely intercellular or close to the intercellular junctions and have been ascribed to agonist-induced *endothelial cell contraction* causing separation of such junctions. An alternative, or additional, mechanism for the formation of such gaps is that they are formed by *intracellular transcytoplasmic* channels—close and perhaps connecting to junctions *(transcytosis)*.[9] Whatever the explanation, the process seems to be mediated by agonist receptor–induced intracellular pathways involving phosphorylation of cytoplasmic and perijunctional contractile and cytoskeletal proteins in endothelial cells.[10]
- *Cytoskeletal reorganization (endothelial retraction)*: An apparently different mechanism of reversible leakage, also resulting in endothelial gaps, can be induced in vitro by cytokine mediators (such as interleukin-1 [IL-1], tumor necrosis factor [TNF],[11] and interferon-γ [IFN-γ]), hypoxia, and sublethal injury to endothelial cells. The endothelial cells undergo a structural reorganization of the cytoskeleton, such that endothelial cells retract from one another. In contrast to the histamine effect, the response is somewhat delayed (4 to 6 hours) and long-lived (24 hours or more). How frequently this mechanism accounts for vascular leakage in vivo is still uncertain.
- *Increased transcytosis* across the endothelial cytoplasm: This is is another potential mechanism of increased permeability. Transcytosis occurs across channels consisting of clusters of interconnected, uncoated vesicles and vacuoles called the *vesiculovacuolar organelle*, many of which are located close to intercellular junctions. Certain factors, for example, vascular endothelial growth factor (VEGF) (Chapter 4), appear to cause vascular leakage by increasing the number and perhaps the size of these channels.[9] As noted earlier, it has been claimed that this is also a path of increased permeability induced by histamine and most chemical mediators.

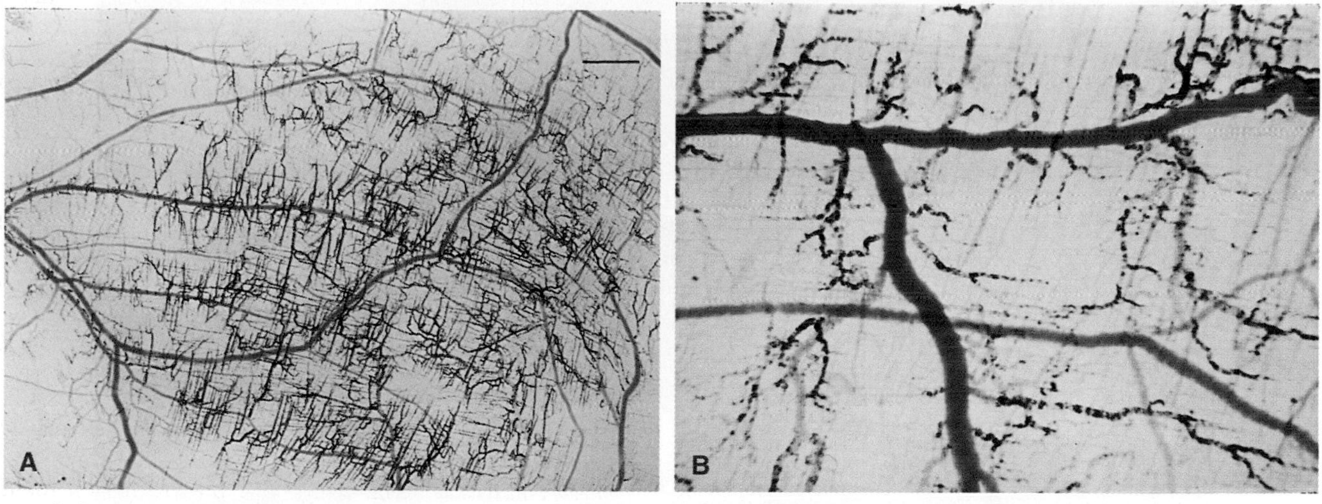

Figure 3–5

A and *B*, Vascular leakage as induced by most chemical mediators. This is a laminar muscle of the rat (cremaster), fixed, cleared in glycerin, and examined unstained by transillumination. One hour before sacrifice, bradykinin was injected over this muscle and colloidal carbon was given intravenously. Plasma, loaded with carbon, escapes, but most of the carbon particles were retained by the basement membrane of the leaking vessels, with the result that these became "labeled" in black. Note that not all the vessels leak—only the venules. In *B*, a higher power, the capillary network is very faintly visible in the background. (Courtesy of Dr. Guido Majno.)

- *Direct endothelial injury, resulting in endothelial cell necrosis and detachment*:[12] This effect is usually encountered in necrotizing injuries and is due to direct damage to the endothelium by the injurious stimulus, as, for example, by severe burns or lytic bacterial infections. In most instances, leakage starts immediately after injury and is sustained at a high level for several hours until the damaged vessels are thrombosed or repaired. The reaction is known as the *immediate sustained response. All levels of the microcirculation are affected, including venules, capillaries, and arterioles.* Endothelial cell detachment is often associated with platelet adhesion and thrombosis.
- *Delayed prolonged leakage* is a curious but relatively common type of increased permeability that *begins after a delay of 2 to 12 hours, lasts for several hours or even days, and involves venules as well as capillaries.* Such leakage is caused, for example, by mild-to-moderate thermal injury, x-radiation or ultraviolet radiation, and certain bacterial toxins. A late-appearing sunburn is a good example of a delayed reaction. The mechanism for such leakage is unclear. It may result from the direct effect of the injurious agent, leading to delayed cell damage (perhaps by apoptosis), or the effect of cytokines causing endothelial retraction, as described earlier.
- *Leukocyte-mediated endothelial injury*: Leukocytes adhere to endothelium relatively early in inflammation. As seen subsequently, such leukocytes may be activated in the process, releasing toxic oxygen species and proteolytic enzymes, which then cause endothelial injury or detachment—resulting in increased permeability. In acute inflammation, this form of injury is largely restricted to vascular sites, such as venules and pulmonary and glomerular capillaries, where leukocytes adhere to the endothelium.
- *Leakage from new blood vessels*. As described later in Chapter 4, during repair, endothelial cells proliferate and form new blood vessels, an important process called *angiogenesis*. New vessel sprouts remain leaky until endothelial cells differentiate and form intercellular junctions. In addition, certain factors that cause angiogenesis (e.g., VEGF) also increase vascular permeability,[9] and endothelial cells in foci of angiogenesis have increased density of receptors for vasoactive mediators.[8] All these factors account for the edema characteristic of healing inflammation (Chapter 4).

Although these mechanisms are separable, all may play a role in response to one stimulus. For example, in various stages of a thermal burn, leakage results from chemically mediated endothelial contraction, direct and leukocyte-dependent injury, and new regenerating capillaries when the injury begins to heal. This accounts for the life-threatening loss of fluid in severely burned patients.

Cellular Events: Leukocyte Extravasation and Phagocytosis

A critical function of inflammation is the delivery of leukocytes to the site of injury. Leukocytes ingest offending agents, kill bacteria and other microbes, and degrade necrotic tissue and foreign antigens. Leukocytes may also prolong inflammation and induce tissue damage by releasing enzymes, chemical mediators, and toxic oxygen radicals.

The sequence of events in the journey of leukocytes from the lumen to the interstitial tissue, called extravasation, can be divided into the following steps:

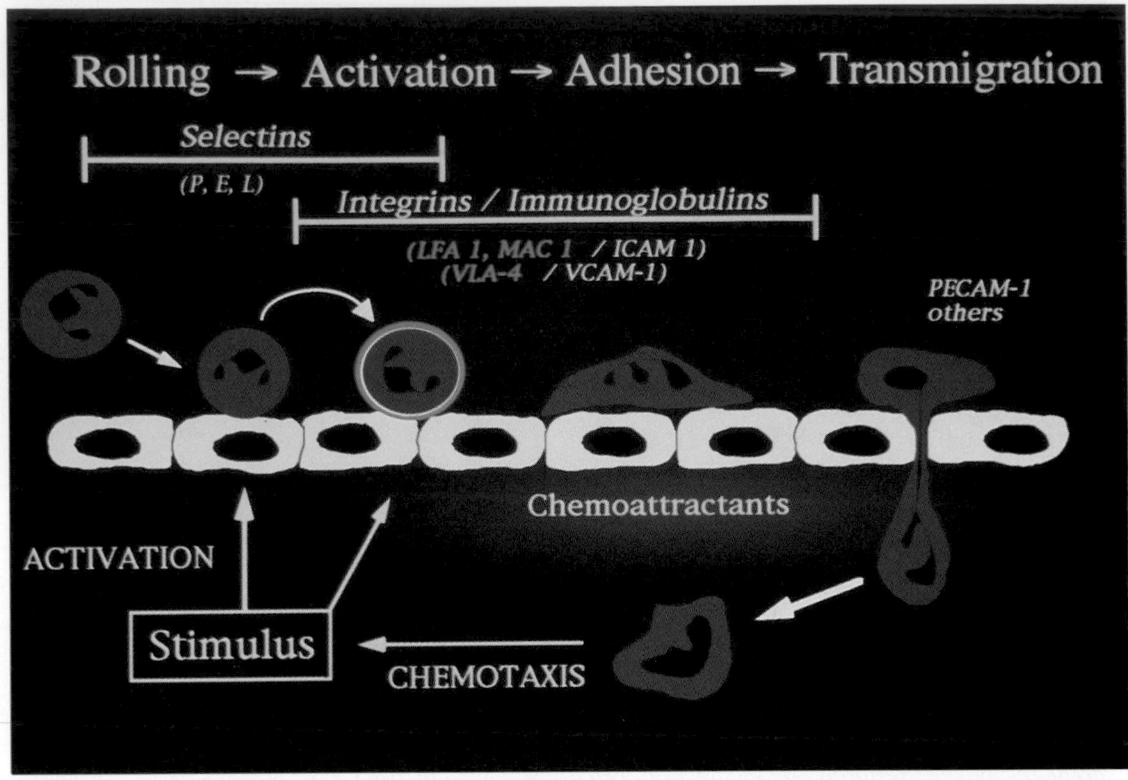

Figure 3–6

Sequence of leukocytic events in inflammation, shown here for neutrophils. The leukocytes first roll, then become activated and adhere to endothelium, then transmigrate across the endothelium, pierce the basement membrane, and migrate toward chemoattractants emanating from the source of injury. Note the roles of selectins in rolling; chemoattractants in activating the neutrophils to increase avidity of integrins (in green); ICAM-1 and VCAM-1 in firm adhesion; and PECAM-1 in transmigration.

1. In the lumen: margination, rolling, and adhesion
2. Transmigration across the endothelium (also called *diapedesis*)
3. Migration in interstitial tissues toward a chemotactic stimulus (Fig. 3–6)

In normally flowing blood in venules, erythrocytes are confined to a central axial column, displacing the leukocytes toward the wall of vessel[13] (Fig. 3–7). Because blood flow slows early in inflammation (as a result of the increased vascular permeability), hemodynamic conditions

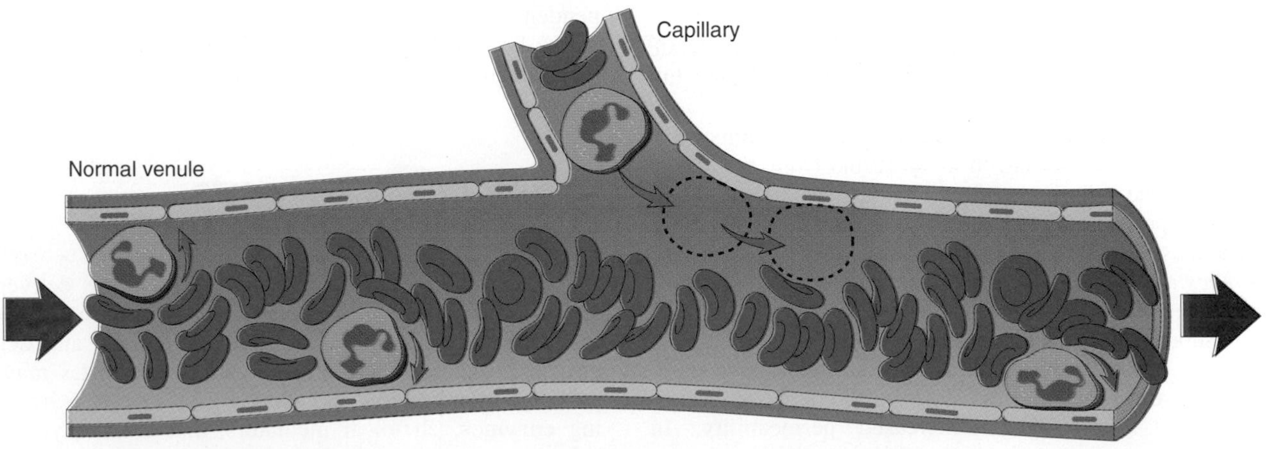

Figure 3–7

Laminar blood flow maintains leukocytes against the venular wall. (Modified and redrawn from Majno G, Joris I: Cells, Tissues, and Disease. Principles of General Pathology. Cambridge, MA, Blackwell Science, 1966.)

change (wall shear stress decreases), and more white cells assume a peripheral position along the endothelial surface. This process of leukocyte accumulation is called *margination*. Subsequently, individual and then rows of leukocytes tumble slowly along the endothelium and adhere transiently (a process called *rolling*), finally coming to rest at some point where they adhere firmly (resembling "pebbles or marbles over which a stream runs without disturbing them"). In time, the endothelium can be virtually lined by white cells, an appearance called *pavementing*. After firm adhesion, leukocytes insert pseudopods into the junctions between the endothelial cells, squeeze through interendothelial junctions, and assume a position between the endothelial cell and the basement membrane. Eventually, they traverse the basement membrane and escape into the extravascular space. Neutrophils, monocytes, lymphocytes, eosinophils, and basophils all use the same pathway. We now examine the molecular mechanisms of each of the steps.

ADHESION AND TRANSMIGRATION

It is now clear that leukocyte adhesion and transmigration are determined largely by the binding of complementary adhesion molecules on the leukocyte and endothelial surfaces and that chemical mediators—chemoattractants and certain cytokines—affect these processes by modulating the surface expression or avidity of such adhesion molecules.[13, 14] The adhesion receptors involved belong to four molecular families—the *selectins*, the *immunoglobulins*, the *integrins*, and *mucin-like glycoproteins*. The most important of these are shown in Table 3–1.

Selectins, so-called because they are characterized by an extracellular N-terminal domain related to sugar-binding mammalian lectins, consist of E-selectin (CD62E, previously known as ELAM-1), which is confined to endothelium; P-selectin (CD62P, previously called GMP140 or PADGEM), present in endothelium and platelets; and L-selectin (CD62L, previously known by many names, including LAM-1), which decorates most leukocyte types. Selectins bind, through their lectin domain, to sialylated forms of oligosaccharides (e.g., sialylated Lewis X), which themselves are covalently bound to various *mucin-like glycoproteins* (GlyCAM-1, PSGL-1, ESL-1, and CD34).

The *immunoglobulin* family molecules include two *endothelial* adhesion molecules: ICAM-1 (intercellular adhesion molecule 1) and VCAM-1 (vascular cell adhesion molecule 1). Both of these molecules interact with *integrins* found on leukocytes.

Integrins are transmembrane-adhesive heterodimeric glycoproteins, made up of α and β chains that also function as receptors for the extracellular matrix (Chapter 4). The principal integrin receptors for ICAM-1 are the β integrins LFA-1 and MAC-1 (CD11a/CD18 and CD11b/CD18), and those for VCAM-1 are the integrins $\alpha_4\beta_1$ (VLA-4) and $\alpha_4\beta_7$.

How are these molecules modulated to induce leukocyte adhesion in inflammation? There are a number of mechanisms, dependent on the duration of inflammation, the type of inflammatory stimulus, and blood flow conditions (Fig. 3–8).

1. *Redistribution of adhesion molecules to the cell surface* (Fig. 3–8*A*): P-selectin, for example, is normally present in the membrane of specific intracytoplasmic endothelial granules, called *Weibel-Palade bodies*. On stimulation by mediators such as histamine, thrombin, and platelet-activating factor (PAF), P-selectin is rapidly redistributed to the cell surface, where it can bind the leukocytes.[15] This process occurs within minutes in flowing blood and serves to deliver preformed adhesion molecules in short order to the surface. Studies suggest that this process may be particularly important in early leukocyte *rolling* on endothelium.
2. *Induction of adhesion molecules on endothelium*: Some inflammatory mediators, particularly cytokines (IL-1 and TNF), induce the synthesis and surface expression of endothelial adhesion molecules (Fig. 3–8*B*). This process requires new protein synthesis and begins usually after a delay of some 1 or 2 hours.[16] E-selectin, for example, which is not present on normal endothelium,

Table 3–1. ENDOTHELIAL/LEUKOCYTE ADHESION MOLECULES

Endothelial Molecule	Leukocyte Receptor	Major Role
P-selectin	Sialyl-Lewis X PSGL-1	Rolling (neutrophils, monocytes, lymphocytes)
E-selectin	Sialyl-Lewis X ESL-1, PSGL-1	Rolling, adhesion to activated endothelium (neutrophils, monocytes, T cells)
ICAM-1	CD11/CD18 (integrins) (LFA-1, Mac-1)	Adhesion, arrest, transmigration (all leukocytes)
VCAM-1	$\alpha4\beta1$ (VLA4) (integrins) $\alpha4\beta7$ (LPAM-1)	Adhesion (eosinophils, monocytes, lymphocytes)
GlyCam-1 CD34	L-selectin	Lymphocyte homing to high endothelial venules Neutrophil, monocyte rolling

ICAM-1 and VCAM-1 belong to the immunoglobulin family of proteins; ESL-1, E-selectin ligand 1; PSGL-1, P-selectin glycoprotein ligand 1.

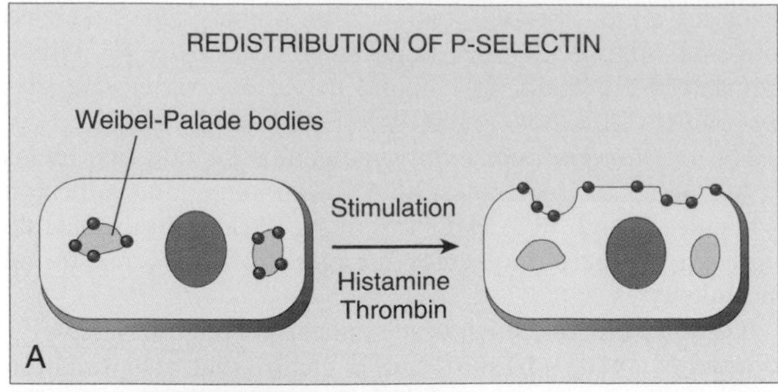

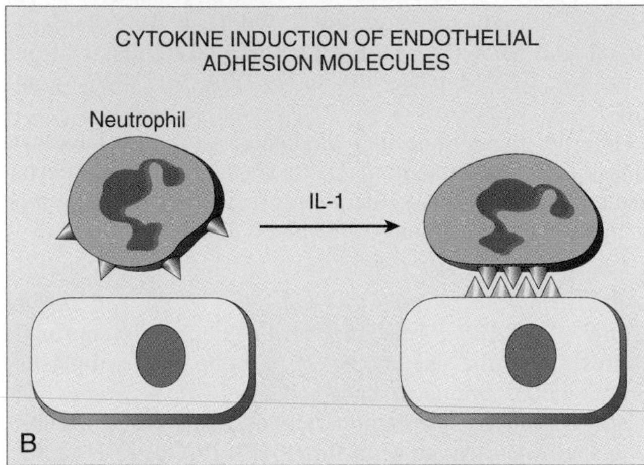

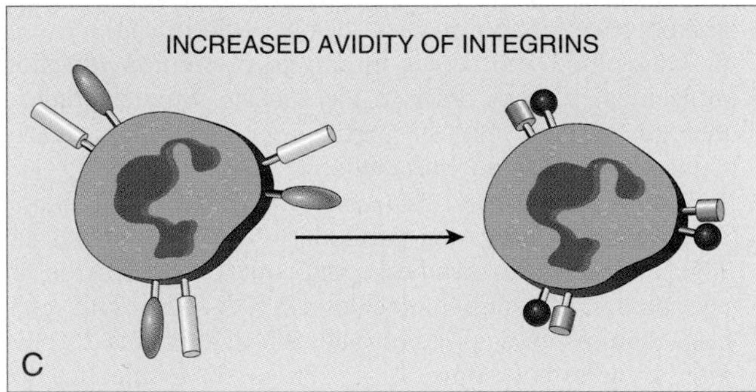

Figure 3–8 ■

Three mechanisms of mediating leukocyte endothelial adhesion. *A*, Redistribution of P-selectin. *B*, Cytokine activation of endothelium. *C*, Increased binding avidity of integrins (see text).

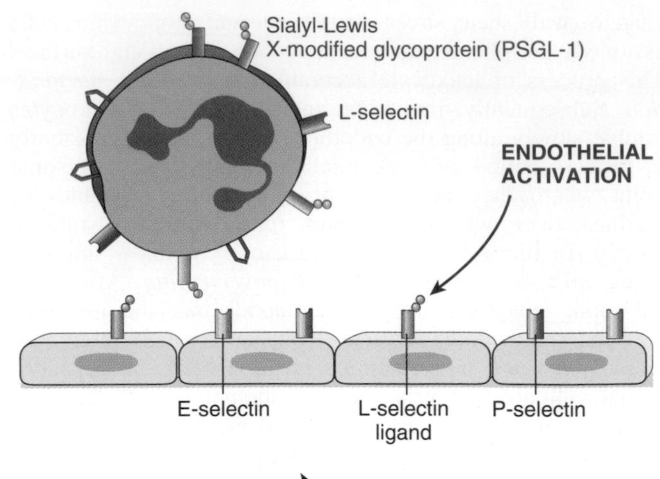

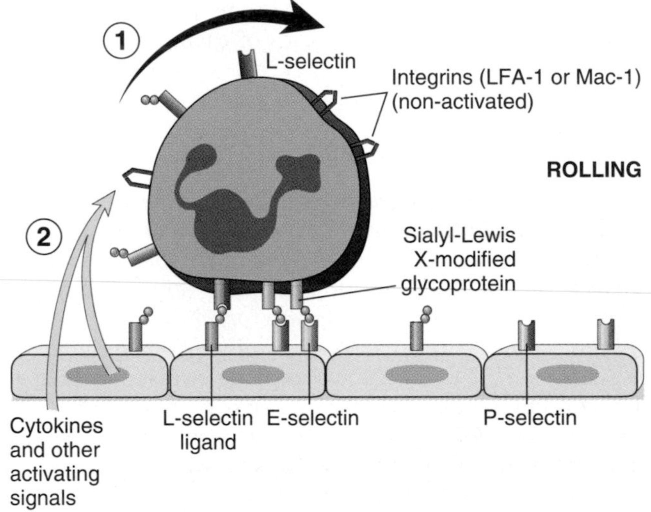

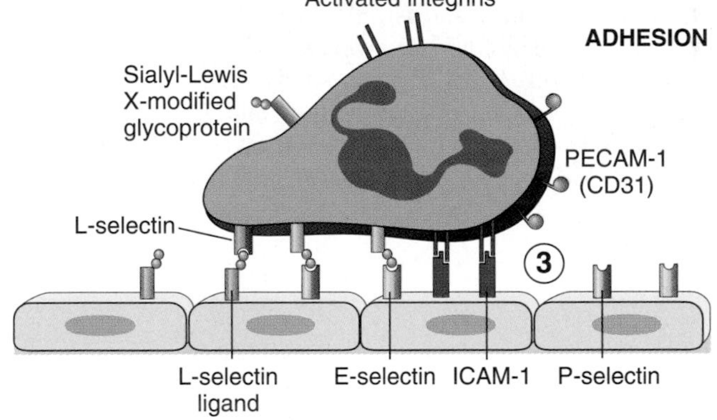

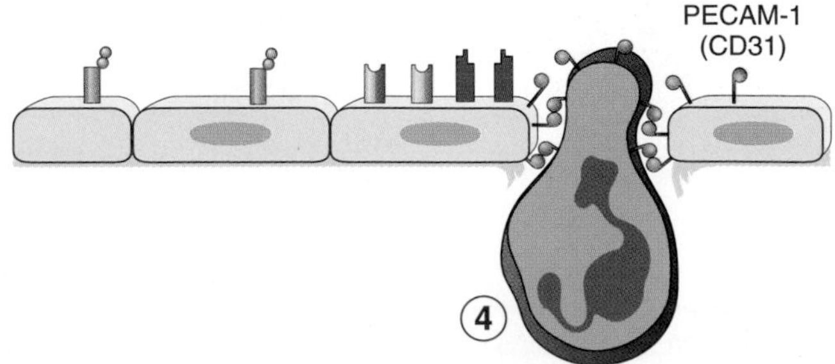

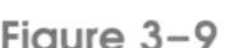

Figure 3–9 ■

Molecules mediating various steps of neutrophil extravasation in endothelial-neutrophil interaction. *Top, Endothelial activation:* Inflammatory mediators have upregulated the expression of E- and P-selectins on the endothelial cell. *Rolling*—E- and P-selectins bind sialyl-Lewis X on specific ligands, such as PSGL-1 and ESL-1, while L-selectin on the leukocytes binds carbohydrate moieties on ligand expressed on the endothelial cell. *Firm adhesion*—The leukocytes become activated by chemokines and increase the avidity of their $\beta 2$ integrins for ICAM-1 expressed by endothelial cells. *Bottom, Transmigration*—leukocytes pass between adjacent endothelial cells, using PECAM-1 and other molecules. The colored balls represent sugar moieties and the various receptors are consistently color coded.

is induced by IL-1 and TNF and mediates the adhesion of neutrophils, monocytes, and certain lymphocytes by binding to its receptors. The same cytokines also increase the expression of ICAM-1 and VCAM-1, which are present at low levels in normal endothelium.

3. *Increased avidity of binding* (Fig. 3–8*C*): This mechanism is most relevant to the binding of integrins. For example, LFA-1 is present on leukocytes—neutrophils, monocytes, and lymphocytes—but does not adhere to its ligand ICAM-1 on endothelium. To become firmly adherent, the neutrophils need to be activated such that LFA-1 is converted from a state of low-affinity binding to high-affinity binding toward ICAM-1, owing to a conformational change in the integrin molecule. The principal agents causing such leukocyte activation are chemotactic agents (including the chemokines, discussed later) made by endothelium or other cells emanating from the site of injury. During inflammation, the increased affinity of LFA-1 on the activated leukocyte, coupled with the increased ICAM-1 expression on endothelium induced by cytokines, sets the stage for strong LFA-1/ICAM-1 binding. The LFA-1/ICAM-1 interaction causes *firm adhesion* to the endothelium and appears also to be necessary for the subsequent *transmigration across* the endothelium.

Based on such studies, a currently accepted scenario for neutrophil adhesion and transmigration in acute inflammation postulates the following steps (Fig. 3–9)[17, 18]: (1) *endothelial activation*—mediators present at the inflammatory sites increase the expression of E-selectins and P-selectins; (2) *rolling*—there is initial rapid and relatively loose adhesion, resulting from interactions between the selectins and their carbohydrate ligands; (3) *firm adhesion*—the leukocytes are then activated by chemokines or other agents to increase the avidity of their integrins; and (4) *transmigration*—this is mediated by interactions between ICAM-1/integrins as well as PECAM-1 on leukocytes and endothe-

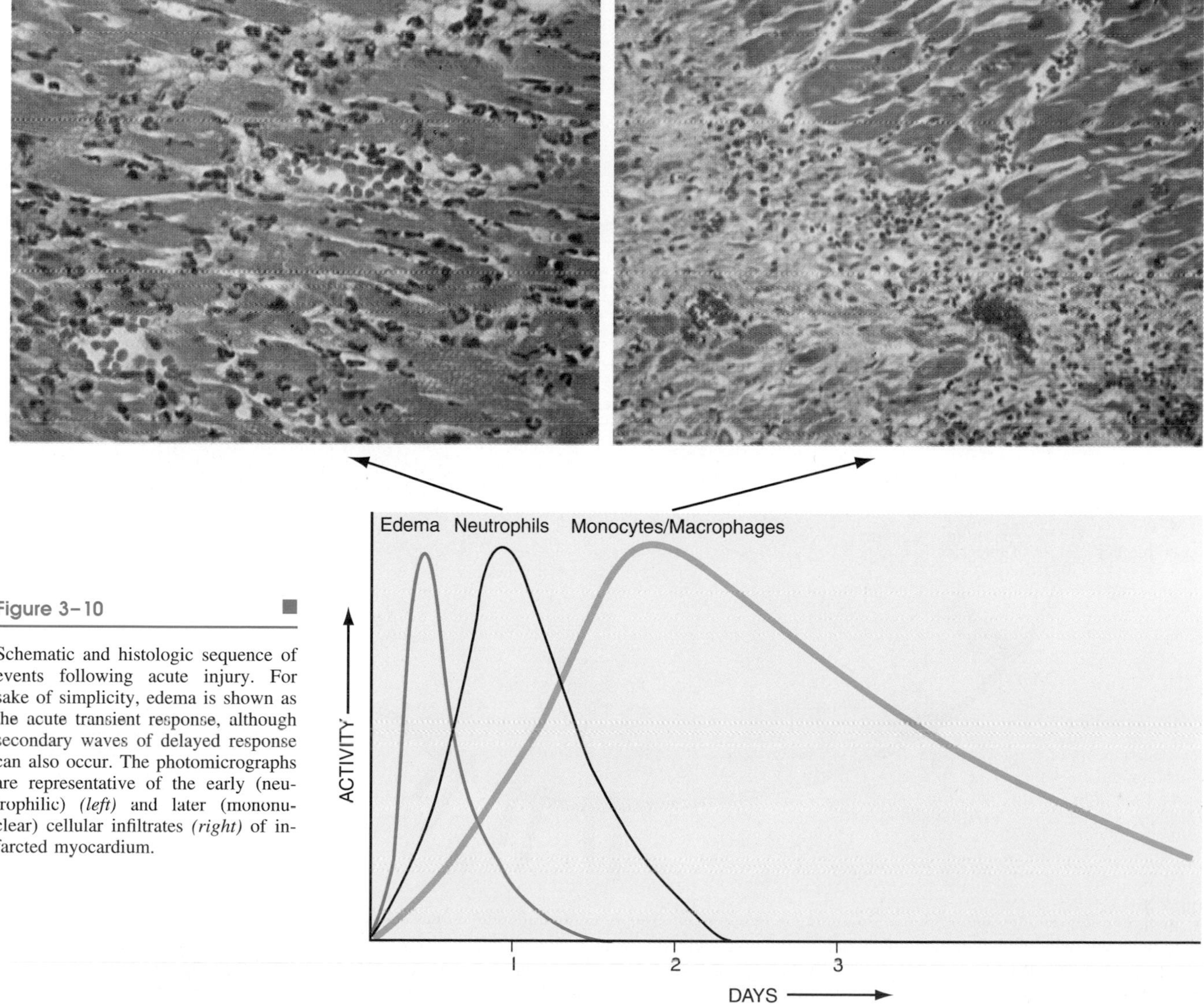

Figure 3–10

Schematic and histologic sequence of events following acute injury. For sake of simplicity, edema is shown as the acute transient response, although secondary waves of delayed response can also occur. The photomicrographs are representative of the early (neutrophilic) *(left)* and later (mononuclear) cellular infiltrates *(right)* of infarcted myocardium.

lial cells (see later). Neutrophils, monocytes, eosinophils, and various types of lymphocytes use different (but overlapping) molecules for rolling and adhesion, and their adhesivity can be modulated by the state of activation of the leukocyte and endothelium.[18]

The most telling proof of the importance of adhesion molecules is the existence of clinical genetic deficiencies in the leukocyte adhesion proteins, which are characterized by impaired leukocyte adhesion and recurrent bacterial infections. In *leukocyte adhesion deficiency type 1*, patients have a defect in the biosynthesis of the β_2 chain shared by LFA-1 and Mac-1 integrins.[19] *Leukocyte adhesion deficiency type 2* is caused by absence of sialyl-Lewis X, the ligand for E-selectin, owing to a generalized defect in fucose metabolism.[20] In addition, antibodies to adhesion molecules abrogate leukocyte extravasation in experimental models of acute inflammation,[21] and transgenic mice deficient in these molecules show a compromise in leukocyte rolling and extravasation.[22]

Although *intracellular* (through the endothelial cell cytoplasm) emigration has been described in an experimental model,[22a] transmigration occurs largely through the intercellular junctions. Certain homophilic adhesion molecules (i.e., adhesion molecules that bind to each other) present in

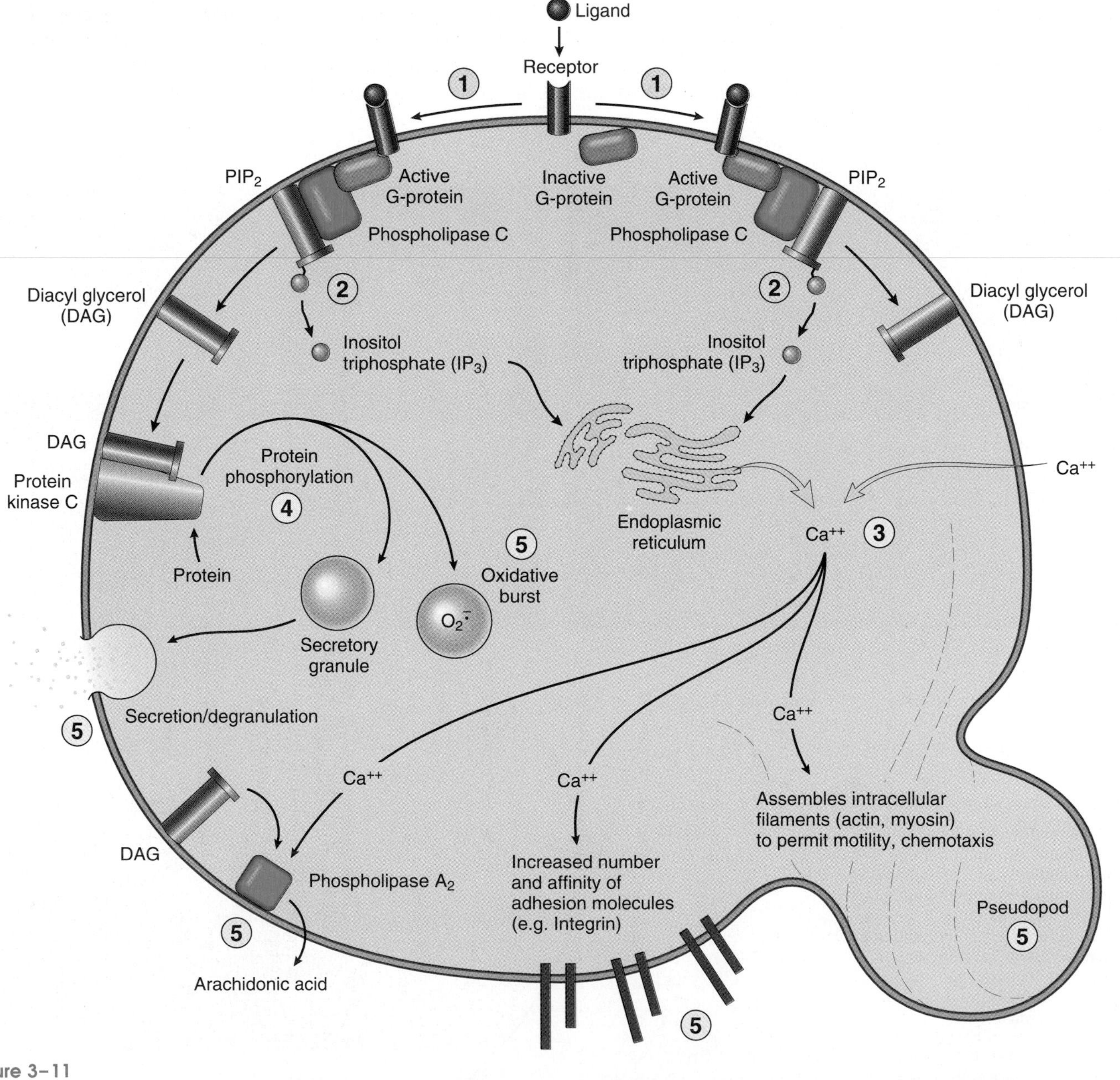

Figure 3–11

Biochemical events in leukocyte activation. The key events are (1) receptor-ligand binding, (2) phospholipase-C activation, (3) increased intracellular calcium, and (4) activation of protein kinase C. The biologic activities (5) resulting from leukocyte activation include chemotaxis, modulation of adhesion molecules, elaboration of arachidonic acid metabolites, secretion/degranulation, and the oxidative burst. PIP_2, phosphatidylinositol bisphosphate.

the intercellular junction of endothelium are involved. One of these is a member of the immunoglobulin gene superfamily called *PECAM-1* (platelet endothelial cell adhesion molecule) or CD31.[23, 23a] Antibodies or soluble forms of this molecule inhibit transmigration in vitro and in experimental animal models.[23a] *Leukocyte diapedesis, similar to increased vascular permeability, occurs predominantly in the venules* (except in the lungs, where it also occurs in capillaries). After traversing the endothelium, leukocytes are transiently retarded in their journey by the continuous basement membrane but eventually pierce it, probably by secreting collagenases that degrade the basement membrane.

The type of emigrating leukocyte varies with the age of the inflammatory lesion and with the type of stimulus. In most forms of acute inflammation, *neutrophils predominate in the inflammatory infiltrate during the first 6 to 24 hours, then are replaced by monocytes in 24 to 48 hours* (Fig. 3–10). The sequence can best be explained by the induction or activation of different adhesion molecule pairs or specific chemotactic factors in different phases of inflammation. In addition, short-lived neutrophils undergo apoptosis and disappear after 24 to 48 hours, whereas monocytes survive longer. There are exceptions to this pattern of cellular exudation, however. In certain infections, for example, those produced by *Pseudomonas* organisms, neutrophils predominate over 2 to 4 days; in viral infections, lymphocytes may be the first cells to arrive; in some hypersensitivity reactions, eosinophilic granulocytes may be the main cell type.

CHEMOTAXIS

After extravasation, leukocytes emigrate in tissues toward the site of injury by a process called *chemotaxis*, defined most simply as locomotion oriented along a chemical gradient. All granulocytes, monocytes, and, to a lesser extent, lymphocytes respond to chemotactic stimuli with varying rates of speed.

Both exogenous and endogenous substances can act as chemoattractants. The most common *exogenous* agents are *bacterial products*. Some of these are peptides that possess an *N*-formyl-methionine terminal amino acid. Others are lipid in nature. *Endogenous* chemical mediators, which are detailed later, include (1) *components of the complement system*, particularly C5a; (2) *products of the lipoxygenase pathway*, mainly leukotriene B_4 (LTB_4); and (3) *cytokines*, particularly those of the chemokine family (e.g., IL-8).

How does the leukocyte *see* (or *smell*) the chemotactic agents, and how do these substances induce directed cell movement? Although not all the answers are known, several important steps and second messengers are recognized (Fig. 3–11) (Chapter 4).[24] Binding of chemotactic agents to specific receptors on the cell membranes of leukocytes results in activation of phospholipase C (mediated by unique G-proteins), leading to the hydrolysis of phosphatidylinositol-4,5-biphosphate (PIP_2) to inositol-1,4,5 triphosphate (IP_3) and diacylglycerol (DAG) and the release of calcium, first from intracellular stores and subsequently from the influx of extracellular calcium. The increased cytosolic calcium triggers the assembly of contractile elements responsible for cell movement.

The leukocyte moves by extending a pseudopod (lamellipod) that pulls the remainder of the cell in the direction of extension, just as an automobile with front-wheel drive is pulled by the wheels in front (Fig. 3–12). The interior of the pseudopod consists of a branching network of filaments composed of *actin* as well as the contractile protein *myosin*. Locomotion involves rapid assembly of actin monomers into linear polymers at the pseudopod's leading edge, cross-linking of filaments, followed by disassembly of such filaments away from the leading edge.[25] These complex events are controlled by the effects of calcium ions and phosphoinositol on a number of actin-regulating proteins, such as *filamin, gelsolin, profilin,* and *calmodulin*. These components interact with actin and myosin in the pseudopod to produce contraction.

Leukocytes migrating in tissues encounter complex patterns of multiple chemoattractant signals, some endogenous (e.g., chemokines) and some derived from the injurious target (e.g., bacterial products). How does the leukocyte solve such a difficult navigation problem and arrive at the correct extravascular location? Leukocytes appear to migrate in a step-by-step manner in response to one agonist after another, their position being determined by the pattern of attractant *receptors* they express, and the sequence of chemokine *gradients* they encounter. In addition, the target-derived chemotactins override the host-derived gradients, helping to guide movement to the initiating stimulus.[26]

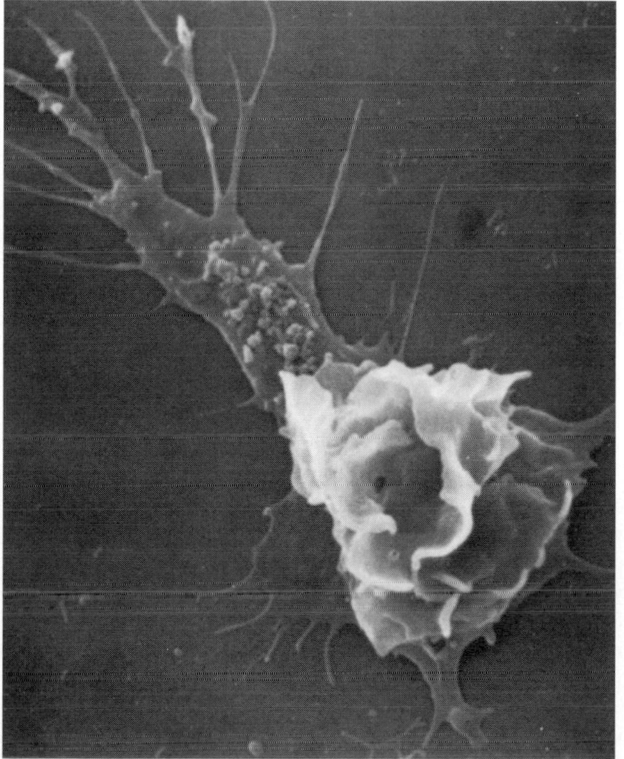

Figure 3–12 ■

Scanning electron micrograph of a moving leukocyte in culture showing a pseudopod *(upper left)* and a trailing tail. (Courtesy of Dr. Morris J. Karnovsky, Harvard Medical School, Boston.)

LEUKOCYTE ACTIVATION

In addition to stimulating locomotion, many chemotactic factors, particularly when in high concentrations, induce other responses in the leukocytes, referred to under the rubric of *leukocyte activation* (see Fig. 3–11). Such responses, which can also be induced by phagocytosis and antigen-antibody complexes, include the following:

- *Production of arachidonic acid metabolites* from phospholipids, owing to activation of phospholipase A_2 by DAG and increased intracellular calcium.
- *Degranulation and secretion of lysosomal enzymes and activation of the oxidative burst* (see discussion under phagocytosis): These two processes are induced by DAG-mediated activation of protein kinase. Activation of intracellular phospholipase D by the increased calcium influx contributes to the sustained DAG accumulation.
- *Modulation of leukocyte adhesion molecules*: Certain chemoattractants cause increased surface expression and, as stated earlier, increased adhesive avidity of the LFA-1 integrin, allowing firm adhesion of activated neutrophils to ICAM-1 on endothelium. In contrast, neutrophils shed L-selectin from their surface, making them less adhesive to the L-selectin ligand on endothelium.

Another phenomenon in leukocyte activation is *priming*, denoting an increased rate and extent of leukocyte activation by exposure to a mediator that itself causes little activation. The cytokine TNF, in particular, markedly increases leukocyte activation by other chemotactic agents, accounting for its powerful in vivo effects, described later in this chapter.

PHAGOCYTOSIS

Phagocytosis and the release of enzymes by neutrophils and macrophages constitute two of the major benefits derived from the accumulation of leukocytes at the inflammatory focus. Phagocytosis involves three distinct but interrelated steps (Fig. 3–13*A*): (1) *recognition* and *attachment* of the particle to be ingested by the leukocyte; (2) its *engulfment*, with subsequent formation of a phagocytic vacuole; and (3) *killing* or *degradation* of the ingested material.[27]

Recognition and Attachment

On occasion, neutrophils and macrophages recognize and engulf bacteria or extraneous matter (e.g., latex beads) in the absence of serum. Most microorganisms, however, are not recognized until they are coated by naturally occurring factors called *opsonins*, which bind to specific receptors on the leukocytes. Opsonization of particles such as bacteria markedly enhances the efficiency of phagocytosis. The major opsonins are (1) the *Fc fragment of immunoglobulin G (IgG)*, presumably naturally occurring antibody against the ingested particle, (2) *C3b*, the so-called *opsonic fragment of C3* (and its stable form *C3bi*), generated by activation of complement by immune or nonimmune mechanisms, as described later and (3) carbohydrate-binding proteins (lectins) of plasma called *collectins*, which bind to microbial cell walls (e.g., mannose-binding protein) and are involved in innate immunity. The corresponding receptors on leukocytes are FcγR, which recognize the Fc fragment of IgG; *complement receptors 1, 2,* and *3* (*CR1, 2, 3*), which interact with C3b and C3bi; and C1q receptors, which bind to the collectins.[26a] *CR3,* which recognizes *C3bi, is a particularly important receptor; it is identical with the β_2 integrin-Mac-1 (CD11b),* which is involved in adhesion to endothelium. It binds certain bacteria by recognizing bacterial lipopolysaccharides, without the intervention of antibody or complement, accounting for so-called *nonopsonic phagocytosis.* CR3/Mac-1 also binds the extracellular matrix components fibronectin and laminin. In addition to engaging the ligand, signals from the FcγRs are involved in metabolic activation of the phagocytes, increasing subsequent intracellular degradation of ingested material, as well as the release of proteases by these cells.

Engulfment

Binding of the opsonized particle to the FcγR is sufficient to trigger engulfment, which is markedly enhanced in the presence of complement receptors. Binding to the C3 receptors alone, however, is not followed by engulfment, unless such receptors are activated either by simultaneous binding to extracellular fibronectin and laminin or by certain cytokines. During engulfment, extensions of the cytoplasm (pseudopods) flow around the object to be engulfed, eventually resulting in complete enclosure of the particle within a phagosome created by the cytoplasmic membrane of the cell. The limiting membrane of this phagocytic vacuole then fuses with the limiting membrane of a lysosomal granule, resulting in discharge of the granule's contents into the phagolysosome (Fig. 3–13*A*). In the course of this action, the neutrophil and the monocyte become progressively degranulated.

Many of the biochemical events involved in phagocytosis and degranulation are similar to those described for chemotaxis (see Fig. 3–11). The process is associated with receptor-ligand binding, phospholipase C activation, DAG and IP_3 production, protein kinase C activation, and increased concentration of cytosolic calcium, the last two acting as second messengers to initiate the cellular events.

Killing or Degradation

The ultimate step in phagocytosis of bacteria is killing and degradation. *Bacterial killing is accomplished largely by oxygen-dependent mechanisms* (Fig. 3–13*B*).[28] Phagocytosis stimulates a burst in oxygen consumption, glycogenolysis, increased glucose oxidation via the hexose-monophosphate shunt, and production of reactive oxygen metabolites.

The generation of oxygen metabolites is due to the rapid activation of an oxidase (NADPH oxidase), which oxidizes NADPH (reduced nicotinamide-adenine dinucleotide phosphate) and, in the process, reduces oxygen to superoxide anion ($O_2^{\bar{\cdot}}$).

$$2O_2 + e^- \xrightarrow[\text{NADPH oxidase}]{} 2O_2^{\bar{\cdot}} + NADP^+ + H^+$$

Superoxide is then converted into H_2O_2, mostly by spontaneous dismutation:

$$2O_2^{\bar{\cdot}} + 2H^+ \longrightarrow H_2O_2 + O_2$$

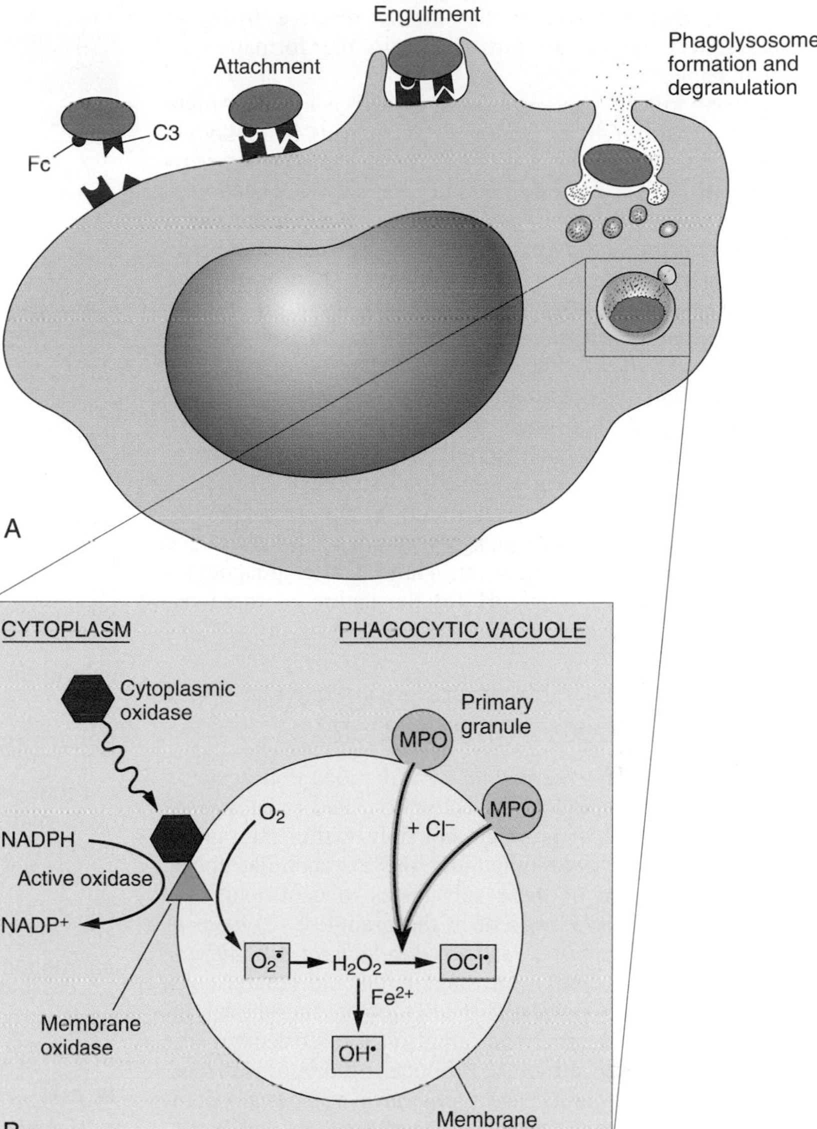

Figure 3–13

A, Phagocytosis of a particle (e.g., bacterium) involves attachment and binding of Fc and C3b to receptors on the leukocyte membrane, engulfment, and fusion of granules *(in red)* with phagocytic vacuoles, followed by degranulation. Note that during phagocytosis, granule contents may be released extracellularly. In innate immunity, collectins also serve as opsonins. *B*, Summary of oxygen-dependent bactericidal mechanisms within the phagocytic vacuole, as described in the text.

The NADPH oxidase is a multiprotein enzyme complex consisting of at least seven proteins.[29] In resting neutrophils, these NADPH oxidase protein components are separated into plasma membrane and cytoplasmic compartments. During assembly and activation of the oxidase, the cytosolic protein components translocate to the plasma membrane or phagosomal membrane, where they assemble to form the functional enzyme complex (Fig. 3–13*B*). Thus, the *hydrogen peroxide is produced within the lysosome*. By segregating the oxidase components into different cellular locations, phagocytes are able to prevent inappropriate activation of the oxidase system and control the timing of the respiratory burst. The phagocyte NADPH oxidase complex is an essential component of the immune response and is also involved in nonspecific tissue damage associated with many inflammatory diseases, as shown subsequently.

The quantities of H_2O_2 produced in the phagolysosome are insufficient to induce effective killing of bacteria. However, the azurophilic granules of neutrophils contain the enzyme *myeloperoxidase* (MPO) which, in the presence of a halide such as Cl^-, converts H_2O_2 to HOCl. The latter is an antimicrobial agent that destroys bacteria by *halogenation* (in which the halide is bound covalently to cellular constituents) or by oxidation of proteins and lipids (lipid peroxidation). *The H_2O_2-MPO-halide system is the most efficient bactericidal system in neutrophils.* A similar mechanism is also effective against fungi, viruses, protozoa, and helminths. Most of the H_2O_2 is eventually broken down by catalase into H_2O and O_2, and some is destroyed by the action of glutathione oxidase. The dead microorganisms are then degraded by the action of lysosomal hydrolases.

MPO-deficient leukocytes are capable of killing bacteria (albeit more slowly than control cells), by virtue of the formation of superoxide, hydroxyl radicals, and singlet oxygen (Fig. 3–13). Recall that hydrogen peroxide can also be further reduced to the highly reactive hydroxyl radical (·OH), which, in turn, leads to the formation of water (Chapter 1).

Bacterial killing can also occur by *oxygen-independent mechanisms,* through the action of substances in leukocyte granules. These include *bactericidal permeability increasing protein* (BPI), a highly cationic granule-associated protein that causes phospholipase activation, phospholipid degradation, and increased permeability in the outer membrane of the microorganisms; *lysozyme*, which hydrolyzes the muramic acid-*N*-acetyl-glucosamine bond, found in the glycopeptide coat of all bacteria; *lactoferrin*, an iron-binding protein present in specific granules; *major basic protein*, a cationic protein of eosinophils, which has limited bactericidal activity but is cytotoxic to many parasites; and *defensins*, cationic arginine-rich granule peptides that are cytotoxic to microbes (and certain mammalian cells).[30]

After killing, acid hydrolases found in azurophil granules degrade the bacteria within phagolysosomes. The pH of the phagolysosome drops to between 4 and 5 after phagocytosis, this being the optimal pH for the action of these enzymes.

RELEASE OF LEUKOCYTE PRODUCTS AND LEUKOCYTE-INDUCED TISSUE INJURY

The metabolic and membrane perturbations that occur in leukocytes during chemotaxis, activation, and phagocytosis result in the release of products not only within the phagolysosome, but also potentially into the extracellular space. The most important of these substances in neutrophils are (1) *lysosomal enzymes*, present in the granules; (2) *oxygen-derived active metabolites*; and (3) *products of arachidonic acid metabolism*, including prostaglandins and leukotrienes. These products are powerful mediators of endothelial injury and tissue damage and amplify the effects of the initial inflammatory stimulus. Products of monocytes/macrophages and other leukocyte types have additional potentially harmful products, which are described in the discussion of chronic inflammation. Thus, if persistent and unchecked, the leukocyte infiltrate itself becomes the offender,[31] and leukocyte-dependent tissue injury underlies many acute and chronic human diseases (Table 3–2). This fact becomes evident in the discussion of the specific disorders thoughout this book.

The ways by which lysosomal granules and enzymes are secreted are diverse. Release may occur if the phagocytic vacuole remains transiently open to the outside before complete closure of the phagolysosome (*regurgitation during feeding*). In cells exposed to potentially ingestible materials, such as immune complexes, on flat surfaces (e.g., glomerular basement membrane), attachment of immune complexes to the leukocyte triggers membrane movement, but, because of the flat surface, phagocytosis does not occur, and lysosomal enzymes are released into the medium (*frustrated phagocytosis*). Lysosomal hydrolases may also be released during *surface phagocytosis*, a mechanism by which phagocytes facilitate ingestion of bacteria and other foreign material by trapping it against a resistant surface. *Cytotoxic release* occurs after phagocytosis of potentially membranolytic substances, such as urate crystals. In addition, there is some evidence that certain granules, particularly the specific (secondary) granules of neutrophils, may be directly secreted by *exocytosis*.[32] After phagocytosis, neutrophils rapidly undergo *apoptotic cell death* and are either ingested by macrophages or are cleared by lymphatics.[33] Such phagocytosis-induced cell death is dependent on the presence of the integrin Mac-1 (CD11b) on the surface of neutrophils, adding to the important role of this molecule in the events of acute inflammation.[34]

Table 3–2. CLINICAL EXAMPLES OF LEUKOCYTE-INDUCED INJURY

Acute	Chronic
Acute respiratory distress syndrome	Arthritis
Acute transplant rejection	Asthma
Asthma	Atherosclerosis
Glomerulonephritis	Chronic lung disease
Reperfusion injury	Chronic rejection
Septic shock	Others
Vasculitis	

DEFECTS IN LEUKOCYTE FUNCTION

From the preceding discussion, it is obvious that leukocytes play a cardinal role in host defense. Not surprisingly, therefore, defects in leukocyte function, both genetic and acquired, lead to increased vulnerability to infections (Table 3–3). Impairments of virtually every phase of leukocyte function—from adherence to vascular endothelium to microbicidal activity—have been identified, and the existence of clinical genetic deficiencies in each of the critical steps in the process has been described. These include the following:

- *Defects in leukocyte adhesion*: We have previously mentioned the genetic deficiencies in leukocyte adhesion molecules (LAD types 1 and 2). LAD type 1 is characterized by recurrent bacterial infections and impaired wound healing. In these patients, there is a deficiency of β_2 integrins (CD18), which results in abnormal neutrophil adhesion, spreading, phagocytosis, and generation of the oxidative burst.[19] LAD type 2 is clinically milder than LAD type 1 but is also characterized by recurrent bacterial infections. The disorder results from an absence of a carbohydrate (sialyl-Lewis X), the ligand on neutrophils that is required for binding to the selectins expressed by cytokine-activated endothelium.[20] The defect is attributed to mutations in the fucosyl transferase that makes the carbohydrate moiety.
- *Defects in phagocytosis*: One such disorder is *Chédiak-Higashi syndrome*, an autosomal recessive condition characterized by neutropenia (decreased numbers of neutrophils), defective degranulation, and delayed microbial killing. The neutrophils (and other leukocytes) have *giant granules*, which can be readily seen in peripheral blood smears and which are thought to result from aberrant organelle fusion.[35] In this syndrome, there is reduced transfer of lysosomal enzymes to phagocytic vac-

Table 3-3. DEFECTS IN LEUKOCYTE FUNCTIONS

Disease	Defect
Genetic	
Leukocyte adhesion deficiency 1	• β chain of CD11/CD18 integrins
Leukocyte adhesion deficiency 2	• Sialylated oligosaccharide (receptor for selectin)
Neutrophil-specific granule deficiency	• Absence of neutrophil-specific granules • Defective chemotaxis
Chronic granulomatous disease X-linked	• Decreased oxidative burst • NADPH oxidase (membrane component)
Autosomal recessive	• NADPH oxidase (cytoplasmic components)
Myeloperoxidase deficiency	• Absent MPO-H_2O_2 system
Chédiak-Higashi syndrome	• Membrane-associated protein involved in organelle membrane docking and fusion
Acquired	
Thermal injury, diabetes, malignancy, sepsis, immunodeficiencies	• Chemotaxis
Hemodialysis, diabetes mellitus	• Adhesion
Leukemia, anemia, sepsis, diabetes, neonates, malnutrition	• Phagocytosis and microbicidal activity

Modified from Gallin JI: Disorders of phagocytic cells. In Gallin JI, et al (eds): Inflammation: Basic Principles and Clinical Correlates, 2nd ed. New York, Raven Press, 1992, pp 860, 861.

uoles (causing susceptibility to infections), melanocytes (leading to albinism), cells of the nervous system (associated with nerve defects), and platelets (generating bleeding disorders). The identification of a candidate gene suggests that the defect in the disorder is in a membrane-associated protein, which is involved in organelle membrane docking and fusion.[35] This could explain the inability to secrete lysosomal components into phagosomes or outside the cell. The secretion of lytic granules by cytotoxic T cells is also affected, explaining the severe immunodeficiency seen in the disorder.

- *Defects in microbicidal activity*: The importance of oxygen-dependent bacterial mechanisms is shown by the existence of a group of congenital disorders in bacterial killing called *chronic granulomatous disease*, which render patients susceptible to recurrent bacterial infection. Chronic granulomatous disease results from *inherited defects in the genes encoding several components of NADPH oxidase*, which generates superoxide. The most common variants are an *X-linked defect* in one of the plasma membrane-bound components (gp91phox) and *autosomal recessive* defects in the genes encoding two of the cytoplasmic components (p47phox and p67-phox).[29]

Although individually rare, these genetic disorders underscore the importance of the complex series of leukocyte events that must occur in vivo after invasion by microorganisms.

Summary of the Acute Inflammatory Response

The vascular phenomena are characterized by increased blood flow to the injured area, resulting mainly from arteriolar dilation and opening of capillary beds. Increased vascular permeability results in the accumulation of protein-rich extravascular fluid, which forms the exudate. Plasma proteins leave the vessels, most commonly through widened interendothelial cell junctions of the venules or by direct endothelial cell injury. The leukocytes, initially predominantly neutrophils, adhere to the endothelium via adhesion molecules, transmigrate across the endothelium, and migrate to the site of injury under the influence of chemotactic agents. Phagocytosis of the offending agent follows, which may lead to the death of the microorganism. During chemotaxis and phagocytosis, activated leukocytes may release toxic metabolites and proteases extracellularly, potentially causing tissue damage.

CHEMICAL MEDIATORS OF INFLAMMATION

Having described the events in acute inflammation, we can now turn to a discussion of the chemical mediators that account for the events. Many mediators have been identified. While the multitude may have survival value for the organism (and also for investigators searching for mediators and pharmaceutical companies for new drugs), they are most difficult for students to remember. Here we review general principles and highlight some of the more important mediators.

- *Mediators originate either from plasma or from cells* (Fig. 3-14). Plasma-derived mediators (e.g., complement) are present in plasma in *precursor forms* that *must be activated*, usually by a series of proteolytic cleavages, to acquire their biologic properties. Cell-derived mediators are normally *sequestered in intracellular granules* that need to be secreted (e.g., histamine in mast cell granules) or *are synthesized de novo* (e.g., prostaglandins, cytokines) in response to a stimulus. The major cellular sources are platelets, neutrophils, monocytes/macrophages, and mast cells, but mesenchymal cells (endothelium, smooth muscle, fibroblasts) and most epithelia can also be induced to elaborate some of the mediators.
- Most mediators perform their biologic activity by initially *binding to specific receptors on target cells*. Some, however, have direct enzymatic activity (e.g., lysosomal proteases) or mediate oxidative damage (e.g., oxygen metabolites).
- *A chemical mediator can stimulate the release of mediators by target cells themselves*. These secondary mediators may be identical or similar to the initial mediators but may also have opposing activities. They provide mechanisms for amplifying—or in certain instances counteracting—the initial mediator action.
- Mediators can act on one or few target cell types, have

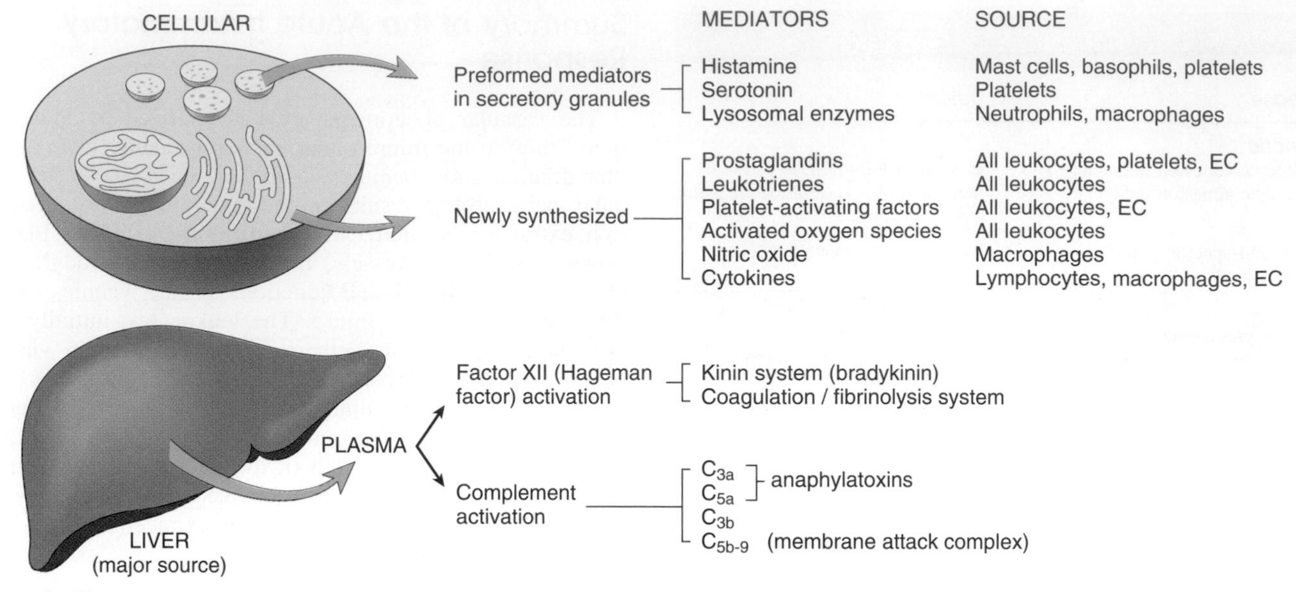

Figure 3–14

Chemical mediators of inflammation. EC, endothelial cells.

widespread targets, or may even have differing effects, depending on cell and tissue types.

- *Once activated and released from the cell, most of these mediators are short-lived.* They quickly decay (e.g., arachidonic acid metabolites) or are inactivated by enzymes (e.g., kininase inactivates bradykinin), or they are otherwise scavenged (e.g., antioxidants scavenge toxic oxygen metabolites) or inhibited (e.g., complement inhibitors). There is thus a system of checks and balances in the regulation of mediator actions.
- *Most mediators have the potential to cause harmful effects.*

We now discuss some of the more important mediators.

Vasoactive Amines

The two amines, histamine and serotonin, are especially important because they are available from preformed stores and are among the first mediators to be released during inflammation.

HISTAMINE

Histamine is widely distributed in tissues, the richest source being the mast cells that are normally present in the connective tissue adjacent to blood vessels (Fig. 3–15). It is also found in blood basophils and platelets. Preformed histamine is present in mast cell granules and is released by mast cell degranulation in response to a variety of stimuli: (1) physical injury such as trauma, cold, or heat; (2) immune reactions involving binding of antibodies to mast cells (Chapter 7); (3) fragments of complement called *anaphylatoxins* (C3a and C5a); (4) histamine-releasing proteins derived from leukocytes; (5) neuropeptides (e.g., substance P); and (6) cytokines (IL-1, IL-8).

In humans, histamine causes dilation of the arterioles and increases vascular permeability of the venules (it, however, *constricts* large arteries). It is considered to be the principal mediator of the immediate phase of increased vascular permeability, causing venular gaps, as we have seen. It acts on the microcirculation mainly via H_1 receptors.

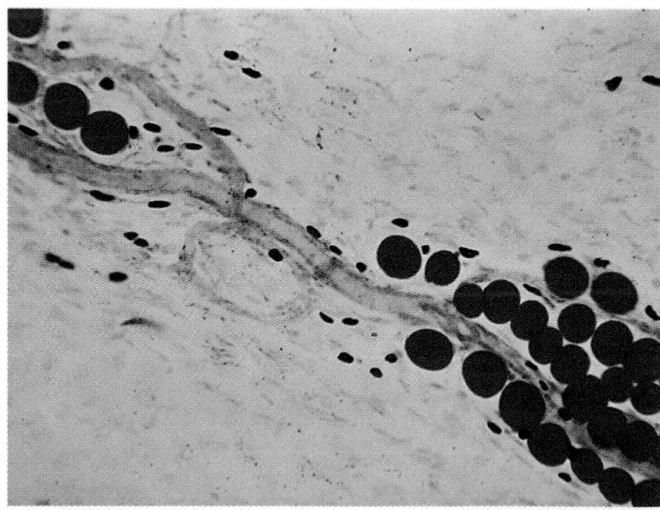

Figure 3–15

A flat spread of omentum showing mast cells around blood vessels and in the interstitial tissue. Stained with metachromatic stain to identify the mast cell granules. The red structures are fat globules stained with fat stain. (Courtesy of Dr. G. Majno.)

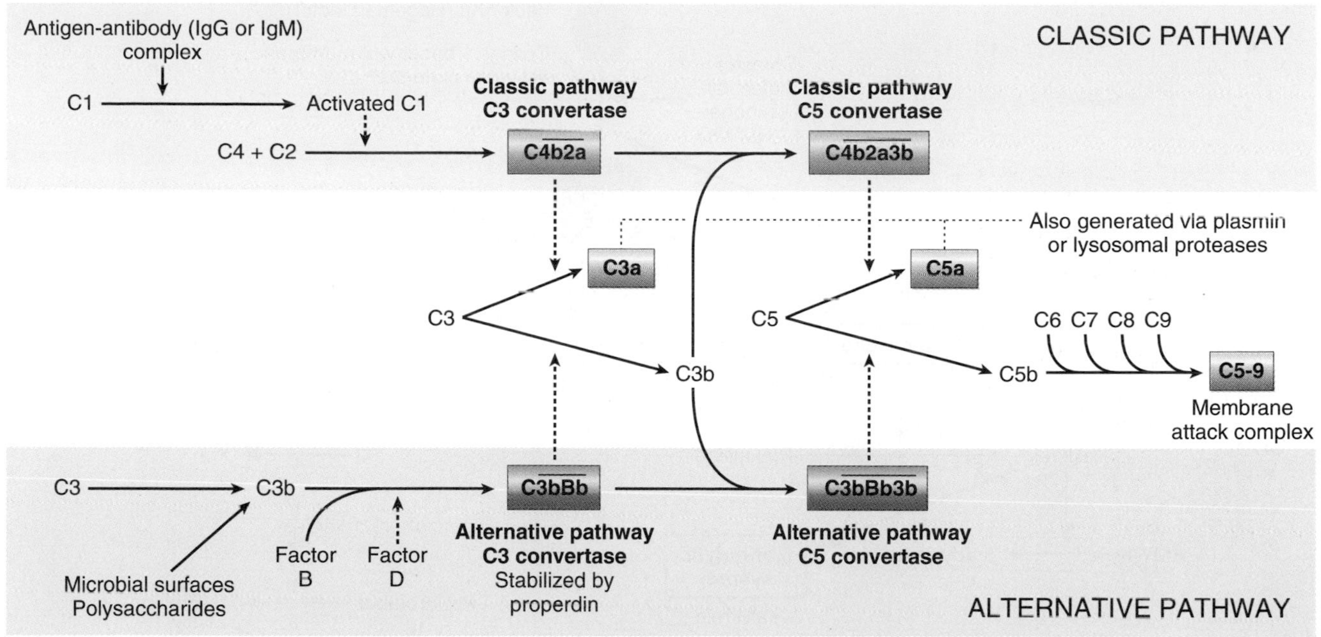

Figure 3–16

Overview of complement activation pathways. The classic pathway is initiated by C1 binding to antigen-antibody complexes, and the alternative pathway is initiated by C3b binding to various activating surfaces, such as microbial cell walls. The C3b involved in alternative pathway initiation may be generated in several ways, including spontaneously, by the classic pathway, or by the alternative pathway itself (see text). Both pathways converge and lead to the formation of inflammatory complement mediators (C3a and C5a) and the membrane attack complex. *Not shown is activation by collectins (the lectin pathway, see text).* In this figure, bars over the letter designations of complement components indicate enzymatically active forms, and dashed lines indicate proteolytic activities of various components. (Modified from Abbas AK, et al: Cellular and Molecular Immunology, 3rd ed. Philadelphia, WB Saunders, 1997.)

SEROTONIN

Serotonin (5-hydroxytryptamine) is a second preformed vasoactive mediator with actions similar to those of histamine. It is present in platelets and enterochromaffin cells and in mast cells in rodents but not humans.

Release of serotonin (and histamine) from *platelets* is stimulated when platelets aggregate after contact with collagen, thrombin, adenosine diphosphate (ADP), and antigen-antibody complexes. Platelet aggregation and release are also stimulated by platelet-activating factor (PAF) derived from mast cells during IgE-mediated reactions. In this way, the platelet release reaction results in increased permeability during immunologic reactions. As discussed later, PAF itself has many inflammatory properties.

Plasma Proteases

A variety of phenomena in the inflammatory response are mediated by three interrelated plasma-derived factors: the complement, kinin, and clotting systems (Figs. 3–16 and 3–17).

COMPLEMENT SYSTEM

The complement system consists of 20 component proteins (together with their cleavage products), which are found in greatest concentration in plasma. This system functions in both innate and adaptive immunity for defense against microbial agents, culminating in lysing microbes by the so-called membrane attack complex (MAC).[29a] In the process, a number of complement components are elaborated that cause increased vascular permeability, chemotaxis, and opsonization (Fig. 3–16).[36]

Complement components present as inactive forms in plasma are numbered C1 through C9. Although we do not go into the detailed molecular events of the activation of the *complement cascade*, a brief review of the salient features is helpful. The most critical step in the elaboration of the biologic functions of complement is the activation of the third component, C3. Cleavage of C3 can occur by the so-called *classic pathway*, which is triggered by fixation of C1 to antibody (IgM or IgG) combined with antigen, or through the *alternative pathway*, which can be triggered by microbial surfaces (e.g., endotoxins), aggregated Ig's, complex polysaccharides, cobra venom, and so forth. The alternative pathway involves the participation of a distinct set of serum components called the *properdin system* (properdin P, factors B and D). In addition, *the collectins,* described in the discussion of opsonins, bind to carbohydrate-containing proteins on bacteria and viruses and activate complement largely via early components of the classical pathway—C1r, C1s *(the lectin pathway).* Whichever pathway is involved, *C3 convertase* splits C3 into two critical fragments—C3a, which is released, and C3b. C3b then

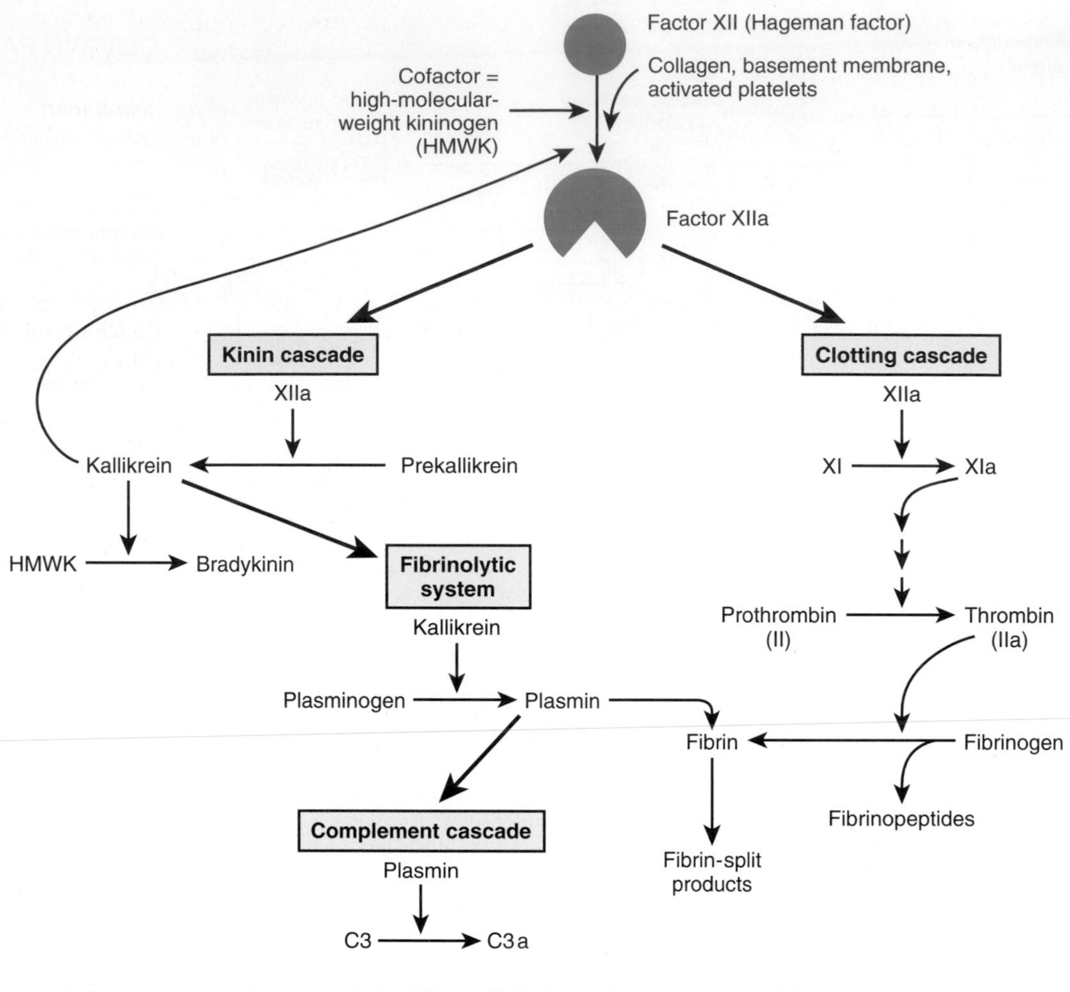

Figure 3–17

Interrelationships between the four plasma mediator systems triggered by activation of factor XII (Hageman factor).

binds to the previously generated fragments to form *C5 convertase*, which interacts with C5 to release C5a and initiate the assembly of the MAC (C5 through C9). MAC causes lysis by initial hydrophobic binding to the lipid bilayer of target cells, eventually forming cylindrical transmembrane channels.

The biologic functions of the complement system fall into two general categories: cell lysis by the MAC, as we have discussed, and the biologic effects of the proteolytic fragments of complement. Complement-derived factors affect a variety of phenomena in acute inflammation:

- *Vascular phenomena*: *C3a, C5a*, and, to a small extent, *C4a* (called *anaphylatoxins*) are the split products of the corresponding complement components (Fig. 3–16). They increase vascular permeability and cause vasodilation mainly by releasing histamine from mast cells. C5a also activates the lipoxygenase pathway of arachidonic acid (AA) metabolism in neutrophils and monocytes, causing further release of inflammatory mediators.
- *Leukocyte adhesion, chemotaxis, and activation*: *C5a* is a powerful chemotactic agent for neutrophils, monocytes, eosinophils, and basophils. It also increases the adhesion of leukocytes to endothelium by activating the leukocytes and increasing the avidity of surface integrins to their endothelial ligand.
- *Phagocytosis*: *C3b* and *C3bi*, when fixed to the bacterial cell wall, act as opsonins and favor phagocytosis by neutrophils and macrophages, which bear cell surface receptors for C3b.

Among the complement components, C3 and C5 are the most important inflammatory mediators. Their significance is further enhanced by the fact that, in addition to the mechanisms already discussed, *C3 and C5 can be activated by several proteolytic enzymes present within the inflammatory exudate*. These include plasmin and lysosomal enzymes released from neutrophils (discussed later in this chapter). Thus, the chemotactic effect of complement and the complement-activating effects of neutrophils can set up a self-perpetuating cycle of neutrophil emigration.

The *complement assembly mechanism is closely controlled by protein inhibitors*.[37] The presence of these inhibitors in the host cell membrane helps to distinguish the host from most microbes and protects the host against inappropriate cell lysis. Because of these regulatory mechanisms, a balance is achieved that results in effective destruction of foreign organisms but prevention of damage to host cells. These regulatory mechanisms include the following:

- *Regulation of C3 and C5 convertases*: As we have seen, the formation of C3 convertase and the generation of C3b is the central feature of both classic and alternative pathways. It is not surprising that a majority of the regulatory proteins are directed at controlling these activities. These regulators function by enhancing the dissociation (decay acceleration) of the convertase complex (e.g., decay-accelerating factor [DAF]), or by proteolytically cleaving C3b (e.g., factor I).
- *Binding of active complement components* by specific proteins in the plasma: The first step in the classic pathway, in which C1 binds to an immune complex, is blocked by a specific inhibitor called *C1 inhibitor* (C1INH). Excessive complement activation is also prevented by a number of proteins that act at the level of MAC formation (e.g., CD59, also called *membrane inhibitor of reactive lysis*).

The importance of each of these inhibitors can be inferred from the study of patients with deficiencies in these proteins. For example, *paroxysmal nocturnal hemoglobinuria* is a disease in which cells lack the ability to express phosphatidylinositol-linked membrane proteins, including DAF. Paroxysmal nocturnal hemoglobinuria is characterized by recurrent bouts of intravascular hemolysis resulting from complement-mediated lysis of red blood cells, leading to chronic hemolytic anemia (Chapter 14). Deficiency of C1INH is associated with the syndrome of *hereditary angioneurotic edema*, characterized by episodic edema accumulation in the skin and extremities as well as in the laryngeal and intestinal mucosa, provoked by emotional stress or trauma.

KININ SYSTEM

The kinin system generates vasoactive peptides from plasma proteins called *kininogens* by specific proteases called *kallikreins*.[38] The kinin system results in the ultimate release of the vasoactive nonapeptide *bradykinin*, a potent agent that increases vascular permeability. *Bradykinin also causes contraction of smooth muscle, dilation of blood vessels, and pain when injected into the skin.* These effects are similar to those of histamine. The cascade that eventually produces kinin is shown in Figure 3–17. It is triggered by activation of Hageman factor (factor XII of the intrinsic clotting pathway; see later) by contact with negatively charged surfaces, such as collagen and basement membranes. A fragment of factor XII (prekallikrein activator, or factor XIIa) is produced, and this converts plasma *prekallikrein* into an active proteolytic form, the enzyme *kallikrein*. The latter cleaves a plasma-glycoprotein precursor, *high molecular-weight kininogen*, to produce *bradykinin* (high-molecular-weight kininogen also acts as a cofactor or catalyst in the activation of Hageman factor). The action of bradykinin is short-lived because it is quickly inactivated by an enzyme called *kininase*. Any remaining kinin is inactivated during passage of plasma through the lung by angiotensin-converting enzyme. *Of importance is that kallikrein itself is a potent activator of Hageman factor, allowing for autocatalytic amplification of the initial stimulus.* Kallikrein has chemotactic activity, and it also directly converts C5 to C5a.

CLOTTING SYSTEM

The clotting system and inflammation are intimately connected processes. The clotting system is divided into two pathways that converge, culminating in the activation of thrombin and the formation of fibrin (Fig. 3–17) (Chapter 5).[39] The intrinsic clotting pathway is a series of plasma proteins that can be activated by Hageman factor, a protein synthesized by the liver that circulates in an inactive form until it encounters collagen or basement membrane or activates platelets (as occurs at the site of endothelial injury). Factor XII then undergoes a conformational change (becoming factor XIIa), exposing an active serine center that can subsequently cleave protein substrates and activate a variety of mediator systems (see later). Two specific components of the activated coagulation system serve as links between coagulation and inflammation:

1. *Thrombin*: Activation of the clotting system results in the activation of thrombin (factor IIa) from precursor prothrombin (factor II), which, in turn, cleaves circulating soluble fibrinogen to generate an insoluble fibrin clot. During this conversion, *fibrinopeptides* are formed, which induce increased vascular permeability and chemotactic activity for leukocytes. *Thrombin* also has inflammatory properties, including causing increased leukocyte adhesion and fibroblast proliferation (see Fig. 5–9).
2. *Factor Xa*: The intrinsic and extrinsic coagulation pathways converge at the point where factor X is converted to factor Xa (see Fig. 5–10). This coagulation protease, by binding to effector cell protease receptor-1, functions as a mediator of acute inflammation,[40] causing increased vascular permeability and leukocyte exudation.

At the same time that factor XIIa is inducing clotting, it can also activate the *fibrinolytic system*. This cascade counterbalances clotting by cleaving fibrin, thereby solubilizing the fibrin clot. The fibrinolytic system contributes to the vascular phenomena of inflammation in several ways (Fig. 3–17). Plasminogen activator (released from endothelium, leukocytes, and other tissues) cleaves plasminogen, a plasma protein that binds to the evolving fibrin clot to generate *plasmin*, a multifunctional protease. Plasmin is important in lysing fibrin clots, but in the context of inflammation it also cleaves C3 to produce C3 fragments, and it degrades fibrin to form *fibrin split products*, which may have permeability-inducing properties. Plasmin can also activate Hageman factor, which can trigger multiple cascades (Fig. 3–17), amplifying the response.

From this discussion of the plasma protease systems activated by the kinin, complement, and clotting systems, a few general conclusions can be drawn:

- *Bradykinin, C3a, and C5a (as mediators of increased vascular permeability)*; *C5a (as the mediator of chemotaxis)*; and *thrombin* (which has effects on many cell types) are the most likely to be important in vivo.
- *C3* and *C5* can be generated by four different groups of influences: (1) classic immunologic reactions; (2) alternative complement pathway activation; (3) lectin pathway proteins; and (4) agents with little immunologic specificity, such as plasmin, kallikrein, and some serine proteases found in normal tissue.
- *Activated Hageman factor (factor XIIa)* initiates four systems involved in the inflammatory response: (1) the *kinin system*, which produces vasoactive kinins; (2) the *clotting system*, which induces formation of thrombin, fibrinopeptides, and factor X, all three of which have inflammatory properties; (3) the *fibrinolytic system*, which produces plasmin and degrades the fibrin; and (4) the *complement system*, which produces anaphylatoxins. Some of the products of this initiation—particularly kallikrein—can, by feedback, activate Hageman factor, resulting in profound amplification of the effects of the initial contact.

Arachidonic Acid (AA) Metabolites: Prostaglandins, Leukotrienes, and Lipoxins

When cells are activated by diverse stimuli, their membrane lipids are rapidly remodeled to generate biologically active lipid mediators that serve as intracellular or extracellular signals. Products derived from the metabolism of AA affect a variety of biologic processes, including inflammation and hemostasis. They are best thought of as *autocoids*, or local short-range hormones, which are formed rapidly, exert their effects locally, then either decay spontaneously or are destroyed enzymatically.[41]

AA is a 20-carbon polyunsaturated fatty acid (5,8,11,14-eicosatetraenoic acid) that is derived directly from dietary sources or by conversion from the essential fatty acid *linoleic acid.* It does not occur free in the cell but is normally esterified in membrane phospholipids, particularly in the carbon 2 position of phosphatidylcholine, phosphatidylinositol, and phosphatidyl ethanolamine. It is released from membrane phospholipids through the activation of cellular phospholipases (e.g., phospholipase A_2) by mechanical, chemical, and physical stimuli or by other mediators (e.g., C5a). AA metabolites, also called *eicosanoids*, are synthesized by two major classes of enzymes: cyclooxygenases (prostaglandins and thromboxanes) and lipoxygenases (leukotrienes and lipoxins) (Fig. 3–18). Eicosanoids can mediate virtually every step of inflammation (Table 3–4). They can be found in inflammatory exudates, and synthesis is increased at sites of inflammation. Structurally distinct agents that suppress cyclooxygenase activity (aspirin, nonsteroidal anti-inflammatory drugs [NSAIDs]) also inhibit inflammation in vivo. The intracellular sites at which the enzymes act to produce the eicosanoid mediators include specialized domains, known as *lipid bodies*, which contain all of the principal eicosanoid-generating enzymes and form rapidly in response to agents such as PAF (see later). It is thought that compartmentalization of eicosanoid formation at lipid bodies provides a pool of arachidonate that could be used to produce the mediators without affecting other cellular membranes.[42]

- The *cyclooxygenase pathway*, mediated by two different enzymes (COX1 and COX2), leads to the generation of *prostaglandins*. Prostaglandins are divided into series based on structural features as coded by a letter (PGD, PGE, PGF, PGG, and PGH) and a subscript numeral (e.g., 1, 2), which indicates the number of double bonds in the compound. The most important ones in inflammation are PGE_2, PGD_2, $PGF_{2\alpha}$, PGI_2 (prostacyclin), and TxA_2 (thromboxane), each of which is derived by the action of a specific enzyme. Some of these enzymes have restricted tissue distribution. For example, platelets contain the enzyme thromboxane synthetase, and hence TxA_2 is the major product in these cells. TxA_2, a potent platelet-aggregating agent and vasoconstrictor, is itself unstable and rapidly converted to its inactive form TxB_2. Vascular endothelium lacks thromboxane synthetase but possesses prostacyclin synthetase, which leads to the formation of prostacyclin (PGI_2) and its stable end product $PGF_{1\alpha}$. Prostacyclin is a vasodilator, a potent inhibitor of platelet aggregation, and also markedly potentiates the permeability-increasing and chemotactic effects of other mediators. Thromboxane-prostacyclin imbalance has been implicated as an early event in thrombus formation in coronary and cerebral blood vessels. The opposing roles of TxA_2 and PGI_2 in hemostasis are further discussed in Chapter 5.

The prostaglandins are also involved in the pathogenesis of *pain* and *fever* in inflammation. PGE_2 is hyperalgesic in that it makes the skin hypersensitive to painful stimuli.[43] It causes a marked increase in pain produced by intradermal injection of suboptimal concentrations of histamine and bradykinin and interacts with cytokines in causing fever during infections (described later). PGD_2 is the major metabolite of the cyclooxygenase pathway in mast cells; along with PGE_2 and $PGF_{2\alpha}$ (which are more widely distributed), it causes vasodilation and potentiates edema formation.

- In the *lipoxygenase pathway*, the initial products are generated by three different lipoxygenases (LO), which are present in only a few types of cells. 5-lipoxygenase (5-LO) is the predominant enzyme in neutrophils. On cell activation, 5-LO translocates to the nuclear membrane and interacts with a membrane-associated regulatory protein, termed *5-LO-activating protein (FLAP)*, to form the active enzyme complex. The main product, 5-HETE, which is chemotactic for neutrophils, is converted into a family of compounds collectively called *leukotrienes*. *LTB_4* is a potent chemotactic agent and activator of neutrophil functional responses, such as aggregation and adhesion of leukocytes to venular endothelium, generation of oxygen free radicals, and release of lysosomal enzymes. The cysteinyl-containing leukotrienes C_4, D_4, and E_4 (*LTC_4*, *LTD_4*, and *LTE_4*) cause

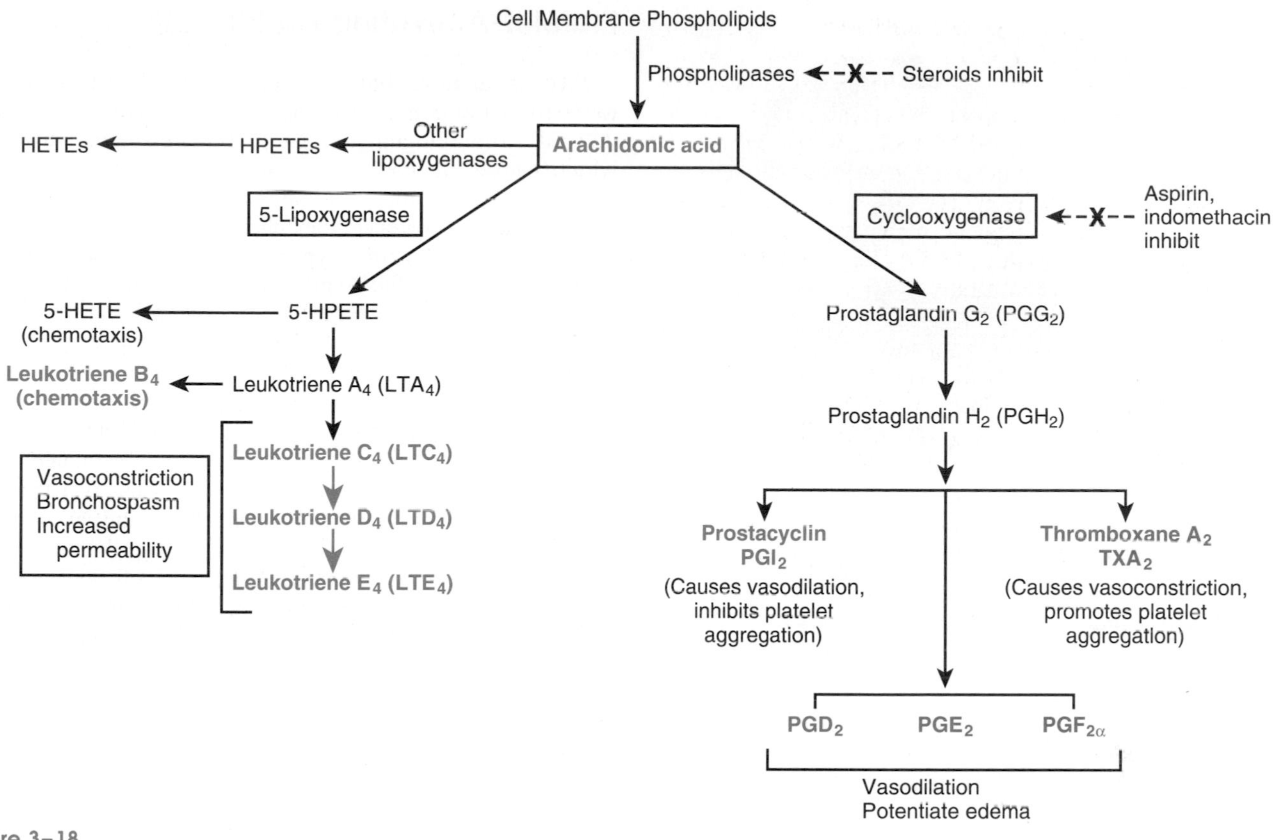

Figure 3–18

Generation of arachidonic acid metabolites and their roles in inflammation.

intense vasoconstriction, bronchospasm, and increased vascular permeability. The vascular leakage, as with histamine, is restricted to venules.

Cell-cell interactions are important in the biosynthesis of leukotrienes. AA products can pass from one cell type to another, and different cell types can cooperate with each other to generate eicosanoids *(transcellular biosynthesis).* In this way, cells that are not capable of generating a particular class of eicosanoid can produce these mediators from intermediates generated in other cells, thus expanding the array and quantities of eicosanoids produced at sites of inflammation. One example of transcellular biosynthesis is the generation of *lipoxins.*

Table 3–4. INFLAMMATORY ACTIONS OF EICOSANOIDS

Action	Metabolite
Vasoconstriction	• Thromboxane A_2, leukotrienes C_4, D_4, E_4
Vasodilation	• PGI_2, PGE_1, PGE_2, PGD_2
Increased vascular permeability	• Leukotrienes C_4, D_4, E_4
Chemotaxis, leukocyte adhesion	• Leukotriene B_4, HETE, lipoxins

- *Lipoxins* are the most recent addition to the family of bioactive products generated from AA, and transcellular biosynthetic mechanisms are key to their production. Platelets alone cannot form lipoxins, but when they interact with leukocytes they can form the metabolites from neutrophil-derived intermediates. Lipoxins A_4 and B_4 (LXA_4, LXB_4) are generated by the action of platelet 12-lipoxygenase on neutrophil LTA_4 (Fig. 3–19). Cell-cell contact enhances transcellular metabolism, and blocking adhesion inhibits lipoxin production.

  Lipoxins have a number of proinflammatory and anti-inflammatory actions. They inhibit neutrophil chemotaxis and adhesion but stimulate monocyte adhesion.[44] LXA_4 stimulates vasodilation and attenuates the actions of LTC_4-stimulated vasoconstriction. There is an inverse relationship between the amount of lipoxin and leukotriene formed, suggesting that the lipoxins may be endogenous negative regulators of leukotriene action.[45]

There are many targets along the eicosanoid biosynthetic pathways at which anti-inflammatory therapy can be directed:

- *Aspirin* and *NSAIDs*, such as indomethacin or ibuprofen, inhibit cyclooxygenase and thus inhibit prostaglandin

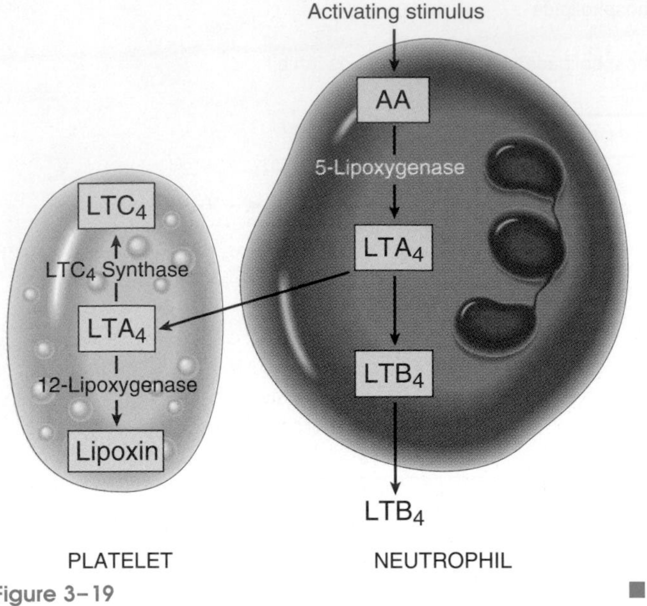

Figure 3–19

Biosynthesis of leukotrienes and lipoxins by cell-cell interaction. Activated neutrophils generate LTB_4 from arachidonic acid–derived LTA_4 by the action of 5-lipoxygenase, but they do not possess LTC_4-synthase activity and consequently do not produce LTC_4. In contrast, platelets cannot form LTC_4 from endogenous substrates, but they can generate LTC_4 and lipoxins from neutrophil-derived LTA_4. (Courtesy of Dr. C. Serhan, Brigham and Women's Hospital.)

synthesis. 5-LO, however, is not affected by these anti-inflammatory agents, and inhibitors of this enzyme are a major target for drug discovery. Pharmacologic agents that block the association of 5-LO with its membrane-bound activating protein (FLAP) inhibit leukotriene production and hold some promise as drugs.[46]

- *Glucocorticoids*, which are powerful anti-inflammatory agents, may act by down-regulating the expression of specific target genes, including COX2, genes encoding proinflammatory cytokines (such as IL-1 and TNF-α), and nitric oxide synthase (iNOS) (see later). Glucocorticoids also *up-regulate* genes that encode potent anti-inflammatory proteins, such as lipocortin 1. Lipocortin 1 inhibits release of AA from membrane phospholipids.[47]
- Another approach to manipulate inflammatory responses has been to modify the intake and content of dietary lipids using *fish oil*. Variations in AA metabolism may account for some of the beneficial effects of fish oil. The basis for this approach is that leukotrienes from fatty acids found in fish oil (e.g., *linoleic acid*) are less potent than those derived from the AA found in most animal or vegetable fat. The fish oil fatty acids serve as poor substrates for conversion to active metabolites of the cyclooxygenase and, particularly, the lipoxygenase series. The replacement of AA at membrane storage sites in phospholipid by dietary fish oil derivatives results in a shift in agonist-induced formation of leukotrienes to less potent forms.[48]

Platelet-Activating Factor

PAF is another bioactive phospholipid-derived mediator.[49] Its name comes from its initial discovery as a factor derived from antigen-stimulated, IgE-sensitized basophils, which causes platelet aggregation and release but is now known to have multiple inflammatory effects. Chemically, PAF is acetyl-glyceryl-ether-phosphorylcholine (AGEPC), or a phospholipid with a typical glycerol backbone, a long-chain fatty acid in the A position, an unusually short chain substituent in the B location, and a phosphatidylcholine moiety (Fig. 3–20). The original long-chain fatty acid in the B position is removed by phospholipase A_2 then acetylated by acetyltransferase to form PAF.

PAF mediates its effects via a single G protein–coupled receptor (Chapter 4), and its effects are regulated by a family of inactivating PAF acetylhydrolases. A variety of cell types, including platelets, basophils (and mast cells), neutrophils, monocytes/macrophages, and endothelial cells, can elaborate PAF, in both secreted and cell-bound forms. In addition to platelet stimulation, PAF causes vasoconstriction and bronchoconstriction, and at extremely low concentrations it induces vasodilation and increased venular permeability with a potency 100 to 10,000 times greater than that of histamine. PAF also causes increased leukocyte adhesion to endothelium (by enhancing leukocyte integrin binding), chemotaxis, degranulation, and the oxidative burst. Thus, PAF can elicit most of the cardinal features of inflammation. PAF also boosts the synthesis of other mediators, particularly eicosanoids, by leukocytes and other cells.

A role for PAF in vivo is supported by the ability of synthetic PAF receptor antagonists to inhibit inflammation in some experimental models. It has been shown that tobacco smoke in experimental animals generates a group of oxidized PAF derivatives, which stimulate interactions between platelets, leukocytes, and endothelial cells and thus augment the inflammatory and thrombogenic consequences of this dangerous habit (Chapter 10).[50]

SOURCES	MAJOR INFLAMMATORY ACTIONS
Mast cells/basophils	Increased vascular permeability
Neutrophils	Leukocyte aggregation
Monocytes/macrophages	Leukocyte adhesion
Endothelium	Leukocyte priming/chemotaxis
Platelets	Platelet activation
Others	Stimulation of other mediators (LT, $O_2^{\bar{\cdot}}$)

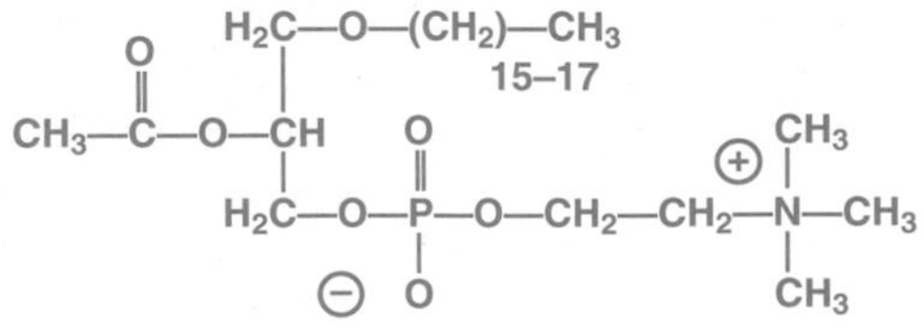

PLATELET-ACTIVATING FACTOR

Figure 3–20

Structure, sources, and main inflammatory actions of platelet-activating factor. LT, leukotrienes.

Cytokines and Chemokines

Cytokines are proteins produced by many cell types (principally activated lymphocytes and macrophages, but also endothelium, epithelium, and connective tissue cells) that modulate the function of other cell types. Long known to be involved in cellular immune responses, these products have additional effects that play important roles in both acute and chronic inflammation. They are discussed further in Chapter 7. Here we review general properties of cytokines and focus on those involved in inflammation.

TERMS AND DEFINITIONS

Cytokines generated by mononuclear phagocytes are often called *monokines*, and those by activated lymphocytes are referred to as *lymphokines*. Additionally, both monocytes and macrophages produce cytokines, such as *colony-stimulating factors (CSFs)*, which stimulate the growth of immature leukocytes in the bone marrow. *Interleukins* represent a broad family of cytokines that are made by hematopoietic cells and act primarily on leukocytes. *Chemokines* are cytokines that share the ability to stimulate leukocyte movement (chemokinesis) and directed movement (chemotaxis) and are particularly important in inflammation. Many classic *growth factors* (Chapter 4) act as cytokines, and conversely many cytokines have growth-promoting properties.

GENERAL PROPERTIES AND FUNCTIONAL CLASSES

Cytokines are produced during immune and inflammatory responses, and secretion of these mediators is transient and closely regulated. Many cell types produce multiple cytokines. The proteins are pleotropic in that they can act on different cell types. Cytokine effects are often redundant, and these proteins can influence the synthesis or action of other cytokines. They are multifunctional in that an individual cytokine may have both positive and negative regulatory actions. Cytokines mediate their effects by binding to specific receptors on target cells, and the expression of cytokine receptors can be regulated by a variety of exogenous and endogenous signals. For some responsive cells, cytokines stimulate cell proliferation, acting as traditional growth factors. The diversity of functions of cytokines as mediators of interactions between cells demonstrates the importance of *context* in cytokine action.

Although many cytokines have multiple functions, cytokines can be grouped into five classes, depending on their major function or on the nature of the target cell.[51]

- *Cytokines that regulate lymphocyte function*: These cytokines regulate lymphocyte activation, growth, and differentiation. Within this category are IL-2 and IL-4, which favor lymphocyte growth, as well as IL-10 and TGF-β, which are negative regulators of immune responses (Chapter 7).
- *Cytokines involved with natural immunity*: This group of cytokines includes two major inflammatory cytokines, TNF-α and IL-1β; type I interferons (IFN-α and IFN-β); and IL-6.
- *Cytokines that activate inflammatory cells*: These cytokines activate macrophages during cell-mediated immune responses and include IFN-γ, TNF-α, TNF-β (lymphotoxin), IL-5, IL-10, and IL-12.
- *Chemokines*: This group of cytokines are characterized by chemotactic activity for various leukocytes and are described in more detail presently.
- *Cytokines that stimulate hematopoiesis*: These mediate immature leukocyte growth and differentiation. Examples include IL-3, IL-7, c-*kit* ligand, granulocyte-macrophage CSF, macrophage CSF, granulocyte CSF, and stem cell factor.

INTERLEUKIN-1 AND TUMOR NECROSIS FACTOR

The major cytokines that mediate inflammation are IL-1 and TNF (α and β). *IL-1* and *TNF* share many biologic properties.[52, 53] IL-1 and TNF-α are produced by activated macrophages, TNF-β (previously known as *lymphotoxin*) by activated T cells, and IL-1 by many other cell types as well. Their secretion can be stimulated by endotoxin, immune complexes, toxins, physical injury, and a variety of inflammatory processes. Similar to growth factors (Chapter 4), they can act on the same cell that produces them (an *autocrine* effect); on cells in the immediate vicinity, as in lymph nodes and joint spaces (a *paracrine* effect); or systematically, as with any other hormone (an *endocrine* effect). Their most important actions in inflammation are their effects on endothelium, leukocytes, and fibroblasts and induction of the systemic acute-phase reactions (Fig. 3–21). In endothelium, they induce a spectrum of changes—mostly regulated at the level of gene transcription—referred to as *endothelial activation*.[16] In particular, they induce the synthesis of endothelial adhesion molecules and chemical mediators—including other cytokines, chemokines, growth factors, eicosanoids, and nitric oxide (NO); production of enzymes associated with matrix remodeling; and increases in the surface thrombogenicity of the endothelium.[54] TNF also causes aggregation and *priming* of neutrophils, leading to augmented responses of these cells to other mediators and the release of proteolytic enzymes from mesenchymal cells, thus contributing to tissue damage. The effects of these cytokines on fibroblasts are relevant to fibrosis and are discussed later.

IL-1 and TNF (as well as IL-6) also induce the systemic *acute-phase responses* associated with infection or injury, including fever; loss of appetite; the production of slow-wave sleep; the release of neutrophils into the circulation; the release of adrenocorticotropic hormone (ACTH) and corticosteroids; and, particularly with regard to TNF, the hemodynamic effects of septic shock—hypotension, de-

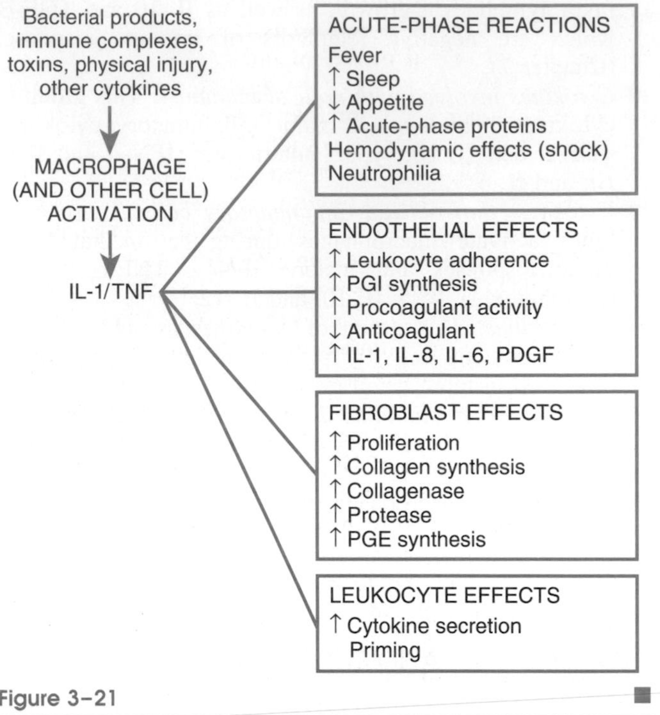

Figure 3–21

Major effects of interleukin-1 (IL-1) and tumor necrosis factor (TNF) in inflammation.

creased vascular resistance, increased heart rate, and decreased blood pH (described in Chapter 5).

TNF-α has a key role in the normal *control of body mass*. In obesity, the physiologic action of TNF-α as a signal to control food intake is impaired (Chapter 10). In cachexia, a pathologic state characterized by weight loss and anorexia that accompanies some infections and neoplastic diseases, there is an overproduction of TNF-α.[55]

CHEMOKINES

Chemokines are a superfamily of small (8 to 10 kD) proteins that act primarily as activators and chemoattractants for specific types of leukocytes and have similarities in their amino acid sequences,[56] namely, they share patterns of paired cysteine repeats and two internal disulfide bridges. They are classified into four major classes, which have relatively distinct biologic activities, according to the arrangement of the conserved cysteine (C) residues of the mature proteins (Table 3–5):

- *C-X-C or α chemokines* have one amino acid residue separating the first two conserved cysteine residues. The C-X-C chemokines act primarily on neutrophils. *IL-8* is typical of this group. It is secreted by activated macrophages, endothelial cells, and other cell types and causes activation and chemotaxis of neutrophils, with limited activity on monocytes and eosinophils. Its most important inducers are other cytokines, mainly IL-1 and TNF-α.[57]
- *C-C or β chemokines* have the first two conserved cysteine residues adjacent. The C-C chemokines, which include *monocyte chemoattractant protein* (MCP-1), *eotaxin, macrophage inflammatory protein-1α* (MIP-1α), and *RANTES* (regulated and normal T cell expressed and secreted), generally attract monocytes, eosinophils, basophils, and lymphocytes but not neutrophils. Although most of the chemokines in this class have overlapping properties, eotaxin selectively recruits eosinophils.[58]
- *C or γ chemokines* lack two (the first and third) of the four conserved cysteines. The C chemokines (e.g., lymphotactin) are relatively specific for lymphocytes.[59]
- *CX_3C chemokines* are a recently described fourth class of cytokines. *Fractalkine* exists as a membrane-bound glycoprotein that has the CX_3C chemokine domain positioned on top of an extended mucin-like stalk. This chemokine exists in two forms: The cell surface–bound protein can be induced on endothelial cells by inflammatory cytokines and promotes strong adhesion of monocytes and T cells, and a soluble form, derived by proteolysis of the membrane-bound protein, has potent chemoattractant activity for the same cells.[60] It is thus both an adhesion molecule and a chemotactic agent. A single receptor mediates both activities in target cells.[61]

In addition to their roles in regulating leukocyte recruitment and activation, chemokines act on stromal cells such as fibroblasts and smooth muscle cells as well as hematopoietic progenitor cells. Chemokines can also bind to components of the extracellular matrix, such as cell surface proteoglycans (Chapter 4). Immobilization of chemokines is thought to be important for maintaining the chemotactic gradients needed for leukocyte recruitment and migration into the tissues.

Chemokines mediate their activities by binding to G protein–linked cell surface receptors. These receptors (called CXCR, or CCR) contain seven transmembrane loops and are called *serpentine* receptors (Chapter 4).[62] The various CXCRs and CCRs usually exhibit overlapping ligand specificities, and leukocytes generally express more than one receptor type. As discussed in Chapter 7, chemokine receptors (CXCR-4, CCR-5) act as viral coreceptors for a viral envelope glycoprotein of human immunodeficiency virus (HIV-1) resulting in binding and entry of the virus into CD4-positive lymphocytes.

Table 3–5. SELECTED INFLAMMATORY CELLS AND THEIR CHEMOKINES

Target Cell	Important Chemokines
Neutrophils	IL-8, Groα, β, γ, others
Monocytes	MIP-1α, MIP-1β, MCP-1, 2, 3
Eosinophils	Eotaxin
Lymphocytes	Lymphotaxin
Basophils	IL-8, MIP-1α, MCP-1,3, RANTES

Nitric Oxide

NO, a pleiotropic mediator of inflammation, was first discovered as a factor released from endothelial cells that caused vasodilation by relaxing vascular smooth muscle—endothelium-derived relaxing factor.[63] NO is a soluble gas that is produced not only by endothelial cells, but also by macrophages and specific neurons in the brain. NO acts in a paracrine manner on target cells through induction of cyclic guanosine monophosphate (GMP), which, in turn, initiates a series of intracellular events leading to a response, such as the relaxation of vascular smooth muscle cells. Since the in vivo half-life of NO is only a matter of seconds, the gas acts only on cells in close proximity to where it is produced. Such a localized activity accounts for the specificity of its actions. NO readily complexes with thiol groups on proteins, forming more stable adducts (S-nitrosoproteins) that have been implicated in some of NO's actions.

NO is synthesized from L-arginine, molecular oxygen, NADPH, and other cofactors by the enzyme nitric oxide synthase (NOS).[64] There are three different types of NOS—endothelial (eNOS), neuronal (nNOS), and cytokine inducible (iNOS) (Fig. 3–22)—which exhibit two patterns of expression. eNOS and nNOS are *constitutively* expressed at low levels and can be activated rapidly by an increase in cytoplasmic calcium ions in the presence of calmodulin. Influx of calcium into these cells leads to a rapid production of NO. iNOS, in contrast, is induced when macrophages are activated by cytokines (e.g., TNF-α, IFN-γ) or other agents; no intracellular increase in calcium is required.

NO plays an important role in vascular function during inflammatory responses. As discussed earlier, NO is a potent vasodilator. Proof of the importance of eNOS in maintaining vascular tone comes from finding that mice lacking the corresponding gene are hypertensive.[65] In addition to vascular smooth muscle relaxation, NO plays other important roles in inflammation. It reduces platelet aggregation and adhesion (Chapter 5), inhibits several features of mast cell–induced inflammation, and serves as a regulator of leukocyte recruitment. Blocking NO production under normal conditions promotes leukocyte rolling and adhesion in postcapillary venules, and delivery of exogenous NO reduces leukocyte recruitment in acute inflammatory processes. *Thus, overproduction of NO from iNOS is an endogenous compensatory mechanism that reduces leukocyte recruitment in inflammatory responses.* Abnormalities in endothelial production of NO occur in atherosclerosis, diabetes, and hypertension (Chapter 12). As will be discussed later, iNOS production of NO by activated macrophages is involved in the *pathogenesis of septic shock*[66] (Chapter 5).

NO also acts in the *host's response to infection.* Evidence supporting the biologic importance of NO-related antimicrobial activity includes the following:[67] (1) Reactive species derived from NO synthase possess antimicrobial activity; (2) interactions occur between NO and reactive oxygen species, leading to the formation of multiple antimicrobial metabolites (e.g., peroxynitrite [$OONO^-$], S-nitrosothiols [RSNO], and nitrogen dioxide [$NO_2\cdot$]), each with distinct stability, compartmentalization, and reactivity, but share the ability to damage microbial DNA protein and lipids; (3) production of NO is increased during host defense; and (4) genetic inactivation of iNOS enhances mi-

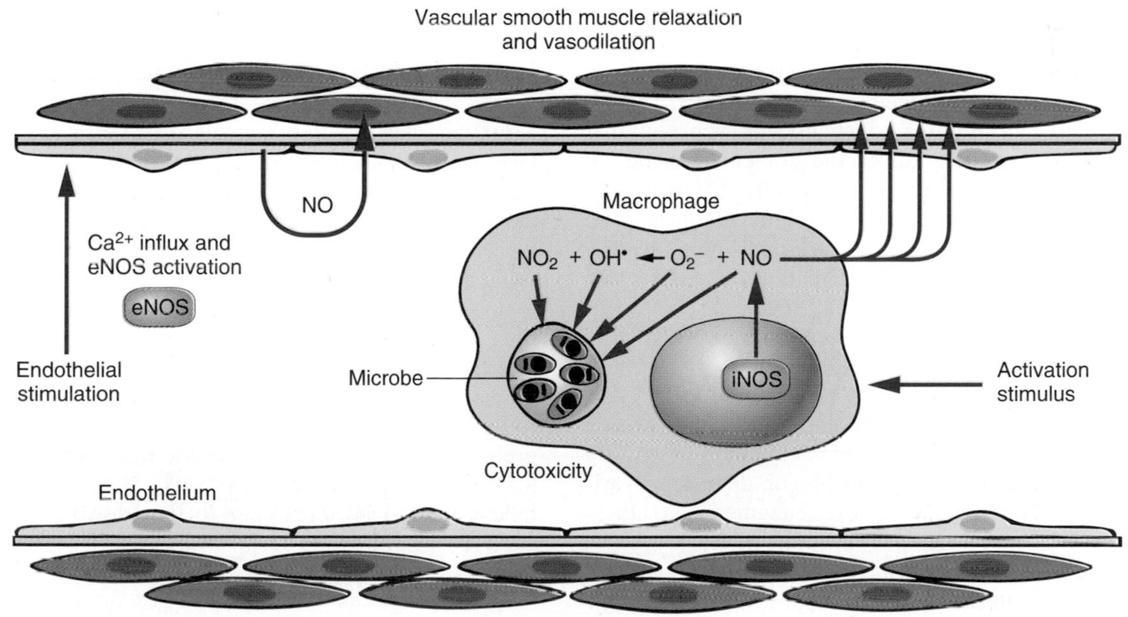

Figure 3–22

Two types of nitric oxide (NO) synthesis in endothelium *(left)* and macrophages *(right).* NO causes vasodilation, and NO free radicals are cytotoxic to microbial and mammalian cells. NOS, nitric oxide synthase.

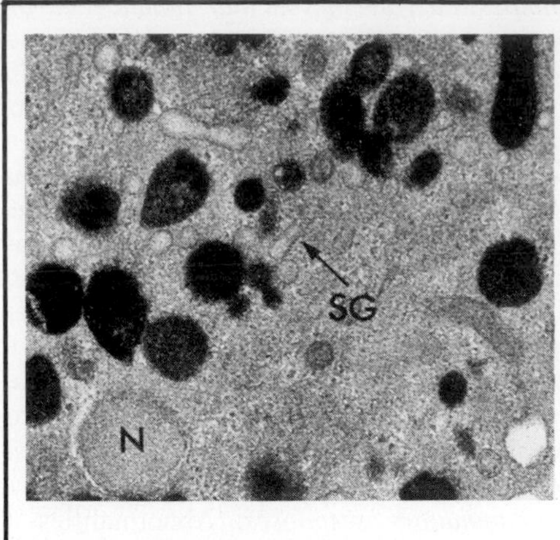

SPECIFIC GRANULES
- Lactoferrin
- Lysozyme
- Alkaline phosphatase
- Type IV collagenase
- Leukocyte adhesion molecules
- Plasminogen activation
- Phospholipase A_2

AZUROPHIL GRANULES
- Myeloperoxidase
- Lysozyme ← Bactericidal factors
- Cationic proteins
- Acid hydrolases
- Elastase
- Nonspecific collagenase
- BPI
- Defensins
- Cathepsin G
- Phospholipase A_2

Figure 3–23

Ultrastructure of neutrophil granules stained for peroxidase activity and their constituents. The large peroxidase-containing granules are the azurophil granules; the smaller peroxidase-negative ones are the specific granules (SG). N, portion of nucleus; BPI, bactericidal permeability increasing protein.

crobial replication in experimental animal models.[66] High levels of NO production by a variety of cells appear to limit the replication of bacteria, helminths, protozoa, and viruses (as well as tumor cells), at the risk of *potential inflammatory damage* to host cells and tissues.

Lysosomal Constituents of Leukocytes

Neutrophils and monocytes contain lysosomal granules, which when released may contribute to the inflammatory response. *Neutrophils* exhibit two main types of granules (Fig. 3–23). The smaller *specific* (or secondary) granules contain lysozyme, collagenase, gelatinase, lactoferrin, plasminogen activator, histaminase, and alkaline phosphatase. The large *azurophil* (or primary) granules contain myeloperoxidase, bactericidal factors (lysozyme, defensins), acid hydrolases, and a variety of neutral proteases (elastase, cathepsin G, nonspecific collagenases, proteinase 3).[69] Both types of granules can empty into phagocytic vacuoles that form around engulfed material, or the contents can be released after cell death. There are, however, differences in the mobilization of specific and azurophil granules. The specific granules are secreted *extracellularly* more readily and by lower concentrations of agonists, while the more potentially destructive azurophil granules release their contents primarily within the phagosome and require high levels of agonists to be released extracellularly.[32]

Acid proteases degrade proteins at an acid pH. Their most likely action is to degrade bacteria and debris *within* the phagolysosomes, in which an acid pH is readily reached. *Neutral proteases* are capable of degrading various extracellular components. These enzymes can attack collagen, basement membrane, fibrin, elastin, and cartilage, resulting in the tissue destruction characteristic of purulent and deforming inflammatory processes. Neutral proteases can also cleave C3 and C5 directly, releasing anaphylatoxins, and release a kinin-like peptide from kininogen. *Monocytes* and *macrophages* also contain acid hydrolases, collagenase, elastase, phospholipase, and plasminogen activator. These may be particularly active in chronic inflammatory reactions.

Lysosomal constituents thus have numerous effects. The initial leukocytic infiltration, if unchecked, can potentiate further increases in vascular permeability, chemotaxis, and tissue damage. These harmful proteases, however, are held in check by a system of *antiproteases* in the serum and tissue fluids. Foremost among these is *α_1-antitrypsin,* which is the major inhibitor of neutrophilic elastase. A deficiency of these inhibitors may lead to sustained action of leukocyte proteases, as is the case in patients with α_1-antitrypsin deficiency (Chapter 16). *α_2-Macroglobulin* is another antiprotease found in serum and various secretions.

Oxygen-Derived Free Radicals

Oxygen-derived free radicals may be released extracellularly from leukocytes after exposure to chemotactic agents, immune complexes, or a phagocytic challenge. Their production is dependent, as we have seen, on the activation of the NADPH oxidative system. Superoxide anion ($O_2^{\cdot-}$), hydrogen peroxide (H_2O_2), and hydroxyl radical ($OH^{\cdot}$) are the major species produced within the cell, and these metabolites can combine with NO to form other reactive nitrogen intermediates. Extracellular release of low levels of these potent mediators can increase the expression of chemokines (e.g., IL-8), cytokines, and endothelial leukocyte adhesion molecules, amplifying the cascade that elicits the inflammatory response.[70] At higher levels, release of these potent mediators can be *damaging* to the host.[68] They are implicated in the following responses:

- *Endothelial cell damage, with resultant increased vascular permeability*: Adherent neutrophils, when activated, not only produce their own toxic species, but also stimulate xanthine oxidation in endothelial cells themselves, thus elaborating more superoxide.

- *Inactivation of antiproteases,* such as α_1-antitrypsin: This leads to unopposed protease activity, with increased destruction of extracellular matrix.
- *Injury to other cell types* (tumor cells, red cells, parenchymal cells).

Serum, tissue fluids, and target cells possess *antioxidant mechanisms* that protect against these potentially harmful oxygen-derived radicals. These antioxidants have been discussed in Chapter 1, but to repeat, they include (1) the copper-containing serum protein *ceruloplasmin*; (2) the iron-free fraction of serum, *transferrin*; (3) the enzyme *superoxide dismutase*, which is found or can be activated in a variety of cell types; (4) the enzyme *catalase*, which detoxifies H_2O_2; and (5) *glutathione peroxidase*, another powerful H_2O_2 detoxifier. Thus, the influence of oxygen-derived free radicals in any given inflammatory reaction depends on the *balance* between the production and the inactivation of these metabolites by cells and tissues.

Neuropeptides

Neuropeptides, similar to the vasoactive amines and the eicosanoids, previously discussed, play a role in the initiation of an inflammatory response. The small peptides, such as *substance P* and neurokinin A, belong to a family of tachykinin neuropeptides in the central and peripheral nervous systems. Nerve fibers containing substance P are prominent in the lung and gastrointestinal tract. Substance P has many biologic functions, including the transmission of pain signals, regulation of blood pressure, and stimulation of secretion by immune and endocrine cells, but is notable as a powerful mediator of increased vascular permeability.[71] It acts by binding to a G protein–coupled receptor bearing seven transmembrane domains (NK-1R). The functional relevance of substance P in inflammation was demonstrated in mice lacking the corresponding receptor. After a stimulus that incited pulmonary capillary leakage and infiltration of inflammatory cells in the lungs of normal mice, the receptor-deficient animals had no response.[72]

Summary of Chemical Mediators of Acute Inflammation

Table 3–6 summarizes the major actions of the principal mediators. When Lewis suggested the existence of histamine, one mediator was clearly not enough. Now, we are wallowing in them! Yet, from this menu of substances we can tentatively extract a few mediators that may be relevant in vivo (Table 3–7). For increased vascular permeability, histamine; the anaphylatoxins (C3a and C5a); the kinins; leukotrienes C, D, and E; PAF; and substance P are almost certainly involved, at least early in the course of inflammation. For chemotaxis, complement fragment C5a, lipoxygenase products (LTB_4), other chemotactic lipids, and chemokines are the most likely protagonists. Also, the important role of prostaglandins in vasodilation, pain, and fever and in potentiating edema cannot be denied. IL-1 and TNF are involved with endothelial-leukocyte interactions and with acute-phase reactions. Lysosomal products and oxygen-derived radicals are the most likely candidates as causes of the ensuing tissue destruction. NO is involved in

Table 3–6. SUMMARY OF MEDIATORS OF ACUTE INFLAMMATION

		Action		
Mediator	**Source**	***Vascular Leakage***	***Chemotaxis***	***Other***
Histamine and serotonin	Mast cells, platelets	+	−	
Bradykinin	Plasma substrate	+	−	Pain
C3a	Plasma protein via liver	+	−	Opsonic fragment (C3b)
C5a	Macrophages	+	+	Leukocyte adhesion, activation
Prostaglandins	Mast cells, from membrane phospholipids	Potentiate other mediators	−	Vasodilation, pain, fever
Leukotriene B_4	Leukocytes	−	+	Leukocyte adhesion, activation
Leukotriene C_4, D_4, E_4	Leukocytes, mast cells	+	−	Bronchoconstriction, vasoconstriction
Oxygen metabolites	Leukocytes	+	−	Endothelial damage, tissue damage
PAF	Leukocytes, mast cells	+	+	Bronchoconstriction, leukocyte priming
IL-1 and TNF	Macrophages, other	−	+	Acute phase reactions, endothelial activation
Chemokines	Leukocytes, others	−	+	Leukocyte activation
Nitric oxide	Macrophages, endothelium	+	+	Vasodilation, cytotoxicity

Table 3–7. MOST LIKELY MEDIATORS IN INFLAMMATION

Vasodilation
Prostaglandins
Nitric oxide
Increased vascular permeability
Vasoactive amines
C3a and C5a (through liberating amines)
Bradykinin
Leukotrienes C_4, D_4, E_4
PAF
Substance P
Chemotaxis, leukocyte activation
C5a
Leukotriene B_4
Chemokines
Bacterial products
Fever
IL-1, IL-6, TNF
Prostaglandins
Pain
Prostaglandins
Bradykinin
Tissue damage
Neutrophil and macrophage lysosomal enzymes
Oxygen metabolites
Nitric oxide

vasodilation, regulation of leukocyte influx, and cytotoxicity.

Outcomes of Acute Inflammation

The discussion of mediators completed the basic description of the relatively uniform pattern of the inflammatory reaction encountered in most injuries. *Although hemodynamic, permeability, and white cell changes have been described sequentially and may be initiated in this order, all these phenomena in the fully evolved reaction to injury are concurrent in a seemingly chaotic but remarkably organized multi-ring circus. As might be expected, many variables may modify this basic process, including the nature and intensity of the injury, the site and tissue affected, and the responsiveness of the host. In general, however, acute inflammation may have one of four outcomes* (Fig. 3–24):

1. *Complete resolution*: In a perfect world, all inflammatory reactions, once they have succeeded in neutralizing the injurious stimulus, should end with restoration of the site of acute inflammation to normal. This is called *resolution* and is the usual outcome when the injury is limited or short-lived or when there has been little tissue destruction and the damaged parenchymal cells can regenerate. Resolution involves neutralization or spontaneous decay of the chemical mediators, with subsequent return of normal vascular permeability, cessation of leukocytic infiltration; death (largely by apoptosis) of neutrophils; and finally removal of edema fluid and protein, leukocytes, foreign agents, and necrotic debris from the site (Fig. 3–25). Lymphatics and phagocytes play a role in these events, as shown subsequently.
2. *Abscess formation*: This occurs particularly in infections with pyogenic organisms.
3. *Healing by connective tissue replacement (fibrosis)*: This occurs after substantial tissue destruction, when the inflammatory injury occurs in tissues that do not regenerate, or when there is abundant fibrin exudation. When the fibrinous exudate in tissue or serous cavities (pleura, peritoneum) cannot be adequately resorbed, connective tissue grows into the area of exudate, converting it into a mass of fibrous tissue—a process also called *organization.*
4. Progression of the tissue response to *chronic inflammation* (discussed next): This may follow acute inflammation, or the response may be chronic almost from the onset. Acute-to-chronic transition occurs when the acute inflammatory response cannot be resolved, owing either to the persistence of the injurious agent or to some interference in the normal process of healing. For example, bacterial infection of the lung may begin as a focus of acute inflammation (pneumonia), but its failure to resolve may lead to extensive tissue destruction and formation of a cavity in which the inflammation continues to smolder, leading eventually to a chronic lung abscess. Another example of chronic inflammation with a persisting stimulus is peptic ulcer of the duodenum or stomach. Peptic ulcers may persist for months or years

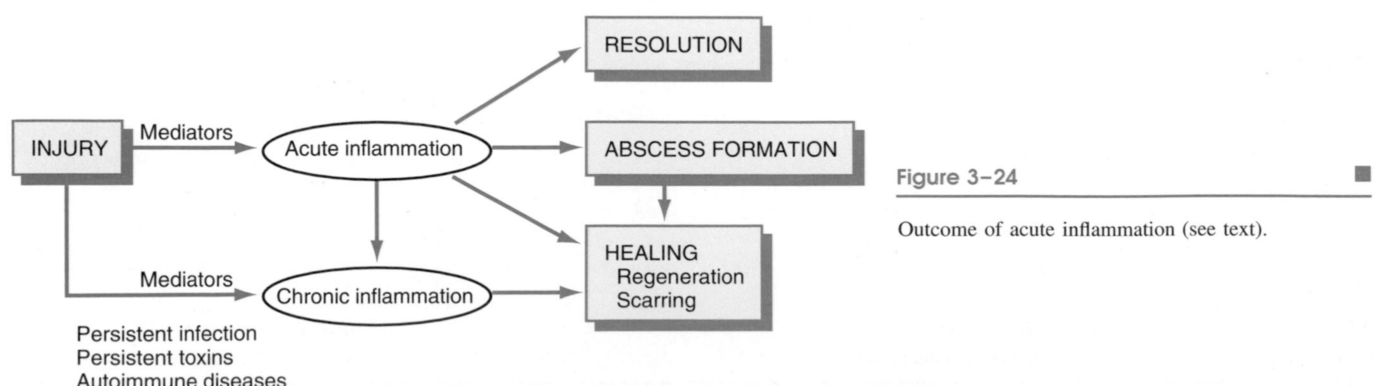

Figure 3–24

Outcome of acute inflammation (see text).

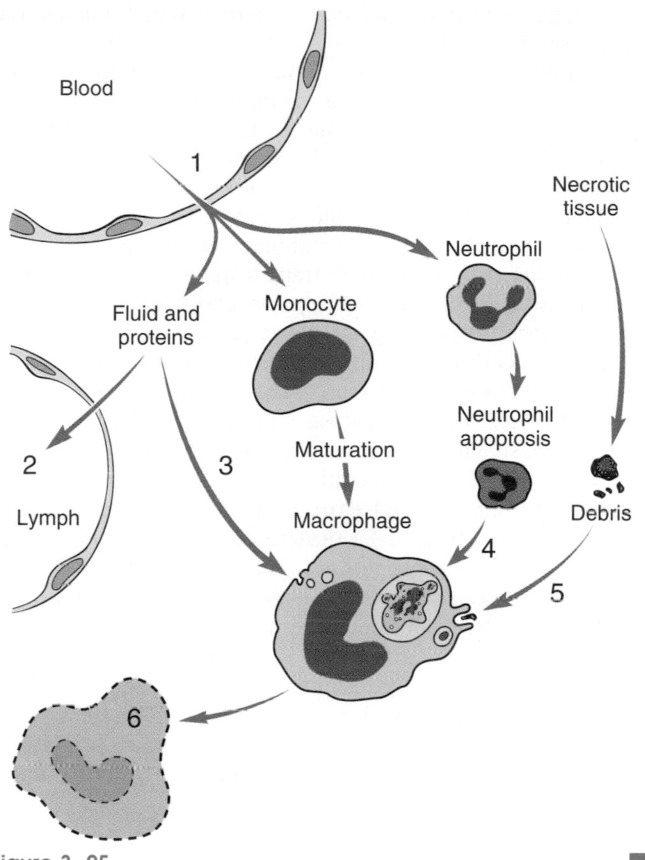

Figure 3–25

Events in the resolution of inflammation: (1) return to normal vascular permeability; (2) drainage of edema fluid and proteins into lymphatics or (3) by pinocytosis into macrophages; (4) phagocytosis of apoptotic neutrophils; (5) necrotic debris by macrophages; and (6) disposal of macrophages. Note the central role of macrophages in resolution. (Modified from Haslett C, Henson PM: In Clark R, Henson PM (eds): The Molecular and Cellular Biology of Wound Repair. New York, Plenum Press, 1996.)

and, as seen subsequently, are manifested by both acute and chronic inflammatory reactions.

CHRONIC INFLAMMATION

Definition and Causes

Although difficult to define precisely, *chronic inflammation* is considered to be *inflammation of prolonged duration* (weeks or months) *in which active inflammation, tissue destruction, and attempts at repair are proceeding simultaneously.* Although it may follow acute inflammation, as described earlier, chronic inflammation frequently begins insidiously, as a low-grade, smoldering, often asymptomatic response. This latter type of chronic inflammation includes some of the most common and disabling human diseases, such as rheumatoid arthritis, atherosclerosis, tuberculosis, and chronic lung diseases. Chronic inflammation arises under the following settings:

- *Persistent infections* by certain microorganisms, such as tubercle bacilli, *Treponema pallidum* (causative organism of syphilis), and certain fungi: These organisms are of low toxicity and evoke an immune reaction called *delayed hypersensitivity* (Chapter 7). The inflammatory response sometimes takes a specific pattern called a *granulomatous reaction* (discussed later).
- *Prolonged exposure to potentially toxic agents, either exogenous or endogenous*: An example of an exogenous agent is particulate silica, a nondegradable inanimate material that when inhaled for prolonged periods results in an inflammatory lung disease called *silicosis* (Chapter 16). *Atherosclerosis* (Chapter 12) is thought to be a chronic inflammatory process of the arterial wall induced, at least in part, by endogenous toxic plasma lipid components.
- *Autoimmunity*: Under certain conditions, immune reactions are set up against the individual's own tissues, leading to *autoimmune diseases* (Chapter 7). In these diseases, autoantigens evoke a self-perpetuating immune reaction that results in several common chronic inflammatory diseases, such as rheumatoid arthritis and lupus erythematosus. In all of these settings, immune reactions play an important role.

Histologic Features

In contrast to acute inflammation, which is manifested by vascular changes, edema, and largely neutrophilic infiltration, *chronic inflammation is characterized by*:

- *Infiltration with mononuclear cells, which include macrophages, lymphocytes, and plasma cells*, a reflection of a persistent *reaction to injury.*
- *Tissue destruction*, largely induced by the inflammatory cells.
- Attempts at *healing by connective tissue replacement of damaged tissue*, accomplished by proliferation of small blood vessels (*angiogenesis*) and, in particular, *fibrosis* (Fig. 3–26). Because angiogenesis and fibrosis are also components of wound healing and repair, they are discussed more fully in Chapter 4.

Mononuclear Infiltration: Cells and Mechanisms

The *macrophage* is the prima donna of chronic inflammation, and we begin our discussion with a brief review of its biology.[73] *Macrophages* are but one component of the *mononuclear phagocyte system* (Fig. 3–27). The mononuclear phagocyte system consists of closely related cells of bone marrow origin, including blood monocytes, and tissue macrophages. The latter are diffusely scattered in the connective tissue or clustered in organs such as the liver

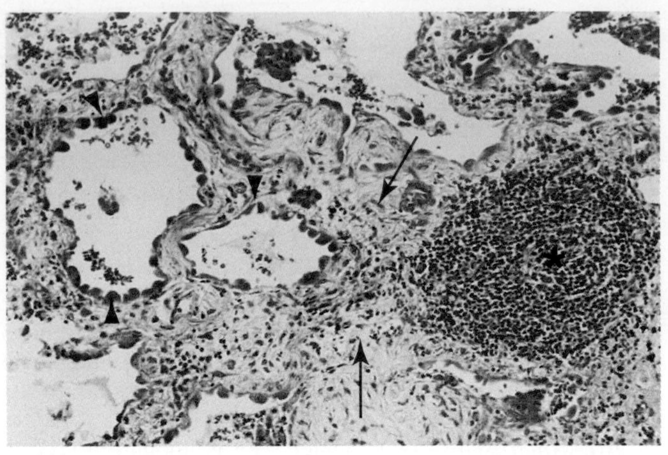

Figure 3–26

Chronic inflammation in the lung, showing all three characteristic histologic features: (1) collection of chronic inflammatory cells (*), (2) destruction of parenchyma (normal alveoli are replaced by spaces lined by cuboidal epithelium, *arrowheads*), and (3) replacement by connective tissue (fibrosis, *arrows*).

(Kupffer cells), spleen and lymph nodes (sinus histiocytes), and lungs (alveolar macrophages). All arise from a common precursor in the bone marrow, which gives rise to blood monocytes. From the blood, monocytes migrate into various tissues and transform into macrophages. The half-life of blood monocytes is about 1 day, whereas the life span of tissue macrophages is several months. The journey from bone marrow stem cell to tissue macrophage is regulated by a variety of growth and differentiation factors, cytokines, adhesion molecules, and cellular interactions (Chapters 7 and 15).

As discussed previously, monocytes begin to emigrate relatively early in acute inflammation, and within 48 hours they constitute the predominant cell type. Extravasation of monocytes is governed by the same factors that are involved in neutrophil emigration, that is, adhesion molecules and chemical mediators with chemotactic and activating properties.[11, 16, 19] When the monocyte reaches the extravascular tissue, it undergoes transformation into a larger phagocytic cell, the *macrophage*. In addition to performing phagocytosis, macrophages have the potential of being *activated*, a process that results in increased cell size, increased levels of lysosomal enzymes, more active metabolism, and greater ability to phagocytose and kill ingested microbes. Activation signals include cytokines (e.g., IFN-γ) secreted by sensitized T lymphocytes, bacterial endotoxins, other chemical mediators, and extracellular matrix proteins such as fibronectin (Fig. 3–28). After activation, the *macrophages secrete a wide variety of biologically active products* that, if unchecked, result in the tissue injury and fibrosis characteristic of chronic inflammation (Fig. 3–28).

In short-lived inflammation, if the irritant is eliminated, macrophages eventually disappear (either dying off or making their way into the lymphatics and lymph nodes). In chronic inflammation, macrophage accumulation persists, mediated by different mechanisms, each predominating in different types of reactions (Fig. 3–29):

1. *Continued recruitment of monocytes from the circulation*, which results from the steady expression of adhesion molecules and chemotactic factors:[74] This is numerically the most important source for macrophages. Chemotactic stimuli for monocytes include C5a; chemo-

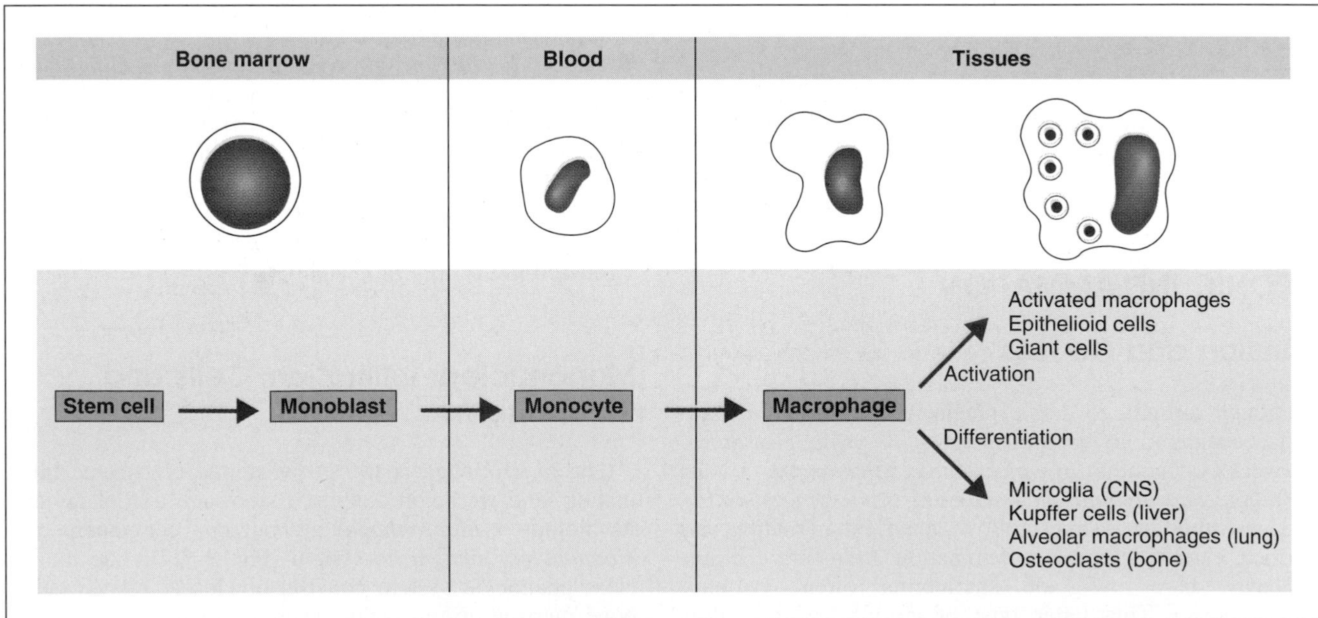

Figure 3–27

Maturation of mononuclear phagocytes. (From Abbas AK, et al: Cellular and Molecular Immunology, 3rd ed. Philadelphia, WB Saunders, 1997.)

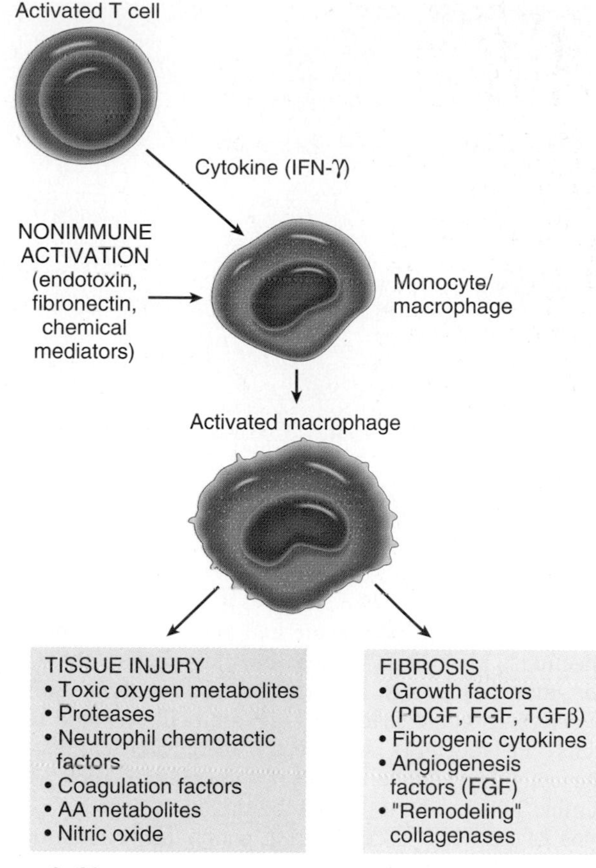

Figure 3–28

Two stimuli for macrophage activation. Activation of macrophages via cytokines from immune-activated T cells (interferon gamma) or by nonimmunologic stimuli such as endotoxin. The products made by activated macrophages that also mediate tissue injury and fibrosis are indicated. AA, arachidonic acid; PDGF, platelet-derived growth factor; FGF, fibroblast growth factor; TGFβ, transforming growth factor β.

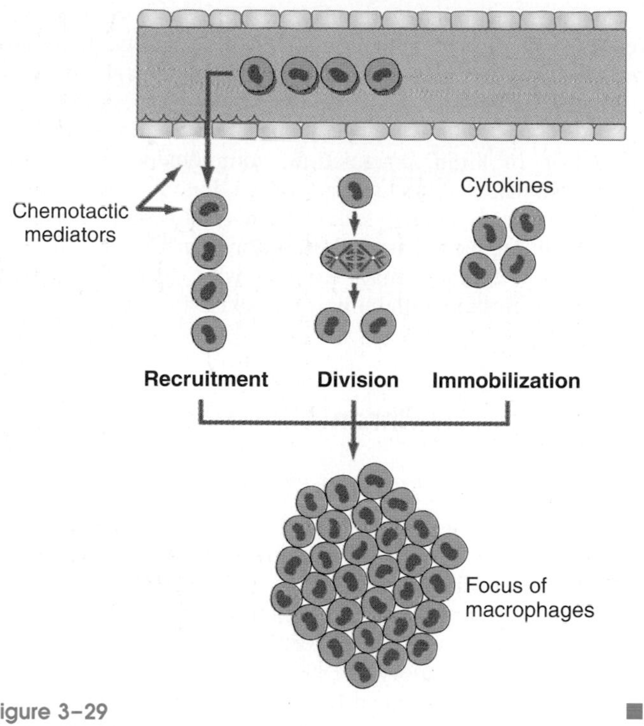

Figure 3–29

Three mechanisms for macrophage accumulation. The most important is continued recruitment from the microcirculation. (Adapted from Ryan G, Majno G: Inflammation. Kalamazoo, MI, Upjohn, 1977.)

kines produced by activated macrophages, lymphocytes, and other cell types (e.g., MCP-1); certain growth factors, such as platelet-derived growth factor and TGF-β; fragments from the breakdown of collagen and fibronectin; and fibrinopeptides. Each of these may play a role under given circumstances; for example, chemokines are almost certainly involved during delayed-hypersensitivity immune reactions.

2. *Local proliferation of macrophages* after their emigration from the bloodstream: Once thought to be an unusual event, macrophage proliferation is now known to occur prominently in atheromatous plaques (Chapter 12).
3. *Immobilization of macrophages* within the site of inflammation: Certain cytokines (macrophage inhibitory factor) and oxidized lipids (Chapter 12) can cause such immobilization.

The macrophage is a central figure in chronic inflammation because of the great number of substances the activated macrophage can produce (Table 3–8). Some of these are toxic to cells (e.g., oxygen and NO metabolites) or extracellular matrix (proteases); some cause influx of other cell types (e.g., cytokines, chemotactic factors); and still others cause fibroblast proliferation, collagen deposition, and angiogenesis (e.g., growth factors). This impressive arsenal of mediators makes macrophages powerful allies in the body's defense against unwanted invaders, but the same weaponry can also induce considerable tissue destruction when macrophages are inappropriately activated. Thus, *tissue destruction is one of the hallmarks of chronic inflammation.*

Table 3–8. PRODUCTS RELEASED BY MACROPHAGES

Enzymes
Neutral proteases
Elastase
Collagenase
Plasminogen activator
Acid hydrolases
Phosphatases
Lipases
Plasma proteins
Complement components (e.g., C1 to C5, properdin)
Coagulation factors (e.g., factors V, VIII, tissue factor)
Reactive metabolites of oxygen
Eicosanoids
Cytokines, chemokines (IL-1, TNF, IL-8)
Growth factors (PDGF, EGF, FGF, TGF-β)
Nitric oxide

As noted, continued tissue damage is one of the main features of chronic inflammation, and a variety of inflammatory cell products contribute to such damage. In addition, necrotic tissue itself can perpetuate the inflammatory cascade through a variety of mechanisms, including the activation of kinin, coagulation, complement and fibrinolytic systems, and the release of mediators from dead or dying passenger leukocytes.[75] The diversity of mechanisms by which ongoing tissue destruction can activate the inflammatory cascade may explain why features of both acute and chronic inflammation coexist in certain circumstances.

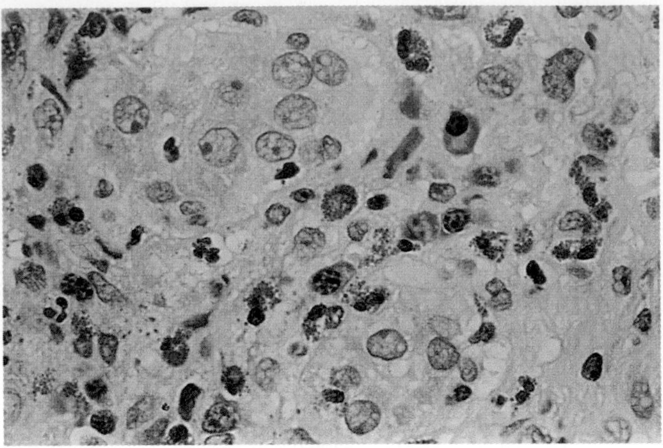

Figure 3–31

A focus of inflammation showing numerous eosinophils.

Other Cells in Chronic Inflammation

Other cell types present in chronic inflammation include lymphocytes, plasma cells, mast cells, and eosinophils:

- *Lymphocytes* are mobilized in both antibody-mediated and cell-mediated immune reactions and, for reasons largely unknown, in non–immune-mediated inflammation. Lymphocytes of different types (T, B) or states (activated or memory T cell) use various adhesion molecule pairs (predominantly $\alpha_4\beta_1$/VCAM-1 and ICAM-1/LFA-1) and chemokines (e.g., RANTES, lymphotactin) to migrate into inflammatory sites. They have a reciprocal relationship to macrophages in chronic inflammation (Fig. 3–30). Lymphocytes can be activated by contact with antigen. Activated lymphocytes produce *lymphokines*, and one of these, IFN-γ, is a major stimulator of monocytes and macrophages. Cytokines from activated macrophages (*monokines*), in turn, activate lymphocytes, which themselves also produce inflammatory mediators—setting the stage for persistence of the inflammatory response (Chapter 7). *Plasma cells* produce antibody directed either against persistent antigen in the inflammatory site or against altered tissue components.
- *Mast cells* are widely distributed in connective tissues and participate in both acute and persistent inflammatory reactions. Mast cells express on their surface the receptor that binds the Fc portion of the IgE antibody (FcϵRI). In acute reactions, IgE antibodies bound to the cells' Fc receptors specifically recognize antigen, and the cells degranulate and release mediators, such as histamine and products of AA oxidation (Chapter 7). This type of response occurs during anaphylactic reactions to foods, insect venom, or drugs, frequently with catastrophic results. When properly regulated, this response can benefit the host. Specific types of parasite infections are associated with increased levels of IgE and activation of mast cells. These cells can participate in more persistent inflammatory responses by elaborating cytokines such as TNF-α, which augments leukocyte infiltration at the site of the response.
- *Eosinophils* are also characteristic of immune reactions mediated by IgE and of parasitic infections (Fig. 3–31). The recruitment of eosinophils involves extravasation from the blood and tissue homing by processes similar to those for other leukocytes. As already seen, the direction of the targeting process is dependent on *eotaxin*, a member of the C-C family of chemokines.[58] Eotaxin is unusual among this class of chemokines in that it binds to only one receptor (CCR-3), which is expressed only by eosinophils.[76] Eotaxin has the ability selectively to prime eosinophils for chemotaxis, to direct their migration, and to activate inflammatory activity in the cells attracted. Eosinophils have granules that contain *major basic protein*, a highly cationic protein that is toxic to parasites but also causes lysis of mammalian epithelial cells. They may thus be of benefit in parasitic infections but contribute to tissue damage in immune reactions.[77]

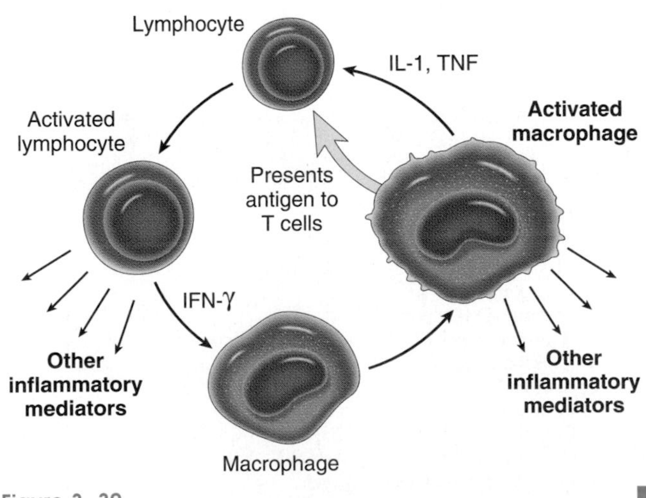

Figure 3–30

Macrophage-lymphocyte interactions in chronic inflammation. Activated lymphocytes and macrophages influence each other and also release inflammatory mediators that affect other cells.

Although neutrophils are the hallmark of acute inflammation, many forms of chronic inflammation, lasting for months, continue to show large numbers of neutrophils, induced either by the persistent bacteria or by mediators produced by macrophages or necrotic cells. In chronic bacterial inflammation of bone (osteomyelitis), a neutrophilic

Table 3–9. EXAMPLES OF GRANULOMATOUS INFLAMMATIONS

Disease	Cause	Tissue Reaction
Tuberculosis	• *Mycobacterium tuberculosis*	Noncaseating tubercle (granuloma prototype): a focus of epithelioid cells, rimmed by fibroblasts, lymphocytes, histiocytes, occasional Langhans giant cell; caseating tubercle: central amorphous granular debris, loss of all cellular detail; acid-fast bacilli
Leprosy	• *Mycobacterium leprae*	Acid-fast bacilli in macrophages; granulomas and epithelioid types
Syphilis	• *Treponema pallidum*	Gumma: microscopic to grossly visible lesion, enclosing wall of histiocytes; plasma cell infiltrate; center cells are necrotic without loss of cellular outline
Cat scratch disease	• Gram-negative bacillus	Rounded or stellate granuloma containing central granular debris and recognizable neutrophils; giant cells uncommon

exudate can persist for many months. Neutrophils are also important in the chronic damage induced in lungs by smoking and other stimuli (Chapter 16).

Granulomatous Inflammation

Granulomatous inflammation is a distinctive pattern of chronic inflammatory reaction in which the predominant cell type is an activated macrophage with a modified epithelial-like (epithelioid) appearance. It is encountered in a relatively few but widespread chronic immune and infectious diseases. Its genesis is firmly linked to immune reactions and thus is described in more detail in Chapter 7. Tuberculosis is the archetype of the granulomatous diseases, but sarcoidosis, cat-scratch disease, lymphogranuloma inguinale, leprosy, brucellosis, syphilis, some mycotic infections, berylliosis, and reactions of irritant lipids are also included (Table 3–9). Recognition of the granulomatous pattern in a biopsy specimen is important because of the limited number of possible conditions that cause it and the significance of the diagnoses associated with the lesions.

A granuloma is a focal area of granulomatous inflammation. It consists of a microscopic aggregation of macrophages that are transformed into epithelium-like cells surrounded by a collar of mononuclear leukocytes, principally lymphocytes and occasionally plasma cells. In the usual hematoxylin and eosin preparations, the epithelioid cells have a pale pink granular cytoplasm with indistinct cell boundaries, often appearing to merge into one another. The nucleus is less dense than that of a lymphocyte, is oval or elongate, and may show folding of the nuclear membrane. Older granulomas develop an enclosing rim of fibroblasts and connective tissue. Frequently, but not invariably, epithelioid cells fuse to form *giant cells* in the periphery or sometimes in the center of granulomas. These giant cells may attain diameters of 40 to 50 μm. They comprise a large mass of cytoplasm containing 20 or more small nuclei arranged either peripherally (Langhans-type giant cell) or haphazardly (foreign body–type giant cell) (Fig. 3–32).

There are two types of granulomas, which differ in their pathogenesis. *Foreign body granulomas* are incited by relatively inert foreign bodies. Typically, foreign body granulomas form when material such as talc (associated with intravenous drug abuse) (Chapter 10), sutures, or other fibers are large enough to preclude phagocytosis by a single macrophage and do not incite either an inflammatory or an immune response. Epithelioid cells and giant cells are apposed to the surface and encompass the foreign body. The foreign material can usually be identified in the center of the granuloma, particularly if viewed with polarized light, in which it appears refractile.

Immune granulomas are caused by insoluble particles that are capable of inducing a cell-mediated immune response (Chapter 7). This type of immune response does not necessarily produce granulomas but does so when the inciting agent is poorly soluble or particulate. In these responses, macrophages engulf the foreign material and process and present some of it to appropriate T lymphocytes, causing them to become activated. The responding T cells produce cytokines, such as IL-2, which activates other T cells perpetuating the response, and IFN-γ, which is important in transforming macrophages into epithelioid cells and multinucleate giant cells. Granulomas are not static. Cytokines have been implicated not only in the formation, but also in the maintenance of granulomas.[75]

The prototype for the immune granuloma is that caused by the bacillus of tuberculosis. In this disease, the granuloma is referred to as a *tubercle* and is *classically charac-*

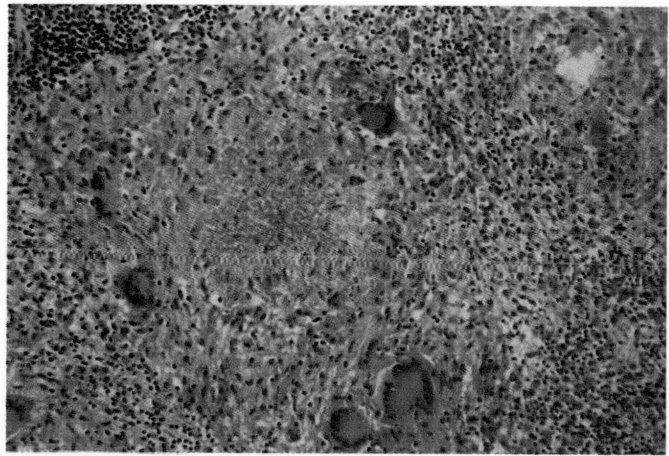

Figure 3–32

Typical tuberculous granuloma showing an area of central necrosis, epithelioid cells, multiple Langhans-type giant cells, and lymphocytes.

terized by the presence of central caseous necrosis (Fig. 3–32). In contrast, caseating necrosis is rare in other granulomatous diseases. The morphologic patterns in the various granulomatous diseases may be sufficiently different to allow reasonably accurate diagnosis by an experienced pathologist (see Table 3–8); however, there are so many atypical presentations that it is always necessary to identify the specific etiologic agent by special stains for organisms (e.g., acid-fast stains for tubercle bacilli), by culture methods (e.g., in tuberculosis, fungal disease), and by serologic studies (e.g., in syphilis). In sarcoidosis, the etiologic agent is unknown (Chapter 16).

In summary, granulomatous inflammation is a specific type of chronic inflammatory reaction characterized by accumulations of modified macrophages (epithelioid cells) and initiated by a variety of infectious and noninfectious agents. The presence of poorly digestible irritants, T cell–mediated immunity to the irritant, or both appears to be necessary for granuloma formation.

Lymphatics in Inflammation

The system of lymphatics and lymph nodes filters and *polices* the extravascular fluids. Together with the *mononuclear phagocyte system*, it represents a secondary line of defense that is called into play whenever a local inflammatory reaction fails to contain and neutralize injury.

Lymphatics are extremely delicate channels that are difficult to visualize in ordinary tissue sections because they readily collapse. They are lined by continuous, thin endothelium with loose, overlapping cell junctions; scant basement membrane; and no muscular support except in the larger ducts. Lymph flow in inflammation is increased and helps drain the edema fluid from the extravascular space. Because the junctions of lymphatics are loose, lymphatic fluid eventually equilibrates with extravascular fluid. Not only fluid, but also leukocytes and cell debris may find their way into lymph. Valves are present in collecting lymphatics, allowing lymph content to flow only proximally. Delicate fibrils, attached at right angles to the walls of the lymphatic vessel, extend into the adjacent tissues and serve to maintain patency of the lymphatic channels.

In severe injuries, the drainage may transport the offending agent, be it chemical or bacterial. The lymphatics may become secondarily inflamed (*lymphangitis*), as may the draining lymph nodes (*lymphadenitis*). Therefore, it is not uncommon in infections of the hand, for example, to observe red streaks along the entire arm up to the axilla following the course of the lymphatic channels, accompanied by painful enlargement of the axillary lymph nodes. The nodal enlargement is usually caused by hyperplasia of the lymphoid follicles as well as by hyperplasia of the phagocytic cells lining the sinuses of the lymph nodes. This constellation of nodal histologic changes is termed *reactive* or *inflammatory lymphadenitis*.

The secondary barriers sometimes contain the spread of the infection, but in some instances they are overwhelmed, and the organisms drain through progressively larger channels and gain access to the vascular circulation, thus inducing a *bacteremia*. The phagocytic cells of the liver, spleen, and bone marrow constitute the next line of defense, but in massive infections, bacteria seed distant tissues of the body. The heart valves, meninges, kidneys, and joints are favored sites of implantation for blood-borne organisms, and in such a fashion endocarditis, meningitis, renal abscesses, and septic arthritis may develop.

MORPHOLOGIC PATTERNS IN ACUTE AND CHRONIC INFLAMMATION

The severity of the reaction, its specific cause, and the particular tissue and site involved all introduce morphologic variations in the basic patterns of acute and chronic inflammation (Fig. 3–33).

Serous Inflammation

Serous inflammation is marked by the outpouring of a thin fluid that, depending on the size of injury, is derived from either the blood serum or the secretions of mesothelial cells lining the peritoneal, pleural, and pericardial cavities (called *effusion*). The skin blister resulting from a burn or viral infection represents a large accumulation of serous fluid, either within or immediately beneath the epidermis of the skin (Fig. 3–33*A*).

Fibrinous Inflammation

With more severe injuries and the resulting greater vascular permeability, larger molecules such as fibrin pass the vascular barrier. A fibrinous exudate develops when the vascular leaks are large enough or there is a procoagulant stimulus in the interstitium (e.g., cancer cells). A fibrinous exudate is characteristic of inflammation in body cavities, such as the pericardium and pleura. Histologically, fibrin appears as an eosinophilic meshwork of threads or sometimes as an amorphous coagulum (Fig. 3–33*B*). Fibrinous exudates may be removed by fibrinolysis and other debris by macrophages. This process, called *resolution*, may restore normal tissue structure, but when the fibrin is not removed, it may stimulate the ingrowth of fibroblasts and blood vessels and thus lead to scarring. Conversion of the fibrinous exudate to scar tissue (*organization*) within the pericardial sac leads either to opaque fibrous thickening of the pericardium and epicardium in the area of exudation or, more often, to the development of fibrous strands that bridge the pericardial space.

Suppurative or Purulent Inflammation

Suppurative or purulent inflammation is characterized by the production of large amounts of pus or purulent exudate consisting of neutrophils, necrotic cells, and edema fluid. Certain organisms (e.g., staphylococci) produce this local-

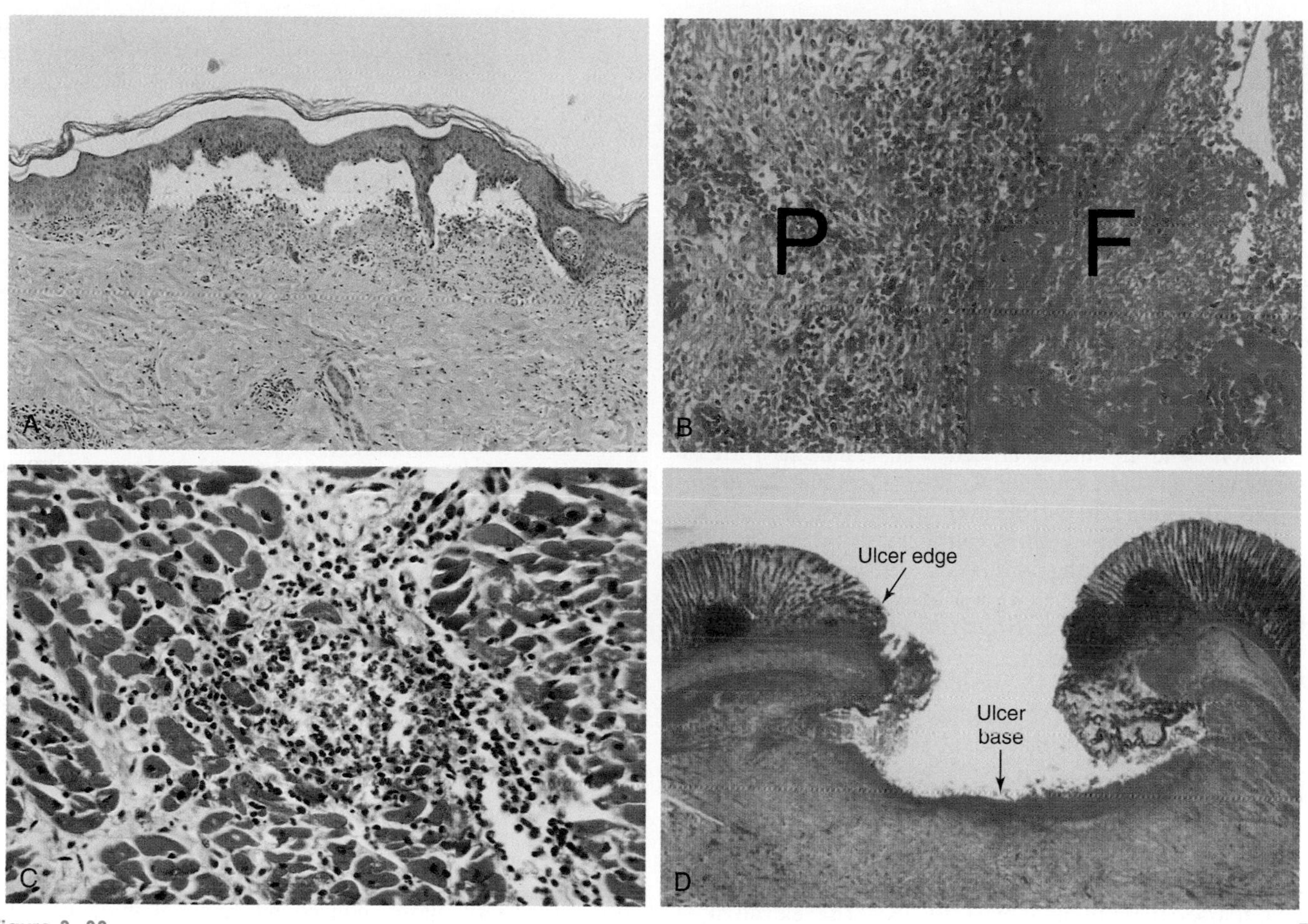

Figure 3–33

Histologic patterns of acute inflammation. *A*, Serous inflammation. Low-power view of a cross-section of a skin blister showing the epidermis separated from the dermis by a focal collection of serous effusion. *B*, Fibrinous inflammation. A pink meshwork of fibrin exudate (F) *(on the right)* overlies the pericardial surface (P). *C*, Suppurative inflammation. A bacterial abscess in the myocardium. *D*, Ulceration. Low-power cross-section of a duodenal ulcer crater with an acute inflammatory exudate in the base.

ized suppuration and are therefore referred to as *pyogenic* (pus-producing) bacteria. A common example of an acute suppurative inflammation is acute appendicitis. *Abscesses are focal localized collections of purulent inflammatory tissue* caused by suppuration buried in a tissue, an organ, or a confined space. They are produced by deep seeding of pyogenic bacteria into a tissue (Fig. 3–33*C*). Abscesses have a central region that appears as a mass of necrotic white cells and tissue cells. There is usually a zone of preserved neutrophils about this necrotic focus, and outside this region vascular dilation and parenchymal and fibroblastic proliferation occur, indicating the beginning of repair. In time, the abscess may become walled off by connective tissue that limits further spread.

Ulcers

An ulcer is a local defect, or excavation, of the surface of an organ or tissue that is produced by the sloughing (shedding) of inflammatory necrotic tissue (Fig. 3–33*D*). Ulceration can occur only when an inflammatory necrotic area exists on or near the surface. It is most commonly encountered in (1) inflammatory necrosis of the mucosa of the mouth, stomach, intestines, or genitourinary tract and (2) subcutaneous inflammations of the lower extremities in older persons who have circulatory disturbances that predispose to extensive necrosis. Ulcerations are best exemplified by peptic ulcer of the stomach or duodenum. During the acute stage, there is intense polymorphonuclear infiltration and vascular dilation in the margins of the defect. With chronicity, the margins and base of the ulcer develop fibroblastic proliferation; scarring; and the accumulation of lymphocytes, macrophages, and plasma cells.

SYSTEMIC EFFECTS OF INFLAMMATION

Anyone who has suffered a severe sore throat or a respiratory infection has experienced the systemic manifestations of acute inflammation. Fever is one of the most prominent of such manifestations, especially when an inflammation is associated with infection. Fever depends on humoral signals from the body. It is coordinated by the hypothalmus and involves the orchestration of a wide range of endocrine, autonomic, and behavioral responses.[78] The components of this so-called *acute-phase reaction* include

- *Endocrine and metabolic*: Secretion of acute-phase proteins by the liver (including C-reactive protein [CRP], serum amyloid A [SAA], serum amyloid P [SAP], complement, and coagulation proteins); increased production of glucocorticoids, activating a stress response; and decreased secretion of vasopressin, thus reducing the volume of body fluid required to be warmed.

  CRP, SAA, and *SAP* are proteins with a unique pentagonal disc structure that, like the collectins, described earlier, bind to microbial cell walls, and may act as opsonins and fix complement. They also bind chromatin, possibly aiding in the clearing of necrotic cell nuclei. Their serum concentrations can increase several hundred fold during inflammation. Their effects are beneficial during acute inflammation, but as we shall see (Chapter 7), cause *secondary amyloidosis* in chronic inflammation.
- *Autonomic*: A redirection in blood flow from cutaneous to deep vascular beds, to minimize heat loss through the skin; increased pulse and blood pressure; and decreased sweating.
- *Behavioral*: Rigors (shivering), chills (search for warmth), anorexia, somnolence, and malaise.

The principal manifestation of fever is an elevation of body temperature, usually by 1 to 4°C. The elevation in temperature by even a few degrees may improve the efficiency of leukocyte killing and probably impairs the replication of many offending microorganisms.

Cytokines play a key role in signaling a fever. *IL-1, IL-6, and TNF-α are* produced by leukocytes (and other cell types) in response to infectious agents or immunologic and toxic reactions and are released into the circulation. *IL-1 acts directly and also by inducing IL-6*, which has essentially similar effects in producing the acute-phase reactions. Among the cytokines, IL-1, IL-6, TNF-α, and the interferons can cause fever, thus functioning as primary endogenous pyrogens.[79] Peripheral cytokines signal the brain through four mechanisms to cause fever: (1) They can enter the brain through regions lacking a blood-brain barrier (specialized areas along the cerebral ventricular surface); (2) they can cross the blood-brain barrier by specific transport mechanisms; (3) they can transmit a signal to the brain via the vagus nerve; and (4) they can activate brain vasculature stimulating release of mediators such as prostaglandins (PGE), NO, or cytokines (IL-1β), which act on brain parenchymal cells. The specific mechanism employed may depend on the conditions. For example, in a mild inflammatory response, when peripheral cytokine levels are low, the cytokine signal may be transmitted by the vagus nerve. In contrast, during more significant sepsis, circulating cytokine levels are high, and the vascular route to brain activation becomes more prominent. Once generated, the signal is transmitted from the anterior through the posterior hypothalamus to the vasomotor center to induce the responses (Fig. 3–34).

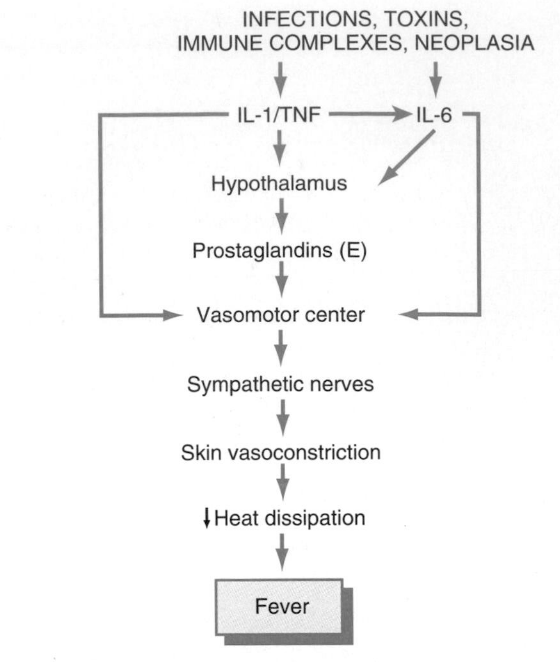

Figure 3–34

Mechanism of fever (see text).

Leukocytosis is a common feature of inflammatory reactions, especially those induced by bacterial infection. The leukocyte count usually climbs to 15,000 or 20,000 cells/ml, but sometimes it may reach extraordinarily high levels of 40,000 to 100,000 cells/ml. These extreme elevations are referred to as *leukemoid reactions* because they are similar to the white cell counts obtained in leukemia. The leukocytosis occurs initially because of *accelerated release* of cells from the bone marrow postmitotic reserve pool (caused by IL-1 and TNF) and is associated with a rise in the number of more immature neutrophils in the blood (*shift to the left*). Prolonged infection, however, also induces proliferation of precursors in the bone marrow, caused by increased production of CSFs. This stimulation of CSF production is also mediated by IL-1 and TNF. (See also discussion of leukocytosis in Chapter 15.)

Most bacterial infections induce *neutrophilia*, but infectious mononucleosis, mumps, and German measles are exceptions and produce a leukocytosis by virtue of an absolute increase in the number of lymphocytes (*lymphocytosis*). In an additional group of disorders, which includes bronchial asthma, hay fever, and parasitic infestations, there is an absolute increase in the number of eosinophils, creating an *eosinophilia*.

Certain infections (typhoid fever and infections caused by viruses, rickettsiae, and certain protozoa) are associated with a decreased number of circulating white cells (*leukopenia*). Leukopenia is also encountered in infections that overwhelm patients debilitated by disseminated cancer or rampant tuberculosis.

Although our discussion of the molecular and cellular events in acute and chronic inflammation is concluded, we still need to consider the changes induced by the body's attempts to heal the damage, the process of *repair*. As described next in Chapter 4, the repair begins almost as soon as the inflammatory changes have started and involves several processes, including cell proliferation, differentiation, and extracellular matrix deposition.

REFERENCES

1. Majno G: The Healing Hand: Man and Wound in the Ancient World. Cambridge, Harvard University Press, 1975.
2. Weissman G: Inflammation: historical perspectives. In Gallin JI, et al (eds): Inflammation: Basic Principles and Clinical Correlates, 2nd ed. New York, Raven Press, 1992, pp 5–13.
3. Hunter J: A Treatise of the Blood, Inflammation, and Gunshot Wounds, Vol 1. London, J Nicoli, 1794.
4. Cohnheim J: Lectures in General Pathology (Translated by AD McKee, from the second German edition, Vol 1). London, New Sydenham Society, 1889.
5. Heifets L: Centennial of Metchnikoff's discovery. J Reticuloendothel Soc 31:381, 1982.
6. Majno G, Palade GE: Studies on inflammation: I. the effect of histamine and serotonin on vascular permeability: an electron microscopic study. J Biophys Biochem Cytol 11:571, 1961.
7. Majno G, et al: Studies on inflammation: II. the site of action of histamine and serotonin along the vascular tree: a topographic study. J Biophys Biochem Cytol 11:607, 1961.
8. Bowden JJ, et al: Substance P (NK1) receptor immunoreactivity on endothelial cells of the rat tracheal mucosa. Am J Physiol 270:404, 1996.
9. Feng D, et al: Vesiculo-vacuolar organelles and the regulation of venule permeability to macromolecules by vascular permeability factor, histamine and serotonin. J Exp Med 183:1981, 1996.
10. Lampugnani MG, Dejana E: Interendothelial junctions: structure, signalling and functional roles. Curr Opin Cell Biol 9:674, 1997.
11. Brett J, et al: Tumor necrosis factor/cachectin increases permeability of endothelial cell monolayers by a mechanism involving regulatory G proteins. J Exp Med 169:1977, 1989.
12. Cotran RS, Briscoe DM: Endothelial cells in inflammation. In Kelley W, et al (eds): Textbook of Rheumatology, 5th ed. Philadelphia, WB Saunders, 1997, pp 183–198.
13. Lipowsky HH: Leukocyte margination and deformation in postcapillary venules. In Granger DN, Schmid-Schonbein GW (eds): Physiology and Pathophysiology of Leukocyte Adhesion. New York, Oxford University Press, 1996, pp 130–147.
14. Springer TA: Traffic signals for lymphocyte circulation and leukocyte migration: the multistep paradigm. Cell 76:301, 1994.
15. McEver RP: Perspectives series: cell adhesion in vascular biology: role of PSGL-1 binding to selectins in leukocyte recruitment. J Clin Invest 100:485, 1997.
16. Pober JS, Cotran RS: Overview: the role of endothelial cells in inflammation. Transplantation 50:537, 1990.
17. Travis JT: Biotech gets a grip on cell adhesion. Science 26:906, 1993.
18. Butcher EC: Leukocyte-endothelial cell recognition: three or more steps to diversity and sensitivity. Cell 67:1033, 1991.
19. Arnaout AM: Leukocyte adhesion molecule deficiency. Immunol Rev 114:145, 1990.
20. Etzioni A, et al: Brief report: recurrent severe infections caused by a novel leukocyte adhesion deficiency. N Engl J Med 327:1789, 1992.
21. Carlos TM, Harlan JM: Leukocyte-endothelial adhesion molecules. Blood 84:2068, 1994.
22. Cotran RS, Mayadas TN: Endothelial adhesion molecules in health and disease. Pathol Biol 46:164, 1998.

22a. Feng D, et al: Neutrophils emigrate from venules by a transendothelial pathway in response to FMLP. J Exp Med 187:903, 1998.

23. Muller WA: The role of PECAM 1 in leukocyte emigration. In Pearson JD (ed): Vascular Adhesion Molecules and Inflammation. Basel, Switzerland, Birkhauser Publishing (in press).

23a. Liao F, et al: Soluble domain 1 of platelet-endothelial cell adhesion molecule (PECAM) is sufficient to block transendothelial migration in vitro and in vivo. J Exp Med 185:1349, 1997.

24. Snyderman R, Uhuig RJ: Chemoattractant stimulus-response coupling. In Gallin JI, et al (eds): Inflammation: Basic Principles and Clinical Correlates, 2nd ed. New York, Raven Press, 1992, pp 421–441.
25. Stossel TP: On the crawling of animal cells. Science 260:1045, 1993.
26. Foxman EF, et al: Multistep navigation and the combinatorial control of leukocyte chemotaxis. J Cell Biol 139:1349–1360, 1997.
27. Moxley G, Ruddy S: Immune complexes and complement. In Kelley WN, et al (eds): Textbook of Rheumatology, 5th ed. Philadelphia, WB Saunders, 1997, pp 228–240.

27a. Reid KB, et al: Complement component C1 and the collectins: parallels between routes of acquired and innate immunity. Immunol Today 19:56–59, 1998.

28. Klebanoff SJ: Oxygen metabolites from phagocytes. In Gallin JI, et al (eds): Inflammation: Basic Principles and Clinical Correlates, 2nd ed. New York, Raven Press, 1992, pp 541–589.
29. DeLeo FR, Quinn MT: Assembly of the phagocyte NADPH oxidase: molecular interaction of the oxidase proteins. J Leukoc Biol 60:677–691, 1996.
30. Martin E, Gantz T, Lehrer RI: Defensins and other endogenous peptide antibiotics of vertebrates. J Leukoc Biol 58:128–136, 1995.
31. Jaeschke H, Smith CW: Mechanisms of neutrophil-induced parenchymal injury. J Leukoc Biol 61:647–653, 1997.
32. Tapper H: The secretion of preformed granules by macrophages and neutrophils. J Leukoc Biol 59:613–622, 1996.
33. Coxon A, et al: A novel role for the $\beta2$ integrin, CD11b/CD18, in neutrophil apoptosis: a homeostatic mechanism in inflammation. Immunity 5:653, 1996.
34. Savill J: Apoptosis in resolution of inflammation. J Leukoc Biol 61: 325, 1997.
35. Ramsay M: Protein trafficking violations. Nat Genet 14:242–245, 1996.
36. Morgan BP: Physiology and pathophysiology of complement: progress and trends. Crit Rev Clin Lab Sci 32:265–298, 1995.
37. Morgan BP: Complement regulatory molecules: application to therapy and transplantation. Immunol Today 16:257–259, 1995.
38. Margolius HS: Kallikreins and kinins: some unanswered questions about system characteristics and roles in human disease. Hypertension 26:221–229, 1995.
39. Carmeliet P, Collen D: Molecular genetics of the fibrinolytic and coagulation systems in haemostasis, thrombogenesis, restenosis and atherosclerosis. Curr Opin Lipidol 8:118–125, 1997.
40. Cirino G, et al: Factor Xa as an interface between coagulation and inflammation. J Clin Invest 99:2446–2451, 1997.
41. Serhan CN, et al: Lipid mediator networks in cell signaling: update and impact of cytokines. FASEB J 10:1147–1158, 1996.
42. Bozza PT, et al: Eosinophil lipid bodies: specific, inducible intracellular sites for enhanced eicosanoid formation. J Exp Med 186:909, 1997.
43. Dray A: Inflammatory mediators of pain. Br J Anaesth 75:125–131, 1995.
44. Maddox JF: Lipoxin B4 regulates human monocyte/neutrophil adherence and motility. FASEB J 12:487, 1998.
45. Brady HR, et al: Potential vascular roles for lipoxins in "stop programs" of host defense and inflammation. Trends Cardiovasc Med 5: 186–192, 1995.
46. Serhan CN: Lipoxins and novel aspirin-triggered lipoxins: a jungle of cell-cell interactions or a therapeutic opportunity? Prostaglandins 53: 107–137, 1997.
47. Buckingham JC, Flower RJ: Lipocortin 1: a second messenger of glucocorticoid action in the hypothalamo-pituitary-adrenocortical axis. Mol Med Today 3:296–302, 1997.
48. Rossetti RG: Oral administration of unsaturated fatty acids: effects on human peripheral blood T lymphocyte proliferation. J Leukoc Biol 62:438–443, 1997.
49. Pinckard RN, et al: Structural and (patho)physiological diversity of PAF. Clin Rev Allergy 12:329–359, 1994.
50. FitzGerald GA: Cigarettes and the wages of sn-2: oxidized species of PAF in smoking hamsters. J Clin Invest 99:2300–2301, 1997.

51. Abbas AK, et al: Cellular and Molecular Immunology, 3rd ed. Philadelphia, WB Saunders, 1997, pp 249–277.
52. Dinarello CA: Biologic basis for interleukin-1 in disease. Blood 87: 2095–2147, 1996.
53. Beutler B: TNF, immunity and inflammatory disease: lessons of the past decade. J Invest Med 43:227–235, 1995.
54. Bevilacqua MP: Endothelial-leukocyte adhesion molecules. Ann Rev Immunol 11:767–804, 1993.
55. Argiles JM, et al: Journey from cachexia to obesity by TNF. FASEB J 11:743–751, 1997.
56. Adams DH, Lloyd AR: Chemokines: leukocyte recruitment and activation cytokines. Lancet 349:490–495, 1997.
57. Kunkel SL, et al: Chemokines and their role in human disease. Agents Actions 46(suppl):11, 1995.
58. Teixeira MM, et al: Chemokine-induced eosinophil recruitment. Evidence of a role for endogenous eotaxin. J Clin Invest 100: 1657, 1997.
59. Kelner GS, et al: Lymphotactin: a cytokine that represents a new class of chemokine. Science 266:1395–1399, 1994.
60. Bazan JF, et al: A new class of membrane bound chemokine with a CX3C motif. Nature 385:640, 1997.
61. Imai T, et al: Identification and molecular characterization of fractalkine receptor CX3CR1, which mediates both leukocyte migration and adhesion. Cell 91:521, 1997.
62. Premack BA, Schall TJ: Chemokine receptors: gateways to inflammation and infection. Nat Med 2:1174–1178, 1996.
63. Furchgott RF, Zawadzki JV: The obligatory role of endothelial cells in the relaxation of arterial smooth muscle by acetylcholine. Nature 288:373, 1980.
64. Nathan C: Inducible nitric oxide synthase. J Clin Invest 100:2417, 1997.
65. Huang PL, et al: Hypertension in mice lacking the gene for endothelial nitric oxide synthase. Nature 377:239–242, 1995.
66. MacMicking JD, et al: Nitric oxide and macrophage function. Annu Rev Immunol 15:323, 1997.
67. Fang FC: Mechanisms of nitric oxide-related antimicrobial activity. J Clin Invest 99:2818–2825, 1997.
68. Ward PA, et al: Oxygen radicals, inflammation and tissue injury. Free Radic Biol Med 5:403, 1988.
69. Venge P, et al: Neutrophils and eosinophils. In Kelley WN, et al (eds): Textbook of Rheumatology, 5th ed. Philadelphia, WB Saunders, 1997, pp 146–160.
70. Remick DG, Villarete L: Regulation of cytokine gene expression by reactive oxygen and reactive nitrogen intermediates. J Leukoc Biol 59:471–475, 1996.
71. Colten HR, Krause JE: Pulmonary inflammation—a balancing act. N Engl J Med 336:1094–1096, 1997.
72. Bozic CR, et al: Neurogenic amplification of immune complex inflammation. Science 273:1722–1725, 1996.
73. Thomas R, Lipsky PE: Monocytes and macrophages. In Kelley WN, et al (eds): Textbook of Rheumatology, 5th ed. Philadelphia, WB Saunders, 1997, pp 128–146.
74. Lluscinskas FW, Gimbrone MA Jr: Endothelial-dependent mechanisms in chronic inflammatory leukocyte recruitment. Annu Rev Med 47:413–421, 1996.
75. Majno G, Joris I: Cells, Tissues, and Disease: Principles of General Pathology. Cambridge, MA, Blackwell Science, 1996, pp 429–463.
76. Ponath PD, et al: Molecular cloning and characterization of a human eotaxin receptor expressed selectively on eosinophils. J Exp Med 183: 2437–2448, 1996.
77. Boyce JA: The pathobiology of eosinophilic inflammation. Allergy Asthma Proc 18:293–300, 1997.
78. Saper CB, Breder CD: The neurologic basis of fever. N Engl J Med 330:1880–1886, 1994.
79. Licinio J, Wong M: Interleukin 1β and fever. Nat Med 2:1314–1315, 1996.

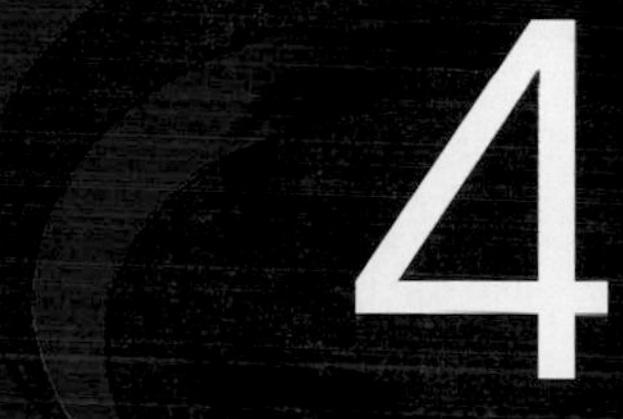

4 Tissue Repair: Cellular Growth, Fibrosis, and Wound Healing

CONTROL OF NORMAL CELL GROWTH

CELL CYCLE AND PROLIFERATIVE POTENTIAL

MOLECULAR EVENTS IN CELL GROWTH

Cell Surface Receptors

Receptors With Intrinsic Kinase Activity

Receptors Without Intrinsic Catalytic Activity

G Protein–Linked Receptors

Signal Transduction Systems

Mitogen-Activated Protein Kinase Pathway

Phosphoinositide-3-Kinase Pathway

Inositol-Lipid Pathway

Cyclic Adenosine Monophosphate Pathway

JAK/STAT Pathway

Stress-Activated Signaling Pathway

Transcription Factors

CELL CYCLE AND THE REGULATION OF CELL DIVISION

Cyclins and Cyclin-Dependent Kinases

Checkpoints

GROWTH INHIBITION

GROWTH FACTORS

EXTRACELLULAR MATRIX AND CELL-MATRIX INTERACTIONS

COLLAGEN

ELASTIN, FIBRILLIN, AND ELASTIC FIBERS

ADHESIVE GLYCOPROTEINS AND INTEGRINS

MATRICELLULAR PROTEINS

PROTEOGLYCANS AND HYALURONAN

SUMMARY OF CELL GROWTH AND DIFFERENTIATION

REPAIR BY CONNECTIVE TISSUE (FIBROSIS)

ANGIOGENESIS

Growth Factors and Receptors

Extracellular Matrix Proteins as Regulators of Angiogenesis

FIBROSIS (FIBROPLASIA)

Fibroblast Proliferation

Extracellular Matrix Deposition

TISSUE REMODELING

WOUND HEALING

HEALING BY FIRST INTENTION (WOUNDS WITH OPPOSED EDGES)

HEALING BY SECOND INTENTION (WOUNDS WITH SEPARATED EDGES)

WOUND STRENGTH

LOCAL AND SYSTEMIC FACTORS THAT INFLUENCE WOUND HEALING

PATHOLOGIC ASPECTS OF WOUND REPAIR

OVERVIEW OF THE INFLAMMATORY-REPARATIVE RESPONSE

The body's ability to replace injured or dead cells and to repair tissues after inflammation is critical to survival. A variety of injurious agents—at the same time that they create havoc within the cell—set in motion a series of events that serve not only to contain the damage, but also to prepare the nonlethally injured cells for the replication necessary to replace the dead cells. We have seen, for example, how the initiation of apoptosis may delete cells bearing damaged DNA (which may be potentially harmful to the organism). Injurious stimuli also

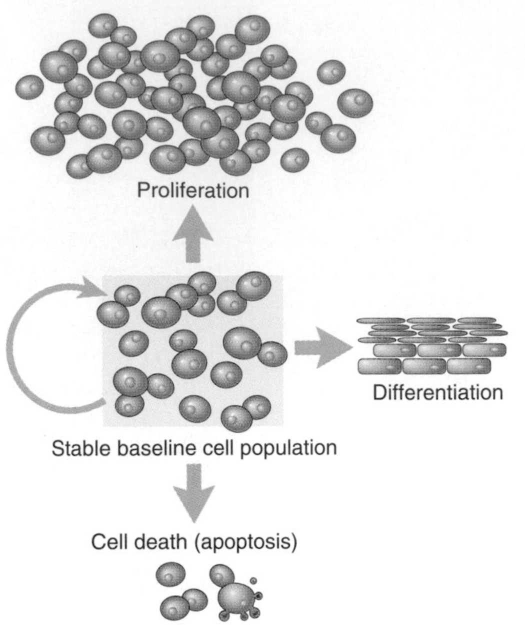

Figure 4–1

Mechanisms regulating cell populations. Cell numbers can be altered by increased or decreased rates of cell death (apoptosis) or by changes in the rates of proliferation or differentiation. (Modified from McCarthy NJ, et al: Apoptosis in the development of the immune system: growth factors, clonal selection and bcl-2. Cancer Metastasis Rev 11:157, 1992.)

trigger the activation of genes that are involved in cell replication.

Repair of tissues involves two distinct processes: (1) *regeneration,* denoting the replacement of injured cells by cells of the same type, sometimes leaving no residual trace of the previous injury, and (2) *replacement by connective tissue,* called *fibroplasia* or *fibrosis,* which leaves a permanent scar. In most instances, both processes contribute to repair. In addition, both regeneration and fibroplasia are determined by essentially similar mechanisms involving cell migration, proliferation, and differentiation as well as cell-matrix interactions. The latter are particularly important. The orderly regeneration of the epithelial tissue of the skin and viscera requires the presence of the basement membrane (BM). This specialized extracellular matrix (ECM) functions as an extracellular scaffold for accurate regeneration of preexisting structures. Maintenance of BM integrity provides for the specificity of cell type and polarity and influences cell migration and growth.

In adult tissues, the size of a population of cells is determined by the rates of cell proliferation, differentiation, and death by apoptosis.[1] Figure 4–1 depicts these relationships and shows that increased cell numbers may result from either increased proliferation or decreased cell death. The impact of *differentiation* depends on the circumstance under which it occurs. The progeny of stem cells in the bone marrow, for example, may divide several times but eventually become terminally differentiated and cannot multiply further. Replication of differentiated cells occurs in certain adult tissues; for example, after partial hepatectomy, liver cell division continues until the signals for such division are abrogated (Chapter 2). Apoptosis is induced by a variety of physiologic and pathologic stimuli and is controlled by a number of genes (Chapter 1).

In this chapter, we first review the major mechanisms involved in the regulation of cell growth, including the important interactions between cells and the ECM. We then examine in detail the process of fibroplasia—the replacement of injured cells by connective tissue. Finally, we discuss wound healing as an important clinical example of both regeneration and fibroplasia.

CONTROL OF NORMAL CELL GROWTH

Cell proliferation can be stimulated by injury, cell death, and mechanical deformation of tissues. It is key in *regeneration.* Cell replication is controlled largely by chemical factors in the microenvironment, which either stimulate or inhibit cell proliferation. An excess of stimulators or a deficiency of inhibitors leads to net growth and, in the case of cancer, uncontrolled growth. Growth can be accomplished by shortening the cell cycle, but the most important factors are those that recruit resting or quiescent cells into the cell.[2]

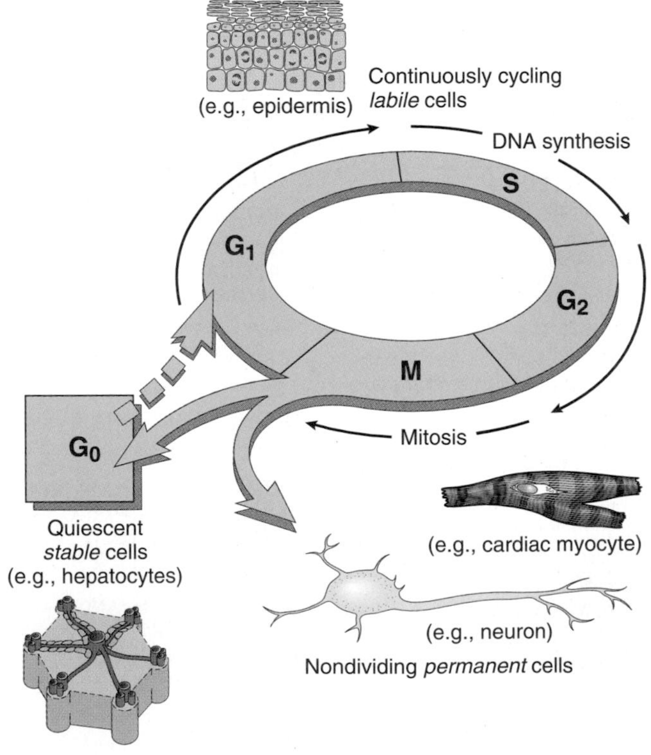

Figure 4–2

Cell populations and cell cycle phases. Constantly dividing labile cells continuously cycle from one mitosis to the next. Nondividing permanent cells have exited the cycle and are destined to die without further division. Quiescent stable cells in G_0 are neither cycling nor dying and can be induced to re-enter the cell cycle by an appropriate stimulus.

Cell Cycle and Proliferative Potential

The cells of the body are divided into three groups on the basis of their proliferative capacity and their relationship to the cell cycle. The cell growth cycle consists of G_1 (presynthetic), *S* (DNA synthesis), G_2 (premitotic), and *M* (mitotic) phases (Fig. 4–2). Quiescent cells are in a physiologic state called G_0. With the exception of tissues composed primarily of nondividing cells, most mature tissues consist of some combination of continuously dividing cells, quiescent cells that occasionally enter into the cell cycle, and nondividing cells.

- *Continuously dividing cells* (also called *labile cells*) follow the cell cycle from one mitosis to the next and continue to proliferate throughout life, replacing cells that are continuously being destroyed. Tissues that contain labile cells include surface epithelia, such as stratified squamous surfaces of the skin, oral cavity, vagina, and cervix; the lining mucosa of all the excretory ducts of the glands of the body (e.g., salivary glands, pancreas, biliary tract); the columnar epithelium of the gastrointestinal tract and uterus; and the transitional epithelium of the urinary tract and cells of the bone marrow and hematopoietic tissues. In most of these tissues, regeneration is derived from a population of *stem cells,* which have an unlimited capacity to proliferate and whose progeny may undergo various streams of differentiation.
- *Quiescent* (or *stable*) *cells* normally demonstrate a low level of replication; however, these cells can undergo rapid division in response to stimuli and are thus capable of reconstituting the tissue of origin. They are considered to be in G_0 but can be stimulated into G_1. In this category are the parenchymal cells of virtually all the glandular organs of the body, such as the liver, kidneys, and pancreas; mesenchymal cells, such as fibroblasts and smooth muscle; and vascular endothelial cells. The regenerative capacity of stable cells is best exemplified by the ability of the liver to regenerate after hepatectomy and after toxic, viral, or chemical injury.

Although labile and stable cells are capable of regeneration, it does not necessarily follow that there will be restitution of normal structure. *The underlying supporting stroma of the parenchymal cells—particularly the BMs—is necessary for organized regeneration, forming a scaffold for the replicating parenchymal cells.* When BMs are disrupted, cells may proliferate in a haphazard fashion and produce disorganized masses of cells bearing no resemblance to the original arrangement. To use the liver as an example, the hepatitis virus destroys parenchymal cells without injuring the more resistant connective tissue cells, or framework, of the liver lobule. Thus, after viral hepatitis, regeneration of liver cells may completely reconstitute the liver lobule. By contrast, a liver abscess that destroys hepatocytes and the connective tissue framework is followed by scarring.

The *connective tissue and mesenchymal cells* (fibroblasts, endothelial cells, smooth muscle cells, chondrocytes, and osteocytes) are quiescent in adult mammals. All proliferate in response to injury, however, and fibroblasts in particular proliferate widely, constituting the connective tissue response to inflammation (see later section on wound healing).

- *Nondividing (permanent) cells* have left the cell cycle and cannot undergo mitotic division in postnatal life. To this group belong most nerve cells and the skeletal and cardiac muscle cells. *Neurons* destroyed in the central nervous system are permanently lost. They are replaced by the proliferation of the central nervous system supportive elements, the glial cells. The situation is somewhat more complicated with respect to the neurons of the peripheral nerves, as detailed in Chapter 29. *Skeletal muscle* does have some regenerative capacity, and most of the regeneration appears to occur from transformation of the satellite cells found attached to the endomysial sheaths. If the ends of severed muscle fibers are closely

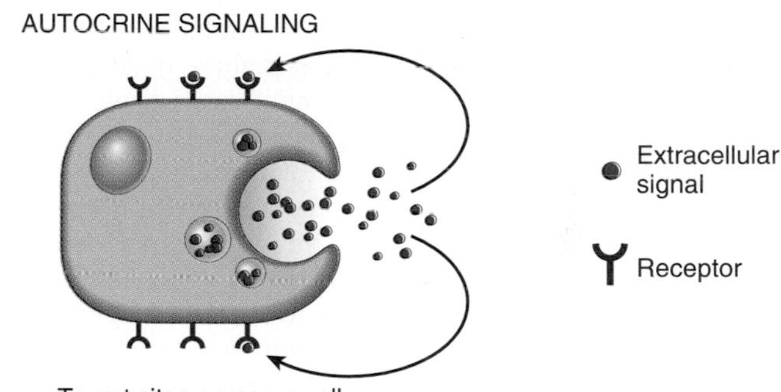

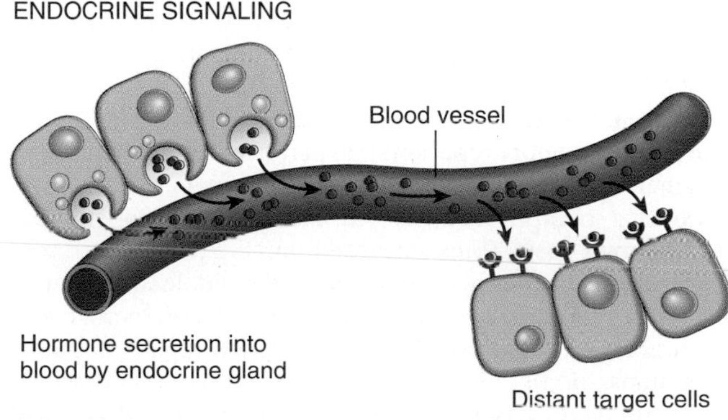

Figure 4–3

General patterns of intercellular signaling (see text). (Modified from Lodish H, et al. (eds): Molecular Cell Biology, 3rd ed. New York, WH Freeman, 1995, p 855. © 1995 by Scientific American Books. Used with permission of WH Freeman and Company.)

juxtaposed, muscle regeneration in mammals can be excellent, but this is a condition that can rarely be attained under practical conditions. As to *cardiac muscle,* it is fair to state that if cardiac muscle has regenerative capacity, it is limited, and most large injuries to the heart are followed by connective tissue scarring. Scarring regularly follows myocardial infarction in humans.

Molecular Events in Cell Growth

Molecular events in cell growth are complex and involve an increasing array of intercellular pathways and molecules, but they are important because it is now clear that aberrations in such pathways may underlie the uncontrolled growth in cancer as well as abnormal cellular responses in a variety of diseases. This section outlines different general types of signaling systems and cell surface receptors, then examines in some detail several intracellular transduction pathways, in which the binding of signaling molecules to cell surface receptors leads to activation of particular transcription factors and changes in gene expression. The explosion in understanding of these molecular events has stemmed largely from the discovery that growth factors induce cell proliferation by affecting the expression of genes involved in normal growth control pathways, the so-called *protooncogenes*. The expression of these genes is tightly regulated during normal growth and regeneration. Alterations in the structure of such protooncogenes can convert them into *oncogenes*, which contribute to uncontrolled cell growth characteristic of cancer; thus, normal and abnormal cellular proliferation follow similar pathways.[3] Oncogenes are discussed in detail in Chapter 8, Neoplasia.

There are three general schemes of intercellular signaling—autocrine, paracrine, or endocrine—based on the distance over which the signal acts.[4] Additionally, some membrane-bound proteins present on one cell can interact directly with receptors on an adjacent cell (Fig. 4–3).

- *Autocrine signaling*: Cells respond to the signaling substances that they themselves secrete. Several polypeptide growth factors (or cytokines) (Chapter 3) can act in this manner. When the same cell produces a growth factor and the corresponding receptor, an *autocrine loop* can be established. Autocrine growth regulation plays a role in compensatory epithelial hyperplasia (e.g., hepatic regeneration) and, particularly, in tumors. Tumor cells frequently overproduce growth factors that can stimulate their own growth and proliferation.
- *Paracrine signaling*: A cell produces molecules that affect only a target cell in close proximity. Paracrine stimulation is common in connective tissue repair of healing wounds, in which a factor produced by one cell type (a macrophage) has its growth effect on adjacent cells usually of a different cell type (e.g., a fibroblast).
- *Endocrine signaling*: Hormones are synthesized by cells of endocrine organs and act on target cells distant from their site of synthesis being usually carried by the blood.

CELL SURFACE RECEPTORS

Cell growth is initiated by the binding of a signaling agent, most commonly a growth factor, to a specific receptor. Receptor proteins can be located on the cell surface of the target cell or found in either the cytoplasm or the nucleus. A receptor protein has binding specificity for particular ligands, and the resulting receptor ligand complex initiates a specific cellular response.

Three major classes of cell surface receptors are important for cell growth (Fig. 4–4). On ligand binding, they deliver signals to the nucleus by using a variety of signal transduction pathways. Some pathways are more or less unique to one family of receptors, whereas others are shared. We first describe the receptors and then their connections to signaling molecules.

Receptors With Intrinsic Kinase Activity

Receptors with intrinsic kinase activity have an extracellular domain for ligand binding; a single transmembrane region; and a cytosolic domain, which can have either tyrosine kinase activity or, less commonly, serine/threonine. For example, epidermal growth factor (EGF), fibroblast growth factor (FGF), and platelet-derived growth factor (PDGF) bind to receptors with intrinsic *tyrosine kinase* activity. Many such growth factors are dimeric proteins, contain two regions for receptor binding, and form stable receptor dimers by simultaneously binding two receptors (Fig. 4–5). *Dimerization* of the receptors is followed by receptor *autophosphorylation*, a process in which one receptor molecule phosphorylates the other in the dimer.[5] Receptor autophosphorylation creates binding sites for a series of cytosolic proteins endowed with *src* homology 2 (SH2) domains, which are recruited to phosphorylated tyrosine residues on the activated receptor. Such cytosolic proteins include (1) a series of adapter proteins, which couple the receptor to the *ras* signaling pathway; (2) components of the phosphoinositide-3-kinase (PI-3-kinase) pathway; (3) phospholipase C-γ in the protein kinase C pathway; and (4) members of the *src* family of tyrosine kinases (Fig. 4–5). Collectively, these four systems, in turn, generate a cascade of responses that ultimately signal irreversible commitment of the cell to enter S phase of the cell cycle. Some of these pathways also provide unique signals that stimulate cellular responses other than growth.

Receptors Without Intrinsic Catalytic Activity

Receptors without intrinsic catalytic activity have an extracellular domain for ligand binding; a single transmembrane region; and a cytosolic domain, which directly associates with and activates one or more *cytosolic* protein tyrosine kinases, which, in turn, phosphorylate the receptor (Fig. 4–4). Because receptors for many *cytokines* (Chapter 3) fall into this category, this group of receptors is sometimes referred to as the *cytokine receptor superfamily*.[6]

G Protein–Linked Receptors

All G protein–linked receptors contain seven transmembrane loops and are frequently called *seven-spanning receptors*. Although not closely linked to the regulation of cell growth, this class of receptors is associated with a variety of important functions. For example, receptors for the inflammatory chemokines (Chapter 3) as well as the hormones epinephrine and glucagon are in this class. Ligand binding activates a signal transducing G protein complex, which, in turn, activates an effector system that generates intracellular second messengers (Fig. 4–6).[7]

SIGNAL TRANSDUCTION SYSTEMS

Signal transduction is the process by which extracellular signals are detected and converted into intracellular signals, which, in turn, generate specific cellular responses. Signal transduction systems are typically arranged as networks of sequential protein kinases; the most important ones involved in the regulation of cell growth are the mitogen-activated protein kinase (MAP kinase), PI-3-kinase, inositol-lipid (IP_3), cyclic adenosine monophosphate (cAMP), the JAK/STAT signaling system (Fig. 4–4), and the stress kinase system.

Mitogen-Activated Protein Kinase Pathway

The MAP kinase system is particularly important in signaling by growth factors. As we have seen, ligand binding by a receptor tyrosine kinase results in autophosphorylation of the receptor and binding of adapter proteins, such as GRB2 and SOS (Fig. 4–5). These ultimately lead to activation of the Ras protein. Ras belongs to the guanosine triphosphatase (GTPase) superfamily of proteins that cycle between active and inactive forms.[8] The inactive Ras is in the guanosine diphosphate (GDP) binding form, which is converted by activation to the active GTP form, initiating a cascade of distal kinases, which culminates in changes in gene expression. Activation of Ras is counteracted by another protein called GAP (GTPase activating protein), which switches Ras to the inactive GDP form. Mutant forms of Ras, which bind but cannot hydrolyze GTP, are permanently fixed in the *on* state and are associated with increased cell proliferation seen in many types of human cancer (Chapter 8). Activated Ras binds to another protein, Raf, which binds to and phosphorylates MEK, a member of the family of kinases collectively called *MAP kinases.*[9] The distal MAP kinase (ERK) translocates into the nucleus, where it phosphorylates specific transcription factors, such as c-*jun* and c-*fos*, which, in turn, activate gene expression. *The net result of this pathway is activation of a protein phosphorylation cascade, which amplifies the signal and stimulates quiescent cells to enter the growth cycle.*

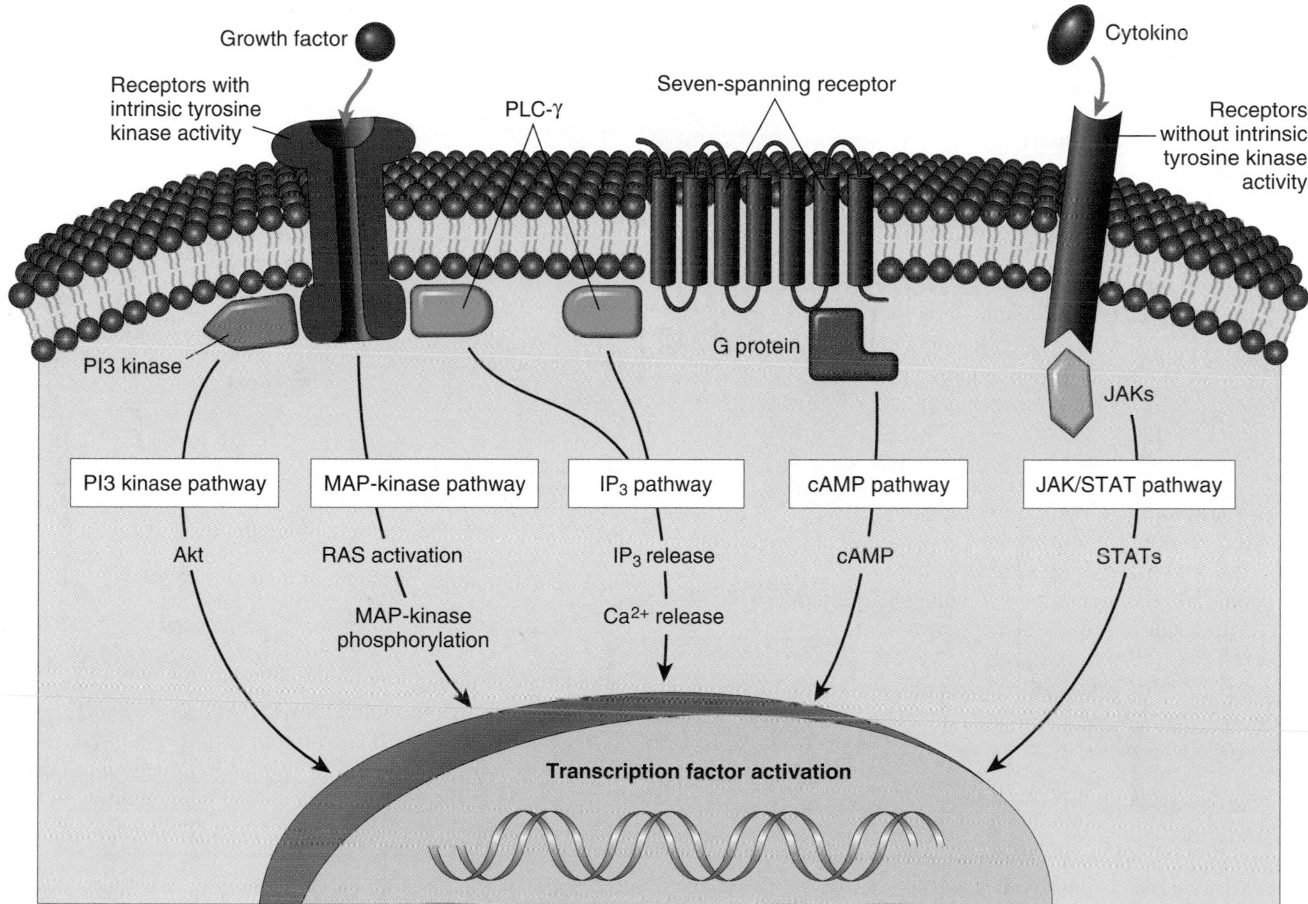

Figure 4–4

Simplified overview of the major types of cell surface receptors and the principal signal transduction pathways (see text). Signaling events from the tyrosine kinase and seven transmembrane receptors are outlined in more detail in Figures 4–5 and 4–6.

Phosphoinositide-3-Kinase Pathway

Although many growth factors act by binding to receptor tyrosine kinases, they do not all convey the same signals. For example, growth factors can differ in their ability to generate signals for cell proliferation and cell survival. The uncoupling of these events may be explained by differing ability of these growth factors to recruit and activate efficiently the PI-3-kinase pathway (Fig. 4–4).[10] This kinase generates membrane-associated lipid mediators (such as phosphatidylinositol-3,4-bisphosphate), which act as second messengers to recruit and activate a series of intracellular kinases, for example, *Akt*. The activity of these kinases eventually leads to cellular responses that are correlated with cellular survival, such as phosphorylation of glycogen synthase kinase 3 and increased glycogen synthesis.[11]

Inositol-Lipid Pathway

The IP_3 signaling system can be coupled to either tyrosine kinase or seven-spanning G protein–linked receptors causing activation of a G protein (G_o or G_q), which then activates phospholipase Cγ (Fig. 4–6). Phospholipase Cγ, in turn, cleaves phosphatidylinositol-4,5-bisphosphate (PIP_2) to inositol 1,4,5-triphosphate (IP_3) and 1,3-diacylglycerol (DAG).[12] The IP_3 then diffuses in the cytoplasm and associates with IP_3-sensitive calcium channels in the membrane of the endoplasmic reticulum, causing release of calcium stores. DAG and calcium also activate protein kinase C, which then phosphorylates a variety of cellular components important in cell growth and metabolism.

Cyclic Adenosine Monophosphate Pathway

Binding of hormones, such as epinephrine and glucagon, or chemokines to seven-spanning receptors is coupled through G proteins to activation of adenylate cyclase and generation of the second messenger cAMP (Fig. 4–4). Elevated levels of cAMP activate protein kinase A, which, through a series of intermediate steps, stimulates expression of target genes.[13]

JAK/STAT Pathway

As discussed earlier, members of the cytokine receptor superfamily lack intrinsic kinase activity. After ligand binding, the receptor associates with and activates one or more protein kinases present in the cytosol (Fig. 4–4), designated Janus kinases (JAKs).[14] The JAKs phosphorylate the receptors as well as downstream proteins designated

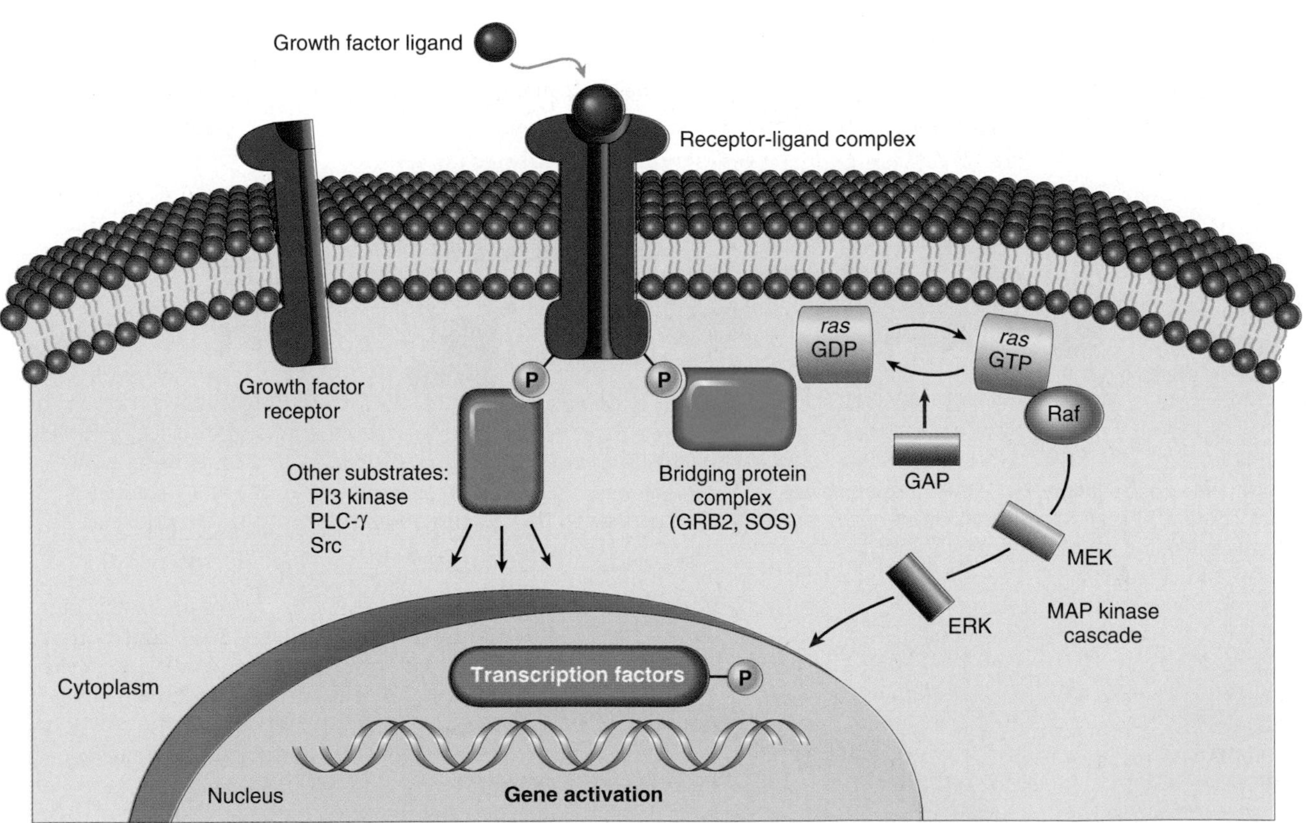

Figure 4–5

Signaling from tyrosine kinase receptors. Binding of a growth factor causes the receptor to dimerize and autophosphorylate tyrosine residues. Binding of adapter (or bridging) proteins (e.g., GRB2 and SOS) couple the receptor in inactive Ras. Cycling of Ras between its inactive and active forms is regulated by GAP. Activated Ras interacts with and activates Raf. This kinase then phosphorylates a component of the MAP kinase signaling pathway, MEK, which then phosphorylates ERK (MAP kinase). Activated MAP kinase phosphorylates other cytoplasmic proteins and nuclear transcription factors generating cellular responses. The phosphorylated tyrosine kinase receptor can also bind other components, such as PI-3 kinase, which activates distinct signaling systems.

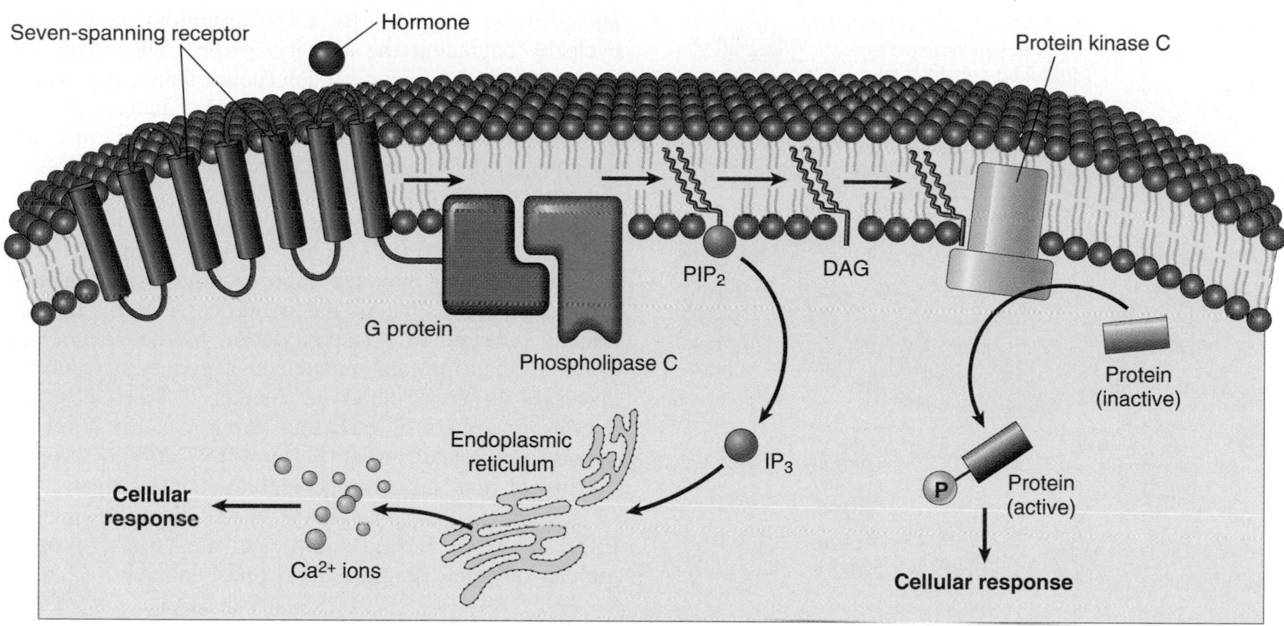

Figure 4–6

The inositol-lipid (IP_3) signaling pathway. Binding of a ligand to a seven transmembrane receptor activates a G protein, which in turn activates phospholipase C. This enzyme then cleaves phosphatidylinositol 4,5-bisphosphate (PIP_2) to inositol 1,4,5-triphosphate (IP_3) and 1,2-diacylglycerol (DAG). DAG activates protein kinase C, which phosphorylates a series of proteins altering cell function. The IP_3 diffuses through the cytoplasm and interacts with membrane channels in the endoplasmic reticulum, causing release of calcium ions and cellular responses.

STATs (signal transducers and activators of transcription). *In general, the JAK/STAT system, like stress activated kinases,*[15] *mediates functional as opposed to proliferative responses.*

TRANSCRIPTION FACTORS

The signal transduction systems just described transfer information to the nucleus where specific changes occur in the regulation of gene expression. This regulation is frequently achieved at the level of transcription of genes, and the latter is controlled by regulatory factors known as *transcription factors*, which then have a vital role in controlling cell growth. Transcription factors exhibit a modular structure composed of specific types of domains—including domains for DNA binding and for transcriptional regulation (regulatory domain). The DNA binding domain permits the factor to bind specifically to short-sequence motifs of DNA by distinct molecular mechanisms (e.g., homeodomain, zinc finger).[16] The regulatory domain allows the protein either to increase (an activation domain) or to decrease (a repression domain) transcription. Transcription factors are phosphorylated by specific proximal kinases, and such phosphorylation can change the subcellular localization of the transcription factor or its affinity for DNA, which, in turn, alters gene expression.[17] Among the transcription factors regulating cell proliferation are a number of proto-oncogenes, in which mutations may be associated with tumors (c-*myc*), and various types of tumor-suppressor genes (or antioncogenes), such as p53 and the retinoblastoma gene (Chapter 8). Transcription factors are also involved in the regulation of the cell cycle itself.

Cell Cycle and the Regulation of Cell Division

Thus far, we have examined the molecular pathways stimulated by growth factors. But what are the mechanisms that control the passage of cells through specific phases of the cell cycle and the orchestration of events leading to cell division? It is now clear that two types of molecular controls regulate such events: (1) a cascade of *protein phosphorylation* pathways involving a group of proteins called *cyclins* and (2) a set of *checkpoints* that monitor completion of the molecular events and, if necessary, delay progression to the next phase of the cycle.

CYCLINS AND CYCLIN-DEPENDENT KINASES

The entry and progression of cells through the cell cycle are controlled by changes in the levels and activities of *cyclins*. The levels of several of the cyclins (termed *A*, *B*, and *E*) peak during specific phases of the cell cycle, then are rapidly degraded as the cell enters the next phase of the cell cycle.[18] Cyclins perform their functions by forming complexes with a group of constitutively expressed proteins called *cyclin-dependent kinases (CDKs).*[19] Different combinations of cyclins and CDKs are associated with each of the important transitions in the cell cycle. The cyclin B/CDK1 function, which controls the transition from G_2 to M is analyzed in some detail in Fig. 4–7*A*.[20] As the cell moves into G_2, cyclin B is synthesized, and it binds to constitutive CDK1, creating the cyclin B/CDK1 complex, whose activity is necessary for cells to enter M phase. The

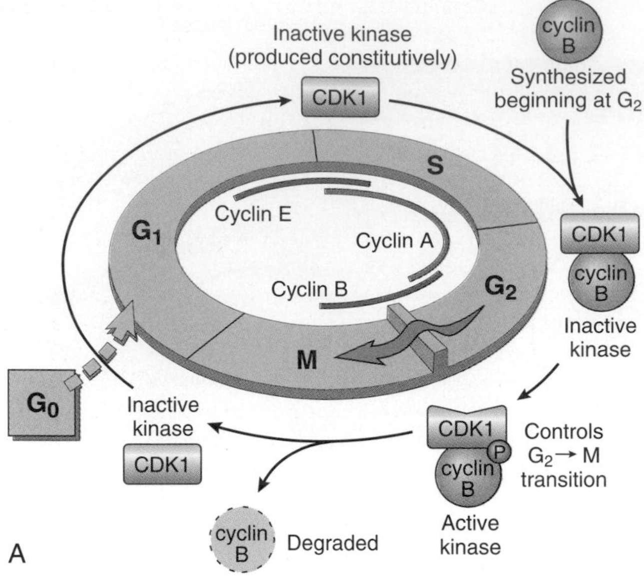

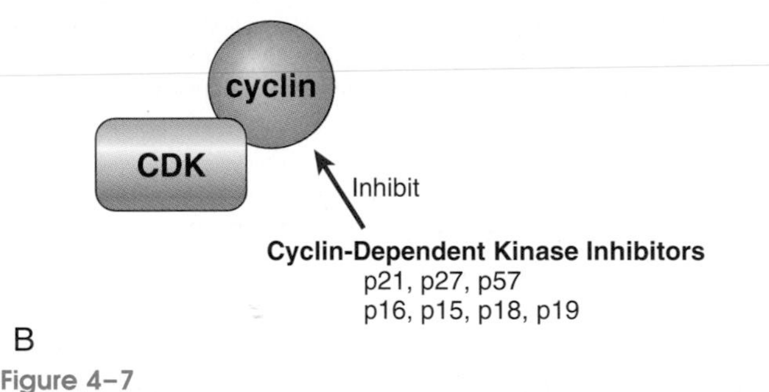

Figure 4–7

Schematic illustrating the role of cyclins, cyclin-dependent kinases, and inhibitors in regulating the cell cycle.

A, In the depicted example, the regulation of CDK1 kinase activity by cyclin B is illustrated. Binding of newly synthesized cyclin B to inactive CDK1 kinase at the beginning of G_2 results in a complex that can be activated by phosphorylation. This active kinase complex then phosphorylates a number of proteins important in regulating the G_2 to M transition. After mitosis, the cyclin B dissociates from the complex and is degraded, leaving the inactive CDK1 kinase, which can re-enter the cycle at the next G_2 stage. (Adapted from Dr. Anindya Dutta, Brigham and Women's Hospital, Boston, MA.)

B, Regulation of cyclin-dependent kinases, some of the inhibitors of which are listed. (Adapted from Elledge SJ: Cell cycle checkpoints: preventing an identity crisis. Science 274:1664, 1996.)

complex is activated by phosphorylation, and the active kinase then phosphorylates a variety of proteins involved in mitosis, DNA replication, depolymerization of the nuclear lamina, and mitotic spindle formation. After mitotic division, the relevant cyclins (in this case, cyclin B) are degraded by the *ubiquitin-proteasome pathway*.[21] In this pathway, proteins are first conjugated to the small protein cofactor *ubiquitin*, and the modified protein is specifically recognized and degraded within the *proteasome*, a large multisubunit proteolytic complex (Chapter 2).

In addition to synthesis and degradation, the active CDK complexes are regulated by binding of *CDK inhibitors*, such as p21 and p27, as well as by other kinases and phosphatases (Fig. 4–7*B*).[22] The inhibitors control the cell cycle by balancing the activity of the CDKs. The interaction of these opposing signals helps determine whether a cell progresses through the cell cycle. Changes in the levels of these inhibitors, as may occur in some tumors (Chapter 8) or possibly in aging cells (Chapter 2), can alter the normal progression of the cell cycle.

The G_1-S interface is another important intersection in the cell cycle. At this point, the cell commits either to replication of the genome or to quiescence or differentiation (or both).[23] One of the major controls on this transition is the state of phosphorylation of the *retinoblastoma protein*, Rb, a protein mutated in a variety of cancers and discussed in great detail in Chapter 8. Normally, Rb sequesters members of *E2F* transcription factor family in an inactive complex during G_0 and G_1. As G_1 progresses, cyclins of the D class accumulate and activate specific CDKs, which hyperphosphorylate Rb, disrupting binding to E2F. Activated E2F, in turn, activates transcription of a number of genes required for S phase entry.

CHECKPOINTS

Checkpoints represent a second mode of cell cycle regulation and provide a *surveillance mechanism* for ensuring that critical transitions occur in the correct order and that important events are completed with fidelity. C*heckpoints* sense problems in DNA replication, DNA repair, and chromosome segregation.[24] When checkpoints are activated, for example, by damaged or underreplicated DNA, signals are sent to the cell cycle machinery that arrest the cell cycle. By delaying progression through the cell cycle, checkpoints provide more time for repair and diminish the possibility of mutations. Checkpoint systems cause cell cycle arrest either by promoting inhibitory pathways or by inhibiting activating pathways (Fig. 4–7*B*). For example, the most common tumor-suppressor gene, *p53*, is activated in response to DNA damage and inhibits the cell cycle by increasing expression of the CDK inhibitor, *p21*. It follows that loss of checkpoints may result in genomic instability, as has been seen in certain hereditary cancer syndromes and at early stages of the evolution of normal cells into cancer cells (Chapter 8).

Growth Inhibition

The other side of the coin in cellular growth control is growth inhibition. The existence of growth inhibitory signals that maintain the integrity of a tissue has been suspected for decades from observations that populations of cells in culture or in vivo can limit one another's growth. *Contact inhibition* of growth in confluent cultures is one such manifestation of growth inhibition. There is also in vivo evidence for growth suppression. After partial hepatectomy, for example, cells stop multiplying when the liver has attained its normal preoperative size and configuration, suggesting the action of inhibitory signals.

The molecular mechanisms of growth inhibition are similar to those of growth stimulation and intertwine along their intercellular routes. A good example of a growth inhibitory signaling system involves the polypeptide growth factor transforming growth factor-β (TGF-β), described later. TGF-β signals through cell surface receptors with serine/threonine kinase activity.[25] The activated receptor phosphorylates its own cytoplasmic domain as well as substrate proteins, known as SMADs.[26] TGF-β inhibits cell cycle progression into S phase by affecting the function of both transcription factors and cell cycle control proteins. For example, it increases the expression of a CDK inhibitor (p27), which decreases CDK2 activity and also results in diminished phosphorylation of Rb protein in late G_1 phase.[27] Hypophosphorylated Rb in turn represses transcription of genes that are normally expressed at S phase, resulting in growth inhibition (Chapter 8).

Growth Factors

Having reviewed the molecular events in cell growth, we can now turn to a description of specific polypeptide growth factors. Some of the growth factors act on a variety of cell types, whereas others have relatively specific targets. Growth factors also have effects on cell locomotion, contractility, and differentiation—effects that may be as important to repair and wound healing as the growth-promoting effects. Table 4–1 lists some of the most important growth factors. Here we review only those that have broad targets and seem to be involved in general pathologic processes. More specific growth factors are alluded to in other sections of the book.

1. *EGF/TGF-α*: EGF was first discovered by its ability to cause precocious tooth eruption and eyelid opening in newborn mice.[28] EGF binds to a receptor (c-*erb* B1) with tyrosine kinase activity, followed by the signal transduction events described earlier.[29] EGF is mitogenic for a variety of epithelial cells and fibroblasts in vitro and causes hepatic cell division in vivo. It is widely distributed in tissue secretions and fluids, such as sweat, saliva, urine, and intestinal contents. TGF-α was initially extracted from sarcoma virus–transformed cells and was thought to be involved in transformation of normal cells to cancer. TGF-α has extensive homology with EGF, binds to the EGF receptor, and produces most of the biologic activities of EGF.
2. *PDGF*: PDGF is a family of several closely related 30-kD dimers consisting of two chains designated *A* and *B*. All three isoforms of PDGF (AA, AB, and BB) are secreted and are biologically active. The PDGF isoforms exert their effects by binding to two cell surface receptors, designated α and β, that have different ligand specificities.[30] PDGF is stored in the platelet α granules and released on platelet activation. It can also be produced by a variety of cells, including activated macrophages, endothelial cells, smooth muscle cells as well as many tumor cells. PDGF causes both migration and proliferation of fibroblasts, smooth muscle cells, and monocytes and has other proinflammatory properties as well. Transgenic animals that are deficient in either the A or B chain of PDGF show defects in the migration and proliferation of connective tissue cells,[31] suggesting that PDGF plays a special role in these processes.
3. *FGFs*: This is a family of growth factors of which acidic FGF (aFGF, or FGF-1) and basic FGF (bFGF or FGF-2) are the best characterized.[32] FGF-1 and FGF-2 are about 18 kD and are made by a variety of cells. Released FGF can associate with heparan sulfate in the ECM, which serves as a reservoir for growth factors controlling cell proliferation. FGF is recognized by a family of cell surface receptors that have intrinsic tyrosine kinase activity after ligand-induced activation. A large number of functions are attributed to FGFs, including roles in the following:
   - *New blood vessel formation (angiogenesis)*: bFGF, in particular, has the ability to induce all the steps necessary for new blood vessel formation both in vivo and in vitro, as we shall see.
   - *Wound repair*: FGFs participate in macrophage, fibroblast, and endothelial cell migration in the damaged tissue and migration of epithelium to form new epidermis (Chapter 3).
   - *Development*: FGFs play a role in skeletal muscle development and in lung maturation. For example, FGF-6 and its receptor induce myoblast proliferation and suppress myocyte differentiation, providing a supply of proliferating myocytes. bFGF is also thought to transform mesoderm to angioblasts during embryogenesis.
   - *Hematopoiesis*: FGFs have been implicated in two aspects of hematopoiesis—development of specific lineages of blood cells and development of bone marrow stroma.
4. *Vascular endothelial growth factor (VEGF)*: VEGF, also called *vascular permeability factor*, is a family of designated VEGF, VEGF-B, VEGF-C, and placental growth factor (PIGF) that promote blood vessel formation in

Table 4–1. GROWTH FACTORS

- Epidermal growth factor (EGF) family
  - EGF
  - Transforming growth factor-α (TGFα)
- Platelet-derived growth factor (PDGF)
- Fibroblast growth factor (FGF)
  - Basic
  - Acidic
- Transforming growth factor β-(TGF) family
  - TGF-β
  - Bone morphogenic proteins
  - Activins, others
- Vascular endothelial growth factors (VEGF)
- Angiopoietins (Ang)
- Insulin-like growth factors (IGF)
- Hepatocyte growth factor (HGF)
- Connective tissue growth factor (CTGF)
- Myeloid colony-stimulating factors (CSFs)
  - Granulocyte-macrophage CSF (GM-CSF)
  - Granulocyte CSF (G-CSF)
  - Macrophage CSF (M-CSF)
  - Erythropoietin
- Cytokines
  - Interleukins
  - Tumor necrosis factor (TNF)
  - Interferons α, β
- Nerve growth factor (NGF)

early development (*vasculogenesis*) and have a central role in the growth of new blood vessels (*angiogenesis*).[33] Members of the VEGF family have distinct functions. VEGF promotes angiogenesis in cancer, chronic inflammatory states, and healing wounds and is discussed in detail later in this chapter. VEGF-C induces specific lymphatic endothelial proliferation and hyperplasia of the lymphatic vasculature.[34]

5. *TGF-β and related growth factors*: TGF-β belongs to a family of homologous polypeptides that includes three major isoforms of TGF-β (TGF-β-1, TGF-β-2, TGF-β-3) and factors of such wide-ranging functions as bone morphogenetic proteins, activins, inhibins, and müllerian inhibiting substance. TGF-β-1 is the most widespread in distribution in mammals.[35] It is a homodimeric protein of approximately 25 kD, produced by a variety of different cell types, including platelets, endothelial cells, lymphocytes, and macrophages. Native TGF-βs are synthesized as precursor proteins, which are proteolytically cleaved to yield the growth factor and a second *latent* component.[36] After secretion, activation must occur to release the biologically active dimer from the latent portions of the molecule. In contrast to most other growth-related polypeptides, TGF-β functions both as an inhibitory and a stimulatory factor. TGF-β is a *growth inhibitor* to most epithelial cell types in culture. Its effects on fibroblasts and smooth muscle cells depend on concentration and culture conditions. In low concentrations, it induces the synthesis and secretion of PDGF and is thus indirectly mitogenic. In high concentrations, it is growth inhibitory, owing to its ability to inhibit the expression of PDGF receptors. TGF-β also stimulates fibroblast chemotaxis and the production of collagen and fibronectin by cells, while inhibiting collagen degradation by decreasing proteases and increasing protease inhibitors. *All these effects favor fibrogenesis,* and there is increasing evidence that TGF-β is involved in the development of fibrosis in a variety of chronic inflammatory conditions.
6. *Cytokines*: Although the cytokines have important functions as mediators of inflammation and immune responses (Chapters 3 and 7), these proteins can be placed into the larger functional group of polypeptide growth factors, since many of them have growth-promoting activities to a variety of cells.

EXTRACELLULAR MATRIX AND CELL-MATRIX INTERACTIONS

Cells grow, move, and differentiate in intimate contact with the ECM, and there is overwhelming evidence that the matrix critically influences these cell functions.[37] This section discusses those aspects of ECM structure and function that are most relevant to cell growth.

The ECM is secreted locally and assembles into a network in the spaces surrounding cells. It forms a significant proportion of the volume of any tissue and consists of the macromolecules outside of the cells. The ECM subserves many functions.[38] For example, the matrix proteins sequester molecules such as water to provide turgor to soft tissues or minerals to provide rigidity to skeletal tissues and provide a reservoir for growth factors controlling cell proliferation. ECM also provides a substratum for cells to adhere, migrate, and proliferate and can directly influence the form and function of cells. The degradation of ECM accompanies morphogenesis and wound healing as well as tumor invasion and metastasis.

Three groups of macromolecules are physically associated to form the ECM: (1) *fibrous structural proteins*, such as the collagens and elastins; (2) a diverse group of *adhesive glycoproteins*, including fibronectin and laminin; and (3) a gel of proteoglycans and hyaluronan. These macromolecules assemble into two general organizations: *interstitial matrix* and *BM (basal membrane)*. The interstitial matrix is present in spaces between epithelial, endothelial, and smooth muscle cells and in connective tissue. It consists of fibrillar (types I, III, V) and nonfibrillar collagen, elastin, fibronectin, proteoglycans, hyaluronate, and other components. BMs are produced by epithelial and mesenchymal cells and are closely associated with the cell surface. They consist of a network of amorphous nonfibrillar collagen (mostly type IV), laminin, heparan sulfate, proteoglycan, and other glycoproteins.[39]

Collagen

Collagen is the most common protein in the animal world, providing the extracellular framework for all multicellular organisms. Without collagen, a human being would be reduced to a clump of cells, interconnected by a few neurons. The *collagens* are composed of a triple helix of three polypeptide α chains, having a gly-x-y repeating sequence.[40] About 30 α chains form at least 14 distinct collagen types (Table 4–2). Types I, II, and III are the *interstitial* or *fibrillar collagens* and are the most abundant. Types IV, V, and VI are nonfibrillar (or amorphous) and are present in interstitial tissue and BMs.

The main steps in collagen synthesis are shown in Figure 4–8. After synthesis on ribosomes, the α chains are subjected to a number of enzymatic modifications, including hydroxylation of proline and lysine residues, providing collagen with its characteristic high content of hydroxyproline (about 10%). Vitamin C is required for hydroxylation of the collagen propeptide, a requirement that explains inadequate wound healing in vitamin C deficiency (scurvy) (Chapter 10). After the modifications, the procollagen chains align and form the triple helix. At this stage, the procollagen molecule is still soluble and contains N-terminal and C-terminal propeptides. During or shortly after secretion from the cell, procollagen peptidases clip the terminal propeptide chains, promoting formation of fibrils, often called *tropocollagen.* A defect in collagen structure can result in failure of aminoprotease to cleave procollagen and defective fiber formation, as seen in Ehlers-Danlos type VII (Chapter 6). Accompanying fibril formation is the oxidation of specific lysine and hydroxylysine residues by the extracellular enzyme lysyl oxidase. This results in *cross-linkages* between α chains of adjacent molecules stabilizing the array that is characteristic of collagen. *Cross-*

Table 4–2. MAJOR TYPES OF COLLAGEN

Type	Characteristics	Distribution
I	Bundles of banded fibers with high tensile strength	Skin (80%), bone (90%), tendons, most other organs
II	Thin fibrils; structural protein	Cartilage (50%), vitreous humor
III	Thin fibrils; pliable	Blood vessels, uterus, skin (10%)
IV	Amorphous	All basement membranes
V	Amorphous/fine fibrils	2–5% of interstitial tissues, blood vessels
VI	Amorphous/fine fibrils	Interstitial tissues
VII	Anchoring filament	Dermal-epidermal junction
VIII	Probably amorphous	Endothelium-Descemet membrane
IX	Possible role in maturation of cartilage	Cartilage

linking is a major contributor to the tensile strength of collagen.

Elastin, Fibrillin, and Elastic Fibers

Tissues such as blood vessels, skin, uterus, and lung require elasticity for their function. Although tensile strength is provided by members of the collagen family, the ability of these tissues to recoil is provided by elastic fibers.[41] These fibers can stretch to several times their length and then return to their original size after release of the tension. Morphologically, elastic fibers consist of a central core surrounded by a peripheral microfibrillar network. The central core is made largely of *elastin*, a 70-kD protein. Substantial amounts of elastin are found in the

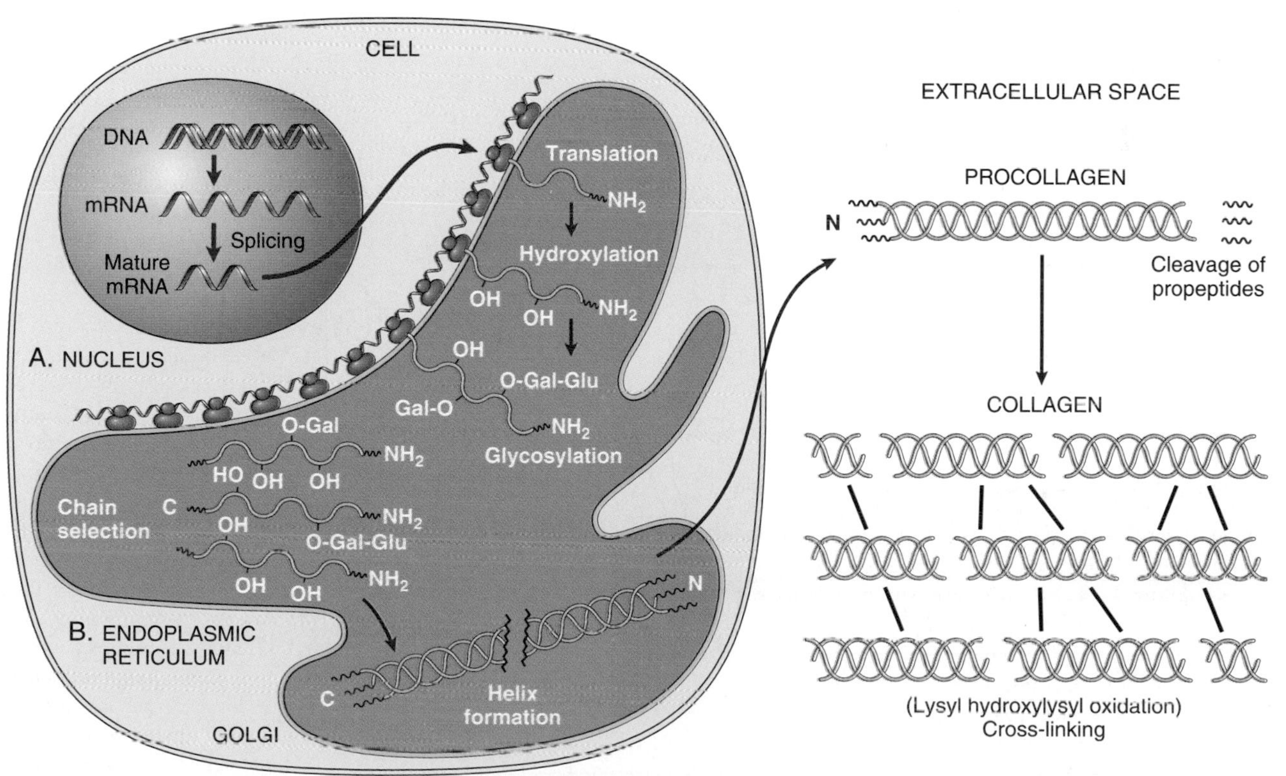

Figure 4–8

Steps in collagen synthesis (see text).

walls of large blood vessels, such as the aorta, and in the uterus, skin, and ligaments. Similar to collagen, one third of the residues of elastin are glycine, and it is rich in proline and alanine; in contrast to collagen, it contains little hydroxyproline and no hydroxylysine residues. Mature elastin contains cross-links that regulate its elasticity.

The peripheral microfibrillar network that surrounds the core consists largely of *fibrillin,* a 350-kD secreted glycoprotein, which associates either with itself or with other components of the ECM.[42] The microfibrils serve as scaffolding for deposition of elastin and the assembly of elastic fibers. Inherited defects in fibrillin result in formation of abnormal elastic fibers in a fairly common familial disorder, Marfan syndrome, manifested by changes in the cardiovascular system (aortic dissection) and skeleton (Chapter 6).

Adhesive Glycoproteins and Integrins

Adhesive glycoproteins and integrins are structurally diverse proteins whose major property is their ability to bind with other ECM components, on the one hand, and with specific integral cell membrane proteins on the other. *They thus link ECM components to one another and to cells.* We focus on two of the adhesive proteins, laminin and fibronectin, and the integrin family of cell surface receptors; the latter have an important role in assembling signaling complexes at sites of contact between cells and ECM.

Fibronectin is a multifunctional adhesive protein whose primary role is to attach cells to a variety of matrices. It is a large (approximately 450 kDa) glycoprotein consisting of two chains held together by disulfide bonds (Fig. 4–9*A*).[43] Associated with cell surfaces, BMs, and pericellular matrices, fibronectin is produced by fibroblasts, monocytes, endothelial cells, and other cells. Fibronectin binds to a number of ECM components (including collagen, fibrin, and proteoglycans) via specific domains and to cells via receptors that recognize the specific amino acid sequence of the tripeptide arginine-glycine-aspartic acid (abbreviated RGD). The RGD recognition element plays a key role in cell-matrix adhesion. Fibronectin is thought to be directly involved in attachment, spreading, and migration of cells. In addition, it serves to enhance the sensitivity of certain cells, such as capillary endothelial cells, to the proliferative effects of growth factors.

Laminin is the most abundant glycoprotein in BMs. This family of matrix proteins are large (about 820 kD), heterotrimeric cross-shaped structures that span the basal lamina and bind, on the one hand, with specific receptors on the surface of cells and, on the other, with matrix components, such as collagen type IV and heparan sulfate (Fig. 4–9*B*).[44] Laminin is also believed to mediate cell attachment to connective tissue substrates; in culture, it alters the growth, survival, morphology, differentiation, and motility of various cell types. In endothelial cell cultures exposed to FGF, laminin causes alignment of endothelial cells and subsequent capillary tube formation, a critical event in angiogenesis. Other ECMs can also induce capillary tube formation. Laminin and fibronectin, similar to many of the components of the ECM, bind to members of the integrin receptor family.

Integrins are the major family of cell surface receptors that mediate cellular attachment to the ECM. Specific clas-

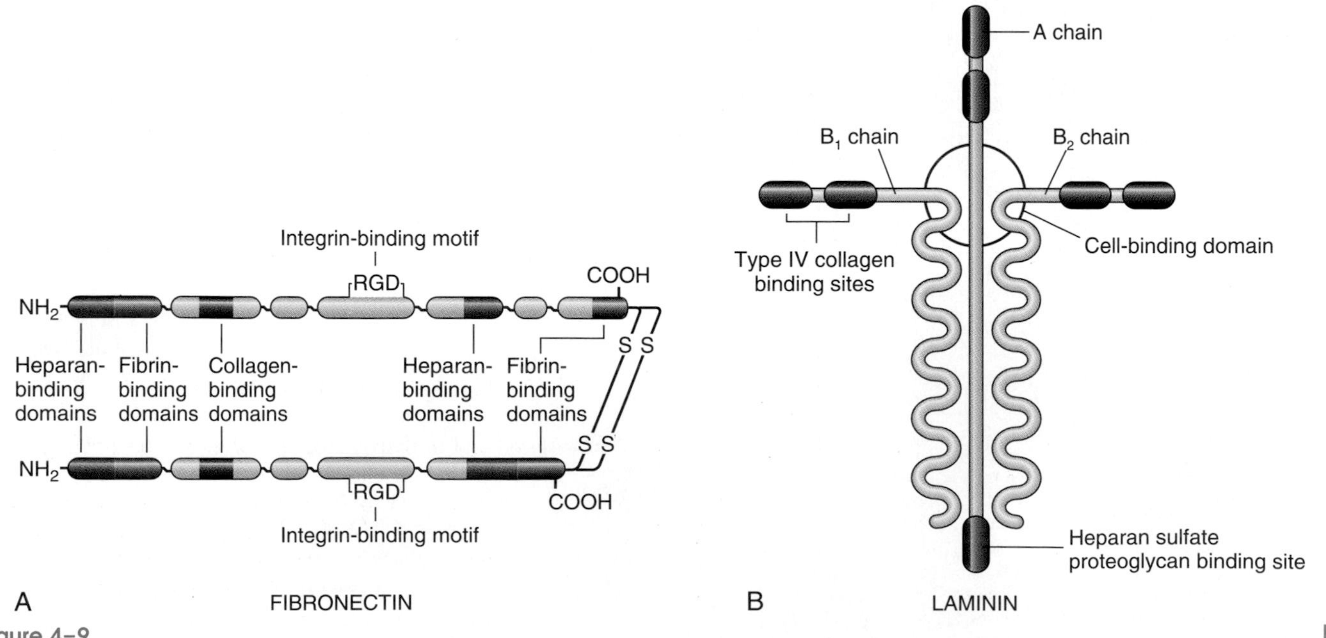

Figure 4–9

The fibronectin molecule (*A*) consists of a dimer held together by S-S bonds. Note the various domains that bind to extracellular matrix and the cell-binding domain containing an arginine-glycine-aspartic acid (RGD) sequence. The cross-shaped laminin (*B*) molecule spans basement membranes and has extracellular matrix (ECM)– and cell-binding domains.

ses of integrins also mediate important cell-cell interactions involved in leukocyte adhesion (Chapter 3). Many integrins are widely expressed, and most cells have more than one integrin on the cell surface. The importance of the integrins is underscored by the crucial functions they play in a wide variety of biologic processes. For example, their role in adhesion makes them key components in leukocyte extravasation (Chapter 3), platelet aggregation (Chapter 5), developmental processes, and wound healing. Additionally, some cells require adhesion to proliferate, and lack of attachment through integrins to an ECM induces apoptosis.

Integrins are transmembrane glycoproteins made up of α and β chains (Fig. 4–10).[45] There are 14 types of α subunits and 8 types of β subunits, generating at least 20 integrin heterodimers. A single β chain can interact with a series of α chains producing integrins that can bind different matrix components. The extracellular domains of the integrins bind to many components in the ECM (e.g., fibronectin, laminin, and some of the collagens) by recognizing the RGD sequence discussed earlier.

Integrin receptors are important both in organizing the actin cytoskeleton of cells and in transduction of signals from the ECM to the cell interior. Integrin receptor engagement by ECM components leads to clustering of the receptors and formation of *focal adhesions*, where integrins link to intracellular cytoskeletal complexes.[46] The proteins that colocalize with integrins in focal adhesions include talin, vinculin, α-actinin, tensin, and paxillin. Once assembled, the integrin-cytoskeletal complexes function similar to activated receptors, and recruit components of the intracellular signaling systems. The subsequent molecular pathways that link ECM proteins to the control of cell growth and differentiation are less clear than those that are involved in cell stimulation by growth factors, described earlier. It is likely, however, that receptors for growth factors and different ECM molecules may share common intracellular pathways, including activation of the MAP kinase, PI-3-kinase, and protein kinase C pathways.

The mechanical linkage between the integrin receptors and the cytoskeletal signaling system may be a mechanism by which cells convert mechanical force into biochemical signals. The *tensegrity* hypothesis suggests that stress applied to the ECM would be transmitted via integrin receptors and a "tensed" cytoskeleton throughout the cell and even into the nucleus, where changes in gene expression occur.[47] The precise molecular connections that provide a discrete path for mechanical signal transfer through cells are now under investigation.

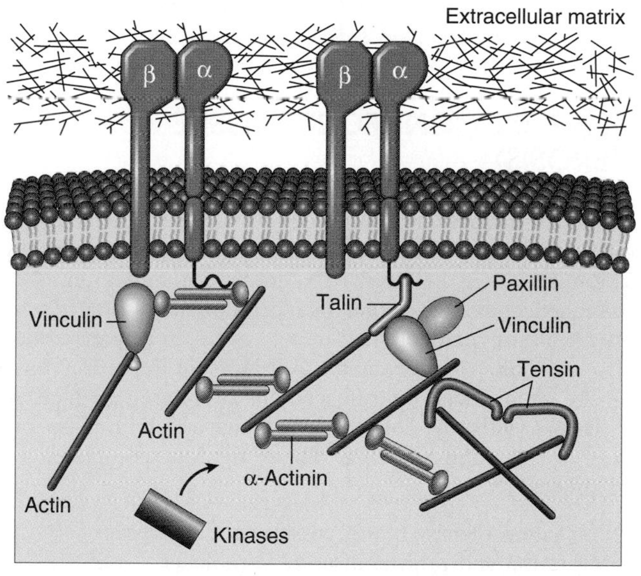

Figure 4–10

Integrins and integrin-mediated signaling events at focal contact sites. The integrins mediate assembly of a signaling complex and redistribution of the cytoskeleton. Each heterodimeric integrin receptor consists of an alpha and a beta chain and is shown interacting with the extracellular matrix. These protein complexes include talin, actin, α-actinin, vinculin, paxillin, and tensin. Ligand occupancy also causes the focal accumulation of a series of signaling molecules and kinases. These complexes generate signals that activate a series of intracellular signaling systems, including the MAP kinase pathway. (Adapted from Hynes RO: Integrins: versatility, modulation and signaling in cell adhesion. Cell 69:11, 1992; and Clark EA, Brugge JS: Integrins and signal transduction pathways: the road taken. Science 268:233, 1995.)

Matricellular Proteins

Matricellular proteins are a newly defined class of secreted proteins that do not function as structural components of the ECM but interact with matrix proteins, cell surface receptors, or other molecules (such as growth factors, cytokines, or proteases) that interact, in turn, with the cell surface. Although diversity of function is inherent in the matricellular proteins, the group shares the ability to disrupt cell-matrix interactions. This family of adapter proteins includes (1) *SPARC* (secreted protein acidic and rich in cysteine), also known as *osteonectin*, which contributes to tissue remodeling in response to injury and functions as an angiogenesis inhibitor[48]; (2) the *thrombospondins*, a family of large multifunctional proteins, some of which, similar to SPARC, also inhibit angiogenesis[49]; (3) *osteopontin*, which was discussed in Chapter 2 because of its potential role in regulating calcification,[50] but which also serves as a mediator of leukocyte migration; and (4) the *tenacin* family members, which are large multimeric proteins involved in morphogenesis and in modulating cell adhesion.[51]

Proteoglycans and Hyaluronan

Proteoglycans and hyaluronan compose the third general type of component in the ECM. *Proteoglycans* consist of a core protein linked to one or more polysaccharides called *glycosaminoglycans*.[52] These are long repeating polymers of specific disaccharides in which one (or both) contains a sulfate residue. Proteoglycans are remarkable in their diversity. A specific ECM may contain several different core proteins, each of which contains different glycosaminoglycans. Proteoglycans are named according to the structure of their principal repeating disaccharide. Some of the most common are heparan sulfate, chondroitin sulfate, and der-

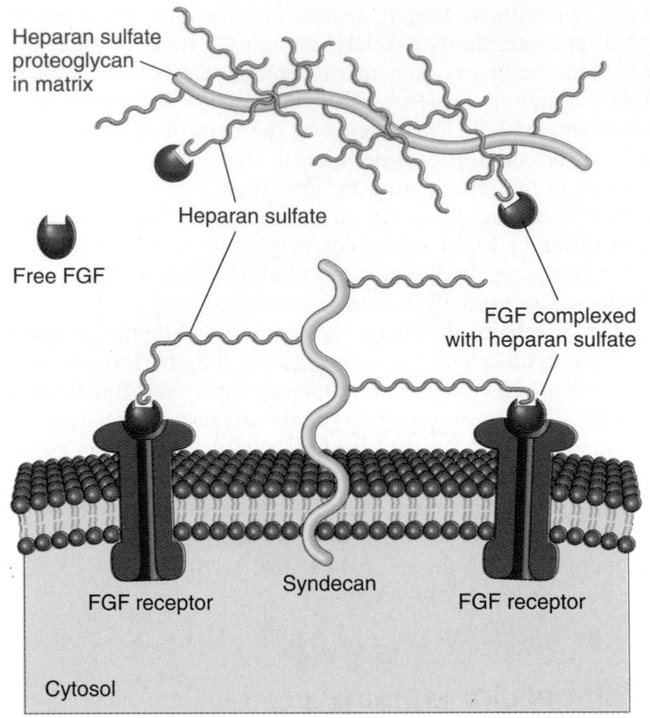

Figure 4–11

Syndecan is a cell surface proteoglycan. Its core protein spans the plasma membrane and contains three heparan sulfate chains and two chondroitin sulfate chains *(not shown)*. The proteoglycans can modulate the activity of fibroblast growth factor (FGF). Free FGF binds poorly to the FGF receptor. Binding of FGF to the heparan sulfate chains like those on syndecan allows FGF to bind efficiently to its receptor. Binding of FGF to heparan sulfate in the ECM protects FGF and forms a reservoir of the growth factor. (Modified from Lodish H, et al [eds]: Molecular Cell Biology, 3rd ed. New York. WH Freeman, 1995, p 1143. © 1995 by Scientific American Books. Used with permission of WH Freeman and Company.)

matan sulfate. They have diverse roles in regulating connective tissue structure and permeability.

Proteoglycans can also be integral membrane proteins and are thus modulators of cell growth and differentiation. For example, in the *syndecan* family, the core protein spans the plasma membrane and contains a short cytosolic domain as well as a long external domain to which a small number of heparan sulfate chains are attached.[53] Syndecan binds collagen, fibronectin, and thrombospondin in the ECM and can modulate the activity of growth factors. For example, binding of FGF to the heparan sulfate chains in syndecan facilitates FGF to binding to its receptor (Fig. 4–11). Syndecan associates with actin cytoskeleton and has been shown to maintain the morphology of epithelial sheets.

Hyaluronan is found in the ECM of many cells. It is a huge molecule that consists of many repeats of a simple disaccharide stretched end-to-end. Hyaluronan serves as a ligand for core proteins such as cartilage link protein, aggrecan, and versican and is often the backbone for large proteoglycan complexes.[54] It also associates with cell surface receptors that regulate cell proliferation and migration, such as CD44. Hyaluronan binds a large amount of water, forming a viscous hydrate gel, which gives connective tissue turgor pressure and an ability to resist compression forces. Because of its ability to bind water and serve as a ligand, this remarkable ECM component helps provide resilience as well as a lubricating feature to many types of connective tissue, notably that found in the cartilage in joints. Hyaluronan is also found in the matrix of cells that are migrating and proliferating, where it inhibits cell-cell adhesion and facilitates cell migration.

Summary of Cell Growth and Differentiation

Cell growth and differentiation involve the cellular integration of multiple signals. Some of these signals are derived from polypeptide growth factors, cytokines, and growth inhibitors. Others are derived from components in the ECM and proceed through integrin-dependent signaling pathways. Although unique pathways may be activated by specific types of receptors, cross-talk between the signaling systems integrates the signals controlling cell proliferation and other cellular events. Figure 4–12 is a model of the interactions between growth factors, ECM, and cell responses.

This concludes the discussion of the control of cell growth by growth factors and interactions with the ECM. We now proceed to discussion of the process of fibrosis—the replacement of parenchyma by connective tissue.

REPAIR BY CONNECTIVE TISSUE (FIBROSIS)

Tissue destruction, with damage to both parenchymal cells and *stromal framework*, occurs in necrotizing inflammation and is a hallmark of chronic inflammation. As a consequence, repair cannot be accomplished solely by regeneration of parenchymal cells, even in organs whose cells are able to regenerate. Attempts at repairing tissue damage then occur by replacement of nonregenerated parenchymal cells by connective tissue, which in time produces *fibrosis* and *scarring*. There are four components to this process:

1. Formation of new blood vessels (angiogenesis)
2. Migration and proliferation of fibroblasts
3. Deposition of ECM
4. Maturation and organization of the fibrous tissue, also known as *remodeling*

Repair begins early in inflammation. Sometimes as early as 24 hours after injury, if resolution has not occurred, fibroblasts and vascular endothelial cells begin proliferating to form (by 3 to 5 days) a specialized type of tissue that is the hallmark of healing, called *granulation tissue*. The term derives from its pink, soft, granular appearance on the surface of wounds, but it is the histologic features that are

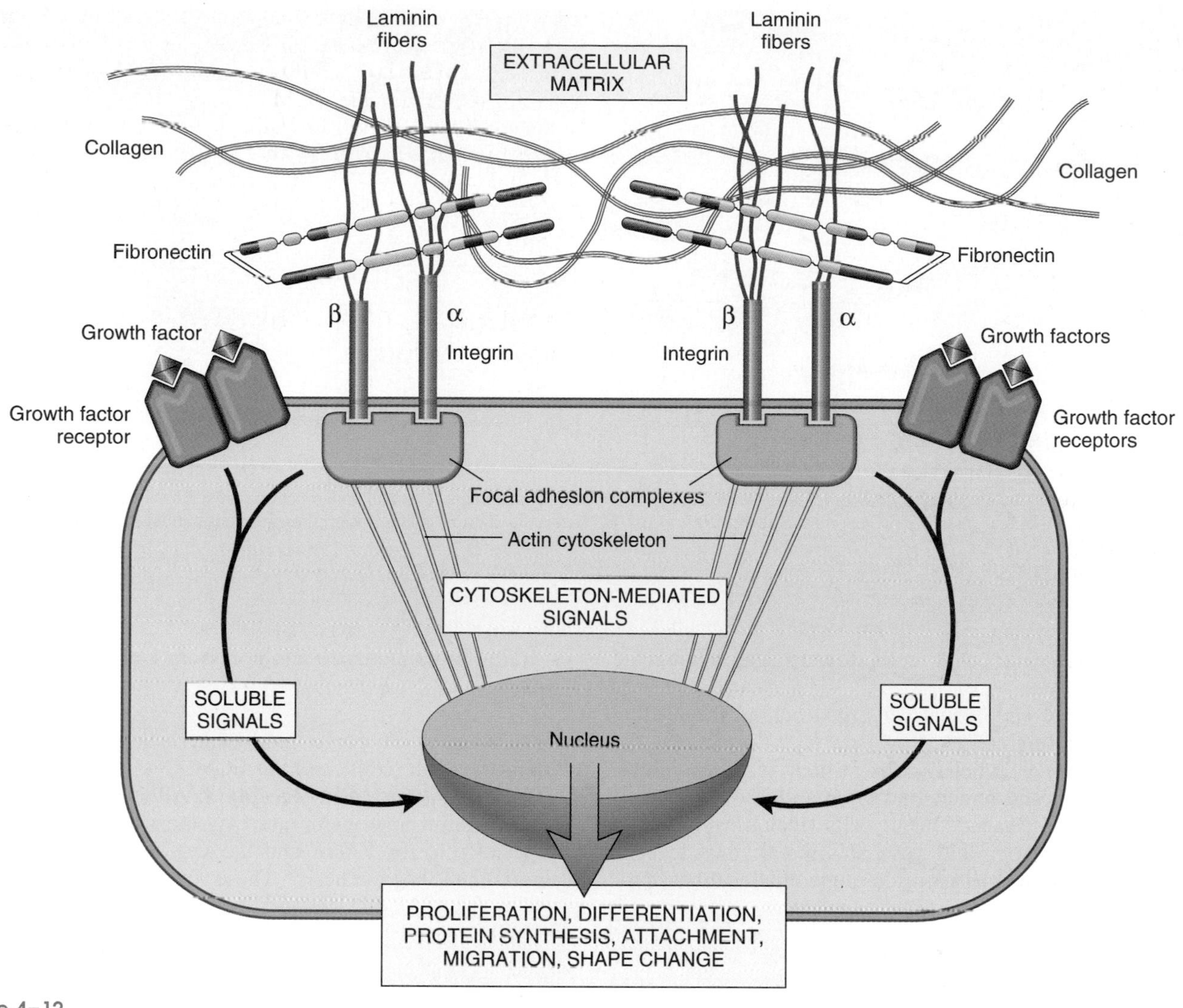

Figure 4–12

Schematic showing the mechanisms by which ECM (e.g., fibronectin and laminin) and growth factors can influence cell growth, motility, differentiation, and protein synthesis. Integrins bind ECM and interact with the cytoskeleton at focal adhesion complexes (protein aggregates that include vinculin, α-actinin, and talin). This can initiate the production of intracellular messengers, or can directly mediate nuclear signals. Cell surface receptors for growth factors also initiate second signals. Collectively, these are integrated by the cell to yield various responses, including changes in cell growth, locomotion, and differentiation.

characteristic: *the formation of new small blood vessels (angiogenesis) and the proliferation of fibroblasts* (Fig. 4–13). These new vessels are leaky, allowing the passage of proteins and red cells into the extravascular space. *Thus, new granulation tissue is often edematous.*

We next discuss mechanisms underlying each one of the components of fibrosis.

Angiogenesis

Blood vessels are assembled by two processes: *vasculogenesis,* in which a primitive vascular network is established during embryonic development from endothelial cell precursors called *angioblasts*; and *angiogenesis*, or *neovascularization*, in which preexisting vessels send out capillary buds or sprouts to produce new vessels.[55] Because angiogenesis is an important process, critical to chronic inflammation and fibrosis, to tumor cell growth, and to the formation of collateral circulation, much work has been done to understand the mechanisms controlling formation of new blood vessels.[56] Both proangiogenic (to increase blood vessels when needed) and antiangiogenic (to block pathologic angiogenesis) therapies are now being explored.

A series of steps are needed in the development of a new capillary vessel during angiogenesis (Fig. 4–14):

- Proteolytic degradation of the BM of the parent vessel to allow formation of a capillary sprout and subsequent cell migration

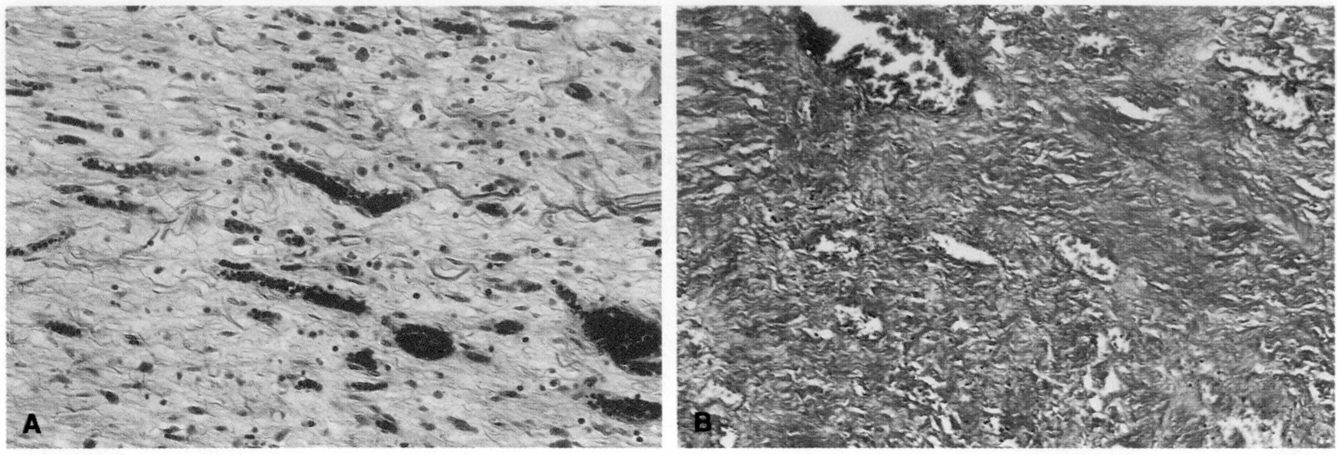

Figure 4–13

A, Granulation tissue showing numerous blood vessels, edema, and a loose ECM containing occasional inflammatory cells. This is a trichrome stain that stains collagen blue; minimal mature collagen can be seen at this point. *B*, Trichrome stain of mature scar, showing dense collagen, with only scattered vascular channels.

- Migration of endothelial cells toward the angiogenic stimulus
- Proliferation of endothelial cells, just behind the leading front of migrating cells
- Maturation of endothelial cells, which includes inhibition of growth and remodeling into capillary tubes
- Recruitment of periendothelial cells (including pericytes for small capillaries and vascular smooth muscle cells for larger vessels) to support the endothelial tubes, providing a maintenance and accessory cell function for the vessel

All these steps are controlled by interactions among growth factors, vascular cells, and the ECM.

Growth Factors and Receptors. Although many growth factors exhibit angiogenic activity, most evidence points to a special role for *VEGF* and the *angiopoietins* in vasculogenesis and angiogenesis. These factors are secreted by

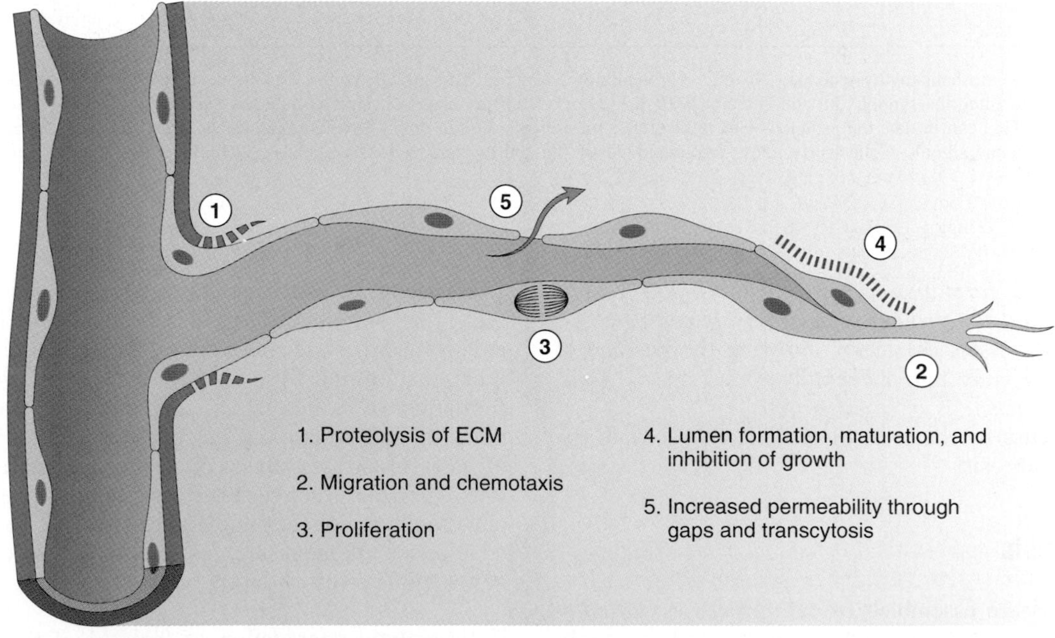

Figure 4–14

Steps in the process of angiogenesis (see text). (Modified from Motamed K, Sage EH: Regulation of vascular morphogenesis by SPARC. Kidney Int 51: 1383, 1997.)

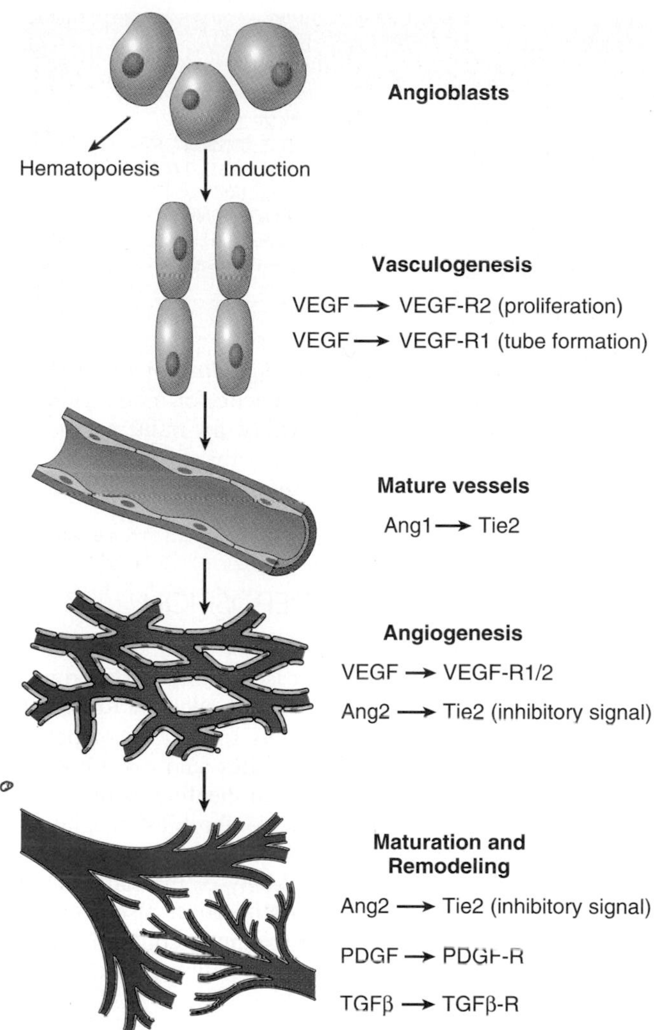

Figure 4–15 ■

Regulation of vascular morphogenesis by receptor tyrosine kinases and their ligands. The establishment of blood vessels during development, or vasculogenesis, requires the interaction of VEGF with VEGF-R2 to induce the proliferation of endothelial cells. VEGF binding to VEGF-R1 stimulates formation of capillary tubes. In mature vessels, Ang1 binding to Tie2 recruits and maintains the association of periendothelial supporting cells (e.g., pericytes, smooth muscle cells), stabilizing a newly formed blood vessel. At sites of angiogenesis and vessel remodeling, Ang2 provides a negative signal that causes vessel structures to become loosened, reducing endothelial cell contacts with the matrix and with supporting cells. This allows access to angiogenic inducers (and inhibitors). Other growth factors, such as platelet-derived growth factor (PDGF) and transforming growth factor β (TGF-β), and their corresponding receptors (PDGF-R and TGF-βR), are also important for proper vascular maturation and remodeling. (Modified from Risau W: Mechanisms of angiogenesis. Nature 386:671, 1997; and Hanahan D: Signaling vascular morphogenesis and maintenance. Science 277:48, 1997.)

many mesenchymal and stromal cells, but their receptors—all of which have tyrosine kinase activity—are largely restricted to endothelium. They contribute to vascular development in embryogenesis and to angiogenesis in adults. A model (Fig. 4–15) for their sequential actions, derived largely from studies in embryos,[57] is as follows: In early vascular development, VEGF binds to one of its receptors (VEGF-R2) on *angioblasts* and induces the formation and proliferation of endothelial cells. Subsequently, VEGF binding to a second distinct receptor (VEGF-R1) induces tube formation characteristic of capillaries. The further progression of angiogenesis appears to be controlled by the angiopoietins (Ang1 and Ang2). Ang1 interacts with a receptor on endothelial cells, called Tie2, to recruit a set of periendothelial cells, which serve to *stabilize* newly formed vessels.[58] The Ang1/Tie2 interaction mediates vessel maturation from simple endothelial tubes into more elaborate vascular structures and helps maintain endothelial quiescence. Ang2, in contrast, also interacting with Tie2, has the opposite effect, loosening endothelial cells such that they become either more responsive to stimulation by growth factors such as VEGF or, in the absence of VEGF, more responsive to inhibitors of angiogenesis.[59] A telling proof of the importance of these molecules is the existence of a genetic disorder, characterized by venous malformations, that is caused by mutations in Tie2.[60] In addition, transgenic mice that are deficient in these molecules show alterations in vasculogenesis and angiogenesis.

bFGF is a powerful angiogenic factor, but VEGF emerges as the most important growth factor in adult tissues undergoing physiologic angiogenesis (e.g., proliferating endometrium) and in the pathologic angiogenesis seen in chronic inflammation, wound healing, tumors, and such conditions as retinopathy of prematurity (retrolental fibroplasia) (Chapter 31). VEGF expression is stimulated by certain cytokines and growth factors (e.g., TGF-β, PDGF, TGF-α) and, notably, by tissue hypoxia, which has long been associated with angiogenesis (Table 4–3).[33] Other growth factors, such as PDGF and TGF-β, and their corre-

Table 4–3. VASCULAR ENDOTHELIAL GROWTH FACTOR (VEGF)

Proteins	Family members: VEGF, VEGF-B, VEGF-C, PIGF Dimeric glycoprotein with multiple isoforms Targeted mutations in VEGF resulted in defective vasculogenesis and angiogenesis
Production	Expressed at low levels in a variety of adult tissues and at higher levels in a few sites, such as podocytes in the glomerulus and cardiac myocytes
Inducing agents	Hypoxia TGF-β PDGF TGF-α
Receptors	VEGF-R1 VEGF-R2 Restricted to endothelial cells Targeted mutations in the receptors resulted in lack of vasculogenesis
Functions	Promotes angiogenesis Increases vascular permeability Stimulates endothelial cell migration Stimulates endothelial cell proliferation VEGF-C selectively induces hyperplasia of lymphatic vasculature Up-regulates endothelial expression of plasminogen activator, plasminogen activator inhibitor-1, tissue factor, and interstitial collagenase

sponding receptors (PDGF-R and TGF-βR) are also important for proper vascular maturation and remodeling (Fig. 4–15).

Extracellular Matrix Proteins as Regulators of Angiogenesis. A key component of angiogenesis is the motility and directed migration of endothelial cells. These processes are controlled by several classes of proteins, including *integrins*, especially $\alpha_v\beta_3$, which is critical for the formation and maintenance of newly formed blood vessels[61]; *matricellular proteins*, including thrombospondin 1, SPARC, and tenascin C, which destabilize cell-matrix interactions and therefore promote angiogenesis[49]; and *proteases*, such as the plasminogen activators and matrix metalloproteases, discussed subsequently, which are important in remodeling events during endothelial invasion. Additionally, these proteases cleave extracellular proteins producing cleavage products that regulate angiogenesis.[62] For example, *endostatin* is a small fragment of a specific type of collagen that inhibits endothelial proliferation and angiogenesis.[63]

Fibrosis (Fibroplasia)

Fibrosis or fibroplasia occurs within the granulation tissue framework of new blood vessels and loose ECM that initially form at the repair site. Two processes are involved in fibrosis: (1) *emigration and proliferation of fibroblasts in the site of injury* and (2) *deposition of ECM* by these cells.

FIBROBLAST PROLIFERATION

Granulation tissue contains numerous newly formed blood vessels. As discussed previously, VEGF promotes angiogenesis but also is responsible for a marked increase in vascular permeability. The latter activity leads to increased deposition of plasma proteins, such as fibrinogen and plasma fibronectin, in the ECM and provides a provisional stroma for fibroblast (and endothelial cell) ingrowth. Migration of fibroblasts to the site of injury and their subsequent *proliferation* are triggered by multiple growth factors, including TGF-β, PDGF, EGF, FGF, and the so-called fibrogenic cytokines, interleukin-1 (IL-1) and TNF-α. The sources of these growth factors include platelets and a variety of inflammatory cells as well as activated endothelium. Macrophages, for example, are important cellular constituents of granulation tissue, responsible for clearing extracellular debris, fibrin, and other foreign material at the site of repair. These cells also elaborate TGF-β, PDGF, and bFGF and therefore promote fibroblast migration and proliferation. If the appropriate chemotactic stimuli are present, mast cells, eosinophils, and lymphocytes may be increased in number. Each of these can contribute directly or indirectly to fibroblast migration and proliferation. Of the growth factors involved in inflammatory fibrosis, TGF-β appears to be the most important because of the multitude of effects that favor fibrous tissue deposition. TGF-β is produced by most of the cells in granulation tissue and causes *fibroblast migration and proliferation, increased synthesis of collagen and fibronectin, and decreased degradation of ECM by metalloproteinases* (discussed later). TGF-β is also chemotactic for monocytes and causes angiogenesis in vivo, possibly by inducing macrophage influx. TGF-β expression is increased in tissues in a number of chronic fibrotic diseases in humans and experimental animals.

Table 4–4. GROWTH FACTORS IN WOUND HEALING

Monocyte chemotaxis	PDGF, FGF, TGF-β
Fibroblast migration	PDGF, EGF, FGF, TGF-β, TNF
Fibroblast proliferation	PDGF, EGF, FGF, TNF
Angiogenesis	VEGF, Ang, FGF
Collagen synthesis	TGF-β, PDGF, TNF
Collagenase secretion	PDGF, FGF, EGF, TNF, TGF-β inhibits

EXTRACELLULAR MATRIX DEPOSITION

As repair progresses, the number of proliferating endothelial cells and fibroblasts decreases. Fibroblasts progressively become more synthetic and deposit increased amounts of ECM. Fibrillar collagens form a major portion of the connective tissue in repair sites and are important for the development of strength in healing wounds. As described later, collagen synthesis by fibroblasts begins relatively early (days 3 to 5) and continues for several weeks, depending on the size of wound. Many of the same growth factors that regulate fibroblast proliferation also stimulate ECM synthesis (Table 4–4). For example, collagen synthesis is enhanced by several factors, including growth factors (PDGF, FGF, TGF-β) and cytokines (IL-1, IL-4), which are secreted by leukocytes and fibroblasts in healing wounds. *Net collagen accumulation, however, depends not only on synthesis, but also on collagen degradation* (discussed later). Ultimately the granulation tissue scaffolding is converted into a scar composed of spindle-shaped fibroblasts, dense collagen, fragments of elastic tissue, and other ECM components. As the scar matures, vascular regression continues, eventually transforming the richly vascularized granulation tissue into a pale, avascular scar.

Tissue Remodeling

The replacement of granulation tissue with a scar involves transitions in the composition of the ECM. Some of the growth factors that stimulate synthesis of collagen and other connective tissue molecules also modulate the synthesis and activation of *metalloproteinases*, enzymes that serve to degrade these ECM components. The net result of ECM *synthesis* versus *degradation* results in *remodeling* of the connective tissue framework—an important feature of both chronic inflammation and wound repair.

Degradation of collagen and other ECM proteins is achieved by a family of *matrix metalloproteinases*, which are dependent on zinc ions for their activity[64] (Fig. 4–16).

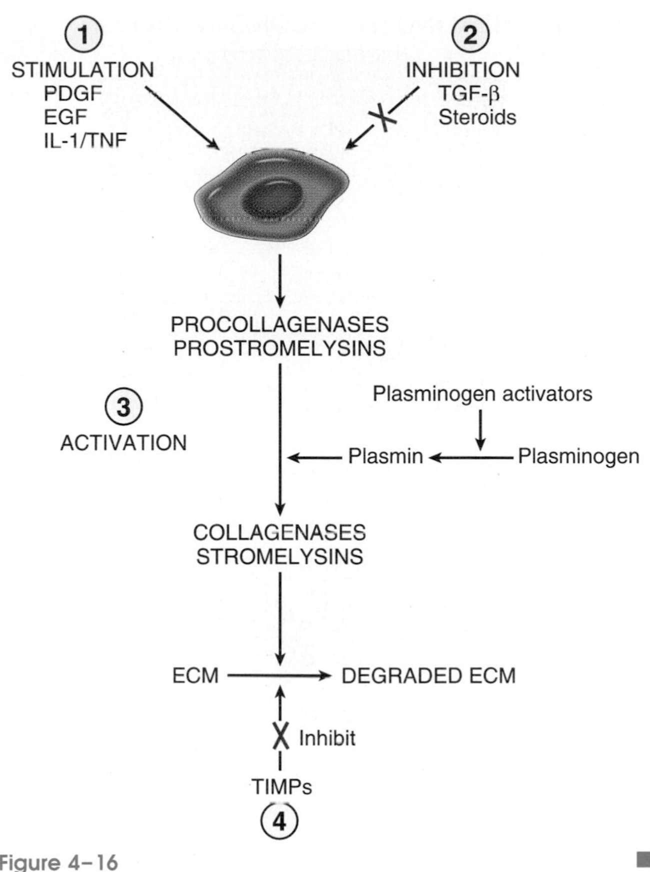

Figure 4–16

Matrix metalloproteinase regulation. The four mechanisms shown include (1) regulation of synthesis by a variety of growth factors or cytokines, (2) inhibition of synthesis by corticosteroids or TGF-β, (3) regulation of the activation of the secreted but inactive precursors, and (4) blockade of the enzymes by specific tissue inhibitors of metalloproteinase (TIMP). (Modified from Matrisian LM: Metalloproteinases and their inhibitors in matrix remodeling. Trends Genet 6:122, 1990, with permission from Elsevier Science.)

(These should be distinguished from neutrophil elastase, cathepsin G, kinins, plasmin, and other important proteolytic enzymes mentioned earlier that can also degrade ECM components, but they are *serine proteinases, not metalloenzymes.*) Metalloproteinases consist of *interstitial collagenases*, which cleave the fibrillar collagen types I, II, and III; *gelatinases* (or *type IV collagenases*), which degrade amorphous collagen as well as fibronectin; *stromelysins*, which act on a variety of ECM components, including proteoglycans, laminin, fibronectin, and amorphous collagens; and the family of *membrane-bound matrix metalloproteinases (MBMM)*, which are cell surface–associated proteases.[65] These enzymes are produced by several cell types (fibroblasts, macrophages, neutrophils, synovial cells, and some epithelial cells), and their secretion is induced by certain stimuli, including growth factors (PDGF, FGF), cytokines (IL-1, TNF-α), phagocytosis, and physical stress. It is inhibited by TGF-β and steroids. Collagenases cleave collagen under physiologic conditions, cutting the triple helix into two unequal fragments, which are then susceptible to digestion by other proteases. This is potentially harmful to the organism, but the enzyme is elaborated in a latent (procollagenase) form that needs to be activated by chemicals, such as HOCl· (produced, as you recall, during the oxidative burst of leukocytes) and proteases (plasmin).

Once formed, activated matrix metalloproteinases are rapidly inhibited by a family of specific *tissue inhibitors of metalloproteinase (TIMP)* which are produced by most mesenchymal cells,[66] thus preventing uncontrolled action of these proteinases (Fig. 4–16). Collagenases and their inhibitors have been shown to be spatially and temporally regulated in healing wounds. They are essential in the debridement of injured sites and in the remodeling of connective tissue necessary to repair the defect.

WOUND HEALING

Wound healing is a complex but orderly phenomenon involving a number of processes:[67]

- *Induction of an acute inflammatory process by the initial injury*
- *Regeneration of parenchymal cells*
- *Migration and proliferation of both parenchymal and connective tissue cells*
- *Synthesis of ECM proteins*
- *Remodeling of connective tissue and parenchymal components*
- *Collagenizaton and acquisition of wound strength*

The mechanisms underlying most of these events have already been discussed and involve the mediators of acute inflammation (Chapter 3); the role of growth factors; cell-ECM interactions in cell migration, proliferation, and differentiation; and the mechanisms of angiogenesis and fibrosis, outlined earlier in this chapter. We discuss wound healing in the skin to illustrate the general principles of wound healing that apply to all tissues.[68] Each organ, however, as we see in later chapters, contains specialized cells that provide some organ specificity to the healing response.

Healing by First Intention (Wounds With Opposed Edges)

The least complicated example of wound repair is the healing of a clean, uninfected surgical incision approximated by surgical sutures (Fig. 4–17). Such healing is referred to as *primary union* or *healing by first intention.* The incision causes death of a limited number of epithelial cells and connective tissue cells as well as disruption of epithelial BM continuity. The narrow incisional space immediately fills with clotted blood containing fibrin and blood cells; dehydration of the surface clot forms the well-known scab that covers the wound.

Within 24 hours, neutrophils appear at the margins of the incision, moving toward the fibrin clot. The epidermis at its cut edges thickens *as a result of mitotic activity of basal cells*, and within 24 to 48 hours, spurs of epithelial

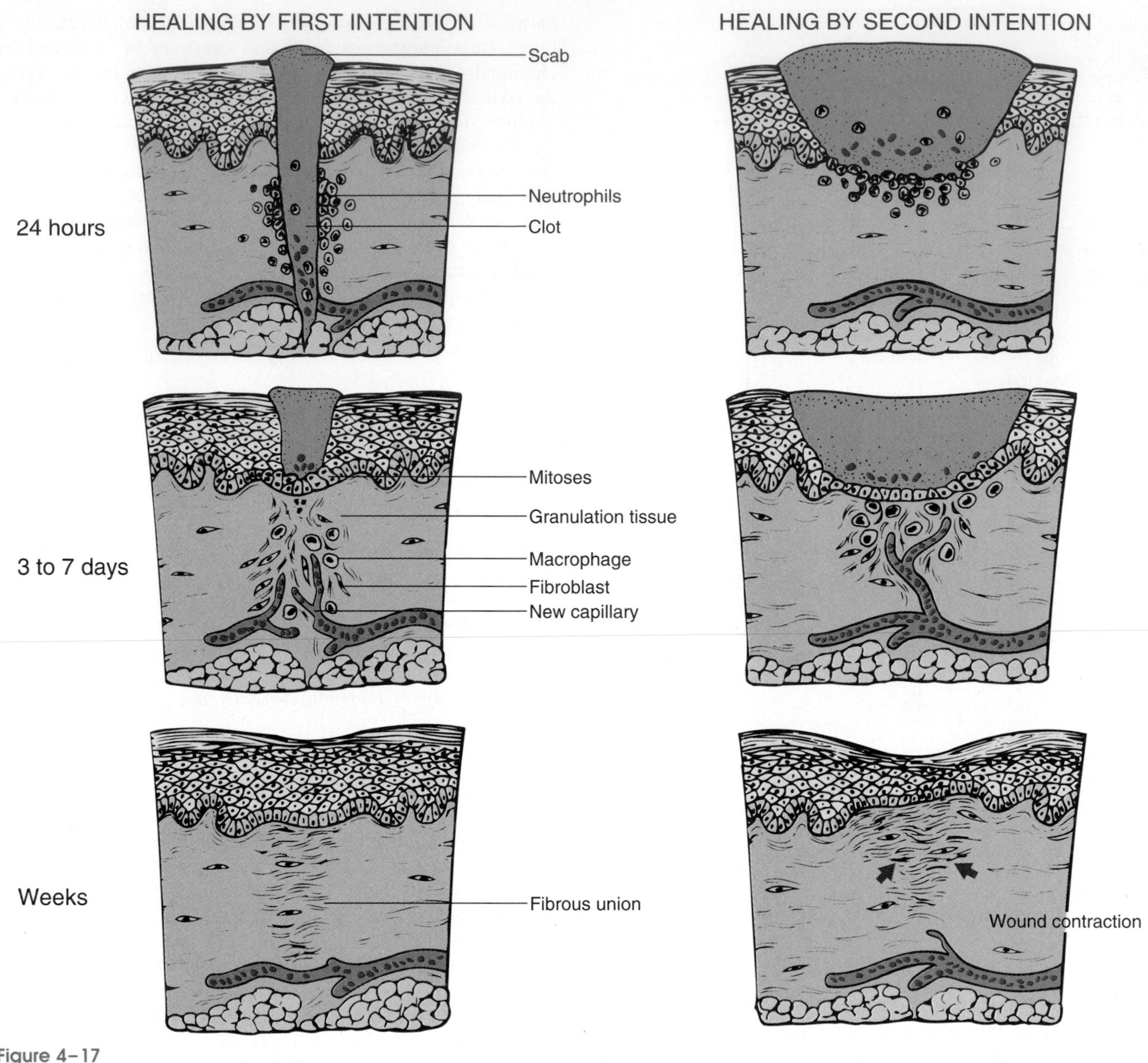

Figure 4–17

Steps in wound healing by first intention *(left)* and second intention *(right).* In the latter, the resultant scar is much smaller than the original wound owing to wound contraction.

cells from the edges both migrate and grow along the cut margins of the dermis, depositing BM components as they move. They fuse in the midline beneath the surface scab, thus producing a continuous but thin epithelial layer.

By day 3, the neutrophils have been largely replaced by macrophages. *Granulation tissue* progressively invades the incision space. Collagen fibers are now present in the margins of the incision, but at first these are vertically oriented and do not bridge the incision. Epithelial cell proliferation continues, thickening the epidermal covering layer.

By day 5, the incisional space is filled with granulation tissue. Neovascularization is maximal. Collagen fibrils become more abundant and begin to bridge the incision. The epidermis recovers its normal thickness, and differentiation of surface cells yields a mature epidermal architecture with surface keratinization.

During the second week, there is continued accumulation of collagen and proliferation of fibroblasts. The leukocytic infiltrate, edema, and increased vascularity have largely disappeared. At this time, the long process of blanching begins, accomplished by the increased accumulation of collagen within the incisional scar, accompanied by regression of vascular channels.

By the end of the first month, the scar comprises a cellular connective tissue devoid of inflammatory infiltrate, covered now by intact epidermis (Fig. 4–17). The dermal appendages that have been destroyed in the line of the incision are permanently lost. Tensile strength of the wound increases thereafter, but it may take months for the wounded area to obtain its maximal strength. Although most skin lesions heal efficiently, the end product may not be functionally perfect. Epidermal appendages do not regenerate, and there remains a dense connective tissue scar in place of the mechanically efficient meshwork of collagen in the unwounded dermis.

Healing by Second Intention (Wounds With Separated Edges)

When there is more extensive loss of cells and tissue, as occurs in infarction, inflammatory ulceration, abscess formation, and surface wounds that create large defects, the reparative process is more complicated (Fig. 4–17). *The common denominator in all these situations is a large tissue defect that must be filled.* Regeneration of parenchymal cells cannot completely reconstitute the original architecture. Abundant granulation tissue grows in from the margin to complete the repair. This form of healing is referred to as *secondary union* or *healing by second intention.* Secondary healing differs from primary healing in several respects:

1. Inevitably, large tissue defects initially have more fibrin and more necrotic debris and exudate that must be removed. Consequently the *inflammatory reaction is more intense.*
2. *Much larger amounts of granulation tissue are formed.* When a large defect occurs in deeper tissues, such as in a viscus, granulation tissue with its numerous scavenger white cells bears the full responsibility for its closure because drainage to the surface cannot occur.
3. Perhaps the feature that most clearly differentiates primary from secondary healing is the phenomenon of *wound contraction,* which occurs in large surface wounds. Large defects in the skin of a rabbit are reduced in approximately 6 weeks to 5 to 10% of their original size, largely by contraction. Contraction has been ascribed, at least in part, to the presence of *myofibroblasts*—altered fibroblasts that have the ultrastructural characteristics of smooth muscle cells.

Whether a wound heals by primary or secondary intention is determined by the nature of the wound, rather than by the healing process itself.

Wound Strength

We now turn to the questions of how long it takes for a skin wound to achieve its maximal strength, and which substances contribute to this strength. When sutures are removed, usually at the end of the first week, wound strength is approximately 10% of the strength of unwounded skin, but it increases rapidly over the next 4 weeks. This rate of increase then slows at approximately the third month after the original incision and then reaches a plateau at about 70 to 80% of the tensile strength of unwounded skin, which may persist for life. The recovery of tensile strength results from increased collagen synthesis exceeding collagen degradation during the first 2 months and from structural modifications of collagen fibers (cross-linking, increased fiber size), when collagen synthesis ceases at later times.

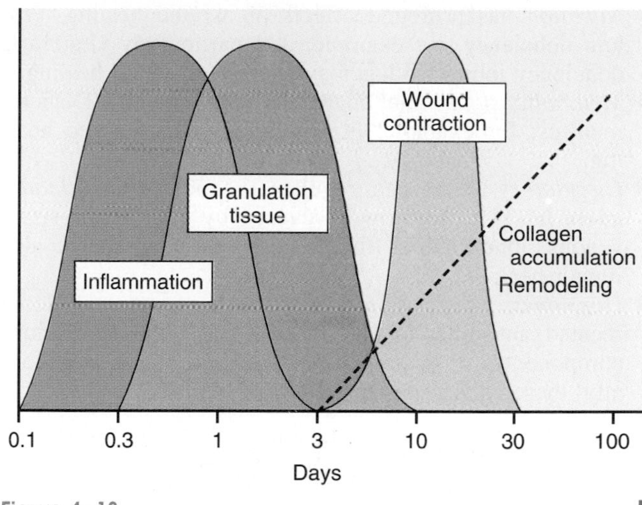

Figure 4–18 ■

Orderly phases of wound healing. (Modified from Clark RA: In Goldsmith LA (ed): Physiology, Biochemistry and Molecular Biology of the Skin, 2nd ed., Vol I. New York, Oxford University Press, 1991, p 577.)

To summarize, the healing wound, as a prototype of tissue repair, is a dynamic and changing process (Fig. 4–18). The early phase is one of inflammation, followed by a stage of fibroplasia, followed by tissue remodeling and scarring. Different mechanisms occurring at different times trigger the release of chemical signals that modulate the orderly migration, proliferation, and differentiation of cells and the synthesis and degradation of ECM proteins. These proteins, in turn, directly affect cellular events and modulate cell responsiveness to soluble growth factors. The magic behind the seemingly precise orchestration of these events under normal conditions remains beyond our grasp but almost certainly lies in the regulation of specific soluble mediators and their receptors on particular cells; cell-matrix interactions; and a controlling effect of physical factors, including forces generated by changes in cell shape.

Local and Systemic Factors That Influence Wound Healing

We have discussed the usual manifestations of repair, and we reviewed the orderly healing of wounds in normal persons. But these processes are modified by a number of known influences and some unknown ones, frequently impairing the quality and adequacy of both inflammation and repair. These influences include both *systemic and local host factors*. Systemic factors include the following:

- *Nutrition* has profound effects on wound healing. Protein deficiency, for example, and particularly vitamin C deficiency inhibit collagen synthesis and retard healing.
- *Metabolic status* can change wound healing. Diabetes mellitus, for example, is associated with delayed healing.
- *Circulatory status* can regulate wound healing. *Inadequate blood supply* usually caused by arteriosclerosis or venous abnormalities that retard venous drainage also impair healing.
- *Hormones*, such as *glucocorticoids*, have well-documented anti-inflammatory effects that influence various components of inflammation and fibroplasia; additionally, these agents inhibit collagen synthesis.

Local factors that influcence healing include the following:

- *Infection* is the single most important cause of delay in healing.
- *Mechanical factors*, such as early motion of wounds, can delay healing.
- *Foreign bodies*, such as unnecessary sutures or fragments of steel, glass, or even bone, constitute impediments to healing.
- *Size, location, and type of wound influence healing.* Wounds in richly vascularized areas, such as the face, heal faster than those in poorly vascularized ones, such as the foot. As we have discussed, small injuries produced intentionally heal faster than larger ones caused by blunt trauma.

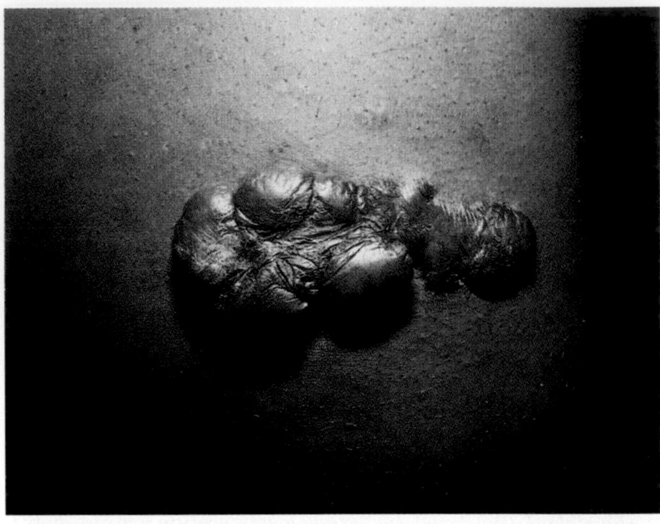

Figure 4–19

Keloid. (From Murphy GF, Herzberg AJ: Atlas of Dermatopathology. Philadelphia, WB Saunders, 1996, p 219.)

Pathologic Aspects of Wound Repair

Complications in wound healing can arise from abnormalities in any of the basic repair processes. These aberrations can be grouped into three general categories: (1) *deficient scar formation*, (2) *excessive formation of the repair components*, and (3) *formation of contractures.* Examples of each of these types of healing abnormalities are discussed.

Inadequate formation of granulation tissue or assembly of a scar can lead to two types of complications: *wound dehiscence* and *ulceration*. Dehiscence or rupture of a wound is most common after abdominal surgery and is due to increased abdominal pressure. This mechanical stress on the abdominal wound can be generated by vomiting, coughing, or ileus. Wounds can ulcerate because of inadequate vascularization during healing. For example, lower extremity wounds in individuals with atherosclerotic peripheral vascular disease typically ulcerate (Chapter 12). Nonhealing wounds also form in areas devoid of sensation. These neuropathic ulcers are occasionally seen in patients with diabetic peripheral neuropathy (Chapters 20 and 29).

Excessive formation of the components of the repair process can also complicate wound healing. Aberrations of growth may occur even in what may begin initially as normal wound healing. The accumulation of excessive amounts of collagen may give rise to a raised tumorous scar known as a *keloid,* or *hypertrophic scar* (Fig. 4–19). Keloid formation appears to be an individual predisposition, and for reasons unknown this aberration is somewhat more common in blacks. The mechanisms of keloid formation are still unknown. Another deviation in wound healing is the formation of excessive amounts of granulation tissue, which protrudes above the level of the surrounding skin and in fact blocks re-epithelialization. This has been called *exuberant granulation* (or, with more literary fervor, *proud flesh*). Excessive granulations must be removed by cautery or surgical excision to permit restoration of the continuity of the epithelium. Finally (fortunately rarely), incisional scars or traumatic injuries may be followed by exuberant proliferations of fibroblasts and other connective tissue elements that may, in fact, recur after excision. Called *desmoids*, or *aggressive fibromatoses*, these lie in the interface between benign proliferations and malignant (though low-grade) tumors. The line between the benign hyperplasias characteristic of repair and neoplasia is frequently finely drawn (Chapter 8).

Contraction in the size of a wound is an important part in the normal healing process. An exaggeration of this process is called a *contracture* and results in deformities of the wound and the surrounding tissues. Contractures are particularly prone to develop on the palms, the soles, and the anterior aspect of the thorax. Contractures are commonly seen after serious burns and can compromise the movement of joints.

The mechanisms underlying the fibroplasia of wound repair—cell proliferation, cell-cell interactions, cell-matrix interactions, and ECM deposition—are similar to those that occur in the chronic inflammatory fibrosis of such diseases as rheumatoid arthritis, lung fibrosis, and hepatic cirrhosis. In contrast to orderly wound healing, however, the diseases are associated with persistence of initial stimuli for fibroplasia or the development of immune and autoimmune reactions. In such reactions, lymphocyte-monocyte interactions sustain the synthesis and secretion of growth factors and fibrogenic cytokines, proteolytic enzymes, and other biologically active molecules. Collagen degradation

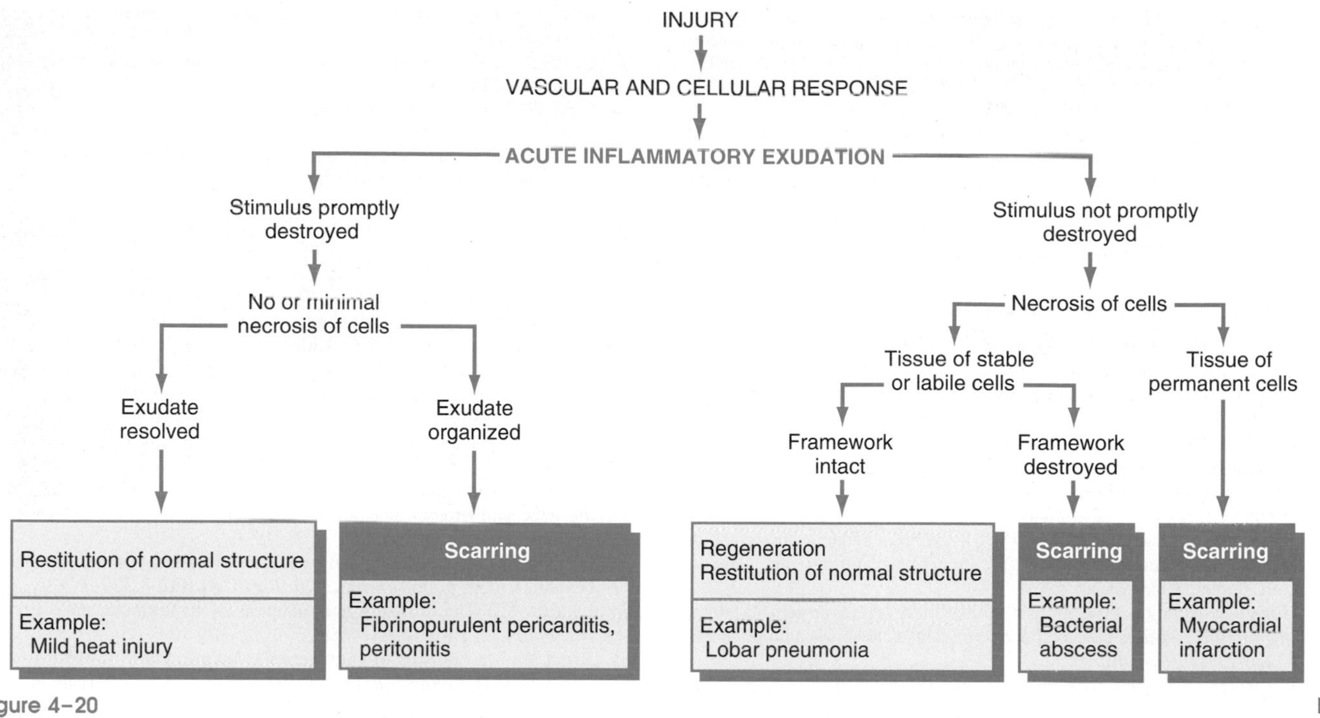

Figure 4–20

Pathways of reparative responses after acute inflammatory injury.

by collagenases, for example, which is important in the normal remodeling of healing wounds, causes much of the joint destruction in rheumatoid arthritis (Chapter 28).

OVERVIEW OF THE INFLAMMATORY-REPARATIVE RESPONSE

This concludes the discussion, begun in Chapter 1, of cellular and tissue injury, the reaction to such injury by the inflammatory process (Chapter 3), and the events underlying repair of injured cells and tissue by regeneration or fibrosis. At this point, a backward look may help relate the multitude of changes that occur simultaneously or sequentially in various forms of injury and the subsequent inflammatory repair process. Figure 4–20 offers an overview of the possible pathways. This schema reemphasizes certain important concepts. Not all injuries result in permanent damage; some are resolved with almost perfect return of normal structure and function. More often, the injury and inflammatory response result in residual scarring. Although it is functionally imperfect, the scarring provides a permanent patch that permits the residual parenchyma more or less to continue functioning. Sometimes, however, the scar itself is so large or so situated that it may cause permanent dysfunction, as in a healed myocardial infarct. In this case, the fibrous tissue not only represents a loss of preexisting contractile muscle, but also constitutes a permanent burden to the overworked residual muscle. Not shown in the figure are the pathways to chronic inflammation, which are described in Chapter 3. In chronic inflammation, persistent injury commonly results in tissue destruction and scarring.

The processes of inflammation and repair underscore the remarkable capacity of the human body to restore itself, far surpassing any device made by humans.

REFERENCES

1. McCarthy NJ, et al: Apoptosis in the development of the immune system: growth factors, clonal selection, and bcl-2. Cancer Metastasis Rev 11:157, 1992.
2. Baserga R: The Biology of Cell Reproduction. Cambridge, MA, Harvard University Press, 1985.
3. Hunter T: Oncoprotein networks. Cell 86:333, 1997.
4. Sporn MB, Roberts AB: Autocrine secretion—10 years later. Ann Intern Med 117:408, 1992.
5. Marshall CJ: Specificity of receptor tyrosine kinase signaling: transient versus sustained extracellular signal-regulated kinase activation. Cell 80:179, 1995.
6. Ihle JN: Cytokine receptor signalling. Nature 377:591, 1995.
7. Neer EJ: Heterotrimeric G proteins: organizers of transmembrane signals. Cell 80:249, 1995.
8. Macara IG, et al: The ras superfamily of GTPases. FASEB J 10:625, 1996.
9. Seger R, Krebs EG: The MAPK signaling cascade. FASEB J 9:726, 1995.
10. Carpenter CL, Cantley LC: Phosphatidylinositol kinases. Curr Opin Cell Biol 8:153, 1996.
11. Hemmings BA: Akt signaling: linking membrane events to life and death decisions. Science 275:628, 1997.
12. Berridge ME: Inositol triphosphate and calcium signaling. Nature 361:315, 1993.
13. Montminy MR: Transcriptional regulation by cAMP. Annu Rev Biochem 66:807, 1997.

14. Darnell JE: STATs and gene regulation. Science 277:1630, 1997.
15. Kyriakis JM, Avruch J: Sounding the alarm: protein kinase cascades activated by stress and inflammation. J Biol Chem 271:24313, 1996.
16. Tjian R, Maniatis T: Transcriptional activation: a complex puzzle with few easy pieces. Cell 77:5, 1994.
17. Hill CS, Treisman R: Transcriptional regulation by extracellular signals: mechanisms and specificity. Cell 80:199, 1995.
18. Hunter T, Pines J: Cyclins and cancer: II. Cyclin D and CDK inhibitors come of age. Cell 89:573, 1994.
19. Morgan DO: Principles of CDK regulation. Nature 274:131, 1995.
20. Nasmyth K: Viewpoint: putting the cell cycle in order. Science 274: 1643, 1996.
21. King RW, et al: How proteolysis drives the cell cycle. Science 274: 1652, 1996.
22. Sherr CJ, Roberts JM: Inhibitors of mammalian G1 cyclin-depdendent kinases. Genes Dev 9:1149, 1995.
23. Sherr CJ: Cancer cell cycles. Science 274:1672, 1996.
24. Elledge SJ: Cell cycle checkpoints: preventing an identity crisis. Science 274:1664, 1996.
25. Massague J: TGFβ signaling: receptors, transducers and Mad proteins. Cell 85:947, 1996.
26. Wrana J, Pawson T: Mad about SMADs. Nature 388:28, 1997.
27. Polyak K, et al: Cloning of $p27^{Kip1}$, a cyclin-dependent kinase inhibitor and a potential mediator of extracellular antimitogenic signals. Cell 78:59, 1994.
28. Cohen S: Isolation of a mouse submaxillary gland protein accelerating incisor eruption and eyelid opening in a newborn animal. J Biol Chem 237:1555, 1962.
29. Carpenter G, Cohen S: Epidermal growth factor. J Biol Chem 265: 7709, 1990.
30. Heldin C-H: Structural and functional studies of platelet-derived growth factor. EMBO J 11:4251, 1992.
31. Betsholtz C, Raines EW: Platelet-derived growth factor: a key regulator of connective tissue cells in embryogenesis and pathogenesis. Kidney Int 51:1361, 1997.
32. Friesel RE, Maciag T: Molecular mechanisms of angiogenesis: fibroblast growth factor signal transduction. FASEB J 9:919, 1995.
33. Dvorak HF, et al: Vascular permeability factor/vascular endothelial growth factor, microvascular hyperpermeability, and angiogenesis. Am J Pathol 146:1029, 1995.
34. Jeltsch M, et al: Hyperplasia of lymphatic vessels in VEGF-C transgenic mice. Science 276:1423, 1997.
35. Roberts AB, Sporn MB: The transforming growth factors-β. In Sporn MD, Roberts AB (eds): Handbook of Experimental Pharmacology: Peptide Growth Factors and Their Receptors. New York, Springer-Verlag, 1990, p 419.
36. Munger JS, et al: Latent transforming growth factor-β: structural features and mechanisms of activation. Kidney Int 51:1376, 1997.
37. Vernon RB, Sage EH: Between molecules and morphology: Extracellular matrix and creation of vascular form. Am J Pathol 147:873, 1995.
38. Hay ED (ed): Cell Biology of Extracellular Matrix, 2nd ed. New York, Plenum Press, 1991.
39. Yurchenco PD, O'Rear JJ: Basal lamina assembly. Curr Opin Cell Biol 6:674, 1994.
40. Prockop DJ, Kivirikko KI: Collagens: molecular biology, diseases and potentials for therapy. Ann Rev Biochem 64:403, 1995.
41. Rosenbloom J, et al: Extracellular matrix 4: the elastic fiber. FASEB J 7:1208, 1993.
42. Reinhardt DP: The structure and function of fibrillin. Ciba Found Symp 192:128, 1995.
43. Potts JR, Campbell ID: Fibronectin structure and assembly. Curr Opin Cell Biol 6:648, 1994.
44. Timpl R, Brown JC: The laminins. Matrix Biol 14:275, 1994.
45. Hynes RO: Integrins: versatility, modulation and signaling in cell adhesion. Cell 69:11, 1992.
46. Clark EA, Brugge JS: Integrins and signal transduction pathways: the road taken. Science 268:233, 1995.
47. Wang N, et al: Mechanotransduction across the cell surface and through the cytoplasm. Science 260:1124, 1993.
48. Motamed K, Sage EH: Regulation of vascular morphogenesis by the matricellular protein SPARC. Kidney Int 51:1383, 1997.
49. Bornstein P: Diversity of function is inherent in matricellular proteins: an appraisal of thrombospondin 1. J Cell Biol 130:503, 1995.
50. Rodan GA: Osteopontin overview. Ann N Y Acad Sci 760:1, 1995.
51. Chiquet-Ehrismann R: Tenascins, a growing family of ECM proteins. Experentia 51:853, 1995.
52. Iozzo R: Proteoglycans of the extracellular environment: clues from the gene and protein side offer novel perpectives in molecular diversity and function. FASEB J 10:598, 1996.
53. Bernfield M, et al: Biology of syndecans: a family of transmembrane heparan sulfate proteoglycans. Ann Rev Cell Biol 8:365, 1992.
54. Laurent TC: The structure and function of hyaluronan: an overview. Immunol Cell Biol 74:A1, 1996.
55. Risau W: Mechanisms of angiogenesis. Nature 386:671, 1997.
56. Folkman J, D'Amore PA: Blood vessel formation: what is its molecular basis. Cell 87:1153, 1996.
57. Hanahan D: Signaling vascular morphogenesis and maintenance. Science 277:48, 1997.
58. Davis S, et al: Isolation of angiopoietin-1, a ligand for the TIE2 receptor by secretion-trap expression cloning. Cell 87:1161, 1996.
59. Maisonpierre PC, et al: Angiopoietin-2, a natural antagonist for Tie2 that disrupts in vivo angiogenesis. Science 277:55, 1997.
60. Vikkula M, et al: Vascular dysmorphogenesis caused by an activating mutation in the receptor tyrosine kinase TIE2. Cell 87:1181, 1996.
61. Brooks PC, et al: Requirement of vascular integrin $\alpha v\beta 3$ for angiogenesis. Science 264:569, 1994.
62. Sage EH: Pieces of eight: bioactive fragments of extracellular proteins as regulators of angiogenesis. Trends Cell Biol 7:182, 1997.
63. O'Reilly MS, et al: Endostatin: an endogenous inhibitor of angiogenesis and tumor growth. Cell 88:277, 1997.
64. Goetzl EJ: Matrix metalloproteinases in immunity. J Immunol 156:1, 1996.
65. Turner AJ, Tanzawa K: Mammalian membrane metalloproteinases. FASEB J 11:355, 1997.
66. Stetler-Stevenson WG: Dynamics and matrix turnover during pathologic remodeling of the ECM. Am J Pathol 148:1345, 1996.
67. Clark RAF (ed): The Molecular and Cellular Biology of Wound Repair. New York, Plenum, 1996.
68. Martin P: Wound healing—aiming for perfect skin regeneration. Science 276:75, 1997.

Hemodynamic Disorders, Thrombosis, and Shock

Richard N. Mitchell and Ramzi S. Cotran

EDEMA
HYPEREMIA AND CONGESTION
HEMORRHAGE
HEMOSTASIS AND THROMBOSIS
NORMAL HEMOSTASIS
Endothelium
Antithrombotic Properties
Prothrombotic Properties
Platelets
Coagulation Cascade
THROMBOSIS
DISSEMINATED INTRAVASCULAR COAGULATION
EMBOLISM
PULMONARY THROMBOEMBOLISM
SYSTEMIC THROMBOEMBOLISM
FAT EMBOLISM
AIR EMBOLISM
AMNIOTIC FLUID EMBOLISM
INFARCTION
TYPES OF INFARCTS
FACTORS THAT INFLUENCE DEVELOPMENT OF AN INFARCT
SHOCK

The health and well-being of cells and tissue depends not only on an intact circulation to deliver oxygen, but also on normal fluid homeostasis. This chapter reviews the major disturbances involving hemodynamics and the maintenance of blood flow. The pathologies include edema, vascular congestion, hemorrhage, thrombosis, embolism, infarction, and shock. All may be precipitated by abnormalities in either blood supply or fluid balance and result in severe morbidity or even mortality. Pulmonary edema, for example, occurring when there is increased hydrostatic pressure in the lung vasculature, may be the terminal complication of ischemic or valvular heart disease. Similarly, hemorrhage and shock may be the fatal sequelae of injury as diverse as trauma or infection. Thrombosis, embolism, and infarction underlie three of the most important causes of morbidity and mortality in Western society: myocardial infarction, pulmonary embolism, and cerebrovascular accident (stroke). Thus, the hemodynamic disorders described in this chapter are important in a wide spectrum of human disease.

EDEMA

Approximately 60% of lean body weight is water, two thirds of which is intracellular with the remainder in the extracellular compartments, mostly as interstitial fluid (only about 5% of total body water is in blood plasma). The term *edema* signifies increased fluid in the interstitial tissue spaces. In addition, depending on the site, fluid collections in the different body cavities are variously designated *hydrothorax, hydropericardium,* and *hydroperitoneum* (the last is more commonly called *ascites*). *Anasarca* ia a severe and generalized edema with profound subcutaneous tissue swelling.

Table 5–1 lists the pathophysiologic categories of edema. The noninflammatory causes are described in further detail subsequently; the mechanisms of inflammatory edema, largely related to local increases in vascular permeability, are described in Chapter 3.

In general, the opposing effects of vascular hydrostatic pressure and plasma colloid osmotic pressure are the major factors that govern movement of fluid between vascular and interstitial spaces. Normally, any outflow of fluid into the interstitium from the arteriolar end of the microcirculation is nearly balanced by inflow at the venular end; a small leftover amount of interstitial fluid is usually removed by the lymphatics. Either increased capillary pressure or diminished colloid osmotic pressure can result in increased interstitial fluid (Fig. 5–1). As extravascular fluid accumulates in either case, the increased tissue hydrostatic pressure and plasma colloid osmotic pressure eventually achieve a new equilibrium, and water reenters the venules. Excess interstitial edema fluid is removed by lymphatic drainage, ultimately returning to the bloodstream via the thoracic duct (Fig. 5–1); clearly, lymphatic obstruction (e.g., due to scarring or tumor) can also impair fluid removal and cause edema. Finally, a primary retention of sodium (and its obligatory associated water) in renal disease also results in edema.

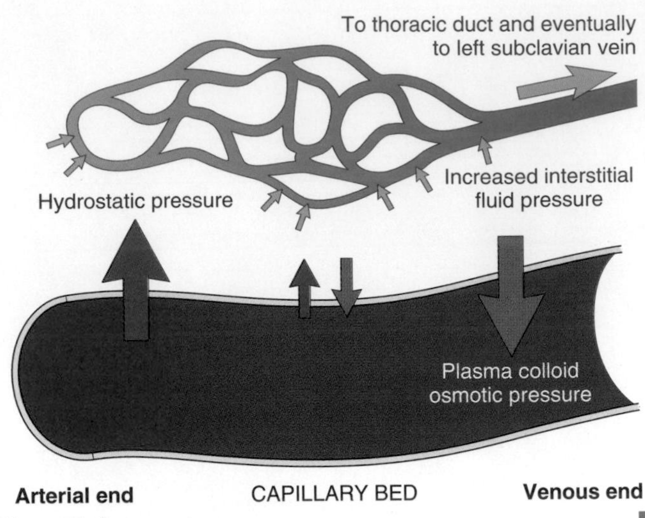

Figure 5–1

Factors affecting fluid balance across capillary walls. Capillary hydrostatic and osmotic forces are normally balanced so that there is no *net* loss or gain of fluid across the capillary bed. However, *increased* hydrostatic pressure or *diminished* plasma osmotic pressure leads to a net accumulation of extravascular fluid (*edema*). As the interstitial fluid pressure increases, tissue lymphatics remove much of the excess volume, eventually returning it to the circulation via the thoracic duct. If the ability of the lymphatics to drain tissue is exceeded, persistent tissue edema results.

Table 5–1. PATHOPHYSIOLOGIC CATEGORIES OF EDEMA

Increased Hydrostatic Pressure
Impaired venous return
Congestive heart failure
Constrictive pericarditis
Ascites (liver cirrhosis)
Venous obstruction or compression
Thrombosis
External pressure (e.g., mass)
Lower extremity inactivity with prolonged dependency
Arteriolar dilation
Heat
Neurohumoral dysregulation
Reduced Plasma Osmotic Pressure (Hypoproteinemia)
Protein-losing glomerulopathies (nephrotic syndrome)
Liver cirrhosis (ascites)
Malnutrition
Protein-losing gastroenteropathy
Lymphatic Obstruction
Inflammatory
Neoplastic
Postsurgical
Postirradiation
Sodium Retention
Excessive salt intake with renal insufficiency
Increased tubular reabsorption of sodium
Renal hypoperfusion
Increased renin-angiotensin-aldosterone secretion
Inflammation
Acute inflammation
Chronic inflammation
Angiogenesis

Modified from Leaf A, Cotran RS: Renal Pathophysiology, 3rd ed. New York, Oxford University Press, 1985, p 146. Used by permission of Oxford University Press, Inc.

The edema fluid occurring in hydrodynamic derangements is typically a protein-poor *transudate,* with a specific gravity below 1.012. Conversely, because of increased vascular permeability, inflammatory edema is a protein-rich *exudate,* with a specific gravity usually over 1.020.

Increased Hydrostatic Pressure

- *Local increases* in hydrostatic pressure may result from impaired venous outflow. For example, *deep venous thrombosis* in the lower extremities leads to edema, which is restricted to the affected leg.
- *Generalized increases* in venous pressure, with resulting systemic edema, occur most commonly in *congestive heart failure* (Chapter 13) affecting right ventricular cardiac function. Although increased venous hydrostatic pressure is important, the pathogenesis of cardiac edema is more complex (Fig. 5–2). Congestive heart failure is associated with reduced cardiac output and therefore reduced renal perfusion. Renal hypoperfusion, in turn, triggers the renin-angiotensin-aldosterone axis, inducing sodium and water retention by the kidneys *(secondary aldosteronism).* This process is putatively designed to increase intravascular volume and thereby improve cardiac output (via the Frank-Starling law) with restoration of normal renal perfusion. If the failing heart cannot increase cardiac output, however, the extra fluid load results only in increased venous pressure and eventually edema.[1] Unless cardiac output is restored or renal water

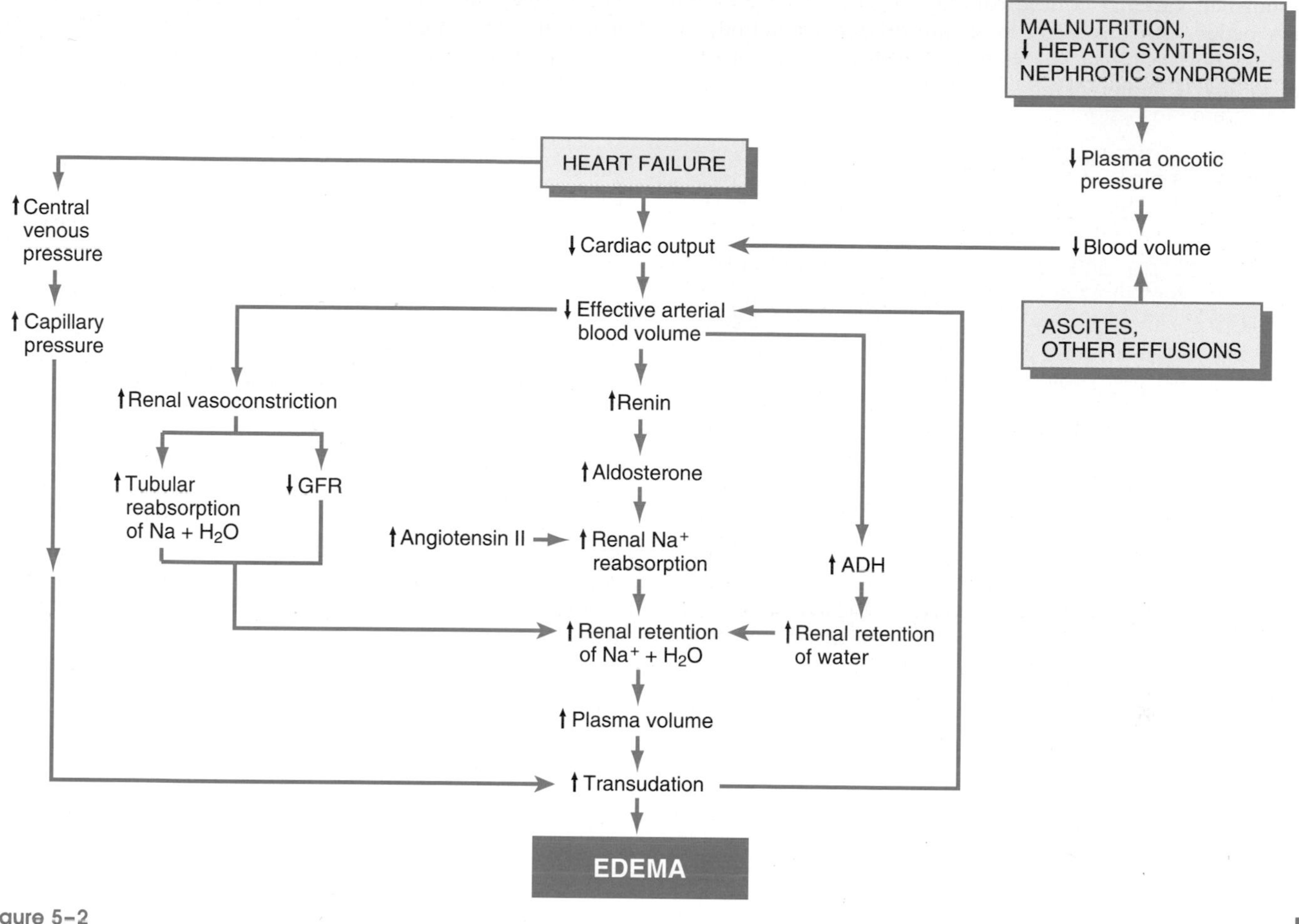

Figure 5–2

Sequence of events leading to systemic edema in heart failure, or with reduced plasma osmotic pressure, as in the nephrotic syndrome. ADH, antidiuretic hormone; GFR, glomerular filtration rate.

retention is reduced (e.g., by salt restriction, diuretics, or aldosterone antagonists), a cycle of renal fluid retention and worsening edema ensues. Although discussed here in the context of edema in congestive heart failure, salt restriction, diuretics, and aldosterone antagonists may also be used to manage generalized edema arising from a variety of other causes.

Reduced Plasma Osmotic Pressure. Reduced plasma osmotic pressure can result from excessive loss or reduced synthesis of albumin, the serum protein most responsible for maintaining colloid osmotic pressure. An important cause of albumin loss is the *nephrotic syndrome* (Chapter 21), characterized by a leaky glomerular capillary wall and generalized edema. Reduced albumin synthesis occurs in the setting of diffuse liver pathology (e.g., cirrhosis) (Chapter 19) or as a consequence of protein malnutrition (Chapter 10). In each case, reduced plasma osmotic pressure leads to a net movement of fluid into the interstitial tissues and a resultant plasma volume contraction. Predictably, with reduced intravascular volume, renal hypoperfusion with secondary aldosteronism follows. The retained salt and water cannot correct the plasma volume deficit because the primary defect of low serum proteins persists. As with congestive heart failure, edema precipitated by *hypoproteinemia* is exacerbated by secondary salt and fluid retention.

Lymphatic Obstruction. Impaired lymphatic drainage and consequent *lymphedema* is usually localized; it can result from inflammatory or neoplastic obstruction. For example, the parasitic infection *filariasis* often causes massive lymphatic and lymph node fibrosis in the inguinal region. The resulting edema of the external genitalia and lower limbs is so extreme it is called *elephantiasis.* Cancer of the breast may be treated by removal or irradiation (or both) of the breast and the associated axillary lymph nodes. The resection of the lymphatic channels as well as scarring related to the surgery and radiation can result in severe edema of the arm.

Sodium and Water Retention. Sodium and water retention are clearly contributory factors in several forms of edema; however, salt retention may also be a primary cause of edema. Increased salt, with the obligate accompanying water, causes *both* increased hydrostatic pressure (owing to expansion of the intravascular fluid volume) and diminished vascular colloid osmotic pressure. Salt retention may occur with any acute reduction of renal function, including *poststreptococcal glomerulonephritis* and *acute renal failure* (Chapter 21).

MORPHOLOGY OF EDEMA. Edema is most easily recognized grossly; microscopically, edema fluid generally manifests only as subtle cell swelling, with clearing and separation of the extracellular matrix elements. Although any organ or tissue in the body may be involved, edema is most commonly encountered in subcutaneous tissues, the lungs, and the brain. Severe, generalized edema is called **anasarca.**

Subcutaneous edema may have different distributions depending on the cause. It can be diffuse or may be relatively more conspicuous at the sites of highest hydrostatic pressures. In the latter case, the edema distribution is typically influenced by gravity and is termed **dependent. Edema of the dependent parts of the body** (e.g., the legs when standing, the sacrum when recumbent) **is a prominent feature of congestive heart failure, particularly of the right ventricle.** Edema as a result of **renal dysfunction** or **nephrotic syndrome** is generally more severe than cardiac edema and **affects all parts of the body equally.** It may, however, be initially manifest in tissues with a loose connective tissue matrix, such as the eyelids, causing **periorbital edema.** Finger pressure over substantially edematous subcutaneous tissue displaces the interstitial fluid and leaves a finger-shaped depression, so-called **pitting edema.**

Pulmonary edema is a common clinical concern (Chapter 16) most typically in the setting of left ventricular failure but also occurring in renal failure, adult respiratory distress syndrome (Chapter 16), pulmonary infections, and hypersensitivity reactions. The lungs are two to three times their normal weight, and sectioning reveals frothy, blood-tinged fluid representing a mixture of air, edema fluid, and extravasated red blood cells.

Edema of the brain may be localized to sites of injury (e.g., abscess or neoplasm) or may be generalized, as in encephalitis, hypertensive crises, or obstruction to the brain's venous outflow. Trauma may result in local or generalized edema depending on the nature and extent of the injury. With generalized edema, the brain is grossly swollen with narrowed sulci and distended gyri showing signs of flattening against the unyielding skull (Chapter 30).

Clinical Correlation. Effects of edema may range from merely annoying to fatal. Subcutaneous tissue edema in cardiac or renal failure is important primarily because it signals underlying disease; however, when significant, it can impair wound healing or the clearance of infection. Pulmonary edema can cause death by interfering with normal ventilatory function. Not only does fluid collect in the alveolar septa around capillaries and impede oxygen diffusion, but also edema fluid in the alveolar spaces creates a favorable environment for bacterial infection. Brain edema is serious and can be rapidly fatal; if severe, brain substance can *herniate* (push out) through, for example, the foramen magnum, or the brain stem vascular supply can be compressed. Either condition can injure the medullary centers and cause death.

HYPEREMIA AND CONGESTION

The terms *hyperemia* and *congestion* indicate a local increased volume of blood in a particular tissue. *Hyperemia* is an *active process* resulting from augmented tissue inflow because of arteriolar dilation, as in skeletal muscle during exercise, or at sites of inflammation. The affected tissue is redder because of the engorgement with oxygenated blood. *Congestion* is a *passive process* resulting from impaired outflow from a tissue. It may occur systemically, as in cardiac failure, or may be local, resulting from an isolated venous obstruction. The tissue has a blue-red color *(cyanosis),* particularly as worsening congestion leads to accumulation of deoxygenated hemoglobin in the affected tissues.

Congestion of capillary beds is closely related to the development of edema, so that congestion and edema commonly occur together. In long-standing congestion, called *chronic passive congestion,* the stasis of poorly oxygenated blood causes chronic hypoxia, which can result in parenchymal cell degeneration or death, sometimes with microscopic scarring. Capillary rupture at these sites of chronic congestion may also cause small foci of hemorrhage; breakdown and phagocytosis of the red cell debris can eventually result in small clusters of hemosiderin-laden macrophages.

MORPHOLOGY. Cut surfaces of hyperemic or congested tissues are hemorrhagic and wet. Microscopically, **acute pulmonary congestion** is characterized by alveolar capillaries engorged with blood; there may be associated alveolar septal edema or focal intra-alveolar hemorrhage (or both). In **chronic pulmonary congestion,** the septa have become thickened and fibrotic, and the alveolar spaces may contain numerous hemosiderin-laden macrophages **(heart failure cells).** In **acute hepatic congestion,** the central vein and sinusoids are distended with blood, and there may even be central hepatocyte degeneration; the periportal hepatocytes are relatively better oxygenated because of their proximity to hepatic arterioles and therefore experience less severe hypoxia, typically developing only fatty change. In **chronic passive congestion of the liver,** the central regions of the hepatic lobules

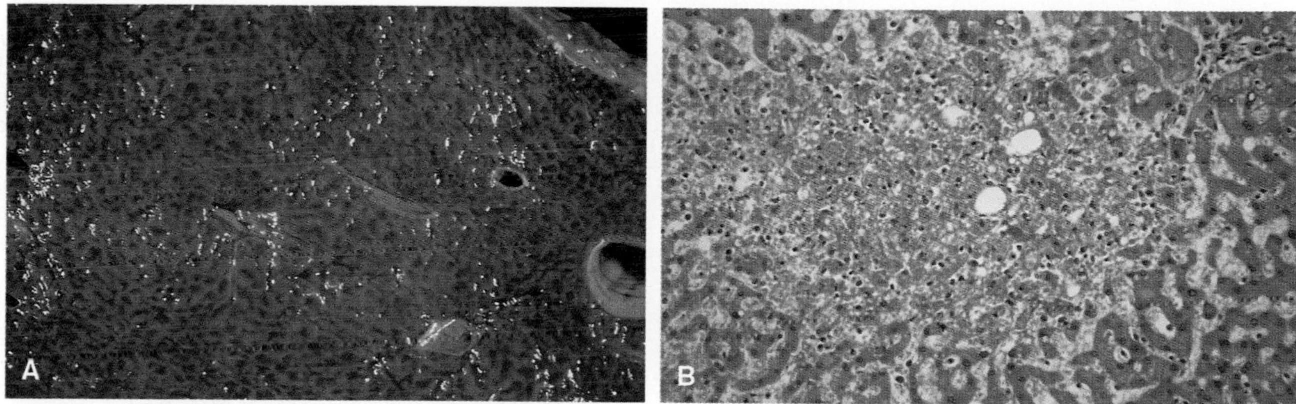

Figure 5–3

Liver with chronic passive congestion and hemorrhagic necrosis. *A*, Central areas are red and slightly depressed compared with the surrounding tan viable parenchyma, forming the so-called "nutmeg liver" pattern. *B*, Centrilobular necrosis with degenerating hepatocytes, hemorrhage, and acute inflammation. (Courtesy of Dr. James Crawford, Department of Pathology, Yale University Medical School, New Haven, CT.)

are grossly red-brown and slightly depressed (owing to a loss of cells) and are accentuated against the surrounding zones of uncongested tan liver **(nutmeg liver)** (Fig. 5–3*A*). Microscopically, there is evidence of **centrilobular necrosis** with hepatocyte dropout and hemorrhage including hemosiderin-laden macrophages (Fig. 5–3*B*). In severe, long-standing hepatic congestion (most commonly associated with heart failure), there may even be grossly evident hepatic fibrosis **(cardiac cirrhosis)**. Because the central portion of the hepatic lobule is the last to receive blood, centrilobular necrosis can also occur whenever there is reduced hepatic blood flow (including shock from any cause); there need not be previous hepatic congestion.

HEMORRHAGE

Hemorrhage generally indicates extravasation of blood because of vessel rupture. As described previously, capillary bleeding can occur under conditions of chronic congestion, and an increased tendency to hemorrhage from usually insignificant injury is seen in a wide variety of clinical disorders collectively called *hemorrhagic diatheses* (Chapter 14). Rupture of a large artery or vein, however, is almost always due to vascular injury, including trauma, atherosclerosis, or inflammatory or neoplastic erosion of the vessel wall.

- Hemorrhage may be external or may be enclosed within a tissue; the accumulation is referred to as a *hematoma.* Hematomas may be relatively insignificant (as in a

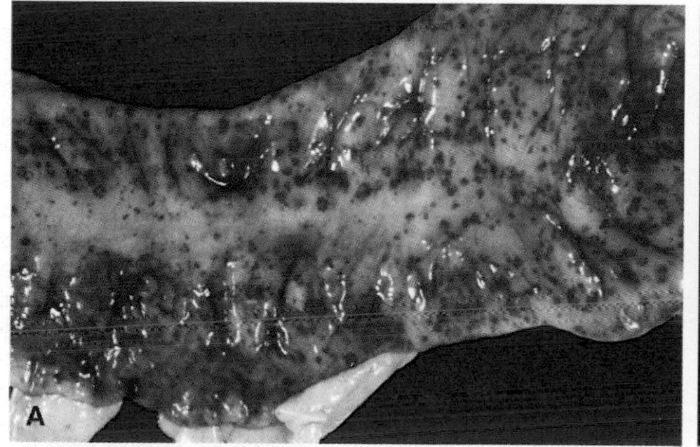

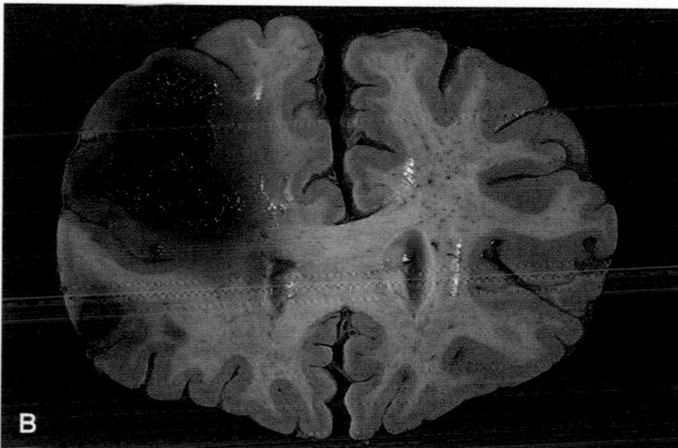

Figure 5–4

A, Punctate petechial hemorrhages of the colonic mucosa, seen here as a consequence of thrombocytopenia. *B*, Fatal intracerebral bleed. Even relatively inconsequential volumes of hemorrhage in a critical location, or into a closed space (such as the cranium), can have fatal outcomes.

bruise) or may accumulate sufficient blood to cause death (e.g., a massive retroperitoneal hematoma resulting from rupture of a dissecting aortic aneurysm can be fatal; Chapter 12).

- Minute 1- to 2-mm hemorrhages into skin, mucous membranes, or serosal surfaces are called *petechiae* (Fig. 5–4*A*) and are typically associated with locally increased intravascular pressure, low platelet counts *(thrombocytopenia),* defective platelet function (as in uremia), or clotting factor deficits.
- Slightly larger (≥3 mm) hemorrhages are called *purpura* and may be associated with similar pathologies as well as trauma, local vascular inflammation *(vasculitis),* or increased vascular fragility (e.g., in amyloidosis).
- Larger (>1 to 2 cm) subcutaneous hematomas (i.e., bruises) are called *ecchymoses* and are typical after trauma but may be exacerbated by any of the aforementioned conditions. The erythrocytes in these local hemorrhages are degraded and phagocytosed by macrophages; the hemoglobin (red-blue color) is then enzymatically converted into bilirubin (blue-green color) and eventually into hemosiderin (gold-brown), accounting for the characteristic color changes in a hematoma.
- Large accumulations of blood in one or another of the body cavities are called *hemothorax, hemopericardium, hemoperitoneum,* or *hemarthrosis.* Patients with extensive hemorrhages occasionally develop jaundice from the massive breakdown of red cells and systemic release of bilirubin.

The clinical significance of hemorrhage depends on the volume and rate of blood loss. Rapid removal of up to 20% of the blood volume or slow losses of even larger amounts may have little impact in healthy adults; greater losses, however, may result in *hemorrhagic (hypovolemic) shock* (discussed later). The site of hemorrhage is also important; bleeding that would be trivial in the subcutaneous tissues may cause death if located in the brain (Fig. 5–4*B*) because the skull is unyielding and bleeding there can result in increased intracranial pressure and herniation (Chapter 30). Finally, loss of iron and subsequent iron-deficiency anemia become a consideration in chronic or recurrent external blood loss (e.g., peptic ulcer or menstrual bleeding). In contrast, when red cells are retained, as in hemorrhage into body cavities or tissues, the iron can be reused for hemoglobin synthesis.

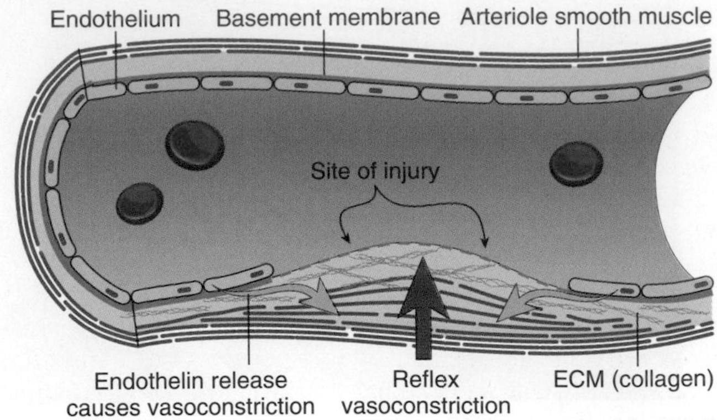

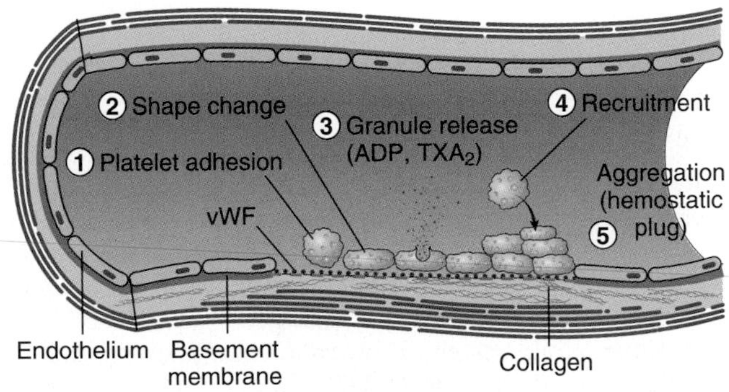

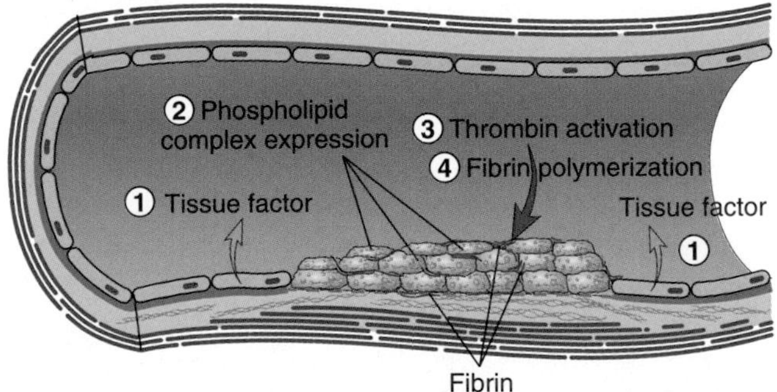

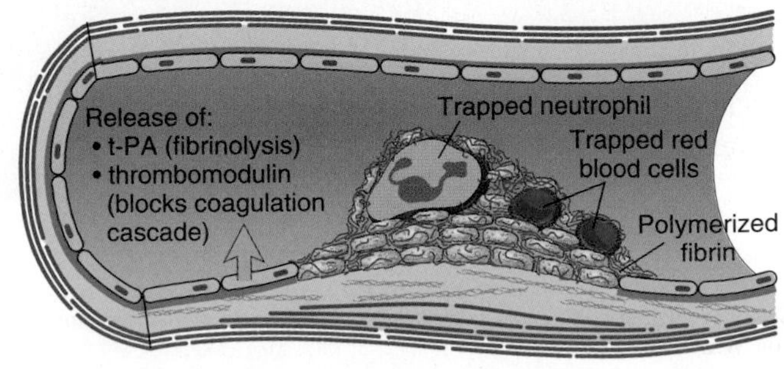

Figure 5–5

Diagrammatic representation of the normal hemostatic process. *A,* After vascular injury, local neurohumoral factors induce a transient vasoconstriction. *B,* Platelets adhere to exposed extracellular matrix (ECM) via von Willebrand factor (vWF), and are activated, undergoing a shape change and granule release; released adenosine diphosphate (ADP) and thromboxane A_2 (TXA_2) lead to further platelet aggregation to form the primary hemostatic plug. *C,* Local activation of the coagulation cascade (involving tissue factor and platelet phospholipids) results in fibrin polymerization, "cementing" the platelets into a definitive secondary hemostatic plug. *D,* Counter-regulatory mechanisms, such as release of tissue type plasminogen activator (t-PA) (fibrinolytic) and thrombomodulin (interfering with the coagulation cascade), limit the hemostatic process to the site of injury.

HEMOSTASIS AND THROMBOSIS

Normal hemostasis is the result of a set of well-regulated processes that accomplish two important functions: (1) They maintain blood in a fluid, clot-free state in normal vessels, and (2) they are poised to induce a *rapid and localized hemostatic plug* at a site of vascular injury. The pathologic opposite to hemostasis is *thrombosis;* it can be considered an inappropriate activation of normal hemostatic processes, such as formation of a blood clot *(thrombus)* in uninjured vasculature or thrombotic occlusion of a vessel after relatively minor injury. Both hemostasis and thrombosis depend on three general components—the *vascular wall, platelets,* and the *coagulation cascade.* The following discussion begins with normal hemostasis and concludes with a description of the components that regulate normal coagulation processes.

Normal Hemostasis

The general sequence of events in hemostasis at the site of vascular injury is shown in Figure 5–5.[2]

- After initial injury, there is a brief period of arteriolar vasoconstriction, largely attributable to *reflex neurogenic mechanisms* and augmented by the local secretion of factors such as *endothelin* (a potent endothelium-derived vasoconstrictor). The effect is transient, however, and bleeding would resume if not for activation of the platelet and coagulation systems (Fig. 5–5*A*).
- Endothelial injury exposes highly thrombogenic subendothelial extracellular matrix, which allows platelets to adhere and become *activated,* that is, undergo a shape change and release secretory granules. Within minutes, the secreted products have recruited additional platelets to form a *hemostatic plug;* this is the process of *primary hemostasis* (Fig. 5–5*B*).
- *Tissue factor,* a membrane-bound procoagulant factor synthesized by endothelium, is also exposed at the site of injury. It acts in conjunction with the secreted platelet factors to activate the coagulation cascade, culminating in the activation of *thrombin.* In turn, thrombin converts circulating soluble fibrinogen to insoluble *fibrin* resulting in local fibrin deposition. Thrombin also induces further platelet recruitment and granule release. This sequence, *secondary hemostasis,* takes longer than the initial platelet plug (Fig. 5–5*C*).
- Polymerized fibrin and platelet aggregates form a solid, *permanent plug* to prevent any further hemorrhage. At this stage, counterregulatory mechanisms (e.g., tissue plasminogen activator [t-PA]) are set into motion to restrict the hemostatic plug to the site of injury (Fig. 5–5*D*).

These events are now discussed in greater detail.

ENDOTHELIUM

Endothelial cells modulate several, frequently opposing, aspects of normal hemostasis. On one hand, they normally possess antiplatelet, anticoagulant, and fibrinolytic properties; on the other hand, after injury or activation, they are capable of exerting *procoagulant functions* (Fig. 5–6). Endothelium may be activated by infectious agents, hemodynamic factors, plasma mediators, and, most significantly,

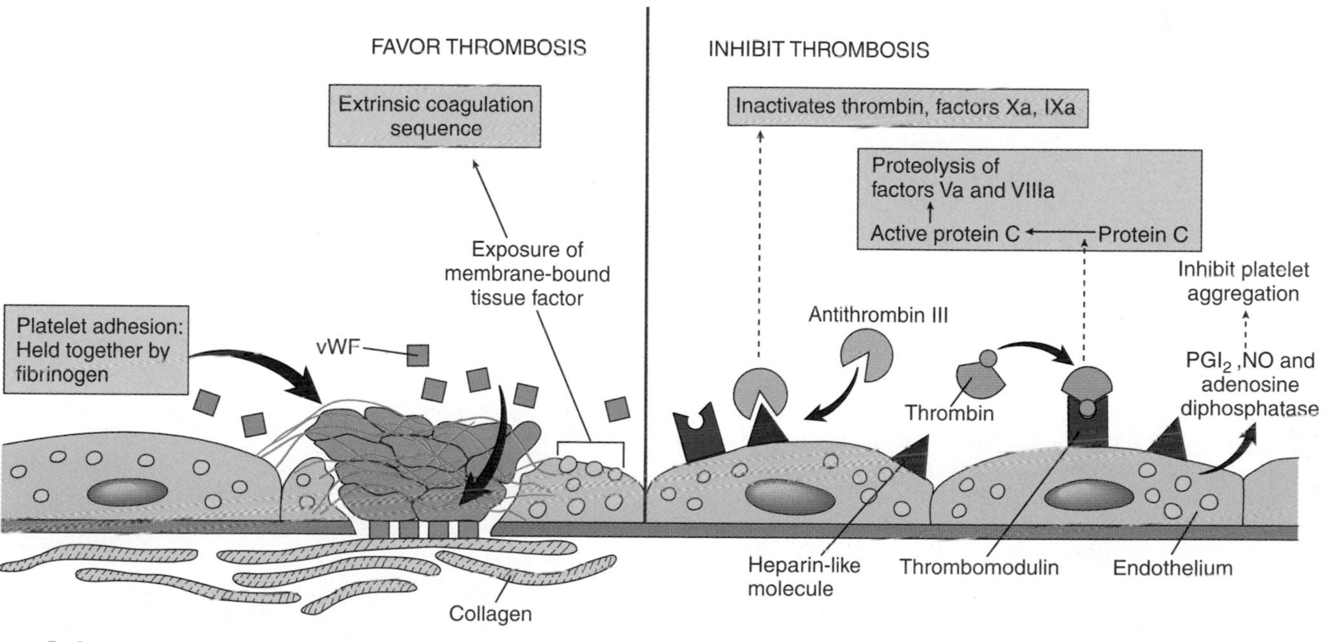

Figure 5–6

Schematic illustration of some of the pro- and anticoagulant activities of endothelial cells. Not shown are the pro- and antifibrinolytic properties. vWF, von Willebrand factor; PGI_2, prostacyclin; NO, nitric oxide.

cytokines (Chapter 3). The balance between endothelial antithrombotic and prothrombotic activities critically determines whether thrombus formation, propagation, or dissolution occurs.[3,4]

Antithrombotic Properties

- *Antiplatelet:*[3] At the most basic level, intact endothelium prevents platelets and plasma coagulation factors from meeting the highly thrombogenic subendothelial extracellular matrix. Nonactivated platelets do not adhere to the endothelium, a property intrinsic to endothelial plasma membrane. If platelets do become activated after focal endothelial injury, they are specifically inhibited from adhering to the surrounding uninjured endothelium by endothelial prostacyclin (PGI_2) and nitric oxide (Chapter 3). Both mediators are potent vasodilators and inhibitors of platelet aggregation; their synthesis by endothelial cells is stimulated by a number of factors (e.g., adenosine diphosphate [ADP], thrombin, and various cytokines) produced during coagulation. Endothelial cells also express adenosine diphosphatase, which degrades ADP and thereby inhibits platelet aggregation.
- *Anticoagulant:* Anticoagulants are mediated by (1) membrane-associated heparin-like molecules and (2) thrombomodulin, a specific thrombin receptor (Fig. 5–6). The *heparin-like molecules* act indirectly; they are cofactors allowing *antithrombin III* to inactivate thrombin, factor Xa, and several other coagulation factors (see later).[3] *Thrombomodulin* also acts indirectly; it binds to thrombin, converting it from a procoagulant to an anticoagulant capable of activating *protein C.* Activated protein C, in turn, inhibits clotting by proteolytic cleavage of factors Va and VIIIa; it requires protein S, synthesized by endothelial cells, as a cofactor.[5]
- *Fibrinolytic:* Endothelial cells synthesize t-PA, promoting fibrinolytic activity to clear fibrin deposits from endothelial surfaces (see Fig. 5–5*D*).[4]

Prothrombotic Properties

While endothelial cells have activities that can limit blood clotting, they can also be prothrombotic, affecting platelets, coagulation proteins, and the fibrinolytic system. Recall that endothelial injury leads to adhesion of platelets to the underlying extracellular matrix; this is facilitated by endothelial production of *von Willebrand factor (vWF),* an essential cofactor for platelet binding to collagen and other surfaces. Endothelial cells are also induced by bacterial endotoxin or by cytokines (e.g., tumor necrosis factor [TNF] or interleukin 1 [IL-1]) to synthesize *tissue factor,* which, as we will see subsequently, activates the extrinsic clotting cascade. By binding activated factors IXa and Xa, endothelial cells further augment the catalytic activities of these coagulation factors. Finally, endothelial cells also secrete *inhibitors of plasminogen activator (PAIs),* which depress fibrinolysis.[6]

Intact endothelial cells serve primarily to inhibit platelet adherence and blood clotting. Injury or activation of endothelial cells, however, results in a procoagulant phenotype that augments local clot formation.

PLATELETS

Platelets play a central role in normal hemostasis.[7] When circulating, they are membrane-bound smooth discs expressing a number of glycoprotein receptors of the integrin family on their surfaces. Platelets contain two specific types of granules. *Alpha granules* express the adhesion molecule P-selectin on their membranes (Chapter 3) and contain fibrinogen, fibronectin, factor V and vWF, platelet factor 4 (a heparin-binding chemokine), platelet-derived growth factor (PDGF), and transforming growth factor-β (TGF-β). The other granules are *dense bodies* or *δ granules,* which contain adenine nucleotides (ADP and adenosine triphosphate [ATP]), ionized calcium, histamine, serotonin, and epinephrine.

After vascular injury, platelets encounter extracellular matrix constituents, which are normally sequestered beneath an intact endothelium; these include collagen (most important), proteoglycans, fibronectin, and other adhesive glycoproteins. On contact with extracellular matrix, platelets undergo three general reactions: (1) adhesion and shape change, (2) secretion (release reaction), and (3) aggregation (see Fig. 5–5*B*).

- *Platelet adhesion* to extracellular matrix is mediated largely via interactions with vWF, which acts as a bridge between platelet surface receptors (e.g., glycoprotein Ib) and exposed collagen (Fig. 5–7).[8] Although adhesion to extracellular matrix also occurs directly via platelet collagen receptors and interactions with fibronectin, the vWF-glycoprotein Ib interaction is uniquely important in that it is the only known way to stabilize the initial platelet adhesion against the high shear forces

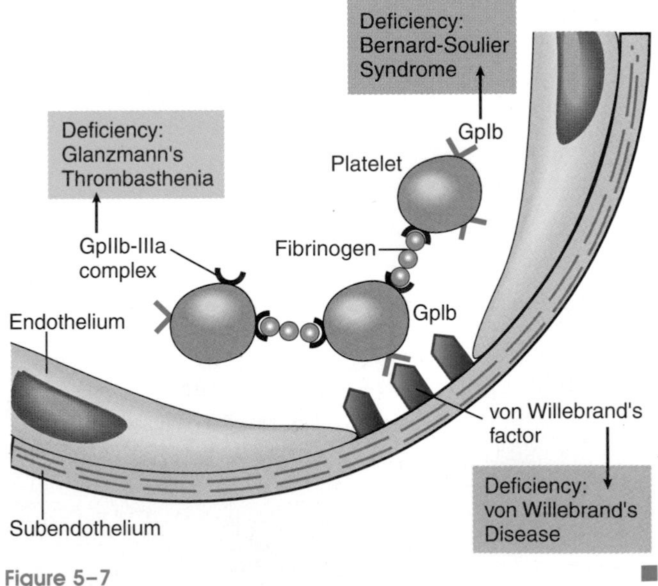

Figure 5–7

Platelet adhesion and aggregation. Von Willebrand's factor functions as an adhesion bridge between subendothelial collagen and the GpIb platelet receptor. Aggregation involves linking platelets via fibrinogen bridges bound to the platelet GpIIb-IIIa receptors.

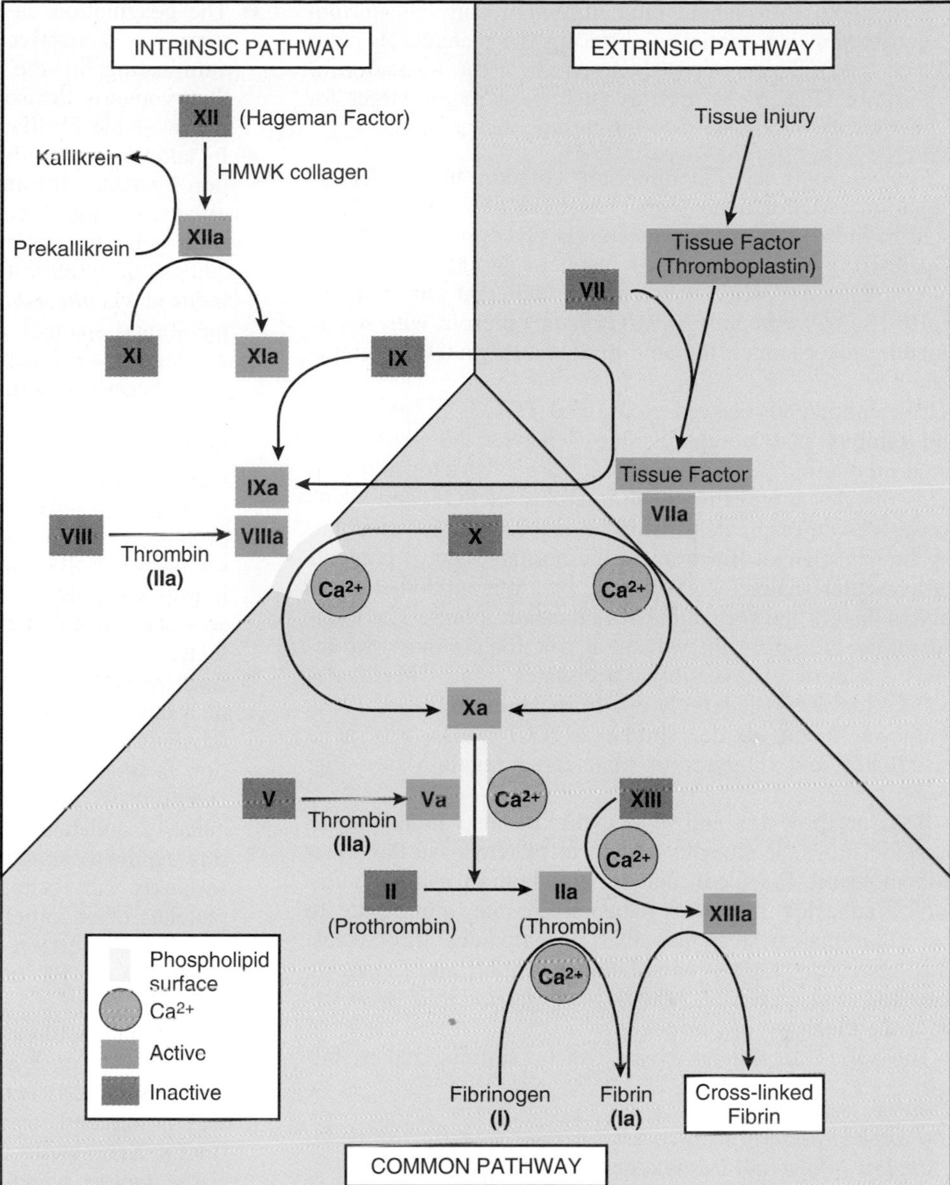

Figure 5–8 ■

The coagulation cascade. Note the common link between the intrinsic and extrinsic pathways at the level of factor IX activation. Factors in red boxes represent inactive molecules; activated factors are indicated with a lower case "a" and a green box. PL, phospholipid surface; HMWK, high-molecular-weight kininogen. Not shown are the anticoagulant inhibitory pathways (see Figs. 5-6 and 5-11).

of flowing blood. Thus, genetic deficiency of vWF (von Willebrand disease; Chapter 14) or of its glycoprotein Ib receptor (Bernard-Soulier syndrome) results in defective platelet adhesion and bleeding disorders.

- *Secretion (release reaction)* of the contents of both types of granules occurs soon after adhesion. The process is initiated by binding of agonists to platelet surface receptors followed by an intracellular protein phosphorylation cascade. The release of the dense body contents is especially important because calcium is required in the coagulation cascade, and ADP is a potent mediator of *platelet aggregation* (platelets adhering to other platelets; see later). ADP also augments further ADP release from other platelets. Finally, platelet activation leads to the surface expression of a *phospholipid complex,* which provides a critical nucleation site for calcium and factor binding in the *intrinsic clotting pathway* (see later).
- *Platelet aggregation* follows adhesion and secretion. Besides ADP, the vasoconstrictor platelet product thromboxane A_2 (TXA_2) (Chapter 3) also stimulates platelet aggregation. ADP and TXA_2 set up an autocatalytic reaction leading to build-up of an enlarging platelet aggregate, the *primary hemostatic plug.* This primary aggregation is reversible, but with activation of the coagulation cascade, *thrombin* is generated. Thrombin binds to a platelet surface receptor and with ADP and TXA_2 results in further aggregation. This is followed by *platelet contraction,* creating an irreversibly fused mass of platelets *(viscous metamorphosis)* constituting the definitive *secondary hemostatic plug.* At the same time

throughout the platelet plug, thrombin converts fibrinogen to *fibrin,* essentially mortaring the platelets in place (see later). Thrombin is thus central in the formation of thrombi (Fig. 5–8) and, as such, is a major target for therapeutic modulation of the thrombotic process.[9]

Fibrinogen is also an important cofactor in platelet aggregation; ADP-activated platelets bind fibrinogen, which, in turn, links with other platelets via glycoprotein receptors (GpIIb-IIIa) to generate large platelet aggregates (see Fig. 5–7). Patients with congenitally deficient or inactive GpIIb-IIIa *(Glanzmann thrombasthenia)* present with severe bleeding disorders attributable to defective platelet aggregation.[10]

The endothelial-derived eicosanoid PGI_2 is a vasodilator and inhibits platelet aggregation, whereas the platelet-derived eicosanoid TXA_2 is a potent vasoconstrictor and activates platelet aggregation. The interplay of PGI_2 and TXA_2 constitutes an exquisitely balanced mechanism for modulating human platelet function: In the normal state, it prevents intravascular platelet aggregation, but after endothelial injury, it favors the formation of hemostatic plugs. The clinical utility of aspirin in patients at risk for coronary thrombosis—aspirin irreversibly acetylates and inactivates cyclooxygenase—is largely due to its ability to block TXA_2 synthesis. Nitric oxide, similar to PGI_2, also acts as a vasodilator and inhibitor of platelet aggregation (see Fig. 5–5).

Both erythrocytes and leukocytes are also found in hemostatic plugs; leukocytes adhere to platelets via the adhesion molecule P-selectin and to endothelium using a number of adhesion receptors (Chapter 3); they contribute to the inflammatory response that accompanies thrombosis. Thrombin also directly stimulates neutrophil and monocyte adhesion and generates chemotactic *fibrin split products* from the cleavage of fibrinogen.

The series of platelet events can be summarized as follows:

1. *Platelets adhere to extracellular matrix at sites of endothelial injury and become activated.*
2. *On activation, they secrete granule products (e.g., ADP) and synthesize TXA_2.*
3. *Platelets also expose phospholipid complexes important in the intrinsic coagulation pathway.*
4. *Injured or activated endothelial cells expose tissue factor, which triggers the extrinsic coagulation cascade.*
5. *Released ADP stimulates formation of a primary hemostatic plug, which is eventually converted (via ADP, thrombin, and TXA_2) into a larger definitive secondary plug.*
6. *Fibrin deposition stabilizes and anchors the aggregated platelets.*

COAGULATION CASCADE

The coagulation cascade constitutes the third component of the hemostatic process and is a major contributor to thrombosis. The details are schematically presented in Figure 5–8; only general principles are discussed.[2]

- The coagulation cascade is essentially a series of conversions of inactive proenzymes to activated enzymes, culminating in the formation of thrombin. Thrombin then converts the soluble plasma protein *fibrinogen* into the insoluble fibrillar protein *fibrin.*
- In addition to catalyzing the final steps in the coagulation cascade, thrombin also exerts a wide variety of effects on the local vasculature and inflammation; it even actively participates in limiting the extent of the hemostatic process (Fig. 5–9). Most of these effects are induced via *thrombin receptors,* which are seven transmembrane spanner proteins coupled to G proteins; the mechanism of receptor activation is extremely interesting. The amino terminal extracellular end of the thrombin receptor is clipped by the proteolytic activity of thrombin; this generates a tethered peptide, which then binds to the rest of the receptor and causes the conformational changes necessary to activate the associated G protein. Thus, the interaction of thrombin and its receptor is essentially a catalytic process, which explains the impressive potency of even relatively small numbers of activated thrombin molecules in eliciting downstream effects.[9]
- Each reaction in the pathway results from the assembly of a complex composed of an *enzyme* (activated coagulation factor), a *substrate* (proenzyme form of coagulation factor), and a *cofactor* (reaction accelerator). These components are typically assembled on a *phospholipid complex* and held together by *calcium ions.* Thus, clotting tends to remain localized to sites where such an assembly can occur (e.g., on the surface of activated platelets or endothelium).[11] Two such reactions—the sequential conversion of factor X to Xa and then II (prothrombin) to IIa (thrombin)—are illustrated in Figure 5–10.
- Traditionally, blood coagulation pathways are divided into *extrinsic* and *intrinsic* pathways, converging where factor X is activated (see Fig. 5–8). The intrinsic pathway is initiated in vitro by activation of Hageman factor (factor XII), while the extrinsic pathway is activated by *tissue factor,* a cellular lipoprotein exposed at sites of tissue injury.[12] Such a division, however, is only an artifact of in vitro testing; there are, in fact, interconnections between the two pathways. For example, a tissue factor–factor VIIa complex also activates factor IX in the *intrinsic pathway* (see Fig. 5–8).[2]
- Once activated, the coagulation cascade must be restricted to the local site of vascular injury to prevent clotting of the entire vascular tree. Besides restricting factor activation to sites of exposed phospholipids, clotting is also regulated by three types of natural anticoagulants: (1) Antithrombins (e.g., antithrombin III) inhibit the activity of thrombin and other serine proteases—factors IXa, Xa, XIa, and XIIa. Antithrombin III is activated by binding to heparin-like molecules on endothelial cells; hence the clinical usefulness of administering heparin to minimize thrombosis (see Fig. 5–6). (2) *Proteins C and S* are two vitamin K–dependent proteins characterized by their ability to inactivate factors Va and VIIIa. The activation of protein C by thrombomodulin

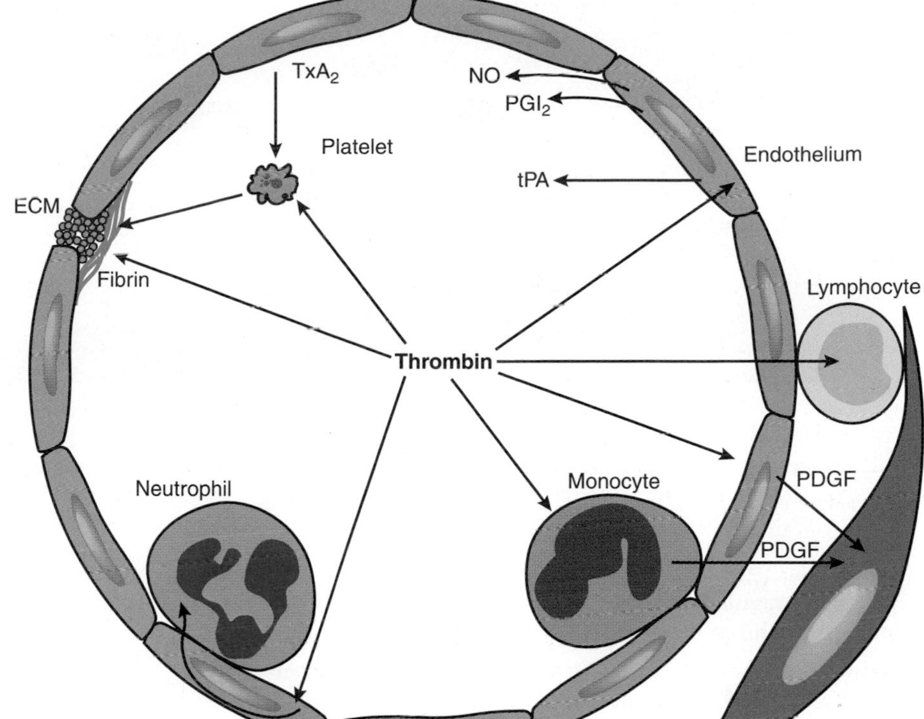

Figure 5–9 ■

The central roles of thrombin in hemostasis and cellular activation. In addition to a critical function in generating cross-linked fibrin (via cleavage of fibrinogen to fibrin and activation of factor XIII), thrombin also directly induces platelet aggregation and secretion (e.g., of TXA_2). Thrombin also activates endothelium to generate leukocyte adhesion molecules and a variety of fibrinolytic (t-PA), vasoactive (NO, PGI_2), or cytokine (PDGF) mediators. Likewise, mononuclear inflammatory cells may be activated by the direct actions of thrombin. ECM, extracellular matrix; NO, nitric oxide; PDGF, platelet-derived growth factor; PGI_2, prostacyclin; TXA_2, thromboxane A_2; t-PA, tissue type plasminogen activator. See Fig. 5-6 for additional anticoagulant modulators of thrombin activity, such as antithrombin III and thrombomodulin. (Modified with permission from Shaun Coughlin, MD, PhD, Cardiovascular Research Institute, University of California at San Francisco.)

was described earlier (see Fig. 5–6). (3) Plasmin, derived from enzymatic activation of the circulating precursor *plasminogen,* breaks down fibrin and interferes with its polymerization (Fig. 5–11). The resulting *fibrin split products* (so-called *fibrin degradation products*) can also act as weak anticoagulants. As a clinical aside, elevated levels of these fibrin split products (the fibrin split product characteristically measured by clinical laboratories is the fibrin *d-dimer*) are helpful in diagnosing abnormal thrombotic states, such as disseminated intra-

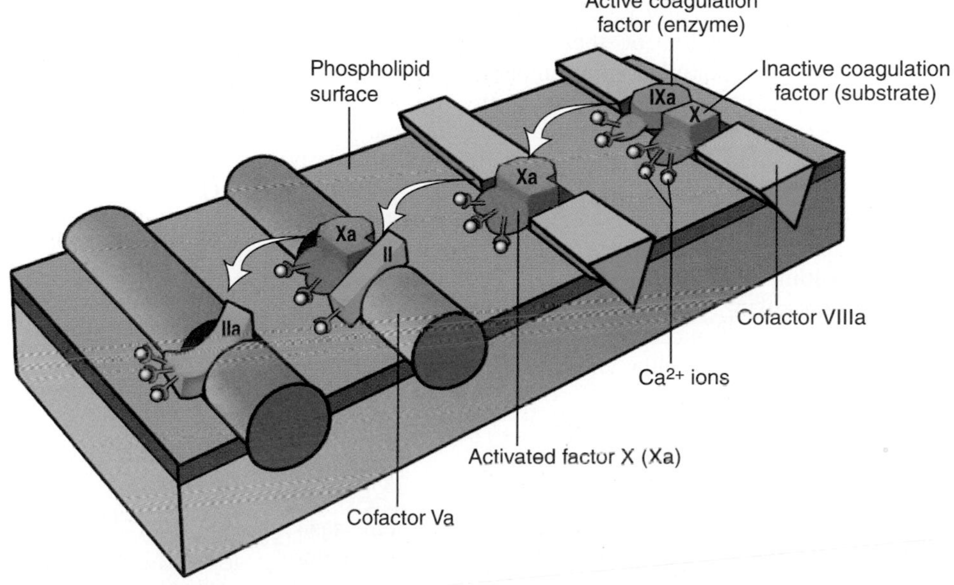

Figure 5–10 ■

Schematic illustration of the conversion of factor X to factor Xa, which in turn converts factor II (prothrombin) to factor IIa (thrombin). The initial reaction complex consists of an enzyme (factor IXa), a substrate (factor X), and a reaction accelerator (factor VIIIa), which are assembled on the phospholipid surface of platelets. Calcium ions hold the assembled components together and are essential for reaction. Activated factor Xa then becomes the enzyme part of the second adjacent complex in the coagulation cascade, converting the prothrombin substrate (II) to thrombin IIa, with the cooperation of the reaction accelerator factor Va. (Modified from Mann KG: Clin Lab Med 4:217, 1984.)

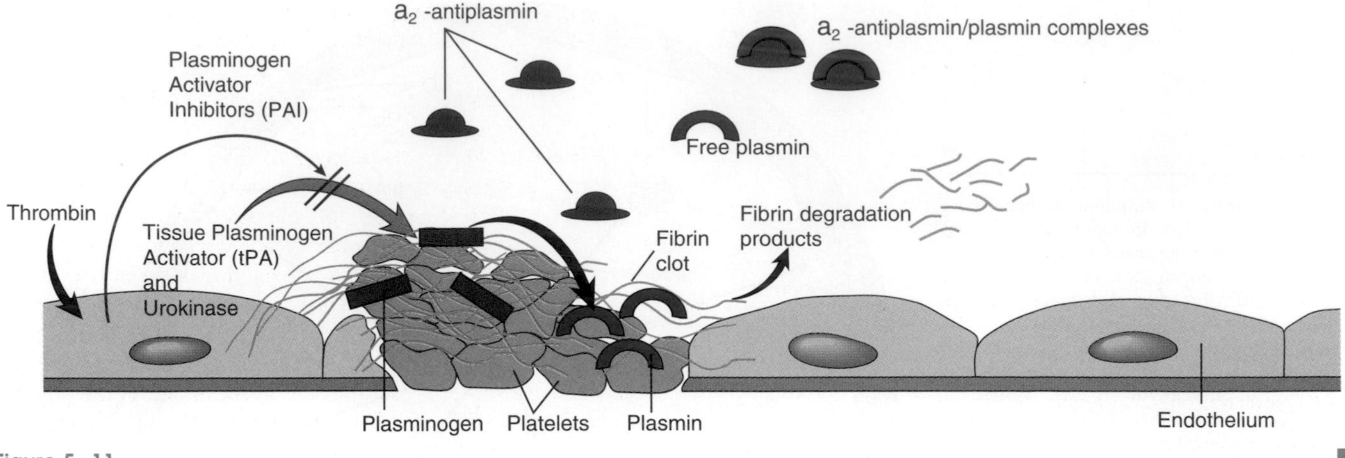

Figure 5–11

The fibrinolytic system, illustrating the plasminogen activators and inhibitors.

vascular coagulation (DIC), deep venous thrombosis, or pulmonary thromboembolism (described in detail later).

Plasminogen is proteolytically cleaved to plasmin either by a factor XII–dependent pathway or by two distinct groups of plasminogen activators (PAs) (Fig. 5–11). The first is the *urokinase-like PA (u-PA),* present in plasma and various tissues and capable of activating plasminogen in the fluid phase. Plasmin, in turn, can convert the inactive pro-urokinase precursor to the active u-PA molecule, thus creating an amplification loop. The second kind of PA is the *tissue-type PA (t-PA);* the primary physiologic activator, t-PA is synthesized principally by endothelial cells and is most active when attached to fibrin. The affinity for fibrin makes t-PA a much more useful therapeutic reagent since it targets the fibrinolytic enzymatic activity to sites of recent clotting.[4] Plasminogen can also be activated by the bacterial product, streptokinase, which may have some significance in certain bacterial infections.

- Although plasmin can also degrade fibrinogen, its functional activity is usually restricted to sites of thrombosis by some combination of the following three mechanisms: (1) t-PA activates plasminogen most effectively when bound to fibrin meshwork, (2) any free plasmin in the circulation is rapidly bound and neutralized by α_2-plasmin inhibitor, and (3) t-PA activity is blocked by *PA inhibitor (PAI)* (Fig. 5–11).
- Endothelial cells modulate the coagulation/anticoagulation balance by releasing PAIs; these block fibrinolysis by inhibiting t-PA binding to fibrin, and confer an overall procoagulant effect. The PAIs are increased by thrombin as well as certain cytokines and probably play a role in the intravascular thrombosis accompanying severe inflammation.[13–15]

Thrombosis

Having discussed the components of normal hemostasis, we now turn our attention to the dysregulation that underlies pathologic thrombus formation.

Pathogenesis. Three primary influences predispose to thrombus formation, the so-called *Virchow's triad:* (1) endothelial injury, (2) stasis or turbulence of blood flow, and (3) blood hypercoagulability (Fig. 5–12).

Endothelial Injury. This is the dominant influence and by itself can lead to thrombosis. Endothelial injury is particularly important in thrombus formation in the heart and arterial circulation, for example, within the cardiac chambers when there has been endocardial injury (e.g., myocardial infarction or valvulitis), over ulcerated plaques in severely atherosclerotic arteries, or at sites of traumatic or inflammatory vascular injury *(vasculitis).* Injury may occur from hemodynamic stress associated with hypertension, turbulent flow over scarred valves, or bacterial endotoxins. Even subtle influences, such as homocystinuria, hypercholesterolemia, radiation, or products absorbed from cigarette smoke, may be sources of endothelial injury. Regardless of

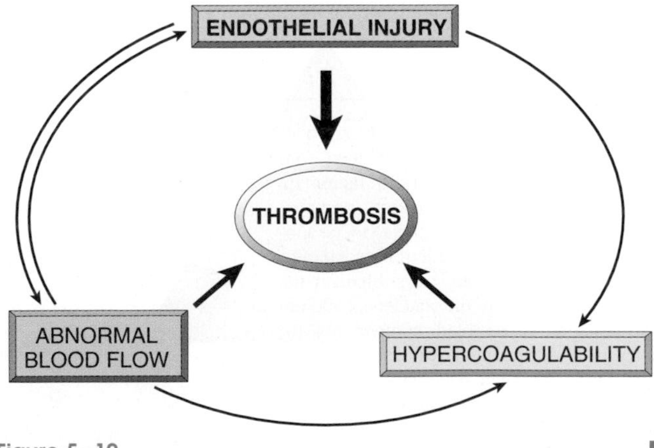

Figure 5–12

Virchow's triad in thrombosis. Endothelial integrity is the single most important factor. Note that injury to endothelial cells can affect local blood flow and/or coagulability; abnormal blood flow (stasis or turbulence), in turn, can cause endothelial injury. The factors may act independently or may combine to cause thrombus formation.

Table 5–2. HYPERCOAGULABLE STATES

Primary (Genetic)
Mutations in factor V
Antithrombin III deficiency
Proteins C or S deficiency
Fibrinolysis defects
Homocysteinemia
Allelic variations in prothrombin levels
Secondary (Acquired)
High risk for thrombosis
Prolonged bed rest or immobilization
Myocardial infarction
Tissue damage (surgery, fracture, burns)
Cancer
Prosthetic cardiac valves
Disseminated intravascular coagulation
Heparin-induced thrombocytopenia
Antiphospholipid antibody syndrome (lupus anticoagulant syndrome)
Lower risk for thrombosis
Atrial fibrillation
Cardiomyopathy
Nephrotic syndrome
Hyperestrogenic states
Oral contraceptive use
Sickle cell anemia
Smoking

the cause of endothelial damage, the end results include exposure of subendothelial collagen (and other platelet activators), adherence of platelets, exposure of tissue factor, and local depletion of prostacyclin and PA (see Figs. 5–5 and 5–6).

Alterations in Normal Blood Flow. *Turbulence* contributes to arterial and cardiac thrombosis by causing endothelial injury or dysfunction as well as by forming countercurrents and local pockets of stasis; *stasis* is a major factor in the development of venous thrombi.[16] Normal blood flow is *laminar,* that is, the cellular elements flow centrally in the vessel lumen, separated from the endothelium by a slower moving clear zone of plasma. Stasis and turbulence therefore (1) disrupt laminar flow and bring platelets into contact with the endothelium; (2) prevent dilution by fresh flowing blood of activated clotting factors; (3) retard the inflow of clotting factor inhibitors and permit the build-up of thrombi; and (4) promote endothelial cell activation, predisposing to local thrombosis, leukocyte adhesion, and a variety of other endothelial cell effects.[17]

Turbulence and stasis clearly contribute to thrombosis in a number of clinical settings. *Ulcerated atherosclerotic plaques* not only expose subendothelial extracellular matrix, but also are sources of local turbulence. Abnormal aortic and arterial dilations called *aneurysms* cause local stasis and are favored sites of thrombosis (Chapter 13). Myocardial infarctions not only have associated endothelial injury, but also have regions of noncontractile myocardium, adding an element of stasis in the formation of mural thrombi. Mitral valve stenosis (e.g., after rheumatic heart disease) results in left atrial dilation. In conjunction with atrial fibrillation, a dilated atrium is a site of profound stasis and a prime location for thrombus development. *Hyperviscosity syndromes* (such as polycythemia; Chapter 14) cause small vessel stasis; the deformed red cells in *sickle cell anemia* (Chapter 14) cause vascular occlusions, with the resulting stasis predisposing to thrombosis.

Hypercoagulability. Hypercoagulability contributes less frequently to thrombotic states but is nevertheless an important (and interesting) component in the equation. It is loosely defined as any alteration of the coagulation pathways that predisposes to thrombosis and can be divided into *primary* (genetic) and *secondary* (acquired) disorders (Table 5–2).[18]

Of the inherited causes of hypercoagulability, mutations in the factor V gene are the most common; somewhere between 2 and 15% of the white population carry a factor V mutation (called the *Leiden mutation,* after the city in the Netherlands where it was first discovered) resulting in a substitution of glutamine for the normal arginine residue at position 506 of factor V. Among patients with recurrent deep venous thrombosis, the carrier frequency is considerably higher, approaching 60% in some series. Mutant factor V Leiden cannot be inactivated by cleavage at the usual arginine residue and is therefore resistant to the anticoagulant effect of activated protein C. As a result, an important antithrombotic counter-regulatory pathway in these patients is no longer active.

Individuals with primary hypercoagulable states associated with an inherited lack of anticoagulants (e.g., antithrombin III, protein C, or protein S) typically present with venous thrombosis and recurrent thromboembolism in adolescence or early adult life. Although these hereditary disorders are uncommon, the basis of the thrombotic tendencies is well understood. More recently, hereditarily elevated levels of homocysteine have been found to contribute to arterial and venous thromboses (and to the development of atherosclerosis; Chapter 12), perhaps via inhibitory effects on antithrombin III and endothelial thrombomodulin.[19] A single nucleotide change (G to A transition) in the 3′-untranslated region of the prothrombin gene is a fairly common allele (1 to 2% of the population) that is associated with elevated prothrombin levels and an almost three-fold increased risk of venous thromboses.[20]

The pathogenesis of the thrombotic diathesis in a number of common clinical settings is more complicated and multifactorial. In some situations (e.g., cardiac failure or trauma), factors such as stasis or vascular injury may be most important. In other cases (e.g., oral contraceptive use and the hyperestrogenic state of pregnancy), hypercoagulability may be partly caused by increased hepatic synthesis of many coagulation factors and reduced synthesis of antithrombin III[21]; heterozygosity for factor V Leiden may also be an underlying contributory component in many series. In disseminated cancers, release of procoagulant tumor products predisposes to thrombosis.[22] The hypercoagulability seen with advancing age may be due to increasing platelet aggregation and reduced PGI_2 release by endothelium. Smoking and obesity promote hypercoagulability by unknown mechanisms.

Among the acquired causes of thrombotic diatheses, the so-called *heparin-induced thrombocytopenia syndrome* and *antiphospholipid antibody syndrome* (previously called the *lupus anticoagulant syndrome*) deserve special mention.

- *Heparin-induced thrombocytopenia syndrome:* This syndrome is seen in upwards of 5% of the population and occurs when administration of unfractionated heparin preparations results in the generation of circulating antibodies that bind a heparin platelet factor 4 complex. This antibody then binds to complexes of platelet factor 4 and heparin-like molecules present on the surface of platelets or endothelium, eventually resulting in platelet activation or endothelial cell injury. In either case, the result is a prothrombotic state.[23] To circumvent this problem, specially manufactured low-molecular-weight heparin preparations, which retain anticoagulant activity but do not interact with platelets (and have the additional advantage of a prolonged serum half-life), have been advocated.
- *Antiphospholipid antibody syndrome:*[24,25] This syndrome refers to a cluster of heterogeneous clinical manifestations—including multiple thromboses—associated with the presence of high titers of serum antibodies directed against anionic phospholipids (e.g., cardiolipin). More accurately, the antibodies are directed to plasma protein epitopes that are unveiled by binding to such phospholipids. In vitro these antibodies interfere with the assembly of phospholipid complexes and thus inhibit coagulation. In contrast, the antibodies in vivo induce a *hypercoagulable* state. The antibodies are being increasingly recognized as possible culprits in a number of thrombotic states; for example, approximately 20% of patients with a recent stroke were found to have anticardiolipin antibodies, versus none in age-matched controls without stroke.[24]

Patients with antiphospholipid antibody syndrome fall into two categories: Many have a well-defined autoimmune disease, such as systemic lupus erythematosus (hence the previous designation of lupus anticoagulant syndrome; Chapter 7).[26–28] The rest show no evidence of lupus and exhibit only the manifestations of a hypercoagulable state. Occasionally the syndrome can occur in association with certain drugs or infections. The presence of anticardiolipin antibodies may also yield a false-positive serologic test for syphilis because the antigen in the standard tests (e.g., Venereal Disease Research Laboratory, VDRL) is embedded in cardiolipin. How antiphospholipid antibodies lead to hypercoagulability is not clear, but possible explanations include direct platelet activation, inhibition of PGI_2 production by endothelial cells, or interference in protein C synthesis or activity. Although antiphospholipid antibodies are associated with thrombotic diatheses, they have also been identified in 5 to 15% of apparently normal individuals and may therefore be necessary but not sufficient to cause full-blown antiphospholipid antibody syndrome.

Individuals with the antiphospholipid antibody syndrome present with a wide variety of clinical manifestations, typically characterized by *recurrent venous* or *arterial thrombi,* but also *repeated miscarriages, cardiac valvular vegetations,* or *thrombocytopenia.* Venous thromboses occur most commonly in deep leg veins, but renal, hepatic, and retinal veins are also susceptible. Arterial thromboses typically occur in the cerebral circulation, but coronary, mesenteric, and renal arterial occlusions have also been described. Depending on the vascular bed involved, the clinical presentations may be protean and can vary from pulmonary embolism from a lower extremity venous thrombus to pulmonary hypertension (from recurrent subclinical pulmonary emboli) to stroke, bowel infarction, or renovascular hypertension.[27] Fetal loss is attributable to antibody-mediated inhibition of t-PA activity necessary for trophoblastic invasion of the uterus. Antiphospholipid antibody syndrome is also a cause of renal microangiopathy, resulting in renal failure owing to multiple capillary and arterial thromboses (Chapter 21).

Patients with antiphospholipid antibody syndrome are at increased risk of a fatal event (upwards of 7% in one series of patients with lupus erythematosus, particularly with arterial thromboses or thrombocytopenia). Current treatment includes anticoagulation therapy (aspirin, heparin, and Coumadin), prednisone for recurrent miscarriages, and immunosuppression in refractory cases.[26,27]

MORPHOLOGY OF THROMBI. Thrombi may develop anywhere in the cardiovascular system: within the cardiac chambers; on valve cusps; or in arteries, veins, or capillaries. They are of variable size and shape, depending on the site of origin and the circumstances leading to their development. Arterial or cardiac thrombi usually begin at a site of endothelial injury (e.g., atherosclerotic plaque) or turbulence (vessel bifurcation); venous thrombi characteristically occur in sites of stasis. An area of attachment to the underlying vessel or heart wall, frequently firmest at the point of origin, is characteristic of all thromboses. Arterial thrombi tend to grow in a retrograde direction from the point of attachment, whereas venous thrombi extend in the direction of blood flow (i.e., toward the heart). The propagating tail may not be well attached and, particularly in veins, is prone to fragmentation, creating an **embolus.**

When formed in the heart or aorta, thrombi may have grossly (and microscopically) apparent laminations called **lines of Zahn;** these are produced by alternating pale layers of platelets admixed with some fibrin and darker layers containing more red cells. Lines of Zahn are significant only in that they imply thrombosis at a site of blood flow; in veins or in smaller arteries, the laminations are typically not as apparent, and, in fact, thrombi formed in the sluggish venous flow usually resemble statically coagulated blood (similar to blood clotted in a test tube). Nevertheless, careful evaluation generally reveals irregular, somewhat ill-defined laminations.

When arterial thrombi arise in heart chambers or in the aortic lumen, they are usually adherent to the wall of the underlying structure and are termed **mural thrombi.** Abnormal myocardial contraction (arrhythmias, dilated cardiomyopa-

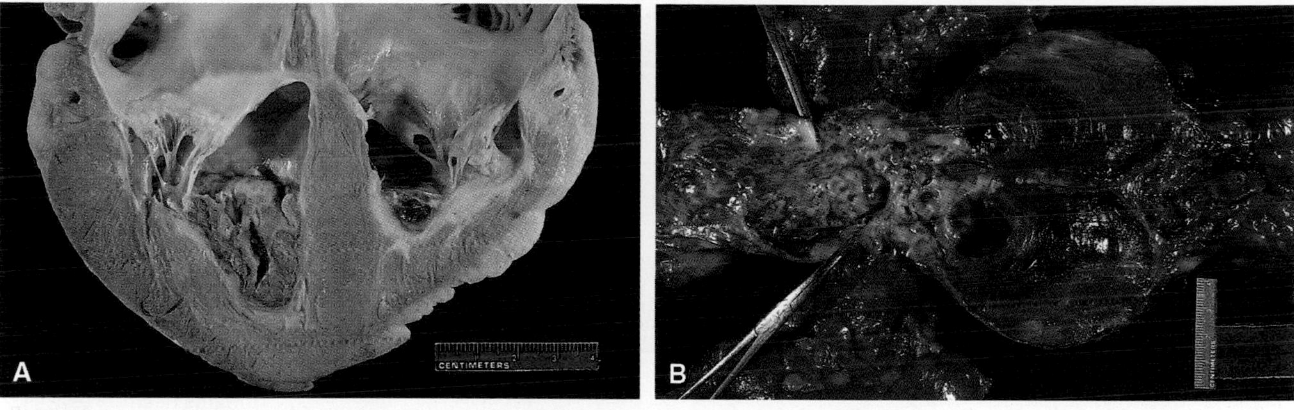

Figure 5–13

Mural thrombi. *A*, Thrombus in the left and right ventricular apices, overlying a white fibrous scar. *B*, Laminated thrombus in a dilated abdominal aortic aneurysm.

thy, or myocardial infarction) leads to cardiac mural thrombi (Fig. 5–13*A*), while ulcerated atherosclerotic plaque and aneurysmal dilation are the precursors of aortic thrombus formation (Fig. 5–13*B*).

Arterial thrombi are usually **occlusive;** the most common sites, in descending order, are coronary, cerebral, and femoral arteries. The thrombus is usually superimposed on an atherosclerotic plaque, although other forms of vascular injury (vasculitis, trauma) may be involved. The thrombi are typically firmly adherent to the injured arterial wall and are gray-white and friable, composed of a tangled mesh of platelets, fibrin, erythrocytes, and degenerating leukocytes.

Venous thrombosis, or **phlebothrombosis,** is almost invariably occlusive; the thrombus often creates a long cast of the vein lumen. Because these thrombi form in a relatively static environment, they tend to contain more enmeshed erythrocytes and are therefore known as **red,** or **stasis, thrombi. Phlebothrombosis most commonly affects the veins of the lower extremities (90% of cases).** Less commonly, venous thrombi may develop in the upper extremities, periprostatic plexus, or the ovarian and periuterine veins; under special circumstances, they may be found in the dural sinuses, the portal vein, or the hepatic vein. At autopsy, postmortem clots may be confused for venous thrombi. Postmortem clots are gelatinous with a dark red dependent portion where red cells have settled by gravity and a yellow *chicken fat* supernatant; they are usually not attached to the underlying wall. In contrast, red thrombi are more firm, almost always have a point of attachment, and on transection reveal vague strands of pale gray fibrin.

Under special circumstances, thrombi may form on heart valves. Bacterial or fungal blood-borne infections may establish a foothold, leading to valve damage and the development of large thrombotic masses or **vegetations (infective endocarditis;** Chapter 13). Sterile vegetations can also develop on noninfected valves in patients with hypercoagulable states, so-called **nonbacterial thrombotic endocarditis** (Chapter 13). Less commonly, noninfective, **verrucous (Libman-Sacks) endocarditis** attributable to elevated levels of circulating immune complexes may occur in patients with systemic lupus erythematosus (Chapter 7).

Fate of the Thrombus. If a patient survives the immediate effects of a thrombotic vascular obstruction, thrombi undergo some combination of the following four events in the ensuing days to weeks (Fig. 5–14):

1. *Propagation:* The thrombus may accumulate more platelets and fibrin (propagate), eventually leading to vessel obstruction.
2. *Embolization:* Thrombi may dislodge and travel to other sites in the vasculature.
3. *Dissolution:* Thrombi may be removed by fibrinolytic activity.
4. *Organization and recanalization:* Thrombi may induce inflammation and fibrosis *(organization)* and may eventually become *recanalized,* that is, may reestablish vascular flow, or may be incorporated into a thickened vascular wall.

Propagation and embolization are discussed further later. As for dissolution, activation of the fibrinolytic pathways can lead to rapid shrinkage and even total lysis of *recent* thrombi. With older thrombi, extensive fibrin polymerization renders the thrombus substantially more resistant to proteolysis, and lysis is ineffectual. This is important because therapeutic infusions of fibrinolytic agents such as t-PA (e.g., for pulmonary thromboemboli or coronary thrombosis) are likely to be effective only for a short time after thrombi form.

Inferior vena cava

Iliac vein

Thrombosed vein

Propagation towards heart

Resolution

Embolization to lungs

Organized and incorporated into wall

Organized and recanalized

Figure 5–14

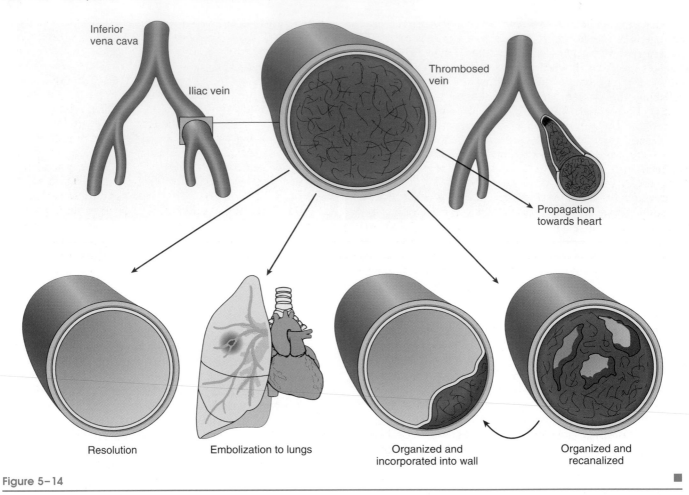

Potential outcomes of venous thrombosis.

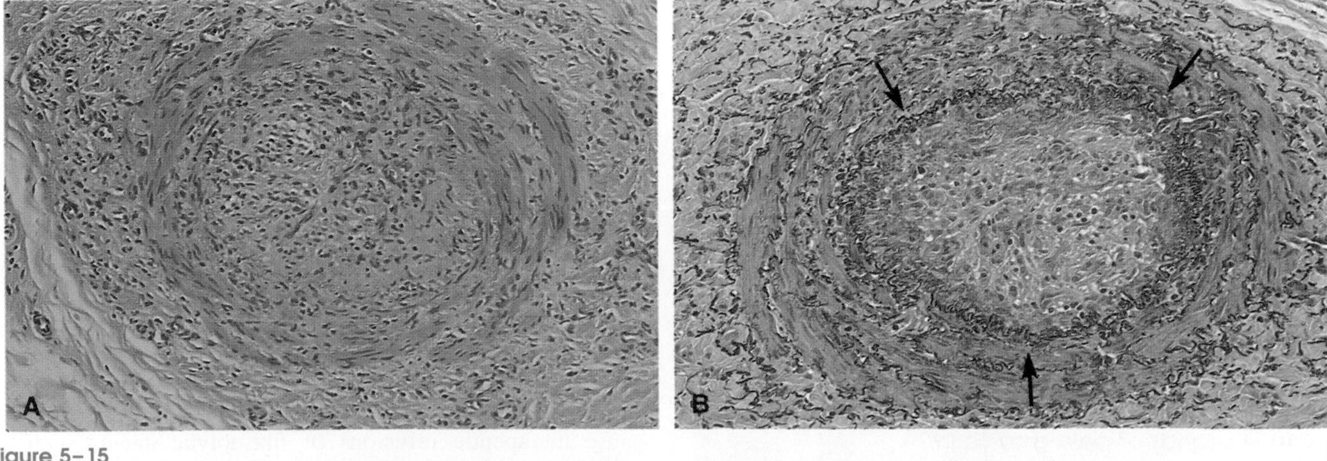

Figure 5–15

Low-power view of a thrombosed artery. *A*, H&E-stained section. *B*, Stain for elastic tissue. The original lumen is delineated by the internal elastic lamina (*arrows*) and is totally filled with organized thrombus, now punctuated by a number of recanalized channels.

Older thrombi tend to become *organized.* This refers to the ingrowth of endothelial cells, smooth muscle cells, and fibroblasts into the fibrin-rich thrombus. In time, capillary channels are formed, which may anastomose to create conduits from one end of the thrombus to the other, reestablishing to some extent the continuity of the original lumen. This *recanalization* (Fig. 5–15) may eventually convert the thrombus into a vascularized mass of connective tissue, which is incorporated as a subendothelial swelling of the vessel wall. With time and contraction of the mesenchymal cells, only a fibrous lump may remain to mark the original thrombus site. Occasionally, instead of organizing, the center of a thrombus undergoes enzymatic digestion, presumably as a result of the release of lysosomal enzymes from trapped leukocytes and platelets. This is particularly likely in large thrombi within aneurysmal dilations or the cardiac chambers. If bacterial seeding occurs, such degraded thrombus is an ideal culture medium, resulting, for example, in a so-called *mycotic aneurysm* (Chapter 12).

Clinical Correlation. Thrombi are significant because (1) *they cause obstruction of arteries and veins,* and (2) *they are possible sources of emboli.* The significance of each depends on where the thrombus occurs. Thus, while venous thrombi may cause congestion and edema in vascular beds distal to an obstruction, a far graver consequence is that thrombi, most frequently those occurring in deep leg veins, are responsible for a major cause of death, pulmonary embolization. Conversely, although arterial thrombi can embolize, their role in vascular obstruction (e.g., in causing myocardial or cerebral infarctions) is much more important.

Venous Thrombosis (Phlebothrombosis). The great preponderance of venous thrombi occur in either the superficial or the deep veins of the leg.[29] Superficial thrombi usually occur in the saphenous system, particularly when there are varicosities. Such thrombi may cause local congestion, and swelling, pain, and tenderness along the course of the involved vein but only rarely embolize. Nevertheless, the local edema and impaired venous drainage do predispose the involved overlying skin to infections from slight trauma and to the development of *varicose ulcers. Deep thrombi* in the larger leg veins at or above the knee (e.g., popliteal, femoral, and iliac veins) are more serious because they may embolize. Although they may cause local pain and distal edema, the venous obstruction may be rapidly offset by collateral bypass channels. Consequently, deep vein thromboses are entirely asymptomatic in *approximately 50% of affected patients* and are recognized only in retrospect after they have embolized.

Deep venous thrombosis may occur with stasis and in a variety of hypercoagulable states as described earlier (Table 5–2). Congestive heart failure is an obvious reason for stasis in the venous circulation. Trauma, surgery, and burns usually result in reduced physical activity, injury to vessels, release of procoagulant substances from tissues, and reduced t-PA activity. Many factors act in concert to predispose to thrombosis in the puerperal and postpartum states. Besides the potential for amniotic fluid embolization at the time of delivery, late pregnancy and the postpartum period are associated with hypercoagulability. Tumor-associated procoagulant release is largely responsible for the increased risk of evanescent thromboses seen in disseminated cancers, giving rise to the pattern known as *migratory thrombophlebitis* (*Trousseau syndrome*). Regardless of the specific clinical setting, advanced age, bed rest, and immobilization increase the risk of deep venous thrombosis; reduced physical activity diminishes the milking action of muscles in the lower leg and so slows venous return.

Arterial Thrombosis. *Myocardial infarction* may be associated with dyskinetic contraction of the myocardium as well as damage to the adjacent endocardium, providing a site for the origin of a mural thrombus (see Fig. 5–13*A*). *Rheumatic heart disease* may result in mitral valve stenosis, followed by left atrial dilation; concurrent atrial fibrillation augments atrial blood stasis. *Atherosclerosis* is a major initiator of thromboses, related to abnormal vascular flow and loss of endothelial integrity (see Fig. 5–13*B*). In addition to the obstructive consequences, cardiac and aortic mural thrombi can also embolize peripherally. Virtually any tissue may be affected, but the brain, kidneys, and spleen are prime targets because of their large flow volume.

While we clearly understand a number of conditions that predispose to thrombosis, the phenomenon remains somewhat unpredictable. It continues to occur at a distressingly high frequency in healthy, ambulatory individuals without apparent provocation or underlying pathology.

Disseminated Intravascular Coagulation (DIC)

A variety of disorders ranging from obstetric complications to advanced malignancy may be complicated by DIC, the sudden or insidious onset of widespread fibrin thrombi in the microcirculation. Although these thrombi are not usually visible on gross inspection, they are readily apparent microscopically and can cause diffuse circulatory insufficiency, particularly in the brain, lungs, heart, and kidneys. With the development of the multiple thrombi, there is a rapid concurrent consumption of platelets and coagulation proteins (hence the synonym *consumption coagulopathy*); at the same time, fibrinolytic mechanisms are activated, and as a result an initially thrombotic disorder can evolve into a serious bleeding disorder. *DIC is not a primary disease but rather a potential complication of any condition associated with widespread activation of thrombin.*[30] It is discussed in greater detail along with other bleeding diatheses in Chapter 14.

EMBOLISM

An embolus is a detached intravascular solid, liquid, or gaseous mass that is carried by the blood to a site distant from its point of origin. Virtually 99% of all emboli represent some part of a dislodged thrombus, hence the commonly used term *thromboembolism.* Rare forms of emboli include droplets of fat, bubbles of air or nitrogen, atherosclerotic debris *(cholesterol emboli),* tumor fragments, bits of bone marrow, or foreign bodies such as bullets. Unless otherwise specified, however, embolism should be considered to be thrombotic in origin. Inevitably, emboli lodge in vessels too small to permit further passage, resulting in partial or complete vascular occlusion. The potential consequence of such thromboembolic events is the ischemic necrosis of distal tissue, known as *infarction.* Depending on the site of origin, emboli may lodge anywhere in the vascular tree; the clinical outcomes are best understood from the standpoint of whether emboli lodge in the pulmonary or systemic circulations.

Pulmonary Thromboembolism

Pulmonary embolism has an incidence of 20 to 25 per 100,000 hospitalized patients.[31] Although the rate of fatal pulmonary emboli (as assessed at autopsy) has declined from 6% to 2% over the last 25 years,[32] pulmonary embolism still causes about 200,000 deaths per year in the United States. In more than 95% of instances, venous emboli originate from deep leg vein thrombi above the level of the knee as described previously. They are carried through progressively larger channels and usually pass through the right side of the heart into the pulmonary vasculature. Depending on the size of the embolus, it may occlude the main pulmonary artery, impact across the bifurcation *(saddle embolus),* or pass out into the smaller, branching arterioles (Fig. 5–16). Frequently, there are multiple emboli, perhaps sequentially or as a shower of smaller emboli from a single large mass; in general, *the patient who has had one pulmonary embolus is at high risk of having more.* Rarely, an embolus may pass through an interatrial or interventricular defect to gain access to the systemic circulation *(paradoxical embolism).* A more complete discussion of pulmonary emboli is presented in Chapter 16; an overview is offered here.[33,34]

- Most pulmonary emboli (60 to 80%) are clinically silent because they are small. With time, they undergo organization and are incorporated into the vascular wall (see Fig. 5–14); in some cases, organization of the thromboembolus leaves behind a delicate, bridging fibrous *web.*
- Sudden death, right heart failure *(cor pulmonale),* or cardiovascular collapse occurs when 60% or more of the pulmonary circulation is obstructed with emboli.
- Embolic obstruction of medium-sized arteries may result in pulmonary hemorrhage but usually does not cause pulmonary infarction because of the dual blood flow into the area from the bronchial circulation. A similar embolus in the setting of left-sided cardiac failure (i.e., with sluggish bronchial artery flow), however, may result in a large infarct.
- Embolic obstruction of small end-arteriolar pulmonary branches usually does result in associated infarction.
- Multiple emboli over time may cause pulmonary hypertension with right heart failure.

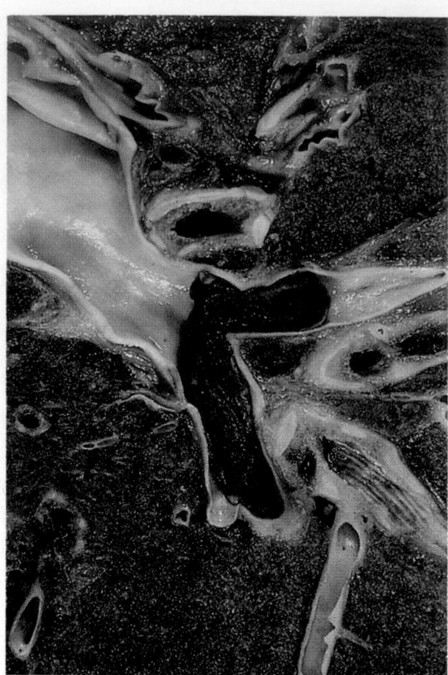

Figure 5–16

Large embolus derived from a lower extremity deep venous thrombosis, and now impacted in a pulmonary artery branch.

Systemic Thromboembolism

Systemic thromboembolism refers to emboli traveling within the arterial circulation. Most (80%) arise from intracardiac mural thrombi, two thirds of which are associated with left ventricular wall infarcts and another quarter with dilated left atria (e.g., secondary to rheumatic valvular disease; Chapter 13). The remainder largely originate from aortic aneurysms, thrombi on ulcerated atherosclerotic plaques, or fragmentation of a valvular vegetation (Chapter 13), while only a small fraction are due to *paradoxical emboli;* 10 to 15% of systemic emboli are of unknown origin. In contrast to venous emboli, which tend to lodge primarily in one vascular bed (the lung), arterial emboli can travel to a wide variety of sites; the site of arrest depends on the point of origin of the thromboembolus and the volume of blood flow through the downstream tissues. The major sites for arteriolar embolization are the lower extremities (75%) and the brain (10%), with the intestines, kidneys, spleen, and upper extremities involved to a lesser extent. The consequences of systemic emboli depend on any collateral vascular supply in the affected tissue, the tissue's vulnerability to ischemia, and the caliber of the vessel occluded; in general, however, arterial emboli cause infarction of tissues in the distribution of the obstructed vessel.

Fat Embolism

Microscopic fat globules may be found in the circulation after fractures of long bones (which have fatty marrows) or, rarely, in the setting of soft tissue trauma and burns. Presumably the fat is released by marrow or adipose tissue injury and enters the circulation by rupture of the marrow vascular sinusoids or of venules. Although *traumatic fat embolism occurs in some 90% of individuals with severe skeletal injuries* (Fig. 5–17), *less than 10% of such patients have any clinical findings. Fat embolism syndrome* typically begins 1 to 3 days after injury, with sudden onset of tachypnea, dyspnea, and tachycardia. Besides pulmonary insufficiency, the syndrome is characterized by neurologic symptoms, including irritability and restlessness, which can progress to delirium or coma. A diffuse petechial rash in nondependent areas (occurring in the absence of thrombocytopenia) is seen in 20 to 50% of cases and is useful in establishing a diagnosis. Patients may also present with thrombocytopenia, presumably caused by platelets adhering to the myriad fat globules and being removed from the circulation; anemia may result as a consequence of erythrocyte aggregation and hemolysis. In its full-blown form, the syndrome is fatal in up to 10% of cases.

The pathogenesis of fat emboli syndrome probably involves both mechanical obstruction and biochemical injury.[35,36] Initially, microemboli of neutral fat cause occlusion of pulmonary or cerebral microvasculature, further exacerbated by local platelet and erythrocyte aggregation. Subsequently, free fatty acids released from neutral fat globules cause local toxic injury to endothelium; platelet activation and recruitment of granulocytes (with free radical, protease, and eicosanoid release; Chapter 3) complete the vascular assault. Because lipids are dissolved out of tissue preparations by the solvents routinely used in paraffin embedding, the microscopic demonstration of fat microglobules (i.e., in the absence of accompanying marrow) typically requires specialized techniques, including frozen sections and fat stains.

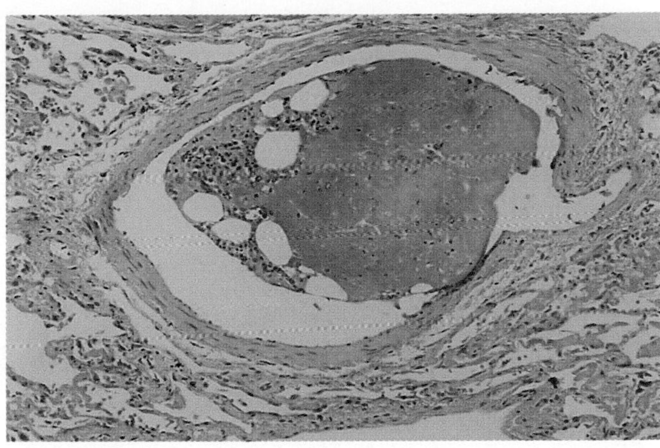

Figure 5–17

Bone marrow embolus in the pulmonary circulation. The cleared vacuoles represent marrow fat that is now impacted in a distal vessel along with the cellular hematopoietic precursors.

Air Embolism

Gas bubbles within the circulation can obstruct vascular flow (and cause distal ischemic injury) almost as readily as thrombotic masses. Air may enter the circulation during obstetric procedures or as a consequence of chest wall injury. Generally, in excess of 100 cc is required to have a clinical effect; the bubbles act like physical obstructions and may coalesce to form frothy masses sufficiently large to occlude major vessels.[35,37]

A particular form of gas embolism, called *decompression sickness,* occurs when individuals are exposed to sudden changes in atmospheric pressure.[38] Scuba and deep sea divers, underwater construction workers, and individuals in unpressurized aircraft in rapid ascent are all at risk. When air is breathed at high pressure (e.g., during a deep sea dive), increased amounts of gas (particularly nitrogen) become dissolved in the blood and tissues. If the diver then ascends (depressurizes) too rapidly, the nitrogen expands in the tissues and bubbles out of solution in the blood to form gas emboli.

Acutely, the formation of painful gas bubbles within skeletal muscles and supporting tissues in and about joints is responsible for what is called *the bends.* Gas emboli may also induce focal ischemia in a number of tissues, including brain and heart. In the lungs, edema, hemorrhages, and focal atelectasis or emphysema may appear, leading to respiratory distress, the so-called *chokes.* Treatment of gas embolism consists of placing the individual in a compression chamber where the barometric pressure may be raised, thus forcing the gas bubbles back into solution. Subsequent slow decompression of the individual, it is hoped, allows gradual resorption and exhalation of the gases so that obstructive bubbles will not reform. A more chronic form of decompression sickness is called *caisson disease,* in which persistence of gas emboli in the skeletal system leads to multiple foci of ischemic necrosis; the more common sites are the heads of the femurs, tibia, and humeri.

Amniotic Fluid Embolism

Amniotic fluid embolism is a grave but uncommon (1 in 50,000 deliveries) complication of labor and the immediate postpartum period. It has a mortality rate in excess of 80%, and as other obstetric complications (e.g., eclampsia, pulmonary embolism) have been better controlled, amniotic fluid embolism has become a major cause of maternal mortality. The onset is characterized by sudden severe dyspnea, cyanosis, and hypotensive shock, followed by seizures and coma. If the patient survives the initial crisis, pulmonary edema typically develops, along with (in half the patients) DIC, owing to release of thrombogenic substances from amniotic fluid.[35,39]

The underlying cause is the infusion of amniotic fluid (and all of its contents) into the maternal circulation via a tear in the placental membranes and rupture of uterine veins. The classic findings are therefore the presence in the pulmonary microcirculation of epithelial squamous cells shed from fetal skin, lanugo hair, fat from vernix caseosa, and mucin derived from the fetal respiratory or gastrointestinal tract. There is also marked pulmonary edema and changes of *diffuse alveolar damage* (Chapter 16) as well as systemic fibrin thrombi indicative of DIC.

INFARCTION

An infarct is an area of ischemic necrosis caused by occlusion of either the arterial supply or the venous drainage in a particular tissue. Tissue infarction is a common and extremely important cause of clinical illness. In the United States, more than half of all deaths are caused by cardiovascular disease, and most of these are attributable to myocardial or cerebral infarction. Pulmonary infarction is a common complication in a number of clinical settings, bowel infarction is frequently fatal, and ischemic necrosis of the extremities (gangrene) is a serious problem in the diabetic population.

Nearly 99% of all infarcts result from thrombotic or embolic events, and almost all result from arterial occlusion. Occasionally, infarction may also be caused by other mechanisms, such as local vasospasm, expansion of an atheroma owing to hemorrhage within a plaque, or extrinsic compression of a vessel (e.g., by tumor). Other uncommon causes include twisting of the vessels (e.g., in testicular torsion or bowel volvulus), compression of the blood supply by edema or by entrapment in a hernial sac, or traumatic rupture of the blood supply. Although venous thrombosis may cause infarction, it more often merely induces venous obstruction and congestion. Usually, bypass channels then rapidly open, providing some outflow from the area, which, in turn, improves the arterial inflow. Infarcts caused by venous thrombosis are more likely in organs with a single venous outflow channel, such as the testis and ovary.

TYPES OF INFARCTS. Infarcts are classified on the basis of their color (reflecting the amount of hemorrhage) and the presence or absence of microbial infection. Therefore, infarcts may be either *red (hemorrhagic)* or *white (anemic)* and may be either *septic* or *bland.*

- *Red infarcts* occur (1) with venous occlusions (such as in ovarian torsion); (2) in loose tissues (such as lung), which allow blood to collect in the infarcted zone; (3) in tissues with dual circulations (e.g., lung and small intestine), permitting flow of blood from the unobstructed vessel into the necrotic zone (although, obviously, such perfusion is not sufficient to rescue the ischemic tissues); (4) in tissues that were previously congested because of sluggish venous outflow; and (5) when flow is reestablished to a site of previous arterial occlusion and necrosis (e.g., fragmentation of an occlusive embolus or angioplasty of a thrombotic lesion) (Fig. 5–18*A*).
- *White infarcts* occur with arterial occlusions or in solid organs (such as heart, spleen, and kidney), where the solidity of the tissue limits the amount of hemorrhage that can seep into the area of ischemic necrosis from adjoining capillary beds (Fig. 5–18*B*).

All infarcts tend to be wedge-shaped, with the occluded vessel at the apex and the periphery of the organ forming the base; when the base is a serosal surface, there is often an overlying fibrinous exudate. The lateral margins may be irregular, reflecting the pattern of vascular supply from adjacent vessels. At the outset, all infarcts are poorly defined and slightly hemorrhagic. The margins of both types of infarcts tend to become better defined with time by a narrow rim of hyperemia attributable to inflammation at the edge of the lesion.

In solid organs, the relatively few extravasated red cells are lysed, with the released hemoglobin remaining in the form of hemosiderin. Thus, white infarcts typically become progressively more pale and sharply defined with time (Fig. 5–18*B*). In spongy organs, by comparison, the hemorrhage is too extensive to permit the lesion ever to become pale (Fig. 5–18*A*). Over the course of a few days, it does, however, become more firm and brown, reflecting the development of hemosiderin pigment.

The dominant histologic characteristic of infarction is *ischemic coagulative necrosis* (Chapter 1). If the vascular occlusion has occurred shortly (minutes to hours) before the death of the patient, no demonstrable histologic changes may be evident; if the patient survives even 12 to 18 hours, the only change present may be hemorrhage.

An inflammatory response begins to develop along the margins of infarcts within a few hours and is usually well defined within 1 or 2 days. Inflammation at these sites is incited by the necrotic material; given sufficient time, there is gradual degradation of the dead tissue with phagocytosis of the cellular debris by neutrophils and macrophages. Eventually the inflammatory response is followed by a reparative response beginning in the preserved margins (Chapter 3). In stable or labile tissues, some parenchymal regeneration may occur at the periphery where the underlying stromal architecture has been spared. Most infarcts, however, are ultimately replaced by scar tissue (Fig. 5–19). The brain is an exception to these generalizations; similar to other causes of cell death, ischemic injury in the central nervous system results in *liquefactive necrosis* (Chapter 1).

Septic infarctions may develop when embolization occurs by fragmentation of a bacterial vegetation from a heart valve or when microbes seed an area of necrotic tissue. In these cases, the infarct is converted into an *abscess,* with a corre-

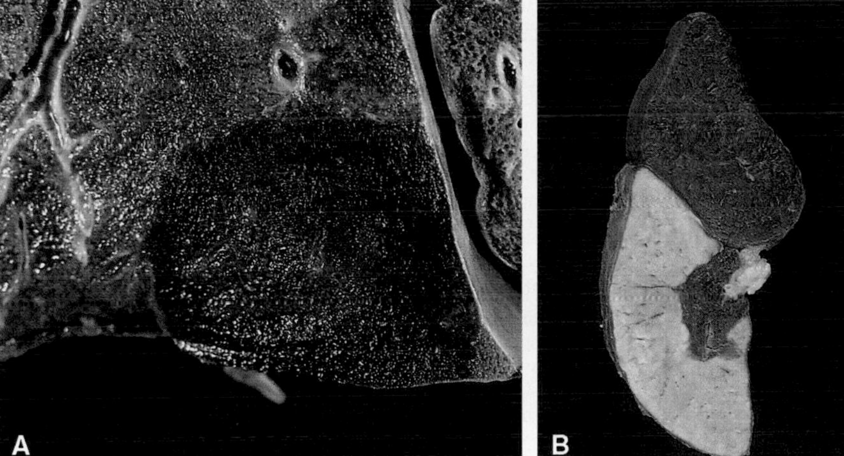

Figure 5–18

Examples of infarcts. *A*, Hemorrhagic, roughly wedge-shaped pulmonary infarct. *B*, Sharply demarcated white infarct in the spleen.

spondingly greater inflammatory response. The eventual sequence of organization, however, follows that pattern already described.

Factors That Influence Development of an Infarct

The consequences of a vascular occlusion can range from no or minimal effect, all the way up to death of a tissue or even the individual. *The major determinants include (1) the nature of the vascular supply, (2) the rate of development of the occlusion, (3) the vulnerability of a given tissue to hypoxia, and (4) the blood oxygen content.*

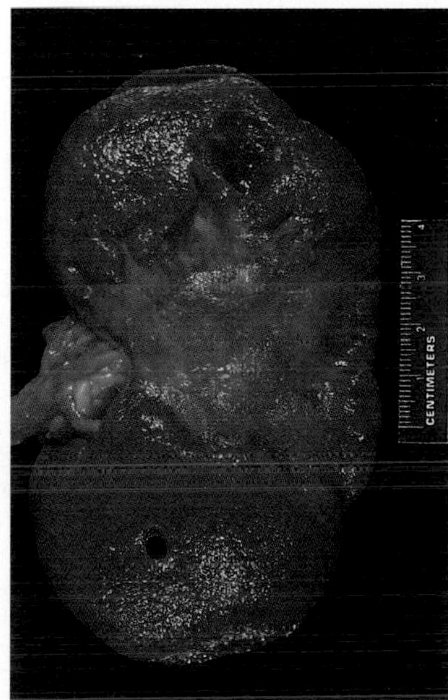

Figure 5–19

Remote kidney infarct, now replaced by a large fibrotic cortical scar.

- *Nature of the vascular supply:* The availability of an alternative blood supply is the most important factor in determining whether occlusion of a vessel will cause damage. Lungs, for example, have a dual pulmonary and bronchial artery blood supply; thus, obstruction of a small pulmonary arteriole has no effect in an otherwise healthy individual with an intact bronchial circulation. Similarly, liver, with the dual hepatic artery and portal vein circulation, is relatively insensitive to local occlusion, as is the hand and forearm owing to the double arterial supply through the radial and ulnar arteries. In contrast, renal and splenic circulations are end arterial, and obstruction of such vessels generally causes infarction.
- *Rate of development of occlusion:* Slowly developing occlusions are less likely to cause infarction since they provide time for the development of alternative perfusion pathways. For example, small interarteriolar anastomoses, normally with minimal functional flow, interconnect the three major coronary arteries in the heart. If one of the coronaries is only slowly occluded (i.e., by an encroaching atherosclerotic plaque), flow within this *collateral circulation* may increase sufficiently to prevent infarction, even though the major coronary artery is eventually occluded.
- *Vulnerability to hypoxia:* The susceptibility of a tissue to hypoxia influences the likelihood of infarction. Neurons undergo irreversible damage when deprived of their blood supply for only 3 to 4 minutes. Myocardial cells, although hardier than neurons, are also quite sensitive and die after only 20 to 30 minutes of ischemia. In contrast, fibroblasts within myocardium are viable even after many hours of ischemia (Chapter 13).
- *Oxygen content of blood:* The partial pressure of oxygen in blood also determines the outcome of vascular occlusion. Partial flow obstruction of a small vessel in an anemic or cyanotic patient might lead to tissue infarction, whereas it would be without effect under conditions of normal oxygen tension. In this way, congestive heart failure, with compromised flow *and ventilation,* could cause infarction in the setting of an otherwise inconsequential blockage.

Table 5–3. THREE MAJOR TYPES OF SHOCK

Type of Shock	Clinical Examples	Principal Mechanisms
Cardiogenic	Myocardial infarction Ventricular rupture Arrhythmia Cardiac tamponade Pulmonary embolism	Failure of myocardial pump owing to intrinsic myocardial damage, extrinsic pressure, or obstruction to outflow
Hypovolemic	Hemorrhage Fluid loss, e.g., vomiting, diarrhea, burns, or trauma	Inadequate blood or plasma volume
Septic	Overwhelming microbial infections Endotoxic shock Gram-positive septicemia Fungal sepsis Superantigens	Peripheral vasodilation and pooling of blood; endothelial activation/injury; leukocyte-induced damage; disseminated intravascular coagulation; activation of cytokine cascades

SHOCK

Shock, or *cardiovascular collapse,* is the final common pathway for a number of potentially lethal clinical events, including severe hemorrhage, extensive trauma or burns, large myocardial infarction, massive pulmonary embolism, or microbial sepsis. Regardless of the underlying pathology, *shock constitutes systemic hypoperfusion owing to reduction either in cardiac output or in the effective circulating blood volume.* The end results are *hypotension, followed by impaired tissue perfusion and cellular hypoxia.* Although the hypoxic and metabolic effects of hypoperfusion initially cause only reversible cellular injury, persistence of the shock state eventually causes irreversible tissue injury and can culminate in the death of the patient.

Shock may be grouped into three general categories (Table 5–3). The mechanisms underlying cardiogenic and hypovolemic shock are fairly straightforward; essentially, they involve *low cardiac output.* Septic shock, by comparison, is substantially more complicated and is discussed in further detail subsequently.

- *Cardiogenic shock* results from myocardial pump failure. This may be caused by intrinsic myocardial damage (infarction), ventricular arrhythmias, extrinsic compression (cardiac tamponade; Chapter 13), or outflow obstruction (e.g., pulmonary embolism).
- *Hypovolemic shock* results from loss of blood or plasma volume. This may be caused by hemorrhage, fluid loss from severe burns, or trauma.
- *Septic shock* is caused by systemic microbial infection. Most commonly, this occurs in the setting of gram-negative infections *(endotoxic shock)* but can also occur with gram-positive and fungal infections.

Less commonly, shock may occur in the setting of anesthetic accident or spinal cord injury *(neurogenic shock),* owing to loss of vascular tone and peripheral pooling of blood. *Anaphylactic shock,* initiated by a generalized IgE-mediated hypersensitivity response, is associated with systemic vasodilation and increased vascular permeability (Chapter 6). In these instances, widespread vasodilation causes a sudden increase in the vascular bed capacitance, which is not adequately filled by the normal circulating blood volume. Hypotension, tissue hypoperfusion, and cellular anoxia are the outcome.

Pathogenesis of Septic Shock. Septic shock has a 25 to 75% mortality rate, ranking first among the causes of death in intensive care units and accounting for some 100,000 deaths annually in the United States. Moreover, the reported incidence of sepsis syndromes is increasing dramatically (e.g., greater than twofold increase was seen between 1979 and 1987), in part owing to improved life support for high-risk patients, increasing invasive procedures, and growing numbers of immunocompromised hosts (secondary to chemotherapy, immunosuppression, or human immunodeficiency virus [HIV]).[40] Septic shock results from spread and expansion of an initially localized infection (e.g., abscess, peritonitis, pneumonia) into the bloodstream.

Most cases of septic shock (approximately 70%) are caused by endotoxin-producing gram-negative bacilli (Chapter 9), hence the term *endotoxic shock.* Endotoxins are bacterial wall lipopolysaccharides (LPS) released when the

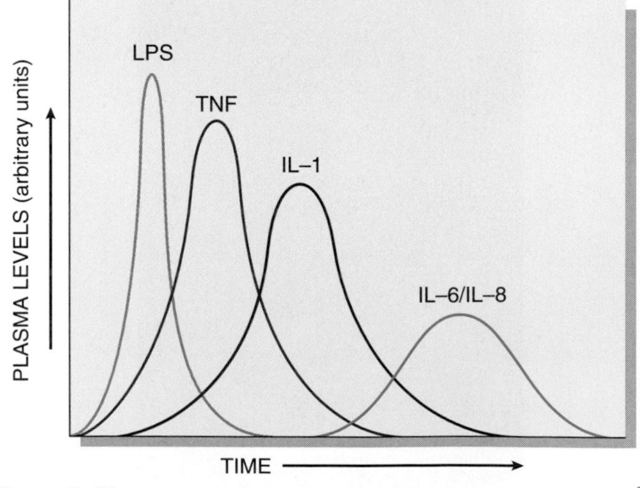

Figure 5–20

Cytokine cascade in sepsis. After release of lipopolysaccharide (LPS), there are successive waves of tumor necrosis factor (TNF), interleukin-1 (IL-1), and IL-6 secretion. (Modified from Abbas AK, et al: Cellular and Molecular Immunology, 3rd ed. Philadelphia, WB Saunders, 1997.)

cell walls are degraded (e.g., in an inflammatory response). LPS consists of a toxic fatty acid *(lipid A)* core and a complex polysaccharide coat (including O antigens) unique to each bacterial species. Analogous molecules in the walls of gram-positive bacteria and fungi can also elicit septic shock.

All of the cellular and resultant hemodynamic effects of septic shock may be reproduced by injection of LPS alone. LPS binds as a complex with a circulating blood protein to CD14 molecules on leukocytes (especially monocytes and macrophages), endothelial cells, and other cell types. Depending on the dosage, the LPS-binding protein complex can then directly activate vascular wall cells and leukocytes or initiate a cascade of cytokine mediators, which propagates the pathologic state.[41–43]

At low doses, LPS predominantly serves to activate monocytes and macrophages, with effects presumably intended to enhance their ability to eliminate invading bacteria. LPS can also directly activate complement, which likewise contributes to local bacterial eradication. The mononuclear phagocytes respond to LPS by producing TNF, which, in turn, induces IL-1 synthesis. TNF and IL-1 both act on endothelial cells to produce further cytokines (e.g., IL-6 and IL-8) as well as induce adhesion molecules (Chapter 3). Thus, the initial release of LPS results in a circumscribed cytokine cascade (Fig. 5–20) doubtless intended to enhance the *local* acute inflammatory response and improve clearance of the infection.

With moderately severe infections, and therefore with higher levels of LPS (and a consequent augmentation of the cytokine cascade), cytokine-induced secondary effectors (e.g., nitric oxide and platelet-activating factor; Chapter 3) become significant. In addition, systemic effects of TNF and IL-1 may begin to be seen; these include fever and increased synthesis of acute phase reactants (Chapter 3; Fig. 5–21). LPS at higher doses also results in endothelial

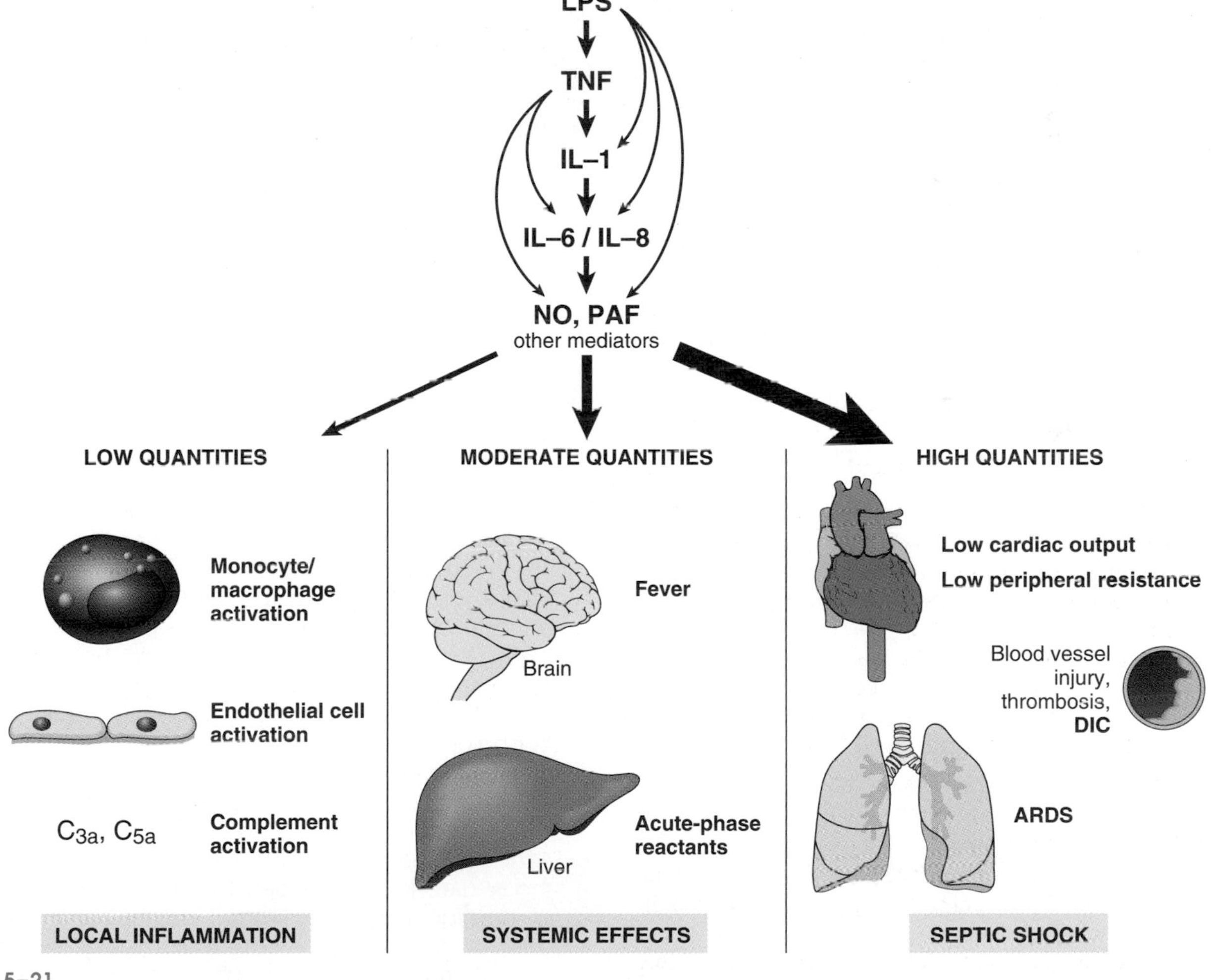

Figure 5–21

Effects of lipopolysaccharide (LPS) and secondarily-induced effector molecules. LPS initiates the cytokine cascade described in Figure 5-20; in addition, LPS and the various factors can directly stimulate down-stream cytokine production, as indicated. Secondary effectors that become important include nitric oxide (NO) and platelet-activating factor (PAF). At low levels, only local inflammatory effects are seen. With moderate levels, more systemic events occur in addition to the local vascular effects. At high concentrations, the syndrome of septic shock is seen. DIC, disseminated intravascular coagulation; ARDS, adult respiratory distress syndrome. (Modified from Abbas AK, et al: Cellular and Molecular Immunology, 3rd ed. Philadelphia, WB Saunders, 1997.)

cell injury, which, in turn, triggers the coagulation cascade. Finally, at still higher levels of LPS, the syndrome of septic shock supervenes (Fig. 5–21); the same cytokine and secondary mediators now at high levels result in

- Systemic vasodilation (hypotension)
- Diminished myocardial contractility
- Widespread endothelial injury and activation, causing systemic leukocyte adhesion and pulmonary alveolar capillary damage (*adult respiratory distress syndrome;* Chapter 16)
- Activation of the coagulation system, culminating in DIC

The hypoperfusion resulting from the combined effects of widespread vasodilation, myocardial pump failure, and DIC induces *multiorgan system failure* affecting the liver, kidneys, and central nervous system, among others (also called *systemic inflammatory response syndrome*).[41,42] Unless the underlying infection (and LPS overload) is rapidly brought under control, the patient usually dies. In some experimental models, soluble CD14 or antibodies to LPS-binding protein, antibodies or antagonists to IL-1 or TNF (or their receptors), or pharmacologic inhibitors of various secondary mediators (e.g., nitric oxide or prostaglandins) have demonstrated some efficacy in protecting against septic shock; these reagents have not yet proved to be of significant clinical benefit in human disease.[42–44]

An interesting group of bacterial proteins called *superantigens* also cause a syndrome similar to septic shock. (These include *toxic shock syndrome toxin-1* produced by staphylococci and responsible for the *toxic shock syndrome*).[45] Superantigens are polyclonal T-lymphocyte activators, which induce systemic inflammatory cytokine cascades similar to those occurring down-stream in septic shock. Their actions can result in a variety of clinical manifestations ranging from a diffuse rash to vasodilation, hypotension, and death.[46]

Stages of Shock. Shock is a progressive disorder that, if uncorrected, leads to death. Unless the insult is massive and rapidly lethal (e.g., a massive hemorrhage from a ruptured aortic aneurysm), shock tends to evolve through three general (albeit somewhat artificial) phases. A brief discussion here can help to integrate the sequential pathophysiologic and clinical events in the progression of shock. These have been documented most clearly in hypovolemic shock but are common to other forms as well:

1. An initial *nonprogressive phase* during which reflex compensatory mechanisms are activated and perfusion of vital organs is maintained
2. A *progressive stage* characterized by tissue hypoperfusion and onset of worsening circulatory and metabolic imbalances including acidosis
3. An *irreversible stage* that sets in after the body has incurred cellular and tissue injury so severe that even if the hemodynamic defects are corrected, survival is not possible

In the early *nonprogressive phase* of shock, a *variety of neurohumoral mechanisms* help maintain cardiac output and blood pressure. These include baroreceptor reflexes, release of catecholamines, activation of the renin-angiotensin axis, antidiuretic hormone release, and generalized sympathetic stimulation. The net effect is *tachycardia, peripheral vasoconstriction, and renal conservation of fluid.* Cutaneous vasoconstriction, for example, is responsible for the characteristic coolness and pallor of skin in well-developed shock (although septic shock may initially cause cutaneous *vasodilation* and thus present with warm, flushed skin). Coronary and cerebral vessels are less sensitive to this compensatory sympathetic response and thus maintain relatively normal caliber, blood flow, and oxygen delivery to their respective vital organs.

If the underlying causes are not corrected, shock passes imperceptibly to the *progressive phase, during which there is widespread tissue hypoxia.* In the setting of persistent oxygen deficit, intracellular aerobic respiration is replaced by anaerobic glycolysis with excessive production of lactic acid. The resultant metabolic *lactic acidosis lowers the tissue pH and blunts the vasomotor response;* arterioles dilate, and blood begins to pool in the microcirculation. Peripheral pooling not only worsens the cardiac output, but also puts endothelial cells at risk for developing anoxic injury with subsequent DIC. With widespread tissue hypoxia, vital organs are affected and begin to fail; *clinically the patient may become confused, and the urinary output declines.*

Unless there is intervention, the process eventually enters an irreversible stage. Widespread cell injury is reflected in lysosomal enzyme leakage, further aggravating the shock state. Myocardial contractile function worsens in part because of nitric oxide synthesis. If ischemic bowel allows intestinal flora to enter the circulation, endotoxic shock may be superimposed. At this point, *the patient has complete renal shutdown owing to acute tubular necrosis* (Chapter 21), and despite heroic measures, the downward clinical spiral almost inevitably culminates in death.

MORPHOLOGY. The cellular and tissue changes induced by shock are essentially those of hypoxic injury (Chapter 1); since shock is characterized by **failure of multiple organ systems,** the cellular changes may appear in any tissue. Nevertheless, they are particularly evident in brain, heart, lungs, kidneys, adrenals, and gastrointestinal tract.

The **brain** may develop so-called ischemic encephalopathy, discussed in Chapter 30. The **heart** may undergo focal or widespread coagulation necrosis or may exhibit subendocardial hemorrhage or **contraction band necrosis** (Chapter 13). Although these changes are not diagnostic of shock (i.e., they may also be seen in the setting of cardiac reperfusion after irreversible injury or after administration of catecholamines), they are usually much more extensive in the setting of shock. The **kidneys** typically exhibit extensive tubular ischemic injury **(acute tubular necrosis;** Chapter 21), so that oliguria, anuria, and electrolyte disturbances constitute major clinical problems. The **lungs** are seldom affected in pure hypovolemic shock because they are resistant to hypoxic injury. When shock is caused by bacterial sepsis or trauma, however, changes of diffuse alveolar damage (Chapter 16) may appear, the so-called **shock lung.** The **adrenal** changes in shock are those seen in all forms of stress; essentially, there is cortical cell lipid depletion. This does not reflect adrenal exhaustion but rather conversion of the relatively inactive vacuolated cells to metabolically active cells that use stored lipids for the synthesis of steroids. The **gastrointestinal tract** may suffer patchy mucosal hemorrhages and necroses, referred to as **hemorrhagic enteropathy.** The **liver** may develop fatty change and, with severe perfusion deficits, central hemorrhagic necrosis (Chapter 19).

With the exception of neuronal and myocyte loss, virtually all of these tissue changes may revert to normal if the patient survives. Most patients with irreversible changes owing to severe shock succumb before the tissues can recover.

Clinical Course. The clinical manifestations depend on the precipitating insult. In hypovolemic and cardiogenic shock, *the patient presents with hypotension; a weak, rapid pulse; tachypnea; and cool, clammy, cyanotic skin.* In septic shock, however, *the skin may initially be warm and flushed because of peripheral vasodilation.* The original threat to life stems from the underlying catastrophe that precipitated the shock state (e.g., the myocardial infarct, severe hemorrhage, or uncontrolled bacterial infection). Rapidly, however, the cardiac, cerebral, and pulmonary changes secondary to the shock state materially worsen the problem. Eventually, electrolyte disturbances and metabolic acidosis also exacerbate the situation. If the patient survives the initial complications, he or she enters *a second phase dominated by renal insufficiency* and marked by a progressive fall in urine output as well as severe fluid and electrolyte imbalances.

The prognosis varies with the origin of shock and its duration. Thus, 80 to 90% of young, otherwise healthy patients with hypovolemic shock survive with appropriate management, whereas cardiogenic shock associated with extensive myocardial infarction and gram-negative shock carry mortality rates of up to 75%, even with the best care currently available.

REFERENCES

1. Abraham WT, Schrier RW: Body fluid volume regulation in health and disease. Adv Intern Med 39:23, 1994.
2. Rick RL, Murano G: Physiology of hemostasis. Clin Lab Med 14: 677, 1994.
3. Wu KK, Thiagarajan P: Role of endothelium in thrombosis and hemostasis. Ann Rev Med 47:315, 1996.
4. Lijnen HR, Collen D: Endothelium in hemostasis and thrombosis. Prog Cardiovasc Dis 39:343, 1997.
5. Tans G, et al: Regulation of thrombin formation by activated protein C: effect of the factor V Leiden mutation. Semin Hematol 34:244, 1997.
6. Lijnen HR, Collen D: Mechanisms of physiological fibrinolysis. Baillieres Clin Haematol 8:277, 1995.
7. Packham MA: Roles of platelets in thrombosis and hemostasis. Can J Physiol Pharmacol 72:278, 1994.
8. Cruz MA, et al: Interaction of the von Willebrand factor (vWF) with collagen: localization of the primary collagen-binding site by analysis of recombinant vWF A domain polypeptides. J Biol Chem 270: 10822, 1995.
9. Harker LA, et al: Antithrombotic strategies targeting thrombin activities, thrombin receptors, and thrombin generation. Thromb Haemostas 78:736, 1997.
10. Caen JP, Rosa JP: Platelet-vessel wall interaction: from bedside to molecules. Thromb Haemost 74:18, 1995.
11. Hoffman M, et al: Cellular interactions in hemostasis. Haemostasis 26 (suppl 1):12, 1996.
12. Semeraro N, Colucci M: Tissue factor in health and disease. Thromb Haemost 78:759, 1997.
13. Esmon CT: Possible involvement of cytokines in diffuse intravascular coagulation and thrombosis. Baillieres Clin Haematol 7:453, 1994.
14. Wiman B: Plasminogen activator inhibitor 1 (PAI-1) in plasma: its role in thrombotic disease. Thromb Haemost 74:71, 1995.
15. Levi M, et al: The cytokine-mediated imbalance between coagulant and anticoagulant mechanisms in sepsis and endotoxaemia. Eur J Clin Invest 27:3, 1997.
16. Pearson TA, et al: Epidemiology of thrombotic-hemostatic factors and their associations with cardiovascular disease. Am J Clin Nutr 65 (suppl 5):S1674, 1997.
17. Resnick N, Gimbrone MA Jr: Hemodynamic forces are complex regulators of endothelial gene expression. FASEB J 9:874, 1995.
18. Macik BG, Ortel TL: Clinical and laboratory evaluation of the hypercoagulable states. Clin Chest Med 16:375, 1995.
19. Harpel PC, et al: Homocysteine and hemostasis: pathogenic mechanisms predisposing to thrombosis. J Nutr 126 (suppl 4):1285S, 1996.
20. Poort SR, et al: A common genetic variation in the 3′-untranslated region of the prothrombin gene is associated with elevated plasma prothrombin levels and an increase in venous thrombosis. Blood 88: 3698, 1996.
21. Lidegaard O, Milsom I: Oral contraceptives and thrombotic diseases: impact of new epidemiological studies. Contraception 53:135, 1996.
22. Green KB, Silverstein RL: Hypercoagulability in cancer. Hematol Oncol Clin North Am 10:499, 1996.
23. Aster RH: Heparin induced thrombocytopenia and thrombosis. N Engl J Med 332:1374, 1995.
24. Chakravarty K, et al: Antibody to cardiolipin in stroke: association with mortality and functional recovery in patients without systemic lupus erythematosus. QJM 79:397, 1991.
25. Ames P et al: Clinical and therapeutic aspects of the antiphospholipid syndrome. Lupus 4:S23, 1995.
26. Shapiro SS: The lupus anticoagulant/antiphospholipid syndrome. Ann Rev Med 47:533, 1996.
27. Petri M: Pathogenesis and treatment of the antiphospholipid antibody syndrome. Med Clin North Am 81:151, 1997.
28. Drenkard C, et al: Influence of the antiphospholipid syndrome in the survival of patients with systemic lupus erythematosus. J Rheumatol 21:1067, 1994.
29. Rosendaal FR: Risk factors for venous thrombosis: prevalence, risk, and interactions. Semin Hematol 34:171, 1997.
30. Hardaway RM, Williams CH: Disseminated intravascular coagulation: an update. Compr Ther 22:737, 1996.
31. Perrier A: Noninvasive diagnosis of pulmonary embolism. Haematologica 82:328, 1997.
32. Cohen AT, et al: The changing pattern of venous thromboembolic disease. Haemostasis 26:65, 1996.
33. Goldhaber SZ: Venous thrombosis: prevention, treatment, and relationship to paradoxical embolus. Cardiol Clin 12:505, 1994.
34. Cina G, et al: Epidemiology, pathophysiology and natural history of venous thromboembolism. Rays 21:315, 1996.
35. Dudney TM, Elliot CG: Pulmonary embolism from amniotic fluid, fat, and air. Prog Cardiovasc Dis 36:447, 1994.
36. Johnson MJ, Lucas GL: Fat embolism syndrome. Orthopedics 19:41, 1996.
37. King MB, Harmon KR: Unusual forms of pulmonary embolism. Clin Chest Med 3:561, 1994.

38. Madsen J, et al: Diving physiology and pathophysiology. Clin Physiol 14:597, 1994.
39. Martin RW: Amniotic fluid embolism. Clin Obstet Gynecol 39:101, 1996.
40. Hoffman WD, et al: Anti-endotoxin therapies in septic shock. Ann Intern Med 120:771, 1994.
41. Parrillo JE: Mechanisms of disease: pathogenetic mechanisms of septic shock. N Engl J Med 328:1471, 1993.
42. Ognibene FO: Pathogenesis and innovative treatment of septic shock. Adv Intern Med 42:313, 1997.
43. Glauser MP: The inflammatory cytokines: new developments in the pathophysiology and treatment of septic shock. Drugs 52 (suppl 2):9, 1996.
44. Natanson C: Anti-inflammatory therapies to treat sepsis and septic shock: a reassessment. Crit Care Med 25:1095, 1997.
45. Johnson HM, et al: Superantigens: structure and relevance to human disease. Proc Soc Exp Biol Med 212:99, 1996.
46. Stevens DL: The toxic shock syndromes. Infect Dis Clin North Am 10:727, 1996.

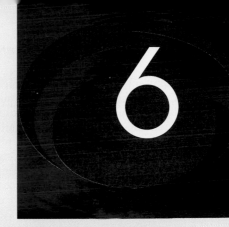

6 Genetic Disorders

MUTATIONS

MENDELIAN DISORDERS

TRANSMISSION PATTERNS OF SINGLE-GENE DISORDERS

Autosomal Dominant Disorders

Autosomal Recessive Disorders

X-Linked Disorders

BIOCHEMICAL AND MOLECULAR BASIS OF SINGLE-GENE (MENDELIAN) DISORDERS

Enzyme Defects and Their Consequences

Defects in Receptors and Transport Systems

Alterations in Structure, Function, or Quantity of Nonenzyme Proteins

Genetically Determined Adverse Reactions to Drugs

DISORDERS ASSOCIATED WITH DEFECTS IN STRUCTURAL PROTEINS

Marfan Syndrome

Ehlers-Danlos Syndromes

DISORDERS ASSOCIATED WITH DEFECTS IN RECEPTOR PROTEINS

Familial Hypercholesterolemia

DISORDERS ASSOCIATED WITH DEFECTS IN ENZYMES

Lysosomal Storage Diseases

Tay-Sachs Disease (GM_2 Gangliosidosis: Hexosaminidase α-Subunit Deficiency)

Niemann-Pick Disease: Types A and B

Gaucher Disease

Mucopolysaccharidoses

Glycogen Storage Diseases (Glycogenoses)

Alkaptonuria (Ochronosis)

DISORDERS ASSOCIATED WITH DEFECTS IN PROTEINS THAT REGULATE CELL GROWTH

Neurofibromatosis: Types 1 and 2

DISORDERS WITH MULTIFACTORIAL INHERITANCE

NORMAL KARYOTYPE

CYTOGENETIC DISORDERS

CYTOGENETIC DISORDERS INVOLVING AUTOSOMES

Trisomy 21 (Down Syndrome)

Other Trisomies

Chromosome 22q11 Deletion Syndrome

CYTOGENETIC DISORDERS INVOLVING SEX CHROMOSOMES

Klinefelter Syndrome

XYY Syndrome

Turner Syndrome

Multi-X Females

Hermaphroditism and Pseudohermaphroditism

SINGLE-GENE DISORDERS WITH NONCLASSIC INHERITANCE

TRIPLET REPEAT MUTATIONS—FRAGILE X SYNDROME

Other Diseases With Unstable Nucleotide Repeats

MUTATIONS IN MITOCHONDRIAL GENES—LEBER HEREDITARY OPTIC NEUROPATHY

GENOMIC IMPRINTING

Prader-Willi Syndrome and Angelman Syndrome

GONADAL MOSAICISM

MOLECULAR DIAGNOSIS

DIAGNOSIS OF GENETIC DISEASES

DIRECT GENE DIAGNOSIS

INDIRECT DNA DIAGNOSIS: LINKAGE ANALYSIS

Genetic disorders are far more common than is widely appreciated. The lifetime frequency of genetic diseases is estimated to be 670 per 1000.[1] Included in this figure are not only the "classic" genetic disorders but also cancer and cardiovascular diseases, the two most common causes of death in the Western world. Both of these have major genetic components. Cardiovascular diseases, such as atherosclerosis and hypertension, result from complex interactions of genes and environment, and most cancers are now known to result from an accumulation of mutations in somatic cells (Chapter 8).

The genetic diseases encountered in medical practice

represent only the tip of the iceberg, that is, those with less extreme genotypic errors permitting full embryonic development and live birth. It is estimated that 50% of spontaneous abortuses during the early months of gestation have a demonstrable chromosomal abnormality; there are, in addition, numerous smaller detectable errors and many others still beyond our range of identification. About 1% of all newborn infants possess a gross chromosomal abnormality, and approximately 5% of individuals under the age of 25 years develop a serious disease with a significant genetic component. How many more mutations remain hidden?

The answer to this question may be available in the not-too-distant future because of the Human Genome Project. By the year 2005, this project aims to obtain the complete sequence of the 3 billion base pairs of human DNA. Included in this pool of nucleotides is the genetic code for the approximately 100,000 human genes and their regulatory elements. This multinational effort will elucidate the "genetic architecture" of humans and generate the biologist's periodic table.[2]

Much of the progress in medical genetics has resulted from the spectacular advances in molecular biology, involving recombinant DNA technology. The details of these techniques are well known and are not repeated here. Some examples, however, of the impact of recombinant DNA technology on medicine are worthy of attention.

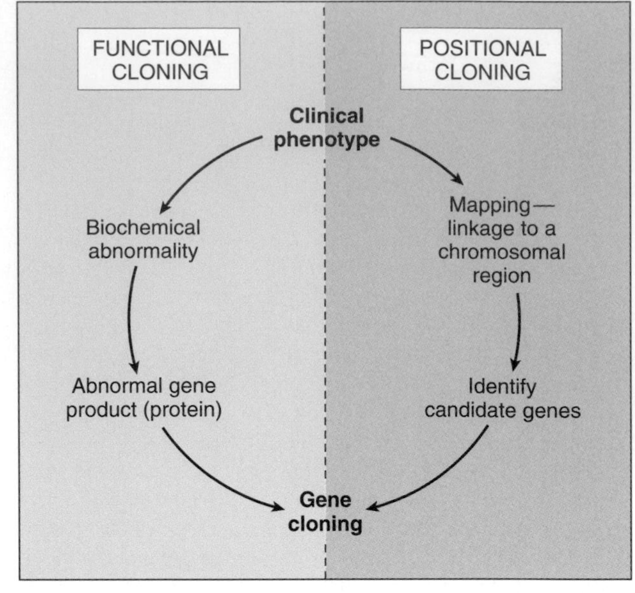

Figure 6–1

Schematic illustration of the strategies employed in functional and positional cloning. Functional cloning begins with relating the clinical phenotype to biochemical-protein abnormalities, followed by isolation of the mutant gene. Positional cloning, also called candidate gene approach, begins by mapping and cloning the disease gene by linkage analysis, without any knowledge of the gene product. Identification of the gene product and the mechanism by which it produces the disease follows the isolation of the mutant gene.

- *Molecular basis of human disease*: Two general strategies have been used to isolate and characterize involved genes (Fig. 6–1). The *functional cloning*, or *classic*, approach has been successfully used to study a variety of inborn errors of metabolism, such as phenylketonuria and disorders of hemoglobin synthesis. Common to these genetic diseases is a knowledge of the abnormal gene product and the corresponding protein. When the affected protein is known, a variety of methods can be employed to isolate the normal gene, to clone it, and ultimately to determine the molecular changes that affect the gene in patients with the disorder. Because in many common single-gene disorders, such as cystic fibrosis, there was no clue to the nature of the defective gene product, an alternative strategy called *positional cloning*, or the "candidate gene," approach had to be employed. This strategy initially ignores the biochemical clues from the phenotype and relies instead on mapping the disease phenotype to a particular chromosome location. This mapping is accomplished if the disease is associated with a distinctive cytogenetic change (e.g., fragile X syndrome, discussed later) or by linkage analysis. In the latter, the approximate location of the gene is determined by linkage to known "marker genes" that are in close proximity to the disease locus. Once the region in which the mutant gene lies has been localized within reasonably narrow limits, the next step is to clone several pieces of DNA from the relevant segment of the genome. Expression of the cloned DNA in vitro, followed by identification of the protein products, can then be used to identify the aberrant protein encoded by the mutant genes. This approach has been used successfully in several diseases, such as cystic fibrosis, neurofibromatosis, Duchenne muscular dystrophy (a hereditary disorder characterized by progressive muscle weakness), polycystic kidney disease, and Huntington disease.

  Another powerful tool for studying the molecular pathogenesis of human diseases—both genetic and acquired—involves creation of rodent (mouse, rat) models of the disease. Two types of mutant mice can be created: transgenic and gene knockout.[3, 4] In transgenic mice, a molecularly cloned human DNA is introduced into the germ line of suitable mice by injecting it into the ovum. The transgenic progeny express the human DNA and often manifest the human disease. For example, mice transgenic for human c-*myc*, a cancer-associated gene, develop tumors, thus providing a mouse model for carcinogenesis (Chapter 8). In the other type of mouse model, both of the copies of a mouse gene are "knocked out" by replacing the normal genes with inactive genes. Thus, for example, both alleles of the low-density lipoprotein (LDL)–receptor gene can be deleted, and the resultant LDL-receptor knockout mice develop hypercholesterolemia and atherosclerosis, mimicking the human disease familial hypercholesterolemia (see later).
- *Production of human biologically active agents*: An array of ultrapure biologically active agents can now be produced in virtually unlimited quantities by inserting the requisite gene into bacteria or other suitable cells in tissue culture. Some examples of genetically engineered products already in clinical use include tissue plasminogen activator for the treatment of thrombotic states,

growth hormone for the treatment of deficiency states, erythropoietin to reverse the anemia of renal disease, and myeloid growth and differentiation factors (granulocyte macrophage colony-stimulating factor, granulocyte colony-stimulating factor) to enhance production of monocytes and neutrophils in states of poor marrow function.

- *Gene therapy*: The goal of treating genetic diseases by transfer of somatic cells transfected with the normal gene, although not yet attained, is on the horizon. Much interest is focused on transplantation of patients' hematopoietic stem cells that have been transfected with the cloned normal gene. The first attempts at human gene therapy have been undertaken in patients with immunodeficiency resulting from a lack of the enzyme adenosine deaminase (ADA). The expression of the transferred ADA gene in lymphoid cells restores enzyme levels in vivo, thereby reversing the state of immunoincompetence that characterizes ADA-deficient patients. In another strategy, being tested in patients with cystic fibrosis, the normal gene is delivered to the somatic cells by way of a harmless viral vector.[5]
- *Disease diagnosis*: Molecular probes are proving to be extremely useful in the diagnosis of both genetic and nongenetic (e.g., infectious) diseases. The diagnostic applications of recombinant DNA technology are detailed at the end of this chapter.

With this background of developments in human genetics, we can turn next to the time-honored classification of human diseases into three categories: (1) those environmentally determined, (2) those genetically determined, and (3) those in which both environmental and genetic factors play a role. Obesity might appear to be representative of the first category; however, even here, with the discovery of genes that control satiety and energy metabolism (Chapter 10), it is evident that overnutrition—and all disorders to a greater or lesser degree—is conditioned by the genotype. Into the third category just mentioned fall many of the important diseases of humans, such as peptic ulcer, diabetes mellitus, atherosclerosis, schizophrenia, and most cancers, in which clearly both nature and nurture play significant roles.

It is beyond the scope of this book to review normal human genetics. It is beneficial to review some fundamental concepts that have bearing on the understanding of genetic diseases. First, however, several commonly used terms are clarified—*hereditary*, *familial*, and *congenital*. Hereditary disorders, by definition, are derived from one's parents and are transmitted in the germ line through the generations and therefore are familial. The term *congenital* simply implies "born with." Some congenital diseases are not genetic, as, for example, congenital syphilis. Not all genetic diseases are congenital; patients with Huntington disease, for example, begin to manifest their condition only after the twenties or thirties.

MUTATIONS

A *mutation* may be defined as a permanent change in the DNA. Mutations that affect the germ cells are transmitted to the progeny and may give rise to inherited diseases. Mutations that arise in somatic cells understandably do not cause hereditary diseases but are important in the genesis of cancers and some congenital malformations.

Based on the extent of genetic change, mutations may be classified into three categories.[6] *Genome mutations* involve loss or gain of whole chromosomes, giving rise to monosomy or trisomy. *Chromosome mutations* result from rearrangement of genetic material and give rise to visible structural changes in the chromosome. Mutations involving

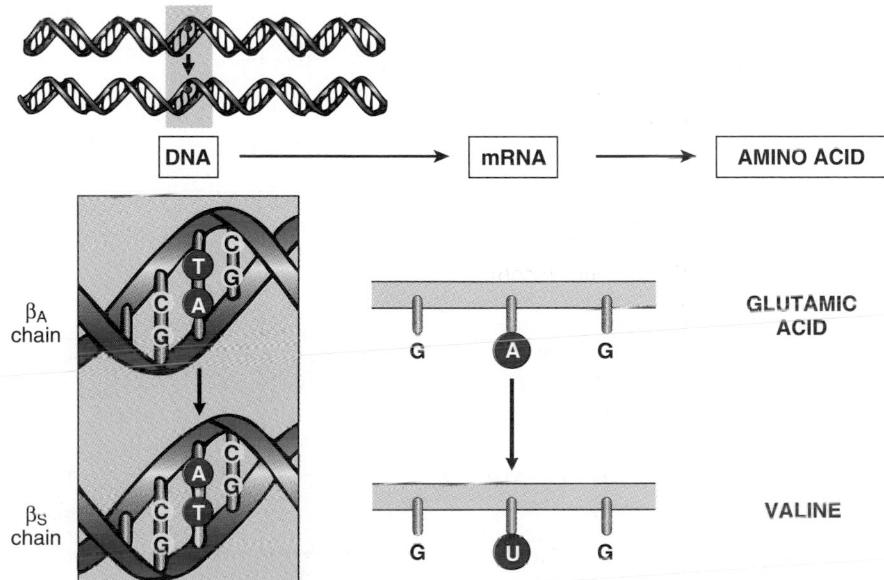

Figure 6–2

Schematic illustration of a point mutation resulting from a single base pair change in the DNA. In the example shown, a CTC to CAC change alters the meaning of the genetic code (GAG to GUG in the opposite strand), leading to replacement of glutamic acid by valine in the polypeptide chain. This change, affecting the sixth amino acid of the normal β-globin (β_A) chain, converts it to sickle β-globin (β_S).

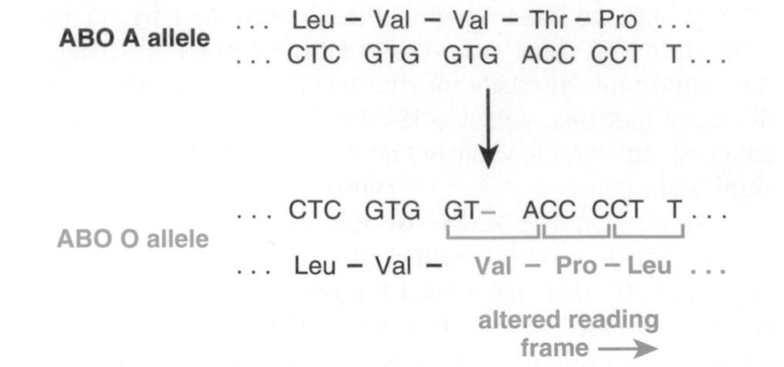

ABO A allele ... Leu – Val – Val – Thr – Pro ...
... CTC GTG GTG ACC CCT T...

... CTC GTG GT– ACC CCT T...
ABO O allele
... Leu – Val – Val – Pro – Leu ...
altered reading frame →

Figure 6–3

Single-base deletion at the ABO (glycosyltransferase) locus, leading to a frameshift mutation responsible for the O allele. (From Thompson MW, et al: Thompson and Thompson Genetics in Medicine, 5th ed. Philadelphia, WB Saunders, 1991, p 134.)

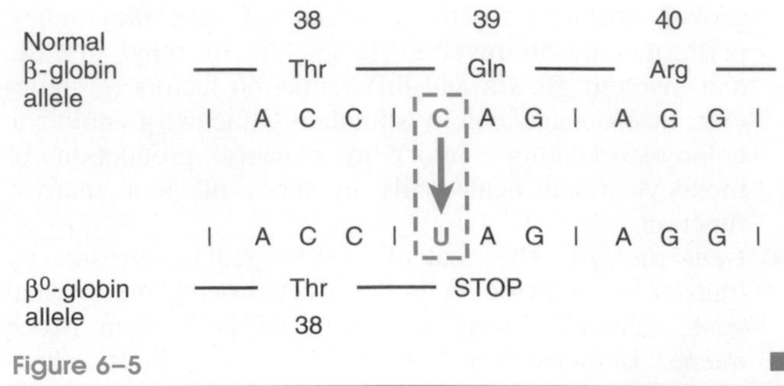

Figure 6–5

Point mutation leading to premature chain termination. Partial mRNA sequence of the β-globin chain of hemoglobin showing codons for amino acids 38 to 40. A point mutation (C→U) in codon 39 changes glutamine (Gln) codon to a stop codon, and hence protein synthesis stops at the 38th amino acid.

changes in the number or structure of chromosomes are transmitted only infrequently because most are incompatible with survival. The vast majority of mutations associated with hereditary diseases are submicroscopic *gene mutations.* These may result in partial or complete deletion of a gene or, more often, affect a single base. For example, a single nucleotide base may be *substituted* by a different base, resulting in a *point mutation* (Fig. 6–2). Less commonly, one or two base pairs may be *inserted* into or *deleted* from the DNA, leading to alterations in the reading frame of the DNA strand; hence these are referred to as *frameshift* mutations (Figs. 6–3 and 6–4). The consequences of mutations are varied, depending on several factors, including the type of mutation and the genomic site affected by it. Details of specific mutations and their effects are discussed along with the relevant disorders throughout this text. Here we briefly review some general principles relating to the effects of gene mutations.

- *Point mutations within coding sequences*: A point mutation (single base substitution) may alter the code in a triplet of bases and lead to the replacement of one amino acid by another in the gene product. Because these mutations alter the meaning of the genetic code, they are often termed *missense mutations.* An excellent example of this type is the sickle mutation affecting the β-globin chain of hemoglobin (Chapter 14). Here the nucleotide triplet CTC (or GAG in messenger RNA [mRNA]), which codes for glutamic acid, is changed to CAC (or GUG in mRNA), which codes for valine (see Fig. 6–2). This single amino acid substitution alters the physicochemical properties of hemoglobin, giving rise to sickle cell anemia. Besides producing an amino acid substitution, a point mutation may change an amino acid codon to a chain terminator, or *stop codon* (*nonsense mutation*). Taking again the example of β-globin, a point mutation affecting the codon for glutamine (CAG) creates a stop codon (UAG) if U is substituted for C (Fig. 6–5). This change leads to premature termination of β-globin gene translation, and the resulting short peptide is rapidly degraded. The affected individuals lack β-globin chains and develop a severe form of anemia called β^0-thalassemia (Chapter 14).
- *Mutations within noncoding sequences*: Deleterious effects may also result from mutations that do not involve the exons. As is well known, transcription of DNA is initiated and regulated by promoter and enhancer sequences that are found down-stream or up-stream of the gene. Point mutations or deletions involving these regulatory sequences may interfere with binding of transcription factors and thus lead to a marked reduction in or total lack of transcription. Such is the case in certain forms of hereditary hemolytic anemias. In addition, point mutations within introns lead to defective splicing of intervening sequences. This, in turn, interferes with normal processing of the initial mRNA transcripts and results in a failure to form mature mRNA transcripts. Therefore, translation cannot take place, and the gene product is not synthesized.

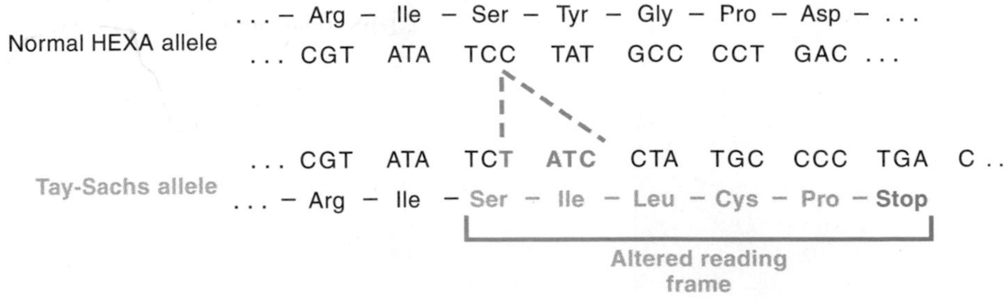

Normal HEXA allele ...– Arg – Ile – Ser – Tyr – Gly – Pro – Asp – ...
... CGT ATA TCC TAT GCC CCT GAC ...

Tay-Sachs allele ... CGT ATA TCT ATC CTA TGC CCC TGA C ...
... – Arg – Ile – Ser – Ile – Leu – Cys – Pro – Stop
Altered reading frame

Figure 6–4

Four-base insertion in the hexosaminidase A gene in Tay-Sachs disease, leading to a frameshift mutation. This mutation is the major cause of Tay-Sachs disease in Ashkenazi Jews. (From Thompson MW, et al: Thompson and Thompson Genetics in Medicine, 5th ed. Philadelphia, WB Saunders, 1991, p 135.)

- *Deletions and insertions*: Small deletions or insertions involving the coding sequence lead to alterations in the reading frame of the DNA strand; hence they are referred to as *frameshift mutations* (see Figs. 6–3 and 6–4). If the number of base pairs involved is three or a multiple of three, frameshift does not occur (Fig. 6–6); instead an abnormal protein missing one or more amino acids is synthesized.
- *Trinucleotide repeat mutations*: Trinucleotide repeat mutations belong to a special category because these mutations are characterized by amplification of a sequence of three nucleotides. Although the specific nucleotide sequence that undergoes amplification differs in various disorders, almost all affected sequences share the nucleotides guanine (G) and cytosine (C). For example, in fragile X syndrome, prototypical of this category of disorders, there are 250 to 4000 tandem repeats of the sequence CGG within a gene called *FMR-1*. In normal populations, the number of repeats is small, averaging 29. It is believed that expansions of the trinucleotide sequences prevent normal expression of the FMR-1 gene, thus giving rise to mental retardation. Another distinguishing feature of trinucleotide repeat mutations is that they are dynamic (i.e., the degree of amplification increases during gametogenesis). These features, discussed in greater detail later, influence the pattern of inheritance and the phenotypic manifestations of the diseases caused by this class of mutations.

To summarize, mutations can interfere with protein synthesis at various levels. Transcription may be suppressed with gene deletions and point mutations involving promoter sequences. Abnormal mRNA processing may result from mutations affecting introns or splice junctions, or both. Translation is affected if a stop codon (chain termination mutation) is created within an exon. Finally, some point mutations may lead to the formation of an abnormal protein without impairing any step in protein synthesis.

Mutations occur spontaneously during the process of DNA replication. Certain environmental influences, such as radiation, chemicals, and viruses, increase the rate of so-called spontaneous mutations. Because the mutagenic potential of environmental agents is linked to their role in carcinogenesis, they are discussed in Chapter 8, Neoplasia.

Against this background, we now turn our attention to the three major categories of genetic disorders: (1) disorders related to mutant genes of large effect, (2) diseases with multifactorial (polygenic) inheritance, and (3) chromosomal disorders. The first category includes many relatively uncommon conditions, such as storage disorders and inborn errors of metabolism, all resulting from single-gene mutations of large effect. Because most of these follow the classic mendelian patterns of inheritance, they are also referred to as *mendelian disorders*. The second category includes some of the most common diseases of humans, such as hypertension and diabetes mellitus. They are called *multifactorial* because they are influenced by both genetic and environmental factors. The genetic component involves the additive result of multiple genes of small effect; the environmental contribution may be small or large, and in some cases, it is required for the expression of disease. The third category includes diseases that result from genomic or chromosomal mutations and are therefore associated with numerical or structural changes in chromosomes.

```
              — Ile — Ile — Phe — Gly — Val —
Normal DNA   ... T ATC ATC TTT GGT GTT ...

                        ΔF508
CF DNA       ... T ATC AT–  ––T GGT GTT ...
              — Ile — Ile ——————— Gly — Val —
```

Figure 6–6

Three-base deletion in the common cystic fibrosis (CF) allele results in synthesis of a protein that is missing amino acid 508 (phenylalanine). Because the deletion is a multiple of three, this is not a frameshift mutation. (From Thompson MW, et al: Thompson and Thompson Genetics in Medicine, 5th ed. Philadelphia, WB Saunders, 1991, p 135.)

To these three well-known categories must be added a heterogeneous group of *single-gene disorders with nonclassic patterns of inheritance*. This group includes disorders resulting from triplet repeat mutations, those arising from mutations in mitochondrial DNA, and those in which the transmission is influenced by genomic imprinting or gonadal mosaicism. Diseases within this group are caused by mutations in single genes, but they do not follow the mendelian pattern of inheritance. These are discussed later in this chapter.

MENDELIAN DISORDERS

All mendelian disorders are the result of expressed mutations in single genes of large effect. It is not necessary to detail Mendel's laws here, as every student in biology, and possibly every garden pea, has learned about them at an early age. Only some comments of medical relevance are made.

The number of mendelian disorders known has grown to monumental proportions. In a recent edition of his book, *Mendelian Inheritance in Man*, McKusick[7] has listed more than 5000 disorders.* It is estimated that every individual is a carrier of five to eight deleterious genes. Most of these are recessive and therefore do not have serious phenotypic effects. About 80 to 85% of these mutations are familial. The remainder represent new mutations acquired de novo by an affected individual.

Some autosomal mutations produce partial expression in the heterozygote and full expression in the homozygote. Sickle cell anemia is caused by substitution of normal hemoglobin (HbA) by hemoglobin S (HbS). When an individual is homozygous for the mutant gene, all the hemoglobin is of the abnormal HbS type, and even under normal atmospheric pressures of oxygen, the disorder is fully expressed (i.e., sickling deformity of all red cells and hemolytic anemia). In the heterozygote, only a proportion of the hemoglobin is HbS (the remainder being HbA), and therefore red cell sickling and possibly hemolysis occur

*An online version of this book is available on the World Wide Web (http://www.ncbi.nlm.nih.gov/Omim/).

only when there is exposure to lowered oxygen tension. This is referred to as the *sickle cell trait* to differentiate it from full-blown sickle cell anemia.

Although gene expression is usually described as dominant or recessive, in some cases, both of the alleles of a gene pair may be fully expressed in the heterozygote—a condition called *codominance.* Histocompatibility and blood group antigens are good examples of codominant inheritance.

A single mutant gene may lead to many end effects, termed *pleiotropism*, and, conversely, mutations at several genetic loci may produce the same trait (*genetic heterogeneity*). Sickle cell anemia may serve as an example of pleiotropism. In this hereditary disorder, not only does the point mutation in the gene give rise to HbS, which predisposes the red cells to hemolysis, but also the abnormal red cells tend to cause a logjam in small vessels, inducing, for example, splenic fibrosis, organ infarcts, and bone changes. The numerous differing end-organ derangements all are related to the primary defect in hemoglobin synthesis. On the other hand, profound childhood deafness, an apparently homogeneous clinical entity, results from any of 16 different types of autosomal recessive mutations. Recognition of genetic heterogeneity not only is important in genetic counseling, but also is relevant in the understanding of the pathogenesis of some common disorders, such as diabetes mellitus.

Transmission Patterns of Single-Gene Disorders

Mutations involving single genes typically follow one of three patterns of inheritance: autosomal dominant, autosomal recessive, and X-linked. The general rules that govern the transmission of single-gene disorders are well known and are not repeated here. Only a few salient features are summarized. Single-gene disorders with nonclassic patterns of inheritance are described later.

AUTOSOMAL DOMINANT DISORDERS

Autosomal dominant disorders are manifested in the heterozygous state, so at least one parent of an index case is usually affected; both males and females are affected, and both can transmit the condition. When an affected person marries an unaffected one, every child has one chance in two of having the disease. In addition to these basic rules, autosomal dominant conditions are characterized by the following:

- With every autosomal dominant disorder, some patients do not have affected parents. Such patients owe their disorder to new mutations involving either the egg or the sperm from which they were derived. Their siblings are neither affected nor at increased risk for developing the disease. The proportion of patients who develop the disease as a result of a new mutation is related to the effect of the disease on reproductive capability. If a disease markedly reduces reproductive fitness, most cases would be expected to result from new mutations. Many new mutations seem to occur in germ cells of relatively older fathers.
- Clinical features can be modified by reduced penetrance and variable expressivity. Some individuals inherit the mutant gene but are phenotypically normal. This is referred to as *reduced penetrance.* Penetrance is expressed in mathematical terms: Thus, 50% penetrance indicates that 50% of those who carry the gene express the trait. In contrast to penetrance, if a trait is seen in all individuals carrying the mutant gene but is expressed differently among individuals, the phenomenon is called *variable expressivity.* For example, manifestations of neurofibromatosis type 1 range from brownish spots on the skin to multiple skin tumors and skeletal deformities. The mechanisms underlying reduced penetrance and variable expressivity are not fully understood, but they most likely result from effects of other genes or environmental factors that modify the phenotypic expression of the mutant allele. For example, the phenotype of a patient with sickle cell anemia (resulting from mutation at the β-globin locus) is influenced by the genotype at the α-globin locus because the latter influences the total amount of hemoglobin made (Chapter 14). The influence of environmental factors is exemplified by familial hypercholesterolemia. The expression of the disease in the form of atherosclerosis is conditioned by the dietary intake of lipids (see later).
- In many conditions, the age at onset is delayed: symptoms and signs do not appear until adulthood (as in Huntington disease).

The biochemical mechanisms of autosomal dominant disorders are best considered in the context of the nature of the mutation and the type of protein affected. Most mutations lead to the reduced production of a gene product or give rise to an inactive protein. The effect of such *loss of function mutations* depends on the nature of the protein affected. If the mutation affects an enzyme protein, the heterozygotes are usually normal. Because up to 50% loss of enzyme activity can be compensated for, mutation in genes that encode enzyme proteins do not manifest an autosomal dominant pattern of inheritance. By contrast, two major categories of nonenzyme proteins are affected in autosomal dominant disorders:

1. Those involved in regulation of complex metabolic pathways that are subject to feedback inhibition: Membrane receptors such as the LDL receptor provide one such example; in familial hypercholesterolemia, discussed in detail later, a 50% loss of LDL receptors results in a secondary elevation of cholesterol that, in turn, predisposes to atherosclerosis in affected heterozygotes.
2. Key structural proteins, such as collagen and cytoskeletal elements of the red cell membrane (e.g., spectrin): The biochemical mechanisms by which a 50% reduction in the levels of such proteins results in an abnormal phenotype are not fully understood. In some cases, especially when the gene encodes one subunit of a multimeric protein, the product of the mutant allele can interfere with the assembly of a functionally normal multimer. For example, the collagen molecule is a tri-

Table 6–1. AUTOSOMAL DOMINANT DISORDERS

System	Disorder
Nervous	Huntington disease Neurofibromatosis* Myotonic dystrophy Tuberous sclerosis
Urinary	Polycystic kidney disease
Gastrointestinal	Familial polyposis coli
Hematopoietic	Hereditary spherocytosis Von Willebrand disease
Skeletal	Marfan syndrome* Ehlers-Danlos syndrome (some variants)* Osteogenesis imperfecta Achondroplasia
Metabolic	Familial hypercholesterolemia* Acute intermittent porphyria

* Discussed in this chapter. Other disorders listed are discussed in appropriate chapters of this book.

mer in which the three collagen chains are arranged in a helical configuration. Each of the three collagen chains in the helix must be normal for the assembly and stability of the collagen molecule. Even with a single mutant collagen chain, normal collagen trimers cannot be formed, and hence there is a marked deficiency of collagen. In this instance, the mutant allele is called *dominant negative* because it impairs the function of a normal allele. This effect is illustrated by some forms of osteogenesis imperfecta, characterized by marked deficiency of collagen and severe skeletal abnormalities (Chapter 28).

Less common than loss of function mutations are *gain of function* mutations. As the name indicates, in this type of mutation, the protein product of the mutant allele acquires properties not normally associated with the wild-type protein. The transmission of disorders produced by gain of function mutations is almost always autosomal dominant, as illustrated by Huntington disease (Chapter 30). In this disease, the trinucleotide repeat mutation affecting the Huntington gene (see later) gives rise to an abnormal protein. The mutant huntingtin protein is toxic to neurons, and hence even heterozygotes develop neurologic deficit.

To summarize, two types of mutations and two categories of proteins are involved in the pathogenesis of autosomal dominant diseases. The more common loss of function mutations affect regulatory proteins and subunits of mulitmeric structural proteins, the latter acting through a dominant negative effect. Gain of function mutations are less common; they endow normal proteins with toxic properties and hence affect the function of other proteins encoded by the mutant gene.

Table 6–1 lists common autosomal dominant disorders. Many are discussed more logically in other chapters. A few conditions not considered elsewhere are discussed later in this chapter as examples of important genetic principles.

AUTOSOMAL RECESSIVE DISORDERS

Autosomal recessive inheritance is the single largest category of mendelian disorders. Because autosomal recessive disorders result only when both alleles at a given gene locus are mutants, such disorders are characterized by the following features: (1) The trait does not usually affect the parents, but siblings may show the disease; (2) siblings have one chance in four of being affected (i.e., the recurrence risk is 25% for each birth); and (3) if the mutant gene occurs with a low frequency in the population, there is a strong likelihood that the proband is the product of a consanguineous marriage. In contrast to those of autosomal dominant diseases, the following features generally apply to most autosomal recessive disorders:

- The expression of the defect tends to be more uniform than in autosomal dominant disorders.
- Complete penetrance is common.
- Onset is frequently early in life.
- Although new mutations for recessive disorders do occur, they are rarely detected clinically. Since the individual with a new mutation is an asymptomatic heterozygote, several generations may pass before the descendants of such a person mate with other heterozygotes and produce affected offspring.
- In many cases, enzyme proteins are affected by a loss of function. In heterozygotes, equal amounts of normal and defective enzyme are synthesized. Usually the natural "margin of safety" ensures that cells with half their usual complement of the enzyme function normally.

Autosomal recessive disorders include almost all inborn errors of metabolism. The various consequences of enzyme deficiencies are discussed later. The more common of these conditions are listed in Table 6–2. Most are presented elsewhere; a few prototypes are discussed later in this chapter.

Table 6–2. AUTOSOMAL RECESSIVE DISORDERS

System	Disorder
Metabolic	Cystic fibrosis Phenylketonuria Galactosemia Homocystinuria Lysosomal storage diseases* α_1-Antitrypsin deficiency Wilson disease Hemochromatosis Glycogen storage diseases*
Hematopoietic	Sickle cell anemia Thalassemias
Endocrine	Congenital adrenal hyperplasia
Skeletal	Ehlers-Danlos syndrome (some variants)* Alkaptonuria*
Nervous	Neurogenic muscular atrophies Friedreich ataxia Spinal muscular atrophy

* Discussed in this chapter. Many others are discussed throughout the text.

X-LINKED DISORDERS

All sex-linked disorders are X-linked, almost all X-linked recessive. The only gene assigned with certainty to the Y chromosome is the determinant for testes; males with mutations affecting the Y-linked genes involved in spermatogenesis are usually infertile, and hence there is no Y-linked inheritance. As discussed later, a few additional genes with homologs on the X chromosome have been mapped to the Y chromosome, but no disorders resulting from mutations in such genes have been described.

X-linked recessive inheritance accounts for a small number of well-defined clinical conditions. The Y chromosome, for the most part, is not homologous to the X, and so mutant genes on the X are not paired with alleles on the Y. Thus, the male is said to be *hemizygous* for X-linked mutant genes, so these disorders are expressed in the male. Other features that characterize these disorders are as follows:

- An affected male does not transmit the disorder to his sons, but all daughters are carriers. Sons of heterozygous women have, of course, one chance in two of receiving the mutant gene.
- The heterozygous female usually does not express the full phenotypic change because of the paired normal allele. Because of the random inactivation of one of the X chromosomes in the female, however, females have a variable proportion of cells in which the mutant X chromosome is active. Thus, it is remotely possible for the normal allele to be inactivated in most cells, permitting full expression of heterozygous X-linked conditions in the female. Much more commonly, the normal allele is inactivated in only some of the cells, and thus the heterozygous female expresses the disorder partially. An illustrative condition is *glucose-6-phosphate dehydrogenase (G6PD) deficiency.* Transmitted on the X chromosome, this enzyme deficiency, which predisposes to red cell hemolysis in patients receiving certain types of drugs (Chapter 14), is expressed principally in males. In the female, a proportion of the red cells may be derived from marrow cells with inactivation of the normal allele. Such red cells are at the same risk for undergoing hemolysis as are the red cells in the hemizygous male. Thus, the female is not only a carrier of this trait, but also is susceptible to drug-induced hemolytic reactions. Because the proportion of defective red cells in heterozygous females depends on the random inactivation of one of the X chromosomes, however, the severity of the hemolytic reaction is almost always less in heterozygous women than in hemizygous men. Most of the X-linked conditions listed in Table 6–3 are covered elsewhere in the text.

Table 6–3. X-LINKED RECESSIVE DISORDERS

System	Disease
Musculoskeletal	Duchenne muscular dystrophy
Blood	Hemophilia A and B Chronic granulomatous disease Glucose-6-phosphate dehydrogenase deficiency
Immune	Agammaglobulinemia Wiskott-Aldrich syndrome
Metabolic	Diabetes insipidus Lesch-Nyhan syndrome
Nervous	Fragile X syndrome*

* Discussed in this chapter.

There are only a few *X-linked dominant* conditions. They are caused by dominant disease alleles on the X chromosome. These disorders are transmitted by an affected heterozygous female to half her sons and half her daughters and by an affected male parent to all his daughters but none of his sons, if the female parent is unaffected. Vitamin D–resistant rickets is an example of this type of inheritance.

Biochemical and Molecular Basis of Single-Gene (Mendelian) Disorders

Mendelian disorders result from alterations involving single genes. The genetic defect may lead to the formation of an abnormal protein or a reduction in the output of the gene product. As mentioned earlier, mutations may affect protein synthesis by affecting transcription, mRNA processing, or translation. The phenotypic effects of a mutation may result directly, from abnormalities in the protein encoded by the mutant gene, or indirectly, owing to interactions of the mutant protein with other normal proteins. For example, all forms of Ehlers-Danlos syndrome (EDS) (described later) are associated with abnormalities of collagen. In some forms (e.g., type IV), there is a mutation in one of the collagen genes, whereas in others (e.g., type VI), the collagen genes are normal, but there is a mutation in the gene that encodes lysyl hydroxylase, an enzyme essential for the cross-linking of collagen. In these patients, collagen weakness is secondary to a deficiency of lysyl hydroxylase.

Virtually any type of protein may be affected in single-gene disorders and by a variety of mechanisms (Table 6–4). To some extent, the pattern of inheritance of the disease is related to the kind of protein affected by the mutation, as was discussed earlier and is reiterated subsequently. For the purposes of this discussion, the mechanisms involved in single-gene disorders can be classified into four categories: (1) *enzyme defects and their consequences*; (2) *defects in membrane receptors and transport systems*; (3) *alterations in the structure, function, or quantity of nonenzyme proteins*; and (4) *mutations resulting in unusual reactions to drugs.*

ENZYME DEFECTS AND THEIR CONSEQUENCES

Mutations may result in the synthesis of a defective enzyme with reduced activity or in a reduced amount of a normal enzyme. In either case, the consequence is a metabolic block. Figure 6–7 provides an example of an enzyme reaction in which the substrate is converted by intracellular

Table 6–4. BIOCHEMICAL AND MOLECULAR BASIS OF SOME MENDELIAN DISORDERS

Protein Type/Function	Example	Molecular Lesion	Disease
Enzyme	Phenylalanine hydroxylase	Splice site mutation: reduced amount	Phenylketonuria
	Hexosaminidase	Splice site mutation or frameshift mutation with stop codon: reduced amount	Tay-Sachs disease
	Adenosine deaminase	Point mutations: abnormal protein with reduced activity	Severe combined immunodeficiency
Enzyme inhibitor	α_1-Antitrypsin	Missense mutations: impair secretion from liver to serum	Emphysema and liver disease
Receptor	Low-density lipoprotein receptor	Deletions, point mutations: reduction of synthesis, transport to cell surface, or binding to low-density lipoprotein	Familial hypercholesterolemia
	Vitamin D receptor	Point mutations: failure of normal signaling	Vitamin D–resistant rickets
Transport			
Oxygen	Hemoglobin	Deletions: reduced amount	α-Thalassemia
		Defective mRNA processing: reduced amount	β-Thalassemia
		Point mutations: abnormal structure	Sickle cell anemia
Ions	Cystic fibrosis transmembrane conductance regulator	Deletions and other mutations	Cystic fibrosis
Structural			
Extracellular	Collagen	Deletions or point mutations cause reduced amount of normal collagen or normal amounts of mutant collagen	Osteogenesis imperfecta; Ehlers-Danlos syndromes
	Fibrillin	Missense mutations	Marfan syndrome
Cell membrane	Dystrophin	Deletion with reduced synthesis	Duchenne/Becker muscular dystrophy
	Spectrin, ankyrin, or protein 4.1	Heterogeneous	Hereditary spherocytosis
Hemostasis	Factor VIII	Deletions, insertions, nonsense mutations, and others: reduced synthesis or abnormal factor VIII	Hemophilia A
Growth regulation	Rb protein	Deletions	Hereditary reinoblastoma
	Neurofibromin	Heterogeneous	Neurofibromatosis type 1

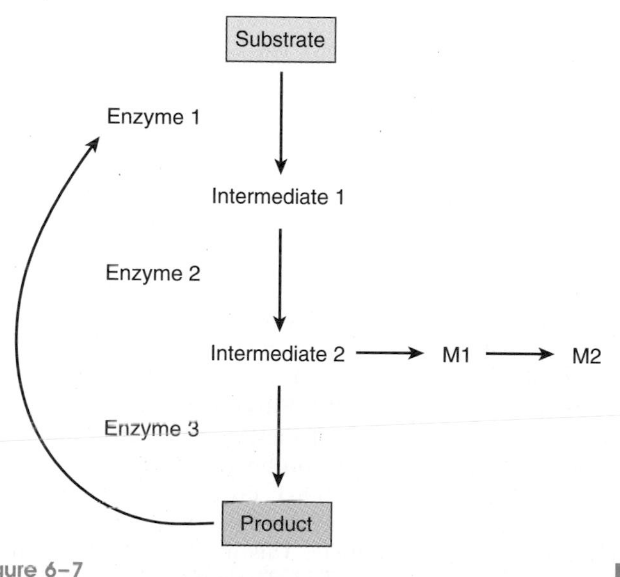

Figure 6–7

Scheme of a possible metabolic pathway in which a substrate is converted to an end product by a series of enzyme reactions. M1, M2, products of a minor pathway.

enzymes, denoted as 1, 2, and 3, into an end product through intermediates 1 and 2. In this model, the final product exerts feedback control on enzyme 1. A minor pathway producing small quantities of M_1 and M_2 also exists. The biochemical consequences of an enzyme defect in such a reaction may lead to three major consequences:

1. *Accumulation of the substrate*, depending on the site of block, may be accompanied by accumulation of one or both intermediates. Moreover, an increased concentration of intermediate 2 may stimulate the minor pathway and thus lead to an excess of M_1 and M_2. Under these conditions, tissue injury may result if the precursor, the intermediates, or the products of alternative minor pathways are toxic in high concentrations. For example, in galactosemia, the deficiency of galactose-1-phosphate uridyltransferase (Chapter 10) leads to the accumulation of galactose and consequent tissue damage. A deficiency of phenylalanine hydroxylase (Chapter 10) results in the accumulation of phenylalanine. Excessive accumulation of complex substrates within the lysosomes as a result of deficiency of degradative enzymes is responsible for a group of diseases generally referred to as *lysosomal storage diseases*.
2. *An enzyme defect can lead to a metabolic block and a decreased amount of end product* that may be necessary

for normal function. For example, a deficiency of melanin may result from lack of tyrosinase, which is necessary for the biosynthesis of melanin from its precursor, tyrosine. This results in the clinical condition called *albinism*. If the end product is a feedback inhibitor of the enzymes involved in the early reactions (in Fig. 6–7, it is shown that the product inhibits enzyme 1), the deficiency of the end product may permit overproduction of intermediates and their catabolic products, some of which may be injurious at high concentrations. A prime example of a disease with such an underlying mechanism is the Lesch-Nyhan syndrome (Chapter 28).

3. *Failure to inactivate a tissue-damaging substrate* is best exemplified by α_1-antitrypsin (α_1-AT) deficiency. Patients who have an inherited deficiency of serum α_1-AT are unable to inactivate neutrophil elastase in their lungs. Unchecked activity of this protease leads to destruction of elastin in the walls of lung alveoli, leading eventually to pulmonary emphysema (Chapter 16).

DEFECTS IN RECEPTORS AND TRANSPORT SYSTEMS

Many biologically active substances have to be actively transported across the cell membrane. This transport is generally achieved by one of two mechanisms—by receptor-mediated endocytosis or by a transport protein. A genetic defect in a receptor-mediated transport system is exemplified by familial hypercholesterolemia, in which reduced synthesis or function of LDL receptors leads to defective transport of LDL into the cells and secondarily to excessive cholesterol synthesis by complex intermediary mechanisms. In cystic fibrosis, the transport system for chloride ions in exocrine glands, sweat ducts, lungs, and pancreas is defective. By mechanisms not fully understood, impaired chloride transport leads to serious injury to the lungs and pancreas (Chapter 10).

ALTERATIONS IN STRUCTURE, FUNCTION, OR QUANTITY OF NONENZYME PROTEINS

Genetic defects resulting in alterations of nonenzyme proteins often have widespread secondary effects, as exemplified by sickle cell disease. The hemoglobinopathies, sickle cell disease being one, all of which are characterized by defects in the structure of the globin molecule, best exemplify this category. In contrast to the hemoglobinopathies, the thalassemias result from mutations in globin genes that affect the amount of globin chains synthesized. Thalassemias are associated with reduced amounts of structurally normal α-globin or β-globin chains (Chapter 14). Other examples of genetically defective structural proteins include collagen, spectrin, and dystrophin, giving rise to osteogenesis imperfecta (Chapter 28), hereditary spherocytosis (Chapter 14), and muscular dystrophies (Chapter 29).

GENETICALLY DETERMINED ADVERSE REACTIONS TO DRUGS

Certain genetically determined enzyme deficiencies are unmasked only after exposure of the affected individual to certain drugs. This special area of genetics, called *pharmacogenetics*, is of considerable clinical importance.[8] The classic example of drug-induced injury in the genetically susceptible individual is associated with a deficiency of the enzyme G6PD. Under normal conditions, G6PD deficiency does not result in disease, but on administration, for example, of the antimalarial drug primaquine, a severe hemolytic anemia results (Chapter 14).

With this overview of the biochemical basis of single gene disorders, we now consider selected examples grouped according to the underlying defect.

Disorders Associated With Defects in Structural Proteins

Several diseases caused by mutations in genes that encode structural proteins are listed in Table 6–4. Many are discussed elsewhere in the text. Only Marfan syndrome and Ehlers-Danlos syndromes are discussed here because they affect connective tissue and hence involve multiple organ systems.

MARFAN SYNDROME

Marfan syndrome is a *disorder of the connective tissues of the body, manifested principally by changes in the skeleton, eyes, and cardiovascular system.*[9] Its prevalence is estimated to range from 1 in 10,000 to 1 in 20,000. Approximately 70 to 85% of the cases are familial and transmitted by autosomal dominant inheritance. The remainder are sporadic and arise from new mutations.

Pathogenesis. Marfan syndrome results from an inherited defect in an extracellular glycoprotein called *fibrillin*. As alluded to in Chapter 4, fibrillin is the major component of microfibrils found in the extracellular matrix. These fibrils form a scaffolding on which tropoelastin is deposited to form elastic fibers. Although microfibrils are widely distributed in the body, they are particularly abundant in the aorta, ligaments, and ciliary zonules of the lens where they support the lens; these tissues are prominently affected in Marfan syndrome.

Fibrillin occurs in two homologous forms, fibrillin-1 and fibrillin-2, encoded by two separate genes, FBN1 and FBN2, mapped to chromosomes 15q21 and 5q3, respectively. Mutations of FBN1 underlie Marfan syndrome; mutations of the related FBN2 gene are less common, and they give rise to *congenital contractural arachnodactyly*, an autosomal dominant disorder characterized by skeletal abnormalities. Mutational analysis has revealed more than 70 distinct mutations of the FBN1 gene in patients with Marfan syndrome.[10] Most of these are missense mutations that give rise to abnormal fibrillin-1. It is believed that in heterozygotes mutant fibrillin-1 disrupts the assembly of normal microfibrils, presumably by interacting with the products of the normal allele. This mechanism of action, as discussed previously, is called *dominant negative*. The importance of fibrillin-1 in maintaining the structural integrity of the extracellular matrix has been confirmed by the generation of FBN1 knockout mice. These mice develop structural changes in the aorta that are similar to those seen in Marfan syndrome.[11]

MORPHOLOGY. Skeletal abnormalities are the most striking feature of Marfan syndrome. Typically the patient is unusually tall with exceptionally long extremities and long, tapering fingers and toes. Because the tall stature is contributed largely by the lower segment of the body, the ratio of the upper segment (top of the head to the pubis) to the lower segment (top of pubic ramus to the floor) is significantly lower than the norm for the age, race, and gender. The joint ligaments in the hands and feet are lax, suggesting that the patient is double-jointed; typically the thumb can be hyperextended back to the wrist. The head is commonly dolichocephalic (long-headed) with bossing of the frontal eminences and prominent supraorbital ridges. Because Abraham Lincoln possessed many of these physical characteristics, it is strongly suspected that he had Marfan syndrome. A variety of spinal deformities may appear, including kyphosis, scoliosis, or rotation or slipping of the dorsal or lumbar vertebrae. The chest is classically deformed, presenting either pectus excavatum (deeply depressed sternum) or a pigeon-breast deformity.

The **ocular changes** take many forms. Most characteristic is bilateral subluxation or dislocation (usually outward and upward) of the lens, referred to as **ectopia lentis**. This abnormality is so uncommon in persons who do not have this genetic disease that the finding of bilateral ectopia lentis should raise the suspicion of Marfan syndrome.

Cardiovascular lesions are the most life-threatening features of this disorder. The two most common lesions are mitral valve prolapse and, of greater importance, dilation of the ascending aorta owing to cystic medionecrosis. Histologically the changes in the media are virtually identical to those found in cystic medionecrosis not related to Marfan syndrome (see section on aortic dissection, Chapter 13). **Loss of medial support results in progressive dilation of the aortic valve ring and the root of the aorta, giving rise to severe aortic incompetence.** Weakening of the media also predisposes to an intimal tear, which may initiate an intramural hematoma that cleaves the layers of the media to produce aortic dissection. After cleaving the aortic layers for considerable distances, sometimes back to the root of the aorta or down to the iliac arteries, the hemorrhage often ruptures through the aortic wall. Such a calamity is the cause of death in 30 to 45% of these individuals.

Although mitral valve lesions are more frequent, they are clinically less important than aortic lesions. Loss of connective tissue support in the mitral valve leaflets makes them soft and billowy, creating the so-called floppy valve (Chapter 13). Valvular lesions, along with lengthening of the chordae tendineae, frequently give rise to mitral regurgitation. Similar changes may affect the tricuspid and, rarely, the aortic valves. Echocardiography greatly enhances the ability to detect the cardiovascular abnormalities and is therefore extremely valuable in the diagnosis of Marfan syndrome. The great majority of deaths are caused by rupture of aortic dissections, followed in importance by cardiac failure.

Although the lesions just described typify Marfan syndrome, it must be emphasized that there is great variation in the clinical expression of this genetic disorder. Patients with prominent eye or cardiovascular changes may have few skeletal abnormalities, whereas others with striking changes in body habitus have no eye changes. Although variability in clinical expression may be seen within a family, interfamilial variability is much more common and extensive. Because of such variations, clinical diagnosis of Marfan syndrome must be based on well-defined diagnostic criteria.[12]

To account for the variable expression of the Marfan defect, it has been hypothesized that Marfan syndrome may be genetically heterogeneous. With one exception, however, all studies to date point to mutations in the FBN1 gene, on chromosome 15q21.1, as the cause of this disease.[13] Thus, variable expressivity is best explained on the basis of allelic mutations within the same locus. Because so many different mutations of the FBN1 gene have been detected in different Marfan families, direct gene diagnosis of this disorder is not feasible. Presymptomatic detection, however, is possible by restriction fragment length polymorphism (RFLP) analysis. The principles underlying these two methods of DNA-based diagnosis are described later.

EHLERS-DANLOS SYNDROMES

Ehlers-Danlos syndromes (EDS) comprise a clinically and genetically heterogeneous group of disorders that result from some defect in collagen synthesis or structure.[14] Other disorders resulting from mutations affecting collagen synthesis include osteogenesis imperfecta (Chapter 28), Alport syndrome (Chapter 21), and epidermolysis bullosa (Chapter 27).

The mode of inheritance of EDS encompasses all three mendelian patterns. This should not be surprising because biosynthesis of collagen is a complex process that can be disturbed by genetic errors that may affect any one of the numerous structural collagen genes or enzymes necessary for post-transcriptional modifications of collagen. Because abnormalities of collagen are fundamental in the pathogenesis of EDS, collagen structure and synthesis should be reviewed (Chapter 4). There are at least 14 genetically distinct collagen types, having somewhat characteristic tissue distribution.[15] As we see subsequently, to some extent the clinical heterogeneity and variable modes of transmission of EDS can be explained on the basis of the specific collagen type involved and the nature of the molecular defects.

On the basis of clinical manifestations and the pattern of inheritance, at least 10 variants of EDS have been recognized. It is beyond the scope of this book to discuss each variant individually, and the interested reader is referred to several excellent reviews for such details.[15] Instead, we first summarize the important clinical features that are common to most variants and then correlate some of the clinical manifestations with the underlying molecular defects in collagen synthesis or structure.

As might be expected, tissues rich in collagen, such as skin, ligaments, and joints, are frequently involved in most variants of EDS. Because the abnormal collagen fibers lack adequate tensile strength, *skin is hyperextensible, and the joints are hypermobile.* These features permit grotesque contortions, such as bending the thumb backward to touch the forearm and bending the knee forward to create almost a right angle. It is believed that most contortionists have one of the EDS. A predisposition to joint dislocation, however, is one of the prices paid for this virtuosity. *The skin is extraordinarily stretchable, extremely fragile, and vulnerable to trauma.* Minor injuries produce gaping defects, and surgical repair or any surgical intervention is accomplished with great difficulty because of the lack of normal tensile strength. *The basic defect in connective tissue may lead to serious internal complications.* These include rupture of the colon and large arteries (EDS type IV), ocular fragility with rupture of cornea and retinal detachment (EDS type VI), and diaphragmatic hernia (EDS type I).

The biochemical and molecular bases of these abnormalities are known in only a few forms of EDS. These are described briefly because they offer some insights into the perplexing clinical heterogeneity of EDS. Perhaps the best characterized is *type VI, the most common autosomal recessive form of EDS.* It results from mutations in the gene encoding lysyl hydroxylase, an enzyme necessary for hydroxylation of lysine residues during collagen synthesis. Affected patients have markedly reduced levels of this enzyme. Because hydroxylysine is essential for the cross-linking of collagen fibers, a deficiency of lysyl hydroxylase results in the synthesis of collagen that lacks normal structural stability. Only collagen types I and III are affected in this disorder; the hydroxylation of collagen types II, IV, and V is normal. The molecular basis of this difference in hydroxylation is not clear.

Type IV EDS results from abnormalities of type III collagen. This form is genetically heterogeneous because at least three distinct types of mutations affecting the pro $\alpha1$ gene for collagen type III can give rise to this variant. Some affect the rate of synthesis of pro $\alpha1$ (III) chains, others affect the secretion of type III procollagen, and still others lead to the synthesis of structurally abnormal type III collagen. Some mutant alleles behave as dominant negatives (see discussion under autosomal dominant disorders) and thus produce severe phenotypic effects. These molecular studies provide a rational basis for the pattern of transmission and clinical features that are characteristic of this variant. First, because EDS IV results from mutations involving a structural protein (rather than an enzyme protein), an autosomal dominant pattern of inheritance would be expected. Second, because blood vessels and intestines are known to be rich in collagen type III, an abnormality of this collagen is consistent with severe defects (e.g., spontaneous rupture) in these organs.

In EDS type VII, the fundamental defect is in the conversion of type I procollagen to collagen. This step in collagen synthesis involves cleavage of noncollagen peptides at the N-terminal and C-terminal of the procollagen molecule. This is accomplished by N-terminal–specific and C-terminal–specific peptidases. *The defect in the conversion of procollagen to collagen in type VII EDS has been traced to mutations that affect one of the two type I collagen genes (i.e., $\alpha1$ [I] or $\alpha2$ [I]).* As a result, structurally abnormal pro $\alpha1$ (I) or pro $\alpha2$ (I) chains that resist cleavage of N-terminal peptides are formed. In patients with a single mutant allele, only 50% of the type I collagen chains are abnormal, but because these chains interfere with the formation of normal collagen helices, heterozygotes manifest the disease.

Finally, *EDS type IX* is worthy of brief mention because it illustrates how trace metals can affect connective tissues. The primary defect in this variant involves copper metabolism. These patients have high levels of copper within the cells, but serum copper and ceruloplasmin levels are low. The molecular basis of this disorder has been traced to a mutation involving a copper-binding protein. The effect of this mutation is to reduce the activity of the copper-dependent enzyme lysyl oxidase, which is essential for cross-linking of collagen and elastin fibers. Because the genes that encode the copper-binding protein map to the X chromosome, this variant of EDS (in contrast to most others) is inherited as an X-linked recessive trait.

To summarize, the common thread in EDS is some abnormality of collagen. These disorders, however, are extremely heterogeneous. At the molecular level, a variety of defects, varying from mutations involving structural genes for collagen to those involving enzymes that are responsible for post-transcriptional modifications of mRNA, have been detected. Such molecular heterogeneity results in the expression of EDS as a clinically heterogeneous disorder with several patterns of inheritance.

Disorders Associated With Defects in Receptor Proteins

FAMILIAL HYPERCHOLESTEROLEMIA

Familial hypercholesterolemia is a "receptor disease" that is the consequence of a *mutation in the gene encoding the receptor for low-density lipoprotein (LDL), which is involved in the transport and metabolism of cholesterol.* As a consequence of receptor abnormalities, there is a loss of feedback control and elevated levels of cholesterol that induce premature atherosclerosis, leading to a greatly increased risk of myocardial infarction.[16]

Familial hypercholesterolemia is possibly the most frequent mendelian disorder. Heterozygotes with one mutant gene, representing about 1 in 500 individuals, have from birth a twofold to threefold elevation of plasma cholesterol level, leading to tendinous xanthomas and premature atherosclerosis in adult life (Chapter 12). Homozygotes, having a double dose of the mutant gene, are much more severely affected and may have fivefold to sixfold elevations in plasma cholesterol levels. These individuals develop skin xanthomas and coronary, cerebral, and peripheral vascular atherosclerosis at an early age. Myocardial infarction may develop before the age of 20 years. Large-scale studies have found that familial hypercholesterolemia is present in 3 to 6% of survivors of myocardial infarction.

An understanding of this disorder requires that we briefly review the normal process of cholesterol metabolism and transport. Approximately 7% of the body's cholesterol circulates in the plasma, predominantly in the form of LDL. As might be expected, the level of plasma cholesterol is influenced by its synthesis and catabolism. Figure 6–8 illustrates that the liver plays a crucial role in both these processes. The first step in this complex sequence is the secretion of very-low-density lipoproteins (VLDL) by the liver into the bloodstream. VLDL particles are rich in triglycerides, although they do contain lesser amounts of cholesteryl esters. When a VLDL particle reaches the capillaries of adipose tissue or muscle, it is cleaved by lipoprotein lipase, a process that extracts most of the triglycerides. The resulting molecule, called *intermediate-density lipoprotein (IDL)*, is reduced in triglyceride content and enriched in cholesteryl esters, but it retains two of the three apoproteins (B-100 and E) present in the parent VLDL particle (Fig. 6–8). After release from the capillary endothelium, the IDL particles have one of two fates. Approximately 50% of newly formed IDL is rapidly taken up by the liver through a receptor-mediated transport. The receptor responsible for the binding of IDL to liver cell membrane recognizes both apoprotein B-100 and apoprotein E. It is called the *LDL receptor*, however, because it is also involved in the hepatic clearance of LDL, as described later. In the liver cells, IDL is recycled to generate VLDL. The IDL particles not taken up by the liver are subjected to further metabolic processing that removes most of the remaining triglycerides and apoprotein E, yielding the cholesterol-rich LDL. *It should be emphasized that IDL is the immediate and major source of plasma LDL.* There appear to be two mechanisms for removal of LDL from plasma, one mediated by an LDL receptor and the other by a receptor for oxidized LDL (scavenger receptor), described later. Although many cell types, including fibroblasts, lymphocytes, smooth muscle cells, hepatocytes, and adrenocortical cells, possess high-affinity LDL receptors, approximately 70% of the plasma LDL appears to be cleared by the liver, using a relatively sophisticated transport process (Fig. 6–9). The first step involves binding of LDL to cell surface receptors, which are clustered in specialized regions of the plasma membrane called *coated pits*. After binding, the coated pits containing the receptor-bound LDL are internalized by invagination to form coated vesicles, after which they migrate within the cell to fuse with the lysosomes. Here the LDL dissociates from the receptor, which is recycled to the surface. In the lysosomes, the LDL molecule is enzymatically degraded; the apoprotein part is hydrolyzed to amino acids, whereas the cholesteryl esters are broken down to free cholesterol. This free cholesterol, in turn, crosses the lysosomal membrane to enter the cytoplasm, where it is used for membrane synthesis and as a regulator of cholesterol homeostasis. Three separate processes are affected by the released intracellular cholesterol, as follows:

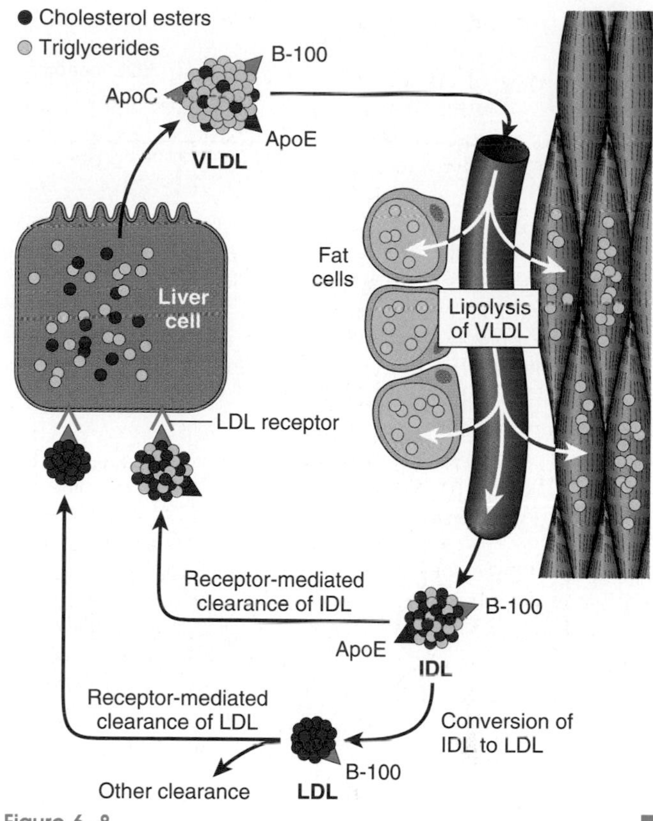

Figure 6–8

Schematic illustration of low-density lipoprotein (LDL) metabolism and the role of liver in its synthesis and clearance. Lipolysis of very-low-density lipoprotein (VLDL) by lipoprotein lipase in the capillaries releases triglycerides, which are then stored in fat cells and used as a source of energy in skeletal muscles.

- Cholesterol *suppresses* cholesterol synthesis within the cell by inhibiting the activity of the enzyme 3-hydroxy-3-methylglutaryl coenzyme A (HMG CoA) reductase, which is the rate-limiting enzyme in the synthetic pathway.
- Cholesterol *activates* the enzyme acyl-coenzyme A:cholesterol acyltransferase, favoring esterification and storage of excess cholesterol.
- Cholesterol *suppresses* the synthesis of LDL receptors, thus protecting the cells from excessive accumulation of cholesterol.

As mentioned earlier, familial hypercholesterolemia results from mutations in the gene specifying the receptor for LDL. Heterozygotes with familial hypercholesterolemia possess only 50% of the normal number of high-affinity LDL receptors because they have only one normal gene. As a result of this defect in transport, the catabolism of LDL by the receptor-dependent pathways is impaired, and the plasma level of LDL increases approximately twofold. Homozygotes have virtually no normal LDL receptors in

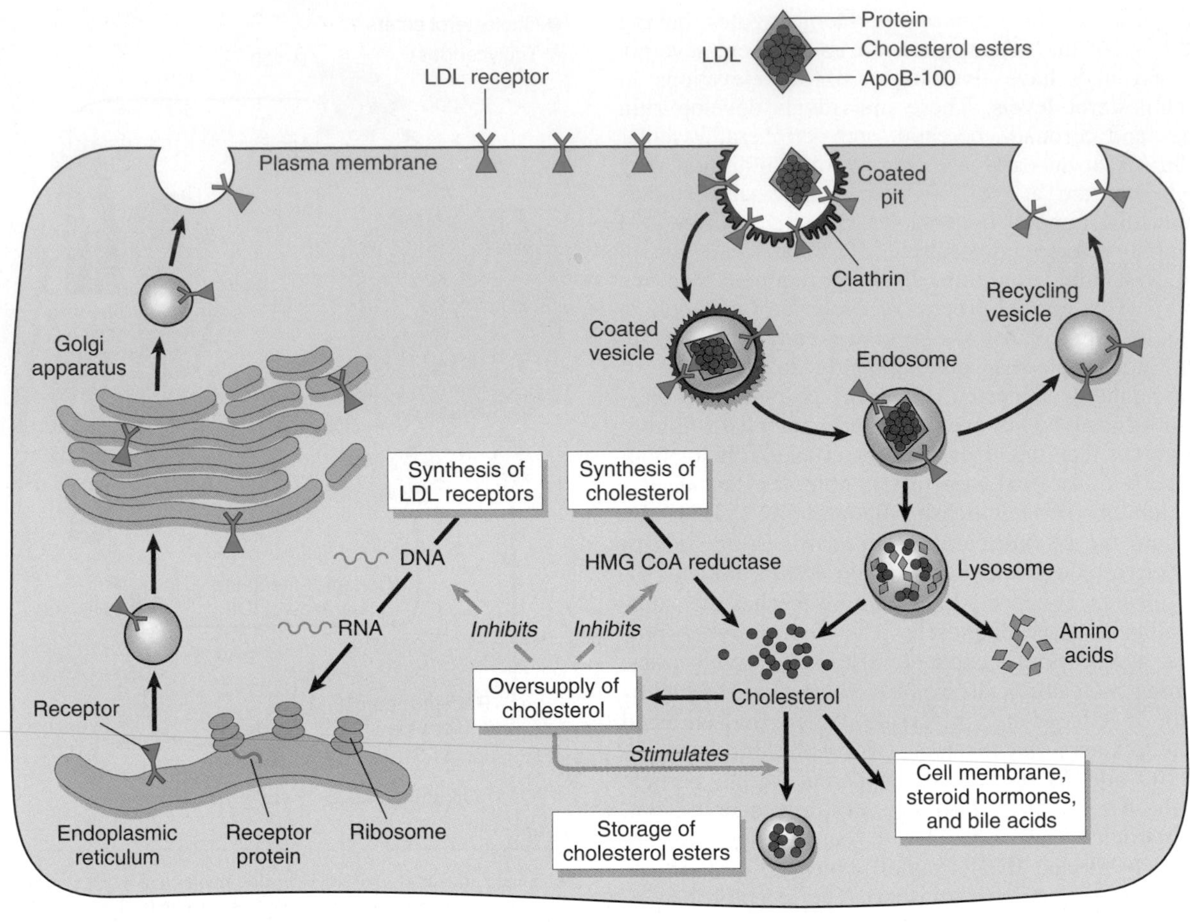

Figure 6–9

The LDL receptor pathway and regulation of cholesterol metabolism.

their cells and have much higher levels of circulating LDL. In addition to defective LDL clearance, both the homozygotes and heterozygotes have increased synthesis of LDL. The mechanism of increased synthesis that contributes to hypercholesterolemia also results from a lack of LDL receptors (see Fig. 6–8). Recall that IDL, the immediate precursor of plasma LDL, also uses hepatic LDL receptors (apoprotein B-100 and E receptors) for its transport into the liver. In familial hypercholesterolemia, impaired IDL transport into the liver secondarily diverts a greater proportion of plasma IDL into the precursor pool for plasma LDL.

The transport of LDL via the scavenger receptor appears to occur at least in part into the cells of the mononuclear phagocyte system. Monocytes and macrophages have receptors for chemically altered (e.g., acetylated or oxidized) LDL. Normally the amount of LDL transported along this scavenger receptor pathway is less than that mediated by the LDL receptor-dependent mechanisms. In the face of hypercholesterolemia, however, there is a marked increase in the scavenger receptor-mediated traffic of LDL cholesterol into the cells of the mononuclear phagocyte system and possibly the vascular walls. This increase is responsible for the appearance of xanthomas and contributes to the pathogenesis of premature atherosclerosis.

The molecular genetics of familial hypercholesterolemia have proven to be extremely complex. The human LDL receptor gene, located on chromosome 19, is extremely large, with 18 exons and 5 domains that span a distance of about 45 kb. More than 150 mutations, including insertions, deletions, and missense and nonsense mutations, involving the LDL receptor gene have been identified. These can be classified into five groups (Fig. 6–10): *Class I mutations* are relatively uncommon, and they lead to a complete failure of synthesis of the receptor protein (null allele). *Class II mutations* are fairly common; they encode receptor proteins that accumulate in the endoplasmic reticulum because they cannot be transported to the Golgi complex. *Class III mutations* affect the LDL-binding domain of the receptor; the encoded proteins reach the cell surface but fail to bind LDL or do so poorly. *Class IV mutations* encode proteins that are synthesized and transported to the cell surface efficiently. They bind LDL normally, but they fail to localize in coated pits, and hence the bound LDL is not internalized. *Class V mutations* encode proteins that are expressed on the cell surface, can bind LDL, and can be internalized; however, the acid-dependent dissociation of the receptor and the bound LDL fails to occur. Such receptors are trapped in the endosome, where they are degraded, and hence they fail to recycle to the cell surface.

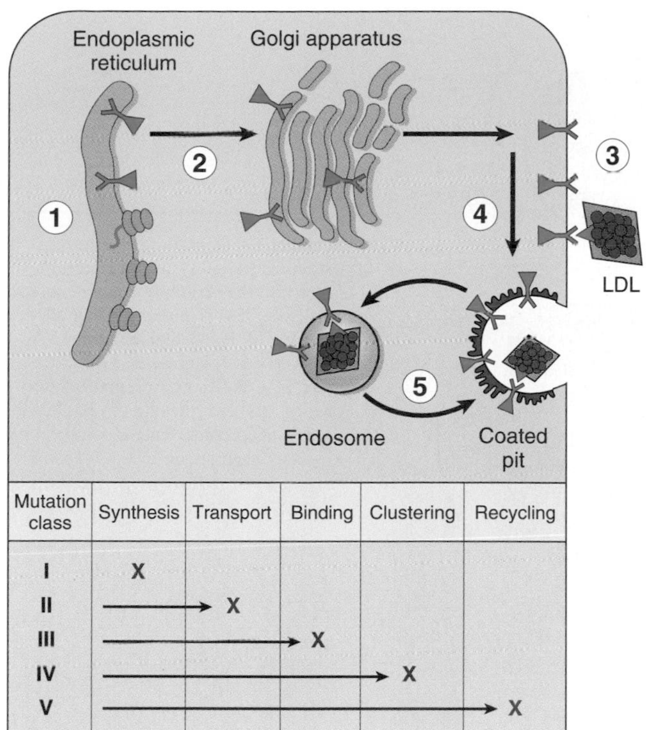

Mutation class	Synthesis	Transport	Binding	Clustering	Recycling
I	X				
II	——→	X			
III	———	——→	X		
IV	———	———	——→	X	
V	———	———	———	——→	X

Figure 6–10 ■

Classification of LDL receptor mutations based on abnormal function of the mutant protein. These mutations disrupt the receptor's synthesis in the endoplasmic reticulum transport to the Golgi complex, binding of apoprotein ligands, clustering in coated pits, and recycling in endosomes. Each class is heterogeneous at the DNA level. (Modified with permission from Hobb HH, et al: The LDL receptor locus in familial hypercholesterolemia: mutational analysis of a membrane protein. Annu Rev Genet 24:133–170, 1990. © 1990 by Annual Reviews.)

The discovery of the critical role of LDL receptors in cholesterol homeostasis has led to the rational design of drugs that lower plasma cholesterol by increasing the number of LDL receptors.[17] One strategy that has proven to be successful is based on the ability of certain drugs (statins) to suppress intracellular cholesterol synthesis by inhibiting the enzyme HMG CoA reductase. This, in turn, allows greater synthesis of LDL receptors (see Fig. 6–9). Efforts are also underway to develop gene therapy for this disorder. Towards this end LDL receptor knockout mice have been generated and like patients with familial hypercholesterolemia, they have elevated cholesterol and accelerated atherosclerosis.[18] Delivery of intact LDL receptor genes via viral vectors lowers cholesterol levels, thus providing a useful model for gene therapy.

Disorders Associated With Defects in Enzymes

LYSOSOMAL STORAGE DISEASES

Lysosomes are key components of the "intracellular digestive tract." They contain a battery of hydrolytic enzymes, which have two special properties. First, they can function in the acid milieu of the lysosomes. Second, these enzymes constitute a special category of secretory proteins that, in contrast to most others, are destined for secretion not into the extracellular fluids but into an intracellular organelle. This latter characteristic requires special processing within the Golgi apparatus, which is reviewed briefly. Similar to all other secretory proteins, lysosomal enzymes (or acid hydrolases, as they are sometimes called) are synthesized in the endoplasmic reticulum and transported to the Golgi apparatus. Within the Golgi complex, they undergo a variety of post-translational modifications, of which one is worthy of special note. This modification involves the attachment of terminal mannose-6-phosphate groupings to some of the oligosaccharide side chains. The phosphorylated mannose residues may be viewed as an "address label" that is recognized by specific receptors found on the inner surface of the Golgi membrane. Lysosomal enzymes bind to these receptors and are thereby segregated from the

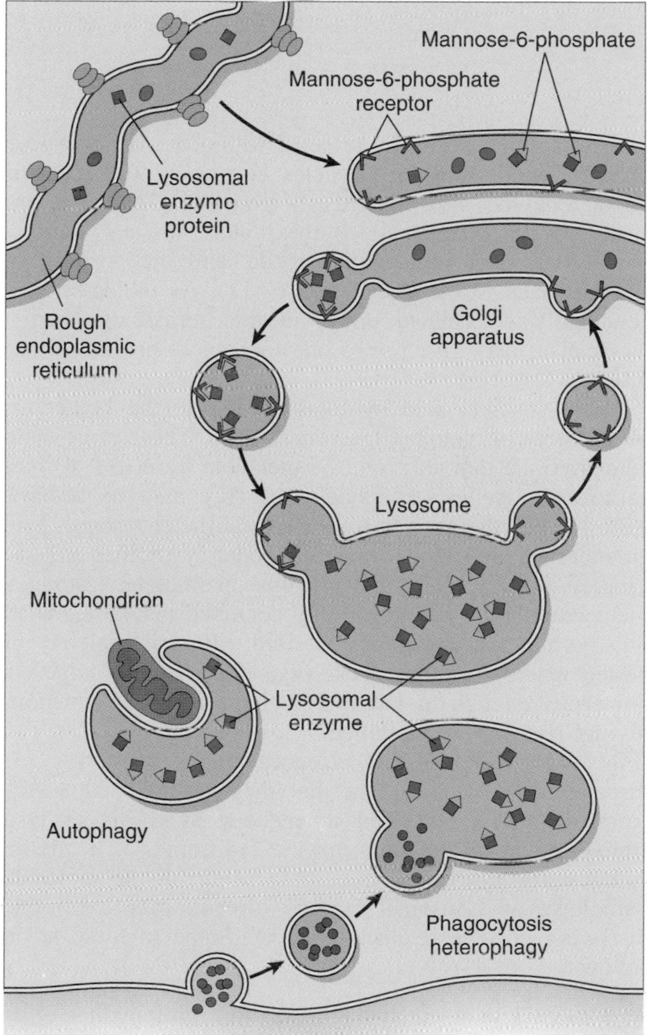

Figure 6–11 ■

Synthesis and intracellular transport of lysosomal enzymes.

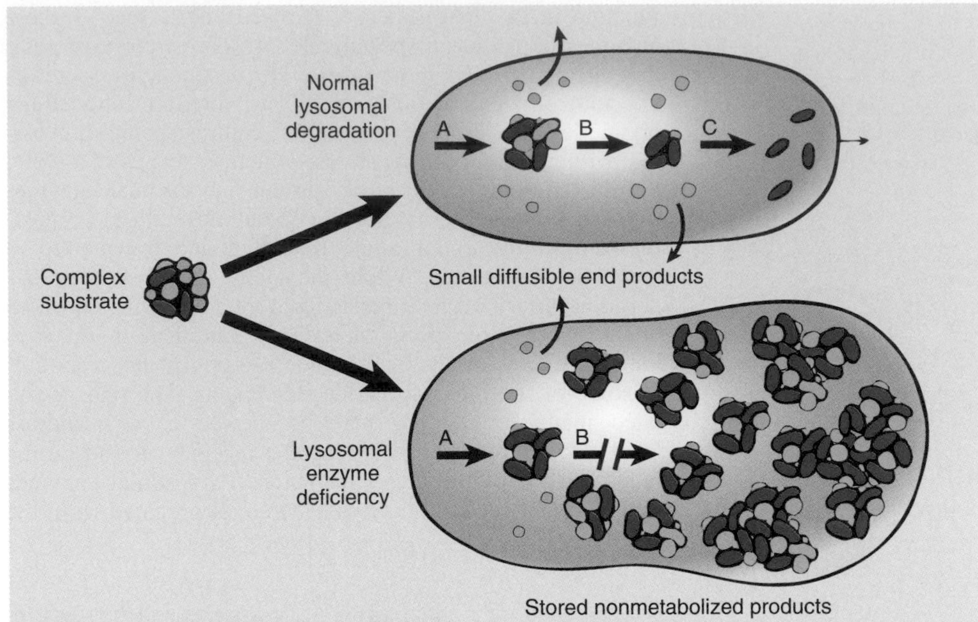

Figure 6–12 ■

Schematic diagram illustrating the pathogenesis of lysosomal storage diseases. In the example shown, a complex substrate is normally degraded by a series of lysosomal enzymes (A, B, and C) into soluble end products. If there is a deficiency or malfunction of one of the enzymes (e.g., B), catabolism is incomplete and insoluble intermediates accumulate in the lysosomes.

numerous other secretory proteins within the Golgi. Subsequently, small transport vesicles containing the receptor-bound enzymes are pinched off from the Golgi and proceed to fuse with the lysosomes. Thus, the enzymes are targeted to their intracellular abode, and the vesicles are shuttled back to the Golgi (Fig. 6–11). As indicated later, genetically determined errors in this remarkable sorting mechanism may give rise to one form of lysosomal storage disease.

The lysosomal acid hydrolases catalyze the breakdown of a variety of complex macromolecules. These large molecules may be derived from the metabolic turnover of intracellular organelles (autophagy), or they may be acquired from outside the cells by phagocytosis (heterophagy). With an inherited deficiency of a functional lysosomal enzyme, catabolism of its substrate remains incomplete, leading to the accumulation of the partially degraded insoluble metabolite within the lysosomes. Stuffed with incompletely digested macromolecules, these organelles become large and numerous enough to interfere with normal cell functions, giving rise to the so-called *lysosomal storage disorders* (Fig. 6–12). When this category of diseases was first discovered, it was thought that they resulted exclusively from mutations that lead to reduced synthesis of lysosomal enzymes ("missing enzyme syndromes"). In the ensuing years, however, research focusing on the molecular pathology of lysosomal storage diseases has led to the discovery of several other defects.[19] Some of these are as follows:

- Synthesis of a catalytically inactive protein that cross-reacts immunologically with the normal enzyme: Thus, by immunoassays the enzyme levels appear to be normal.
- Defects in post-translational processing of the enzyme protein: Included in this category is a failure to attach the mannose-6-phosphate "marker," the absence of which prevents the enzyme from following its correct path to the lysosome. Instead the enzyme is secreted outside the cell.
- Lack of an enzyme activator or protector protein.
- Lack of a substrate activator protein: In some instances, proteins that react with the substrate to facilitate its hydrolysis may be missing or defective.
- Lack of a transport protein required for egress of the digested material from the lysosomes.

It should be evident, therefore, that the concept of lysosomal storage disorders has to be expanded to include the lack of any protein essential for the normal function of lysosomes.

Several distinctive and separable conditions are included among the lysosomal storage diseases (Table 6–5). In general, the distribution of the stored material, and hence the organs affected, is determined by two interrelated factors: (1) the site where most of the material to be degraded is found and (2) the location where most of the degradation normally occurs. *For example, brain is rich in gangliosides, and hence defective hydrolysis of gangliosides, as occurs in GM_1 and GM_2 gangliosidoses, results primarily in storage within neurons and neurologic symptoms.* Defects in degradation of mucopolysaccharides affect virtually every organ because mucopolysaccharides are widely distributed in the body. Because cells of the mononuclear phagocyte system are especially rich in lysosomes and are involved in the degradation of a variety of substrates, organs rich in phagocytic cells, such as the spleen and liver, are frequently enlarged in several forms of lysosomal storage disorders. The ever-expanding number of lysosomal storage diseases can be divided into rational categories based on the biochemical nature of the accumulated metabolite, thus creating such subgroups as the *glycogenoses,*

Table 6–5. LYSOSOMAL STORAGE DISEASES

Disease	Enzyme Deficiency	Major Accumulating Metabolites
Glycogenosis		
Type 2—Pompe disease	α-1,4-Glucosidase (lysosomal glucosidase)	Glycogen
Sphingolipidoses		
GM_1 gangliosidosis	GM_1 ganglioside β-galactosidase	GM_1 ganglioside, galactose containing oligosaccharides
Type 1—infantile, generalized		
Type 2—juvenile		
GM_2 gangliosidosis		
Tay-Sachs disease	Hexosaminidase-α subunit	GM_2 ganglioside
Sandhoff disease	Hexosaminidase-β subunit	GM_2 ganglioside, globoside
GM_2 gangliosidosis, variant AB	Ganglioside activator protein	GM_2 ganglioside
Sulfatidoses		
Metachromatic leukodystrophy	Arylsulfatase A	Sulfatide
Multiple sulfatase deficiency	Arylsulfatases A, B, C; steroid sulfatase; iduronate sulfatase, heparan N-sulfatase	Sulfatide, steroid sulfate, heparan sulfate, dermatan sulfate
Krabbe disease	Galactosylceramidase	Galactocerebroside
Fabry disease	α-Galactosidase A	Ceramide trihexoside
Gaucher disease	Glucocerebrosidase	Glucocerebroside
Niemann-Pick disease: types A and B	Sphingomyelinase	Sphingomyelin
Mucopolysaccharidoses (MPS)		
MPS I H (Hurler)	α-L-Iduronidase	Dermatan sulfate, heparan sulfate
MPS II (Hunter)	L-Iduronosulfate sulfatase	
Mucolipidoses (ML)		
I-cell disease (ML II) and pseudo-Hurler polydystrophy	Deficiency of phosphorylating enzymes essential for the formation of mannose-6-phosphate recognition marker; acid hydrolases lacking the recognition marker cannot be targeted to the lysosomes but are secreted extracellularly	Mucopolysaccharide, glycolipid
Other diseases of complex carbohydrates		
Fucosidosis	α-Fucosidase	Fucose-containing sphingolipids and glycoprotein fragments
Mannosidosis	α-Mannosidase	Mannose-containing oligosaccharides
Aspartylglycosaminuria	Aspartylglycosamine amide hydrolase	Aspartyl-2-deoxy-2-acetamido-glycosylamine
Other lysosomal storage diseases		
Wolman disease	Acid lipase	Cholesterol esters, triglycerides
Acid phosphate deficiency	Lysosomal acid phosphatase	Phosphate esters

sphingolipidoses (lipidoses), mucopolysaccharidoses (MPS), and *mucolipidoses* (Table 6–5). Only one among the many glycogenoses results from a lysosomal enzyme deficiency, and so this family of storage diseases is considered later. Only the most common disorders among the remaining groups are considered here.

Tay-Sachs Disease (GM_2 Gangliosidosis: Hexosaminidase α-Subunit Deficiency)

GM_2 gangliosidoses are a group of three lysosomal storage diseases caused by an inability to catabolize GM_2 gangliosides. Degradation of GM_2 gangliosides requires three polypeptides encoded by three separate loci (Fig. 6–13). The phenotypic effects of mutations affecting these genes are fairly similar because they result from accumulation of GM_2 gangliosides. The underlying enzyme defect, however, is different for each. Tay-Sachs disease, the most common form of GM_2 gangliosidosis, results from mutations that affect the α-subunit locus on chromosome 15 and cause a severe deficiency of hexosaminidase A. This disease is especially prevalent among Jews, particularly among those of Eastern European (Ashkenazic) origin, in whom a carrier rate of 1 in 30 has been reported.[20]

MORPHOLOGY. The hexosaminidase A is absent from virtually all the tissues that have been examined, including leukocytes and plasma, and so GM_2 ganglioside accumulates in many tissues (e.g., heart, liver, spleen), but the involvement of neurons in the central and autonomic nervous systems and retina dominates the clinical picture. On histologic examination, the neurons are ballooned with cytoplasmic vacuoles, each of which constitutes a markedly distended lysosome filled with gangliosides (Fig. 6–14*A*). Stains for fat such as oil red O and Sudan black B are positive. With the electron microscope, several types of cytoplasmic inclusions can be visualized, the most prominent being whorled configurations within lysosomes composed of onion-skin layers of membranes (Fig. 6–14*B*). In time, there is progressive

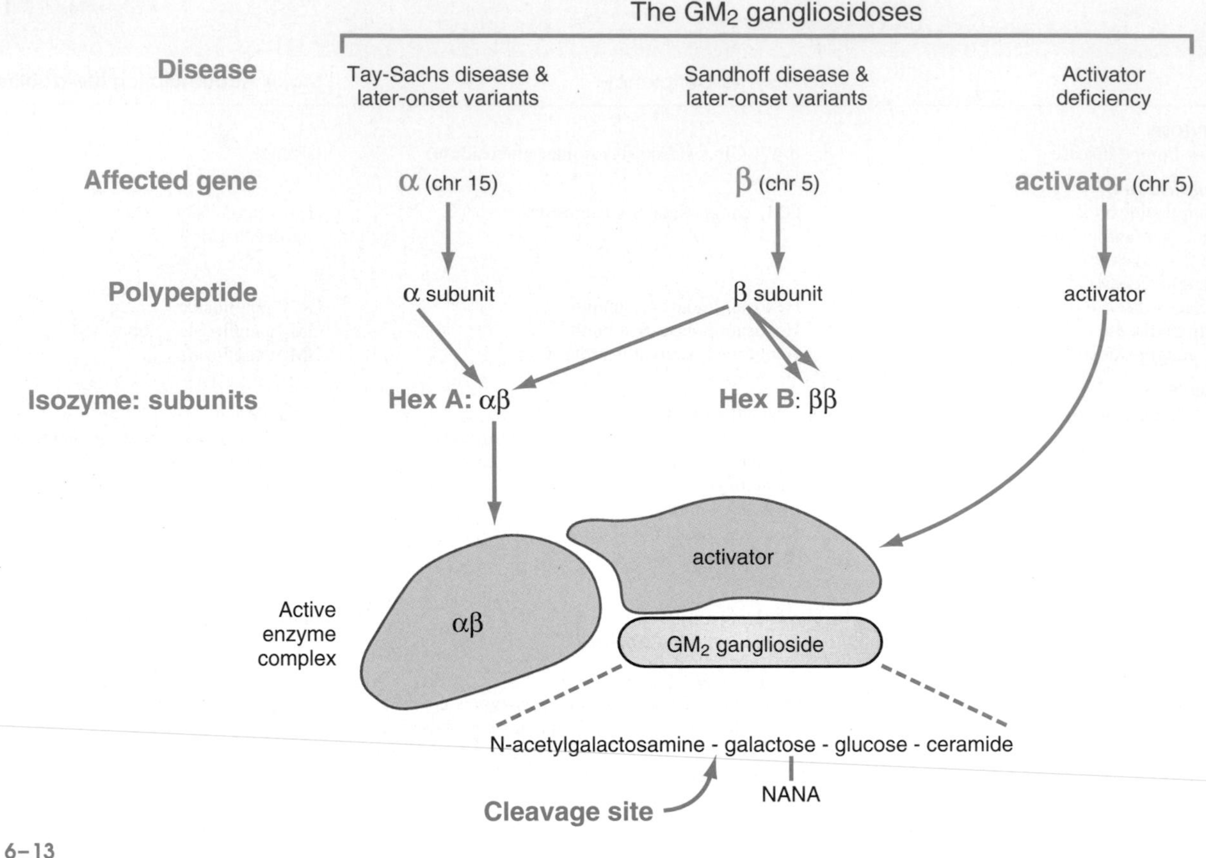

Figure 6–13

The three-gene system required for hexosaminidase A activity and the diseases that result from defects in each of the genes. The function of the activator protein is to bind the ganglioside substrate and present it to the enzyme. (Modified from Sandhoff K, et al: The GM_2 gangliosidoses. In Scriver CR, et al (eds): The Metabolic Basis of Inherited Disease, 6th ed. New York, McGraw-Hill, 1989, p 1824.)

destruction of neurons, proliferation of microglia, and accumulation of complex lipids in phagocytes within the brain substance. A similar process occurs in the cerebellum as well as in neurons throughout the basal ganglia, brain stem, spinal cord, and dorsal root ganglia and in the neurons of the autonomic nervous system. The ganglion cells in the retina are similarly swollen with GM_2 ganglioside, particularly at the margins of the macula. A **cherry-red spot** thus appears in the macula, representing accentuation of the normal color of the macular choroid contrasted with the pallor produced by the swollen ganglion cells in the remainder of the retina. This finding is characteristic of Tay-Sachs disease and other storage disorders affecting the neurons.

More than 30 alleles have been identified at the α-subunit locus, each associated with a variable degree of enzyme deficiency and hence with variable clinical manifestations. The most frequent allele carries a 4 base pair insertion in the coding sequence, causing the formation of a stop codon down-stream. These patients have a profound deficiency of hexosaminidase A. The affected infants appear normal at birth but begin to manifest signs and symptoms at about 6 months of age. There is relentless motor and mental deterioration, beginning with motor incoordination, mental obtundation leading to muscular flaccidity, blindness, and increasing dementia. Sometime during the early course of the disease, the characteristic, but not pathognomonic, cherry-red spot appears in the macula of the eye grounds in almost all patients. Over the span of 1 or 2 years, a complete, pathetic vegetative state is reached, followed by death at 2 to 3 years of age.

Antenatal diagnosis and carrier detection are possible by enzyme assays and DNA-based analysis.[21] The clinical features of the two other forms of GM_2 gangliosidosis (see Fig. 6–13), Sandhoff disease, resulting from β-subunit defect, and GM_2 activator deficiency, are similar to those of Tay-Sachs disease.

Niemann-Pick Disease: Types A and B

Niemann-Pick disease types A and B refers to two related disorders that are characterized by lysosomal accumulation of sphingomyelin resulting from an inherited deficiency of sphingomyelinase. In the past, these two condi-

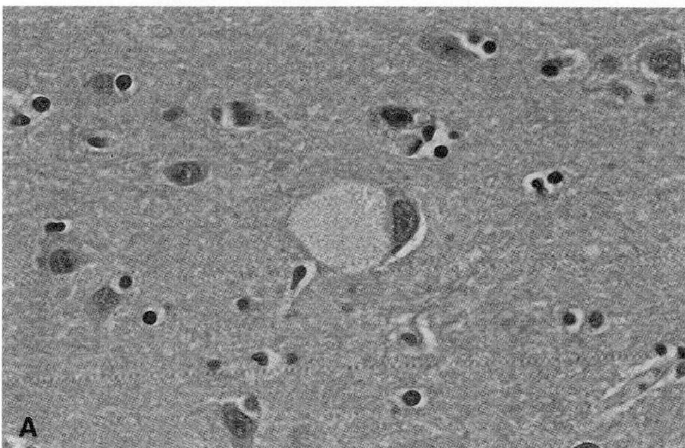

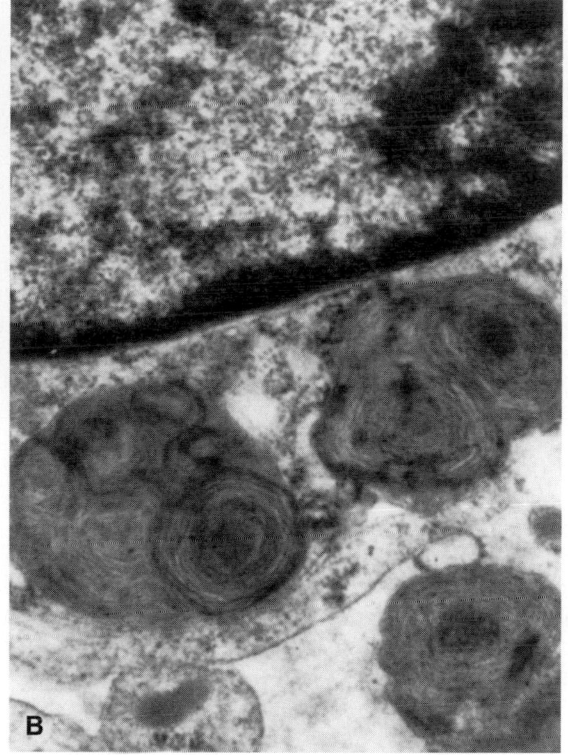

Figure 6–14

Ganglion cells in Tay-Sachs disease. *A*, Under the light microscope, a large neuron has obvious lipid vacuolation. (Courtesy of Dr. Arthur Weinberg, Department of Pathology, University of Texas, Southwestern Medical Center, Dallas, TX.) *B*, A portion of a neuron under the electron microscope shows prominent lysosomes with whorled configurations. Part of the nucleus is shown above. (Electron micrograph courtesy of Dr. Joe Rutledge, University of Texas Southwestern Medical Center, Dallas, TX.)

tions were grouped with an unrelated disorder, called *Niemann-Pick disease type C*.[22] In the latter type, there is a primary defect in intracellular cholesterol esterification and transport. The mutant gene, localized to 18q11-12, has been cloned, but the molecular basis of the disturbance in cholesterol metabolism is not known.[23] All types are rare, so our discussion is confined largely to sphingomyelinase-deficient, type A variant, representing 75 to 80% of all cases. *This is the severe infantile form with extensive neurologic involvement, marked visceral accumulations of sphingomyelin, and progressive wasting and early death within the first 3 years of life.* To provide a perspective on the differences between the variants of Niemann-Pick disease, we need only point out that in type B, for example, patients have organomegaly but generally no central nervous system involvement. They usually survive into adulthood. As with Tay-Sachs disease, types A and B Niemann-Pick disease are common in Ashkenazi Jews.

MORPHOLOGY. In the classic infantile type A variant, a missense mutation causes almost complete deficiency of sphingomyelinase. Sphingomyelin is a ubiquitous component of cellular (including organellar) membranes, and so the enzyme deficiency blocks degradation of the lipid, resulting in its progressive accumulation within lysosomes, particularly within cells of the mononuclear phagocyte system. Affected cells become enlarged, sometimes to 90 mm in diameter, secondary to the distention of lysosomes with sphingomyelin and cholesterol. Innumerable small vacuoles of relatively uniform size are created, imparting a foaminess to the cytoplasm (Fig. 6–15). In frozen sections of fresh tissue, the vacuoles stain for fat with Sudan black B and oil red O. Electron microscopy confirms that the vacuoles are engorged secondary lysosomes that often contain membranous cytoplasmic bodies resembling concentric

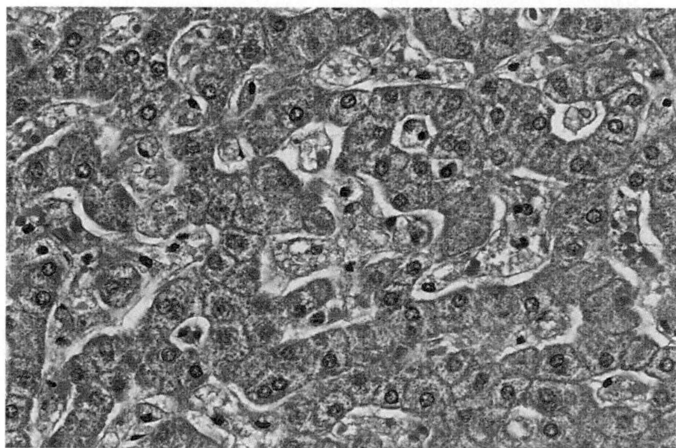

Figure 6–15

Niemann-Pick disease in liver. The hepatocytes and Kupffer cells have a foamy, vacuolated appearance owing to deposition of lipids. (Courtesy of Dr. Arthur Weinberg, Department of Pathology, University of Texas Southwestern Medical Center, Dallas, TX.)

lamellated myelin figures. Sometimes the lysosomal configurations take the form of parallel palisaded lamellae, creating so-called zebra bodies.

The lipid-laden phagocytic foam cells are widely distributed in the spleen, liver, lymph nodes, bone marrow, tonsils, gastrointestinal tract, and lungs. The involvement of the spleen generally produces massive enlargement, sometimes to 10 times its normal weight, but the hepatomegaly is usually not quite so striking. The lymph nodes are generally moderately to markedly enlarged throughout the body.

Involvement of the brain and eye deserves special mention. In brain, the gyri are shrunken and the sulci widened. The neuronal involvement is diffuse, affecting all parts of the nervous system. Vacuolation and ballooning of neurons constitute the dominant histologic change, which in time leads to cell death and loss of brain substance. A retinal cherry-red spot similar to that seen in Tay-Sachs disease is present in about one third to one half of affected individuals. Its origin is similar to that described in Tay-Sachs disease except that the accumulated metabolite is sphingomyelin.

Clinical manifestations may be present at birth but almost certainly become evident by 6 months of age. Infants typically have a protuberant abdomen because of the hepatosplenomegaly. Once the manifestations appear, they are followed by progressive failure to thrive, vomiting, fever, and generalized lymphadenopathy as well as progressive deterioration of psychomotor function. Death comes as a release, usually within the first or second year of life.

The diagnosis is established by biochemical assays for sphingomyelinase activity in liver or bone marrow biopsy. The sphingomyelinase gene has been cloned, and hence individuals affected with types A and B as well as carriers can be detected by DNA probe analysis.

Gaucher Disease

Gaucher disease refers to a cluster of autosomal recessive disorders resulting from mutations in the gene encoding glucocerebrosidase.[24] This disease is the most common lysosomal storage disorder. The affected gene encodes glucocerebrosidase, an enzyme that normally cleaves the glucose residue from ceramide. As a result, glucocerebroside accumulates principally in the phagocytic cells of the body but in some forms also in the central nervous system. Glucocerebrosides are continually formed from the catabolism of glycolipids derived mainly from the cell membranes of senescent leukocytes and erythrocytes. Three clinical subtypes of Gaucher disease have been distinguished. The most common, accounting for 99% of cases, is called *type I*, or the chronic non-neuronopathic form. In this type, *storage of glucocerebrosides is limited to the mononuclear phagocytes throughout the body without involving the brain. Splenic and skeletal involvements dominate this pattern of the disease.* It is found principally in Jews of European stock. Patients with this disorder have reduced but detectable levels of glucocerebrosidase activity. Longevity is shortened but not markedly. Type II, or acute neuronopathic, Gaucher disease is the *infantile acute cerebral pattern. This infantile form has no predilection for Jews. In these patients, there is virtually no detectable glucocerebrosidase activity in the tissues.* Hepatosplenomegaly is also seen in this form of Gaucher disease, but the clinical picture is dominated by progressive central nervous system involvement, leading to death at an early age. A third pattern, type III, is sometimes distinguished, intermediate between types I and II. These patients are usually juveniles and have the systemic involvement characteristic of type I but have progressive central nervous system disease that usually begins in the teens or twenties. These specific patterns run within families, resulting from different allelic mutations in the structural gene for the enzyme.

MORPHOLOGY. The glucocerebrosides accumulate in massive amounts within phagocytic cells throughout the body in all forms of Gaucher disease. The distended phagocytic cells, known as **Gaucher cells,** are found in the spleen, liver, bone marrow, lymph nodes, tonsils, thymus, and Peyer patches. Similar cells may be found in both the alveolar septa and the air spaces in the lung. In contrast to the lipid storage diseases already discussed, Gaucher cells rarely appear vacuolated but instead have a fibrillary type of cytoplasm likened to crumpled tissue paper (Fig. 6–16). Gaucher cells are often enlarged, sometimes up to 100 μm in diameter, and have one or more dark, eccentrically placed nuclei. Periodic acid–Schiff (PAS) staining is usually intensely positive. With the electron microscope, the fibrillary cytoplasm can be resolved as elongated, distended lysosomes, containing the stored lipid in stacks of bilayers.[25]

The accumulation of Gaucher cells produces a variety of gross anatomic changes. The spleen is enlarged in the type I variant, sometimes up to 10 kg. It may appear uniformly pale or have a mottled surface owing to focal accumulations of Gaucher cells. The lymphadenopathy is mild to moderate and is body-wide. The accumulations of Gaucher cells in the bone marrow may produce small focal areas of bone erosion or large, soft, gray tumorous masses that cause skeletal deformities or destroy sufficient bone to give rise to fractures. In patients with cerebral involvement, Gaucher cells are seen in the Virchow-Robin spaces, and arterioles are surrounded by swollen adventitial cells. There is no storage of lipids in the neurons, yet neurons appear shriveled and are progressively destroyed. It is suspected that the lipids that accumulate in the phagocytic cells around blood vessels are in some manner toxic to neural tissue.

The clinical course of Gaucher disease depends on the clinical subtype. In the type I pattern, symptoms and signs

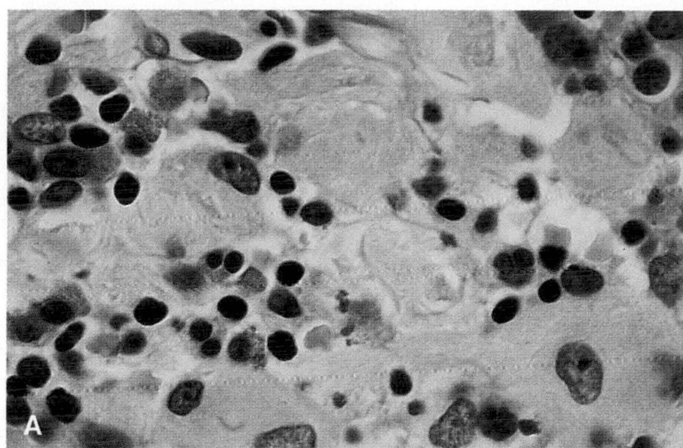

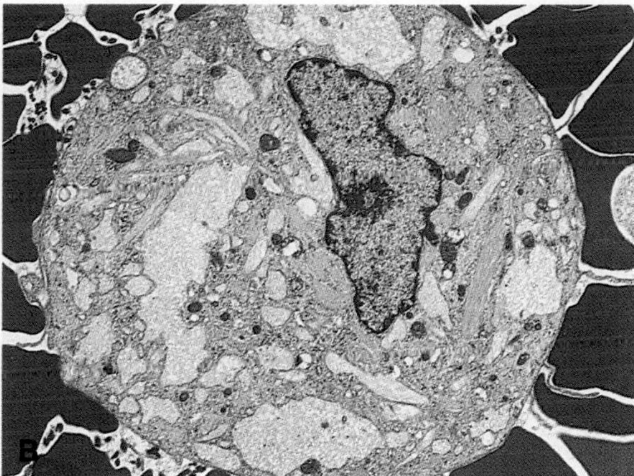

Figure 6–16

Gaucher disease involving the bone marrow. *A*, Gaucher cells with abundant lipid-laden granular cytoplasm. *B*, Electron micrograph of Gaucher cells with elongated distended lysosomes. (Courtesy of Dr. Mathew Frieze, Department of Pathology, University of Texas Southwestern Medical Center, Dallas, TX.)

first appear in adult life and are related to splenomegaly or bone involvement. Most commonly, there is pancytopenia or thrombocytopenia secondary to hypersplenism. Pathologic fractures and bone pain occur if there has been extensive expansion of the marrow space. Although the disease is progressive in the adult, it is compatible with long life. In types II and III, central nervous system dysfunction, convulsions, and progressive mental deterioration dominate, although organs such as the liver, spleen, and lymph nodes are also affected.

The diagnosis of homozygotes can be made by measurement of glucocerebrosidase activity in peripheral blood leukocytes or in extracts of cultured skin fibroblasts. Because there is substantial overlap between the enzyme levels in normals and heterozygotes, such assays are not reliable for carrier detection. In principle, detection of specific mutations can be used for detecting heterozygotes. Because more than 30 allelic mutations can cause Gaucher disease, however, it is not possible to use a single genetic test.

As with all lysosomal storage diseases, the treatment of Gaucher disease is difficult. Replacement therapy with recombinant enzymes is effective but extremely expensive. Because the fundamental defect resides in mononuclear phagocytic cells originating from marrow stem cells, bone marrow transplantation has been attempted. In the future, attempts will be directed toward correction of the enzyme defect by transfer of the normal glucocerebrosidase gene into the patient's cells. A mouse model of Gaucher disease has been produced by targeted disruption (gene knockout) of the murine glucocerebrosidase gene.[26] This animal model may prove useful in designing gene therapy for Gaucher disease.

Mucopolysaccharidoses

The mucopolysaccharidoses (MPS) are a group of closely related syndromes that result from genetically determined deficiencies of lysosomal enzymes involved in the degradation of mucopolysaccharides (glycosaminoglycans). Chemically, mucopolysaccharides are long-chain complex carbohydrates that are linked with proteins to form proteoglycans. They are abundant in the ground substance of connective tissue. The glycosaminoglycans that accumulate in MPS are dermatan sulfate, heparan sulfate, keratan sulfate, and chondroitin sulfate.[27] The enzymes involved in the degradation of these molecules cleave terminal sugars from the polysaccharide chains disposed along a polypeptide or core protein. When there is a block in the removal of a terminal sugar, the remainder of the polysaccharide chain is not further degraded, and thus these chains accumulate within lysosomes in various tissues and organs of the body. Severe somatic and neurologic changes result.

Several clinical variants of MPS, classified numerically from MPS I to MPS VII, have been described, each resulting from the deficiency of one specific enzyme. All the MPS except one are inherited as autosomal recessive traits; the exception, called *Hunter syndrome*, is an X-linked recessive. Within a given group (e.g., MPS I, characterized by a deficiency of α-l-iduronidase), subgroups exist that result from different mutant alleles at the same genetic locus. Thus, the severity of enzyme deficiency and the clinical picture even within subgroups are often different.

In general, MPS are progressive disorders, characterized by involvement of multiple organs, including liver, spleen, heart, and blood vessels. Most are associated with *coarse facial features, clouding of the cornea, joint stiffness*, and *mental retardation.* Urinary excretion of the accumulated mucopolysaccharides is often increased.

MORPHOLOGY. The accumulated mucopolysaccharides are generally found in mononuclear phagocytic cells, endothelial cells, intimal smooth muscle cells, and fibroblasts throughout the body. Common sites of involvement are thus the spleen, liver, bone marrow, lymph nodes, blood vessels, and heart.

Microscopically, affected cells are distended and have apparent clearing of the cytoplasm to create so-called balloon cells. The cleared cytoplasm can be resolved as numerous minute vacuoles, which, with the electron microscope, can be visualized as swollen lysosomes filled with a finely granular PAS-positive material that can be identified biochemically as mucopolysaccharide. Similar lysosomal changes are found in the neurons of those syndromes characterized by central nervous system involvement. In addition, however, some of the lysosomes in neurons are replaced by lamellated zebra bodies similar to those seen in Niemann-Pick disease. **Hepatosplenomegaly, skeletal deformities, valvular lesions, and subendothelial arterial deposits, particularly in the coronary arteries and lesions in the brain, are common threads that run through all the MPS.** In many of the more protracted syndromes, coronary subendothelial lesions lead to myocardial ischemia. Thus, myocardial infarction and cardiac decompensation are important causes of death.

Of the seven recognized variants, only two well-characterized syndromes are described briefly here. *Hurler syndrome*, also called MPS I H, results from a deficiency of α-l-iduronidase. It is one of the most severe forms of MPS. Affected children appear normal at birth but develop hepatosplenomegaly by 6 to 24 months. Their growth is retarded, and, as in other forms of MPS, they develop coarse facial features and skeletal deformities. Death occurs by 6 to 10 years of age and is often due to cardiovascular complications. *Hunter syndrome*, also called MPS II, differs from Hurler syndrome in mode of inheritance (X-linked), absence of corneal clouding, and milder clinical course.

GLYCOGEN STORAGE DISEASES (GLYCOGENOSES)

A number of genetic syndromes have been identified that result from some metabolic defect in the synthesis or catabolism of glycogen. The best understood and most important category includes the *glycogen storage diseases*, resulting from a hereditary deficiency of one of the enzymes involved in the synthesis or sequential degradation of glycogen. Depending on the tissue or organ distribution of the specific enzyme in the normal state, *glycogen storage in these disorders may be limited to a few tissues, may be more widespread while not affecting all tissues, or may be systemic in distribution.*[28]

The significance of a specific enzyme deficiency is best understood from the perspective of the normal metabolism of glycogen (Fig. 6–17). As is well known, glycogen is a storage form of glucose. Glycogen synthesis begins with the conversion of glucose to glucose-6-phosphate by the action of a hexokinase (glucokinase). A phosphoglucomutase then transforms the glucose-6-phosphate to glucose-1-phosphate, which, in turn, is converted to uridine diphosphoglucose. A highly branched, large polymer is then built up (molecular weight up to 100 million), containing up to 10,000 glucose molecules linked together by α-1,4-glucoside bonds. The glycogen chain and branches continue to be elongated by the addition of glucose molecules mediated by glycogen synthetases. During degradation, distinct phosphorylases in the liver and muscle split glucose-1-phosphate from the glycogen until about four glucose residues remain on each branch, leaving a branched oligosaccharide called *limit dextrin*. This can be further degraded only by the debranching enzyme. In addition to these major pathways, glycogen is also degraded in the lysosomes by acid maltase. If the lysosomes are deficient in this enzyme, the glycogen contained within them is not accessible to degradation by cytoplasmic enzymes such as phosphorylases.

On the basis of specific enzyme deficiencies and the resultant clinical pictures, glycogenoses have traditionally been divided into a dozen or so syndromes designated by roman numerals, and the list continues to grow. Rather than describing each syndrome, we offer a more manageable classification that is based on the pathophysiology of these disorders.[29] According to this approach, glycogenoses can be divided into three major subgroups.

- *Hepatic forms*: As is well known, the liver is a key player in glycogen metabolism. It contains enzymes that synthesize glycogen for storage and ultimately break it down into free glucose, which is then released into the blood. An inherited deficiency of hepatic enzymes that are involved in glycogen metabolism therefore leads not only to the storage of glycogen in the liver, but also to a reduction in blood glucose level (hypoglycemia) (Fig. 6–18). Deficiency of the enzyme glucose-6-phosphatase (von Gierke disease, or type I glycogenosis) is a prime example of the hepatic-hypoglycemic form of glycogen storage disease (Table 6–6). Other examples include lack of liver phosphorylase and debranching enzyme, both involved in the breakdown of glycogen (see Fig. 6–17). In all of these cases, glycogen is stored in many organs, but the *hepatic enlargement and hypoglycemia dominate the clinical picture.*[30]
- *Myopathic forms*: In the striated muscles, as opposed to the liver, glycogen is used predominantly as a source of energy. This is derived by glycolysis, which leads ultimately to the formation of lactate (see Fig. 6–18). If the enzymes that fuel the glycolytic pathway are deficient, glycogen storage occurs in the muscles and is associated with muscular weakness owing to impaired energy production. Examples in this category include deficiencies of muscle phosphorylase (McArdle disease, or type V glycogenosis), muscle phosphofructokinase (type VII glycogen storage disease), and several others. *Typically, patients with the myopathic forms present with muscle cramps after exercise and a failure of exercise-induced rise in blood lactate levels owing to a block in glycolysis.*[31]
- Glycogen storage diseases associated with (1) deficiency of α-glucosidase (acid maltase) and (2) lack of branching enzyme do not fit into the hepatic or myopathic

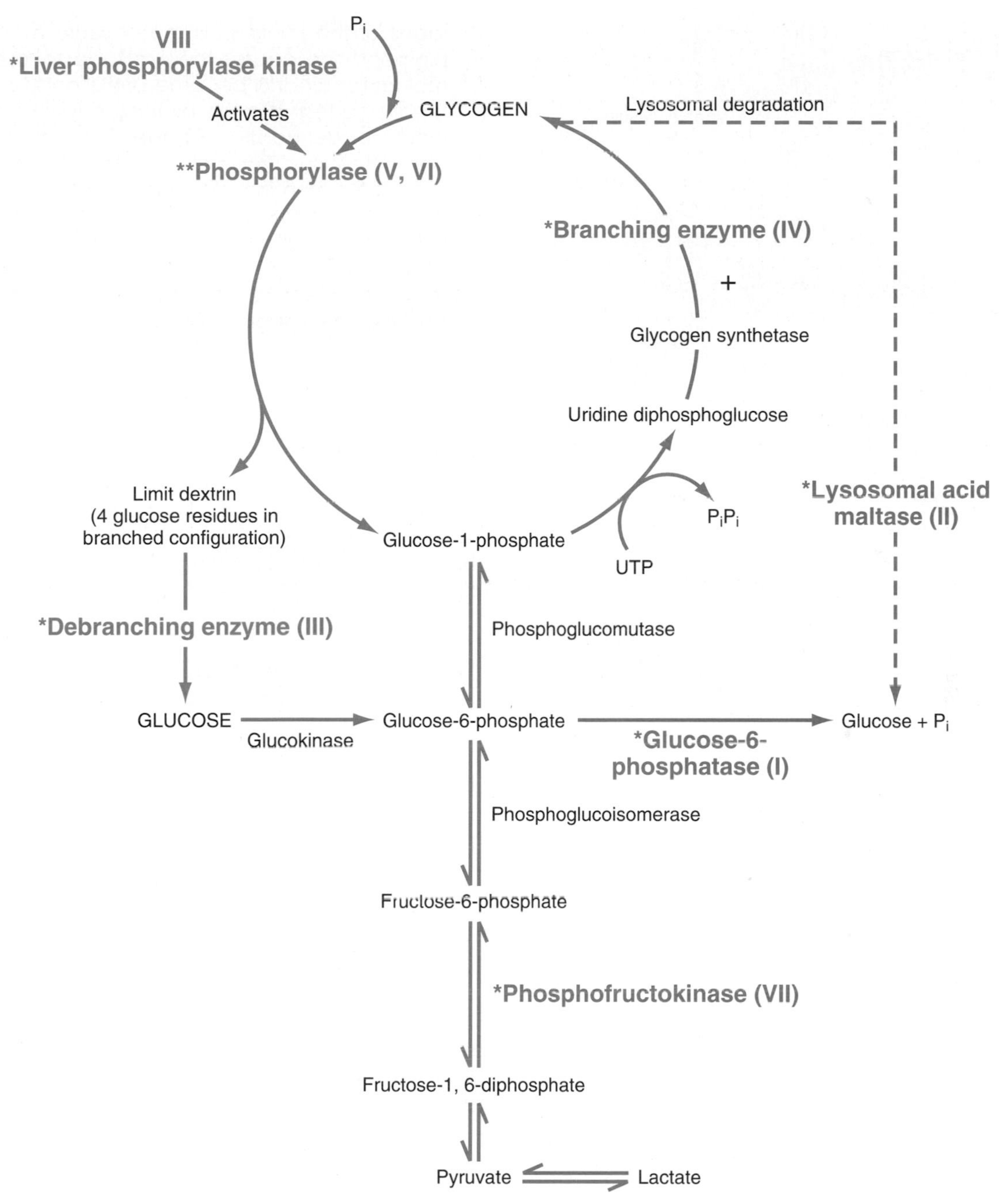

Figure 6–17

Pathways of glycogen metabolism. Asterisks mark the enzyme deficiencies associated with glycogen storage diseases. Roman numerals indicate the type of glycogen storage disease associated with the given enzyme deficiency. Types V and VI result from deficiencies of muscle and liver phosphorylases, respectively. (Modified from Hers H, et al: Glycogen storage diseases. In Scriver CR, et al (eds): The Metabolic Basis of Inherited Disease, 6th ed. New York, McGraw-Hill, 1989, p 425.)

categories just described. They are associated with glycogen storage in many organs and death early in life. Acid maltase is a lysosomal enzyme, and hence its deficiency leads to lysosomal storage of glycogen (type II glycogenosis, or Pompe disease) in all organs, but cardiomegaly is most prominent (Fig. 6–19). Brancher glycogenosis (type IV) is associated with widespread deposition of an abnormal form of glycogen with detrimental effects on the brain, heart, skeletal muscles, and liver.

The principal features of some important examples from each of the aforementioned three categories are summa-

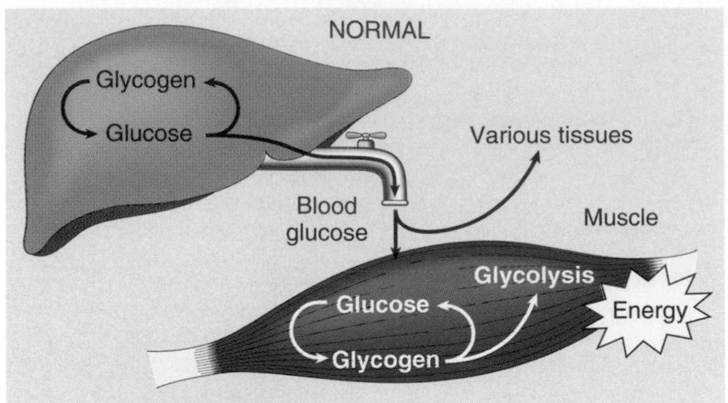

GLYCOGEN STORAGE DISEASE—HEPATIC TYPE

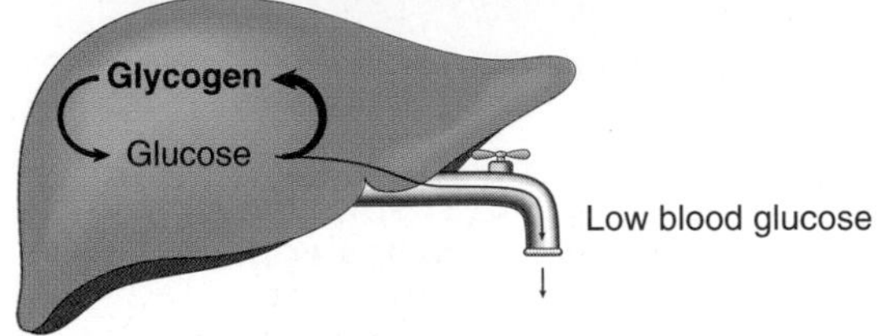

GLYCOGEN STORAGE DISEASE—MYOPATHIC TYPE

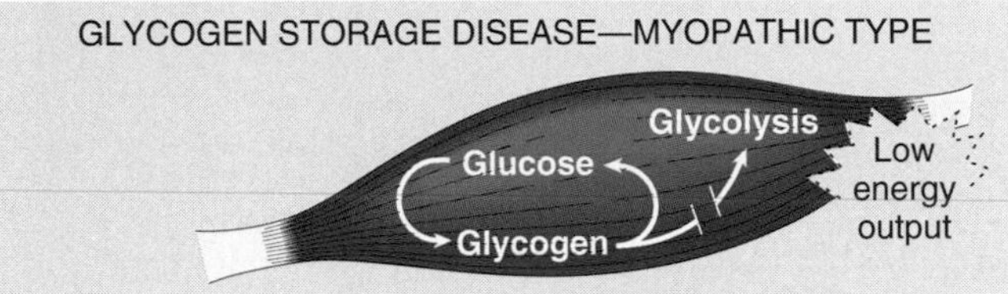

Figure 6–18

Top, Simplified schema of normal glycogen metabolism in the liver and skeletal muscles. *Middle*, Effects of an inherited deficiency of hepatic enzymes involved in glycogen metabolism. *Bottom*, Consequences of a genetic deficiency in the enzymes that metabolize glycogen in skeletal muscles.

rized in Table 6–6. Details of other forms may be found in specialized texts.[32]

ALKAPTONURIA (OCHRONOSIS)

Alkaptonuria, the first human inborn error of metabolism to be discovered, was recognized by Garrod. It is an autosomal recessive disorder in which *the lack of homogentisic oxidase blocks the metabolism of phenylalanine-tyrosine at the level of homogentisic acid.* Thus, homogentisic acid accumulates in the body. A large amount is excreted, imparting a black color to the urine if allowed to stand and undergo oxidation.[33] The gene encoding homogentisic oxidase, mapped to 3q21, was cloned in 1996,[34] 64 years after the initial description of the disease by Garrod.

MORPHOLOGY. The retained homogentisic acid selectively binds to collagen in connective tissues, tendons, and cartilage, imparting to these tissues a blue-black pigmentation (**ochronosis**) most evident in the ears, nose, and cheeks. **The most serious consequences of ochronosis, however, stem from deposits of the pigment in the articular cartilages of the joints.** In some obscure manner, the pigmentation causes the cartilage to lose its normal resiliency and become brittle and fibrillated.[35] Wear-and-tear erosion of this abnormal cartilage leads to denudation of the subchondral bone, and often tiny fragments of the fibrillated cartilage are driven into the underlying bone, worsening the damage. The vertebral column, particularly the intervertebral disc, is the prime site of attack, but later the knees, shoulders, and hips may be affected. The small joints of the hands and feet are usually spared.

Although the metabolic defect is present from birth, the degenerative arthropathy develops slowly and usually does not become clinically evident until the thirties. Although it is not life-threatening, it may be severely crippling. The disability may be as extreme as that encountered in the severe forms of osteoarthritis (Chapter 28) of the elderly, but in alkaptonuria the arthropathy occurs at a much earlier age.

Disorders Associated With Defects in Proteins That Regulate Cell Growth

Normal growth and differentiation of cells is regulated by two classes of genes: protooncogenes and tumor-suppressor genes, whose products promote or restrain cell growth (Chapters 4 and 8). It is now well established that mutations in these two classes of genes are important in the pathogenesis of tumors. In the vast majority of cases, cancer-causing mutations affect somatic cells and hence are not passed in the germ line. In approximately 5% of all cancers, however, mutations transmitted through the germ line contribute to the development of cancer. Most familial cancers are inherited in an autosomal dominant fashion, but a few recessive disorders have also been described. This subject is discussed in greater detail in Chapter 8. Here we provide an example of two common familial neoplasms.

NEUROFIBROMATOSIS: TYPES 1 AND 2

Neurofibromatoses comprise two autosomal dominant disorders, affecting approximately 100,000 people in the United States. They are referred to as *neurofibromatosis type 1* (previously called *von Recklinghausen disease*) and *neurofibromatosis type 2* (previously called *acoustic neurofibromatosis*). Although there is some overlap in clinical features, these two entities are genetically distinct.[36]

Neurofibromatosis-1 is a relatively common disorder, with a frequency of almost 1 in 3000. Although approximately 50% of the patients have a definite family history consistent with autosomal dominant transmission, the remainder appear to represent new mutations. In familial cases, the expressivity of the disorder is extremely variable, but the penetrance is 100%. Neurofibromatosis-1 has three major features: (1) *multiple neural tumors (neurofibromas) dispersed anywhere on or in the body*; (2) *numerous pig-*

Table 6–6. PRINCIPAL SUBGROUPS OF GLYCOGENOSES

Clinicopathologic Category	Specific Type	Enzyme Deficiency	Morphologic Changes	Clinical Features
Hepatic type	Hepatorenal—von Gierke disease (type I)	Glucose-6-phosphatase	Hepatomegaly—intracytoplasmic accumulations of glycogen and small amounts of lipid; intranuclear glycogen Renomegaly—intracytoplasmic accumulations of glycogen in cortical tubular epithelial cells	In untreated patients: failure to thrive, stunted growth, hepatomegaly, and renomegaly. Hypoglycemia due to failure of glucose mobilization, often leading to convulsions. Hyperlipidemia and hyperuricemia resulting from deranged glucose metabolism; many patients develop gout and skin xanthomas. Bleeding tendency due to platelet dysfunction. With treatment most survive and develop late complications, e.g,, hepatic adenomas.
Myopathic type	McArdle syndrome (type V)	Muscle phosphorylase	Skeletal muscle only—accumulations of glycogen predominant in subsarcolemmal location	Painful cramps associated with strenuous exercise. Myoglobinuria occurs in 50% of cases. Onset in adulthood (>20 y old). Muscular exercise fails to raise lactate level in venous blood. Compatible with normal longevity
Miscellaneous types	Generalized glycogenosis—Pompe disease (type II)	Lysosomal glucosidase (acid maltase)	Mild hepatomegaly—ballooning of lysosomes with glycogen creating lacy cytoplasmic pattern Cardiomegaly—glycogen within sarcoplasm as well as membrane-bound Skeletal muscle—similar to heart (see Cardiomegaly)	Massive cardiomegaly, muscle hypotonia, and cardiorespiratory failure within 2 y. A milder adult form with only skeletal muscle involvement presenting with chronic myopathy

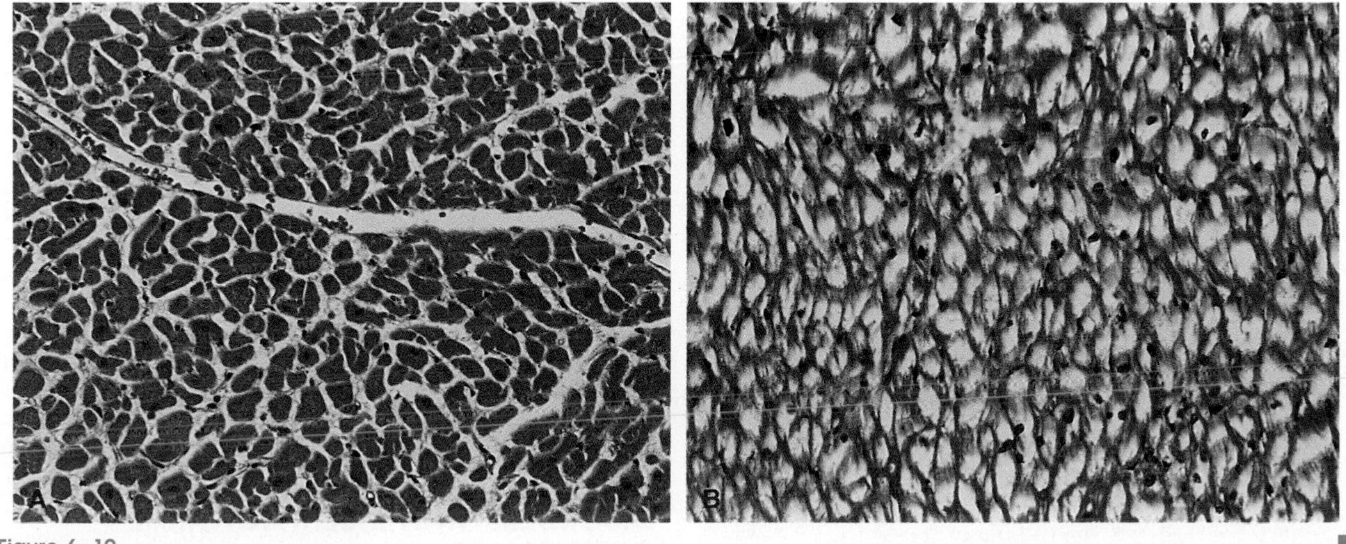

Figure 6–19

Pompe disease (glycogen storage disease type II). *A*, Normal myocardium with abundant eosinophilic cytoplasm. *B*, Patient with Pompe disease (same magnification) showing the myocardial fibers full of glycogen seen as clear spaces. (Courtesy of Dr. Trace Worrell, Department of Pathology, University of Texas Southwestern Medical Center, Dallas, TX.)

mented skin lesions, some of which are café au lait spots; and (3) *pigmented iris hamartomas, also called Lisch nodules*. A bewildering assortment of other abnormalities (cited later) may accompany these cardinal manifestations.

MORPHOLOGY. The neurofibromas arise within or are attached to nerve trunks anywhere in the skin, including the palms and soles, as well as in every conceivable internal site, including the cranial nerves. Three types of neurofibromas are found in individuals with neurofibromatosis-1: cutaneous, subcutaneous, and plexiform. **Cutaneous**, or dermal, neurofibromas are soft, sessile, or pedunculated lesions that vary in number from a few to many hundreds. **Subcutaneous neurofibromas** grow just beneath the skin; they are firm, round masses that are often painful. The cutaneous and subcutaneous neurofibromas may be less than 1 cm in diameter; moderate-sized pedunculated lesions; or huge, multilobar pendulous masses, 20 cm or more in greatest diameter. The third variant, referred to as **plexiform neurofibroma**, diffusely involves subcutaneous tissue and contains numerous tortuous, thickened nerves; the overlying skin is frequently hyperpigmented. These may grow to massive proportions, causing striking enlargement of a limb or some other body part. Similar tumors may occur internally, and in general the deeply situated lesions tend to be large. Microscopically, neurofibromas reveal proliferation of all the elements in the peripheral nerve, including neurites, Schwann cells, and fibroblasts. Typically, these components are dispersed in a loose, disorderly pattern, often in a loose, myxoid stroma. Elongated, serpentine Schwann cells predominate, with their slender, spindle-shaped nuclei. The loose and disorderly architecture helps differentiate these neural tumors from schwannomas. The latter, composed entirely of Schwann cells, virtually never undergo malignant transformation, whereas plexiform neurofibromas become malignant in about 5% of patients with neurofibromatosis-1.[37] Malignant transformation is most common in the large plexiform tumors attached to major nerve trunks of the neck or extremities. The superficial lesions, despite their size, rarely become malignant.

The cutaneous pigmentations, the second major component of this syndrome, are present in more than 90% of patients. Most commonly, they appear as light brown **café au lait** macules, with generally smooth borders, often located over nerve trunks. They are usually round to ovoid, with their long axes parallel to the underlying cutaneous nerve. Although normal individuals may have a few café au lait spots, it is a clinical maxim that when six or more spots greater than 1.5 cm in diameter are present in an adult, the patient is likely to have neurofibromatosis-1.

Lisch nodules (pigmented hamartomas in the iris) are present in more than 94% of patients who are 6 years old or older. They do not produce any symptoms but are helpful in establishing the diagnosis.

A wide range of associated abnormalities has been reported in these patients. Perhaps most common (seen in 30 to 50% of patients) are skeletal lesions, which take a variety of forms, including (1) erosive defects owing to contiguity of neurofibromas to bone, (2) scoliosis, (3) intraosseous cystic lesions, (4) subperiosteal bone cysts, and (5) pseudoarthrosis of the tibia. Patients with neurofibromatosis-1 have a twofold to fourfold greater risk of developing other tumors, especially Wilms' tumors, rhabdomyosarcomas, meningiomas, optic gliomas, and pheochromocytomas. Affected children are at increased risk of developing chronic myeloid leukemia.

Although some patients with this condition have normal intelligence quotients (IQs), there is an unmistakable tendency for reduced intelligence. When neurofibromas arise within the gastrointestinal tract, intestinal obstruction or gastrointestinal bleeding may occur. Narrowing of a renal artery by a tumor may induce hypertension. Owing to variable expression of the gene, the range of clinical presentations is almost limitless, but ultimately the diagnosis rests on the concurrence of multiple café au lait spots and multiple skin tumors. The neurofibromatosis-1 (NF-1) gene has been mapped to chromosome 17q11.2. It encodes a protein called *neurofibromin*, which down-regulates the function of the *p21 ras* oncoprotein (see section on oncogenes, Chapter 8). NF-1 therefore belongs to the family of tumor-suppressor genes.

Neurofibromatosis-2 is an autosomal dominant disorder in which patients develop a range of tumors, most commonly bilateral acoustic schwannomas and multiple meningiomas. Gliomas, typically ependymomas of the spinal cord, also occur in these patients. Many individuals with neurofibromatosis-2 also have non-neoplastic lesions, which include nodular ingrowth of Schwann cells into the spinal cord (schwannosis), meningioangiomatosis (a proliferation of meningeal cells and blood vessels that grows into the brain), and glial hamartia (microscopic nodular collections of glial cells at abnormal locations, often in the superficial and deep layers of the cerebral cortex). Café au lait spots are present, but Lisch nodules in the iris are not found. This disorder is much less common than neurofibromatosis-1, having a frequency of 1 in 40,000 to 50,000.

The NF-2 gene, located on chromosome 22q12, is also a tumor-suppressor gene. As further discussed in Chapter 8, the product of the NF-2 gene called merlin shows structural similarity to a series of cytoskeletal proteins.[38] The protein is widely distributed throughout tissues, and its function remains uncertain.

DISORDERS WITH MULTIFACTORIAL INHERITANCE

As pointed out earlier, the multifactorial disorders result from the combined actions of environmental influences and two or more mutant genes having additive effects. The genetic component exerts a dosage effect—the greater the number of inherited deleterious genes, the more severe the expression of the disease. Because environmental factors significantly influence the expression of these genetic disorders, the term *polygenic inheritance* should not be used.

A number of normal phenotypic characteristics are governed by multifactorial inheritance, such as hair color, eye color, skin color, height, and intelligence. These characteristics exhibit a continuous variation in population groups, producing the standard bell-shaped curve of distribution. Environmental influences, however, significantly modify the phenotypic expression of multifactorial traits. For example, certain subsets of diabetes mellitus have many of the features of a multifactorial disorder. It is well recognized clinically that individuals often first manifest this disease after weight gain. Thus, obesity as well as other environmental influences unmasks the diabetic genetic trait. Nutritional influences may cause even monozygous twins to achieve different heights. The culturally deprived child cannot achieve his or her full intellectual capacity.

The following features characterize multifactorial inheritance. These have been established for the multifactorial inheritance of congenital malformations and, in all likelihood, obtain for other multifactorial diseases.[39]

- *The risk of expressing a multifactorial disorder is conditioned by the number of mutant genes inherited. Thus, the risk is greater in sibs of patients having severe expressions of the disorder. For example, the risk of cleft lip in the sibs of an index case is 2.5% if the cleft lip is unilateral but 6% if it is bilateral. Similarly, the greater the number of affected relatives, the higher is the risk for other relatives.*
- *The rate of recurrence of the disorder (in the range of 2 to 7%) is the same for all first-degree relatives (i.e., parents, sibs, and offspring) of the affected individual. Thus, if parents have had one affected child, the risk that the next child will be affected is between 2 and 7%. Similarly, there is the same chance that one of the parents will be affected.*
- *The likelihood that both identical twins will be affected is significantly less than 100% but is much greater than the chance that both nonidentical twins will be affected. Experience has proven, for example, that the frequency of concordance for identical twins is in the range of 20 to 40%.*
- *The risk of recurrence of the phenotypic abnormality in subsequent pregnancies depends on the outcome in previous pregnancies. When one child is affected, there is up to a 7% chance that the next child will be affected, but after two affected sibs, the risk rises to about 9%.*
- *Expression of a multifactorial trait may be continuous (lack a distinct phenotype, e.g., height) or discontinuous (with a distinct phenotype, e.g., diabetes mellitus). In the latter, disease is expressed only when the combined influences of the genes and environment cross a certain threshold. In the case of diabetes, for example, the risk of phenotypic expression increases when the blood glucose levels go above a certain level.*

Assigning a disease to this mode of inheritance must be done with caution. It depends on many factors but first on familial clustering and the exclusion of mendelian and chromosomal modes of transmission. A range of levels of severity of a disease is suggestive of multifactorial inheritance, but, as pointed out earlier, variable expressivity and reduced penetrance of mendelian mutant genes may also account for this phenomenon. Because of these problems, sometimes it is difficult to distinguish between mendelian and multifactorial inheritance.

In contrast to the mendelian disorders, many of which are uncommon, the multifactorial group includes some of the most common ailments to which humans are heir (Table 6–7). Most of these disorders are described in appropriate chapters elsewhere in this book.

Table 6–7. MULTIFACTORIAL DISORDERS

Disorder	Chapter
Cleft lip or cleft palate (or both)	Chapter 17
Congenital heart disease	Chapter 13
Coronary heart disease	Chapter 13
Hypertension	Chapter 12
Gout	Chapter 28
Diabetes mellitus	Chapter 20
Pyloric stenosis	Chapter 18

NORMAL KARYOTYPE

As is well known, human somatic cells contain 46 chromosomes; these comprise 22 homologous pairs of autosomes and two sex chromosomes, XX in the female and XY in the male. The study of chromosomes—karyotyping—is the basic tool of the cytogeneticist. The usual procedure of producing a chromosome spread is to arrest mitosis in dividing cells in metaphase by the use of colchicine and then to stain the chromosomes. In a metaphase spread, the individual chromosomes take the form of two chromatids connected at the centromere. A karyotype is a standard arrangement of a photographed or imaged stained metaphase spread in which chromosome pairs are arranged in order of decreasing length.

A variety of staining methods that allow identification of each individual chromosome on the basis of a distinctive and reliable pattern of alternating light and dark bands along the length of the chromosome have been developed. The one most commonly employed uses a Giemsa stain and is hence called *G banding*. A normal male karyotype with G banding is illustrated in Figure 6–20. With G banding, approximately 400 to 800 bands per haploid set can be detected. The resolution obtained by banding techniques can be dramatically improved by obtaining the cells in prophase. The individual chromosomes appear markedly elongated, and up to 1500 bands per karyotype may be recognized. The use of these banding techniques permits certain identification of each chromosome as well as delin-

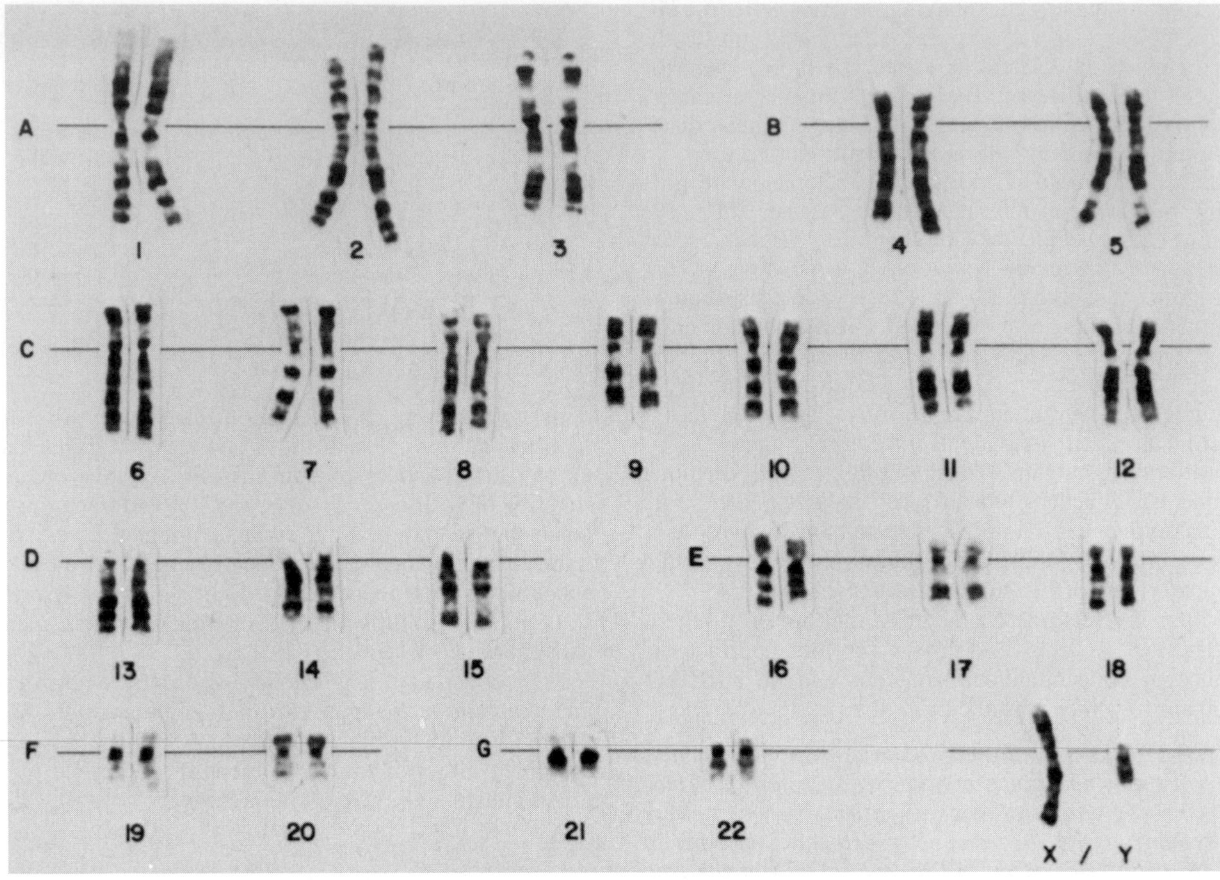

Figure 6–20

Normal male karyotype with G banding. (Courtesy of Dr. Nancy Schneider, Department of Pathology, University of Texas Southwestern Medical Center, Dallas, TX.)

eation of precise breakpoints and other subtle alterations, to be described later.

Before this discussion of the normal karyotype is concluded, reference must be made to commonly used cytogenetic terminology. Karyotypes are usually described using a shorthand system of notations. In general, the following order is used: Total number of chromosomes is given first, followed by the sex chromosome complement, and finally the description of any abnormality. For example, a male with trisomy 21 is designated *47,XY,+21*. Some of the notations denoting structural alterations of chromosomes are described along with the abnormalities in a later section. Here we should mention that the short arm of a chromosome is designated *p* (for petit), and the long arm is referred to as *q* (the next letter of alphabet). In a banded karyotype, each arm of the chromosome is divided into two or more regions by prominent bands. The regions are numbered (e.g., 1, 2, 3) from the centromere outward. Each region is further subdivided into bands and subbands, and these are ordered numerically as well (Fig. 6–21). Thus, the notation *Xp21.2* refers to a chromosomal segment located on the short arm of the X chromosome, in region 2, band 1, and sub-band 2.

Fluorescence In Situ Hybridization. Fluorescence in situ hybridization (FISH) has become an important adjunct to routine karyotyping and has greatly expanded the power of cytogenetic analysis.[40] A major limitation of karyotyping is that it is applicable only to cells that are dividing or can be induced to divide in vitro. This problem can be overcome with DNA probes that recognize chromosome-specific sequences. Such probes are labeled with fluorescent dyes and applied to interphase nuclei. The probe binds to its complementary sequence on the chromosome and thus labels the specific chromosome that can then be visualized under a fluorescent microscope (Fig. 6–22). Thus, FISH can be used to enumerate chromosomes in interphase nuclei. The application of FISH is not limited to interphase nuclei, however. By using DNA probes that are specific for defined regions of the chromosomes, FISH can be used to demonstrate subtle microdeletions and complex translocations not readily detectable by routine karyotyping (Fig. 6–23). In addition to its diagnostic utility, FISH has also provided a powerful tool to map newly isolated genes of clinical interest. Novel DNA sequences are labeled with a fluorescent dye and then applied to a metaphase spread. The DNA binds to its complementary sequence and thus betrays the localization of the gene to a specific site. Chromosome painting is an extension of FISH, whereby whole

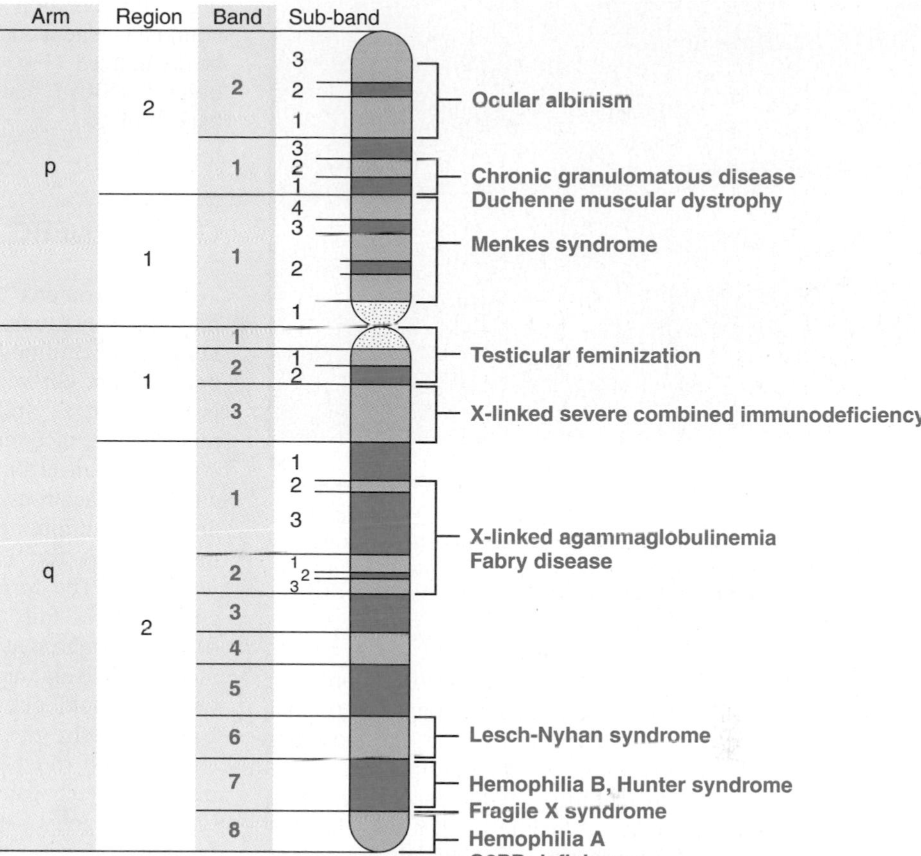

Figure 6-21 ■

Details of a banded karyotype of the X chromosome (also called "idiogram"). Note the nomenclature of arms, regions, bands, and sub-bands. On the right side, the approximate locations of some genes that cause disease are indicated.

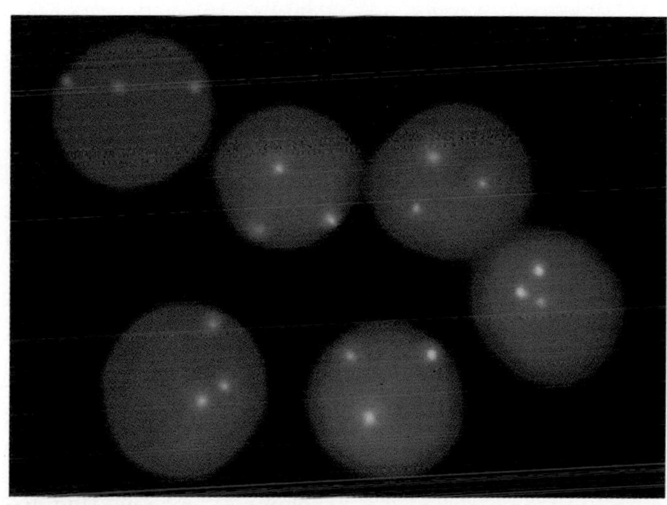

Figure 6-22 ■

Fluorescent in situ hybridization (FISH). Interphase nuclei of a childhood hepatic cancer (hepatoblastoma) stained with a fluorescent DNA probe that hybridizes to chromosome 20. Under ultraviolet light, each nucleus reveals three bright yellow fluorescent dots representing three copies of chromosome 20. Normal diploid cells (*not shown*) have two fluorescent dots. (Courtesy of Dr. Vijay Tonk, Department of Pathology, University of Texas Southwestern Medical Center, Dallas, TX.)

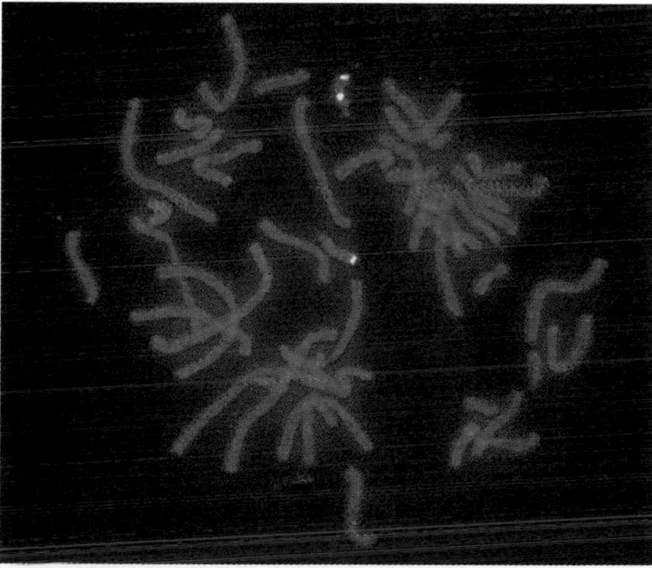

Figure 6-23 ■

FISH. A metaphase spread in which two fluorescent probes, one for the terminal ends of chromosome 22 and the other for the D22S75 locus that maps to chromosome 22, have been used. The terminal ends of the two chromosomes 22 have been labeled. One of the two chromosomes does not stain with the probe for the D22S75 locus, indicating a microdeletion in this region. This deletion gives rise to the 22q11 deletion syndrome described on p. 173. (Courtesy of Dr. Nancy Schneider, Department of Pathology, University of Texas Southwestern Medical Center, Dallas, TX.)

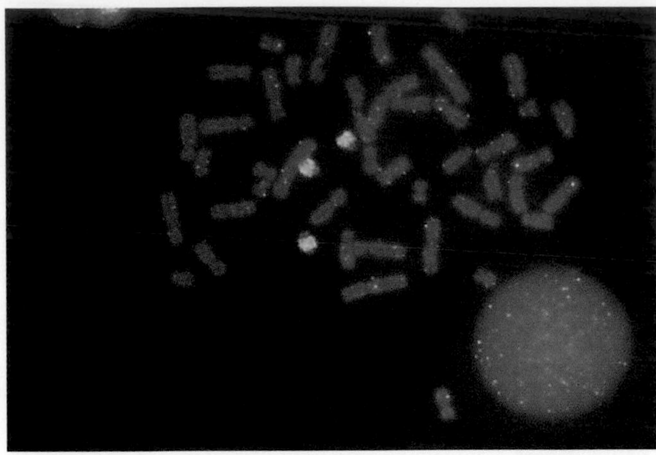

Figure 6–24

Chromosome painting with a library of chromosome 22–specific DNA probes. The presence of three fluorescent chromosomes indicates that the patient has trisomy 22. (Courtesy of Dr. Charleen M. Moore, The University of Texas Health Science Center at San Antonio, San Antonio, TX.)

chromosomes can be labeled with a series of fluorescent DNA probes that bind to multiple sites along a particular chromosome (Fig. 6–24). The number of chromosomes that can be *detected simultaneously* by chromosome painting is limited by the availability of fluorescent dyes that excite different wavelengths of visible light. Thus, chromosome painting cannot be used to visualize all 46 human chromosomes simultaneously. This hurdle has been overcome by the introduction of spectral karyotyping.[41] By using a combination of five fluorochromes and appropriate computer-generated signals, the entire human genome can be visualized (Fig. 6–25). So powerful is spectral karyotyping (SKY) that it might well be called "spectacular karyotyping."

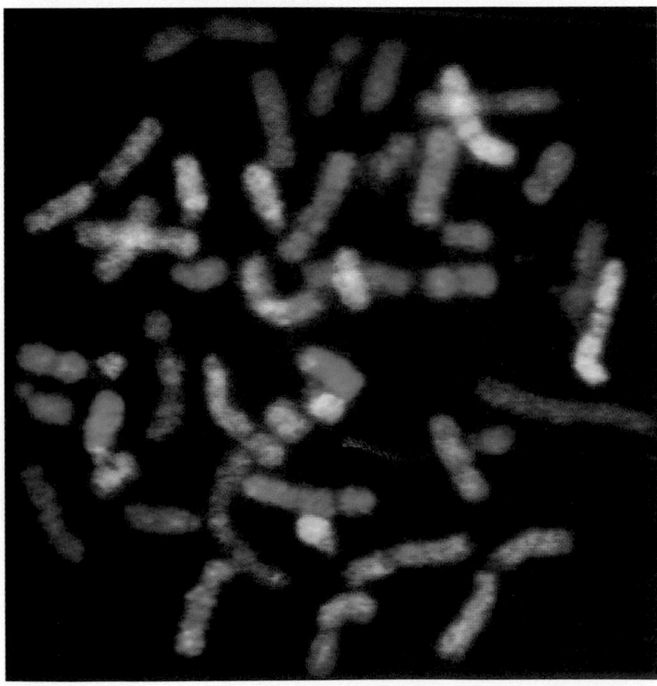

Figure 6–25

Spectral karyotype. (Courtesy of Dr. Janet D. Rowley, University of Chicago Medical Center, Chicago, IL.)

CYTOGENETIC DISORDERS

The aberrations underlying cytogenetic disorders (chromosome mutations) may take the form of an abnormal number of chromosomes or alterations in the structure of one or more chromosomes. The normal chromosome count is expressed as 46,XX for the female and 46,XY for the male. Any exact multiple of the haploid number is called *euploid.* If an error occurs in meiosis or mitosis, however, and a cell acquires a chromosome complement that is not an exact multiple of 23, it is referred to as *aneuploidy*. The usual causes for aneuploidy are *nondisjunction* and *anaphase lag*. The former occurs when a homologous pair of chromosomes fails to disjoin at the first meiotic division, or the two chromatids fail to separate either at the second meiotic division or in somatic cell divisions, resulting in two aneuploid cells. When nondisjunction occurs during gametogenesis, the gametes formed have either an extra chromosome (n+1) or one less chromosome (n−1). Fertilization of such gametes by normal gametes results in two types of zygotes—trisomic (2n+1) or monosomic (2n−1). In anaphase lag, one homologous chromosome in meiosis or one chromatid in mitosis lags behind and is left out of the cell nucleus. The result is one normal cell and one cell with monosomy. As seen subsequently, monosomy or trisomy involving the sex chromosomes, or even more bizarre aberrations, are compatible with life and are usually associated with variable degrees of phenotypic abnormalities. *Monosomy involving an autosome generally represents loss of too much genetic information to permit live birth or even embryogenesis, but a number of autosomal trisomies do permit survival.* With the exception of trisomy 21, all yield severely handicapped infants who almost invariably die at an early age.

Occasionally, *mitotic errors in early development give rise to two or more populations of cells in the same individual*, a condition referred to as *mosaicism.* Mosaicism can result from mitotic errors during the cleavage of the fertilized ovum or in somatic cells. Mosaicism affecting the sex chromosomes is relatively common. In the division of the fertilized ovum, an error may lead to one of the daughter cells receiving three sex chromosomes, whereas the other receives only one, yielding, for example, a 45,X/47,XXX mosaic. All descendent cells derived from each of these precursors thus have either a 47,XXX count or a 45,X count. Such a patient is a mosaic variant of Turner syndrome, with the extent of phenotypic expression dependent on the number and distribution of the 45,X cells. If the error occurs at a later cleavage, the mosaic has three populations of cells, with some possessing the normal 46,XX complement (i.e., 45,X/46,XX/47,XXX). Repeated mitotic errors may lead to many populations of cells.

Autosomal mosaicism appears to be much less common

than that involving the sex chromosomes. An error in an early mitotic division affecting the autosomes usually leads to a nonviable mosaic with autosomal monosomy. Rarely, the loss of a nonviable cell line in embryogenesis is tolerated, yielding a mosaic (e.g., 46,XY/47,XY,+21). Such a patient is a trisomy 21 mosaic with partial expression of Down syndrome, depending on the proportion of cells expressing the trisomy.

A second category of chromosomal aberrations is associated with changes in the structure of chromosomes. To be visible by routine banding techniques, a fairly large amount of DNA (approximately 4 million base pairs), containing several genes, must be involved. The resolution is much higher with FISH. Structural changes in chromosomes usually result from chromosome breakage followed by loss or rearrangement of material. Such alterations occur spontaneously at a low rate that is increased by exposure to environmental mutagens, such as chemicals and ionizing radiations. In addition, several rare autosomal recessive genetic disorders—Fanconi anemia, Bloom syndrome, and ataxia-telangiectasia—are associated with such a high level of chromosomal instability that they are known as *chromosome-breakage syndromes*. As discussed later, in Chapter 8, there is a significantly increased risk of cancers in all these conditions. In the following section, we briefly review the more common forms of alterations in chromosome structure and the notations used to signify them.

Deletion refers to loss of a portion of chromosome (Fig. 6–26). It may be terminal or interstitial. Terminal deletions result from a single break in the arm of a chromosome, producing a fragment with no centromere, which is then lost at the next cell division. One can specify in which region and at what band the break and deletion has occurred, as, for example, *46,XY,del(16)(p14)*, meaning a break point in region 1 band 4 of the short arm of chromosome 16. Interstitial deletions occur when there are two breaks in the chromosome followed by loss of the region between the breaks.

A *ring chromosome* is a special form of deletion. It is produced when a deletion occurs at both ends of a chromosome with fusion of the damaged ends (Fig. 6–26). If significant genetic material is lost, phenotypic abnormalities result. This might be expressed as *46,XY,r(14)*. Ring chromosomes do not behave normally in meiosis or mitosis and usually result in serious consequences.

Inversion refers to a rearrangement that involves two breaks within a single chromosome with inverted reincorporation of the segment (Fig. 6–26). Such an inversion involving only one arm of the chromosome is known as *paracentric*. If the breaks are on opposite sides of the centromere, it is known as *pericentric*. Inversions are perfectly compatible with normal development.

Isochromosome formation results when one arm of a chromosome is lost and the remaining arm is duplicated, resulting in a chromosome consisting of two short arms only or of two long arms (Fig. 6–26). An isochromosome has genetic information that is morphologically identical in both arms. The most common isochromosome present in live births involves the long arm of the X and is designated *i(X)(q10)*. The Xq isochromosome is associated with

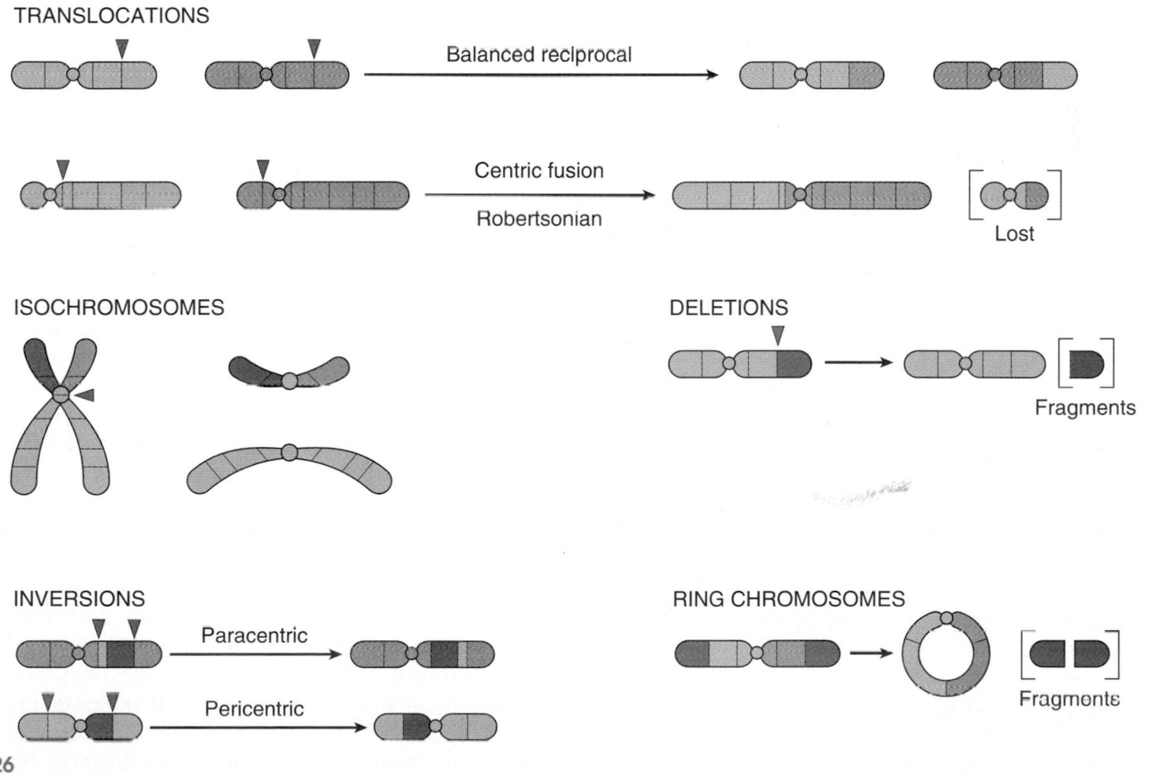

Figure 6–26

Types of chromosomal rearrangements.

monosomy for genes on the short arm of X and with trisomy for genes on the long arm of X.

In *translocation*, a segment of one chromosome is transferred to another (Fig. 6–26). In one form, called *balanced reciprocal translocation*, there are single breaks in each of two chromosomes, with exchange of material. Such a translocation might not be disclosed without banding techniques. A balanced reciprocal translocation between the long arm of chromosome 2 and the short arm of chromosome 5 would be written *46,XX,t(2;5)(q31;p14)*. This individual has 46 chromosomes with altered morphology of one of the chromosomes 2 and one of the chromosomes 5. Because there has been no loss of genetic material, the individual is phenotypically normal. A balanced translocation carrier, however, is at increased risk for producing abnormal gametes. For example, in the case cited above, a gamete containing one normal chromosome 2 and a translocated chromosome 5 may be formed. Such a gamete would be unbalanced because it would not contain the normal complement of genetic material. Subsequent fertilization by a normal gamete would lead to the formation of an abnormal (unbalanced) zygote, resulting in spontaneous abortion or birth of a malformed child. The other important pattern of translocation is called a *robertsonian translocation* (or centric fusion), a translocation between two acrocentric chromosomes. Typically the breaks occur close to the centromeres of each chromosome. Transfer of the segments then leads to one very large chromosome and one extremely small one. Usually the small product is lost (Fig. 6–26); however, it carries so little genetic information that this loss is compatible with a normal phenotype, and robertsonian translocation between two chromosomes is encountered in 1 in 1000 apparently normal individuals. The significance of this form of translocation also lies in the production of abnormal progeny, as discussed later with Down syndrome.

Many more numerical and structural aberrations are described in specialized texts, and the number of abnormal karyotypes encountered in genetic diseases increases with each passing month. As pointed out earlier, the clinically detected chromosome disorders represent only the "tip of the iceberg." It is estimated that approximately 7.5% of all conceptions have a chromosomal abnormality, most of which are not compatible with survival or live birth. Thus, chromosome abnormalities are identified in 50% of early spontaneous abortuses and in 5% of stillbirths and infants who die in the immediate postnatal period. Even in liveborn infants, the frequency is approximately 0.5 to 1.0%. It is beyond the scope of this book to discuss most of the clinically recognizable chromosomal disorders. Hence we focus attention on those few that are most common.

Cytogenetic Disorders Involving Autosomes

TRISOMY 21 (DOWN SYNDROME)

Down syndrome is the most common of the chromosomal disorders and a major cause of mental retardation. In the United States, the incidence in newborns is about 1 in 700. Approximately 95% of affected individuals have trisomy 21, so their chromosome count is 47 (Fig. 6–27); most others have normal chromosome numbers, but the extra chromosomal material is present as a translocation. As mentioned earlier, the most common cause of trisomy and therefore of Down syndrome is meiotic nondisjunction. The parents of such children have a normal karyotype and are normal in all respects.

Maternal age has a strong influence on the incidence of trisomy 21. It occurs once in 1550 live births in women under the age of 20 years, in contrast to 1 in 25 live births for mothers over 45 years of age.[6] The correlation with maternal age suggests that in most cases the meiotic nondisjunction of chromosome 21 occurs in the ovum. Studies in which DNA polymorphisms were used to trace the parental origin of chromosome 21 have revealed that in 95% of the cases with trisomy 21 the extra chromosome is of maternal origin.[42, 43] Although many hypotheses have been advanced, the reason for the increased susceptibility of the ovum to nondisjunction remains unknown.

In about 4% of all cases of Down syndrome, the extra chromosomal material derives from the presence of a robertsonian translocation of the long arm of chromosome 21 to another acrocentric chromosome (e.g., 22 or 14). Because the fertilized ovum already possesses two normal autosomes 21, the translocated material provides the same triple gene dosage as in trisomy 21. Such cases are frequently (but not always) familial, and the translocated chromosome is inherited from one of the parents (usually the mother), who is a carrier of a robertsonian translocation, for example, a mother with karyotype 45,XX,der(14;21)(q10;q10). Theoretically the carrier parent has a one in three chance of bearing a live child with Down syndrome; however, the observed frequency of affected children in such cases is much lower. The reasons for this discrepancy are not well understood. In those cases in which neither parent is a carrier of the translocation, the rearrangement occurs during gametogenesis.

Approximately 1% of Down syndrome patients are mosaics, usually having a mixture of cells with 46 and 47 chromosomes. This mosaicism results from mitotic nondisjunction of chromosome 21 during an early stage of embryogenesis. Symptoms in such cases are variable and milder, depending on the proportion of abnormal cells. Clearly, *in cases of translocation or mosaic Down syndrome, maternal age is of no importance*.

The diagnostic clinical features of this condition (Fig. 6–28) are usually readily evident, even at birth. The flat facial profile, oblique palpebral fissures, and epicanthic folds account for the older designations "mongolism" and "mongolian idiocy." Down syndrome is a leading cause of mental retardation. The mental retardation is severe; approximately 80% of those afflicted have an IQ of 25 to 50. Ironically, these severely disadvantaged children may have a gentle, shy manner and may be more easily directed than their more fortunate siblings, not burdened with extra chromosomes. It should be pointed out that some mosaics with Down syndrome have mild phenotypic changes and may even have normal or near-normal intelligence. In addition to the phenotypic abnormalities and the mental retardation already noted, some other clinical features are worthy of note.

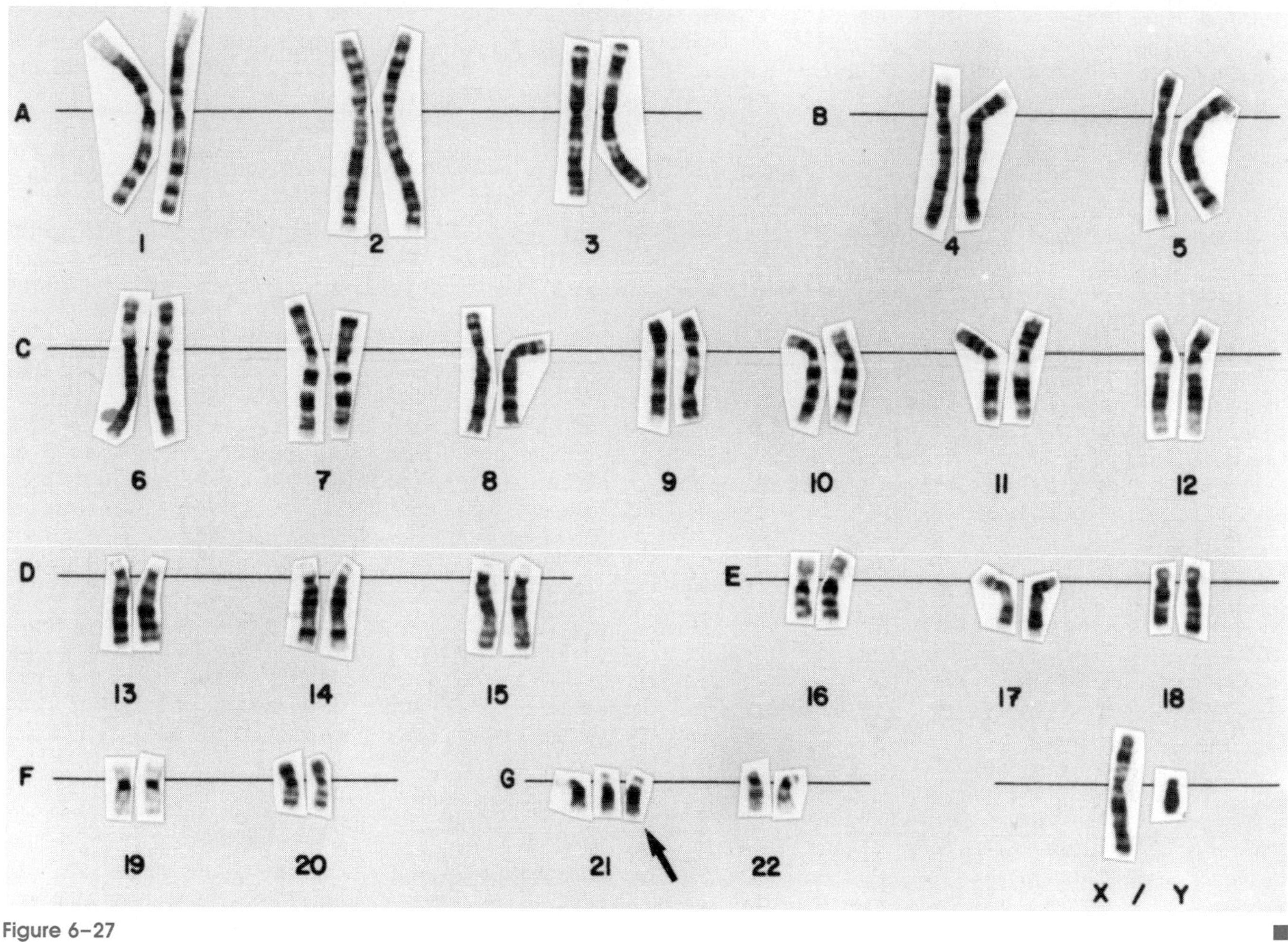

Figure 6–27

G-banded karyotype of a male with trisomy 21. (Courtesy of Dr. Nancy Schneider, University of Texas Southwestern Medical Center, Dallas, TX.)

- Approximately 40% of the patients have congenital heart disease, most commonly defects of the endocardial cushion, including ostium primum, atrial septal defect, atrioventricular valve malformations, and ventricular septal defects. Cardiac problems are responsible for the majority of the deaths in infancy and early childhood. Several other congenital malformations, including atresias of the esophagus and small bowel, are also noted.[44]
- Children with trisomy 21 have a 10-fold to 20-fold increased risk of developing acute leukemia. Both acute lymphoblastic leukemias and acute myelogenous leukemias occur. The relative distribution of these two types of leukemia is similar for children with and without Down syndrome.
- Virtually all patients with trisomy 21 older than 40 years of age develop neuropathologic changes characteristic of Alzheimer disease, a degenerative disorder of the brain.[45]
- Patients with Down syndrome have abnormal immune responses that predispose them to serious infections, particularly of the lungs, and to thyroid autoimmunity. Although several abnormalities, affecting mainly T-cell subsets, have been reported, the cellular basis of immunologic disturbances is not clear.[46]

Despite all these problems, improved medical care has increased the longevity of patients with trisomy 21. Currently more than 80% survive to age 30 or beyond.

Although the karyotype and clinical features of trisomy 21 have been known for decades, little is known about the molecular basis of Down syndrome. Advances in gene mapping, however, have begun to penetrate the mystery.[47] By a careful study of patients with the translocation variant of Down syndrome who exhibit partial trisomy 21, it has been determined that the region of chromosome 21 that is required for the expression of the facial, neurologic, and cardiovascular changes is limited to the 21q22.2 and 21q22.3 region. Genes located within this "obligate Down syndrome region" must be critical to the pathogenesis of the Down syndrome phenotype, but their identity remains unknown.

OTHER TRISOMIES

A variety of other trisomies, involving chromosomes 8, 9, 13, 18, and 22, have been described. Only trisomy 18 (Edwards syndrome) and trisomy 13 (Patau syndrome) are common enough to merit brief mention here. As noted in

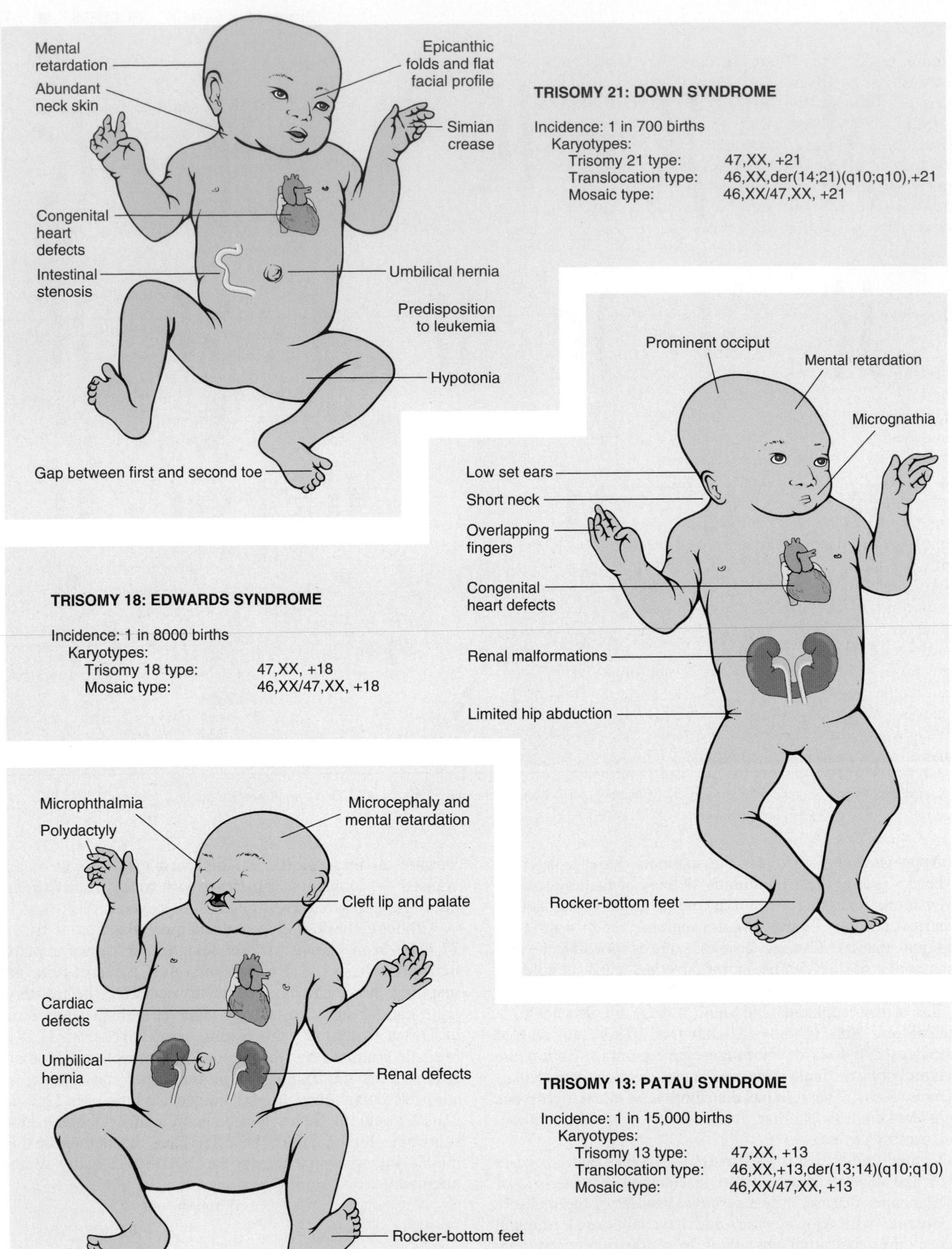
Mental retardation
Epicanthic folds and flat facial profile
Abundant neck skin
Simian crease
Congenital heart defects
Intestinal stenosis
Umbilical hernia
Predisposition to leukemia
Hypotonia
Gap between first and second toe
TRISOMY 21: DOWN SYNDROME
Incidence: 1 in 700 births
Karyotypes:
Trisomy 21 type: 47,XX, +21
Translocation type: 46,XX,der(14;21)(q10;q10),+21
Mosaic type: 46,XX/47,XX, +21
Prominent occiput
Mental retardation
Micrognathia
Low set ears
Short neck
Overlapping fingers
Congenital heart defects
Renal malformations
Limited hip abduction
Rocker-bottom feet
TRISOMY 18: EDWARDS SYNDROME
Incidence: 1 in 8000 births
Karyotypes:
Trisomy 18 type: 47,XX, +18
Mosaic type: 46,XX/47,XX, +18
Microphthalmia
Polydactyly
Microcephaly and mental retardation
Cleft lip and palate
Cardiac defects
Umbilical hernia
Renal defects
Rocker-bottom feet
TRISOMY 13: PATAU SYNDROME
Incidence: 1 in 15,000 births
Karyotypes:
Trisomy 13 type: 47,XX, +13
Translocation type: 46,XX,+13,der(13;14)(q10;q10)
Mosaic type: 46,XX/47,XX, +13

Figure 6–28

Clinical features of karyotypes of selected autosomal trisomies.

Figure 6–28, they share several karyotypic and clinical features with trisomy 21. Thus, most cases result from meiotic nondisjunction and therefore carry a complete extra copy of chromosome 18 or 13. As in Down syndrome, an association with increased maternal age is also noted. In contrast to trisomy 21, however, the malformations are much more severe and wide-ranging. As a result, only rarely do these infants survive beyond the first year of life. Most succumb within a few weeks to months.

CHROMOSOME 22q11 DELETION SYNDROME

Chromosome 22q11 deletion syndrome encompasses a spectrum of disorders that result from a small deletion of band 11 on the long arm of chromosome 22.[48] The clinical features of this syndrome include congenital heart defects, abnormalities of the palate, facial dysmorphism, developmental delay, and variable degrees of T-cell immunodeficiency and hypocalcemia. Previously, these clinical features were considered to represent two different disorders—*DiGeorge syndrome* and *velocardiofacial syndrome*. Patients with DiGeorge syndrome have thymic hypoplasia, with resultant T-cell immunodeficiency (Chapter 7), parathyroid hypoplasia giving rise to hypocalcemia, a variety of cardiac malformations affecting the outflow tract, and mild facial anomalies. The clinical features of the so-called velocardiofacial syndrome include facial dysmorphism (prominent nose, retrognathia), cleft palate, cardiovascular anomalies, and learning disabilities. Less frequently, these patients also have immunodeficiency. Until recently the overlapping clinical features of these two conditions (e.g., cardiac malformations, facial dysmorphology) were not appreciated; it was only after these two apparently unrelated syndromes were found to be associated with a similar cytogenetic abnormality that the clinical overlap came into focus. With this realization, the acronym CATCH 22 (*c*ardiac *a*bnormality/*a*bnormal facies, *T*-cell deficit owing to thymic hypoplasia, *c*left palate, *h*ypocalcemia owing to hypoparathyroidism resulting from *22*q11 deletion) was coined to describe this condition. Although convenient for memorizing the clinical features of the 22q11 deletion syndrome, this mnemonic should best be avoided because it seems disrespectful to the patients.

The diagnosis of this condition may be suspected on clinical grounds but can be established only by detection of the deletion by FISH probes (see Fig. 6–23). By using this method, approximately 90% of those previously diagnosed as having DiGeorge syndrome and 60% of those with the velocardiofacial syndrome have a deletion of 22q11. Thirty per cent of patients with conotruncal cardiac defects but no other features of this syndrome also reveal deletions of the same chromosomal region.

The molecular basis of this syndrome is not known. The size of the deleted region is large enough (approximately 1.5 megabases) to include many genes. The clinical heterogeneity, with predominant immunodeficiency in some cases (DiGeorge syndrome) and predominant dysmorphology and cardiac malformations in other cases, probably reflects the variable position and size of the deleted segment from this genetic region. Several genes, including some that are homologous to *Drosophila* and yeast transcription factors and to *Drosophila* embryonic segmentation, have been localized in the deleted segment, but no single gene has emerged as the culprit so far.

Cytogenetic Disorders Involving Sex Chromosomes

The genetic diseases associated with karyotypic changes involving the sex chromosomes are far more common than those related to autosomal aberrations. Furthermore, imbalances (excess or loss) of sex chromosomes are much better tolerated than are similar imbalances of autosomes. In large part, this latitude relates to two factors that are peculiar to the sex chromosomes: (1) lyonization or inactivation of all but one X chromosome and (2) the small amount of genetic material carried by the Y chromosome. We discuss these features briefly to aid our understanding of sex chromosomal disorders.

In 1961, Lyon[49] outlined the X-inactivation, or what is commonly known as the Lyon, hypothesis. It states that (1) *only one of the X chromosomes is genetically active*, (2) *the other X of either maternal or paternal origin undergoes heteropyknosis and is rendered inactive*, (3) *inactivation of either the maternal or paternal X occurs at random among all the cells of the blastocyst on or about the 16th day of embryonic life*, and (4) *inactivation of the same X chromosome persists in all the cells derived from each precursor cell.* Thus, the great preponderance of normal females are in reality mosaics and have two populations of cells, one with an inactivated maternal X and the other with an inactivated paternal X. Herein lies the explanation of why females have the same dosage of X-linked active genes as have males. The inactive X can be seen in the interphase nucleus as a darkly staining small mass in contact with the nuclear membrane known as the *Barr body* or *X chromatin.* Barr bodies are present in all somatic cells of normal females, but they are most readily demonstrated in smears of buccal squamous epithelial cells.

Although the basic tenets of the Lyon hypothesis have stood the test of time, several modifications have been made. For example, at first it was thought that all the genes on the inactive X are "shut off." More recent molecular studies have revealed that many genes escape X inactivation. It is believed that at least some of the genes that are expressed from both X chromosomes are important for normal growth and development. This notion is supported by the fact that patients with monosomy of the X chromosome (Turner syndrome: 45,X) have severe somatic and gonadal abnormalities. If a single dose of X-linked genes were sufficient, no detrimental effect would be expected in such cases. Furthermore, although one X chromosome is inactivated in all cells during embryogenesis, it is selectively reactivated in germ cells before the first meiotic division. Thus, it seems that both X chromosomes are required for normal oogenesis.

With respect to the Y chromosome, it is well known that this chromosome is both necessary and sufficient for male development. *Regardless of the number of X chromosomes, the presence of a single Y determines the male sex.* The gene that dictates testicular development (*Sry*: sex-determining region Y gene) has been located on its distal short arm.[50] In addition, there is increasing evidence that some genes on the long arm of Y are essential for spermatogenesis.[51] With this background, we review some features that are common to all sex chromosome disorders.

- *In general, they induce subtle, chronic problems relating to sexual development and fertility.*
- *They are often difficult to diagnose at birth, and many are first recognized at the time of puberty.*
- *In general, the higher the number of X chromosomes, in both male and female, the greater the likelihood of mental retardation.*

The most important disorders arising in aberrations of sex chromosomes are described briefly here.

KLINEFELTER SYNDROME

Klinefelter syndrome is best defined as male hypogonadism that occurs when there are two or more X chromosomes and one or more Y chromosomes. It is one of the most frequent forms of genetic disease involving the sex chromosomes as well as one of the most common causes of hypogonadism in the male. The incidence of this condition is approximately 1 in 850 live male births. It can rarely be diagnosed before puberty, particularly because the testicular abnormality does not develop before early puberty. Most patients have a distinctive body habitus with an increase in length between the soles and the pubic bone, which creates the appearance of an elongated body. Also characteristic are eunuchoid body habitus with abnormally long legs; small atrophic testes often associated with a small penis; and lack of such secondary male characteristics as deep voice, beard, and male distribution of pubic hair. Gynecomastia may be present. The mean IQ is somewhat lower than normal, but mental retardation is uncommon. This typical pattern is not seen in all cases, the only consistent finding being hypogonadism. Plasma gonadotropin levels, particularly follicle-stimulating hormone (FSH), are consistently elevated, whereas testosterone levels are variably reduced. Mean plasma estradiol levels are elevated by an as yet unknown mechanism. The ratio of estrogens and testosterone determines the degree of feminization in individual cases.

Klinefelter syndrome is the principal cause of reduced spermatogenesis and male infertility. In some patients, the testicular tubules are totally atrophied and replaced by pink, hyaline, collagenous ghosts. In others, apparently normal tubules are interspersed with atrophic tubules. In some patients, all tubules are primitive and appear embryonic, consisting of cords of cells that never developed a lumen or progressed to mature spermatogenesis. Leydig cells appear prominent, owing to the atrophy and crowding of tubules.

The classic pattern of Klinefelter syndrome is associated with a 47,XXY karyotype (82% of cases). This complement results from nondisjunction during the meiotic divisions in one of the parents. Maternal nondisjunction at the first meiotic division accounts for a little more than half of the cases. Most of the remaining result from nondisjunction during the first paternal meiotic division. There is no phenotypic difference between those who receive the extra X chromosome from their father and those who receive it from their mother. Maternal age is increased in the cases associated with errors in oogenesis. In addition to this classic karyotype, approximately 15% of patients with Klinefelter syndrome have been found to have a variety of mosaic patterns, most of them being 46,XY/47,XXY. Other patterns are 47,XXY/48,XXXY and variations on this theme. Rare individuals have also been found to possess 48,XXXY or 49,XXXXY karyotypes. Such polysomic X individuals have further physical abnormalities, including cryptorchidism, hypospadias, more severe hypoplasia of the testes, and skeletal changes, such as prognathism and radioulnar synostosis.

XYY SYNDROME

Supernumerary Y chromosomes may be found in the male, giving rise to 47,XYY, or even greater Y polysomy. Approximately 1 in 1000 live-born males has one of these karyotypes. Nearly all are phenotypically normal, but the individuals frequently are excessively tall and may be susceptible to severe acne. From present data, it appears that the intelligence of these individuals is in the normal range.

The impact of extra Y chromosomes on behavior is uncertain and controversial. These karyotypes have been identified with increased frequency among inmates of penal institutions. The behavioral difficulties take the form of antisocial (not violent), delinquent, impulsive acting-out disorders. From more recent studies, it appears that only about 1 to 2% of individuals with XYY phenotypes exhibit such deviant behavior; the overwhelming majority are no more antisocial than their peers who have fewer Y chromosomes.

TURNER SYNDROME

Turner syndrome results from complete or partial monosomy of the X chromosome and is characterized primarily by hypogonadism in phenotypic females.[52] It is the most common sex chromosome abnormality in females.

With routine cytogenetic methods, three types of karyotypic abnormalities are seen in patients with Turner syndrome. Approximately 57% are missing an entire X chromosome, resulting in a 45,X karyotype. Of the remaining, approximately one third (approximately 14%) have structural abnormalities of the X chromosomes, and two thirds (approximately 29%) are mosaics. The net effect of structural abnormalities is to produce partial monosomy of the X chromosome. In the order of frequency, the structural abnormalities of the X chromosome include (1) deletion of the small arm, resulting in the formation of an isochromosome of the long arm, 46,X,i(X)(q10); (2) deletion of portions of both long and short arms, resulting in the formation of a ring chromosome, 46,X,r(X); and (3) deletion of portions of the short or long arm, 46X,del(Xq) or 46X,del(Xp). The mosaic patients have a 45,X cell line along with one or more karyotypically normal or abnormal cell types. Examples of karyotypes that mosaic Turner females may have are the following: (1) 45,X/46,XX; (2) 45,X/46,XY; (3) 45,X/47,XXX; or (4) 45,X/46,X,i(X)(q10). Studies suggest that the prevalence of mosaicism in Turner syndrome is much higher than the 30% detected by conventional cytogenetic studies. With the use of more sensitive techniques, including FISH and polymerase chain reaction (PCR), and analysis of more than one cell type (e.g., peripheral blood and fibroblasts), the prevalence of mosaic Turner syndrome increases to 75%.[52] Because 99% of 45,X conceptuses are nonviable, many authorities believe that there are no truly nonmosaic Turner syndrome patients. This issue, however, remains controversial. Nevertheless, it is important to appreciate the karyotypic heterogeneity associated with Turner syndrome because it is responsible for significant variations in phenotype. In patients who are truly 45,X, or in whom the proportion of 45,X cells is high, the phenotypic changes are more severe than in those who have readily detectable mosaicism. The latter may have an almost normal appearance and may present only with primary amenorrhea.

The most severely affected patients generally present during infancy with edema (owing to lymph stasis) of the dorsum of the hand and foot and sometimes swelling of the nape of the neck. The latter is related to markedly distended lymphatic channels, producing a so-called cystic hygroma (Chapter 11). As these infants develop, the swellings subside but often leave bilateral neck webbing and persistent looseness of skin on the back of the neck. Congenital heart disease is also common, particularly preductal coarctation of the aorta and bicuspid aortic valve. Cardiovascular abnormalities are the single most important cause of increased mortality in children with Turner syndrome.

The principal clinical features in the adolescent and adult are illustrated in Figure 6–29. At puberty, there is failure to develop normal secondary sex characteristics. The genitalia remain infantile, breast development is inadequate, and there is little pubic hair. The mental status of these patients is usually normal, but a few may exhibit some retardation. Of particular importance in establishing the diagnosis in the adult is the shortness of stature (rarely exceeding 150 cm in height) and the amenorrhea. *Turner syndrome is the single most important cause of primary amenorrhea*, accounting for approximately one third of the cases. For reasons not quite clear, approximately 50% of patients develop autoantibodies directed to the thyroid gland, and up to one half of these develop clinically manifest hypothyroidism. Equally mysterious is the presence of glucose intolerance, obesity, and insulin resistance in a minority of patients. The last mentioned is significant be-

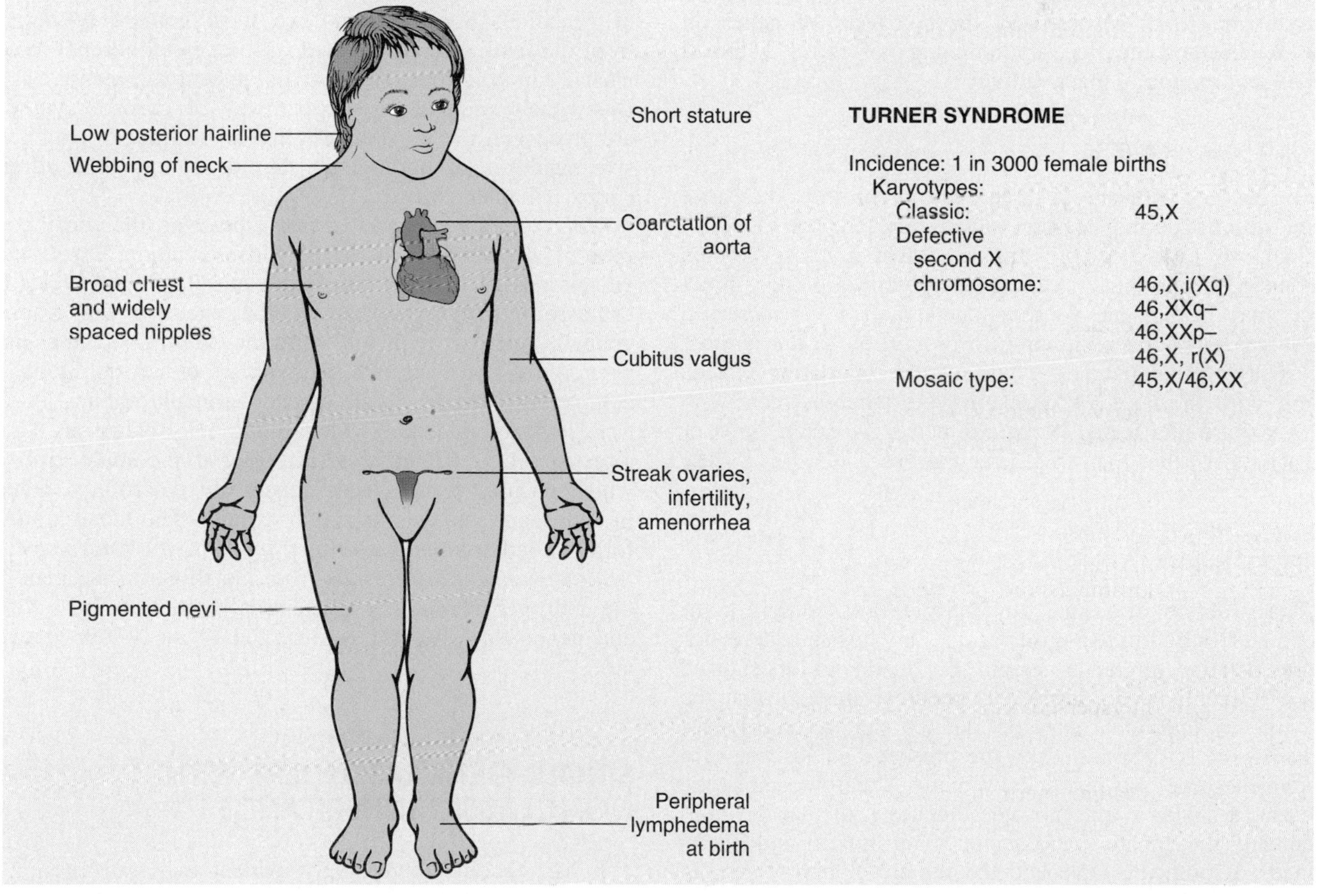

Figure 6–29

Clinical features and karyotypes of Turner syndrome.

cause therapy with growth hormone, commonly used in these patients, worsens insulin resistance.

The molecular pathogenesis of Turner syndrome is not completely understood, but studies have begun to shed some light.[53] As mentioned earlier, both X chromosomes are active during oogenesis and are essential for normal development of the ovaries. During normal fetal development, ovaries contain as many as 7 million oocytes. The oocytes gradually disappear so that by menarche their numbers have dwindled to a mere 400,000, and when menopause occurs fewer than 10,000 remain. In Turner syndrome, fetal ovaries develop normally early in embryogenesis, but the absence of the second X chromosome leads to an accelerated loss of oocytes, which is complete by the age of 2 years. In a sense, therefore, "menopause occurs before menarche," and the ovaries are reduced to atrophic fibrous strands, devoid of ova and follicles (*streak ovaries*). Because patients with Turner syndrome also have other (nongonadal) abnormalities, it follows that some genes for normal growth and development of somatic tissues must also reside on the X chromosome. Studies indicate that a locus important for normal stature maps to the short arm of X chromosome. Gene(s) at this locus are among those that remain active on both copies of the X chromosome in normal females (see earlier). If some X-linked genes are required in diploid dosage for normal somatic development, then how do males develop normally with only one copy of the X chromosome? This apparent paradox has been resolved by the discovery of genes on the Y chromosome that are homologs of those X-linked genes that escape X-inactivation.

MULTI-X FEMALES

Karyotypes with one to three extra X chromosomes have been described and are not uncommon, being found in about 1 in 1200 newborn females. Most of these women are entirely normal. A variety of random findings, however, may be present. As mentioned, there is an increased tendency to mental retardation in proportion to the number of extra X chromosomes. Thus, mental retardation is seen in all with the 49,XXXXX karyotype, whereas most with 47,XXX are unaffected. Some women have amenorrhea or occasionally other menstrual irregularities.

HERMAPHRODITISM AND PSEUDOHERMAPHRODITISM

The problem of sexual ambiguity is exceedingly complex, and only limited observations are possible here; for more details, reference should be made to specialized texts.[54] It will be no surprise to medical students that the sex of an individual can be defined on several levels. *Genetic sex* is determined by the presence or absence of a Y chromosome. No matter how many X chromosomes are present, a single Y chromosome dictates testicular development and the genetic male gender. The initially indifferent gonads of both the male and the female embryos have an inherent tendency to feminize, unless influenced by Y chromosome–dependent masculinizing factors. *Gonadal sex* is based on the histologic characteristics of the gonads. *Ductal sex* depends on the presence of derivatives of the müllerian or wolffian ducts. *Phenotypic*, or *genital*, *sex* is based on the appearance of the external genitalia. Sexual ambiguity is present whenever there is disagreement among these various criteria for determining sex.

The term true hermaphrodite implies the presence of both ovarian and testicular tissue. In contrast, a pseudohermaphrodite represents a disagreement between the phenotypic and gonadal sex (i.e., a female pseudohermaphrodite has ovaries but male external genitalia; a male pseudohermaphrodite has testicular tissue but female-type genitalia).

True hermaphroditism, implying the presence of both ovarian and testicular tissue, is an extremely rare condition. In some cases, there is a testis on one side and an ovary on the other, whereas in other cases, there may be combined ovarian and testicular tissue, referred to as *ovotestes*. The karyotype is 46,XX in 50% of patients; of the remaining, approximately equal numbers have 46,XY and 45,X/XY karyotypes. The pathogenesis of 46,XX hermaphrodites is mysterious because they seem to lack Y chromosome–derived DNA, even by molecular analysis.

Female pseudohermaphroditism is much less complex. The genetic sex in all cases is XX, and the development of the gonads (ovaries) and internal genitalia is normal. Only the external genitalia are ambiguous or virilized. The basis of female pseudohermaphroditism is excessive and inappropriate exposure to androgenic steroids during the early part of gestation. Such steroids are most commonly derived from the fetal adrenal affected by congenital adrenal hyperplasia, which is transmitted as an autosomal recessive trait. Biosynthetic defects in the pathway of cortisol synthesis are present in these cases, which lead secondarily to excessive synthesis of androgenic steroids by the fetal adrenal cortex (Chapter 26).

Male pseudohermaphroditism represents the most complex of all disorders of sexual differentiation. These individuals possess a Y chromosome, and thus their gonads are exclusively testes, but the genital ducts or the external genitalia are incompletely differentiated along the male phenotype. Their external genitalia are either ambiguous or completely female. Male pseudohermaphroditism is extremely heterogeneous, with a multiplicity of causes. Common to all is defective virilization of the male embryo, which usually results from genetically determined defects in androgen synthesis or action or both. The most common form, called *complete androgen insensitivity syndrome (testicular feminization)*, results from mutations in the gene for the androgen receptor. This gene is located at Xq11-Xq12, and hence this disorder is inherited as an X-linked recessive.

SINGLE-GENE DISORDERS WITH NONCLASSIC INHERITANCE

It has become increasingly evident that transmission of certain single-gene disorders does not follow classic mendelian principles. This group of disorders can be classified into four categories:

- Diseases caused by triplet-repeat mutations
- Disorders caused by mutations in mitochondrial genes
- Disorders associated with genomic imprinting
- Disorders associated with gonadal mosaicism

Clinical and molecular features of some single-gene diseases that exemplify nonclassic patterns of inheritance are described next.

Triplet Repeat Mutations—Fragile X Syndrome

Fragile X syndrome is the prototype of diseases in which the mutation is characterized by a long repeating sequence of three nucleotides. Although the specific nucleotide sequence that undergoes amplification differs in the dozen or so disorders included in this group, in most cases the affected sequences share the nucleotides guanine (G) and cytosine (C). In the ensuing discussion, we consider the clinical features and inheritance pattern of the fragile X syndrome, to be followed by the causative molecular lesion. The remaining disorders in this group are discussed later, in this chapter and elsewhere in the text.

With a frequency of 1 in 1550 for affected males, *fragile X syndrome is the second most common genetic cause of mental retardation, after Down syndrome.* It is an X-linked disorder characterized by an inducible cytogenetic abnormality in the X chromosome and an unusual mutation within the familial mental retardation-1 (FMR-1) gene. The cytogenetic alteration is seen as a discontinuity of staining or as a constriction in the long arm of the X chromosome when cells are cultured in folate-deficient medium. Because it appears that the chromosome is "broken" at this locale, it is referred to as a *fragile site* (Fig. 6–30). The affected males are *mentally retarded,* with an IQ in the range of 20 to 60. They express a characteristic physical phenotype that includes a *long face with a large mandible, large everted ears,* and *large testicles (macro-orchidism).* Hyperextensible joints, a high arched palate, and mitral valve prolapse noted in some patients mimic a connective tissue disorder. These and other physical abnormalities described in this condition, however, are not always present and, in some cases, are quite subtle. *The only distinctive feature that can be detected in at least 90% of postpubertal males with fragile-X syndrome is macro-orchidism.*[55]

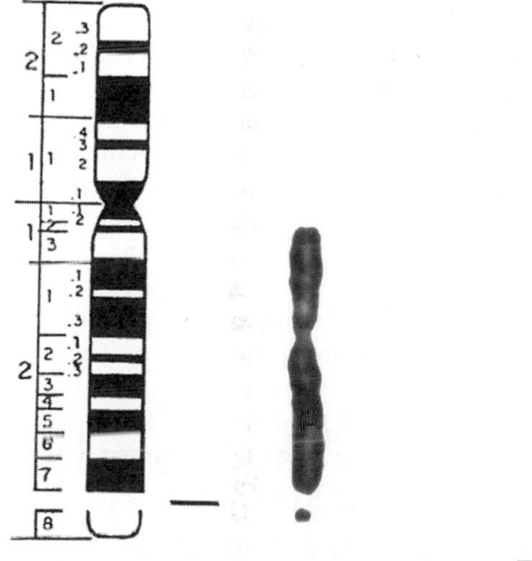

Figure 6–30

Fragile X, seen as discontinuity of staining. (Courtesy of Dr. Patricia Howard-Peebles, University of Texas Southwestern Medical Center, Dallas, TX.)

As with all X-linked diseases, fragile X syndrome affects males. Analysis of several pedigrees, however, reveals some patterns of transmission not typically associated with other X-linked recessive disorders (Fig. 6–31). These include the following:

- *Carrier males*: Approximately 20% of males who by pedigree analysis and by molecular tests are known to carry a fragile X mutation are clinically and cytogenetically normal. Because carrier males transmit the trait through all their daughters (phenotypically normal) to affected grandchildren, they are called *transmitting males.*
- *Affected females*: Approximately 50% of carrier females are affected (i.e., mentally retarded), a number much higher than that in other X-linked recessive disorders.
- *Risk of phenotypic effects*: Risk depends on the position of the individual in the pedigree. For example, brothers of transmitting males are at a 9% risk of having mental retardation, whereas grandsons of transmitting males incur a 40% risk. This positional risk is sometimes referred to as Sherman's paradox.
- *Anticipation*: This refers to the observation that clinical features of fragile X worsen with each successive generation, as if the mutation becomes increasingly deleterious as it is transmitted from a man to his grandsons and great-grandsons.

These unusual patterns perplexed geneticists for years, but molecular studies have finally begun to unravel the complexities of this condition.[56–58] The first breakthrough came when linkage studies localized the mutation responsible for this disease to Xq27.3, within the cytogenetically abnormal region. Within this region lies the FMR-1 gene, characterized by multiple tandem repeats of the nucleotide sequence CGG in its 5′ untranslated region. In the normal population, the number of CGG repeats is small, ranging from 6 to 46 (average 29). The presence of clinical symptoms and a cytogenetically detectable fragile site seem related to the extent of amplification of the CGG repeats. Thus, normal transmitting males and carrier females carry 50 to 230 CGG repeats. Expansions of this size are called *premutations.* In contrast, affected individuals have an extremely large expansion of the repeat region (230 to 4000 repeats, or *full mutations*). Full mutations are believed to arise by further amplification of the CGG repeats seen in premutations. How this process takes place is quite peculiar. Carrier males transmit the repeats to their progeny with small changes in repeat number. When the premutation is passed on by a carrier female, however, there is a high probability of a dramatic amplification of the CGG repeats, leading to mental retardation in most of male offspring and 50% of female offspring. Thus, *it appears that during the process of oogenesis, but not in spermatogene-*

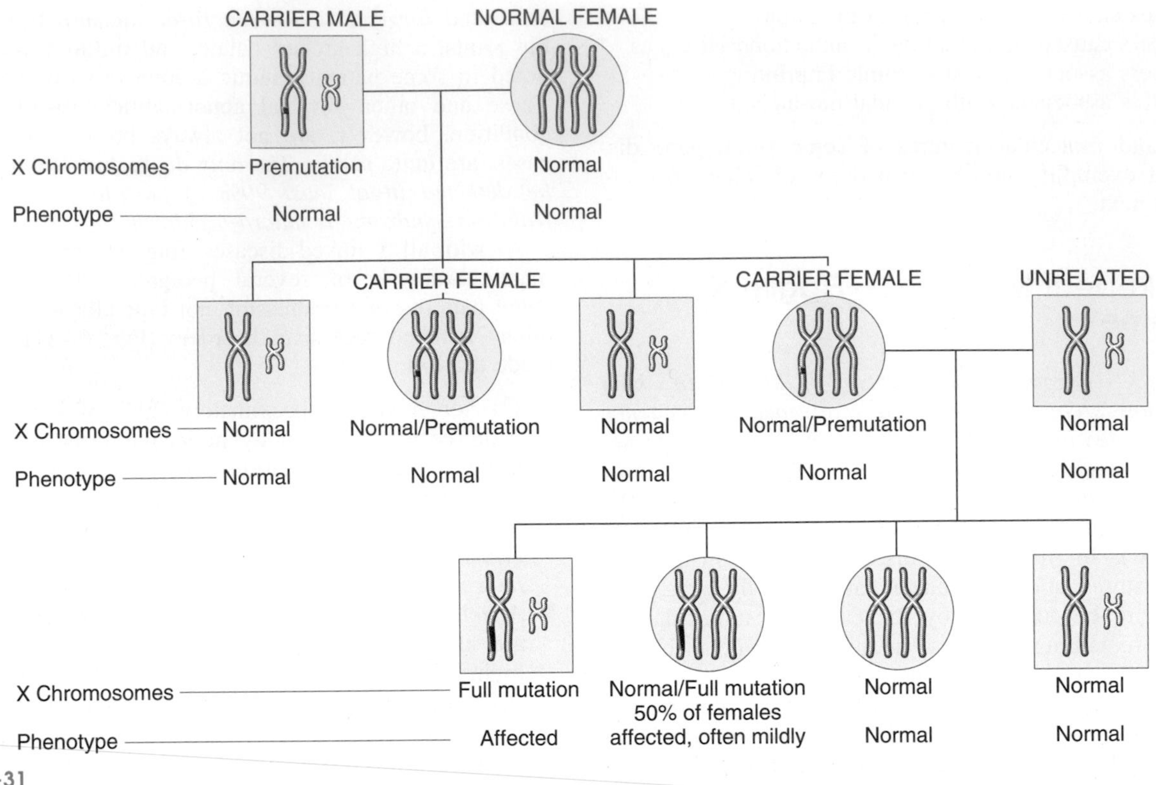

Figure 6–31

Fragile X pedigree. Note that in the first generation all sons are normal and all females are carriers. During oogenesis in the carrier female, premutation expands to full mutation; hence in the next generation, all males who inherit the X with full mutation are affected. However, only 50% of females who inherit the full mutation are affected, and only mildly. (Courtesy of Dr. Nancy Schneider, Department of Pathology, University of Texas Southwestern Medical Center, Dallas, TX.)

sis, premutations can be converted to mutations by triplet repeat amplification. This explains Sherman's paradox; that is, the likelihood of mental retardation is much higher in grandsons than in brothers of transmitting males because grandsons incur the risk of inheriting a premutation from their grandfather that is amplified to a "full mutation" in their mothers' ova. By comparison, brothers of transmitting males, being "higher up" in the pedigree, are less likely to have a full mutation. These molecular details also provide a satisfactory explanation of anticipation—a phenomenon observed by clinical geneticists but not believed by molecular geneticists until triplet repeat mutations were identified. Why only 50% of the females with full mutation are clinically affected is not clear. Presumably in those clinically affected, there is unfavorable lyonization (i.e., there is a higher frequency of cells in which the X chromosome carrying the mutation is active).

The molecular basis of mental retardation and other somatic manifestations is not entirely clear, but it appears related to a loss of function of the FMR-1 gene. As mentioned earlier, the normal FMR-1 gene contains up to 46 CGG repeats in its 5′ untranslated region. When the trinucleotide repeats in the FMR-1 gene exceed approximately 230, the DNA of the entire 5′ region of the gene becomes abnormally methylated. Methylation also extends up-stream into the promoter region of the gene, resulting in transcriptional suppression of FMR-1. The resulting absence of the FMR protein is believed to cause the phenotypic changes. This hypothesis is supported by the observation that FMR-1 knockout mice exhibit certain features of the fragile X syndrome, such as enlarged testes and learning deficits.[59] Although the importance of the FMR-1 gene in the causation of the fragile X syndrome is established, the function of the encoded FMR protein is not known. This cytoplasmic protein is widely expressed in normal tissues, but higher levels of FMR-1 transcripts are found in the brain and testis, suggesting that it may play an important role in these tissues.

Until recently, cytogenetic demonstration of the fragile X (see Fig. 6–29) was the only method of laboratory diagnosis. Polymerase chain reaction–based diagnosis, however, is now the method of choice. With Southern blot analysis, distinction between premutations and mutations can be made prenatally as well as postnatally. Hence, this technique is valuable not only for establishing the diagnosis, but also for genetic counseling. These techniques are described later.

OTHER DISEASES WITH UNSTABLE NUCLEOTIDE REPEATS

The discovery in 1991 of expanding trinucleotide repeats as a cause of fragile X syndrome was a landmark in human genetics. Since then, the origins of at least a dozen human diseases (Table 6–8) have been traced to a similar type of mutation,[60] and the number continues to grow. All

Table 6–8. SELECTED DISEASES ASSOCIATED WITH UNSTABLE REPEAT EXPANSIONS

Repeat Sequence	Disease	Transmission	Protein Affected
Expansions Affecting Noncoding Regions			
CGG	Fragile X syndrome	XD	FMR-1
CTG	Myotonic dystrophy	AD	Myotonin protein kinase
GAA	Friedreich ataxia	AR	Frataxin
GC rich 12 mer	Progressive myoclonus epilepsy	AR	Cystastatin B
Expansions Affecting Coding Regions			
CAG	Spinobulbar muscular atrophy (Kennedy disease)	XR	Androgen receptor
CAG	Huntington disease	AD	Huntingtin
CAG	Spinocerebellar ataxia type 1	AD	Ataxin 1
CAG	Dentorubropallidolusian atrophy	AD	Atrophin

disorders discovered so far are associated with neurodegenerative changes.[61] Some general principles that apply to these diseases are as follows:

- The causative mutations are associated with the expansion of a stretch of nucleotides. Initially, it was thought that the involved nucleotide sequences occurred as triplets and that they shared the nucleotides G and C. This is certainly true of most disorders in this group (Table 6–8), but exceptions have been found. In Friedreich ataxia, the affected sequence is GAA; in progressive myoclonus epilepsy, the expansion is made up of a 12 base pair motif, rather than the usual 3 base pairs (Fig. 6–32). Thus, it may no longer be accurate to call these conditions "trinucleotide repeat disorders."
- In all cases, the mutations impair gene function by an expansion of the repeats. In general, above a certain threshold, which varies in different conditions, the expansions are unstable; thus, as illustrated with the fragile X syndrome, premutations consisting of 50 to 230 repeats tend to expand further and are converted to mutations; these, in turn, interfere with the normal expression or function of the gene. The proclivity to expand depends strongly on the sex of the transmitting parent. In the fragile X syndrome, expansions occur during oogenesis, but in Huntington disease, they occur during spermatogenesis.
- From a mechanistic standpoint, the mutations can be divided into two groups. In the first group are disorders such as the fragile X syndrome and myotonic dystrophy; they are caused by mutations that affect noncoding regions of the genes, such as promoters and introns. This secondarily leads to reduced transcription or translation (or both) of the gene, thus producing loss of function mutations. In the second group, the expansions occur in the exons and usually involve CAG repeats. The affected genes are transcribed, but apparently the protein products acquire new properties whereby they bind to and interfere with the function of other nonmutant proteins. This mechanism is exemplified by Huntington disease, in which the abnormal huntingtin (the gene product) binds to and inactivates huntingtin-associated proteins. Because these mutations endow new properties on the gene product, they fall in the category of gain of function mutations.

Mutations in Mitochondrial Genes—Leber Hereditary Optic Neuropathy

As is well known, the vast majority of genes are located on chromosomes in the cell nucleus. Mendelian inheritance applies to such genes. There exist several mitochondrial genes, however, that are inherited in quite a different manner.[62] *A feature unique to mitochondrial DNA (mtDNA) is maternal inheritance.* This peculiarity results from the fact that ova contain mitochondria within their abundant cyto-

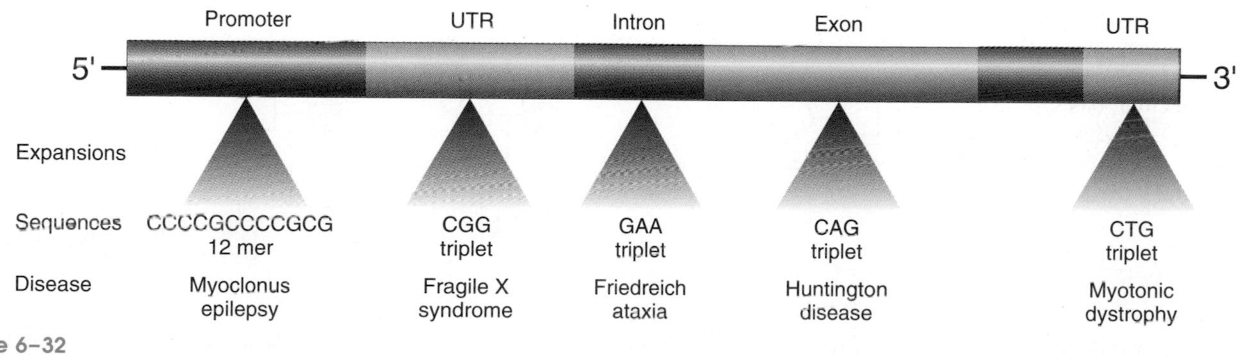

Figure 6–32

Sites of expansion and the affected sequence in selected diseases caused by nucleotide repeat mutations. UTR, untranslated region.

plasm, whereas spermatozoa contain few, if any, mitochondria. Hence, the mtDNA complement of the zygote is derived entirely from the ovum. Thus, mothers transmit mtDNA to all their offspring—male and female; however, daughters but not sons transmit the DNA further to their progeny (Fig. 6–33). Several other features apply to mitochondrial inheritance.[63]

- Because mtDNA encodes enzymes involved in oxidative phosphorylation, mutations affecting these genes exert their deleterious effects primarily on the organs most dependent on oxidative phosphorylation. These include the central nervous system, skeletal muscle, cardiac muscle, liver, and kidneys.
- During cell division, mitochondria and their contained DNA are randomly distributed to the daughter cells. Thus, when a cell containing normal and mutant mtDNA divides, the proportion of the normal and mutant mtDNA in daughter cells is extremely variable. Therefore, the expression of disorders resulting from mutations in mtDNA is quite variable.

As mentioned earlier, many diseases associated with mitochondrial inheritance affect the neuromuscular system. All are rare, and hence only one—Leber hereditary optic neuropathy—is described briefly. This is a neurodegenerative disease that manifests itself as progressive bilateral loss of central vision. Visual impairment is first noted between 15 and 35 years of age, and it leads, in due course, to blindness. Cardiac conduction defects and minor neurologic manifestations have also been observed in some families.[64]

Genomic Imprinting

As is well known, we all inherit two copies of each gene, carried on homologous maternal and paternal chromosomes. It is generally assumed that there is no difference between the genes derived from the mother or the father. Recent studies have challenged this notion, and there is accumulating evidence that, at least with respect to some genes, there are functional differences between the paternal gene and the maternal gene. These differences result from an epigenetic process, called *imprinting*. In most cases, *imprinting selectively inactivates either the maternal or paternal allele*. Thus, *maternal imprinting* refers to transcriptional silencing of the maternal allele, whereas *paternal imprinting* implies that the paternal allele is inactivated. Imprinting occurs in the ovum or the sperm, before fertilization, and then is stably transmitted to all somatic cells through mitosis.[65] As is often the case in medicine, genomic imprinting is best illustrated by considering two uncommon genetic disorders: Prader-Willi syndrome and Angelman syndrome.

PRADER-WILLI SYNDROME AND ANGELMAN SYNDROME

Prader-Willi syndrome is characterized by mental retardation, short stature, hypotonia, obesity, small hands and feet, and hypogonadism. In 50 to 60% of cases, an interstitial deletion of band q12 in the long arm of chromosome 15, del(15)(q11q13), can be detected. In many patients without a detectable cytogenetic abnormality, FISH analysis reveals smaller deletions within the same region. *It is striking that in all cases the deletion affects the paternally derived chromosome 15.* In contrast with the Prader-Willi syndrome, patients with the phenotypically distinct Angelman syndrome are *born with a deletion of the same chromosomal region derived from their mothers.* Patients with Angelman syndrome are also mentally retarded, but in addition they present with ataxic gait, seizures, and inappropriate laughter. Because of their laughter and ataxia, they are also called "happy puppets." A comparison of these two syndromes clearly demonstrates the *parent of origin* effects on gene function.

The molecular basis of these two syndromes can be understood in the context of imprinting (Fig. 6–34). It is believed that a gene or set of genes on maternal chromosome 15 is imprinted (and hence silenced), and thus the only functional allele(s) are provided by the paternal chromosome. When these are lost as a result of a deletion, the patient develops Prader-Willi syndrome. Conversely, a second group of distinct genes that also map to the same

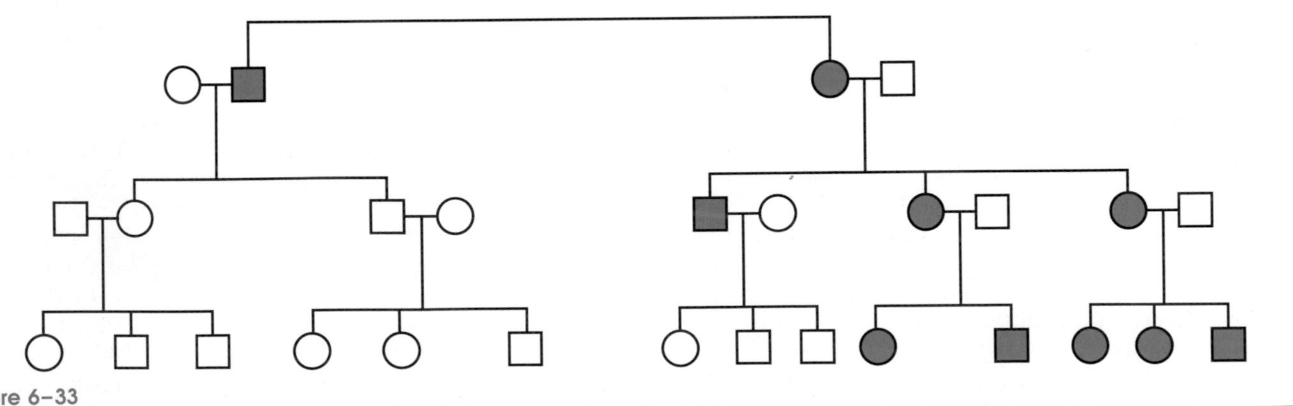

Figure 6–33

Pedigree of Leber optic neuropathy, a disorder caused by mutation in mitochondrial DNA. Note that all progeny of an affected male are normal, but all children, male and female, of the affected female manifest disease.

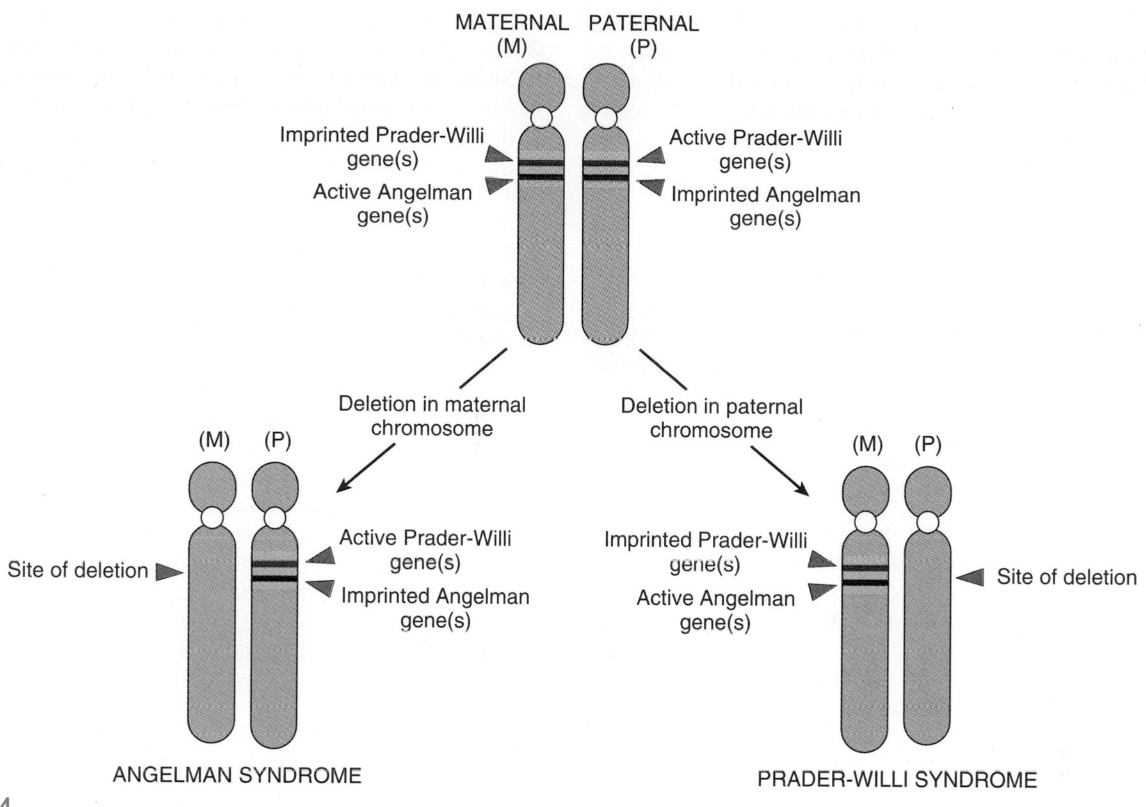

Figure 6–34

Diagrammatic representation of Prader-Willi and Angelman syndromes.

region of chromosome 15 is imprinted on the paternal chromosome. Only the maternally derived allele(s) of these genes are normally active. Deletion of these maternal genes on chromosome 15 gives rise to the Angelman syndrome. Molecular studies of cytogenetically normal patients with the Prader-Willi syndrome have revealed that in some cases both of the structurally normal chromosome 15's are derived from the mother. Inheritance of both chromosomes of a pair from one parent is called *uniparental disomy.* The net effect is the same (i.e., the patient does not have a functional set of genes from the [nonimprinted] paternal chromosome 15). Angelman syndrome, as might be expected, can also result from uniparental disomy of paternal chromosome 15.

The molecular basis of imprinting is still not clear. Because methylation of DNA is known to affect gene expression, it is strongly suspected that imprinting is associated with differential patterns of DNA methylation. Regardless of the mechanism, it is believed that the marking of paternal and maternal chromosomes occurs during gametogenesis, and thus it seems that from the moment of conception some chromosomes remember where they came from.

The importance of imprinting is not restricted to rare chromosomal disorders. Parent-of-origin effects have been identified in a variety of inherited diseases, such as Huntington disease and myotonic dystrophy and in tumorigenesis.[66] As discussed in Chapter 8, many cancers arise by loss of both copies of the so-called tumor-suppressor genes. This may occur by mutational inactivation of both alleles or alternatively by functional loss of one gene copy through imprinting and the inactivation of the other copy by a mutation.

Gonadal Mosaicism

It was mentioned earlier that with every autosomal dominant disorder some patients do not have affected parents. In such patients, the disorder results from a new mutation in the egg or the sperm from which they were derived; as such, their siblings are neither affected nor at increased risk of developing the disease. This is not always the case, however. In some autosomal dominant disorders, exemplified by osteogenesis imperfecta, phenotypically normal parents have more than one affected child. This clearly violates the laws of mendelian inheritance. Studies indicate that gonadal mosaicism may be responsible for such unusual pedigrees.[67] Gonadal mosaicism results from a mutation that occurs postzygotically during early (embryonic) development. If the mutation affects only cells destined to form the gonads, the gametes carry the mutation, but the somatic cells of the individual are completely normal. Such an individual is said to exhibit *germ line* or *gonadal mosaicism.* A phenotypically normal parent who has germ line mosaicism can transmit the disease-causing mutation to the offspring through the mutant gamete. Because the progenitor cells of the gametes carry the mutation, there is a definite possibility that more than one child of such a parent would be affected. Obviously the likelihood of such an occurrence depends on the proportion of germ cells carrying the mutation.

MOLECULAR DIAGNOSIS

Medical applications of recombinant DNA technology have come of age. With the rapid transfer of technology from "the bench to the bedside," it is now clear that DNA probes can be powerful tools for the diagnosis of human disease, both genetic and acquired.[68] Molecular diagnostic techniques have found application in virtually all areas of medicine. These include the following:

- Detection of inherited mutations that underlie the development of genetic diseases either prenatally or after birth
- Detection of acquired mutations that underlie the development of neoplasms
- Accurate diagnosis and classification of neoplasms, especially those that originate in the hematopoietic system
- Diagnosis of infectious diseases, including human immunodeficiency virus (HIV) disease
- Determination of relatedness and identity in transplantation, paternity testing, and forensic medicine

In the next section, we briefly review the diagnostic applications of molecular techniques as they relate to genetic disorders.

DIAGNOSIS OF GENETIC DISEASES

Diagnosis of genetic diseases requires examination of genetic material (i.e., chromosomes and genes). Hence, two general methods are employed: cytogenetic analysis and molecular analysis. Cytogenetic analysis requires karyotyping.

Prenatal chromosome analysis should be offered to all patients who are at risk of cytogenetically abnormal progeny. It can be performed on cells obtained by amniocentesis, on chorionic villus biopsy, or on umbilical cord blood. Some important indications are the following:

- Advanced maternal age (>34 years) because of greater risk of trisomies
- A parent who is a carrier of a balanced reciprocal translocation, robertsonian translocation, or inversion (in these cases the gametes may be unbalanced, and hence the progeny would be at risk for chromosomal disorders)
- A previous child with a chromosomal abnormality
- A parent who is a carrier of an X-linked genetic disorder (to determine fetal sex)

Postnatal chromosome analysis is usually performed on peripheral blood lymphocytes. Indications are as follows:

- Multiple congenital anomalies
- Unexplained mental retardation or developmental delay
- Suspected aneuploidy (e.g., features of Down syndrome)
- Suspected unbalanced autosome (e.g., Prader-Willi syndrome)
- Suspected sex chromosomal abnormality (e.g., Turner syndrome)
- Suspected fragile X syndrome
- Infertility (to rule out sex chromosomal abnormality)
- Multiple spontaneous abortions (to rule out the parents as carriers of balanced translocation; both partners should be evaluated)

Many genetic diseases are caused by subtle changes in individual genes that cannot be detected by karyotyping. Traditionally the diagnosis of single-gene disorders has depended on the identification of abnormal gene products (e.g., mutant hemoglobin or enzymes) or their clinical effects, such as anemia or mental retardation (e.g., phenylketonuria). Now it is possible to identify mutations at the level of DNA and offer gene diagnosis for several mendelian disorders. The use of recombinant DNA technology for the diagnosis of inherited diseases has several distinct advantages over other techniques:

- It is remarkably sensitive. The amount of DNA required for diagnosis by molecular hybridization techniques can be readily obtained from 100,000 cells. Furthermore, the use of PCR allows several million-fold amplification of DNA or RNA, making it possible to use as few as 100 cells or 1 cell for analysis. Tiny amounts of whole blood or even dried blood can supply sufficient DNA for PCR amplification.
- DNA-based tests are not dependent on a gene product that may be produced only in certain specialized cells (e.g., brain) or expression of a gene that may occur late in life. Because virtually all cells of the body of an affected individual contain the same DNA, each postzygotic cell carries the mutant gene.

These two features have profound implications for the prenatal diagnosis of genetic diseases because a sufficient number of cells can be obtained from a few milliliters of amniotic fluid or from a biopsy of chorionic villus that can be performed as early as the first trimester.

There are two distinct approaches to the diagnosis of single-gene diseases by recombinant DNA technology: direct detection of mutations and indirect detection based on linkage of the disease gene with a harmless "marker gene."

Direct Gene Diagnosis

McKusick, an eminent geneticist, has appropriately called direct gene diagnosis the *diagnostic biopsy of the human genome*. Such diagnosis depends on the detection of an important qualitative change in the DNA.[69] There are several methods of direct gene diagnosis.

- One technique relies on the fact that some mutations alter or destroy certain restriction sites on DNA; this occurs in the gene encoding factor V. This protein is

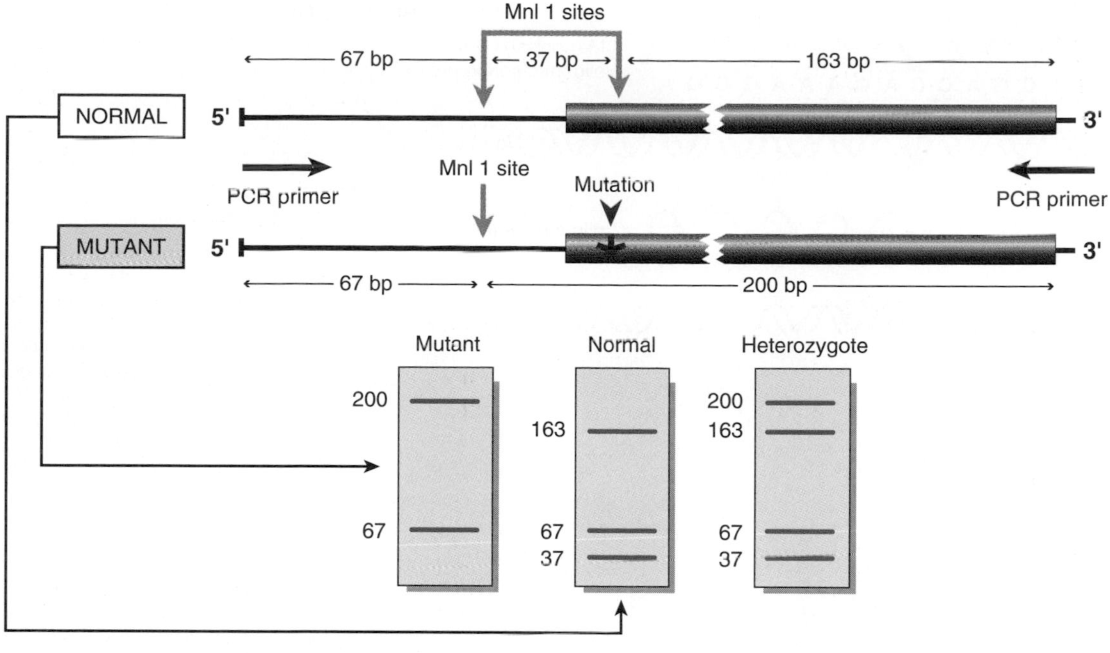

Figure 6–35

Direct gene diagnosis: detection of coagulation factor V mutation by polymerase chain reaction (PCR) analysis. A G→A substitution in an exon destroys one of the two MnlI restriction sites. The mutant allele therefore gives rise to two, rather than three, fragments by PCR analysis.

involved in the coagulation pathway (Chapter 5), and a mutation affecting the factor V gene is the most common cause of inherited predisposition to thrombosis. Exon 10 of the factor V gene and the adjacent intron have two MnlI restriction sites. A G→A mutation within the exon destroys one of the two MnlI sites (Fig. 6–35). To detect the mutant gene, two primers that bind to the 3′ and 5′ prime ends of the normal sequence are designed. By using appropriate DNA polymerases and thermal cycling, the DNA betweeen the primers is greatly amplified, producing millons of copies of the DNA between the two primer sites. The amplified normal DNA and patient's DNA are then digested with the MnlI enzyme. Under these conditions, the normal DNA yields three fragments (67 base pairs, 37 base pairs, and 163 base pairs long); by contrast, the patient's DNA yields only two products, an abnormal fragment that is 200 base pairs and a normal fragment that is 67 base pairs long. These DNA fragments can be readily resolved by polyacrylamide gel electrophoresis and then visualized after staining with ethidium bromide under ultraviolet light.

- Allele-specific oligonucleotide hybridization is another technique for direct gene diagnosis that is used when the mutation does not alter the cutting sites of any known restriction enzymes. An illustrative example is that of α_1-AT deficiency, which in many cases is associated with a single G→A change in exon 5 of the α_1-AT gene, producing the so-called Z allele (Chapter 16). At first, the control DNA and the patient's DNA are amplified by using primers that flank the mutation site (Fig. 6–36). Each amplified DNA sample is applied twice in the form of a dot (hence the name "dot blot") on an appropriate filter paper. Two oligonucleotides that have at their center the single base by which the normal and mutant genes differ are synthesized and radiolabeled. These allele-specific oligonucleotides are then allowed to hybridize with the dotted control and patient DNA (Fig. 6–36). The oligonucleotide containing the sequence of the normal gene hybridizes with both the normal and the mutant DNA, but hybridization to the mutant DNA is unstable owing to the single base pair mismatch. Thus, under stringent conditions of hybridization, the labeled normal probe produces a strong autoradiographic signal with amplified DNA from a normal individual, no signal in the DNA amplified from a patient homozygous for the mutant gene, and a faint signal with DNA from a heterozygote. With the probe containing the mutant sequence, the pattern of hybridization is reversed. Of course, heterozygotes react with both probes because they carry one normal and one mutant gene.
- Mutations that affect the length of DNA (e.g., deletions or expansions) can also be detected by PCR analysis. As discussed earlier, several diseases, such as the fragile X syndrome, are associated with trinucleotide repeats. Figure 6–37 reveals how PCR analysis can be used to detect this mutation. Two primers that flank the region affected by trinucleotide repeats are used to amplify the intervening sequences. Because there are large differences in the number of repeats, the size of the PCR products obtained from the DNA of normal individuals, or those with premutation, is quite different. These size differences are revealed by differential migration of the amplified DNA products on a gel. Currently the full mutation cannot be detected by PCR analysis because the affected segment of DNA is too large for conven-

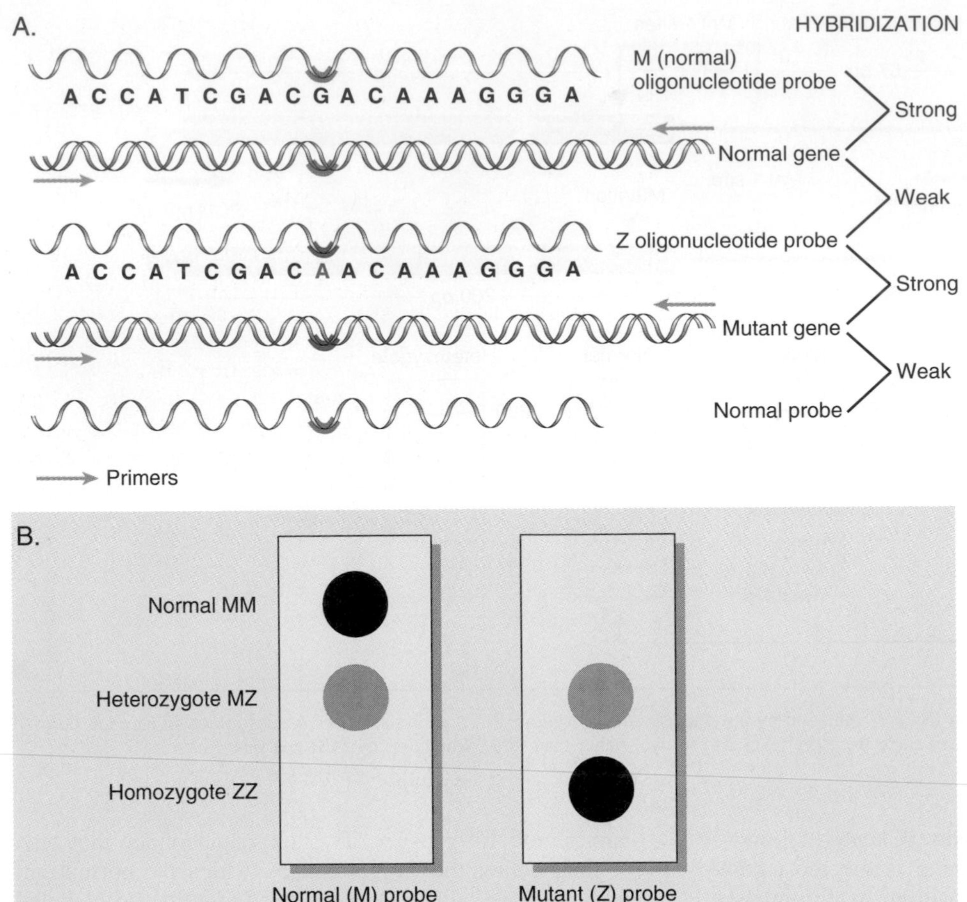

Figure 6–36 ■

Direct gene diagnosis by using PCR and an allele-specific oligonucleotide probe. *A*, A G→A change converts a normal α_1-antitrypsin allele (allele M) to a mutant (Z) allele. Two synthetic oligonucleotide probes, one corresponding in sequence to the normal allele (M probe) and the other corresponding to the mutant allele (Z probe), are lined up against normal and mutant genes, and expected patterns of hybridization are indicated on the right: the arrows indicate primers used to amplify the normal or mutant DNA. *B*, The PCR products from normal individuals, those heterozygous for the Z allele or homozygous for the Z allele, are applied to filter papers in duplicate, and each spot is hybridized with radiolabeled M or Z probe. A dark spot indicates that the probe is bound to the DNA.

tional PCR. In such cases, a Southern blot analysis of genomic DNA has to be performed.

Indirect DNA Diagnosis: Linkage Analysis

Direct gene diagnosis is possible only if the mutant gene and its normal counterpart have been identified and cloned and their nucleotide sequences are known. In a large number of genetic diseases, including some that are relatively common, information about the gene sequence is lacking. Therefore, alternative strategies must be employed to track the mutant gene on the basis of its linkage to detectable genetic markers. In essence, one has to determine whether a given fetus or family member has inherited the same relevant chromosomal region(s) as a previously affected family member. It follows therefore that the success of such a strategy depends on the ability to distinguish the chromosome that carries the mutation from its normal homologous counterpart. This is accomplished by exploiting naturally occurring variations or polymorphisms in DNA sequences. Such polymorphisms can be grouped into two general categories: site polymorphisms and length polymorphisms.

- *Site polymorphisms* are also called *restriction fragment length polymorphisms (RFLPs)*. Examination of DNA from any two persons reveals variations in the DNA sequences involving approximately one nucleotide in every 200 to 500 base pair stretches. Most of these variations occur in noncoding regions of the DNA and are hence phenotypically silent; however, these single base pair changes may abolish or create recognition sites for restriction enzymes, thereby altering the length of DNA fragments produced after digestion with certain restriction enzymes. Using appropriate DNA probes that hybridize with sequences in the vicinity of the polymorphic sites, it is possible to detect the DNA fragments of different lengths by Southern blot analysis. To summarize, *RFLP* refers to variation in fragment length between individuals that results from DNA sequence polymorphisms.

With this background, we can discuss how RFLPs can be used in gene tracking. Figure 6–38 illustrates the principle of RFLP analysis. In this example of an autosomal recessive disease, both of the parents are heterozygote carriers and the children are normal, are carriers, or are affected. In the illustrated example, the normal chromosome (A) has two restriction sites, 7.6 kb apart, whereas chromosome B, which carries the mutant gene, has a DNA se-

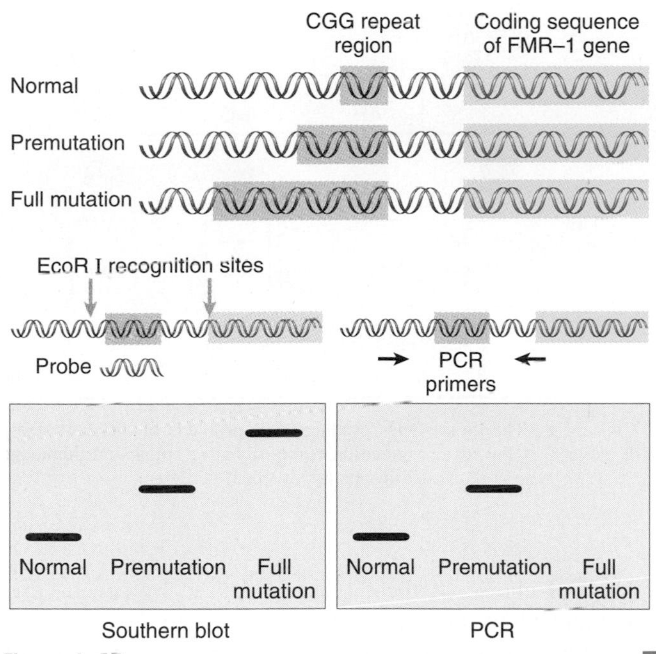

Figure 6–37

Diagnostic application of PCR and Southern blot analysis in fragile X syndrome. With PCR, the differences in the size of CGG repeat between normal and premutation give rise to products of different sizes and mobility. With a full mutation, the region between the primers is too large to be amplified by conventional PCR. In Southern blot analysis the DNA is cut by enzymes that flank the CGG repeat region, and is then probed with a complementary DNA that binds to the affected part of the gene. A single small band is seen in normal males, a higher-molecular-weight band in males with premutation, and a very large (usually diffuse) band in those with the full mutation.

quence polymorphism resulting in the creation of an additional (third) restriction site for the same enzyme. Note that the additional restriction site has not resulted from the mutation but from a naturally occurring polymorphism. When DNA from such an individual is digested with the appropriate restriction enzyme and probed with a cloned DNA fragment that hybridizes with a stretch of sequences between the restriction sites, the normal chromosome yields a 7.6 kb band, whereas the other chromosome (carrying the mutant gene) produces a smaller, 6.8 kb, band. Thus, on Southern blot analysis, two bands are noted. It is possible by this technique to distinguish family members who have inherited both normal chromosomes from those who are heterozygous or homozygous for the mutant gene. Polymerase chain reaction followed by digestion with the appropriate restriction enzyme and gel electrophoresis can also be used to detect RFLPs if the target DNA is of the size that can be amplified by conventional PCR.

- *Length polymorphisms*: Human DNA contains short repetitive sequences of noncoding DNA. Because the number of repeats affecting such sequences varies greatly between different individuals, the resulting *length polymorphisms* are quite useful for linkage analysis. These polymorphisms are often subdivided on the basis of their length into *microsatellite* repeats and *minisatellite* repeats. Microsatellites are usually less than 1 kb and are characterized by a repeat size of 2 to 6 base pairs. Minisatellite repeats, by comparison, are larger (1 to 3 kb), and the repeat motif is usually 15 to 70 base pairs. It is important to note that the number of repeats, both in microsatellites and minisatellites, is extremely variable within a given population, and hence these stretches of DNA can be used quite effectively to distinguish different chromosomes (Fig. 6–39*A*). Figure 6–39*B* illustrates how microsatellite polymorphisms can be

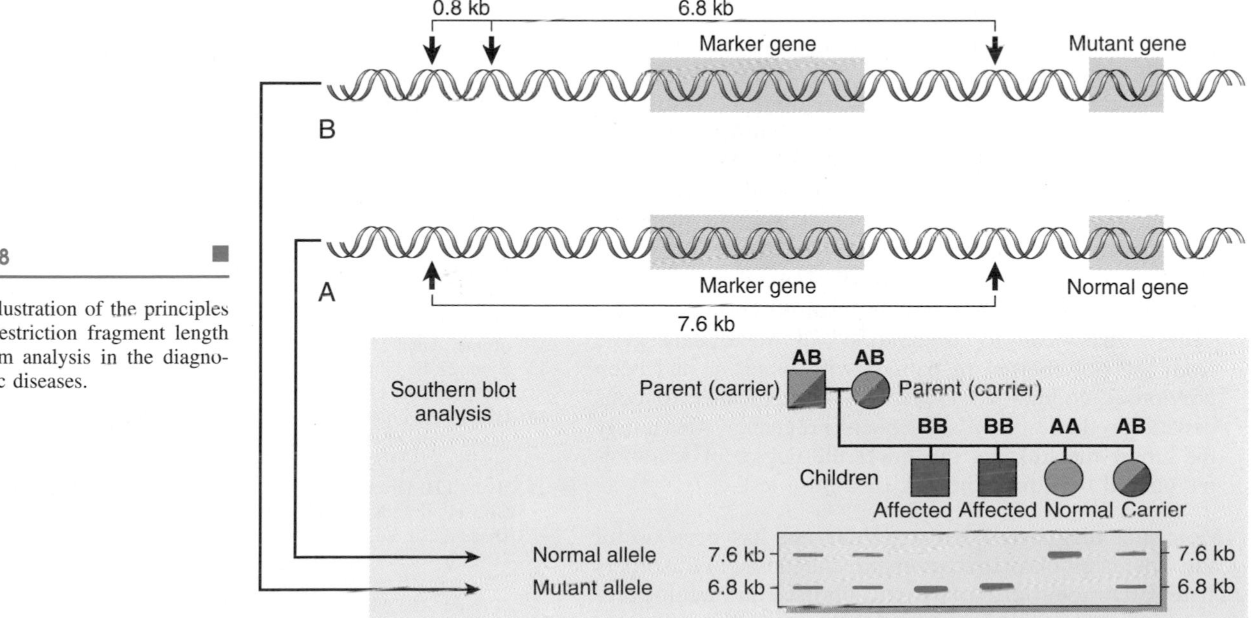

Figure 6–38

Schematic illustration of the principles underlying restriction fragment length polymorphism analysis in the diagnosis of genetic diseases.

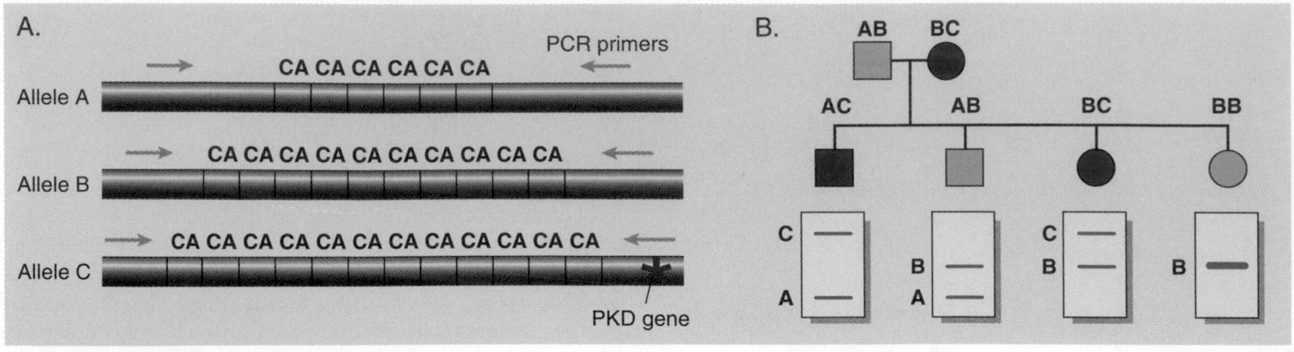

Figure 6–39

Schematic diagram of DNA polymorphisms resulting from a variable number of CA repeats. The three alleles produce PCR products of different sizes, thus identifying their origins from specific chromosomes. In the example depicted, allele C is linked to a mutation responsible for autosomal dominant polycystic kidney disease (PKD). Application of this to detect progeny carrying the disease gene is illustrated in one hypothetical pedigree.

used to track the inheritance of autosomal dominant polycystic kidney disease (PKD). In this case, allele C, which produces a larger PCR product than allele A or B, carries the disease-related gene. Hence all individuals who carry the C allele are affected. Microsatellites have assumed great importance in linkage studies and hence in the development of the human genome map. Currently, linkage to all human chromosomes can be identified by microsatellite polymorphisms.[70, 71]

Because in linkage studies the mutant gene itself is not identified, certain limitations listed below become apparent:

1. For diagnosis, several relevant family members must be available for testing. With an autosomal recessive disease, for example, a DNA sample from a previously affected child is necessary to determine the polymorphism pattern that is associated with the homozygous genotype.
2. Key family members must be heterozygous for the polymorphism (i.e., the two homologous chromosomes must be distinguishable for the polymorphic site). Because there can be only two variations of restriction sites (i.e., presence or absence of the restriction site), this is an important limitation of RFLPs. Microsatellite polymorphisms have multiple alleles and hence much greater chances of heterozygosity. These are therefore much more useful than restriction site polymorphism.
3. Normal exchange of chromosomal material between homologous chromosomes (recombination) during gametogenesis may lead to "separation" of the mutant gene from the polymorphism pattern with which it had been previously coinherited. This may lead to an erroneous genetic prediction in a subsequent pregnancy. Obviously the closer the linkage, the lower the degree of recombination and the lower the risk of a false test.

Molecular diagnosis by linkage analysis has been useful in the antenatal or presymptomatic diagnosis of disorders such as Huntington disease, cystic fibrosis, and adult polycystic kidney disease. In general, when a disease gene is identified and cloned, direct gene diagnosis becomes the method of choice. If the disease is caused by several different mutations in a given gene (e.g., fibillin-1; see earlier), however, direct gene diagnosis is not feasible, and linkage analysis remains the preferred method.

REFERENCES

1. Rimoin DL, et al: Nature and frequency of genetic disease. In Rimoin DL, et al (eds): Emery and Rimoin's Principles and Practice of Medical Genetics, 3rd ed. New York, Churchill Livingstone, 1997, p 32.
2. Lander ES: The new genomics—global views of biology. Science 274:536, 1996.
3. Shuldiner AR: Transgenic animals. N Engl J Med 334:653, 1996
4. Majzoub JA, et al: Knockout mice. N Engl J Med 334:904, 1996
5. Blau H, Khavari P: Gene therapy: problems, prospects. Nat Med 3: 612, 1997.
6. Thompson MW, et al: Thompson and Thompson Genetics in Medicine, 5th ed. Philadelphia, WB Saunders, 1991, p 116.
7. McKusick VA: Mendelian Inheritance in Man, 11th ed. Baltimore, Johns Hopkins University Press, 1994.
8. Price Evans DA: Phamacogenetics. In Rimoin DL, et al (eds): Emery and Rimoin's Principles and Practice of Medical Genetics, 3rd ed. New York, Churchill Livingstone, 1997, p 455.
9. Pyeritz RE: Marfan syndrome and other disorders of fibrillin. In Rimoin DL, et al (eds): Emery and Rimoin's Principles and Practice of Medical Genetics, 3rd ed. New York, Churchill Livingstone, 1997, p, 1027.
10. Dietz HC, Pyeritz RE: Mutations in the human gene for fibrillin-1 (FBN-1) in the Marfan syndrome. Hum Mol Genet 4:1799, 1995.
11. Pereira L, et al: Targeting of fibrillin-1 recapitulates the vascular phenotype of Marfan syndrome in the mouse. Nat Genet 17:218, 1997.
12. De Paepe A, et al: Revised diagnostic ciriteria for the Marfan syndrome. Am J Med Genet 62:417, 1996.
13. Ramirez F: Fibrillin mutations in Marfan syndrome and related phenotypes. Curr Opin Genet Dev 6:309, 1996.
14. Byers PH: Ehlers-Danlos syndrome: recent advances and current understanding of the clinical and genetic heterogeneity. J Invest Dermatol 103:475, 1994.
15. Byers PH: Disorders of collagen biosynthesis and structure. In Scriver CR, et al (eds): The Metabolic and Molecular Basis of Inherited Disease, 7th ed. New York, McGraw-Hill Health Profession Division, 1995, p 4029.
16. Goldstein JL, et al: Familial hypercholesterolemia. In Scriver CR, et al (eds): The Metabolic and Molecular Basis of Inherited Disease, 7th ed. New York, McGraw-Hill Health Profession Division, 1995, p 1981.

17. Illingworth DR, Sexton GJ: Hypocholesterolemic effects of mevinolin in patients with heterozygous familial hypercholesterolemia. J Clin Invest 74:1972, 1984.
18. Ishibashi S, et al: Massive xanthomatosis and atherosclerosis in cholesterol-fed low-density lipoprotein receptor-negative mice. J Clin Invest 93:885, 1994.
19. Tager JM: Inborn errors of cellular organelles: an overview. J Inherit Metab Dis 10(suppl 1):3, 1987.
20. Rutledge SL, Percy AK: Gangliosidoses and related lipid storage diseases. In Rimoin DL, et al (eds): Emery and Rimoin's Principles and Practice of Medical Genetics, 3rd ed. New York, Churchill Livingstone, 1997, p 2105.
21. Triggs-Raine BL, et al: Screening for carriers of Tay-Sachs disease among Ashkenazi Jews: a comparison of DNA-based and enzyme-based tests. N Engl J Med 323:6, 1990.
22. Weisz B, et al: Niemann-Pick disease: newer classification based on genetic mutations of the disease. Adv Pediatr 41:415, 1994.
23. Carstea ED, et al: Niemann-Pick C1 disease gene: homology to mediators of cholesterol homeostasis. Science 277:228, 1997.
24. Grabowski GA, et al: Gaucher disease: a prototype for molecular medicine. Crit Rev Oncol Hematol 23:25, 1996.
25. Lee RE, et al: Gaucher's disease: clinical, morphologic, and pathogenetic considerations. Pathol Annu 12:309, 1977.
26. Tybulewicz VLJ, et al: Animal model of Gaucher's disease from targeted disruption of mouse glucocerebrosidase gene. Nature 357: 407, 1992.
27. Spranger J: Mucopolysaccharidoses. In Rimoin DL, et al (eds): Emery and Rimoin's Principles and Practice of Medical Genetics, 3rd ed. New York, Churchill Livingstone, 1997, p 2071.
28. DiMauro S, et al: Biochemistry and molecular genetics of human glycogenosis: an overview. Muscle Nerve 3:S10–7, 1995.
29. Chen Y-T: Glycogen storage diseases. In Fauci AS, et al (eds.): Harrison's Principles of Internal Medicine, 14th ed. New York, McGraw-Hill, 1998, p 2176.
30. Lee PJ, Leonard JV: The hepatic glycogen storage diseases—problems beyond childhood. J Inherit Metab Dis 18:462, 1995.
31. Bartram C, et al: McArdle disease—muscle glycogen phosphorylase deficiency. Biochim Biophys Acta 1272:1, 1995.
32. Chen Y-T, Burchell A: Glycogen storage diseases. In Scriver CR, et al (eds): The Metabolic and Molecular Basis of Inherited Disease, 7th ed. New York, McGraw-Hill Health Profession Division, 1995, p 935.
33. Van Offel JF, et al: The clinical manifestations of ochronosis: a review. Acta Clin Belg 50:358, 1995.
34. Fernandez-Canon JM, et al: The molecular basis of alkaptonuria. Nat Genet 14:19, 1996.
35. Gaines JJ Jr: The pathology of alkaptonuric ochronosis. Hum Pathol 20:40, 1989.
36. Zwarthoff EC: Neurofibromatosis and associated tumor suppressor genes. Path Res Pract 192:647, 1996.
37. Ricardi VM, Eichner JE: Neurofibromatosis: Phenotype, Natural History and Pathogenesis. Baltimore, Johns Hopkins University Press, 1986, p 115.
38. Gusella JF, et al: Neurofibromatosis 2: loss of Merlin's protective spell. Curr Opin Genet Dev 6:87, 1996.
39. Nelson K, Holmes LB: Malformations due to presumed spontaneous mutations in newborn infants. N Engl J Med 320:19, 1989.
40. Mark HFL, et al: Current applications of molecular cytogenetic technologies. Ann Clin Lab Sci 27:47, 1997.
41. Schrock E, et al: Multicolor spectral karyotyping of human chromosomes. Science 273:494, 1996.
42. Hernandez D, Fisher EMC: Down syndrome genetics: unravelling a multifactorial disorder. Hum Mol Genet 5:1411, 1996.
43. Mutton D, et al: Cytogenetic and epidemiologic findings in Down syndrome, England and Wales 1989 to 1993. National Down Syndrome Cytogenetic Register and the Association of Clinical Cytogeneticists. J Med Genet 33:387, 1996.
44. Kallen B, et al: Major congenital malformations in Down syndrome. Am J Med Genet 65:160, 1996.
45. Cork LC: Neuropathology of Down syndrome and Alzheimer disease. Am J Med Genet 7(suppl):282, 1990.
46. Ugazio AG, et al: Immunology of Down syndrome: a review. Am J Med Genet 7(suppl):204, 1990.
47. Korenberg JR, et al: Down syndrome: toward a molecular definition of the phenotype. Am J Med Genet 7(suppl):91, 1990.
48. Thomas JA, Graham JM Jr: Chromosome 22q11 deletion syndrome: an update and review for the primary pediatricians. Clin Pediatr 36: 253, 1997.
49. Lyon MF: Epigenetic inheritance in man. Trends Genet 9:123, 1993.
50. Goodfellow PH, Lovell-Badge R: SRY and sex determination in mammals. Ann Rev Genet 27:71, 1993.
51. Pryor JL, et al: Microdeletions in the Y chromosome of infertile men. N Engl J Med 336:534, 1997.
52. Saeger P: Turner syndrome. N Engl J Med 335:1749, 1996.
53. Chu CE, Conner JM: Molecular biology of Turner syndrome. Arch Dis Child 72:285, 1995.
54. Grumbach MM, Conte FA: Disorders of sex differentiation. In Wilson JD, Foster DW (eds): Williams Textbook of Endocrinology, 8th ed. Philadelphia, WB Saunders, 1992, p 853.
55. Maddalena A, et al: Fragile X-syndrome. In Rosenberg RN, et al (eds): The Molecular and Genetic Basis of Neurologic Diseases, 2nd ed. Boston, Butterworth & Heinemann, 1997, p 81.
56. Ashley CT, Warren ST: Trinucleotide repeat expansion and human disease. Ann Rev Genet 29:703, 1995.
57. Timchenko LT, Caskey CT: Trinucleotide repeat disorders in humans: discussions of mechanisms and medical issues. FASEB J 10:1589, 1996.
58. Warren ST: Trinucleotide repetition and fragile X syndrome. Hosp Pract 32:73, 1997.
59. Consortium Dutch-Belgium: Fragile X: FMR-1 knockout mice: a model to study fragile X mental retardation. Cell 78:23, 1994.
60. Mandel JL: Breaking the rule of three. Nature 386:767, 1997.
61. Rosenberg RN: DNA-triplet repeat and neurologic disease. N Engl J Med 335:1222, 1996.
62. Johns DR: The other human genome: mitochondrial DNA and disease. Nat Med 2:1065, 1996.
63. Wallace DC: Mitochondrial DNA in aging and disease. Sci Am 277: 40, 1997.
64. Brown MD, et al: Leber's hereditary optic neuropathy: a model for mitochondrial neurodegenerative diseases. FASEB J 6:2791, 1992.
65. Loland M: Parental imprinting and human disease. Ann Rev Genet 30:173, 1997.
66. Squire J, Weksberg R: Genomic imprinting in tumors. Semin Cancer Biol 7:41, 1996.
67. Bernards A, Gusella JF: The importance of genetic mosaicism in human disease. N Engl J Med 331:1447, 1994.
68. Shikata H, et al: DNA-based diagnostics in the study of heritable and acquired disorders. J Lab Clin Med 125:421, 1995.
69. Ferrari M, et al: Molecular diagnosis of genetic diseases. Clin Biochem 29:201, 1996.
70. Koreth J, et al: Microsatellites and PCR genomic analysis. J Pathol 178:239, 1996.
71. Collins FS: Sequencing the human genome. Hosp Pract 32:35, 1997.

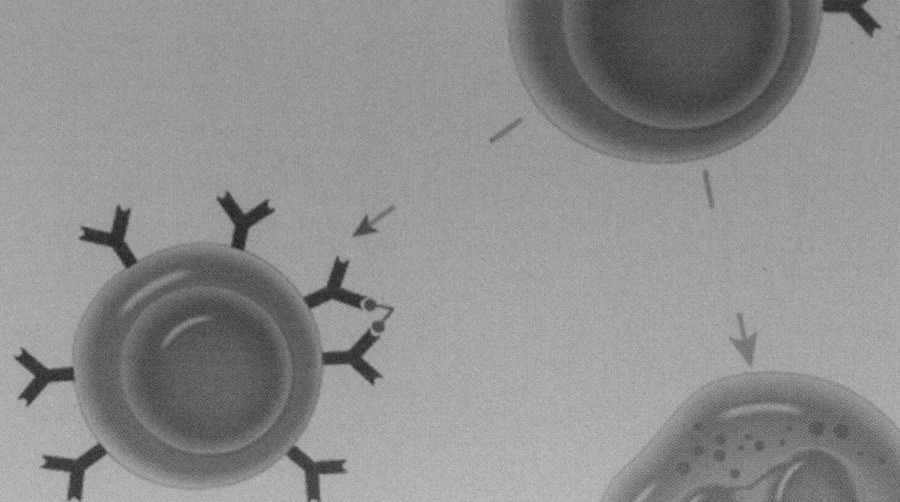

7

Diseases of Immunity

GENERAL FEATURES OF THE IMMUNE SYSTEM
CELLS OF THE IMMUNE SYSTEM
T Lymphocytes
B Lymphocytes
Macrophages
Dendritic Cells
Natural Killer Cells
CYTOKINES: MESSENGER MOLECULES OF THE IMMUNE SYSTEM
General Properties of Cytokines
STRUCTURE AND FUNCTION OF HISTOCOMPATIBILITY ANTIGENS
HLA and Disease Association
DISORDERS OF THE IMMUNE SYSTEM
MECHANISMS OF IMMUNOLOGIC TISSUE INJURY (HYPERSENSITIVITY REACTIONS)
Type I Hypersensitivity (Anaphylactic Type)
Systemic Anaphylaxis
Local Anaphylaxis
Type II Hypersensitivity
Complement-Dependent Reactions
Antibody-Dependent Cell-Mediated Cytotoxicity
Antibody-Mediated Cellular Dysfunction
Type III Hypersensitivity (Immune Complex Mediated)
Systemic Immune Complex Disease
Local Immune Complex Disease (Arthus Reaction)
Type IV Hypersensitivity (Cell Mediated)
Delayed-Type Hypersensitivity
T Cell–Mediated Cytotoxicity
Transplant Rejection
Mechanisms Involved in Rejection
Methods of Increasing Graft Survival
Transplantation of Other Solid Organs
Transplantation of Hematopoietic Cells
AUTOIMMUNE DISEASES
Immunologic Tolerance
Mechanisms of Autoimmune Diseases
Failure of Peripheral Tolerance
Genetic Factors in Autoimmunity
Microbial Agents in Autoimmunity
Systemic Lupus Erythematosus
Sjögren Syndrome
Systemic Sclerosis (Scleroderma)
Inflammatory Myopathies
Mixed Connective Tissue Disease
Polyarteritis Nodosa and Other Vasculitides
IMMUNOLOGIC DEFICIENCY SYNDROMES
Primary Immunodeficiencies
X-Linked Agammaglobulinemia of Bruton
Common Variable Immunodeficiency
Isolated IgA Deficiency
Hyper IgM Syndrome
DiGeorge Syndrome (Thymic Hypoplasia)
Severe Combined Immunodeficiency Diseases
Immunodeficiency With Thrombocytopenia and Eczema (Wiskott-Aldrich Syndrome)
Genetic Deficiencies of the Complement System
Acquired Immunodeficiency Syndrome
AMYLOIDOSIS

GENERAL FEATURES OF THE IMMUNE SYSTEM

Although vital to survival, the immune system is similar to the proverbial two-edged sword. On the one hand, immunodeficiency states render humans easy prey to infections and possibly tumors; on the other hand, a hyperactive immune system may cause fatal disease, as in the case of an overwhelming allergic reaction to the sting of a bee. In yet another series of derangements, the immune system may lose its normal capacity to distinguish self from non-self, resulting in the emergence of immunity against one's own tissues and cells (autoimmunity). This chapter considers diseases caused by too little immunity as well as those resulting from too much immunologic reactivity. We also consider amyloidosis, a disease in which an abnormal protein, derived in some cases from fragments of immunoglobulins, is deposited in tissues. First, we review some advances in the understanding of lymphocyte biology, then a brief description of the histocompatibility genes is given because their products are relevant to several immunologically mediated diseases and to the rejection of transplants.

Cells of the Immune System

T LYMPHOCYTES

As is well known, cellular immunity is mediated by thymus-derived (T) lymphocytes. In the blood, T cells constitute 60 to 70% of peripheral lymphocytes. *T lymphocytes are also found in the paracortical areas of lymph nodes and periarteriolar sheaths of the spleen.* Each T cell is genetically programmed to recognize a specific cell-bound antigen by means of an antigen-specific T-cell receptor (TCR).[1] In approximately 95% of T cells, the TCR consists of a disulfide-linked heterodimer made up of an α and a β polypeptide chain (Fig. 7–1), each having a variable (antigen-binding) and a constant region. In a minority of peripheral blood T cells, another type of TCR, composed of γ and δ polypeptide chains, is found. The TCR γ/δ cells tend to aggregate at epithelial interfaces, such as the mucosa of the respiratory and gastrointestinal tracts. Both the α/β and the γ/δ TCRs are noncovalently linked to a cluster of five polypeptide chains, referred to as the CD3 molecular complex. The CD3 proteins are nonvariable. They do not bind antigen but are involved in the transduction of signals into the T cell after it has bound the antigen. TCR diversity is generated by somatic rearrangement of the genes that encode the α, β, γ, and δ TCR chains. As might be expected, every somatic cell has TCR genes from

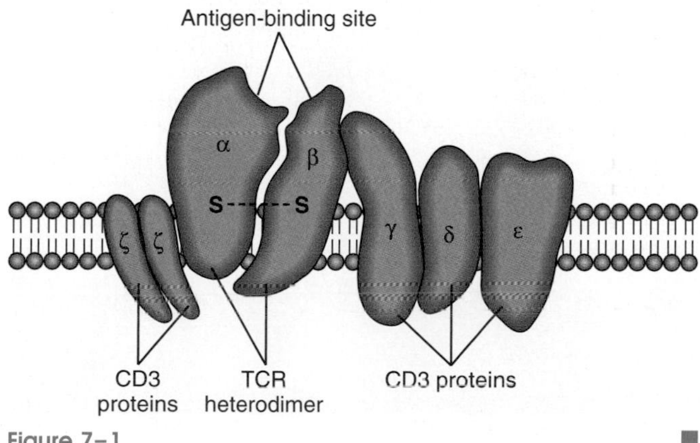

Figure 7–1

The T-cell receptor (TCR) complex: schematic illustration of TCR and TCRα and TCRβ polypeptide chains linked to the CD3 molecular complex.

the germ line. During ontogeny, somatic rearrangements of these genes occur only in T cells; hence the *demonstration of TCR gene rearrangements by Southern blot analysis is a molecular marker of T-lineage cells.* Such analyses are used in classification of lymphoid malignancies (Chapter 15). Furthermore, because each T cell has a unique DNA rearrangement (and hence a unique TCR), it is possible to distinguish polyclonal (non-neoplastic) T-cell proliferations from monoclonal (neoplastic) T-cell proliferations.

In addition to CD3 proteins, T cells express a variety of other nonpolymorphic function–associated molecules, including CD4, CD8, and many so-called accessory molecules, such as CD2, CD11a, CD28, and CD40 ligand. Of these, CD4 and CD8 are particularly important. They are expressed on two mutually exclusive subsets of T cells. CD4 is expressed on approximately 60% of mature CD3+ T cells, whereas CD8 is expressed on about 30% of T cells. These T-cell membrane-associated glycoproteins serve as coreceptors in T-cell activation. During antigen presentation, CD4 molecules bind to the nonpolymorphic portions of class II major histocompatibility complex (MHC) molecules expressed on antigen-presenting cells (Fig. 7–2). In contrast, CD8 molecules bind to class I MHC molecules. Because of these properties, CD4+ helper T cells can recognize antigen only in the context of class II MHC antigens, whereas the CD8+ cytotoxic T cells recognize cell-bound antigens only in association with class I MHC antigens. It is now well established that T cells need two signals for activation. Signal 1 is provided when the TCR is engaged by the appropriate MHC-bound antigen. The coreceptors CD4 and CD8 enhance this signal. Signal 2 is delivered by the interaction of the CD28 molecule on T cells with the costimulatory molecules B7-1 and B7-2 expressed on antigen-presenting cells (Fig. 7–2). The importance of costimulation by this pathway is attested to by the fact that, in the absence of signal 2, the T cells undergo apoptosis or become unreactive.[2]

The CD4+ and CD8+ T cells perform distinct but somewhat overlapping functions. The CD4+ T cell can be viewed as a master regulator—the conductor of a symphony orchestra, so to speak. By secreting soluble factors (cytokines), CD4+ T cells influence the function of virtually all other cells of the immune system, including other T cells, B cells, macrophages, and natural killer (NK) cells. The central role of CD4+ T cells is tragically illustrated when the human immunodeficiency virus (HIV) cripples the immune system by selective destruction of this T-cell subset. In recent years, two functionally different populations of CD4+ helper cells have been recognized.[3] The T-helper-1 (T_H1) subset synthesizes and secretes interleukin-2 (IL-2) and interferon-γ (IFN-γ) but not IL-4 or IL-5, whereas T_H2 cells produce IL-4 and IL-5 but not IL-2 or IFN-γ. This distinction is significant because the cytokines secreted by these subsets have different effects on other immune cells. In general, the T_H1 subset is involved in facilitating delayed hypersensitivity, macrophage activation, and synthesis of IgG2b antibodies. The T_H2 subset aids in the synthesis of other classes of antibodies, including IgE. The CD8+ T cells, similar to CD4+ T cells, can secrete cytokines, primarily of the T_H1 type, but they mediate their functions primarily by acting as cytotoxic cells.

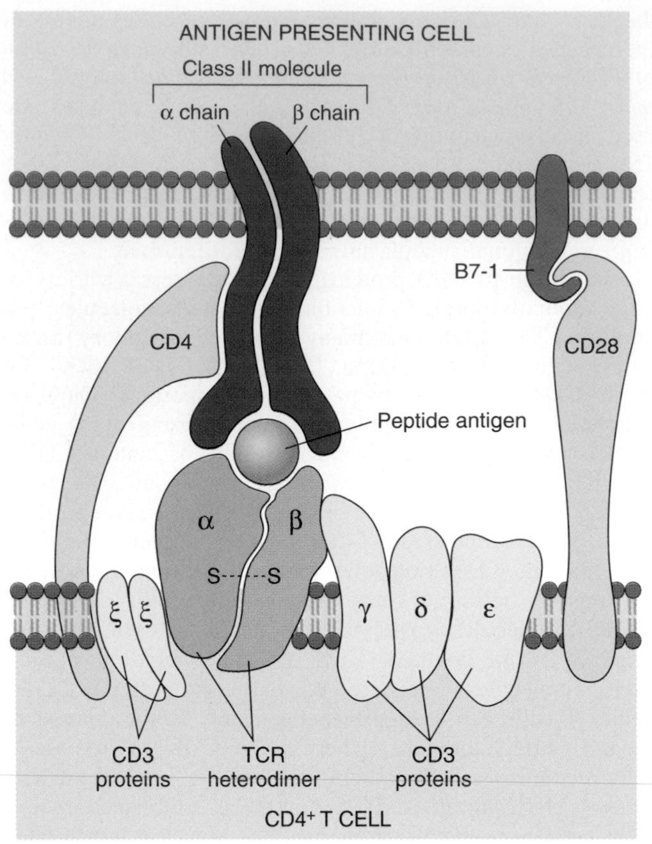

Figure 7–2

Schematic representation of antigen recognition by CD4+ T cells. Note that the T-cell receptor (TCR heterodimer) recognizes a peptide fragment of antigen bound to the major histocompatibility complex (MHC) class II molecule. The CD4 molecule binds to the nonpolymorphic portion of the class II molecule. The interaction between the TCR and the MHC-bound antigen provides signal 1 for T-cell activation. Signal 2 is provided by the interaction of the CD28 molecule with the costimulatory molecules (B7-1 and B7-2) expressed on antigen presenting cell.

B LYMPHOCYTES

B lymphocytes constitute 10 to 20% of the circulating peripheral lymphocyte population. They are also present in bone marrow; peripheral lymphoid tissues such as lymph nodes, spleen, or tonsils; and extralymphatic organs, such as the gastrointestinal tract. In lymph nodes, they are found in the superficial cortex. In the spleen, they are found in the white pulp. At both sites, they are aggregated in the form of lymphoid follicles, which on activation develop pale-staining germinal centers (Fig. 7–3).

On antigenic stimulation, B cells form plasma cells that secrete immunoglobulins, which, in turn, are the mediators of humoral immunity. B cells recognize antigen via the B-cell antigen receptor complex. Immunoglobulin M (IgM), present on the surface of all B cells, constitutes the antigen-binding component of the B-cell receptor. As with T cells, each B-cell receptor has a unique antigen specificity, derived, in part, from somatic rearrangements of immunoglobulin genes. *Thus, the presence of rearranged immunoglobulin genes in a lymphoid cell is used as a molecular marker of B-lineage cells.* In addition to membrane IgM, the B-cell antigen receptor complex contains a heterodimer of nonpolymorphic transmembrane proteins: Igα and Igβ. Similar to the CD3 proteins of the TCR, Igα and Igβ do not bind antigen but are essential for signal transduction through the receptor. B cells also express several other nonpolymorphic molecules that are essential for B-cell function. These include complement receptors, Fc receptors, and CD40. It is worthy of note that complement receptor-2 (CD21) is also the receptor for the Epstein-Barr virus (EBV), and hence B cells are readily infected by EBV. The CD40 molecule, a member of the tumor necrosis factor (TNF)–receptor family, plays an important role in the interaction of T helper cells and B cells. Activated T helper cells express CD40 ligand, which specifically binds to CD40 expressed on B cells. This interaction is essential for B-cell maturation and secretion of IgG, IgA, and IgE antibodies.[4] Patients with mutations in the CD40 ligand have an immunodeficiency called *X-linked hyper-IgM syndrome*, described later.

MACROPHAGES

Macrophages are a part of the mononuclear phagocyte system, and, as such, their origin, differentiation, and role in inflammation are discussed in Chapter 3. Here we need only to emphasize that macrophages play important roles both in the induction and in the effector phase of immune responses.

- First, they are required to process and present antigen to immunocompetent T cells. T cells (in contrast to B cells) cannot be activated by soluble antigens; therefore, presentation of processed, membrane-bound antigens by macrophages or other antigen-presenting cells (e.g., dendritic cells and B cells) is obligatory for induction of cell-mediated immunity.
- Macrophages are important effector cells in certain forms of cell-mediated immunity, such as the delayed

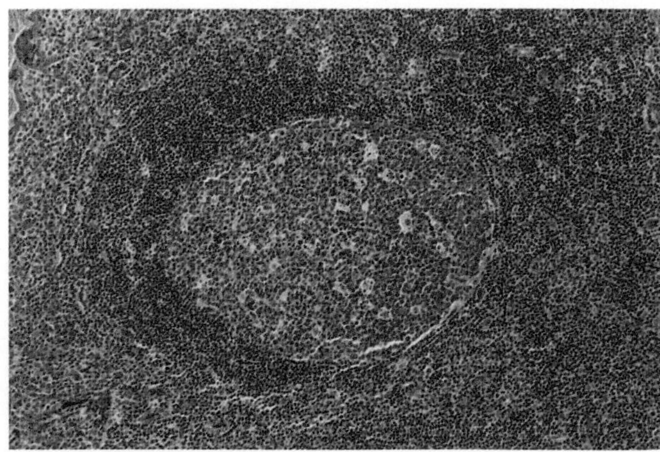

Figure 7–3

Lymph node cortex showing a lymphoid follicle, the B cell–containing area. (Courtesy of Dr. Jon Aster, Brigham and Women's Hospital, Boston, MA.)

hypersensitivity reaction. As mentioned earlier, macrophage activation is facilitated by cytokines, such as IFN-γ produced by the T_H1 subset of CD4+ cells. Such activation enhances the microbicidal properties of macrophages and augments their ability to kill tumor cells.

- Macrophages are also important in the effector phase of humoral immunity. As discussed in Chapter 3, macrophages phagocytose microbes that are opsonized (coated) by IgG or C3b.

DENDRITIC CELLS

There are two types of cells with dendritic morphology that are functionally quite different. Both have numerous fine dendritic cytoplasmic processes, from which they derive their name. One type is called *interdigitating dendritic cells*, or just *dendritic cells*.[4a] These cells are nonphagocytic, and they express high levels of MHC class II molecules as well as the costimulatory molecules B7-1 and B7-2. Thus, they are ideally suited for presenting antigens to CD4+ T cells and are believed to be the most potent antigen-presenting cells for naive T cells. Dendritic cells are widely distributed. They are found in lymphoid tissue and in the interstitium of many nonlymphoid organs, such as the heart and lungs. Similar cells within the epidermis have been called *Langerhans cells*. The other type of cells with dendritic morphology are present in the germinal centers of lymphoid follicles in the spleen and lymph nodes and are hence called *follicular dendritic cells*. These cells bear Fc receptors for IgG and hence can trap antigen bound to antibodies. Such cells play a role in ongoing immune response and are discussed later in the section on acquired immunodeficiency syndrome (AIDS).

NATURAL KILLER CELLS

Natural killer (NK) cells make up approximately 10 to 15% of the peripheral blood lymphocytes and do not bear T-cell receptors or cell surface immunoglobulins. Morphologically, NK cells are somewhat larger than small lymphocytes, and they contain abundant azurophilic granules (Fig. 7–4). Hence, they are also called *large granular lymphocytes*. NK cells are endowed with an innate ability to lyse a variety of tumor cells, virally infected cells, and some normal cells, *without previous sensitization*. These cells are believed to be a part of the *natural* (as opposed to adaptive) immune system that may be the first line of defense against neoplasms or viral infections. Although they share some surface markers with T cells (e.g., CD2), NK cells do not rearrange T-cell receptor genes and are CD3 negative. Two cell surface molecules, CD16 and CD56, are widely used to identify NK cells. Of these, CD16 is of functional significance. It represents the Fc receptor for IgG and hence endows NK cells with another function—the ability to lyse IgG-coated target cells. This phenomenon, known as *antibody-dependent cell-mediated cytotoxicity* (ADCC), is described in greater detail later. NK cells express two types of receptors on their cell membrane. One type activates NK cell killing by recognizing ill-defined molecules on target cells; the other type inhibits the lytic pathway by recognition of self class I MHC molecules. These class I–recognizing receptors on NK cells are biochemically distinct from T-cell receptors. It is believed that NK cells are inhibited from killing normal cells because all nucleated normal cells express self class I MHC molecules. If virus infection or neoplastic transformation perturbs or reduces the expression of class I molecules, inhibitory signals delivered to NK cells are interrupted, and lysis occurs (Fig. 7–5). NK cells also secrete cytokines, such as TNF-α and granulocyte macrophage colony-stimulating factor (GM-CSF), and are believed to be an important source of IFN-γ. Through these soluble mediators, NK cells can influence T- and B-cell function. IFN-γ, in particular, favors the differentiation of T_H1 cells. Thus, activation of NK cells early in the immune response can favor induction of delayed hypersensitivity and secretion of opsonizing (IgG2b) antibodies by promoting the differentiation of T_H1 cells. The lytic activity of NK cells is greatly augmented by the cytokines IL-2 and IL-15. Hence these cytokines may be used to augment the tumoricidal activity of NK cells in vivo.

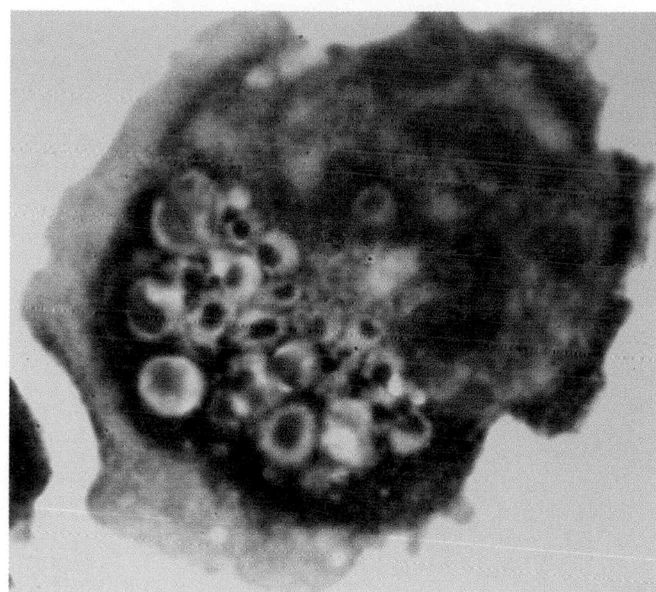

Figure 7–4

A highly activated natural killer cell with abundant cytoplasmic granules. (Courtesy of Dr. Noelle Williams, Department of Pathology, University of Texas Southwestern Medical School, Dallas, TX.)

Cytokines: Messenger Molecules of the Immune System

The induction and regulation of the immune responses involve multiple interactions among lymphocytes, monocytes, inflammatory cells (e.g., neutrophils), and endothelial cells. Many such interactions are cognitive and so depend on cell-to-cell contact; however, many interactions and effector functions are mediated by short-acting soluble mediators, called *cytokines*. This term includes the previously designated lymphokines (lymphocyte derived); monokines

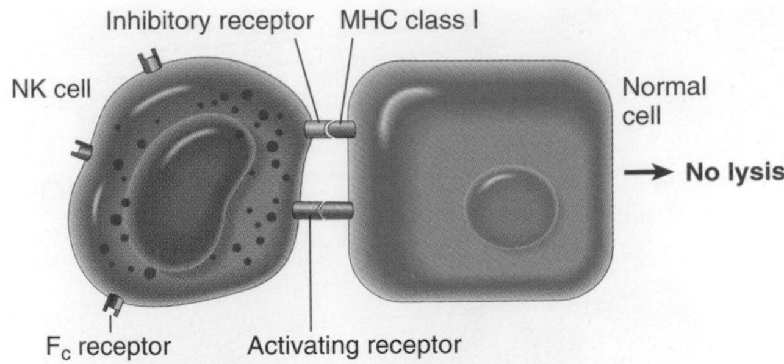

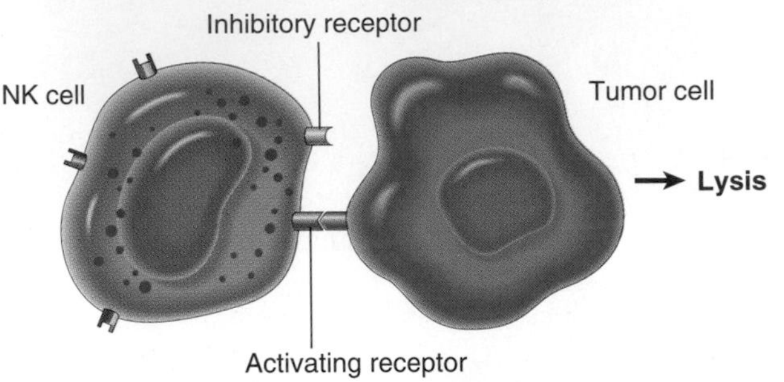

Figure 7–5

Schematic representation of NK cell receptors and killing. Normal cells are not killed because inhibitory signals from normal MHC class I molecules override activating signals. In tumor cells, or virus-infected cells, reduced expression or alteration of MHC molecules interrupts the inhibitory signals, allowing activation of NK cells and lysis of target cells.

(monocyte derived); and several other polypeptides that regulate the immunologic, inflammatory, and reparative host responses. Most cytokines have a wide spectrum of effects, and some are produced by several different cell types.

The currently well-characterized and molecularly cloned cytokines are not listed here because any such list would soon be dwarfed by the torrent of new cytokines being isolated and reported every day. Instead, we classify the currently known cytokines into five categories and list some of their general properties:

- Cytokines that mediate natural immunity. Included in this group are IL-1, TNF-α, type 1 interferons, and IL-6. Certain of these cytokines (e.g., interferons) protect against viral infections, whereas others (e.g., IL-1, TNF-α, IL-6) initiate nonspecific inflammatory responses.
- Cytokines that regulate lymphocyte growth, activation, and differentiation. Within this category are IL-2, IL-4, IL-5, IL-12, IL-15, and transforming growth factor-β (TGF-β). Although some, such as IL-2 and IL-4, favor lymphocyte growth and differentiation, others, such as IL-10 and TGF-β, down-regulate immune responses.
- Cytokines that activate inflammatory cells. In this category are IFN-γ, TNF-α, lymphotoxin (TNF-β), and migration inhibitory factor. Most of these cytokines serve to activate the functions of nonspecific effector cells.
- Cytokines that affect leukocyte movements are also called *chemokines* (Chapter 3). They occur in two structurally distinct subfamilies, referred to as *C-C* and *C-X-C* chemokines, on the basis of the position of cysteine (c) residues. The C-X-C chemokines are produced by activated macrophages and tissue cells (e.g., endothelium), whereas the C-C chemokines are produced largely by T cells. IL-8 is an important C-X-C chemokine, whereas monocyte chemotactic proteins and monocyte inflammatory proteins exemplify C-C chemokines.[5]
- Cytokines that stimulate hematopoiesis. Many cytokines derived from lymphocytes or stromal cells stimulate the growth and production of new blood cells by acting on hematopoietic progenitor cells. Several members of this family are called *colony-stimulating factors* (CSFs) because they were initially detected by their ability to promote the in vitro growth of hematopoietic cell colonies from the bone marrow. Some members of this group (e.g., GM-CSF and G-CSF) act on committed progenitor cells, whereas others, exemplified by stem cell factor (c-kit ligand), act on pluripotent stem cells.

This subdivision of cytokines into functional groups, although convenient, is somewhat arbitrary because, as noted subsequently, many cytokines, such as IL-1, TNF-α, and IFN-γ, are pleiotropic in their effects.

GENERAL PROPERTIES OF CYTOKINES

- Many individual cytokines are produced by several different cell types. For example, IL-1 and TNF-α can be produced by virtually any cell.
- The effects of cytokines are pleiotropic: They act on many cell types. For example, IL-2, initially discovered as a T-cell growth factor, is known to affect the growth and differentiation of B cells and NK cells as well.
- Cytokines induce their effects in three ways: (1) They act on the same cell that produces them (*autocrine* effect), such as occurs when IL-2 produced by activated T cells promotes T-cell growth; (2) they affect other cells in their vicinity (*paracrine* effect), as occurs when IL-7 produced by marrow stromal cells promotes the differentiation of B-cell progenitors in the marrow; and (3) they affect many cells systemically (*endocrine* effect), the best examples in this category being IL-1 and TNF-α, which produce the acute-phase response during inflammation.
- Cytokines mediate their effects by binding to specific high-affinity receptors on their target cells. For example, IL-2 activates T cells by binding to high-affinity IL-2 receptors (IL-2R). Blockade of the IL-2R by specific antireceptor monoclonal antibodies prevents T-cell activation. This observation provides a means by which T-cell activation, when undesirable (as in transplant rejection), may be controlled.

The knowledge gained about cytokines has practical therapeutic ramifications. First, by regulating cytokine production or action, it may be possible to control the harmful effects of inflammation or tissue-damaging immune reactions. Second, recombinant cytokines can be administered to enhance immunity against cancer or microbial infections (immunotherapy). Both of these avenues are currently being pursued on an experimental basis in humans.

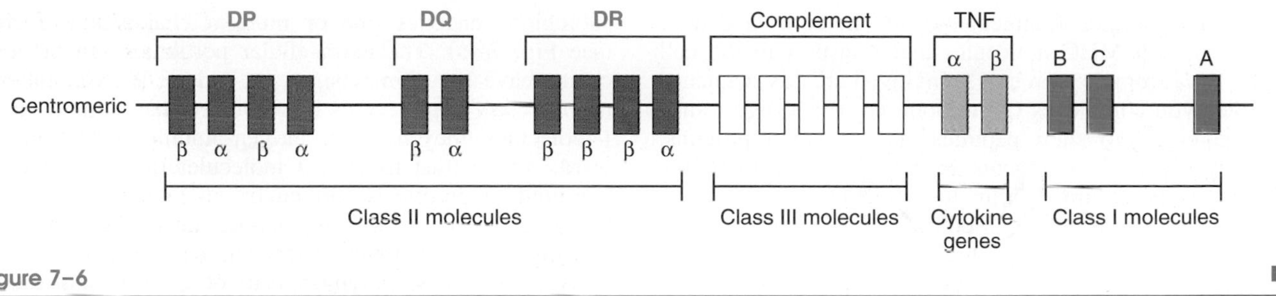

Figure 7–6

Schematic representation of the HLA complex and its subregions. The relative distances between various genes and regions are not drawn to scale.

Structure and Function of Histocompatibility Antigens

Although originally identified as antigens that evoke rejection of transplanted organs, histocompatibility molecules are now known to be extremely important for the induction and regulation of the immune response and for certain nonimmunologic functions. *The principal physiologic function of the cell surface histocompatibility molecules is to bind peptide fragments of foreign proteins for presentation to appropriate antigen-specific T cells.* Recall that T cells (in contrast to B cells) can recognize only membrane-bound antigens, and hence histocompatibility antigens are critical to the induction of T-cell immunity. The histocompatibility molecules and the corresponding genes are complex in structure and are still incompletely understood. Here we summarize only the salient features of human histocompatibility antigens, primarily to facilitate understanding of their role in rejection of organ transplants and in disease susceptibility. Several genes code for histocompatibility antigens, but those that code for the most important transplantation antigens are clustered on a small segment of chromosome 6. This cluster constitutes the human MHC and is also known as the *human leukocyte antigen* (HLA) complex (Fig. 7–6) because MHC-encoded antigens were initially detected on the white cells. The HLA system is highly polymorphic. This, as we see subsequently, constitutes a formidable barrier in organ transplantation.

On the basis of their chemical structure, tissue distribution, and function, the MHC gene products are classified into three categories. Class I and class II genes encode cell surface glycoproteins, and class III genes encode components of the complement system (Chapter 3). The last mentioned, as is well known, are soluble proteins; they are not discussed in this section.

Class I antigens are expressed on all nucleated cells and platelets. They are encoded by three closely linked loci, designated HLA-A, HLA-B, and HLA-C (Fig. 7–6). Each of these molecules is a heterodimer, consisting of a polymorphic α, or heavy, chain (44-kD) linked noncovalently to a smaller (12-kD) nonpolymorphic peptide called β_2-microglobulin. The latter is not encoded within the MHC. The extracellular region of the heavy chain is divided into three domains: α_1, α_2, and α_3 (Fig. 7–7). Crystal structure of class I molecules has revealed that the α_1 and α_2 domains contain a cleft, or groove, where peptides bind to the MHC molecule. Biochemical analyses of several different class I alleles have revealed that almost all polymorphic residues line the sides or the base of the peptide-binding groove. As a result, *different class I alleles bind to different peptide fragments.* In general, class I MHC molecules bind to those peptides that are derived from proteins, such as viral antigens, synthesized within the cell. The

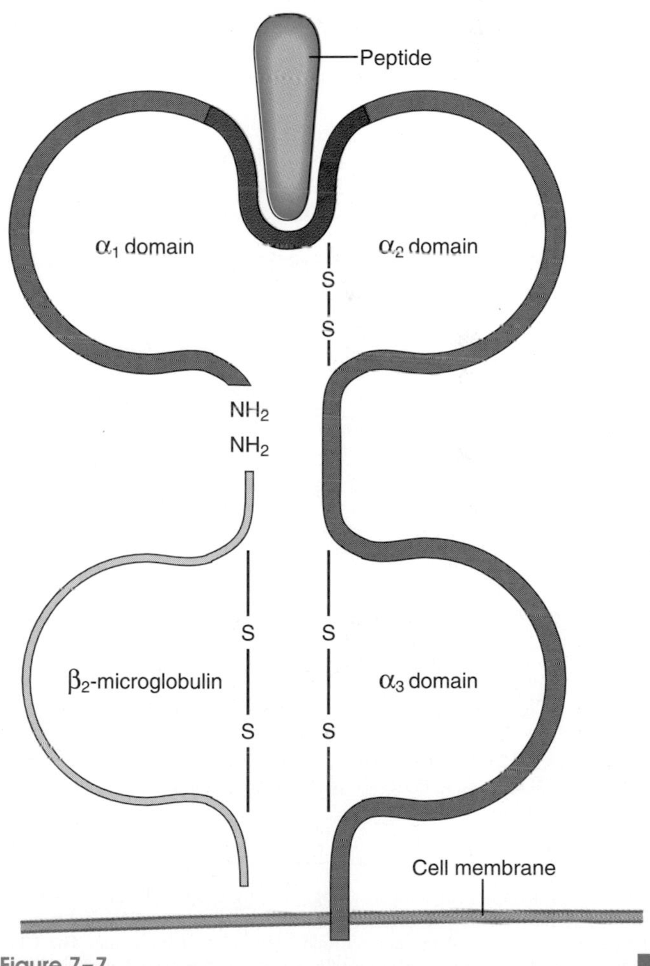

Figure 7–7

Schematic diagram of HLA class I molecule.

generation of peptide fragments within the cells, and their association with MHC molecules and transport to the cell surface, is a complex process.[6] Involved in this sequence are proteolytic complexes (proteosomes), which digest antigenic proteins into short peptides, and transport proteins, which ferry peptide fragments from the cytoplasm to the endoplasmic reticulum. Within the endoplasmic reticulum, peptides bind to the antigen-binding cleft of newly synthesized class I heavy chains, which then associate with β_2-microglobulin to form a stable trimer that is transported to the cell surface for presentation to the CD8+ cytotoxic T lymphocytes (Fig. 7–8). In this interaction, the TCR recognizes the MHC-peptide complex, and the CD8 molecule, acting as a coreceptor, binds to the nonpolymorphic, α_3, domain of the class I heavy chain. CD8+ cytotoxic T cells can recognize viral (or other) peptides only if presented as a complex with self class I antigens. In the eyes of T cells, self MHC molecules are those that they "grew up with" during maturation within the thymus. Because one of the important functions of CD8+ T cells is to eliminate virus-infected T cells, it makes good sense to have widespread expression of class I HLA antigens.

Class II antigens are coded for in a region called *HLA-D*, which has three subregions: HLA-DP, HLA-DQ, and HLA-DR. Each class II molecule is a heterodimer consisting of a noncovalently associated α chain and β chain. Both chains are polymorphic, and each of three HLA-D subregions encodes one or more α chains and β chains (see Fig. 7–6). The extracellular portions of the α and β chains have two domains: α_1, α_2 and β_1, β_2. Crystal structure of class II molecules has revealed that, similar to class I molecules, they have an antigen-binding cleft facing outward.[7] In contrast to class I molecules, however, the antigen-binding groove is formed by an interaction of the α_1 and β_1 domains of both the chains, and it is in this portion that most class II alleles differ. Thus, it seems that, as with class I molecules, polymorphism of class II molecules is associated with differential binding of antigenic peptides. The nature of peptides that bind to class II molecules is different from that of peptides that bind to class I molecules. In general, class II molecules present exogenous antigens (e.g., extracellular microbes, soluble proteins) that are first internalized and processed in the endosomes or lysosomes. Peptides resulting from proteolytic cleavage then associate with class II heterodimers assembled in the endoplasmic reticulum. Finally, the peptide-MHC complex is transported to the cell surface,[8] where it can be recognized by CD4+ helper T cells. In this interaction, the CD4 molecule acts as the coreceptor. Because CD4+ T cells can recognize antigens only in the context of self class II molecules, they are referred to as *class II restricted.* In contrast to class I antigens, the tissue distribution of MHC class II molecules is largely restricted to antigen-presenting cells (macrophages, dendritic cells, and B cells). Expression of class II molecules can be induced on several other cell types, however, including endothelial cells and fibroblasts, by the action of IFN-γ.

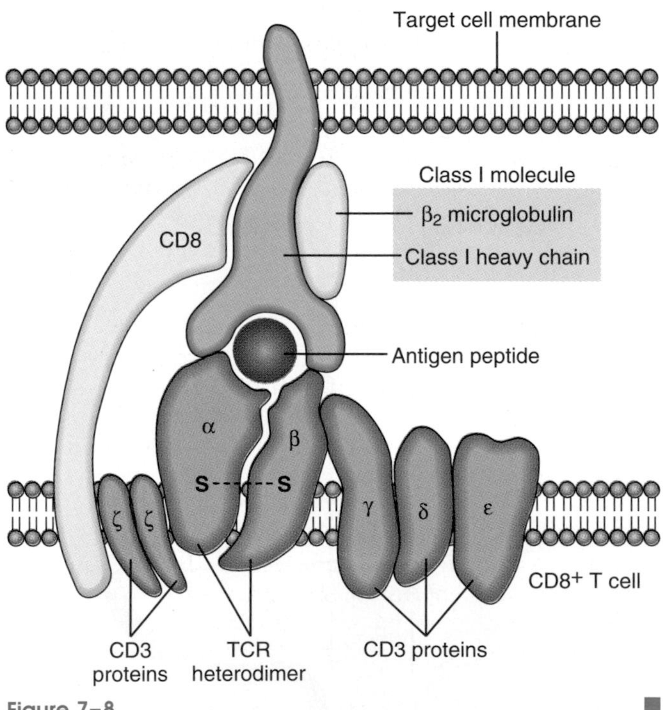

Figure 7–8

Schematic illustration of antigen recognition by CD8 + T cells. Note that the T-cell receptor (TCR heterodimer) recognizes a complex formed by the peptide fragment of the antigen and MHC class I molecule. The CD8 molecule binds to the nonpolymorphic portion of the class I molecule and thus acts as an accessory structure during antigen recognition.

The role of class II antigens in the induction of helper T cells has an important bearing on the genetic regulation of the immune response. How class II molecules regulate immune responses is not entirely clear, but there are two plausible mechanisms:

- One possibility rests on the fact that different antigenic peptides bind to different class II gene products. It follows that an individual mounts a vigorous immune response against an antigen only if he or she inherits the gene(s) for those class II molecule(s) that can bind the nominal antigen and present it to helper T cells. The consequences of inheriting a given class II gene depend on the nature of the antigen bound by the class II molecule. For example, if the antigen was a peptide from ragweed pollen, the individual would be genetically prone to type I hypersensitivity disease. An inherited capacity to bind a bacterial peptide may provide resistance to disease by evoking an antibody response or perhaps induce an autoimmune response if the antibody cross-reacts with normal tissues (see later).
- The other possibility is related to the role of MHC molecules in shaping the T-cell repertoire. During intrathymic differentiation, only T cells that can recognize self MHC molecules are selected for export to the periphery (see later discussion of immunologic tolerance). Thus, the type of MHC molecules that T cells encounter during their differentiation influences the functional capacity of mature peripheral T cells.

Table 7–1. ASSOCIATION OF HLA WITH DISEASE

Disease	HLA Allele	Relative Risk
Ankylosing spondylitis	B27	87.4
Postgonococcal arthritis	B27	14.0
Acute anterior uveitis	B27	14.6
Rheumatoid arthritis	DR4	5.8
Chronic active hepatitis	DR3	13.9
Primary Sjögren syndrome	DR3	9.7
Insulin-dependent diabetes	DR3	5.0
	DR4	6.8
	DR3/DR4	14.3
21-Hydroxylase deficiency	BW47	15.0

HLA AND DISEASE ASSOCIATION

A variety of diseases have been found to be associated with certain HLA types (Table 7–1). The best known is the association between ankylosing spondylitis and HLA-B27; individuals who possess this antigen have a 90-fold greater chance (relative risk) of developing the disease than those who are negative for HLA-B27. The diseases that show association with HLA can be broadly grouped into the following categories: (1) *inflammatory diseases,* including ankylosing spondylitis and several postinfectious arthropathies, all associated with HLA-B27; (2) *inherited errors of metabolism,* such as 21-hydroxylase deficiency (HLA-BW47); and (3) *autoimmune diseases,* including autoimmune endocrinopathies, associated with alleles at the DR locus. The mechanisms underlying these associations are not fully understood. In some cases (e.g., 21-hydroxylase deficiency), the linkage results from the fact that the relevant disease-associated gene, in this case the gene for 21-hydroxylase, maps within the HLA complex. In the case of immunologically mediated disorders, it seems likely that the role of HLA class II molecules in regulating the immunoresponsiveness may be relevant. One may speculate therefore that an association between certain autoimmune diseases and HLA-DR antigens may result from an exaggerated or inappropriate immune response to autoantigens.

DISORDERS OF THE IMMUNE SYSTEM

Having reviewed some fundamentals of basic immunology, we can now turn to general disorders of the immune system and some specific immunologic diseases. These are discussed under four broad headings: (1) *hypersensitivity reactions*, which give rise to immunologic injury in a variety of diseases, discussed throughout this book; (2) *autoimmune diseases*, which are caused by immune reactions against self; (3) *immunologic deficiency syndromes*, which result from relatively distinct, genetically determined or acquired defects in some components of the normal immune response; and (4) *amyloidosis*, a poorly understood disorder having immunologic association.

Mechanisms of Immunologic Tissue Injury (Hypersensitivity Reactions)

Humans live in an environment teeming with substances capable of producing immunologic responses. Contact with antigen leads not only to induction of a protective immune response, but also to reactions that can be damaging to tissues. Exogenous antigens occur in dust, pollens, foods, drugs, microbiologic agents, chemicals, and many blood products used in clinical practice. The immune responses that may result from such exogenous antigens take a variety of forms, ranging from annoying but trivial discomforts, such as itching of the skin, to potentially fatal disease, such as bronchial asthma. The various reactions produced are called *hypersensitivity reactions*, and these can be initiated either by the interaction of antigen with humoral antibody or by cell-mediated immune mechanisms.

Tissue-damaging immune reactions may be evoked not only by exogenous antigens, but also by those that are intrinsic to the body (endogenous). Many of the most important immune diseases are caused by antigens intrinsic to humans. Some antiself immune reactions are triggered by homologous antigens that differ among humans with different genetic backgrounds. Transfusion reactions and graft rejection are examples of immunologic disorders evoked by homologous antigens. Another category of disorders, those incited by autologous antigens, constitutes the important group of autoimmune diseases (discussed later). These diseases appear to arise because of the emergence of immune responses against self-antigens.

Hypersensitivity diseases can be classified on the basis of the immunologic mechanism that mediates the disease (Table 7–2). This approach is of value in clarifying the manner in which the immune response ultimately causes tissue injury and disease.

- In *type I disease*, the immune response releases vasoactive and spasmogenic substances that act on vessels and smooth muscle and proinflammatory cytokines that recruit inflammatory cells.
- In *type II disorders*, humoral antibodies participate directly in injuring cells by predisposing them to phagocytosis or lysis.
- *Type III disorders* are best remembered as *immune complex diseases*, in which humoral antibodies bind antigens and activate complement. The fractions of complement then attract neutrophils, which produce tissue damage by release of lysosomal enzymes and generation of toxic free radicals.
- *Type IV disorders* involve tissue injury in which cell-mediated immune responses with sensitized T lymphocytes are the cause of the cellular and tissue injury.

Prototypes of each of these immune mechanisms are presented in the following sections.

Table 7–2. MECHANISMS OF IMMUNOLOGICALLY MEDIATED DISORDERS

Type	Prototype Disorder	Immune Mechanism
I Anaphylactic type	Anaphylaxis, some forms of bronchial asthma	Formation of IgE (cytotropic) antibody → immediate release of vasoactive amines and other mediators from basophils and mast cells followed by recruitment of other inflammatory cells
II Cytotoxic type	Autoimmune hemolytic anemia, erythroblastosis fetalis, Goodpasture syndrome	Formation of IgG, IgM → Binds to antigen on target cell surface → phagocytosis of target cell or lysis of target cell by C8,9 fraction of activated complement or antibody-dependent cellular cytotoxicity
III Immune complex disease	Arthus reaction, serum sickness, systemic lupus erythematosus, certain forms of acute glomerulonephritis	Antigen-antibody complexes → activated complement → attracted neutrophils → release of lysosomal enzymes and other toxic moieties
IV Cell-mediated (delayed) hypersensitivity	Tuberculosis, contact dermatitis, transplant rejection	Sensitized T lymphocytes → release of lymphokines and T cell–mediated cytotoxicity

TYPE I HYPERSENSITIVITY (ANAPHYLACTIC TYPE)

Type I hypersensitivity may be defined as a rapidly developing immunologic reaction occurring within minutes after the combination of an antigen with antibody bound to mast cells or basophils in individuals previously sensitized to the antigen. It may occur as a systemic disorder or as a local reaction. The systemic reaction usually follows an intravenous injection of an antigen to which the host has already become sensitized. Often within minutes, a state of shock is produced, which is sometimes fatal. Local reactions depend on the portal of entry of the allergen and take the form of localized cutaneous swellings (skin allergy, hives), nasal and conjunctival discharge (allergic rhinitis and conjunctivitis), hay fever, bronchial asthma, or allergic gastroenteritis (food allergy). Many local type I hypersensitivity reactions have two well-defined phases: the *initial response*, characterized by vasodilation, vascular leakage, and, depending on the location, smooth muscle spasm or glandular secretions. These changes usually become evident within 5 to 30 minutes after exposure to an allergen and tend to subside in 60 minutes. In many instances (e.g., allergic rhinitis and bronchial asthma), a *second, late-phase* reaction sets in 2 to 8 hours later without additional exposure to antigen and lasts for several days. This late-phase reaction is characterized by more intense infiltration of tissues with eosinophils, neutrophils, basophils, monocytes, and CD4+ T cells as well as tissue destruction in the form of mucosal epithelial cell damage.

Because mast cells and basophils are central to the development of type I hypersensitivity, we first review some of their salient characteristics and then discuss the immune mechanisms that underlie this form of hypersensitivity.[9] Mast cells are bone marrow–derived cells that are widely distributed in the tissues. They are found predominantly near blood vessels and nerves and in subepithelial sites, where local type I reactions tend to occur. Mast cell cytoplasm contains membrane-bound granules that possess a variety of biologically active mediators. In addition, mast cell granules contain acidic proteoglycans that bind basic dyes such as toluidine blue. Because the stained granules often acquire a color that is different from that of the native dye, they are referred to as *metachromatic* granules. As is detailed next, mast cells and basophils are activated by the cross-linking of high-affinity IgE Fc receptors; in addition, mast cells may also be triggered by several other stimuli, such as complement components C5a and C3a (anaphylatoxins), both of which act by binding to their receptors on the mast cell membrane. Other mast cell secretagogues include macrophage-derived cytokines (e.g., IL-8), some drugs such as codeine and morphine, mellitin (present in bee venom), and physical stimuli (e.g., heat, cold, sunlight). Basophils are similar to mast cells in many respects, including the presence of cell-surface IgE Fc receptors as well as cytoplasmic granules. In contrast to mast cells, however, basophils are not normally present in tissues but rather circulate in the blood in extremely small numbers. Similar to other granulocytes, they can be recruited to inflammatory sites.

In humans, type I reactions are mediated by IgE antibodies. The differentiation of IgE-secreting B cells is highly dependent on the induction of CD4+ helper T cells of the T_H2 type (Fig. 7–9). Hence, T_H2 cells are pivotal in the pathogenesis of type I hypersensitivity.[10] The first step in the synthesis of IgE is the presentation of the antigen (also called *allergen*) to precursors of T_H2 cells by antigen-presenting dendritic cells. The newly minted T_H2 cells produce a cluster of cytokines, including IL-3, IL-4, IL-5, and GM-CSF. Of these, IL-4 is absolutely essential for turning on the IgE-producing B cells and for sustaining the development of T_H2 cells. IL-3, IL-5, and GM-CSF promote the survival of eosinophils, which as we discuss subsequently, are important effectors of type I hypersensitivity. IgE antibodies have a strong tendency to attach to mast cells and basophils, which possess high-affinity receptors for the Fc portion of IgE. *When a mast cell or basophil, armed with cytophilic IgE antibodies, is re-exposed to the specific allergen, a series of reactions takes place, leading eventually to the release of a variety of powerful mediators responsible for the clinical expression of type I hypersensitivity reactions.* In the first step in this sequence, antigen (allergen) is bound to the IgE antibodies previously attached to the mast cells. In this process, multivalent antigens bind to

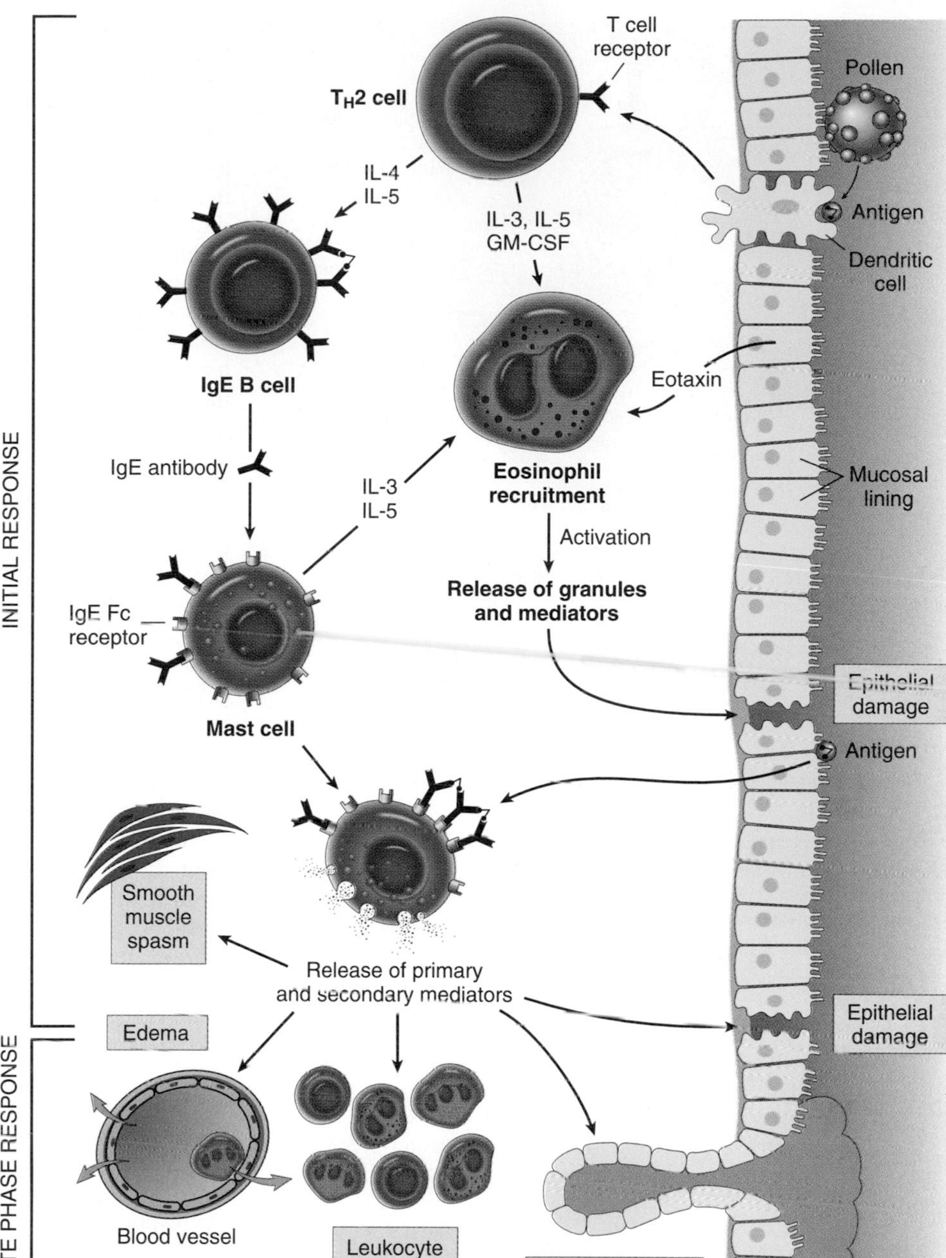

Figure 7–9

Pathogenesis of type I hypersensitivity reaction. T_H2, T-helper type 2 CD4 cells. Late-phase response is dominated by leukocyte infiltration and tissue injury.

more than one IgE molecule and cause cross-linkage of adjacent IgE antibodies. The bridging of IgE molecules activates signal transduction pathways from the cytoplasmic portion of the IgE Fc receptors. These signals initiate two parallel and interdependent processes (Fig. 7–10)—one leading to *mast cell degranulation with discharge of preformed (primary) mediators* and the other involving *de novo synthesis and release of secondary mediators, such as arachidonic metabolites.* These mediators are directly responsible for the initial, sometimes explosive, symptoms of type I hypersensitivity, and they also set into motion the events that lead to the late-phase response.[10a]

Primary Mediators. Primary mediators contained within mast cell granules can be divided into four categories:[11]

- *Biogenic amines*: These include histamine and adenosine. Histamine causes intense bronchial smooth muscle contraction; increased vascular permeability; and increased secretion by nasal, bronchial, and gastric glands. Adenosine enhances mast cell mediator release, causes bronchoconstriction, and inhibits platelet aggregation.
- *Chemotactic mediators*: These include eosinophil chemotactic factor and neutrophil chemotactic factor.
- *Enzymes*: These are contained in the granule matrix and include proteases (chymase, tryptase) and several acid

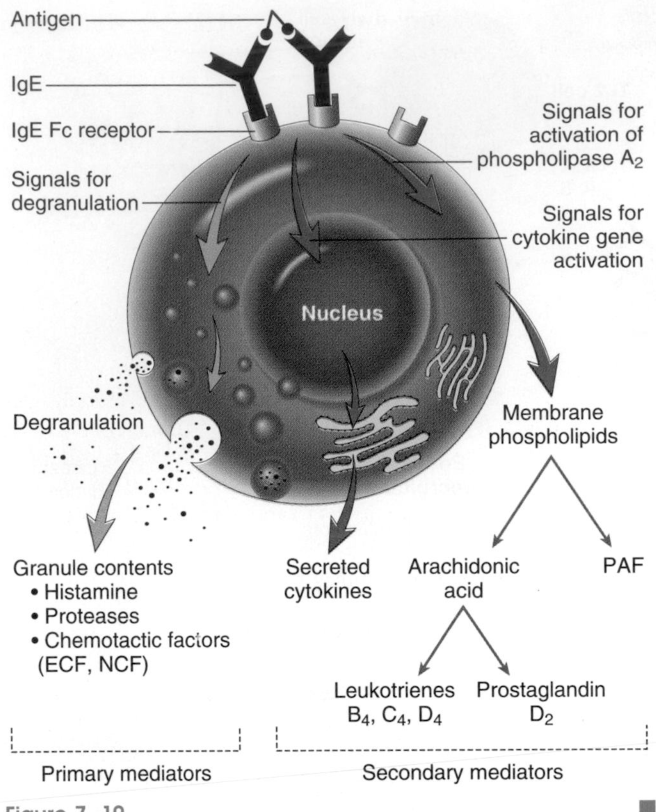

Figure 7–10

Activation of mast cells in type I hypersensitivity and release of their mediators. ECF, eosinophil chemotactic factor; NCF, neutrophil chemotactic factor; PAF, platelet-activating factor.

hydrolases. The enzymes lead to the generation of kinins and activated components of complement (e.g., C3a) by acting on their precursor proteins.

- *Proteoglycans*: These include heparin, a well-known anticoagulant, and chondroitin sulfate. The proteoglycans serve to package and store the other mediators in the granules.

Secondary Mediators. Secondary mediators include two classes of compounds: (1) lipid mediators and (2) cytokines. The lipid mediators are generated by sequential reactions in the mast cell membranes that lead to activation of phospholipase A_2, an enzyme that acts on membrane phospholipids to yield *arachidonic acid.* This is the parent compound from which leukotrienes and prostaglandins are derived by the 5-lipoxygenase and cyclooxygenase pathways (Chapter 3).

- *Leukotrienes*: Leukotrienes are extremely important in the pathogenesis of type I hypersensitivity. *Leukotrienes C_4 and D_4* are the most potent vasoactive and spasmogenic agents known. On a molar basis, they are several thousand times more active than histamine in increasing vascular permeability and causing bronchial smooth muscle contraction. *Leukotriene B_4* is highly chemotactic for neutrophils, eosinophils, and monocytes.
- *Prostaglandin D_2*: This is the most abundant mediator derived by the cyclooxygenase pathway in mast cells. It causes intense bronchospasm as well as increased mucus secretion.
- *Platelet-activating factor*: Platelet-activating factor (PAF) (Chapter 3) is a secondary mediator that causes platelet aggregation, release of histamine, bronchospasm, increased vascular permeability, and vasodilation. In addition, it has important proinflammatory actions. PAF is chemotactic for neutrophils and eosinophils. At higher concentrations, it activates the newly elicited inflammatory cells, causing them to aggregate and degranulate. Because of its ability to recruit and activate inflammatory cells, it is considered important in the initiation of the late-phase response. Although its production is also triggered by the activation of phospholipase A_2, it is not a product of arachidonic acid metabolism.
- *Cytokines*: These polypeptides play an important role in the pathogenesis of type I hypersensitivity reactions because of their ability to recruit and activate inflammatory cells. Mast cells are believed to produce a variety of cytokines, including TNF-α, IL-1, IL-3, IL-4, IL-5, IL-6, and GM-CSF, as well as chemokines, such as macrophage inflammatory protein (MIP)-1α and MIP-1β.[9] Many of these cytokines are produced by T_H2 cells as well, and as mentioned earlier they promote IgE secretion and eosinophil accumulation. In addition, mast cell–derived TNF-α is an important mediator of the inflammatory response seen at the site of allergic inflammation. It may be recalled that TNF-α is a potent cytokine that can attract neutrophils and eosinophils, favor their transmigration through the vasculature, and activate them in the tissues (Chapter 3). Inflammatory cells that accumulate at the sites of type I hypersensitivity reactions are additional sources of cytokines and of histamine-releasing factors that cause further mast cell degranulation.

A variety of chemotactic, vasoactive, and spasmogenic compounds mediate type I hypersensitivity reactions (Table 7–3). Some, such as histamine and leukotrienes, are released rapidly from sensitized mast cells and are believed to be responsible for the intense immediate reactions characterized by edema, mucus secretion, and smooth muscle spasm; many others, exemplified by leukotrienes, PAF, TNF-α, and cytokines, set the stage for the late-phase response by recruiting additional leukocytes, basophils, neutrophils, and eosinophils. Not only do these inflammatory cells release additional waves of mediators (including cytokines), but they also cause epithelial cell damage. Epithelial cells themselves are not passive bystanders in this reaction; they can also produce soluble mediators, such as IL-6, IL-8, and GM-CSF.[12]

Among the cells that are recruited in the late-phase reaction, *eosinophils* are particularly important.[13] Their survival in tissues is favored by IL-3, IL-5, and GM-CSF. These cytokines, as mentioned earlier, are derived from T_H2 cells and mast cells. The chemokines eotaxin and RANTES promote eosinophil chemotaxis. They are released from activated epithelial cells under the influence of mediators such as TNF-α. The armamentarium of eosinophils is as extensive as that of mast cells, and in addition they produce

Table 7–3. SUMMARY OF THE ACTION OF MAST CELL MEDIATORS IN TYPE I HYPERSENSITIVITY

Action	Mediator
Cellular infiltration	Cytokines, e.g., TNF-α Leukotriene B_4 Eosinophil chemotactic factor of anaphylaxis Neutrophil chemotactic factor of anaphylaxis PAF
Vasoactive (vasodilation, increased vascular permeability)	Histamine PAF Leukotrienes C_4, D_4, E_4 Neutral proteases that activate complement and kinins Prostaglandin D_2
Smooth muscle spasm	Leukotrienes C_4, D_4, E_4 Histamine Prostaglandins PAF

PAF, platelet activating factor.

major basic protein and eosinophil cationic protein, which are toxic to epithelial cells. Activated eosinophils and other leukocytes also produce leukotriene C_4 and PAF and directly activate mast cells to release mediators. Thus, *the recruited cells amplify and sustain the inflammatory response without additional exposure to the triggering antigen.* It is now believed that this late-phase inflammatory response is a major cause of symptoms in type I hypersensitivity disorders, such as allergic asthma. Therefore, treatment requires the use of broad-spectrum anti-inflammatory reagents, such as steroids.

To summarize, type I hypersensitivity is a complex disorder resulting from an IgE-mediated triggering of mast cells and subsequent accumulation of inflammatory cells at sites of antigen deposition. These events are regulated in large part by the induction of T_H2-type helper T cells that promote synthesis of IgE and accumulation of inflammatory cells, particularly eosinophils. The clinical features result from release of mast cell mediators as well as the accumulation of an eosinophil-rich inflammatory exudate. With this consideration of the basic mechanisms of type I hypersensitivity, we turn to some conditions that are important examples of IgE-mediated disease.

Systemic Anaphylaxis

In humans, systemic anaphylaxis may occur after administration of heterologous proteins (e.g., antisera), hormones, enzymes, polysaccharides, and drugs (such as the antibiotic penicillin).[14] The severity of the disorder varies with the level of sensitization. The shock dose of antigen, however, may be exceedingly small, as, for example, the tiny amounts used in ordinary skin testing for various forms of allergies. Within minutes after exposure, itching, hives, and skin erythema appear, followed shortly thereafter by a striking contraction of respiratory bronchioles and the appearance of respiratory distress. Laryngeal edema results in hoarseness. Vomiting, abdominal cramps, diarrhea, and laryngeal obstruction follow, and the patient may go into shock and even die within the hour. It is obvious that the effects of anaphylaxis must always be borne in mind when a therapeutic agent is administered. Although patients at risk can generally be identified by a previous history of some form of allergy, the absence of such a history does not preclude the possibility of an anaphylactic reaction.

Local Anaphylaxis

Local anaphylaxis reactions are exemplified by so-called atopic allergy. The term *atopy* implies a genetically determined predisposition to develop localized anaphylactic reactions to inhaled or ingested allergens. About 10% of the population suffers from allergies involving localized anaphylactic reactions to extrinsic allergens, such as pollen, animal dander, house dust, fish, and the like. Specific diseases include urticaria, angioedema, allergic rhinitis (hay fever), and some forms of asthma, all discussed elsewhere in this book. Of interest is the familial predisposition to the development of this type of allergy. A positive family history of allergy is found in 50% of atopic individuals. The basis of familial predisposition is not clear, but studies in patients with asthma reveal linkage to several loci, some of which map near the genes whose products regulate the IgE response.[15] Candidate genes have been mapped to 5q31, where genes for the cytokines IL-3, IL-4, IL-5, IL-9, IL-13, and GM-CSF are located; linkage has also been noted to 6p, close to the HLA complex.[16] Atopic individuals tend to have higher serum IgE levels, as compared with the general population. Perhaps in those genetically prone to develop allergies, environmental antigens preferentially activate the T_H2 pathway. Such genetic predisposition can be clearly demonstrated in experimental animals exposed to helminth infections.

TYPE II HYPERSENSITIVITY

Type II hypersensitivity is mediated by antibodies directed toward antigens present on the surface of cells or other tissue components. The antigenic determinants may be intrinsic to the cell membrane, or they may take the form of an exogenous antigen, such as a drug metabolite, adsorbed on the cell surface. In either case, the hypersensitivity reaction results from the binding of antibodies to normal or altered cell-surface antigens. Three different antibody-dependent mechanisms involved in this type of reaction are depicted in Figure 7–11 and described next.

Complement-Dependent Reactions

There are two mechanisms by which antibody and complement may mediate type II hypersensitivity: direct lysis and opsonization. In the first pattern, antibody (IgM or IgG) reacts with an antigen present on the surface of the cell, causing activation of the complement system and resulting in the assembly of the membrane attack complex that disrupts membrane integrity by "drilling holes" through the lipid bilayer. In the second pattern, the cells become susceptible to phagocytosis by fixation of antibody or C3b fragment to the cell surface (opsonization). This

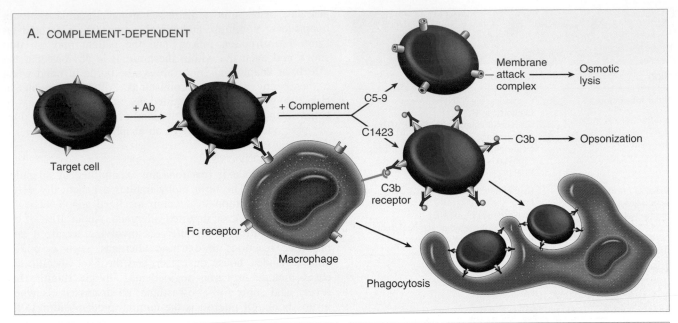

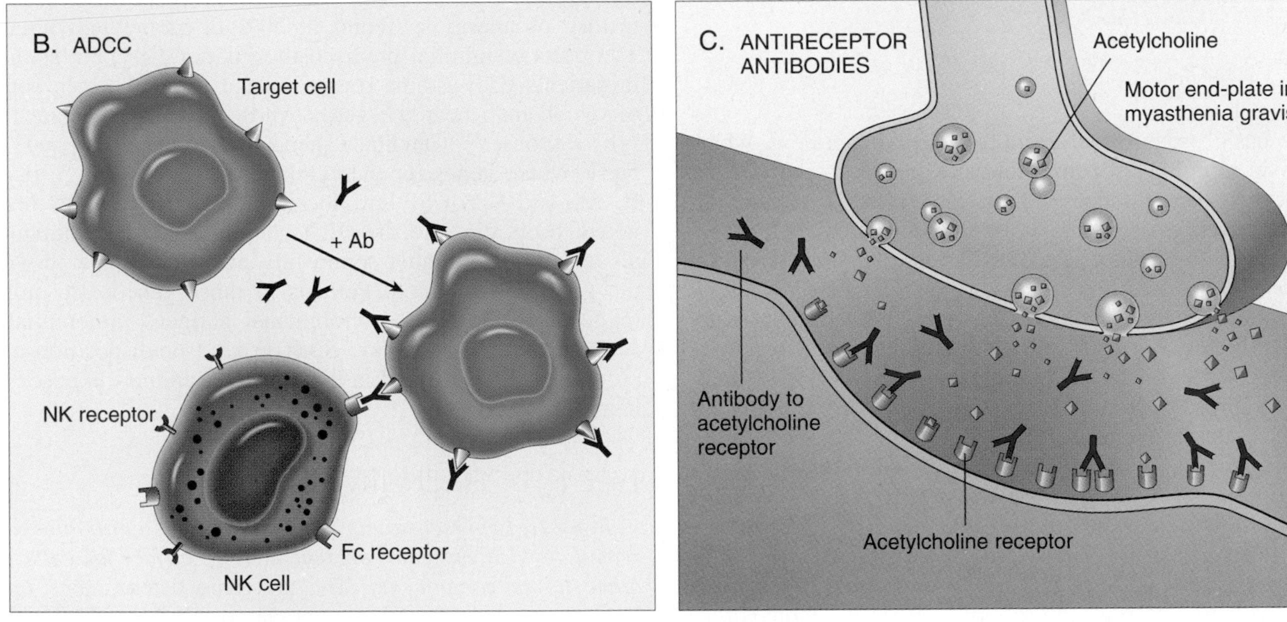

Figure 7–11

Schematic illustration of three different mechanisms of antibody-mediated injury in type II hypersensitivity. *A*, Complement-dependent reactions that lead to lysis of cells or render them susceptible to phagocytosis. *B*, Antibody-dependent cell-mediated cytotoxicity (ADCC). IgG-coated target cells are killed by cells that bear Fc receptors for IgG (e.g., NK cells, macrophages). *C*, Antireceptor antibodies disturb the normal function of receptors. In this example, acetylcholine receptor antibodies impair neuromuscular transmission in myasthenia gravis.

form of type II hypersensitivity most commonly involves blood cells—red blood cells, white blood cells, and platelets—but the antibodies can also be directed against extracellular tissue (e.g., glomerular basement membrane in anti–glomerular basement membrane nephritis) (Chapter 21). Clinically, such reactions occur in the following situations: (1) *transfusion reactions*, in which cells from an incompatible donor react with autochthonous antibody of the host; (2) *erythroblastosis fetalis*, in which there is an antigenic difference between the mother and the fetus, and antibodies (of the IgG class) from the mother cross the placenta and cause destruction of fetal red cells; (3) *autoimmune hemolytic anemia, agranulocytosis*, or *thrombocytopenia*, in which individuals produce antibodies to their own blood cells, which are then destroyed; (4) *pemphigus vulgaris*, in which antibodies against desmosomes disrupt intercellular junctions in epidermis, leading to the formation of skin vesicles; and (5) *certain drug reactions*, in which antibodies are produced that react with the drug, which may be complexed to red cell antigen.

Table 7–4. SELECTED EXAMPLES OF TYPE II HYPERSENSITIVITY DISORDERS

Disease	Clinical Features	Antibody Specificity
Goodpasture syndrome	Nephritis and lung hemorrhages (Chapters 16 and 21)	Type IV collagen in basement membranes of glomeruli and lung alveoli
Bullous pemphigoid	Skin vesicles (Chapter 27)	Epidermal basement membrane proteins
Pernicious anemia	Megaloblastic anemia (Chapter 14)	Intrinsic factor and gastric parietal cells
Vasculitides (many forms)	Varied (Chapter 12)	Neutrophil cytoplasmic antibodies
Thrombotic phenomena	Varied (Chapter 12)	Antiphospholipid antibodies
Acute rheumatic fever	Carditis (Chapter 13)	Antibodies against streptococcal antigens cross-react with heart

Antibody-Dependent Cell-Mediated Cytotoxicity

This form of antibody-mediated cell injury does not involve fixation of complement but instead requires the cooperation of leukocytes. The target cells, coated with low concentrations of IgG antibody, are killed by a variety of *nonsensitized* cells that have Fc receptors. The latter bind to the target by their receptors for the Fc fragment of IgG, and *cell lysis proceeds without phagocytosis.* ADCC may be mediated by monocytes, neutrophils, eosinophils, and NK cells. Although in most instances, IgG antibodies are involved in ADCC, in certain cases (e.g., eosinophil-mediated cytotoxicity against parasites), IgE antibodies are used. ADCC may be relevant to the destruction of targets too large to be phagocytosed, such as parasites or tumor cells, and it may also play some role in graft rejection.

Antibody-Mediated Cellular Dysfunction

In some cases, antibodies directed against cell surface receptors impair or dysregulate function without causing cell injury or inflammation. For example, in myasthenia gravis, antibodies reactive with acetylcholine receptors in the motor end plates of skeletal muscles impair neuromuscular transmission and therefore cause muscle weakness. The converse (i.e., antibody-mediated stimulation of cell function) is noted in Graves disease. In this disorder, antibodies against the thyroid-stimulating hormone receptor on thyroid epithelial cells stimulate the cells, resulting in hyperthyroidism. Some additional examples of type II hypersensitivity disorders are listed in Table 7–4.

TYPE III HYPERSENSITIVITY (IMMUNE COMPLEX MEDIATED)

Type III hypersensitivity reaction is induced by antigen-antibody complexes that produce tissue damage as a result of their capacity to activate the complement system. The toxic reaction is initiated when antigen combines with antibody, whether within the circulation (circulating immune complexes) or at extravascular sites where antigen may have been deposited (in situ immune complexes). Some forms of glomerulonephritis in which immune complexes are formed in situ after initial implantation of the antigen on the glomerular basement membrane are discussed in Chapter 21. Complexes formed in the circulation produce damage, particularly as they localize within blood vessel walls or when they are trapped in filtering structures, such as the renal glomerulus. *The mere formation of antigen-antibody complexes in the circulation does not imply the presence of disease*; immune complexes are formed during many immune responses and represent a normal mechanism of antigen removal. The factors that determine whether the immune complexes formed in circulation will be pathogenic are not fully understood, but some possible influences are discussed later.

Two general types of antigens cause immune complex–mediated injury: (1) The antigen may be *exogenous*, such as a foreign protein, a bacterium, or a virus, but (2) under some circumstances, the individual can produce antibody against self components—*endogenous antigens* (Table 7–5). The latter can be trace components present in the blood or, more commonly, antigenic components in cells and tissues. Immune complex–mediated diseases can be *generalized*, if immune complexes are formed in the circulation and are deposited in many organs, or *localized* to particular organs, such as the kidney (glomerulonephritis), joints (arthritis), or the small blood vessels of the skin if the complexes are formed and deposited locally (the local Arthus reaction). These two patterns are considered separately.

Table 7–5. SOME ANTIGENS ASSOCIATED WITH IMMUNE COMPLEX DISORDERS

Antigens		Clinical Manifestations
Exogenous		
Infectious agents		
Bacteria:	Streptococci	Glomerulonephritis, infective endocarditis
	Yersinia enterocolitica	Arthritis
	Treponema pallidum	Glomerulonephritis
Viruses:	Hepatitis B	Polyarteritis nodosa
	Cytomegalovirus	
Parasites:	*Plasmodium* sp.	Glomerulonephritis
	Schistosoma sp.	
Fungi:	*Actinomycetes*	Farmer's lung
Drugs or chemicals		
Foreign serum (antithymocyte globulin)		Serum sickness
Quinidine		Hemolytic anemia
Heroin		Glomerulonephritis
Endogenous		
Nuclear antigens		Systemic lupus erythematosus
Immunoglobulins		Rheumatoid arthritis
Tumor antigens		Glomerulonephritis

Systemic Immune Complex Disease

Acute serum sickness is the prototype of a systemic immune complex disease; it was at one time a frequent sequela to the administration of large amounts of foreign serum (e.g., horse antitetanus serum) used for passive immunization. It is now seen infrequently and in different clinical settings. For example, serum sickness may occur after administration of horse antithymocyte globulin for treatment of aplastic anemia or antibiotic therapy for microbial diseases.[17]

For the sake of discussion, the pathogenesis of systemic immune complex disease can be resolved into three phases: (1) *formation of antigen-antibody complexes in the circulation* and (2) *deposition of the immune complexes in various tissues, thus initiating* (3) *an inflammatory reaction in dispersed sites throughout the body* (Fig. 7–12). The *first phase* is initiated by the introduction of antigen into the circulation and its interaction with immunocompetent cells, resulting in the formation of antibodies. Approximately 5 days after serum injection, antibodies directed against the serum components are produced; these react with the antigen still present in the circulation to form antigen-antibody complexes. In the *second phase*, antigen-antibody complexes formed in the circulation are deposited in various tissues. The factors that determine whether immune complex formation will lead to tissue deposition and disease are not fully understood, but two possible influences are the size of the immune complexes and the functional status of the mononuclear phagocyte system:

- Large complexes formed in great antibody excess are rapidly removed from the circulation by the mononuclear phagocyte system cells and are therefore relatively harmless. The most pathogenic complexes are of small or intermediate size (formed in slight antigen excess), circulate longer, and bind less avidly to phagocytic cells.
- Because the mononuclear phagocyte system normally filters out the circulating immune complexes, its overload or intrinsic dysfunction increases the probability of persistence of immune complexes in circulation and tissue deposition.

In addition, several other factors, such as charge of the immune complexes (anionic versus cationic), valency of the antigen, avidity of the antibody, affinity of the antigen to various tissue components, three-dimensional (lattice) structure of the complexes, and hemodynamic factors, influence their tissue deposition. Because most of these influences have been investigated with reference to deposition of immune complexes in the glomeruli, they are discussed further in Chapter 21. In addition to the renal glomeruli, the favored sites of immune complex deposition are joints, skin, heart, serosal surfaces, and small blood vessels.

For complexes to leave the microcirculation and deposit within or outside the vessel wall, an increase in vascular permeability must occur. This is believed to occur when immune complexes bind to inflammatory cells through their Fc or C3b receptors and trigger release of vasoactive mediators as well as permeability-enhancing cytokines. Once complexes are deposited in the tissues, they initiate an acute inflammatory reaction (*phase three*). During this phase (approximately 10 days after antigen administration), clinical features such as fever, urticaria, arthralgias, lymph node enlargement, and proteinuria appear.

Wherever complexes deposit, the tissue damage is similar (Fig. 7–12). Two mechanisms are believed to operate:

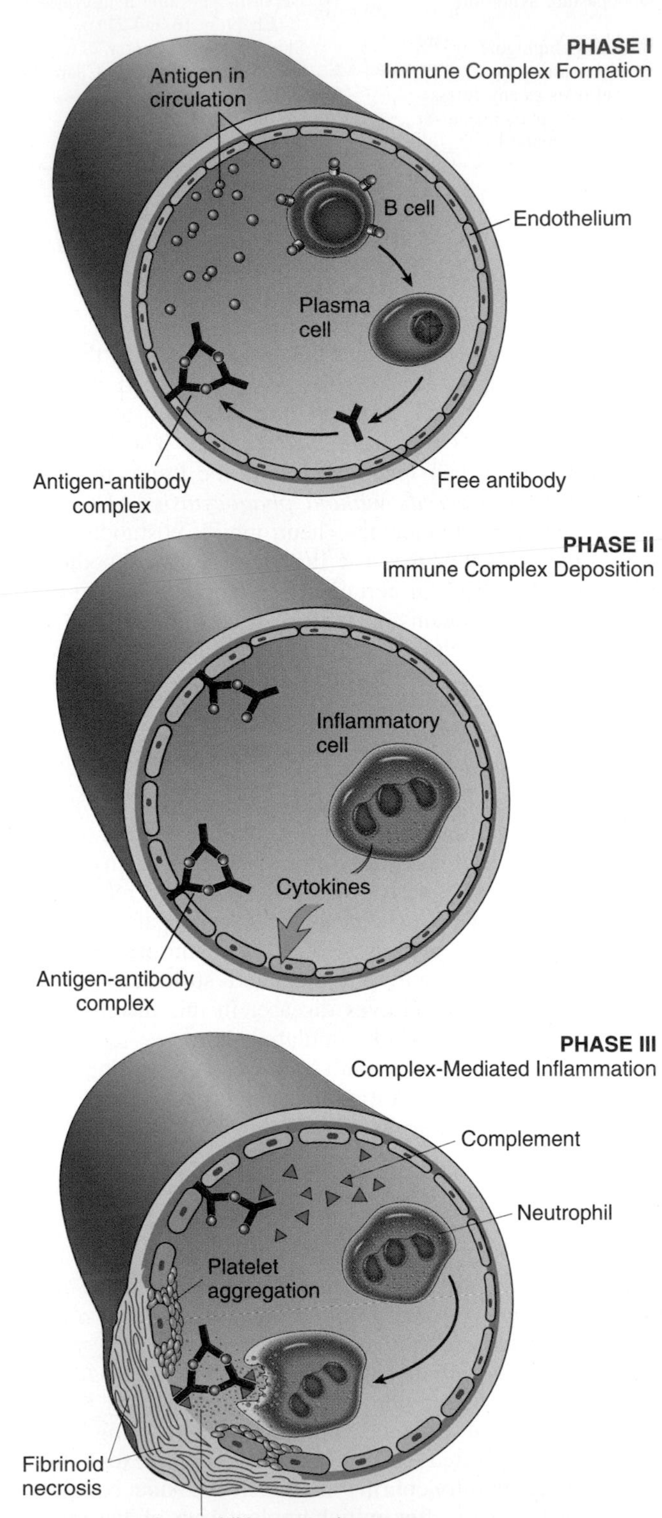

Figure 7–12

Schematic illustration of the three sequential phases in the induction of systemic type III (immune complex) hypersensitivity.

(1) activation of the complement cascade and (2) activation of neutrophils and macrophages through their Fc receptors. Each of these is described next. As discussed in Chapter 3, complement activation has several proinflammatory effects:

- Release of C3b, the opsonin that promotes phagocytosis of particles and organisms
- Production of chemotactic factors, which direct the migration of polymorphonuclear leukocytes and monocytes (C5 fragments, C5b67)
- Release of anaphylatoxins (C3a and C5a), which increase vascular permeability and cause contraction of smooth muscle
- Formation of membrane attack complex (C5-9), causing cell membrane damage or even cytolysis

Neutrophils and macrophages can be activated by immune complexes even in the absence of complement. These cells have Fc receptors for IgG and therefore can bind to the Fc portion of the antigen-complexed IgG. When several Fc receptor molecules are so occupied by aggregates of immune complexes, the inflammatory cells are activated.

With either scenario, phagocytosis of antigen-antibody complexes by leukocytes drawn in by the chemotactic factors results in the release or generation of a variety of additional proinflammatory substances, including prostaglandins, vasodilator peptides, and chemotactic substances, as well as several lysosomal enzymes, including proteases capable of digesting basement membrane, collagen, elastin, and cartilage. Tissue damage is also mediated by free oxygen radicals produced by activated neutrophils. Immune complexes have several other effects: They cause aggregation of platelets and activate Hageman factor; both of these reactions augment the inflammatory process and initiate the formation of microthrombi (Fig. 7–13). The resultant pathologic lesion is termed *vasculitis* if it occurs in blood vessels, *glomerulonephritis* if it occurs in renal glomeruli, *arthritis* if it occurs in the joints, and so on.

It is clear from the foregoing that complement-fixing antibodies (i.e., IgG and IgM) induce these lesions. Because IgA can activate complement by the alternate pathway, IgA-containing complexes may also induce tissue injury. The important role of complement in the pathogenesis of the tissue injury is supported by the observation that experimental depletion of serum complement levels greatly reduces the severity of the lesions, as does depletion of neutrophils. *During the active phase of the disease, consumption of complement decreases the serum levels.*

MORPHOLOGY. The morphologic consequences of immune complex injury are dominated by acute necrotizing vasculitis, with deposits of fibrinoid and intense neutrophilic exudation permeating the entire arterial wall, similar to the changes that we describe for polyarteritis nodosa (Fig. 7–14). Affected glomeruli are hypercellular because of swelling and proliferation of endothelial and mesangial cells, accompanied by neutrophilic and monocytic infiltration. **The complexes can be seen on immunofluorescence microscopy as granular lumpy deposits of immunoglobulin and complement** and on electron microscopy as electron dense deposits along the glomerular basement membrane (see Figs. 7–26 and 7–27).

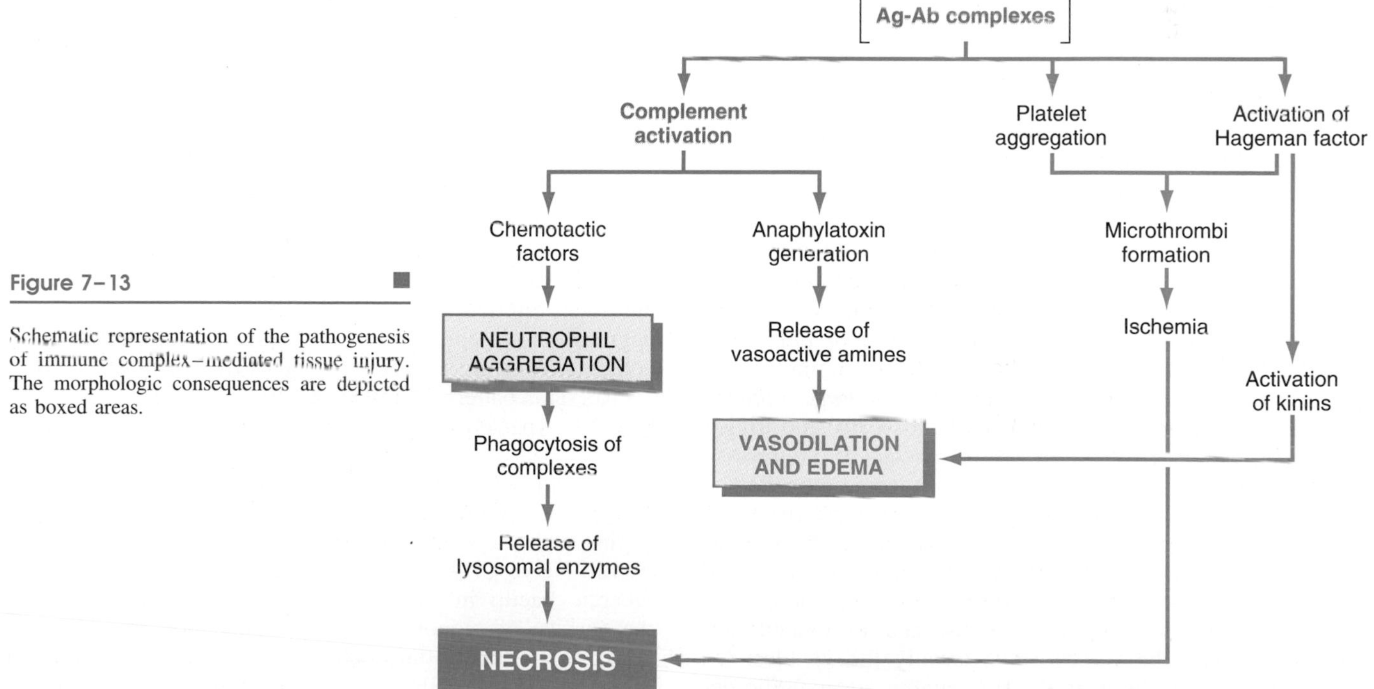

Figure 7–13

Schematic representation of the pathogenesis of immune complex–mediated tissue injury. The morphologic consequences are depicted as boxed areas.

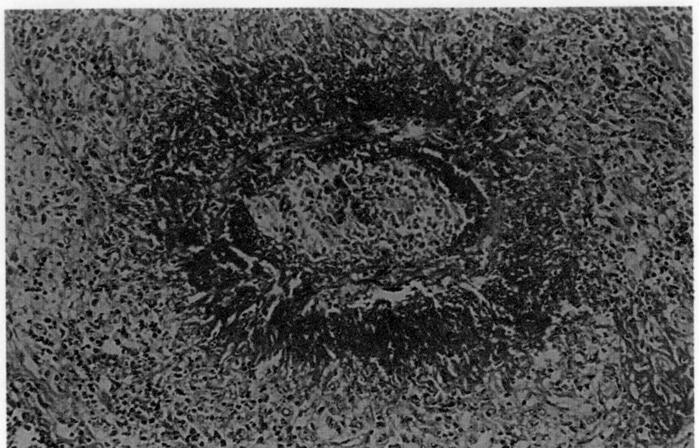

Figure 7–14

Immune complex vasculitis. The necrotic vessel wall is replaced by smudgy, pink "fibrinoid" material. (Courtesy of Dr. Trace Worrell, Department of Pathology, University of Texas Southwestern Medical School, Dallas, TX.)

If the disease results from a single large exposure to antigen (e.g., acute poststreptococcal glomerulonephritis and acute serum sickness), all lesions tend to resolve, owing to catabolism of the immune complexes. A *chronic form of serum sickness* results from repeated or prolonged exposure to an antigen. Continuous antigenemia is necessary for the development of chronic immune complex disease because, as stated earlier, complexes in antigen excess are the ones most likely to be deposited in vascular beds. This occurs in several human diseases, such as systemic lupus erythematosus (SLE), which is associated with persistent exposure to autoantigens. Often, however, despite the fact that the morphologic changes and other findings suggest immune complex disease, the inciting antigens are unknown. Included in this category are rheumatoid arthritis, polyarteritis nodosa, membranous glomerulonephritis, and several other vasculitides.

Local Immune Complex Disease (Arthus Reaction)

The Arthus reaction is defined as a localized area of tissue necrosis resulting from acute immune complex vasculitis, usually elicited in the skin. The reaction can be produced experimentally by intracutaneous injection of antigen in *an immune animal having circulating antibodies against the antigen.* Because of the excess of antibodies, as the antigen diffuses into the vascular wall, large immune complexes are formed, which precipitate locally and trigger the inflammatory reaction already discussed. In contrast to IgE-mediated type I reactions, which appear immediately, the Arthus lesion develops over a few hours and reaches a peak 4 to 10 hours after injection, when it can be seen as an area of visible edema with severe hemorrhage followed occasionally by ulceration. Immunofluorescent stains disclose complement, immunoglobulins, and fibrinogen precipitated within the vessel walls, usually the venules. On light microscopy, these produce a smudgy eosinophilic deposit that obscures the underlying cellular detail, an appearance termed *fibrinoid necrosis* of the vessels (Fig. 7–14). Rupture of these vessels may produce local hemorrhages, but more often the vascular lumens undergo thrombosis, adding an element of local ischemic injury.

TYPE IV HYPERSENSITIVITY (CELL MEDIATED)

The cell-mediated type of hypersensitivity is initiated by specifically sensitized T lymphocytes. It includes the classic *delayed-type hypersensitivity reactions initiated by CD4 T cells and direct cell cytotoxicity mediated by CD8 T cells.* It is the principal pattern of immunologic response not only to a variety of intracellular microbiologic agents, particularly *Mycobacterium tuberculosis,* but also to many viruses, fungi, protozoa, and parasites. So-called contact skin sensitivity to chemical agents and graft rejection are other instances of cell-mediated reactions. Two forms of type IV hypersensitivity are described next.

Delayed-Type Hypersensitivity

The classic example of delayed hypersensitivity is the *tuberculin reaction,* which is produced by the intracutaneous injection of tuberculin, a protein-lipopolysaccharide component of the tubercle bacillus. In a previously sensitized individual, reddening and induration of the site appear in 8 to 12 hours, reach a peak in 24 to 72 hours, and thereafter slowly subside. Morphologically, delayed-type hypersensitivity is characterized by the accumulation of mononuclear cells around small veins and venules, producing a perivascular "cuffing." There is an associated increased microvascular permeability caused by mechanisms similar to those in other forms of inflammation (Chapter 3). Not unexpectedly, there is an escape of plasma proteins, giving rise to dermal edema and deposition of fibrin in the interstitium. The latter appears to be the main cause of induration, which is characteristic of delayed hypersensitivity skin lesions. In fully developed lesions, the lymphocyte-cuffed venules show marked endothelial hypertrophy and, in some cases, hyperplasia. Immunoperoxidase staining of the lesions reveals a preponderance of CD4 (helper) T lymphocytes (Fig. 7–15).

With certain persistent or nondegradable antigens, such as tubercle bacilli, the initial perivascular lymphocytic infiltrate is replaced by macrophages over a period of 2 or 3 weeks. The accumulated macrophages often undergo a morphologic transformation into epithelium-like cells and are then referred to as *epithelioid cells.* A microscopic aggregation of epithelioid cells, usually surrounded by a collar of *lymphocytes, is referred to as a granuloma* (Fig. 7–16). This pattern of inflammation that is characteristic of type IV hypersensitivity is called *granulomatous inflammation.*

The sequence of cellular events in delayed hypersensitivity can be exemplified by the tuberculin reaction, which begins with the first exposure of the individual to tubercle bacilli. Naive CD4 T cells recognize peptides derived from tubercle bacilli in association with class II molecules on the surface of monocytes or epidermal dendritic (Langerhans) cells. This initial encounter drives the differentiation of naive CD4 T cells to T_H1 cells. The induction of T_H1

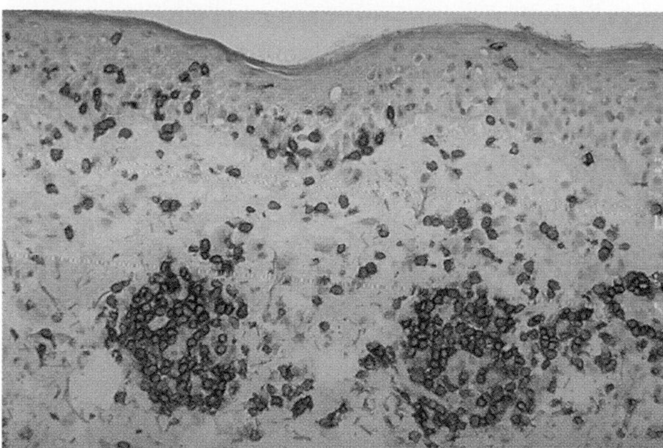

Figure 7–15

Delayed hypersensitivity in the skin. Immunoperoxidase staining reveals a predominantly perivascular cellular infiltrate that marks positively with anti-CD4 antibodies. (Courtesy of Dr. Louis Picker, Department of Pathology, University of Texas Southwestern Medical School, Dallas, TX.)

cells is of signal importance because the expression of delayed hypersensitivity depends in large part on the cytokines secreted by T_H1 cells. Why certain antigens preferentially induce the T_H1 response is not entirely clear, but the cytokine milieu in which naive CD4 T cells are activated seems to be relevant,[3] as discussed subsequently. Some of the sensitized T_H1 cells so formed enter the circulation and remain in the memory pool of T cells for long periods, sometimes years. On intracutaneous injection of tuberculin in an individual previously exposed to tubercle bacilli, the memory T_H1 cells interact with the antigen on the surface of antigen-presenting cells and are activated (i.e., they undergo blast transformation and proliferation). These changes are accompanied by the secretion of the T_H1 type cytokines, which are responsible for the expression of delayed-type hypersensitivity (Fig. 7–17). Cytokines most relevant to this reaction and their actions are as follows:

- IL-12, a cytokine produced by macrophages, is critical for the induction of the T_H1 response and hence delayed hypersensitivity. On initial encounter with a microbe, the resting macrophages attempt to phagocytose and kill the organism. The resting macrophages are not particularly adept at these functions. Nevertheless, this interaction leads to the production of IL-12, which, in turn, drives the differentiation of naive CD4+ helper cells (also called T_H0 cells) to T_H1 cells. These, in turn, produce other cytokines, listed below. IL-12 is also a potent inducer of IFN-γ secretion by T cells and NK cells. IFN-γ further augments the differentiation of T_H1 cells.
- IFN-γ has many effects and is an extremely important mediator of delayed-type hypersensitivity. It is a powerful activator of macrophages, causing further secretion of IL-12. Activated macrophages are altered in several ways: Their ability to phagocytose and kill microorganisms is markedly augmented; they express more class II molecules on the surface, thus facilitating further antigen presentation; their capacity to kill tumor cells is enhanced; and they secrete several polypeptide growth factors, such as platelet-derived growth factor and TGF-β, that stimulate fibroblast proliferation and augment

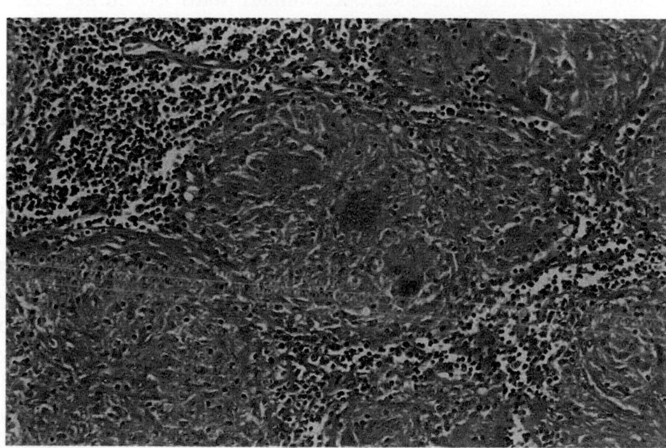

Figure 7–16

A section of a lymph node shows several granulomas, each made up of an aggregate of epithelioid cells and surrounded by lymphocytes. The granuloma in the center shows several multinucleate giant cells. (Courtesy of Dr. Trace Worrell, Department of Pathology, University of Texas Southwestern Medical School, Dallas, TX.)

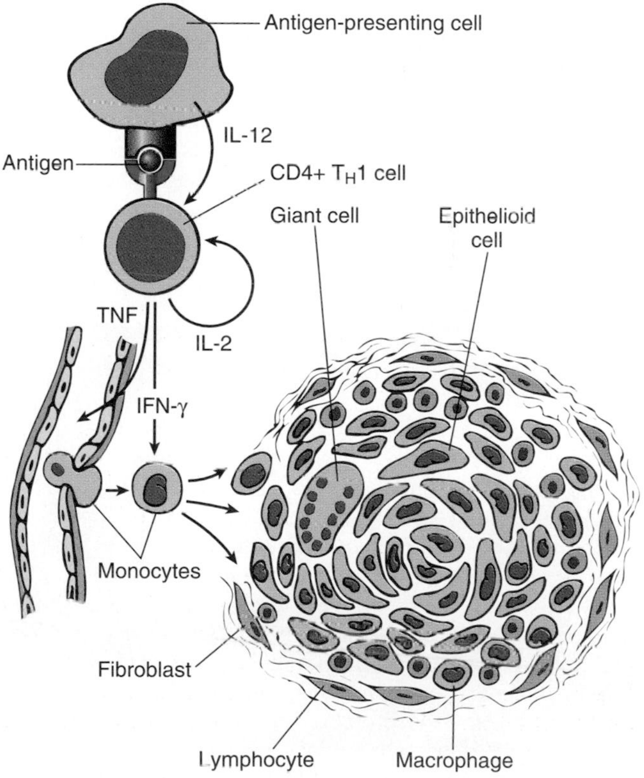

Figure 7–17

Schematic illustration of the events that give rise to the formation of granuloma in type IV hypersensitivity reactions. Note the role played by T cell–derived cytokines.

collagen synthesis. Thus activated, macrophages serve to eliminate the offending antigen, and if the activation is sustained, fibrosis results.

- IL-2 causes autocrine and paracrine proliferation of T cells, which accumulate at sites of delayed hypersensitivity; included in this infiltrate are some antigen-specific CD4+ T_H1 cells and many more bystander T cells activated by IL-2.
- TNF-α and lymphotoxin are two cytokines that exert important effects on endothelial cells: (1) increased secretion of prostacyclin, which, in turn, favors increased blood flow by causing local vasodilation; (2) increased expression of E-selectin (Chapter 3), an adhesion molecule that promotes attachment of the passing lymphocytes and monocytes; and (3) induction and secretion of low-molecular-weight chemotactic factors such as IL-8. Together, all these changes in the endothelium facilitate the extravasation of lymphocytes and monocytes at the site of the delayed hypersensitivity reaction. The process by which T cells and monocytes exit the vasculature is generally similar to that described for neutrophils in Chapter 3. Involved is initial rolling on the endothelium, followed by up-regulation of integrins and firm adhesion, and, ultimately, transmigration through the vessel wall.

This type of hypersensitivity is a major mechanism of defense against a variety of intracellular pathogens, including mycobacteria, fungi, and certain parasites, and may also be involved in transplant rejection and tumor immunity. In addition to its beneficial, protective role, delayed-type hypersensitivity can also be a cause of disease. *Contact dermatitis* is a common example of tissue injury resulting from delayed hypersensitivity. It is evoked by coming in contact with urshiol, the antigenic component of poison ivy or poison oak, and manifests in the form of a vesicular dermatitis (Fig. 7–18). The basic mechanism is similar to that described for tuberculin sensitivity. On reexposure to the plants, the sensitized CD4+ cells of the T_H1 type first accumulate in the dermis, then migrate toward the antigen within the epidermis. Here they release cytokines that damage keratinocytes, causing separation of these cells and formation of an intraepidermal vesicle (Fig. 7–18). In this form of delayed hypersensitivity, there is evidence that, in addition to CD4+ cells, some CD8+ cells may also be involved. In certain other forms of delayed hypersensitivity reactions, especially those that follow viral infections, cytokine-producing CD8+ cells may be the dominant effector cells.

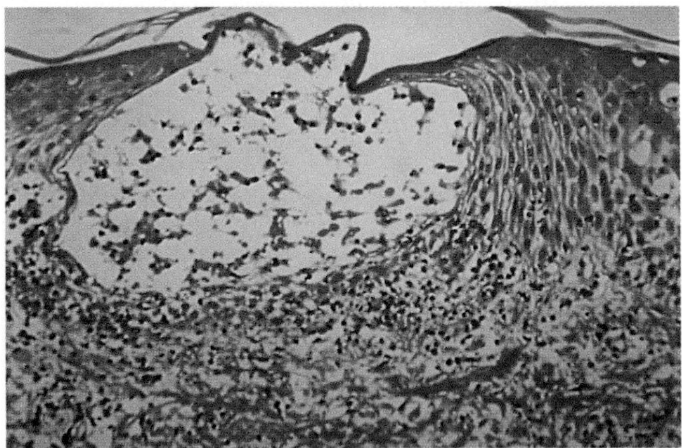

Figure 7–18 ■

Contact dermatitis showing an epidermal blister (vesicle) with dermal and epidermal mononuclear infiltrates. (Courtesy of Dr. Louis Picker, Department of Pathology, University of Texas Southwestern Medical School, Dallas, TX.)

T Cell–Mediated Cytotoxicity

In this variant of type IV hypersensitivity, sensitized CD8+ T cells kill antigen-bearing target cells. Such effector cells are called *cytotoxic T lymphocytes* (CTLs). CTLs, directed against cell surface histocompatibility antigens, play an important role in graft rejection, to be discussed next. They also play a role in resistance to virus infections. In a virus-infected cell, viral peptides associate with the class I molecules within the cell, and the two are transported to the cell surface in the form of a complex. It is this complex that is recognized by the TCR of cytotoxic CD8+ T lymphocytes. The lysis of infected cells before viral replication is completed leads, in due course, to the elimination of the infection. It is believed that many tumor-associated antigens (Chapter 8, Neoplasia) may also be similarly presented on the cell surface. CTLs therefore may also be involved in tumor immunity.

Much has been learned about the mechanisms by which CTLs kill their targets, and this knowledge may be of value in therapeutic modulation of T cell–mediated cytotoxicity in the settings of some autoimmune diseases. Two principal mechanisms of T cell–mediated damage have been discovered: (1) perforin-granzyme-dependent killing and (2) Fas-Fas ligand-dependent killing.[18] Perforins and granzymes are soluble mediators contained in the lysosome-like granules of CTLs. As its name indicates, perforin can perforate the plasma membranes of the target cells that are under attack by CD8+ lymphocytes. At first, CD8+ T cells come in close contact with the target cells; this is followed by polymerization of the perforin molecules and their insertion into the target cell membranes, thus "drilling holes" into the membrane. These pores allow water to enter the cells, thus causing osmotic lysis. The lymphocyte granules also contain a series of proteases called *granzymes*, which are delivered into the target cells via the perforin-induced pores. Once within the cell, granzymes activate apoptosis of the target cells (Chapter 1). Fas-dependent killing also induces apoptosis of the target cells but by a different mechanism. Activated CTLs express Fas-ligand, a molecule with homology to TNF-α, that can bind to Fas expressing target cells. This interaction leads to apoptosis by mechanisms discussed in Chapter 1.

TRANSPLANT REJECTION

Transplant rejection is discussed here because it appears to involve several of the hypersensitivity reactions discussed earlier. One of the goals of present-day immunologic research is successful transplantation of tissues in humans without immunologic rejection. Although the surgical expertise for the transplantation of skin, kidneys, heart, lungs, liver, spleen, bone marrow, and endocrine organs is now well in hand, it outpaces thus far the ability to confer on the recipient permanent acceptance of foreign grafts.

Mechanisms Involved in Rejection

Graft rejection depends on recognition by the host of the grafted tissue as foreign. The antigens responsible for such rejection in humans are those of the major histocompatibility antigen (HLA) system. *Rejection is a complex process in which both cell-mediated immunity and circulating antibodies play a role*; moreover, the relative contributions of these two mechanisms to rejection vary among grafts and are often reflected in the histologic features of the rejected organs.

T Cell–Mediated Reactions. The critical role of T cells in transplant rejection has been documented both in humans and in experimental animals. How do T lymphocytes cause graft destruction? Both activation of CD8 CTLs and delayed hypersensitivity reactions triggered by activated CD4 helper cells seem to be involved. The cellular and molecular basis of allorecognition by host T cells is not entirely clear. Two somewhat distinct but not mutually exclusive pathways, called direct and indirect, have been proposed.[19]

- In the so-called *direct pathway,* T cells of the transplant recipient recognize allogeneic MHC molecules on the surface of an antigen-presenting cell of the donor (Fig. 7–19). It is believed that interstitial dendritic cells carried in the donor organs are the most important immunogens because they not only richly express class I and II HLA molecules, but also are endowed with costimulatory molecules (e.g., B7-1). The T cells of the host encounter the dendritic cells within the grafted organ or after these cells migrate to the draining lymph nodes. Both the CD4+ and the CD8+ T cells of the transplant recipient are involved in this reaction. The CD4 helper T-cell subset is triggered into proliferation by recognition of the allogeneic class II specificities. At the same time, precursors of CD8 CTLs (prekiller T cells), which bear receptors for class I HLA antigens, differentiate into mature CTLs. This process of differentiation is complex and incompletely understood. Among other factors, it is dependent on the release of cytokines, such as IL-2, IL-4, and IL-5, from CD4+ cells (Fig. 7–19). Once mature CTLs are generated, they lyse the grafted tissue by mechanisms already discussed. In addition to the specific cytotoxic T cells, lymphokine-secreting CD4 T cells are also generated by sensitization, and they are believed to play an extremely important role in graft rejection. As in delayed hypersensitivity reactions, cytokines derived from the activated CD4 T cells cause increased vascular permeability and local accumulation of mononuclear cells (lymphocytes and macrophages).
- In the so-called *indirect pathway* of allorecognition, recipient T lymphocytes recognize antigens of the graft donor after they are presented by the recipient's own antigen-presenting cells. This involves the uptake and processing of the MHC molecules shed from the grafted organ by host antigen-presenting cells. The peptides derived from the donor tissue are presented in the antigen-binding groove of the host's own MHC molecules. This indirect pathway is similar to the physiologic processing and presentation of other foreign (e.g., microbial) antigens. By contrast, the direct recognition of allogeneic MHC molecules seems paradoxic to the rules of self MHC restriction. It has been explained by assuming that allogeneic MHC molecules, with their bound peptides, in some manner mimic the determinants recognized by self MHC-restricted T cells. The structural basis of such mimicry is not entirely clear.

Antibody-Mediated Reactions. Although there is little doubt that T cells are pivotal in the rejection of organ transplants, antibodies evoked against alloantigens can also mediate rejection. This process can take two forms. *Hyperacute rejection occurs when preformed antidonor antibodies are present in the circulation of the recipient.* Such antibodies may be present in a recipient who has already rejected a kidney transplant. Multiparous women who develop anti-HLA antibodies against paternal antigens shed from the fetus may also have preformed antibodies to grafts taken from their husbands or children. Prior blood transfusions from HLA-nonidentical donors can also lead to presensitization because platelets and white cells are particularly rich in HLA antigens. In such circumstances, rejection occurs immediately after transplantation because the circulating antibodies react with and deposit rapidly on the vascular endothelium of the grafted organ. Complement fixation occurs, and an Arthus-type reaction follows. With the current practice of crossmatching, that is, testing recipient's serum for antibodies against donor's lymphocytes, hyperacute rejection is no longer a significant clinical problem.

In recipients not previously sensitized to transplantation antigens, exposure to the class I and class II HLA antigens of the donor may evoke antibodies, as depicted in Figure 7–19. The antibodies formed by the recipient may cause injury by several mechanisms, including complement-dependent cytotoxicity, antibody-dependent cell-mediated cytolysis, and the deposition of antigen-antibody complexes. *The initial target of these antibodies in rejection appears to be the graft vasculature.* Thus, antibody-dependent rejection phenomena in the kidney are reflected histologically by a vasculitis, sometimes referred to as *rejection vasculitis.*

MORPHOLOGY OF REJECTION REACTIONS. On the basis of the morphology and the underlying mechanism, **rejection reactions are classified as hyperacute, acute, and chronic.[20] The morphologic changes in these patterns are described as they relate to renal transplants.[21]** Similar changes are encountered in any other vascularized organ transplant.

Hyperacute Rejection. This form of rejection occurs within minutes or hours after transplantation and can sometimes be recognized by the surgeon just after the graft vasculature is anastomosed to the recipient's. In contrast to the nonre-

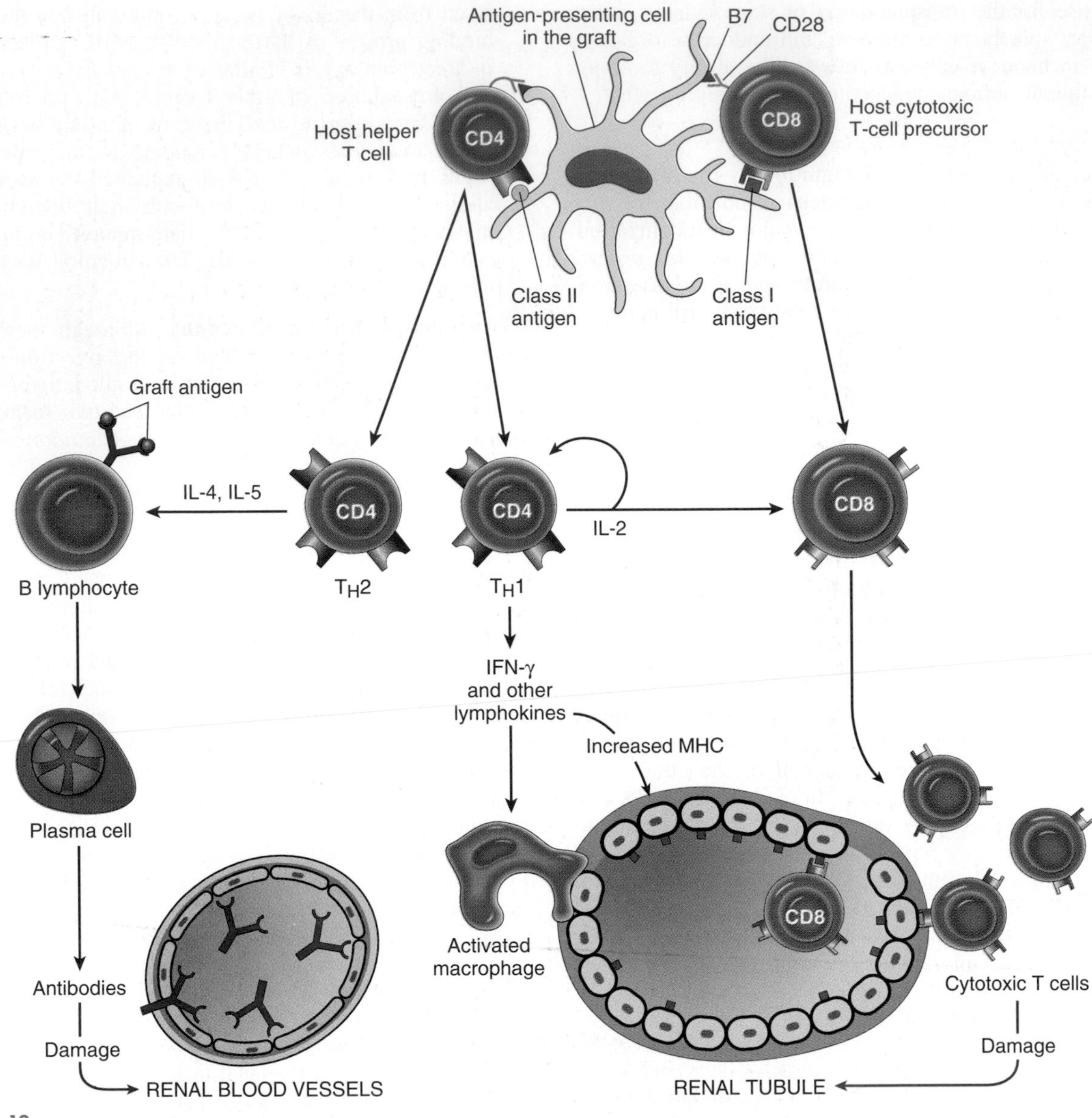

Figure 7–19

Schematic representation of the events that lead to the destruction of histoincompatible grafts. Donor class I and class II antigens along with B7 molecules are recognized by CD8+ cytotoxic T cells and CD4+ helper T cells, respectively, of the host. The interaction of the CD4+ cells with peptides presented by class II antigens leads to proliferation of T_H1-type CD4+ cells and the release of interleukin 2 (IL-2) from the cells. IL-2 further augments the proliferation of CD4+ cells and also provides helper signals for the differentiation of class I–specific CD8+ cytotoxic cells. In addition, activation of T_H2-type CD4+ cells generates a variety of other soluble mediators (lymphokines) that promote B-cell differentiation. The T_H1 cells also participate in the induction of a local delayed hypersensitivity reaction. Eventually, several mechanisms converge to destroy the graft: (1) lysis of cells that bear class I antigens by CD8+ cytotoxic T cells, (2) antigraft antibodies produced by sensitized B cells, and (3) nonspecific damage inflicted by macrophages and other cells that accumulate as a result of the delayed hypersensitivity reaction.

jecting kidney graft, which rapidly regains a normal pink coloration and normal tissue turgor and promptly excretes urine, a hyperacutely rejecting kidney rapidly becomes cyanotic, mottled, and flaccid and may excrete a mere few drops of bloody urine. The histologic lesions are characteristic of the classic Arthus reaction. There is a rapid accumulation of neutrophils within arterioles, glomeruli, and peritubular capillaries. Immunoglobulin and complement are deposited in the vessel wall, and electron microscopy discloses early endothelial injury together with fibrin-platelet thrombi. **These early lesions point to an antigen-antibody reaction at the level of vascular endothelium.** Subsequently, these changes become diffuse and intense, the glomeruli undergo thrombotic occlusion of the capillaries, and fibrinoid necrosis occurs in arterial walls. The kidney cortex then undergoes outright infarction (necrosis), and such nonfunctioning kidneys are removed.

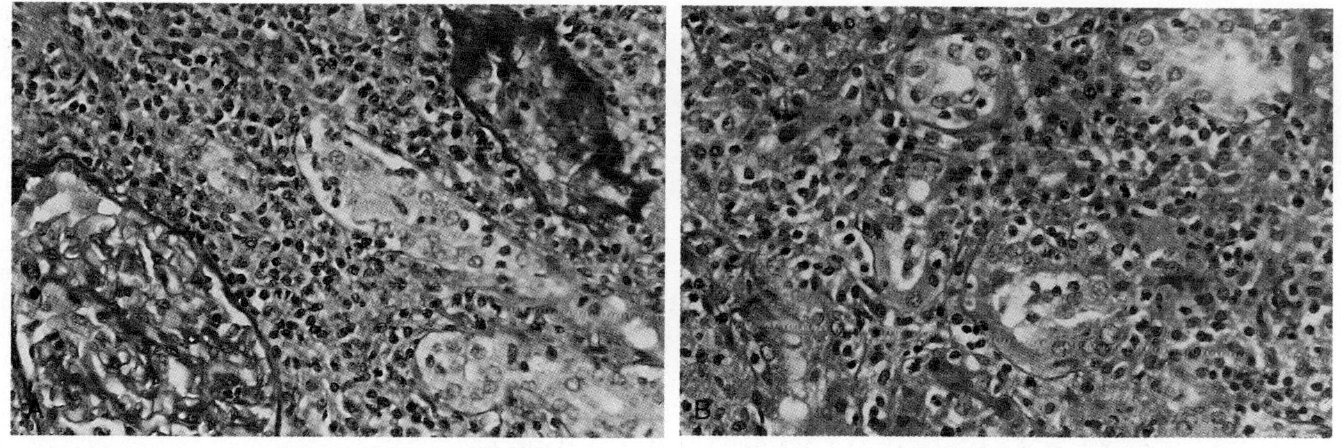

Figure 7–20

Acute cellular rejection of a renal allograft. *A*, An intense mononuclear cell infiltrate occupies the space between the glomerulus *(bottom left)* and the tubules. *B*, Tubules, highlighted by the basement membrane, undergoing destruction by invading lymphocytes. (Courtesy of Dr. Ihsan Housini, Department of Pathology, University of Texas Southwestern Medical School, Dallas, TX.)

Acute Rejection. This may occur within days of transplantation in the untreated recipient or may appear suddenly months or even years later, after immunosuppression has been employed and terminated. As suggested earlier, acute graft rejection is a combined process in which both cellular and humoral tissue injuries play parts. In any one patient, one or the other mechanism may predominate. Histologically, humoral rejection is associated with vasculitis, whereas cellular rejection is marked by an interstitial mononuclear cell infiltrate.

Acute cellular rejection is most commonly seen within the initial months after transplantation and is heralded by an elevation of serum creatinine level followed by clinical signs of renal failure. Histologically, there may be extensive interstitial mononuclear cell infiltration and edema as well as mild interstitial hemorrhage (Fig. 7–20*A*). As might be expected, immunoperoxidase staining reveals both CD4+ and CD8+ lymphocytes. In many cases, IL-2 receptors, which appear on activated T cells, can be demonstrated. Glomerular and peritubular capillaries contain large numbers of mononuclear cells that may also invade the tubules, causing focal tubular necrosis (Fig. 7–20*B*). In addition to causing tubular damage, CD8+ cells may also injure vascular endothelial cells, causing a so-called endothelitis. This form of cell-mediated vascular damage is limited to the endothelium and is distinct from the antibody-mediated vasculitis described later. The affected vessels have swollen endothelial cells, and at places the lymphocytes can be seen between the endothelium and the vessel wall. The recognition of cellular rejection is important because, in the absence of an accompanying arteritis, patients promptly respond to immunosuppressive therapy. Cyclosporine, a widely used immunosuppressive drug, is also nephrotoxic, and hence the histologic changes resulting from cyclosporine may be superimposed.

Acute rejection vasculitis is mediated primarily by antidonor antibodies, and hence it is manifested primarily by damage to the blood vessels. This may take the form of necrotizing vasculitis with endothelial cell necrosis; neutrophilic infiltration; deposition of immunoglobulins, complement, and fibrin; and thrombosis. Such lesions are associated with extensive necrosis of the renal parenchyma. In many cases, the vasculitis is less acute and is characterized by marked thickening of the intima by proliferating fibroblasts, myocytes, and foamy macrophages (Fig. 7–21). The resultant narrowing of the arterioles may cause infarction

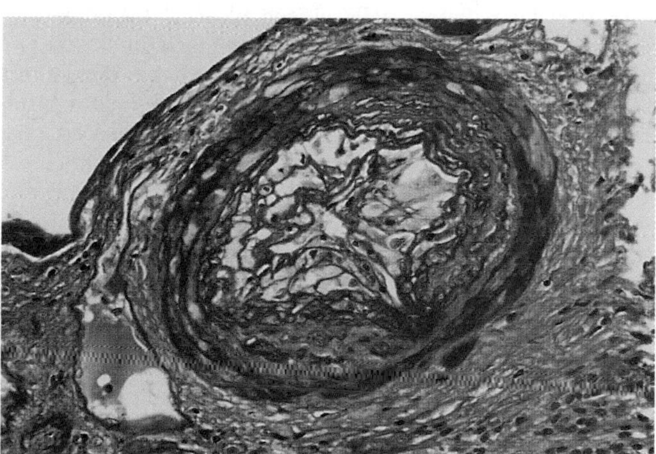

Figure 7–21

Antibody-mediated damage to the blood vessel in a renal allograft. The blood vessel is markedly thickened, and the lumen is obstructed by proliferating fibroblasts and foamy macrophages. (Courtesy of Dr. Ihsan Housini, Department of Pathology, University of Texas Southwestern Medical School, Dallas, TX.)

or renal cortical atrophy. The proliferative vascular lesions mimic arteriosclerotic thickening and are believed to be caused by cytokines that cause growth of vascular smooth muscles.

Chronic Rejection. Because most instances of acute graft rejection are more or less controlled by immunosuppressive therapy, chronic changes are commonly seen in the renal allograft. Patients with chronic rejection present clinically with a progressive rise in serum creatinine level over a period of 4 to 6 months. Chronic rejection is dominated by vascular changes, interstitial fibrosis, and loss of renal parenchyma. The **vascular changes** consist of dense intimal fibrosis, principally in the cortical arteries, the lesion probably being the end stage of the proliferative arteritis described previously. These vascular lesions result in renal ischemia, manifested by glomerular loss, interstitial fibrosis and tubular atrophy, and shrinkage of the renal parenchyma. Together with the vascular lesions, chronically rejecting kidneys usually have interstitial mononuclear cell infiltrates containing large numbers of plasma cells and numerous eosinophils.

Methods of Increasing Graft Survival

Because HLA antigens are the major targets in transplant rejection, minimization of the HLA disparity between the donor and the recipient would be expected to influence graft survival.[22] In the case of intrafamilial (related donor) kidney transplants, a markedly beneficial effect of matching for class I antigens has been observed. In cadaver renal transplants, matching for HLA class I antigens (HLA-A and HLA-B) has at best a modest effect on graft acceptance. Additional matching for class II antigens (HLA-DR) results in a definite improvement in graft survival. In all likelihood, this benefit is derived because class II antigen-reactive CD4+ helper cells, which play an important role in the induction of both cellular and humoral immunity, are not triggered. Even HLA-matched unrelated donors are likely to differ from the host at one or more minor histocompatibility antigens. These antigens are formed by peptides derived from polymorphic proteins other than those encoded by HLA complex. They evoke a weak or slower rejection reaction that, nevertheless, necessitates the use of immunosuppression.

Except in the case of identical twins, who are obviously matched for all possible histocompatibility antigens, *immunosuppressive therapy* is a practical necessity in all other donor-recipient combinations.[23] At present, drugs such as azathioprine, steroids, cyclosporine, antilymphocyte globulins, and monoclonal anti-T cell antibodies (e.g., monoclonal anti-CD3) are employed. Cyclosporine suppresses T cell–mediated immunity by inhibiting activation of cytokine genes, in particular, the gene for IL-2. Although immunosuppression has produced significant gains in terms of graft survival, immunosuppressive therapy is similar to the proverbial double-edged sword. The price paid in the form of increased susceptibility to opportunistic fungal, viral, and other infections is not small. These patients are also at increased risk for developing EBV-induced lymphomas, human papillomavirus–induced squamous cell carcinomas, and Kaposi sarcoma (KS) (Chapter 13). To circumvent the untoward effects of immunosuppression, much effort is devoted to induce donor-specific tolerance in host T cells. One strategy being pursued in experimental animals is to prevent host T cells from receiving costimulatory signals from donor dendritic cells during the initial phase of sensitization. This can be accomplished by interrupting the interaction between the B7 molecules on the dendritic cells of the graft donor with the CD28 receptors on host T cells, as, for example, by administration of antibodies that bind to CD28 receptors. This, as discussed earlier, interrupts the second signal for T-cell activation and renders the T cells anergic or induces their apoptosis.

Transplantation of Other Solid Organs

In addition to the kidney, a variety of organs, such as the liver (Chapter 19), heart (Chapter 13), lungs, and pancreas, are also transplanted. Transplantations of the liver and the heart are now performed at most major medical centers in the United States. In contrast to the case with kidney transplantation, no effort is made to match HLA antigens of the donor and host. Because the transplanted liver or heart has to fit snugly into the space previously occupied by the host organ, the size and availability of the donor organ is of major importance, and it takes precedence over HLA match. Furthermore, the window of time during which donor liver and heart remain viable is too short for tissue typing by routinely available methods. The rejection reaction against heart and liver transplants is not as vigorous as might be expected from the degree of HLA disparity. The molecular basis of this "privilege" is not totally understood. Furthermore, with effective immunosuppression, the rejection reactions can be greatly reduced.

Transplantation of Hematopoietic Cells

Use of hematopoietic cell transplants for hematologic malignancies, certain nonhematologic cancers, aplastic anemias, and certain immunodeficiency states is increasing. Transplantation of genetically engineered hematopoietic stem cells is also likely to be useful for somatic cell gene therapy. Hematopoietic stem cells are usually obtained from the bone marrow but may also be harvested from peripheral blood after they are mobilized from the bone marrow by administration of hematopoietic growth factors. Several features distinguish allogeneic bone marrow transplants from solid organ transplants. In most of the conditions in which bone marrow transplantation is indicated, the recipient is irradiated with lethal doses either to destroy the malignant cells (e.g., leukemias) or to create a graft bed (aplastic anemias). Two major problems arise in allogeneic bone marrow transplantation: graft-versus-host (GVH) disease and transplant rejection.

GVH disease occurs in any situation in which immunologically competent cells or their precursors are transplanted into immunologically crippled recipients. GVH disease occurs most commonly in the setting of allogeneic bone marrow transplantation but may also follow transplantation of solid organs rich in lymphoid cells (e.g., the liver) or following transfusion of unirradiated blood.

Recipients of bone marrow transplants are immunodeficient because of either primary disease or prior treatment of the disease with drugs or irradiation. When such recipients receive normal bone marrow cells from allogeneic donors, the immunocompetent T cells derived from the donor marrow recognize the recipient's HLA antigens as *foreign* and react against them. With sensitization, antirecipient CD4+ and CD8+ T cells are generated.

Acute GVH disease occurs within days to weeks after allogeneic bone marrow transplantation. Although any organ may be affected, predominant manifestations result from the involvement of the *immune system and epithelia of skin, liver, and intestines.* Affected individuals are profoundly immunosuppressed and are easy prey to infections. Although they may be infected by many different types of organisms, infection with cytomegalovirus is particularly important. This usually results from activation of previously silent infection. Cytomegalovirus-induced pneumonitis can be a fatal complication. Involvement of skin in GVH is manifested by a generalized rash leading to desquamation in severe cases. Destruction of small bile ducts gives rise to jaundice, and mucosal ulceration of the gut results in bloody diarrhea. Despite considerable tissue damage, the affected tissues are not heavily infiltrated by lymphocytes. It is believed that in addition to direct cytotoxicity by CD8+ T cells, considerable damage is inflicted by cytokines released by the sensitized donor T cells.

Chronic GVH disease may follow the acute syndrome or may occur insidiously. These patients have extensive cutaneous injury, with destruction of skin appendages and fibrosis of the dermis. The changes may resemble systemic sclerosis (discussed later). Chronic liver disease manifested by cholestatic jaundice is also frequent. Damage to the gastrointestinal mucosa may cause esophageal strictures. The immune system is devastated, with involution of the thymus and depletion of lymphocytes in the lymph nodes. Not surprisingly, the patients experience recurrent and life-threatening infections. The apparent autoimmunity is postulated to result from the failure of the irradiated and damaged thymus to delete potentially *autoreactive* T cells that develop from the donor stem cells.

Because GVH disease is mediated by T lymphocytes contained in the donor bone marrow, depletion of donor T cells before transfusion virtually eliminates GVH disease. This protocol, however, has proved to be a mixed blessing: GVH disease is ameliorated, but the incidence of graft failures and the recurrence of disease in leukemic patients increases. It seems that the multifaceted T cells not only mediate GVH, but also are required for engraftment of the transplanted marrow stem cells and control of leukemic cells. The latter, called *graft-versus-leukemia* effect, can be quite dramatic. Deliberate induction of graft-versus-leukemia effect by infusion of allogeneic T cells is being tested in the treatment of chronic myelogenous leukemia if the patient appears to relapse after bone marrow transplantation.

The mechanisms responsible for rejection of allogeneic bone marrow transplants are poorly understood. It seems to be mediated by NK cells and T cells that survive in the irradiated host. NK cells react against allogeneic stem cells because the latter are lacking self MHC class I molecules and hence fail to deliver the inhibitory signal to NK cells.[24] Host T cells react to donor MHC antigens by a mechanism similar to the reactions against solid tissue grafts.

In addition to allogeneic bone marrow transplants, there is also increasing use of autologous stem cell transplants. These are performed in selected patients with solid tumors if the bone marrow is not involved by the malignancy. The stem cells are usually harvested from the peripheral blood and cryopreserved. The patient is then subjected to intense chemotherapy at doses that destroy not only the tumor but also hematopoietic stem cells. After this, the cryopreserved autologous stem cells are infused into the patient to restore the hematopoietic system. Such "stem cell rescue" allows treatment with doses of anti-cancer agents that would cause death due to hematopoietic failure. Because the stem cells are of host origin, the complications of allogeneic bone marrow transplants are not seen in the setting of autologous transplants. This form of treatment is being evaluated in patients with aggressive breast cancer and in patients with certain lymphomas.

Autoimmune Diseases

The evidence is now compelling that an immune reaction against *self-antigens*—autoimmunity—is the cause of certain diseases in humans. A growing number of diseases have been attributed to autoimmunity (Table 7–6), but in many the evidence is not firm. Autoantibodies can be found in the serum of a remarkably large number of apparently normal individuals, particularly in older age groups. Furthermore, innocuous autoantibodies are also formed after damage to tissue and may serve a physiologic role in the removal of tissue breakdown products.

How, then, does one define *pathologic* autoimmunity? Ideally, at least three requirements should be met before a

Table 7–6. AUTOIMMUNE DISEASES

Single Organ or Cell Type	Systemic
Probable	***Probable***
Hashimoto thyroiditis	Systemic lupus erythematosus
Autoimmune hemolytic anemia	Rheumatoid arthritis
Autoimmune atrophic gastritis of pernicious anemia	Sjögren syndrome
Autoimmune encephalomyelitis	Reiter syndrome
Autoimmune orchitis	***Possible***
Goodpasture syndrome*	Inflammatory myopathies
Autoimmune thrombocytopenia	Systemic sclerosis (scleroderma)
Insulin-dependent diabetes mellitus	Polyarteritis nodosa
Myasthenia gravis	
Graves disease	
Possible	
Primary biliary cirrhosis	
Chronic active hepatitis	
Ulcerative colitis	
Membranous glomerulonephritis	

* Target is basement membrane of glomeruli and alveolar walls.

disorder is categorized as truly due to autoimmunity: (1) the presence of an autoimmune reaction, (2) clinical or experimental evidence that such a reaction is *not secondary* to tissue damage but is of primary pathogenetic significance, and (3) the absence of another well-defined cause of the disease. These requirements are met in only a few diseases, such as SLE and autoimmune blood dyscrasias.

The autoimmune disorders form a spectrum on one end of which are conditions in which autoantibodies are directed against a single organ or tissue, therefore resulting in localized tissue damage. A classic example is insulin-dependent diabetes mellitis, in which the antibodies have absolute specificity for β cells of the pancreatic islets. At the other end of the spectrum is SLE, in which a diversity of antibodies directed against DNA, platelets, red cells, and protein-phospholipid complexes results in widespread lesions throughout the body. In the middle of the spectrum falls Goodpasture syndrome, in which antibodies to basement membranes of lung and kidney induce lesions and symptoms in these organs. It is obvious that autoimmunity implies loss of self-tolerance, and the question arises as to how this happens. Before we look for answers to this question, we review the mechanisms of immunologic tolerance and self-tolerance.

IMMUNOLOGIC TOLERANCE

Immunologic tolerance is a state in which the individual is incapable of developing an immune response to a specific antigen. Self-tolerance refers to lack of responsiveness to an individual's antigens, and obviously it underlies our ability to live in harmony with our own cells and tissues. Several mechanisms, albeit not well understood, have been postulated to explain the tolerant state.[25, 26, 26a] They can be broadly classified into two groups: *central tolerance* and *peripheral tolerance*. Each of these is considered briefly.

- *Central tolerance*: This refers to clonal deletion of self-reactive T and B lymphocytes during their maturation in the central lymphoid organs (i.e., thymus for T cells and the bone marrow for B cells). Clonal deletion of developing intrathymic T cells has been extensively investigated. Experiments with transgenic mice provide abundant evidence that T lymphocytes that bear receptors for self-antigens undergo apoptosis within the thymus during the process of T-cell maturation. It is proposed that many autologous protein antigens are processed and presented by thymic antigen-presenting cells in association with self MHC molecules. The developing T cells that express high-affinity receptors for such self-antigens are *negatively selected*, or deleted, and therefore the peripheral T-cell pool is lacking or deficient in self-reactive cells (Fig. 7–22). What triggers apoptosis in self-reactive T cells is not entirely clear. Although developing thymocytes express high levels of Fas, until recently, the Fas-Fas ligand pathway of apoptosis was not considered important in clonal deletion. Studies suggest, however, that Fas-mediated cell death does occur during negative selection in the thymus.[27] As with T cells, clonal deletion is also operative in B cells. When developing B cells encounter a membrane-bound antigen within the bone marrow, they undergo apoptosis.[26] Clonal deletion of self-reactive lymphocytes, however, is far from perfect. Many self-antigens are not present in the thymus, and hence T cells bearing receptors for such autoantigens escape into the periphery. There is similar "slippage" in the B-cell system as well. B cells that bear receptors for a variety of self-antigens, including thyroglobulin, collagen, and DNA, can be found in the peripheral blood of healthy individuals.
- *Peripheral tolerance*: Those self-reactive T cells that escape intrathymic negative selection can inflict tissue injury unless they are deleted or muzzled in the peripheral tissues. Several "back-up" mechanisms that silence such potentially autoreactive T cells are known to exist.[28] They include the following:

1. *Clonal deletion by activation-induced cell death*: One of the mechanisms to prevent uncontrolled T-cell activation during a normal immune response involves apoptotic death of activated T cells by the Fas-Fas ligand system. Lymphocytes as well as many other cells express Fas (CD95), a member of the TNF-receptor family. Its expression is up-regulated in antigen-activated T cells. The ligand for Fas (Fas L), a membrane protein that is structurally homologous to the cytokine TNF, is expressed chiefly on activated T lymphocytes. The engagement of Fas by Fas L, coexpressed on activated T cells, dampens the immune response by inducing apoptosis of activated T cells. In all likelihood, such activation-induced cell death also underlies the peripheral deletion of autoreactive T cells. It is believed that those self-antigens that are abundant in peripheral tissues cause repeated and persistent stimulation of self-antigen–specific T cells, leading eventually to their elimination via Fas-mediated apoptosis (Fig. 7–22). The importance of this mechanism in the peripheral deletion of autoreactive T cells is highlighted by two strains of mice that are natural "knockouts" of Fas or Fas L. The so-called *lpr* mice have a mutation in the Fas gene, whereas the *gld* mice are born with defective Fas L. Mice of both of these strains develop severe autoimmune disease resembling human SLE. (In contrast to SLE, however, these mice also suffer from generalized lymphoproliferation.)
2. *Clonal anergy*: This refers to prolonged or irreversible functional inactivation of lymphocytes, induced by encounter with antigens under certain conditions. We discussed earlier that activation of antigen-specific T cells requires two signals: recognition of peptide antigen in association with self MHC molecules on the surface of antigen-presenting cells and a set of second costimulatory signals provided by antigen-presenting cells. To initiate second signals, certain T cell–associated molecules, such as CD28, must bind to their ligands (called *B7-1* and *B7-2*) on antigen-presenting cells. If the antigen is presented by cells that do not bear the CD28 ligand, a negative signal is delivered, and the cell becomes anergic (Fig. 7–22). Such a cell then fails to be activated even if the

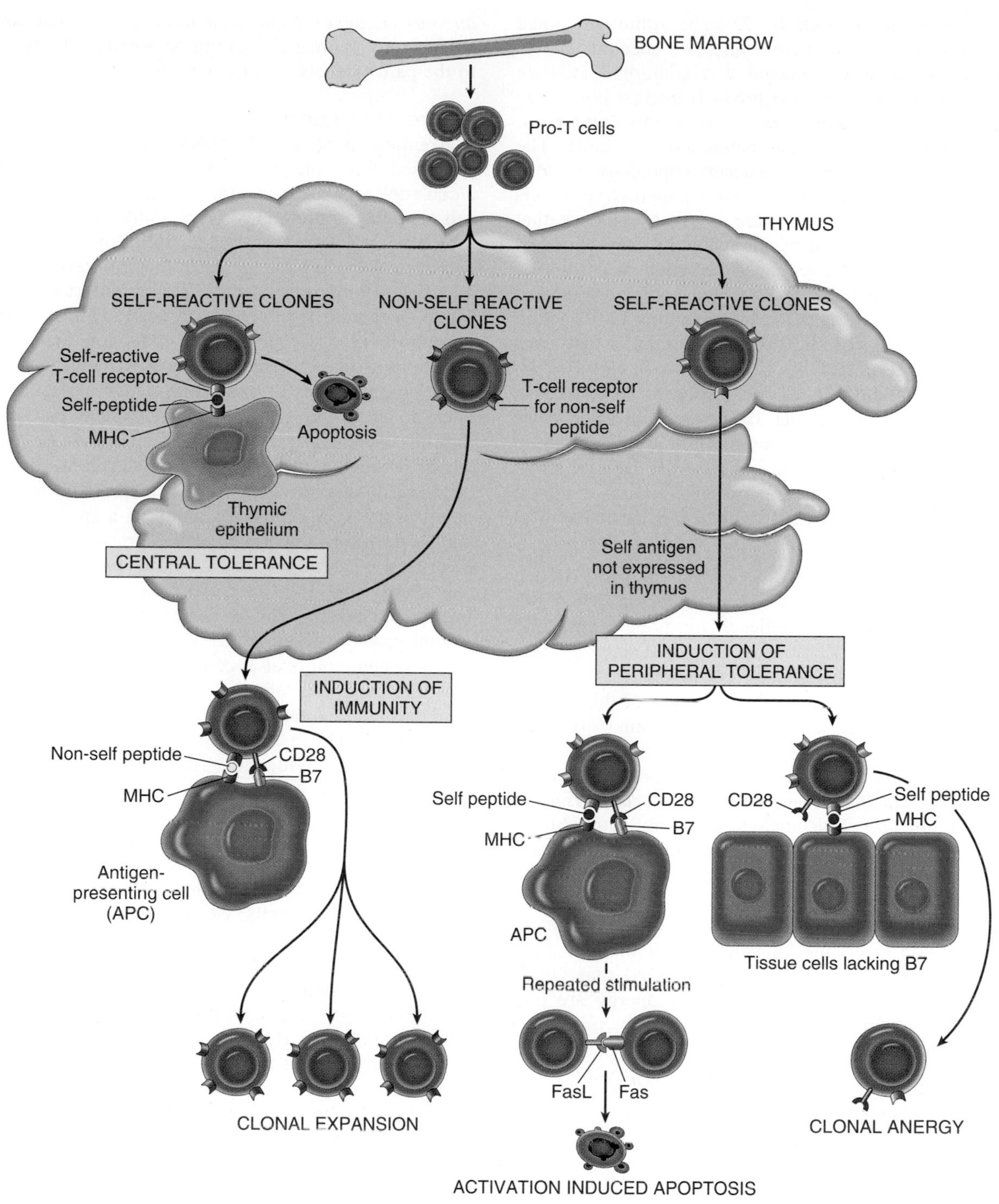

Figure 7–22

Schematic illustration of the mechanisms involved in central and peripheral tolerance.

relevant antigen is presented by competent antigen-presenting cells (e.g., macrophages, dendritic cells) that can deliver costimulation. Because costimulatory molecules are not expressed or are weakly expressed on most normal tissues, the encounter between autoreactive T cells and their specific self-antigens leads to clonal anergy. Clonal anergy affects B cells in the tissues as well. It is believed that if B cells encounter antigen in the absence of specific helper T cells, the antigen-receptor complex is down-regulated, and such cells never re-express their immunoglobulin receptors. Understandably, such cells are unable to respond to subsequent antigenic stimulation. In addition to antigen-induced loss of surface immunoglobulin receptors, other mechanisms of B-cell anergy are also postulated to exist.

3. *Peripheral suppression by T cells*: Although clonal deletion and anergy are the primary mechanisms of self-tolerance, it is believed that additional fail-safe mechanisms must also exist. Much interest is focused on suppressor T cells with the ability to down-regulate the function of other autoreactive T cells. The molecular mechanisms by which suppressor T cells recognize antigens and exert their suppressive effects have remained elusive. There is some evidence that peripheral suppression of autoreactivity may be mediated, in part, by the regulated secretion of cytokines. CD4+ T cells of the T_H2 type have been implicated in mediating self-tolerance by regulating the function of pathogenic T_H1 type cells. Certainly, cytokines produced by T_H2 cells (e.g., IL-4, IL-10, and TGF-β) can down-modulate the T_H1 response. As evidence, targeted disruption of the TGF-β gene in mice gives rise to inflammatory lesions that are similar to those seen in many autoimmune diseases.[29] Despite these tantalizing data, there is at present no firm evidence that self-antigens normally induce a selective T_H2 response.

Prevention of autoimmunity is so vital to survival that several mechanisms have evolved to protect us from our "protectors." There is firm evidence for both central and peripheral clonal deletion as well as clonal anergy; their relative importance in maintaining self-tolerance is not established and may well vary with the nature of the autoantigen (e.g., abundance, expression in thymus). Because helper T cells are critical control elements for both cellular and humoral immunity, *tolerance of self-reactive T cells is extremely important for prevention of autoimmune diseases.* Most self-antigens are T dependent; therefore, autoantibody formation may be prevented by tolerance of hapten-specific B cells or the relevant helper T cells or both. Because in experimental models T cells are more readily tolerized, especially with low doses of antigen, it is believed that T-cell tolerance is a major mechanism for prevention of autoreactivity. Lymphocytes (both T and B cells) that "leak" through the barriers of clonal deletion or anergy are perhaps restrained by suppressor mechanisms.

MECHANISMS OF AUTOIMMUNE DISEASES

Although it would be attractive to explain all autoimmune diseases by a single mechanism, it is now clear that there are a number of ways by which tolerance can be bypassed, thus terminating a previously unresponsive state to autoantigens. More than one defect might be present in each disease, and the defects vary from one disorder to the other. Furthermore, the pathogenesis of autoimmunity appears to involve immunologic, genetic, and microbial factors interacting through complicated mechanisms that are poorly understood. Here we discuss the initiating immunologic mechanisms, then the role of genetic and microbial factors is reviewed briefly.

The initiating mechanisms in autoimmunity can best be discussed in terms of those discussed for tolerance. Of the two major forms of tolerance, central and peripheral, *there is no convincing evidence of breakdown of central tolerance as a cause of autoimmunity.* Several mechanisms exist whereby failure of peripheral tolerance may contribute to the pathogenesis of autoimmune diseases.

Failure of Peripheral Tolerance

Breakdown of T-Cell Anergy. In an earlier section, we discussed that potentially autoreactive T cells that escape clonal deletion are rendered anergic when they encounter self-antigens expressed on costimulator-deficient antigen-presenting cells in the tissues. It follows that such T-cell anergy may be broken if these antigen-presenting cells can be induced to express costimulatory molecules such as B7-1 and to secrete cytokines such as IL-12 that stimulate the generation of T_H1 cells. Such induction may occur after infections with resultant tissue necrosis and local inflammation. Up-regulation of the costimulator molecule B7-1 has been noted in the central nervous system of patients with multiple sclerosis, a presumed autoimmune disease in which T cells attack the myelin sheath of the nerve fibers.[30] Similar induction of B7-1 expression has also been noted in the synovium of patients with rheumatoid arthritis and in the skin of patients with psoriasis. An elegant demonstration of autoimmunity resulting from breakdown in T-cell anergy has been noted in transgenic mouse models of insulin-dependent (type I) diabetes mellitus. In this model, a viral protein driven by the insulin promoter is expressed as a transgene on islet β cells. Because the transgenic mice are born with this antigen, for all practical purposes this viral protein is treated as a "self-antigen," and there is no autoimmune response against it. If the transgenic mice are made to express both the viral protein and B7-1 under the insulin promoter, however, coexpression of the viral antigen and B7-1 on the pancreatic β cells occurs. This breaks down peripheral tolerance, and T cell–mediated injury to the islet cells occurs. Presumably, in the transgenic mice expressing only the viral antigen on the islet cells, the antigen-specific T cells were rendered anergic owing to lack of costimulation, but in the double transgenic mice, the expression of B7-1 led to the activation of anergic T cells by provision of the costimulatory signals. These observations open the exciting possibility of immunologic manipulations aimed at interrupting the costimulatory signals for treatment of autoimmune diseases.

Failure of Activation-Induced Cell Death. We discussed earlier how persistent activation of potentially autoreactive T cells may lead to their apoptosis by the Fas-Fas ligand system. It follows therefore that defects in this pathway of apoptosis may allow persistence and proliferation of autoreactive T cells in the peripheral tissues. In support of this hypothesis, mice with genetic defects in Fas or Fas L develop chronic autoimmune diseases accompanied by massive lymphoid proliferation. The autoimmune disease in these mice resembles SLE. There are differences as well, however, the most striking of which is the absence of the severe lymphoid proliferation in patients with SLE. Furthermore, thus far, no patients with SLE have been found to have mutations in the Fas or Fas L genes. There may, however, be other subtle defects in activation-induced cell death that may contribute to human autoimmune disease. These remain to be discovered.

Failure of T Cell–Mediated Suppression. The idea that loss of regulatory or *suppressor* T cells that can limit the function of autoreactive T and B cells can lead to autoimmunity is quite attractive. This notion has been difficult to prove, however, in large part because of the difficulty in the isolation and identification of antigen-specific regulatory T cells. Studies suggest that a special type of antigen-specific CD4+ T cell that secretes IL-10, but not other T_H2 cell-derived cytokines (e.g., IL-4), can be isolated from both mice and humans. This type of CD4+ T cell can suppress antigen-specific proliferation of other T cells and, quite importantly, prevent autoimmune colitis in a mouse model.[31] Whether loss of such regulatory T cells contributes to human autoimmunity is under investigation.

Molecular Mimicry. Some infectious agents share epitopes with self-antigens. An immune response against such microbes may produce tissue-damaging reactions against the cross-reacting self-antigen. It is well known that rheumatic heart disease sometimes follows streptococcal infection because an antibody to streptococcal M protein cross-reacts with cardiac glycoproteins. Molecular mimicry or cross-reactions may also apply to T-cell epitopes. The most compelling evidence supporting this concept has come from studies with myelin basic protein–reactive T cell clones derived from patients with multiple sclerosis.[32] These clones could also react with peptides derived from a variety of nonself proteins, including many derived from viruses. Some of the viral peptides seemed to react even more strongly with the T cells than with the myelin basic protein–derived peptides.[32]

Polyclonal Lymphocyte Activation. As mentioned earlier, tolerance in some cases is maintained by clonal anergy. Autoimmunity may occur if such self-reactive but anergic clones are stimulated by antigen-independent mechanisms. Several microorganisms and their products are capable of causing polyclonal (i.e., antigen nonspecific) activation of B cells. The best investigated among these is bacterial lipopolysaccharide (endotoxin), which can induce mouse lymphocytes to form anti-DNA, antithymocyte, and anti–red cell antibodies in vitro. In addition, certain other bacterial products can bind to and activate a large pool of CD4+ T cells in an antigen-independent manner. They do so by binding to class II MHC molecules on antigen-presenting cells and the β chains of the T-cell receptor (TCR), outside the antigen-binding groove. Because they stimulate all T cells that express a certain set or family of the Vβ TCRs, they are called *superantigens.* It is proposed that among the T cells activated by superantigens, some may be reactive to self-antigens, and thus autoimmunity may result from arousal of such cells. Such a mechanism may contribute to the pathogenesis of type I diabetes, at least in some cases.[33]

Release of Sequestered Antigens. Regardless of the exact mechanism by which self-tolerance is achieved (clonal deletion or anergy), it is clear that induction of tolerance requires interaction between the antigen and the immune system. Thus, any self-antigen that is completely sequestered during development is likely to be viewed as foreign if introduced into the circulation, and an immune response develops. Spermatozoa and ocular antigens fall into this category. Post-traumatic uveitis and orchitis after vasectomy probably result from immune responses against antigens normally sequestered in the eye and the testis. The mere release of antigens is not sufficient to cause autoimmunity; the inflammation associated with the tissue injury is essential for the up-regulation of costimulatory pathways that are critical for the induction of an immune response.

Exposure of Cryptic Self and Epitope Spreading. In recent years, it has been recognized that molecular sequestration of antigens is much more common than anatomic sequestration.[34] It is believed that each self protein has relatively few antigenic determinants (epitopes) that are effectively processed and presented to T cells. During development, most T cells capable of reacting to such dominant epitopes are either deleted in the thymus or rendered anergic in the periphery. By contrast, a large number of self-determinants are not readily recognized by the immune system, and hence T cells specific for such "cryptic" self-epitopes are not deleted. It follows that such T cells could cause autoimmune diseases if the cryptic epitopes are somehow presented to them in an immunogenic form. The molecular basis of epitope crypticity and the unmasking of such epitopes is not fully understood.[35] Several factors could be responsible for rendering an epitope cryptic, including the available amount of the determinant, its ability to be processed by antigen-presenting cells, and the availability of costimulatory factors. Thus, it is postulated that *regardless of the initial trigger of an autoimmune response (e.g., infection with a cross-reacting microbe, release of a sequestered antigen, failure of suppressor T cells), the progression and chronicity of the autoimmune response is maintained by recruitment of autoreactive T cells that recognize normally cryptic self-determinants.* The induction of such autoreactive T cells is sometimes referred to as *epitope spreading* because the immune response "spreads" to determinants that were initially not recognized. There is compelling evidence for the role of epitope spreading in the pathogenesis of a murine model of multiple sclerosis,[36] type I diabetes, and SLE.

Genetic Factors in Autoimmunity

There is little doubt that genetic factors determine the frequency and the nature of autoimmune diseases.[37] This conclusion is based on several lines of evidence: (1) familial clustering of several human autoimmune diseases, such as SLE, autoimmune hemolytic anemia, and autoimmune thyroiditis; (2) linkage of several autoimmune diseases with HLA, especially class II, antigens[38]; and (3) induction of autoimmune disease in HLA-B27 transgenic rats.[39] In humans, this HLA molecule is strongly associated with certain autoimmune diseases, such as ankylosing spondylitis (Chapter 28). Rats carrying the human HLA-B27 transgene develop ankylosing spondylitis and several other autoimmune disorders. This provides direct evidence for regulation of autoimmunity by a human MHC gene.

The precise mechanism by which certain genes predispose to autoimmunity is not clear, but attention is focused on the relationship of autoimmunity to class II MHC molecules. At least two mechanisms can explain this association:

- CD4+ helper cells are triggered by peptide antigens bound to class II MHC molecules. A class II allele that can bind to a given self-antigen may facilitate an autoimmune response. Molecular analyses of class II antigens have provided support for this hypothesis. The majority of patients with rheumatoid arthritis (an autoimmune disease of joints; Chapter 28) carry the HLA-DR4 or HLA-DR1, or both alleles. These two alleles share a common stretch of four amino acids located in the antigen-binding cleft of the DR molecule. Thus, the association between rheumatoid arthritis and certain DR molecules may be explained by the capacity of these DR molecules to bind an arthritogenic antigen, which, in turn, activates CD4+ T cells.
- Another possibility involves the effect of MHC class II molecules on the T-cell repertoire of the individual. It is postulated that MHC antigens influence the clonal deletion of potentially autoreactive T cells within the thymus. Because clonal deletion in the thymus is based on high-affinity binding of the T-cell receptors with self-antigens presented by class II molecules, it follows that if a given MHC allele presents an autoantigen poorly, the relevant autoreactive T-cell clone may not be deleted. Individuals who inherit such class II molecules may therefore be at increased risk for developing autoimmunity.

Despite the association between MHC class II genes and several autoimmune diseases, it must be remembered that many patients with the susceptibility-related MHC gene never develop any disease, and, conversely, individuals without the relevant MHC gene can develop the disease. It follows that expression of a particular MHC gene is but one factor that can facilitate induction of autoimmunity. Furthermore, microsatellite-based scans of the human genome have detected several non–MHC-linked loci that confer susceptibility to autoimmune diseases such as type I diabetes and SLE. The genes at these loci have not been identified but could include genes that regulate apoptosis or encode proteins that regulate immunity, such as cytokines and their receptors and costimulatory molecules.

Microbial Agents in Autoimmunity

A variety of microbes, including bacteria, mycoplasmas, and viruses, have been implicated in triggering autoimmunity at one time or another. Microbes may trigger autoimmune reactions in several ways, many of which were mentioned previously and are summarized below[40]:

- Viruses and other microbes may share cross-reacting epitopes with self-antigens. In addition to previously mentioned examples, cross-reactions between certain coxsackieviruses and the islet cell antigen glutamic acid decarboxylase are worthy of note.
- Microbial infections with resultant tissue necrosis and inflammation can cause up-regulation of costimulatory molecules on resting antigen-presenting cells in tissue, thus favoring a breakdown of T-cell anergy. In addition, the inflammatory response may facilitate presentation of cryptic antigens and thus induce epitope spreading.
- Superantigens and other microbial products (e.g., lipopolysaccharidase) can activate a large pool of T and B cells, some of which may be autoreactive.

There is no dearth of possible and some plausible mechanisms by which infectious agents may participate in the pathogenesis of autoimmunity. At present, however, there is no evidence that clearly implicates any microbe in the causation of human autoimmune diseases.

Against this background, we can proceed to discuss the consequences of the loss of self-tolerance, that is, autoimmune diseases. As stated earlier, the autoimmune diseases of humans range from those in which the target is a single tissue, such as the autoimmune hemolytic anemias and thyroiditis, to those in which a host of self-antigens evoke a constellation of reactions against many organs and systems. In this chapter, we deal principally with those presumed autoimmune diseases that are primarily of a systemic nature, and we leave most single-tissue diseases to specific chapters throughout the book. For reference, however, Table 7–6 lists both systemic and organ-specific autoimmune disorders.

SYSTEMIC LUPUS ERYTHEMATOSUS

Systemic lupus erythematosus (SLE) is the classic prototype of the multisystem disease of autoimmune origin, characterized by a bewildering array of autoantibodies, particularly antinuclear antibodies (ANAs). *Acute or insidious in its onset, it is a chronic, remitting and relapsing, often febrile illness characterized principally by injury to the skin, joints, kidney, and serosal membranes.* Virtually every other organ in the body, however, may also be affected. The clinical presentation of SLE is so variable that the American Rheumatism Association developed criteria for diagnosis of this disorder (Table 7–7). SLE is a fairly common disease, with a prevalence that may be as high as 1 in 2500 in certain populations.[41] Similar to most autoimmune diseases, SLE is predominantly a disease of women, with a frequency of 1 in 700 among women of childbearing age and a female-to-male ratio of 9:1. By comparison, the female-to-male ratio is only 2:1 for disease developing during childhood or after the age of 65. The disease is more common and severe in American black women (1 in 245). Although SLE usually arises in the twenties and thirties, it may become manifest at any age, even in early childhood.

Etiology and Pathogenesis. The cause of SLE remains unknown, but the existence of a seemingly limitless number of antibodies in these patients against self-constituents indicates that the *fundamental defect in SLE is a failure of the regulatory mechanisms that sustain self-tolerance.* Antibodies have been identified against an array of nuclear and cytoplasmic components of the cell that are neither organ nor species specific. In addition, a third group of antibodies is directed against cell surface antigens of blood elements. Apart from their value in the diagnosis and management of patients with SLE, these antibodies are of major pathogenetic significance, as, for example, in the immune complex–mediated glomerulonephritis so typical of this disease.[42]

ANAs are directed against several nuclear antigens and

Table 7–7. 1997 REVISED CRITERIA FOR CLASSIFICATION OF SYSTEMIC LUPUS ERYTHEMATOSUS*

Criterion	Definition
1. Malar rash	Fixed erythema, flat or raised, over the malar eminences, tending to spare the nasolabial folds
2. Discoid rash	Erythematous raised patches with adherent keratotic scaling and follicular plugging; atrophic scarring may occur in older lesions
3. Photosensitivity	Skin rash as a result of unusual reaction to sunlight, by patient history or physician observation
4. Oral ulcers	Oral or nasopharyngeal ulceration, usually painless, observed by a physician
5. Arthritis	Nonerosive arthritis involving two or more peripheral joints, characterized by tenderness, swelling, or effusion
6. Serositis	Pleuritis—convincing history of pleuritic pain or rub heard by a physician or evidence of pleural effusion, or Pericarditis—documented by electrocardiogram or rub or evidence of pericardial effusion
7. Renal disorder	Persistent proteinuria >0.5 g/dl or >3+ if quantitation not performed, or Cellular casts—may be red blood cell, hemoglobin, granular, tubular, or mixed
8. Neurologic disorder	Seizures—in the absence of offending drugs or known metabolic derangements, e.g., uremia, ketoacidosis, or electrolyte imbalance, or Psychosis—in the absence of offending drugs or known metabolic derangements, e.g., uremia, ketoacidosis, or electrolyte imbalance
9. Hematologic disorder	Hemolytic anemia—with reticulocytosis, or Leukopenia—$<4.0 \times 10^9$/L (4000/mm^3) total on two or more occasions, or Lymphopenia—$<1.5 \times 10^9$/L (1500/mm^3) on two or more occasions, or Thrombocytopenia—$<100 \times 10^9$/L (100×10^3/mm^3) in the absence of offending drugs
10. Immunologic disorder	Anti-DNA antibody to native DNA in abnormal titer, or Anti-Sm—presence of antibody to Sm nuclear antigen, or Positive finding of antiphospholipid antibodies based on (1) an abnormal serum level of IgG or IgM anticardiolipin antibodies, (2) a positive test for lupus anticoagulant using a standard test, or (3) a false-positive serologic test for syphilis known to be positive for at least 6 months and confirmed by negative *Treponema pallidum* immobilization or fluorescent treponemal antibody absorption test
11. Antinuclear antibody	An abnormal titer of antinuclear antibody by immunofluorescence or an equivalent assay at any point in time and in the absence of drugs known to be associated with drug-induced lupus syndrome

* The proposed classification is based on 11 criteria. For the purpose of identifying patients in clinical studies, a person is said to have systemic lupus erythematosus if any 4 or more of the 11 criteria are present, serially or simultaneously, during any interval of observation.

From Tan EM, et al: The revised criteria for the classification of systemic lupus erythematosus. Arthritis Rheum 25:1271, 1982; and Hochberg, MC: Updating the American College of Rheumatology revised criteria for the classification of systemic lupus erythematosus. Arthritis Rheum 40:1725, 1997.

can be grouped into four categories:[43, 43a] (1) *antibodies to DNA*, (2) *antibodies to histones*, (3) *antibodies to nonhistone proteins bound to RNA*, and (4) *antibodies to nucleolar antigens.* Table 7–8 lists several ANAs and their association with SLE as well as with other autoimmune diseases to be discussed later. Several techniques are used to detect ANAs. Clinically the most commonly used method is indirect immunofluorescence, which detects a variety of nuclear antigens, including DNA, RNA, and proteins (collectively called *generic ANAs*). The pattern of nuclear fluorescence suggests the type of antibody present in the patient's serum. Four basic patterns are recognized:

- *Homogeneous or diffuse nuclear staining* usually reflects antibodies to chromatin, histones, and, occasionally, double-stranded DNA.
- *Rim or peripheral staining* patterns are most commonly indicative of antibodies to double-stranded DNA.
- *Speckled pattern* refers to the presence of uniform or variable-sized speckles. This is one of the most commonly observed patterns of fluorescence and therefore the least specific. It reflects the presence of antibodies to non-DNA nuclear constituents. Examples include Sm antigen, ribonucleoprotein (RNP), and SS-A and SS-B reactive antigens (Table 7–8).
- *Nucleolar pattern* refers to the presence of a few discrete spots of fluorescence within the nucleus and represents antibodies to nucleolar RNA. This pattern is reported most often in patients with systemic sclerosis.

The fluorescence patterns are not absolutely specific for the type of antibody, and because many autoantibodies may be present, combinations of patterns are frequent. *The immunofluorescence test for ANA is positive in virtually every patient with SLE; hence this test is sensitive, but it is not specific because patients with other autoimmune diseases also frequently score positive* (Table 7–8). *Furthermore, approximately 5 to 15% of normal individuals have low titers of these antibodies.* The incidence increases with age.

Detection of antibodies to specific nuclear antigens requires specialized techniques. Of the numerous nuclear antigen-antibody systems,[44] some that are clinically useful are listed in Table 7–8. *Antibodies to double-stranded DNA and the so-called Smith (Sm) antigen are virtually diagnostic of SLE.*

There is some, albeit imperfect, correlation between the presence or absence of certain ANAs and clinical manifestations. For example, high titers of double-stranded DNA antibodies are usually associated with active renal disease. Conversely the risk of nephritis is low if anti-SS-B antibodies are present.[45]

In addition to ANAs, lupus patients have a host of other autoantibodies. Some are directed against elements of the blood, such as red cells, platelets, and lymphocytes; others are directed against proteins complexed to phospholipids. In recent years, there has been much interest in these so-called antiphospholipid antibodies.[46] They are present in 40 to 50% of lupus patients. Although initially believed to be directed against anionic phospholipids, they are actually

Table 7–8. ANTINUCLEAR ANTIBODIES IN VARIOUS AUTOIMMUNE DISEASES

		Disease, % Positive					
Nature of Antigen	**Antibody System**	***SLE***	***Drug-Induced LE***	***Systemic Sclerosis —Diffuse***	***Limited Scleroderma —CREST***	***Sjögren Syndrome***	***Inflammatory Myopathies***
Many nuclear antigens (DNA, RNA, proteins)	Generic ANA (indirect IF)	>95	>95	70–90	70–90	50–80	40–60
Native DNA	Anti–double-stranded DNA	40–60	<5	<5	<5	<5	<5
Histones	Antihistone	50–70	>95	<5	<5	<5	<5
Core proteins of small nuclear ribonucleoprotein particles (Smith antigen)	Anti-Sm	20–30	<5	<5	<5	<5	<5
Ribonucleoprotein (U1RNP)	Nuclear RNP	30–40	<5	15	10	<5	<5
RNP	SS-A(Ro)	30–50	<5	<5	<5	70–95	10
RNP	SS-B(La)	10–15	<5	<5	<5	60–90	<5
DNA topoisomerase I	Scl-70	<5	<5	28–70	10–18	<5	<5
Centromeric proteins	Anticentromere	<5	<5	22–36	90	<5	<5
Histidyl-t-RNA synthetase	Jo-1	<5	<5	<5	<5	<5	25

Boxed entries indicate high correlation.
SLE, systemic lupus erythematosus; LE, lupus erythematosus; ANA, antinuclear antibodies; RNP, ribonucleoprotein.

directed against plasma proteins complexed to phospholipids. A variety of protein substrates have been implicated, including prothrombin, annexin V, β_2-glycoprotein I, protein S, and protein C. *Antibodies against the phospholipid-β_2-glycoprotein complex also bind to cardiolipin antigen, used in syphilis serology, and therefore lupus patients may have a false-positive test result for syphilis.* Some of these antibodies interfere with in vitro clotting tests, such as partial thromboplastin time. Therefore, these antibodies are sometimes referred to as *lupus anticoagulant.* Despite having a circulating anticoagulant that delays clotting in vitro, these patients have complications associated with a *pro*coagulant state.[47] They have venous and arterial thromboses, which may be associated with recurrent spontaneous miscarriages and focal cerebral or ocular ischemia. This constellation of clinical features, in association with the lupus anticoagulant, is referred to as the *antiphospholipid antibody syndrome.* The pathogenesis of thrombosis in these patients is unknown. Proposed mechanisms include direct endothelial cell injury, antibody-mediated platelet activation, and inhibition of endogenous anticoagulants such as protein C. Some patients develop these autoantibodies and the clinical syndrome without associated SLE. They are said to have the primary antiphospholipid syndrome (Chapter 5).

Given the presence of all these autoantibodies, we still know little about the mechanism of their emergence. Three converging lines of investigation hold center stage today: genetic predisposition, some nongenetic (environmental) factors, and a fundamental abnormality in the immune system.

Genetic Factors. SLE is a complex genetic trait with contribution from MHC and multiple non-MHC genes. The evidence that supports a genetic predisposition takes many forms.[48]

- Family members have an increased risk of developing SLE.
- Up to 20% of clinically unaffected first-degree relatives reveal autoantibodies and other immunoregulatory abnormalities.
- There is a higher rate of concordance (24%) in monozygotic twins when compared with dizygotic twins (1 to 3%).[49] Monozygotic twins who are discordant for SLE have similar patterns and titers of autoantibodies. These data suggest that the genetic makeup regulates the formation of autoantibodies, but the expression of the disease (i.e., tissue injury) is influenced by nongenetic (possibly environmental) factors.
- Studies of HLA associations further support the concept

that MHC genes regulate production of specific autoantibodies, rather than conferring a generalized predisposition to SLE. Specific polymorphisms of the HLA-DQ locus have been linked to the production of anti-double-stranded DNA, anti-Sm, and antiphospholipid antibodies.[50] In addition, there is considerable evidence that multiple non-MHC genes are also involved in the pathogenesis of SLE. Genome-wide linkage studies using microsatellite markers have revealed linkage with at least 12 non-MHC loci in murine models of lupus. Identification of the genes at these loci and their human counterparts is currently in progress.[48]

- Some lupus patients (approximately 6%) have inherited deficiencies of early complement components, such as C2 or C4. Lack of complement presumably impairs removal of circulating immune complexes by the mononuclear phagocyte system, thus favoring tissue deposition.

Nongenetic Factors. There are many indications that, in addition to genetic factors, several *environmental* or nongenetic factors must be involved in the pathogenesis of SLE. The clearest example comes from the observation that *drugs* such as hydralazine, procainamide, and D-penicillamine can induce an SLE-like response in humans.[43] Exposure to *ultraviolet light* is another environmental factor that exacerbates the disease in many individuals. How ultraviolet light acts is not entirely clear, but it is strongly suspected of modulating the immune response. For example, it induces keratinocytes to produce IL-1, a factor known to influence the immune response. *Sex hormones* seem to exert an important influence on the occurrence and manifestations of SLE. During the reproductive years, the frequency of SLE is 10 times greater in women than in men, and exacerbation has been noted during normal menses and pregnancy.

Immunologic Factors. With all the immunologic findings in SLE patients, there can be little doubt that some fundamental derangement of the immune system is involved in the pathogenesis of SLE. Although a variety of immunologic abnormalities affecting both T cells and B cells have been detected in patients with SLE,[51] it has been difficult to relate any one of them to the causation of this disease. For years, it had been thought that an intrinsic B-cell hyperactivity is fundamental to the pathogenesis of SLE. Polyclonal B-cell activation can be readily demonstrated in patients with SLE and in murine models of this disease. Molecular analyses of anti-double-stranded DNA antibodies, however, strongly suggest that pathogenic autoantibodies are not derived from polyclonally activated B cells. Instead, it appears that the production of tissue-damaging antibodies is driven by self-antigens and results from an oligoclonal B-cell response not dissimilar to the response to foreign antigens. The pathogenic anti-DNA antibodies isolated from patients are cationic, a feature associated with deposition in renal glomeruli, whereas the anti-DNA antibodies produced by polyclonally activated B cells are anionic and nonpathogenic. These observations have shifted the onus of driving the autoimmune response squarely on helper T cells. Based on these findings, a model for the pathogenesis of SLE (Fig. 7–23) has been proposed. SLE is a heterogeneous disease, however, and as mentioned earlier, the production of different autoantibodies is regulated by distinct genetic factors. Hence, there may well be distinct immunoregulatory disturbances in patients with different genetic backgrounds and autoantibody profiles.[42]

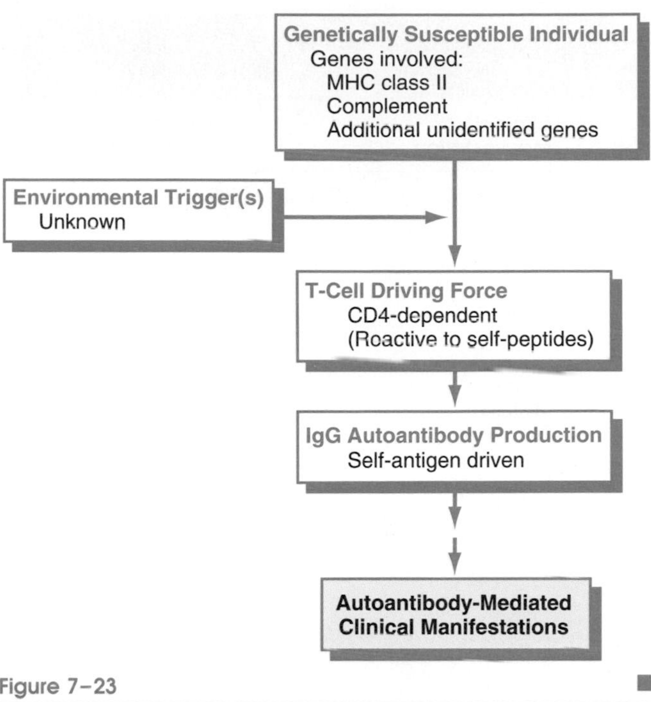

Figure 7–23

Model for the pathogenesis of systemic lupus erythematosus. (Modified from Kotzin BL: Systemic lupus erythematosus. Cell 65:303, 1996. Copyright 1996, Cell Press.)

Regardless of the exact sequence by which autoantibodies are formed, they are clearly the mediators of tissue injury. *Most of the visceral lesions are mediated by immune complexes (type III hypersensitivity).* DNA-anti-DNA complexes can be detected in the glomeruli and small blood vessels. Low levels of serum complement and granular deposits of complement and immunoglobulins in the glomeruli further support the immune complex nature of the disease. *Autoantibodies against red cells, white cells, and platelets mediate their effects via type II hypersensitivity.* There is no evidence that ANAs, which are involved in immune complex formation, can penetrate intact cells. If cell nuclei are exposed, however, the ANAs can bind to them. In tissues, nuclei of damaged cells react with ANAs, lose their chromatin pattern, and become homogeneous, to produce so-called lupus erythematosus (LE) bodies or hematoxylin bodies. Related to this phenomenon is the LE cell, which is readily seen in vitro. Basically the LE cell is any phagocytic leukocyte (neutrophil or macrophage) that has engulfed the denaturated nucleus of an injured cell. Sometimes LE cells are found in pericardial or pleural effusions in patients.

The demonstration of LE cells in vitro involves the microscopic examination of white cells. If the withdrawn

Table 7–9. CLINICAL MANIFESTATIONS OF SYSTEMIC LUPUS ERYTHEMATOSUS

Clinical Manifestation	Prevalence in Patients, %
Hematologic	100
Arthritis	90
Skin	85
Fever	83
Fatigue	81
Weight loss	63
Renal	50
Central nervous system	50
Pleurisy	46
Myalgia	33
Pericarditis	25
Gastrointestinal	21
Raynaud phenomenon	20
Ocular	15
Peripheral neuropathy	14

blood is agitated, a sufficient number of leukocytes can be damaged, thus exposing their nuclei to ANAs. The binding of ANAs to nuclei denatures them, and subsequent fixation of complement renders antibody-coated nuclei strongly chemotactic for phagocytic cells. With new techniques for detection of ANAs, however, this test is now largely of historical interest.

To summarize, SLE appears to be a complex disorder of multifactorial origin resulting from interactions among genetic, hormonal, and environmental factors acting in concert to cause activation of helper T cells and B cells that results in the secretion of several species of autoantibodies. In this complex web, each factor may be necessary but not enough for the clinical expression of the disease; the relative importance of various factors may vary from individual to individual.

MORPHOLOGY. The morphologic changes in SLE are extremely variable, reflecting the variability of the clinical manifestations and the course of the disease in individual patients. The constellation of clinical, serologic, and morphologic changes is essential for diagnosis (see Table 7–7). The frequency of individual organ involvement is shown in Table 7–9. The most characteristic lesions result from the deposition of immune complexes and are found in the blood vessels, kidneys, connective tissue, and skin.

An acute necrotizing vasculitis involving small arteries and arterioles may be present in any tissue.[52] The arteritis is characterized by fibrinoid deposits in the vessel walls. In chronic stages, vessels undergo fibrous thickening with luminal narrowing.

Kidney. On light microscopic examination, the kidney appears to be involved in 60 to 70% of cases, but if immunofluorescence and electron microscopy are included in the examination of biopsy material, almost all cases of SLE show some renal abnormality.[53] According to the World Health Organization (WHO) morphologic classification of lupus nephritis, five patterns are recognized: (1) normal by light, electron, and immunofluorescent microscopy (class I), which is quite rare; (2) mesangial lupus glomerulonephritis (class II); (3) focal proliferative glomerulonephritis (class III); (4) diffuse proliferative glomerulonephritis (class IV); and (5) membranous glomerulonephritis (class V). None of these patterns is specific for lupus.

Mesangial lupus glomerulonephritis is the mildest of the lesions and is seen in patients who have minimal clinical manifestations, such as mild hematuria or transient proteinuria. It occurs in approximately 20% of patients. There is a slight-to-moderate increase in the intercapillary mesangial matrix as well as in the number of mesangial cells. Despite the mild histologic changes, **granular mesangial deposits of immunoglobulin and complement are always present.** Such deposits presumably reflect the earliest change because filtered immune complexes accumulate primarily in the mesangium. The other changes to be described are usually superimposed on the mesangial changes.

Focal proliferative glomerulonephritis is seen in about 20% of initial biopsy specimens of these patients. As the name implies, this is a focal lesion, affecting usually fewer than 50% of the glomeruli and generally only portions of each glomerulus. Typically, one or two tufts in an otherwise normal glomerulus exhibit swelling and proliferation of endothelial and mesangial cells, infiltration with neutrophils, and sometimes fibrinoid deposits and in-

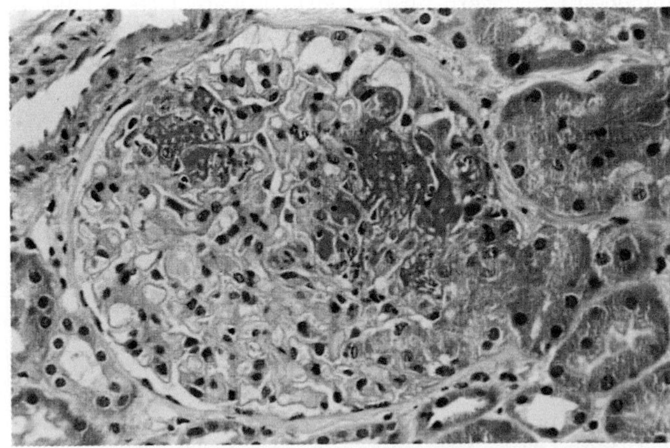

Figure 7–24

Lupus nephritis. There are two focal necrotizing lesions at 11 and 2 o'clock. (H&E stain.) (Courtesy of Dr. Helmut Rennke, Department of Pathology, Brigham and Women's Hospital, Boston, MA.)

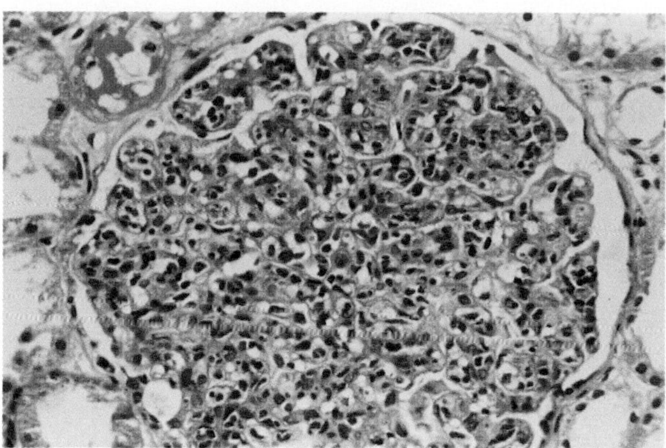

Figure 7–25 ■

Lupus nephritis, diffuse proliferative type. Note the marked increase in cellularity throughout the glomerulus. (H&E stain.) (Courtesy of Dr. Helmut Rennke, Department of Pathology, Brigham and Women's Hospital, Boston, MA.)

tracapillary thrombi (Fig. 7–24). Focal lesions are associated with hematuria and proteinuria. In some patients, the nephritis progresses to diffuse proliferative disease.

Diffuse proliferative glomerulonephritis is the most serious of the renal lesions in SLE, occurring in 40 to 50% of patients who undergo biopsy. Anatomic changes are dominated by proliferation of endothelial, mesangial, and sometimes epithelial cells (Fig. 7–25), producing in some cases epithelial crescents that fill the Bowman space (Chapter 21). The presence of fibrinoid necrosis and hyaline thrombi indicates active disease. Most or all glomeruli are involved in both kidneys, and the entire glomerulus is almost always affected. Patients with diffuse lesions are usually overtly symptomatic, showing microscopic or gross hematuria as well as proteinuria that is severe enough to cause the nephrotic syndrome in more than 50% of patients. Hypertension and mild-to-severe renal insufficiency are also common.

Membranous glomerulonephritis occurs in 15% of patients and is a designation given to glomerular disease in which the principal histologic change consists of widespread thickening of the capillary walls. The lesions are similar to those encountered in idiopathic membranous glomerulonephritis, described more fully in Chapter 21. Patients with this histologic change almost always have severe proteinuria with the nephrotic syndrome.

All four types are thought to have the same general pathogenetic mechanism (i.e., the deposition of DNA-anti-DNA complexes within the glomeruli). These complexes are believed to form in situ (i.e., the DNA is deposited first on the basement membrane, followed by anti-DNA antibody). Granular deposits of immunoglobulin and complement are regularly present in the mesangium alone or along the entire basement membrane and sometimes massively throughout the entire glomerulus (Fig. 7–26). Why this same pathogenetic mechanism produces such different histologic lesions (and clinical manifestations) in different patients is not entirely clear.

Electron microscopy demonstrates electron-dense immune complexes that may be mesangial, intramembranous, subepithelial, or subendothelial in location: (1) All histologic types show large amounts of deposits in the mesangium; (2) in membranous glomerulonephritis (class V), the deposits are predominantly between the basement membrane and the visceral epithelial cell (subepithelial), a location similar to that of deposits in other types of membranous nephropathy; and (3) subendothelial deposits (between the endothelium and the basement membrane) are most commonly seen in the diffuse proliferative variety (Fig. 7–27). When extensive, subendothelial deposits create a peculiar thickening of the capillary wall, which can be seen by means of light microscopy as a **wire loop** lesion (Fig. 7–28). Such wire loops are often found in the diffuse proliferative type of glomerulonephritis (class IV) but can also be present in the focal (class III) and membranous types (class V). They usually reflect active disease and generally indicate a poor prognosis.

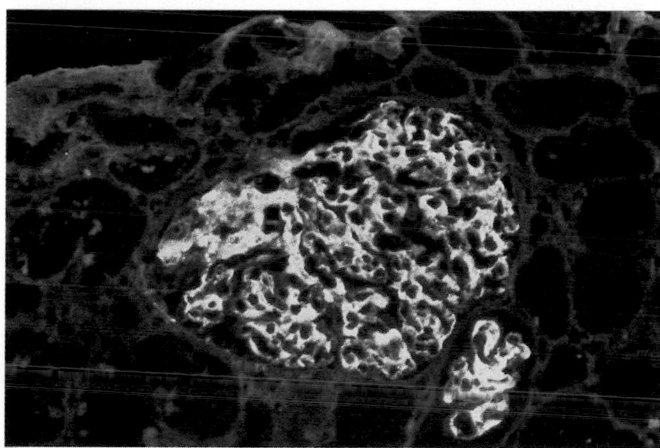

Figure 7–26 ■

Immunofluorescence micrograph stained with fluorescent anti-IgG from a patient with diffuse proliferative lupus nephritis. One complete glomerulus and part of another one are seen. Note the mesangial and capillary wall deposits of IgG. (Courtesy of Dr. Helmut Rennke, Department of Pathology, Brigham and Women's Hospital, Boston, MA.)

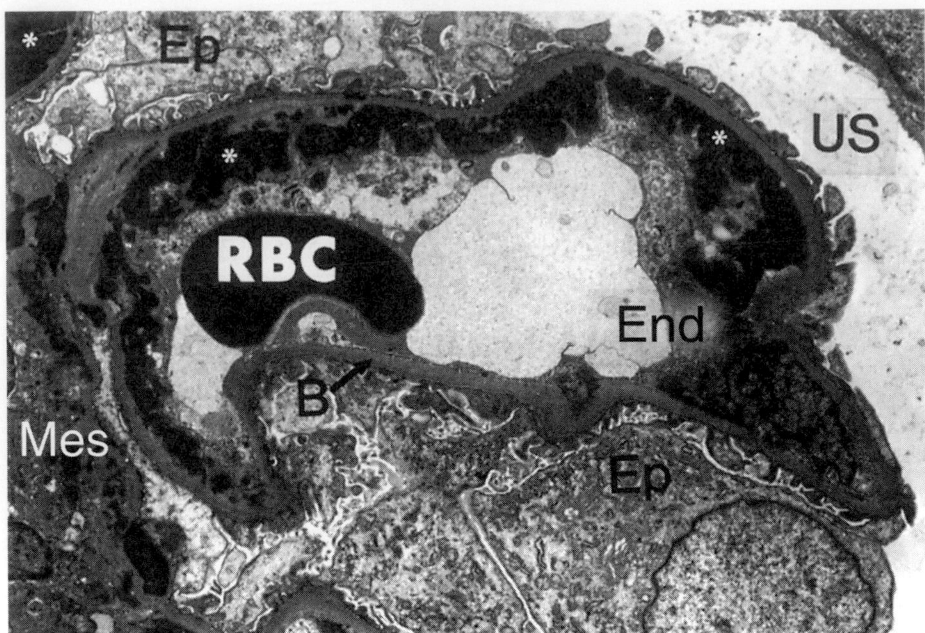

Figure 7–27

Electron micrograph of a renal glomerular capillary loop from a patient with systemic lupus erythematosus nephritis. Subendothelial dense deposits correspond to "wire loops" seen by light microscopy. End, endothelium; Mes, mesangium; Ep, epithelial cell with foot processes; RBC, red blood cell in capillary lumen; B, basement membrane; US, urinary space; *, electron-dense deposits in subendothelial location. (Courtesy of Dr. Edwin Eigenbrodt, Department of Pathology, University of Texas Southwestern Medical School, Dallas, TX.)

Changes in the **interstitium and tubules are also frequently present in patients with SLE,** especially in association with diffuse proliferative glomerulonephritis. In a few cases, tubulointerstitial lesions may be the dominant abnormality. As we shall see in Chapter 21, granular deposits composed of immunoglobulin and complement similar to those seen in glomeruli are present in the tubular basement membranes in about 50% of patients with SLE, a pattern indicative of so-called tubular immune complex disease.

Skin. The skin is involved in the majority of patients. Characteristic erythema affects the facial **butterfly** area (bridge of the nose and cheeks) in approximately 50% of patients, but a similar rash may also be seen on the extremities and trunk. Urticaria, bullae, maculopapular lesions, and ulcerations also occur. **Exposure to sunlight incites or accentuates the erythema.** Histologically the involved areas show liquefactive degeneration of the basal layer of the epidermis together with edema at the dermal junction (Fig. 7–29). In the dermis, there is variable edema and perivascular mononuclear infiltrates. Vasculitis with fibrinoid necrosis of the vessels may be prominent. Immunofluorescence microscopy shows deposition of immunoglobulin and complement along the dermoepidermal junction (Fig. 7–29). Similar deposits may be present in uninvolved skin. The presence of immunoglobulin and complement at the dermoepidermal junction is not diagnostic of SLE because similar deposits are sometimes seen in the skin of patients with scleroderma or dermatomyositis.

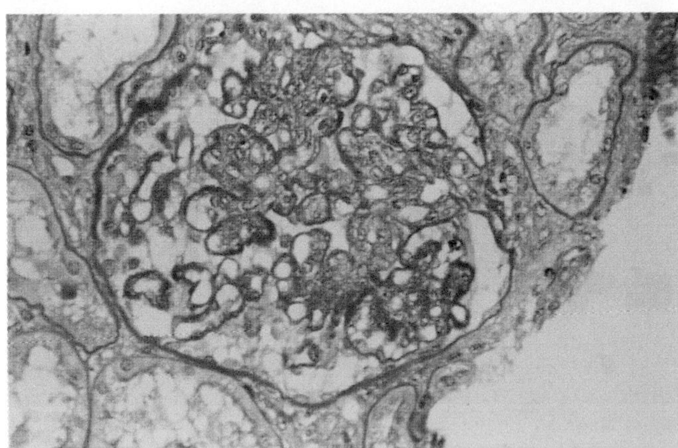

Figure 7–28

Lupus nephritis showing a glomerulus with several "wire loop" lesions representing extensive subendothelial deposits of immune complexes. (Periodic acid–Schiff [PAS] stain.) (Courtesy of Dr. Helmut Rennke, Department of Pathology, Brigham and Women's Hospital, Boston, MA.)

Joints. Joint involvement is frequent, the typical lesion being a nonerosive synovitis with little deformity. The latter fact distinguishes this arthritis from that seen in rheumatoid disease. In the acute phases of arthritis in SLE, there is exudation of neutrophils and fibrin into the synovium and a perivascular mononuclear cell infiltrate in the subsynovial tissue.

Central Nervous System. The pathologic basis of central nervous system symptoms is not entirely clear. It has often been ascribed to acute vasculitis with resultant focal neurologic symptoms. Histologic studies, however, of the nervous system in patients with neuropsychiatric manifestations of

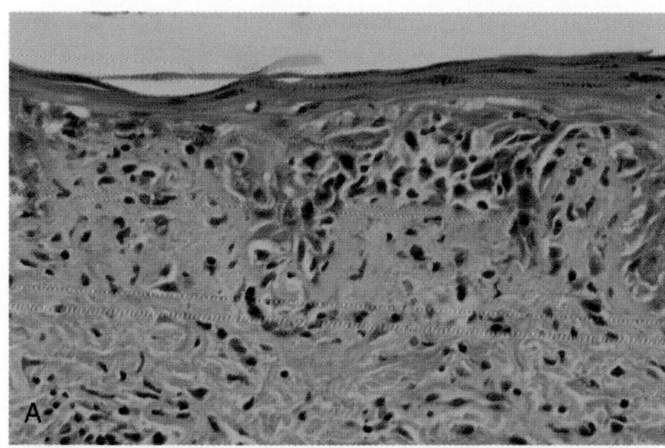

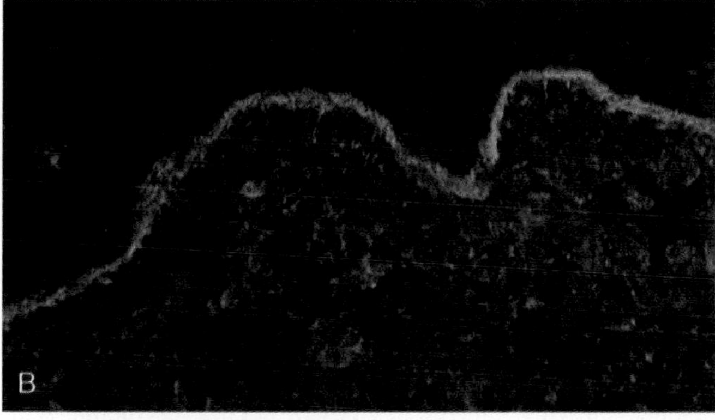

Figure 7–29

Systemic lupus erythematosus involving the skin. *A*, An H&E-stained section shows liquefactive degeneration of the basal layer of the epidermis and edema at the dermoepidermal junction. (Courtesy of Dr. Jag Bhawan, Boston University School of Medicine, Boston, MA.) *B*, An immunofluorescence micrograph stained for IgG reveals deposits of immunoglobulin along the dermoepidermal junction. (Courtesy of Dr. Richard Sontheimer, Department of Dermatology, University of Texas Southwestern Medical School, Dallas, TX.)

SLE fail to reveal significant vasculitis. Instead, noninflammatory occlusion of small vessels by intimal proliferation is sometimes noticed. These changes are believed to result from damage to the endothelium by antiphospholipid antibodies. In addition, studies suggest that antibodies against a synaptic membrane protein may play a role in the pathogenesis of central nervous system symptoms.[54]

Pericarditis and Other Serosal Cavity Involvement. Inflammation of the serosal lining membranes may be acute, subacute, or chronic. During the acute phases, the mesothelial surfaces are sometimes covered with fibrinous exudate. Later they become thickened, opaque, and coated with a shaggy fibrous tissue that may lead to partial or total obliteration of the serosal cavity.

Cardiovascular system involvement is manifested primarily in the form of pericarditis. Symptomatic or asymptomatic pericardial involvement is present in the vast majority of patients. Myocarditis, manifested as nonspecific mononuclear cell infiltration, may also be present but is less common. It may cause resting tachycardia and electrocardiographic abnormalities. Subtle or overt valvular abnormalities, detected readily by echocardiography, are fairly common in SLE. They affect mainly the mitral and aortic valves and are manifested as diffuse valve thickening that may be associated with dysfunction (stenosis or regurgitation).[55] Valvular endocarditis may occur, but it is clinically insignificant. In the era before the widespread use of steroids, so-called Libman-Sacks endocarditis was more common. This **nonbacterial verrucous endocarditis** takes the form of single or multiple irregular, 1- to 3-mm warty deposits on any valve in the heart, distinctively on **either surface of the leaflets** (i.e., on the surface exposed to the forward flow of the blood or on the underside of the leaflet) (Fig. 7–30). By comparison, the vegetations in infective endocarditis are considerably larger, and those in rheumatic heart disease (Chapter 13) are smaller and confined to the lines of closure of the valve leaflets.

An increasing number of patients have clinical evidence of coronary artery disease (angina, myocardial infarction) owing to coronary atherosclerosis. This complication is noted particularly in young patients with long-standing disease and especially in those who have been treated with corticosteroids. The pathogenesis of accelerated

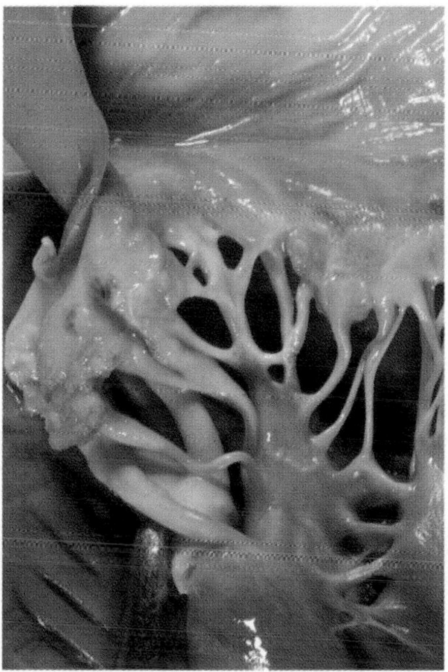

Figure 7–30

Libman-Sacks endocarditis of the mitral valve in lupus erythematosus. The vegetations attached to the margin of the thickened valve leaflet are easily seen. (Courtesy of Dr. Fred Schoen, Department of Pathology, Brigham and Women's Hospital, Boston, MA.)

coronary atherosclerosis is unclear but is probably multifactorial. The traditional risk factors, including hypertension, obesity, and hyperlipidemia, are more common in patients with lupus than in control populations. Glucocorticoid treatment induces a dyslipoproteinemia; immune complexes may damage the endothelium and promote atherosclerosis.[56]

Spleen. The spleen may be moderately enlarged. Capsular thickening is common, as is follicular hyperplasia. Plasma cells are usually numerous in the pulp and can be shown to contain immunoglobulins of the IgG and IgM types by fluorescence microscopy. The central penicilliary arteries show thickening and perivascular fibrosis, producing so-called onion-skin lesions.

Lungs. Pleuritis and pleural effusions are the most common pulmonary manifestations, affecting almost 50% of patients. Less commonly, there is evidence of alveolar injury in the form of edema and hemorrhage. In some cases, there is chronic interstitial fibrosis. None of these changes is specific for SLE.

Other Organs and Tissues. Acute vasculitis may be seen in the portal tracts of the liver accompanied by lymphocytic infiltrates, creating nonspecific portal triaditis. LE, or hematoxylin, bodies in the bone marrow may be strongly indicative of SLE. Lymph nodes may be enlarged and contain hyperactive follicles as well as plasma cells, changes that are indicative of B-cell activation.

Clinical Course. It should be evident from Tables 7–6 and 7–7 that SLE is a multisystem disease, and as such it is highly variable in its clinical presentation.[57] Typically the patient is a young woman with a butterfly rash over the face, fever, pain but no deformity in one or more peripheral joints (feet, ankles, knees, hips, fingers, wrists, elbows, shoulders), pleuritic chest pain, and photosensitivity. In many patients, however, the presentation of SLE is subtle and puzzling, taking forms such as a febrile illness of unknown origin, abnormal urinary findings, or joint disease masquerading as rheumatoid arthritis or rheumatic fever. ANAs can be found in virtually 100% of patients. ANAs, however, can also be found in patients with other autoimmune disorders (see Table 7–8). *As mentioned earlier, antibodies against double-stranded DNA and Sm antigen are virtually diagnostic of SLE.* A variety of clinical findings may point toward renal involvement, including hematuria, red cell casts, proteinuria, and, in some cases, the classic nephrotic syndrome (Chapter 21). Laboratory evidence of some hematologic derangement is seen in virtually every case, but in some patients, anemia or thrombocytopenia may be the presenting manifestation as well as the dominant clinical problem. In still others, mental aberrations, including psychosis or convulsions, may constitute prominent clinical problems. Patients with SLE are also prone to infections, presumably because of their underlying immune dysfunction and treatment with immunosuppressive drugs.[58]

The course of the disease is variable and almost unpredictable. Rare acute cases result in death within weeks to months. More often, with appropriate therapy, the disease is characterized by flare-ups and remissions spanning a period of years or even decades. During acute flare-ups, increased formation of immune complexes and the accompanying complement activation often result in hypocomplementemia. Disease exacerbations are usually treated by corticosteroids or other immunosuppressant drugs. Even without therapy, in some patients, the disease may run a benign course with skin manifestations and mild hematuria for years. The outcome has improved significantly, and an approximately 90% 5-year and 80% 10-year survival can be expected. *The most common causes of death are renal failure and intercurrent infections, followed by diffuse central nervous system disease.* Coronary artery disease is also becoming an important cause of death. Patients treated with steroids and immunosuppressive drugs incur the usual risks associated with such therapy.

As mentioned earlier, involvement of skin along with multisystem disease is fairly common in SLE. In addition, two syndromes have been recognized in which the cutaneous involvement is the most prominent or exclusive feature.

Chronic Discoid Lupus Erythematosus. Chronic discoid lupus erythematosus is a disease in which the skin manifestations may mimic SLE, but systemic manifestations are rare.[59] It is characterized by the presence of skin plaques showing varying degrees of edema, erythema, scaliness, follicular plugging, and skin atrophy surrounded by an elevated erythematous border. The face and scalp are usually affected, but widely disseminated lesions occasionally occur. The disease is usually confined to the skin, but 5 to 10% of patients with discoid lupus erythematosus develop multisystem manifestations after many years. Conversely, some patients with SLE may have prominent discoid lesions in the skin. Approximately 35% of patients show a positive ANA test, but *antibodies to double-stranded DNA are rarely present.* Immunofluorescence studies of skin biopsy specimens show the same deposition of immunoglobulin and C3 at the dermoepidermal junction that is seen in SLE.

Subacute Cutaneous Lupus Erythematosus. This condition also presents with predominant skin involvement and can be distinguished from chronic discoid lupus erythematosus by several criteria. It is characterized by widespread but superficial and nonscarring lesions and mild systemic disease. Furthermore, there is a strong association with antibodies to the SS-A antigen and with the HLA-DR3 genotype. Thus, the term *subacute cutaneous lupus erythematosus* seems to define a group intermediate between SLE and lupus erythematosus localized only to skin.[60]

Drug-Induced Lupus Erythematosus. A lupus erythematosus–like syndrome develops in patients receiving a variety of drugs, including hydralazine (given for hypertension), procainamide, isoniazid, and D-penicillamine, to name only a few of the many therapeutic agents that have been implicated.[61] Many are associated with the development of ANAs, but most do not have symptoms of lupus erythematosus. For example, 80% of the patients receiving procainamide are positive for ANAs, but only one third of these manifest clinical symptoms, such as arthralgias, fever, and serositis. *Although multiple organs are affected, renal and central nervous system involvement is distinctly uncommon.* As compared with idiopathic SLE, there are serologic and genetic differences as well. Anti-double-stranded DNA antibodies are rare, but there is an *extremely high frequency of antihistone antibodies.* Persons with the HLA-DR4 antigen are at a greater risk of developing lupus erythematosus after administration of hydralazine. The disease remits after withdrawal of the offending drug.

SJÖGREN SYNDROME

Sjögren syndrome is a clinicopathologic entity characterized by dry eyes (keratoconjunctivitis sicca) and dry mouth (xerostomia) resulting from immunologically mediated destruction of the lacrimal and salivary glands. It occurs as an isolated disorder (primary form), also known as the *sicca syndrome*, or more often in association with another autoimmune disease (secondary form). Among the associated disorders, rheumatoid arthritis is the most common, but some patients have SLE, polymyositis, scleroderma, vasculitis, mixed connective tissue disease, or thyroiditis.

Etiology and Pathogenesis. As discussed in the description of morphology, the decrease in tears and saliva (sicca syndrome) is the result of *lymphocytic infiltration* and fibrosis of the lacrimal and salivary glands. The infiltrate contains predominantly activated CD4+ helper T cells and some B cells, including plasma cells that secrete antibody locally.[62] About 75% of patients have rheumatoid factor regardless of whether coexisting rheumatoid arthritis is present or not. ANAs are detected in 50 to 80% of patients. A host of other organ-specific and non–organ-specific antibodies have also been identified. Most important, however, are antibodies directed against two RNP antigens, SS-A (Ro) and SS-B (La) (see Table 7–8), which can be detected in up to 90% of patients by highly sensitive techniques. These antibodies are thus considered serologic markers of this disease. Those with high titers of antibodies to SS-A are more likely to have extraglandular manifestations, such as cutaneous vasculitis and nephritis.[45] These autoantibodies are also present in a smaller percentage of patients with SLE and hence are not diagnostic of Sjögren syndrome.

As with other autoimmune diseases, Sjögren syndrome shows association with certain HLA alleles. Studies of whites and blacks suggest linkage of the primary form with HLA-B8, HLA-DR3, and DRW52 as well as HLA-DQA1 and HLA-DQB1 loci; in patients with anti-SS-A or anti-SS-B antibodies, specific alleles of HLA-DQA1 and HLA-DQB1 are frequent. This suggests, as in SLE, that inheritance of certain class II molecules predisposes to the development of these two autoantibodies.

Despite the plethora of antibodies, there is no evidence that they cause primary tissue injury. As with SLE, Sjögren syndrome is in all likelihood initiated by CD4+ T cells. Molecular analysis of the T-cell receptors of the infiltrating CD4+ cells indicates that some of the T cells expand clonally, suggesting antigen-driven stimulation.[63] The nature of the autoantigen(s) recognized by these T cells is still mysterious. Evidence suggests that a cytoskeletal protein called α-fodrin is a candidate autoantigen.[64]

How autoimmune reactions are initiated is equally uncertain. Much attention has focused on viruses as potential etiologic agents.[65] There is some circumstantial evidence linking EBV, the perennial culprit, to the causation of Sjögren syndrome. More compelling, however, is the association of two human retroviruses, human immunodeficiency virus type 1 (HIV-1) and human T-cell lymphotropic virus type 1 (HTLV-1). A small proportion of individuals infected with HIV-1 or HTLV-1 develop a clinical picture and pathologic changes that are virtually identical to those seen in Sjögren syndrome. Whether these viruses also play a role in the pathogenesis of Sjögren syndrome in patients who do not have other manifestations of such viral infection is not entirely clear. Molecular footprints of the HTLV-1 genome have been noted in some, but not all, cases of Sjögren syndrome. The mechanisms by which viruses can induce autoimmunity, including molecular mimicry and epitope spreading, were discussed earlier.

MORPHOLOGY. As mentioned earlier, lacrimal and salivary glands are the major targets of the disease, although other exocrine glands, including those lining the respiratory and gastrointestinal tracts and the vagina, may also be involved. The earliest histologic finding in both the major and the minor salivary glands is **periductal and perivascular lymphocytic infiltration.**[62] Eventually the lymphocytic infiltrate becomes extensive (Fig. 7–31), and in the larger salivary glands, lymphoid follicles with germinal centers may be seen. The ductal lining epithelial cells may show hyperplasia, thus obstructing the ducts. Later, there is atrophy of the acini, fibrosis, and hyalinization and, still later in the course, atrophy and replacement of parenchyma with fat. In some cases, the lymphoid infiltrate may be so intense as to give the appearance of a lymphoma; however, the benign appearance of the lymphocytes, the heterogeneous population of cells, and the preservation of lobular architecture of the gland differentiate the lesions from those of lymphoma.

The lack of tears leads to drying of the corneal epithelium, which becomes inflamed, eroded, and ulcerated; the oral mucosa may atrophy, with inflammatory fissuring and ulceration; and dryness and crusting of the nose may lead to ulcerations and even perforation of the nasal septum. In approximately 25% of cases, extraglandular tissues, such as kidneys, lungs, skin, central nervous system, and muscles, are also involved. These are more common in patients with high titers of anti-SS-A antibodies. **In contrast to SLE, glomerular lesions are extremely rare in Sjögren syndrome.** Defects of tubular function, however, including renal tubular acidosis, uricosuria, and phosphaturia, are often seen and are associated

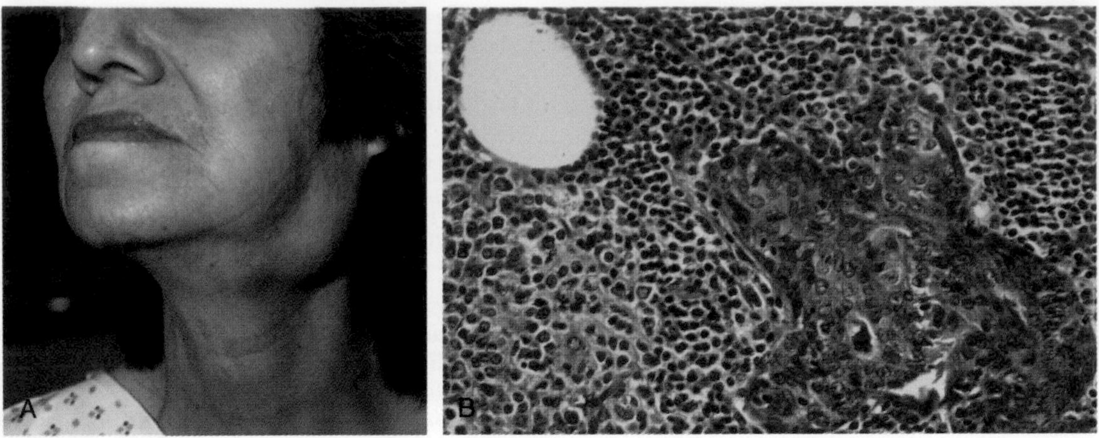

Figure 7–31

Sjögren's syndrome. *A*, Enlargement of the salivary gland. (Courtesy of Dr. Richard Sontheimer, Department of Dermatology, University of Texas Southwestern Medical School, Dallas, TX.) *B*, The histologic view shows intense lymphocytic and plasma cell infiltration with ductal epithelial hyperplasia. (Courtesy of Dr. Dennis Burns, Department of Pathology, University of Texas Southwestern Medical School, Dallas, TX.)

histologically with a **tubulointerstitial nephritis** (Chapter 21).

Clinical Manifestations. Approximately 90% of patients with Sjögren syndrome are women between the ages of 35 and 45 years.[66] As might be expected, symptoms result from inflammatory destruction of the exocrine glands. The keratoconjunctivitis produces blurring of vision, burning, and itching, and thick secretions accumulate in the conjunctival sac. The xerostomia results in difficulty in swallowing solid foods, a decrease in the ability to taste, cracks and fissures in the mouth, and dryness of the buccal mucosa. Parotid gland enlargement is present in half the patients; dryness of the nasal mucosa, epistaxis, recurrent bronchitis, and pneumonitis are other symptoms. Manifestations of extraglandular disease include synovitis, diffuse pulmonary fibrosis, and peripheral neuropathy. The 60% of patients who have an accompanying autoimmune disorder, such as rheumatoid arthritis, also have the symptoms and signs of that disorder.

The combination of lacrimal and salivary gland inflammatory involvement was once called *Mikulicz disease.* The name has now been replaced, however, by *Mikulicz syndrome*, broadened to include lacrimal and salivary gland enlargement of whatever cause. Sarcoidosis, leukemia, lymphoma, and other tumors likewise produce Mikulicz syndrome. Thus, *biopsy of the lip (to examine minor salivary glands) is essential for the diagnosis of Sjögren syndrome.*

The lymph nodes of patients with Sjögren syndrome show not only enlargement, but also a pleomorphic infiltrate of cells with frequent mitoses. In the early stages of the disease, the B cells, responding presumably to several autoantigens, are polyclonal. Clear-cut non-Hodgkin lymphomas, however, mostly of the B-cell type, have developed in the salivary glands and lymph nodes in some patients, and it is believed that patients with Sjögren syndrome have an approximately 40-fold higher risk of developing lymphoid malignancies. Presumably, polyclonal B cell activation within the glands and lymph nodes sets the stage for eventual emergence of a neoplastic, monoclonal B-cell population. These tumors are referred to as *marginal zone lymphomas* (Chapter 15).

SYSTEMIC SCLEROSIS (SCLERODERMA)

Although the term *scleroderma* is ingrained in the literature through common usage, this disease is better named *systemic sclerosis* because it is characterized by excessive fibrosis *throughout the body.* The skin is most commonly affected, but the gastrointestinal tract, kidneys, heart, muscles, and lungs also are frequently involved. In some patients, the disease appears to remain confined to the skin for many years, but in the majority, it progresses to visceral involvement with death from renal failure, cardiac failure, pulmonary insufficiency, or intestinal malabsorption. In recent years, the clinical heterogeneity of systemic sclerosis has been recognized by classifying the disease into two major categories:[67] (1) *diffuse scleroderma*, characterized by widespread skin involvement at onset, with rapid progression and early visceral involvement, and (2) *localized scleroderma*, associated with relatively limited skin involvement often confined to fingers, forearms, and face. Visceral involvement occurs late; hence the clinical course is relatively benign. Because of the somewhat higher incidence of *c*alcinosis, *R*aynaud phenomenon, *e*sophageal dysmotility, *s*clerodactyly, and *t*elangiectasia, these patients are sometimes said to have the *CREST syndrome*. Several other variants and related conditions, such as eosinophilic fasciitis, are far less frequent and are not described here.

Etiology and Pathogenesis. Systemic sclerosis is a disease of unknown cause. Excessive deposition of collagen, the hallmark of systemic sclerosis, results from multiple interacting factors that ultimately lead to the production of a variety of fibroblast growth factors and vascular endothelial injury. Both immunologic derangements and vascular abnormalities play a role in fibrogenesis.[68, 69]

Although systemic sclerosis is characterized by widespread fibrosis, there is no evidence for a primary defect in fibroblasts or collagen. *There seems to be a general consensus among experts that fibrosis is secondary to abnormal activation of the immune system.*[70] It is proposed that CD4+ T cells responding to an as yet unidentified antigen accumulate in the skin and release cytokines that recruit inflammatory cells, including mast cells and macrophages. In the skin and other affected tissues, the accumulated T cells and other inflammatory cells release a variety of mediators, such as histamine, heparin, IL-1, IL-2, IL-4, TNF-α, PDGF, and TGF-β. Several of these mediators, including TGF-β, IL-4, and PDGF, can cause transcriptional up-regulation of genes that encode collagen and other extracellular matrix proteins (e.g., fibronectin) in fibroblasts.[71] In support of this hypothesis, activated CD4+ T cells can be found in the skin of many patients with systemic sclerosis. As previously discussed in Sjögren syndrome, the molecular analysis of their T-cell receptors suggests that the accumulated CD4+ cells are oligoclonal, and their expansion is antigen driven. The possibility that the immune system may be playing a role in the pathogenesis of systemic sclerosis is further supported by the finding that several features of this disease (including the cutaneous sclerosis) are found in chronic GVH disease, a disorder that results from activation of T cells.

Microvascular disease is consistently present early in the course of systemic sclerosis. Intimal fibrosis is evident in 100% of digital arteries of patients with systemic sclerosis. Capillary dilation as well as destruction is also common. Nailfold capillary loops are distorted early in the course of disease, and later they disappear. Thus, there is unmistakable morphologic evidence of microvascular injury. Telltale signs of endothelial injury (increased levels of von Willebrand factor) and increased platelet activation (increased percentage of circulating platelet aggregates) have also been noted. It is postulated that soluble mediators released by immune-inflammatory cells inflict damage on microvascular endothelium. Some studies suggest that granzyme A, a protease released from activated CD8+ T cells, causes endothelial injury. Repeated cycles of endothelial injury followed by platelet aggregation lead to release of platelet factors (e.g., PDGF, TGF-β) that trigger periadventitial fibrosis. Activated or injured endothelial cells themselves may release PDGF and factors chemotactic for fibroblasts. Eventually, widespread narrowing of the microvasculature leads to ischemic injury as well. Whether endothelial injury can also be initiated by toxic effects of environmental triggers remains uncertain but cannot be definitively excluded.

Although T cell–mediated fibrogenesis and vascular injury are believed to be important in the pathogenesis of systemic sclerosis, there is abundant evidence for inappropriate activation of humoral immunity as well. Virtually all patients have ANAs that react with a variety of intranuclear targets.[72] Two ANAs more or less unique to systemic sclerosis have been described. One of these, directed against *DNA topoisomerase* I (anti-Scl 70), is highly specific. Depending on the ethnic group and the assay, it is present in 28 to 70% of patients with diffuse systemic sclerosis. Patients who have this antibody are more likely to have pulmonary fibrosis and peripheral vascular disease. The other, an *anticentromere antibody*, is found in 22 to 36% of patients with this disease.[73] The detection of anticentromere antibody is somewhat less specific for systemic sclerosis, being also found in 9 to 30% of patients with primary biliary cirrhosis. More importantly, 96% of those with the anticentromere antibody (including those with biliary cirrhosis) have the CREST syndrome. Hence this antibody, in contrast to the anti-DNA topoisomerase antibody, is restricted largely to patients with limited systemic sclerosis. *It is rare to have both antibodies in the same patient.*

To summarize, systemic sclerosis is associated with excessive fibrosis, changes in the microvasculature, and a variety of immunologic abnormalities. Although the antigens that trigger the (auto-)immune response have not been identified, it has been postulated that immunologic mechanisms lead to fibrosis by elaborating cytokines that activate fibroblasts or by inflicting damage on the small blood vessels, or by both (Fig. 7–32).

MORPHOLOGY. Virtually all organs may be involved in systemic sclerosis.[74] The prominent changes occur in the skin, alimentary tract, mus-

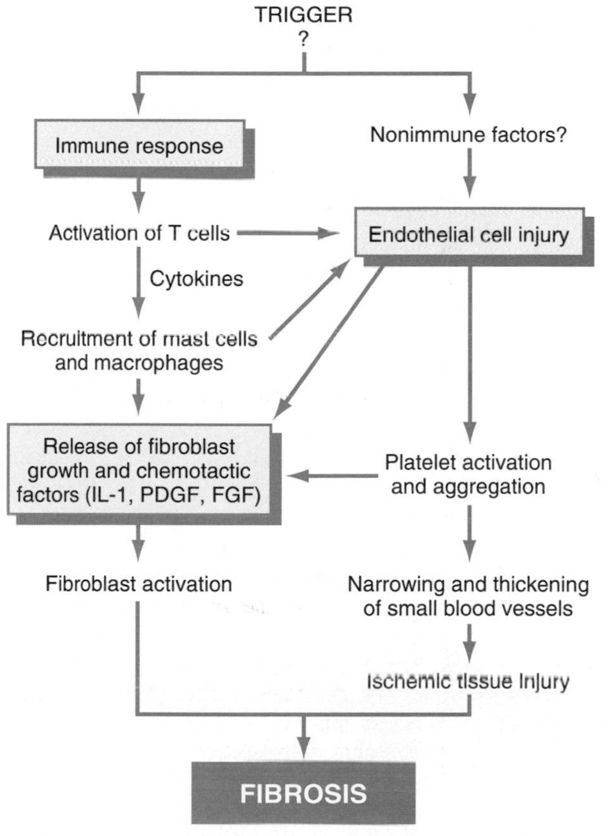

Figure 7–32 ■

Schematic illustration of the possible mechanisms leading to systemic sclerosis.

culoskeletal system, and kidney, but lesions also are often present in the blood vessels, heart, lungs, and peripheral nerves.

Skin. A great majority of patients have diffuse, sclerotic atrophy of the skin, which usually begins in the fingers and distal regions of the upper extremities and extends proximally to involve the upper arms, shoulders, neck, and face. In the early stages, affected skin areas are somewhat edematous and have a doughy consistency. Histologically, there are edema and perivascular infiltrates containing CD4+ T cells, together with swelling and degeneration of collagen fibers, which become eosinophilic. Capillaries and small arteries (150 to 500 μm in diameter) may show thickening of the basal lamina, endothelial cell damage, and partial occlusion. With progression, the edematous phase is replaced by progressive fibrosis of the dermis, which becomes tightly bound to the subcutaneous structures. There is marked increase of compact collagen in the dermis along with thinning of the epidermis, loss of rete pegs, atrophy of the dermal appendages, and hyaline thickening of the walls of dermal arterioles and capillaries (Fig. 7–33). Focal and sometimes diffuse subcutaneous calcifications may develop, especially in patients with the CREST syndrome. In advanced stages, the fingers take on a tapered, clawlike appearance with limitation of motion in the joints, and the face becomes a drawn mask. Loss of blood supply may lead to cutaneous ulcerations and to atrophic changes in the terminal phalanges (Fig. 7–34). Sometimes the tips of the fingers undergo autoamputation.

Alimentary Tract. The alimentary tract is affected in approximately 90% of patients. Progressive atrophy and collagenous fibrous replacement of the muscularis may develop at any level of the gut but are most severe in the esophagus. The lower two thirds of the esophagus often develops a rubber-hose inflexibility. The associated dysfunction of the lower esophageal sphincter gives rise to gastroesophageal reflux and its complications, including Barrett metaplasia (Chapter 18) and strictures. The mucosa is thinned and may be ulcerated, and there is excessive collagenization of the lamina propria and submucosa. Loss of villi and microvilli in the small bowel is the anatomic basis for the malabsorption syndrome sometimes encountered.

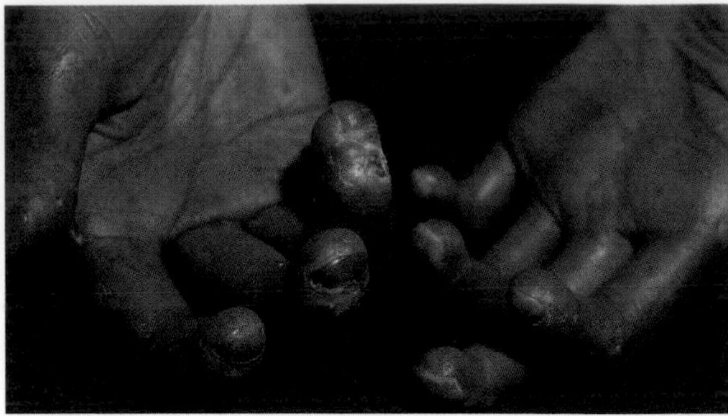

Figure 7–34

Advanced systemic sclerosis. The extensive subcutaneous fibrosis has virtually immobilized the fingers, creating a clawlike flexion deformity. Loss of blood supply has led to cutaneous ulcerations. (Courtesy of Dr. Richard Sontheimer, Department of Dermatology, University of Texas Southwestern Medical School, Dallas, TX.)

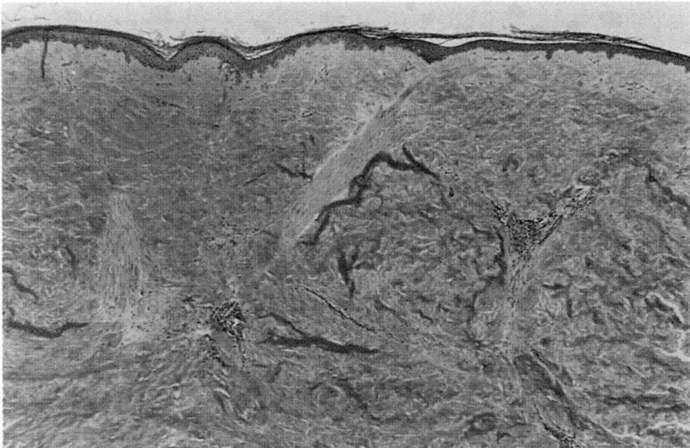

Figure 7–33

Systemic sclerosis. Note the extensive deposition of dense collagen in the dermis with virtual absence of appendages and thinning of epidermis. (Courtesy of Dr. Trace Worrell, Department of Pathology, University of Texas Southwestern Medical School, Dallas, TX.)

Musculoskeletal System. Inflammation of the synovium, associated with hypertrophy and hyperplasia of the synovial soft tissues, is common in the early stages; fibrosis later ensues. It is evident that these changes are closely reminiscent of rheumatoid arthritis, but joint destruction is not common in systemic sclerosis. In a small subset of patients (approximately 10%), inflammatory myositis indistinguishable from polymyositis may develop.

Kidneys. Renal abnormalities occur in two thirds of patients with systemic sclerosis. The most prominent are those in the vessel walls. Interlobular arteries (150 to 500 μm in diameter) show intimal thickening as a result of deposition of mucinous or finely collagenous material, which stains histochemically for glycoprotein and acid mucopolysaccharides. There is also concentric proliferation of intimal cells. These changes may resemble those seen in malignant hypertension, but it has been stressed that in scleroderma the alterations are restricted to vessels 150 to 500 μm in diameter and are not always associated with hypertension. Hypertension, however, occurs in 30% of patients with scleroderma, and in 20% it takes an ominously malignant course (malignant hypertension). In hypertensive patients, vascular alterations are more pronounced and are often associated with fibrinoid necrosis involving the arterioles together with thrombosis and infarction. When this occurs, it becomes difficult to differentiate the lesions of scleroderma from those of other types of malignant hypertension (Chapter 21). Such patients often die of renal failure, which accounts for about 50% of deaths in patients with this disease. There are no specific glomerular changes.

Lungs. The lungs are involved in more than 50% of patients with systemic sclerosis. This involvement may manifest as pulmonary hypertension and interstitial fibrosis. Pulmonary hypertension with associated vascular changes may be noted, with or without coexistent pulmonary fibrosis. Pulmonary vasospasm, secondary to pulmonary vascular endothelial dysfunction, is considered important in the pathogenesis of pulmonary hypertension. Pulmonary fibrosis, when present, is indistinguishable from that seen in idiopathic pulmonary fibrosis (Chapter 16). Hence systemic sclerosis must be considered in the differential diagnosis of diffuse pulmonary interstitial disease as well as pulmonary hypertension.

Heart. Pericarditis with effusion and myocardial fibrosis, along with thickening of intramyocardial arterioles, occurs in one third of the patients. Clinical myocardial involvement, however, is less common.

Clinical Course. Systemic sclerosis is primarily a disease of women (female-to-male ratio, 3:1) with a peak incidence in the 50- to 60-year age group. It must be apparent from the described anatomic changes that systemic sclerosis shares many features with SLE, with rheumatoid arthritis (described in Chapter 28), and with polymyositis (see later under Inflammatory Myopathies). Its distinctive features are the striking cutaneous changes. Raynaud phenomenon, manifested as episodic vasoconstriction of the arteries and arterioles of the extremities, precedes all other symptoms in 70% of cases. Dysphagia attributable to esophageal fibrosis and its resultant hypomotility is present in more than 50% of patients. Eventually, destruction of the esophageal wall leads to atony and dilation, especially at its lower end. Abdominal pain, intestinal obstruction, or malabsorption syndrome with weight loss and anemia reflect involvement of the small intestine. Respiratory difficulties owing to the pulmonary fibrosis may result in right-sided cardiac dysfunction, and myocardial fibrosis may cause either arrhythmias or cardiac failure. Mild proteinuria occurs in up to 70% of patients, but rarely is the proteinuria so severe as to cause a nephrotic syndrome. The most ominous manifestation is malignant hypertension, with the subsequent development of fatal renal failure, but in its absence progression of the disease may be slow. The disease tends to be more severe in blacks, especially black women.

As mentioned earlier, the CREST syndrome is seen in some patients with limited systemic sclerosis. It is characterized by *c*alcinosis, *R*aynaud phenomenon, *e*sophageal dysfunction, *s*clerodactyly, *t*elangiectasia, and the presence of anticentromere antibodies. Patients with the CREST syndrome have relatively limited involvement of skin, often confined to fingers, forearms, and face, and calcification of the subcutaneous tissues. Raynaud phenomenon and involvement of skin are the initial manifestations and often the only manifestations for several years. Involvement of the viscera, including esophageal lesions, pulmonary hypertension, and biliary cirrhosis, occurs late, and in general the patients live longer than those with systemic sclerosis with its diffuse visceral involvement at the outset.

INFLAMMATORY MYOPATHIES

Inflammatory myopathies comprise an uncommon, heterogeneous group of disorders characterized by immunologically mediated injury and inflammation of mainly the skeletal muscles. Three relatively distinct disorders, *dermatomyositis, polymyositis,* and *inclusion-body myositis*, are included in this category.[75] These may occur alone or with other immune-mediated diseases, particularly systemic sclerosis. The distinctive clinical features of each disorder are presented first to facilitate discussion of pathogenesis and morphologic changes.

Dermatomyositis. As the name indicates, patients with dermatomyositis have involvement of the skin as well as the skeletal muscles. Dermatomyositis may occur in children or adults and is characterized by a distinctive skin rash that may accompany or precede the onset of muscle disease. The *classic rash takes the form of a lilac or heliotrope discoloration of the upper eyelids with periorbital edema* (Fig. 7–35*A*). It is often accompanied by a scaling erythematous eruption or dusky red patches over the knuckles, elbows, and knees (Grotton lesions). *Muscle weakness* is slow in onset, is bilaterally symmetric, and *typically affects the proximal muscles first.* Thus, tasks such as getting up from a chair and climbing steps become increasingly difficult. Fine movements controlled by distal muscles are affected late in the disease. Dysphagia resulting from involvement of oropharyngeal and esophageal muscles is present in one third of the patients. Extramuscular manifestations, including interstitial lung disease, vasculitis, and myocarditis, may be present in some cases. As compared with the normal population, adults with dermatomyositis have a higher risk of developing visceral cancers. The magnitude of the risk is uncertain. According to different studies, 6 to 45% of patients with dermatomyositis have cancer.

Polymyositis. In this inflammatory myopathy, the pattern of symmetric proximal muscle involvement is similar to that seen in dermatomyositis. *It differs from dermatomyositis by the lack of cutaneous involvement and its occurrence mainly in adults*. There is a slight but statistically insignificant increase in the risk of developing visceral cancers. Similar to dermatomyositis, there may be inflammatory involvement of heart, lungs, and blood vessels.

Inclusion-Body Myositis. This is the most recently identified inflammatory myopathy. In contrast with the other two entities, inclusion-body myositis begins with the *involvement of distal muscles*, especially extensors of the knee (quadriceps) and flexors of the wrists and fingers.

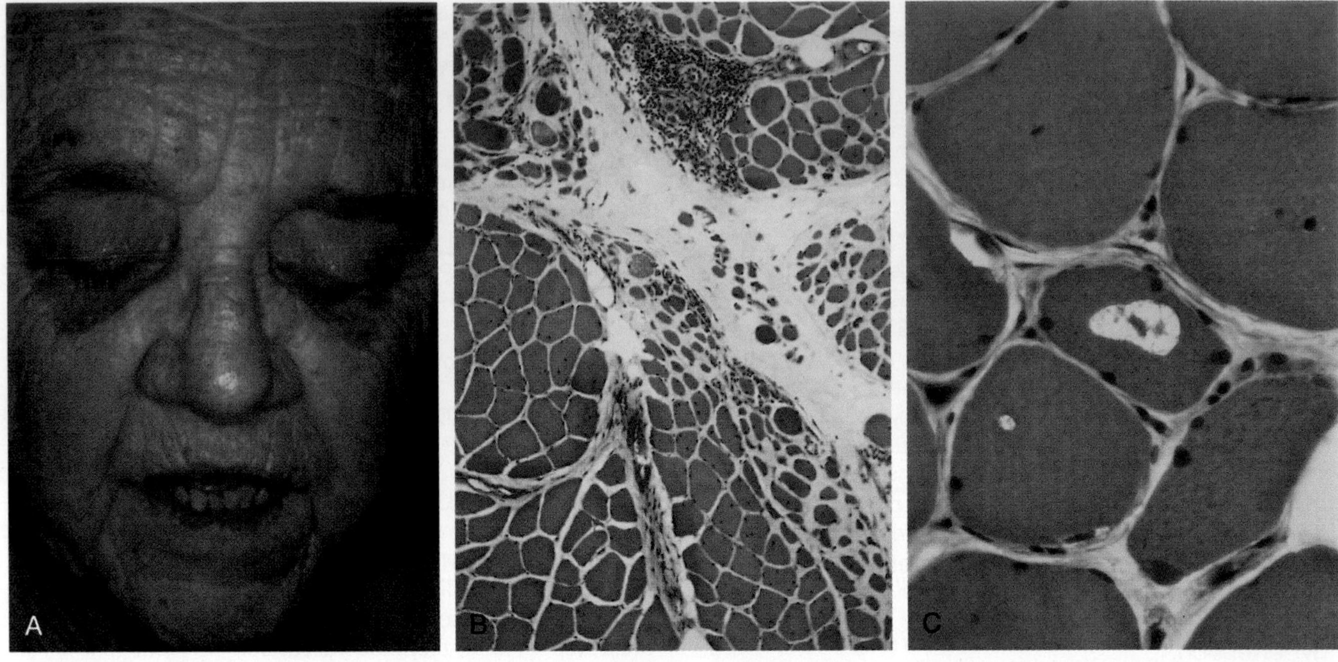

Figure 7–35

A, Dermatomyositis. Note the rash affecting the eyelids. *B*, Dermatomyositis. The histologic appearance of muscle shows perifascicular inflammation and atrophy. *C*, Inclusion body myositis showing a vacuole within a myocyte. (Courtesy of Dr. Dennis Burns, Department of Pathology, University of Texas Southwestern Medical School, Dallas, TX.)

Furthermore, muscle weakness may be *asymmetric*. This is an insidiously developing disorder that typically affects individuals over the age of 50 years.

Etiology and Pathogenesis. The cause of inflammatory myopathies is unknown, but the tissue injury seems to be mediated by immunologic mechanisms.[76] In dermatomyositis, capillaries seem to be the principal targets. The microvasculature is attacked by antibodies and complement, giving rise to foci of ischemic myocyte necrosis. This hypothesis is supported by the presence of C5b-9 membrane attack complex in small blood vessels. Such deposition precedes inflammation and destruction of muscle fibers. B cells and CD4+ T cells are present within the muscle, but there is a paucity of lymphocytes within the areas of myofiber injury. CD4+ T cells presumably provide helper function for immunoglobulin secretion by B cells. Polymyositis, in contrast, seems to be caused by cell-mediated injury. CD8+ cytotoxic T cells and macrophages are seen near damaged muscle fibers, and the expression of HLA class I molecules is increased on the sarcolemma of normal fibers. As discussed earlier, cytotoxic CD8+ T cells recognize antigens only when presented by class I MHC molecules. The pathogenesis of inclusion-body myositis is less clear. As in polymyositis, CD8+ cytotoxic T cells are found in the muscle, but in contrast to the other two forms of myositis, immunosuppressive therapy is not beneficial.

How and why autoreactive B cells and T cells develop is as mysterious in the inflammatory myopathies as it is in other presumed autoimmune diseases. Similar to other diseases in this category, ANAs are present in a variable number of cases, regardless of the clinical category (Table 7–8). The specificities of the autoantibodies are quite varied,[77] but those directed against tRNA synthetases seem to be more or less specific for inflammatory myopathies. One such antibody, referred to as anti-Jo-1, is noted in 15 to 25% of all patients within this group. Although the pathogenetic significance of this antibody is unknown, its presence is a marker of coexisting interstitial pulmonary fibrosis. This antibody may be present in dermatomyositis or polymyositis.

MORPHOLOGY. The histologic features of the individual forms of myositis are quite distinctive and are described separately.

Dermatomyositis. The inflammatory infiltrates in dermatomyositis are located predominantly around small blood vessels and in the perimysial connective tissue. Typically a few layers of atrophic fibers are present at the periphery of fascicles. Perifascicular atrophy is sufficient for diagnosis even if the inflammation is mild or absent (Fig. 7–35*B*). Quantitative analyses reveal a dramatic reduction in the intramuscular capillaries, believed to result from vascular endothelial injury and fibrosis. The perifascicular atrophy is most likely related to a relative state of hypoperfusion of this region of muscle fascicles. In addition, there are several nonspecific changes indicative of muscle fiber necrosis and regeneration.

Polymyositis. In this condition, caused by direct injury to the myofibers by CD8+ T cells, the inflammatory cells are found in the endomysium. Lymphoid cells can be seen to surround and invade healthy muscle fibers. Both necrotic and regenerating fibers are present. There is no evidence of vascular Injury.

Inclusion-Body Myositis. The diagnostic finding in this form of myositis is the presence of rimmed vacuoles (Fig. 7–35C). The vacuoles are present within myocytes, and they are marked by basophilic granules at their periphery. In addition, the vacuolated fibers also contain amyloid deposits that reveal typical staining with Congo Red (see later). Under the electron microscope, tubular filamentous inclusions are seen in the cytoplasm and the nucleus. The pattern of the inflammatory cell infiltrate is similar to that seen in polymyositis.

The diagnosis of myositis is based on clinical symptoms, electromyography, levels of muscle-related enzymes in serum, and biopsy. In a patient with muscle weakness, electromyography allows distinction between inflammatory muscle disease and diseases of neurons and receptors. As might be expected, muscle injury is associated with elevated serum levels of creatine kinase. Biopsy is required for definitive diagnosis.

MIXED CONNECTIVE TISSUE DISEASE

The term *mixed connective tissue disease* is sometimes used to describe the disease seen in a group of patients who are identified clinically by the coexistence of features suggestive of SLE, polymyositis, and systemic sclerosis and *serologically by high titers of antibodies to RNP particle-containing U1 RNP.*[78] Two other factors have been considered important in lending distinctiveness to mixed connective tissue disease—the paucity of renal disease and an extremely good response to corticosteroids, both of which could be considered as indicative of a good long-term prognosis.

Mixed connective tissue disease may present with arthritis, swelling of the hands, Raynaud phenomenon, abnormal esophageal motility, myositis, leukopenia and anemia, fever, lymphadenopathy, and hypergammaglobulinemia. These manifestations suggest SLE, polymyositis, and systemic sclerosis. Because of these overlapping features, it is not entirely clear whether mixed connective tissue disease constitutes a distinct disease or is a heterogeneous mixture of subsets of SLE, systemic sclerosis, and polymyositis.[79] Most authorities believe that mixed connective tissue disease is not a specific disorder.

POLYARTERITIS NODOSA AND OTHER VASCULITIDES

Polyarteritis nodosa belongs to a group of diseases characterized by necrotizing inflammation of the walls of blood vessels and showing strong evidence of an immunologic pathogenetic mechanism. The general term *noninfectious necrotizing vasculitis* differentiates these conditions from those due to direct infection of the blood vessel wall (such as occurs in the wall of an abscess) and serves to emphasize that any type of vessel may be involved—arteries, arterioles, veins, or capillaries.

Noninfectious necrotizing vasculitis is encountered in many clinical settings. A detailed classification and description of vasculitides is presented in Chapter 12, Diseases of the Blood Vessels, where the immunologic mechanisms are also discussed.

Immunologic Deficiency Syndromes

The immunologic deficiency syndromes are experiments of nature that allow insights into the complexities of the human immune system. Nowhere has the relevance of the individual components of immunologic function been more distinctly shown than when genetically determined deficiencies of single components have given rise to distinctive disorders. Many of the important concepts of immunology either arose from or were confirmed by the study of clinical examples of specific immunodeficiencies.

Immunodeficiencies can be divided into the primary immunodeficiency disorders, which are almost always genetically determined, and secondary immunodeficiency states, arising as complications of infections; malnutrition; aging; or side effects of immunosuppression, irradiation, or chemotherapy for cancer and other autoimmune diseases. Here we briefly discuss some of the more important primary immunodeficiencies, to be followed by a more detailed description of AIDS, the most devastating example of secondary immunodeficiency.

PRIMARY IMMUNODEFICIENCIES

Most primary immunodeficiency diseases are genetically determined and affect specific immunity (i.e., humoral and cellular) or nonspecific host defense mechanisms mediated by complement proteins and cells such as phagocytes or NK cells. Defects in specific immunity are often subclassified on the basis of the primary component involved (i.e., B cells or T cells); however, in view of the extensive interactions between T and B lymphocytes, these distinctions are not clear-cut (Fig. 7–36). In particular, T-cell defects almost always lead to impaired antibody synthesis, and hence isolated deficiencies of T cells are usually indistinguishable from combined deficiencies of T and B cells. Although originally thought to be quite rare, some forms, such as IgA deficiency, are common, and collectively they are a significant health problem, especially in children. Most primary immunodeficiencies manifest themselves in infancy, between 6 months and 2 years of life, and they are noted because of the susceptibility of infants to recurrent infections. The nature of infecting organisms depends to some extent on the nature of the underlying defect, as summarized in Table 7–10. Detailed classification of the primary immunodeficiencies according to the suggested cellular defect may be found in the WHO report on immunodeficiency and in other specialized sources.[80] Defects of phagocytes were discussed in Chapter 3. Here we present

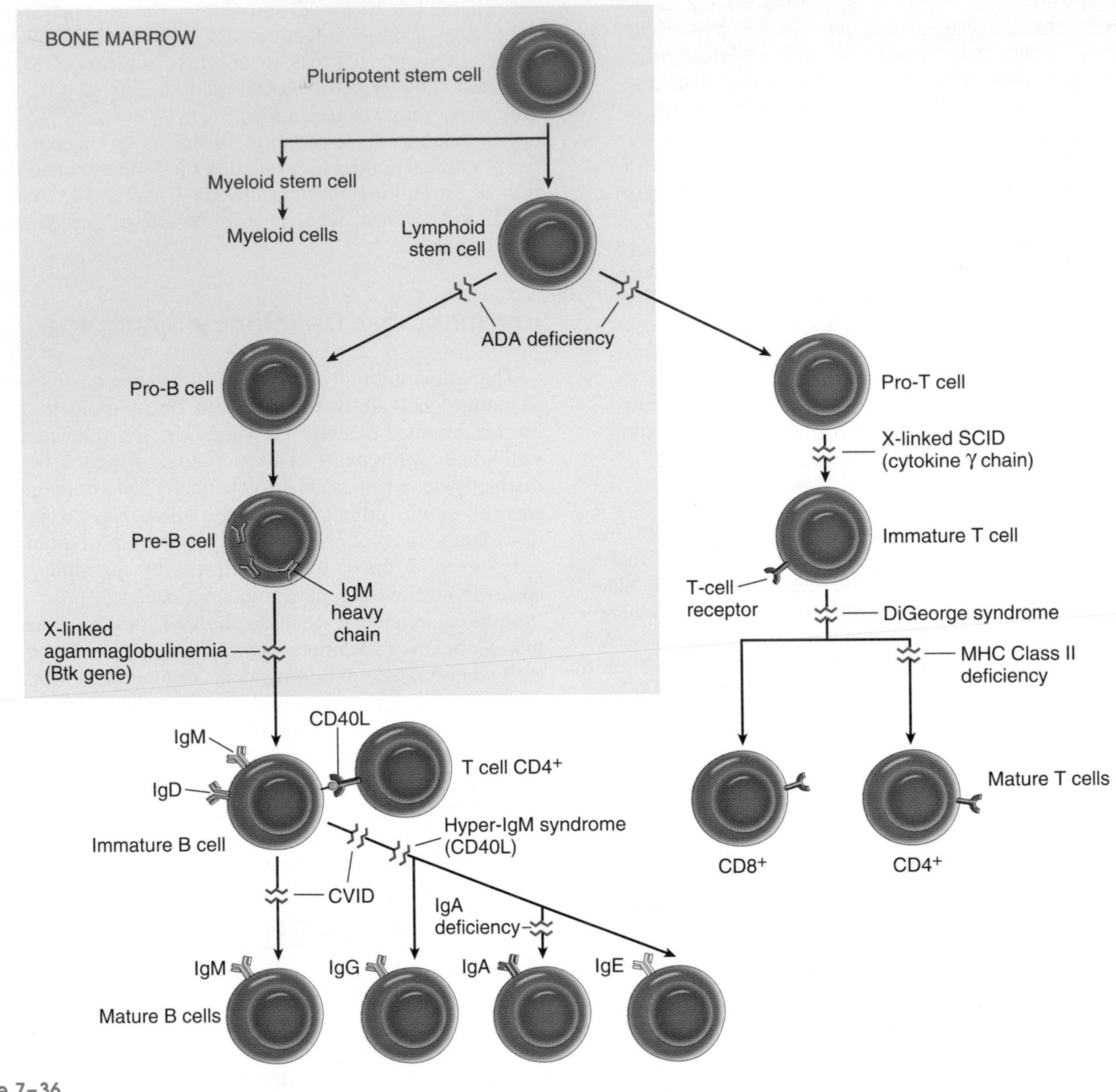

Figure 7–36

Simplified scheme of lymphocyte development and sites of block in primary immunodeficiency diseases. The affected genes are indicated in parentheses for some of the disorders. ADA, adenosine deaminase; CD40L, CD40 ligand; CVID, common variable immunodeficiency; SCID, severe combined immunodeficiency.

selected examples of other immunodeficiencies. We begin with isolated defects in B cells, followed by a discussion of combined immunodeficiencies and defects in complement proteins. Finally, Wiskott-Aldrich syndrome, a complex disorder affecting lymphocytes as well as platelets, is presented.

X-Linked Agammaglobulinemia of Bruton

Bruton disease is one of the more common forms of primary immunodeficiency.[81] It is *characterized by the failure of B-cell precursors (pro-B cells and pre-B cells) to differentiate into B cells.* During normal B-cell differentiation in the bone marrow, the immunoglobulin heavy-chain genes are rearranged first, followed by rearrangement of the light chains. In Bruton agammaglobulinemia, B-cell maturation stops after the rearrangement of heavy-chain genes. Because light chains are not produced, the complete immunoglobulin molecule containing heavy and light chains cannot be assembled and transported to the cell membrane. Free heavy chains can be found in the cytoplasm. This block in differentiation is due to mutations in a cytoplasmic tyrosine kinase, appropriately called *Bruton tyrosine kinase (btk).* Protein tyrosine kinases are known to be involved in signal transduction, and it is believed that *btk* is critical for transducing signals that drive pro-B cells to pre-B cells and pre-B cells to mature B cells. The *btk*

Table 7–10. EXAMPLES OF INFECTIOUS AGENTS IN DIFFERENT TYPES OF IMMUNE DEFICIENCIES

Pathogen Type	T-Cell Defect	B-Cell Defect	Granulocyte Defect	Complement Defect
Bacteria	Bacterial sepsis	Streptococci, staphylococci, *Haemophilus*	Staphylococci, *Pseudomonas*	Neisserial infections, other pyogenic bacterial infections
Viruses	Cytomegalovirus, Epstein-Barr virus, severe varicella, chronic infections with respiratory and intestinal viruses	Enteroviral encephalitis		
Fungi and parasites	*Candida, Pneumocystis carinii*	Severe intestinal giardiasis	*Candida, Nocardia, Aspergillus*	
Special features	Aggressive disease with opportunistic pathogens, failure to clear infections	Recurrent sinopulmonary infections, sepsis, chronic meningitis		

From Puck JM: Primary immunodeficiency diseases. JAMA 278:1835, 1997. Copyright 1997, American Medical Association.

gene maps to the long arm of the X chromosome at Xq21.2-22.

As an X-linked disease, this disorder is seen almost entirely in males, but sporadic cases have been described in females. *It usually does not become apparent until about 6 months of age, when maternal immunoglobulins are depleted.* In most cases, recurrent bacterial infections of the respiratory tract, such as acute and chronic pharyngitis, sinusitis, otitis media, bronchitis, and pneumonia, call attention to the underlying immune defect. Almost always the causative organisms are *Haemophilus influenzae, Streptococcus pneumoniae,* or *Staphylococcus aureus.* These organisms are cleared by phagocytosis for which antibodies are opsinins. Because antibodies are important for neutralizing infectious viruses during their passage through the bloodstream, these patients are also susceptible to certain viral infections, especially those caused by enteroviruses, such as echovirus, poliovirus, and coxsackievirus. These viruses infect the gastrointestinal tract, and from here they can disseminate to the nervous system via the blood. Thus, immunization with live poliovirus carries the risk of paralytic poliomyelitis, and echovirus can cause fatal encephalitis. For similar reasons, *Giardia lamblia*, an intestinal protozoon that is normally resisted by secreted IgA, causes persistent infections in these cases. In general, however, most viral, fungal, and protozoal infections are handled normally owing to intact T cell–mediated immunity. Approximately 35% of children develop arthritis that clears with restorative immunoglobulin therapy. This arthritis is believed to be infectious in origin, caused in some cases by *Mycoplasma* infection. The classic form of this disease has the following characteristics:

- B cells are absent or remarkably decreased in the circulation, and the serum levels of all classes of immunoglobulins are depressed. Precursors of B cells that express the B-lineage marker CD19 but not membrane immunoglobulin (pre-B cells) are found in normal numbers in bone marrow.
- Germinal centers of lymph nodes, Peyer's patches, the appendix, and tonsils are underdeveloped or rudimentary.
- There is remarkable absence of plasma cells throughout the body.
- T cell–mediated reactions are entirely normal.

Autoimmune diseases, such as SLE and dermatomyositis, occur with increased frequency in patients with this disease. The basis for this association is not known. The treatment of Bruton agammaglobulinemia is replacement therapy with immunoglobulins. In the past, most of the patients succumbed to infection in infancy or early childhood. Prophylactic intravenous immunoglobulin therapy allows most individuals to reach adulthood.

Common Variable Immunodeficiency

This relatively common but poorly defined derangement represents a heterogeneous group of disorders. *The feature common to all patients is hypogammaglobulinemia, generally affecting all the antibody classes but sometimes only IgG.*[82] The diagnosis of common variable immunodeficiency is based on exclusion of other well-defined causes of decreased antibody synthesis.

As might be expected in a heterogeneous group of disorders, both sporadic and inherited forms of the disease occur. In familial forms, there is no single pattern of inheritance. In some patients, linkage with unidentified gene(s) within the HLA complex has been noted. Relatives of such patients have a high incidence of selective IgA deficiency (see later). These studies suggest that at least in some cases, selective IgA deficiency and common variable immunodeficiency may represent different expressions of a common genetic defect in antibody synthesis. The basis of immunoglobulin deficiency in common variable immunodeficiency is varied, but it is distinct from that in X-linked agammaglobulinemia. In contrast to the latter, most patients with common variable immunodeficiency have normal or near-normal numbers of B cells in the blood and lymphoid tissues. These B cells, however, are not able to differentiate into plasma cells.

The molecular basis of abnormal B-cell differentiation is incompletely understood. According to some authorities, there is no evidence of any intrinsic B-cell defects.[82] Rather, there are several different defects in the ability of

T cells to send appropriate maturational and activation signals to B cells. According to others, some patients have intrinsic B-cell defects as well as abnormalities of T cell–mediated regulation of B cells.[83] The reported differences in the mechanisms of the B-cell defect further attest to the heterogeneity of this condition.

The clinical manifestations of common variable immunodeficiency are those of antibody deficiency, and hence they resemble those of X-linked agammaglobulinemia. Thus, the patients typically present with recurrent sinopulmonary pyogenic infections. In addition, about 20% of patients present with recurrent herpesvirus infections. Serious enterovirus infections causing meningoencephalitis may also occur. Patients are also prone to the development of persistent diarrhea caused by *G. lamblia.* In contrast to X-linked agammaglobulinemia, however, common variable immunodeficiency affects both sexes equally, and the onset of symptoms is later—in childhood or adolescence. Histologically the B-cell areas of the lymphoid tissues (i.e., lymphoid follicles in nodes, spleen, and gut) are hyperplastic. The enlargement of B-cell areas probably reflects defective immunoregulation, that is, B cells can proliferate in response to antigen, but because antibody production is impaired, the normal feedback inhibition by IgG is absent.

These patients have a high frequency of autoimmune diseases (approximately 20%), including rheumatoid arthritis, pernicious anemia, and hemolytic anemia. The risk of lymphoid malignancy is also increased, particularly in women. A 50-fold increase in gastric cancer has also been noted. All these features suggest widespread defects in immunoregulation.

Isolated IgA Deficiency

Isolated IgA deficiency is a common immunodeficiency. In the United States, it occurs in about 1 in 600 individuals of European descent.[84] It is far less common in blacks and Asians. Affected individuals have extremely low levels of *both serum and secretory IgA.* It may be familial or acquired in association with toxoplasmosis, measles, or some other viral infection. The association of IgA deficiency with common variable immunodeficiency and their linkage to HLA genes was mentioned earlier. It is generally believed that most individuals with this disease are completely asymptomatic. Because IgA is the major immunoglobulin in external secretions, mucosal defenses are weakened, and infections occur in the respiratory, gastrointestinal, and urogenital tracts. Symptomatic patients commonly present with recurrent sinopulmonary infections and diarrhea. It is now apparent that some individuals previously classified as having selective IgA deficiency are also deficient in IgG_2 and IgG_4 subclasses of IgG. This group of patients is particularly prone to developing infections. In addition, IgA-deficient patients have a high frequency of respiratory tract allergy and a variety of autoimmune diseases, particularly SLE and rheumatoid arthritis. The basis of the increased frequency of autoimmune and allergic diseases is not known. Because secretory IgA normally acts as a mucosal barrier against foreign proteins and antigens, it could be speculated that unregulated absorption of foreign protein antigens triggers abnormal immune responses in vivo.

The basic defect is in the differentiation of IgA B lymphocytes. The molecular basis of this defect, however, is still elusive.[84] In most patients, the number of IgA-positive B cells is normal, but only a few of these cells can be induced to transform into IgA plasma cells in vitro. Serum antibodies to IgA are found in approximately 40% of the patients. Whether this finding is of any etiologic significance is unknown, but it has important clinical implications. When transfused with blood containing normal IgA, some of these patients develop severe, even fatal, anaphylactic reactions.

Hyper IgM Syndrome

Hyper IgM syndrome was originally thought to be a B-cell disorder because the *affected patients make IgM antibodies but are deficient in their ability to produce IgG, IgA, and IgE antibodies.* It is now known that this is a T-cell disorder in which functionally abnormal T cells fail to induce B cells to make antibodies of isotypes other than IgM. To understand the molecular basis of this disorder, it is essential to review the mechanisms responsible for the formation of antibodies of different isotypes. In an immune response to protein antigen, IgM and IgD antibodies are produced first, followed by the sequential formation of IgG, IgA, and IgE antibodies. This orderly appearance of antibody types during a normal immune response is called *isotype switching*. The ability of IgM-producing B cells to turn on the transcription of genes that encode other immunoglobulin isotypes depends on soluble (cytokines) and contact-mediated signals from CD4+ T cells. Involved in this process is physical interaction between the CD40 molecules in B cells and CD40 ligands (CD40L) expressed on activated T cells. Thus, mutations in either CD40L or CD40 prevent the T-cell and B-cell interaction necessary for isotype switching, and the patients develop this type of immunodeficiency. In approximately 70% of the cases, the mutations affect the gene for CD40L that maps to Xq26. These patients have the X-linked form of the disease. In the remaining patients, the precise mutations have not been fully characterized but are believed to affect CD40 or other B-cell molecules in the CD40 signaling pathway.

Clinically, male patients with the X-linked form of the hyper-IgM syndrome present with recurrent pyogenic infections because the level of opsonizing IgG antibodies is low. In addition, they are also susceptible to *Pneumocystis carinii* pneumonia, suggesting that there is a defect in T cell–mediated immunity as well. In keeping with this, studies suggest that CD40-CD40L interactions play a central role in many cellular interactions, including those essential for the development of cytotoxic T cells[85] and activation of macrophages. Defects in T cell–mediated signaling of macrophages can induce susceptibility to organisms such as *P. carinii.*

The serum of patients with this syndrome contains normal or elevated levels of IgM and IgD but no IgA or IgE and extremely low levels of IgG. The number of B and T cells is normal. Many of the IgM antibodies react with elements of blood, giving rise to autoimmune hemolytic anemia, thrombocytopenia, and neutropenia. In older patients, there may be uncontrolled proliferation of IgM-producing plasma cells with infiltrations of the gastrointestinal tract. Although the proliferating B cells are polyclonal, extensive infiltration may lead to death.

DiGeorge Syndrome (Thymic Hypoplasia)

DiGeorge syndrome is an example of a T-cell deficiency that derives from failure of development of the third and fourth pharyngeal pouches. The latter give rise to the thymus, the parathyroids, some of the clear cells of the thyroid, and the ultimobranchial body. Thus, these patients have a variable loss of T cell–mediated immunity (owing to hypoplasia or lack of the thymus), tetany (owing to lack of the parathyroids), and congenital defects of the heart and great vessels. In addition, the appearance of the mouth, ears, and facies may be abnormal. Absence of cell-mediated immunity is reflected in low levels of circulating T lymphocytes and a poor defense against certain fungal and viral infections. Plasma cells are present in normal numbers in lymphoid tissues, but the thymic-dependent paracortical areas of the lymph nodes and the periarteriolar sheaths of the spleen are depleted. Immunoglobulin levels may be normal or reduced, depending on the severity of the T-cell deficiency.

Patients with *partial* DiGeorge syndrome, who have an extremely small but histologically normal thymus, have also been recorded. T-cell function improves with age in these children, so that by 5 years of age, many have no T-cell deficit. In those with a complete absence of thymus, transplantation of fetal thymus may be of benefit.

DiGeorge syndrome is not a familial disorder. It results from the deletion of some unidentified genes that map to chromosome 22q11.[86] This deletion is seen in 90% of patients, and DiGeorge syndrome is now considered a component of the 22q11 deletion syndrome, as discussed in greater detail in Chapter 6.

Severe Combined Immunodeficiency Diseases

Severe combined immunodeficiency disease (SCID) represents a constellation of genetically distinct syndromes, all having in common variable defects in both humoral and cell-mediated immune responses. Affected infants present with prominent thrush (oral candidiasis), extensive diaper rash, and failure to thrive. Some patients develop a morbilliform rash shortly after birth owing to transplacental transfer of maternal T cells that cause graft-versus-host disease. Patients with SCID are extremely susceptible to recurrent, severe infections by a wide range of pathogens, including *Candida albicans, P. carinii, Pseudomonas,* cytomegalovirus, varicella, and a whole host of bacteria. Without bone marrow transplantation, death occurs within the first year of life. Despite the common clinical manifestations, the underlying defects are quite different and in many cases unknown. The so-called classic form, initially described in Swiss infants and believed to result from a defect in the common lymphoid stem cell, is extremely uncommon (Fig. 7–36). More commonly, the SCID defect resides in the T-cell compartment, with a secondary impairment of humoral immunity. The T-cell defects may occur at any stage of the T-cell differentiation and activation pathway.

The most common form, accounting for 50 to 60% of cases, is X-linked, and hence SCID is more common in boys than in girls. The genetic defect in the X-linked form is a mutation in the common γ chain subunit (γc) of several cytokine receptors. This transmembrane protein is part of the signal transducing components of the receptors for IL-2, IL-4, IL-7, IL-9, IL-11, and IL-15. As a result of this mutation, the lymphoid progenitor cells in patients with X-linked SCID fail to be stimulated by these cytokines, and in effect there is a functional deficiency of all these growth factors. Because many of these cytokines are required for lymphoid development, X-linked SCID is associated with a profound defect in the earliest stages of T-cell development and late stages of B-cell development. Not surprisingly, T-cell numbers are greatly reduced, and although B cells are normal in number, antibody synthesis is greatly impaired because of lack of T-cell help.

The remaining cases of SCID are inherited as autosomal recessives. The most common cause of autosomal recessive SCID is a deficiency of the enzyme adenosine deaminase (ADA). Although the mechanisms by which ADA deficiency causes SCID are not entirely clear, it has been proposed that deficiency of ADA leads to accumulation of deoxyadenosine and its derivatives (e.g., deoxy-ATP), which are particularly toxic to immature lymphocytes,[87] especially those of T lineage. Hence there may be a greater reduction in the number of T lymphocytes than of B lymphocytes. Patients with ADA deficiency have been treated with bone marrow transplantation and, more recently, with gene therapy. The ADA gene may be introduced into the patient's bone marrow cells before reinfusion. Alternatively, T cells harvested from the patient's peripheral blood are expanded in vitro, transfected with the ADA gene, then returned to the patient. This experimental form of therapy has met with some success.[88]

Several other less common causes of autosomal recessive SCID have been discovered, as follows:[89]

- Mutations in recombinase activating genes prevent the somatic gene rearrangements essential for the assembly of T-cell receptors and immunoglobulin genes. This blocks the development of T and B cells.
- An intracellular kinase called *Jak 3* is essential for signal transduction through the common cytokine receptor γ chain (that is mutated in X-linked SCID). Mutations of Jak 3 therefore have the same effects as mutations in the γ chain. The difference between these two forms of SCID is in their patterns of inheritance.
- Mutations that impair the expression of class II MHC molecules prevent the development of CD4+ T cells. Class II MHC molecules present antigen to CD4+ T cells, and during T-cell development in the thymus, CD4 T-cell development depends on interaction with MHC class II molecules expressed on thymic epithelium. CD4+ T cells provide help to other T cells as well as B cells, and hence MHC class II deficiency is associated with combined immunodeficiency. The genetic defect in these cases does not lie in MHC genes but transcription factors that regulate their expression.

The histologic findings in SCID depend on the underlying defect. In the two most common forms (ADA deficiency and γc mutation), the thymus is small and devoid of lymphoid cells. In the ADA-negative SCID, remnants of

Hassall corpuscles can be found, whereas in the X-linked recessive SCID, the thymus contains lobules of undifferentiated epithelial cells resembling fetal thymus.[90] In either case, other lymphoid tissues are hypoplastic as well, with marked depletion of T-cell areas and in some cases both T-cell and B-cell zones.

Currently, bone marrow transplantation is the mainstay of treatment, but with the elucidation of genetic defects, specific gene therapy is on the horizon.

Immunodeficiency With Thrombocytopenia and Eczema (Wiskott-Aldrich Syndrome)

Wiskott-Aldrich syndrome has been deemed "curious," "enigmatic," or "confusing" because its immunologic defects are so difficult to explain. *It is an X-linked recessive disease characterized by thrombocytopenia, eczema, and a marked vulnerability to recurrent infection, ending in early death.* The thymus is morphologically normal, at least early in the course of the disease, but there is progressive secondary depletion of T lymphocytes in the peripheral blood and in the paracortical (thymus-dependent) areas of the lymph nodes, with variable loss of cellular immunity. Patients do not make antibodies to polysaccharide antigens, and the response to protein antigens is poor. IgM levels in the serum are low, but levels of IgG are usually normal. Paradoxically the levels of IgA and IgE are often elevated. Patients are also prone to developing malignant lymphomas. The Wiskott-Aldrich syndrome maps to Xp11.23, where the disease gene called *Wiskott-Aldrich syndrome protein* is located. This multifunctional protein is involved in maintaining the integrity of the cytoskeleton as well as signal transduction.[91] How this protein is responsible for normal lymphocyte and platelet function is unclear. The only treatment is bone marrow transplantation.

Genetic Deficiencies of the Complement System

The various components of the complement system play a critical role in inflammatory and immunologic responses. Hereditary deficiencies have been described for virtually all components of the complement system and two of the inhibitors.[92] A deficiency of C2 is the most common of all. With a deficiency of C2 or the other components of the classic pathway (i.e., C1 [C1q,r, or s], C2, or C4), there is some increased susceptibility to infections, but the dominant manifestation is an increased incidence of an SLE-like disease. Presumably the alternative complement pathway is adequate for the control of most infections. The basis of an increase in the incidence of SLE is not fully understood. One possibility is that in the absence of complement proteins antigen-antibody complexes are not cleared well by the monocyte-macrophage system, and hence they deposit in tissues. Alternatively, there may be linkage disequilibrium between complement genes and other disease-associated genes that also map within the HLA region. The deficiency of components of the alternative pathway (properdin and factor D) is rare. It is associated with recurrent pyogenic infections. The C3 component of complement is required for both the classic and alternative pathways, and hence a deficiency of this protein gives rise to serious and recurrent pyogenic infections. There is also increased incidence of immune complex–mediated glomerulonephritis. The terminal components of complement C5, 6, 7, 8, and 9 are required for the assembly of the membrane attack complex involved in the lysis of organisms. With a deficiency of these late-acting components, there is increased susceptibility to recurrent neisserial (gonococcal and meningococcal) infections, reflecting the importance of bacterial lysis in the defense against *Neisseria*.

A deficiency of C1 inhibitor gives rise to hereditary angioedema. This autosomal dominant disorder is more common than complement deficiency states.[93] The C1 inhibitor is a protease inhibitor whose target enzymes are C1r and C1s of the complement cascade, factor XII of the coagulation pathway, and the kallikrein system. As discussed in Chapter 3, these pathways are closely linked, and their unregulated activation can give rise to vasoactive peptides such as bradykinin. Although the exact nature of the bioactive compound produced in hereditary angioedema is uncertain, these patients have episodes of edema affecting skin and mucosal surfaces such as the larynx and the gastrointestinal tract. This may result in life-threatening asphyxia or nausea, vomiting, and diarrhea after minor trauma or emotional stress. Acute attacks of hereditary angioedema can be treated with C1 inhibitor concentrates prepared from human plasma.

ACQUIRED IMMUNODEFICIENCY SYNDROME

AIDS is a *retroviral disease characterized by profound immunosuppression that leads to opportunistic infections, secondary neoplasms, and neurologic manifestations.* The magnitude of this modern plague is truly staggering. By the end of 1997, more than 600,000 cases of AIDS had been reported in the United States. Of these, about 60% had died, and, despite dramatic improvements in drug therapy, the true mortality rate is likely to approach 100%. In the United States, AIDS is the leading cause of death in men between 25 and 44 years of age, and it is the third leading cause of death in women in this age group.[94] Although initially recognized in the United States, AIDS is a global problem. According to United Nations estimates, by the end of the year 2000 about 40 million people will be infected with HIV, the causative agent of AIDS; of these, more than 90% will be in developing countries.[95, 95a] Because of the magnitude of the AIDS problem, there has been an explosion of new knowledge relating to HIV and its remarkable ability to cripple host defenses. So rapid is the pace of research on the molecular biology and immunology of HIV that any review of this rapidly changing field is destined to be out of date by the time it is published. It is with this humbling realization that an attempt is made here to summarize the currently available data on the epidemiology, cause, pathogenesis, and clinical features of HIV infection.

Epidemiology. Although AIDS was first described in the United States, and the United States has the majority of the reported cases, AIDS has now been reported from more than 193 countries around the world, and the pool of HIV-infected persons in Africa and Asia is large and expanding. Epidemiologic studies in the United States have identified five groups of adults at risk for developing AIDS. The case distribution in these groups is as follows:

- *Homosexual or bisexual men* constitute by far the largest group, accounting for 57% of the reported cases. This includes 6% who were intravenous drug abusers as well. Transmission of AIDS in this category is on the decline: Currently, fewer than 50% of new cases can be attributed to male homosexual contacts.
- *Intravenous drug abusers* with no previous history of homosexuality compose the next largest group, representing about 25% of all patients. They represent the majority of all cases among heterosexuals.
- *Hemophiliacs,* especially those who received large amounts of factor VIII concentrates before 1985, make up 0.8% of all cases.
- *Recipients of blood and blood components* who are not hemophiliacs but who received transfusions of HIV-infected whole blood or components (e.g., platelets, plasma) account for 1.2% of patients. (Organs obtained from HIV-infected donors can also transmit AIDS.)
- *Heterosexual contacts* of members of other high-risk groups (chiefly intravenous drug abusers) constitute 10% of the patient population.
- In approximately 6% of cases, the risk factors cannot be determined.

The epidemiology of AIDS is quite different in children under the age of 13 years. Close to 2% of all AIDS cases occur in this pediatric population. In this group, more than 90% have resulted from transmission of the virus from mother to child (discussed later). The remaining 10% are hemophiliacs and others who received blood or blood products before 1985.

It should be apparent from the preceding discussion that transmission of HIV occurs under conditions that facilitate exchange of blood or body fluids containing the virus or virus-infected cells. Hence the three major routes of transmission are *sexual contact, parenteral inoculation,* and *passage of the virus from infected mothers to their newborns.*

Sexual transmission is clearly the predominant mode of infection worldwide, accounting for about 75% of all cases of HIV transmission.[96] Because the majority of patients in the United States are homosexual or bisexual men, most sexual transmission has occurred among homosexual men. The virus is carried in the semen, both within the lymphocytes and in the cell-free state, and it enters the recipient's body through abrasions in rectal mucosa. Hence receptive anal intercourse increases the probability of infection. Viral transmission occurs in two ways: (1) direct inoculation into the blood vessels breached by trauma and (2) into Langerhans cells within the mucosa. Heterosexual transmission, although initially of less quantitative importance in the United States, is globally the most common mode by which HIV is spread. In the past few years, even in the United States, *the rate of increase of heterosexual transmission has outpaced transmission by other means.* Such spread is occurring most rapidly in female sex partners of male intravenous drug abusers. As such, the number of women with AIDS is rising rapidly. In contrast to the US experience, heterosexual transmission is the dominant mode of HIV infection in Asia and Africa.

In addition to male-to-male and male-to-female transmission, there is evidence supporting female-to-male transmission. HIV is present in vaginal secretions and cervical cells of infected women. In the United States, this form of heterosexual spread, however, is approximately 20-fold less efficient than male-to-female transmission. By contrast, in Thailand, the risk of female-to-male transmission is much higher. This is believed to be related to the predominance of a different strain of the causative virus in Thailand. All forms of sexual transmission of HIV are aided and abetted by coexisting sexually transmitted diseases, especially those associated with genital ulceration. In this regard, syphilis, chancroid, and herpes are particularly important. Other sexually transmitted diseases, including gonorrhea and chlamydia, are also cofactors for HIV transmission. In these genital inflammatory states, there is greater concentration of the virus in seminal fluid, in part owing to increased numbers of inflammatory cells in the semen.

Parenteral transmission of HIV has occurred in three groups of individuals: intravenous drug abusers, hemophiliacs who received factor VIII concentrates, and random recipients of blood transfusion. Of these three, intravenous drug abusers constitute by far the largest group. Transmission occurs by sharing of needles, syringes, and other paraphernalia contaminated with HIV-containing blood. This group occupies a pivotal position in the AIDS epidemic because it represents the principal link in the transmission of HIV to other adult populations through heterosexual activity.

Transmission of HIV by transfusion of blood or blood products, such as lyophilized factor VIII concentrates, has been virtually eliminated. This happy outcome resulted from three public health measures: screening of donated blood and plasma for antibody to HIV, heat treatment of clotting factor concentrates, and screening of donors on the basis of history. There persists, however, an extremely small risk of acquiring AIDS through transfusion of seronegative blood because a recently infected individual may be antibody negative. Currently, this risk is estimated to be 1 in 493,000 per unit of blood transfused.[97] Because it is now possible to detect HIV-associated p24 antigens in the blood before the development of humoral antibodies, this small risk is likely to decrease even further.

As alluded to earlier, *mother-to-infant transmission* is the major cause of pediatric AIDS. Infected mothers can transmit the infection to their offspring by three routes: (1) in utero by transplacental spread, (2) during delivery through an infected birth canal, and (3) after birth by ingestion of breast milk. Of these, transmission during birth (intrapartum) and in the immediate period thereafter (peripartum) is considered to be the most common mode in the United States. The reported transmission rates vary from 7% to 49% in different parts of the world. In most North American locales, the rate for perinatal transmission is about 25%. Higher risk of transmission is associated with high maternal viral load and low CD4+ T cell counts as well as chorioamnionitis.[98]

Because of the uniformly fatal outcome of AIDS, much concern has arisen in the lay public and among health care workers regarding spread of HIV infection outside the high-risk groups. Extensive studies indicate that *HIV infec-*

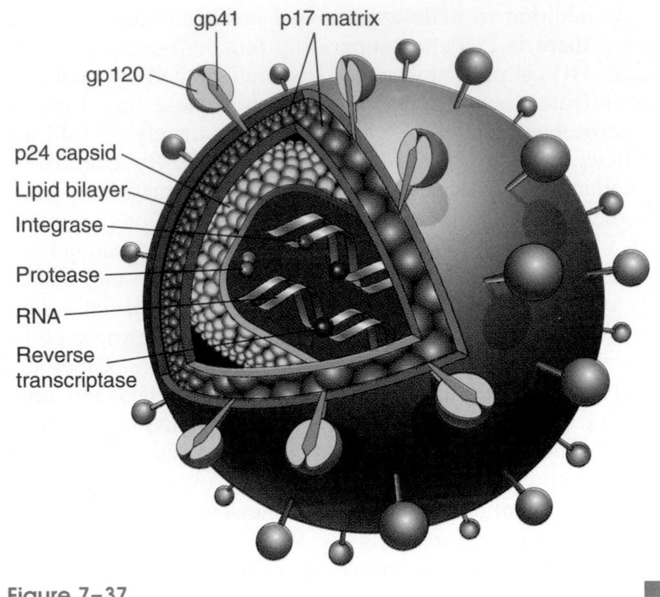

Figure 7–37

Schematic illustration of an HIV-1 virion. The viral particle is covered by a lipid bilayer that is derived from the host cell.

tion cannot be transmitted by casual personal contact in the household, workplace, or school. No convincing evidence for spread by insect bites has been obtained. Regarding transmission of HIV infection to health care workers, an extremely small but definite risk seems to be present. Seroconversion has been documented after accidental needle-stick injury or exposure of nonintact skin to infected blood in laboratory accidents. After such accidents, the risk of seroconversion is believed to be about 0.3%.[99] By comparison, approximately 30% of those accidentally exposed to hepatitis B–infected blood become seropositive.[100] Although much publicized and a cause of justifiable concern, the transmission of AIDS from an infected health care provider to a patient is extremely rare. There is currently only one such case of suspected transmission: from a dentist to his patient.

Etiology. There is little doubt that AIDS is caused by HIV, a nontransforming human retrovirus belonging to the lentivirus family.[101] Included in this group are feline immunodeficiency virus, simian immunodeficiency virus, visna virus of sheep, and the equine infectious anemia virus.[102]

Two genetically different but related forms of HIV, called *HIV-1* and *HIV-2*, have been isolated from patients with AIDS. HIV-1 is the most common type associated with AIDS in the United States, Europe, and Central Africa, whereas HIV-2 causes a similar disease principally in West Africa. Although distinct, HIV-1 and HIV-2 share some antigens. Specific tests for HIV-2, however, are now available, and blood collected for transfusion is routinely screened for HIV-2 seropositivity. The ensuing discussion relates primarily to HIV-1 and diseases caused by it, but it is generally applicable to HIV-2 as well.

Similar to most retroviruses, the HIV-1 virion is spherical and contains an electron-dense, cone-shaped core surrounded by a lipid envelope derived from the host cell membrane.[103] The virus core contains (1) the major capsid protein p24, (2) nucleocapsid protein p7/p9, (3) two copies of genomic RNA, and (4) the three viral enzymes (protease, reverse transcriptase, and integrase). p24 is the most readily detected viral antigen and, as such, is the target for the antibodies that are used for the diagnosis of HIV infection in the widely used enzyme-linked immunosorbent assay (ELISA). The viral core is surrounded by a matrix protein called *p17*, which lies underneath the virion envelop (Fig. 7–37). Studding the viral envelope are two viral glycoproteins, gp 120 and gp 41, which are critical for HIV infection of cells. The HIV-1 proviral genome contains the *gag, pol,* and *env* genes, which code for various viral proteins. The products of the *gag* and *pol* genes are translated initially into large precursor proteins that must be cleaved by the viral protease to yield the mature proteins. The highly effective anti-HIV-1 protease inhibitor drugs thus prevent viral assembly by inhibiting the formation of mature viral proteins (Fig. 7–38).

In addition to these three standard retroviral genes, HIV contains several other genes, including *tat, rev, vif, nef, vpr,* and *vpu,* that regulate the synthesis and assembly of infectious viral particles. The product of the *tat* (transactivator) gene, for example, is critical for virus replication. The *tat* protein functions by causing a 1000-fold increase in the transcription of viral genes; thus it increases virus replication. Similar to *tat, rev* is also essential for HIV-1 replication, but it exerts its effects at a post-transcriptional level by regulating the transport of viral mRNAs from the nucleus to the cytoplasm. The products of the *vpu* and *vif* genes act late in the viral life cycle and seem to be essential for the budding of virions from infected cells (*vpu*) and for endowing the cell-free virus with the ability to infect other cells (*vif*). The *vpr* gene seems to help increase virus production by several different mechanisms. It allows nondividing cells such as macrophages to be infected by HIV[104]; more strikingly, it causes cell cycle arrest in the G2 phase of cell cycle, during which the viral long terminal repeat (LTR) is most active, thus maximizing virus protection.[105]

Finally, the *nef* protein appears to be essential for the development of progressive HIV infection in vivo. Strains of simian immunodeficiency virus that have mutations in the *nef* gene do not cause AIDS in monkeys. Similarly, in rare instances, humans transfused with blood tainted with a *nef*-defective HIV-1 strain displayed exceptionally low viral burden and did not develop AIDS many years after infection. The mechanism by which *nef* exerts its effects on AIDS pathogenesis is not clear. One report suggests that *nef* causes expression of FasL on infected cells, thus causing apoptosis of Fas-expressing CTLs. It has also been reported that the *nef* protein down-regulates the expression of MHC class I molecules in HIV-infected T cells. Because CD8+ cytotoxic T cells can recognize viral antigens only when presented by MHC class I molecules, such down-regulation can prevent the recognition and lysis of HIV-infected target cells. In this manner, *nef* may help evade immunologically mediated resistance against HIV infection.[106, 107] From this review of the functions of HIV-1 genes, it should be apparent that the products of regulatory

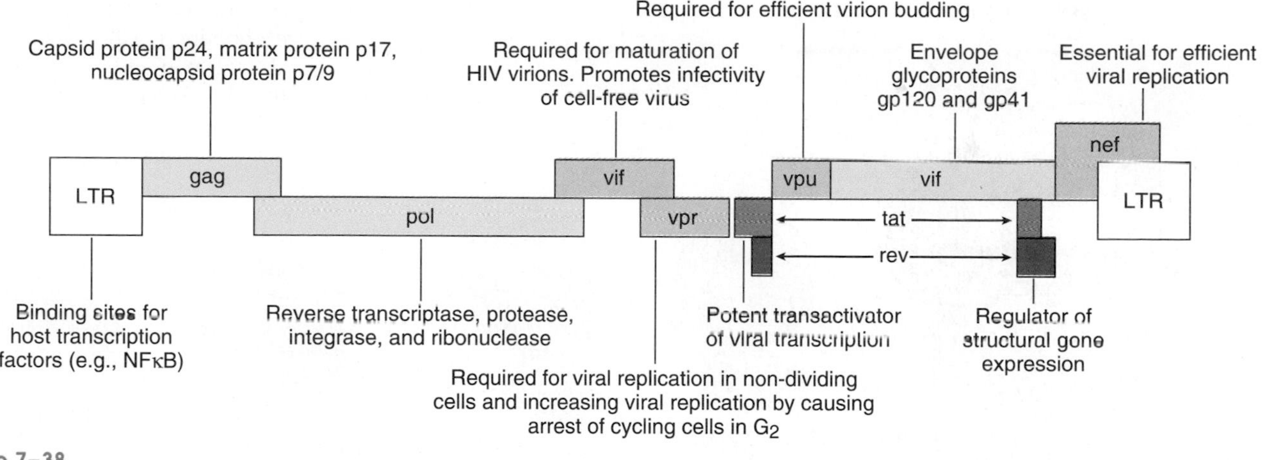

Figure 7–38

HIV proviral genome. Several viral genes and their corresponding functions are illustrated. The genes outlined in red are unique to HIV; others are shared by all retroviruses.

genes are important for the pathogenicity of HIV, and hence there is considerable interest in developing therapeutic agents that can block the action of these genes.[108]

Molecular analysis of different HIV-1 isolates has revealed considerable variability in certain parts of their genome. Most variations are clustered in certain regions of the envelope glycoproteins. Because the immune response against HIV-1 is targeted against its envelope, such variability poses problems for the development of a single vaccine. On the basis of genetic analysis, HIV-1 can be divided into two groups, designated *M* (major) and *O* (outlier). Group M viruses are the most common form worldwide, and they are further divided into several subtypes or clades, designated A through J. Various subtypes differ in their geographic distribution; for example, subtype B is the most common form in western Europe and the United States, whereas subtype E is the most common clade in Thailand. It is thought that the mode of transmission of different subtypes is different. For example, subtype E is spread predominantly by heterosexual contact (male-to-female), presumably because of its ability to infect subepithelial dendritic cells in the vagina. By contrast, subtype B, the most common form in the United States, grows in these cells poorly and is believed to be transmitted by infection of monocytes and lymphocytes in the blood.

Pathogenesis. There are two major targets of HIV: the immune system and the central nervous system. The effects of HIV infection on each of these two are discussed separately.

Immunopathogenesis of HIV Disease. Profound immunosuppression, primarily affecting cell-mediated immunity, is the hallmark of AIDS. This results chiefly from infection of and a severe loss of CD4+ T cells as well as an impairment in the function of surviving helper T cells. As discussed later, macrophages and dendritic cells are also targets of HIV infection. We first describe the mechanisms involved in the viral entry into T cells and macrophages and the life cycle of the virus within cells. This is followed by a more detailed review of the interaction between HIV and its cellular targets.

There is abundant evidence that the *CD4 molecule is, in fact, a high-affinity receptor for HIV*. This explains the selective tropism of the virus for CD4+ T cells and other CD4+ cells, particularly monocytes/macrophages and Langerhans cells/dendritic cells. Binding to CD4 is not sufficient for infection, however. HIV gp120 must also bind to other cell surface molecules (coreceptors) for entry into the cell. Two cell surface molecules, CCR5 and CXCR4, receptors for β-chemokines and α-chemokines (Chapter 3), serve this role.[109] Molecular details of this fatal handshake between HIV glycoproteins and their cell surface receptors have been uncovered in elegant detail and are important to understand because they may provide the basis of anti-HIV therapy. As illustrated in Figure 7–39, the HIV envelope contains two glycoproteins, surface gp120 that is noncovalently attached to transmembrane gp41. The initial step in infection is the binding of the gp120 envelope glycoprotein to CD4 molecules. This binding leads to an important conformational change that results in the formation of a new recognition site on gp120 for the coreceptors CCR5 or CXCR4. The next step involves conformational changes in the gp41; these changes result in the insertion of a fusion peptide at the tip of gp41 into the cell membrane of the target T cells or macrophages.[110] After fusion, the virus core containing the HIV genome enters the cytoplasm of the cell. There is strong evidence that HIV binding to its coreceptors is important in the pathogenesis of AIDS. First, chemokines, occupying their receptors, sterically hinder HIV infection of cells in culture. Thus, the level of chemokines in the microenvironment surrounding HIV and its target cells may influence the efficiency of viral infection in vivo. Second, individuals who inherit two defective copies of the CCR5 receptor gene are resistant to the development of AIDS, despite repeated exposure to HIV in vivo.[111] The frequency of those who are homozygous for the protective CCR5 mutation is about 1% in white Americans, whereas 18 to 20% of individuals are heterozygotes. The latter are

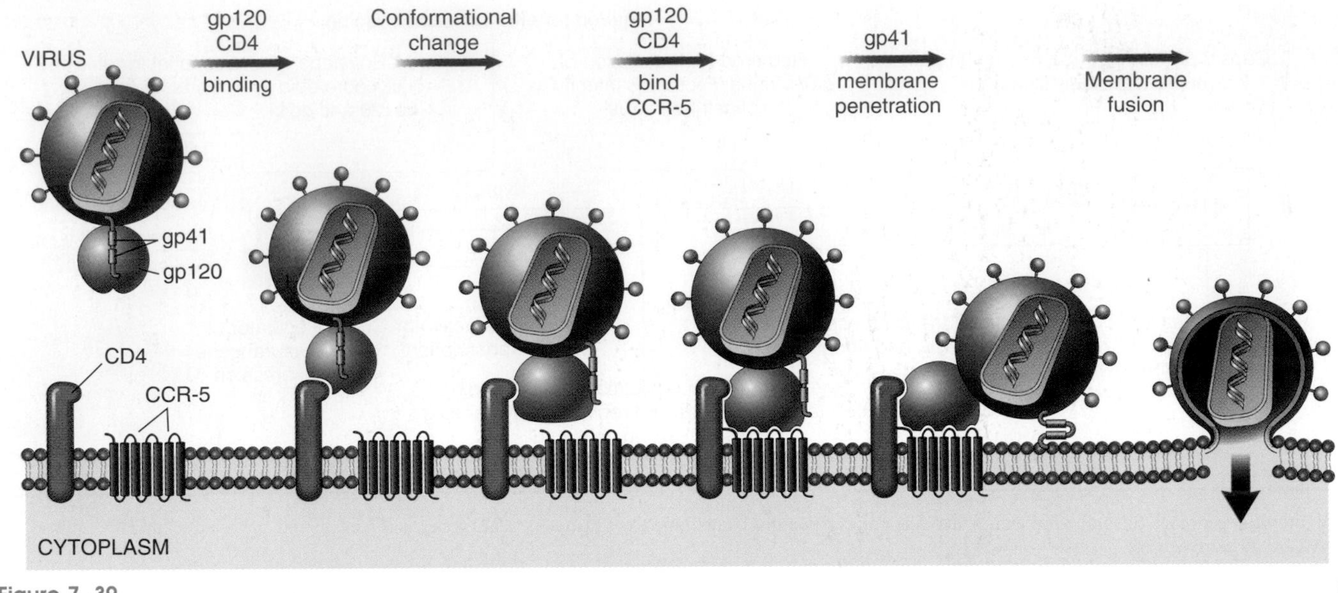

Figure 7–39

Molecular basis of HIV entry into host cells. Interactions with CD4 and CCR5 coreceptor are illustrated. (Adapted with permission from Wain-Hobson S: HIV. One on one meets two. Nature 384:117, 1996. Copyright 1996, Macmillam Magazines Limited.)

not protected from AIDS, but the onset of their disease is somewhat delayed. No homozygotes for the mutation have been found in African or East Asian populations.

The discovery of coreceptors for HIV infection has also solved previously puzzling observations of HIV tropism. It has been known for some time that HIV strains can be classified into two groups on the basis of their ability to infect macrophages and CD4+ T cells. Macrophage-tropic (M-tropic) strains, their name notwithstanding, can infect both monocytes/macrophages and freshly isolated peripheral blood T cells (but not in vitro propagated T-cell lines). By contrast, the T-cell tropic strains can infect only T cells, both freshly isolated and retained in culture. This selectivity is based on coreceptor usage; M-tropic strains use CCR5, the β-chemokine receptor, whereas T-tropic strains bind to the CXCR4 α-chemokine receptor. Because CCR5 is expressed on both monocytes and T cells, they succumb to infection by M-tropic strains; CXCR4 is expressed on T cells but not on monocytes/macrophages, and hence T cells but not macrophages are susceptible to infection with T-tropic strains. Primary T cells (freshly isolated) express both CCR5 and CXCR4 and hence can be infected by either of the two viral types. In approximately 90% of cases, HIV is transmitted by M-tropic strains, and hence early in the course of HIV infection, patients harbor mainly M-tropic strains. Over the course of infection, however, T-tropic viruses gradually accumulate; these are especially virulent and cause the final rapid phase of disease progression.[112] Because the ability to bind the coreceptors resides in the gp120 protein of the viral envelope, it follows that there must be molecular differences between the gp120 molecule of M-tropic and T-tropic HIV. Such is the case; further, it is thought that during the course of HIV infection M-tropic strains evolve into T-tropic strains, owing to mutations in genes that encode gp120. The resultant transition in the ability of the virus to bind CXCR4 but not CCR5 is probably important in the pathogenesis of AIDS because T-tropic (i.e., CXCR4-tropic) viruses are particularly adept at depleting T cells. Why M-tropic viruses are more efficient in transmitting AIDS is not entirely clear. Studies provide two possible explanations. First, Langerhans cells within the mucosal epithelium richly express CCR5 but do not express CXCR4, thus avoiding infection by T-tropic viruses. Second, binding of M-tropic strains to CCR5 on T cells signals these cells to make chemotactic factors for other T cells, thus increasing the population of potential targets in the vicinity of an infected T cell. Envelope glycoproteins of T-tropic viruses do not cause such activation of T-cell signals after binding to CXCR4.[113]

Because of the significance of HIV-coreceptor interaction in the pathogenesis of AIDS, investigators are searching for ways to prevent this interaction.[114] One of the more innovative strategies has involved targeting genetically engineered rhabdoviruses to HIV-infected cells. The natural envelope of these viruses is replaced by one that carries human CD4 and CXRC4. When mixed with HIV-infected cells, they fuse with the membranes of the HIV-infected cells because the latter express gp120/41 complex during viral budding. Because rhabdoviruses lyse mammalian cells, an engineered rhabdovirus that has gained access to the HIV-infected cell kills it. Quite appropriately, this "strategy" has been called "fighting HIV-1's fire with fire."[115] Whether such "viraceuticals" will be useful in vivo remains to be seen. With this review of viral entry into cells, we proceed now to the remainder of the HIV life cycle.

Once internalized, the viral genome undergoes reverse transcription, leading to formation of cDNA (proviral DNA). In quiescent T cells, HIV cDNA may remain in the cytoplasm in a linear episomal form. In dividing T cells, the cDNA circularizes, enters the nucleus, and is then integrated into the host genome. After this integration, the provirus may remain locked into the chromosome for months or years, and hence the infection may become latent. Alternatively, proviral DNA may be transcribed, with the formation of complete viral particles that bud from the cell membrane. Such productive infection, when associated with extensive viral budding, leads to cell death (Fig. 7–40). It is important to note that although HIV-1

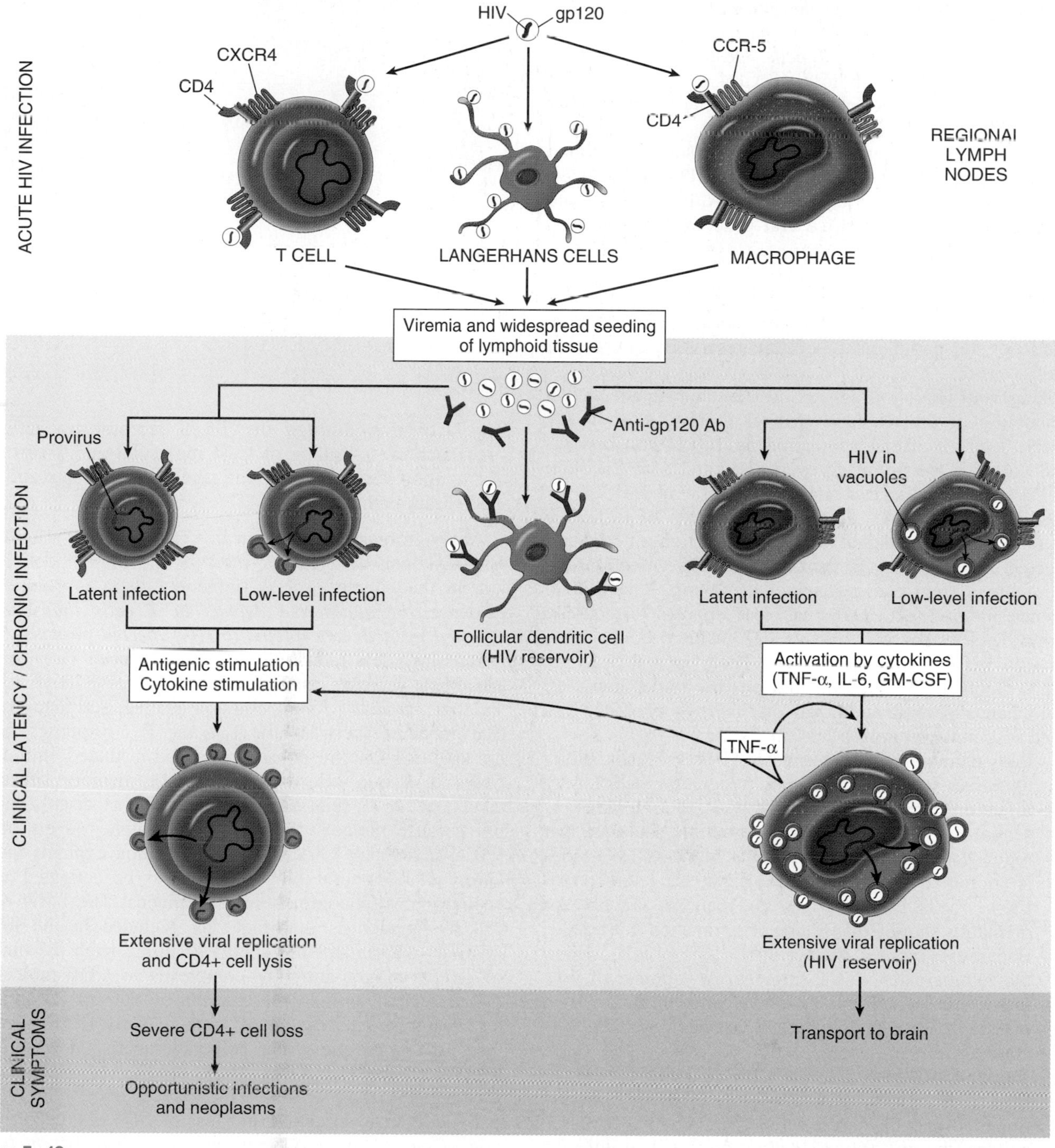

Figure 7–40

Pathogenesis of HIV-1 infection. Initially, HIV-1 infects T cells and macrophages directly or is carried to these cells by Langerhans cells. Viral replication in the regional lymph nodes leads to viremia and widespread seeding of lymphoid tissue. The viremia is controlled by the host immune response *(not shown)* and the patient then enters a phase of clinical latency. During this phase, viral replication in both T cells and macrophages continues unabated, but there is some immune containment of virus *(not illustrated)*. There continues a gradual erosion of CD4 + cells by productive infection (or other mechanisms, *not shown*). When the numbers of CD4 + cells that are destroyed cannot be replenished, CD4 + cell numbers decline and the patient develops clinical symptoms of full-blown AIDS. Macrophages are also parasitized by the virus early; they are not lysed by HIV-1 and they transport the virus to tissues, particularly the brain.

can infect resting T cells, the initiation of proviral DNA transcription (and hence productive infection) occurs only when the infected cell is activated by an exposure to antigens or cytokines. It is obvious therefore that physiologic stimuli that promote activation and growth of normal T cells lead to the death of HIV-infected T cells.

It might be surmised from the preceding discussion that productive infection of T cells is the mechanism by which HIV causes lysis of CD4+ T cells. Despite the relentless, and eventually profound, loss of CD4+ cells from the peripheral blood, however, there is a relative paucity of productively infected T cells in circulation. These observations have spawned many hypotheses (some described later) that attempt to explain the loss of CD4+ T cells by mechanisms other than direct cytolysis. Although this issue is not completely resolved, several observations are pertinent.

- Early in the course of disease, HIV colonizes the lymphoid organs (spleen, lymph nodes, tonsils). These, and not the peripheral blood, are reservoirs of infected cells.
- Using anti-HIV-1 drugs as probes and mathematical modeling of the resultant changes in virus titer, it has been determined that approximately 100 billion new viral particles are produced every day, and 1 to 2 billion CD4+ T cells die each day.[116] These viral and CD4+ cell turnover studies suggest that the loss of CD4+ T cells can be accounted for by destruction of HIV-infected T cells. Early in the course of HIV infection, the immune system can regenerate the dying T cells, and hence the rate of CD4+ cell loss appears deceptively low. This masks the massive cell death occurring primarily in the lymphoid tissues. There is not complete agreement among investigators on this issue, however, and hence several additional mechanisms of CD4+ T-cell loss have been proposed, including
  1. Loss of immature precursors of CD4+ T cells, either by direct infection of thymic progenitor cells or by infection of accessory cells that secrete cytokines essential for CD4+ T-cell differentiation. The idea that reduced production may underlie loss of CD4+ cells is supported by the observation that the telomeres of CD4+ cells from HIV-infected patients are not appreciably shorter than those of uninfected controls.[117] Because telomeres shorten every time a cell divides, the telomere length can provide an estimate of how many times a cell has divided over its lifetime. With massive CD4+ cell death and compensatory regeneration, telomere length would be expected to have shortened (Chapter 2).
  2. Fusion of infected and uninfected cells, with formation of syncytia (giant cells) (Fig. 7–41). In tissue culture, the gp120 expressed on productively infected cells binds to CD4 molecules on uninfected T cells, followed by cell fusion. Fused cells develop *ballooning* and usually die within a few hours. This property of syncytia formation is confined to the T-tropic HIV-1.
  3. Apoptosis of uninfected CD4+ T cells by binding of soluble gp120 to the CD4 molecule, followed by activation through the T-cell receptor by antigens; such cross-linking of CD4 molecules and T-cell activation leads to aberrant signaling and activation of death pathways.

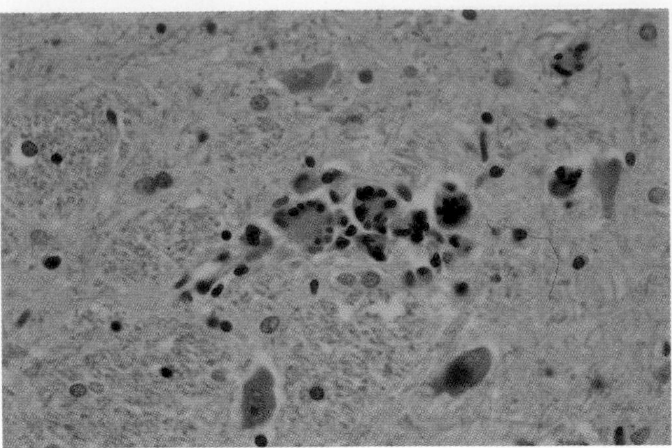

Figure 7–41

HIV infection showing the formation of giant cells in the brain. (Courtesy of Dr. Dennis Burns, Department of Pathology, University of Texas Southwestern Medical School, Dallas, TX.)

Although marked reduction in CD4+ T cells, a hallmark of AIDS, can account for most of the immunodeficiency late in the course of HIV infection, there is compelling evidence for *qualitative defects in T cells that can be detected even in asymptomatic HIV-infected persons.* Such defects include a reduction in antigen-induced T-cell proliferation, a decrease in T_H1 type responses relative to the T_H2 type, defects in intracellular signaling, and many more. The imbalance between the T_H1 and T_H2 responses favors humoral immune responses over cell-mediated immunity. There is also a selective loss of the memory subset of CD4+ helper T cells early in the course of disease, possibly because memory T cells express higher levels of the HIV-1 coreceptor CCR5. This observation explains the inability of peripheral blood T cells to be activated when challenged with common recall antigens. The basis of T-cell dysfunction is multifactorial. Included in the list of possible mechanisms are anergy resulting from the binding of gp120 antigen-antibody complexes to CD4 molecules, impairment of antigen presentation by anti-gp120 antibodies that cross-react with and bind to class II HLA molecules on antigen-presenting cells, and anergy of large numbers of T cells resulting from binding of HIV-derived superantigens to β chains of T-cell receptors.

In addition to infection and loss of CD4+ T cells, *infection of monocytes and macrophages is also extremely important in the pathogenesis of HIV infection.* Similar to T cells, the majority of the *macrophages that are infected by HIV are found in the tissues and not in peripheral blood.* A relatively high frequency (10 to 50%) of productively infected macrophages is detected in certain tissues, such as brain and lungs. Several aspects of HIV infection of macrophages need to be emphasized:[118]

- Although cell division is requisite for replication of most retroviruses, HIV-1 can infect and multiply in terminally differentiated nondividing macrophages. This property of HIV-1 is dependent on the HIV-1 *vpr* gene. The *vpr* protein allows nuclear targeting of the HIV preintegration complex through the nuclear pore.
- Infected macrophages bud relatively small amounts of virus from the cell surface, but these cells contain large numbers of virus particles located exclusively in intracellular vacuoles. Despite the fact that macrophages allow viral replication, in contrast to CD4+ T cells, they are quite resistant to the cytopathic effects of HIV.
- Macrophages, in all likelihood, act as gatekeepers of infection. Recall that in more than 90% of cases, HIV infection is transmitted by M-tropic strains. The more virulent T-tropic strains that evolve later in the course of HIV infection are inefficient in transmitting HIV. This suggests that the initial infection of macrophages or dendritic cells may be important in the pathogenesis of HIV disease.

HIV infection of macrophages has three important implications. First, monocytes and macrophages represent a veritable virus factory and reservoir, whose output remains largely protected from host defenses. Second, macrophages provide a safe vehicle for HIV to be transported to various parts of the body, particularly the nervous system. Third, in late stages of HIV infection, when the CD4+ T-cell numbers decline greatly, macrophages may be the major site of continued viral replication.[119]

In contrast to tissue macrophages, the number of monocytes in circulation infected by HIV is low; yet there are unexplained functional defects that have important bearing in host defense. These defects include impaired microbicidal activity, decreased chemotaxis, decreased secretion of IL-1, inappropriate secretion of TNF-α, and, most important, poor capacity to present antigens to T cells.

Studies have documented that, in addition to macrophages, two types of *dendritic cells* are also important targets for the initiation and maintenance of HIV infection: mucosal and follicular dendritic cells. It is thought that mucosal dendritic cells, also called *Langerhans cells, capture the virus and transport it to regional lymph nodes*, where CD4+ T cells are infected.[120] Whether the virus infects the dendritic cells or is carried on the dendritic processes is uncertain. *Follicular dendritic cells in the germinal centers of lymph nodes are, similar to macrophages, important reservoirs* of HIV. Although some follicular dendritic cells are infected by HIV, most virus particles are found on the surface of their dendritic processes. Follicular dendritic cells have receptors for the Fc portion of immunoglobulins, and hence they trap HIV virions coated with anti-HIV antibodies.[121] The antibody-coated virons localized to follicular dendritic cells retain the ability to infect CD4+ T cells as they traverse the intricate meshwork formed by the dendritic processes of the follicular dendritic cells. *To summarize, CD4+ T cells, macrophages, and follicular dendritic cells contained in the lymphoid tissues are the major sites of HIV infection and persistence.*

Low-level chronic or latent infection of T cells and macrophages is an important feature of HIV infection. Early in the course of this infection, only rare CD4+ T cells in the blood or lymph nodes express infectious virus, whereas in the lymph nodes, up to 30% can be demonstrated by polymerase chain reaction to harbor the HIV genome. It is widely believed that integrated provirus, without virus expression (latent infection), can remain in the cells for months to years. Even with potent antiviral therapy, which practically sterilizes the peripheral blood, latent virus lurks within the CD4+ cells in the lymph nodes. According to some estimates, 0.05% of resting CD4+ T cells in the lymph nodes are latently infected. Because these CD4+ T cells are memory T cells, they are long-lived, with a life span of months to years.[122] Completion of the viral life cycle in latently infected cells occurs only after cell activation, which in the case of CD4+ T cells results in cell lysis. To understand the molecular basis of release from latency, we must briefly consider the events that are associated with activation of CD4+ helper T cells. It is well known that antigen-induced or mitogen-induced activation of T cells is associated with transcription of genes encoding the cytokine IL-2 and its receptor (IL-2R). At the molecular level, this is accomplished in part by the induction of a nuclear binding factor called NF-kB (nuclear factor kB). In resting T cells, NF-kB is sequestered in the cytoplasm in a complex with members of the I-kB family. Cellular activation by antigen or cytokines (e.g., TNF-α, IL-1, IL-2) induces cytoplasmic kinases that release the NF-kB from the grasp of I-kB, allowing its translocation to the nucleus. In the nucleus, NF-kB binds to enhancer sequences (kB sites) within the promoter regions of several genes, including those of cytokines that are expressed in immunologically activated cells.[123] The long terminal repeat (LTR) sequences that flank the HIV genome also contain similar kB sites that can be triggered by the same nuclear regulatory factors. Imagine now a latently infected CD4+ cell that encounters an environmental antigen. Induction of NF-kB in such a cell (a physiologic response) activates the transcription of HIV proviral DNA (a pathologic outcome) and leads ultimately to the production of virions and to cell lysis. Furthermore, TNF-α, a cytokine produced by activated macrophages, also leads to transcriptional activation of HIV-mRNA by production of nuclear factors that bind to kB-enhancer elements of HIV. The production of HIV-1 by macrophages is up-regulated by other proinflammatory cytokines, such as TNF-α, TNF-β, IFN-γ, IL-6, and GM-CSF as well. Many of these cytokines are produced during a normal immune response. Of these, TNF-α, produced by macrophages, is particularly important because it can act in both an autocrine and a paracrine manner (see Fig. 7–40). Anti-inflammatory cytokines, such as IL-10, inhibit HIV-1 replication by down-regulating the production of HIV-inducing cytokines. Thus, it seems that HIV thrives when the host macrophages and T cells are physiologically activated, an act that can be best described as "subversion from within." Such activation in vivo may result from antigenic stimulation, especially by other infecting microorganisms, such as cytomegalovirus, EBV, hepatitis B virus, and *M. tuberculosis*. The life style of most HIV-infected patients in the United States places them at increased risk for recurrent exposure to other sexually transmitted diseases, and in Africa, socioeconomic conditions probably impose a higher burden of chronic microbial infections. It is easy to visualize how in patients with AIDS a vicious cycle of cell destruction may be set up. The multiple infections to which these patients are prone because of diminished helper T-cell function lead to increased production of proinflammatory cytokines, which, in turn, stimulate more HIV production, followed by infection and loss of additional CD4+ T cells.

Although much attention has been focused on T cells and macrophages because they can be infected by HIV, patients with AIDS also display profound abnormalities of B-cell function. Paradoxically, these patients have hypergammaglobulinemia and circulating immune complexes owing to polyclonal B-cell activation. This may result from multiple interacting factors, such as infection with cytomegalovirus and EBV, both of which are polyclonal B-cell activators; gp41 itself can promote B-cell growth and differentiation, and HIV-infected macrophages produce increased amounts of IL-6, which favors activation of B cells. *Despite the presence of spontaneously activated B cells, patients with AIDS are unable to mount an antibody response to a new antigen.* This could be due, in part, to lack of T-cell help, but antibody responses against T-independent antigens are also suppressed, and hence there may be other defects in B cells as well. Impaired humoral immunity renders these patients prey to disseminated infections caused by encapsulated bacteria, such as *S. pneumoniae* and *H. influenzae,* both of which require antibodies for effective opsonization.

CD4+ T cells play a pivotal role in regulating the immune response: They produce a plethora of cytokines, such as IL-2, IL-4, IL-5, IFN-γ, macrophage chemotactic factors, and hematopoietic growth factors (e.g., GM-CSF). Therefore, loss of this "master cell" has ripple effects on virtually every other cell of the immune system, as illustrated in Figure 7–42 and summarized in Table 7–11.

Pathogenesis of Central Nervous System Involvement. The pathogenesis of neurologic manifestations deserves special mention because, in addition to the lymphoid system, the nervous system is a major target of HIV infection.[124] Macrophages and cells belonging to the monocyte and macrophage lineage (microglia) are the predominant cell types in the brain that are infected with HIV. Hence it is widely believed that HIV is carried into the brain by infected monocytes. In keeping with this, the HIV isolates from the brain are almost exclusively M-tropic. The mechanism of HIV-induced damage of the brain, however, remains obscure. Because neurons are not infected by HIV, and the extent of neuropathologic changes is often less than might be expected from the severity of neurologic symptoms, most workers believe that neurologic deficit is caused indirectly by viral products and soluble factors pro-

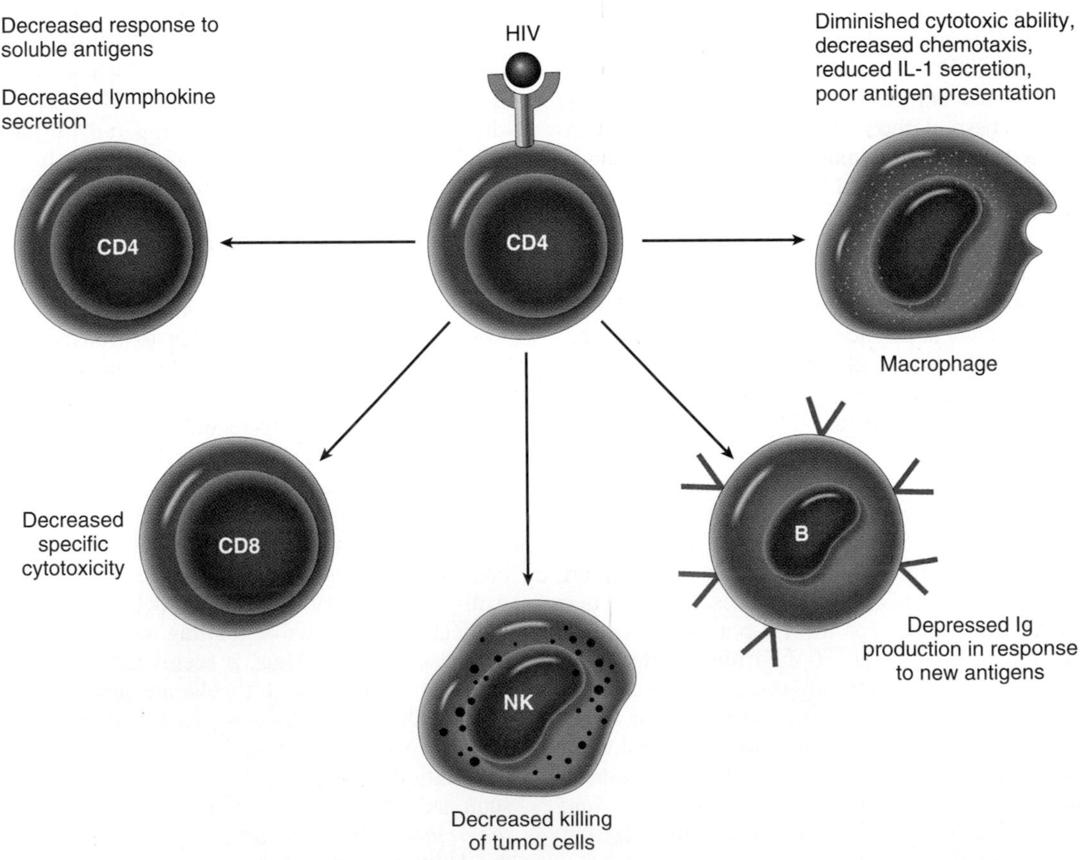

Figure 7–42

The multiple effects of loss of CD4 + T cells as a result of HIV infection.

Table 7–11. MAJOR ABNORMALITIES OF IMMUNE FUNCTION IN AIDS

Lymphopenia
Predominantly due to selective loss of the CD4+ helper-inducer T-cell subset; inversion of CD4 : CD8 ratio
Decreased T-Cell Function In Vivo
Preferential loss of memory T cells
Susceptibility to opportunistic infections
Susceptibility to neoplasms
Decreased delayed-type hypersensitivity
Altered T-Cell Function In Vitro
Decreased proliferative response to mitogens, alloantigens, and soluble antigens
Decreased specific cytotoxicity
Decreased helper function for pokeweed mitogen-induced B-cell immunoglobulin production
Decreased IL-2 and IFN-γ production
Polyclonal B-Cell Activation
Hypergammaglobulinemia and circulating immune complexes
Inability to mount de novo antibody response to a new antigen
Refractoriness to the normal signals for B-cell activation in vitro
Altered Monocyte or Macrophage Functions
Decreased chemotaxis and phagocytosis
Decreased HLA class II antigen expression
Diminished capacity to present antigen to T cells
Increased spontaneous secretion of IL-1, TNF-α, IL-6

duced by macrophages/microglia. Included among the soluble factors are the usual culprits, such as IL-1, TNF-α, and IL-6. In addition, nitric oxide induced in neuronal cells by gp41 has also been implicated.[125] Direct damage of neurons by soluble HIV gp120 has also been postulated. According to some investigators, these diverse soluble neurotoxins act by triggering excessive entry of Ca^{2+} into the neurons through their action on glutamate-activated ion channels that regulate intracellular calcium.[126]

Table 7–12. PHASES OF HIV INFECTION AND CORRESPONDING CDC CLASSIFICATION CATEGORIES

Phase	CDC Classification
Early, acute	Group I: Acute infection
Middle, chronic	Group II: Asymptomatic infection
	Group III: Persistent generalized lymphadenopathy
Final, crisis	Group IV
	Subgroup A: Constitutional disease
	Subgroup B: Neurologic disease
	Subgroup C: Secondary infection
	Subgroup D: Secondary neoplasm
	Subgroup E: Other conditions

CDC, Centers for Disease Control.

Natural History of HIV Infection. The course of HIV infection can be best understood in terms of an interplay between HIV and the immune system. *Three phases reflecting the dynamics of virus-host interaction can be recognized:* (1) an *early, acute phase*; (2) a *middle, chronic phase*; and (3) a *final, crisis phase* (Fig. 7–43).[127] The four clinical subgroups of HIV infection proposed by the Centers for Disease Control (CDC) can reasonably be assigned to the three phases of infection (Table 7–12). We first present the cardinal features of the three phases of HIV infection and their associated clinical syndromes then recount the sequential virologic and immunologic findings during the course of HIV infection.

The *early, acute phase* represents the initial response of an immunocompetent adult to HIV infection. It is characterized initially by a high level of virus production, viremia, and *widespread seeding of the lymphoid tissues.* The

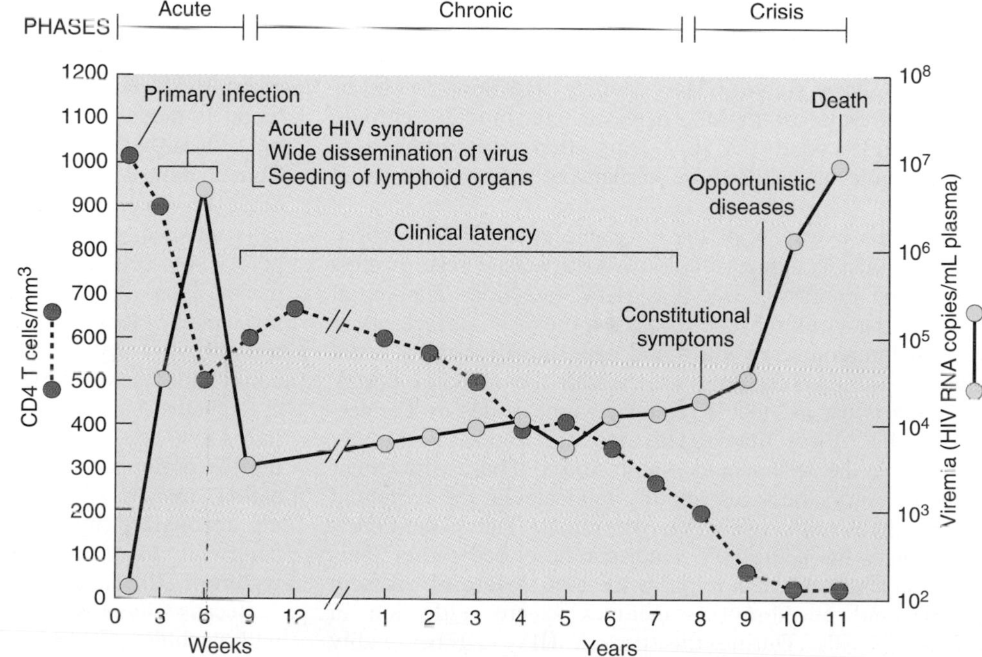

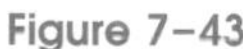
Figure 7–43

Typical course of HIV infection. During the early period after primary infection, there is widespread dissemination of virus and a sharp decrease in the number of CD4 + T cells in peripheral blood. An immune response to HIV ensues, with a decrease in viremia followed by a prolonged period of clinical latency. During this period, viral replication continues. The CD4 + T-cell count gradually decreases during the following years, until it reaches a critical level below which there is a substantial risk of opportunistic diseases. (Redrawn from Fauci AS, Lane HC: Human immunodeficiency virus disease: AIDS and related conditions. In Fauci AS, et al (eds): Harrison's Principles of Internal Medicine, 14th ed. New York, McGraw-Hill, 1997, p 1791.)

initial infection, however, is readily controlled by the development of an antiviral immune response. Clinically, this phase is associated with a self-limited acute illness that develops in 50 to 70% of adults infected with HIV. The symptoms are nonspecific and include, most frequently, sore throat, myalgias, fever, weight loss, and fatigue. Other clinical features, such as rash, cervical adenopathy, diarrhea, and vomiting, may also occur. They develop 3 to 6 weeks after infection and resolve spontaneously 2 to 4 weeks later.[128]

The *middle, chronic phase* represents a stage of relative containment of the virus, associated with a period of clinical latency. The immune system is largely intact, but *there is continuous HIV replication, predominantly in the lymphoid tissues, which may last for several years.* Patients are either asymptomatic (CDC group II) or develop persistent generalized lymphadenopathy (CDC group III). In addition, many patients have minor opportunistic infections, such as thrush and herpes zoster. Thrombocytopenia may also be noted (Chapter 14). Persistent lymphadenopathy with significant constitutional symptoms (fever, rash, fatigue) reflects the onset of immune system decompensation, escalation of viral replication, and onset of the *crisis* phase.

The *final, crisis phase* is characterized by a breakdown of host defense, a dramatic increase in plasma virus, and clinical disease. Typically the patient presents with long-lasting fever (>1 month), fatigue, weight loss, and diarrhea; the CD4+ cell count is reduced below 500 cells/μl. After a variable period, serious opportunistic infections, secondary neoplasms, or clinical neurologic disease (grouped under the rubric *AIDS-defining conditions*) supervene, and the patient is said to have developed AIDS. In addition, according to current guidelines of the CDC, any HIV-infected person with fewer than 200 CD4+ T cells/μl is considered to have AIDS.

In the absence of treatment, most but not all patients with HIV infection progress to AIDS after a chronic phase lasting from 7 to 10 years. Exceptions to this typical course are exemplified by long-term nonprogressors and by rapid progressors. Nonprogressors are defined as HIV-1–infected individuals who remain asymptomatic for 10 years or more, with stable CD4+ counts and low levels of plasma viremia. In rapid progressors, the middle, chronic phase is telescoped to 2 to 3 years after primary infection. The possible basis for these variant outcomes is discussed later.

With this overview of the three phases of HIV infection, we can consider some details of host-parasite relationships during the course of a typical HIV infection. The initial entry of the virus may be through a mucosal surface, as in vaginal intercourse or via blood exposure (breach in rectal mucosa, intravenous drug use). From the mucosal portal, the virus is carried to the regional lymph nodes by Langerhans cells. Virus inoculated into the blood is rapidly cleared by the spleen and lymph nodes. Thus, with either mode of entry, the virus initially replicates in the lymphoid organs then spills over into the blood. The patient now experiences the acute HIV syndrome described earlier. This phase is characterized initially by high levels of virus in plasma and an abrupt, sometimes severe, reduction in CD4+ T cells. During this period, HIV can be readily isolated from the blood, and there are high levels of HIV p24 antigen in serum. Soon, however, a virus-specific immune response develops, evidenced by seroconversion (usually within 3 to 7 weeks of presumed exposure) and, more importantly, by the development of virus-specific CD8+ cytotoxic T cells. *HIV-specific cytotoxic T cells are detected in blood at about the time viral titers begin to fall and are most likely responsible for the containment of HIV infection.*[129] As viral replication abates, CD4+ T cells return to near-normal numbers, signaling the end of the early acute phase. Although plasma viremia declines, there is widespread dissemination and seeding of the virus, especially in the lymphoid organs. With the formation of anti-HIV antibodies, immune complexes containing virions are trapped by follicular dendritic cells in the germinal centers. As discussed earlier, both latent and replicating HIV can be found in CD4+ T cells and macrophages within the lymph nodes, and viral particles are readily detected on the surface of follicular dendritic cells.

The viral load at the end of the acute phase is a reflection of the equilibrium reached between the virus and the host after the initial battle, and in a given patient it remains fairly stable for several years. This level of steady-state viremia, or the viral "set-point," is an extremely important predictor of the rate of progression of HIV disease. In one study, only 8% of patients with a viral load of less than 4350 copies of viral mRNA/mm^3 progressed to full-blown AIDS in 5 years, whereas 62% of those with a viral load of greater than 36,270 copies had developed AIDS in the same period.[130] From a practical standpoint, therefore, *the extent of viremia, measured as HIV-1 RNA, is the best surrogate marker of HIV disease progression and is of great clinical value in the management of patients with HIV infection.*[131]

Regardless of the viral burden, during the middle or chronic phase, there is a continuing battle between HIV and the host immune system. The CD8+ cytotoxic T-cell response remains activated, and extensive viral and CD4+ cell turnover continues. As emphasized earlier, however, because of the immense regeneration capacity of the immune system, a large proportion of the lost CD4+ cells is replenished. Thus, the decline in the CD4+ cell count in blood is modest. After an extended and variable period of time, there begins a gradual erosion of the CD4+ T cells. Concomitant with the loss of CD4+ T cells, host defenses begin to wane, and the proportion of the surviving CD4+ cells infected with HIV increases, as does the viral burden per CD4+ cell. Not unexpectedly, HIV spillover into the plasma increases. How the HIV escapes immune control is not entirely clear. CD8+ cytotoxic T cells presumably control the virus by lysing virus-infected CD4+ cells before completion of viral life cycle. CD8+ T cells also secrete C-C chemokines, such as MIP-1, that can block viral entry into CD4+ cells by occupying the CCR5 coreceptor. During the prolonged chronic phase, with extensive viral replication, mutant HIV virions whose envelope proteins are not recognized by cytotoxic T cells emerge. This could contribute to escape from immune containment, but the picture is still quite murky.[132]

Because the loss of immune containment is associated with declining CD4+ cell counts, the CDC classification of

HIV infection stratifies patients into three categories on the basis of CD4+ cell counts: CD4+ greater than or equal to 500 cells/μl, 200 to 499 cell/μl, and fewer than 200 cells/μl. Patients in the first group are generally asymptomatic; counts below 500 are associated with early symptoms, and a decline of CD4+ levels below 200 is associated with severe immunosuppression. For clinical management, CD4+ counts are an important adjunct to HIV viral load measurements. The significance of these two measurements, however, is slightly different: Whereas CD4+ cell counts indicate where the patient's disease is at the time of measurement, the viral load provides information regarding the direction in which the disease is headed.

It should be evident from our discussion that in each of the three phases of HIV infection, viral replication continues to occur. Even in the clinical latent phase, before the severe decline in CD4+ cell count, there is extensive turnover of the virus. In other words, *HIV infection lacks a phase of true microbiologic latency*, that is, a phase during which *all* the HIV is in the form of proviral DNA, and no cell is productively infected. Therefore, antiretroviral therapy must be commenced early in the course of disease, before clinical symptoms appear.

Before this discussion of the virus-host relationship is ended, some comments on those patients who are considered long-term nonprogressors are in order. Individuals in this group remain asymptomatic for long periods of time (10 years), have low levels of viremia, and have stable CD4+ cell counts. Patients with such an uncommon clinical course have attracted great attention in the hope that their study may shed light on host and viral factors that influence disease progression. Studies to date suggest that this group is heterogeneous with respect to the factors that influence the course of the disease. In a small subset of nonprogressors, the infecting HIV had deletions or mutations in the *nef* gene, suggesting that *nef* proteins are critical to disease progression. In most cases, the viral isolates do not show any qualitative abnormalities. In all cases, there is evidence of vigorous anti-HIV immune response. These patients have high levels of HIV-specific cytotoxic CD8+ cells, and these levels are maintained over the course of infection. It is not clear whether the robust CD8+ response is the cause or consequence of the slow progression. Further studies, it is hoped, will provide the answers to this and other questions critical to disease progression.

Clinical Features. The clinical manifestations of HIV infection can be readily surmised from the foregoing discussion. They range from a mild acute illness to severe disease. Because the salient clinical features of the acute early and chronic middle phases of HIV infection were described earlier, here we summarize the clinical manifestations of the terminal phase, commonly known as AIDS.

In the United States, the typical adult patient with AIDS presents with fever, weight loss, diarrhea, generalized lymphadenopathy, multiple opportunistic infections, neurologic disease, and, in many cases, secondary neoplasms. The infections and neoplasms listed in Table 7–13 are included in the surveillance definition of AIDS.[133]

Opportunistic infections account for approximately 80% of deaths in patients with AIDS. Their spectrum is constantly changing, as a result of improvements in prophylaxis and the increasing life span of HIV-infected individuals. A brief summary of selected opportunistic infections is provided here. Extensive reviews on the subject are available.[134]

Table 7–13. AIDS-DEFINING OPPORTUNISTIC INFECTIONS AND NEOPLASMS FOUND IN PATIENTS WITH HIV INFECTION

Infections

Protozoal and Helminthic Infections

Cryptosporidiosis or isosporidiosis (enteritis)
Pneumocytosis (pneumonia or disseminated infection)
Toxoplasmosis (pneumonia or CNS infection)

Fungal Infections

Candidiasis (esophageal, tracheal, or pulmonary)
Cryptococcosis (CNS infection)
Coccidioidomycosis (disseminated)
Histoplasmosis (disseminated)

Bacterial Infections

Mycobacteriosis (atypical, e.g., *M. avium-intracellulare,* disseminated or extrapulmonary; *M. tuberculosis,* pulmonary or extrapulmonary)
Nocardiosis (pneumonia, meningitis, disseminated)
Salmonella infections, disseminated

Viral Infections

Cytomegalovirus (pulmonary, intestinal, retinitis, or CNS infections)
Herpes simplex virus (localized or disseminated)
Varicella-zoster virus (localized or disseminated)
Progressive multifocal leukoencephalopathy

Neoplasms

Kaposi sarcoma
B-cell non-Hodgkin lymphomas
Primary lymphoma of the brain
Invasive cancer of uterine cervix

CNS, central nervous system.

Pneumonia caused by the opportunistic fungus *P. carinii* (representing reactivation of a prior latent infection) is the presenting feature in about 20% of cases, and approximately 50% of AIDS patients develop this infection at some time during the course of their illness. The risk of developing this infection is extremely high in individuals with fewer than 200 CD4+ cells/μl. In recent years, there has been a substantial decline in the incidence of this infection because of the development of effective prophylaxis. An increasing number of patients present with an opportunistic infection other than *P. carinii* pneumonia. Among the most common pathogens are *Candida*, cytomegalovirus, atypical and typical mycobacteria, *Cryptococcus neoformans*, *Toxoplasma gondii*, *Cryptosporidium*, herpes simplex virus, papovaviruses, and *Histoplasma capsulatum.*[135]

Candidiasis is the most common fungal infection in patients with AIDS. *Candida* infection of the oral cavity (thrush) and esophagus are the two most common clinical manifestations of candidiasis in HIV-infected patients. In asymptomatic HIV-infected individuals, oral candidiasis is a sign of immunologic decompensation, and it often heralds the transition to AIDS. Invasive candidiasis is not common in patients with AIDS, and it usually occurs when there is drug-induced neutropenia or use of indwelling catheters. *Cytomegalovirus* may cause disseminated disease, although, more commonly, it affects the eye and gastrointestinal tract. Chorioretinitis occurs in approximately 25% of patients, whereas gastrointestinal disease, seen in about 10% of cases, manifests as esophagitis and colitis, the latter associated with multiple mucosal ulcerations. Cytomegalovirus retinitis occurs almost exclusively in patients with CD4+ cell counts below 50/mm^3. Disseminated bacterial infection with *atypical mycobacteria* (mainly *M. avium-intracellulare*) also occurs late, in the setting of severe immunosuppression. Approximately 40% of patients with AIDS have clinical evidence of disseminated infection, but the incidence at autopsy approaches 80%. Coincident with the AIDS epidemic, the incidence of tuberculosis has risen dramatically.[136] Patients with AIDS have reactivation of latent pulmonary disease as well as outbreaks of primary infection.[137] In contrast to infection with atypical mycobacteria, *M. tuberculosis* manifests itself early in the course of AIDS. As with tuberculosis in other settings, the infection may be confined to lungs or may involve multiple organs. The pattern of expression depends on the degree of immunosuppression; dissemination is more common in patients with very low CD4+ cell counts. Most worrisome are reports indicating that a growing number of isolates are resistant to multiple drugs.

Cryptococcosis occurs in about 10% of AIDS patients. Among fungal infections that prey on HIV-infected individuals, it is second only to candidiasis. As in other settings with immunosuppression, meningitis is the major clinical manifestation of cryptococcosis. In contrast to *Cryptococcus*, *T. gondii*, another frequent invader of the central nervous system in AIDS, causes encephalitis and is responsible for 50 to 60% of all mass lesions in the central nervous system. JC virus, a human papovavirus, is another important cause of central nervous system infections in HIV-infected patients. It causes progressive multifocal leukoencephalopathy (Chapter 30). *Herpes simplex virus infection* is manifested by mucocutaneous ulcerations involving the mouth, esophagus, external genitalia, and perianal region. *Persistent diarrhea*, so common in patients with AIDS, is often caused by infections with protozoans such as *Cryptosporidium*, *Isospora belli*, or microsporidia. These patients have chronic, profuse, watery diarrhea with massive fluid loss. Diarrhea may also result from infection with enteric bacteria, such as *Salmonella* and *Shigella*, as well as *M. avium-intracellulare*. Depressed humoral immunity renders AIDS patients susceptible to severe, recurrent bacterial pneumonias.

Patients with AIDS have a high incidence of certain tumors, especially Kaposi sarcoma (KS), non-Hodgkin lymphoma, and cervical cancer in women.[138] The basis of the increased risk of malignancy is multifactorial: profound defects in T-cell immunity, dysregulated B-cell and monocyte functions, and multiple infections with known (e.g., human herpesvirus type 8, EBV, human papillomavirus) and unknown viruses.

KS, a vascular tumor that is otherwise rare in the United States, is the most common neoplasm in patients with AIDS. The morphology of KS and its occurrence in patients not infected with HIV is discussed in Chapter 12. At the onset of the AIDS epidemic, up to 40% of the reported cases had KS, but in recent years there has been a definite decline in its incidence. There are several peculiar features of this tumor in patients with AIDS. It is far more common in homosexual or bisexual men than in intravenous drug abusers or patients belonging to other risk categories. The lesions can arise early, before the immune system is compromised, or in advanced stages of HIV infections. There is still some uncertainty regarding the nature of the proliferating cells and whether the lesions represent an exuberant hyperplasia or a neoplasm. The lesions contain spindle cells that share features with endothelial cells and smooth muscle cells and are in all likelihood primitive mesenchymal cells that can form vascular channels. Studies indicate that these cells are monoclonal in origin, even in patients with multicentric lesions, indicating therefore that KS is a neoplasm.[139]

Although the cause and pathogenesis of KS are still not clear, a model that favors *a complex web of interaction between a sexually transmitted infectious agent, altered expression and response to cytokines, and modulation of cell growth by HIV gene products is currently favored.*[138, 140] Each of these three is considered individually, followed by a schema that incorporates the role of all three cofactors (Fig. 7–44).

Both epidemiologic and molecular studies support the role of an infectious agent in the causation of KS. The high rate of KS in homosexual men relative to patients with parenterally acquired HIV infection points to a sexually transmitted agent.[140a] The decline in the incidence of KS is in keeping with the decline of AIDS in homosexual men. The observation that KS is much more common in women who have sex with bisexual men than in other women with AIDS is also consistent with sexual transmission. The discovery in 1994 that a novel type of human herpesvirus is present in KS lesions has bolstered the case for a viral cofactor in the pathogenesis of KS lesions. The genomic sequences of this herpesvirus, aptly labeled *KS herpesvirus* (KSHV), are found in virtually all KS lesions, including those that occur in HIV-negative populations. DNA of KSHV, also called human herpesvirus type 8, is also found in a rare type of body cavity–based B-cell lymphoma that occurs in HIV-infected patients. Approximately 50% of the circulating B cells in patients with KS also harbor the KSHV. Although the association of this virus with KS is firmly established, its precise role in the causation of these tumors is much less clear. A study of the viral genes of KSHV has revealed that it encodes homologs of several human genes that can participate in cell proliferation. These include the cytokine IL-6, the chemokine MIP-1α, a G-protein coupled chemokine receptor, cyclin D, and bc1-2.[141–143] The virally encoded IL-6, similar to human IL-6, is mitogenic for spindle cells in the lesions, and the chemokine receptor encoded by the virus binds to IL-8 with high affinity. IL-8 is mitogenic for endothelial cells and promotes angiogenesis. As is discussed in greater detail in Chapter 8, bc1-2 is an antiapoptosis gene, and cyclin D regulates the transition from G1 to S phase of cell cycle. In addition to the virally encoded

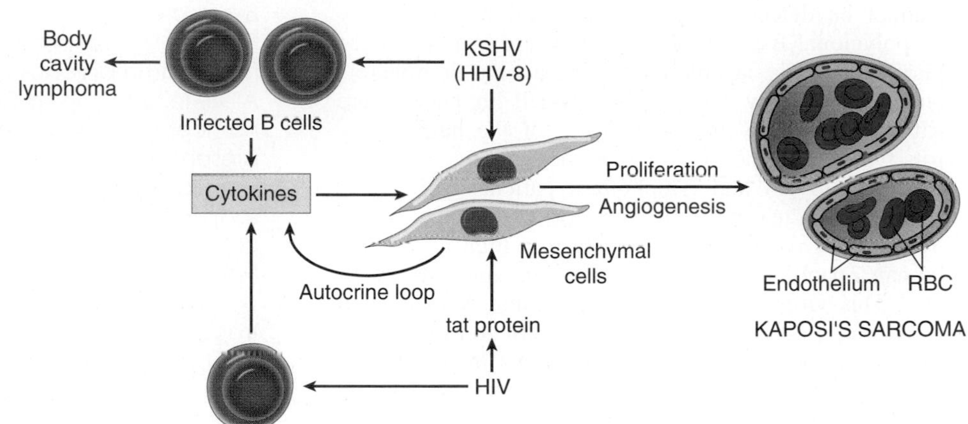

Figure 7–44 ■

Proposed role of HIV, KSHV (HHV-8), and cytokines in the pathogenesis of Kaposi sarcoma. Cytokines are produced by the mesenchymal cells infected by KSHV, by B cells infected by KSHV, or by HIV-infected CD4+ cells.

growth-promoting factors, KS cells produce a variety of other cytokines, including TNF-α, IL-1, IL-6, GM-CSF, basic fibroblast growth factor, and oncostatin M. These mediators stimulate the growth of spindle cells in an autocrine and paracrine fashion. What drives the production of these cytokines is not entirely clear. Perhaps infection with KSHV endows the mesenchymal cells to secrete these factors; KS herpesvirus–infected B cells within the lesions could also be the source of these mediators. There is some evidence that HIV-encoded transactivating (tat) protein also plays a role in the proliferation of spindle cells. Although there is no HIV in the KS cells, HIV-infected CD4+ cells produce soluble *tat* that can bind to integrins on the surface of KS cells. This stimulates them to proliferate and to produce proinflammatory and angiogenic cytokines. Mice transgenic for the HIV-*tat* gene also develop KS-like vascular lesions, albeit transiently. It should be remembered that KS can develop in HIV-negative individuals (Chapter 12), hence HIV or its products are not obligatory for the development of all forms of KS.

To summarize, KS is composed of mesenchymal cells that form blood vessels; the proliferation of these cells is driven by a variety of cytokines and growth factors that are derived from the tumor cells themselves and from HIV-infected T cells. KS herpesvirus–infected B cells may also contribute to the cytokine soup. What triggers the outpouring of this mitogenic brew is not clear, but it seems linked to infection of the tumor cells by KS herpesvirus.

Clinically the AIDS-associated KS is quite different from the sporadic form (Chapter 12). In HIV-infected individuals, the tumor is generally widespread, affecting the skin, mucous membranes, gastrointestinal tract, lymph nodes, and lungs. These tumors also tend to be more aggressive than classic KS.

With prolonged survival, the number of AIDS patients who develop non-Hodgkin lymphoma has increased steadily. It is currently believed that approximately 6% of all patients with AIDS develop lymphoma during their lifetime. Thus, the risk of developing non-Hodgkin lymphoma is approximately 120-fold greater than in the general population. In contrast to KS, immunodeficiency is firmly implicated as the central predisposing factor. It appears that patients with CD4+ cell counts below 50/mm^3 incur an extremely high risk.[138]

AIDS-related lymphomas can be divided into three groups on the basis of their location: systemic, primary central nervous system, and body cavity–based lymphomas.[144] Systemic lymphomas involve lymph nodes as well as extranodal, visceral sites; they constitute 80% of all AIDS-related lymphomas. Central nervous system is the most common extranodal site affected, followed by gastrointestinal tract and, less commonly, virtually any other location, including the orbit, salivary glands, and lungs. The vast majority of these lymphomas are aggressive B-cell tumors that present in an advanced stage (Chapter 15). In addition to being commonly involved by systemic non-Hodgkin lymphomas, central nervous system is also the primary site of lymphomatous involvement in 20% of HIV-infected patients who develop lymphomas. Primary central nervous system lymphoma is 1000 times more common in patients with AIDS than in the general population. The third category of AIDS-related lymphomas is rare but has an unusual distribution. It grows exclusively in body cavities in the form of pleural, peritoneal, and pericardial effusions.

The pathogenesis of AIDS-associated B-cell lymphomas probably involves sustained polyclonal B-cell activation, followed by the emergence of monoclonal or oligoclonal B-cell populations. It is believed that during the frenzy of proliferation, some clones undergo somatic mutations and neoplastic transformation (Chapter 8). There is morphologic evidence of B-cell activation in lymph nodes, and it is believed that such triggering of B cells is multifactorial.[145] Patients with AIDS have high levels of several cytokines, some of which, including IL-6, are important growth factors for B cells. In addition, there seems to be a role for EBV, known to be a polyclonal mitogen for B cells. The EBV genome is found in approximately 50% of the systemic B-cell lymphomas and in virtually all lymphomas primary in the central nervous system. Other evidence of EBV infection includes oral hairy leukoplakia (white projections on the tongue), believed to result from EBV-driven squamous cell proliferation of the oral mucosa (Chapter 17). In cases in which molecular footprints of EBV infection cannot be detected, other viruses and microbes may initiate polyclonal B-cell proliferation. There is no evidence that HIV by itself is capable of causing neoplastic transformation. The rare body cavity–based B-cell lymphomas are uniformly associated with the presence of the human herpesvirus type 8 genome, discussed earlier.

In addition to KS and lymphomas, patients with AIDS also have an increased occurrence of carcinoma of the uterine cervix. This is most likely due to a high prevalence of human papillomavirus infection in patients with AIDS.[146] This virus is believed to be intimately associated with squamous cell carcinoma of the cervix and its precursor lesions, cervical dysplasia and carcinoma in situ (Chapters 8 and 24). Human papillomavirus–associated cervical dysplasia is ten times more common in HIV-infected women as compared with uninfected women attending family planning clinics. Hence it is recommended that gynecologic examination be part of a routine work-up of HIV-infected women.

A large variety of other neoplasms, including Hodgkin disease and T-cell lymphomas, have been reported in patients with AIDS. It is not clear, however, whether the incidence of these tumors is increased with HIV infection.

Involvement of the central nervous system is a common and important manifestation of AIDS. *Ninety per cent of patients demonstrate some form of neurologic involvement at autopsy, and 40 to 60% have clinically manifest neurologic dysfunction.* Importantly, in some patients, neurologic manifestations may be the sole or earliest presenting feature of HIV infection. In addition to opportunistic infections and neoplasms, several virally determined neuropathologic changes occur. These include a self-limited meningoencephalitis occurring at the time of seroconversion, aseptic meningitis, vacuolar myelopathy, peripheral neuropathies, and, most commonly, a progressive encephalopathy designated clinically as the *AIDS-dementia complex* (Chapter 30).

MORPHOLOGY. The anatomic changes in the tissues (with the exception of lesions in the brain) are neither specific nor diagnostic. In general, the pathologic features of AIDS are those characteristic of widespread opportunistic infections, KS, and lymphoid tumors. Most of these lesions are discussed elsewhere because they also occur in patients who do not have HIV infection. To appreciate the distinctive nature of lesions in the central nervous system, they are discussed in the context of other disorders affecting the brain. Here we concentrate on changes in the lymphoid organs.

Biopsy specimens from enlarged lymph nodes in the early stages of HIV infection reveal a **marked follicular hyperplasia.**[147] The enlarged follicles have irregular, sometimes serrated borders, and they are present not only in the cortex, but also in the medulla and may even extend outside the capsule. The mantle zones that surround the follicles are markedly attenuated, and hence the germinal centers seem to merge with the interfollicular area. These changes, affecting primarily the B-cell areas of the node, are the morphologic reflections of the polyclonal B-cell activation and hypergammaglobulinemia seen in patients with AIDS. In addition to B-cell expansion within germinal centers, activated monocytoid B cells are present within and around the sinusoids and trabecular blood vessels. Under the electron microscope and by in situ hybridization, HIV particles can be detected within the germinal centers. Here they seem to be concentrated on the villous processes of follicular dendritic cells, presumably trapped in the form of immune complexes. During the early phase of HIV infection, viral DNA can be found within the nuclei of CD4+ T cells located predominantly in the follicular mantle zone. With disease progression, the frenzy of B-cell proliferation subsides and gives way to a pattern of severe follicular involution. The follicles are depleted of cells, and the **organized network of follicular dendritic cells is disrupted.** The germinal centers may even become hyalinized. During this advanced stage, viral burden in the nodes is reduced, in part because of the disruption of the follicular dendritic cells. These "burnt-out" lymph nodes are atrophic and small and may harbor numerous opportunistic pathogens. Because of profound immunosuppression, the inflammatory response to infections both in the lymph nodes and at extranodal sites may be sparse or atypical. For example, mycobacteria may not evoke granuloma formation because CD4+ cells are deficient. In the empty-looking lymph nodes and in other organs, the presence of infectious agents may not be readily apparent without the application of special stains. As might be expected, lymphoid depletion is not confined to the nodes; in later stages of AIDS, spleen and thymus also appear to be "wastelands." Non-Hodgkin lymphomas, involving the nodes as well as extranodal sites, such as the liver, gastrointestinal tract, and bone marrow, are primarily high-grade diffuse B-cell neoplasms (Chapter 15).

Since the emergence of AIDS in 1981, the concerted efforts of epidemiologists, immunologists, and molecular biologists have resulted in spectacular advances in understanding of this disorder. Despite all this progress, however, the prognosis of patients with AIDS remains dismal. Approximately 12 million people had succumbed to the disease worldwide by the end of 1997. Although the mortality rate has begun to decline in the United States as a result of the use of potent combinations of antiretroviral drugs, the treated patients still carry viral DNA in their lymphoid tissues. Can there be a cure with persistent virus?[148a] Although a considerable effort has been mounted to develop a vaccine, many hurdles remain to be crossed before vaccine-based prophylaxis or treatment becomes a reality. Molecular analyses have revealed an alarming degree of polymorphism in viral isolates from different patients; this renders the task of producing a vaccine remark-

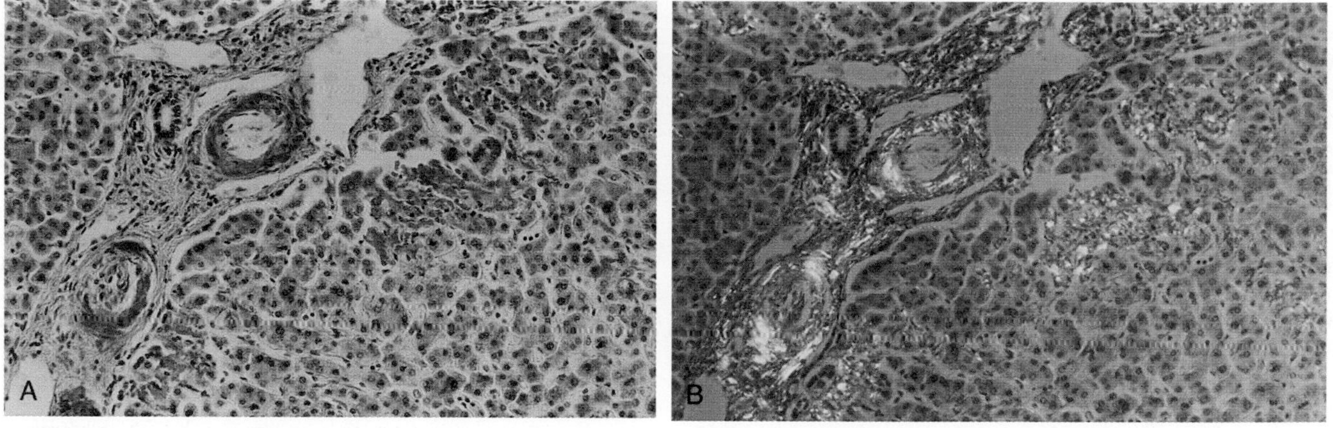

Figure 7–45

Amyloidosis. *A*, A section of the liver stained with Congo red reveals pink-red deposits of amyloid in the walls of blood vessels and along sinusoids. *B*, Note the yellow-green birefringence of the deposits when observed by polarizing microscope. (Courtesy of Dr. Trace Worrell and Sandy Hinton, Department of Pathology, University of Texas Southwestern Medical School, Dallas TX.)

ably difficult. This task is further complicated by the fact that the nature of the protective immune response is not yet fully understood. At present, therefore, prevention and effective public health measures remain the mainstay in the fight against AIDS.

Amyloidosis

Immunologic mechanisms are suspected of contributing to a large number of diseases in addition to those already described in this chapter. Some of the entities are discussed in the chapters dealing with individual organs and systems. Amyloidosis is described here. There is strong evidence that in most patients some derangement in the immune apparatus underlies this disease, and as a systemic disease it cannot be assigned to any single organ or system.

Amyloid is a pathologic proteinaceous substance, deposited between cells in various tissues and organs of the body in a wide variety of clinical settings. Because amyloid deposition appears so insidiously and sometimes mysteriously, its clinical recognition ultimately depends on morphologic identification of this distinctive substance in appropriate biopsy specimens. *With the light microscope and standard tissue stains, amyloid appears as an amorphous, eosinophilic, hyaline, extracellular substance that, with progressive accumulation, encroaches on and produces pressure atrophy of adjacent cells.* To differentiate amyloid from other hyaline deposits (e.g., collagen, fibrin), a variety of histochemical techniques, described later, are used. Perhaps most widely used is the Congo red stain, which under ordinary light imparts a pink or red color to tissue deposits, but far more dramatic and specific is the green birefringence of the stained amyloid when observed by polarizing microscopy (Fig. 7–45).

Despite the fact that all deposits have a uniform appearance and tinctorial characteristics, *it is quite clear that amyloid is not a chemically distinct entity.* There are three major and several minor biochemical forms. These are deposited by several different pathogenetic mechanisms, and therefore amyloidosis *should not be considered a single disease; rather it is a group of diseases having in common the deposition of similar-appearing proteins.*[148] At the heart of the morphologic uniformity is the remarkably uniform physical organization of amyloid protein, which we consider first. This is followed by a discussion of the chemical nature of amyloid.

Physical Nature of Amyloid. By electron microscopy, amyloid is seen to be made up largely of nonbranching fibrils of indefinite length and a diameter of approximately 7.5 to 10 nm. This electron microscopic structure is identical in all types of amyloidosis. X-ray crystallography and infrared spectroscopy demonstrate a characteristic cross β-pleated sheet conformation (Fig. 7–46). This conformation

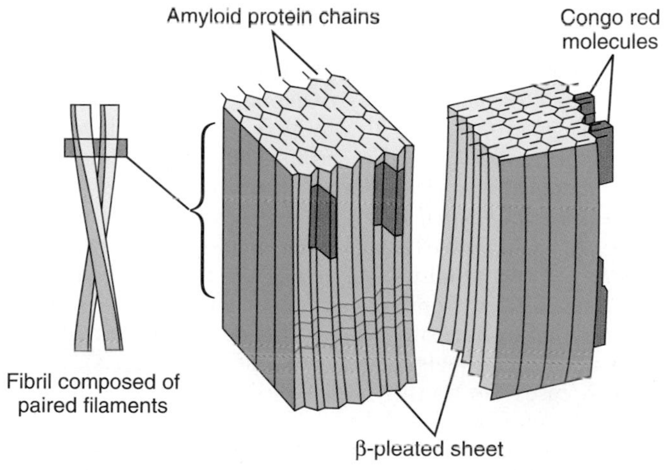

Figure 7–46

Structure of an amyloid fibril, depicting the beta-pleated sheet structure and binding sites for the Congo red dye, which is used for diagnosis of amyloidosis. (Modified from Glenner GG: Amyloid deposit and amyloidosis. The β-fibrilloses. N Engl J Med 52:148, 1980. By permission of The New England Journal of Medicine.)

is seen regardless of the clinical setting or chemical composition and is responsible for the distinctive staining and birefringence of Congo red–stained amyloid. In addition to amyloid fibrils, other minor components are always present in amyloid. These include serum amyloid P component, proteoglycans, and highly sulfated glycosaminoglycans. These nonproteinaceous substances are presumably derived from the connective tissue in which amyloid is deposited.

Chemical Nature of Amyloid. Approximately 95% of the amyloid material consists of fibril proteins, the remaining 5% being the P component and other glycoproteins. *Of the 15 biochemically distinct forms of amyloid proteins that have been identified, three are most common:* (1) *AL (amyloid light chain) is derived from plasma cells (immunocytes) and contains immunoglobulin light chains,* (2) *AA (amyloid-associated) is a unique nonimmunoglobulin protein synthesized by the liver,*[149] and (3) *Aβ amyloid is found in the cerebral lesion of Alzheimer disease* and is hence discussed in greater detail in Chapter 30.

The two noncerebral amyloid proteins are deposited in distinct clinicopathologic settings. The AL protein is made up of complete immunoglobulin light chains, the NH_2-terminal fragments of light chains, or both. Most of the AL proteins analyzed are composed of λ light chains (particularly λ VI type) or their fragments, but in some cases κ chains have been identified. As might be expected, the amyloid fibril protein of the AL type is produced by immunoglobulin-secreting cells, and their deposition is associated with some form of monoclonal B cell proliferation.

The second major class of amyloid fibril protein (AA) does not have structural homology to immunoglobulins. It has a molecular weight of 8500 and consists of 76 amino acid residues. The AA protein is found in those clinical settings described as *secondary amyloidosis.* AA fibrils are derived from a larger (12,000 daltons) precursor in the serum called SAA (serum amyloid–associated) protein that is synthesized in the liver and circulates in association with the HDL3 subclass of lipoproteins. Several other biochemically distinct proteins have been found in amyloid deposits in a variety of clinical settings.

- *Transthyretin* (TTR) is a normal serum protein that binds and transports thyroxine and retinol, hence the name *trans-thy-retin.* It was previously called *prealbumin* because it precedes serum albumin on serum electrophoresis. *A mutant form of transthyretin (and its fragments) is deposited in a group of genetically determined disorders referred to as familial amyloid polyneuropathies.*[150] Amyloid transthyretin (ATTR) deposited in the tissues differs from its normal counterpart by a single amino acid. Transthyretin is also deposited in the heart of aged individuals (senile systemic amyloidosis), but in such cases the transthyretin molecule is structurally normal.
- *β_2-microglobulin,* a component of the MHC class I molecules and a normal serum protein, has been identified as the amyloid fibril subunit (Aβ_2m) in amyloidosis that complicates the course of patients on *long-term hemodialysis.* Aβ_2m fibers are structurally similar to normal β_2m protein.
- *β-amyloid protein* (Aβ), not to be confused with β_2-microglobulin, is a 4000-dalton peptide that constitutes the core of cerebral plaques found in Alzheimer disease as well as the amyloid deposited in walls of cerebral blood vessels in patients with Alzheimer disease. The Aβ protein is derived from a much larger transmembrane glycoprotein, called *amyloid precursor protein* (APP).

In addition to the foregoing, amyloid deposits derived from diverse precursors such as hormones (procalcitonin) and keratin have also been reported.

The P component, a glycoprotein, is distinct from the amyloid fibrils but is closely associated with them in all forms of amyloidosis. It has a striking structural homology to C-reactive protein, a well-known acute-phase reactant. The serum P component has an affinity for amyloid fibrils, and it may be necessary for tissue deposition. Its presence in amyloid is responsible for staining with periodic acid–Schiff (PAS), which led early observers to believe that amyloid was a saccharide.

Classification of Amyloidosis. According to devoted "amyloidologists," who congregate every few years to discuss their favorite protein, amyloid should be classified based on its constituent chemical fibrils into categories such as AL, AA, and ATTR and not based on clinical syndromes.[151] Because a given biochemical form of amyloid (e.g., AA) may be associated with amyloid deposition in diverse clinical settings, we follow a combined biochemical-clinical classification for our discussion (Table 7–14). Amyloid may be *systemic* (generalized), involving several organ systems, or it may be *localized,* when deposits are limited to a single organ, such as the heart. As should become evident, several different biochemical forms of amyloid are encompassed by such a segregation.

On clinical grounds, the systemic, or generalized, pattern is subclassified into *primary amyloidosis,* when associated with some immunocyte dyscrasia, or *secondary amyloidosis,* when it occurs as a complication of an underlying chronic inflammatory or tissue destructive process. *Hereditary* or familial amyloidosis constitutes a separate, albeit heterogeneous group, with several distinctive patterns of organ involvement.

Immunocyte Dyscrasias With Amyloidosis (Primary Amyloidosis). Amyloid in this category is usually systemic in distribution and is of the AL type. With approximately 1275 to 3200 new cases every year in the United States, this is the most common form of amyloidosis. In many of these cases, the patients have some form of plasma cell dyscrasia. Best defined is the occurrence of systemic amyloidosis in 5 to 15% of patients with multiple myeloma, a form of plasma cell neoplasia characterized by multiple osteolytic lesions throughout the skeletal system (Chapter 15). The malignant B cells characteristically synthesize abnormal amounts of a single specific immunoglobulin (monoclonal gammopathy), producing an M (myeloma) protein spike on serum electrophoresis. In addition to the synthesis of whole immunoglobulin molecules, only the light chains (referred to as Bence Jones protein) of either the κ or the λ variety may be elaborated and found in the serum. By virtue of the small molecular size of the Bence Jones protein, it is frequently excreted in the urine. Almost

Table 7–14. CLASSIFICATION OF AMYLOIDOSIS

Clinicopathologic Category	Associated Diseases	Major Fibril Protein	Chemically Related Precursor Protein
Systemic (Generalized) Amyloidosis			
Immunocyte dyscrasias with amyloidosis (primary amyloidosis)	Multiple myeloma and other monoclonal B-cell proliferations	AL	Immunoglobulin light chains, chiefly λ type
Reactive systemic amyloidosis (secondary amyloidosis)	Chronic inflammatory conditions	AA	SAA
Hemodialysis-associated amyloidosis	Chronic renal failure	$A\beta_2m$	β_2-microglobulin
Hereditary amyloidosis			
Familial Mediterranean fever	—	AA	SAA
Familial amyloidotic neuropathies (several types)	—	ATTR	Transthyretin
Systemic senile amyloidosis	—	ATTR	Transthyretin
Localized Amyloidosis			
Senile cerebral	Alzheimer disease	$A\beta$	APP
Endocrine			
Medullary carcinoma of thyroid	—	A Cal	Calcitonin
Islet of Langerhans	Type II diabetes	AIAPP	Islet amyloid peptide
Isolated atrial amyloidosis	—	AANF	Atrial natriuretic factor

all the patients with myeloma who develop amyloidosis have Bence Jones proteins in the serum or urine, or both, but a great majority of myeloma patients who have free light chains do not develop amyloidosis. Clearly, therefore, *the presence of Bence Jones proteins, although necessary, is by itself not enough to produce amyloidosis.* We discuss later the other factors, such as the type of light chain produced (*amyloidogenic potential*) and the subsequent handling (possibly degradation) that may have a bearing on whether Bence Jones proteins are deposited as amyloid.

The great majority of patients with AL amyloid do not have classic multiple myeloma or any other overt B-cell neoplasm; such cases have been traditionally classified as primary amyloidosis because their clinical features derive from the effects of amyloid deposition without any other associated disease. In virtually all such cases, however, monoclonal immunoglobulins or free light chains, or both, can be found in the serum or urine. Most of these patients also have a modest increase in the number of plasma cells in the bone marrow, which presumably secrete the precursors of AL protein. Clearly, these patients have an underlying B-cell dyscrasia in which production of an abnormal protein, rather than production of tumor masses, is the predominant manifestation. Whether the condition of most of these patients would evolve into multiple myeloma if they lived long enough can only be a matter for speculation.

Reactive Systemic Amyloidosis. The amyloid deposits in this pattern are systemic in distribution and are composed of AA protein. This category was previously referred to as *secondary amyloidosis* because it is secondary to the associated inflammatory condition. The feature common to most of the conditions associated with reactive systemic amyloidosis is protracted breakdown of cells resulting from a wide variety of infectious and noninfectious chronic inflammatory conditions. At one time, tuberculosis, bronchiectasis, and chronic osteomyelitis were the most important underlying conditions, but with the advent of effective antimicrobial chemotherapy, the importance of these conditions has diminished. More commonly now, reactive systemic amyloidosis complicates rheumatoid arthritis, other connective tissue disorders such as ankylosing spondylitis, and inflammatory bowel disease, particularly regional enteritis and ulcerative colitis. Among these, the most frequent associated condition is rheumatoid arthritis. Amyloidosis is reported to occur in approximately 3% of patients with rheumatoid arthritis and is clinically significant in one half of those affected. Heroine abusers who inject the drug subcutaneously also have a high occurrence rate of generalized AA amyloidosis. The chronic skin infections associated with "skin-popping" of narcotics seem to be responsible for amyloidosis in this group of patients. Reactive systemic amyloidosis may also occur in association with non–immunocyte-derived tumors, the two most common being renal cell carcinoma and Hodgkin disease.

Hemodialysis-Associated Amyloidosis. Patients on long-term hemodialysis for renal failure develop amyloidosis owing to deposition of β_2-microglobulin. This protein is present in high concentrations in the serum of patients with renal disease and is retained in circulation because it cannot be filtered through the cuprophane dialysis membranes. In some series, as many as 60 to 80% of the patients on long-term dialysis developed amyloid deposits in the synovium, joints, and tendon sheaths.[152]

Heredofamilial Amyloidosis. A variety of familial forms of amyloidosis have been described. Most of them are rare and occur in limited geographic areas. The most common and best studied is an autosomal recessive condition called *familial Mediterranean fever.* This is a febrile disorder of unknown cause characterized by attacks of fever accompanied by inflammation of serosal surfaces, including peritoneum, pleura, and synovial membrane. This disorder is encountered largely in individuals of Armenian, Sephardic Jewish, and Arabic origins. It is associated with widespread tissue involvement indistinguishable from reactive systemic amyloidosis. The amyloid fibril proteins are made up of AA proteins, suggesting that this form of amyloidosis is related to the recurrent bouts of inflammation that characterize this disease. The gene for familial Mediterranean fever has been cloned, and its product is called pyrin; although its exact function is not known, it has been suggested that pyrin is responsible for regulating acute inflammation, presumably by inhibiting the function of neutrophils. With a mutation in this gene, minor traumas unleash a vigorous, tissue-damaging inflammatory response.[153]

In contrast to familial Mediterranean fever, a group of autosomal dominant familial disorders is characterized by deposition of amyloid predominantly in the nerves—peripheral and autonomic.[154] These familial amyloidotic polyneuropathies have been described in different parts of the world. For example, neuropathic amyloidosis has been identified in individuals in Portugal, Japan, Sweden, and the United States. As mentioned previously, in all of these genetic disorders, the fibrils are made up of mutant transthyretins (ATTR).

Localized Amyloidosis. Sometimes amyloid deposits are limited to a single organ or tissue without involvement of any other site in the body. The deposits may produce grossly detectable nodular masses or be evident only on microscopic examination. Nodular (tumor-forming) deposits of amyloid are most often encountered in the lung, larynx, skin, urinary bladder, tongue, and the region about the eye. Frequently, there are infiltrates of lymphocytes and plasma cells in the periphery of these amyloid masses, raising the question of whether the mononuclear infiltrate is a response to the deposition of amyloid or instead is responsible for it. At least in some cases, the amyloid consists of AL protein and may therefore represent a localized form of immunocyte-derived amyloid.

Endocrine Amyloid. Microscopic deposits of localized amyloid may be found in certain endocrine tumors, such as medullary carcinoma of the thyroid gland, islet tumors of the pancreas, pheochromocytomas, and undifferentiated carcinomas of the stomach, and in the islets of Langerhans in patients with type II diabetes mellitus. In these settings, the amyloidogenic proteins seem to be derived either from polypeptide hormones (medullary carcinoma) or from unique proteins (e.g., islet amyloid polypeptide [IAPP]).

Amyloid of Aging. Several well-documented forms of amyloid deposition occur with aging.[155] *Senile systemic amyloidosis* refers to the systemic deposition of amyloid in elderly patients (usually in their seventies and eighties). Because of the dominant involvement and related dysfunction of the heart, this form was previously called *senile cardiac amyloidosis*. Those who are symptomatic present with a restrictive cardiomyopathy and arrhythmias. The amyloid in this form is composed of the normal transthyretin molecule. In addition to the sporadic senile systemic amyloidosis, another form, affecting, predominantly, the heart, that results from the deposition of a mutant form of transthyretin has also been recognized. Approximately 4% of the black population in the United States is a carrier of the mutant allele, and cardiomyopathy has been identified in both homozygous and heterozygous patients. The precise prevalance of patients with this mutation who develop clinically manifest cardiac disease is not known.[156]

Pathogenesis. Although the precursors of virtually all amyloid proteins have been identified, several aspects of their origins still are not clear. In reactive systemic amyloidosis, it appears that long-standing tissue destruction and inflammation lead to elevated SAA levels (Fig. 7–47). SAA is synthesized by the liver cells under the influence of cytokines such as IL-6 and IL-1; however, increased production of SAA by itself is not sufficient for the deposition of amyloid. Elevation of serum SAA levels is common to inflammatory states but in most instances does not lead to amyloidosis. There are two possible explanations for this. According to one view, SAA is normally degraded to soluble end products by the action of monocyte-derived enzymes. Conceivably, individuals who develop amyloidosis have an enzyme defect that results in incomplete breakdown of SAA, thus generating insoluble AA mole-

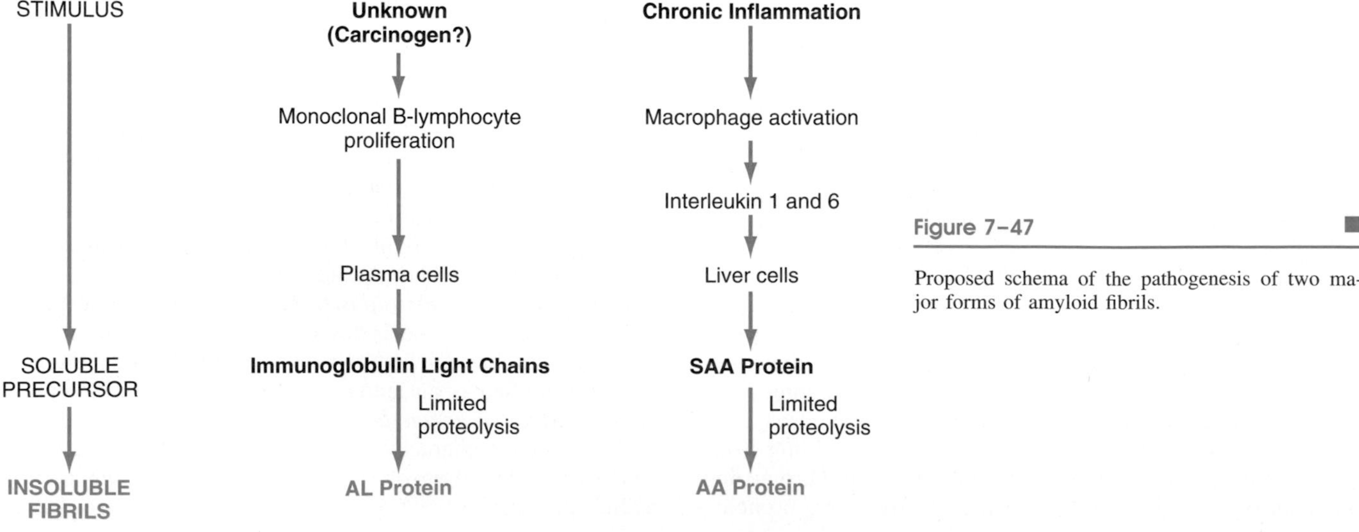

Figure 7–47

Proposed schema of the pathogenesis of two major forms of amyloid fibrils.

cules. Alternatively a genetically determined structural abnormality in the SAA molecule itself renders it resistant to degradation by monocytes. In the case of immunocyte dyscrasias, there is an excess of immunoglobulin light chains, and amyloid can be derived by proteolysis of immunoglobulin light chains in vitro. Again, defective degradation has been invoked, and perhaps particular light chains are resistant to complete proteolysis.

In contrast to the two examples already cited, in familial amyloidosis the deposition of transthyretins as amyloid fibrils does not result from overproduction of transthyretins. It has been proposed that genetically determined alterations of structure render the transthyretins prone to abnormal aggregation and proteolysis.

The cells involved in the conversion of the precursor proteins into the fibrils are not fully characterized, but macrophages seem to be the most likely candidates.

MORPHOLOGY. There are no consistent or distinctive patterns of organ or tissue distribution of amyloid deposits in any of the categories cited. Nonetheless a few generalizations can be made. Amyloidosis secondary to chronic inflammatory disorders tends to yield the most severe systemic involvements. Kidneys, liver, spleen, lymph nodes, adrenals, and thyroid as well as many other tissues are classically involved. Although immunocyte-associated amyloidosis cannot reliably be distinguished from the secondary form by its organ distribution, more often it involves the heart, kidney, gastrointestinal tract, peripheral nerves, skin, and tongue.

Macroscopically the affected organs are often enlarged and firm and have a waxy appearance. If the deposits are sufficiently large, painting the cut surface with iodine imparts a yellow color that is transformed to blue violet after application of sulfuric acid.

As noted earlier, the histologic diagnosis of amyloid is based almost entirely on its staining characteristics. The most commonly used staining technique employs the dye Congo red, which under ordinary light imparts a pink or red color to amyloid deposits. Under polarized light, the Congo red–stained amyloid shows a green birefringence (see Fig. 7–43). This reaction is shared by all forms of amyloid and is due to the cross-β-pleated configuration of amyloid fibrils. Confirmation can be obtained by electron microscopy. AA, AL, and transthyretin amyloid can be distinguished in histologic sections by specific immunohistochemical staining. Because the pattern of organ involvement in different clinical forms of amyloidosis is variable, each of the major organ involvements is described separately.

Kidney. Amyloidosis of the kidney is the most common and potentially the most serious form of organ involvement. In most reported series of patients with amyloidosis, renal amyloidosis is the major cause of death. On gross inspection, the kidney may appear normal in size and color, or it may be enlarged. In advanced cases, it may be shrunken and contracted owing to vascular narrowing induced by the deposition of amyloid within arterial and arteriolar walls.

Histologically the amyloid is deposited primarily in the glomeruli, but the interstitial peritubular tissue, arteries, and arterioles are also affected. The glomerular deposits first appear as subtle thickenings of the mesangial matrix, accompanied usually by uneven widening of the basement membranes of the glomerular capillaries. In time, the mesangial depositions and the deposits along the basement membranes cause capillary narrowing and distortion of the glomerular vascular tuft. With progression of the glomerular amyloidosis, the capillary lumens are obliterated, and the obsolescent glomerulus is flooded by confluent masses or interlacing broad ribbons of amyloid (Fig. 7–48).

Spleen. Amyloidosis of the spleen may be inapparent grossly or may cause moderate to marked splenomegaly (up to 800 gm). For completely mysterious reasons, one of two patterns of deposition is seen. In one, the deposit is largely limited to the splenic follicles, producing tapioca-like granules on gross inspection, designated **sago spleen.** Histologically the entire follicle may be replaced in advanced cases. In the other pattern, the amyloid appears to spare the follicles and instead involves the walls of the splenic sinuses and connective tissue framework in the red pulp. Fusion of the early deposits gives rise to large, maplike areas of amyloidosis, creating what has been designated the **lardaceous** spleen.

Liver. The deposits may be grossly inapparent or may cause moderate to marked hepatomegaly. The amyloid appears first in the space of Disse then progressively encroaches on adjacent he-

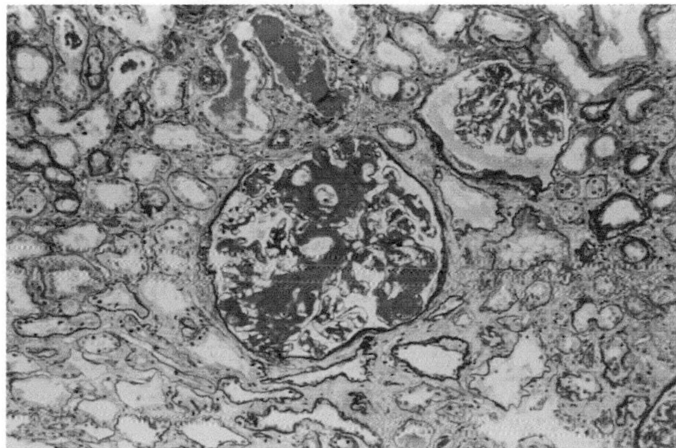

Figure 7–48

Amyloidosis of the kidney. The glomerular architecture is almost totally obliterated by the massive accumulation of amyloid.

patic parenchymal cells and sinusoids. In time, deformity, pressure atrophy, and disappearance of hepatocytes occur, causing total replacement of large areas of liver parenchyma. Vascular involvement and Kupffer cell depositions are frequent. Normal liver function is usually preserved despite sometimes quite severe involvement of the liver.

Heart. Amyloidosis of the heart may occur in any form of systemic amyloidosis, much more commonly in persons with immunocyte-derived disease. It is also the major organ involved in senile systemic amyloidosis. The heart may be enlarged and firm, but more often it shows no significant changes on cross-section of the myocardium. Histologically the deposits begin in focal subendocardial accumulations and within the myocardium between the muscle fibers. Expansion of these myocardial deposits eventually causes pressure atrophy of myocardial fibers (Fig. 7–49). In most cases, the deposits are separated and widely distributed, but when they are subendocardial, the conduction system may be damaged, accounting for the electrocardiographic abnormalities noted in some patients.

Other Organs. Amyloidosis of other organs is generally encountered in systemic disease. The adrenals, thyroid, and pituitary are common sites of involvement. In the adrenals, the intercellular deposits begin adjacent to the basement membranes of the cortical cells, usually first in the zona glomerulosa. With progression, large sheets of amyloid may replace considerable amounts of the cortical parenchyma. Similar patterns are seen in the thyroid and pituitary. The gastrointestinal tract may be involved at any level, from the oral cavity (gingiva, tongue) to the anus. The early lesions mainly affect blood vessels but eventually extend to involve the adjacent areas of the submucosa, muscularis, and subserosa.

Nodular depositions in the tongue may cause macroglossia, giving rise to the designation **tumor-forming amyloid of the tongue**. The respiratory tract may be involved focally or diffusely from the larynx down to the smallest bronchioles. As mentioned earlier, a distinct chemical form of amyloid has been found in the brain of patients with Alzheimer disease. It involves so-called plaques as well as blood vessels (Chapter 30). Amyloidosis of peripheral and autonomic nerves is a feature of several familial amyloidotic neuropathies. Depositions of amyloid in patients on long-term hemodialysis are most prominent in the carpal ligament of the wrist, resulting in compression of the median nerve (carpal tunnel syndrome). These patients may also have extensive amyloid deposition in the joints.

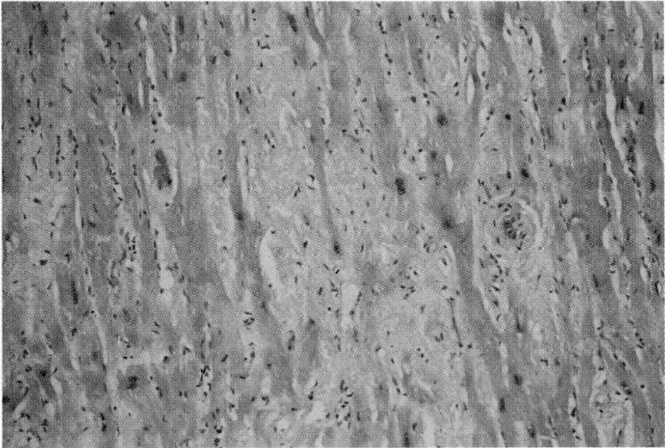

Figure 7–49

Cardiac amyloidosis. The atrophic myocardial fibers are separated by structureless, pink-staining amyloid.

Clinical Correlation. Amyloidosis may be found as an unsuspected anatomic change, having produced no clinical manifestations, or it may cause death. The symptoms depend on the magnitude of the deposits and on the particular sites or organs affected. Clinical manifestations at first are often entirely nonspecific, such as weakness, weight loss, lightheadedness, or syncope. Somewhat more specific findings appear later and most often relate to renal, cardiac, and gastrointestinal involvement.

Renal involvement gives rise to proteinuria and is an important cause of the nephrotic syndrome (Chapter 21). Progressive obliteration of glomeruli in advanced cases ultimately leads to renal failure and uremia. *Cardiac amyloidosis* may present as an insidious congestive heart failure. The most serious aspects of cardiac amyloidosis are the conduction disturbances and arrhythmias that may prove fatal. Occasionally, cardiac amyloidosis produces a restrictive pattern of cardiomyopathy and masquerades as chronic constrictive pericarditis (Chapter 13). *Gastrointestinal amyloidosis* may be entirely asymptomatic, or it may present in a variety of ways. Amyloidosis of the tongue may cause sufficient enlargement and inelasticity to hamper speech and swallowing. Depositions in the stomach and intestine may lead to malabsorption, diarrhea, and disturbances in digestion.

The diagnosis of amyloidosis depends on demonstration of amyloid deposits in tissues. The most common sites biopsied are the kidney, when renal manifestations are present, or rectal or gingival tissues in patients suspected of having systemic amyloidosis. Examination of abdominal fat aspirates stained with Congo red is an extremely useful technique for the diagnosis of systemic amyloidosis. In suspected cases of immunocyte-associated amyloidosis, serum and urine protein electrophoresis and immunoelectrophoresis should be performed. Bone marrow aspirates in such cases often show plasmacytosis even in the absence of overt multiple myeloma.

The prognosis for patients with generalized amyloidosis is poor. Those with immunocyte-derived amyloidosis (not including multiple myeloma) have a median survival of 2 years after diagnosis. Patients with myeloma-associated amyloidosis have a poorer prognosis.[157] The outlook for patients with reactive systemic amyloidosis is somewhat better and depends to some extent on the control of the underlying condition. Resorption of amyloid after treatment of the associated condition has been reported, but this is a rare occurrence.

REFERENCES

1. Weiss A: Structure and function of the T cell antigen receptor. J Clin Invest 86:1015, 1990.
2. Reiser H, Stadecker MJ: Costimulatory B7 molecules in the pathogenesis of infection and autoimmune diseases. N Engl J Med 335: 1369, 1996.
3. Abbas AK, et al: Functional diversity of helper T lymphocytes. Nature 383:787, 1996.
4. Clarke LB, Noelle RJ: CD40 and its ligand. Adv Immunol 63:43, 1996.
4a. Banchereau J, Steinman RM: Dendritic cells and the control of immunity. Nature 392:245, 1998.
5. Luster AD: Chemokines—chemotactic cytokines that mediate inflammation. N Engl J Med 338:436, 1998.
6. Monaco JJ: A molecular model of MHC class-I-restricted antigen processing. Immunol Today 13:173, 1992.
7. Brown JH: Three-dimensional structure of the human class II histocompatibility antigen HLA-DR1. Nature 364:33, 1993.
8. Neefjes JJ, Ploegh HL: Intracellular transport of MHC class II molecules. Immunol Today 13:179, 1992.
9. Costa JJ, et al: The cells of the allergic response: mast cells, basophils, and eosinophils. JAMA 278:1815, 1997.
10. Baraniuk JN: Pathogenesis of allergic rhinitis. J Allergy Clin Immunol 99:5763, 1997.
10a. Howarth PH: ABC of allergies. Pathogenic mechanisms: a rational basis for treatment. BMJ 316:758, 1998.
11. Borish L, Joseph B: Inflammation and allergic response. Med Clin North Am 76:765, 1992.
12. Krishna MT, et al: Molecular mediators of asthma. Hosp Pract 31: 115, 1996.
13. Desreumax P, Capron M: Eosinophils in allergic reactions. Curr Opin Inmmunol 8:790, 1996.
14. Bochner BS, Lichtenstein LM: Anaphylaxis. N Engl J Med 324: 1785, 1991.
15. Daniels SE, et al: A genome-wide search for quantitative trait loci underlying asthma. Nature 383:247, 1996.
16. Holgate ST: Asthma genetics: waiting to exhale. Nat Genet 15:227, 1997.
17. Martin J, Abbot G: Serum sickness like illness and antimicrobials in children. N Z Med J 108:123, 1995.
18. Liu C, et al: Lymphocyte-mediated cytolysis. N Engl J Med 335: 1651, 1996.
19. Sayegh MH, Turka LA: The role of T-cell costimulatory activation pathways in transplant rejection. N Engl J Med 338:1813, 1998.
20. VanBuskirk AM, et al: Transplantation immunology. JAMA 278: 1993, 1997.
21. Pardo-Mindan FJ, et al: Pathology of renal transplantation. Semin Diagn Pathol 9:185, 1992.
22. Takemoto S, et al: Survival of nationally shared, HLA-matched kidney transplants from cadaveric donors. N Engl J Med 327:834, 1992.
23. Lu CY, et al: Prevention and treatment of renal allograft rejection: new therapeutic approaches and new insights into established therapies. J Am Soc Nephrol 4:1239, 1993.
24. Kumar V, et al: Role of murine NK cells and their receptors in hybrid resistance. Curr Opin Immunol 9:52, 1997.
25. Miller JFAP, Basten A: Mechanisms of tolerance to self. Curr Opin Immunol 8:815, 1996.
26. Cornall RJ, et al: The regulation of self-reactive B cells. Curr Opin Immunol 7:804, 1995.
26a. Parijs LV, Abbas AK: Homeostasis and self-tolerance in the immune system: turning lymphocytes off. Science 280:243, 1998.
27. Winoto A: Cell death in the regulation of immune responses. Curr Opin Immunol 9:365, 1997.
28. Kruisbeek AM, Amsen D: Mechanisms underlying T cell tolerance. Curr Opin Immunol 8:233, 1996.
29. Shull M, et al: Targeted disruption of the mouse transforming growth factor-b1 gene results in multifocal inflammatory disease. Nature 359:693, 1992.
30. Tivol EA, et al: Costimulation and autoimmunity. Curr Opin Immunol 8:822, 1996.
31. Groux H, et al: A CD4+ T cell subset inhibits antigen-specific T-cell responses and prevents colitis. Nature 389:737, 1997.
32. Barnaba V, Sinigaglia F: Molecular mimicry and T cell-mediated autoimmune disease. J Exp Med 185:1529, 1997.
33. Benoist C, Mathis D: Autoimmune diabetes: retrovirus as trigger, precipitator or marker? Nature 388:833, 1997.
34. Theofilopoulos AN: The basis of autoimmunity: Part I. mechanisms of aberrant self recognition. Imunol Today 16:90, 1995.
35. Lanzavecchia A: How can cryptic epitopes trigger autoimmunity? J Exp Med 181:1945, 1995.
36. Vanderlugt CJ, Miller SD: Epitope spreading. Curr Opin Immunol 8: 831, 1996.
37. Theofilopoulos AN: The basis of autoimmunity: Part II. Genetic predisposition. Immunol Today 16:150, 1995.
38. Dalton TA, Bennett JC: Autoimmune diseases and the major histocompatibility complex: therapeutic implications. Am J Med 92:183, 1992.
39. Hammer RE, et al: Spontaneous inflammatory disease in transgenic rats expressing HLA-B27 and human beta 2m: an animal model of HLA-B27-associated human disorders. Cell 63:1099, 1990.
40. Steinman L, Conlon P: Viral damage and breakdown of self-tolerance. Nat Med 3:1085, 1997.
41. Michet CJ Jr, et al: Epidemiology of SLE and other connective tissue diseases in Rochester, Minnesota, 1950 through 1979. Mayo Clin Proc 60:105, 1985.
42. Kotzin BL: Systemic lupus erythematosus. Cell 85:303, 1996.
43. Kotzin AL, O'Dell JR: Systemic lupus erythematosus. In Frank MM, et al (eds): Samter's Immunologic Diseases, 5th ed. Boston, Little, Brown, 1995, p 667.
43a. Hahn BH: Antibodies to DNA. N Engl J Med 338:1359, 1998.
44. Hietarinta M, Lassila O: Clinical significance of antinuclear antibodies in systemic rheumatic diseases. Ann Med 28:283, 1996.
45. Hang LM, Nakamura RM: Current concepts and advances in clinical laboratory testing for autoimmune diseases. Crit Rev Clin Lab Sci 34:275, 1997.
46. Galli M, et al: Antiphospholipid antibodies: predictive value of laboratory tests. Thromb Hemost 78:75, 1997.
47. Shapiro SS: The lupus anticoagulant-antibody syndrome. Ann Rev Med 47:533, 1996.
48. Kotzin BL: Susceptibility loci for lupus: guiding light from murine models? J Clin Invest 99:557, 1997.
49. Deapen D, et al: A revised estimate of twin concordance in SLE. Arthritis Rheum 35:311, 1992.
50. Schur PH: Genetics of SLE. Lupus 4:425, 1995.
51. Tsokos GC: Lymphocyte abnormalities in human lupus. Clin Immunol Immunopathol 63:7, 1992.
52. Belmart HM, Abramson SB: Pathology and pathogenesis of vascular injury in SLE. Arthritis Rheum 39:9, 1996.
53. Pollak VE, Pirani CL: Lupus nephritis. In Wallace DJ, Hahn BH (eds): Dubois' Lupus Erythematosus, 4th ed. Philadelphia, Lea & Febiger, 1993, p 525.
54. Moore PM, Lisak RP: Systemic lupus erythematosus: immunopathogenesis of neurologic dysfunction. Springer Semin Immunopathol 17:43, 1995.
55. Roldan CA, et al: An echocardiographic study of valvular heart disease associated with SLE. N Engl J Med 335:1424, 1996.
56. Boumpas DT, et al: Systemic lupus erythematosus: emerging concepts. Ann Intern Med 122:940, 1995.
57. Rasaratnam I, Ryan PFJ: Systemic lupus erythematosus. Med J Aust 166:266, 1997.
58. Iliopoulos AG, Toskos GC: Immunopathogenesis and spectrum of infection in SLE. Semin Arthritis Rheum 25:318, 1996.
59. Donnelly AM, et al: Discoid lupus erythematosus. Australas J Dermatol 36:3, 1995.
60. Sontheimer R: Subacute cutaneous lupus erythematosus. Clin Dermatol 3:58, 1985.

61. Yung RL, Richardson BC: Drug-induced lupus. Rheum Dis Clin North Am 20:61, 1994.
62. Fox RI, Kang HI: Pathogenesis of Sjogren syndrome. Rheum Dis Clin North Am 18:517, 1992.
63. Sumida T, et al: TCR in Sjogren syndrome. Br J Rheumatol 36:622, 1997.
64. Haneji N, et al: Identification of a-fodrin as a candidate autoantigen in primary Sjogren syndrome. Science 276:604, 1997.
65. Venables PJW, Rigby SP: Viruses in the etiopathogenesis of Sjogren syndrome. J Rheumatol 24(suppl 50):3, 1997.
66. Manthorpe R, et al: Primary Sjogren syndrome: diagnostic criteria, clinical features, and disease activity. J Rheumatol 24(suppl 50):8, 1997.
67. Geppert T: Southwestern Internal Medicine Conference: Clinical features, pathogenic mechanisms, and new developments in the treatment of systemic sclerosis. Am J Med Sci 299:193, 1990.
68. White B: Immunopathogenesis of systemic sclerosis. Rheum Dis Clin North Am 22:695, 1996.
69. LeRoy EC: Systemic sclerosis: a vascular perspective. Rheum Clin North Am 22:675, 1996.
70. Furst DE, Clements PJ: Hypothesis for the pathogenesis of systemic sclerosis. J Rheumatol 24(suppl 48):53, 1997.
71. Jimenez SA, et al: Pathogenesis of scleroderma: collagen. Rheum Dis Clin North Am 22:647, 1996.
72. Okano Y: Antinuclear antibody in systemic sclerosis. Rheum Dis Clin North Am 22:709, 1996.
73. Rothfield N: Autoantibodies in scleroderma. Rheum Dis Clin North Am 18:483, 1992.
74. Mitchell H, et al: Scleroderma and related conditions. Med Clin North Am 81:129, 1997.
75. Amato AA, Barohn RJ: Idiopathic inflammatory myopathies. Neurol Clin 15:615, 1997.
76. Dalakas M, Sivakumar K: The immunopathologic and inflammatory differences between dermatomyositis, polymyositis, and sporadic inclusion body myositis. Curr Opin Neurol 9:235, 1996.
77. Targoff IN: Autoantibodies in polymyositis. Rheum Dis Clin North Am 18:455, 1992.
78. Lundberg I, Hedfors E: Clinical course of patients with anti-RNP antibodies: a prospective study of 32 patients. J Rheumatol 18:1511, 1991.
79. Citera G, et al: Mixed connective tissue disease: fact or fiction. Lupus 4:255, 1995.
80. World Health Organization Scientific Group: Primary immunodeficiency diseases. Clin Exp Immunol 109(suppl):1, 1997.
81. Ochs HD, Smith CID: X-linked agammaglobulinemia: a clinical and molecular analysis. Medicine 75:287, 1996.
82. Rosen FS, et al: The primary immunodeficiencies. N Engl J Med 333:431, 1995.
83. Sneller MC (moderator): New insights into common variable immunodeficiency. Ann Intern Med 118:720, 1993.
84. Burrows PD, Cooper MD: IgA deficiency. Adv Immunol 65:245, 1997.
85. Lanzavecchia A: Licence to kill. Nature 393:413, 1998.
86. Thomas JA, Graham JM Jr: Chromosome 22q11 deletion syndrome: an update and review for primary pediatricians. Clin Pediatr 36:253, 1997.
87. Resta R, Thompson LF: SCID: the role of adenosine deaminase deficiency. Immunol Today 18:371, 1997.
88. Blaese RM, et al: T-lymphocyte directed gene therapy for ADA-SCID: initial trial result after 4 years. Science 270:475, 1995.
89. Puck JM: Primary immunodeficiency diseases. JAMA 278:1635, 1997.
90. Huber, J, et al: Pathology of congenital immunodeficiencies. Semin Diagn Pathol 9:31, 1992.
91. Featherstone C: Research News. The many faces of WAS protein. Science 275:27, 1997.
92. Frank MM: Complement in disease: inherited and acquired complement deficiencies. In Frank MM, et al (eds): Samter's Immunologic Diseases, 52nd ed. Boston, Little, Brown, 1995, p 487.
93. Acardi M, Agostoni A: Hereditary angioedema. N Engl J Med 334: 1666, 1996.
94. Update: mortality attributable to HIV infection among persons aged 25–44 years—United States, 1994. MMWR 45:121, 1996.
95. Quinn TC: Global burden of the HIV pandemic. Lancet 348:99, 1996.
95a. Balter M: Global program struggles to stem the flood of new cases. Science 280:1863, 1998.
96. Royce RA, et al: Sexual transmission of HIV. N Engl J Med 336: 1072, 1997.
97. Schreiber GB, et al: The risk of transfusion-associated viral infections. N Engl J Med 334:1685, 1996.
98. Wizinia AA, et al: Pediatric HIV infection. Med Clin North Am 80: 1309, 1996.
99. Cardo DM, et al: A case control study of HIV seroconversion in health care workers after percutaneous exposure. N Engl J Med 337: 1485, 1997.
100. Geberding JL, et al: Risk of transmitting the human immunodeficiency virus to health care workers exposed to patients with AIDS and AIDS-related conditions. J Infect Dis 156:1, 1987.
101. O'Brien J, Goedert JJ: HIV causes AIDS: Koch's postulates fulfilled. Curr Opin Immunol 8:613, 1996.
102. Hardy WD: The human immunodeficiency virus. Med Clin North Am 80:1239, 1996.
103. Barre-Sinoussi F: HIV as the cause of AIDS. Lancet 348:31, 1996.
104. Emerman M: HIV-1 and the cell cycle. Curr Biol 6:1096, 1996.
105. Goh WC, et al: HIV-1 vpr increases viral expression by manipulation of the cell cycle: a mechanism for selection of vpr in vivo. Nat Med 4:65, 1998.
106. Johnson RP: Upregulation of Fas ligand by Simian immunodeficiency virus: a nef-arious mechanism of immune evasion. J Exp Med 186:1, 1997.
107. Collins KL, et al: HIV-1 nef protein protects infected primary cells against killing by cytotoxic T lymphocytes. Nature 391:397, 1998.
108. Miller RH, Sarver N: HIV accessory proteins as therapeutic targets. Nat Med 4:389, 1997.
109. Doms RW, Peiper SC: Unwelcomed guests with master keys: how HIV uses chemokine receptors for cellular entry. Virology 235:179, 1997.
110. Binley J, Moore JP: The viral mousetrap. Nature 387:346, 1997.
111. O'Brien SJ, Dean M: In search of AIDS resistance genes. Sci Am 277:46,1997.
112. Moore JP: Coreceptors: implications for HIV pathogenesis and therapy. Science 276:51, 1997.
113. Graziosi C, Pantaleo G: The multifaceted personality of HIV. Nat Med 3:1318, 1997.
114. Research News. Exploiting the HIV-chemokine nexus. Science 275: 1261, 1997.
115. Nolan G: Harnessing viral devices or pharmaceuticals: fighting HIV-1's fire with fire. Cell 90:821,1997.
116. Ho D: Dynamics of HIV-1 replication in vivo. J Clin Invest 99: 2505, 1997.
117. Wolthers KC, et al: T cell telomere length in HIV-1 infection: no evidence for increased CD4+ T cell turnover. Science 274:1543, 1996.
118. Research News. HIV's other immune system targets: macrophages. Science 24:1464, 1997.
119. Orenstein JM, Wahl SM: Macrophages as a source of HIV during opportunistic infections. Science 276:2857, 1997.
120. Knight SC, Patterson S: Bone-marrow derived dendritic cells, infection with human immunodeficiency virus, and immunopathology. Ann Rev Immunol 15:593, 1997.
121. Embretson J, et al: Massive covert infection of helper T lymphocytes and macrophages by HIV during the incubation period of AIDS. Nature 362:359, 1993.
122. Wain-Hobson S: Down or out in blood and lymph? Nature 387:123, 1997.
123. Cohen OJ, et al: Host factors in the pathogenesis of HIV disease. Immunol Rev 159:31, 1997.
124. Glass JD, Johnson RT: Human immunodeficiency virus and the brain. Ann Rev Neurosci 19:1, 1996.
125. Adamson DC, et al: Immunologic NO synthetase: elevation in severe AIDS dementia and induction by HIV gp41. Science 274:1917, 1996.
126. Dewhurst S, et al: Neuropathogenesis of AIDS. Mol Med Today 2: 16, 1996.

127. Pantaleo G, et al: The immunopathogenesis of human immunodeficiency virus infection. N Engl J Med 328:327, 1993.
128. Shacker T, et al: Clinical and epidemiologic features of primary HIV infection. Ann Intern Med 125:257, 1996.
129. Musey L, et al: Cytotoxic T cell responses, viral load and disease progression in early human immunodeficiency virus type 1 infection. N Engl J Med 337:1306, 1997.
130. Mellors JW, et al: Prognosis in HIV-1 infection predicted by the quantity of virus in plasma. Science 272:1167, 1996.
131. Sage MS: Use of HIV viral load in clinical practice: back to the future. Ann Intern Med 126:983, 1997.
132. McMichael AJ, Phillips RE: Escape of human immunodeficiency virus from immune control. Ann Rev Immunol 15:271, 1997.
133. Centers for Disease Control and Prevention: 1993 revised classification system and expanded surveillance definition for AIDS among adolescents and adults. MMWR 41(RR-17):1, 1992.
134. Gold JWM, et al (eds): Management of the HIV-infected patient: Part II. Med Clin North Am 81:299, 1997.
135. Kessler HA, et al: AIDS: Part II. Dis Mon 38:695, 1992.
136. Markowitz N, et al: Incidence of tuberculosis in the United States among HIV-infected persons. Ann Intern Med 126:123, 1997.
137. Telzak EE: Tuberculosis and human immunodeficiency virus infection. Med Clin North Am 81:345, 1997.
138. Nasti G, et al: Malignant tumors and AIDS. Biomed Pharmacother 51:243, 1997.
139. Rabkin CS, et al: Monoclonal origin of multicenter KS lesions. N Engl J Med 336:988, 1997.
140. Kroll MH, Shandera WX: AIDS-associated Kaposi's sarcoma. Hosp Pract 33:85, 1998.
140a. Martin JN, et al: Sexual transmission and natural history of human herpesvirus 8 infection. N Engl J Med 338:948, 1998.
141. Murphy PM: Pirated genes in KS. Nature 385:296, 1997
142. Nicholas J, et al: KS-associated human herpes virus-8 encodes homologs of macrophage inflammatory protein-1, and interleukin-6. Nat Med 3:287, 1997.
143. Boshoff C: Coupling herpesvirus to angiogenesis. Nature 391:24, 1998.
144. Knowles DM: Molecular pathology of acquired immunodeficiency syndrome-related non-Hodgkin's lymphoma. Semin Diagn Pathol 14: 87, 1997.
145. Levine R: Lymphoma in the setting of human immunodeficiency virus infection. In Canellos GP, et al (eds): The Lymphomas. Philadelphia, WB Saunders, 1998, p 507.
146. Shah KV: Human papillomavirus and anogenital cancers. N Engl J Med 337:1386, 1997.
147. Knowles DM, Chadburn A: Lymphadenopathy and the lymphoid neoplasms associated with the acquired immune deficiency syndrome. In Knowles DM (ed): Neoplastic Hematopathology. Baltimore, Williams & Wilkins, 1992, p 773.
148. Shah KV. Human papillomavirus and anogenital cancers. N Engl J Med 337:1386, 1997.
148a. Ho DD: Toward HIV eradication or remission: the tasks ahead. Science 280:1866, 1998.
149. Belloti V, Merlini G: Current concepts in the pathogenesis of systemic amyloidosis. Nephrol Dial Transplant 2(suppl 9):53, 1996.
150. Codho T: Familial amyloid polyneuropathy: new developments in genetics and treatment. Curr Opin Neurol 9:355, 1996.
151. Buxbaum J: The amyloidosis. Mt Sinai Med J 63:16, 1996.
152. Campistol JM, Argiles A: Dialysis-related amyloidosis: visceral involvement and protein constitutents. Nephrol Dial Transplant 11(suppl 3):142, 1996.
153. Kastner DL: Familial Mediterranean fever: the genetics of inflammation. Hosp Pract 33:131, 1998.
154. Benson MD: Inherited amyloidosis. J Med Genet 28:73, 1991.
155. Cornwell GG, et al: The age related amyloids: a growing family unique biochemical substances. J Clin Pathol 48:984, 1995.
156. Jacobson DR, et al: Variant sequence transthyretin (isoleucin 122) in late onset cardiac amyloidosis in black Americans. N Engl J Med 336:466, 1997.
157. Kyle RA, Gertz MA: Systemic amyloidosis. Crit Rev Oncol Hematol 10:49, 1990.

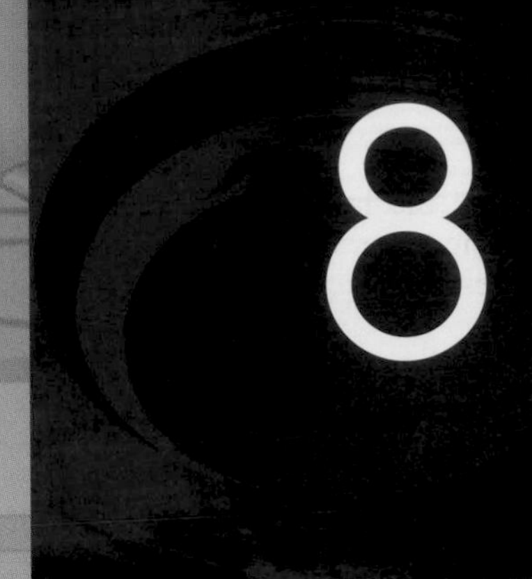

Neoplasia

DEFINITIONS

NOMENCLATURE

CHARACTERISTICS OF BENIGN AND MALIGNANT NEOPLASMS

DIFFERENTIATION AND ANAPLASIA

RATE OF GROWTH

LOCAL INVASION

METASTASIS

- Pathways of Spread

EPIDEMIOLOGY

CANCER INCIDENCE

GEOGRAPHIC AND ENVIRONMENTAL FACTORS

AGE

HEREDITY

ACQUIRED PRENEOPLASTIC DISORDERS

MOLECULAR BASIS OF CANCER

ONCOGENES AND CANCER

- Protein Products of Oncogenes
- Activation of Oncogenes

CANCER-SUPPRESSOR GENES

- Protein Products of Tumor-Suppressor Genes

GENES THAT REGULATE APOPTOSIS

GENES THAT REGULATE DNA REPAIR

TELOMERES AND CANCER

MOLECULAR BASIS OF MULTISTEP CARCINOGENESIS

KARYOTYPIC CHANGES IN TUMORS

BIOLOGY OF TUMOR GROWTH

KINETICS OF TUMOR CELL GROWTH

TUMOR ANGIOGENESIS

TUMOR PROGRESSION AND HETEROGENEITY

MECHANISMS OF INVASION AND METASTASIS

- Invasion of Extracellular Matrix
- Vascular Dissemination and Homing of Tumor Cells
- Molecular Genetics of Metastases

CARCINOGENIC AGENTS AND THEIR CELLULAR INTERACTIONS

CHEMICAL CARCINOGENESIS

- Steps Involved in Chemical Carcinogenesis
- Initiation of Carcinogenesis
- Promotion of Carcinogenesis
- Carcinogenic Chemicals

RADIATION CARCINOGENESIS

- Ultraviolet Rays
- Ionizing Radiation

VIRAL AND MICROBIAL CARCINOGENESIS

- DNA Oncogenic Viruses
- RNA Oncogenic Viruses
- *Helicobacter pylori*

HOST DEFENSE AGAINST TUMORS—TUMOR IMMUNITY

TUMOR ANTIGENS

ANTITUMOR EFFECTOR MECHANISMS

IMMUNOSURVEILLANCE

CLINICAL FEATURES OF TUMORS

EFFECTS OF TUMOR ON HOST

- Local and Hormonal Effects
- Cancer Cachexia
- Paraneoplastic Syndromes

GRADING AND STAGING OF TUMORS

LABORATORY DIAGNOSIS OF CANCER

In the United States each year, well over 1 million individuals learn for the first time that they have some type of cancer. Many of these tumors can be cured. Nonetheless, according to American Cancer Society estimates, cancer caused approximately 564,000 deaths in 1998, accounting for about 23% of all deaths.[1] Only cardiovascular diseases cause more deaths. Some good news, however, has also emerged from the most recent statistics: For the first time in the last half century, cancer mortality has declined in each of the years from 1991 to 1995. Thus, there is progress, but the problem is still overwhelming. The discussion that follows deals with both benign tumors and cancers; the latter receive more attention. The focus is on the basic morphologic and behavioral characteristics and present understanding of the molecular basis of carcinogenesis. We also discuss the interactions of the tumor with the host and the host response to tumor. Although the discussion of therapy is beyond the scope of this chapter, with many forms of malignancy, notably the leukemias and lymphomas, there are now dramatic improvements in 5-year survival rates. A greater proportion of cancers are being cured or arrested today than ever before.

DEFINITIONS

Neoplasia literally means "new growth," and the new growth is a *neoplasm*. The term *tumor* was originally applied to the swelling caused by inflammation. Neoplasms also may induce swellings, but by long precedent, the non-neoplastic usage of *tumor* has passed into limbo; thus, the term is now equated with neoplasm. *Oncology* (Greek *oncos* = tumor) is the study of tumors or neoplasms. *Cancer is the common term for all malignant tumors.* Although the ancient origins of this term are somewhat uncertain, it probably derives from the Latin for crab, *cancer*—presumably because a cancer "adheres to any part that it seizes upon in an obstinate manner like the crab."

Although all physicians know what they mean when they use the term *neoplasm*, it has been surprisingly difficult to develop an accurate definition. The eminent British oncologist Willis[2] has come closest: "A neoplasm is an abnormal mass of tissue, the growth of which exceeds and is uncoordinated with that of the normal tissues and persists in the same excessive manner after cessation of the stimuli which evoked the change." To this characterization we might add that the abnormal mass is purposeless, preys on the host, and is virtually autonomous. It preys on the host insofar as the growth of the neoplastic tissue competes with normal cells and tissues for energy supplies and nutritional substrate. Inasmuch as these masses may flourish in a patient who is wasting away, they are to a degree autonomous. Later it becomes evident that such autonomy is not complete. All neoplasms ultimately depend on the host for their nutrition and vascular supply; many forms of neoplasia require endocrine support.

NOMENCLATURE

All tumors, benign and malignant, have two basic components: (1) proliferating neoplastic cells that constitute their *parenchyma* and (2) *supportive stroma* made up of connective tissue and blood vessels. Although parenchymal cells represent the proliferating "cutting edge" of neoplasms and so determine their nature, the growth and evolution of neoplasms are critically dependent on their stroma. An adequate stromal blood supply is requisite, and the stromal connective tissue provides the framework for the parenchyma. In some tumors, the stromal support is scant, and so the neoplasm is soft and fleshy. Sometimes the parenchymal cells stimulate the formation of an abundant collagenous stroma—referred to as *desmoplasia.* Some tumors, for example, some cancers of the female breast, are stony hard or scirrhous. The nomenclature of tumors is, however, based on the parenchymal component.

Benign Tumors. In general, benign tumors are designated by attaching the suffix *-oma* to the cell of origin. Tumors of mesenchymal cells generally follow this rule. For example, a benign tumor arising from fibroblastic cells is called a *fibroma.* A cartilaginous tumor is a *chondroma*, and a tumor of osteoblasts is an *osteoma.* In contrast, nomenclature of benign epithelial tumors is more complex. They are variously classified, some based on their cells of origin, others on microscopic architecture, and still others on their macroscopic patterns.

Adenoma is the term applied to the benign epithelial neoplasm that forms glandular patterns as well as to the tumors derived from glands but not necessarily reproducing glandular patterns. On this basis, a benign epithelial neoplasm that arises from renal tubular cells growing in the form of numerous tightly clustered small glands would be termed an *adenoma*, as would a heterogeneous mass of adrenal cortical cells growing in no distinctive pattern. Benign epithelial neoplasms producing microscopically or macroscopically visible finger-like or warty projections from epithelial surfaces are referred to as *papillomas* (Fig. 8–1). Those that form large cystic masses, as in the ovary, are referred to as *cystadenomas.* Some tumors produce papillary patterns that protrude into cystic spaces and are called *papillary cystadenomas*. When a neoplasm, benign or malignant, produces a macroscopically visible projection above a *mucosal* surface and projects, for example, into the gastric or colonic lumen, it is termed a *polyp* (Fig. 8–2). The term *polyp* preferably is restricted to benign tumors. Malignant polyps are better designated *polypoid cancers*.

Malignant Tumors. The nomenclature of malignant tumors essentially follows the same schema used for benign neoplasms, with certain additions. *Malignant tumors arising in mesenchymal tissue are usually called sarcomas*

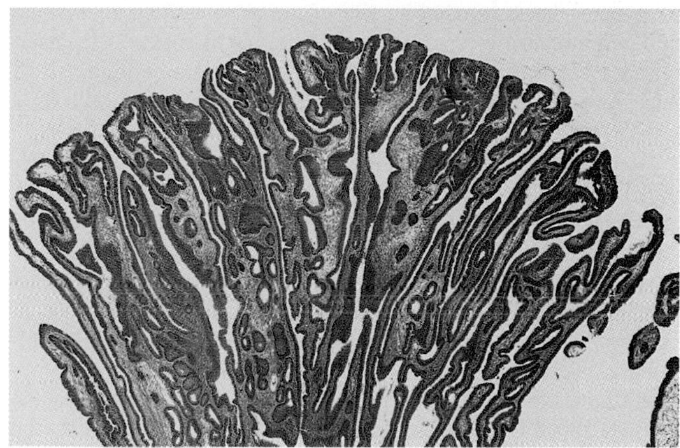

Figure 8–1

Papilloma of the colon with finger-like projections into the lumen. (Courtesy of Dr. Trace Worrell, Department of Pathology, University of Texas Southwestern Medical School, Dallas, TX.)

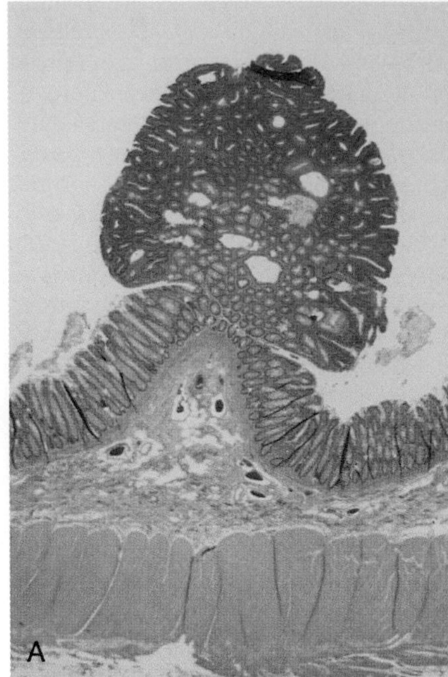

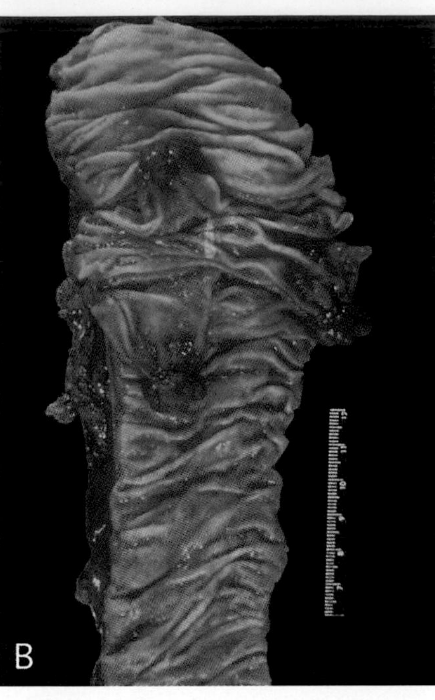

Figure 8–2

Colonic polyp. *A,* This benign glandular tumor (adenoma) is projecting into the colonic lumen and is attached to the mucosa by a distinct stalk. *B,* Gross appearance of several colonic polyps.

(Greek *sar* = fleshy) because they have little connective tissue stroma and so are fleshy (e.g., fibrosarcoma, liposarcoma, and leiomyosarcoma for smooth muscle cancer and rhabdomyosarcoma for a cancer that differentiates toward striated muscle). Malignant neoplasms of epithelial cell origin, derived from any of the three germ layers, are called *carcinomas.* Thus, cancer arising in the epidermis of ectodermal origin is a carcinoma, as is a cancer arising in the mesodermally derived cells of the renal tubules and the endodermally derived cells of the lining of the gastrointestinal tract. Carcinomas may be further qualified. One with a glandular growth pattern microscopically is termed an *adenocarcinoma,* and one producing recognizable squamous cells arising in any epithelium of the body is termed a *squamous cell carcinoma.* It is further common practice to specify, when possible, the organ of origin (e.g., a renal cell adenocarcinoma or bronchogenic squamous cell carcinoma). Not infrequently, however, a cancer is composed of undifferentiated cells and must be designated merely as a poorly differentiated or undifferentiated malignant tumor.

In most neoplasms, benign and malignant, the parenchymal cells bear a close resemblance to each other, as though all were derived from a single cell, as we know to be the case with cancers. Infrequently, divergent differentiation of a single line of parenchymal cells creates what are called *mixed tumors.* The best example is the *mixed tumor of salivary gland origin.* These tumors contain epithelial components scattered within a myxoid stroma that sometimes contains islands of apparent cartilage or even bone (Fig. 8–3). All these elements, it is believed, arise from epithelial and myoepithelial cells of salivary gland origin; thus the preferred designation of these neoplasms is *pleomorphic adenoma.* The great majority of neoplasms, even mixed tumors, are composed of cells representative of a single germ layer. The *teratoma,* in contrast, is made up of a variety of parenchymal cell types representative of more than one germ layer, usually all three. They arise from totipotential cells and so are principally encountered in the gonads, although, rarely, they occur in sequestered primitive cell rests elsewhere. These totipotential cells differentiate along various germ lines, producing, for example, tissues that can be identified as skin, muscle, fat, gut epithelium, tooth structures, and, indeed, any tissue of the body. A particularly common pattern is seen in the ovarian *cystic teratoma* (dermoid cyst), which differentiates princi-

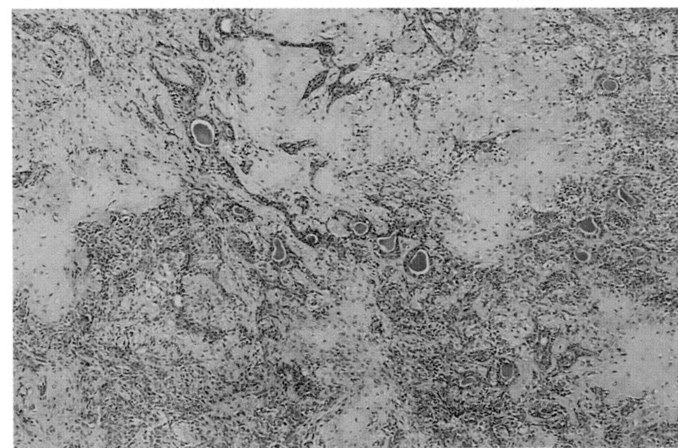

Figure 8–3

This mixed tumor of the parotid gland contains epithelial cells forming ducts and myxoid stroma that resembles cartilage. (Courtesy of Dr. Trace Worrell, Department of Pathology, University of Texas Southwestern Medical School, Dallas, TX.)

pally along ectodermal lines to create a cystic tumor lined by skin replete with hair, sebaceous glands, and tooth structures (Fig. 8–4).

The nomenclature of the more common forms of neoplasia is presented in Table 8–1. It is evident from this compilation that there are some inappropriate but deeply entrenched usages. For generations, carcinomas of melanocytes have been called *melanomas*, although correctly they should be referred to as melanocarcinomas. Analogously, carcinomas of testicular origin are stubbornly called *seminomas*. Other instances are encountered in which innocent designations belie ugly behavior. The converse is also true when ominous terms are applied to usually trivial lesions. An ectopic rest of normal tissue is sometimes called a *choristoma*—as, for example, a rest of adrenal cells under the kidney capsule. Occasionally a pancreatic nodular rest in the mucosa of the small intestine may mimic a neoplasm, providing some partial justification for the use of a term that implies a tumor. Analogously, aberrant differentiation may produce a mass of disorganized but mature specialized cells or tissue indigenous to the particular site, referred to as a *hamartoma*. Thus, a hamartoma in the lung may contain islands of cartilage, blood vessels, bronchial-type structures, and lymphoid tissue. Sometimes the lesion is purely cartilaginous or purely angiomatous. Although these might be construed as benign neoplasms, the complete resemblance of the tissue to normal cartilage or blood vessels and the occasional admixture of other elements favor a hamartomatous origin. In any event, the hamartoma is totally benign.

Table 8–1. NOMENCLATURE OF TUMORS

Tissue of Origin	Benign	Malignant
Composed of One Parenchymal Cell Type		
Mesenchymal tumors		
Connective tissue and derivatives	Fibroma	Fibrosarcoma
	Lipoma	Liposarcoma
	Chondroma	Chondrosarcoma
	Osteoma	Osteogenic sarcoma
Endothelial and related tissues		
Blood vessels	Hemangioma	Angiosarcoma
Lymph vessels	Lymphangioma	Lymphangiosarcoma
Synovium		Synovial sarcoma
Mesothelium		Mesothelioma
Brain coverings	Meningioma	Invasive meningioma
Blood cells and related cells		
Hematopoietic cells		Leukemias
Lymphoid tissue		Malignant lymphomas
Muscle		
Smooth	Leiomyoma	Leiomyosarcoma
Striated	Rhabdomyoma	Rhabdomyosarcoma
Epithelial tumors		
Stratified squamous	Squamous cell papilloma	Squamous cell or epidermoid carcinoma
Basal cells of skin or adnexa		Basal cell carcinoma
Epithelial lining		
Glands or ducts	Adenoma	Adenocarcinoma
	Papilloma	Papillary carcinoma
	Cystadenoma	Cystadenocarcinoma
Respiratory passages		Bronchogenic carcinoma
		Bronchial adenoma (carcinoid)
Neuroectoderm	Nevus	Malignant melanoma
Renal epithelium	Renal tubular adenoma	Renal cell carcinoma
Liver cells	Liver cell adenoma	Hepatocellular carcinoma
Urinary tract epithelium (transitional)	Transitional cell papilloma	Transitional cell carcinoma
Placental epithelium (trophoblast)	Hydatidiform mole	Choriocarcinoma
Testicular epithelium (germ cells)		Seminoma
		Embryonal carcinoma
More Than One Neoplastic Cell Type—Mixed Tumors, Usually Derived From One Germ Layer		
Salivary glands	Pleomorphic adenoma (mixed tumor of salivary origin)	Malignant mixed tumor of salivary gland origin
Breast	Fibroadenoma	Malignant cystosarcoma phyllodes
Renal anlage		Wilms tumor
More Than One Neoplastic Cell Type Derived From More Than One Germ Layer—Teratogenous		
Totipotential cells in gonads or in embryonic rests	Mature teratoma, dermoid cyst	Immature teratoma, teratocarcinoma

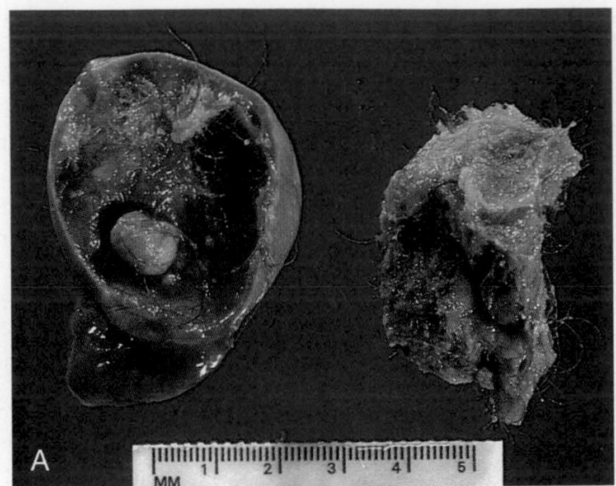

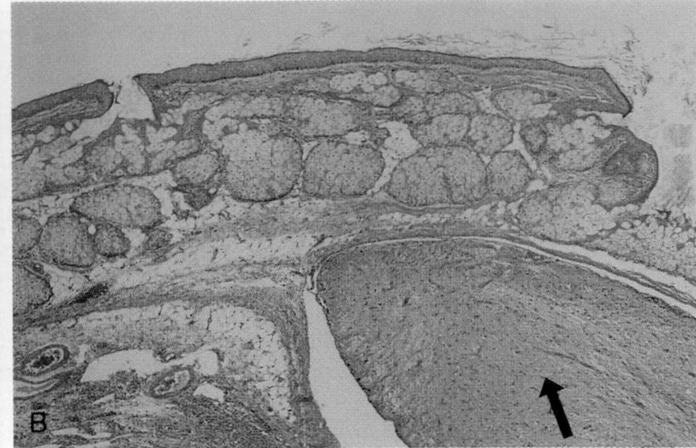

Figure 8-4

A, Gross appearance of an opened cystic teratoma of the ovary. Note the presence of hair, sebaceous material, and tooth. *B*, A microscopic view of a similar tumor shows skin, sebaceous glands, fat cells, and a tract of neural tissue *(arrow)*.

The nomenclature of tumors is important because specific designations have specific clinical implications. The historically sanctified term *seminoma* connotes a form of carcinoma that tends to spread to lymph nodes along the iliac arteries and aorta. Further, these tumors are extremely radiosensitive and can be eradicated by radiotherapy; thus few patients with seminomas die of the neoplasm. By contrast, the embryonal carcinoma of the testis is not radiosensitive and tends to invade locally beyond the confines of the testis and spread throughout the body. There also are other varieties of testicular neoplasms, and so the designation *cancer of the testis* tells little of its clinical significance.

CHARACTERISTICS OF BENIGN AND MALIGNANT NEOPLASMS

In the great majority of instances, the differentiation of a benign from a malignant tumor can be made morphologically with considerable certainty; sometimes, however, a neoplasm defies categorization. It has been said, "All tumors need not of necessity be either benign or malignant." Certain anatomic features may suggest innocence, whereas others point toward cancerous potential. Ultimately, all morphologic diagnosis is subjective and constitutes prediction of the future course of a neoplasm. Occasionally, this prediction is confounded by a marked discrepancy between the morphologic appearance of a tumor and its biologic behavior: An innocent face may mask an ugly nature. Such deception or ambiguity, however, is not the rule; in general, there are criteria by which benign and malignant tumors can be differentiated, and they behave accordingly. These differences can conveniently be discussed under the following headings: (1) differentiation and anaplasia, (2) rate of growth, (3) local invasion, and (4) metastasis.

Differentiation and Anaplasia

The terms *differentiation* and *anaplasia* apply to the parenchymal cells of neoplasms. *Differentiation refers to the extent to which parenchymal cells resemble comparable normal cells, both morphologically and functionally.* Well-differentiated tumors are thus composed of cells resembling the mature normal cells of the tissue of origin of the neoplasm (Fig. 8–5). Poorly differentiated or undifferentiated tumors have primitive-appearing, unspecialized cells. *In general, benign tumors are well differentiated* (Fig. 8–6). The neoplastic cell in a benign smooth muscle tumor—a leiomyoma—so closely resembles the normal cell as to make it impossible to recognize it as a tumor cell on high-power examination. Only the massing of these cells

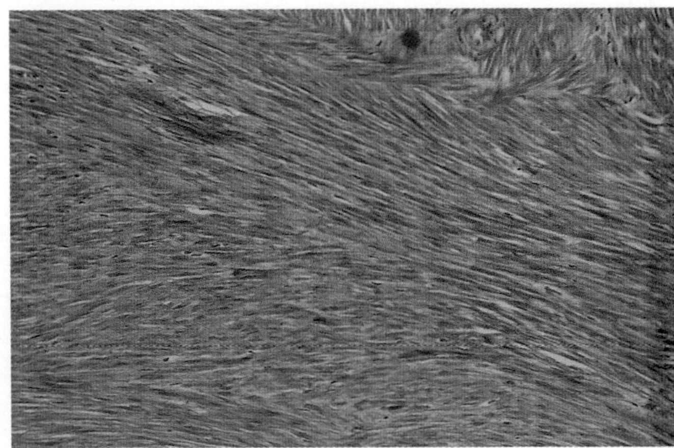

Figure 8-5

Leiomyoma of the uterus. This benign, well-differentiated tumor contains interlacing bundles of neoplastic smooth muscle cells that are virtually identical in appearance to normal smooth muscle cells in the myometrium.

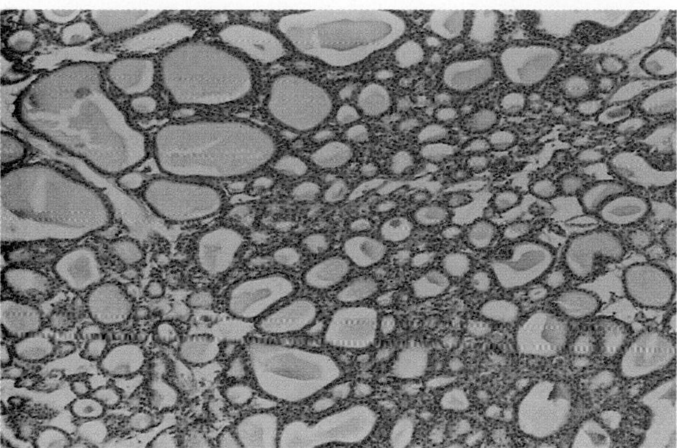

Figure 8–6

Benign tumor (adenoma) of the thyroid. Note the normal-looking (well-differentiated), colloid-filled thyroid follicles. (Courtesy of Dr. Trace Worrell, Department of Pathology, University of Texas Southwestern Medical School, Dallas, TX.)

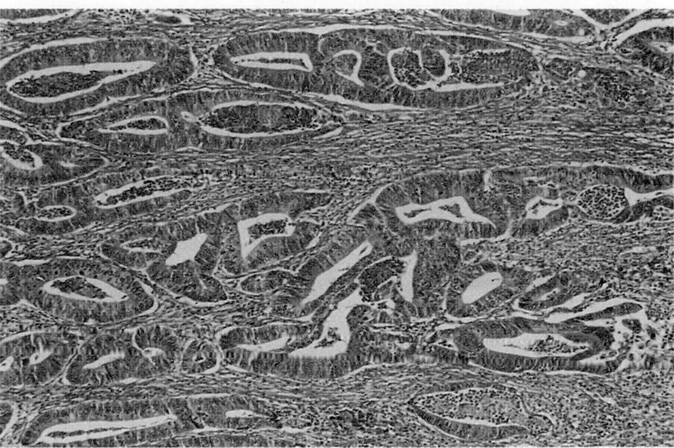

Figure 8–7

Malignant tumor (adenocarcinoma) of the colon. Note that compared with the well-formed and normal-looking glands characteristic of a benign tumor (see Fig. 8–6), the cancerous glands are irregular in shape and size and do not resemble the normal colonic glands. This tumor is considered differentiated because gland formation can be seen. The malignant glands have invaded the muscular layer of the colon. (Courtesy of Dr. Trace Worrell, Department of Pathology, University of Texas Southwestern Medical School, Dallas, TX.)

into a nodule discloses the tumorous nature of the lesion. One may get so close to the tree that one loses sight of the forest.

Malignant neoplasms, in contrast, range from well differentiated to undifferentiated. Malignant neoplasms composed of undifferentiated cells are said to be anaplastic. Lack of differentiation, or *anaplasia*, is considered a hallmark of malignant transformation. Literally, anaplasia means "to form backward," implying a reversion from a high level of differentiation to a lower level. There is substantial evidence, however, that cancers arise from stem cells present in all specialized tissues. The well-differentiated cancer (Fig. 8–7) evolves from maturation or specialization of undifferentiated cells as they proliferate, whereas the undifferentiated malignant tumor derives from proliferation without maturation of the transformed cells. Lack of differentiation then is not the consequence of dedifferentiation.

Lack of differentiation, or anaplasia, is marked by a number of morphologic and functional changes. Both the cells and the nuclei characteristically display *pleomorphism*—variation in size and shape (Fig. 8–8). Cells may be found that are many times larger than their neighbors, and other cells may be extremely small and primitive appearing. Characteristically the nuclei contain an abundance of DNA and are extremely dark staining (*hyperchromatic*). The nuclei are disproportionately large for the cell, and the nuclear-to-cytoplasmic ratio may approach 1:1 instead of the normal 1:4 or 1:6. The nuclear shape is usually extremely variable, and the chromatin is often coarsely clumped and distributed along the nuclear membrane. Large nucleoli are usually present in these nuclei.

As compared with benign tumors and some well differentiated malignant neoplasms, undifferentiated tumors usually possess large numbers of mitoses, reflecting the higher proliferative activity of the parenchymal cells. *The presence of mitoses, however, does not necessarily indicate that a tumor is malignant or that the tissue is neoplastic.* Many normal tissues exhibiting rapid turnover, such as bone marrow, have numerous mitoses, and non-neoplastic proliferations such as hyperplasias contain many cells in mitosis. More important as a morphologic feature of malignant neoplasia are atypical, bizarre mitotic figures sometimes producing tripolar, quadripolar, or multipolar spindles (Fig. 8–9).

Another feature of anaplasia is the formation of *tumor giant cells*, some possessing only a single huge polymorphic nucleus and others having two or more nuclei. These giant cells are not to be confused with inflammatory Lang-

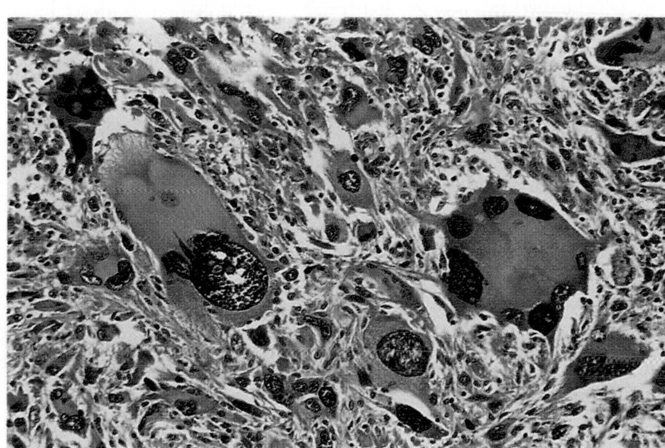

Figure 8–8

Anaplastic tumor of the skeletal muscle (rhabdomyosarcoma). Note the marked cellular and nuclear pleomorphism, hyperchromatic nuclei, and tumor giant cells. (Courtesy of Dr. Trace Worrell, Department of Pathology, University of Texas Southwestern Medical School, Dallas, TX.)

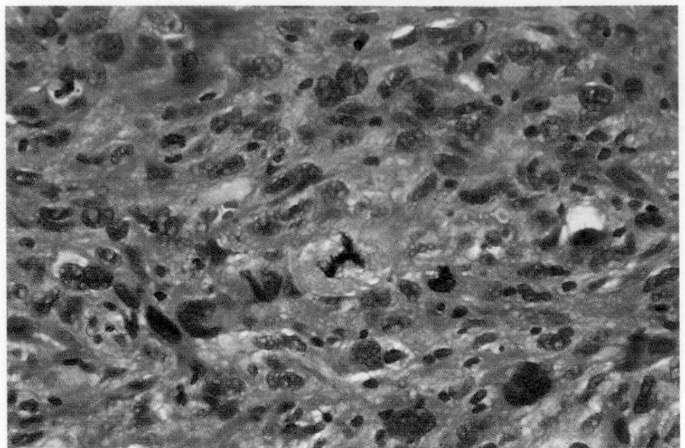

Figure 8-9

High-power detail of anaplastic tumor cells to show cellular and nuclear variation in size and shape. The prominent cell in the center field has an abnormal tripolar spindle.

hans or foreign body giant cells, which possess many small, normal-appearing nuclei. In the cancer giant cell, the nucleus is hyperchromatic and is large in relation to the cell. In addition to the cytologic abnormalities described here, the *orientation of anaplastic cells is markedly disturbed (i.e., they lose normal polarity).* Sheets or large masses of tumor cells grow in an anarchic, disorganized fashion. Although these growing cells obviously require a blood supply, often the vascular stroma is scant, and in many anaplastic tumors, large central areas undergo ischemic necrosis. As mentioned at the outset, malignant tumors differ widely in the extent to which their morphologic appearance deviates from the norm. On one end of the spectrum are the extremely undifferentiated, anaplastic tumors, and at the other end are cancers that bear striking resemblance to their tissues of origin. Certain well-differentiated adenocarcinomas of the thyroid, for example, may form normal-appearing follicles, and some squamous cell carcinomas contain cells that do not differ cytologically from normal squamous epithelial cells (Fig. 8–10). Thus, the morphologic diagnosis of malignancy in well-differentiated tumors may sometimes be quite difficult. In between the two extremes lie tumors that are loosely referred to as *moderately well differentiated.*

Before we leave the subject of differentiation and anaplasia, we should discuss *dysplasia*, a term that literally means disordered growth. Dysplasia is encountered principally in the epithelia, and it is characterized by a constellation of changes that include *a loss in the uniformity of the individual cells as well as a loss in their architectural orientation.* Dysplastic cells also exhibit considerable pleomorphism (variation in size and shape) and often possess deeply stained (hyperchromatic) nuclei, which are abnormally large for the size of the cell. Mitotic figures are more abundant than usual, although almost invariably they conform to normal patterns. Frequently the mitoses appear in abnormal locations within the epithelium. Thus, in dysplastic stratified squamous epithelium, mitoses are not confined to the basal layers and may appear at all levels and even in surface cells. There is considerable architectural anarchy. For example, the usual progressive maturation of tall cells in the basal layer to flattened squames on the surface may be lost and replaced by a disordered scrambling of dark basal-appearing cells. When dysplastic changes are marked and involve the entire thickness of the epithelium, the lesion is considered a preinvasive neoplasm and is referred to as *carcinoma in situ* (Fig. 8–11). Although dysplastic changes are often found adjacent to foci of invasive carcinoma and in long-term studies of cigarette smokers, epithelial dysplasia almost invariably antedates the appearance of cancer, *dysplasia does not necessarily progress to cancer.* Mild-to-moderate changes that do not involve the entire thickness of epithelium may be reversible, and with removal of the putative inciting causes, the epithelium may revert to normal.

Turning to the functional differentiation of neoplastic cells, as you might presume, the better the differentiation of the cell, the more completely it retains the functional capabilities found in its normal counterparts. Thus, benign neoplasms and well-differentiated carcinomas of endocrine glands frequently elaborate the hormones characteristic of their origin. Well-differentiated squamous cell carcinomas of the epidermis elaborate keratin, just as well-differentiated hepatocellular carcinomas elaborate bile. Highly anaplastic undifferentiated cells, whatever their tissue of origin, come to resemble each other more than the normal cells from which they have arisen. In some instances, however, unanticipated functions emerge. Some tumors may elaborate fetal proteins (antigens) not produced by the comparable cells in the adult. Analogously, carcinomas of nonendocrine origin may assume hormone synthesis to produce so-called ectopic hormones. For example, bronchogenic carcinomas may produce adrenocorticotropic hormone, parathyroid-like hormone, insulin, and glucagon as

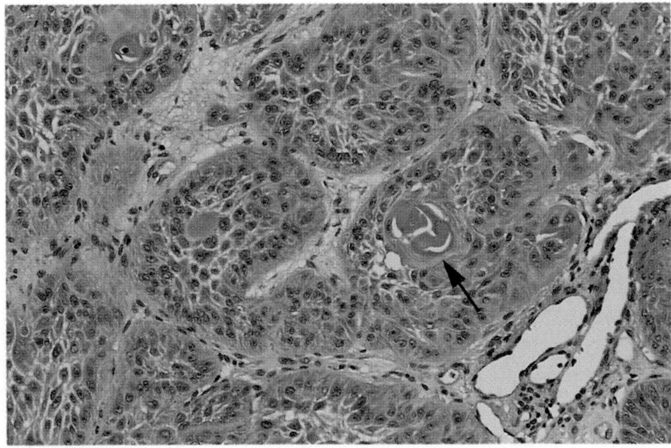

Figure 8-10

Well-differentiated squamous cell carcinoma of the skin. The tumor cells are strikingly similar to normal squamous epithelial cells, with intercellular bridges and nests of keratin pearls *(arrow).* (Courtesy of Dr. Trace Worrell, Department of Pathology, University of Texas Southwestern Medical School, Dallas, TX.)

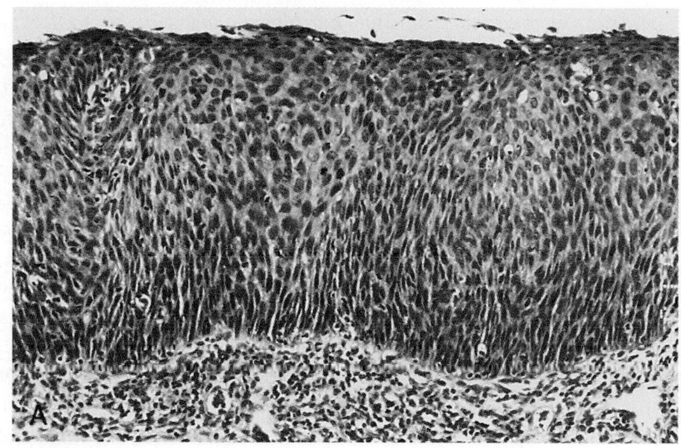

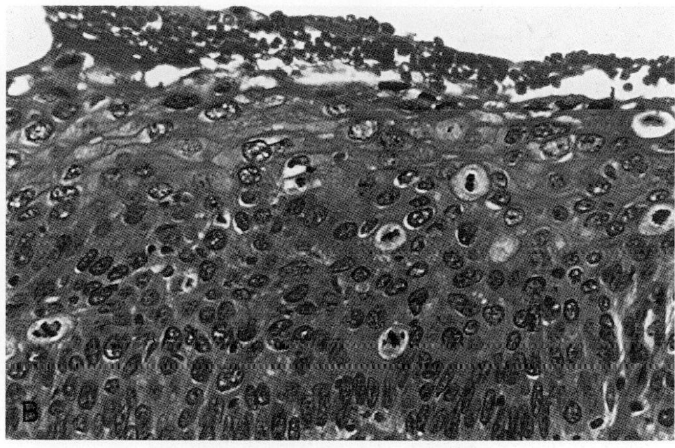

Figure 8–11 ■

A, Carcinoma in situ. This low-power view shows that the entire thickness of the epithelium is replaced by atypical dysplastic cells. There is no orderly differentiation of squamous cells. The basement membrane is intact and there is no tumor in the subepithelial stroma. *B*, A high-power view of another region shows failure of normal differentiation, marked nuclear and cellular pleomorphism, and numerous mitotic figures extending toward the surface. The basement membrane (below) is not seen in this section.

well as others. More is said about these phenomena later. *Despite exceptions, the more rapidly growing and the more anaplastic a tumor, the less likely it is that there will be specialized functional activity. The cells in benign tumors are almost always well differentiated and resemble their normal cells of origin; the cells in cancer are more or less differentiated, but some loss of differentiation is always present.*

Rate of Growth

The generalization can be made that *most benign tumors grow slowly over a period of years, whereas most cancers grow rapidly, sometimes at an erratic pace,* and eventually spread and kill their hosts. Such an oversimplification, however, must be extensively qualified. Some benign tumors have a higher growth rate than malignant tumors. Moreover, the rate of growth of benign as well as malignant neoplasms may not be constant over time. Factors such as hormone dependence, adequacy of blood supply, and likely unknown influences may affect their growth. For example, leiomyomas (benign smooth muscle tumors) of the uterus are common. Not infrequently, repeated clinical examination of women bearing such neoplasms over the span of decades discloses no significant increase in size. After the menopause, the neoplasms may atrophy and later be found to be replaced largely by collagenous, sometimes calcified, tissue. Leiomyomas frequently enter a growth spurt during pregnancy. These neoplasms to some extent depend on the circulating levels of steroid hormones, particularly estrogens.

In general, *the growth rate of tumors correlates with their level of differentiation, and thus most malignant tumors grow more rapidly than do benign lesions.* There is, however, a wide range of behavior. Some malignant tumors grow slowly for years then suddenly increase in size virtually under observation, explosively disseminating to cause death within a few months of discovery. It is believed that such behavior results from the emergence of an aggressive subclone of transformed cells. At the other extreme are those that grow more slowly than benign tumors and may even enter periods of dormancy lasting for years. On occasion, cancers have been observed to decrease in size and even spontaneously disappear, but the handful of "miracles" fills only a small volume. To examine this variable behavior more closely, we consider what is known about the life history of cancer, including the cell kinetics of cancer growth and the influences that modify the growth of malignant tumors, in a later section.

Local Invasion

Nearly all benign tumors grow as cohesive expansile masses that remain localized to their site of origin and do not have the capacity to infiltrate, invade, or metastasize to distant sites, as do malignant tumors. Because they grow and expand slowly, they usually develop a rim of compressed connective tissue, sometimes called a fibrous *capsule*, that separates them from the host tissue. This capsule is derived largely from the stroma of the native tissue as the parenchymal cells atrophy under the pressure of expanding tumor. Such encapsulation tends to contain the benign neoplasm as a discrete, readily palpable, and easily movable mass that can be surgically enucleated (Figs. 8–12 and 8–13). Although a well-defined cleavage plane exists around most benign tumors, in some it is lacking. Thus, hemangiomas (neoplasms composed of tangled blood vessels) are often unencapsulated and may appear to permeate the site in which they arise (commonly the dermis of the skin).

The growth of cancers is accompanied by progressive infiltration, invasion, and destruction of the surrounding tissue. In general, they are poorly demarcated from the

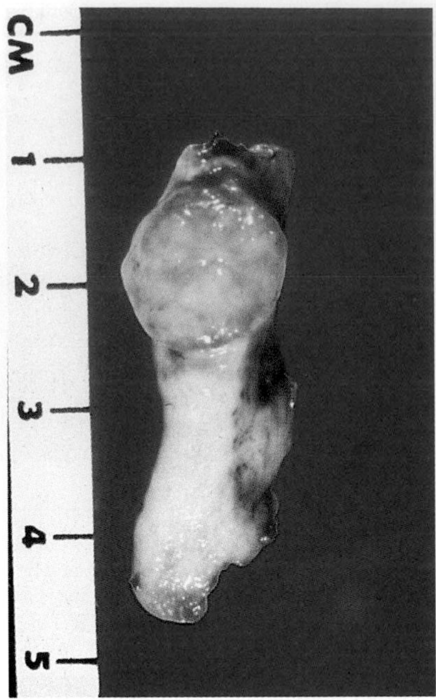

Figure 8–12

Fibroadenoma of the breast. The tan-colored, encapsulated small tumor is sharply demarcated from the whiter breast tissue.

surrounding normal tissue, and a well-defined cleavage plane is lacking (Figs. 8–14 and 8–15). Slowly expanding malignant tumors, however, may develop an apparently enclosing fibrous capsule and may push along a broad front into adjacent normal structures. Histologic examination of such apparently encapsulated masses almost always discloses tiny crablike feet penetrating the margin and infiltrating the adjacent structures.

Most malignant tumors are obviously invasive and can be expected to penetrate the wall of the colon or uterus, for example, or fungate through the surface of the skin. They recognize no normal anatomic boundaries. Such invasiveness makes their surgical resection difficult, and even if the tumor appears well circumscribed, it is necessary to remove a considerable margin of apparently normal tissues about the infiltrative neoplasm. *Next to the development of metastases, invasiveness is the most reliable feature that differentiates malignant from benign tumors.* We noted earlier that some cancers seem to evolve from a preinvasive stage referred to as *carcinoma in situ.* This is best illustrated by carcinoma of the uterine cervix (Chapter 24). *In situ cancers display the cytologic features of malignancy without invasion of the basement membrane.* They may be considered one step removed from invasive cancer, and with time, most penetrate the basement membrane and invade the subepithelial stroma.

Metastasis

Metastases are tumor implants discontinuous with the primary tumor. *Metastasis unequivocally marks a tumor as malignant because benign neoplasms do not metastasize.* The invasiveness of cancers permits them to penetrate into blood vessels, lymphatics, and body cavities, providing the opportunity for spread. *With few exceptions, all cancers can metastasize.* The major exceptions are most malignant neoplasms of the glial cells in the central nervous system, called *gliomas*, and basal cell carcinomas of the skin. Both are highly invasive forms of neoplasia (the latter being known in the older literature as *rodent ulcers* because of their invasive destructiveness), but they rarely metastasize. It is evident then that the properties of invasion and metastasis are separable.

In general, the more aggressive, the more rapidly growing, and the larger the primary neoplasm, the greater the likelihood that it will metastasize or already has metastasized. There are innumerable exceptions, however. Small, well-differentiated, slowly growing lesions sometimes metastasize widely, and, conversely, some rapidly growing lesions remain localized for years. No judgment can be made about the probability of metastasis from pathologic examination of the primary tumor. Many factors relating to both invader and host are involved, as is pointed out later.

Approximately 30% of newly diagnosed patients with solid tumors (excluding skin cancers other than melanomas) present with metastases. Metastatic spread strongly reduces the possibility of cure; hence short of prevention of cancer, no achievement would confer greater benefit on patients than methods to prevent distant spread.

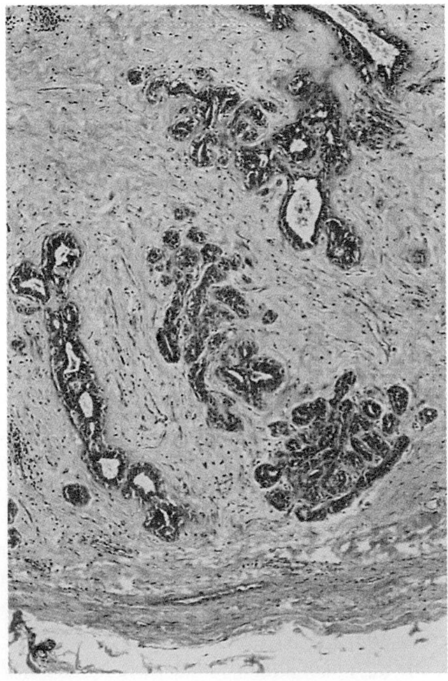

Figure 8–13

Microscopic view of fibroadenoma of the breast seen in Figure 8–12. The fibrous capsule *(below)* sharply delimits the tumor from the surrounding tissue. (Courtesy of Dr. Trace Worrell, Department of Pathology, University of Texas Southwestern Medical School, Dallas, TX.)

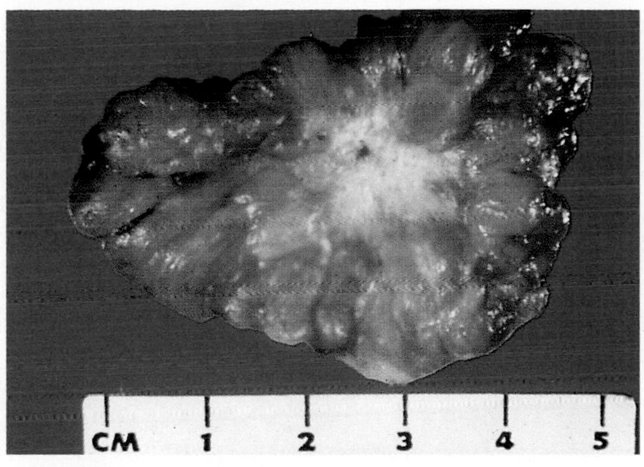

Figure 8–14

Cut section of an invasive ductal carcinoma of the breast. The lesion is retracted, infiltrating the surrounding breast substance, and would be stony hard on palpation.

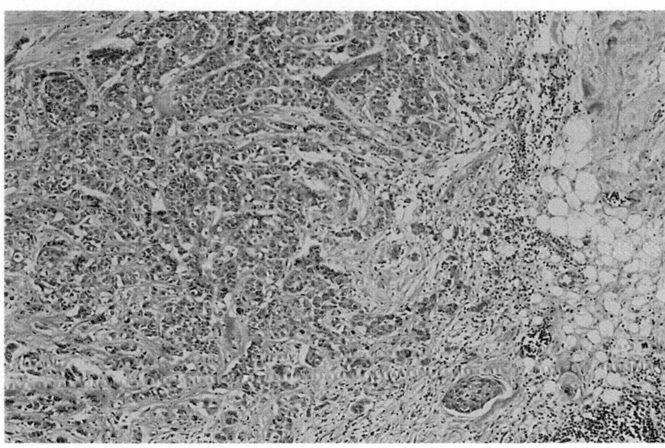

Figure 8–15

The microscopic view of breast carcinoma seen in Figure 8–14 illustrates the invasion of breast stroma and fat by nests and cords of tumor cells (compare with Fig. 8–13). The absence of a well-defined capsule should be noted. (Courtesy of Dr. Trace Worrell, Department of Pathology, University of Texas Southwestern Medical School, Dallas, TX.)

PATHWAYS OF SPREAD

Dissemination of cancers may occur through one of three pathways: (1) direct seeding of body cavities or surfaces, (2) lymphatic spread, and (3) hematogenous spread. Although direct transplantation of tumor cells, as for example on surgical instruments, may theoretically occur, it is rare and, in any event, an artificial mode of dissemination that is not discussed further. Each of the three major pathways is described separately.

Seeding of Body Cavities and Surfaces. Seeding of body cavities and surfaces may occur whenever a malignant neoplasm penetrates into a natural "open field." Most often involved is the peritoneal cavity, but any other cavity—pleural, pericardial, subarachnoid, and joint space—may be affected. Such seeding is particularly characteristic of carcinomas arising in the ovaries, when, not infrequently, all peritoneal surfaces become coated with a heavy layer of cancerous glaze. Remarkably the tumor cells may remain confined to the surface of the coated abdominal viscera without penetrating into the substance. Sometimes mucus-secreting ovarian and appendiceal carcinomas fill the peritoneal cavity with a gelatinous neoplastic mass referred to as *pseudomyxoma peritonei.*

Lymphatic Spread. Transport through lymphatics is the most common pathway for the initial dissemination of carcinomas (Fig. 8–16), but sarcomas may also use this route. The emphasis on lymphatic spread for carcinomas and hematogenous spread for sarcomas is misleading because ultimately there are numerous interconnections between the vascular and the lymphatic systems. *The pattern of lymph node involvement follows the natural routes of drainage.* Because carcinomas of the breast usually arise in the upper outer quadrants, they generally disseminate first to the axillary lymph nodes. Cancers of the inner quadrant may drain through lymphatics to the nodes within the chest along the internal mammary arteries. Thereafter the infraclavicular and supraclavicular nodes may become involved. Carcinomas of the lung arising in the major respiratory passages metastasize first to the perihilar tracheobronchial and mediastinal nodes. Local lymph nodes, however, may be bypassed—"skip metastasis"—because of venous-lymphatic

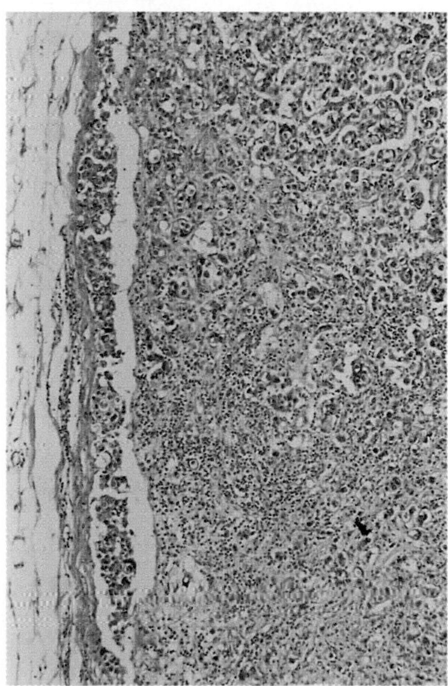

Figure 8–16

Axillary lymph node with metastatic breast carcinoma. The subcapsular sinus *(left)* is distended with tumor cells. Nests of tumor cells have also invaded the subcapsular cortex. (Courtesy of Dr. Trace Worrell, Department of Pathology, University of Texas Southwestern Medical School, Dallas, TX.)

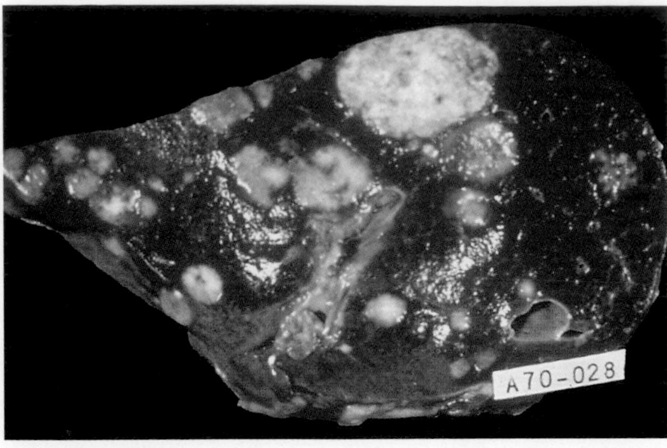

Figure 8–17

A liver studded with metastatic cancer.

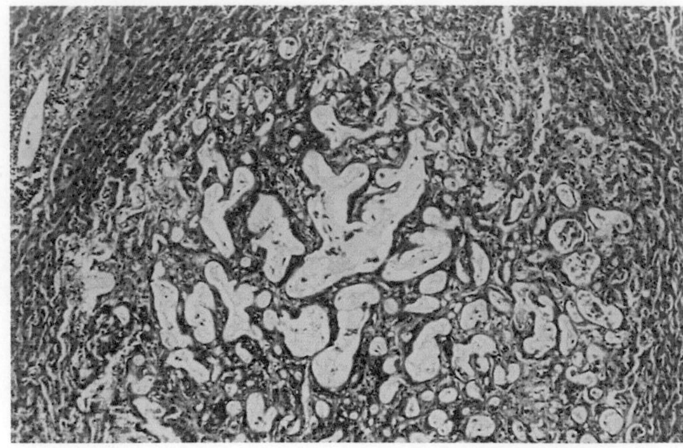

Figure 8–18

Microscopic view of liver metastasis. A pancreatic adenocarcinoma has formed a metastatic nodule in the liver. (Courtesy of Dr. Trace Worrell, Department of Pathology, University of Texas Southwestern Medical School, Dallas, TX.)

anastomoses or because inflammation or radiation has obliterated channels.

In many cases, the regional nodes serve as effective barriers to further dissemination of the tumor, at least for a time. Conceivably the cells, after arrest within the node, may be destroyed. A tumor-specific immune response may participate in this cell destruction. Drainage of tumor cell debris or tumor antigens, or both, also induces reactive changes within nodes. Thus, enlargement of nodes may be caused by (1) the spread and growth of cancer cells or (2) reactive hyperplasia (Chapter 15). Therefore, *nodal enlargement in proximity to a cancer does not necessarily mean dissemination of the primary lesion.*

Hematogenous Spread. Hematogenous spread is typical of sarcomas but is also used by carcinomas. Arteries, with their thicker walls, are less readily penetrated than are veins. Arterial spread, however, may occur when tumor cells pass through the pulmonary capillary beds or pulmonary arteriovenous shunts or when pulmonary metastases themselves give rise to additional tumor emboli. In such arterial spread, a number of factors (to be discussed) condition the patterns of distribution of the metastases. With venous invasion, the blood-borne cells follow the venous flow, draining the site of the neoplasm. Understandably the liver and lungs are most frequently involved secondarily in such hematogenous dissemination (Figs. 8–17 and 8–18). All portal area drainage flows to the liver, and all caval blood flows to the lungs. Cancers arising in close proximity to the vertebral column often embolize through the paravertebral plexus, and this pathway is probably involved in the frequent vertebral metastases of carcinomas of the thyroid and prostate.

Certain cancers have a propensity for invasion of veins. Renal cell carcinoma often invades the branches of the renal vein and then the renal vein itself to grow in a snakelike fashion up the inferior vena cava, sometimes reaching the right side of the heart. Hepatocellular carcinomas often penetrate portal and hepatic radicles to grow within them into the main venous channels. Remarkably, such intravenous growth may not be accompanied by widespread dissemination. Histologic evidence of penetration of small vessels at the site of the primary neoplasm is obviously an ominous feature. Such changes, however, must be

Table 8–2. COMPARISONS BETWEEN BENIGN AND MALIGNANT TUMORS

Characteristics	Benign	Malignant
Differentiation/anaplasia	Well differentiated; structure may be typical of tissue of origin	Some lack of differentiation with anaplasia; structure is often atypical
Rate of growth	Usually progressive and slow; may come to a standstill or regress; mitotic figures are rare and normal	Erratic and may be slow to rapid; mitotic figures may be numerous and abnormal
Local invasion	Usually cohesive and expansile well-demarcated masses that do not invade or infiltrate surrounding normal tissues	Locally invasive, infiltrating the surrounding normal tissues; sometimes may be seemingly cohesive and expansile
Metastasis	Absent	Frequently present; the larger and more undifferentiated the primary, the more likely are metastases

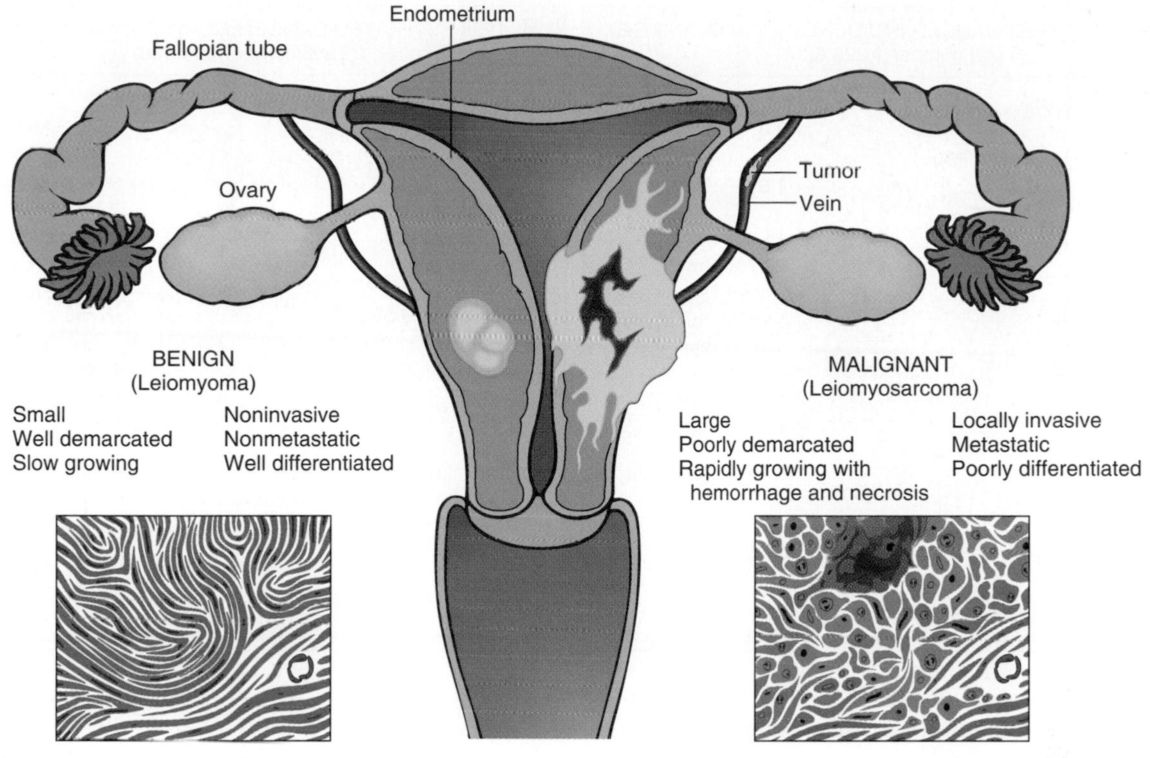

Figure 8–19

Comparison between a benign tumor of the myometrium (leiomyoma) and a malignant tumor of similar origin (leiomyosarcoma).

viewed guardedly because, for reasons discussed later, they do not indicate the inevitable development of metastases.

The differential features discussed in this overview of the specific characteristics of benign and malignant tumors are summarized in Table 8–2 and Figure 8–19. With this background on the structure and behavior of neoplasms, we now discuss the origin of tumors, starting with insights gained from the epidemiology of cancer and followed by the molecular basis of transformation.

EPIDEMIOLOGY

Because cancer is a disorder of cell growth and behavior, its ultimate cause has to be defined at the cellular and subcellular levels. Study of cancer patterns in populations, however, can contribute substantially to knowledge about the origins of cancer. For example, the concept that chemicals can cause cancer arose from the astute observations of Sir Percival Pott, who related the increased incidence of scrotal cancer in chimney sweeps to chronic exposure to soot. Thus, major insights into the cause of cancer can be obtained by epidemiologic studies that relate particular environmental, racial (possibly hereditary), and cultural influences to the occurrence of malignant neoplasms. In addition, certain diseases associated with an increased risk of developing cancer can provide insights into the pathogenesis of malignancy. Therefore, in the following discussion, we first summarize the overall incidence of cancer to provide an insight into the magnitude of the cancer problem, then review a number of factors relating to both the patient and the environment that influence predisposition to cancer.

Cancer Incidence

In some measure, an individual's likelihood of developing a cancer is expressed by national incidence and mortality rates. For example, residents of the United States have about a one in five chance of dying of cancer. There were, it is estimated, about 564,000 deaths from cancer in 1998, representing 23% of all mortality.[1] These data do not include an additional 1 million, for the most part readily curable, nonmelanoma cancers of the skin and 100,000 cases of carcinoma in situ, largely of the uterine cervix but also of the breast. The major organ sites affected and overall frequency are cited in Figure 8–20.

The age-adjusted death rates (number of deaths per 100,000 population) for many forms of cancer have significantly changed over the years (Fig. 8–21). Many of the temporal comparisons are noteworthy. Over the last 50 years, in men, the overall cancer death rate has significantly increased, whereas in women, it has fallen slightly. The increase in men can be largely attributed to lung cancer. The improvement in women is mainly attributable to a

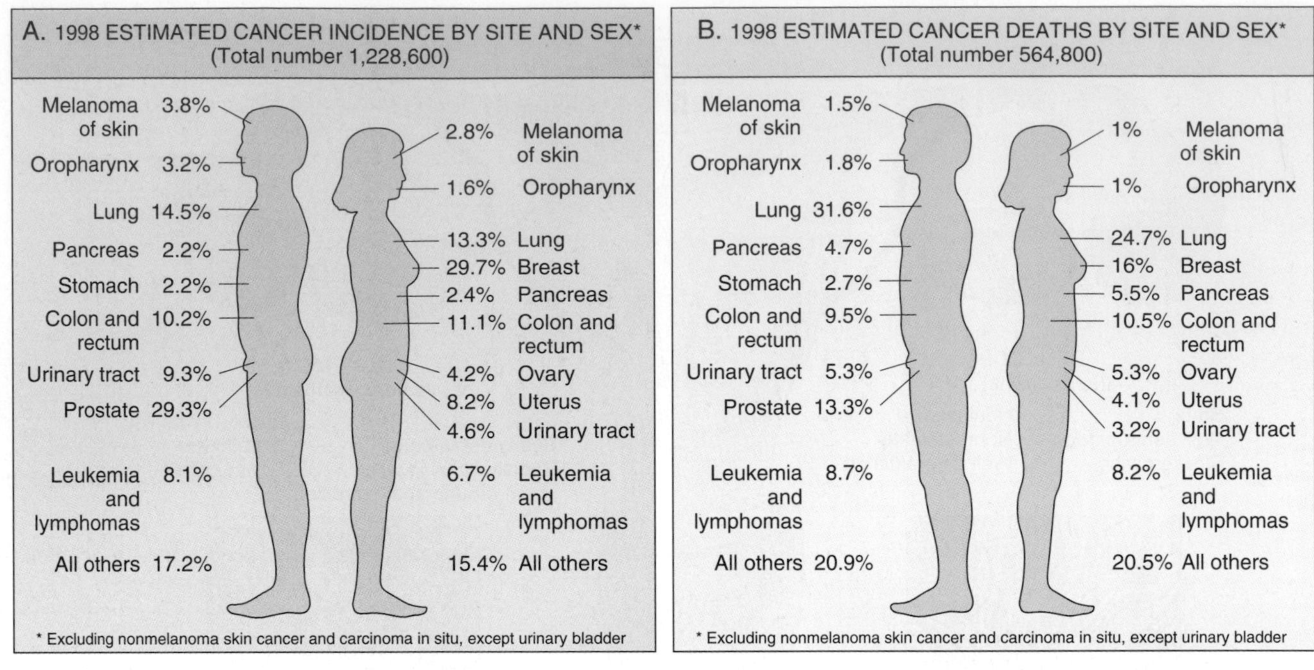

Figure 8–20

Cancer incidence and mortality by site and sex. (Adapted from Landis SH, et al: Cancer statistics. CA 48:6, 1998.)

Figure 8–21

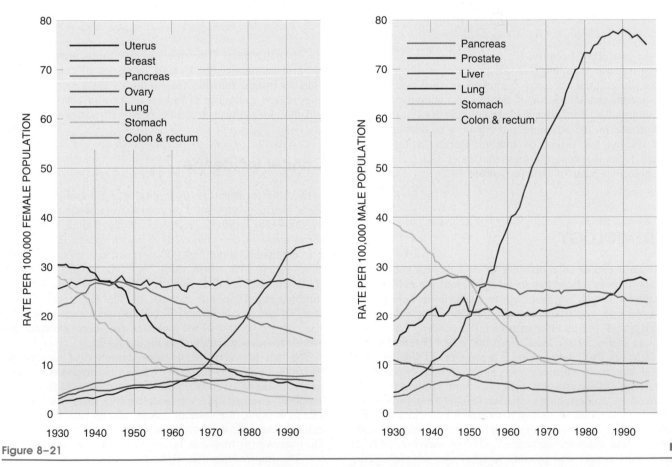

Age-adjusted cancer death rates for selected sites in the United States. (Adapted from Landis SH, et al: Cancer statistics. CA 48:6, 1998.)

significant decline in death rates from cancers of the uterus, stomach, and liver and notably carcinoma of the cervix, one of the frequent forms of malignant neoplasia in women. Striking is the alarming increase in deaths from carcinoma of the lung in both sexes. Although the deaths from lung cancer have begun to decline in men, the curve in women continues to point upward—a consequence of the increasing use of cigarettes by women. In women, carcinomas of the breast are about 2.5 times more frequent than those of the lung. Because of a striking difference in the cure rates of these two cancers, however, bronchogenic carcinoma has become the leading cause of cancer deaths in women. The decline in the number of deaths caused by uterine, including cervical, cancer probably relates to earlier diagnosis and more cures made possible by the Papanicolaou (Pap) smear. Much more mysterious is the downward trend in deaths from stomach and liver carcinomas. This trend may be due to a decrease in some dietary carcinogens.

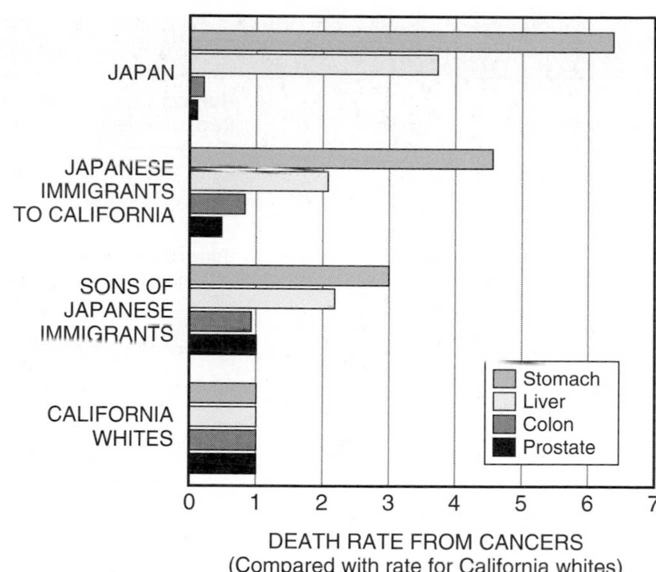

Figure 8–22

The change in incidence of various cancers with migration from Japan to the United States provides evidence that the occurrence of cancers is related to components of the environment that differ in the two countries. The incidence of each kind of cancer is expressed as the ratio of the death rate in the population being considered to that in a hypothetical population of California whites with the same age distribution; the death rates for whites are thus defined as 1. The death rates among immigrants and immigrants' sons tend consistently toward California norms. (From Cairns J: The cancer problem. In Readings from Scientific American—Cancer Biology. New York, WH Freeman, 1986, p 13. © 1975 by Scientific American, Inc. All rights reserved.)

Geographic and Environmental Factors

Remarkable differences can be found in the incidence and death rates of specific forms of cancer around the world. For example, the death rate for stomach carcinoma in both men and women is seven to eight times higher in Japan than in the United States. In contrast, the death rate from carcinoma of the lung is slightly more than twice as great in the United States as in Japan, and in Belgium it is even higher than in the United States. Skin cancer deaths, largely caused by melanomas, are six times more frequent in New Zealand than in Iceland, which is probably attributable to differences in sun exposure. Although racial predispositions cannot be ruled out, it is generally believed that most of these geographic differences are the consequence of environmental influences. This is best brought out by comparing mortality rates for Japanese immigrants to the United States and Japanese born in the United States of immigrant parents (Nisei) with those of long-term residents of both countries. Figure 8–22 indicates that cancer mortality rates for first-generation Japanese immigrants are intermediate between those of natives of Japan and natives of California, and the two rates come closer with each passing generation. This points strongly to environmental and cultural factors rather than genetic predisposition. There is no paucity of environmental factors: They are found in the ambient environment, in the workplace, in food, and in personal practices.

The carcinogenicity of ultraviolet (UV) rays and many drugs is discussed in a later section. Asbestos, vinyl chloride, and 2-naphthylamine can serve as examples of occupational hazards, and many others are listed in Table 8–3; the risks may be incurred in lifestyle and personal exposures (e.g., dietary influences). Overall, mortality data indicate that persons more than 25% overweight have a higher death rate from cancer than do their slimmer counterparts. Alcohol abuse alone increases the risk of carcinomas of the oropharynx (excluding lip), larynx, and esophagus and, through the intermediation of alcoholic cirrhosis, carcinoma of the liver. Smoking, particularly of cigarettes, has been implicated in cancer of the mouth, pharynx, larynx, esophagus, pancreas, and bladder but most significantly is responsible for about 77% of lung cancer among men and 43% among women (Chapter 10). Cigarette smoking has been called the single most important environmental factor contributing to premature death in the United States. Alcohol and tobacco together multiply the danger of incurring cancers in the upper aerodigestive tract. The risk of cervical cancer is linked to age at first intercourse and the number of sex partners. These associations point to a possible causal role for venereal transmission of cervical viral infections. It begins to appear that everything one does to gain a livelihood or for pleasure is fattening, immoral, illegal, or, even worse, oncogenic.

Age

Age is an important influence on the likelihood of being afflicted with cancer. Most carcinomas occur in the later years of life (≥55 years). Each age group has its own predilection to certain forms of cancer, as is evident in Tables 8–4 and 8–5. Here the striking increase in mortality from cancer in the age group 55 to 74 years should be noted. The decline in deaths in the 75-year-and-over group

Table 8–3. OCCUPATIONAL CANCERS

Agents or Groups of Agents	Human Cancer Site for Which Reasonable Evidence Is Available	Typical Use or Occurrence
Arsenic and arsenic compounds	Lung, skin, hemangiosarcoma	Byproduct of metal smelting. Component of alloys, electrical and semiconductor devices, medications and herbicides, fungicides, and animal dips
Asbestos	Lung, mesothelioma; gastrointestinal tract (esophagus, stomach, large intestine)	Formerly used for many applications because of fire, heat, and friction resistance; still found in existing construction as well as fire-resistant textiles, friction materials (i.e., brake linings), underlayment and roofing papers, and floor tiles
Benzene	Leukemia, Hodgkin disease	Principal component of light oil. Although use as solvent is discouraged, many applications exist in printing and lithography, paint, rubber, dry cleaning, adhesives and coatings, and detergents. Formerly widely used as solvent and fumigant
Beryllium and beryllium compounds	Lung	Missile fuel and space vehicles. Hardener for lightweight metal alloys, particularly in aerospace applications and nuclear reactors
Cadmium and cadmium compounds	Prostate	Uses include yellow pigments and phosphors. Found in solders. Used in batteries and as alloy and in metal platings and coatings
Chromium compounds	Lung	Component of metal alloys, paints, pigments, and preservatives
Ethylene oxide	Leukemia	Ripening agent for fruits and nuts. Used in rocket propellant and chemical synthesis, in fumigants for foodstuffs and textiles, and in sterilants for hospital equipment
Nickel compounds	Nose, lung	Nickel plating. Component of ferrous alloys, ceramics, and batteries. Byproduct of stainless steel arc welding
Radon and its decay products	Lung	From decay of minerals containing uranium. Can be serious hazard in quarries and underground mines
Vinyl chloride	Angiosarcoma, liver	Refrigerant. Monomer for vinyl polymers. Adhesive for plastics. Formerly inert aerosol propellant in pressurized containers

Modified from Stellman JM, Stellman SD: Cancer and workplace CA 46:70, 1996.

Table 8–4. REPORTED DEATHS FOR THE FIVE LEADING CANCER SITES FOR MALES BY AGE, UNITED STATES, 1994

All Ages	Under 15 yr	15–34 yr	35–54 yr	55–74 yr	75+ yr
All sites* 280,465	All sites 919	All sites 3570	All sites 29,296	All sites 140,843	All sites 105,826
Lung and bronchus 91,825	Leukemia 299	Leukemia 728	Lung and bronchus 8684	Lung and bronchus 54,381	Lung and bronchus 28,597
Prostate 34,902	Brain and ONS 254	Non-Hodgkin lymphoma 471	Colon and rectum 2703	Colon and rectum 13,574	Prostate 22,712
Colon and rectum 28,471	Endocrine system 111	Brain and ONS 452	Non-Hodgkin lymphoma 1828	Prostate 11,789	Colon and rectum 11,972
Pancreas 12,920	Non-Hodgkin lymphoma 61	Colon and rectum 221	Brain and ONS 1655	Pancreas 6896	Pancreas 4557
Non-Hodgkin lymphoma 11,280	Soft tissue 49	Soft tissue 204	Pancreas 1431	Non-Hodgkin lymphoma 5002	Leukemia 4207

* *All sites* excludes basal and squamous cell skin cancers and in situ carcinomas except urinary bladder.
ONS, other nervous system.
Data source: Vital Statistics of the United States, 1997.

Table 8–5. REPORTED DEATHS FOR THE FIVE LEADING CANCER SITES FOR FEMALES BY AGE, UNITED STATES, 1994

All Ages	Under 15 yr	15–34 yr	35–54 yr	55–74 yr	75+ yr
All sites* 253,845	All sites 711	All sites 3226	All sites 31,135	All sites 112,203	All sites 106,565
Lung and bronchus 57,535	Leukemia 251	Breast 564	Breast 9548	Lung and bronchus 32,098	Lung and bronchus 19,793
Breast 43,644	Brain and ONS 193	Leukemia 394	Lung and bronchus 5516	Breast 18,705	Colon and rectum 16,074
Colon and rectum 28,936	Endocrine system 87	Cervix (uterus) 322	Colon and rectum 2115	Colon and rectum 10,596	Breast 14,827
Pancreas 13,914	Bones and joints 39	Brain and ONS 307	Ovary 1892	Ovary 6457	Pancreas 7150
Ovary 13,500	Soft tissue 36	Non-Hodgkin lymphoma 231	Cervix (uterus) 1676	Pancreas 5863	Non-Hodgkin lymphoma 5086

* *All sites* excludes basal and squamous cell skin cancers and in situ carcinomas except urinary bladder.
ONS, other nervous system.
Data source: Vital Statistics of the United States, 1997.

merely reflects the dwindling population reaching this age. Also to be noted is that children under the age of 15 are not spared. Cancer accounts for slightly more than 10% of all deaths in this group in the United States and is second only to accidents. Acute leukemia and neoplasms of the central nervous system are responsible for approximately 60% of these deaths. The common neoplasms of infancy and childhood include neuroblastoma, Wilms tumor, retinoblastoma, acute leukemias, and rhabdomyosarcomas. These are discussed in Chapter 11 and elsewhere in the text.

Heredity

One frequently asked question is: "My mother and father both died of cancer. Does that mean I am doomed to get it?" Based on current knowledge, the answer must be carefully qualified.[3] The evidence now indicates that for a large number of types of cancer, including the most common forms, there exist not only environmental influences, but also hereditary predispositions. For example, lung cancer is in most instances clearly related to cigarette smoking, yet mortality from lung cancer has been shown to be four times greater among nonsmoking relatives (parents and siblings) of lung cancer patients than among nonsmoking relatives of controls. Hereditary forms of cancers can be divided into three categories (Table 8–6).

Inherited Cancer Syndromes. Inherited cancer syndromes include several well-defined cancers in which inheritance of a single mutant gene greatly increases the risk of developing a tumor. The predisposition to these tumors shows an autosomal dominant pattern of inheritance. Childhood retinoblastoma is the most striking example in this category. Approximately 40% of retinoblastomas are familial. Carriers of this gene have a 10,000-fold increased risk of developing retinoblastoma, usually bilateral. They also have a greatly increased risk of developing a second cancer, particularly osteogenic sarcoma. As is discussed later, a *cancer-suppressor* gene has been implicated in the pathogenesis of this tumor. Familial adenomatous polyposis (FAP) is another hereditary disorder marked by an extraordinarily high risk of cancer. Individuals who inherit the autosomal dominant mutation have at birth, or soon thereafter, innumerable polypoid adenomas of the colon and in virtually 100% of cases are fated to develop a carcinoma of the colon by age 50.

There are several features that characterize inherited cancer syndromes:

- In each syndrome, tumors involve specific sites and tis-

Table 8–6. INHERITED PREDISPOSITION TO CANCER

Inherited Cancer Syndromes (Autosomal Dominant)
Inherited predisposition indicated by strong family history of uncommon cancer and/or associated marker phenotype
- Familial retinoblastoma
- Familial adenomatous polyps of the colon
- Multiple endocrine neoplasia syndromes
- Neurofibromatosis types 1 and 2
- Von Hippel–Lindau syndrome

Familial Cancers
Evident familial clustering of cancer but role of inherited predisposition may not be clear in an individual case
- Breast cancer
- Ovarian cancer
- Colon cancers other than familial adenomatous polyps

Autosomal Recessive Syndromes of Defective DNA Repair
- Xeroderma pigmentosum
- Ataxia-telangiectasia
- Bloom syndrome
- Fanconi anemia

Modified from Ponder BAJ: Inherited predisposition to cancer. Trends Genet 6:213, 1990.

sues. For example, in the multiple endocrine neoplasia (MEN) syndrome type 2, thyroid, parathyroid, and adrenals are involved. There is no increase in predisposition to cancers in general.

- Tumors within this group are often associated with a specific marker phenotype. For example, there may be multiple benign tumors in the affected tissue, as occurs in familial polyposis of the colon and in MEN. Sometimes, there are abnormalities in tissue that are not the target of transformation (e.g., Lisch nodules and café-au-lait spots in neurofibromatosis type 1; Chapter 6).
- As in other autosomal dominant conditions, both incomplete penetrance and variable expressivity are noted.

Familial Cancers. Virtually all the common types of cancers that occur sporadically have also been reported to occur in familial forms. Examples include carcinomas of colon, breast, ovary, and brain. Features that characterize familial cancers include early age at onset, tumors arising in two or more close relatives of the index case, and sometimes multiple or bilateral tumors. Familial cancers are not associated with specific marker phenotypes. For example, in contrast to the familial adenomatous polyp syndrome, familial colonic cancers do not arise in preexisting benign polyps. The transmission pattern of familial cancers is not clear. In general, sibs have a relative risk between 2 and 3. Segregation analyses of large families usually reveals that predisposition to the tumors is dominant, but multifactorial inheritance cannot be easily ruled out. As discussed later, certain familial cancers can be linked to the inheritance of mutant genes. Examples include linkage of BRCA-1 and BRCA-2 genes to familial breast and ovarian cancers.

Autosomal Recessive Syndromes of Defective DNA Repair. Besides the dominantly inherited precancerous conditions, a small group of autosomal recessive disorders is collectively characterized by chromosomal or DNA instability. One of the best studied examples is xeroderma pigmentosum, in which DNA repair is defective. This and other familial disorders of DNA instability are described in a later section.

It is impossible to estimate the contribution of heredity to the fatal burden of human cancer. The best "guesstimates," however, suggest that no more than 5 to 10% of all human cancers are included in the three categories just listed. What can be said about the influence of heredity on the large preponderance of malignant neoplasms? It could be argued that they are entirely or largely of environmental origin. There is increasing realization, however, that lack of family history does not preclude a genetic hereditary component. For example, if a dominant cancer-susceptibility gene has low penetrance, familial cases are uncommon. Furthermore, the genotype can significantly influence the likelihood of developing environmentally induced cancers. It is likely that inherited variations (polymorphisms) of enzymes that metabolize procarcinogens to their active carcinogenic forms (see Initiation of Carcinogenesis) may well influence the susceptibility to cancer. Of interest in this regard are genes that encode the cytochrome P-450 enzymes. As discussed later under Chemical Carcinogenesis, polymorphism at one of the P-450 loci confers inherited susceptibility to lung cancers in cigarette smokers. More such correlations are likely to be found, and it is suspected that genetic predisposition contributes to many, if not most, spontaneous tumors of humans.

Acquired Preneoplastic Disorders

The only certain way of avoiding cancer is not to be born; to live is to incur the risk. The risk is greater than average, however, under many circumstances, as is evident from the predisposing influences discussed earlier. Certain clinical conditions are also important. Because cell replication is involved in cancerous transformation, regenerative, hyperplastic, and dysplastic proliferations are fertile soil for the origin of a malignant neoplasm. There is a well-defined association between certain forms of endometrial hyperplasia and endometrial carcinoma and between cervical dysplasia and cervical carcinoma (Chapter 24). The bronchial mucosal metaplasia and dysplasia of habitual cigarette smokers are ominous antecedents of bronchogenic carcinoma. About 80% of hepatocellular carcinomas arise in cirrhotic livers, which are characterized by active parenchymal regeneration (Chapter 19). Other examples could be offered, but although these settings constitute important predispositions, in the great majority of instances they are not complicated by neoplasia.

Certain non-neoplastic disorders—*the chronic atrophic gastritis of pernicious anemia; solar keratosis of the skin; chronic ulcerative colitis; and leukoplakia of the oral cavity, vulva, and penis*—have such a well-defined association with cancer that they have been termed *precancerous conditions*. This designation is somewhat unfortunate because in the great majority of instances no malignant neoplasm emerges. Nonetheless, the term persists because it calls attention to the increased risk. Analogously, certain forms of benign neoplasia also constitute precancerous conditions. The villous adenoma of the colon, as it increases in size, develops cancerous change in up to 50% of cases. It might be asked: Is there not a risk with all benign neoplasms? Although some risk may be inherent, a large cumulative experience indicates that *most benign neoplasms do not become cancerous*. Nonetheless, numerous examples could be offered of cancers arising, albeit rarely, in benign tumors: for example, a leiomyosarcoma beginning in a leiomyoma, and carcinoma appearing in long-standing pleomorphic adenomas. Generalization is impossible because each type of benign neoplasm is associated with a particular level of risk ranging from virtually never to frequently. Only follow-up studies of large series of each neoplasm can establish the level of risk, and always the question remains: Was the tumor an indolent form of cancer from the outset, or was there a malignant focus in the benign tumor?

MOLECULAR BASIS OF CANCER

It could be justifiably argued that the proliferation of literature on the molecular basis of cancer has outpaced the growth of even the most malignant of tumors! Understandably, therefore, it is easy to get lost in the growing forest of information. We list some fundamental principles before delving into the details of the genetic basis of cancer.

- *Nonlethal genetic damage lies at the heart of carcinogenesis.* Such genetic damage (or mutation) may be acquired by the action of environmental agents, such as chemicals, radiation, or viruses, or it may be inherited in the germ line. The genetic hypothesis of cancer implies that a tumor mass results from the clonal expansion of a single progenitor cell that has incurred the genetic damage (i.e., tumors are monoclonal). This expectation has been realized in most tumors that have been analyzed. Clonality of tumors is assessed quite readily in women who are heterozygous for polymorphic X-linked markers, such as the enzyme glucose-6-phosphate dehydrogenase (G6PD) or X-linked restriction fragment length polymorphisms. The principle underlying such an analysis is illustrated in Figure 8–23.
- *Three classes of normal regulatory genes—the growth-promoting protooncogenes, the growth-inhibiting cancer-suppressor genes (antioncogenes), and genes that regulate programmed cell death, or apoptosis—are the principal targets of genetic damage.* Mutant alleles of protooncogenes are considered dominant because they transform cells despite the presence of their normal counterpart. In contrast, both normal alleles of the tumor-suppressor genes must be damaged for transformation to occur, so this family of genes is sometimes referred to as *recessive oncogenes.* Genes that regulate apoptosis may be dominant, as are protooncogenes, or they may behave as cancer-suppressor genes.
- In addition to the three classes of genes mentioned earlier, a fourth category of genes, those that regulate repair of damaged DNA, is also pertinent in carcinogenesis. *The DNA repair genes affect cell proliferation or survival indirectly by influencing the ability of the organism to repair nonlethal damage in other genes, including protooncogenes, tumor-suppressor genes, and genes that regulate apoptosis.* A disability in the DNA repair genes can predispose to mutations in the genome and hence to neoplastic transformation. Both alleles of DNA repair genes must be inactivated to induce such genomic instability; in this sense, DNA repair genes may also be considered as tumor-suppressor genes.
- *Carcinogenesis is a multistep process at both the phenotypic and the genetic levels.* A malignant neoplasm has several phenotypic attributes, such as excessive growth, local invasiveness, and the ability to form distant metastases. These characteristics are acquired in a stepwise fashion, a phenomenon called *tumor progression.* At the molecular level, progression results from accumulation of genetic lesions that in some instances are favored by defects in DNA repair.

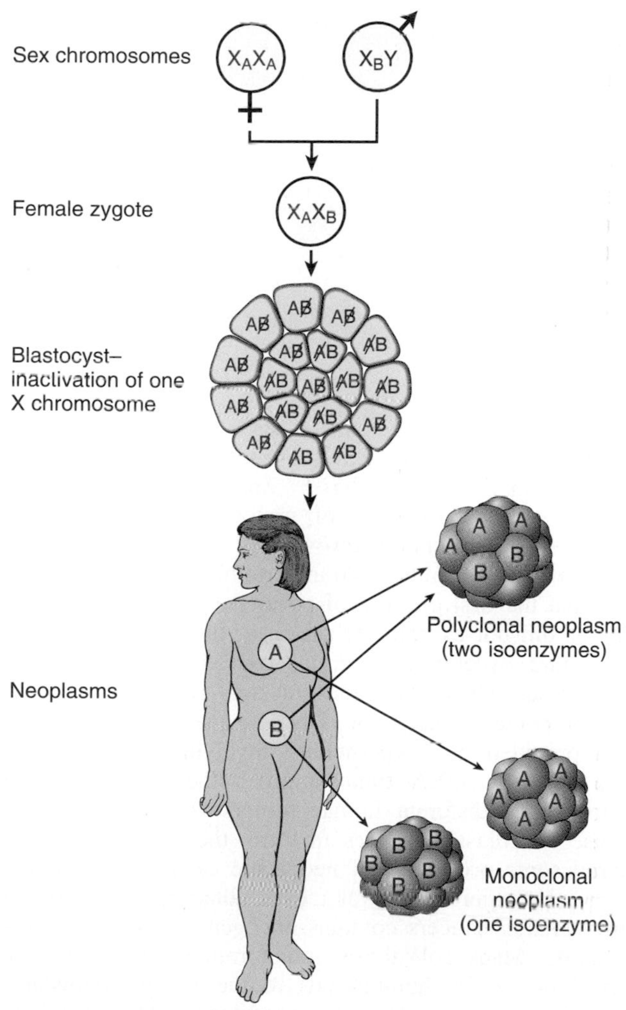

Figure 8–23

Diagram depicting the use of X-linked isoenzyme cell markers as evidence of the monoclonality of neoplasms. Because of random X inactivation, all females are mosaics with two cell populations (with G6PD isoenzyme A or B in this case). When neoplasms that arise in women who are heterozygous for X-linked markers are analyzed, they are made up of cells that contain the active maternal (X_A) or the paternal (X_B) X chromosome but not both.

With this overview (Fig. 8–24), we now address in some detail the molecular pathogenesis of cancer then discuss the carcinogenic agents that inflict genetic damage.

Oncogenes and Cancer

Oncogenes, or cancer-causing genes, are derived from *protooncogenes*, cellular genes that promote normal growth and differentiation. As often happens in science, the discovery of protooncogenes was not straightforward. These cellular genes were first discovered as "passengers" within the genome of *acute transforming retroviruses*, by the Nobel Laureates Varmus and Bishop. These retroviruses cause rapid induction of tumors in animals and can also transform animal cells in vitro. Molecular dissection of their genomes revealed the presence of unique transforming sequences (viral oncogenes [v-*oncs*]) not found in the genomes of nontransforming retroviruses. Most surprisingly, molecular hybridization revealed that the v-*onc* sequences were almost identical to sequences found in the normal

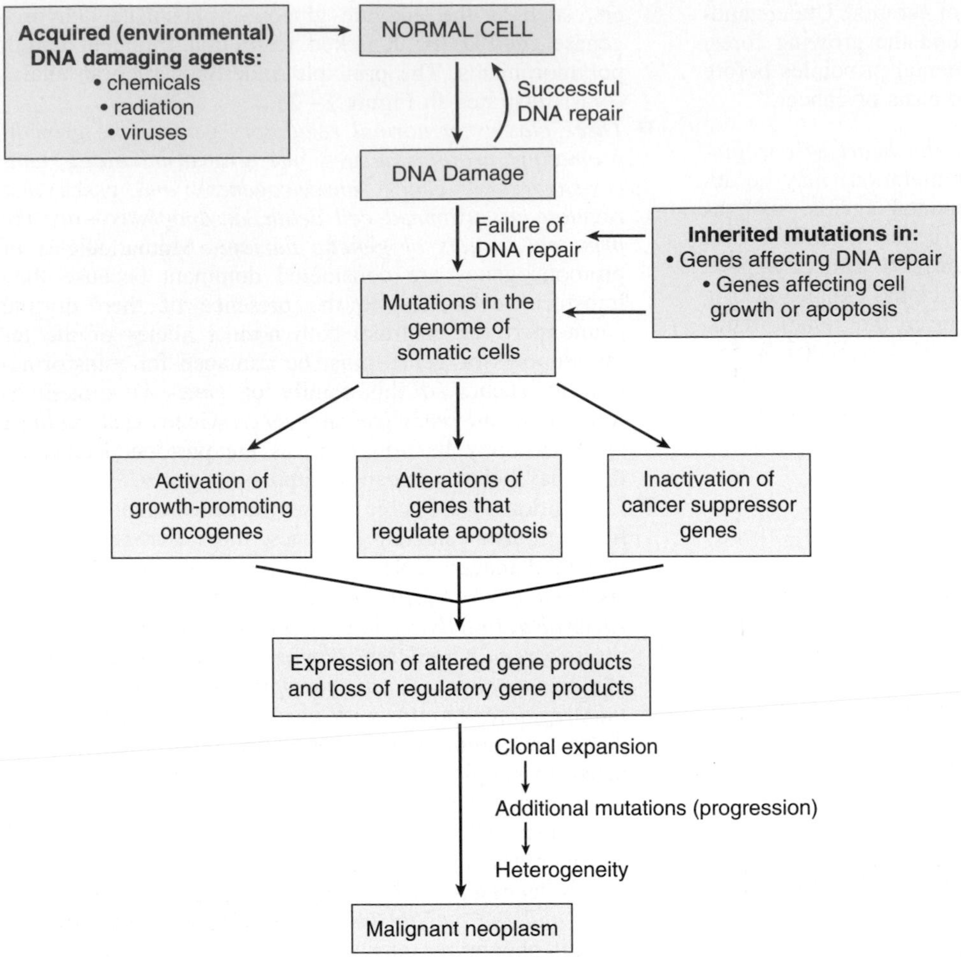

Figure 8–24

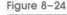

Flow chart depicting a simplified scheme of the molecular basis of cancer.

cellular DNA. From this evolved the concept that during evolution, retroviral oncogenes were *transduced* (captured) by the virus through a chance recombination with the DNA of a (normal) host cell that had been infected by the virus. Because they were discovered initially as *viral genes*, protooncogenes are named after their viral homologs. Each v-*onc* is designated by a three-letter word that relates the oncogene to the virus from which it was isolated. Thus, the v-*onc* contained in *fe*line *s*arcoma virus is referred to as v-*fes*, whereas the oncogene in *si*mian *s*arcoma virus is called v-*sis*. The corresponding protooncogenes are referred to as *fes* and *sis* by dropping the prefix.

v-*oncs* are not present in several cancer-causing RNA viruses. One such example is a group of so-called slow transforming viruses that cause leukemias in rodents after a long latent period. The mechanism by which they cause neoplastic transformation implicates protooncogenes. Molecular dissection of the cells transformed by these leukemia viruses has revealed that the proviral DNA is always found to be integrated (inserted) near a protooncogene. One consequence of proviral insertion near a protooncogene is to induce a structural change in the cellular gene, thus converting it into a cellular oncogene (c-*onc*). Alternatively, strong retroviral promoters inserted in the vicinity of the protooncogenes lead to dysregulated expression of the cellular gene. This mode of protooncogene activation is called *insertional mutagenesis*.

Although the study of transforming animal retroviruses provided the first glimpse of protooncogenes, these investigations did not explain the origin of human tumors, which (with rare exceptions) are not caused by infection with retroviruses. Hence the question was raised: Do nonviral tumors contain oncogenic DNA sequences? The answer was provided by experiments involving DNA-mediated gene transfer (DNA transfection). When DNA extracted from several different human tumors was transfected into mouse fibroblast cell lines in vitro, the recipient cells acquired some properties of neoplastic cells. The conclusion from such experiments was inescapable: DNA of spontaneously arising cancers contains oncogenic sequences, or oncogenes. Many of these transforming sequences have turned out to be homologous to the *ras* protooncogenes that are the forbears of v-*oncs* contained in Harvey (H) and Kirsten (K) sarcoma viruses. Others, such as the c-*erb B2* oncogene, represent novel transforming sequences that have never been detected in retroviruses. *To summarize, protooncogenes may become oncogenic by retroviral transduction (v-oncs) or by influences that alter their behavior in situ, thereby converting them into cellular oncogenes (c-oncs).* Two questions follow: (1) What are the functions of oncogene products? (2) How do the normally "civilized" protooncogenes turn into "enemies within"? These issues are discussed next.

PROTEIN PRODUCTS OF ONCOGENES

Oncogenes encode proteins called *oncoproteins*, which resemble the normal products of protooncogenes, with the exception that (1) oncoproteins are devoid of important regulatory elements, and (2) their production in the transformed cells does not depend on growth factors or other external signals. To aid in the understanding of the nature and functions of oncoproteins, it is necessary to review briefly the sequence of events that characterize normal cell proliferation. (These are discussed in more detail in Chapter 4.) Under physiologic conditions, cell proliferation can be readily resolved into the following steps:

- The binding of a growth factor to its specific receptor on the cell membrane
- Transient and limited activation of the growth factor receptor, which, in turn, activates several signal-transducing proteins on the inner leaflet of the plasma membrane
- Transmission of the transduced signal across the cytosol to the nucleus via second messengers
- Induction and activation of nuclear regulatory factors that initiate DNA transcription
- Entry and progression of the cell into the cell cycle, resulting ultimately in cell division

With this background, we can readily identify oncogenes and oncoproteins as altered versions of their normal counterparts and group them on the basis of their role in the signal transduction cascade and cell cycle regulation (Table 8–7).[4, 5]

Growth Factors. A number of polypeptide growth factors that stimulate proliferation of normal cells have been described (Chapter 4), and many are suspected to play a role in tumorigenesis.[6] Mutations of genes that encode growth factors can render them oncogenic. Such is the case with the protooncogene c-*sis*, which encodes the β chain of platelet-derived growth factor (PDGF). This oncogene was first discovered in the guise of the viral oncogene contained in v-*sis*. Subsequently, several human tumors, especially astrocytomas and osteosarcomas, have been found to produce PDGF. Furthermore, it appears that the same tumors also express receptors for PDGF and are hence subject to autocrine stimulation. Although an autocrine loop is considered to be an important element in the pathogenesis of several tumors, in most instances the growth factor gene itself is not altered or mutated. More commonly, products

Table 8–7. SELECTED ONCOGENES, THEIR MODE OF ACTIVATION, AND ASSOCIATED HUMAN TUMORS

Category	Protooncogene	Mechanism	Associated Human Tumor
Growth Factors			
PDGF-B chain	*sis*	Overexpression	Astrocytoma Osteosarcoma
Fibroblast growth factors	*hst*-1	Overexpression	Stomach cancer
	int-2	Amplification	Bladder cancer Breast cancer Melanoma
Growth Factor Receptors			
EGF-receptor family	*erb*-B1	Overexpression	Squamous cell carcinomas of lung
	erb-B2	Amplification	Breast, ovarian, lung, and stomach cancers
	erb-B3	Overexpression	Breast cancers
CSF-1 receptor	*fms*	Point mutation	Leukemia
	*ret**	Point mutation	Multiple endocrine neoplasia 2A and B. Familial medullary thyroid carcinoma
		Rearrangement	Sporadic papillary carcinomas of thyroid
Proteins Involved in Signal Transduction			
GTP-binding	*ras*	Point mutations	A variety of human cancers, including lung, colon, pancreas; many leukemias
Nonreceptor tyrosine kinase	*abl*	Translocation	Chronic myeloid leukemia Acute lymphoblastic leukemia
Nuclear Regulatory Proteins			
Transcriptional activators	*myc*	Translocation	Burkitt lymphoma
	N-*myc*	Amplification	Neuroblastoma Small cell carcinoma of lung
	L-*myc*	Amplification	Small cell carcinoma of lung
Cell Cycle Regulators			
Cyclins	cyclin D	Translocation	Mantle cell lymphoma
		Amplification	Breast, liver, esophageal cancers
Cyclin-dependent kinase	CDK4	Amplification or point mutation	Glioblastoma, melanoma, sarcoma

PDGF, platelet-derived growth factor; EGF, epidermal growth factor; CSF, colony-stimulating factor; GTP, guanosine triphosphate.
**ret* protooncogene is a receptor for glial cell line-derived neurotrophic factor.

of other oncogenes such as *ras* (that lie along the signal transduction pathway) cause overexpression of growth factor genes, thus forcing the cells to secrete large amounts of growth factors, such as transforming growth factor-α (TGF-α). This growth factor is related to epidermal growth factor (EGF) and induces proliferation by binding to the EGF receptor. TGF-α is often detected in carcinomas that express high levels of EGF receptors.

In addition to c-*sis,* a group of related oncogenes that encode homologs of fibroblast growth factors (FGFs) (e.g., *hst*-1 and *int*-2) is activated in several gastrointestinal and breast tumors; bFGF, a member of the fibroblast growth factor family, is expressed in human melanomas but not in normal melanocytes. Small cell lung carcinomas produce bombesin-like peptides that stimulate their proliferation.

Despite extensive documentation of growth factor–mediated autocrine stimulation of transformed cells, increased growth factor production is not sufficient for neoplastic transformation. Extensive cell proliferation, in all likelihood, contributes to the malignant phenotype by increasing the risk of spontaneous or induced mutations in the cell population.

Growth Factor Receptors. The next group in the sequence of signal transduction involves growth factor receptors, and, not surprisingly, several oncogenes that encode growth factor receptors have been found. To understand how mutations affect the function of these receptors, it should be recalled that several growth factor receptors are transmembrane proteins with an external ligand-binding and a cytoplasmic tyrosine kinase domain (Chapter 4). In the normal forms of these receptor tyrosine kinases, the kinase activity is *transiently* activated by binding of their specific growth factors, followed rapidly by receptor dimerization and tyrosine phosphorylation of several substrates that are a part of the mitotic cascade. *The oncogenic versions of these receptors are associated with persistent dimerization and activation without binding to the growth factor.* Hence the mutant receptors deliver continuous mitogenic signals to the cell.

Growth factor receptors are activated in human tumors by several mechanisms. These include mutations, gene rearrangements, and overexpression. The *ret* protooncogene, a receptor tyrosine kinase, exemplifies oncogenic conversion via mutations and gene rearrangements.[7] The *ret* protein is a receptor for the glial cell line–derived neurotrophic factor that is normally expressed in neuroendocrine cells, such as parafollicular C cells of the thyroid, adrenal medulla, and parathyroid cell precursors. Point mutations in the *ret* protooncogene are associated with dominantly inherited MEN types 2A and 2B and familial medullary thyroid carcinoma (Chapter 26). In MEN 2A, point mutations in the extracellular domain cause constitutive dimerization and activation, whereas in MEN 2B, point mutations in the cytoplasmic catalytic domain activate the receptor. In all these familial tumors, the affected individuals inherit the *ret* mutation in the germ line. By contrast, sporadic papillary carcinomas of the thyroid are associated with somatic rearrangements of the *ret* gene. In these tumors, the tyrosine kinase domain of the *ret* gene is juxtaposed with one of four different partner genes. The fused genes encode hybrid proteins in which the tyrosine kinase domain is constitutively activated, and hence the cell is led to believe that the *ret* receptor is being continuously activated by its ligand. Oncogenic conversions by mutations and rearrangements have also been noted with other growth factor receptor genes. In myeloid leukemias, point mutations that activate c-*fms*, the gene encoding the colony-stimulating factor 1 (CSF-1) receptor, have been detected. In certain chronic myelomonocytic leukemias with the t(12;9) translocation, the entire cytoplasmic domain of the PDGF receptor is fused with a segment of the ETS family transcription factor, resulting in permanent dimerization of the PDGF receptor.

Far more common than mutations of these protooncogenes is overexpression of the normal forms of growth factor receptors. Three members of the EGF receptor family are the ones most commonly involved.[8] The normal form of c-*erb B1*, the EGF receptor gene, is overexpressed in up to 80% of squamous cell carcinomas of the lung and, less commonly, in carcinomas of the urinary bladder, gastrointestinal tract, and astrocytomas. In some cases, increased receptor expression results from gene amplification. In most others, the molecular basis of increased receptor expression is not fully known. In contrast, the c-*erb B2* gene (also called c-*neu*), the second member of the EGF receptor family, is amplified in a high percentage of human adenocarcinomas arising within the breast, ovary, lung, stomach, and salivary glands. A third member of the EGF receptor family, c-*erb B3*, is also overexpressed in breast cancers. It might be suspected that tumors that overexpress the growth factor receptors, such as c-*erb B2*, would be exquisitely sensitive to the growth-promoting effects of a small amount of growth factors and hence likely to be more aggressive. This hypothesis is supported by the observation that high levels of c-*erb B2* protein on breast cancer cells are a harbinger of poor prognosis.

Signal-Transducing Proteins. Several examples of oncoproteins that mimic the function of normal cytoplasmic signal-transducing proteins have been found. Most such proteins are strategically located on the inner leaflet of the plasma membrane, where they receive signals from outside the cell (e.g., by activation of growth factor receptors) and transmit them to the cell's nucleus. Biochemically the signal-transducing proteins are heterogeneous. The best and most well studied example of a signal transducing oncoprotein is the *ras* family of guanine triphosphate (GTP)–binding proteins. This is discussed next.

The *ras* proteins were discovered initially in the form of viral oncogenes. Approximately 10 to 20% of all human tumors contain mutated versions of *ras* proteins.[9] In some tumors (e.g., carcinomas of the colon, pancreas, and thyroid), the incidence of *ras* mutation is even higher. *Mutation of the* ras *gene is the single most common abnormality of dominant oncogenes in human tumors.* Several studies indicate that *ras* plays an important role in mitogenesis induced by growth factors. For example, blockade of *ras* function by microinjection of specific antibodies blocks the proliferative response to EGF, PDGF, and CSF-1. Normal *ras* proteins are tethered to the cytoplasmic aspect of plasma membrane, and they flip back and forth between an activated, signal-transmitting form and an inactive, quiescent state. In the inactive state, *ras* proteins bind guanosine diphosphate (GDP); when cells are stimulated by growth factors or other receptor-ligand interactions, *ras* becomes activated by exchanging GDP for GTP (Fig. 8–25). The activated *ras*, in turn, excites the MAP kinase pathway by recruiting the cytosolic protein raf-1. The MAP kinases so activated target nuclear transcription factors and thus promote mitogenesis. In normal cells, the activated signal-transmitting stage of *ras* protein is transient because its intrinsic GTPase activity hydrolyzes GTP to GDP, thereby returning *ras* to its quiescent ground state.

The orderly cycling of the *ras* protein depends on two reactions: (1) nucleotide exchange (GDP by GTP), which activates *ras* protein, and (2) GTP hydrolysis, which converts the GTP-bound, active *ras* to the GDP-bound, inactive form.[10, 11] Both these processes are enzymatically regulated. The removal of GDP and its replacement by GTP during *ras* activation is catalyzed by a family of guanine nucleotide releasing proteins that are recruited to the cytosolic aspect of activated growth factor receptors by adapter proteins. Much more importantly, the GTPase activity intrinsic to normal *ras* proteins is dramatically accelerated by GTPase-activating proteins (GAPs). These widely distributed proteins bind to the active *ras* and augment its GTPase activity by more than 1000-fold, leading to rapid hydrolysis of GTP to GDP and termination of signal transduction. Thus, GAPs function as "brakes" that prevent uncontrolled *ras* activity. The response to this braking action of GAPs seems to falter when mutations affect the *ras* gene. *Mutant ras proteins bind GAP, but their GTPase activity fails to be augmented.* Hence the mutant proteins are "trapped" in their excited GTP-bound form, causing, in turn, a pathologic activation of the mitogenic signaling pathway. The importance of GTPase activation in normal growth control is underscored by the fact that a disabling mutation of neurofibromin (NF-1), a GTPase-activating protein, is also associated with neoplasia (see Cancer-Suppressor Genes).

Recent studies have revealed that, in addition to its role in transducing growth factor–initiated activating signals, *ras* is also involved in the regulation of cell cycle. As detailed later, the passage of cells from G_0 to the S phase is modulated by a series of proteins called *cyclins* and *cyclin-dependent kinases (CDKs)*. *ras*, it seems, controls the levels of CDKs by unknown mechanisms.[12]

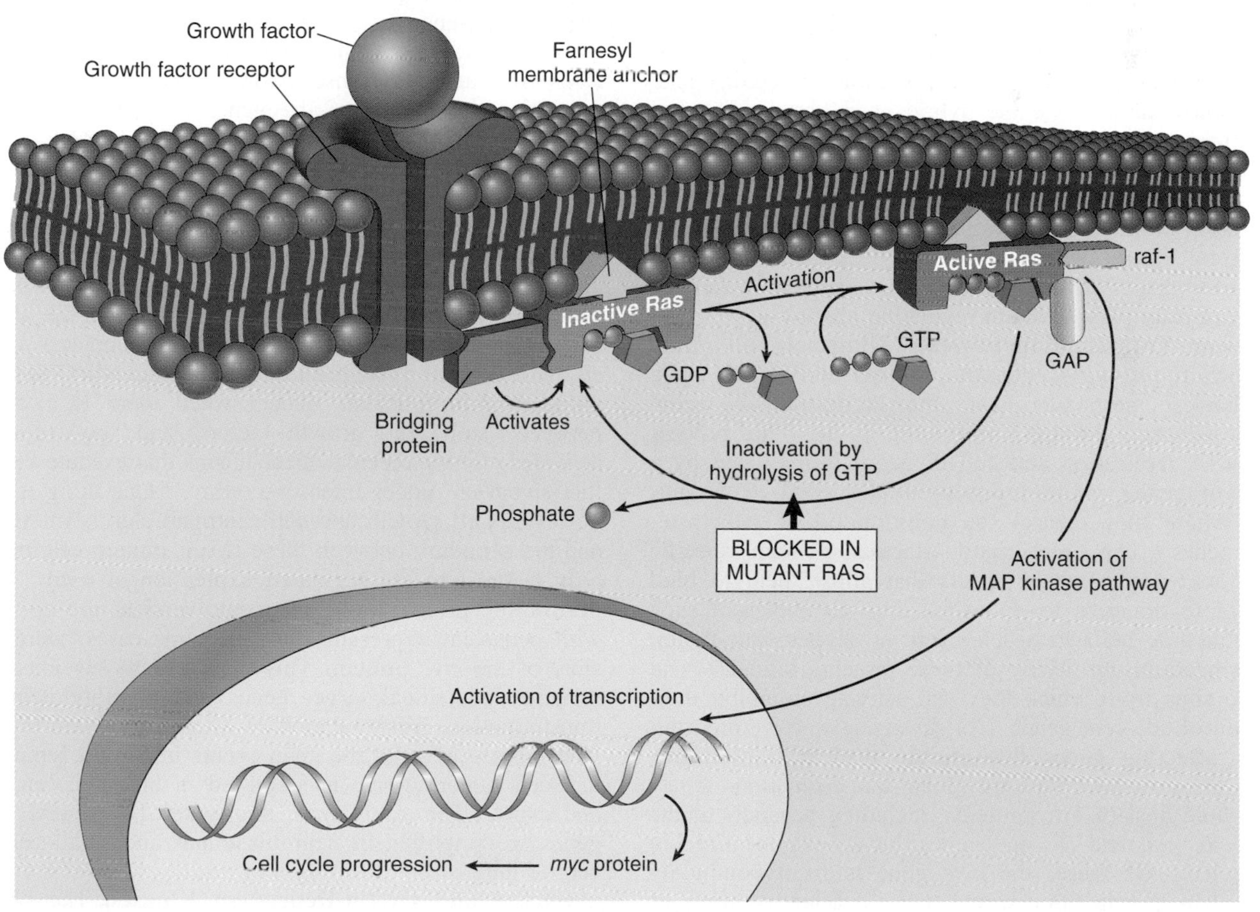

Figure 8–25

Model for action of *ras* genes. When a normal cell is stimulated through a growth factor receptor, inactive (GDP bound) *ras* is activated to a GTP-bound state. Activated *ras* recruits *raf*-1 and stimulates the MAP-kinase pathway to transmit growth-promoting signals to the nucleus. The mutant *ras* protein is permanently activated because of inability to hydrolyze GTP, leading to continuous stimulation of cells without any external trigger. The anchoring of *ras* to the cell membrane by the farnesyl moiety is essential for its action.

Because *ras* is mutated so often in human cancers, much effort has been devoted to devising means by which the activity of renegade *ras* can be controlled. To block *ras* activity, researchers have taken advantage of the fact that to receive activating signals from growth factor receptors, *ras* must be anchored under the cell membrane close to the cytoplasmic domain of the growth factor receptors. Such anchoring is made possible by attachment of an isoprenyl lipid group to the *ras* molecule by the enzyme *farnesyl transferase*. The *farnesyl* moiety forms the bridge between *ras* and the lipid membrane. Inhibitors of *farnesyl transferase* can disable *ras* by preventing its normal localization. Such drugs seem to have activity in animal models of tumors and are likely to be tested in humans.[13]

In addition to *ras*, several nonreceptor-associated tyrosine kinases also function in the signal transduction pathways. Mutant forms of nonreceptor-associated tyrosine kinases that have acquired transforming potential are commonly found in the form of v-*oncs* in animal retroviruses (e.g., v-*abl*, v-*src,* v-*fyn,* v-*fes,* and many others). With the exception of c-*abl*, however, they are rarely activated in human tumors. The *abl* protooncogene has tyrosine kinase activity, which is dampened by negative regulatory domains. In chronic myeloid leukemia and some acute lymphoblastic leukemias, however, this activity is unleashed because the c-*abl* gene is translocated from its normal abode on chromosome 9 to chromosome 22; here it fuses with part of the *bcr* (*b*reak-point *c*luster *r*egion) gene on chromosome 22, and the hybrid gene has potent tyrosine kinase activity. The molecular pathways activated by the *bcr-c-abl* hybrid gene are poorly understood. There is accumulating evidence that the *abl* gene acts not only in the growth-promoting pathway, but also in pathways that control cell death. New evidence suggests that c-*abl*, similar to *p53* (discussed later), is activated after DNA damage and hence may play a role in regulating apoptosis.[14, 15]

Nuclear Transcription Proteins. Ultimately, all signal transduction pathways enter the nucleus and impact on a large bank of responder genes that orchestrate the cells' orderly advance through the mitotic cycle. This process (i.e., DNA replication and cell division) is regulated by a family of genes whose products are localized to the nucleus, where they control the transcription of growth-related genes. The transcription factors contain specific amino acid sequences or motifs that allow them to bind DNA or to dimerize for DNA binding. Examples of such motifs include helix-loop-helix, leucine zipper, zinc-finger, and homeodomains. Many of these proteins bind DNA at specific sites from which they can activate or inhibit transcription of adjacent genes. Not surprisingly, therefore, mutations affecting genes that encode nuclear transcription factors are associated with malignant transformation.

A whole host of oncoproteins, including products of the *myc, myb, jun,* and *fos* oncogenes, have been localized to the nucleus. Of these, the *myc* gene is most commonly involved in human tumors, and hence a brief overview of its function is warranted.[16] The c-*myc* protooncogene is expressed in virtually all eukaryotic cells and belongs to the immediate early growth response genes, which are rapidly induced when quiescent cells receive a signal to divide. After a transient increase of c-*myc* mRNA, the expression declines to a basal level. The importance of c-*myc* in cell proliferation is underscored by experiments in which specific inhibition of c-*myc* expression by antisense oligonucleotides prevents the entry of cells into the S phase.

The molecular basis of c-*myc* function in cell replication is not entirely clear, but some general principles have emerged. After translation, the c-*myc* protein is rapidly translocated to the nucleus. Either before or after transport to the nucleus, it forms a heterodimer with another protein, called *max.* The *myc-max* heterodimer binds to specific DNA sequences (termed *E-boxes*) and is a potent transcriptional activator. Mutations that impair the ability of *myc* to bind to DNA or to *max* also abolish its oncogenic activity. In addition to forming a heterodimer with *myc*, the *max* protein can also form homodimers that are transcriptionally inactive. Furthermore, *mad*, another member of the *myc* superfamily of transcriptional regulators, can also bind *max* to form a dimer. The *mad-max* heterodimer functions as a transcription repressor. Thus, the emerging theme seems to be that the degree of transcriptional activation by c-*myc* is regulated not only by the levels of *myc* protein, but also by the abundance and availability of *max* and *mad* proteins. In this network, *myc-max* favors proliferation, whereas *mad-max* inhibits cell growth. *mad* may therefore be considered an antioncogene (or tumor-suppressor gene).[17] Although there is little doubt that *myc-max* heterodimers bind to DNA and activate transcription, it has been difficult to determine the nature of the genes that obey their commands.[18] Several candidates have emerged, including genes for ornithine decarboxylase (necessary for DNA synthesis), certain CDKs (regulating cell cycle, see later), and eIF2-α (a rate-limiting enzyme for protein translation).

It is becoming increasingly evident that *myc* not only controls cell growth, but also it can drive cell death by apoptosis. Thus, when *myc* activation occurs in the absence of survival signals (growth factors), cells undergo apoptosis. This deviation has been dubbed the "conflict" model. It proposes that apoptosis occurs when there is a conflict between "stop" (no growth factors) and "go" (c-*myc* is activated). The molecular mechanisms that execute the conflict signal are under intense scrutiny.[19] One thing is clear, however: Cell growth and cell death are closely interlinked, and the boundary between these two is quite precarious.

In contrast to the regulated expression of c-*myc* during normal cell proliferation, oncogenic versions are associated with persistent expression, and in some cases overexpression, of the *myc* protein. This may lead to sustained transcription of critical target genes and possibly neoplastic transformation. Dysregulation of c-*myc* expression resulting from translocation of the gene occurs in Burkitt lymphoma, a B-cell tumor; c-*myc* is amplified in breast, colon, lung, and many other carcinomas; the related N-*myc* and L-*myc* genes are amplified in neuroblastomas and small cell cancers of lung.

Cyclins and Cyclin-Dependent Kinases. The ultimate outcome of all growth-promoting stimuli is the entry of quiescent cells into the cell cycle. As discussed in Chapter 4, the orderly progression of cells through the various phases of cell cycle is orchestrated by cyclins and cyclin-dependent kinases (CDKs) and their inhibitors. Mutations in genes that encode these cell cycle regulators have been found in several human cancers.

To understand the cancer-associated derangements in cell cycle, it is essential to review the normal functions and regulation of these proteins. Cyclin-dependent kinases drive the cell cycle by phosphorylating critical target proteins that are required for progression of the cells to the next phase of the cell cycle (Fig. 8–26). Cyclin-dependent kinases are expressed constitutively during the cell cycle but in an inactive form. They are activated by phosphorylation after binding to another family of proteins, called *cyclins*. By contrast with CDKs, cyclins are synthesized during specific phases of the cell cycle, and their function is to activate the CDKs. On completion of this task, cyclin levels decline rapidly. While cyclins arouse the CDKs, their inhibitors, of which there are several, silence the CDKs and thus exert another level of control over the cell cycle. Although each phase of the cell cycle circuitry is carefully monitored, the transition from G_1 to S is an extremely important checkpoint in the cell cycle clock because once cells cross this barrier they are committed to progress into S phase.[20] When a cell receives growth-promoting signals, the synthesis of D type cyclins that bind CDK4 and CDK6 is stimulated in the early part of G_1. Later in the G_1 phase of cell cycle, the synthesis of E cyclin is stimulated, which, in turn, binds to CDK2. The cyclin D/CDK4, CDK6, and cyclin E/CDK2 complexes phosphorylate the retinoblastoma protein (pRb) (Fig. 8–27). This is a critical reaction, for as we discuss later, underphosphorylated pRb binds to the E2F family of transcription factors. Phosphorylation of pRb unshackles the E2F proteins, and they, in turn, activate the transcription of several genes whose products are essential for progression through the S phase. These include DNA polymerases, thymidine kinase, dihydrofolate reductase, and many others. Further progress of cells from the S phase into the G_2 phase is facilitated by up-regulation of cyclin A, which binds to CDK2 and to CDK1. The targets phosphorylated by cyclin A/CDK2, CDK1 are not fully known. Early in the G_2 phase, B cyclin takes over. By forming complexes with CDK1, it helps the cell move from G_2 to M. The cyclin B/CDK1 complex phosphorylates a variety of proteins required for mitosis.

The activity of CDKs is regulated by two families of CDK inhibitors (CDKIs). One family of CDKIs, composed of three proteins, called *p21, p27,* and *p57,* inhibits the CDKs broadly, whereas the other family of CDKI has selective effects on cyclin D/CDK4 and cyclin D/CDK6. The four members of this family (p15, p16, p18, p19) are sometimes called *INK4* proteins (because they are *IN*hibitors of CD*K4* and CDK6).

With this background, it is easy to appreciate that mutations that dysregulate the activity of cyclins and CDKs would favor cell proliferation. Indeed, mishaps affecting the expression of cyclin D or CDK4 seem to be a common event in neoplastic transformation. The cyclin D genes are overexpressed in many cancers, including those affecting the breast, esophagus, and liver, and in a subset of lymphomas. Amplification of the CDK4 gene occurs in melanomas, sarcomas, and glioblastomas. Mutations affecting cy-

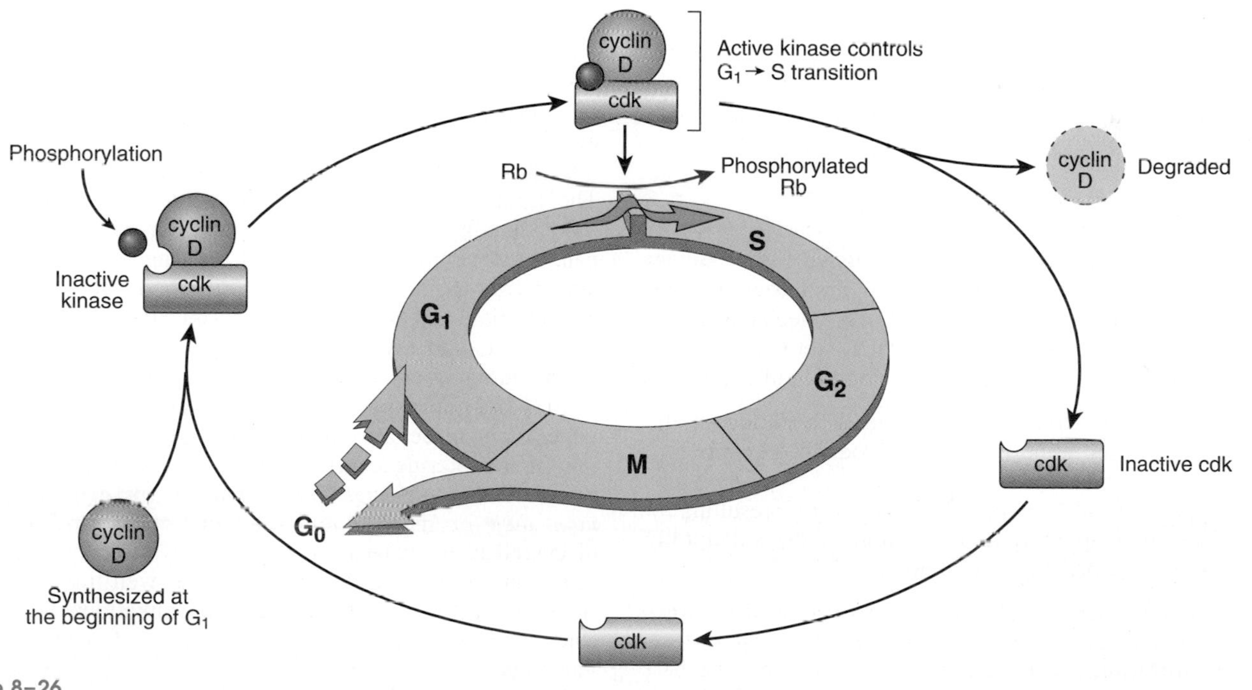

Figure 8–26

Schematic illustrating the role of cyclins and cyclin-dependent kinases (CDKs) in regulating the cell cycle. In the depicted example, inactive CDK is constitutively expressed; it is activated by binding to cyclin D, which is synthesized in G_1. The activated CDK allows the cell to cross the $G_1 \rightarrow S$ checkpoint by phosphorylating retinoblastoma *(Rb)* protein. After the cell enters the S phase, cyclin D is degraded, returning CDK to the inactive state.

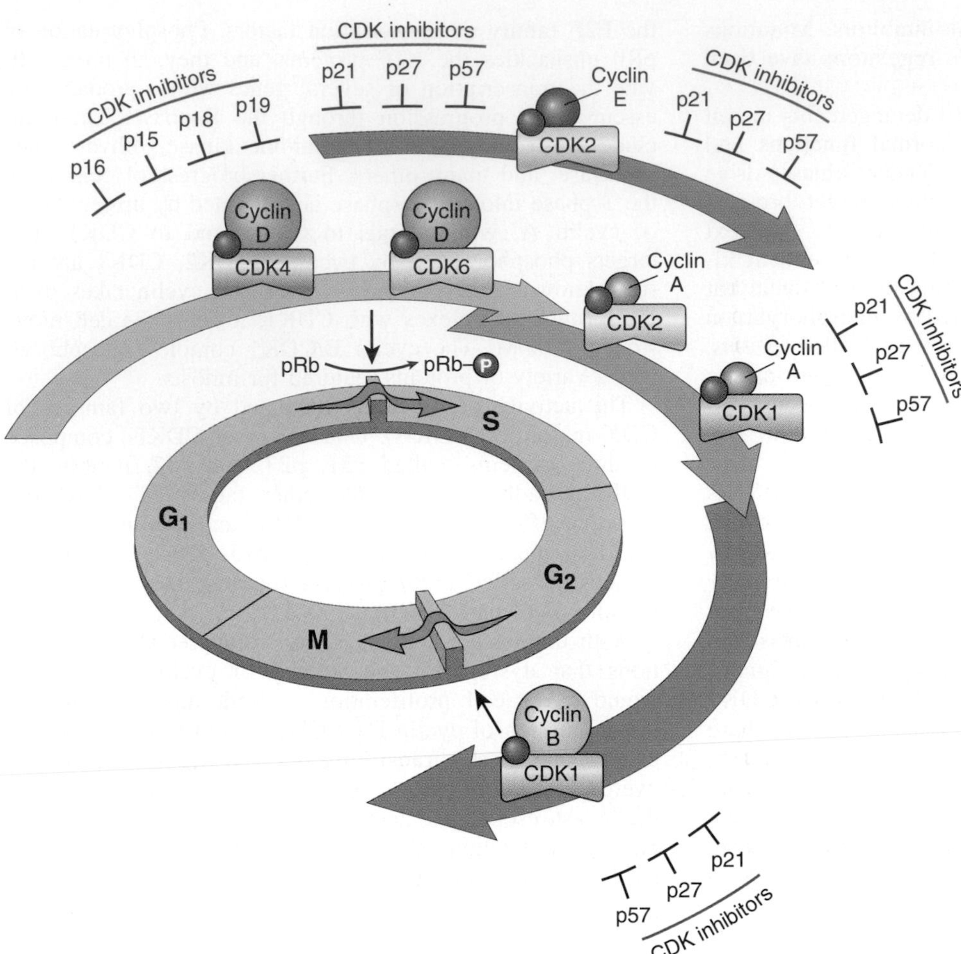

Figure 8–27 ■

Schematic illustration of the role of cyclins, CDKs, and cyclin-dependent kinase inhibitors (CDKIs) in regulating the cell cycle. The shaded arrows represent the phases of cell cycle during which specific cyclin/CDK complexes are active. As illustrated, cyclin D/CDK4, cyclin D/CDK6, and cyclin E/CDK2 regulate the $G_1 \rightarrow S$ transition by phosphorylation of the *Rb* protein (pRb). Cyclin A/CDK2 and cyclin A/CDK1 are active in the S phase. Cyclin B/CDK1 is essential for the $G_2 \rightarrow M$ transition. Two families of CDK inhibitors, so-called INK4 inhibitors composed of p16, p15, p18, and p19, act on cyclin D/CDK4 and cyclin D/CDK6. The other family of three inhibitors, p21, p27, and p57, can inhibit all CDKs.

clin B and cyclin E and other CDKs also occur in certain malignant neoplasms, but they are much less frequent than those affecting cyclin D/CDK4.

ACTIVATION OF ONCOGENES

In the preceding section, we discussed how mutant forms of protooncogenes may provide gratuitous growth-stimulating signals. Next we focus on mechanisms by which protooncogenes are transformed into oncogenes. This is brought about by two broad categories of changes:

- Changes in the structure of the gene, resulting in the synthesis of an abnormal gene product (oncoprotein) having an aberrant function
- Changes in regulation of gene expression, resulting in enhanced or inappropriate production of the structurally normal growth-promoting protein

We can now discuss the specific lesions that lead to structural and regulatory changes that affect protooncogenes.

Point Mutations. The *ras* oncogene represents the best example of activation by point mutations. Several distinct mutations have been identified, all of which dramatically reduce the GTPase activity of the *ras* proteins. Most of them involve codon 12. As mentioned in an earlier section, the intrinsic GTPase activity of normal *ras* proteins is augmented greatly by GAPs; in contrast, the GTPase activity of mutant *ras* proteins is poorly stimulated by GAPs. The mutant *ras* thus remains in the active GTP-bound form.

A large number of human tumors carry *ras* mutations. The frequency of such mutations varies with different tumors, but in some types it is high. For example, 90% of pancreatic adenocarcinomas and cholangiocarcinomas contain a *ras* point mutation, as do about 50% of colon, endometrial, and thyroid cancers and 30% of lung adenocarcinomas and myeloid leukemias. In general, carcinomas have mutations of K-*ras*, whereas hematopoietic tumors bear N-*ras* mutations. *ras* mutations are infrequent or even nonexistent in certain other cancers, particularly those arising in the uterine cervix or breast. It should be obvious therefore that *although ras mutations are extremely common, their presence is not essential for carcinogenesis.* As discussed later, there are many pathways to cancer, and *ras* mutations happen to lie on one of the well-traveled roads. In addition to *ras*, activating point mutations have been found in the c-*fms* gene in some cases of acute myeloid leukemia.

Chromosomal Rearrangements. Two types of chromosomal rearrangements can activate protooncogenes— translocations and inversions. Of these, chromosomal translocations are much more common. Translocations can activate protooncogenes in two ways:

1. In lymphoid tumors, specific translocations result in overexpression of protooncogenes by placing them under the regulatory elements of the immunoglobulin or T-cell receptor loci.
2. In many hematopoietic tumors, the translocations allow normally unrelated sequences from two different chromosomes to recombine and form hybrid genes that encode growth-promoting chimeric proteins.

Translocation-induced overexpression of a protooncogene is best exemplified by Burkitt lymphoma. All such tumors carry one of three translocations, each involving chromosome 8q24, where the c-*myc* gene has been mapped, as well as one of the three immunoglobulin gene-carrying chromosomes. At its normal locus, the expression of the *myc* gene is tightly controlled and is expressed only during certain stages of the cell cycle (Chapter 4). In Burkitt lymphoma, the most common form of translocation results in the movement of the c-*myc*-containing segment of chromosome 8 to chromosome 14q band 32 (Fig. 8–28). This places c-*myc* close to the immunoglobulin heavy-chain (IgH) gene. The molecular mechanisms of the translocation-associated activation of c-*myc* are variable, as are the precise breakpoints within the gene. In some cases, the translocation renders the c-*myc* gene subject to relentless stimulation by the adjacent enhancer element of the immunoglobulin gene. In others, the translocation causes mutations in the regulatory sequences of the *myc* gene. In all instances, the coding sequences of the gene remain intact, and the c-*myc* gene is constitutively expressed at high levels. The invariable presence of the translocated c-*myc* gene in Burkitt lymphomas attests to the importance of c-*myc* overexpression in the pathogenesis of this tumor.

The immunoglobulin heavy chain locus is involved in translocation-mediated overexpression of several other genes as well. In mantle cell lymphoma, the cyclin D1 gene on chromosome 11q32 is overexpressed by juxtaposition to the IgH locus on 14q32. In follicular lymphoma, a t(14;18)(q32;q21) translocation causes activation of the *bcl-2* gene (described later). Not unexpectedly, all these tumors in which the immunoglobulin gene is involved are of B-cell origin. In an analogous situation, overexpression of several protooncogenes in T-cell tumors results from translocations affecting the T-cell antigen receptor locus. The affected oncogenes are diverse, but in most cases, similar to c-*myc*, they encode nuclear transcription factors.

The Philadelphia chromosome, characteristic of chronic myeloid leukemia and a subset of acute lymphoblastic leukemias, provides the prototypic example of an oncogene formed by fusion of two separate genes. In these cases, a reciprocal translocation between chromosomes 9 and 22 relocates a truncated portion of the protooncogene c-*abl* (from chromosome 9) to the *bcr* on chromosome 22. The hybrid c-*abl-bcr* gene encodes a chimeric protein that has tyrosine kinase activity (Fig. 8–28). Although the translocations are cytogenetically identical in chronic myeloid leukemia and acute lymphoblastic leukemias, they differ at the molecular level. In chronic myeloid leukemia, the chimeric protein has a molecular weight of 210 kD, whereas in the more aggressive acute leukemias, a slightly different, 180-kD, *abl-bcr* fusion protein is formed.

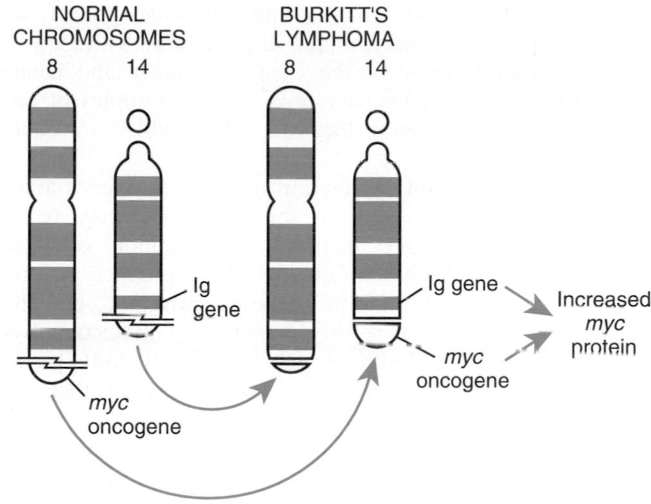

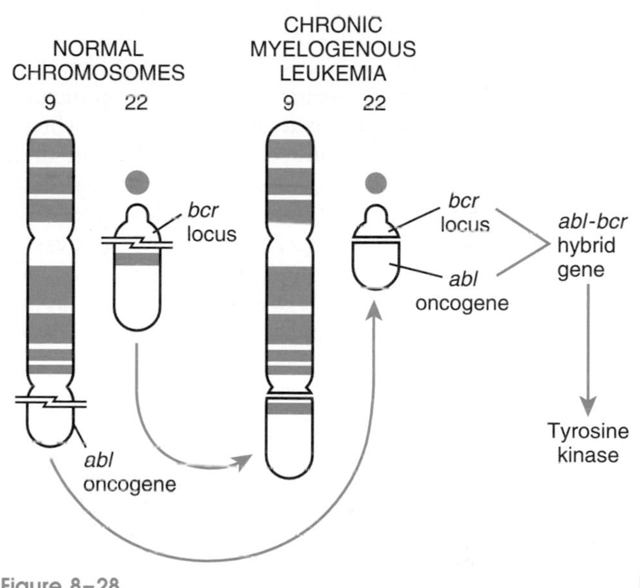

Figure 8–28

The chromosomal translocation and associated oncogenes in Burkitt lymphoma and chronic myelogenous leukemia.

Gene fusions often involve transcription factors.[21] One such transcription factor, encoded by the *MLL* (myeloid, lymphoid leukemia) gene on 11q23, is known to be involved in 25 different translocations with several different partner genes, some of which themselves encode a transcription factor. The *MLL* gene is involved in approximately 5 to 10% of all acute leukemias. It encodes the mammalian homolog of the Drosophila *trithorax* (*trx*) gene and is believed to regulate the expression of homeobox (*Hox*) genes in hematopoietic progenitor cells. In addition to hemopoietic neoplasms, many sarcomas have specific translocations that result in the formation of chimeric genes encoding transcription factors.[22] The *Ewing Sarcoma* (*EWS*) gene at 22q12, first described in the t(11;22)(q24;12) translocation of Ewing sarcoma, is translocated in several types of sarcomas. *EWS* is itself a transcription factor, and all of its partner genes analyzed so far also encode a transcription factor. In Ewing tumor, for example, the *EWS* gene fuses with the *FL-1* gene; the resultant chimeric EWS-FL-1 protein is a transactivator of the c-*myc* promoter and hence can cause overexpression of c-*myc*. Some examples of oncogene activation by translocation are provided in Table 8–8.

Gene Amplification. Activation of protooncogenes associated with overexpression of their products may result from reduplication and manifold amplification of their DNA sequences. Such amplification may produce several hundred copies of the protooncogene in the tumor cell. The amplified genes can be readily detected by molecular hybridization with the appropriate DNA probe. In some cases, the amplified genes produce cytogenetic changes that can be identified microscopically. Two mutually exclusive patterns are seen: multiple small, chromosome-like structures called *double minutes* (dms) or *homogeneous staining regions* (HSRs). The latter derive from the assembly of amplified genes into new chromosomes; because these regions containing amplified genes lack a normal banding pattern, they appear homogeneous in a G-banded karyotype (Fig. 8–29). The most interesting cases of amplification involve N-*myc* in neuroblastoma and c-*erb B2* in breast cancers. These genes are amplified in 30 to 40% of these two tumors, and in both settings this amplification is associated with poor prognosis.[23] Similarly, amplification of L-*myc* and N-*myc* correlates strongly with disease progression in small cell cancer of the lung. Other genes frequently amplified include c-*myc* (breast, ovarian, and lung carcinomas) and cyclin D (breast carcinomas and several squamous cell carcinomas).

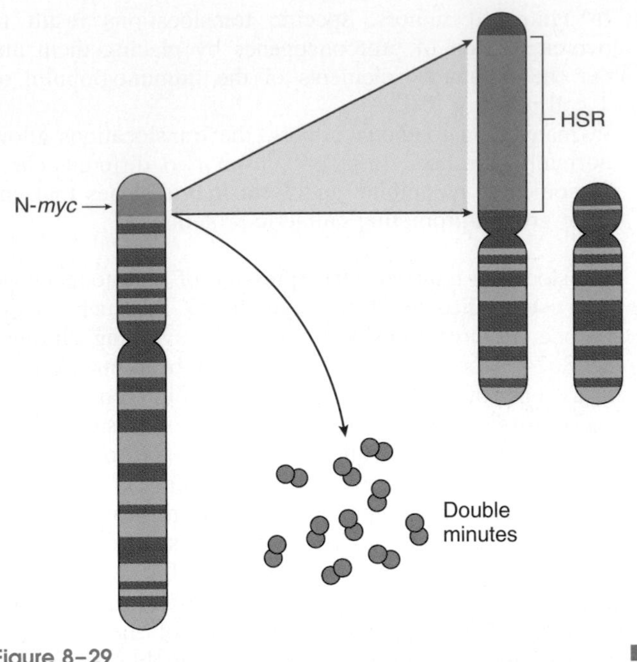

Figure 8–29

Amplification of the N-*myc* gene in human neuroblastomas. The N-*myc* gene, normally present on chromosome 2p, becomes amplified and is seen either as extra chromosomal double minutes or as a chromosomally integrated, homogeneous staining region. The integration involves other autosomes, such as 4, 9, or 13. (Modified from Brodeur GM: Molecular correlates of cytogenetic abnormalities in human cancer cells: implications for oncogene activation. In Brown EB (ed): Progress in Hematology, Vol 14, Orlando, FL, Grune & Stratton, 1986, pp 229–256.)

Table 8–8. SELECTED EXAMPLES OF ONCOGENES ACTIVATED BY TRANSLOCATION

Malignancy	Translocation	Affected Genes
Chronic myeloid leukemia	(9;22)(q34;q11)	Abl 9q34 *bcr* 22q11
Acute leukemias (AML and ALL)	(4;11)(q21;q23)	AF4 4q21 MLL 11q23
	(6;11)(q27;q23)	AF6 6q27 MLL 11q23
Burkitt lymphoma	(8;14)(q24;q32)	c-*myc* 8q24 IgH 14q32
Mantle cell lymphoma	(11;14)(q13;q32)	Cyclin D 11q13 IgH 14q32
Follicular lymphoma	(14;18)(q32;q21)	IgH 14q32 *bcl*-2 18q21
T-cell acute lymphoblastic leukemia	(8;14)(q24;q11)	c-*myc* 8q24 TCR-α 14q11
	(10;14)(q24;q11)	*Hox* 11 10q24 TCR-α 14q11
Ewing sarcoma	(11;22)(q24;q12)	FL-1 11q24 EWS 22q12
Melanoma of soft parts	(12;22)(q13;q12)	ATF-1 12q13 EWS 22q12

Underlined genes are involved in multiple translocations.
AML, acute myeloid leukemia; ALL, acute lymphoblastic leukemia.

Cancer-Suppressor Genes

While protooncogenes encode proteins that promote cell growth, the products of tumor-suppressor genes apply brakes to cell proliferation. In a sense, the term *tumor-suppressor genes* is a misnomer because the physiologic function of these genes is to regulate cell growth, not to prevent tumor formation. Because the loss of these genes is a key event in many, possibly all, human tumors and because their discovery resulted from the study of tumors, the names tumor suppressor and antioncogene persist.

Similar to many discoveries in medicine, the cancer-suppressor genes were discovered by studying rare diseases, in this case retinoblastoma, a tumor that affects about 1 in 20,000 infants and children. Approximately 60% of retinoblastomas are sporadic, and the remaining 40% are familial, with the predisposition to develop the tumor being transmitted as an autosomal dominant trait. To explain the familial and sporadic occurrence of an apparently identical tumor, Knudson proposed his now famous "two-hit" hypothesis of oncogenesis. He suggested that in hereditary cases, one genetic change ("first hit") is inherited from an affected parent and is therefore present in all somatic cells of the body, whereas the second mutation "second hit" occurs in one of the many retinal cells (which already carry the first mutation). In sporadic cases, however, both mutations (hits) occur somatically within a single retinal cell, whose progeny then form the tumor. Knudson's hypothesis has been amply substantiated by cytogenetic and molecular studies and can now be formulated in more precise terms:

- The mutations required to produce retinoblastoma involve the *Rb* gene, located on chromosome 13q14. In some cases, the genetic damage is large enough to be visible in the form of a deletion of 13q14.
- Both normal alleles of the *Rb* locus must be inactivated (two hits) for the development of retinoblastoma (Fig. 8–30). In familial cases, children are born with one normal and one defective copy of the *Rb* gene. They lose the intact copy in the retinoblasts through some form of somatic mutation (point mutation, interstitial deletion of 13q14, or even complete loss of the normal chromosome 13). In sporadic cases, both normal *Rb* alleles are lost by somatic mutation in one of the retinoblasts. The end result is the same: A retinal cell that has lost both normal copies of the *Rb* gene gives rise to cancer.
- Patients with familial retinoblastoma are also at greatly increased risk of developing osteosarcoma and some other soft tissue sarcomas. Furthermore, inactivation of the *Rb* locus has been noted in several other tumors, including adenocarcinoma of the breast, small cell carcinoma of the lung, and bladder carcinoma. Thus the loss of *Rb* genes has implications beyond the development of retinoblastoma.

At this point, we should clarify some terminology. A child carrying an inherited mutant *Rb* allele in all somatic cells is perfectly normal (except for the increased risk of developing cancer). Because such a child is heterozygous at the *Rb* locus, it implies that heterozygosity for the *Rb* gene does not affect cell behavior. *Cancer develops when the cell becomes homozygous for the mutant allele or, put another way, loses heterozygosity for the normal Rb gene. Because the Rb gene is associated with cancer when both normal copies are lost, it is sometimes referred to as a recessive cancer gene.*

The *Rb* gene stands as a paradigm for several other genes that act similarly. For example, one or more genes on the short arm of chromosome 11 play a role in the formation of Wilms tumor, hepatoblastoma, and rhabdomyosarcoma. Consistent and nonrandom loss of heterozygosity has provided important clues to the location of several cancer-suppressor genes. A list of selected tumor-suppressor genes is provided in Table 8–9. A discussion of their function follows.

PROTEIN PRODUCTS OF TUMOR-SUPPRESSOR GENES

The signals and signal-transducing pathways for growth inhibition are much less well understood than those for growth promotion. Nevertheless, it is reasonable to assume that, similar to mitogenic signals, growth inhibitory signals originate outside the cell and use receptors, signal transducers, and cell cycle and nuclear transcription regulators to accomplish their effects. The tumor-suppressor genes seem to encode various components of this growth inhibitory pathway. We begin our discussion from the inside out, with those tumor-suppressor genes that control the cell

Table 8–9. SELECTED TUMOR-SUPPRESSOR GENES INVOLVED IN HUMAN NEOPLASMS

Subcellular Location	Gene	Function	Tumors Associated with Somatic Mutations	Tumors Associated with Inherited Mutations
Cell surface	TGF-β receptor	Growth inhibition	Carcinomas of colon	Unknown
	E-cadherin	Cell adhesion	Carcinoma of stomach, breast	Familial gastric cancer
Under plasma membrane	NF-1	Inhibition of *ras* signal transduction	Schwannomas	Neurofibromatosis type I and sarcomas
Cytoskeleton	NF-2	Unknown	Schwannomas and meningiomas	Neurofibromatosis type II; acoustic schwannomas and meningiomas
Cytosol	APC	Inhibition of signal transduction	Carcinomas of stomach, colon, pancreas; melanoma	Familial adenomatous polyposis coli; colon cancer
Nucleus	*Rb*	Regulation of cell cycle	Retinoblastoma; osteosarcoma; carcinomas of breast, colon, lung	Retinoblastomas, osteosarcoma
	p53	Regulation of cell cycle and apoptosis in response to DNA damage	Most human cancers	Li-Fraumeni syndrome; multiple carcinomas and sarcomas
	WT-1	Nuclear transcription	Wilms tumor	Wilms tumor
	p16(INK4a)	Regulation of cell cycle by inhibiting cyclin-dependent kinases	Pancreatic, esophageal cancers	Malignant melanoma
	BRCA-1	DNA repair		Carcinomas of female breast and ovary
	BRCA-2	DNA repair		Carcinomas of male and female breast

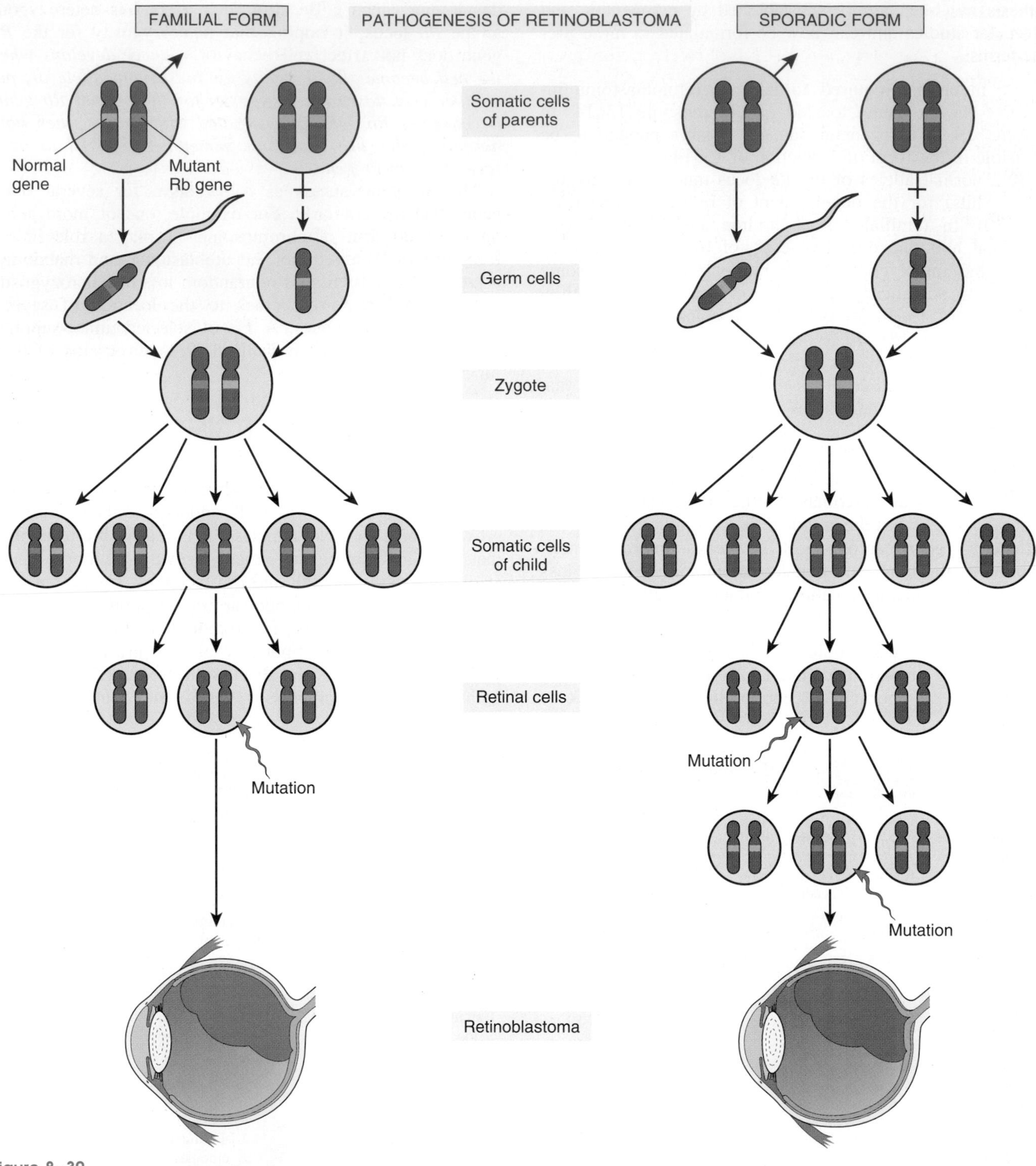

Figure 8–30

Pathogenesis of retinoblastoma. Two mutations of the Rb locus on chromosome 13q14 lead to neoplastic proliferation of the retinal cells. In the familial form, all somatic cells inherit one mutant Rb gene from a carrier parent. The second mutation affects the Rb locus in one of the retinal cells after birth. In the sporadic form, on the other hand, both mutations at the Rb locus are acquired by the retinal cells after birth.

cycle and nuclear transcription, because they hold the key to cell division.

Molecules That Regulate Nuclear Transcription and Cell Cycle. Ultimately, all positive and negative signals converge on the nucleus, where decisions to divide or not to divide are made. In keeping with this, products of several tumor-suppressor genes (*Rb*, *WT-1*, and *p53*) are localized to the nucleus.

Rb Gene. Much is known about the *Rb* gene because this was the first tumor-suppressor gene discovered.[24, 25] pRb, the product of the *Rb* gene, is a nuclear phosphoprotein that plays a key role in regulating the cell cycle. It is expressed in every cell type examined, where it exists in an active underphosphorylated and an inactive hyperphosphorylated state. In its active state, pRb serves as a brake on the advancement of cells from the G_1 to the S phase of the cell cycle. When the cells are stimulated by growth factors, the *Rb* protein is inactivated by phosphorylation (pRb-P), the brake is released, and the cells transverse the $G_1 \rightarrow S$ checkpoint. Once the cells enter S phase, they are committed to divide without additional growth factor stimulation. During the ensuing M phase, the phosphate groups are removed from pRb by cellular phosphatases, thus regenerating the dephosphorylated form of pRb.

The molecular basis of this braking action has been unraveled in elegant detail.[20] *Quiescent cells (in G_0 or early G_1) contain the active hypophosphorylated form of pRb. In this state, pRb prevents cell replication by binding, and possibly sequestering, the E2F family of transcription factors.* When the quiescent cells are stimulated by growth factors, the concentrations of the D and E cyclins (see earlier) goes up, and the resultant activation of cyclin D/CDK4, cyclin D/CDK6, and cyclin E/CDK2 leads to phosphorylation of pRb (Fig. 8–31). The hyperphosphorylated form of pRb releases the E2F transcription factors. The released E2F proteins then form heterodimers with the DP family of proteins (Fig. 8–31) and activate the transcription of several target genes. E2F-DNA binding sites have been identified in the regulatory region of a number of genes whose products are required for the S phase of cell cycle. The exact workings of the pRb-E2F nexus in regulating the $G_1 \rightarrow S$ transition are not entirely clear. According to one view, hypophosphorylated pRb prevents the activation of E2F-responsive genes by physical sequestration of

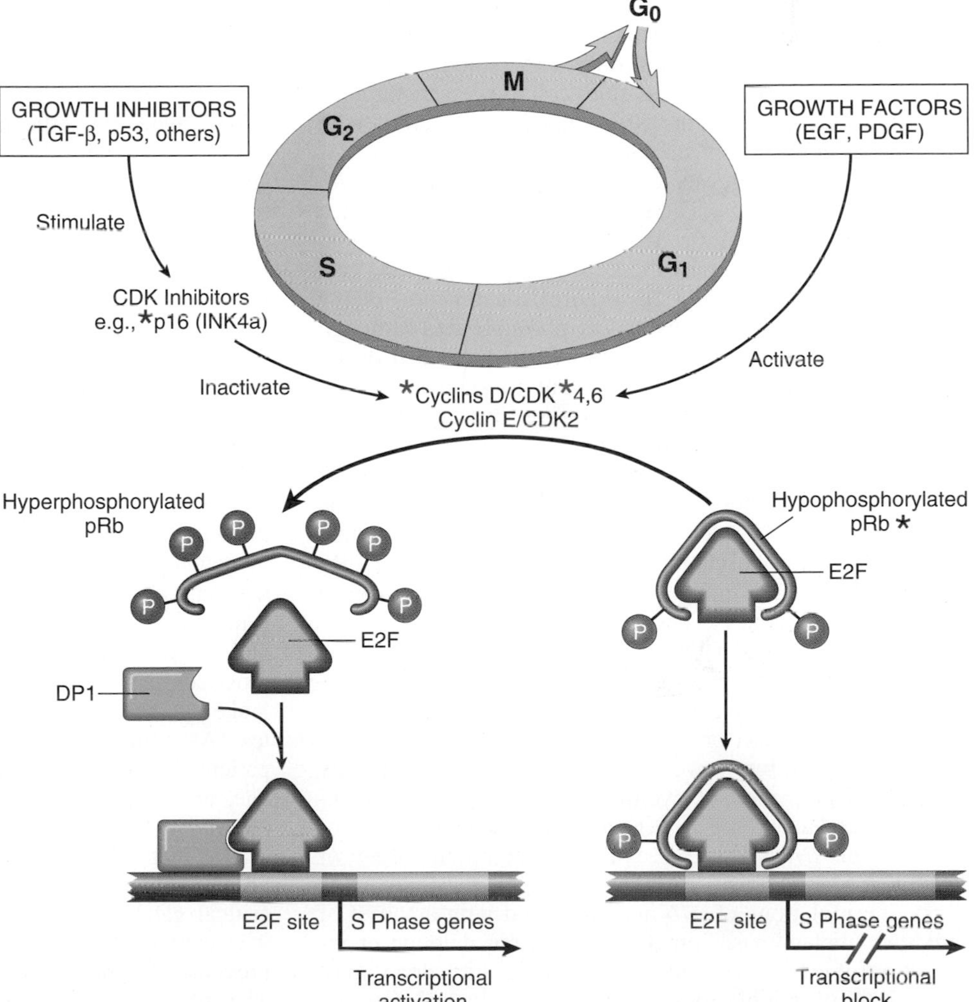

Figure 8–31 ■

The role of pRb in regulating the $G_1 \rightarrow S$ checkpoint of cell cycle. Hypophosphorylated pRb complexed to the E2F transcription factors binds to DNA and inhibits transcription of genes whose products are required for the S phase of the cell cycle. When pRb is phosphorylated by the cyclin D/CDK4, 6, and cyclin E/CDK2 complexes, it releases E2F. The latter then activates transcription of S-phase genes. The phosphorylation of pRb is inhibited by CDK inhibitors because they inactivate cyclin/CDK complexes. Virtually all cancer cells show dysregulation of the $G_1 \rightarrow S$ checkpoint owing to mutation in one of four genes that regulate the phosphorylation of pRb; these genes (*Rb*, CDK4, cyclin D, and *p16*) are indicated by an asterisk.

E2F proteins. More recent evidence suggests that hypophosphorylated pRb is not a mere sponge that holds back E2F from its target genes; rather the pRb-E2F complex binds to DNA and actively inhibits the transcription of the S phase genes.[26] Regardless of the precise mechanism by which pRb regulates the function of E2F, it is clear that *the state of pRb phosphorylation is a critical determinant of cell cycle progression.*

It should be obvious from this discussion that if the *Rb* protein is absent (owing to gene deletions) or its ability to regulate E2F transcription factors is derailed by mutations, the molecular brakes on the cell cycle are released, and the cells move blithely into the S phase. The mutations of *Rb* genes found in tumors are localized to a region, called the "*Rb* pocket," that is involved in binding to E2F.

It was mentioned previously that germ line loss or mutations of the *Rb* gene predispose to occurrence of retinoblastomas and to a lesser extent osteosarcomas. Furthermore, somatically acquired mutations have been described in glioblastomas, small cell carcinomas of lung, breast cancers, and bladder carcinomas. Given the presence of pRb in every cell and its importance in cell cycle control, two questions arise: (1) Why do patients with germ line mutation of the *Rb* locus develop only retinoblastomas? (2) Why are inactivating mutations of pRb not much more common in human cancer? The basis for the occurrence of tumors restricted to the retina in patients who inherit one defective allele of *Rb* is not fully understood, but some clues have emerged from the study of mice with targeted disruption of the *Rb* locus. $Rb^{-/-}$ mice die in utero with evidence of apoptosis in their nervous system and hematopoietic cells. This suggests that homozygous loss of the *Rb* gene triggers apoptosis. There is evidence that unrestrained action of E2F proteins (as would occur with loss of both *Rb* alleles) not only drives the cell cycle, but also triggers apoptosis. This action of E2F requires the function of the *p53* gene (see later). It thus seems plausible that although in most tissues, homozygous loss of *Rb* induces cell death, the retinoblasts are relatively resistant to such apoptosis-inducing effect. In these cells, therefore, dysregulated E2F gives rise to neoplastic proliferation.

With respect to the second question (i.e., why the loss of *Rb* is not much more common in human tumors), the answer is much simpler: Mutations in other genes that control pRb phosphorylation can mimic the effect of pRb loss; such genes are mutated in many cancers that seem to have normal *Rb* genes. Thus, for example, mutational activation of cyclin D or CDK4 would favor cell proliferation by facilitating pRb phosphorylation. As previously discussed, cyclin D is overexpressed in many tumors because of gene amplification or translocation. Mutational inactivation of CDK inhibitors would also drive the cell cycle by unregulated activation of cyclins and CDKs. One such inhibitor, encoded by the *p16* gene (also called *in*hibitor of *k*inase *4* or *INK4a*) is an extremely common target of deletion or mutational inactivation in human tumors.[26a] Germ line mutations of *p16* are associated with a subset of hereditary melanomas. Somatically acquired deletion or inactivation of *p16* is seen in 75% of pancreatic carcinomas; 40 to 70% of glioblastomas; 50% of esophageal cancers; and 20% of non–small cell lung carcinomas, soft tissue sarcomas, and bladder cancers. Thus, *the emerging paradigm is that loss of normal cell cycle control is central to malignant transformation and that at least one of the four key regulators of cell cycle (p16, cyclin D, CDK4, Rb) is mutated in the vast majority of human cancers.*[5] In cells that harbor mutations in p16, cyclin D, or CDK4, the function of the *Rb* gene is disrupted even if the Rb gene itself is not mutated. Several other pathways of cell growth regulation, some to be discussed in more detail later, also converge on pRb (Fig. 8–31).

- TGF-β induces inhibition of cellular proliferation. This effect of TGF-β is induced, at least in part, by up-regulation of the CDK inhibitors *p27* and *p15.*
- The transforming proteins of several oncogenic animal and human DNA viruses seem to act, in part, by neutralizing the growth inhibitory activities of *pRb.* SV40 and polyoma virus large T antigens, adenoviruses EIA protein, and human papillomavirus (HPV) E7 protein all bind to the hypophosphorylated form of *pRb.* The binding occurs in the same *pRb* pocket that normally sequesters E2F transcription factors. Thus, the *pRb* protein, unable to bind the E2F transcription factors, is functionally deleted, and the transcription factors are free to cause cell cycle progression.
- The *p53* gene, a well-known tumor-suppressor gene, described next, exerts its growth-inhibiting effects at least in part by up-regulating the synthesis of the CDK inhibitor *p21.*

p53 *gene.* p53, the other well-studied tumor-suppressor gene, is located on chromosome 17p13.1, and it is the single most common target for genetic alteration in human tumors. *A little over 50% of human tumors contain mutations in this gene.* Homozygous loss of the *p53* gene is found in virtually every type of cancer, including carcinomas of the lung, colon, and breast—the three leading causes of cancer deaths. In most cases, the inactivating mutations affecting both *p53* alleles are acquired in somatic cells. Less commonly, some individuals inherit a mutant *p53* allele. As with the *Rb* gene, inheritance of one mutant allele predisposes individuals to develop malignant tumors because only one additional "hit" is needed to inactivate the second, normal, allele. Such individuals, said to have the *Li-Fraumeni syndrome*, have a 25-fold greater chance of developing a malignant tumor by age 50 compared with the general population.[27] In contrast to patients who inherit a mutant *Rb* allele, the spectrum of tumors that develop in patients with the Li-Fraumeni syndrome is quite varied; the most common types of tumors are sarcomas, breast cancer, leukemia, brain tumors, and carcinomas of the adrenal cortex. As compared with sporadic tumors, those that afflict patients with the Li-Fraumeni syndrome occur at a younger age, and a given individual may develop multiple primary tumors.

The fact that *p53* mutations are common in a variety of human tumors suggests that the *p53* protein serves as a critical gatekeeper against the formation of cancer. Indeed, it is evident that *p53* acts as a "molecular policeman" that prevents the propagation of genetically damaged cells.[28] The *p53* protein is localized to the nucleus, and when called into action, it functions primarily by controlling the transcription of several other genes. Under physiologic conditions, *p53* has a short half-life (20 minutes), presumably because of ubiquitin-mediated proteolysis, and hence, in contrast to pRb, it does not police the normal cell cycle. *p53* is called in to apply emergency brakes, however, when DNA is damaged by irradiation, UV light, or mutagenic chemicals. With such an assault on genetic material, there are dramatic changes in the otherwise sleepy *p53* (Fig. 8–32). Through poorly understood mechanisms, there is a rapid increase in *p53* levels and activation of *p53* as a transcription factor. The accumulated wild-type *p53* binds to DNA and stimulates transcription of several genes that mediate the two major effects of *p53*: cell-cycle arrest and apoptosis. *p53*-induced cell cycle arrest occurs late in the G_1 phase and is caused by the *p53*-dependent transcription of the CDK inhibitor *p21*. The *p21* gene, as discussed earlier, inhibits the cyclin/CDK complexes and thus prevents the phosphorylation of *pRb* necessary for cells to enter the S phase. Such a pause in cell cycling is welcome because it allows the cells time to repair the DNA damage inflicted by the mutagenic agent. *p53* also helps in this process directly by inducing the transcription of *GADD45* (*G*rowth *A*rrest and *D*NA *D*amage), a protein involved in DNA repair. GADD45 also assists in G_1 arrest by unknown mechanisms. If the DNA damage is repaired successfully, quite ingeniously, *p53* activates a gene called *mdm2*, whose product binds to and down-regulates *p53*, thus relieving the cell cycle block. If during the pause in cell division the DNA damage cannot be successfully repaired, normal *p53*, perhaps as a last-ditch effort, sends the cell to the graveyard by inducing the activation of apoptosis-inducing genes. *bax* and IGF-BP3 are the two *p53*-responsive genes that carry the cell death commands of *p53*. *bax*, as we discuss later, binds to and antagonizes the apoptosis-inhibiting protein *bcl*-2. IGF-BP3 binds to the receptor of the insulin-like growth factor (IGF) and presumably induces apoptosis by blocking IGF-mediated intracellular signaling. It should be emphasized that transcriptional activation of downstream genes, such as *p21*, GADD45, and *bax*, is central to the normal functioning of

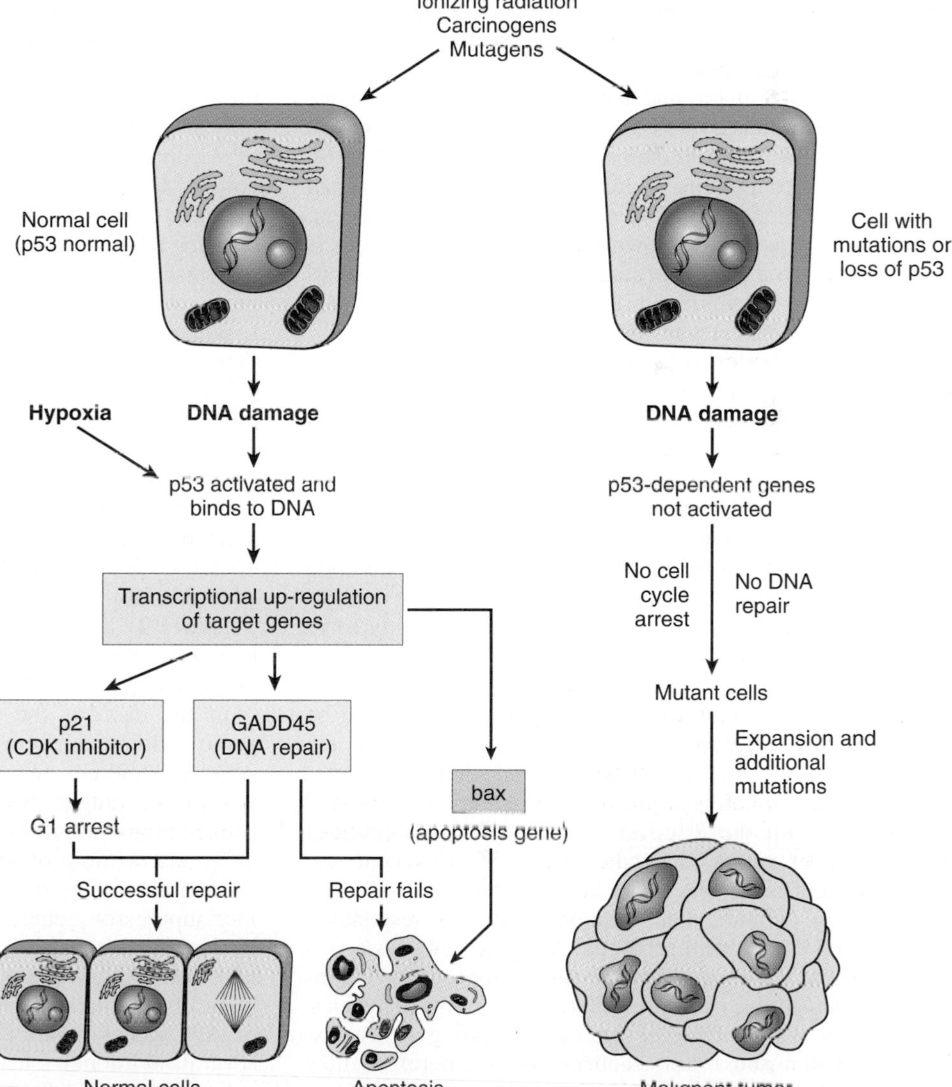

Figure 8–32 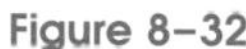

The role of *p53* in maintaining the integrity of the genome. Activation of normal *p53* by DNA-damaging agents or by hypoxia leads to cell cycle arrest in G_1 and induction of DNA repair, by transcriptional up-regulation of the cyclin-dependent kinase inhibitor *p21*, and the GADD45 genes, respectively. Successful repair of DNA allows cells to proceed with the cell cycle; if DNA repair fails, *p53*-induced activation of the *bax* gene promotes apoptosis. In cells with loss or mutations of *p53*, DNA damage does not induce cell cycle arrest or DNA repair, and hence genetically damaged cells proliferate, giving rise eventually to malignant neoplasms.

p53. In keeping with this notion, the most common mutations that disable *p53* affect its DNA-binding domain, thus preventing the *p53*-dependent transcription of genes. Whether *p53* also mediates some of its effects by protein-protein interactions is considered quite likely, but this is not fully understood.

To summarize, p53 senses DNA damage by unknown mechanisms and assists in DNA repair by causing G_1 arrest and inducing DNA repair genes. A cell with damaged DNA that cannot be repaired is directed by p53 to undergo apoptosis (Fig. 8–32). *In view of these activities, p53 has been rightfully called a "guardian of the genome." With homozygous loss of p53, DNA damage goes unrepaired, mutations become fixed in dividing cells, and the cell turns onto a one-way street leading to malignant transformation.*

Yet another mechanism by which normal *p53* may prevent tumor growth has been discovered recently. It seems that, in addition to DNA damage, hypoxia can also stimulate the activation of normal *p53*.[29] As discussed in more detail later, tumor angiogenesis is critical to the growth of tumor cells. Tumor cells that are hypoxic undergo apoptosis if they have normal copies of the *p53* gene. If the *p53* gene is mutated, however, the hypoxic tumor cells are resistant to apoptosis. Thus, hypoxia selects for cells in which the *p53* gene is inactive, and propagation of *p53*-deficient cells is favored.

In addition to somatic and inherited mutations, *p53* gene functions can be inactivated by other mechanisms. As with pRb, the transforming proteins of several DNA viruses, including the E6 protein of human papillomaviruses, can bind to and degrade *p53*. The cellular *p53*-binding protein, *mdm2*, which normally down-regulates *p53* activity, is overexpressed in a subset of human soft tissue sarcomas as a result of gene amplification. By promoting rapid degradation of *p53*,[30] *mdm2* acts as an oncogene.

The ability of *p53* to control apoptosis in response to DNA damage has some practical therapeutic implications. Radiation and chemotherapy, the two common modalities of cancer treatment, mediate their effects by inducing DNA damage and subsequent apoptosis. It follows that tumors that retain normal *p53* genes are more likely to respond to such therapy than tumors that carry mutant *p53*. Such is the case with testicular teratocarcinomas[31] and childhood acute lymphoblastic leukemias. By contrast, tumors such as lung cancers and colorectal cancers, which frequently carry *p53* mutations, are relatively resistant to chemotherapy and radiotherapy.

In closing this discussion of the *p53* gene, it should be pointed out that for almost 20 years after its discovery, the *p53* gene was the only known gene of its kind, both structurally and functionally. In late 1997, this situation changed dramatically with the discovery of the *p73* gene (dubbed the big brother of *p53*). Located on 1p36, this gene encodes a protein that bears many similarities to *p53*. It has a DNA-binding domain that resembles the corresponding region of *p53*, and similar to the latter it can cause cell cycle arrest as well as apoptosis under appropriate conditions.[32, 33] Deletions of 1p36, where the *p73* gene resides, are common in a variety of tumors, including neuroblastoma and colon and breast cancers. Much interest is now focused on this missing relative of the *p53* gene.

BRCA-1 and BRCA-2 Genes. BRCA-1, on chromosome 17q12-21, and BRCA-2, on chromosome 13q12-13, are two recently discovered tumor-suppressor genes that are associated with the occurrence of breast and several other cancers. As with other tumor-suppressor genes, individuals who inherit mutations of BRCA-1 or BRCA-2 are highly susceptible to the development of breast cancer. With germ line mutations of the BRCA-1 gene, there is, in addition, a substantially higher risk of epithelial ovarian cancers and a slightly increased risk of prostate and colon cancers. Likewise, mutations in the BRCA-2 gene increase the risk of developing cancers of the male breast, ovary, and, possibly, prostate, pancreas, and larynx.[34] Approximately 5 to 10% of breast cancers are familial, and mutations in BRCA-1 and BRCA-2 account for 80% of the familial cases. Mutations of BRCA-1 and BRCA-2 are rarely found in sporadic breast cancer. Thus, it seems that, in contrast to many other tumor-suppressor genes (*Rb*, *p53*, NF-1) associated with heritable cancer syndromes, neither of the two BRCA genes is associated with the development of nonfamilial (sporadic) forms of breast cancer.

The functions of BRCA-1 and BRCA-2 are not fully defined. Protein products of both genes are localized to the nucleus and are believed to be involved in transcriptional regulation. Some data suggest that BRCA-1 and BRCA-2 are involved in DNA repair. This conclusion is based on the observation that the BRCA-1 and BRCA-2 proteins interact with Rad 51, a protein implicated in the regulation of recombination and double-stranded DNA repair.[35] According to this view, mutations in BRCA genes, similar to mutations in other DNA repair genes (see later), do not directly regulate cell growth; rather they predispose to errors in DNA replication, thus leading to mutations in other genes that directly affect cell cycle and cell growth. This hypothesis is not entirely consistent with the observation that, similar to *p53*, BRCA-1 can negatively regulate the cell cycle by transcriptional activation of the CDK inhibitor *p21*.[36] These complexities are currently under active investigation.

Molecules That Regulate Signal Transduction. Down-regulation of growth-promoting signals is another potential area in which products of tumor-suppressor genes may be operative. The products of the NF-1 gene and the APC gene fall into this category. Germ line mutations at the NF-1 (17q11.2) and the APC (5q21) loci are associated with benign tumors that are precursors of carcinomas that develop later.

In the case of the APC (*a*denomatous *p*olyposis *c*oli) gene, individuals born with one mutant allele invariably develop hundreds or even thousands of adenomatous polyps in the colon during their teens or twenties (familial adenomatous polyposis [FAP]; Chapter 18). Almost invariably, one or more of these polyps undergo malignant transformation, giving rise to colon cancer. As with other tumor-suppressor genes, both copies of the APC gene must be lost for tumor development. When this occurs, adenomas form. This conclusion is supported by the development of colonic adenomas in mice, with targeted disruption of APC genes in the colonic mucosa.[37] As discussed later, several additional mutations must occur for cancers to develop in adenomas (see p. 296). In addition to cancers arising in the setting of FAP, the majority (70 to 80%) of nonfamilial colorectal carcinomas and sporadic adenomas also show homozygous loss of the APC gene, thus firmly implicating APC loss in the pathogenesis of colonic tumors.

The molecular basis of APC action and the basis of its tumor-suppressor activity have been learned by the study of homologous genes in the fruitfly *Drosophila* and the amphibian *Xenopus*.[38] The APC protein is located in the cytoplasm, where it interacts with several other intracellular proteins, including β-catenin, a protein that can enter the nucleus and activate transcription of growth-promoting genes. *An important function of the APC protein is to cause degradation of β-catenin, thus maintaining low levels of the latter in the cytoplasm.* Inactivation of APC gene, and the consequent loss of APC protein, increases the cellular levels of β-catenin, which, in turn, translocates to the nucleus and up-regulates cellular proliferation. Thus, APC is a negative regulator of β-catenin signaling.[39] The importance of the APC-β-catenin signaling pathway in tumorigenesis is attested to by the fact that in those colonic cancers that have normal APC genes, β-catenin levels are elevated because mutations in β-catenin render it refractory to the degrading action of APC.[40] Dysregulation of the APC-β-catenin pathway is not restricted to colon cancers; mutations in either APC or β-catenin have also been found in nearly 30% of melanoma cell lines. Both β-catenin and APC have other cellular partners as well, suggesting that their normal functions extend beyond the regulation of β-catenin signaling. Of interest, β-catenin binds to the cytoplasmic aspect of E-cadherin, a cell surface protein that maintains intercellular adhesiveness. Cancer cells have reduced adhesiveness, resulting possibly from defects in the cadherin-catenin axis.

The NF-1 gene behaves similar to the APC gene. Individuals who inherit one mutant allele develop numerous benign neurofibromas, presumably as a result of inactivation of the second copy of the NF-1 gene. This condition is called *neurofibromatosis type 1* (Chapter 6). Some of the neurofibromas later develop into neurofibrosarcomas. Children with neurofibromatosis-1 also are at increased risk of developing acute myeloid leukemia.[41] The function of neurofibromin, the protein product of the NF-1 gene, is to regulate signal transduction via the *ras* protein (see earlier). Recall that the *ras* protein, involved in transmitting growth-promoting signals, flips back and forth between GDP-binding (inactive) and GTP-binding (active) states. Neurofibromin is a GTPase activating protein that facilitates conversion of active *ras* to inactive *ras*. With a loss of NF-1, *ras* is trapped in an active, signal-emitting state.

Cell Surface Receptors. Several types of molecules expressed on the cell surface can regulate cell growth and behavior. Such molecules include receptors for growth-inhibitory factors, such as TGF-β, and proteins that regulate cellular adhesions, such as the cadherins. The binding of TGF-β to its receptors up-regulates transcription of growth-inhibitory genes. It mediates this effect, in part, by stimulating the synthesis of cyclin-dependent kinase (CDK) inhibitors. These block the cell cycle by inhibiting the actions of cyclin/CDK complexes. Mutations of the TGF-β receptor and its signaling pathway have been discovered in many cancers. For example, the gene encoding a TGF-β receptor is inactivated in approximately 15% of colon cancers; similarly, SMAD2 and SMAD4 genes, which encode proteins in the TGF-β growth-inhibitory pathway, are also deleted or inactivated in certain colon and pancreatic cancers.[42]

Cadherins are a family of glycoproteins that act as glues between epithelial cells. Loss of cadherins can favor the malignant phenotype by allowing easy disaggregation of cells, which can then invade locally or metastasize. Reduced cell surface expression of E-cadherin has been noted in many types of cancers, including those that arise in the esophagus, colon, breast, ovary, and prostate.[43] Furthermore, loss of E-cadherin is causally related to the transition of an adenoma to a carcinoma in a mouse model of pancreatic β-cell tumors.[43a] Recent studies indicate that like many other tumor-suppressor genes, germ line mutations of the E-cadherin gene can predispose to familial gastric carcinoma.[43b] The molecular basis of reduced E-cadherin expression is varied. In a small proportion of cases, there are mutations in the E-cadherin gene (located on 16q); in other cancers, E-cadherin expression is reduced secondary to mutations in the catenin genes. Catenins, as discussed earlier, bind to the intracellular portion of cadherins and stabilize their expression.

*D*eleted in *c*olon *c*arcinoma (*DCC*) is a gene located on chromosome 18q21. Because this chromosome region is frequently deleted in human colon and rectum carcinomas, the DCC gene has been considered a candidate tumor-suppressor gene. Its structure resembles other cell surface molecules that are involved in cell-to-cell and cell-to-matrix interactions; hence it was proposed that the DCC gene may regulate cell growth and differentiation by integrating signals from the cell's environment. Study of DCC knockout mice, however, has raised serious doubts regarding the likelihood of DCC being a tumor-suppressor gene. Instead, it appears that DCC is a cell surface receptor important in axonal growth.[44] Thus, it seems that some other gene in close linkage with DCC on chromosome 18q21 is the real culprit for carcinogenesis.

Other Tumor-Suppressor Genes. There is little doubt that many more tumor-suppressor genes remain to be discovered. Often, their location is suspected by the detection of consistent sites of chromosomal deletions or by loss-of-heterozygosity studies. Some of the tumor-suppressor genes of unknown function that are associated with well-defined clinical syndromes are briefly described below:

- *NF-2 gene*: Germ line mutations in the NF-2 gene predispose to the development of neurofibromatosis type 2. As discussed in Chapter 6, patients with NF-2 develop bilateral schwannomas of the acoustic nerve. In addition, somatic mutations affecting both alleles of NF-2 have also been found in sporadic meningiomas and ependymomas. The product of the NF-2 gene, called *merlin*, shows a great deal of homology with the red cell membrane cytoskeletal protein 4.1 (Chapter 14).[45] Merlin binds, on one hand, to actin and, on the other hand, to CD44, a transmembrane protein that is involved in cell-matrix interactions; how loss of merlin leads to transformation is not known.
- *VHL*: Germ line mutations of the *V*on *H*ippel–*L*indau

(*VHL*) gene on chromosome 3p are associated with hereditary renal cell cancers, pheochromocytomas, hemangioblastomas of the central nervous system, retinal angiomas, and renal cysts. Mutations of the VHL gene have also been noted in sporadic renal cell cancers (Chapter 21). The VHL protein regulates transcription elongation by RNA polymerase. How this function is related to tumorigenesis is not understood at present.

- *PTEN*: *P*hosphatase and *ten*sin homolog, deleted on chromosome 10 gene (*PTEN*), mapped on chromosome 10q23, is frequently deleted in many human cancers, including glioblastomas, prostate cancer, endometrial cancer, and breast cancer. The structure of this gene suggests that it may negatively regulate cell interactions with extracellular matrix by dephosphorylating undefined substrates.[46, 46a]
- *WT-1*: WT-1 gene, located on chromosome 11p13, is associated with the development of *W*ilms *t*umor. Both inherited and sporadic forms of Wilms tumor occur, and mutational inactivation of the WT-1 locus has been seen in both forms. The WT-1 protein is a transcriptional regulator that presumably inhibits transcription of growth-promoting genes. In addition to WT-1, Wilms tumor is also associated with two other genes, one located on 11p15 and the other at a site not linked to chromosome 11 (Chapter 11).

Genes That Regulate Apoptosis

For many years, oncogenes and cancer-suppressor genes held center stage in the understanding of the molecular basis of tumorigenesis. Although they act quite differently, ultimately genes belonging to both of these classes regulate cell proliferation. It is now appreciated that genes that prevent or induce programmed cell death are also important variables in the cancer equation.[47] A large family of genes that regulate apoptosis has been identified.[48] Mercifully for nonexperts, these genes can be remembered as a series of three-letter words beginning with *b*. The first antiapoptotic gene identified, *bcl-2* is a member of a large family of homodimerizing and heterodimerizing proteins, some of which inhibit apoptosis (such as *bcl-2* itself and *bcl-xL*), whereas others (such as *bax*, *bad*, and *bcl-xS*) favor programmed cell death.

The discovery of *bcl-2*, the prototypic gene in this category, began with the observation that approximately 85% of B-cell lymphomas of the follicular type (Chapter 15) carry a characteristic t(14;18)(q32;q21) translocation. Recall that 14q32, the site where immunoglobulin heavy-chain genes are found, is also involved in Burkitt lymphoma. Juxtaposition of this transcriptionally active locus with *bcl-2* (located at 18q21) causes overexpression of the *bcl-2* protein. *By mechanisms not yet clear, overexpression of bcl-2 protects lymphocytes from apoptosis and allows them to survive for long periods; thus there is a steady accumulation of B lymphocytes, resulting in lymphadenopathy and marrow infiltration.* Because *bcl-2* overexpressing lymphomas arise in large part from reduced cell death rather than explosive cell proliferation, they tend to be indolent (slow growing) compared with most other lymphomas. Supporting the role of *bcl-2* in lymphomagenesis is the observation that mice transgenic for *bcl-2* develop B-cell lymphomas. Not only is the function of *bcl-2* unusual, but also its location is different from most cancer-associated genes. It is localized on the outer leaflet of the mitochondrial membrane, the endoplasmic reticulum, and the nuclear membrane. The mitochondrial location of *bcl-2* and other members of the *bcl-2* family may have bearing on the functioning of these genes.

The biochemical basis of *bcl-2* action, also discussed in Chapter 1, is not entirely clear. Apoptosis is the end point of a cascade of molecular events that are initiated by several stimuli and lead ultimately to the activation of proteolytic enzymes responsible for cell death. The *bcl-2* family of proteins regulates the activation of these proteolytic enzymes (caspases). How, precisely, the *bcl-2* family members influence the activation of caspases is under intense scrutiny. The following represents an outline of the current thinking on the action of *bcl-2*.[49–51] (In this rapidly moving field, however, hypotheses are proposed and rejected more rapidly than the growth of highly malignant tumors!)

- In many models of apoptosis, release of cytochrome C from the mitochondria appears to be a critical step in the chain of events that lead to apoptosis. One function of the released cytochrome C seems to be to assist in the activation of the proteolytic enzyme caspase 9.[52]
- Located strategically on the outer mitochondrial membranes, *bcl-2* and its partners are believed to regulate the exit of cytochrome C from the mitochondrion to the cytoplasm. How exactly this transit of cytochrome C is regulated is not entirely clear, but there is some evidence that *bax*, a proapoptotic member of the *bcl-2* family, forms a channel in the mitochondrial membrane that allows the exit of cytochrome C (and hence apoptosis), whereas *bcl-2* blocks the channel-forming activity of *bax*.
- The proapoptotic and antiapoptotic members of the *bcl-2* family act as a rheostat in regulating programmed cell death. The ratio of death antagonists (*bcl-2, bcl-xL*) to agonists (*bax, bcl-xS*, *bad, bid*) determines whether a cell will respond to an apoptotic stimulus (Fig. 8–33). This rheostat is operated, at least in part, by competitive dimerization between various family members. Thus, whereas *bcl-2* homodimers favor cell survival (possibly by displacing the channel-forming *bax* from the mitochondrial membrane), *bax* homodimers favor apoptosis. It follows that factors that regulate the transcription of *bcl-2* family members can influence apoptosis. As previously discussed, the proapoptotic action of the tumor-suppressor gene *p53* seems to be mediated by up-regulation of the *bax* gene. In keeping with this notion, up-regulation of *bax* in *bax*-transgenic mice suppresses tumor growth by promoting apoptosis.[53]

Finally, although the *bcl-2* family of genes plays an important role in regulating apoptosis, at least two other cancer-associated genes are also intimately connected with apoptosis: the *p53* gene and the protooncogene c-*myc*. The molecular mechanisms of cell death induced by these two intersect with the *bcl-2* pathways. Activation of *p53*, as discussed previously, up-regulates *bax* synthesis and hence

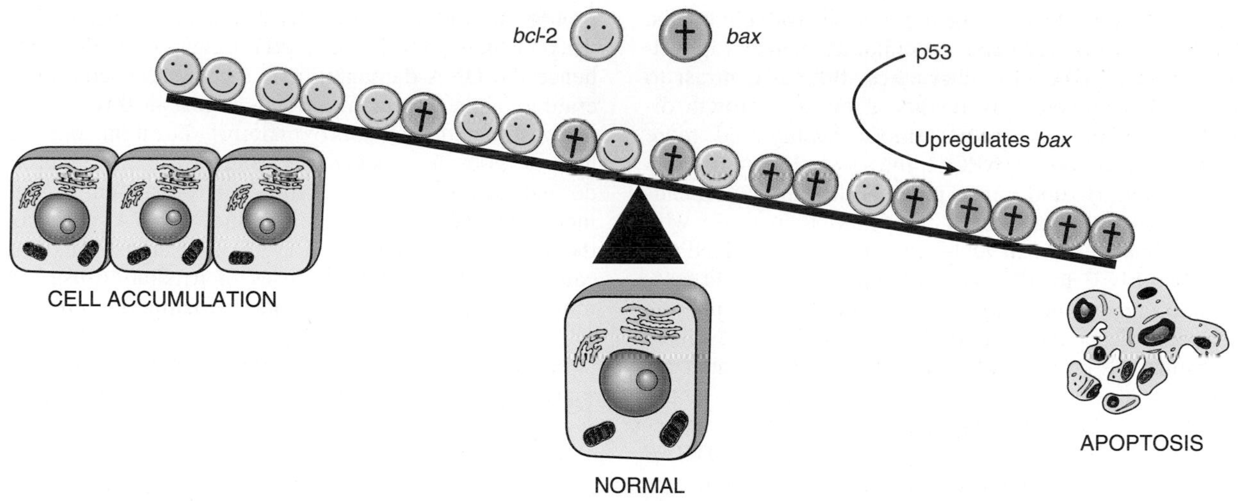

Figure 8–33

Regulation of cell death by *bcl*-2, *bax,* and *p53. bcl*-2 dimers favor cell accumulation by inhibiting apoptosis; *bax* dimers favor apoptosis. The apoptosis-inducing effect of normal *p53* genes is mediated in part by increasing the synthesis of *bax* protein.

counteracts the antiapoptotic action of *bcl-2.* c-*myc* induces apoptosis when cells are driven by c-*myc* activation, but growth is restricted by the limited availability of growth factors in the milieu. When confronted by such conflicting signals, the cells are programmed to die by up-regulation of *p53* and other undefined signals. Overexpression of *bcl-2* can rescue cells from c-*myc*-initiated apoptosis. Thus, it appears that *myc* and *bcl-2* may collaborate in tumorigenesis: c-*myc* triggers proliferation, and *bcl-2* prevents cell death, even if growth factors become limiting. This is one of many examples in which two or more cancer genes cooperate in giving rise to cancer.

Genes That Regulate DNA Repair

Humans literally swim in a sea of environmental carcinogens. Although exposure to naturally occurring DNA-damaging agents, such as ionizing radiation, sunlight, and dietary carcinogens, is common, cancer is a relatively rare outcome of such encounters. This happy state of affairs results from the ability of normal cells to repair DNA damage and thus prevent mutations in genes that regulate cell growth and apoptosis. In addition to possible DNA damage from environmental agents, the DNA of normal dividing cells is also susceptible to alterations resulting from errors that occur spontaneously during DNA replication. Such mistakes, if not repaired promptly, can also push the cells along the slippery slope of neoplastic transformation. The importance of DNA repair in maintaining the integrity of the genome is highlighted by several inherited disorders in which genes that encode proteins involved in DNA repair are defective. *Those born with such inherited mutations of DNA repair proteins are at a greatly increased risk of developing cancer.* Several examples are discussed next.

The role of DNA repair genes in predisposition to cancer is illustrated dramatically by the *h*ereditary *non*polyposis colon cancer (*HNPCC*) syndrome. This disorder is characterized by familial carcinomas of the colon affecting predominantly the cecum and proximal colon (Chapter 18). In contrast to the carcinomas in patients with germ line APC mutations, the cancers in HNPCC do not arise in adenomatous polyps. There are several types of DNA damage, and, correspondingly, there are many forms of DNA repair. HNPCC results from defects in genes involved in DNA mismatch repair. When a strand of DNA is replicating, mismatch repair genes act as "spell checkers." Thus, for example, if there is an erroneous pairing of G with T, rather than the normal A with T, the mismatch repair genes correct the defect.[54] Without these proofreaders, errors slowly accumulate in several genes, including protooncogenes and tumor-suppressor genes. *DNA repair genes themselves are not oncogenic, but they allow mutations in other genes during the process of normal cell division.*

Cells with such defects in DNA repair are said to have the *replication error* (RER) phenotype, which can be readily documented by examination of microsatellite sequences in the tumor cell DNA. Microsatellites are tandem repeats of one to six nucleotides scattered throughout the genome (Chapter 6). Microsatellite sequences of an individual are fixed for life and are the same in every tissue. With errors in mismatch repair, there are expansions and contractions of these repeats in tumor cells, creating alleles not found in normal cells of the same patient. Such *microsatellite instability* is a hallmark of defective mismatch repair. Of the various DNA mismatch repair genes, at least four are involved in the pathogenesis of HNPCC. Germ line mutations in hMSH2 (2p16) account for tumor development in 50% of the families with HNPCC. In roughly 30% of HNPCC cases, the mutation affects the hMLH1 gene, on chromosome 3p21. The remaining 20% of cases have mutations in hPMS1 and hPMS2 and other mismatch repair genes.[55] Each affected individual inherits one defective copy of one of the several DNA mismatch repair genes and acquires the "second hit" in the colonic epithelial cells. Thus, DNA repair genes behave similar to cancer-suppressor genes in their mode of inheritance, but, in contrast to tumor-suppressor genes, they do not affect cell growth directly. Because mutations occur more readily and more rapidly in patients with HNPCC, the evolution of tumors occurs more rapidly, and hence patients develop colon cancers at a much younger age (<50 years) than those who do not have any defects in DNA repair. Although HNPCC accounts for only 2 to 4% of all colonic cancers, microsatellite instability can be detected in about 15% of sporadic colon cancers. It is likely that these sporadic cases have somatic mutations in other genes that affect mismatch repair. The growth-regulating genes that are mutated in patients with HNPCC have not yet been completely characterized but include those that encode receptors for TGF-β and the apoptosis-inducing protein *bax*. As discussed earlier, loss of TGF-β receptors nullifies the growth-inhibiting action of TGF-β, and mutations in the *bax* gene dysregulate apoptosis. It is likely that the genomic instability resulting from loss of mismatch repair genes also affects many other cancer-associated genes. Although mismatch errors in DNA replication can occur in any dividing cell, carcinomas occur mainly in the proximal colon in those with HNPCC. In some families, there is also an associated increase in endometrial and ovarian cancers, but, quite mysteriously, most other tissues are spared.

Patients with another inherited disorder, xeroderma pigmentosum, are at increased risk for the development of cancers of the skin exposed to the UV light contained in sun rays. The basis of this disorder is also defective DNA repair. UV light causes cross-linking of pyrimidine residues, thus preventing normal DNA replication. Such DNA damage is repaired by the nucleotide excision repair system (discussed later). Several proteins and genes are involved in nucleotide excision repair, and an inherited loss of any one can give rise to xeroderma pigmentosum.

In addition to the examples mentioned earlier, a group of autosomal recessive disorders comprising Bloom syndrome, ataxia telangiectasia, and Fanconi anemia are characterized by hypersensitivity to other DNA-damaging agents, such as ionizing radiation (Bloom syndrome and ataxia telangiectasia), or DNA cross-linking agents, such as nitrogen mustard (Fanconi anemia). Their phenotype is complex and includes, in addition to predisposition to cancer, other features such as neural symptoms (ataxia telangiectasia), anemia (Fanconi anemia), and developmental defects (Bloom syndrome).[56]

Patients with *ataxia telangiectasia* (AT) have a complex phenotype, characterized by gradual loss of Purkinje cells in the cerebellum, immunodeficiency, acute sensitivity to ionizing radiation, and profound susceptibility to lymphoid malignancies. For a while, it was thought that ataxia telangiectasia is genetically heterogeneous, but the AT gene has been cloned, and this disorder results from mutation in a single gene. All the functions of the AT gene have not yet been elucidated, but it seems quite likely that the AT protein acts as a sensor of DNA damage caused by ionizing radiation. After such damage, the *p53* gene is activated, and this causes cell cycle arrest in G_1. It seems that the AT protein recognizes DNA damage and then signals the *p53* protein into action.[57] In cells lacking the normal AT genes, the *p53*-induced delay in the cell cycle does not occur, and hence the DNA-damaged cells are liable to continue proliferating. There is much current interest in this gene because it is estimated that approximately 1% of the population is heterozygous and hence a carrier. Although heterozygotes do not develop cancers, they are presumed to be at an increased risk for radiation-induced DNA damage. It is therefore speculated that they may be at risk of developing cancers after exposure to doses of irradiation used in common radiologic procedures such as mammography.

Telomeres and Cancer

In the discussion of cellular aging (Chapter 2), it was pointed out that after a fixed number of divisions, normal cells become arrested in a terminally nondividing state, known as cellular senescence. How normal cells can "count" their divisions is not known, but it has been noted that with each cell division there is some shortening of specialized structures, called *telomeres*, at the ends of chromosomes. Once the telomeres are shortened beyond a certain point, the loss of telomere function leads to end-to-end chromosome fusion and cell death. Thus, telomere shortening is believed to be a clock that counts cell divisions. In germ cells, telomere shortening is prevented by the sustained function of the enzyme telomerase, thus explaining the ability of these cells to self-replicate extensively. This enzyme is absent from most somatic cells, and hence they suffer progressive loss of telomeres. A recent study has shown that introduction of telomerase into normal human cells causes considerable extension of their life span,[58] thus supporting the hypothesis that telomerase loss is causally associated with loss of replication ability. If loss of telomerase is the basis of the finite life span of cells, how do cancer cells continue to divide indefinitely? The telomerase hypothesis of cellular aging would predict that in addition to the loss of normal growth regulatory influences, cancer cells must find a way to prevent telomere shortening. An obvious mechanism to accomplish this might be to reactivate telomerase. Indeed, telomerase activity has been detected in the vast majority of human tumors,[59] and in those that lack telomerase, other telomere-lengthening mechanisms have been found.[60] It could be hypothesized therefore that telomere shortening is a tumor-suppressive mechanism. This intriguing notion is now under active investigation.

Molecular Basis of Multistep Carcinogenesis

The notion that malignant tumors arise from a protracted sequence of events is supported by epidemiologic, experimental, and molecular studies. Many eons ago, before oncogenes and antioncogenes had infiltrated the scientific literature, cancer epidemiologists had suggested that the age-associated increase in cancers could best be explained by postulating that five or six independent steps were required for tumorigenesis. This idea received initial support from experimental models of chemical carcinogenesis in which the process of tumor formation could be divided into distinct steps, such as initiation and promotion. The study of oncogenes and tumor-suppressor genes has provided a firm molecular footing for the concept of multistep carcinogenesis:[61]

- DNA transfection experiments reveal that no single oncogene (e.g., *myc, ras*) can fully transform cells in vitro but that together *ras* and *myc* can transform fibroblasts. Such cooperation is required because each oncogene is specialized to induce part of the phenotype necessary for full transformation. In this example, *ras* oncogene induces cells to secrete growth factors and enables them to grow without anchorage to a normal substrate (anchorage independence), whereas *myc* oncogene renders cells more sensitive to growth factors and immortalizes cells. As mentioned earlier, *myc* and *bcl-2* also cooperate in neoplastic transformation.
- *Every human cancer that has been analyzed reveals multiple genetic alterations involving activation of several oncogenes and loss of two or more cancer-suppressor genes.* Each of these alterations represents a crucial step in the progression from a normal cell to a malignant tumor. A dramatic example of incremental acquisition of the malignant phenotype is documented by the study of colon carcinoma.[61, 62] These lesions evolve through a series of morphologically identifiable stages: colon epithelial hyperplasia followed by formation of adenomas that progressively enlarge and ultimately undergo malignant transformation (Chapter 18). The proposed molecular correlates of this adenoma-carcinoma sequence are illustrated in Figure 8–34. According to this scheme, inactivation of the APC tumor-suppressor gene occurs first, followed by activation of *ras* and, ultimately, loss of some unidentified tumor-suppressor gene on 18q and loss of *p53* genes.

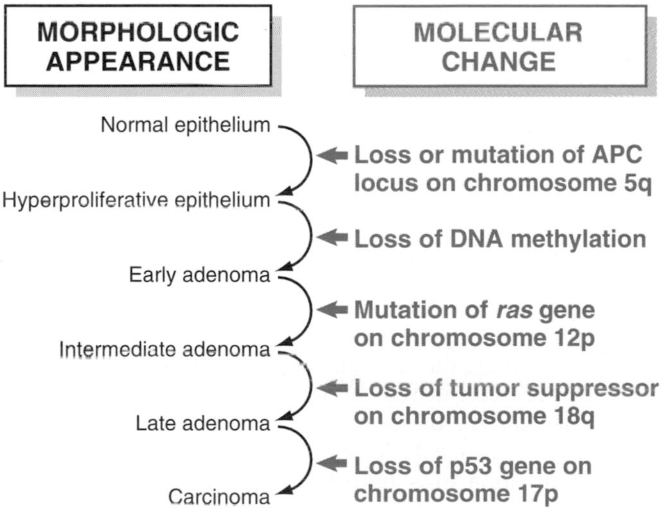

MORPHOLOGIC APPEARANCE	MOLECULAR CHANGE
Normal epithelium	
	Loss or mutation of APC locus on chromosome 5q
Hyperproliferative epithelium	
	Loss of DNA methylation
Early adenoma	
	Mutation of *ras* gene on chromosome 12p
Intermediate adenoma	
	Loss of tumor suppressor on chromosome 18q
Late adenoma	
	Loss of p53 gene on chromosome 17p
Carcinoma	

Figure 8–34

Molecular model for the evolution of colorectal cancers through the adenoma-carcinoma sequence. (Based on studies of Fearon ER, Vogelstein B: A genetic model of colorectal carcinogenesis. Cell 61:759, 1990. Copyright 1990, Cell Press.)

Given the fact that multiple mutations are essential for the development of cancer, one might ask whether the specific order of mutations is also important. Contrary to earlier beliefs, it is now thought that the temporal sequence of mutations does determine the propensity of tumor development. Thus, in the case of colon cancer, APC inactivation is considered an important first step for carcinogenesis, and this mutation is present in the earliest neoplastic lesions (adenomas). Furthermore, although mice with targeted disruption of the APC gene develop multiple colonic adenomas, those with homozygous deletions of the *p53* gene develop many tumors but not colon carcinomas. This suggests that *p53* mutations play a role in the progression (but not initiation) of colonic cancer.

Genes such as APC that seem to regulate the entry into the multistep carcinogenesis pathway have been called "gatekeeper" genes.[63] These genes directly regulate the growth of tumors. According to this view, each cell type has only one (or few) gatekeeper genes, and thus even if a given gatekeeper gene is inactivated in every somatic cell, there is a specific tissue distribution of cancer (Fig. 8–35). In support of this hypothesis, germ line mutations of the *Rb*, NF-1, VHL, or APC genes give rise to retinoblastomas, schwannomas, renal cell cancer, and colon cancer. In contrast to gatekeeper genes, those that affect genomic stability are called "caretaker" genes. In this category are mismatch repair genes and other putative DNA repair genes, such as BRCA-1 and BRCA-2. Inactivation of these genes does not promote tumor initiation directly. Instead, loss of caretaker genes results in increased mutation of all genes, including gatekeeper genes. Thus, in patients with germ line mutations of caretaker genes (such as DNA mismatch repair genes), three subsequent somatic events are required for cancer initiation: inactivation of the other (normal) caretaker allele followed by mutational inactivation of both copies of a gatekeeper gene. By comparison, those who inherit one defective copy of a gatekeeper gene require only one more somatic event for cancer initiation (Fig. 8–35). Thus, although patients with germ line mutations of either the gatekeeper or caretaker genes are at a higher-than-normal risk of developing cancer, the relative risk is much greater in those born with a defective copy of a gatekeeper gene.

This distinction between gatekeepers and caretakers is of some practical importance. If this hypothesis is correct, tumors associated with defective caretaker genes might respond to treatments that inflict the kind of DNA damage that is normally repaired by the caretaker gene. As an example, breast cancer cells that arise as a result of inherited mutation in BRCA-2 would be killed by γ-irradiation because normal BRCA-2 and its partner, Rad 51, are involved in repairing irradiation-induced damage. By contrast, cells in sporadic breast cancer with no inactivation of BRCA-2 are likely to be less sensitive to irradiation because they would retain the BRCA-2-mediated capacity to repair DNA damage caused by irradiation. Whether this is the case remains to be tested, but it is certain that such molecular insights into the causation of cancer are likely to

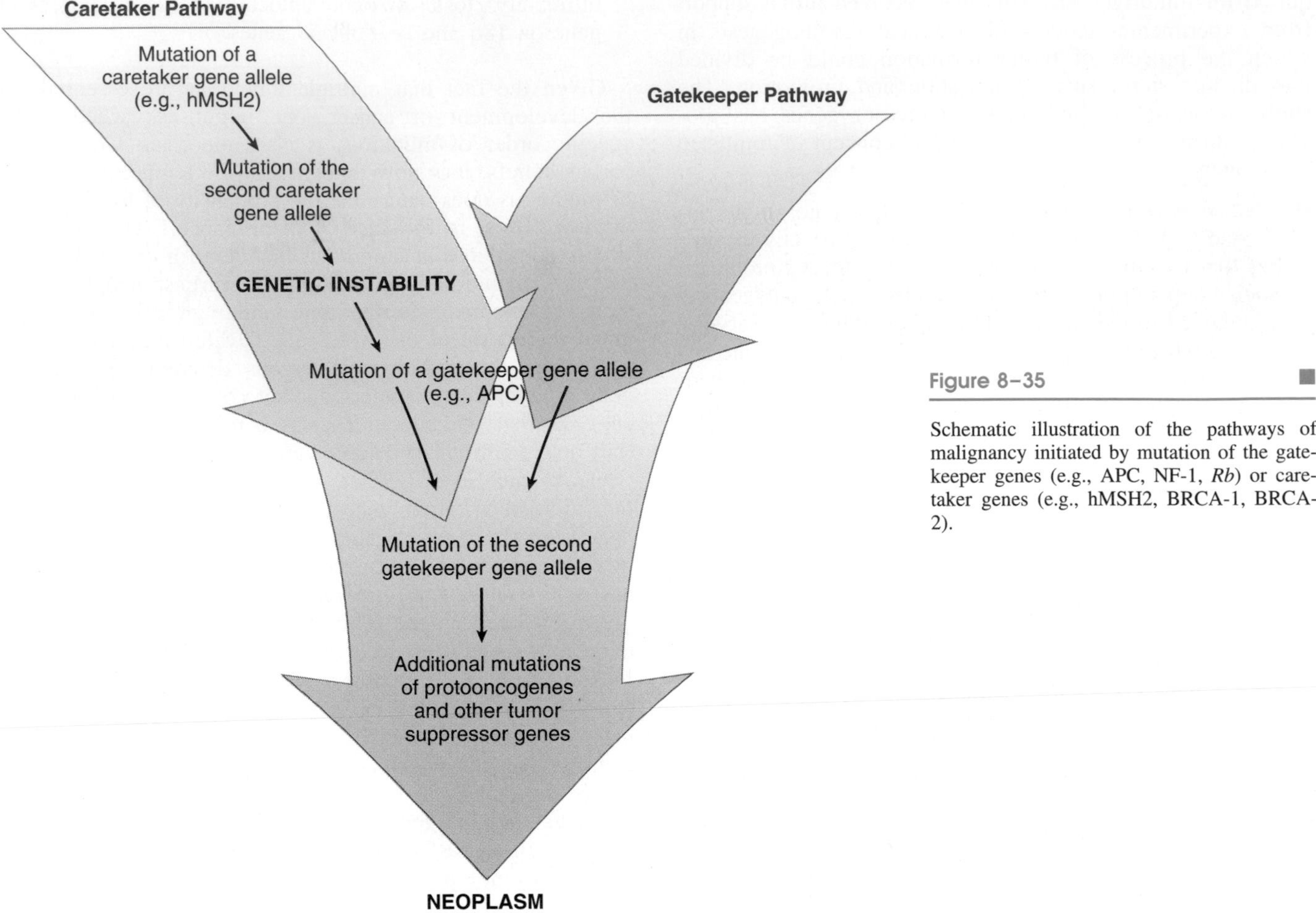

Figure 8–35

Schematic illustration of the pathways of malignancy initiated by mutation of the gatekeeper genes (e.g., APC, NF-1, *Rb*) or caretaker genes (e.g., hMSH2, BRCA-1, BRCA-2).

have an impact on therapy in the future. Figure 8–36 summarizes the possible functions and subcellular locations of genes that are altered in malignant tumors.

Karyotypic Changes in Tumors

The genetic damage that activates oncogenes or inactivates tumor-suppressor genes may be subtle (e.g., point mutations) or be large enough to be detected in a karyotype. In certain neoplasms, karyotypic abnormalities are nonrandom and common. Specific abnormalities have been identified in most leukemias and lymphomas and in an increasing number of nonhematopoietic tumors. The common types of nonrandom structural abnormalities in tumor cells are (1) balanced translocations, (2) deletions, and (3) cytogenetic manifestations of gene amplification. In addition, whole chromosomes may be gained or lost.

The study of chromosomal changes in tumor cells is important on two accounts. First, molecular cloning of genes in the vicinity of chromosomal breakpoints or deletions has been extremely useful in identification of oncogenes (e.g., *bcl*-2, c-*abl*) and tumor-suppressor genes (e.g., APC, *Rb*). Second, certain karyotypic abnormalities are specific enough to be of diagnostic value, and in some cases they are predictive of clinical course. Several examples of karyotypic changes were provided in the discussion of carcinogenesis. Many others are described with later considerations of specific forms of neoplasia.

BIOLOGY OF TUMOR GROWTH

The natural history of most malignant tumors can be divided into four phases: (1) malignant change in the target cell, referred to as *transformation*; (2) *growth* of the transformed cells; (3) local *invasion*; and (4) distant *metastases.* In this sequence, the molecular basis of transformation has already been considered. Next we discuss the factors that affect the growth of transformed cells and, last, the biochemical and molecular basis of invasion and metastasis.

The formation of a tumor mass by the clonal descendants of a transformed cell is a complex process that is influenced by many factors. Some, such as doubling time of tumor cells, are intrinsic to the tumor cells, whereas others, such as angiogenesis, represent host responses elicited by tumor cells or their products. The multiple factors

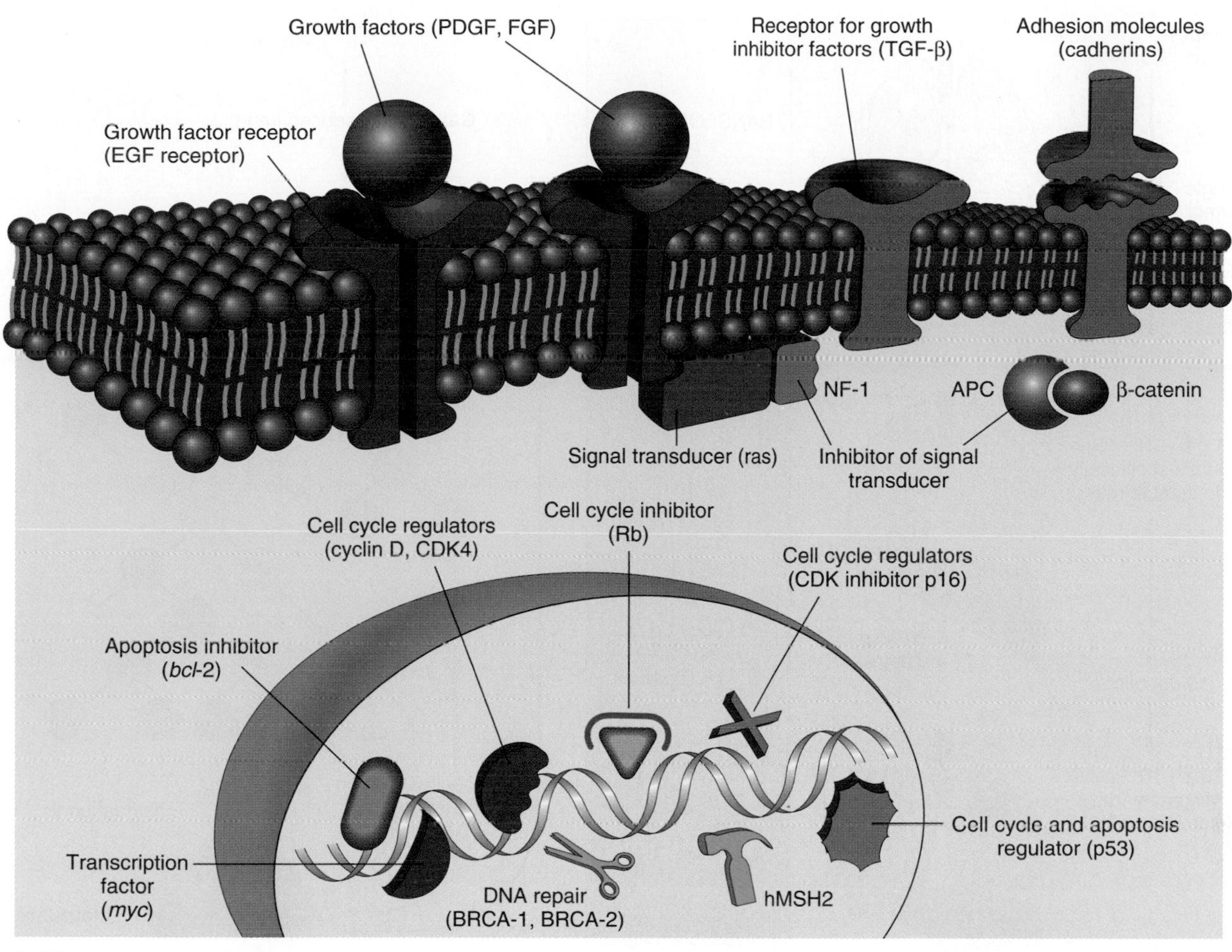

Figure 8–36

Subcellular localization and functions of major classes of cancer-associated genes. The protooncogenes are colored red, cancer suppressor genes blue, DNA repair genes green, and genes that regulate apoptosis purple.

that influence tumor growth are considered under three headings: (1) kinetics of tumor cell growth, (2) tumor angiogenesis, and (3) tumor progression and heterogeneity.

Kinetics of Tumor Cell Growth

One can begin the consideration of tumor cell kinetics by asking the question: How long does it take to produce a clinically overt tumor mass? It can be readily calculated that the original transformed cell (approximately 10 μ in diameter) must undergo at least 30 population doublings to produce 10^9 cells (weighing approximately 1 gm), which is the smallest clinically detectable mass. In contrast, only 10 further doubling cycles are required to produce a tumor containing 10^{12} cells (weighing approximately 1 kg), which is usually the maximal size compatible with life (Fig. 8–37). These are minimal estimates, based on the assumption that all descendants of the transformed cell retain the ability to divide and that there is no loss of cells from the replicative pool. This concept of tumor as a "pathologic dynamo" is not entirely correct, as we discuss subsequently.[64] Nevertheless, this calculation highlights an extremely important concept about tumor growth: *By the time a solid tumor is clinically detected, it has already completed a major portion of its life cycle.* This, as we see subsequently, is a major impediment in the treatment of cancer. First, however, we examine the veracity of the assumption that a malignant tumor is a pathologic dynamo—a mass of rapidly and relentlessly dividing cells. To resolve this issue, it is necessary to address the following questions that relate to tumor cell kinetics:

- What is the doubling time of tumor cells?
- What is the fraction of tumor cells that are in the replicative pool?
- What is the rate at which cells are shed and lost in the growing lesion?

Because cell cycle controls exerted by *Rb*, *p53*, and cyclins are deranged in most tumors, tumor cells can be triggered into cycle more readily and without the usual restraints. The dividing cells, however, do not complete the

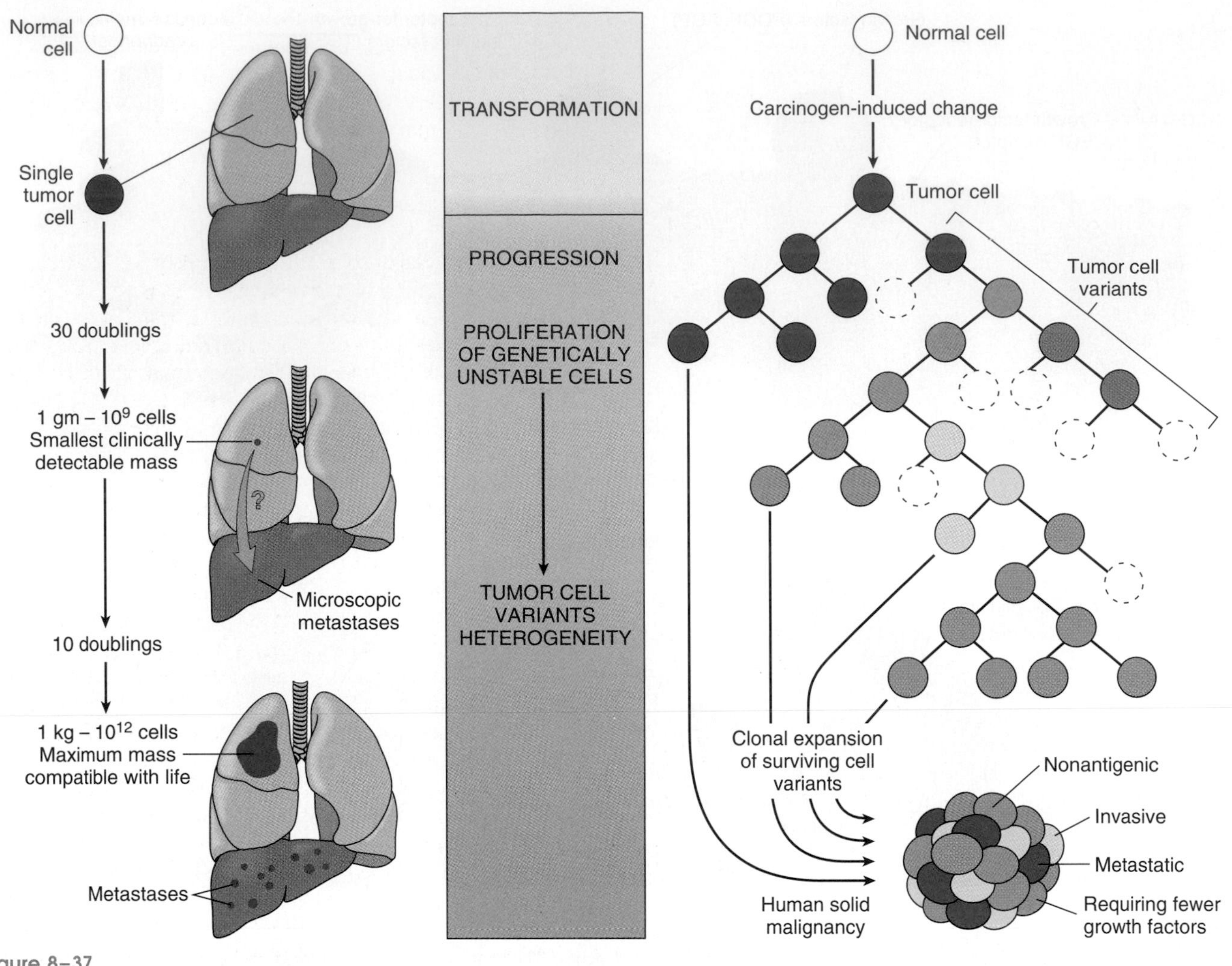

Figure 8–37

Biology of tumor growth. The left panel depicts minimal estimates of tumor cell doublings that precede the formation of a clinically detectable tumor mass. It is evident that by the time a solid tumor is detected, it has already completed a major portion of its life cycle as measured by cell doublings. The right panel illustrates clonal evolution of tumors and generation of tumor cell heterogeneity. New subclones arise from the descendants of the original transformed cell, and with progressive growth the tumor mass becomes enriched for those variants that are more adept at evading host defenses and are likely to be more aggressive. (Adapted from Tannock IF: Biology of tumor growth. Hosp Pract 18:81, 1983.)

cell cycle more rapidly than normal cells. In reality, total cell cycle time for many tumors is equal to or longer than that of corresponding normal cells. *Thus, it can be safely concluded that growth of tumors is not commonly associated with a shortening of cell cycle time.*

The proportion of cells within the tumor population that are in the proliferative pool is referred to as the *growth fraction.* Clinical and experimental studies suggest that during the early, submicroscopic phase of tumor growth, the vast majority of transformed cells are in the proliferative pool (Fig. 8–38). As tumors continue to grow, cells leave the replicative pool in ever-increasing numbers owing to shedding or lack of nutrients, by differentiating, and by reversion to G_0. Most cells within cancers remain in the G_0 or G_1 phase. Thus, by the time a tumor is clinically detectable, most cells are not in the replicative pool. Even in some rapidly growing tumors, the growth fraction is approximately 20%.

Ultimately the progressive growth of tumors and the rate at which they grow are determined by the *excess of cell production over cell loss.* In some tumors, especially those with a relatively high growth fraction, the imbalance is large, resulting in more rapid growth than in those in which cell production exceeds cell loss by only a small margin.

There are several important conceptual and practical lessons to be learned from these studies of tumor cell kinetics:

- The rate of tumor growth depends on the growth fraction and the degree of imbalance between cell production and cell loss. Some leukemias and lymphomas and

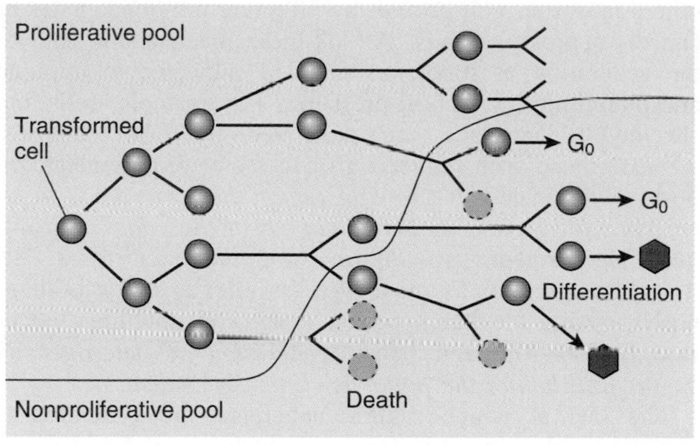

Figure 8–38

Schematic representation of tumor growth. As the cell population expands, a progressively higher percentage of tumor cells leaves the replicative pool by reversion of G_0, differentiation, and death.

certain lung cancers (small cell carcinoma) have a relatively high growth fraction, and their clinical course is rapid. By comparison, many common tumors such as cancers of the colon and breast have low growth fractions, and cell production exceeds cell loss by only about 10%; they tend to grow at a much slower pace.

- The growth fraction of tumor cells has a profound effect on their susceptibility to cancer chemotherapy. Because most anticancer agents act on cells that are in cell cycle, it is not difficult to imagine that a tumor that contains 5% of all cells in the replicating pool will be slow growing but relatively refractory to treatment with drugs that kill dividing cells. Paradoxically, otherwise aggressive tumors (such as certain lymphomas) that contain a large pool of dividing cells literally melt away with chemotherapy, and even cures may be effected. One strategy employed in the treatment of tumors with low growth fraction (e.g., cancer of colon, breast) is first to shift tumor cells from G_0 into the cell cycle. This can be accomplished by debulking the tumor with surgery or radiation. The surviving tumor cells tend to enter the cell cycle and thus become susceptible to drug therapy. Such considerations form the basis of combined modality treatment.

We can now return to the question posed earlier: How long does it take for one transformed cell to produce a clinically detectable tumor containing 10^9 cells? If every one of the daughter cells remained in cell cycle and no cells were shed or lost, we could anticipate the answer to be 90 days (30 population doublings, with a cell cycle time of 3 days; see Fig. 8–37). In reality, *the latent period before which a tumor becomes clinically detectable is quite unpredictably long, probably years, emphasizing once again that human cancers are diagnosed only after they are fairly advanced in their life cycle.* After they become clinically detectable, the average volume-doubling time for such common killers as cancer of the lung and colon is about 2 to 3 months. As might be anticipated from the discussion of the variables that affect growth rate, however, the range of doubling time values is extremely broad, varying from less than 1 month for some childhood cancers to more than 1 year for certain salivary gland tumors. Cancer is indeed an unpredictable disorder.

Tumor Angiogenesis

Factors other than cell kinetics modify the rate of tumor growth. Most important among these is blood supply. Tumors cannot enlarge beyond 1 to 2 mm in diameter or thickness unless they are vascularized. Presumably the 1- to 2-mm zone represents the maximal distance across which oxygen and nutrients can diffuse from blood vessels. Beyond this size, the tumor fails to enlarge without vascularization because hypoxia induces apoptosis by activation of *p53* (see earlier). Neovascularization has a dual effect on tumor growth: Perfusion supplies nutrients and oxygen, and newly formed endothelial cells stimulate the growth of adjacent tumor cells by secreting polypeptides such as insulin-like growth factors, PDGF, GM-CSF, and IL-1.[65] Angiogenesis is requisite not only for continued tumor growth, but also for metastasis. Without access to the vasculature, the tumor cells cannot metastasize. Hence *angiogenesis is a necessary biologic correlate of malignancy.*[66] In keeping with this, several studies have revealed a correlation between the extent of angiogenesis (microvessel density) and the probability of metastases in melanomas and cancers of the breast, lung, colon, and prostate.[67] In some of these cancers (breast, prostate), vessel density has proven to be a significant prognostic indicator.

How do growing tumors develop a blood supply? Several studies indicate that tumors contain factors that are capable of effecting the entire series of events involved in the formation of new capillaries (Chapter 4). Tumor-associated angiogenic factors may be produced by tumor cells or may be derived from inflammatory cells (e.g., macrophages) that infiltrate tumors. Of the dozen or so tumor-associated angiogenic factors, the two most important are vascular endothelial growth factor (VEGF) and basic fibroblast growth factor (bFGF). The mechanisms whereby bFGF and VEGF cause angiogenesis were discussed in Chapter 4. These two are commonly expressed in a wide variety of tumor cells, and elevated levels can be detected in the serum and urine of a significant fraction of cancer patients. The clinical utility of these surrogate markers of angiogenesis in predicting clinical course and prognosis of cancer is under investigation.

Recent studies suggest that tumor cells not only produce angiogenic factors, but also induce antiangiogenesis molecules. Tumor growth is thus controlled by the balance between angiogenic factors and those that inhibit angiogenesis. Antiangiogenesis factors, such as thrombospondin-1, may be produced by the tumor cells themselves, or their production may be induced by tumor cells. To the latter category belong angiostatin, endostatin, and vasculostatin. These three potent angiogenesis inhibitors are derived by proteolytic cleavage of plasminogen, collagen, and transthyretin, respectively.

Experimental and clinical data indicate that early in their growth most human tumors do not induce angiogenesis. They exist in situ without developing a blood supply for months to years, then, presumably owing to the accumulation of mutations, some cells within the small tumor switch to an angiogenic phenotype. The molecular basis of the angiogenic switch is not entirely clear but may involve increased production of angiogenic factors or loss of angiogenesis inhibitors.[68] Wild-type *p53* gene seems to inhibit angiogenesis by inducing the synthesis of the antiangiogenic molecule thrombospondin-1. With mutational inactivation of both *p53* alleles (a common event in many cancers), the levels of thrombospondin-1 drop precipitously, thus tilting the balance in favor of angiogenic factors. It is suspected that there is another tumor-suppressor gene located on 16p that also inhibits angiogenesis, presumably by regulating the balance of angiogenic and antiangiogenic factors.

Because angiogenesis is critical for the growth and spread of tumors, much attention is focused on the use of angiogenesis inhibitors as adjuncts to other forms of therapy.[69] Success has been achieved in treating fairly large tumors in mice by administration of endostatin.[70] Results of ongoing clinical trials in humans are eagerly awaited.

Tumor Progression and Heterogeneity

It is well established that over a period of time many tumors become more aggressive and acquire greater malignant potential. In some instances (e.g., colon cancer; Chapter 18), there is an orderly progression from preneoplastic lesions to benign tumors and, ultimately, invasive cancers. This phenomenon is referred to as tumor *progression.* Careful clinical and experimental studies reveal that increasing malignancy (e.g., accelerated growth, invasiveness, and ability to form distant metastases) is often acquired in an incremental fashion. *This biologic phenomenon is related to the sequential appearance of subpopulations of cells that differ with respect to several phenotypic attributes, such as invasiveness, rate of growth, metastatic ability, karyotype, hormonal responsiveness, and susceptibility to antineoplastic drugs. Thus, despite the fact that most malignant tumors are monoclonal in origin, by the time they become clinically evident, their constituent cells are extremely heterogeneous.* At the molecular level, tumor progression and associated heterogeneity most likely result from multiple mutations that accumulate independently in different cells, thus generating subclones with different characteristics.

What predisposes the original transformed cell to additional genetic damage is not entirely clear. Many investigators believe that transformed cells are genetically unstable. Such instability may result, for example, from the loss of *p53*. As discussed earlier, inherited or acquired mutations in the so-called caretaker genes that regulate DNA repair may also contribute to genomic instability. These and other unidentified factors render tumor cells prone to a high rate of random, spontaneous mutations during clonal expansion (see Fig. 8–37). Some of these mutations may be lethal; others may spur cell growth by affecting protooncogenes or cancer-suppressor genes. All of these mechanisms lead to the generation of subclones that are subjected to immune and nonimmune selection pressures. For example, cells that are highly antigenic are destroyed by host defenses, whereas those with reduced growth factor requirements are positively selected. *A growing tumor therefore tends to be enriched for those subclones that "beat the odds" and are adept at survival, growth, invasion, and metastases.* Although progression is most obvious after a tumor is diagnosed, during the latent period many cell doublings occur (see Fig. 8–37), and hence *generation of heterogeneity begins well before the tumor is clinically evident.*

The rate at which mutant subclones are generated is quite variable. In some tumors, such as osteosarcomas, metastatic subclones are already present when the patient first presents to the physician. In others, typified by certain salivary gland tumors, aggressive subclones develop late and infrequently. Knowledge of such biologic differences is of obvious importance to the clinical potential of cancers and to the management of cancer patients.

Mechanisms of Invasion and Metastasis

Invasion and metastasis are biologic hallmarks of malignant tumors. They are the major cause of cancer-related morbidity and mortality and hence the subjects of intense scrutiny. For tumor cells to break loose from a primary mass, enter blood vessels or lymphatics, and produce a secondary growth at a distant site, they must go through a series of steps that are summarized in Figure 8–39. Each step in this sequence is subject to a multitude of influences, and hence at any point in the sequence the breakaway cell may not survive. Studies in mice reveal that although millions of cells are released into the circulation each day from a primary tumor, only a few metastases are produced. What then is the basis of the apparent inefficiency of this process? To understand this, it must be recalled that cells within a tumor are heterogeneous with respect to metastatic potential; only certain subclones possess the right combination of gene products to complete all the steps outlined in Figure 8–39. For the purpose of discussion, the metastatic cascade can be divided into two phases: (1) invasion of the extracellular matrix and (2) vascular dissemination and homing of tumor cells.

INVASION OF EXTRACELLULAR MATRIX

As is well known, tissues are organized into a series of compartments separated from each other by two types of extracellular matrix: basement membranes and interstitial connective tissue. Although organized differently, each of these components of extracellular matrix is made up of collagens, glycoproteins, and proteoglycans. A review of Figure 8–39 reveals that tumor cells must interact with the extracellular matrix at several stages in the metastatic cascade. A carcinoma must first breach the underlying base-

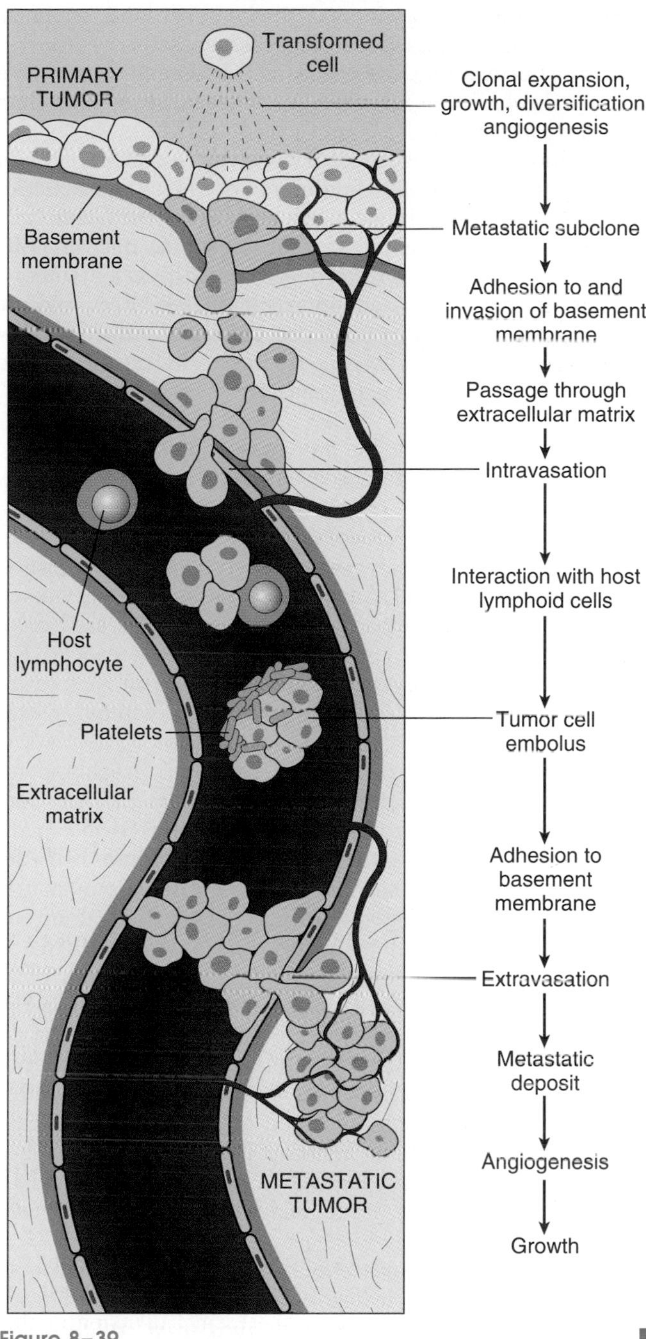

Figure 8–39 ■

The metastatic cascade. Schematic illustration of the sequential steps involved in the hematogenous spread of a tumor.

ment membrane, then traverse the interstitial connective tissue, and ultimately gain access to the circulation by penetrating the vascular basement membrane. This cycle is repeated when tumor cell emboli extravasate at a distant site. Invasion of the extracellular matrix is an active process that can be resolved into several steps:

1. Detachment ("loosening up") of the tumor cells from each other
2. Attachment to matrix components
3. Degradation of extracellular matrix
4. Migration of tumor cells

Normal cells are neatly glued to each other and their surroundings by a variety of adhesion molecules. Of these, the cadherin family of transmembrane glycoproteins is of particular importance.[71] Epithelial (E) cadherins mediate homotypic adhesions in epithelial tissue, thus serving to keep the epithelial cells together. In several epithelial tumors, including adenocarcinomas of the colon and breast, there is a down-regulation of E-cadherin expression. Presumably, this down-regulation reduces the ability of cells to adhere to each other and facilitates their detachment from the primary tumor and their advance into the surrounding tissues. E-cadherins are linked to the cytoskeleton by a family of proteins called *catenins*, which lie under the plasma membrane. The normal function of E-cadherin is dependent on its linkage to catenins. In some tumors, E-cadherin is normal, but its expression is reduced because of mutations in the gene for a catenin.[72]

To penetrate the surrounding extracellular matrix, the tumor cells must first adhere to the matrix components (Fig. 8–40). There is substantial evidence that receptor-mediated attachment of tumor cells to laminin and fibronectin is important for invasion and metastasis. Normal epithelial cells express high-affinity receptors for basement membrane laminin that are polarized to their basal surface. In contrast, some carcinoma cells have many more receptors, and they are distributed all around the cell membrane. Much more important, there seems to be a correlation between the invasiveness and the density of laminin receptors in carcinomas of the breast and colon.[72] In addition to laminin-specific receptors, tumor cells also express integrins that can serve as receptors for many components of the extracellular matrix, including fibronectin, laminin, collagen, and vitronectin.[73] As with laminin receptors, there seems to be a correlation between the expression of certain integrins (e.g., $\alpha_4\beta_1$ integrin [VLA-4]) on melanoma cells and their ability to metastasize. Such a relationship, however, is not universal, and hence it is likely that tumor cells use several different mechanisms to adhere to extracellular matrix.

After attachment to the components of the basement membrane or interstitial extracellular matrix, tumor cells must create passageways for migration. Invasion of the matrix is not due merely to passive growth pressure but requires active enzymatic degradation of the extracellular matrix components.[72] Tumor cells secrete proteolytic enzymes themselves or induce host cells (e.g., stromal fibroblasts and infiltrating macrophages) to elaborate proteases. The activity of these proteases is tightly regulated by antiproteases. At the invading edge of tumors, the balance between proteases and antiproteases is tilted in favor of proteases. Three classes of proteases have been identified: the serine, cysteine, and matrix metalloproteinases (MMP). Type IV collagenase is an MMP (MMP-2) that cleaves type IV collagen of epithelial and vascular basement membranes. Liotta and Kohn[74] have provided compelling evidence supporting the role of type IV collagenase in tumor cell invasion:

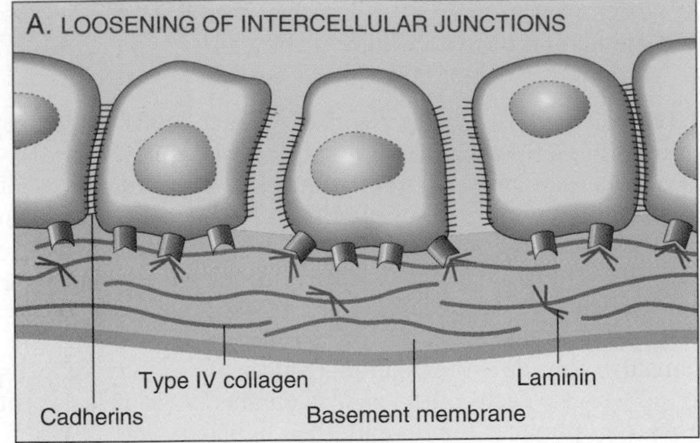

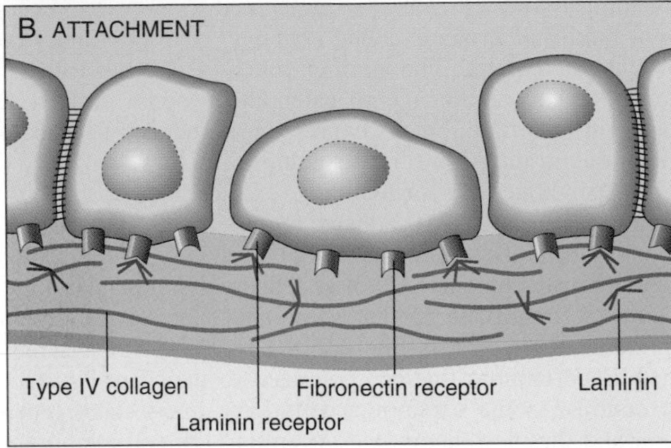

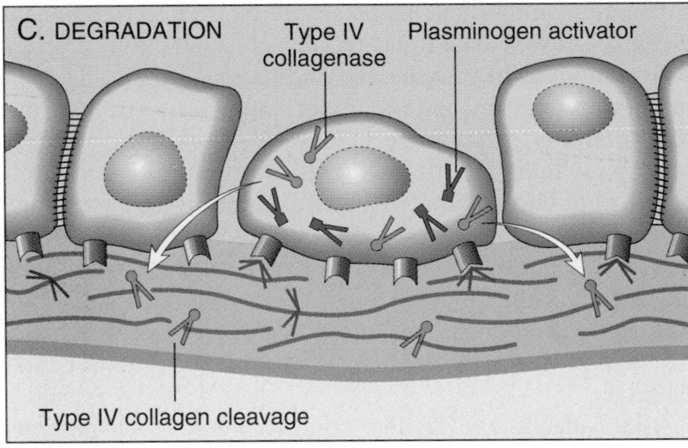

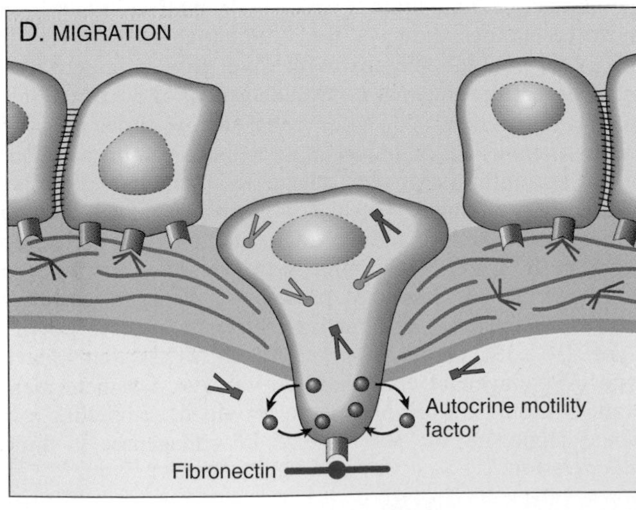

- Several invasive carcinomas, melanomas, and sarcomas contain high levels of type IV collagenase.
- In situ lesions and adenomas of breast and colon have much lower levels of type IV collagenase content than do invasive lesions.
- Inhibition of collagenase activity by transfection with the gene for tissue inhibitors of metalloproteinases (TIMP) greatly reduces metastases in experimental animals.[75] TIMP overexpression in transgenic mice inhibits the growth and progression of virally induced tumors. Thus, it seems that metalloproteinase inhibitors may be of value in the treatment of cancer. Synthetic compounds with such activity are being tested as therapeutic agents in certain forms of cancer.

Cathepsin D (a cysteine proteinase) and urokinase-type plasminogen activator (a serine proteinase) are also important in the degradation of extracellular matrix.[76] These enzymes act on a large variety of substrates, including fibronectin, laminin, and protein cores of proteoglycans. Levels of these enzymes are elevated in several animal and human tumors. Levels of cathepsin D in the tumor cells and serum seem to be prognostic in patients with breast cancer. Patients with elevated levels, presumably harboring more invasive tumors, fare less well than those without elevations.[77]

Locomotion is the next step of invasion, propelling tumor cells through the degraded basement membranes and zones of matrix proteolysis. Migration seems to be mediated by two categories of molecules: (1) tumor cell–derived motility factors, and (2) cleavage products of matrix components (e.g., collagen, laminin). In the first group are several autocrine motility factors and thymosin β15. In normal prostatic epithelium or epithelium of benign prostatic hyperplasia, β15 thymosin is not expressed; it is up-regulated in prostate cancer cells. Further, the extent of β15 thymosin up-regulation correlates with metastatic potential of prostatic cancers.[78] Another motility factor, called *hepatocyte growth factor*, is found at the interface of cancer cells and extracellular matrix. The *met* protooncogene encodes the receptor for hepatocyte growth factor, and its expression is markedly up-regulated in a number of cancers.

While the most obvious effect of matrix destruction is to create a passage for invasion by tumor cells, *cleavage products of matrix components, derived from collagen and proteoglycans, have growth-promoting, angiogenic, and chemotactic activities.* The latter may promote the migration of tumor cells into the loosened extracellular matrix. Some investigators believe that an important role of matrix metalloproteinases (discussed earlier) is to generate, from

Figure 8–40

A to *D*, Schematic illustration of the sequence of events in the invasion of epithelial basement membranes by tumor cells. Tumor cells detach from each other because of reduced adhesiveness, and cells then attach to the basement membrane via the laminin receptors and secrete proteolytic enzymes, including type IV collagenase and plasminogen activator. Degradation of the basement membrane and tumor cell migration follow.

the extracellular matrix, factors that promote tumor growth and motility.[75]

VASCULAR DISSEMINATION AND HOMING OF TUMOR CELLS

Once in circulation, tumor cells are particularly vulnerable to destruction by natural and adaptive immune defenses. The details of tumor immunity are considered later. Suffice it to say that natural killer cells seem to be particularly important in controlling hematogenous spread of tumors.

Within the circulation, tumor cells tend to aggregate in clumps. This is favored by homotypic adhesions among tumor cells as well as heterotypic adhesion between tumor cells and blood cells, particularly platelets (see Fig. 8–39). Formation of platelet-tumor aggregates seems to enhance tumor cell survival and implantability.[79] Arrest and extravasation of tumor emboli at distant sites involve adhesion to the endothelium, followed by egress through the basement membrane. Involved in these processes are adhesion molecules (integrins, laminin receptors) and proteolytic enzymes, discussed earlier. Of particular interest is an adhesion molecule called *CD44*, which is expressed on normal T lymphocytes and is used by these cells to migrate to selective sites in the lymphoid tissue. Such migration is accomplished by the binding of CD44 to hyaluronate on high endothelial venules. There is some evidence to suggest that up-regulation of CD44 expression on colonic and some other cancers favors metastasis. Other studies indicate that variant forms of CD44 are correlated with malignant transformation. Although it is attractive to postulate that tumor cells with high levels of CD44 are likely to be adept at extravascular dissemination, this hypothesis is not yet fully supported.[80]

The site at which circulating tumor cells leave the capillaries to form secondary deposits is related, in part, to the anatomic localization of the primary tumor. Many observations, however, suggest that natural pathways of drainage do not wholly explain the distributions of metastases. For example, prostatic carcinoma preferentially spreads to bone, bronchogenic carcinomas tend to involve the adrenals and the brain, and neuroblastomas spread to the liver and bones. Such organ tropism may be related to the following three mechanisms:[81]

1. Because the first step in extravasation is adhesion to the endothelium, tumor cells may express adhesion molecules whose ligands are expressed preferentially on the endothelial cells of the target organ.
2. Some target organs may liberate chemoattractants that tend to recruit tumor cells to the site. Examples include insulin-like growth factors I and II.
3. In some cases, the target tissue may be an unpermissive environment—unfavorable soil, so to speak, for the growth of tumor seedlings. For example, inhibitors of proteases could prevent the establishment of a tumor colony.

Despite the foregoing considerations, however, the precise localization of metastases cannot be predicted with any form of cancer. Evidently, many tumors have not read textbooks of pathology.

MOLECULAR GENETICS OF METASTASES

Are there oncogenes or tumor-suppressor genes that elicit metastases as their principal or sole contribution to tumorigenesis? This question is of more than academic interest because if altered forms of certain genes promote or suppress the metastatic phenotype, their detection in a primary tumor may have prognostic as well as therapeutic implications. At present, no single "metastasis gene" has been found. Some have argued that because metastatic cells must acquire multiple properties (e.g., expression of adhesion receptors, production of collagenases, motility factors), no single genetic alteration is likely to render a cell metastasis-prone.[82] It could be argued, however, that genes that encode E-cadherin, or tissue inhibitors of metalloproteinases, should be considered "metastasis-suppressor genes." Loss of their activity would reduce cell adhesiveness and promote proteolysis of the extracellular matrix. A variety of approaches are being used to identify candidate metastasis-suppressor genes. One such method involves subtractive hybridization of cDNA libraries obtained from metastatic tumor cell lines and their nonmetastatic but transformed counterparts. This led to the discovery of *nm23*. In murine models, the expression of *nm23* is high in lines with low metastatic potential and is reduced tenfold in lines with high metastatic ability. In a series of human breast cancers, *nm23* levels were highest in tumors that had three or fewer involved nodes and were uniformly low in tumors that had extensive nodal metastases. This correlation has not been upheld in other types of cancer, however, and hence the status of *nm23* as a suppressor of metastasis remains uncertain. Two other candidates have been described: the *KAI-1* and *KiSS* genes. Located on chromosome 11p11-2, the KAI-1 gene suppresses metastasis of human prostate cancer cells in animal models. KAI-1 is expressed in normal prostate but not in metastatic prostate cancer. Transfer of chromosome 11, containing the KAI-1 gene, suppresses the metastatic ability but not tumorigenicity of prostate cancer cells. The KiSS-1 gene, also on human chromosome 11, functions in an analogous manner in human malignant melanoma. The functions of these interesting genes are not yet known but are likely to be related to regulation of some critical step in the metastasis cascade.

CARCINOGENIC AGENTS AND THEIR CELLULAR INTERACTIONS

A large number of agents cause genetic damage and induce neoplastic transformation of cells. They fall into the following categories: (1) chemical carcinogens; (2) radiant energy; and (3) oncogenic microbes, chiefly viruses. Radiant energy and certain chemical carcinogens are documented causes of cancer in humans, and the evidence linking certain viruses to human cancers grows ever stronger. Each group of agents is considered separately, but several may act in concert or synergize the effects of others.

Chemical Carcinogenesis

Although John Hill earlier called attention to the association of "immoderate use of snuff" and the development of "polypusses" (polyps), we owe largely to Sir Percival Pott our awareness of the potential carcinogenicity of chemical agents. Pott astutely related the increased incidence of scrotal skin cancer in chimney sweeps to chronic exposure to soot. A few years later, based on this observation, the Danish Chimney Sweeps Guild ruled that its members must bathe daily. No public health measure since that time has so successfully controlled a form of cancer! Over the succeeding two centuries, hundreds of chemicals have been shown to transform cells in vitro and to be carcinogenic in animals. Some of the most potent (e.g., the polycyclic aromatic hydrocarbons) have been extracted from fossil fuels or are products of incomplete combustions. Some are synthetic products created by industry or for the study of chemical carcinogenesis. Some are naturally occurring components of plants and microbial organisms. Most important, a significant number (including, ironically, some medical drugs) have been strongly implicated in the causation of cancers in humans.

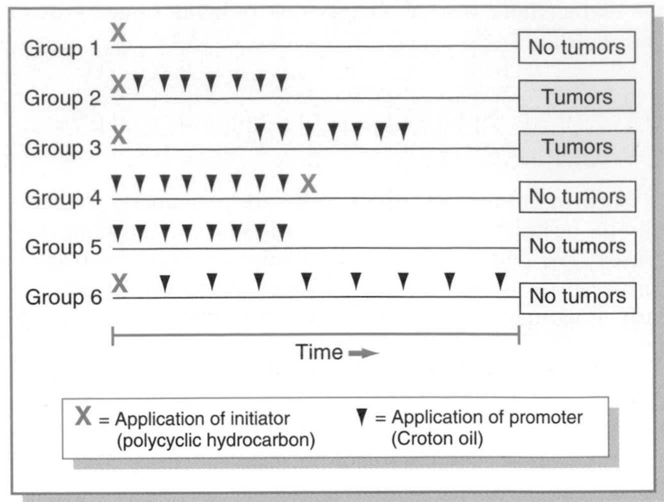

Figure 8–41

Experiments demonstrating the initiation and promotion phases of carcinogenesis in mice. Group 2: application of promoter repeated at twice-weekly intervals for several months; group 3: application of promoter delayed for several months and then applied twice weekly; group 6: promoter applied at monthly intervals.

STEPS INVOLVED IN CHEMICAL CARCINOGENESIS

It was discussed earlier that carcinogenesis is a multistep process. This is most readily demonstrated in experimental models of chemical carcinogenesis, in which cancer induction can be broadly divided into two stages: initiation and promotion.[83] The classic experiments that allowed the distinction between initiation and promotion were performed on mouse skin and are outlined in Figure 8–41. The following concepts relating to the initiation-promotion sequence have emerged from these experiments:

- Initiation results from exposure of cells to an appropriate dose of a carcinogenic agent (initiator); an initiated cell is in some manner altered, rendering it likely to give rise to a tumor (groups 2 and 3). Initiation alone, however, is not sufficient for tumor formation (group 1).
- Initiation causes permanent DNA damage (mutations). It is therefore rapid and irreversible and has "memory." This is illustrated by group 3, in which tumors were produced even if the application of the promoting agent was delayed for several months after a single application of the initiator.
- *Promoters can induce tumors in initiated cells, but they are nontumorigenic by themselves* (group 5). Furthermore, tumors do not result when the promoting agent is applied before, rather than after, the initiating agent (group 4). This indicates that, *in contrast to the effects of initiators, the cellular changes resulting from the application of promoters do not affect DNA directly and are reversible.* As discussed later, promoters render cells susceptible to additional mutations by causing cellular proliferation.
- That the effects of promoters are reversible is further documented in group 6, in which tumors failed to develop in initiated cells if the time between multiple applications of the promoter was sufficiently extended.

Although the concepts of initiation and promotion have been derived largely from experiments involving induction of skin cancer in mice, these stages are also discernible in the development of cancers of the liver, urinary bladder, breast, colon, and respiratory tract. With this brief overview of the two major steps in carcinogenesis, we can examine initiation and promotion in more detail, following the outline in Figure 8–42.[84]

INITIATION OF CARCINOGENESIS

Chemicals that initiate carcinogenesis are extremely diverse in structure and include both natural and synthetic products (Table 8–10). They fall into one of two categories: (1) *direct-acting* compounds, which do not require chemical transformation for their carcinogenicity, and (2) *indirect-acting* compounds or *procarcinogens,* which require metabolic conversion in vivo to produce *ultimate carcinogens* capable of transforming cells. All direct-acting and ultimate carcinogens have one property in common: *They are highly reactive electrophiles* (have electron-deficient atoms) *that can react with nucleophilic (electron-rich) sites in the cell.* These reactions are nonenzymatic and result in the formation of covalent adducts (addition products) between the chemical carcinogen and a nucleotide in DNA. The electrophilic reactions may attack several electron-rich sites in the target cells, including DNA, RNA, and proteins, thus sometimes producing lethal damage. In initiated cells, the interaction is obviously nonlethal, and, as should be evident, DNA is the primary target.

Metabolic Activation of Carcinogens. Except for the

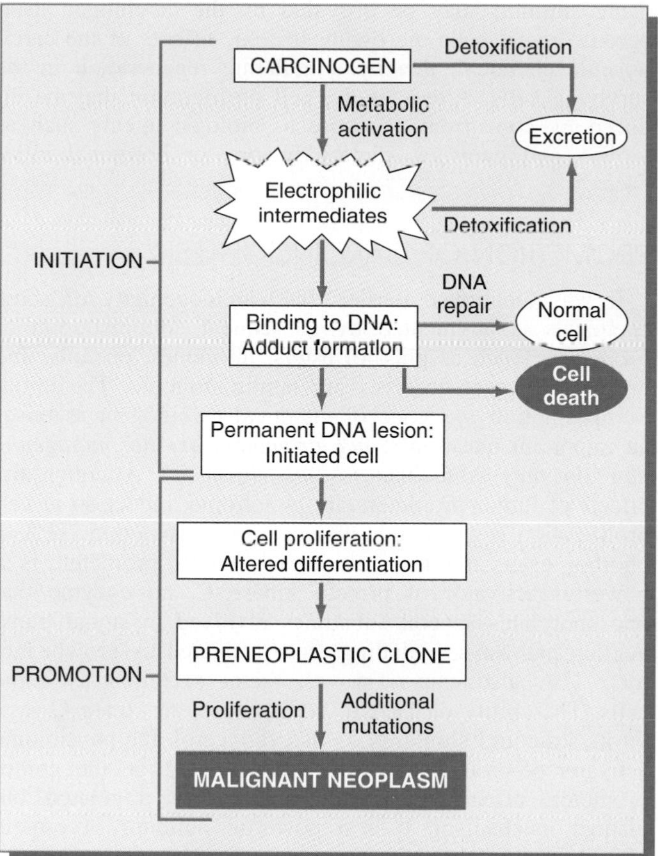

Figure 8–42

General schema of events in chemical carcinogenesis. Note that promoters cause clonal expansion of the initiated cell, thus producing a preneoplastic clone. Futher proliferation induced by the promoter or other factors causes accumulation of additional mutations and emergence of a malignant tumor.

Table 8–10. MAJOR CHEMICAL CARCINOGENS

Direct-Acting Carcinogens

Alkylating Agents
β-Propiolactone
Dimethyl sulfate
Diepoxybutane
Anticancer drugs (cyclophosphamide, chlorambucil, nitrosoureas, and others)

Acylating Agents
1-Acetyl-imidazole
Dimethylcarbamyl chloride

Procarcinogens that Require Metabolic Activation

Polycyclic and Heterocyclic Aromatic Hydrocarbons
Benz(a)anthracene
Benzo(a)pyrene
Dibenz(a,h)anthracene
3-Methylcholanthrene
7,12-Dimethylbenz(a)anthracene

Aromatic Amines, Amides, Azo Dyes
2-Naphthylamine (β-naphthylamine)
Benzidine
2-Acetylaminofluorene
Dimethylaminoazobenzene (butter yellow)

Natural Plant and Microbial Products
Aflatoxin B_1
Griseofulvin
Cycasin
Safrole
Betel nuts

Others
Nitrosamine and amides
Vinyl chloride, nickel, chromium
Insecticides, fungicides
Polychlorinated biphenyls

few direct-acting alkylating and acylating agents that are intrinsically electrophilic, most chemical carcinogens require metabolic activation for conversion into ultimate carcinogens. Other metabolic pathways may lead to the inactivation (detoxification) of the procarcinogen or its derivatives. Thus, *the carcinogenic potency of a chemical is determined not only by the inherent reactivity of its electrophilic derivative, but also by the balance between metabolic activation and inactivation reactions.*[85]

Most of the known carcinogens are metabolized by cytochrome P-450–dependent mono-oxygenases. The genes that encode these enzymes are quite polymorphic, and the activity and inducibility of these enzymes have been shown to vary among different individuals. Because these enzymes are essential for the activation of procarcinogens, the susceptibility to carcinogenesis is regulated in part by polymorphisms in the genes that encode these enzymes. A few examples suffice to illustrate this important concept. The product of the P-450 gene, CYP1A1, metabolizes polycyclic aromatic hydrocarbons such as benz(o)pyrene. Approximately 10% of the white population has a highly inducible form of this enzyme that is associated with an increased risk of lung cancer in smokers.[86] Light smokers with the susceptible genotype of CYP1A1 have a sevenfold higher risk of developing lung cancer as compared with smokers without the permissive genotype. As another example, the enzyme glutathione-*S*-transferase (GST), involved in the detoxification of polycyclic aromatic hydrocarbons, is also polymorphic; in about 50% of whites, this locus is entirely deleted, and hence these individuals incur a higher risk of lung and bladder cancer but only if exposed to tobacco smoke. Not all variations in the activation or detoxification of carcinogens are genetically determined. Age, sex, and nutritional status also determine the internal dose of toxicants and hence determine the likelihood of chemical carcinogens.[85]

Molecular Targets of Chemical Carcinogens. Because malignant transformation results from mutations that affect oncogenes, cancer-suppressor genes, and genes that regulate apoptosis, it comes as no surprise that the vast majority of initiating chemicals are mutagenic. Their mutagenic potential has been investigated, most commonly using the *Ames test.* This test uses the ability of a chemical to induce mutations in the bacterium *Salmonella typhimurium.* The vast majority (70 to 90%) of known chemical carcinogens score positive in the Ames test. Conversely, most but not all chemicals that are mutagenic in vitro are carcinogenic in vivo. Because of the high correlation between mutagenicity and carcinogenicity, the Ames test is frequently used to screen chemicals for their carcinogenic potential.

That DNA is the primary target for chemical carcinogens seems fairly well established, but there is no single or unique alteration that can be associated with initiation of chemical carcinogenesis. Nevertheless, the interaction of each chemical carcinogen with the DNA is not completely random, and each class of carcinogens tends to produce a limited pattern of DNA damage. Thus, the presence of certain types of DNA damage in human tumors can provide molecular clues to their causation. This is exemplified by the study of mutations in the *ras* and *p53* genes, as discussed subsequently. It should be emphasized that carcinogen-induced changes in DNA do not necessarily lead to initiation because several forms of DNA damage can be repaired by cellular enzymes. It is likely that environmentally induced insults to DNA are far more common than is the occurrence of cancer. This is illustrated by the rare hereditary disorder xeroderma pigmentosum, which is associated with a defect in DNA repair and a greatly increased vulnerability to skin cancers caused by UV light and some chemicals (see Radiation Carcinogenesis).

Although virtually any gene may be targeted by chemical carcinogens, *ras* mutations are particularly common in several chemically induced tumors in rodents. Molecular analyses of mutant *ras* genes isolated from such tumors reveal that the change in nucleotide sequence is precisely that predicted from the known sites of reaction of the carcinogen with specific bases in DNA. Thus, it seems that each carcinogen produces a molecular "fingerprint" that can link specific chemicals with their mutational effects.[87] A telling example of this phenomenon is provided by the study of hepatocellular carcinomas. In certain parts of China and Africa, hepatocellular carcinoma has been linked to the ingestion of the fungal metabolite aflatoxin B1, whereas in other regions of the world, it follows chronic hepatitis B virus infection. In all cases, there is mutation of the *p53* gene. In areas where aflatoxin B1 exposure is high, the *p53* gene of the tumor cells shows a characteristic G:C→T:A transversion in codon 249 (called *249^{ser}p53* mutation). By contrast, in liver tumors in areas where aflatoxin contamination of food is not a risk factor, the 249^{ser}*p53* mutation is uncommon; instead, there is a diverse spectrum of other *p53* mutations.[88] These and other similar observations strongly support the notion that molecular fingerprinting of tumors can provide clues to the identity of initiating agents.

Initiated Cell. In the preceding sections, we noted that unrepaired alterations in the DNA are essential first steps in the process of initiation. *For the change to be heritable, the damaged DNA template must be replicated. Thus, for initiation to occur, carcinogen-altered cells must undergo at least one cycle of proliferation, so that the change in DNA becomes fixed, or permanent.* In the liver, many chemicals are activated to reactive electrophiles, yet most of them do not produce cancers unless the liver cells proliferate within 72 to 96 hours of the formation of DNA adducts. In tissues that are normally quiescent, the mitogenic stimulus may be provided by the carcinogen itself because many cells die owing to toxic effects of the carcinogenic chemical, thereby stimulating regeneration in the surviving cells. Alternatively, cell proliferation may be induced by concurrent exposure to biologic agents such as viruses and parasites, dietary factors, or hormonal influences.[89]

PROMOTION OF CARCINOGENESIS

It was mentioned earlier that carcinogenicity of some chemicals is augmented by subsequent administration of *promoters* (such as phorbol esters, hormones, phenols, and drugs) that by themselves are nontumorigenic. The initiation-promotion sequence of chemical carcinogenesis raises an important question: *Since promoters are not mutagenic, how do they contribute to tumorigenesis?* Although the effects of tumor promoters are pleiotropic, induction of cell proliferation is a sine qua non of tumor promotion. TPA, a phorbol ester and the best-studied tumor promoter, is a powerful activator of protein kinase C, an enzyme that phosphorylates several substrates involved in signal transduction pathways, including those activated by growth factors. TPA also causes growth factor secretion by some cells. The ability of TPA to activate protein kinase C rests on its structural similarity to diacylglycerol, the physiologic activator of protein kinase C. Okadoic acid, another tumor promoter, affects signal transduction by a related but distinct mechanism. It is a powerful inhibitor of protein phosphatases and hence prevents dephosphorylation of substrates that promote signal transduction in their phosphorylated form.

No single genetic change is sufficient for neoplastic transformation. Thus, while the application of an initiator may cause the mutational activation of an oncogene such as *ras*, it can at best give rise to a preneoplastic or hyperplastic lesion. Subsequent application of promoters leads to proliferation and clonal expansion of initiated (mutated) cells. Initiated cells respond differently to promoters than normal cells and hence expand selectively. Such cells (especially after *ras* activation) have reduced growth factor requirements and may also be less responsive to growth inhibitory signals in their extracellular milieu. Forced to proliferate, the initiated clone of cells suffers additional mutations, developing eventually into a malignant tumor. Thus, the process of tumor promotion includes multiple steps: proliferation of preneoplastic cells, malignant conversion, and eventually tumor progression (see p. 302).

The concept that sustained cell proliferation increases the risk of mutagenesis and hence neoplastic transformation is also applicable to human carcinogenesis. For example, pathologic hyperplasia of the endometrium (Chapter 24) and increased regenerative activity that accompanies chronic liver cell injury are associated with the development of cancer in these organs.

CARCINOGENIC CHEMICALS

Before closing this discussion on chemical carcinogenesis, we briefly describe some initiators (Table 8–10) and promoters of chemical carcinogenesis, with special emphasis on those that have been linked to cancer development in humans.

Direct-Acting Alkylating Agents. These agents are activation independent, and in general they are weak carcinogens. Nonetheless, they are important because many therapeutic agents (e.g., cyclophosphamide, chlorambucil, busulfan, melphalan, and others) fall into this category. These are used as anticancer drugs but have been documented to induce lymphoid neoplasms, leukemia, and other forms of cancer. Some alkylating agents, such as cyclophosphamide, are also powerful immunosuppressive agents and are therefore used in treatment of immunologic disorders, including rheumatoid arthritis and Wegener granulomatosis. Although the risk of induced cancer with these agents is low, judicious use of them is indicated. Alkylating agents appear to exert their therapeutic effects by interacting with and damaging DNA, but it is precisely these actions that render them also carcinogenic.

Polycyclic Aromatic Hydrocarbons. These agents represent some of the most potent carcinogens known. They require metabolic activation and can induce tumors in a wide variety of tissues and species. Painted on the skin, they cause skin cancers; injected subcutaneously, they evoke sarcomas; introduced into a specific organ, they cause cancers locally. The polycyclic hydrocarbons are of particular interest as carcinogens because they are produced in the combustion of tobacco, particularly with cigarette smoking, and may well contribute to the causation of lung cancer and bladder cancer.[90] They are also produced from animal fats in the process of broiling meats and are present in smoked meats and fish.

Aromatic Amines and Azo Dyes. The carcinogenicity of most aromatic amines and azo dyes is exerted mainly in the liver, where the "ultimate carcinogen" is formed by the intermediation of the cytochrome P-450 oxygenase systems. Thus, fed to rats, acetylaminofluorene and the azo dyes induce hepatocellular carcinomas but not cancers of the gastrointestinal tract. An agent implicated in human cancers, β-naphthylamine, is an exception. In the past, it has been responsible for a 50-fold increased incidence of bladder cancer in heavily exposed workers in aniline dye and rubber industries.[91] After absorption, it is hydroxylated into an active form then detoxified by conjugation with glucuronic acid. When excreted in the urine, the nontoxic conjugate is split by the urinary enzyme glucuronidase to release the electrophilic reactant again, thus inducing bladder cancer. Regrettably, humans are one of the few species to possess the urinary glucuronidase. Some of the azo dyes were developed to color food (e.g., butter yellow to give margarine the appearance of butter and scarlet red to impart the seductive coloration of certain foods such as maraschino cherries). These dyes are now federally regulated in the United States because of the fear that they may be dangerous to humans.

Naturally Occurring Carcinogens. Among the several known chemical carcinogens produced by plants and microorganisms, the potent hepatic carcinogen aflatoxin B1 is most important. It is produced by some strains of *Aspergillus flavus* that thrive on improperly stored grains and peanuts. A strong correlation has been found between the dietary level of this hepatocarcinogen and the incidence of hepatocellular carcinoma in some parts of Africa and the Far East. Infection with hepatitis B virus has also been strongly correlated with this cancer, and when exposure to both of these agents occurs, the aflatoxin and the virus collaborate in the production of this form of neoplasia.

Nitrosamines and Amides. These carcinogens are of interest because of the possibility that they are formed in the gastrointestinal tract of humans and so may contribute to the induction of some forms of cancer, particularly gastric carcinoma. They are derived in the stomach from the reaction of nitrostable amines and nitrate used as a preservative, which is converted to nitrites by bacteria. Such concerns have led many to shun processed food containing nitrate preservatives.

Miscellaneous Agents. Scores of other chemicals have been indicted as carcinogens. Only a few that represent important industrial hazards were listed earlier in Table 8–3 and are briefly mentioned here. Occupational exposure to *asbestos* has been associated with an increased incidence of bronchogenic carcinomas, mesotheliomas, and gastrointestinal cancers, as discussed in Chapter 16. Concomitant cigarette smoking heightens the risk of bronchogenic carcinoma manyfold. *Vinyl chloride* is the monomer from which the polymer polyvinyl chloride is fabricated. It was first identified as a carcinogen in animals, but investigations soon disclosed a scattered incidence of the extremely rare hemangiosarcoma of the liver among workers exposed to this chemical. *Chromium, nickel*, and other metals, when volatilized and inhaled in industrial environments, have caused cancer of the lung. Skin cancer associated with arsenic is also well established. Similarly, there is reasonable evidence that many insecticides, such as aldrin, dieldrin, and chlordane and the polychlorinated biphenyls, are carcinogenic in animals (Chapter 10).

Promoters of Chemical Carcinogenesis. Certain promoters may contribute to cancers in humans. It has been argued that promoters are at least as important as initiating chemicals because cells initiated by exposure to environmental carcinogens are innocuous unless subjected to repeated assault by promoters. Tumor promotion may occur after exposure to exogenous agents, such as cigarette smoke or viral infections that cause tissue damage and reactive hyperplasia. Perhaps more serious, because they are difficult to control, are endogenous promoters such as hormones and bile salts. Hormones such as estrogens serve in animals as promoters of liver tumors. The prolonged use of diethylstilbestrol is implicated in the production of postmenopausal endometrial carcinoma and in the causation of vaginal cancer in offspring exposed in utero (Chapter 24). Intake of high levels of dietary fat has been associated with increased risk of colon cancer. This may be related to an increase in synthesis of bile acids, which have been shown to act as promoters in experimental models of colon cancer.

Radiation Carcinogenesis

Radiant energy, whether in the form of the UV rays of sunlight or as ionizing electromagnetic and particulate radiation, can transform virtually all cell types in vitro and induce neoplasms in vivo in both humans and experimental animals. UV light is clearly implicated in the causation of skin cancers, and ionizing radiations of medical, occupational, and atomic bomb origins have produced a variety of forms of malignant neoplasia. Although the contribution of radiation to the total human burden of cancer is probably small, the well-known latency of radiant energy and its cumulative effect require extremely long periods of observation and make it difficult to ascertain its total significance. Only now, decades later, an increased incidence of breast cancer has become apparent among women exposed during childhood to the atomic bomb.[92] Moreover, its possible additive or synergistic effects on other potential carcinogenic influences add yet another dimension. The effects of UV light on DNA differ somewhat from those of ionizing radiations. Because the cellular and molecular effects of ionizing radiation are discussed in Chapter 10, the present discussion focuses in large part on the carcinogenic effects of UV rays.

ULTRAVIOLET RAYS

There is ample evidence from epidemiologic studies that *UV rays* derived from the sun induce an increased incidence of squamous cell carcinoma, basal cell carcinoma, and possibly malignant melanoma of the skin.[93] The degree of risk depends on the type of UV rays, the intensity of exposure, and the quantity of light-absorbing "protective mantle" of melanin in the skin. Persons of European origin who have fair skin that repeatedly gets sunburned but stalwartly refuses to tan and who live in locales receiving a great deal of sunlight (e.g., Queensland, Australia, close to the equator) have the highest incidence of skin cancers. The UV portion of the solar spectrum can be divided into three wavelength ranges: UVA (320 to 400 nm), UVB (280 to 320 nm), and UVC (200 to 280 nm). Of these, UVB is believed to be responsible for the induction of cutaneous cancers. UVC, although a potent mutagen, is not considered significant because it is filtered out by the ozone shield around the earth (hence the concern about ozone depletion).

UV rays have a number of effects on cells, including inhibition of cell division, inactivation of enzymes, induction of mutations, and in sufficient dosage, killing of cells. *The carcinogenicity of UVB light is attributed to its formation of pyrimidine dimers in DNA.* This type of DNA damage is repaired by the nucleotide excision repair (NER) pathway. There are five steps in NER: (1) recognition of the DNA lesion, (2) incision of the damaged strand on both sites of the lesion, (3) removal of the damaged oligonucleotide, (4) synthesis of a nucleotide patch, and (5) its ligation. This process requires the products of at least 20 genes. It is postulated that with excessive sun exposure, the capacity of the NER pathway is overwhelmed, and hence some DNA damage remains unrepaired. This leads to large transcriptional errors and, in some instances, cancer. The importance of the NER pathway of DNA repair is most graphically illustrated by a study of patients with the hereditary disorder *xeroderma pigmentosum.* This autosomal recessive disorder is characterized by extreme photosensitivity, a 2000-fold increased risk of skin cancer in sun-exposed skin and, in some cases, neurologic abnormalities. The molecular basis of the degenerative changes in sun-exposed skin and occurrence of cutaneous tumors rests on inherited inability to repair UV-induced DNA damage. Xeroderma pigmentosum is genetically heterogeneous—with at least seven different variants. Each of these is caused by a mutation in one of several genes involved in NER.[94]

As with other carcinogens, UVB also causes mutations in oncogenes and tumor-suppressor genes. In particular, mutant forms of the *ras* and *p53* genes have been detected both in human skin cancers and in UVB-induced cancers in mice. These mutations occur mainly at dipyridimine sequences within the DNA, thus implicating UVB-induced genetic damage in the causation of skin cancers. In animal models, *p53* mutations occur early after exposure to UVB, before the appearance of tumors, and hence it has been proposed that *p53* mutations may provide a molecular marker for prior solar exposure in skin.[95]

IONIZING RADIATION

Electromagnetic (x-rays, γ rays) and particulate (α particles, β particles, protons, neutrons) radiations are all carcinogenic. The evidence is so voluminous that a few examples suffice.[96] Many of the pioneers in the development of roentgen rays developed skin cancers. Miners of radioactive elements in central Europe and the Rocky Mountain region of the United States have suffered a tenfold increased incidence of lung cancers. Most telling is the follow-up of survivors of the atomic bombs dropped on Hiroshima and Nagasaki. Initially, there was a marked increase in the incidence of leukemias—principally acute and chronic myelocytic leukemia—after an average latent period of about 7 years. Subsequently the incidence of many solid tumors with longer latent periods (e.g., breast, colon, thyroid, and lung) has increased.

Even therapeutic irradiation has been documented to be carcinogenic. Thyroid cancers have developed in approximately 9% of those exposed during infancy and childhood to head and neck radiation. The previous practice of treating a form of arthritis of the spine known as ankylosing spondylitis with therapeutic irradiation has yielded a 10- to 12-fold increase in the incidence of leukemia years later.

Finally, the residents of the Marshall Islands were exposed on one occasion to accidental fallout from a hydrogen bomb test that contained thyroid-seeking radioactive iodines. As many as 90% of the children under the age of 10 years on Rongelap Island developed thyroid nodules within 15 years, and about 5% of these nodules proved to be thyroid carcinomas. A marked increase in the incidence of thyroid cancer has also been noted in areas exposed to the fallout from the nuclear power plant accident in Chernobyl.[97] It is evident that radiant energy—whether absorbed in the pleasant form of sunlight, through the best intentions of a physician, or by tragic exposure to an atomic bomb blast—has awesome carcinogenic potential.

In humans, there is a hierarchy of vulnerability to radiation-induced cancers. Most frequent are the leukemias except for chronic lymphocytic leukemia, which, for unknown reasons, almost never follows radiation injury.

Cancer of the thyroid follows closely but only in the young. In the intermediate category are cancers of the breast, lungs, and salivary glands. In contrast, skin, bone, and the gastrointestinal tract are relatively resistant to radiation-induced neoplasia, even though the gastrointestinal mucosal cells are vulnerable to the cell-killing effects of radiation, and the skin is in the pathway of all external radiation. Nonetheless, the physician dare not forget: *Any* cell can be transformed into a cancer cell by sufficient exposure to radiant energy.

Viral and Microbial Carcinogenesis

A large number of DNA and RNA viruses have proved to be oncogenic in a wide variety of animals, ranging from amphibia to primates, and the evidence grows stronger that certain forms of human cancer are of viral origin. In the following discussion, the better characterized and most intensively studied human oncogenic viruses are presented first. This is followed by a brief account of the association between infection by the bacterium *Helicobacter pylori* and gastric lymphoma.

DNA ONCOGENIC VIRUSES

Several DNA viruses have been associated with the causation of cancer in animals. Some, such as adenoviruses, cause tumors only in laboratory animals, whereas others, such as the bovine papillomaviruses, cause benign as well as malignant neoplasms in their natural hosts. Of the various human DNA viruses, four (papillomaviruses, Epstein-Barr virus [EBV], hepatitis B virus [HBV], and Kaposi sarcoma herpesvirus [KSHV]) are of particular interest because they have been implicated in the causation of human cancer. KSHV was discussed in Chapter 7. Before we discuss the role of the other three viruses in carcinogenesis, a few general comments relating to transformation by DNA viruses are offered:

- Transforming DNA viruses form stable associations with the host cell genome. The integrated virus is unable to complete its replicative cycle because the viral genes essential for completion of replication are interrupted during integration of viral DNA.
- Those viral genes that are transcribed early (early genes) in the viral life cycle are important for transformation. They are expressed in transformed cells.

Human Papillomavirus. Approximately 70 genetically distinct types of HPV have been identified. Some types (e.g., 1, 2, 4, and 7) definitely cause benign squamous papillomas (warts) in humans. Human papillomaviruses have been implicated in the genesis of several cancers, particularly squamous cell carcinoma of the cervix and anogenital region. In addition, human papillomaviruses have been linked to the causation of oral and laryngeal cancers.[98]

Epidemiologic studies suggest that carcinoma of the cervix is caused by a sexually transmitted agent, and HPV is a prime suspect. DNA sequences of HPV types 16 and 18 and, less commonly, types 31, 33, 35, and 51 are found in approximately 85% of invasive squamous cell cancers and their presumed precursors (severe dysplasias and carcinoma in situ). In contrast to cervical cancers, genital warts with low malignant potential are associated with distinct HPV types, predominantly HPV-6 and HPV-11 ("low-risk" types).

Molecular analyses of HPV-associated carcinomas and benign genital warts reveal differences that may be pertinent to the transforming activity of these viruses. In benign warts and in preneoplastic lesions, the HPV genome is maintained in an episomal (nonintegrated) form, whereas in cancers, the viral DNA is usually integrated into the host cell genome. This suggests that integration of viral DNA is important in malignant transformation. Although the site of viral integration in host chromosomes is random (the viral DNA is found at different locations in different cancers), the pattern of integration is clonal, that is, the site of integration is identical within all cells of a given cancer. This would not be expected if HPV were merely a passenger that infects cells after transformation. Furthermore, the site at which the viral DNA is interrupted in the process of integration is fairly constant: It is almost always within the E1/E2 open reading frame of the viral genome. Because the E2 region of the viral DNA normally represses the transcription of the E6 and E7 early viral genes, its interruption causes overexpression of the E6 and E7 proteins of HPV-16 and HPV-18.[99] The oncogenic potential of HPV-16 and HPV-18 can be related to these two early viral gene products.[100, 101] The E7 protein binds to the underphosphorylated form of the tumor-suppressor protein pRb and displaces the E2F transcription factors that are normally bound by pRb; the E6 protein binds to and facilitates the degradation of the *p53* gene product. The affinity of these viral proteins for the products of tumor-suppressor genes differs depending on the oncogenic potential of HPV. E6 and E7 proteins derived from high-risk human papillomaviruses (types 16, 18, and 31) bind to pRb and *p53* with high affinity, whereas the E6 and E7 gene products of low-risk human papillomaviruses (types 6 and 11) bind with low affinity. Thus, it seems that the *E6 and E7 proteins of the high-risk HPV disable two important tumor-suppressor proteins that regulate the cell cycle* (see earlier). In HPV-induced tumors, *p53* mutations are extremely uncommon, presumably because loss of *p53* function is accomplished by the E6 oncoprotein.

That the E6-p53 interaction is important in the pathogenesis of cervical cancers is supported by recent studies in which the relationship between p53 polymorphisms and risk of developing this cancer was investigated. It has been reported that one particular allele of p53 with an arginine rather than a proline at a certain position is much more susceptible to degradation by E6. Correspondingly, individuals with the "arginine form" of p53 have a seven-fold higher risk of developing cervical cancer than those who do not possess this allele of p53.[101]

Although these observations implicate certain HPV types in the pathogenesis of human cancer, when human keratinocytes are transfected with DNA from HPV 16, 18, or 31 in vitro they are immortalized, but they do not form tumors in experimental animals. Cotransfection with a mutated *ras* gene results in full malignant transformation. Thus, it seems most likely that infection with HPV acts as an initiating event and that additional somatic mutations are essential for malignant transformation. The occurrence of such changes is facilitated by cigarette smoking, coexisting microbial infections, dietary deficiencies, and hormonal changes, all of which have been implicated as cofactors in the pathogenesis of cervical cancers.

Epstein-Barr Virus. EBV, a member of the herpes family, has been implicated in the pathogenesis of four types of human tumors: the African form of Burkitt lymphoma; B-cell lymphomas in immunosuppressed individuals, particularly in those with human immunodeficiency virus (HIV) infection and organ transplantation; some cases of Hodgkin disease; and nasopharyngeal carcinomas.[102, 103] These neoplasms are reviewed elsewhere in this book, and therefore only their association with EBV is discussed here.

EBV infects epithelial cells of the oropharynx and B lymphocytes. It gains entry into B cells via the CD21 molecule, which is expressed on all B cells. Within B lymphocytes, the linear genome of EBV circularizes to form an episome in the cell nucleus. The infection of B cells is latent; that is, there is no replication of the virus, and the cells are not killed. The latently infected B cells are immortalized and acquire the ability to propagate indefinitely in vitro. The molecular basis of B-cell immortalization by EBV is complex.[104] In contrast to HPV, there is no convincing evidence that tumor-suppressor genes are targeted for inactivation by EBV. Instead, it appears that several viral genes dysregulate the normal proliferative and survival signals in latently infected cells.[104a] For example, the latent membrane protein-1 (LMP-1) prevents apoptosis of B cells by up-regulating the expression of *bcl*-2, and it activates growth-promoting pathways that are normally triggered by T cell–derived signals. Thus, LMP-1 can induce both cell growth and cell survival. The importance of LMP-1 in mediating the effects of EBV is further highlighted by the observation that expression of LMP-1 in rodent cell lines can render them immortal and, in some cases, tumorigenic; in transgenic mice, LMP-1 expression in the skin gives rise to hyperplasia and abnormal keratin expression. Similarly the EBV-encoded EBNA-2 gene transactivates several host genes, including cyclin D and members of the *src* family.[105] EBNA-2 also activates the transcription of LMP-1. Thus, it seems that several viral genes collaborate to render B cells immortal. With this brief review of EBV infection, we turn to its role in the causation of B-cell tumors.

Burkitt lymphoma is a neoplasm of B lymphocytes that is the most common childhood tumor in Central Africa and New Guinea. A morphologically identical lymphoma occurs sporadically throughout the world. The association between African Burkitt lymphoma and EBV is quite strong:

- More than 90% of African tumors carry the EBV genome.
- One hundred per cent of the patients have elevated antibody titers against viral capsid antigens.
- Serum antibody titers against viral capsid antigens are correlated with the risk of developing the tumor.

Although these data strongly support the idea that EBV is intimately involved in the causation of Burkitt lymphoma, several other observations suggest that additional factors must also be involved. *(1)* EBV infection is not limited to the geographic locales where Burkitt lymphoma is found. EBV is a ubiquitous virus that asymptomatically infects almost all adults worldwide. *(2)* EBV is known to cause infectious mononucleosis, a self-limited disorder (Chapter 9) in which B cells are infected. *(3)* The EBV genome can be found in only 15 to 20% of cases of Burkitt lymphoma outside Africa, but both the endemic (African) and the sporadic cases of Burkitt lymphoma have a t(8;14) or, less commonly, variant translocations that lead to dysregulated expression of the c-*myc* oncogene. *(4)* Although EBV infection immortalizes B cells in vitro, these cells do not form tumors when injected into immunosuppressed mice in vivo. There are significant differences in the patterns of viral gene expression in EBV-transformed (but not tumorigenic) B-cell lines and Burkitt lymphoma cells. For instance, the tumor cells do not express several viral-encoded membrane proteins that are known to be targeted by host cytotoxic T cells.

It appears therefore that EBV serves as one factor in the multistep development of Burkitt lymphoma (Fig. 8–43).[106] In normal individuals, EBV infection is readily controlled by effective immune responses directed against viral antigens expressed on the cell membranes, and hence the vast majority of infected individuals remain asymptomatic or develop self-limited infectious mononucleosis. In regions of Africa where Burkitt lymphoma is endemic, poorly understood cofactors (e.g., chronic malaria) favor sustained proliferation of B cells immortalized by EBV. The actively dividing B-cell population is at increased risk for developing mutations, such as the t(8;14) translocation, that juxtapose c-*myc* with one of the immunoglobulin gene loci. This provides growth advantage to the affected cell owing to activation of c-*myc*. One of the EBV-encoded proteins, EBNA-1, activates the machinery for rearrangement of immunoglobulin genes. This activity may increase the likelihood of a t(8;14) translocation and the resultant c-*myc* activation. Overexpression of the c-*myc* oncogene by itself is not sufficient for malignant transformation. In all likelihood, it represents one of multiple steps in lymphomagenesis. Additional mutations, possibly affecting the N-*ras* oncogene, occur in the B cells immortalized by EBV. Together these changes lead to the emergence of a monoclonal B-cell neoplasm. According to this view, EBV itself is not directly oncogenic, but by acting as a polyclonal B-cell mitogen, it sets the stage for the acquisition of the t(8;14) translocation and other mutations, which ultimately release the cells from normal growth regulation. Concurrent with these changes, there is alteration in viral gene expression as well, such that the display of antigens that could be recognized by cytotoxic T cells is reduced.

The role played by host immune response in controlling EBV-transformed B cells is illustrated dramatically by the occurrence of B-cell lymphomas in immunosuppressed patients. Some patients with acquired immunodeficiency syndrome (AIDS) and those who receive long-term immunosuppressive therapy for preventing allograft rejection present with multifocal B-cell tumors within lymphoid tissue or in the central nervous system. These tumors are polyclonal at the outset but can develop into monoclonal proliferations. The expression of viral antigens such as

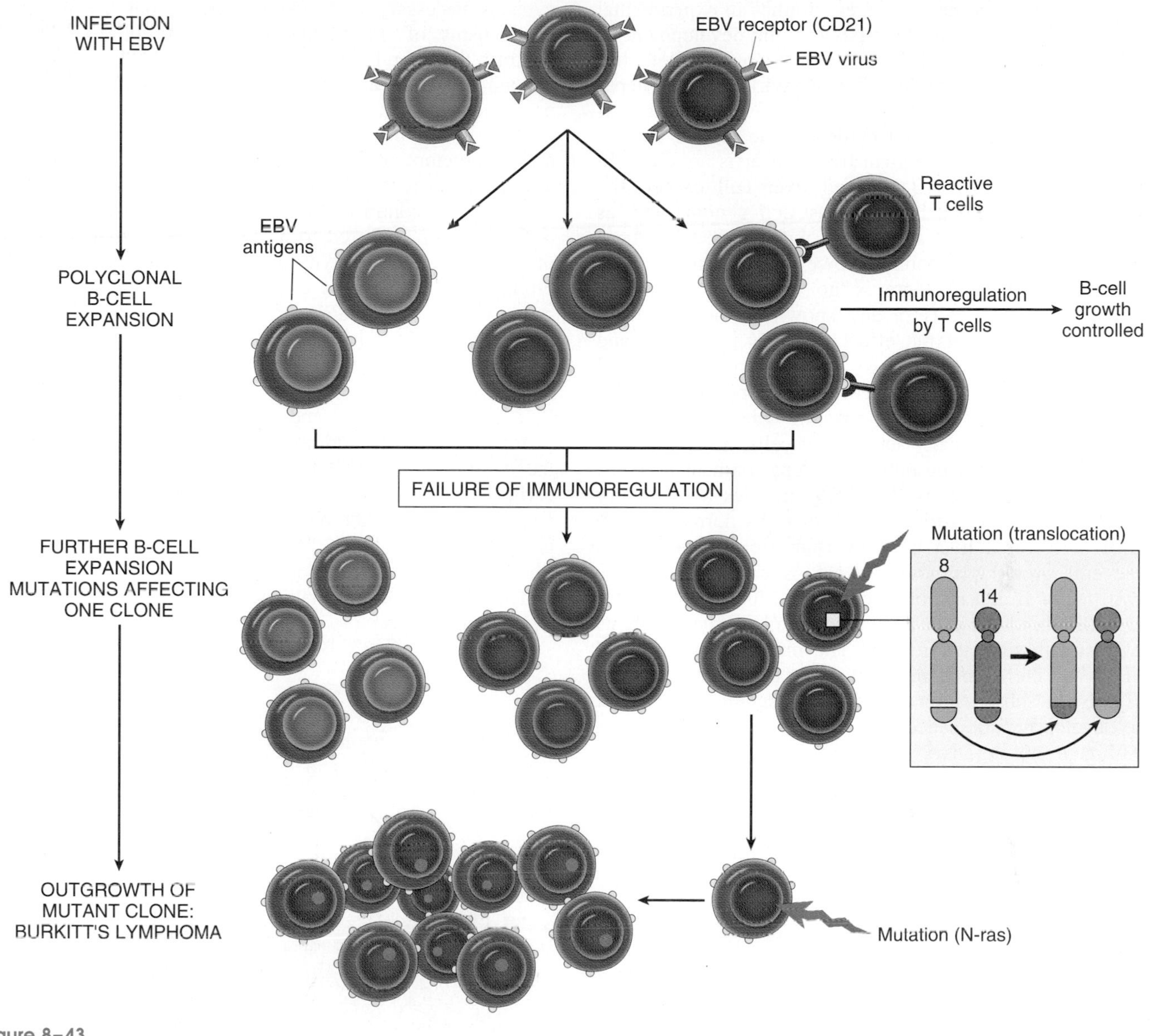

Figure 8–43

Schema depicting the possible evolution of Epstein-Barr virus (EBV)–induced Burkitt lymphoma.

LMP-1 remains high on these cells, and hence these tumors seem to represent the in vivo counterparts of the B-cell lines immortalized by EBV infection in vitro. That the growth of these EBV-driven cells is sensitive to immunologic regulation is evident from the observation that in some cases the tumors regress after relaxation of immunosuppressive therapy.

Nasopharyngeal carcinoma is the other tumor associated with EBV infection. This tumor is endemic in Southern China, in some parts of Africa, and in Arctic Eskimos. In contrast to Burkitt lymphoma, 100% of nasopharyngeal carcinomas obtained from all parts of the world contain EBV DNA.[107] The viral integration in the host cells is clonal, thus ruling out the possibility that EBV infection occurred after tumor development. In addition, antibody titers to viral capsid antigens are greatly elevated, and in endemic areas patients develop IgA antibodies before the appearance of the tumor. The 100% correlation between EBV and nasopharyngeal carcinoma suggests that EBV plays a role in the genesis of this tumor, but (as with Burkitt tumor) the restricted geographic distribution indicates that genetic or environmental cofactors, or both, also contribute to its cause.[108] The relationship of EBV with the pathogenesis of Hodgkin disease is discussed in Chapter 15.

Hepatitis B Virus. Epidemiologic studies strongly suggest a close association between HBV infection and the occurrence of liver cancer (Chapter 19). HBV is endemic in countries of the Far East and Africa, and correspondingly these areas have the highest incidence of hepatocellular carcinoma. For example, in Taiwan, those who are infected with HBV have a greater than 200-fold increased risk of developing liver cancer as compared with uninfected individuals in the same area. Studies in experimental animals also support a role for HBV in the development of liver cancer. Although HBV infection is restricted to humans and chimpanzees, related hepadnaviruses cause hepatocellular cancers in woodchucks. Despite compelling epidemiologic and experimental evidence, the precise role of HBV in the causation of human liver cancer is not clear. In virtually all cases of HBV-related liver cell cancer, the viral DNA is integrated into the host cell genome and, as with HPV, the tumors are clonal with respect to these insertions. The HBV genome, however, does not encode any oncoproteins, and there is no consistent pattern of integration in the vicinity of any known protooncogene. It is likely therefore that the effect of HBV is indirect and possibly multifactorial.[109] *(1)* By causing chronic liver cell injury and accompanying regenerative hyperplasia, HBV expands the pool of cells at risk for subsequent genetic changes. In the mitotically active liver cells, mutations may arise spontaneously or be inflicted by environmental agents, such as dietary aflatoxins. *(2)* HBV encodes a regulatory element called *HBx protein*, which disrupts normal growth control of infected liver cells by transcriptional activation of several growth-promoting genes, such as insulin-like growth factor II and receptors for insulin-like growth factor I. *(3)* HBx binds to *p53* and appears to interfere with its growth-suppressing activities.[110] The important role played by HBx in the pathogenesis of liver cell cancer is buttressed by the observation that mice transgenic for the HBx gene develop hepatic cancers.

Although not a DNA virus, hepatitis C virus is also strongly linked to the pathogenesis of hepatocellular carcinoma. As with hepatitis B virus, the epidemiologic evidence of an association with hepatitis C virus is compelling. In the case of hepatitis C virus, the role of this virus in the pathogenesis of liver cancer seems to be limited to its ability to cause chronic liver cell injury and the accompanying regeneration. The mitotically active liver, presumably, provides a fertile soil for mutations.

RNA ONCOGENIC VIRUSES

Although the study of animal retroviruses has provided spectacular insights into the molecular basis of cancer, only one human retrovirus, human T-cell leukemia virus type 1 (HTLV-1), is firmly implicated in the causation of cancer.

Human T-Cell Leukemia Virus Type 1. HTLV-1 is associated with a form of T-cell leukemia/lymphoma that is endemic in certain parts of Japan and the Caribbean basin but is found sporadically elsewhere, including the United States. Similar to the AIDS virus, HTLV-1 has tropism for $CD4^+$ T cells, and hence this subset of T cells is the major target for neoplastic transformation. Human infection requires transmission of infected T cells via sexual intercourse, blood products, or breast-feeding. Leukemia develops in only about 1% of the infected individuals after a long latent period of 20 to 30 years. In addition to leukemia, HTLV-1 is associated with a demyelinating neurologic disorder called *tropical spastic paraparesis* (Chapter 30) and possibly some forms of uveitis and arthritis in endemic areas.[111]

There is little doubt that HTLV-1 infection of T lymphocytes is necessary for leukemogenesis, but the molecular mechanisms of transformation are not entirely clear. In contrast to several murine retroviruses, HTLV-1 does not contain a v-*onc*, and no consistent integration next to a protooncogene has been discovered. In leukemic cells, however, viral integration shows a clonal pattern. The genomic structure of HTLV-1 reveals the *gag, pol, env*, and long terminal repeat (LTR) regions typical of other retroviruses, but, in contrast to other leukemia viruses, it contains another region, referred to as *tax*. It seems that the secrets of its transforming activity are locked in the *tax* gene. The product of this gene is essential for viral replication because it stimulates transcription of viral mRNA by acting on the 5′ LTR. It is now established that the *tax* protein can also activate the transcription of several host cell genes, including c-*fos*, c-*sis*, genes encoding the cytokine IL-2 and its receptor, and the gene for myeloid growth factor GM-CSF. In addition, *tax* prevents the formation of the complex between CDK4 and its inhibitor $p16^{INK}$ (see earlier), and thus the cell cycle becomes dysregulated. From these and other observations, the following scenario is emerging (Fig. 8–44): HTLV-1 infection stimulates proliferation of T cells. This is brought about by the *tax* gene, which turns on genes that encode a T-cell growth factor, IL-2, and its receptor, setting up an autocrine system for

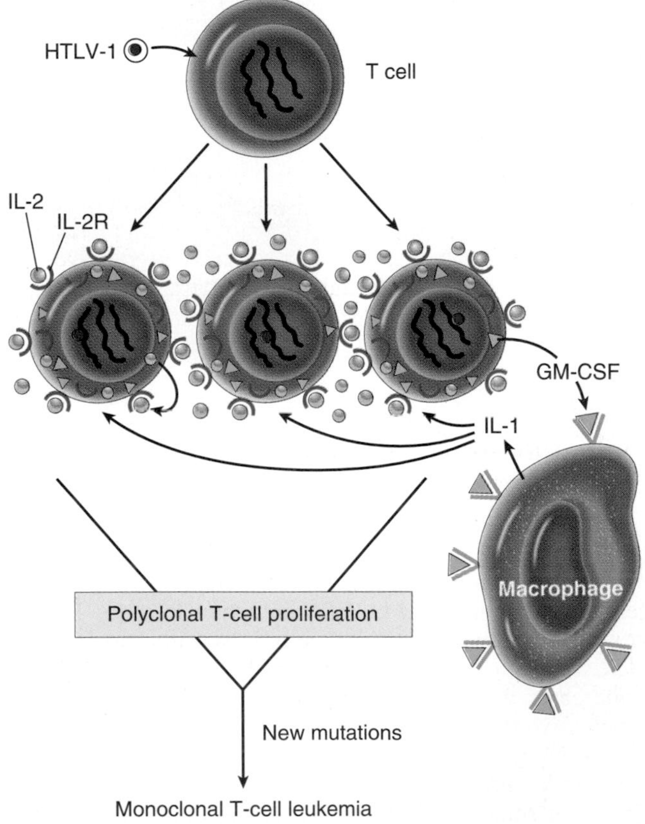

Figure 8–44

Pathogenesis of human T-cell leukemia virus type 1 (HTLV-1)–induced T-cell leukemia/lymphoma. HTLV-1 infects many T cells and initially causes polyclonal proliferation by autocrine and paracrine pathways. Ultimately, a monoclonal T-cell leukemia/lymphoma results when one proliferating T cell suffers additional mutations.

proliferation. At the same time, a paracrine pathway is activated by the increased production of GM-CSF. This myeloid growth factor, by acting on neighboring macrophages, induces increased secretion of other T-cell mitogens, such as IL-1. Initially the T-cell proliferation is polyclonal because the virus infects many cells. The proliferating T cells are at increased risk of secondary transforming events (mutations), which lead ultimately to the outgrowth of a monoclonal neoplastic T-cell population whose growth is independent of IL-2.[112] The transforming function of the *tax* gene is supported by the occurrence of tumors in *tax*-transgenic mice.

HELICOBACTER PYLORI

There is accumulating evidence linking gastric infection with the bacterium *H. pylori* to the causation of gastric lymphomas and gastric carcinomas. The association is stronger with B-cell lymphoma of the stomach than with carcinomas. This relationship has been established by epidemiologic studies as well as by detection of *H. pylori* infection in the vast majority of cases of gastric lymphomas. Furthermore, treatment of *H. pylori* with antibiotics results in regression of the lymphoma in most cases. Because the tumors arise in mucosa-associated lymphoid tissue (MALT), they sometimes are called *MALTomas*. The B cells that give rise to these tumors normally reside in the marginal zones of lymphoid follicles and hence the alternative name of *marginal zone lymphoma* (Chapter 15). It is thought that chronic infection with *H. pylori* leads to the generation of *H. pylori*–reactive T cells, which, in turn, activate a polyclonal population of B cells by secreting soluble factors. With time, a monoclonal but still T cell–dependent population of proliferating B cells emerges. Presumably, such monoclonal B-cell proliferation subsides when the antigenic stimulus for T cells is removed by antibiotic treatment. Eventually, proliferating B cells accumulate mutations and become T cell independent.[113]

HOST DEFENSE AGAINST TUMORS—TUMOR IMMUNITY

Neoplastic transformation, as we have discussed, results from a series of genetic alterations, some of which may result in the expression of cell surface antigens that are seen as nonself by the immune system. The idea that tumors are not entirely self was conceived by Ehrlich, who proposed that immune-mediated recognition of autologous tumor cells may be a positive mechanism capable of eliminating transformed cells. Subsequently, Thomas and Burnet formalized this concept by coining the term *immune surveillance* to refer to recognition and destruction of nonself tumor cells on their appearance. The fact that cancers occur suggests that immune surveillance is imperfect; however, because some tumors escape such policing does not preclude the possibility that others may have been aborted. It is necessary therefore to explore certain questions about tumor immunity: What is the nature of tumor antigens? What host effector systems may recognize tumor cells? Is antitumor immunity effective against spontaneous neoplasms? Can immune reactions against tumors be exploited for immunotherapy?

Tumor Antigens

Antigens that elicit an immune response have been demonstrated in many experimentally induced tumors and in some human cancers. They can be broadly classified into two categories: *tumor-specific antigens* (TSAs), which are present only on tumor cells and not on any normal cells, and *tumor-associated antigens* (TAAs), which are present on tumor cells and also on some normal cells.

TSAs were initially demonstrated in chemically induced tumors of rodents. In experimental model systems, tumor antigenicity is usually assessed by (1) the ability of an animal to resist a live tumor implant after previous immunization with live or killed tumor cells, (2) the ability of tumor-free host animals to resist challenge when infused with sensitized T cells from a tumor-immunized syngeneic donor, and (3) the demonstration in vitro of tumor cell destruction by cytotoxic CD8+ T cells derived from a tumor-immunized animal. By these methods, it has been found that many chemically induced tumors express "private" or "unique" antigens not shared by other (histologically identical) tumors induced by the same chemical, even in the same animal.

The identity of TSAs in experimentally induced tumors and their existence on human tumors remained elusive until the molecular basis of T-cell recognition was understood. With the realization that T-cell receptors recognize peptides bound to the antigen-binding cleft of major histocompatibility complex (MHC) molecules (Chapter 7), it became evident that *TSAs that evoke a cytotoxic T-cell response must be derived from peptides that are uniquely present within tumor cells and presented on the cell surface by class I MHC molecules.* What is the nature of proteins that give rise to tumor-specific antigens? How tumor specific are the human tumor antigens recognized by T cells? The answers to these questions are now becoming available, and it is clear that human tumors do express antigens that can be recognized by autologous T cells. Some such antigens are truly tumor specific, whereas many others are expressed on some normal cells as well. The TSAs and TAAs recognized by T cells are illustrated in Figure 8–45 and discussed next.[114]

Tumor-Specific Shared Antigens. These antigens are encoded by genes that are silent in virtually all normal adult tissues but expressed in a number of tumors of various histologic types. Prototype antigens of this group are those encoded by the *MAGE* family of genes. Testis is the only normal organ in which MAGE proteins are present; however, because male germ cells do not express HLA molecules, the MAGE antigens cannot be expressed on their cell surface. Thus, for all practical purposes, these antigens are tumor specific. In contrast to the TSAs of chemically induced mouse tumors, discussed previously, these antigens are not unique to each tumor; instead the

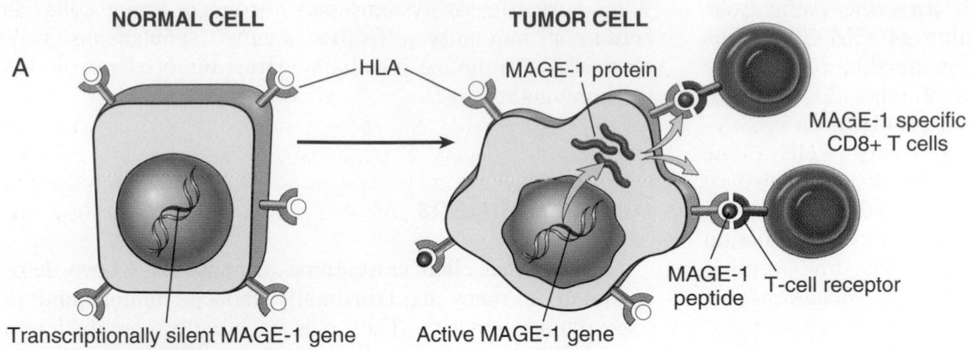

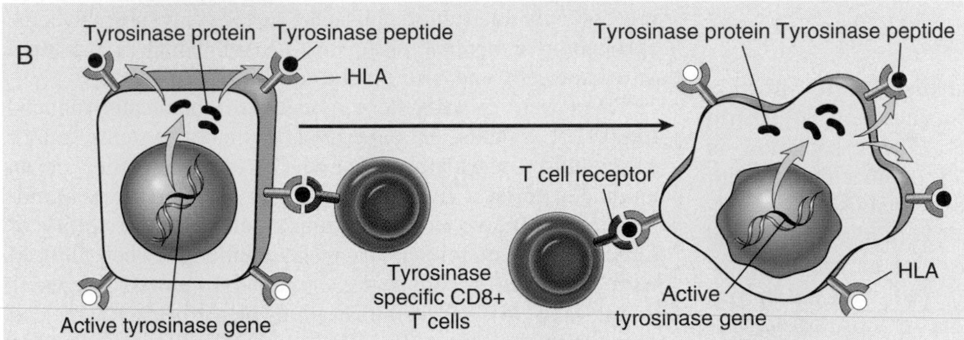

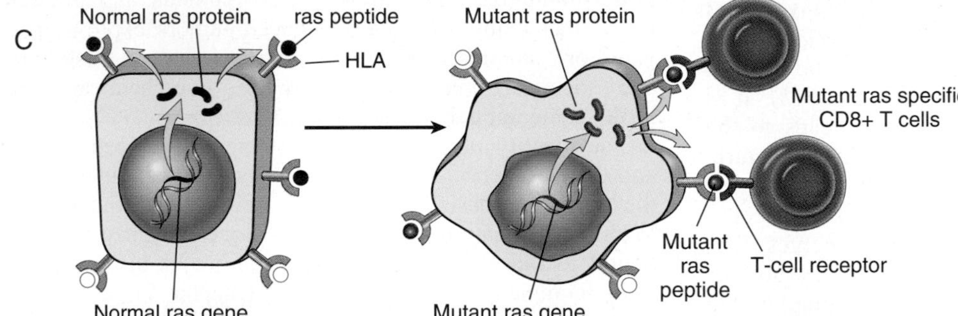

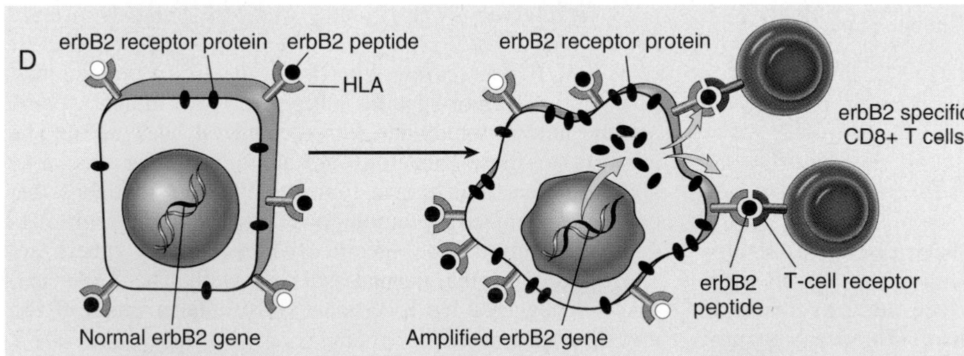

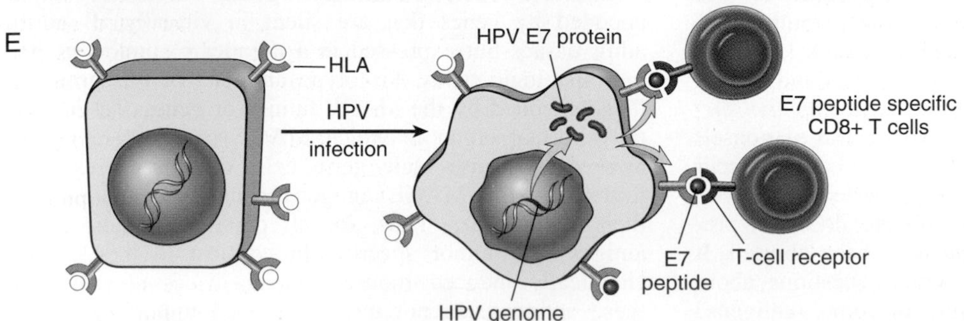

Figure 8-45

Molecular mechanisms underlying the formation of tumor antigens recognized by CD8+ T cells.

same antigen is shared by many different types of tumors. For example, the MAGE-1 antigen (melanoma antigen-1), discovered initially in melanomas and expressed on 37% of these tumors, is also expressed in carcinomas of lung, liver, stomach, esophagus, and urinary bladder. In each of these tumors, a peptide derived from the MAGE-1 protein is bound to HLA-A1 and presented on the tumor surface to specific CD8+ T cells. Currently, at least 12 MAGE genes mapped to chromosome Xq have been identified. Similar antigens, called *GAGE, BAGE*, and *RAGE*, have also been detected in several human tumors. Similar to the MAGE family of genes, the BAGE and GAGE genes are expressed only in testis, and the RAGE gene is expressed only in HLA-negative retinal cells. Why these genes are selectively expressed in tumor cells is not known. There are no tumor-associated mutations in these genes. Because the MAGE antigens are shared by many different types of tumors, they are attractive targets for immunotherapy. For example, it may be possible to administer MAGE antigens in an immunogenic form to cancer patients, with the idea of boosting their MAGE-specific T cells.

Mucins are another type of protein that can give rise to TSAs. In some pancreatic, ovarian, and breast carcinomas, peptides derived from abnormally glycosylated cell-surface mucins can be recognized by cytotoxic T cells. In normal cells, the mucin is heavily glycosylated, but in these cancers certain peptide repeats are unmasked by underglycosylation.[115] The cytotoxic T cells that recognize these peptides are, for all practical purposes, tumor specific because in normal cells these epitopes are hidden by the carbohydrate cover.

Tissue-Specific Antigens. Antigens in this category are shared by tumor cells and their normal untransformed counterparts. For example, both normal melanocytes and melanomas express tyrosinase. Peptides derived from this enzyme protein, presented on the cell surface by HLA class I molecules, can be recognized by specific cytotoxic T cells. Such T cells can destroy the tumor cells as well as normal epidermal melanocytes. In some patients, spontaneous regression of the melanoma is accompanied by local areas of depigmentation, as if both the tumor and the normal melanocytes were destroyed by cytotoxic T cells. Because melanocytes are also present in the eye and the brain, active immunization against tyrosinase-derived peptides must be considered carefully.

Antigens Resulting From Mutations. Antigens in this category are derived from those regions of protooncogenes and tumor-suppressor genes that are mutated in tumor cells. Because such mutations are present only in tumor cells, the T cells directed against the products of mutant proteins are highly tumor specific. It has been possible to generate cytotoxic T cells against several such antigens, including peptides derived from mutated *p53*, K-*ras*, CDK4, and the *bcr-c-abl* gene product. There is no evidence that immune responses against such antigens occur spontaneously in vivo.

Overexpressed Antigens. This class of semi–tumor-specific antigens comprises proteins encoded by genes that are not mutated but are overexpressed in tumors. To this category belongs the c-*erbB2* (or *neu*) protein, which is overexpressed in 30% of breast and ovarian carcinomas. Although this protein is also present in normal ovarian and breast cells, its expression is generally below the threshold level required for recognition by cytotoxic T cells.

Viral Antigens. Antigens derived from oncogenic viruses could also be recognized by T cells. The best example in humans is peptides derived from the E7 protein of HPV-16. Because this virus is present in many cervical carcinomas, the cytotoxic T cells can lyse the cancer cells.

Other Tumor Antigens. Several other TAAs are normal self proteins that do not evoke an immune response in humans and are of little functional significance in tumor rejection. Serologic detection of these antigens is nevertheless of value in the diagnosis of certain tumors, and antibodies raised against them can be useful for immunotherapy. Some examples follow.

Oncofetal antigens, or embryonic antigens, are normally expressed in developing (embryonic) tissues but not in normal adult tissues. Their expression in some types of cancer cells is presumably due to derepression of genetic programs. The two best examples of oncofetal antigens—α-fetoprotein (AFP) and carcinoembryonic antigen (CEA)—are described later.

Differentiation antigens are peculiar to the differentiation state at which cancer cells are arrested. For example, CD10 (CALLA antigen), an antigen expressed in early B lymphocytes, is expressed in B-cell leukemias and lymphomas. Similarly, prostate-specific antigen is expressed on normal as well as cancerous prostatic epithelium. Both serve as useful differentiation markers in the diagnosis of lymphoid and prostatic cancers.

Antitumor Effector Mechanisms

Both cell-mediated and humoral immunity can have antitumor activity. The cellular effectors that mediate immunity were described in Chapter 7, so it is necessary here only to characterize them briefly (Fig. 8–46):

- *Cytotoxic T lymphocytes*: The role of specifically sensitized cytotoxic T cells in experimentally induced tumors is well established. In humans, they play a protective role against virus-associated neoplasms (e.g., EBV-induced Burkitt lymphoma and HPV-induced tumors). In addition, the presence of HLA-restricted cytotoxic T cells within several human tumors suggests a wider role for protective T-cell immunity. In many cases, these tumor-infiltrating lymphocytes are directed against the T cell–defined tumor antigens discussed earlier. The tumor-infiltrating lymphocytes can be harvested and expanded in vitro and reinfused into the autologous host. Such adoptive immunotherapy has met with some success. Further refinements include transfection of cytokine genes into tumor-infiltrating lymphocytes to potentiate their antitumor effects.
- *Natural killer cells*: Natural killer cells are lymphocytes that are capable of destroying tumor cells without prior sensitization. After activation with IL-2, natural killer cells can lyse a wide range of human tumors, including many that appear to be nonimmunogenic for T cells.

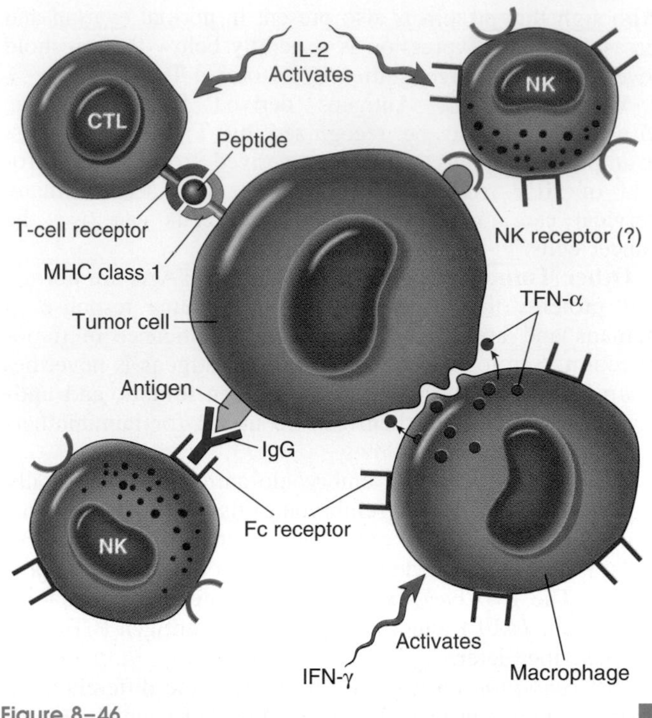

Figure 8–46

Cellular effectors of antitumor immunity and some cytokines that modulate antitumor activities. The nature of antigens recognized by T cells is depicted in Figure 8–45.

Thus, natural killer cells may provide the first line of defense against many tumors. Natural killer cells have been found to be effective against a variety of tumors in experimental animals. These cells are most effective against tumors that have reduced levels of class I MHC molecules because class I molecules inhibit natural killer cell cytotoxicity by engaging inhibitory receptors expressed on natural killer cells (Chapter 7). Thus, class I–deficient tumor cells that escape T-cell recognition may succumb to natural killer cells. Adoptive immunotherapy with in vitro expanded and activated human natural killer cells has met with limited success. In addition to direct lysis of tumor cells, natural killer cells can also participate in antibody-dependent cellular cytotoxicity (ADCC) (Chapter 7).

- *Macrophages*: Activated macrophages exhibit somewhat selective cytotoxicity against tumor cells in vitro. T cells and natural killer cells may collaborate with macrophages in antitumor reactivity because interferon-γ (IFN-γ), a T cell–derived and natural killer cell–derived cytokine, is a potent activator of macrophages. These cells may kill tumors by mechanisms similar to those used to kill microbes (e.g., production of reactive oxygen metabolites) or by secretion of tumor necrosis factor-α (TNF-α). In addition to its many other effects, this cytokine is lytic for several tumor cells.
- *Humoral* mechanisms may also participate in tumor cell destruction by two mechanisms: activation of complement and induction of ADCC by natural killer cells.

IMMUNOSURVEILLANCE

Given the host of possible and potential antitumor mechanisms, is there any evidence that they operate in vivo to prevent emergence of neoplasms? The strongest argument for the existence of immunosurveillance is the increased frequency of cancers in immunodeficient hosts. About 5% of persons with congenital immunodeficiencies develop cancers, about 200 times the expected prevalence. Analogously, immunosuppressed transplant recipients and patients with AIDS have more malignancies. Most (but not all) of these neoplasms are lymphomas, often immunoblastic B-cell lymphomas. Particularly illustrative is the rare X-linked recessive immunodeficiency disorder termed *XLP*.[116] When affected boys develop an EBV infection, it does not take the usual self-limited form of infectious mononucleosis but in the vast majority of cases evolves into a fatal form of infectious mononucleosis. Approximately 25% of XLP patients develop malignant lymphoma.

Most cancers occur in persons who do not suffer from any overt immunodeficiency. It is evident then that *tumor cells must develop mechanisms to escape* or evade the immune system in immunocompetent hosts. Several such mechanisms may be operative.[117]

- *Selective outgrowth of antigen-negative variants*: During tumor progression, strongly immunogenic subclones may be eliminated.
- *Loss or reduced expression of histocompatibility antigens*: Tumor cells may fail to express normal levels of HLA class I molecules, thereby escaping attack by cytotoxic T cells. Such cells, however, may trigger natural killer cells.
- *Lack of costimulation*: It may be recalled that sensitization of T cells requires two signals, one by foreign peptide presented by MHC and the other by costimulatory molecules (Chapter 7); although tumor cells may express peptide antigens with class I molecules, they often do not express costimulatory molecules. This not only prevents sensitization, but also it may render T cells anergic or, worse, cause them to undergo apoptosis. To bypass this problem, attempts are being made to immunize patients with autologous tumor cells that have been transfected with the gene for the costimulatory molecule B7-1. In another approach, autologous dendritic cells expanded in vitro and pulsed with tumor antigens (e.g., MAGE-1) are infused into cancer patients. Because dendritic cells express high levels of costimulatory molecules, it is expected that such immunization will evoke the formation of antitumor T cells.
- *Immunosuppression*: Many oncogenic agents (e.g., chemicals and ionizing radiation) suppress host immune responses. Tumors or tumor products may also be immunosuppressive. For example, TGF-β, secreted in large quantities by many tumors, is a potent immunosuppressant. In some cases, the immune response induced by the tumor (e.g., activation of suppressor T cells) may itself inhibit tumor immunity.
- *Apoptosis of cytotoxic T cells*: Some melanomas and hepatocellular carcinomas express Fas ligand. These tumors kill Fas-expressing T lymphocytes that come in

contact with them, thus eliminating tumor-specific T cells.[118, 119]

Thus, it seems that there is no dearth of mechanisms by which tumor cells can outwit the host and thrive despite an intact immune system.

Although the increased occurrence of tumors in immunodeficient hosts supports the existence of immunosurveillance, the strongest argument against the concept of immunosurveillance also derives from the study of immunosuppressed patients. The most common forms of cancers in immunosuppressed and immunodeficient patients are lymphomas, notably immunoblastic B-cell lymphomas, which could be the consequence of abnormal immunoproliferative responses to microbes such as EBV or to the various therapeutic agents administered to these patients. Significantly, an increased incidence of the most common forms of cancer—lung, breast, gastrointestinal tract—and multiple neoplasms might be anticipated in immunologic cripples but does not occur.

CLINICAL FEATURES OF TUMORS

Neoplasms are essentially parasites. Some cause only trivial mischief, but others are catastrophic. All tumors, even benign ones, may cause morbidity and mortality. Moreover, every new growth requires careful appraisal lest it be cancerous. This differential comes into sharpest focus with lumps in the female breast. Both cancers and many benign disorders of the female breast present as palpable masses. In fact, benign lesions are more common than cancers. Although clinical evaluation may suggest one or the other, "the only unequivocally benign breast mass is the excised and anatomically diagnosed one." This is equally true of all neoplasms. There are, however, instances when adherence to this dictum must be tempered by clinical judgment. Subcutaneous lipomas, for example, are quite common and readily recognized by their soft, yielding consistency. Unless they are uncomfortable, subject to trauma, or aesthetically disturbing, small lesions are often merely observed for significant increase in size. A few other examples might be cited, but it suffices that *with a few exceptions, all masses require anatomic evaluation.* Besides the concern malignant neoplasms arouse, even benign ones may have many adverse effects. The sections that follow consider (1) the effects of a tumor on the host, (2) the grading and clinical staging of cancer, and (3) the laboratory diagnosis of neoplasms.

Effects of Tumor on Host

Obviously, cancers are far more threatening to the host than benign tumors are. Nonetheless, both types of neoplasia may cause problems because of (1) location and impingement on adjacent structures, (2) functional activity such as hormone synthesis, (3) bleeding and secondary infections when they ulcerate through adjacent natural surfaces, and (4) initiation of acute symptoms caused by either rupture or infarction. Any metastasis has the potential to produce these same consequences. Cancers may also be responsible for cachexia (wasting) or paraneoplastic syndromes.

LOCAL AND HORMONAL EFFECTS

An example of disease related to critical location is the pituitary adenoma. Although benign and possibly not productive of hormone, expansile growth of the tumor can destroy the remaining pituitary and thus lead to serious endocrinopathy. Analogously, cancers arising within or metastatic to an endocrine gland may cause an endocrine insufficiency by destroying the gland. Neoplasms in the gut, both benign and malignant, may cause obstruction as they enlarge. Infrequently the peristaltic pull telescopes the neoplasm and its affected segment into the downstream segment, producing an obstructing intussusception (Chapter 18).

Neoplasms arising in endocrine glands may produce manifestations by elaboration of hormones. Such functional activity is more typical of benign tumors than of cancers, which may be sufficiently undifferentiated to have lost such capability. A benign β-cell adenoma of the pancreatic islets less than 1 cm in diameter may produce sufficient insulin to cause fatal hypoglycemia. In addition, nonendocrine tumors may elaborate hormones or hormone-like products and give rise to paraneoplastic syndromes (discussed later). The erosive destructive growth of cancers or the expansile pressure of a benign tumor on any natural surface, such as the skin or mucosa of the gut, may cause ulcerations, secondary infections, and bleeding. Melena (blood in the stool) and hematuria, for example, are characteristic of neoplasms of the gut and urinary tract. Neoplasms, benign as well as malignant, may then cause problems in varied ways, but all are far less common than the cachexia of malignancy.

CANCER CACHEXIA

Patients with cancer commonly suffer progressive loss of body fat and lean body mass accompanied by profound weakness, anorexia, and anemia. This wasting syndrome is referred to as *cachexia*. The origins of cancer cachexia are obscure. There is little doubt, however, that cachexia is not caused by the nutritional demands of the tumor. Cancers rarely grow as rapidly as the fetus, yet many a postpartum mother, when getting on the scale, laments that she did not suffer just a bit of "cachexia." Current evidence indicates that cachexia results from the action of soluble factors such as cytokines produced either by the tumor or by the host in response to the tumor.

Clinically, anorexia is a common problem in patients with cancer, even in those who do not have mechanical obstruction caused by gastrointestinal tumors. Reduced food intake has been related to abnormalities in taste and central control of appetite, but reduced intake alone is not sufficient to explain the cachexia of malignancy. In patients with cancer, calorie expenditure often remains high, and basal metabolic rate is increased despite reduced food intake. By contrast, in starvation, there is an adaptational lowering of metabolic rate.[120] Furthermore, in cancer cachexia, there is equal loss of fat and muscle, whereas in starvation the muscle mass is relatively preserved at the expense of fat stores. The basis of these metabolic abnormalities is not fully understood. Many of the changes associated with cancer cachexia, including loss of appetite and alterations in fat metabolism, are mimicked by the administration of TNF-α in experimental animals. It is suspected therefore that TNF-α, produced by macrophages or possibly some tumor cells, is a mediator of the wasting syndrome that accompanies cancer.[121] Other cytokines, such as IL-1 and IFN-γ, synergize with TNF-α. In addition to these cytokines, there is evidence for the existence of other soluble factors that increase the catabolism of muscle and adipose tissue by acting directly on fat and muscle protein. A protein-mobilizing factor has been isolated from the serum of both animals and humans with cancer cachexia. Quite remarkably, injections of purified preparations of this factor into healthy mice causes rapid weight loss, without any reduction in food intake.[122] Thus, it seems that several soluble factors collaborate in contributing to malnutrition in cancer patients. Identification and neutralization of such factors may help ameliorate cancer cachexia.

PARANEOPLASTIC SYNDROMES

Symptom complexes in cancer-bearing patients that cannot readily be explained, either by the local or distant spread of the tumor or by the elaboration of hormones indigenous to the tissue from which the tumor arose, are known as *paraneoplastic syndromes.* These occur in about 10% of patients with malignant disease. Despite their relative infrequency, paraneoplastic syndromes are important to recognize:[123]

- First, they may represent the earliest manifestation of an occult neoplasm.
- Second, in affected patients, they may represent significant clinical problems and may even be lethal.
- Third, they may mimic metastatic disease and therefore confound treatment.

A classification of paraneoplastic syndromes and their presumed origins is presented in Table 8–11. A few comments on some of the more common and interesting syndromes follow.

The *endocrinopathies* are frequently encountered paraneoplastic syndromes.[124] Because the native cells giving rise to the cancer are not of endocrine origin, the functional activity is referred to as *ectopic hormone production.* Among the endocrinopathies, Cushing syndrome is the most common. Approximately 50% of the patients with this endocrinopathy have carcinoma of the lung, chiefly the small cell type. It is caused by excessive production of adrenocorticotropic hormone (ACTH) or ACTH-like peptides. The precursor of ACTH is a large molecule known as proopiomelanocortin (POMC). Lung cancer patients with Cushing syndrome have elevated serum levels of POMC as well as ACTH. The former is not found in serum of patients with a pituitary source of excess ACTH.

Hypercalcemia is probably the most common paraneoplastic syndrome, and conversely, overtly symptomatic hypercalcemia is most often related to some form of cancer rather than to hyperparathyroidism. Two general processes are involved in cancer-associated hypercalcemia: (1) osteolysis induced by cancer, whether primary in bone, such as multiple myeloma, or metastatic to bone from any primary lesion, and (2) the production of calcemic humoral substances by extraosseous neoplasms. *Hypercalcemia owing to skeletal metastases is not a paraneoplastic syndrome.*

Several humoral factors have been associated with paraneoplastic hypercalcemia of malignancy.[124] Perhaps the most important is a molecule related to, but distinct from, parathyroid hormone (PTH). The so-called parathyroid hormone–related protein (PTHrP) resembles the native hormone only in its amino terminus. It shares several biologic actions with PTH and acts by binding to the PTH receptor. In contrast to PTH, PTHrP is produced by many normal tissues, including keratinocytes, muscles, bone, and ovary. The amounts produced by normal cells, however, are small. It is thought to regulate calcium transport in lactating breast and across the placenta. In addition to PTHrP, several other factors, such as IL-1, TGF-α, TNF-α, and dihydroxyvitamin D, have also been implicated in causing the hypercalcemia of malignancy. Tumors most often associated with paraneoplastic hypercalcemia are carcinomas of the breast, lung, kidney, and ovary. The most common lung neoplasm associated with hypercalcemia is the squamous cell bronchogenic carcinoma, rather than small cell cancer of the lung (more often associated with endocrinopathies).

The *neuromyopathic paraneoplastic syndromes* take diverse forms, such as peripheral neuropathies, cortical cerebellar degeneration, a polymyopathy resembling polymyositis, and a myasthenic syndrome similar to *myasthenia gravis.* The cause of these syndromes is poorly understood. In some cases, antibodies, presumably induced against tumor cells that cross-react with neuronal cells, have been detected. It is postulated that some neural antigens are ectopically expressed by visceral cancers. For some unknown reason, the immune system recognizes these antigens as foreign and mounts an immune response.[125]

Acanthosis nigricans is characterized by gray-black patches of verrucous hyperkeratosis on the skin. This disorder occurs rarely as a genetically determined disease in juveniles or adults. In addition, particularly in those over the age of 40, the appearance of such lesions is associated in about 50% of cases with some form of cancer. Sometimes the skin changes appear before discovery of the cancer.[126]

Hypertrophic osteoarthropathy, is encountered in 1 to 10% of patients with bronchogenic carcinomas. Rarely, other forms of cancer are involved. This disorder is characterized by *(1) periosteal new bone formation primarily at the distal ends of long bones, metatarsals, metacarpals, and proximal phalanges,* (2) *arthritis of the adjacent joints, and (3) clubbing of the digits.* Although the osteoarthropathy is seldom seen in noncancer patients, clubbing of the fingertips may be encountered in liver diseases, diffuse lung disease, congenital cyanotic heart disease, ulcerative colitis, and other disorders. The cause of hypertrophic osteoarthropathy is unknown.

Several *vascular and hematologic manifestations* may appear in association with a variety of forms of cancer. As mentioned in the earlier discussion of thrombosis (Chapter

Table 8–11. PARANEOPLASTIC SYNDROMES

Clinical Syndromes	Major Forms of Underlying Cancer	Causal Mechanism
Endocrinopathies		
Cushing syndrome	Small cell carcinoma of lung Pancreatic carcinoma Neural tumors	ACTH or ACTH-like substance
Syndrome of inappropriate antidiuretic hormone secretion	Small cell carcinoma of lung; intracranial neoplasms	Antidiuretic hormone or atrial natriuretic hormones
Hypercalcemia	Squamous cell carcinoma of lung Breast carcinoma Renal carcinoma Adult T-cell leukemia/lymphoma Ovarian carcinoma	Parathyroid hormone related peptide, TGF-α, TNF-α, IL-1
Hypoglycemia	Fibrosarcoma Other mesenchymal sarcomas Hepatocellular carcinoma	Insulin or insulin-like substance
Carcinoid syndrome	Bronchial adenoma (carcinoid) Pancreatic carcinoma Gastric carcinoma	Serotonin, bradykinin, ?histamine
Polycythemia	Renal carcinoma Cerebellar hemangioma Hepatocellular carcinoma	Erythropoietin
Nerve and Muscle Syndromes		
Myasthenia	Bronchogenic carcinoma	Immunologic
Disorders of the central and peripheral nervous systems	Breast carcinoma	
Dermatologic Disorders		
Acanthosis nigricans	Gastric carcinoma Lung carcinoma Uterine carcinoma	?Immunologic, ?secretion of epidermal growth factor
Dermatomyositis	Bronchogenic, breast carcinoma	?Immunologic
Osseous, Articular, and Soft Tissue Changes		
Hypertrophic osteoarthropathy and clubbing of the fingers	Bronchogenic carcinoma	Unknown
Vascular and Hematologic Changes		
Venous thrombosis (Trousseau phenomenon)	Pancreatic carcinoma Bronchogenic carcinoma Other cancers	Tumor products (mucins that activate clotting)
Nonbacterial thrombotic endocarditis	Advanced cancers	Hypercoagulability
Anemia	Thymic neoplasms	Unknown
Others		
Nephrotic syndrome	Various cancers	Tumor antigens, immune complexes

ACTH, adrenocorticotropic hormone; TGF, transforming growth factor; TNF, tumor necrosis factor; IL, interleukin.

5), *migratory thrombophlebitis* (Trousseau syndrome) may be encountered in association with deep-seated cancers, most often with carcinomas of the pancreas or lung. Disseminated intravascular coagulation may complicate a diversity of clinical disorders (Chapter 14). Acute disseminated intravascular coagulation is most commonly associated with acute promyelocytic leukemia and prostatic adenocarcinoma. Bland, small, nonbacterial fibrinous vegetations sometimes form on the cardiac valve leaflets (more often on left-sided valves), particularly in patients with advanced mucin-secreting adenocarcinomas. These lesions, called *nonbacterial thrombotic endocarditis*, are described further in Chapter 13. The vegetations are potential sources of emboli that can further complicate the course of cancer.

Grading and Staging of Tumors

Comparison of end results of various forms of cancer treatment, particularly between clinics, requires some degree of comparability of the neoplasms being assayed. To this end, systems have been derived to express, at least in semiquantitative terms, the level of differentiation, or *grade*, and extent of spread of a cancer within the patient, or *stage*, as parameters of the clinical gravity of the disease.

Grading of a cancer is based on the degree of differentiation of the tumor cells and the number of mitoses within the tumor as presumed correlates of the neoplasm's aggressiveness. Thus, cancers are classified as grades I to IV with increasing anaplasia. Criteria for the individual grades vary with each form of neoplasia and so are not detailed here, but all attempt, in essence, to judge the extent to which the tumor cells resemble or fail to resemble their normal counterparts. Although histologic grading is useful, the correlation between histologic appearance and biologic behavior is less than perfect. In recognition of this problem and to avoid spurious quantification, it is common practice to characterize a particular neoplasm in descriptive terms, for example, well-differentiated, mucin-secreting adenocarcinoma of the stomach, or highly undifferentiated, retroperitoneal malignant tumor—probably sarcoma. In general, with a few exceptions, such as soft tissue sarcomas, grading of cancers has proved of less clinical value than has staging.

The staging of cancers is based on the size of the primary lesion, its extent of spread to regional lymph nodes, and the presence or absence of blood-borne metastases. Two major staging systems are currently in use, one developed by the Union Internationale Contre Cancer (UICC) and the other by the American Joint Committee (AJC) on Cancer Staging. The UICC employs a so-called *TNM system*—*T* for primary tumor, *N* for regional lymph node involvement, and *M* for metastases. The TNM staging varies for each specific form of cancer, but there are general principles. With increasing size, the primary lesion is characterized as T1 to T4. T0 is added to indicate an in situ lesion, N0 would mean no nodal involvement, whereas N1 to N3 would denote involvement of an increasing number and range of nodes. M0 signifies no distant metastases, whereas M1 or sometimes M2 indicates the presence of blood-borne metastases and some judgment as to their number.

The AJC employs a somewhat different nomenclature and divides all cancers into stages 0 to IV, incorporating within each of these stages the size of the primary lesion as well as the presence of nodal spread and distant metastases. The use of these systems of staging and additional details are described later in the consideration of specific tumors. It merits emphasis here, however, that staging of neoplastic disease has assumed great importance in the selection of the best form of therapy for the patient. Indeed, staging has proved to be of greater clinical value than grading.

Laboratory Diagnosis of Cancer

Every year the approach to laboratory diagnosis of cancer becomes more complex, more sophisticated, and more specialized. For virtually every neoplasm mentioned in this text, a number of subcategories have been characterized by the experts; we must walk, however, before we can run. Each of the following sections attempts to present the state-of-the-art, avoiding details of method.

Histologic and Cytologic Methods. The laboratory diagnosis of cancer is, in most instances, not difficult. The two ends of the benign-malignant spectrum pose no problems; however, in the middle lies a "no man's land" where wise men tread cautiously. This issue was sufficiently emphasized earlier; here the focus is on the roles of the clinician (often a surgeon) and the pathologist in facilitating the correct diagnosis.

Clinicians tend to underestimate the important contributions they make to the diagnosis of a neoplasm. Clinical data are invaluable for optimal pathologic diagnosis. Radiation changes in the skin or mucosa can be similar to cancer. Sections taken from a healing fracture can mimic remarkably an osteosarcoma. Moreover the laboratory evaluation of a lesion can be only as good as the specimen made available for examination. It must be adequate, representative, and properly preserved. Several sampling approaches are available: (1) excision or biopsy, (2) needle aspiration, and (3) cytologic smears. When excision of a small lesion is not possible, selection of an appropriate site for biopsy of a large mass requires awareness that the margins may not be representative and the center largely necrotic. Analogously with disseminated lymphoma (involving many nodes), those in the inguinal region draining large areas of the body often have reactive changes that may mask neoplastic involvement. Appropriate preservation of the specimen is obvious, yet it involves such actions as prompt immersion in a usual fixative (e.g., formalin solution) or instead preservation of a portion in a special fixative (e.g., glutaraldehyde) for electron microscopy or prompt refrigeration to permit optimal hormone or receptor analysis. Requesting "quick-frozen section" diagnosis is sometimes desirable, for example, in determining the nature of a breast lesion or in evaluating the margins of an excised cancer to ascertain that the entire neoplasm has been removed. This method allows sectioning of a "quick-frozen" sample and permits histologic evaluation within minutes. In experienced, competent hands, frozen-section diagnosis is highly accurate, but there are particular instances in which the better histologic detail provided by the more time-consuming routine methods is needed—for example, when extremely radical surgery, such as the amputation of an extremity, may be indicated. Better to wait a day or two despite the drawbacks than to perform inadequate or unnecessary surgery.

Fine-needle aspiration of tumors is another approach that is widely used. The procedure involves aspirating cells and attendant fluid with a small-bore needle, followed by cytologic examination of the stained smear. This method is used most commonly for the assessment of readily palpable lesions in sites such as the breast, thyroid, lymph nodes, and, with the aid of a special needle, the prostate. Modern imaging techniques enable the method to be extended to lesions in deep-seated structures, such as pelvic lymph nodes. Fine-needle aspiration is less invasive and more rapidly performed than are needle biopsies. In experienced hands, it is an extremely reliable, rapid, and useful technique.

Cytologic (Pap) smears provide yet another method for

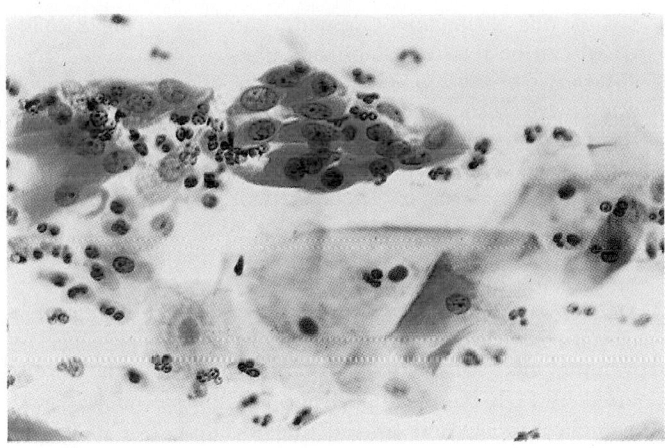

Figure 8–47

A normal cervicovaginal smear shows large, flattened squamous cells and groups of metaplastic cells; interspersed are some neutrophils. There are no malignant cells. (Courtesy of Dr. P. K. Gupta, Department of Pathology and Laboratory Medicine, University of Pennsylvania Medical Center, Philadelphia, PA.)

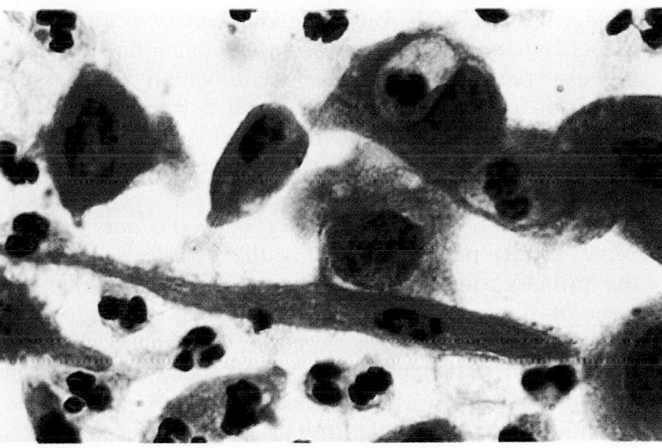

Figure 8–48

An abnormal cervicovaginal smear shows numerous malignant cells that have pleomorphic, hyperchromatic nuclei; interspersed are some normal polymorphonuclear leukocytes. (Courtesy of Dr. P. K. Gupta, Department of Pathology and Laboratory Medicine, University of Pennsylvania Medical Center, Philadelphia, PA.)

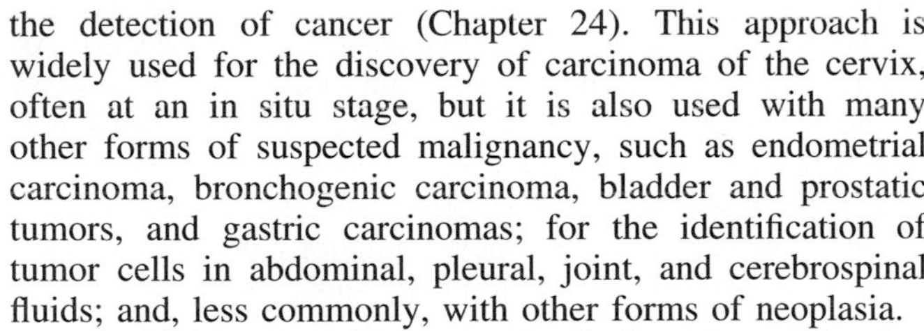

the detection of cancer (Chapter 24). This approach is widely used for the discovery of carcinoma of the cervix, often at an in situ stage, but it is also used with many other forms of suspected malignancy, such as endometrial carcinoma, bronchogenic carcinoma, bladder and prostatic tumors, and gastric carcinomas; for the identification of tumor cells in abdominal, pleural, joint, and cerebrospinal fluids; and, less commonly, with other forms of neoplasia.

As pointed out earlier, cancer cells have lowered cohesiveness and exhibit a range of morphologic changes encompassed by the term *anaplasia*. Thus, shed cells can be evaluated for the features of anaplasia indicative of their origin in a cancer (Figs. 8–47 and 8–48). In contrast to the histologist's task, judgment here must be rendered based on individual cell cytology or (at most, perhaps) on that of a clump of a few cells without the supporting evidence of architectural disarray, loss of orientation of one cell to another, and (perhaps most important) evidence of invasion. This method permits differentiation among normal, dysplastic, and cancerous cells and in addition permits the recognition of cellular changes characteristic of carcinoma in situ. The gratifying control of cervical cancer is the best testament to the value of the cytologic method.

Although histology and exfoliative cytology remain the most commonly used methods in the diagnosis of cancer, new techniques are being constantly added to the tools of the surgical pathologist. Some, such as immunocytochemistry, are already well established and widely used; others, including molecular methods, are rapidly finding their way into the "routine" category. Only some highlights of these diagnostic modalities are presented.

Immunocytochemistry. The availability of specific monoclonal antibodies has greatly facilitated the identification of cell products or surface markers. Some examples of the utility of immunohistochemistry in the diagnosis or management of malignant neoplasms follow.[127]

■ *Categorization of undifferentiated malignant tumors*: In many cases, malignant tumors of diverse origin resemble each other because of poor differentiation. These tumors are often quite difficult to distinguish on the basis of routine hematoxylin and eosin–stained tissue sections. For example, certain anaplastic carcinomas, malignant lymphomas, melanomas, and sarcomas may look quite similar, but they must be accurately identified because their treatment and prognosis are different. Antibodies against intermediate filaments have proved to be of value in such cases because tumor cells often contain intermediate filaments characteristic of their cell of origin. For example, the presence of keratin, detected by immunohistochemistry, points to an epithelial origin (carcinoma) (Fig. 8–49), whereas desmin is specific for neoplasms of muscle cell origin.

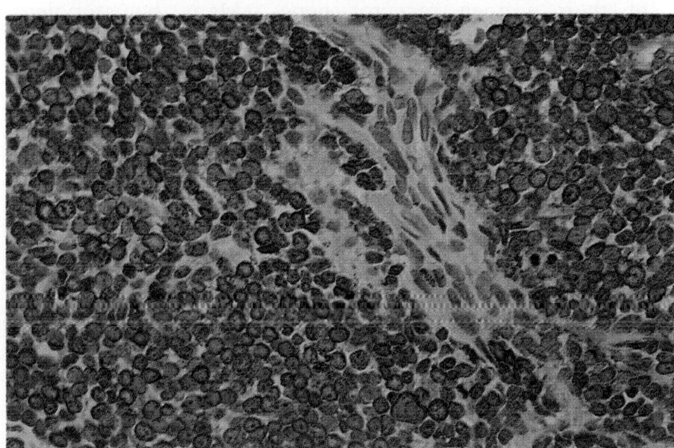

Figure 8–49

Antikeratin immunoperoxidase stain of an undifferentiated tumor. The dark brown staining of keratin indicates an epithelial origin of this tumor (carcinoma).

- *Categorization of leukemias and lymphomas*: Immunocytochemistry (in conjunction with immunofluorescence) has also proved useful in the identification and classification of tumors arising from T and B lymphocytes and from mononuclear-phagocytic cells. Monoclonal antibodies directed against various lymphohematopoietic cells are listed in Chapter 15.
- *Determination of site of origin of metastatic tumors*: Many cancer patients present with metastases. In some, the primary site is obvious or readily detected on the basis of clinical or radiologic features. In cases in which the origin of the tumor is obscure, immunohistochemical detection of tissue-specific or organ-specific antigens in a biopsy specimen of the metastatic deposit can lead to the identification of the tumor source. For example, prostate-specific antigen and thyroglobulin are markers of tumors of the prostate and thyroid, respectively.
- *Detection of molecules that have prognostic or therapeutic significance*: Immunohistochemical detection of hormone (estrogen/progesterone) receptors in breast cancer cells is of prognostic and therapeutic value because these cancers are susceptible to antiestrogen therapy (Chapter 25). In general, receptor-positive breast cancers have a better prognosis. Protein products of oncogenes such as *c-erbB2* in breast cancers can also be detected by immunostaining. Breast cancers with overexpression of *c-erbB2* protein have a poor prognosis.

Molecular Diagnosis. Several examples of molecular techniques—some established, others emerging—have been applied for diagnosis or in some cases predicting behavior of tumors.[128]

- *Diagnosis of malignant neoplasms*: Although molecular methods are not the primary modality of cancer diagnosis, they are of considerable value in selected cases. Molecular techniques are useful in differentiating benign (polyclonal) proliferations of T or B cells from malignant (monoclonal) proliferations. As discussed in Chapter 7, it is possible to identify monoclonal T-cell and B-cell proliferations on the basis of clonal rearrangement of their antigen receptor genes. Many hematopoietic neoplasms (leukemias and lymphomas) are associated with specific translocations that activate oncogenes. Detection of such translocations, usually by routine cytogenetic analysis or by FISH technique (Chapter 6), is often extremely helpful in diagnosis. In some cases, molecular techniques can reveal translocations or other rearrangements that fail to be detected by cytogenetics. Thus, for example, the detection of *bcr-c-abl* transcripts by polymerase chain reaction (PCR) provides precise diagnosis of chronic myeloid leukemia, even in cases that appear to be negative by cytogenetics. Molecular detection of translocations is also of particular value in the diagnosis of certain sarcomas (Chapter 28) because chromosome preparations are often difficult to obtain from solid tumors. For example, many sarcomas of childhood, so-called round blue cell tumors (Chapter 11), can be difficult to distinguish from each other on the basis of morphology. Using sensitive PCR-based assays for the specific translocations, however, the diagnosis of one such tumor, Ewing sarcoma [t(11;22)(q24;q12)] can be readily established.[129]
- *Prognosis of malignant neoplasms*: Certain genetic alterations are associated with poor prognosis, and hence their detection allows stratification of the patients for therapy. As an example, amplification of the N-*myc* gene and deletions of 1p bode poorly for patients with neuroblastoma. These can be detected by routine cytogenetics in about 30% of affected cases; the remaining can be detected by FISH or PCR assays.
- *Detection of minimal residual disease*: After treatment of patients with leukemia or lymphoma, the presence of minimal disease or the onset of relapse can be monitored by PCR-based amplification of unique nucleic acid sequences generated by the translocation. For example, detection of *bcr-c-abl* transcripts by PCR gives a measure of the residual leukemia cells in treated patients with chronic myeloid leukemia. Similarly, detection of specific K-*ras* mutations in stool samples of patients previously treated for colon cancer can alert to the possible recurrence of the tumor. The clinical importance of minimal disease that is detected only by PCR remains to be established, and several studies addressing this issue are in progress.
- *Diagnosis of hereditary predisposition to cancer*: As was discussed earlier, germ line mutations in several cancer-suppressor genes, including BRCA1, BRCA2, and the RET protooncogene, are associated with an extremely high risk of developing specific cancers. Thus, detection of carriers of these mutations in family members of affected patients or in those at high risk of carrying the mutation has become important. Such analysis usually requires detection of a specific mutation (e.g., RET gene) or sequencing of the entire gene (e.g., BRCA1). The latter is necessitated when several different cancer-associated mutations are known to exist. Although the detection of mutations in such cases is relatively straightforward, the ethical issues surrounding such presymptomatic diagnosis are complex.

Several other diagnostic applications of recombinant DNA technology are cited with the discussion of specific tumors.

Flow Cytometry. Flow cytometry can rapidly and quantitatively measure several individual cell characteristics, such as membrane antigens and the DNA content of tumor cells. Identification of cell surface antigens by flow cytometry is widely used in the classification of leukemias and lymphomas (Chapter 15). Flow cytometric detection of ploidy is applied to specimens from a variety of sources, such as fresh-frozen surgical biopsy specimens (from which nuclei can be extracted), pleural or peritoneal effusions associated with cancer, bone marrow aspirations, and cells obtained by irrigation of the urinary bladder. A relationship between abnormal DNA content and prognosis is becoming apparent for a variety of malignancies. In general, aneuploidy seems to be associated with poorer prognosis in early-stage breast cancer, carcinoma of the urinary bladder, lung cancer, colorectal cancer, and prostate cancer.

Tumor Markers. Tumor markers are biochemical indicators of the presence of a tumor. They include cell surface antigens, cytoplasmic proteins, enzymes, and hormones. In

Table 8–12. SELECTED TUMOR MARKERS

Markers	Associated Cancers
Hormones	
Human chorionic gonadotropin	Trophoblastic tumors, nonseminomatous testicular tumors
Calcitonin	Medullary carcinoma of thyroid
Catecholamine and metabolites	Pheochromocytoma and related tumors
Ectopic hormones	See Paraneoplastic Syndromes in Table 8–11
Oncofetal Antigens	
α-fetoprotein	Liver cell cancer, nonseminomatous germ cell tumors of testis
Carcinoembryonic antigen	Carcinomas of the colon, pancreas, lung, stomach, and breast
Isoenzymes	
Prostatic acid phosphatase	Prostate cancer
Neuron-specific enolase	Small cell cancer of lung, neuroblastoma
Specific Proteins	
Immunoglobulins	Multiple myeloma and other gammopathies
Prostate-specific antigen	Prostate cancer
Mucins and Other Glycoproteins	
CA-125	Ovarian cancer
CA-19-9	Colon cancer, pancreatic cancer
CA-15-3	Breast cancer

clinical practice, however, the term usually refers to a molecule that can be detected in plasma or other body fluids.[130] *Tumor markers cannot be construed as primary modalities for the diagnosis of cancer.* Their main utility in clinical medicine has been as a laboratory test to support the diagnosis. Some tumor markers are also of value in determining the response to therapy and in indicating relapse during the follow-up period.

A host of tumor markers have been described, and new ones appear every year. Only a few have stood the test of time and proved to have clinical usefulness. The application of several markers, listed in Table 8–12, is considered with specific forms of neoplasia discussed in other chapters, so only two widely used examples suffice here.

Carcinoembryonic antigen (CEA), normally produced in embryonic tissue of the gut, pancreas, and liver, is a complex glycoprotein that is elaborated by many different neoplasms. Depending on the serum level adopted as a significant elevation, it is variously reported to be positive in 60 to 90% of colorectal, 50 to 80% of pancreatic, and 25 to 50% of gastric and breast carcinomas. Much less consistently, elevated CEA has been described in other forms of cancer. CEA elevations have also been reported in many benign disorders, such as alcoholic cirrhosis, hepatitis, ulcerative colitis, Crohn disease, and others. Occasionally, levels of this antigen are elevated in apparently healthy smokers. Thus, *CEA assays lack both specificity and the sensitivity required for the detection of early cancers.* Preoperative CEA levels have some bearing on prognosis because the level of elevation is correlated with body burden of tumor. In colon cancer, the levels correlate with the widely used Dukes grading system (Chapter 18). In patients with CEA-positive colon cancers, the presence of elevated CEA levels 6 weeks after therapy indicates residual disease. Recurrence is indicated by a rising CEA level, with an increase in tumor marker level often preceding clinically detectable disease. Serum CEA is also useful in monitoring the treatment of metastatic breast cancer.

Alpha-fetoprotein (AFP) is another well-established tumor marker (Chapters 19 and 23). This glycoprotein is synthesized normally early in fetal life by the yolk sac, fetal liver, and fetal gastrointestinal tract. Abnormal plasma elevations are encountered in adults with cancer arising principally in the liver and germ cells of the testis. Elevated plasma AFP is also found less regularly in carcinomas of the colon, lung, and pancreas. Similar to CEA, nonneoplastic conditions, including cirrhosis, toxic liver injury, hepatitis, and pregnancy (especially with fetal distress or death), also may cause minimal to moderate plasma elevations of AFP. Although there is then some problem with specificity, marked elevations of the plasma AFP level have proved to be a useful indicator of hepatocellular carcinomas and germ cell tumors of the testis. AFP levels decline rapidly after surgical resection of liver cell cancer or treatment of germ cell tumors. Serial post-therapy measurements of AFP (and human chorionic gonadotropin) levels in patients with germ cell tumors of the testis provide a sensitive index of response to therapy and recurrence.

REFERENCES

1. Landis SH, et al: Cancer statistics, 1998. Cancer J Clin 48:6, 1998.
2. Willis RA: The Spread of Tumors in the Human Body. London, Butterworth & Co, 1952.
3. Ponder BAJ: Genetic predisposition to cancer. In Holland JF, et al (eds): Cancer Medicine, 4th ed. Baltimore, Williams & Wilkins, 1997, p 245.
4. Weinberg RA: How cancer arises. Sci Am 275:62, 1996.
5. Hunter T: Oncoprotein networks. Cell 88:333, 1997.
6. Pusztal L, et al: Growth factors: Regulation of normal and neoplastic growth. J Pathol 169:191, 1993.
7. Komminoth P: The RET protooncogene in medullary and papillary thyroid carcinoma: molecular features, pathophysiology and clinical implications. Virchow Arch 431:1, 1997.

8. Salomon DS, et al: Epidermal growth factor-related peptides and their receptors in human malignancies. Crit Rev Hematol Oncol 19: 183, 1995.
9. deVries JE, et al: p21^{ras} in carcinogenesis. Pathol Res Pract 192:658, 1996.
10. Waldmann V, Robes HM: What's new in Ras genes? Pathol Res Pract 192:883, 1996.
11. McCormick F: Ras signalling and NF-1. Curr Opin Genet Dev 5:51, 1995.
12. Leone G, et al: Myc and Ras collaborate in inducing accumulation of active cyclin E/cdk2 and E2F. Nature 387:422, 1997.
13. Baringa M: News. From benchtop to bedside. Science 278:1036, 1997.
14. Brown L, McCarty N: A sense-able response. Nature 387:450, 1997.
15. Sanchez-Garcia I, Martin-Zonca D: Regulation of bcl-2 gene expression by *bcr-c-abl* is mediated by *ras*. J Mol Biol 267:225, 1997.
16. Koskinen PJ, Alitalo K: Role of *myc* amplification and overexpression in cell growth, differentiation, and death. Semin Cancer Biol 4: 3, 1993.
17. Desborats L, et al: Myc: a single gene controls both proliferation and apoptosis in mammalian cells. Experientia 52:1123, 1996.
18. Grandori C, Eisenman RN: Myc target genes. Trends Biochem Sci 22:177, 1997.
19. Green DR: A myc-induced apoptosis pathway surface. Science 278: 1246, 1997.
20. Sherr CJ: Cancer cell cycle. Science 274:1672, 1996.
21. Look A: Oncogenic transcription factors in human acute leukemias. Science 278:1059, 1997.
22. Sorenson PBH, Triche JJ: Gene fusions encoding transcription factors in solid tumors. Semin Cancer Biol 7:3, 1996.
23. Schwab M: Amplification of N-*myc* as a prognostic marker for patients with neuroblastoma. Semin Cancer Biol 4:13, 1993.
24. Kaelin WG: Recent insights into the functions of the retinoblastoma susceptibility gene product. Cancer Invest 15:243, 1997.
25. Lin S-CJ: Genes in the *Rb* pathway and their knockout in mice. Semin Cancer Biol 7:279, 1996.
26. DePinho RA: The cancer-chromatin connection. Nature 391:533, 1998.
26a. Clurman BE, Groudine M: The CDKN2A tumor suppressor locus—a tale of two proteins. N Engl J Med 338:910,1998.
27. Evans SC, Lozono G: The Li-Fraumeni syndrome: an inherited susceptibility to cancer. Mol Med Today 3:390, 1997.
28. Levine AJ: *p53*, the cellular gatekeeper for growth and division. Cell 88:323, 1997.
29. Graeber AJ, et al: Hypoxia-mediated selection of cells with diminished apoptotic potential in solid tumors. Nature 379:88, 1996.
30. Haupt Y, et al: Mdm2 promotes the rapid degradation of *p53*. Nature 387:296, 1997.
31. Chresta CM, Hickman JA: Oddball *p53* in testicular tumors. Nat Med 2:745, 1996.
32. Oren M: Lonely no more: *p53* finds its kin in a tumor-suppressor haven. Cell 90:829, 1997.
33. Jost CA, et al: *p73* is a human *p53*-related protein that can induce apoptosis. Nature 389:191, 1997.
34. Gayther SA, Ponder AJ: Mutations of the BRCA-1 and BRCA-2 genes and possibilities for predictive testing. Mol Med Today 3:168, 1997.
35. Brugarolos J, Jacks T: Double indemnity: *p53*, BRCA and cancer. Nat Med 3:721, 1997.
36. Somasundaram K, et al: Arrest of the cell cycle by the tumor-suppressor BRCA-1 requires the CDK inhibitor *p21*$^{WAF-1/CiP1}$. Nature 389:187, 1997.
37. Shibata H, et al: Rapid colorectal adenoma formation initiated by conditional targeting of the APC gene. Science 278:120, 1997.
38. Gumbiner BM: Carcinogenesis: A balance between β-catenin and APC. Curr Biol 7:R443, 1997.
39. Fearon ER: Human cancer syndromes: Clues to the origin and nature of cancer. Science 278:1043, 1997.
40. Peifer M: β-catenin as oncogene: The smoking gun. Science 275: 1752, 1997.
41. Side L, et al: Homozygous inactivation of the NF-1 gene in bone marrow cells from children with neurofibromatosis type-1 and malignant myeloid disorders. N Engl J Med 336:1713, 1997.
42. Heldin CH, et al: TGF-β signaling from cell membrane to nucleus through SMAD proteins. Nature 390:465, 1997.
43. Shiozaki H, et al: E-cadherin mediated adhesion system in cancer cells. Cancer 77(suppl):1605, 1996.
43a. Perl A-K, et al: A causal role for E-cadherin in transition from adenoma to carcinoma. Nature 392:190, 1998.
43b. Guilford P, et al: E-cadherin germline mutations in familial gastric cancer. Nature 392:402, 1998.
44. Fazeli A, et al: Phenotype of mice lacking functional Deleted in colorectal cancer (DCC) gene. Nature 386:796, 1997.
45. Zwarthoff EC: Neurofibromatosis and associated tumor-suppressor genes. Pathol Res Pract 192:647, 1996.
46. Li J, et al: PTEN, a putative protein tyrosine phosphatase gene mutated in human brain, breast, and prostate cancer. Science 275: 1943, 1997.
46a. Tamura M, et al: Inhibition of cell migration, spreading, and focal adhesions by tumor suppressor PTEN. Science 280:1614, 1998.
47. Wyllie AH: Apoptosis and carcinogenesis. Eur J Cell Biol 73:189, 1997.
48. McDonnell TJ, et al: Importance of the *bcl-2* family in cell death regulation. Experientia 52:1008, 1996.
49. Reed JC: Double indemnity for proteins of the bcl-2 family. Nature 387:773, 1997.
50. Hengartner MO: Death cycle and Swiss army knives. Nature 391: 441, 1998.
51. Kroemer G: The protooncogene bcl-2 and its role in regulating apoptosis. Nat Med 3:614, 1997.
52. Reed JC: Cytochrome C: can't live with it—can't live without it. Cell 91:559, 1997.
53. Yin C, et al: Bax suppresses tumorigenesis and stimulates apoptosis in vivo. Nature 385:637, 1997.
54. Marra G, Boland CR: DNA repair and colorectal cancer. Gastroenterol Clin North Am 25:755, 1996.
55. Papadopoulos N, Lindblom A: Molecular basis of HNPCC: mutations of MMR genes. Hum Mut 10:89, 1997.
56. Friedberg EC, et al: DNA Repair and Mutagenesis. Washington, ASM Press, 1995, p 663.
57. Lavin MF, Shiloh Y: The genetic defect in ataxia-telangiectasia. Ann Rev Immunol 15:177, 1997.
58. Bodnar AG, et al: Extension of life-span by introduction of telomerase into normal human cells. Science 279:349, 1998.
59. Baccheti S, Counter CM: Telomeres and telomerase in human cancer. Int J Oncol 7:423, 1995.
60. Bryan TM, et al: Evidence for an alternative mechanism for maintaining telomere length in human tumors and tumor-derived lines. Nat Med 3:1271, 1997.
61. Kinzler KW, Vogelstein B: Lessons from hereditary colorectal cancer. Cell 87:159, 1996.
62. Hoops TC, Traber PG: Molecular pathogenesis of colorectal cancer. Hematol Oncol Clin North Am 11:609, 1997.
63. Kinzler KW, Vogelstein B: Gatekeeper and caretakers. Nature 386: 761, 1997.
64. Tannock IF: Cell proliferation. In Tannock IF, Hill RP (eds): The Basic Science of Oncology, 2nd ed. New York, McGraw-Hill, 1992, p 154.
65. Rak J, et al: Reciprocal paracrine interaction between tumor cells and endothelial cells: the 'angiogenesis progression' hypothesis. Eur J Cancer 32A:2438, 1996.
66. Pluda JM: Tumor-associated angiogenesis: mechanisms, clinical implications, and therapeutic strategies. Semin Oncol 24:203, 1997.
67. Folkman J: Angiogenesis. In Holland JF, et al (eds): Cancer Medicine, 4th ed. Baltimore, Williams & Wilkins, 1997, p 181.
68. Hanahan D, Folkman J: Patterns and emerging mechanisms of the angiogenic switch during tumorigenesis. Cell 86:353, 1996.
69. Baringa M: Designing therapies that target tumor blood vessels. Science 275:482, 1997.
70. Boehm T, et al: Antiangiogenic therapy of experimental cancer does not induce acquired drug resistance. Nature 390:404, 1997.
71. Jiang WG: E-cadherin and its associated proteins, catenins, cancer invasion and metastasis. Br J Surg 83:437, 1996.
72. Price JT, et al: Biochemistry of cancer dissemination. Crit Rev Biochem Mol Biol 32:175, 1997.
73. Ziober BL, et al: Laminin-binding integrins in tumor progression and metastasis. Semin Cancer Biol 7:119, 1996.

74. Liotta LA, Kohn EC: Invasion and metastasis. In Holland JF, et al (eds): Cancer Medicine, 4th ed. Baltimore, Williams & Wilkins, 1997, p 165.
75. Chambers AF, Matrisian LM: Changing view of the role of matrix metalloproteinases in metastasis. J Natl Cancer Inst 89:1260, 1997.
76. Andreasen PA, et al: The urokinase-type plasminogen activator system in cancer metastasis: a review. Int J Cancer 72:1, 1997.
77. Garcia M, et al: Biologic and clinical significance of cathepsin D in breast cancer metastasis. Stem Cells 14:642, 1996.
78. Bao L, et al: Thymosin β15: a novel regulator of tumor cell motility upregulated in metastatic prostatic cancer. Nat Med 2:1322, 1996.
79. Tuszynski GP: Adhesive proteins and hematogenous spread of cancer. Acta Hematol 97:29, 1997.
80. Sy M-S, et al: CD44 as a marker in human cancers. Curr Opin Oncol 9:108, 1997.
81. Rusciano D, Burger M: Why do cancer cells metastasize into particular organs. Bioessays 14:185, 1992.
82. Fidler IJ, Radinsky R: Search for genes that suppress cancer metastasis. J Natl Cancer Inst 88:1700, 1996.
83. Tennant R, et al: Chemical carcinogenesis. In Franks LM, Teich NM (eds): An Introduction to the Cellular and Molecular Biology of Cancer, 3rd ed. Oxford, Oxford University Press, 1997, p 106.
84. Weston A, Harris CC: Chemical carcinogenesis. In Holland JF, et al (eds): Cancer Medicine, 4th ed. Baltimore, Williams & Wilkins, 1997, p 261.
85. Perera FP: Environment and cancer: who are susceptible? Science 278:1068, 1997.
86. Vineis P: Molecular epidemiology: low dose carcinogens and genetic susceptibility. Int J Cancer 71:1, 1997.
87. Yuspa SH, Shields PG: Etiology of cancer: chemical factors. In DeVita VT, et al (eds): Cancer: Principles and Practice of Oncology, 5th ed. Philadelphia, Lippincott-Raven, 1997, p 185.
88. Montesano R, et al: Hepatocellular carcinoma: from gene to public health. J Natl Cancer Inst 89:1844, 1997.
89. Cohen SM, Ellwein LB: Genetic errors, cell proliferation, and carcinogenesis. Cancer Res 51:6493, 1991.
90. Mastrangelo G, et al: Polycyclic aromatic hydrocarbons and cancer in man. Environ Health Perspect 104:1166, 1996.
91. Kleinfeld M, et al: Bladder tumors in a coal tar dye plant. Ind Med Surg 35:570, 1966.
92. Rauth AM: Radiation carcinogenesis. In Tannock IF, Hill RP (eds): The Basic Science of Oncology, 2nd ed. New York, McGraw-Hill, 1992, p 119.
93. Cleaver JE, Mitchell DL: Ultraviolet radiation carcinogenesis. In Holland JF, et al (eds): Cancer Medicine, 4th ed. Baltimore, Williams & Wilkins, 1997, p 307.
94. Boulikas T: Xeroderma pigmentosum and molecular cloning of DNA repair genes. Anticancer Res 16:693, 1996.
95. Ananthaswamy HN, et al: Sunlight and skin cancer: inhibition of *p53* mutations in UV-irradiated mouse skin by sunscreens. Nat Med 3:510, 1997.
96. Adams GE, Cox R: Radiation carcinogenesis. In Franks LM, Teich NM (eds): Introduction to the Cellular and Molecular Biology of Cancer, 3rd ed. Oxford, Oxford University Press, 1997, p 130.
97. Stsjazhko VA, et al: Childhood thyroid cancer since accident at Chernobyl. BMJ 310:801, 1995.
98. zur Hausen H: Papillomavirus infections—a major cause of human cancers. Biochim Biophys Acta 1288:F55, 1996.
99. Vousden K: Interaction of HPV transforming proteins with products of tumor-suppressor genes. FASEB J 7:872, 1993.
100. Huibregtse JM, Beaudenon SL: Mechanism of HPV E6 protein in cellular transformation. Semin Cancer Biol 7:317, 1996.
101. zur Hausen H. Papillomavirus and p53. Nature 393:217, 1998.
102. Purtillo DT, et al: Epstein-Barr virus-associated lymphoproliferative disorders. Lab Invest 67:5, 1992.
103. Straus SE, et al: Epstein-Barr virus infections: biology, pathogenesis, and management. Ann Intern Med 118:45, 1993.
104. Oudejons JJ, et al: Epstein-Barr virus and its possible role in the pathogenesis of B cell lymphomas. Crit Rev Oncol Hematol 25:127, 1997.
104a. Rickinson AB: Epstein Barr virus action in vivo. N Engl J Med 338:1461, 1998.
105. Knecht H, et al: Epstein-Barr virus oncogenesis. Crit Rev Oncol Hematol 26:177, 1997.
106. Su I-J: The role of Epstein-Barr virus in lymphoid malignancies. Crit Rev Oncol Hematol 26:25, 1997.
107. Vasef MA: Nasopharyngeal carcinoma with emphasis on its relationship to Epstein-Barr virus. Ann Otol Rhinol Laryngol 106:348, 1997.
108. Raab-Traub N: Epstein-Barr virus and nasopharyngeal carcinoma. Semin Cancer Biol 3:297, 1992.
109. Sung MW: Hepatitis viruses. In Holland JF, et al (eds): Cancer Medicine, 4th ed. Baltimore, Williams & Wilkins, 1997, p 375.
110. Feitelson MA, Duan L-X: Hepatitis B virus x antigen in the pathogenesis of chronic infections and development of hepatocellular carcinoma. Am J Pathol 150:1141, 1997.
111. Uchiyama T: Human T cell leukemia virus type I (HTLV-1) and human disease. Ann Rev Immunol 15:15, 1997.
112. Ressler S, et al: Cellular transformation by human T-cell leukemia virus type 1. FEMS Microb Lett 140:99, 1996.
113. Vanagunas A: Eradication of *Helicobacter pylori* and regression of B-cell lymphoma. Biomed Pharmacother 51:156, 1997.
114. Van den Eynde BJ, van der Bruggen P: T cell-defined tumor antigens. Curr Opin Immunol 9:684, 1997.
115. Taylor-Papadimitriou J, Finn OJ: Biology, biochemistry and immunology of carcinoma-associated mucins. Immunol Today 18:105, 1997.
116. Purtillo DT, et al: Epstein-Barr virus-associated lymphoproliferative disorders. Lab Invest 67:5, 1992.
117. Shu S, et al: Tumor immunology. JAMA 278:1972, 1997.
118. Hahne M, et al: Melanoma cell expression of Fas (Apo-1/CD95) ligand: implications of tumor immune escape. Science 274:1363, 1996.
119. Strand S, et al: Lymphocyte apoptosis induced by CD95 (Apo-1/Fas) ligand-expressing tumor cells—a mechanism of immune evasion? Nat Med 2:1361, 1996.
120. Tisdale MJ: Biology of cachexia. J Natl Cancer Inst 89:1763, 1997.
121. Beutler B: Cytokines and cancer cachexia. Hosp Pract 28:45, 1993.
122. Todorov P, et al: Characterization of a cancer cachectic factor. Nature 379:739, 1996.
123. Nathanson L, Hall TC: Introduction: paraneoplastic syndromes. Semin Oncol 24:265, 1997.
124. Odell WD: Endocrine/metabolic syndromes of cancer. Semin Oncol 24:299, 1997.
125. Dalmau JO, Posner JB: Paraneoplastic syndromes affecting the nervous system. Semin Oncol 24:318, 1997.
126. Cohen PR, Kurzock R: Mucocutaneous paraneoplastic syndromes. Semin Oncol 24:334, 1997.
127. Connolly JL, et al: Principles of cancer pathology. In Holland J, et al (eds): Cancer Medicine, 4th ed. Baltimore, Williams & Wilkins, 1997, p 533.
128. Sklar JL, Costa JC: Principles of cancer management: molecular pathology. In DeVita VT, et al (eds): Cancer: Principles and Practice of Oncology, 5th ed. Philadelphia, Lippincott-Raven, 1997, p 259.
129. Sheer D, Squire J: Clinical application of genetic rearrangements in cancer. Semin Cancer Biol 7:25, 1996.
130. Pamies RJ, Crawford DR: Tumor markers: an update. Med Clin North Am 80:185, 1996.

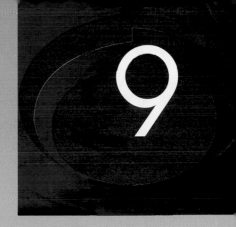

Infectious Diseases

John Samuelson

GENERAL PRINCIPLES OF MICROBIAL PATHOGENESIS

HISTORY

NEW AND EMERGING INFECTIOUS DISEASES

CATEGORIES OF INFECTIOUS AGENTS

- Prions
- Viruses
- Bacteriophages, Plasmids, Transposons
- Bacteria
- Chlamydiae, Rickettsiae, Mycoplasmas
- Fungi
- Protozoa
- Helminths
- Ectoparasites

TRANSMISSION AND DISSEMINATION OF MICROBES

- Host Barriers to Infection
- Spread and Dissemination of Microbes
- Release and Transmission of Microbes

HOW MICROORGANISMS CAUSE DISEASE

- Mechanisms of Viral Injury
- Mechanisms of Bacteria-Induced Tissue Injury

IMMUNE EVASION BY MICROBES

SPECIAL TECHNIQUES FOR DIAGNOSING INFECTIOUS AGENTS

SPECTRUM OF INFLAMMATORY RESPONSES TO INFECTION

- Suppurative (Polymorphonuclear) Inflammation
- Mononuclear and Granulomatous Inflammation
- Cytopathic-Cytoproliferative Inflammation
- Necrotizing Inflammation
- Chronic Inflammation and Scarring

RESPIRATORY INFECTIONS

VIRAL RESPIRATORY INFECTIONS

- Rhinoviruses
- Influenza Viruses

BACTERIAL RESPIRATORY INFECTIONS

- *Haemophilus influenzae* Infection
- Tuberculosis *(Mycobacterium tuberculosis)*

FUNGAL RESPIRATORY INFECTIONS

- Histoplasmosis
- Coccidioidomycosis

GASTROINTESTINAL INFECTIONS

BARRIERS TO INFECTION OF THE GUT

VIRAL ENTERITIS AND DIARRHEA

BACTERIAL ENTERITIS

- *Shigella* Bacillary Dysentery
- *Campylobacter* Enteritis
- *Yersinia* Enteritis

SALMONELLOSIS AND TYPHOID FEVER

CHOLERA

PARASITIC INTESTINAL INFECTIONS

AMEBIASIS

GIARDIASIS

SEXUALLY TRANSMITTED DISEASES

HERPESVIRUS INFECTIONS

CHLAMYDIAL INFECTIONS

GONORRHEA

SYPHILIS

TRICHOMONIASIS

GRAM-POSITIVE PYOGENIC BACTERIAL INFECTIONS

STAPHYLOCOCCAL INFECTIONS

STREPTOCOCCAL INFECTIONS

CLOSTRIDIAL INFECTIONS

NON–SPORE-FORMING ANAEROBIC INFECTIONS

- Septic Abortion, Salpingitis, and Periodontal Abscesses *(Prevotella)*

INFECTIONS OF CHILDHOOD AND ADOLESCENCE

MEASLES

MUMPS

INFECTIOUS MONONUCLEOSIS (EPSTEIN-BARR VIRUS)

POLIOVIRUS INFECTION

VARICELLA-ZOSTER INFECTION (CHICKENPOX AND SHINGLES)

WHOOPING COUGH

DIPHTHERIA

OPPORTUNISTIC AND AIDS-ASSOCIATED INFECTIONS

INFECTIONS ASSOCIATED WITH NEUTROPENIA AND HELPER T-CELL DEPLETION

CYTOMEGALIC INCLUSION DISEASE

PSEUDOMONAS INFECTION

LEGIONNAIRES DISEASE

LISTERIOSIS

CANDIDIASIS

CRYPTOCOCCOSIS

ASPERGILLOSIS

MUCORMYCOSIS

PNEUMOCYSTIS PNEUMONIA

CRYPTOSPORIDIUM AND *CYCLOSPORA* INFECTIONS

TOXOPLASMOSIS

TROPICAL, ZOONOTIC, AND VECTOR-BORNE INFECTIONS

DENGUE FEVER

RICKETTSIAL INFECTIONS

TRACHOMA

LEPROSY

PLAGUE

RELAPSING FEVER

LYME DISEASE

MALARIA

BABESIOSIS

LEISHMANIASIS

AFRICAN TRYPANOSOMIASIS

CHAGAS DISEASE

TRICHINELLOSIS

HOOKWORM

CYSTICERCOSIS AND HYDATID DISEASE

SCHISTOSOMIASIS

LYMPHATIC FILARIASIS

ONCHOCERCIASIS

GENERAL PRINCIPLES OF MICROBIAL PATHOGENESIS

Despite improved living conditions, widespread vaccination, and availability of effective antibiotics, infectious diseases continue to take a heavy toll in the United States among persons with acquired immunodeficiency syndrome (AIDS), debilitated with chronic disease, or treated with immunosuppressive drugs. In developing countries, unsanitary living conditions and malnutrition contribute to a massive burden of infectious disease that kills more than 10 million persons each year.[1] Most of these deaths are among children, who suffer respiratory and diarrheal infections caused by viruses and bacteria.

Table 9–1. TWELVE MAJOR DISCOVERIES IN MICROBIAL PATHOGENESIS

Year	Investigator	Discovery
1796	Jenner	Vaccination against smallpox
1843	Holmes	Discovery of the iatrogenic nature of "black death of childbirth"
1865	Pasteur	Proof of germ theory and the beginning of modern biology
1882	Koch	Criteria for proof of causality in infectious disease
1884	Mechnikov	Description of phagocytosis by macrophages
1902	Ross	Identification of mosquito vector for *Plasmodium falciparum* malaria
1906	Ehrlich	Description of chemotherapeutic agents
1908	Ellerman and Bang	Viral oncogenesis in chickens
1933	Lancefield	Serotyping of organisms and association of bacterial clones with disease
1945	Avery	Identification of DNA as genetic material and the start of the molecular biology revolution
1949	Enders	Culture of viruses and production of the poliovirus vaccine
1983	Montagnier and Gallo	Identification of HIV as cause of AIDS

History

Table 9–1 presents in chronologic sequence 12 major breakthroughs in our understanding of infectious diseases and their causes, selected with the intent of providing a historical perspective for the concepts of microbial pathogenesis to be discussed here. Jenner's discovery in 1796 that milkmaids working with cows were resistant to smallpox paved the way to our understanding of cross-reactive immunity. Vaccinia virus (cowpox) induces immune reactions that neutralize subsequent infection with the much more virulent variola virus of smallpox. Because of a heroic vaccination campaign by the World Health Organization (WHO) and others, *smallpox is the first and only disease of humans that has been eradicated from the earth.* Now the WHO has a worldwide vaccination campaign to eliminate poliovirus, first cultured by Enders in 1949.

Oliver Wendell Holmes, who named anesthesia (and was father of the renowned Supreme Court justice), noted that puerperal infections of women after childbirth ("the black death of childbirth") were associated with particular physicians who attended the delivery. This first example of iatrogenic infections, now known to be caused by *Staphylococcus*, led to recommendations that physicians wash their hands *before and after* delivery and persuaded most middle-class women to have their children at home. Pasteur demonstrated that infectious illnesses were caused by particular bacteria, many of which could be eliminated by moderate heating (pasteurization) of milk and other liquids.

Koch's postulates established criteria for linking a specific microorganism to a specific disease: (1) the organism is regularly found in the lesions of the disease, (2) the organism can be isolated as single colonies on solid medium, (3) inoculation of this culture causes lesions in an experimental animal, and (4) the organism can be recovered from lesions in the animals. Lancefield's system of classifying bacteria by their surface antigens greatly facilitated the linkage of particular bacteria to specific illnesses. In the past decade, the revolution in molecular biology has led to a molecular form of Koch's postulates, which links a particular trait of an organism to a particular disease process[2]: (1) the phenotype or trait should be associated with virulent strains of the organism and not with avirulent strains; (2) specific inactivation of the gene associated with virulence—for example, by replacing the normal (called the wild type) gene with a changed or mutant gene—should lead to a measurable decrease in pathogenicity; (3) replacement of the mutant gene with the wild type gene should restore full pathogenicity to the organism.

Mechnikov's discovery (1884) of the process of phagocytosis, whereby leukocytes ingest foreign particles, initiated the study of white cells and cell-mediated immunity in the protection against infection.[3] Ross's demonstration in Egypt of the mosquito as vector to malaria led to a series of public health interventions against mosquitoes including draining of swamps, widespread use of insecticides, and insecticide-impregnated bed nets, presently advocated by the WHO. Ehrlich described antimicrobial "silver bullets," including emetine against amebae, long before the discovery of penicillin by Fleming in 1928 and the development of antibiotics during and after World War II. Ellerman and Bang identified viral causes of cancer, which include hepatitis B virus (HBV) and liver cancer, Epstein-Barr virus (EBV) and lymphoma, human T-cell lymphotropic virus type I (HTLV-I) and leukemia, and human herpesvirus 8 (HHV-8) and Kaposi sarcoma. These are described in Chapter 8.

Avery's demonstration of DNA as the genetic material determining the capsule of virulent pneumococci began the molecular biologic revolution. The identification of human immunodeficiency virus (HIV) as the cause of AIDS, the devastating pandemic of the late 20th century, has led to effective methods of screening donor blood, numerous new concepts in viral pathogenesis, and dramatic advances in antiviral drugs. The entire genome has recently been sequenced from numerous microbes including *Escherichia coli*, *Haemophilus influenzae*, *Helicobacter pylori*, and *Saccharomyces cerevisiae* (bakers' yeast).[4, 5] These genome sequences reveal all possible proteins that each organism may make, demonstrate how some genes are organized into expression groups or operons, and suggest possible targets for new antimicrobial drugs. By themselves, however, these gene sequences cannot reveal mechanisms of pathogenesis, which must be identified by experiment, nor do they identify surface proteins that might be used as vaccine candidates.

New and Emerging Infectious Diseases

Although infectious diseases such as leprosy have been known since biblical times and parasitic schistosomes have been demonstrated in Egyptian mummies, a surprising number of new infectious agents are described each year[6] (Table 9–2). The causes of some infections with significant morbidity and mortality (e.g., *Helicobacter* gastritis, hepatitis B and hepatitis C, rotavirus diarrhea, and legionnaires pneumonia) were previously unrecognized, because the infectious agent was difficult to culture.[7] Some new infectious agents (e.g., Ebola virus, Hantavirus, and "flesh-eating bacteria" that cause streptococcal toxic shock syndrome) are newsworthy for their lethality, even though they are rare or infect persons in faraway places.[8] Other infectious agents may be genuinely new to humans (e.g., HIV that causes AIDS and *Borrelia burgdorferi* that causes Lyme disease) or may be secondary to severe immunosuppression caused by AIDS (e.g., cytomegalovirus [CMV], HHV-8, *Mycobacterium avium-intracellulare*, *Pneumocystis carinii*, and *Cryptosporidium parvum*).

Table 9–2. SOME RECENTLY RECOGNIZED INFECTIOUS AGENTS

1973	Rotavirus	Infantile diarrhea
1975	*Cryptosporidium parvum*	Acute and chronic diarrhea
1977	Ebola virus	Epidemic hemorrhagic fever
	Hantaan virus	Hemorrhagic fever with renal disease
	Legionella pneumophila	Legionnaires pneumonia
	Campylobacter jejuni	Enteritis
1980	HTLV-I	T-cell lymphoma or leukemia
1981	*Staphylococcus aureus*	Toxic shock syndrome
1982	HTLV-II	Hairy cell leukemia
	Escherichia coli O157:H7	Hemorrhagic colitis and hemolytic-uremic syndrome
	Borrelia burgdorferi	Lyme disease
1983	HIV	AIDS
	Helicobacter pylori	Chronic gastritis
1985	*Enterocytozoon bieneusi*	Chronic diarrhea
1988	HHV-6	Roseola subitum
	Hepatitis E	Enterically transmitted hepatitis
1989	Hepatitis C	Non-A, non-B hepatitis
	Ehrlichia chaffeensis	Human ehrlichiosis
1992	*Vibrio cholerae* O139	New epidemic cholera strain
	Bartonella henselae	Cat-scratch disease
1993	*Encephalitozoon cuniculi*	Opportunistic infections
1995	HHV-8	Kaposi sarcoma in AIDS

Adapted from Lederberg J: Infectious disease as an evolutionary paradigm. Emerg Infect Dis 3:417, 1997.

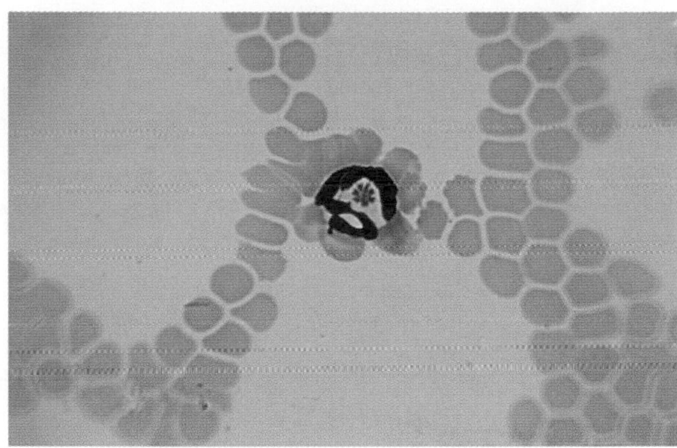

Figure 9–1

Asterisk-shaped inclusion body of *Ehrlichia,* cause of human granulocytic ehrlichiosis, within a neutrophil. (Courtesy of Dr. Sam Telford, Harvard School of Public Health.)

The patterns of disease caused by the new infectious agents may vary dramatically depending on geography: AIDS has been predominantly (but not exclusively) a disease of homosexuals and drug abusers in the United States and Western countries, while AIDS in Africa is predominantly a heterosexual disease that is much more frequent in areas where men remain uncircumcised. Changes in the environment occasionally drive rates of infectious diseases: reforestation of the eastern part of the United States has led to massive increases in deer and mice, which carry the ticks that transmit Lyme disease, babesiosis, and ehrlichiosis (Fig. 9–1). Failure of DDT to control mosquitoes that transmit malaria, in association with the development of drug-resistant parasites, has dramatically increased the morbidity and mortality of *Plasmodium falciparum* in Asia, Africa, and Latin America. Similarly, the development of new drug-resistant *Mycobacterium tuberculosis*, *Neisseria gonorrhoeae*, *Staphylococcus aureus*, and *Enterococcus faecium* has changed the treatment of these infections.

In discussing the mechanisms of infectious disease, two separate but interrelated aspects must be considered: (1) the specific properties of the organisms causing the infection and (2) the host response to the infectious agents. This chapter begins with a review of the categories of infectious agents and a discussion of the mechanisms by which these organisms cause disease. These general principles are then illustrated with a selection of major human infectious diseases, organized by the organ system involved or the groups of patients frequently infected and including descriptions of the lesions caused by each organism.[9, 10] Detailed discussions of many other infectious diseases are presented elsewhere in this book (e.g., viral hepatitis in Chapter 19; pneumococcal pneumonia in Chapter 16; and HIV infection and AIDS in Chapter 7).

Categories of Infectious Agents

Infectious agents that can enter the human host (endoparasites) belong to a wide range of classes and vary in

Table 9–3. CLASSES OF HUMAN ENDOPARASITES AND THEIR HABITATS

Taxonomic Class	Size	Site of Propagation	Sample Species and Its Disease	
Viruses	20–30 nm	Obligate intracellular	Poliovirus	Poliomyelitis
Chlamydiae	200–100 nm	Obligate intracellular	*Chlamydia trachomatis*	Trachoma
Rickettsiae	300–1200 nm	Obligate intracellular	*Rickettsia prowazekii*	Typhus fever
Mycoplasmas	125–350 nm	Extracellular	*Mycoplasma pneumoniae*	Atypical pneumonia
Bacteria, spirochetes, mycobacteria	0.8–15 μm	Cutaneous	*Staphylococcus epidermidis*	Wound infection
		Mucosal	*Vibrio cholerae*	Cholera
		Extracellular	*Streptococcus pneumoniae*	Pneumonia
		Facultative intracellular	*Mycobacterium tuberculosis*	Tuberculosis
Fungi imperfecti	2–200 μm	Cutaneous	*Trichophyton* sp.	Tinea pedis (athlete's foot)
		Mucosal	*Candida albicans*	Thrush
		Extracellular	*Sporothrix schenckii*	Sporotrichosis
		Facultative intracellular	*Histoplasma capsulatum*	Histoplasmosis
Protozoa	1–50 μm	Mucosal	*Giardia lamblia*	Giardiasis
		Extracellular	*Trypanosoma gambiense*	Sleeping sickness
		Facultative intracellular	*Trypanosoma cruzi*	Chagas disease
		Obligate intracellular	*Leishmania donovani*	Kala-azar
Helminths	3 mm–10 m	Mucosal	*Enterobius vermicularis*	Oxyuriasis
		Extracellular	*Wuchereria bancrofti*	Filariasis
		Intracellular	*Trichinella spiralis*	Trichinosis

size from the nucleic acid–free prion to 2-nm poliovirus to 10-m tapeworms (Table 9–3). In addition, several classes of arthropods are ectoparasites, that is, cause damage only through the skin.

PRIONS

Prions, which are apparently composed only of a modified host protein, cause transmissible spongiform encephalopathies including kuru (associated with human cannibalism), Creutzfeldt-Jakob disease (associated with corneal transplants),[11] bovine spongiform encephalopathy (better known as mad cow disease), and atypical Creutzfeldt-Jakob disease transmitted to humans from bovine spongiform encephalopathy. They are discussed in detail in Chapter 30.

VIRUSES

All viruses depend on host cell metabolism for their replication, that is, are obligate intracellular parasites (Table 9–4). They are classified by the nucleic acid content of their core (DNA or RNA) and by the shape of their protein coat or capsid, which can be spherical if capsid proteins form an icosahedron or cylindrical if they form a helix. Many of the more than 400 viral species known to inhabit humans do not cause any disease, but some are frequent causes of acute illness (e.g., colds, influenza). Others are capable of lifelong latency and of long-term reactivation (herpesviruses) or may give rise to chronic disease (e.g., HBV). Together, viral pathogens account for a major share of all human infections. Different viral species can give rise to the same clinical picture (e.g., upper respiratory infection; see section on viral respiratory infections); conversely, a single virus can cause different lesions depending on host age or immune status (e.g., CMV). Further, the same virus may definitely cause one disease (e.g., coxsackievirus B and inflammatory cardiac disease) and be implicated in another (type I diabetes).[12]

BACTERIOPHAGES, PLASMIDS, TRANSPOSONS

These are mobile genetic elements that encode bacterial virulence factors (e.g., adhesins, toxins, or enzymes that confer antibiotic resistance). They can infect bacteria and incorporate themselves into their genome (e.g., toxin genes of *Vibrio cholerae* and *Shigella flexneri*), thus converting an otherwise harmless bacterium into a virulent one or an antibiotic-sensitive organism into a resistant one. Exchange of these elements between bacterial strains and species therefore endows the recipients with a survival advantage or with the capacity to cause disease, or both.

BACTERIA

Bacterial cells are prokaryotes that lack nuclei and endoplasmic reticulum. Their cell walls are relatively rigid, composed either of two phospholipid bilayers with a peptidoglycan layer sandwiched in between (gram-negative species) or of a single bilayer covered by peptidoglycan (gram-positive bacteria) (Table 9–5 and Fig. 9–2). Bacteria synthesize their own DNA, RNA, and proteins but

Table 9–4. HUMAN VIRAL DISEASES AND THEIR PATHOGENS

Viral Pathogen	Virus Family	Genomic Type	Disease Expression
Respiratory			
Adenovirus	Adenoviridae	DS DNA	Upper and lower respiratory tract infections, conjunctivitis, diarrhea
Echovirus	Picornaviridae	SS RNA*	Upper respiratory tract infection, pharyngitis, rash
Rhinovirus	Picornaviridae	SS RNA*	Upper respiratory tract infection
Coxsackievirus	Picornaviridae	SS RNA*	Pleurodynia, herpangina, hand-foot-and-mouth disease
Coronavirus	Coronaviridae	SS RNA*	Upper respiratory tract infection
Influenza viruses A, B	Orthomyxoviridae	SS RNA†,‡	Influenza
Parainfluenza virus 1–4	Paramyxoviridae	SS RNA†	Upper and lower respiratory tract infections, croup
Respiratory syncytial virus	Paramyxoviridae	SS RNA†	Bronchiolitis, pneumonia
Digestive			
Mumps virus	Paramyxoviridae	SS RNA†	Mumps, pancreatitis, orchitis
Rotavirus	Reoviridae	DS RNA‡	Childhood diarrhea
Norwalk agent	Caliciviridae	SS RNA	Gastroenteritis
Hepatitis A virus	Picornaviridae	SS RNA*	Acute viral hepatitis
Hepatitis B virus	Hepadnaviridae	DS DNA	Acute or chronic hepatitis
Hepatitis D virus	Viroid-like	SS RNA	With HBV, acute or chronic hepatitis
Hepatitis C virus	Flaviviridae	SS RNA	Acute or chronic hepatitis
Hepatitis E virus	Norwalk-like	SS RNA	Enterically transmitted hepatitis
Systemic With Skin Eruptions			
Measles virus	Paramyxoviridae	SS RNA†	Measles (rubeola)
Rubella virus	Togaviridae	SS RNA*	German measles (rubella)
Parvovirus	Parvoviridae	SS DNA	Erythema infectiosum, aplastic anemia
Vaccinia virus	Poxviridae	DS DNA	Smallpox vaccine
Varicella-zoster virus	Herpesviridae	DS DNA	Chickenpox, shingles
Herpes simplex virus 1	Herpesviridae	DS DNA	"Cold sore"
Herpes simplex virus 2	Herpesviridae	DS DNA	Genital herpes
Systemic With Hematopoietic Disorders			
Cytomegalovirus	Herpesviridae	DS DNA	Cytomegalic inclusion disease
Epstein-Barr virus	Herpesviridae	DS DNA	Infectious mononucleosis
HTLV-I	Retroviridae	SS RNA§	Adult T-cell leukemia; tropical spastic paraparesis
HTLV-II	Retroviridae	SS RNA§	Role still uncertain
HIV-1 and HIV-2	Retroviridae	SS RNA§	AIDS
Arboviral and Hemorrhagic Fevers			
Dengue virus 1–4	Togaviridae	SS RNA*	Dengue, hemorrhagic fever
Yellow fever virus	Togaviridae	SS RNA*	Yellow fever
Colorado tick fever virus	Reoviridae (Orbivirus)	SS RNA‡	Colorado tick fever
Regional hemorrhagic fever viruses	Arenaviridae	SS RNA†,‡	Bolivian, Argentinian, Lassa fever
	Bunyaviridae	SS RNA†,‡	Crimean-Congo, Hantaan, sandfly fever
	Filoviridae?	SS RNA	Ebola, Marburg disease
	Hantavirus	SS RNA	Korean, U.S. pneumonia
Warty Growths			
Papillomavirus	Papovaviridae	DS DNA	Condyloma; cervical carcinoma
Molluscum virus	Poxviridae	DS DNA	Molluscum contagiosum
Central Nervous System			
Poliovirus	Picornaviridae	SS RNA*	Poliomyelitis
Rabiesvirus	Rhabdoviridae	SS RNA†	Rabies
JC virus	Papovaviridae	DS DNA	Progressive multifocal leukoencephalopathy (opportunistic)
Arboviral encephalitis viruses	Togaviridae	SS RNA*	Eastern, Western, Venezuelan, St. Louis, California group
	Bunyaviridae	SS RNA†,‡	

*Positive-sense genome (nucleotide sequences directly translated).
†Negative-sense genome (complementary to positive-sense strand).
‡Segmented genome.
§DNA step required in retroviral replication.

Table 9–5. BACTERIAL, SPIROCHETAL, AND MYCOBACTERIAL DISEASES

Clinical or Microbiologic Category	Species	Frequent Disease Presentations
Infections by pyogenic cocci	*Staphylococcus aureus, S. epidermidis*	Abscess, cellulitis, pneumonia, septicemia
	Streptococcus pyogenes, β-hemolytic	Upper respiratory tract infection, erysipelas, scarlet fever, septicemia
	Streptococcus pneumoniae (pneumococcus)	Lobar pneumonia, meningitis
	Neisseria meningitidis (meningococcus)	Cerebrospinal meningitis
	Neisseria gonorrhoeae (gonococcus)	Gonorrhea
Gram-negative infections, common	**Escherichia coli* **Klebsiella pneumoniae* **Enterobacter (Aerobacter) aerogenes* **Proteus* spp. *(P. mirabilis, P. morgagni)* **Serratia marcescens* **Pseudomonas* spp. *(P. aeruginosa)*	Urinary tract infection, wound infection, abscess, pneumonia, septicemia, endotoxemia, endocarditis
	Bacteroides sp. *(B. fragilis)*	Anaerobic infection
	Legionella spp. *(L. pneumophila)*	Legionnaires disease
Gram-negative infections, rare	*Klebsiella rhinoscleromatis, K. ozaenae*	Rhinoscleroma, ozena
	Haemophilus ducreyi	Chancroid (soft chancre)
	Calymmatobacterium donovani	Granuloma inguinale
	Bartonella bacilliformis	Carrión disease (Oroya fever)
Contagious childhood bacterial diseases	*Haemophilus influenzae*	Meningitis, upper and lower respiratory tract infections
	Bordetella pertussis	Whooping cough
	Corynebacterium diphtheriae	Diphtheria
Enteropathic infections	Enteropathogenic *E. coli* *Shigella* sp. *Vibrio cholerae* *Campylobacter fetus, C. jejuni* *Yersinia enterocolitica* *Salmonella* spp. (1000 strains)	Invasive or noninvasive gastroenterocolitis, some with septicemia
	Salmonella typhi	Typhoid fever
Clostridial infections	*Clostridium tetani*	Tetanus (lockjaw)
	Clostridium botulinum	Botulism (paralytic food poisoning)
	Clostridium perfringens, C. septicum	Gas gangrene, necrotizing cellulitis
	**Clostridium difficile*	Pseudomembranous colitis
Zoonotic bacterial infections	*Bacillus anthracis*	Anthrax (malignant pustule)
	**Listeria monocytogenes*	*Listeria* meningitis, listeriosis
	Yersinia pestis	Bubonic plague
	Francisella tularensis	Tularemia
	Brucella melitensis, B. suis, B. abortus	Brucellosis (undulant fever)
	Pseudomonas mallei, P. pseudomallei	Glanders, melioidosis
	Leptospira spp. (many groups)	Leptospirosis, Weil disease
	Borrelia recurrentis	Relapsing fever
	Borrelia burgdorferi	Lyme borreliosis
	Bartonella henselae	Cat-scratch disease; bacillary angiomatosis
	Spirillum minus, Streptobacillus moniliformis	Rat-bite fever
Human treponemal infections	*Treponema pallidum*	Venereal, endemic syphilis (bejel)
	Treponema pertenue	Yaws (frambesia)
	Treponema carateum (T. herrejoni)	Pinta (carate, mal del pinto)
Mycobacterial infections	**Mycobacterium tuberculosis, M. bovis* (Koch bacillus)	Tuberculosis
	M. leprae (Hansen bacillus)	Leprosy
	**M. kansasii, M. avium, M. intracellulare*	Atypical mycobacterial infections
	M. ulcerans	Buruli ulcer
Actinomycetaceae	**Nocardia asteroides*	Nocardiosis
	Actinomyces israelii	Actinomycosis

*Important opportunistic infections.

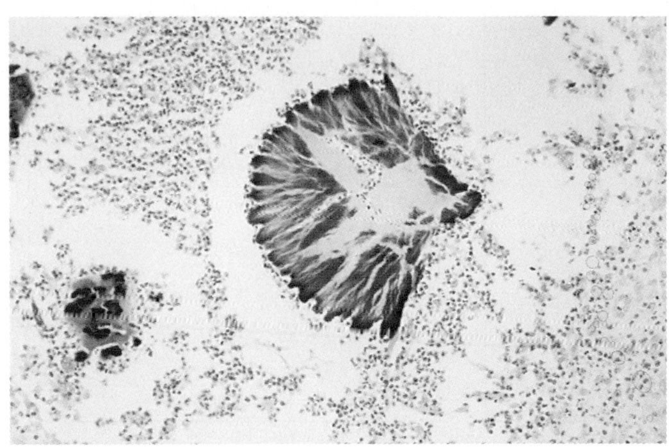

Figure 9–2

Actinomyces, a filamentous bacterium, within an airway (periodic acid–Schiff [PAS] stain).

depend on the host for favorable growth conditions. Some thrive mainly on the body's surface layers; normal persons carry 10^{12} bacteria on the skin, including *Staphylococcus epidermidis* and *Propionibacterium acnes,* the agent responsible for adolescent pimples. Normally, 10^{14} bacteria reside inside the gastrointestinal tract, 99.9% of which are anaerobic, including *Bacteroides* species. Many bacterial pathogens invade host tissue and are capable of extracellular division (e.g., pneumococcus) or of both extracellular and intracellular division (e.g., *Mycobacterium tuberculosis*). Next to viruses, bacteria are the most frequent and diverse class of human pathogens and include many of the major pathogens discussed in this chapter and elsewhere throughout the text.

CHLAMYDIAE, RICKETTSIAE, MYCOPLASMAS

These infectious agents are grouped together because they are similar to bacteria in that they divide by binary fission and are susceptible to antibiotics but lack certain structures (e.g., mycoplasmas lack a cell wall) or metabolic capabilities (e.g., chlamydiae lack adenosine triphosphate [ATP] synthesis). Chlamydiae, which are frequent causes of genitourinary infections, conjunctivitis, and respiratory infections of newborn infants, are discussed with the sexually transmitted diseases.

Most rickettsiae are transmitted by insect vectors, including lice (epidemic typhus), ticks (Rocky Mountain spotted fever [RMSF], Q fever, and ehrlichiosis), and mites (scrub typhus).[13] Rickettsiae are obligate intracellular agents that replicate in the cytoplasm of endothelial cells (see section on vector-borne infections). By injuring the endothelial cells, rickettsiae cause a hemorrhagic vasculitis often visible as a rash but may also cause a transient pneumonia or hepatitis (Q fever) or injure the central nervous system and cause death (RMSF and epidemic typhus).

Mycoplasmas and the closely related genus *Ureaplasma* are the tiniest free-living organisms known (125 to 300 nm). *Mycoplasma pneumoniae* spreads from person to person by aerosols, binds to the surface of epithelial cells in the airways by an adhesin called P1, and causes an atypical pneumonia characterized by peribronchiolar infiltrates of lymphocytes and plasma cells (Chapter 16). Ureaplasmas are transmitted venereally and may cause nongonococcal urethritis.

FUNGI

Fungi possess thick, ergosterol-containing cell walls and grow as perfect, sexually reproducing forms in vitro and as imperfect forms in vivo, which include budding yeast cells and slender tubes (hyphae) (Figs. 9–3 and 9–4). Some produce spores, which are resistant to extreme environmental conditions, whereas hyphae may produce fruiting bodies called *conidia.* Some fungal species, for example, those of the *Tinea* group causing "athlete's foot," are confined to the superficial layers of the human skin; other "dermatophytes" preferentially damage the hair shafts or nails. Certain fungal species invade the subcutaneous tissue, causing abscesses or granulomas, as happens in sporotrichosis and in tropical mycoses. Deep fungal infections can spread systemically, destroying vital organs in immunocompromised hosts, whereas these fungal lesions heal spontaneously or remain latent in otherwise normal hosts. Some deep fungal species are limited to a particular geographic region (e.g., *Coccidioides, Histoplasma,* and *Blastomyces).* Opportunistic fungi *(Candida, Aspergillus, Mucor),* by contrast, are ubiquitous contaminants colonizing the normal human skin or gut without causing illness. Only in immunosuppressed individuals do opportunistic fungi give rise to life-threatening infections. In addition, AIDS patients, late in their course, are frequent victims of the opportunistic fungus-like organism *Pneumocystis carinii.*

PROTOZOA

Parasitic protozoa are single-celled organisms endowed with motility, pliable plasma membranes, and complex cytoplasmic organelles (Table 9–6). The flagellate *Tricho-*

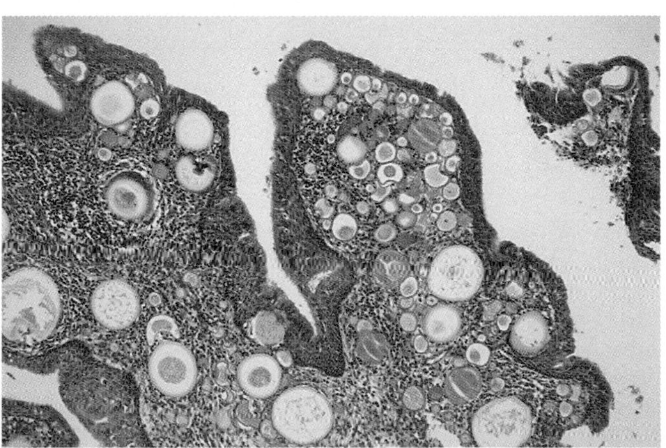

Figure 9–3

Skin with massive infiltrate of *Rhinosporidium,* a tropical fungus.

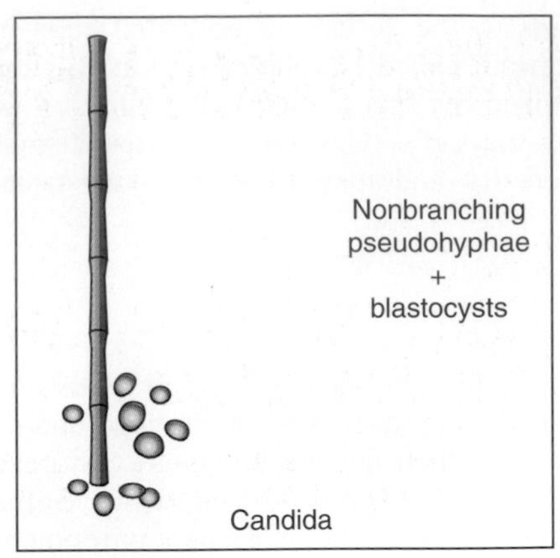

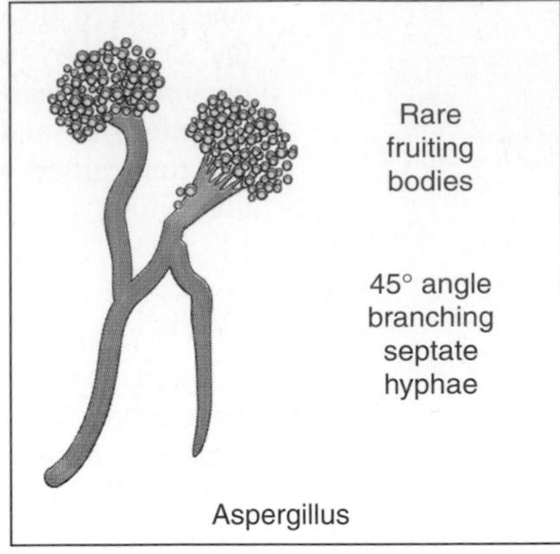

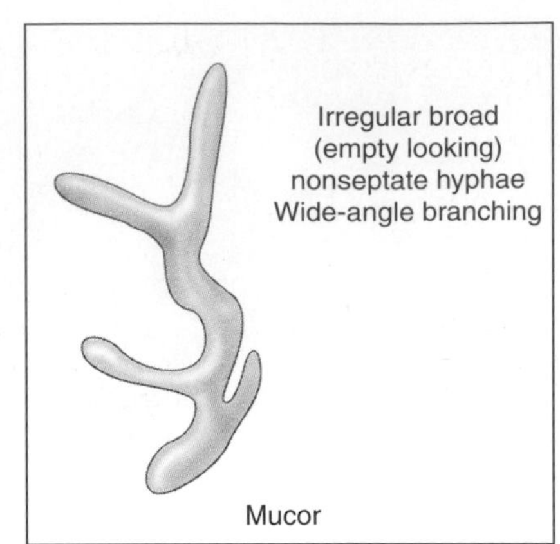

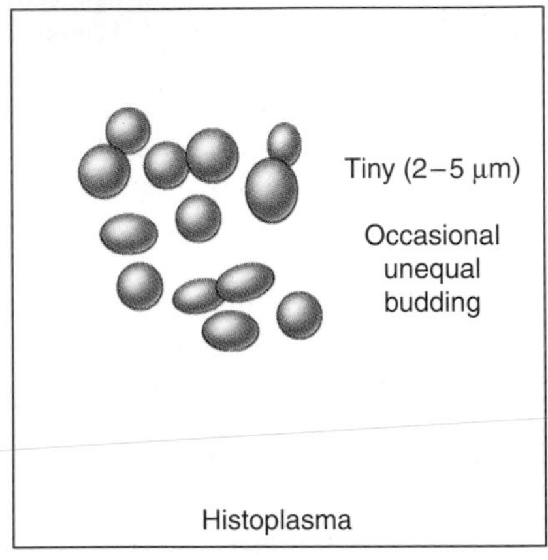

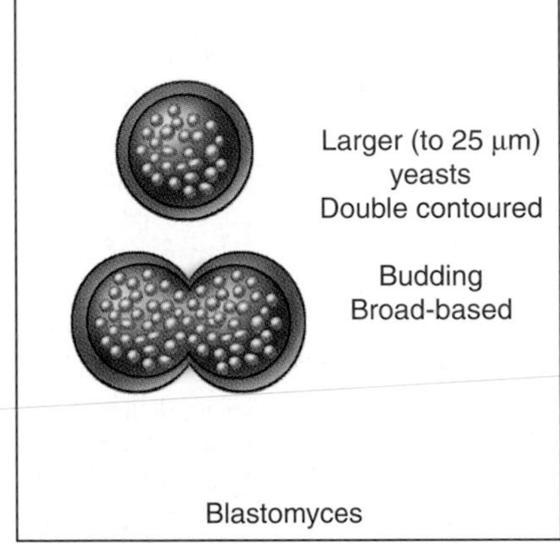

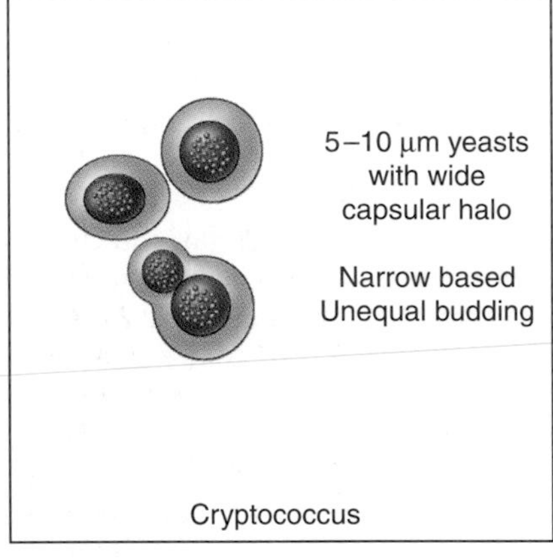

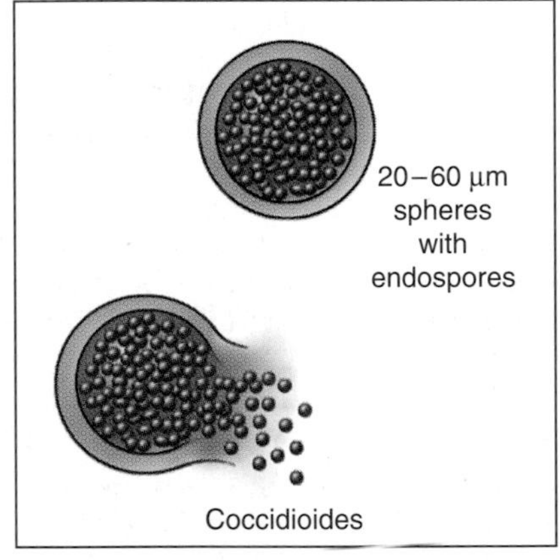

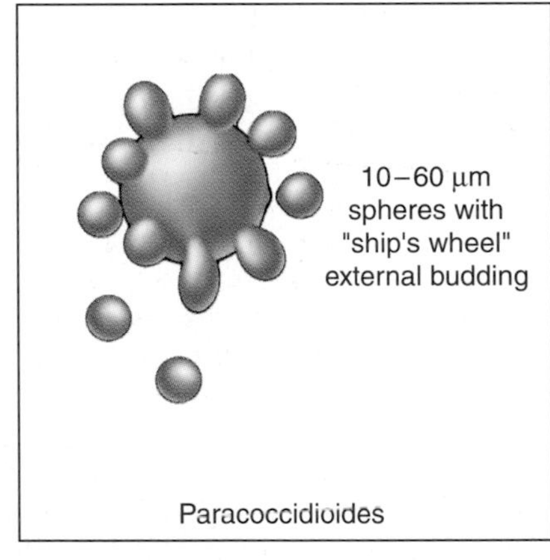

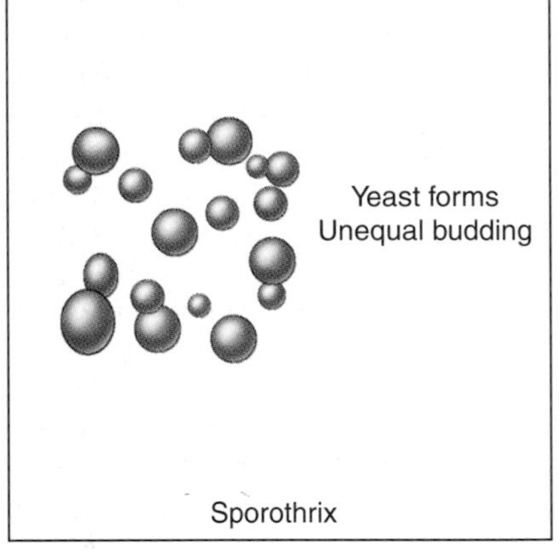

Figure 9–4

Characteristic tissue forms of fungi.

monas vaginalis is transmitted sexually from person to person. The intestinal protozoa (e.g., *Entamoeba histolytica* and *Giardia lamblia*) are spread by the fecal-oral route. Blood-borne protozoa (e.g., *Plasmodium* species, *Trypanosoma* species, and *Leishmania* species) are transmitted by blood-sucking insects, in which they undergo a complex succession of life stages before being passed to new human hosts (Fig. 9–5). *Toxoplasma gondii* is acquired either by contact with oocyst-shedding kittens or by eating cyst-ridden, undercooked meat.

HELMINTHS

Parasitic worms are highly differentiated multicellular organisms. Their life cycles are complex; most alternate between sexual reproduction in the definitive host and asexual multiplication in an intermediary host or vector. Thus, depending on parasite species, humans may harbor either adult worms (e.g., *Ascaris*) or immature stages (e.g., *Toxocara canis*) or asexual larval forms (e.g., *Echinococcus*). Adult worms, once resident in humans, do not multiply in

Table 9–6. PROTOZOA PATHOGENIC FOR HUMANS

Species	Order	Form, Size	Disease
Luminal or Epithelial			
Entamoeba histolytica	Amebae	Trophozoite 15–50 μm	Amebic dysentery; liver abscess
Balantidium coli	Ciliates	Trophozoite 50–100 μm	Colitis
Naegleria fowleri	Ameboflagellates	Trophozoite 10–20 μm	Meningoencephalitis
Acanthamoeba sp.	Ameboflagellates	Trophozoite 15–30 μm	Meningoencephalitis or ophthalmitis
Giardia lamblia	Mastigophora	Trophozoite 11–18 μm	Diarrheal disease, malabsorption
Isospora belli	Coccidia	Oocyst 10–20 μm	Chronic enterocolitis or malabsorption or both
Cryptosporidium sp.	Coccidia	Oocyst 5–6 μm	
Enterocytozoon bieneusi	Microsporida	Spore	Diarrhea in AIDS patients
Trichomonas vaginalis	Mastigophora	Trophozoite 10–30 μm	Urethritis, vaginitis
Bloodstream			
Plasmodium vivax	Hemosporidia	Trophozoites, schizonts, gametes (all small and inside red cells)	Benign tertian malaria
Plasmodium ovale	Hemosporidia		Benign tertian malaria
Plasmodium malariae	Hemosporidia		Quartan malaria
Plasmodium falciparum	Hemosporidia		Malignant tertian malaria
Babesia microti, B. bovis	Hemosporidia	Trophozoites inside red cells	Babesiosis
Trypanosoma brucei, T. rhodesiense, T. gambiense	Hemoflagellates	Trypomastigote 14–33 μm	African sleeping sickness
Intracellular			
Trypanosoma cruzi	Hemoflagellates	Trypomastigote 20 μm	Chagas disease
Leishmania donovani	Hemoflagellates	Amastigote 2 μm	Kala-azar
Leishmania tropica, L. mexicana, L. braziliensis	Hemoflagellates	Amastigote 2 μm	Cutaneous and mucocutaneous leishmaniasis
Toxoplasma gondii	Coccidia (eimeriae)	Tachyzoite 4–6 μm (cyst larger)	Toxoplasmosis

number but generate eggs or larvae destined for the next phase of the cycle. An exception is *Strongyloides,* the larvae of which can become infective inside the gut and cause overwhelming autoinfection in immunosuppressed persons. There are two important consequences of the lack of replication of adult worms: (1) disease is often caused by inflammatory responses to the eggs or larvae rather than to the adults (e.g., schistosomiasis) and (2) disease is in proportion to the number of organisms that have infected the individual (e.g., 10 hookworms cause little disease, whereas 1000 hookworms cause severe anemia by consuming 100 ml of blood per day). Fortunately, most persons in endemic areas harbor few worms and are free of disease, and only a minority are heavily infected and ill.

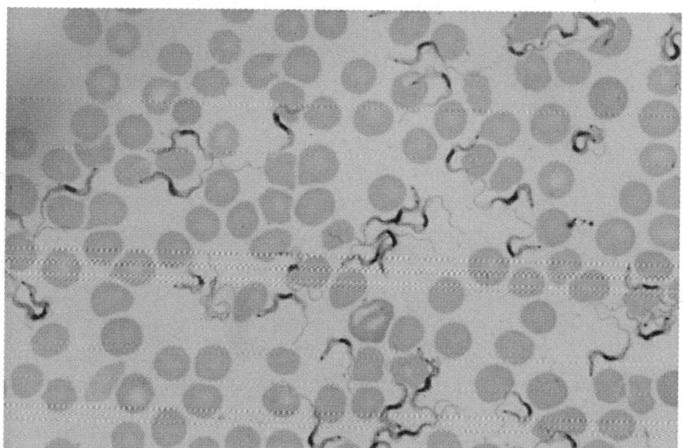

Figure 9–5

Slender bloodstream parasites of African sleeping sickness.

Parasitic worms are of three classes. The first class, *roundworms* (nematodes), is characterized by a collagenous tegument and a nonsegmented structure. These include *Ascaris,* hookworms, and *Strongyloides* among the intestinal worms and the filariae and *Trichinella* among the tissue invaders. The second class, *flatworms* (cestodes), comprises gutless worms, whose head (scolex) sprouts a ribbon of flat segments (proglottids) covered by an absorptive tegument. This class includes the pork, beef, and fish tapeworms and the cystic tapeworm larvae (cysticerci and hydatid cysts). The third class, *flukes* (trematodes), which are primitive leaflike worms with syncytial integument, includes the oriental liver and lung flukes and the blood-dwelling schistosomes, discussed later.

ECTOPARASITES

Ectoparasites are arthropods (lice, ticks, bedbugs, fleas) that attach to and live on the skin. In addition, skin lesions can be caused by the stings of mosquitoes and bees. Scabies is an example of severe dermatitis elicited by mites burrowing into the stratum corneum (Chapter 27). Skin nodules caused by burrowing botfly larvae are intensely inflamed and eosinophil enriched. In addition, attached ar-

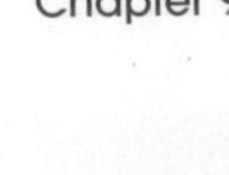

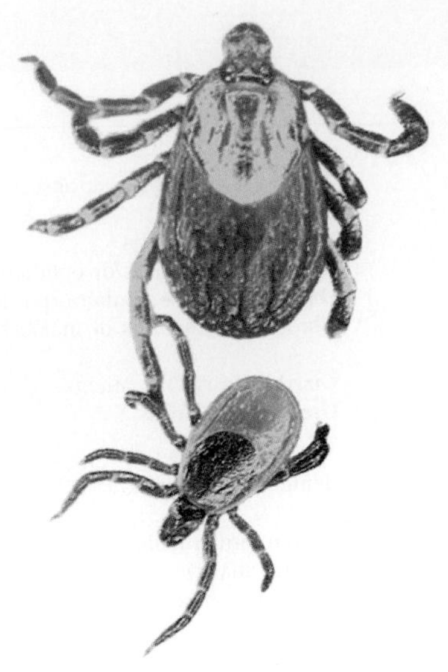

Figure 9–6

Tiny deer tick *(bottom)*, which transmits Lyme disease and *Babesia* and *Ehrlichia* organisms, contrasted with a larger dog tick *(top)*, which is not thought to transmit human infections. (Courtesy of Dr. F.R. Matuschka, Free University of Berlin, Germany.)

thropods can be vectors for other pathogens that make characteristic skin lesions, for example, the expanding erythematous plaque caused by the Lyme disease spirochete *Borrelia burgdorferi*, which is transmitted by deer ticks (Fig. 9–6).

Transmission and Dissemination of Microbes

HOST BARRIERS TO INFECTION

The first and most formidable barriers to infection are the intact host skin and mucosal surfaces and their secretory-excretory products.[14] For example, lysozyme secreted by the tear glands degrades the peptidoglycans of bacterial cell walls and protects the eyes from infection. Acid gastric juice is lethal for some enteric pathogens; for example, normal volunteers do not become infected by *Vibrio cholerae* unless they are fed 10^{11} organisms. In contrast, *Shigella* and *Giardia* are relatively resistant to acid, and less than 100 organisms of each species is infective. In general, skin infections in normal persons tend to arise in damaged sites, that is, wounds, cuts, or burns, and can be caused by resident bacteria of relatively low virulence. In contrast, infections transmitted by the respiratory, gastrointestinal, or genitourinary route generally require virulent organisms capable of damaging or penetrating normal mucosal barriers. Host barriers to infection of the respiratory tracts, gastrointestinal tract, and skin are discussed in the sections devoted to these organs.

SPREAD AND DISSEMINATION OF MICROBES

Once implanted, microbes spread on the surface of moist and warm mucosae faster than on cool and dry skin. Some of the superficial pathogens stay confined to the lumen of hollow viscera (e.g., cholera); others adhere to or proliferate exclusively in or on epithelial cells (e.g., papillomaviruses, dermatophytes). A variety of pathogenic bacteria, fungi, and helminths are invasive pathogens by virtue of their motility or ability to secrete lytic enzymes (e.g., streptococcal hyaluronidase, schistosome proteases). Microbial spread initially follows tissue planes of least resistance, for example, along aponeurotic compartments. Spread through serosal cavities (pleura, peritoneum, meninges) is particularly fast and dangerous. Microbes may also ascend the lymphatics from their entry site to the regional nodes and hence into the bloodstream (Fig. 9–7). Thus, untreated staphylococcal infections may progress from a localized abscess or furuncle to regional lymphadenitis followed by bacteremia, endocarditis, or formation of multiple pyemic abscesses in distant metastatic sites (brain, kidney, bone). Depending on microbial species, secondary foci of infection, established through the bloodstream, take the form of abscesses or granulomas. They can be single and large (a solitary abscess or tuberculoma) or multiple and tiny, the size of millet seeds (e.g., miliary tuberculosis or *Candida* microabscesses). Viruses may propagate from cell to cell by fusion or axonal transport (e.g., poliovirus), but like other intracellular pathogens (e.g., tubercle bacilli), they can enter the bloodstream and be carried to distant sites by migratory macrophages (HIV-1) or by circulating red cells (Colorado tick fever virus).

- *The major manifestations of infectious disease may arise at sites distant from those of parasite entry.* For example, chickenpox and measles viruses enter through the airways but manifest themselves first as rashes; poliovirus is ingested and multiplies inside the gut wall before proceeding to viremic invasion and killing of motor neurons. Several helminth parasites (e.g., hookworm) enter the skin as penetrating larvae but complete their migratory cycle and maturation inside the gut.
- Bloodstream invasion by sporadic low-virulence or nonvirulent microbes is a common event but is quickly suppressed by the normal host defenses. By contrast, sustained bloodstream invasion with dissemination of pathogens, that is, viremia, bacteremia, fungemia, or parasitemia, is a serious insult and manifests itself by fever, low arterial pressure, and multiple other systemic "septic" signs and symptoms. Massive bloodstream invasion by bacteria or their endotoxins can rapidly become fatal, even for previously healthy individuals.
- *The placental-fetal route is an important mode of transmission* (Chapter 11). When infectious organisms reach the pregnant uterus through the cervical orifice or the bloodstream and are able to traverse the placenta, severe damage to the fetus may result. Bacterial or mycoplasmal placentitis may cause premature delivery or stillbirth. *Treponema pallidum* infecting the mother breaches the placenta by the end of the second trimester and

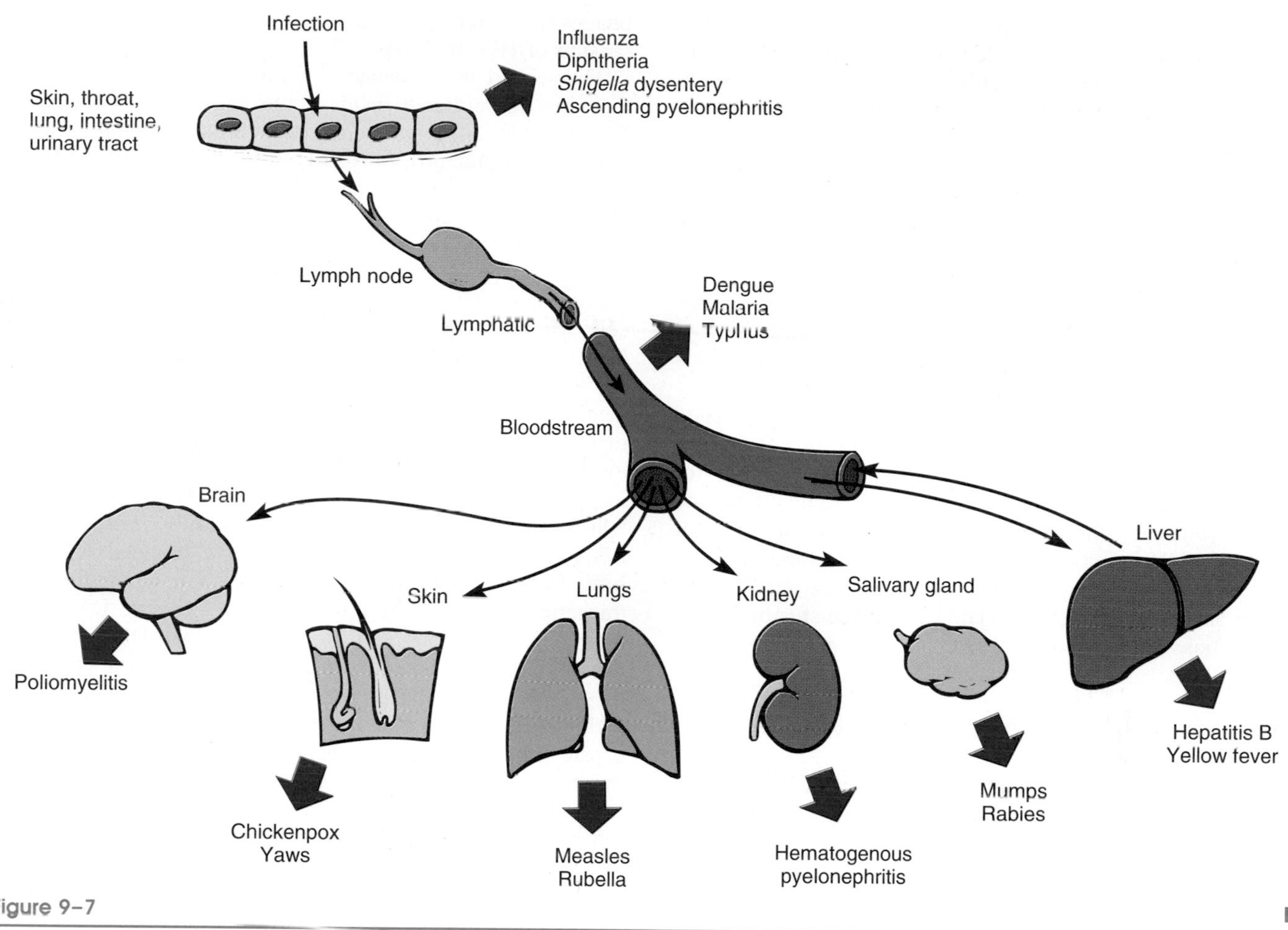

Figure 9–7

Routes of entry, dissemination, and release of microbes from the body. (Adapted from Mims CA: The Pathogenesis of Infectious Disease, 4th ed. San Diego, CA, Academic Press, 1996.)

causes manifestations of congenital syphilis in the infant, ranging from dental deformities to stillbirth. By contrast, transmission of maternal viruses or of *Toxoplasma* infections is most dangerous during early pregnancy and can result in flagrant systemic disease of the fetus (e.g., CMV), fetal maldevelopment, deafness, and congenital heart disease (e.g., rubella). Central nervous system damage is particularly common in the so-called TORCH *(Toxoplasma,* rubella, CMV, herpesviruses, and other) infections (Chapter 11). The same agents can also cause more subtle mental retardation or learning disabilities during childhood. Fetuses infected late during pregnancy or during passage through the birth canal and infants receiving virus through maternal milk usually fare better than those infected during early embryonal life; their lesions may resemble those of adult patients. Maternal transmission of HIV results in opportunistic infections in 50% of untreated children during the first year of life. Maternal transmission of HBV is common in third world countries and among the drug addicted. Such children are at high risk for liver cancer later during adult life.

RELEASE AND TRANSMISSION OF MICROBES

For transmission to occur, microbial pathogens must be able to leave the host organism. Depending on the location of infection, release may be accomplished by skin shedding, mucosal contact, coughing, sneezing, shouting, or voiding of urine or feces. Microbes directly transmissible from person to person by contact or aerosol (e.g., measles or chickenpox) are termed *contagious.* Viruses infecting the salivary glands (e.g., herpesviruses, mumps viruses) are released principally by kissing or spitting. Other pathogens are infective mainly by prolonged intimate or mucosal contact, as occurs during sexual transmission (e.g., HIV-1, herpes simplex virus [HSV-2], papillomaviruses, chlamydiae, syphilis). Bacteria and fungi transmitted by the respiratory route are infective only when lesions are open to the airways (e.g., pulmonary tuberculosis). Many pathogens, from viruses to helminths, are transmitted by the fecal-oral route, that is, by ingestion of stool-contaminated food or water. Water-borne viruses involved in epidemic outbreaks include hepatitis A and E viruses, poliovirus, and rotavirus.[15] To ensure transmission, organisms may form spores, protozoan cysts, or thick-shelled helminth eggs, which can survive in a cool and dry environment. Alternatively, some enteric pathogens are shed for long periods by asymptomatic carrier hosts (e.g., salmonellae).

Transmission of microbes from skin to insect occurs during feeding, either because the pathogen circulates in the blood or because it resides in the skin. Some parasitic helminths shed eggs that gain access to new hosts by larval skin penetration rather than by oral intake (e.g., hookworms, schistosomes). Higher parasite phyla, that is, protozoa and helminths, have evolved complex transmission cycles involving a chain of intermediary and vector hosts bearing successive developmental parasite stages.

Transmission of pathogens by the various routes listed occurs not only from human to human but also from animal to human (e.g., field mice are the "reservoir hosts" for Lyme disease) and vice versa. Diseases of this type are termed *zoonotic infections.* By contrast, transmission of HBV and HIV infections through blood and blood products is frequently caused by human agency, that is, needle sharing by addicts, virus-contaminated blood transfusions, cuts, needle-sticks, and other accidents.

How Microorganisms Cause Disease

Infectious agents establish infection and damage tissues in three ways:

- They can contact or enter host cells and directly cause cell death.
- They may release endotoxins or exotoxins that kill cells at a distance, release enzymes that degrade tissue components, or damage blood vessels and cause ischemic necrosis.
- They induce host cellular responses that, although directed against the invader, may cause additional tissue damage, including suppuration, scarring, and hypersensitivity reactions. Thus, the defensive responses of the host are a two-edged sword: they are necessary to overcome the infection but at the same time directly contribute to tissue damage.

Here we describe some of the particular mechanisms whereby viruses and bacteria damage host tissues.

MECHANISMS OF VIRAL INJURY

Viruses damage host cells by entering the cell and replicating at the host's expense. Viral tropism—the tendency to infect some cells but not others—is in part caused by the binding of specific viral surface proteins to particular host cell surface receptor proteins, many of which have known functions. For example, EBV binds to the complement receptor on macrophages (CD2), rabies virus binds to the acetylcholine receptor on neurons, and rhinoviruses bind to the adhesion protein intercellular adhesion molecule 1 (ICAM-1) on mucosal cells. HIV, the cause of AIDS, binds to two different proteins on target cells,[16, 17] the CD34 protein on lymphocytes (but also present on macrophages and glial cells) and chemokine receptors on macrophages and microglia—CCR5, CCR3, or CCR2b (see discussion of HIV in Chapter 7).

The second major cause of viral tropism is the ability of the virus to replicate inside some cells but not in others. For example, JC papovavirus, which causes leukoencephalopathy (Chapter 30), is restricted to oligodendroglia in the central nervous system because the promoter and enhancer DNA sequences upstream from the viral genes are active in glial cells but not in neurons or endothelial cells.

Once attached, the entire virion or a portion containing the genome and essential polymerases *penetrates* into the cell cytoplasm by one of three ways: (1) translocation of the entire virus across the plasma membrane, (2) fusion of the viral envelope with the cell membrane, or (3) receptor-mediated endocytosis of the virus and fusion with endosomal membranes. Within the cell, the virus uncoats, separating its genome from its structural components and losing its infectivity. Viruses then replicate with use of enzymes, which are distinct for each virus family. For example, RNA polymerase is used by negative-stranded RNA viruses to generate positive-stranded mRNA, whereas reverse transcriptase is used by retroviruses to generate DNA from their RNA template and to integrate that DNA into the host genome. Viruses also use host enzymes for viral synthesis, which may be present in some differentiated tissues and not in others. Newly synthesized viral genomes and capsid proteins are then assembled into progeny virions in the nucleus or cytoplasm and are released directly (unencapsulated viruses) or bud through the plasma membrane (encapsulated viruses). In some cases (e.g., measles virus), viruses use actin filaments to transport them to the surface of host cells.[18]

Viral infection can be *abortive,* with incomplete viral replicative cycle; *latent,* in which the virus (e.g., herpes zoster) persists in a cryptic state within the dorsal root ganglia and then presents as painful shingles; or *persistent*, in which virions are synthesized continuously with or without altered cell function (e.g., hepatitis B).

Viruses kill host cells in a number of ways (Fig. 9–8):

- Viruses inhibit host cell DNA, RNA, or protein synthesis. For example, poliovirus inactivates cap-binding protein, which is essential for protein synthesis directed by capped host cell mRNAs, while allowing protein synthesis from uncapped poliovirus mRNAs.
- Viral proteins insert into the host cell's plasma membrane and directly damage its integrity or promote cell fusion (HIV, measles virus, and herpesviruses).
- Viruses replicate efficiently and lyse host cells (e.g., liver cells by yellow fever virus, and neurons by poliovirus).
- Viral proteins on the surface of the host cells are recognized by the immune system, and the host lymphocytes attack the virus-infected cells. For example, acute liver failure during hepatitis B infection may be accelerated by Fas ligands on cytotoxic T lymphocytes, which bind to Fas receptors on the surface of hepatocytes and induce apoptosis in target cells[19] (Chapter 1). Respiratory syncytial virus, a major cause of lower respiratory infections in infants, causes release of cytokines interleukin (IL)–4 and IL-5 from T_H2 type cells, which induce

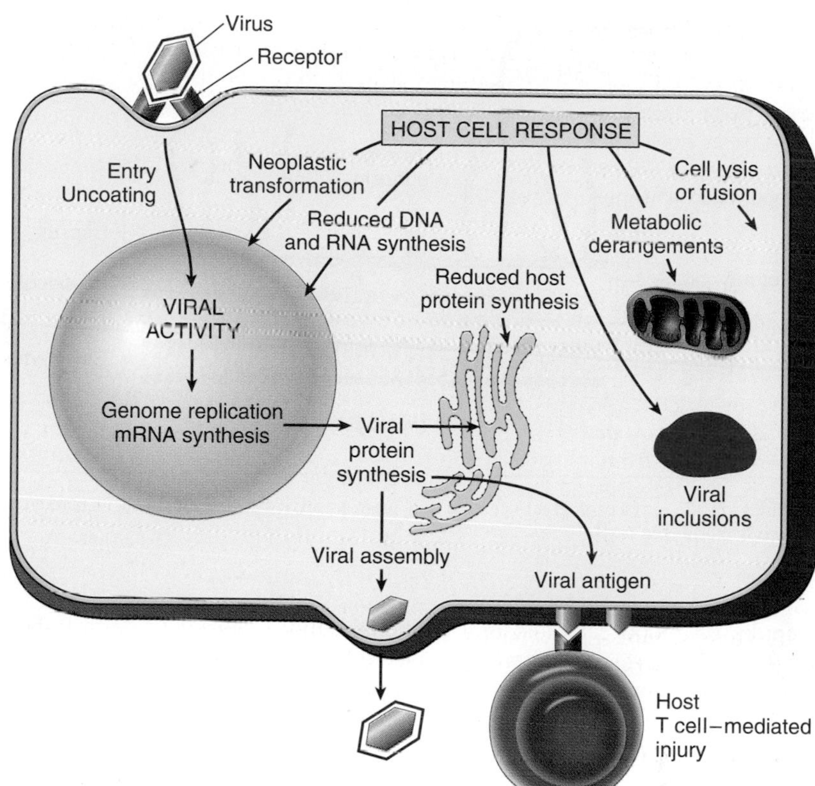

Figure 9–8

Mechanisms by which viruses cause injuries to cells.

mast cell activation and eosinophil accumulation and result in asthma[20] (Chapter 16).

- Viruses damage cells involved in host antimicrobial defense, leading to secondary infections. For example, viral damage to respiratory epithelium allows subsequent pneumonias caused by pneumococcus or *Haemophilus,* and HIV depletes CD4+ helper lymphocytes, which normally suppress opportunistic bacterial infections.
- Viral killing of one cell type causes the death of other cells that depend on them. For example, poliovirus causes motor neuron injury and atrophy of distal skeletal muscle supplied by such neurons.
- *Slow virus infections* (e.g., subacute sclerosing panencephalitis caused by measles virus) culminate in severe progressive disease after a long latency period.
- In addition to causing cell injury, viruses induce *cell proliferation and transformation* (e.g., HBV, human papillomavirus, or EBV), which result in neoplastic growth. The mechanisms of viral transformation are numerous[21] and are discussed in Chapter 8.

MECHANISMS OF BACTERIA-INDUCED INJURY

Bacterial Virulence. Bacterial damage to host tissues depends on their ability to adhere to host cells, invade cells and tissues, and deliver toxic moieties. These virulence properties are determined by a multitude of genes and gene products.

There are both similarities and differences in genes expressed by virulent and avirulent bacteria. For example, most of the genes necessary for virulence of *Salmonella typhi*, the cause of typhoid fever, are also present in nonpathogenic *E. coli.*[22] These "housekeeping" virulence genes encode proteins involved in nutrient assimilation, toxin transport, and, most important, gene regulation. In addition, virulent *Salmonella* or *Shigella* have numerous genes encoding proteins involved in host recognition and invasion, which are absent in avirulent *E. coli*. Such genes are sometimes called "pathogenicity islands," because they are *physically* associated—for example, a *Shigella* plasmid (circular DNA) encodes Shiga toxin and other adherence proteins,[23] which are expressed coordinately. Adherence and toxin genes of *Vibrio cholerae* are induced together by iron deprivation, while sets of *Salmonella* genes are coordinately expressed when the bacterium enters the acidic environment within the macrophage phagolysosome. Finally, a pathogenicity island called *cag* encoding a vacuolating toxin may convert *Helicobacter pylori* from an avirulent commensal bacterium into a gastritis-producing pathogen.[24] Important virulence genes of *intracellular* bacteria, which are induced by contact with host cells, encode proteins involved in so-called type III intracellular secretion systems, which deliver bacterial proteins directly into the host cell cytosol.[25]

Bacterial Adhesins. Bacterial adhesins that bind bacteria to host cells are limited in type but have a broad range of host cell specificity. The *fibrillae* covering the surface of gram-positive cocci such as *Streptococcus* are composed of M protein and lipoteichoic acids[26] (Fig. 9–9). *Lipoteichoic acids* are hydrophobic and bind to the surface of all eukaryotic cells, although with a higher affinity to particular

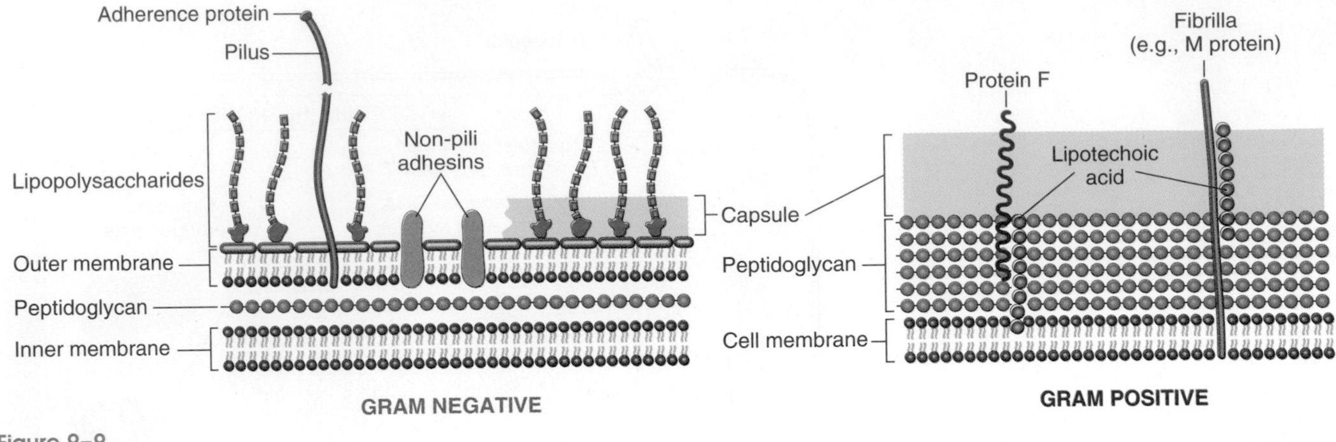

Figure 9–9

Molecules on the surface of gram-negative and gram-positive bacteria involved in pathogenesis. Not shown is the type 3 secretory apparatus of gram-negative bacteria (see text).

receptors on blood cells and oral epithelial cells. *Fimbriae* or *pili* on the surface of gram-negative rods and cocci are nonflagellar filamentous structures composed of repeating subunits. Pili mediate binding of the phagemid carrying cholera toxin genes, which integrates into the *Vibrio* chromosome in the same way that retroviruses integrate into the chromosomes of infected host cells.[27] Other pili such as those on *Neisseria gonorrhoeae* mediate adherence of bacteria to host cells (Fig. 9–10). The base of the subunit that anchors the pili to the bacterial cell wall is similar for widely divergent bacteria. At the tips of the pili are minor protein components that determine to which host cells the microbes will attach (bacterial tropism). In *E. coli,* these minor proteins are antigenically distinct and are associated with particular infections. For example, type I proteins bind mannose and cause urinary tract infections, type P proteins

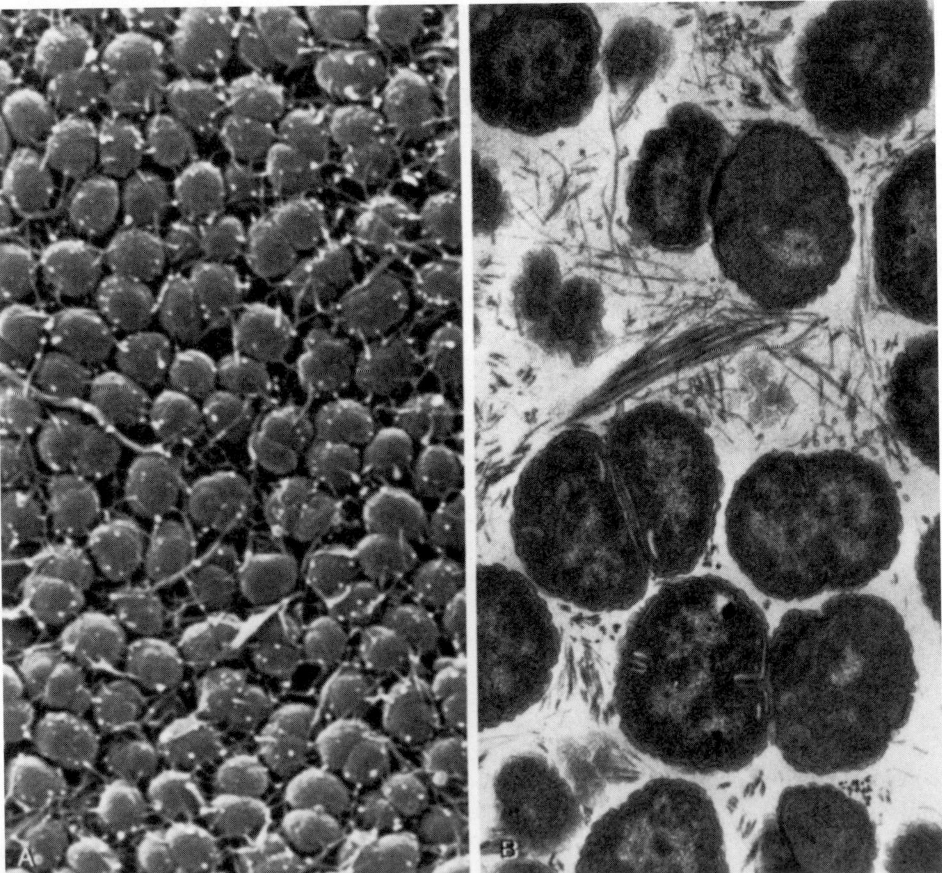

Figure 9–10

Gonococcal culture showing pili, as seen by scanning microscopy (*A*), and in clusters, as seen by transmission electron microscopy (*B*). (Courtesy of Dr. John Swanson, Rocky Mountain Laboratories, Hamilton, MT.)

bind galactose and cause pyelonephritis, and type S proteins bind sialic acid and cause meningitis. A single bacterium can express more than one type of pili as well as nonpilar adhesins.

In contrast to viruses, which can infect a broad range of host cells, facultative *intracellular* bacteria infect mainly epithelial cells *(Shigella* and enteroinvasive *E. coli),* macrophages (*Mycobacterium tuberculosis* and *Mycobacterium leprae, Legionella pneumophila,* and *Yersinia),* or both cell types *(Salmonella typhi* and *Listeria monocytogenes).*

- Entry into macrophages is for the most part directed by receptors that recognize antibodies or complement on the surface of bacteria (Chapter 3). In addition, certain organisms such as *Mycobacterium* and *Legionella* inhibit the acidification that normally occurs when the endosome fuses with the lysosome and thus protect from lysosomal digestion. Many bacteria (e.g., *Mycobacterium avium)* can replicate within macrophages in the absence of a host immune response (e.g., lepromatous leprosy), but activated macrophages kill these bacteria and slow or suppress the infection.
- Entry into epithelial cells is dependent on an interaction between a bacterial surface and epithelial cell receptors, which stimulate host signaling pathways and subsequent cytoskeletal rearrangements. Many bacteria attach to integrins. For example, *Legionella* and *M. tuberculosis* bind to CR3, the cell receptor for complement iC3b. Some intracellular bacteria use a hemolysin to escape from the endocytic vacuole into the cytoplasm.[28] Once in the cytoplasm, certain bacteria *(Shigella* and *E. coli)* inhibit host protein synthesis, rapidly replicate, and lyse the host cells. Others such as *L. monocytogenes*, a cause of opportunistic meningitis infections, use host actin filaments to propel the bacteria within the cell.

Bacterial Endotoxin. Bacterial endotoxin is a lipopolysaccharide that is a structural component in the outer cell wall of gram-negative bacteria. Lipopolysaccharide is composed of a long-chain fatty acid anchor (lipid A) connected to a core sugar chain, both of which are the same in all gram-negative bacteria. Attached to the core sugar is a variable carbohydrate chain (O antigen), which is used to serotype and discriminate different bacteria. Most biologic activities of lipopolysaccharide, including the induction of fever, macrophage activation, and B-cell mitogenicity, come from lipid A and the core sugars and are mediated by induction of host cytokines, including tumor necrosis factor (TNF) and IL-1 (Chapters 3 and 5).[29]

Bacterial Exotoxins. Bacteria secrete a variety of enzymes (hemolysins, hyaluronidases, coagulases, fibrinolysins) that act on their respective substrates in vitro, but their role in human disease remains presumptive. In contrast, *the role of bacterial exotoxins is well established, and the molecular mechanisms of most of their actions are known.* The mechanism of action of diphtheria toxin, for example, is well understood.[30] The toxin is composed of fragment B, which is at the carboxyl end of the molecule and is essential for attachment to host cells, and fragment A, which is at the amino end and linked to fragment B by a disulfide bridge (Fig. 9–11). Bound diphtheria toxin enters the acidic endosome of cells, where it fuses with the

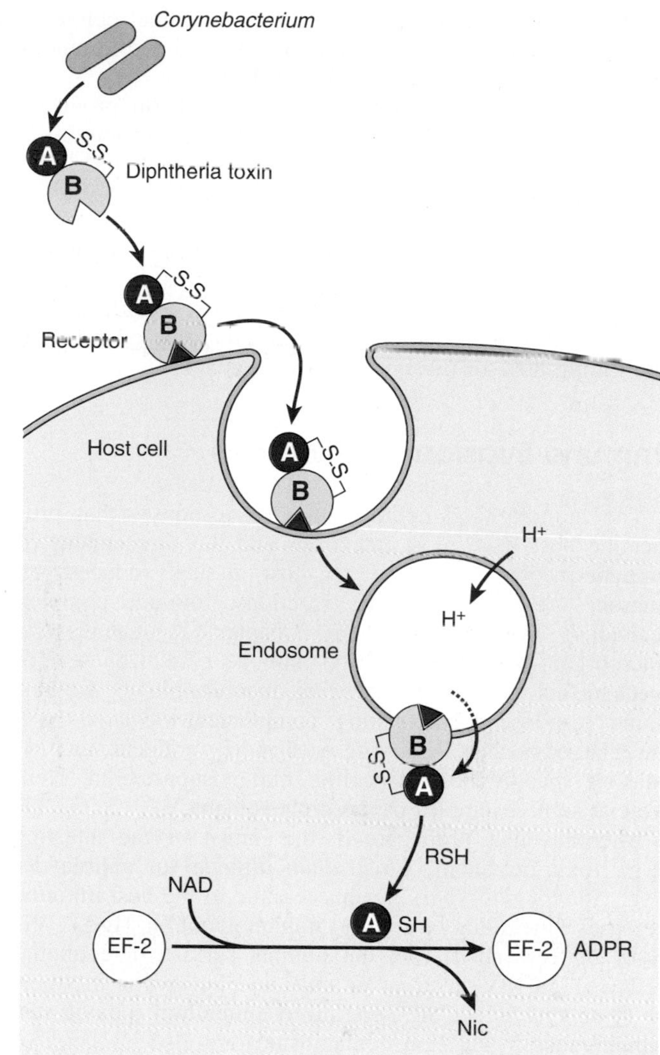

Figure 9–11

Inhibition of cellular protein synthesis by diphtheria toxin. (Adapted from Collier RJ: Corynebacteria. In Davis BD, et al [eds]: Microbiology, 3rd ed. New York, Harper & Row, 1990.)

endosomal membrane and enters the cell cytoplasm. There the disulfide bond of the toxin is broken, releasing the enzymatically active fragment A that catalyzes the covalent transfer of adenosine diphosphate (ADP)–ribose from nicotinamide adenine dinucleotide (NAD) to EF-2; the latter, a ribosomal *elongation factor* involved in protein synthesis, is thus inactivated. One molecule of diphtheria toxin can kill a cell by ADP-ribosylating more than a million EF-2 molecules. Diphtheria toxin creates a layer of dead cells in the throat, on which *Corynebacterium diphtheriae* outgrows competing bacteria. Subsequently, wide dissemination of diphtheria toxin causes the characteristic neural and myocardial dysfunction of diphtheria.

The heat-labile enterotoxins of *V. cholerae* and of *E. coli* also have an A-B structure and are ADP-ribosyltransferases, but these enzymes catalyze transfer from NAD to the guanyl nucleotide–dependent regulatory component of adenylate cyclase.[31] This generates excess cyclic adenosine monophosphate (cAMP), which causes intestinal epithelial cells to secrete isosmotic fluid, resulting in voluminous diarrhea and loss of water and electrolytes.

Another well-understood toxin is the α toxin produced by the gram-positive anaerobic *Clostridium perfringens,* the agent of gas gangrene. The α toxin is a lecithinase that disrupts plasma membranes of erythrocytes, leukocytes, and endothelial cells, resulting in tissue injury.

Finally and regrettably, toxin-producing bacteria, particularly spore-formers that may be transmitted by aerosols (e.g., *Bacillus anthracis* that makes anthrax toxin), are the agents of choice for biologic terrorism, capable of infecting and killing 80% of persons in a single attack.[32]

Immune Evasion by Microbes

The humoral and cellular immune responses that protect the host from most infections and the mechanisms of immune-mediated damage to host tissues induced by microbes (e.g., anaphylactic reactions, immune complex reactions) are discussed in Chapter 7. Conversely, microorganisms can escape the immune system by several mechanisms, including (1) being inaccessible to the immune response, (2) resisting complement-mediated lysis and phagocytosis, (3) varying or shedding antigens, and (4) causing specific or nonspecific immunosuppression. Here we cite some examples of these phenomena.

Microbes that propagate in the lumen of the intestine (e.g., toxin-producing *Clostridium difficile*) or gallbladder (e.g., *Salmonella typhi*) are inaccessible to the host immune defenses, including secretory immunoglobulin (IgA). Viruses that are shed from the luminal surface of epithelial cells (e.g., CMV in urine or milk and poliovirus in stool) or those that infect the keratinized epithelium (poxviruses, which cause molluscum contagiosum) are also inaccessible to the host humoral immune system. Some organisms establish infections by rapidly invading host cells before the host humoral response becomes effective (e.g., malaria sporozoites entering liver cells; *Trichinella* and *Trypanosoma cruzi* entering skeletal or cardiac muscles). Some larger parasites (e.g., the larvae of tapeworms) form cysts in host tissues that are covered by a dense fibrous capsule that walls them off from host immune responses.

Viruses have numerous means for circumventing the host immune response, including (1) blocking complement activation (e.g., vaccinia) or using complement receptors to enter B lymphocytes (e.g., EBV), (2) inhibiting interferon-induced antiviral responses (e.g., adenovirus, EBV, and HIV), (3) blocking production of cytokines or response to cytokines (cowpox, adenovirus, and HBV), (4) suppressing major histocompatibility complex (MHC) class I (e.g., adenovirus), and (5) reducing B-cell activation (e.g., EBV).[33] Many of these effects are mediated by viral homologs of host regulatory proteins (e.g., a serpin homolog of myxoma virus inhibits urokinase and plasminogen activator and so reduces inflammation).

The carbohydrate capsule on the surface of all the major pathogens that cause pneumonia or meningitis (pneumococcus, meningococcus, *Haemophilus)* makes them more virulent by shielding bacterial antigens and preventing phagocytosis of the organisms by neutrophils. *Pseudomonas* bacteria secrete a leukotoxin that kills neutrophils. Some *E. coli* have K antigens that prevent activation of complement by the alternative pathway and lysis of the cells. Conversely, some gram-negative bacteria have long polysaccharide O antigens, which bind host antibody and activate complement at such distance from the bacterial cells that the organisms fail to lyse. Staphylococci are covered by protein A molecules that bind the Fc portion of the antibody and so inhibit phagocytosis. *Neisseria, Haemophilus,* and *Streptococcus* all secrete proteases that degrade antibodies.

Table 9–7. PATHOGENS WITH SIGNIFICANT ANTIGENIC VARIATION

Rhinoviruses	Colds
Influenza virus	Influenza
Neisseria gonorrhoeae	Gonorrhea
Borrelia hermsii	Relapsing fever
Borrelia burgdorferi	Lyme disease
Trypanosoma brucei	African sleeping sickness
Giardia lamblia	Giardiasis
Plasmodium falciparum	Severe malaria

Viral infection evokes neutralizing *antibodies* that prevent viral attachment, penetration, or uncoating. This highly specific immunity is the basis of antiviral vaccination, but it cannot protect against viruses with many antigenic variants (e.g., rhinoviruses or influenza viruses) (Table 9–7). Pneumococci are capable of more than 80 permutations of their capsular polysaccharides, so in repeated infection the host is unlikely to recognize the new serotype. *Neisseria gonorrhoeae* have pilar (attachment) proteins composed of a constant region and a hypervariable region. The latter allows *Neisseria* to change its antigens during infection and prevent immune clearance. Similarly, the spirochete *Borrelia recurrentis* causes a relapsing fever by repeatedly switching its surface antigens before each successive clone is eliminated by the host, while the Lyme disease borreliae use similar mechanisms to vary their outer membrane proteins.[34] Successive clones of African trypanosomes also vary their major surface antigen to escape host antibody responses. Nearly 5% of the genome of *Plasmodium falciparum*, the cause of severe malaria, are *var* genes that encode variable proteins present on knobs on the surface of infected red cells.[35] Cercariae of *Schistosoma mansoni* shed parasite antigens that are recognized by host antibodies or activate complement by the alternative pathway, within minutes of penetrating the skin. Finally, viruses that infect lymphocytes (HIV and EBV) directly damage the host immune system and cause opportunistic infections (AIDS).

Special Techniques for Diagnosing Infectious Agents

Some infectious agents or their products can be directly observed in hematoxylin and eosin–stained sections (e.g.,

Table 9–8. SPECIAL TECHNIQUES FOR DIAGNOSING INFECTIOUS AGENTS

Gram stain	Most bacteria
Acid-fast stain	Mycobacteria, nocardiae (modified)
Silver stains	Fungi, legionellae, pneumocystis
Periodic acid–Schiff	Fungi, amebae
Mucicarmine	Cryptococci
Giemsa	Campylobacteria, leishmaniae, malaria parasites
Antibody probes	Viruses, rickettsiae
Culture	All classes
DNA probes	Viruses, bacteria, protozoa

the inclusion bodies formed by CMV and herpesvirus; bacterial clumps, which usually stain blue; *Candida* and *Mucor,* among the fungi; most protozoans; and all helminths). Many infectious agents, however, are best visualized by special stains that identify organisms on the basis of particular characteristics of their cell walls or coat—Gram, acid-fast, silver, mucicarmine, and Giemsa stains—or after labeling with specific antibody probes (Table 9–8). Regardless of the staining technique, organisms are usually best visualized at the advancing edge of a lesion rather than at its center, particularly if there is necrosis. Because these morphologic techniques cannot define species of organisms, determine drug sensitivity, or identify virulence characteristics, cultures of lesional tissue are performed. DNA probes identify microbes that grow slowly in culture (mycobacteria or CMV) or do not culture at all (hepatitis B and C viruses). DNA sequence analysis has been used to classify bacteria that have never been cultured, including those that cause Whipple disease (a gram-positive actinobacterium related to *Actinomyces* and *Streptomyces*[36]) and bacillary angiomatosis (genus *Bartonella).* Finally, molecular biologic techniques to distinguish viruses, bacteria, and parasites have revolutionized epidemiologic studies of infectious agents in the hospitals and in the environment.[37]

Regardless of the method of microbial identification, the final step in diagnosis of infectious pathogens is correlation of the suspect organism with the lesion caused and the signs and symptoms produced.

Spectrum of Inflammatory Responses to Infection

In contrast to the vast molecular diversity of microbes, the patterns of tissue responses to these agents are limited. At the microscopic level, therefore, many pathogens produce identical reaction patterns, and few features are unique or pathognomonic of each agent. Moreover, it is the interaction between the microorganism and the host that determines the histologic features of the inflammatory response. Thus, in a profoundly neutropenic host, pyogenic bacteria, which normally evoke vigorous leukocyte responses, may cause rapid tissue necrosis with little leukocyte exudation. Similarly, in a normal patient, *M. tuberculosis* causes well-formed granulomas with few mycobacteria present, whereas in an AIDS patient, the same mycobacteria multiply profusely in macrophages, which fail to coalesce into granulomas.

Organisms induce five major patterns of tissue reaction.

SUPPURATIVE (POLYMORPHONUCLEAR) INFLAMMATION

Suppurative inflammation is characterized by increased vascular permeability and leukocytic infiltration, predominantly of neutrophils (Fig. 9–12). The neutrophils are attracted to the site of infection by release of chemoattractants from the rapidly dividing, "pyogenic" bacteria that evoke this response, mostly extracellular gram-positive cocci and gram-negative rods. The bacterial chemoattractants include secreted bacterial peptides, which contain *N*-formylmethionine residues at their amino termini that are recognized by specific receptors on neutrophils. Alternatively, bacteria attract neutrophils indirectly by releasing endotoxin that stimulates macrophages to secrete IL-1 or TNF or by cleaving complement into chemoattractant peptides. Massing of neutrophils results in the formation of pus. The sizes of exudative lesions vary from tiny microabscesses formed in multiple organs in bacterial septicemia to diffuse involvement of entire lobes of the lung in pneumococcal infections. How destructive the lesions are depends on their location and the organism involved. For example, pneumococci spare alveolar walls, whereas staphylococci and *Klebsiella* species destroy them and form abscesses. Bacterial pharyngitis heals without sequelae, whereas untreated acute bacterial inflammation of a joint can destroy it in a few days.

MONONUCLEAR AND GRANULOMATOUS INFLAMMATION

Diffuse, predominantly mononuclear interstitial infiltrates occur in response to viruses, intracellular bacteria, spirochetes, intracellular parasites, or helminths. Which mononuclear cell predominates within the inflammatory lesion depends on the host immune response to the organism. For

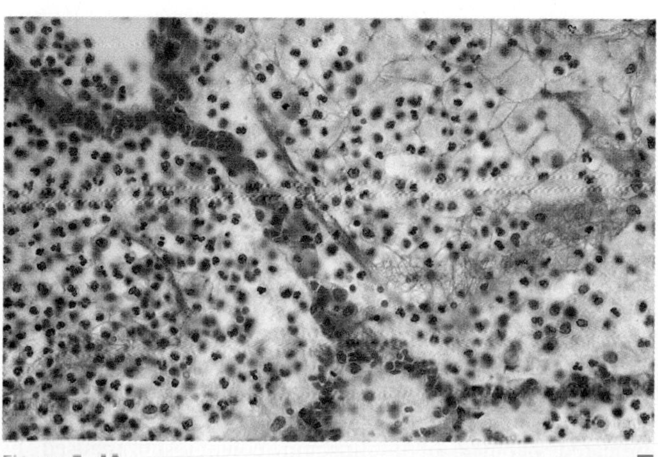

Figure 9–12

Pneumococcal pneumonia. Note the intra-alveolar polymorphonuclear exudate and intact alveolar septa.

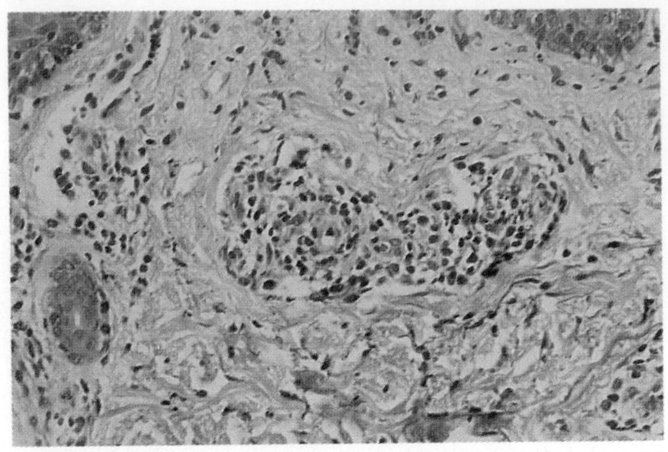

Figure 9–13

Secondary syphilis in the dermis with perivascular lymphoplasmacytic infiltrate and endothelial proliferation.

example, mostly plasma cells are seen in the chancres of primary syphilis, mostly lymphocytes with active HBV infection or Lyme disease or in viral infections of the brain (Fig. 9–13). These lymphocytes reflect cell-mediated immunity against the pathogen or the pathogen-infected cells. *Granulomatous inflammation* occurs when aggregates of altered macrophages form, sometimes around a central necrotic focus, or fuse together to form giant cells (Chapter 3). These distinctive lesions are usually evoked by relatively slowly dividing infectious agents (e.g., *M. tuberculosis* or *Histoplasma)* or by those of relatively large size (e.g., schistosome eggs) in the presence of T cell–mediated immunity. At the other extreme, macrophages may become filled with organisms, as occurs in *M. avium* infections in AIDS patients, who can mount no immune response to the organisms. For *M. leprae* and for cutaneous *leishmaniasis,* some individuals mount a strong immune response so their lesions contain few organisms, few macrophages, and many lymphocytes, whereas other individuals with a weak immune response have lesions with many organisms, many macrophages, and few lymphocytes.

CYTOPATHIC-CYTOPROLIFERATIVE INFLAMMATION

These reactions are characteristic of virus-mediated damage to individual host cells in the absence of host inflammatory response. Some viruses replicate within cells and make viral aggregates that are visible as inclusion bodies (e.g., CMV or adenovirus) or induce cells to fuse and form polykaryons (e.g., measles virus or herpesviruses). Focal cell damage may cause epithelial cells to become discohesive and form blisters (e.g., herpes; Fig. 9–14). Viruses can also cause epithelial cells to proliferate and form unusual individual and aggregate morphologic lesions (e.g., venereal warts caused by human papillomavirus or the umbilicated papules of molluscum contagiosum caused by poxviruses). Finally, viruses can cause dysplastic changes and cancers in epithelial cells and lymphocytes as discussed in Chapter 8.

NECROTIZING INFLAMMATION

Clostridium perfringens and other organisms that secrete strong toxins cause such rapid and severe tissue damage that cell death is the dominant feature. Because so few inflammatory cells are involved, these lesions resemble ischemic necrosis with disruption or loss of basophilic nuclear staining and preservation of cellular outlines. Similarly, the parasite *Entamoeba histolytica* causes colonic ulcers and liver abscesses characterized by extensive tissue destruction with liquefactive necrosis, in the absence of a prominent inflammatory infiltrate. By entirely different mechanisms, viruses can cause necrotizing inflammation when host cell damage is particularly widespread and severe, as exemplified by total destruction of the temporal lobes of the brain by herpesvirus or the liver by HBV.

CHRONIC INFLAMMATION AND SCARRING

The final common pathway of many infections is chronic inflammation, which may lead either to complete healing or to extensive scarring. For some organisms that are relatively inert, the exuberant scarring response is a major cause of dysfunction (e.g., the "pipe-stem" fibrosis of the liver caused by schistosome eggs or the constrictive fibrous pericarditis in tuberculosis) (Fig. 9–15).

These patterns of tissue reaction are useful as working tools in analyzing microscopic features of infective processes, but they rarely appear in pure form because they frequently overlap. For example, a cutaneous lesion of leishmaniasis may contain two separate histopathologic regions: a central ulcerated area filled with neutrophils and a peripheral region containing a mixed infiltrate of lymphocytes and mononuclear cells, where the leishmanial parasites are located. The lung of an AIDS patient may be infected with CMV that causes cytolytic changes and *Pneumocystis* that causes interstitial inflammation. Similar patterns of inflammation can also be seen in tissue responses to physical or chemical agents and in inflammatory diseases of unknown cause.

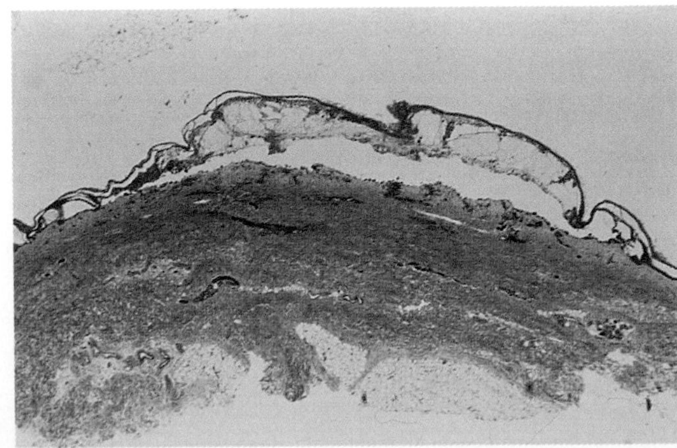

Figure 9–14

Herpesvirus blister in mucosa (see Fig. 9–28 for viral inclusions).

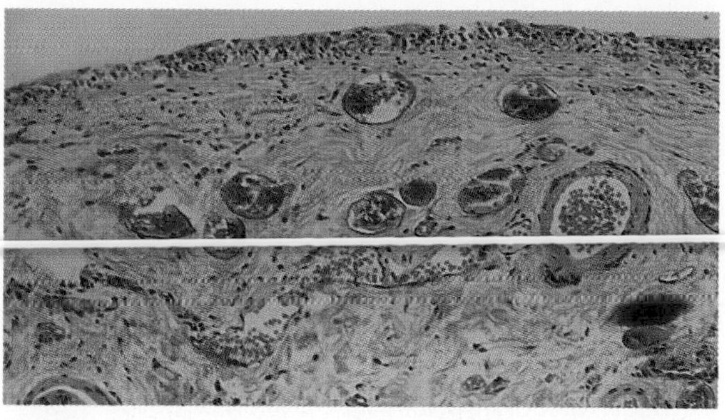

Figure 9–15

Schistosoma haematobium infection of the bladder with numerous calcified eggs and extensive scarring.

This concludes our discussion of the general principles in the pathogenesis and pathology of infectious disease. We now turn to brief descriptions of specific infections as they affect different organ systems and distinct populations of patients. In each of these categories, we begin with viral infections, followed by bacterial, fungal, or parasitic diseases. In this discussion, we emphasize *pathogenetic mechanisms* and *pathologic changes,* rather than details of clinical features, which are available in clinical textbooks.

RESPIRATORY INFECTIONS

Each city inhabitant inhales some 10,000 microorganisms per day, including potentially pathogenic viruses, bacteria, and fungi. Most of the larger inhaled microbes are trapped in the mucociliary blanket of the upper air passages. Those that manage to reach the trachea are either coughed up or pushed backward toward the throat by ciliary action, then swallowed and cleared. Only particles 5 μm or smaller in size reach the alveoli, where they are attacked and interiorized by alveolar macrophages or by neutrophils attracted to the site by cytokines. This normal clearing system (Chapter 16) is efficient, but mucociliary action can be impaired by smoking, by viscous secretions in cystic fibrosis, by aspiration of acid stomach contents, or by the trauma of intubation. Some respiratory viruses (e.g., influenza viruses) possess hemagglutinins, which attach to epithelial surface carbohydrates and thus prevent mucociliary clearance. Others also have neuraminidases, which degrade respiratory mucus and thereby prevent viral entrapment. Some respiratory bacterial pathogens (e.g., *Haemophilus* and *Bordetella*) elaborate toxins that paralyze mucosal cilia. *Mycobacterium tuberculosis,* in contrast, gains its foothold in normal alveoli because of its resistance to killing by nonactivated macrophages.

Viral Respiratory Infections

Viral respiratory disorders are the most frequent and least preventable of all infectious diseases and range in severity from the discomforting but self-limited common cold to life-threatening pneumonias. Moreover, viral infections damage bronchial epithelium and obstruct airways and so may lead to superinfection with bacteria, including pneumococcus, *Staphylococcus,* and *Haemophilus.* Of the many viruses capable of causing upper respiratory infections (rhinitis, sinusitis, otitis media, pharyngitis, and tonsillitis) and lower respiratory infections (laryngotracheobronchitis, bronchiolitis, interstitial pneumonia, and pleuritis), *rhinovirus* and *influenza virus* are the most important and the best studied.

RHINOVIRUSES

Rhinovirus accounts for 60% of common colds. The other causes are coronavirus (15%), influenza viruses, parainfluenza virus, respiratory syncytial virus, adenovirus, and enterovirus (each 1% to 10% of colds). In addition, atypical bacteria (e.g., *Mycoplasma pneumoniae* and *Chlamydia pneumoniae*) may give similar symptoms.[38]

Rhinoviruses are members of the picornavirus family (small RNA viruses), which includes poliovirus, hepatitis A virus, and coxsackievirus. Rhinoviruses have a single-stranded RNA genome, surrounded by an unencapsulated, icosahedral capsid composed of four proteins that vary in their antigenicity and account for more than 100 serotypes.[39] There is a cleft, or "canyon," in the rhinovirus surface, inaccessible to antibody, that does not vary among immunotypes and is the presumed site of attachment of the virus to host cells. *The human rhinovirus receptor is ICAM-1 (CD54),*[40] a member of the immunoglobulin gene superfamily (Fig. 9–16). The site of binding of rhinovirus on the ICAM-1 molecule is the same as that used by the leukocyte adhesion molecule LFA-1, the integrin on the surface of lymphocytes that mediates T lymphocyte–specific, antigen-specific responses and leukocyte emigration into inflammatory sites (Chapter 3).

Rhinoviruses infect humans and higher primates, who have ICAM-1 on their epithelial cells. The infection is

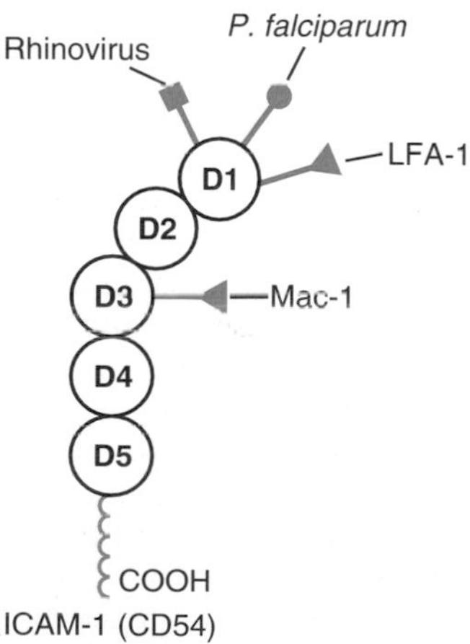

Figure 9–16

ICAM-1, a multifunctional receptor, binds to rhinovirus, *Plasmodium falciparum,* and integrins LFA-1 and Mac-1. D1 and D5 are Ig domains of the molecule.

confined to the upper respiratory tract because the viruses grow best at 33 to 35°C. The injury to epithelial cells is relatively slight, but inflammatory mediators such as bradykinins cause the excessive mucous secretions characteristic of the common cold. Rhinoviruses induce serotype-specific IgG and IgA antibodies, which prevent reinfection with the same rhinovirus but not with other serotypes.

INFLUENZA VIRUSES

Influenza viruses are larger and more complex than rhinoviruses. The genome of influenza virus is composed of eight helices of single-stranded RNA, each encoding a single gene and each bound by a nucleoprotein that determines the type of influenza virus (A, B, or C). The spherical surface of influenza virus is a lipid bilayer (envelope) containing the viral hemagglutinin and neuraminidase, which determine the subtype of the virus (H1–H3; N1 or N2). The rod-shaped hemagglutinin binds to sialic acid–containing proteins and lipids on host cells and mediates the entry of the virus into the endosome.[41] When the endosome fuses with the lysosome and becomes acidified, the viral hemagglutinin undergoes pH-dependent conformational changes, becoming spearlike and injecting the virus into the cytosol. The neuraminidase forms a mushroom-like projection on the viral surface and, by removing sialic acids, may be important in the release of viruses from host cells. Host antibodies to the hemagglutinin and neuraminidase prevent and ameliorate, respectively, future infection with the influenza virus. Two mechanisms account for the clearance of primary influenza virus infection: cytotoxic T cells kill virus-infected cells, and an intracellular anti-influenza protein (called Mx1) is induced in macrophages by the cytokines interferon-α and interferon-β.[42]

Influenza viruses of type A infect humans, pigs, horses, and birds and are the major cause of pandemic and epidemic influenza infections. A single subtype of influenza virus A predominates throughout the world at a given time.[43] Epidemics of influenza occur through mutations of the hemagglutinin and neuraminidase that allow the virus to escape most host antibodies *(antigenic drift)*. Pandemics, which are longer and more widespread than epidemics, may occur when both the hemagglutinin and the neuraminidase are replaced through recombination of RNA segments with those of animal viruses, making all individuals susceptible to the new influenza virus (*antigenic shift*). Recent polymerase chain reaction analysis of influenza virus from the lungs of a soldier who died in the 1918 influenza pandemic that killed 20 million people worldwide identified a swine influenza virus belonging to the same family of influenza viruses causing illness today.[44] Influenza virus types B and C, which do not show antigenic drift or shift, infect mostly children, who develop antibodies against reinfection in a manner similar to chickenpox, mumps, and other childhood viral illnesses. Rarely, influenza virus may cause interstitial myocarditis or, after aspirin therapy, Reye syndrome (Chapter 19).

MORPHOLOGY. Viral upper respiratory infections are marked by mucosal hyperemia and swelling with a predominantly lymphomonocytic and plasmacytic infiltration of the submucosa accompanied by overproduction of mucous secretions. The swollen mucosa and viscid exudate may plug the nasal channels, sinuses, or eustachian tubes and lead to suppurative secondary bacterial infection. Virus-induced tonsillitis with enlargement of the lymphoid tissue within Waldeyer ring is frequent in children, although lymphoid hyperplasia is not usually associated with suppuration or abscess formation, such as is encountered with streptococci or staphylococci.

In **laryngotracheobronchitis** and **bronchiolitis,** there is vocal cord swelling and abundant mucous exudation. Impairment of bronchociliary function invites bacterial superinfection with more marked suppuration. Plugging of small airways may give rise to focal lung atelectasis. In the more severe bronchiolar involvement, widespread plugging of secondary and terminal airways by cell debris, fibrin, and inflammatory exudate may, when prolonged, cause organization and fibrosis, resulting in obliterative bronchiolitis and permanent lung damage. Viral pneumonias, like bacterial pneumonias, take a variety of anatomic forms, which are described in Chapter 16.

Bacterial Respiratory Infections

Bacterial pneumonias are some of the most common bacterial infections in humans and are particularly important because they are most frequently cited as the *immediate cause* of death in hospitalized patients. Almost any type of virulent bacterial species can cause pneumonia, and the pathogenesis and pathology of the most common pneumonias are described in detail in Chapter 16. Here we cover only infections caused by *Haemophilus influenzae* and *Mycobacterium tuberculosis.*

HAEMOPHILUS INFLUENZAE INFECTION

H. influenzae is a pleomorphic, gram-negative organism that is a major cause of life-threatening acute lower respiratory tract infections and meningitis in young children. *H. influenzae* is an ubiquitous colonizer of the pharynx, where it exists in two forms — encapsulated (5%) and unencapsulated (95%). The encapsulated *H. influenzae* dominates the unencapsulated forms by secreting an antibiotic called haemocin that kills the unencapsulated *H. influenzae.*[45] Although there are six serotypes of the encapsulated form (a to f), type b, which has a polyribosephosphate capsule, is the most frequent cause of severe invasive disease. Nonencapsulated forms, however, may also spread along the surface of the upper respiratory tract and produce otitis media (infection of the middle ear), sinusitis, and bronchopneumonia.

Pili on the surface of *H. influenzae* mediate adherence of the organisms to the respiratory epithelium.[46] In addition, *H. influenzae* secretes a factor that disorganizes ciliary beating and a protease that degrades IgA, the major class of antibody secreted into the airways. Survival of *H. influenzae* in the bloodstream correlates with the presence of the capsule, which, like that of pneumococcus, prevents opsonization by complement and phagocytosis by host cells. Antibodies against the capsule protect the host from *H. influenzae* infection, so the capsular polysaccharide b is incorporated in a vaccine for children against *H. influenzae*. In *H. influenzae* meningitis, a lipopolysaccharide endotoxin induces leukocyte chemotaxis and leukocytosis, and a cell wall peptidoglycan damages the vascular endothelium and disrupts the blood-brain barrier.

MORPHOLOGY. *H. influenzae* respiratory infections range from trivial involvement of the pharynx, middle ear, sinuses, or tonsils, which resemble viral upper respiratory infections, to severe febrile bacteremic illnesses that may be resistant to routine antibiotics. Acute epiglottitis and related involvement are more frequently caused by *H. influenzae* than by any other pathogen. The uvula, epiglottic folds, and vocal cords swell rapidly and may suffocate the child within less than 24 hours if an open airway is not promptly established.

H. influenzae **pneumonia,** which may follow a viral respiratory infection, is a pediatric emergency and has a high mortality rate. Descending laryngotracheobronchitis results in airway obstruction as the smaller bronchi are plugged by dense, fibrin-rich exudate of polymorphonuclear cells, similar to that seen in pneumococcal pneumonias. Pulmonary consolidation is usually lobular and patchy but may be confluent and involve the entire lung lobe.

Before a vaccine became widely available, *H. influenzae* was a common cause of suppurative meningitis in children up to 5 years of age. *H. influenzae* also causes an acute, purulent conjunctivitis (pinkeye) in children and, in predisposed older patients, may cause septicemia, endocarditis, pyelonephritis, cholecystitis, and suppurative arthritis.

TUBERCULOSIS *(MYCOBACTERIUM TUBERCULOSIS)*

M. tuberculosis infects about one third of the world's population and kills about 3 million patients each year and so is the single most important infectious cause of death on earth.[47] With alleviation of overcrowding, which causes the spread of *M. tuberculosis,* and with the introduction of effective antibiotics in the 1950s, the United States and Western countries enjoyed a long decline in the rates of *M. tuberculosis* infections and deaths until the mid-1980s. Since that time, tuberculosis has been increasing here and in Europe and especially in Africa, in part because *M. tuberculosis* frequently and dramatically infects persons with AIDS. These individuals, who have a diminished T cell–mediated resistance to *M. tuberculosis* (see later), develop disease at much higher rates than do healthy persons, have more abundant pulmonary disease, and are more likely to transmit *M. tuberculosis* to others. In addition, multidrug-resistant *M. tuberculosis* has appeared among AIDS patients, threatening close contacts and health care workers. Because mycobacteria grow 20 to 100 times slower than other bacteria, it takes 4 to 6 weeks to obtain a colony of *M. tuberculosis* for drug sensitivity studies. Resistance to the best antimycobacterial drugs—rifampin and isoniazid—is caused by mutations in the RNA polymerase and catalase, respectively.[48] Tuberculosis is discussed further in Chapter 16. Here, we review general aspects of etiology and pathogenesis and review the morphology of only selected features of the disease.

Etiology and Pathogenesis. Mycobacteria are aerobic, non–spore-forming, nonmotile bacilli with a waxy coat that causes them to retain the red dye when treated with acid ("red snappers") in the acid-fast stains. Two species of *Mycobacterium* cause tuberculosis: *M. tuberculosis* and *M. bovis*. *M. tuberculosis* is transmitted by inhalation of infective droplets coughed or sneezed into the air by a patient with tuberculosis. *M. bovis* is transmitted by milk from diseased cows and first produces intestinal or tonsillar lesions. In developed countries, control of *M. bovis* in dairy herds and pasteurization of milk have virtually eradicated this organism. *M. avium* and *M. intracellulare,* two closely related mycobacteria, have no virulence in normal hosts but cause disseminated infections in 15% to 24% of patients with AIDS.[49] *M. leprae* is the cause of leprosy, discussed later in this chapter.

M. tuberculosis pathogenicity is related to its ability to escape killing by macrophages and induce delayed type hypersensitivity.[50] This has been attributed to several components of the *M. tuberculosis* cell wall. First is *cord factor,* a surface glycolipid that causes *M. tuberculosis* to grow in serpentine cords in vitro. Virulent strains of *M. tuberculosis* have cord factor on their surface, whereas avirulent strains do not, and injection of purified cord factor into mice induces characteristic granulomas. Second, *lipoarabinomannan (LAM),* a major heteropolysaccharide similar in structure to the endotoxin of gram-negative bacteria, inhibits macrophage activation by interferon-γ. LAM also induces macrophages to secrete TNF-α, which causes fever, weight loss, and tissue damage, and IL-10, which suppresses mycobacteria-induced T-cell proliferation (Chapter 7). Third, *complement* activated on the surface of mycobacteria may opsonize the organism and facilitate its uptake by the macrophage complement receptor CR3 (Mac-1 integrin) without triggering the respiratory burst necessary to kill the organisms. Fourth, a highly immunogenic 65-kD *M. tuberculosis heat-shock protein* is similar to human heat-shock proteins (Chapter 1) and may have a role in autoimmune reactions induced by *M. tuberculosis.*

M. tuberculosis resides in phagosomes, which are not acidified into lysosomes.[51] Inhibition of acidification has been associated with urease secreted by mycobacteria and with uptake of mycobacteria by complement- or mannose-binding receptors rather than Fc receptors.

The development of cell-mediated, or type IV, hypersensitivity to the tubercle bacillus probably explains the organism's destructiveness in tissues and also the emergence of resistance to the organisms. On the initial exposure to the organism, the inflammatory response is nonspecific, resembling the reaction to any form of bacterial invasion. Within 2 or 3 weeks, coincident with the appearance of a positive skin reaction, the reaction becomes granulomatous and the centers of granulomas become caseous, forming typical "soft tubercles." The sequence of events that follow an initial lung infection is outlined in Figure 9–17. The pattern of host response depends on whether the infection represents a *primary* first exposure to the organism or *secondary* reaction in an already sensitized host.

Primary Infection. The primary phase of *M. tuberculosis* infection begins with inhalation of the mycobacteria and ends with a T cell–mediated immune response that induces hypersensitivity to the organisms and controls 95% of infections. Most often in the periphery of one lung, inhaled *M. tuberculosis* is first phagocytosed by alveolar macrophages and transported by these cells to hilar lymph nodes. Naive macrophages are unable to kill the mycobacteria, which multiply, lyse the host cell, infect other macrophages, and sometimes disseminate through the blood to other parts of the lung and elsewhere in the body. After a few weeks, T cell–mediated immunity demonstrable by a positive purified protein derivative (PPD) test reaction develops. Mycobacteria-activated T cells interact with macrophages in three ways. First, CD4+ helper T cells secrete interferon-γ, which activates macrophages to kill intracellular mycobacteria through reactive nitrogen intermediates, including NO, NO_2, and HNO_3. This is associated with the formation of epithelioid cell granulomas

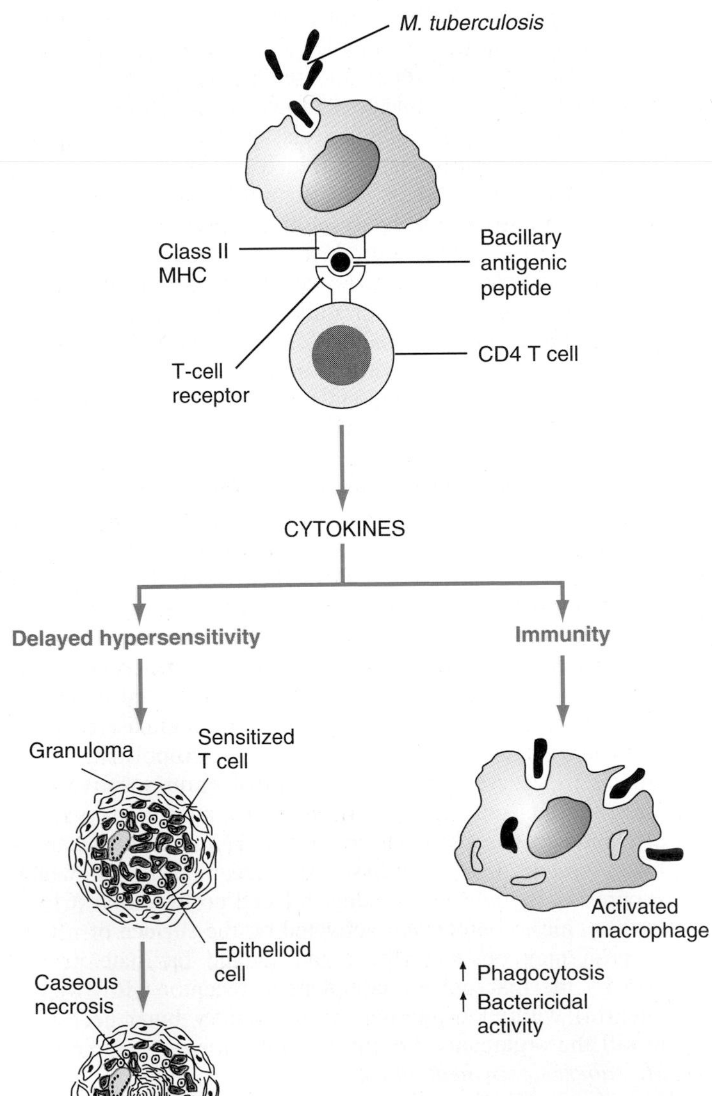

Figure 9–17

Tuberculosis: the dual consequences of macrophage activation and sensitization.

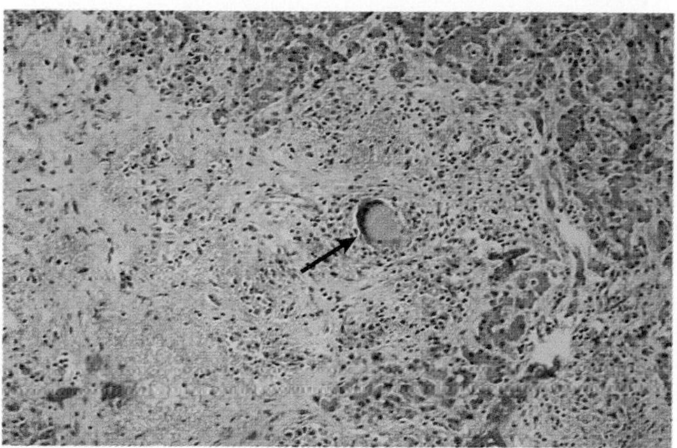

Figure 9–18

Granuloma caused by *Mycobacterium tuberculosis* in the liver with central caseation and giant cells *(arrow).*

(Chapter 3) and clearance of the mycobacteria. Second, CD8+ suppressor T cells lyse macrophages infected with mycobacteria through a Fas-independent, granule-dependent reaction and kill mycobacteria.[52] Third, CD4−CD8− (double-negative) T cells lyse macrophages in a Fas-dependent manner, without killing mycobacteria. Lysis of macrophages results in the formation of caseating granulomas (delayed type hypersensitivity reactions; Fig. 9–18). Direct toxicity of the mycobacteria to the macrophages may contribute to the necrotic caseous centers. Mycobacteria cannot grow in this acidic, extracellular environment lacking in oxygen, and so the mycobacterial infection is controlled. The ultimate residuum of the primary infection is a calcified scar in the lung parenchyma and in the hilar lymph node, together referred to as the *Ghon complex* (Chapter 16).

Secondary and Disseminated Tuberculosis. Some individuals become reinfected with mycobacteria, reactivate dormant disease, or progress directly from the primary mycobacterial lesions into disseminated disease. This may be because the strain of mycobacterium is particularly virulent or the host is particularly susceptible. In mice, susceptibility to mycobacterial (as well as *Salmonella* and *Leishmania)* infection is determined by an autosomal dominant gene called *Bcg,* which encodes a membrane transport protein.[53] Whether the protein acts at the level of the plasma membrane or interferes with bacterial killing in the phagolysosome is unclear. Granulomas of secondary tuberculosis most often occur in the apex of the lungs but may be widely disseminated in the lungs, kidneys, meninges, marrow, and other organs. These granulomas, which fail to contain the spread of the mycobacterial infection, are the major cause of tissue damage in tuberculosis and are a reflection of delayed type hypersensitivity. Two special features of secondary tuberculosis are *caseous necrosis* and *cavities*; necrosis may cause rupture into blood vessels, spreading mycobacteria throughout the body, and break into airways, releasing infectious mycobacteria in aerosols.

MORPHOLOGY. The histopathology of primary and secondary pulmonary tuberculosis is described in Chapter 16. **Miliary tuberculosis** refers to hematogenous dissemination of tuberculous lesions throughout the body. The term miliary is descriptive of the small, yellow-white lesions that resemble millet seeds fed to birds and are present in the lungs and systemic organs. Certain tissues are relatively resistant to tuberculous infection, so it is rare to find tubercles in the heart, striated muscle, thyroid, and pancreas. In certain instances, hematogenously spread organisms are destroyed in all tissues but persist in only one organ (isolated end-organ disease). This occurrence is most frequent in the lungs, cervical lymph nodes (scrofula), meninges (tuberculous meningitis), kidneys, adrenals, bones (tuberculous osteomyelitis), fallopian tubes, and epididymis. In vertebral tuberculosis (Pott disease), long fistulas may form along the psoas muscle to open and drain into the groin region.

M. tuberculosis ***and*** **M. avium-intracellulare** ***Lesions in AIDS.*** Mycobacterial infection in patients with AIDS can take three forms, depending on the degree of immunosuppression. (1) In developing countries, where *M. tuberculosis* infection is frequent, HIV-infected individuals often have primary and secondary *M. tuberculosis* infection with the usual, well-formed granulomas composed of epithelioid cells, Langerhans giant cells, and lymphocytes. In these lesions, acid-fast mycobacteria are few and often difficult to find. (2) When HIV-positive patients develop AIDS and are moderately immunosuppressed (less than 200 CD4+ helper T cells/mm^3), *M. tuberculosis* infection is frequently caused by reactivation or by exposure to new mycobacteria. Because HIV infects both T cells and macrophages, defects in the host immune response to *M. tuberculosis* may be secondary to the failure of helper T cells to secrete lymphokines that activate macrophages to kill mycobacteria or the failure of HIV-infected and mycobacteria-infected macrophages to respond to lymphokines. The relative increase in the number of CD8+ cytotoxic T cells may also cause macrophage destruction in the *M. tuberculosis* lesions. On histologic examination, granulomas are less well formed, are more frequently necrotic, and contain more abundant acid-fast organisms. Neutrophils may be present where tuberculous cavities have eroded into the airways. Although the sputum is positive for acid-fast organisms in 31% to 82% of patients with AIDS, only 33% of patients are reactive to PPD. Extrapulmonary tuberculosis occurs in 70% of such patients, involving lymph nodes, blood, central nervous system, and bowel. Despite the severity of *M. tuberculosis* infection in AIDS patients, treatment with multiple drugs clears all but the multidrug-resistant organisms. (3) Opportunistic infection with *M. avium-*

intracellulare occurs in severely immunosuppressed patients (less than 60 CD4+ cells/mm^3). Most infections with these organisms originate in the gastrointestinal tract, although some begin in the lung. *M. avium-intracellulare* infections are usually widely disseminated throughout the reticuloendothelial systems, causing enlargement of involved lymph nodes, liver, and spleen. There may be a yellowish pigmentation to these organs secondary to the large number of *M. avium-intracellulare* present in swollen macrophages (as many as 10^{10} organisms per gram of tissue) (Fig. 9–19). Granulomas, lymphocytes, and tissue destruction are rare.

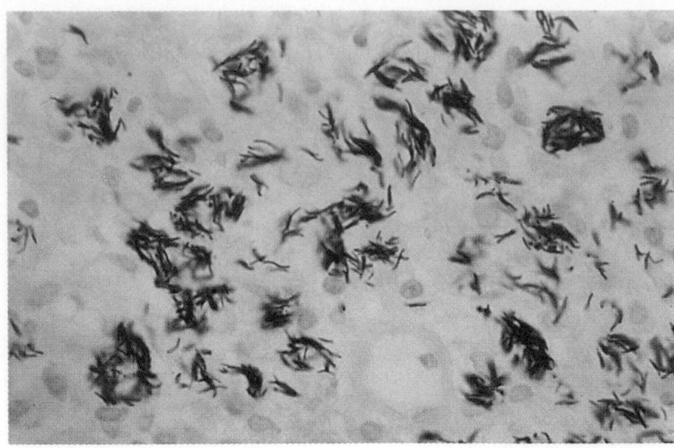

Figure 9–19

Mycobacterium avium infection in a patient with AIDS, showing massive infection with acid-fast organisms. (Courtesy of Dr. Arlene Sharpe, Brigham and Women's Hospital, Boston, MA.)

Fungal Respiratory Infections

Histoplasmosis and *coccidioidomycosis* are discussed together because (1) both are granulomatous diseases of the lungs that may resemble tuberculosis, (2) both are caused by fungi that are thermally dimorphic in that they grow as hyphae that produce spores at environmental temperatures but grow as yeasts (spherules or ellipses) at body temperature within the lungs, and (3) each fungus is geographic in that it causes disease primarily among persons living along the Ohio and Mississippi rivers and in the Caribbean *(Histoplasma)* and in the Southwest and Far West of the United States and in Mexico *(Coccidioides).*

HISTOPLASMOSIS

Histoplasma capsulatum infection is acquired by inhalation of dust particles from soil contaminated with bird or bat droppings that contain small spores (microconidia), the infectious form of the fungus. Like *M. tuberculosis, H. capsulatum* is an intracellular parasite of macrophages. The clinical presentations and morphologic lesions of histoplasmosis also strikingly resemble those of tuberculosis, including (1) a self-limited and often latent primary pulmonary involvement, which may result in coin lesions on chest radiography; (2) chronic, progressive, secondary lung disease, which is localized to the lung apices and causes cough, fever, and night sweats; (3) localized lesions in extrapulmonary sites, including mediastinum, adrenals, liver, or meninges; and (4) a widely disseminated involvement, particularly in immunosuppressed patients. Differentiation of histoplasmosis from tuberculosis is made by eliciting a delayed type hypersensitivity response to skin injection of a fungal lysate (histoplasmin test, similar to the tuberculin test) or by identifying the fungus in lung, lymph node, or bone marrow biopsy specimens in patients with disseminated histoplasmosis.

Unopsonized *Histoplasma* conidia (infectious form) and yeasts (tissue form) bind to the β chain of the integrin receptors. Proteins involved in differentiation of *Histoplasma* may be important for pathogenesis and are potential targets for new antifungal drugs.[54] *Histoplasma* yeasts are phagocytosed by the unstimulated macrophages, multiply within the phagolysosome, and lyse the host cells. *Histoplasma* infections are controlled by helper T cells that recognize fungal cell wall antigens and heat-shock proteins and subsequently secrete interferon-γ that activates macrophages to kill intracellular yeasts. In addition, *Histoplasma* induces macrophages to secrete TNF-α, which stimulates other macrophages to kill *Histoplasma.* Lacking cellular immunity, patients with AIDS are susceptible to disseminated infection with *Histoplasma,* which is a major opportunistic pathogen in this disease.

MORPHOLOGY. In the lungs of otherwise healthy adults, *Histoplasma* infections produce epithelioid cell granulomas, which usually undergo coagulative necrosis and coalesce to produce large areas of consolidation but may also liquefy to form cavities. With spontaneous or drug control of the infection, these lesions undergo fibrosis and calcification. Histologic differentiation from tuberculosis, sarcoidosis, and coccidioidomycosis requires identification of the 2- to 5-μm thin-walled yeast forms (stained with methenamine silver) that may persist in tissues for years.

In **chronic histoplasmosis,** gray-white granulomas are usually present in the apices of the lungs with retraction and thickening of the pleura and in the hilar nodes (Fig. 9–20). Further progression involves more and more of the lung parenchyma, with cavity formation less frequent than in tuberculosis.

In **fulminant disseminated histoplasmosis,** which occurs in immunosuppressed individuals, epithelioid cell granulomas are not formed, but instead there are focal accumulations of mononuclear phagocytes filled with fungal yeasts throughout the tissues and organs of the body. The overloading of the reticuloendothelial system with macrophages stuffed with organisms resembles that found in severe cases of visceral leishmaniasis (Fig. 9–21), described later.

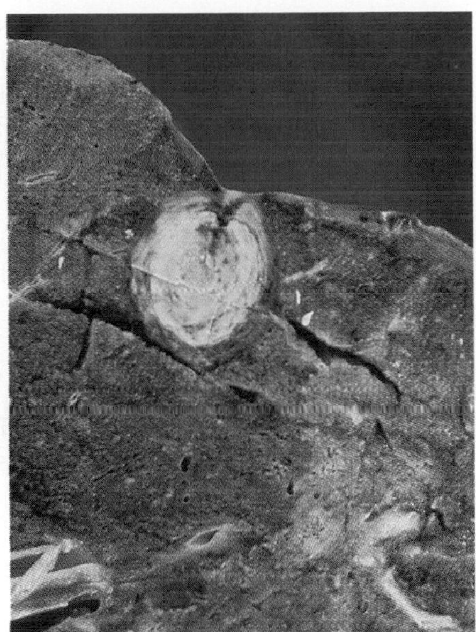

Figure 9–20

Laminated *Histoplasma* granuloma of the lung.

COCCIDIOIDOMYCOSIS

Almost everyone who inhales the spores of *Coccidioides immitis* becomes infected and develops a delayed type hypersensitivity to the fungus, so that more than 80% of persons in endemic areas of the Southwest and western United States have a positive skin test reaction. Indeed, increases in populations in the West and in construction that mobilize the spores have caused *Coccidioides* to be classified as a re-emerging pathogen.[55] One reason for the high rate of infectivity by *C. immitis* is that infective arthroconidia, when ingested by alveolar macrophages, block fusion of the phagosome and lysosome and so resist intracellular killing. As is the case with *Histoplasma,* most primary infections with *C. immitis* are asymptomatic, but 10% of persons have lung lesions, fever, cough, and pleuritic pains, accompanied by erythema nodosum or erythema multiforme (the San Joaquin Valley fever complex). Less than 1% of persons develop disseminated *C. immitis* infection, which frequently involves the skin and meninges.

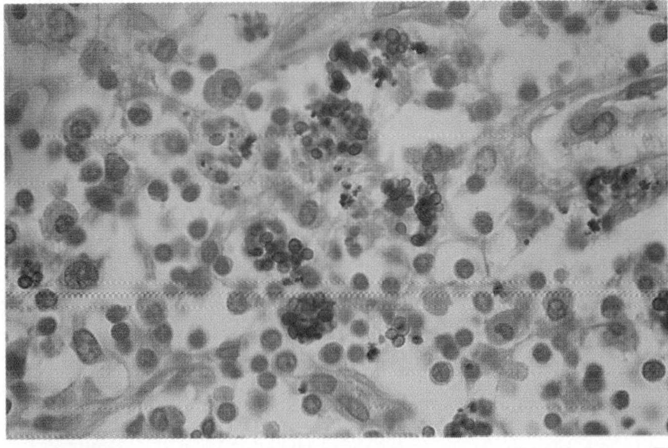

Figure 9–21

Histoplasma capsulatum yeast forms fill phagocytes in a lymph node of a patient with disseminated histoplasmosis.

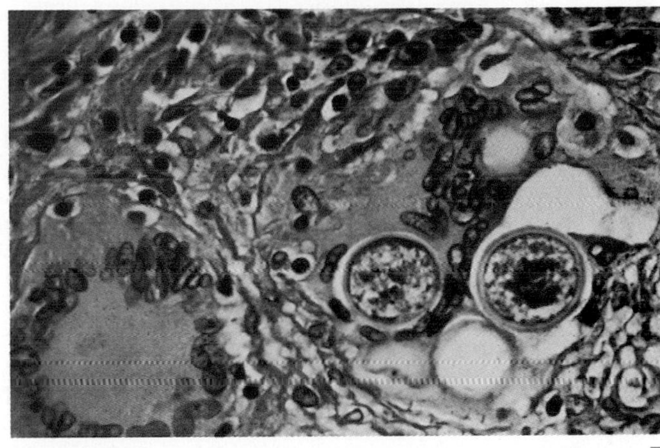

Figure 9–22

Coccidioidomycosis with an intact spherule and a ruptured spherule releasing endospores.

MORPHOLOGY. The primary and secondary lung lesions of *C. immitis* are similar to the granulomatous lesions of *Histoplasma.* Within macrophages or giant cells, *C. immitis* is present as thick-walled, nonbudding spherules 20 to 60 μm in diameter, often filled with small endospores (Fig. 9–22). A pyogenic reaction is superimposed when the spherules rupture to release the endospores, which are not infectious. In contrast, infectious *C. immitis* boxcar-like arthrospores produced in culture are easily detached and disseminated by air, so extreme caution is needed in handling this fungus in the laboratory. Rare progressive *C. immitis* disease involves the lungs, meninges, skin, bones, adrenals, lymph nodes, spleen, or liver. At all these sites, the inflammatory response may be purely granulomatous, pyogenic, or mixed. Purulent lesions dominate in patients with diminished resistance and with widespread dissemination.

GASTROINTESTINAL INFECTIONS

The clinicopathologic features of gastrointestinal infections are discussed in Chapter 18; in this chapter, attention is directed largely to pathogenetic mechanisms.

Barriers to Infection of the Gut

Most gastrointestinal pathogens are transmitted by food or drink contaminated with fecal material. Exposure can therefore be reduced by sanitary disposal of waste and vermin, clean drinking water, hand washing, and thorough cooking of food. Where hygiene fails, diarrheal disease becomes rampant.

Normal defenses against ingested pathogens include (1) acid gastric juice, (2) the viscous mucous layer covering the gut, (3) lytic pancreatic enzymes and bile detergents, and (4) secreted IgA antibodies. IgA antibodies are made by B cells located in mucosa-associated lymphoid tissues (MALT), which are covered by a single layer of epithelial specialized cells called M cells. M cells are important for transport of antigen to MALT and for binding or uptake of numerous gut pathogens including poliovirus, enteropathic *Escherichia coli, Vibrio cholerae, Salmonella typhi,* and *Shigella flexneri*.[56]

Pathogenic organisms must compete for nutrients with abundant commensal bacteria resident in the lower gut, and all gut microbes are intermittently expelled by defecation. Host defenses are weakened by low gastric acidity, by antibiotics that unbalance the normal bacterial flora, by stalled peristalsis, or by mechanical obstruction. Most enveloped viruses are killed by the digestive juices, but non-enveloped ones may be resistant (e.g., the hepatitis A virus, rotaviruses, reoviruses, and Norwalk agents). Rotaviruses directly damage the intestinal epithelial cells they infect, whereas reoviruses pass through mucosal M cells into the bloodstream without any detectable local cell injury.

Enteropathogenic bacteria elicit gastrointestinal disease by a variety of mechanisms. (1) While growing on contaminated food, certain staphylococcal strains release powerful enterotoxins that, on ingestion, cause food poisoning symptoms without any bacterial multiplication in the gut. (2) *V. cholerae* and toxigenic *E. coli* multiply inside the mucous layer overlying the gut epithelium and release exotoxins that cause the gut epithelium to secrete excessive volumes of watery diarrhea. (3) By contrast, *Shigella, Salmonella,* and *Campylobacter* invade and damage the intestinal mucosa and lamina propria and so cause ulceration, inflammation, and hemorrhage, clinically manifested as dysentery. Bacterial invasion, which probably occurs to a small degree at all times, is greatly accelerated when certain bacteria overgrow within the lumen, intestinal mucosal injury occurs, or normal immune defenses are compromised.[57] (4) *S. typhi* passes from the damaged mucosa through Peyer patches and mesenteric lymph nodes and into the bloodstream, resulting in a systemic infection.

Fungal infection of the gastrointestinal tract occurs mainly in immunologically compromised patients. *Candida* shows a predilection for stratified squamous epithelium, causing oral thrush or membranous esophagitis, but may also disseminate to the stomach, lower gastrointestinal tract, and systemic organs.

The cyst forms of intestinal protozoa are essential for their transmission because cysts resist stomach acid. In the gut, cysts convert to motile trophozoites and attach to sugars on the intestinal epithelia through surface lectins. Thereafter, there is wide species variation. *Giardia lamblia* attaches to the epithelial brush border, whereas cryptosporidia are taken up by enterocytes, in which they form gametes and spores. *Entamoeba histolytica* causes contact-mediated cytolysis analogous to that of cytotoxic T lymphocytes by releasing a channel-forming pore protein that depolarizes and kills its cellular prey. In this manner, the colonic mucosa is ulcerated and invaded. Intestinal helminths, as a rule, cause disease only when they are present in large numbers or in ectopic sites, for example, by obstructing the gut or invading and damaging the bile ducts *(Ascaris).* Hookworms may cause iron deficiency anemia by chronic loss of blood sucked from intestinal villi; the fish tapeworm *Diphyllobothrium* competes with and can deplete its host of vitamin B_{12}, giving rise to an illness resembling pernicious anemia. Finally, the larvae of several helminth parasites pass through the gut briefly on their way toward another organ habitat; for example, *Trichinella* larvae preferentially encyst in muscle, *Echinococcus* larvae in the liver or lung.

Viral Enteritis and Diarrhea

Acute, self-limited infectious diarrhea, which is a major cause of morbidity among children, is most frequently caused by enteric viruses, including rotaviruses, Norwalk-like viruses, coronaviruses, adenoviruses, and astroviruses. In infants, infectious diarrhea may cause severe dehydration and metabolic acidosis, which may result in hospitalization in developed countries and death in developing countries.

Rotavirus, which is an encapsulated virus with a segmented double-stranded RNA genome, is the major cause of diarrhea in infants.[7] Rotaviruses invade and destroy mature host epithelial cells in the middle and upper villus. Viral diarrhea is caused by a decreased absorption of sodium and water from the bowel lumen, in contrast to toxin-mediated bacterial diarrheas, which are caused by increased secretion from host epithelial cells. Because secretory immunity to rotavirus surface antigens develops, older children and adults are resistant to infection. These antirotavirus antibodies are present in mother's milk, so rotavirus infection is most frequent at the time of weaning. Although rotaviruses were initially diagnosed in the stool by electron microscopy, these viruses are now identified by enzyme-linked immunosorbent assays.[58]

Norwalk-like viruses, which are small icosahedral viruses containing a single-stranded RNA genome, cause epidemic gastroenteritis with diarrhea, nausea, and vomiting among children. *Coronaviruses* are pleomorphic enveloped viruses that have large club-shaped projections (crowns). Coronaviruses cause diarrhea and upper respiratory tract infections and are usually endemic rather than epidemic. *Enteric adenoviruses,* distinguished from adenoviruses that cause respiratory disease by their failure to grow easily in culture, are the second leading cause of diarrhea among infants.

MORPHOLOGY. Although the enteric viruses are genetically and morphologically different from each other, the lesions they cause in the intestinal tract are similar.[59] There is a blunting and destruction of the villus epithelial cells, which contain viruses visible by electron microscopy or immunofluorescence staining. There is secondary hyperplasia of the mucosal crypts and a mixed inflammatory infiltrate of the lamina propria.

Bacterial Enteritis

SHIGELLA BACILLARY DYSENTERY

Dysentery refers to diarrhea with abdominal cramping and tenesmus in which loose stools contain blood, pus, and mucus. Bacillary dysentery, which results in as many as 500,000 deaths among children in developing countries each year, is caused by *Shigella dysenteriae, Shigella flexneri, Shigella boydii,* and *Shigella sonnei* as well as certain O type enterotoxic *E. coli.* (Amebic dysentery is caused by the protozoan parasite *Entamoeba histolytica*, discussed later in this chapter). *Shigella* species are gram-negative facultative anaerobes, which infect only humans. *S. flexneri* is the major cause of bacillary dysentery in endemic locations of poor hygiene, including large regions of the developing world and institutions in the developed world. Epidemic shigellosis occurs when individuals consume uncooked foods at picnics or other events.

Pathogenesis. Transmission is fecal-oral and is remarkable for the small number of organisms that may cause disease (10 ingested organisms cause illness in 10% of volunteers, and 500 organisms cause disease in 50% of volunteers). *Shigella* bacteria invade the intestinal mucosal cells but do not usually go beyond the lamina propria. *Shigella* invasion genes, which are carried on a plasmid, are the same as those that are part of the chromosome of *S. typhi.*[60] Dysentery is caused when the bacteria escape the epithelial cell phagolysosome, multiply within the cytoplasm, and destroy host cells. Shiga toxin causes hemorrhagic colitis and hemolytic-uremic syndrome by damaging endothelial cells in the microvasculature of the colon and the glomeruli, respectively (Chapter 21). Shiga toxin binds to globo glycolipids on host endothelial cells and blocks protein synthesis by cleaving the 28S ribosomal RNA.[61] In addition, chronic arthritis secondary to *S. flexneri* infection in HLA-B27 individuals, called Reiter syndrome, may be caused by a bacterial antigen that cross-reacts with the HLA-B27 host protein.

MORPHOLOGY. In severe bacillary dysentery, the colonic mucosa becomes hyperemic and edematous; enlargement of the lymphoid follicles creates small, projecting nodules. Within the course of 24 hours, a fibrinosuppurative exudate first patchily, then diffusely covers the mucosa and produces a dirty gray to yellow pseudomembrane (Fig. 9–23). The inflammatory reaction within the intestinal mucosa builds up, the mucosa becomes soft and friable, and irregular superficial ulcerations appear. If the infection is severe, large tracts may be denuded, leaving only islands of preserved mucosa.

On histologic examination, there is a predominantly mononuclear leukocytic infiltrate within the lamina propria, but the surfaces of the ulcers are covered with an acute, suppurative, neutrophilic reaction accompanied by congestion, marked edema, fibrin deposition, and thromboses of small vessels. As the disease progresses, the ulcer margins are transformed into active granulation tissue. When the disease remits, this granulation tissue fills the defect, and the ulcers heal by regeneration of the mucosal epithelium.

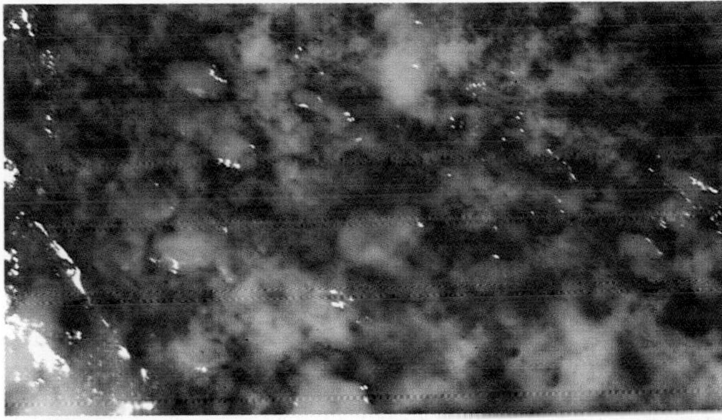

Figure 9–23 ■

Close-up of a gross specimen showing colonic mucosa in *Shigella* colitis with erythema, ulceration, and pseudomembrane formation (white plaques).

CAMPYLOBACTER ENTERITIS

This comma-shaped, flagellated, gram-negative organism was once classified with the vibrios. Only when special culture conditions permitted its isolation did it become apparent that *Campylobacter* was an important cause of chronic gastritis, enterocolitis, and septicemia in humans that had frequently been missed by routine cultures for enterobacteria. The role of *Helicobacter pylori,* previously called *Campylobacter,* in gastritis and peptic ulceration is discussed in detail in Chapter 18; here our attention is directed to the enteritis. Currently in the United States, *Campylobacter jejuni* is responsible for twice the enteric disease of *Salmonella* and four times that of *Shigella.*[62] Most infections with *Campylobacter* are sporadic and are associated with ingestion of improperly cooked chicken, which is frequently contaminated with both *Campylobacter* and *Salmonella.* Sporadic infections may also be associated with contact with infected dogs. Outbreaks of *Campylobacter* are usually associated with unpasteurized milk or contaminated water.

Pathogenesis. Flagella of *Campylobacter,* which give the organism its comma shape and motility, are necessary for the bacterium to penetrate mucus covering epithelial surfaces. Invasiveness is strain dependent and dependent on intact host cell signal transduction pathways.[63] For example, invasion of *Campylobacter* into host cells is blocked when host trimeric G proteins or phosphatidylinositol 3-kinase is inhibited. Three clinical outcomes of *Campylobacter* infection are possible: (1) diarrhea, which is independent of invasion; (2) dysentery with blood and mucus in the stool as bacteria disrupt the epithelium; and (3) enteric fever when bacteria proliferate within the lamina propria and mesenteric lymph nodes. Postinfectious complications of *Campylobacter* infections include reactive arthritis in HLA-B27 persons, as has been described for *Shigella,* as well as Guillain-Barré syndrome, a demyelinating disease of peripheral nerves described in Chapter 29.

MORPHOLOGY. Inflammation may involve the gut from the jejunum to the anus. In invasive infection, the colonic mucosa appears friable or superficially eroded on proctoscopy. By light microscopy, hyperemia, edema, and inflammatory infiltrates of neutrophils, lymphocytes, and plasma cells are seen. There may be colonic crypt abscesses and ulcerations resembling those of chronic ulcerative colitis. In the small bowel, there is some decrease in the crypt-villus ratio.

YERSINIA ENTERITIS

Yersinia enterocolitica and *Yersinia pseudotuberculosis* are gram-negative facultative intracellular bacteria related to *Yersinia pestis,* which causes epidemic plague (see later). *Y. enterocolitica* and *Y. pseudotuberculosis* cause fecal-orally transmitted ileitis and mesenteric lymphadenitis, which may lead to significant postinfectious autoimmune sequelae including arthritis, erythema nodosum, and glomerulonephritis.

Y. pseudotuberculosis has a variety of molecules on its surface involved in attachment to and phagocytosis by host epithelial cells, including a protein called invasin, which binds to host cell β_1 integrins that also bind fibronectin and collagen.[64] A second *Yersinia* attachment protein called Ail, which is present on most enteric bacteria, may also confer resistance to complement. Multiplication of *Y. enterocolitis* and *Y. pestis* within host cells depends on the presence of a virulence plasmid or pathogenicity island called Yop.[65] Yop encodes a type III secretion apparatus and numerous proteins that disrupt normal host cell signal transduction pathways including a serine-threonine kinase and a protein tyrosine phosphatase.[66]

MORPHOLOGY. *Y. enterocolitica* and *Y. pseudotuberculosis* most frequently involve the distal ileum and colon, although they can cause pharyngitis and tonsillitis. The ulcerative intestinal lesions resemble those of typhoid fever, although there may also be a diffuse enteritis with villus shortening, crypt hyperplasia, and mucosal microabscesses. Within submucosal tissues, yersiniae produce microabscesses rimmed by activated macrophages, which resemble the stellate granulomas of lymphogranuloma venereum and cat-scratch disease.

Salmonellosis and Typhoid Fever

Salmonellae are flagellated, gram-negative bacteria that cause a self-limited food-borne and water-borne gastroenteritis (*Salmonella enteritidis, Salmonella typhimurium,* and others) or a life-threatening systemic illness marked by fever *(Salmonella typhi).* In the United States, *Salmonella* species cause approximately 500,000 reported cases of food poisoning, and many cases go unreported. Because *Salmonella* species (other than *S. typhi*) infect most commercially raised chickens and many cows, the major sources of *Salmonella* in the United States are feces-contaminated meat and chicken that are insufficiently washed and cooked. In contrast, humans are the only host of *S. typhi,* which is shed in the feces, urine, vomitus, and oral secretions by acutely ill persons and in the feces by chronic carriers without overt disease. Therefore, typhoid fever is a disease largely of developing countries where sanitary conditions are insufficient to stop its spread. Typhoid fever is a protracted disease that is associated with bacteremia, fever, and chills during the first week; widespread reticuloendothelial involvement with rash, abdominal pain, and prostration in the second week; and ulceration of Peyer patches with intestinal bleeding and shock during the third week.

Pathogenesis. Salmonellae invade intestinal epithelial cells as well as tissue macrophages.[67] Invasion of intestinal epithelial cells is controlled by invasion genes that are induced by the low oxygen tension found in the gut. These genes encode proteins involved in adhesion and in recruitment of host cytoskeletal proteins that internalize the bacterium. Similarly, intramacrophage growth is important in pathogenicity, and this seems to be mediated by bacterial genes that are induced by the acid pH within the macrophage phagolysosome.[68, 69]

MORPHOLOGY. Lesions induced by *S. enteritidis* or *S. typhimurium* are limited to the ileum and colon and include erosion of the epithelium and mixed inflammation in the lamina propria. Variable numbers of polymorphonuclear neutrophils are found in the stools, depending on the severity of the infections. *S. typhi* causes proliferation of phagocytes with enlargement of reticuloendothelial and lymphoid tissues throughout the body. Peyer patches in the terminal ileum become sharply delineated, plateau-like elevations up to 8 cm in diameter, with enlargement of draining mesenteric lymph nodes. In the second week, the mucosa over the swollen lymphoid tissue is shed, resulting in oval ulcers with their long axes in the direction of bowel flow. On microscopic examination, macrophages containing bacteria, red blood cells (erythrophagocytosis), and nuclear debris form small nodular aggregates in Peyer patches. Intermingled with the phagocytes are lymphocytes and plasma cells, whereas neutrophils are present near the ulcerated surface. The **spleen** is enlarged, soft, and bulging, with uniformly pale red pulp, obliterated follicular markings, and prominent sinus histiocytosis and reticuloendothelial proliferation. The **liver** shows small, randomly scattered foci of parenchymal necrosis in which the hepatocytes are replaced by a phagocytic mononuclear cell aggregate, called a typhoid nodule (Fig. 9–24). These distinctive nodules also occur in the bone marrow and lymph nodes. **Gallbladder** colonization, which may be associated with gallstones, causes a chronic carrier state.

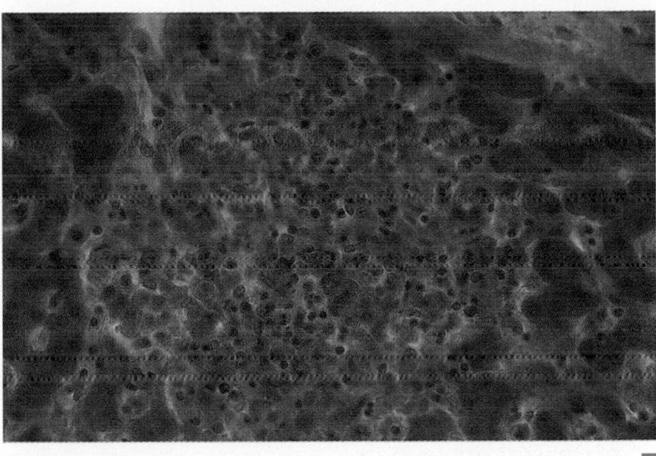

Figure 9–24

Typhoid nodule in the liver of a patient with systemic infection by *Salmonella typhi.*

Cholera

Vibrio cholerae are comma-shaped, gram-negative bacteria that have been the cause of seven great long-lasting epidemics (pandemics) of diarrheal disease. Many of these pandemics begin in the Ganges Valley of India and Bangladesh, which is never free from cholera, and then move east. Although there are 140 serotypes of *V. cholerae*, until recently only the O1 serotype was associated with severe diarrhea. Beginning in 1992, a new *V. cholerae* serotype (O139, also known as Bengal) has been associated with severe, watery diarrhea.[70]

Pathogenesis. The vibrios never invade the epithelium but instead remain within the lumen and secrete enterotoxin, which is encoded by a virulence phage.[27] Flagellar proteins involved in motility and attachment are necessary for efficient bacterial colonization as has been described for *Campylobacter.* (This is in contrast to *Shigella* species and certain *E. coli* strains, which are nonmotile and yet invasive.) The *Vibrio* hemagglutinin, which is a metalloprotease, is important for detachment of *Vibrio* from epithelial cells, analogous to the neuraminidase of influenza virus described earlier.

The secretory diarrhea characteristic of the disease is caused by release of an enterotoxin, called cholera toxin, that is nearly identical to *E. coli* enterotoxin[71] (Fig. 9–25). Cholera toxin is composed of five binding peptides B and a catalytic peptide A. The peptides B bind to carbohydrates on GM_1 ganglioside on the surface of epithelial cells of the small intestines. Within the cell, the disulfide bond linking the two fragments of peptide A (A1 and A2) is cleaved, and catalytic peptide A1 interacts with 20-kD cytosolic G proteins called ADP-ribosylation factors. ADP-ribosylation factors and guanosine triphosphate (GTP) increase the activity of cholera toxin, which ADP-ribosylates a 49-kD G protein (called $G_{s\alpha}$) that in turn stimulates adenylate cyclase. ADP-ribosylated $G_{s\alpha}$ is permanently in an active GTP-bound state (similar to activated *ras* mutants described in Chapter 8), resulting in persistent activation of adenylate cyclase, high levels of intracellular cAMP, and massive secretion of chloride, sodium, and water. Because the effects of cholera toxin are abrogated by inhibitors of serotonin, the intestinal nervous system may also be involved in the action of the cholera toxin. The reabsorptive function of the large intestine is overwhelmed, and

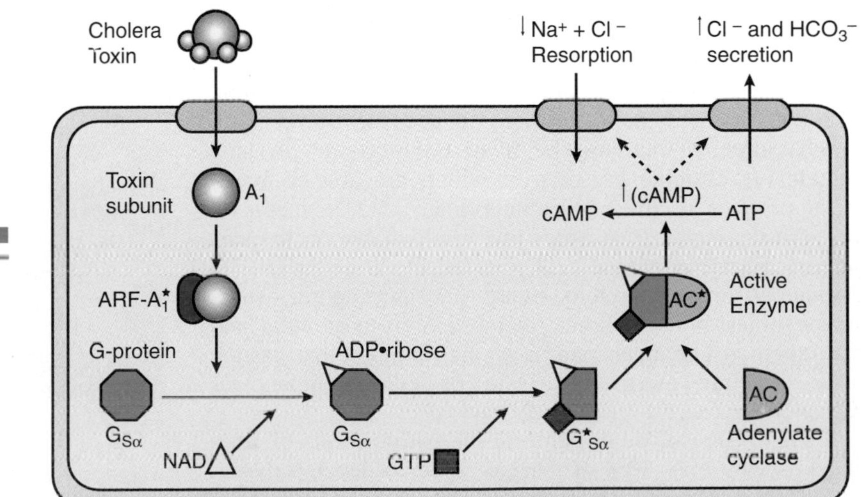

Figure 9–25

Mechanism of action of cholera toxin.

liters of dilute "rice-water" diarrhea containing flecks of mucus but few leukocytes are produced. Because overall absorption in the gut remains intact, oral formulas can replace massive sodium, chloride, and bicarbonate and fluid losses and reduce the mortality rate from 50% to less than 1%.

MORPHOLOGY. *V. cholerae* bacteria do not invade the gut mucosa and consequently cause minor histopathologic changes that underestimate the physiologic damage caused by the secreted toxin. There is usually congestion of the mucosal lamina propria, moderate infiltration of mononuclear inflammatory cells, and hyperplasia of Peyer patches.

PARASITIC INTESTINAL INFECTIONS

Amebiasis

Pathogenesis. The protozoan *Entamoeba histolytica* infects approximately 500 million persons in developing countries, such as India, Mexico, and Colombia, resulting in approximately 40 million cases of dysentery and liver abscess.[72] *E. histolytica* cysts, which have a chitin wall and four nuclei, are the infectious form because they are resistant to gastric acid. In the colonic lumen, cysts release trophozoites, the ameboid form, that reproduce under anaerobic conditions without harming the host. Because the parasites lack mitochondria or Krebs cycle enzymes, amebae are obligate fermenters of glucose to ethanol. Metronidazole, the best drug to treat invasive infections with entamoebae (as well as other parasites such as *Giardia* and trichomonads), targets ferredoxin-dependent pyruvate oxidoreductase, an enzyme critical in such fermentation that is present in these organisms but is absent in humans. Remarkably, the genes encoding the fermentation enzymes of amebae appear to derive from an anaerobic bacterial endosymbiont, which is different from the bacterium from which mammalian mitochondria derive.[73]

Amebae cause dysentery—bloody diarrhea, intestinal pain, fever—when they attach to the colonic epithelium, lyse colonic epithelial cells, and invade the bowel wall. Ameba proteins that may be involved in tissue invasion include (1) cysteine proteinases, which are able to break down proteins of the extracellular matrix; (2) a lectin on the parasite surface that binds to carbohydrates on the surface of colonic epithelial cells and red blood cells; and (3) a channel-forming protein called the amebapore, which makes holes in the plasma membrane of host cells and lyses them.[74] The amebapore is a small peptide that has the same structure as the NK-lysin of killer lymphocytes (Chapter 7).

A major unresolved question in the pathogenesis of amebiasis is why only 10% of persons infected develop dysentery. One explanation is the existence of two genetically distinct forms of amebae: *E. histolytica* that causes disease and *Entamoeba dispar* that does not.[75] The cysts of virulent and nonvirulent amebae have a similar structure in stool, but the presence of trophozoites containing ingested red blood cells is indicative of tissue invasion by virulent *E. histolytica* parasites.

MORPHOLOGY. Amebiasis most frequently involves the cecum and ascending colon, followed in order by the sigmoid, rectum, and appendix. In severe full-blown cases, however, the entire colon is involved. Amebae can mimic the appearance of macrophages because of their comparable size and large number of vacuoles; the parasites, however, have a smaller nucleus, which contains a large karyosome (Fig. 9–26). Amebae invade the crypts of the colonic glands, burrow through the tunica propria, and are halted by the muscularis mucosae. There the amebae fan out laterally to create a flask-shaped ulcer with a narrow neck and broad base. As the lesion progresses, the overlying surface mucosa is deprived of its blood supply and sloughs. The earliest amebic lesions show neutrophilic infiltrates in the mucosa, which later develop into ulcers that contain few host inflammatory cells and areas of extensive liquefactive necrosis. The mucosa between ulcers is often normal or mildly inflamed. An uncommon lesion is the **ameboma,** a napkin-like constrictive lesion, which represents a focus of profuse granulation tissue response to the parasites and is sometimes mistaken for a colonic tumor.

In about 40% of patients with amebic dysentery, parasites penetrate portal vessels and embolize to the liver to produce solitary, or less often multiple, discrete abscesses, some exceeding 10 cm in diameter. **Amebic liver abscesses** have a scant inflammatory reaction at their margins and a shaggy fibrin lining. Because of hemorrhage into

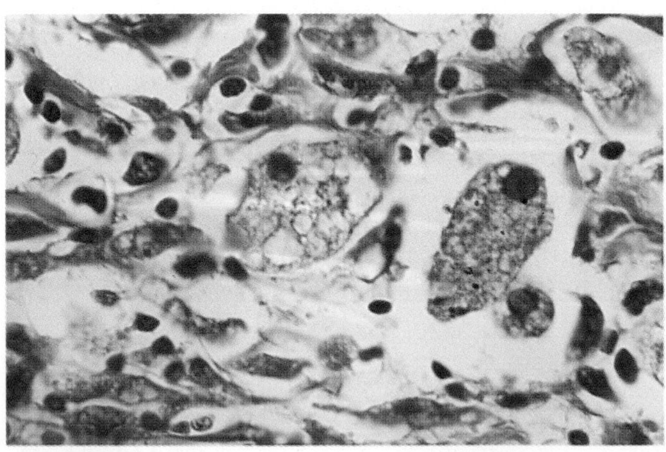

Figure 9–26

Amebiasis of the colon with a portion of three *Entamoeba histolytica* trophozoites.

the cavities, the abscesses are sometimes filled with a chocolate-colored, odorless, pasty material likened to anchovy paste. Secondary bacterial infection may make these abscesses purulent. As the amebic abscesses enlarge, they produce pain by pressing on the liver capsule and can be visualized with ultrasound examination. Amebic liver abscesses are treated with drainage and drugs or with drugs alone. Rarely, amebic abscesses reach the lung and the heart by direct extension or spread through the blood into the kidneys and brain.

Giardiasis

Giardia lamblia is the most prevalent pathogenic intestinal protozoan worldwide.[76] Infection may be subclinical or may cause acute or chronic diarrhea, steatorrhea, or constipation. Because *Giardia* cysts are not killed by chlorine, *Giardia* is endemic in public water supplies that are not filtered through sand and in streams accessed by campers.

Pathogenesis. In the United States, *Giardia* infections are especially frequent in institutions for the retarded and in daycare centers. *Giardia,* like *Entamoeba,* ferments glucose, lacks mitochondria, and exists in two forms: (1) a dormant but infectious cyst spread by the fecal-oral route from person to person (as well as beavers to persons) and (2) trophozoites that multiply in the intestinal lumen. Transition from trophozoites to cysts is signaled by decreases in availability of cholesterol as *Giardia* moves from duodenum to jejunum.[77] In contrast to *Entamoeba, Giardia* trophozoites have two nuclei rather than one, are flagellated, reside in the duodenum rather than the colon, adhere to but do not invade intestinal epithelial cells, and so cause diarrhea rather than dysentery.

Giardia trophozoites adhere to sugars on intestinal epithelial cells through a parasite lectin that is activated when it is cleaved by proteases, which are plentiful in the lumen of the duodenum. Tight contact between the parasite and the epithelial cell is made by a sucker-like disc, composed of cytoplasmic tubulin and unique intermediate filaments called *giardins.* Although *Giardia* does not secrete toxin, it contains a cysteine-rich surface protein that resembles diarrhea-causing toxins secreted by certain snakes.[78] Antibody-mediated immunity, including secretory IgA, is important in resistance to *Giardia* because agammaglobulinemic individuals are severely affected by the parasite. Immunity to *Giardia,* however, is limited by the parasite's ability to vary its major surface proteins into antigenically distinct forms, encoded by more than 50 different genes.[79]

MORPHOLOGY. In stool smears, *G. lamblia* trophozoites are pear shaped and binucleate, resembling a cartoonist's drawing of a ghost. Duodenal biopsy specimens are often teeming with sickle-shaped trophozoites, which are tightly bound by the concave attachment disc to the villus surface of the epithelial cells (Fig. 9–27). Although the intestinal morphology may range from virtually normal to markedly abnormal, most commonly *Giardia* causes clubbing of villi, a decreased villus-crypt ratio, and a mixed inflammatory infiltrate of the lamina propria. The brush borders of the absorptive cells are irregular, and sometimes there is virtual absence of villi, resembling the atrophic stage of gluten-induced enteropathy (Chapter 18). *Giardia* in individuals with immunoglobulin deficiencies causes follicular hypertrophy of the mucosal lymphoid tissue.

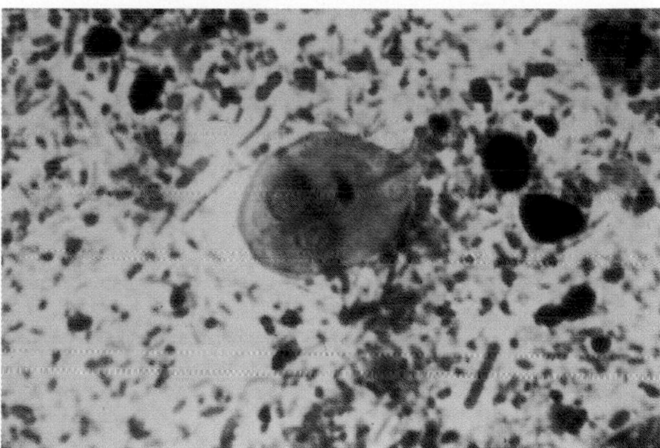

Figure 9–27

Binucleate *Giardia lamblia* trophozoite in stool. (Courtesy of Dr. Anita Zaidi, Department of Infectious Diseases, Children's Hospital, Boston, MA.)

SEXUALLY TRANSMITTED DISEASES

Although the classic sexually transmitted diseases gonorrhea, syphilis, and chlamydial infection have been greatly reduced in some segments of Western societies, these diseases are increasing at epidemic rates among certain urban populations in the United States.[80] Worldwide pandemics of HIV (Chapter 7) and HBV (Chapter 19) remain uncontrolled and involve adults of both sexes and children of infected mothers. In addition, viruses spread by intimate contact include those that cause oral and genital sores (HSV-1 and HSV-2), infectious mononucleosis (EBV), and opportunistic congenital infections in infants with AIDS (CMV) (Table 9–9).

Herpesvirus Infections

Herpesviruses are large encapsulated viruses that have a double-stranded DNA genome that encodes approximately 70 proteins. Nine types of herpesviruses, belonging to three groups, have been isolated from humans: *neurotropic α-group viruses,* including HSV-1, HSV-2, and varicella-zoster virus (VZV); *lymphotropic β-group viruses,* including CMV, human herpesvirus 6 (which causes exanthema subi-

Table 9–9. SEXUALLY TRANSMITTED INFECTIOUS DISEASES

Causal Agent	Disease Manifestations
Exclusively or Regularly Transmitted by Sexual Contact	
■ *Viral*	
HIV-1, HIV-2	AIDS
HSV-1, HSV-2	Herpes lesions
Papillomaviruses	Condyloma, cervical neoplasia
■ *Chlamydial, Mycoplasmal*	
Chlamydia trachomatis (L type)	Lymphogranuloma venereum
Chlamydia trachomatis	Nongonorrheal urethritis, cervicitis
Ureaplasma urealyticum	Nongonorrheal urethritis, cervicitis
■ *Bacterial*	
Neisseria gonorrhoeae	Gonorrhea
Treponema pallidum	Syphilis (lues venerea)
Haemophilus ducreyi	Chancroid
Calymmatobacterium donovani	Granuloma inguinale
■ *Protozoal*	
Trichomonas vaginalis	Trichomoniasis
■ *By Arthropod*	
Phthirus pubis	Pediculosis pubis (crabs)
Transmissible Sexually or by Other Means	
■ *Viral*	
Cytomegalovirus, hepatitis B virus, Epstein-Barr virus, molluscum contagiosum virus	Hepatitis, mononucleosis, warts
■ *Bacterial*	
Group B streptococci; gram-negative bacilli	Neonatal sepsis, cystitis
■ *Fungal*	
Candida	Thrush, vaginitis
■ *Protozoal*	
Entamoeba histolytica	Colitis, liver abscess

tum, a benign rash of infants), and human herpesvirus 7 (which is not yet associated with a specific disease); and γ-*group viruses*—EBV and HHV-8, the apparent cause of Kaposi sarcoma. In addition, herpesvirus simiae is an Old World monkey virus that resembles HSV-1 and may cause fatal neurologic disease in animal handlers. Here we discuss the lesions induced by HSV-1 and HSV-2.

Natural History of HSV-1 and HSV-2 Infections. HSV-1 and HSV-2 are genetically similar and cause a similar set of primary and recurrent infections.[81] Both viruses replicate in the skin and the mucous membranes at the site of entrance of the virus (oropharynx or genitals), where they cause vesicular lesions of the epidermis and infect the neurons that innervate these locations. Within the nucleus of host epithelial cells, HSV-encoded proteins form a replication compartment where viral DNA is made and capsid proteins are attached. In immunocompetent hosts, primary HSV infection resolves in a few weeks, although herpesviruses remain latent in the nerve cells. Latency is operationally defined as the inability to recover infectious particles from disrupted cells that harbor the virus, although viral DNA and a few viral mRNAs may be identified by molecular methods.[82] Reactivation of HSV-1 and HSV-2 may occur repeatedly with or without symptoms and results in the spread of virus from the neurons to the skin or to mucous membranes.

In addition to causing cutaneous lesions, HSV-1 is the major infectious cause of corneal blindness in the United States, secondary to stromal conjunctivitis; such inflammation appears to be immune mediated because it responds to corticosteroids, and the lesions show numerous mononuclear cells surrounding keratinocytes.[83] HSV-1 is also the major cause of fatal sporadic encephalitis in the United States when viruses spread to the brain, particularly the temporal lobes. In addition, neonates and individuals with decreased cellular immunity secondary to AIDS or chemotherapy may suffer disseminated herpesvirus infections.

MORPHOLOGY. All HSV lesions are marked by formation of large, pink to purple (Cowdry type A) intranuclear inclusions that contain intact and disrupted virions and push darkly stained host cell chromatin to the edges of the nucleus (Fig. 9–28). Although cell and nuclear size increase only slightly, herpesvirus produces inclusion-bearing multinucleated syncytia, which are diagnostic in smears of blister fluid.

HSV-1 and HSV-2 cause lesions ranging from self-limited cold sores and gingivostomatitis to life-threatening disseminated visceral infections and encephalitis. **Fever blisters or cold sores** favor the facial skin around mucosal orifices (lips, nose), where their distribution is frequently bilateral and independent of skin dermatomes. Intraepithelial vesicles (blisters), which are formed by intracellular edema and ballooning degeneration of epidermal cells, frequently burst and crust over, but some may result in superficial ulcerations.

Gingivostomatitis, which is usually encountered in children, is caused by HSV-1. It is a vesicular eruption extending from the tongue to the retropharynx and causing cervical lymphadenopathy.

Genital herpes is characterized by vesicles on the genital mucous membranes as well as on the external genitalia that are rapidly converted into

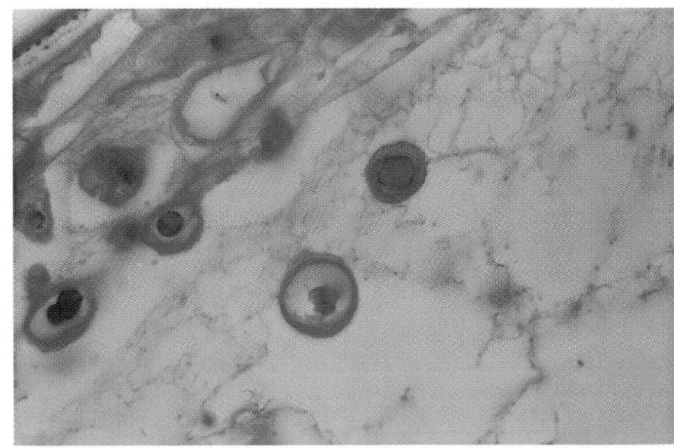

Figure 9–28

High-power view of cells from the blister in Fig. 9–14 showing glassy intranuclear herpes simplex inclusion bodies.

superficial ulcerations, rimmed by an inflammatory infiltrate. HSV-2 is transmitted to neonates during passage through the birth canal of infected mothers. Although HSV-2 disease in the neonate may be mild, it is more often fulminating with generalized lymphadenopathy, splenomegaly, and necrotic foci throughout the lungs, liver, adrenals, and central nervous systems.

Two forms of **corneal lesions** are caused by HSV. **Herpes epithelial keratitis** shows typical virus-induced cytolysis of the superficial epithelium and is sensitive to antiviral drugs. In contrast, **herpes stromal keratitis** shows infiltrates of mononuclear cells around keratinocytes and endothelial cells, leading to neovascularization, scarring, opacification of the cornea, and eventual blindness. This is an immunologic reaction to the HSV infection and responds to corticosteroid therapy.

Herpes simplex encephalitis is described in Chapter 30.

Disseminated skin and visceral herpes infections are usually encountered in hospitalized patients with some form of underlying cancer or under immunosuppressive treatment. **Kaposi varicelliform eruption** is a generalized vesiculating involvement of the skin, whereas **eczema herpeticum** is characterized by confluent, pustular, or hemorrhagic blisters, often with bacterial superinfection and viral dissemination to internal viscera. **Herpes esophagitis** is frequently complicated by superinfection with bacteria or fungi. **Herpes bronchopneumonia,** which may be introduced with an airway inserted through oral herpes lesions, is often necrotizing, and **herpes hepatitis** may cause liver failure.

As described in Chapter 8, HHV-8 is implicated in the pathogenesis of **Kaposi sarcoma.**[84]

Chlamydial Infections

Chlamydia trachomatis is an obligate intracellular pathogen of columnar epithelial cells that causes venereal urethritis, lymphogranuloma venereum, and trachoma (Table 9–10). Closely related, *Chlamydia pneumoniae* and *Chlamydia psittaci* cause mild and severe pneumonias, respectively. *C. trachomatis* causes more than a half-million reported cases of nongonorrheal urethritis in the United States each year, which are more frequently symptomatic in men than in women. In some men, *C. trachomatis* infection causes *Reiter syndrome,* a triad of conjunctivitis, polyarthritis, and genital infection. *Lymphogranuloma venereum* is caused by a specific strain of *C. trachomatis* and results in granulomatous inflammation of the inguinal and rectal lymph nodes. Infants born to mothers with *C. trachomatis* cervicitis may develop inclusion conjunctivitis or neonatal pneumonia. Trachoma or chronic keratoconjunctivitis, a leading global cause of blindness, is a disease of poverty and overcrowding, transmitted from eye to eye by aerosols or by hand contact.[85]

Pathogenesis. Chlamydiae exist in two forms: elementary bodies, which never divide but are infectious, and reticulate bodies, which multiply within host cells but are not infectious.[86] Elementary bodies have a cell wall that is made rigid by disulfide bonds rather than cross-linked peptidoglycans found in most bacteria, and thus *chlamydiae are not susceptible to penicillin.* They have adhesins on their surface, which bind to microvilli on host columnar epithelial cells. Depending on the *Chlamydia* species and type of host cell, organisms enter host cells through endosomes or phagosomes. Within endosome-bound inclusion bodies that fail to fuse with host lysosomes, elementary bodies transform to reticulate bodies and multiply to as many as 500 organisms per host cell. Because chlamydiae are unable to synthesize ATP, the organisms induce host cell mitochondria (which make ATP) to closely appose the inclusion body. Reticulate bodies then transform back to elementary bodies, which cause bursting of host cells, infecting neighboring cells.

MORPHOLOGY. Inclusions of chlamydial forms in epithelial cells are best seen with fluorescent anti-*Chlamydia* antibodies. Chlamydial urethritis or cervicitis may also be diagnosed by culture on McCoy cells and by molecular biologic methods, which are the most sensitive.[87]

Lymphogranuloma venereum causes a small epidermal vesicle at the site of infection on the genitalia. The vesicle ulcerates and oozes a neu-

Table 9–10. HUMAN CHLAMYDIAL DISEASES AND SPECIES

Species and Serotype	Diseases	Transmission
Chlamydia psittaci	Ornithosis (psittacosis)	Aspiration of bird-contaminated particles
Chlamydia pneumoniae	Mild pneumonia	Aerosols (person to person)
Chlamydia trachomatis		
A, B, Ba, C	Trachoma	Repeated contact, fomites, insects
D, E, F, G, H, I, J, K	Inclusion conjunctivitis	Birth canal infection (infants)
		Sexual contact, swimming (adults)
	Nongonorrheal urethritis	Sexual contact
	Postgonorrheal urethritis	Sexual contact
	Proctitis, pharyngitis, cervicitis, arthritis	Sexual contact
L1, L2, L3	Lymphogranuloma venereum	Sexual contact

trophilic exudate. At the base of this ulcer, there is a zone of chronic, often granulomatous inflammation. In addition, lymphogranuloma venereum causes rapid swelling of the inguinal, pelvic, and rectal lymph nodes by a mixture of suppurative and granulomatous inflammation. Irregular, stellate abscesses form when granulomas with suppurative centers fuse. These abscesses are rimmed by a layer of epithelioid macrophages and resemble lesions seen in cat-scratch disease. Later lesions in lymphogranuloma venereum show fewer granulomas, plasma cell infiltrates, and increasing fibrosis.

Inclusion conjunctivitis is a self-limited disease of infants born to mothers with cervical infections with *C. trachomatis.* The conjunctivae are hyperemic and edematous and show a monocytic infiltrate.

C. psittaci is excreted from infected birds and inhaled with dust particles. Although human infection may be asymptomatic or mild, *C. psittaci* also causes a severe pneumonia, also known as ornithosis. Lethal generalized disease, most frequent during epidemics, is marked by focal areas of necrosis in the liver and spleen and diffuse mononuclear infiltrates in the kidneys, heart, and (sometimes) brain.

Gonorrhea

Gonorrhea is caused by *Neisseria gonorrhoeae,* a pyogenic, encapsulated, gram-negative diplococcus. There are nearly 700,000 reported cases of gonorrheal urethritis in the United States each year, but *N. gonorrhoeae* can also cause pharyngitis or proctitis, depending on sexual practices. In men, the gonococcus may result in urethral strictures and chronic infections of the epididymis, prostate, and seminal vesicles. Infection of the fallopian tubes in women (salpingitis) may result in scars, which increase rates of sterility and ectopic pregnancy or lead to chronic infections with anaerobic bacteria (see also Chapter 24). Gonococcal bacteremia leads to an arthritis-dermatitis syndrome, whereas conjunctivitis may appear in adults from autoinoculation. *N. gonorrhoeae* is genetically similar to *Neisseria meningitidis,* which causes meningitis (Chapter 30), bacteremia, and in fatal cases diffuse intravascular coagulation (DIC) with the Waterhouse-Friderichsen syndrome (Chapter 26).[88]

Pathogenesis. *N. gonorrhoeae* is a facultative intracellular pathogen that binds to and invades epithelial cells. Important cell binding sites include vitronectin and syndecan (a proteoglycan receptor), while internalization is dependent on rearrangements in host cell actin filaments.[89] Bacteria bind through adhesins or pili, which show antigenic variation on the basis of intragenomic recombination and recombination after incorporation of exogenous DNA from lysed gonococci. Internalization is based on a second set of adhesins that show antigenic variation by genetic mechanisms different from those of pili.[90] Capsular polysaccharides contribute to virulence by inhibiting phagocytosis in the absence of antigonococcal antibodies. Pathogenic neisseriae secrete a protease that cleaves IgA. In addition, neisseriae release peptidoglycans and endotoxins, which induce host cell secretion of TNF-α that may cause shock and multisystem failure. Damage to the epithelial cells of the fallopian tubes by *N. gonorrhoeae* may also be mediated by TNF-α.[91]

MORPHOLOGY. All gonococcal lesions show exudative and purulent reactions followed by granulation tissue formation, plasma cell infiltration, and fibrosis. Gonococci in men cause a mucopurulent discharge from an edematous and inflamed urethral meatus 2 to 7 days after exposure. If untreated, suppurative inflammation with focal abscesses spreads to the posterior urethra, epididymis, prostate, and seminal vesicles. Chronic inflammation may lead to urethral strictures and sterility.

In women, urethral inflammation is less prominent, whereas abscesses frequently cause bulging of Bartholin and Skene glands. Gonococcal cervicitis results in few sequelae, whereas salpingitis may seal the fallopian tubes, which become massively distended with pus and may be left severely scarred. Tubo-ovarian abscesses and pelvic peritonitis (pelvic inflammatory disease) result from further extension and may create multiple adhesions and points of blockage of the oviducts (see also Chapter 24).

Syphilis

Treponema pallidum is the microaerophilic spirochete that causes syphilis, a systemic venereal disease with multiple clinical presentations, thus designated *the great impostor.* Other closely related treponemas cause yaws *(Treponema pertenue),* pinta *(Treponema carateum),* and periodontal disease *(Treponema denticola).* Like the *Borrelia* spirochetes of Lyme disease and relapsing fever, described later, *T. pallidum* organisms have an axial periplasmic flagellum wound around a slender, helical protoplasm, all of which are covered by a unit membrane called the outer sheath. *T. pallidum* spirochetes cannot be cultured but are detectable by silver stains, darkfield examination, and immunofluorescence techniques. Sexual intercourse is the usual mode of transmission. Transplacental transmission of *T. pallidum* occurs readily, and active disease during pregnancy results in congenital syphilis.

Clinical Features of Syphilis (Fig. 9–29). The *primary stage* of syphilis, occurring approximately 3 weeks after contact with an infected individual, features a single firm, nontender, raised, red lesion (*chancre*) located at the site of treponemal invasion on the penis, cervix, vaginal wall, or anus. Although spirochetes seed the body by hematogenous spread, the chancre heals in a few weeks with or without therapy. The *secondary stage* of syphilis, which occurs 2

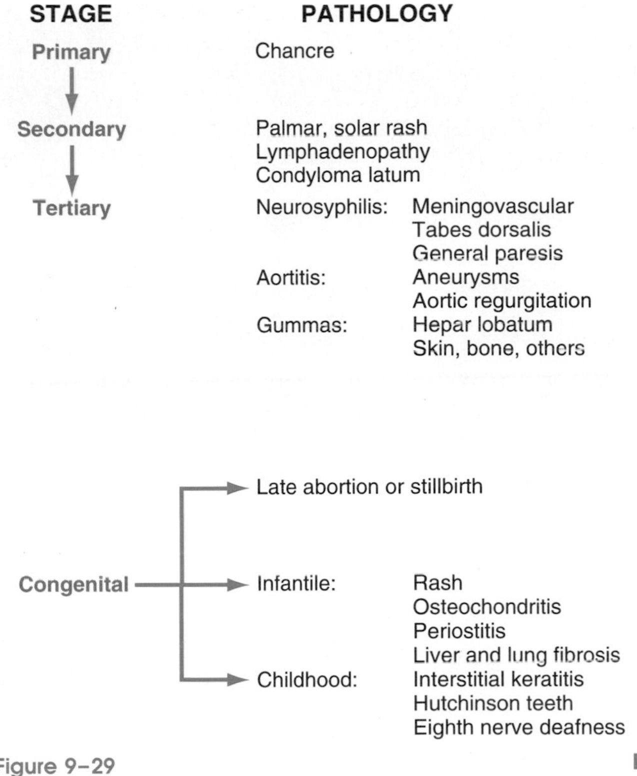

Figure 9–29

Protean manifestations of syphilis.

to 10 weeks after the primary chancre, is characterized by a diffuse rash, particularly of the palms and soles, that may be accompanied by white oral lesions, fever, lymphadenopathy, headache, and arthritis. These lesions as well resolve spontaneously. The *tertiary stage,* which occurs years after the primary lesion, is characterized either by active inflammatory lesions of the aorta, heart (Chapter 13), and central nervous system (Chapter 30) or by quiescent lesions (*gummas*) involving the liver, bones, and skin. Congenital syphilis is described subsequently.

Pathogenesis. Whatever the stage of the disease and location of the lesions, the histologic hallmarks of syphilis are obliterative endarteritis and plasma cell–rich mononuclear infiltrates. The endarteritis is secondary to the binding of spirochetes to endothelial cells, mediated by fibronectin molecules bound to the surface of the spirochetes.[92] The mononuclear infiltrates reflect an immunologic response. In animal models, a delayed type hypersensitivity response is more important than antibodies are in limiting the initial localized infection. The antibodies may be against spirochete-specific antigens (the basis of treponemal serologic tests) or against antigens that cross-react with host molecules (the basis of nontreponemal tests, including the Wassermann and Venereal Disease Research Laboratory tests). Host humoral and cellular immune responses may prevent the formation of a chancre on subsequent infections with *T. pallidum* but are insufficient to clear the spirochetes. This may be because the outer membrane of syphilis spirochetes contains 100-fold less proteins than usual gram-negative bacteria and so is lacking antigens.[93] Alternatively, treponeme escape from host immune responses may be secondary to down-regulation of helper T cells of the T_H1 class.[94]

MORPHOLOGY. In primary syphilis, a chancre occurs on the penis or scrotum of 70% of men and on the vulva or cervix of 50% of women. The chancre is a slightly elevated, firm, reddened papule, up to several centimeters in diameter, that erodes to create a clean-based shallow ulcer. The contiguous induration creates a button-like mass directly subjacent to the eroded skin, providing the basis of the designation hard chancre (Fig. 9–30). On histologic examination, the chancre contains an intense infiltrate of plasma cells, with scattered macrophages and lymphocytes and an obliterative endarteritis (see Fig. 9–13). Treponemes are visible with silver stains or immunofluorescence techniques at the surface of the ulcer. The regional nodes are usually enlarged and may show nonspecific acute or chronic lymphadenitis, plasma cell–rich infiltrates, or focal epithelioid granulomas.

In **secondary syphilis,** widespread mucocutaneous lesions involve the oral cavity, palms of the hands, and soles of the feet. The rash is frequently macular, with discrete red-brown spots less than 5

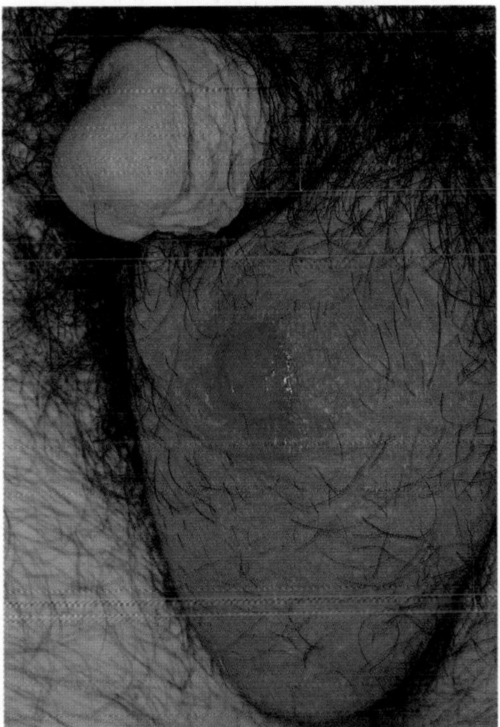

Figure 9–30

Syphilitic chancre in the scrotum (see Fig. 9–13 for the histopathology of syphilis). (Courtesy of Dr. Richard Johnson, Beth Israel-Deaconess Hospital.)

mm in diameter, but may be follicular, pustular, annular, or scaling. Reddened mucous patches in the mouth or vagina contain the most organisms and are the most infectious. Papular lesions in the region of the penis or vulva form 2- to 3-cm elevated red-brown plaques, which are called **condylomata lata** (not to be confused with venereal warts, which are called condylomata acuminata (Chapter 23)). Histologically, the lesions of secondary syphilis show the same plasma cell infiltrate and obliterative endarteritis as the primary chancre, although the inflammation is often less intense.

Tertiary syphilis occurs years after the initial infection and most frequently involves the aorta (80% to 85%); the central nervous system (5% to 10%); and the liver, bones, and testes (gummas). **Aortitis** is manifested by aortic aneurysms in which there is inflammatory scarring of the tunica media, widening and incompetence of the aortic valve ring, and narrowing of the mouths of the coronary ostia (Chapter 13). **Neurosyphilis** takes one of several forms, designated meningovascular syphilis, tabes dorsalis, and general paresis (Chapter 30). **Syphilitic gummas** are white-gray and rubbery, occur singly or multiply, and vary in size from microscopic defects resembling tubercles to large tumor-like masses. They occur in most organs but particularly in skin, subcutaneous tissue, bone, and joints. In the liver, scarring as a result of gummas may cause a distinctive hepatic lesion known as hepar lobatum (Fig. 9–31). On histologic examination, the gummas contain a center of coagulated, necrotic material and margins composed of plump or palisaded macrophages and fibroblasts surrounded by large numbers of mononuclear leukocytes, chiefly plasma cells. Treponemes are scant in these gummas and are difficult to demonstrate.

Congenital syphilis is most severe when the mother's infection is recent. Because treponemes do not invade the placental tissue or the fetus until the fifth month of gestation, syphilis causes late abortion, stillbirth, or death soon after delivery, or it may persist in latent form to become apparent only during childhood or adult life. In **perinatal and infantile syphilis,** a diffuse rash develops, which differs from that of the acquired secondary stage in that there is extensive sloughing of the epithelium, particularly on the palms, soles, and skin about the mouth and anus. These lesions teem with spirochetes. **Syphilitic osteochondritis and periostitis** affect all bones, although lesions of the nose and lower legs are most distinctive. Destruction of the vomer causes collapse of the bridge of the nose and, later on, the characteristic saddle nose deformity. Periostitis of the tibia leads to excessive new bone growth on the anterior surfaces and anterior bowing, or saber shin. There is also widespread disturbance in endochondral bone formation. The epiphyses become widened as the cartilage overgrows, and cartilage is found as displaced islands within the metaphysis.

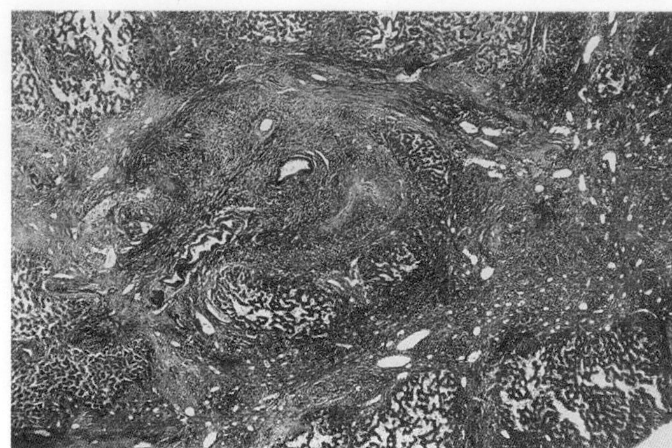

Figure 9–31

Trichrome stain of liver shows liver gumma (scar), stained blue, which is caused by tertiary syphilis (also known as hepar lobatum). Compare with nodules of alcoholic cirrhosis (Chapter 19).

The **liver** is often severely affected in congenital syphilis. Diffuse fibrosis permeates lobules to isolate hepatic cells into small nests, accompanied by the characteristic white cell infiltrate and vascular changes. Gummas are occasionally found in the liver, even in early cases. The **lungs** may be affected by a diffuse interstitial fibrosis. In the syphilitic stillborn, the lungs appear as pale, airless organs (pneumonia alba). The generalized spirochetemia may lead to diffuse interstitial inflammatory reactions in virtually any other organ of the body (e.g., the pancreas, kidneys, heart, spleen, thymus, endocrine organs, and central nervous system).

The late-occurring form of congenital syphilis is distinctive for the **triad of interstitial keratitis, Hutchinson teeth, and eighth nerve deafness.** Eye changes consist of interstitial keratitis and choroiditis with abnormal pigment production causing a spotted retina. The dental changes involve the incisor teeth, which are small and shaped like a screwdriver or a peg, often with notches in the enamel (Hutchinson teeth). Eighth nerve deafness and optic nerve atrophy develop secondary to meningovascular syphilis.

Trichomoniasis

Trichomonas vaginalis, a sexually transmitted anaerobic, flagellated protozoan parasite, infects some 3 million new persons each year. *T. vaginalis* is the simplest of all protozoan parasites: there is only a trophozoite form, which adheres to and causes superficial lesions of the mucosal

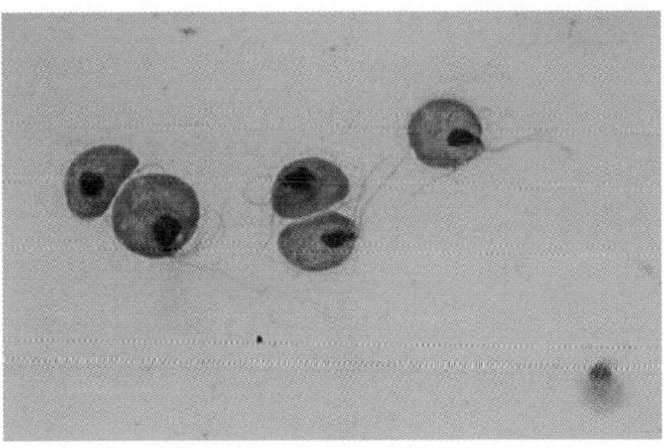

Figure 9–32

Flagellated trophozoites of *Trichomonas vaginalis.*

surfaces of the male and female genital tracts but fails to invade host tissues. *T. vaginalis* infection in women is often associated with loss of acid-producing Döderlein bacilli, may be asymptomatic, but frequently causes itching and a profuse watery vaginal discharge. It is exacerbated by menstruation and by pregnancy. Urethral colonization by *T. vaginalis* causes urinary frequency and dysuria. *T. vaginalis* infection of men is mostly asymptomatic but may result in nongonococcal urethritis and rarely prostatitis. Infants infected with *T. vaginalis* during the birth process spontaneously clear the parasites in a few weeks.

Like *Giardia* and *Entamoeba,* trichomonads live in an anaerobic lumen and are obligate fermenters. Trichomonads have a modified mitochondrion, called the hydrogenosome, in which mitochondrial enzymes of oxidative phosphorylation are replaced by anaerobic fermentation enzymes.[95]

MORPHOLOGY. Trichomonads cause a spotty reddening and edema of the affected mucosa, sometimes with small blisters or papules, referred to as strawberry mucosa. On histologic examination, the mucosa and superficial submucosa are infiltrated by lymphocytes, plasma cells, and polymorphonuclear leukocytes. The discharge is rarely purulent, as in gonorrheal or chlamydial infection. The turnip-shaped trichomonads are best seen in fresh preparations diluted with warm saline, where they are rapidly motile, or in Giemsa-stained smears (Fig. 9–32).

GRAM-POSITIVE PYOGENIC BACTERIAL INFECTIONS

Staphylococcal Infections

Staphylococcus aureus organisms are pyogenic, nonmotile, gram-positive cocci that tend to form grapelike clusters. Staphylococci cause a myriad of skin lesions (boils, carbuncles, impetigo, and scalded skin) and also cause pharyngitis, pneumonia, endocarditis, food poisoning, and toxic shock syndrome (Fig. 9–33). Here we review the general characteristics of *S. aureus* infection. Specific organ infections are described in other chapters. *S. aureus* is the major cause of infection of patients with severe burns and surgical wounds and is second only to *E. coli* as a cause of hospital-acquired infections. *Staphylococcus epidermidis,* a species that is related to *S. aureus,* causes opportunistic infections in catheterized patients, patients with prosthetic cardiac valves, and drug addicts. Most staphylococci lack a capsule, and so these cocci are typed by their ability to be infected by bacteriophages. In addition, staphylococci are distinguished by their large number of plasmids, which encode enzymes involved in antibiotic resistance and other virulence factors.

Pathogenesis. *S. aureus* and other virulent staphylococci possess a multitude of virulence factors, which include surface proteins involved in adherence, secreted enzymes that degrade proteins, and secreted toxins that damage host cells. Expression of many of these virulence factors (pathogenicity island) is controlled by an autoinducing peptide that is secreted by the bacteria.[96] This positive feedback loop may accelerate release of toxins from the same strain of staphylococci but may inhibit other strains of staphylococci that have slightly different receptors for the autoinducing peptide.

S. aureus has, on its surface, receptors for fibrinogen (called clumping factor), fibronectin, and vitronectin and uses these molecules as a bridge to bind to host endothelial cells.[97] *S. aureus* has a laminin receptor that is similar to metastatic tumor cells and allows bacteria to bind to host extracellular matrix proteins and invade host tissues. Staphylococci infecting prosthetic valves and catheters have an exopolysaccharide capsule that allows them to attach to the artificial materials and to resist host cell phagocytosis. The lipase of *S. aureus* degrades lipids on the skin surface, and its expression is correlated with the ability of the bacteria to produce skin abscesses. Staphylococci also have protein A on their surface, which binds the Fc portion of immunoglobulins.

S. aureus produces multiple hemolytic toxins, including α toxin, which is a pore-forming protein that intercalates into the plasma membrane of host cells and depolarizes them[98]; β toxin, a sphingomyelinase; and δ toxin, which is an amphipathic (detergent-like) peptide. Staphylococcal γ-hemolysin and leukocidin lyse erythrocytes and leukocytes, respectively.

S. aureus enterotoxins are associated with food poisoning and appear to act by stimulating emetic receptors in the abdominal viscera and so cause vomiting and diarrhea. In addition, *S. aureus* enterotoxins are superantigens.[99] They bind to macrophage MHC class II molecules at a conserved site away from the hypervariable groove and then to the side of the T-cell receptor β chain, rather than to its variable face that recognizes conventionally processed antigens bound to the MHC. This leads to massive stimulation of host T cells and release of cytokines, which mediate the systemic effects of *S. aureus* enterotoxin.

Exfoliative toxins of *S. aureus* are associated with the staphylococcal *scalded skin syndrome,* in which cells in the

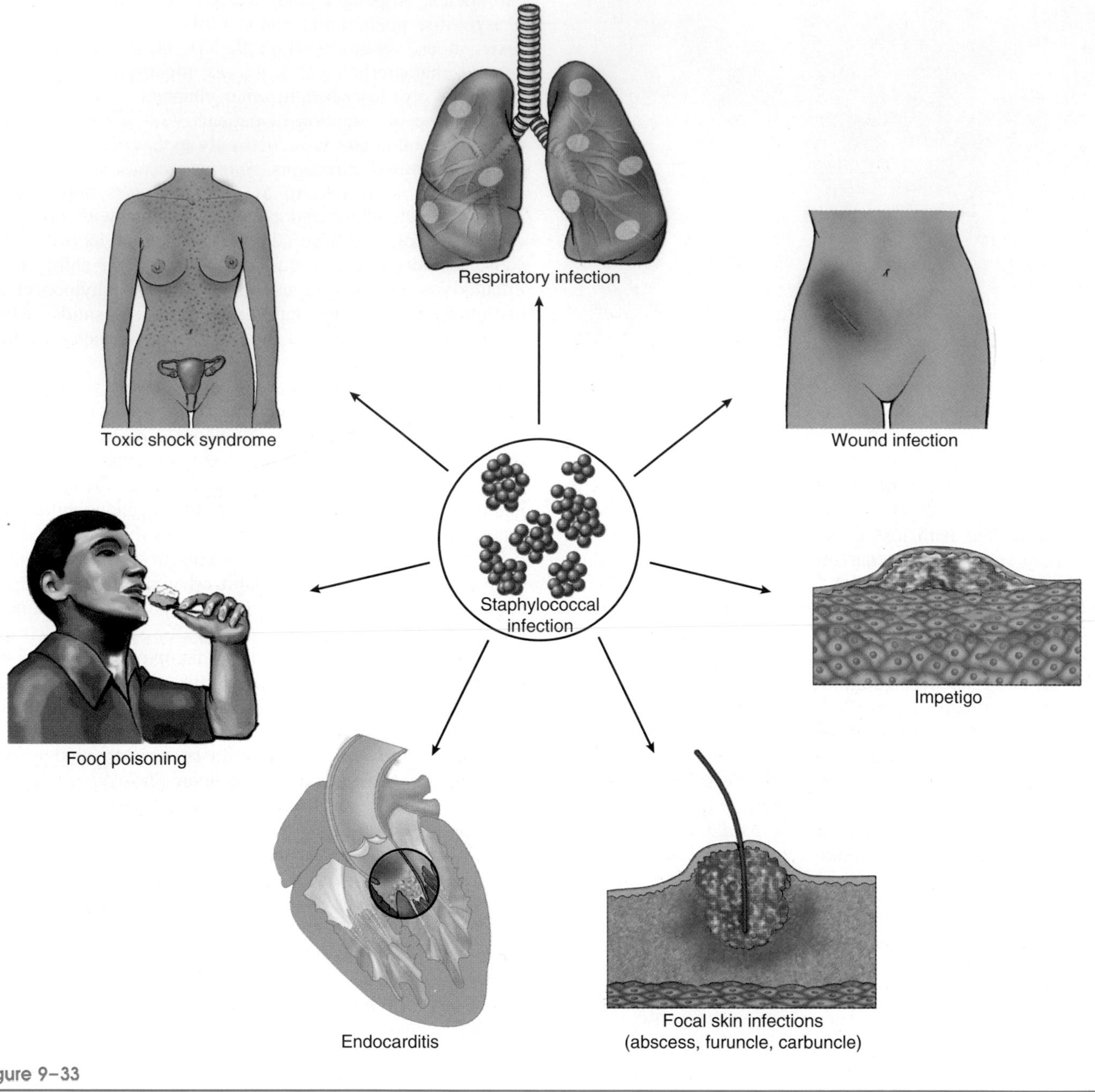

Figure 9–33

The many consequences of staphylococcal infection.

granular layer of the epidermis detach from each other and form skin blisters. Toxic shock syndrome toxin (TSST-1) is secreted by *S. aureus* colonizing the vagina of women using tampons and causes shock by mechanisms similar to those of *S. aureus* enterotoxins, which it resembles in structure.[100]

MORPHOLOGY. Whether the lesion is located in the skin, lungs, bones, or heart valves, *S. aureus* causes pyogenic inflammation that is distinctive for its local destructiveness. Excluding impetigo, which is a staphylococcal or streptococcal infection restricted to the superficial epidermis, staphylococcal skin infections are centered around the hair follicles.

A **furuncle,** or **boil,** is a focal suppurative inflammation of the skin and subcutaneous tissue, either solitary or multiple, or recurrent in successive crops. Furuncles are most frequent in moist, hairy areas, such as the face, axillae, groin, legs, and submammary folds. Beginning in a single hair follicle, a boil develops into a growing and deepening abscess that eventually "comes to a head" by thinning and rupturing the overlying skin. A **carbuncle** is associated with deeper suppuration that spreads laterally beneath the deep subcutaneous fascia and then burrows superficially to erupt in multiple adjacent skin sinuses. Carbuncles typically appear beneath the skin of the upper back and posterior neck, where fascial planes favor their spread. Persistent abscess formation of apocrine gland regions, most frequently of the axilla, is known as **hidradenitis suppurativa.** Those of the nail bed **(paronychia)** or on the palmar side of the fingertips **(felons)** are exquisitely painful. They may follow trauma or embedded splinters and, if deep enough, destroy the bone of the terminal phalanx or detach the fingernail.

Staphylococcal lung infections (Fig. 9–34), which are frequently opportunistic, have a polymorphonuclear infiltrate similar to that of pneumococcus (see Fig. 9–12) but are much more destructive of lung tissues.

Staphylococcal scalded skin syndrome, also called **Ritter disease,** is a toxin-mediated, exfoliative dermatitis that most frequently occurs in children with staphylococcal infections of the nasopharynx or skin. In staphylococcal scalded skin syndrome, there is a sunburn-like rash that spreads over the entire body and forms fragile bullae that lead to partial or total skin loss. The intraepithelial split in staphylococcal scalded skin syndrome is in the granulosa layer, distinguishing it from toxic epidermal necrolysis, or Lyell disease, which is secondary to drug hypersensitivity and causes splitting at the epidermal-dermal junction (Chapter 27).

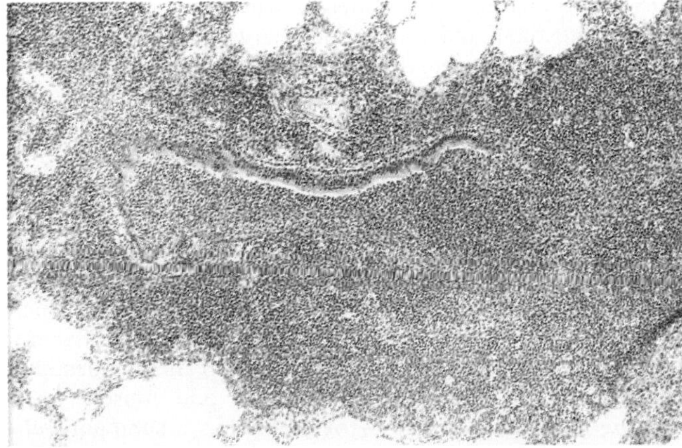

Figure 9–34

Staphylococcal abscess of the lung with extensive neutrophilic infiltrate and destruction of the alveoli (contrast with Fig. 9–12).

Streptococcal Infections

Streptococci are facultative anaerobic gram-positive cocci that grow in pairs or chains and cause a myriad of suppurative infections of the skin, oropharynx, lungs, and heart valves and also cause poststreptococcal syndromes, including rheumatic fever (Chapter 13), immune complex glomerulonephritis (Chapter 21), and erythema nodosum (Chapter 27). Most streptococci are β-hemolytic and are typed according to their surface (Lancefield) antigens. *Streptococcus pyogenes* (group A) causes pharyngitis, scarlet fever, erysipelas, impetigo, rheumatic fever, and glomerulonephritis; *Streptococcus agalactiae* (group B) causes neonatal sepsis and urinary tract infections; and *Enterococcus faecalis* (group D) causes endocarditis and urinary tract infections. *Streptococcus viridans,* which is α-hemolytic and thus green on blood agar plates, comprises a group of untypable variants that can cause endocarditis (Chapter 13). *Streptococcus pneumoniae* (pneumococcus) is typed by its capsular antigens and is the major cause of community-acquired pneumonia in the United States and a major cause of bacterial meningitis among adults. Finally, *Streptococcus mutans* is the major cause of dental caries.

Pathogenesis. As is the case with many other microbes, multiple virulence-associated genes of *Streptococcus* are coregulated in response to environmental stimuli. These include M protein, a surface protein that prevents bacteria from being phagocytosed, and a complement C5a peptidase, which degrades this chemotactic peptide.[26] Streptococci also have surface molecules, including lipoteichoic acid, that bind to the host extracellular matrix protein laminin, and pneumococci have a polysaccharide capsule that prevents phagocytosis.[101] Pneumolysin, which is also found in *Listeria monocytogenes*, is a cytosolic bacterial protein released on disruption of streptococci.[102] Pneumolysin inserts into target cell membranes and lyses them (like amebapore). Pneumolysin also activates the classical pathway of complement, reducing complement available for opsonization of bacteria. Streptococci secrete a phage-encoded pyrogenic exotoxin that causes fever and rash in scarlet fever. *S. mutans* produces caries by metabolizing sucrose to lactic acid (which causes demineralization of tooth enamel) and by secreting high-molecular-weight glucans that promote aggregation of bacteria and plaque formation.[103] Poststreptococcal autoimmune diseases of the heart (rheumatic fever) may result from antistreptococcal M protein antibodies that cross-react with cardiac myosin.[104] Finally, streptococci have been referred to as flesh-eating bacteria, secondary to an exfoliating skin condition, which is a rare complication of infection by group A streptococci.[105]

MORPHOLOGY. Streptococcal infections are characterized by diffuse interstitial neutrophilic infiltrates with minimal destruction of host tissues. The skin lesions caused by streptococci (furuncles, carbuncles, and impetigo) resemble those of staphylococci, although there is less tendency to form discrete abscesses.

Erysipelas is most common among middle-aged persons in warm climates and is caused by exotoxins released chiefly from group A and occasionally group C streptococci. It is characterized by rapidly spreading, erythematous cutaneous swelling that may begin on the face or, less frequently, on the body or an extremity. The rash has a sharp, well-demarcated, serpiginous border and may form a "butterfly" distribution on the face (Fig. 9–35). On histologic examination, there is a diffuse, acute edematous, neutrophilic, interstitial reaction in the dermis and epidermis extending into the subcutaneous tissues. The leukocytic infiltration is more intense about vessels and the skin adnexa. Microabscesses may be formed, but tissue necrosis is usually minor.

Streptococcal pharyngitis, which is the major antecedent of poststreptococcal glomerulonephritis (Chapter 21), is marked by edema, epiglottic swelling, and punctate abscesses of the tonsillar crypts, sometimes accompanied by cervical lymphadenopathy. With extension of the pharyngeal infection, there may be encroachment on the airways, especially if there is peritonsillar or retropharyngeal abscess formation **(quinsy sore throat)**. On microscopic examination, these lesions show vasodilation, spreading edema, and intense diffuse neutrophilic exudation, often with a liberal admixture of mononuclear phagocytes.

Pneumococci are important causes of lobar pneumonia (described in Chapter 16 and pictured in Figure 9–12).

Scarlet fever, associated with streptococcal group A pharyngitis and tonsillitis, is most frequent between the ages of 3 and 15 years. It is manifested by a punctate erythematous rash that is most abundant over the trunk and inner aspects of the arms and legs. The face is also involved, but usually a small area about the mouth remains relatively unaffected to produce a circumoral pallor. On microscopic examination, there is a characteristic acute, edematous, neutrophilic inflammatory reaction within the affected tissues (i.e., the oropharynx, skin, and lymph nodes). The inflammatory involvement of the epidermis is usually followed by hyperkeratosis of the skin, which accounts for the scaling during defervescence.

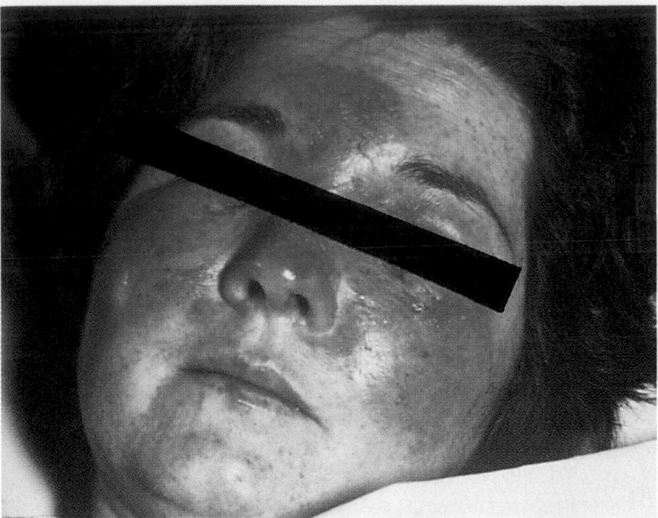

Figure 9–35

Streptococcal erysipelas.

Clostridial Infections

Clostridium species are gram-positive bacilli that grow under anaerobic conditions and produce spores that are frequently present in the soil. There are four types of *Clostridium* that cause human disease:

1. *Clostridium perfringens (welchii), Clostridium septicum,* and other species invade traumatic and surgical wounds and cause an anaerobic cellulitis or myonecrosis *(gas gangrene),* contaminate illegal abortions and cause uterine myonecrosis, cause mild food poisoning, and infect the small bowel of ischemic or neutropenic patients to produce severe sepsis.
2. *Clostridium tetani* proliferates in puncture wounds and in the umbilical stump of newborn infants in developing countries and releases a potent neurotoxin, called tetanospasmin, that causes convulsive contractions of skeletal muscles (lockjaw).
3. *Clostridium botulinum* grows in inadequately sterilized canned foods and releases a potent neurotoxin that blocks synaptic release of acetylcholine and causes a severe paralysis of respiratory and skeletal muscles (botulism).
4. *Clostridium difficile* overgrows other intestinal flora in antibiotic-treated patients, releases multiple toxins, and causes pseudomembranous colitis (Chapter 18).

Severe trauma, gross contamination, and delayed surgical debridement all contribute to high rates of gas gangrene during wars. In peacetime, 50% of the severe *C. perfringens* infections follow accidents, whereas the other 50% follow intestinal and gallbladder surgery. Tetanus toxoid (formalin-fixed neurotoxin) is part of the DPT (diphtheria, pertussis, and tetanus) immunizations given to children that has greatly decreased the incidence of tetanus in the United States and in developing countries.

Pathogenesis. Clostridia release collagenase and hyaluronidase that degrade extracellular matrix proteins and contribute to bacterial invasiveness, but their most powerful virulence factors are the many toxins they produce. *C. perfringens* secretes 12 toxins, the most important of which is *α toxin.*[106] The α toxin is a phospholipase C that degrades lecithin, a major component of cell membranes, and so destroys red blood cells, platelets, and muscle cells, *causing myonecrosis.* The α toxin also has a sphingomyelinase activity that contributes to nerve sheath damage. The *θ toxin* binds cholesterol and forms a membrane-destabilizing pore that causes leukocyte lysis, explaining the paucity of polymorphonuclear leukocytes in the lesions of gas gangrene. The *β toxin* is a major cause of enteritis in sheep, calves, and pigs and causes food poisoning in malnourished persons who eat the meat of infected animals. *Enterotoxin* forms pores in the target epithelial cell membranes and lyses the cells and is the major cause of *C. perfringens* food poisoning.

The *C. tetani* neurotoxin, like those of *C. botulinum*, is composed of a light chain, which is catalytic, and a heavy chain, which is necessary for toxin specificity and cell targeting.[107] Tetanus toxin is bound by gangliosides on peripheral nerves, transported to the nucleus within the axon, released, and taken up by inhibitory neurons. There tetanus toxin, which is a protease, cleaves synaptobrevin, the major transmembrane protein of the synaptic vesicles of the inhibitory neurons. Secretion of inhibitory neurotransmitters, which normally control muscle spasms, is blocked, leading to the tetanal contractions.

C. botulinum makes numerous extremely potent neurotoxins, which are released when the organisms die and autolyse. Botulinum toxins act at the peripheral nerve endings, where they are bound, cleaving either synaptobrevin (as described for tetanus toxin) or synapse-associated proteins, called SNAP-25 and syntaxin. Toxin-infected neurons are unable to release acetylcholine at the neuromuscular junction and at the synaptic ganglia and parasympathetic motor end-plates of the autonomic nervous system, leading to descending paralysis from the cranial nerves down to the extremities.

C. difficile produces *toxin A,* which is an enterotoxin and a potent chemoattractant for granulocytes, and *toxin B,* a cytotoxin, which causes distinctive cytopathic effects in cultured cells and is used in the diagnosis of *C. difficile* infections. Both toxins are part of a pathogenicity island, which is absent from the chromosomes of nonpathogenic strains of *C. difficile*.[108]

MORPHOLOGY. **Clostridial cellulitis**, which originates in wounds, can be differentiated from infection caused by pyogenic cocci by its foul odor, its thin discolored exudate, and the relatively prompt and wide tissue destruction. On microscopic examination, the amount of tissue necrosis is disproportionate to the number of neutrophils and gram-positive bacteria present (Fig. 9–36). Clostridial cellulitis, which often has granulation tissue at its borders, is treatable by debridement and antibiotics.

In contrast, **clostridial gas gangrene** is life threatening and is characterized by marked edema and enzymatic necrosis of involved muscle cells 1 to 3 days after injury. An extensive fluid exudate, which is lacking in inflammatory cells, causes swelling of the affected region and the overlying skin, forming large, bullous vesicles that rupture. Gas bubbles caused by bacterial fermentations appear within the gangrenous tissues. As the infection progresses, the inflamed muscles become soft, blue-black, friable, and semifluid as a result of the massive proteolytic action of the released bacterial enzymes. On microscopic examination, there is severe **myonecrosis**, extensive hemolysis, and marked vascular injury, with thrombosis. *C. perfringens* is also associated with dusk-colored, wedge-shaped infarcts in the small bowel, particularly of neutropenic patients. Regardless of the location of the source, when *C. perfringens* disseminates hematogenously, there is widespread formation of gas bubbles. Despite the severe neurologic damage caused by botulinum and tetanus toxins, the neuropathologic changes are subtle and nonspecific.

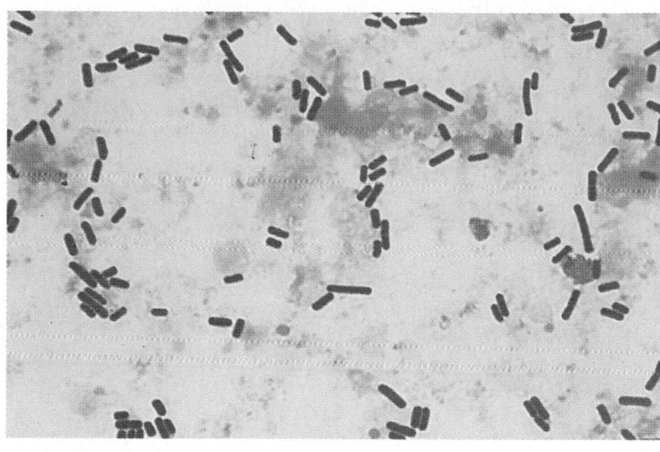

Figure 9–36 ■

Boxcar-shaped gram-positive *Clostridium perfringens* in gangrenous tissue.

Non–Spore-Forming Anaerobic Infections

SEPTIC ABORTION, SALPINGITIS, AND PERIODONTAL ABSCESSES (*PREVOTELLA*)

Anaerobic non–spore-forming bacteria are the most frequent commensal organisms in the gastrointestinal tract (99.9%), female genitals, mouth, and skin.[109] These organisms include gram-negative bacilli *(Bacteroides, Prevotella,* and *Fusobacterium),* gram-positive bacilli *(Actinomyces* and *Propionibacterium acnes*), and gram-positive cocci *(Peptostreptococcus).* In contrast to the spore-forming anaerobes (*Clostridium* species), the non–spore-forming anaerobes do not secrete toxins. Instead, these organisms are for the most part opportunistic pathogens, causing acne in the oil-laden pores of adolescents *(Propionibacterium),* intra-abdominal abscesses secondary to surgery or perforation (*Bacteroides fragilis* and others), septic abortion, salpingitis, and periodontal abscesses *(Prevotella).*

MORPHOLOGY. *Prevotella,* alone or in association with aerobic organisms, is found in abscesses and phlegmons mostly above the diaphragm (e.g., in the floor of the mouth, the retropharynx, and even the lung and brain). *B. fragilis* is typically a cause of, or a participant in, intra-abdominal and retroperitoneal sepsis and in pelvic peritonitis of women beyond their 20s; sometimes it infects surgical abdominal wounds. It may also be present in lung abscesses. In all these lesions, the pus is often discolored and foul smelling, especially in lung abscesses, and the suppuration is often poorly walled off. Otherwise, these lesions pathologically resemble those of the common pyogenic infections.

INFECTIONS OF CHILDHOOD AND ADOLESCENCE

With the exception of EBV, the cause of infectious mononucleosis, all of the infectious agents described here are now in theory preventable by vaccination. Still these viruses and bacteria, which are among the best studied, cause not infrequent miniepidemics in the United States and are responsible for considerable morbidity and mortality in the developing world, where vaccination rates are still regrettably low.

Measles

Measles (rubeola) virus is the cause of 1.5 million deaths per year among third world children, who by reasons of poor nutrition are 10 to 1000 times more likely to die of measles pneumonia than are Western children.[110] In the United States, the incidence of measles has decreased dramatically since 1963, when a measles vaccine was licensed. However, epidemics of measles affecting as many as 10,000 children still occur among unvaccinated individuals and among vaccinated individuals who did not develop protective immunity (primary vaccine failure).[111]

Pathogenesis. Measles virus is an RNA virus of the paramyxovirus family that includes mumps, respiratory syncytial virus (the major cause of lower respiratory infections in infants), and parainfluenza virus (the cause of croup). There is only one strain of measles virus. It has an envelope that contains a hemagglutinin that binds to many host cells by CD46, a complement regulatory protein that inactivates C3 convertases.[112] Measles virus is spread by respiratory droplets and multiplies within upper respiratory epithelial cells and mononuclear cells, including B and T lymphocytes and macrophages. A transient viremia spreads the measles virus throughout the body and may cause croup, pneumonia, diarrhea with protein-losing enteropathy, keratitis with scarring and blindness, encephalitis, and hemorrhages ("black measles"). Most children, however, develop T cell–mediated immunity to measles virus that controls the viral infection and produces the measles rash, a hypersensitivity reaction to viral antigens in the skin. The rash does not occur in patients with deficiencies in cell-mediated immunity but does occur in agammaglobulinemic patients. Antibody-mediated immunity to measles virus protects against reinfection. Subacute sclerosing panencephalitis (described in Chapter 30) and measles inclusion body encephalitis (in immunocompromised individuals) are rare late complications of measles caused by hypermutated, "defective" viruses that cannot produce matrix or envelope proteins.[113]

MORPHOLOGY. The blotchy, reddish brown rash of measles virus infection on the face, trunk, and proximal extremities is produced by dilated skin vessels, edema, and a moderate, nonspecific, mononuclear perivascular infiltrate. Ulcerated mucosal lesions in the oral cavity near the opening of Stensen ducts (the pathognomonic Koplik spots) are marked by necrosis, neutrophil exudate, and neovascularization. The lymphoid organs typically have marked follicular hyperplasia, large germinal centers, and randomly distributed multinucleate giant cells, called Warthin-Finkeldey cells, which have eosinophilic nuclear and cytoplasmic inclusion bodies. These are pathognomonic of measles and are also found in the lung and sputum (Fig. 9–37). The milder forms of measles pneumonia show the same peribronchial and interstitial mononuclear infiltration seen in other nonlethal viral infections. In severe or neglected cases, bacterial superinfection may be a cause of death.

Mumps

The mumps vaccine reduced the incidence of mumps by 99% in the United States, but outbreaks still occur among schoolchildren in states that lack mumps immunization laws.[114] Mumps virus causes a transient inflammation of the parotid glands and, less often, of the testes, pancreas,

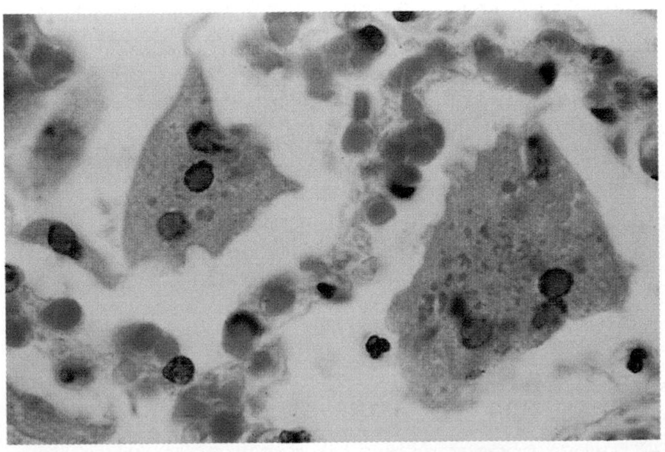

Figure 9–37

Measles giant cells in the lung. Note the glassy eosinophilic intranuclear inclusions.

and central nervous system. Mumps virus is similar in structure to measles virus except that the large glycoprotein on its surface has both hemagglutinin and neuraminidase activities. Mumps viruses are spread by respiratory droplets and multiply within upper respiratory epithelial cells, salivary glands, and T cells in lymph nodes. A transient viremia spreads the mumps virus to other glands and the central nervous system through the choroid plexus. Mumps virus is a rare cause of aseptic meningitis and encephalitis.

MORPHOLOGY. In mumps parotitis, which is bilateral in 70% of cases, affected glands are enlarged, have a doughy consistency, and are moist, glistening, and reddish brown on cross-section. On microscopic examination, the gland interstitium is edematous and diffusely infiltrated by histiocytes, lymphocytes, and plasma cells that compress acini and ducts. Neutrophils and necrotic debris may fill the ductal lumen and cause focal damage to the ductal epithelium.

In **mumps orchitis**, testicular swelling may be marked, caused by edema, mononuclear cell infiltration, and focal hemorrhages. Because the testis is tightly contained within the tunica albuginea, parenchymal swelling may compromise the blood supply and cause areas of infarction. Sterility, when it occurs, is caused by scars and atrophy of the testis after resolution of viral infection.

In the enzyme-rich pancreas, lesions may be destructive, causing parenchymal and fat necrosis and polymorphonuclear cell infiltration. Mumps encephalitis causes perivenous demyelinization and perivascular mononuclear cuffing.

Infectious Mononucleosis (Epstein-Barr Virus)

Infectious mononucleosis is a benign, self-limited lymphoproliferative disease caused by EBV, a γ-group herpesvirus. Infectious mononucleosis is characterized by fever, generalized lymphadenopathy, splenomegaly, sore throat, and the appearance in the blood of atypical activated T lymphocytes (mononucleosis cells). Some patients develop hepatitis, meningoencephalitis, and pneumonitis. Infectious mononucleosis occurs principally in late adolescents or young adults (it delights in college students) among upper socioeconomic classes in developed nations. In the rest of the world, primary infection with EBV occurs in childhood, is usually asymptomatic, and confers immunity to subsequent reinfection.

Pathogenesis. EBV is transmitted by close human contact, frequently with the saliva during kissing. An EBV envelope glycoprotein binds to CD21 protein, the complement receptor CR2[115] (Chapter 3) present on epithelial cells and B cells. The virus enters the cytoplasm of epithelial cells by directly fusing with the plasma membrane and of B cells by fusing with endosomal membranes. The virus initially penetrates nasopharyngeal, oropharyngeal, and salivary epithelial cells (Fig. 9–38). Simultaneously, it spreads to underlying lymphoid tissue and, more specifically, to B lymphocytes. Infection of B cells may take one of two forms. In a minority of B cells, there is productive infection with lysis of infected cells and release of virions that reinfect oropharyngeal epithelium and persist as a subclinical productive infection. Thus, the agent is shed in the saliva. In most B cells, however, the virus associates with the host cell genome, giving rise to latent infection. B cells that harbor the EBV genome undergo polyclonal activation and proliferation. Two EBV proteins, EBNA2 and latent membrane protein 1 (LMP-1), are associated with such B-cell immortalization.[116] LMP-1 appears to act by binding to a host cell protein called tumor necrosis factor receptor–associated factor, which is involved in signal transduction and activation of B lymphocytes. B cells then disseminate in the circulation and secrete antibodies with several specificities, including the well-known heterophil anti–sheep red blood cell antibodies used for the diagnosis of infectious mononucleosis.

A normal immune response is important in controlling the proliferation of EBV-infected B cells and suppressing cell-free virus. Early in the course of the infection, IgM antibodies are formed against viral capsid antigens; later, IgG antibodies are formed that persist for life. IgA antibodies prevent infection of B cells but increase infectivity of EBV for epithelial cells.[117] More important in the control of polyclonal B-cell proliferation are cytotoxic CD8+ T cells and natural killer cells. Curiously, however, a large number of activated T cells with the phenotypic attributes of suppressor cells are also generated. They are not specific for EBV-infected B cells, so their role in recovery from EBV infection is not clear. Together with the virus-specific cytotoxic T cells, these suppressor T cells appear in the circulation as *atypical lymphocytes*, so characteristic of this disease. In otherwise healthy persons, the fully developed humoral and cellular responses to EBV act as brakes on viral shedding, limiting the number of infected B cells rather than eliminating them. Latent EBV remains in a few B cells as well as in oropharyngeal epithelial cells and, as described in Chapter 8, is associated with the development of Burkitt lymphoma and nasopharyngeal carcinoma, respectively. In Burkitt lymphoma, there is a characteristic 8:14 translocation in which the c-*myc* oncogene is placed into the immunoglobulin heavy chain expression region (Fig. 9–38).

MORPHOLOGY. The major alterations involve the blood, lymph nodes, spleen, liver, central nervous system, and, occasionally, other organs. The **peripheral blood** shows absolute lymphocytosis with a total white cell count between 12,000 and 18,000 cells/ml, more than 60% of which are lymphocytes. Many of these are large, **atypical lymphocytes**, 12 to 16 μm in diameter, characterized by an abundant cytoplasm containing multiple clear vacuolations and an oval, indented, or

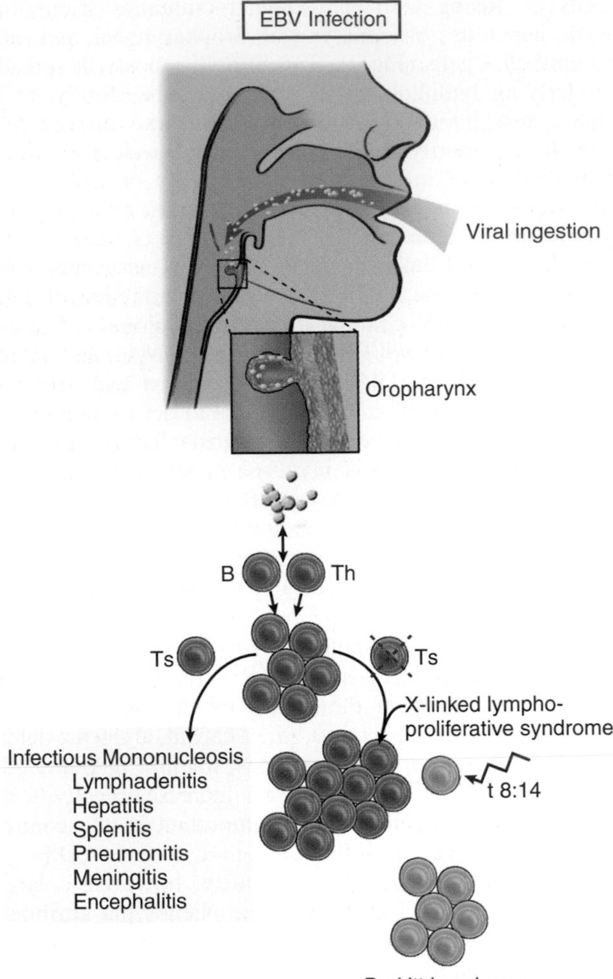

Figure 9–38

Pathways of transmission of the Epstein-Barr virus. In an individual with normal immune function, infection leads to mononucleosis. In the setting of cellular immunodeficiency (e.g., the X-linked immunodeficiency syndrome), proliferation of infected B cells is uncontrolled and may eventuate in B-cell neoplasms. One secondary genetic event that collaborates with Epstein-Barr virus (EBV) to cause B-cell transformation is a balanced 8;14 chromosomal translocation, which is seen in Burkitt's lymphoma. EBV has also been implicated in the pathogenesis of nasopharyngeal carcinoma, Hodgkin's disease, and certain other rare non-Hodgkin's lymphomas. T_h, T helper cell; T_c, cytotoxic T cell.

folded nucleus (Fig. 9–39). These atypical lymphocytes, most of which bear T-cell markers, are usually sufficiently distinctive to permit the diagnosis from examination of a peripheral blood smear.

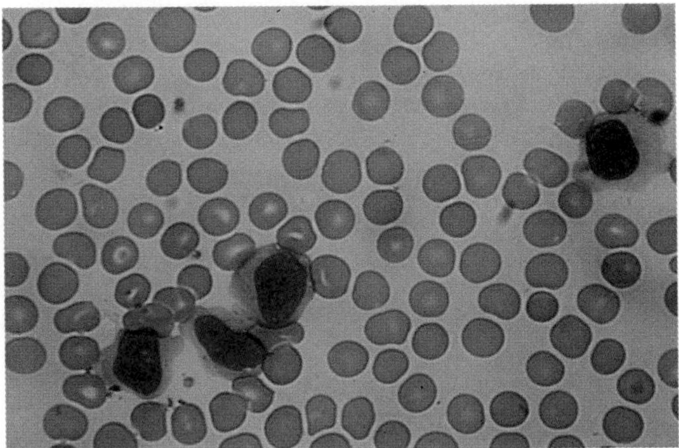

Figure 9–39

Atypical lymphocytes in infectious mononucleosis.

The **lymph nodes** are typically discrete and enlarged throughout the body, principally in the posterior cervical, axillary, and groin regions. On histologic examination, the lymphoid tissue is flooded by atypical lymphocytes, which occupy the paracortical (T-cell) areas. There is, in addition, some B-cell reaction, with enlargement of follicles. Although the underlying architecture is usually preserved, it may be blurred by intense lymphoproliferation. Cells resembling Reed-Sternberg cells may also occasionally be found in the nodes. Together these features sometimes make it difficult to distinguish the nodal morphology from that seen in malignant lymphomas, particularly Hodgkin disease. Differentiation then depends on recognition of the atypical lymphocytes. Similar changes commonly occur in the tonsils and lymphoid tissue of the oropharynx.

The **spleen** is enlarged in most cases, weighing between 300 and 500 gm. It is usually soft and fleshy, with a hyperemic cut surface. The histologic changes are analogous to those of the lymph nodes, showing a heavy infiltration of atypical lymphocytes, which may result either in prominence of the splenic follicles or in some blurring of the architecture. These spleens are especially vulnerable to rupture, possibly resulting in part from infiltration of the trabeculae and capsule by the lymphocytes.

Liver function is almost always transiently impaired to some degree, although hepatomegaly is at most moderate. On histologic examination, atypical lymphocytes are seen in the portal areas and sinusoids, and scattered, isolated cells or foci of parenchymal necrosis filled with lymphocytes may be present. This histologic picture may be difficult to distinguish from that of viral hepatitis.

The **central nervous system** may show congestion, edema, and perivascular mononuclear infiltrates in the leptomeninges. Myelin degeneration and destruction of axis cylinders have been described in the peripheral nerves.

Although infectious mononucleosis classically presents with fever, sore throat, lymphadenitis, and the other features mentioned earlier, often it is more aberrant in behavior. It may present with little or no fever and only malaise, fatigue, and lymphadenopathy, raising the specter of leukemia-lymphoma; as a fever of unknown origin without significant lymphadenopathy or other localized findings; as hepatitis that is difficult to differentiate from one of the hepatotropic viral syndromes; or as a febrile rash resembling rubella. *Ultimately, the diagnosis depends on the following findings (in increasing order of specificity): (1) lymphocytosis with the characteristic atypical lymphocytes in the peripheral blood, (2) a positive heterophil reaction (monospot test), and (3) specific antibodies for EBV antigens (viral capsid antigens, early antigens, or Epstein-Barr nuclear antigen).* In most patients, infectious mononucleosis resolves within 4 to 6 weeks, but sometimes the fatigue lasts longer. One or more complications occasionally supervene. They may involve virtually any organ or system in the body. Perhaps most common is marked hepatic dysfunction with jaundice, elevated hepatic enzyme levels, disturbed appetite, and rarely even liver failure. Other complications involve the nervous system, kidneys, bone marrow, lungs, eyes, heart, and spleen (splenic rupture has been fatal). A more serious complication in those suffering from some form of immunodeficiency, such as AIDS, or receiving immunosuppressive therapy (perhaps after transplantation) is that the polyclonal B-cell proliferation may run amok, leading to death. True monoclonal B-cell lymphomas have also appeared, sometimes preceded by polyclonal lymphoproliferation. These unfortunate consequences were described in a family suffering from an X-linked recessive T-cell defect, and so the condition has been designated Duncan disease or X-linked lymphoproliferation syndrome.

Poliovirus Infection

Poliovirus is a spherical, unencapsulated RNA virus of the enterovirus family. Other members of the family cause childhood diarrhea as well as rashes (coxsackievirus A), conjunctivitis (enterovirus 70), viral meningitis (coxsackieviruses and echovirus), myopericarditis (coxsackievirus B), and jaundice (hepatitis A virus). It is also similar in structure to the rhinoviruses that cause the common cold. The 7500-bp genome encodes four structural proteins, two proteases, and an RNA-dependent RNA polymerase. There are three major strains of poliovirus, each of which is included in the Salk formalin-fixed (killed) vaccine and the Sabin oral, attenuated (live) vaccine.[118] These vaccines, which have nearly eliminated poliovirus from the Western hemisphere, may be used to rid polio from the earth, because the poliovirus, like smallpox virus, infects people but not other animals, is only briefly shed, and is effectively prevented by immunization.[119]

Poliovirus, like other enteroviruses, first infects tissues in the oropharynx, is secreted into the saliva and swallowed, and then multiplies in the intestinal mucosa and lymph nodes, causing a transient viremia and fever. The species specificity of poliovirus for humans is determined by particular amino acid residues that are present in the human receptor, which has numerous immunoglobulin-like domains, but are absent in the homologous mouse protein.[120] In 1 of 100 infected persons, poliovirus invades the central nervous system and replicates in motor neurons of the spinal cord (spinal poliomyelitis) or brain stem (bulbar poliomyelitis). Although it is clear that antivirus antibodies control the disease in most cases, it is not known why some individuals fail to control the virus. Virus spread to the nervous system may be secondary to viremia or by retrograde transport of the virus along axons of motor neurons.[121] Rare cases of poliomyelitis that occur after vaccination are caused by mutations of the attenuated viruses to wild type forms. The neuropathology of poliovirus infection is described in Chapter 30.

Varicella-Zoster Infection (Chickenpox and Shingles)

Two conditions—chickenpox and shingles—are caused by VZV. Chickenpox is an uncomfortable and often scarring childhood illness and a major cause of lost workdays by parents; shingles, caused by VSV reactivation, is a source of morbidity in elderly and immunosuppressed persons.[122] Like HSV, VZV infects mucous membranes, skin, and neurons and causes a self-limited primary infection in immunocompetent individuals. In contrast to HSV, VZV is transmitted in epidemic fashion by aerosols, disseminates hematogenously, and causes widespread vascular skin lesions. VZV primarily infects satellite cells around neurons in the dorsal root ganglia and may recur many years after the primary infection, causing shingles. Localized recurrences of VZV are most frequent and painful in dermatomes innervated by the trigeminal ganglia, where VZV is most likely to exist in a state of latency. One reason that VZV recurs less frequently than HSV is that the genes involved in reactivation in HSV are missing in VSV.[123] In addition, immune surveillance may prevent VZV recur-

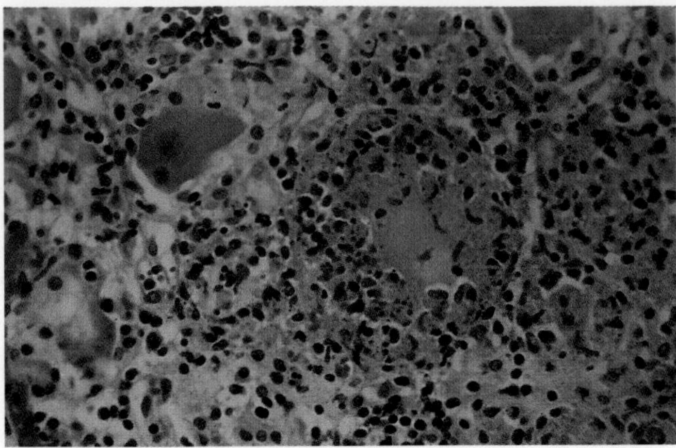

Figure 9–40

Dorsal root ganglion with varicella-zoster virus infection. Note the ganglion cell necrosis and associated inflammation. (Courtesy of Dr. James Morris, Radcliffe Infirmary, Oxford, England.)

rences because shingles occurs most frequently in immunosuppressed or elderly persons.

MORPHOLOGY. The **chickenpox** rash occurs approximately 2 weeks after respiratory infection and travels in multiple waves centrifugally from the torso to the head and extremities. Each lesion progresses rapidly from a macule to a vesicle, which resembles "a dewdrop on a rose petal." On histologic examination, chickenpox vesicles contain intranuclear inclusions of the epithelial cells identical to those of HSV-1 (see Figs. 9–14 and 9–28). After a few days, most chickenpox vesicles rupture, crust over, and heal by regeneration, leaving no scars, whereas traumatic rupture of some vesicles with bacterial superinfection may lead to destruction of the basal epidermal layer and residual scarring.

Shingles occurs when VZVs, which have long remained latent in the dorsal root ganglia after a previous chickenpox infection, are activated and infect sensory nerves that carry viruses to one or more dermatomes. There VZVs cause vesicular lesions, differentiated from chickenpox by the often intense itching, burning, or sharp pain because of the simultaneous radiculoneuritis. This pain is especially strong when the trigeminal nerves are involved; rarely, the geniculate nucleus is involved, causing facial paralysis (Ramsay Hunt syndrome). In the sensory ganglia, there is a dense, predominantly mononuclear infiltrate, with herpetic intranuclear inclusions within neurons and their supporting cells (Fig. 9–40). VZV also causes interstitial pneumonia, encephalitis, transverse myelitis, and necrotizing visceral lesions, particularly in immunosuppressed patients.

Whooping Cough

Whooping cough, caused by the gram-negative coccobacillus *Bordetella pertussis,* is an acute, highly communicable illness characterized by violent coughing paroxysms followed by a loud inspiratory "whoop." Although the DPT vaccine, which contains heat-killed *B. pertussis* bacteria, has greatly reduced the prevalence of whooping cough in the United States, *B. pertussis* infects tens of millions of children and causes hundreds of thousands of deaths annually in the developing world. Because the classical pertussis vaccine causes pain at the site of injection and fever, present efforts are to produce a peptide vaccine containing filamentous hemagglutinin and inactivated toxin.[124]

Pathogenesis. *B. pertussis* colonizes the brush border of the bronchial epithelium and also invades macrophages. Conditions in the upper respiratory tract induce *B. pertussis* to coordinately produce numerous virulence factors, including a hemagglutinin, fimbriae, pertussis toxin, and an adenylate cyclase–hemolysin toxin.[125] The filamentous hemagglutinin binds to carbohydrates on the surface of respiratory epithelial cells as well as to CR3 (Mac-1) integrins on macrophages. Pertussis toxin is an exotoxin composed of five distinct peptides, including a catalytic peptide S1 that shows homology with the catalytic peptides of cholera toxin and *E. coli* heat-labile toxin.[126] Like cholera toxin, pertussis toxin ADP-ribosylates and inactivates guanine nucleotide–binding proteins, so that these G proteins no longer transduce signals from host plasma membrane receptors. Other *B. pertussis* toxins include a hemolysin important in early colonization, a bacterial lipopolysaccharide that has endotoxin activity, and a small peptidoglycan toxin that competes for 5-hydroxytryptamine sites on respiratory epithelial cells. Together these toxins reduce the number of ciliated respiratory epithelial cells and decrease the quantity of cilia per cell.

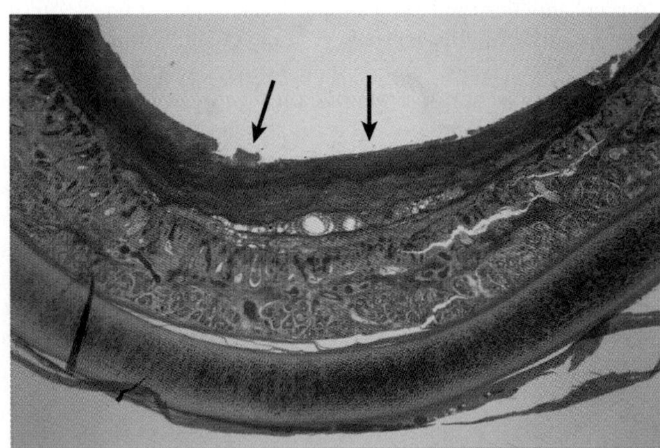

Figure 9–41

Whooping cough showing bacilli *(arrows)* covering the cilia of bronchial columnar epithelial cells.

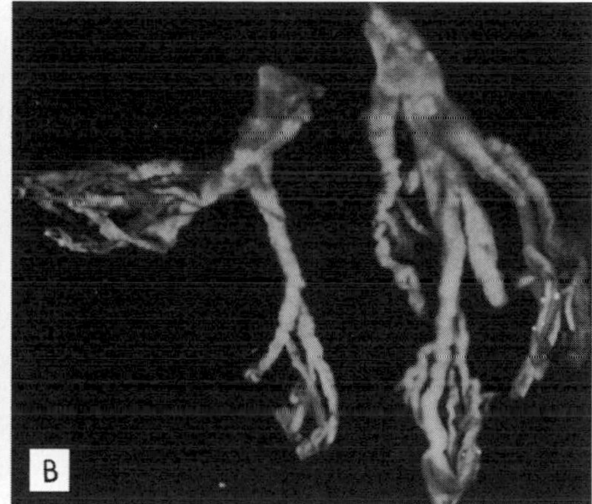

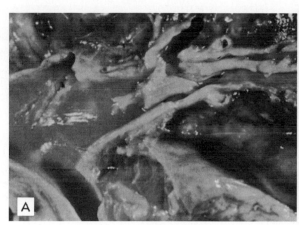

Figure 9–42

Membrane of diphtheria lying within a transverse bronchus (*A*) and forming a perfect cast (removed from the lung) of the branching respiratory tree (*B*).

MORPHOLOGY. *Bordetella* bacteria cause a laryngotracheobronchitis that in severe cases features bronchial mucosal erosion, hyperemia, and copious mucopurulent exudate (Fig. 9–41). Unless superinfected, the lung alveoli remain open and intact. In parallel with a striking peripheral lymphocytosis (up to 90%), there is hypercellularity and enlargement of the mucosal lymph follicles and peribronchial lymph nodes.

Diphtheria

Diphtheria is caused by a slender gram-positive rod, *Corynebacterium diphtheriae,* that is passed from person to person through aerosols or skin shedding. *C. diphtheriae* causes a range of illnesses: asymptomatic carriage; skin lesions in neglected wounds of combat troops in the tropics; and a life-threatening syndrome that includes formation of a tough pharyngeal membrane and toxin-mediated damage to the heart, nerves, and other organs. In contrast to *Bordetella* and other bacteria, *C. diphtheriae* has only one toxin, which is encoded by a lysogenic phage and described in detail previously. Inclusion of diphtheria toxoid (formalin-fixed toxin) in the childhood vaccines does not prevent colonization with *C. diphtheriae* but protects immunized individuals from the lethal effects of released toxin. Recent large outbreaks of diphtheria in the former Soviet Union resulted from decreased vaccination rates, socioeconomic instability, and a deteriorating health infrastructure.[127]

MORPHOLOGY. Inhaled *C. diphtheriae* proliferate at the site of attachment on the mucosa of the nasopharynx, oropharynx, larynx, or trachea but also form satellite lesions in the esophagus or lower airways. Release of exotoxin causes necrosis of the epithelium, accompanied by an outpouring of a dense fibrinosuppurative exudate. The coagulation of this exudate on the ulcerated necrotic surface creates a tough, dirty gray to black, superficial membrane (Fig. 9–42). Neutrophilic infiltration in the underlying tissues is intense and is accompanied by marked vascular congestion, interstitial edema, and fibrin exudation. When the membrane sloughs off its inflamed and vascularized bed, bleeding and asphyxiation may occur. With control of the infection, the membrane is coughed up or removed by enzymatic digestion, and the inflammatory reaction subsides.

Although the bacterial invasion remains localized, generalized reticuloendothelial hyperplasia of the spleen and lymph nodes ensues owing to the absorption of soluble exotoxin into the blood. The exotoxin may cause fatty myocardial change with isolated myofiber necrosis, polyneuritis with degeneration of the myelin sheaths and axis cylinders, and (less commonly) fatty change and focal necroses of parenchymal cells in the liver, kidneys, and adrenals.

OPPORTUNISTIC AND AIDS-ASSOCIATED INFECTIONS

Infections Associated With Neutropenia and Helper T-Cell Depletion

Infections that are usually innocuous or dormant in normal individuals appear with increased frequency in "altered" hosts with genetic or acquired immunodeficiencies. Such opportunistic infections occur in particular in patients receiving cytotoxic and immunosuppressive therapy for tumors, in recipients of tissue transplants, in patients with autoimmune disease, and most dramatically in patients with AIDS (Chapter 7). Viral, bacterial, fungal, and parasitic infections all fall into this category, and we discuss some of the more important examples.

Cytomegalic Inclusion Disease

CMV is a β-group herpesvirus that causes an asymptomatic or mononucleosis-like infection in healthy individuals. CMV, however, can also cause devastating systemic infections in neonates and in immunosuppressed patients. CMV is spread by (1) intrauterine transmission, (2) perinatal transmission at childbirth, (3) mother's milk, (4) respiratory droplets, (5) semen and vaginal fluid, (6) blood transfusions (in about 5% of blood donors, the circulating leukocytes contain latent CMV), and (7) transplantation of virus-infected grafts from a donor with a latent infection.[128] In immunocompetent individuals, CMV infects and remains latent in white blood cells. In immunocompromised patients, CMV causes esophagitis, colitis, hepatitis, pneumonitis, renal tubulitis, chorioretinitis, and meningoencephalitis. In patients with AIDS, CMV pneumonitis is almost always accompanied by *Pneumocystis carinii,* which determines the outcome of infection. In contrast, CMV causes an interstitial pneumonitis in recipients of autologous marrow transplants, which is usually not complicated by *P. carinii* infection and appears to be facilitated by graft-versus-host reactions.[129]

Although 90% of CMV-infected neonates have no sequelae, full-blown congenital CMV infection resembles erythroblastosis fetalis. Affected infants manifest a hemolytic form of anemia, jaundice, thrombocytopenic, purpura, hepatosplenomegaly (due to extramedullary hematopoiesis), pneumonitis, deafness, chorioretinitis, and extensive brain damage. At least half the infants with such severe disease die; some of the survivors are mentally retarded.

MORPHOLOGY. The lesions caused by disseminated CMV infection in the newborn and in immunosuppressed patients are similar and so are described together. Cells infected with CMV are markedly enlarged, with large purple intranuclear inclusions surrounded by a clear halo and smaller basophilic cytoplasmic inclusions (Fig. 9–43). Disseminated CMV causes focal necrosis with minimal inflammation in virtually any organ but most often in the salivary glands, kidneys, liver, lungs, gut, pancreas, thyroid, adrenals, and brain. Cytomegalic inclusions are present in both endothelial and epithelial cells and are most abundant in the renal tubular epithelium, hepatocytes, and lining cells of portal bile ducts. In the lung, CMV also infects alveolar epithelial cells, macrophages, and endothelial cells and causes an interstitial pneumonitis with intra-alveolar edema, proteinaceous exudate, and focal hyaline membranes. CMV causes sharply punched-out ulcerations in the small and large intestines.

CMV encephalitis is most frequent in congenital infections, in which there are focal acute inflammatory changes with inclusion-bearing giant cells distributed in a narrow band in the subependymal and subpial tissue as well as necrotic lesions irregularly scattered in the cerebrum. CMV lesions are often located about the lateral ventricles, aqueduct, and fourth ventricle and may become calcified. CMV chorioretinitis can occur alone or together with other organ involvements and is a frequent cause of blindness in patients with AIDS.

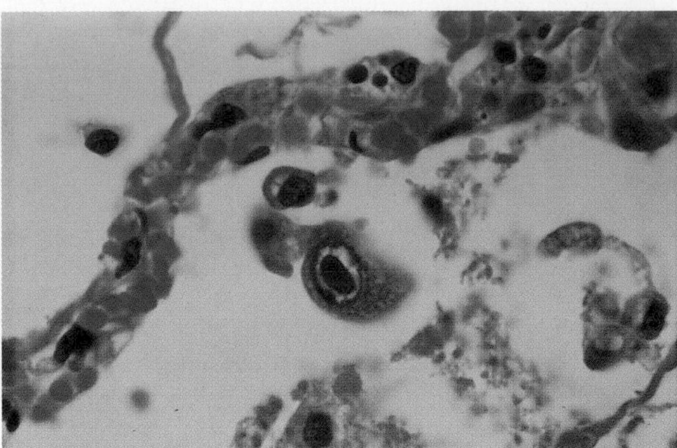

Figure 9–43

Cytomegalovirus: distinct nuclear and ill-defined cytoplasmic inclusions in the lung. (Courtesy of Dr. Arlene Sharpe.)

Pseudomonas Infection

Pseudomonas aeruginosa is an opportunistic gram-negative bacterium that is a frequent, deadly pathogen of patients with cystic fibrosis, severe burns, or neutropenia.[130] Most patients with cystic fibrosis die of pulmonary failure secondary to chronic infection with *P. aeruginosa.* In addition, a related bacterium called *Burkholderia cepacia*, which may be transmitted between cystic fibrosis patients, causes an acute necrotizing pneumonia and fever, which may be fatal. Although gram-positive cocci are most frequently present soon after extensive skin burns, *P. aeruginosa* eventually predominates, spreads locally, and causes sepsis. *P. aeruginosa* is the third leading cause of hospital-acquired infections (after *S. aureus* and *E. coli*); it has been cultured from washbasins, respirator tubing, nursery cribs, and even antiseptic-containing bottles.

P. aeruginosa also causes corneal keratitis in wearers of contact lenses, endocarditis and osteomyelitis in intravenous drug abusers, external otitis (swimmer's ear) in normal individuals, and severe external otitis in diabetics.

Pathogenesis. *P. aeruginosa* has coregulated pili and

adherence proteins that mediate adherence to epithelial cells and lung mucin as well as an endotoxin that causes the symptoms and signs of gram-negative sepsis. *Pseudomonas* also has a number of virulence factors that are distinctive. (1) *Pseudomonas* bacteria in the lungs of patients with cystic fibrosis form colonies on a biofilm composed of a mucoid exopolysaccharide called *alginate*. Alginate, which is similar to that of seaweed, covers the bacteria and protects them from antibacterial antibodies, complement, and phagocytes. (2) The organisms secrete *exotoxin A*, which is similar in structure to diphtheria toxin and, like diphtheria toxin, inhibits protein synthesis by ADP-ribosylating EF-2, a ribosomal G protein.[131] (3) *P. aeruginosa* elaborates *exoenzyme S*, which ADP-ribosylates small G proteins, including p21^{ras}, and so may interfere with host cell growth. (4) The organisms also secrete a phospholipase C that lyses red blood cells and degrades pulmonary surfactant and an elastase that degrades IgGs and extracellular matrix proteins and so may be important in tissue invasion and destruction of the cornea in keratitis. (5) Finally, *P. aeruginosa* produces iron-containing compounds that are extremely toxic to endothelial cells and so may cause the vascular lesions characteristic of this infection.[132]

MORPHOLOGY. *Pseudomonas* pneumonia, particularly in the altered host, is the prototype of **necrotizing inflammation**, distributing through the terminal airways in a fleur-de-lis pattern, with striking whitish necrotic centers and red hemorrhagic peripheral areas. On microscopic examination, masses of organisms cloud the host tissue with a bluish haze, concentrating in the wall of blood vessels, where host cells undergo coagulation necrosis and nuclei fade away (Fig. 9–44). This picture of gram-negative vasculitis accompanied by thrombosis and hemorrhage, although not pathognomonic, is highly suggestive of *P. aeruginosa*.

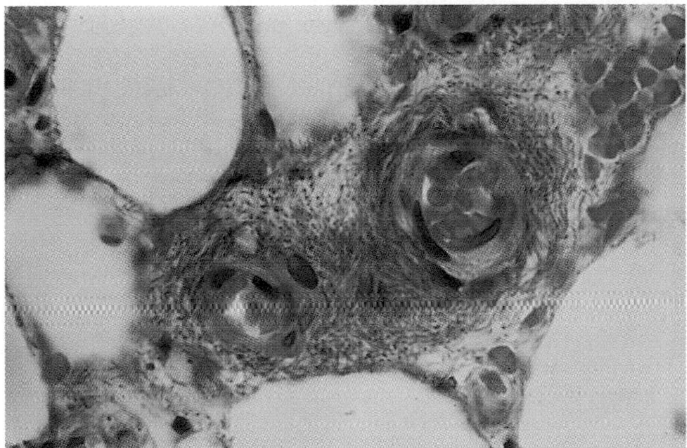

Figure 9–44

Pseudomonas vasculitis in which masses of organisms form a perivascular blue haze.

Bronchial obstruction caused by mucous plugging and *P. aeruginosa* infection are characteristic of cystic fibrosis. Despite antibiotic treatment and the host immune response against the bacteria, chronic *P. aeruginosa* infection results in bronchiectasis and pulmonary fibrosis (Chapter 16).

In skin burns, *P. aeruginosa* proliferates widely, penetrating deeply into the veins to induce massive bacteremias. Well-demarcated necrotic and hemorrhagic skin lesions of oval shape often arise during these bacteremias, called **ecthyma gangrenosum**. DIC is a frequent complication of bacteremia.

Legionnaires Disease

When a lethal pneumonia struck a group of participants at the 1976 convention of the American Legion in Philadelphia, the microbe hunt that ensued led to a hitherto unknown gram-negative bacterial pathogen, *Legionella pneumophila*.[133] Although *L. pneumophila* was not a new pathogen and had caused at least one outbreak of fever in Pontiac, Michigan, in 1968, the bacterium had been missed because the organisms demand culture on special media and are visible in tissue sections only after silver staining. *L. pneumophila* is resistant to chlorine, and epidemic foci have been associated with aerosols from cooling systems of buildings. The same *L. pneumophila* bacterium causes a mild, self-limited fever (Pontiac fever) in otherwise healthy individuals or a severe pneumonia (legionnaires disease) in smokers, the elderly, individuals with chronic lung disease, and immunosuppressed patients.

L. pneumophila is unique among bacteria because it is a facultative intracellular parasite of macrophages and of the aquatic protozoa *Hartmannella vermiformis* and *Tetrahymena pyriformis*. *L. pneumophila* bacteria enter the macrophage in two ways: (1) in nonimmune serum, complement-coated bacteria bind to macrophage CR1 and CR3 complement receptors and are engulfed by pseudopods; and (2) when coated with anti–*L. pneumophila* antibodies, bacteria bind the macrophage Fc receptors and enter by conventional "zipper" phagocytosis. Within the macrophage, *L. pneumophila* fails to induce a respiratory burst; the organisms block phagosome fusion with the lysosome, multiply, and eventually lyse the host cell. A 24-kD protein on the surface of the bacteria (called macrophage infectivity potentiator) is necessary for growth in the macrophages and protozoa and for infectivity in animal models.[134]

MORPHOLOGY. *Legionella* species produce a multifocal pneumonia of fibrinopurulent type that is initially nodular but may become confluent or lobar. The lesions are focused on the alveoli and distal bronchioles, with sparing of the proximal bronchioles and bronchi. A high ratio of mononuclear phagocytes to neutrophils is characteristic, with many destroyed phagocytes at the center of the lesions (leukocytoclasis), surrounded by intact macrophages. Silver-stained bacteria are copious in the leukocytoclastic areas and are also present locally inside large, bubbly-appearing macrophages and in hilar lymph nodes. Secondary inflammation of the walls of small pulmonary arteries and veins is often intense and accompanied by thrombosis. Abscesses are frequent but tend to be small and rarely confluent. These destructive lesions explain the tendency toward organization and scarring.

Listeriosis

Listeria monocytogenes is a gram-positive, motile facultative intracellular bacterium that causes severe food-borne infections.[135] Miniepidemics of *Listeria* have been linked to dairy products, chicken, and hotdogs. Pregnant women, their neonates, and immunosuppressed persons (e.g., transplant recipients or AIDS patients) are particularly susceptible to severe *Listeria* infection. In pregnant women (and sheep and cattle), *Listeria* causes an amnionitis that may result in abortion, stillbirth, or neonatal sepsis. In neonates, *Listeria* may cause disseminated disease (granulomatosis infantiseptica) and an exudative meningitis, also found in immunosuppressed adults.

Listeria has on its surface leucine-rich proteins called *internalins*, which bind to E-cadherin on host epithelial cells and induce phagocytosis of the bacterium.[136] *Listeria* then escape from the phagosome and multiply in the cytosol[137] and use ActA proteins on their surfaces to polymerize host actin and move the bacterium to cell surface filopodia, which break off and release bacteria. Naive macrophages, which internalize *Listeria* through C3 activated on the bacterial surface, fail to kill the bacterium. In contrast, activated macrophages, which depend on cell-mediated immunity, phagocytose and kill the bacterium.

MORPHOLOGY. In acute human infections, *L. monocytogenes* evokes an exudative pattern of inflammation with numerous neutrophils. The **meningitis** it causes is macroscopically and microscopically indistinguishable from that caused by other pyogens. The finding of gram-positive, mostly intracellular bacillary rods in the cerebrospinal fluid (CSF) is virtually diagnostic. More varied lesions may be encountered in neonates and predisposed adults. Focal abscesses alternate with grayish or yellow nodules representing necrotic amorphous basophilic tissue debris. These can occur in any organ, including the lung, liver, spleen, and lymph nodes. In infections of longer duration, macrophages appear in large numbers, eventually to dispose of the necrotic remnants, but true epithelioid cell granulomas are rare. Infants born live with *Listeria* sepsis often have a papular red rash over the extremities, and listerial abscesses can be seen in the placenta. A smear of the meconium will disclose the gram-positive organisms.

Candidiasis

Candida species, which are part of the normal flora of the skin, mouth, and gastrointestinal tract, are the most frequent cause of human fungal infections. (The most common is *C. albicans.*) These infections vary from superficial lesions in healthy persons to disseminated infections in neutropenic patients. *Candida* grow as yeast forms, tandem arrays of elongated forms without hyphae (pseudohyphae), and true hyphae with septa. All may be mixed together in the same tissue, and all are stained with Gram, periodic acid–Schiff, or methenamine silver stain. *Candida* grows best on warm, moist surfaces and so frequently causes vaginitis (particularly during pregnancy), diaper rash, and oral thrush. Dishwashers, diabetics, and burn patients are also particularly susceptible to superficial candidiasis. Chronic mucocutaneous candidiasis occurs in persons with AIDS, in individuals with inherited or iatrogenic defects in T cell–mediated immunity, and in persons with polyendocrine deficiencies (hypoparathyroidism, hypoadrenalism, and hypothyroidism). Severe disseminated candidiasis is associated with neutropenia secondary to chronic granulomatous disease, leukemia, anticancer therapy, or immunosuppression after transplantation. *Candida* is directly introduced into the blood by intravenous lines, catheters, peritoneal dialysis, cardiac surgery, or intravenous drug abuse. Although the course of candidal sepsis is less rampant than that of bacterial sepsis, disseminated *Candida* eventually causes shock and DIC.

Pathogenesis. *Candida* has molecules on its surface that mediate its adherence to tissues, including (1) a receptor homologous to the human CR3 integrin, which binds arginine–glycine–aspartic acid (RGD) groups on iC3b, fibrinogen, fibronectin, and laminin; (2) a lectin that binds sugars on epithelial cells; and (3) mannose-containing proteins that bind to lectin-like molecules on epithelial cells.[138] Other virulence-associated factors include secreted aspartyl proteinase, which may be involved in tissue invasion by degrading extracellular matrix proteins, and secreted adenosine, which blocks neutrophil oxygen radical production and degranulation.[139] Finally, the transition from yeast to hyphal forms is important to fungal virulence because hyphae appear to spear their way out of cells, which engulf them.[140]

MORPHOLOGY. *Candida* infections of the oral cavity (thrush) and vagina produce superficial white patches or large, almost fluffy membranes that are easily detached, leaving a reddened, irritated underlying surface. Spread of oral candidiasis, as by a nasogastric tube, may lead to similar lesions in the esophagus (Fig. 9–45). *Candida* also causes cutaneous eczematoid lesions in

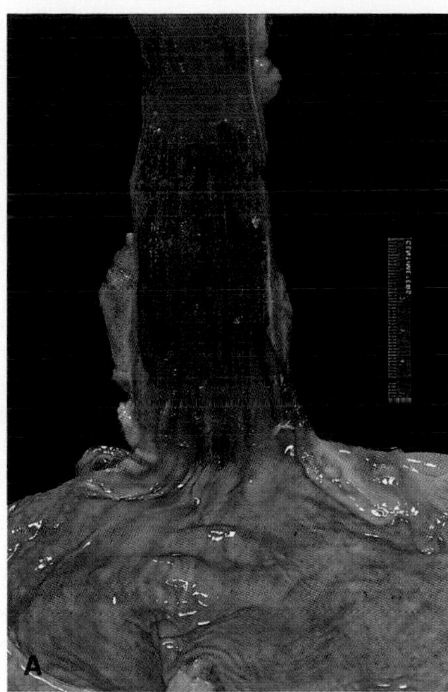

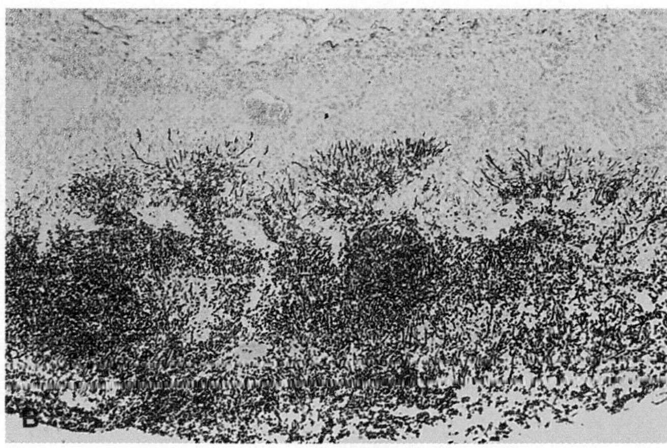

Figure 9–45

A, Severe candidiasis of the distal esophagus. *B*, Silver stain of a section of the same lesion reveals the dense mat of *Candida*.

moist areas of the skin (i.e., between the fingers and toes and in inguinal creases, inframammary folds, and the anogenital region). On microscopic examination, these lesions contain acute and chronic inflammation with microabscesses, but in their chronic states, granulomatous reactions may develop. Sometimes hypersensitivity dermal reactions develop in sites remote from the infections, and these lesions are known as **candidids** or **id reactions.**

Severe, invasive candidiasis associated with immunosuppression or with phagocyte depletion involves the **kidney** in 90% of cases, causing multiple microabscesses in both the cortex and the medulla. On microscopic examination, the yeast or pseudohyphal forms of the fungus occupy the center of the lesion, with a surrounding area of necrosis and polymorphonuclear infiltrate. Some fungal cells may be found inside glomerular capillary loops. *Candida* right-sided **endocarditis**, resulting from direct inoculation of the fungi into the bloodstream, most often in drug addicts, gives rise to large, friable vegetations that frequently break off into emboli. In the lungs, lesions are extensive and polymorphous and often are hemorrhagic and infarct-like owing to fungal invasion of vascular walls. Meningitis, intracerebral abscesses, hepatic abscesses, enteritis, endophthalmitis, multiple subcutaneous abscesses, arthritis, and osteomyelitis are some of the other presentations of disseminated candidiasis. In any of these locations, the fungus may evoke little or no inflammatory reaction, cause the usual suppurative response, or occasionally produce granulomas.

Cryptococcosis

Cryptococcus neoformans is an encapsulated yeast that can cause meningoencephalitis in normal individuals but more frequently in patients with AIDS, leukemia, lymphoma, systemic lupus erythematosus, Hodgkin disease, or sarcoidosis and in transplant recipients. Many of these patients receive high-dose corticosteroids, a major risk factor for *Cryptococcus* infection.

Pathogenesis. *C. neoformans* is present in the soil and in bird (particularly pigeon) droppings and infects patients when it is inhaled. Three properties of *C. neoformans* are associated with virulence: (1) the capsular polysaccharide, a surface molecule that stains bright red with mucicarmine in tissues, stains negative in India ink preparations in CSF, and can be detected with antibody-coated beads in the CSF; (2) resistance to killing by alveolar macrophages; and (3) production of phenol oxidase[141]; this enzyme consumes host epinephrine in the synthesis of fungal melanin, thus protecting the fungi from the epinephrine oxidative system present in the host nervous system. One reason that *C. neoformans* preferentially infects the brain may be that the CSF lacks alternative pathway complement components (present in serum) that bind to the carbohydrate capsule and facilitate phagocytosis and killing by polymorphonuclear cells.

MORPHOLOGY. Although the lung is the primary site of localization, pulmonary infection with *C. neoformans* is usually mild and asymptomatic, even while the fungus is spreading to the central nervous system. *C. neoformans,* however, may form a solitary pulmonary granuloma similar to the

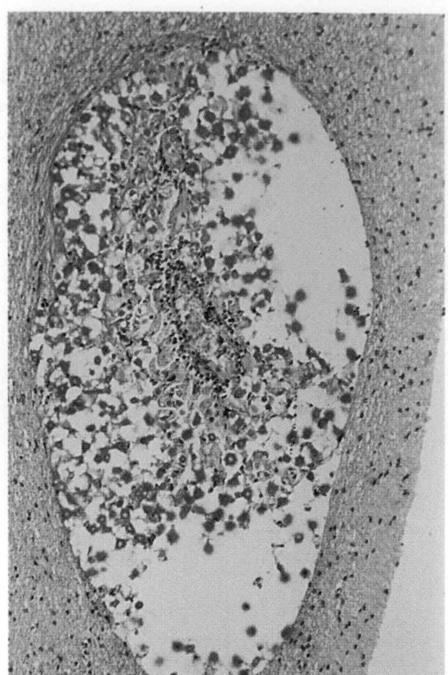

Figure 9–46

Mucicarmine stain of cryptococci (staining red) in a Virchow-Robin perivascular space of the brain (soap-bubble lesion).

coin lesions caused by *Histoplasma*. The major pathologic change of *C. neoformans* is in the central nervous system, including the meninges, cortical gray matter, and basal nuclei. The tissue response to cryptococci is extremely variable. In immunosuppressed patients, organisms may evoke virtually no inflammatory reaction, so gelatinous masses of fungi grow in the meninges or in small cysts within the gray matter (soap-bubble lesions; Fig. 9–46) as though in a culture medium. In nonimmunosuppressed patients or in those with protracted disease, the fungi induce a chronic granulomatous reaction composed of macrophages, lymphocytes, and foreign body type giant cells. Neutrophils and suppuration may also occur, as well as a rare granulomatous arteritis of the circle of Willis. In severely immunosuppressed persons, *C. neoformans* may disseminate widely to the skin, liver, spleen, adrenals, and bones.

Aspergillosis

Aspergillus is an ubiquitous mold that causes allergies (brewer's lung) in otherwise healthy persons and serious *sinusitis, pneumonia,* and *fungemia* in neutropenic persons. Molecular epidemiologic studies of *Aspergillus* isolated from opportunistic infections show many different strains of *Aspergillus,* suggesting that characteristics of the host are more important than characteristics of the fungi.[142]

Pathogenesis. Sialic acid moieties on the surface bind extracellular matrix proteins laminin and fibrinogen.[143] *Aspergillus* species secrete three toxins that may be important in human disease. The carcinogen *aflatoxin* is made by *Aspergillus* species growing on the surface of peanuts and may be a major cause of liver cancer in Africa (Chapter 10).[144] *Restrictocin* and *mitogillin* are ribotoxins that inhibit host cell protein synthesis by degrading mRNAs.[145] In addition, mitogillin is a potent inducer of IgE and so may be involved in host allergic responses to *Aspergillus.* Sensitization to the *Aspergillus* spores produces an allergic alveolitis by inducing type III and type IV hypersensitivity reactions (Chapter 16). *Allergic bronchopulmonary aspergillosis,* which is associated with hypersensitivity arising from superficial colonization of the bronchial mucosa and often occurs in asthmatic patients, may eventually result in chronic obstructive lung disease.

MORPHOLOGY. Colonizing aspergillosis (aspergilloma) implies growth of the fungus in pulmonary cavities with minimal or no invasion of the tissues. The cavities usually result from preexisting tuberculosis, bronchiectasis, old infarcts, or abscesses. Proliferating masses of fungal hyphae called fungus balls form brownish masses lying free within the cavities. The surrounding inflammatory reaction may be sparse, or there may be chronic inflammation and fibrosis. Patients with aspergillomas usually have recurrent hemoptysis.

Invasive aspergillosis is an opportunistic infection confined to immunosuppressed and debilitated hosts. The primary lesions are usually in the lung, but widespread hematogenous dissemination with involvement of the heart valves, brain, and kidneys is common. The pulmonary lesions take the form of necrotizing pneumonia with sharply delineated, rounded, gray foci with hemorrhagic borders, often referred to as **target lesions**. Aspergillus forms fruiting bodies (particularly in cavities) and septate filaments, 5 to 10 μm thick, branching at acute angles (40 degrees) (Fig. 9–47). *Aspergillus* has a tendency to invade blood vessels, and thus areas of hemorrhage and infarction are usually superimposed on the necrotizing, inflammatory tissue reactions. Rhinocerebral *Aspergillus* infection in immunosuppressed individuals resembles that caused by Phycomycetes (e.g., mucormycosis).

Mucormycosis

Mucormycosis is an opportunistic infection of neutropenic persons and ketoacidotic diabetics caused by "bread mold fungi," including *Mucor, Absidia, Rhizopus,* and *Cunninghamella,* which are collectively referred to as the Phycomycetes. These fungi, which are widely distributed in

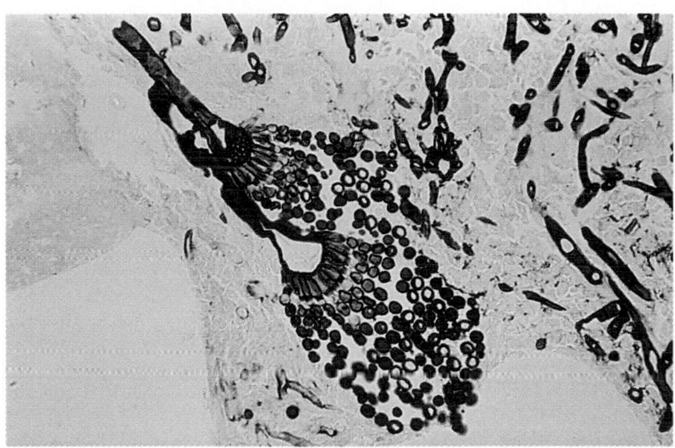

Figure 9–47

Aspergillus colony showing fruiting body and septate hyphae in the nasal septum (silver stain).

nature and cause no harm to immunocompetent individuals, infect immunosuppressed patients somewhat less frequently than do *Candida* or *Aspergillus*.

MORPHOLOGY. The three primary sites of *Mucor* invasion are the nasal sinuses, lungs, and gastrointestinal tract, depending on whether the spores (widespread in dust and air) are inhaled or ingested. In diabetics, the fungus may spread from nasal sinuses to the orbit, and brain, giving rise to **rhinocerebral mucormycosis**. The Phycomycetes cause local tissue necrosis, invade arterial walls, and penetrate the periorbital tissues and cranial vault. Meningoencephalitis follows, sometimes complicated by cerebral infarctions when fungi invade arteries and induce thrombosis. Phycomycetes form nonseptate, irregularly wide (6 to 50 μm) fungal hyphae with frequent right-angle branching, which are readily demonstrated in the necrotic tissues by hematoxylin and eosin or special fungal stains (Fig. 9–48).

Lung involvement with *Mucor* may be secondary to rhinocerebral disease, or it may be primary in patients with hematologic neoplasms. The lung lesions combine areas of hemorrhagic pneumonia with vascular thrombi and distal infarctions.

Pneumocystis Pneumonia

Pneumocystis carinii is a ubiquitous organism that produces no disease in normal individuals but causes a severe pneumonia in most patients with AIDS and in children with protein-calorie malnutrition.[37] *Pneumocystis* pneumonia is frequently the first diagnosed opportunistic infection in HIV-1–infected persons and is a leading cause of death in AIDS. *Pneumocystis* is diagnosed by the demonstration of 4- to 6-μm cup-shaped or boat-shaped cysts in bronchoalveolar lavage fluid, sputum, or transbronchial biopsy specimen stained by silver, Giemsa, or toluidine blue stain. Aggressive treatment with pentamidine and with folic acid inhibitors greatly reduces the morbidity caused by *Pneumocystis* in AIDS but often fails to clear the infection and is complicated by adverse drug reactions.[146]

P. carinii was long considered a protozoan parasite because of its multiple forms, including one that is trophozoite-like. However, studies have strongly suggested that *P. carinii* is a fungus on the basis of properties of its cell wall, the paucity of its intracellular organelles, and phylogenetic analysis of its small-subunit ribosomal RNA sequence.[147] Inhaled *P. carinii* attach to type 1 alveolar epithelial cells and multiply within the alveolar space. In mice with severe combined immunodeficiency, which lack B and T cells but have normal macrophages, resistance to *P. carinii* infection is transferred by either CD4+ helper T cells or hyperimmune serum.[148] In HIV-1–infected persons, *P. carinii* infection occurs when the CD4+ helper T cells fall below 200 cells/mm^3, and anti–*P. carinii* antibodies appear to have no effect on host resistance to the organisms.

MORPHOLOGY. *P. carinii* causes a diffuse or patchy pneumonia. Affected lungs are airless, red, and beefy. On histologic examination, the alveolar spaces are filled by a foamy, amorphous

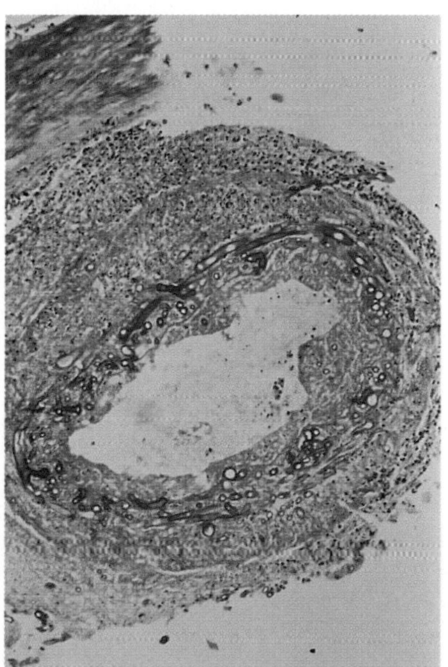

Figure 9–48

PAS stain of mucormycosis showing hyphae, which have an irregular width and right-angle branching, invading an artery wall.

material resembling proteinaceous edema fluid, composed of proliferating parasites and cell debris (Fig. 9–49). Usually there is an accompanying mild interstitial inflammatory reaction, with widening of the septa, protein and fibrin exudation, pneumocyte proliferation, escape of red cells, and formation of hyaline membranes. Frequently, there is concurrent infection by opportunistic bacteria, fungi, or viruses, especially CMV, which may overshadow the pathologic changes caused by *P. carinii.*

Cryptosporidium and *Cyclospora* Infections

Cryptosporidium parvum is a coccidian protozoan parasite (family that includes malaria and *Toxoplasma* parasites) that has long been known to cause diarrhea in cattle. Cryptosporidia have recently been shown to cause a transient watery diarrhea in normal children and a chronic, debilitating diarrhea in patients with AIDS.[149] This is in contrast to *Entamoeba* and *Giardia,* which have an increased incidence among homosexual men but do not cause increased disease in patients with AIDS. *C. parvum* oocytes are not killed by chlorine and are incompletely removed by filtration through sand, so that some 400,000 people in Milwaukee in 1993 suffered diarrhea with cryptosporidia after drinking contaminated municipal water.

C. parvum has a complicated life cycle that includes infectious, environmentally resistant oocysts resembling those of *Entamoeba* and *Giardia* as well as asexual sporozoites and merozoites and sexual gametes that resemble malaria parasites.[150] Sporozoites have a lectin on their surface that mediates adherence to intestinal and colonic epithelial cells. Malabsorption and a secretory diarrhea occur when sporozoites disrupt the microvilli and enter the cytoplasm of epithelial cells. Cryptosporidia also enter M cells and macrophages in underlying Peyer patches. Although both normal persons and patients with AIDS produce antiparasite IgAs, intact T cell–mediated immunity (lacking in AIDS) appears to be necessary for clearing the parasites.[151]

Cyclospora cayetanensis is another coccidian parasite that was associated with cases of diarrhea in 20 states in 1996.[152] The cause of the *Cyclospora* outbreak was contaminated Guatemalan raspberries, suggesting the importance of careful washing of imported fruits and vegetables before they are consumed raw.

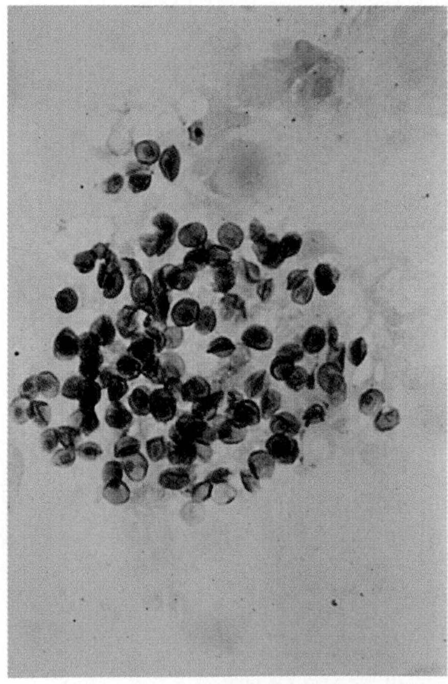

Figure 9–49 ■

Silver stain of cup-shaped *Pneumocystis carinii* organisms within a sputum sample from an AIDS patient.

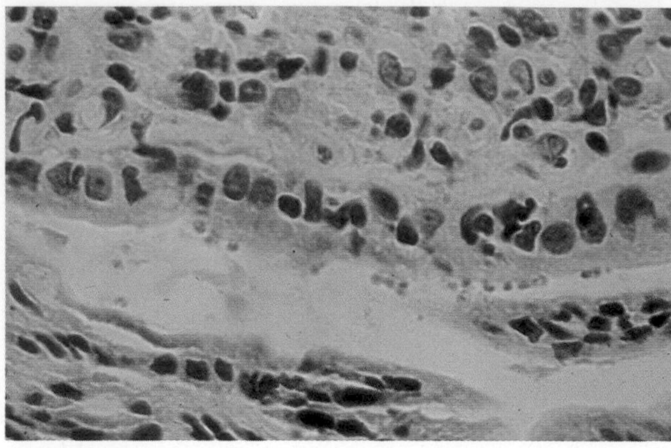

Figure 9–50 ■

Blue cryptosporidia lining the edge of colonic epithelial cells.

MORPHOLOGY. Cryptosporidia adhere to the apical brush border of absorptive gut epithelia, enveloped by a host cell membrane (Fig. 9–50). There is mixed inflammation of the lamina propria. Cryptosporidia shed in the stool are best visualized after staining with a modified acid-fast stain.

Toxoplasmosis

Toxoplasma gondii is a coccidian protozoan parasite that commonly causes subclinical infection or mild lymphadenopathy in normal persons yet produces severe opportunistic infections in infants in utero and patients with AIDS, both of whom lack intact cell-mediated immune systems.[153]

Life Cycle and Pathogenesis. *Toxoplasma* infects a wide range of animals, but human infections are predominantly caused by one strain.[154] Sexual reproduction occurs only in the intestinal epithelium of the cat, but humans can be infected either by ingesting oocysts from cat feces or incompletely cooked lamb or pork; the latter contains

Toxoplasma cysts filled with intracystic organisms called bradyzoites. Entering through the gut, *T. gondii* spreads systemically and penetrates into any type of host cell, a unique property of this parasite. Bow-shaped *T. gondii* tachyzoites spread from cell to cell until T cell–mediated immunity develops and macrophages are activated to kill the intracellular parasites. One strong inducer of T cell–mediated immunity may be a superantigen of *Toxoplasma,* which, like that of staphylococci that causes toxic shock, binds directly to receptors on many T cells and causes release of large quantities of interferon-γ.[155] Some *T. gondii* cysts containing bradyzoites, however, remain dormant for years in muscle and visceral cells.

After primary *T. gondii* infection of the mother during the first trimester of pregnancy, disseminated and often fatal parasitemias occur in 25% of fetuses. *T. gondii* tachyzoites travel through the placenta into the fetus and destroy the developing heart, brain, and lung tissues. Congenital infection with *T. gondii* is also the most common cause of chorioretinitis in the United States, which may result in blindness in one or both eyes. In patients with AIDS, *Toxoplasma* reactivated from dormant cysts causes encephalitis, which frequently produces mass lesions. Iatrogenic immunosuppression in organ transplant patients results in toxoplasmosis from (1) reactivation of the cysts within the grafted kidney, heart, liver, or lungs or (2) the recipient's own tissues after bone marrow graft.

T. gondii is able to infect all types of cells because the parasites bind the extracellular matrix protein laminin to their surface, in turn attaching to laminin receptors on the surface of host cells. While bacterial invasion of epithelial cells is dependent on host actin, invasion of host cells by *Toxoplasma* is dependent on parasite actin.[156] During host cell penetration, *Toxoplasma* releases numerous proteins from its secretory organelles.[157] This route of entry of the *T. gondii* parasites appears to be important in preventing acidification, because organisms covered with antiparasite antibodies and entering host cells by Fc receptors enter acidified vacuoles.

MORPHOLOGY. In otherwise normal adults, *Toxoplasma* causes lymphadenitis characterized by follicular hyperplasia; focal proliferation of transformed, histiocytoid B cells; and scattered accumulations of enlarged, epithelioid type macrophages, which do not form well-defined granulomas. Lesions are more frequent in young women than in men, posterior cervical lymph nodes are most often affected, and the diagnosis can be confirmed by serologic titers to *Toxoplasma* antigens or by staining for parasite antigens by immunohistochemical techniques.

In **neonatal toxoplasmosis**, destructive lesions of the central nervous system are composed of microglial nodules containing many tachyzoites located about the ventricles and aqueduct, which may be obstructed and so cause hydrocephalus. These lesions are often accompanied by extensive central nervous system necrosis, vascular thrombosis, and intense inflammation. In addition, the liver, heart, lungs, and adrenals may become necrotic.

In ***Toxoplasma* chorioretinitis**, destruction of the retina by tachyzoites is accompanied by a granulomatous reaction in the choroid and sclera. Central nervous system involvement with *Toxoplasma* is discussed and illustrated in Chapter 30.

TROPICAL, ZOONOTIC, AND VECTOR-BORNE INFECTIONS

This section describes a diverse collection of infectious diseases caused by viruses, rickettsiae, bacteria, and parasites. They fall into three groups. The first are diseases prevalent predominantly in the tropics that are transmitted by an arthropod vector (dengue fever, plague, malaria, kala-azar, African sleeping sickness, and river blindness). The second are tropical infectious diseases associated with poor living conditions (e.g., *M. leprae* or hookworm) or poor sanitation (tapeworm, *Trichinella,* and schistosomes). The third are arthropod-borne infections of temperate climates, including RMSF, ehrlichiosis, Lyme disease, and babesiosis.

Dengue Fever

Dengue fever is caused by an arthropod-borne virus (arbovirus) of the Flavivirus family group, which also includes those that cause Eastern encephalitis and yellow fever (see Table 9–4). Dengue fever is considered an emerging infectious disease because its incidence is increasing in Central America and Mexico with failure to control its mosquito vector, *Aedes aegypti,* which is also capable of transmitting malaria parasites.[158]

Dengue virus infection causes systemic infection with two important components. First, there is a transient bone marrow suppression, which may lead to neutropenia at the same time as the fever.[159] Second, in persons previously exposed to dengue virus, antiviral antibodies may enhance the uptake of virus into host cells and cause shock and death.[160] This ironic exacerbation of disease by antibodies may make development of vaccines to dengue virus more difficult than to measles virus, poliovirus, and hepatitis B virus.

Hemorrhagic dengue causes a DIC-like syndrome. Deaths associated with dengue virus infection, which are more frequent in children, are caused by hemorrhages in the lungs and the cerebrum.

Rickettsial Infections

Rickettsiae are vector-borne obligate intracellular bacteria that cause epidemic typhus *(Rickettsia prowazekii),* scrub typhus *(Rickettsia tsutsugamushi),* and spotted fevers (*Rickettsia rickettsii* and others) (see Table 9–10).[161] In contrast,

Q fever, which is caused by the related organism *Coxiella burnetii* and produces pneumonia and fever, is transmitted by aerosols. *Ehrlichia chaffeensis,* a newly discovered intracellular organism related to the rickettsiae, causes an acute febrile illness similar to the spotted fevers, but without a rash.[13] It is tick transmitted and may predominantly affect neutrophils or macrophages. Epidemic typhus, which is transmitted from person to person by body lice, is particularly associated with wars and human suffering, when persons are forced to live in close contact without changing clothes (e.g., a 1996 outbreak in a Burundi prison).[162] Scrub typhus, transmitted by chiggers, was a major problem for U.S. soldiers in the Pacific in World War II and in Vietnam. RMSF, transmitted to humans by rodent and dog ticks, is most frequent in the southeastern and southwestern United States. Rickettsiae of RMSF enter the skin with the bite or with scratching of the skin covered with insect feces.

Pathogenesis. Regardless of the route of infection, rickettsiae predominantly infect endothelial and vascular smooth muscle cells, causing a vasculitis that may be complicated by thrombi and hemorrhages. Rickettsiae have an endotoxin but lack secreted toxins. In addition, *R. rickettsii* activates host kallikrein and kinins and so causes local clotting. Rickettsiae bind to cholesterol-containing receptors, are endocytosed into phagolysosomes, escape into the cytosol, and multiply until they burst the cells. Antibody-dependent and cell-dependent immunity may prevent reinfection with rickettsiae but may not prevent reactivation of typhus after many years, which is referred to as Brill-Zinsser disease. Instead, T lymphocyte–mediated immunity is most important for clearing rickettsiae.[163] One effect of cellular immunity may be release of cytokines that induce nitric oxide–mediated, antirickettsial activity, not dissimilar to that described for activated macrophages.[164] Rickettsial infections are diagnosed by immunostaining of organisms or by detection of antibodies in the serum. Against this background, we can turn to the morphology of rickettsial infections with particular emphasis on typhus fever and RMSF.

MORPHOLOGY. ***Typhus Fever.*** In milder cases, the gross changes are limited to a rash and small hemorrhages incident to the vascular lesions. In more severe cases, there may be areas of necrosis of the skin with gangrene of the tips of the fingers, nose, earlobes, scrotum, penis, and vulva. In such cases, irregular ecchymotic hemorrhages may be found internally, principally in the brain, heart muscle, testes, serosal membrane, lungs, and kidneys.

The most prominent microscopic changes are the small-vessel lesions that underlie the rash and the focal areas of hemorrhage and inflammation in the various organs and tissues affected. Endothelial proliferation and swelling in the capillaries, arterioles, and venules may narrow the lumina of these vessels. Surrounding the involved vessels, a cuff of inflammatory mixed leukocytes is usually present. The vascular lumina are sometimes thrombosed, but necrosis of the vessel wall is unusual in typhus compared with RMSF. It is the vascular thromboses that lead to the gangrenous necroses of the skin and other structures. In the brain, characteristic typhus nodules are composed of focal microglial proliferations mixed with leukocytes (Fig. 9–51).

Rocky Mountain Spotted Fever. An eschar at the site of the tick bite followed by a hemorrhagic rash that extends over the entire body, including the palms of the hands and soles of the feet, is the hallmark of RMSF. The vascular lesions that underlie the rash often lead to acute necrosis, fibrin extravasation, and thrombosis of the small blood vessels, including arterioles (Fig. 9–52). In severe RMSF, foci of necrotic skin are thus induced, particularly on the fingers, toes, elbows, ears, and scrotum. Vascular necrosis and thrombosis are far more frequent with RMSF than with typhus and may mimic the necrotizing vasculitis of the collagen vascular diseases. Despite frequent local thrombi, systemic DIC is rare, even in the most severe cases. The perivascular inflammatory response is similar to that of typhus, particularly in the brain, skeletal muscle, lungs, kidneys, testes, and heart muscle. The vascular necroses in the brain may involve larger vessels and produce focal areas of ischemic demyelinization or microinfarcts. A pneumonitis of primary rickettsial origin is present in severely affected patients and often predisposes to a secondary bacterial infection.

Other Rickettsial Infections. *Coxiella* **infections (Q fever)** mainly involve the lungs, producing an interstitial pneumonitis that resembles viral pneumonia. In severe cases, small granulomas may appear in the spleen, liver, and bone marrow along with focal perivascular inflammatory infiltrates.

Scrub typhus, or mite-borne infection, is usually a milder version of typhus fever. The rash is usually

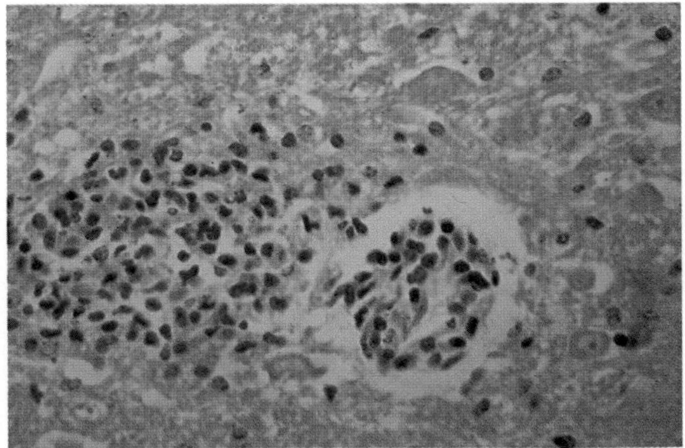

Figure 9–51

Typhus nodule in the brain.

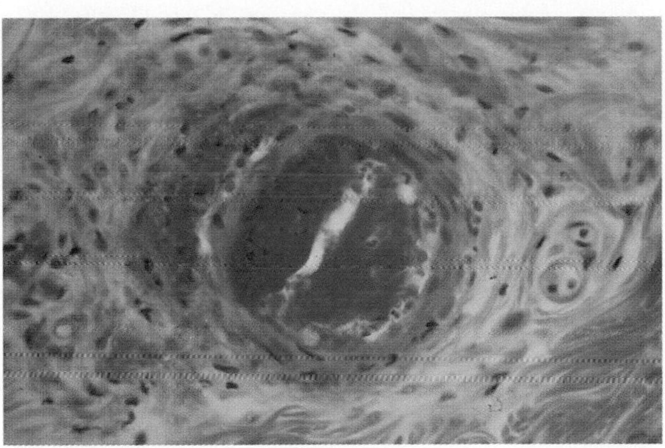

Figure 9–52

Rocky Mountain spotted fever with a thrombosed vessel and vasculitis.

transitory or may not appear. Vascular necrosis or thrombosis is rare, but there may be a prominent inflammatory lymphadenopathy.

Trachoma

Trachoma is a chronic suppurative eye disease manifested by follicular keratoconjunctivitis and caused by subtypes of *Chlamydia trachomatis* (Table 9–11). It is the leading infectious cause of blindness worldwide, causing 6 million cases of vision impairment and 3 million cases of blindness.[165] *Progressive trachoma is seen mostly in dry and sandy regions and among poor people and nomads,* where the infection is acquired during childhood. Trachoma is transmitted by direct human contact, by contaminated particles (fomites), and possibly by flies.

Infections can be either self-limiting or progressive; the progressive type begins with a suppurative stage to deeper tissue involvement, with lymphoplasmacytic infiltration and the formation of lymphoid follicles. Numerous cytokines are released including TNF-α, transforming growth factor-β, interferon-γ, and IL-2.[166] The upper limbus of the cornea and the upper tarsal plate tend to be most severely involved by epithelial hyperplasia and follicular hypertrophy. Soon, the conjunctiva ulcerates, and penetration into the cornea leads to pannus formation, fibroblast ingrowth, scarring, and eventual blindness. The scarring also hampers closure of the eyelids, in turn promoting bacterial superinfection. Furrowing of the mucosa overlying the tarsal plate and pitting of the upper rim of the limbus are characteristic late deformities of trachoma.

Leprosy

Leprosy, or Hansen disease, is a slowly progressive infection caused by *Mycobacterium leprae,* affecting the skin and peripheral nerves and resulting in disabling deformities. *M. leprae* is for the most part contained within the skin, but leprosy is likely to be transmitted from person to

Table 9–11. RICKETTSIAL DISEASES AND PATHOGENS

Disease	Geography	Agent	Transmission	Distinctive Features
Typhus Group (No Eschar)				
Epidemic typhus	Worldwide (war, famine)	*R. prowazekii*	Louse feces	Endothelial infection; centrifugal type rash
Brill-Zinsser disease	That of epidemic typhus	*R. prowazekii*	Late reactivation	Those of epidemic typhus, but generally milder
Flying squirrel typhus	Southeastern United States	*R. prowazekii*	Fleas, lice of flying squirrel	Similar to epidemic typhus, but mortality is lower
Murine typhus	Worldwide (rat-related)	*R. typhi (R. mooseri)*	Rat flea feces	Similar to epidemic typhus, but mortality is lower
Spotted Fever Group				
Rocky Mountain spotted fever	North and South America	*R. rickettsii*	Tick bite	Endothelia and vascular smooth muscle infected; rash is centripetal; eschar rarely seen
Boutonneuse fever	Mediterranean, India	*R. conorii*	Tick bite	Prominent eschar, tache noire
North Asian and Queensland tick typhus	USSR, China Australia	*R. sibirica* *R. australis*	Tick bite	Both diseases are typical spotted fevers commonly with eschar
Rickettsialpox	United States, USSR, Korea, Africa	*R. akari*	Mite bite	Prominent eschar, papulovesicular rash (milder than RMSF)
Other				
Scrub typhus	East Asia, Pacific	*R. tsutsugamushi*	Chigger bite	Frequent eschar and lymphadenopathy
Q fever	Worldwide	*Coxiella burnetti*	Droplet inhalation	No eschar or rash; fever, pneumonia, ring granuloma
Ehrlichiosis	Not yet fully known	*Ehrlichia sennetsu, E. canis*	Tick bite	Fever, lymphadenopathy, no eschar or rash

person through aerosols from lesions in the upper respiratory tract. Inhaled *M. leprae,* like *M. tuberculosis,* is taken up by alveolar macrophages, disseminates through the blood, but grows only in relatively cool tissues of the skin and extremities. Despite its low communicability, leprosy remains endemic among an estimated 10 to 15 million people living in poor tropical countries.

Pathogenesis. *M. leprae* is an acid-fast obligate intracellular organism that does not grow in culture but can be grown in the armadillo. It grows more slowly than other mycobacteria and grows best at 32 to 34°C, the temperature of the human skin and the core temperature of armadillos. Like *M. tuberculosis, M. leprae* secretes no toxins, but its virulence is based on properties of its cell wall. The cell wall is similar enough to that of *M. tuberculosis* that immunization to bacille Calmette-Guérin alone confers 50% protection against *M. leprae* infection. Further immunization may work as an adjuvant to treatment with antimycobacterial drugs.[167] Cell-mediated immunity is reflected by delayed type hypersensitivity reactions to dermal injections of a bacterial extract called *lepromin.* A 10-kD heat-shock protein of *M. leprae* is an important antigen recognized by the cellular immune system.[168]

Leprosy is a bipolar disease, determined by the host cellular immune response. Two forms of the disease occur, depending on whether the host mounts a T cell–mediated immune response *(tuberculoid leprosy)* or is anergic *(lepromatous leprosy).* Patients with *tuberculoid leprosy* form granulomas similar to those seen in tuberculosis, containing epithelioid macrophages, giant cells, and few surviving mycobacteria (paucibacillary disease). The 48-hour lepromin skin test reaction is strongly positive. At the circumference of the granulomas are CD4+ type 1 helper T cells that like mouse T_H1 cells secrete IL-2 and interferon-γ.[169] There are also a few CD8+ lymphocytes in the center of the tuberculoid leprosy lesions. Damage to the nervous system occurs and granulomas form in the nerve sheaths.

In contrast, patients with *lepromatous leprosy* lack T cell–mediated immunity, are anergic to lepromin, and have diffuse lesions containing foamy macrophages stuffed with large numbers of mycobacteria (multibacillary disease). Lepromatous leprosy lesions lack CD4+ type 1 T cells at their margins but instead contain many CD8+ suppressor T cells in a diffuse pattern. The CD8+ suppressor T cells secrete IL-10, which inhibits helper T cells and may mediate the anergy seen in lepromatous leprosy. These CD8+ suppressor T cells also secrete IL-4, which induces antibody production by B cells. The antibody is not protective, and indeed the formation of antigen-antibody complexes in lepromatous leprosy leads to erythema nodosum leprosum, a life-threatening vasculitis and glomerulonephritis. In lepromatous leprosy, damage to the nervous system comes from widespread invasion of the mycobacteria into Schwann cells and into endoneural and perineural macrophages. Because of the diffuse, parasite-filled lesions, patients with lepromatous leprosy are more infectious than are those with tuberculoid leprosy.

Preliminary studies of the genetic basis of human responsiveness to *M. leprae* shed some light on why leprosy runs varying courses in different persons.[170] Individuals who recognized certain *M. leprae* antigens and had no disease showed different alleles at the human *Bcg* locus than did those who were anergic and had multibacillary disease. The mouse *bcg* gene controls responses to intracellular bacteria and parasites (see earlier).[53] Particular polymorphisms in T-cell receptor genes also correlated with presence of multibacillary or paucibacillary disease.

MORPHOLOGY. Tuberculoid leprosy begins with localized skin lesions that are at first flat and red but enlarge and develop irregular shapes with indurated, elevated, hyperpigmented margins and depressed pale centers (central healing). Neuronal involvement dominates tuberculoid leprosy as nerves become enclosed within granulomatous inflammatory reactions and, if small enough (e.g., the peripheral twigs), are destroyed (Fig. 9–53). Nerve degeneration causes skin anesthesias and skin and muscle atrophy that render the patient liable to trauma of the affected parts, with the development of indolent skin ulcers. Contractures, paralyses, and autoamputation of fingers or toes may ensue. Facial nerve involvement can lead to paralysis of the lids, with keratitis and corneal ulcerations. On microscopic examination, all sites of involvement disclose granulomatous lesions closely resembling hard tubercles, and bacilli are almost never found. Because leprosy pursues an extremely slow course, spanning decades, most patients die with leprosy rather than of it.

Lepromatous (anergic) leprosy involves the skin, peripheral nerves, anterior eye, upper airways (down to the larynx), testes, hands, and feet. The vital organs and central nervous system are rarely affected, presumably because the core temperature is too high for growth of *M. leprae.* Lepromatous lesions contain large aggregates of lipid-laden macrophages (lepra cells), often filled with masses of acid-fast bacilli (globi; Fig. 9–54). Macular, papular, or nodular lesions form on the face, ears, wrists, elbows, and knees. With progression, the nodular lesions coalesce to yield a distinctive leonine facies. Most skin lesions are hypoesthetic or anesthetic. Lesions in the nose may cause persistent inflammation and bacilli-laden discharge. The peripheral nerves, particularly the ulnar and peroneal nerves where they approach the skin surface, are symmetrically invaded with mycobacteria, with minimal inflammation. Loss of sensation and trophic changes in the hands and feet follow the nerve lesions. Lymph nodes show aggregation of foamy histiocytes in the paracortical (T-cell) areas, with enlargement of germinal centers. In advanced disease, aggregates of macrophages are also present in the splenic red pulp and the liver. The testes are usually extensively involved, with destruction of the seminiferous tubules and consequent sterility.

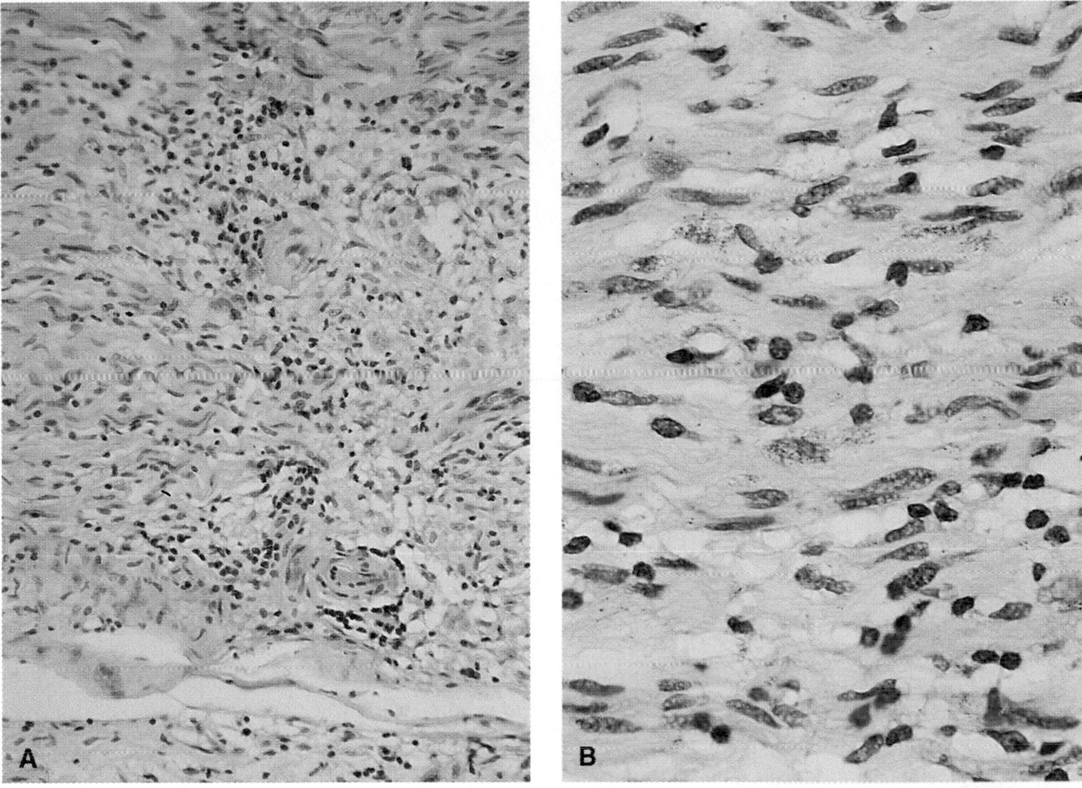

Figure 9–53

Leprosy. *A*, Peripheral nerve. Note the inflammatory cell infiltrates in the endoneural and epineural compartments. *B*, A cell within the endoneurium contains acid-fast positive lepra bacilli. (Courtesy of E.P. Richardson Jr. and U. De Girolami, Harvard Medical School.)

Plague

Yersinia pestis is a gram-negative facultative intracellular bacterium that is transmitted by flea bites or by aerosols and causes a highly invasive, frequently fatal systemic infection called *plague.* Plague, also named Black Death, caused three great pandemics that killed an estimated 100 million persons in Egypt and Byzantium in the 6th century; one quarter of Europe's population in the 14th and 15th centuries; and tens of millions in India, Burma, and China at the beginning of the 20th century.[171] Currently, wild rodents in the western United States are infected with *Y. pestis,* which is rarely transmitted to humans. Most cases of plague occur in urban foci in Southeast Asia, where rats are the reservoir of infection.[172] *Y. enterocolitica* and *Y. pseudotuberculosis* are genetically similar to *Y. pestis;* these bacteria cause fecal-orally transmitted ileitis and mesenteric lymphadenitis, as described earlier.

Y. pestis makes a plasmid-encoded secreted protease that activates plasminogen and cleaves complement C3 at a specific site.[173] This secreted protease is essential for spread of the bacteria from the local site of inoculation and inflammation into the bloodstream, so mutant bacteria lacking this protease are 1 million times less virulent to mice when inoculated into the skin.

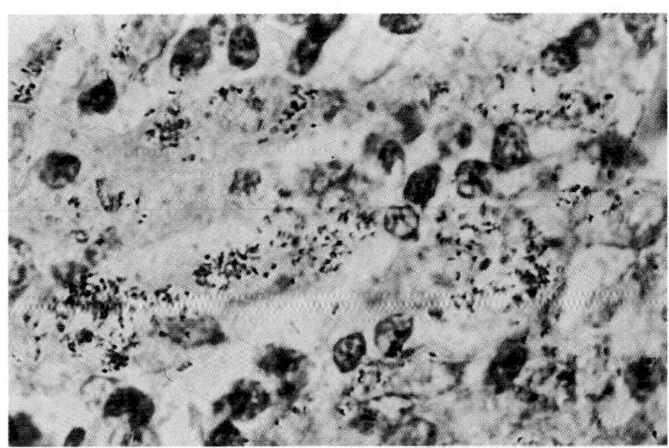

Figure 9–54

Lepromatous leprosy. Acid-fast bacilli (red snappers) proliferate in the macrophages.

MORPHOLOGY. Plague causes lymph node enlargement (bubo), pneumonia, or sepsis, all with a striking neutrophilia. The distinctive histologic features include (1) massive proliferation of the organisms, (2) early appearance of protein-rich and polysaccharide-rich effusions with few inflammatory cells but with marked tissue swelling, (3) necrosis of tissues and blood vessels with hemorrhage and thrombosis, and (4) neutrophilic infiltrates that accumulate adjacent to necrotic areas as healing begins.

In **bubonic plague**, the site of entry is usually on the legs and is marked by a small pustule or ulceration. The nodes of drainage enlarge dramatically within a few days and become soft, pulpy, and plum colored and may infarct or rupture through the skin. In **pneumonic plague**, there is a severe, confluent, hemorrhagic, and necrotizing bronchopneumonia, often with fibrinous pleuritis. In **septicemic plague**, lymph nodes throughout the body as well as reticuloendothelial organs develop foci of necrosis. Fulminating bacteremias also induce DIC with widespread hemorrhages and thrombi.

Relapsing Fever

Relapsing fever is caused by helical *Borrelia spirochetes (B. recurrentis),* which are transmitted from person to person by body lice or from animals to humans by soft ticks. Louse-transmitted *Borrelia,* associated with overcrowding due to poverty or war, caused multiple large epidemics in Africa, Eastern Europe, and Russia in the first half of the 20th century, infecting 15 million persons and killing 5 million, and is still a problem in some developing countries.

In both lice- and tick-transmitted borreliosis, there is a 1- to 2-week latent period after the bite as the spirochetes multiply in the serum. Clinical infection is heralded by shaking chills, fever, headache, and fatigue, followed by DIC and multiorgan failure. Cytokines include TNF-α. Spirochetes are cleared from the blood by anti-*Borrelia* antibodies that target a single major surface protein called the variable major protein.[174] After a few days, bacteria bearing a different surface antigen reach high densities in the blood, and symptoms return until a second set of host antibodies clears these organisms. Other infectious agents that change surface molecules in response to antibodies, which is called *antigenic variation,* are listed in Table 9–7. The lessening severity of successive attacks of relapsing fever and its spontaneous cure in many untreated patients have been attributed to the limited genetic repertoire of *Borrelia,* enabling the host to build up cross-reactive as well as clone-specific antibodies. Antibiotic treatment of *Borrelia* infections may cause a massive release of endotoxin, resulting in a dangerous rise in temperature with rigors, fall in blood pressure, and leukopenia (the Jarisch-Herxheimer reaction).[175] Because reactions to endotoxin are mediated by host TNF-α, anti-TNF antibodies can protect patients from the Jarisch-Herxheimer reaction.

MORPHOLOGY. In fatal louse-borne disease, the spleen is moderately enlarged (300 to 400 gm) and contains focal necroses and miliary collections of leukocytes, including neutrophils, and numerous borreliae. There is congestion and hypercellularity of the red pulp with erythrophagocytosis. The liver may also be enlarged and congested with prominent Kupffer cells and septic foci. Scattered hemorrhages resulting from DIC may be found in serosal and mucosal surfaces, skin, and viscera. Pulmonary bacterial superinfection is a frequent complication.

Lyme Disease

Lyme disease, named for the Connecticut town where in the mid-1970s there was an epidemic of arthritis associated with skin erythema, is caused by the spirochete *Borrelia burgdorferi.* Lyme disease, transmitted from rodents to people by tiny hard deer ticks (see Fig. 9–6), is the major arthropod-borne disease currently in the United States and is also frequent in Europe and Japan. In the eastern United States, the incidence of Lyme disease is now increasing because of reforestation, which has occurred during the last 75 years, allowing large increases in numbers of white-tailed deer and field mice that are necessary for transmission of Lyme spirochetes. Indeed, in endemic areas such as coastal areas of Massachusetts, as many as 50% of ticks are infected with *Borrelia,* and ticks may also be infected with *Ehrlichia* (discussed before) and *Babesia* (discussed later). In the Chesapeake Bay region and parts of the Southeast, a second somewhat less virulent *Borrelia* spirochete may be transmitted by the Lone Star ticks.[176]

Clinical Stages and Their Pathogenesis. As in another major spirochetal disease, syphilis, clinical disease caused by Lyme spirochetes involves multiple organ systems and is usually divided into three stages.[177] In *stage 1* (Fig. 9–55) at the site of the tick bite, spirochetes multiply and spread within the dermis, causing an expanding area of

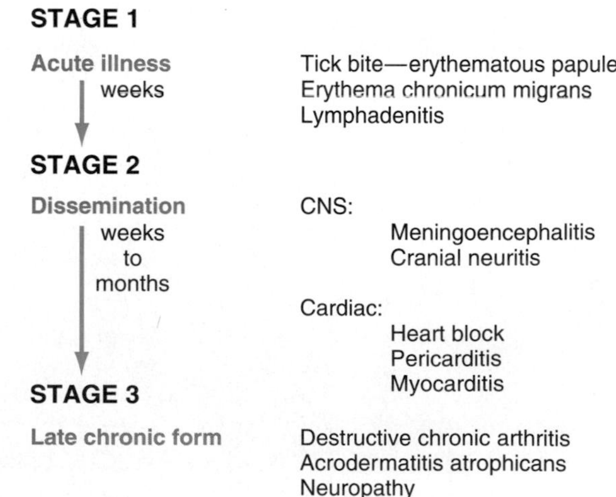

Figure 9–55

Clinical stages of Lyme disease.

redness, often with an indurated or pale center. This skin lesion, called *erythema chronicum migrans,* may be accompanied by fever and lymphadenopathy but usually disappears in a few weeks' time. In *stage 2, the early disseminated stage,* spirochetes spread hematogenously throughout the entire body and cause secondary annular skin lesions, lymphadenopathy, migratory joint and muscle pain, cardiac arrhythmias, and meningitis often with cranial nerve involvement. In untreated patients, antibodies develop to spirochete flagellar proteins and to two major outer membrane proteins. These antibodies are useful for serodiagnosis of *Borrelia* infection, and recombinant outer membrane proteins are included in a Lyme disease vaccine. Antibody-covered *Borrelia* are phagocytosed by macrophages by means of the same coiling process used in the uptake of *Legionella, Trypanosoma,* and *Leishmania.* Some spirochetes, however, escape host antibody and T-cell responses by sequestering themselves in the central nervous system or (as intracellular forms) within endothelial cells.[178] Lyme borreliae bind to galactocerebroside, a glycolipid component of myelin. *Borrelia* may also induce inflammatory cytokines within the central nervous system, including IL-6 and TNF-α. In *stage 3, the late disseminated stage,* 2 or 3 years after the initial bite, Lyme borreliae cause a chronic arthritis sometimes with severe damage to large joints and an encephalitis that varies from mild to debilitating. The host immune response is out of proportion to the scant number of organisms detectable and may be caused by host cell reaction to spirochete heat-shock proteins that cross-react with host tissues.[179]

MORPHOLOGY. Skin lesions caused by *B. burgdorferi* are characterized by edema and a lymphocytic plasma cell infiltrate. In early Lyme arthritis, the synovium resembles that of early rheumatoid arthritis, with villous hypertrophy, lining cell hyperplasia, and abundant lymphocytes and plasma cells in the subsynovium. A distinctive feature of Lyme arthritis is an arteritis, with onionskin-like lesions resembling those seen in lupus (Chapter 7). In late Lyme disease, there may be extensive erosion of the cartilage in large joints. In Lyme meningitis, the CSF is hypercellular, shows a marked lymphoplasmacytic infiltrate, and contains anti-spirochete IgGs.

Malaria

Malaria caused by the intracellular protozoan parasite *Plasmodium falciparum* is a worldwide infection that affects 100 million and kills 1 to 1.5 million persons per year and so is the major parasitic cause of death. *P. falciparum* and the three other malaria parasites that infect humans *(P. vivax, P. ovale, P. malariae)* are transmitted by more than a dozen species of *Anopheles* mosquitoes widely distributed throughout Africa, Asia, and Latin America. The wide geographic distribution of malaria is due to the failure of a massive campaign from the 1950s to 1980s to eradicate malaria. This campaign produced mosquitoes that are resistant to DDT and malathion and *P. falciparum* parasites resistant to chloroquine and pyrimethamine. Some of the molecular mechanisms for parasite resistance to these drugs have recently been determined.[180]

P. vivax and *P. malariae* cause mild anemia and, in rare instances, splenic rupture and nephrotic syndrome. Acute *P. falciparum* infections produce high parasitemias, severe anemia, cerebral symptoms, renal failure, pulmonary edema, and death. Therefore, the focus of the discussion that follows is on the pathologic process caused by *P. falciparum.*

Life Cycle and Pathogenesis. Malaria sporozoites, the stage transmitted by mosquito bites, have a single antigen on their surface that is an important vaccine candidate.[181] Sporozoites are released into the blood and within minutes attach to and invade liver cells by binding to the hepatocyte receptor for the serum proteins thrombospondin and properdin, located on the basolateral surface of hepatocytes (Fig. 9–56).[182] The binding is accomplished because of the presence of sporozoite surface proteins that contain a domain homologous to the binding domain of thrombospondin. Within liver cells, malaria parasites multiply rapidly, so as many as 30,000 merozoites (asexual, haploid blood forms) are released when the hepatocyte ruptures. The HLA-B53–associated resistance to *P. falciparum* infections exhibited by many Africans appears to be caused by the ability of HLA-B53 to present liver stage–specific malaria antigens to cytotoxic T cells, which then kill malaria-infected hepatocytes.[183]

Once released, *P. falciparum* merozoites bind by a parasite lectin-like molecule to sialic residues on glycophorin molecules on the surface of red blood cells. (*P. vivax* merozoites bind by a homologous lectin to the Duffy antigens on red blood cells, so many Africans who are Duffy-negative are resistant to this parasite.) The merozoites release multiple proteases from a special organelle called the *rhoptry,* also found, as we have seen, in *Toxoplasma, Cryptosporidium,* and *Babesia* parasites. Within the red blood cells, the parasites multiply in a membrane-bound digestive vacuole, hydrolyzing hemoglobin through secreted enzymes that include an aspartate protease homologous to that of HIV, which is the target of new anti-AIDS drugs.[184] Individuals with the sickle cell trait are resistant to malaria because their red blood cells sickle when parasitized and so are removed by the spleen. Although most malaria parasites within the red blood cells develop into merozoites, rupture the cell, and then infect new red blood cells, some parasites develop into sexual forms called *gametocytes* that infect the mosquito when it takes its blood meal.

As the malaria parasites mature within red blood cells, they change morphologic appearance from ring to schizont form and secrete proteins that form 100-nm bumps on the red blood cell surface, called *knobs.* Malaria proteins on the surface of the knobs, called *sequestrins,* are encoded by *var* genes, so called because they exhibit antigenic variation (see earlier).[35] Sequestrins bind to endothelial cells by ICAM-1, the thrombospondin receptor, and the glycophorin CD46 and so cause malaria-infected red blood cells to be

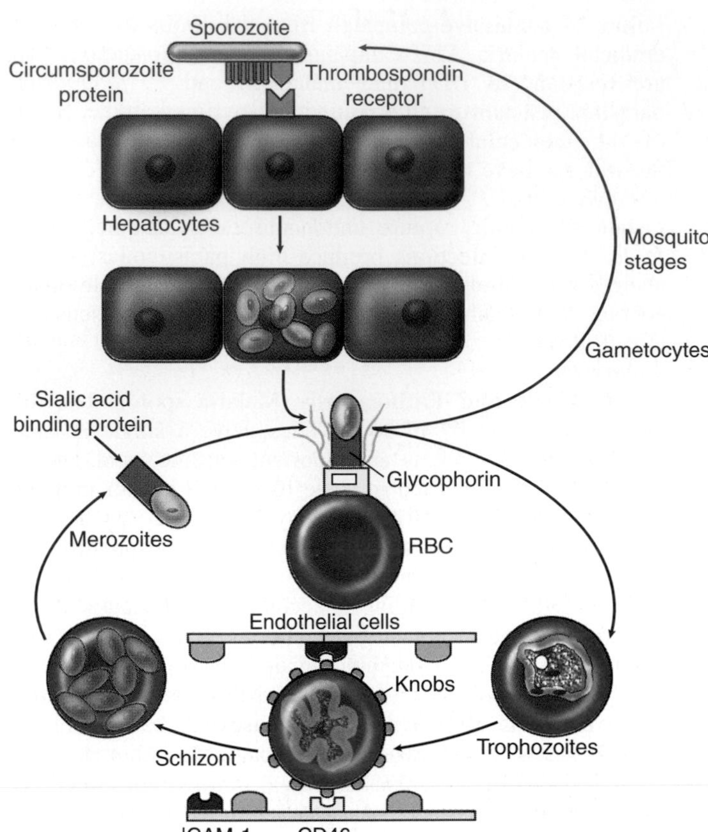

Figure 9–56

Life cycle of *Plasmodium falciparum.* (Drawn by Dr. Jeffrey Joseph, Beth Israel-Deaconess Hospital, Boston.)

removed from circulation[185] (Fig. 9–56). In this way, red blood cells containing immature ring forms of the parasite, which are flexible and can pass through the spleen, circulate in the blood, whereas red blood cells containing mature schizonts, which are more rigid, avoid sequestration in the spleen. In addition, sequestrin causes red blood cells to bind to and form rosettes with uninfected red blood cells.

Cerebral involvement by *P. falciparum,* which causes as many as 80% of deaths in children, is due to adhesion of the *P. falciparum* parasites to endothelial cells within the brain. Patients with cerebral malaria have increased amounts of ICAM-1, thrombospondin receptor, and CD46 on their cerebral endothelial cells (perhaps activated by cytokines such as TNF) to which the malaria-infected red blood cells bind.

MORPHOLOGY. *P. falciparum* infection initially causes congestion and enlargement of the **spleen**, which may eventually exceed 1000 gm in weight. Parasites are present within red blood cells, and there is increased phagocytic activity of the reticuloendothelial cells. In chronic malaria infection, the spleen becomes increasingly fibrotic and brittle, with a thick capsule and fibrous trabeculae. The parenchyma is gray or black because of phagocytotic cells containing granular, brown-black, faintly birefringent hemozoin pigment. In addition, macrophages with engulfed parasites, red blood cells, and debris are numerous.

The **liver** becomes progressively enlarged and pigmented with progression of malaria. Kupffer cells are heavily laden with malarial pigment, parasites, and cellular debris, while some pigment is also present in the parenchymal cells. Pigmented phagocytic cells may be found dispersed throughout the bone marrow, lymph nodes, subcutaneous tissues, and lungs. The kidneys are often enlarged and congested with a dusting of pigment in the glomeruli and hemoglobin casts in the tubules.

In **malignant cerebral malaria** caused by *P. falciparum,* brain vessels are plugged with parasitized red cells, each cell containing dots of hemozoin pigment (Fig. 9–57). About the vessels, there are ring hemorrhages that are probably related to local hypoxia incident to the vascular stasis and small focal inflammatory reactions (called malarial or Dürck granulomas). With more severe hypoxia, there is degeneration of neurons, focal ischemic softening, and occasionally scant inflammatory infiltrates in the meninges.

Nonspecific focal hypoxic lesions in the **heart** may be induced by the progressive anemia and circulatory stasis in chronically infected patients. In some, the myocardium shows focal interstitial infiltrates. Finally, in the nonimmune patient, pulmonary edema or shock with DIC may cause

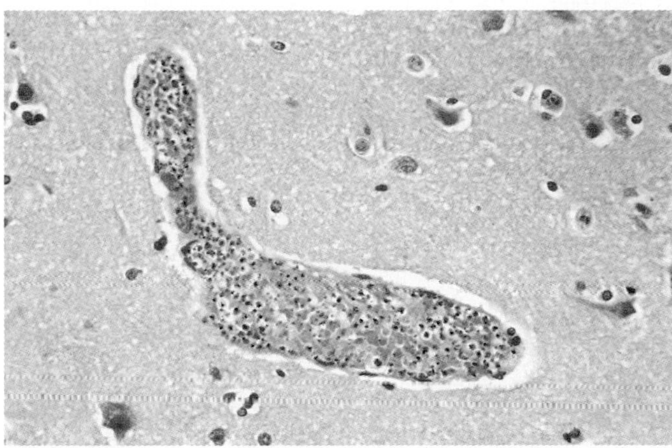

Figure 9–57

P. falciparum–infected red cells marginating within a vein in cerebral malaria.

death, sometimes in the absence of other characteristic lesions.

Babesiosis

Babesia microti is a malaria-like protozoan transmitted by the same deer ticks that carry Lyme disease.[186] Babesiae parasitize red blood cells and cause fever and hemolytic anemia. The symptoms are mild except in debilitated or splenectomized individuals, who develop severe and fatal parasitemias. Splenectomized persons may also be infected by *Babesia bovis*, which causes an economically important disease in cattle (Texas cattle fever).

MORPHOLOGY. In blood smears, *Babesia* resemble *P. falciparum* ring stages, although they lack hemozoin pigment (Fig. 9–58). They form characteristic tetrads, which are diagnostic if found. The level of *B. microti* parasitemia is a good indication of the severity of infection: 1% in mild cases and up to 30% in splenectomized persons, who also show marked erythrophagocytosis associated with the red cell destruction. In fatal cases, the anatomic findings are related to shock and hypoxia and include jaundice, hepatic necrosis, acute renal tubular necrosis, adult respiratory distress syndrome, hemolysis, and visceral hemorrhages.

Leishmaniasis

Leishmaniasis is a chronic inflammatory disease of the skin, mucous membranes, or viscera caused by obligate intracellular, kinetoplastid protozoan parasites transmitted through the bite of infected sandflies. Leishmaniasis is endemic throughout the Middle East, South Asia, Africa, and Latin America, so that numerous American soldiers were infected with *Leishmania* during operation Desert Storm.[187] Leishmaniasis may also be epidemic, as is tragically the case in southern Sudan, where tens of thousands of persons have died of visceral leishmaniasis. Finally, leishmanial infection, like that with other intracellular organisms (mycobacteria, *Histoplasma, Toxoplasma,* and trypanosomes), is exacerbated by AIDS.

Pathogenesis. The infective stage of *Leishmania* is a slender, flagellated parasite released into the host dermis along with the sandfly saliva, which potentiates parasite infectivity.[188] How far the amastigotes spread throughout the body is determined by the *Leishmania* species. Cutaneous disease is caused by *Leishmania major* and *Leishmania aethiopica* in the Old World and *Leishmania mexicana* and *Leishmania braziliensis* in the New World; mucocutaneous disease (also called espundia) is caused by *L. braziliensis;* and visceral disease involving the liver and spleen is caused by *Leishmania donovani* in the Old World and *Leishmania chagasi* in the New World. One explanation for the tropism of *Leishmania* appears to be temperature, because parasites that cause visceral disease grow at 37°C in vitro, whereas parasites that cause mucocutaneous disease grow only at 34°C.

Leishmaniae are phagocytosed by macrophages, and acidity within the phagolysosome induces them to transform into round amastigotes that lack flagella but contain a single large mitochondrion-like structure called the kinetoplast.[189] *Leishmania* amastigotes are the only protozoan parasites that survive and reproduce in macrophage phagolysosomes, which have a pH of 4.5. Amastigotes are protected from the intravacuolar acid by a proton-transporting ATPase, which maintains the intracellular parasite pH at 6.5. *Leishmania* parasites also have on their surface two abundant glycoconjugates anchored to lipid anchors, which appear to be important for their virulence.[190] The first, *lipophosphoglycans,* are glycolipids that form a dense glycocalyx and bind C3b or iC3b. Organisms resist lysis

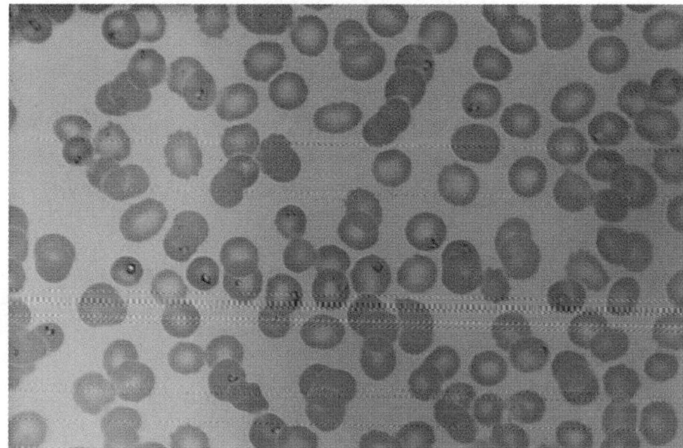

Figure 9–58

Babesia microti–filled erythrocytes.

by complement C5–C9, however, and are phagocytosed by macrophages through complement receptors CR1 (LFA-1) and CR3 (Mac-1 integrin). Lipophosphoglycans may also protect the parasites within the phagolysosomes by scavenging oxygen radicals and by inhibiting lysosomal enzymes. The second glycoconjugate, *gp63,* is a zinc-dependent proteinase that cleaves complement and some lysosomal antimicrobial enzymes.

As is the case with *M. leprae* infection, the severity of disease caused by *Leishmania* is determined by the host immune response. Hosts with parasite-specific, cell-mediated immunity control the infection or make granulomas with few parasites present, whereas anergic hosts have diffuse lesions composed of macrophages stuffed with parasites. *Leishmania* parasites are cleared from the body by cell-mediated immune mechanisms, which is reflected by a positive, delayed type hypersensitivity reaction to extracts of *Leishmania* injected into the skin *(leishmanin test).* Parasite-specific CD4+ helper T lymphocytes of the T_H1 class may secrete interferon-γ, which along with TNF-α secreted by other macrophages activates phagocytes to kill the parasites through toxic metabolites of oxygen or nitric acid (or both).[191] In contrast, down-regulation of the immune response that leads to anergy and progressive disease may be caused by parasite-specific CD4+ helper T cells of the T_H2 class that secrete IL-4, which inhibits macrophage activation by interferon-γ and inhibits secretion of TNF-α.

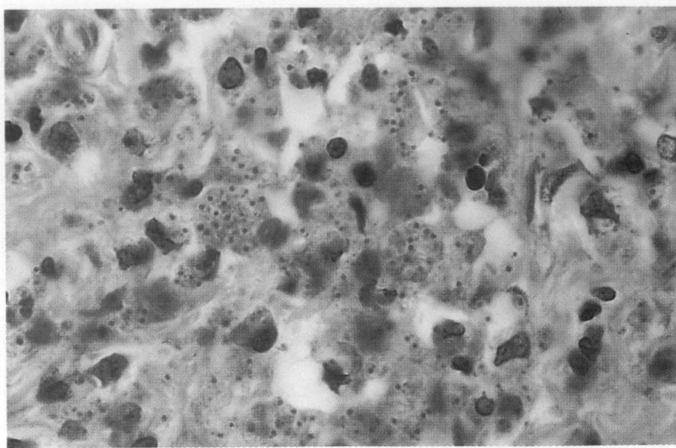

Figure 9–59

Leishmania donovani parasites within the macrophages of a lymph node in visceral leishmaniasis (kala-azar).

MORPHOLOGY. *Leishmania* species produce four different lesions in humans: visceral, cutaneous, mucocutaneous, and diffuse cutaneous. In **visceral leishmaniasis**, *L. donovani* or *L. chagasi* parasites invade macrophages throughout the reticuloendothelial system and cause severe systemic disease marked by hepatosplenomegaly, lymphadenopathy, pancytopenia, fever, and weight loss. The spleen may weigh as much as 3 kg, and the lymph nodes may measure 5 cm in diameter. Phagocytic cells are enlarged and filled with *Leishmania,* many plasma cells are present, and the normal architecture of the spleen is obscured (Fig. 9–59). In the late stages, the liver becomes increasingly fibrotic. Phagocytic cells crowd the bone marrow and may also be found in the lungs, gastrointestinal tract, kidneys, pancreas, and testes. Often there is hyperpigmentation of the skin in the extremities, which is why the disease is called kala-azar or "black fever" in Hindi. In the kidneys, there may be an immune complex–mediated mesangioproliferative glomerulonephritis and in advanced cases amyloid deposition. The overloading of the reticuloendothelial system with parasites predisposes the patients to bacterial infections, the usual cause of death. Hemorrhages related to thrombocytopenia may also be fatal.

Cutaneous leishmaniasis, caused by *L. major, L. mexicana,* and *L. braziliensis,* is a relatively mild, localized disease consisting of a single ulcer on exposed skin. The lesion (often called *tropical sore*) begins as an itching papule surrounded by induration, changes into a shallow and slowly expanding ulcer with irregular borders, and usually heals by involution within 6 months without treatment. On microscopic examination, the lesion is granulomatous, usually with many giant cells and few parasites.

Mucocutaneous leishmaniasis, caused by *L. braziliensis,* is found only in the New World. Moist, ulcerating, or nonulcerating lesions, which may be disfiguring, develop in the larynx and at the mucocutaneous junctions of the nasal septum, anus, or vulva. On microscopic examination, there is a mixed inflammatory infiltrate with parasite-containing histiocytes in association with lymphocytes and plasma cells. Later the tissue reaction becomes granulomatous, and the number of parasites declines. Eventually, the lesions remit and scar, although reactivation may occur after long intervals by mechanisms not currently understood.

Diffuse cutaneous leishmaniasis is a rare form of dermal infection, thus far found only in Ethiopia and adjacent East Africa and in Venezuela, Brazil, and Mexico. Diffuse cutaneous leishmaniasis begins as a single skin nodule, which continues spreading until the entire body is covered by bizarre nodular lesions. These lesions, which resemble keloids or large verrucae, are frequently confused with the nodules of lepromatous leprosy, so patients may be incorrectly sent to leprosaria. The lesions do not ulcerate but contain vast aggregates of foamy macrophages stuffed with leishmania. Patients are usually anergic not only to leishmanin but also to other skin antigens, and the lesions often respond poorly to treatment.

African Trypanosomiasis

African trypanosomes are kinetoplastid parasites that proliferate as extracellular forms in the blood and cause sustained or intermittent fevers, lymphadenopathy, splenomegaly, progressive brain dysfunction (sleeping sickness), cachexia, and death. *Trypanosoma rhodesiense* infection is often acute and virulent. Its tsetse fly vector prefers the savanna plains of East Africa. *Trypanosoma gambiense* infection tends to be chronic and occurs most frequently in the West African bush. *Trypanosoma brucei brucei,* to which humans have become refractory on the basis of a high-density lipoprotein that is toxic to parasites, ravages cattle and sheep over millions of square miles of East Africa.[192]

Pathogenesis. African trypanosomes are covered by a single, abundant, glycolipid-anchored protein called the variable surface glycoprotein (VSG).[193] As parasites increase in numbers in the bloodstream, the host produces antibodies to the VSG, which, in association with phagocytes, kill most of the organisms, causing a spike of fever. A small number of parasites, however, undergo a genetic rearrangement and produce a different VSG on their surface and so escape the host immune response for a while. These successor clones multiply until the host recognizes their VSG and kills them, allowing another clone with a new VSG to take over. In this way, African trypanosomes cause waves of fever before they finally break down the host defenses and invade the central nervous system. A second important way in which the parasites trick the host immune system is by secreting a lymphocyte-triggering factor that binds to CD8 molecules on suppressor T cells and causes these cells to secrete interferon-γ, which is a strong stimulator of growth of the parasites.[194] The precise mechanisms of tissue injury are unknown, although antigen-antibody complexes and release of lysosomal enzymes from degenerating phagocytes may be involved.

MORPHOLOGY. A large, red, rubbery chancre forms at the site of the insect bite, where large numbers of parasites are surrounded by a dense, largely mononuclear, inflammatory infiltrate. With chronicity, the lymph nodes and spleen enlarge owing to hyperplasia and infiltration by lymphocytes, plasma cells, and macrophages, which are filled with killed parasites. Trypanosomes, which are small and difficult to visualize, concentrate in capillary loops, such as the choroid plexus and glomeruli. When parasites breach the blood-brain barrier and invade the central nervous system, a leptomeningitis extends into the perivascular Virchow-Robin spaces, and eventually a demyelinating panencephalitis occurs. Plasma cells containing glycoprotein globules are frequent and are referred to as **flame cells** or **Mott cells.** Chronic disease leads to progressive cachexia, and patients, devoid of energy and normal mentation, waste away.

Chagas Disease

Trypanosoma cruzi is a kinetoplastid, intracellular protozoan parasite that causes American trypanosomiasis or Chagas disease, the most frequent cause of heart failure in Brazil and neighboring Latin American countries. *T. cruzi* infections are exacerbated by AIDS, which regrettably is rapidly increasing among homosexual and heterosexual populations in Brazil. *T. cruzi* parasites are transmitted from person to person by "kissing bugs" (triatomids), which hide in the cracks of rickety houses, feed on the sleeping inhabitants, and pass infectious parasites in the feces; the infectious parasites enter the host through damaged skin or through mucous membranes. At the site of skin entry, there may be a transient, erythematous nodule called a *chagoma.*

Pathogenesis. *T. cruzi* has on its surface a homolog of the human complement regulatory protein decay-accelerating factor (DAF).[195] Like human DAF, the parasite homolog is anchored by means of a glycosyl phosphatidylinositol linkage, binds C3b, and inhibits C3 convertase formation and alternative pathway complement activation.

At least two different proteins on the surface of *T. cruzi* are involved in parasite entry into macrophages and other cells. The first, a parasite *trans-sialidase,* removes host cell sialic residues and transfers them to a parasite surface protein, which binds to host cells.[196] The second, a protein called *penetrin,* on the surface of *T. cruzi* binds extracellular matrix proteins, heparin, heparan sulfate, and collagen and mediates invasion of the parasites into host cells. *T. cruzi* avoids killing by macrophages by rapidly moving from the lysosome into the host cell cytosol. Two parasite proteins are again involved. (1) A parasite *neuraminidase* removes sialic acids from host proteins lining the lysosomes and so destabilizes this organelle. (2) Stimulated by acid pH within the lysosome, parasites release *hemolysins* that form pores in and disrupt the lysosomal membranes.[197] Parasites reproduce as rounded amastigotes in the cytoplasm of host cells and then develop flagella, burst host cells, enter the bloodstream, and penetrate smooth, skeletal, and heart muscles or infect kissing bugs when the insects take a blood meal.

In acute Chagas disease, which is mild in most individuals, cardiac damage results from direct invasion of myocardial cells by the organisms and from the consequent inflammatory changes. Rarely, acute Chagas patients present with high parasitemia, fever, or progressive cardiac dilation and failure, often with generalized lymphadenopathy or splenomegaly. In *chronic Chagas disease,* which occurs in 20% of infected patients 5 to 15 years after initial infection, the mechanism of cardiac and digestive tract damage is controversial; it appears to result from an autoimmune response induced by *T. cruzi* parasites, which are still present in small numbers. The striking inflammatory infiltration of the myocardium may be induced by the scant number of organisms present, as is the case in mycobacterial granulomas (see earlier).[198] Alternatively, parasites may induce an autoimmune response, such that antibodies and T cells react with parasite proteins and cross-react with host myocardial and nerve cells, lymphocytes, and extracellular proteins such as laminin. Damage to myocardial cells and to conductance pathways causes a dilated cardiomyopathy and cardiac arrhythmias, whereas damage to the myenteric plexus causes dilated colon and esophagus. Autoimmune damage in an experimental mouse model is mediated by CD4+ helper T cells.[199]

MORPHOLOGY. In lethal acute myocarditis, the changes are diffusely distributed throughout the heart. Clusters of leishmanial forms cause swelling of individual myocardial fibers and create intracellular pseudocysts. There is focal myocardial cell necrosis accompanied by extensive, dense, acute interstitial inflammatory infiltration throughout the myocardium (Chapter 13), and there is often four-chamber cardiac dilation.

In **chronic Chagas disease,** which has been treated by cardiac transplantation, the heart is typically dilated, rounded, and increased in size and weight. Often there are mural thrombi that in about half of autopsy cases have given rise to pulmonary or systemic emboli or infarctions. On histologic examination, interstitial and perivascular inflammatory infiltration is composed of lymphocytes, plasma cells, and monocytes and is heaviest in the right bundle branch of the cardiac conduction system. There are scattered foci of myocardial cell necrosis and interstitial fibrosis, especially toward the apex of the left ventricle, which may undergo aneurysmal dilation and thinning. In the Brazilian endemic foci, as many as half of the patients with lethal carditis also have dilation of the esophagus or colon, apparently related to damage to the intrinsic innervation of these organs. At the late stages, however, when such changes appear, parasites cannot be found within these ganglia.

Trichinellosis

Trichinella spiralis is a nematode parasite that is acquired by ingestion of improperly cooked meat from pigs that have themselves been infected by eating *T. spiralis*–infected rats or pork. In the United States, the number of *T. spiralis*–infected pigs was reduced from 11% to 0.5% from 1950 to 1968, with a consequent decrease in *T. spiralis* infection at autopsy from 16% to 4%. Still, trichinosis is widespread where undercooked pork is eaten.

In the human gut, *T. spiralis* parasites develop into adults that mate and release larvae, which penetrate into the tissues. Larvae disseminate hematogenously and penetrate muscle cells, causing fever, myalgias, marked eosinophilia, and periorbital edema. Much less commonly, patients develop dyspnea (because of invasion of the diaphragm), encephalitis, and cardiac failure. In striated skeletal muscle, *T. spiralis* larvae become intracellular parasites, increase dramatically in size, and modify the host muscle cell (referred to as the nurse cell) so that it loses its striations, gains a collagenous capsule, and develops a plexus of new blood vessels around itself.[200] The nurse cell–parasite complex is largely asymptomatic and may exist for years before it calcifies. Antibodies to larval antigens, which include an immunodominant carbohydrate epitope called tyvelose, may reduce reinfection and are useful for serodiagnosis of infections.[201] Although eosinophils are numerous, their precise role is uncertain, because mice depleted of eosinophils with antibodies to IL-5, the lymphokine that stimulates eosinophils, are not more susceptible to primary infection or reinfection with *T. spiralis.*

MORPHOLOGY. During the invasive phase of trichinosis, cell destruction can be widespread but is rarely lethal. In the **heart,** there is a patchy interstitial myocarditis characterized by many eosinophils and giant cells. The myocarditis may lead to scarring. Larvae do not encyst and are difficult to identify, because they die and disappear. In the **lungs,** trapped larvae cause focal edema and hemorrhages, sometimes with an allergic eosinophilic infiltrate. In the **central nervous system,** larvae cause a diffuse lymphocytic and eosinophilic infiltrate, with focal gliosis in and about small capillaries of the brain.

T. spiralis preferentially encysts in striated skeletal muscles with the richest blood supply, including the diaphragm; the extraocular eye; and the laryngeal, deltoid, gastrocnemius, and intercostal muscles (Fig. 9–60). Coiled larvae are approximately 1 mm long and are surrounded by membrane-bound vacuoles within nurse cells, which in turn are surrounded by new blood vessels and a lymphocytic and plasmacytic infiltrate. This infiltrate is greatest around dying parasites, which eventually calcify and leave behind characteristic scars useful for retrospective diagnosis of trichinosis.

Hookworm

Hookworms, primarily *Ancylostoma duodenale* and *Necator americanus*, infect the small intestines of nearly 1 billion persons, mostly in developing countries in the tropics, and cause anemia sufficient to exsanguinate 1.5 million persons each day.[202] Hookworm eggs are passed in the

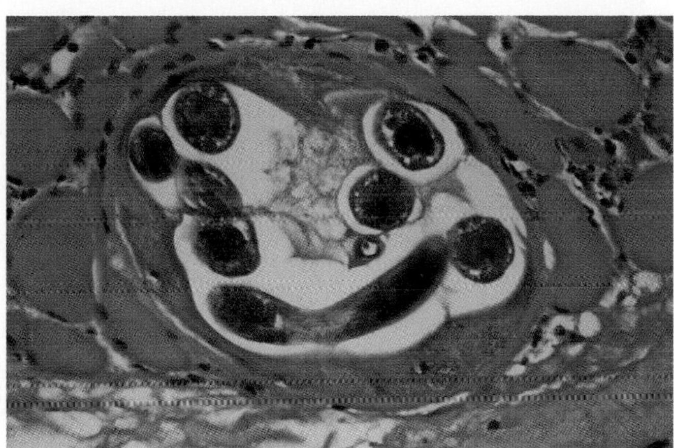

Figure 9–60

Coiled *Trichinella spiralis* larva within a skeletal muscle cell.

feces, hatch in the soil, and infect persons through the skin. Larvae pass through the blood to the lungs, where they escape into alveoli and are coughed up and swallowed. Larvae mature into adults, which attach to the intestinal wall with large teeth and suck the blood of the host. *Ancylostoma,* which consumes 0.2 ml of blood per day per worm, causes severe anemia (resulting in lethargy, weakness, and sometimes death) because individuals may be infected with more than 100 worms. This illustrates the principle alluded to earlier in this chapter that the severity of infections caused by helminths, which do not divide within the host, is proportional to the number of infecting worms. Further, individuals infected with *Ancylostoma* are frequently malnourished and iron deficient, exacerbating their anemia. *Necator,* which consumes only one tenth as much blood as *Ancylostoma,* causes less anemia.

Important virulence factors secreted by hookworms are (1) an anticoagulant protein called AcAP that inactivates clotting factor Xa, (2) antioxidants that inhibit nitric oxide and other reactive oxygen radicals, (3) an anticholinesterase to inhibit intestinal neurons, and (4) hyaluronidase that breaks down host tissues.[203] Rather than target drugs against these proteins, vaccines are being developed to induce inhibitory antibodies.[204]

Cysticercosis and Hydatid Disease

Taenia solium and *Echinococcus granulosus* are cestode parasites (tapeworms) that invade into tissues and cause cysticercus and hydatid infections, respectively. Depending on the route of infection, *T. solium* produces either mild abdominal symptoms, caused by a solitary adult tapeworm in the gut lumen, or convulsions, increased intracranial pressure, and mental disturbances caused by *T. solium* cysts in brain tissue. Adult tapeworms are derived from the ingestion of undercooked pork that contains *T. solium* cysticerci. *T. solium* tapeworms, which may be many inches long, attach to the intestinal wall by hooklike scolices and release proglottid segments with thousands of eggs in the feces each day. When eggs are ingested, the larvae hatch, penetrate the gut wall, disseminate hematogenously, and encyst in the central nervous system, causing cerebral cysticercosis. *T. solium* cysts secrete a protein called antigen B, which binds collagen and the first component of complement, thus inhibiting initiation of the classical complement pathway.[205]

Hydatid disease is caused by ingestion of tapeworm eggs in dog feces, which hatch in the duodenum and invade into the liver, lungs, or bones.[206] Unilocular cysts caused by *E. granulosus,* which also infects sheep, are most common. Multilocular cysts caused by *Echinococcus multilocularis,* which also infects rodents, or *Echinococcus vogeli,* which infects pacas, are less common.

MORPHOLOGY. Cysticerci may be found in any organ, but preferred locations include the brain, muscles, skin, and heart. Cerebral symptoms depend on the precise location of the cysts, which includes the meninges, gray and white matter, sylvian aqueduct, and ventricular foramina. The cysts are ovoid and white to opalescent, rarely exceeding 1.5 cm, and contain an invaginated scolex with hooklets that are bathed in clear cyst fluid (Fig. 9–61). The cyst wall is more than 100 μm thick, is rich in glycoproteins, and evokes little host reaction when it is intact. When cysts degenerate, however, there is inflammation, followed by focal scarring, and calcifications, which may be visible by radiography.

About two thirds of human *E. granulosus* cysts are found in the liver, 5% to 15% in the lung, and the rest in bones and brain or other organs. In the various organs, the larvae lodge within the capil-

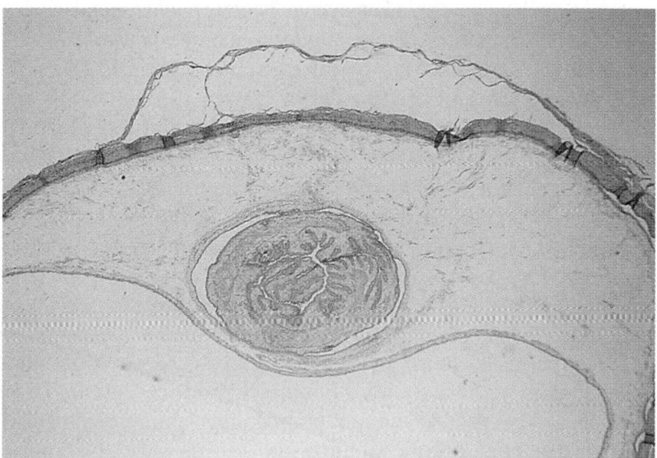

Figure 9–61

Portion of a cysticercus cyst.

laries and first incite an inflammatory reaction composed principally of mononuclear leukocytes and eosinophils. Many such larvae are destroyed, but others encyst. The cysts begin at microscopic levels and progressively increase in size, so that in 5 years or more they may have achieved dimensions more than 10 cm in diameter. Enclosing an opalescent fluid is an inner, nucleated, germinative layer and an outer, opaque, non-nucleated layer. The outer non-nucleated layer is distinctive and has innumerable delicate laminations as though made up of many layers of gelatin. Outside this opaque layer, there is a host inflammatory reaction that produces a zone of fibroblasts, giant cells, and mononuclear and eosinophilic cells. In time, a dense fibrous capsule forms. When these cysts have been present for about 6 months, daughter cysts develop within them. These appear first as minute projections of the germinative layer that develop central vesicles and thus form tiny brood capsules. Scolices of the worm develop on the inner aspects of these brood capsules and separate from the germinative layer to produce a fine, sandlike sediment within the hydatid fluid.

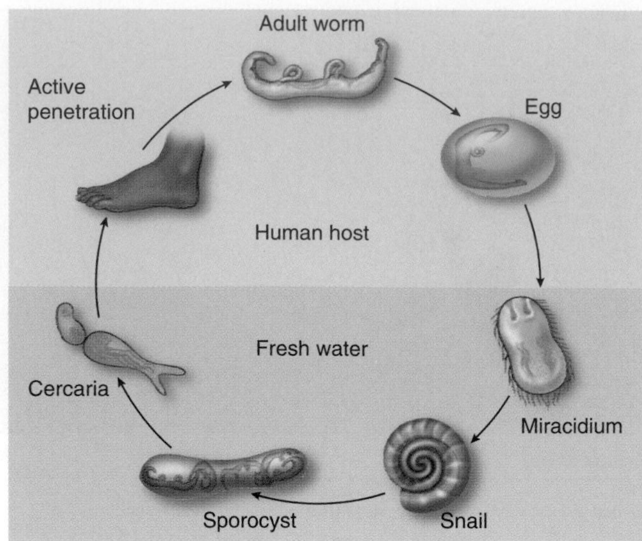

Figure 9–62

Schistosomal life cycle.

Schistosomiasis

Schistosomiasis is the most important helminth disease, infecting approximately 200 million persons and killing approximately 250,000 annually. Most of the mortality comes from hepatic granulomas and fibrosis, caused by *Schistosoma mansoni* in Latin America, Africa, and the Middle East and *Schistosoma japonicum* and *Schistosoma mekongi* in East Asia. In addition, *Schistosoma haematobium,* found in Africa, causes hematuria and granulomatous disease of the bladder, resulting in chronic obstructive uropathy.

Life Cycle. Schistosomiasis is transmitted by freshwater snails that live in the slow-moving water of tropical rivers, lakes, and irrigation ditches, which ironically link agricultural development with spread of schistosomiasis (Fig. 9–62). Infectious schistosome larvae swim through fresh water and penetrate human skin with the aid of powerful proteolytic enzymes that degrade the keratinized layer. Within the skin, schistosome larvae shed a surface glycocalyx that protects the organisms from osmotic shock; this glycocalyx, however, activates complement by the alternative pathway and is recognized by many human antischistosome antibodies. *Schistosomes* migrate into the peripheral vasculature, traverse to the lung, and settle in the portal or pelvic venous system, where they develop into adult male and female schistosomes. Females produce hundreds of eggs per day, around which granulomas and fibrosis form, the major pathologic manifestation in schistosomiasis. Some schistosome eggs are passed from the portal veins through the intestinal wall into the colonic lumen, are shed with the feces, and release into freshwater miracidia that infect the snails to complete the life cycle.

Pathogenesis. *S. mansoni* eggs cause liver disease in multiple ways. First, substances released from schistosome eggs are directly hepatotoxic, because lesions do occur in mice with severe combined immunodeficiency lacking both B and T cells.[207] Second, carbohydrate antigens from eggs induce macrophage accumulation and granuloma formation, mediated by TNF and T_H1 and T_H2 helper cells.[208] T_H2 helper T cells are responsible for the eosinophilia, mastocytosis, and high levels of serum IgE in human schistosomiasis, because these cells secrete IL-4, which induces IgE synthesis by B cells; IL-3 and IL-4, which stimulate mastocytosis; and IL-5, which is a growth factor for eosinophils. Resistance to reinfection by schistosomes after treatment correlates with IgE levels, whereas eosinophil major basic protein may destroy larval schistosomula. Third, eggs release factors that stimulate lymphocytes to secrete a fibrogenic lymphokine that stimulates fibroblast proliferation and portal fibrosis.[209] This exuberant fibrosis, which is out of proportion to the injury caused by the eggs and granulomas, occurs in 5% of persons infected with schistosomes and causes severe portal hypertension, esophageal varices, and ascites, the hallmarks of severe schistosomiasis.

MORPHOLOGY. In mild *S. mansoni* or *S. japonicum* **infections,** white, pinhead-sized granulomas are scattered throughout the gut and liver. The center of the granuloma is the schistosome egg, which contains a miracidium; this degenerates over time and calcifies. The granulomas are composed of macrophages, lymphocytes, neutrophils, and eosinophils; the last-mentioned are distinctive for helminth infections (Fig. 9–63). The liver is darkened by regurgitated heme-derived pigments from the schistosome gut, which like malaria pigments are iron-negative and accumulate in Kupffer cells and splenic macrophages.

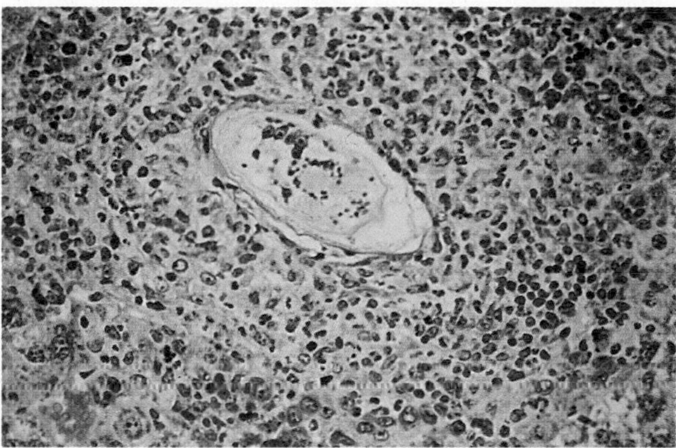

Figure 9–63

Schistosoma mansoni granuloma with a miracidium-containing egg *(center)* and numerous scattered eosinophils.

In severe *S. mansoni* or *S. japonicum* infections, inflammatory patches or pseudopolyps may form in the colon. The surface of the liver is bumpy, whereas cut surfaces reveal granulomas and a widespread fibrous portal enlargement without distortion of the intervening parenchyma by regenerative nodules. Because these fibrous triads resemble the stem of a clay pipe, the lesion is named *pipe-stem fibrosis* (Fig. 9–64). Many of these portal triads lack a vein lumen, causing presinusoidal portal hypertension and severe congestive splenomegaly, esophageal varices, and ascites. Schistosome eggs, diverted to the lung through portal collaterals, may produce granulomatous pulmonary arteritis with intimal hyperplasia, progressive arterial obstruction, and ultimately heart failure (cor pulmonale). On histologic examination, arteries in the lungs show disruption of the elastica layer by granulomas and scars, luminal organizing thrombi, and angiomatoid lesions similar to those of idiopathic pulmonary hypertension (Chapter 16). Patients with hepatosplenic schistosomiasis also have an increased frequency of mesangioproliferative or membranous glomerulopathy (Chapter 21), in which glomeruli contain deposits of immunoglobulin and complement but rarely schistosome antigen.

In *S. haematobium* infection, bladder inflammatory patches due to massive egg deposition and granulomas appear early and, when they erode, cause hematuria (see Fig. 9–15). Later the granulomas calcify and develop a "sandy" appearance, which if severe may line the wall of the bladder and cause a dense concentric rim (calcified bladder) on x-ray films. The most frequent complication of *S. haematobium* infection is inflammation and fibrosis of the ureteral walls, leading to obstruction, hydronephrosis, and chronic pyelonephritis. There is also an association between urinary schistosomiasis and squamous carcinoma of the bladder (Chapter 22).

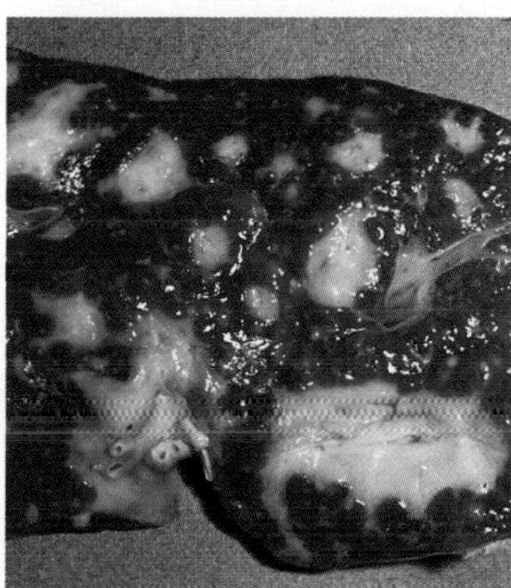

Figure 9–64

Pipe-stem fibrosis of the liver due to chronic *Schistosoma japonicum* infection.

Lymphatic Filariasis

Lymphatic filariasis is transmitted by mosquitoes and is caused by two closely related nematodes, *Wuchereria bancrofti* and *Brugia malayi,* which are responsible for 90% and 10%, respectively, of the 90 million infections worldwide. In endemic areas, which include parts of Latin America, sub-Saharan Africa, and Southeast Asia, filariasis causes a spectrum of diseases, including (1) asymptomatic microfilaremia, (2) chronic lymphadenitis with swelling of the dependent limb or scrotum (elephantiasis), and (3) tropical pulmonary eosinophilia. As is the case with leprosy and leishmanial infections, some of the different disease manifestations caused by lymphatic filariae may be understood in the context of varying patterns of host T-cell responses to the parasites.[210]

Pathogenesis. Infective larvae released by mosquitoes into the tissues during the blood meal develop within lymphatic channels into adult males and females, which mate and release microfilariae that enter into the bloodstream. Experiments in nude mice suggest that adult filariae secrete factors that, by themselves, are capable of causing lymphatic dilation, lymphedema, and elephantiasis. In contrast, microfilariae, even in massive numbers in microfilaremic hosts, are not directly toxic to the host.

In chronic lymphatic filariasis, damage to the lymphatics is caused directly by the adult parasites and by a T_H1 helper T cell–mediated immune response, which forms granulomas around the adult parasites. Microfilariae are absent from the bloodstream, secondary to immune damage to the adults and to microfilariae.

In contrast, there is a *hypoimmune response* to circulating parasites in microfilaremic individuals, associated with filaria-specific T_H2 helper cells that down-regulate T_H1

cells and inhibit granuloma formation.[211] Because most microfilaremic individuals come from areas endemic with filariasis, there is speculation that the hypoimmune response is caused by prenatal exposure to parasite antigens that may tolerize the host.

Finally, there is an *IgE-mediated hypersensitivity* to microfilariae in *tropical pulmonary eosinophilia.* Both IgE and eosinophils may be secondary to secretion of IL-4 and IL-5, respectively, by filaria-specific T_H2 helper T cells. Tropical pulmonary eosinophilia results in restrictive lung disease, discussed in Chapter 16.

MORPHOLOGY. Chronic filariasis is characterized by persistent lymphedema of the scrotum, penis, vulva, leg, or arm (Fig. 9–65). Frequently, there is hydrocele and lymph node enlargement. In severe and long-lasting infections, chylous weeping of the enlarged scrotum may ensue, or a chronically swollen leg may develop tough subcutaneous fibrosis and epithelial hyperkeratosis, termed **elephantiasis.** Elephantoid skin shows dilation of the dermal lymphatics with widespread lymphocytic infiltrates and focal cholesterol deposits; the epidermis is thickened and hyperkeratotic. Adult filarial worms—live, dead, or calcified—are present in the scrotal draining lymphatics or nodes, surrounded by (1) mild or no inflammation, (2) an intense eosinophilia with hemorrhage and fibrin (recurrent filarial funiculoepididymitis), or (3) granulomas not dissimilar to those found in mycobacterial infections. Organization of the endolymphatic exudate results in polypoid infoldings of the vessels with persisting eosinophilic and lymphocytic infiltrates. In time, hydrocele fluid, which often contains cholesterol crystals, red cells, and hemosiderin, induces thickening and calcification of the tunica vaginalis.

Lung involvement by microfilariae is marked by eosinophilia caused by circulating antimicrofilarial IgEs that trigger mast cell degranulation (tropical eosinophilia) or by dead microfilariae surrounded by stellate, hyaline, eosinophilic precipitates embedded in small epithelioid granulomas (Meyers-Kouvenaar bodies). Typically, these patients lack any other manifestations of filarial disease.

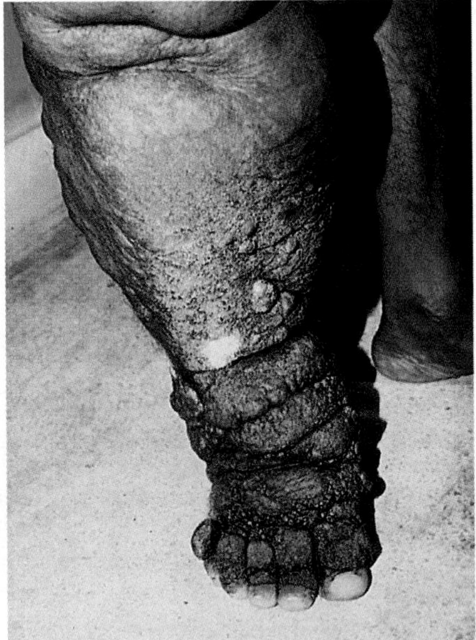

Figure 9–65

Filariasis of the leg. (Courtesy of Dr. Willy Piessens, Harvard School of Public Health.)

Onchocerciasis

Onchocerca volvulus, a filarial nematode transmitted by black flies, has been a major cause of blindness in equatorial Africa, where the parasite once infected 20 million persons. Recently, an aggressive campaign of ivermectin treatment has dramatically reduced the incidence of *Onchocerca* infection and may lead to eradication of this disease in some areas.[212]

Adult *O. volvulus* parasites mate in the dermis, where they are surrounded by a mixed infiltrate of host cells that produces a characteristic subcutaneous nodule *(onchocercoma).* The major pathologic process, however, which includes blindness and chronic pruritic dermatitis, is caused by large numbers of microfilariae, released by females, that accumulate in the skin and in the eye chambers. *Punctate keratitis* is caused by inflammation around a degenerating microfilaria. It is sometimes accentuated by treatment with antifilarial drugs (Mazzotti reaction), resulting in blindness. Damage to the retina, which is disproportionate to the number of parasites in the posterior eye chamber, is probably caused by release of host cytokines including IL-12.[213]

MORPHOLOGY. Severe infection with *O. volvulus* causes chronic, itchy dermatitis with focal darkening or loss of pigment and scaling referred to as leopard, lizard, or elephant skin. Foci of epidermal atrophy and elastic fiber breakdown may alternate with areas of hyperkeratosis, hyperpigmentation with pigment incontinence, dermal atrophy, and fibrosis. The subcutaneous onchocercoma is composed of a fibrous capsule surrounding adult worms and a mixed chronic inflammatory infiltrate that includes fibrin, neutrophils, eosinophils, lymphocytes, and giant cells (Fig. 9–66). The progressive eye lesions begin with punctate keratitis along with small, fluffy opacities of the cornea caused by degenerating microfilariae, which evoke an eosinophilic infiltrate. This is followed by a sclerosing keratitis that opacifies the cornea, beginning at the scleral limbus. Microfilariae in the anterior chamber cause iridocyclitis and glaucoma, whereas involvement of the choroid and retina results in atrophy and loss of vision.

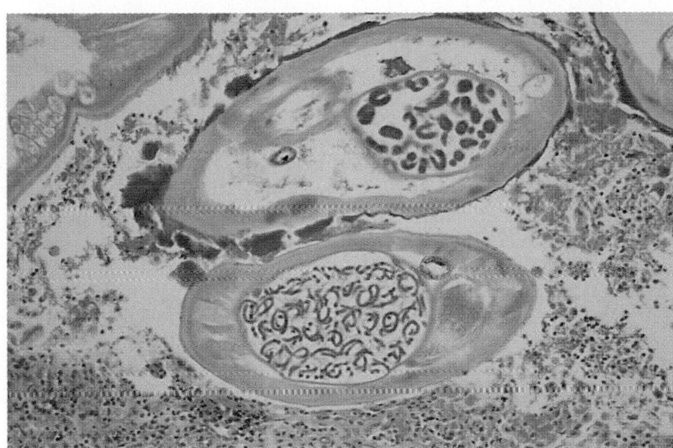

Figure 9–66 ■

Gravid female of *Onchocerca volvulus* in a subcutaneous fibrous nodule.

The extraordinary contributions of Dr. Franz von Lichtenberg to previous editions of this chapter, which include many of the descriptions of the lesions and most of the photomicrographs, are acknowledged here, with deepest appreciation.

REFERENCES

1. Murray CJ, Lopez AD: Global mortality, disability, and the contribution of risk factors: Global Burden of Disease Study. Lancet 349: 1436, 1997.
2. Falkow S: Molecular Koch's postulates applied to microbial pathogenicity. Rev Infect Dis 10:S274, 1988.
3. Brown H: Ilya Mechnikov and his studies on comparative inflammation. Proc Soc Exp Biol Med 209:99, 1995.
4. Tomb J-F, et al: The complete genome sequence of the gastric pathogen *Helicobacter pylori*. Nature 388:539, 1997.
5. Blattner FR, et al: The complete genome sequence of *Escherichia coli* K-12. Science 277:1453, 1997.
6. Lederberg J: Infectious disease as an evolutionary paradigm. Emerg Infect Dis 3:417, 1997.
7. Greenberg HB, et al: Rotavirus pathology and pathophysiology. Curr Top Microbiol Immunol 185:255, 1994.
8. Le Guenno B, et al: Isolation and partial characterization of a new strain of Ebola virus. Lancet 345:1271, 1995.
9. von Lichtenberg F: Pathology of Infectious Disease. New York, Raven Press, 1991.
10. O'Connor DH, et al: Pathology of Infectious Diseases. Stanford, CT, Appleton & Lange, 1996.
11. Horwich AL, Weissman JS: Deadly conformations—protein misfolding in prion disease. Cell 89:499, 1997.
12. Tracey S, et al: Genetics of coxsackievirus B cardiovirulence and inflammatory heart muscle disease. Trends Microbiol 4:175, 1996.
13. Walker DH, Tumler JS: Emergence of the ehrlichioses as human health problems. Emerg Infect Dis 2:18, 1996.
14. Mims CA: The Pathogenesis of Infectious Disease, 4th ed. San Diego, CA, Academic Press, 1996.
15. Metcalf TG, et al: Environmental virology: from detection of virus in sewage and water by isolation to identification by molecular biology—a trip of over 50 years. Annu Rev Microbiol 49:461, 1995.
16. Chan DC, et al: Core structure of gp41 from the HIV envelope glycoprotein. Cell 89:263, 1997.
17. Liu R, et al: Homozygous defect in HIV-1 coreceptor accounts for resistance of some multiply-exposed individuals to HIV-1 infection. Cell 86:367, 1996.
18. Cudmore S, et al: Viral manipulations of the actin cytoskeleton. Trends Microbiol 5:142, 1997.
19. Kondo T, et al: Essential roles of the Fas ligand in the development of hepatitis. Nat Med 3:409, 1997.
20. Graham BS: Immunological determinants of disease caused by respiratory syncytial virus. Trends Microbiol 4:293, 1996.
21. Gillet G, Brun G: Viral inhibition of apoptosis. Trends Microbiol 4: 312, 1996.
22. Groisman EA, Ochman H: How *Salmonella* became a pathogen. Trends Microbiol 5:343, 1997.
23. Hale TL: Genetic basis of virulence in *Shigella* species. Microbiol Rev 55:206, 1991.
24. Covacci A, et al: Did inheritance of a pathogenicity island modify the virulence of *Helicobacter pylori?* Trends Microbiol 5:205, 1997.
25. Lee CA: Type III secretion systems: machines to deliver bacterial proteins into eukaryotic cells? Trends Microbiol 5:148, 1997.
26. Fischetti VA: Streptococcal M protein. Sci Am 264:58, 1991.
27. Waldor MK, Mekalanos JJ: Lysogenic conversion by a filamentous phage encoding cholera toxin. Science 272:1910, 1996.
28. Marra A, Isberg R: Common entry mechanisms. Bacterial pathogenesis. Curr Biol 6:1084, 1996.
29. Brandtzaeg P: Significance and pathogenesis of septic shock. Curr Top Microbiol Immunol 216:16, 1996.
30. Choe S, et al: The crystal structure of diphtheria toxin. Nature 357: 216, 1992.
31. Sears CL, Kaper JB: Enteric bacterial toxins: mechanisms of action and linkage to intestinal secretion. Microbiol Rev 60:167, 1996.
32. Kaufman AF, et al: The economic impact of a bioterrorist attack: are prevention and postattack intervention programs justfiable? Emerg Infect Dis 3:83, 1997.
33. Smith GL: Virus strategies for evasion of the host response to infection. Trends Microbiol 2:81, 1994.
34. Zhang J-R, et al: Antigenic variation in Lyme disease borreliae by promiscuous recombination of VMP-like sequences. Cell 89:275, 1997.
35. Su X-Z, et al: The large diverse gene family *var* encodes proteins involved in cytoadherence and antigenic variation of *Plasmodium falciparum*–infected erythrocytes. Cell 82:89, 1995.
36. Relman DA, et al: Identification of the uncultured bacillus of Whipple's disease. N Engl J Med 327:293, 1992.
37. Beard CB, Navin TR: Molecular epidemiology of *Pneumocystis carinii* pneumonia. Emerg Infect Dis 2:147, 1996.
38. Johnston SL: Problems and prospects of developing effective therapy for common cold viruses. Trends Microbiol 5:58, 1997.
39. Rossman MG, Johnson JE: Icosahedral virus structure. Annu Rev Biochem 58:533, 1989.
40. Staunton DE, et al: The arrangement of the immunoglobulin-like domains of ICAM-1 and the binding sites for LFA-1 and rhinovirus. Cell 61:243, 1990.
41. Bullough PA, et al: Structure of influenza haemagglutinin at the pH of membrane fusion. Nature 371:37, 1994.
42. Arnheiter H, et al: Transgenic mice with intracellular immunity to influenza virus. Cell 62:51, 1990.
43. Gorman OT, et al: Evolutionary processes in influenza viruses: divergence, rapid evolution, and stasis. Curr Top Microbiol Immunol 176:75, 1992.
44. Taubenberger JK, et al: Initial genetic characterization of the 1918 "Spanish" influenza virus. Science 275:1739, 1997.
45. Roche RJ, Moxon ER: Phenotypic variation of carbohydrate surface antigens and the pathogenesis of *Haemophilus influenzae* infections. Trends Microbiol 3:304, 1995.
46. Gilsdorf JR, et al: Role of pili in *Haemophilus influenzae* adherence and colonization. Infect Immun 65:2997, 1997.
47. Bloom BR, Murray CJL: Tuberculosis: commentary on a reemergent killer. Science 257:1055, 1992.
48. Heym B, et al: Mechanisms of drug resistance in *Mycobacterium tuberculosis*. Curr Top Microbiol Immunol 215:49, 1996.
49. Long EG, et al: Model for pathogenesis of *Mycobacterium avium*. Ann N Y Acad Sci 797:255, 1996.
50. Quinn FD, et al: Virulence determinants of *Mycobacterium tuberculosis*. Curr Top Microbiol Immunol 215:131, 1996.
51. Clemens DL: Characterization of the *Mycobacterium tuberculosis* phagosome. Trends Microbiol 4:113, 1996.

52. Stenger S, et al: Differential effects of cytolytic T cell subsets on intracellular infection. Science 276:1684, 1997.
53. Vidal SM, et al: Natural resistance to infection with intracellular parasites: isolation of a candidate for *Bcg*. Cell 73:469, 1993.
54. Maresca B, et al: Morphological transition in the human fungal pathogen *Histoplasma capsulatum*. Trends Microbiol 2:110, 1994.
55. Kirkland TN, Fierer J: Coccidioidomycosis: a reemerging infectious disease. Emerg Infect Dis 2:192, 1996.
56. Neutra MR, et al: Antigen sampling across epithelial barriers and induction of mucosal immune responses. Annu Rev Immunol 14: 275, 1996.
57. Berg RD: Bacterial translocation from the gastrointestinal tract. Trends Microbiol 3:149, 1995.
58. Burke B, Desselberger U: Rotavirus pathogenicity. Virology 218: 299, 1996.
59. Hall GA: Comparative pathology of infection by novel diarrhea viruses. Ciba Found Symp 128:192, 1987.
60. Hermant D, et al: Functional conservation of the *Salmonella* and *Shigella* effectors of entry into epithelial cells. Mol Microbiol 17: 781, 1995.
61. Lingwood CA: Role of verotoxin receptors in pathogenesis. Trends Microbiol 4:147, 1996.
62. Allos BM, Blaser MJ: *Campylobacter jejuni* and the expanding spectrum of related infections. Clin Infect Dis 20:1092, 1995.
63. Wooldridge KG, Ketley JM: *Campylobacter*–host cell interactions. Trends Microbiol 5:96, 1997.
64. Isberg RR: Uptake of enteropathogenic *Yersinia* by mammalian cells. Curr Top Microbiol Immunol 209:1, 1996.
65. Cornelis GR, Wolf-Watz H: The *Yersinia* Yop virulon: a bacterial system for subverting eukaryotic cells. Mol Microbiol 23:861, 1997.
66. Galyov EE, et al: A secreted protein kinase of *Y. pseudotuberculosis* is an indispensible virulence determinant. Nature 361:730, 1993.
67. Jones BB, Falkow S: Salmonellosis: host immune responses and bacterial virulence determinants. Annu Rev Immunol 14:533, 1996.
68. Alpuche Aranda CM, et al: *Salmonella typhimurium* activates gene transcription within acidified macrophage phagosomes. Proc Natl Acad Sci USA 89:10079, 1992.
69. Mahan MJ, et al: Selection of bacterial virulence genes that are specifically induced in host tissues. Science 259:686, 1993.
70. Mooi FR, Bik EM: The evolution of epidemic *Vibrio cholerae* strains. Trends Microbiol 5:161, 1997.
71. Spangler BD: Structure and function of cholera toxin and the related *Escherichia coli* heat-labile enterotoxin. Microbiol Rev 56:622, 1992.
72. Ravdin JI: Amebiasis. State-of-the-art clinical article. Clin Infect Dis 20:1453, 1995.
73. Rosenthal B, et al: Evidence for the bacterial origin of genes encoding fermentation enzymes of the amitochondriate protozoan parasite *Entamoeba histolytica*. J Bacteriol 179:3736, 1997.
74. Leippe M: Amoebapores. Parasitol Today 13:178, 1997.
75. Diamond LS, Clark CG: A redescription of *Entamoeba histolytica* Schaudinn, 1903 (emended Walker, 1911) separating it from *Entamoeba dispar* Brumpt, 1925. J Eukaryot Microbiol 40:340, 1993.
76. Adam RD: The biology of *Giardia* spp. Microbiol Rev 55:706, 1991.
77. Lujan HD, et al: Cholesterol starvation induces differentiation of the intestinal parasite *Giardia lamblia*. Proc Natl Acad Sci USA 93: 7628, 1996.
78. Upcroft P, et al: Telomeric organization of a variable and inducible toxin gene family in the ancient eukaryote *Giardia duodenalis*. Genome Res 7:37, 1997.
79. Mowatt MR, et al: Size heterogeneity among antigenically related *Giardia lamblia* variant-specific surface proteins is due to differences in tandem repeat copy number. Infect Immun 62:1213, 1994.
80. Aral SO, Holmes KK: Sexually transmitted diseases in the AIDS era. Sci Am 264:62, 1991.
81. Stanbury LR: Pathogenesis of herpes simplex virus infection and animal models for its study. Curr Top Microbiol Immunol 179:15, 1992.
82. Croen KD, Straus SE: Varicella-zoster virus latency. Annu Rev Microbiol 45:265, 1991.
83. Doymaz MZ, Rouse BT: Immunopathology of herpes simplex virus infections. Curr Top Microbiol Immunol 179:121, 1992.
84. Offerman MK: HHV-8: a new herpesvirus associated with Kaposi's sarcoma. Trends Microbiol 4:383, 1996.
85. Thylefors B, et al: Global data on blindness. Bull World Health Organ 73:115, 1995.
86. Moulder JW: Interaction of chlamydiae and host cells in vitro. Microbiol Rev 55:143, 1991.
87. Black CM: Current methods of laboratory diagnosis of *Chlamydia trachomatis* infections. Clin Microbiol Rev 10:160, 1997.
88. Olyhoek T, et al: Clonal population structure of *Neisseria meningitidis* serogroup A isolated from epidemics and pandemics between 1915 and 1983. Rev Infect Dis 9:665, 1987.
89. Gomez-Duarte OG, et al: Binding of vitronectin to opa-expressing *Neisseria gonorrhoeae* mediates invasion of HeLa cells. Infect Immun 65:3857, 1997.
90. Seifert HS: Questions about gonococcal pilus phase- and antigenic variation. Mol Microbiol 21:433, 1996.
91. McGee ZA, et al: Local induction of tumor necrosis factor as a molecular mechanism of mucosal damage by gonococci. Microb Pathog 12:333, 1992.
92. Thomas DD, et al: Enhanced levels of attachment of fibronectin-primed *Treponema pallidum* to extracellular matrix. Infect Immun 52:736, 1986.
93. Blanco DR, et al: Surface antigens of the syphilis spirochete and their potential as virulence determinants. Emerg Infect Dis 3:11, 1997.
94. Fitzgerald TJ: The Th_1/Th_2-like switch in syphilitic infection: is it detrimental? Infect Immun 60:3475, 1992.
95. Bradley PJ, et al: Targeting and translocation of proteins into the hydrogenosome of the protist *Trichomonas:* similarities with mitochondrial protein import. EMBO J 16:3484, 1997.
96. Ji G, et al: Bacterial interference caused by autoinducing peptide variants. Science 276:2027, 1997.
97. Foster TJ, McDevitt D: Surface-associated proteins of *Staphylococcus aureus*: their possible roles in virulence. FEMS Microbiol Lett 118:199, 1994.
98. Kaneko J, et al: Sequential binding of staphylococcal gamma-hemolysin to human erythrocytes and complex formation of the hemolysin on the cell surface. Biosci Biotech Biochem 61:846, 1997.
99. Swaminathan S, et al: Crystal structure of staphylococcal enterotoxin B, a superantigen. Nature 359:801, 1992.
100. See RH, Chow AW: Microbiology of toxic shock syndrome. Rev Infect Dis 11:S55, 1989.
101. Johnston RB: Pathogenesis of pneumococcal pneumonia. Rev Infect Dis 13:S509, 1991.
102. Paton JC: The contribution of pneumolysin to the pathogenicity of *Streptococcus pneumoniae*. Trends Microbiol 4:103, 1996.
103. Loeche WJ: Role of *Streptococcus mutans* in human dental decay. Microbiol Rev 50:353, 1986.
104. Cunningham MW, et al: Cytotoxic and viral neutralizing antibodies cross-react with streptococcal M protein, enteroviruses, and human cardiac myosin. Proc Natl Acad Sci USA 89:1320, 1992.
105. Stevens DL: The toxins of group A streptococcus, the flesh eating bacteria. Immunol Invest 26:129, 1997.
106. Songer JG: Bacterial phospholipases and their role in virulence. Trends Microbiol 5:156, 1997.
107. Linial M: Bacterial neurotoxins—a thousand years later. Isr J Med Sci 31:591, 1995.
108. Hammond GA, et al: Transcriptional analysis of the toxigenic element of *Clostridium difficile*. Microb Pathog 22:143, 1997.
109. Brook I: Encapsulated anaerobic bacteria in synergistic infections. Microbiol Rev 50:452, 1986.
110. Weiss R: Measles battle loses potent weapon. Science 258:546, 1992.
111. Hutchins S: Measles outbreaks in the United States, 1987 through 1990. Pediatr Infect Dis J 15:31, 1996.
112. Hsu EC, et al: Artificial mutations and natural variations in the CD46 molecules from human and monkey cells define regions important for measles virus binding. J Virol 71:6144, 1997.
113. Cattaneo R, Billeter MA: Mutations and A/I hypermutations in measles virus persistent infections. Curr Top Microbiol Immunol 176:63, 1992.
114. van Loon FP, et al: Mumps surveillance—United States, 1988–1993. MMWR CDC Surveill Summ 44:1, 1995.

115. Birkenbach M, et al: Characterization of an Epstein-Barr virus receptor on human epithelial cells. J Exp Med 176:1405, 1992.
116. Izumi KM, et al: The Epstein-Barr virus LMP1 amino acid sequence that engages tumor necrosis factor receptor associated factors is critical for primary B lymphocyte growth transformation. Proc Natl Acad Sci USA 94:1447, 1997.
117. Sixbey JW, Yao Q-Y: Immunoglobulin A–induced shift of Epstein-Barr virus tissue tropism. Science 255:1578, 1992.
118. Minor PD: The molecular biology of polioviruses vaccines. J Gen Virol 73:3065, 1992.
119. Dowdle WR, Birmingham ME: The biologic principles of poliovirus eradication. J Infect Dis 175:S286, 1997.
120. Nomoto A, et al: Tissue tropism and species specificity of poliovirus infection. Trends Microbiol 2:47, 1994.
121. Racaniello VR, et al: Poliovirus biology and pathogenesis. Curr Top Microbiol Immunol 206:305, 1996.
122. White CJ: Varicella-zoster virus vaccine. Clin Infect Dis 24:753, 1997.
123. Steiner I: Human herpes viruses latent infection in the nervous system. Immunol Rev 152:157, 1996.
124. Cherry JD: Historical review of pertussis and the classical vaccine. J Infect Dis 174:S259, 1996.
125. Beier D, et al: Signal transduction and virulence regulation in *Bordetella pertussis*. Microbiologia 12:185, 1996.
126. Gierschik P: ADP-ribosylation of signal-transducing guanine nucleotide–binding proteins by pertussis toxin. Curr Top Microbiol Immunol 175:69, 1992.
127. Hardy IR, et al: Current situation and control strategies for resurgence of diphtheria in newly independent states of the former Soviet Union. Lancet 347:1739, 1996.
128. Sinzger C, Jahn G: Human cytomegalovirus cell tropism and pathogenesis. Intervirology 39:302, 1996.
129. Grundy JE: Virologic and pathogenetic aspects of cytomegalovirus infections. Rev Infect Dis 12:S711, 1990.
130. Govan JRW, Deretic V: Microbial pathogenesis in cystic fibrosis: mucoid *Pseudomonas aeruginosa* and *Burkholderia cepacia*. Microbiol Rev 60:539, 1996.
131. Kreitman RJ, Pastan I: Targeting *Pseudomonas* exotoxin to hematologic malignancies. Semin Cancer Biol 6:297, 1995.
132. Britigan BE, et al: Interaction of the *Pseudomonas aeruginosa* secretory products pyocyanin and pyochelin generates hydroxyl radical and causes synergistic damage to endothelial cells. J Clin Invest 90: 2187, 1992.
133. Stout JE, Yu VL: Legionellosis. N Engl J Med 337:682, 1997.
134. Cianciotto NP, Fields BS: *Legionella pneumophila mip* gene potentiates intracellular infection of protozoa and human macrophages. Proc Natl Acad Sci USA 89:5188, 1992.
135. Southwick FS, Purich DL: Intracellular pathogenesis of listeriosis. N Engl J Med 334:770, 1996.
136. Mengaud J, et al: E-cadherin is the receptor for internalin, a surface protein required for entry of *L. monocytogenes* into epithelial cells. Cell 84:923, 1996.
137. Dramsi S, et al: Molecular and genetic determinants involved in invasion of mammalian cells by *Listeria monocytogenes*. Curr Top Microbiol Immunol 209:61, 1996.
138. Calderone RA, Braun PC: Adherence and receptor relationships of *Candida albicans*. Microbiol Rev 55:1, 1991.
139. Sanglard D, et al: A triple deletion of the secreted aspartyl proteinase genes SAP4, SAP5, and SAP6 of *Candida albicans* causes attenuated virulence. Infect Immun 65:3539, 1997.
140. Kohler JR, Fink GR: *Candida albicans* strains heterozygous and homozygous for mutations in mitogen-activated protein kinase signaling components have defects in hyphal development. Proc Natl Acad Sci USA 93:13223, 1996.
141. Kozel TR: Virulence factors of *Cryptococcus neoformans*. Trends Microbiol 3:295, 1995.
142. Debeaupuis JP, et al: Genetic diversity among clinical and environmental isolates of *Aspergillus fumigatus*. Infect Immun 65:3080, 1997.
143. Bouchara JP, et al: Sialic acid–dependent recognition of laminin and fibrinogen by *Aspergillus fumigatus* conidia. Infect Immun 65:2717, 1997.
144. Prieto R, et al: Identification of aflatoxin biosynthesis genes by genetic complementation in an *Aspergillus flavus* mutant lacking the aflatoxin gene cluster. Appl Environ Microbiol 62:3567, 1996.
145. Arruda LK, et al: *Aspergillus fumigatus* allergen I, a major IgE-binding protein, is a member of the mitogillin family of cytotoxins. J Exp Med 172:1529, 1990.
146. Simonds RJ, et al: Preventing *Pneumocystis carinii* pneumonia in persons infected with human immunodeficiency virus. Clin Infect Dis 21:S44, 1995.
147. Edman JC, et al: Ribosomal RNA sequence shows *Pneumocystis carinii* to be a member of the fungi. Nature 334:519, 1988.
148. Roths JB, Sidman CL: Both immunity and hyperresponsiveness to *Pneumocystis carinii* result from transfer of CD4+ but not CD8+ T cells into severe combined immunodeficiency mice. J Clin Invest 90: 673, 1992.
149. Steiner TS, et al: Protozoal agents: what are the dangers for the public water supply? Annu Rev Med 48:329, 1997.
150. Guerrant RL: Cryptosporidiosis: an emerging, highly infectious threat. Emerg Infect Dis 3:51, 1997.
151. McDonald V, et al: Immune responses to *Cryptosporidium muris* and *Cryptosporidium parvum* in adult immunocompetent or immunocompromised (nude and SCID) mice. Infect Immun 60:3325, 1992.
152. Herwaldt BL, Ackers ML: An outbreak in 1996 of cyclosporiasis associated with imported raspberries. N Engl J Med 336:1548, 1997.
153. Ambrose-Thomas P, Pelloux H: Toxoplasmosis—congenital and in immunocompromised patients: a parallel. Parasitol Today 9:61, 1993.
154. Howe DK, et al: Determination of genotypes of *Toxoplasma gondii* strains isolated from patients with toxoplasmosis. J Clin Microbiol 35:1411, 1997.
155. Sher A, et al: Induction and regulation of host cell–mediated immunity by *Toxoplasma gondii*. Ciba Found Symp 195:95, 1995.
156. Dobrowolski JM, Sibley LD: *Toxoplasma* invasion of mammalian cells is powered by the actin cytoskeleton of the parasite. Cell 84: 933, 1996.
157. Carruthers VB, Sibley LD: Sequential protein secretion from three distinct organelles of *Toxoplasma gondii* accompanies invasion of human fibroblasts. Eur J Cell Biol 73:114, 1997.
158. Monath TP: Dengue: the risk to developed and developing countries. Proc Natl Acad Sci USA 91:2395, 1994.
159. La Russa VF, Innis BL: Mechanisms of dengue virus–induced bone marrow suppression. Baillieres Clin Haematol 8:249, 1995.
160. Morens DM: Antibody-dependent enhancement of infection and the pathogenesis of viral disease. Clin Infect Dis 19:500, 1994.
161. Walker DH, Dumler JS: Emerging and reemerging rickettsial diseases. N Engl J Med 331:1651,1994.
162. Bise G, Coninx R: Epidemic typhus in a prison in Burundi. Trans R Soc Trop Med Hyg 91:133, 1997.
163. Feng H, et al: Role of T lymphocyte subsets in immunity to spotted fever group rickettsiae. J Immunol 158:5314, 1997.
164. Walker DH, et al: Cytokine-induced, nitric oxide–dependent, intracellular antirickettsial activity of mouse endothelial cells. Lab Invest 76:129, 1997.
165. Ranson MK, Evans TG: The global burden of trachomatous visual impairment: I. Assessing prevalence. Int Ophthalmol 19:261, 1995.
166. Bobo L, et al: Evidence for a predominant proinflammatory conjunctival cytokine response in individuals with trachoma. Infect Immun 64:3273, 1996.
167. Rada E, et al: A longitudinal study of immunologic reactivity in leprosy patients treated with immunotherapy. Int J Lepr Other Mycobact Dis 62:552, 1994.
168. Kim J, et al: Determinants of T cell reactivity to the *Mycobacterium leprae* GroES homologue. J Immunol 159:335, 1997.
169. Yamamura M, et al: Defining protective responses to pathogens: cytokine profiles in leprosy lesions. Science 254:277, 1991.
170. Kaur G, et al: Association of polymorphism at *COL3A* and *CTLA4* loci on chromosome 2q31–33 with the clinical phenotype and in-vitro CMI status in healthy and leprosy subjects: a preliminary study. Hum Genet 100:43, 1997.
171. Cravens G, Marr JS: The Black Death. New York, Ballantine Books, 1977.
172. Perry RD, Fetherston JD: *Yersinia pestis*—etiologic agent of plague. Clin Microbiol Rev 10:35, 1997.
173. Sodeinde OA, et al: A surface protease and the invasive character of plague. Science 258:1004, 1992.

174. Barbour AG, et al: Variable antigen genes of the relapsing fever agent *Borrelia hermsii* are activated by promoter addition. Mol Microbiol 5:489, 1991.
175. Fekade D, et al: Prevention of Jarisch-Herxheimer reactions by treatment with antibodies against tumor necrosis factor alpha. N Engl J Med 335:311, 1996.
176. Armstrong PM, et al: A new *Borrelia* infecting Lone Star ticks. Lancet 347:67, 1996.
177. Evans J: Lyme disease. Curr Opin Rheumatol 9:328, 1997.
178. Garcia-Monco JC, Benach JL: Mechanisms of injury in Lyme neuroborreliosis. Semin Neurol 17:57, 1997.
179. Sigal LH: Lyme disease: a review of aspects of its immunology and immunopathogenesis. Annu Rev Immunol 15:63, 1997.
180. Goldberg DE, et al: Probing the chloroquine resistance locus of *Plasmodium falciparum* with a novel class of multidentate metal(III) coordination complexes. J Biol Chem 272:6567, 1997.
181. Stoute JA, et al: A preliminary evaluation of a recombinant circumsporozoite protein vaccine against *Plasmodium falciparum* malaria. N Engl J Med 336:86, 1997.
182. Cerami C: The basolateral domain of the hepatocyte plasma membrane bears receptors for the circumsporozoite protein of *Plasmodium falciparum* sporozoites. Cell 70:1021, 1992.
183. Hill AVS, et al: Molecular analysis of the association of HLA-B53 and resistance to severe malaria. Nature 360:434, 1992.
184. Francis SE, et al: Characterization of native falcipain, an enzyme involved in *Plasmodium falciparum* hemoglobin degradation. Mol Biochem Parasitol 83:189, 1996.
185. Crabb BS, et al: Targeted gene disruption shows that knobs enable malaria-infected red cells to cytoadhere under physiological shear stress. Cell 89:287, 1997.
186. Boustani MR, Gelfand JA: Babesiosis. Clin Infect Dis 22:611, 1996.
187. Magill AJ: Epidemiology of the leishmaniases. Dermatol Clin 13: 505, 1995.
188. Titus RG, Ribeiro JMC: Salivary gland lysates from the sandfly *Lutzomyia longipalpis* enhance *Leishmania* infectivity. Science 239: 1306, 1988.
189. Zilberstein D, Shapira M: The role of pH and temperature in the development of *Leishmania* parasites. Annu Rev Microbiol 48:449, 1994.
190. Beverley SM, Turco SJ: Identification of genes mediating lipophosphoglycan biosynthesis by functional complementation of *Leishmania donovani* mutants. Ann Trop Med Parasitol 89S:11, 1995.
191. Reiner SL, Locksley RM: The regulation of immunity to *Leishmania major*. Annu Rev Immunol 13:151, 1995.
192. Hajduk SL, et al: Human high density lipoprotein killing of African trypanosomes. Annu Rev Microbiol 48:139, 1994.
193. Carrington M, Boothroyd J: Implications of conserved structural motifs in disparate trypanosome surface proteins. Mol Biochem Parasitol 81:119, 1996.
194. Ollson T, et al: CD8 is critically involved in lymphocyte activation by a *T. brucei brucei*–released molecule. Cell 72:715, 1993.
195. Norris KA, et al: Characterization of a *Trypanosoma cruzi* C3 binding protein with functional and genetic similarities to the human complement regulatory protein, decay-accelerating factor. J Immunol 147:2240, 1993.
196. Pereira ME, et al: Invasive phenotype of *Trypanosoma cruzi* restricted to a population expressing *trans*-sialidase. Infect Immun 64: 3884, 1996.
197. Rodriguez A, et al: Host cell invasion by trypanosomes requires lysosomes and microtubule/kinesin–mediated transport. J Cell Biol 134:349, 1996.
198. Tarleton RL, et al: "Autoimmune rejection" of neonatal heart transplants in experimental Chagas disease is a parasite-specific response to infected host tissue. Proc Natl Acad Sci USA 94:3932, 1997.
199. Van Voorhis WC, et al: Molecular mimicry by *Trypanosoma cruzi:* the F1–160 epitope that mimics mammalian nerve can be mapped to a 12–amino acid peptide. Proc Natl Acad Sci USA 88:5993, 1991.
200. Polvere RI, et al: *Trichinella spiralis*: synthesis of type IV and type VI collagen during nurse cell formation. Exp Parasitol 86:191, 1997.
201. Ortega-Pierres MG, et al: Workshop on a detailed characterization of *Trichinella spiralis* antigens: a platform for future studies on antigens and antibodies to this parasite. Parasite Immunol 18:273, 1996.
202. Hotez PJ: Hookworm infection. Sci Am 272:68, 1995.
203. Stassens P, et al: Anticoagulant repertoire of the hookworm *Ancylostoma caninum.* Proc Natl Acad Sci USA 93:2149, 1996.
204. Hotez PJ, et al: Molecular approaches to vaccinating against hookworm disease. Pediatr Res 40:515, 1996.
205. LaClette JP, et al: Paramyosin inhibits complement C1. J Immunol 148:124, 1992.
206. Clarkson MJ: Hydatid disease. J Med Microbiol 46:24, 1997.
207. Amiri P, et al: Tumour necrosis factor alpha restores granulomas and induces parasite egg-laying in schistosome-infected SCID mice. Nature 356:604, 1992.
208. Velupillai P, et al: B-1 cell (CD5+B220+) outgrowth in murine schistosomiasis is genetically restricted and is largely due to activation by polylactosamine sugars. J Immunol 158:338, 1997.
209. Prakash S, Wyler DJ: Fibroblast stimulation in schistosomiasis. J Immunol 148:3583, 1992.
210. Ottesen EA: Wellcome Trust Lecture: Infection and disease in lymphatic filariasis: an immunological perspective. Parasitology 104: S71, 1992.
211. Sartono E, et al: Specific T cell unresponsiveness in human filariasis: diversity in underlying mechanisms. Parasite Immunol 17:587, 1995.
212. Boussinesq M, et al: *Onchocerca volvulus:* striking decrease in transmission in the Vina Valley (Cameroon) after eight annual large scale ivermectin treatments. Trans R Soc Trop Med Hyg 91:82, 1997.
213. Pearlman E, et al: IL-12 exacerbates helminth-mediated corneal pathology by augmenting inflammatory cell recruitment and chemokine expression. J Immunol 158:827, 1997.

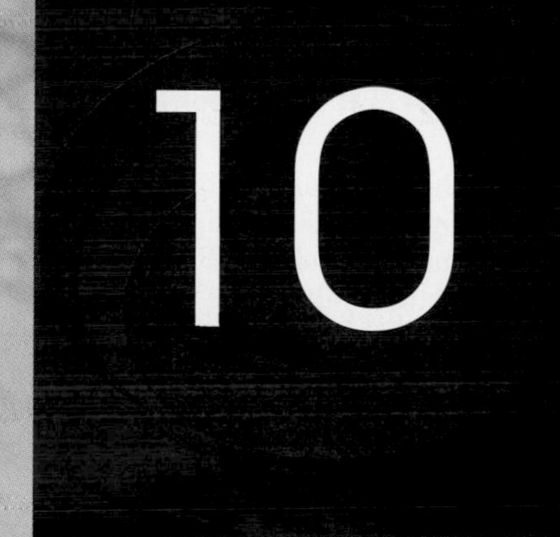

Environmental and Nutritional Pathology

Agnes B. Kane and Vinay Kumar

HUMANS AND THE ENVIRONMENT
RECOGNITION OF OCCUPATIONAL AND ENVIRONMENTAL DISEASES
MECHANISMS OF TOXICITY
COMMON ENVIRONMENTAL AND OCCUPATIONAL EXPOSURES
PERSONAL EXPOSURES
Tobacco Use
Alcohol Abuse
Drug Abuse
THERAPEUTIC DRUGS
Exogenous Estrogens and Oral Contraceptives
Acetaminophen
Aspirin (Acetylsalicylic Acid)
OUTDOOR AIR POLLUTION
INDOOR AIR POLLUTION
INDUSTRIAL EXPOSURES
Volatile Organic Compounds
Polycyclic Aromatic Hydrocarbons
Plastics, Rubber, and Polymers
Metals
AGRICULTURAL HAZARDS
NATURAL TOXINS
RADIATION INJURY
Ionizing Radiation
Ultraviolet Radiation
Electromagnetic Fields
PHYSICAL ENVIRONMENT
Mechanical Force
Thermal Injuries
Electrical Injuries
Injuries Related to Changes in Atmospheric Pressure
FOOD AND NUTRITION
FOOD SAFETY: ADDITIVES AND CONTAMINANTS
NUTRITIONAL DEFICIENCIES
Protein-Energy Malnutrition
Anorexia Nervosa and Bulimia
Vitamin Deficiencies
Mineral Deficiencies
OBESITY
DIET AND SYSTEMIC DISEASES
CHEMOPREVENTION OF CANCER

HUMANS AND THE ENVIRONMENT

Environmental and occupational health encompasses the diagnosis, treatment, and prevention of injuries and illnesses resulting from exposure to exogenous chemical or physical agents. Such exposure may occur in the workplace, or people may voluntarily expose themselves to these hazards, for example, by abusing drugs or ethanol and smoking cigarettes. These personal habits may lead to involuntary exposure of fetuses and infants to drugs, ethanol, or environmental tobacco smoke.

People are often confused about the magnitude of the potential adverse health effects of exogenous physical and chemical agents. There is widespread concern about the potential chronic or delayed effects of exposure to low levels of contaminants in air, water, and food, and hence patients frequently seek advice and information from their health care professionals about the risk of disease associated with specific environmental and occupational exposures. This chapter provides a basic foundation in the most important diseases associated with environmental and occupational exposures, emphasizing the mechanisms leading to these diseases. This framework will help physicians to recognize and treat injuries and illness resulting from environmental and occupational exposures and to educate their patients about the risks of these exposures.[1]

Recognition of Occupational and Environmental Diseases

Accidents, illness, and premature deaths caused by occupational exposures affect 120 million workers in the United States. The annual number of fatal workplace injuries was about 10,000 in 1992: 40% were caused by transportation accidents, 20% were due to assaults and physical violence, 10% were caused by falls, 5% were caused by electrocutions, and 5% were caused by explosions and fires. Nonfatal injuries were estimated at 13,247 million; 6 million of these injuries resulted in disability. The economic cost of these occupational injuries is estimated to be $145 billion.[2] The incidence of nonfatal injuries is highest among construction workers, followed by people employed in agriculture, forestry, fishing, and manufacturing. In addition to injuries, occupational exposures contribute to a wide range of illnesses, including cancer and cardiovascular and cerebrovascular diseases, leading to premature death (Table 10–1). It is estimated that in 1992, 862,000 new cases of occupational illnesses occurred; these resulted in 60,300 premature deaths, with an estimated economic cost of $25 billion. The total costs of occupational injuries and illnesses are greater than the costs associated with the treatment of acquired immunodeficiency syndrome (AIDS) and Alzheimer disease.

The magnitude and extent of illness related to environmental exposures are difficult to ascertain. The Environmental Protection Agency estimates that more than 60,000 chemicals are currently used in the United States; approximately 1500 are pesticides and 5500 are food additives that affect our water and food supplies. Although not all of these chemicals have been tested, 600 have produced cancer in at least one rodent species.[2] Industrial chemicals, production byproducts, and metals are commonly detected at hazardous waste sites (Table 10–2). It is estimated that 4 million people live within 1 mile of 785 heavily contaminated sites that are slated for clean-up ("superfund sites").

Table 10–1. ESTIMATED OCCUPATIONAL DISEASE MORTALITY IN THE UNITED STATES IN 1992

Cause of Death	Number of Deaths	Percentage Attributed to Occupation
Cancer	517,090	6–10
Cardiovascular and cerebrovascular disease	101,846	5–10
Chronic respiratory disease	91,541	10
Pneumoconioses	1,136	100
Nervous system disease	26,936	1–3
Renal disease	22,957	1–3

From Leigh JP, et al: Occupational injury and illness in the United States. Estimates of costs, morbidity, and mortality. Arch Intern Med 157:1557, 1997.

Table 10–2. COMMON CHEMICALS AT HAZARDOUS WASTE SITES

Chemical	Number of Sites
Metals	564
Volatile organic compounds	518
Polycyclic aromatic hydrocarbons	187
Polychlorinated biphenyls	162
Phthalate ester plasticizers	106
Pesticides	82
Dioxins	47

From Mitchell FL: Hazardous waste. In Rom WH (ed): Environmental and Occupational Medicine, 2nd ed. Boston, Little, Brown, 1992, p 1275.

Up to 1.8 million workers are employed at hazardous waste sites.[3]

There is considerable difference in the magnitudes of exposure in the occupational and environmental settings. Occupational exposures affect a defined cohort of workers who are exposed to chemicals in the range of parts per million (ppm); by contrast, environmental exposures to these same chemicals in the air, water, or hazardous waste sites may be in the parts per billion (ppb) or parts per trillion (ppt) range. The health effects of such chronic, low-level exposures are unknown.

In the United States, four regulatory agencies determine exposure limits for environmental and occupational hazards: the Environmental Protection Agency, the Food and Drug Administration, the Occupational Safety and Health Administration, and the Consumer Products Safety Commission. The Environmental Protection Agency regulates exposure to pesticides, toxic chemicals, water and air pollutants, and hazardous wastes. The Food and Drug Administration regulates drugs, medical devices, food additives, and cosmetics. The Occupational Safety and Health Administration mandates that employers (including hospitals and physicians) provide safe working conditions for employees. All other products sold for use in homes, schools, or recreation are regulated by the Consumer Products Safety Commission.

Physicians should be familiar with current approaches used by regulatory agencies in the United States and be prepared to explain the strengths and limitations of the scientific evidence in nontechnical terms. Unfortunately, the perception of risk by the public may differ from the risk determined by scientists. For example, estimated annual fatalities related to tobacco smoking predicted by technical experts (150,000) varied widely from the number of fatalities predicted by college students (2400). Physicians can help patients identify specific environmental and occupational hazards that may cause adverse health effects, educate them about the nature and magnitude of these risks, and encourage behaviors that reduce these risks.[4]

Mechanisms of Toxicity

Toxicology is the scientific discipline that studies the detection, effects, and mechanisms of action of poisons and toxic chemicals. Toxicity is a relative phenomenon that depends on the inherent structure and properties of a chemical and on its dose. Dose-response curves are typically generated in laboratory animals exposed to various amounts of a chemical. A typical dose-response curve for acute toxicity is illustrated in Figure 10–1. In this example, a measurable response occurs at a dose of 0.1 mg/kg; this is defined as the *threshold dose.* To the left of this dose, at subthreshold levels, there is no measurable response. For this chemical, this is the *no observed effect level* and can be considered a safe dose. This information is used to establish a daily or annual *threshhold limit value* or *permissible exposure level* for occupational exposures. Frequently, a plateau is reached at higher doses; this is defined as the *ceiling effect.*[5] It is uncertain whether carcinogens show a threshold effect or whether the dose-response curve should be extrapolated linearly to zero.[6]

Despite the inherent limitations of toxicity testing in animals, several important toxicologic principles have been established by this experimental approach. Exogenous chemicals are absorbed after ingestion, inhalation, or skin contact, then distributed to various organs (Fig. 10–2). Chemicals are frequently metabolized, often by multiple pathways, to products that may be more or less toxic than the parent chemical. One or more of these products then interacts with the target macromolecule, resulting in a toxic effect.[7] The site of toxicity is frequently the site where metabolism or excretion of toxic metabolites occurs. The dose administered (external dose) may not be the same as the *biologic effective dose* delivered to the target organ and target macromolecule.

The basic principles of xenobiotic metabolism with some specific examples are discussed next.

- *Most xenobiotics are lipophilic;* this property facilitates their transport in the bloodstream by lipoproteins and penetration through lipid membranes.
- Lipophilic toxicants are metabolized to hydrophilic metabolites in two steps (Fig. 10–3). In *phase I reactions,* a polar functional group is added to the parent compound. These are frequently oxidation reactions that produce reactive, electrophilic intermediates as a primary metabolite. This metabolite may be eliminated or it may participate in *phase II reactions.* These reactions produce conjugation products with endogenous substrates that are more water soluble and more readily excreted.
- *There are genetic variations in the level of activity of these xenobiotic-metabolizing enzymes.* For example, the mixed function oxidase system, or cytochrome P-450–dependent monooxygenase system (P-450), has multiple isozymes. Cytochrome P-450 enzymes are involved in detoxification of endogenous hormones and natural products as well as in activation of xenobiotics to reactive intermediates or ultimate carcinogens. The cytochrome P-450 gene *CYP1A1* is induced by polycyclic aromatic hydrocarbons present in tobacco smoke.[8] Smokers who have inherited alleles of the *CYP1A1* gene that confer higher activity and increased inducibility of this enzyme may be at higher risk of developing lung cancer[9] (Chapter 8). Glutathione-*S*-transferases are enzymes involved in detoxification of xenobiotic metabolites by conjugation to glutathione. People with inherited GSTM1 deficiency (null phenotype) may be at increased risk for lung, bladder, and colon cancers.[9]
- Multiple pathways may be involved in metabolism of a chemical toxicant. Predominance of one pathway over

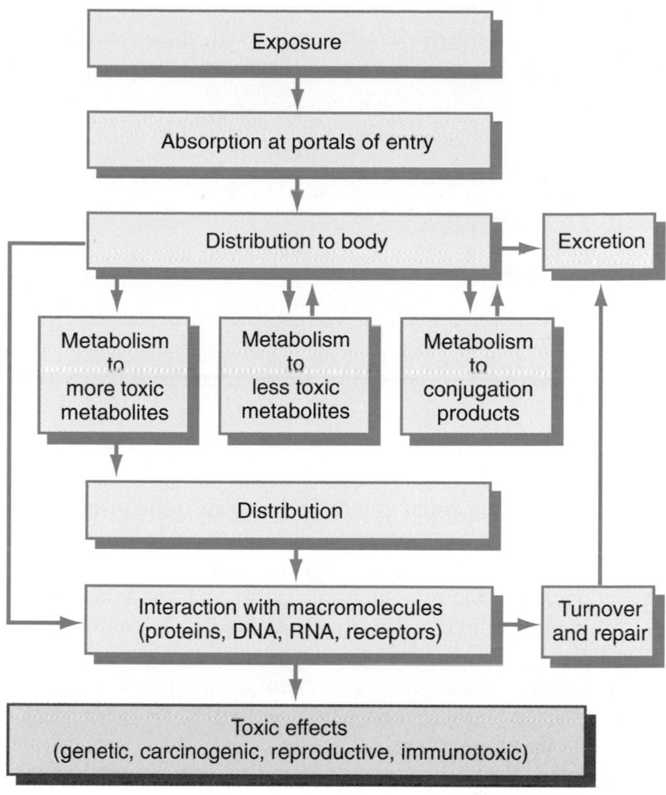

Figure 10–2

Absorption and distribution of toxicants. (From Hodgson E, Levi PE: Absorption and distribution of toxicants. In Hodgson E, Levi PE (eds): A Textbook of Modern Toxicology. Stamford, CT, Appleton & Lange, 1997, p 52.)

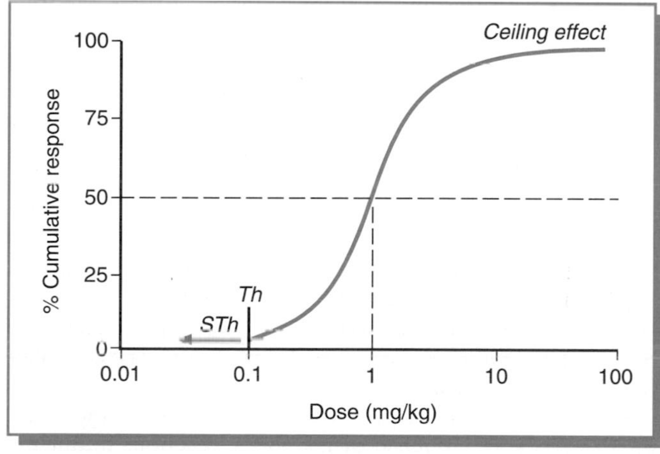

Figure 10–1

The dose-response curve for acute chemical toxicity. Th, threshold dose; STh, subthreshold levels. (From Hughes WW. Essentials of Environmental Toxicology: The Effects of Environmentally Hazardous Substances on Human Health. Washington, DC, Taylor & Francis, 1996, p 33.)

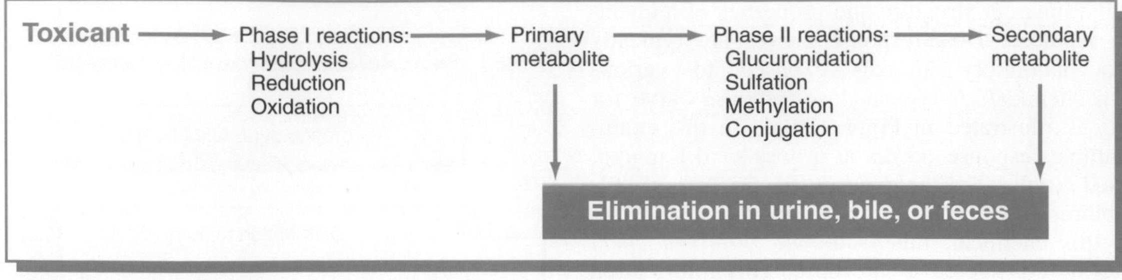

Figure 10–3

Biotransformation of lipophilic toxicants to hydrophilic metabolites. (Adapted from Hodgson E: Metabolism of toxicants. In Hodgson E, Levi PE (eds): A Textbook of Modern Toxicology. Stamford, CT, Appleton & Lange, 1997, p 57.)

another may account for differences in toxicity and carcinogenicity assays between different species, sexes, and age groups.

- Endogenous factors such as nutritional and hormonal status alter enzyme activities involved in xenobiotic metabolism.
- Exogenous factors (e.g., chemicals, drugs, ethanol, stress) can induce or inhibit activities of xenobiotic-metabolizing enzymes.
- Other repair pathways may modify the interaction between the ultimate metabolite and target macromolecule, resulting in increased or decreased sensitivity to the toxic and carcinogenic effects of xenobiotics.

With this background of the principles of xenobiotic metabolism, we now examine some biochemical pathways that are involved in the processing of toxic chemicals using specific examples that are relevant to human disease. Each of the two phases of xenobiotic metabolism is discussed separately. The most important phase I reactions are

1. *Cytochrome P-450–dependent monooxygenase system.* This system, located in the smooth endoplasmic reticulum, is composed of a heme protein (cytochrome P-450); NADPH–P-450 reductase, which transfers electrons from the reduced form of nicotinamide adenine dinucleotide phosphate (NADPH) to cytochrome P-450; and phosphatidylcholine. The activity of this system is highest in the liver, followed by the skin, lung, and gastrointestinal mucosa. Different P-450 isozymes have different tissue distributions; these isozymes show preferential activity toward different substrates. An example of activation of a xenobiotic by cytochrome P-450 is metabolism of benzo[a]pyrene to a secondary metabolite that binds covalently to DNA and causes lung and skin tumors (Fig. 10–4*A*). Benzo[a]pyrene is one of several chemical carcinogens present in cigarette smoke.
2. *Flavin-containing monooxygenase system.* This is also located in the smooth endoplasmic reticulum in the liver. As shown in Figure 10–4*A*, it oxidizes nicotine in cigarette smoke as well as other amines.
3. *Peroxidase-dependent cooxidation.* This reaction is catalyzed by prostaglandin-H synthase, an enzyme involved in arachidonic acid metabolism. It is located in the smooth endoplasmic reticulum with high activity in seminal vesicles, kidneys, and the urinary bladder. It is involved in the metabolism of 2-naphthylamine, a chemical found in synthetic dyes that is associated with an increased risk of bladder cancer (Fig. 10–4).

All of these oxidative reactions may generate oxygen free radicals as byproducts. Some of the primary metabolites are also highly reactive radicals with unpaired electrons (e.g., nitrogen- and carbon-centered radicals derived from 2-naphthylamine; Fig. 10–4). As discussed in Chapter 1, our cells have multiple defense mechanisms against free radicals, including enzymes such as superoxide dismutases, catalase, and glutathione reductase. Vitamins C and E, as well as beta-carotene, also serve as endogenous antioxidants. Reduced glutathione is a major defense mechanism against oxygen free radicals and toxic metabolites of xenobiotics. Xenobiotic metabolism may lead to depletion of cellular reduced glutathione in the setting of (1) cysteine or selenium deficiency, the two cofactors required for glutathione synthetase, or (2) excessive redox cycling of chemicals such as the herbicide paraquat (Fig. 10–4*A*). This compound undergoes cyclic oxidation and reduction in the lungs, resulting in generation of excess reactive oxygen species that cause acute lung injury and pulmonary edema. Oxidant stress occurs when endogenous free radical defense mechanisms are overwhelmed.

As mentioned earlier, the products of phase I reactions are often conjugated with endogenous substrates to yield water-soluble end products that can be excreted from the body. Examples of such phase II reactions are as follows:

1. *Glucuronidation.* An alternative pathway for metabolism of naphthylamine is oxidation by cytochrome P-450 followed by glucuronidation in the liver. The secondary glucuronide metabolite is excreted in the urine. Under the acidic conditions in the urine, it gives rise to the ultimate carcinogen, *N*-hydroxy-2-naphthylamine (Fig. 10–4*B*). This sequence of metabolic reactions ultimately leads to an increased incidence in cancer of the urinary bladder in workers exposed to synthetic dyes.
2. *Biomethylation.* Inorganic mercury, usually in the form of $HgCl_2$, causes necrosis of the proximal convoluted tubules of the kidneys. Occupational exposure to inor-

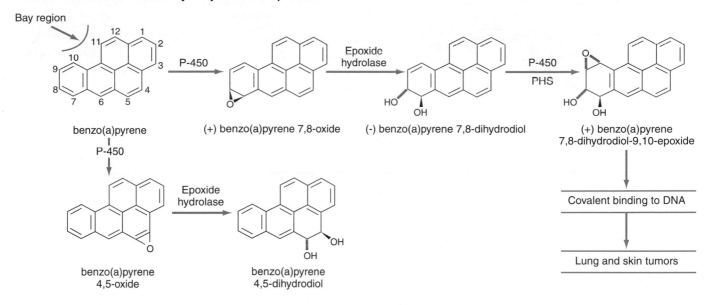

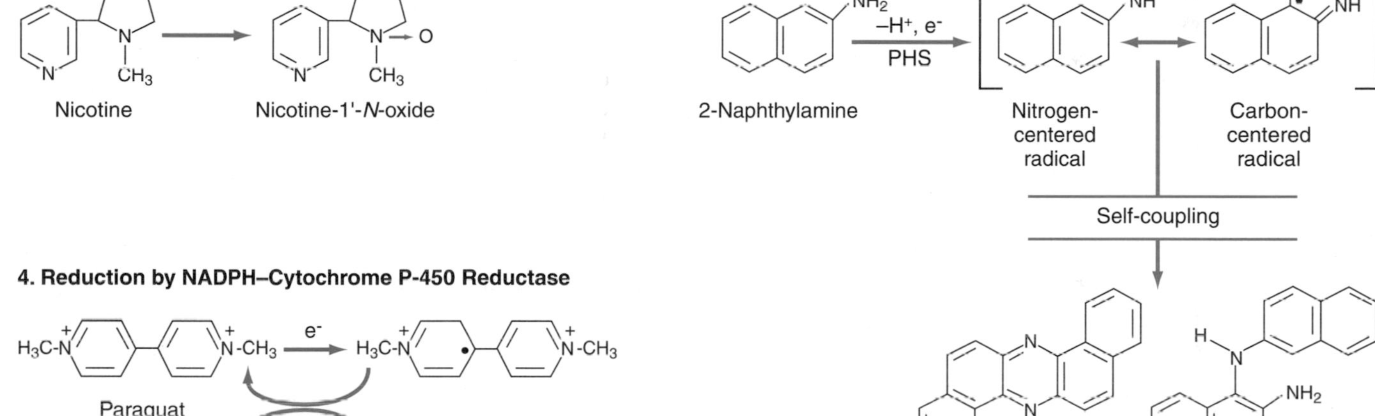

Figure 10–4

A, Xenobiotic metabolism: phase I reactions. FMO, flavin-containing monooxygenase; PHS, prostaglandin-H synthases.

Illustration continued on following page

ganic mercury compounds usually occurs in industries that manufacture germicides, fungicides, electronics, and plastics. Mercury can be methylated by aquatic microorganisms that are subsequently ingested by herbivorous fish (Fig. 10–4*B*). These fish are ingested by carnivorous fish, which may be eaten by humans. This is an example of *bioaccumulation* of a toxic chemical in the environment. The tragic consequences of human exposure to methylmercury were realized in the 1950s and 1960s after an epidemic of poisoning in Minamato, Japan. Industrial discharge of mercury into a bay resulted in bioaccumulation of this toxicant a million-fold in fish. People who ingested these fish developed delayed paralysis and death. Methylmercury is more easily absorbed from the gastrointestinal tract than is inorganic mercury and readily crosses the blood-brain barrier and the placenta. The fetus is especially susceptible to methylmercury; the consequences of maternal exposure are fetal brain damage, mental retardation, and death. Dimethyl mercury is even more toxic; it can be absorbed via the skin or inhaled and can lead to severe neurotoxicity and death.[9a]

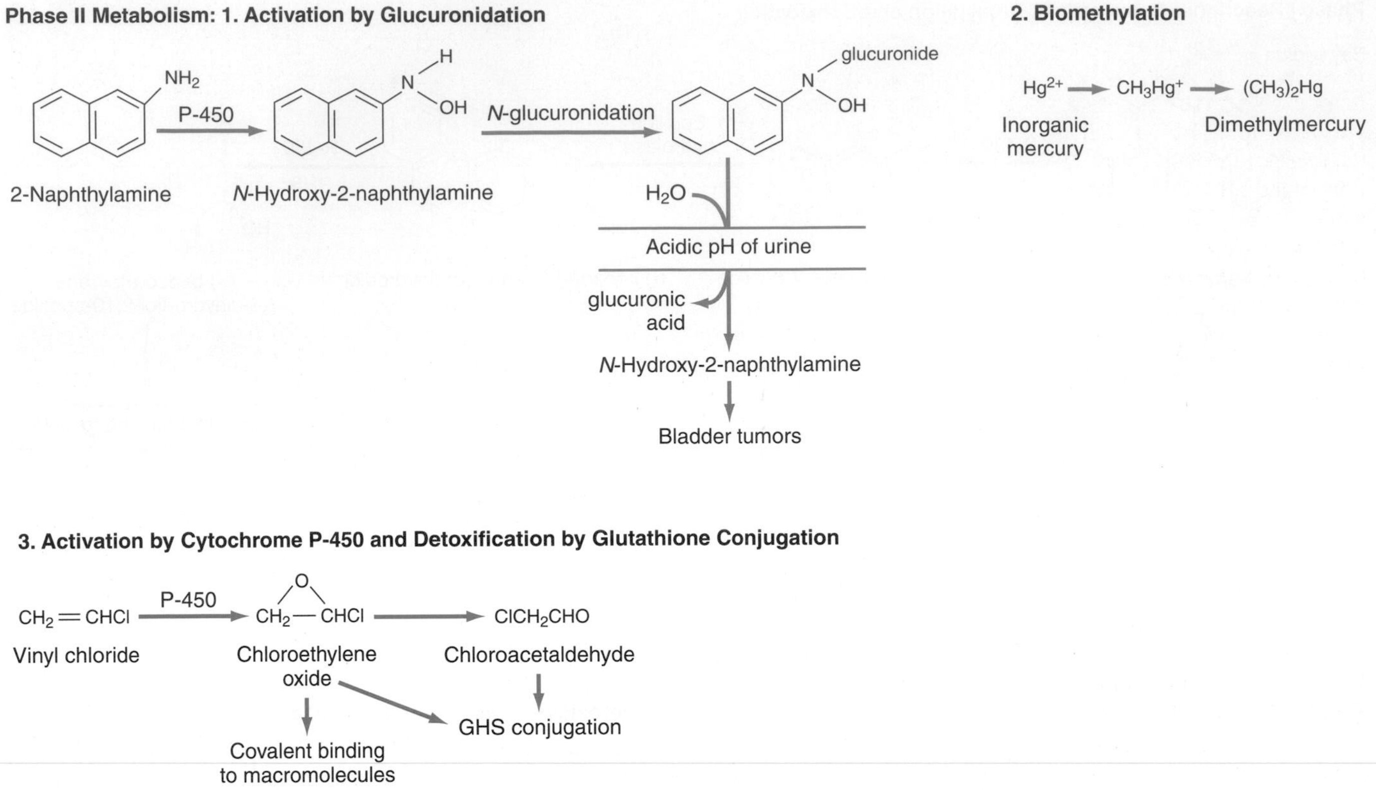

Phase II Metabolism: 1. Activation by Glucuronidation

2-Naphthylamine → (P-450) → *N*-Hydroxy-2-naphthylamine → (*N*-glucuronidation) → N-glucuronide, OH → (H_2O; Acidic pH of urine; glucuronic acid) → *N*-Hydroxy-2-naphthylamine → Bladder tumors

2. Biomethylation

Hg^{2+} → CH_3Hg^+ → $(CH_3)_2Hg$

Inorganic mercury ... Dimethylmercury

3. Activation by Cytochrome P-450 and Detoxification by Glutathione Conjugation

$CH_2{=}CHCl$ (Vinyl chloride) → (P-450) → CH_2—$CHCl$ with O bridge (Chloroethylene oxide) → $ClCH_2CHO$ (Chloroacetaldehyde) → GHS conjugation

Chloroethylene oxide → Covalent binding to macromolecules; Chloroethylene oxide → GHS conjugation

B

Figure 10–4 *Continued*

B, Xenobiotic metabolism: phase II reactions (see text for details). (Adapted from Parkinson A: Biotransformation of xenobiotics. In Klaasen CD (ed): Casarett and Doull's Toxicology: The Basic Science of Poisons, 5th ed. New York, McGraw-Hill, 1996, pp 113–186; and Hodgson E, Levi PE (eds): A Textbook of Modern Toxicology. Stamford, CT, Appleton & Lange, 1997, pp 57, 95.)

3. *Glutathione conjugation.* A common pathway for detoxification of primary metabolites is conjugation to reduced glutathione; these water-soluble secondary metabolites are readily excreted in the bile and urine. Vinyl chloride monomer is widely used in the manufacture of plastics, and it can cause angiosarcoma of the liver in exposed workers. Vinyl chloride is activated to a reactive intermediate by cytochrome P-450 in the liver. This intermediate can bind covalently to cellular macromolecules or be metabolized to chloroacetaldehyde and conjugated to reduced glutathione and excreted (Fig. 10–4*B*).

COMMON ENVIRONMENTAL AND OCCUPATIONAL EXPOSURES

Personal Exposures

TOBACCO USE

Use of tobacco products, including cigarettes, cigars, pipes, and snuff, is associated with more mortality and morbidity than any other personal, environmental, or occupational exposure. Tobacco use is estimated to contribute to 390,000 premature deaths per year in the United States and is associated with 10 million cases of chronic diseases, especially cardiovascular and pulmonary diseases.[10]

Beginning in World War I, annual cigarette consumption increased in men, followed by women, reaching a peak of 4336 cigarettes per capita in 1963. After the Surgeon General's Advisory Committee report, released in 1964, concluded that cigarette smoking is one of the most important risk factors for lung cancer, per capita consumption of cigarettes declined to 3196 in 1987. Unfortunately, smoking among teenagers is still quite common, especially teenage girls. Whereas smoking is a major risk factor for lung cancer, it can also interact with other environmental and occupational exposures in an additive or synergistic fashion. The most important example of such synergism is the increase in risk of lung cancer in cigarette smokers exposed to asbestos.[10]

Mainstream cigarette smoke inhaled by the smoker is composed of a particulate phase and a gas phase; tar is the total particulate phase without water or nicotine. There are 0.3 to 3.3 billion particles per milliliter of mainstream smoke and more than 4000 constituents, including 43 known carcinogens. Examples of the organ-specific carcinogens found in tobacco smoke and snuff are listed in Table 10–3. In addition to these chemical carcinogens, cigarette smoke contains carcinogenic metals such as arsenic, nickel, cadmium, and chromium; potential promoters such as acetaldehyde and phenol; irritants such as nitrogen dioxide and formaldehyde; cilia toxins such as hydrogen cyanide; and carbon monoxide. Carbon monoxide is a colorless, odorless gas produced during incomplete combustion of fossil fuels or tobacco. It has 200 times higher affinity for hemoglobin than oxygen does and impairs release of oxygen from hemoglobin. Thus, carbon monoxide exposure decreases the delivery of oxygen to peripheral tissues. Carbon monoxide also binds to other heme-containing proteins such as myoglobin and cytochrome oxidase. Nicotine is an important constituent of cigarette smoke. It is an alkaloid that readily crosses the blood-brain barrier and stimulates nicotine receptors in the brain. It is also responsible for the acute pharmacologic effects associated with tobacco use that are most likely mediated by catecholamines: increased heart rate and blood pressure, increased coronary artery blood flow, increased contractility and cardiac output, and mobilization of free fatty acids. Nicotine is responsible for tobacco addiction.

The inhaled agents in cigarette smoke may act directly on the mucous membranes, may be swallowed in saliva, or may be absorbed into the bloodstream from the abundant alveolar capillary bed. By various routes of delivery, the constituents of cigarette smoke act on distant target organs and cause a variety of systemic diseases, listed in Table 10–4. The greatest number of deaths attributable to cigarette smoking are due to lung cancer, ischemic heart disease, and chronic obstructive lung disease. Lung cancer is caused by multiple carcinogens and promoters in cigarette smoke. As described in Chapter 16, specific preneoplastic changes are found in the tracheobronchial lining of cigarette smokers. These cellular changes are dose related, and the incidence of lung cancer is directly related to the number of cigarettes smoked. Cessation of smoking reduces, but does not completely eliminate, the risks of lung cancer[11] as well as coronary artery disease over time. It is estimated that 30% of all cancer deaths and up to 90% of all lung cancer deaths are attributable to cigarette smoking. Cigarette smoking is a multiplicative risk factor with hypertension and hypercholesterolemia for development of coronary artery disease and arteriosclerosis. It is also a multiplicative risk factor for acute myocardial infarction and stroke in women who take oral contraceptives. Smoking may contribute to cardiac arrest by increasing platelet adhesion and aggregation, triggering arrhythmia, and by causing an imbalance between the demand for oxygen and supply to the myocardium. Smokers also suffer from increased morbidity due to acute respiratory tract infections, including influenza, and acute and chronic sinusitis. Ciliatoxins in cigarette smoke impair tracheobronchial clearance, and many of the gas phase constituents of smoke are direct irritants of the respiratory epithelium. The pathogenesis of chronic obstructive lung disease associated with cigarette smoking is discussed in Chapter 16.

Table 10–4. DEATHS PER YEAR ATTRIBUTABLE TO CIGARETTE SMOKING IN THE UNITED STATES

Cause of Death	Number of Deaths	Percentage of Deaths*
Cancer		
Trachea, lung, bronchus	123,000	90
Larynx	3,600	82
Lip, oral cavity, pharynx	5,500	92
Esophagus	7,600	80
Bladder and urinary tract	7,800	50
Cervix	1,400	30
Pancreas	8,000	30
Stomach	2,800	20
Ischemic heart disease	108,200	27
Cardiac arrest	13,700	37
Cerebrovascular disease	26,300	12
Arteriosclerosis	8,200	29
Chronic respiratory disease	62,800	90

* This refers to the fraction of deaths caused by the listed diseases that are attributed to cigarette smoking. For example, 90% of all deaths due to cancer of the trachea, lung, and bronchus are believed to be smoking related.

From Becker CG: Tobacco abuse. In Craighead JE (ed): Pathology of Environmental and Occupational Disease. St. Louis, Mosby–Year Book, 1996, p 229.

The fetus is especially vulnerable to the consequences of maternal smoking. Even 10 cigarettes per day can cause fetal hypoxia; fetal carboxyhemoglobin levels are higher than maternal levels. The consequences of fetal hypoxia are low birth weight, prematurity, and increased incidence of spontaneous abortion; serious complications at the time of delivery include premature rupture of the membranes, placenta previa, and abruptio placentae, as described in Chapter 11.

Cigarette smoking is especially hazardous in the workplace. Smokers have higher rates of accidental injuries, especially fires, and cigarette smoke may act as a vector to transport other hazardous agents into the lungs, such as radon gas in miners. Similar to asbestos exposure, cigarette smoke is synergistic with radon decay products in causing lung cancer. Cigarette smoke exacerbates bronchitis, asthma, and pneumoconiosis associated with exposure to silica, coal dust, grain dust, cotton dust, and welding fumes.

Tobacco use also increases the prevalence of peptic ulcers; smoking impairs healing of ulcers and increases the likelihood of recurrence. Smoking may also increase pyloric reflux and decrease bicarbonate secretion from the pancreas.

Table 10–3. ORGAN-SPECIFIC CARCINOGENS IN TOBACCO SMOKE

Organ	Carcinogen
Lung, larynx	Polycyclic aromatic hydrocarbons 4-(Methylnitrosoamino)-1-(3-pyridyl)-1-butanone (NNK) Polonium 210
Esophagus	*N'*-Nitrosonornicotine (NNN)
Pancreas	NNK (?)
Bladder	4-Aminobiphenyl, 2-naphthylamine
Oral cavity (smoking)	Polycyclic aromatic hydrocarbons, NNK, NNN
Oral cavity (snuff)	NNK, NNN, polonium 210

From Szczesny LB, Holbrook JH: Cigarette smoking. In Rom WH (ed): Environmental and Occupational Medicine, 2nd ed. Boston, Little, Brown, 1992, p 1211.

In addition to the health hazards of mainstream tobacco smoke, there are risks associated with exposure to side-stream smoke, also called passive smoking or environmental tobacco smoke (ETS). In 1986, two reports issued by the National Research Council and the Surgeon General concluded that ETS increases the risk of lung cancer, ischemic heart disease, and acute myocardial infarction.[12] The Environmental Protection Agency classified ETS as a known human carcinogen in 1992. ETS is especially hazardous for infants and young children. Maternal smoking increases the incidence of sudden infant death syndrome. Young children in households of cigarette smokers suffer from an increased incidence of respiratory and ear infections and exacerbation of asthma.

ALCOHOL ABUSE

Ethanol is the most widely used and abused agent throughout the world. There are 15 to 20 million alcoholics in the United States; approximately 100,000 deaths in the United States are attributed to alcohol abuse per year, with an economic cost of $100 to $130 billion.[13] Ethanol is ingested in alcoholic beverages such as beer, wine, and distilled spirits. A blood alcohol concentration of 100 mg/dl is the legal definition for drunk driving in many states. Approximately 3 ounces (44 ml) of ethanol is required to produce this blood alcohol level in a 70-kg person. This is equivalent to 12 ounces of fortified wine, 8 bottles of beer (12 ounces each), or 6 ounces of 100-proof whiskey. In occasional drinkers, a blood alcohol level of 200 mg/dl produces inebriation, with coma, death, and respiratory arrest at 300 to 400 mg/dl. Habitual drinkers can tolerate blood alcohol levels up to 700 mg/dl. This metabolic tolerance is partially explained by a fivefold to tenfold induction of the cytochrome P-450 xenobiotic-metabolizing enzyme CYP2E1. Such induction increases the metabolism of ethanol as well as that of other drugs and chemicals, including cocaine and acetaminophen. Although no specific receptor for ethanol has been identified, chronic use results in psychologic and physical dependence. The biologic basis for ethanol addiction is unknown, although genetic factors may be involved.

Ethanol is metabolized to acetaldehyde by alcohol dehydrogenase in the gastric mucosa and liver, and by cytochrome P-450 (CYP2E1) and catalase in the liver (Fig. 10–5). Acetaldehyde is converted to acetic acid by aldehyde dehydrogenase. There are genetic polymorphisms in aldehyde dehydrogenase that affect ethanol metabolism; approximately 50% of Chinese, Vietnamese, and Japanese people have reduced activity of this enzyme due to a point mutation that converts glutamine to lysine at amino acid 487. These ethnic groups also rapidly convert ethanol to acetaldehyde, which builds up and triggers a facial flushing syndrome. Women have lower levels of gastric alcohol dehydrogenase activity than men do; therefore, they may develop higher blood alcohol levels than men after drinking the same quantity of ethanol.[13]

The metabolism of ethanol is directly responsible for most of its toxic effects. In addition to its acute action as a central nervous system depressant, chronic ethanol use can cause a wide range of systemic effects (Table 10–5). Some of these chronic effects can be attributed to specific vita-

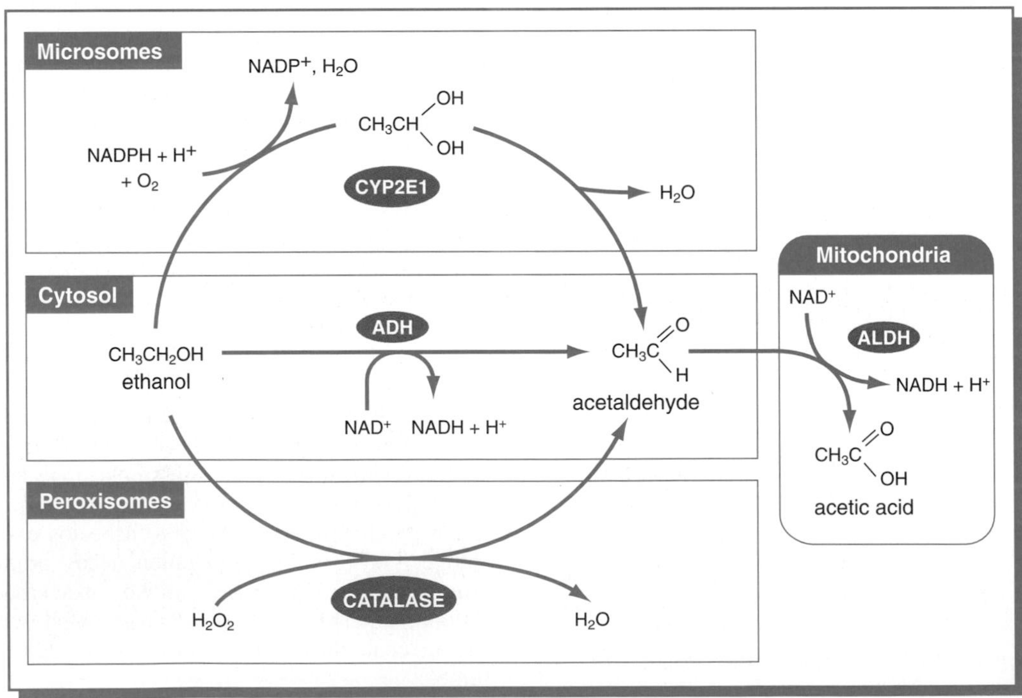

Figure 10–5

Metabolism of ethanol. ADH, alcohol dehydrogenase; ALDH, aldehyde dehydrogenase. (From Parkinson A: Biotransformation of xenobiotics. In Klassen CD (ed): Casarett and Doull's Toxicology: The Basic Science of Poisons, 5th ed. New York, McGraw-Hill, 1996, p 128.)

Table 10–5. MECHANISMS OF DISEASE CAUSED BY ETHANOL ABUSE

Organ System	Lesion	Mechanism
Liver	Fatty change Acute hepatitis Alcoholic cirrhosis	Toxicity
Nervous system	Wernicke syndrome Korsakoff syndrome Cerebellar degeneration Peripheral neuropathy	Thiamine deficiency Toxicity and thiamine deficiency Nutritional deficiency Thiamine deficiency
Cardiovascular system	Cardiomyopathy Hypertension	Toxicity Vasopressor
Gastrointestinal tract	Gastritis Pancreatitis	Toxicity Toxicity
Skeletal muscle	Rhabdomyolysis	Toxicity
Reproductive system	Testicular atrophy Spontaneous abortion	? ?
Fetal alcohol syndrome	Growth retardation Mental retardation Birth defects	Toxicity

From Rubin E: Alcohol abuse. In Craighead JE (ed): Pathology of Environmental and Occupational Disease. St. Louis, Mosby–Year Book, 1996, p 249; and Lewis DD, Woods SE: Fetal alcohol syndrome. Am Fam Physician 50:1025, 1994.

min deficiencies; for example, damage to the peripheral and central nervous systems is related to thiamine deficiency, whereas others result from direct toxicity. The effects of ethanol on various organ systems are discussed next.

Liver. Ethanol can cause fatty change, acute alcoholic hepatitis, and cirrhosis. *Fatty change* is an acute, reversible manifestation of ethanol ingestion. In chronic alcoholism, fat accumulation can cause massive enlargement of the liver. The biochemical mechanisms responsible for fat accumulation in hepatocytes are the following:

- Catabolism of fat by peripheral tissues is increased, and there is increased delivery of free fatty acids to the liver.
- Metabolism of ethanol in the cytosol and of its derivative, acetaldehyde, in the mitochondria converts the oxidized form of nicotinamide adenine dinucleotide (NAD^+) to the reduced form (NADH); an excess of NADH over NAD stimulates lipid biosynthesis.
- Oxidation of fatty acids by mitochondria is decreased.
- Acetaldehyde forms adducts with tubulin and impairs function of microtubules, resulting in decreased transport of lipoproteins from the liver.

Acute alcoholic hepatitis is another potentially reversible form of liver injury (Chapter 19). Although fatty change is asymptomatic except for liver enlargement, alcoholic hepatitis can produce fever, liver tenderness, and jaundice. On histologic examination, there are focal areas of hepatocyte necrosis and cell injury manifest by fat accumulation and alcoholic hyalin or Mallory bodies. Neutrophils accumulate around foci of necrosis (Fig. 10–6). Alcoholic hepatitis is a direct toxic effect of ethanol. It is believed to be mediated by mitochondrial injury, depletion of reduced glutathione by acetaldehyde, and increased generation of reactive oxygen species by induced cytochrome P-450 activity. Acetaldehyde-protein adducts may also serve as neoantigens and stimulate an immune response. Hepatocellular necrosis, as well as fibrosis, begin around the central vein, suggesting that hypoxia may contribute to this injury. With chronic ethanol use, 10% to 15% of alcoholics develop irreversible liver damage or *alcoholic cirrhosis.* This is characterized by a hard, shrunken liver with formation of micronodules of regenerating hepatocytes surrounded by dense bands of collagen (Fig. 10–7). Alcoholic cirrhosis is a serious, potentially fatal disease accompanied by weakness, muscle wasting, ascites, gastrointestinal hemorrhage, and coma. Perisinusoidal fibrosis occurs initially, with deposition of collagen by perisinusoidal stellate cells (Ito cells)

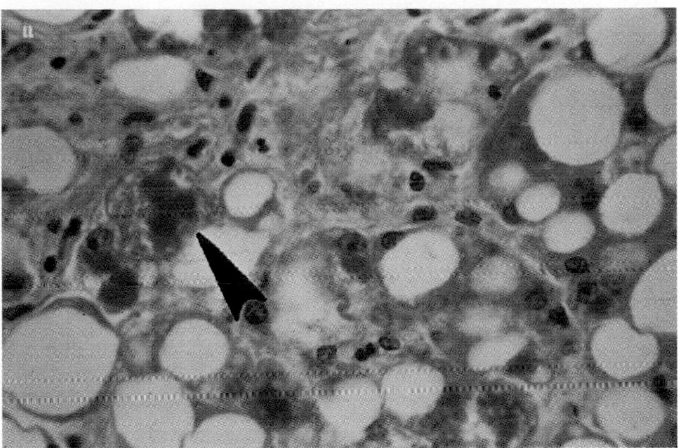

Figure 10–6

Acute alcoholic hepatitis. The liver cells show cytoplasmic accumulation of fat and hyaline *(arrow).* A scattered inflammatory infiltrate is present. (MEDCOM © 1976.)

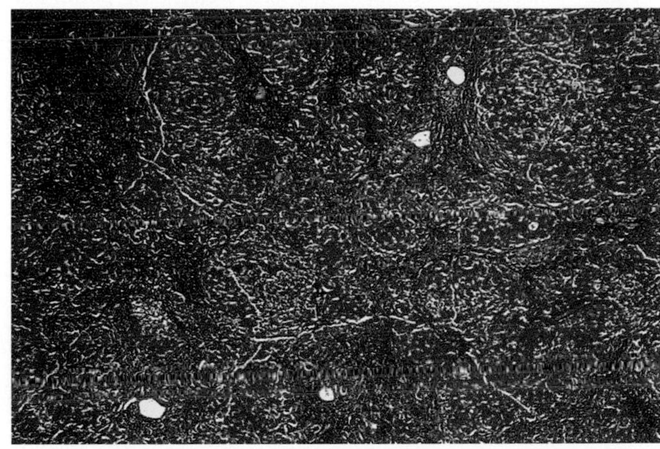

Figure 10–7

Micronodular cirrhosis is a late complication of chronic alcoholism (Masson trichrome stain). The liver architecture is distorted by regenerating nodules of hepatocytes surrounded by dense bands of fibrous tissue that stain blue. (Courtesy of Dr. Steve Kroft, Department of Pathology, Southwestern Medical School, Dallas, TX.)

in the spaces of Disse. Stimulation of collagen synthesis by Ito cells may be caused by direct toxic effect of ethanol or its metabolites, or it may be mediated by cytokines. Patients with cirrhosis have depleted liver stores of α-tocopherol, which increases their vulnerability to oxidative injury.

Nervous System. The acute depressive effects and addiction produced by ethanol are hypothesized to be related to fluidization of membrane phospholipids and altered signal transduction. A deficiency of thiamine is common in chronic alcoholics. Chronic thiamine deficiency contributes to degeneration of nerve cells, reactive gliosis, and atrophy of the cerebellum and peripheral nerves. It produces the ataxia, disturbed cognition, ophthalmoplegia, and nystagmus characteristic of *Wernicke syndrome.* Some alcoholics with poor nutrition develop severe memory loss characteristic of Korsakoff syndrome; this is believed to result from a combination of toxicity and thiamine deficiency. These effects are discussed further under thiamine deficiency, later in this chapter and in Chapter 30.

Cardiovascular System. Chronic ethanol abuse can cause cardiomyopathy, a degenerative disease of the heart muscle, resulting in dilation of the heart (Chapter 13). The exact mechanism responsible for myocardial injury and altered contractility is unknown, although it is most likely due to direct toxicity rather than thiamine deficiency. Hypertension is also more common in chronic alcoholics, secondary to the vasopressor effects of ethanol triggered by increased release of catecholamines. Paradoxically, moderate consumers (one to two drinks per day) show a protective effect of ethanol on the cardiovascular system. At this level of consumption, drinkers show increased levels of high-density lipoprotein and decreased platelet aggregation.

Gastrointestinal Tract. Acute gastritis is a direct toxic effect of ethanol use (Chapter 18). Chronic users are vulnerable to acute and chronic pancreatitis, which may lead to destruction of pancreatic acini and islets. Pancreatic acinar destruction leads to impaired intestinal absorption of nutrients and contributes to vitamin deficiencies.

Skeletal Muscle. Direct ethanol toxicity can also injure skeletal muscles, leading to muscle weakness, pain, and breakdown of myoglobin.

Reproductive System. Chronic ethanol use leads to testicular atrophy and decreased fertility in both men and women. Women who drink alcohol also have an increased risk of spontaneous abortion. The mechanisms responsible for these adverse reproductive effects are unknown.

Fetal Alcohol Syndrome. A tragic consequence of maternal ethanol consumption at levels of only one drink per day is the fetal alcohol syndrome, first recognized in 1968. This syndrome is characterized by growth and developmental defects, including microcephaly; facial dysmorphology; and malformations of the brain, cardiovascular system, and genitourinary system (Chapter 11). This is the most common type of preventable mental retardation in the United States and it affects at least 1200 children per year.[14] The pathogenesis of fetal alcohol syndrome is not entirely clear. It is hypothesized that acetaldehyde, a metabolite of ethanol (see Fig. 10–5), crosses the placenta and damages the fetal brain. Altered prostaglandin release and altered placental blood flow cause fetal hypoxia and growth retardation.[15]

Ethanol and Cancer. Use of alcoholic beverages is associated with an increased incidence of cancer of the oral cavity, pharynx, esophagus, liver, and possibly the breast. Although ethanol is not a direct-acting carcinogen, one of its metabolites, acetaldehyde, may act as a tumor promoter.[16] Induction of cytochrome P-450 metabolizing enzymes by ethanol may enhance metabolic activation of other carcinogens and increase oxidative stress. Chronic ethanol use causes increased degradation of retinol by the liver, and resultant vitamin A deficiency may be associated with an increased incidence of cancer.

Two other chemicals, *methanol* and *ethylene glycol,* may be ingested accidentally or used as inexpensive substitutes for ethanol. They are metabolized by alcohol dehydrogenase, but more slowly than ethanol, resulting in initial symptoms of intoxication, followed by toxic effects after several hours or days. *Methanol* is metabolized to formaldehyde and formic acid, resulting in metabolic acidosis, dizziness, vomiting, blurred vision or blindness, and respiratory depression. Methanol has been proposed as a gasoline additive or substitute, but there is concern that chronic inhalation of methanol-containing fumes may cause central nervous system depression. The lethal dose of *ethylene glycol* is only 1.4 ml/kg; it is metabolized by alcohol dehydrogenase to aldehydes, glycolate, oxalate, and lactate. If a person survives the initial toxicity, acute renal failure may occur several days later because of obstruction of the kidney tubules by calcium oxalate crystals. Acute methanol or ethylene glycol poisoning is treated by administration of ethanol, which slows the production of toxic metabolites.

DRUG ABUSE

Drug abuse, addiction, and overdose are serious public health problems. More than 2 million people in the United States are addicted to cocaine. Some of the abused drugs are available only by prescription, but they are readily available through a black market. Others, such as amphetamines and marijuana, are easily synthesized or extracted from plants. Commonly abused drugs can be classified as central nervous system depressants, stimulants, narcotics, or hallucinogens, as summarized in Table 10–6.

Central Nervous System Depressants. Ethanol is the most widely abused central nervous system depressant, as discussed before. Barbiturates are circulated illegally and are known as downers. They induce sedation and decrease anxiety. Tolerance develops rapidly, causing drug users to increase the dose. Simultaneous use of barbiturates and ethanol is potentially lethal, causing coma and cardiopulmonary arrest. Chronic use of barbiturates induces cytochrome P-450 activity, increasing the metabolism of drugs such as dicumarol, tetracycline, digoxin, and oral contraceptives. Barbiturates have been replaced by safer sedatives such as diazepam (Valium), a member of the benzodiazepines. These drugs have a wider margin of safety and infrequently produce addiction or tolerance. At high doses, these sedatives can cause drowsiness, dizziness, and coma, but they do not induce cytochrome P-450 activity.

Central Nervous System Stimulants. Cocaine is an alkaloid extracted from the leaves of *Erythroxylon coca.* The leaves have been chewed by South American Indians for

Table 10-6. COMMON DRUGS OF ABUSE

Central nervous system depressants	Ethanol Barbiturates Benzodiazepines
Central nervous system stimulants	Cocaine Amphetamine
Narcotics	Morphine Meperidine Propoxyphene
Hallucinogens	Marijuana Mescaline Psilocybin Dimethyltryptamine Lysergic acid diethylamide Phencyclidine

Adapted from Hodgson E: Introduction to toxicology. In Hodgson E, Levi PE (eds): A Textbook of Modern Toxicology. Stamford, CT, Appleton & Lange, 1997, p 1; and Levi PE: Classes of toxic chemicals. In Hodgson E, Levi PE (eds): A Textbook of Modern Toxicology. Stamford, CT, Appleton & Lange, 1997, p 229.

two centuries to relieve fatigue and hunger. Cocaine abuse is a serious public health problem. Beginning in the 1960s, cocaine sniffing and smoking of freebase cocaine (also called "crack" because of the sound it produces when heated) have escalated in the United States. Cocaine produces a rapid "high" of short duration characterized by euphoria, increased energy, and stimulation. Chronic abuse can also cause insomnia, increased anxiety, paranoia, and hallucinations. *Acute overdose produces seizures, cardiac arrhythmias, and respiratory arrest;* these usually occur after intravenous injection or smoking of crack. Cocaine readily crosses the blood-brain barrier, where it blocks the reuptake of dopamine from central nervous system synapses. In the periphery, it blocks reuptake of epinephrine and norepinephrine, resulting in excess catecholamine stimulation (Fig. 10–8).[17] This induces systemic vasoconstriction; *chronic use of cocaine is associated with hypertension, strokes, and sudden death.* Cocaine also induces premature atherosclerosis and coronary artery spasm; these effects are accentuated by concurrent cigarette smoking.[18] The fetus is particularly at risk: decreased blood flow to the placenta causes fetal hypoxia resulting in increased spontaneous abortion, abruptio placentae, and hemorrhages in newborn infants.[17] Metabolites of cocaine can be detected in at least 6% of newborn infants; these babies show evidence of neurologic impairment and a diminished response to external stimuli. Cocaine addiction is a complex problem with economic, social, and health implications. As with all drug and ethanol addictions, treatment requires behavioral and pharmacologic approaches, with variable rates of success. A novel therapeutic approach has been developed using

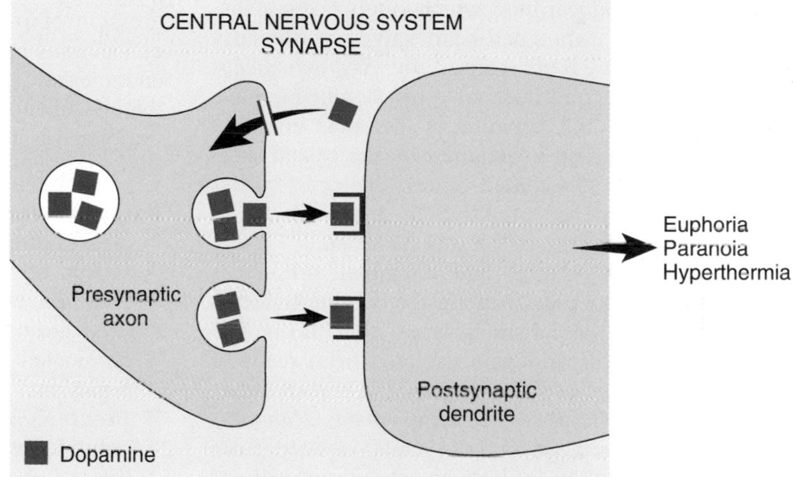

Figure 10–8

Effects of cocaine on neurotransmitters. Cocaine inhibits the reuptake of the neurotransmitters dopamine and norepinephrine in the central and peripheral nervous systems.

passive transfer of an anticocaine monoclonal antibody. This cocaine vaccine produced a long-lasting antibody response in mice that diminished delivery of cocaine to the brain.[19]

Amphetamines are also potent central nervous system stimulants. Overdose causes sweating, tremors, restlessness, and confusion that may progress to delirium, convulsions, cardiac arrhythmias, coma, and death. Amphetamines can induce fetal malformations and withdrawal symptoms in the neonate. The molecular basis of addiction to these central nervous system stimulants is unknown; there may be an underlying abnormality in the dopamine D_4 receptor.[20] These addictive drugs also cause short-term adaptive changes in intracellular signal transduction pathways in the brain that may contribute to tolerance and withdrawal symptoms.[21]

Narcotics. These drugs are prescribed to relieve pain, but they also cause sedation and altered mood. Opiates can be isolated from opium or synthesized from morphine. Heroin and codeine are morphine derivatives. Intravenous heroin abuse induces suppression of anxiety, sedation, mood changes, nausea, and respiratory depression. Chronic abuse induces tolerance as well as psychologic dependence. Overdose can cause convulsions, cardiorespiratory arrest, and death. All intravenous drug users are susceptible to serious infections. The four sites most commonly affected are the skin and subcutaneous tissue, heart valves, liver, and lungs. In a series of addicts admitted to the hospital, more than 10% had endocarditis, which often takes a distinctive form involving right-sided heart valves, particularly the tricuspid. Most cases are caused by *Staphylococcus aureus,* but fungi and a multitude of other organisms have also been implicated. Viral hepatitis is the most common infection among addicts and is acquired by the casual sharing of dirty needles. In the United States, this practice has also led to a high incidence of AIDS in drug addicts, an incidence second only to that in homosexual men.

Hallucinogens. Both natural and chemical substances have hallucinogenic properties. Among the natural hallucinogens are the alkaloid mescaline, isolated from the peyote cactus, which is chewed; psilocybin, isolated from seeds of the morning glory flower or sacred teonanacatl mushrooms; and marijuana, isolated from the hemp plant, *Cannabis sativa.* The active ingredient in marijuana, isolated from the leaves and flowers, or in hashish, the resin isolated from the plants, is Δ^9-tetrahydrocannabinol (THC). Smoking rapidly delivers THC to the brain, producing a state of relaxation and heightened sensation. Intoxication impairs cognitive and motor functions. Chronic marijuana smoking may induce lung damage similar to that caused by tobacco smoke; however, it is not carcinogenic.

Phencyclidine (PCP) was formerly used as an anesthetic; it is now available as a street drug and is ingested, smoked, or snorted. Drug users experience inebriation, disorientation, and numbness. PCP characteristically induces nystagmus. High doses can induce coma lasting a few hours up to 10 days. Lysergic acid diethylamide (LSD) is a potent synthetic drug usually taken orally. It is absorbed rapidly and produces psychic effects, visual illusions, and altered perception for up to 12 hours. In high doses, LSD can cause death.

Therapeutic Drugs

Adverse drug reactions refer to untoward effects of drugs that are given in conventional therapeutic settings. These reactions are extremely common in the practice of medicine. Table 10–7 lists common pathologic findings in adverse drug reactions and the drugs most frequently involved. Because they are widely used, estrogens and oral contraceptives are discussed in more detail. In addition, because acetaminophen and aspirin, commonly used as nonprescription drugs, are important causes of accidental or intentional overdose, they also merit additional comment. Sedatives and hypnotic and anxiolytic agents are also important causes of drug injury, but injury associated with their use is usually in the context of abuse.

EXOGENOUS ESTROGENS AND ORAL CONTRACEPTIVES

Estrogens and oral contraceptives are discussed separately because (1) estrogens for postmenopausal syndrome may be given alone and are usually natural estrogens, and (2) oral contraceptives contain synthetic estrogens, always with progesterone.

Exogenous Estrogens. Estrogen therapy, once used primarily for the distressing symptoms of menopause, is currently also used widely in postmenopausal women, with or without added progesterones, to prevent or slow the progression of osteoporosis (Chapter 28). Given the fact that endogenous hyperestrinism increases the risk of developing endometrial carcinoma and, probably, breast carcinoma, there is understandable concern about the use of exogenous estrogens as therapeutic agents.[22] Current data support the following adverse effects of estrogen therapy:

- *Endometrial carcinoma.* Unopposed estrogen therapy increases the risk of endometrial carcinoma threefold to sixfold after 5 years of use and more than tenfold after 10 years, compared with the risk in women who had not used hormones. This risk is drastically reduced or even eliminated when progestins are added to the therapeutic regimen.
- *Breast carcinoma.* Although some studies continue to point to an increased risk of this form of cancer with the use of unopposed estrogen (i.e., for postmenopausal replacement), the weight of the evidence suggests that the increased risk is small, if any, and is not influenced by the addition of progestins to the formulation (Chapter 25).
- *Thromboembolism.* Although estrogen therapy might be expected to increase the risk of this complication because synthetic estrogens stimulate the production of coagulation factors by the liver, statistics have not borne this out. This happy outcome is perhaps related to the more frequent use of natural estrogens, which appear to be less thrombogenic than synthetic estrogens.
- *Cardiovascular disease.* Myocardial infarction and stroke are among the leading causes of death in postmenopausal women, and hence there is considerable interest in the effects of estrogens on the incidence of cardiovascular disease. Estrogens tend to elevate the

Table 10–7. SOME COMMON ADVERSE DRUG REACTIONS AND THEIR AGENTS

Reaction	Major Offenders
Blood Dyscrasias (feature of almost half of all drug-related deaths)	
Granulocytopenia, aplastic anemia, pancytopenia	Antineoplastic agents, immunosuppressives, and chloramphenicol
Hemolytic anemia, thrombocytopenia	Penicillin, methyldopa, quinidine
Cutaneous	
Urticaria, macules, papules, vesicles, petechiae, exfoliative dermatitis, fixed drug eruptions	Antineoplastic agents, sulfonamides, hydantoins, many others
Cardiac	
Arrhythmias	Theophylline, hydantoins
Cardiomyopathy	Doxorubicin, daunorubicin
Renal	
Glomerulonephritis	Penicillamine
Acute tubular necrosis	Aminoglycoside antibiotics, cyclosporine, amphotericin B
Tubulointerstitial disease with papillary necrosis	Phenacetin, salicylates
Pulmonary	
Asthma	Salicylates
Acute pneumonitis	Nitrofurantoin
Interstitial fibrosis	Busulfan, nitrofurantoin, bleomycin
Hepatic	
Fatty change	Tetracycline
Diffuse hepatocellular damage	Halothane, isoniazid, acetaminophen
Cholestasis	Chlorpromazine, estrogens, contraceptive agents
Systemic	
Anaphylaxis	Penicillin
Lupus erythematosus syndrome (drug-induced lupus)	Hydralazine, procainamide
Central Nervous System	
Tinnitus and dizziness	Salicylates
Acute dystonic reactions and parkinsonian syndrome	Phenothiazine antipsychotics
Respiratory depression	Sedatives

level of high-density lipoprotein (HDL) and reduce the level of low-density lipoprotein (LDL). This lipid profile is protective against the development of atherosclerosis. Progestins, on the other hand, tend to lower HDL and elevate LDL, which counters the estrogen effect. Epidemiologic studies of the role of estrogens have shown a 40% to 50% decrease in the risk of ischemic heart disease in women who received postmenopausal estrogen therapy, compared with those who did not receive estrogens. The general consensus seems to be that unopposed estrogens are likely to be beneficial. The addition of sequential progestins does not alter the benefit of estrogen regimens. The risk of strokes seems unaltered by estrogen therapy.

Oral Contraceptives. Although oral contraceptives have been in use for more than 30 years, and despite innumerable analyses of their effects, experts continue to disagree about their safety and adverse effects. These drugs nearly always contain a synthetic estradiol and variable amounts of a progestin (combined oral contraceptives), but a few preparations contain only progestins. Currently, prescribed oral contraceptives contain smaller amounts of estrogens (<50 μg/day) and are clearly associated with fewer side effects than were earlier formulations. Hence, the results of epidemiologic studies must be interpreted in the context of the dosage. Nevertheless, there is reasonable evidence to support the following conclusions about the effects of these drugs.[23, 24]

- *Breast carcinoma.* The issue of breast cancer risk is controversial. Despite the disagreements, the prevailing opinion is that there is a slight increase in breast cancer risk when combined oral contraceptives are used by women younger than 45 years, particularly nulliparous women younger than 25 years. For women older than 45 years, the risk, if any, is negligible.
- *Endometrial cancer.* There is no increased risk, and oral contraceptives probably exert a protective effect.
- *Cervical cancer.* Oral contraceptives carry some increased risk, which is correlated with duration of use. More recent studies suggest that the increased risk may be more strongly correlated with life style than with the drug (Chapter 24).
- *Ovarian cancer.* Oral contraceptives protect against ovarian cancer; the longer they are used, the greater the protection, and this protection persists for some time after use stops.
- *Thromboembolism.* The oral contraceptives used in the past (>50 μg estrogens) were clearly associated with an increased risk of venous thrombosis and pulmonary thromboembolism because of increased hepatic synthesis of coagulation factors and reduced levels of antithrom-

bin III. Data with the newer (second-generation) formulations (<50 μg estrogens) suggest that the overall risk is much less, especially in women younger than 35 years who do not smoke and do not have other predisposing influences such as diabetes. More recently, third-generation oral contraceptives, which combine low-dose estrogens with synthetic progestins, have been introduced because the synthetic progestins affect LDL and HDL levels to a lesser extent than natural progestins do and hence the risk of acute myocardial infarction is reduced.[25] However, unexpectedly, the third-generation oral contraceptives confer a higher risk of venous thrombosis than do second-generation oral contraceptives. Furthermore, there is an even greater risk of venous thrombosis in users who are carriers of a mutation in factor V.[26] As stated earlier (Chapter 5), the carrier rate of the factor V mutation is fairly high (2% to 15%) in whites. With all of these potential complications, the risks and benefits of these newest oral contraceptives are under careful scrutiny.

- *Hypertension.* Even the newer low-estrogen formulations of oral contraceptives cause a slight increase in blood pressure. The effect is more marked in older women with a family history of hypertension.
- *Cardiovascular disease.* As discussed, estrogens and progestins have opposing effects on HDL and LDL levels. The overall effect on the levels of these lipoproteins seems to depend on the preparations used, particularly the dose of progestin in the formulation. There is considerable uncertainty regarding the risk of atherosclerosis and myocardial infarction in users of oral contraceptives. This stems from the fact that several variables (e.g., the estrogen content of the formulation; the age of the women studied; and the presence or absence of other risk factors for atherosclerosis, especially smoking) can influence the outcome of epidemiologic studies. Recent evidence seems to absolve oral contraceptives: it appears that nonsmoking, healthy women younger than 45 years who use the newer low-estrogen formulations do not incur an increased risk of ischemic heart disease. Conversely, young women smokers who use the pill are ten times more likely to suffer myocardial infarction than are users who do not smoke.
- *Hepatic adenoma.* There is a well-defined association between the use of oral contraceptives and this rare benign hepatic tumor, especially in older women who have used oral contraceptives for prolonged periods.
- *Gallbladder disease.* The slightly increased risk found with older formulations is not seen with the newer ones.

Obviously, the pros and cons of oral contraceptives use must be viewed in the context of their wide applicability and acceptance as a form of contraception that protects against unwanted pregnancies with their attendant hazards.

ACETAMINOPHEN

When taken in large doses, this widely used nonprescription analgesic and antipyretic causes *hepatic necrosis.* The window between the usual therapeutic dose (0.5 gm) and the toxic dose (15 to 25 gm) is large, however, and the drug is ordinarily safe. Toxicity begins with nausea, vomiting, diarrhea, and sometimes shock, followed in a few days by evidence of jaundice; with serious overdosage, liver failure ensues, with centrilobular necrosis that may extend to the entire lobule. Some patients show evidence of concurrent renal and myocardial damage.

ASPIRIN (ACETYLSALICYLIC ACID)

Overdose may result from accidental ingestion by young children; in adults, overdose is frequently suicidal. The major untoward consequences are metabolic with few morphologic changes. At first respiratory alkalosis develops, followed by metabolic acidosis that often proves fatal before anatomic changes can appear. Ingestion of as little as 2 to 4 gm by children or 10 to 30 gm by adults may be fatal, but survival has been reported after doses five times larger.

Chronic aspirin toxicity (salicylism) may develop in persons who take 3 gm or more daily, the dose required to treat chronic inflammatory conditions. Chronic salicylism is manifested by headache, dizziness, ringing in the ears (tinnitus), difficulty hearing, mental confusion, drowsiness, nausea, vomiting, and diarrhea. The central nervous system changes may progress to convulsions and coma. The morphologic consequences of chronic salicylism are varied. Most often there is an acute erosive gastritis (Chapter 18), which may produce overt or covert gastrointestinal bleeding and lead to gastric ulceration. A bleeding tendency may appear concurrently with chronic toxicity, because aspirin acetylates platelet cyclooxygenase and blocks the ability to make thromboxane A_2, an activator of platelet aggregation. Petechial hemorrhages may appear in the skin and internal viscera, and bleeding from gastric ulcerations may be exaggerated.

Proprietary analgesic mixtures of aspirin and phenacetin or its active metabolite, acetaminophen, when taken for a span of years, have caused renal papillary necrosis, referred to as *analgesic nephropathy* (Chapter 21).

Outdoor Air Pollution

Air pollution is a serious problem in the United States and many other industrialized countries. In the United States, the Environmental Protection Agency, is charged with identification and regulation of pollutants in the ambient air that may cause adverse health effects. The current National Ambient Air Quality Standards for six pollutants are listed in Table 10–8. Despite these federal and state regulations, many cities and regions in the United States currently do not meet these primary standards. Epidemiologic research, human clinical studies, and animal toxicologic studies continue to provide evidence for adverse health effects of ambient air pollutants, even at exposure levels below the current standards. The major sources of ambient air pollutants are

- *Combustion of fossil fuels.* These are divided into mobile sources such as motor vehicles, stationary sources such as power plants and factories, and other sources

Table 10–8. NATIONAL AMBIENT AIR QUALITY STANDARDS AND NUMBER OF PEOPLE AT RISK

Pollutant	Primary Standard	Millions of People Exposed to Pollutants Above Primary Standard
Ozone	0.08 ppm maximum daily 1 hr average	69.7
Nitrogen dioxide	0.053 ppm annual arithmetic mean	8.9
Sulfur dioxide	0.03 ppm annual arithmetic mean	5.2
Particulates	15 μg/m³ annual arithmetic mean	21.5
Carbon monoxide	9 ppm maximum 8 hr annually	19.9
Lead	1.5 μg/m³ maximum quarterly average	14.7

From Bascom R, et al: Health effects of outdoor air pollution. Am J Respir Crit Care Med 153:3, 477, 1996.

such as barbecues and fireplaces. Tailpipe emissions from motor vehicles are a complex mixture of carbon monoxide, oxides of nitrogen, hydrocarbons, diesel exhaust particles, and other particulates including lead oxide from tetraethyl lead contained in leaded gasoline.

- *Photochemical reactions.* Oxides of nitrogen and hydrocarbons interact in the atmosphere to produce ozone (O_3) as a secondary pollutant.
- *Power plant emissions.* These release sulfur dioxide (SO_2) and particulates into the atmosphere. Coal and oil contain sulfur, leading to atmospheric formation of sulfates. Automobiles release oxides of nitrogen, leading to atmospheric formation of nitrates. Aerosolized acid sulfates contribute to acid rain.
- *Waste incinerators, industry, smelters.* These point sources release acid aerosols, metals, and organic compounds that may be hazardous for human health. One example of the numerous hazardous chemicals emitted by these sources is methyl isocyanate that was accidentally released at Bhopal in India in 1984, resulting in 3000 deaths due to pulmonary edema. Some of the air toxins, such as polycyclic aromatic hydrocarbons, are known carcinogens.[27]

Lungs are the major target of common outdoor air pollutants; especially vulnerable are children, asthmatics, and people with chronic lung or heart disease, as summarized in Table 10–9. The serious toxicity associated with lead exposure is discussed subsequently under Industrial Exposures. The major air pollutants and the mechanisms responsible for their adverse health effects are summarized briefly.[27]

Ozone. Ozone is a major component of smog that accompanies summer heat waves over much of the United States. Exposure of exercising children and adults to as little as 0.08 ppm produces cough, chest discomfort, and inflammation in the lungs. Asthmatics are especially sensitive and require more frequent visits to emergency rooms and more hospitalizations during smog episodes. It is not known whether these acute changes lead to chronic, irreversible lung injury. Ozone is highly reactive and oxidizes polyunsaturated lipids to hydrogen peroxide and lipid aldehydes. These products act as irritants and induce release of inflammatory mediators, cause increased epithelial permeability and reactivity of the airways, and decrease ciliary clearance. The highest inhaled dose is delivered at the bronchoalveolar junction; however, ozone also causes inflammation of the upper respiratory tract.

Nitrogen Dioxide. Oxides of nitrogen include NO and NO_2. These have lower reactivity than ozone. Nitrogen dioxide dissolves in water in the airways to form nitric and nitrous acids, which damage the airway epithelial lining. Children and patients with asthma have increased susceptibility to nitrogen dioxide; there is a wide variation in individual responses to this pollutant.

Sulfur Dioxide. This pollutant is highly soluble in water; it is absorbed in the upper and lower airways, where it releases H^+, HSO_3^- (bisulfite), and $SO_3^=$ (sulfite), which cause local irritation.

Acid Aerosols. Primary combustion products of fossil fuels are emitted by tall smoke stacks at high altitudes and are transported by air. In the atmosphere, sulfur and nitrogen dioxide are oxidized to sulfuric acid and nitric acid, respectively, which are dissolved in water droplets or ad-

Table 10–9. HEALTH EFFECTS OF OUTDOOR AIR POLLUTANTS

Pollutant	Populations at Risk	Effects
Ozone	Healthy adults and children	Decreased lung function Increased airway reactivity Lung inflammation
	Athletes, outdoor workers	Decreased exercise capacity
	Asthmatics	Increased hospitalizations
Nitrogen dioxide	Healthy adults Asthmatics Children	Increased airway reactivity Decreased lung function Increased respiratory infection
Sulfur dioxide	Healthy adults	Increased respiratory symptoms
	Patients with chronic lung disease Asthmatics	Increased mortality Increased hospitalization Decreased lung function
Acid aerosols	Healthy adults	Altered mucociliary clearance
	Children	Increased respiratory infections
	Asthmatics	Decreased lung function Increased hospitalizations
Particulates	Children	Increased respiratory infections Decreased lung function
	Patients with chronic lung or heart disease	Excess mortality
	Asthmatics	Increased attacks

From Bascom R, et al: Health effects of outdoor air pollution. Am J Respir Crit Care Med 153:3, 477, 1996.

sorbed to particulates. These acid aerosols are irritants to the airway epithelium and alter mucociliary clearance. Asthmatics have decreased lung function and increased hospitalizations when exposed to acid aerosols, although there is a wide variation in airway responses.

Particulates. As discussed in Chapter 16, the deposition and clearance of particulates inhaled into the lungs depend on their size. Ambient particulates are highly heterogeneous in size and in chemical composition. It is uncertain which characteristics of ambient particulates contribute to their adverse health effects. According to some animal toxicology studies, ultrafine particulates (less than 0.05 μm in aerodynamic diameter) are more hazardous.[28] The mechanisms responsible for increased morbidity and mortality associated with exposure of sensitive populations to particulates are unknown; it is suspected that they may be related to free radical generation at the surface of fine particles.

Indoor Air Pollution

Rising energy costs during the last 20 years have led to increased insulation and decreased ventilation of homes that elevates the level of indoor air pollutants. The health hazards of environmental tobacco smoke have already been discussed. Other sources of indoor air pollutants are gas cooking stoves and furnaces, wood stoves, construction materials, furniture, radon, allergens associated with pets, dust mites, and fungal spores and bacteria. The major categories of indoor air pollutants and their health effects are summarized in Table 10–10 and discussed briefly next.[29]

Carbon Monoxide. This odorless, colorless gas is a byproduct of combustion produced from burning gasoline, oil, coal, wood, and natural gas. It is also a major pollutant in tobacco smoke, and its untoward effects were discussed earlier along with cigarette smoking. Here we should note that carbon monoxide levels in ambient air should not exceed 9 ppm (see Table 10–8); however, indoor levels of 2 to 4 ppm have been measured in homes during the winter. Such carbon monoxide pollution of indoor air can reduce exercise capacity and aggravate myocardial ischemia. Higher levels can cause poisoning manifested as headaches, dizziness, loss of motor control, and coma. Approximately 900 accidental deaths due to asphyxia are caused by indoor carbon monoxide pollution each year in the United States.

Table 10–10. HEALTH EFFECTS OF INDOOR AIR POLLUTANTS

Pollutant	Populations at Risk	Effects
Carbon monoxide	Adults and children	Acute poisoning
Nitrogen dioxide	Children	Increased respiratory infections
Wood smoke	Children	Increased respiratory infections
Formaldehyde	Adults and children	Eye and nose irritation, asthma
Radon	Adults and children	Lung cancer
Asbestos fibers	Maintenance and abatement workers	Lung cancer; mesothelioma
Manufactured mineral fibers	Maintenance and construction workers	Skin and airway irritation
Bioaerosols	Adults and children	Allergic rhinitis, asthma

Data from Lambert WE, Samet JM: Indoor air pollution. In Harber P, et al (eds): Occupational and Environmental Respiratory Disease. St. Louis, Mosby–Year Book, 1996, p 784; and Menzies D, Bourbeau J: Building-related illnesses. N Engl J Med 337:1524, 1997.

Nitrogen Dioxide. Gas stoves and kerosene space heaters can raise indoor levels of nitrogen dioxide to 20 to 40 ppm in homes; this is several orders of magnitude higher than outdoor air levels. Children are more susceptible to the untoward effects of nitrogen dioxide. It impairs lung defenses and is hence associated with increased respiratory infections.

Wood Smoke. This is a complex mixture of nitrogen oxides, particulates, and polycyclic aromatic hydrocarbons. High concentrations of wood smoke in poorly ventilated homes can increase the incidence of respiratory infections in children.

Formaldehyde. This highly soluble, volatile chemical has been used in the manufacture of many consumer products, including textiles, pressed wood, furniture, and urea formaldehyde foam insulation. Although indoor levels are usually less than 1 ppm, it can cause acute irritation of the eyes and upper respiratory tract and exacerbation of asthma. Formaldehyde is frequently emitted with acrolein and acetaldehyde, which may have additive or synergistic irritant effects. Additional volatile organic compounds that may be present at low levels in indoor air include benzene, tetrachloroethylene, polycyclic aromatic hydrocarbons, and chloroform. The potential for toxicity or carcinogenicity at these exposure levels is low, although occupational exposure to these volatile compounds can be hazardous. Formaldehyde at high doses (6 to 14 ppm) has produced nasal tumors in rats.[30]

Radon. Radon, a radioactive gas, is a decay product of uranium widely distributed in the soil. Radon gas emanating from the earth is prevalent in homes. Indoor levels of radon average around 1.5 pCi/L; approximately 4% of homes have an annual average level greater than 4 pCi/L. Radon gas is inhaled into the lungs; its decay products emit alpha radiation, which has been associated with lung cancer in miners. According to some estimates, the low levels found in indoor air account for 10,000 lung cancers per year in the United States.[31]

Asbestos Fibers. Homes and public buildings built before the 1970s in the United States contain asbestos insulation, pipe covers, ceiling tiles, and flooring. If these materials are nonfriable and undisturbed, low levels of fibers can be measured in indoor air. Maintenance and abatement workers who repair or remove asbestos-containing materials are at risk for lung cancer and mesothelioma if they do not use respirators.[32]

Manufactured Mineral Fibers. Fiberglass has been widely used as an asbestos substitute for home insulation. Low levels of these fibers can be measured in indoor air. The exposures measured during installation of fiberglass are at least two orders of magnitude lower than the threshold dose required to produce lung tumors in rats.[33] Maintenance and construction workers can develop skin and lung irritation when using these materials.[34]

Bioaerosols. Aerosolization of bacteria responsible for *Legionella* pneumonia has been associated with contaminated heating and cooling systems in public buildings (Chapter 9). More common hazards in indoor air are allergens associated with pets, dust mites, cockroaches, fungi, and molds. These allergens cause allergic rhinitis and exacerbate asthma.[34]

The etiology of the so-called *sick building syndrome,* or *multiple chemical sensitivity syndrome,* is less clear. In some cases, high levels of one or more of these indoor air pollutants may be responsible. In most cases, poor ventilation is at fault.[34]

Industrial Exposures

For centuries, physicians have recognized that occupational exposures contribute to human disease. The Ancient Greek physicians Hippocrates, Pliny, and Celsus described respiratory symptoms associated with mining that they defined as *phthisis.*[35] In the early part of the 20th century, Alice Hamilton, considered the mother of occupational medicine in the United States, investigated numerous cases of occupational illnesses resulting from exposure to lead, phosphorus, mercury, benzene, and carbon disulfide and established occupational medicine as an academic discipline in the United States.

The spectrum of human diseases associated with occupational exposures is summarized in Table 10–11. Almost all organ systems can be affected, resulting in acute toxicity or irritation, hypersensitivity reactions, chronic toxicity, fibrosis, and cancer. The chronic effects of occupational exposures are complex; they include degenerative changes in the nervous system, reproductive dysfunction, lung fibrosis, and cancer. The mechanisms responsible for these effects are not well understood. Some examples of acute and chronic diseases resulting from occupational exposures and potential hazards of environmental exposures are discussed in the following sections.

VOLATILE ORGANIC COMPOUNDS

Large volumes of organic solvents and vapors are used in industry and in homes. These chemicals are known as volatile organic compounds (VOCs). They are used in manufacturing, degreasing, and dry cleaning and as components of paint removers and aerosol sprays. VOCs and petroleum products such as kerosene, mineral oil, and turpentine are stored in underground tanks. Surface spills and leakage from storage tanks can cause contamination of underground water supplies. In general, high levels of exposure encountered in industry cause headache, dizziness, and liver or kidney toxicity. At lower levels of exposure, there is concern about potential carcinogenicity and adverse reproductive effects. Some VOCs and their adverse effects are described next.

Aliphatic Hydrocarbons. These compounds are the most widely used industrial solvents and dry cleaning agents. All of these chemicals are readily absorbed through the lungs, skin, and gastrointestinal tract. In addition to acute central nervous system depression, they can cause liver and kidney toxicity. Common examples of these chemicals are chloroform and carbon tetrachloride; both are carcinogenic in rodents. Methylene chloride, another such

Table 10–11. HUMAN DISEASES ASSOCIATED WITH OCCUPATIONAL EXPOSURES

Organ	Effect	Toxicant
Cardiovascular system	Heart disease	Carbon monoxide, lead, solvents, cobalt, cadmium
Respiratory system	Nasal cancer	Isopropyl alcohol, wood dust
	Lung cancer	Radon, asbestos, silica, bis(chloromethyl)ether, nickel, arsenic, chromium, mustard gas
	Chronic obstructive lung disease	Grain dust, coal dust, cadmium
	Hypersensitivity	Beryllium, isocyanates
	Irritation	Ammonia, sulfur oxides, formaldehyde
	Fibrosis	Silica, asbestos, cobalt
Nervous system	Peripheral neuropathies	Solvents, acrylamide, methyl chloride, mercury, lead, arsenic, DDT
	Ataxic gait	Chlordane, toluene, acrylamide, mercury
	Central nervous system depression	Alcohols, ketones, aldehydes, solvents
	Cataracts	Ultraviolet radiation
Urinary system	Toxicity	Mercury, lead, glycol ethers, solvents
	Bladder cancer	Naphthylamines, 4-aminobiphenyl, benzidine, rubber products
Reproductive system	Male infertility	Lead, phthalate plasticizers
	Female infertility	Cadmium, lead
	Teratogenesis	Mercury, polychlorinated biphenyls
Hematopoietic system	Leukemia	Benzene, radon, uranium
Skin	Folliculitis and acneiform dermatosis	Polychlorinated biphenyls, dioxins, herbicides
	Cancer	Ultraviolet radiation
Gastrointestinal tract	Liver angiosarcoma	Vinyl chloride

Adapted from Leigh JP, et al: Occupational injury and illness in the United States. Estimates of costs, morbidity, and mortality. Arch Intern Med 157:1557, 1997; Mitchell FL: Hazardous waste. In Rom WN (ed): Environmental and Occupational Medicine, 2nd ed. Boston, Little, Brown, 1992, p 1275; and Levi PE: Classes of toxic chemicals. In Hodgson E, Levi PE (eds): A Textbook of Modern Toxicology, Stamford, CT, Appleton & Lange, 1997, p 229.

chemical, is used in paint removers and aerosols. In enclosed areas, high concentrations can be reached because it is highly volatile. Methylene chloride is metabolized by cytochrome P-450 to carbon dioxide and carbon monoxide. Carbon monoxide can form carboxyhemoglobin, causing respiratory depression and death. Perchloroethylene and related compounds are widely used in the dry cleaning industry. Acute exposure causes central nervous system depression, confusion, dizziness, impaired gait, and nausea. Repeated exposures may cause dermatitis. Perchloroethylene is a potential human carcinogen.

Petroleum Products. Gasoline, kerosene, mineral oil, and turpentine are highly volatile and are a common cause of poisoning in children. Inhalation of these vapors causes dizziness, incoordination, and central nervous system depression.

Aromatic Hydrocarbons. Benzene, toluene, and xylene are widely used solvents in the rubber and shoe industries and in printing and paper-coating. Although toluene and xylene are not carcinogenic, inhalation of benzene is hazardous because it can cause bone marrow toxicity, aplastic anemia, and acute leukemia. Benzene is metabolized by the cytochrome P-450 system in liver, producing benzoquinone and muconaldehyde. These metabolic products are believed to cause bone marrow toxicity.

POLYCYCLIC AROMATIC HYDROCARBONS

Polycyclic aromatic hydrocarbons are among the most potent chemical carcinogens (Chapter 8). The carcinogenicity of these compounds was recognized in 1775, with the description of scrotal cancer in English chimney sweeps exposed to soot. A variety of polycyclic aromatic hydrocarbons characterized by three or more fused benzene rings are produced by combustion of fossil fuels; high-temperature processing of coke, coal, and crude oil; and iron and steel foundries. Benzo[a]pyrene is the prototype of polycyclic aromatic hydrocarbons. As described earlier, it is metabolized by cytochrome P-450, prostaglandin H synthetase, and epoxide hydrolase, an inducible microsomal enzyme in the liver. Activated epoxide intermediates bind to DNA; these adducts have been used as markers of polycyclic aromatic hydrocarbon exposure. Occupational exposure to polycyclic aromatic hydrocarbons is associated with an increased risk of lung and bladder cancers.[36] Cigarette smoking is another important source of benzo[a]pyrene. Mutations in the *p53* tumor-suppressor gene found in lung cancers associated with cigarette smoking are most commonly G:C → T:A transversions. This mutational spectrum is consistent with metabolism of benzo[a]pyrene to reactive intermediates that attack deoxyguanines on the nontranscribed DNA strand.[9]

PLASTICS, RUBBER, AND POLYMERS

Millions of tons of synthetic plastics, rubber, and polymers are produced throughout the world. These products are then fabricated into latex fabrics, pipe, cables, flooring, home and recreational products, medical products, and containers. In 1974, occupational exposure to vinyl chloride monomers used to produce polyvinyl chloride resins was found to be associated with angiosarcoma of the liver. Vinyl chloride is a colorless gas that is flammable and explosive. Before the polymerization step in the manufacturing of polyvinyl chloride, it can be absorbed through the skin or lungs. Vinyl chloride is metabolized by the cytochrome P-450 system in the liver to chloroacetaldehyde. This metabolite covalently binds to DNA and is mutagenic. Exposure of rubber workers to 1,3-butadiene was recently shown to be associated with an increased risk of leukemia. Plastics are widely used in consumer products, including food and beverage containers. Public exposure to plasticizers, such as phthalate esters, and to additives such as bisphenol-A raises concern about potential adverse reproductive effects of these synthetic chemicals. Phthalate esters have been shown to induce testicular injury in rats, and bisphenol-A mimics the proliferative effects of estrogen.

METALS

Occupational exposure to metals in mining and manufacturing is associated with acute and chronic toxicity, as well as carcinogenicity, as summarized in Table 10–12.[37] Occupational as well as environmental exposure to lead continues to be a serious public health problem. Agricultural exposure to arsenic-containing pesticides is discussed subsequently. The pulmonary effects of beryllium are described in Chapter 16. The health effects of inorganic and organic mercury were discussed earlier in this chapter under Mechanisms of Toxicity. The untoward effects of some of the remaining metals listed in Table 10–12 are described here.

Lead. Epidemics of lead poisoning in the Middle Ages were due to fortification of wine and drinking beverages from lead-glazed containers. Lead was recognized clinically as an occupational hazard in 1839. More than 4 million tons of lead are produced each year for use in batteries, alloys, exterior red lead paint, and ammunition. Workers employed in these industries as well as in mining, smelting, spray painting, recycling, and radiator repair are exposed to lead. In some countries, tetraethyl lead is still used as a gasoline additive, thus polluting the air. Inhalation is the most important route of occupational exposure. Environmental sources of lead are urban air due to use of leaded gasoline, soil contaminated with exterior lead paint, the water supply due to lead plumbing, and house dust in homes with interior lead paint. Consumers may be exposed to lead-glazed ceramics, lead solder in food and soft drink cans, and illegally produced alcoholic beverages (moonshine in southeastern United States). Lead ingested in this manner is absorbed through the gastrointestinal tract. Intestinal absorption of lead is enhanced by calcium, iron, or zinc deficiency; compared with adults, the absorption is greater in children and infants and hence they are particularly vulnerable to lead toxicity.[38] Absorbed lead is mainly (80% to 85%) taken up by bone and developing teeth in children; the blood accumulates 5% to 10%, and the remainder is distributed throughout the soft tissues. Lead clears rapidly from blood, but that deposited in bones has a half-life of 30 years.[39] Thus, presence of lead in blood indicates recent exposure and it does not allow the determi-

Table 10–12. TOXIC AND CARCINOGENIC METALS

Metal	Disease	Occupation
Lead	Renal toxicity Anemia, colic Peripheral neuropathy Insomnia, fatigue Cognitive deficits	Battery and ammunition workers, foundry workers, spray painting, radiator repair
Mercury	Renal toxicity Muscle tremors, dementia Cerebral palsy Mental retardation	Chlorine-alkali industry
Arsenic	Cancer of skin, lung, liver	Miners, smelters, oil refinery workers, farm workers
Beryllium	Acute lung irritant Chronic lung hypersensitivity ? Lung cancer	Beryllium refining, aerospace manufacturing, ceramics
Cobalt and tungsten carbide	Lung fibrosis Asthma	Toolmakers, grinders, diamond polishers
Cadmium	Renal toxicity ? Prostate cancer	Battery workers, smelters, welders, soldering
Chromium	Cancer of lung and nasal cavity	Pigment workers, smelters, steel workers
Nickel	Cancer of lung and nasal sinuses	Smelters, steel workers, electroplating

Adapted from Levi PE: Classes of toxic chemicals. In Hodgson E, Levi PE (eds): A Textbook of Modern Toxicology. Stamford, CT, Appleton & Lange, 1997, p 229; and Sprince NL: Hard metal disease. In Rom WN (eds): Environmental and Occupational Medicine, 2nd ed. Boston, Little, Brown, 1992, p 791.

nation of total body burden. The toxicity of lead is related to its multiple biochemical effects:

- *High affinity for sulfhydryl groups.* The most important enzymes inhibited by lead due to this mechanism are involved in heme biosynthesis: δ-aminolevulinic acid dehydratase and ferroketolase. These enzymes are involved in the incorporation of iron into the heme molecule, and hence patients develop hypochromic anemia.
- *Competition with calcium ions.* As a divalent cation, lead competes with calcium and is stored in bone. It also interferes with nerve transmission and brain development.
- *Inhibition of membrane-associated enzymes.* Lead inhibits 5′-nucleotidase activity and sodium-potassium ion pumps, leading to decreased survival of red blood cells (hemolysis), renal damage, and hypertension.
- *Impaired metabolism of 1,25-dihydroxyvitamin D.* This is the active metabolite of vitamin D.[37]

Lead contributes to multiple chronic health effects, illustrated in Figure 10–9. *Injury to the central and peripheral nervous systems* causes headache, dizziness, memory deficits, and decreased nerve conduction velocity. *Blood changes* occur early and are characteristic. Because lead interferes with heme biosynthesis, it causes a microcytic hypochromic anemia; punctate basophilic stippling of erythrocytes is characteristic. There is also an element of hemolysis because lead inhibits membrane-associated red cell enzymes. Because lead inhibits incorporation of iron into heme, the iron is displaced, and zinc protoporphyrin is formed. Thus, an elevated blood level of zinc protoporphyrin or its product, free erythrocyte protoporphyrin, is an important indicator of lead poisoning. *Gastrointestinal symptoms* include colic and anorexia.[37] The kidneys are a major route of excretion of lead. Acutely, there is *damage to the proximal tubules,* with intranuclear lead inclusions and clinical evidence of renal tubule dysfunction. Chronically, lead can cause diffuse interstitial fibrosis, gout, and renal failure. Even in the absence of overt clinical symptoms of kidney damage, lead causes hypertension.[39] Lead can cause infertility in men due to testicular injury; failure of implantation of the fertilized ovum can occur in women.[37]

Infants and children are especially vulnerable to lead toxicity. It is estimated that more than 10% of preschool children in urban areas have blood lead levels greater than 15 μg/dl. Even at this level, intellectual impairment as measured by IQ scores, behavioral abnormalities, and learning deficits have been described. Lead exposure begins in utero because lead may be mobilized from the maternal skeleton during pregnancy and readily crosses the placental barrier. Similar to neurotoxicity caused by methylmercury, the developing nervous system of the fetus and infants is extremely susceptible to lead toxicity.[38]

Cobalt and Tungsten Carbide. Cutting tools, metal grinders, polishers, and drilling equipment are fabricated from tungsten carbide with cobalt as a binder. Workers who use these tools or work in related industries can develop asthma and interstitial lung fibrosis (called hard metal disease). Asthma and lung injury appear to be caused by cobalt, although lung damage may be exacerbated by metal mixtures.

Cadmium. Occupational exposure to cadmium occurs near mines and smelters; this metal is also used in paint pigments, alloys, solder, electroplating, and batteries. Acute effects are lung edema and irritation. Chronic toxicity affects the kidney. Cadmium induces the synthesis of metal-

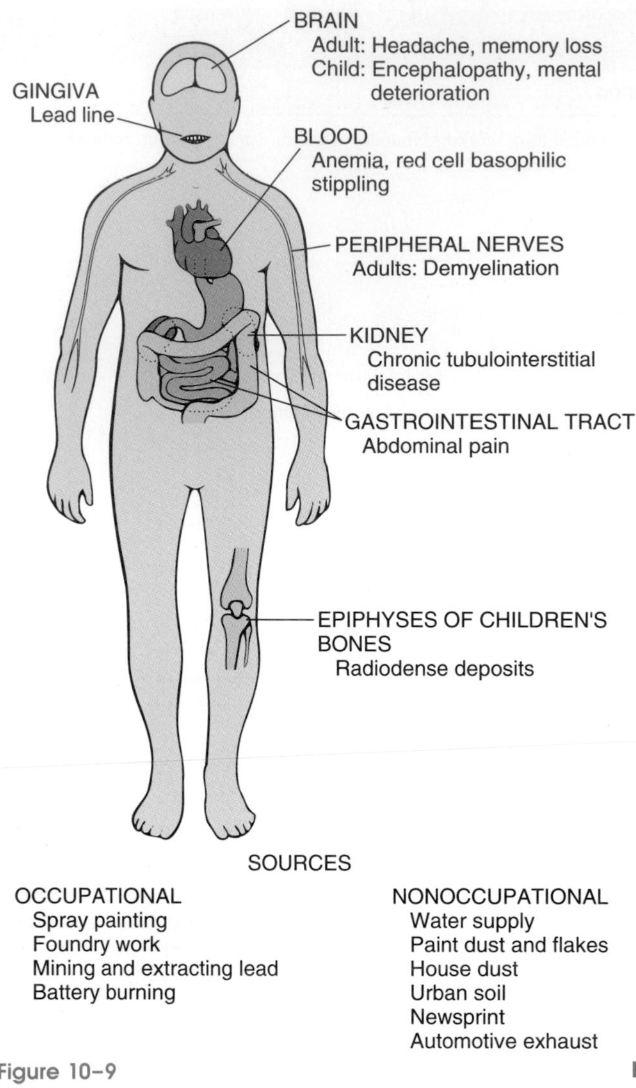

Figure 10–9

Consequences of lead exposure.

lothionein, a metal-binding protein, in the liver and kidney. When this defense mechanism is overwhelmed, cadmium damages the proximal convoluted tubules, causing proteinuria.

Chromium. Occupational exposure to chromium occurs in mining and smelting. Chromium is also used in stainless steel, pigments, and alloys. Hexavalent chromium is readily absorbed across cell membranes; it is reduced to trivalent chromium, leading to generation of free radicals and DNA damage. Chromium is an important occupational carcinogen.

Nickel. Topical exposure to metals that contain nickel frequently causes contact dermatitis. Metallic nickel is widely used in industry in steels and alloys, batteries, fuel cells, electroplating, and ceramics. Nickel is also recycled from scrap metal and is emitted from waste incinerators, power plants, and cigarette smoke. The major route of occupational exposure is by inhalation. Particulate nickel compounds are carcinogenic; they enter target cells after phagocytosis, with release of nickel ions intracellularly. Nickel ions can catalyze the generation of reactive oxygen species, increase endogenous generation of oxidants, and form DNA-protein cross-links. Nickel appears to damage heterochromatin selectively and can inactivate tumor-suppressor genes by hypermethylation.[40]

Agricultural Hazards

Although agricultural productivity has been improved by the use of fertilizers and pesticides, the use of these chemicals is not an unalloyed blessing. They cause disease in those exposed to them, particularly farmers. However, the potential health hazards of pesticides extend beyond the farming community because pesticide residues are found on foods and they contaminate soil and water supplies. Environmental contamination is a threat to wildlife; some pesticides undergo bioaccumulation and persist in wildlife and humans for decades. Bioaccumulation and biopersistence are characteristic of organochlorines, such as DDT (dichlorodiphenyltrichloroethane), and dioxins, such as TCDD (2,3,7,8-tetrachlorodibenzo-*p*-dioxin). There is considerable controversy about the adverse health effects of these persistent pesticides and their metabolites, especially concerning their relationship to breast cancer[41, 42] and to reproductive abnormalities.[43]

Agricultural pesticides are divided into five categories, depending on the target pest: insecticides, herbicides, fungicides, rodenticides, and fumigants (Table 10–13). All pesticides are toxic to some plant or rodent species; at higher doses, they can also be toxic to farm animals, pets, and humans. In general, herbicides used to control weeds have low acute toxicity for mammals; fungicides are characterized as moderately toxic. Acute toxicity of insecticides for mammals ranges from low to high. Fumigants used to eliminate insects from enclosed spaces and rodenticides are highly toxic. Whereas the acute toxicity of agricultural pesticides is well known and safe exposure limits for humans have been established, the chronic toxicity of these chemicals is less certain, especially after exposure to low doses in food residues or in the soil or water. For example, DDT was widely used as an insecticide in the 1940s and 1950s because it has low acute toxicity for humans. However, DDT persists in the environment and accumulates in the food chain. Birds that ingested DDT-contaminated insects and fish suffered reproductive defects. DDT and its major metabolite, DDE (1,1-dichloro-2,2-bis(*p*-chlorophenyl) ethylene), accumulate in fat tissue and have been detected in human milk. Organochlorines, as well as industrial chemicals such as polychlorinated biphenyls (PCBs), are weakly estrogenic. Some of these chemicals are carcinogenic in rodents and cause reproductive dysfunction in amphibians, birds, and fish.[41] Although an epidemiologic study did not find increased levels of DDE or PCBs in women with breast cancer compared with matched controls subjects,[42] there is still concern that these persistent organochlorines, other potentially estrogenic pesticides, and natural phytoestrogens in plants such as soybeans may have adverse reproductive effects in humans.[43, 44] The mechanisms of action of these xenoestrogens, alone or in combination, in the development of cancer and in reproductive dysfunction is unknown.[43]

Table 10–13. HEALTH EFFECTS OF AGRICULTURAL PESTICIDES

Category	Example	Effect
Insecticides	Organochlorines	Neurotoxicity; hepatotoxicity
	DDT	
	Chlordane	
	Lindane	
	Methoxychlor	
	Organophosphates	Neurotoxicity; delayed neuropathy
	Parathion	
	Diazinon	
	Malathion	
	Carbamates	Neurotoxicity (reversible)
	Aldicarb	
	Carbaryl	
	Botanical agents	Paresthesia; lung irritant; allergic dermatitis
	Nicotine	
	Pyrethrins	
	Rotenone	
Herbicides	Arsenic compounds	Hyperpigmentation, gangrene; anemia; sensory neuropathy; cancer
	Dinitrophenols	Hyperthermia; sweating
	Chlorophenoxy herbicides	
	2,4-D and 2,4,5-T	? Lymphoma; sarcoma
	TCDD	Fetotoxicity; immunotoxicity; cancer
	Paraquat	Acute lung injury
	Atrazine	? Cancer
	Alachlor	? Cancer
Fungicides	Captan	? Reproductive toxicity
	Maneb	
	Benomyl	
Rodenticides	Fluoroacetate	Cardiac and respiratory failure
	Warfarin	Hemorrhage
	Strychnine	Respiratory failure
Fumigants	Carbon disulfide	Cardiac toxicity
	Ethylene dibromide	Neurotoxicity
	Phosphine	Lung edema, brain damage
	Chloropicrin	Eye irritation, lung edema, arrhythmias

Adapted from Hodgson E: Introduction to toxicology. In Hodgson E, Levi PE (eds): A Textbook of Modern Toxicology. Stamford, CT, Appleton & Lange, 1997, p 1; and Levi PE: Classes of toxic chemicals. In Hodgson E, Levi PE (eds): A Textbook of Modern Toxicology. Stamford, CT, Appleton & Lange, 1997, p 229.

The major health effects of the most common agricultural pesticides are summarized in Table 10–13. Selected examples are discussed here.

Organochlorines, such as DDT, have low acute toxicity for humans; however, they bioaccumulate and persist in the environment and in fat tissue. These chemicals are absorbed through the skin, gastrointestinal tract, and lungs. As alluded to earlier, the role of DDT and its metabolites as an endocrine disrupting agent is controversial. *Chlordane* is representative of cyclodienes that are used to control termites and other soil insects. Acute toxicity causes hypothermia, tremor, and convulsions. Chlordane also causes immune dysfunction and may act as a nongenotoxic carcinogen. These effects may contribute to the increased incidence of lymphoma observed in some farm workers. *Lindane* is an isomer of benzene hexachloride that is used to control lice and scabies, as a wood preservative, and as a household fumigant. It has been reported to cause immune dysfunction and reproductive problems in women.

Organophosphates are irreversible inhibitors of cholinesterases resulting in abnormal transmission at peripheral and central nerve endings. These chemicals are absorbed through the skin, gastrointestinal tract, and lungs. Up to 40% of farm workers in the United States show measurable inhibition of red blood cell or plasma cholinesterase activity; fatalities have been reported from organophosphate exposure. *Carbamates* are reversible inhibitors of cholinesterase that produce acute neurotoxic effects similar to those of organophosphate insecticides. Carbaryl (Sevin) is potentially mutagenic and teratogenic because it poisons the mitotic spindle.

Among *herbicides,* the dioxin TCDD has received much attention. During the Vietnam War, the defoliant agent orange was contaminated with TCDD. A chemical factory explosion in Seveso, Italy, in 1976 caused local environmental contamination and human exposure to TCDD, resulting in chloracne and an increased incidence of leukemia, lymphoma, and sarcomas. TCDD and structurally similar dioxins are also produced in the paper pulp industry using chlorine bleach and by waste incinerators. Low doses of dioxin are present in our food, soil, and water. In some laboratory animals, TCDD is highly toxic, immunosuppressive, teratogenic, and carcinogenic. The sensitivity of some strains of laboratory mice to dioxin is linked to the aryl

Table 10-14. NATURAL TOXINS

Category	Example	Source	Effect
Mycotoxins	Ergot alkaloids	*Claviceps* fungi	Gangrene, convulsions, abortion
	Aflatoxins	*Aspergillus flavus*	Liver cancer
	Tricothecenes	*Fusarium, Trichoderma*	Diarrhea, ataxia
Phytotoxins	Cycasin	Cycad flour	Amyotrophic lateral sclerosis
	Monocrotaline	*Senecio* plants	Hepatitis
	Safrole	Black pepper; oil of Sassafras	Cancer
	Solanine	Solanaceae plants (potato)	Neurotoxin
Animal toxins	Venoms	Snakes	Cardiotoxin, neurotoxin
		Bees	Direct toxicity, cardiotoxin
	Saxitoxin	Dinoflagellates	Neurotoxin, paralysis
	Ciguatoxin	Dinoflagellates	Paresthesia, paresis, vomiting, diarrhea
	Tetrodotoxin	Puffer fish	Neurotoxin, shock

From Hodgson E: Introduction to toxicology. In Hodgson E, Levi PE (eds): A Textbook of Modern Toxicology. Stamford, CT, Appleton & Lange, 1997, p 1.

hydrocarbon hydroxylase receptor.[45] TCDD can induce liver cytochrome P-450 enzyme activity, increase estrogen metabolism, and interfere with development of the male reproductive tract. TCDD also decreases thyroxine levels in adult rats. Extrapolation of these multiple adverse effects observed in laboratory animals to low-dose exposure of humans is difficult.[43]

Rodenticides are highly toxic chemicals with restricted use. The major health threat is death from suicidal or accidental ingestion.

Natural Toxins

In addition to manufactured pesticides, potent toxins and carcinogens are present in the natural environment, as summarized in Table 10-14. These mycotoxins and phytotoxins may contaminate foods. For example, cycad flour is used in arid climates. This plant contains the toxin cycasin (methylazoxymethanol β-glucoside). If the plant and seeds are cut into small pieces, soaked in water, and dried, the toxin is leached. However, if these precautions are not followed, a degenerative neurologic disorder (amyotrophic lateral sclerosis) is produced by ingestion of cycasin. Animal toxins can be ingested by eating fish, snails, or mollusks. The most common poisoning results from eating tropical fish and snails that have ingested dinoflagellates containing ciguatoxin. Ciguatera poisoning can be severe and occurs in the South Pacific and the Caribbean. Paralytic shellfish poisoning occurs in North America after eating mollusks that have ingested dinoflagellates that contain saxitoxin. Aflatoxin B_1 is produced by fungi that contaminate peanuts, corn, and cottonseed. It is a potent carcinogen that contributes to the high incidence of liver cancer in some regions of Africa and the Far East (Chapters 8 and 19).

Radiation Injury

Radiation is energy distributed across the electromagnetic spectrum as waves (long wavelengths, low frequency) or particles (short wavelengths, high frequency). The types, frequencies, and biologic effects of electromagnetic radiation are summarized in Table 10-15. Approximately 80% of radiation is derived from natural sources, including cosmic radiation, ultraviolet light, and natural radioisotopes, especially radon gas. The remaining 20% is derived from manufactured sources that include instruments used in medicine and dentistry, consumer products that emit radiowaves or microwaves, and nuclear power plants. The potentially catastrophic effects of radiation are most vividly illustrated by the effects of nuclear explosions. The atomic bombs dropped on Hiroshima and Nagasaki in 1945 not only caused acute injury and death but also increased incidence of various cancers among the survivors. There are numerous historical incidents that document the deleterious effects of therapeutic radiation. For example, early in the 20th century, American radiologists experienced an increased incidence of aplastic anemia and neoplasms of the skin, brain, and hematopoietic system. Children who were treated with radiation for an enlarged thymus or benign skin lesions between 1910 and 1959 suffered from an increased incidence of thyroid abnormalities, thyroid tumors, and leukemias and lymphomas. Exposure of the fetus to radiation can produce mental retardation, congenital anomalies, leukemia, and solid tumors. Investigation of these deliberate or accidental exposures to radiation led to an understanding of the relationship between the dose and

Table 10-15. IONIZING AND NONIONIZING ELECTROMAGNETIC RADIATION

Frequency (Hz)	Radiation	Biologic Effects
1-50	Electric power	?
10^6-10^{11}	Radio waves and radar	Thermal effects, cataracts
10^9-10^{10}	Microwaves	Lens opacities
10^{11}-10^{14}	Infrared	Cataracts
10^{15}	Visible light	Retinal burns (lasers)
10^{15}-10^{18}	Ultraviolet light	Skin burns, cancer
10^{18}-10^{20}	X-rays and gamma rays	Acute and delayed injury; cancer
10^{27}	Cosmic radiation	?

timing of radiation and the acute and chronic health effects. However, in general, these historical exposures were higher than radiation currently received by the general population from natural and manufactured sources, by patients undergoing diagnostic procedures such as mammography or chest radiography, and by nuclear power plant workers. Despite our understanding of the health effects of high doses of radiation, the potential adverse effects of low doses are controversial. Furthermore, accidents at nuclear power plants in Windscale, England, in 1957, at Three Mile Island in Pennsylvania in 1979, and at Chernobyl in 1986 in the former Soviet Union perpetuate public anxiety about excess cancers associated with the medical, commercial, and military uses of radioactivity.

Electromagnetic radiation characterized by long wavelengths and low frequencies is described as *nonionizing radiation.* Electric power, radio waves and microwaves, infrared, and ultraviolet light are examples of nonionizing radiation. They produce vibration and rotation of atoms in biologic molecules. Radiation energy of short wavelengths and high frequency can ionize biologic target molecules and eject electrons. X-rays, gamma rays, and cosmic rays are forms of *ionizing radiation.* Ionizing radiation can be in the form of electromagnetic waves, such as x-rays produced by a roentgen tube or gamma rays emitted from natural sources, or particles that are released by natural decay of radioisotopes or by artificial acceleration of subatomic particles. *Particulate radiation* is classified by the type of particles emitted: alpha particles, beta particles or electrons, protons, neutrons, mesons, or deuterons. The energy of these particles is measured in million electron volts (MeV). Radioisotopes decay by emission of alpha or beta particles or by capture of electrons. In the case of radon gas, unstable daughter nuclei are produced that subsequently disintegrate, releasing alpha particles. Alpha particles consist of two neutrons and two protons: they have strong ionizing power but low penetration because of their large size. In contrast, beta particles are electrons emitted from the nucleus of an atom; these have weaker ionizing power but higher penetration than alpha particles. The decay of radioisotopes is expressed by the *curie* (Ci), 3.7×10^{10} disintegrations per second, or the *becquerel* (Bq), 1 disintegration per second. The rate of decay of radioisotopes is usually expressed as the ($t_{1/2}$) and ranges from a few seconds to centuries. Internal deposition of radioisotopes with long half-lives is especially dangerous because it results in continuous release of radioactive particles and gamma rays. For example, radium was used to paint watch dials and treat cancer in the first half of the 20th century; its long half-life of 1638 years and ability to be concentrated in the skeleton result in delayed appearance of bone tumors.

IONIZING RADIATION

The dose of ionizing radiation is measured in several units:

- *roentgen:* unit of charge produced by x-rays or gamma rays that ionize a specific volume of air.
- *rad:* the dose of radiation that will produce absorption of 100 ergs of energy per gram of tissue; 1 gm of tissue exposed to 1 roentgen of gamma rays is equal to 93 ergs.
- *gray* (Gy): the dose of radiation that will produce absorption of 1 joule of energy per kilogram of tissue; 1 Gy corresponds to 100 rad.
- *rem:* the dose of radiation that causes a biologic effect equivalent to 1 rad of x-rays or gamma rays.
- *sievert* (Sv): the dose of radiation that causes a biologic effect equivalent to 1 Gy of x-rays or gamma rays; 1 Sv corresponds to 100 rem.[46]

These measurements do not directly quantify energy transferred per unit of tissue and therefore do not predict the biologic effects of radiation. The following terms provide a better approximation of such information.

- *Linear energy transfer* (LET) expresses energy loss per unit of distance traveled as electron volts per micrometer. This value depends on the type of ionizing radiation. LET is high for alpha particles, less so for beta particles, and even less for gamma rays and x-rays. Thus, alpha and beta particles penetrate short distances and interact with many molecules within that short distance. Gamma rays and x-rays penetrate deeply but interact with relatively few molecules per unit distance. It should be evident that if equivalent amounts of energy entered the body in the form of alpha and gamma radiation, the alpha particles would induce heavy damage in a restricted area, whereas gamma rays would dissipate energy over a longer course and produce considerably less damage per unit of tissue.
- *Relative biologic effectiveness* (RBE) is simply a ratio that represents the relationship of the LETs of various forms of irradiation to cobalt gamma rays and megavolt x-rays, both of which have an RBE of unity (1).

In addition to the physical properties of the radioactive material and the dose, the biologic effects of ionizing radiation depend on several factors:

- Dose rate: a single dose can cause greater injury than divided or fractionated doses that allow time for cellular repair.
- Since DNA is the most important subcellular target of ionizing radiation, rapidly dividing cells are more radiosensitive than quiescent cells. Hematopoietic cells, germ cells, gastrointestinal epithelium, squamous epithelium, endothelial cells, and lymphocytes are highly susceptible to radiation injury; bone, cartilage, muscle, and peripheral nerves are more resistant.
- A single dose of external radiation administered to the whole body is more lethal than regional doses with shielding. For example, the median lethal dose (LD_{50}) of ionizing radiation is 2.5 to 4.0 Gy (250 to 400 rad), whereas doses of 40 to 70 Gy (4000 to 7000 rad) can be delivered in a fractionated manner during several weeks for cancer therapy.
- Cells in the G_2 and mitotic phases of the cell cycle are most sensitive to ionizing radiation; different cell types differ in the extent of their adaptive and reparative responses.

- Since ionizing radiation produces oxygen-derived radicals from the radiolytic cleavage of water (Chapter 1), cell injury induced by x-rays and gamma rays is enhanced by hyperbaric oxygen. Halogenated pyrimidines can also increase radiosensitivity to tumor cells. Conversely, free radical scavengers and antioxidants protect against radiation injury.

Cellular Mechanisms of Radiation Injury. The acute effects of ionizing radiation range from overt necrosis at high doses (>10 Gy), killing of proliferating cells at intermediate doses (1 to 2 Gy), and no histopathologic effect at doses less than 0.5 Gy.[46] Subcellular damage does occur at these lower doses, primarily targeting DNA; however, most cells show adaptive and reparative responses to low doses of ionizing radiation. If cells undergo extensive DNA damage or if they are unable to repair this damage, they enter apoptosis. Surviving cells may show delayed effects of radiation injury: mutations, chromosome aberrations, and genetic instability. These genetically damaged cells may become malignant; tissues with rapidly proliferating cell populations are especially susceptible to the carcinogenic effects of ionizing radiation. Most cancers induced by ionizing radiation have occurred after doses greater than 0.5 Gy. Acute cell death, especially of vascular endothelial cells, can cause delayed organ dysfunction several months or years after radiation exposure. In general, this delayed injury is caused by a combination of atrophy of parenchymal cells, ischemia due to vascular damage, and fibrosis. Acute and delayed effects of ionizing radiation are listed in Table 10–16, and their mechanisms are described next.

Acute Effects. Ionizing radiation can produce a variety of lesions in DNA, including DNA-protein cross-links, cross-linking of DNA strands, oxidation and degradation of bases, cleavage of sugar-phosphate bonds, and single-stranded or double-stranded DNA breaks. This damage may be produced directly by particulate radiation, x-rays, or gamma rays or indirectly by oxygen-derived free radicals or soluble products derived from peroxidized lipids.[47] Even relatively low doses of ionizing radiation (less than 0.5 Gy) induce alterations in gene expression in some target cell populations. These changes include increased expression of the c-*fos,* c-*jun,* and c-*myc* protooncogenes, induction of cytokines such as tumor necrosis factor (TNF)–α, and antioxidant defense enzymes such as manganese superoxide dismutase. Free radicals generated directly or indirectly by exposure to ionizing radiation may produce oxidant stress that activates transcription factors (such as NF-κB) that increase gene expression.[48] DNA damage itself stimulates expression of several genes involved in DNA repair, cell cycle arrest, and apoptosis. As discussed in Chapter 8, the tumor-suppressor gene *p53* is activated after many different forms of DNA damage. The p53 protein recognizes DNA damage and becomes activated and stabilized by posttranslational mechanisms. Depending on the dose of ionizing radiation and the target cell, p53 acts as a transcription factor to induce several downstream effector genes.[49] The end-points resulting from activation of this p53-mediated DNA damage response are discussed in Chapter 8. Briefly, activation of p53 induces cell cycle arrest, DNA repair, and, in some cases, apoptosis.

Fibrosis. An important delayed complication of ionizing radiation, usually at doses used for cancer therapy, is replacement of normal parenchymal tissue by fibrosis, resulting in scarring and loss of function. These fibrotic changes may be secondary to acute necrosis of parenchymal cells in organs that cannot regenerate or to ischemic injury caused by vascular damage. In addition, ionizing radiation administered to the breast tissue or lungs of rodents induces expression of cytokines and growth factors that persist for weeks after the initial exposure.[50, 51] In the lungs of rats, alveolar macrophages show increased production of interleukin-1, TNF-α, and interleukin-4. Irradiated alveolar macrophages also have increased expression of platelet-derived growth factor, basic fibroblast growth factor, and transforming growth factor-β.[51] As described in Chapter 4, these cytokines and growth factors play important roles in wound healing and collagen deposition by fibroblasts.

Carcinogenesis. Occupational or accidental exposures to ionizing radiation produce an increased incidence of various types of cancer, including skin cancers, leukemia, osteogenic sarcomas, and lung cancer. There is usually a latent period of 10 to 20 years before appearance of these cancers. In survivors of the atomic blasts at Hiroshima and

Table 10–16. ACUTE INJURY AND DELAYED COMPLICATIONS CAUSED BY IONIZING RADIATION

Organ	Acute Injury	Delayed Complications
Bone marrow	Atrophy	Hypoplasia, leukemia
Skin	Erythema	Atrophy of epidermis and fibrosis of dermis; cancer
Heart	—	Interstitial fibrosis
Lung	Edema, endothelial and epithelial cell death	Interstitial and intra-alveolar fibrosis; cancer
Gastrointestinal tract	Edema, mucosal ulcers	Ulcers; fibrosis; strictures; adhesions; cancer
Liver	Veno-occlusive disease	Cirrhosis; liver tumors
Kidney	Vasodilation	Cortical atrophy, interstitial fibrosis
Urinary bladder	Mucosal erosion	Submucosal fibrosis; cancer
Brain	Edema, necrosis	Necrosis of white matter, gliosis; brain cancer
Testis	Necrosis	Tubular atrophy
Ovary	Atresia of follicles	Stromal fibrosis
Thyroid	—	Hypothyroidism; cancer
Breast	—	Fibrosis; cancer
Thymus, lymph nodes	Atrophy	Lymphoma

Table 10–17. CLINICAL FEATURES OF THE ACUTE RADIATION SYNDROME

Category	Whole-Body Dose (rem)	Symptoms	Prognosis
Subclinical	<200	Mild nausea and vomiting Lymphocytes <1500/mm³	100% survival
Hematopoietic	200–600	Intermittent nausea and vomiting Petechiae, hemorrhage Maximum neutrophil and platelet depression in 2 wk Lymphocytes <1000/mm³	Infections May require bone marrow transplant
Gastrointestinal	600–1000	Nausea, vomiting, diarrhea Hemorrhage and infection in 1–3 wk Severe neutrophil and platelet depression Lymphocytes <500/mm³	Shock and death in 10–14 days even with replacement therapy
Central nervous system	>1000	Intractable nausea and vomiting Confusion, somnolence, convulsions Coma in 15 min–3 hr Lymphocytes absent	Death in 14–36 hr

Nagasaki, all types of leukemias were especially common, with the exception of chronic lymphocytic leukemia. Exposure of children to irradiation causes an increased incidence of breast and thyroid cancers as well as gastrointestinal and urinary tract tumors. The nuclear power accident at Chernobyl in 1986 caused more than 50 deaths, with estimated exposures of 50 to 300 rad. More than 20,000 people were exposed up to 40 rem. As early as 1990, an increased incidence of thyroid cancer was seen in exposed children. Approximately 2 million people living near Three Mile Island were exposed to low doses of 100 mrem in 1979; no adverse effects have yet been reported. Workers in the nuclear energy industry and in health care and research are exposed annually to doses ranging from 1 to 9 mSv. The annual maximal permissible exposure level for these workers is 50 mSv or 1 rem. There is uncertainty about the potential carcinogenic risk at these low exposures because the shape of the dose-response curve is unknown.

The mechanisms responsible for the delayed carcinogenic effects of ionizing radiation are not completely understood. The latent period between acute exposure to ionizing radiation and the delayed appearance of cancer may be due to a phenomenon called *induced genetic instability.* Quantitative analysis of mutation rates in irradiated cells in culture shows that mutations continue to be expressed in surviving cells after several generations. Accumulation of these delayed mutations may be the result of persistent DNA lesions that are not repaired or due to an epigenetic mechanism, such as altered methylation at CpG sites or shortening of telomeres. Delayed chromosome aberrations are also observed after exposure to ionizing radiation, especially in human lymphocytes.[52] These mechanisms may be responsible for induction of secondary cancers, especially leukemias in cancer patients treated with radiation therapy.[53]

Clinical Manifestations of Exposure to Ionizing Radiation

Acute, Whole-Body Exposure. Whole-body irradiation is potentially lethal; the clinical manifestations are dose dependent and described as the *acute radiation syndrome* or *radiation sickness.* On the basis of calculated doses delivered in nuclear reactor accidents or the atomic bombing of Japan, the LD_{50} at 60 days for humans exposed to a single dose of x-rays or gamma radiation is 2.5 to 4.0 Gy (250 to 400 rad). Depending on the dose, four clinical syndromes are produced: a subclinical or prodromal syndrome, hematopoietic syndrome, gastrointestinal syndrome, or central nervous system syndrome. These are summarized in Table 10–17. The acute symptoms are manifestations of the high sensitivity of rapidly proliferating tissues, such as the lymphohematopoietic cells and gastrointestinal epithelium, to acute radiation-induced necrosis or apoptosis (Fig. 10–10). If the patient survives the acute radiation syndrome, sublethally injured cells may repair the radiation damage, and the necrotic or apoptotic cells may be replaced by the progeny of more radioresistant stem cells.

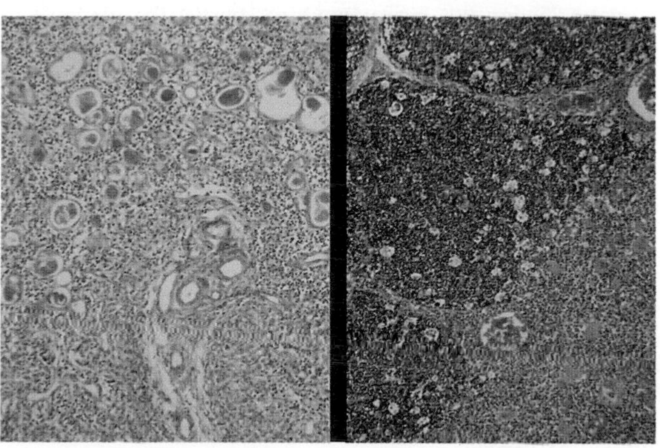

Figure 10–10

Atrophy of the thymus gland after exposure to ionizing radiation. The right panel shows a normal thymus with deeply staining cortex and pale staining medulla; the left panel shows depletion of lymphocytes with preservation of (pink, concentric) Hassall corpuscles. (American Registry of Pathology © 1990.)

Radiation Therapy. External radiation is delivered to malignant neoplasms at fractionated doses up to 40 to 70 Gy (4000 to 7000 rad), with shielding of adjacent normal tissues. Radiation therapy, especially when it is delivered to the chest or abdomen, can cause acute radiation sickness and neutrophil and platelet depression. These patients may experience transient fatigue, vomiting, and anorexia that may require reduction of the dose. Acutely, radiation therapy may shrink the tumor mass and relieve pain or compression of adjacent tissues. Unfortunately, cancer patients treated with radiation therapy may develop sterility, a secondary malignant neoplasm, or delayed radiation injury (described later).[53]

Growth and Developmental Abnormalities. The developing fetus and young children are highly sensitive to growth and developmental abnormalities induced by ionizing radiation. Four susceptible phases can be defined:

- Preimplantation embryo. Before implantation, irradiation of the mother can be lethal to the embryo.
- Critical stages of organogenesis. From the time of implantation until 9 weeks of gestation, exposure of the mother even to diagnostic radiation can produce a wide range of congenital malformations. This is the period of maximal growth and differentiation in the developing fetus, when it is most susceptible to a wide range of teratogenic agents, as discussed in Chapter 11.
- Fetal period. From 9 weeks of gestation until birth, functional abnormalities of the central nervous system and reproductive systems may be produced by maternal irradiation. The reproductive organs may be underdeveloped. Mental retardation affected offspring of Japanese mothers who were exposed to the atomic bomb in the first trimester of pregnancy. Newborns exposed to irradiation in utero have an increased incidence of childhood leukemia and brain tumors.
- Postnatal period. In infants and young children exposed to radiation, bone growth and maturation may be retarded. Development of the central nervous system, eyes, and teeth may also be perturbed. Although external radiation has been shown to shorten the life span of rodents, it is controversial whether ionizing radiation accelerates the process of aging in humans.

Heritable Mutations. *Drosophila* and laboratory mice show heritable mutations and chromosome abnormalities when exposed to ionizing radiation. Although chromosome aberrations have been demonstrated in the peripheral blood lymphocytes of atomic bomb survivors and radiation workers, there is no evidence so far that radiation-induced mutations have been transmitted to future generations. Geneticists are concerned, however, that recessive mutations induced by radiation may be accumulating in the human population. In addition, there are no dose-response data for the frequency of mutations induced by ionizing radiation in human germ cells.[46]

Delayed Radiation Injury. Months or years after irradiation, delayed complications, other than carcinogenesis, may occur. Radiation damage to the heart, lungs, central nervous system, or kidneys can be life-threatening. Infertility can occur in men or women. Cataracts can impair vision, and excess connective tissue can cause intestinal obstruction. Fibrous strictures and chronic ulcers may affect the skin, gastrointestinal tract, urinary bladder, and vagina. Chronic vascular insufficiency and excess connective tissue also complicate subsequent surgical procedures. Wound healing is impaired, and infections are more common. Unfortunately, cancer patients who received fractionated doses of radiation may also suffer from these delayed complications. The following are most vulnerable sites of delayed radiation injury:

- Blood vessels. After an initial inflammatory reaction that may be accompanied by necrosis of endothelial cells (Fig. 10–11), blood vessels in the field of irradiation show subintimal fibrosis, fibrosis of the muscle wall, degeneration of the internal elastic lamina, and severe narrowing of the lumen (Fig. 10–12). Capillaries may become thrombosed and obliterated or ectatic. The organs supplied by these damaged vessels will show ischemic changes, atrophy, and fibrosis.

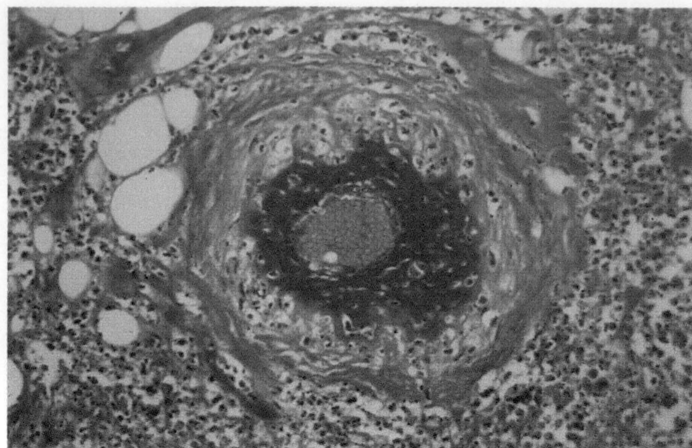

Figure 10–11

Acute vascular injury with fibrinoid necrosis and edema after exposure to ionizing radiation. (American Registry of Pathology © 1990.)

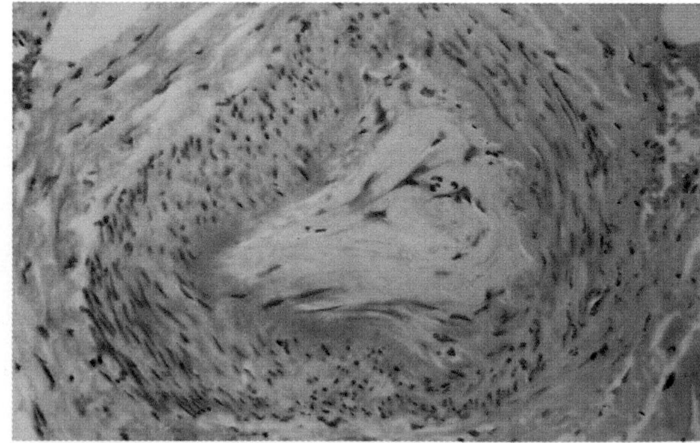

Figure 10–12

Chronic vascular injury with subintimal fibrosis occluding the lumen. (American Registry of Pathology © 1990.)

- Skin. Hair follicles and the epidermis are sensitive to acute radiation-induced injury. Desquamation can occur that is replaced by atrophic epidermis with hyperkeratosis, hyperpigmentation, and hypopigmentation. The subcutaneous vessels may be weakened and dilated; they are surrounded by dense bands of collagen in the dermis (Fig. 10–13). Impaired healing, increased susceptibility to infection, and ulceration may occur. These changes are called *radiation dermatitis.* As described earlier, skin cancer, especially basal cell and squamous cell carcinomas, may occur as long as 20 years after exposure.
- Heart. Radiotherapy delivered to the chest for malignant lymphoma, lung cancer, or breast cancer may damage the heart and pericardium. Fibrosis of the pericardium can cause constrictive pericarditis (Fig. 10–14). Less commonly, radiation-induced injury of capillaries and the coronary arteries can cause myocardial ischemia and fibrosis.
- Lungs. The lungs are highly susceptible to radiation-induced injury, leading to acute lung injury and delayed radiation pneumonitis. Delayed injury causes dyspnea, chronic cough, and diminished lung function. This is caused by intra-alveolar and interstitial fibrosis. Both internal and external irradiation increase the incidence of lung cancer; this effect is synergistic with cigarette smoking. In addition to carcinogenic chemicals, cigarette smoke contains two radionuclides: lead 210 and polonium 210. Underground miners are exposed to radon 222, which increases their risk of developing lung cancer. Lung cancers that develop in underground miners have a characteristic mutation (G → T) at codon 249 of the *p53* tumor-suppressor gene.[54]
- Kidneys and urinary bladder. The kidneys are moderately susceptible to radiation-induced injury. Delayed peritubular fibrosis, vascular damage, and hyalinization of glomeruli develop gradually, leading to hypertension and atrophy. The urinary bladder is sensitive to radiation injury, with acute necrosis of the epithelium followed by submucosal fibrosis, contracture, bleeding, and ulceration. Tumors of the bladder and kidney have been reported in Japanese atomic bomb survivors and in women irradiated for treatment of cervical carcinoma.
- Gastrointestinal tract. Esophagitis, gastritis, enteritis, colitis, and proctitis can result from irradiation. These are associated with exfoliation of the epithelial mucosa, susceptibility to infection, and loss of electrolytes and fluid. Delayed injury to small blood vessels causes chronic ischemia, ulceration and atrophy of the mucosa, and fibrosis that can cause strictures and obstruction.
- Breast. Diagnostic doses of ionizing radiation administered during adolescence increase the incidence of breast cancer after 15 to 20 years. Radiotherapy for breast cancer causes a dense, fibrotic reaction with extreme pleomorphism of epithelial cells (Fig. 10–15).

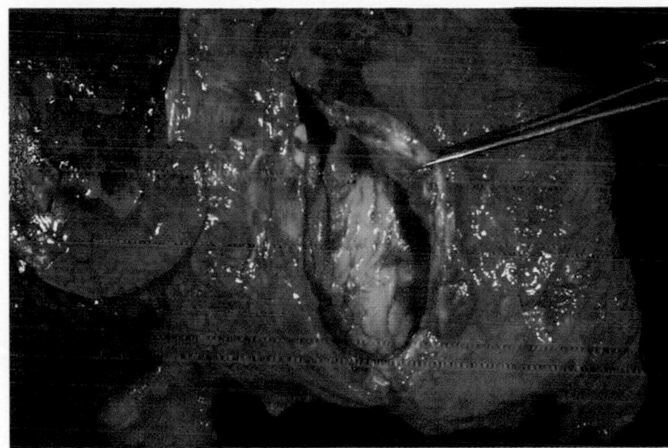

Figure 10–14

Extensive mediastinal fibrosis after radiotherapy for carcinoma of the lung. Note the markedly thickened pericardium. (From the teaching collection of the Department of Pathology, Southwestern Medical School, Dallas, TX.)

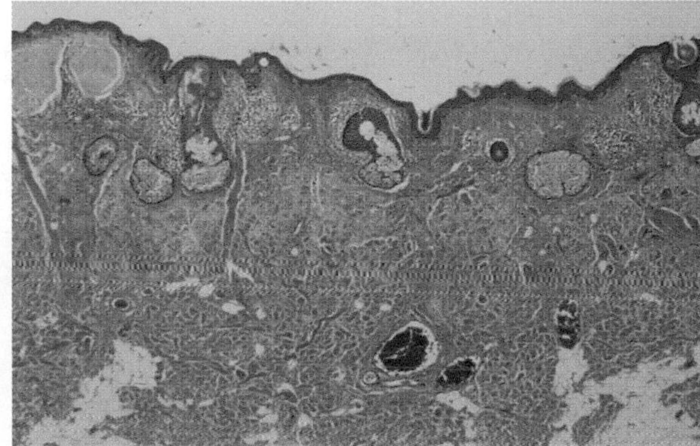

Figure 10–13

Chronic radiation dermatitis with atrophy of the epidermis, dermal fibrosis, and telangiectasia of the subcutaneous blood vessels. (American Registry of Pathology © 1990.)

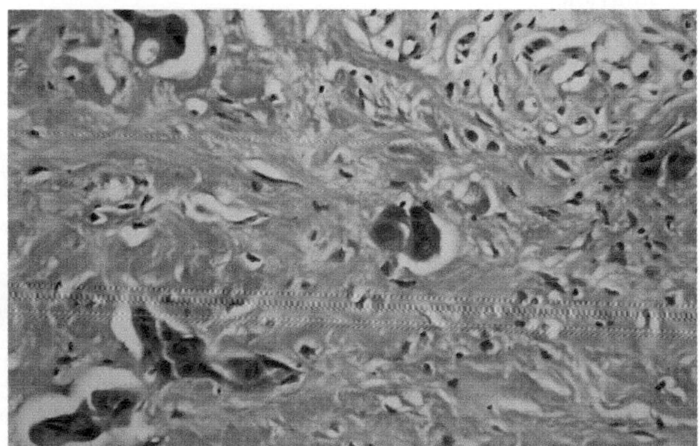

Figure 10–15

Radiation fibrosis of the breast stroma after radiotherapy for infiltrating ductal carcinoma. The nests of remaining tumor cells are pleomorphic and multinucleated. (American Registry of Pathology © 1990.)

- Ovary and testis. The spermatogonia are extremely sensitive to irradiation; even low doses may cause suppression of meiosis and infertility. Blood vessels may be obliterated and the seminiferous tubules become fibrotic, leaving the Sertoli cells and interstitial Leydig cells intact. Ovarian follicles degenerate acutely after irradiation; usually a few primordial oocytes and their follicular epithelium remain scattered in a fibrous stroma.
- Eyes and central nervous system. The lens is sensitive to ionizing radiation, and hence radiation gives rise to cataracts; the retinal and ciliary arteries may also be damaged. The brain may show focal necrosis and demyelination of the white matter. Irradiation of the spinal cord can damage small blood vessels, leading to necrosis, demyelination, and paraplegia. This is called *transverse myelitis.*

ULTRAVIOLET RADIATION

Solar radiation spans the spectrum of wavelengths between 200 and 4000 nm, including ultraviolet, visible, and infrared radiation. Ultraviolet radiation is divided into ultraviolet A (UVA), ultraviolet B (UVB), and ultraviolet C (UVC); 3% to 5% of the total solar radiation that penetrates the earth's surface is ultraviolet radiation. Ozone in the atmosphere is an important protective agent against ultraviolet radiation because it completely absorbs all UVC and partially absorbs UVB. Chlorofluorocarbons, used commercially as propellants, as solvents, and in refrigerators and air conditioners, interact with and deplete ozone. Such depletion is predicted to contribute to an increase in UVB and possibly UVC exposure, thus triggering a 2% to 4% increase in the incidence of skin cancers. Some protection from the effects of UV light is afforded by window glasses: they absorb UVB radiation, but transmit UVA radiation. Sunblocks and sunscreens offer greater protection because they absorb or block UVB and UVA to variable degrees. There are two major health effects of ultraviolet radiation: premature aging of the skin and skin cancer (Table 10–18). The carcinogenic effects of ultraviolet light are discussed in Chapter 8. Here we focus on other effects of ultraviolet radiation.

The acute effects of UVA and UVB are short-lived and reversible. They include erythema, pigmentation, and injury to Langerhans cells and keratinocytes in the epidermis. The kinetics and chemical mediators of these reactions differ in response to UVA and UVB. Depending on the intensity and length of exposure, erythema, edema, and acute inflammation are mediated by release of histamine from mast cells in the dermis and synthesis of arachidonic acid metabolites. The cytokine interleukin-1 is also induced by UVB exposure. UVA produces oxidation of melanin with transient, immediate darkening, especially in individuals with darker skin. Tanning induced by UVA and UVB is due to a delayed increase in the number of melanocytes, elongation and extension of dendritic processes, and transfer of melanin to keratinocytes. Tanning induced by UVB is protective against subsequent exposures; tanning induced by UVA provides limited protection. Both UVA and UVB deplete Langerhans cells and thus reduce the processing of antigens in the epidermis. UVB causes apoptosis of keratinocytes in the epidermis, resulting in dyskeratotic, sunburn cells.[55]

Repeated exposures to ultraviolet radiation give rise to changes in the skin that are characteristic of premature aging (e.g., wrinkling, solar elastosis, and irregularities in pigmentation). In contrast to ionizing radiation that increases deposition of collagen in the dermis, ultraviolet radiation causes degenerative changes in elastin and collagen, leading to wrinkling, increased laxity, and a leathery appearance. These connective tissue alterations accumulate over time and are largely irreversible. They are caused by increased expression of the elastin gene, increased expression of matrix metalloproteinases that degrade collagen, and induction of a tissue inhibitor of matrix metalloproteinase. The end result of these changes in connective tissue enzymes is degradation of type I collagen fibrils and disorganization and degeneration of the dermal connective tissue[56] (Fig. 10–16).

Skin damage induced by UVB is believed to be caused by generation of reactive oxygen species and by damage to endogenous chromophores such as melanin. Ultraviolet radiation also damages DNA, resulting in the formation of pyrimidine dimers between adjacent pyrimidines on the same DNA strand. Other forms of DNA damage, for example, formation of pyrimidine-pyrimidone (6-4) photoproducts, single-stranded breaks, and DNA-protein cross-links, are also noted.[55] A unique spectrum of mutations has been

Table 10–18. ACUTE AND DELAYED EFFECTS OF ULTRAVIOLET RADIATION

Radiation	Wavelength (nm)	Acute Effects	Delayed Effects
UVA	320–400	Erythema 8–48 hr Depletion of Langerhans cells Pigment darkening Dermal inflammation	Tanning ? Skin cancer
UVB	290–320	Erythema 3–24 hr Apoptosis of keratinocytes Depletion of Langerhans cells	Tanning Solar elastosis Premature aging Actinic keratosis Skin cancer
UVC	200–290		? Skin cancer

From Rosen CF: Ultraviolet radiation. In Craighead JE (ed): Pathology of Environmental and Occupational Disease. St. Louis, Mosby–Year Book, 1996, p 193.

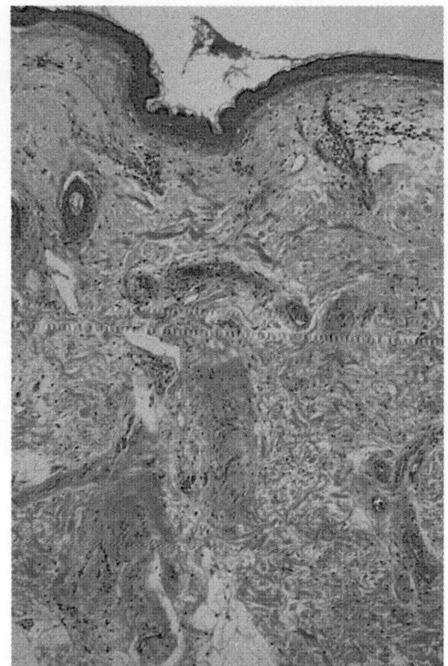

Figure 10–16

Solar elastosis with basophilic degeneration of the connective tissue in the upper layer of the dermis. (American Registry of Pathology © 1990.)

identified in premalignant and malignant skin lesions in humans, involving adjacent pyrimidine bases in *p53:* C → T or CC → TT double-base substitutions. This observation provides strong evidence for an etiologic role of ultraviolet light in induction of skin cancer.[57]

Exposure to UV radiation induces a series of molecular changes collectively referred to as the ultraviolet response pathway. The triggering of this pathway involves activation of the *ras* signal transduction with activation of mitogen-activated protein kinases and induction of cellular protooncogenes and other genes involved in cell proliferation.[58] This effect is believed to be independent of DNA damage. Subsequently, thymidine dinucleotides produced by ultraviolet radiation activate the *p53* pathway in a manner analogous to DNA breaks produced by ionizing radiation.[59] Thus, exposure to ultraviolet radiation can induce a protective cellular response leading to DNA repair, cell cycle arrest, or apoptosis, depending on the intensity of exposure and the target cell. The importance of DNA repair as a defense mechanism against skin cancer is illustrated by increased susceptibility of patients with xeroderma pigmentosum to ultraviolet light–induced skin cancers (Chapter 8).

ELECTROMAGNETIC FIELDS

Nonionizing electromagnetic fields range from less than 1 cycle/second (Hertz or Hz) for DC power lines up to 100 GHz for long-distance microwaves and radar.[60] There is public concern that residential exposure to ambient 50- to 60-Hz magnetic fields is a health threat that may contribute to an increased incidence of leukemia in children. However, epidemiologic studies have failed to establish a significant relationship between the usual levels of residential magnetic fields and an increased incidence of childhood leukemia.[61] Workers may be exposed to more intense magnetic fields; for example, welders and electricians may experience tenfold higher exposures at work than at home. Epidemiologic studies of highly exposed workers are contradictory. A few studies have reported an increased incidence in leukemia, brain cancer, and breast cancer in men with high occupational exposures.[60] However, animal studies and in vitro cellular assays do not provide any mechanistic evidence for a causal relationship between exposure to magnetic fields and cancer.[60, 62]

Physical Environment

Human injury, death, and disability remain a major public health problem in modern industrialized societies. Among people up to the age of 34 years, injuries are the most common cause of death, accounting for 151,000 fatalities per year in the United States. Among unintentional injuries, deaths due to motor vehicles are most numerous, followed by falls, especially among the elderly. Intentional injuries (homicides and suicides) caused 56,000 deaths in 1994: firearms were used in 72% of homicides and in 60% of suicides (Table 10–19). Identification of risk factors and their prevention are important for the prevention of such

Table 10–19. UNINTENTIONAL DEATHS, HOMICIDES, AND SUICIDES IN THE UNITED STATES IN 1994

Cause	Unintentional Deaths	Homicides	Suicides
Motor vehicle	42,000		390
Occupant	34,000		110
Pedestrian	6,000		280
Motorcyclist	1,800		
Bicycle	800		
Fall	14,000	25	720
Fire or scalding	4,000	200	170
Drowning	4,000	52	380
Poisoning	9,000	48	5,300
Firearm	1,400	18,000	19,000
Other	16,000	6,800	5,000

From Rivara FP, et al: Injury prevention. N Engl J Med 337:543, 613, 1997.

injuries. Physicians and health care personnel play an important role in educating their patients about potential risk factors and in encouraging active preventive strategies. For example, motor vehicles are a major cause of injury: approximately 40% of deaths resulting from motor vehicle accidents involve ethanol. Physicians can discourage their patients from drinking and driving and encourage the use of seat belts, air bags, and safety seats for infants and children. Violence, in association with use of firearms, drug and alcohol use, and physical and mental abuse, is a major concern in the United States. Restricting access to guns is vital, especially in homes with young children and adolescents.[63]

Injuries caused by physical environment, resulting from human activities as well as from external forces, can be divided into four categories: mechanical force, heat and cold, electrical injuries, and high altitudes.

MECHANICAL FORCE

Mechanical force may inflict soft tissue injuries, bone injuries, and head injuries. Injuries of the bones and of the head are considered in Chapter 30. Soft tissue injuries can be superficial, involving mainly the skin, or deep, associated with visceral damage. The skin injuries can be further described as follows.

Abrasion. This type of skin injury represents basically a scrape, in which the superficial epidermis is torn off by friction or force (Fig. 10–17). Regeneration without scarring usually occurs promptly unless infection complicates the process.

Laceration Versus Incision. A laceration is an irregular tear in the skin produced by overstretching. It may be linear or stellate, depending on the tearing force. Typical of a laceration are the bridging strands of fibrous tissue or blood vessels across the wound, not seen in an incision (Fig. 10–18). The immediate margins of the laceration are frequently hemorrhagic and traumatized. In contrast, an incision is made by a sharp cutting object, such as a knife (scalpel) or a piece of glass. The margins of the incision are usually relatively clean, and there are no bridging strands of tissue. The incision, in contrast with the laceration, can usually be neatly approximated by sutures, leaving little or no scar. Deep tissues and organs may sustain lacerations from an external blow with or without apparent superficial injury. For example, when the unrestrained body impacts on the steering wheel in a head-on collision, the liver or spleen may sustain fatal lacerations.

Contusion. This is an injury caused by a blunt force that damages small blood vessels and causes interstitial bleeding, usually without disruption of the continuity of the tissue (Fig. 10–19). With superficial contusions, the bleeding is usually evident almost at once, but with deeper

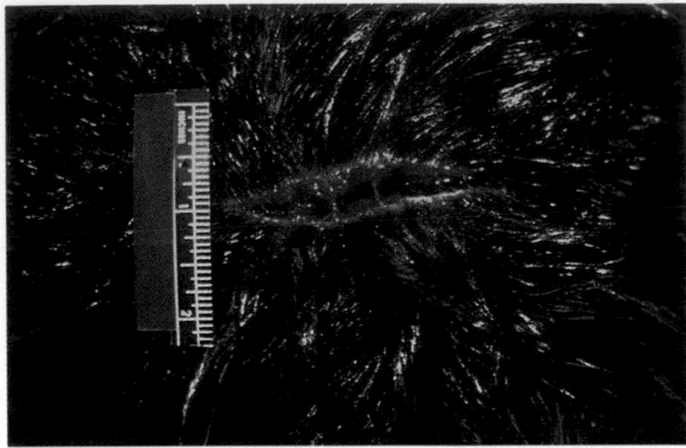

Figure 10–18

Laceration of the scalp. The bridging strands of the fibrous tissue are evident. (From the teaching collection of the Department of Pathology, Southwestern Medical School, Dallas, TX.)

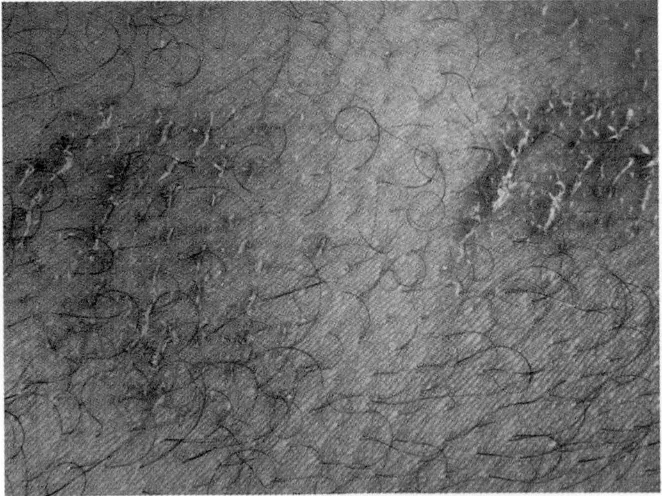

Figure 10–17

Abrasion. Note the superficial tears in the epidermis. There is bleeding under the skin as well. (From the teaching collection of the Department of Pathology, Southwestern Medical School, Dallas, TX.)

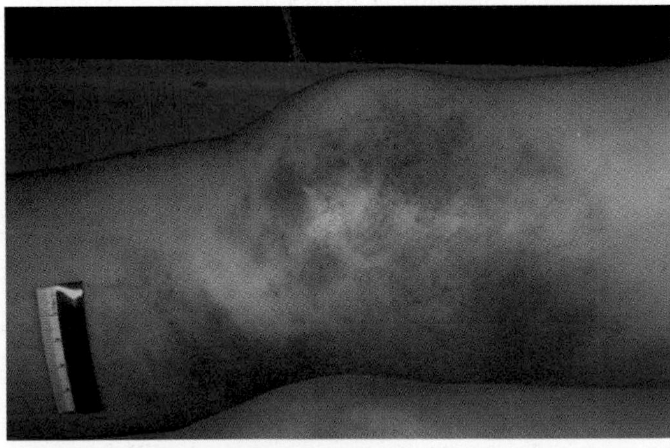

Figure 10–19

Contusion resulting from blunt trauma. The skin is intact but there is hemorrhage in subcutaneous vessels, producing extensive discoloration. (From the teaching collection of the Department of Pathology, Southwestern Medical School, Dallas, TX.)

contusions, of skeletal muscle, for example, the bleeding may not be evident for many hours and may leave only swelling and tenderness at the site. Older individuals with small-vessel fragility may sustain extensive hematomas at contused sites.

Gunshot Wounds. Injuries of this nature fall largely into the domain of forensic pathology, a specialty dealing with trauma and medicolegal issues. The character of a gunshot wound at entry and exit and the extent of injury depend on the type of gun used (handgun or rifle) and on a large number of variables, including the caliber of the bullet, the type of ammunition, the distance of the firearm from the body, the locus of the injury, the trajectory of the missile (at right angles to the skin or oblique), and the gyroscopic stability of the bullet (the presence or absence of wobbling or tumbling).

With handguns held at close range (within a foot of the skin surface), there is a gray-black discoloration about the wound of entrance (fouling) produced by the heat, smoke, and burned powder deposits exiting with the bullet from the muzzle. In addition, there may be discrete, larger particles of unburned powder producing a halo of stippling about the entrance wound, the diameter of which depends on the distance of the gun from the body. When firearms are held more than a foot away, but within 3 feet, there may be only stippling without fouling. At greater distances, neither is present (Fig. 10–20). In general, the perforating cutaneous wound is slightly smaller than the diameter of the bullet and has a narrow enclosing rim of abrasion. When the trajectory of the bullet is angled into the skin, the abrasion is asymmetric, having its greatest width at the margin closest to the origin of the bullet. Depending on the size and velocity of the bullet and the distance between the target and the muzzle to the firearm, when the skin is closely applied to underlying bone as in the scalp, entering gas may elevate the overlying skin and, in some instances, produce stellate lacerations about the perforating wound. Similarly, large-caliber, high-velocity missiles, after penetrating the skin and subcutaneous tissues, may traverse internal organs and, by their mass and velocity, cause extending massive lacerations through the liver or other viscera. In contrast, smaller, low-velocity bullets, even though they penetrate the organ, may produce only fairly restricted burrowing or through-and-through tracts with limited surrounding injury.

Cutaneous exit wounds are generally more irregular than wounds of entrance, because in passing through the tissues, the bullet almost inevitably develops a wobbling trajectory. In fact, with high-velocity rifle bullets, the exit wound may be considerably larger than the entrance wound. The margins of the wound may be everted, and there is no fouling or stippling and, often, little surrounding abrasion. To the experienced eye, it is evident that gunshot wounds tell a story.

THERMAL INJURIES

Both excess heat and excess cold are important causes of injury. Burns are all too common and are discussed first; a brief discussion of hyperthermia and hypothermia follows.

Thermal Burns. In the United States, burns cause 5000 deaths per year and result in the hospitalization of more than ten times that many persons. Many victims are children, who are often scalded by hot liquids. Fortunately, marked decreases have been seen in both mortality rates and length of hospitalizations since the 1970s. This improved prognosis results from a better understanding of the systemic effects of massive burns and discoveries of better ways to prevent wound infection and facilitate healing of skin surfaces.

The clinical significance of burns depends on the following important factors:

- Depth of the burn
- Percentage of body surface involved
- Possible presence of internal injuries from inhalation of hot and toxic fumes

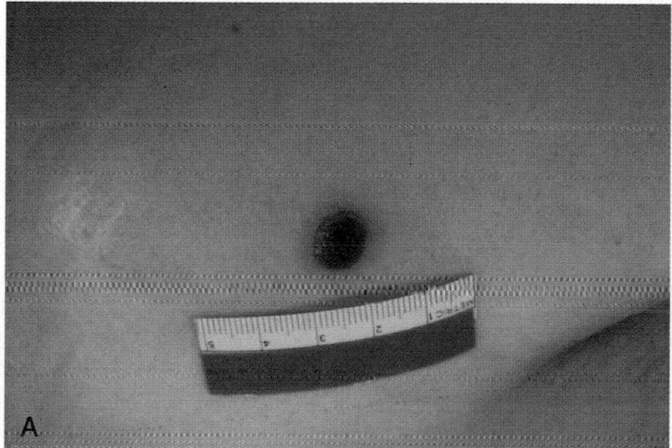

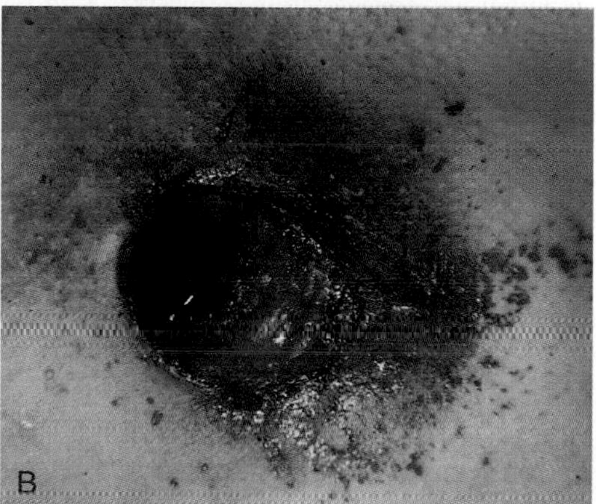

Figure 10–20

A, Gunshot wound of entry from a long distance. (From the teaching collection of the Department of Pathology, Southwestern Medical School, Dallas, TX.) *B*, An entry gunshot wound at close range revealing the prominent black discoloration produced by unburned powder, heat, and smoke as well as the more peripheral stippling resulting from larger particles of unburned powder. (Courtesy of George Katsas, MD, Forensic Pathologist, Boston, MA.)

- Promptness and efficacy of therapy, especially fluid and electrolyte management and prevention or control of wound infections

A *full-thickness burn* involves total destruction of the epidermis and dermis, with loss of the dermal appendages that would have provided cells for epithelial regeneration. Both *third-* and *fourth-degree burns* are in this category. In *partial-thickness burns,* at least the deeper portions of the dermal appendages are spared. Partial-thickness burns include *first-degree burns* (epithelial involvement only) and *second-degree burns* (both epidermis and superficial dermis).

MORPHOLOGY. On gross inspection, full-thickness burns are white or charred, dry, and anesthetic (because of nerve ending destruction); depending on the depth, partial-thickness burns are pink or mottled with blisters and are painful. On histologic examination, devitalized tissue demonstrates coagulative necrosis; adjacent vital tissue quickly develops inflammatory changes with an accumulation of inflammatory cells and marked exudation.

Despite continuous improvement in therapy, any burn exceeding 50% of the total body surface, whether superficial or deep, is grave and potentially fatal. With burns of more than 20% of the body surface, there is a rapid shift of body fluids into the interstitial compartments, both at the burn site and systematically, which can result in hypovolemic shock (Chapter 5). The mechanisms include an increase in local interstitial osmotic pressure (from release of osmotically active constituents of dying cells) and both neurogenic and mediator-induced increases in vascular permeability. Because protein from the blood is lost into interstitial tissue, generalized edema, including pulmonary edema, may become severe if fluids used for volume replacement are not osmotically active.

Another important consideration in patients with burns is the degree of *injury to the airways and lungs.* Inhalation injury is frequent in persons trapped in burning buildings and may result from the direct effect of heat on the mouth, nose, and upper airways or from the inhalation of toxic components in smoke. Water-soluble gases such as chlorine, sulfur oxides, and ammonia may react with water to form acids or alkalis, particularly in the upper airways, to produce inflammation and swelling, which may lead to partial or complete airway obstruction. Lipid-soluble gases such as nitrous oxide and products of burning plastics are more likely to reach deeper airways, producing pneumonitis. Unlike shock, which develops within hours, pulmonary manifestations may not develop for 24 to 48 hours. Thus, the initial absence of respiratory symptoms does not necessarily imply that there has been no respiratory injury.

Secondary *burn infection* is an important complication in all burn patients who have lost epidermis. Organ system failure resulting from burn sepsis continues to be the leading cause of death in burned patients. The burn site is ideal for growth of microorganisms; the serum and debris provide nutrients, and the burn injury compromises blood flow, blocking effective inflammatory responses. The most common offender is the opportunist *Pseudomonas aeruginosa,* but antibiotic-resistant strains of other common hospital-acquired bacteria, such as *S. aureus,* and fungi, particularly *Candida* species, may also be involved. Furthermore, cellular and humoral defenses against infections are compromised, and both lymphocyte and phagocyte functions are impaired. Direct bacteremic spread and release of toxic substances such as endotoxin from the local site exert dire consequences. Pneumonia or septic shock with renal failure and the acute respiratory distress syndrome (Chapter 16) are the most common serious sequelae. Aggressive, early debridement of burn wounds is designed not only to provide a clean, vascular surface on which wound repair can proceed but also to provide phagocytes ready access to infecting microorganisms. Topical antibiotics may help, but burn infection continues to be an important problem.

Another important pathophysiologic effect of burns is the *development of a hypermetabolic state* with excess heat loss and an increased need for nutritional support. It is estimated that when more than 40% of the body surface is burned, the resting metabolic rate may approach twice normal. The consequence is breakdown of tissue, which may result in loss of essential protein stores, reaching lethal proportions comparable to starvation within several weeks. Thus, it is essential to keep the patient's room temperature elevated to reduce body heat loss and to implement appropriate nutritional supplementation.

Hyperthermia. Prolonged exposure to elevated ambient temperatures can result in heat cramps, heat exhaustion, and heat stroke.

- *Heat cramps* result from loss of electrolytes through sweating. Cramping of voluntary muscles, usually in association with vigorous exercise, is the hallmark. Heat-dissipating mechanisms are able to maintain normal core body temperature.
- *Heat exhaustion* is probably the most common heat syndrome. Its onset is sudden, with prostration and collapse, and it results from a failure of the cardiovascular system to compensate for hypovolemia, secondary to water depletion. After a period of collapse, which is usually brief, equilibrium is spontaneously re-established.
- *Heat stroke* is associated with high ambient temperatures and high humidity. Thermoregulatory mechanisms fail, sweating ceases, and core body temperature rises. Body temperatures of 112° to 113°F have been recorded in some terminal cases. Clinically, a rectal temperature of 106°F or higher is considered a grave prognostic sign, and the mortality rate for such patients exceeds 50%. The underlying mechanism is marked generalized peripheral vasodilation with peripheral pooling of blood and a decreased effective circulating blood volume. Necrosis of the muscles and myocardium may occur. Arrhythmias, disseminated intravascular coagulation, and other systemic effects are common. Elderly persons, in-

dividuals undergoing intense physical stress (including young athletes and military recruits), and persons with cardiovascular disease are prime candidates for heat stroke.

Hypothermia. Prolonged exposure to low ambient temperature leads to hypothermia, a condition seen all too frequently in homeless persons. Lowering of body temperature is hastened by high humidity in cold, wet clothing and dilation of superficial blood vessels as a result of the ingestion of alcohol. At about 90°F, loss of consciousness occurs, followed by bradycardia and atrial fibrillation at lower core temperatures.

Local Reactions. Chilling or freezing of cells and tissues causes injury in two ways:

1. Direct effects are probably mediated by physical dislocations within cells and high salt concentrations incident to the crystallization of the intracellular and extracellular water.
2. Indirect effects are exerted by circulatory changes. Depending on the rate at which the temperature drops and the duration of the drop, slowly developing chilling may induce vasoconstriction and increased permeability, leading to edematous changes. Such changes are typical of "trench foot." Atrophy and fibrosis may follow. Alternatively, with sudden sharp drops in temperature that are persistent, the vasoconstriction and increased viscosity of the blood in the local area may cause ischemic injury and degenerative changes in peripheral nerves. In this situation, only after the temperature begins to return toward normal do the vascular injury and increased permeability with exudation become evident. However, during the period of ischemia, hypoxic changes and infarction of the affected tissues may develop (e.g., gangrene of toes or feet).

ELECTRICAL INJURIES

The passage of an electric current through the body may be without effect; may cause sudden death by disruption of neural regulatory impulses, producing, for example, cardiac arrest; or may cause thermal injury to organs interposed in the pathway of the current. Many variables are involved, but most important are the resistance of the tissues to the conductance of the electric current and the intensity of the current. The greater the resistance of tissues, the greater the heat generated. Although all tissues of the body are conductors of electricity, their resistance to flow varies inversely with their water content. Dry skin is particularly resistant, but when skin is wet or immersed in water, its resistance is greatly decreased. Thus, an electric current may cause only a surface burn of dry skin but may cause death by disruption of regulatory pathways when it is transmitted through wet skin, producing, for example, ventricular fibrillation or respiratory paralysis without injury to the skin.

The thermal effects of the passage of the electric current depend on its intensity. High-intensity current, such as lightning coursing along the skin, produces linear arborizing burns known as lightning marks. Sometimes intense current is conducted around the victim (so-called flash-over), blasting and disrupting the clothing but doing little injury. When lightning is transmitted internally, it may produce sufficient heat and steam to explode solid organs, fracture bones, or char areas of organs. Focal hemorrhages from rupture of small vessels may be seen in the brain. Sometimes, death is preceded by violent convulsions related to brain damage. Less intense voltage may heat, coagulate, or rupture vessels and cause hemorrhages or, in solid organs such as the spleen and kidneys, cause infarctions or ruptures.

INJURIES RELATED TO CHANGES IN ATMOSPHERIC PRESSURE

Depending on the direction of change (increase or decrease) in atmospheric pressure, its rate of development, and the magnitude of change, four syndromes can be produced:

- High-altitude illness
- Blast injury
- Air or gas embolism
- Decompression disease—also know as caisson disease—which is sometimes referred to as barotrauma

High-Altitude Illness. As is well known, this is encountered in mountain climbers in the rarefied atmosphere encountered at altitudes above 4000 m. The lowered oxygen tension produces progressive mental obtundation and may be accompanied by poorly understood increased capillary permeability with systemic and, in particular, pulmonary edema.

Blast Injury. This form of injury obviously implies a violent increase in pressure either in the atmosphere (air blast) or in water (immersion blast). With *air blast,* the compression wave impinges on the side toward the explosion and so may collapse the thorax or violently compress the abdomen, with rupture of internal organs. The pressure wave may enter the airways and damage the alveoli. The following wave of decreased pressure, with its sudden expansion of the abdomen and thorax, may rupture the intestines or lungs. In *immersion blast,* the pressure is supplied to the body from all sides, inducing injuries similar to those of air blast.

Air or Gas Embolism. This may occur as a complication of scuba diving, mechanical positive-pressure ventilatory support, and hyperbaric oxygen therapy and only rarely as a manifestation of decompression disease (see next). Common to all these settings is an abnormal increase in intra-alveolar air or gas pressure, leading to tearing of tissue with entrance of air into the interstitium and small blood vessels. Pulmonary, mediastinal, and subcutaneous emphysema may result, and in some instances, the coalescence of numerous small air or gas emboli that gain access to the arterial circulation may lead acutely to stroke-like syndromes or a myocardial ischemic episode. Either the neurologic or the myocardial embolism may cause sudden death.

Decompression (Caisson) Disease. As the name implies, this disorder is encountered in deep-sea divers and underwater workers who spend long periods in caissons or tunnels, under increased atmospheric pressure. The injury, encountered with too rapid decompression, is a function of Henry's law, which in essence states that the solubility of a gas in a liquid (e.g., blood) is proportional to the partial pressure of that gas in the environment. As the underwater depth and consequent atmospheric pressure increase, larger and larger amounts of oxygen and accompanying gases (nitrogen or helium) dissolve in the blood and tissue fluids. Once the ascent begins (decompression), the dissolved gases come out of solution and form minute bubbles in the bloodstream and tissues. Coalescence of these bubbles produces even larger masses capable of becoming significant emboli in the bloodstream. The oxygen bubbles are soluble in blood and tissues and so redissolve. The nitrogen and helium dissolve only slowly. Periarticular bubbles produce the *bends.* Bubbles formed within the lung or gaseous emboli give rise to respiratory difficulties, with severe substernal pain referred to as the *chokes.* Various central nervous system manifestations may appear, ranging from headache and visual disturbances to behavioral disorientation. Involvement of the inner ear may produce vertigo and the *staggers.* All these manifestations may appear within hours of the too rapid ascent, but skeletal manifestations—*caisson disease of bone*—may sometimes appear days later. This takes the form of foci of aseptic necrosis, typically of femoral and humeral heads, and medullary foci, particularly in the lower femur and upper tibia, attributed to embolic occlusion of the vascular supply.

FOOD AND NUTRITION

Food Safety: Additives and Contaminants

Food is essential for life, yet it contains numerous natural constituents and additives that may threaten human health. This mixture of natural compounds and chemical additives is the most complex and variable environmental exposure that humans experience. A wide range of chemicals are natural constituents of foods, including carcinogens such as safrole in nutmeg and parsley and estragole in basil and fennel. Coffee contains more than 200 compounds, including tannins that are carcinogenic. Natural pesticides are also found in plants, for example, 5- and 8-methoxypsoralen in celery, parsnips, and parsley.[64] Some scientists contend that natural plant pesticides and carcinogens are a greater threat to humans than are agricultural pesticide residues or industrial toxicants. Food may be contaminated by natural toxicants or microorganisms, for example, the liver carcinogen aflatoxin B_1 or the deadly botulin toxin. Contamination with pathogenic viruses and bacteria continues to threaten public health. Hepatitis A virus, *Salmonella enteritidis, Escherichia coli, Listeria monocytogenes, Campylobacter,* and *Cryptosporidium* are common examples of food-borne infections. Additional toxicants can be generated in foods during preservation or preparation. Broiling meat produces oxidized fats, pyrolysis products of amino acids, and carcinogenic polycyclic aromatic hydrocarbons. Foods preserved by smoking or by nitrate and nitrite additives may contain precursors of *N*-nitrosamines. These chemicals are potent carcinogens in many animal species, producing cancers of the mouth, esophagus, larynx, liver, and kidney.[64]

Additional chemicals are added to foods either directly (chemical sweeteners, preservatives, food colors) or indirectly. Indirect additives include residues of drugs or hormones fed to animals, agricultural pesticides, industrial contaminants, and residues from food packaging. Low levels of metals such as mercury and lead, PCBs, and chlorinated hydrocarbons are present in our food supply. Other metals, such as arsenic and cadmium, may be natural contaminants of water and soil in some geographic locations. The Food and Drug Administration monitors the levels of pesticides, metals, and industrial contaminants in food samples in the United States. The level of some contaminants such as dieldrin approach the acceptable daily intake that has been established as a safe threshold dose. Despite the considerable concern about additives and contaminants, regulation of their content in food is complicated by the detection limit of potential carcinogens, reliance on toxicologic assays using high doses of chemicals in rodents, and uncertainties in extrapolation of risk for humans under lifetime exposures at low doses.[64]

Nutritional Deficiencies

Although the potential health hazards associated with food additives and contaminants are of concern, much more significant are the global health problems associated with inadequate nutrition. In third world countries, undernutrition or protein-energy malnutrition continues to be common; and in industrialized societies, the most frequent diseases (atherosclerosis, cancer, diabetes, and hypertension) have all been linked to some form of dietary impropriety.

An adequate diet should provide (1) energy, in the form of carbohydrates, fats, and proteins; (2) essential (as well as non-essential) amino acids and fatty acids to be used as building blocks for synthesis of structural and functional proteins and lipids; and (3) vitamins and minerals, which function as coenzymes or hormones in vital metabolic pathways or, as in the case of calcium and phosphate, as important structural components. In *primary malnutrition,* one or all of these components are missing from the diet. By contrast, in *secondary,* or *conditional, malnutrition,* the supply of nutrients is adequate, but malnutrition may result from nutrient malabsorption, impaired nutrient use or storage, excess nutrient losses, or increased need for nutrients.

In developing nations, the incidence of overt hunger is high, and the incidence of more subtle forms of undernutrition is even higher. Vitamin A deficiencies are rampant in certain parts of Africa, iodine deficiencies occur in regions where iodized salt is not available, and iron deficiency is often seen in infants fed exclusively milk diets. Thus, ignorance about the nutritional value of foods also plays an important role in malnutrition. In the United States, the National Research Council recommends daily allowances for protein, vitamins, and minerals for healthy adults, specifying ranges for both men and women. These standards represent the scientifically based general consensus of the safe (not minimal) amounts of each nutrient necessary to maintain good health. Debates continue as to optimal levels of fat and fiber to prevent cardiovascular disease and cancer, and this subject is briefly discussed later.

Affluent societies are not immune to a significant incidence of undernutrition. The following listing of common causes in the United States highlights this point:

- *Ignorance and poverty.* Homeless persons, aged individuals, and children of the poor demonstrate effects of protein energy malnutrition as well as trace nutrient deficiencies. Even the affluent may fail to recognize that infants, adolescents, and pregnant women have increased nutritional needs.
- *Chronic alcoholism.* Alcoholics may sometimes suffer protein energy malnutrition but are more frequently deficient in several vitamins, especially thiamine, pyridoxine, folate, and vitamin A, owing to a combination of dietary deficiency, defective gastrointestinal absorption, abnormal nutrient use and storage, increased metabolic needs, and an increased rate of loss. A failure to recognize the likelihood of thiamine deficiency in chronic alcoholics may result in irreversible brain damage (e.g., Korsakoff psychosis, discussed later).
- *Acute and chronic illnesses.* The basal metabolic rate becomes accelerated in many illnesses (in patients with extensive burns, it may double), resulting in an increased daily requirement for all nutrients. Failure to appreciate this fact can compromise recovery.
- *Self-imposed dietary restriction.* Anorexia nervosa, bulimia nervosa, and less overt eating disorders affect a large population who are concerned about body image or suffer from an unreasonable fear of cardiovascular disease.

Other, less common causes of malnutrition include the malabsorption syndromes, genetic diseases, specific drug therapies (which block uptake or use of particular nutrients), and total parenteral nutrition.

In the sections that follow, we barely skim the surface of nutritional disorders. Included in the discussion are protein energy malnutrition, deficiencies of most of the vitamins and trace minerals, obesity, and a brief overview of the relationships of diet to atherosclerosis and cancer. Several other nutrients and nutritional issues are discussed in the context of specific disorders throughout the text.

PROTEIN-ENERGY MALNUTRITION

Severe protein-energy malnutrition (PEM) is a disastrous disease. It is far too common in third world countries, where up to 25% of children may be affected; in these countries, it is a major factor in the high death rates among children younger than 5 years.

PEM refers to a *range of clinical syndromes* characterized by an inadequate dietary intake of protein and calories to meet the body's needs. From a functional standpoint, there are two protein compartments in the body: the *somatic protein compartment,* represented by the skeletal muscles; and the *visceral protein compartment,* represented by protein stores in the visceral organs, primarily the liver. These two compartments are regulated differently, and as we shall see, the somatic compartment is affected more severely in marasmus, and the visceral compartment is depleted more severely in kwashiorkor. Before the clinical presentations of the two polar forms of severe malnutrition (marasmus and kwashiorkor) are discussed, some comments are made on the clinical assessment of undernutrition and some of its general metabolic characteristics.

The diagnosis of PEM is obvious in its most severe forms; in mild to moderate forms, the usual approach is to compare the body weight for a given height with standard tables; other parameters are also helpful, including evaluation of fat stores, muscle mass, and serum proteins. With a loss of fat, the major storage form of energy, the thickness of skinfolds (which includes skin and subcutaneous tissue) is reduced. If the somatic protein compartment is catabolized, the resultant reduction in muscle mass is reflected by reduced circumference of the midarm. Measurement of serum proteins (albumin, transferrin, and others) provides a measure of the adequacy of the visceral protein compartment.

The most common victims of PEM worldwide are children. A child whose weight falls to less than 80% of normal is considered malnourished. When the level falls to 60% of normal weight for sex and age, the child is considered to have *marasmus.* A marasmic child suffers growth retardation and loss of muscle. The loss of muscle mass results from catabolism and depletion of the somatic protein compartment. This seems to be an adaptational response that serves to provide the body with amino acids as a source of energy. Interestingly, the visceral protein compartment, which is presumably more precious and critical for survival, is depleted only marginally, and hence *serum albumin levels are either normal or only slightly reduced.* In addition to muscle proteins, subcutaneous fat is also mobilized and used as a fuel. With such losses of muscle and subcutaneous fat, the *extremities are emaciated;* by comparison, the head appears too large for the body. Anemia and manifestations of multivitamin deficiencies are present, and there is evidence of *immune deficiency,* particularly of T cell–mediated immunity. Hence, concurrent infections are usually present, and they impose an additional stress on an already weakened body.

Kwashiorkor occurs when protein deprivation is relatively greater than the reduction in total calories. This is the most common form seen in African children who have been weaned (often too early, owing to the arrival of another child) and are subsequently fed an exclusively carbohydrate diet. The prevalence of kwashiorkor is also high in impoverished countries of Southeast Asia. Less severe forms may occur worldwide in persons with chronic diarrheal states in which protein is not absorbed or in those with conditions in which chronic protein loss occurs (e.g., protein-losing enteropathies, the nephrotic syndrome, or after extensive burns).

Kwashiorkor is a more severe form of malnutrition than marasmus. Unlike marasmus, marked protein deprivation is associated with severe loss of the visceral protein compart-

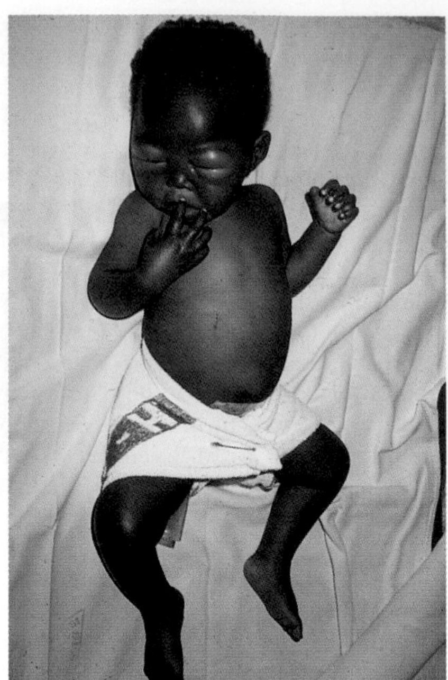

Figure 10–21

Kwashiorkor. The infant shows generalized edema, seen in the form of puffiness of the face, arms, and legs.

ment, and the resultant hypoalbuminemia gives rise to generalized or dependent edema (Fig. 10–21). The weight of children with severe kwashiorkor is typically 60% to 80% of normal. However, the true loss of weight is masked by the increased fluid retention (edema). In further contrast to marasmus, there is relative sparing of subcutaneous fat and muscle mass. The modest loss of these compartments may also be masked by edema. Children with kwashiorkor have characteristic *skin lesions,* with alternating zones of hyperpigmentation, areas of desquamation, and hypopigmentation, giving a "flaky paint" appearance. *Hair changes* include overall loss of color or alternating bands of pale and darker hair, straightening, line texture, and loss of firm attachment to the scalp. Other features that differentiate kwashiorkor from marasmus include an enlarged, *fatty liver* (resulting from reduced synthesis of carrier proteins) and a tendency to develop early apathy, listlessness, and loss of appetite. As in marasmus, other vitamin deficiencies are likely to be present, as are *defects in immunity* and *secondary infections.* The latter add to the catabolic state, thus setting up a vicious circle. Marasmus and kwashiorkor are two ends of a spectrum, and considerable overlap exists.

Secondary PEM is not uncommon in chronically ill or hospitalized patients within the United States. Both marasmus-like and kwashiorkor-like syndromes (with intermediate forms) may develop. Table 10–20 summarizes the secondary forms of these two syndromes.

Secondary PEM is a common complication in advanced cancer patients and in patients with AIDS. The malnutrition in these settings is sometimes called cachexia. Individuals with chronic gastrointestinal disease and elderly patients who are weak and bedridden may show physical signs of protein and energy malnutrition: (1) depletion of subcutaneous fat in the arms, chest wall, shoulders, or metacarpal regions; (2) wasting of the quadriceps femoris and deltoid muscles; and (3) ankle or sacral edema. Bedridden or hospitalized malnourished patients have an increased risk of infection, sepsis, impaired wound healing, and death after surgery.[65] The biochemical mechanisms responsible for secondary PEM in patients with cachexia are complex. In contrast to patients with anorexia nervosa, described next, patients with cachexia show loss of fat as well as muscle mass that may occur before a decrease in appetite. Cachectic patients show increased expenditure of resting energy; in contrast, in chronic starvation, the basal metabolic rate is decreased. Cytokines produced by the host during sepsis, for example, or by tumors have been postulated to be involved in cachexia: TNF-α, interleukin-1, interleukin-6, and interferon-γ. In addition, as discussed in Chapter 8, lipid- and protein-mobilizing factors have been isolated from animals and people with cancer cachexia.[66]

MORPHOLOGY. The central anatomic changes in PEM are (1) growth failure; (2) peripheral edema in kwashiorkor; and (3) loss of body fat and atrophy of muscle, more marked in marasmus.

Table 10–20. COMPARISON OF SEVERE MARASMUS-LIKE AND KWASHIORKOR-LIKE SECONDARY PROTEIN-ENERGY MALNUTRITION

Syndrome	Clinical Setting	Time Course	Clinical Features	Laboratory Findings	Prognosis
Marasmus-like protein-energy malnutrition	Chronic illness (e.g., chronic lung disease, cancer)	Months	History of weight loss Muscle wasting Absent subcutaneous fat	Normal or mildly reduced serum proteins	Variable; depends on underlying disease
Kwashiorkor-like protein-energy malnutrition	Acute, catabolic illness (e.g., severe trauma, burns, sepsis)	Weeks	Normal fat and muscle Edema Easily pluckable hair	Serum albumin <2.8 gm/dl	Poor

Modified from Bennett JC, Plum F (eds): Cecil Textbook of Medicine, 20th ed. Philadelphia, WB Saunders, 1996, p 1156.

The **liver** in kwashiorkor, but not in marasmus, is enlarged and fatty: superimposed cirrhosis is rare.

In kwashiorkor (rarely in marasmus), the **small bowel** shows a decrease in the mitotic index in the crypts of the glands, associated with mucosal atrophy and loss of villi and microvilli. In such cases, concurrent loss of small intestinal enzymes occurs, most often manifested as disaccharidase deficiency. Hence, infants with kwashiorkor initially may not respond well to a full-strength, milk-based diet. With treatment, the mucosal changes are reversible.

The **bone marrow** in both kwashiorkor and marasmus may be hypoplastic, mainly because of decreased numbers of red cell precursors. How much of this derangement is due to a deficiency of protein and folates or to reduced synthesis of transferrin and ceruloplasmin is uncertain. Thus, anemia is usually present, most often hypochromic microcytic anemia, but a concurrent deficiency of folates may lead to a mixed microcytic-macrocytic anemia.

The **brain** in infants who are born to malnourished mothers and who suffer PEM during the first 1 or 2 years of life has been reported by some observers to show cerebral atrophy, a reduced number of neurons, and impaired myelinization of the white matter, but there is no universal agreement on the validity of these findings.

Many **other changes** may be present, including (1) thymic and lymphoid atrophy (more marked in kwashiorkor than in marasmus): (2) anatomic alterations induced by intercurrent infections, particularly with all manner of endemic worms and other parasites; and (3) deficiencies of other required nutrients, such as iodine and vitamins.

ANOREXIA NERVOSA AND BULIMIA

Anorexia nervosa is self-induced starvation, resulting in marked weight loss; bulimia is a condition in which the patient binges on food and then induces vomiting. These eating disorders occur primarily in previously healthy young women who have developed an obsession with attaining thinness.

The clinical findings in anorexia nervosa are generally similar to those in severe PEM. In addition, effects on the endocrine system are prominent. *Amenorrhea,* resulting from decreased secretion of gonadotropin-releasing hormone (and subsequent decreased secretion of luteinizing hormone and follicle-stimulating hormone), is so common that its presence is a diagnostic feature for the disorder. Other common findings, related to decreased thyroid hormone release, include cold intolerance, bradycardia, constipation, and changes in the skin and hair. The skin becomes dry and scaly and may be yellow because of excess carotene in the blood. Body hair may be increased but is usually fine and pale (lanugo). Bone density is decreased, most likely owing to low estrogen levels, which mimic the postmenopausal acceleration of osteoporosis. As expected with severe PEM, anemia, lymphopenia, and hypoalbuminemia may be present. A major complication of anorexia nervosa is an increased susceptibility to cardiac arrhythmia and sudden death, resulting in all likelihood from hypokalemia.

In bulimia, binge eating is the norm. Huge amounts of food, principally carbohydrates, are ingested, only to be followed by induced vomiting. Although menstrual irregularities are common, amenorrhea occurs in less than 50% of bulimia patients, probably because weight and gonadotropin levels are maintained near normal. The major medical complications relate to continual induced vomiting and include (1) electrolyte imbalances (hypokalemia), which predispose the patient to cardiac arrhythmias; (2) pulmonary aspiration of gastric contents; and (3) esophageal and cardiac rupture.

VITAMIN DEFICIENCIES

Thirteen vitamins are necessary for health; four—A, D, E, and K—are fat soluble, and the remainder are water soluble. The distinction between fat- and water-soluble vitamins is important, because although fat-soluble vitamins are more readily stored in the body, they are likely to be poorly absorbed in gastrointestinal disorders of fat malabsorption (Chapter 18). Small amounts of some vitamins can be synthesized endogenously—vitamin D from precursor steroids; vitamin K and biotin by the intestinal microflora; and niacin from tryptophan, an essential amino acid—but the rest must be supplied in the diet. A deficiency of vitamins may be primary (dietary in origin) or secondary (because of disturbances in intestinal absorption, transport in the blood, tissue storage, or metabolic conversion). In the following sections, the major vitamins, together with their well-defined deficiency states, are discussed individually (with the exception of B_{12} and folate, which are discussed in Chapter 14), beginning with the fat-soluble vitamins. However, deficiencies of a single vitamin are uncommon, and the expression of a deficiency of a combination of vitamins may be submerged in concurrent PEM. A summary of all the essential vitamins, along with their functions and deficiency syndromes, is presented in Table 10–21.

Vitamin A. Vitamin A is actually a group of related natural and synthetic chemicals that exert a hormone-like activity or function.[67] The relationship of some important members of this group is presented in Figure 10–22. *Retinol,* perhaps the most important form of vitamin A, is the transport form and, as the retinol ester, also the storage form. It is oxidized in vivo to the aldehyde *retinal* (the form used in visual pigment) and the acid *retinoic acid.* Important dietary sources of vitamin A are animal derived (e.g., liver, fish, eggs, milk, butter). Yellow and leafy green vegetables such as carrots, squash, and spinach supply large amounts of carotenoids, many of which are pro-vitamins that can be metabolized to active vitamin A in vivo; the most important of these is beta-carotene. A widely used term, *retinoids,* refers to both natural and synthetic chemicals that are structurally related to vitamin A but do not necessarily have vitamin A activity.

Table 10–21. VITAMINS: MAJOR FUNCTIONS AND DEFICIENCY SYNDROMES

Vitamin	Functions	Deficiency Syndromes
Fat-Soluble		
Vitamin A	A component of visual pigment Maintenance of specialized epithelia Maintenance of resistance to infection	Night blindness, xerophthalmia, blindness Squamous metaplasia Vulnerability to infection, particularly measles
Vitamin D	Facilitates intestinal absorption of calcium and phosphorus and mineralization of bone	Rickets in children Osteomalacia in adults
Vitamin E	Major antioxidant; scavenges free radicals	Spinocerebellar degeneration
Vitamin K	Cofactor in hepatic carboxylation of procoagulants—factors II (prothrombin), VII, IX, and X; and protein C and protein S	Bleeding diathesis
Water-Soluble		
Vitamin B_1 (thiamine)	As pyrophosphate, is coenzyme in decarboxylation reactions	Dry and wet beriberi, Wernicke syndrome, ?Korsakoff syndrome
Vitamin B_2 (riboflavin)	Converted to coenzymes flavin mononucleotide and flavin adenine dinucleotide, cofactors for many enzymes in intermediary metabolism	Ariboflavinosis, cheilosis, stomatitis, glossitis, dermatitis, corneal vascularization
Niacin	Incorporated into nicotinamide adenine dinucleotide (NAD) and NAD phosphate involved in a variety of redox reactions	Pellagra—three "D's": dementia, dermatitis, diarrhea
Vitamin B_6 (pyridoxine)	Derivatives serve as coenzymes in many intermediary reactions	Cheilosis, glossitis, dermatitis, peripheral neuropathy
Vitamin B_{12}	Requisite for normal folate metabolism and DNA synthesis Maintenance of myelinization of spinal cord tracts	Combined system disease (megaloblastic pernicious anemia and degeneration of posterolateral spinal cord tracts)
Vitamin C	Serves in many oxidation-reduction (redox) reactions and hydroxylation of collagen	Scurvy
Folate	Essential for transfer and use of 1-carbon units in DNA synthesis	Megaloblastic anemia, neural tube defects
Pantothenic acid	Incorporated in coenzyme A	No nonexperimental syndrome recognized
Biotin	Cofactor in carboxylation reactions	No clearly defined clinical syndrome

As with all fats, the digestion and absorption of carotenes and retinoids require bile, pancreatic enzymes, and some level of antioxidant activity in the food. *Retinol,* whether derived from ingested esters or from beta-carotene (through an intermediate oxidation step involving retinal), is transported in chylomicrons to the liver for esterification and storage. More than 90% of the body's vitamin A reserves is stored in the liver, predominantly in the perisinusoidal stellate (Ito) cells. In normal persons who consume an adequate diet, these reserves are sufficient for at least 6 months' deprivation. *Retinoic acid,* on the other hand, can be absorbed unchanged; it represents a small fraction of vitamin A in the blood and is active in epithelial differentiation and growth but not in the maintenance of vision.

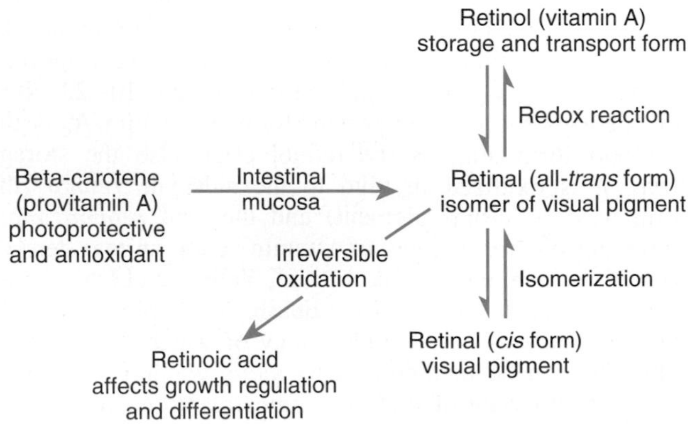

Figure 10–22

Interrelationships of retinoids and their major functions.

When dietary intake of vitamin A is inadequate, the retinol esters in the liver are mobilized, and released retinol is then bound to a specific retinol-binding protein, synthesized in liver. The uptake of retinol by the various cells of the body is dependent on surface receptors specific for retinol-binding protein, rather than receptors specific for the retinol. Retinol is transported across the cell membrane, where it binds to a cellular retinol-binding protein, and the retinol-binding protein is released back into the blood.

Function. In humans, the best-defined functions of vitamin A are as follows:

- Maintaining normal vision in reduced light
- Potentiating the differentiation of specialized epithelial cells, mainly mucus-secreting cells
- Enhancing immunity to infections, particularly in children

In addition, the retinoids, beta-carotene, and some related carotenoids have been shown to function as photoprotective and antioxidant agents.

The *visual process* involves four forms of vitamin A–containing pigments: rhodopsin in the rods, the most light-sensitive pigment and therefore important in reduced light, and three iodopsins in cone cells, each responsive to specific colors in bright light. The synthesis of rhodopsin from retinol involves (1) oxidation to all-*trans*-retinal, (2) isomerization to 11-*cis*-retinal, and (3) interaction with the rod protein opsin to form rhodopsin. When a photon of light impinges on the dark-adapted retina, rhodopsin undergoes a sequence of configurational changes to ultimately yield all-*trans*-retinal and opsin. In the process, a nerve impulse is generated (by changes in membrane potential) that is transmitted by neurons from the retina to the brain. During dark adaptation, some of the all-*trans*-retinal is reconverted to 11-*cis*-retinal, but most is reduced to retinol and lost to the retina, dictating the need for continuous input of retinol.

Vitamin A plays an important role in the orderly *differentiation of mucus-secreting epithelium;* when a deficiency state exists, the epithelium undergoes squamous metaplasia and differentiation to a keratinizing epithelium. The mechanism is not precisely understood; but in cell culture systems, retinoic acid (retinol is much less potent) regulates the gene expression of a number of cell receptors and secreted proteins, including receptors for growth factors.

Vitamin A plays some role in *host resistance to infections.* This beneficial effect of vitamin A seems to derive in part from its ability to stimulate the immune system, possibly through the formation of a recently discovered metabolite called *14-hydroxyretinol.* In addition, it appears that during infections, the bioavailability of vitamin A is reduced. The acute-phase response that accompanies many infections reduces the formation of retinol-binding protein in the liver, resulting in depression of circulating retinol levels, which in turn leads to reduced tissue availability of vitamin A. In keeping with this, supplements of the vitamin during the course of infections such as measles dramatically improves the clinical outcome.

Deficiency State. Vitamin A deficiency occurs worldwide either on the basis of general undernutrition or as a conditioned deficiency among individuals having some cause for malabsorption of fats. One of the earliest manifestations of vitamin A deficiency is impaired vision, particularly in reduced light (night blindness). Because vitamin A and retinoids are involved in maintaining the differentiation of epithelial cells, persistent deficiency gives rise to a series of changes, the most devastating of which occur in the eyes. Collectively, the ocular changes are referred to as *xerophthalmia* (dry eye). First, there is dryness of the conjunctivae (xerosis) as the normal lacrimal and mucus-secreting epithelium is replaced by keratinized epithelium. This is followed by the build-up of keratin debris in small opaque plaques (Bitot spots) and, eventually, erosion of the roughened corneal surface with softening and destruction of the cornea (keratomalacia) and total blindness.

In addition to the ocular epithelium, the epithelium lining the upper respiratory passages and urinary tract is replaced by keratinizing squamous cells (squamous metaplasia). Loss of the mucociliary epithelium of the airways predisposes to secondary pulmonary infections, and desquamation of keratin debris in the urinary tract predisposes to renal and urinary bladder stones. Hyperplasia and hyperkeratinization of the epidermis with plugging of the ducts of the adnexal glands may produce follicular or papular dermatosis. The pathologic effects of vitamin A deficiency are summarized in Figure 10–23.

Another serious consequence of avitaminosis A is immune deficiency. This impairment of immunity leads to higher mortality rates from common infections such as measles, pneumonia, and infectious diarrhea. In parts of the world where vitamin A deficiency is endemic, dietary supplements reduce mortality by 20% to 30%.

Vitamin A Toxicity. Both short- and long-term excess of vitamin A may produce toxic manifestations, a point of some concern because of the megadoses being popularized by certain health food stores. The clinical consequences of acute hypervitaminosis A include headache, vomiting, stupor, and papilledema, symptoms also suggestive of brain tumor. Chronic toxicity is associated with weight loss, nausea, and vomiting; dryness of the mucosa of the lips; bone and joint pain; hyperostosis; and hepatomegaly with parenchymal damage and fibrosis. Although synthetic retinoids used for the treatment of acne are not associated with the complications listed, their use in pregnancy should be avoided owing to a well-established increase in the incidence of congenital malformations (Chapter 11).

Vitamin D. The major function of vitamin D is the *maintenance of normal plasma levels of calcium and phosphorus.* In this capacity, it is required for the prevention of bone diseases (rickets in growing children whose epiphyses have not already closed and osteomalacia in adults) and of hypocalcemic tetany. With respect to tetany, vitamin D maintains the correct concentration of ionized calcium in the extracellular fluid compartment required for normal neural excitation and relaxation of muscle. Insufficient ionized calcium in the extracellular fluid results in continuous excitation of muscle, leading to the convulsive state, hypocalcemic tetany. Our attention here is focused on the function of vitamin D in the regulation of serum calcium levels.

Metabolism of Vitamin D. Humans have two possible sources of vitamin D: endogenous synthesis in the skin, and diet. There are large amounts of the precursor 7-dehydrocholesterol in the skin; ultraviolet light in sunlight converts it to vitamin D_3. Depending on the skin's level of melanin pigmentation, which absorbs ultraviolet light, and the amount of exposure to sunlight, about 80% of the vitamin D needed can be endogenously derived. The remainder must be obtained from dietary sources such as deep-sea fish, plants, and grains. In plant sources, vitamin D is present in its precursor form (ergosterol), which is converted to vitamin D_2 in the body. In many countries, various foods are fortified with vitamin D_2.[68] Since D_3 and D_2 undergo identical metabolic transformations and have

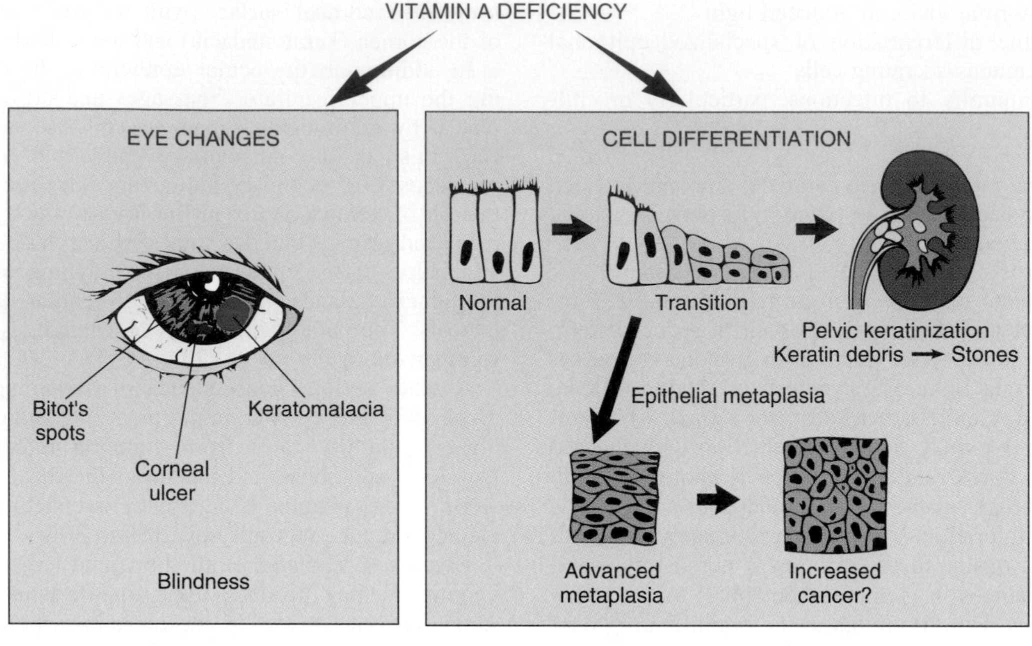

Figure 10–23

Vitamin A deficiency: its major consequences in the eye, in the production of keratinizing metaplasia of specialized epithelial surfaces, and its possible role in potentiating neoplasia.

identical functions, both are hereafter referred to as vitamin D.

The metabolism of vitamin D can be outlined as follows:

1. Absorption of vitamin D in the gut or synthesis from precursors in the skin
2. Binding to a plasma α_1-globulin (D-binding protein) and transport to liver
3. Conversion to 25-hydroxyvitamin D, 25(OH)D, by 25-hydroxylase in the liver
4. Conversion of 25(OH)D to $1,25(OH)_2D$ by α_1-hydroxylase in the kidney; *biologically this is the most active form of vitamin D*

The production of $1,25(OH)_2D$ by the kidney is regulated by three mechanisms:

1. In a feedback loop, increased levels of $1,25(OH)_2D$ down-regulate synthesis of this metabolite by inhibiting the action of α_1-hydroxylase, and decreased levels have the opposite effect.
2. Hypocalcemia stimulates secretion of parathyroid hormone (PTH), which in turn augments the conversion of 25(OH)D to $1,25(OH)_2D$ by activating α_1-hydroxylase.
3. Hypophosphatemia directly activates α_1-hydroxylase and thus increases formation of $1,25(OH)_2D$.

Functions of Vitamin D. $1,25(OH)_2D$, the biologically active form of vitamin D, is best regarded as a steroid hormone. Like other steroid hormones, it acts by binding to a high-affinity receptor that is widely distributed. However, the essential function of vitamin D—the maintenance of normal plasma levels of calcium and phosphorus—involves actions on the intestines, bones, and kidneys. The active form of vitamin D

- Stimulates intestinal absorption of calcium and phosphorus
- Collaborates with PTH in the mobilization of calcium from bone
- Stimulates the PTH-dependent reabsorption of calcium in the distal renal tubules

How $1,25(OH)_2D$ stimulates intestinal absorption of calcium and phosphorus is still somewhat unclear. The weight of evidence favors the view that it binds to epithelial receptors, activating the synthesis of calcium transport proteins. The increased absorption of phosphorus is independent of the effects on calcium transport.

The effects of vitamin D on bone depend on the plasma levels of calcium. On the one hand, with hypocalcemia, $1,25(OH)_2D$ collaborates with PTH in the resorption of calcium and phosphorus from bone to support blood levels. On the other hand, vitamin D is required for normal mineralization of epiphyseal cartilage and osteoid matrix. It is still not clear how the resorptive function is mediated, but direct activation of osteoclasts is ruled out. It is more likely that vitamin D favors differentiation of osteoclasts from their precursors (monocytes). The precise details of mineralization of bone when vitamin D levels are adequate are also uncertain. It is widely believed that the main function of vitamin D is to maintain calcium and phosphorus at supersaturated levels in the plasma. However, vitamin D–mediated increases in the synthesis of the calcium-binding proteins osteocalcin and osteonectin in the osteoid matrix may also play a role.

Equally unclear is the role of vitamin D in renal reabsorption of calcium. PTH is clearly necessary, but it is believed that vitamin D is also. There is no substantial

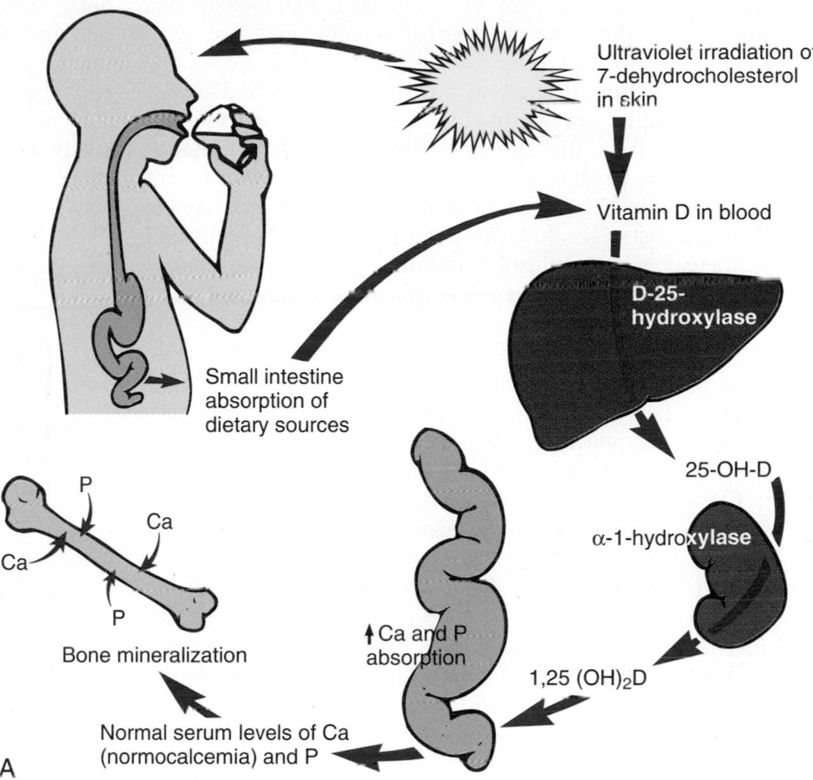

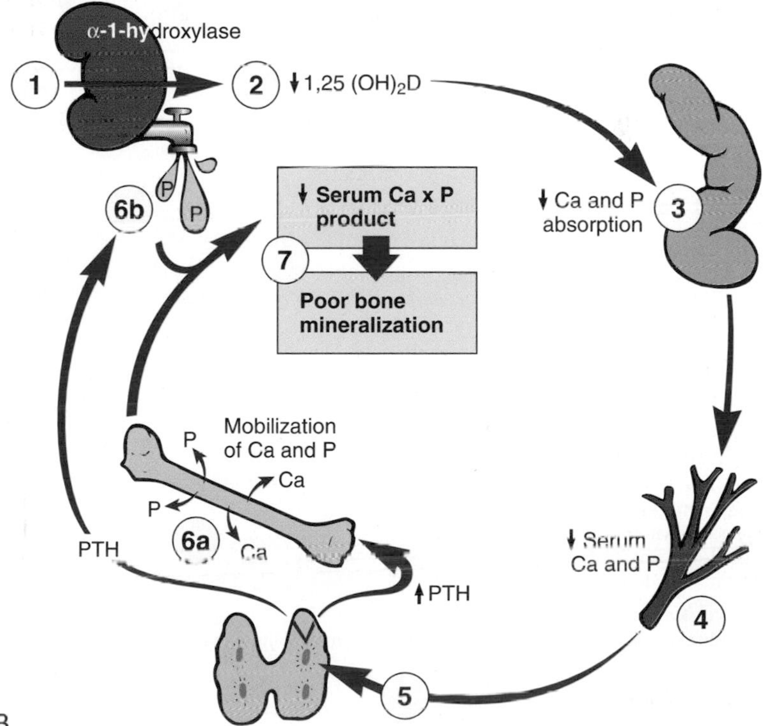

Figure 10–24

A, Schema of normal vitamin D metabolism. *B,* Vitamin D deficiency. There is inadequate substrate for the renal hydroxylase (1), yielding a deficiency of 1,25 $(OH)_2D$ (2), and deficient absorption of calcium and phosphorus from the gut (3), with consequent depressed serum levels of both (4). The hypocalcemia activates the parathyroid glands (5), causing mobilization of calcium and phosphorus from bone (6a). Simultaneously, the parathyroid hormone (PTH) induces wasting of phosphate in the urine (6b) and calcium retention. Consequently, the serum levels of calcium are normal or nearly normal but the phosphate is low; hence, mineralization is impaired (7).

evidence that vitamin D participates in renal reabsorption of phosphorus. An overview of the normal metabolism of vitamin D and the consequences of a deficiency are depicted in Figure 10–24.

Deficiency States. Rickets in growing children and osteomalacia in adults are worldwide skeletal diseases; but in developed countries, they rarely occur as a result of dietary deficiencies. Both forms of skeletal disease may result from deranged vitamin D absorption or metabolism or, less commonly, from disorders that affect the function of vitamin D or disturb calcium or phosphorus homeostasis. A summary of the causes of rickets and osteomalacia is given in Table 10–22.

Whatever the basis, a deficiency of vitamin D tends to cause hypocalcemia. When hypocalcemia occurs, PTH production is increased, which (1) activates renal α_1-hydroxylase, thus increasing the amount of active vitamin D and calcium absorption; (2) mobilizes calcium from bone; (3) decreases renal calcium excretion; and (4) increases renal excretion of phosphate. Thus, the serum level of calcium is restored to nearly normal, but hypophosphatemia persists, and so mineralization of bone is impaired.

An understanding of the morphologic changes in rickets and osteomalacia is facilitated by a brief summary of normal bone development and maintenance. The development of flat bones in the skeleton involves intramembranous ossification, while the formation of long tubular bones reflects endochondral ossification. With intramembranous bone formation, mesenchymal cells differentiate directly into osteoblasts, which synthesize the collagenous osteoid matrix on which calcium is deposited. In contrast, with endochondral ossification, growing cartilage at the epiphyseal plates is provisionally mineralized and then progressively resorbed and replaced by osteoid matrix, which undergoes mineralization to create bone (Fig. 10–25*B*).

Table 10–22. PREDISPOSING CONDITIONS FOR RICKETS OR OSTEOMALACIA

Inadequate Synthesis or Dietary Deficiency of Vitamin D
Inadequate exposure to sunlight
Limited dietary intake of fortified foods
Poor maternal nutrition
Dark skin pigmentation

Decreased Absorption of Fat-Soluble Vitamin D
Cholestatic liver disease
Pancreatic insufficiency
Biliary tract obstruction
Celiac sprue
Extensive small bowel disease

Derangements in Vitamin D Metabolism
Increased degradation of vitamin D and 25(OH)D
  Induction of cytochrome P-450 enzymes (phenytoin, phenobarbital, rifampin)
Impaired synthesis of 25(OH)D
  Diffuse liver disease
Decreased synthesis of 1,25$(OH)_2$D
  Advanced renal disease
  Inherited deficiency of renal α_1-hydroxylase (vitamin D–dependent rickets type I)

End-Organ Resistance to 1,25$(OH)_2$D
Inherited absence of or defective receptors for acute metabolite of vitamin D (vitamin D–dependent rickets type II)

Phosphate Depletion
Poor absorption of phosphate due to chronic use of antacids—binding by aluminum hydroxide
Excess renal tubule excretion of phosphate (X-linked hypophosphatemic rickets)

MORPHOLOGY. The basic derangement in both rickets and osteomalacia is an excess of unmineralized matrix. The changes that occur in the growing bones of children with rickets, however, are complicated by inadequate provisional calcification of epiphyseal cartilage deranging endochondral bone growth. The following sequence ensues in rickets:

- Overgrowth of epiphyseal cartilage due to inadequate provisional calcification and failure of the cartilage cells to mature and disintegrate
- Persistence of distorted, irregular masses of cartilage, many of which project into the marrow cavity (Fig. 10–25*A*)
- Deposition of osteoid matrix on inadequately mineralized cartilaginous remnants
- Disruption of the orderly replacement of cartilage by osteoid matrix, with enlargement and lateral expansion of the osteochondral junction
- Abnormal overgrowth of capillaries and fibroblasts in the disorganized zone because of microfractures and stresses on the inadequately mineralized, weak, poorly formed bone
- Deformation of the skeleton due to the loss of structural rigidity of the developing bones

The conformation of the gross skeletal changes depends on the severity of the rachitic process, its duration, and in particular the stresses to which individual bones are subjected. During the nonambulatory stage of infancy, the head and chest sustain the greatest stresses. The softened occipital bones may become flattened, and the parietal bones can be buckled inward by pressure; with the release of the pressure, elastic recoil snaps the bones back into their original positions **(craniotabes).** An excess of osteoid produces **frontal bossing** and a **squared appearance to the head.** Deformation of the chest results from overgrowth of cartilage or osteoid tissue at the costochondral junction, producing the **"rachitic rosary."** The weakened metaphyseal areas of the ribs are subject to the pull of the respiratory muscles and thus bend inward, creating anterior protrusion of the sternum **(pigeon breast deformity).** The inward pull at the margin of the diaphragm creates **Harrison** groove, girdling the thoracic cavity at the lower margin of the rib cage. The

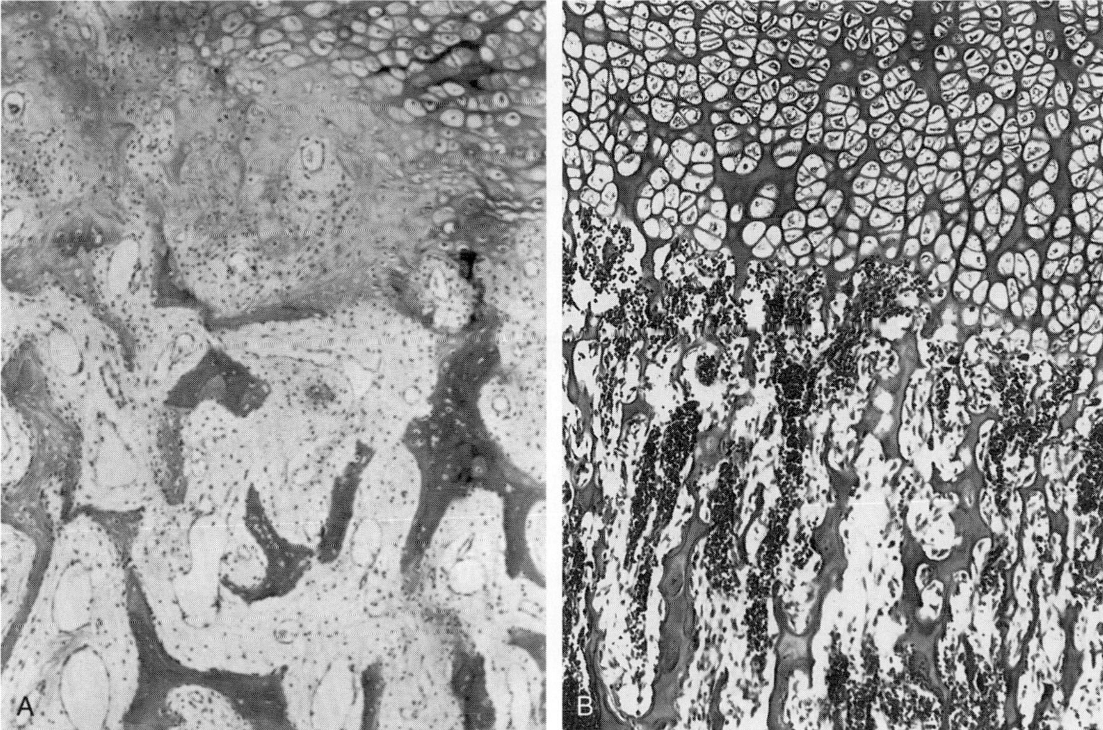

Figure 10–25

A, Detail of a rachitic costochondral junction. The palisade of cartilage is lost. Some of the trabeculae are old, well-formed bone, but the paler ones consist of uncalcified osteoid. *B,* For comparison, normal costochondral function from a young child demonstrates the orderly transition from cartilage to new bone formation.

pelvis may become deformed. When an ambulating child develops rickets, deformities are likely to affect the spine, pelvis, and long bones (e.g., tibia), causing, most notably, **lumbar lordosis** and **bowing of the legs** (Fig. 10–26).

In adults, the lack of vitamin D deranges the normal bone remodeling that occurs throughout life. The newly formed osteoid matrix laid down by osteoblasts is inadequately mineralized, thus producing the excess of persistent osteoid characteristic of **osteomalacia**. Although the contours of the bone are not affected, the bone is weak and vulnerable to gross fractures or microfractures, which are most likely to affect vertebral bodies and femoral necks.

On histologic examination, the unmineralized osteoid can be visualized as a thickened layer of matrix (which stains pink in hematoxylin and eosin preparations) arranged about the more basophilic, normally mineralized trabeculae.

Persistent failure of mineralization in adults leads eventually to loss of skeletal mass, referred to as *osteopenia.* It is then difficult to differentiate osteomalacia from other osteopenias such as osteoporosis (Chapter 28). Osteoporo-

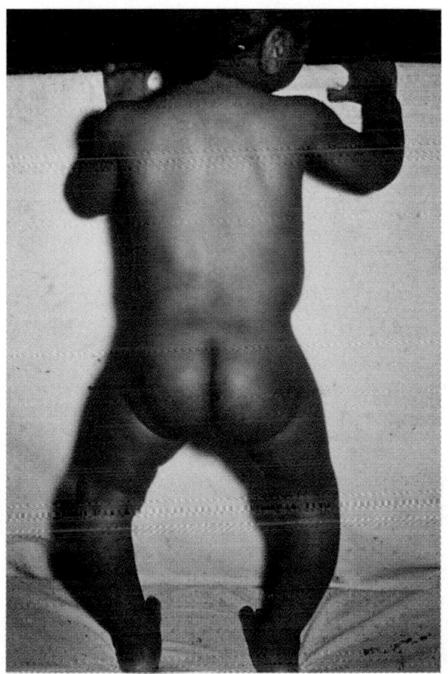

Figure 10–26

Rickets. The bowing of legs in a toddler due to the formation of poorly mineralized bones is evident.

sis, unlike osteomalacia, results from reduced production of osteoid, the protein matrix of the bone. Studies suggest that vitamin D may also be essential for preventing demineralization of bones. In certain familial forms of osteoporosis, the defect has been localized to the vitamin D receptor. It appears that certain genetically determined variants of the vitamin D receptor are associated with an accelerated loss of bone minerals with aging.

Vitamin E. A group of eight closely related fat-soluble compounds—four tocopherols and four tocotrienols—all exhibit vitamin E biologic activity, but α-tocopherol is the most active and the most widely available. Vitamin E is abundant in so many foods—vegetables, grains, nuts and their oils, dairy products, fish, and meat—that a diet sufficient to sustain life is unlikely to be insufficient in vitamin E. The absorption of tocopherols, as of all fat-soluble vitamins, requires normal biliary tract and pancreatic function. After absorption, vitamin E is transported in the blood in the form of chylomicrons, which rapidly equilibrate with the plasma lipoproteins, mainly LDLs. Unlike vitamin A, which is stored predominantly in the liver, vitamin E accumulates throughout the body, mostly in fat depots but also in liver and muscle.

This essential nutrient is one of a group of *antioxidants that serve to scavenge free radicals formed in redox reactions throughout the body*[69] (Chapter 1). It plays a role in termination of free radical–generated lipid peroxidation chain reactions, particularly in cellular and subcellular membranes that are rich in polyunsaturated lipids. This action complements that of selenium, which, as a constituent of glutathione peroxidase, also metabolizes peroxides before they cause membrane damage. For reasons that are not clear, the nervous system is a particular target of vitamin E deficiency. Although the basis for this affinity is not entirely clear, it is speculated that neurons with long axons are particularly vulnerable because of their large membrane surface area. Mature red cells may also be vulnerable to vitamin E deficiency because they are at risk for oxidative injury imposed by the generation of superoxide radicals during oxygenation of hemoglobin.

Hypovitaminosis E resulting from a deficient diet is uncommon in the Western world and occurs almost exclusively in association with (1) fat malabsorption that accompanies cholestasis, cystic fibrosis, and primary small intestinal disease; (2) infant low birth weight with immature liver and gastrointestinal tract; (3) abetalipoproteinemia, a rare autosomal recessive disorder in which transport of vitamin E is abnormal because the apoprotein B component of chylomicrons, LDLs, and very-low-density lipoproteins (VLDLs) is not synthesized; and (4) rare autosomal recessive syndrome of impaired vitamin E metabolism.

MORPHOLOGY. The anatomic changes found in the nervous system depend on the duration and severity of the deficiency state. Most consistent is **degeneration of the axons in the posterior columns of the spinal cord, with focal accumulation of lipopigment and loss of nerve cells in the dorsal root ganglia, attributed to a dying-back type of axonopathy.** Myelin degeneration in sensory axons of peripheral nerves may also be present, and in more marked cases, degenerative changes in the spinocerebellar tracts may occur as well. In occasional cases, features of both primary and denervation muscle disease have been observed in skeletal muscle.

Vitamin E–deficient erythrocytes are more susceptible to oxidative stress and have a shorter half-life in the circulating blood.

The neurologic manifestations of vitamin E deficiency are depressed or, more often, absent tendon reflexes: ataxia; dysarthria; loss of position and vibration sense; and loss of pain sensation. Muscle weakness is also common. In addition, there may be impaired vision and disorders of eye movement, sometimes progressing to total ophthalmoplegia. Anemia is not a feature of the deficiency state in adults but is often found in premature infants and is probably multifactorial in origin.

In closing, attention should be drawn to the ongoing interest in the possible protective effects of vitamin E against atherosclerosis and cancer, the two most common causes of death in the United States. In the case of atherosclerosis, it is suggested that vitamin E may inhibit atheroma formation by reducing the oxidation of LDL (Chapter 12); in the context of cancer, the antioxidant effect is postulated to reduce mutagenesis. However, to date, epidemiologic studies designed to assess the protective role of vitamin E in these two conditions remain inconclusive.[70]

Vitamin K. Vitamin K is a required cofactor for a liver microsomal carboxylase that is necessary to convert glutamyl residues in certain protein precursors to γ-carboxyglutamates.[71] *Clotting factors VII, IX, and X and prothrombin all require carboxylation of glutamate residues for functional activity.* Carboxylation provides calcium-binding sites and thus allows calcium-dependent interaction of these clotting factors with a phospholipid surface involved in the generation of thrombin (Chapter 5). In addition, activation of anticoagulant proteins C and S also requires glutamate carboxylation. In recent years, a diverse group of proteins with no connection to coagulation have also been found to be vitamin K dependent. Such proteins have been found in a wide variety of tissues, including kidney, bone, placenta, and lung. As with the proteins involved in coagulation, vitamin K serves to facilitate carboxylation of glutamyl residues in these other proteins as well. Of particular interest is osteocalcin, a noncollagenous protein secreted by osteoblasts; as with the coagulation proteins, γ-carboxylation of osteocalcin facilitates binding to calcium. Thus, *it appears that vitamin K may favor calcification of bone proteins.* Hence, much interest is focused on delineating the role of vitamin K in bone metabolism.

In the course of the reaction of vitamin K with its substrate proteins, its active (reduced) form is oxidized to an epoxide but then is promptly reduced back by a liver epoxide reductase. Thus, in a healthy liver, vitamin K is efficiently recycled, and the daily dietary requirement is low. Furthermore, endogenous intestinal bacterial flora readily synthesize the vitamin. Nevertheless, there is a small but definite need for exogenous vitamin, which fortunately is widely available in the usual Western diet. Deficiency usually occurs (1) in fat malabsorption syndromes, particularly with biliary tract disease, as with the other fat-soluble vitamins; (2) after destruction of the endogenous vitamin K–synthesizing flora, particularly with ingestion of broad-spectrum antibiotics; (3) in the neonatal period, when liver reserves are small, the bacterial flora is not yet developed, and the level of vitamin K in breast milk is low; and (4) in diffuse liver disease, even in the presence of normal vitamin K stores, because hepatocyte dysfunction interferes with the synthesis of the vitamin K–dependent coagulation factors. In patients with thromboembolic disease, therapeutically desirable vitamin K deficiency is induced by coumarin anticoagulants (e.g., warfarin). These agents block the activity of liver epoxide reductase and thereby prevent regeneration of reduced vitamin K.

The major consequence of vitamin K deficiency (or of inefficient use of vitamin K by the liver) is the development of a *bleeding diathesis.* In neonates, it causes hemorrhagic disease of the newborn. Its most serious manifestation is intracranial hemorrhage, but bleeding may occur at any site, including skin, umbilicus, and viscera. The estimated 3% prevalence of vitamin K–dependent bleeding diathesis among neonates warrants routine prophylactic vitamin K therapy for all newborns. However, in normal full-term infants, by 1 week of age, endogenous flora provide sufficient vitamin K to correct any lingering deficit. In adults suffering from vitamin K deficiency or decreased synthesis of vitamin K–dependent factors, a bleeding diathesis may occur, characterized by *hematomas, hematuria, melena, ecchymoses,* and *bleeding from the gums.*

Thiamine. Thiamine is widely available in the diet, although refined foods such as polished rice, white flour, and white sugar contain little. During absorption from the gut, thiamine undergoes phosphorylation to produce thiamine pyrophosphate, the functionally active coenzyme form of the vitamin. Thiamine pyrophosphate has three major functions: (1) it regulates oxidative decarboxylation of α-keto acids, leading to the synthesis of adenosine triphosphate; (2) it acts as a cofactor for transketolase in the pentose phosphate pathway; and (3) in a little-understood manner, it maintains neural membranes and normal nerve conduction (chiefly of peripheral nerves).

In underdeveloped countries where a large part of the scant diet consists of polished rice, as occurs in many areas of Southeast Asia, thiamine deficiency sometimes develops. In developed countries, clinically evident thiamine deficiency, although uncommon on a strictly dietary basis, *affects as many as one fourth of chronic alcoholics admitted to general hospitals.* A thiamine deficiency state may also result from the pernicious vomiting of pregnancy or from debilitating illnesses that impair the appetite, predispose to vomiting, or cause protracted diarrhea. Because a subclinical deficiency state may be converted to overt disease by extended intravenous glucose therapy or refeeding of chronically malnourished persons (particularly alcoholics), care must be taken that adequate amounts of thiamine are administered concurrently.

The major targets of thiamine deficiency are the peripheral nerves, the heart, and the brain, so persistent thiamine deficiency gives rise to three distinctive syndromes:

- A polyneuropathy (dry beriberi)
- A cardiovascular syndrome (wet beriberi)
- Wernicke-Korsakoff syndrome

Typically, these three syndromes appear in this sequence, but on occasion the deficiency manifests as only one of them. The *polyneuropathy is usually symmetric and takes the form of a nonspecific peripheral neuropathy with myelin degeneration* and disruption of axons involving motor, sensory, and reflex arcs. It usually first appears in the legs, but it may also extend to the arms, so classically these patients present with toedrop, footdrop, and wristdrop. The progressive sensory loss is accompanied by muscle weakness and hyporeflexia or areflexia.

Beriberi heart disease (wet beriberi) is associated with peripheral vasodilation, leading to more rapid arteriovenous shunting of blood, high-output cardiac failure, and eventually peripheral edema. The heart may be normal, have subtle changes, or be markedly enlarged and globular (owing to four-chamber dilation), with pale, flabby myocardium. The dilation thins the ventricular walls. Mural thrombi are often present, particularly in the dilated atria.

In protracted severe deficiency states, most often encountered in chronic alcoholics in the Western world, Wernicke-Korsakoff syndrome may appear. It usually develops against a background of peripheral neuropathy and cardiac insufficiency, but in some instances it is the only manifestation of thiamine deficiency. The details of this syndrome are presented in Chapter 30. Briefly, Wernicke encephalopathy is marked by ophthalmoplegia; nystagmus; ataxia of gait and stance; and derangement of mental function, characterized by global confusion, apathy, listlessness, and disorientation. Korsakoff psychosis takes the form of serious impairment of remote recall (retrograde amnesia), inability to acquire new information, and confabulation. Wernicke encephalopathy and Korsakoff psychosis are not distinct syndromes but rather are successive stages of a single central nervous system disease that have the same pathophysiologic substrate.

The central nervous system lesions affect *the mamillary bodies, the periventricular regions of the thalamus, the floor of the fourth ventricle, and the anterior region of the cerebellum.* There are hemorrhages and degenerative changes in the neurons (Chapter 30). The three major syndromes of thiamine deficiency are summarized in Figure 10–27.

Riboflavin. Riboflavin is a critical component of the coenzymes flavin mononucleotide and flavin adenine dinucleotide, which participate in a wide range of oxidation-reduction reactions. In addition, flavin in covalent linkage is incorporated into succinic dehydrogenase and monoamine oxidase as well as into other mitochondrial enzymes. It is widely distributed in meat, dairy products, and vegetables as free riboflavin or riboflavin phosphate and is absorbed in the upper gastrointestinal tract.

Ariboflavinosis still occurs as a primary deficiency state among persons in economically deprived and developing countries. Under such circumstances, it is frequently ac-

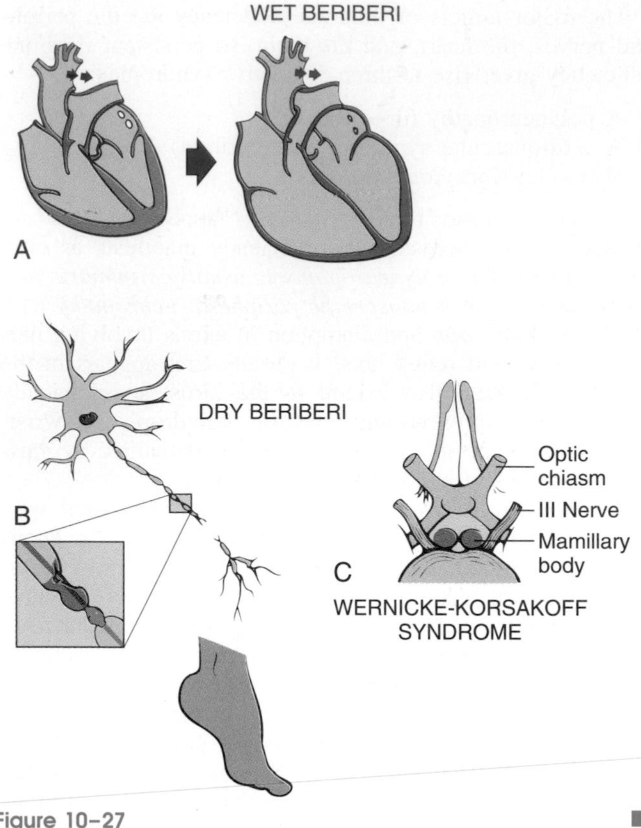

Figure 10–27

A, The flabby, four-chambered, dilated heart of wet beriberi. *B,* The peripheral neuropathy with myelin degeneration leading to footdrop, wristdrop, and sensory changes in dry beriberi. *C,* Hemorrhages into the mamillary bodies in the Wernicke-Korsakoff syndrome.

companied by deficiencies of other vitamins and proteins. In industrialized nations, a deficiency is most likely to be encountered in alcoholics and in persons who have chronic infections, advanced cancer, or other debilitating diseases.

MORPHOLOGY. Ariboflavinosis is associated with changes at the angles of the mouth (known as cheilosis or cheilitis), glossitis, and ocular and skin changes.

Cheilosis is usually the first and most characteristic sign of this deficiency state. It begins as areas of pallor at the angles of the mouth. Later, cracks or fissures may appear, radiating from the corners of the mouth, which tend to become secondarily infected.

With **glossitis,** the **tongue** becomes atrophic, taking on a magenta hue strongly resembling the red-blue coloration of cyanosis.

The **eye change** is a superficial interstitial keratitis. In the earlier stages, the superficial layers of the cornea are invaded by capillaries. Interstitial inflammatory infiltration and exudation follow, producing opacities and sometimes ulcerations of the corneal surface.

A greasy, scaling **dermatitis** over the nasolabial folds may extend into a butterfly distribution to involve the cheeks and skin about the ears. Scrotal and vulvar lesions are common. In well-defined cases, atrophy of the skin may also develop. Erythroid hypoplasia in the **bone marrow** is typically present but is usually not marked.

Niacin. Niacin is the generic designation for nicotinic acid and its functionally active derivatives (e.g., nicotinamide). In the form of nicotinamide, it is an essential component of two coenzymes, nicotinamide adenine dinucleotide (NAD) and nicotinamide adenine dinucleotide phosphate (NADP), both of which play central roles in cellular intermediary metabolism. NAD functions as a coenzyme for a variety of dehydrogenases involved in the metabolism of fat, carbohydrate, and amino acids. NADP participates in a variety of dehydrogenation reactions, particularly in the hexose-monophosphate shunt of glucose metabolism.

Niacin can be derived from the diet or may be synthesized endogenously. It is widely available in grains, legumes, and seed oils and in much smaller quantities in meats. In some grains, it is present in bound form and therefore not absorbable; the niacin in maize (corn), in particular, is bound, so the niacin deficiency syndrome *pellagra* has appeared with unexpected frequency among native populations that subsist largely on maize. Niacin can also be synthesized endogenously from tryptophan. Thus, pellagra may result from either a niacin or a tryptophan deficiency. *In industrialized countries, pellagra is encountered sporadically (usually in combination with other vitamin deficiencies), principally among alcoholics and persons suffering from chronic debilitating illnesses.* It may also occur with protracted diarrheal states, with diets that are grossly deficient in protein, and with long-term administration of drugs such as isoniazid and 6-mercaptopurine.

In pharmacologic doses, nicotinic acid lowers plasma LDL levels by reducing hepatic synthesis of VLDL, and hence it is used in the treatment of hypercholesterolemia.

MORPHOLOGY. The term **pellagra,** strictly speaking, refers to rough skin. The clinical syndrome, however, is classically identified by most clinicians by the "three Ds": dermatitis, diarrhea, and dementia.

Dermatitis is usually bilaterally symmetric and is found mainly on exposed areas of the body. The changes at first comprise redness, thickening, and roughening of the skin, which may be followed by extensive scaling and desquamation, producing fissures and chronic inflammation (Fig. 10–28). Similar lesions may occur in the mucous membranes of the mouth and vagina.

Diarrhea is caused by atrophy of the columnar epithelium of the gastrointestinal tract mucosa,

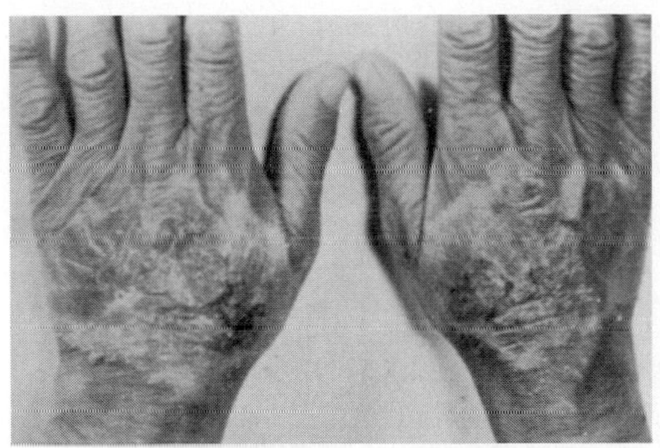

Figure 10–28

The sharply demarcated, characteristic scaling dermatitis of pellagra.

followed by submucosal inflammation. Atrophy may be followed by ulceration.

Dementia results from degeneration of the neurons in the brain, accompanied by degeneration of the corresponding tracts in the spinal cord. The spinal cord lesions bear a close resemblance to the posterior column alterations observed in pernicious anemia.

Pyridoxine (Vitamin B_6). A primary, clinically overt deficiency of vitamin B_6 is rare in humans, but subclinical conditioned deficiency states, paradoxically, are thought to be common. Three naturally occurring substances—pyridoxine, pyridoxal, and pyridoxamine—together with the phosphate forms of each possess vitamin B_6 activity and are generically referred to as *pyridoxine.* All are equally active metabolically, and all are converted in the tissues to the coenzyme form, pyridoxal 5-phosphate. This coenzyme participates as a cofactor for a large number of enzymes involved in transaminations, carboxylations, and deaminations in the metabolism of lipids and amino acids and in the immune response.

Vitamin B_6 is present in virtually all foods; however, food processing may destroy pyridoxine and in the past was responsible for severe deficiency in infants fed poorly controlled dried milk preparations. Secondary hypovitaminosis B_6 is produced most often by long-term use of any of a variety of drugs that act as pyridoxine antagonists. These include isoniazid (used to treat tuberculosis), estrogens, and penicillamine. Alcoholics are also prone to develop vitamin B_6 deficiency because acetaldehyde, an alcohol metabolite, enhances pyridoxine degradation. Pregnancy is associated with increased demand. Thus, pyridoxine supplementation is required in these conditions.

Clinical findings in vitamin B_6–deficient patients resemble those seen in patients with riboflavin and niacin deficiency. Patients may have seborrheic dermatitis, cheilosis, glossitis, peripheral neuropathy, and sometimes convulsions.

Vitamin C (Ascorbic Acid). A deficiency of vitamin C leads to the development of scurvy, characterized principally by bone disease in growing children and hemorrhages and healing defects in both children and adults. Unlike some other vitamins, ascorbic acid cannot be synthesized endogenously, and therefore humans are dependent on intake with food. Ascorbic acid is present in milk and some animal products (liver, fish) and is abundant in a variety of fruits and vegetables. All but the most restricted diets provide adequate amounts of vitamin C.

With the abundance of ascorbic acid in many foods, scurvy has ceased to be a global problem, although it is sometimes encountered even in affluent populations as a conditioned deficiency, particularly among elderly individuals, persons who live alone, and alcoholics—all groups that often have erratic and inadequate eating patterns. Scurvy occasionally appears in patients undergoing peritoneal dialysis and hemodialysis and among food faddists. Tragically, the condition sometimes appears in infants who are maintained on formulas of processed milk without supplementation.

Ascorbic acid functions in a variety of biosynthetic pathways by accelerating hydroxylation and amidation reactions. The most clearly established *function of vitamin C is the activation of prolyl and lysyl hydroxylases from inactive precursors, providing for hydroxylation of procollagen.* Inadequately hydroxylated precursors cannot acquire a stable helical configuration and cannot be adequately cross-linked, so they are poorly secreted from the fibroblast. Those that are secreted lack tensile strength, are more soluble, and are more vulnerable to enzymatic degradation. Collagen, which normally has the highest content of hydroxyproline, is most affected, particularly in blood vessels, accounting for the predisposition to hemorrhages in scurvy. In addition, it appears that a deficiency of vitamin C leads to *suppression of the rate of synthesis of collagen peptides,* independent of an effect on proline hydroxylation.

While the role of vitamin C in collagen synthesis has been known for many decades, it is only in relatively recent years that its antioxidant properties have been recognized. Vitamin C can scavenge free radicals directly in aqueous phases of the cell and can act indirectly by regenerating the antioxidant form of vitamin E. Thus, vitamins E and C act in concert. It is because of these synergistic actions that both of these vitamins have attracted interest as agents that may retard atherosclerosis by reducing the oxidation of LDL (Chapter 12).

MORPHOLOGY. Scurvy in a growing child is far more dramatic than in an adult. **Hemorrhages** constitute one of the most striking features. Because the defect in collagen synthesis results in inadequate support of the walls of capillaries and venules, purpura and ecchymoses often appear in the skin and in the gingival mucosa. Furthermore, the loose attachment of the periosteum to bone, together with the vascular wall defects, leads to extensive **subperiosteal hematomas** and **bleeding into joint spaces** after minimal trauma. Retrobulbar, subarachnoid, and intracerebral hemorrhages may prove fatal.

Skeletal changes may also develop in infants and children. The primary disturbance is in the

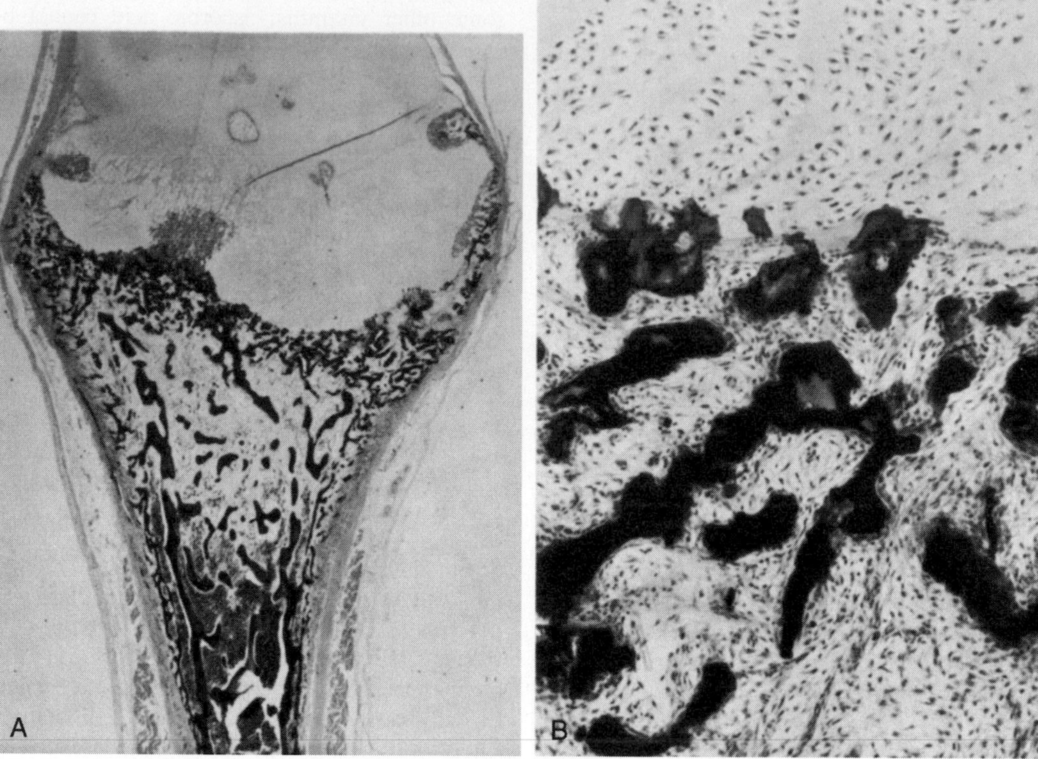

Figure 10–29

A, Longitudinal section of a scorbutic costochondral junction with widening of the epiphyseal cartilage and projection of masses of cartilage into the adjacent bone. *B,* Detail of a scorbutic costochondral junction. The orderly palisade is totally destroyed. There is dense mineralization of the spicules but no evidence of newly formed osteoid.

formation of osteoid matrix, rather than in mineralization or calcification, such as occurs in rickets. In scurvy, the palisade of cartilage cells is formed as usual and is provisionally calcified. However, there is insufficient production of osteoid matrix by osteoblasts. Resorption of the cartilaginous matrix then fails or slows; as a consequence, there is cartilaginous overgrowth, with long spicules and plates projecting into the metaphyseal region of the marrow cavity, and sometimes widening of the epiphysis (Fig. 10–29). The scorbutic bone yields to the stresses of weight bearing and muscle tension, with bowing of the long bones of the lower legs and abnormal depression of the sternum with outward projection of the ends of the ribs. The bone changes in adults are similar to those in children, with decreased formation of osteoid matrix, but deformation does not occur.

In severely scorbutic children and adults, **gingival swelling, hemorrhages,** and **secondary bacterial periodontal infection** are common. A distinctive **perifollicular, hyperkeratotic, papular rash** that may be ringed by hemorrhage often appears. **Wound healing and localization of focal infections are impaired** because of the derangement in collagen synthesis. Anemia is common, resulting from bleeding and from a secondary decrease in iron absorption (Chapter 14). The major features of scurvy are summarized in Figure 10–30.

Folate. Marginal body stores and inadequate dietary intake contribute to folate deficiency throughout the world. Folates are essential cofactors in nucleic acid synthesis; the conversion of 5-methyltetrahydrofolate to tetrahydrofolate requires vitamin B_{12}. Therefore, deficiency of either folate or vitamin B_{12} results in megaloblastic anemia. Rapidly dividing cells in the fetus are especially vulnerable to folate deficiency. The requirement for folate, similar to that of pyridoxine, is increased in pregnancy. Poor diet during the first trimester of pregnancy has been shown to be associated with an increased incidence of neural tube defects in the fetus. Folate supplements have been shown to decrease the risk of neural tube defects.[72]

Folate is found in whole-wheat flour, beans, nuts, liver, and green leafy vegetables. It is heat labile and depleted in cooked and processed foods. In the United States, it is estimated that 15% to 20% of adults have low serum folate. In developing countries that rely on diets based on corn with few fresh vegetables, folate deficiency is more common. Even in those people with adequate diets, oral contraceptives, anticonvulsants, ethanol, and cigarette smoking interfere with folate absorption and metabolism. Chronic diseases such as intestinal malabsorption and metastatic cancer are also associated with folate deficiency.[72]

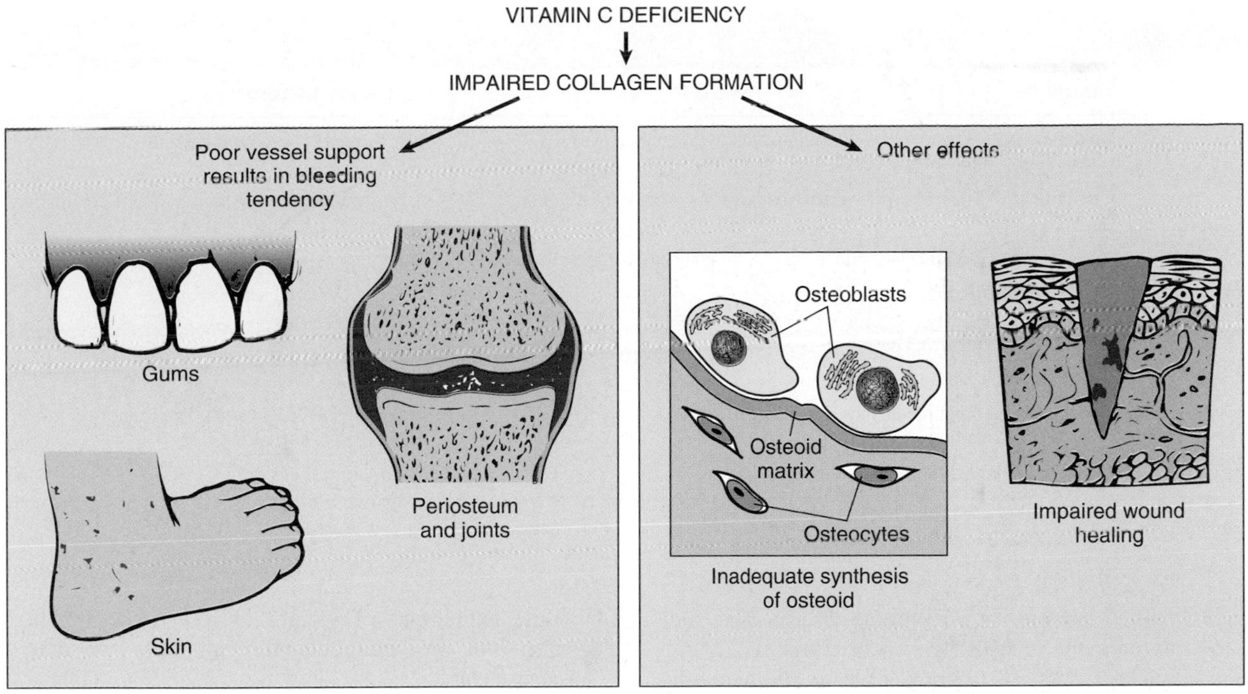

Figure 10–30

The major consequences of vitamin C deficiency.

Combined folate and vitamin B_{12} deficiency has been postulated to contribute to the development of colon cancer. The following mechanisms have been proposed: (1) altered DNA methylation; (2) accumulation of cells in S phase with increased susceptibility in induction of DNA damage; and (3) perturbations of nucleotide pools that impair DNA synthesis and repair.[72]

The consequences of vitamin B_{12} deficiency and pernicious anemia are described in Chapter 14. In contrast to folate deficiency, vitamin B_{12} deficiency is associated with myelin degeneration in both sensory and motor pathways of the spinal cord as described in Chapter 30.

MINERAL DEFICIENCIES

A number of minerals are essential for health. Calcium and phosphorus are required in large amounts and are considered in the discussion of vitamin D. Trace elements are metals that occur at concentrations smaller than 1 μg per gram of wet tissue. *Of the various trace elements found in the body, only five—iron, zinc, copper, selenium, and iodine—have been associated with well-characterized deficiency states.* In theory, a deficiency of a trace element might occur for many of the same reasons as a vitamin deficiency does, but three influences are particularly relevant: (1) inadequate supplementation in preparations used for total parenteral nutrition, (2) interference with absorption by dietary constituents, and (3) inborn errors of metabolism leading to abnormalities of trace metal absorption. Dietary interference as a mechanism was first noted among inhabitants of Egypt and Iran who subsisted largely on unrefined cereals; sufficient phytic acid and fiber were present in the diet to bind and block zinc absorption. Genetic malabsorption syndromes involving a trace element are rare. In one, failure to synthesize metallothionein (a metal-binding protein) in intestinal mucosal cells blocks absorption of both copper and zinc.

Table 10–23 provides brief comments on the role of several trace elements in health and disease. Additional comments are offered only for zinc and selenium deficiency.

Zinc Deficiency. A lack of zinc is unusual because it is reasonably abundant in meats, fish, shellfish, whole-grain cereals, and legumes. Most cases of zinc deficiency have been related to either total parenteral nutrition unsupplemented by zinc or the aforementioned rare genetic syndrome that interferes with absorption.

The essential features of zinc deficiency are (1) a distinctive rash, most often around the eyes, nose, mouth, anus, and distal parts, called *acrodermatitis enteropathica* (Fig. 10–31); (2) anorexia, often accompanied by diarrhea; (3) growth retardation in children; (4) impaired wound healing; (5) hypogonadism with diminished reproductive capacity; (6) altered immune function; (7) impaired night vision related to altered vitamin A metabolism; (8) depressed mental function; and (9) an increased incidence of congenital malformations in infants of zinc-deficient mothers. Zinc deficiency should be suspected in any case of obscure growth retardation or infertility associated with a distinctive rash (acrodermatitis enteropathica). Oral zinc supplementation is promptly curative.

Selenium Deficiency. Selenium, like vitamin E, protects

Table 10–23. FUNCTIONS OF TRACE METALS AND DEFICIENCY SYNDROMES

Nutrient	Functions	Deficiency Syndromes
Iron	Essential component of hemoglobin as well as a number of iron-containing metalloenzymes	Hypochromic microcytic anemia
Zinc	Component of enzymes, principally oxidases	Acrodermatitis enteropathica, growth retardation, infertility
Iodine	Component of thyroid hormone	Goiter and hypothyroidism
Selenium	Component of glutathione peroxidase	Myopathy, rarely cardiomyopathy
Copper	Component of cytochrome c oxidase, dopamine β-hydroxylase, tyrosinase, lysyl oxidase, and unknown enzyme involved in cross-linking keratin	Muscle weakness, neurologic defects, hypopigmentation, abnormal collagen cross-linking
Manganese	Component of metalloenzymes, including oxidoreductases, hydrolases, and lipases	No well-defined deficiency syndrome
Fluoride	Mechanism unknown	Dental caries

against oxidative damage of membrane lipids. The deficiency of this element is well known in China as *Keshan disease,* which presents as a congestive cardiomyopathy, mainly in children and young women. It results from a markedly low level of the metal in soil, water, and food.

Obesity

Obesity is epidemic in the United States. Approximately 25% of the U.S. population older than the age of 20 is clinically obese.[72a] Because it is highly correlated with an increased incidence of several diseases, it is important to define and recognize it, to understand its causes, and to be able to initiate appropriate measures to prevent it or to treat it.

How does one measure fat accumulation? There are several highly technical ways to approximate the measurement, but for practical considerations, the following ones are commonly used:

- Some expression of weight in relation to height, especially the measurement referred to as the *body mass index* (BMI)
- Skinfold measurements
- Various body circumferences, particularly the ratio of the waist to hip circumference

The BMI, expressed in kilograms per square meter, is closely correlated to body fat. A BMI of approximately 25 kg/m^2 is considered normal. It is generally agreed that a 20% excess in body weight (BMI greater than 27 kg/m^2) imparts a health risk. This is illustrated in Figure 10–32. Note that in this figure, a BMI below 20 kg/m^2 is also associated with an increased mortality rate. This may be related to smoking and its attendant risks, because smoking is known to decrease appetite and, subsequently, the BMI.

The untoward effects of obesity are related not only to the total body weight but also to the distribution of the

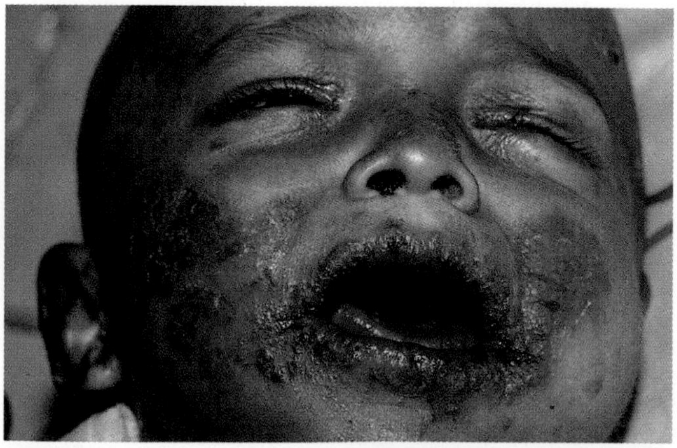

Figure 10–31

Zinc deficiency with hemorrhagic dermatitis around the mouth and eyes.

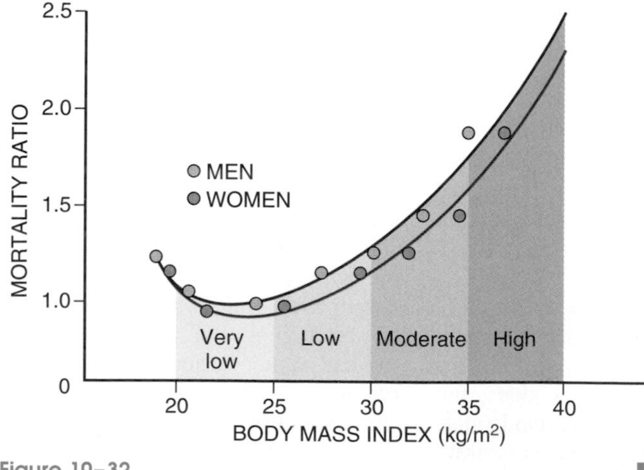

Figure 10–32

Mortality ratios for men and women at different levels of body mass index. (Data from Lew EA, Garfinkel L: Variations in mortality by weight among 750,000 men and women. J Chronic Dis 32:563, 1979.)

stored fat. Central or visceral obesity, in which fat accumulates in the trunk and in the abdominal cavity (in the mesentery and around viscera), is associated with a much higher risk for several diseases than is excess accumulation of fat diffusely in subcutaneous tissue.

The etiology of obesity is complex and incompletely understood. However, simply put, *obesity is a disorder of energy balance. When food-derived energy chronically exceeds energy expenditure, the excess calories are stored as triglycerides in adipose tissue.* The two sides of the energy equation, intake and expenditure, are finely regulated by neural and hormonal mechanisms. In most individuals, when food intake increases, so does the consumption of calories, and vice versa. Hence, body weight is maintained within a narrow range for many years. Apparently, this fine balance is maintained by an internal set-point, or "lipostat," that can sense the quantity of the energy stores (adipose tissue) and appropriately regulate the food intake as well as the energy expenditure. The molecular nature of the lipostat remained obscure for many years, but starting in 1994, a series of breathtaking discoveries changed the picture.

A simplified scheme of the current understanding of neurohumoral mechanisms involved in weight control is illustrated in Figure 10–33 and described here. It is now established that adipocytes communicate with the hypothalamic centers that control appetite and energy expenditure by secreting a polypeptide hormone called leptin.[73] Leptin acts as an antiobesity factor, a notion that is buttressed by the studies of mice with mutations in the leptin gene. Leptin-deficient (*ob/ob*) mice are massively obese; the administration of leptin reduces their food intake and increases energy expenditure, thus tending to ameliorate obesity. Leptin mediates its effects by binding to and activating leptin receptors in the hypothalamus. In experimental animals, triggering of the leptin receptor inhibits appetite and increases energy expenditure, physical activity, and production of heat. Thermogenesis is controlled, at least in part, by leptin receptor–mediated hypothalamic signals that increase the release of norepinephrine from sympathetic nerve endings in the adipose tissue. The fat cells express β_3-adrenergic receptors that, when stimulated by norepinephrine, cause fatty acid hydrolysis and also uncouple energy production from storage. Thus, the fats are literally burned, and the energy so produced is dissipated as heat. There are other catabolic effects mediated by leptin, all transduced by its hypothalamic receptor, which in turn

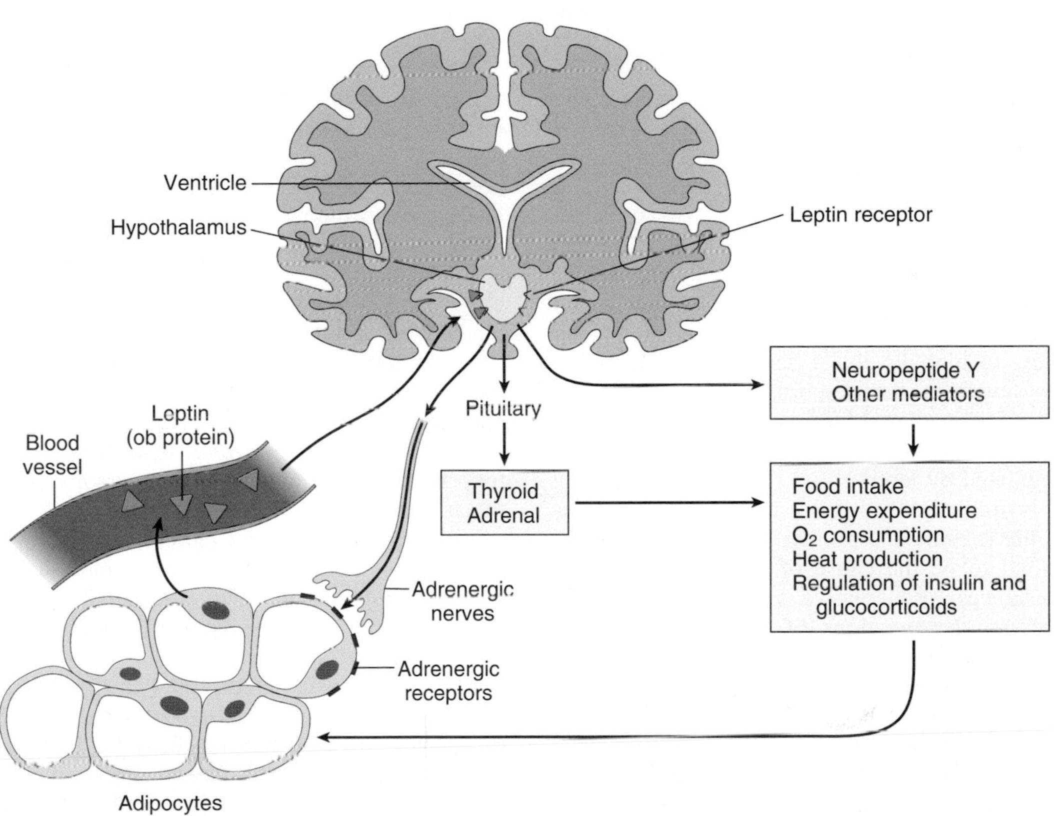

Figure 10–33

The hormonal and neural circuits that regulate body weight. Adipocytes secrete a hormone called leptin (also called *ob* protein) in response to nutritional status (available fat stores) and hormones such as insulin and glucocorticoids. Leptin is transported to the hypothalamus through the circulation, where it binds to the leptin receptor. This interaction regulates energy balance by affecting satiety (food intake) and energy expenditure. Leptin decreases the synthesis and secretion of the appetite stimulant neurotransmitter neuropeptide Y. In addition, through neuronal pathways, the activation of leptin receptor in the hypothalamus increases the release of norepinephrine from sympathetic nerve terminals that innervate adipose tissue. Norepinephrine binds to the β_3-adrenergic receptors on fat cells and leads to increased metabolism of fatty acids and dissipation of the energy as heat. (Modified from Scott J: New chapter for the fat controller. Nature 379:113, 1996. Reprinted with permission from Nature. Copyright 1996 Macmillan Magazines Limited.)

communicates with other endocrine glands through the hypothalamic-pituitary axis. The role of the leptin–leptin receptor system in the regulation of body weight is also supported by the observation that mutant mice lacking leptin receptors are massively obese.[74] Unlike the case with leptin-deficient (*ob/ob*) mice, the obesity in leptin receptor–deficient (*db/db*) mice cannot be corrected by leptin administration. Indeed, leptin levels are markedly elevated in *db/db* mice. In these mice, obesity occurs because the leptin-mediated afferent signals impinging on the hypothalamus fail to regulate appetite and energy expenditure.

Because the uncoupling of the leptin–leptin receptor system can give rise to obesity in mice, much interest is focused on the effectors of leptin action in the hypothalamus. Prominent among the hypothalamic mediators of leptin signaling is neuropeptide Y (NPY). This polypeptide increases appetite and inhibits sympathetic activity and the production of heat, thus favoring weight gain. It is postulated that leptin deficiency causes obesity by increasing the production of NPY, and conversely, signaling through the leptin receptor inhibits the synthesis of NPY. Despite compelling data for a role of NPY as the mediator of leptin action, animals genetically engineered to lack NPY do not have abnormalities in feeding behavior, and leptin is still effective in these NPY knockout mice. Thus, it seems that leptin must have other targets in the hypothalamus,[75] and additional effector pathways that are regulated by leptin have been discovered.

On the basis of these studies in rodents, it is highly likely that dysfunction of the leptin system plays a role in human obesity. However, to date, obesity caused by mutational inactivation of the leptin gene has been found in only few humans.[75a] By contrast, a great majority of obese humans have a high level of plasma leptin, indicating that there is some form of leptin resistance. Such resistance may be at the level of transport of leptin into the central nervous system. That such a defect exists is supported by the fact that despite high levels of serum leptin in obese individuals, the levels in the cerebrospinal fluid are not proportionately increased. In addition to defective transport, there may be abnormalities in hypothalamic pathways that are normally regulated by leptin.

Although it is unlikely that gross mutations that completely disrupt the action of leptin or its downstream targets will be found to be the cause of human obesity (except in rare instances), nonablative variations that cause subtle alterations in the functions of genes in the leptin pathway could well be responsible for obesity. Because the storage of fat in the body is regulated over a long time, even a 5% to 10% difference in the activity of a gene such as leptin could result in obesity during a period of years. Thus, polymorphisms in genes implicated in animal models of obesity are currently being investigated. Before closing this discussion about leptin, it should be mentioned that, in addition to its role in regulating body fat, leptin is also required for initiation of puberty and secondary sexual characteristics.[75a] These effects of leptin are also mediated via the hypothalamic-pituitary axis.

Despite the rarity of well-defined genetic syndromes of obesity in humans, there is little doubt that genetic influences play an important role in weight control. Support comes from a study in which identical twins, reared apart, had a remarkable concordance in the degree of obesity. However, as with all complex traits, obesity is not merely a genetic disease. There are definite environmental factors[72a]; the prevalence of obesity in Asians who immigrate to the United States is much higher than in those who remain in their native land. These changes in all likelihood result from changes in the type and amount of dietary intake. After all, even with bad genes, obesity would not occur without intake of food!

Obesity, particularly *central obesity, increases the risk for a number of conditions,*[76] including diabetes, hypertension, hypertriglyceridemia, low HDL cholesterol (Chapter 12), and possibly coronary artery disease. The mechanisms underlying these associations are complex and likely to be interrelated. Obesity, for instance, is associated with *insulin resistance* and hyperinsulinemia, important features of non–insulin-dependent, or type II, diabetes, and weight loss is associated with improvement (Chapter 20). It has been speculated that excess insulin, in turn, may play a role in the retention of sodium, expansion of blood volume, production of excess norepinephrine, and smooth muscle proliferation that are the hallmarks of hypertension. Regardless of whether these pathogenic mechanisms are actually operative, *the risk of developing hypertension among previously normotensive persons increases proportionately with weight.*

Obese persons are likely to have hypertriglyceridemia and a low HDL cholesterol value, and these factors may increase the risk of *coronary artery disease* in the *very* obese. The association between obesity and heart disease is not straightforward, and such linkage as there may be relates more to the associated diabetes and hypertension than to weight.

Cholelithiasis (gallstones) is six times more common in obese than in lean subjects. The mechanism is mainly an increase in total body cholesterol, increased cholesterol turnover, and augmented biliary excretion of cholesterol in the bile, which in turn predisposes to the formation of cholesterol-rich gallstones (Chapter 19).

Hypoventilation syndrome is a constellation of respiratory abnormalities in very obese persons. It has been called the *pickwickian syndrome,* after the fat lad who was constantly falling asleep in Charles Dickens' *Pickwick Papers.* Hypersomnolence, both at night and during the day, is characteristic and is often associated with apneic pauses during sleep, polycythemia, and eventual right-sided heart failure.

Marked adiposity predisposes to the development of degenerative joint disease (*osteoarthritis*). This form of arthritis, which typically appears in older persons, is attributed in large part to the cumulative effects of wear and tear on joints. It is reasonable to assume that the greater the body burden of fat, the greater the trauma to joints with passage of time.

The relationship between *obesity and stroke* is unclear, and opposing views can be found in the literature. According to some, the true relationship is between stroke and hypertension, not between stroke and obesity (i.e., obese patients who are not hypertensive are not at higher risk for stroke).

Equally controversial is the relationship between *obesity and cancer,* particularly cancers arising in the endometrium and breast. Here the problem is complicated by the role of particular foods, such as animal fats, which may be independently associated with cancer and obesity. Nevertheless, it seems that obese women are at a higher risk of developing endometrial cancer than are lean women in the same age group. This relationship may be indirect; high estrogen levels are associated with increased risk of endometrial cancer (Chapter 24), and obesity is known to raise estrogen levels. With breast cancer, the data are controversial. It seems that in postmenopausal women who live in countries with a moderate or low risk of breast cancer (e.g., Japan), central obesity is associated with an increased risk of breast cancer. Again, the role of sex hormones is a confounding factor.

Diet and Systemic Diseases

The problems of undernutrition and overnutrition, as well as specific nutrient deficiencies, have been discussed; however, the composition of the diet, even in the absence of any of these problems, may make a significant contribution to the causation and progression of a number of diseases. A few examples suffice here.

Currently one of the most important and controversial issues is the contribution of diet to atherogenesis. The central question is, Can dietary modification—specifically, reduction in the consumption of cholesterol and saturated animal fats (e.g., eggs, butter, beef)—reduce serum cholesterol levels and prevent or retard the development of atherosclerosis (most importantly, coronary heart disease)? The average adult in the United States consumes an inordinate amount of fat and cholesterol daily, with a ratio of saturated fatty acids to polyunsaturated fatty acids of about 3:1. Lowering the level of saturates to the level of the polyunsaturates effects a 10% to 15% reduction in serum cholesterol level within a few weeks. Vegetable oils (e.g., corn and safflower oils) and fish oils contain polyunsaturated fatty acids and are good sources of such cholesterol-lowering lipids. Fish oil fatty acids belonging to the omega-3, or n-3, family have more double bonds than do the omega-6, or n-6, fatty acids found in vegetable oils. Substitution of a portion of the saturated fat with a fish oil for a 4-week period has been shown to effect a substantial reduction in serum levels of triglycerides and VLDLs but can result in increased LDL cholesterol levels. A study of Dutch men whose usual daily diet contained 30 gm of fish revealed a substantially lower frequency of death from coronary heart disease than that among comparable control subjects. Thus, although dietary modification can affect heart disease, currently there are insufficient data to suggest that long-term supplementation of food with omega-3 fatty acids is of benefit in reducing coronary artery disease.

There are other examples of the effect of diet on disease:

- Hypertension is beneficially affected by restricting sodium intake.
- Dietary fiber, or roughage, resulting in increased fecal bulk, has a preventive effect against diverticulosis of the colon.
- People who consume diets that contain abundant fresh fruits and vegetables with limited intake of meats and processed foods have a lower risk of myocardial infarction. One mechanism that may explain these epidemiologic observations is the association of hyperhomocysteinemia with increased intake of meats and decreased intake of vitamin B_6, vitamin B_{12}, and folate. Excess levels of homocysteine are hypothesized to contribute to atherosclerosis (Chapter 12).[77]
- Calorie restriction has been convincingly demonstrated to increase life span in experimental animals. The basis of this striking observation is not clear. It seems, however, that in such animals, the age-related decline in immunologic functions is modest, and the animals are more resistant to experimental carcinogenesis.
- Even lowly garlic has been touted to protect against heart disease (and also, alas, kisses), although research has yet to prove this effect unequivocally.

Chemoprevention of Cancer

Epidemiologic studies have provided evidence that populations who consume large quantities of fruits and vegetables in their diets have a lower risk of cancer. It is hypothesized that carotenoids that are converted to vitamin A in the liver and intestine may be important in the primary chemoprevention of cancer.[78] The following mechanisms are proposed for the anticarcinogenic effects of carotenoids and retinoids:

- Retinoic acid promotes differentiation of mucus-secreting epithelial tissues. Supplementation of the diet with beta-carotene and retinol is hypothesized to reverse squamous metaplasia and preneoplastic lesions in the respiratory tract of cigarette smokers and workers exposed to asbestos.[79]
- Fruits and vegetables provide antioxidants such as beta-carotene, vitamins C and E, and selenium that would prevent oxidative damage to DNA.
- Vitamin A can enhance immune responses; other retinoids may modulate inflammatory reactions that are potential sources of reactive oxygen and nitrogen intermediates.[80]

Clinical trials using beta-carotene and retinyl palmitate as primary preventive agents against lung cancer were terminated because the participants showed an excess of lung cancers and increased mortality.[79] On the other hand, 13-*cis* retinoic acid was effective in prevention of secondary squamous cell carcinomas of the head and neck region.[80] These apparently conflicting results are not easily explained; however, there are multiple chemical forms of retinoids that alter gene expression, cell proliferation, differentiation, and apoptosis by binding to six different nuclear receptors. Some retinoids are associated with significant toxicity, including dry skin, conjunctivitis, and hypertriglyceridemia. Until the biochemical and molecular mechanisms of action of individual retinoids and other antioxidants are understood, it is unwise to recommend dietary supplements for the primary chemoprevention of cancer. However, a diet rich in fruits, vegetables, and unprocessed grains that is low in fat and animal protein has been associated with a decreased risk of cardiovascular disease and some types of cancer.[78]

High animal fat intake combined with low fiber intake has been implicated in the causation of colon cancer. The most convincing explanation of these associations is as follows: high fat intake increases the level of bile acids in the gut, which in turn modifies intestinal flora, favoring the growth of microaerophilic bacteria. The bile acids or bile acid metabolites produced by these bacteria might serve as carcinogens or promoters. The protective effect of a high-fiber diet might relate to (1) increased stool bulk and decreased transit time, which decrease the exposure of mucosa to putative offenders, and (2) the capacity of certain fibers to bind carcinogens and thereby protect the mucosa. Attempts to document these theories in clinical and experimental studies have, on the whole, led to contradictory results.

Thus, we must conclude that despite many tantalizing trends and proclamations by "diet gurus," to date there is no definite proof that diet can cause or protect against cancer. Nonetheless, concern persists that carcinogens lurk in things as pleasurable as a juicy steak and rich ice cream.

REFERENCES

1. Newman LS: Occupational illness. N Engl J Med 333:1128, 1995.
2. Leigh JP, et al: Occupational injury and illness in the United States. Estimates of costs, morbidity, and mortality. Arch Intern Med 157:1557, 1997.
3. Mitchell FL: Hazardous waste. In Rom WN (ed): Environmental and Occupational Medicine, 2nd ed. Boston, Little, Brown, 1992, p 1275.
4. Bresnitz EA, et al: Hazard and risk communication and public policy. In Harber PH, et al (eds): Occupational and Environmental Respiratory Disease. St. Louis, Mosby, 1996, p 938.
5. Hodgson E: Introduction to toxicology. In Hodgson E, Levi PE (eds): A Textbook of Modern Toxicology. Stamford, CT, Appleton & Lange, 1997, p 1.
6. Rhomberg L: Risk assessment and the use of information on underlying biologic mechanisms: a perspective. Mutat Res 365:175, 1996.
7. Hodgson E, Levi PE: Absorption and distribution of toxicants. In Hodgson E, Levi PE (eds): A Textbook of Modern Toxicology. Stamford, CT, Appleton & Lange, 1997, p 27.
8. Guengerich FP: Catalytic selectivity of human cytochrome P450 enzymes: relevance to drug metabolism and toxicity. Toxicol Lett 70:133, 1994.
9. Perera FP: Environment and cancer: who are susceptible? Science 278:1068, 1997.
9a. Nierenberg DW, et al: Delayed cerebellar disease and death after accidental exposure to dimethylmercury. N Engl J Med 338:1672, 1998.
10. Szczesny LB, Holbrook JH: Cigarette smoking. In Rom WH (ed): Environmental and Occupational Medicine, 2nd ed. Boston, Little, Brown, 1992, p 1211.
11. Wistuba II, et al: Molecular damage in the bronchial epithelium of current and former smokers. J Natl Cancer Inst 89:1366, 1997.
12. Hanrahan JP, Weiss ST: Environmental tobacco smoke. In Harber PH, et al (eds): Occupational and Environmental Respiratory Disease. St. Louis, Mosby, 1996, p 767.
13. Lieber CS: Medical disorders of alcoholism. N Engl J Med 333:1058, 1995.
14. Lewis DD, Woods SE: Fetal alcohol syndrome. Am Fam Physician 50:1025, 1994.
15. Shibley IA Jr, Pennington SN: Metabolic and mitotic changes associated with the fetal alcohol syndrome. Alcohol Alcohol 32:423, 1997.
16. Harris EL: Association of oral cancers with alcohol consumption: exploring mechanisms. J Natl Cancer Inst 89:1656, 1997.
17. Gawin FH, Ellinwood EH Jr: Cocaine and other stimulants: actions, abuse, and treatment. N Engl J Med 318:1173, 1988.
18. Isner JM, et al: Acute cardiac events temporally related to cocaine abuse. N Engl J Med 315:1438, 1986.
19. Fox BS, et al: Efficacy of a therapeutic cocaine vaccine in rodent models. Nat Med 2:1129, 1996.
20. Rubinstein M, et al: Mice lacking dopamine D_4 receptors are supersensitive to ethanol, cocaine, and methamphetamine. Cell 90:991, 1997.
21. Nestler EJ, Aghajanian GK: Molecular and cellular basis of addiction. Science 278:58, 1997.
22. Lupulescu A: Estrogen use and cancer incidence: a review. Cancer Invest 13:287, 1995.
23. Samsioe G: Coagulation and anticoagulation effects of contraceptive steroids. Am J Obstet Gynecol 170:1523, 1994.
24. Bagshaw S: The combined oral contraceptive risks and adverse effects in perspective. Drug Safety 12:91, 1995.
25. Lewis MA, et al: Third generation oral contraceptives and risk of myocardial infarction: an international case-control study. BMJ 312:88, 1996.
26. Weiss N: Third generation oral contraceptives: how risky? Lancet 346:1570, 1995.
27. Bascom R, et al: Health effects of outdoor air pollution. Am J Respir Crit Care Med 153:3, 477, 1996.
28. Oberdorster G, et al: Association of particulate air pollution and acute mortality: involvement of ultrafine particles? Inhalation Toxicol 7:111, 1995.
29. Lambert WE, Samet JM: Indoor air pollution. In Harber P, et al (eds): Occupational and Environmental Respiratory Disease. St. Louis, Mosby, 1996, p 784.
30. Morgan KT: A brief review of formaldehyde carcinogenesis in relation to rat nasal pathology and human health risk assessment. Toxicol Pathol 25:291, 1997.
31. Samet JM: Indoor radon exposure and lung cancer: risky or not?—all over again. J Natl Cancer Inst 89:4, 1997.
32. Asbestos in Public and Commercial Buildings: A Literature Review and Synthesis of Current Knowledge. Cambridge, MA, Health Effects Institute–Asbestos Research, 1991, pp 1–10.
33. Fayerweather WE, et al: Quantitative risk assessment for a glass fiber insulation product. Regul Toxicol Pharmacol 267:103, 1997.
34. Menzies D, Bourbeau J: Building-related illnesses. N Engl J Med 337:1524, 1997.
35. Corn JK: History of occupational and environmental respiratory disease. In Harber P, et al (eds): Occupational and Environmental Respiratory Disease. St. Louis, Mosby, 1996, p 2.
36. Mastrangelo G, et al: Polycyclic aromatic hydrocarbons and cancer in man. Environ Health Perspect 104:1166, 1996.
37. Fischbein A: Occupational and environmental lead exposure. In Rom WN (ed): Environmental and Occupational Medicine, 2nd ed. Boston, Little, Brown, 1992, p 735.
38. Goyer RA: Results of lead research: prenatal exposure and neurological consequences. Environ Health Perspect 104:1050, 1996.
39. Loghman-Adham M: Renal effects of environmental and occupational lead exposure. Environ Health Perspect 105:928, 1997.
40. Costa M, et al: Molecular mechanisms of nickel carcinogenesis. Environ Health Perspect 102(Suppl 3):127, 1994.
41. Wolff MS, et al: Breast cancer and environmental risk factors: epidemiology and experimental findings. Annu Rev Pharmacol Toxicol 36:573, 1996.
42. Hunter DJ, et al: Plasma organochlorine levels and the risk of breast cancer. N Engl J Med 337:1253, 1997.
43. Peterson RE, et al: Environmental endocrine disruptors. In Boekelheide K, et al (eds): Reproductive and Endocrine Toxicology, Vol 10. New York, Elsevier Science, 1977, p 181.
44. Ashby J, et al: The challenge posed by endocrine-disrupting chemicals. Environ Health Perspect 105:164, 1997.
45. Huff J, et al: Carcinogenicity of TCDD: Experimental, mechanistic, and epidemiologic evidence. Annu Rev Pharmacol Toxicol 34:343, 1994.
46. Upton AC: Ionizing radiation. In Craighead JE (ed): Pathology of Environmental and Occupational Disease. St. Louis, Mosby, 1996, p 205.

47. Narayanan PK, et al: α Particles initiate biological production of superoxide anions and hydrogen peroxide in human cells. Cancer Res 57:3963, 1997.
48. Janssen YMW, et al: Cell and tissue responses to oxidative damage. Lab Invest 69:261, 1993.
49. Smith ML, Fornace AJ Jr: Mammalian DNA damage-inducible genes associated with growth arrest and apoptosis. Mutat Res 340:109, 1996.
50. Ehrhart EJ, et al: Latent transforming growth factor $\beta 1$ activation in situ: quantitative and functional evidence after low dose γ-irradiation. FASEB J 11:1991, 1997.
51. Büttner C, et al: Local production of interleukin-4 during radiation-induced pneumonitis and pulmonary fibrosis in rats: macrophages as a prominent source of interleukin-4. Am J Respir Cell Mol Biol 17:315, 1997.
52. Murnane JP: Role of induced genetic instability in the mutagenic effects of chemicals and radiation. Mutat Res 367:11, 1996.
53. Smith MA, et al: The secondary leukemias: challenges and research directions. J Natl Cancer Inst 88:407, 1996.
54. Greenblatt MS, et al: Mutations in the *p53* tumor suppressor gene: clues to cancer etiology and molecular pathogenesis. Cancer Res 54: 4855, 1994.
55. Rosen CF: Ultraviolet radiation. In Craighead JE (ed): Pathology of Environmental and Occupational Disease. St. Louis, Mosby, 1996, p 193.
56. Fisher GJ, et al: Pathophysiology of premature skin aging induced by ultraviolet light. N Engl J Med 337:1419, 1997.
57. Tommasi S, et al: Sunlight induces pyrimidine dimers preferentially at 5-methylcytosine bases. Cancer Res 57:4727, 1997.
58. Smith ML, Fornance AJ Jr: p53-mediated protective responses to UV irradiation. Proc Natl Acad Sci USA 94:12255, 1997.
59. Eller MS, et al: Enhancement of DNA repair in human skin cells by thymidine dinucleotides: evidence for a p53-mediated mammalian SOS response. Proc Natl Acad Sci USA 94:12627, 1997.
60. Cleary SF: Electromagnetic energy. In Craighead JE (ed): Pathology of Environmental and Occupational Disease. St. Louis, Mosby, 1996, p 215.
61. Linet MS, et al: Residential exposure to magnetic fields and acute lymphoblastic leukemia in children. N Engl J Med 337:1, 1997.
62. Valberg PA, et al: Can low-level 50/60 Hz electric and magnetic fields cause biological effects? Radiat Res 148:2, 1997.
63. Rivara FP, et al: Injury prevention. N Engl J Med 337:543, 613, 1997.
64. Rodricks JV, Jackson BA: Food constituents and contaminants. In Lippmann M (ed): Environmental Toxicants: Human Exposures and Their Health Effects. New York, Van Nostrand Reinhold, 1992, p 266.
65. Detsky AL, et al: Is this patient malnourished? JAMA 271:54, 1994.
66. Tisdale MJ: Biology of cachexia. J Natl Cancer Inst 89:1763, 1997.
67. Bates CJ: Vitamin A. Lancet 345:31, 1995.
68. Fraser DR: Vitamin D. Lancet 345:104, 1995.
69. Meydani M: Vitamin E. Lancet 345:170, 1995.
70. Greenberg ER, Sporn MB: Antioxidant vitamins, cancer, and cardiovascular disease. N Engl J Med 334:1189, 1998.
71. Shearer MJ: Vitamin K. Lancet 345:229, 1995.
72. Branda RF: Folic acid deficiency. In Craighead JM (ed): Pathology of Environmental and Occupational Disease. St. Louis, Mosby, 1996, p 170.
72a. Hill JO, Peters JC: Environmental contributions to the obesity epidemic. Science 280:1371, 1998.
73. Hirsch J, Leibel RL: The genetics of obesity. Hosp Pract 33:55, 1998.
74. Leibel RL, et al: The molecular genetics of rodent single gene obesities. J Biol Chem 272:31937, 1997.
75. Flier JS, Maratos-Flier E: Obesity and hypothalamus: novel peptides, new pathways. Cell 92:437, 1998.
75a. O'Rahilly S: Life without leptin. Nature 392:330, 1998.
76. Jung RT: Obesity as a disease. Br Med Bull 53:307, 1997.
77. McCully KS: Homocysteine and vascular disease. Nat Med 2:386, 1996.
78. Hong WK, Sporn MB: Recent advances in chemoprevention of cancer. Science 278:1073, 1997.
79. Omenn GS, et al: Risk factors for lung cancer and for intervention effects in CARET, the beta-carotene and retinol efficacy trial. J Natl Cancer Inst 88:1550, 1996.
80. Khuri FR, et al: Molecular epidemiology and retinoid chemoprevention of head and neck cancer. J Natl Cancer Inst 89:199, 1997.

Diseases of Infancy and Childhood

Deborah Schofield and Ramzi S. Cotran

BIRTH WEIGHT AND GESTATIONAL AGE
INTRAUTERINE GROWTH RETARDATION
IMMATURITY OF ORGAN SYSTEMS
Lungs
Kidneys
Brain
Liver
APGAR SCORE
BIRTH INJURIES
CONGENITAL MALFORMATIONS
DEFINITIONS
CAUSES OF MALFORMATIONS
Genetic Causes
Environmental Causes
Multifactorial Causes
MECHANISMS OF MALFORMATIONS
PERINATAL INFECTIONS
TRANSCERVICAL (ASCENDING) INFECTIONS
TRANSPLACENTAL (HEMATOLOGIC) INFECTIONS
ONSET OF SEPSIS
NEONATAL RESPIRATORY DISTRESS SYNDROME (RDS)
ERYTHROBLASTOSIS FETALIS—HEMOLYTIC DISEASE OF THE NEWBORN
INBORN ERRORS OF METABOLISM AND OTHER GENETIC DISORDERS
PHENYLKETONURIA
GALACTOSEMIA
CYSTIC FIBROSIS (MUCOVISCIDOSIS)
SUDDEN INFANT DEATH SYNDROME
TUMORS AND TUMOR-LIKE LESIONS OF INFANCY AND CHILDHOOD
BENIGN TUMORS AND TUMOR-LIKE LESIONS
MALIGNANT TUMORS
Incidence and Types
Neuroblastoma and Ganglioneuroma
Wilms' Tumor

Children are not merely little adults, and the diseases they get are not merely variants of adult diseases. Many childhood conditions are unique to, or at least take distinctive forms in, this stage of life and so are discussed separately in this chapter. Diseases originating in the perinatal period are important in that they account for significant morbidity and mortality in the United States. As would be expected, the chances for survival of live-born infants improves with each passing week. The mortality rate in the first week of life is more than 10 times greater than in the second week. This striking differential represents, at least in part, a triumph of improved medical care. Better prenatal care, more effective methods of monitoring the condition of the fetus, and judicious resort to cesarean section before term when there is evidence of fetal distress all contribute to bringing onto this "mortal coil" live-born infants who in past years might have been stillborn. These infants represent an increased number of *high-risk* infants. Nonetheless, the infant mortality rate in the United States has shown a decline from a level of 20.0 deaths per 1000 population in 1970 to about 7.5 in 1995.[1] Although the death rate has continued to decline for all infants, American blacks continue to have more than twice (14.9 deaths per 1000) that of American whites (6.3 deaths per 1000). In addition, the infant mortality rate of the United States ranks 21st among industrialized countries. Variations on the reporting of events among countries, however, may account for much of the differences. For example, birth weight–specific mortality rates are as low in the United States as in any other country in the world.

Each stage of development of the infant and child is prey to a somewhat different group of disorders. The data available permit a survey of four time spans: (1) the neonatal period (the first 4 weeks of life), (2) infancy (the first year of life), (3) 1 to 4 years of age, and (4) 5 to 14 years of age. The single most hazardous period of life is unquestionably the neonatal period. Never again is the individual confronted with more dramatic challenges than in the transition from dependent, intrauterine existence to independent, postnatal life. From the moment the umbilical cord is severed, the circulation through the heart and lungs is radically rerouted. Respiratory function must take over the role of oxygenation of the blood. Maintenance of body temperature and other homeostatic constants must now be borne alone by the fledgling organism. All these adaptations render the neonate particularly vulnerable. The number of deaths within the first year of life is almost twice as great as the number of deaths occurring in children ages 1 to 14 years.

The major causes of death in infancy and childhood are cited in Table 11–1. Congenital anomalies, disorders relating to short gestation and low birth weight, and sudden infant death syndrome (SIDS) represent the leading causes of death in the first 12 months of life. Once the infant survives the first year of life, the outlook brightens measurably. In the next two age groups—1 to 4 years and 5 to 14 years—injuries resulting from accidents have become the leading cause of death (Table 11–1). Among the natural diseases, in order of importance, congenital anomalies and malignant neoplasms assume major significance. It would appear then that, in a sense, life is an obstacle course. For the great majority, the obstacles are surmounted or, even better, bypassed. We now take a closer look at the specific conditions encountered during the various stages of infant and child development.

Table 11–1. CAUSES OF DEATH AND AGE

Causes*	Rate†
Under 1 Year: All Causes	752.4
Perinatal conditions	
Disorders related to short gestation and unspecified low birth weight	
Respiratory distress syndrome	
Conditions related to maternal complications of pregnancy	
Conditions related to complications of placenta, cord, and membranes	
Intrauterine hypoxia and birth asphyxia	
Congenital anomalies	
Sudden infant death syndrome	
Infections and pneumonia	
Accidents and adverse effects	
1–4 Years: All Causes	40.4
Accidents and adverse effects	
Congenital anomalies	
Malignant neoplasms	
Homicide and legal intervention	
Diseases of the heart‡	
5–14 Years: All Causes	22.1
Accidents and adverse effects	
Malignant neoplasms	
Homicide and legal intervention	
Congenital anomalies	
Suicide	
15–24 Years: All Causes	98.5
Accidents and adverse effects	
Homicide	
Suicide	
Malignant neoplasms	
Diseases of the heart	

*Causes are listed in decreasing order of frequency. Causes and rates for infants and children up to 14 years of age are preliminary 1995 statistics.[1] Causes and rates for children aged 15 to 24 years are sex-averaged, provisional 1994 statistics (Singh GK, et al: Annual summary of births, marriages, divorces, and deaths: United States, 1994. Monthly Vital Statistics Report 43:26, 1995).

†Rates are expressed per 100,000 population.

‡Excludes congenital heart disease.

BIRTH WEIGHT AND GESTATIONAL AGE

Infants born before completion of the normal gestation period have higher morbidity and mortality rates than full-term infants. The vital organs of preterm infants are immature and therefore unable to adapt readily to early extrauterine existence. Infants who have failed to complete normal intrauterine growth weigh less than full-term infants, and in the past, premature infants were defined as those having a birth weight of less than 2500 gm. It is inaccurate, however, to define prematurity by birth weight alone because weight is only one of several measures of intrauterine growth. For example, an infant weighing 2300 gm and born at 34 weeks of gestation is likely to be physiologically immature and therefore at greater risk for suffering the consequences of organ system immaturity (e.g., respiratory distress syndrome [RDS] or transient hyperbilirubinemia) than a full-term infant also weighing 2300 gm but with corresponding functional maturity of most organ systems. Therefore, a system of classification that takes into account both gestational age and birth weight has been adopted. Infants are classified as being

- *Appropriate for gestational age (AGA)*
- *Small for gestational age (SGA)*
- *Large for gestational age (LGA)*

Infants whose birth weight falls between the 10th and the 90th percentiles for a given gestational age are considered AGA, whereas those who fall above or below these norms are classified as LGA or SGA. With respect to gestational age, infants born before 37 or 38 weeks are considered *preterm*, whereas those delivered after the 42nd week are considered *post-term.* The usefulness of this classification system is illustrated in Figure 11–1, which graphically depicts the correlation among gestational age, birth weight, and risk of perinatal mortality. For example, an AGA 1500-gm infant born at 32 weeks of gestation has a mortality risk of up to 20%, whereas an SGA, 700-gm

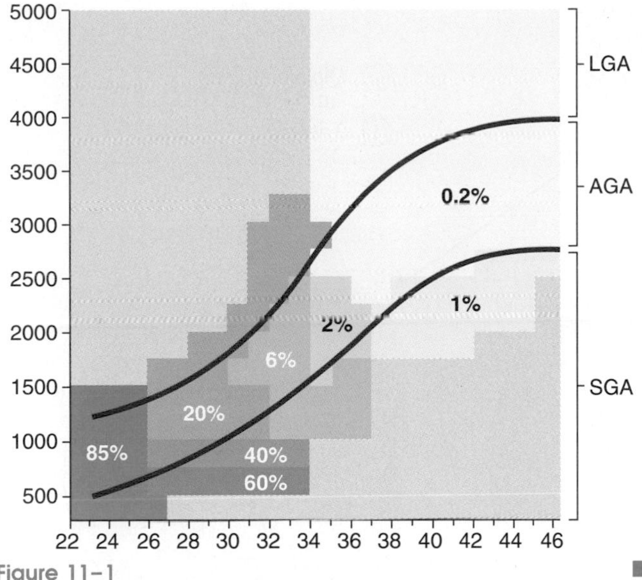

Figure 11-1

Neonatal mortality risk based on actual data from 14,413 live births at the University of Colorado Health Sciences Center from 1974 to 1980. Differentially shaded areas correspond to different mortality risks. For example, an infant born at 36 weeks of gestation and weighing 1250 gm has a mortality risk of 6%. If the same infant weighs 3000 gm, the risk of mortality falls to 0.2%. (Redrawn from Koops B, et al: Neonatal mortality risk in relation to birth weight and gestational age: update. J Pediatr 101: 969, 1982.)

infant born at a similar gestational age has a mortality risk of about 60%. The variation in mortality (and morbidity) rates seen in these different birth weight/gestational age groups is a reflection of the different and distinctive diseases with which these infants are afflicted. We briefly discuss the group of infants that are SGA because prematurity and low birth weight are factors accounting for a significant proportion of perinatal mortality.

Intrauterine Growth Retardation

It is generally accepted that at least one third of infants who weigh less than 2500 gm are born at term and that they are therefore undergrown rather than immature. Hence, intrauterine growth retardation (IUGR) commonly underlies SGA. Significant IUGR (usually asymmetric) is occasionally present in an infant whose weight falls above the 5th to 10th percentile for age. IUGR can be detected before delivery by ultrasonographic measurement of various fetal parameters, such as biparietal diameter, head circumference, abdominal circumference, femur length (as an indicator of fetal length), head-to-abdominal circumference ratio, femur length-to-abdominal circumference ratio, and total intrauterine volume. Although in a significant percentage of infants with IUGR the cause is unknown, those factors known to result in IUGR can be divided into three main groups: fetal, placental, and maternal.

- *Fetal*: Fetal factors are those that intrinsically reduce growth potential of the fetus despite an adequate supply of nutrients from the mother. Prominent among such fetal conditions are *chromosomal disorders*, *congenital anomalies*, and *congenital infections*.[2] Chromosomal abnormalities may be detected in up to 17% of fetuses sampled for IUGR and in up to 66% of fetuses with documented ultrasonographic malformations.[3] Among the first group, the abnormalities include triploidy (7%), trisomy 18 (6%), trisomy 21 (1%), trisomy 13 (1%), and a variety of deletions and translocations (2%). *Fetal infection* should be considered in all infants with IUGR. Those most commonly responsible for IUGR are cytomegalovirus, rubella, syphilis, and toxoplasmosis. Infants who are SGA because of fetal factors are usually characterized by symmetric growth retardation (also referred to as *proportionate IUGR*), meaning that all organ systems are similarly affected.[4]
- *Placental*: During the third trimester of pregnancy, vigorous fetal growth places particularly heavy demands on the uteroplacental supply line. Therefore, the adequacy of placental growth in the preceding midtrimester is extremely important, and *uteroplacental insufficiency is an important cause of growth retardation.* This insufficiency may result from *umbilical-placental vascular anomalies* (such as single umbilical artery, abnormal cord insertion, placental hemangioma), *placental abruption, placenta previa, placental thrombosis and infarction, placental infection*, or *multiple gestations* (Chapter 24). In some cases, the placenta may be small without any detectable underlying cause.

  Placental causes of IUGR tend to result in asymmetric (or disproportionate) growth retardation of the fetus with relative sparing of the brain. Physiologically, this general type of IUGR is viewed as a down regulation of growth in the latter half of gestation because of limited availability of nutrients or oxygen.[5]

  Confined placental mosaicism is a more recently discovered cause of IUGR[6] and has been documented in up to 2% of viable pregnancies studied by chorionic villus sampling at 9 to 11 weeks' gestation. Chromosomal mosaicism, in general, results from viable genetic mutations occurring after zygote formation. Depending on the developmental timing and cell of origin of the mutation, variable forms of chromosomal mosaicism result. For example, genetic mutations occurring at the time of the first or second postzygotic division result in generalized constitutional mosaicism of the fetus and placenta. Conversely, if the mutation occurs later and within dividing trophoblast or extraembryonic progenitor cells of the inner cell mass (approximately 90% of the time), a genetic abnormality limited to the placenta results confined placental mosaicism (Fig. 11-2). The phenotypic consequences of such placental mosaicism depend on both the specific cytogenetic abnormality and the percentage of cells involved. Chromosomal trisomies, in particular trisomy 7, are the most frequent abnormality documented.
- *Maternal*: By far the most common factors associated with SGA infants are maternal because many conditions affecting the mother's health result in decreased placental blood flow. Vascular diseases, such as *toxemia* and *chronic hypertension*, are often the underlying cause. The list of other maternal conditions associated with

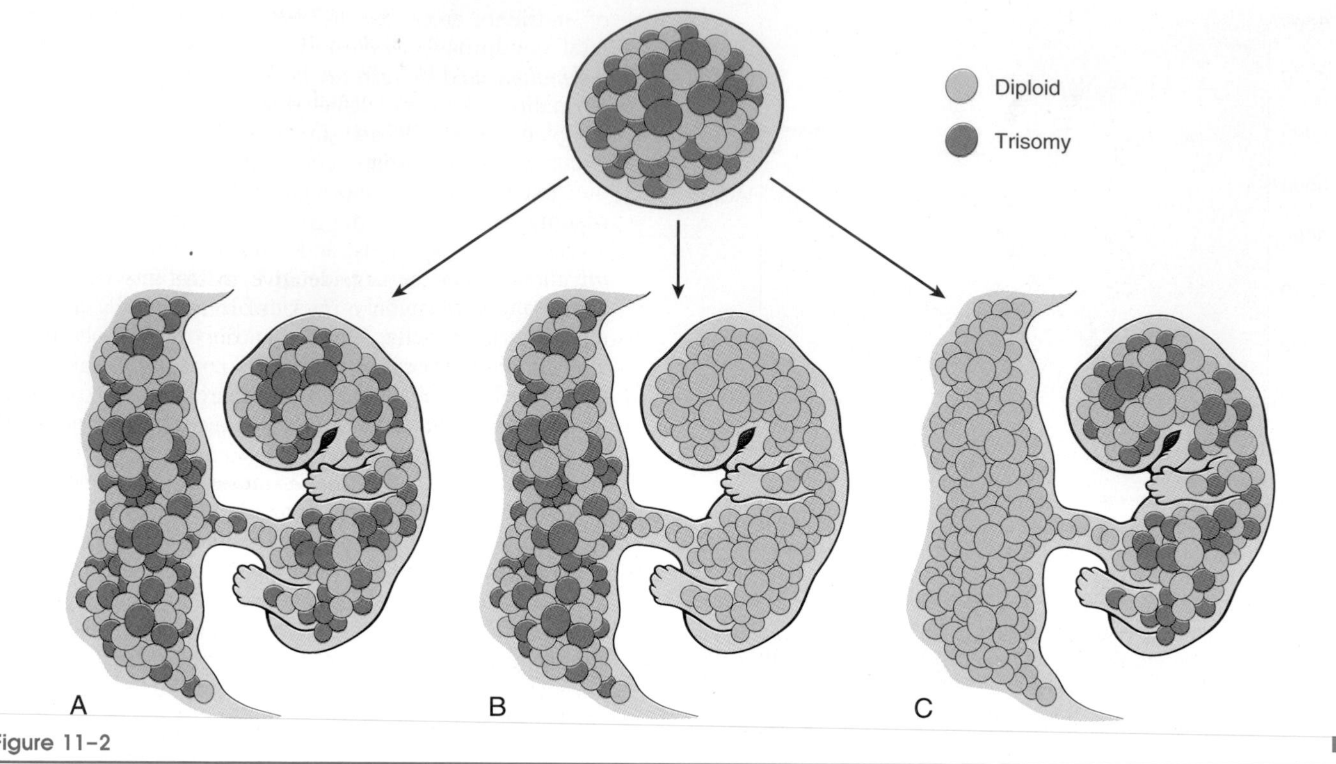

Figure 11–2

Diagrammatic representation of constitutional chromosomal mosaicism. *A*, Generalized. *B*, Confined to the placenta. *C*, Confined to the embryo. (Modified and redrawn from Kalousek DK: Confined placental mosaicism and intrauterine development. Pediatr Pathol 10:69, 1990.)

SGA infants is long,[7] but some of the avoidable factors worth mentioning are maternal *narcotic abuse, alcohol intake,* and *heavy cigarette smoking. Drugs* causing IUGR include both classic teratogens, such as antimetabolites, and some commonly administered therapeutic agents, such as phenytoin (Dilantin). *Maternal malnutrition* (in particular, prolonged hypoglycemia) may also affect fetal growth, but the association between SGA infants and the nutritional status of the mother is complex.

The SGA infant faces a difficult course, not only in the perinatal period, while struggle for survival is the main objective, but also in childhood and adult life. Depending on the underlying cause of IUGR and, to a lesser extent, the degree of prematurity, there is a significant risk of morbidity in the form of a major handicap, cerebral dysfunction, learning disability, or hearing and visual impairment.

Immaturity of Organ Systems

A major problem confronting the preterm infant regardless of birth weight is the functional and sometimes structural immaturity of various organs. Those who are also SGA are the most seriously handicapped. Because immaturity may be the direct cause of death in early preterm infants and significantly biases the probable outcome in others, it is appropriate to consider the features of immaturity of the more vital organs.

LUNGS

During the first half of fetal life, the development of the lungs consists essentially of the formation of a system of branching tubes from the foregut that eventually give rise to the trachea, bronchi, and bronchioles. The alveoli begin to differentiate only at approximately the seventh month of gestation. They are at first imperfectly formed, with thick walls, large amounts of interlobular and intralobular connective tissue, and a cuboidal epithelium. The vascularization is buried within this connective tissue and is not in immediate contact with the alveolar spaces (Fig. 11–3). Between the 26th and 32nd weeks of gestation, the cuboidal epithelium shows transition to the flat, type I alveolar epithelial cells as well as type II cells that contain lamellar bodies (Chapter 16). Further maturation of the lungs leads to reduction in the interstitial tissues and increasing numbers of capillaries. Even at full term, however, the alveoli are small and the septa are considerably thicker than in the adult. Development of alveoli continues after birth, and the full adult complement of alveoli is reached at about 8 years of age.

The immature lungs are grossly unexpanded, red, and meaty. The alveolar spaces are incompletely expanded and often lined by cuboidal epithelium and usually contain pink proteinaceous precipitate and occasional squamous epithe-

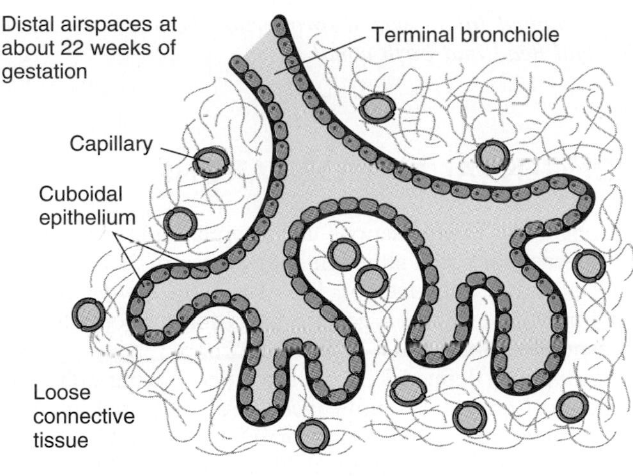

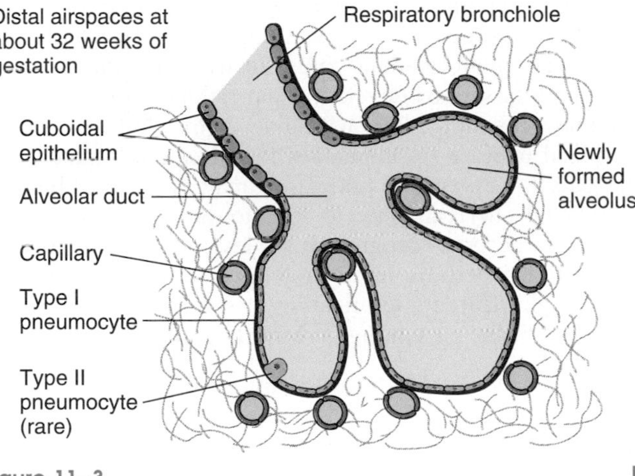

Figure 11–3

Schematic diagrams of fetal lung maturation.

lial cells. The presence of large amounts of amniotic debris, such as squames, lanugo hair, and mucus, usually indicates prenatal respiratory distress.

KIDNEYS

In the preterm infant, the formation of glomeruli is incomplete. Primitive glomeruli can be seen in the subcapsular zone. These structures have an organoid, glandular appearance imparted by the presence of cuboidal cells in the parietal and visceral layers of Bowman capsule. The deeper glomeruli are well formed, however, and renal function is adequate to permit survival.

BRAIN

The brain is also incompletely developed in the preterm infant. The surface is relatively smooth and devoid of the typical convolutions found in the cerebral hemispheres of the adult. The brain substance is soft, gelatinous, and easily torn. There is poorly developed myelination of the nerve fibers. To the best of present knowledge, despite this underdevelopment, the vital brain centers are sufficiently developed, even in the very immature infant, to sustain normal central nervous system function. Homeostasis is not perfect, however, and the preterm infant has difficulty in maintaining a constant normal level of temperature and has poor vasomotor control, irregular respirations, muscular inertia, and feeble sweating.

LIVER

The liver, although large relative to the size of the preterm infant, suffers from lack of physiologic maturity. Some of this increase in size is due to persistence of extramedullary hematopoiesis in this organ. Many or most of the functions of the liver are marginally adequate to carry out the demands placed on them. Almost all newborns and particularly those of low birth weight have a transient period of *physiologic jaundice* within the first postnatal week. This jaundice stems from both breakdown of fetal red cells and inadequacy of the biliary excretory function of liver cells.

Apgar Score

The Apgar score, devised by Virginia Apgar, represents a clinically useful method of evaluating the physiologic condition and responsiveness of newborn infants and hence their chances of survival.[8] Table 11–2 indicates the five parameters to be scored and how they are quantitated. The newborn infant may be evaluated at 1 minute or at 5 minutes. A total score of 10 indicates an infant in the best possible condition. The correlation between the Apgar score and the mortality during the first 28 days of life is impressive. Infants with a 5-minute Apgar score of 0 to 1 have a 50% mortality within the first month of life. This

Table 11–2. EVALUATION OF THE NEWBORN INFANT*

Sign	0	1	2
Heart rate	Absent	Below 100	Over 100
Respiratory effort	Absent	Slow, irregular	Good, crying
Muscle tone	Limp	Some flexion of extremities	Active motion
Response to catheter in nostril (tested after oropharynx is clear)	No response	Grimace	Cough or sneeze
Color	Blue, pale	Body pink, extremities blue	Completely pink

*Sixty seconds after the complete birth of the infant (disregarding removal of the cord and placenta), the five objective signs are evaluated and each is given a score of 0, 1, or 2. A total score of 10 indicates an infant in the best possible condition.

Modified from Apgar V: A proposal for a new method of evaluation of the newborn infant. Anesth Analg 32:260, 1953.

drops to 20% with a score of 4 and to almost 0% when the score is 7 or better.[9] Despite the established value of the Apgar score in predicting perinatal morbidity, particularly in normal-birth-weight infants, it is not a reliable indicator of long-term neurologic morbidity.[10]

BIRTH INJURIES

Birth injuries constitute important causes of illness or death in infants as well as in children during the first years of life. No infant is immune to birth injury, although the risk and type of injury vary from the LGA infant to the preterm AGA or SGA infant. These injuries most commonly involve the head, skeletal system, liver, adrenals, and peripheral nerves. Considering the violent expulsive forces to which the fragile fetus is exposed, it is quite surprising that birth injuries are so relatively uncommon.

Morbidity associated with birth injury may be acute (e.g., that due to fractures) or the result of later-appearing sequelae (e.g., after damage to nerves or the brain). The distribution of injuries in a large municipal hospital, in descending order of frequency, is as follows:[11] clavicular fracture, facial nerve injury, brachial plexus injury, intracranial injury, humeral fracture, and lacerations. Not surprisingly, LGA infants are at greater risk for birth injury, in particular those involving the skeletal system and peripheral nerves. We briefly discuss only injuries involving the head because they are the most ominous.[12]

Intracranial hemorrhage is the most common important birth injury. These hemorrhages are generally thought to be related to excessive molding of the head or sudden pressure changes in its shape as it is subjected to the pressure of forceps or sudden precipitate expulsion. Prolonged labor, hypoxia, hemorrhagic disorders, or intracranial vascular anomalies are important predispositions. The hemorrhage may arise from tears in the dura or from rupture of vessels that traverse the brain. The substance of the brain may be torn or bruised, leading to intraventricular hemorrhages or bleeding into the brain substance. Whatever their origin, intracranial hemorrhages are of great importance because they cause sudden increases in intracranial pressure; damage to the brain substance; herniation of the medulla or base of the brain into the foramen magnum; and serious, frequently fatal depression of function of the vital medullary centers.

Caput succedaneum and *cephalhematoma* are so common, even in normal uncomplicated births, that they hardly merit the designation *birth injury*. The first refers to progressive accumulation of interstitial fluid in the soft tissues of the scalp, giving rise to a usually circular area of edema, congestion, and swelling at the site where the head begins to enter the lower uterine canal. Hemorrhage may occur into the scalp, producing a cephalhematoma. Both forms of injury are of little clinical significance and are important only insofar as *they must be differentiated from skull fractures with attendant hemorrhage and edema. In approximately 25% of cephalhematomas, there is an underlying skull fracture. Such skull fractures may occur in cases of precipitate delivery, inappropriate use of forceps, or prolonged labor with disproportion between the size of the fetal head and birth canal.*

CONGENITAL MALFORMATIONS

Congenital malformations are morphologic defects that are present at birth, although they may not become clinically apparent until later in life. The term *congenital* does not imply or exclude a genetic basis for malformations. It is estimated that about 3% of newborns have a *major malformation*, defined as a malformation having either cosmetic or functional significance.[13] As indicated in Table 11–1, they are a major cause of infant mortality, affecting 20 to 25% of infants dying in the perinatal period. Moreover, they continue to be a significant cause of illness, disability, and death throughout the early years of life. In a real sense, malformations found in live-born infants represent the less serious developmental failures in embryogenesis that are compatible with live birth. Perhaps 20% of fertilized ova are so anomalous that they are blighted from the outset. Less severe anomalies may be compatible with early fetal survival, only to lead to spontaneous abortion. As they become progressively less severe, a level is reached that permits more prolonged intrauterine survival, with some disorders terminating in stillbirth and those still less significant permitting live birth despite the handicaps imposed.

Definitions

Before proceeding, we define some of the terms used for various kinds of errors in morphogenesis—*malformations, deformations, disruptions, sequences,* and *syndromes.*

- *Malformations* represent intrinsic abnormalities occurring during the developmental process. Malformations may present in several patterns. Some, such as congenital heart defects and anencephaly (absence of brain), involve single body systems, whereas in other cases multiple malformations involving many organs may coexist. Malformations are further discussed shortly.
- *Deformations*, in contrast to malformations, arise later in fetal life and represent an alteration in form or structure resulting from *mechanical factors*. They usually manifest as abnormalities in shape, form, or position of the body and, in general, are associated with much less risk of recurrence in subsequent siblings. *Uterine constraint* is the most common underlying factor in infants born with deformations. Constraint is partially due to the fact that between the 35th and 38th weeks of gestation, the rapidly increasing growth of the fetus outpaces the growth of the uterus, while there is a relative decrease in the amount of amniotic fluid (which normally acts as a cushion). Thus, even the normal fetus is subjected to some form of uterine constraint. Several factors increase the likelihood of excessive compression of the fetus resulting in deformations. *Maternal factors* include first pregnancy, small uterus, malformed (bicornuate) uterus,

and leiomyomas. *Fetal* or *placental factors* include oligohydramnios, multiple fetuses, and abnormal fetal presentation. An example of a deformation is clubfeet, often a component of Potter sequence, described subsequently.

- *Disruptions*, the third main error in morphogenesis, result from secondary destruction of or interference with an organ or body region that was previously normal in development. Disruptions may be caused by either extrinsic factors or internal interferences, such as vascular insults, and are not heritable. *Amniotic bands*, resulting from rupture of the amnion during fetal development, may compress, attach to, or encircle parts of the developing fetus and are the classic example of a disruption (Fig. 11–4).
- A *sequence* is a pattern of cascade anomalies. Approximately half of the time, malformations occur as single anomalies. In the remaining cases, multiple congenital anomalies are recognized. In some instances, the constellation of anomalies may be explained by a single, localized aberration in organogenesis (malformation, disruption, or deformation) leading to secondary effects in other organs.

A good example of a sequence is the *oligohydramnios* (or *Potter*) *sequence* (Fig. 11–5). Oligohydramnios (decreased amniotic fluid) may be caused by a variety of unrelated maternal, placental, or fetal abnormalities. Chronic leakage of amniotic fluid because of rupture of the amnion, uteroplacental insufficiency resulting from maternal hypertension or severe toxemia, and renal agenesis in the fetus (as fetal urine is a major constituent of amniotic fluid) all are causes of oligohydramnios. The fetal compression associated with significant oligohydramnios, in turn, results in a classic phenotype in the newborn infant, including flattened facies and positional abnormalities of the hands and feet (Fig. 11–6). The hips may be dislocated. Growth of the chest wall and

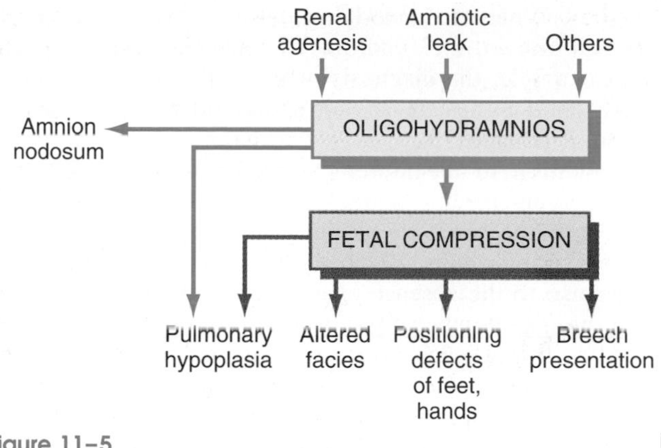

Figure 11–5

Schematic diagram of the pathogenesis of the oligohydramnios sequence.

the contained lungs is also compromised so that the lungs are frequently hypoplastic, occasionally to the degree that they are the cause of fetal demise. Nodules in the amnion (*amnion nodosum*) are frequently present.

- A *syndrome* is a constellation of congenital anomalies, believed to be pathologically related, that, in contrast to a sequence, *cannot* be explained on the basis of a single, localized, initiating defect.

Syndromes are most often caused by a single etiologic agent, such as a viral infection or specific chromosomal abnormality, that simultaneously affects several

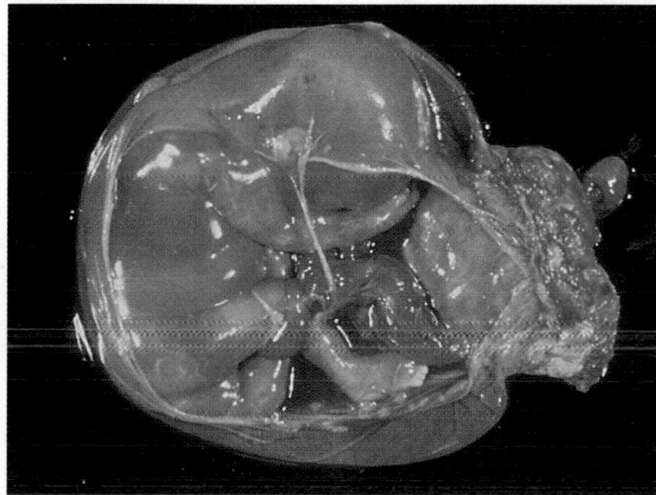

Figure 11–4

Amniotic band syndrome. Note the placenta at the right of the diagram and the band of amnion extending from the top portion of the amniotic sac to encircle the leg of the fetus. (Courtesy of Dr. Theonia Boyd, Children's Hospital of Boston.)

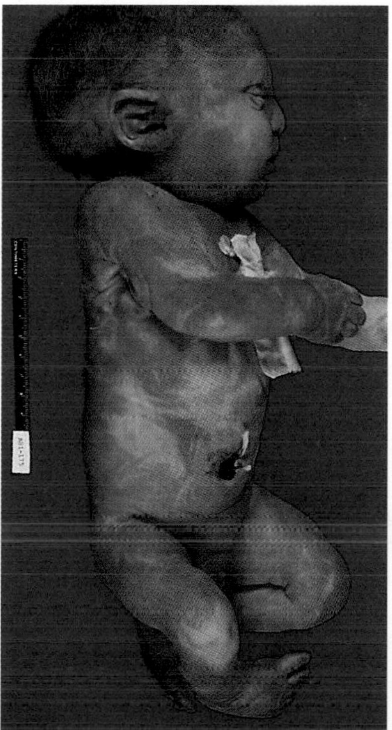

Figure 11–6

Infant with oligohydramnios sequence. Note the flattened facial features and deformed right foot (talipes equinovarus).

tissues. When the underlying cause of the condition becomes known, the syndrome is referred to as a *disease*. For example, the diagnosis of neurofibromatosis is made in a child with café au lait spots and multiple neurofibromas (Chapter 6).

- In addition to the aforementioned global definitions, a few organ-specific terms should be defined. *Agenesis* refers to the complete absence of an organ and its associated primordium. A closely related term, *aplasia*, refers also to the absence of an organ but owing to failure of the developmental anlage to develop. *Atresia* describes the absence of an opening, usually of a hollow visceral organ, such as the trachea and intestine. *Hypoplasia*, or incomplete development or underdevelopment of an organ with decreased numbers of cells, is a less severe form of aplasia, whereas *hyperplasia* refers to the converse, that is, overdevelopment of an organ associated with increased numbers of cells. An abnormality in an organ or a tissue as a result of an increase or a decrease in the size (rather than the number) of individual cells defines *hypertrophy* or *hypotrophy*. Finally, *dysplasia*, in the context of malformations (versus neoplasia) describes an abnormal organization of cells.

Table 11–3. CAUSES OF CONGENITAL MALFORMATIONS IN HUMANS

Cause	Malformed Live Births (%)
Genetic	
Chromosomal aberrations	10–15
Mendelian inheritance	2–10
Environmental	
Maternal/placental infections	2–3
Rubella	
Toxoplasmosis	
Syphilis	
Cytomegalovirus	
Human immunodeficiency virus (HIV)	
Maternal disease states	6–8
Diabetes	
Phenylketonuria	
Endocrinopathies	
Drugs and chemicals	1
Alcohol	
Folic acid antagonists	
Androgens	
Phenytoin	
Thalidomide	
Warfarin	
13-*cis*-retinoic acid	
Others	
Irradiation	1
Multifactorial (Multiple Genes ± Environment)	20–25
Unknown	40–60

Adapted from Stevenson RE, et al (eds): Human Malformations and Related Anomalies. New York, Oxford University Press, 1993, p 115.

Causes of Malformations

At one time, it was believed that the presence of a visible, external malformation was divine punishment for wickedness, a belief that occasionally jeopardized the mother's life. Although we are learning a great deal about some of the molecular bases of malformations, the exact cause remains unknown in at least half of the cases. The common causes of malformations can be grouped into three major categories: genetic, environmental, and multifactorial (Table 11–3).

GENETIC CAUSES

Malformations that are known to be genetic in origin can be divided into two groups:

- Those associated with karyotypic aberrations
- Those arising from single gene mutations

A third group is suspected of resulting from *multifactorial inheritance*, a term that implies the interaction of two or more genes of small effect with environmental factors, and is discussed separately.

Virtually all the *chromosomal syndromes* (Chapter 6) are characterized by congenital anomalies. Karyotypic abnormalities are present in approximately 10 to 15% of liveborn infants with congenital malformations, but only one approaches a birth frequency of 1 in 1000 total births—trisomy 21 (Down syndrome). Next in order of frequency are Klinefelter syndrome, Turner syndrome, and trisomy 13 (Patau syndrome). The remaining chromosomal syndromes associated with malformations are far rarer. *The great preponderance of these cytogenetic aberrations arise as defects in gametogenesis and so are not familial.* There are, however, several transmissible chromosomal abnormalities, for example, the translocation form of Down syndrome, which is passed from one generation to the next, thus constituting a familial pattern of structural abnormalities.

Single gene mutations of large effect may underlie major malformations, which, as expected, follow mendelian patterns of inheritance.[14, 15] Of these, approximately 90% are inherited in an autosomal dominant or recessive pattern, while the remainder segregate in an X-linked pattern. Although these genetic aberrations account for a relatively small percentage of birth defects, much research effort has been devoted to their discovery. Among these rare entities are the relatively less serious limb malformations: polydactyly (increased numbers of digits), syndactyly (deformed digits), and brachydactyly (short digits). Some of these, as seen subsequently, are caused by mutations in HOX genes. There is still some question, however, about the mode of transmission of others, and multifactorial inheritance cannot be excluded. In a few anomalies, such as holoprosencephaly (Chapter 30), mutations in more than one gene may result in a similar phenotype. In addition, there are a number of malformation syndromes in which multiple anomalies occur in disorders having mendelian modes of transmission, for example, Marfan syndrome and the mucopolysaccharidoses (Chapter 6).

ENVIRONMENTAL CAUSES

Environmental influences, such as viral infections, drugs, and irradiation, to which the mother was exposed during pregnancy may induce malformations in the fetus and infant.[16] As discussed later, many agents known to be carcinogenic postnatally are teratogenic to the fetus.

- *Viruses*: Many viruses have been implicated in causing malformations, including the agents responsible for rubella, cytomegalic inclusion disease, herpes simplex, varicella-zoster infection, influenza, mumps, human immunodeficiency virus (HIV), and enterovirus infections. Among these, the rubella virus and cytomegalovirus are the most extensively investigated. With all viruses, the gestational age at which the infection occurs in the mother is critically important. *The at-risk period for rubella infection extends from shortly before conception to the 16th week of gestation*, the hazard being greater in the first 8 weeks than in the second 8 weeks. The incidence of malformations is reduced from 50% to 20% to 7% if infection occurs in the first, second, or third month of gestation. The fetal defects are varied, but the major triad comprises cataracts, heart defects (persistent ductus arteriosus, pulmonary artery hypoplasia or stenosis, ventricular septal defect, tetralogy of Fallot), and deafness, referred to as *rubella syndrome*.

  Intrauterine infection with cytomegalovirus, mostly asymptomatic, is the most common fetal viral infection.[17] This viral disease is considered in detail in Chapter 9; *the highest at-risk period is the second trimester of pregnancy*. Because organogenesis is largely completed by the end of the first trimester, congenital malformations occur less frequently than in rubella; nevertheless, the effects of virus-induced injury on the formed organs are often severe. Involvement of the central nervous system is a major feature, and the most prominent clinical changes are mental retardation, microcephaly, deafness, and hepatosplenomegaly.
- *Drugs and other chemicals*: A variety of drugs and chemicals have been suspected to be teratogenic, but perhaps fewer than 1% of congenital malformations are caused by these agents. The list includes thalidomide, folate antagonists, androgenic hormones, alcohol, anticonvulsants, warfarin (oral anticoagulant), and 13-*cis*-retinoic acid used in the treatment of severe acne. For example, *thalidomide*, once used as a tranquilizer in Europe, caused an extremely high frequency (50 to 80%) of limb abnormalities in exposed fetuses. *Alcohol*, perhaps the most widely used agent today, is a teratogen. Affected infants show growth retardation, microcephaly, atrial septal defect, short palpebral fissures, maxillary hypoplasia, and several other minor anomalies. These together are labeled the *fetal alcohol syndrome*.[18]
- *Radiation*: In addition to being mutagenic and carcinogenic, radiation is teratogenic. Exposure to heavy doses of radiation during the period of organogenesis leads to malformations, such as microcephaly, blindness, skull defects, spina bifida, and other deformities. Such exposure occurred in the past when radiation was used to treat cervical cancer.

MULTIFACTORIAL CAUSES

The genetic and environmental factors just discussed account for no more than half of human congenital malformations. The causes of the vast majority of birth defects, including some relatively common disorders such as cleft lip and cleft palate, remain unknown. In these malformations, it would appear that inheritance of a certain number of mutant genes and their interaction with the environment is required before the disorder is expressed. In the case of congenital dislocation of the hip, for example, depth of the acetabular socket and laxity of the ligaments are believed to be genetically determined, whereas a significant environmental factor is believed to be frank breech position in utero, with hips flexed and knees extended. The approximate frequency of some common malformations in the United States is presented in Table 11–4. Both temporal and regional variability are common in the reporting of many malformations. For example, between 1979 and 1989, there was a mean annual per cent decrease in the incidence of anencephaly of 6.4 and a mean annual increase in the incidence of atrial septal defect of 22.0.[19]

Mechanisms of Malformations

The pathogenesis of congenital malformations is complex and still poorly understood, but certain general principles of developmental pathology are relevant regardless of the etiologic agent.

The timing of the prenatal teratogenic insult has an important impact on the occurrence and the type of malformation produced (Fig. 11–7).[13] The intrauterine development of humans can be divided into two phases: (1) the embryonic period occupying the first 9 weeks of pregnancy and (2) the fetal period terminating at birth. In the *early embryonic period* (first 3 weeks after fertilization), an injurious agent damages either enough cells to cause death and abortion or only a few cells, presumably allowing the embryo to recover without developing defects. *Between the third and the ninth weeks, the embryo is extremely suscep-*

Table 11–4. APPROXIMATE FREQUENCY OF THE MORE COMMON CONGENITAL MALFORMATIONS IN THE UNITED STATES

Malformation	Frequency Per 10,000 Total Births
Clubfoot without central nervous system anomalies	25.7
Patent ductus arteriosus	16.9
Ventricular septal defect	10.9
Cleft lip with or without cleft palate	9.1
Spina bifida without anencephalus	5.5
Congenital hydrocephalus without anencephalus	4.8
Anencephalus	3.9
Reduction deformity (musculoskeletal)	3.5
Rectal and intestinal atresia	3.4

Adapted from James LM: Maps of birth defects occurrence in the U.S., birth defects monitoring program (BDMP)/CPHA, 1970–1987. Teratology 48:551, 1993.

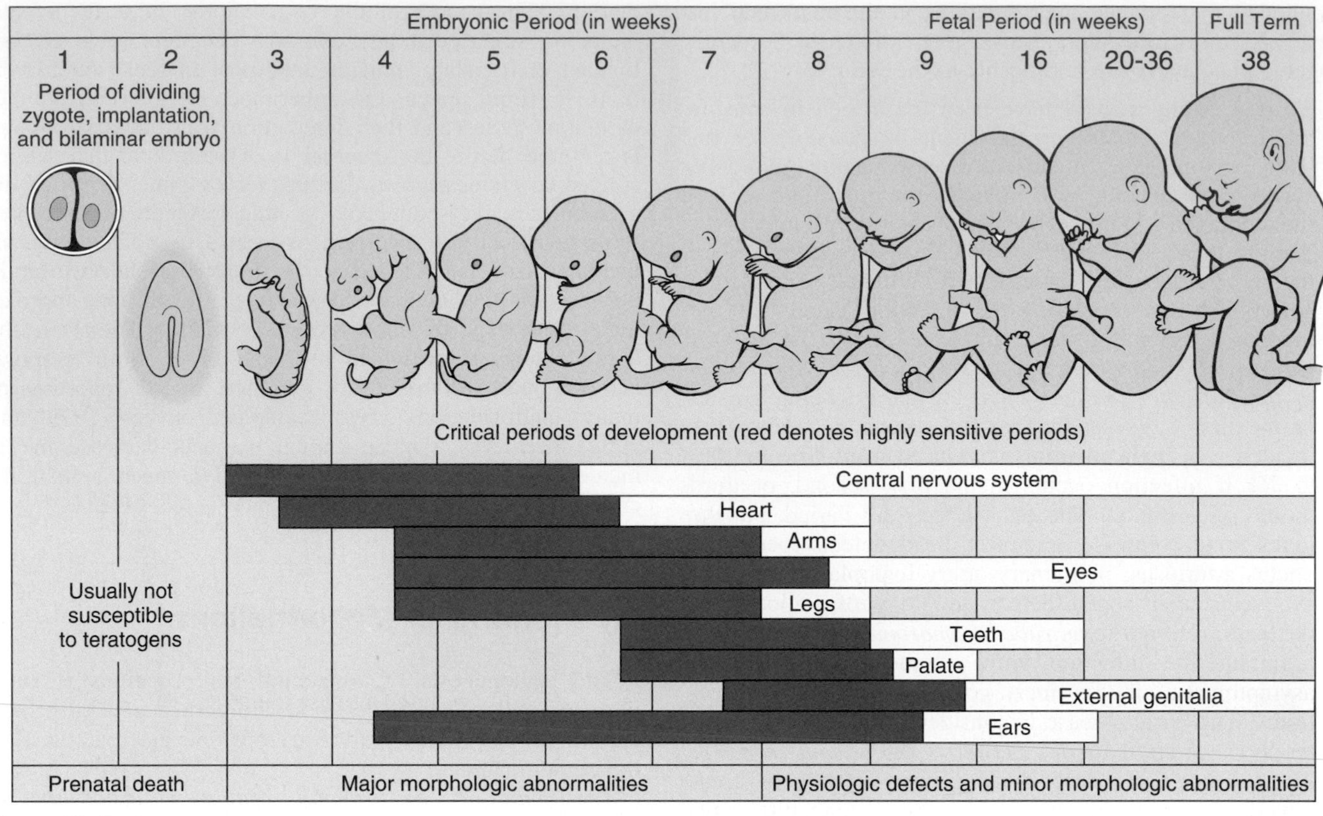

Figure 11–7

Critical periods of development for various organ systems and the resultant malformations. (Modified and redrawn from Moore KL: The Developing Human, 5th ed. Philadelphia, WB Saunders, 1993, p 156.)

tible to teratogenesis, and the peak sensitivity during this period is between the fourth and the fifth weeks. During this period, organs are being created out of the germ cell layers. The *fetal period* that follows organogenesis is marked chiefly by the further growth and maturation of the organs, with greatly reduced susceptibility to teratogenic agents. Instead the fetus is susceptible to growth retardation or injury to already formed organs. It is therefore possible for a given agent to produce different malformations if exposure occurs at different times of gestation.

Teratogens and genetic defects may act at several levels involved in normal morphogenesis. These include the following:[14]

- Proper *cell migration* to predetermined locations that influence the development of other structures
- *Cell proliferation*, which determines the size and form of embryonic organs
- *Cellular interactions* among tissues derived from different structures (e.g., ectoderm, mesoderm), which affect the differentiation of one or both of these tissues
- *Cell-matrix associations*, which affect growth and differentiation
- *Programmed cell death (apoptosis)*, which, as we have seen, allows orderly organization of tissues and organs during embryogenesis (Chapter 1)
- *Hormonal influences* and *mechanical forces*, which affect morphogenesis at many levels

These events are influenced, during development, by the same growth regulatory molecules (e.g., growth factors), cell-matrix interactions, signal transduction pathways, and genes (e.g., apoptosis-associated genes) that are discussed in Chapters 1 through 4 and that are involved in wound healing and neoplasia. For example, the transforming growth factor-β (TGF-β) family includes, in addition to TGF-β-1, TGF-β-2, and TGF-β-3 described earlier, molecules that induce mesoderm (activin), influence bone morphogenesis (bone morphogenetic protein), and cause inhibition of müllerian duct development.[20] There are an increasing number of examples in which spontaneous or experimentally induced aberrations in growth factors are associated with congenital malformations. There is an association, for example, between rare mutations of TGF-α and cleft palate,[21] and mutations in some of the TGF-β family genes cause malformations in mice.[20] Another dramatic example is the role of the Wilms' tumor gene (WT-1), which is a tumor-suppressor gene that acts as a transcriptional repressor after growth factor stimulation (Chapter 8; see also later in this chapter). The WT-1 gene is expressed at critical times of urogenital development. Mutations in WT-1 are associated with urogenital malformations, and deletion of the gene in transgenic mice causes renal agenesis (absent kidneys).[22] Similarly, genetically engineered mice with aberrations or deficiencies in fibronectin or some of the integrins either die as embryos or are born with congenital defects.[23] Teratogens may disrupt cell migrations. For example, in experimental animals, disturbance in collagen-matrix formation by cadmium produces major craniofacial anomalies because the migration of neural crest cells is inhibited. Anticonvulsant drugs impair the appropriate differentiation of the mesenchyme and give rise to cleft palate in rodents.

Since many congenital malformations reflect failure of normal *morphogenesis* during development, it is reasonable to expect that alterations of genes that control these events might cause birth defects. Two such classes of genes deserve special mention.

- *Homeobox genes*: Classes of genes known to be important in embryonic patterning include those that contain conserved regions involved in transcriptional regulation. One such class, *the HOX genes*, were first identified from study of the *Drosophila* mutant, *antennapedia*, in which legs appear in the position normally occupied by the antennae. HOX genes have a 180 nucleotide motif, dubbed the *homeobox*, which has DNA-binding properties and is conserved between species as divergent as insects and humans. In vertebrates, *these genes have been implicated in the patterning of limbs, vertebrae, and craniofacial structures*. Introduction of altered Hox genes in transgenic mice, embryonic exposure to chemical agents known to increase or decrease expression of HOX genes, mutations, and experimental deletion of those genes (*knockouts*) produce malformations concordant with their presumed role in embryonic patterning.[24] In humans, mutations of HOX D-13 cause synpolydactyly (extra digits) in heterozygous individuals,[21] and mutations of HOX A-13 cause brachydactyly (short digits) and uterine malformations.[25a]

Homeobox genes themselves are regulated by upstream genes and interact with down-stream target genes. Up-stream regulators of HOX genes are also implicated in teratogenesis.[26] For example, the vitamin A (retinol) derivative, *all-trans-retinoic acid*, is essential for normal development, and its absence during embryogenesis results in a constellation of malformations affecting multiple organ systems, including the eyes, genitourinary system, cardiovascular system, diaphragm, and lungs (Fig. 11–8, *left*).[27] Conversely, *retinoic acid itself is a known human teratogen*. Infants born to mothers treated with retinoic acid for severe acne have a predictable phenotype (*retinoic acid embryopathy*), including central nervous system, cardiac, and craniofacial defects (Fig. 11–8, *right*).[28] In animals, retinoic acid exposure produces reproducible changes in HOX gene expression and causes a wide range of structural congenital malformations, the nature of which is determined by the dosage and timing of exposure.[29] The precise mechanisms by which retinoic acid interacts with these genes in a normal embryo and the manner by which malformations are caused are unclear. One scenario (Fig. 11–8, *center*) is that the latter is related to differential temporal and spatial expression of nuclear retinoic acid receptors (RAR; RXR) and cellular retinoic acid–binding proteins

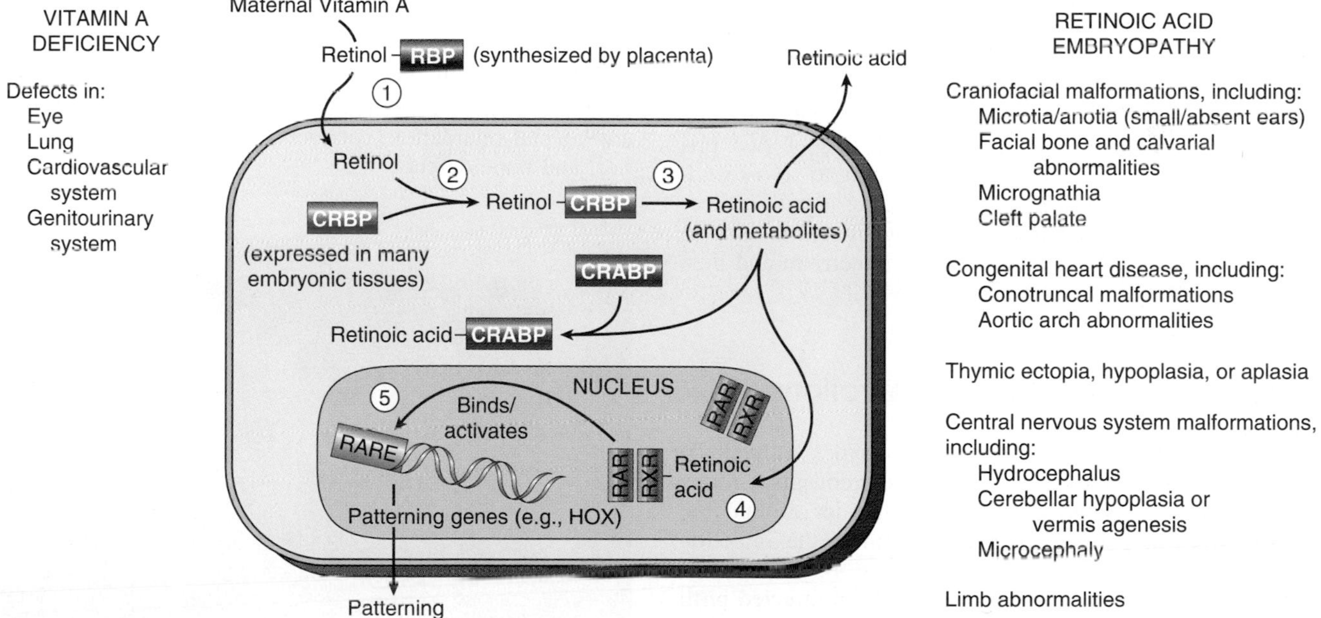

Figure 11–8

Schematic representation of the postulated role of retinoic acid in normal development, the general features of its deficiency (vitamin A deficiency) (*left*), and retinoic acid embryopathy (*right*). *1*, Retinol in the maternal circulation is bound by retinol-binding protein (RBP), which is synthesized by the placenta and enters the fetal circulation. *2*, Once in fetal cells, retinol is bound by cytoplasmic retinol-binding protein (CRBP), which *(3)* regulates the conversion to retinoic acid and metabolites. The retinoic acid either remains in the cytoplasm (bound to cytoplasmic/cellular retinoic acid–binding protein [CRABP]) or *(4)* enters the nucleus, where it is bound to nuclear retinoic acid receptors (RAR, RXR). The retinoic acid–receptor complex acts as a transcriptional regulator of various patterning genes (e.g., HOX) that have the appropriate retinoic acid response element (RARE). Expression of the binding proteins and receptors in various tissues and at various times during embryogenesis may be a mechanism of selectively modulating the action of retinoic acid. This differential expression may also explain the pattern of abnormalities seen in vitamin A deficiency and retinoic acid embryopathy.

(CRABP), which determine the activity of retinoic acid receptor complexes as transcriptional regulators of HOX genes (Fig. 11–8, *center*).[30]

- *PAX genes*: Another family of developmental genes are the PAX genes, which are characterized by a 384 base pair sequence—the *paired box*. Similar to the HOX genes, the PAX genes are highly conserved throughout evolution[31]; they encode for DNA-binding proteins and are therefore believed to be transcription factors. In contrast to HOX genes, however, their expression patterns suggest that they act singly, rather than in a temporal or spatial combination. Mutations in two of the PAX genes cause human malformations. PAX-3 is mutated in Waardenburg syndrome, characterized by congenital pigment abnormalities and deafness, and PAX-6 mutations may cause congenital absence of the iris—aniridia. Parenthetically, PAX genes may function also as protooncogenes, in that their overexpression is associated with tumorigenesis. Translocations involving PAX 3 and 7 have been identified in the majority of alveolar rhabdomyosarcomas, and a translocation involving PAX 5 is observed in a subset of lymphomas. PAX 2 is believed to be involved in a subset of patients with Wilms' tumors and plays an important role in renal development.[32]

PERINATAL INFECTIONS

Infections of the embryo, fetus, and neonate are manifested in a variety of ways and are mentioned as etiologic factors in Chapter 9, Infectious Disease, and numerous other sections within this chapter. Here we discuss only the general routes and timing of infections. In general, fetal and perinatal infections are acquired via one of two primary routes—*transcervically* (also referred to as *ascending*) or *transplacentally* (*hematologic*). Occasionally, infections occur by a combination of the two routes in that an ascending microorganism infects the endometrium and then the fetal bloodstream via the chorionic villi.

Transcervical (Ascending) Infections

Most bacterial and a few viral (e.g., herpes simplex II) infections are acquired by way of the cervicovaginal route. Such infections may be acquired in utero or around the time of birth. In general, the fetus acquires the infection either by inhaling infected amniotic fluid into the lungs shortly before birth or by passing through an infected birth canal during delivery. Preterm birth of these infants is not uncommon and may be related either to damage and rupture of the amniotic sac as a direct consequence of the inflammation or to the induction of labor associated with a release of prostaglandins by the infiltrating neutrophils. Chorioamnionitis of the placental membranes and *funisitis* (inflammation of the umbilical cord) are usually demonstrable, although the presence or absence and severity of chorioamnionitis does not necessarily correlate with the severity of the fetal infection. In the fetus infected via inhalation of amniotic fluid, pneumonia, sepsis, and meningitis are the most common sequelae.

Transplacental (Hematologic) Infections

Most parasitic and viral infections and a few bacterial infections (i.e., *Listeria*, *Treponema*) gain access to the fetal bloodstream transplacentally via the chorionic villi. This hematogenous transmission may occur at any time during gestation or occasionally, as may be the case with hepatitis B and HIV, at the time of delivery via maternal-to-fetal transfusion. [33] The clinical manifestations of these infections are highly variable, depending largely on the gestational timing and microorganism involved.

Some infections, such as those with *parvovirus B19* (which causes *fifth disease* in the mother), may induce spontaneous abortion, stillbirth, hydrops fetalis, and congenital anemia.[34] While the virus can bind to different cell types, replication occurs only in erythroid cells, and diagnostic viral cytopathic effect can be recognized in late erythroid progenitor cells of infected infants (Fig. 11–9).

TORCH infections are caused by toxoplasma (*T*), rubella (*R*), cytomegalovirus (*C*), herpesvirus (*H*), and a number of other (*O*) bacterial and viral agents. They are grouped together because they may evoke similar clinical and pathologic manifestations. The latter include fever, encephalitis, chorioretinitis, hepatosplenomegaly, pneumonitis, myocarditis, hemolytic anemia, and vesicular or hemorrhagic skin lesions. Such infections occurring early in gestation may also cause chronic sequelae in the child, including growth and mental retardation, cataracts, congenital cardiac anomalies, and bone defects.

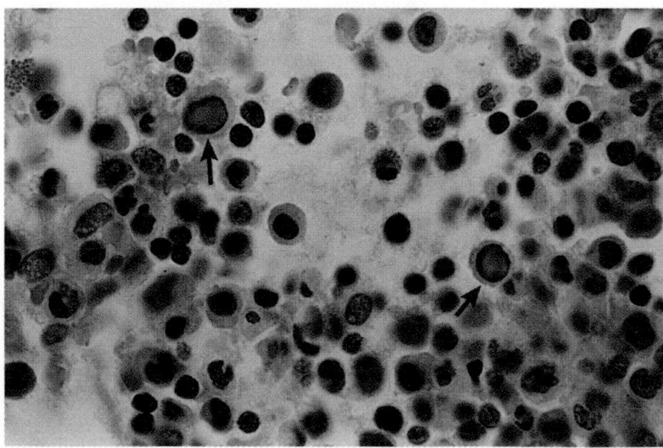

Figure 11–9

Bone marrow from an infant infected with parvovirus B19. The arrows point to two erythroid precursors with large homogeneous intranuclear inclusions and a surrounding peripheral rim of residual chromatin.

Onset of Sepsis

Perinatal infections can also be grouped clinically by whether they tend to result in *early-onset* versus *late-onset* sepsis. Most cases of early-onset sepsis are acquired at or shortly before birth and tend to result in clinical signs and symptoms of pneumonia, sepsis, and occasionally meningitis within 4 or 5 days of life. Group B streptococcus is the most common organism isolated in early-onset sepsis and is also the most common cause of bacterial meningitis.[35] Infections with *Listeria* and *Candida* require a latent period between the time of microorganism inoculation and the appearance of clinical symptoms and present as late-onset sepsis.

NEONATAL RESPIRATORY DISTRESS SYNDROME (RDS)

There are many causes of respiratory distress in the newborn, including excessive sedation of the mother, fetal head injury during delivery, aspiration of blood or amniotic fluid, and intrauterine hypoxia brought about by coiling of the umbilical cord about the neck. The most common cause, however, is RDS, also known as *hyaline membrane disease* because of the formation of *membranes* in the peripheral airspaces of infants who succumb to this condition. Approximately 60,000 cases of RDS are reported each year in the United States, with annual deaths totaling 5000.

In untreated infants (not receiving surfactant), RDS presents in a stereotyped fashion, characterized by the following characteristic clinical setting. The infant is almost always preterm and AGA, and there are strong, but not invariable, associations with diabetes in the mother and with delivery by cesarean section. Resuscitation may be necessary at birth, but usually within a few minutes rhythmic breathing and normal color are reestablished. Soon afterward, often within 30 minutes, breathing becomes more difficult, there is retraction of the lower ribs and sternum on inspiration, and an expiratory grunt becomes audible. Over the span of the next few hours, the respiratory distress becomes worse, and cyanosis becomes evident. Fine rales can now be heard over both lung fields. A chest x-ray film at this time usually reveals uniform minute reticulogranular densities, producing a so-called ground-glass picture. At first, the administration of oxygen to the infant lessens the cyanosis; during the next 12 to 24 hours, recovery may ensue, but in the full-blown condition the respiratory distress persists, cyanosis increases, and even the administration of 80% oxygen by a variety of ventilatory methods fails to improve the situation. Flaccidity, unresponsiveness, and periods of apnea may now appear and may presage death. If therapy staves off death for the first 3 or 4 days, however, the infant has an excellent chance of recovery.[36]

Etiology and Pathogenesis. Immaturity of the lungs is the most important subsoil on which this condition develops. It may be encountered in full-term infants but is much less frequent than in those "born before their time into this breathing world."[37] The incidence of RDS is inversely proportional to gestational age. It occurs in about 60% of infants born at less than 28 weeks of gestation, 15 to 20% of those born between 32 and 36 weeks of gestation, and less than 5% of those born after 37 weeks of gestation.[38]

The *fundamental defect in RDS is a deficiency of pulmonary surfactant.* As described in Chapter 16, surfactant consists predominantly of dipalmitoyl phosphatidylcholine, smaller amounts of phosphatidylglycerol, and at least two proteins that are thought to be important for normal surfactant function in vivo.[39] Surfactant reduces surface tension within the alveoli so that less pressure is required to hold alveoli open, and it maintains alveolar expansion by varying surface tension with alveolar size. It is synthesized by type II alveolar cells most abundantly after the 35th week of gestation in the fetus. At birth, the first breath of life requires high inspiratory pressures to expand the lungs. With normal levels of surfactant, the lungs retain up to 40% of the residual air volume after the first breath; thus, subsequent breaths require far lower inspiratory pressures. With a deficiency of surfactant, the lungs collapse with each successive breath, and so infants must work as hard with each successive breath as they did with the first. The problem of *stiff* atelectatic lungs is compounded by the *soft* thoracic wall that is pulled in as the diaphragm descends. Progressive atelectasis and reduced lung compliance then lead to a train of events as depicted in Figure 11–10, resulting in a protein-rich, fibrin-rich exudation into the alveolar spaces with the formation of hyaline membranes. The fibrin-hyaline membranes constitute barriers to gas exchange, leading to carbon dioxide retention and hypoxemia. The hypoxemia itself further impairs surfactant synthesis, and a vicious cycle ensues.

Surfactant synthesis is modulated by a variety of hormones and growth factors, including cortisol, insulin, prolactin, and thyroxine. The role of glucocorticoids is particularly important. Corticosteroids induce the formation of surfactant lipids and apoprotein in fetal lung.[40] Surfactant synthesis can be suppressed by the compensatory high blood levels of insulin in infants of diabetic mothers, which counteracts the effects of steroids. This may explain, in part, why infants of diabetic mothers have a higher risk of developing RDS.

MORPHOLOGY. The lungs are distinctive on gross examination. Although of normal size, they are solid, airless, and reddish purple similar to the color of the liver, and they usually sink in water. Microscopically, atelectatic alveoli are poorly developed, and those that are present are collapsed. When the infant dies early in the course of the disease, necrotic cellular debris is present in the terminal bronchioles and alveolar ducts. Later the necrotic material becomes incorporated within eosinophilic hyaline membranes lining the respiratory bronchioles, alveolar ducts, and random alveoli, mostly the proximal alveoli (Fig. 11–11). The membranes are largely made up of fi-

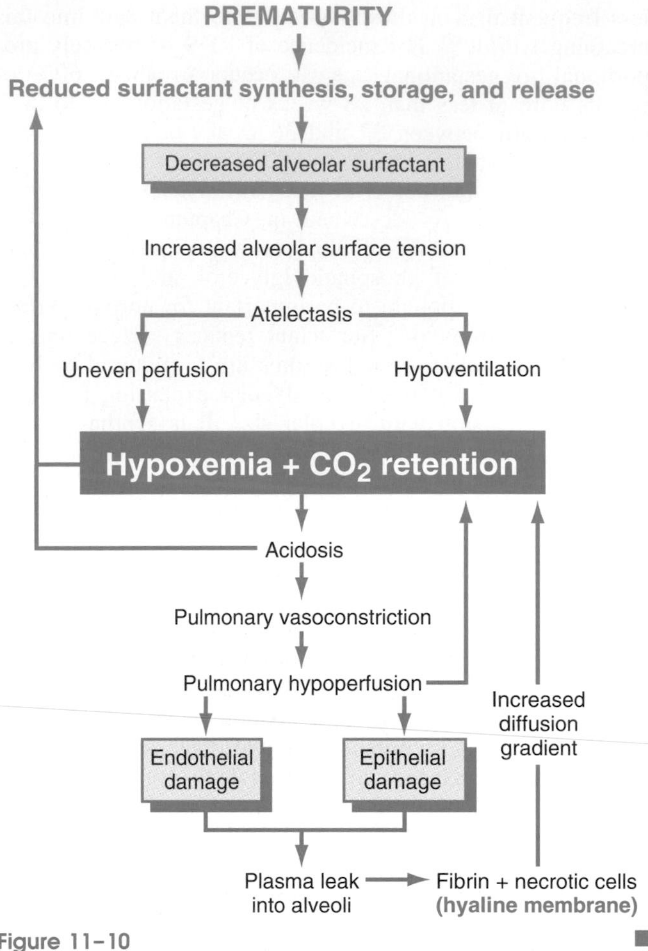

Figure 11–10

Schematic outline of the pathophysiology of the respiratory distress syndrome (see text).

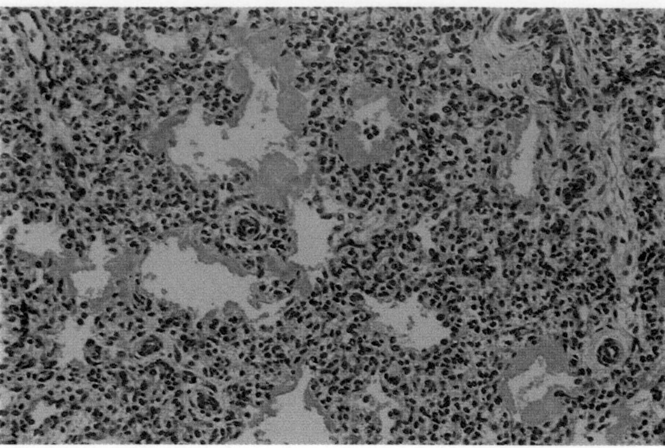

Figure 11–11

Hyaline membrane disease. There is alternating atelectasis and dilation of the alveoli. Note the eosinophilic thick hyaline membranes lining the dilated alveoli.

brinogen and fibrin admixed with cell debris derived chiefly from necrotic type II pneumocytes. The sequence of events that leads to the formation of hyaline membranes is depicted in Figure 11–10. There is a remarkable paucity of neutrophilic inflammatory reaction associated with these membranes. The lesions of hyaline membrane disease are never seen in stillborn infants or in liveborn infants who die within a few hours of birth.

In infants who survive more than 48 hours, reparative changes occur in the lungs. The alveolar epithelium proliferates under the surface of the membrane, which may be desquamated into the airspace, where it may undergo partial digestion or phagocytosis by macrophages.

Clinical Course. Although a classic clinical presentation before the era of treatment with exogenous surfactant was described earlier, the actual clinical course and prognosis for neonatal RDS vary, dependent on the maturity and birth weight of the infant and the promptness of institution of therapy. A major thrust in the control of RDS focuses on prevention, either by delaying labor until the fetal lung reaches maturity or by inducing maturation of the lung in the fetus at risk. Critical to these objectives is the ability to assess fetal lung maturity accurately. Because pulmonary secretions are discharged into the amniotic fluid, analysis of amniotic fluid phospholipids provides a good estimate of the level of surfactant in the alveolar lining. Prophylactic administration of exogenous surfactant at birth to extremely premature infants (gestational age <26 to 28 weeks) and symptomatic administration of surfactant to older premature infants have been shown to be extremely beneficial, such that it is now uncommon for infants to die of acute RDS.[41, 42] In addition, antenatal corticosteroids decrease neonatal morbidity and mortality when administered to mothers with threatened premature delivery at 24 to 34 weeks' gestation.[43] Once the infant is born, the cornerstone of treatment is the delivery of surfactant replacement therapy and oxygen, usually accomplished by a variety of ventilatory assistance methods, including high-frequency ventilation.

In uncomplicated cases, recovery begins to occur within 3 or 4 days. Therapy carries with it the now well-recognized hazard of *oxygen toxicity*, however, caused by oxygen-derived free radicals. High concentrations of oxygen administered for prolonged periods cause two well-known complications: *retrolental fibroplasia* (also called *retinopathy of prematurity*) *in the eyes* and *bronchopulmonary dysplasia*. The retinopathy has been ascribed to changes in expression of vascular endothelial growth factor, which also serves as a survival factor for endothelial cells and causes angiogenesis (Chapter 4). Vascular endothelial growth factor is markedly decreased during hyperoxia, causing endothelial cell apoptosis, but increases after return to room air—inducing the retinal vessel proliferation characteristic of the lesions in the retina[44] (Chapter 31).

Clinically, *bronchopulmonary dysplasia* is defined as oxygen dependence at 28 days of age and is characterized by persistence of respiratory distress for up to 3 to 6 months or more. Pathologically, the more severe forms of bronchopulmonary dysplasia present with airway epithelial hyperplasia and squamous metaplasia, alveolar wall thickening, and peribronchial as well as interstitial fibrosis. If oxygen toxicity is avoided, as is usually the case in current clinical settings, and the infant can be kept alive for about 3 or 4 days, recovery of infants of 31 weeks' gestation or more can be anticipated without permanent sequelae. Bronchopulmonary dysplasia persists as a major problem among infants of very low birth weight, however, with the incidence exceeding 50% of infants less than 1000 gm. Because of the morbidity associated with the prolonged use of high concentrations of oxygen, alternative methods of ventilation are now being used, especially high-frequency ventilation, extracorporeal membrane oxygenation, and liquid ventilation by perfluorochemical fluids that act as a medium for respiratory gas exchange.[45]

Infants who recover from RDS are at increased risk for developing a variety of other complications as well. Most important among these are *patent ductus arteriosus, intraventricular hemorrhage,* and *necrotizing enterocolitis.* Thus, although current high technology saves many infants with RDS, it also brings to the surface the exquisite fragility of the immature neonate.

ERYTHROBLASTOSIS FETALIS—HEMOLYTIC DISEASE OF THE NEWBORN

Erythroblastosis fetalis is defined as a hemolytic disease in the newborn caused by blood-group incompatibility between mother and child. When the fetus inherits red cell antigenic determinants from the father that are foreign to the mother, a maternal immune reaction may occur, leading to hemolytic disease in the infant. Basic to such a phenomenon are leakage of fetal red cells into the maternal circulation and, in turn, transplacental passage of maternal antibodies into the fetus. Any of the numerous red cell antigenic systems may theoretically be involved, but the major antigens known to induce clinically significant immunologic disease are the ABO and certain of the Rh antigens. The incidence of Rh erythroblastosis in urban populations has declined remarkably, owing largely to the current methods of preventing Rh immunization in at-risk mothers. Successful prophylaxis of this disorder has resulted directly from an understanding of its pathogenesis.

Etiology and Pathogenesis. The underlying basis of erythroblastosis fetalis is the immunization of the mother by blood group antigens on fetal red cells and the free passage of antibodies from the mother through the placenta to the fetus. Fetal red cells may reach the maternal circulation during the last trimester of pregnancy, when the cytotrophoblast is no longer present as a barrier, or during childbirth itself. The mother thus becomes sensitized to the foreign antigen.

Of the numerous antigens included in the Rh system, only the D antigen is the major cause of Rh incompatibility. Several factors influence the immune response to Rh-positive fetal red cells that reach the maternal circulation.

- Concurrent ABO incompatibility protects the mother against Rh immunization because the fetal red cells are promptly coated by isohemagglutinins and removed from the maternal circulation.
- The antibody response depends on the dose of immunizing antigen; hence, hemolytic disease develops only when the mother has experienced a significant transplacental bleed (more than 1 ml of Rh-positive red cells).
- The istotype of the antibody is important because immunoglobulin G (IgG) (but not immunoglobulin M [IgM]) antibodies can cross the placenta. The initial exposure to Rh antigen evokes the formation of IgM antibodies, so Rh disease is uncommon with the first pregnancy. Subsequent exposure during a second or third pregnancy generally leads to a brisk IgG antibody response.

The incidence of maternal Rh isoimmunization has significantly decreased since the use of Rhesus immune globulin (RhIg) containing anti-D antibodies. Administration of RhIg at 28 weeks and within 72 hours of delivery to Rh-negative mothers significantly decreases the risk for hemolytic disease in Rh-positive neonates and in subsequent pregnancies. Moreover, antenatal identification and management of the at-risk fetus have been greatly facilitated by amniocentesis and the advent of chorionic villus and fetal blood sampling. In addition, cloning of the Rh D gene has resulted in efforts to determine fetal Rh status using maternal blood. When identified, cases of severe intrauterine hemolysis may be treated by fetal intravascular transfusions via the umbilical cord and early delivery.[46]

The pathogenesis of fetal hemolysis caused by maternal/fetal ABO incompatibility is slightly different than that caused by differences in the Rh antigens. ABO incompatibility occurs in approximately 20 to 25% of pregnancies, but laboratory evidence of hemolytic disease occurs only in 1 in 10 of such infants, and the hemolytic disease is severe enough to require treatment in only 1 in 200 cases. Several factors account for this. First, most anti-A and anti-B antibodies are of the IgM type and hence do not cross placenta. Second, neonatal red cells express blood group antigens A and B poorly. Third, many cells other than red cells express A and B antigens and thus sop up some of the transferred antibody. ABO hemolytic disease occurs almost exclusively in infants born to group O mothers because some have IgG anti-A and anti-B antibodies without obvious sensitization. There is no effective protection against ABO reactions.

There are two consequences of excessive destruction of red blood cells in the neonate (Fig. 11–12). One is *anemia*, and the other is the accumulation of bilirubin (*jaundice*). The severity of these changes varies considerably, however, depending on the degree of hemolysis and the maturity of the infant organ systems. Extramedullary hematopoiesis in the liver and spleen may suffice to maintain normal red cell levels if the hemolysis is mild. If the hemolytic reaction is marked, anemia associated with jaundice and the presence of unconjugated bilirubin occurs.

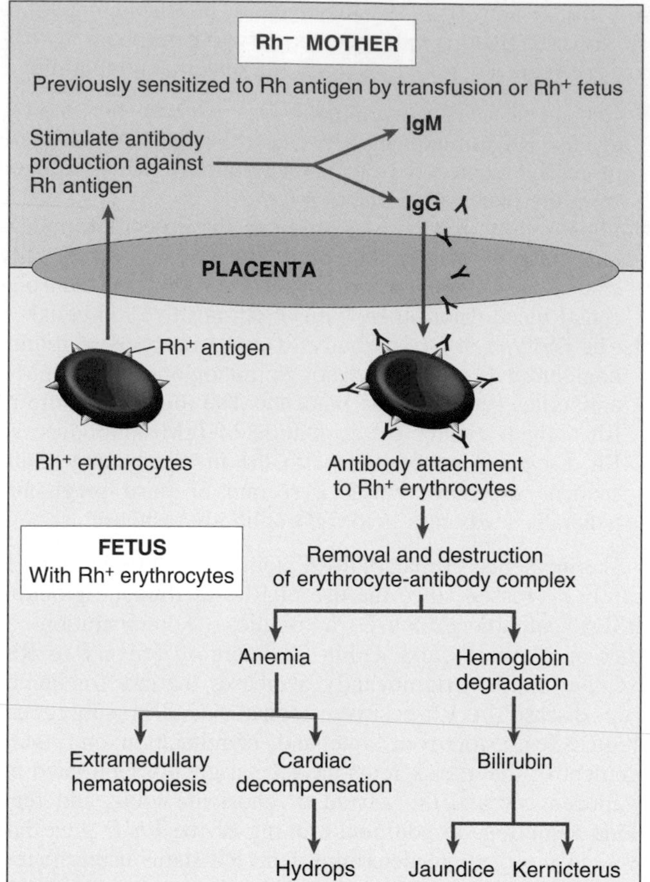

Figure 11–12

Pathogenesis of erythroblastosis fetalis (see text).

Because unconjugated bilirubin is water insoluble and has an affinity for lipids, it binds to lipids in the brain owing to the poorly developed blood-brain barrier in the infant, resulting in serious damage to the central nervous system, termed *kernicterus.* In addition, the anemia may be associated with hypoxic injury to the heart and liver, resulting in circulatory and hepatic failure and edema. If severe, plasma protein levels may drop to as low as 2.0 to 2.5 gm/dl because of reduced hepatic synthesis. *This decrease in oncotic pressure within the circulation, combined with a secondary increase in venous capillary pressure owing to cardiac failure, results in generalized edema and ascites* (anasarca). This latter condition is referred to as *hydrops fetalis.*[47]

The list of disorders reported to be associated with *hydrops fetalis* is extensive, including both immune (as in the case of erythroblastosis fetalis) and nonimmune conditions. Because of the remarkable success achieved in the prevention of Rh hemolytic disease, greater than 90% of cases have a nonimmunologic basis. These include structural anomalies and hamartomas of the fetus, chromosomal abnormalities, inherited metabolic disease, and intrauterine infection (Table 11–5). In addition, approximately 10% of cases of nonimmune hydrops may be related to monozygous twin pregnancies and twin-twin transfusion occurring through anastomoses between the two circulations.

Table 11–5. GENERAL CAUSES OF NONIMMUNE HYDROPS FETALIS*

General Cause	Estimated %
Cardiovascular	17–35
Malformations	
Tachyarrhythmia	
High-output failure	
Chromosomal	13.5–15.7
45,X	
Trisomy 21	
Hematologic	4.2–12
Pulmonary	3–6
Cystic adenomatoid malformation	
Diaphragmatic hernia	
Multiple malformation syndrome	3–15
Twin-twin transfusion	3–10.3
Infection	1.5–5.3
Cytomegalovirus	
Bacteria	
Toxoplasmosis	
Skeletal dysplasia	3–4
Gastrointestinal	2–3.7
Urogenital	2.2–3
Tumors	2.5–3
Metabolic disorders	1
Idiopathic	15.5–40

*Only some of the most common entities under major categories are listed as examples. Adapted from Machin GA: Hydrops revisited: literature review of 1,414 cases published in the 1980s. Am J Med Genet 34:366, 1989.

MORPHOLOGY. The anatomic findings in erythroblastosis fetalis vary with the severity of the hemolytic process. Infants may be stillborn, die within the first few days, or recover completely. In its mildest form, the anemia may be only slight, and the child may survive without further complication. More severe hemolysis gives rise to jaundice and other features associated with hemolytic anemias. In some cases, **hydrops fetalis** develops. In most cases, the liver and spleen are enlarged, the degree depending on the severity of the hemolytic processes and the compensatory extramedullary erythropoiesis.

The most serious threat in erythroblastosis is central nervous system damage known as **kernicterus.**[48] In jaundiced infants, the unconjugated bilirubin appears to be particularly toxic to the brain (Chapter 31). The brain is enlarged and edematous and, when sectioned, is found to have a bright yellow pigmentation (kernicterus), particularly in the basal ganglia, thalamus, cerebellum, cerebral gray matter, and spinal cord. The precise level of bilirubin that induces kernicterus is unpredictable, but neural damage rarely occurs if the serum bilirubin concentration is below 20 mg/dl. At lower levels, premature infants especially are at risk.

Histologically the diagnosis of erythroblastosis fetalis depends on the identification of abnormally increased erythropoietic activity in the infant. The red cell series in the marrow is hyperactive, and extramedullary hematopoiesis is almost invariably present in the liver (Fig. 11–13), spleen, and possibly other tissues, such as the lymph nodes, kidneys, lungs, and even the heart. This hematopoietic activity is sufficiently striking to account for increased numbers of reticulocytes, normoblasts, and erythroblasts in the circulating blood. Evidence of subcutaneous and visceral edema is present in the hydrops syndrome along with fluid in the peritoneal, pleural, and pericardial cavities.

Clinical Features. The clinical manifestations of erythroblastosis vary with the severity of the disease and can be predicted from the preceding discussion. Minimally affected infants display pallor, possibly accompanied by hepatosplenomegaly (to which may be added jaundice with more severe hemolytic reactions), whereas the most gravely ill neonates present with intense jaundice, widespread edema, and signs of neurologic involvement in the pattern referred to as *hydrops fetalis*. These latter infants may be supported by a variety of measures, including phototherapy (visual light oxidizes toxic unconjugated bilirubin to harmless, readily excreted, water-soluble dipyrroles) and, in severe cases, total exchange transfusion of the infant. Administration of high-dose intravenous immunoglobulin may also play an important role, although specific details regarding optimal dosage and timing of this therapy still need to be determined.[49]

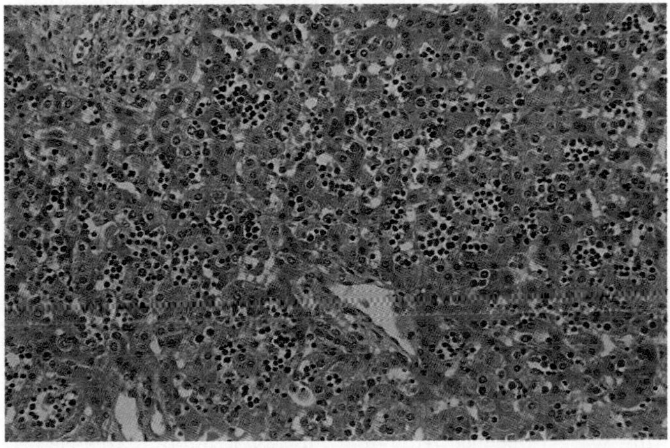

Figure 11–13

Numerous islands of extramedullary hematopoiesis (small blue cells) are scattered among mature hepatocytes in this infant with erythroblastosis fetalis.

INBORN ERRORS OF METABOLISM AND OTHER GENETIC DISORDERS

The number of well-characterized genetic disorders resulting in inborn errors of metabolism is constantly increasing and is beyond the scope of this chapter. Most of these conditions are rare. Some were discussed in Chapter 6. Three additional metabolic genetic defects, phenylketonuria (PKU), galactosemia, and cystic fibrosis, are selected for discussion here. PKU and galactosemia are reviewed because their early diagnosis (via neonatal screening programs)[50] is particularly important as institution of an appropriate dietary regimen can prevent early death or mental retardation in surviving patients. Cystic fibrosis is included because it is one of the most common, potentially lethal diseases occurring in whites. Neonatal screening for cystic fibrosis remains a controversial topic, with the benefits and risks much less clear than in the other two diseases.

Phenylketonuria

There are several variants of PKU, an inborn error of metabolism. The most common form, referred to as *classic PKU*, is quite common in persons of Scandinavian descent and is distinctly uncommon in blacks and Jews.

Homozygotes with this autosomal recessive disorder classically have a severe lack of phenylalanine hydroxylase, leading to hyperphenylalaninemia and PKU. Affected infants are normal at birth but within a few weeks develop a rising plasma phenylalanine level, which in some way impairs brain development. Usually by 6 months of life severe mental retardation becomes evident; fewer than 4% of untreated PKU children have intelligence quotient values greater than 50 or 60. About one third of these children are never able to walk, and two thirds cannot talk. Seizures, other neurologic abnormalities, decreased pigmentation of hair and skin, and eczema often accompany the mental retardation in untreated children. Hyperphenylalaninemia and the resultant mental retardation can be avoided by restriction of phenylalanine intake early in life. Hence, a number of screening procedures are routinely used for detection of PKU in the immediate postnatal period.

Many clinically normal female PKU patients who were treated with diet early in life have now reached childbearing age. Most of them have discontinued dietary treatment and have marked hyperphenylalaninemia. Seventy-five per cent to 90% of children born to such women are mentally retarded and microcephalic, and 15% have congenital heart disease, even though the infants themselves are heterozygotes. This syndrome, termed *maternal PKU*,[51] results from the teratogenic effects of phenylalanine or its metabolites that cross the placenta and affect specific fetal organs during development. The presence and severity of the fetal anomalies directly correlate with the maternal phenylalanine level, so *it is imperative that maternal dietary restriction of phenylalanine is initiated before conception and continues throughout the pregnancy.*

The biochemical abnormality in PKU is an inability to

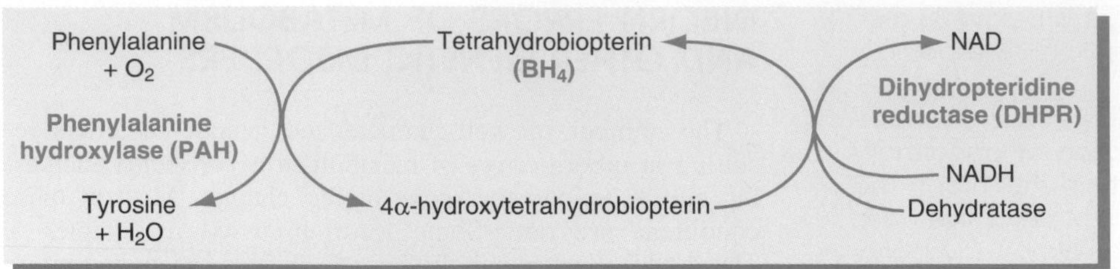

Figure 11-14

The phenylalanine hydroxylase system.

convert phenylalanine into tyrosine. In normal children, less than 50% of the dietary intake of phenylalanine is necessary for protein synthesis. The rest is irreversibly converted to tyrosine by a complex hepatic phenylalanine hydroxylase system (Fig. 11–14), which has several components in addition to the enzyme phenylalanine hydroxylase. Although neonatal hyperphenylalaninemia can be caused by deficiencies in any of these components, 98 to 99% of cases are attributable to abnormalities in phenylalanine hydroxylase. With a block in phenylalanine metabolism owing to lack of phenylalanine hydroxylase, minor shunt pathways come into play, yielding phenylpyruvic acid, phenyllactic acid, phenylacetic acid, and *o*-hydroxyphenylacetic acid, which are excreted in large amounts in the urine in PKU. Some of these abnormal metabolites are excreted in the sweat, and phenylacetic acid in particular imparts a strong musty or mousy odor to affected infants. It is believed that excess phenylalanine or its metabolites contribute to the brain damage in PKU.

At the molecular level, several mutant alleles of the phenylalanine hydroxylase gene have been identified. Each mutation induces a particular alteration in the enzyme resulting in a corresponding quantitative effect on residual enzyme activity ranging from complete absence to 50% of normal values. The degree of hyperphenylalaninemia and clinical phenotype is inversely related to the amount of residual enzyme activity. Infants with mutations resulting in a lack of phenylalanine hydroxylase activity present with the classic features of PKU, while those with up to 6% residual activity present with milder disease. Moreover, some mutations result in only modest elevations of phenylalanine levels, and the affected children have no neurologic damage. This latter condition, referred to as *benign hyperphenylalaninemia* or *mild PKU*, is important to recognize because the individuals may well test *positive* in screening tests but do not develop the stigmata of classic PKU. Measurement of serum phenylalanine levels differentiates benign hyperphenylalaninemia and PKU.[52]

Although dietary restriction of phenylalanine is relatively successful in reducing or preventing the mental retardation associated with PKU, there are problems with long-term compliance (resulting in a decline in mental or behavioral status) and nutritional imbalances involving trace minerals, fatty acids, and lipids. Investigations into the potential role of somatic gene therapy as alternative treatment for these patients show some promise, as adenovirus-mediated transfer and transient expression of a functional recombinant phenylalanine hydroxylase gene have been accomplished in animal systems.[53] As alluded to earlier, a number of variant forms of PKU have been identified, resulting from deficiencies of enzymes other than phenylalanine hydroxylase. For instance, some patients lack dihydropteridine reductase (Fig. 11–14). Similar to those with classic PKU, they are also unable to metabolize phenylalanine, but in addition they have associated abnormalities of tyrosine and tryptophan metabolism, since dihydropteridine reductase is required for hydroxylation of these two amino acids. The concomitant impairment of tyrosine and tryptophan hydroxylation leads to disturbance in the synthesis of neurotransmitters, and neurologic damage is not arrested despite normalization of phenylalanine levels. Although they account for a small minority of patients with hyperphenylalaninemia, *it is clinically important to recognize these PKU variants because they cannot be treated by dietary control of phenylalanine levels.*

Galactosemia

Galactosemia is an autosomal recessive disorder of galactose metabolism. Normally, lactose, the major carbohydrate of mammalian milk, is split into glucose and galactose in the intestinal microvilli by lactase. Galactose is then converted to glucose in three steps (Fig. 11–15). *Two variants of galactosemia have been identified. In the more common variant, there is a total lack of galactose-1-phosphate uridyl transferase involved in reaction 2. The rare variant arises from a deficiency of galactokinase, involved in reaction 1.* Because galactokinase deficiency leads to a milder form of the disease not associated with mental retardation, it is not considered in this discussion. As a result of the transferase lack, galactose-1-phosphate accumulates in many locations, including the liver, spleen, lens of the eye, kidneys, heart muscle, cerebral cortex, and erythrocytes. Alternative metabolic pathways are activated, leading to the production of galactitol, which also accumulates in the tissues. Heterozygotes may have a mild deficiency but are spared the clinicomorphologic consequences of the homozygous state.

The clinical picture is variable, probably reflecting the heterogeneity of mutations in the galactose-1-phosphate uridyl transferase gene leading to galactosemia.[54] The liver, eyes, and brain bear the brunt of the damage. The early-to-develop *hepatomegaly* is due largely to fatty change, but in time widespread scarring that closely resembles the cirrhosis of alcohol abuse may supervene (Fig. 11–16). *Opacification of the lens (cataracts)* develops, probably because the lens absorbs water and swells as galactitol, produced by alternative metabolic pathways, accumulates and increases its tonicity. *Nonspecific alterations appear in the*

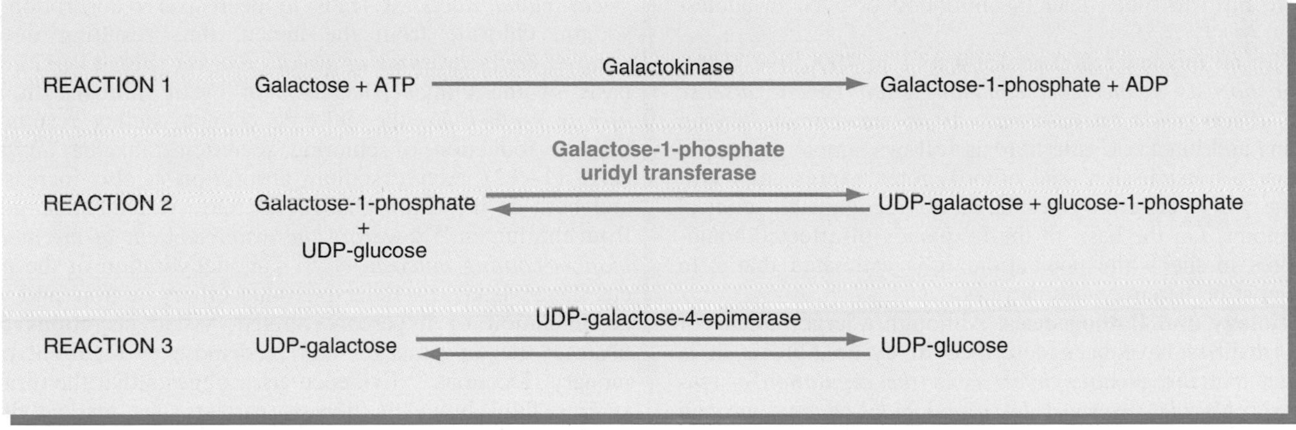

Figure 11–15

Pathways of galactose metabolism.

central nervous system, including loss of nerve cells, gliosis, and edema, particularly in the dentate nuclei of the cerebellum and the olivary nuclei of the medulla. Similar changes may occur in the cerebral cortex and white matter.

There is still no clear understanding of the mechanism of injury to the liver and brain. Toxicity has been imputed to galactose-1-phosphate. Alternatively, galactitol has been indicted as the toxic product. It is also possible that the abnormal galactose metabolism interferes with the formation of galactose-containing cerebral lipids.

Almost from birth these infants *fail to thrive. Vomiting* and *diarrhea* appear within a few days of milk ingestion. *Jaundice* and *hepatomegaly* usually become evident during the first week of life and may seem to be a continuation of the physiologic jaundice of the newborn. The *cataracts* develop within a few weeks, and within the first 6 to 12 months of life mental retardation may be detected. Even in untreated infants, the mental deficit is usually not as severe as that with PKU. Accumulation of galactose and galactose-1-phosphate in the kidney impairs amino acid transport, resulting in aminoaciduria. There is an increased frequency of fulminant *Escherichia coli* septicemia.

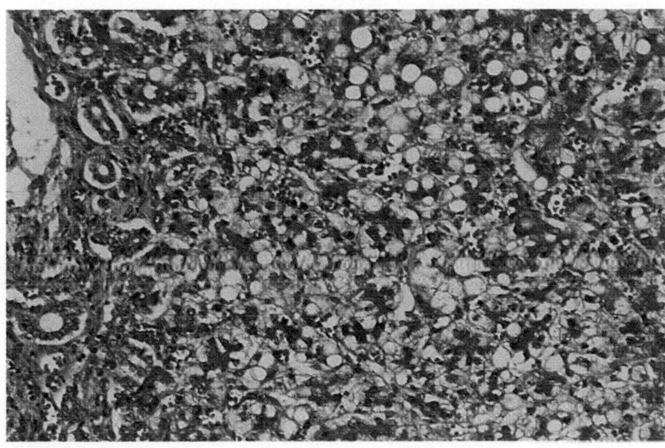

Figure 11–16

Galactosemia. The liver shows extensive fatty change and a delicate fibrosis. (Courtesy of Dr. Wesley Tyson, The Children's Hospital, Denver, CO.)

The diagnosis of galactosemia can be suspected by the demonstration in the urine of a reducing sugar other than glucose, but tests that directly identify the deficiency of the transferase in leukocytes and erythrocytes are more reliable. Antenatal diagnosis is possible by the assay of galactose-1-phosphate uridyl transferase activity in cultured amniotic fluid cells or determination of galactitol level in amniotic fluid supernatant. *Many of the clinical and morphologic changes of galactosemia can be prevented or ameliorated by early removal of galactose from the diet for at least the first 2 years of life.* Control instituted soon after birth prevents the cataracts and liver damage and permits almost normal development. Even with dietary restrictions, however, it is now well established that older patients are frequently affected by a speech disorder and gonadal failure and, less commonly, by an ataxic condition. The pathogenesis of these long-term sequelae is unclear, although elevated levels of galactitol and galactonate that are present (despite dietary compliance) may be partially responsible.[55]

Cystic Fibrosis (Mucoviscidosis)

Among the genetic pediatric disorders, cystis fibrosis is the most important. It is common and often fatal in childhood and young adult life.[56] It is fundamentally a *widespread disorder in epithelial transport affecting fluid secretion in exocrine glands and the epithelial lining of the respiratory, gastrointestinal, and reproductive tracts.* In many infants, this disorder leads to abnormally viscid mucous secretions, which obstruct organ passages, resulting in most of the clinical features of this disorder, for example, recurrent pulmonary infections leading to chronic lung disease, pancreatic insufficiency, steatorrhea, malnutrition, hepatic cirrhosis, intestinal obstruction, and male infertility. These manifestations may appear at any point in life from before birth to much later in childhood or even in adolescence.

With an incidence of 1 in 1500 to 1 in 4000 live births, *cystic fibrosis is the most common lethal genetic disease that affects white populations.* It is uncommon among Asians and blacks. Cystic fibrosis follows simple autosomal recessive transmission, and homozygotes express this syndrome fully. Heterozygotes have no recognizable clinical symptoms. On the basis of the frequency of affected homozygotes in the white population, it is estimated that 2 to 4% must be heterozygous carriers.

Etiology and Pathogenesis. Although a large number of abnormalities have been described in cystic fibrosis, it is agreed that *the primary defect is in the regulation of epithelial chloride transport by a chloride channel protein encoded by the cystic fibrosis gene.* In normal duct epithelia, chloride is transported by plasma membrane channels (*chloride channels*). Opening of these channels is mediated by agonist-induced increases in cyclic adenosine monophosphate (cAMP), followed by activation of a protein kinase A that phosphorylates the channel.[57] The impact of this defect in chloride transport differs in various tissues. In *sweat gland ducts,* it leads to decreased reabsorption of sodium chloride from the lumen, thus resulting in *increased concentrations of sweat chloride* (Fig. 11–17), the basis of the clinical diagnosis of cystic fibrosis. In the *airway epithelium*, the chloride channel defect results in loss or reduction of chloride secretion into the airways (Fig. 11–17). Active sodium absorption is also increased, and both of these ion changes increase water reabsorption from the lumen,[58] *lowering the water content of the mucus blanket coating mucosal cells.* This dehydration of the mucus layer leads to defective mucociliary action and the accumulation of hyperconcentrated, viscid secretions that obstruct the air passages and predispose to recurrent pulmonary infections.[59] Evidence also suggests that the airway surface fluid in cystic fibrosis patients has markedly reduced activity of antibacterial endogenous substances (e.g., defensins)[60]—possibly related to its increased salt content—which contributes to the susceptibility to infection.[61]

The cystic fibrosis gene is located on chromosome 7 (band q31–32),[62] *and as noted, encodes chloride channel protein.*[63] The protein, named *CFTR* (cystic fibrosis transmembrane conductance regulator), has two transmembrane

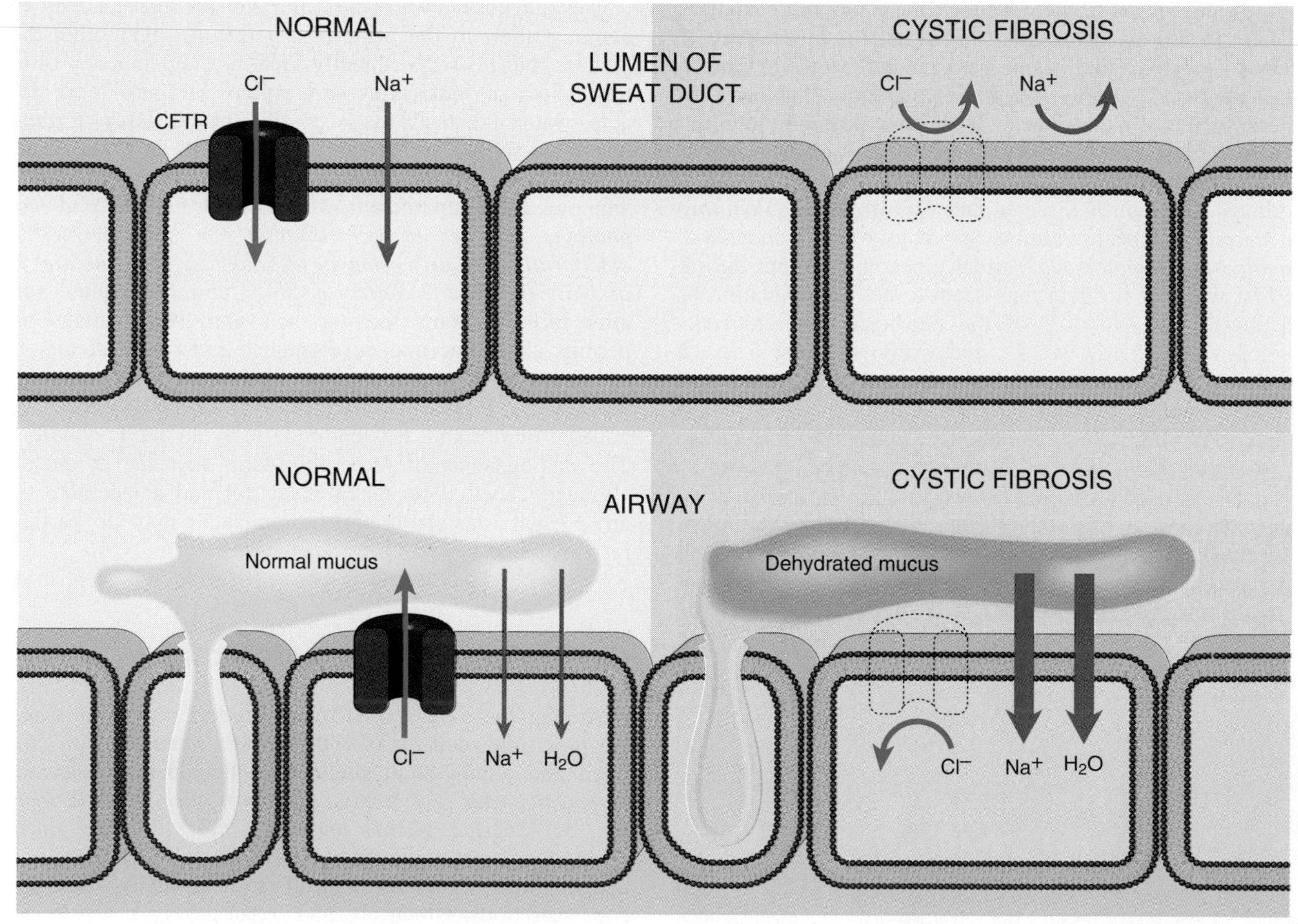

Figure 11–17

Chloride channel defect in the sweat duct (*top*) causes increased chloride and sodium concentration in sweat. In the airway (*bottom*), cystic fibrosis patients have decreased chloride secretion and increased sodium and water reabsorption leading to dehydration of the mucous layer coating epithelial cells, defective mucociliary action, and mucous plugging of airways. There is also evidence that airway surface fluid in cystic fibrosis is deficient in antibacterial activity.

domains, two nucleotide binding domains, and a regulatory domain (R domain) that contains protein kinase A and C phosphorylation sites (Fig. 11–18). The two transmembrane domains form a channel through which chloride passes. At least 550 mutations of the cystic fibrosis gene have been identified. Commercial probes currently available test for only 70 of these mutations, although these account for greater than 90% of the abnormal genes.[64] The most common cystic fibrosis gene abnormality is a deletion of three nucleotides coding for phenylalanine at amino acid position 508 (ΔF508).[65] The ΔF508 mutation results in defective processing of the protein from the endoplasmic reticulum to the Golgi apparatus; the protein does not become fully folded and glycosylated and is instead degraded before it reaches the cell surface (Fig. 11–18, *bottom*; see also Chapter 2). Other mutations affect the synthesis of CFTR, nucleotide binding domains, and the R domains required for phosphorylation of CFTR, or the membrane-spanning domains essential for conduction.

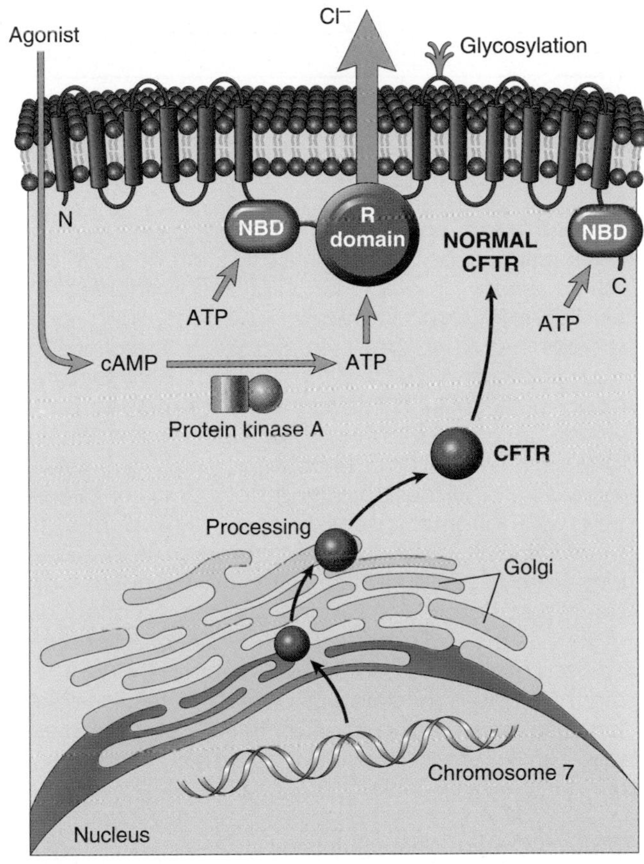

Figure 11–18

Top, Normal cystic fibrosis transmembrane conductance regulator (CFTR) structure and activation. CFTR consists of two transmembrane domains, two nucleotide-binding domains (NBD), and a regulatory R domain. Agonists (e.g., acetylcholine) bind to epithelial cells and increase cAMP, which activates protein kinase A, the latter phosphorylating the CFTR at the R domain, resulting in opening of the chloride channel. *Bottom*, CFTR from gene to protein. The most common mutation in the CFTR gene results in defective protein folding in the Golgi/ER and degradation of CFTR before it reaches the cell surface. Other mutations affect synthesis of CFTR, nucleotide-binding and R domains, and membrane-spanning domains.

Reliable prediction of clinical outcome based on the genotype is not yet possible for most mutations, and there is a great deal of variability in the magnitude of pulmonary disease within similar genotypes. Defects in additional chloride channels or in transport of other ions as well or involvement of alternative pathogenetic mechanisms may account for these discrepancies. There is a correlation, however, between the percentage of normal residual CFTR function and the presence of disease in various organs (Fig. 11–19).[65] On one end of the spectrum is virtual absence of membrane CFTR (as is the case with the homozygous ΔF508 mutation)—patients present with pancreatic insufficiency and variable degrees of pulmonary compromise.[65] On the opposite end are patients with relatively normal chloride transport (as is the case with some mutations involving the membrane-spanning domain); these patients have the mildest forms of cystic fibrosis and may present as congenital absence of the vas deferens and male sterility or certain isolated pulmonary diseases, such as allergic pulmonary aspergillosis.[66]

Secondary pathogenetic mechanisms play a role in cystic fibrosis. In the lung, for example, defective mucociliary action because of deficient hydration of the mucus results in inability of the airways to clear bacteria (Chapter 16). *Pseudomonas aeruginosa* species, in particular, colonize the lower respiratory tract, first intermittently and then chronically. Concurrent viral infections predispose to such colonization. In chronic infections, *Pseudomonas* species express abundant amounts of *alginate*, endowing the organisms with mucoid growth into microcolonies that are protected from antibodies or antibiotics, thus favoring persistence of the infection. Antibody and cell-mediated reactions induced by the organisms then result in further tissue destruction that characterizes the lung lesions in cystic fibrosis.

MORPHOLOGY. The anatomic changes are highly variable and depend on which glands are affected and on the severity of this involvement. In some infants, the disease is quite mild and does not seriously disturb their growth and development, and they readily survive into adolescence or adulthood. In others, the pancreatic involvement is severe and impairs intestinal absorption because of the pancreatic achylia, and so malabsorption, inanition, and stunted development not only seriously hamper life, but also shorten survival. In others, the mucus secretion defect leads to defective mucociliary action, obstruction of bronchi and bronchioles, and crippling fatal pulmonary infections (Fig. 11–20). Thus, cystic fibrosis may be compatible with long life or may cause death in infancy. Significantly the sweat glands, producing a watery secretion, are morphologically unaffected.

Pancreatic abnormalities are present in approximately 85 to 90% of patients. In the milder cases, there may be only accumulations of mucus in the small ducts with some dilation of the exocrine glands. In more advanced cases, usually seen in

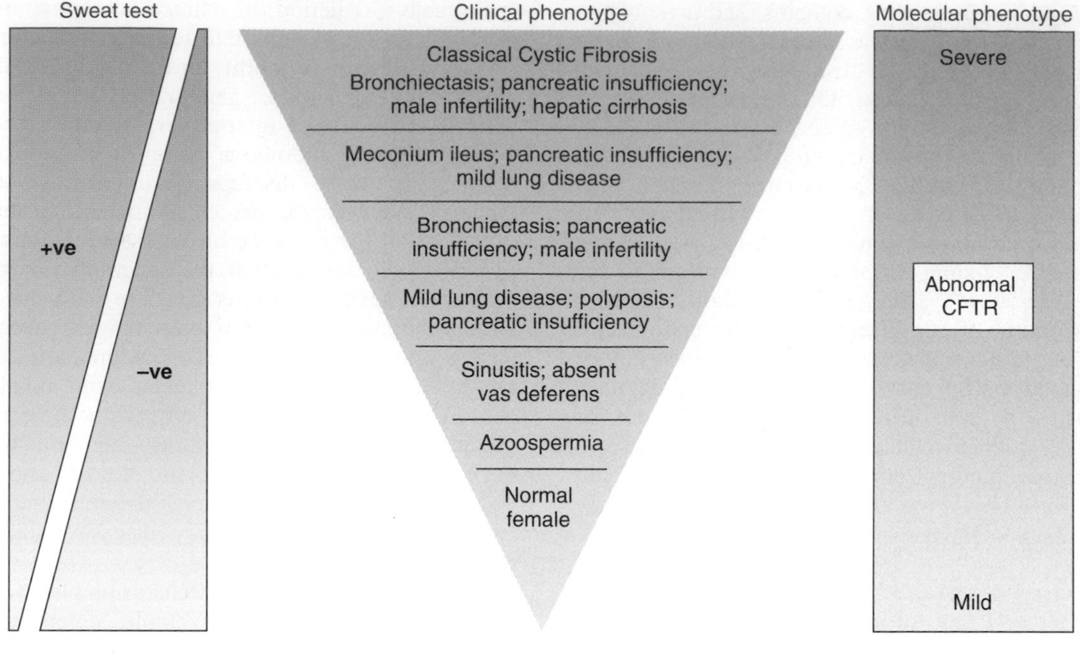

Figure 11–19

The many clinical manifestations of mutations in the cystic fibrosis gene, from most severe to asymptomatic. (Redrawn from Wallis C: Diagnosing cystic fibrosis: blood, sweat, and tears. Arch Dis Child *76*:85, 1997.)

older children or adolescents, the ducts are totally plugged, causing atrophy of the exocrine glands and progressive fibrosis (Fig. 11–21). Total atrophy of the exocrine portion of the pancreas may occur, leaving only the islets within a fibrofatty stroma. The total loss of pancreatic exocrine secretion impairs fat absorption, and so avitaminosis A may contribute to squamous metaplasia of the lining epithelium of the ducts in the pancreas, which are already injured by the inspissated mucus secretions. Thick viscid plugs of mucus may also be found in the small intestine of infants. Sometimes these cause small bowel obstruction, known as **meconium ileus.**

The **liver involvement** follows the same basic pattern. Bile canaliculi are plugged by mucinous material. When this is of long duration, biliary cirrhosis (Chapter 19) with its diffuse hepatic nodularity may develop. Such severe hepatic involvement is encountered in only approximately 5% of patients.

The **salivary glands** are frequently involved, with histologic changes similar to those described in the pancreas: progressive dilation of ducts, squamous metaplasia of the lining epithelium, and glandular atrophy followed by fibrosis.

The **pulmonary changes** are seen in almost every case and are the most serious complications of this disease. These stem from the viscous mucus secretions of the submucosal glands of the respiratory tree with secondary obstruction and infection of the air passages. The bronchioles are often distended with thick mucus associated with marked hyperplasia and hypertrophy of the mucus-secreting cells. Superimposed infections give rise to severe chronic bronchitis and bronchiectasis (Chapter 16). In many instances, lung abscesses develop. *Staphylococcus aureus* and *P. aeruginosa* are the two most common organisms responsible for lung infections. As mentioned previously, a mucoid form of *P. aeruginosa* is particularly frequent and causes chronic reactions. Even more sinister is the increasing frequency of infection with another pseudomonad, *Pseudomonas cepacia.* This opportunistic bacterium is particularly hardy, and infection with this organism has been associated with fulminant illness. A variety of other morphologic changes may be present; important among these is **the obstruction of the epididymis and vas deferens, which is responsible for azoospermia and infertility in 95% of the males who survive to adulthood.**

Clinical Course. Few childhood diseases are as protean as cystic fibrosis in clinical manifestations. The symptoms are extremely varied and range from mild to severe, from onset at birth to onset years later, and from involvement of one organ system to involvement of many. Approximately 5 to 10% of the cases come to clinical attention at birth or soon after because of an attack of meconium ileus. More commonly, manifestations of malabsorption (e.g., large, foul stools; abdominal distention; and poor weight gain) appear during the first year of life. The faulty fat absorption may induce deficiency states of the fat-soluble vitamins, resulting in manifestations of avitaminosis A, D, or

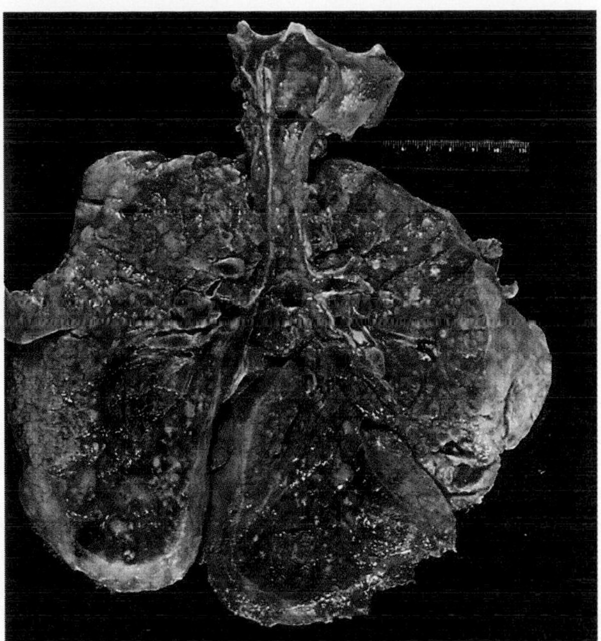

Figure 11–20 ■

Lungs of a patient dying of cystic fibrosis. There is extensive mucous plugging and dilation of the tracheobronchial tree. The pulmonary parenchyma is consolidated by a combination of both secretions and pneumonia—the green color associated with *Pseudomonas* infections. (Courtesy of Dr. Eduardo Yunis, Children's Hospital of Pittsburgh.)

K. If the child survives these hazards, pulmonary problems, such as chronic cough, persistent lung infections, obstructive pulmonary disease, and cor pulmonale, may make their appearance.

In most cases, the diagnosis of cystic fibrosis is based on persistently elevated sweat electrolyte concentrations (often the mother makes the diagnosis because her infant tastes salty) and characteristic clinical findings (gastrointestinal or pulmonary) or a family history.[66] A minority of patients with cystic fibrosis have a normal or near-normal sweat test. Therefore, in patients with suggestive clinical findings or family history (or both), genotyping may be warranted.

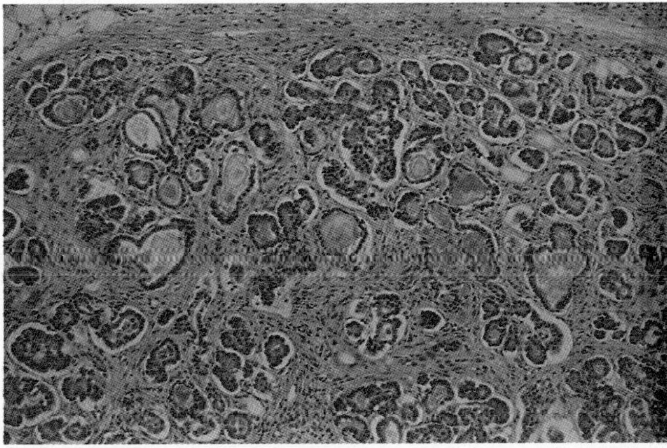

Figure 11–21 ■

Mild to moderate cystic fibrosis changes in the pancreas. The ducts are dilated and plugged with eosinophilic mucin, and the parenchymal glands are atrophic and replaced by fibrous tissue.

Recurrent pulmonary infections are responsible for 80 to 90% of the deaths in patients with cystic fibrosis. Advances in treatment include both improved control of infections and the viable option of bilateral lung (or lobar), heart-lung, liver, pancreas, or liver-pancreas transplantation. Children and adolescents undergoing bilateral lung transplantation have overall survival rates around 70%.[67] These improvements in management mean that more patients are now surviving to adulthood; the median life expectancy approaches 30 years and continues to increase. There are new reports suggesting an increased risk of digestive tract cancer in patients with cystic fibrosis.[68] These cancers affect the entire gastrointestinal system, the biliary tract, liver, and pancreas. The pathenogenesis of such cancers is unclear.

Cloning of the cystic fibrosis gene raises hope for eventual gene therapy. In vitro, it has been possible to correct the chloride defect in epithelial cells of cystic fibrosis patients efficiently by adenoviral transfer of the CFTR gene. Although currently unattainable, it may be possible with time to devise strategies for efficient transfer of the gene in vivo.[69]

SUDDEN INFANT DEATH SYNDROME

A panel convened by the National Institute of Child Health and Human Development defined *SIDS* as "the sudden death of an infant under 1 year of age which remains unexplained after a thorough case investigation, *including performance of a complete autopsy, examination of the death scene, and review of the clinical history.*"[70] An aspect of SIDS that is not stressed in the definition is that the infant usually dies while asleep, hence the pseudonyms of *crib death* or *cot death.*

Incidence and Epidemiology. SIDS is estimated to account for about 6000 deaths annually in the United States. As infantile deaths owing to nutritional problems and microbiologic infections have come under control in countries with higher standards of living, SIDS has assumed greater importance and in many countries, including the United States, is the most common cause of mortality in postnatal infants. Around the world, it causes from 1 to 5 deaths per 1000 live births.

Approximately 90% of all SIDS deaths occur during the first 6 months of life, most between the ages of 2 and 4 months. This narrow window of peak susceptibility is a unique characteristic that is independent of other risk factors (to be described) and the geographic locale. Most of these infants die at home, usually during the night after a period of sleep. Only rarely is the catastrophic event observed, but even when seen it is reported that the apparently healthy infant suddenly turns blue, stops breathing, and becomes limp without emitting a cry or struggling.

Most have had minor manifestations of an upper respiratory infection preceding the fatal event. The term *near-SIDS* has been applied to those infants who could be resuscitated after such an episode. Although this term is diagnostically imprecise and many such infants have definable underlying diseases, some of the apparently normal *near-misses* have been reported to succumb later to SIDS.

The circumstances surrounding SIDS have been explored in great detail, and it is generally accepted that it is a multifactorial condition, with variable contributing factors in an individual victim.[71] These factors may be attributable to the mother, infant, or environment. Among the potential environmental factors are a prone sleeping position and thermal stress. Results of studies from Europe, Australia, New Zealand, and the United States showed clearly increased risk in infants who sleep in a prone position, prompting the American Academy of Pediatrics to recommend placing healthy infants on their back or side when laying them down to sleep.[72] Population-based studies have also suggested that heavy wrapping and overnight heating may be risk factors for SIDS,[73] possibly related to developmental changes in thermoregulation between 8 and 16 weeks of age. A composite of other maternal and fetal factors associated with an increased risk of SIDS are summarized in Table 11–6. A number of these factors are features of infant deaths in general.

MORPHOLOGY. At autopsy, a variety of findings have been reported.[74] They are usually subtle and of uncertain significance and are not present in all cases. Within the respiratory system, there may be some histologic evidence of recent infection (correlating with the clinical symptoms), although the changes are generally considered not to be of lethal significance. The central nervous system shows astrogliosis of the brain stem. Nonspecific findings include frequent persistence of hepatic extramedullary hematopoiesis and periadrenal brown fat and an increased volume of adrenal chromaffin cells. It is tempting to speculate that many of these findings relate to chronic hypoxemia, retardation of normal development, and chronic stress. An increase in the thickness of small pulmonary arteries, cardiac right ventricular hypertrophy, and histologic abnormalities in the myocardial conduction system (in particular, the bundle of His and the sinoatrial node) have been reported by some authors, although the observations have not been confirmed by others. Finally, petechiae in the pleura and epicardium as well as pulmonary congestion and edema compatible with hypoxic death are often found, but these could be agonal changes. Thus, autopsy fails to provide a clear cause of death, and this may well be related to the possibility that SIDS is not a single entity.

Table 11–6. FACTORS ASSOCIATED WITH SUDDEN INFANT DEATH SYNDROME

Maternal	Infant
Young (<20 years of age)	Prematurity
Unmarried	Low birth weight
Short intergestational intervals	Male sex
Low socioeconomic group	Product of a multiple birth
Smoking	Not the first sibling
Drug abuse (e.g., methadone)	SIDS in a prior sibling
Risk greater for American blacks than whites (?socioeconomic)	

Pathogenesis. Although the cause of SIDS remains unknown, it is now thought that SIDS is a heterogeneous entity sometimes caused by specific disorders. For example, a *deficiency in medium-chain acyl-coenzyme A dehydrogenase* is present in some infants clinically presenting with sudden, unexpected death. It has been estimated that approximately 10% of SIDS cases are due to an inborn error in metabolism.

As to "idiopathic" SIDS, there is currently agreement on two issues. One is that some of the events thought to occur in SIDS, such as *apnea* and *abnormal temperature control*, are related to the other neonatal risk factors cited, including prematurity and birth weight. The other is that the underlying pathophysiology in many cases may originate in utero. It is postulated that there is a group of infants with subtle developmental abnormalities who are subsequently at risk for sudden death during the first 6 months of life, a time when integration of numerous, complex autonomic functions is being accomplished. Because of the finding of astrogliosis in the brain stem, as well as the importance of this area in integrating cardiopulmonary function and arousal mechanisms, some of the studies focus on abnormalities in this region,[75] and particularly in the arcuate nucleus.[76, 76a] According to this scenario, a developmental delay may be a critical abnormality in the pathophysiology of SIDS.

As mentioned at the outset, it is likely that SIDS is a heterogeneous, multifactorial disorder. Thus, it might be expected that further investigations will allow an increasing number of patients to be moved from the *unexplained* to the *explained* category, permitting fewer *maybe's*.

TUMORS AND TUMOR-LIKE LESIONS OF INFANCY AND CHILDHOOD

Only 2% of all malignant tumors occur in infancy and childhood; nonetheless, cancer (including leukemia) is the leading cause of death from disease in the United States in children over the age of 4 and up to 14 years of age. Neoplastic disease accounts for approximately 9% of all deaths in this cohort; only accidents cause significantly more deaths. Benign tumors are even more common than cancers. Most benign tumors are of little concern, but on occasion they cause serious disease by virtue of their location or rapid increase in size.

It is sometimes difficult to segregate, on morphologic grounds, true tumors or neoplasms from tumor-like lesions in the infant and child. In this context, two special categories of tumor-like lesions have been created.

The term *heterotopia* (or *choristoma*) is applied to microscopically normal cells or tissues that are present in abnormal locations. Examples of heterotopias include a rest of pancreatic tissue found in the wall of the stomach or small intestine or a small mass of adrenal cells found in the kidney, lungs, ovaries, or elsewhere. The heterotopic rests are usually of little significance, but they can be confused clinically with neoplasms. Rarely, they are sites of origin of true neoplasms, producing the paradox of an adrenal carcinoma arising in the ovary.

The term *hamartoma* refers to an excessive but focal overgrowth of cells and tissues native to the organ in which it occurs. Although the cellular elements are mature and identical to those found in the remainder of the organ, they do not reproduce the normal architecture of the surrounding tissue. Hamartomas can be thought of as the linkage between malformations and neoplasms—the line of demarcation between a hamartoma and a benign neoplasm is frequently tenuous and is variously interpreted. Hemangiomas; lymphangiomas; rhabdomyomas of the heart; adenomas of the liver; and developmental cysts within the kidneys, lungs, or pancreas are interpreted by some as hamartomas and by others as true neoplasms. The frequency of these lesions in infancy and childhood and their clinical behavior give credence to the belief that many are developmental aberrations. Their unequivocally benign histology, however, does not preclude bothersome and rarely life-threatening clinical problems in some cases.

Benign Tumors and Tumor-Like Lesions

Reference has already been made to the difficulty in distinguishing benign tumors from hamartomas. Benign neoplasms are far more common in infancy and childhood than are cancers. Virtually any tumor may be encountered, but within this wide array hemangiomas, lymphangiomas, fibrous lesions, and teratomas deserve special mention. They are described in greater detail in appropriate chapters, but here a few comments are made about their special features in childhood.

- *Hemangiomas*: Hemangiomas (Chapter 12) are the most common tumors of infancy. Architecturally, they do not differ from those encountered in adults. In children, most are located in the skin, particularly on the face and scalp, where they produce flat-to-elevated, irregular, red-blue masses; some of the flat, larger lesions (considered by some to represent vascular ectasias) are referred to as *port-wine stains*. Hemangiomas may enlarge along with the growth of the child, but in many instances they spontaneously regress (Fig. 11–22). In addition to their cosmetic significance, they can represent one facet of the hereditary disorder, von Hippel–Lindau disease (Chapter 21). Rarely, vascular tumors, particularly those in the liver and soft tissues, become malignant.
- *Lymphatic tumors*: A wide variety of lesions are of lymphatic origin. Some of them—*lymphangiomas*—are hamartomatous or neoplastic in origin, whereas others appear to represent abnormal dilations of preexisting lymph channels known as *lymphangiectasis*. The *lymphangiomas* are usually characterized by cystic and cavernous spaces. Lesions of this nature may occur on the skin but, more important, are encountered in the deeper regions of the neck, axilla, mediastinum, retroperitoneal tissue, and elsewhere. Although histologically benign, they tend to increase in size after birth, both by the collection of fluid and by the budding of preexisting spaces. In this manner, they may encroach on vital structures, such as those in the mediastinum or nerve trunks in the axilla, to constitute clinical problems. *Lymphangiectasis*, in contrast, usually presents as a diffuse swelling of part or all of an extremity; considerable

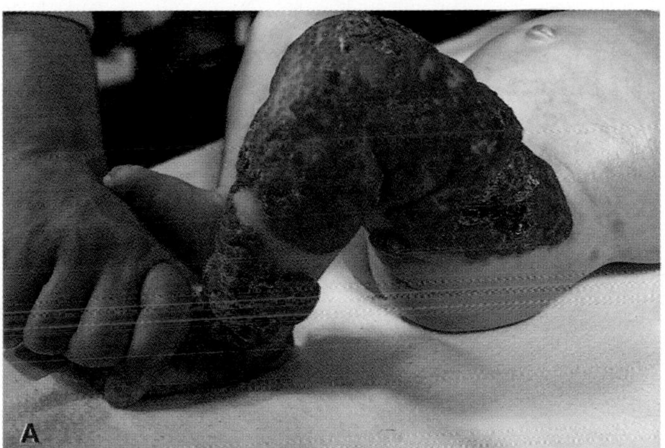

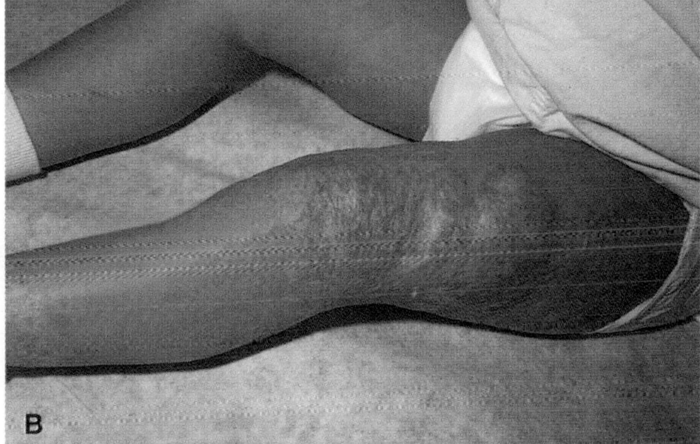

Figure 11–22

Congenital capillary hemangioma at birth (*A*) and at 2 years of age (*B*) after spontaneous regression. (Courtesy of Dr. Eduardo Yunis, Children's Hospital of Pittsburgh.)

distortion and deformation may result as a consequence of the spongy, dilated subcutaneous and deeper lymphatics. The lesion is not progressive, however, and does not extend beyond its original location. Nonetheless, it gives rise to difficult corrective cosmetic problems.

- *Fibrous tumors*: Fibrous tumors occurring in infants and children range from sparsely cellular proliferations of spindle-shaped cells (designated as *fibromatosis*) to richly cellular lesions indistinguishable from fibrosarcomas occurring in adults. Biologic behavior cannot be predicted based on histology alone, however, because some of the lesions (including the cellular fibromatoses or infantile fibrosarcomas) may spontaneously regress. In some of these soft tissue fibrous lesions, a variable proportion of the cells acquire a moderate amount of pink cytoplasm and express muscle-specific actin. These *myofibromatoses* present in infants and younger children, and although usually solitary, they may be multifocal, involving any organ. Solitary lesions are benign, but multifocal lesions may result in significant morbidity and mortality when they involve vital organs.
- *Teratomas*: Teratomas (Chapter 8) illustrate the relationship of histologic maturity to biologic behavior. They may occur as benign, well-differentiated cystic lesions or as solid malignant (immature) teratomas. They exhibit two peaks in incidence: the first at approximately 2 years of age and the second in late adolescence or early adulthood. The first peak represents congenital neoplasms; the later-occurring lesions may also be of prenatal origin but more slowly growing. *Most teratomas of infancy and childhood arise in the sacrococcygeal region.* Other sites include the testis (Chapter 23), ovaries (Chapter 24), and various midline locations, such as the mediastinum, retroperitoneum, and head and neck.

Sacrococcygeal teratomas occur in 1 in 20,000 to 40,000 live births, four times more frequently in girls than in boys (Fig. 11–23). Occasionally diagnosed by prenatal imaging studies, these tumors may be associated with nonimmune hydrops fetalis or polyhydramnios and, depending on their size, may necessitate cesarean section delivery. In view of the overlap in the mechanisms underlying teratogenesis and oncogenesis, it is interesting that approximately 10% of sacrococcygeal teratomas are associated with congenital anomalies, primarily defects of the hindgut and cloacal region and other midline defects (meningocele, spina bifida), not believed to be due to the local effects of the tumor. Approximately 75% of these tumors are histologically mature (Chapter 24) with a benign course, and about 12% are unmistakably malignant (containing endodermal sinus tumor) and lethal. The remainder are designated as immature teratomas, and their malignant potential correlates with the amount of immature tissue elements present. Most of the benign teratomas are encountered in younger infants (<4 months), whereas children with malignant lesions tend to be somewhat older.

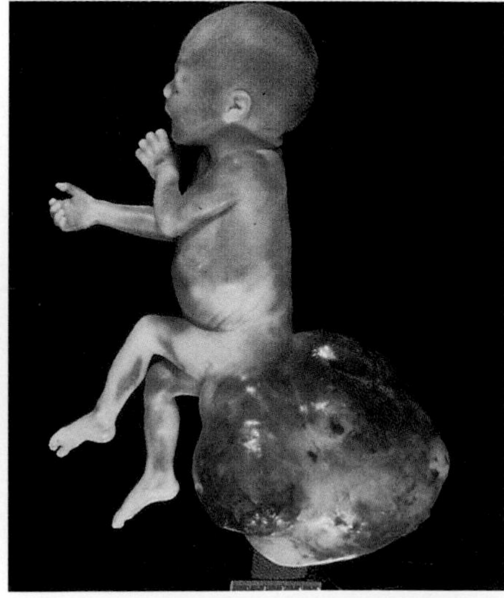

Figure 11–23

Sacrococcygeal teratoma. Note the size of the lesion compared with that of the infant.

Malignant Tumors

Cancers of infancy and childhood differ biologically and histologically from their counterparts occurring later in life. The main differences, some of which have already been alluded to, include the following:

- Incidence and type of tumor[77]
- Relatively frequent demonstration of a close relationship between abnormal development (teratogenesis) and tumor induction (oncogenesis)
- Prevalence of underlying familial or genetic aberrations
- Tendency of fetal and neonatal malignancies to regress spontaneously or cytodifferentiate[78]
- Improved survival or cure of many childhood tumors, so that more attention is now being paid to minimizing the adverse delayed effects of chemotherapy and radiotherapy in survivors, including the development of second malignancies

INCIDENCE AND TYPES

The most frequent childhood cancers arise in the hematopoietic system, nervous tissue (including the central and sympathetic nervous system, adrenal medulla, and retina), soft tissues, bone, and kidney. This is in sharp contrast to adults, in whom the skin, lung, breast, prostate, and colon are the most common sites of tumors.

Neoplasms that exhibit sharp peaks in incidence in children younger than 10 years of age include (1) leukemia (principally acute lymphoblastic leukemia); (2) neuroblastoma; (3) Wilms' tumor; (4) hepatoblastoma; (5) retinoblastoma; (6) rhabdomyosarcoma; (7) teratoma; (8) Ewing sarcoma; and, finally, posterior fossa neoplasms—principally (9) juvenile astrocytoma, (10) medulloblastoma, and (11) ependymoma. Other forms of cancer are also common in childhood but do not have the same striking early peak. The age distribution of these cancers is roughly indicated in Table 11–7. Within this large array, leukemia alone

Table 11–7. COMMON MALIGNANT NEOPLASMS OF INFANCY AND CHILDHOOD

0 to 4 Years	5 to 9 Years	10 to 14 Years
Leukemia	Leukemia	
Retinoblastoma	Retinoblastoma	
Neuroblastoma	Neuroblastoma	
Wilms' tumor		
Hepatoblastoma	Hepatocarcinoma	Hepatocarcinoma
Soft tissue sarcoma (especially rhabdomyosarcoma)	Soft tissue sarcoma	Soft tissue sarcoma
Teratomas		
Central nervous system tumors	Central nervous system tumors	
	Ewing sarcoma	
	Lymphoma	Osteogenic sarcoma
		Thyroid carcinoma
		Hodgkin disease

accounts for more deaths in children younger than 15 years of age than all of the other tumors collectively.

Histologically, many of the malignant pediatric neoplasms are unique. In general, they tend to have a more primitive (embryonal) rather than pleomorphic-anaplastic microscopic appearance and frequently exhibit features of organogenesis specific to the site of tumor origin. Because of this latter characteristic, these tumors are frequently designated by the suffix *-blastoma*, for example, nephroblastoma (Wilms' tumor), hepatoblastoma, and neuroblastoma.

Owing to their primitive histologic appearance, many childhood tumors have been collectively referred to as *small round blue cell tumors*. These are characterized by sheets of cells with small, round nuclei. The differential diagnosis of such tumors includes neuroblastoma, lymphoma, rhabdomyosarcoma, Ewing sarcoma (peripheral neuroectodermal tumor), and occasionally Wilms' tumor. Rendering a definitive diagnosis is usually possible on histologic examination alone, but, when necessary, clinical and radiographic findings combined with ancillary studies, such as chromosome analysis, immunoperoxidase stains, and electron microscopy, are used. The diagnostic features associated with the more common childhood neoplasms are summarized in Table 11–8. Two of these tumors are particularly illustrative and are discussed here: neuroblastoma and Wilms' tumor. The remaining tumors are discussed in their respective organ-specific chapters.

Neuroblastoma and Ganglioneuroma

Neuroblastoma is one of the most common childhood solid tumors and is the most common tumor diagnosed in infants less than 1 year of age. Approximately 500 new cases are diagnosed each year.[79] Alone, it accounts for at least 15% of all childhood cancer deaths, although the 5-year survival rate has improved from 25% in the early 1960s to almost 60% in the late 1980s.[80] There are different clinicobiologic subsets of neuroblastoma, ranging from those that rarely kill, however hopeless the clinical situation may appear to be, to those that rapidly cause death despite all therapeutic efforts. Although the vast majority of tumors occur sporadically, familial occurrence has been rarely noted.

MORPHOLOGY. In childhood, about 25 to 35% of neuroblastomas arise in the adrenal medulla. The remainder occur anywhere along the sym-

Table 11–8. GENETIC AND OTHER USEFUL MARKERS OF SMALL ROUND CELL TUMORS OF CHILDHOOD

Tumor Type	Genetic Markers	Other Diagnostically Useful Features
Neuroblastoma	■ 1p deletion*, N-*myc* amplification* DNA hyperdiploidy†	■ Clinical elevation in level of urinary catecholamines Neurosecretory granules by electron microscopy
Ewing sarcoma/PNET	■ t(11;22)‡, t(21;22), t(7;22)	■ MIC2 gene expression
Rhabdomyosarcoma	■ t(2;13)‡*, t(1;13)—alveolar rhabdomyosarcoma[78a] ■ Chromosome 11p deletion—embryonal rhabdomyosarcoma	■ Desmin or actin expression Alternating thick and thin filaments by electron microscopy
Burkitt lymphoma	■ t(8;14)‡	■ B cell; most commonly expressing IgM, κ light chains
Lymphoblastic lymphoma/acute lymphoblastic leukemia	■ DNA hyperdiploidy† Various translocations, including t(9;22)*	■ T cell markers (Chapter 15)
Wilms' tumor	■ 11p13 deletion/mutation 11p15.5 deletion/mutation 16q13 deletion	
Retinoblastoma	■ 13q14 deletion/mutation	
Medulloblastoma	■ Isochromosome 17q	

*Generally associated with a poorer prognosis.
†Generally associated with a better prognosis.
‡Most common translocation.
PNET, peripheral neuroectodermal tumor.

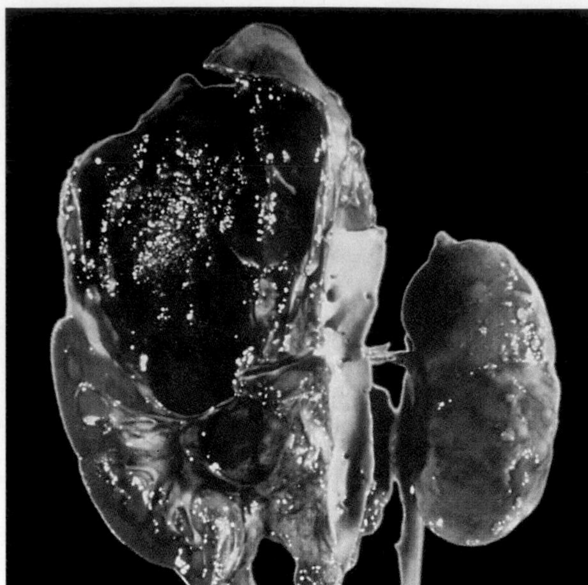

Figure 11–24

Adrenal neuroblastoma in a 6-month-old child. The hemorrhagic, partially encapsulated tumor has displaced the opened left kidney and is impinging on the aorta and left renal artery. (Courtesy of Dr. Arthur Weinberg, University of Texas Southwestern Medical School, Dallas, TX.)

pathetic chain, with the second most common location being the paravertebral region of the posterior mediastinum. Closely following is the paravertebral region in the lower abdomen, but tumors may arise in numerous other sites, including the pelvis and neck and within the brain. By contrast, rare neuroblastomas in adults are found in the head, neck, and legs.

Macroscopically, neuroblastomas range in size from minute nodules (the **in situ lesions**) to large masses more than 1 kg in weight (Fig. 11–24). In situ neuroblastomas are reported to be 40 times more frequent than overt tumors. The great preponderance of these lesions spontaneously regress leaving only a focus of fibrosis or calcification in the adult. Some clinically overt neuroblastomas have regressed or, alternatively, have undergone differentiation and maturation into a relatively benign ganglioneuroma. Some neuroblastomas are sharply demarcated and may appear encapsulated, but others are far more infiltrative and invade surrounding structures, such as the kidneys, renal vein, and vena cava, and envelop the aorta. On transection, they are composed of soft, gray, **brainlike** tissue. Larger tumors have areas of necrosis, cystic softening, and hemorrhage. Occasionally, foci of calcification can be palpated.

Histologically, most neuroblastomas are composed of small, primitive-appearing cells with dark nuclei, scant cytoplasm, and poorly defined cell borders growing in solid sheets. Such tumors may be difficult to differentiate from other **small, blue, round cell tumors**. In characteristic lesions, rosettes (Homer-Wright pseudorosettes) can be found in which the tumor cells are arranged about a central space filled with fibrillar extensions of the cells (Fig. 11–25). The number of mitotic/karyorrhectic cells and the amount of schwannian stroma present may be used to help classify a tumor as having either **favorable** or **unfavorable** histology.[81] Certain neuroblastomas reveal some level of differentiation. Clusters of scattered larger cells resembling ganglion cells and characterized by more abundant cytoplasm, large vesicular nuclei, and a prominent nucleolus may be present in tumors composed largely of primitive neuroblasts. Even better-differentiated lesions may contain many more ganglion cells. In the most well-differentiated lesions, comprised of ganglion cells and Schwann cells, neuroblasts are no longer present, and the neoplasm merits the diagnosis of **ganglioneuroma**.

Metastases, when they develop, appear early and widely. In addition to local infiltration and lymph node spread, there is a pronounced tendency to spread through the bloodstream to involve the liver, lungs, and bones. A staging system for this tumor is as follows:

- Stage I: Tumor confined to the organ of origin
- Stage II: Tumor extends in continuity beyond organ of origin but does not cross the midline; ipsilateral lymph nodes may or may not be involved.
- Stage III: Tumor extends in continuity beyond the midline; ipsilateral beyond the midline, ipsilateral lymph nodes may or may not be involved.
- Stage IV: Metastatic disease to the viscera, distal lymph nodes, soft tissue, and skeleton
- Stage IV-S (Special): Small adrenal tumors and extensive disease infiltrating the liver, skin, or

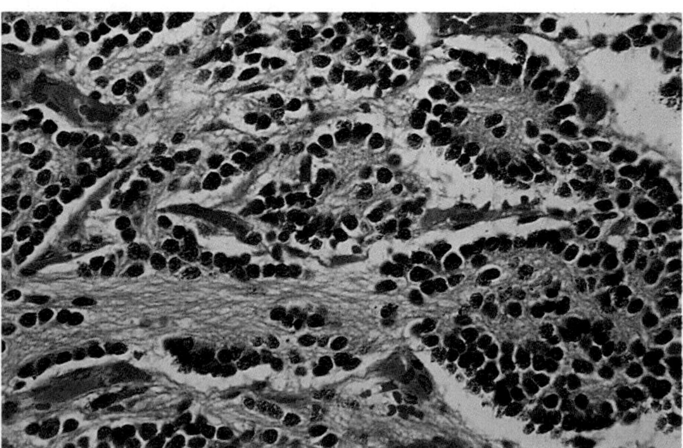

Figure 11–25

Adrenal neuroblastoma. This tumor is composed of small cells embedded in a finely fibrillar matrix.

bone marrow (without evidence of bony destruction)

The staging system is of particular importance with neuroblastomas, as becomes evident subsequently.

Clinical Course and Biologic Features. In young children, under 2 years of age, neuroblastomas generally present with large abdominal masses, fever, and possibly weight loss. In older children, they may not come to attention until metastases produce manifestations, such as bone pain, respiratory symptoms, or gastrointestinal complaints. Proptosis and ecchymosis may also be present because the periorbital region is a common metastatic site. The course of these neoplasms is extremely variable, and, as indicated earlier, there appear to be distinctive subsets based on many variables.

- *Age* and *stage* are important determinants of outcome. Infants younger than 1 year of age have an excellent prognosis regardless of the stage of the neoplasm. Most often in this age group, the neoplasms are stage I or II. At this early age, even when metastases are present, in about half the spread is limited to the liver, bone marrow, and skin (stage IV-S), and such infants have at least an 80% 5-year survival with only minimal therapy. Even when the dissemination is more widespread in the first year of life, the survival is greater than 50%. At this age with stages I or II, therapy yields a 95 to 98% survival. Children older than 1 year of age with stages III and IV tumor have only a 10% survival despite all forms of treatment.
- Ploidy of the tumor cells correlates with outcome. The hyperdiploid or near-triploid tumors occurring in infants have a particularly good prognosis, whereas the near-diploid tumors occurring at any age tend to have an unfavorable outcome. The overall DNA content tends to correlate with cytogenetic findings in that structural chromosomal abnormalities (deletions, translocations, amplification) are much more common in the diploid tumors or those hyperdiploid tumors occurring in older patients.
- Deletion of the distal short arm of chromosome 1 in the region of band p36 (determined either karyotypically or by loss of heterozygosity) is the most characteristic cytogenetic abnormality in neuroblastomas and has been demonstrated in 70 to 80% of tumors with a diploid or near-diploid content of DNA. The loss of genetic material implies that a tumor-suppressor gene in this region may be important in the evolution of this subset of tumors. Tumors with chromosome 1 deletions have a worse prognosis. Deletions involving the long arm of chromosome 14 are present in 25 to 50% of neuroblastomas and may also be associated with more aggressive tumor behavior.
- Amplification of N-*myc* oncogene is karyotypically manifest as double minutes or homogeneously staining regions and is present in about 25% of primary tumors (Fig. 11–26). Up to 300 copies of N-*myc* have been observed in some tumors; the greater the number of copies, the greater the number of double minutes and homogeneously staining regions and the worse the prognosis. N-*myc* amplification tends to occur in advanced stage tumors with chromosome 1p deletions.
- The differentiation and regression of neuroblastomas appear to be at least partially affected by nerve growth factor and its high-affinity receptor, Trk A. High levels of expression of the Trk A gene are associated with a favorable outcome and almost always occur in tumors lacking N-*myc* amplification.

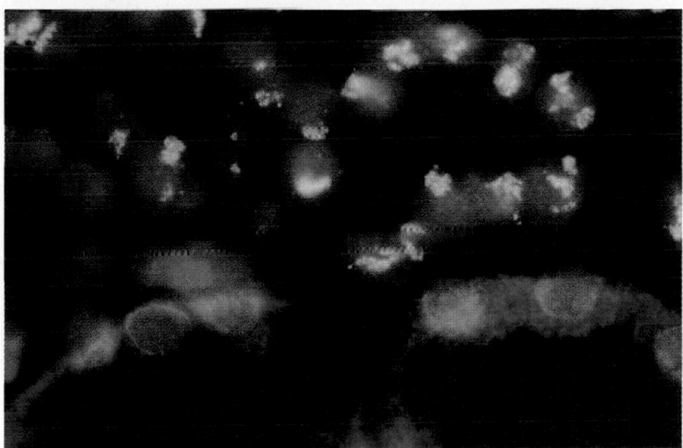

Figure 11–26 ■

Fluorescence in situ hybridization using a fluorescein-labeled cosmid probe for N-*myc* on a tissue section. Note the neuroblastoma cells on the upper half of the photo with large areas of staining (yellow-green); this corresponds to amplified N-*myc* in the form of homogeneously staining regions. Renal tubular epithelial cells in the lower half of the photograph show no nuclear staining and background (green) cytoplasmic staining. (Courtesy of Dr. Timothy Triche, Children's Hospital, Los Angeles, CA.)

In general, based on many of the aforementioned factors, neuroblastomas can be classified into three groups.[82, 83] The first group is characterized by a hyperdiploid or near-triploid content of DNA and high levels of Trk A expression in the absence of N-*myc* amplification and chromosome 1p deletions. These tumors tend to occur in infants with low stage (I, II, or IV-S) disease, and the cure rate is greater than 90%. The second group is characterized by a near-diploid or tetraploid DNA content, absence of N-*myc* amplification, frequent chromosome 1p deletions, and usually low levels of Trk A expression. These tumors tend to occur in older patients with more advanced stage (III or IV) and are slowly progressive with a cure rate of 25 to 50%. The third and final group of neuroblastomas has multiple unfavorable features and is associated with the worst prognosis and a cure rate of less than 5%. These neuroblastomas tend to occur in children between 1 and 5 years of age with advanced stage disease and are characterized by N-*myc* amplification, usually in the presence of a diploid or tetraploid DNA content, chromosome 1p deletions, and minimal Trk A expression.

Wilms' Tumor

Wilms' tumor is the most common primary renal tumor of childhood, usually diagnosed between the ages of 2 and

5 years. Its biology and histology illustrate many of the important concepts of childhood neoplasia: the relationship between malformations and neoplasia, premalignant lesions and the two-hit theory of oncogenesis, the similarity between tumor and developmental histology, and the potential for treatment modalities to affect prognosis and outcome dramatically.

Pathogenesis and Genetics. The risk of Wilms' tumor is increased in association with at least three recognizable groups of congenital malformations exhibiting aberrations in at least two distinct chromosomal loci.[84]

- The first group of patients have the *WAGR syndrome* characterized by *a*niridia, *g*enital anomalies, and mental *r*etardation and have a 33% chance of developing *W*ilms' tumor. Studies of these patients led to the identification of an autosomal dominant gene for aniridia within band p13 on chromosome 11. Slightly proximal to this, also within band p13, is the Wilms' tumor–associated gene, WT-1 (Table 11–9) (Chapter 8). Many infants with WAGR syndrome have a sporadic deletion of genetic material at 11p13 that includes both of these loci. The development of Wilms' tumor in these patients frequently correlates with the presence of nonsense or frameshift mutation in the second WT-1 allele. Approximately 5% of patients with sporadic Wilms' tumors appear to have mutations in WT-1. It has already been noted in the discussion of congenital malformations that the WT-1 protein is expressed within the kidney and gonads of the developing human fetus and that transgenic mice lacking both copies of the WT-1 locus have renal agenesis.
- A second group of patients at risk for Wilms' tumor have the *Denys-Drash syndrome*, which is characterized by gonadal dysgenesis (male pseudohermaphroditism) and nephropathy leading to renal failure. The majority of these patients develop Wilms' tumors. As in patients with WAGR, the genetic abnormality in these children has also been mapped to chromosome 11, p13. In patients with Denys-Drash syndrome, however, the genetic abnormality is a dominant negative missense mutation in the WT-1 gene that affects its DNA-binding properties, rather than a deletion. There may be some clinical overlap between these two groups of patients, depending on the size and nature of the 11p13 deletion or mutation.
- Clinically distinct from these previous two groups of patients but also having an increased risk of developing Wilms' tumor are those children with *Beckwith-Wiedemann syndrome*, characterized by enlargement of body organs, hemihypertrophy, renal medullary cysts, and abnormal large cells in adrenal cortex (adrenal cytomegaly). The genetic locus that is involved in these patients is in band p15.5 of chromosome 11 distal to the WT-1 locus. The function of this second Wilms' tumor gene (WT-2) is unknown. Selected loss of maternal alleles in this group of patients with Wilms' tumors, combined with the demonstration of uniparental paternal disomy for 11p15.5 in sporadic cases of Beckwith-Wiedemann syndrome, indicates a role for *genomic imprinting* at the WT-2 locus.[85] In addition, patients with Beckwith-Wiedemann syndrome are also at increased risk for developing hepatoblastoma, adrenocortical tumors, rhabdomyosarcomas, and pancreatic tumors.

A few familial cases of Wilms' tumors not associated with identifiable deletions or mutations involving either the WT-1 or the WT-2 gene suggest that there may be another locus that plays a role in some tumors (WT-3), but it remains unknown.

Related to the molecular genetic and corresponding heterogeneity of Wilms' tumor is the recognition of a *premalignant* or precursor lesion in many of these cases—*nephroblastomatosis.* This term refers to multicentric or diffuse foci of immature nephrogenic elements within areas of otherwise non-neoplastic kidney parenchyma.[86] Recognition of this lesion is important because its presence implies a substantially increased risk of developing a Wilms' tumor.

Table 11–9. WILMS' TUMOR–ASSOCIATED GENE WT-1

Location	■ Chromosome 11p13
Protein/function	■ Transcription factor
Embryonic expression	■ Early Intermediate mesoderm Mesenchyme of metanephros Epithelial cells of nephric tubules Later Mesothelium, spinal cord, brain, spleen Derivatives of urogenital ridge
Developmental anomalies	■ WT-1 homozygous deletion Renal and gonadal agenesis, incomplete mesothelium (mice) Heterozygous gross deletions WAGR syndrome: *W*ilms' tumor susceptibility, *a*niridia, *g*enitourinary malformations, mental *r*etardation Dominant missense point mutations Denys-Drash syndrome: ambiguous genitalia, streak gonads, renal failure, increased susceptibility to Wilms' tumor
Cancer	■ Wilms' tumor

MORPHOLOGY. Grossly, Wilms' tumor tends to present as a large, solitary, well-circumscribed mass, although 10% are either bilateral or multicentric at the time of diagnosis. On cut section, the tumor is soft, homogeneous, and tan to gray with occasional foci of hemorrhage, cyst formation, and necrosis (Fig. 11–27).

Microscopically, Wilms' tumors are characterized by recognizable attempts to recapitulate different stages of nephrogenesis. The classic triphasic combination of blastemic, stromal, and epithelial cell types is observed in the vast majority of lesions, although the percentage of each component is variable (Fig. 11–28). Epithelial **differentiation** is usually in the form of abortive tubules or glomeruli. Stromal cells are usually fibrocytic or myxoid in nature, although skeletal muscle **differ-**

Figure 11–27

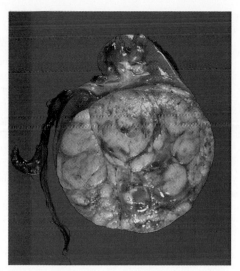

Wilms' tumor in the lower pole of the kidney with the characteristic tan to gray color and well-circumscribed margins.

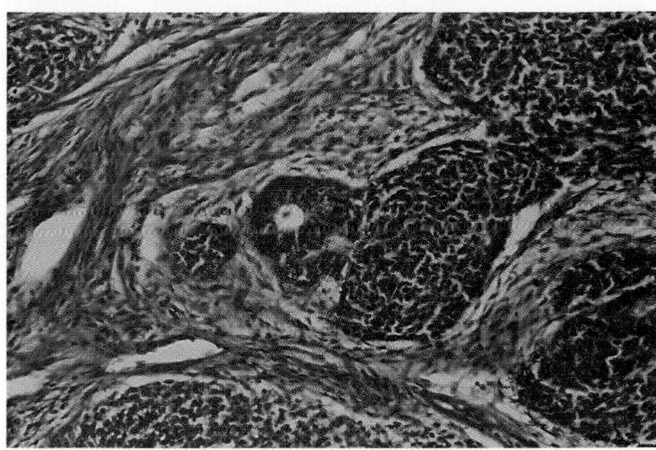

Figure 11–28

Triphasic histology of Wilms' tumor with a stromal, less cellular area on the left, spindle-shaped cells, and epithelial (one clear tubule in the center) and blastemic (tightly packed blue cells) elements. (Courtesy of Dr. Charles Timmons, Department of Pathology, University of Texas Southwestern Medical School, Dallas TX.)

entiation is not uncommon. Rarely, other heterologous elements are identified, including squamous or mucinous epithelium, smooth muscle, adipose tissue, cartilage, and osteoid and neurogenic tissue. Wilms' tumors are histologically heterogeneous—the percentage of each of the three components is variable within a given tumor and may correlate with tumor aggressiveness. For example, most tumors comprised predominantly of epithelial elements tend to present as stage I (confined to the kidney), whereas most tumors comprised primarily of blastema present as stage III or IV. Another histologic marker of tumor biology is anaplasia, defined as the presence of cells with large, hyperchromatic, pleomorphic nuclei and abnormal mitoses. Approximately 5% of tumors contain foci of anaplasia, a feature that appears to correlate with resistance to therapy and is therefore particularly important in tumors not amenable to complete surgical resection.[87]

Clinical Features. Most children with Wilms' tumors present with a large abdominal mass that may be unilateral or, when very large, may extend across the midline and down into the pelvis. Hematuria, pain in the abdomen after some traumatic incident, intestinal obstruction, and appearance of hypertension are other patterns of presentation. In a considerable number of these patients, pulmonary metastases are present at the time of primary diagnosis.

Up to the mid-1960s, the 5-year survival rate of these patients was low (10 to 40%), a tragedy rendered the more poignant because of the age of the patients. The combined use of chemotherapy, radiotherapy, and surgery, however, has produced dramatic results in patients whose lesions were previously thought to be inoperable. Most large centers now report 90% long-term survival rates if the tumors are available for primary treatment with the three modalities mentioned. Even recurrences can be successfully treated.

Along with the increased survival of patients with Wilms' tumor have come reports of an increased relative risk of developing second primary tumors. Although many of these tumors can be attributed to therapy, studies of families of these patients suggest a possible association of Wilms' tumor with bone and soft tissue sarcomas, leukemia and lymphomas, brain tumors, and genitourinary tumors.[88]

REFERENCES

1. Guyer B, et al: Annual summary of vital statistics—1995. Pediatrics 98:1007, 1996.
2. Palo P, Erkkola R: Risk factors and deliveries associated with preterm, severely small for gestational age fetuses. Am J Perinatol 10:88, 1993.
3. Soothill PW, et al: Diagnosis of intrauterine growth retardation and its fetal and perinatal consequences. Acta Paediatr 399(suppl):55, 1994.
4. Pearce JK, Campbell S: Intrauterine growth retardation. Birth Defects 21:109, 1985.
5. Clapp JF: The clinical significance of asymmetric intrauterine growth retardation. Pediatr Ann 25:223, 1996.
6. Kalousek D: Confined placental mosaicism and intrauterine development. Pediatr Pathol 10:69, 1990.
7. Levene MI, Dubowitz V: Intrauterine growth retardation. In Stern L, Vert P (eds): Neonatal Medicine. New York, Masson Publishing USA, 1987, p 107.
8. Apgar V: A proposal for a new method of evaluation of the newborn infant. Curr Res Anesth Analg 32:260, 1953.
9. Drage JS, Berendes H: Apgar scores and outcome of the newborn. Pediatr Clin North Am 13:635, 1966.
10. Jepson HA, et al: The Apgar score: evolution, limitations, and scoring guidelines. Birth 18:83, 1991.
11. Gresham EL: Birth trauma. Pediatr Clin North Am 22:317, 1975.
12. Andre M, Vert P: Birth injury. In Stern L, Vert P (eds): Neonatal Medicine. New York, Masson Publishing USA, 1987, p 176.

13. Shepard TH: Human teratogenicity. Adv Pediatr 33:225, 1986.
14. Jones KL (ed): Smith's Recognizable Patterns of Human Malformation, 5th ed. Philadelphia, WB Saunders, 1997.
15. Winter RM: Analysing human developmental abnormalities. BioEssays 18:965, 1996.
16. Stevenson RE: The environmental basis of human anomalies. In Stevenson RE, et al (eds): Human Malformations and Related Anomalies, Vol 1. New York, Oxford University Press, 1993.
17. Beckman DA, Brent RL: Mechanism of known environmental teratogens: drugs and chemicals. Clin Perinatol 13:649, 1986.
18. Jones KL: The fetal alcohol syndrome. Growth Genet Horm 4:1, 1988.
19. Edmonds LD, et al: Temporal trends in the birth prevalence of selected congenital malformations in the birth defects monitoring program/commission on professional and hospital activities, 1979–1989. Teratology 48:647, 1993.
20. Lyons KM, Hogan BLM: The DVR gene family in embryonic development. In Robertson LJ, et al (eds): Cell-Cell Signaling in Vertebrate Development. New York, Academic Press, 1993.
21. Ardinger HH, et al: Association of genetic variation in TGFX gene in the cleft lip and palate. Am J Hum Genet 45:348, 1990.
22. Kreidberg JA, et al: WT-1 is required for early kidney development. Cell 74:679, 1993.
23. George E, et al: Defects in mesoderm, neural tube, and vascular development in mouse embryos lacking fibronectin. Development 119:1079, 1993.
24. Goodman FR, et al: Synpolydactyly phenotypes correlate with size of expansions in HOXD13 polyalanine tract. Proc Natl Acad Sci 94: 7458, 1997.
25. Murugaki Y, et al: Altered growth and branching patterns in synpolydactyly caused by mutations in HOXD13. Science 272:548, 1996.
25a. Mortlock DP, Innis JW: Mutation of HOXA13 in hand-foot-genital syndrome. Nature Genet 15:179, 1997.
26. Tabin C: Retinoids, homeobox genes, and genetic factors. Cell 66: 199, 1991.
27. Morriss-Kay GM, et al: Embryonic development and pattern formation. FASEB J 10:961, 1996.
28. Lammer EJ, et al: Retinoic acid embryopathy. N Engl J Med 313: 837, 1985.
29. Kessel M: Respecification of vertebral identities by retinoic acid. Development 115:487, 1992.
30. Marshall H, et al: Retinoids and *Hox* genes. FASEB J 10:969, 1996.
31. Mansouri A, et al: Pax genes and their roles in cell differentiation and development. Curr Opin Cell Biol 8:851, 1996.
32. Dressler GR: *Pax-2*, kidney development and oncogenesis. Med Pediatr Oncol 27:440, 1996.
33. Kuhn L, et al: Mother-to-infant HIV transmission: timing, risk factors and prevention. Paediatr Perinat Epidemiol 9:1, 1995.
34. Heegaard ED, et al: Parvovirus: the expanding spectrum of disease. Acta Paediatr 84:109, 1995.
35. Greenough A: Neonatal infections. Curr Opin Pediatr 8:6, 1996.
36. Stark AR, Frantz ID: Respiratory distress syndrome. Pediatr Clin North Am 33:533, 1986.
37. Editorial: Born before their time into this breathing world. BMJ 2: 1403, 1976.
38. Oh W, Stern L: Respiratory diseases of the newborn. In Stern L, Vert P (eds): Neonatal Medicine. New York, Masson Publishing USA, 1987, p 395.
39. Jobe AH: Lung development, surfactant, and respiratory distress syndrome. Acta Paediatr Jpn 32:1, 1990.
40. Ballard PL, et al: Regulation of pulmonary surfactant apoprotein SP28-36 gene in fetal human lung. Proc Natl Acad Sci U S A 83: 9527, 1986.
41. Ishisaka DY: Exogenous surfactant use in neonates. Ann Pharmacother 30:389, 1996.
42. Sun B: Use of surfactant in pulmonary disorders in full-term infants. Curr Opin Pediatr 8:113, 1996.
43. NIH Consensus Conference: Effect of corticosteroids for fetal maturation on perinatal outcomes. JAMA 273:413, 1995.
44. Stone J, et al: Role of VEGF and astrocyte degeneration in the genesis of retinopathy of prematurity. Invest Ophthalmol Vis Sci 37: 290, 1996.
45. Shaffer TH, et al: Liquid ventilation: an alternative ventilation strategy management of neonatal respiratory distress. Eur J Pediatr 155(suppl 2):S30, 1996.
46. Gollin YG, et al: Management of the Rh-sensitized mother. Clin Perinatol 22:544, 1995.
47. Norton ME: Nonimmune hydrops fetalis. Semin Perinatol 18:321, 1994.
48. Harper RG, et al: Kernicterus. Clin Perinatol 7:75, 1980.
49. Peterec SM: Management of neonatal Rh disease. Clin Perinatol 22: 561, 1995.
50. Allen DB, et al: Newborn screening: principles and practice. Adv Pediatr 43:231, 1996.
51. Levy HL, et al: Maternal phenylketonuria: a metabolic teratogen. Teratology 53:176, 1996.
52. Guttler F, et al: Mutations in the phenylalanine hydroxylase gene: genetic determinants for the phenotypic variability of hyperphenylalaninemia. Acta Paediatr 407(suppl):49, 1994.
53. Eisensmith RC, et al: Somatic gene therapy for phenylketonuria and other hepatic deficiencies. J Inherit Metab Dis 19:412, 1996.
54. Holton JB: Galactosaemia: pathogenesis and treatment. J Inherit Metab Dis 19:3, 1996.
55. Segal S: Galactosemia unsolved. Eur J Pediatr 154(suppl 2):S97–S102, 1995.
56. Davis PB: Cystic fibrosis from bench to bedside. N Engl J Med 325: 757, 1991.
57. Sperra TJ, Collins FS: The molecular basis of cystic fibrosis. Annu Rev Med 44:133, 1993.
58. Jiaug C, et al: Altered fluid transport across airway epithelium in cystic fibrosis. Science 262:424, 1993.
59. Koch C, Hoiby N: Pathogenesis of cystic fibrosis. Lancet 341:1065, 1993.
60. Goldman MJ, et al: Human β-defensin is a salt sensitive antibiotic in lung that is inactivated by cystic fibrosis. Cell 88:553, 1997.
61. Wine JJ: A sensitive defense: salt and cystic fibrosis. Nat Med 3:494, 1997.
62. Rommens JM, et al: Identification of the cystic fibrosis gene: cloning and characterization of the complementary DNA. Science 245:1066, 1989.
63. Tsui LC, Durie P: Genotype and phenotype in cystic fibrosis. Hosp Pract 32:115, 1997.
64. Stern RC: The diagnosis of cystic fibrosis. N Engl J Med 336:487, 1997.
65. Kerem E, Kerem B: Genotype-phenotype correlations in cystic fibrosis. Pediatr Pulmonol 22:387, 1996.
66. Wallis C: Diagnosing cystic fibrosis: blood, sweat, and tears. Arch Dis Child 76:85, 1997.
67. Noyes BE, et al: Lung and heart-lung transplantation in children. Pediatr Pulmonol 23:39, 1997.
68. Neglia JP, et al: The risk of cancer among patients with cystic fibrosis. N Engl J Med 332:494, 1995.
69. Wanger JA, Gardner P: Toward cystic fibrosis gene therapy. Ann Rev Med 48:203, 1997.
70. Willinger M, et al: Defining the sudden infant death syndrome (SIDS): deliberations of an expert panel convened by the National Institute of Health and Human Development. Pediatr Pathol 11:677, 1991.
71. Hoffman JH, et al: Risk factors for SIDS: results of the National Institute of Child Health and Human Development SIDS Cooperative Epidemiologic Study. Ann N Y Acad Sci 533:13, 1988.
72. Willinger M, et al: Infant sleep position and risk for sudden infant death syndrome: report of meeting held January 13 and 14, 1994, National Institutes of Health, Bethesda, MD. Pediatrics 93:814, 1994.
73. Fleming PJ, et al: Understanding and preventing sudden infant death syndrome. Curr Opin Pediatr 6:158, 1994.
74. Valdes-Dapena M: The sudden infant death syndrome: pathologic findings. Clin Perinatol 19:701, 1992.
75. Becker LE: Neural maturational delay as a link in the chain of events leading to SIDS. Can J Neurol Sci 17:361, 1990.
76. Kinney HC, et al: Decreased muscarinic receptor binding in the arcuate nucleus in sudden infant death syndrome. Science 269:1446, 1995.
76a. Panigrahy A, et al: Decreased kainate receptor binding in the arcuate nucleus of the sudden infant death syndrome. J Neuropathol Exper Neurol 56:1253, 1997.
77. Isaacs H Jr: Perinatal (congenital and neonatal) neoplasms: a report of 110 cases. Pediatr Pathol 3:165, 1985.

78. Bolande RP: Models and concepts derived from human teratogenesis and oncogenesis in early life. J Histochem Cytochem 32:878, 1984.

78a. Kelly KM, et al: Common and variant gene fusions predict distinct clinical phenotypes in rhabdomyosarcoma. J Clin Oncol 15:1831, 1997.

79. Matthay KK: Neuroblastoma: a clinical challenge and biologic puzzle. CA Cancer J Clin 45:179, 1995.

80. Wingo PA, et al: Cancer statistics, 1995. CA Cancer J Clin 45:8, 1995.

81. Shimada H: Tumors of the neuroblastoma group. Pathol State Art Rev 2:43, 1993.

82. Brodeur GM: Molecular basis for heterogeneity in human neuroblastomas. Eur J Cancer 31A:505, 1995.

83. Treuner J, et al: Neuroblastoma mass screening: the arguments for and against. Eur J Cancer 31A:565, 1995.

84. Grundy P, et al: An overview of the clinical and molecular genetics of Wilms' tumor. Med Pediatr Oncol 27:394, 1996.

85. Moulton T, et al: Genomic imprinting and Wilms' tumor. Med Pediatr Oncol 27:476, 1996.

86. Beckwith JB, et al: Nephrogenic rests, nephroblastomatosis, and the pathogenesis of Wilms' tumor. Pediatr Pathol 10:1, 1990.

87. Beckwith JB, et al: Histological analysis of aggressiveness and responsiveness in Wilms' tumor. Med Pediatr Oncol 27:422, 1996.

88. Birch JM et al: Epidemiologic features of Wilms' tumor. Hematol Oncol Clin North Am 9:1157, 1995.

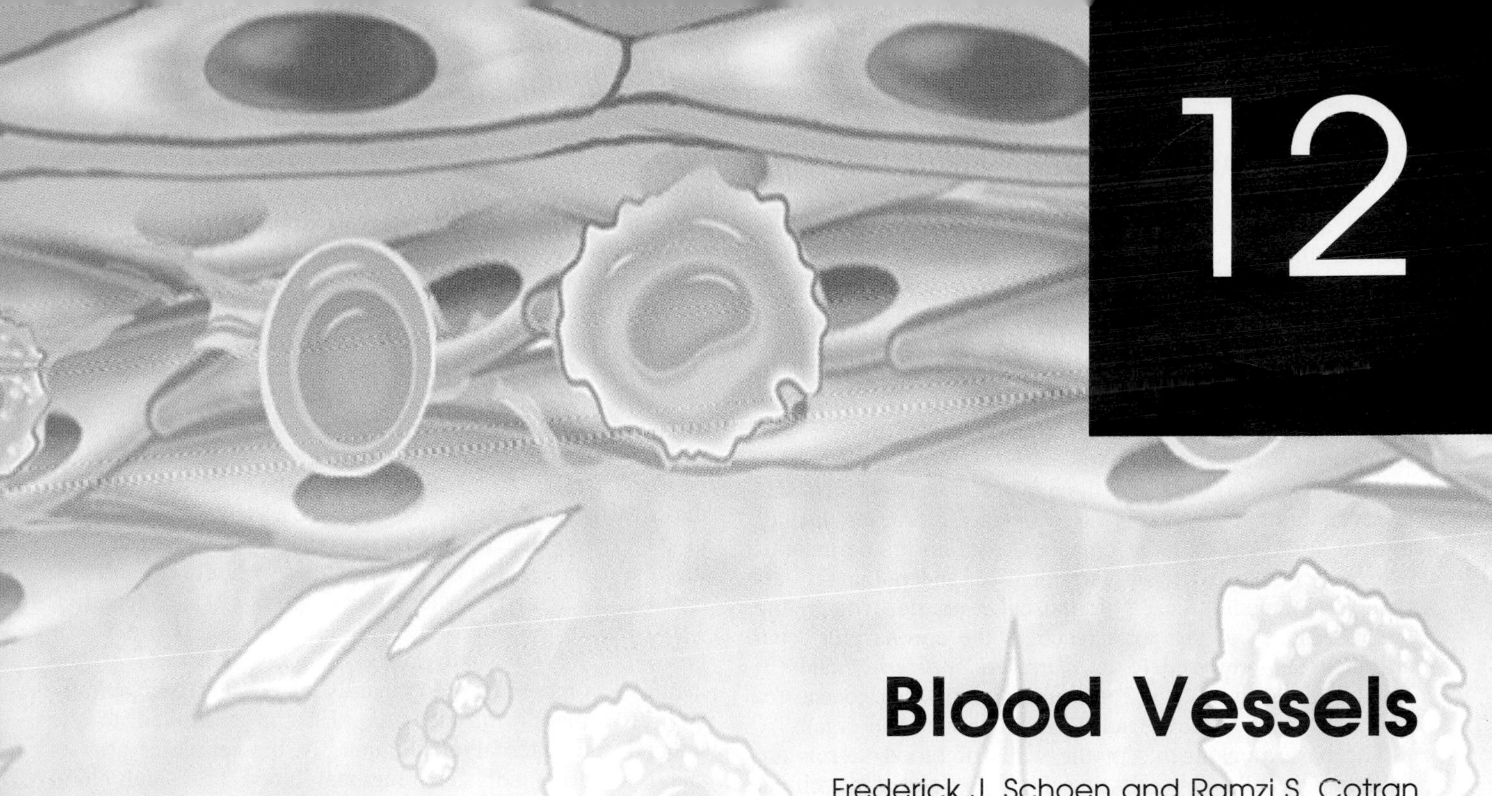

Blood Vessels

Frederick J. Schoen and Ramzi S. Cotran

NORMAL VASCULATURE

VASCULAR WALL CELLS AND THEIR RESPONSE TO INJURY

ENDOTHELIAL CELLS

ENDOTHELIAL DYSFUNCTION AND ENDOTHELIAL ACTIVATION

VASCULAR SMOOTH MUSCLE CELLS

INTIMAL THICKENING—A RESPONSE TO VASCULAR INJURY

VASCULAR DISEASES

CONGENITAL ANOMALIES

Arteriovenous Fistula

ATHEROSCLEROSIS

Clinical Significance

Epidemiology and Risk Factors

Pathogenesis

Clinical Features and Prevention

HYPERTENSIVE VASCULAR DISEASE

Hypertension

INFLAMMATORY DISEASE—THE VASCULITIDES

Giant Cell (Temporal) Arteritis

Takayasu Arteritis

Polyarteritis Nodosa (Classic)

Kawasaki Syndrome (Mucocutaneous Lymph Node Syndrome)

Microscopic Polyangiitis (Microscopic Polyarteritis, Hypersensitivity or Leukocytoclastic Angiitis)

Wegener Granulomatosis

Thromboangiitis Obliterans (Buerger Disease)

Vasculitis Associated With Other Disorders

Infectious Arteritis

RAYNAUD DISEASE

ANEURYSMS AND DISSECTION

Abdominal Aortic Aneurysms

Syphilitic (Luetic) Aneurysms

Aortic Dissection (Dissecting Hematoma)

VEINS AND LYMPHATICS

Varicose Veins

Thrombophlebitis and Phlebothrombosis

Obstruction of Superior Vena Cava (Superior Vena Caval Syndrome)

Obstruction of Inferior Vena Cava (Inferior Vena Caval Syndrome)

Lymphangitis and Lymphedema

TUMORS

Benign Tumors and Tumor-like Conditions

Hemangioma

Lymphangioma

Glomus Tumor (Glomangioma)

Vascular Ectasias

Bacillary Angiomatosis

Intermediate-Grade (Borderline Low-Grade Malignant) Tumors

Kaposi Sarcoma

Hemangioendothelioma

Malignant Tumors

Angiosarcoma

Hemangiopericytoma

PATHOLOGY OF THERAPEUTIC INTERVENTIONS IN VASCULAR DISEASE

Balloon Angioplasty and Related Techniques

Vascular Replacement

Coronary Artery Bypass Graft Surgery

Vascular disorders are responsible for more morbidity and mortality than any other category of human disease. Vascular abnormalities cause clinical disease by two principal mechanisms:

- *Narrowing* or *completely obstructing* the lumens of vessels, either progressively (e.g., by atherosclerosis) or precipitously (e.g., by thrombosis), often inducing downstream deficiency of blood flow to the tissue perfused by that vessel
- *Weakening* of the walls of vessels, leading to dilation or rupture

NORMAL VASCULATURE

The architecture of the vasculature varies with and reflects distinct functional requirements at different locations. To withstand the pulsatile and higher blood pressures in arteries, arterial walls are generally thicker than their venous counterparts. Arterial wall thickness gradually diminishes as the vessels become smaller, but the ratio of wall thickness to lumen diameter becomes greater. Veins have a larger overall diameter, a larger lumen, and a thinner wall than corresponding arteries.

Arteries are divided into three types, based on their size and structural features: (1) large or elastic arteries, including the aorta and its large branches (e.g., aorta and innominate, subclavian, common carotid, iliac, and pulmonary arteries); (2) medium-sized or muscular arteries comprising other branches of the aorta (such as the coronary or renal arteries), also referred to as *distributing arteries*; and (3) small arteries (usually <2 mm in diameter) that course, for the most part, within the substance of tissues and organs.

The basic constituents of the walls of blood vessels are endothelial cells, smooth muscle cells, and extracellular matrix, including elastic elements, collagen, and proteoglycans. They are arranged in concentric layers—the *intima* (adjacent to the lumen), *media*, and *adventitia* (externally)—most clearly defined in the larger vessels (Fig. 12–1). In normal arteries, the intima is composed of the lining endothelial cells with minimal underlying subendothelial connective tissue. It is separated from the media by a dense elastic membrane called the *internal elastic lamina*. The outer limit of the media of most arteries is marked by a well-defined *external elastic lamina*. In the large and medium-sized arteries, the smooth muscle cell layers of the media near the vessel lumen depend primarily on direct diffusion of oxygen from the vessel lumen for their nutritional needs. Diffusion is facilitated by holes (*fenestrations*) in the internal elastic membrane. Because diffusion from the lumen provides inadequate oxygen to the outer portion of the media in the large and medium-sized vessels, small arterioles arising from outside the vessel perforate the external elastic membrane and send vascular twigs into the outer one half to two thirds of the media. These vessels that nourish the vascular walls are called *vasa vasorum* (literally *vessels of the vessels*). External to the media is the adventitia, a layer of investing connective tissue in which nerve fibers and the vasa vasorum are dispersed.

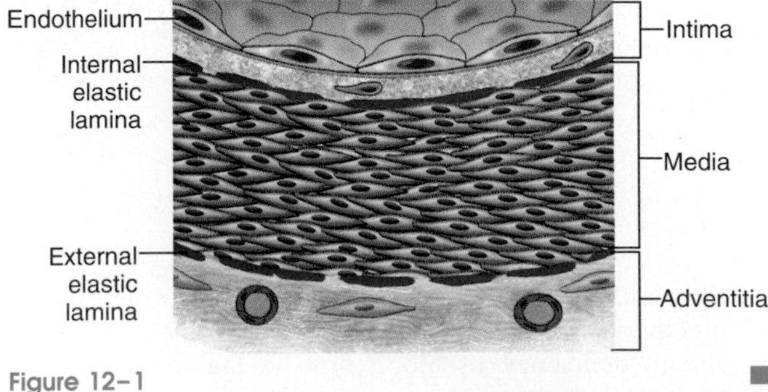

Figure 12–1

Diagrammatic representation of the main components of the vascular wall, seen here in a muscular artery.

The relative amount and configuration of the basic constituents vary along the arterial system owing to local adaptations to mechanical or metabolic needs. In the *elastic arteries*, the media is rich in elastic fibers, disposed in fairly compact layers separated by and alternating with layers of smooth muscle cells. The elastic components of the aorta allow it to expand during systole, thereby storing some of the energy of each heartbeat. Following and in between cardiac contractions during the diastolic phase of the cardiac cycle, elastic recoil of the vascular wall propels blood through the peripheral vascular system. During aging, the aorta loses elasticity, and these vessels expand less readily, particularly when blood pressure is increased. Thus, the arteries of older individuals often become progressively tortuous and dilated. In *muscular arteries*, the media is composed predominantly of circularly or spirally arranged smooth muscle cells. Elastin is limited to the internal and external membranes. In the muscular arteries and arterioles (see later), regional blood flow and blood pressure are regulated by changes in lumen size through smooth muscle cell contraction (*vasoconstriction*) or relaxation (*vasodilation*), controlled in part by the autonomic nervous system and in part by local metabolic factors and cellular interactions.

Arterioles are the smallest branches of the arteries (generally 20 to 100 μm in diameter). Changes in the state of contraction of the medial smooth muscle of arterioles cause dramatic adjustments in lumen diameter that regulate systemic arterial blood pressure and significantly influence blood flow distribution among the various capillary beds. Because the resistance of a blood vessel to fluid flow is inversely proportional to the fourth power of the diameter (i.e., halving the diameter increases resistance 16-fold), small changes in the lumen size of small blood vessels can have a profound flow-limiting effect. Thus, *arterioles are the principal points of physiologic resistance to blood flow, inducing a sharp reduction in pressure and velocity and a change from pulsatile to steady flow.* Moreover, small arteries and arterioles bear the brunt of blood pressure elevations; abnormal stresses alter their structure, with important consequences detailed later.

Some pathologic lesions involve arteries of a characteristic size range. For example, *atherosclerosis* affects largely elastic and muscular arteries, *hypertension* affects primarily small muscular arteries and arterioles, and specific types of vasculitis are associated with certain vascular segments.

Capillaries are approximately the diameter of a red blood cell (7 to 8 μm) and have thin walls. Since many capillaries arise from each arteriole, the capillary bed has a large total cross-sectional area, and blood flow is quite slow, analogous to the decrease in flow rate seen at the wide regions of a river. Lined by endothelial cells, capillaries are supported on the outside by a thin basement membrane, and the media is absent. Slow flow, high surface area, and thin walls only one cell thick render capillaries ideally suited to the rapid exchange of diffusible substances between blood and tissue.

The structure of capillaries varies at different sites, particularly in the degree of continuity of endothelium and basement membrane. Muscle, heart, lung, skin, and nervous system capillaries have a *continuous endothelial layer.* In contrast, in endocrine glands, renal glomeruli, and some vessels of the gastrointestinal tract, the endothelium is fenestrated, which allows more rapid transport of larger molecules and fluid (e.g., hormones or the glomerular filtrate) than do capillaries with a continuous endothelium. Some capillary vascular channels (called *sinusoids*) have a discontinuous endothelium with partial or no basement membrane, as in the liver, spleen, and bone marrow, facilitating the passage of cells across the walls.

Blood returning to the heart from capillary beds flows initially into the *postcapillary venules* then sequentially through collecting venules and small, medium, and large veins. Postcapillary venules are an important point of interchange between the lumen of the vessels and the surrounding tissues. For example, because the pressure in the venules is lower than that in the capillary bed as well as lower than interstitial tissue pressure, fluid can enter the circulation from the tissue surrounding the venules. Moreover, both vascular leakage and leukocytic exudation occur preferentially in venules in many types of inflammation (Chapter 3).

Veins are large-caliber but thin-walled vessels with a poorly defined internal elastic membrane and media not as well developed as that of arteries. Veins collectively have a large capacity; approximately two thirds of systemic blood is in the venous circulation. Veins have relatively poor support and are predisposed to irregular dilation, compression, and easy penetration by tumors and inflammatory processes. Reversed flow is prevented by the valves found in many veins, particularly those in the extremities in which blood flows against gravity.

Lymphatics are thin-walled, endothelium-lined channels devoid of blood cells that serve as a drainage system for returning interstitial tissue fluid to the blood. They also constitute an important pathway for disease dissemination, however, through transport of bacteria and tumor cells to distant sites.

VASCULAR WALL CELLS AND THEIR RESPONSE TO INJURY

The main cellular components of the walls of blood vessels are *endothelial cells* and *smooth muscle cells* (Fig. 12–2). Both play an important role in vascular pathology.

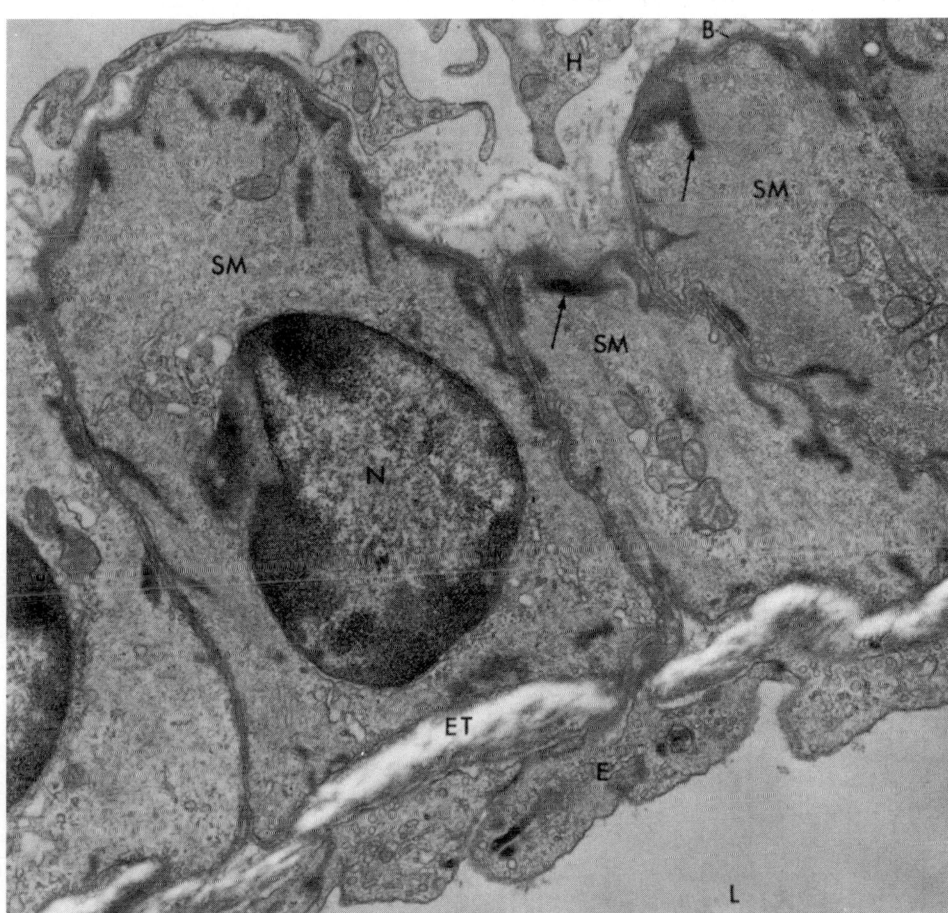

Figure 12–2

Wall of a small artery in the myocardium. Continuous endothelium (E) is separated from the smooth muscle layer (SM) by a thin internal elastic membrane (ET)—unstained. Note the peripheral bands in the medial smooth muscle cells (*arrows*) and the prominent external basement membrane (B). L, lumen; H, perivascular fibroblast; N, nucleus.

Endothelial Cells

Endothelial cells form a monolayer that lines the entire vascular system (the *endothelium*). Their structural and functional integrity is fundamental to the maintenance of vessel wall homeostasis and circulatory function. Endothelial cells are polygonal, elongated cells that have many pinocytotic vesicles and form junctional complexes with their neighbors. They uniquely contain *Weibel-Palade bodies*, 0.1-μm-wide, 3-μm-long membrane-bound structures that represent the storage organelle for von Willebrand factor (vWF). Endothelial cells are identified immunohistochemically with antibody to vWF (also called factor VIII–related antigen) and other endothelial antigens such as CD31.

Vascular endothelium is a versatile multifunctional tissue having many synthetic and metabolic properties (Table 12–1). Endothelial cells (1) serve as a semipermeable membrane, controlling the transfer of small and large molecules into the arterial wall and through the walls of capillaries and venules; (2) maintain the nonthrombogenic blood-tissue interface by regulating thrombosis, thrombolysis, and platelet adherence (Chapter 5); (3) modulate vascular tone and blood flow; (4) metabolize hormones; (5) regulate immune and inflammatory reactions, largely by controlling leukocyte interactions with the vessel wall; (6) modify lipoproteins in the artery wall; and (7) regulate the growth of other cell types, particularly smooth muscle cells. Thus, the endothelium is an active participant in the interaction between blood and tissues. Moreover, besides contributing to the formation of thrombi, endothelial injury is critical to the initiation of atherosclerosis and the vascular effects of hypertension and other disorders.

Table 12–1. ENDOTHELIAL CELL PROPERTIES AND FUNCTIONS

Maintenance of permeability barrier	Modulation of blood flow and vascular reactivity
Elaboration of anticoagulant and antithrombotic molecules	Vasoconstrictors: endothelin, ACE
Prostacyclin	Vasodilators: NO/EDRF, prostacyclin
Thrombomodulin	Regulation of inflammation and immunity
Plasminogen activator	IL-1, IL-6, IL-8
Heparin-like molecules	Adhesion molecules
Elaboration of prothrombotic molecules	Histocompatibility antigens
von Willebrand factor (factor VIII-vWF)	Regulation of cell growth
Tissue factor	Growth stimulators: PDGF, CSF, FGF
Plasminogen activator inhibitor	Growth inhibitors: heparin, TGF-β
Extracellular matrix production (collagen, proteoglycans)	Oxidation of LDL

ACE, angiotensin-converting enzyme (AI → AII); NO/EDRF, nitric oxide/endothelium-derived relaxing factor; IL, interleukin; PDGF, platelet-derived growth factor; CSF, colony-stimulating factor; FGF, fibroblast growth factor; TGF-β, transforming growth factor-β; LDL, low-density lipoprotein.

Endothelial Dysfunction and Endothelial Activation

Endothelial cells can respond to various abnormal stimuli by adjusting some of the constitutive functions listed in Table 12–1 and by expressing newly acquired (induced) properties. The term endothelial dysfunction is often used to describe several types of potentially reversible changes in the functional state of endothelial cells that occur in response to environmental stimuli.[1] Some of these changes, arbitrarily termed *endothelial stimulation*, denote rapid (within minutes), reversible responses that are independent of new protein synthesis. Examples are the endothelial cell changes induced by histamine, serotonin, and other vasoactive mediators that cause increased vascular permeability, inhibition of the release of endothelial cell–derived nitric oxide, and the redistribution of the adhesive glycoprotein P-selectin on stimulation by thrombin or histamine (Chapter 3). Others, termed *endothelial activation*, reflect alterations in gene expression and protein synthesis and may require hours or even days to occur.

Endothelial activation is emerging as a critical process in the pathogenesis of vascular diseases because it is induced by stimuli known to contribute to vascular injury and results in responses that influence the initiation and evolution of vascular lesions (Fig. 12–3).[2, 3] *Inducers* of endothelial activation include cytokines and bacterial products, which cause inflammatory injury and septic shock (Chapter 3); hemodynamic stresses and lipid products, critical to the pathogenesis of atherosclerosis (see later); advanced glycosylation end products (important in diabetes, Chapter 20) as well as viruses, complement components, and hypoxia. Activated endothelial cells, in turn, elaborate adhesion molecules (Chapter 3), other cytokines and chemokines, growth factors, vasoactive molecules that result either in vasoconstriction or in vasodilation, major histocompatibility complex (MHC) molecules, procoagulant and

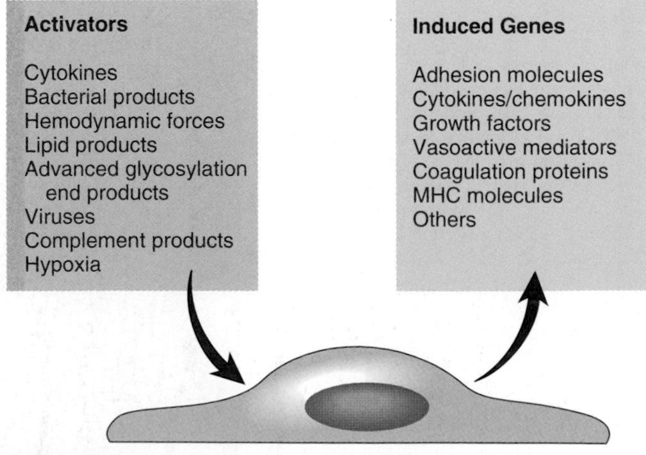

Figure 12–3

Endothelial activation: causes (activators) and consequences (induced genes).

anticoagulant moieties, and a variety of other gene products with biologic activity. The molecular regulation of such important responses is now under intensive study. One pathway that appears to mediate expression of many genes during endothelial activation is the transcription factor *nuclear factor* κB (NF-κB)/IκB system of transcriptional factors (Chapters 1, 2). Several of the activators of endothelial cells have in common the ability to generate *oxidative stress*, which is known to activate the NF-κB pathway.

Vascular Smooth Muscle Cells

Vascular smooth muscle cells are capable of many functions, including vasoconstriction and dilation in response to normal or pharmacologic stimuli; synthesis of collagen, elastin, and proteoglycans; elaboration of growth factors and cytokines; and migration to the intima and proliferation. As the predominant cellular element of the vascular media, smooth muscle cells constitute an important element of not only normal vascular repair, but also pathologic processes such as atherosclerosis. Resting vascular smooth muscle cells are spindle shaped, with single, elongated nuclei, resembling fibroblasts. The contractile function of smooth muscle cells is mediated by cytoplasmic filaments that contain actin and myosin.

The migratory and proliferative activity of smooth muscle cells is physiologically regulated by growth promoters and inhibitors. Promoters include platelet-derived growth factor (PDGF) derived from platelets as well as endothelial cells and macrophages, basic fibroblast growth factor (bFGF), and interleukin (IL) 1. Inhibitors include heparan sulfates, nitric oxide/endothelial-derived relaxing factor (NO/EDRF); interferon-γ (IFN-γ), and transforming growth factor-β (TGF-β).

Intimal Thickening—A Response to Vascular Injury

Vascular injury stimulates smooth muscle cell growth by disrupting the physiologic balance between inhibition and stimulation. Reconstitution of the damaged vascular wall, including endothelium, comprises a physiologic healing response with the formation of a *neointima*, involving (1) smooth muscle cell migration from the media to the intima, (2) subsequent multiplication of intimal cells, and (3) synthesis and deposition of extracellular matrix (Fig. 12–4). Injuries that cause only focal endothelial loss without frank denudation can often be repaired by migration and proliferation of neighboring endothelial cells. A more extensive or chronic injury to the smooth muscle cells of the media induces a more complex repair sequence.[2]

During the healing response, smooth muscle cells undergo changes that resemble dedifferentiation.[3] Smooth muscle cells migrating from the media to the intima lose the capacity to contract, gain the capacity to divide, and increase the synthesis of extracellular matrix molecules, often designated a shift from the *contractile* phenotype to the *proliferative-synthetic* phenotype. Structurally, there is a decrease in the thick, myosin-containing filaments and an increase in the amount of organelles involved with protein synthesis, such as rough endoplasmic reticulum and Golgi apparatus. Marked proliferation can be induced by injury. Although only a rare smooth muscle cell is dividing in the normal arterial wall, approximately 15 to 40% of cells have undergone mitosis within 48 hours after experimental arterial injury.[4] Intimal smooth muscle cells may return to a nonproliferative state when either the overlying endothelial layer is reestablished after acute injury or the chronic stimulation ceases.

An exaggerated healing response constitutes *intimal thickening*, which can cause stenosis or occlusion of small and medium-sized blood vessels or vascular grafts. Such a scenario contributes to many well-known, important clinical vascular disorders in which the initial injurious stimulus varies from predominantly mechanical (e.g., restenosis after angioplasty) to predominantly immunologic (e.g., transplant arteriosclerosis) to multifactorial (e.g., atherosclerosis).[5]

VASCULAR DISEASES

Vascular disease primarily affect arteries, and of these, the most prevalent and clinically significant problem is

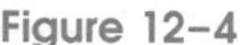

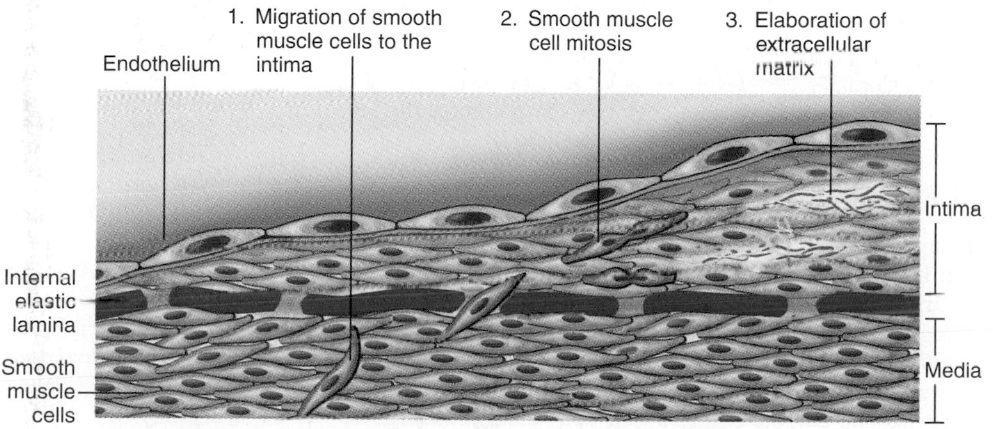

Figure 12–4 ■

Schematic mechanism for intimal thickening, emphasizing smooth muscle cell migration to, and proliferation and extracellular matrix elaboration in, the intima. (Modified and redrawn from Schoen FJ: Interventional and Surgical Cardiovascular Pathology: Clinical Correlations and Basic Principles. Philadelphia, WB Saunders, 1989, p 254.)

atherosclerosis. Hypertension, vascular inflammatory disease, and other less common arterial disorders may also be responsible for considerable disability and even death. Venous disorders, such as varicose veins, are also frequently encountered in clinical practice, but diseases of veins are more noteworthy for the disability they produce than for their importance as causes of death. Phlebothrombosis, however, may lead to death by pulmonary thromboembolism. Diseases of arteries, veins, and lymphatics are discussed separately.

Congenital Anomalies

Rarely symptomatic, aberrations of the usual anatomic pattern of branching and anastomosing are of particular importance in surgical operative technique; prior recognition of the deviation avoids the risk of disrupting an unexpected vessel. Among the other diverse congenital vascular anomalies, two others have importance: *developmental* or *berry aneurysm* and *arteriovenous fistulas* or *aneurysms.* Berry aneurysms involve cerebral vessels and are discussed in Chapter 30.

ARTERIOVENOUS FISTULA

Abnormal communications between arteries and veins usually arise as developmental defects, from rupture of an arterial aneurysm into the adjacent vein, from penetrating injuries that pierce the walls of artery and vein and produce an artificial communication, or from inflammatory necrosis of adjacent vessels. The connection between artery and vein may consist of a well-formed vessel, a vascular channel formed by the canalization of a thrombus, or an aneurysmal sac. Rare and usually small, such lesions may be of clinical significance because they short-circuit blood from the arterial to the venous side, causing the heart to pump additional volume, sometimes inducing cardiac failure (high-output failure). Moreover, they can rupture and cause hemorrhage, especially in the brain. In contrast, intentionally created arteriovenous fistulas are used to provide vascular access for long-term hemodialysis.

Atherosclerosis

Arteriosclerosis literally means *hardening of the arteries*; more accurately, however, it is a generic term for three patterns of vascular disease that have in common thickening and loss of elasticity of arterial walls:

- The dominant pattern is *atherosclerosis*, characterized by the formation of intimal fibrous plaques that often have a central grumous core rich in lipid. It is discussed first.
- Of much less clinical importance is the second morphologic form of atherosclerosis, *Mönckeberg medial calcific sclerosis*, characterized by calcific deposits in medium-sized muscular arteries in persons older than 50 years. The calcifications, which occasionally undergo ossification, take the form of irregular medial plates or discrete transverse rings; they create a nodularity on palpation and are readily visualized radiographically. Although these medial lesions do not encroach on the vessel lumen, arteries so affected may also develop atherosclerosis.
- Disease of small arteries and arterioles (*arteriolosclerosis*) is the third pattern. The two anatomic variants, hyaline and hyperplastic, cause thickening of vessel walls with luminal narrowing that may induce downstream ischemic injury. Arteriolosclerosis is most often associated with hypertension and diabetes mellitus and thus is described later in the section on hypertension.

CLINICAL SIGNIFICANCE

Atherosclerosis is characterized by intimal lesions called *atheromas* or *fibrofatty plaques* that protrude into the lumen, weaken the underlying media, and undergo a series of complications. Atherosclerosis overwhelmingly contributes to more mortality—approximately half or more of all deaths—and serious morbidity in the Western world than any other disorder. Global in distribution, it has reached epidemic proportions in economically developed societies.

Despite the ongoing health impact of atherosclerosis-related disease, significant progress has been made over the last decades in the United States and elsewhere. Between 1963 (the peak year) and 1995, there was an approximately 50% decrease in the death rate from ischemic heart disease and a 70% decrease in death from strokes, a reduction in mortality that has increased the average life expectancy in the United States by 5 years.[6] The basis for this trend has been attributed to (1) prevention of atherosclerosis through changes in living habits, including reduced cigarette smoking, altered dietary habits with reduced consumption of cholesterol and other saturated animal fats, and control of hypertension; (2) improved methods of treatment of myocardial infarction and other complications of ischemic heart disease; and (3) prevention of recurrences in patients who have previously suffered serious atherosclerosis-related clinical events.

Atherosclerosis primarily affects elastic arteries (e.g., aorta, carotid and iliac arteries) and large and medium-sized muscular arteries (e.g., coronary and popliteal arteries). The disease often begins in childhood, but symptoms are not usually evident until middle age or later when the arterial lesions precipitate organ injury (Fig. 12–5). Although any organ or tissue in the body may be so involved, *symptomatic atherosclerotic disease is most often localized to the arteries supplying the heart, brain, kidneys, lower extremities, and small intestine. Myocardial infarction (heart attack), cerebral infarction (stroke), and aortic aneurysms are the major consequences of this disease. Thus, epidemiologic data on atherosclerosis are expressed largely in terms of the incidence of or the number of deaths caused by ischemic heart disease* (Chapter 13). Atherosclerosis also takes a toll through other consequences of acutely or chronically diminished arterial perfusion, *such as gangrene of the legs, mesenteric occlusion, sudden cardiac death, chronic ischemic heart disease, and ischemic encephalopathy.*

Atheromas are focal and sparsely distributed at first, but

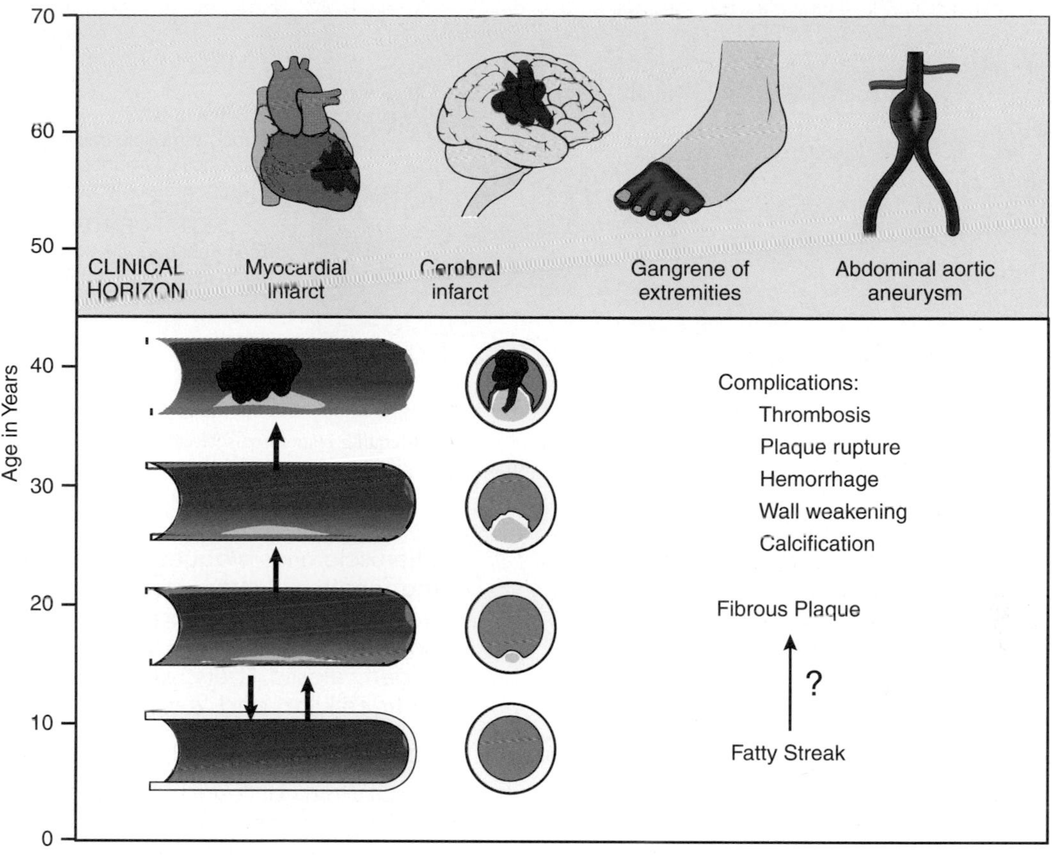

Figure 12–5

Natural history of atherosclerosis. Plaques usually develop slowly and insidiously over many years, beginning in childhood or shortly thereafter. As described in the text, they may progress from a fatty streak to a fibrous plaque and then to a complicated plaque that is likely to lead to clinical effects. (Modified from McGill HC Jr, et al: Natural history of human atherosclerotic lesions. In Sandler M, Bourne GH (eds): Atherosclerosis and Its Origin. New York, Academic Press, 1963, p 42; Wissler RW. Principles of the pathogenesis of atherosclerosis. In Braunwald E (ed): Heart Disease, Philadelphia, WB Saunders, 1984, p 1183.)

as the disease advances, they become more numerous, sometimes covering the entire circumference of severely affected arteries. Consequently, in small arteries, atheromas are themselves occlusive, compromising blood flow to distal organs and causing ischemic injury. Moreover, as seen in Chapter 13, plaques can undergo disruption and precipitate thrombi that further obstruct blood flow. In large arteries, they are destructive, encroaching on the subjacent media and weakening the affected vessel wall, causing aneurysms or rupture, or favoring thrombosis. In addition, extensive atheromas are friable, often yielding emboli into the distal circulation supplied by both the descending and the ascending aorta.[7]

MORPHOLOGY. The key processes in atherosclerosis are intimal thickening and lipid accumulation, producing the characteristic atheromatous plaques. As the principal cause of arterial narrowing in adults, these lesions are described first. Discussed subsequently is the **fatty streak,** present nearly universally in children and important mainly as a possible precursor of the atheromatous plaque.

***Atheromatous Plaque.* The basic lesion consists of a raised focal plaque within the intima, having a core of lipid (mainly cholesterol and cholesterol esters) and a covering fibrous cap** (Fig. 12–6). Also called **fibrous, fibrofatty, lipid, or fibrolipid plaques,** atheromatous plaques appear white to whitish yellow and impinge on the lumen of the artery. They vary in size from approximately 0.3 to 1.5 cm in diameter but sometimes coalesce to form larger masses (Fig. 12–7). On section, the superficial portion of these lesions at the luminal surface tends to be firm and white (the **fibrous cap**) and the deep portions yellow or whitish yellow and soft. The centers of larger plaques may contain a yellow, grumous debris, hence the term **atheroma,** an alternative name for atherosclerotic plaque derived from the Greek word for gruel.

The distribution of atherosclerotic plaques in humans is characteristic. The abdominal aorta is

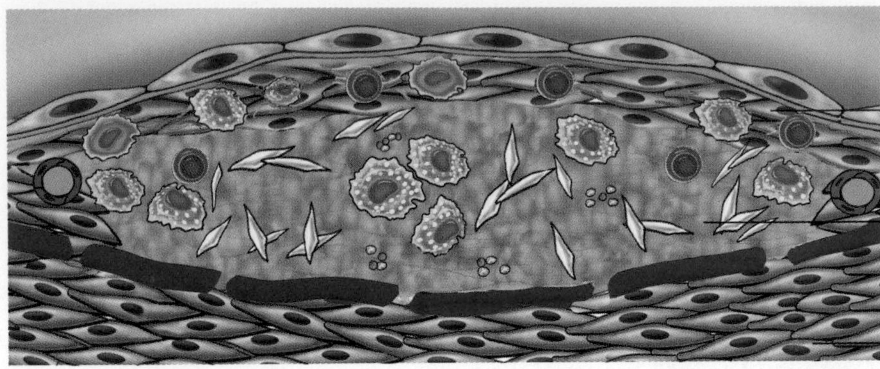

Figure 12–6

Major components of well-developed atheromatous plaque: fibrous cap composed of proliferating smooth muscle cells, macrophages, lymphocytes, foam cells, and extracellular matrix. The necrotic core consists of cellular debris, extracellular lipid with cholesterol crystals, and foamy macrophages.

usually much more involved than the thoracic aorta, and aortic lesions tend to be much more prominent around the origins (ostia) of its major branches. In descending order (after the lower abdominal aorta), the most heavily involved vessels are the coronary arteries, the popliteal arteries, the descending thoracic aorta, the internal carotid arteries, and the vessels of the circle of Willis. Vessels of the upper extremities are usually spared, as are the mesenteric and renal arteries except at their ostia. Nevertheless, in an individual case, the severity of atherosclerosis in one artery does not predict the severity in another. Atherosclerotic lesions usually involve the arterial wall only partially around its circumference (**eccentric** lesions) and are patchy and variable along the vessel length.

Atherosclerotic plaques have three principal components: (1) cells, including smooth muscle cells, macrophages, and other leukocytes; (2) **connective tissue extracellular matrix, including collagen, elastic fibers, and proteoglycans;** and (3) **intracellular and extracellular lipid deposits** (see Fig. 12–6). These three components occur in varying proportions in different plaques, giving rise to a spectrum of lesions. Typically the superficial fibrous cap is composed of smooth muscle cells with a few leukocytes and relatively dense connective tissue; a cellular area beneath and to the side of the cap (the **shoulder**), consisting of a mixture of macrophages, smooth muscle cells, and T lymphocytes; and a deeper necrotic core, in which there is a disorganized mass of lipid material, cholesterol clefts, cellular debris, lipid-laden

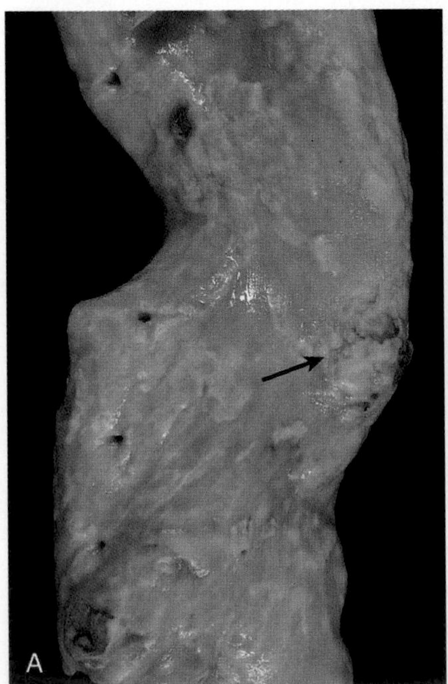

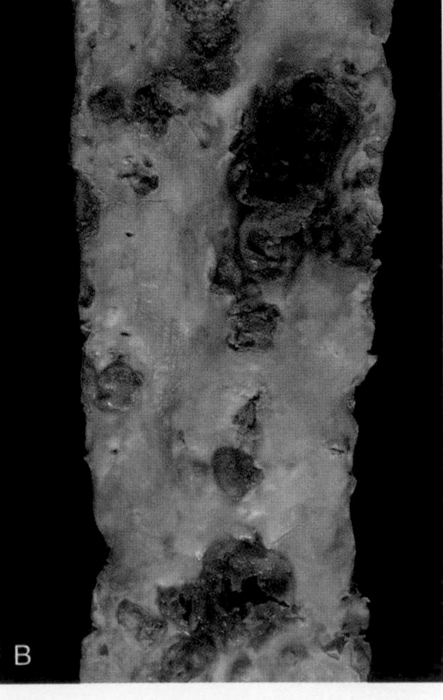

Figure 12–7

Gross views of atherosclerosis in the aorta. *A*, Mild atherosclerosis composed of fibrous plaques, one of which is denoted by the arrow. *B*, Severe disease with diffuse and complicated lesions.

foam cells, fibrin, thrombus in various stages of organization, and other plasma proteins (Fig. 12–8). The lipid is primarily cholesterol and cholesterol esters. Foam cells predominantly derive from blood monocytes (to become macrophages), but smooth muscle cells can also imbibe lipid to become foam cells. Finally, particularly around the periphery of the lesions, there is usually evidence of neovascularization (proliferating small blood vessels).

Common in adults and not considered atherosclerosis is a diffuse lipid-free thickening of the intima of the coronary arteries to a width approximately equal to that of the media, a normal response of the vessel wall to hemodynamic stimuli.

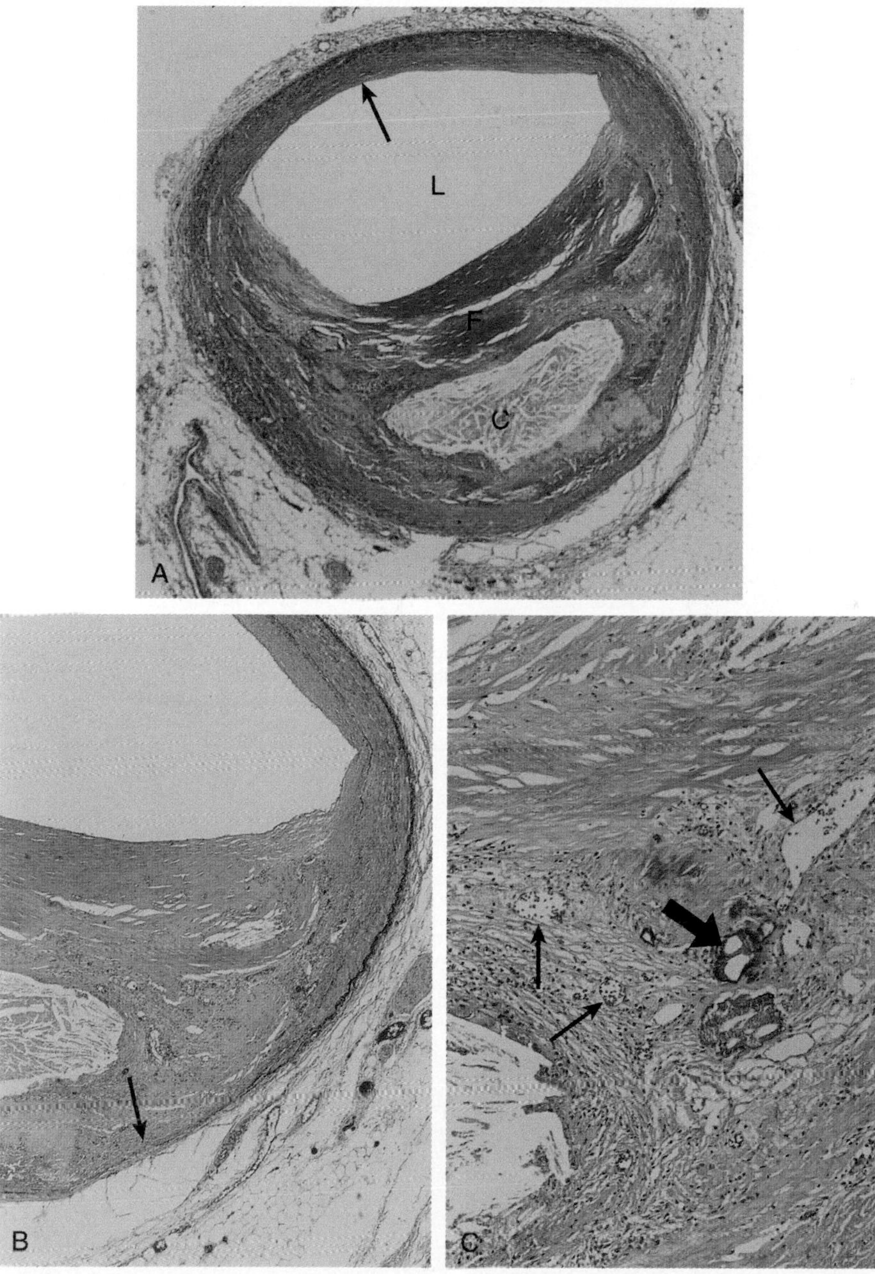

Figure 12–8 ■

Histologic features of atheromatous plaque in the coronary artery. *A*, Overall architecture demonstrating a fibrous cap (F) and a central lipid core (C) with typical cholesterol clefts. The lumen (L) has been moderately narrowed. Note the plaque-free segment of the wall (*arrow*). In this section, collagen has been stained blue (Masson trichrome stain). *B*, Higher-power photograph of a section of the plaque shown in *A*, stained for elastin (black) demonstrating that the internal and external elastic membranes are destroyed and the media of the artery is thinned under the most advanced plaque (*arrow*). *C*, Higher-magnification photomicrograph at the junction of the fibrous cap and core showing scattered inflammatory cells, calcification (*broad arrow*), and neovascularization (*small arrows*).

Variations of the histologic features of plaques involve the relative numbers of smooth muscle cells and macrophages and the amount and distribution of collagen and lipid. Typical atheromas contain relatively abundant lipid. Nevertheless, many so-called fibrous plaques are composed mostly of smooth muscle cells and fibrous tissue. In advanced atherosclerosis, the fatty atheroma may be converted to a fibrous scar.

The **complicated lesion** of atherosclerosis, defined by the following changes, has the most clinical significance:

- Almost always, atheromas in advanced disease undergo patchy or massive **calcification.** Arteries may become virtual pipe stems, and the aorta may assume an eggshell brittleness. Patients with high coronary artery calcium appear to be at increased risk for coronary events. Using calcification as a marker, new technologies such as computed tomography and intravascular ultrasound may provide an accurate noninvasive approach to diagnosis.[8,9]
- Focal **rupture** or gross **ulceration,** or both, of the luminal surface of atheromatous plaques may result in exposure of highly thrombogenic substances that induce thrombus formation (see Fig. 13–3) or discharge of debris into the bloodstream, producing microemboli (**cholesterol emboli** or **atheroemboli**).
- **Hemorrhage** into a plaque may occur, especially in the coronary arteries, from rupture of either the overlying fibrous cap or the thin-walled capillaries that vascularize the plaque. A contained hematoma may induce plaque rupture.
- Superimposed **thrombosis,** the most feared complication, usually occurs on disrupted lesions (those with rupture, ulceration, erosion, or

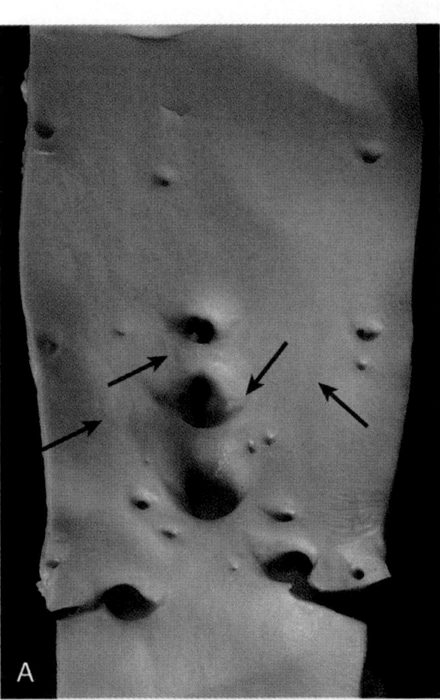

Figure 12–9

Fatty streak—a collection of foam cells in the intima. *A*, Aorta with fatty streaks (*arrows*), associated largely with the ostia of branch vessels. *B*, Close-up photograph of fatty streaks from the aorta of an experimental hypercholesterolemic rabbit shown after staining with Sudan red, a lipid-soluble dye, again illustrating the relationship of the lesions to the two-branch vessel ostia. *C*, Photomicrograph of fatty streak in an experimental hypercholesterolemic rabbit, demonstrating intimal macrophage-derived foam cells (*arrow*). (*B* and *C* courtesy of Myron I. Cybulsky, MD, University of Toronto, Canada.)

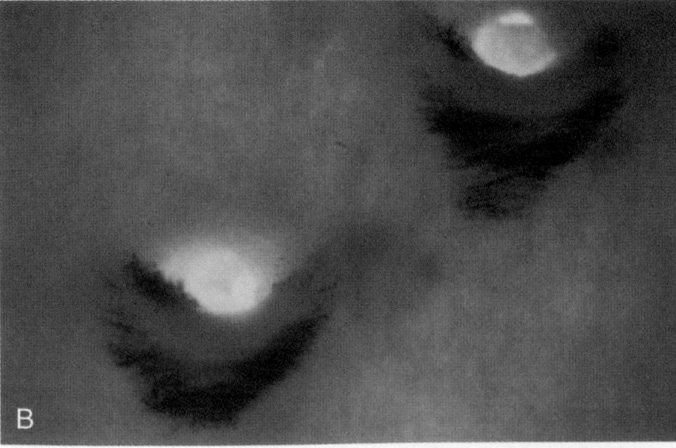

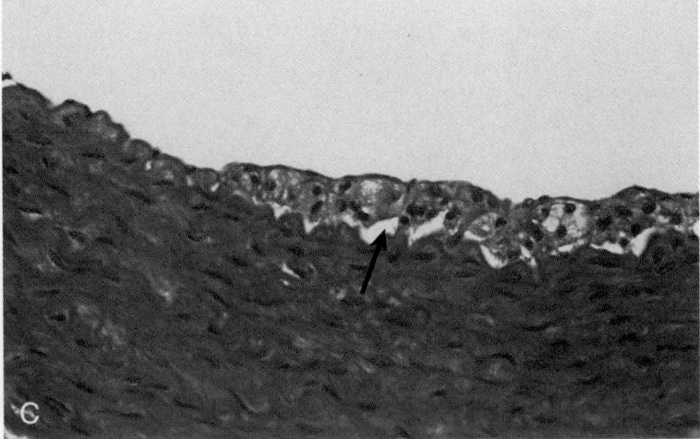

hemorrhage). Thrombi may partially or completely occlude the lumen; they may become incorporated within the intimal plaque by organization.

- Although atherosclerosis is initially an intimal disease, in severe cases, particularly in large vessels, the underlying media undergoes considerable atrophy with loss of elastic tissue (Fig. 12–8*B*), causing sufficient weakness to permit **aneurysmal dilation**, discussed later.

Fatty Streak. Fatty streaks are not significantly raised and thus do not cause any disturbance in blood flow. They may be precursors, however, of the more ominous atheromatous plaques. The streaks begin as multiple yellow; flat spots (**fatty dots**) less than 1 mm in diameter that coalesce into elongated streaks; 1 cm long or longer. Fatty streaks (Fig. 12–9) are composed of lipid-filled foam cells with T lymphocytes and extracellular lipid present in smaller amounts than in plaques.

Fatty streaks appear in the aortas of some children younger than 1 year of age and all children older than 10 years, regardless of geography, race, sex, or environment. Coronary fatty streaks are less common than aortic but begin to form in adolescence, and they occur at the same anatomic sites that are later prone to develop plaques.[10] They subsequently decrease in number as atherosclerotic plaques become more prevalent.

The relationship of fatty streaks to atherosclerotic plaques is complex. Fatty streaks are related to the known risk factors of atherosclerosis in adults (especially serum lipoprotein cholesterol concentrations and smoking), and some experimental evidence supports the concept of the evolution of fatty streaks into plaques. Fatty streaks, however, often occur in areas of the vasculature that are not particularly susceptible to developing atheromas later in life. Moreover, they frequently affect individuals in geographic locales and populations in which atherosclerotic plaque is uncommon. Thus, although fatty streaks may be precursors of plaques, not all fatty streaks are destined to become fibrous plaques or more advanced lesions.

An American Heart Association classification divides atherosclerotic lesions into six types, beginning with isolated foam cells (**fatty dots**) through stages of fatty streaks, atheromas, and fibroatheromas, to the complicated lesions (Fig. 12–10).[11]

Having examined the characteristic morphology of plaques and fatty streaks, we now discuss risk factors and pathogenesis.

EPIDEMIOLOGY AND RISK FACTORS

Atherosclerosis is virtually ubiquitous among the populations of North America, Europe, Australia, New Zealand, Russia, and other developed nations. In contrast, judged by the number of deaths attributable to ischemic heart disease (including myocardial infarction), it is much less prevalent in Central and South America, Africa, and Asia. For example, the mortality rate for ischemic heart disease in the United States is among the highest in the world and six

Nomenclature and main histology	Sequences in progression	Main growth mechanism	Earliest onset	Clinical correlation
Type I (initial) lesion Isolated macrophage foam cells	I	Growth mainly by lipid accumulation	From first decade	Clinically silent
Type II (fatty streak) lesion Mainly intracellular lipid accumulation	II			
Type III (intermediate) lesion Type II changes and small extracellular lipid pools	III		From third decade	
Type IV (atheroma) lesion Type II changes and core of extracellular lipid	IV			Clinically silent or overt
Type V (fibroatheroma) lesion Lipid core and fibrotic layer, or multiple lipid cores and fibrotic layers, or mainly calcific, or mainly fibrotic	V	Accelerated smooth muscle and collagen increase	From fourth decade	
Type VI (complicated) lesion Surface defect, hematoma-hemorrhage, thrombus	VI (from IV or V)	Thrombosis, hematoma		

Figure 12–10 ■

American Heart Association classification of human atherosclerotic lesions from the fatty dot (type I) to the complicated type VI lesion. The diagram also includes growth mechanisms and clinical correlations. (Modified from Stary HC, et al: A definition of advanced types of atherosclerotic lesions and a histological classification of atherosclerosis. Circulation 92:1355, 1995.)

times higher than that in Japan. Japanese who migrate to the United States and adopt US life styles and dietary customs acquire the predisposition to atherosclerotic diseases typical of the American population.

The prevalence and severity of the disease among individuals and groups—and therefore the age when it is likely to cause tissue or organ injury—are related to a number of factors, some constitutional and therefore immutable but others acquired and potentially capable of control. The risk factors that predispose to atherosclerosis and resultant ischemic heart disease have been identified by means of a number of prospective studies in well-defined population groups, most notably the Framingham (Massachusetts) Study and the Multiple Risk Factor Intervention Trial (MRFIT) (Table 12–2 and Fig. 12–11).[12, 13] The constitutional factors include age, sex, and genetics.

Age. Age is a dominant influence. Although atherosclerosis is not usually clinically evident until middle age or later, when the arterial lesions precipitate organ injury, it is a slowly progressive disease that begins in childhood and develops slowly over decades.[14] Death rates from ischemic heart disease rise with each decade even into advanced age. For example, from age 40 to age 60, there is a greater than fivefold increase in the incidence of myocardial infarction.

Sex. Other factors being equal, men are much more prone to atherosclerosis and its consequences than women. Myocardial infarction and other complications of atherosclerosis are uncommon in premenopausal women unless they are predisposed by diabetes or some form of hyperlipidemia or severe hypertension. Between ages 35 and 55 years, the mortality rate of ischemic heart disease for white women is one fifth that for white men. After menopause, the incidence of atherosclerosis-related diseases increases, probably owing to a decrease in natural estrogen levels. The frequency of myocardial infarction becomes the same in both sexes by the sixties to seventies. Some protection against atherosclerosis is afforded by postmenopausal hormone replacement therapy,[15] which is associated with a more favorable lipid profile and improved function of the endothelium.[16]

Genetics. The well-established familial predisposition to atherosclerosis and ischemic heart disease is most likely polygenic. In some instances, it relates to familial clustering of other risk factors, such as hypertension or diabetes, whereas in others it involves well-defined hereditary genetic derangements in lipoprotein metabolism that result in excessively high blood lipid levels, such as familial hypercholesterolemia (Chapter 6).

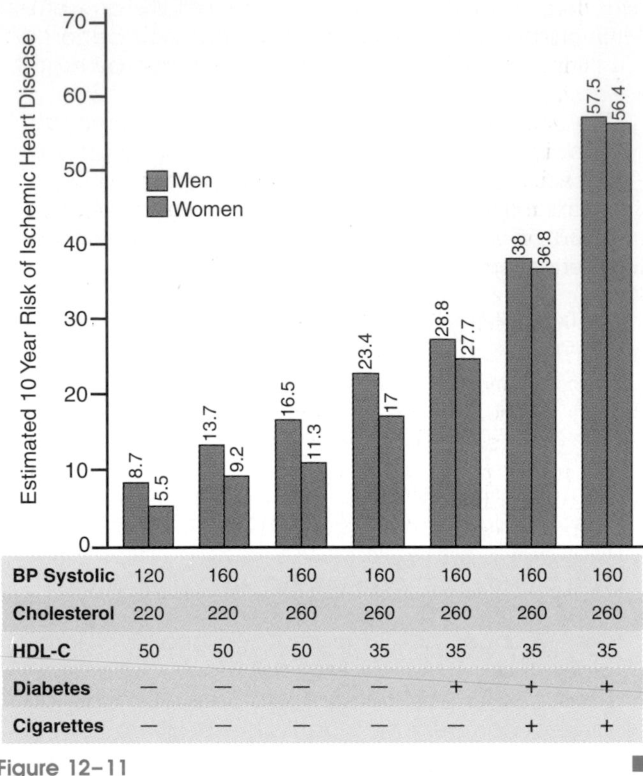

Figure 12–11

Estimated 10-year risk of coronary heart disease according to various combinations of risk factor levels. (From Kannel WB, et al: An update on coronary risk factors. Med Clin North Am 79:951, 1995.)

Although the aforementioned factors are unchangeable in an individual, *other risk factors, particularly diet, life style, and personal habits, are to a large extent potentially reversible.* The four major well-accepted modifiable conditions are hyperlipidemia, hypertension, cigarette smoking, and diabetes, but a variety of other factors are being uncovered. We shall discuss the most important separately.

Hyperlipidemia. Hyperlipidemia is acknowledged to be a major risk factor for atherosclerosis. Most of the evidence specifically implicates *hypercholesterolemia*; hypertriglyceridemia plays a less significant role, but its effect may be greater in women than men. The major component of the total serum cholesterol that is associated with increased risk is low-density lipoprotein (LDL) cholesterol. In contrast, there is an inverse relationship between symptomatic atherosclerosis and high-density lipoprotein (HDL) level; *thus, the higher the levels of HDL, the lower is the risk of ischemic heart disease.* HDL is believed to mobilize cholesterol from developing and existing atheroma and transport it to the liver for excretion in the bile. Thus, HDL participates in reverse transport of cholesterol, thereby earning its designation as the *good cholesterol.* There is thus great interest in dietary, pharmacologic, and

Table 12–2. RISK FACTORS FOR ATHEROSCLEROSIS

Major	Lesser, Uncertain, or Nonquantitated
Nonmodifiable	Obesity
Increasing age	Physical inactivity
Male gender	Stress (*type A* personality)
Family history	Homocysteine
Genetic abnormalities	Postmenopausal estrogen deficiency
Potentially Controllable	High carbohydrate intake
Hyperlipidemia	Alcohol
Hypertension	Lipoprotein(a)
Cigarette smoking	Hardened (trans) unsaturated fat intake
Diabetes	*Chlamydia pneumoniae*

behavioral methods of lowering serum LDL and raising serum HDL. Exercise and moderate consumption of ethanol both raise the HDL level, whereas obesity and smoking lower it.

The various classes of blood lipids are transported as lipoproteins complexed to specific apoproteins (Chapter 6). Apoproteins have many functions, among them activating or inhibiting particular enzymes, facilitating transmembrane transport of certain lipoproteins, and serving as ligands to high-affinity cellular receptors that guide the lipoproteins to specific sites of catabolism.

Dyslipoproteinemias result either from genetic mutations that yield defective apolipoproteins (Table 12–3) or from some other underlying disorder, such as the nephrotic syndrome, alcoholism, hypothyroidism, or diabetes mellitus. Four types of lipoprotein abnormalities are frequently found in the population (and one or more are present in many myocardial infarction survivors): (1) increased LDL cholesterol levels, (2) decreased HDL cholesterol levels, (3) increased chylomicron remnants and intermediate-density lipoprotein (IDL), and (4) increased levels of an abnormal lipoprotein Lp(a) (see later).

The major evidence implicating hypercholesterolemia in the genesis of atherosclerosis includes the following:

- Genetic defects in lipoprotein metabolism causing hyperlipoproteinemia are associated with accelerated atherosclerosis (Table 12–3).[17] For example, homozygous familial hypercholesterolemia often results in myocardial infarction before age 20 years. Familial hypercholesterolemia is caused by defects in the LDL receptor, leading to inadequate hepatic uptake of LDL and markedly increasing circulating LDL (Chapter 6). In another syndrome, increased LDL levels are due to the presence of a genetically variant apoprotein (apo) E that fails to bind properly to the LDL receptor. This defect has been traced to a single amino acid substitution (i.e., arginine to cysteine at residue 158) in the receptor binding site of the apo E molecule, which reduces binding activity to 1 to 2% of normal. Mutations producing defective apo B-100 cause similar binding abnormalities, resulting in increased serum LDL. There is also evidence that genetic polymorphisms in apolipoproteins or other proteins important to cholesterol metabolism (e.g., cholesterol ester transfer protein) contribute to atherosclerosis susceptibility and progression in the general population.[18]
- Other genetic or acquired disorders (e.g., diabetes mellitus, hypothyroidism) that cause hypercholesterolemia lead to premature and severe atherosclerosis.
- The major lipids in atheromas (plaques) are cholesterol and cholesterol esters derived from the plasma.
- Many large-scale epidemiologic analyses have demonstrated a significant correlation between the severity of atherosclerosis as judged by the mortality rate from ischemic heart disease and the levels of total plasma cholesterol or LDL, the lipoprotein moiety richest in cholesterol. No single level of plasma cholesterol identifies those at risk. The higher the level, the higher the risk, although the risk rises more steeply once a plateau level of approximately 200 mg/dl is exceeded (5.2 mmol/liter). Atherosclerotic events are uncommon with total serum cholesterol levels below 150 mg/dl.
- High-cholesterol diets can produce atherosclerotic plaques in experimental animals, including nonhuman primates, that are nearly identical to those observed in human disease.
- When levels of serum cholesterol are lowered by diet or drugs, the rate of progression of atherosclerotic disease is slowed, some atherosclerotic plaques regress, and the risk of cardiovascular events is reduced.[19] Cholesterol lowering increases overall survival and reduces risk of atherosclerosis-related events in patients with established coronary heart disease with elevated[20] or average[21] cholesterol levels as well as in patients with hypercholesterolemia but without overt atherosclerosis-related disease.[22]

Table 12–3. HYPERLIPOPROTEINEMIAS AND THEIR GENETIC BASIS

Electrophoretic Phenotype	Increased Lipoprotein Class(es)	Increased Lipid Class(es)	Relative Frequency (%)	Known Underlying Genetic Defects	Atherogenicity
I	Chylomicrons	Triglycerides	<1	Mutation in lipoprotein lipase gene	None
IIa	LDL	Cholesterol	10	Mutation in LDL receptor gene or in apolipoprotein B gene	+++
IIb	LDL and VLDL	Cholesterol and triglycerides	40	Mutation in LDL receptor gene or in apoliprotein B gene	+++
III	Remnants (chylomicrons) and IDL	Triglycerides and cholesterol	<1	Mutation in apoliprotein E gene	+++
IV	VLDL	Triglycerides	45	Mutation in lipoprotein lipase gene	+
V	VLDL and chylomicrons	Triglycerides and cholesterol	5	Mutation in apolipoprotein CII gene or in lipoprotein lipase gene	+

LDL, low-density lipoprotein; VLDL, very-low-density lipoprotein; IDL, intermediate-density lipoprotein.

- Transgenic mice deficient in apo E and with other genetic abnormalities of lipid metabolism develop atherosclerosis with cholesterol feeding.[23] Such models also emphasize the combined effects of genes and environmental influences in atherogenesis.
- High dietary intake of cholesterol and saturated fats, such as those present in egg yolk, animal fats, and butter, raises the plasma cholesterol level. Conversely a diet low in cholesterol and low in the ratio of saturated to polyunsaturated fats lowers plasma cholesterol levels. Paradoxically, persons in Greenland and Japan have low rates of ischemic heart disease despite a high dietary fat consumption in the form of fish, possibly owing to the high content of omega-3 fatty acids abundant in fish oils. Such fatty acids have a number of potentially antiatherogenic effects, including lowering of plasma LDL, increasing vasodilation, and reducing platelet aggregation (Chapter 3).[24] Dietary replacement of saturated fats with monounsaturated or polyunsaturated fats and omega-3 fatty acids derived from fish remains controversial, however.[25] Moreover, there is now good evidence that hardened (trans) unsaturated fats produced by artificial hydrogenation of polyunsaturated vegetable fats and used in baked goods and margarine may adversely affect cholesterol profiles and contribute to ischemic heart disease.[26]

Hypertension. Hypertension is a major risk factor for atherosclerosis at all ages, but after age 45 years hypertension is a stronger risk factor than hypercholesterolemia. Men at age 45 to 62 whose blood pressure exceeds 169/95 mm Hg have a more than fivefold greater risk of ischemic heart disease than those with blood pressures of 140/90 mm Hg or lower. Both systolic and diastolic levels are important in increasing risk. In the MRFIT study, increased death rates were associated with systolic blood pressure greater than 110 mm Hg and diastolic pressure greater than 70 mm Hg. Antihypertensive therapy reduces the incidence of atherosclerosis-related diseases, particularly strokes and ischemic heart disease.[27]

Cigarette Smoking. Cigarette smoking is not only a well-established risk factor in men, but also is thought to account for the relatively recent increase in the incidence and severity of atherosclerosis in women. When one or more packs of cigarettes are smoked per day for several years, the death rate from ischemic heart disease increases by up to 200%. Cessation of smoking approximately halves this increased risk.

Diabetes Mellitus. Diabetes mellitus induces hypercholesterolemia and a markedly increased predisposition to atherosclerosis. Other factors being equal, the incidence of myocardial infarction is twice as high in diabetics as in nondiabetics. There is also an increased risk of strokes and, even more striking, perhaps a 100-fold increased risk of atherosclerosis-induced gangrene of the lower extremities. In the absence of diabetes, atherosclerotic gangrene of the lower extremities is uncommon. The complex mechanisms of increased atherosclerosis in diabetes are discussed in Chapter 20.

Elevated Plasma Homocysteine. *Homocystinuria* refers to a group of rare inborn errors of metabolism resulting in high levels of circulating homocysteine (>100 μmol/liter) and urinary homocysteine. Patients with this condition have premature vascular disease, and it had been postulated since the 1960s that elevated levels of homocysteine may be a risk factor for atherosclerosis.[28] Recent clinical and epidemiologic studies have indeed shown a more general relationship between total serum homocysteine levels and coronary artery disease, peripheral vascular disease, stroke, or venous thrombosis. There is evidence that homocysteine may cause endothelial dysfunction, through formation of reactive oxygen species that, as we shall see, play an important role in atherogenesis. It also interferes with the vasodilator and antithrombotic functions of nitric oxide.[29] Hyperhomocystinemia can potentially be caused by low folate and vitamin B intake, and evidence suggests that folate and vitamins B_6 and B_{12} ingestion beyond conventional dietary recommendations reduces cardiovascular disease in women.[30]

Factors Affecting Hemostasis and Thrombosis. Epidemiologic evidence also indicates that several markers of hemostatic and thrombotic function, in addition to homocysteine level, are potent predictors of risk for major atherosclerotic events, including myocardial infarction and stroke. Such markers include those related primarily to fibrinolysis, such as elevated levels of plasminogen activator inhibitor-1 such as (PAI-1) and inflammation, such as plasma fibrinogen and C-reactive protein (CRP). For example, plasma concentration of CRP, a marker for systemic inflammation, predicts the risk of myocardial infarction and stroke.[31] Reduction of incidence of first myocardial infarction associated with the use of aspirin appears to be directly related to the level of CRP.

Lipoprotein Lp(a) is an altered form of LDL that contains the apo B-100 portion of the LDL linked to apo A, itself a large glycoprotein molecule with a high degree of structural homology to plasminogen (a key protein in fibrinolysis). Some but not all epidemiologic studies have shown a correlation between increased blood levels of Lp(a) and coronary and cerebrovascular disease, independent of the level of total cholesterol or LDL. Lp(a) has several potential atherogenic effects, including lipid accumulation, endothelial cell modulation, smooth muscle cell proliferation, and control of plaque neovascularization.[32]

Assessment of hemostatic and thrombotic factors may prove useful in identifying individuals at increased risk for cardiovascular morbidity and mortality. Moreover, such associations emphasize the role of thrombosis and chronic inflammation in the initiation and progression of atherosclerosis as well as the conversion of stable atherosclerotic plaque to an unstable and potentially occlusive lesion.

Other Factors. Other factors associated with a less pronounced or difficult-to-quantitate risk include lack of exercise, competitive, stressful life style with *type A* personality behavior, and unrestrained weight gain (largely because obesity induces hypertension, diabetes, hypertriglyceridemia, and decreased HDL). Epidemiologic data also indicate a protective role for moderate intake of alcohol.[33]

Multiple risk factors may impose more than an additive effect (Fig. 12–11). Two risk factors increase the risk approximately fourfold. When three risk factors are present (e.g., hyperlipidemia, hypertension, and smoking), the rate

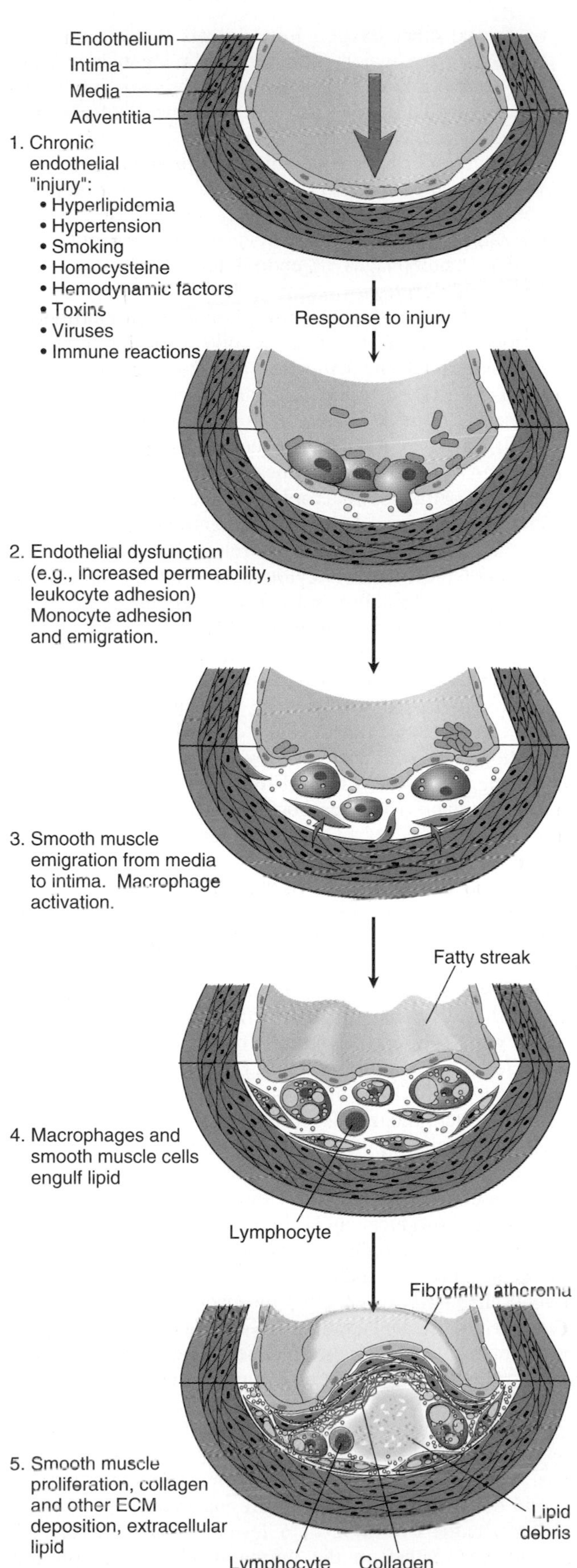

of myocardial infarction is seven times greater than when none are present. The converse is equally important: Atherosclerosis may develop in the absence of any apparent risk factors, so even those who live "the prudent life" and have no apparent genetic predispositions are not immune to this killer disease. Many patients with ischemic heart disease do not have a risk factor profile that would predict severe atherosclerosis. This fact dramatically emphasizes the significant gaps in our knowledge. Moreover, demonstration of an epidemiologic association with a risk factor does not necessarily prove a pathogenetic (causal) relationship. For these reasons and because of the overall importance of atherosclerosis, its causes and pathogenesis remain subjects of lively speculation and controversy.

PATHOGENESIS

The overwhelming importance of atherosclerosis has stimulated enormous efforts to discover its cause. Historically, two hypotheses for atherogenesis were dominant: One emphasized cellular proliferation in the intima as a reaction to insudation of plasma proteins and lipids from the blood, whereas the other postulated that organization and repetitive growth of thrombi resulted in plaque formation. The contemporary view of the pathogenesis of atherosclerosis incorporates elements of both older theories and accommodates the risk factors previously discussed. This concept, called the *response to injury hypothesis, considers atherosclerosis to be a chronic inflammatory response of the arterial wall initiated by some form of injury to the endothelium* (Fig. 12–12).[34] Central to this thesis are the following events:

- The development of focal regions of *chronic endothelial injury*, usually subtle, with resultant endothelial dysfunction, such as increased endothelial permeability and increased leukocyte adhesion
- Insudation of *lipoproteins* into the vessel wall, mainly LDL with its high cholesterol content and also very-low-density lipoprotein (VLDL), and modification of such lipoproteins by *oxidation*
- Adhesion of *blood monocytes* (and other leukocytes) to the endothelium, followed by migration of monocytes into the intima and their transformation into *macrophages* and *foam cells*
- Adhesion of *platelets* to focal areas of denudation (when present) or to adherent leukocytes
- Release of factors from activated platelets, macrophages, or vascular cells that cause *migration of smooth muscle cells* from media into the intima

Figure 12–12

Processes in the response to injury hypothesis. *1*, Normal. *2*, Endothelial injury with adhesion of monocytes and platelets (the latter to denuded endothelium). *3*, Migration of monocytes (from the lumen) and smooth muscle cells (from the media) into the intima. *4*, Smooth muscle cell proliferation in the intima. *5*, Well-developed plaque.

- *Proliferation of smooth muscle cells* in the intima and elaboration of extracellular matrix, leading to *accumulation of collagen and proteoglycans*
- *Enhanced accumulation of lipids* both within cells (macrophages and smooth muscle cells) and extracellularly

We shall now consider these events in some detail.

Role of Endothelial Injury. Chronic or repetitive endothelial injury is the cornerstone of the response-to-injury hypothesis. Endothelial injury induced in experimental animals by mechanical denudation, hemodynamic forces, immune complex deposition, irradiation, and chemicals causes intimal thickening and, in the presence of high-lipid diets, typical atheromas. *Early human lesions, however, develop at sites of morphologically intact endothelium.* Thus, nondenuding endothelial dysfunction and activation are more important in the human disease—these are manifested by increased endothelial permeability, enhanced leukocyte adhesion, and alterations in expression of a number of endothelial gene products (see Fig. 12–3). For example, endothelial adhesion molecules such as intercellular adhesion molecule-1 (ICAM-1) and vascular cell adhesion molecule-1 (VCAM-1) (Chapter 3) are expressed in the luminal endothelium overlying developing plaques[35, 36] and are thought to mediate the adhesion of circulating monocytes and lymphocytes during their entry into plaque.

What initiates endothelial dysfunction in early atherosclerosis? Endotoxins, hypoxia, products derived from cigarette smoke, specific endothelial toxins such as homocysteine, and possibly viruses or other infectious agents may be involved. However, it is currently thought that the two important determinants of endothelial alterations, perhaps acting in concert, are (1) the *hemodynamic disturbances that accompany normal circulatory function* and (2) *the adverse effects of hypercholesterolemia.*

In support of a hemodynamic effect is the well-defined tendency for plaques to occur at ostia of exiting vessels, branch points, and along the posterior wall of the descending and abdominal aorta. It is thought that turbulent flow patterns with variable levels of shear stress cause focal areas of endothelial dysfunction and predispose to the development of lesions at these sites. Alteration of shear stress associated with disturbed flow induces numerous endothelial genes with potential proinflammatory and proatherogenic activities, including cytokines, adhesion molecules, and coagulation proteins, and can cause increased endothelial permeability and cell turnover and enhanced receptor-mediated LDL endocytosis.[37]

Additionally, based on in vitro studies, it has been postulated that the laminar shear stresses typically encountered in *lesion-protected areas* of the arterial vasculature induce endothelial genes whose products (such as the antioxidant superoxide dismutase) actually *protect* from the development of lesions.[37] These so-called *atheroprotective* genes could explain the nonrandom localization of early atherosclerotic lesions.

Role of Lipids. The mechanisms by which hyperlipidemia contributes to atherogenesis include the following:

- Chronic hyperlipidemia, particularly hypercholesterolemia, may itself impair endothelial function. This is thought to occur through increased production of superoxide and other oxygen free radicals that deactivate nitric oxide, the major endothelial-relaxing factor. Oxidative stress, as we have seen, also activates NF-κB and the endothelial gene expression of numerous biologically active molecules (see Fig. 12–3).
- With chronic hyperlipidemia, lipoproteins accumulate within the intima at sites of increased endothelial permeability.
- Oxidative modification of lipid by free radicals generated in macrophages or endothelial cells in the arterial wall yields *oxidized (modified) LDL.*[38] Oxidized LDL, in turn, has the following effects that may contribute to lesion formation: (1) It is readily ingested by macrophages through the *scavenger receptor*, which is distinct from the LDL receptor (Chapter 6), thus forming foam cells; (2) it is chemotactic for circulating monocytes; (3) it increases monocyte adhesion, largely through the induction of endothelial adhesion molecules; (4) it inhibits the motility of macrophages already in lesions, thus favoring the recruitment and retention of macrophages in plaques; (5) it stimulates release of growth factors and cytokines; (6) it is cytotoxic to endothelial cells and smooth muscle cells; and (7) it is immunogenic, inducing the production of antibodies to oxidized lipoproteins.

The concept that hyperlipidemia leads to lesion formation through oxidative stress on the endothelium is consistent with experimental and clinical studies showing protection from atherosclerosis by antioxidant vitamins (betacarotene and vitamin E) and by drugs that reduce generation of oxidants (e.g., probucol).[39] Moreover, cholesterol-lowering and antioxidant therapy improve clinical measures of endothelial dysfunction.[40]

Role of Macrophages. Monocytes adhere to endothelium early in atherosclerosis via the specific endothelial adhesion molecules induced on the surface of activated endothelial cells described previously. Monocytes then migrate between endothelial cells to localize subendothelially. There they become transformed into macrophages and avidly engulf lipoproteins, largely oxidized LDL, to become foam cells. Oxidized LDL is chemotactic to monocytes and immobilizes macrophages at sites where it accumulates. Macrophages also proliferate in the intima. If the injury is denuding, platelets also adhere to the endothelium.

Macrophages have a multifactorial role in the progression of atherosclerotic lesions, owing to their large number of secretory products and biologic activities (Chapter 4). For example, macrophages produce IL-1 and tumor necrosis factor (TNF), which increase adhesion of leukocytes; several chemokines generated by macrophages (e.g., monocyte chemoattractant protein-1 [MCP-1]) may further recruit leukocytes into the plaque. Macrophages produce toxic oxygen species that also cause oxidation of the LDL in the lesions, and they elaborate growth factors that may contribute to smooth muscle cell proliferation. T lymphocytes (both CD4+ and CD8+) are also present in atheromas, but the precise stimuli for their recruitment and their role in the evolution of lesions are uncertain.

Early in the evolution of a lesion, smooth muscle cells migrate and gather in the intima, where they proliferate, and some take up lipids also to be transformed into foam cells. As long as the hypercholesterolemia persists, monocyte adhesion, subendothelial migration of smooth muscle cells, and accumulation of lipids within the macrophages and smooth muscle cells continue, eventually yielding aggregates of foam cells in the intima, which are apparent macroscopically as *fatty streaks*. Should the hypercholesterolemia be ameliorated, however, these fatty streaks may regress.

Role of Smooth Muscle Proliferation. *If the hypercholesterolemia (or other inciting event) persists, smooth muscle cell proliferation and extracellular matrix deposition in the intima continue and are the major processes that convert a fatty streak into a mature fibrofatty atheroma, accounting for the progressive growth of atherosclerotic lesions.* Arterial smooth muscle cells synthesize collagen, elastin, and glycoproteins. Several growth factors have been implicated in the proliferation of smooth muscle cells: PDGF, which is released by platelets adherent to the focus of endothelial injury, macrophages, endothelial cells, smooth muscle cells; FGF; and TGF-α. Smooth muscle proliferation is modulated by inhibitors, including heparin-like molecules present in endothelial cells and smooth muscle cells or TGF-β derived from endothelial cells or macrophages.

Progression of Lesions. At an early stage of atherogenesis, the intimal plaque represents a central aggregation of foam cells of macrophage and smooth muscle cell origin, some of which may have died and released extracellular lipid and cellular debris surrounded by smooth muscle cells. With progression, the cellular-fatty atheroma is modified by further deposition of collagen and proteoglycans. Connective tissue is particularly prominent on the intimal aspect, where it produces the *fibrous cap*. Thus evolves the fully mature fibrofatty atheroma. Some atheromas undergo additional cellular proliferation and connective tissue formation to yield *fibrous plaques*. Others retain a central core of lipid-laden cells and fatty debris. Plaques often undergo disruption with superimposed thrombus, and this sequence is often associated with catastrophic clinical events (Chapter 13). Should the patient survive, the thrombus may organize, thereby contributing to plaque enlargement.

Other Factors in Atherogenesis

Oligoclonality of Lesions. *The development of the atheromatous plaque could also be explained if smooth muscle cell proliferation were in fact the primary event.* For example, the *monoclonal hypothesis* of atherogenesis, put forth in 1977, was based on the observation that some human plaques are monoclonal or at most oligoclonal. One interpretation of such oligoclonality is that plaques may be equivalent to benign neoplastic growths, perhaps induced by an exogenous chemical (e.g., cholesterol or some of its oxidized products) or an oncogenic virus. More recent data indicate that the monoclonal populations result from patches of preexisting (developmental) clones of cells.[41]

Infection. There is current interest in whether infectious processes could contribute to atherosclerosis.[42] In animals, certain viruses (e.g., the agent of Marek disease in chickens) can cause plaques in the aorta. Viruses can cause vasculitis (see later),[43] and both herpesvirus and cytomegalovirus have been detected in human atheromatous plaques.[44] Recently *Chlamydia pneumoniae* has been demonstrated in atherosclerotic plaques but not in normal arteries. It has been suggested that this infectious organism incites a chronic inflammatory process that contributes to atheroma formation. Antibiotic therapy appropriate for *C. pneumoniae* reduces recurrent clinical events in patients with ischemic heart disease.[45] The association of *Chlamydia* and atherosclerosis will undoubtedly be the subject of continued scrutiny.

Figure 12–13 *summarizes the major proposed mechanisms of atherogenesis. This scheme considers atherosclerosis as a chronic inflammatory response of the vascular wall to a variety of events that are initiated early in life. Multiple mechanisms contribute to plaque formation and progression, including endothelial dysfunction, monocyte adhesion and infiltration, lipid accumulation and oxidation, smooth muscle proliferation, extracellular matrix deposition, and thrombosis.*

CLINICAL FEATURES AND PREVENTION

As noted, the clinical features of atherosclerosis are those of its complications (thrombosis, calcification, aneurysmal dilatation) and the distal ischemic events (in the heart, brain, lower extremities, and other organs). Owing to such consequences of atherosclerosis, intensive efforts are underway to devise means to reduce its toll. These involve *primary prevention* programs, aimed at either delaying atheroma formation or causing regression of established lesions in persons who have never suffered a serious complication and *secondary prevention* programs, intended to prevent recurrence of events such as myocardial infarction.

As detailed earlier, there is ample justification for the following recommendations for primary prevention by virtue of risk factor modification: abstention from or cessation of cigarette smoking; control of hypertension; weight reduction by control of total caloric intake coupled with increased exercise; moderation of alcohol consumption; and, most importantly, lowering total and LDL blood cholesterol levels while increasing HDL. Moreover, several lines of evidence suggest that risk factor examination and prevention directed at modification of risk should begin in childhood:[46, 47]

- Pediatric epidemiology programs and pathologic studies have established that atherosclerotic coronary artery disease begins in childhood.
- Cardiovascular risk factors in children are predictive of adult levels and have distinct ethnic and sex differences that relate to adult heart disease.
- Serum lipoprotein cholesterol concentrations and smoking are important determinants of the early stages of atherosclerosis noted at autopsy in adolescents and young adults.

Secondary prevention programs based on attempts not only to lower blood lipid levels (discussed earlier), but also to prevent thrombotic complications using antiplatelet drugs[48] have successfully reduced the frequency of recurrent myocardial infarcts and strokes.

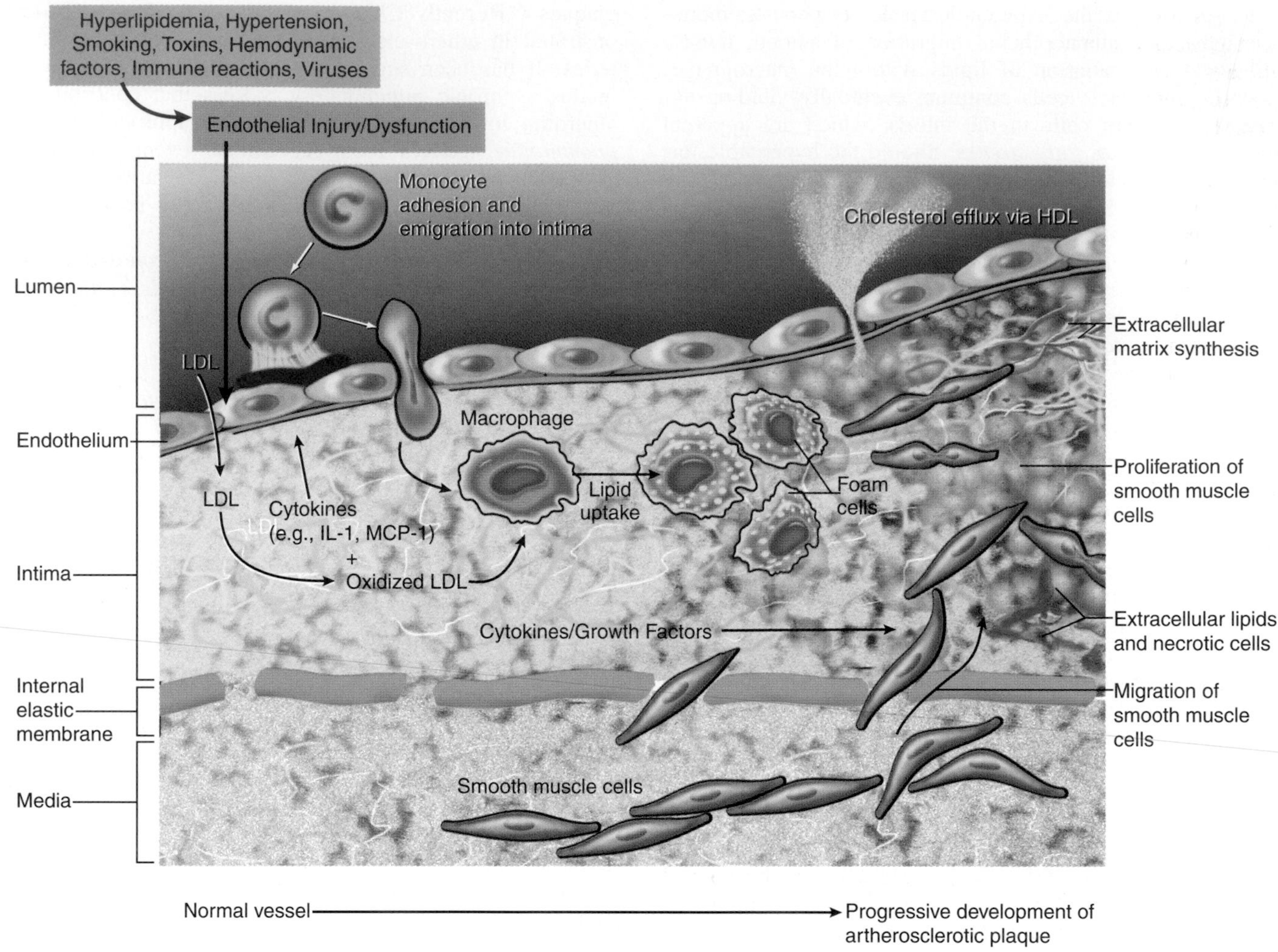

Figure 12–13

Schematic diagram of a hypothetical sequence of cell-level events and cellular interactions in atherosclerosis. Hyperlipidemia and other risk factors are thought to cause endothelial injury, resulting in adhesion of platelets and monocytes and release of growth factors, including platelet-derived growth factor (PDGF), which lead to smooth muscle cell migration and proliferation. Smooth muscle cells produce large amounts of extracellular matrix, including collagen and proteoglycans. Foam cells of atheromatous plaques are derived from both macrophages and smooth muscle cells—from macrophages via the very-low-density lipoprotein (VLDL) receptor and low-density lipoprotein (LDL) modifications recognized by scavenger receptors (e.g., oxidized LDL), and from smooth muscle cells by less certain mechanisms. Extracellular lipid is derived from insudation from the vessel lumen, particularly in the presence of hypercholesterolemia, and also from degenerating foam cells. Cholesterol accumulation in the plaque should be viewed as reflecting an imbalance between influx and efflux, and it is possible that high-density lipoprotein (HDL) helps clear cholesterol from these accumulations.

Hypertensive Vascular Disease

Elevated blood pressure (*hypertension*) affects both the function and the structure of blood vessels, largely small muscular arteries and arterioles. In this section, we discuss the mechanisms of normal blood pressure control, the possible mechanisms of hypertension, and the pathologic changes in the vasculature associated with the disorder.

HYPERTENSION

A common health problem with widespread and sometimes devastating consequences, elevated blood pressure often remains asymptomatic until late in its course.[49] Hypertension is one of the most important risk factors in both coronary heart disease and cerebrovascular accidents and may also lead to cardiac hypertrophy with heart failure (hypertensive heart disease), aortic dissection, and renal failure. The detrimental effects of blood pressure increase continuously as the pressure rises. There is no rigidly defined threshold of blood pressure above which an individual is considered at risk for the complications of hypertension and below which an individual is safe. Nevertheless, a sustained diastolic pressure greater than 90 mm Hg or a sustained systolic pressure in excess of 140 mm Hg is considered to constitute hypertension (Table 12–4). By these criteria, screening programs reveal that 25% of persons in the general population are hypertensive. The prevalence increases with age. Black individuals are affected by hypertension about twice as often as whites and seem more vulnerable to is complications. Reduction of blood pressure has striking effects on incidence and death rates from ischemic heart disease, heart failure, and stroke.

Table 12–5 lists the major causes of hypertension. *About 90 to 95% of hypertension is idiopathic and apparently primary (essential hypertension). Of the remaining 5 to 10%, most is secondary to renal disease or, less often, to narrowing of the renal artery, usually by an atheromatous plaque (renovascular hypertension).* Infrequently, secondary hypertension is the result of diseases related to the adrenal glands, such as primary aldosteronism, Cushing syndrome, and pheochromocytoma, or other disorders (Table 12–5).

In most cases, hypertension remains at a modest level and fairly stable over years to decades and, unless a myocardial infarction, heart failure, or cerebrovascular accident supervenes, is compatible with long life. About 5% of hypertensive persons show a rapidly rising blood pressure, which, if untreated, leads to death within 1 or 2 years. This is called *accelerated* or *malignant hypertension.* The full-blown clinical syndrome of malignant hypertension includes severe hypertension (diastolic pressure >120 mm Hg), renal failure, and retinal hemorrhages and exudates, with or without papilledema. This form of hypertension may develop in previously normotensive persons but more often is superimposed on preexisting hypertension, either essential or secondary.

The blood pressure level in any individual is a complex trait that is determined by the interaction of multiple genetic, environmental, and demographic factors. It should not be surprising therefore that multiple mechanisms play a role in hypertension. These mechanisms constitute aberrations of the normal physiologic regulation of blood pressure.

Regulation of Normal Blood Pressure. *The magnitude of the arterial pressure depends on two fundamental hemodynamic variables: cardiac output* and *total peripheral resistance* (Fig. 12–14). Cardiac output is influenced by blood volume, which is greatly dependent on body sodium. Thus, sodium homeostasis is central to blood pressure regulation.[50] Total peripheral resistance is predominantly determined at the level of the arterioles and depends on lumen size, itself dependent on the thickness of the arteriolar wall and the effects of neural and hormonal influences that either constrict or dilate these vessels. Normal vascular tone depends on the competition between vasoconstricting influences (including angiotensin II, catecholamines, thromboxane, leukotrienes, and endothelin) and vasodilators (in-

Table 12–5. TYPES OF HYPERTENSION (SYSTOLIC AND DIASTOLIC)

Essential Hypertension

Secondary Hypertension

Renal
- Acute glomerulonephritis
- Chronic renal disease
- Polycystic disease
- Renal artery stenosis
- Renal vasculitis
- Renin-producing tumors

Endocrine
- Adrenocortical hyperfunction (Cushing syndrome, primary aldosteronism, congenital adrenal hyperplasia, licorice ingestion)
- Exogenous hormones (glucocorticoids, estrogen [including oral contraceptives], sympathomimetics, tyramine-containing foods, monoamine oxidase inhibitors)
- Pheochromocytoma
- Acromegaly
- Hypothyroidism (Myxedema)
- Hyperthyroidism (Thyrotoxicosis)
- Pregnancy-induced

Cardiovascular
- Coarctation of aorta
- Polyarteritis nodosa
- Increased intravascular volume
- Increased cardiac output
- Rigidity of the aorta

Neurologic
- Psychogenic
- Increased intracranial pressure
- Sleep apnea
- Acute stress, including surgery

Table 12–4. CLASSIFICATION OF BLOOD PRESSURE IN ADULTS

Category	Systolic (mm Hg)	Diastolic (mm Hg)
Normal	<130	<85
High normal	130–139	85–89
Hypertension		
Stage 1 (mild)	140–159	90–99
Stage 2 (moderate)	160–179	100–109
Stage 3 (severe)	180–209	110–119
Stage 4 (very severe)	>210	>120

Per: The fifth report on the Joint National Committee on Detection, Evaluation and Treatment of High Blood Pressure (JNC V). Arch Intern Med 153:154, 1993. From Kaplan NM: Systemic hypertension: mechanisms and diagnosis. In Braunwald E (ed): Heart Disease, 5th ed. Philadelphia, WB Saunders, 1997, p 807.

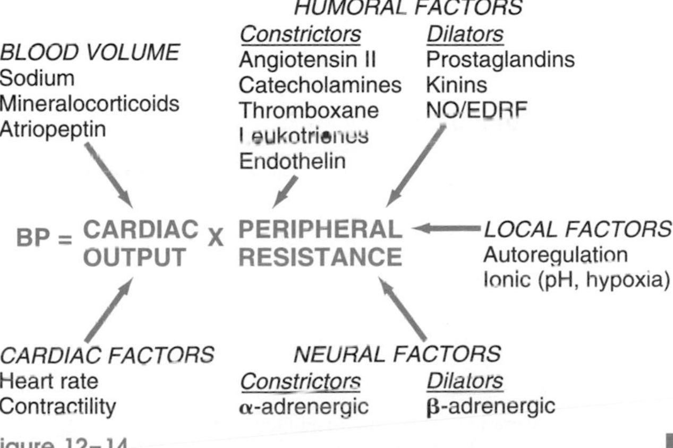

Figure 12–14

Blood pressure regulation. NO/EDRF, nitric oxide–endothelium-derived relaxing factor.

cluding kinins, prostaglandins, and nitric oxide). Certain metabolic products (such as lactic acid, hydrogen ions, and adenosine) and hypoxia can also function as local vasodilators. Resistance vessels also exhibit *autoregulation*, a process by which increased blood flow to such vessels induces vasoconstriction, an adaptive mechanism that protects against hyperperfusion of tissues.

The kidneys play an important role in blood pressure regulation, and there is considerable evidence that renal dysfunction is essential for the development and maintenance of both essential and secondary hypertension.[51]

- The kidney influences both peripheral resistance and sodium homeostasis, and the renin-angiotensin system appears central to these influences. Renin elaborated by the juxtaglomerular cells of the kidney transforms *plasma angiotensinogen* to *angiotensin I*, and the latter is converted to *angiotensin II* by angiotensin-converting enzyme (ACE) (Fig. 12–15). Angiotensin II alters blood pressure by increasing both peripheral resistance and blood volume. The former effect is achieved largely by its ability to cause vasoconstriction through direct action on vascular smooth muscle, the latter by stimulation of aldosterone secretion, which increases distal tubular reabsorption of sodium and thus of water.
- The kidney produces a variety of vasodepressor or antihypertensive substances that presumably counterbalance the vasopressor effects of angiotensin. These include the prostaglandins, a urinary kallikrein-kinin system, platelet-activating factor, and nitric oxide.
- When blood volume is reduced, the *glomerular filtration rate* (GFR) falls; this, in turn, leads to increased reabsorption of sodium by proximal tubules in an attempt to conserve sodium and expand blood volume.
- *GFR-independent natriuretic factors*, including atrial natriuretic factor (ANF), a peptide secreted by heart atria in response to volume expansion, inhibit sodium reabsorption in distal tubules and cause vasodilation. Abnormalities in these renal mechanisms are implicated in the pathogenesis of secondary hypertension in a variety of renal diseases, but they also play important roles in essential hypertension.

Pathogenesis of Essential Hypertension. *Arterial hypertension occurs when changes develop that alter the relationship between blood volume and total peripheral resistance.* For many of the secondary forms of hypertension, these factors are reasonably well understood, as, for example, in so-called *renovascular hypertension*. In this condition, renal artery stenosis causes decreased glomerular flow

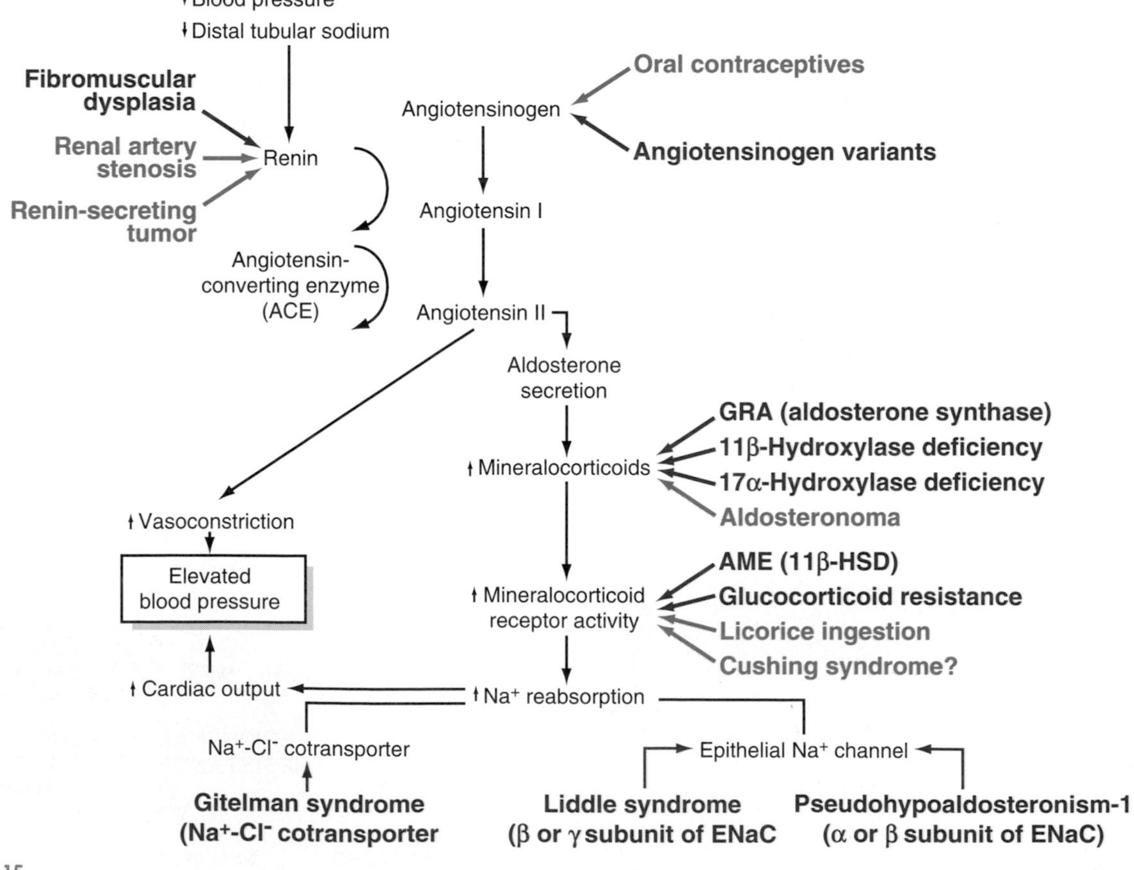

Figure 12–15

Blood pressure variation in the renin-angiotensin system. Components of the systemic renin-angiotensin system are shown in black. Genetic disorders that affect blood pressure by altering activity of this pathway are shown in red; arrows indicate sites in the pathway altered by mutation. Genes that are mutated in these disorders are indicated in parentheses. Acquired disorders that alter blood pressure through effects on this pathway are shown in blue. ENaC, epithelial sodium channel. (Modified with permission from Lifton RP: Molecular genetics of human blood pressure variation. Science 272:676, 1996. Copyright 1996, American Association for the Advancement of Science.)

and pressure in the afferent arteriole of the glomerulus and induces renin secretion by the juxtaglomerular cells. This initiates angiotensin II–induced vasoconstriction; increased peripheral resistance; and, through the aldosterone mechanism, increased sodium reabsorption and increased blood volume. Similarly, in pheochromocytoma, a tumor of the adrenal medulla (Chapter 26), catecholamines produced by tumor cells cause episodic vasoconstriction and thus induce hypertension.

Genetic Factors. It is now thought that essential hypertension results from an interaction of genetic and environmental factors that affect cardiac output, peripheral resistance, or both. A generally accepted concept is that blood pressure (similar to height and weight) is a continuously distributed variable and that essential hypertension is one extreme of this distribution rather than a distinct disease. *Genetic factors* clearly play a role in determining blood pressure levels, as evidenced by studies comparing blood pressure in monozygotic and dizygotic twins, studies of familial aggregation of hypertension comparing the blood pressure of biologic and adoptive siblings, and adoption studies. Although single-gene disorders can be responsible for hypertension in unusual cases (see later), it is unlikely that a mutation at a single gene locus is a major cause of essential hypertension. It is more likely that essential hypertension is a polygenic and heterogeneous disorder (Chapter 6)[52] in which the combined effect of mutations or polymorphisms at several gene loci influence blood pressure.

Single-gene disorders are known to cause relatively rare forms of hypertension through several mechanisms (Fig. 12–15). These include:[53]

- Gene defects in enzymes involved in *aldosterone metabolism* (e.g., aldosterone synthase, 11β-hydroxylase, 17α-hydroxylase). These lead to an adaptive increase in secretion of aldosterone, increased salt and water resorption, plasma volume expansion, and ultimately hypertension.
- Mutations in proteins that affect sodium reabsorption. For example, mutations in an epithelial sodium channel protein lead to increased distal tubular reabsorption of sodium induced by aldosterone, resulting in a moderately severe form of salt-sensitive hypertension called *Liddle syndrome*).

Inherited variations in blood pressure may also depend on the cumulative effects of allelic forms of several genes that affect blood pressure. For example, predisposition to essential hypertension has been associated with heterogeneity of the genes encoding components of the renin angiotensin system: there is an association of hypertension with polymorphisms in both the angiotensinogen locus and the angiotensin II type I receptor locus.[54] Genetic variants in the renin-angiotensin system may contribute to the known racial differences in blood pressure regulation.

Environmental Factors. Environmental factors are thought to contribute to expression of the genetic determinants of increased pressure. The role of environment is illustrated by the lower incidence of hypertension in Chinese people living in China as compared with persons of Chinese descent living in the United States. Stress, obesity, smoking, physical inactivity, and heavy consumption of salt have all been implicated as exogenous factors in hypertension. As will be emphasized later, the evidence linking the level of dietary sodium intake with the prevalence of hypertension in different population groups is particularly impressive. In both of the major pathways for hypertension to be discussed—primary renal and primary vascular defects—heavy sodium intake augments the hypertension.

Mechanisms. What then is the primary defect in essential hypertension? Two overlapping pathways are proposed.

Renal Retention of Excess Sodium. The studies on the single-gene disorders and renin-angiotensin system genes discussed previously have been interpreted to favor the hypothesis that defects in renal sodium homeostasis are the primary cause of hypertension (Fig. 12–16, *left*). Such scenarios suggest the existence of genetic factors that result in reduced renal sodium excretion—in the presence of normal arterial pressure—as the initiating event. Decreased sodium excretion leads to an increase in fluid volume and a high cardiac output. In the face of increasing cardiac output, peripheral vasoconstriction occurs (as a result of autoregulation) to prevent the overperfusion of tissues that would ensue from an unchecked increase in cardiac output. Autoregulation leads to increased peripheral resistance, however, and along with it an elevation of blood pressure. At the higher setting of blood pressure, enough additional sodium can be excreted by the kidneys to equal intake and prevent fluid retention. Thus, an altered but steady state of sodium excretion is achieved (*resetting of pressure natriuresis*) but at the expense of stable increases in blood pressure. The evidence supporting the importance of sodium homeostasis in hypertension is as follows:

- Rise in blood pressure with age is directly correlated with increasing levels of sodium intake.
- People who consume little sodium have little or no hypertension, but when they consume more sodium, hypertension appears.
- Genetically predisposed animals given sodium loads develop hypertension.
- Some individuals given large sodium loads over short periods develop an increase in vascular resistance and blood pressure.
- Increased sodium is present in the vascular tissue and blood cells of most hypertensives.
- Sodium restriction lowers blood pressure in most people.
- Diuretics act as effective antihypertensive drugs by promoting excretion of sodium.

Vasoconstriction and Vascular Hypertrophy. An alternative hypothesis implicates increased peripheral resistance as the primary cause of hypertension. Such increased resistance is caused either by factors that induce functional vasoconstriction or by stimuli that induce structural changes in the vessel wall (i.e., hypertrophy, remodeling, and hyperplasia of smooth muscle cells), leading to a thickened wall and narrowed lumen, or by both effects. Vasoconstrictive influences may consist of (1) behavioral or neurogenic factors, as exemplified by the reduction of blood pressure achieved by meditation (the *relaxation response*); (2) increased release of vasoconstrictor agents (e.g., renin, catecholamines, endothelin); or (3) increased sensitivity of vascular smooth muscle to constricting agents. It has been suggested that such increased sensitivity is caused by a primary, possibly genetic defect in transport of sodium and calcium across the smooth muscle cell membrane, leading to increased intracellular calcium and contraction of smooth muscle cells. In this scenario, such vasoconstrictive influences, if exerted chronically or repeatedly, may themselves cause structural thickening of the resistance vessels, thus perpetuating increased blood pressure. Certain vasoconstrictors (e.g., angiotensin II) also function as growth factors, causing smooth muscle hypertrophy, hyperplasia, and matrix deposition. Conversely, there is evidence that structural changes in the vessel wall may occur early in hypertension, *preceding* rather than being strictly secondary to the vasoconstriction. Such evidence has led to a hypothesis that genetic or environmentally induced defects in intracellular signaling in smooth muscle cells affect cell cycle genes and ion fluxes that modulate both smooth cell growth and increased vascular tone, resulting in wall thickening and vasoconstriction, respectively (Fig. 12–16, *right*).

To summarize, essential hypertension is a complex disorder that almost certainly has more than one cause. It may be initiated by environmental factors (e.g., stress, salt intake, estrogens), which affect the variables that control blood pressure in the genetically predisposed individual. Although the susceptibility genes for essential hypertension are currently unknown, they may well include genes that govern responses to an increased renal sodium load, levels of pressor substances, such as angiotensin II, reactivity of vascular smooth muscle to pressor agents, or smooth muscle cell growth. In established hypertension, both increased cardiac output and increased peripheral resistance contribute to the increased pressure (Fig. 12–16).

Vascular Pathology. Hypertension accelerates atherogenesis and causes changes in the structure of the walls of blood vessels that potentiate both aortic dissection and cerebrovascular hemorrhage. In addition, hypertension is associated with two forms of small blood vessel disease: hyaline arteriolosclerosis and hyperplastic arteriolosclerosis (Fig. 12–17). Both lesions are related to elevations of blood pressure, but other causes may also be involved.

MORPHOLOGY.

Hyaline Arteriolosclerosis. This condition is encountered frequently in elderly patients, whether normotensive or hypertensive, but it is more generalized and more severe in patients with hypertension. Common in diabetes, it forms part of the microangiography characteristic of diabetic disease (see Chapter 20). Whatever the clinical setting, the vascular lesion consists of a homogenous, pink, hyaline thickening of the walls of arterioles with loss of underlying structural detail and with narrowing of the lumen.

It is believed that the lesions reflect leakage of plasma components across vascular endothelium and increasing extracellular matrix production by smooth muscle cells. Presumably the chronic hemodynamic stress of hypertension or a metabolic stress in diabetes accentuates endothelial injury, thus resulting in leakage and hyaline deposition (Fig. 12–17*a*). The narrowing of the arteriolar lumens causes impairment of the blood supply to affected organs, particularly well exemplified in the kidneys. Thus, **hyaline arteriolosclerosis is a major morphologic characteristic of benign nephrosclerosis,** in which the arteriolar narrowing causes diffuse renal ischemia and symmetric shrinking of the kidneys (Chapter 21).

Hyperplastic Arteriolosclerosis. The hyperplastic type of arteriolosclerosis is generally related to more acute or severe elevations of blood pres-

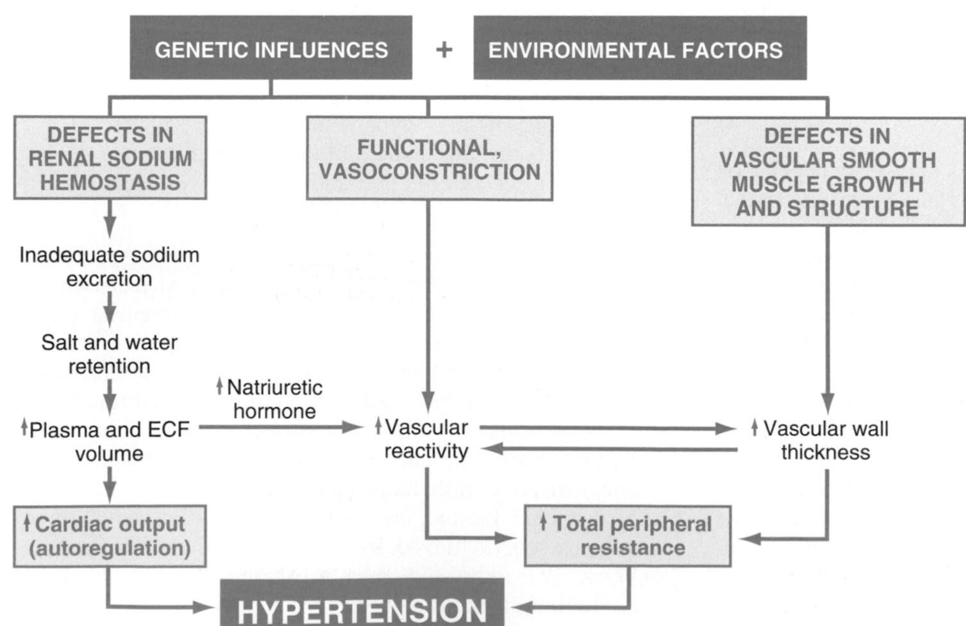

Figure 12–16

Hypothetical scheme for the pathogenesis of essential hypertension, implicating genetic defects in renal excretion of sodium, functional regulation of vascular tone, and structural regulation of vascular caliber. Environmental factors, especially increased salt intake, potentiate the effects of genetic factors. The resultant increase in cardiac output and peripheral resistance contributes to hypertension. ECF, extracellular fluid.

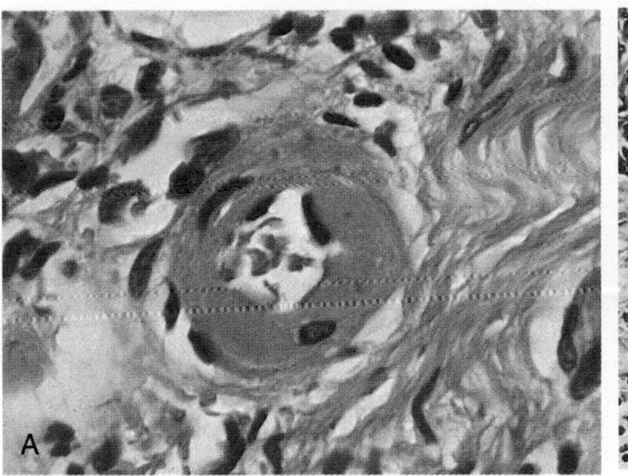

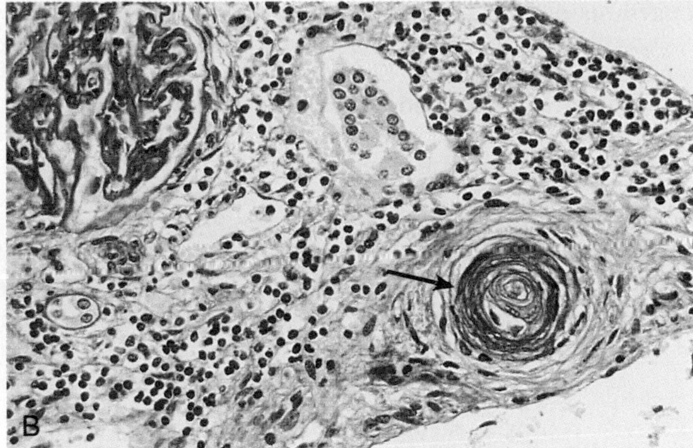

Figure 12–17 ■

Vascular pathology in hypertension. *A*, Hyaline arteriolosclerosis. The arteriolar wall is hyalinized and the lumen is markedly narrowed. *B*, Hyperplastic arteriolosclerosis (onionskinning) causing luminal obliteration (*arrow*), with secondary ischemic changes, manifested by wrinkling of the glomerular capillary vessels at the upper left (periodic acid–Schiff [PAS] stain). (Courtesy of Helmut Rennke, MD, Brigham and Women's Hospital, Boston, MA.)

sure and is therefore characteristic of but not limited to malignant hypertension (diastolic pressures usually >110 mm Hg). This form of arteriolar disease can be identified with the light microscope by virtue of its onion-skin, concentric, laminated thickening of the walls of arterioles with progressive narrowing of the lumens (Fig. 12–17*B*). With the electron microscope, the laminations consist of smooth muscle cells and thickened and reduplicated basement membrane. Frequently, these hyperplastic changes are accompanied by deposits of fibrinoid and acute necrosis of the vessel walls, referred to as **necrotizing arteriolitis**. The arterioles in all tissues throughout the body may be affected, but the favored site is the kidney (Chapter 21).

Inflammatory Disease—The Vasculitides

Inflammation of the walls of vessels, called *vasculitis*, is encountered in diverse diseases and clinical settings. Vessels of any type in virtually any organ can be affected; this leads to a wide spectrum of clinical manifestations, which often includes constitutional signs and symptoms, such as fever, myalgias, arthralgias, and malaise. The two most common mechanisms of vasculitis are immune-mediated inflammation and direct invasion of vascular walls by infectious pathogens (Table 12–6). Infections can indirectly induce a noninfectious vasculitis, for example, by generating immune complexes or triggering cross-reactivity. In a particular patient, it is critical to distinguish between directly infectious and immunologic mechanisms because the treatment approaches differ widely; for example, the immunosuppressive therapy appropriate for immune-mediated vasculitis would be potentially harmful for infectious vasculitis. Moreover, physical and chemical injury, such as irradiation, mechanical trauma, and toxins, can also cause vascular damage. In such cases, one or a relatively few vessels may be affected, as, for example, in a localized area of infection, irradiation, or mechanical trauma.

Table 12–6. CLASSIFICATION OF VASCULITIS BASED ON PATHOGENESIS

Direct Infection
- Bacterial (e.g., *Neisseria*)
- Rickettsial (e.g., Rocky Mountain spotted fever)
- Spirochetal (e.g., syphilis)
- Fungal (e.g., aspergillosis, mucormycosis)
- Viral (e.g., herpes zoster-varicella)

Immunologic
- Immune complex mediated
  - Infection induced (e.g., hepatitis B and C virus)
  - Henoch-Schönlein purpura
  - SLE and rheumatoid arthritis
  - Drug induced
  - Cryoglobulinemia
  - Serum sickness
- Antineutrophil cytoplasmic autoantibody (ANCA) mediated
  - Wegener granulomatosis
  - Microscopic polyangiitis (microscopic polyarteritis)
  - Churg-Strauss syndrome
- Direct antibody attack mediated
  - Goodpasture syndrome (anti-GBM antibodies)
  - Kawasaki disease (antiendothelial antibodies)
- Cell mediated
  - Allograft organ rejection
- Inflammatory bowel disease
- Paraneoplastic vasculitis

Unknown
- Giant cell (temporal) arteritis
- Takayasu arteritis
- Polyarteritis nodosa (classic polyarteritis nodosa)

GBM, glomerular basement membrane.
Data from Jennette JC, Falk RJ: Update on the pathobiology of vasculitis. In Schoen FJ, Gimbrone MA (eds): Cardiovascular Pathology: Clinicopathologic Correlations and Pathogenetic Mechanisms. Baltimore, Williams & Wilkins, 1995, p 156; and Jennette JC, Falk RJ: Small-vessel vasculitis. N Engl J Med 1337:1512, 1997.

Pathogenesis of Non-Infectious Vasculitis. Most noninfectious vasculitides appear to be initiated by one of several immunologic mechanisms. Such processes often induce relatively distinctive clinicopathologic entities, in which the vasculitis is widespread. Of these so-called *systemic necrotizing vasculitides*, several types affect the aorta and medium-sized vessels; most affect vessels smaller than arteries, such as arterioles, venules, and capillaries (designated *small vessel vasculitis*).[55, 56]

Immune Complexes. The evidence for involvement of immune complexes in vasculitides can be summarized as follows:

- The vascular lesions resemble those found in experimental immune complex–mediated conditions, such as the local Arthus phenomenon and serum sickness. Immune reactants and complement can be detected in the serum or vessels of patients with vasculitis. For example, DNA–anti-DNA complexes are present in the vascular lesions of systemic lupus erythematosus–associated vasculitis; IgG, IgM, and complement in cryoglobulinemic vasculitis; and a number of other antigens in isolated cases.
- Hypersensitivity to drugs causes approximately 10% of vasculitic skin lesions. Some, such as penicillin conjugate serum proteins, whereas others such as streptokinase are foreign proteins; both can lead to vascular deposits of immune complexes.
- The most impressive evidence comes from vasculitis associated with viral infections, particularly hepatitis. There is a high incidence of hepatitis B antigen (HBsAg) and HBsAg–anti-HBsAg immune complexes in the serum and, with complement, in the vascular lesions of some patients with vasculitis, particularly those with large vessel polyarteritis nodosa and less commonly in those with membranous or membranoproliferative glomerulonephritis or leukocytoclastic vasculitis.[57] Importantly, immunosuppressive treatment results in a remission of the vasculitis but perpetuates the hepatitis B virus infection. Chronic hepatitis C virus (HCV) infection leads to glomerulonephritis, in which HCV/RNA and cryoprecipitates containing anti-HCV antibodies are detected in glomeruli.

Whether complexes accrue in vessel walls by deposition from the circulation, by in situ formation, or by a combination of these mechanisms is not known (Chapter 21). Moreover, many small vessel vasculitides show a paucity of vascular immune deposits,[58] and therefore other mechanisms have been sought for these so-called *pauci-immune* vasculitides.

Antineutrophil Cytoplasmic Antibodies. Serum from many patients with vasculitis in small vessels reacts with cytoplasmic antigens in neutrophils, indicating the presence of *antineutrophil cytoplasmic autoantibodies* (ANCA). ANCA comprise a heterogeneous group of autoantibodies against enzymes mainly found within the azurophil or primary granules in neutrophils but also found in the lysosomes of monocytes and in endothelial cells.[59] ANCA can be detected in serum by immunofluorescent microscopy of ethanol-fixed neutrophils and by immunochemical assays. Two main patterns of immunofluorescent staining distinguish different ANCA types. One ANCA type shows cytoplasmic localization of the staining (c-ANCA), and the most common target antigen is proteinase 3 (PR-3), a neutrophil granule constituent. The second type shows perinuclear staining (p-ANCA) and is usually specific for myeloperoxidase (MPO). Either ANCA specificity may occur in a patient with ANCA-associated small vessel vasculitis, but c-ANCA (PR-3 specificity) are typically found in Wegener granulomatosis and p-ANCA (MPO specificity) are found in most cases of microscopic polyangiitis and Churg-Strauss syndrome. Approximately 10% of patients with these disorders, however, do not demonstrate ANCA by typical assays.

ANCA serve as useful quantitative diagnostic markers for these disorders, and their discovery has led to segregation of a group of these disorders as the *ANCA-associated vasculitides*.[60, 61] The close association between ANCA titers and disease activity, particularly c-ANCA in Wegener granulomatosis, suggests that they may be important in the pathogenesis of this disease, but the precise mechanisms by which ANCA induce injury are unknown. One scenario currently being pursued postulates the following events:

- An autoimmune process of yet uncertain cause and mechanism initiates the formation of ANCA.
- Proinflammatory cytokines produced during an infection, by malignancy, or possibly triggered by drugs induce surface expression of the ANCA target antigens PR-3 and MPO on susceptible cells, thereby making them accessible to the respective antibodies.
- Binding of circulating ANCA to these antigens leads to neutrophil degranulation and endothelial cell injury with subsequent vascular damage.

Other Mechanisms. Antibodies to endothelial cells, perhaps induced by defects in immune regulation, may predispose to certain vasculitides, such as those associated with systemic lupus erythematosus and Kawasaki disease. Additionally, in Goodpasture syndrome the glomerulitis and pneumonitis are caused by anti–glomerular basement membrane antibodies. Finally, there is experimental evidence that certain viruses (e.g., herpes, coxsackievirus) may cause vasculitis by immune mechanisms involving T-cell action and γ-interferon.[43]

Classification. The systemic vasculitides are classified on the basis of the size of the involved blood vessels, the anatomic site and histologic characteristics of the lesion, and the clinical manifestations. There is considerable clinical and pathologic overlap among these disorders. The nomenclature used here is that developed at the Chapel Hill Consensus Conference on the Nomenclature of Systemic Vasculitides (Table 12–7 and Fig. 12–18),[62] and the sequence of entities discussed follows that in Table 12–7.

GIANT CELL (TEMPORAL) ARTERITIS

Giant cell (temporal) arteritis, the most common of the vasculitides, is an acute and chronic, often granulomatous, inflammation of medium-sized and small arteries. It affects

Table 12–7. CLASSIFICATION AND CHARACTERISTICS OF VASCULITIS*

Large Vessel Vasculitis†	
Giant cell (temporal) arteritis	Granulomatous arteritis of the aorta and its major branches, with a predilection for the extracranial branches of the carotid artery. *Often involves the temporal artery. Usually occurs in patients older than 50 and often is associated with polymyalgia rheumatica*
Takayasu arteritis	Granulomatous inflammation of the aorta and its major branches. *Usually occurs in patients younger than 50*
Medium-Sized Vessel Vasculitis‡	
Polyarteritis nodosa (classic polyarteritis nodosa)	Necrotizing inflammation of medium-sized or small arteries without glomerulonephritis or vasculitis in arterioles, capillaries, or venules
Kawasaki disease	Arteritis involving large, medium-sized, and small arteries and associated with mucocutaneous lymph node syndrome. *Coronary arteries are often involved. Aorta and veins may be involved. Usually occurs in children*
Small Vessel Vasculitis§	
Wegener granulomatosis‖	Granulomatous inflammation involving the respiratory tract and necrotizing vasculitis affecting small to medium-sized vessels (e.g., capillaries, venules, arterioles, and arteries). *Necrotizing glomerulonephritis is common*
Churg-Strauss syndrome‖	Eosinophil-rich and granulomatous inflammation involving the respiratory tract and necrotizing vasculitis affecting small to medium-sized vessels associated with asthma and blood eosinophilia
Microscopic polyangiitis (microscopic polyarteritis)‖	Necrotizing vasculitis with few or no immune deposits affecting small vessels (i.e., capillaries, venules, or arterioles). *Necrotizing arteritis involving small and medium-sized arteries may be present. Necrotizing glomerulonephritis is common. Pulmonary capillaritis often occurs*
Henoch-Schönlein purpura	Vasculitis with IgA-dominant immune deposits affecting small vessels (i.e., capillaries, venules, or arterioles). *Typically involves skin, gut, and glomeruli and associated with arthralgias or arthritis*
Essential cryoglobulinemic vasculitis	Vasculitis with cryoglobulin immune deposits affecting small vessels (i.e., capillaries, venules, or arterioles) and associated with cryoglobulins in serum. *Skin and glomeruli are often involved*
Cutaneous leukocytoclastic angiitis	Isolated cutaneous leukocytoclastic angiitis without systemic vasculitis or glomerulonephritis

*Note that some small and large vessel vasculitides may involve medium-sized arteries, but large and medium-sized vessel vasculitides do not involve vessels smaller than arteries.

†Aorta and its largest branches to extremities and head and neck.

‡Main visceral arteries and their branches.

§Arterioles, venules, capillaries (occasionally small arteries).

‖Strongly associated with antineutrophil cytoplasmic autoantibodies (ANCA), predominantly cytoplasmic (antiproteinase 3) ANCA in Wegener and perinuclear (antimyeloperoxidase) ANCA in microscopic polyangiitis and Churg-Strauss syndrome.

Modified from Jennette JC, et al: Nomenclature of systemic vasculitides: the proposal of an international consensus conference. Arthritis Rheum 37:187, 1994.

principally the arteries in the head—especially the temporal arteries—but also the vertebral and ophthalmic arteries. The latter may lead to blindness. In other expressions of this disorder, lesions have been found in arteries throughout the body, and in some cases the aortic arch has been involved to produce so-called *giant cell aortitis.*

MORPHOLOGY. Characteristically, short segments of one or more affected arteries develop **nodular thickenings with reduction of the lumen,** possibly to a slitlike orifice, which may become thrombosed. Histologically, two patterns are seen. In the more common variant, there is **granulomatous inflammation** of the inner half of the media centered on the internal elastic membrane marked by a mononuclear infiltrate, multinucleate giant cells of both foreign body and Langerhans type, and fragmentation of the internal elastic lamina (Fig. 12–19). In the other, less common pattern, granulomas are rare or absent, and there is only a nonspecific panarteritis with a mixed inflammatory infiltrate composed largely of lymphocytes and macrophages admixed with some neutrophils and eosinophils but no giant cells. Occasionally in this variant, there is some fibrinoid necrosis. The later healed stage of both of these patterns reveals only collagenous thickening of the vessel wall; organization of the luminal thrombus sometimes transforms the artery into a fibrous cord.

Giant cells are present in only two thirds of cases of temporal arteritis, and many histologic sections may have to be examined before one is detected. In the healed phase, the artery has considerable scarring that may be difficult to distinguish from aging changes.

Pathogenesis. The cause of this relatively common disease remains unknown. The morphologic alterations suggest an immunologic reaction against a component of the arterial wall, such as elastin. On the basis of the granulomatous nature of the inflammation, association with certain human leukocyte DR antigens (HLA-DR), and the response to corticosteroid therapy, T cell–mediated injury is suspected. These concepts are supported by experiments in which temporal artery segments from patients with giant cell arteritis were inserted into immunodeficient mice; selective proliferation of T cells in the grafted arteries suggested recognition of a locally expressed antigen.[63]

Clinical Features. The disease is most common in older individuals and rare before the age of 50. Clinically, it begins with only vague constitutional symptoms—fever, fatigue, weight loss—without localizing signs or symptoms, but in most instances there is facial pain or headache, which is severe, sometimes unilateral, and often most intense along the course of the superficial temporal artery. The vessel itself may be nodular and painful to palpation. More serious are ocular symptoms, which appear quite abruptly in about half of patients and range from diplopia

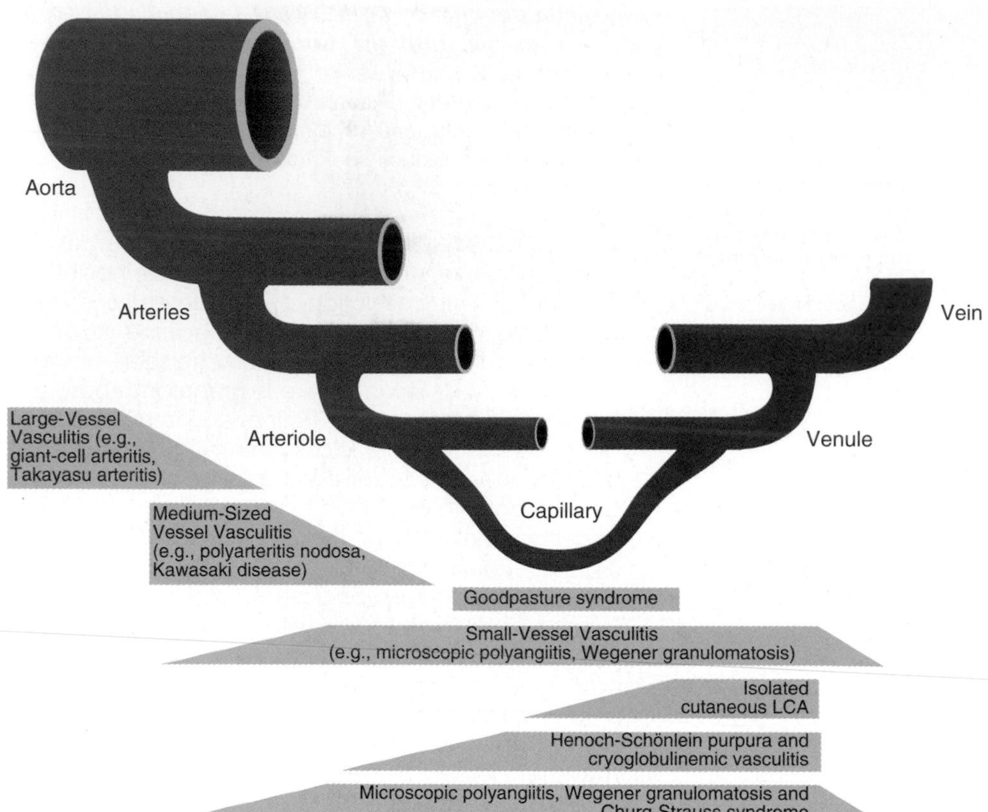

Figure 12–18

Diagrammatic representation of the preferred site of the vasculature involved by the major forms of vasculitis. The widths of the trapezoids indicate the frequencies of involvement of various portions. Note that large-, medium-, and small-vessel vasculitis affects arteries, but only small-vessel vasculitis involves vessels smaller than arteries. LCA, leukocytoclastic angiitis. (From Jennette JC, Falk RJ: Small-vessel vasculitis. N Engl J Med 337:1512, 1997. Copyright © 1997, Massachusetts Medical Society. All rights reserved.)

to transient or permanent complete vision loss. Because treatment with anti-inflammatory agents is remarkably effective, there is urgency in establishing the diagnosis promptly. The diagnosis depends on biopsy and histologic confirmation, but because of the segmental nature of the involvement, adequate biopsy requires at least a 2- to 3-cm length of artery, and a negative biopsy result does not rule out the condition.

Approximately one third of biopsies of the temporal artery are negative in patients with classic manifestations of this disease, and it must be assumed that the lesions were focal and missed on biopsy. In the absence of morphologic confirmation, it is often necessary to institute therapy on clinical grounds alone. Involvement of visceral vessels may give rise to manifestations of myocardial ischemia, gastrointestinal disturbances, or neurologic derangements.

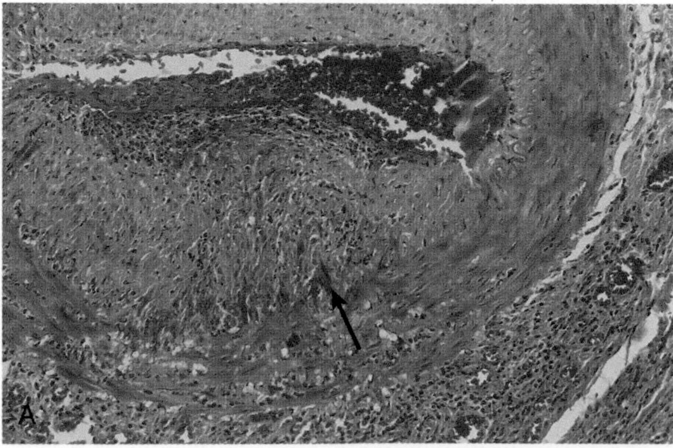

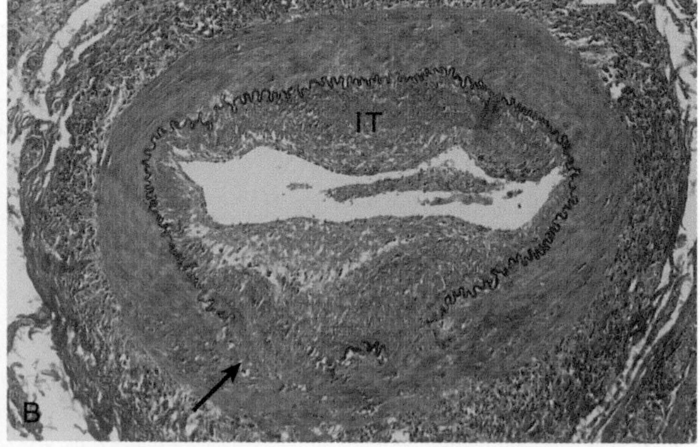

Figure 12–19

Temporal (giant cell) arteritis. *A*, H&E stain of giant cells at the degenerated internal elastic membrane in active arteritis. *B*, Elastic tissue stain demonstrating focal destruction of internal elastic membrane (*arrow*) and intimal thickening (IT) characteristic of long-standing or healed arteritis.

TAKAYASU ARTERITIS

Takayasu arteritis is a granulomatous vasculitis of medium and larger arteries that was described in 1908 by Takayasu as a *clinical syndrome characterized principally by ocular disturbances and marked weakening of the pulses in the upper extremities (pulseless disease), related to fibrous thickening of the aortic arch with narrowing or virtual obliteration of the origins or more distal portions of the great vessels arising in the arch* (Fig. 12–20). It has been reported in most areas of the world, including the United States. The illness is seen predominantly in women younger than 40 years old. The cause and pathogenesis are unknown, although immune mechanisms are suspected.

MORPHOLOGY. Although Takayasu arteritis classically involves the aortic arch, in one third of cases, it also affects the remainder of the aorta and its branches and often the pulmonary arteries. The gross morphologic changes comprise, in most cases, irregular thickening of the aortic or branch vessel wall with intimal wrinking (Fig. 12–20*A* and *B*) When the aortic arch is involved, the orifices of the major arteries to the upper portion of the body may be markedly narrowed or even obliterated by intimal thickening, accounting for the designation **pulseless disease.** The coronary and renal arteries may be similarly affected. Sometimes the lesions extend for some distance into the aortic branches and in half of cases involve the pulmonary arteries. Histologically the early changes consist of an adventitial mononuclear infiltrate with perivascular cuffing of the vasa vasocrum. Later, there may be intense mononuclear inflammation in the media, in some cases accompanied by granulomatous changes, replete with giant cells and patchy necrosis of the media (Fig. 12–20*C*). The morphologic changes of Takayasu arteritis may be indistinguishable from those in giant cell (temporal) arteritis.[64] Thus, distinctions among active giant cell lesions of the aorta are based largely on clinical data, including the age of the patient. Moreover, the description Takayasu arteritis is currently being used widely to designate most giant cell lesions of the aorta in young patients. As the disease runs its course or after treatment with steroids, the inflammatory reaction is predominantly marked by collagenous fibrosis involving all layers of the vessel wall but particularly the intima, accompanied by lymphocytic infiltration. When the root of the aorta is affected, it may undergo dilation, producing aortic valve insufficiency. Narrowing of the coronary ostia may lead to myocardial infarction.

Clinical Features. The salient clinical features include weakening of the pulses and markedly lower blood pressure in the upper extremities with coldness or numbness of the fingers; ocular disturbances, including visual defects, retinal hemorrhages, and total blindness; hypertension; and various neurologic deficits, ranging from dizziness and focal weakness to complete hemiparesis. Involvement of the more distal aorta may lead to claudication of the legs and of cranial vessels, leading to visual disturbances and neurologic manifestations. Involvement of pulmonary arteries may lead to pulmonary hypertension and manifestations of

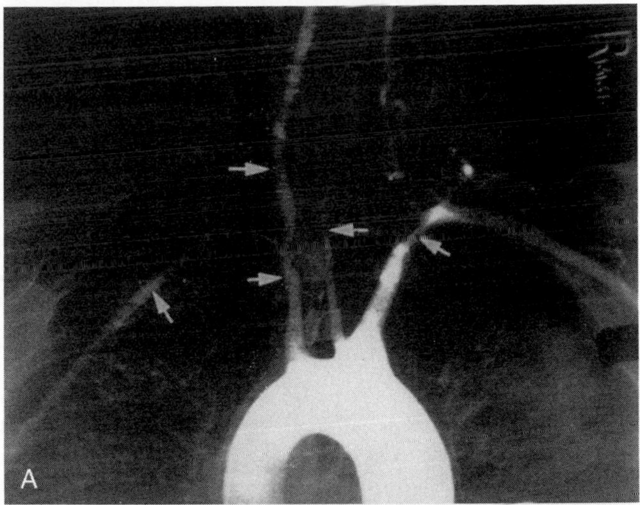

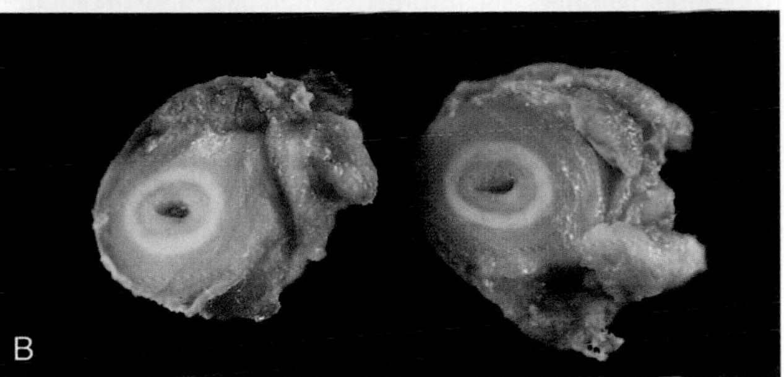

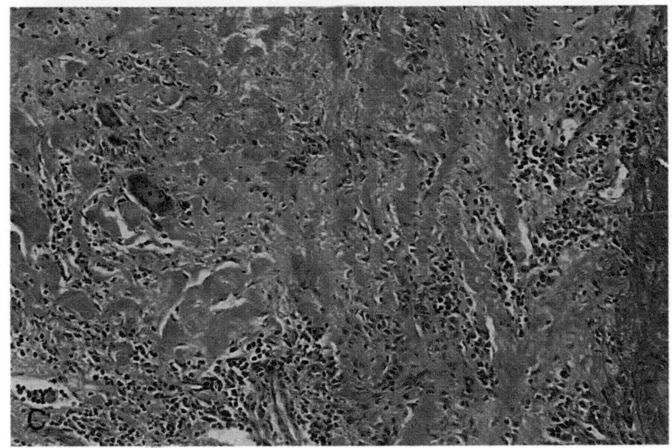

Figure 12–20

Takayasu arteritis. *A*, Aortic arch angiogram showing narrowing of brachiocephalic, carotid, and subclavian arteries (*arrows*). *B*, Gross photograph of two cross-sections of the right carotid artery taken at the autopsy of the patient shown in *A*, demonstrating marked intimal thickening with minimal residual lumen. *C*, Histologic view of active Takayasu aortitis, illustrating destruction of the arterial media by mononuclear inflammation with giant cells.

cor pulmonale. The course of the disease is variable. In some persons, there is rapid progression, but in others a quiescent stage is reached in 1 or 2 years, permitting long-term survival, albeit sometimes with visual or neurologic deficits. The course of the disease is quite variable.

POLYARTERITIS NODOSA (CLASSIC)

Polyarteritis nodosa is a systemic vasculitis manifested by transmural necrotizing inflammation of small or medium-sized muscular arteries, typically involving renal and visceral vessels and sparing the pulmonary circulation. Neither glomerulonephritis nor vasculitis of arterioles, capillaries, or venules is present. The involvement is peculiarly focal, random, and episodic. It often produces irregular aneurysmal dilation, nodularity, and vascular obstruction and sometimes infarctions. To differentiate this disorder from other similar vasculitides, which are now thought to be distinct entities, the term *classic* is sometimes added to the designation.

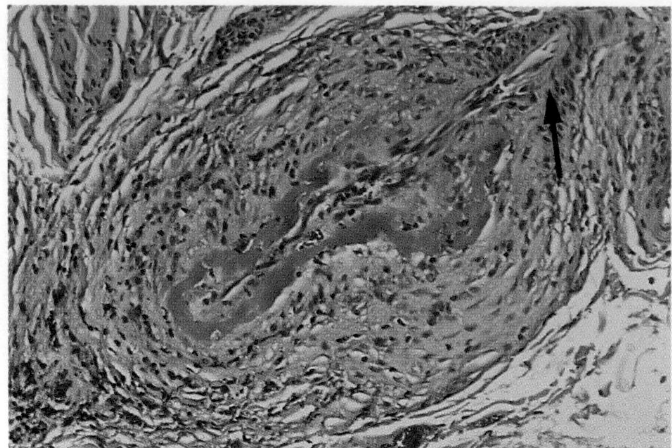

Figure 12–21

Polyarteritis nodosa. Polyarteritis nodosa with segmental fibrinoid necrosis and thrombotic occlusion of the lumen of this small artery. Note that part of the vessel wall at the upper right (*arrow*) is uninvolved. (Courtesy of Sid Murphree, MD, Department of Pathology, University of Texas Southwestern Medical School, Dallas, TX.)

MORPHOLOGY. In classic cases, polyarteritis nodosa involves **arteries of medium to small size in any organ,** with the possible exception of the lung. The distribution of lesions, in descending order of frequency is kidneys, heart, liver, and gastrointestinal tract, followed by pancreas, testes, skeletal muscle, nervous system, and skin. Individual lesions are sharply segmental, may involve only a portion of the vessel circumference, and have a predilection for branching points and bifurcations. Segmental erosion with weakening of the arterial wall owing to the inflammatory process may cause aneurysmal dilation or localized rupture that is perceived clinically as a palpable nodule and can be demonstrated by arteriography. Impairment of perfusion causing ulcerations, infarcts, ischemic atrophy, or hemorrhages in the area supplied by these vessels may provide the first clue to the existence of the underlying disorder. Sometimes, however, the lesions are exclusively microscopic and produce no gross changes.

Histologically the vasculitis during the acute phase is characterized by **transmural inflammation of the arterial wall** with a heavy infiltrate of neutrophils, eosinophils, and mononuclear cells, frequently accompanied by fibrinoid necrosis of the inner half of the vessel wall (Fig. 12–21). Typically the inflammatory reaction permeates the adventitia. The lumen may become thrombosed. In some lesions, only a portion of the circumference is affected, leaving segments of normal arterial wall juxtaposed to areas of vascular inflammation. At a later stage, the acute inflammatory infiltrate begins to disappear and is replaced by fibrous thickening of the vessel wall accompanied by a mononuclear infiltrate. The fibroblastic proliferation may extend into the adventitia, contributing to the firm nodularity that sometimes marks the lesions. At a still later stage, all that remains is marked fibrotic thickening of the affected vessel, devoid of significant inflammatory infiltration. **Particularly characteristic of polyarteritis nodosa is that all stages of activity may coexist in different vessels or even within the same vessel.** Thus, whatever the inflammatory insult, it is apparently recurrent and strangely haphazard.

Clinical Course. Classic polyarteritis nodosa is a disease of young adults, although it may occur in children and older individuals. The course may be acute, subacute, or chronic and is frequently remittent, with long symptom-free intervals. Because the vascular involvement is widely scattered, the clinical signs and symptoms of this disorder may be varied and puzzling. The most common manifestations are malaise, fever of unknown cause, and weight loss; hypertension, usually developing rapidly; abdominal pain and melena (bloody stool) owing to vascular lesions in the alimentary tract; diffuse muscular aches and pains; and peripheral neuritis, which is predominantly motor. Renal involvement is one of the prominent manifestations of polyarteritis nodosa and a major cause of death. Because small vessel involvement is absent, however, there is no glomerulonephritis. About 30% of patients with polyarteritis nodosa have hepatitis B antigen in their serum. Unlike microscopic polyarteritis (microscopic polyangiitis, see later), classic polyarteritis nodosa has little association with ANCA.

The diagnosis can usually be definitely established by the identification of necrotizing arteritis on tissue biopsy specimens, particularly *medium-sized* arteries of clinically involved tissue, such as kidney and nodular skin lesions. Angiography shows vascular aneurysms or occlusions of main visceral arteries in 50% of cases. Untreated, the disease is fatal in most cases, either during an acute fulminant attack or after a protracted course, but therapy with corticosteroids and cyclophosphamide results in remissions or cures in 90%. Effective treatment of the hypertension is a prerequisite for a favorable prognosis.

KAWASAKI SYNDROME (MUCOCUTANEOUS LYMPH NODE SYNDROME)

Kawasaki syndrome is an arteritis involving large, medium-sized, and small arteries (often the coronary arteries) that is associated with the mucocutaneous lymph node syndrome, usually in young children and infants (80% younger than 4 years old). The acute illness is manifested by fever, conjunctival and oral erythema and erosion, edema of the hands and feet, erythema of the palms and soles, a skin rash often with desquamation, and enlargement of cervical lymph nodes. It is usually self-limited.[65] Epidemic in Japan, the disease has also been reported in Hawaii and increasingly in the United States. Approximately 20% of patients develop cardiovascular sequelae, with a range of severity from asymptomatic vasculitis of the coronary arteries, coronary artery ectasia, or aneurysm formation to giant coronary artery aneurysms (7 to 8 mm) with rupture or thrombosis, myocardial infarction, or sudden death. Kawasaki syndrome is the leading cause of acquired heart disease in children in the United States. Acute fatalities occur in approximately 1% of patients owing to coronary arteritis with superimposed thrombosis or ruptured coronary artery aneurysm. Pathologic changes outside the cardiovascular system are rarely significant.

Pathogenesis. The cause of the condition is unknown, but there is evidence that the vasculitis is based on an immunoregulatory defect characterized by T-cell and macrophage activation, secretion of cytokines, polyclonal B-cell hyperactivity, and the formation of autoantibodies to endothelial and smooth muscle cells, leading to acute vasculitis. The nature of the initiating antigen remains unknown, but it is currently speculated that in genetically susceptible persons, a variety of common infectious agents (most likely viral) may trigger the sequence of changes described.

MORPHOLOGY. Although the vasculitis resembles that of polyarteritis nodosa, with necrosis and pronounced inflammation affecting the entire thickness of the vessel wall, fibrinoid necrosis is usually less prominent in Kawasaki syndrome. Coronary artery lesions range from severe destruction of all constituents of the wall by a segmental necrotizing process, with moderate fibrinoid changes and dense infiltrate of inflammatory cells, to mild changes involving the intima only.[66] The acute phase eventually begins to subside spontaneously or in response to treatment, but it is during this subsiding phase that the acute vasculitis of the coronary arteries often leads to aneurysm formation and sometimes associated thrombosis with myocardial infarction.

MICROSCOPIC POLYANGIITIS (MICROSCOPIC POLYARTERITIS, HYPERSENSITIVITY OR LEUKOCYTOCLASTIC VASCULITIS)

While classic polyarteritis nodosa is restricted to arteries, this type generally affects arterioles, capillaries, and venules, although in unusual cases arteries may be involved. Moreover, in contrast to polyarteritis nodosa, in a single patient, all lesions tend to be of the same age, and ANCA are present in the majority of cases. The lesions are thought to represent a hypersensitivity reaction, and it involves the skin, mucous membranes, lungs, brain, heart, gastrointestinal tract, kidneys, and muscle. Necrotizing glomerulonephritis (90% of patients) and pulmonary capillaritis are particularly common. The major resultant clinical features are hemoptysis, hematuria, and proteinuria; bowel pain or bleeding; and muscle pain or weakness. In many cases, the lesions are limited to the skin (*cutaneous leukocytoclastic vasculitis*). Cutaneous vasculitis (Chapter 27) is manifested by palpable purpura. In many cases, reaction to an antigen such as drugs (e.g., penicillin), microorganisms (e.g., streptococci), heterologous proteins, and tumor antigens can be traced as the precipitating cause, but *there are few or no immune deposits in this type of vasculitis.*

MORPHOLOGY. The lesions of microscopic polyangiitis are often histologically similar to those of polyarteritis nodosa, **but muscular and large arteries are usually spared.** Thus, macroscopic infarcts similar to those seen in polyarteritis nodosa are uncommon. Histologically, segmental fibrinoid necrosis of the media may be present, but in some the change is limited to infiltration with neutrophils, which become fragmented as they follow the vessel wall **(leukocytoclasia).** The term **leukocytoclastic angiitis** is given to such lesions, most commonly found in postcapillary venules (Fig. 12–22). Immunoglobulins and complement components may be present in the vascular lesions of the skin, especially if these are examined within 24 hours of development, but in general there is a paucity of immunoglobulin demonstrable by immunofluorescence microscopy **(pauci-immune injury).**

Clinical Features. Greater than 80% of patients have ANCA, most often p-ANCA. Most patients with isolated cutaneous vasculitis respond well simply to removal of the offending agent, but those with systemic disease may develop organ failure unless treated.

Small vessel vasculitis may also appear in distinct diseases, including Henoch-Schönlein purpura, essential mixed cryoglobulinemia, and certain connective tissue disorders, and associated with malignancy. They are discussed with the specific entities elsewhere in this book. ANCA are usually not present.

In *allergic granulomatosis and angiitis* (the Churg-

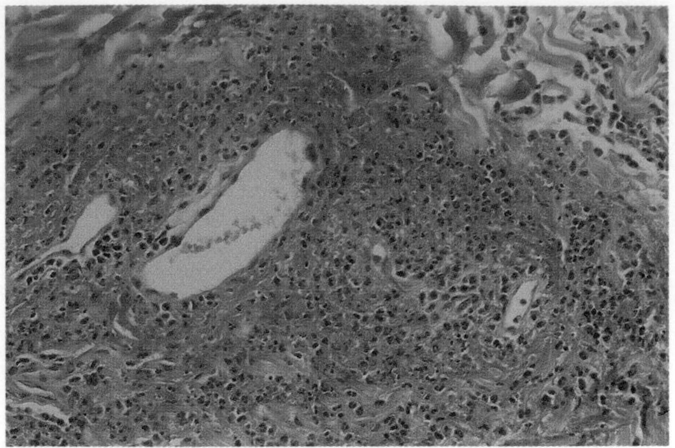

Figure 12–22

Leukocytoclastic vasculitis in a skin biopsy showing fragmentation of neutrophil nuclei in and around vessel walls. (Courtesy of Scott Granter, MD, Brigham and Women's Hospital, Boston, MA.)

Strauss syndrome), the vascular lesions may be histologically identical to those of classic polyarteritis nodosa and microscopic polyangiitis. There is a strong association, however, with allergic rhinitis, bronchial asthma, and eosinophilia. Vessels in the lung, heart, spleen, peripheral nerves, and skin are frequently involved by intravascular and extravascular granulomas, and infiltration of vessels and perivascular tissues by eosinophils is striking. Severe renal disease is infrequent. Coronary arteritis and myocarditis are the principal causes of morbidity and mortality. p-ANCA are present in 70% of patients.

WEGENER GRANULOMATOSIS

Wegener granulomatosis is a necrotizing vasculitis characterized by the triad of (1) *acute necrotizing granulomas* of the upper respiratory tract (ear, nose, sinuses, throat), the lower respiratory tract (lung), or both; (2) *focal necrotizing or granulomatous vasculitis* affecting small to medium-sized vessels (e.g., capillaries, venules, arterioles, and arteries), most prominent in the lungs and upper airways but affecting other sites as well; and (3) renal disease in the form of focal or necrotizing, often crescentic, glomerulitis.[67] Some patients who do not manifest the full triad are said to have *limited* Wegener granulomatosis, in which the kidneys are unaffected and the involvement is restricted to the respiratory tract. Men are affected somewhat more often than women, at an average age of about 40 years.

Pathogenesis. The striking resemblance to polyarteritis nodosa and serum sickness suggests that Wegener granulomatosis may represent some form of hypersensitivity, possibly to an inhaled infectious or other environmental agent, but this is unproved. Immune complexes have been seen in the glomeruli and vessel walls in occasional patients. The presence of granulomas and dramatic response to immunosuppressive therapy also strongly suggest an immunologic mechanism, perhaps of the cell-mediated type. c-ANCA are present in the serum in 90% of patients with active generalized disease, and this appears to be a good marker for disease activity. During treatment, a rising titer of c-ANCA suggests a relapse; most patients in remission have a negative test, or the titer falls significantly.

MORPHOLOGY. Morphologically the upper respiratory tract lesions range from inflammatory sinusitis resulting from the development of **mucosal granulomas** to **ulcerative lesions of the nose, palate, or pharynx, rimmed by necrotizing granulomas and accompanying vasculitis.** In the lungs, dispersed focal necrotizing granulomas may coalesce to produce nodules that may undergo cavitation. Microscopically the granulomas reveal a geographic pattern of necrosis rimmed by lymphocytes, plasma cells, macrophages, and variable numbers of giant cells. In association with such lesions, there is a **necrotizing or granulomatous vasculitis** of small and sometimes larger arteries and veins (Fig. 12–23). Almost identical with those of the acute phase of PAN, these lesions often contain granulomas, which may be within, adjacent to, or clearly separated from the vessel wall. These areas are generally surrounded by a zone of fibrolastic proliferation with giant cells and leukocytic infiltrate and may become cavitary creating a more than superficial resemblance to a tubercle. Thus, the major pathologic differential is mycobacterial or fungal infection. Lesions may ultimately undergo progressive fibrosis and organization.

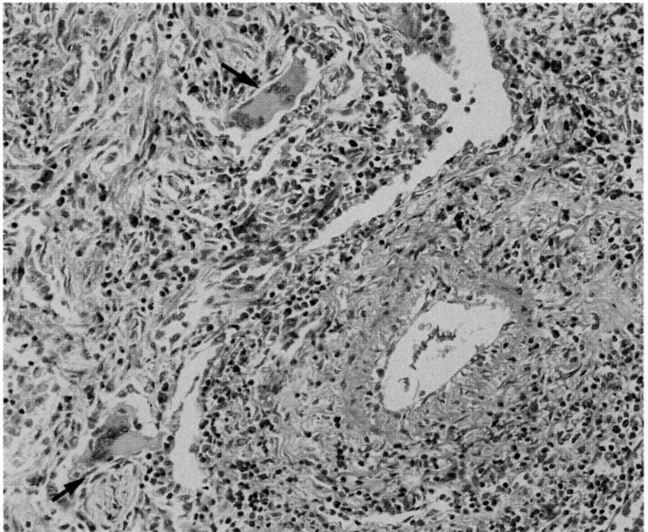

Figure 12–23

Wegener granulomatosis. There is inflammation (vasculitis) of a small artery along with adjacent granulomatous inflammation, in which epithelioid cells and giant cells (*arrows*) can be seen. (Courtesy of Sid Murphree, MD, Department of Pathology, University of Texas Southwestern Medical School, Dallas, TX.)

The renal lesions are of two types (Chapter 21). In milder forms or early in the disease, there is acute focal proliferation and necrosis in the glomeruli, with thrombosis of isolated glomerular capillary loops (focal necrotizing glomerulonephritis). More advanced glomerular lesions are characterized by diffuse necrosis, proliferation, and crescent formation (crescentic glomerulonephritis). Patients with focal lesions may have only hematuria and proteinuria responsive to therapy, whereas those with diffuse disease can develop rapidly progressive renal failure.

Clinical Features. The peak incidence is in the forties. Typical clinical features include persistent pneumonitis with bilateral nodular and cavitary infiltrates (95%), chronic sinusitis (90%), mucosal ulcerations of the nasopharynx (75%), and evidence of renal disease (80%). Other features include skin rashes, muscle pains, articular involvement, mononeuritis or polyneuritis, and fever. Untreated, the course of the disease is malignant; 80% of patients die within 1 year. When the diagnosis is established, appropriate therapy (i.e., immunosuppressive drugs, cyclophosphamide, possibly prednisone, and sometimes antibacterial drugs) produces a gratifying response in most patients, with only occasional relapses.

Sometimes difficult to differentiate from Wegener granulomatosis is a condition called *lymphomatoid granulomatosis*, characterized by pulmonary infiltration by nodules of lymphoid and plasmacytoid cells, often with cellular atypia. Although these infiltrates invade vessels, giving the histologic appearance of a vasculitis, they do not constitute a true vasculitis. About one third of patients eventually show similar lesions in the kidneys, liver, brain, and other organs. Lymphomatoid granulomatosis probably represents an evolving lymphoproliferative disorder because up to 50% develop a lymphoid malignancy, most commonly non-Hodgkin lymphoma.

THROMBOANGIITIS OBLITERANS (BUERGER DISEASE)

Thromboangiitis obliterans (*Buerger disease*) is a distinctive disease characterized by segmental, thrombosing, acute and chronic inflammation of medium-sized and small arteries, principally the tibial and radial arteries and sometimes secondarily extending to veins and nerves of the extremities.[68] The condition had occurred almost exclusively in men who were heavy cigarette smokers. There has been an increase in reported cases in women, probably reflecting increases in smoking by women in the past several decades. Buerger disease begins before the age of 35 years in most patients and before 20 years in some. Buerger disease often leads to vascular insufficiency.

The relationship to cigarette smoking is one of the most consistent aspects of this disorder, and most patients show hypersensitivity to intradermally injected tobacco extracts. Several possibilities have been postulated for this association, including direct endothelial cell toxicity induced by or hypersensitivity to some tobacco products. There is an increased prevalence of the human leukocyte antigens-A9 and HLA-B5 in these patients, and the condition is far more common in Israel, Japan, and India than in the United States and Europe, all of which hints at genetic influences.

MORPHOLOGY. Thromboangiitis obliterans is characterized by **sharply segmental acute and chronic vasculitis of medium-sized and small arteries** with secondary spread to contiguous veins and nerves. Often the vascular supply to the extremities, upper as well as lower, is affected. By contrast, atherosclerosis affects predominantly the larger arteries, mostly those in the lower extremities. Microscopically acute and chronic inflammation permeates the arterial walls, accompanied by thrombosis of the lumen, which may undergo organization and recanalization. Characteristically the thrombus contains small microabscesses marked by a central focus of neutrophils surrounded by granulomatous inflammation (Fig. 12–24).

Clinical Features. The early manifestations are a superficial nodular phlebitis, cold sensitivity of the Raynaud type (see later) in the hands, and pain in the instep of the foot induced by exercise (so-called *instep claudication*). In contrast to the insufficiency caused by atherosclerosis, in Buerger disease the insufficiency tends to be accompanied by severe pain, even at rest, related undoubtedly to the neural involvement. Chronic ulcerations of the toes, feet, or fingers may appear, perhaps followed in time by frank gangrene. Abstinence from cigarette smoking in the early stages of the disease often brings dramatic relief from further attacks.

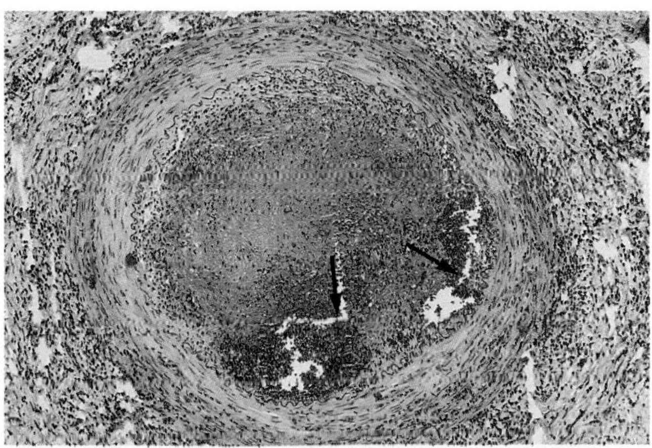

Figure 12–24 ■

Thromboangiitis obliterans (Buerger disease). The lumen is occluded by a thrombus containing two abscesses (*arrows*). The vessel wall is infiltrated with leukocytes.

VASCULITIS ASSOCIATED WITH OTHER DISORDERS

Vasculitis may sometimes be associated with an underlying disorder, such as an immunologic connective tissue disease, a malignancy, or systemic illnesses such as mixed cryoglobulinemia and Henoch-Schönlein purpura. Usually of the hypersensitivity angiitis pattern, it may resemble classic polyarteritis nodosa in some cases. Of the *connective tissue disorders*, rheumatoid arthritis and systemic lupus erythematosus, as pointed out earlier, commonly manifest a vasculitis (Fig. 12–25). *Rheumatoid vasculitis* usually affects small and medium-sized arteries in multiple organs and may thereby result in life-threatening visceral infarction but also may cause a clinically significant aortitis.[69] It occurs predominantly after long-standing rheumatoid arthritis in patients who also exhibit rheumatoid nodules, hypocomplementemia, and high titers of rheumatoid factor. *Malignancies* associated with vasculitis are commonly of the lymphoproliferative type.

INFECTIOUS ARTERITIS

Localized arteritis is most frequently caused by the direct invasion of infectious agents—usually bacteria or fungi, particularly aspergillosis and mucormycosis. Vascular lesions frequently accompany bacterial pneumonia or occur adjacent to caseous tuberculous reactions, in the neighborhood of abscesses, or in the superficial cerebral vessels in cases of meningitis. Much less commonly, they arise from the hematogenous spread of bacteria, in cases of septicemia or embolization from infective endocarditis. Vascular infections may weaken the arterial wall and result in the formation of a *mycotic aneurysm* (see later).

Clinically, infectious arteritis may be important on several counts. By inducing thrombosis, it adds an element of infarction to tissues that are already the seat of an inflammatory reaction and worsen the initial infection. In bacterial meningitis, for example, inflammation of the superficial vessels of the brain may predispose to vascular thromboses, with subsequent infarction of the brain substance and extension of the subarachnoid infection into the brain tissue.

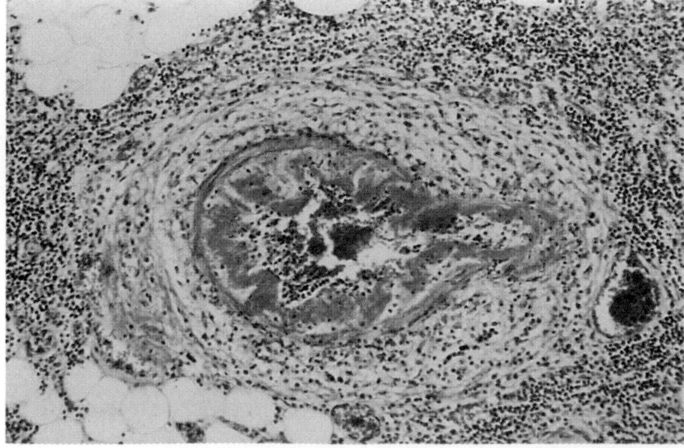

Figure 12–25

Vasculitis with fibrinoid necrosis in a patient with active systemic lupus erythematosus.

Raynaud Disease

Raynaud disease refers to paroxysmal pallor or cyanosis of the digits of the hands or feet and infrequently the tips of the nose or ears (acral parts). It is caused by intense vasospasm of local small arteries or arterioles, principally of young, otherwise healthy women. Characteristically the fingers change color in the sequence white, blue, red. *No organic changes are present in the arterial walls except late in the course, when intimal proliferation can appear.* Of uncertain cause, Raynaud disease reflects an exaggeration of normal central and local vasomotor responses to cold or emotion. The course of Raynaud disease is usually benign, but long-standing, chronic cases can have atrophy of the skin, subcutaneous tissues, and muscles. Ulceration and ischemic gangrene are rare.

In contrast, *Raynaud phenomenon* refers to arterial insufficiency of the extremities *secondary to the arterial narrowing induced by various conditions, including systemic lupus erythematosus, progressive systemic sclerosis (scleroderma), atherosclerosis, or Buerger disease* (see earlier). Raynaud phenomenon may be the first manifestation of any of these conditions.

Aneurysms and Dissection

An *aneurysm* is a *localized abnormal dilation of a blood vessel that occurs most commonly in the aorta or the heart.* Aneurysms can be either *true* or *false*. A *true aneurysm* is bounded by generally complete but often attenuated arterial wall components. The blood within a true aneurysm remains within the confines of the circulatory system. Atherosclerotic, syphilitic, and congenital vascular aneurysms and the typical left ventricular aneurysm that can follow a myocardial infarction are of this type. In contrast, a *false aneurysm* (also called *pseudoaneurysm*) is an extravascular hematoma that communicates with the intravascular space (thus a *pulsating hematoma*). The vascular wall has been breached, and the external wall of the aneurysmal sac consists of only outer arterial layers, perivascular tissue, or blood clot. A leak at the junction (*anastomosis*) of a vascular graft with a natural artery produces this type of lesion. *Arterial dissections*, usually of the aorta (sometimes called *dissecting aneurysms*), arise when blood enters the wall of the artery, dissecting between its layers and creating a cavity within the vessel wall itself.

The two most important causes of true aortic aneurysms are atherosclerosis and cystic medial degeneration, but any vessel may be affected by a wide variety of disorders that weaken arterial walls, including congenital defects, infections (mycotic aneurysms), syphilis, trauma (traumatic aneurysms or arteriovenous aneurysms), or systemic diseases. Arterial aneurysms can also be caused by vascular immunologic injury, as in polyarteritis nodosa, Kawasaki syndrome, and other vasculitides; trauma leading to arteriovenous aneurysms; or congenital defects, such as that producing *berry* aneurysms (Chapter 30).

Infection of a major artery that weakens its wall is called a *mycotic aneurysm.* A mycotic aneurysm can be either *true* or *false*; thrombosis and rupture are possible complications. Mycotic aneurysms may originate (1) at the site of sticking of a dislodged septic embolus within a vessel, usually as a complication of infective endocarditis; (2) as an extension of an adjacent suppurative process; or (3) by circulating organisms directly infecting the arterial wall.

Aneurysms are often classified by macroscopic shape and size. *Saccular* aneurysms are essentially spherical (involving only a portion of the vessel wall) and vary in size 5 up to 20 cm in diameter, often partially or completely filled by thrombus. A *fusiform* aneurysm is a gradual, progressive dilation of the complete circumference of the vessel. Fusiform aneurysms vary in diameter (up to 20 cm) and in length; many involve the entire ascending and transverse portions of the aortic arch, whereas others may involve large segments of the abdominal aorta or even the iliacs. These shapes, however, are not specific for any disease or clinical manifestations.

ABDOMINAL AORTIC ANEURYSMS

Atherosclerosis, the most frequent cause of aneurysms, causes arterial wall thinning through medial destruction secondary to plaque that originates in the intima. *Atherosclerotic aneurysms most frequently occur in the abdominal aorta (abdominal aortic aneurysm)*, but the common iliac arteries, the arch, and descending parts of the thoracic aorta can be involved.

MORPHOLOGY. Abdominal aortic aneurysms are usually positioned below the renal arteries and above the bifurcation of the aorta (Fig. 12–26). Abdominal aortic aneurysms take the form of saccular (balloon-like), cylindroid, or fusiform swellings, sometimes up to 15 cm in greatest diameter and of variable length (up to 25 cm). As would be expected, at these sites there is severe complicated atherosclerosis, which destroys the underlying tunica media and thus weakens the aortic wall. Mural thrombus frequency is found within the aneurysmal sac. In saccular forms, the thrombus may completely fill the outpouching. The elongated fusiform or cylindroid patterns more often have layers of mural thrombus that only partially fill the dilation. Occasionally the aneurysm may affect the origins of the renal, superior, and inferior mesenteric arteries, either by involving these vessels directly or by narrowing or occluding their ostia with mural thrombi. Not infrequently, they are accompanied by smaller fusiform or saccular dilations of the iliac arteries. The aneurysm often contains atheromatous ulcers covered by mural thrombi, with consequent thinning and destruction of the media, prime sites for the formation of atheroemboli that can lodge in the vessels of the kidneys or lower extremities.

Two variants of abdominal aortic aneurysm merit special mention. **Inflammatory abdominal aneurysms** are characterized by dense periaortic fibrosis containing an abundant lymphoplasmacytic inflammatory reaction with many macrophages and often giant cells.[70] Their cause is uncertain. **Mycotic abdominal aneurysms** are atherosclerotic abdominal aortic aneurysms that have become infected by deposition of circulating organisms in the wall, particularly in bacteremia from a primary *Salmonella* gastroenteritis. In such cases, suppuration further destroys the media, potentiating rapid dilation and rupture.

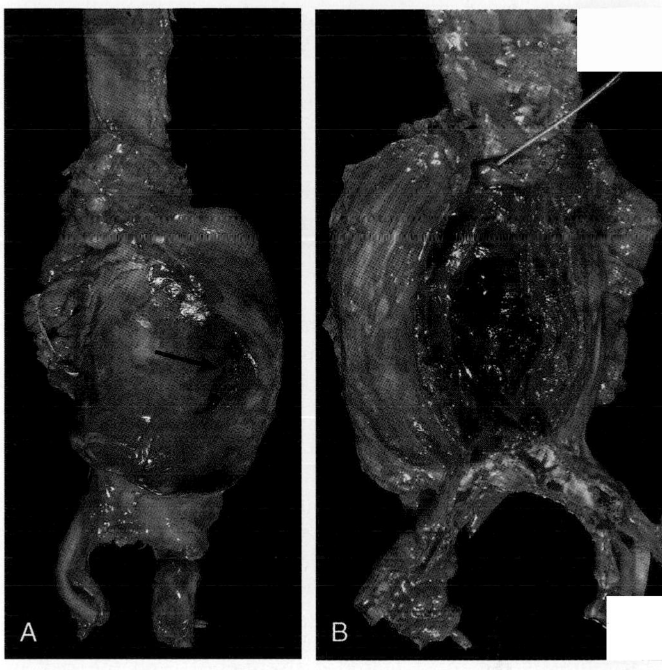

Figure 12–26

Gross photographs of an abdominal aortic aneurysm that ruptured. *A*, External view of the large aneurysm; the rupture site is indicated by the arrow. *B*, Opened view with the location of the rupture tract indicated by a probe. The wall of the aneurysm is exceedingly thin and the lumen is filled by a large quantity of layered but largely unorganized thrombus.

Pathogenesis. Atherosclerosis is a major cause of abdominal aortic aneurysms, but other factors contribute to aneurysm formation in this and other sites.[71] Abdominal aortic aneurysms rarely develop before the age of 50 and are much more common in men. Aortic aneurysms have been shown to be familial—beyond the familial and genetic predisposition to atherosclerosis or hypertension. As discussed subsequently in the section on Marfan syndrome and dissecting aneurysms, genetic defects in structural components of the aorta can themselves produce aneurysms and dissections. It has been postulated that subtle defects in a connective tissue component responsible for the strength of blood vessels could provide a particularly susceptible substrate on which atherosclerosis or hypertension, or both, could act to weaken the aortic wall.[72, 73]

There is also evidence that matrix metalloproteinases (MMPs) and plasminogen activators, which degrade extracellular matrix (ECM) (Chapter 4), contribute to aneurysm formation.[74]

Clinical Course. The clinical consequences of abdominal aortic aneurysms depend primarily on their location and size. They give rise to clinical symptoms and recognition by various effects:[75]

- Rupture into the peritoneal cavity or retroperitoneal tissues with massive or fatal hemorrhage
- Occlusion of a branch vessel by either direct pressure or mural thrombus formation, particularly of the iliac, renal, mesenteric, or vertebral branches that supply the spinal cord
- Embolism from the atheroma or mural thrombus
- Impingement on an adjacent structure, such as compression of a ureter or erosion of vertebrae
- Presentation as an abdominal mass (often palpably pulsating) that simulates a tumor

Rupture is the most feared consequence, and the risk is directly related to the size of the aneurysm. It varies from about 2% for a small abdominal aortic aneurysm (<4 cm) to 5 to 10% per year or greater for aneurysms larger than 5 cm. Thus, large aneurysms are usually surgically replaced by prosthetic grafts. Timely surgery is critical; operative mortality for unruptured aneurysms is approximately 5%, whereas emergency surgery after rupture carries a mortality rate of more than 50%. Patients with aneurysms are also at significantly increased risk for other complications of atherosclerosis, such as ischemic heart disease and other cardiovascular disease.

SYPHILITIC (LUETIC) ANEURYSMS

The tertiary stage of syphilis shows a predilection for the cardiovascular and nervous systems. With better control and treatment of syphilis in its early stages, these involvements are becoming less common. The *obliterative endarteritis* characteristic of tertiary syphilis may involve small vessels in any part of the body, but it is clinically most devastating when it affects the vasa vasorum of the aorta. This complication, thoracic aortitis, can lead to aneurysmal dilation of the aorta and aortic annulus characteristic of full-blown cardiovascular syphilis.

MORPHOLOGY. The development of aneurysms is based on the medial destruction characteristic of tertiary syphilis. Inflammatory involvement begins in the adventitia of the aorta, particularly involving the vasa vasorum with the production of **obliterative endarteritis** rimmed by an infiltrate of lymphocytes and plasma cells. The narrowing of the lumens of the vasa causes **ischemic injury of the aortic media**, with patchy uneven loss of the medial elastic fibers and muscle cells followed by inflammation and scarring. With destruction of the media, the aorta loses its elastic support and tends to become dilated, producing a syphilitic aneurysm. Aortic dissection is unusual owing to medial scarring. Contraction of fibrous scars may lead to wrinkling of intervening segments of aortic intima, called **tree-barking.** Luetic involvement of the aorta favors the development of superimposed atherosclerosis inducing sometimes florid atheromatosis of the aortic root (an unusual location for **garden variety** atherosclerosis), which can envelop and occlude the coronary ostia. **Even when these aneurysms are complicated by atherosclerosis, their location in the thorax tends to distinguish them from typical atherosclerotic aneurysms, which rarely affect the aortic arch and never involve the root of the aorta.**

Luetic aortitis may also cause aortic valve ring dilation, resulting in valvular insufficiency through circumferential stretching of the value cusps and widening of the commissures between the cusps. Over the course of time, the regurgitant turbulence produces thickening and rolling of the free margins, worsening the valvular incompetence. As a consequence, the left ventricular wall undergoes volume overload hypertrophy, sometimes producing a massively enlarged heart (that can reach 1000 gm, about three times normal weight), descriptively referred to as **cor bovinum (cow's heart)**.

Clinical Features. Whether of luetic or atherosclerotic origin, thoracic aortic enlargements can give rise to signs and symptoms referable to (1) encroachment on mediastinal structures, (2) respiratory difficulties owing to encroachment on the lungs and airways, (3) difficulty in swallowing owing to compression of the esophagus, (4) persistent cough owing to irritation of or pressure on the recurrent laryngeal nerves, (5) pain caused by erosion of bone (i.e., ribs and vertebral bodies), (6) cardiac disease as the aortic aneurysm leads to aortic valve dilation with valvular insufficiency or narrowing of the coronary ostia causing myocardial ischemia, and (7) rupture of the aneurysm. Most patients with syphilitic aneurysms die of heart failure as a result of aortic valvular incompetence.

AORTIC DISSECTION (DISSECTING HEMATOMA)

Aortic dissection is a catastrophic illness characterized by dissection of blood in between and along the laminar planes of the media, with the formation of a blood-filled channel within the aortic wall—a dissecting intramural hematoma (Fig. 12–27)*—that often ruptures, causing massive hemorrhage. In contrast to atherosclerotic and syphilitic aneurysms, aortic dissection is not usually associated with marked dilation of the aorta.* For this reason, the older term *dissecting aneurysm* is discouraged. Aortic dissection occurs principally in two groups of patients: One is most commonly men 40 to 60 years of age, in whom hypertension is almost invariably an antecedent (>90% of

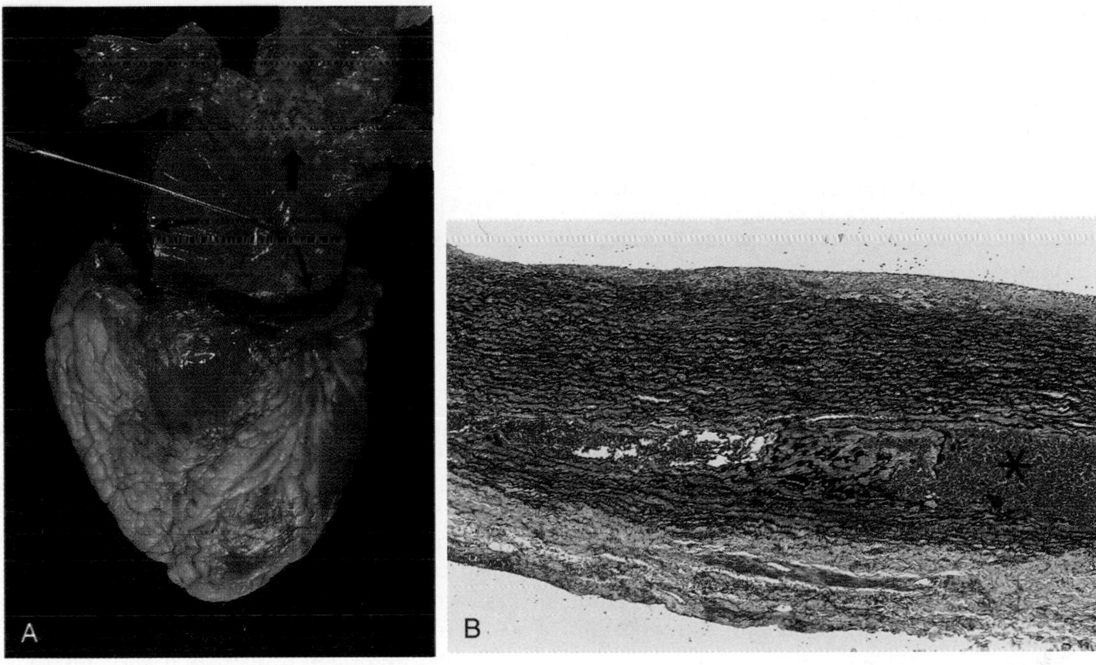

Figure 12–27

A, Gross photograph of proximal aortic dissection demonstrating a small, oblique intimal tear (demarcated by the probe), allowing blood to enter the media, creating an intramural hematoma (*narrow arrows*). Note that the intimal tear has occurred in a region largely free from atherosclerotic plaque, and that propagation of the intramural hematoma is arrested at a site more distally where atherosclerosis begins (*broad arrow*). *B*, Histologic view of the dissection demonstrating an aortic intramural hematoma (*asterisk*). Aortic elastic layers black and blood red in this section, stained with Movat stain.

cases of dissection). The second major group of patients, usually younger, has a systemic or localized abnormality of connective tissue that affects the aorta (e.g., Marfan syndrome, discussed subsequently and in Chapter 6). Dissection can also be a complication of arterial cannulation (e.g., during diagnostic catheterization or cardiopulmonary bypass). Rarely, for unknown reasons, aortic, coronary arterial, or other vascular dissection occurs during pregnancy. Dissection is unusual in the face of substantial atherosclerosis, probably owing to the obstruction to an ongoing dissecting hematoma caused by medial scarring.

MORPHOLOGY. There is usually, but not always, an **intimal tear** that extends into but not through the media of the ascending aorta, usually within 10 cm of the aortic valve (Fig. 12–27*A*). Presumably, this is the origin of dissection. Such tears are usually transverse or oblique, 1 to 5 cm length, with sharp, jagged edges. The dissection can extend proximally toward the heart as well as distally along the aorta to variable distances, sometimes all the way into the iliac and femoral arteries. The dissecting hematoma spreads characteristically along the laminar planes of the aorta, usually approximately between the middle and outer thirds (Fig. 12–27*B*). In some instances, the blood reruptures into the lumen of the aorta, producing second or distal intimal tear and a new vascular channel within the media of the aortic wall that connects the proximal and distal intimal tears. It is assumed that in these "double-barreled" aortas, the two intimal tears have permitted the establishment of through-and-through blood flow in the aortic wall and thus averted a fatal extra-aortic hemorrhage. In the course of time, such false channels may become endothelialized.

The most common cause of death is rupture of the dissection into any of the three major body cavities (i.e., pericardial, pleural, or peritoneal). Other vascular complications that frequently correlate with clinical manifestations include extension of the dissection into the great arteries of the neck or into the coronary, renal, mesenteric, or iliac arteries, causing critical vascular obstruction. Retrograde dissection into the aortic root can cause disruption of the aortic valvular apparatus. Thus, common clinical manifestations include cardiac tamponade, aortic insufficiency, and myocardial infarction; compression of spinal arteries may cause transverse myelitis.

The most frequent preexisting histologically detectable lesion is **cystic medial degeneration (CMD)**. Sometimes called **cystic medial necrosis** (an inaccurate term because true necrosis is not present), the lesions consist of elastic tissue fragmentation and separation of the elastic and fibromuscular elements of the tunica media by small cleftlike or cystic spaces filled with amorphous extracellular matrix. Ultimately, there may be large-scale loss of elastic laminae (Fig. 12–28). Inflammation is absent. Cystic medial degeneration of the aorta is frequently found in patients with Marfan syndrome, but those with hypertension have variable nonspecific changes in aortic wall histology ranging from mild fragmentation of elastic tissue (the most common and easily recognized abnormality) to overt CMD. **CMD is frequently found incidentally at autopsy of patients who are free from dissection,** increasing in severity with age and possibly the presence of hypertension.

Pathogenesis. Hypertension is clearly the major risk factor overall, but its contribution to CMD is uncertain. Indeed, there is not a good correlation between dissection and the presence of CMD, and CMD is not critical to the development of dissection.

Some dissections are related to inherited connective tissue disorders, most prominently Marfan syndrome, an autosomal dominant disease caused by mutations in the fibrillin gene and characterized by skeletal, cardiovascular, and ocular manifestations (Chapter 6). Serious cardiovascular complications of Marfan syndrome include aortic dissection, dilation of the aortic root (called *annuloaortic ectasia*), and mitral valve prolapse and frequently cause premature death of persons with this disorder. The cause of dissections not associated with hypertension and genetic disorders is often unknown.

Regardless of the underlying cause, the trigger for intimal tear and intramural aortic hemorrhage is also unknown in most cases of dissection. Nevertheless, once the tear has occurred, hypertension enhances hematoma progression within the vessel wall. Aggressive antihypertensive therapy is thus effective in limiting an evolving dissection.

Clinical Course. The risk and nature of serious complications of dissection depend strongly on the level of the aorta affected. Thus, aortic dissections are generally classified into two types:

- The more common (and dangerous) *proximal* lesions, involving either the ascending portion only or both the ascending and the descending aorta (types I and II of DeBakey's classification, often collectively called *type A*)
- *Distal lesions not involving the ascending part* and usually beginning distal to the subclavian artery (DeBakey type III, often called type B) (Fig. 12–29)

The classic clinical symptoms of aortic dissection are the sudden onset of excruciating pain, usually beginning in the anterior chest, radiating to the back, and moving downward as the dissection progresses. This intense pain can be readily confused with that of acute myocardial infarction. The antemortem diagnosis of aortic dissection and the differentiation of the various types are based largely on aortic angiography, but the noninvasive techniques, two-dimensional cardiac ultrasound (especially transesophageal echocardiography), computed tomography, and magnetic resonance imaging, are increasingly useful.[76]

At one time, aortic dissection was almost invariably fatal, but the prognosis has markedly improved. The development of surgical procedures involving plication of the aortic wall and the early institution of intensive antihypertensive therapy permit salvage of 65 to 75% of patients with dissections.

Veins and Lymphatics

Varicose veins and phlebothrombosis and thrombophlebitis together account for at least 90% of clinical venous disease. In general, varicose veins have narrowing or abnormal dilation with subsequent incompetence of the venous valves causing venous stasis. Thrombosis may occur, but embolism is rare. In contrast, pulmonary embolism and

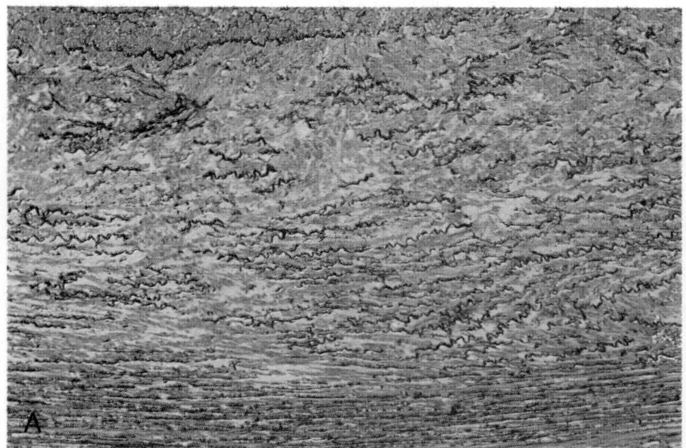

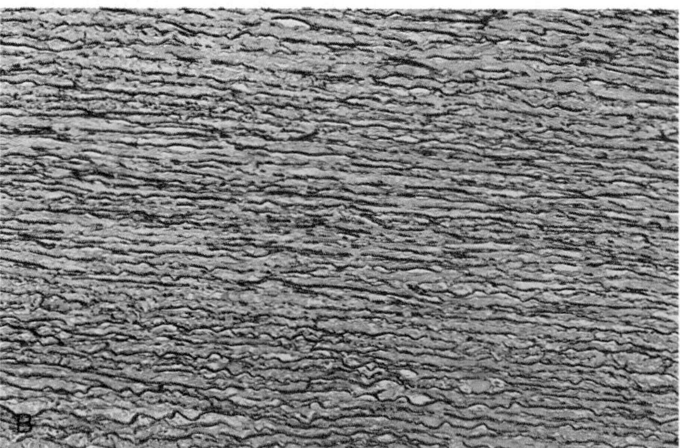

Figure 12–28

Cystic medial degeneration. *A*, Cross-section of aortic media with marked elastin fragmentation and formation of areas devoid of elastin that resemble cystic spaces, from a patient with Marfan syndrome. *B*, Normal aortic media for comparison, showing the regular layered pattern of elastic tissue. In both *A* and *B* the tissue section is stained to highlight elastin as black.

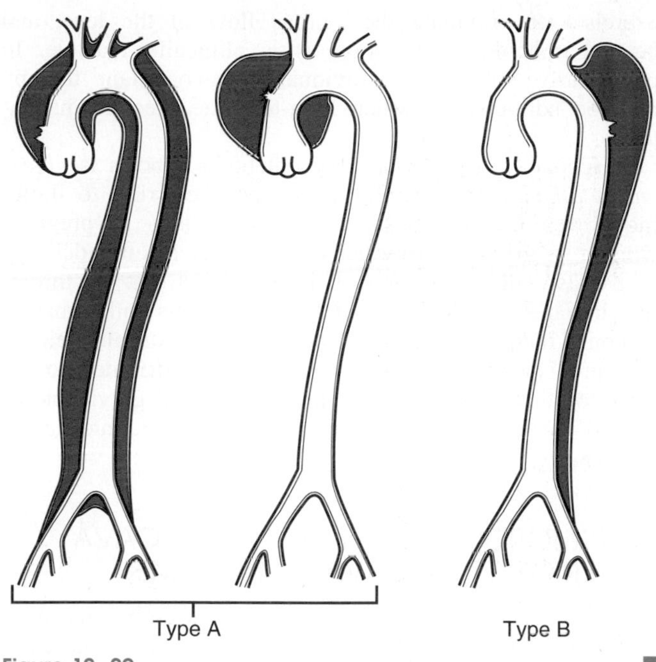

Figure 12–29

Classification of dissection into types A and B. Type A (proximal) involves the ascending aorta, whereas type B (distal) does not.

infarction are potential serious sequelae of thrombophlebitis.

VARICOSE VEINS

Varicose veins are abnormally dilated, tortuous veins produced by prolonged, increased intraluminal pressure and, to a lesser extent, by loss of support of the vessel wall. The *superficial veins* of the leg are the preponderant site of involvement (Fig. 12–30). The most important influence on intraluminal venous blood pressure is posture; when the legs are dependent for long periods of time, venous pressures in these sites are markedly elevated (up to ten times normal). Therefore, occupations that require long periods of standing and long automobile or airplane rides frequently lead to marked venous stasis and pedal edema, even in normal individuals with essentially normal veins (*simple orthostatic edema*).

It is estimated that 15 to 20% of the general population eventually develop varicose veins in the lower legs.[77] The condition is much more common over age 50, in obese persons, and in women, a reflection of the elevated venous pressure in the lower legs caused by pregnancy. A *familial tendency* toward the development of varicosities earlier in life is postulated to be due to defective development of the walls of veins.

MORPHOLOGY. Veins affected by varicosities are dilated, tortuous, elongated and scarred. There is marked variation in the thickness of the wall, with thinning at the points of maximal dilation. Intraluminal thrombosis and valvular deformities (thickening, rolling, and shortening of the cusps) are frequently discovered when these vessels are opened. Microscopically the changes consist of variations in the thickness of the vein wall caused by dilation on the one hand and by compensatory hypertrophy of the smooth muscle and subintimal fibrosis on the other hand. Frequently, there is elastic tissue degeneration and spotty calcifications within the media **(phlebosclerosis).**

Clinical Course. Varicose dilation of veins renders the valves incompetent and leads to venous stasis, congestion, edema, and thrombosis. *Despite thrombosis of superficial varicose veins, embolism is rare. This is in sharp contrast to the relatively frequent thromboembolism that arises from thrombosed deep veins* (see subsequently), in which contraction of surrounding muscles tends to milk the contents loose from their attachments to the vein walls. Distention of the superficial leg veins is often painful, but most patients have no symptoms until marked venous stasis and edema develop. *Some of the most disabling sequelae are the development of persistent edema in the extremity and trophic changes in the skin that lead to stasis dermatitis and ulcerations.* Because of the impaired circulation, the tissues of the affected part are extremely vulnerable to injury. Wounds and infections heal slowly or tend to become chronic *varicose ulcers*.

Attention should be called to two special sites of varix formation. Varicosities occur in the esophagus, in patients who have cirrhosis of the liver and its attendant portal hypertension (Chapter 19). Rupture of an *esophageal varix* leading to upper gastrointestinal hemorrhage may be more

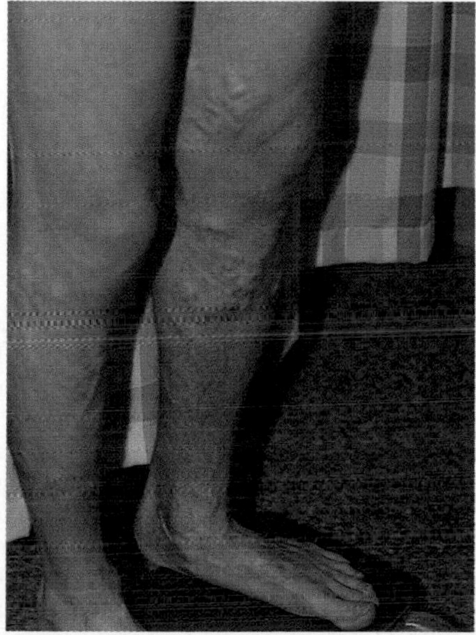

Figure 12–30

Varicose veins of the leg. (Courtesy of Magruder C. Donaldson, MD, Brigham and Women's Hospital, Boston, MA.)

serious than the primary liver disease itself. *Hemorrhoids* result from varicose dilation of the hemorrhoidal plexus of veins at the anorectal junction. The causative mechanism is presumed to be prolonged pelvic congestion resulting, for example, from repeated pregnancies or chronic constipation and straining at stools. Hemorrhoids not only are uncomfortable, but also may be a source of bleeding. Sometimes they thrombose, and in this distended state, they are prone to painful ulceration.

THROMBOPHLEBITIS AND PHLEBOTHROMBOSIS

Thrombophlebitis and *phlebothrombosis* are two designations for venous thrombosis. Predisposing factors have already been considered in the general discussion of thrombosis (Chapter 5). It need simply be reemphasized now that *cardiac failure, neoplasia, pregnancy, obesity, postoperative state, and prolonged bed rest or immobilization are the most important clinical predispositions.* Genetic hypercoagulability syndromes can also be associated with venous thrombosis.[78]

The deep leg veins account for more than 90% of cases of thrombophlebitis.[79] The periprostatic venous plexus in men and the pelvic veins in women are additional sites for the appearance of thrombi. Also, the large veins in the skull and the dural sinuses are possible sites of thrombosis when these channels become inflamed by bacterial infections of the meninges, middle ears, or mastoids. Similarly, infections in the abdominal cavity, such as peritonitis, acute appendicitis, acute salpingitis, and pelvic abscesses, may lead to inflammation and thrombosis of the portal vein or its tributaries.

Thrombi in the legs tend, on the whole, to arise insidiously and to produce in the early stages few, if any, signs or symptoms. Local manifestations, including edema distal to the occluded vein, dusky cyanosis, dilation of superficial veins, heat, tenderness, redness, swelling, and pain, may be absent in a bedridden patient. In some cases, however, pain can be elicited by pressure over affected veins, squeezing the calf muscles, or forced dorsiflexion of the foot (Homan sign). Several noninvasive methods (iodine-labeled fibrinogen, ultrasonography, plethysmography) aid in the diagnosis, but venous angiography may have to be performed in some cases to establish the presence of deep vein thrombosis.

Not infrequently, the first manifestation of thrombophlebitis is the development of an embolic episode. Pulmonary embolism is a common and serious clinical problem. In patients with cancer, particularly adenocarcinomas of the pancreas, colon, or lung, hypercoagulability occurs as a paraneoplastic syndrome (Chapter 8). The resultant venous thromboses have a tendency to appear spontaneously in one site, only to disappear and be followed by thromboses in other veins, giving rise to the entity referred to as *migratory thrombophlebitis (Trousseau sign).* Because of the clinical settings in which phlebothrombosis appears, pulmonary embolization often constitutes the final mortal blow to those already gravely ill. To avoid venous thrombi, cardiac, postpartum, cancer, and postoperative patients are urged to move about constantly in bed, perform muscle exercises to stimulate the venous flow in the legs, and become ambulatory as soon as is clinically feasible. In particularly vulnerable individuals, anticoagulant therapy may be administered when long-term bed rest is mandatory.

A special variant of primary phlebothrombosis is *phlegmasia alba dolens* (painful white leg), referring to iliofemoral venous thrombosis occurring usually in pregnant women in the third trimester or immediately after delivery (aptly also called *milk leg*). It is postulated that the thrombus initiates a phlebitis, and the perivenous inflammatory response induces lymphatic blockage with painful swelling. The predisposition to thrombosis here is attributed to the stasis of flow caused by the pressure of the gravid uterus and to the development of a hypercoagulable state during pregnancy.

OBSTRUCTION OF SUPERIOR VENA CAVA (SUPERIOR VENA CAVAL SYNDROME)

The *superior vena caval syndrome* is usually caused by neoplasms that compress or invade the superior vena cava, most commonly a primary bronchogenic carcinoma or mediastinal lymphoma. Occasionally, other lesions, such as an aortic aneurysm, may impinge on the superior vena cava. Regardless of the cause, the consequent obstruction produces a distinctive clinical complex manifested by dusky cyanosis and marked dilation of the veins of the head, neck, and arms. Commonly the pulmonary vessels are also compressed, and consequently respiratory distress may develop.

OBSTRUCTION OF INFERIOR VENA CAVA (INFERIOR VENA CAVAL SYNDROME)

Analogous to the superior vena caval syndrome, the inferior vena caval syndrome may be caused by many of the same processes. Neoplasms may either compress or penetrate the walls of the inferior vena cava, or a thrombus from the femoral or iliac vein may propagate upward. Moreover, certain neoplasms, particularly hepatocellular carcinoma and renal cell carcinoma, show a striking tendency to grow within the lumens of the veins, extending ultimately into the inferior vena cava. As would be anticipated, obstruction to the inferior vena cava induces marked edema of the legs, distention of the superficial collateral veins of the lower abdomen, and, when the renal veins are involved, massive proteinuria.

LYMPHANGITIS AND LYMPHEDEMA

Disorders of the lymphatic channels fall into two categories: primary diseases, which are extremely uncommon, and secondary processes, which develop in association with inflammation or cancer. Bacterial infections may spread into and through the lymphatics to create acute inflammatory involvement in these channels (*lymphangitis*). The most common etiologic agents are the group A β-hemolytic streptococci, although any virulent pathogen may be responsible for an acute lymphangitis. Anatomically the affected lymphatics are dilated and filled with an exudate, chiefly of neutrophils and histiocytes, that usually extends through the wall into the perilymphatic tissues and may in severe cases produce cellulitis or focal abscesses. Clinically, lymphangitis is recognized by painful subcutaneous red streaks that extend along the course of lymphatics, with painful enlargement of the regional lymph nodes, which often have acute lymphadenitis. If the lymph nodes fail to block the spread of bacteria, spillage into the venous system can initiate a bacteremia or septicemia.

Occlusion of lymphatic drainage is followed by the abnormal accumulation of interstitial fluid in the affected part, referred to as *obstructive lymphedema*. Lymphatic blockage is most commonly secondary to (1) spread of malignant tumors obstructing either the lymphatic channels or the regional lymph nodes, (2) radical surgical procedures with removal of regional groups of lymph nodes (e.g., the axillary dissection of radical mastectomy), (3) postirradiation fibrosis, (4) filariasis, and (5) postinflammatory thrombosis and scarring. *Chylous ascites, chylothorax*, and *chylopericardium* are caused by rupture of obstructed, dilated lymphatics into the peritoneum, pleural cavity, and pericardium. Almost invariably, this is due to obstruction of lymphatics by an infiltrating tumor mass.

In contrast, *primary lymphedema* may occur as an isolated congenital defect (simple congenital lymphedema), or it may be familial, in which case it is known as *Milroy disease* or *heredofamilial congenital lymphedema*. A third form of primary lymphedema, known as *lymphedema praecox*, appears between the ages of 10 and 25 years, usually in females. Of unknown cause, this disorder begins in one or both feet, and the edema slowly accumulates throughout life so that the involved extremity may swell to many times its normal size; the process may extend upward to affect the trunk. Although the size of the limb may produce some disability, serious complications such as superimposed infection or chronic ulcerations may also occur.

The morphologic changes of lymphedema consist of dilation of lymphatics up to the points of obstruction, accompanied by increases of interstitial fluid. Persistence of the edema leads to an increase of subcutaneous interstitial fibrous tissue, with consequent enlargement of the affected part, brawny induration, *peau d'orange* appearance of the skin, and skin ulcers.

Tumors

Tumors of the blood and lymphatic vessels constitute a spectrum from the benign hemangiomas (some of which are regarded as hamartomatous), to intermediate lesions that are locally aggressive but infrequently metastasize, to relatively rare, highly malignant angiosarcomas (Table 12–8).[80] In addition, congenital or developmental malformations, such as those that occur in the Sturge-Weber syndrome, may present as tumor-like lesions, as do some nonneoplastic reactive vascular proliferations, such as *bacillary angiomatosis*. For these reasons, vascular masses are difficult to categorize clinically and histologically. Neoplasms of this group display endothelial cell differentiation (e.g., hemangioma, lymphangioma, angiosarcoma) or appear to be derived from cells that support or invest blood vessels (e.g., glomus tumor, hemangiopericytoma). Here we describe only those lesions that are common or clinically important. These occur outside the vascular system per se, in soft tissues and viscera. Primary tumors of the large vessels, such as aorta, pulmonary artery, and vena cava are extremely rare, most being connective tissue sarcomas.

Table 12–8. CLASSIFICATION OF VASCULAR TUMORS AND TUMOR-LIKE CONDITIONS

Benign Neoplasms, Developmental and Acquired Conditions
Hemangioma
  Capillary hemangioma
  Cavernous hemangioma
  Pyogenic granuloma (lobular capillary hemangioma)
Lymphangioma
  Simple (capillary) lymphangioma
  Cavernous lymphangioma (cystic lymphangioma)
Glomus tumor
Vascular ectasias
  Nevus flammeus
  Spider telangiectasia (arterial spider)
  Hereditary hemorrhagic telangiectasis (Osler-Weber-Rendu disease)
Reactive vascular proliferations
  Bacillary angiomatosis

Intermediate-Grade Neoplasms
Kaposi sarcoma
Hemangioendothelioma

Malignant Neoplasms
Angiosarcoma
Hemangiopericytoma

Although in most cases well-differentiated benign hemangioma can be readily distinguished from an anaplastic high-grade angiosarcoma, the line dividing benign from malignant vascular tumors is poorly defined but is in general based on the following criteria:

- Benign tumors produce readily recognized vascular channels filled with blood cells or, in the case of lymphatics, with transudate. The lining of the channels is usually a monolayer of normal endothelial cells, without atypia.
- Malignant tumors are more solidly cellular with cytologic anaplasia, including mitotic figures, and usually do not form well-organized vessels.

The endothelial derivation of neoplastic proliferations that do not form distinct vascular lumens can usually be confirmed by immunohistochemical demonstration of endothelial cell-specific markers such as CD31 or vWF.

Analysis of genetic vascular malformations and tumor-like lesions has provided insights into the mechanisms underlying these disorders. For example, hereditary hemorrhagic telangiectasia (Osler-Rendu-Weber syndrome, described later), in which localized capillary dilation causes arterial blood to be shunted directly into postcapillary venules, has been shown to be caused by mutations in two TGF-β binding proteins, including the endothelial protein endoglin,[81] suggesting that TGF-β signaling pathways are crucial for development of normal capillary beds. Moreover, developmental venous abnormalities have been associated with genetic mutations in TIE2, the tyrosine kinase receptor for angiopeptin involved in vasculogenesis (discussed in Chapter 4).[82]

BENIGN TUMORS AND TUMOR-LIKE CONDITIONS

Hemangioma

As neoplasms characterized by an increased number of normal or abnormal vessels, *hemangiomas* (*angiomas*) may be difficult to distinguish with certainty from malformations or hamartomas (Fig. 12–31). Hemangiomas are most commonly localized; however, some involve large segments of the body, such as an entire extremity, for which the term *angiomatosis* is applied. The majority are superficial lesions, often of the head or neck, but they may occur internally, with nearly one third in the liver. Malignant transformation occurs rarely if at all.

Hemangiomas are extremely common, particularly in infancy and childhood, constituting 7% of all benign tumors. Most benign pediatric angiomas—capillary and cavernous—are present from birth and expand along with the growth of the child. Nevertheless, many of the capillary lesions regress spontaneously at or before puberty. There are several histologic and clinical variants.

Capillary Hemangioma. *Capillary hemangiomas*, the largest single group, are composed of blood vessels that resemble capillaries—narrow, thin-walled, and lined by relatively thin endothelium. Usually occurring in the skin, subcutaneous tissues, and mucous membranes of the oral cavities and lips, they may also occur in internal viscera, such as the liver, spleen, and kidneys. The *strawberry type* of capillary hemangioma (juvenile hemangiomas) of the skin of newborns is extremely common (1 in 200 births) and may be multiple. They grow rapidly in the first few months, begin to fade when the child is 1 to 3 years old, and regress by age 7 in 75 to 90% of cases.

MORPHOLOGY. Varying in size from a few millimeters up to several centimeters in diameter, lesions are bright red to blue, level with the surface of the skin or slightly elevated, and usually have an intact covering epithelium (Fig. 12–31*A*). Occasionally, pedunculated lesions are formed, attached by a broad-to-slender stalk. Histologically,

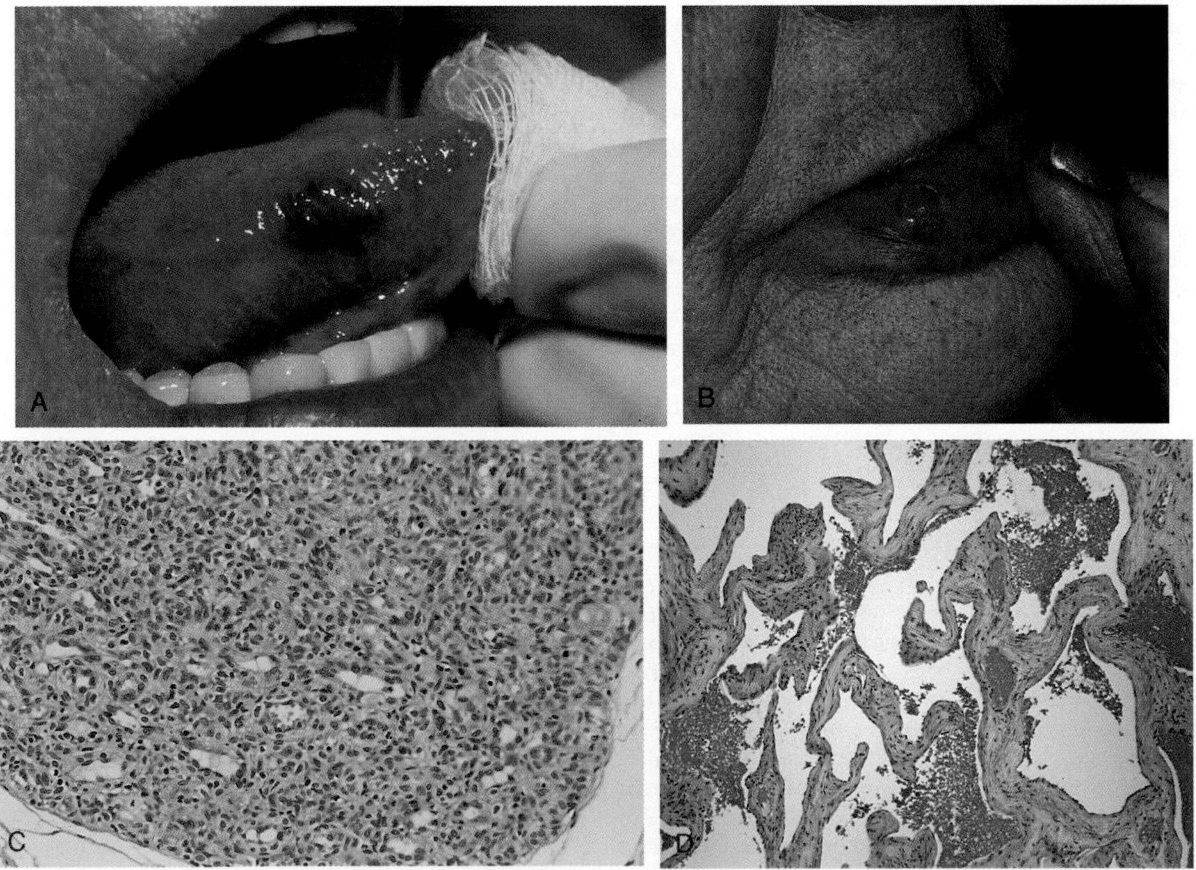

Figure 12–31

Hemangiomas. *A*, Hemangioma of the tongue. *B*, Pyogenic granuloma of the lip. *C*, Juvenile capillary hemangioma. *D*, Cavernous hemangioma. (*A* and *B* courtesy of John Sexton, MD, Beth Israel Hospital, Boston MA; *C* courtesy of Christopher D.M. Fletcher, MD, Brigham and Women's Hospital, Boston, MA; *D* courtesy of Thomas Rogers, MD, University of Texas Southwestern Medical School, Dallas, TX.)

capillary hemangiomas are usually lobulated but unencapsulated aggregates of closely packed, thin-walled capillaries, usually blood-filled and lined by a flattened endothelium, separated by scant connective tissue stroma (Fig. 12–31*C*). The lumens may be partially or completely thrombosed and organized. Rupture of vessels causes scarring and accounts for the hemosiderin pigment occasionally found.

Cavernous Hemangioma. Less common than the capillary variety, *cavernous hemangiomas* are distinguished by the formation of large, dilated vascular channels. Although they share age and anatomic distribution, they are usually larger, are less circumscribed, and more frequently involve deep structures than capillary hemangiomas.

MORPHOLOGY. Grossly the usual cavernous hemangioma is a red-blue; soft, spongy mass 1 to 2 cm in diameter. Quite rarely, giant forms occur that affect large subcutaneous areas of the face, extremities, or other regions of the body. Histologically the mass is sharply defined but not encapsulated and made up of large, cavernous vascular spaces, partly or completely filled with blood separated by a scant connective tissue stroma (Fig. 12–31*D*). Intravascular thrombosis with associated dystrophic calcification is common.

In most situations, hemangiomas are of little clinical significance; however, they can be a cosmetic disturbance owing to their vulnerability to traumatic ulceration and bleeding. Moreover, when picked up in internal organs by computed tomography or magnetic resonance imaging scans, they must be differentiated from more ominous lesions. Those in the brain are most threatening, since they may cause pressure symptoms or rupture. In one rare systemic entity, *von Hippel–Lindau disease* (discussed in Chapters 21 and 30), cavernous hemangiomas occur within the cerebellum or brain stem and eye grounds, along with similar angiomatous lesions or cystic neoplasms in the pancreas and liver and other visceral neoplasms.

Pyogenic Granuloma (Lobular Capillary Hemangioma). Pyogenic granuloma is a polypoid form of capillary hemangioma that occurs as a rapidly growing exophytic red nodule attached by a stalk to the skin and gingival or oral mucosa, which bleeds easily and is often ulcerated (Fig. 12–31*B*). Perhaps one third of lesions develop after trauma, growing rapidly to reach a maximal size of 1 to 2 cm within a few weeks. The proliferating capillaries are often accompanied by extensive edema and an acute and chronic inflammatory infiltrate, especially when ulcerated, yielding a striking resemblance on histologic examination to exuberant granulation tissue and sometimes suggesting an infectious cause. Recurrence occurs infrequently as a solitary nodule or as satellite nodules. *Pregnancy tumor* (granuloma gravidarum) is a pyogenic granuloma occurring in the gingiva of 1% of pregnant women that regresses after delivery. These lesions, similar to the spider telangiectasias discussed subsequently, emphasize the yet poorly understood role of estrogen in vascular growth and proliferation under certain circumstances.

Lymphangioma

Lymphangiomas are the lymphatic analogue of the hemangiomas of blood vessels.

Simple (Capillary) Lymphangioma. Simple (capillary) lymphangiomas are masses, composed of small lymphatic channels, that tend to occur subcutaneously in the head and neck region and in the axilla. Rarely, they are found in the trunk, within internal organs, or in the connective tissue in and about the abdominal or thoracic cavities. On body surfaces, they are slightly elevated or sometimes pedunculated lesions, 1 to 2 cm in diameter. Histologically, they are composed of a network of endothelium-lined lymph spaces that can be *differentiated from capillary channels only by the absence of blood cells*. These tumors are clinically benign.

Cavernous Lymphangioma (Cystic Hygroma). These benign lymphatic tumors are composed of cavernous lymphatic spaces and therefore are analogous to the cavernous hemangioma. Almost invariably occurring in children in the neck or axilla and only rarely retroperitoneally, they occasionally achieve considerable size, up to 15 cm in diameter. Such large masses may fill the axilla or produce gross deformities in and about the neck. The tumors are made up of massively dilated cystic spaces lined by endothelial cells and separated by a scant intervening connective tissue stroma, which often contain lymphoid aggregates. The margins of the tumor are not discrete, and these lesions are not encapsulated. Their removal can therefore be difficult.

Glomus Tumor (Glomangioma)

A *glomus tumor* is a biologically benign but often exquisitely painful tumor that arises from the modified smooth muscle cells of the glomus body, a specialized arteriovenous anastomosis that is involved in thermoregulation. Glomus tumors may be located anywhere in the skin (or soft tissue and sometimes in the gastrointestinal tract) but *are most commonly found in the distal portion of the digits*, especially under the fingernails. Excision is curative.

MORPHOLOGY. Grossly the lesions are usually small (<1 cm in diameter), slightly elevated, rounded, red-blue, and firm nodules, which may appear as minute foci of fresh hemorrhage under the nail. Histologically; **two components are present**; branching vascular channels separated by a connective tissue stroma that contains the second element—**aggregates, nests, and masses of the specialized glomus cells that typically are arranged around vessels.** Individual cells are usually small, regular in size, and round or cuboidal, with scant cytoplasm and features similar to smooth muscle cells on electron microscopy. Glomangiomas constitute a distinct subgroup that resemble cavernous hemangiomas.

Vascular Ectasias

Vascular ectasias constitute a common group of lesions characterized by localized dilation of preformed vessels. The term *telangiectasis* designates a group of abnormally prominent capillaries, venules, and arterioles that creates a small focal red lesion, usually in the skin or mucous membranes. Telangiectases represent congenital anomalies or acquired exaggerations of preexisting vessels and are not true neoplasms.

Nevus Flammeus. Nevus flammeus, the most common form of ectasia, also known as the *salmon patch*, is the ordinary birthmark. Most commonly on the head and neck, they range in color from light pink to deep purple and are ordinarily flat. Histologically, they show only dilation of vessels in the dermis. The vast majority ultimately fade and regress.

A special form of nevus flammeus, the so-called *port-wine stain*, may grow proportionately with a child, thicken the skin surface, become unsightly, and demonstrate no tendency to fade. Port-wine stains in the distribution of the trigeminal nerve may be associated with the *Sturge-Weber syndrome* (also called *encephalotrigeminal angiomatosis*). An extremely uncommon congenital disorder attributed to faulty development of certain mesodermal and ectodermal elements, this disorder is characterized by venous angiomatous masses in the leptomeninges over the cortex and by ipsilateral port-wine nevi of the face and often associated with mental retardation, seizures, hemiplegia, and radiopacities in the skull. Thus, a large vascular malformation in the face may indicate the presence of more extensive vascular malformation in a child who exhibits some evidence of mental deficiency.

Spider Telangiectasia (Arterial Spider). Another clearly non-neoplastic vascular lesion is the *spider telangiectasia*. It is a more or less radial and often pulsatile array of dilated subcutaneous arteries or arterioles about a central core that blanches with pressure applied to its center. They tend to be on the face, neck, or upper chest and are most frequent in pregnant women and in patients with liver cirrhosis. The hyperestrinism found in these two settings is believed in some way to play a role in the development of these telangiectases.

Hereditary Hemorrhagic Telangiectasia (Osler-Weber-Rendu Disease). In the autosomal dominant *Osler-Weber-Rendu disease*, telangiectases are genetic malformations comprising dilated capillaries and veins present from birth and distributed widely over the skin and mucous membranes of the oral cavity; lips; and respiratory, gastrointestinal, and urinary tracts. Any one of these innumerable lesions may rupture to cause only rarely serious nosebleeds, bleeding into the gut, or hematuria.

Bacillary Angiomatosis

First described in patients with the acquired immunodeficiency syndrome (AIDS), *bacillary angiomatosis* is an opportunistic infection of immunocompromised persons manifest as vascular proliferations that involve skin, bone, brain, and other organs. Along with the closely related vascular lesion of the liver and spleen called *bacillary peliosis*, bacillary angiomatosis is caused by infection with gram-negative bacilli of the *Bartonella* genus, particularly *Bartonella henselae*, the organism that causes cat-scratch disease in immunocompetent persons, and *Bartonella quintana*, the cause of trench fever affecting soldiers during World War I. Difficult to cultivate in the laboratory, these organisms can be demonstrated using molecular methods (polymerase chain reaction and species-specific primers).[83] How these organisms cause the exuberant vessel lesions is unclear.

MORPHOLOGY. Grossly cutaneous bacillary angiomatosis is marked by one to numerous red papules and nodules or rounded subcutaneous masses (Fig. 12–32*A*). Histologically, there is a tumor-like growth pattern with proliferation of capil-

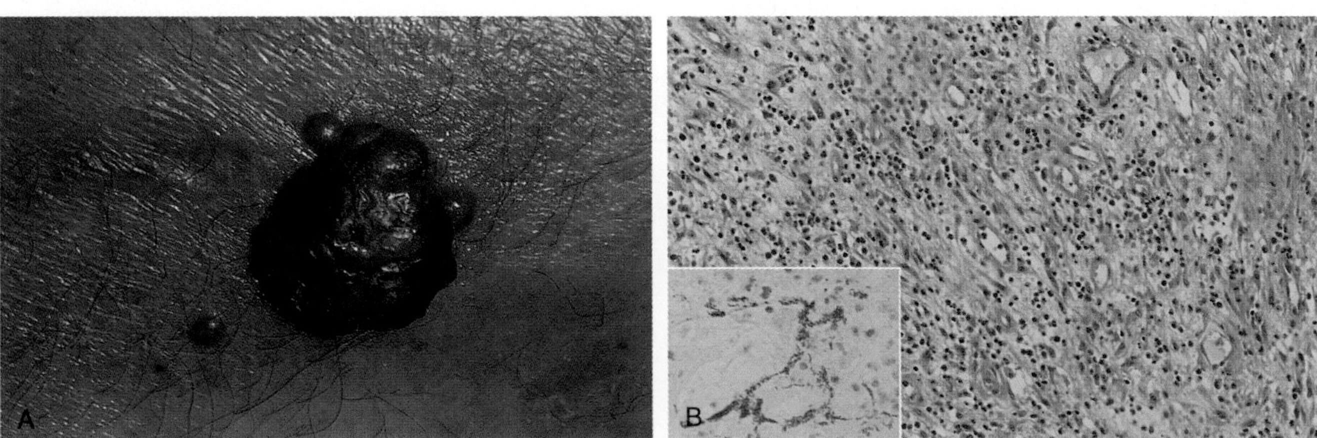

Figure 12–32

Bacillary angiomatosis. *A*, Photograph of a moist, erosive cutaneous lesion. *B*, Histologic appearance with acute neutrophilic inflammation and vascular (capillary) proliferation. *Inset*, Demonstration by modified silver (Warthin-Starry) stain of clusters of tangled bacilli (black). (*A* courtesy of Richard Johnson, MD, Beth Israel Deaconess Medical Center, Boston, MA; *B* and inset courtesy of Scott Granter, MD, Brigham and Women's Hospital, Boston, MA.)

laries having protuberant epithelioid endothelial cells, which have nuclear atypia and mitoses (Fig. 12–32*B*). The key features in differentiating this from pyogenic granuloma, Kaposi sarcoma, or angiosarcoma, which it resembles (see later), include numerous stromal neutrophils, nuclear dust, and granular material that consists of the causative bacteria (Fig. 12–32*C*).

The domestic cat is the principal reservoir of *B. henselae* and the cat flea its vector, whereas the human body louse plays an important role in infection caused by *B. quintana*. Infections with either species are initiated by transmission through traumatic inoculation of the skin and are prevented or cured by macrolide antibiotics (including erythromycin).[84]

INTERMEDIATE-GRADE (BORDERLINE, LOW-GRADE MALIGNANT) TUMORS

Kaposi Sarcoma

Long considered to be an uncommon tumor with an unknown histogenesis, Kaposi sarcoma has come to the forefront because of its frequent occurrence in patients with AIDS. Four forms of the disease are recognized:

- *Chronic*, also called *classic* or *European*, *Kaposi sarcoma*, first described by Kaposi in 1872, occurs primarily (90%) in older men of Eastern European (especially Ashkenazic Jews) or Mediterranean descent but is uncommon in the United States. This form also manifests an association with a second malignant tumor or altered immune state but is not associated with human immunodeficiency virus (HIV). Clinically, chronic Kaposi sarcoma commences with multiple red-to-purple skin plaques or nodules primarily in the distal lower extremities, slowly increasing in size and number and spreading to more proximal sites. Different stages of the disease may be present simultaneously. The tumors frequently remain asymptomatic and localized to the skin and subcutaneous tissue but are locally persistent, with an erratic course of lapses and remissions.
- *Lymphadenopathic*, also called *African* or *endemic*, *Kaposi sarcoma*, is particularly prevalent among young Bantu children of South Africa (same geographic distribution as Burkitt lymphoma), who present with localized or generalized lymphadenopathy and in whom the disease is extremely aggressive. Skin lesions are sparse. Occasionally the virulent form is largely restricted to lymph nodes, sparing the skin but occasionally involving the viscera.
- *Transplant-associated Kaposi sarcoma* occurs several months to a few years postoperatively in some organ transplant recipients who receive high doses of immunosuppressive therapy. Lesions are either localized to the skin or widely metastatic. Skin lesions sometimes regress when immunosuppressive therapy is markedly reduced, but patients who develop internal involvement usually succumb to their disease.
- *AIDS-associated* (*epidemic*) *Kaposi sarcoma* is found in approximately one fourth or more of AIDS patients, most often in homosexual men. Approximately 40% of individuals in this risk group have developed Kaposi sarcoma, compared with 5% of others with AIDS. Diagnosis of the tumor may precipitate the clinical recognition of the syndrome. Cutaneous or AIDS-associated Kaposi sarcoma lesions have no site of predilection, but involvement of lymph nodes and the gut and wide dissemination tend to occur early in the course. Most patients eventually succumb to the opportunistic infectious complications of AIDS rather than directly to the consequences of Kaposi sarcoma. About one third of these patients with Kaposi sarcoma, however, subsequently develop a second malignancy, most often lymphoma.

MORPHOLOGY. The morphology of Kaposi sarcoma is illustrated in Figure 12–33. In the relatively indolent classic disease of older men and sometimes in the other variants, three stages can be identified patch, plaque, and nodule. The **patches** comprise pink-to-red-to-purple solitary or multiple macules that in the classic disease are usually confined to the distal lower extremities or feet (Fig. 12–33*A*). Microscopic examination discloses only dilated perhaps irregular and angulated blood vessels lined by endothelial cells with an interspersed infiltrate of lymphocytes, plasma cells, and macrophages (sometimes containing hemosiderin), lesions difficult to distinguish from granulation tissue. Over time, lesions in the classic disease spread proximally and usually convert into larger, violaceous, **raised plaques** that reveal dermal, dilated, jagged vascular channels lined by somewhat plump spindle cells accompanied by perivascular aggregates of similar spindled cells. Scattered between the vascular channels are red cells, hemosiderin-laden macrophages, lymphocytes, and plasma cells. Pink hyaline globules of uncertain nature may be found in the spindled cells and macrophages. Occasional mitotic figures may be present.

At a still later stage, the lesions may become **nodular** and more distinctly neoplastic and may be composed of sheets of plump, proliferating spindle cells, mostly in the dermis or subcutaneous tissues (Fig. 12–33*D*). Particularly characteristic in this cellular background are scattered small vessels and slitlike spaces that often contain rows of red cells and hyaline droplets. More marked hemorrhage, hemosiderin pigment, lymphocytes, and occasional macrophages may be admixed with this cellular background. Mitotic figures are common as are the round, pink, cytoplasmic globules. The nodular stage is often accompanied by involvement of lymph nodes and of viscera, particularly in the African and AIDS-associated diseases. The progressive gross and microscopic stages of Kaposi sarcoma are summarized schematically in Figure 12–34.

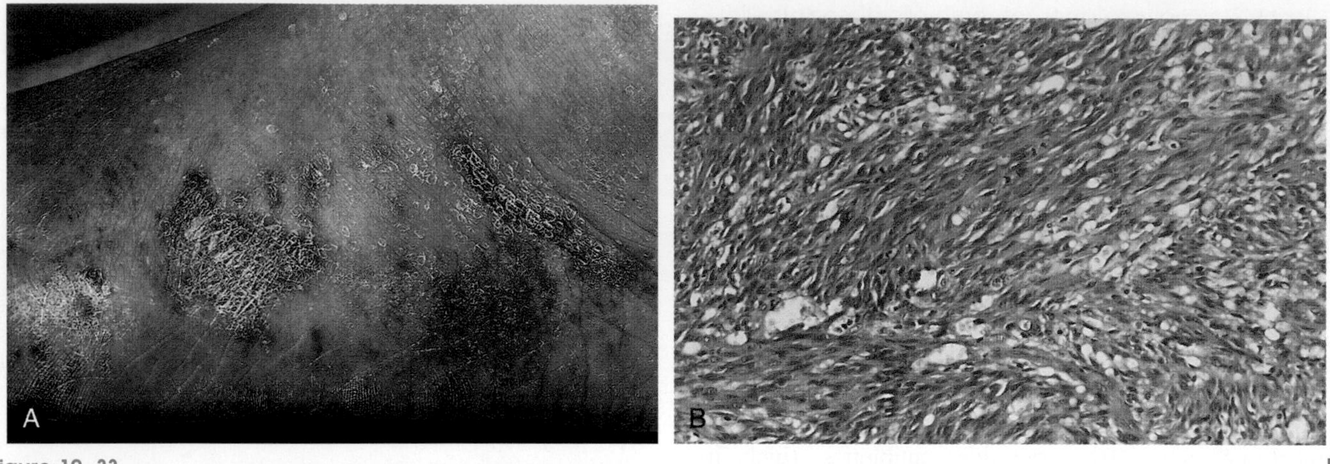

Figure 12–33

Kaposi sarcoma. *A*, Gross photograph illustrating coalescent red-purple macules and plaques of the skin. *B*, Histologic view of the nodular form demonstrating sheets of plump, proliferating spindle cells and vascular spaces. (Courtesy of Christopher D.M. Fletcher, MD, Brigham and Women's Hospital, Boston, MA.)

Pathogenesis. The pathogenesis of Kaposi sarcoma remains uncertain as does the nature of the undifferentiated spindle-shaped tumor cells. Current evidence, however, favors a viral-associated (if not viral-caused) neoplasm of primitive mesenchymal or endothelial cells whose course is greatly influenced by the immune status of the individual. As discussed in Chapter 6, both HIV products and human herpesvirus type 8 may play a major role in inducing these tumors.[85] Additionally, there is considerable evidence that locally produced growth factors or cytokines, acting in a paracrine or autocrine fashion, cause unchecked growth of tumor cells.

Clinical Course. The presentation and natural course of Kaposi sarcoma vary widely and are significantly affected by the clinical setting. Whereas the classic form at the outset is largely restricted to the surface of the body, in the endemic and epidemic subsets, the condition at presentation tends to be more widespread, particularly in persons who

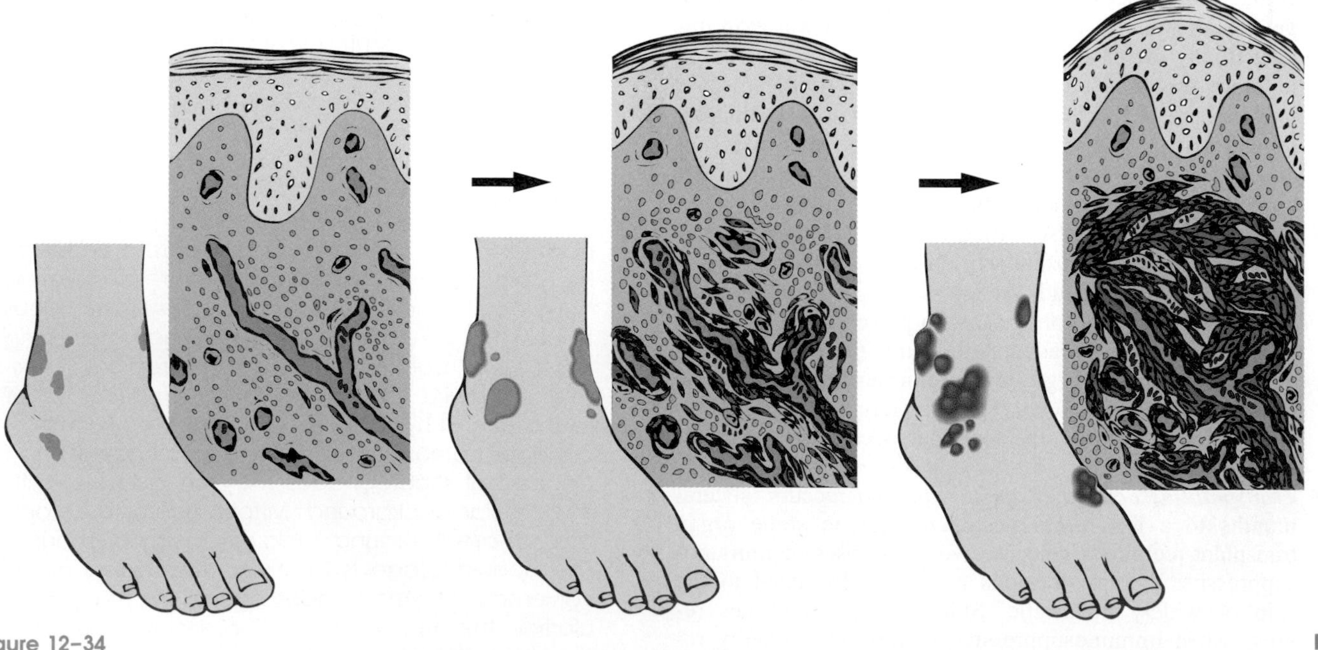

Figure 12–34

Schematic representation of the progressive gross and microscopic stages of Kaposi sarcoma.

have AIDS. Visceral involvement is often present when the cutaneous manifestations appear. Whereas the classic disease is relatively indolent and compatible with long survival, the course of both the endemic and the epidemic patterns may be more aggressive.

Hemangioendothelioma

The term *hemangioendothelioma* is used to denote vascular neoplasms showing histologic features and clinical behavior *intermediate between the benign, well-differentiated hemangiomas and the frankly anaplastic angiosarcomas* (see later). This term encompasses a wide and divergent array of clinical situations, prognosis, and biologic behavior.

Representative of this group is the *epithelioid hemangioendothelioma*, a unique vascular tumor occurring around medium-sized and large veins in the soft tissue of adults. In such tumors, well-defined vascular channels are inconspicuous, and the tumor cells are plump and often cuboidal, thus resembling epithelial cells. The differential diagnosis includes metastatic carcinoma, melanoma, and sarcomas that can assume an epithelioid appearance. Clinical behavior of epithelioid hemangioendothelioma is variable; most are cured by excision, but up to 40% recur, 20 to 30% eventually metastasize, and perhaps 15% of patients die of the tumors. These adverse behavioral characteristics emphasize that clear distinction between intermediate grade and malignant does not exist and that there is a broad morphologic and clinical spectrum between hemangioendothelioma and angiosarcoma.

MALIGNANT TUMORS

Angiosarcoma

Angiosarcomas are malignant endothelial neoplasms (Fig. 12–35) with structure varying from highly differentiated tumors that resemble hemangiomas (*hemangiosarcoma*) to those whose anaplasia makes them difficult to distinguish from malignant epithelial neoplasms, such as carcinoma or melanoma. They occur in both sexes and more often older adults anywhere in the body but most often in the skin, soft tissue, breast, and liver.

Hepatic angiosarcomas are rare but of interest because they are associated with distinct carcinogens, including arsenic (exposure to arsenical pesticides), Thorotrast (a radioactive contrast medium formerly widely used in radiology), and polyvinyl chloride (PVC) (widely used in plastics). The increased frequency of angiosarcomas among workers in the PVC industry is one of the truly well-documented instances of chemical carcinogenesis in humans. With all three agents, there is a long latent period of many years between exposure and the development of tumors.

Angiosarcomas may also arise in the setting of lymphedema, most typically approximately 10 years after radical mastectomy for breast cancer. In such cases, the tumor presumably arises from dilated lymphatic vessels (*lymphangiosarcomas*). Clinically the edematous arm may undergo acute swelling followed by the appearance of subcutaneous nodules, hemorrhage, and skin ulceration. The nodules are frequently multiple, but they later become confluent, forming a large mass. Angiosarcomas may also be induced by radiation in the absence of lymphedema, although both

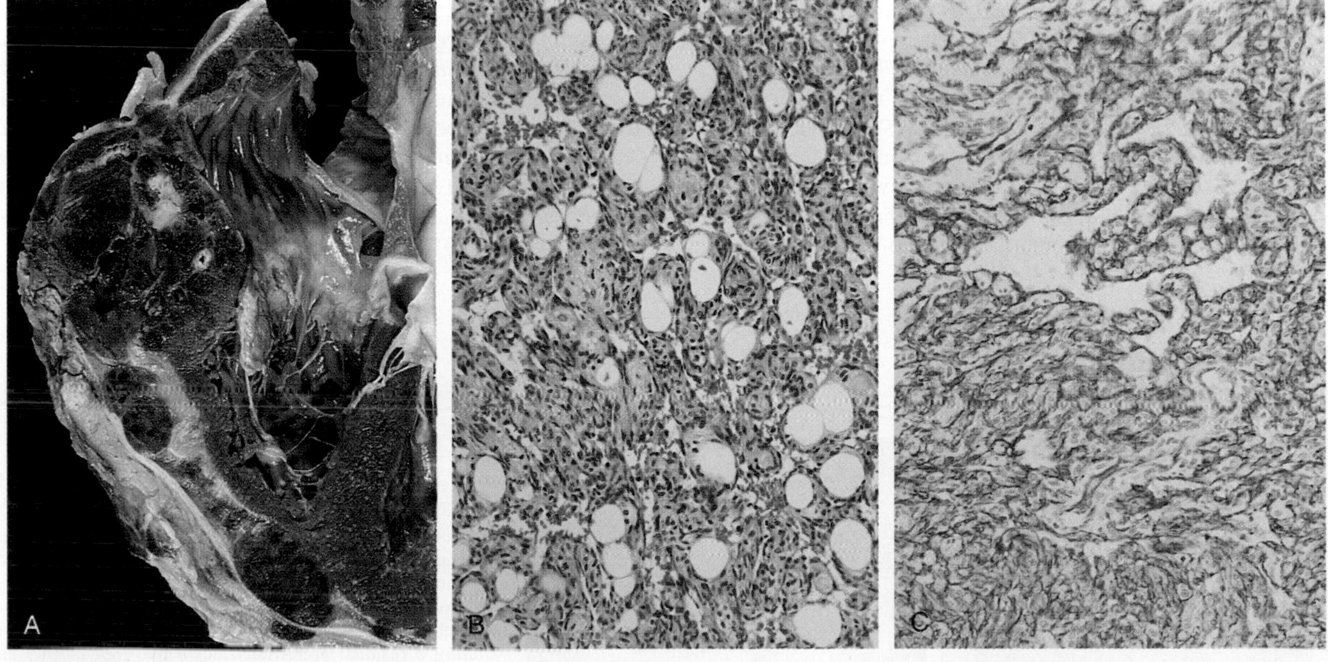

Figure 12–35

Angiosarcoma. *A*, Gross photograph of angiosarcoma of the heart (right ventricle). *B*, Photomicrograph of moderately well differentiated angiosarcoma with dense clumps of irregular, moderate anaplastic cells and distinct vascular lumens. *C*, Positive immunohistochemical staining of angiosarcoma for the endothelial cell marker CD31, proving the endothelial nature of the tumor cells.

factors may be present in some cases after treatment for breast cancer or other neoplasm. Some have been associated with foreign material introduced into the body either iatrogenically or accidentally.

MORPHOLOGY. Grossly, cutaneous angiosarcoma may begin as deceptively small, sharply demarcated, asymptomatic, often multiple red nodules, but eventually most angiosarcomas become large, fleshy masses of pale gray-white soft tissue. The margins blend imperceptibly with surrounding structures. Central softening and areas of necrosis and hemorrhage are frequent.

Microscopically, **all degrees of differentiation of these tumors may be found,** from those that are largely vascular with plump, anaplastic but recognizable endothelial cells producing vascular channels to tumors that are quite undifferentiated produce no definite blood vessels, and are markedly atypical. The more malignant variant tends to have a solid spindle cell appearance.

Clinical Features. Clinically, angiosarcomas have all the usual features of a malignancy, with local invasion and distal metastatic spread. The majority of patients have a poor outcome with few surviving 5 years.

Hemangiopericytoma

Derived from pericytes, the cells normally arranged along capillaries and venules, hemangiopericytoma is a rare neoplasm that may occur as a slowly enlarging, painless mass at any anatomic site but is most common on the lower extremities (especially the thigh) and in the retroperitoneum. Most of these neoplasms are 4 to 8 cm at removal. They consist of numerous branching capillary channels and large gaping sinusoidal spaces surrounded by and enclosed within nests and masses of spindle-shaped cells, which occasionally can be ovoid or even round. Silver impregnation can be used to confirm that these cells are outside the basement membrane of the endothelium and hence are pericytes rather than endothelial cells. The tumors may recur, and as many as 50% metastasize to lungs, bone, and liver. Because many tumors share the vascular pattern of hemangiopericytoma, this is usually a diagnosis of exclusion.

Pathology of Therapeutic Interventions in Vascular Disease

Characteristic morphologic changes are introduced by current modes of therapy of vascular disease, such as balloon angioplasty and vascular replacement, including coronary artery bypass graft surgery. Some key morphologic considerations of each of these and related interventions are discussed briefly.

BALLOON ANGIOPLASTY AND RELATED TECHNIQUES

Balloon angioplasty (dilation of an atheromatous stenosis of an artery by a percutaneously inserted balloon catheter) is being used extensively. Although done in the peripheral arteries in many cases, angioplasty has been studied most extensively after coronary arterial dilation (*percutaneous transluminal coronary angioplasty*). The morphologic effects of angioplasty are demonstrated in Figure 12–36.

The process of balloon dilation of an atherosclerotic vessel characteristically causes plaque fracture, often with accompanying localized hemorrhagic dissection of the adjacent arterial wall (Fig. 12–36*A*).[86] The plaque splits at its weakest point, which is not necessarily the area most severely obstructed. *The key elements of luminal expansion in angioplasty are plaque rupture, medial dissection, and stretching of the media of the dissected segment*, leading to local flow abnormalities and generation of new, potentially thrombogenic blood-contacting surfaces. *Thus, an atherosclerotic plaque after angioplasty is unstable, having many features of the disrupted plaque associated with the acute coronary syndromes and other complications of atherosclerosis* (Chapter 13).

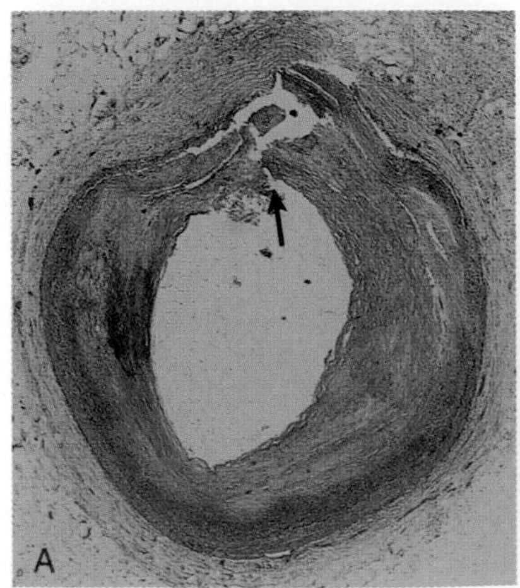

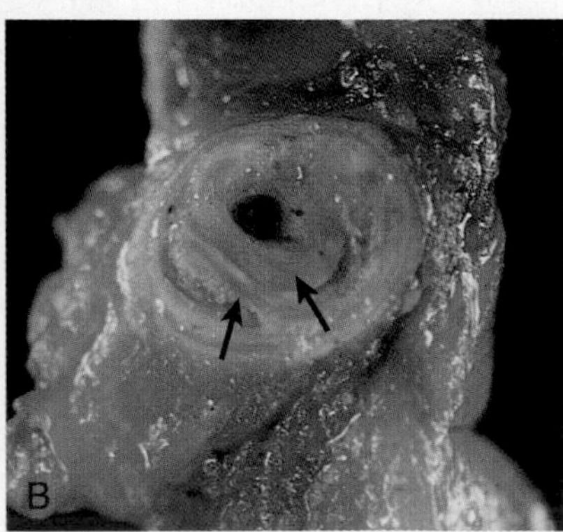

Figure 12–36

Balloon angioplasty. *A*, Coronary artery with recent balloon angioplasty in a low-power photomicrograph showing the split encompassing the intima and media (*arrow*) and partial circumferential wall dissection. *B*, Gross photograph of restenosis after balloon angioplasty demonstrating a residual atherosclerotic plaque (*left arrow*) and a new, glistening proliferative lesion (*right arrow*).

Uncommonly, *abrupt reclosure* follows the angioplasty. This reclosure usually occurs as a result of compression of the lumen by an extensive circumferential or longitudinal dissection or by thrombosis. Nevertheless, most patients improve symptomatically after angioplasty, thereby avoiding the need for aortocoronary bypass graft surgery at that time.

The long-term success of angioplasty is limited by the development of *proliferative restenosis* that occurs in approximately 30 to 50% of patients within the first 4 to 6 months after angioplasty (Fig. 12–36*B*).[87] The factors causing restenosis are complex but probably relate primarily to endothelial cell and smooth muscle cell injury, plaque inflammatory cell elaboration of cytokines and growth factors, local thrombosis, and elastic recoil of the dilated segment.[88] The end result is an occlusive, rapidly progressive fibrous lesion that contains abundant smooth muscle cells and extracellular matrix. This sadly is a relatively frequent complication of a widespread, potentially curative procedure, and a multitude of strategies are now being explored to minimize it.[89]

VASCULAR REPLACEMENT

Many patients now receive synthetic or autologous grafts that replace a segment of vessel or bypass diseased arteries. The clinical performance of a vascular graft depends primarily on its type and location. Large-diameter (10 cm) Dacron grafts in current use function well in high-flow locations such as the aorta. In contrast, small-diameter fabric vascular grafts (6 to 8 mm in diameter) perform less well.

The most widely used small vessel replacements are *autologous saphenous vein* (the patient's own vein, dissected free, reversed in direction, and transplanted to a different site) and *expanded-polytetrafluoroethylene* (essentially a spongy Teflon fabric).[90] Failure of small-diameter vascular prostheses (6 mm diameter) is most frequently due to (1) thrombotic occlusion; (2) intimal fibrous hyperplasia, either generalized (in vein grafts) or primarily at the junction of the graft with the native vasculature (in synthetic grafts) (Fig. 12–37); or occasionally (3) atherosclerosis.

Healing of a vascular graft depends on the migration and proliferation of endothelial cells and smooth muscle cells, derived from adjacent artery at the junction (*anastomosis*). The ability to endothelialize cardiovascular prostheses is limited in humans, and full endothelialization of clinical grafts is unusual. Luminal coverage develops relatively slowly and incompletely; formation of *neointima* (a surface covered by endothelial cells) is generally restricted to a 10- to 15-mm zone near the anastomosis, and the remainder of the graft surface constitutes a *pseudointima* (thrombotic material or cells other than endothelial cells).

Coronary Artery Bypass Graft Surgery

Coronary artery bypass graft surgery (aortocoronary bypass) is one of the most frequently performed major surgical procedures in the United States (>400,000 per year). Bypasses are done using grafts of either autologous reversed saphenous vein or internal mammary artery (usually the left internal mammary artery is used owing to proximity to the heart). Although most patients do well for extended periods after their surgery, many develop late recurrence of symptoms because of either graft occlusion or progression of atherosclerosis in their native coronary arteries distal to the grafts. The long-term patency of saphenous vein grafts is 50% at 10 years, owing to pathologic changes, including thrombosis (usually occurs early), intimal thickening (which usually occurs several months to several years postoperatively), and atherosclerosis in the

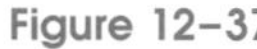

Figure 12–37

Anastomotic hyperplasia at the distal anastomosis of a synthetic femoropopliteal graft. *A*, Angiogram demonstrating constriction (*arrow*). *B*, Photomicrograph demonstrating expanded polytetrafluoroethylene graft (*arrow*) with prominent intimal proliferation and a very small residual lumen (*asterisk*). (*A* courtesy of Anthony D. Whittemore, MD, Brigham and Women's Hospital, Boston, MA.)

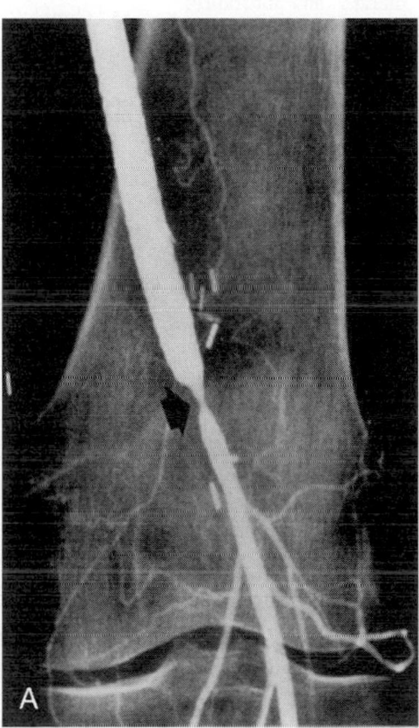

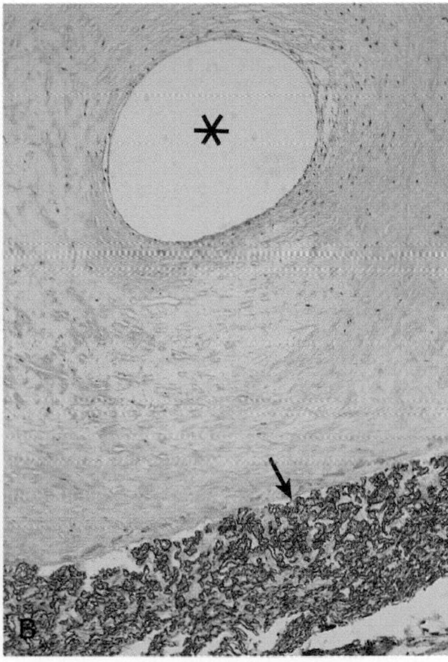

graft, sometimes with superimposed plaque rupture, thrombi, or aneurysms (usually more than 2 to 3 years).[91] In contrast, the internal mammary artery has a greater than 90% patency at 10 years.

REFERENCES

1. Pober J, Cotran RS: Cytokines and endothelial cell biology. Physiol Rev 70:427, 1990.
2. Davies MG, Hagen PO: Pathology of intimal hyperplasia. Br J Surg 81:1254, 1994.
3. Okamoto E, et al: Diversity of the synthetic-state smooth-muscle cells proliferating in mechanically and hemodynamically injured rabbit arteries. Lab Invest 74:120, 1996.
4. Allaire E, Clowes AW: The intimal hyperplastic response. Ann Thorac Surg 64:S38, 1997.
5. Schoen FJ: Interventional and Surgical Cardiovascular Pathology: Clinical Correlations and Basic Principles. Philadelphia, WB Saunders, 1989, p 33.
6. Braunwald E: Cardiovascular medicine at the turn of the millennium: triumphs, concerns, and opportunities. N Engl J Med 337:1360, 1997.
7. Amarenco P, et al: Atherosclerotic disease of the aortic arch and the risk of ischemic stroke. N Engl J Med 331:1474, 1994.
8. Mintz GS, et al: Determinants and correlates of target lesion calcium in coronary artery disease: a clinical, angiographic and intravascular ultrasound study. J Am Coll Cardiol 29:268, 1997.
9. Rumberger JA, et al: Electron beam computed tomography and coronary artery disease: scanning for coronary artery calcification. Mayo Clin Proc 71:369, 1996.
10. Berenson GS, et al: Atherosclerosis of the aorta and coronary arteries and cardiovascular risk factors in persons aged 6 to 30 years and studied at necropsy (The Bogalusa Heart Study). Am J Cardiol 70: 851, 1992.
11. Stary HO, et al: A definition of advanced types of atherosclerotic lesions and a histological classification of atherosclerosis. Circulation 92:1355, 1995.
12. Kannel WB, Wilson PWF: An update on coronary risk factors. Med Clin North Am 79:951, 1995.
13. Neaton JD, Wentworth D: Serum cholesterol, blood pressure, cigarette smoking, and death from coronary heart disease: overall findings and differences by age for 316,099 white men. Arch Intern Med 152: 56, 1992.
14. Strong JP: The natural history of atherosclerosis in childhood. Ann N Y Acad Sci 623:9, 1991.
15. Grodstein F, et al: Postmenopausal hormone therapy and mortality. N Engl J Med 336:1769, 1997.
16. Liebermann EH, et al: Estrogen improves endothelium-dependent, flow-mediated vasodilation in post-menopausal women. Ann Intern Med 121:936, 1994.
17. Dammerman M, Breslow JL: Genetic basis of lipoprotein disorders. Circulation 91:505, 1995.
18. Kuivenhoven JA, et al: The role of a common variant of the cholesteryl ester transfer protein gene in the progression of coronary atherosclerosis. N Engl J Med 338:86, 1998.
19. Gotto AM: Cholesterol management in theory and practice. Circulation 96:4424, 1997.
20. Pedersen TR, et al: Randomised trial of cholesterol lowering in 4444 patients with coronary heart disease: the Scandinavian Simvastatin Survival Study (4S). Lancet 344:1383, 1994.
21. Sacks FM, et al: The effect of pravastatin on coronary events after myocardial infarction in patients with average cholesterol levels. N Engl J Med 335:1001, 1996.
22. Shepard J, et al: Prevention of coronary heart disease with pravastatin in men with hypercholesterolemia. N Engl J Med 333:1301, 1995.
23. Breslow JL: Mouse models of atherosclerosis. Science 272:685, 1996.
24. Schmidt EB, Dyerberg J: Omega-3 fatty acids: current status in cardiovascular medicine. Drugs 47:405, 1994.
25. Ascherio A, et al: Dietary intake of marine n-3 fatty acids, fish intake, and the risk of coronary disease among men. N Engl J Med 332:977, 1995.
26. Hu FB, et al: Dietary fat intake and the risk of coronary heart disease in women. N Engl J Med 337:1491, 1997.
27. SHEP Cooperative Research Group: Prevention of stroke by antihypertensive drug treatment in older persons with isolated systolic hypertension: final results of the Systolic Hypertension in the Elderly Program. JAMA 265:3255, 1991.
28. McCully KS: Vascular pathology of homocysteinemia: implications for the pathogenesis of arteriosclerosis. Am J Pathol 56:111, 1969.
29. Welch GN, Loscalzo J: Homocysteine and atherothrombosis. N Engl J Med 338:1042, 1998.
30. Rimm EB, et al: Folate and vitamin B_6 from diet and supplements in relation to risk of coronary heart disease among women. JAMA 279: 359, 1998.
31. Ridker PM, et al: Inflammation, aspirin, and the risk of cardiovascular disease in apparently healthy men. New Engl J Med 336:973, 1997.
32. Nachman RL: Lipoprotein(a): molecular mischief in the microvasculature. Circulation 96:2485, 1997.
33. Thun J, et al: Alcohol consumption and mortality among middle-aged and elderly U.S. adults. N Engl J Med 337:1705, 1997.
34. Ross R: The pathogenesis of atherosclerosis: a perspective for the 1990s. Nature 362:801, 1993.
35. Cybulsky MI, Gimbrone MA: Endothelial expression of a mononuclear leukocyte adhesion molecule during atherogenesis. Science 251: 788, 1991.
36. O'Brien KD, et al: Neovascular expression of E-selectin, intercellular adhesion molecule-1, and vascular cell adhesion molecule-1 in human atherosclerosis and their relation to intimal leukocyte content. Circulation 93:672, 1996.
37. Gimbrone MA, Nagel T, Topper JN: Biomechanical activation: an emerging paradigm in endothelial adhesion biology. J Clin Invest 99: 1809, 1997.
38. Steinberg D: Oxidative modification of LDL and atherogenesis. Circulation 95:1062, 1997.
39. Treasure CB, et al: Beneficial effects of cholesterol-lowering therapy on the coronary endothelium in patients with coronary artery disease. N Engl J Med 332:481, 1995.
40. Anderson TJ, et al: The effect of cholesterol-lowering and antioxidant therapy on endothelium-dependent coronary vasomotion. N Engl J Med 332:488, 1995.
41. Murry CE, et al: Monoclonality of smooth muscle cells in human atherosclerosis. Am J Pathol 151:697, 1997.
42. Libby P, et al: Roles of infectious agents in atherosclerosis and restenosis: an assessment of the evidence and need for future research. Circulation 96:4095, 1997.
43. Weck KE, et al: Murine γ-herpesvirus 68 causes severe large-vessel arteritis in mice lacking interferon-γ responsiveness: a new model for virus-induced vascular disease. Nat Med 3:1346, 1997.
44. Buja LM: Does atherosclerosis have an infectious etiology? Circulation 94:872, 1996.
45. Gupta S, et al: Elevated *Chlamydia pneumoniae* antibodies, cardiovascular events, and azithromycin in male survivors of myocardial infarction. Circulation 96:404, 1997.
46. Berenson GS, et al: Association between multiple cardiovascular risk factors and atherosclerosis in children and young adults. N Engl J Med 338:1650, 1998.
47. Strong JP: Atherosclerotic lesions: natural history, risk factors, and topography. Arch Pathol Lab Med 116:1268, 1992.
48. Antiplatelet Trialists' Collaboration: Collaborative overview of randomised trials of antiplatelet therapy: I. Prevention of death, myocardial infarction, and stroke by prolonged antiplatelet therapy in various categories of patients. BMJ 308:81, 1994.
49. Kaplan NM: Systemic hypertension: mechanisms and diagnosis. In Braunwald E. (ed): Heart Disease, 5th ed. Philadelphia, WB Saunders, 1997, p 807.
50. Lijnen P: Alterations in sodium metabolism as an etiological model for hypertension. Cardiovasc Drugs Ther 9:377, 1995.
51. Cowley AW, Roman RJ: The role of the kidney in hypertension. JAMA 275:1581, 1996.
52. Hingorani AD, Brown MJ: Identifying the genes for human hypertension. Nephrol Dial Transplant 11:575, 1996.
53. Lifton RP: Molecular genetics of human blood pressure variation. Science 272:676, 1996.
54. Thibonnier M, Schork NJ: The genetics of hypertension. Curr Opin Genet Dev 5:362, 1995.
55. Jennette JC, Falk RJ: Small-vessel vasculitis. N Engl J Med 337: 1512, 1997.

56. Allen NB, Bressler PB: Diagnosis and treatment of the systemic and cutaneous necrotizing vasculitis syndromes. Med Clin North Am 81: 243, 1997.
57. Lee WM: Hepatitis B virus infection. N Engl J Med 337:1733, 1997.
58. Cotran RS, Pober JS: Recent insights into the mechanisms of vascular injury: implications for the pathogenesis of vasculitis. In Simionescu N, Simionescu M (eds): Endothelial Cell Dysfunctions. New York, Plenum Press, 1992, p 183.
59. Gross WL: Antineutrophil cytoplasmic autoantibody testing in vasculitides. Rheum Dis Clin North Am 21:987, 1995.
60. Jennette JC, Falk RJ: Update on the pathobiology of vasculitis. In Schoen FJ, Gimbrone MA (eds): Cardiovascular Pathology: Clinicopathologic Correlations and Pathogenetic Mechanisms. Baltimore, Williams & Wilkins, 1995, p 156.
61. Mayet WJ, Helmreich-Becker I, Buschenfelde KHM: The pathophysiology of anti-neutrophil cytoplasmic antibodies (ANCA) and their clinical relevance. Crit Rev Oncol Hematol 23:151, 1996.
62. Jennette JC, et al: Nomenclature of systemic vasculitides: the proposal of an international consensus conference. Arthritis Rheum 37: 187, 1994.
63. Brack A, et al: Giant cell vasculitis is a T cell-dependent disease. Mol Med 3:350, 1997.
64. Hall S, et al: Takayasu arteritis: a study of 32 North American patients. Medicine 64:89, 1985.
65. Rowley AH, et al: Kawasaki syndrome. Curr Probl Pediatr 21:387, 1991.
66. Naoe S, et al: Kawasaki disease: with particular emphasis on arterial lesions. Acta Pathol Jpn 41:785, 1991.
67. Hoffman GS, et al: Wegener granulomatosis: an analysis of 158 patients. Ann Intern Med 116:488, 1992.
68. Joyce JW: Buerger's disease (thromboangiitis obliterans). Rheum Dis Clin North Am 16:463, 1990.
69. Gravallese EM, et al: Rheumatoid aortitis: a rarely recognized but clinically significant entity. Medicine 68:95, 1989.
70. Sterpetti AV, et al: Inflammatory aneurysms of the abdominal aorta: incidence, pathologic, and etiologic considerations. J Vasc Surg 9: 643, 1989.
71. Patel MI, et al: Current views on the pathogenesis of abdominal aortic aneurysms. J Am Coll Surg 181:371, 1995.
72. Kuivaniemi H, et al: Genetic causes of aortic aneurysms: Unlearning at least part of what the textbooks say. J Clin Invest 88:1441, 1991.
73. Prockop D: Mutations in collagens as a cause of connective tissue diseases. N Engl J Med 326:540, 1992.
74. Knox JB, Sukhova GK, Whittemore AD, Libby P: Evidence for altered balance between matrix metalloproteinases and their inhibitors in human aortic diseases. Circulation 95:205, 1997.
75. Ernst CB: Abdominal aortic aneurysms. N Engl J Med 328:1167, 1993.
76. Cigarra JE, et al: Diagnostic imaging in the evaluation of suspected aortic dissection. N Engl J Med 328:35, 1993.
77. Callam MJ: Epidemiology of varicose veins. Br J Surg 81:167, 1994.
78. Rosen SB, Sturk A: Activated protein C resistance—a major risk factor for thrombosis. Eur J Clin Chem Clin Biochem 35:501, 1997.
79. Weinmann EE, Salzman EW: Deep-vein thrombosis. N Engl J Med 331:1630, 1994.
80. Calonje E, Fletcher CDM: Tumors of blood vessels and lymphatics. In CDM Fletcher (ed): Diagnostic Histopathology of Tumors. New York, Churchill Livingstone, 1995, p 43.
81. Shovlin CL, et al: Characterization of endoglin and identification of novel mutations in hereditary hemorrhagic telangiectasia. Am J Hum Genet 61:68, 1997.
82. Folkman J, D'Amore PA. Blood vessel formation: what is its molecular basis? Cell 87:1153, 1996.
83. Relman DA, et al: The agent of bacillary angiomatosis: an approach to the identification of uncultured pathogens. N Engl J Med 323:1573, 1990.
84. Koehler JE, et al: Molecular epidemiology of bartonella infections in patients with bacillary angiomatosis-pelosis. N Engl J Med 337:1876, 1997.
85. Kemeńy L, et al: Kaposi's sarcoma-associated herpesvirus/human herpesvirus-8: a new virus in human pathology. J Am Acad Dermatol 37:107, 1997.
86. Waller BF, et al: Coronary artery and saphenous vein graft remodeling: a review of histologic findings after various interventional procedures—part IV. Clin Cardiol 19:960, 1996.
87. Gottsauner-Wolf M, et al: Restenosis: an open file. Clin Cardiol 19: 347, 1996.
88. Landzberg BR, et al: Pathophysiology and pharmacological approaches for prevention of coronary artery restenosis following coronary artery balloon angioplasty and related procedures. Prog Cardiovasc Dis 34:361, 1997.
89. Bittl JA: Advances in coronary angioplasty. N Engl J Med 335:1290, 1996.
90. Zdrahala RJ: Small caliber vascular grafts: Part I. state of the art. J Biomater Appl 10:309, 1996.
91. Nwasokwa ON: Coronary artery bypass graft disease. Ann Intern Med 123:528, 1995.

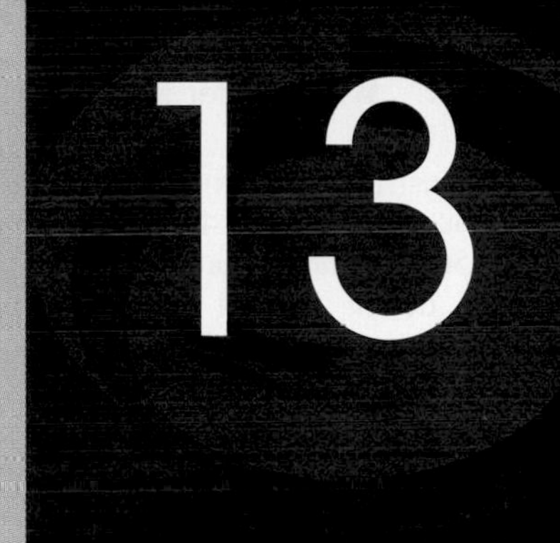

The Heart

Frederick J. Schoen

NORMAL HEART

MYOCARDIUM

BLOOD SUPPLY

VALVES

EFFECTS OF AGING ON THE HEART

PRINCIPLES OF CARDIAC DYSFUNCTION

HEART FAILURE

- Cardiac Hypertrophy: Pathophysiology and Progression to Failure
- Left-Sided Heart Failure
- Right-Sided Heart Failure

TYPES OF HEART DISEASE

ISCHEMIC HEART DISEASE

- Angina Pectoris
- Myocardial Infarction
- Chronic Ischemic Heart Disease
- Sudden Cardiac Death

HYPERTENSIVE HEART DISEASE

- Systemic (Left-Sided) Hypertensive Heart Disease
- Pulmonary (Right-Sided) Hypertensive Heart Disease (Cor Pulmonale)

VALVULAR HEART DISEASE

- Valvular Degeneration Caused by Calcification
  - *Calcific Aortic Stenosis*
  - *Calcification of a Congenitally Bicuspid Aortic Valve*
  - *Mitral Annular Calcification*
- Myxomatous Degeneration of the Mitral Valve (Mitral Valve Prolapse)
- Rheumatic Fever and Rheumatic Heart Disease
- Infective Endocarditis
- Noninfected Vegetations
  - *Nonbacterial Thrombotic Endocarditis*
  - *Endocarditis of Systemic Lupus Erythematosus (Libman-Sacks Disease)*
- Carcinoid Heart Disease
- Complications of Artificial Valves

MYOCARDIAL DISEASE

- Dilated Cardiomyopathy
- Hypertrophic Cardiomyopathy
- Restrictive Cardiomyopathy
- Myocarditis
- Other Specific Causes

PERICARDIAL DISEASE

- Pericardial Effusion and Hemopericardium
- Pericarditis
  - *Acute Pericarditis*
  - *Healed Pericarditis*
- Rheumatoid Heart Disease

NEOPLASTIC HEART DISEASE

- Primary Cardiac Tumors
  - *Myxoma*
  - *Lipoma*
  - *Papillary Fibroelastoma*
  - *Rhabdomyoma*
  - *Sarcoma*
- Cardiac Effects of Noncardiac Neoplasms

CONGENITAL HEART DISEASE

- Left-to-Right Shunts—Late Cyanosis
  - *Atrial Septal Defect*
  - *Ventricular Septal Defect*
  - *Patent Ductus Arteriosus*
  - *Atrioventricular Septal Defect*
- Right-to-Left Shunts—Early Cyanosis
  - *Tetralogy of Fallot*
  - *Transposition of Great Arteries*
  - *Truncus Arteriosus*
  - *Tricuspid Atresia*
  - *Total Anomalous Pulmonary Venous Connection*
- Obstructive Congenital Anomalies
  - *Coarctation of Aorta*
  - *Pulmonary Stenosis and Atresia*
  - *Aortic Stenosis and Atresia*

CARDIAC TRANSPLANTATION

The human heart is a remarkably efficient, durable, and reliable pump that propels more than 6000 liters of blood through the body daily during an individual's lifetime, thereby providing the tissues with a steady supply of vital nutrients and facilitating the excretion of waste products. As might be anticipated, cardiac dysfunction can be associated with devastating physiologic consequences. Heart disease is the predominant cause of disability and death in industrialized nations. In the United States, it currently accounts for about 40% of all postnatal deaths totaling about 750,000 individuals annually and nearly twice the number of deaths caused by all forms of cancer combined. The yearly economic burden of ischemic heart disease (IHD), the most prevalent subgroup, is estimated to be in excess of $100 billion. The major categories of cardiac diseases considered in this chapter include obstructive coronary artery disease (also called *IHD*), heart disease caused by systemic hypertension, heart disease caused by pulmonary diseases (cor pulmonale), valvular heart diseases, primary myocardial diseases, and congenital heart diseases. Pericardial diseases and cardiac neoplasms as well as cardiac transplantation are also briefly discussed. Before considering details of specific conditions, we review salient features of normal anatomy and function as well as the principles of cardiac hypertrophy and failure, the common end points of many different types of heart disease.

NORMAL HEART

The normal heart weight varies with body height and weight; it averages approximately 250 to 300 gm in females and 300 to 350 gm in males. The expected thickness of the free wall of the right ventricle is 0.3 to 0.5 cm and that of the left ventricle 1.3 to 1.5 cm. Increases in cardiac size and weight accompany many forms of heart disease. Greater heart weight or ventricular thickness indicates *hypertrophy*, and an enlarged chamber size implies *dilation*. Wall thickness itself may not be a good measure of increased cardiac mass. For example, an apparently normal (or less than normal) left ventricular thickness may be found in a markedly heavy, hypertrophied heart that has dilated before death. An increase in cardiac weight or size is termed *cardiomegaly*.

Myocardium

Basic to the heart's function is the near-inexhaustible cardiac muscle, the *myocardium*, composed primarily of a collection of branching and anastomosing striated muscle cells (*cardiac myocytes*). They, in turn, have five major components: (1) cell membrane (sarcolemma) and T tubules, for impulse conduction; (2) sarcoplasmic reticulum, a calcium reservoir needed for contraction; (3) contractile elements; (4) mitochondria; and (5) the nucleus. Cardiac muscle cells contain many more mitochondria between myofibrils than skeletal muscle cells (approximately 23% of cell volume versus 2%), reflecting the extreme dependence of cardiac muscle on aerobic metabolism.

The functional intracellular contractile unit of cardiac muscle is a *sarcomere*, an orderly arrangement of thick filaments composed principally of *myosin*, thin filaments containing *actin* as well as the regulatory proteins troponin and tropomyosin. As in skeletal muscle, the ends of each sarcomere are demarcated by a Z-line, to which the thin filaments are anchored. Relative to skeletal muscle, however, cardiac muscle has a more complex structure consisting of individual branching cells, usually containing one spindle-shaped nucleus each and many parallel myofilaments (arrays of sarcomeres in series). Contraction of cardiac muscle occurs by the cumulative effort of sliding of the actin filaments between the myosin filaments toward the center of each sarcomere. The lengths of sarcomeres range from 1.6 to 2.2 μm, depending on the state of contraction. Shorter sarcomeres have considerable overlap of actin and myosin filaments, with consequent reduction in contractile force, whereas longer lengths enhance contractility (Frank-Starling mechanism). Thus, moderate ventricular dilation increases the force of contraction. There is a point, however, with progressive dilation at which effective overlap of the actin and myosin filaments is reduced, and the force of contraction turns sharply downward, as occurs in heart failure.

Because cardiac myocytes are so much larger than the intervening interstitial cells, they account for more than 90% of the volume of the myocardium. Myocytes, however, compose only approximately 25% of the total number of cells in the heart. The remainder are endothelial cells, mostly associated with the rich capillary network, and connective tissue cells. Inflammatory cells are rare and collagen is sparse in normal myocardium.

Reflecting their different functional requirements, atrial myocytes are generally smaller in diameter and less structured than their ventricular counterparts. Some atrial cells also differ from ventricular cells in having distinctive electron dense granules in the cytoplasm called *specific atrial granules*. They are the site of storage of *atrial natriuretic peptide*, a polypeptide synthesized in the atrial muscle cells and secreted into the blood under conditions of atrial pressure elevation and distention. Atrial natriuretic peptide can produce a variety of physiologic effects, including vasodilation, natriuresis, suppression of the renin-angiotensin-aldosterone axis, and a fall in arterial pressure,[1] actions beneficial in pathologic states such as hypertension and congestive heart failure.

Functional integration of myocytes is mediated by structures unique to cardiac muscle called *intercalated discs* that join individual cells, within which specialized intercellular junctions permit both mechanical and ionic coupling. Most importantly, *gap junctions* facilitate synchronous myocyte contraction by providing electrical coupling with relatively unrestricted passage of ions across the membranes of adjoining cells. Gap junctions consist of clusters of plasma membrane channels that directly link the cytoplasmic compartments of neighboring cells. Abnormalities in the spatial distribution of gap junctions and their respective proteins in IHD and myocardial heart disease may contribute to electromechanical dysfunction (arrhythmias).[2]

In addition, specialized excitatory and conducting myocytes within the cardiac conduction system are involved in the regulation of the rate and rhythm of the heart. Components include (1) the sinoatrial (SA) pacemaker of the heart, *the SA node*, located near the junction of the right atrial appendage with the superior vena cava; (2) the *atrioventricular (AV) node*, located in the right atrium along the atrial septum; (3) the *bundle of His*, which courses from the right atrium to the summit of the ventricular septum; and division of the bundle of His into limbs, and (4) the right and left bundle branches that further arborize in the respective ventricles.

Blood Supply

Generating energy almost exclusively by the oxidation of substrates, the heart relies heavily on an adequate flow of oxygenated blood through the coronary arteries. With origins from the aorta immediately distal to the aortic valve, the coronary arteries consist of 5 to 10 cm long, 2 to 4 mm diameter conduits that run along the external surface of the heart (*epicardial coronary arteries*) and smaller vessels that penetrate the myocardium (*intramural arteries*).

The three major epicardial coronary arteries are (1) the left anterior descending (LAD) and (2) the left circumflex (LCX) artery, both arising as branches from a bifurcation of the left (main) coronary artery, and (3) the right coronary artery (RCA). Branches of the LAD are called *diagonals* and *septal perforators*, and those of the LCX are *obtuse marginals*. Most coronary arterial blood flow to the myocardium occurs during ventricular diastole, when the microcirculation is not compressed by the cardiac contraction.

Knowledge of the areas of supply (*perfusion*) of the three major coronary arteries helps correlate sites of vascular obstruction with regions of myocardial infarction. Most commonly, the LAD supplies most of the *apex* of the heart (the rounded point at the distal parts of the ventricles as contrasted with the wide proximal part, the *base*), the anterior wall of the left ventricle, and the anterior two thirds of the ventricular septum. By convention, whichever coronary artery gives rise to the posterior descending branch and thereby perfuses the posterior third of the septum is called *dominant* (although the LAD and LCX collectively perfuse the majority of the left ventricular myocardium—the LAD itself about 50%). In a *right dominant circulation*, present in approximately four fifths of individuals, the circumflex branch of the left coronary artery generally perfuses only the lateral wall of the left ventricle, and the RCA supplies the entire right ventricular free wall and the posterobasal wall of the left ventricle and the posterior third of the ventricular septum. *Thus, occlusions of the right as well as the left coronary arteries can cause left ventricular damage.*

Functionally the right and left coronary arteries behave as end arteries, although anatomically there are numerous intercoronary anastomoses in most hearts (called the *collateral circulation*). Little blood courses through these channels in the normal heart. When one artery is severely narrowed, however, blood flows via collaterals from the high to the low pressure system and causes the channels to enlarge. Progressive dilation of collaterals, stimulated by ischemia (see later), may play a role in providing blood flow to areas of the myocardium otherwise deprived of adequate perfusion. When blood flow is compromised and collateral blood flow is inadequate, however, the subendocardium (myocardium adjacent to the ventricular cavities) represents the area most susceptible to ischemic damage.

Valves

The four cardiac valves function to maintain unidirectional blood flow. During closure, the three cusps of the *semilunar* valves (aortic and pulmonary) overlap along an area (the *lunula*) between the free edge and the closing edge. The coaptation area is substantial; in the aortic valve, for example, the total cuspal area is approximately one third greater than the valve orifice area. Because only the portion of the cusps below the closing edge separates aortic from left ventricular cavity blood, the occasionally occurring defects or fenestrations of the cusp in the lunula usually do not compromise valve competence. Each aortic cusp has a small nodule (*nodule of Arantius*) in the center of the free edge, which facilitates closure. On gross inspection, normal valve cusps appear thin and translucent.

The free margins of the *AV valves* (mitral and tricuspid) are tethered to the ventricular wall by many delicate tendinous cords (*chordae tendineae*), attached to papillary muscles that are contiguous with the underlying ventricular walls. Left ventricular papillary muscles are themselves positioned beneath the commissures and thereby receive cords from two adjacent leaflets. Thus, normal mitral valve competency depends on the coordinated actions of annulus, leaflets, cords, papillary muscles, and associated left ventricular wall (collectively the *mitral apparatus*) acting to maintain leaflet coaptation in the annulus. Tricuspid valve function depends on analogous structures. The function of semilunar valves similarly depends on the integrity and coordinated movements of the cusps and their attachments. Thus, dilation of the aortic root can hinder coaptation of the aortic valve cusps during closure, just as left ventricular dilation or a ruptured cord or papillary muscle can interfere with mitral closure, each resulting in regurgitant flow.

The cardiac valves are lined with endothelium; all have a similar, layered architecture consisting predominantly of a dense collagenous core (*fibrosa*) close to the outflow surface and continuous with valvular supporting structures and loose connective tissue (*spongiosa*) near to the inflow surface.[3] The fibrosa maintains the structural integrity of a valve, and the spongiosa functions as a shock absorber. In general, normal leaflets and cusps have scant blood vessels limited to the proximal portion because they are thin enough to be nourished by diffusion from the heart's blood.

Effects of Aging on the Heart

With an increasing number of persons surviving into their seventies and beyond, knowledge of changes in the cardiovascular system that frequently occur with aging is important. Changes occur in the pericardium, cardiac chambers, valves, epicardial coronary arteries, conduction system, myocardium, and aorta (Table 13–1).[4]

With advancing age, the amount of epicardial fat increases, particularly over the anterior surface of the right ventricle and in the atrial septum. Associated with increasing age and accentuated by systemic hypertension is a

Table 13–1. CHANGES IN THE AGING HEART

Chambers
Increased left atrial cavity size
Decreased left ventricular cavity size
Sigmoid-shaped ventricular septum

Valves
Aortic valve calcific deposits
Mitral valve annular calcific deposits
Fibrous thickening of leaflets
Hooding of mitral leaflets toward the left atrium
Lambl excrescences

Epicardial Coronary Arteries
Tortuosity
Increased cross-sectional luminal area
Calcific deposits
Atherosclerotic plaque

Myocardium (Walls)
Increased mass
Increased subepicardial fat
Brown atrophy
Lipofuscin deposition
Basophilic degeneration
Amyloid deposits

Aorta
Dilated ascending aorta with rightward shift
Elongated (tortuous) thoracic aorta
Sinotubular junction calcific deposits
Elastic tissue fragmentation and collagen accumulation
Atherosclerotic plaque

reduction in the size of the left ventricular cavity, particularly in the base-to-apex dimension. Accompanied by a rightward shift and tortuosity of a dilated ascending aorta, this chamber alteration causes the basal ventricular septum to bend leftward, bulging into the left ventricular outflow tract (termed *sigmoid septum*), and can simulate the obstruction to blood leaving the left ventricle that often occurs with hypertrophic cardiomyopathy (HCM) (discussed later).

Several changes of the valves are noted, including calcification of the mitral annulus and aortic valve, the latter frequently leading to aortic stenosis (see discussion later). In addition, the valves develop fibrous thickening, and the mitral leaflets tend to buckle back toward the left atrium during ventricular systole, simulating a prolapsing (myxomatous) mitral valve (see later). Moreover, many older persons develop small filiform processes (*Lambl excrescences*) on the closure lines of aortic and mitral valves that probably arise from organization of small thrombi on the valve contact margins.

Compared with younger myocardium, elderly myocardium also has fewer myocytes, increased collagenized connective tissue, and, in some individuals, deposition of amyloid. In the muscle cells, lipofuscin deposits (Chapter 1) and *basophilic degeneration*, an accumulation within cardiac myocytes of a gray bluish–appearing byproduct of glycogen metabolism, may be present. Extensive lipofuscin deposition in a small, atrophied heart is often called *brown atrophy*. Although the morphologic changes described are common in elderly patients at necropsy and they may mimic disease, only in a minority are they associated with clinical cardiac dysfunction.

PRINCIPLES OF CARDIAC DYSFUNCTION

Although many diseases can involve the heart and blood vessels,[5, 6] cardiovascular dysfunction results from five principal mechanisms:

1. *Failure of the pump itself*: In the most frequent circumstance, damaged muscle contracts weakly or inadequately, and the chambers cannot empty properly. In some conditions, however, the muscle cannot relax sufficiently.
2. *An obstruction to flow*, owing to a lesion preventing valve opening or otherwise causing increased ventricular chamber pressure (e.g., aortic valvular stenosis, systemic hypertension, or aortic coarctation): This overworks the chamber behind the obstruction.
3. *Regurgitant flow* (e.g., mitral or aortic valvular regurgitation) that causes some of the output from each contraction to reflux backward: This necessarily adds a volume workload on the ventricle.
4. *Disorders of cardiac conduction* (e.g., heart block) or arrhythmias owing to uncoordinated generation of impulses (e.g., ventricular fibrillation): These lead to nonuniform and inefficient contractions of the muscular walls.
5. *Disruption of the continuity of the circulatory system* (e.g., gunshot wound through the thoracic aorta): This permits blood to escape.

Heart Failure

The above-listed abnormalities often culminate in heart failure, an extremely common result of many forms of heart disease. In heart failure, often called *congestive heart failure*, the heart is unable to pump blood at a rate commensurate with the requirements of the metabolizing tissues or can do so only from an elevated filling pressure. Although usually caused by a slowly developing deficit in myocardial contraction, a similar clinical syndrome is present in some patients with heart failure caused by conditions in which the normal heart is suddenly presented with a load that exceeds its capacity or in which ventricular filling is impaired. Congestive heart failure is a common and often recurrent condition with a poor prognosis (mortality of more than 50% in less than 5 years) that is the underlying or contributing cause of death of an estimated 300,000 individuals annually in the United States and for which 2 million individuals are currently being treated. It is the leading discharge diagnosis in hospitalized patients over 65 years of age.

The cardiovascular system acts to maintain arterial pressure and perfusion of vital organs by responding to excessive hemodynamic burden or disturbance in myocardial contractility by a number of mechanisms.[7] The most important are as follows:

- *The Frank-Starling mechanism*, in which the increased preload of dilation helps to sustain cardiac performance by enhancing contractility
- *Myocardial hypertrophy with or without cardiac chamber dilation*, in which the mass of contractile tissue is augmented
- *Activation of neurohumoral systems*, especially (1) release of the neurotransmitter norepinephrine by adrenergic cardiac nerves (which increases heart rate and augments myocardial contractility), (2) activation of the renin-angiotensin-aldosterone system, and (3) release of atrial natriuretic peptide

These adaptive mechanisms may be adequate to maintain the overall pumping performance of the heart at relatively normal levels, but their capacity to sustain cardiac performance may ultimately be exceeded. Most instances of heart failure are the consequence of progressive deterioration of myocardial contractile function (*systolic dysfunction*), as often occurs with ischemic injury, pressure or volume overload, or dilated cardiomyopathy (DCM).[8] The most frequent specific causes are hypertension and IHD (to be discussed subsequently). Sometimes, however, failure results from an inability of the heart chamber to relax, expand, and fill sufficiently during diastole to accommodate an adequate ventricular blood volume (*diastolic dysfunction*), as can occur with massive left ventricular hypertrophy, myocardial fibrosis, deposition of amyloid, or constrictive pericarditis.[9] *Whatever its basis, congestive heart failure is characterized by diminished cardiac output (sometimes called forward failure) or damming back of blood in the venous system (so-called backward failure), or both.*

CARDIAC HYPERTROPHY: PATHOPHYSIOLOGY AND PROGRESSION TO FAILURE

In many pathologic states, the onset of heart failure is preceded by *cardiac hypertrophy*, the compensatory response of the myocardium to increased mechanical work (see later) or trophic signals (e.g., hyperthyroidism through stimulation of β-adrenergic receptors). These stimuli increase the rate of protein synthesis, the amount of protein in each cell, the size of myocytes, the number of sarcomeres and mitochondria, and consequently the mass and size of the heart. The response is also accompanied by selective up-regulation of several immediate early response genes and embryonic forms of contractile and other proteins (Chapter 2). Because adult cardiac myocytes cannot divide, augmentation of myocyte number (*hyperplasia*) cannot occur.

The pattern of hypertrophy reflects the nature of the stimulus. Pressure-overloaded ventricles (e.g., hypertension or aortic stenosis) develop *pressure* (also called *concentric*) *hypertrophy* of the left ventricle, with an increased wall thickness and a normal to reduced cavity diameter. In contrast, volume-overloaded ventricles (e.g., mitral or aortic valve regurgitation) develop hypertrophy accompanied by dilation with increased ventricular diameter (Fig. 13–1). Moreover, as emphasized by Figure 13–1, wall thickness does not necessarily correlate with the pathologic state; despite its increased mass, a heart in which both hypertrophy and dilation has occurred may have increased, decreased, or normal wall thickness.

The extent of hypertrophy varies for different underlying causes. Heart weight usually ranges to 600 gm (up to approximately two times normal) in pulmonary hypertension and IHD; to 800 gm (up to two to three times normal) in systemic hypertension, aortic stenosis, mitral regurgitation,

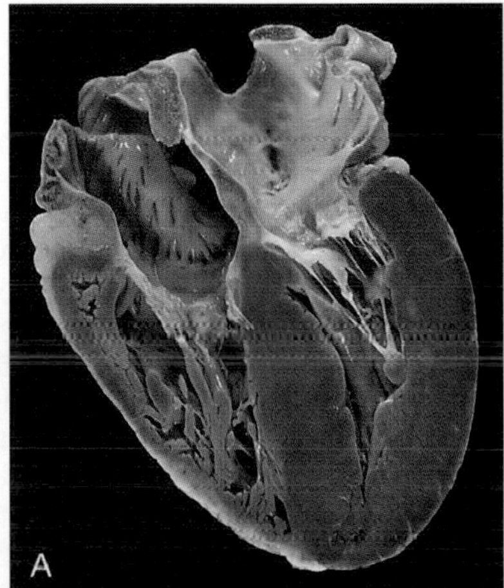

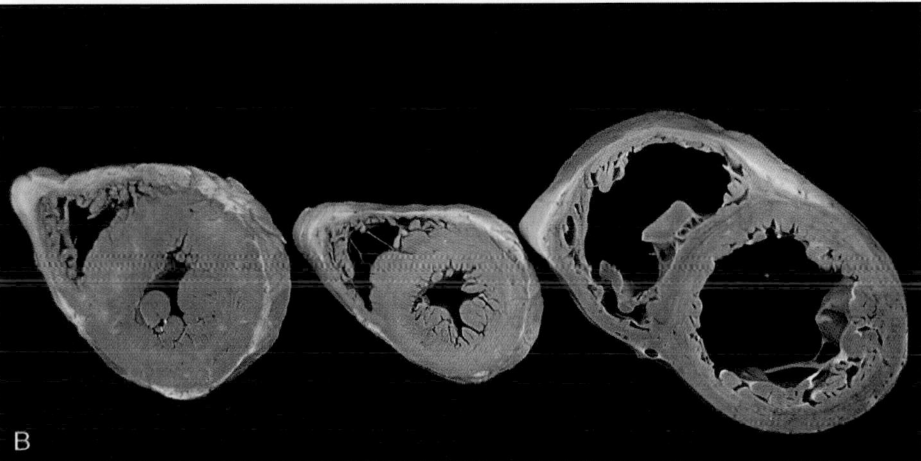

Figure 13–1

Left ventricular hypertrophy. *A*, Pressure hypertrophy due to left ventricular outflow obstruction. The left ventricle is on the lower right in this apical four-chamber view of the heart. *B*, Altered cardiac configuration in left ventricular hypertrophy without and with dilation, viewed in transverse heart sections. Compared with a normal heart *(center)*, the pressure hypertrophied hearts (*left* and in *A*) have increased mass and a thick left ventricular wall, but the hypertrophied and dilated heart *(right)* has increased mass but a diminished wall thickness. (From Edwards WD: Cardiac anatomy and examination of cardiac specimens. In Emmanouilides GC, et al [eds]: Moss and Adams' Heart Disease in Infants, Children, and Adolescents: Including the Fetus and Young Adults, 5th ed. Baltimore, Williams & Wilkins, 1995, p 86.)

or DCM; and to 1000 gm (three or more times normal) in aortic regurgitation or HCM. Hearts weighing more than 1000 gm are rare.

The structural, biochemical, and molecular basis for myocardial contractile failure is obscure in many cases. Nevertheless, in some instances (e.g., myocardial infarction), there is obvious death of myocytes and loss of vital elements of the *pump*; consequently, noninfarcted regions of cardiac muscle are overworked. In contrast, in valvular heart disease, increased pressure or volume work affects the myocardium globally. The increased myocyte size that occurs in cardiac hypertrophy is usually accompanied by decreased capillary density, increased intercapillary distance, and deposition of fibrous tissue.

The molecular and cellular changes in hypertrophied hearts that initially mediate enhanced function may contribute to the development of heart failure.[7, 10] With prolonged hemodynamic overload, gene expression is altered, leading to re-expression of a pattern of protein synthesis analogous to that seen in fetal cardiac development; other changes are analogous to events that occur during mitosis of normally proliferating cells (Chapter 2). Thus, proteins related to contractile elements, excitation-contraction coupling, and energy use may be significantly altered through production of different isoforms that either may be less functional than normal or may be reduced or increased in amount. Alterations of intracellular handling of calcium ions may also contribute to impaired contraction and relaxation.[11] Additional proposed mechanisms potentiating congestive heart failure include reduced adrenergic drive, decreased calcium availability, impaired mitochondrial function, and microcirculatory spasm.

Evidence suggests that loss of myocytes because of apoptosis may contribute to progressive myocardial dysfunction in hypertrophic states.[12] Most often associated with dividing cells, apoptosis may represent an aborted response to pathophysiologic stimuli that reactivate the fetal growth program in cardiac myocytes, presumably because such cells are no longer capable of progressing through the cell cycle to mitosis.

Clearly the geometry, structure, and composition (cells and extracellular matrix) of the hypertrophied heart are not normal. Cardiac hypertrophy then constitutes a tenuous balance between adaptive characteristics (including new sarcomeres) and potentially deleterious structural, biochemical, and molecular alterations (including decreased capillary-to-myocyte ratio; increased fibrous tissue; and synthesis of abnormal, perhaps dysfunctional, proteins). It should not be surprising therefore that sustained cardiac hypertrophy often evolves to cardiac failure. The proposed sequence of initially beneficial and later harmful events in the response to increased cardiac work is summarized in Figure 13–2. Besides predisposing to congestive heart failure, left ventricular hypertrophy is an independent risk factor for cardiac mortality and morbidity, especially for sudden death.[13]

Interestingly, and in contrast to the *pathologic hypertrophy* just discussed, hypertrophy that is induced by regular strenuous exercise (*physiologic hypertrophy*) seems to be an extension of normal growth and have minimal or no deleterious effect.

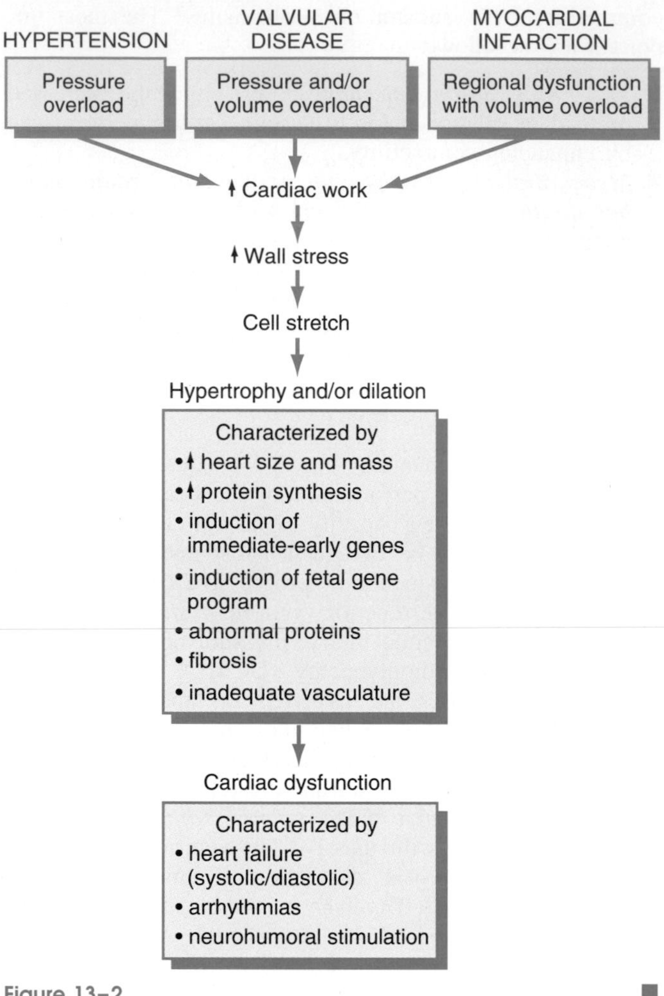

Figure 13–2

Schematic representation of the sequence of events in cardiac hypertrophy and its progression to heart failure, emphasizing cellular and extracellular changes.

Whatever the underlying basis for congestive heart failure, a variety of compensatory mechanisms come into play when the hypertrophied heart can no longer accommodate the increased demand. Eventually, however, the compensatory mechanisms themselves constitute an added burden. Myocardial hypertrophy itself may become increasingly detrimental because of the increased metabolic requirements of the enlarged muscle mass and the increased wall tension, both major determinants of the oxygen consumption of the heart. The other major determinants are heart rate and contractility (inotropic state, or force of contraction).

Ultimately the primary cardiac disease and the superimposed compensatory burdens further encroach on the myocardial reserve. Then begins the downward slide of stroke volume and cardiac output that often ends in death. At autopsy, the hearts of patients having congestive heart failure are generally characterized by increased weight, chamber dilation, and thin walls, with microscopic changes of hypertrophy, but the extent of these changes varies among patients.

The degree of structural abnormality does not always reflect the level of dysfunction, and it may be impossible from morphologic examination of the heart to distinguish a damaged but compensated heart from one that has decompensated. *Moreover, many of the significant adaptations and morphologic changes noted in congestive heart failure are distant from the heart and are produced by the hypoxic and congestive effects of the failing circulation on other organs and tissues.* Thus, congestive heart failure represents a clinical syndrome characterized primarily by findings outside the cardiovascular system—in both *forward* (e.g., poor organ perfusion) and *backward* (pulmonary and peripheral edema) directions, to be discussed subsequently.

To some extent, the right and left sides of the heart act as two distinct anatomic and functional units. Thus, left-sided and right-sided failure can occur independently. Nevertheless, because the cardiovascular system is a closed circuit, failure of one side cannot exist for long without eventually producing excessive strain on the other, terminating in global heart failure. Despite this interdependency, the clearest understanding of the pathologic physiology and anatomy of heart failure is derived from a consideration of each side separately.

LEFT-SIDED HEART FAILURE

As discussed, left-sided heart failure is most often caused by (1) IHD, (2) hypertension, (3) aortic and mitral valvular diseases, and (4) nonischemic myocardial diseases. The morphologic and clinical effects of left-sided congestive heart failure primarily result from progressive damming of blood within the pulmonary circulation and the consequences of diminished peripheral blood flow.

MORPHOLOGY. Except with obstruction at the mitral valve or other processes that restrict the size of the left ventricle, this chamber is usually hypertrophied and often dilated, sometimes quite massively. Secondary enlargement of the left atrium with resultant atrial fibrillation (i.e., uncoordinated, chaotic contraction of the atrium) may either compromise stroke volume or cause blood stasis and possible thrombus formation (particularly in the appendage). A fibrillating left atrium carries an increased risk of embolic stroke. The extracardiac effects of left-sided failure are manifested most prominently in the lungs, although the kidneys and brain may also be affected.

Lungs. Pressure in the pulmonary veins mounts and is ultimately transmitted retrogradely to the capillaries and arteries. The result is pulmonary congestion and edema, with heavy, wet lungs as described in detail in Chapters 5 and 16. It is sufficient to note here that the pulmonary changes include, in sequence, (1) a perivascular and interstitial transudate, particularly in the interlobular septa, responsible for Kerley B lines on x-ray; (2) progressive edematous widening of alveolar septa; and (3) accumulation of edema fluid in the alveolar spaces. Iron-containing proteins in edema fluid and hemoglobin from erythrocytes, which leak from congested capillaries, are phagocytosed by macrophages and converted to hemosiderin. Hemosiderin-containing macrophages in the alveoli (called **siderophages** or **heart failure cells**) denote previous episodes of pulmonary edema.

These anatomic changes produce striking clinical manifestations. **Dyspnea** (breathlessness), usually the earliest and the cardinal complaint of patients in left-sided heart failure, is an exaggeration of the normal breathlessness that follows exertion. With further impairment, there is **orthopnea,** which is dyspnea on lying down that is relieved by sitting or standing. Thus, the orthopneic patient needs to sleep while sitting upright. **Paroxysmal nocturnal dyspnea** is an extension of orthopnea that consists of attacks of extreme dyspnea bordering on suffocation, usually occurring at night. Cough is a common accompaniment of left-sided failure.

Kidneys. Decreased cardiac output causes a reduction in renal perfusion, which activates the renin-angiotensin-aldosterone system, inducing retention of salt and water with consequent expansion of the interstitial fluid and blood volumes. This compensatory reaction can contribute to the pulmonary edema in left-sided heart failure. Salt retention is counteracted by the release of atrial natriuretic peptide through atrial dilation, which acts to decrease excessive blood volume. If the perfusion deficit of the kidney becomes sufficiently severe, impaired excretion of nitrogenous products may cause azotemia, in this instance, **prerenal azotemia** (Chapter 21).

Brain. In far-advanced congestive heart failure, cerebral hypoxia may give rise to **hypoxic encephalopathy** (Chapter 30), with resultant irritability, loss of attention span, and restlessness, which may even progress to stupor and coma.

RIGHT-SIDED HEART FAILURE

Isolated right-sided heart failure occurs in only a few diseases. Usually, it is a secondary consequence of left-sided failure because any increase in pressure in the pulmonary circulation incident to left-sided failure inevitably produces an increased burden on the right side of the heart. The causes of right-sided failure must then include all those that induce left-sided heart failure.

Pure right-sided failure most often occurs with chronic severe pulmonary hypertension and thus is called *cor pulmonale* (see later). In these cases, the right ventricle is burdened by a pressure workload owing to increased resistance within the pulmonary circulation. Hypertrophy and dilation are generally confined to the right ventricle and atrium, although bulging of the ventricular septum to the left can alter the shape of the heart and may cause dysfunction of the left ventricle.

The major morphologic and clinical effects of pure right-sided failure differ from those of left-sided failure in that pulmonary congestion is minimal, whereas engorgement of the systemic and portal venous systems may be pronounced.

MORPHOLOGY. ***Liver and Portal System Drainage.*** The liver is usually increased in size and weight (**congestive hepatomegaly**), and a cut section displays prominent **chronic passive congestion** (see Figs. 5–3 and 19–35). Congested red centers of the liver lobules are surrounded by paler, sometimes fatty, peripheral regions. In some instances, especially when left-sided failure is also present, the severe central hypoxia produces **centrilobular necrosis** along with the sinusoidal congestion. With long-standing severe right-sided cardiac failure, the central areas in time can become fibrotic, creating so-called **cardiac sclerosis** or **cardiac cirrhosis** (Chapter 19).

Right-sided heart failure also leads to elevated pressure in the portal vein and its tributaries. Congestion produces a tense, enlarged spleen (**congestive splenomegaly**). Microscopically, there may be marked sinusoidal dilation. With long-standing congestion, the enlarged spleen may achieve a weight of 300 to 500 gm (normal, approximately 150 gm). Chronic edema of the bowel wall can also occur and in some patients may interfere with absorption of nutrients. In addition, abnormal accumulations of transudate in the peritoneal cavity may give rise to **ascites**.

Kidneys. Congestion of the kidneys is more marked with right-sided heart failure than with left-sided failure, leading to greater fluid retention, peripheral edema, and more pronounced azotemia.

Brain. Symptoms essentially identical to those described in left-sided failure may occur, representing venous congestion and hypoxia of the central nervous system.

Pleural and Pericardial Spaces. Pleural (particularly right) and pericardial effusions may appear. Pleural effusions can range from 100 ml to well over 1 liter. Large effusions can cause partial atelectasis of the corresponding lung.

Subcutaneous Tissues. Peripheral edema of dependent portions of the body, especially ankle (pedal) and pretibial edema, is a hallmark of right-sided failure. In chronically bedridden patients, the edema may be primarily presacral. Generalized massive edema is called **anasarca**.

Thus, the effects of pure left-sided heart failure are largely due to pulmonary congestion and edema. In contrast, respiratory symptoms may be absent or quite insignificant in right-sided failure, in which there is a systemic (and portal) venous congestive syndrome, with hepatic and splenic enlargement, peripheral edema, pleural effusion, and ascites. *In many cases of frank chronic cardiac decompensation, however, the patient presents with the picture of biventricular congestive heart failure, encompassing the clinical syndromes of both right-sided and left-sided heart failure.*

TYPES OF HEART DISEASE

With the introduction to general principles of cardiac functional anatomy and heart failure that has just been presented, we now turn to a discussion of the major forms of heart disease. Five categories of disease account for nearly all cardiac mortality:

1. IHD
2. Hypertensive heart disease (systemic and pulmonary)
3. Valvular heart disease
4. Nonischemic (primary) myocardial disease
5. Congenital heart disease

Because IHD is responsible for 80 to 90% of these deaths, it is discussed first.

Ischemic Heart Disease

IHD is the generic designation for a group of closely related syndromes resulting from myocardial *ischemia*—an imbalance between the supply (perfusion) and demand of the heart for oxygenated blood. Ischemia is characterized by not only insufficiency of oxygen, but also reduced availability of nutrient substrates and inadequate removal of metabolites (Chapter 1). Isolated hypoxemia (i.e., diminished transport of oxygen by the blood) induced by cyanotic congenital heart disease, severe anemia, or advanced lung disease is less deleterious than ischemia because perfusion (including metabolic substrate delivery and waste removal) is maintained.

In more than 90% of cases, the cause of myocardial ischemia is reduction in coronary blood flow because of atherosclerotic coronary arterial obstructions. Thus, IHD is often termed *coronary artery disease* or *coronary heart disease*. In most cases, there is a long period (decades) of silent, slowly progressive, coronary atherosclerosis before these disorders become manifest. Thus, *the syndromes of IHD are only the late manifestations of coronary atherosclerosis that probably began during childhood or adolescence* (Chapter 12).

Certain conditions aggravate ischemia through increase in cardiac energy demand (e.g., hypertrophy), lowered systemic blood pressure (e.g., shock), or hypoxemia. Moreover, increased heart rate not only increases demand through more contractions per unit time, but also decreases supply (by decreasing the length of diastole—when coronary perfusion occurs—relative to systole).

The risk of an individual developing detectable IHD depends in part on the number, distribution, and degree of narrowing by atheromatous plaques. The clinical manifestations of IHD, however, are not strongly predicted by these anatomic observations. Moreover, there is an extraordinarily broad spectrum of the expression of disease from elderly individuals with extensive coronary atherosclerosis who have never had a symptom to the previously asymptomatic young adult in whom modestly obstructive disease comes unexpectedly to medical attention as a result of acute myocardial infarction (MI) or sudden cardiac death. *The reasons for clinical heterogeneity of the disease are complex. However, the often precipitous and variable onset largely depends on the pathologic basis of the so-called acute coronary syndromes of IHD (comprising unstable angina, acute MI and,* for our purposes owing to the frequently similar pathophysiologic basis, *sudden death)—unpredictable and abrupt conversion of a stable atherosclerotic plaque to an unstable, potentially life-threatening atherothrombotic lesion through superficial erosion, ulceration, fissuring, rupture or deep hemorrhage, usually with superimposed thrombosis.* For purposes of simplicity herein, this spectrum of alteration in atherosclerotic lesions is termed either *disruption* or *acute plaque change.* In general, however, the clinical manifestations of IHD can be divided into four syndromes:

1. *MI,* the most important form of IHD, in which the duration and severity of ischemia is sufficient to cause death of heart muscle
2. *Angina pectoris,* of which there are three variants—stable angina, Prinzmetal angina, and unstable angina (the last-mentioned is the most threatening since it is frequently a harbinger of MI)
3. *Chronic ischemic heart disease* with heart failure
4. *Sudden cardiac death*

Epidemiology. IHD in its various forms is the leading cause of death for both men and women in the United States and other industrialized nations. Each year, nearly 500,000 Americans die of IHD. Awesome as these data may be, they represent an improvement over those that prevailed several decades ago. Since 1980, the overall death rate from IHD has fallen in the United States by approximately one third, owing to both (1) *prevention* achieved by modification of determinants of risk, such as smoking, elevated blood cholesterol, hypertension, and a sedentary life style,[14, 15] and (2) *therapeutic advances,* including new medications, coronary care units, thrombolysis for MI, percutaneous transluminal coronary angioplasty (PTCA), intravascular stents, coronary bypass surgery, and improved control of arrhythmias.[16, 17] Additional risk reduction may potentially be associated with maintenance of normal blood glucose levels in diabetic patients, postmenopausal estrogen replacement therapy, lipid lowering and antioxidant therapy, and aspirin prophylaxis in middle-aged men (see Chapter 12). However, the death rate from cardiovascular disease is presently increasing in the United States and worldwide.

Pathogenesis. The dominant influence in the causation of the IHD syndromes is diminished coronary perfusion relative to myocardial demand, owing largely to a complex dynamic interaction among fixed atherosclerotic narrowing of the epicardial coronary arteries, intraluminal thrombosis overlying a disrupted atherosclerotic plaque, platelet aggregation, and vasospasm. The individual elements and their interactions are discussed subsequently.

Role of Fixed Coronary Obstructions. More than 90% of patients with IHD have coronary atherosclerosis, which compromises blood flow (*fixed* obstructions). Most—but not all—have one or more lesions causing at least 75% reduction of the cross-sectional area of at least one of the major epicardial arteries, a threshold of obstruction at which the augmented coronary flow provided by compensatory vasodilation is no longer sufficient to meet even moderate increases in myocardial demand.

Although only a single major coronary epicardial trunk may be affected, more often two or all three—LAD, LCX, RCA—are involved. Clinically significant stenosing plaques may be located anywhere within these vessels but tend to predominate within the first several centimeters of the LAD and LCX and the entire length of the RCA. Sometimes the major secondary epicardial branches are also involved (i.e., diagonal branches of the LAD, obtuse marginal branches of the LCX, or posterior descending branch of the RCA, but atherosclerosis of the intramural branches is rare). *The onset of symptoms and prognosis of IHD, however, depend not only on the extent and severity of fixed, chronic anatomic disease, but also critically on dynamic changes in coronary plaque morphology (to be discussed).*

Role of Acute Plaque Change. In most patients, the myocardial ischemia underlying the acute coronary syndromes—unstable angina, acute MI, and (in many cases) sudden cardiac death—is precipitated by abrupt plaque change followed by thrombosis (Figs. 13–3 and 13–4).[18, 19] *Most often, the initiating event is disruption of previously only partially stenosing plaques with*

- *Hemorrhage into the atheroma,* expanding its volume
- *Rupture or fissuring,* exposing the highly thrombogenic plaque constituents
- *Erosion or ulceration,* exposing the thrombogenic subendothelial basement membrane to blood

Although the factors that trigger these acute alterations in plaque configuration are uncertain, disruption implies an inability of plaque to withstand imposed mechanical stresses. Several extrinsic and intrinsic influences seem important. Adrenergic stimulation can elevate physical stresses on the plaque through systemic hypertension or local vasospasm. The adrenergic stimulation associated with awakening induces a pronounced circadian periodicity for the time of onset of acute MI, with a peak incidence at 6 AM to 12 noon, concurrent with a surge in blood pressure and immediately following heightened platelet reactivity.[20] Aspirin, a drug well known to interfere with platelet function, depresses the morning peak in the incidence of acute MI. Interestingly, an unexpected increase in individuals suffering sudden cardiac death that accompanied the Northridge (Los Angeles) earthquake in 1994 has been attributed to emotional stress-related adrenergic stimulation.[21]

The structure and composition of plaque are dynamic and may contribute to the propensity to disruption.[22, 23] Disrupted lesions characteristically have a markedly eccentric configuration (in which the plaque is not uniform around the vessel circumference), a large soft core of necrotic debris and lipid, a high density of macrophages, and

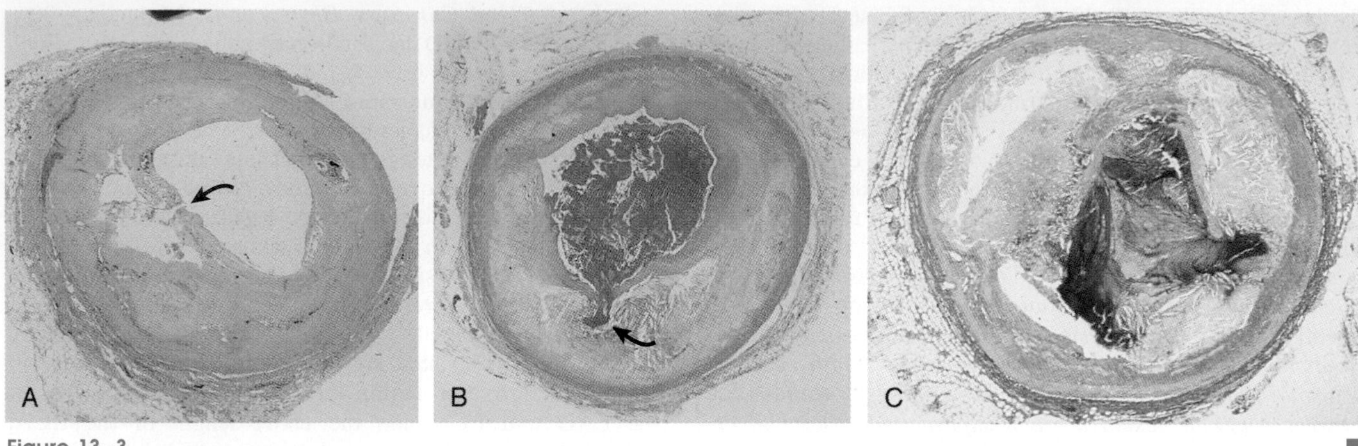

Figure 13–3

Atherosclerotic plaque rupture. *A*, Plaque rupture without superimposed thrombus in a patient who died suddenly. *B*, Acute coronary thrombosis superimposed on an atherosclerotic plaque with focal disruption of the fibrous cap, triggering fatal myocardial infarction. *C*, Massive plaque rupture with superimposed thrombus, also triggering a fatal myocardial infarction (special stain highlighting fibrin in red). In both *A* and *B* an arrow points to the site of plaque rupture. (*B* from Schoen FJ: Interventional and Surgical Cardiovascular Pathology: Clinical Correlations and Basic Principles. Philadelphia, WB Saunders, 1989, p 61.)

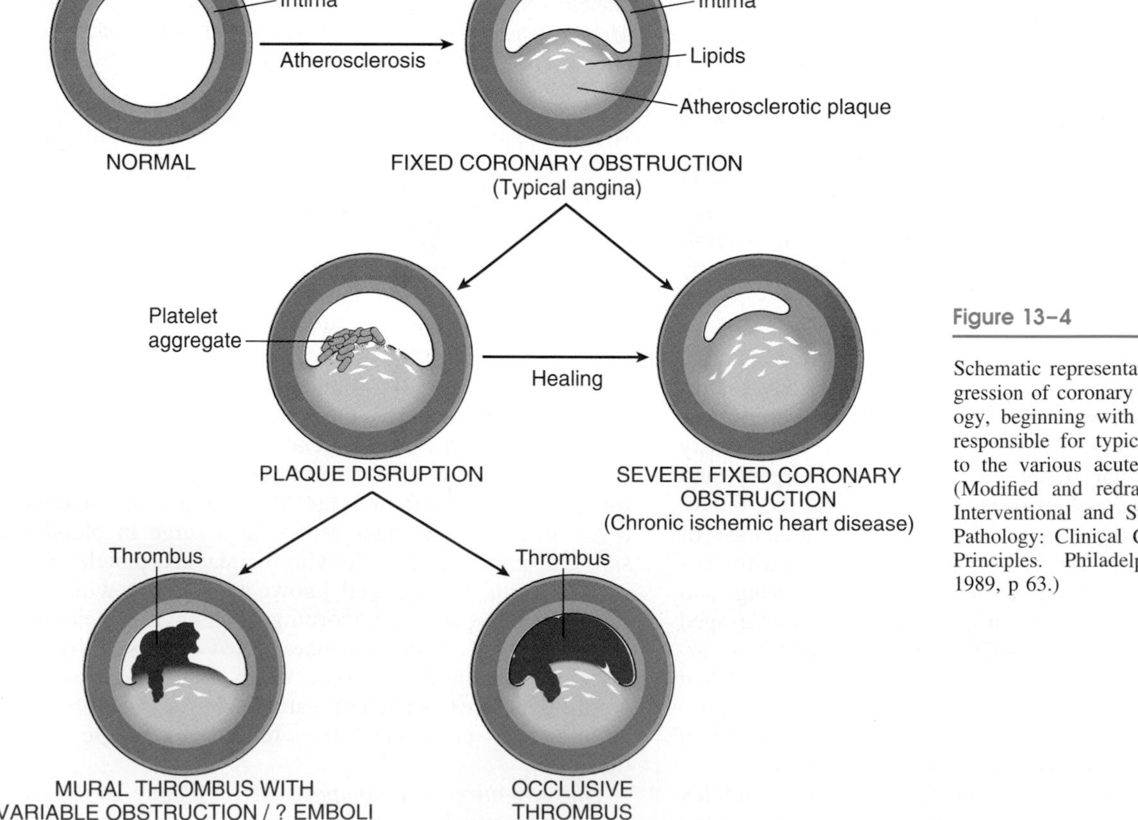

Figure 13–4

Schematic representation of sequential progression of coronary artery lesion morphology, beginning with stable chronic plaque responsible for typical angina and leading to the various acute coronary syndromes. (Modified and redrawn from Schoen FJ: Interventional and Surgical Cardiovascular Pathology: Clinical Correlations and Basic Principles. Philadelphia, WB Saunders, 1989, p 63.)

only a thin fibrous cap. Degradation of collagen, the major structural component of the fibrous cap, may be an important contributor to plaque rupture. Such breakdown involves the action of metalloproteinases, expressed by macrophages in atheroma. Moreover, fissures frequently occur at the junction of the fibrous cap and the adjacent normal plaque-free arterial segment, a location at which the blood flow–inducing mechanical stresses within the plaque are highest.

It is now recognized that the preexisting culprit lesion in patients who develop MI and other acute coronary syndromes is often not a severely stenotic and hemodynamically significant lesion before its acute change. The most dangerous lesions are the moderately stenotic (usually 50 to 75%), lipid-rich atheromas, which are themselves insufficient to induce stable angina before disruption. Thus, a rather large number of now asymptomatic adults in the industrial world have a real but unpredictable risk of a catastrophic coronary event. Several factors underlie this rather disquieting realization. First, an atheroma of moderate size often has a complex configuration with a well-developed soft core capable of disruption. Second, plaques causing obstruction sufficient to limit flow severely may have correspondingly reduced mechanical stresses in their walls, thus making disruption less likely. Third, high-grade but slowly developing occlusions stimulate collateral vessel formation that may protect against infarction. Finally, repetitive nonlethal myocardial ischemia may be protective to infarction by a mechanism yet unknown (termed *preconditioning*—see later).

Accumulating evidence indicates that plaque disruption and the ensuing platelet aggregation and intraluminal thrombosis are common, repetitive, and often clinically silent complications of atheroma. Moreover, healing of subclinical plaque disruption and overlying thrombosis comprises an important mechanism of growth of atherosclerotic lesions.

Role of Coronary Thrombus. As mentioned earlier, partial or total thrombosis associated with a disrupted plaque is critical to the pathogenesis of the acute coronary syndromes. In acute transmural MI, thrombus superimposed on a disrupted but previously only partially stenotic plaque has converted it to a total occlusion (see discussion of transmural versus subendocardial infarction later). In contrast, with unstable angina, acute subendocardial infarction, or sudden cardiac death, the extent of luminal obstruction by thrombosis is usually incomplete. Moreover, in unstable angina, there is a temporal relation between chest pain and generation of thromboxane A_2 and other platelet constituents in the coronary circulation, suggesting that these mediators are available at sites of plaque disruption and transient mural thrombosis to promote further platelet aggregation and vasoconstriction.[24] Factors not related to platelets may augment thrombotic potential, including elevated blood concentrations of fibrinogen, low plasminogen activator inhibitor 1 (an inhibitor of fibrinolysis), and high lipoprotein (a) (a form of low-density lipoprotein that inhibits fibrinolysis).

Mural thrombus can also embolize. Small fragments of thrombotic material in the distal intramyocardial circulation or microinfarcts may be found at autopsy of patients who have had unstable angina. Finally, thrombus is a potent activator of multiple growth-related signals in smooth muscle cells that can contribute to the growth of atherosclerotic lesions (Chapter 12).

Role of Vasoconstriction. Vasoconstriction itself compromises lumen size and can increase the local mechanical forces that can contribute to plaque fracture. Vasoconstriction at sites of atheroma is stimulated by (1) circulating adrenergic agonists, (2) locally released platelet contents, (3) impaired secretion of endothelial cell relaxing factors (e.g., nitric oxide) relative to contracting factors (e.g., endothelin) owing to atheroma-associated endothelial dysfunction, and potentially (4) mediators released from perivascular inflammatory cells (e.g., mast cells).

To summarize, the acute coronary syndromes—acute MI, unstable angina, and often sudden death—share a common pathophysiologic basis in coronary atherosclerotic plaque disruption and associated intraluminal platelet-fibrin thrombus formation (Table 13–2). Stable angina results from an increase in myocardial oxygen demand that outstrips the ability of markedly stenosed coronary arteries to increase oxygen delivery but is not usually associated with plaque disruption. Unstable angina derives from a sudden change in plaque morphology, which induces partially occlusive platelet aggregation or mural thrombus, and vasoconstriction leading to severe but transient reductions in coronary blood flow. In some cases, distal microinfarction occurs secondary to thromboemboli. In MI, acute plaque change induces total thrombotic occlusion. Finally, sudden cardiac death frequently involves a coronary lesion in which disrupted plaque and often partial

Table 13–2. CORONARY ARTERY PATHOLOGY IN ISCHEMIC HEART DISEASE

Syndrome	Stenoses	Plaque Disruption	Plaque-Associated Thrombus
Stable angina	>75%	No	No
Unstable angina	Variable	Frequent	Nonocclusive, often with thromboemboli
Transmural myocardial infarction	Variable	Frequent	Occlusive
Subendocardial myocardial infarction	Variable	Variable	Widely variable, may be absent, partial/complete or lysed
Sudden death	Usually severe	Frequent	Often small platelet aggregates or thrombi and/or thromboemboli

thrombus have led to regional myocardial ischemia that induces a fatal ventricular arrhythmia. Each of these important syndromes is now discussed in detail.

ANGINA PECTORIS

Angina pectoris is a symptom complex of IHD characterized by paroxysmal and usually recurrent attacks of substernal or precordial chest discomfort (variously described as constricting, squeezing, choking, or knifelike) caused by transient (15 seconds to 15 minutes) myocardial ischemia that falls short of inducing the cellular necrosis that defines infarction. There are three overlapping patterns of angina pectoris: (1) stable or typical angina, (2) Prinzmetal or variant angina, and (3) unstable or crescendo angina. They are caused by varying combinations of increased myocardial demand and decreased myocardial perfusion, owing to fixed stenosing plaques, disrupted plaques, vasospasm, thrombosis, platelet aggregation, and embolization. Moreover, it is being increasingly recognized that not all ischemic events are perceived by patients, even though such events may have adverse prognostic implications (*silent ischemia*).

Stable angina, the most common form and therefore called *typical angina pectoris, appears to be caused by the reduction of coronary perfusion to a critical level by chronic stenosing coronary atherosclerosis; this renders the heart vulnerable to further ischemia whenever there is increased demand, such as that produced by physical activity, emotional excitement, or any other cause of increased cardiac workload.* Typical angina pectoris is usually relieved by rest (thereby decreasing demand) or nitroglycerin, a strong vasodilator (which although the coronary arteries are usually maximally dilated by intrinsic regulatory influences also decreases cardiac work by dilating the peripheral vasculature). In particular instances, local vasospasm may contribute to the imbalance between supply and demand.

Prinzmetal variant angina is an uncommon pattern of episodic angina that occurs at rest and has been documented to be due to coronary artery spasm. Usually there is elevation of the ST segment of the electrocardiogram (ECG), indicative of transmural ischemia. Although individuals with this form of angina may well have significant coronary atherosclerosis, the anginal attacks are unrelated to physical activity, heart rate, or blood pressure. Prinzmetal angina generally responds promptly to vasodilators, such as nitroglycerin and calcium channel blockers.

Unstable or *crescendo angina* refers to a pattern of pain that occurs with progressively increasing frequency, is precipitated with progressively less effort, often occurs at rest, and tends to be of more prolonged duration. As discussed earlier, *in most patients, unstable angina is induced by disruption of an atherosclerotic plaque with superimposed partial (mural) thrombosis and possibly embolization or vasospasm (or both).* Although the ischemia that occurs in unstable angina falls precariously short of inducing clinically detectable infarction, unstable angina is a harbinger of subsequent acute MI in many patients. Thus, this syndrome is sometimes referred to as *preinfarction angina.* In the spectrum of IHD, unstable angina lies intermediate between stable angina on the one hand and MI on the other.

MYOCARDIAL INFARCTION

MI, also known as *heart attack*, is overwhelmingly the most important form of IHD and alone is the leading cause of death in the United States and industrialized nations. About 1.5 million individuals in the United States suffer an acute MI annually, and approximately one third of them die. At least 250,000 people a year die of heart attack before they reach the hospital.

Transmural Versus Subendocardial Infarction. Most myocardial infarcts are *transmural*, in which the ischemic necrosis involves the full or nearly full thickness of the ventricular wall in the distribution of a single coronary artery. This pattern of infarction is usually associated with chronic coronary atherosclerosis, acute plaque change, and superimposed, completely obstructive thrombosis (as discussed previously). In contrast, a *subendocardial (nontransmural) infarct* constitutes an area of ischemic necrosis limited to the inner one third or at most one half of the ventricular wall; it may extend laterally beyond the perfusion territory of a single coronary artery. As previously pointed out, the subendocardial zone is normally the least well-perfused region of myocardium and therefore most vulnerable to any reduction in coronary flow. In the majority of subendocardial infarcts, there is diffuse stenosing coronary atherosclerosis and reduction of coronary flow but *neither* plaque disruption *nor* superimposed thrombosis. The two types of infarcts, however, are closely interrelated because, in experimental models, the transmural infarct begins with a zone of subendocardial necrosis that progressively encompasses the full thickness of the ventricular wall (see later). Therefore, a subendocardial infarct can occur as a result of a plaque disruption followed by a coronary thrombus that becomes lysed before myocardial necrosis extends across the major thickness of the wall. Subendocardial infarcts, however, can also result from sufficiently prolonged and severe reduction in systemic blood pressure, as in shock; in cases of global hypotension, resulting subendocardial infarcts are usually circumferential rather than limited to the distribution of a single major coronary artery.

Incidence and Risk Factors. The risk factors for atherosclerosis, the major underlying cause of IHD in general, are discussed in detail in Chapter 12 and are not reiterated here. *MI may occur at virtually any age, but the frequency rises progressively with increasing age and when predispositions to atherosclerosis are present*, such as hypertension, cigarette smoking, diabetes mellitus, genetic hypercholesterolemia, and other causes of hyperlipoproteinemia. Nearly 10% of myocardial infarcts occur in people under age 40 years, and 45% occur in people under age 65. Blacks and whites are affected equally often. Throughout life, men are at significantly greater risk of MI than women, the differential progressively declining with advancing age. *Except for those having some predisposing atherogenic condition, women are remarkably protected against MI during the reproductive years.* The decrease of estrogen after menopause can permit rapid development of coronary heart disease. Epidemiologic evidence strongly suggests that postmenopausal hormone replacement therapy protects women against MI through favorable adjustment of risk factors, albeit with slightly increased risk of breast and endometrial cancer.[25]

Pathogenesis. We now consider the basis for and subsequent consequences of myocardial ischemia, particularly as they relate to the transmural infarct.

Coronary Arterial Occlusion. In nearly all transmural acute myocardial infarcts, a dynamic interaction has occurred among several or all of the following—severe coronary atherosclerosis, acute atheromatous plaque change (such as rupture), superimposed platelet activation, thrombosis, and vasospasm—eventuating in an occlusive intracoronary thrombus overlying a disrupted plaque. In addition, either increased myocardial demand (as with hypertrophy or tachycardia) or hemodynamic compromise (as with a drop in blood pressure) can worsen the situation. Collateral circulation may provide perfusion to ischemic zones from a relatively unobstructed branch of the coronary tree, bypassing the point of obstruction and protecting against the effects of an acute coronary occlusion.

In the typical case of MI, the following sequence of events can be proposed:

- *The initial event is a sudden change in the morphology of an atheromatous plaque* (i.e., disruption)—manifest as intraplaque hemorrhage, erosion or ulceration, or rupture or fissuring.
- Exposed to subendothelial collagen and necrotic plaque contents, *platelets undergo adhesion, aggregation, activation, and release of potent aggregators*, including thromboxane A_2, serotonin, and platelet factors 3 and 4; vasospasm is stimulated.
- Other mediators activate the extrinsic pathway of coagulation and add to the bulk of the thrombus.
- *Frequently within minutes, the thrombus evolves to occlude completely the lumen of the culprit coronary vessel.*

The evidence for this sequence is compelling and derives from (1) autopsy studies of patients dying with acute MI, (2) angiographic studies demonstrating a high frequency of thrombotic occlusion early after MI, (3) both the high success rate of therapeutic thrombolysis and primary angioplasty and the demonstration of residual disrupted atherosclerotic lesions by angiography after thrombolysis. Although coronary angiography performed within 4 hours of the onset of apparent MI shows a thrombosed coronary artery in almost 90% of cases, the observation of occlusion, however, falls to about 60% when angiography is delayed until 12 to 24 hours after onset.[26] Thus, with the passage of time, at least some occlusions appear to clear spontaneously owing to lysis of the thrombus or relaxation of spasm or both. Spontaneous lysis occurring after more than several hours following MI onset is incapable of salvaging substantial useful myocardium.

In approximately 10% of cases, transmural acute MI is not associated with atherosclerotic plaque thrombosis stimulated by disruption. In such situations, other mechanisms may be involved, as follows:

- *Vasospasm*: Isolated, intense, and relatively prolonged, with or without coronary atherosclerosis, perhaps in association with platelet aggregation
- *Emboli*: From the left atrium in association with atrial fibrillation, a left-sided mural thrombus, or vegetative endocarditis, or *paradoxical emboli* from the right side of the heart or the peripheral veins, which cross to the systemic circulation, through a patent foramen ovale, to cause coronary occlusion
- *Unexplained*: In about one third of such cases, the coronary arteries are free of obstruction by angiography. Some such cases may involve unusual diseases of small intramural coronary vessels, hematologic abnormalities such as hemoglobinopathies, or other disorders.

Myocardial Response. The consequence of coronary arterial obstruction is the loss of critical blood supply to the myocardium (Fig. 13–5), *which induces profound functional, biochemical, and morphologic consequences. Occlusion of a major coronary artery results in ischemia and potentially cell death throughout the anatomic region supplied by that artery (called area at risk), most pronounced in the subendocardium. The outcome largely depends on the severity and duration of flow deprivation.*

The principal early biochemical consequence of myocardial ischemia is the cessation of aerobic glycolysis (and therefore onset of anaerobic glycolysis) within seconds, leading to inadequate production of high-energy phosphates (e.g., creatine phosphate and adenosine triphosphate [ATP])

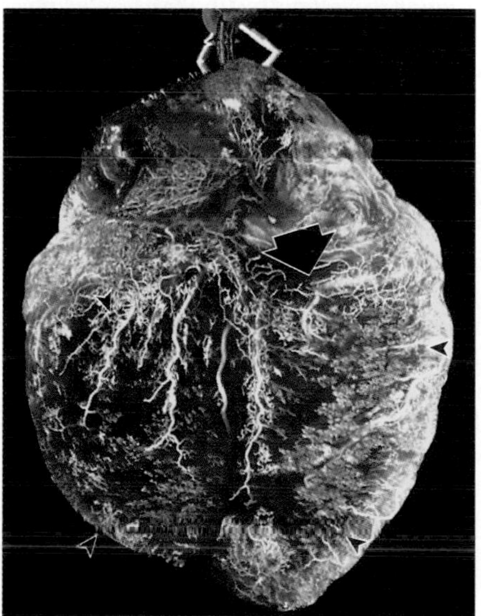

Figure 13–5

Postmortem angiogram demonstrating the posterior aspect of the heart of a patient who died during evolution of acute myocardial infarction. There is total occlusion of the distal right coronary artery by an acute thrombus *(arrow)* and a large zone of myocardial hypoperfusion involving the posterior left and right ventricles *(arrowheads)*. The heart has been fixed by coronary arterial perfusion with glutaraldehyde and cleared with methyl salicylate, followed by intracoronary injection of silicone polymer. Photograph courtesy of Lewis L. Lainey. (From Schoen FJ: Interventional and Surgical Cardiovascular Pathology: Clinical Correlations and Basic Principles. Philadelphia, WB Saunders, 1989, p 60. Courtesy of Lewis L. Lainey.)

and accumulation of potentially noxious breakdown products (e.g., lactic acid). Since myocardial function is exceedingly sensitive to severe ischemia, striking loss of contractility occurs within 60 seconds of onset of ischemia and can precipitate acute heart failure. As detailed in Chapter 1, ultrastructural changes also develop within a few minutes after onset of ischemia (e.g., myofibrillar relaxation, glycogen depletion, cell and mitochondrial swelling). Nevertheless, these early changes are potentially *reversible*, and cell death is not immediate. As demonstrated experimentally in the dog, only severe ischemia lasting at least 20 to 40 minutes or longer leads to irreversible damage (necrosis) of some cardiac myocytes. Ultrastructural evidence of *irreversible* myocyte injury (primary structural defects in the sarcolemmal membrane) develops after 20 to 40 minutes in severely ischemic myocardium (with blood flow of 10% or less of normal).[27] Microvascular injury follows. This time frame is summarized in Table 13–3.

Classic acute MI with extensive damage occurs when the perfusion of the myocardium is reduced severely below its needs for an extended interval (usually hours), causing profound, prolonged ischemia and resulting in permanent loss of function through cell death (typically by coagulation necrosis). In contrast, if restoration of myocardial blood flow (known as reperfusion) follows briefer periods of flow deprivation (less than 20 minutes in the most severely ischemic myocardium), loss of cell viability generally does not result. This provides the rationale for the early detection of acute MI—to permit early therapy such as thrombolysis, establish reperfusion of the area at risk, salvage as much ischemic but not yet dead myocardium as possible, and consequently minimize infarct size.

Myocardial ischemia also contributes to arrhythmias through complex, largely uncertain mechanisms.[28] Sudden death, a leading cause of mortality in IHD patients, is usually due to ventricular fibrillation caused by myocardial irritability induced by ischemia or infarction. Interestingly, studies of resuscitated survivors of *sudden death* show that the majority do not develop acute MI; in such cases, ischemia owing to severe chronic coronary arterial stenosis and, in many cases, acute plaque change with minimal thrombus presumably led directly to the fatal arrhythmia.

Apoptosis is a recently recognized component of the lethal cell injury that follows severe myocardial ischemia. Apoptosis occurs in experimental and human MI.[29, 30]

Table 13–3. APPROXIMATE TIME OF ONSET OF KEY EVENTS IN ISCHEMIC CARDIAC MYOCYTES

Feature	Time
Onset of ATP depletion	Seconds
Loss of contractility	<2 min
ATP reduced	
to 50% of normal	10 min
to 10% of normal	40 min
Irreversible cell injury	20–40 min
Microvascular injury	>1 hr

ATP, adenosine triphosphate.

Apoptotic cell death occurs rapidly after ischemia onset, and novel early therapeutic interventions that inhibit apoptotic events could conceivably promote myocyte preservation during ischemic injury. The relative importance of apoptosis rather than typical coagulation necrosis in clinical infarcts and the roles of ischemia, reperfusion, and other factors in inducing apoptosis are still unclear, however, and are under intense scrutiny.

The progression of ischemic necrosis in the myocardium is summarized in Figure 13–6. Irreversible injury of ischemic myocytes occurs first in the subendocardial zone. With more extended ischemia, a *wavefront* of cell death moves through the myocardium to involve progressively more of the transmural thickness of the ischemic zone. The precise location, size, and specific morphologic features of an acute myocardial infarct depend on the following:

- The location, severity, and rate of development of coronary atherosclerotic obstructions
- The size of the vascular bed perfused by the obstructed vessels
- The duration of the occlusion
- The metabolic/oxygen needs of the myocardium at risk
- The extent of collateral blood vessels
- The presence, site, and severity of coronary arterial spasm
- Other factors, such as alterations in blood pressure, heart rate, and cardiac rhythm

The extent of necrosis is largely complete within 3 to 6 hours in experimental models, involving nearly all of the ischemic myocardial bed at risk supplied by the occluded coronary artery. Progression of necrosis, however, frequently follows a more protracted course in humans (possibly over 6 to 12 hours or longer), in whom the coronary arterial collateral system, often stimulated by chronic ischemia, is better developed and thereby more effective.

MORPHOLOGY. The evolution of the morphologic changes in acute MI and its healing are summarized in Table 13–4. Virtually all transmural infarcts involve at least a portion of the left ventricle (including the ventricular septum). About 15 to 30% of those that affect the posterior free wall and posterior portion of the septum transmurally extend into the adjacent right ventricular wall. Isolated infarction of the right ventricle, however, occurs in only 1 to 3% of cases. Infarction of the atrial wall accompanies a large posterior left ventricular infarct in some cases.

Transmural infarcts usually encompass nearly the entire perfusion zone of the occluded coronary artery. However, almost always there is a narrow rim (approximately 0.1 mm) of preserved subendocardial myocardium sustained by diffusion of oxygen and nutrients from the lumen. The frequencies of critical narrowing (and thrombosis) of each of the three main arterial trunks and the

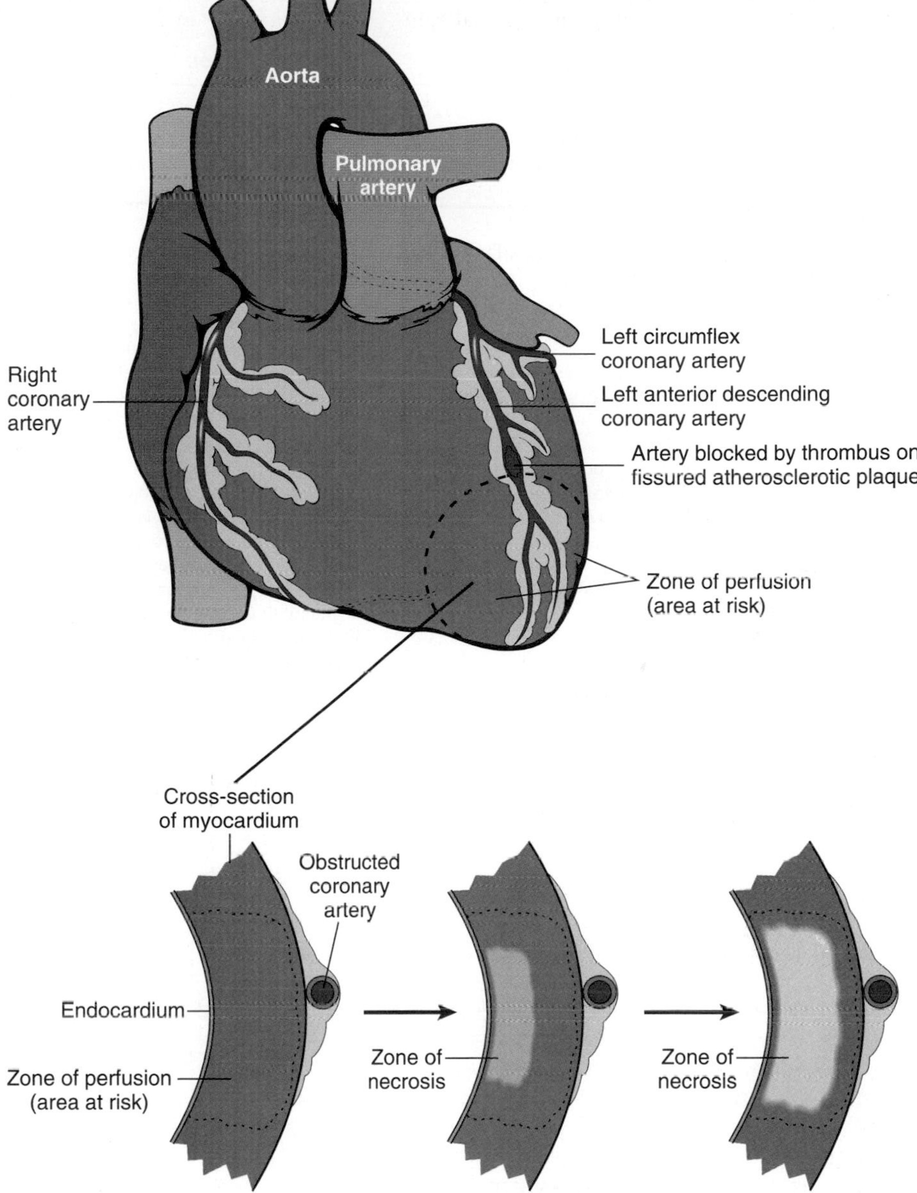

Figure 13–6

Schematic representation of the progression of myocardial necrosis after coronary artery occlusion. Necrosis begins in a small zone of the myocardium beneath the endocardial surface in the center of the ischemic zone. This entire region of myocardium *(dashed outline)* depends on the occluded vessel for perfusion and is the area at risk. Note that a very narrow zone of myocardium immediately beneath the endocardium is spared from necrosis because it can be oxygenated by diffusion from the ventricle.

corresponding sites of myocardial lesions (in the typical right dominant heart) are as follows:

LAD (40 to 50%)	Anterior wall of left ventricle near apex; anterior portion of ventricular septum; apex circumferentially
RCA (30 to 40%)	Inferior-posterior wall of left ventricle; posterior portion of ventricular septum; inferior-posterior right ventricular free wall in some cases
LCX (15 to 20%)	Lateral wall of left ventricle except at apex

Other locations of critical coronary arterial lesions causing infarcts are sometimes encountered, such as the left main coronary artery or the secondary branches (e.g., diagonal branches of the LAD or marginal branches of the LCX). In contrast, stenosing atherosclerosis or thrombosis of a penetrating intramyocardial branch of the coronary arteries is almost never encountered. Occasionally the observation of multiple severe stenoses or thromboses in the absence of myocardial damage suggests that intercoronary collaterals were protective.

Several infarcts of varying age are frequently found in the same heart. Repetitive necrosis of adjacent regions yields progressive **extension** of

Table 13–4. EVOLUTION OF MORPHOLOGIC CHANGES IN MYOCARDIAL INFARCTION

Time	Gross Features	Light Microscope	Electron Microscope
Reversible Injury			
0–½ hr	None	None	Relaxation of myofibrils; glycogen loss; mitochondrial swelling
Irreversible Injury			
½–4 hr	None	Usually none; variable waviness of fibers at border	Sarcolemmal disruption; mitochondrial amorphous densities
4–12 hr	Occasionally dark mottling	Beginning coagulation necrosis; edema; hemorrhage	
12–24 hr	Dark mottling	Ongoing coagulation necrosis; pyknosis of nuclei; myocyte hypereosinophilia; marginal contraction band necrosis; beginning neutrophilic infiltrate	
1–3 days	Mottling with yellow-tan infarct center	Coagulation necrosis, with loss of nuclei and striations; interstitial infiltrate of neutrophils	
3–7 days	Hyperemic border; central yellow-tan softening	Beginning disintegration of dead myofibers, with dying neutrophils; early phagocytosis of dead cells by macrophages at infarct border	
7–10 days	Maximally yellow-tan and soft, with depressed red-tan margins	Well-developed phagocytosis of dead cells; early formation of fibrovascular granulation tissue at margins	
10–14 days	Red-gray depressed infarct borders	Well-established granulation tissue with new blood vessels and collagen deposition	
2–8 wk	Gray-white scar, progressive from border toward core of infarct	Increased collagen deposition, with decreased cellularity	
>2 mo	Scarring complete	Dense collagenous scar	

an individual infarct over a period of days to weeks. Examination of the heart in such cases often reveals a central zone of infarction that is days to weeks older than a peripheral margin of more recent ischemic necrosis. An initial infarct may extend because of retrograde propagation of a thrombus, proximal vasospasm, progressively impaired cardiac contractility that renders flow through moderate stenoses critically insufficient, development of platelet-fibrin microemboli, or appearance of an arrhythmia that impairs cardiac function.

Areas of damage undergo a progressive sequence of changes that consist of typical ischemic coagulative necrosis, followed by inflammation and repair that parallels that occurring after injury at other, noncardiac sites. Thus, the appearance of an infarct at autopsy depends on the duration of survival of the patient after MI.

Early recognition of acute myocardial infarcts by pathologists can be a difficult problem, particularly when death has occurred within a few hours after the onset of symptoms. Myocardial infarcts fewer than 12 hours old are usually inapparent on gross examination. It is often possible, however, to highlight the area of necrosis that first becomes apparent after 2 to 3 hours by immersion of tissue slices in a solution of **triphenyltetrazolium chloride**. This dye imparts a brick-red color to intact, noninfarcted myocardium where the dehydrogenase activity is preserved. Because dehydrogenases are depleted in the area of ischemic necrosis (i.e., they leak out through the damaged cell membranes), an infarcted area is revealed as an unstained pale zone (Fig. 13–7). Subsequently, lesions are often visible grossly. By 12 to 24 hours, the lesion can be identified in routinely fixed gross slices owing to a red-blue hue as a result of stagnated, trapped blood. Progressively thereafter, the infarct becomes a more sharply defined, yellow-tan, somewhat softened area (with inflammatory cells) that by 10 days to 2 weeks is rimmed by a hyperemic zone of highly vascularized granulation tissue. Over the succeeding weeks, the injured region evolves to a fibrous scar.

The histopathologic changes also have a more or less predictable sequence (summarized in Table 13–4 and Fig. 13–8). Using light microscopy of sections stained by routine tissue stains, the typical microscopic changes of coagulative necrosis become detectable variably in the first 4 to 12 hours. *Wavy fibers* may be present at the periphery of the infarct; these changes probably result from the forceful systolic tugs by the viable fibers immediately adjacent to the noncontractile dead fibers, thereby stretching and buckling them. An

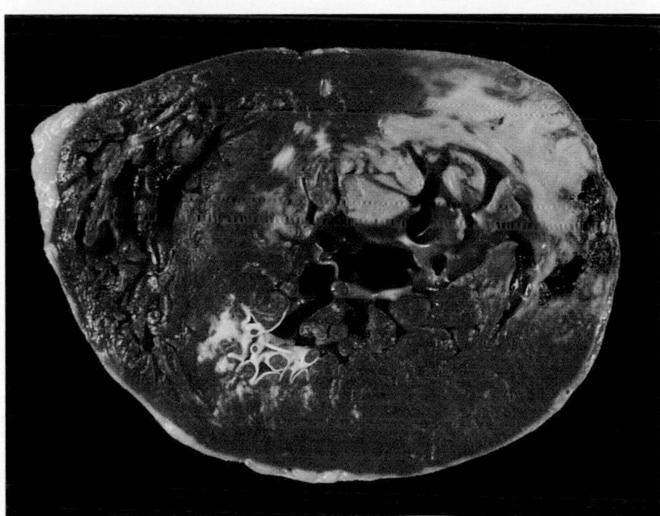

Figure 13–7 ■

Acute myocardial infarct, predominantly of the posterolateral left ventricle, demonstrated histochemically by a lack of staining by the triphenyltetrazolium chloride (TTC) stain in areas of necrosis. The staining defect is due to the enzyme leakage that follows cell death. Note the myocardial hemorrhage at one edge of the infarct that was associated with cardiac rupture, and the anterior scar *(lower left)*, indicative of old infarct. (Specimen oriented with posterior wall at top.)

additional but sublethal ischemic change may be seen in the margins of infarcts: so-called vacuolar degeneration or **myocytolysis**, comprising large vacuolar spaces within cells, probably containing water. This potentially reversible alteration is particularly frequent in the thin zone of viable subendocardial cells. Subendocardial myocyte vacuolization in other contexts may signify severe chronic ischemia.

The necrotic muscle elicits acute inflammation (typically most prominent at 2 to 3 days). Thereafter, macrophages remove the necrotic myocytes (most pronounced at 5 to 10 days), and the damaged zone is progressively replaced by the ingrowth of highly vascularized granulation tissue (most prominent at 2 to 4 weeks), which progressively becomes less vascularized and more fibrous. In most instances, scarring is well advanced by the end of the sixth week, but the efficiency of repair depends on the size of the original lesion. A large infarct may not heal as readily as a small one. Moreover, once a lesion is completely healed, it is impossible to distinguish its age (i.e., an 8-week-old lesion and a 10-year-old lesion can look similar).

The morphology of evolving subendocardial and transmural infarcts is qualitatively similar. By definition, however, the necrosis in subendocardial lesions is limited to the inner third to one half of the left ventricular wall and may be multifocal, cover an arc of the circumference of the left ventricle, or sometimes totally encircle it.

Infarct Modification After Reperfusion by Thrombolysis, Angioplasty, or Coronary Bypass Graft Surgery. Thrombolytic therapy is used in an attempt to dissolve the thrombus that initiated acute MI, to reestablish blood flow to the area at risk for infarction, and possibly to rescue the ischemic (but not yet necrotic) heart muscle. The effectiveness of thrombolysis by streptokinase or tissue-type plasminogen activator is based on the ability of these agents to activate the human fibrinolytic system.

Thrombolysis reestablishes flow through the occluded coronary artery in most cases; early reperfusion can salvage myocardium and thereby limit infarct size, with consequent improvement in both short-term and long-term function and survival.[31] As discussed previously, loss of myocardial viability in infarction is progressive, occurring over a period of at least several hours. Thus, reperfusion of jeopardized myocardium offers an effective approach to restoring the balance between myocardial perfusion and need. The potential benefit clearly is related to the rapidity with which the coronary occlusion is alleviated, and the first 3 to 4 hours after onset of symptoms are critical.

Thrombolysis, however, can at best remove a thrombus occluding a coronary artery; it does not significantly alter the underlying disrupted atherosclerotic plaque that initiated it. In contrast, PTCA not only eliminates a thrombotic occlusion, but also relieves some of the original obstruction caused by the underlying plaque[32] (see earlier).

Severe ischemia does not cause immediate cell death even in the most severely affected regions of myocardium, and not all regions of myocardium are equally ischemic. Therefore, the outcome distal to the occlusion after restoration of flow to previously ischemic myocardium may vary from region to region. Reperfusion of myocardium sufficiently early (within 15 to 20 minutes) after onset of ischemia may prevent all necrosis. Reperfusion after a longer interval may not prevent necrosis but can salvage (i.e., prevent necrosis of) at least some myocytes that would have died with more prolonged or permanent ischemia.

The gross and histologic appearance of an infarct that has been reperfused is illustrated in Figure 13–9. A partially completed then reperfused infarct is hemorrhagic because some vasculature injured during the period of ischemia becomes leaky on restoration of flow. Moreover, disintegration of myocytes that were critically damaged by the preceding ischemia is accentuated or accelerated by reperfusion. Microscopic examination reveals that myocytes already irreversibly injured at the time of reflow often have *necrosis with contraction bands.* Contraction bands are intensely eosinophilic transverse bands composed of closely packed hypercontracted sarcomeres. They are most likely produced by exaggerated contraction of myofibrils at the instant perfusion is reestablished, at which time the internal portions of an already dead cell whose membranes have been damaged by ischemia are exposed to a high concentration of calcium ions from the plasma. Thus, *reperfusion not only salvages reversibly injured cells, but also alters the morphology of tissue with cells already lethally injured at the time of reflow.*

Moreover, despite the potential for myocardial salvage on reperfusion of ischemic myocardium, some small amount of *new* cellular damage may occur that blunts the

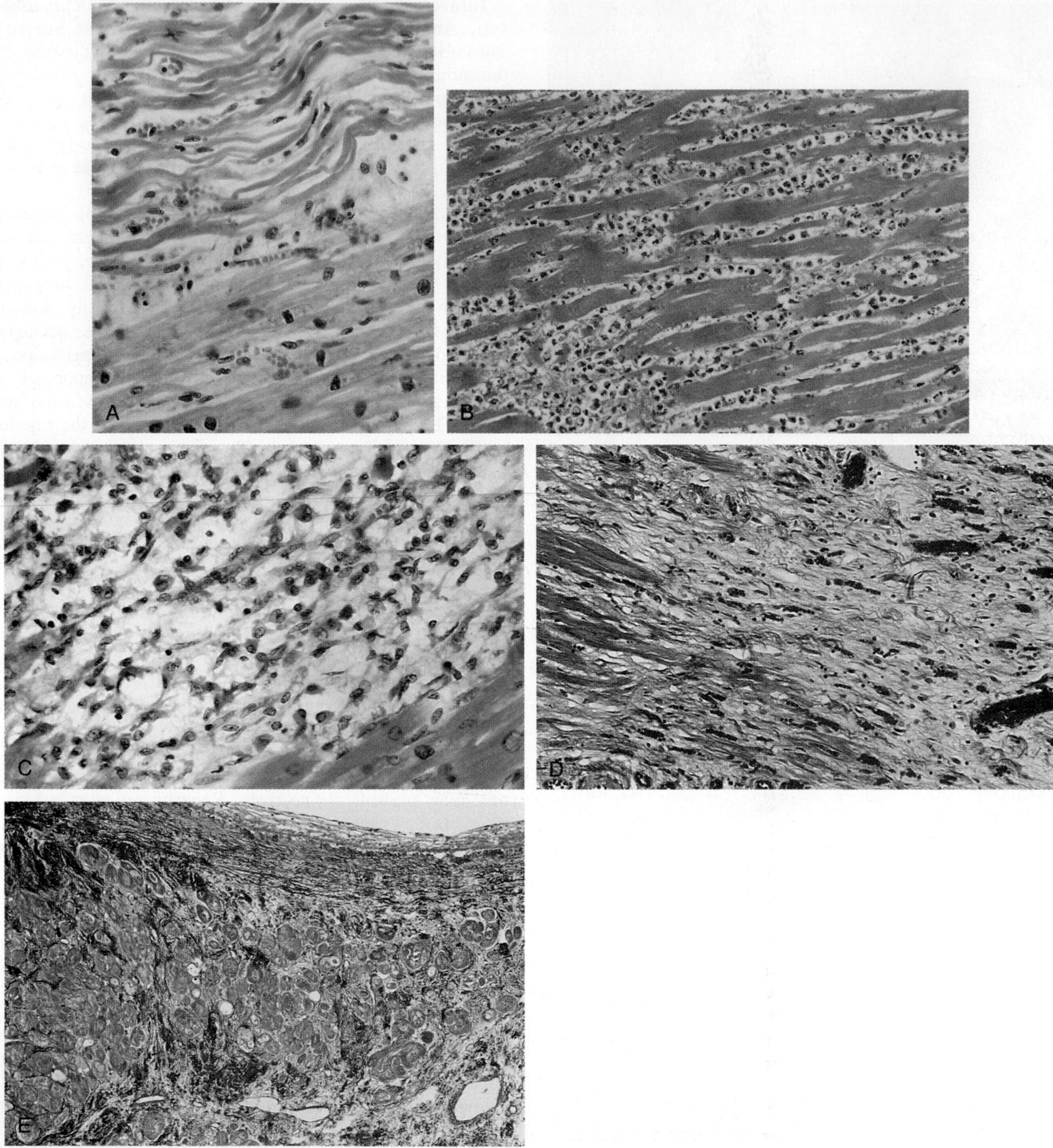

Figure 13–8

Microscopic features of myocardial infarction. *A*, One-day-old infarct showing coagulative necrosis, wavy fibers with elongation, and narrowing, compared with adjacent normal fibers *(lower right)*. Widened spaces between the dead fibers contain edema fluid and scattered neutrophils. *B*, Dense polymorphonuclear leukocytic infiltrate in an area of acute myocardial infarction of 3 to 4 days' duration. *C*, Nearly complete removal of necrotic myocytes by phagocytosis (approximately 7 to 10 days). *D*, Granulation tissue with a rich vascular network and early collagen deposition, approximately 3 weeks after infarction. *E*, Well-healed myocardial infarct with replacement of the necrotic fibers by dense collagenous scar. A few residual cardiac muscle cells are present. (In *D* and *E*, collagen is highlighted as blue in this Masson trichrome stain.)

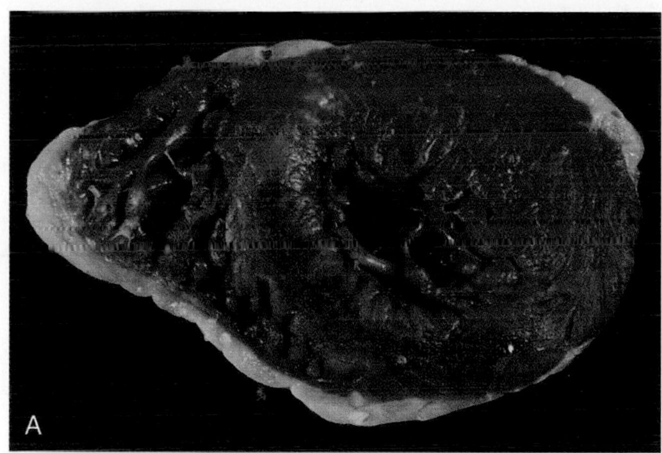

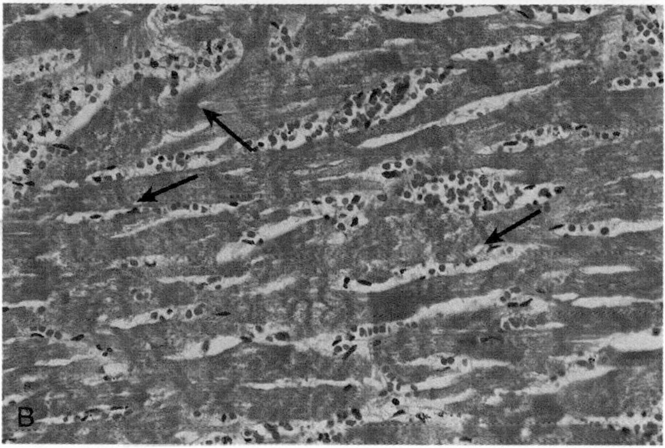

Figure 13–9

Gross and microscopic appearance of myocardium modified by reperfusion. *A*, Large, densely hemorrhagic, anterior wall acute myocardial infarction from a patient with left anterior descending (LAD) artery thrombus treated with streptokinase intracoronary thrombolysis (TTC-stained heart slice). *B*, Myocardial necrosis with hemorrhage and contraction bands, visible as dark bands spanning some myofibers *(arrows)*. This is the characteristic appearance of markedly ischemic myocardium that has been reperfused. (Specimen in *A* oriented with posterior wall up.)

beneficial effect of reperfusion itself (*reperfusion injury*).[33] As discussed in Chapter 1, reperfusion injury is mediated, at least in part, by the generation of oxygen free radicals, but their source is uncertain.

Although most of the viable myocardium existing at the time of reflow ultimately recovers after alleviation of ischemia, critical abnormalities in cellular biochemistry and function of myocytes salvaged by reperfusion may persist for several days (*prolonged postischemic ventricular dysfunction*, or *stunned myocardium*). Myocardium subjected to persistently low flow, or which is repetitively stunned, has chronically depressed function and is said to be *hibernating*.[34] Paradoxically, short-lived transient severe ischemia as might occur in repetitive angina pectoris or silent ischemia may protect the myocardium against a greater subsequent ischemic insult (a phenomenon known as *preconditioning*) by mechanisms that are yet uncertain.[35]

Clinical Features. Patients with MI have rapid, weak pulse and are often diaphoretic. Dyspnea owing to impaired contractility of the ischemic myocardium is common and accompanied by pulmonary congestion and edema. In about 10 to 15% of MI patients, the onset is entirely asymptomatic, and the disease is discovered only later by ECG changes, usually consisting of new Q waves. Such *silent* MIs are particularly common in patients with underlying diabetes mellitus and in elderly patients. *Laboratory evaluation* is based on measurement of release into the circulation of intracellular macromolecules that leak out of fatally damaged myocardial cells through a compromised sarcolemmal membrane.

Creatine kinase (CK) is an enzyme that is highly concentrated in brain, myocardium, and skeletal muscle and composed of two dimers designated *M* and *B*. The isoenzyme CK-MM is derived predominantly from skeletal muscle and heart; CK-BB from brain, lung, and many other tissues; and CK-MB principally from myocardium, although variable amounts of the MB form are also present in skeletal muscle. Total CK activity begins to rise within 2 to 4 hours of onset of MI, peaks at about 24 hours, and returns to normal within approximately 72 hours. The peak is accelerated in patients who have had reperfusion. *Total CK activity is sensitive but not specific* because CK is also elevated in other conditions, such as skeletal muscle injury. Specificity is enhanced by measurement of the CK-MB fraction. CK-MB rises within 4 to 8 hours, peaks at 18 hours, and usually disappears by 48 to 72 hours. *An absence of a change in the levels of CK and CK-MB during the first 2 days of chest pain essentially excludes the diagnosis of MI.* Isoforms of CK-MB may refine the early and specific diagnosis of MI. Lactate dehydrogenase (LDH) is released from cardiac myocytes following injury (but later than CK), and its isoenzymes were previously measured in this context. However, this analysis will likely be superseded by the newer cardiac-specific markers discussed below.

The ideal marker would be an abundant cardiac-specific protein released into the serum following injury in amounts proportional to the extent of injury, and be persistent and inexpensively, rapidly and easily assayed.[36] Troponins are proteins that regulate calcium-mediated contraction of cardiac and skeletal muscle. Troponin I (TnI) and troponin T (TnT) are not normally detectable in the circulation, and different genes encode these proteins in skeletal muscle and myocardium. Therefore, serum elevations are abnormal, and cardiac and skeletal muscle forms can be distinguished by specific antibodies that also permit quantitative immunologic assays. After acute MI, both TnT and TnI levels arise at about the same time as CK-MB. The diagnostic sensitivity of cardiac troponin measurements is similar to that of CK-MB in the early stages. Troponin levels remain elevated for 7 to 10 days after the acute event, however, allowing the diagnosis of acute MI long after CK-MB levels have returned to normal.[37] Other diagnostic modalities, such as echocardiography (for visualization of abnormalities of regional wall motion), radioisotopic studies (such as radionuclide angiography for chamber configuration), perfusion scintigraphy (for regional perfusion), and magnetic resonance imaging (for structural characterization), sometimes provide additional anatomic, biochemical, and functional data.

Consequences and Complications of Myocardial Infarction. Extraordinary progress has been made in the outcome of patients with acute MI. Concurrent with the marked decrease in the overall mortality of IHD since the 1960s, the in-hospital death rate has declined from approximately 30% then to 10 to 13% today overall (and approximately 7% in those receiving aggressive reperfusion therapy). Nevertheless, half of the deaths associated with acute MI occur within 1 hour of onset and these individuals never reach the hospital. Factors associated with a poor prognosis include advanced age, female gender, diabetes mellitus, and a history of previous MI. Nearly three fourths of patients have one or more complications after acute MI, which include the following (some of which are illustrated in Figs. 13–10 and 13–11):

- *Contractile dysfunction: Myocardial infarcts produce abnormalities in left ventricular function approximately proportional to their size.* Most often, there is some degree of left ventricular failure with hypotension, pulmonary vascular congestion, and transudation into the interstitial pulmonary spaces, which may progress to pulmonary edema with respiratory embarrassment. Severe *pump failure (cardiogenic shock)*, which occurs in 10 to 15% of patients after acute MI, generally indicates a large infarct (often greater than 40% of the left ventricle). Cardiogenic shock has a nearly 70% mortality rate and accounts for two thirds of in-hospital deaths.
- *Arrhythmias*: Many patients have *conduction disturbances* or *myocardial irritability* after MI, which undoubtedly is responsible for many of the sudden deaths. MI-associated arrhythmias include sinus bradycardia or tachycardia, ventricular premature contractions or ventricular tachycardia, ventricular fibrillation, or asystole. Owing to the location of portions of the AV conduction system (bundle of His) in the inferoseptal myocardium, infarcts of this region may also be associated with heart block. Prompt intervention by mobile and hospital coronary care units has succeeded in controlling potentially lethal arrhythmias in many patients.
- *Myocardial rupture*: Illustrated in Figure 13–10, the *cardiac rupture syndromes* result from the mechanical weakening that occurs in necrotic and subsequently inflamed myocardium and include (1) *rupture of the ventricular free wall* (most commonly), with hemopericardium and cardiac tamponade and usually fatal; (2) *rupture of the ventricular septum* (less commonly), leading to a left-to-right shunt; and (3) *papillary muscle rupture* (least commonly), resulting in the acute onset of severe mitral regurgitation. Free wall rupture may occur at almost any time after MI but is most frequent approximately 3 to 7 days after onset. Incomplete rupture of the free wall, although rare, results in the formation of a pseudoaneurysm whose wall consists only of thrombus.
- *Pericarditis*: A fibrinous or fibrohemorrhagic pericarditis usually develops about the second or third day after a transmural infarct and usually resolves over time (Fig.

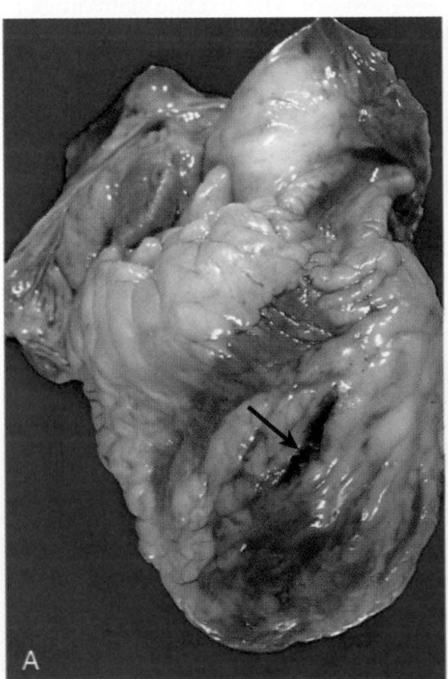

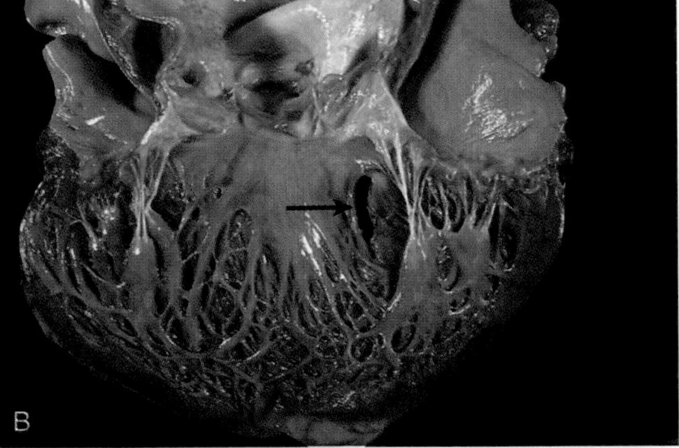

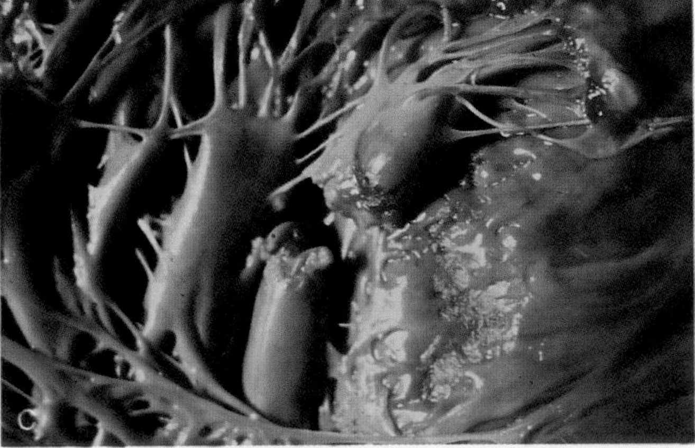

Figure 13–10

Cardiac rupture syndromes complicating acute myocardial infarction. *A*, Anterior myocardial rupture in an acute infarct *(arrow)*. *B*, Rupture of the ventricular septum *(arrow)*. *C*, Complete rupture of a necrotic papillary muscle.

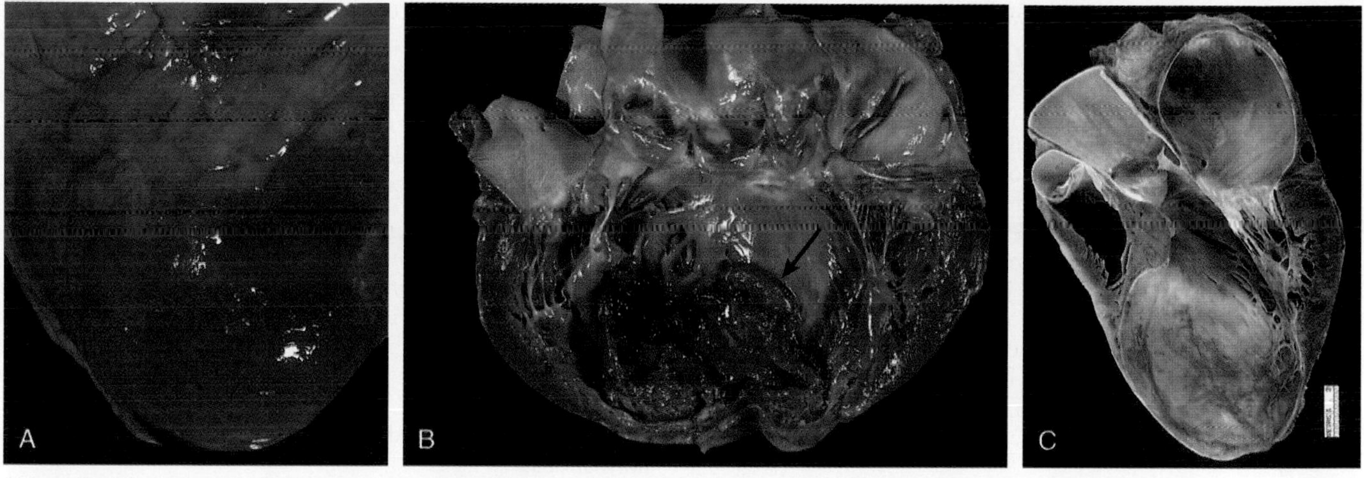

Figure 13–11

Complications of myocardial infarction. *A*, Fibrinous pericarditis, with a dark, roughened epicardial surface overlying an acute infarct. *B*, Early expansion of an anteroapical infarct with wall thinning and mural thrombus *(arrow)*. (From Schoen FJ: Interventional and Surgical Cardiovascular Pathology: Clinical Correlations and Basic Principles. Philadelphia, WB Saunders, 1989.) *C*, Large apical left ventricular aneurysm. The left ventricle is on the right on this apical four-chamber view of the heart. (Courtesy of William D. Edwards, MD, Mayo Clinic, Rochester, MN.)

13–11*A*). Pericarditis is the epicardial manifestation of the underlying myocardial inflammation.

- *Right ventricular infarction*: Although isolated infarction of the right ventricle is unusual, infarction of the right ventricular myocardium often accompanies ischemic injury of the adjacent posterior left ventricle and ventricular septum. A right ventricular infarct of either type can yield serious functional impairment.
- *Infarct extension*: New necrosis may occur adjacent to an existing infarct.
- *Infarct expansion*: Owing to the weakening of necrotic muscle, there may be disproportionate stretching, thinning, and dilation of the infarct region (especially with anteroseptal infarcts), which is often associated with mural thrombus (Fig. 13–11*B*).
- *Mural thrombus*: With any infarct, the combination of a local myocardial abnormality in contractility (causing stasis) with endocardial damage (causing a thrombogenic surface) can foster *mural thrombosis* (Chapter 5) and potentially *thromboembolism*.
- *Ventricular aneurysm*: This is a late complication that most commonly results from a large transmural anteroseptal infarct that heals into a large region of thin scar tissue, which paradoxically bulges during systole (Fig. 13–11*C*). Complications of ventricular aneurysms include mural thrombus, arrhythmias, and heart failure, but rupture of the fibrotic wall rarely occurs.
- *Papillary muscle dysfunction*: Postinfarct mitral regurgitation is most commonly due to early ischemic dysfunction of a papillary muscle and underlying myocardium without rupture and later to papillary muscle fibrosis and shortening or ventricular dilation (see later).
- *Progressive late heart failure*: This is illustrated in Figure 13–11*C* and discussed as chronic ischemic heart disease later.

The propensity toward specific complications and the prognosis after MI depend primarily on infarct size, site, and transmural extent (i.e., the fractional thickness of the myocardial wall that is damaged—subendocardial or transmural). Large transmural infarcts yield a higher probability of cardiogenic shock, arrhythmias, and late congestive heart failure. Patients with anterior transmural infarcts are at greatest risk for rupture, expansion, mural thrombi, and aneurysm and thus have a substantially worse clinical course than those with inferior (posterior) infarcts. In contrast, posterior transmural infarcts are more likely to be complicated by serious conduction blocks, right ventricular involvement, or both. Mural thrombi may form on the endocardial surface of subendocardial infarcts, but pericarditis, rupture, and aneurysms rarely occur.

Multiple dynamic structural changes maintain cardiac output after acute MI. Both the necrotic zone and the noninfarcted segments of the ventricle undergo progressive changes in size, shape, and thickness comprising early wall thinning, healing, hypertrophy and dilation, and late aneurysm formation, collectively termed *ventricular remodeling*.[38] Clearly the initial compensatory hypertrophy of noninfarcted myocardium is hemodynamically beneficial. The adaptive effect of remodeling, however, may be overwhelmed by expansion and ventricular aneurysm or late depression of regional and global contractile function owing to degenerative changes in viable myocardium. Late impairment of ventricular performance may result.

Long-term prognosis after MI depends on many factors, the most important of which are the quality of left ventricular function and the extent of vascular obstructions in vessels that perfuse viable myocardium. The overall total mortality within the first year is about 30%, including those who die before reaching the hospital. Thereafter, there is a 3 to 4% mortality among survivors with each passing year. Attempts to prevent infarction in those who have never experienced MI through control of risk factors (*primary prevention*) or prevent reinfarction in those who have recovered from an acute MI (*secondary prevention*) are under investigation.

CHRONIC ISCHEMIC HEART DISEASE

The designation *chronic IHD* is used here to describe the cardiac findings in patients, often but not exclusively elderly, who develop progressive heart failure as a consequence of ischemic myocardial damage. In most instances, there has been prior MI and sometimes previous aortocoronary bypass graft surgery. Chronic IHD usually constitutes postinfarction cardiac decompensation owing to exhaustion of the compensatory hypertrophy of noninfarcted viable myocardium that is itself in jeopardy of ischemic injury (see earlier discussion of cardiac hypertrophy). In other cases, however, severe obstructive coronary artery disease may be present without acute or healed infarction but with diffuse myocardial dysfunction.

MORPHOLOGY. Hearts from patients with chronic IHD are usually enlarged and heavy, secondary to left ventricular hypertrophy and dilation (Fig. 13–11C). Invariably, there is moderate to severe stenosing atherosclerosis of the coronary arteries and sometimes total occlusions. Discrete, gray-white scars of healed previous infarcts are usually present. The mural endocardium is generally normal except for some superficial, patchy, fibrous thickenings. The major microscopic findings include myocardial hypertrophy, diffuse subendocardial vacuolization, and scars of previous healed infarcts.

The term *ischemic cardiomyopathy* is often used by clinicians to describe chronic IHD. The clinical diagnosis is made largely by the insidious onset of congestive heart failure in patients who have past episodes of MI or anginal attacks. In some individuals, however, progressive myocardial damage is entirely silent, and heart failure is the first indication of chronic IHD. The diagnosis rests largely on the exclusion of other forms of cardiac involvement.

SUDDEN CARDIAC DEATH

Sudden cardiac death strikes down about 300,000 to 400,000 individuals annually in the United States. *Sudden cardiac death* is most commonly defined as unexpected death from cardiac causes early (usually within 1 hour) after or without the onset of symptoms. In the vast majority of cases in adults, sudden cardiac death is a complication and often the first clinical manifestation of IHD. With decreasing age of the victim, the following nonatherosclerotic causes of sudden cardiac death become increasingly probable:[39, 40]

- Congenital structural or coronary arterial abnormalities
- Aortic valve stenosis
- Mitral valve prolapse
- Myocarditis
- Dilated or hypertrophic cardiomyopathy
- Pulmonary hypertension
- Hereditary or acquired abnormalities of the cardiac conduction system
- Isolated hypertrophy, hypertensive or unknown cause: Increased cardiac mass is an independent risk factor for cardiac death; thus some young patients who die suddenly, including athletes, have hypertensive hypertrophy or unexplained increased cardiac mass as the only finding.[13, 39, 40]

The ultimate mechanism of sudden cardiac death is almost always a lethal arrhythmia (e.g., asystole, ventricular fibrillation). Although ischemic injury can impinge on the conduction system and create electromechanical cardiac instability, in most cases the fatal arrhythmia is triggered by electrical irritability of myocardium distant from the conduction system induced by ischemia or other cellular abnormalities.

MORPHOLOGY. Marked coronary atherosclerosis with critical (>75%) stenosis involving one or more of the three major vessels is present in 80 to 90% of victims; only 10 to 20% of cases are of nonatherosclerotic origin. Usually, there are high-grade stenoses (>90%), and acute plaque disruption is common. A healed myocardial infarct is present in about 40%, but in those who were successfully resuscitated from sudden cardiac arrest, new MI is found in only one third or less. Subendocardial myocyte vacuolization indicative of severe chronic ischemia is common.

Hypertensive Heart Disease

Hypertensive heart disease is the response of the heart to the increased demands induced by systemic hypertension. Pulmonary hypertension also causes heart disease and is referred to as *right-sided hypertensive heart disease* or *cor pulmonale*.

SYSTEMIC (LEFT-SIDED) HYPERTENSIVE HEART DISEASE

The minimal criteria for the diagnosis of systemic hypertensive heart disease are the following: (1) *left ventricular hypertrophy (usually concentric) in the absence of other cardiovascular pathology that might have induced it* and (2) *a history or pathologic evidence (see Chapter 12) of hypertension.* The Framingham Heart Study established unequivocally that even mild hypertension (levels only slightly above 140/90 mm Hg), if sufficiently prolonged, induces left ventricular hypertrophy.[41] Approximately 25% of the U.S. population suffers from hypertension of at least this degree. The pathogenesis of hypertension is discussed in Chapter 12. In hypertension, hypertrophy of the heart is an adaptive response to pressure overload, which can lead to myocardial dysfunction, cardiac dilation, congestive heart failure, and sudden death (see section on cardiac hypertrophy earlier).

MORPHOLOGY. Because systemic hypertension induces left ventricular pressure overload, the heart in compensated left-sided hypertensive heart disease is characterized by circumferential hypertrophy without dilation of the left ventricle. The thickening of the left ventricular wall increases the ratio of its wall thickness to radius and increases the weight of the heart disproportionately to the increase in overall cardiac size (Fig. 13–12). The left ventricular wall thickness may exceed 2.0 cm, and the heart weight may exceed 500 g. In time, the increased thickness of the left ventricular wall imparts a stiffness that impairs diastolic filling. This often induces left atrial enlargement.

Microscopically the earliest change of systemic hypertensive heart disease is an increase in transverse myocyte diameters, which may be difficult to appreciate on routine microscopy. At a more advanced stage, the cellular and nuclear enlargement becomes somewhat more prominent and irregular, with variation in cell size among adjacent cells and interstitial fibrosis. The biochemical, molecular, and morphologic changes that occur in hypertensive hypertrophy are similar to those noted in other conditions of myocardial overload.

Compensated systemic hypertensive heart disease may be asymptomatic and suspected only in the appropriate clinical setting by ECG or echocardiographic indications of left ventricular enlargement. As already emphasized, other causes for such hypertrophy must be excluded. In many patients, systemic hypertensive heart disease comes to attention by the onset of atrial fibrillation (owing to left atrial enlargement) or congestive heart failure with cardiac dilation, or both. Depending on the severity of the hypertension, its duration, the adequacy of therapeutic control, and underlying basis, the patient may enjoy normal longevity and die of unrelated causes, may develop progressive IHD owing to the effects of hypertension in potentiating coronary atherosclerosis, may suffer progressive renal damage or cerebrovascular accident, or may experience progressive heart failure or sudden cardiac death. There is substantial evidence that effective control of hypertension can prevent or lead to regression of cardiac hypertrophy and its associated risks.[41]

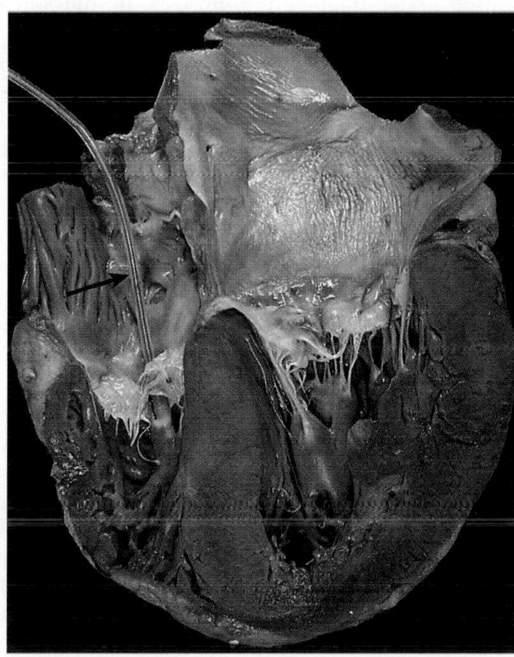

Figure 13–12

Hypertensive heart disease with marked concentric thickening of the left ventricular wall causing reduction in lumen size. The left ventricle is on the right in this apical four-chamber view of the heart. A pacemaker is incidentally present *(arrow)* with the lead terminating in the right ventricle.

PULMONARY (RIGHT-SIDED) HYPERTENSIVE HEART DISEASE (COR PULMONALE)

Cor pulmonale, as pulmonary hypertensive heart disease is frequently called, constitutes right ventricular hypertrophy, dilation, and potentially failure secondary to pulmonary hypertension caused by disorders of the lungs or pulmonary vasculature (Table 13–5) and is the right-sided counterpart of left-sided (systemic) hypertensive heart disease. *Although quite common, right ventricular thickening and dilation caused either by congenital heart diseases or by diseases of the left side of the heart and the resultant pulmonary venous hypertension owing to postcapillary obstruction to blood flow are excluded from this definition of cor pulmonale.*

Based on the suddenness of development of pulmonary

Table 13–5. DISORDERS PREDISPOSING TO COR PULMONALE

Diseases of the Pulmonary Parenchyma
- Chronic obstructive pulmonary disease
- Diffuse pulmonary interstitial fibrosis
- Pneumoconioses
- Cystic fibrosis
- Bronchiectasis

Diseases of Pulmonary Vessels
- Recurrent pulmonary thromboembolism
- Primary pulmonary hypertension
- Extensive pulmonary arteritis (e.g., Wegener granulomatosis)
- Drug-, toxin-, or radiation-induced vascular obstruction
- Extensive pulmonary tumor microembolism

Disorders Affecting Chest Movement
- Kyphoscoliosis
- Marked obesity (pickwickian syndrome)
- Neuromuscular diseases

Disorders Inducing Pulmonary Arterial Constriction
- Metabolic acidosis
- Hypoxemia
- Chronic altitude sickness
- Obstruction to major airways
- Idiopathic alveolar hypoventilation

hypertension, cor pulmonale may be acute or chronic. *Acute cor pulmonale* can follow massive pulmonary embolism. *Chronic cor pulmonale* usually implies right ventricular hypertrophy (and dilation) secondary to prolonged pressure overload owing to obstruction of the pulmonary arteries or arterioles or compression or obliteration of septal capillaries (e.g., owing to primary pulmonary hypertension or emphysema).

MORPHOLOGY. In acute cor pulmonale, there is marked dilation of the right ventricle without hypertrophy. On cross-section, the normal crescent shape of the right ventricle is transformed to a dilated ovoid. In chronic cor pulmonale, the ventricular wall thickens, sometimes up to 1.0 cm or more, and may even come to approximate that of the left ventricle (Fig. 13–13). More subtle stages of right ventricular hypertrophy may be observed as thickening of the muscle bundles in the outflow tract, immediately below the pulmonary valve, or of the moderator band, the muscle bundle that connects the ventricular septum to the anterior right ventricular papillary muscle. Sometimes, there is secondary compression of the left ventricular chamber or tricuspid regurgitation with fibrous thickening of this valve.

Valvular Heart Disease

Valvular involvement by disease causes stenosis, insufficiency (regurgitation), or both. *Stenosis is the failure of a valve to open completely, thereby impeding forward flow. Insufficiency, regurgitation, or incompetence, in contrast, results from failure of a valve to close completely, thereby allowing reversed flow.* These abnormalities can be either *pure,* when only stenosis *or* regurgitation is present, or *mixed,* when both stenosis and regurgitation coexist in the same valve, but one of these defects usually predominates. Dysfunction may affect a single valve (*isolated disease*) or multiple valves (*combined disease*). *Functional regurgitation* results when a valve becomes incompetent owing to ventricular dilation, which causes the right or left ventricular papillary muscles to be pulled down and outward, thereby preventing coaptation of otherwise intact leaflets during systole. Abnormalities of flow often produce abnormal heart sounds known as *murmurs.*

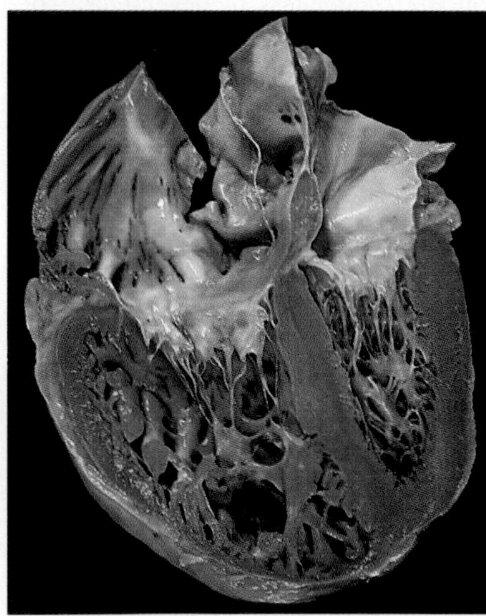

Figure 13–13

Chronic cor pulmonale characterized by a markedly dilated and hypertrophied right ventricle, with thickened free wall and hypertrophied trabeculae (apical four-chamber view of the heart, right ventricle on the left). The shape of the left ventricle (to the right) has been distorted by the right ventricular enlargement. Compare with Figure 13–12.

Valvular dysfunction can vary in degree from slight and physiologically unimportant to severe and rapidly fatal. The clinical consequences depend on the valve involved, the degree of impairment, the rate of its development, and the rate and quality of compensatory mechanisms.[42] For example, sudden destruction of an aortic valve cusp by infection (as in infective endocarditis; see later) may cause rapidly fatal cardiac failure owing to massive regurgitation. In contrast, rheumatic mitral stenosis usually develops over years, and its clinical effects may be remarkably well tolerated. Depending on degree, duration, and cause, valvular stenosis or insufficiency often produces secondary changes in the heart, blood vessels, and other organs, both proximal and distal to the valvular lesion. Most important are the myocardial hypertrophy and pulmonary and systemic changes discussed earlier. Moreover, a patch of endocardial thickening often occurs at the point where a jet lesion impinges, such as the focal endocardial fibrosis in the left atrium secondary to a regurgitant jet of mitral insufficiency.

Valvular abnormalities may be caused by congenital disorders (see later) or by a variety of acquired diseases. Most frequent are acquired stenoses of the mitral and aortic valves, which account for approximately two thirds of all valve lesions. *Valvular insufficiency may result from either intrinsic disease of the valve cusps or damage to or distortion of the supporting structures (e.g., the aorta, mitral annulus, tendinous cords, papillary muscles, ventricular free wall) without primary changes in the cusps. It may appear acutely with infective endocarditis or chronically with leaflet scarring and retraction. In contrast, valvular stenosis almost always is due to a primary cuspal abnormality and is virtually always a chronic process.*

The most important causes of acquired heart valve dysfunction are summarized in Table 13–6 and are discussed in the following sections. In contrast to the many potential causes of valvular insufficiency, only a relatively few mechanisms commonly produce acquired valvular stenosis. The most frequent chronic causes of the major functional valvular lesions are as follows:

- Mitral stenosis—rheumatic heart disease
- Mitral insufficiency—myxomatous degeneration (mitral valve prolapse)
- Aortic stenosis—calcification of anatomically normal and congenitally bicuspid aortic valves

Table 13–6. MAJOR CAUSES OF ACQUIRED HEART VALVE DISEASE

Mitral Valve Disease	Aortic Valve Disease
Mitral Stenosis	***Aortic Stenosis***
Postinflammatory scarring (rheumatic heart disease)	Postinflammatory scarring (rheumatic heart disease)
	Senile calcific aortic stenosis
	Calcification of congenitally deformed valve
Mitral Regurgitation	***Aortic Regurgitation***
Abnormalities of leaflets and commissures	Intrinsic valvular disease
Postinflammatory scarring	Postinflammatory scarring (rheumatic heart disease)
Infective endocarditis	Infective endocarditis
Mitral valve prolapse	Aortic disease
Abnormalities of tensor apparatus	Degenerative aortic dilation
Rupture of papillary muscle	Syphilitic aortitis
Papillary muscle dysfunction (fibrosis)	Ankylosing spondylitis
Rupture of chordae tendineae	Rheumatoid arthritis
Abnormalities of left ventricular cavity and/or annulus	Marfan syndrome
Left ventricular enlargement (myocarditis, dilated cardiomyopathy)	
Calcification of mitral annulus	

Modified from Schoen FJ: Surgical pathology of removed natural and prosthetic valves. Hum Pathol 18:558, 1987.

- Aortic insufficiency—dilation of the ascending aorta, related to hypertension and aging

VALVULAR DEGENERATION CAUSED BY CALCIFICATION

The heart valves are subjected to high repetitive mechanical stresses, particularly at the hinge points of the cusps and leaflets owing to (1) 40 million or more cardiac cycles per year, (2) substantial tissue deformations at each cycle, and (3) transvalvular gradients in the closed phase of approximately 120 mm Hg for the mitral and 80 mm Hg for the aortic valve. It is therefore not surprising that these normally delicate structures can suffer cumulative damage complicated by deposition of calcium phosphate mineral, which may lead to clinically important disease (Chapter 1). The most frequent calcific valvular diseases (Fig. 13–14) are calcific aortic stenosis, calcification of a congenitally bicuspid aortic valve, and mitral annular calcification. Each comprises primarily dystrophic calcification with less prominent lipid deposition and cellular proliferation, a process that is distinct from but with some features of atherosclerosis.[43]

Calcific Aortic Stenosis

Aortic stenosis is the most frequent of all valvular abnormalities; it can be congenital (when the valvular obstruction is present from birth) or acquired. *Acquired aortic stenosis* is usually the consequence of either calcification induced by *wear and tear* of congenitally bicuspid (or unicuspid) valves (see later) or calcification of aortic valves with previous normal anatomy in aged individuals. The overwhelming majority of cases represent age-related degenerative calcification. With the decline in the incidence of rheumatic fever in North America, rheumatic aortic stenosis now accounts for less than 10% of cases of acquired

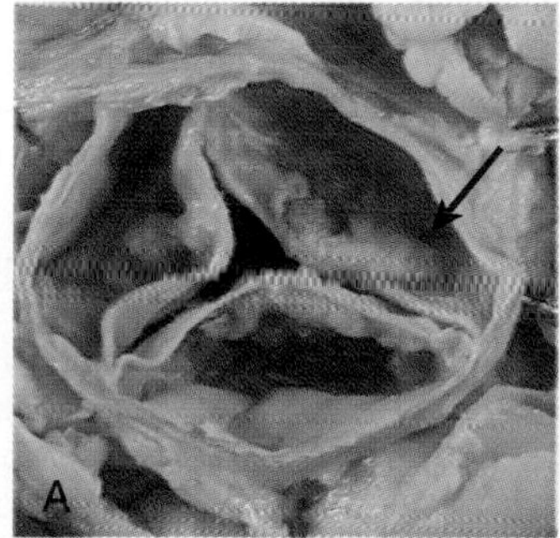

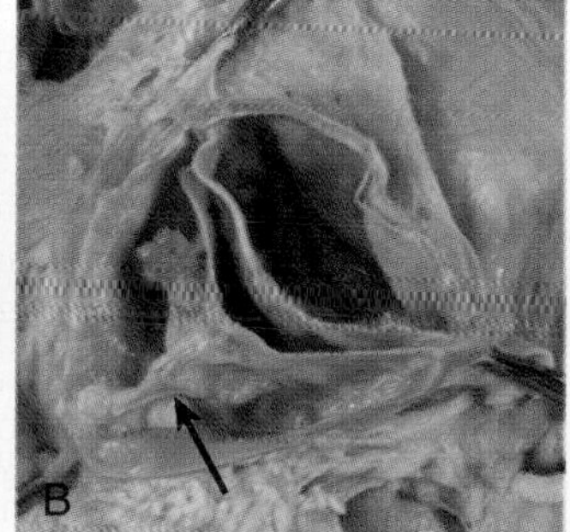

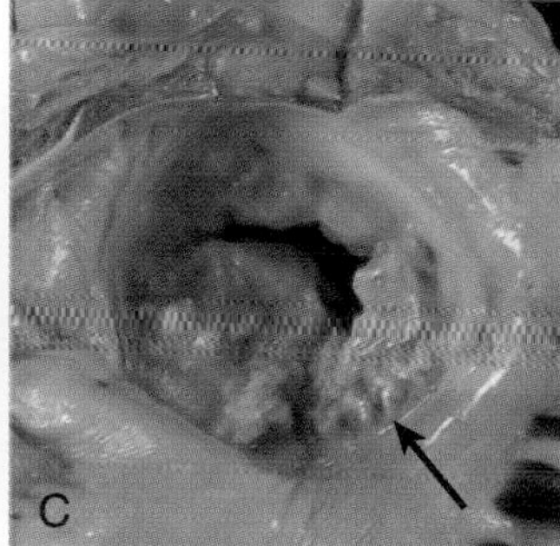

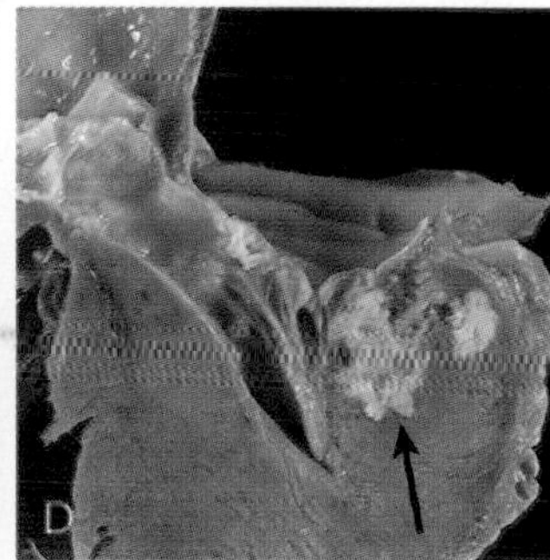

Figure 13–14

Valvular calcific degeneration. *A*, Degenerative calcific aortic stenosis of a previously normal valve having three cusps (viewed from the aortic aspect). Nodular masses of calcium are heaped up within the sinuses of Valsalva *(arrow)*. Note that the commissures are not fused, as in postrheumatic aortic valve stenosis (see Fig. 13–16*E*). *B*, Calcific aortic stenosis occurring on a congenitally bicuspid valve. One cusp has a partial fusion at its center, called a *raphe (arrow)*. *C* and *D*, Mitral annular calcification with calcific nodules at the base (attachment margin) of the anterior mitral leaflet *(arrows)*. C, Left atrial view; *D*, cut section of myocardium.

aortic stenosis. Aortic stenosis comes to clinical attention primarily in individuals in their fifties to sixties with congenitally bicuspid valves (see later) but not until the seventies and eighties with previously normal valves having three cusps; hence the term *senile calcific aortic stenosis* to describe the latter condition.

MORPHOLOGY. The morphologic hallmark of nonrheumatic, calcific aortic stenosis (with either tricuspid or bicuspid valves) is heaped-up calcified masses within the aortic cusps that ultimately protrude through the outflow surfaces into the sinuses of Valsalva, preventing the opening of the cusps. The calcific deposits distort the cuspal architecture, primarily at the bases; the free cuspal edges are usually not involved (Fig. 13–14*A*). The calcific process begins in the valvular fibrosa, at the points of maximal cusp flexion (the margins of attachment), and the microscopic layered architecture is largely preserved. An earlier hemodynamically insignificant stage of the calcification process is called **aortic valve sclerosis.**

Notably, in contrast to rheumatic aortic stenosis (see Fig. 13–16*E*), commissural fusion is usually absent in degenerative aortic stenosis. By the time these changes are seen at surgical resection or postmortem examination, however, the cusps may be fibrosed and thickened and the commissures fused. The mitral valve is generally normal in patients with calcific aortic stenosis, other than mitral annular calcification or direct extension of aortic valve calcific deposits onto the mitral anterior leaflet. In contrast, virtually all patients with rheumatic aortic stenosis have concomitant and characteristic structural abnormalities of the mitral valve (see later).

Clinical Features. In calcific aortic stenosis or calcification of a bicuspid aortic valve, the obstruction to left ventricular outflow leads to a gradually increasing pressure gradient across the calcified valve, which may reach 75 to 100 mm Hg in severe cases. Left ventricular pressure must consequently rise to 200 mm Hg or more in such instances, and cardiac output is maintained by the development of concentric left ventricular (pressure overload) hypertrophy. Eventually as the stenosis worsens, angina or syncope may appear. Angina is probably a consequence of impaired microcirculatory perfusion of the hypertrophied myocardium, but the basis of syncope is poorly understood. Eventually, cardiac decompensation with congestive heart failure may ensue. The onset of such symptoms (angina, syncope, or congestive heart failure) in aortic stenosis heralds the exhaustion of compensatory cardiac hyperfunction and carries a poor prognosis if not treated by surgery, with death, sometimes sudden, occurring in more than 50% of patients within 3 years. Because the rate of development of valvular obstruction varies greatly among patients, noninvasive techniques, such as Doppler echocardiography (which measures flow velocities as well as structure), can be used repetitively to examine the progression of disease with time.

Calcification of a Congenitally Bicuspid Aortic Valve

An estimated 1 to 2% of the population has a congenitally bicuspid aortic valve as an isolated abnormality. The two cusps are usually of unequal size, with the larger cusp having a midline *raphe*, resulting from the incomplete embryologic separation; less frequently the cusps are of the same size and the raphe is absent. Valves that become bicuspid owing to an acquired deformity (e.g., postinflammatory commissural fusion in rheumatic valve disease) have a conjoined cusp containing the fused commissure that is generally twice the size of the nonconjoined cusp. The mitral valve is normal in patients with a congenitally bicuspid aortic valve.

Bicuspid aortic valves are generally neither stenotic nor symptomatic at birth or throughout early life, but they are predisposed to progressive degenerative calcification, similar to that occurring in aortic valves with initially normal anatomy (Fig. 13–14*B*). The raphe that composes the incomplete commissure is frequently a major site of calcific deposits. Once stenosis is present, the clinical course is similar to that described earlier for calcific aortic stenosis. Bicuspid aortic valves may also become incompetent as a result of aortic dilation or cusp prolapse, and they are predisposed to infective endocarditis. They are also associated with aortic coarctation, aneurysm, and dissection, for inexplicable reasons.

Mitral Annular Calcification

Degenerative calcific deposits can develop in the ring (*annulus*) of the mitral valve, visualized on gross inspection as irregular, stony hard, and occasionally ulcerated nodules (2 to 5 mm in thickness) that lie behind the leaflets (Fig. 13–14*C*). The process generally does not affect valvular function. In unusual cases, however, it may lead to regurgitation by interfering with systolic contraction of the mitral valve ring, to stenosis by impairing opening of the mitral leaflets, or to arrhythmias and occasionally sudden death by the calcium deposits penetrating sufficiently deeply to impinge on the AV conduction system. Because ulcerated calcific nodules may provide a site for thrombi that can embolize, some patients with mitral annular calcification have an increased risk of stroke. The calcific nodules can also be the nidus for infective endocarditis. Heavy calcific deposits are sometimes visualized on echocardiography or seen as a distinctive, ringlike opacity on chest radiographs. Mitral annular calcification is most common in women over 60 years of age and individuals with myxomatous mitral valve (see later) or elevated left ventricular pressure (as in systemic hypertension, aortic stenosis, or hypertrophic cardiomyopathy, discussed later).

MYXOMATOUS DEGENERATION OF THE MITRAL VALVE (MITRAL VALVE PROLAPSE)

Myxomatous degeneration of the mitral valve (mitral valve prolapse) is estimated to affect 3% or more of adults in the United States, most often young women, and is considered the most common form of valvular heart disease in the industrialized world. In this valvular abnormality, one or both mitral leaflets are enlarged, hooded, redundant or *floppy*, and *prolapse* or balloon back into the left atrium during systole. Usually an incidental finding on physical examination, *mitral valve prolapse*, as it is known clinically, may lead to serious complications in a small minority of those who are affected.

MORPHOLOGY. The characteristic anatomic change in myxomatous degeneration is intercordal ballooning (hooding) of the mitral leaflets or portions thereof (Fig. 13–15). The affected leaflets are often thick and rubbery. Frequently involved, the tendinous cords are elongated, thinned, and occasionally ruptured. Annular dilation is characteristic, a finding that is rare in other causes of mitral insufficiency. Concomitant involvement of the tricuspid valve is present in 20 to 40% of cases, and the aortic or pulmonic valve (or both) may also be affected. Commissural fusion, which typifies rheumatic heart disease, is absent. Histologically the essential change is attenuation of the fibrosa layer of the valve, on which the structural integrity of the leaflet depends, accompanied by focally marked thickening of the spongiosa layer with deposition of mucoid (myxomatous) material. The collagenous structure of the cords is attenuated.

Secondary changes reflect the stresses and injury incident to the billowing leaflets: (1) fibrous thickening of the valve leaflets, particularly where they rub against each other; (2) linear fibrous thickening of the left ventricular endocardial surface where abnormally long cords snap against it; (3) thickening of the mural endocardium of the left atrium as a consequence of friction-induced injury induced by the prolapsing leaflets; (4) thrombi on the atrial surfaces of the leaflets, particularly in the recesses behind the ballooned

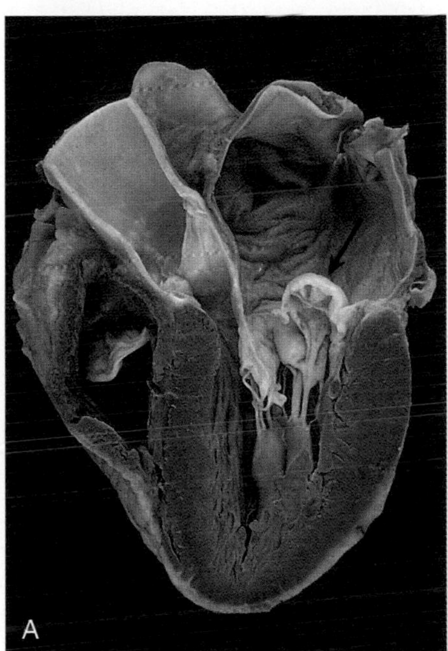

Figure 13–15

Myxomatous degeneration of the mitral valve. *A*, Long axis view of the left ventricle demonstrating hooding with prolapse of the posterior mitral leaflet into the left atrium *(arrow)*. The left ventricle is on the right. (Courtesy of William D. Edwards, MD, Mayo Clinic, Rochester, MN.) *B*, Opened valve showing pronounced hooding of the posterior mitral leaflet with thrombotic plaques at sites of leaflet–left atrium contact *(arrows)*. *C*, Opened valve with pronounced hooding from a patient who died suddenly. Note also the mitral annular calcification.

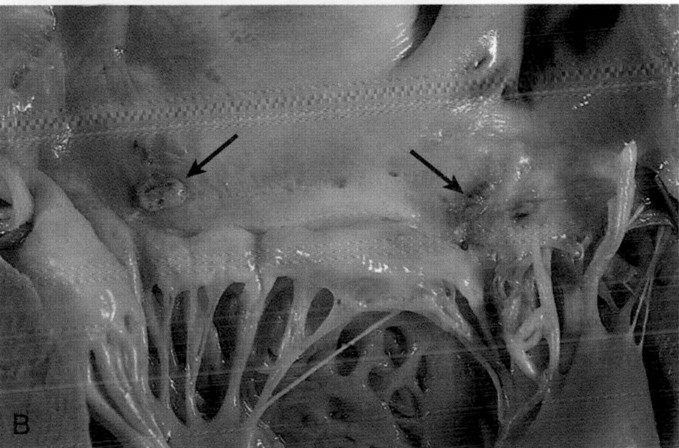

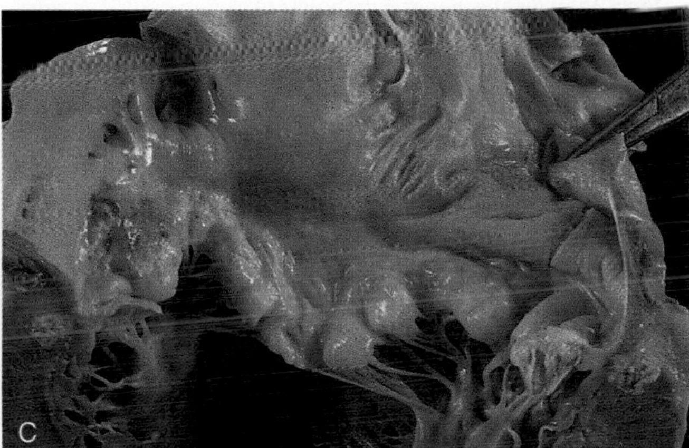

cusps and on the atrial walls they contact; and (5) focal calcifications at the base of the posterior mitral leaflet. Changes of myxomatous degeneration can also occur secondarily in mitral valves having regurgitation due to another cause (e.g., ischemic dysfunction).

Pathogenesis. The basis for the changes within the valve leaflets and associated structures is unknown. Favored is the proposition of a developmental anomaly of connective tissue, because this valvular abnormality is one common feature of Marfan syndrome caused by mutations in the gene encoding fibrillin (Chapter 6) and occasionally occurs with other hereditary disorders of connective tissue. Even in the absence of these well-defined conditions, there are hints of extracardiac systemic structural abnormalities in some individuals with the floppy mitral valve syndrome, such as scoliosis, straight back, and high-arched palate. Subtle defects in structural proteins may predispose connective tissues rich in microfibrils and elastin (such as cardiac valves) to damage by long-standing hemodynamic stress. A fibrillin mutation has been found in a patient with the so-called MASS phenotype (which includes mitral valve prolapse and borderline aortic dilation without dissection as prominent features).[44]

Clinical Features. Most patients with mitral valve prolapse are asymptomatic, and the condition is discovered only on routine examination by the presence of a midsystolic click. It is usually an incidental finding on physical examination but in a small fraction of those affected may lead to serious complications. Auscultation may reveal a midsystolic click or clicks corresponding to snapping or tensing of an everted cusp, scallop, or tendinous cord. The valve may become incompetent, and the mitral regurgitation induces an accompanying late systolic or sometimes holosystolic murmur. Echocardiography reveals varying degrees of mitral valve prolapse. A minority of patients have chest pain mimicking angina, dyspnea, and fatigue or, curiously, psychiatric manifestations, such as depression, anxiety reactions, and personality disorders. Although the great majority of patients with mitral valve prolapse have no untoward effects, approximately 3% develop any of four serious complications:

- *Infective endocarditis*, manyfold more frequent in these patients than in the general population
- *Mitral insufficiency* requiring surgery, either slow onset attributed to leaflet deformity, dilation of the mitral annulus, or cordal lengthening, or sudden owing to cordal rupture
- *Stroke or other systemic infarct*, resulting from embolism of leaflet or atrial wall thrombi
- *Arrhythmias*: Both ventricular and atrial arrhythmias can develop. Sudden death can occur but is uncommon. The mechanism of ventricular arrhythmia is unknown in most cases.

The risk of these complications is higher in men, older patients, and those with either arrhythmias or some mitral regurgitation, as evidenced by holosystolic murmurs and left-sided chamber enlargement.[45]

RHEUMATIC FEVER AND RHEUMATIC HEART DISEASE

Rheumatic fever is an acute, immunologically mediated, multisystem inflammatory disease that occurs a few weeks after an episode of group A (β-hemolytic) streptococcal pharyngitis and often involves the heart. Acute rheumatic carditis, which complicates the active phase of rheumatic fever, may progress to chronic valvular deformities. Rheumatic fever does not follow infections by other strains of streptococci at other sites, such as the skin. The incidence and mortality rate of rheumatic fever have declined remarkably in many parts of the world over the past 30 years owing to improved socioeconomic conditions, rapid diagnosis and treatment of streptococcal pharyngitis, and an unexplained decrease in the virulence of group A streptococci.[46] Nevertheless, in third world countries and in many crowded, economically depressed urban areas in the Western world, rheumatic fever remains an important public health problem. Fortunately, rheumatic fever occurs in only about 3% of patients with group A streptococcal pharyngitis. After an initial attack, however, there is increased vulnerability to reactivation of the disease with subsequent pharyngeal infections.

Rheumatic fever is characterized by a constellation of findings that includes as major manifestations (1) *migratory polyarthritis of the large joints*, (2) *carditis*, (3) *subcutaneous nodules*, (4) *erythema marginatum of the skin*, and (5) *Sydenham chorea—a neurologic disorder with involuntary purposeless, rapid movements.* The diagnosis is established by the so-called Jones criteria: evidence of a preceding group A streptococcal infection, with the presence of either two of the major manifestations just listed or one major and two minor manifestations (nonspecific signs and symptoms, which include fever, arthralgia, or elevated acute-phase reactants). *The most important consequence of rheumatic fever is chronic rheumatic heart disease, characterized principally by deforming fibrotic valvular disease (particularly mitral stenosis), which can produce permanent dysfunction and severe, sometimes fatal, cardiac dysfunction decades later.*

MORPHOLOGY. Key pathologic features of acute rheumatic fever and chronic rheumatic heart disease are summarized in Figure 13–16. **During acute rheumatic fever**, widely disseminated but focal inflammatory lesions are found in various sites. They are most distinctive within the heart where they are called **Aschoff bodies**. They constitute foci of fibrinoid degeneration surrounded by lymphocytes (primarily T cells), occasional plasma cells, and plump macrophages called *Anitschkow cells* (pathognomonic for rheumatic fever). These distinctive cells have abundant amphophilic cytoplasm and central round-to-ovoid nuclei in which the chromatin is disposed in a central, slender, wavy ribbon (hence the designation *caterpillar cells*). Some of the larger altered histiocytes become multinucleated to form Aschoff giant cells.

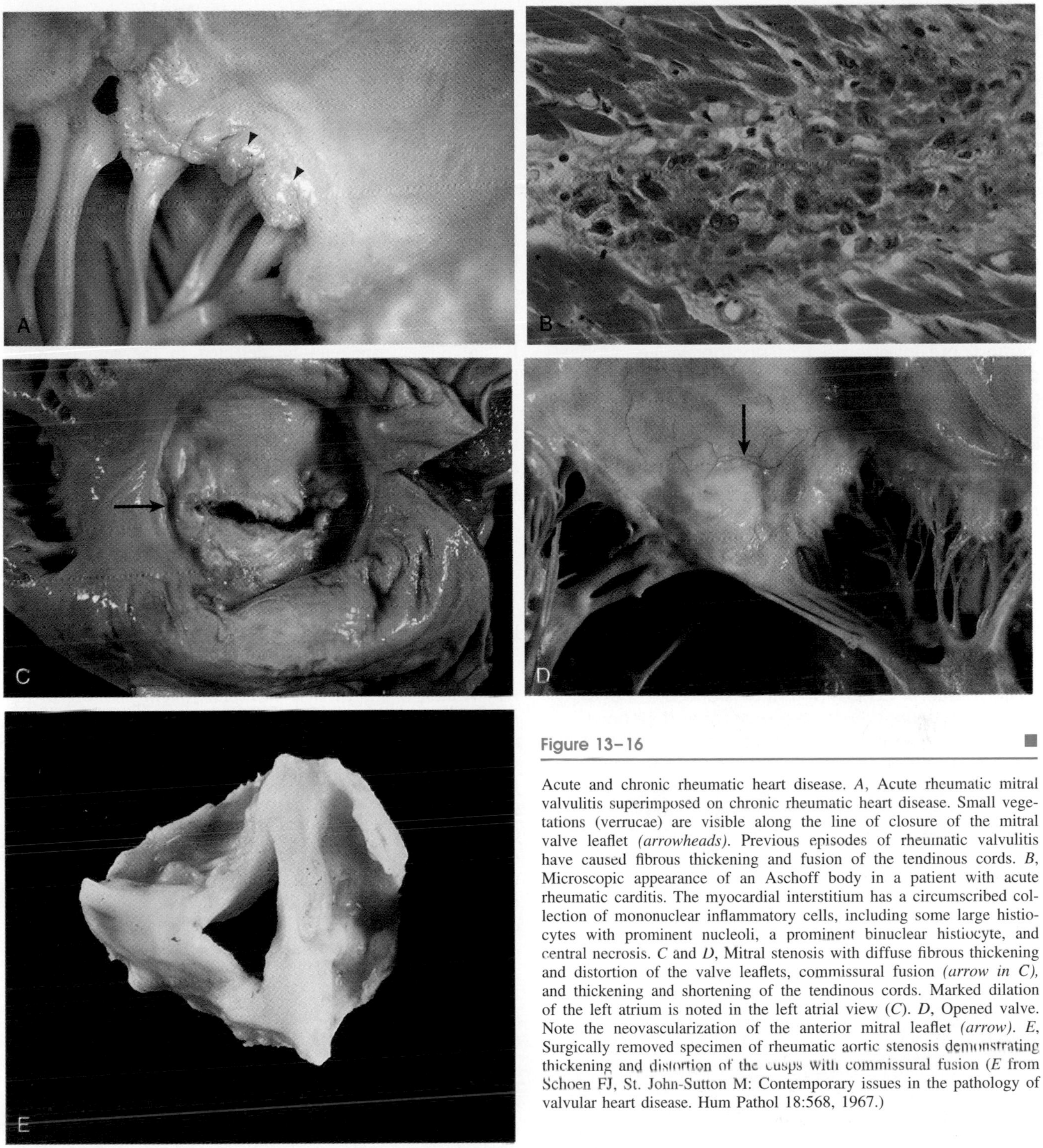

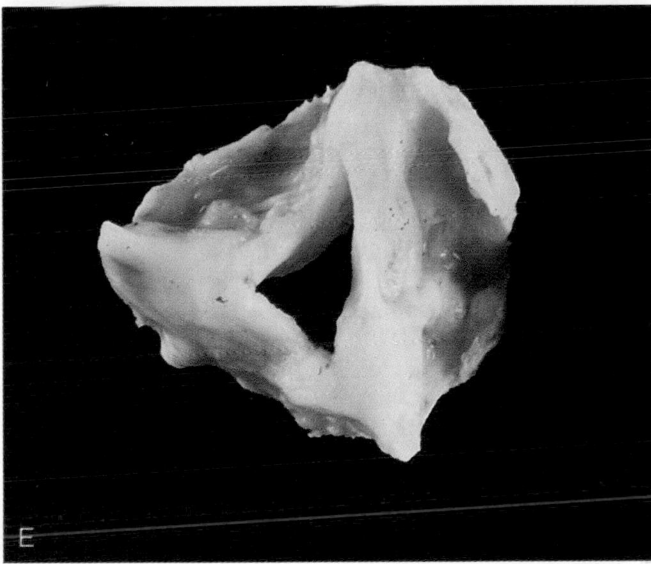

Figure 13–16

Acute and chronic rheumatic heart disease. *A*, Acute rheumatic mitral valvulitis superimposed on chronic rheumatic heart disease. Small vegetations (verrucae) are visible along the line of closure of the mitral valve leaflet *(arrowheads)*. Previous episodes of rheumatic valvulitis have caused fibrous thickening and fusion of the tendinous cords. *B*, Microscopic appearance of an Aschoff body in a patient with acute rheumatic carditis. The myocardial interstitium has a circumscribed collection of mononuclear inflammatory cells, including some large histiocytes with prominent nucleoli, a prominent binuclear histiocyte, and central necrosis. *C* and *D*, Mitral stenosis with diffuse fibrous thickening and distortion of the valve leaflets, commissural fusion *(arrow in C)*, and thickening and shortening of the tendinous cords. Marked dilation of the left atrium is noted in the left atrial view (*C*). *D*, Opened valve. Note the neovascularization of the anterior mitral leaflet *(arrow)*. *E*, Surgically removed specimen of rheumatic aortic stenosis demonstrating thickening and distortion of the cusps with commissural fusion (*E* from Schoen FJ, St. John-Sutton M: Contemporary issues in the pathology of valvular heart disease. Hum Pathol 18:568, 1967.)

During acute rheumatic fever, diffuse inflammation and Aschoff bodies may be found in any of the three layers of the heart—pericardium, myocardium, or endocardium—hence a **pancarditis**. In the pericardium, they are accompanied by a fibrinous or serofibrinous pericardial exudate, described as a *bread-and-butter* pericarditis, which generally resolves without sequelae. The myocardial involvement—**myocarditis**—takes the form of scattered Aschoff bodies within the interstitial connective tissue, often perivascular.

Concomitant involvement of the endocardium and the left-sided valves by inflammatory foci typically comprises fibrinoid necrosis within the cusps or along the tendinous cords on which sit small (1 to 2 mm) vegetations—**verrucae**—along the lines of closure. These irregular, warty projections probably result from the precipitation of fibrin at sites of erosion related to underlying inflammation and fibrinoid degeneration. These acute valvular changes cause little disturbance in cardiac function. Subendocardial lesions, perhaps exacerbated by regurgitant jets, may induce irregular thickenings called **MacCallum plaques**, usually in the left atrium.

Chronic rheumatic heart disease is characterized by organization of the acute inflammation and subsequent deforming fibrosis. In particular, the valvular leaflets become thickened and retracted, causing permanent deformity. **In chronic disease, the mitral valve is virtually always deformed, but involvement of another valve, such as the aortic, may be the most clinically important in some cases. The cardinal anatomic changes of the mitral (or tricuspid) valve are leaflet thickening; commissural fusion; and shortening, thickening, and fusion of the tendinous cords** (Fig. 13–16*C* and *D*). Microscopically, there is diffuse fibrosis and often neovascularization that obliterate the originally layered and avascular leaflet architecture. Aschoff bodies are replaced by fibrous scar; diagnostic forms are rarely seen in surgical specimens or autopsy tissue from patients with chronic rheumatic heart disease at extended intervals after acute rheumatic fever.

Rheumatic heart disease is overwhelmingly the most frequent cause of mitral stenosis (99% of cases). In patients with rheumatic heart disease, the mitral valve alone is involved in 65 to 70% of the cases, mitral and aortic in about 25%; similar but generally less severe fibrous thickenings and stenoses can occur in the tricuspid valve and rarely in the pulmonary. Fibrous bridging across the valvular commissures and calcification create **fish mouth** or **buttonhole** stenoses. With tight mitral stenosis, the left atrium progressively dilates and may harbor mural thrombus either in the appendage or along the wall. The long-standing congestive changes in the lungs may induce pulmonary vascular and parenchymal changes and in time lead to right ventricular hypertrophy. The left ventricle is normal with isolated pure mitral stenosis.

Pathogenesis. It is strongly suspected that *acute rheumatic fever is a hypersensitivity reaction induced by group A streptococci*, but the exact pathogenesis remains uncertain.[47] It is proposed that antibodies directed against the M proteins of certain strains of streptococci cross-react with tissue glycoproteins in the heart, joints, and other tissues. The onset of symptoms usually 2 to 3 weeks after infection and the absence of streptococci from the lesions support the concept that rheumatic fever results from an immune response against the offending bacteria. Because the nature of cross-reacting antigens has been difficult to define, it has also been suggested that the streptococcal infection evokes an autoimmune response against self-antigens. Because only a minority of infected patients develop rheumatic fever, it is suspected that genetic susceptibility regulates the hypersensitivity reaction. The proposed pathogenetic sequence is summarized in Figure 13–17. The chronic sequelae result from progressive fibrosis because of both healing of the acute inflammatory lesions and the turbulence induced by ongoing valvular deformities.

Clinical Features. Acute rheumatic fever occurs from 10 days to 6 weeks after an episode of pharyngitis caused by group A streptococci. Acute rheumatic fever appears most often in children between the ages of 5 and 15 years, but about 20% of first attacks occur in middle to later life. Although pharyngeal cultures for streptococci are negative by the time the illness begins, antibodies to one or more streptococcal enzymes, such as streptolysin O and DNAse B, are present and can be detected in the sera of most patients. The predominant clinical manifestations are those of arthritis and carditis. Far more common in adults than in children, *arthritis* typically begins with migratory polyarthritis accompanied by fever in which one large joint after another becomes painful and swollen for a period of days and then subsides spontaneously, leaving no residual disability. Clinical features related to *acute carditis* include pericardial friction rubs, weak heart sounds, tachycardia, and arrhythmias. The myocarditis may cause cardiac dilation that may evolve to functional mitral valve insufficiency or even heart failure. Overall the prognosis for the primary attack is generally good, and only 1% of patients die from fulminant rheumatic fever.

After an initial attack, there is increased vulnerability to reactivation of the disease with subsequent pharyngeal infections, and the same manifestations are likely to appear with each recurrent attack. Carditis is likely to worsen with each recurrence, and damage is cumulative. Other hazards include embolization from mural thrombi, primarily within the atria or their appendages, and infective endocarditis superimposed on deformed valves. *Chronic rheumatic carditis* usually does not cause clinical manifestations for years or even decades after the initial episode of rheumatic fever. The signs and symptoms of valvular disease depend on which cardiac valve or valves are involved. In addition to various cardiac murmurs, cardiac hypertrophy and dilation, and heart failure, patients with chronic rheumatic heart disease may suffer from arrhythmias (particularly atrial fibrillation in the setting of mitral stenosis), thromboembolic complications, and infective endocarditis. The long-term prognosis is highly variable. In some cases, there is a relentless cycle of valvular deformity yielding hemodynamic abnormality, which begets further deforming fibrosis. Surgical replacement of diseased valves with prosthetic devices has greatly improved the outlook for patients with rheumatic heart disease.

INFECTIVE ENDOCARDITIS

Infective endocarditis, one of the most serious of all infections, is characterized by colonization or invasion of the heart valves, the mural endocardium, or other cardiovascular sites by a microbiologic agent, leading to the formation of bulky, friable *vegetations* composed of thrombotic debris and organisms, often associated with destruc-

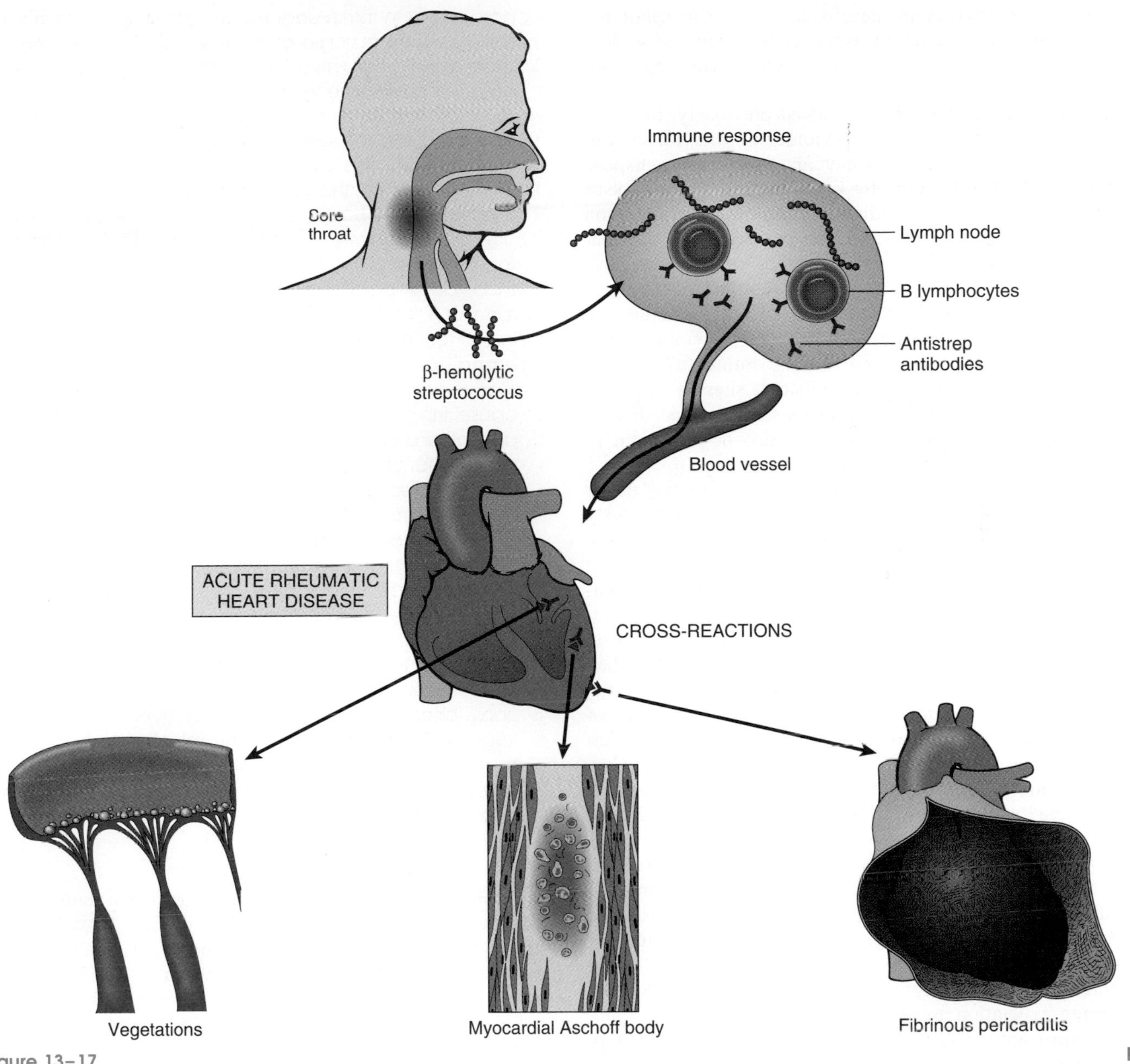

Figure 13–17

The pathogenetic sequence and key morphologic features of acute rheumatic heart disease.

tion of the underlying cardiac tissues. The aorta, aneurysmal sacs, other blood vessels, and prosthetic devices can also become infected. Although fungi, rickettsiae (Q fever), and chlamydiae have at one time or another been responsible for these infections, most cases are bacterial; hence the usual term *bacterial endocarditis.* Prompt diagnosis and effective treatment of endocarditis can significantly alter the outlook for the patient.

Traditionally, endocarditis has been classified on clinical grounds into acute and subacute forms. This subdivision expresses the range of severity of the disease and its tempo, determined in large part by the virulence of the infecting microorganism and the presence of underlying cardiac disease. *Acute endocarditis* describes a destructive, tumultuous infection, frequently of a previously normal heart valve with a highly virulent organism, that leads to death within days to weeks of more than 50% of patients despite antibiotics and surgery. In contrast, organisms of low virulence can cause infection in a previously abnormal heart, particularly on deformed valves. In such cases, the disease may appear insidiously and, even untreated, pursue a protracted course of weeks to months (*subacute endocarditis*). Most patients with subacute infective endocarditis recover after appropriate therapy.

The highly virulent organisms of acute endocarditis tend to produce necrotizing, ulcerative, invasive valvular infections, whereas the lower virulence organisms of subacute disease are less destructive, and the vegetations often show evidence of healing. Both the clinical and the morphologic patterns, however, are points along a spectrum, and a clear delineation between acute and subacute disease does not always exist.

Cause and Pathogenesis. As stated previously, infective endocarditis may develop on previously normal valves, but a variety of cardiac and vascular abnormalities predispose to this form of infection. In years past, rheumatic heart disease was the major contributor, but now more common is myxomatous mitral valve, degenerative calcific valvular stenosis, bicuspid aortic valve (whether calcified or not), and artificial (prosthetic) valves and vascular grafts. Host factors such as neutropenia, immunodeficiency, therapeutic immunosuppression, diabetes mellitus, and alcohol or intravenous drug abuse are predisposing influences. Sterile platelet-fibrin deposits that accumulate at sites of impingement of jet streams caused by preexisting cardiac disease or indwelling vascular catheters may also be important in the development of endocarditis.

The causative organisms differ somewhat in the major high-risk groups. Endocarditis of native but previously damaged or otherwise abnormal valves is caused most commonly (50 to 60% of cases) by α-hemolytic (viridans) streptococci; this is *not* the organism responsible for rheumatic disease discussed earlier. In contrast, the more virulent *Staphylococcus aureus* organisms commonly found on the skin can attack either healthy or deformed valves; they are responsible for 10 to 20% of cases overall and are the major offender in intravenous drug abusers. The roster of the remaining bacteria includes enterococci and the so-called HACEK group (*Haemophilus, Actinobacillus, Cardiobacterium, Eikenella,* and *Kingella*), all commensals in the oral cavity. Prosthetic valve endocarditis is caused most commonly by coagulase-negative staphylococci (e.g., *Staphylococcus epidermidis*). Other agents causing endocarditis include gram-negative bacilli and fungi. In about 10% of all cases of endocarditis, no organism can be isolated from the blood (*culture-negative* endocarditis) because of prior antibiotic therapy, other difficulties in isolation of the offending agent, or deeply embedded organisms within the enlarging vegetation are not released into the blood.

Foremost among the factors predisposing to the development of endocarditis is seeding of the blood with microbes. The portal of entry of the agent into the bloodstream may be an obvious infection elsewhere; a dental or surgical procedure that causes a bacteremia; injection of contaminated material directly into the bloodstream by intravenous drug users; or an occult source from the gut, oral cavity, or trivial injuries. Recognition of predisposing anatomic substrates and clinical conditions causing bacteremia facilitates prevention by appropriate antibiotic prophylaxis.[48]

MORPHOLOGY. Both the subacute and the acute forms of the disease have friable, bulky, and potentially destructive vegetations containing fibrin, inflammatory cells, and bacteria or other organisms, most commonly on the heart valves (Fig. 13–18). The aortic and mitral valves are the most common sites of infection, although the valves of the right side of the heart may also be involved, particularly in intravenous drug abusers. The vegetations may be single or multiple and may involve more than one valve. Vegetations are often destructive and sometimes erode into the underlying myocardium to produce an abscess cavity (**ring abscess**), one of several important complications (Fig. 13–18*B*). The appearance of the vegetations is influenced by the type of organism responsible, the degree of host reaction to the infection, and previous antibiotic therapy. **Fungal endocarditis**, for example, tends to cause larger vegetations than does bacterial infection. In the subacute form of the disease, vegetations are smaller and less often erode or perforate the cusps. **Systemic emboli** may occur at any time because of the friable nature of the vegetations, and they may cause infarcts in the brain, kidneys, myocardium, and other tissues. Because the embolic fragments contain large numbers of virulent organisms, abscesses often develop at the sites of such infarcts (**septic infarcts**).

Microscopically the vegetations of typical subacute infective endocarditis often have granulation tissue at their bases. With the passage of time, fibrosis, calcification, and a chronic inflammatory infiltrate may develop. Figure 13–19 compares the gross appearance of the vegetations of infective endocarditis with those of the valve lesions characterized by noninfective thrombotic vegetations (nonbacterial thrombotic endocarditis (NBTE)) and the endocarditis of systemic lupus erythematosus, called *Libman-Sacks endocarditis* (see later).

Clinical Features. Fever is the most consistent sign of infective endocarditis. With subacute disease, however, particularly in the elderly, fever may be slight or absent, and the only manifestations are sometimes nonspecific fatigue, loss of weight, and a flulike syndrome. Murmurs are present in 90% of patients with left-sided lesions but may merely relate to the preexisting cardiac abnormality predisposing to endocarditis. The previously important clinical findings of petechiae, subungual hemorrhages, and Roth spots in the eyes (secondary to retinal microemboli) have now become uncommon owing to the shortened clinical course of the disease as a result of antibiotic therapy.

In contrast, acute endocarditis has a stormy onset with rapidly developing fever, chills, weakness, and lassitude. Complications generally begin within the first weeks of the onset of the disease. Murmur is common because of the large size of the vegetations or leaflet destruction. Ring abscess is frequent, and the vegetations are also more likely to embolize.

Sometimes complications involving the heart or extracardiac sites call attention to endocarditis. They include the following:

- *Cardiac complications:*
  - Valvular insufficiency or stenosis with cardiac failure
  - Myocardial ring abscess, with possible perforation of

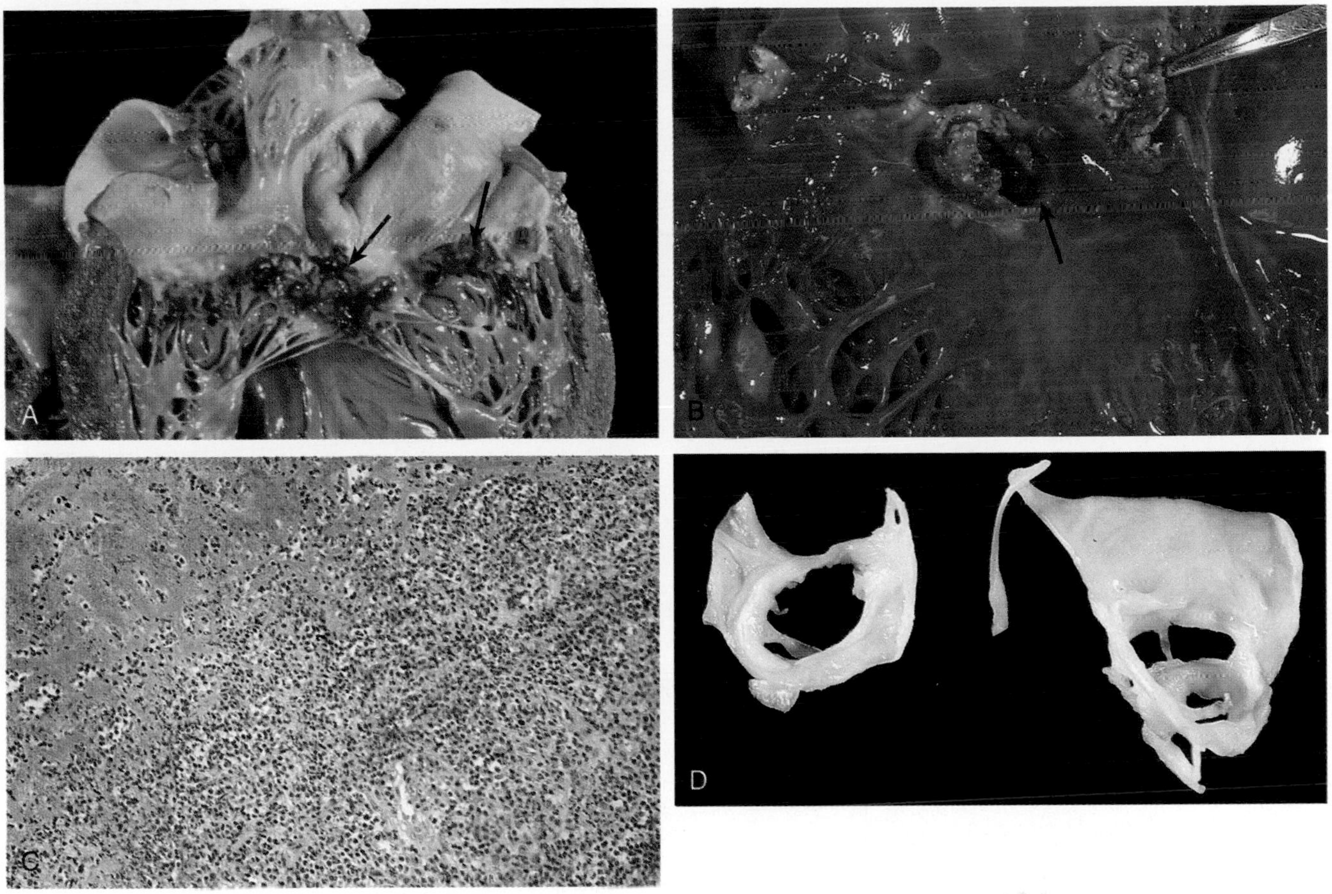

Figure 13–18

Bacterial infective endocarditis. *A*, Endocarditis of the mitral valve (subacute, caused by *Streptococcus viridens*). The irregular, large friable vegetations are denoted by arrows. *B*, Acute endocarditis of a congenitally bicuspid aortic valve (caused by *Staphylococcus aureus*) with severe cuspal destruction and ring abscess *(arrow)*. *C*, Histologic appearance of vegetation of endocarditis with extensive acute inflammatory cells and fibrin. Bacterial organisms were demonstrated by tissue Gram stain. *D*, Gross photograph illustrating healed endocarditis with perforations on bicuspid aortic valve.

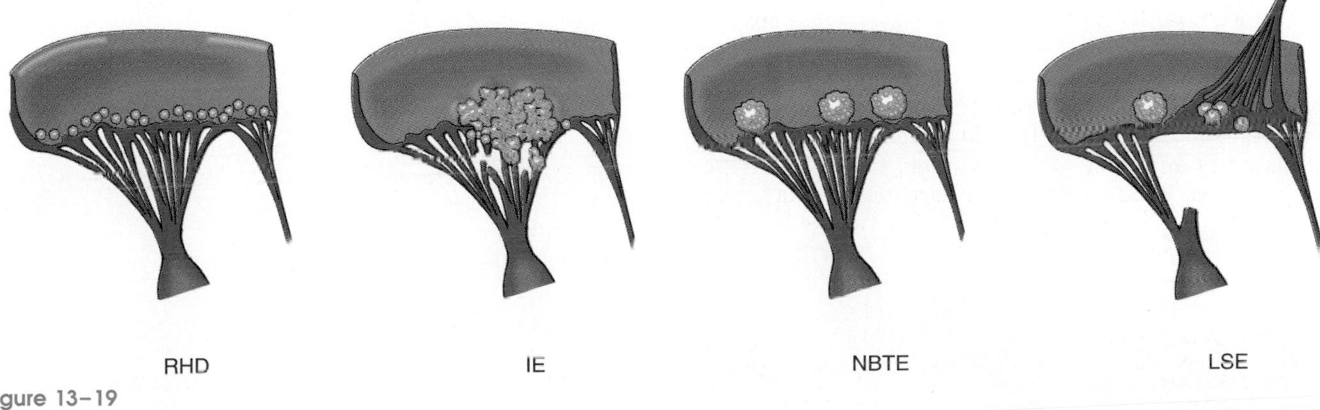

Figure 13–19

Diagrammatic comparison of the lesions in the four major forms of vegetative endocarditis. The rheumatic fever phase of RHD (rheumatic heart disease) is marked by a row of warty, small vegetations along the lines of closure of the valve leaflets. IE (infective endocarditis) is characterized by large, irregular masses on the valve cusps that can extend onto the cords (see Fig. 13–18*A*). NBTE (nonbacterial thrombotic endocarditis) typically exhibits small, bland vegetations, usually attached at the line of closure. One or many may be present (see Fig. 13–20). LSE (Libman-Sacks endocarditis) has small or medium-sized vegetations on either or both sides of the valve leaflets.

aorta, interventricular septum or free wall, or invasion of the conduction system
  - Suppurative pericarditis
  - With endocarditis on artificial valves, partial dehiscence with paravalvular leak
- *Embolic complications*:
  - With left-sided lesions—to the brain (cerebral infarct or abscess, meningitis), heart (MI), spleen (abscess), kidneys (abscess), other sites
  - With right-sided lesions—to the lungs (infarct, abscess, pneumonia)
- *Renal complications:*
  - Embolic infarction
  - Focal and diffuse glomerulonephritis, owing to trapping of antigen-antibody complexes, which may lead to hematuria, albuminuria, or renal failure (Chapter 21)
  - Multiple abscesses—especially with acute staphylococcal endocarditis

Although the diagnosis can be suspected based on the appearance of one or more of the complications mentioned, a positive blood culture is required for confirmation. With repeated blood samples, positive cultures can be obtained in about 90% of cases. As important as the diagnosis of infective endocarditis is its prevention by the prophylactic use of antibiotics in the patient with some form of cardiac anomaly or artificial valve who is about to have a dental, surgical, or other invasive procedure.

NONINFECTED VEGETATIONS

Nonbacterial Thrombotic Endocarditis

NBTE is characterized by the deposition of small masses of fibrin, platelets, and other blood components on the leaflets of the cardiac valves. In contrast to the vegetations of infective endocarditis, discussed previously, *the valvular lesions of NBTE are sterile, do not contain microorganisms, and are only loosely attached to the underlying valve.* NBTE is often encountered in debilitated patients, such as those with cancer or sepsis—hence the previously used term *marantic endocarditis.* Although the local effect on the valves is unimportant, NBTE may achieve clinical significance by producing emboli and resultant infarcts in the brain, heart, or elsewhere.

MORPHOLOGY. NBTE is characterized by the deposition of masses of fibrin and other blood elements on the valve leaflets of either side of the heart, usually on previously normal valves. In contrast to infective endocarditis, the vegetations of NBTE are sterile, nondestructive, noninflammatory, and small (1 to 5 mm) and occur singly or multiply along the line of closure of the leaflets or cusps (Fig. 13–20). Histologically, they are composed of bland thrombus without accompanying inflammatory reaction or induced valve damage. Should the patient survive the underlying disease, organization may occur, leaving delicate strands of fibrous tissue.

Pathogenesis. NBTE frequently occurs concomitantly with venous thromboses or pulmonary embolism, suggesting *a common origin in a hypercoagulable state with systemic activation of blood coagulation such as disseminated intravascular coagulation. This may be related to some underlying disease, such as a cancer* and, in particular, mucinous adenocarcinomas of the pancreas. The striking association with mucinous adenocarcinomas in general may relate to the procoagulant effect of circulating mucin, and thus NBTE can be a part of the Trousseau syndrome. Lesions of NBTE, however, are also seen occasionally in association with non–mucin-producing malignancy, such as acute promyelocytic leukemia, and in other debilitating dis-

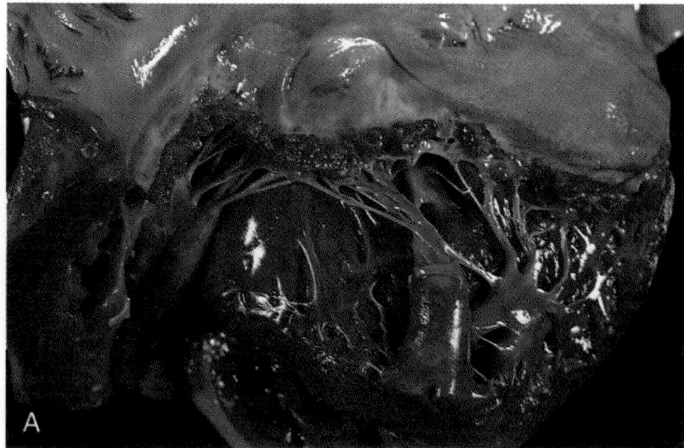

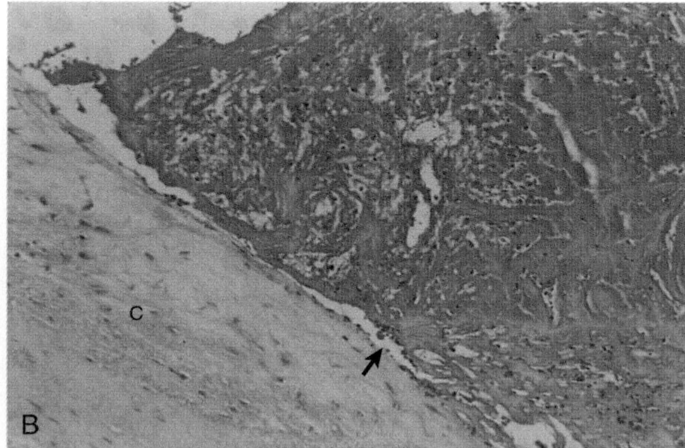

Figure 13–20

Nonbacterial thrombotic endocarditis (NBTE). *A*, Nearly complete row of thrombotic vegetations along the line of closure of the mitral valve leaflets. *B*, Photomicrograph of NBTE showing bland thrombus, with virtually no inflammation in the valve cusp (c) or the thrombotic deposit. The thrombus is only loosely attached to the cusp *(arrow)*.

eases or conditions promoting hypercoagulability (e.g., hyperestrogenic states, extensive burns, or sepsis). Endocardial trauma as from an indwelling catheter is also a well-recognized predisposing condition, and one frequently encounters right-sided valvular and endocardial thrombotic lesions along the track of a Swan-Ganz pulmonary artery catheter.

Endocarditis of Systemic Lupus Erythematosus (Libman-Sacks Endocarditis)

In systemic lupus erythematosus, mitral and tricuspid valvulitis with small, sterile vegetations called *Libman-Sacks endocarditis* is occasionally encountered. Thrombotic heart valve lesions with sterile vegetations or rarely fibrous thickening commonly occur with the antiphospholipid syndrome[49] (Chapter 7). Circulating antiphospholipid antibodies are also commonly associated with venous or arterial thrombosis, recurrent pregnancy loss, or thrombocytopenia. The mitral valve is more frequently involved than the aortic; regurgitation is the usual functional abnormality.

MORPHOLOGY. The lesions are small single or multiple, sterile, granular pink vegetations ranging from 1 to 4 mm in diameter. Frequently the lesions are located on the undersurfaces of the AV valves, but they may be scattered on the valvular endocardium, on the cords, and on the mural endocardium of atria or ventricles. Histologically the verrucae consist of a finely granular, fibrinous eosinophilic material that may contain hematoxylin bodies (the tissue equivalent of the lupus erythematosus cell of the blood and bone marrow; Chapter 7). An intense valvulitis may be present, characterized by fibrinoid necrosis of the valve substance that is often contiguous with the vegetation. Leaflet vegetations can be difficult in some cases to distinguish from those of infectious endocarditis or NBTE. Subsequent fibrosis and serious deformity can result that resemble chronic rheumatic heart disease and require surgery.

CARCINOID HEART DISEASE

Principally involving the endocardium and valves of the right side of the heart, cardiac lesions involve one half of patients with the *carcinoid syndrome*, itself characterized by *episodic flushing of the skin, cramps, nausea, vomiting, and diarrhea* (Chapter 18).

MORPHOLOGY. The cardiovascular lesions associated with the carcinoid syndrome are distinctive, comprising fibrous intimal thickenings on the inside surfaces of the cardiac chambers and valvular leaflets, mainly in the right ventricle and tricuspid and pulmonic valves, and occasionally the major blood vessels (Fig. 13–21). The endocardial plaquelike thickenings are composed predominantly of smooth muscle cells and sparse collagen fibers embedded in an acid mucopolysaccharide-rich matrix material that expands the endocardium. Elastic fibers are not present. Underlying structures are intact, including the valve layers and the subendocardial elastic tissue layer. Occasionally, left-sided lesions are also encountered.

The clinical and pathologic findings relate to the elaboration by carcinoid tumors of a variety of bioactive products, including serotonin (5-hydroxytryptamine), kallikrein, bradykinin, histamine, prostaglandins, and tachykinins. Which of the secretory products induces the syndrome or the cardiac pathology is still not clear, but there is a correlation of the plasma levels of serotonin urinary excretion of the serotonin metabolite 5-hy-

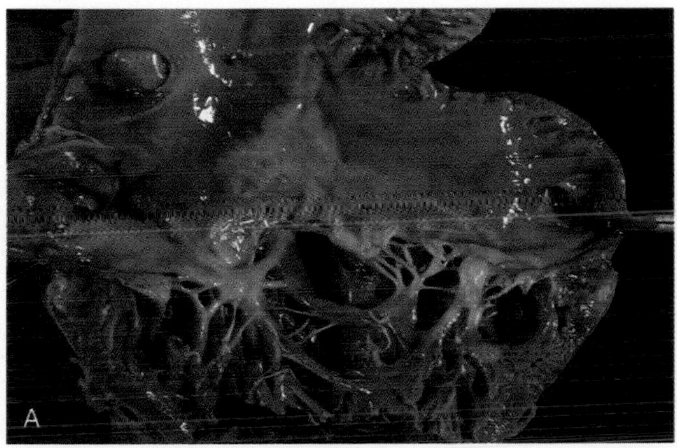

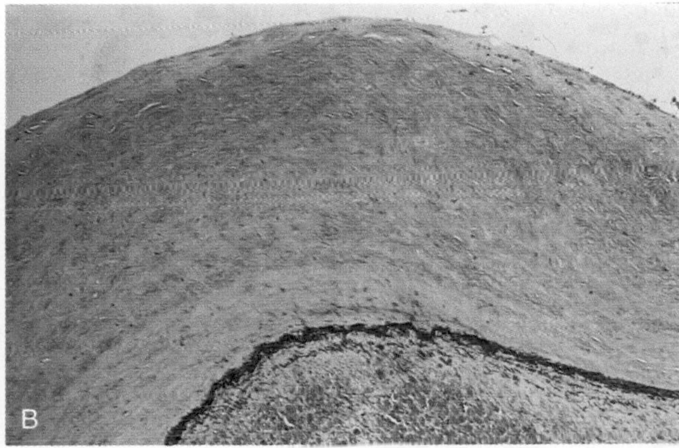

Figure 13–21

Carcinoid heart disease. *A*, Characteristic endocardial fibrotic lesion involving the right ventricle and tricuspid valve. *B*, Microscopic appearance of carcinoid heart disease with intimal thickening. Movat staining shows underlying myocardial elastic tissue as black and acid mucopolysaccharides as blue-green.

droxyindoleacetic acid with the severity of the right-sided heart lesions.[50]

The fact that the cardiac changes are largely right-sided is explained by inactivation of both serotonin and bradykinin in the blood during passage through the lungs by the monoamine oxidase found in the pulmonary vascular endothelium. In the absence of hepatic metastases, gastrointestinal carcinoids (with venous drainage via the portal system) do not usually induce the carcinoid syndrome because there is rapid metabolism of serotonin during passage of blood through the liver. In contrast, carcinoid tumors primary in organs outside of the portal system of venous drainage (e.g., ovary or lung), whose venous drainage bypasses the liver, may induce the syndrome without antecedent hepatic metastases. Left-sided lesions can occur when blood containing the responsible mediator enters the left side of the heart owing to incomplete inactivation of high blood levels or with a pulmonary carcinoid or patent foramen ovale with right-to-left flow.

Rarely, similar left-sided plaques are found in patients who receive methysergide or ergotamine therapy for migraine headaches; these serotonin analogs are metabolized to serotonin as they pass through the pulmonary vasculature. Left-sided valve lesions with pathologic features similar to those seen in the carcinoid syndrome have also been reported to complicate the use of fenfluramine and phentermine (*fen-phen*), appetite suppressants used for the treatment of obesity that may affect systemic serotonin metabolism.[51]

COMPLICATIONS OF ARTIFICIAL VALVES

Replacement of damaged cardiac valves with prostheses has now become a common and often lifesaving mode of therapy.[52] Artificial valves fall primarily into two categories: (1) *Mechanical prostheses* use various rigid, mobile occluders composed of nonphysiologic biomaterials, such as caged balls, tilting discs, or hinged semicircular flaps, and (2) tissue valves are usually *bioprostheses* that consist of chemically treated animal tissue, especially porcine aortic valve tissue, which has been preserved in a dilute glutaraldehyde solution and subsequently mounted on a frame (called a *stent*). Tissue valves are flexible and function somewhat like natural semilunar valves.

Approximately 60% of substitute valve recipients develop a serious prosthesis-related problem within 10 years postoperatively.[53] Although the *frequency* of total prosthetic valve–related events is similar among valve categories, the *nature* of these complications differs among types (Table 13–7 and Fig. 13–22).

Table 13–7. CAUSES OF FAILURE OF CARDIAC VALVE PROSTHESES

- Thrombosis/thromboembolism
- Anticoagulant-related hemorrhage
- Prosthetic valve endocarditis
- Structural deterioration (intrinsic)
  - Wear, fracture, poppet escape, cuspal tear, calcification
- Nonstructural dysfunction
  - Pannus, suture/tissue entrapment, paravalvular leak, disproportion, hemolytic anemia, noise

- *Thromboembolic complications* constituting local obstruction of the prosthesis by thrombus or distant thromboemboli are the major problem with mechanical valves (Fig. 13–22). This problem necessitates long-term anticoagulation in patients with these devices. Moreover, hemorrhagic complications, such as stroke or gastrointestinal bleeding, may arise secondarily in patients who receive long-term anticoagulation.
- *Infective endocarditis* is infrequent but serious. Always with mechanical valves and frequently with bioprostheses, endocarditis is located at the prosthesis-tissue interface, causing a ring abscess, which can eventuate in a paravalvular regurgitant blood leak. In addition, vegetations may directly involve bioprosthetic valvular cusps. The major organisms causing such infections are staphylococcal skin contaminants (e.g., *S. aureus, S. epidermidis*) and streptococci.
- *Structural deterioration* uncommonly causes failure of contemporary mechanical valves. It is a major failure mode of bioprostheses, however, usually with calcification or cuspal tearing, or both, causing secondary regurgitation.
- Other complications include hemolysis induced by high blood shear, mechanical obstruction to flow inherent in all artificial valves, and dysfunction owing to overgrowth by fibrous tissue.

Myocardial Disease

It should be clear from the previous sections that myocardial dysfunction occurs commonly but secondarily in a

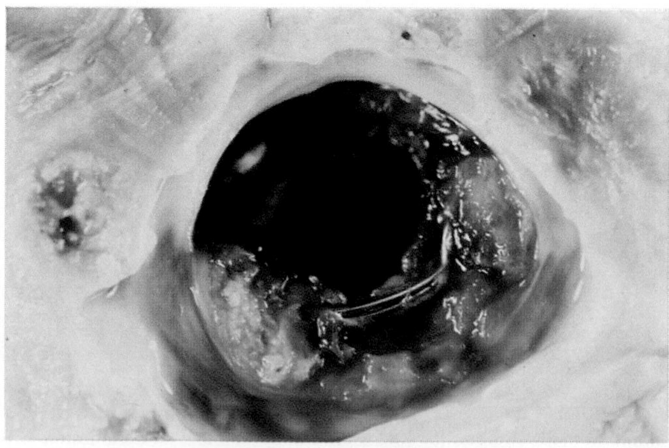

Figure 13–22

Thrombosis of a mechanical prosthetic heart valve.

number of different conditions, such as IHD, hypertension, and valvular heart disease. Far less frequently observed is disease whose cause is intrinsic to the myocardium. Myocardial diseases are a diverse group that includes inflammatory disorders (*myocarditis*), immunologic diseases, systemic metabolic disorders, muscular dystrophies, genetic abnormalities in cardiac muscle cells, and an additional group of diseases of unknown cause.

The term *cardiomyopathy* (literally, heart muscle disease) could be applied to almost any heart disease but by convention is used to describe *heart disease resulting from a primary abnormality in the myocardium.* This definition is somewhat arbitrary and often frustrating as one attempts to wade through various classification schemes,[54, 55] because some authors exclude any myocardial disorder of known cause, while others take a more ecumenical view and include any heart disease manifested by primary myocardial dysfunction. Although chronic myocardial dysfunction owing to ischemia should also be excluded from the cardiomyopathy rubric, the term *ischemic cardiomyopathy* has gained some popularity among clinicians to describe congestive heart failure caused by coronary artery disease.

In many cases, cardiomyopathies are *idiopathic* (i.e., of unknown cause), but in some instances, well-defined myocardial diseases may, in the end, resemble those without known causes, both functionally and structurally. A major advance in understanding of myocardial disease has been the demonstration that specific genetic abnormalities in cardiac energy metabolism or structural and contractile proteins underlie myocardial dysfunction in many patients that previously was considered idiopathic.[57] Thus, etiologic distinctions have become somewhat blurred. Therefore, our discussion herein avoids the controversies associated with classification schemes and emphasizes etiologic and mechanistic considerations in the context of clinicopathologic features.

Without additional data, the clinician encountering a patient with myocardial disease is usually unaware of the cause. The clinical picture is largely determined by one of the following three clinical, functional, and pathologic patterns (Fig. 13–23 and Table 13–8):

- Dilated cardiomyopathy (DCM)
- Hypertrophic cardiomyopathy (HCM)
- Restrictive cardiomyopathy

Among these three categories, the dilated form is most common (90% of cases), and the restrictive is least prevalent. Within the hemodynamic patterns of myocardial dysfunction, there is a spectrum of clinical severity, and overlap of clinical features often occurs between groups. Moreover, each of these patterns can be either idiopathic or due to a specific identifiable cause or secondary to primary extramyocardial disease (Table 13–9).

Endomyocardial biopsies are used widely in the diagnosis and management of patients with myocardial disease and cardiac transplant recipients. Endomyocardial biopsy involves inserting a device (called a *bioptome*) transvenously into the right side of the heart and snipping a small piece of myocardium in its jaws. The resulting pieces of myocardium are examined histologically.

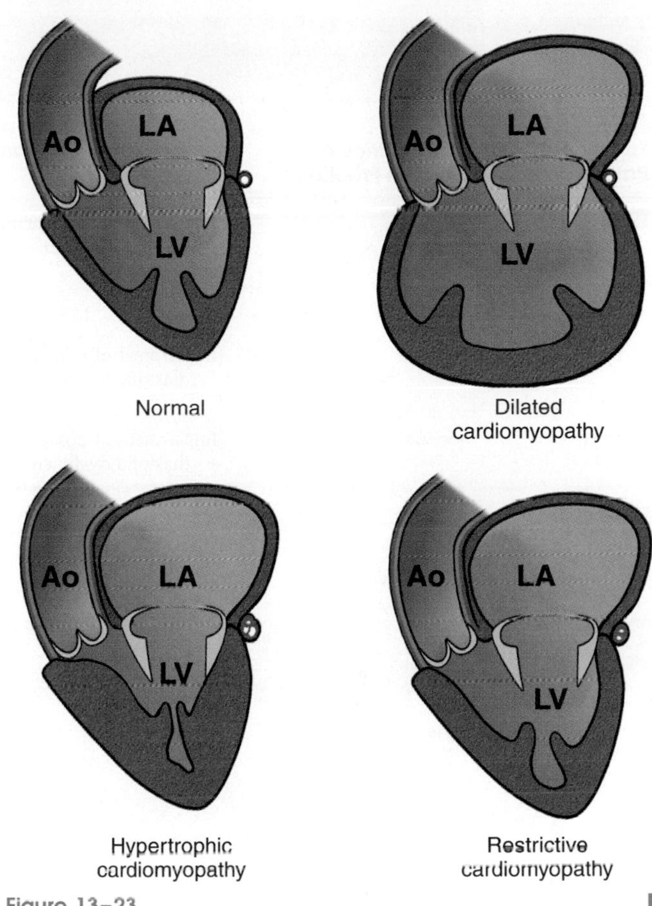

Figure 13–23

Representation of the three distinctive clinical-pathologic-functional forms of myocardial disease.

DILATED CARDIOMYOPATHY

DCM is applied to a form of cardiomyopathy characterized by *progressive cardiac hypertrophy, dilation,* and *contractile (systolic) dysfunction*. It is sometimes called *congestive cardiomyopathy*. This clinicopathologic picture can result from a number of different myocardial insults whose morphology and consequences resemble DCM.

- Myocarditis (see later): *Viral nucleic acids* from coxsackievirus B and other enteroviruses have been detected in the myocardium of some patients, and sequential endomyocardial biopsies have demonstrated progression from myocarditis to DCM in others, suggesting that, in at least some cases, DCM was a consequence of myocarditis.
- Alcohol or other toxicity: *Alcohol abuse* is also strongly associated with the development of DCM, raising the possibility that ethanol toxicity (Chapter 10) or a secondary nutritional disturbance may be the cause of the myocardial injury. Alcohol or its metabolites (especially acetaldehyde) have a direct toxic effect on the myocardium. Nevertheless, a cause-and-effect relationship with alcohol alone remains tenuous, and no morphologic features serve to distinguish *alcoholic cardiomyopathy* from

Table 13–8. CARDIOMYOPATHY AND INDIRECT MYOCARDIAL DYSFUNCTION: FUNCTIONAL PATTERNS AND CAUSES

Functional Pattern	Left Ventricular Ejection Fraction*	Mechanisms of Heart Failure	Causes	Indirect Myocardial Dysfunction (Not Cardiomyopathy)
Dilated	<40%	Impairment of contractility (systolic dysfunction)	Idiopathic; alcohol; peripartum; genetic; myocarditis; hemochromatosis; chronic anemia; doxorubicin (Adriamycin); sarcoidosis	Ischemic heart disease; valvular heart disease; hypertensive heart disease; congenital heart disease
Hypertrophic	50–80%	Impairment of compliance (diastolic dysfunction)	Idiopathic; genetic; Friedreich ataxia; storage diseases; infants of diabetic mothers	Hypertensive heart disease; aortic stenosis
Restrictive	45–90%	Impairment of compliance (diastolic dysfunction)	Idiopathic; amyloidosis; radiation-induced fibrosis	Pericardial constriction

*Normal, approximately 50–65%.

Table 13–9. MAJOR ASSOCIATIONS OF SPECIFIC HEART MUSCLE DISEASE

Cardiac Infections
Viruses
Chlamydiae
Rickettsiae
Bacteria
Fungi
Protozoa

Toxic
Alcohol
Cobalt
Catecholamines
Carbon monoxide
Lithium
Hydrocarbons
Arsenic
Cyclophosphamide
Doxorubicin (Adriamycin) and daunorubicin

Metabolic
Hyperthyroidism
Hypothyroidism
Hypokalemia
Hyperkalemia
Nutritional deficiency (protein, thiamine, other avitaminoses)
Hemochromatosis

Neuromuscular Disease
Friedreich ataxia
Muscular dystrophy
Congenital atrophies

Storage Disorders and Other Depositions
Hunter-Hurler syndrome
Glycogen storage disease
Fabry disease
Amyloidosis

Infiltrative
Leukemia
Carcinomatosis
Sarcoidosis
Radiation-induced fibrosis

Immunologic
Myocarditis (several forms)
Post-transplant rejection

DCM of other etiology. Moreover, chronic alcoholism may be associated with thiamine deficiency, introducing an element of beriberi heart disease (also indistinguishable from DCM) (Chapter 10). In yet other cases, a nonalcoholic *toxic insult* is the cause of the myocardial failure. Particularly important in this last group (as discussed later) is myocardial injury caused by certain chemotherapeutic agents, including doxorubicin (Adriamycin). In the past, cobalt has also caused congestive heart failure.

- Pregnancy-associated: A special form of DCM, termed *peripartum cardiomyopathy*, occurs late in pregnancy or several weeks to months postpartum. The cause of peripartum cardiomyopathy is poorly understood but is probably multifactorial. Pregnancy-associated hypertension, volume overload, nutritional deficiency, other metabolic derangement, or as yet poorly characterized immunologic reaction may be involved.
- Genetic: *Genetic influences* have been documented in some cases, particularly when multiple members of a family are affected. DCM has a familial occurrence in 20 to 30% of cases. Autosomal dominant, autosomal recessive, and X-linked inheritance have all been proposed for particular kindreds. Genetic linkage studies in some families have indicated deletions in the mitochondrial genes causing abnormal oxidative phosphorylation, mutations in genes encoding enzymes involved in β-oxidation of fatty acids, and mutations in the gene for dystrophin. The last-mentioned, as described in Chapter 30, is a cell membrane–based cytoskeletal protein that is thought to play a critical role in linking the internal cytoskeleton with the external basement membrane and is the protein mutated in Duchenne and Becker muscular dystrophies.[58] Some patients and families with dystrophin gene mutations have DCM as their primary clinical feature, suggesting either differences in dystrophin function or control of expression between cardiac and skeletal muscle.

Together, the various known causes account for only a fraction of all cases. In others, the cause is unknown, and they are appropriately designated as idiopathic DCM.

MORPHOLOGY. In DCM, the heart is usually heavy, weighing two to three times normal, and large and flabby, with dilation of all chambers (Fig. 13–24). Nevertheless, because of the wall thinning that accompanies dilation, the ventricular wall thickness may be less than, equal to, or more than normal. Mural thrombi are common and may be a source of thromboemboli. Primary valvular alterations are absent, and mitral or tricuspid regurgitation when present are a result of left ventricular chamber dilation (functional regurgitation). The coronary arteries are usually free of significant narrowing, but any coronary arterial obstructions that do exist are insufficient to explain the degree of cardiac dysfunction.

The histologic abnormalities in idiopathic DCM also are nonspecific and usually do not reflect a specific causative agent. Their severity does not necessarily reflect the degree of dysfunction or the patient's prognosis. Most muscle cells are hypertrophied with enlarged nuclei, but many are attenuated or stretched. Interstitial and endocardial fibrosis of variable degree is present, and small subendocardial scars replace individual cells or groups of cells, probably reflecting healing of previous secondary myocyte ischemic necrosis caused by hypertrophy-induced imbalance between perfusion supply and demand.

Clinical Features. DCM may occur at any age, including in childhood, but it commonly affects those 20 to 60 years old. It presents with slowly progressive congestive heart failure, but patients may slip precipitously from a compensated to a decompensated functional state. In the end stage, patients often have ejection fractions of less than 25% (normal approximately 50 to 65%). Fifty percent of patients die within 2 years, and only 25% survive longer than 5 years. Death is usually attributable to progressive cardiac failure or arrhythmia. Embolism from dislodgment of an intracardiac thrombus may occur. Cardiac transplantation is frequently recommended.

A variant is *arrhythmogenic right ventricular cardiomyopathy* or *arrhythmogenic right ventricular dysplasia*, a sometimes familial disorder that is most commonly associated with right-sided and sometimes left-sided heart failure and various rhythm disturbances, particularly ventricular tachycardia.[59] Sudden death may occur. Morphologically the right ventricular wall is severely thinned because of loss of myocytes, with extensive fatty infiltration and interstitial fibrosis. Although a gene defect was localized on chromosome 14, the pathogenesis remains obscure.

HYPERTROPHIC CARDIOMYOPATHY

HCM is also known by such terms as *idiopathic hypertrophic subaortic stenosis* and *hypertrophic obstructive cardiomyopathy.* It is characterized by *myocardial hypertrophy, abnormal diastolic filling,* and, in about one third of cases, *intermittent left ventricular outflow obstruction.* The heart is heavy, muscular, and *hypercontracting*, in striking contrast to the flabby, *hypocontracting* heart of DCM. HCM is primarily a diastolic rather than systolic disorder.

MORPHOLOGY. The essential feature of HCM is massive myocardial hypertrophy without ventricular dilation (Fig. 13–25). The classic pattern is said

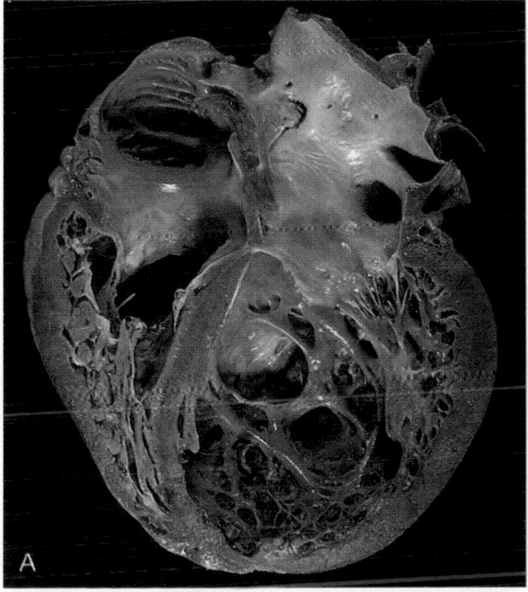

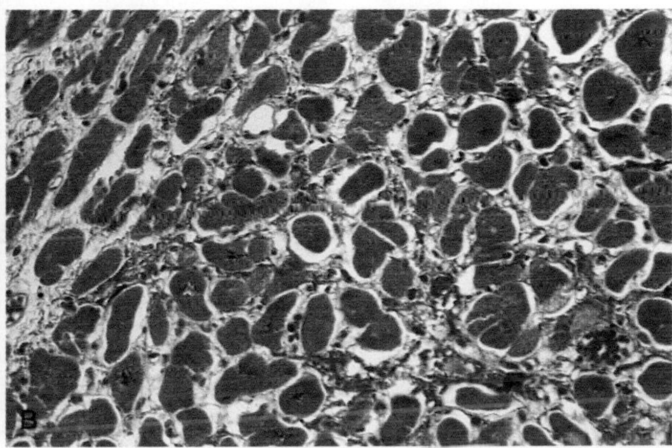

Figure 13–24

Dilated cardiomyopathy. *A*, Gross photograph. Four-chamber dilation and hypertrophy are evident. There is granular mural thrombus at the apex of the left ventricle (on the right in this apical four-chamber view). The coronary arteries were unobstructed. *B*, Histology demonstrating variable myocyte hypertrophy and interstitial fibrosis (collagen is highlighted as blue in this Masson trichrome strain).

to be disproportionate thickening of the ventricular septum as compared with the free wall of the left ventricle (with a ratio >1.3), frequently termed **asymmetric septal hypertrophy**. In about 10% of cases, however, the hypertrophy is symmetric throughout the heart. On cross-section, the ventricular cavity loses its usual round-to-ovoid shape and may be compressed into a **banana-like** configuration by bulging of the ventricular septum into the lumen (Fig. 13–25*A*). Although disproportionate hypertrophy can involve the entire septum, it is usually most prominent in the subaortic region. Also often present are endocardial thickening or mural plaque formation in the left ventricular outflow tract and thickening of the anterior mitral leaflet; both findings are a result of

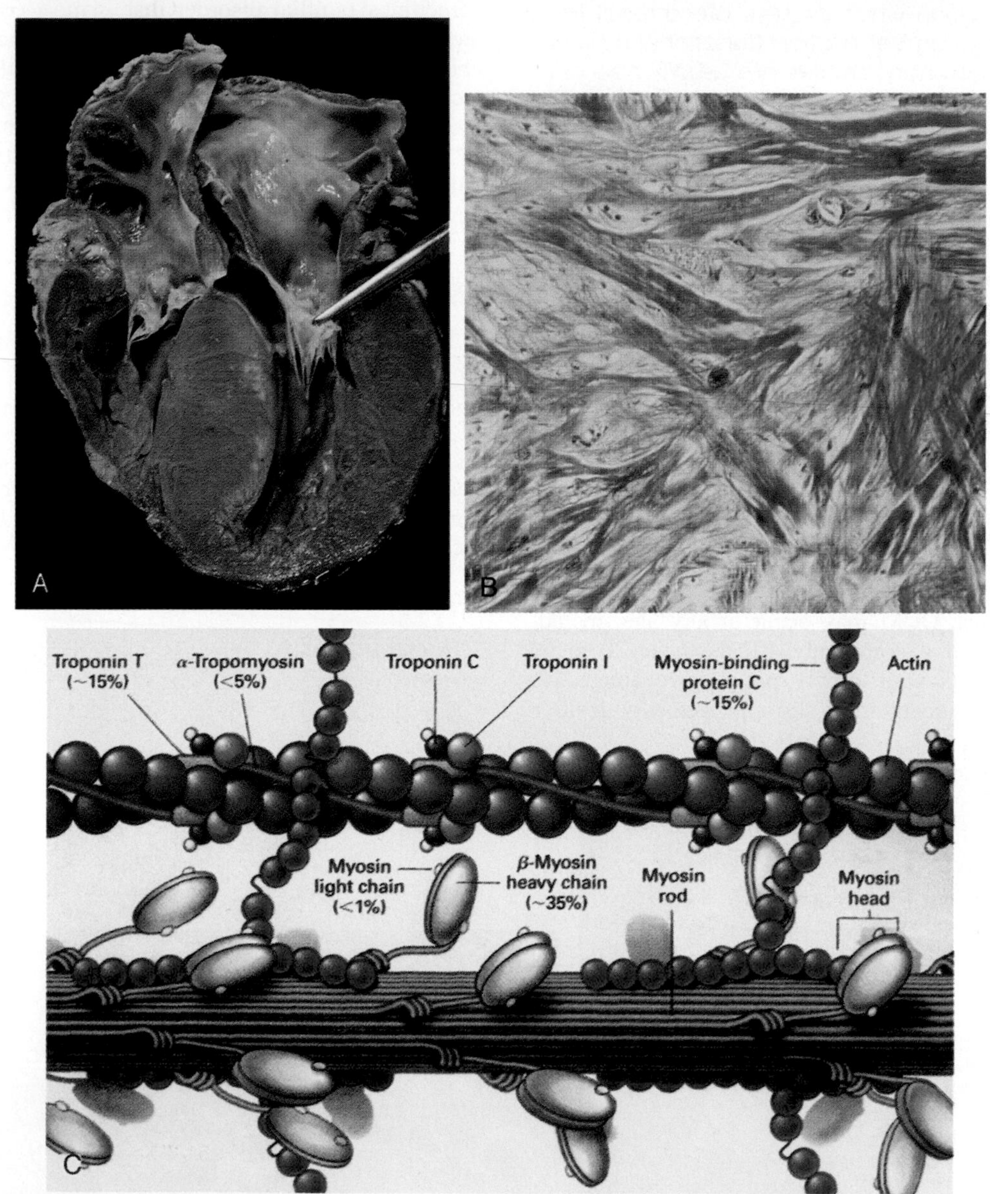

Figure 13–25 ■

Hypertrophic cardiomyopathy. *A*, There is asymmetric hypertrophy of the septal muscle, which bulges into the left ventricular outflow tract, and the left atrium is enlarged. Apical four-chamber view; left ventricle on right. The anterior mitral leaflet has been moved away from the septum to reveal a fibrous endocardial plaque (see text). (From Schoen FJ: Interventional and Surgical Cardiovascular Pathology: Clinical Correlations and Basic Principles. Philadelphia, WB Saunders, 1989, p 180.) *B*, Histologic appearance demonstrating disarray, extreme hypertrophy, and peculiar branching of myocytes as well as interstitial fibrosis (collagen is blue in this Masson trichrome stain). *C*, Structure of the sarcomere of cardiac muscle, highlighting proteins in which mutations cause defective contraction, hypertrophy, and myocyte disarray in hypertrophic cardiomyopathy. The frequency of a particular gene mutation is indicated as a percentage; most common are mutations in β-myosin heavy chain. Normal contraction of the sarcomere involves myosin-actin interaction initiated by calcium binding to troponin C, I, and T and α-tropomyosin. Actin stimulates ATPase activity in the myosin head and produces force along the actin filaments. Myocyte-binding protein C modulates contraction. (From Spirito P, et al: The management of hypertrophic cardiomyopathy. N Engl J Med 336:775, 1997.)

contact of the anterior mitral leaflet with the septum during ventricular systole correlating with the echocardiographic functional left ventricular outflow tract obstruction during midsystole. End-stage ventricular dilation may occur late in a minority of patients.

The most important histologic features of the myocardium in HCM are (1) extensive myocyte hypertrophy to a degree unusual in other conditions, with transverse myocyte diameters frequently more than 40 μm (normal approximately 15 μm); (2) haphazard disarray of bundles of myocytes, individual myocytes, and contractile elements in sarcomeres within cells (**myofiber disarray**); and (3) interstitial and replacement fibrosis (Fig. 13–25*B*).

The two most common diseases that must be distinguished from HCM are amyloidosis and other infiltrative/deposition disorders (see later) and hypertensive heart disease coupled with age-related subaortic septal hypertrophy (see earlier section on hypertensive heart disease). Occasionally, valvular or congenital subvalvular aortic stenosis can also mimic HCM.

Pathogenesis. In contrast to DCM, much is known about the genetic basis of HCM. In approximately half of patients, the disease is familial, and the pattern of transmission is autosomal dominant with variable expression. Remaining cases appear to be sporadic; it is possible that some represent new mutations or are the result of autosomal recessive transmission with reduced gene penetrance. The genetic defects in HCM comprise mutations in any one of four genes that encode proteins of the cardiac contractile elements, the sarcomeres: β-myosin heavy chain (most frequently), cardiac troponin T, α-tropomyosin, and myosin-binding protein C (Fig. 13–25*C*).[60] More than 50 distinct mutations in these proteins have been identified in HCM, and the molecular defect responsible for unrelated cases varies greatly. Although it is clear that these genetic defects are critical to the cause of this entity, the sequence of events leading from mutations to disease is still poorly understood.

Clinical Features. The basic physiologic abnormality is reduced chamber size and poor compliance with reduced stroke volume that results from *impaired diastolic filling of the massively hypertrophied left ventricle.* In addition, there may be dynamic obstruction to the left ventricular outflow, as explained earlier. The limitation of cardiac output and a secondary increase in pulmonary venous pressure cause exertional dyspnea. Auscultation discloses a harsh systolic ejection murmur, caused by ventricular outflow obstruction as the anterior mitral leaflet moves toward the ventricular septum during systole. Owing to the massive hypertrophy, high left ventricular chamber pressure, and potentially abnormal intramural arteries, focal myocardial ischemia commonly results, even in the absence of concomitant coronary artery disease, and thus anginal pain is frequent. The major clinical problems in HCM are atrial fibrillation with mural thrombus formation and possibly embolization, infective endocarditis on the mitral valve, intractable cardiac failure, ventricular arrhythmias, and sudden death. HCM is one of the most common causes of sudden unexplained death in young athletes.

Given the heterogeneous genetic defects, it should not be surprising that the clinical and morphologic features are markedly heterogeneous among affected patients. Many patients are stable over many years of observation, and some improve. Different specific responsible gene mutations carry vastly differing clinical expression and prognosis. For example, the 403 Arg → Gln mutation in the β-myosin heavy chain gene (the most frequent mutation observed) yields severe disease and a high incidence of sudden death; in contrast, the substitution 908 Leu → Val in this same gene is associated with a low incidence of cardiac complications.[61]

Although symptoms are not due solely to thickening of the ventricular septum or obstruction, reduction of the mass of the septum by surgical excision of muscle is occasionally performed. Most patients can be significantly helped by medical therapy that enhances ventricular relaxation.

RESTRICTIVE CARDIOMYOPATHY

Restrictive cardiomyopathy is a disorder characterized by a *primary decrease in ventricular compliance, resulting in impaired ventricular filling during diastole*; the contractile (systolic) function of the left ventricle is usually unaffected.[62] Thus, the functional state can be confused with that of constrictive pericarditis or HCM. Restrictive cardiomyopathy can be idiopathic or associated with distinct diseases that affect the myocardium, principally radiation fibrosis, amyloidosis, sarcoidosis, metastatic tumor, or products of inborn errors of metabolism. These can often be diagnosed during life by endomyocardial biopsy, which often reveals the characteristic features of the disease.

MORPHOLOGY. In idiopathic **restrictive cardiomyopathy**, the ventricles are of approximately normal size or slightly enlarged, the ventricular cavities are not usually dilated, and the myocardium is firm. Biatrial dilation is commonly observed. Microscopically, there is often only patchy or diffuse interstitial fibrosis, which can vary from minimal to extensive. Restrictive cardiomyopathy of identifiable causes (e.g., some of those listed in Table 13–9) has similar gross morphology but disease-specific histology.

Several other restrictive conditions require brief mention. *Endomyocardial fibrosis* is principally a disease of children and young adults in Africa and other tropical areas, characterized by fibrosis of the ventricular endocardium and subendocardium that extends from the apex toward and often involving the tricuspid and mitral valves. The fibrous tissue markedly diminishes the volume and compliance of affected chambers and so induces a restrictive functional defect. Ventricular mural thrombi sometimes develop, and there is a suggestion that the fibrous tissue results from their organization. The cause is unknown.

Loeffler endomyocarditis is also marked by endomyocardial fibrosis typically with large mural thrombi similar to those seen in the tropical disease, but cases are not restricted to a specific geographic area. In addition to the cardiac changes, there is often an eosinophilia or eosinophilic leukemia. The circulating eosinophils generally have measurable structural and functional abnormalities, and many are degranulated. The release of toxic products of eosinophils, especially major basic protein, is postulated to initiate endocardial damage, with subsequent foci of endomyocardial necrosis accompanied by an eosinophilic infiltrate. This damage is followed by scarring of the necrotic area, layering of the endocardium by thrombus, and finally organization of the thrombus. Eosinophilic endomyocardial disease has a poor prognosis, but benefits are reported from surgical endomyocardial stripping.

Endocardial fibroelastosis is an uncommon heart disease of obscure cause characterized by focal or diffuse fibroelastic thickening usually involving the mural left ventricular endocardium. Most common in the first 2 years of life and rarely encountered in adults, it is often accompanied by some form of congenital cardiac anomaly, most often aortic valve obstruction in about one third of all cases. The significance of endocardial fibroelastosis depends on the extent of involvement. When focal, it may have no functional importance; if diffuse, it may be responsible for rapid, progressive cardiac decompensation and death, particularly in children.

Table 13–10. MAJOR CAUSES OF MYOCARDITIS

Infections
Viruses (e.g., coxsackievirus, ECHO, influenza, HIV, cytomegalovirus)
Chlamydiae (e.g., *C. psittaci*)
Rickettsiae (e.g., *R. typhi* typhus fever)
Bacteria (e.g., *Corynebacterium diphtheria, Neisseria meningococcus, Borrelia* Lyme disease)
Fungi (e.g., *Candida*)
Protozoa (e.g., *Trypanosoma* Chagas disease, toxoplasmosis)
Helminths (e.g., trichinosis)

Immune-Mediated Reactions
Postviral
Poststreptococcal (rheumatic fever)
Systemic lupus erythematosus
Drug hypersensitivity (e.g., methyldopa, sulfonamides)
Transplant rejection

Unknown
Sarcoidosis
Giant cell myocarditis

HIV, human immunodeficiency virus.

MYOCARDITIS

Under the category of *myocarditis* are grouped inflammatory processes of the myocardium that result in injury to the cardiac myocytes. The presence of inflammation alone is not diagnostic of myocarditis, however, because inflammatory infiltrates may also be seen as a secondary response in conditions such as ischemic injury. In myocarditis, by contrast, the inflammatory process plays a primary role in the development of myocardial injury.

Cause and Pathogenesis. In the United States, *infections* and particularly *viruses* are the most common cause of myocarditis. *Coxsackieviruses A and B* and other enteroviruses probably account for most of the cases. Other less common etiologic agents include cytomegalovirus, human immunodeficiency virus (HIV), and a host of other agents listed in Table 13–10. Although it is often difficult to isolate the offending virus from the tissues after the onset of clinical symptoms, serologic studies and, more recently, the identification of viral DNA or RNA sequences in the myocardium using gene amplification by polymerase chain reaction may identify the culprit. Whether the viruses are the direct cause of the myocardial injury or they initiate an immune response that cross-reacts with myocardial cells is unclear in most cases.[63] As with hepatitis viruses (Chapter 9), T cells may damage virus-infected myocytes by reacting against viral antigens expressed on the cell membrane.

Nonviral biologic agents are an important cause of myocarditis, particularly direct cardiac infection caused by the protozoa *Trypanosoma cruzi* producing Chagas disease. Although uncommon in the northern hemisphere, Chagas disease affects up to one half of the population in endemic areas of South America, and myocardial involvement is found in approximately 80% of infected individuals.[64] About 10% of patients die during an acute attack; others may enter a chronic immune-mediated phase and develop progressive signs of cardiac insufficiency 10 to 20 years later. Trichinosis is the most common helminthic disease with associated cardiac involvement. Parasitic diseases including toxoplasmosis and bacterial infections including Lyme disease and diphtheria can also cause myocarditis. In the case of diphtheritic myocarditis, toxins released by *Corynebacterium diphtheriae* appear to be responsible for the myocardial injury.

Myocarditis occurs in approximately two thirds of patients with Lyme disease, a systemic illness caused by the bacterial spirochete *Borrelia burgdorferi*, which has dermatologic, neurologic, and rheumatologic manifestations. Lyme myocarditis is usually mild and reversible but occasionally requires a temporary pacemaker for AV block.

Myocarditis occurs in many patients with acquired immunodeficiency syndrome (AIDS).[65] Two types have been identified: (1) inflammation and myocyte damage without a clear causative agent and (2) myocarditis caused directly by HIV or by an opportunistic pathogen. HIV nucleic acid sequences have been detected in some patients who have died of AIDS.[66]

There are also noninfectious causes of myocarditis. Myocarditis can be related to allergic reactions (*hypersensitivity myocarditis*), often to drugs such as antibiotics, diuretics, and antihypertensive agents. Myocarditis can also be associated with systemic diseases of immune origin, such as rheumatic fever, systemic lupus erythematosus, and polymyositis. Cardiac sarcoidosis and rejection of a transplanted heart are also considered forms of myocarditis.

Against this background, we can turn to the anatomic changes seen in the major forms of myocarditis.

MORPHOLOGY. During the active phase of myocarditis, the heart may appear normal or dilated; some hypertrophy may be present. The lesions may be diffuse or patchy. The ventricular myocardium is typically flabby and often mottled by either pale foci or minute hemorrhagic lesions. Mural thrombi may be present in any chamber.

During active disease, myocarditis is most frequently characterized by an interstitial inflammatory infiltrate and by injury (usually focal necrosis) to myocytes adjacent to the inflammatory cells, not typical of ischemic damage (Fig. 13–26).[67] Myocarditis in which the infiltrate is mononuclear and predominantly lymphocytic is most common (Fig. 13–26*A*). Although endomyocardial biopsies are diagnostic in some cases, they can be spuriously negative because inflammatory involvement may be focal or patchy. **Hypersensitivity myocarditis** has interstitial infiltrates, principally perivascular, composed of lymphocytes, macrophages, and a high proportion of eosinophils (Fig. 13–26*B*).

A morphologically distinctive form of myocarditis of uncertain cause and poor prognosis called **giant cell myocarditis** is characterized by a widespread inflammatory cellular infiltrate containing multinucleate giant cells interspersed with lymphocytes, eosinophils, plasma cells, and macrophages and having at least focal but frequently extensive necrosis (Fig. 13–26*C*). The giant cells are of either macrophage or myocyte origin. This variant carries a poor prognosis.[68]

If the patient survives the acute phase of myocarditis, the inflammatory lesions either resolve, leaving no residual changes, or heal by progressive fibrosis, as mentioned earlier.

The myocarditis of **Chagas disease** is rendered distinctive by parasitization of myofibers by trypanosomes accompanied by an inflammatory infiltrate of neutrophils, lymphocytes, macrophages, and occasional eosinophils (Fig. 13–26*D*).

Clinical Features. The clinical spectrum is broad; at one end, the disease is entirely asymptomatic, and such patients

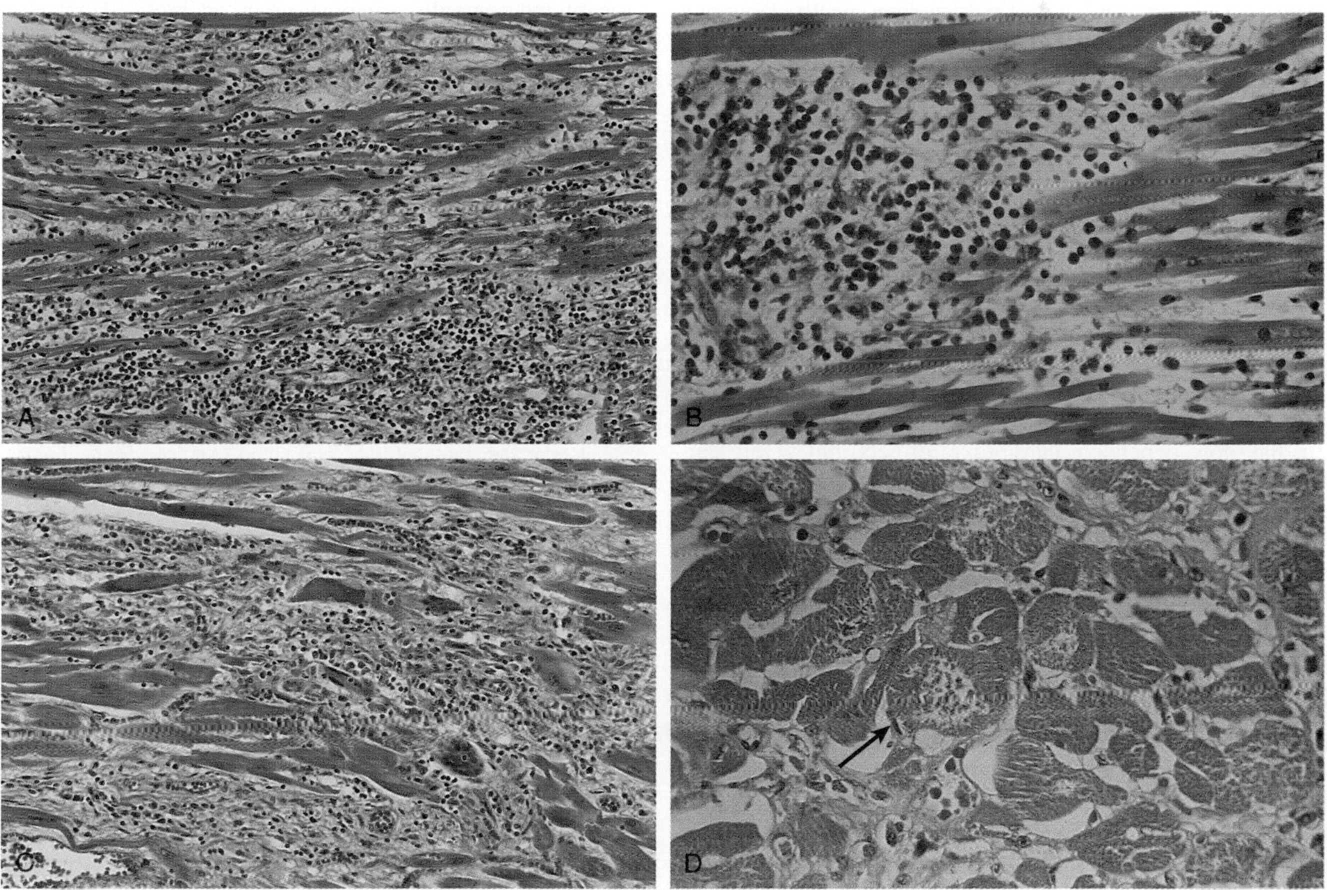

Figure 13–26

Myocarditis. *A*, Lymphocytic myocarditis, with dense mononuclear inflammatory cell infiltrate and associated myocyte injury. *B*, Hypersensitivity myocarditis, characterized by interstitial inflammatory infiltrate composed largely of eosinophils and mononuclear inflammatory cells. *C*, Giant cell myocarditis, with mononuclear inflammatory infiltrate containing lymphocytes and macrophages, with extensive loss of muscle, and multinucleated giant cells, apparently derived from muscle. *D*, Myocarditis of Chagas disease. A myofiber is distended with trypanosomes *(arrow)*. There is a surrounding inflammatory reaction and individual myofiber necrosis.

recover completely without sequelae. At the other extreme is the precipitous onset of heart failure or arrhythmias, occasionally with sudden death. A systolic murmur may appear, indicating functional mitral regurgitation related to dilation of the left ventricle. Between these extremes are the many levels of involvement associated with such symptoms as fatigue, dyspnea, palpitations, precordial discomfort, and fever. The clinical features of myocarditis can mimic those of acute MI. Occasionally, years later, when an attack of myocarditis is forgotten, the patient may be diagnosed as having DCM. Some patients have been observed to progress from unequivocal myocarditis to DCM both clinically and by successive endomyocardial biopsy.

OTHER SPECIFIC CAUSES

Doxorubicin and Other Drugs. The anthracycline chemotherapeutic agents doxorubicin (Adriamycin) and daunorubicin are well-recognized causes of toxic myocardial injury that can cause DCM.[69] The hazard is dose dependent (cardiotoxicity usually requires a total dose >500 mg/m^2) and attributed primarily to lipid peroxidation of myofiber membranes. Many other agents, such as lithium, phenothiazines, chloroquine, and cocaine, have been implicated in myocardial injury and sometimes sudden death. Common threads running throughout the cardiotoxicity of many chemicals and drugs (including diphtheria exotoxin) are myofiber swelling and vacuolization, fatty change, individual cell lysis (myocytolysis), and sometimes patchy foci of necrosis. Electron microscopy usually reveals cytoplasmic vacuolization and lysis of myofibrils, typified by Adriamycin cardiotoxicity. With discontinuance of the toxic agent, these changes may resolve completely, leaving no apparent sequelae. Sometimes, however, nonspecific hypertrophy with interstitial fibrosis or small focal replacement scars remains, and both the physiologic and the morphologic patterns are indistinguishable from those of DCM.

Another chemotherapeutic agent with cardiotoxicity is cyclophosphamide (Cytoxan), which, similar to Adriamycin, has dose-dependent cardiotoxic effects, but severe cardiomyopathy may occur after single high-dose therapy. In contrast to the primary myocyte injury with Adriamycin, the principal insult with cyclophosphamide appears to be vascular, leading to myocardial hemorrhage.

Catecholamines. Foci of myocardial necrosis with contraction bands are frequently observed in patients who have a pheochromocytoma (Chapter 26), with its elaboration of catecholamines. This is considered to be a manifestation of *catecholamine effect* that appears in association with the administration of large doses of vasopressor agents, such as dopamine. Cocaine also causes catecholamine-induced cell damage.[70] The mechanism of catecholamine cardiotoxicity is uncertain, but it appears to relate either to direct toxicity of these agents to cardiac myocytes via calcium overload or to vasoconstriction in the myocardial circulation in the face of an increased heart rate. The mononuclear cell infiltrate is likely a secondary reaction to the foci of myocyte cell death. Similar morphology may be encountered in patients who have recovered from hypotensive episodes or have been resuscitated from a frank cardiac arrest. In such cases, myocyte necrosis results from ischemia followed by reperfusion (see section on IHD), and inflammation follows. Curiously, some patients with intracranial lesions associated with elevated cerebrospinal fluid pressure and neurostimulation also develop focal myocardial necrosis with contraction bands.[71]

Amyloidosis. Cardiac amyloidosis (Chapter 8) may appear along with systemic amyloidosis or may be isolated to the heart, particularly in the aged. Cardiac amyloid deposits may occur in the ventricles (*senile cardiac amyloidosis* [SCA] or systemic senile amyloidosis with cardiac involvement) or be limited to the atria (*isolated atrial amyloidosis*). In SCA, the protein deposits derive from transthyretin (prealbumin), a normal serum protein that normally transports both thyroxine and retinol-binding protein. The cardiac manifestations of SCA may be histologically indistinguishable from those of primary amyloidosis, but SCA can be identified by immunohistochemical staining of tissue with antisera to transthyretin.[72] SCA has a far better prognosis than primary amyloidosis. Although SCA is exclusively a disease of elderly people, mutant forms of transthyretin can accelerate cardiac (and systemic) amyloidosis. For example, the risk of isolated cardiac amyloidosis is four times greater in blacks than whites after the age of 60; 4% of blacks have a gene mutation in which isoleucine is substituted for valine at position 122 (Ile 122) that causes an amyloidogenic/fibrillogenic form of transthyretin (autosomal dominant familial transthyretin amyloidosis).[73] In isolated atrial amyloidosis, the deposits consist of atrial natriuretic peptide. Most frequently, cardiac amyloidosis produces restrictive hemodynamics, but it can be asymptomatic or can be manifested by dilation, arrhythmias, or features mimicking those of ischemic or valvular disease owing to deposits in the interstitium, conduction system, vasculature, and valves.

MORPHOLOGY. Grossly the heart in cardiac amyloidosis varies from normal to firm, rubbery, and noncompliant with thickened walls. Usually the chambers are of normal size, but in some cases they are dilated. Numerous, small semitranslucent nodules resembling sand or drips of wax may be seen at the atrial endocardial surface, particularly on the left. Amyloid deposits are extracellular, and they may occur in the myocardial interstitium, conduction tissue, valves, endocardium, pericardium, and small intramural coronary arteries, and they are highlighted by the classic apple-green birefringence demonstrated by polarization of slides stained with Congo-red. In the interstitium, amyloid deposits often form rings around cardiac myocytes and capillaries. Intramural arteries may have sufficient amyloid in their walls to compress and occlude their lumens.

Iron Overload. *Iron overload* can occur in either hereditary hemochromatosis or hemosiderosis owing to multiple blood transfusions. The heart is identical in each. Patients with iron storage disease present most commonly with a dilated pattern. Iron deposition is more prominent in ventricles than atria and in the working myocardium than in the conduction system. It is thought that iron causes systolic dysfunction by interfering with metal-dependent enzyme systems.

MORPHOLOGY. Grossly the myocardium of the iron-overloaded heart is rust-brown in color but is usually otherwise indistinguishable from that of idiopathic DCM. Microscopically, there is marked accumulation of hemosiderin within cardiac myocytes (contrast with the extracellular deposition of amyloid discussed previously), particularly in the perinuclear region, demonstrable with a Prussian blue stain. This accumulation of hemosiderin is associated with varying degrees of cellular degeneration and replacement fibrosis. Ultrastructurally, cardiac myocytes contain abundant perinuclear siderosomes (iron-containing lysosomes).

Hyperthyroidism and Hypothyroidism. Cardiac manifestations are among the earliest, most consistent features of hyperthyroidism and hypothyroidism and reflect direct and indirect effects of thyroid hormones on the cells of the heart.[74] In *hyperthyroidism* (Chapter 26), tachycardia, palpitations, and cardiomegaly are common; supraventricular arrhythmias occasionally appear. Cardiac failure occurs uncommonly, usually in the elderly superimposed on other cardiac diseases. In *hypothyroidism* (Chapter 26), cardiac output is decreased, with reduced stroke volume and heart rate. Increased peripheral vascular resistance and decreased blood volume result in narrowing of the pulse pressure, prolongation of circulation time, and decreased flow to peripheral tissues. Reduced circulation in the skin accounts for the characteristic cold sensitivity.

MORPHOLOGY. In hyperthyroidism, the gross and histologic features are those of nonspecific hypertrophy. In well-advanced hypothyroidism (myxedema), the heart is flabby, enlarged, and dilated. Histologic features include myofiber swelling with loss of striations and basophilic degeneration, accompanied by interstitial mucopolysaccharide-rich edema fluid. A similar fluid sometimes accumulates within the pericardial sac. To these changes, the term **myxedema heart** has been applied.

Pericardial Disease

Pericardial lesions are almost always associated with disease in other portions of the heart or surrounding structures or secondary to a systemic disorder; isolated pericardial disease is unusual. Despite the large number of causes of pericardial disease, there are relatively few anatomic forms of pericardial involvement.

PERICARDIAL EFFUSION AND HEMOPERICARDIUM

Normally, there is about 30 to 50 ml of thin, clear, straw-colored fluid in the pericardial sac. Under various circumstances, the parietal pericardium undergoes distention by fluid of variable composition (*pericardial effusion*), blood (*hemopericardium*), or pus (*purulent pericarditis*). The consequences depend on the ability of the parietal pericardium to stretch, based on the speed of accumulation and the amount of fluid. Thus, with slowly accumulating effusions of less than 500 ml, the only clinical significance is a characteristic globular enlargement of the heart shadow noted on chest radiograph. In contrast, larger chronic effusions or rapidly developing fluid collections of as little as 200 to 300 ml—for example, in the hemopericardium caused by ruptured MI, traumatic perforation, infective endocarditis, or ruptured aortic dissection—may produce compression of the thin-walled atria and venae cavae or the ventricles themselves, restricting cardiac filling, producing potentially fatal *cardiac tamponade*.

PERICARDITIS

Pericardial inflammation is usually secondary to a variety of cardiac diseases, thoracic or systemic disorders, or metastases from neoplasms arising in remote sites. Primary pericarditis is unusual and almost always of viral origin. The major causes of pericarditis are presented in Table 13–11. Most evoke an acute pericarditis, but a few, such as tuberculosis and fungi, produce chronic reactions. Since it is often impossible from pathologic examination to determine the etiologic basis for the reaction, a morphologic classification follows.

Acute Pericarditis

Serous Pericarditis. Serous inflammatory exudates are characteristically produced by noninfectious inflammations,

Table 13–11. CAUSES OF PERICARDITIS

Infections
Viruses
Pyogenic bacteria
Tuberculosis
Fungi
Other parasites
Presumably Immune-Mediated Reactions
Rheumatic fever
Systemic lupus erythematosus
Scleroderma
Postcardiotomy
Post–myocardial infarction (Dressler) syndrome
Drug hypersensitivity reaction
Miscellaneous
Myocardial infarction
Uremia
After cardiac surgery
Neoplasia
Trauma
Radiation

such as rheumatic fever, systemic lupus erythematosus, scleroderma, tumors, and uremia. An infection in the tissues contiguous to the pericardium, for example, a bacterial pleuritis, may cause sufficient irritation of the parietal pericardial serosa to cause a sterile serous effusion that may progress to serofibrinous pericarditis and ultimately to a frank suppurative reaction.

In some instances, a well-defined viral infection elsewhere—upper respiratory tract, pneumonia, parotitis—antedates the pericarditis and serves as the primary focus of infection. Infrequently, viral pericarditis occurs as an apparent primary involvement, usually in young adults, that may accompany myocarditis (*myopericarditis*).

MORPHOLOGY. Whatever the cause, there is an inflammatory reaction in the epicardial and pericardial surfaces with scant numbers of polymorphonuclear leukocytes, lymphocytes, and histiocytes. Usually the volume of fluid is not large (50 to 200 ml) and accumulates slowly. Dilation and increased permeability of the vessels because of inflammation produces a fluid of high specific gravity and rich protein content. A mild inflammatory infiltrate in the epipericardial fat consisting predominantly of lymphocytes is frequently termed **chronic pericarditis**. Organization into fibrous adhesions rarely occurs.

Fibrinous and Serofibrinous Pericarditis. These two anatomic forms are the *most frequent type of pericarditis* and are composed of serous fluid mixed with a fibrinous exudate. Common causes include acute MI (see Fig. 13–11*A*), the postinfarction (Dressler) syndrome (likely an autoimmune condition, which appears several weeks after an MI), uremia, chest radiation, rheumatic fever, systemic lupus erythematosus, and trauma. A fibrinous reaction also follows routine cardiac surgery.

MORPHOLOGY. In fibrinous pericarditis, the surface is dry, with a fine granular roughening. In serofibrinous pericarditis, an increased inflammatory process induces more and thicker fluid, which is yellow and cloudy owing to contained leukocytes and erythrocytes (which may be sufficient to give a visibly bloody appearance) and often fibrin. As with all inflammatory exudates, **fibrin may be digested with resolution of the exudate, or it may become organized** (Chapter 4).

From the clinical standpoint, *the development of a loud pericardial friction rub is the most striking characteristic of fibrinous pericarditis.* A collection of serous fluid may obliterate the rub by separating the two layers of the pericardium. Pain, systemic febrile reactions, and signs suggestive of cardiac failure may accompany the pathognomonic friction rub.

Purulent or Suppurative Pericarditis. Purulent or suppurative pericarditis almost invariably denotes the invasion of the pericardial space by infective organisms. These organisms may reach the pericardial cavity by several routes: (1) direct extension from neighboring inflammations, such as an empyema of the pleural cavity, lobar pneumonia, mediastinal infections, or extension of a ring abscess through the myocardium or aortic root in infective endocarditis; (2) seeding from the blood; (3) lymphatic extension; or (4) direct introduction during cardiac surgery. Immunosuppression potentiates all of these pathways.

MORPHOLOGY. The exudate ranges from a thin to a creamy pus of up to 400 to 500 ml in volume. The serosal surfaces are reddened, granular, and coated with the exudate (Fig. 13–27). Microscopically, there is an acute inflammatory reaction. Sometimes the inflammatory process extends into surrounding structures to induce a so-called **mediastinopericarditis. Organization is the usual outcome; resolution is infrequent.** Because of the great intensity of the inflammatory response, the organization frequently produces **constrictive pericarditis**, a serious consequence (see later).

The clinical findings in the active phase are essentially the same as those present in fibrinous pericarditis, but signs of systemic infection are usually marked—for example, spiking temperatures, chills, and fever.

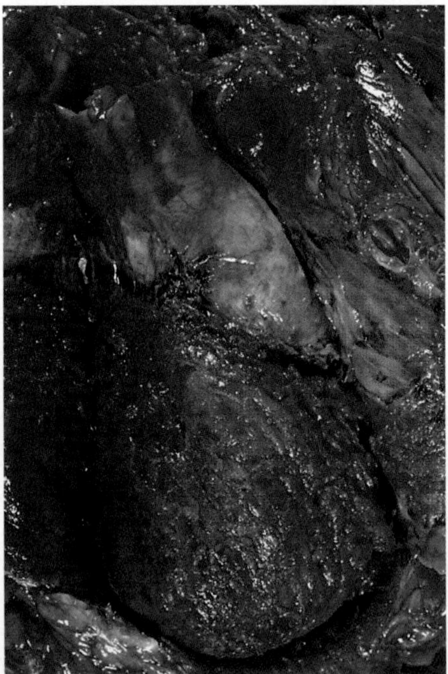

Figure 13–27

Acute suppurative pericarditis as an extension from pneumonia. Extensive purulent exudate is evident in this in situ photograph.

Hemorrhagic Pericarditis. An exudate composed of blood mixed with a fibrinous or suppurative effusion is most commonly caused by tuberculosis or by direct malignant neoplastic involvement of the pericardial space. It may also be found in bacterial infections or in cases of pericarditis occurring in patients with some underlying bleeding diathesis. Hemorrhagic pericarditis often follows cardiac surgery and sometimes is responsible for significant blood loss or even tamponade, requiring a *second-look* operation.

If the underlying cause is a tumor, neoplastic cells may be present in the effusion, so that cytologic examination of fluid removed through a pericardial tap may yield the specific cause. The clinical significance is similar to that of the spectrum of fibrinous or suppurative pericarditis.

Caseous Pericarditis. Caseation within the pericardial sac is, until proved otherwise, tuberculous in origin; infrequently, fungal infections evoke a similar pattern. The pericardium is usually involved by direct spread from tuberculous foci within the tracheobronchial nodes. The anatomic changes are typical of tuberculous infections elsewhere. Caseous pericarditis is rare but is the most frequent antecedent of disabling, fibrocalcific, chronic constrictive pericarditis.

Healed Pericarditis

In some cases, organization merely produces plaquelike fibrous thickenings of the serosal membranes (*soldier's plaque*) or thin, delicate adhesions of obscure origin that are observed fairly frequently at autopsy and rarely cause impairment of cardiac function. In other cases, organization results in complete obliteration of the pericardial sac. This fibrosis yields a delicate, stringy type of adhesion between parietal and visceral pericardium called *adhesive pericarditis*, which rarely hampers or restricts cardiac action. In some cases, however, healed pericarditis can be clinically important, especially when it takes the form of adhesive mediastinopericarditis or constrictive pericarditis.

Adhesive Mediastinopericarditis. Adhesive mediastinopericarditis may follow a suppurative or caseous pericarditis, previous cardiac surgery, or irradiation to the mediastinum. Only rarely is it a sequel to simple fibrinous exudation. The pericardial sac is obliterated, and adherence of the external aspect of the parietal layer to surrounding structures produces a great strain on cardiac function. With each systolic contraction, the heart is pulling not only against the parietal pericardium, but also against the attached surrounding structures. Systolic retraction of the rib cage and diaphragm, pulsus paradoxus, and a variety of other characteristic clinical findings may be observed. *The increased workload causes cardiac hypertrophy and dilation, which may be quite massive in more severe cases, mimicking DCM* (see earlier).

Constrictive Pericarditis. The heart may be encased in a dense, fibrous, or fibrocalcific scar that limits diastolic expansion and seriously restricts cardiac output, resembling restrictive cardiomyopathy. A well-defined history of a previous suppurative, hemorrhagic, or caseous (tuberculous) pericarditis may or may not be present. In constrictive pericarditis, the pericardial space is obliterated, and the heart is surrounded by a dense, adherent layer of scar with or without calcification, often 0.5 to 1.0 cm thick, which can resemble a plaster mold in extreme cases (*concretio cordis*).

Although the signs of cardiac failure may resemble those produced by adhesive mediastinopericarditis, *cardiac hypertrophy and dilation cannot occur because of the dense enclosing scar, and the heart is consequently quiet with reduced output.* The major therapy is surgical removal of the shell of constricting fibrous tissue (*pericardiectomy*).

RHEUMATOID HEART DISEASE

Rheumatoid arthritis is mainly a disorder of the joints, but it is also associated with many nonarticular involvements (e.g., subcutaneous rheumatoid nodules, acute vasculitis, and Felty syndrome; Chapter 28). The heart is also involved in 20 to 40% of cases of severe prolonged rheumatoid arthritis. The most common finding is a fibrinous pericarditis that may progress to fibrous thickening of the visceral and parietal pericardium with dense fibrous adhesions. Rheumatoid inflammatory granulomatous nodules resembling those that occur subcutaneously may also be identifiable below the pericardial surfaces. Much less frequently, rheumatoid nodules involve the myocardium, endocardium, valves of the heart, and root of the aorta. Rheumatoid valvulitis can lead to marked fibrous thickening and secondary calcification of valve cusps, producing changes resembling those of chronic rheumatic valvular disease, but intercommissural adhesion is rarely present.

Neoplastic Heart Disease

Primary tumors of the heart are rare; in contrast, metastatic tumors to the heart occur in about 5% of patients dying of cancer. The most common primary tumors, in descending order of frequency (overall, including adults and children), are myxomas, fibromas, lipomas, papillary fibroelastomas, rhabdomyomas, angiosarcomas, and other sarcomas. The five most common all are benign and account collectively for 80 to 90% of primary tumors of the heart.[75]

PRIMARY CARDIAC TUMORS

Myxoma

Myxomas are the most common primary tumor of the heart in adults (Fig. 13–28).[76] Although they may arise in any of the four chambers or, rarely, on the heart valves, about 90% are located in the atria, with a left-to-right ratio of approximately 4:1 (*atrial myxomas*).

MORPHOLOGY. The tumors are almost always single, but rarely several occur simultaneously. The region of the fossa ovalis in the atrial septum is the favored site of origin. Myxomas range from small (<1 cm) to large (up to 10 cm) sessile or pedunculated masses (Fig. 13–28*A*) that vary from globular hard masses mottled with hemorrhage to soft, translucent, papillary, or villous le-

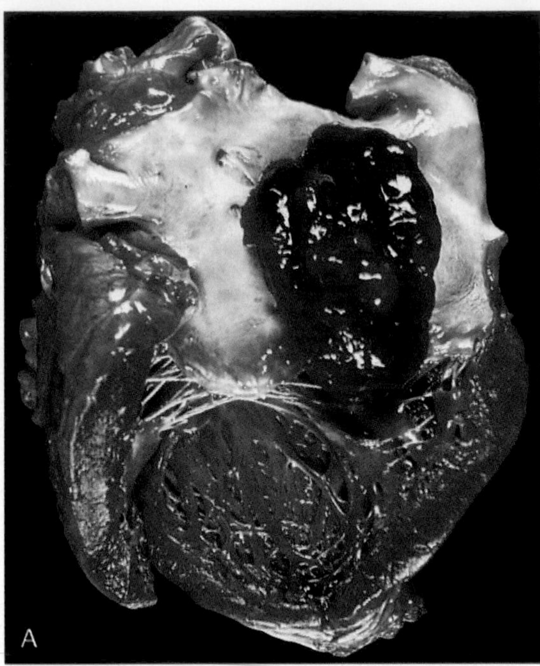

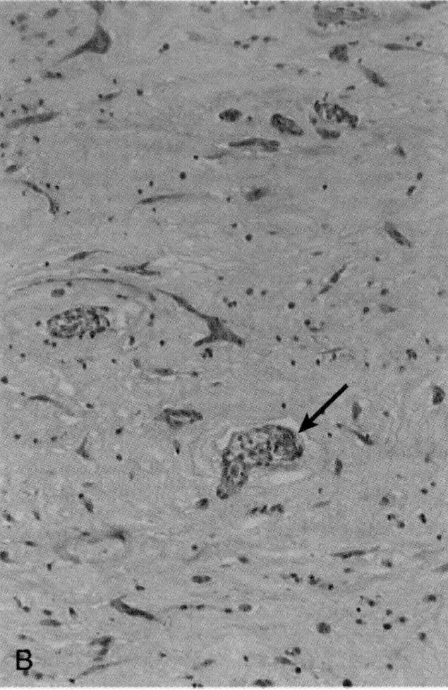

Figure 13–28

Left atrial myxoma. *A*, Gross photograph showing a large pedunculated lesion arising from the region of the fossa ovalis and extending into the mitral valve orifice. *B*, Microscopic appearance, with abundant amorphous extracellular matrix in which are scattered collections of myxoma cells in various groupings, including abnormal vascular formations *(arrow)*.

sions having a gelatinous appearance. The pedunculated form is frequently sufficiently mobile to move into or sometimes through the AV valves during systole, causing intermittent and often position-dependent obstruction. Sometimes, such mobility exerts a **wrecking-ball** effect, causing damage to the valve leaflets.

Histologically, myxomas are composed of stellate or globular myxoma (**lepidic**) cells, endothelial cells, smooth muscle cells, and an undifferentiated form embedded within an abundant acid mucopolysaccharide ground substance and covered on the surface by endothelium (Fig. 13–28*B*). Peculiar structures that variably resemble poorly formed glands or vessels are characteristic. Some hemorrhage and mononuclear inflammation is usually present.

It has long been questioned whether cardiac myxomas are hamartomas or organized thrombi, but the weight of evidence is on the side of benign neoplasia. All the tumor cell types present are thought to derive from differentiation of primitive multipotential mesenchymal cells.

The major clinical manifestations are due to valvular *ball-valve* obstruction, embolization, or a syndrome of constitutional symptoms, such as fever and malaise. Sometimes, fragmentation with systemic embolization calls attention to these lesions. Constitutional symptoms are likely due to the elaboration by some myxomas of the cytokine interleukin-6, a major mediator of the acute-phase response of the systemic inflammatory reaction. Echocardiography provides the opportunity to identify these masses noninvasively. Surgical removal is usually curative, although rarely the neoplasm recurs months to years later.

Approximately 10% of patients with myxoma have a familial cardiac myxoma syndrome (known as *Carney syndrome*) characterized by autosomal dominant transmission, multiple cardiac and often extracardiac (e.g., skin) myxomas, spotty pigmentation, and endocrine overactivity. Therefore, echocardiographic screening of first-degree relatives of myxoma patients may be appropriate.

Lipoma

Lipomas may occur in the subendocardium, subepicardium, or within the myocardium, as localized, poorly encapsulated masses, which may be asymptomatic, can create ball-valve obstructions as with myxomas, or produce arrhythmias. They are most often located in the left ventricle, right atrium, or atrial septum and are not necessarily neoplastic. In the atrial septum, the depositions are called *lipomatous hypertrophy*.

Papillary Fibroelastoma

Papillary fibroelastomas are curious, usually incidental lesions, most often identified at autopsy, but they may embolize.

MORPHOLOGY. Papillary fibroelastomas are generally located on valves, particularly the ventricular surfaces of semilunar valves and the atrial surfaces of AV valves. They constitute a distinctive cluster of hairlike projections up to 1 cm in diameter, covering up to several centimeters in diameter of the endocardial surface. Histologically, they are covered by endothelium, deep to which is myxoid connective tissue containing abundant mucopolysaccharide matrix and elastic fibers. Although called neoplasms, fibroelastomas may represent organized thrombi, similar to the much smaller, usually trivial, **Lambl excrescences** that are frequently found on the aortic valves of older individuals.

Rhabdomyoma

Rhabdomyomas are the most frequent primary tumor of the heart in infants and children and are frequently discovered in the first years of life because of obstruction of a valvular orifice or cardiac chamber.

MORPHOLOGY. Rhabdomyomas are generally small, gray-white myocardial masses up to several centimeters in diameter located on either the left or the right side of the heart, protruding into the ventricular chambers. Histologically, they are composed of a mixed population of cells, the most characteristic of which are large, rounded, or polygonal cells containing numerous glycogen-laden vacuoles separated by strands of cytoplasm running from the plasma membrane to the more or less centrally located nucleus, the so-called **spider cells**. These cells can be shown to have myofibrils. That rhabdomyomas are hamartomas or malformations rather than true neoplasms is supported by a high frequency of tuberous sclerosis (Chapter 28) in patients with cardiac rhabdomyomas (and vice versa).

Sarcoma

Cardiac *angiosarcomas* and other sarcomas are not clinically or morphologically distinctive from their counterparts in other locations (Chapter 28) and so require no further comment here.

CARDIAC EFFECTS OF NONCARDIAC NEOPLASMS

With enhanced patient survival as a result of diagnostic and therapeutic advances, significant cardiovascular effects of noncardiac neoplasms and their therapy are now commonly encountered (Table 13–12). Effects may be due directly to infiltration of tumor tissue, indirectly to circulating mediators, or to tumor therapy.

Carcinomas of the lung and breast, melanomas, leukemias, and lymphomas most frequently involve the heart. Metastases can reach the heart and pericardium by retrograde lymphatic extension (most carcinomas), by hematogenous seeding (many tumors), by direct contiguous extension (primary carcinoma of the lung, breast, or esophagus), or by direct venous extension (tumors of the kidney or liver). Clinical symptoms are most often associated with pericardial spread, by either a pericardial effusion that causes tamponade or sufficient tumor bulk to restrict cardiac filling directly. Myocardial metastases are usually clinically silent or have nonspecific features, such as a generalized defect in ventricular contractility or compliance. Bronchogenic carcinoma or malignant lymphoma may infiltrate the mediastinum extensively, causing encasement, compression, or invasion of the superior vena cava with resultant obstruction to blood coming from the head and upper extremities (*superior vena cava syndrome*). Renal cell carcinoma, because of its high propensity to invade the renal vein, can grow in the lumen of the renal vein into and along the inferior vena cava and occasionally extend into the right atrium blocking venous return to the heart.

Table 13–12. CARDIOVASCULAR EFFECTS OF NONCARDIAC NEOPLASMS

Direct Consequences of Tumor
Pericardial and myocardial metastases
Large vessel obstruction
Pulmonary tumor emboli
Indirect Consequences of Tumor
Nonbacterial thrombotic endocarditis
Carcinoid heart disease
Pheochromocytoma-associated heart disease
Myeloma-associated amyloidosis
Effects of Tumor Therapy
Chemotherapy
Radiation therapy

Modified from Schoen FJ, et al: Cardiac effects of non-cardiac neoplasms. Cardiol Clin 2:657, 1984.

Of the indirect cardiac effects of noncardiac tumors, NBTE, carcinoid heart disease, pheochromocytoma-associated myocardial damage, amyloidosis, and complications of chemotherapy are discussed earlier in this chapter. Radiation used to treat breast, lung, or mediastinal neoplasms can cause pericarditis, pericardial effusion, myocardial fibrosis, and chronic pericardial disorders. Other cardiac effects of radiotherapy include accelerated coronary artery disease and mural and valvular endocardial fibrosis.

Congenital Heart Disease

Congenital heart disease is a general term used to describe abnormalities of the heart or great vessels that are present from birth. Most such disorders arise from faulty embryogenesis during gestational weeks 3 through 8, when major cardiovascular structures develop. The most severe anomalies may be incompatible with intrauterine survival; however, most others are associated with live births. Some may produce manifestations soon after birth, frequently accompanying the change from fetal to postnatal circulatory patterns (with reliance on the lungs, rather than placenta, for oxygenation). Others, however, do not necessarily become evident until adulthood (e.g., aortic coarctation or atrial septal defect [ASD]). Immense strides have been made in the diagnosis and therapy of congenital heart defects, allowing extended survival for many children.[77] Most forms are now amenable to surgical repair with good results.

The population of adults with congenital heart disease is increasing rapidly. This population includes those who have never had cardiac surgery, those who have had reparative cardiac surgery and require no further operation, and those who have had incomplete or palliative surgery. An understanding of their prognosis and potential problems requires consideration of the underlying congenital malformation, the nature and effects of the therapeutic interventions, and the postoperative or postinterventional residual lesions and sequelae.[78] Most important are risk of endocarditis; specific difficulties owing to hyperviscosity; maternal and focal risks associated with childbearing in those with cyanotic congenital disease; and residual pathology after reparative surgery (including abnormal valves; prosthetic patches, valves, and conduits; and an increased risk of arrhythmias).

Incidence. Congenital heart disease is the most common type of heart disease among children. Although figures vary, a generally accepted incidence is 6 to 8 per 1000 live-born, full-term births. The incidence is higher in premature infants and in stillborns. Twelve disorders account for nearly all cases, with approximate frequencies presented in Table 13–13.

Cause and Pathology. The cause of congenital malformations in general was discussed in Chapter 6. Therefore, discussion is confined to factors of particular relevance to congenital cardiac malformations. *Genetic factors* play an obvious role in some cases, as evidenced by the occurrence of familial forms of congenital heart disease and by well-defined associations between certain chromosomal abnormalities (e.g., trisomies 13, 15, 18, and 21 and Turner syndrome) and congenital cardiac malformations. *Environmental factors*, such as congenital rubella infection, are responsible for some additional cases. Overall, however, obvious genetic or environmental influences are identifiable in only about 10% of cases of congenital heart disease, but the understanding of probable genetic links is increasing.[79] For example, a familial ASD disease gene mapping to chromosome 5p and affecting multiple generations of one kindred was recently identified.[80] Multifactorial genetic and environmental factors probably account for the remaining majority of cases in which a cause is not apparent.

Table 13–13. RELATIVE FREQUENCY AND GENDER DISTRIBUTION OF 12 MOST COMMONLY ENCOUNTERED CONGENITAL CARDIAC MALFORMATIONS

Malformation	Relative Frequency (%)	Male-to-Female Ratio
Ventricular septal defect	32	1:1
Atrial septal defect	8	1:2
Patent ductus arteriosus	8	1:2
Tetralogy of Fallot	8	1:1
Pulmonary stenosis	8	1:1
Aortic stenosis or atresia	8	3:1
Coarctation of aorta	6	2:1
Transposition of great arteries	5	2:1
Atrioventricular septal defect	4	1:1
Tricuspid atresia	2	1:1
Total anomalous pulmonary venous connection	2	1:1
Truncus arteriosus	1	1:1
Other	8	—

Modified from Edwards WD: Congenital heart disease. In Damjanov I, Linder J (eds): Anderson's Pathology, 10th ed. St. Louis, Mosby–Year Book, 1996, p 1339.

Clinical Features. *The varied structural anomalies in congenital heart disease fall primarily into three major categories*:

- Malformations causing a *left-to-right shunt*
- Malformations causing a *right-to-left shunt*
- Malformations causing an *obstruction*

A *shunt* is an abnormal communication between chambers or blood vessels. Abnormal channels permit the flow of blood from left to right or the reverse, depending on pressure relationships. When blood from the right side of the heart enters the left side (*right-to-left shunt*), a dusky blueness of the skin and mucous membranes (*cyanosis*) results because there is diminished pulmonary blood flow and poorly oxygenated blood enters the systemic circulation (called *cyanotic congenital heart disease*, the most important examples of which are tetralogy of Fallot, transposition of the great arteries, persistent truncus arteriosus, tricuspid atresia, and total anomalous pulmonary venous connection). Moreover, with right-to-left shunts, bland or septic emboli arising in peripheral veins can bypass the normal filtration action of the lungs and thus directly enter the systemic circulation (*paradoxical embolism*); brain infarction and abscess are potential consequences. Clinical findings frequently associated with severe, long-standing cyanosis include clubbing of the tips of the fingers and toes (*hypertrophic osteoarthropathy*) and polycythemia.

In contrast, left-to-right shunts (such as ASD, ventricular septal defect [VSD], and patent ductus arteriosus [PDA]) increase pulmonary blood flow and are not initially associated with cyanosis. They expose the postnatal normally low-pressure, low-resistance pulmonary circulation to increased pressure or volume (or both), which can result in pulmonary hypertension followed by right ventricular hypertrophy and potentially failure. Shunts associated with increased pulmonary blood flow include ASDs, and shunts associated with both increased pulmonary blood flow and pressure include VSDs and PDA. The muscular pulmonary arteries (<1 mm diameter) first respond to increased pressure by medial hypertrophy and vasoconstriction, which maintains relatively normal distal pulmonary capillary and venous pressures, helping to prevent pulmonary edema. Prolonged pulmonary arterial vasoconstriction, however, stimulates the development of irreversible obstructive intimal lesions. Eventually, pulmonary vascular resistance and pressures increase toward systemic levels, thereby reversing the shunt to right-to-left with unoxygenated blood in the systemic circulation (*late cyanotic congenital heart disease* or *Eisenmenger syndrome*).

Once significant irreversible pulmonary hypertension develops, the structural defects of congenital heart disease are considered irreparable. The secondary pulmonary vascular changes can eventually lead to the patient's death.

This is the rationale for early surgical or nonsurgical intervention.

Some developmental anomalies of the heart produce obstructions to flow because of abnormal narrowings of chambers, valves, or blood vessels. Examples are valvular stenoses (partial obstructions) or *atresias* (complete occlusions) and are called *obstructive congenital heart disease* (e.g., coarctation of the aorta, aortic valvular stenosis, and pulmonary valvular stenosis). In some disorders (e.g., tetralogy of Fallot), an obstruction (pulmonary stenosis) is associated with a shunt (right-to-left through a VSD).

In congenital heart disease, altered hemodynamics usually cause cardiac dilation, hypertrophy, or both. In contrast, a decrease in the volume and muscle mass of a cardiac chamber is called *hypoplasia* if it occurs before birth and *atrophy* if it develops after birth.

LEFT-TO-RIGHT SHUNTS—LATE CYANOSIS

The most commonly encountered left-to-right shunts include ASDs, VSDs, PDA, and AV septal defects (AVSDs) and are shown in Figure 13–29. Note that each is designated by an abbreviation containing the letter *D*.

Atrial Septal Defect

An ASD is an abnormal opening in the atrial septum that allows communication of blood between the left and right atria (not to be confused with a *patent foramen ovale*, present in up to one third of normal individuals, which generally does not permit flow unless right atrial pressures are elevated). ASD is the most common congenital cardiac anomaly that is usually asymptomatic until adulthood (Fig. 13–29*A*).

MORPHOLOGY. The three major types of ASDs, classified according to their location in the septum, are secundum, primum, and sinus venosus. The **secundum ASD**, accounting for approximately 90% of all ASDs, comprises a defect located at and results from a deficient or fenestrated oval fossa near the mid-septum. Most are isolated (not associated with other anomalies). When associated with another defect, such as tetralogy of Fallot, the other defect is usually hemodynamically dominant. The atrial aperture may be of any size and may be single, multiple, or fenestrated. **Primum** anomalies (5% of ASDs) occur adjacent to the AV valves and are usually associated with a cleft anterior mitral leaflet. This combination is known as a **partial AVSD** (see later). **Sinus venosus** defects (5%) are located near the entrance of the superior vena cava. They are commonly accompanied by anomalous connections of right pulmonary veins to the superior vena cava or right atrium.

ASDs result in a left-to-right shunt, largely because pulmonary vascular resistance is considerably less than systemic vascular resistance and because the compliance (distensibility) of the right ventricle is much greater than that of the left. Pulmonary blood flow may be two to four times

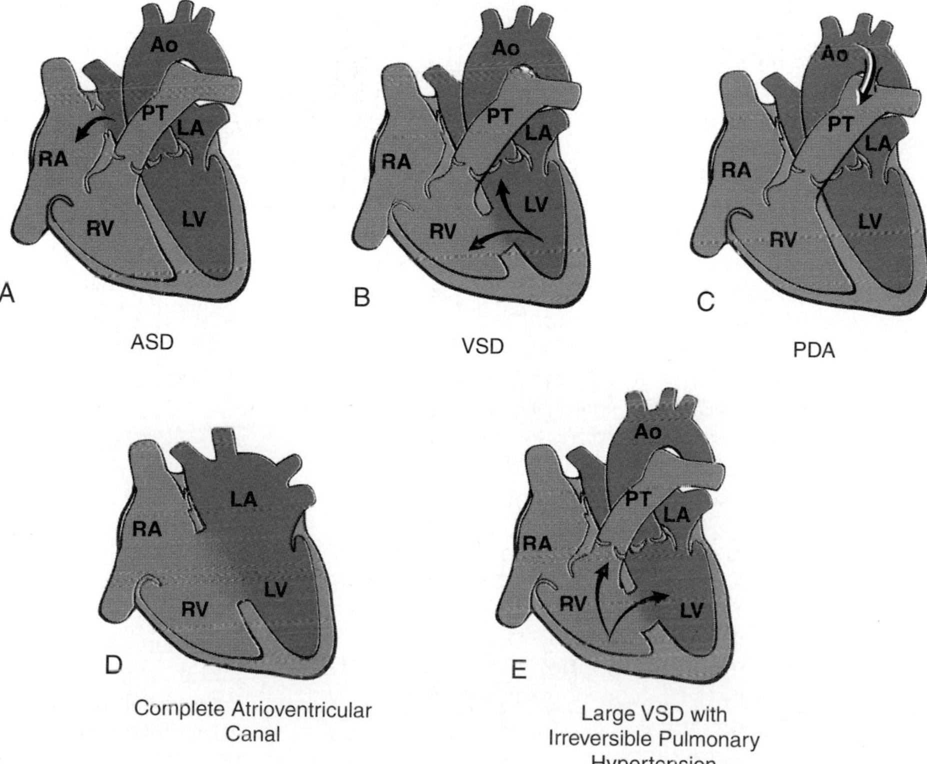

Figure 13–29 ■

Schematic diagram of congenital left-to-right shunts. *A*, Atrial septal defect. *B*, Ventricular septal defect (VSD). The shunt is left to right and the pressures are the same in both ventricles. Pressure hypertrophy of the right ventricle and volume hypertrophy of the left ventricle are present. *C*, Patent ductus arteriosus. *D*, Atrioventricular septal defect. *E*, Large VSD with irreversible pulmonary hypertension. In *E*, the shunt is right to left (shunt reversal) and there is volume and pressure hypertrophy of the right ventricle. Arrows indicate the direction of blood flow. Ao, aorta; RA, right atrium; LA, left atrium; LV, left ventricle; RV, right ventricle; PT, pulmonary trunk. (Courtesy of William D. Edwards, MD, Mayo Clinic, Rochester, MN.)

normal. Although some neonates may be in profound congestive heart failure, most isolated ASDs are well tolerated and usually do not become symptomatic before 30 years of age. A murmur is often present as a result of excessive flow through the pulmonary valve. Eventually, volume hypertrophy of the right atrium and right ventricle may develop.

Irreversible pulmonary hypertension develops in fewer than 10% of subjects with an isolated unoperated ASD. The objectives of surgical closure of an ASD are the reversal of the hemodynamic abnormalities and the prevention of complications, including heart failure, paradoxical embolization, and irreversible pulmonary vascular disease. Mortality is low, and postoperative survival is comparable to that of a normal population.[81]

Ventricular Septal Defect

Incomplete closure of the ventricular septum, allowing free communication between right and left ventricles, is the most common congenital cardiac anomaly (Fig. 13–29*B*). Frequently, VSD is associated with other structural defects, such as tetralogy. About 30% occur as isolated anomalies. Depending on the size of the defect, it may produce difficulties virtually from birth or, with smaller lesions, may not be recognized until later or may even spontaneously close.

MORPHOLOGY. VSDs are classified according to size and location. Most are about the size of the aortic valve orifice. About 90% involve the region of the membranous septum (**membranous VSD**) (Fig. 13–30). The remainder lie below the pulmonary valve (**infundibular VSD**) or within the muscular septum. Although most often single, VSDs in the muscular septum may be multiple (so-called **Swiss-cheese septum**).

The functional significance of a VSD depends on the size of the defect and the presence of other anomalies. About 50% of small muscular VSDs close spontaneously, and the remainder are generally well tolerated for years. Large defects are usually membranous or infundibular, and they generally remain patent and permit a significant left-to-right flow. Right ventricular hypertrophy and pulmonary hypertension are present from birth. Over time, irreversible pulmonary vascular disease develops in virtually all patients with large unoperated VSDs, leading to shunt reversal, cyanosis, and death.

Large defects may become manifest virtually at birth with signs of cardiac failure accompanying the murmur. Surgical closure of asymptomatic VSDs is generally not attempted during infancy, in hope of spontaneous closure. Correction, however, is indicated at age 1 year with large defects, before obstructive pulmonary vascular disease becomes irreversible.

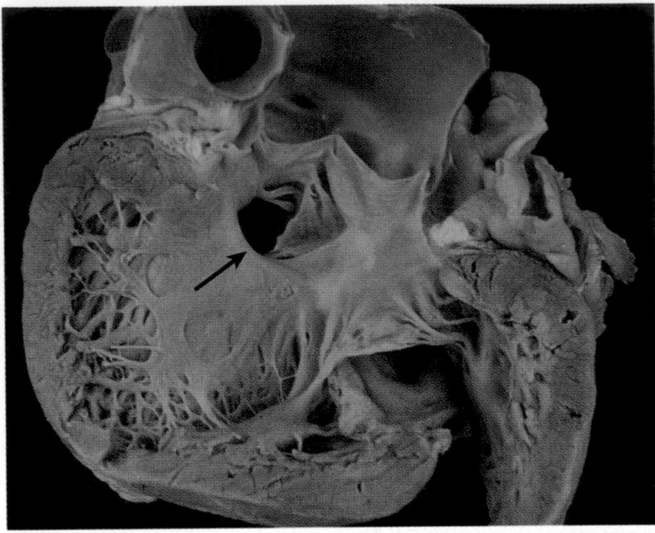

Figure 13–30

Gross photograph of a ventricular septal defect *(arrow)* (membranous type) viewed from the left ventricle. (Courtesy of William D. Edwards, MD, Mayo Clinic, Rochester, MN.)

Patent Ductus Arteriosus

PDA is a persistence after birth of the normal communication between the pulmonary arterial system and the aorta of the fetus (see Fig. 13–29*C*). About 90% of PDAs occur as an isolated anomaly. The remainder are most often associated with VSD, coarctation, or pulmonary or aortic stenosis. The length and diameter of the ductus vary widely.

Most often, PDA does not produce functional difficulties at birth. A narrow ductus may have no effect on growth and development during childhood. Its existence, however, can generally be detected by a continuous harsh murmur, described as *machinery-like*. Because the shunt is at first left-to-right, there is no cyanosis. Obstructive pulmonary vascular disease eventually ensues, however, with ultimate reversal of flow and its associated consequences.

There is general agreement that a PDA should be closed as early in life as is feasible. Preservation of ductal patency (by administering prostaglandin E) may assume great importance in the survival of infants with various forms of congenital heart disease with obstructed pulmonary or systemic blood flow, such as aortic valve atresia. Ironically the ductus may be either life-threatening or lifesaving.

Atrioventricular Septal Defect

AVSDs result from abnormal development of the embryologic AV canal, in which the superior and inferior endocardial cushions fail to fuse adequately, resulting in incomplete closure of the AV septum and inadequate formation of the tricuspid and mitral valves (see Fig. 13–29*D*). The two most common forms are *partial* AVSD (consisting of a primum ASD and a cleft anterior mitral leaflet, causing mitral insufficiency) and *complete* AVSD (consisting of a large combined AVSD and a large common AV valve—essentially a hole in the center of the heart). In the complete form, all four cardiac chambers freely communicate, inducing volume hypertrophy of each. More than one third of all patients with complete AVSD have Down syndrome. Surgical repair is possible.

RIGHT-TO-LEFT SHUNTS—EARLY CYANOSIS

Although a VSD is the most common congenital cardiac malformation, tetralogy of Fallot represents the most common form of *cyanotic* congenital heart disease. Other relatively frequently encountered anomalies in this category include transposition of the great arteries, tricuspid atresia, total anomalous pulmonary venous connection, and truncus arteriosus. For ease of recall, note that each entity begins with the letter *T*. Tetralogy and transposition are illustrated schematically in Figure 13–31.

Tetralogy of Fallot

The four features of the Fallot tetralogy are (1) *VSD*, (2) *obstruction to the right ventricular outflow tract (subpulmonary stenosis)*, (3) *an aorta that overrides the VSD*, and (4) *right ventricular hypertrophy* (Fig. 13–31*A*). All of the features result embryologically from anterosuperior displacement of the infundibular septum. Even untreated, some patients with tetralogy often survive into adult life (large series of patients with this condition showed 10% alive at 20 years and 3% at 40 years). The clinical consequences of tetralogy of Fallot depend primarily on the severity of subpulmonary stenosis.

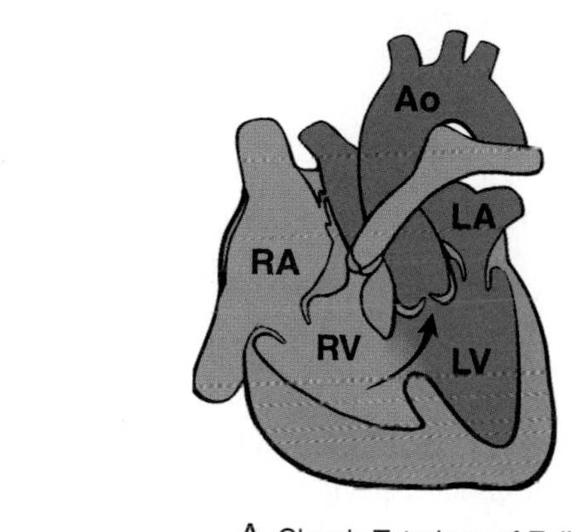

A Classic Tetralogy of Fallot

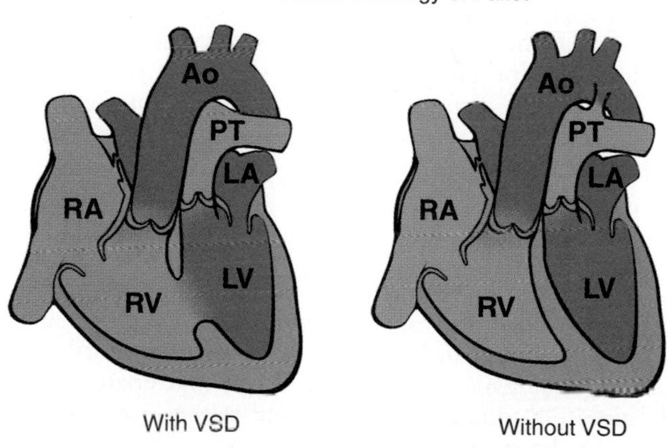

B Complete Transposition

Figure 13–31

Schematic diagram of the most important right-to-left shunts (cyanotic congestive heart disease). *A*, Tetralogy of Fallot. Diagrammatic representation of anatomic variants, indicating that the direction of shunting across the VSD depends on the severity of the subpulmonary stenosis. Arrow indicates the direction of the blood flow. *B*, Transposition of the great vessels with and without VSD. Ao, aorta; LA, left atrium; RA, right atrium; LV, left ventricle; RV, right ventricle; PT, pulmonary trunk (Courtesy of William D. Edwards, MD, Mayo Clinic, Rochester, MN.)

MORPHOLOGY. The heart is often enlarged and may be **boot-shaped** owing to marked right ventricular hypertrophy, particularly of the apical region. The VSD is usually large and approximates the diameter of the aortic orifice. The aortic valve forms its superior border, thereby overriding the defect and both ventricular chambers. The obstruction to right ventricular outflow is most often due to narrowing of the infundibulum (subpulmonary stenosis) but is often accompanied by pulmonary valvular stenosis. Sometimes, there is complete atresia of the pulmonary valve and variable portions of the pulmonary arteries, such that blood flow through a patent ductus or dilated bronchial arteries, or through both, is necessary for survival. Aortic valve insufficiency or ASD may also be present, and a right aortic arch is present in about 25%.

The severity of obstruction to right ventricular outflow determines the direction of blood flow. If the subpulmonary stenosis is mild, the abnormality resembles an isolated VSD, and the shunt may be left-to-right, without cyanosis (so-called *pink tetralogy*). *As the obstruction increases in severity, there is commensurately greater resistance to right ventricular outflow. As it approaches the level of systemic vascular resistance, right-to-left shunting predominates and, along with it, cyanosis (classic tetralogy).* With increasing severity of subpulmonary stenosis, the pulmonary arteries are progressively smaller and thinner walled (hypoplastic), and the aorta is progressively larger in diameter. As the child grows and the heart increases in size, the pulmonary orifice does not expand proportionally, making the obstruction ever worse. Thus, most infants with tetralogy are cyanotic from birth or soon thereafter. The subpulmonary stenosis, however, protects the pulmonary vasculature from pressure overload, and right ventricular failure is rare because the right ventricle is decompressed into the left ventricle and aorta. Complete surgical repair is possible for classic tetralogy but is more complicated for patients with pulmonary atresia and dilated bronchial arteries.

Transposition of Great Arteries

Transposition implies ventriculoarterial discordance, such that the aorta arises from the right ventricle, and the pulmonary artery emanates from the left ventricle (Fig. 13–31*B*). The AV connections are normal (concordant), with right atrium joining right ventricle and left atrium emptying into left ventricle.

The essential embryologic defect in complete transposition is abnormal formation of the truncal and aortopulmonary septa. *The aorta arises from the right ventricle and lies anterior and to the right of the pulmonary artery* (Fig. 13–32); *in contrast, in the normal heart, the aorta is posterior and to the right.* The result is separation of the systemic and pulmonary circulations, a condition incompatible with postnatal life, unless a shunt exists for adequate mixing of blood. Patients with transposition and a VSD (about 35%) have a stable shunt. Those with only a patent foramen ovale or PDA (about 65%), however, have unstable shunts that tend to close and therefore require immediate intervention to create a shunt (such as balloon atrial septostomy) within the first few days of life. Right ventricular hypertrophy becomes prominent as this chamber functions as the systemic ventricle. Concurrently the left ventricle becomes thin-walled (atrophic) as it supports the low-resistance pulmonary circulation.

The outlook for infants with transposition of the great vessels depends on the degree of *mixing* of the blood, the magnitude of the tissue hypoxia, and the ability of the right ventricle to maintain the systemic circulation. Without surgery, most patients die within the first months of life. Currently, most patients undergo a reparative operation (usually entailing transection and *switching* of the great arteries as well as the coronary arteries) during the first several weeks of life.

Truncus Arteriosus

The *persistent truncus arteriosus* anomaly arises from a developmental failure of separation of the embryologic truncus arteriosus into the aorta and pulmonary artery. The result is a single great artery that receives blood from both ventricles, accompanied by an underlying VSD, and that gives rise to the systemic, pulmonary, and coronary circulations. Because blood from the right and left ventricles mixes, there is early systemic cyanosis as well as increased pulmonary blood flow, with the danger of inoperable pulmonary hypertension.

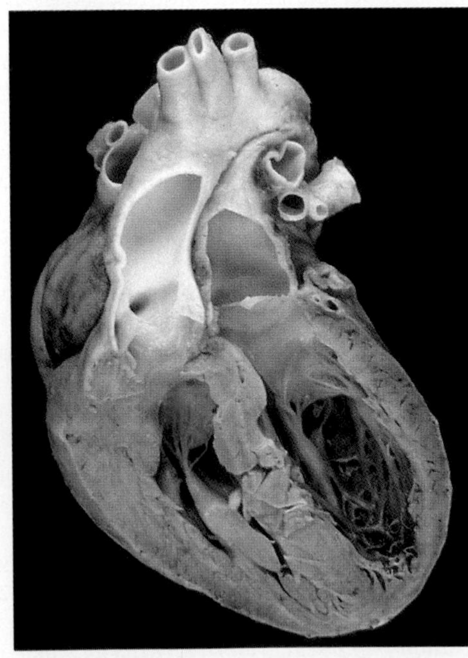

Figure 13–32

Gross photograph showing transposition of the great vessels. The aorta is arising from the right ventricle (at left) and the pulmonary artery from the left ventricle (at right). (Courtesy of William D. Edwards, MD, Mayo Clinic, Rochester, MN.)

Tricuspid Atresia

Complete occlusion of the tricuspid valve orifice is known as *tricuspid atresia.* It results embryologically from unequal division of the AV canal, and thus the mitral valve is larger than normal. This lesion is almost always associated with underdevelopment (hypoplasia) of the right ventricle. The circulation is maintained by a right-to-left shunt through an interatrial communication (ASD or patent foramen ovale). A VSD is also present and affords communication between the left ventricle and the great artery that arises from the hypoplastic right ventricle. Cyanosis is present virtually from birth, and there is a high mortality in the first weeks or months of life.

Total Anomalous Pulmonary Venous Connection

Total anomalous pulmonary venous connection, in which no pulmonary veins directly join the left atrium, results embryologically when the common pulmonary vein fails to develop or becomes atretic, causing primitive systemic venous channels from the lungs to remain patent. Total anomalous pulmonary venous connection usually drains into the left innominate vein or to the coronary sinus. Either a patent foramen ovale or an ASD is always present, allowing pulmonary venous blood to enter the left atrium. Consequences of total anomalous pulmonary venous connection include volume and pressure hypertrophy of the right atrium and right ventricle, and these chambers and the pulmonary trunk are dilated. The left atrium is hypoplastic, but the left ventricle is usually normal in size. Cyanosis may be present, owing to mixing of well-oxygenated and poorly oxygenated blood at the site of anomalous pulmonary venous connection and owing to a large right-to-left shunt at the ASD.

OBSTRUCTIVE CONGENITAL ANOMALIES

Congenital obstruction to blood flow may occur at the level of the heart valves or within a great vessel. Relatively common examples include stenosis of the pulmonary valve, stenosis or atresia of the aortic valve, and coarctation of the aorta. Obstruction can also occur within a chamber, as with subpulmonary stenosis in tetralogy.

Coarctation of Aorta

Coarctation (narrowing, constriction) of the aorta ranks high in frequency among the common structural anomalies. Males are affected twice as often as females, although females with Turner syndrome (Chapter 11) frequently have a coarctation. Two classic forms have been described: (1) an *infantile* form with tubular hypoplasia of the aortic arch proximal to a PDA that is often symptomatic in early childhood and (2) an *adult* form in which there is a discrete ridgelike infolding of the aorta, just opposite the closed ductus arteriosus (ligamentum arteriosum) (Fig. 13–33). Encroachment on the aortic lumen is of variable severity, sometimes leaving only a small channel or at other times producing only minimal narrowing. Clinical manifestations depend almost entirely on the severity of the narrowing and the patency of the ductus arteriosus. Although coarctation may occur as a solitary defect, it is accompanied by a bicuspid aortic valve in 50% of cases and may also be associated with congenital aortic stenosis, ASD, VSD, mitral regurgitation, and Berry aneurysms of the circle of Willis.

Coarctation with a PDA usually leads to manifestations early in life, and indeed it may cause signs and symptoms immediately after birth. Many infants with this anomaly do not survive the neonatal period without surgical intervention. In such cases, the delivery of unsaturated blood through the ductus arteriosus produces cyanosis localized to the lower half of the body.

The outlook is different with *coarctation* without a PDA, unless it is severe. Most of the children are asymptomatic, and the disease may go unrecognized until well into adult life. Typically, there is hypertension in the upper extremities, but there are weak pulses and a lower blood pressure in the lower extremities, associated with manifestations of arterial insufficiency (i.e., claudication and coldness). Particularly characteristic in adults is the development of collateral circulation between the precoarctation arterial branches and the postcoarctation arteries through enlarged intercostal and internal mammary arteries and the radiographically visible erosions (*notching*) of the undersurfaces of the ribs.

With all significant coarctations, murmurs are often present throughout systole, and sometimes a thrill may be present and there is cardiomegaly owing to left ventricular hypertrophy. With uncomplicated coarctation, surgical resection and end-to-end anastomosis or replacement of the affected aortic segment by a prosthetic graft yields excellent results.

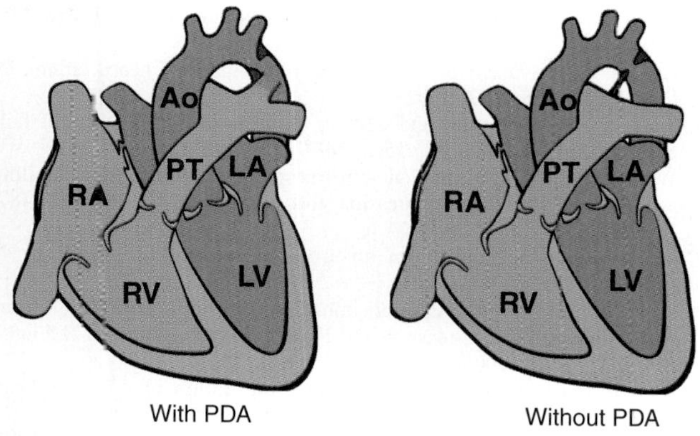

Figure 13–33 ■

Diagram showing coarctation of the aorta with and without persistent ductus arteriosus (PDA). Ao, aorta; LA, left atrium; RA, right atrium; LV, left ventricle; RV, right ventricle; PT, pulmonary trunk. (Courtesy of William D. Edwards, MD, Mayo Clinic, Rochester, MN.)

Pulmonary Stenosis and Atresia

Pulmonary stenosis and atresia, a relatively frequent malformation, constitutes an obstruction at the pulmonary valve, which may be mild to severe. It may occur as an isolated defect or as part of a more complex anomaly—either tetralogy of Fallot or transposition. Right ventricular hypertrophy often develops, and there is sometimes poststenotic dilation of the pulmonary artery owing to jetstream injury to the wall. With coexistent subpulmonary stenosis (as in tetralogy), the high ventricular pressure is not transmitted to the valve, and the pulmonary trunk is not dilated and may, in fact, be hypoplastic. When the valve is entirely atretic, there is no communication between the right ventricle and lungs, and so the anomaly is commonly associated with a hypoplastic right ventricle and an ASD; flow enters the lungs through a PDA. Mild stenosis may be asymptomatic and compatible with long life. The smaller the valvular orifice, the more severe is the cyanosis and the earlier its appearance.

Aortic Stenosis and Atresia

Aortic stenosis and atresia constitute the narrowings and obstructions of the aortic valve present from birth. There are three major types of stenosis: valvular, subvalvular, and supravalvular. With *valvular aortic stenosis*, the cusps may be hypoplastic (small), dysplastic (thickened, nodular), or abnormal in number (acommissural, unicommissural, bicuspid valve). In severe congenital aortic stenosis or atresia, obstruction of the left ventricular outflow tract leads to underdevelopment (hypoplasia) of the left ventricle and ascending aorta. There may be dense, porcelain-like left ventricular endocardial fibroelastosis (see section on restrictive cardiomyopathy). The ductus must be open to allow blood flow to the aorta and coronary arteries. This constellation of findings, called the *hypoplastic left heart syndrome*, is nearly always fatal in the first week of life, when the ductus closes. Less severe degrees of congenital aortic stenosis may be compatible with long survival.

Subaortic stenosis represents either a thickened ring (discrete type) or collar (tunnel type) of dense endocardial fibrous tissue below the level of the cusps. With the exception of coarctation of the aorta and PDA, other associated anomalies are uncommon; aortic stenosis is an isolated lesion in 80% of cases. *Supravalvular aortic stenosis* represents an inherited form of aortic dysplasia in which the ascending aortic wall is greatly thickened, causing luminal constriction. It may be related to a developmental disorder affecting multiple organ systems, including the vascular system, which includes hypercalcemia of infancy (Williams syndrome). Studies suggest that mutations in the elastin gene can cause supravalvular aortic stenosis.[82]

A prominent systolic murmur is usually detectable and sometimes a thrill, which does not distinguish the site of stenosis. Pressure hypertrophy of the left ventricle develops as a consequence of the obstruction to blood flow. In general, congenital stenoses are well tolerated unless severe. Mild stenoses can be managed conservatively with antibiotic prophylaxis and avoidance of strenuous activity, but the threat of sudden death with exertion always looms.

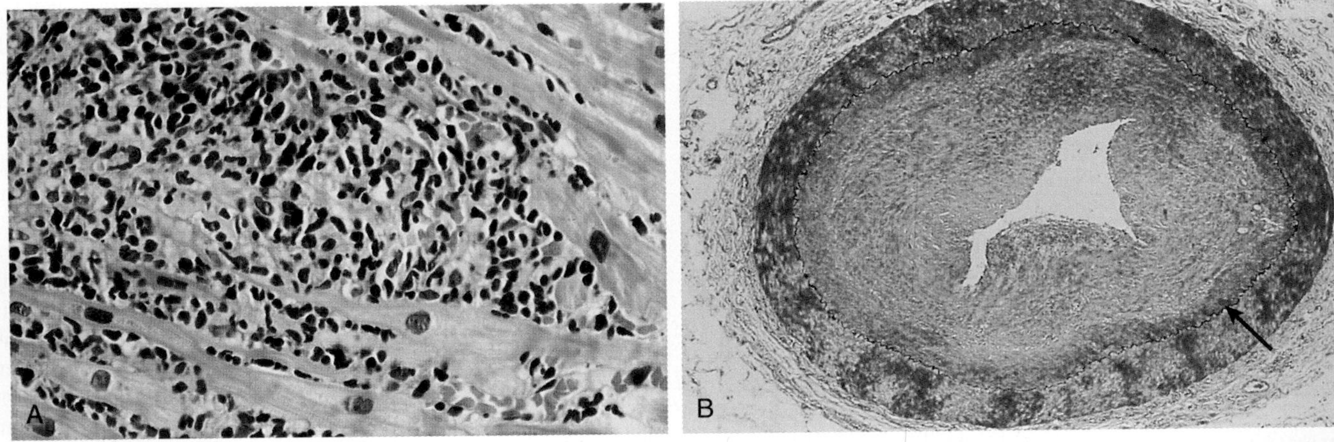

Figure 13–34

Complications of heart transplantation. *A*, Cardiac allograft rejection typified by lymphocytic infiltrate, with associated damage to cardiac myocytes. *B*, Graft coronary arteriosclerosis demonstrating severe diffuse concentric intimal thickening producing critical stenosis. The internal elastic lamina *(arrow)* and media are intact (Movat pentachrome stain, elastin black). (*B* from Salomon RN, et al: Human coronary transplantation-associated arteriosclerosis. Evidence for chronic immune reaction to activated graft endothelial cells. Am J Pathol 138:791, 1991.)

CARDIAC TRANSPLANTATION

Transplantation of cardiac allografts (approximately 2500 per year worldwide)[83] is now frequently performed for severe, intractable heart failure of diverse causes, the two most common of which are DCM and IHD. Three major factors contribute to the widespread success of cardiac transplantation: (1) careful selection of candidates, (2) improved maintenance immunosuppression (including the use of cyclosporin A, along with steroids and azathioprine), and (3) early histopathologic diagnosis of acute allograft rejection by sequential endomyocardial biopsy.

The major complications are illustrated in Figure 13–34. Allograft rejection is a major postoperative problem; scheduled interval endomyocardial biopsy is the only reliable means of diagnosing acute cardiac rejection before substantial myocardial damage (and clinical recognition) has occurred and at a stage that is reversible in the majority of instances. Rejection is characterized by interstitial lymphocytic inflammation that in its more advanced stages damages adjacent myocytes (Fig. 13–34*A*). When myocardial injury is not extensive, the *rejection episode* is usually either self-limited or successfully reversed by increased immunosuppressive therapy. Advanced rejection may be irreversible and fatal.

Other postoperative problems include infection and development of malignancies, particularly lymphomas (generally related to Epstein-Barr virus in the presence of profound chronic therapeutic immunosuppression). The major current limitation to the long-term success of cardiac transplantation is late, progressive, diffuse stenosing intimal thickening of the coronary arteries (*graft vascular disease, graft arteriosclerosis*) (Fig. 13–34*B*). This is a particularly vexing problem because it may lead to silent MI (particularly difficult to diagnose because these patients, with denervated hearts, do not experience chest pain); in this situation, congestive heart failure or sudden death is the usual outcome. Despite these problems, the overall outlook is good, with a 1-year survival of 70 to 80% and 5-year survival of more than 60%.

REFERENCES

1. Christensen G: Cardiovascular and renal effects of atrial natriuretic factor. Scand J Clin Lab Invest 53:203, 1993.
2. Peters NS, et al: Cardiac arrhythmogenesis and the gap junction. J Mol Cell Cardiol 27:37, 1995.
3. Schoen FJ: Aortic valve structure-function correlations: role of elastic fibers no longer a stretch of the imagination. J Heart Valve Dis 6:1, 1997.
4. Duncan AK, et al: Cardiovascular disease in elderly patients. Mayo Clin Proc 71:184, 1996.
5. Silver MD: Cardiovascular Pathology, 2nd ed. New York, Churchill Livingstone, 1996.
6. Braunwald E (ed): Heart Disease: A Textbook of Cardiovascular Medicine, 5th ed. Philadelphia, WB Saunders, 1997.
7. Katz AM: The cardiomyopathy of overload: an unnatural response in the hypertrophied heart. Ann Intern Med 121:363, 1994.
8. Cohn J: The management of chronic heart failure. N Engl J Med 335: 490, 1996.
9. Grossman W: Diastolic dysfunction in congestive heart failure. N Engl J Med 325:1552, 1992.
10. Colucci WS: Molecular and cellular mechanisms of myocardial failure. Am J Cardiol 80(11A):15L, 1997.
11. Wankerl M, Schwartz K: Calcium transport proteins in the nonfailing and failing heart: gene expression and function. J Mol Med 73:487, 1995.
12. Narula J, et al: Apoptosis in myocytes in end-stage heart failure. N Engl J Med 335:1182, 1996.
13. Levy D, et al: Prognostic implications of echocardiographically determined left ventricular mass in the Framingham heart study. N Engl J Med 322:1561, 1990.
14. Rich Edwards JW, et al: The primary prevention of coronary heart disease in women. N Engl J Med 332:1758, 1995.
15. Hennekens CH: Increasing burden of cardiovascular disease: current knowledge and future directions for research on risk factors. Circulation 97:1095, 1998.
16. ACC/AHA guidelines for the management of patients with acute MI. J Am Coll Cardiol 28:1328, 1996.
17. The History and Practice of Coronary Revascularization. Supplement to J Am Coll Cardiol 31:1B, 1998.

18. Burke AP, et al: Coronary risk factors and plaque morphology in men with coronary disease who died suddenly. N Engl J Med 336:1276, 1997.
19. Theroux P, Fuster V: Acute coronary syndromes: unstable angina and non-Q wave myocardial infarction. Circulation 97:1195, 1998.
20. Johnstone MT, et al: The pathophysiology of the onset of morning cardiovascular events. Am J Hypertens 9:22S, 1996.
21. Leor J, et al: Sudden cardiac death triggered by an earthquake. N Engl J Med 334:413, 1996.
22. Libby P: Molecular bases of the acute coronary syndromes. Circulation 91:2844, 1995.
23. Davies MJ: Stability and instability: two faces of coronary arteriosclerosis. Circulation 94:2013, 1996.
24. Ribeiro PA, Shah PM: Unstable angina: new insights into pathophysiologic characteristics, prognosis, and management strategies. Curr Probl Cardiol 21:669, 1996.
25. Goldstein F, et al: Postmenopausal hormone therapy and mortality. N Engl J Med 336:1769, 1997.
26. DeWood MA, et al: Prevalence of total coronary occlusion during the early hours of transmural MI. N Engl J Med 303:897, 1980.
27. Jennings RB, et al: Development of cell injury in sustained acute ischemia. Circulation 82:II-2, 1990.
28. James TN: Complex causes of fatal MI. Circulation 96:1696, 1997.
29. Itoh G, et al: DNA fragmentation of human infarcted myocardial cells demonstrated by the nick end labeling method and DNA agarose gel electrophoresis. Am J Pathol 146:1325, 1995.
30. Kajstura J, et al: Apoptotic and necrotic myocyte cell deaths are independent contributing variables of infarct size in rats. Lab Invest 74:86, 1996.
31. White HD, Van der Werf FJJ: Thrombolysis for acute myocardial infarction. Circulation 97:1632, 1998.
32. Bittl JA: Advances in coronary angioplasty. N Engl J Med 335:1290, 1996.
33. Kloner RA, et al: Medical and cellular implications of stunning, hibernation, and preconditioning. Circulation 97:1848, 1998..
34. Vanoverschelde JL, et al: Chronic myocardial hibernation in humans: from bedside to bench. Circulation 95:1961, 1997.
35. Kloner RA, Yellon D: Does ischemic preconditioning occur in patients? J Am Coll Cardiol 24:1133, 1994.
36. Van der Werf F: Cardiac troponins in acute coronary syndromes. N Engl J Med 335:1388, 1996.
37. Adams JE, et al: Diagnosis of perioperative MI with measurement of cardiac troponin I. N Engl J Med 330:670, 1994.
38. Vaughan DE, Pfeffer MA: Angiotensin converting enzyme inhibitors and cardiovascular remodeling. Cardiovasc Res 28:159, 1994.
39. Wright JN, Salem D: Sudden cardiac death and the "athlete's heart." Arch Intern Med 155:1473, 1995.
40. Liberthson RR: Sudden death from cardiac causes in children and young adults. N Engl J Med 334:1039, 1996.
41. Kannel WB: Blood pressure as a cardiovascular risk factor: prevention and treatment. JAMA 275:1571, 1996.
42. Carabello BA, Crawford FA: Valvular heart disease. N Engl J Med 337:32, 1997.
43. Otto CM, et al: Characterization of the early lesion of "degenerative" valvular aortic stenosis: histological and immunohistochemical studies. Circulation 90:844, 1994.
44. Dietz HC: New insights into the genetic basis of aortic aneurysms. In Schoen FJ, Gimbrone MA Jr (eds): Cardiovascular Pathology: Clinicopathologic Correlations and Pathogenetic Mechanisms. Baltimore, Williams & Wilkins, 1995, p 144.
45. Zuppiroli A, et al: Natural history of mitral valve prolapse. Am J Cardiol 75:1028, 1995.
46. Bronze MS, Dale JB: The reemergence of serious group streptococcal infections and acute rheumatic fever. Am J Med Sci 311:41, 1996.
47. Veasy LG, Hill HR: Immunologic and clinical correlations in rheumatic fever and rheumatic heart disease. Pediatr Infect Dis J 16:400, 1997.
48. Dajani AS, et al: Prevention of bacterial endocarditis: recommendations by the American Heart Association. Circulation 96:358, 1997.
49. Hojnik M, et al: Heart valve involvement (Libman-Sacks endocarditis) in the antiphospholipid syndrome. Circulation 93:1579, 1996.
50. Robiolio PA, et al: Carcinoid heart disease: correlation of high serotonin levels with valvular abnormalities detected by cardiac catheterization and echocardiography. Circulation 92:790, 1995.
51. Connolly HM, et al: Fenfluramine-phentermine associated valvular heart disease: a new observation. N Engl J Med 337:581, 1997.
52. Vongpatanasin W, et al: Prosthetic heart valves. N Engl J Med 355: 407, 1996.
53. Hammermeister KE, et al: A comparison of outcomes in men 11 years after heart-valve replacement with a mechanical valve or bioprosthesis. N Engl J Med 328:1289, 1993.
54. Report of the WHO/ISFC Task Force on the definition and classification of cardiomyopathies. Br Heart J 44:672, 1980.
55. Richardson P, et al: Report of the 1995 World Health Organization/International Society and Federation of Cardiology Task Force on the definition and classification of cardiomyopathies. Circulation 93:841, 1996.
56. Dec GW, Fuster V: Idiopathic dilated cardiomyopathy. N Engl J Med 331:1564, 1994.
57. Keating MT, Sanguinetti MC: Molecular genetic insights into cardiovascular disease. Science 272:681, 1996.
58. Beggs AH: Dystrophinopathy, the expanding phenotype: dystrophin abnormalities in X-linked dilated cardiomyopathy. Circulation 95: 2344, 1997.
59. Basso C, et al: Arrhythmogenic right ventricular cardiomyopathy: dysplasia, dystrophy, or myocarditis? Circulation 94:983, 1996.
60. Spirito P, et al: The management of hypertrophic cardiomyopathy. N Engl J Med 336:775, 1997.
61. Marian AJ, Roberts R: Recent advances in the molecular genetics of hypertrophic cardiomyopathy. Circulation 92:1336, 1995.
62. Kushwaha SS, et al: Restrictive cardiomyopathy. N Engl J Med 336: 267, 1997.
63. Huber SA: Autoimmunity in myocarditis: relevance of animal models. Clin Immunol Immunopathol 83:93, 1997.
64. Morris SA, et al: Pathophysiological insights into the cardiomyopathy of Chagas' disease. Circulation 82:1900, 1990.
65. Michaels AD, et al: Cardiovascular involvement in AIDS. Curr Probl Cardiol 22:109, 1997.
66. Grady WW, et al: Infection of the heart by the human immunodeficiency virus. Am J Cardiol 66:203, 1990.
67. Aretz HT, et al: Myocarditis: a histopathologic definition and classification. Am J Cardiovasc Pathol 1:3, 1986.
68. Cooper LT Jr, et al: Idiopathic giant-cell myocarditis—natural history and treatment. Multicenter Giant Cell Myocarditis Study Group Investigators. N Engl J Med 336:1860, 1997.
69. Shan K, et al: Anthracycline-induced cardiotoxicity. Ann Intern Med 125:47, 1996.
70. Kloner RA, et al: The effects of acute and chronic cocaine use on the heart. Circulation 85:407, 1992.
71. Samuels MA: Neurally induced cardiac damage: definition of the problem. Neurol Clin 11:273, 1993.
72. Kyle RA, et al: The premortem recognition of systemic senile amyloidosis with cardiac involvement. Am J Med 171:395, 1996.
73. Jacobson DR, et al: Variant-sequence transthyretin (isoleucine 122) in late-onset cardiac amyloidosis in black Americans. N Engl J Med 336:466, 1997.
74. Polikar R, et al: The thyroid and the heart. Circulation 87:1435, 1993.
75. Burke A, Virmani R: Tumors of the Heart and Great Vessels, 3rd series, fascicle 16: Atlas of Tumor Pathology. Washington, DC, Armed Forces Institute of Pathology, 1996.
76. Reynen K: Cardiac myxomas. N Engl J Med 333:1610, 1995.
77. Morris CD, Manashe VD: 25-year mortality after surgical repair of congenital heart defect in childhood. JAMA 266:3447, 1991.
78. Edwards WD: Congenital heart disease. In Damjanov I, Linder J (eds): Anderson's Pathology, 10th ed. St. Louis, Mosby, 1996.
79. Payne RM, et al: Toward a molecular understanding of congenital heart disease. Circulation 91:494, 1995.
80. Benson DW, et al: Reduced penetrance, variable expressivity, and genetic heterogeneity of familial atrial septal defects. Circulation 97: 2043, 1998.
81. Murphy JG, et al: Long-term outcome after surgical repair of isolated atrial septal defect. N Engl J Med 323:1645, 1990.
82. Smoot LB: Elastin gene deletions in Williams syndrome. Curr Opin Pediatr 7:698, 1995.
83. O'Connell JB, et al: Cardiac transplantation: recipient selection, donor procurement, and medical follow-up. Circulation 86:1061, 1992.

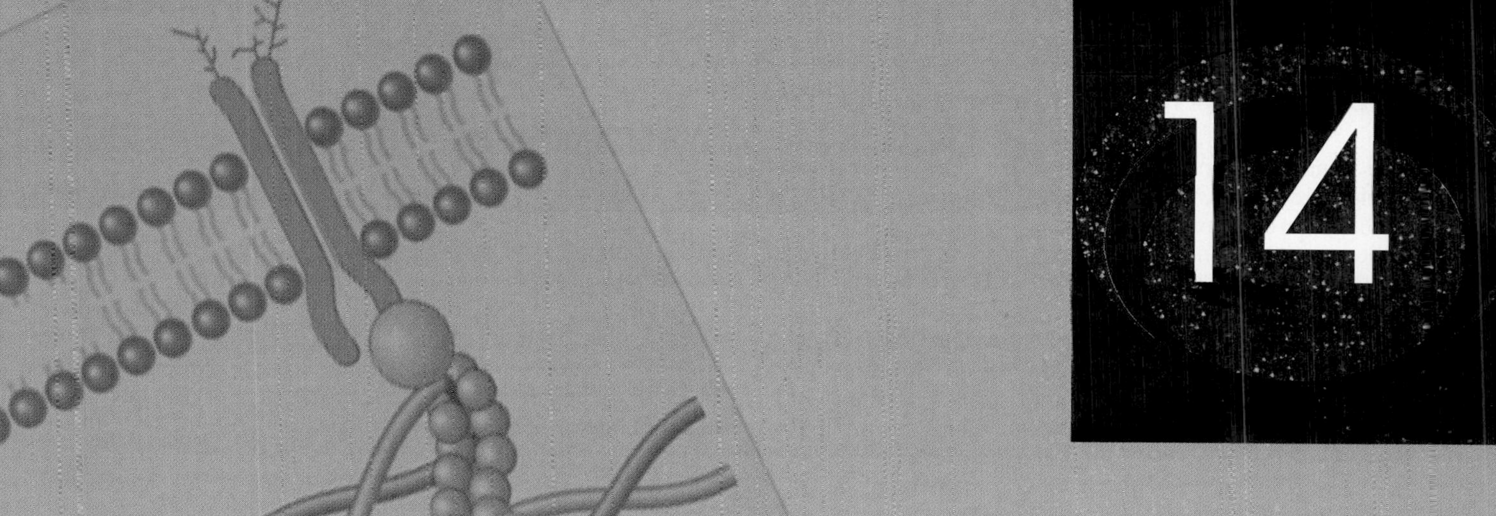

14

Red Cells and Bleeding Disorders

NORMAL DEVELOPMENT OF BLOOD CELLS

ORIGIN AND DIFFERENTIATION OF HEMATOPOIETIC CELLS

ANEMIAS

ANEMIAS OF BLOOD LOSS

Acute Blood Loss

Chronic Blood Loss

HEMOLYTIC ANEMIAS

Hereditary Spherocytosis

Hemolytic Disease Due to Erythrocyte Enzyme Defects: Glucose-6-Phosphate Dehydrogenase Deficiency

Sickle Cell Disease

Thalassemia Syndromes

β-Thalassemias

α-Thalassemias

Paroxysmal Nocturnal Hemoglobinuria

Immunohemolytic Anemia

Hemolytic Anemia Resulting From Trauma to Red Cells

ANEMIAS OF DIMINISHED ERYTHROPOIESIS

Megaloblastic Anemias

Anemias of Vitamin B_{12} Deficiency: Pernicious Anemia

Anemia of Folate Deficiency

Iron Deficiency Anemia

Anemia of Chronic Disease

Aplastic Anemia

Pure Red Cell Aplasia

Other Forms of Marrow Failure

POLYCYTHEMIA

BLEEDING DISORDERS: HEMORRHAGIC DIATHESES

BLEEDING DISORDERS CAUSED BY VESSEL WALL ABNORMALITIES

BLEEDING RELATED TO REDUCED PLATELET NUMBER: THROMBOCYTOPENIA

Idiopathic Thrombocytopenic Purpura (ITP)

Acute Idiopathic Thrombocytopenic Purpura

Drug-Induced Thrombocytopenia

HIV-Associated Thrombocytopenia

Thrombotic Microangiopathies: Thrombotic Thrombocytopenic Purpura and Hemolytic-Uremic Syndrome

BLEEDING DISORDERS RELATED TO DEFECTIVE PLATELET FUNCTIONS

HEMORRHAGIC DIATHESES RELATED TO ABNORMALITIES IN CLOTTING FACTORS

Deficiencies of Factor VIII–vWF Complex

von Willebrand Disease

Hemophilia A (Factor VIII Deficiency)

Hemophilia B (Christmas Disease, Factor IX Deficiency)

DISSEMINATED INTRAVASCULAR COAGULATION (DIC)

The bone marrow, lymph nodes, and spleen are involved in hematopoiesis. These organs and tissues have traditionally been divided into *myeloid tissue,* which includes the bone marrow and the cells derived from it (e.g., erythrocytes, platelets, granulocytes, and monocytes), and *lymphoid tissue,* consisting of thymus, lymph nodes, and spleen. This subdivision is artificial with respect to both the normal physiology of hematopoietic cells and the diseases affecting them. For example, although bone marrow is not the site where most of the mature lymphoid cells are found, it is the source of lymphoid stem cells. Similarly, leukemias, which are neoplastic disorders of the leukocytes, originate within the bone marrow but involve the lymph nodes and spleen quite prominently. Some red cell disorders (hemolytic anemias) result from the formation of autoantibodies, signifying a primary disorder of the lymphocytes. Thus, it is not possible to draw neat lines between diseases involving the myeloid and lymphoid tissues. Recognizing this difficulty, we have somewhat arbitrarily divided diseases of the hematopoietic tissues into two chapters. In the first, we consider diseases of red cells and those affecting hemostasis. In the second, we discuss diseases affecting the leukocytes and the lymph nodes and disorders affecting primarily the spleen and thymus.

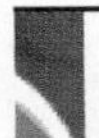

NORMAL

A complete discussion of normal hematopoiesis is beyond our scope, but certain features are helpful to an understanding of the diseases of blood.

NORMAL DEVELOPMENT OF BLOOD CELLS

In the human embryo, clusters of stem cells, called blood islands, appear in the yolk sac in the third week of fetal development.[1] Recent data suggest that hematopoietic stem cells may also arise in the intraembryonic aorta/gonad/mesonephros and that germ cells may give rise to hematopoietic stem cells. At about the third month of embryogenesis, some of these cells migrate to the liver, which then becomes the chief site of blood cell formation until shortly before birth. Beginning in the fourth month of development, hematopoiesis commences in the bone marrow. At birth, all the marrow throughout the skeleton is active and is virtually the sole source of blood cells. In the full-term infant, hepatic hematopoiesis has dwindled to a trickle but may persist in widely scattered small foci, which become inactive soon after birth. Up to the age of puberty, all the marrow throughout the skeleton is red and hematopoietically active. Usually by 18 years of age only the vertebrae, ribs, sternum, skull, pelvis, and proximal epiphyseal regions of the humerus and femur retain red marrow, the remaining marrow becoming yellow, fatty, and inactive. Thus, in adults, only about half of the marrow space is active in hematopoiesis.

Several features of this normal sequence should be emphasized. By the time of birth, the bone marrow is virtually the sole source of all forms of blood cells and a major source of lymphocyte precursors. In the premature infant, foci of hematopoiesis are frequently evident in the liver and, rarely, in the spleen, lymph nodes, or thymus. However, significant postembryonic extramedullary hematopoiesis is abnormal in the full-term infant. With an increased demand for blood cells in the adult, the fatty marrow may become transformed to red, active marrow. Moreover, this is accompanied by increased productive activity throughout the marrow. These adaptive changes are capable of increasing red cell production (erythropoiesis) sevenfold to eightfold. Thus, if the marrow precursor cells are not destroyed by metastatic cancer or irradiation, for example, and necessary substrate is available (e.g., adequate amounts of iron, protein, requisite vitamins), such loss of red cells as may occur in hemolytic disorders produces anemia only when the marrow compensatory mechanisms are outstripped. Under these circumstances, extramedullary hematopoiesis may reappear, first within the liver and then in the spleen and lymph nodes.

Origin and Differentiation of Hematopoietic Cells

There is little doubt that the formed elements of blood—erythrocytes, granulocytes, monocytes, platelets, and lymphocytes—have a common origin in a pluripotent hematopoietic stem cell.[1] This common precursor then gives rise to lymphoid stem cells and the trilineage myeloid stem cells, which are committed to produce lymphocytes and the myeloid cells, respectively (Fig. 14–1). The recently identified lymphoid stem cell gives rise to precursors of T cells (pro–T cells), B cells (pro–B cells), and possibly natural killer (NK) cells.[1a] The details of lymphoid differentiation are not discussed here, but it is worth pointing out that unlike myeloid differentiation, there are no distinctive, morphologically recognizable stages. For definition, reliance must be placed on the detection of differentiation-specific antigens by monoclonal antibodies (Chapter 15). From the multipotent myeloid stem cell arise at least three types of *committed stem cells* capable of differentiating along the erythroid/megakaryocytic, eosinophilic, and granulocyte-macrophage pathways. The committed stem cells have been called colony-forming units (CFU) because they give rise to colonies of differentiated progeny in vitro (Fig. 14–1). From the various committed stem cells are derived intermediate stages and ultimately the morphologically recognizable precursors of the differentiated cell lines, that is, proerythroblasts, myeloblasts, megakaryoblasts, monoblasts, and eosinophiloblasts. These in turn give rise to mature progeny. Since the mature blood elements have a finite life span, it follows that their numbers must be constantly replenished. This can be realized if the stem cells possess the capacity not only to differentiate but also to renew themselves. *Thus, self-renewal is an important property of stem cells.* The pluripotent stem cells have the greatest capacity for self-renewal, but normally most of them are not in cell cycle. As commitment proceeds, self-renewal ability becomes limited, but a greater fraction of the stem cells are found to be in cycle. For example, few trilineage myeloid stem cells are normally in cell cycle, but up to 50% of CFU-GM (the precursors of granulocytes and macrophages) are synthesizing DNA. This suggests that normally the pool of differentiated cells is replenished mainly by the proliferation of restricted stem cells. Although the earliest recognizable precursors (e.g., myeloblasts or proerythro-

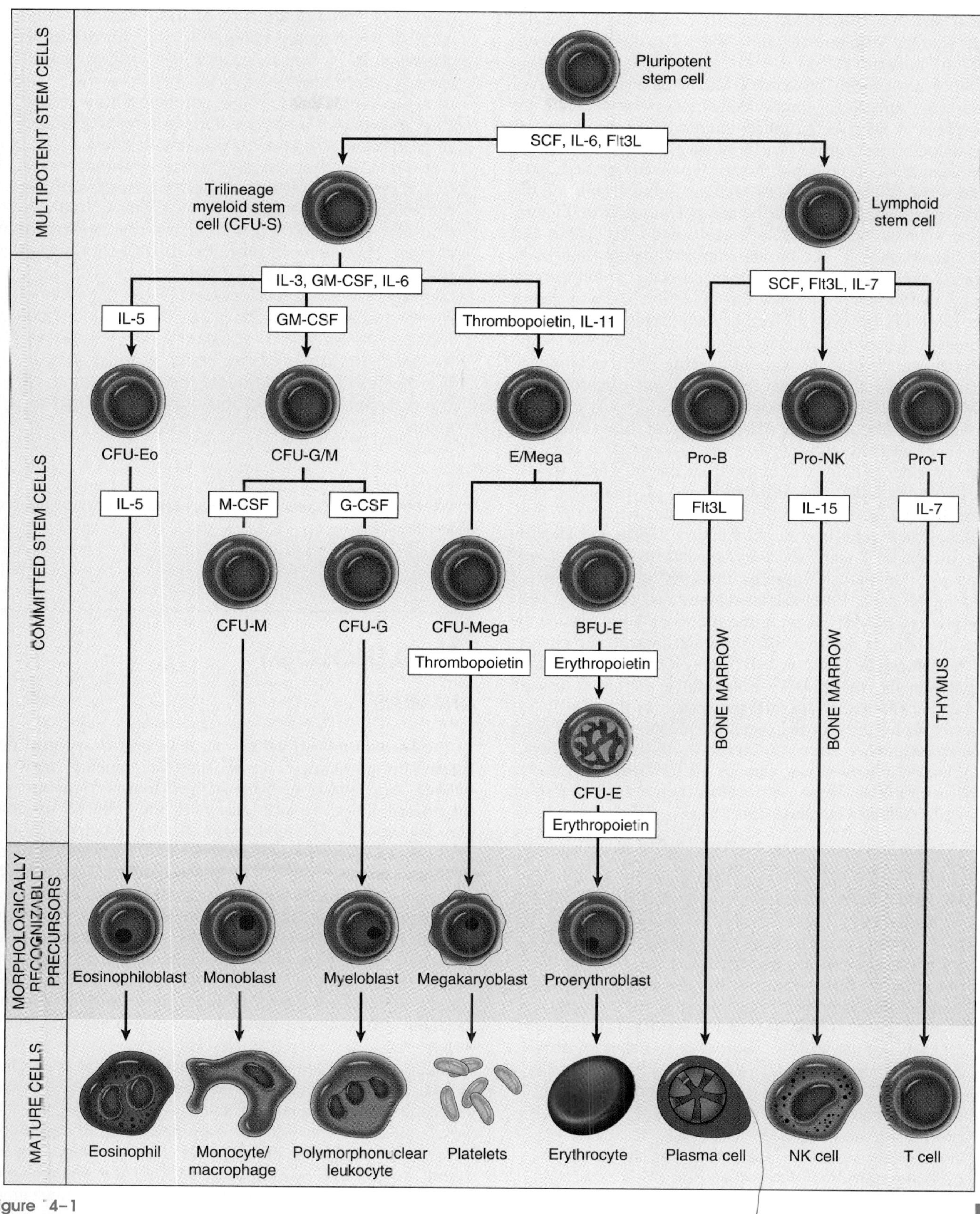

Figure 14–1

Differentiation of hematopoietic cells. SCF, stem cell factor; Flt3L, Flt3 ligand; GM-CSF, granulocyte-macrophage colony-stimulating factor; M-CSF, macrophage colony-stimulating factor; G-CSF, granulocyte colony-stimulating factor. (Modified from Wyngaarden JB, et al [eds]: Cecil Textbook of Medicine, 19th ed. Philadelphia, WB Saunders, 1992, p 820.)

blasts) are in active cell division, they cannot self-replicate; that is, they differentiate and "die." By definition, then, they are not stem cells.

Since most forms of marrow failure or neoplastic disorders (e.g., aplastic anemias, leukemias, polycythemia) are disorders of stem cells, much interest is centered on the physiologic mechanisms that regulate the proliferation and differentiation of progenitor cells. Involved in these processes are soluble factors as well as stromal cells of the bone marrow. Among the hematopoietic growth factors, some, such as stem cell factor (also called c-*kit* ligand) and flt3-ligand (flt3-L), act on the most immature stem cell. Others, such as the granulocyte-macrophage colony-stimulating factor (GM-CSF), act on CFU-GM. Because genes for most of the growth factors have been cloned, large amounts of recombinant proteins can be generated. Some recombinant factors are currently being used to stimulate hematopoiesis. Included in this group are erythropoietin, GM-CSF, G-CSF, and thrombopoietin.

Normal Anatomy and Morphology of Bone Marrow. The bone marrow not only is a reservoir of stem cells but also provides a unique microenvironment in which the orderly proliferation and differentiation of precursor cells takes place. In addition, it regulates the release of fully differentiated cells into the circulation. Under the electron microscope, the marrow cavity appears to be a vast network of thin-walled sinusoids lined by a single layer of endothelial cells. Basement membrane and adventitial cells are present, but they form a discontinuous layer outside the endothelium. In between the sinusoidal network lie clusters of hematopoietic cells and fat cells. Differentiated blood cells enter the sinusoids by transcellular migration through the endothelial cells. That this process is finely regulated is attested to by the fact that when hematopoiesis takes place at extramedullary sites, for example, the spleen (Chapter 15), the peripheral blood contains all forms of abnormal as well as primitive blood cells that do not enter the blood in normal medullary hematopoiesis.

MORPHOLOGY. Although the morphology of the hematopoietic cells within the bone marrow is best studied in smears of marrow aspirates, useful information can also be obtained by studying the histology of bone marrow biopsy specimens. For example, a reasonable estimate of marrow activity may be obtained by examining the ratio of fat cells to hematopoietic elements in bone marrow biopsy samples. In normal adults, this ratio approaches 1:1, but with marrow hypoplasia (e.g., aplastic anemia), the proportion of fat cells is greatly increased, and conversely, fat cells may virtually disappear in diseases characterized by increased hematopoiesis (e.g., hemolytic anemias). When subjected to fixatives and tissue staining methods, the cells of the bone marrow and peripheral blood differ in appearance from those in air-dried Giemsa- or Wright-stained preparations. While the earliest cells of the myeloid and erythroid lineages (myeloblasts, pronormoblasts) can usually be distinguished in stained marrow aspirates, it is extremely difficult, if not impossible, to differentiate in tissue sections the various "blast" forms. Often, tentative identification must be made on the basis of "the company they keep." Thus, a primitive cell found in relation to a focus of granulocytes is likely to be a myeloblast.

The relative proportion of cells in the bone marrow is almost always deranged in diseases of the blood and bone marrow. The marrow normally contains about 60% granulocytes and their precursors; 20% erythroid precursors; 10% lymphocytes and monocytes and their precursors; and 10% unidentified or disintegrating cells. Thus, the normal myeloid to erythroid ratio is 3:1. The dominant cell types in the myeloid compartment include myelocytes, metamyelocytes, and granulocytes. In the erythroid compartment, the dominant forms are polychromatophilic and orthochromic normoblasts.

We now turn to consider the various disorders of the red blood cells.

PATHOLOGY

ANEMIAS

The function of red cells is the transport of oxygen into tissues. In physiologic terms, therefore, anemia may be defined as a reduction in the oxygen transport capacity of the blood. Since in most instances the reduced oxygen-carrying capacity of blood results from a deficiency of red cells, *anemia may be defined as a reduction below normal limits of the total circulating red cell mass.* This value is not easily measured, however, and therefore anemia has been defined as a reduction below normal in the volume of packed red cells, as measured by the hematocrit, or a reduction in the hemoglobin concentration of the blood. It hardly needs pointing out that fluid retention may expand plasma volume and fluid loss may contract plasma volume, creating spurious abnormalities in clinically measured values.

Innumerable classifications of anemia have been proposed. A highly acceptable one based on the underlying mechanism is presented in Table 14–1. Anemias can also be classified on the basis of the appearance of red blood cells in the peripheral blood smear. Factors taken into account in such categorizations are red cell size (normocytic, microcytic, or macrocytic); degree of hemoglobinization, reflected in the color of red cells (normochromic or hypochromic); and several other special features, such as red cell shape. Although these red cell indices are often judged subjectively by the physician, they are also measured objectively and expressed by various terms, as follows:

Table 14-1. CLASSIFICATION OF ANEMIA ACCORDING TO UNDERLYING MECHANISM

Blood Loss
Acute: trauma
Chronic: lesions of gastrointestinal tract, gynecologic disturbances

Increased Rate of Destruction (Hemolytic Anemias)
Intrinsic (intracorpuscular) abnormalities of red cells
Hereditary
Red cell membrane disorders
Disorders of membrane cytoskeleton: spherocytosis, elliptocytosis
Disorders of lipid synthesis: selective increase in membrane lecithin
Red cell enzyme deficiencies
Glycolytic enzymes: pyruvate kinase deficiency, hexokinase deficiency
Enzymes of hexose monophosphate shunt: G6PD, glutathione synthetase
Disorders of hemoglobin synthesis
Deficient globin synthesis: thalassemia syndromes
Structurally abnormal globin synthesis (hemoglobinopathies): sickle cell anemia, unstable hemoglobins
Acquired
Membrane defect: paroxysmal nocturnal hemoglobinuria
Extrinsic (extracorpuscular) abnormalities
Antibody mediated
Isohemagglutinins: transfusion reactions, erythroblastosis fetalis
Autoantibodies: idiopathic (primary), drug-associated, systemic lupus erythematosus, malignant neoplasms, mycoplasmal infection
Mechanical trauma to red cells
Microangiopathic hemolytic anemias: thrombotic thrombocytopenic purpura, disseminated intravascular coagulation
Cardiac traumatic hemolytic anemia
Infections: malaria
Chemical injury: lead poisoning
Sequestration in mononuclear phagocyte system: hypersplenism

Impaired Red Cell Production
Disturbance of proliferation and differentiation of stem cells: aplastic anemia, pure red cell aplasia, anemia of renal failure, anemia of endocrine disorders
Disturbance of proliferation and maturation of erythroblasts
Defective DNA synthesis: deficiency or impaired use of vitamin B_{12} and folic acid (megaloblastic anemias)
Defective hemoglobin synthesis
Deficient heme synthesis: iron deficiency
Deficient globin synthesis: thalassemias
Unknown or multiple mechanisms: sideroblastic anemia, anemia of chronic infections, myelophthisic anemias due to marrow infiltrations

- *Mean cell volume*: the average volume of a red blood cell, expressed in femtoliters (cubic micrometers)
- *Mean cell hemoglobin*: the average content (mass) of hemoglobin per red blood cell, expressed in picograms
- *Mean cell hemoglobin concentration*: the average concentration of hemoglobin in a given volume of packed red blood cells, expressed in grams per deciliter
- *Red blood cell distribution width*: the coefficient of variation of red blood cell volume

Red blood cell indices may be calculated from hematocrit, hemoglobin, and red cell count values, but in most laboratories instruments directly measure or automatically calculate them. Adult reference ranges are shown in Table 14–2. Anemias classified on the basis of morphology and alterations in red cell indices usually correlate with the cause of red cell deficiency. Whatever the nature of anemia, the reduction in red cell mass and oxygen transport, when it is sufficiently severe, leads to certain clinical features.

Table 14-2. ADULT REFERENCE RANGES FOR RED BLOOD CELLS*

	Units	Men	Women
Hemoglobin	gm/dl	13.6–17.2	12.0–15.0
Hematocrit	%	39–49	33–43
Erythrocyte count (RBCs)	$\times 10^6$/mm³	4.3–5.9	3.5–5.0
Reticulocyte count	%	0.5–1.5	
Mean cell volume	μm³	76–100	
Mean corpuscular hemoglobin	pg	27–33	
Mean corpuscular hemoglobin concentration	gm/dl	33–37	
RBC distribution width	—	11.5–14.5	

*Reference ranges vary among laboratories. The reference ranges for the laboratory providing the result should always be used in interpreting a laboratory test result.
RBC, red blood cell.

With significant anemia, the patients appear pale. Weakness, malaise, and easy fatigability are common complaints. The lowered oxygen content of the circulating blood leads to dyspnea on mild exertion. The nails may become brittle and lose their usual convexity to assume a concave spoon shape (koilonychia). Anoxia may cause fatty changes in the liver, myocardium, and kidney. If the fatty changes in the myocardium are sufficiently severe, cardiac failure may develop and compound the respiratory difficulty caused by reduced oxygen transport. On occasion, the myocardial hypoxia manifests itself as angina pectoris, particularly when a preexisting vascular disease has already rendered the myocardium partially ischemic. With acute blood loss and shock, oliguria and anuria may develop in the shock kidney. Central nervous system hypoxia may be evidenced by headache, dimness of vision, and faintness.

Anemias of Blood Loss

ACUTE BLOOD LOSS

The clinical and morphologic reactions to blood loss depend on the rate of hemorrhage and whether the blood is lost externally or internally. With acute blood loss, the alterations reflect principally the loss of blood volume rather than the loss of hemoglobin. Shock and death may follow. If the patient survives, the blood volume is rapidly restored by shift of water from the interstitial fluid compartment. The resulting hemodilution lowers the hematocrit. Reduction in the oxygenation of tissues triggers the production of erythropoietin, and the marrow responds by increasing erythropoiesis. When the blood is lost internally, as into the peritoneal cavity, the iron can be recaptured; but if the blood is lost externally, the adequacy of the red cell recovery may be hampered by iron deficiency when insufficient reserves are present.

Soon after the acute blood loss, the red blood cells appear normal in size and color (normocytic, normochromic). However, as the marrow begins to regenerate, changes occur in the peripheral blood. *Most striking is an increase in the reticulocyte count, reaching 10% to 15% after 7 days.* The reticulocytes are seen as polychromatophilic macrocytes in the usual blood smear. These changes of red cell regeneration can sometimes be mistaken for an underlying hemolytic process. Mobilization of platelets and granulocytes from the marginal pools leads to thrombocytosis and leukocytosis in the period immediately after acute blood loss.

CHRONIC BLOOD LOSS

Chronic blood loss induces anemia only when the rate of loss exceeds the regenerative capacity of the erythroid precursors or when iron reserves are depleted. In addition to chronic blood loss, any cause of iron deficiency such as malnutrition, malabsorption states, or an increased demand above the daily intake as occurs in pregnancy will lead to an identical anemia, discussed later.

Hemolytic Anemias

The hemolytic anemias are characterized by the following features:

- *Shortening of the normal red cell life span, that is, premature destruction of red cells*
- *Accumulation of the products of hemoglobin catabolism*
- *A marked increase in erythropoiesis within the bone marrow,* in an attempt to compensate for the loss of red cells

These and some other general features are briefly discussed before we describe the features of specific hemolytic anemias.

As is well known, the physiologic destruction of senescent red cells takes place within the mononuclear phagocytic cells of the spleen. In hemolytic anemias, too, the premature destruction of red cells occurs predominantly within the mononuclear phagocyte system (extravascular hemolysis). In only a few cases does lysis of red cells within the vascular compartment (intravascular hemolysis) predominate.

Intravascular hemolysis occurs when normal erythrocytes are damaged by mechanical injury, complement fixation to red cells, or exogenous toxic factors. Trauma to red cells may be caused by mechanical cardiac valves or by thrombi within the microcirculation. Complement fixation may occur on antibody-coated cells during transfusion of mismatched blood. Toxic injury is exemplified by falciparum malaria (Chapter 9) and clostridial sepsis.

Whatever the mechanism, *intravascular hemolysis is manifested by (1) hemoglobinemia, (2) hemoglobinuria, (3) methemalbuminemia, (4) jaundice, and (5) hemosiderinuria.* When hemoglobin escapes into the plasma, it is promptly bound by an α_2-globulin (haptoglobin) to produce a complex that prevents excretion into the urine, since the complexes are rapidly cleared by the reticuloendothelial system. *A decrease in serum haptoglobin level is characteristically seen in all cases of intravascular hemolysis.* When the haptoglobin is depleted, the unbound or free hemoglobin is in part rapidly oxidized to methemoglobin, and both hemoglobin and methemoglobin are excreted through the kidneys, imparting a red-brown color to the urine—hemoglobinuria and methemoglobinuria. The renal proximal tubular cells may reabsorb and catabolize much of this filtered hemoglobin, but some passes out with the urine. Within the tubular cells, iron released from the hemoglobin may accumulate, giving rise to hemosiderosis of the renal tubular epithelium. Concomitantly, the heme groups derived from the complexes are catabolized within the mononuclear phagocyte system, leading ultimately to jaundice. In hemolytic anemias, the serum bilirubin is unconjugated and the level of hyperbilirubinemia depends on the functional capacity of the liver as well as on the rate of hemolysis. With a normal liver, the jaundice is rarely severe. Excessive bilirubin excreted by the liver into the gastrointestinal tract leads eventually to increased formation and fecal excretion of urobilin (Chapter 19).

Extravascular hemolysis takes place whenever red cells are injured, are rendered "foreign," or become less deformable. For example, in hereditary spherocytosis, an abnormal membrane cytoskeleton decreases the deformability of the red cell. Analogously, in sickle cell anemia, the abnormal hemoglobin "gels" or "crystallizes" within the erythrocyte, deforming it and reducing its plasticity. Since extreme alterations in shape are required for red cells to navigate the splenic sinusoids successfully, reduced deformability makes the passage difficult and leads to sequestration within the cords, followed by phagocytosis (Fig. 14–2). This is believed to be an important pathogenetic mechanism of extravascular hemolysis in a variety of hemolytic anemias. With extravascular hemolysis, it is obvious that hemoglobinemia, hemoglobinuria, and the related intravascular changes do not appear. However, the catabolism of erythrocytes in the phagocytic cells induces anemia and jaundice that are otherwise indistinguishable from those caused by intravascular hemolysis. Furthermore, since some hemoglobin manages to escape from the phagocytic cells, plasma haptoglobin levels are invariably reduced. The morphologic changes that follow are identical to those in intravascular hemolysis, except that the erythrophagocytosis generally causes hypertrophy of the mononuclear phagocyte system of cells, and this may lead to splenomegaly.

MORPHOLOGY. Certain morphologic changes are standard in the hemolytic anemias, whether they are caused by intravascular or extravascular mechanisms. The anemia and lowered tissue oxygen tension stimulate increased production of erythropoietin, leading to **a marked increase in**

the numbers of normoblasts in the marrow (Fig. 14–3); sometimes the expansion leads to extramedullary hematopoiesis. The accelerated compensatory erythropoiesis leads to a **prominent reticulocytosis in the peripheral blood.** The elevated levels of bilirubin, when it is excreted through the liver, promote the formation of pigment gallstones (cholelithiasis). With chronicity, the phagocytosed red cells or hemoglobin eventually leads to hemosiderosis, usually confined to the mononuclear phagocyte system. Thus, whatever the basis of the hemolysis, when it is sufficiently chronic, a common sequence of morphologic changes may be anticipated.

The hemolytic anemias can be classified in a variety of ways. One has already been suggested, namely, division into intravascular and extravascular hemolytic disorders. However, since the number of disorders with predominantly intravascular hemolysis is limited, this classification is not entirely satisfactory. A pathogenetic classification could be based on whether the underlying cause of red cell destruction is extrinsic (extracorpuscular mechanism) or a defect inherent in the red cell (intracorpuscular defect). These anemias can also be divided into hereditary and acquired disorders. *In general, hereditary disorders are due to intracorpuscular defects and the acquired disorders to extrinsic factors such as autoantibodies.* Each of the classifications has value, but here we follow the intrinsic-extrinsic outline given in Table 14–1, limiting consideration to the more common entities.

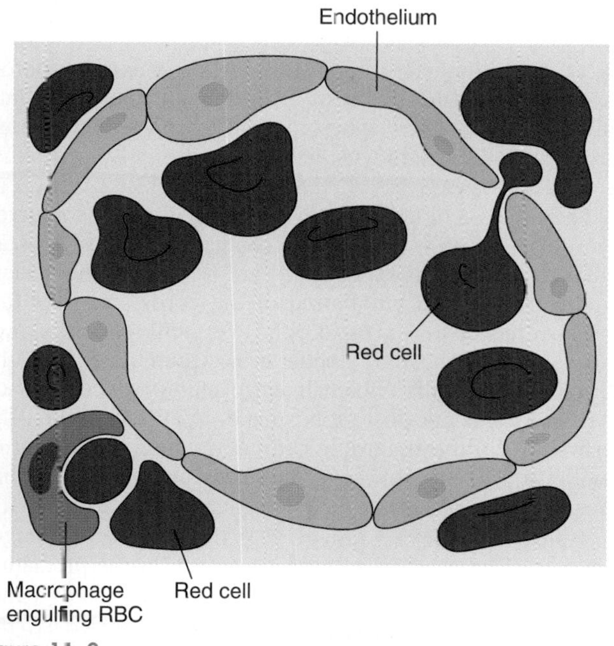

Figure 14–2

Schematic of splenic sinus (electron micrograph). An erythrocyte is in the process of squeezing from the dead into the sinus lumen. Note the degree of deformability required for the red cells to pass through the wall of the sinus.

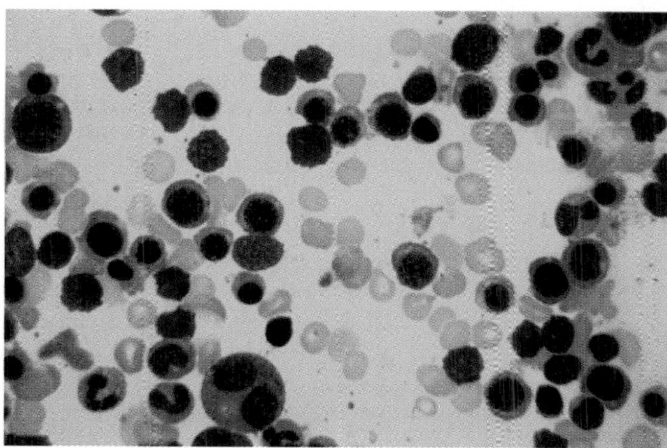

Figure 14–3

Marrow smear from a patient with hemolytic anemia. The marrow reveals many clusters of proliferating normoblasts. (Courtesy of Dr. Steven Kroft, Department of Pathology, University of Texas Southwestern Medical School, Dallas, TX.)

HEREDITARY SPHEROCYTOSIS (HS)

This inherited disorder is characterized by an intrinsic defect in the red cell membrane that renders erythrocytes spheroidal, less deformable, and vulnerable to splenic sequestration and destruction. The prevalence of HS is highest in people of northern European extraction, in whom rates of 1 in 5000 have been reported. In approximately 75% of cases, the inheritance follows an autosomal dominant pattern. The remaining patients have an autosomal recessive form of the disease that is much more severe than the autosomal dominant form.

Molecular Pathology. The spheroidal shape of the erythrocyte appears to result from a fundamental defect in the skeleton of the red cell membrane.[2] Spectrin, the major protein of the membrane cytoskeleton, consists of two polypeptide chains, α and β, which are intertwined (helical) dimers lying "flat" on the cytoplasmic aspect of the cell membrane (Fig. 14–4). The individual spectrin dimers are like segments of an extensive cable network that are linked to each other head to head to form tetramers. Lateral connections between spectrin tetramers are established through actin. The two-dimensional spectrin cable meshwork so formed is tethered to the inner surface of the cell membrane by ankyrin and protein 4.1. Ankyrin forms a bridge between spectrin and the transmembrane ion transporter, called band 3, whereas protein 4.1 connects spectrin to glycophorin A. Together these proteins are responsible for maintenance of the normal shape, strength, and flexibility of the red cell membrane. Although a deficiency of any one of the membrane skeletal proteins could adversely affect the red cells, *a deficiency of spectrin seems to be the most common biochemical abnormality in patients with all forms of HS.* The spectrin content of these cells varies

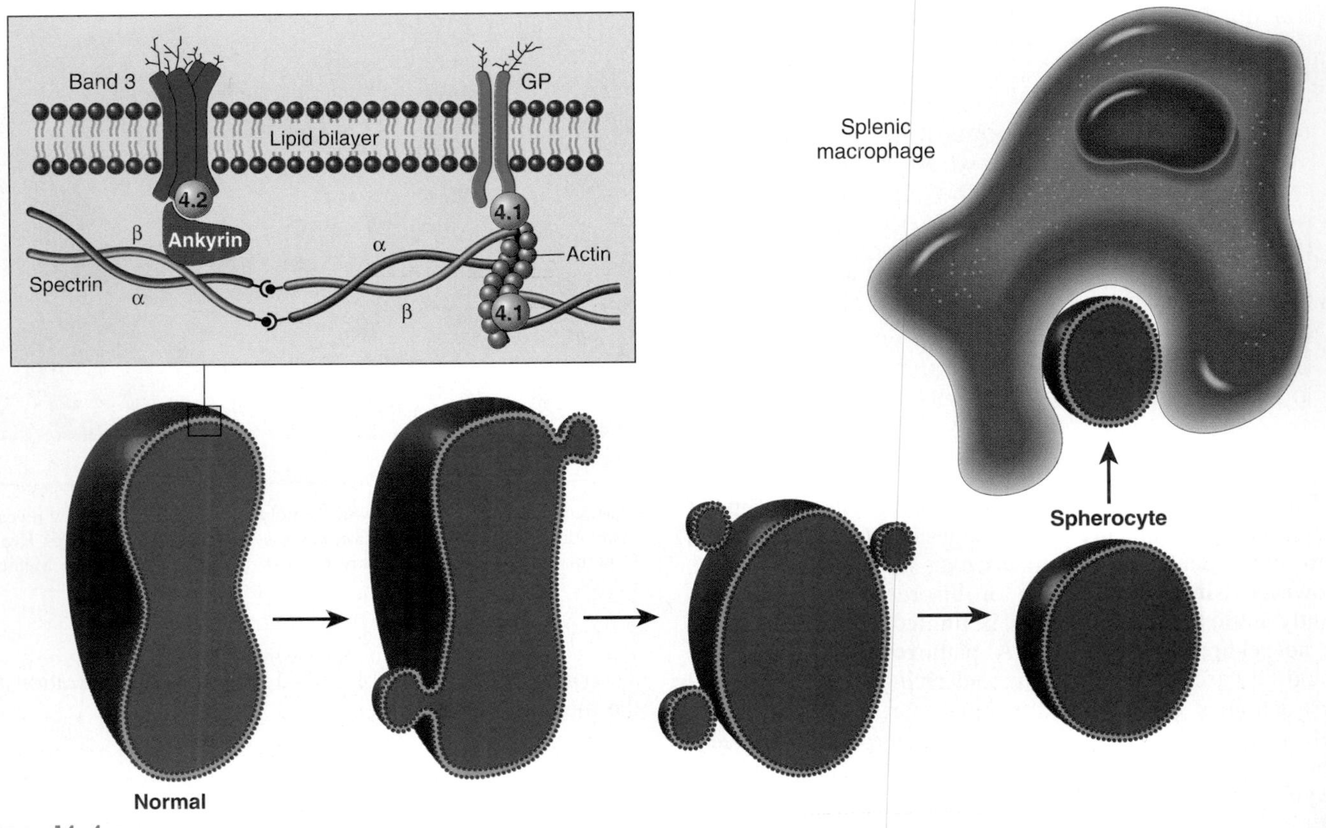

Figure 14–4

Schematic representation of the red cell membrane cytoskeleton and the effects of alterations in the cytoskeletal proteins on the shape of red cells. With mutations that affect the integrity of the membrane cytoskeleton, the normal biconcave erythrocyte loses membrane fragments. To accommodate the loss of surface area, the cell adopts a spherical shape. Such spherocytic cells are less deformable than normal and are therefore trapped in the splenic cords, where they are phagocytosed by macrophages.

from 60% to 90% of normal and correlates closely with the severity of spherocytosis.

The molecular basis of spectrin deficiency is varied, but all of the mutations seen in HS act to diminish "vertical" interactions that serve to connect the membrane cytoskeleton to the overlying lipid bilayer. For example, the common autosomal dominant form of HS is caused most frequently by a *mutation in the ankyrin gene.* The resultant reduced synthesis of ankyrin leads, in turn, to a secondary reduction in the assembly of spectrin on the membrane; thus, these patients have a combined ankyrin and spectrin deficiency.[3] In addition, mutations in the band 3 gene have been detected in approximately 20% of patients with the autosomal dominant form of this disease.[4] A mutation in the α-spectrin gene is found in the uncommon autosomal recessive form of the disease. Regardless of the primary molecular defect, *spectrin deficiency is associated with reduced membrane stability and loss of membrane fragments as the cells are exposed to shear stresses in the circulation* (Fig. 14–4). The resulting reduction in cell surface to volume ratio "forces" the cells to assume the smallest possible diameter for a given volume, namely, a sphere.

Although much remains to be learned about the molecular defects in HS, the travails of the spherocytic red cells are fairly well defined (Fig. 14–5). In the life of the "portly" (and therefore inflexible) spherocyte, the spleen acts as the villain. Red cells must undergo extreme deformation to leave the cords of Billroth and enter the sinusoids. Because of their spheroidal shape and reduced membrane plasticity, spherocytes have great difficulty in leaving the cords. Reduced deformability of spheroidal red cells has been aptly compared with the difficulties encountered by an "obese man attempting to bend at the waist."[5] As an increasing number of spherocytes are trapped in the spleen, the already sluggish circulation of the cords stagnates further, and the environment around the cells becomes progressively more hostile. Lactic acid accumulates and the extracellular pH falls, which in turn inhibits glycolysis and generation of adenosine triphosphate (ATP). Loss of ATP impairs the ability to extrude sodium, adding an element of osmotic injury. Stagnation in the cords also promotes contact with macrophages, which are plentiful, and eventually the hapless spherocytes fall prey to the appetite of phagocytic cells. The cardinal role of the spleen in the premature demise of the spherocytes is proved by the invariably beneficial effect of splenectomy. The spherocytes persist, but the anemia is corrected.

MORPHOLOGY. Perhaps the most outstanding morphologic feature of this disease is the spheroidal shape of the red cells, apparent on smears as

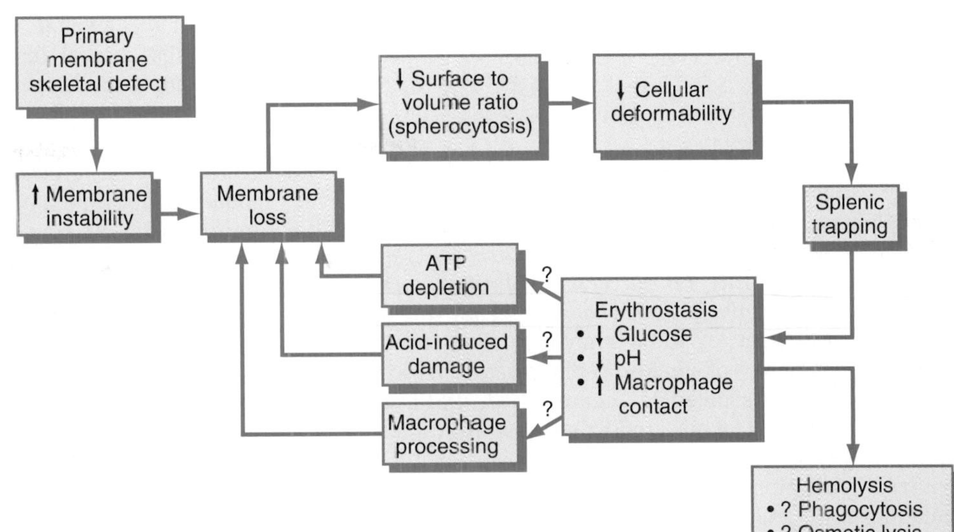

Figure 14–5 ■

Model of the pathophysiology of hereditary spherocytosis. (Adapted from Wyngaarden JB, et al [eds]: Cecil Textbook of Medicine, 19th ed. Philadelphia, WB Saunders, 1992, p 859.)

abnormally small cells lacking their central zone of pallor (Fig. 14–6). Spherocytosis, although distinctive, is not pathognomonic, since it is also seen in autoimmune hemolytic anemias. In addition to reticulocytosis and the general features of all hemolytic anemias, as previously detailed, certain alterations are fairly distinctive. Moderate splenic enlargement is characteristic of HS (500 to 1000 gm); in few other hemolytic anemias is the spleen enlarged as much or as often. It results from marked congestion of the cords of Billroth, leaving the sinuses virtually empty. Erythrophagocytosis can be seen within the congested cords. Typically present are the associated changes found in all hemolytic anemias, including increased erythropoiesis, bone changes, and hemosiderosis. Cholelithiasis (pigment stones) occurs in 40% to 50% of the affected adults.

Clinical Course. The characteristic clinical features are anemia, splenomegaly, and jaundice. The severity of the disease varies greatly from one patient to another.[6] In a minority of patients, HS presents at birth with marked jaundice, requiring exchange transfusion. In 20% to 30% of patients, the disease is largely asymptomatic because the mild red cell destruction is readily compensated for by increased erythropoiesis. In most, however, this compensatory reaction is outpaced and hence the patients have a chronic hemolytic anemia, usually of mild to moderate severity. This more or less stable clinical course may be punctuated by an *aplastic crisis* (triggered usually by a parvovirus infection of the marrow red cell precursors). It is characterized by temporary suppression of red cell production, manifested by sudden worsening of the anemia and the disappearance of reticulocytes from the peripheral blood. Transfusions may be necessary to support the patient, but eventually the crisis remits in most instances. A "hemolytic crisis" resulting from accelerated red cell destruction is seen in some patients, but clinically it is less significant than the aplastic crisis. Gallstones, found in many patients, may also produce symptoms. Diagnosis of HS is based on family history, hematologic findings, and laboratory evidence of spherocytosis manifested by osmotic fragility. In two thirds of the patients, the spherocytes are particularly vulnerable to *osmotic lysis*, induced in vitro by solutions of hypotonic salt, since there is little margin for expansion of red cell volume without rupture. Cellular dehydration, resulting perhaps from membrane injury, is manifested by increased mean cell hemoglobin concentration. This abnormality is seen in most patients with HS.[6] As mentioned earlier, most patients are benefitted by splenectomy.

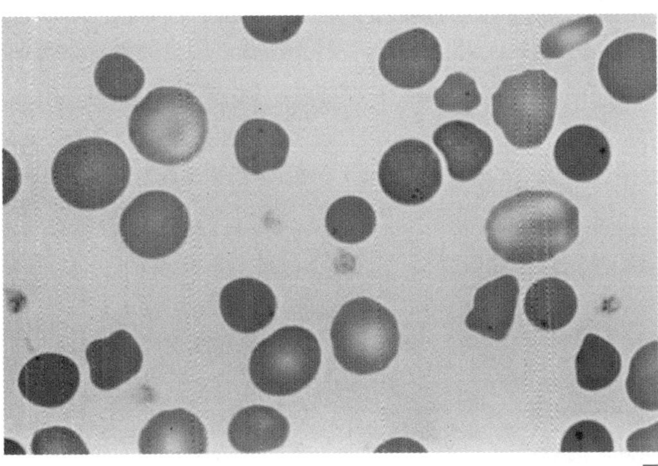

Figure 14–6 ■

Peripheral smear from a patient with hereditary spherocytosis. Note the anisocytosis and several dark-appearing spherocytes with no central pallor. (Courtesy of Dr. Robert W. McKenna, Department of Pathology, University of Texas Southwestern Medical School, Dallas, TX.)

HEMOLYTIC DISEASE DUE TO ERYTHROCYTE ENZYME DEFECTS: GLUCOSE-6-PHOSPHATE DEHYDROGENASE DEFICIENCY

The erythrocyte and its membrane are vulnerable to injury by exogenous and endogenous oxidants. *Abnormalities in the hexose monophosphate shunt or in glutathione metabolism resulting from deficient or impaired enzyme function reduce the ability of red cells to protect themselves against oxidative injuries and lead to hemolytic disease.* The most important of these enzyme derangements is a hereditary deficiency of glucose-6-phosphate dehydrogenase (G6PD) activity. As noted in Figure 14–7, G6PD reduces NADP to NADPH while oxidizing glucose-6-phosphate. NADPH then provides the reducing power that converts oxidized glutathione to reduced glutathione. The reduced glutathione so generated protects against oxidant injury by catalyzing the breakdown of oxidant compounds like H_2O_2.

Several hundred G6PD genetic variants have been identified, but fortunately most evoke no clinical disorder or hemolytic anemia. The most common normal form is called G6PD B. Two variants, designated G6PD A^- and G6PD Mediterranean, lead to clinically significant hemolysis.[7] The A^- type is present in about 10% of American blacks; G6PD Mediterranean, as the name implies, is found largely in populations in the Middle East. The prevalence of such deleterious genes is believed to have been maintained because a deficiency of G6PD protects against malaria due to *Plasmodium falciparum*.[8]

The G6PD variants are grouped into four classes on the basis of the level of enzyme activity, which in turn determines the clinical features. The G6PD A^- variant, associated with a moderate deficiency (10% to 60% of activity), belongs to class III; the Mediterranean form, in which the red cells have less than 10% of normal activity, is considered to be in group II. In both of these, however, the mutation does not impair enzyme synthesis; rather, the stability of the enzyme is affected. Accordingly, the enzyme activity is normal in reticulocytes, but older red cells are markedly deficient. Exposure to oxidants, therefore, induces hemolysis of older red cells but not of younger ones. The recent elucidation of the crystal structure of G6PD has provided insights into the basis of reduced stability. The disease-associated mutations result in a loss of normal folding of the G6PD protein; because the unfolded forms are susceptible to proteolytic degradation, they have a shorter half-life. Thus, G6PD deficiency, along with α_1-antitrypsin deficiency, belongs to a group of diseases in which *defective folding of the proteins* lies at the heart of the disorder.[9]

Inheritance of the mutant gene is X-linked. Thus, the defect is expressed in all erythrocytes of the affected male. In the heterozygous female, two populations of red cells, some deficient, others normal, are present owing to random inactivation of the X chromosomes. It follows that males are more vulnerable to oxidant injury than females are. G6PD deficiency manifests itself in several distinct clinical patterns, the most common of which is hemolysis after exposure to oxidant stress. This may occur after ingestion of certain *drugs* or even more commonly by exposure to oxidant free radicals generated by leukocytes in the course of *infections*. The oxidant drugs implicated in the causation of hemolysis are numerous.[7] They include the antimalarials primaquine and chloroquine, sulfonamides, nitrofurantoins, and others. Some drugs are harmless in those with the milder G6PD A^- variant but cause hemolysis in those who have the Mediterranean variant. Although many infections can trigger hemolysis in patients with G6PD deficiency, particularly important are viral hepatitis, pneumonia, and typhoid fever. Patients with G6PD deficiency may also present with hemolysis after ingestion of fava beans *(favism)* because these legumes generate oxidants, much in the same way as oxidant drugs do. Favism is endemic in the Mediterranean, Middle East, and parts of Africa, understandably in regions where consumption of fava beans is prevalent. Uncommonly, G6PD deficiency presents without known exposure to oxidant stresses in the form of neonatal jaundice or a chronic low-grade hemolytic anemia.

The hemolysis in G6PD deficiency is both intravascular and extravascular; it seems to involve the following sequence. Infection or exposure to oxidants causes oxidation of the sulfhydryl groups of the globin chains. This leads to denaturation of hemoglobin and formation of precipitates (Heinz bodies) that can be seen within the red cells as dark inclusions when they are stained with crystal violet (Fig. 14–8). These precipitates of denatured hemoglobin may damage the membrane sufficiently to cause intravascular hemolysis. In addition, when attached to the cell membrane, Heinz bodies decrease erythrocyte deformability. As the inclusion-bearing red cells pass through the splenic cords, macrophages pluck out the Heinz bodies, giving rise to red cells that appear to have a bite of cytoplasm re-

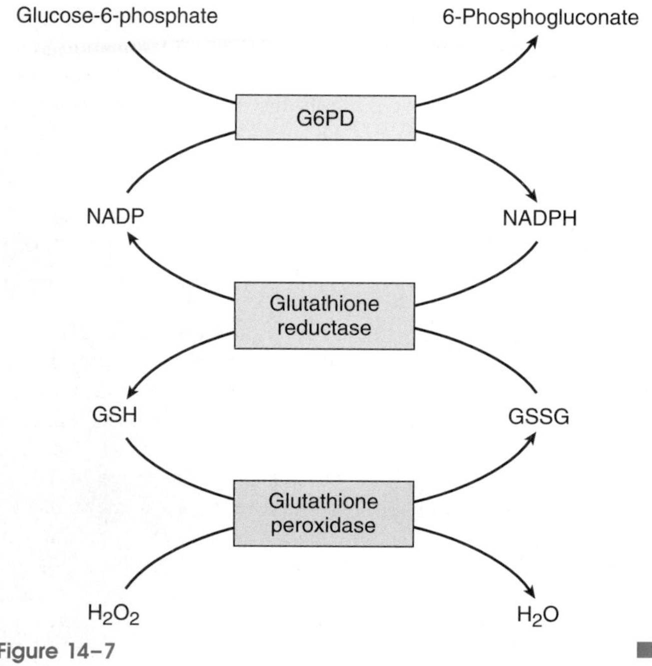

Figure 14–7

The role of glucose-6-phosphate dehydrogenase (G6PD) in the defense against oxidant injury. The disposal of H_2O_2, a potential oxidant, is dependent on the adequacy of reduced glutathione (GSH), which in turn is generated by the action of NADPH. The synthesis of NADPH is dependent on the activity of G6PD. GSSG, oxidized glutathione.

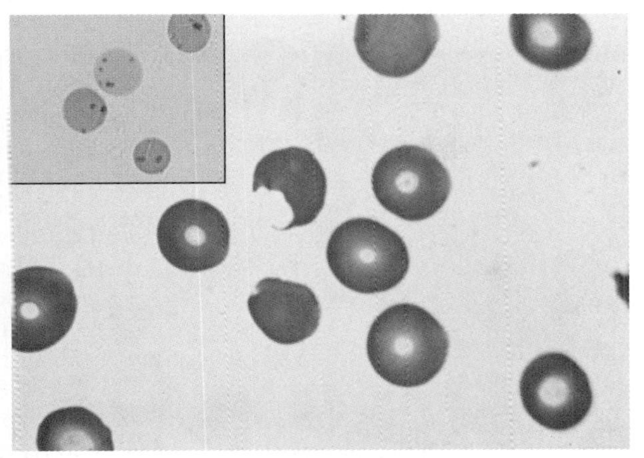

Figure 14–8

Peripheral blood smear from a patient with G6PD deficiency after exposure to an oxidant drug. *Inset,* Red cells with precipitates of denatured globin (Heinz bodies) revealed by supravital staining. As the splenic macrophages pluck out these inclusions, "bite cells" like the one in this smear are produced. (Courtesy of Dr. Robert W. McKenna, Department of Pathology, University of Texas Southwestern Medical School, Dallas, TX.)

moved ("bite cells") (Fig. 14–8). The resultant loss of membrane leads to further membrane damage and simultaneously induces the formation of spherocytes. All these changes predispose the red cells to become trapped in splenic cords and destroyed by erythrophagocytosis.

The clinical features of G6PD deficiency may be surmised from this discussion. Persons with the deficient enzyme usually do not have hemolysis unless they are exposed to the oxidant injuries alluded to before. After a variable lag period of 2 to 3 days, *acute intravascular hemolysis, characterized by hemoglobinemia, hemoglobinuria, and decreased hematocrit levels, is triggered.* Since only senescent red cells are lysed, the episode is *self-limited* and hemolysis stops when only the younger red cells remain in the circulation (despite continued administration of the oxidant drug). Because patients with the Mediterranean variant have much lower levels of G6PD, their anemia is more severe.

The recovery phase is heralded by reticulocytosis, as in the case of other hemolytic anemias. Since hemolytic episodes related to deficiencies of G6PD occur in most patients only when there is oxidant injury, the morphologic changes encountered in most chronic hemolytic anemias are rarely present.

SICKLE CELL DISEASE

Sickle cell disease is the prototype of *hereditary hemoglobinopathies, characterized by the production of a structurally abnormal hemoglobin.* Hemoglobin, as you recall, is a tetramer of four globin chains comprising two pairs of similar chains, each with its own heme group. The hemoglobin in the adult is composed of 96% HbA ($\alpha_2\beta_2$), 3% HbA$_2$ ($\alpha_2\delta_2$), and 1% fetal hemoglobin ($\alpha_2\gamma_2$). The clinically significant hemoglobinopathies result from mutations in the β-globin gene. Sickle cell anemia results from a point mutation that leads to substitution of valine for glutamic acid at the sixth position of the β-globin chain. The resultant hemoglobin, HbS, has abnormal physiochemical properties that lead to sickle cell disease. Several hundred abnormal hemoglobins have been identified in which there is either a point mutation or a deletion in one of the globin chains.

About 8% of black Americans are heterozygous for HbS. If an individual is homozygous for the sickle mutation, almost all the hemoglobin in the erythrocyte is HbS. In the heterozygote, only about 40% is HbS, the remainder being normal hemoglobins. Where malaria is endemic, as many as 30% of black Africans are heterozygous. This frequency may be related in part to the slight protection against falciparum malaria afforded by HbS.

Pathogenesis. *On deoxygenation, the HbS molecules undergo aggregation and polymerization.* This change converts hemoglobin from a freely flowing liquid to a viscous gel, leading ultimately to formation of HbS fibers and resultant distortion of the red cells, which acquire a sickle or holly-leaf shape (Fig. 14–9).

Sickling of red cells is initially a reversible phenomenon; with oxygenation, HbS returns to the depolymerized state. However, with repeated episodes of sickling and unsickling, membrane damage ensues and the cells become irreversibly sickled. These deformed cells retain their abnormal shape even when they are fully oxygenated and despite deaggregation of HbS. The precipitation of HbS fibers also has *deleterious effects on the red cell membrane.* These include defects in membrane phosphorylation and detachment of the cell membrane from the underlying membrane skeleton. Such *secondary membrane damage is seen not only in irreversibly sickled cells but also in normal-appearing cells.* With membrane injury, the red blood cells lose potassium and water and at the same time gain calcium, which normally is rigorously excluded. They have difficulty in maintaining normal intracellular volume, and consequently intracellular hemoglobin concentration increases and the cells become dehydrated and hence dense.[10] These membrane changes are believed to be important in the pathogenesis of microvascular occlusions, described later.

A number of factors affect the rate and degree of sickling.

- *Perhaps most important of all is the amount of HbS and its interaction with the other hemoglobin chains in the cell.* In heterozygotes, approximately 40% of the hemoglobin is HbS, the rest being HbA, which interacts only weakly with HbS during the processes of gelation. Therefore, the heterozygote has little tendency to sickle, except under conditions of severe hypoxia. Such an individual is said to have the *sickle cell trait* and, unless exposed to marked hypoxia, has no hemolysis of red cells and no anemia. In contrast, the homozygote, with virtually undiluted hemoglobin of the S type, has full-blown *sickle cell anemia. Hemoglobins other than the normal HbA, in particular fetal hemoglobin (HbF), profoundly influence the crystallization of HbS and the severity of sickle cell anemia. For example, HbF inhibits the polymerization of HbS*, and hence newborns do not manifest the disease until they are 5 to 6 months of age,

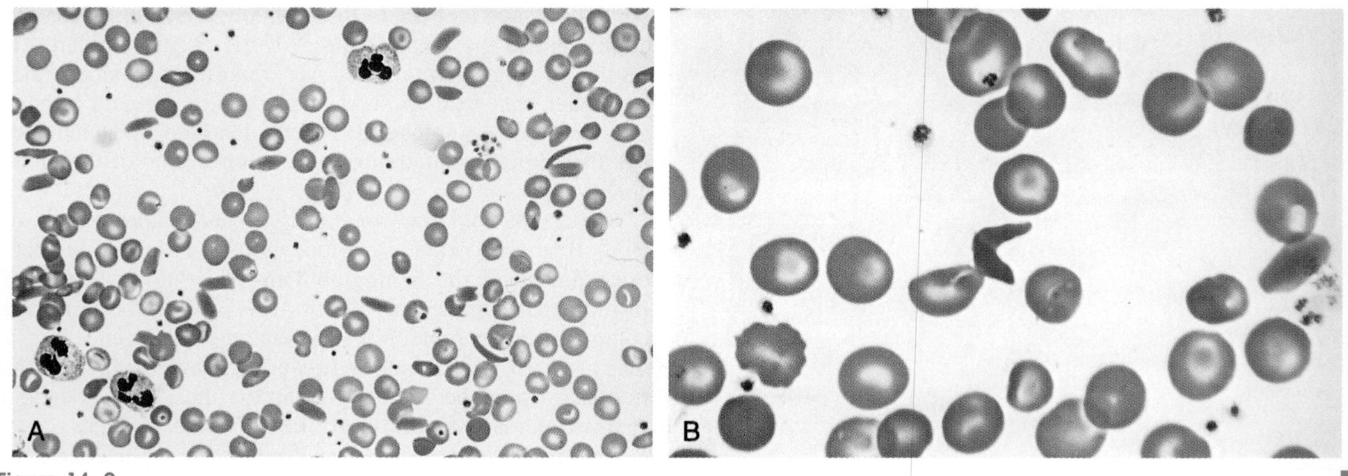

Figure 14–9

Peripheral blood smear from a patient with sickle cell anemia. *A*, Low magnification shows sickle cells, anisocytosis, and poikilocytosis. *B*, Higher magnification shows an irreversibly sickled cell in the center. (Courtesy of Dr. Robert W. McKenna, Department of Pathology, University of Texas Southwestern Medical School, Dallas, TX.)

when the amount of HbF in the cells begins to approach adult levels. *The salutary effect of HbF, as we shall see, has been exploited in developing therapy for sickle cell anemia.* The modulating effect of other hemoglobins is further exemplified by HbC and HbD. These two hemoglobins also have mutations in the β-globin chain, but these mutations are different from the one in HbS. Either of these may be present along with HbS in red cells of a double heterozygote for HbS and the variant globin gene. The carrier rate for HbC in American blacks is about 2% to 3%, giving the likelihood that one in 1250 newborns will be a double heterozygote for HbS and HbC. HbC has a greater tendency to aggregate with HbS than does HbA, and hence those with HbS and HbC (designated *HbSC*) have a more severe disease than do those with HbS and HbA (sickle cell trait).

- *The rate of HbS polymerization is also significantly affected by the hemoglobin concentration per cell,* that is, the mean corpuscular hemoglobin concentration (MCHC). The higher the HbS concentration within the cell, the greater are the chances of contact and interaction between HbS molecules. Thus, *dehydration, which increases the MCHC, greatly facilitates sickling and vascular occlusion* (see later). Conversely, for a given amount of HbS per cell, conditions that decrease the MCHC reduce disease severity. This is most clearly illustrated in patients with homozygous sickle cell anemia and coexistent α-thalassemia. These patients have milder disease because thalassemia is characterized by reduced globin synthesis, which limits the total hemoglobin concentration per cell.
- Finally, *a fall in pH,* by reducing the oxygen affinity of hemoglobin, can increase sickling because it enhances the amount of deoxygenated HbS.

The formation of HbS has two major consequences: (1) a chronic hemolytic anemia and (2) occlusion of small blood vessels, resulting in ischemic tissue damage (Fig. 14–10).

Irreversibly sickled cells have rigid and nondeformable cell membranes and have difficulty in negotiating the splenic sinusoids. They become sequestered in the spleen, where they are destroyed by the mononuclear phagocyte system. Some intravascular hemolysis may also occur because of increased mechanical fragility of the severely damaged cells. *The average red cell survival correlates with the percentage of irreversibly sickled cells in circulation* and is shortened to approximately 20 days. This finding supports the concept that the hemolysis results primarily from the lysis of irreversibly sickled cells.

The pathogenesis of microvascular occlusions, a clinically important component of sickle cell anemia, is much less certain.[11] There is no correlation between the frequency of irreversibly sickled cells and the frequency or severity of ischemic episodes. Hence, it is believed that microvascular occlusion is initiated by cells that contain HbS but are not obviously sickled. In this regard, the abnormalities of red cell membrane, described earlier, are believed to play a role. The altered membranes have an increased expression of adhesion molecules that promote increased adhesiveness of the red cells to the endothelium in vitro; indeed, cells that are not irreversibly sickled are the most adherent to cultured endothelial cells. It is the normal-appearing cells whose cell membranes have been altered by repeated cycles of reversible sickling that adhere to the endothelium and cause narrowing of microvessels. This leads secondarily to trapping of the more rigid, sickled cells and subsequent vaso-occlusion.[12] Even more important, the narrowing increases the time required for the normal-looking red cells to transit the microcirculation. This in turn favors sickling by exposing the HbS contained within these cells to a longer than normal period of relative oxygen lack, thus further aggravating the obstruction.[10]

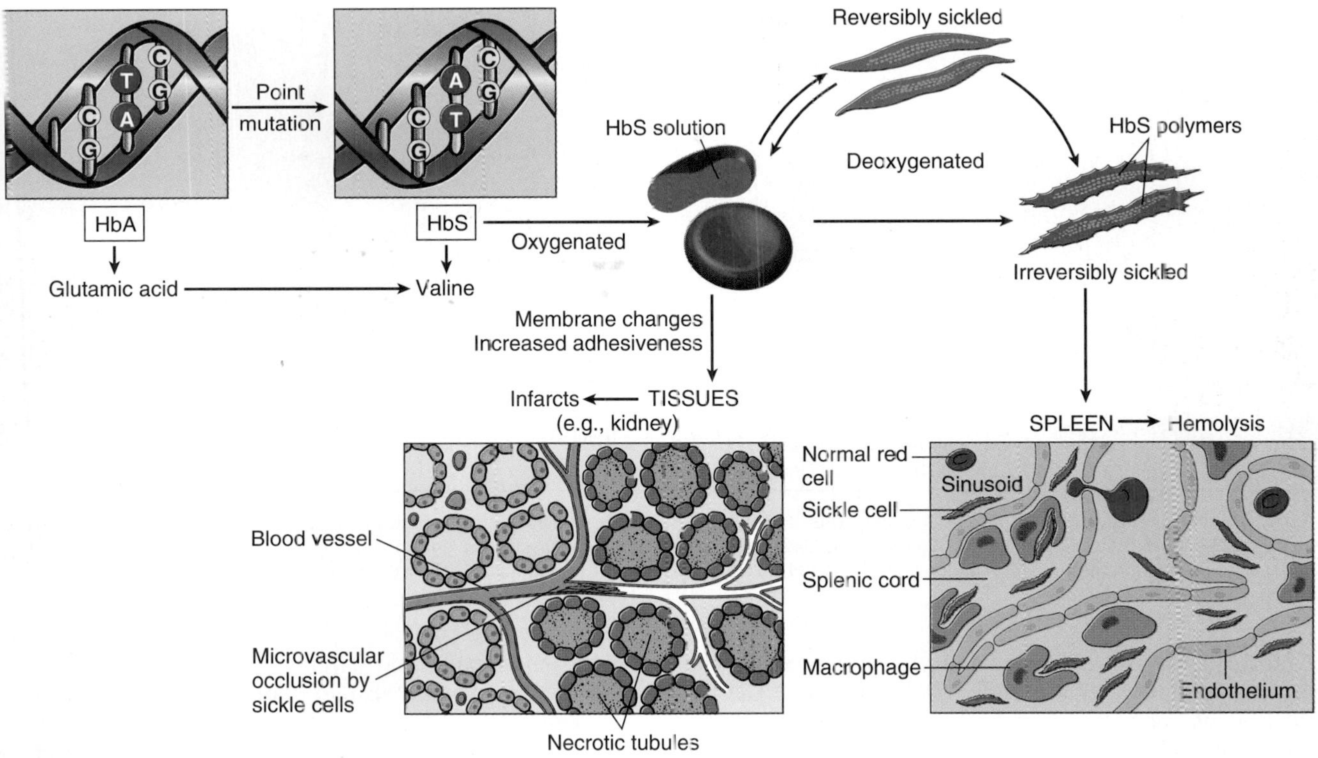

Figure 14–10

Pathophysiology and morphologic consequences of sickle cell anemia.

MORPHOLOGY. The anatomic alterations are based on the following three characteristics of sickle cell anemia: increased destruction of the sickled red cells with the development of anemia, increased release of hemoglobin and formation of bilirubin, and capillary stasis and thrombosis. The consequences of the increased red cell destruction and anemia have already been detailed in the general consideration of all hemolytic anemias. The bone marrow is hyperplastic because of compensatory expansion of the normoblasts. The expansion of the marrow may lead to resorption of bone with secondary new bone formation to produce the roentgenographic appearance in the skull of the "crew haircut." Extramedullary hematopoiesis may appear in the spleen or liver and, rarely, in other sites.

In children, during the early phase of the disease, the spleen is commonly enlarged up to 500 gm. On histologic examination, there is marked congestion of the red pulp, due mainly to the trapping of sickled red cells in the splenic cords and sinuses (Fig. 14–11). This erythrostasis in the spleen leads to thrombosis and infarction or at least to marked tissue hypoxia. Continued scarring causes progressive shrinkage of the spleen so that by adolescence or early adulthood, only a small nubbin of fibrous tissue may be left; this is called **autosplenectomy** (Fig. 14–12). Infarction secondary to vascular occlusions and anoxia occurs also in the bones, brain, kidney, liver, and retina. Thrombotic occlusions have also been described in the pulmonary vessels, and many patients have cor pulmonale. Vascular stagnation in the subcutaneous tissue leads to leg ulcers in adult patients but is rare in children. The increased release of hemoglobin leads to pigment gallstones in some individuals, and all patients develop hyperbilirubinemia during periods of active hemolysis.

Clinical Course. *From the description of the disease to this point, it is evident that these patients are beset with problems stemming from (1) severe anemia, (2) vaso-occlusive complications, and (3) chronic hyperbilirubinemia.*[13] Increased susceptibility to infections is another threat, the basis of which is multifactorial: (1) splenic function is impaired because erythrophagocytosis interferes with the ability of the spleen to clear bacteria; (2) in later stages, total splenic fibrosis removes an important filter of blood-borne microorganisms; and (3) defects in the alternative complement pathway impair opsonization of encapsulated bacteria such as pneumococci and *Haemophilus influenzae*. Septicemia and meningitis caused by these two organisms are the most common causes of death in children with sickle cell anemia.

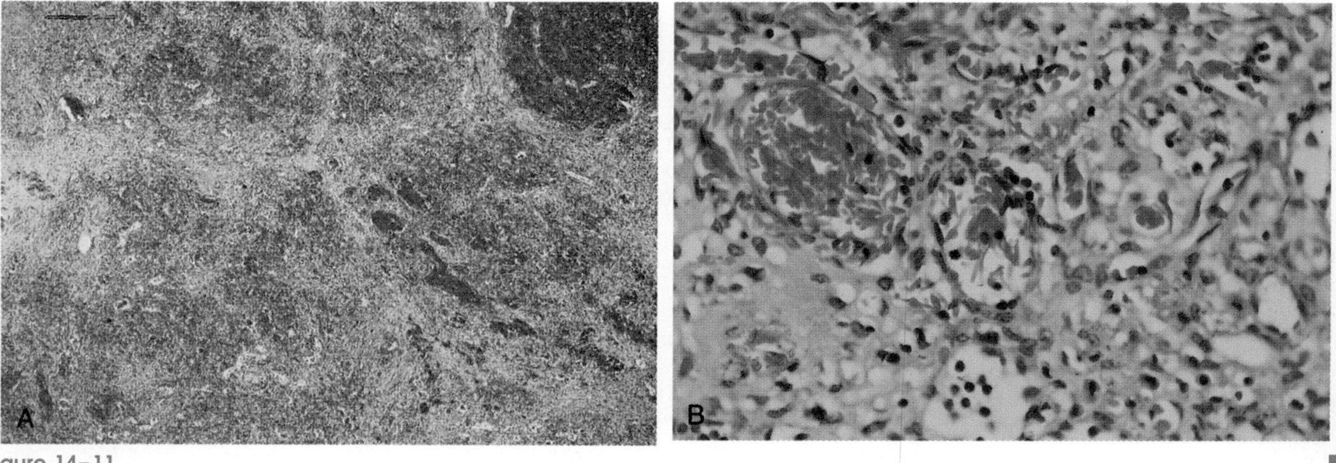

Figure 14–11

A, Spleen in sickle cell anemia (low power). Red pulp with its cords and sinusoids is markedly congested; in between the congested areas, pale areas of fibrosis resulting from ischemic damage are also seen. *B*, Under high power, splenic sinusoids are dilated and filled with sickled red cells. (Courtesy of Dr. Darren Wirthwein, Department of Pathology, University of Texas Southwestern Medical School, Dallas, TX.)

Chronic hemolysis induces a fairly severe anemia, with hematocrit values ranging between 18% and 30%. The hemolysis is associated with striking reticulocytosis and hyperbilirubinemia. Irreversibly sickled cells ranging in frequency from 5% to 15% can usually be seen in the peripheral smear. This protracted course is frequently punctuated by a variety of "crises." *Vaso-occlusive crises,* also called *painful crises,* represent episodes of hypoxic injury and infarction associated with severe pain in the affected region. No predisposing causes can usually be identified, although an association with infection, dehydration, and acidosis (all of which favor sickling) has been noted. Sites most commonly involved by vaso-occlusive episodes are the bones, lungs, liver, brain, spleen, and penis. *In children, painful bone crises are extremely common and often difficult to distinguish from acute osteomyelitis.* They frequently manifest as the *hand-foot syndrome* because of dactylitis of the bones of the hands or feet or both.[14] Similarly, involvement of the lungs may present with fever, cough, chest pain, and a pulmonary infiltrate. This *acute chest syndrome* may also in some cases result from lung infection. Central nervous system hypoxia may produce manifestations of a seizure or stroke. Leg ulcers are an additional reflection of the vaso-occlusive tendency. An *aplastic crisis* represents a temporary cessation of bone marrow activity, usually triggered by parvovirus infection of erythroid progenitor cells. Reticulocytes disappear from the peripheral blood, and there is sudden and rapid worsening of anemia. A so-called *sequestration crisis* may appear in children with splenomegaly. Massive sequestration of deformed red cells leads to rapid splenic enlargement, hypovolemia, and sometimes shock. With transfusion, this can be reversed. Male patients may suddenly develop painful priapism owing to vascular engorgement of the penis. Chronic hypoxia causes a generalized impairment of growth and development as well as organ damage affecting spleen, heart, kidneys, and lungs. Before closing this discussion it must be emphasized that there is great variation in the clinical manifestations of sickle cell anemia. For reasons not entirely clear, some individuals are crippled by repeated vaso-occlusive crises, whereas others have mild symptoms.

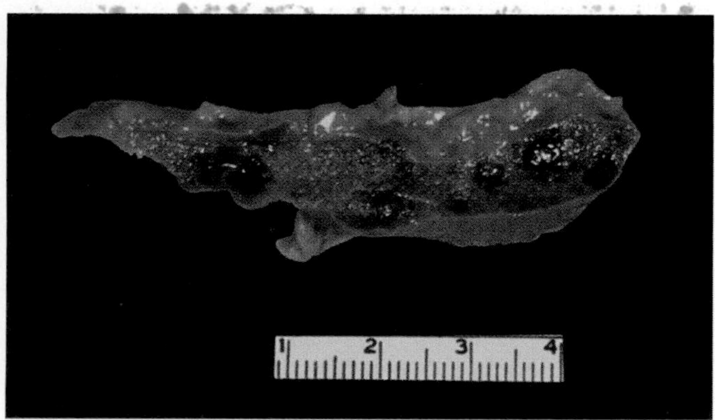

Figure 14–12

Markedly shrunken spleen from a patient with sickle cell anemia. (Courtesy of Drs. Dennis Burns and Darren Wirthwein, Department of Pathology, University of Texas Southwestern Medical School, Dallas, TX.)

Diagnosis is usually readily made from the clinical findings and the appearance of the peripheral blood smear. It can be confirmed by various tests for sickling that, in general, are based on mixing a blood sample with an oxygen-consuming reagent, such as metabisulfite, to induce sickling. Hemoglobin electrophoresis demonstrates HbS on the basis of specific mobility. Prenatal, molecular, diagnosis is possible by analysis of fetal DNA obtained by amniocentesis or chorionic biopsy. The outlook for patients with sickle cell anemia has improved considerably as a result of better supportive care. Approximately 90% of patients survive to the age of 20 years, and close to 50% survive beyond the fifth decade. A major advance in the treatment of sickle cell anemia has resulted from the understanding that HbF retards sickling. Treatment of patients with the cancer therapeutic drug hydroxyurea causes a dramatic increase in the concentration of HbF in the red cells and concomitantly decreases the frequency of vaso-occlusive crises.[15] The mechanism by which this "reawakening" of HbF genes occurs is under active investigation.[16]

THALASSEMIA SYNDROMES

The thalassemia syndromes are a heterogeneous group of mendelian disorders, all characterized by a lack of or decreased synthesis of either the α- or β-globin chain of HbA ($\alpha_2\beta_2$). *β-Thalassemia is characterized by deficient synthesis of the β chain, whereas α-thalassemia is characterized by deficient synthesis of the α chain. The hematologic consequences of diminished synthesis of one globin chain derive not only from the low intracellular hemoglobin (hypochromia) but also from the relative excess of the other chain.* For example, in β-thalassemia, there is an excess of α chains. As a consequence, free α chains tend to aggregate into insoluble inclusions within erythrocytes and their precursors, causing premature destruction of maturing erythroblasts within the marrow *(ineffective erythropoiesis)* as well as lysis of mature red cells in the spleen *(hemolysis)*.

β-Thalassemias

The abnormality common to all β-thalassemias is a total lack of or a reduction in the synthesis of structurally normal β-globin chains with unimpaired synthesis of α chains. However, the clinical severity of the anemia as well as the biochemical and genetic basis of β-globin chain deficiency is varied. We begin our discussion with the molecular lesions in β-thalassemia and then integrate the clinical variants with the underlying molecular defects.

Molecular Pathogenesis. The adult hemoglobin, or HbA, contains two α chains and two β chains. The β chains are coded by two β-globin genes, each located on one of the two chromosomes 11. In contrast, two pairs of functional α-globin genes are located on each chromosome 16.

β-Thalassemia syndromes can be classified into two categories: (1) *β^0-thalassemia,* associated with total absence of β-globin chains in the homozygous state; and (2) *β^+-thalassemia,* characterized by reduced (but detectable) β-globin synthesis in the homozygous state. Sequencing of cloned β-globin genes obtained from thalassemia patients has revealed approximately 100 different mutations responsible for β^0-thalassemia or β^+-thalassemia.[17] Most of these result from point mutations. Unlike in α-thalassemia, to be discussed later, gene deletions are uncommon in β-thalassemia. Details of these mutations and their effects on β-globin synthesis can be found in specialized texts.[18] A few illustrative examples are cited (Fig. 14–13).

- *Promoter region mutations.* Several point mutations within the promoter sequences reduce binding of RNA polymerase and thereby reduce the transcription rate by 75% to 80%. Since some β-globin is synthesized, the patients develop β^+-thalassemia.
- *Chain terminator mutations.* Two types of mutations can cause premature termination of mRNA translation. A point mutation in one of the exons can lead to the formation of a stop codon; in other cases, single nucleotide substitutions or small deletions alter mRNA reading frames and introduce stop codons downstream that terminate protein synthesis (frameshift mutations; see Chapter 6). Premature chain termination by either of these two mechanisms generates nonfunctional fragments of the β-globin gene, leading to β^0-thalassemia.
- *Splicing mutations. Mutations that lead to aberrant splicing are the most common cause of β-thalassemia.* Most of these affect introns, but some have been located within exons. If the mutation alters the normal splice junctions, splicing does not occur, and all of the mRNA formed is abnormal. Unspliced mRNA is degraded within the nucleus, and β^0-thalassemia results. However, some mutations affect the introns at locations away from the normal intron-exon splice junction. These mutations create new sites sensitive to the action of splicing enzymes at abnormal locations—within an intron, for example. Because normal splice sites remain unaffected, both normal and abnormal splicing occurs, giving rise to normal as well as abnormal β-globin mRNA. These patients develop β^+-thalassemia.

Impaired β-globin synthesis contributes to the pathogenesis of anemia by two mechanisms (Fig. 14–14). There is, of course, lack of adequate HbA formation, so that the overall concentration of hemoglobin in the cells (MCHC) is lower and the cells are hypochromic. Much more impor-

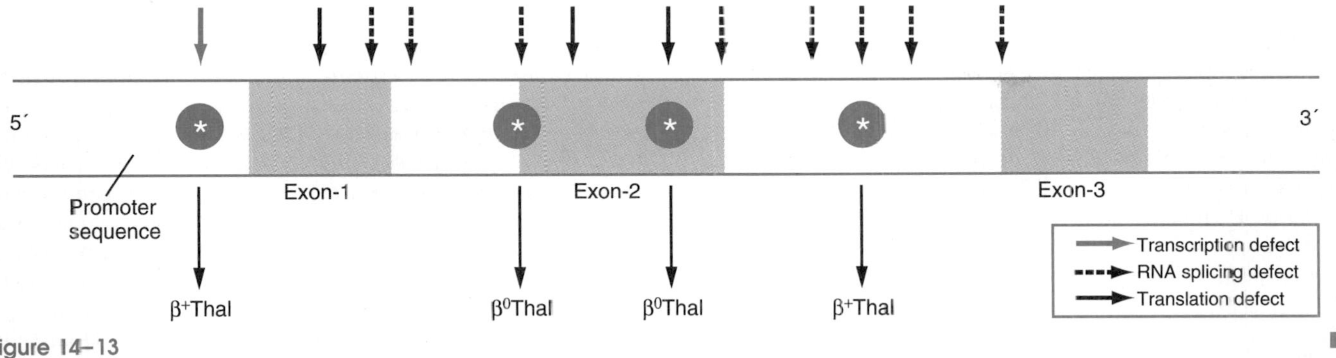

Figure 14–13

Diagrammatic representation of the β-globin gene, and some sites where point mutations giving rise to thalassemia have been localized.

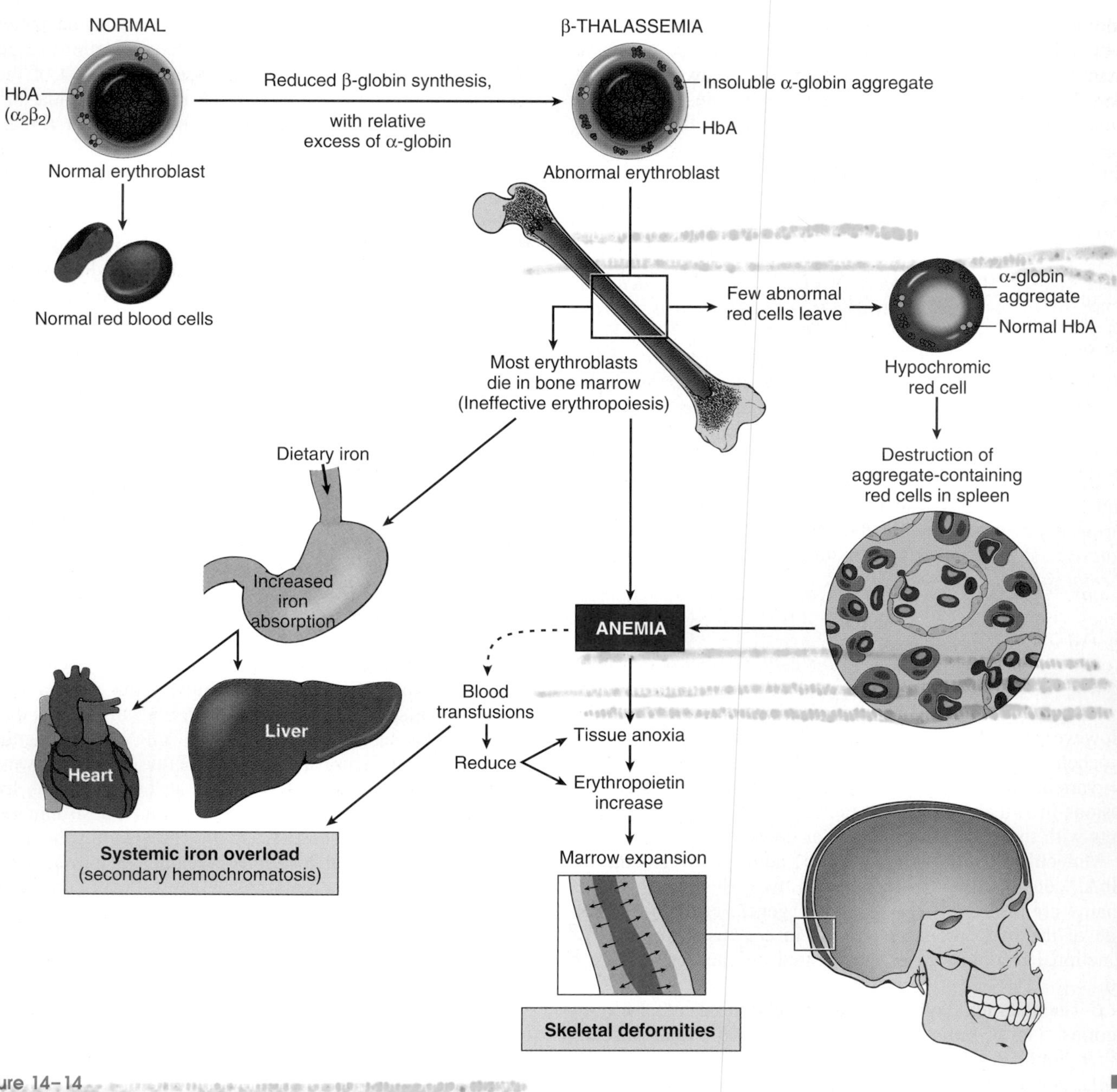

Figure 14–14

Pathogenesis of β-thalassemia major. Note that aggregates of excess α-globin are not visible on routine blood smears. Blood transfusions, on the one hand, correct the anemia and reduce the stimulus for erythropoietin secretion and deformities induced by marrow expansion; on the other hand, they add to the systemic iron overload.

tant is the effect on survival of red cells and their precursors, resulting from an imbalance between α- and β-chain synthesis. Since synthesis of α-globin chains continues unimpaired, most of the chains produced cannot find complementary β chains to bind. The free α chains form highly unstable aggregates that precipitate within the normoblasts in the form of insoluble inclusions. *A variety of untoward effects follow, the most important being cell membrane damage leading to a loss of K^+ and impaired DNA synthesis. The net effect is apoptotic death of red cell precursors within the bone marrow, a phenomenon called ineffective erythropoiesis.*[19] *It is estimated that approximately 70% to 85% of the marrow normoblasts undergo apoptosis in severely affected patients. The inclusion-bearing red cells derived from the precursors that escape intramedullary death are at increased risk for sequestration and destruction in the spleen. The inclusions damage the cell membranes, reduce their plasticity, and render them a "happy meal" for phagocytes in the spleen. The hemolytic component leads to a considerable shortening of red cell survival.*

In severe β-thalassemia, marked anemia produced by ineffective erythropoiesis and hemolysis leads to several additional problems. Erythropoietin secretion is stimulated, which leads to severe erythroid hyperplasia in the bone marrow and often at extramedullary sites. Massive erythropoiesis within the bones invades the bony cortex, impairs bone growth, and produces other skeletal abnormalities, described later. Extramedullary hematopoiesis involves the liver and spleen and in extreme cases produces extraosseous masses in the thorax, abdomen, and pelvis. *Another disastrous effect seen in severe β-thalassemia (as well as in other causes of ineffective erythropoiesis) is excessive absorption of dietary iron.* This, coupled with the iron accumulation due to repeated blood transfusions required by these patients, leads to a severe state of iron overload. Secondary injury to parenchymal organs, particularly the iron-laden liver, often follows and sometimes induces secondary hemochromatosis (Chapter 19).

Clinical Syndromes. The clinical classification of β-thalassemias is based on the severity of the anemia, which in turn is based on the type of genetic defect (β^+ or β^0) as well as the gene dosage (homozygous or heterozygous).[20] In general, individuals who are homozygous for the β-thalassemia genes (β^+/β^+ or β^0/β^0) have severe, transfusion-dependent anemia and are said to have *β-thalassemia major.* The presence of one normal gene in the heterozygotes (β^+/β or β^0/β) usually leads to enough normal β-globin chain synthesis so that the affected individuals are usually asymptomatic with only a mild anemia. This condition is referred to as *β-thalassemia minor* or *β-thalassemia trait.* A third clinical variant is characterized by an intermediate degree of severity, the so-called *β-thalassemia intermedia.* These patients have severe anemia, but not enough to require regular blood transfusions. Genetically, intermedia disorders are heterogeneous and include mild variants of homozygous β^+-thalassemia, some severe variants of heterozygous β-thalassemia (β^0/β or β^+/β), and double heterozygosity for the β^+ and β^0 genes (genotype β^+/β^0). The clinical and morphologic features of thalassemia intermedia are not described separately but may be surmised from the following discussions of thalassemia major and minor.

Thalassemia Major. The β-thalassemia genes are most frequent, and thalassemia major is most common, in Mediterranean countries and parts of Africa and Southeast Asia. In the United States, the incidence is highest in immigrants from these areas. As indicated in Table 14–3, the genotype of these patients is usually β^+/β^+ or β^0/β^0. In some cases, it is β^0/β^+ (double heterozygotes, if the two parents are carriers of β^+ and β^0). With all these genotypes, the anemia is severe and first becomes manifest 6 to 9 months after birth, as hemoglobin synthesis switches from HbF to HbA. In untransfused patients, hemoglobin levels range between 3 and 6 gm/dl. The peripheral blood smear shows severe abnormalities; there is marked anisocytosis (variation in size) with many small and virtually colorless (microcytic, hypochromic) red cells. Abnormal forms, including target cells (so called because the small amount of hemoglobin collects in the center), stippled red cells, and fragmented red cells, are common. Inclusions representing aggregated α chains are removed by the spleen and hence are not visible in peripheral blood. The reticulocyte count is elevated, but because of ineffective erythropoiesis, it is lower than would be predicted from the severity of anemia. Variable numbers of poorly hemoglobinized normoblasts are seen in the peripheral blood. The red cells contain either no HbA at all (β^0/β^0 genotype) or small amounts (β^+/β^+ genotype). HbF is markedly increased and indeed constitutes the major hemoglobin of red cells. HbA_2 levels may be normal, low, or high.

Table 14–3. CLINICAL AND GENETIC CLASSIFICATION OF THALASSEMIAS

Clinical Nomenclature	Genotype	Disease	Molecular Genetics
β-Thalassemias			
Thalassemia major	Homozygous β^0-thalassemia (β^0/β^0) Homozygous β^+-thalassemia (β^+/β^+)	Severe, requires blood transfusions regularly	Rare gene deletions in β^0/β^0 Defects in transcription, processing, or translation of β-globin mRNA
Thalassemia intermedia	β^0/β β^+/β^+	Severe, but does not require regular blood transfusions	
Thalassemia minor	β^0/β β^+/β	Asymptomatic with mild or absent anemia; red cell abnormalities seen	
α-Thalassemias			
Silent carrier	$-\alpha/\alpha\alpha$	Asymptomatic; no red cell abnormality	Gene deletions mainly
α-Thalassemia trait	$--/\alpha\alpha$ (Asian) $-\alpha/-\alpha$ (black African)	Asymptomatic, like β-thalassemia minor	
HbH disease	$--/-\alpha$	Severe, resembles β-thalassemia intermedia	
Hydrops fetalis	$--/--$	Lethal in utero	

MORPHOLOGY. The major morphologic alterations, in addition to those characteristic of all hemolytic anemias, involve the bone marrow and spleen. In the untransfused patient, there is striking expansion of the red marrow, particularly in facial bones, giving rise to thinning of the cortical bone with new bone formation on the external aspect, giving rise to the "crew-cut" appearance on x-rays (Fig. 14–15). Marked hepatosplenomegaly results both from reticuloendothelial cell hyperplasia secondary to active erythrophagocytosis and from extramedullary hematopoiesis. The spleen may weigh up to 1500 gm.

Hemosiderosis and even sometimes secondary hemochromatosis, the two manifestations of iron overload (Chapter 19), are seen in almost all patients. Excess iron deposition results from numerous blood transfusions and increased absorption of dietary iron, the latter secondary to ineffective erythropoiesis. Excess body iron causes damage to several organs, including the heart, liver, and pancreas (Chapter 19).

The clinical course of β-thalassemia major is brief because, unless supported by transfusions, children suffer from growth retardation and die at an early age from the profound effects of anemia. Blood transfusions not only improve the anemia but also suppress secondary features related to excessive erythropoiesis. The clinical manifestations can be deduced largely from the hematologic and morphologic changes. In those who survive long enough, the face becomes overlarge and somewhat distorted. Hepatosplenomegaly is usually present. Cardiac disease resulting from progressive iron overload and secondary hemochromatosis (Chapter 19) is an important cause of death even in patients who can otherwise be supported by blood transfusions. To reduce the amount of iron overload, most patients also receive iron chelators. With transfusions and iron chelation, many patients survive into the third decade, but the overall outlook continues to be grim. Bone marrow transplantation from an HLA-identical sibling is currently the only therapy that offers a cure. Prenatal diagnosis is possible by molecular analysis of DNA.

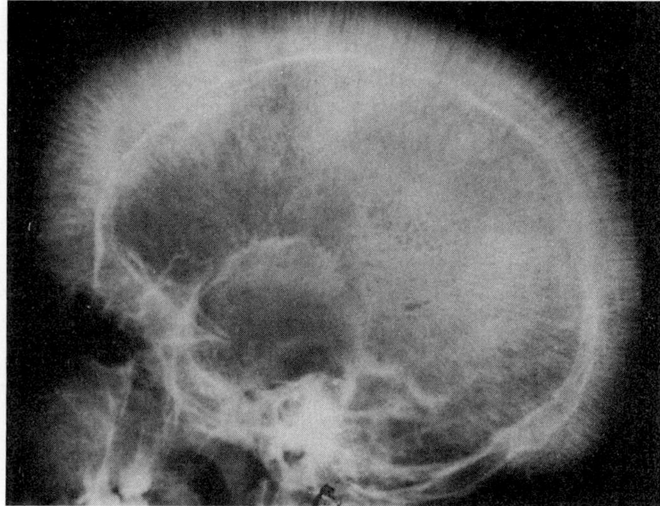

Figure 14–15

Thalassemia: x-ray film of the skull showing new bone formation on the outer table, producing perpendicular radiations characterized as a "crew haircut." (Courtesy of Dr. Jack Reynolds, Department of Radiology, University of Texas Southwestern Medical School, Dallas, TX.)

Thalassemia Minor. This is much more common than thalassemia major and understandably affects the same ethnic groups. In most cases, these patients are heterozygous for the β^+ or β^0 gene. Thalassemia trait is believed to offer resistance against falciparum malaria, accounting for its prevalence in those parts of the world where malaria is endemic. Almost invariably, individuals with the thalassemia trait are asymptomatic, and anemia is mild if it is present. The peripheral blood smear usually shows some abnormalities affecting the red cells, including hypochromia, microcytosis, basophilic stippling, and target cells. Mild erythroid hyperplasia is seen in the bone marrow. A characteristic finding on hemoglobin electrophoresis is an increase in HbA_2, which may constitute 4% to 8% of the total hemoglobin (normal, 2.5% ± 0.3%). HbF levels may be normal or slightly increased. Recognition of β-thalassemia trait is important on two counts: (1) its differentiation from the hypochromic microcytic anemia of iron deficiency and (2) genetic counseling. The importance of differentiating thalassemia trait from iron deficiency lies in the fact that the latter is benefited by iron therapy, whereas the former may be worsened. The distinction can usually be made by measurement of serum iron, total iron-binding capacity, and serum ferritin (see Iron Deficiency Anemia). Hemoglobin electrophoresis is also helpful.

α-Thalassemias

These disorders are characterized by reduced synthesis (α^+-thalassemia) or absent synthesis (α°-thalassemia) of α-globin chains. Since there are normally four α-globin genes, the severity of the clinical syndromes shows a great variation, depending on the number of affected α-globin genes. As in the case of β-thalassemias, the anemia stems both from lack of adequate hemoglobin and from the effects of excess unpaired non−α chains (β, γ, δ). However, the situation is somewhat complicated by the fact that normally different non−α chains are synthesized at different times of development. Thus, in the newborn with α-thalassemia, there is an excess of unpaired γ-globin chains resulting in the formation of γ_4-tetramers called Bart hemoglobin, whereas in adults, the excess β-globin chains aggregate to form tetramers called HbH. Since the non−α chains in general form more soluble and less toxic aggregates than those derived from α chains, the hemolytic anemia and ineffective erythropoiesis tend to be less severe than with β-thalassemias of similar degree of chain imbalance. A variety of molecular lesions have been detected in α-thalassemia. Unlike in β-thalassemia, however, the most common cause of reduced α-chain synthesis seems to be the deletion of α-globin genes.

Clinical Syndromes. These are classified on the basis of the number and position of the α-globin genes deleted, which in turn determine the clinical syndrome. α-Globin genes occur in linked pairs on each of the two chromosomes 16. Each α-globin gene normally contributes approximately 25% of the α-globin chains and may be deleted independently of the other α-globin genes. The terminology of α-thalassemias is best considered along with Table 14–3, in which clinical terms and their genetic equivalents are presented with the salient clinical features. Capsule descriptions follow.

Silent Carrier State. This is characterized by the deletion of a single α-globin gene and a barely detectable reduction in α-globin chain synthesis. These individuals carrying three normal α-globin genes are completely asymptomatic and do not have anemia.

α-Thalassemia Trait. This is characterized by deletion of two α-globin genes. The involved genes may be from the same chromosome (with the other chromosome carrying the two normal genes), or one α-globin gene may be deleted from each of the two chromosomes (Table 14–3). The former genotype is more common among Asian populations, whereas the latter is seen in those of African origin. Both of these genetic patterns produce similar quantitative deficiencies of α-globin chains and therefore are identical clinically, but the position of deleted genes makes a big difference to the likelihood of severe α-thalassemia (HbH disease or hydrops fetalis) in the offspring. As is evident from Table 14–3, in black African populations, in whom the two α genes are deleted from two separate chromosomes, mating of two individuals with the α-thalassemia trait would not result in progeny with HbH disease or hydrops fetalis.

The clinical picture in α-thalassemia trait is identical to that described for β-thalassemia minor, that is, minimal or no anemia and no abnormal physical signs.

Hemoglobin H Disease. This is associated with deletion of three of the four α-globin genes. As already discussed, HbH disease is seen mainly in Asian populations and rarely in those of African origin. With only one normal α-globin gene, the synthesis of α chains is markedly reduced and tetramers of excess β-globin, called HbH, are formed. HbH has extremely high oxygen affinity and therefore is not useful for oxygen exchange. Hence, the patient's anemia appears disproportionate to the level of hemoglobin. Inclusions of HbH can be demonstrated by incubation of red cells with brilliant cresyl blue in vitro. Oxidized HbH is precipitated by this procedure, since it is unable to withstand oxidative stress. This property of HbH is the major cause of anemia, since older red cells with precipitates of oxidized HbH are removed by the spleen. These patients have a moderately severe anemia; the clinical picture resembles that of β-thalassemia intermedia.

Hydrops Fetalis. This is the most severe form of α-thalassemia, resulting from the deletion of all four α-globin genes. In the fetus, excess γ-globin chains form tetramers (hemoglobin Bart) that have extremely high oxygen affinity but are unable to deliver the oxygen to tissues. In the past, severe tissue anoxia associated with this condition invariably led to intrauterine fetal death; with intrauterine transfusion, many such infants can be saved. The fetus shows severe pallor, generalized edema, and massive hepatosplenomegaly similar to that seen in erythroblastosis fetalis (Chapter 11).

PAROXYSMAL NOCTURNAL HEMOGLOBINURIA

Despite its rarity, this disorder has fascinated hematologists because this is the only example of hemolytic anemia in which there is an acquired rather than hereditary defect in the cell membrane. Before we describe the molecular basis of paroxysmal nocturnal hemoglobinuria (PNH), it is instructive to recall that proteins are anchored into the lipid bilayer in one of two ways. Most membrane proteins contain a sequence that allows them to insert into the cell membrane (Fig. 14–16). They are called transmembrane proteins. Some proteins, however, do not possess a membrane-spanning domain; instead, they are anchored into the cell membrane through a phospholipid called glycosylphosphatidylinositol (GPI). *PNH results from a mutation in the phosphatidylinositol glycan A, or PIGA, gene that is essential for the synthesis of the GPI anchor.* The somatic mutation in the *PIGA* gene affects pluripotent stem cells; hence, the clonal progeny of the mutant stem cells (red cells, white cells, platelets) are deficient in all those proteins that are attached to the cell membrane by a GPI anchor.[21] Because several GPI-linked proteins inactivate complement, their absence renders blood cells unusually sensitive to lysis by endogenous complement. Not all blood cells are affected in a patient with PNH; a substantial number are entirely normal, indicating that the mutant clone exists side by side with progeny of normal stem cells. Because PNH is an acquired disorder, there is no evidence for increased incidence within families.

Three GPI-linked proteins that regulate complement activity—decay-accelerating factor, or CD55; membrane inhibitor of reactive lysis, or CD59; and a C8 binding protein—are deficient in PNH. Of these, CD59 is the most important because it limits spontaneous in vivo activation of the alternative complement pathway by rapid inactiva-

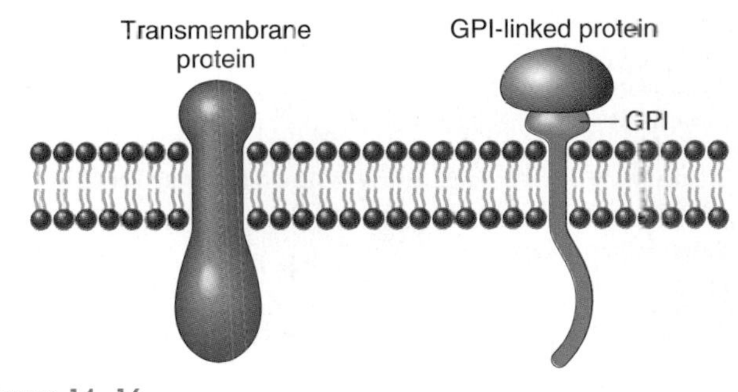

Figure 14–16

Two kinds of membrane proteins: transmembrane and glycosyl phosphatidyl inositol (GPI) linked. The latter are anchored to the cell membrane by glycosyl phospatidyl inositol. In PNH the GPI moiety cannot be synthesized, and therefore the GPI-linked proteins cannot be expressed on the cell membrane.

tion of C3 convertase. These defects are not limited to red blood cells, and therefore platelets and granulocytes are also more sensitive to lysis by complement.

Patients classically have intravascular hemolysis, which is paroxysmal and nocturnal in only 25% of cases. Most of the remaining patients have chronic hemolysis without dramatic hemoglobinuria. During the long course of the disease, hemosiderinuria with loss of iron eventually leads to iron deficiency. The other clinical manifestations include multiple episodes of venous thromboses in the hepatic, portal, or cerebral veins, which are fatal in 50% of cases. The course of this disease is chronic, with a median survival of 10 years. Because PNH is an acquired clonal disorder of stem cells, it sometimes evolves into other stem cell disorders, such as aplastic anemia and acute leukemia.

IMMUNOHEMOLYTIC ANEMIA

Hemolytic anemias in this category are caused by extracorpuscular mechanisms. Although these disorders are commonly referred to as autoimmune hemolytic anemias, the designation *immunohemolytic anemias* is preferred because in some instances the immune reaction is initiated by drug ingestion.[22] The immunohemolytic disorders have been classified in various ways but most commonly on the basis of the specific nature of the antibody involved (Table 14–4).

Whatever the antibody, the differentiation of immunohemolytic anemias from other forms of hemolytic anemia depends on demonstration of the anti–red cell antibodies. The major diagnostic criterion is the Coombs' antiglobulin test, which relies on the capacity of the antibodies prepared in animals against human globulins to agglutinate red cells if these globulins are present on red cell surfaces. The temperature dependence of the autoantibody further helps to specify the type of antibody. Quantitative immunologic methods to measure these autoantibodies directly are now available.

Table 14–4. CLASSIFICATION OF IMMUNE HEMOLYTIC ANEMIAS

Warm Antibody Type

The antibody is of the IgG type, does not usually fix complement, and is active at 37°C.

- *Primary* or idiopathic
- *Secondary* to
  - Lymphomas and leukemias
  - Other neoplastic diseases
  - Autoimmune disorder (particularly systemic lupus erythematosus)
  - Drugs

Cold Agglutinin Type

The antibodies are IgM and are most active in vitro at 0 to 4°C. Antibodies dissociate at 30°C or above. The antibody fixes complement at warmer temperatures, but agglutination of cells by IgM and complement occurs only in the peripheral cool parts of the body.

- *Acute* (mycoplasmal infection, infectious mononucleosis)
- *Chronic*
  - Idiopathic
  - Associated with lymphoma

Cold Hemolysins (Paroxysmal Cold Hemoglobinuria)

IgG antibodies bind to red cells at low temperature, fix complement, and cause hemolysis when the temperature is raised to 30°C.

Warm Antibody Hemolytic Anemia. This is the most common form of immune hemolytic anemia. In about 50% of patients, the condition is idiopathic and primary; in the remaining 50%, there is an underlying predisposing condition (Table 14–4) or some drug exposure to thus produce a secondary form of immune hemolytic anemia. Most of the autoantibodies are of the immunoglobulin (Ig) G class; only sometimes are IgA antibodies found. Most of the red cell destruction in this form of hemolytic disease is not due to intravascular hemolysis.[22] Instead, IgG-coated red cells are bound to Fc receptors on monocytes and splenic macrophages and undergo spheroidal transformation. This process results from a partial loss of the red cell membrane by attempted phagocytosis of the IgG-coated cell. *The spherocytes are then sequestered and removed in the spleen, the major site of red cell destruction in this disorder. Thus, moderate splenomegaly is characteristic of this form of anemia.*

As is the case with most forms of autoimmunity, the cause of autoantibody formation is largely unknown. Surprisingly, in many cases, the antibodies are directed against the Rh blood group antigens. The mechanisms of drug-induced hemolysis are better understood. Two different immunologic mechanisms have been implicated.[23]

- *Hapten model.* The drugs—exemplified by penicillin and cephalosporins—act as a hapten and combine with the red cell membrane to induce antibody directed against the cell-bound drug, resulting in the destructive sequence cited before. This form of hemolytic anemia is usually caused by large intravenous doses of the antibiotic and occurs 1 to 2 weeks after onset of therapy. Whereas the antibodies bind only to the offending drug in penicillin-induced hemolytic anemia, in the other cases, exemplified by quinidine-induced hemolysis, the antibodies recognize a complex of the drug and a membrane protein. In drug-induced hemolytic anemias, the destruction of red cells may occur intravascularly after fixation of complement or extravascularly in the reticuloendothelial system.
- *Autoantibody model.* The drug, such as the antihypertensive agent α-methyldopa, in some manner initiates the production of antibodies that are directed against intrinsic red cell antigens, in particular the Rh blood group antigens. Approximately 10% of patients taking methyldopa develop autoantibodies that can be detected in the Coombs' test. However, only 1% develop clinically significant hemolysis.

Cold Agglutinin Immune Hemolytic Anemia. This form of immune hemolytic anemia is caused by IgM antibodies that bind avidly to red cells at low temperatures (0 to 4°C).[24] Because they agglutinate red cells at low temperatures, they are referred to as cold agglutinins. These antibodies occur *acutely* during the recovery phase of certain infectious disorders, such as mycoplasmal pneumonia and infectious mononucleosis. This form of hemolytic anemia is self-limited and rarely induces clinical manifestations of hemolysis. *Chronic* cold agglutinins occur with lymphoproliferative disorders or as an idiopathic condition. The antibodies produced are monoclonal, suggesting that the underlying basis is similar to that of other monoclonal gammopathies (Chapter 15). The clinical symptoms result from an in vivo agglutination of red cells and fixation of complement in distal body parts, where the temperature may drop to below 30°C. Thus, there may be intravascular hemolysis. In most cases, however, the IgM bound to red cells is released when the cells return to 37°C. This leaves C3, specifically C3b, bound to the cell membrane, making it susceptible to phagocytosis by mononuclear phagocytes in the liver and spleen. The hemolytic anemia is usually of variable severity. In addition, vascular obstruction caused by red cell agglutinates results in pallor, cyanosis of the body parts exposed to cold temperatures, and Raynaud phenomenon (Chapter 12).

Cold Hemolysin Hemolytic Anemia. These autoantibodies are characteristic of the disease *paroxysmal cold hemoglobinuria*, which is noted for acute intermittent massive hemolysis, frequently with hemoglobinuria, after exposure of the affected patient to cold. Lysis is clearly complement dependent. The autoantibodies are IgG in nature and are directed against the P blood group antigen; they attach to the red cells and bind complement at low temperatures. When the temperature is elevated, the hemolytic action is mediated by the activation of the lytic complement cascade. The antibody is also known as the Donath-Landsteiner antibody, previously associated with syphilis. Today, most cases of paroxysmal cold hemoglobinuria follow various infections such as mycoplasmal pneumonia, measles, mumps, and some ill-defined viral and "flu" syndromes. The mechanisms responsible for the production of such autoantibodies are unknown.

HEMOLYTIC ANEMIA RESULTING FROM TRAUMA TO RED CELLS

Red blood cells may be disrupted by physical trauma in a variety of circumstances. *Clinically important are the hemolytic anemias associated with cardiac valve prostheses and with narrowing or obstruction of the vasculature.* Traumatic hemolytic anemia is more severe with artificial, mechanical valves than with bioprosthetic, porcine valves. In patients with prosthetic valves of either type, the red cells are damaged by the shear stresses resulting from the turbulent blood flow and abnormal pressure gradients caused by the valves. Microangiopathic hemolytic anemia, on the other hand, is characterized by mechanical damage to the red cells as they squeeze through abnormally narrowed vessels. The narrowing is most often caused by widespread deposition of fibrin in the small vessels in association with disseminated intravascular coagulation, discussed later in this chapter. Other causes of microangiopathic hemolytic anemia include malignant hypertension, systemic lupus erythematosus, thrombotic thrombocytopenic purpura (TTP), hemolytic-uremic syndrome (HUS), and disseminated cancer. Most of these disorders are discussed elsewhere in this book. It suffices to say that common to all of these disorders is the presence of vascular lesions that predispose the circulating red cells to mechanical injury. The morphologic appearance of red cell fragments (schistocytes) may be striking. Thus, "burr cells," "helmet cells," and "triangle cells" may be seen in the peripheral blood film (Fig. 14–17). Except for TTP and the related HUS, hemolysis is not a major clinical problem in most instances.

Anemias of Diminished Erythropoiesis

Diminished erythropoiesis may result from a deficiency of some vital substrate necessary for red cell formation. Included in this group are anemia of vitamin B_{12} and folate deficiency, characterized by defective DNA synthesis (megaloblastic anemias), and iron deficiency anemias, in which heme synthesis is impaired. Other causes of decreased erythropoiesis include anemia of chronic disease and "marrow stem cell failure," which embraces such conditions as aplastic anemia, pure red cell aplasia, and anemia of renal failure.

MEGALOBLASTIC ANEMIAS

The following discussion attempts first to characterize the major features of these anemias and then to discuss the two principal types of megaloblastic anemia: (1) pernicious anemia, the major form of vitamin B_{12} deficiency anemia, and (2) folate deficiency anemia.

The megaloblastic anemias constitute a diverse group of entities, having in common *impaired DNA synthesis* and distinctive morphologic changes in the blood and bone marrow. As the name implies, the erythroid precursors and

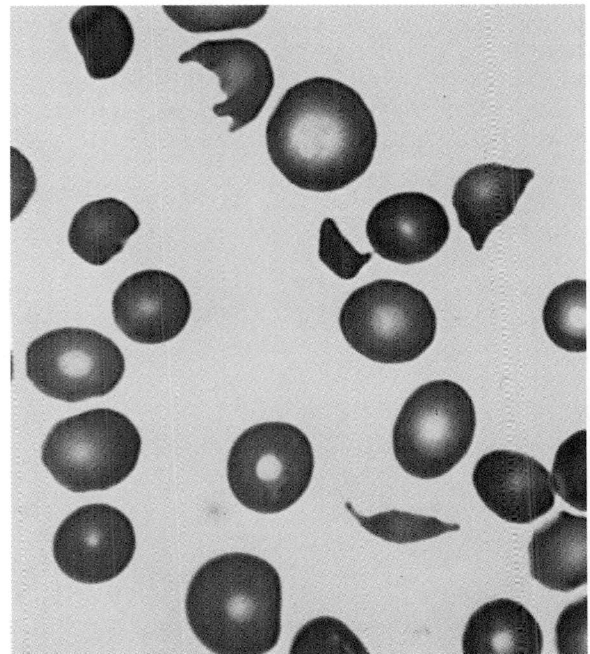

Figure 14–17 ■

Microangiopathic hemolytic anemia. The peripheral blood smear from a patient with hemolytic-uremic syndrome shows several fragmented red cells. (Courtesy of Dr. Robert W. McKenna, Department of Pathology, University of Texas Southwestern Medical School, Dallas, TX.)

erythrocytes are abnormally large, thought to be related to defective cell maturation and division. The precise basis of these changes is not fully understood.

Some of the metabolic roles of vitamin B_{12} and folate are considered later, but for now it suffices that vitamin B_{12} and folic acid are coenzymes in the DNA synthetic pathway. A deficiency of these vitamins or impairment in their use results in defective nuclear maturation due to deranged or inadequate synthesis of DNA. The synthesis of RNA and protein is unaffected, however, so cytoplasmic enlargement is not matched by DNA synthesis, and there is a delay or block in mitotic division. Thus, there appears to be asynchronism between the cytoplasmic maturation and nuclear maturation.

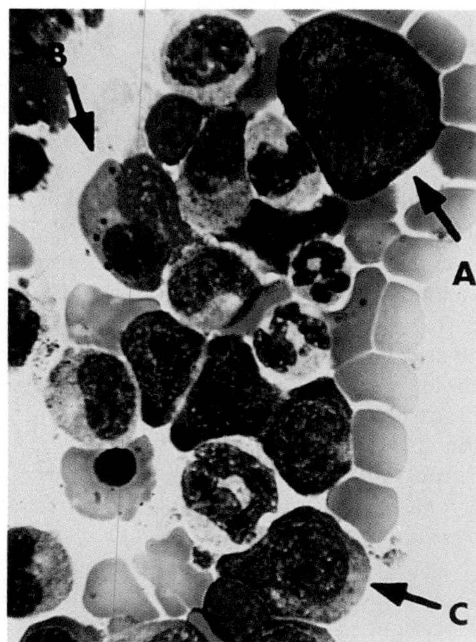

Figure 14–19

Marrow smear from a patient with megaloblastic anemia. *A* to *C*, Megaloblasts in various stages of differentiation. Note that the orthochromatic megaloblast (*B*) is hemoglobinized (as evidenced by cytoplasmic color), but in contrast to an orthochromatic normoblast, the nucleus is not pyknotic. The granulocytic precursors are also large. (Courtesy of Dr. Jose Hernandez, Department of Pathology, University of Texas Southwestern Medical School, Dallas, TX.)

MORPHOLOGY. Certain morphologic features are common to all forms of megaloblastic anemia. The peripheral blood reveals marked variation in the size and shape of red cells (anisocytosis), which are nonetheless normochromic. **Many erythrocytes are macrocytic and oval (macro-ovalocytes), with mean corpuscular volumes above 100 μm^3 (normal, 82 to 92).** Because they are thicker than normal and well filled with hemoglobin, most macrocytes lack the central pallor of normal red cells and may even appear "hyperchromic," but the MCHC is not elevated. The reticulocyte count is lower than normal, and nucleated red cells occasionally appear in the circulating blood with severe anemia. **Neutrophils too are larger than normal (macropolymorphonuclear) and are hypersegmented, that is, have five to six or more nuclear lobules (Fig. 14–18).** The marrow is hypercellular, and the megaloblastic change is detected in all stages of red cell development. The most primitive cells (promegaloblasts) are large, with a deeply basophilic cytoplasm and a distinctive fine chromatin pattern in the nucleus (Fig. 14–19, cell A). The nucleoli are large. As these cells differentiate and begin to acquire hemoglobin, the nucleus retains its finely distributed chromatin and thus fails to undergo the chromatin clumping typical of the normoblast. For example, orthochromatic megaloblasts have a large amount of pink, well-hemoglobinized cytoplasm; but the nucleus, instead of becoming pyknotic, remains relatively large and immature, creating an apparent dissociation between cytoplasmic and nuclear maturation. Because DNA synthesis is impaired in all proliferating cells, the granulocytic precursors also reveal nuclear-cytoplasmic asynchrony, yielding giant metamyelocytes and band forms and hypersegmentation of the neutrophils, as previously mentioned. Megakaryocytes, too, may be abnormally large and have bizarre, multilobate nuclei, but sometimes they appear relatively normal. With increased cellularity, much or all of the normally fatty marrow may be converted to red marrow. The erythroid to myeloid ratio, normally 1:3, may be transformed to 1:1.

Because of these maturational derangements, there is an accumulation of megaloblasts in the bone marrow, yielding too few erythrocytes; hence, the anemia. Two concomitant processes further aggravate the anemia: (1) ineffective erythropoiesis and (2) increased hemolytic destruction of

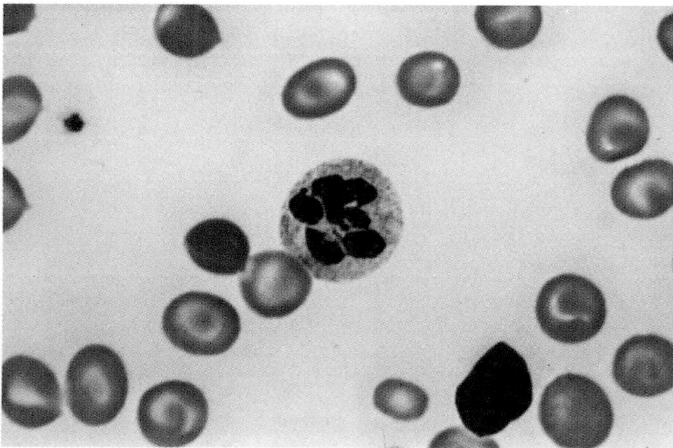

Figure 14–18

A peripheral blood smear from a patient with megaloblastic anemia shows a neutrophil with a six-lobed nucleus (macropolycyte). (Courtesy of Dr. Robert W. McKenna, Department of Pathology, University of Texas Southwestern Medical School, Dallas, TX.)

red cells. Ineffective erythropoiesis results from intramedullary destruction of megaloblasts, which undergo autohemolysis more readily than do normoblasts and are more vulnerable to phagocytosis by mononuclear phagocytic cells in the marrow than are normal erythroid precursors. Premature destruction of granulocytic and platelet precursors also occurs, resulting in leukopenia and thrombocytopenia. The basis of the increased hemolysis of the mature erythrocytes is not entirely clear. Both an intracorpuscular defect, related perhaps to the defective red cells, and a poorly characterized plasma factor are believed to contribute. As in other hemolytic states, accelerated destruction of the red cells may lead to anatomic signs of mild to moderate iron overload after several years (Chapter 19).

Anemias of Vitamin B_{12} Deficiency: Pernicious Anemia

The major causes of megaloblastic anemia are listed in Table 14–5. As mentioned at the outset, pernicious anemia is an important cause of vitamin B_{12} deficiency. *The feature that sets pernicious anemia apart from the other vitamin B_{12} deficiency megaloblastic anemias is the cause of the vitamin B_{12} malabsorption: atrophic gastritis with failure of production of intrinsic factor (IF).*

Table 14–5. CAUSES OF MEGALOBLASTIC ANEMIA

Vitamin B_{12} Deficiency
- Decreased intake
  - Inadequate diet, vegetarianism
- Impaired absorption
  - Intrinsic factor deficiency
    - Pernicious anemia
    - Gastrectomy
  - Malabsorption states
  - Diffuse intestinal disease, e.g., lymphoma, systemic sclerosis
  - Ileal resection, ileitis
  - Competitive parasitic uptake
    - Fish tapeworm infection
  - Bacterial overgrowth in blind loops and diverticula of bowel
- Increased requirement
  - Pregnancy, hyperthyroidism, disseminated cancer

Folic Acid Deficiency
- Decreased intake
  - Inadequate diet—alcoholism, infancy
- Impaired absorption
  - Malabsorption states
  - Intrinsic intestinal disease
  - Anticonvulsants, oral contraceptives
- Increased loss
  - Hemodialysis
- Increased requirement
  - Pregnancy, infancy, disseminated cancer, markedly increased hematopoiesis
- Impaired use
  - Folic acid antagonists

Unresponsive to Vitamin B_{12} or Folic Acid Therapy
- Metabolic inhibitors, e.g., mercaptopurines, fluorouracil, cytosine
- Unexplained disorders
  - Pyridoxine- and thiamine-responsive megaloblastic anemia
  - Acute erythroleukemia (M6) (Di Guglielmo syndrome)

Modified from Beck WS: Megaloblastic anemias. In Wyngaarden JB, Smith LH (eds): Cecil Textbook of Medicine, 18th ed. Philadelphia, WB Saunders, 1988, p 900.

It is well to discuss first the economy of vitamin B_{12} in the body to place pernicious anemia in perspective relative to the other forms of vitamin B_{12} deficiency anemia.

Etiology of Vitamin B_{12} Deficiency. Vitamin B_{12} is a complex organometallic compound known as cobalamin. Under normal circumstances, humans are totally dependent on dietary animal products for their vitamin B_{12} requirement. Microorganisms are the ultimate origin of cobalamin in the food chain. Plants and vegetables contain little cobalamin save that contributed by microbial contamination; strictly vegetarian or macrobiotic diets, then, do not provide adequate amounts of this essential nutrient. The daily requirement is of the order of 2 to 3 mg, and the normal balanced diet contains significantly larger amounts. The reserves in the body, when fully maintained, are sufficient for years.

Absorption of vitamin B_{12} requires IF, which is secreted by the parietal cells of the fundic mucosa along with hydrochloric acid (Fig. 14–20). Initially the vitamin is released from its protein-bound form by the action of pepsin in the acidic environment of the stomach. The liberated vitamin is then bound to salivary vitamin B_{12}–binding proteins called cobalophilins, or R-binders. In the duodenum, R–vitamin B_{12} complexes are broken down by the action of pancreatic proteases, and the released vitamin B_{12} then attaches to IF. In this form, IF–vitamin B_{12} complex is transported to the ileum, where it adheres to IF-specific receptors on the ileal cells. Vitamin B_{12} then traverses the plasma membrane to enter the mucosal cell. It is picked up from the cell by a plasma protein, transcobalamin II, which is capable of delivering it to the liver and other cells of the body, particularly the rapidly proliferating pool in the bone marrow and mucosal lining of the gastrointestinal tract.

With this background, we can consider the various causes of vitamin B_{12} deficiency (Table 14–5). Inadequate diet is obvious but must be present for many years to deplete reserves. The absorption of vitamin B_{12} may be impaired by disruption of any one of the steps outlined earlier. With achlorhydria and loss of pepsin secretion (which occurs in some elderly individuals), vitamin B_{12} is not readily released from its protein-bound form. With gastrectomy and pernicious anemia, IF is not available for transport to the ileum. With loss of exocrine pancreatic function, vitamin B_{12} deficiency occurs because the vitamin cannot be released from the R–vitamin B_{12} complexes. Ileal resection or diffuse ileal disease can remove or damage the site of IF–vitamin B_{12} complex absorption. Tapeworm infestation, by competing for the nutrient, can induce a deficiency state. Under some circumstances, for example, pregnancy, hyperthyroidism, and disseminated cancer, the demand for vitamin B_{12} can be so great as to produce a relative deficiency, even with normal absorption.

Biochemical Functions of Vitamin B_{12}. Two reactions in humans are known to require vitamin B_{12}. *Methylcobalamin is an essential cofactor for the enzyme methionine synthase, involved in the conversion of homocysteine to*

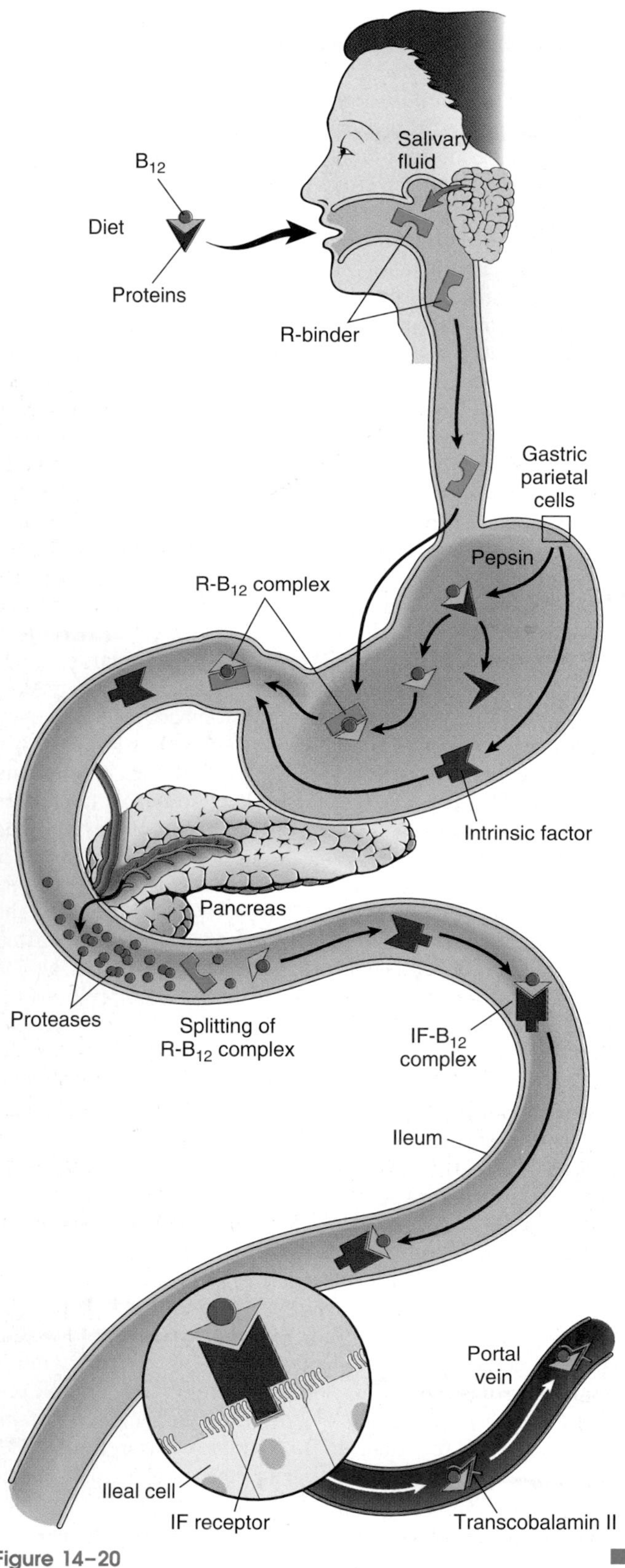

Figure 14–20

Schematic illustration of vitamin B_{12} absorption.

methionine (Fig. 14–21). In the process, methylcobalamin yields its methyl group and is regenerated from N^5-methyltetrahydrofolic acid (N^5-methyl FH_4), the principal form of folic acid in plasma, which is thus converted to tetrahydrofolic acid (FH_4). The FH_4 is crucial, since it is required (through its derivative $N^{5,10}$-methylene FH_4) for the conversion of deoxyuridine monophosphate to deoxythymidine monophosphate, which is an immediate precursor of DNA. It has been postulated that the fundamental cause of impaired DNA synthesis in vitamin B_{12} deficiency is the reduced availability of tetrahydrofolic acid, since most of it is "trapped" as N^5-methyl FH_4.[25] In addition to the trapping of tetrahydrofolic acid in its methylated form, the "internal" folate deficiency resulting from the lack of vitamin B_{12} may also be caused by a failure to synthesize the metabolically active polyglutamate forms of folates.[26] The synthesis of folate polyglutamates requires the single carbon formate groups derived from methionine, which in turn is generated by a vitamin B_{12}–dependent reaction (Fig. 14–21). Whatever the mechanism of internal folate deficiency, *the hypothesis that lack of folate is the proximate cause of anemia in vitamin B_{12} deficiency is supported by the observation that the anemia improves with the administration of folic acid.*

Neurologic complications appear with vitamin B_{12} deficiency but are an even greater enigma.[27] Since the administration of folic acid, which relieves the megaloblastic anemia of vitamin B_{12} deficiency, fails to improve the neurologic deficit, internal folate deficiency must not be involved. It was stated earlier that two reactions are known to require vitamin B_{12}. In addition to the transmethylation reaction discussed previously, cobalamin is involved in the *isomerization of methylmalonyl coenzyme A to succinyl coenzyme A, requiring adenosylcobalamin as a prosthetic*

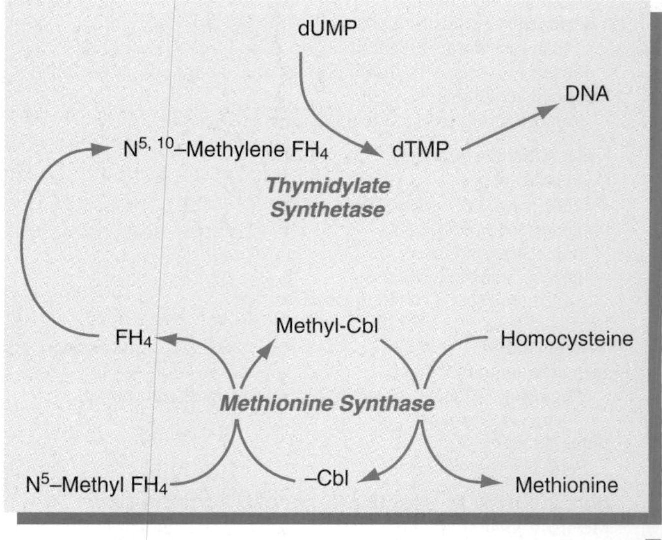

Figure 14–21

Diagram of the relationship between N^5-methyl FH_4, methionine synthase, and thymidylate synthetase. In cobalamin deficiency, folate is sequestered as N^5-methyl FH_4. This ultimately deprives thymidylate synthetase of its folate coenzyme ($N^{5,10}$-methylene FH_4) and thereby impairs DNA synthesis.

group on the enzyme methylmalonyl–coenzyme A mutase. A deficiency of vitamin B_{12} thus leads to increased levels of methylmalonate, excreted in the urine as methylmalonic acid. Interruption of the succinyl pathway with the build-up of increased levels of methylmalonate and propionate (a precursor) could lead to the formation of abnormal fatty acids that may be incorporated into neuronal lipids. This biochemical abnormality may predispose to myelin breakdown and thereby produce some of the neurologic complications of vitamin B_{12} deficiency (Chapter 30).

With this overview of vitamin B_{12} metabolism, we can now turn our attention to pernicious anemia.

Incidence. Although somewhat more prevalent in Scandinavian and "English-speaking" populations, pernicious anemia occurs in all racial groups, including, in the United States, blacks and Hispanics. It is a disease of older age, generally diagnosed in the fifth to eighth decades of life. A genetic predisposition is strongly suspected, but no definable genetic pattern of transmission has been discerned. As discussed next, these patients probably inherit a predisposition to forming autoantibodies.

Pathogenesis. Pernicious anemia is believed to result from immunologically mediated, possibly autoimmune, destruction of gastric mucosa. The resultant *chronic atrophic gastritis* is marked by a loss of parietal cells, a prominent infiltrate of lymphocytes and plasma cells, and nuclear changes in the mucosal cells similar to those found in the erythroid precursors. A number of immunologic reactions are associated with these morphologic changes. *Three types of antibodies are present in many but not all patients with pernicious anemia.* About 75% of patients have the type I antibody that blocks binding of vitamin B_{12} to IF and is referred to as a *blocking antibody*. Type I antibodies are found in both the serum and gastric juice. Type II antibodies prevent binding of IF or IF–vitamin B_{12} complex to its ileal receptor. These immunoglobulins are also found in a large proportion of patients with pernicious anemia. The third type of antibody, present in 85% to 90% of patients, localizes in the microvilli of the canalicular system of the gastric parietal cell, sometimes referred to as *parietal canalicular antibody*. It is directed against the α and β subunits of the gastric proton pump.[28] However, parietal canalicular antibodies are not absolutely specific for pernicious anemia or other autoimmune diseases. They can be found in up to 50% of elderly patients with idiopathic chronic gastritis not associated with pernicious anemia. As discussed next, they most likely result from gastric injury, rather than cause it.

Despite the presence of these autoantibodies, it is not established that they are the primary cause of gastric changes. It is suspected that an autoreactive T-cell response initiates gastric mucosal injury, which then triggers the formation of autoantibodies. These antibodies cause further injury to the epithelium, and after the mass of IF-secreting cells falls below a threshold (and the reserves of stored vitamin B_{12} are depleted), anemia develops. In an animal model of autoimmune gastritis, the disease is mediated by CD4+ T cells, and a pattern of autoantibodies resembling that seen in pernicious anemia develops.[28] The possibility that pernicious anemia is an autoimmune disease is also supported by the well-known association of this disease with autoimmune thyroiditis and adrenalitis. Conversely, patients with other organ-specific autoimmune disease have a predisposition to developing autoantibodies against IF.

MORPHOLOGY. The major specific changes in pernicious anemia are found in the bone marrow, alimentary tract, and central nervous system. The changes in the bone marrow and blood are similar to those described earlier for all megaloblastic anemias.

In the **alimentary system**, abnormalities are regularly found in the tongue and stomach. The tongue is shiny, glazed, and "beefy" **(atrophic glossitis)**. The changes in the stomach are those of diffuse chronic gastritis (Chapter 18). The most characteristic histologic alteration is the atrophy of the fundic glands, affecting both chief cells and parietal cells. The parietal cells are virtually absent. The glandular lining epithelium is replaced by mucus-secreting goblet cells that resemble those lining the large intestine. Such metaplasia is referred to as **intestinalization**. Some of the cells as well as their nuclei may increase to double the normal size. These enlargements presumably reflect the defect in DNA synthesis discussed earlier. As will be seen, patients with pernicious anemia have a higher incidence of gastric cancer. The gastric changes are due to autoimmunity and not to vitamin B_{12} deficiency; hence, parenteral administration of vitamin B_{12} corrects the bone marrow changes, but gastric atrophy and achlorhydria persist.

Central nervous system lesions are found in approximately three quarters of all cases of fulminant pernicious anemia, but in some cases, neuronal involvement may occur in the absence of megaloblastic anemia. **The principal alterations involve the spinal cord, where there is myelin degeneration of the dorsal and lateral tracts**, sometimes followed by loss of axons. These changes give rise to spastic paraparesis, sensory ataxia, and severe paresthesias in the lower limbs. Less frequently, degenerative changes occur in the ganglia of the posterior roots and in the peripheral nerves (Chapter 30). Because both sensory and motor pathways are involved, the term "subacute combined degeneration" or "combined system disease" is sometimes used to designate the neurologic changes associated with vitamin B_{12} deficiency.

Clinical Course. Pernicious anemia is characteristically insidious in onset, so that by the time the patient seeks medical attention, the anemia is usually marked. The usual course is progressive unless it is halted by therapy.

Diagnostic features include (1) a moderate to severe megaloblastic anemia; (2) leukopenia with hypersegmented granulocytes; (3) mild to moderate thrombocytopenia; (4) neurologic changes related to involvement of the postero-

lateral spinal tracts; (5) achlorhydria even after histamine stimulation; (6) inability to absorb an oral dose of cobalamin (assessed by urinary excretion of radiolabeled cyanocobalamin given orally, called the Schilling test); (7) low serum levels of vitamin B_{12}; (8) excretion of methylmalonic acid in the urine; and (9) a striking reticulocytic response and improvement in hematocrit levels after parenteral administration of vitamin B_{12}. Serum antibodies to IF are highly specific for pernicious anemia. Their presence attests to the cause of B_{12} deficiency, rather than the presence or absence of cobalamin deficiency.

The cytologic aberrations in the gastric mucosa are associated with an increased risk of gastric cancer (Chapter 18). With parenteral vitamin B_{12}, the anemia can be cured and the peripheral neurologic changes reversed, or at least halted in their progression, but the changes in the gastric mucosa are unaffected. Overall longevity may be restored virtually to normal.

Anemia of Folate Deficiency

A deficiency of folic acid, more properly pteroylmonoglutamic acid, results in a megaloblastic anemia having the same characteristics as those encountered in vitamin B_{12} deficiency. However, the neurologic changes seen in vitamin B_{12} deficiency do not occur. The prime function of folic acid, specifically tetrahydrofolate (FH_4) derivatives, is to act as an intermediate in the transfer of one-carbon units such as formyl and methyl groups to various compounds (Fig. 14–22). In this process, FH_4 acts as an acceptor of one-carbon fragments from compounds such as serine and formiminoglutamic acid (FIGlu), and the FH_4 derivatives so generated donate the acquired one-carbon fragments for the synthesis of biologically active molecules. FH_4, then, may be viewed as the biologic "middleman" in this trade. The most important metabolic processes dependent on such one-carbon transfers are (1) the synthesis of purines; (2) the synthesis of methionine from homocysteine, a reaction that also requires vitamin B_{12}; and (3) the synthesis of deoxythymidylate monophosphate. In the first two reactions, FH_4 is regenerated from its one-carbon carrier derivatives and is available to accept another one-carbon fragment and re-enter the donor pool. In the synthesis of thymidylate, a dihydrofolate is produced that has to be reduced by dihydrofolate reductase to FH_4 to re-enter the pool. The reductase step is significant, since this enzyme is susceptible to inhibition by various drugs. Among the biologically active molecules whose synthesis is dependent on folates, thymidylate is perhaps the most important. As discussed earlier in relation to pernicious anemia, deoxythymidylate monophosphate is required for DNA synthesis. It should be apparent from our discussion that suppressed synthesis of DNA, the common denominator of folic acid and vitamin B_{12} deficiency, is the immediate cause of megaloblastosis. A clinically insignificant biochemical effect of folate deficiency is the failure to metabolize FIGlu, a breakdown product of histidine. With a deficiency of folate, FIGlu accumulates and is excreted in the urine, providing a useful clinical indicator of folate deficiency.

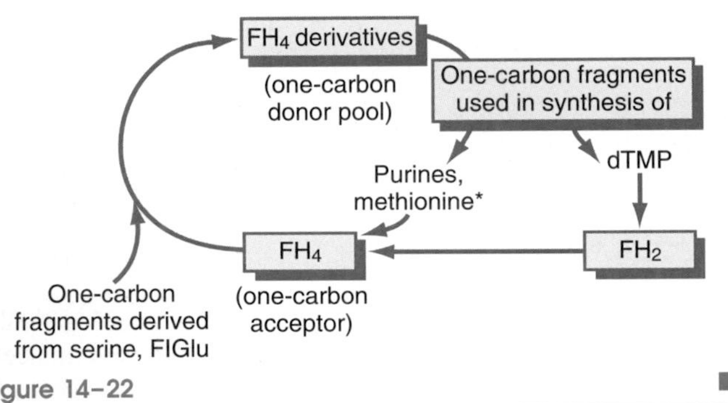

Figure 14–22

Schematic illustration of the role of folate derivatives in the transfer of one-carbon fragments for synthesis of biologic macromolecules. FH_4, tetrahydrofolic acid; FH_2, dihydrofolic acid; FIGlu, formiminoglutamate; dTMP, deoxythymidylate monophosphate. *Synthesis of methionine also requires vitamin B_{12}.

Etiology. Humans are entirely dependent on dietary sources for their folic acid requirement, which is of the order of 50 to 200 mg daily. Most normal diets contain ample amounts, the richest sources being green vegetables such as lettuce, spinach, asparagus, and broccoli. Certain fruits (e.g., lemons, bananas, melons) and animal proteins (e.g., liver) contain lesser amounts. The folic acid in these foods is largely in the form of folylpolyglutamates. *Despite their abundance in raw foods, polyglutamates (depending on the specific form) are sensitive to heat; boiling, steaming, or frying of foods for 5 to 10 minutes may destroy up to 95% of the folate content.* Intestinal conjugases split the polyglutamates into monoglutamates that are readily absorbed in the proximal jejunum. During intestinal absorption, they are modified so that only 5-methyltetrahydrofolate enters the circulation as the normal transport form of folate. The body's reserves of folate are relatively modest, and a deficiency may arise with months of a negative balance. There are three major causes of folic acid deficiency: (1) decreased intake, (2) increased requirements, and (3) impaired use (Table 14–5).

Decreased intake can result from either a nutritionally inadequate diet or impairment of intestinal absorption. A normal daily diet contains folate in excess of the minimal daily adult requirement. Inadequate dietary intakes are almost invariably associated with grossly deficient diets, particularly those lacking vitamins such as the "B group." *Such dietary inadequacies are most frequently encountered in chronic alcoholics, the indigent, and the very elderly.* In alcoholics with cirrhosis, other mechanisms of folate deficiency such as trapping of folate within the liver, excessive urinary loss, and disordered folate metabolism have also been implicated. Under these circumstances, the megaloblastic anemia is often accompanied by general malnutrition and manifestations of other avitaminoses, including cheilosis, glossitis, and dermatitis. Malabsorption syndromes such as nontropical and tropical sprue may lead to inadequate absorption of this nutrient. Similarly, diffuse infiltrative disease of the small intestine (e.g., lymphoma) may impair intestinal absorption. In addition, certain drugs, particularly the anticonvulsant phenytoin and oral contraceptives, impair absorption.

Despite adequate intake of folic acid, a *relative deficiency* can be encountered in states of increased requirement, such as pregnancy, infancy, hematologic derangements associated with hyperactive hematopoiesis (hemolytic anemias), and disseminated cancer. In all these circumstances, the demands of active DNA synthesis render normal intake inadequate.

Folic acid antagonists, such as methotrexate, 6-mercaptopurine, and cyclophosphamide, inhibit dihydrofolate reductase and lead to a deficiency of tetrahydrofolate. With inhibition of folate function, all rapidly growing cells are affected, thus leading to ulcerative lesions within the gastrointestinal tract as well as megaloblastic anemia. Owing to their growth-inhibitory actions, these antimetabolites are used in cancer therapy.

As mentioned at the outset, *the megaloblastic anemia resulting from a deficiency of folic acid is identical to that encountered in vitamin B_{12} deficiency.* Thus, the recognition of folate deficiency requires the demonstration of (1) decreased folate levels in the serum or red cells and (2) increased excretion of FIGlu after an administered dose of histidine.

Although prompt hematologic response heralded by the appearance of a reticulocytosis follows the administration of folic acid, it should be cautioned that even in patients with a vitamin B_{12} deficiency anemia, a similar reticulocytosis may be produced by folic acid therapy. However, folic acid has no effect on the progression of the neurologic changes typical of the vitamin B_{12} deficiency states, and therefore the hematologic response to folate therapy cannot be used to rule out vitamin B_{12} deficiency.

IRON DEFICIENCY ANEMIA

Deficiency of iron is probably the most common nutritional disorder in the world. Although the prevalence of iron deficiency anemia is higher in the developing countries, this form of anemia is also common in the United States,[29] particularly in toddlers, adolescent girls, and women of childbearing age. The factors underlying the iron deficiency differ somewhat in various population groups and can be best considered in the context of normal iron metabolism.

Iron Metabolism. The total body iron content is normally in the range of 2 gm in women and up to 6 gm in men. As indicated in Table 14–6, it is divided into functional and storage compartments. Approximately 80% of the functional iron is found in hemoglobin; myoglobin and iron-containing enzymes such as catalase and the cytochromes contain the rest. The storage pool represented by hemosiderin and ferritin contains approximately 15% to 20% of total body iron. Even healthy young females have substantially smaller stores of iron than do males. They are therefore in much more precarious iron balance and are accordingly more vulnerable to excessive losses or increased demands associated with menstruation and pregnancy.

Table 14–6. IRON DISTRIBUTION IN HEALTHY YOUNG ADULTS (mg)

	Men	Women
Total	3450	2450
Functional		
Hemoglobin	2100	1750
Myoglobin	300	250
Enzymes	50	50
Storage		
Ferritin, hemosiderin	1000	400

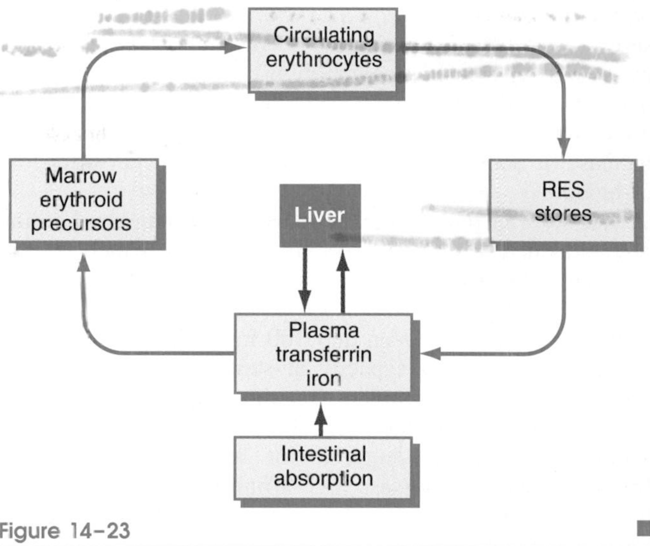

Figure 14–23

The internal iron cycle. In the plasma, iron bound to transferrin is transported to the marrow, where it is transferred to developing red blood cells and incorporated into hemoglobin. The mature red blood cells are released into the circulation and, after 120 days, are ingested by macrophages in the reticuloendothelial system (RES). Here the iron is extracted from hemoglobin and returned to the plasma, completing the cycle. (From Wyngaarden JB, et al [eds]: Cecil Textbook of Medicine 19th ed. Philadelphia, WB Saunders, 1992, p 841.)

All storage of iron is in the form of either ferritin or hemosiderin.[30] *Ferritin is essentially a protein-iron complex* that can be found in all tissues but particularly in liver, spleen, bone marrow, and skeletal muscles. In the liver, most of the ferritin is stored within the parenchymal cells; in other tissues, such as spleen and bone marrow, it is mainly in the mononuclear phagocytic cells. The iron within the hepatocytes is derived from plasma transferrin, whereas the storage iron in the mononuclear phagocytic cells, including that in Kupffer cells, is obtained largely from the breakdown of red blood cells (Fig. 14–23). Within cells, ferritin is located both in the cell sap and in lysosomes, in which the protein shells of the ferritin are degraded and iron is aggregated into *hemosiderin* granules. With the usual cellular stains, hemosiderin appears in cells as golden yellow granules. The iron is chemically reactive, and when hemosiderin is exposed to potassium ferrocyanide (Prussian blue reaction) in tissue sections, the granules turn blue-black. With normal iron stores, only trace amounts of hemosiderin are found in the body, principally in reticuloendothelial cells in the bone marrow, spleen, and liver. In iron-overloaded cells, most of the iron is stored in the form of hemosiderin.

Very small amounts of ferritin normally circulate in the plasma. *Since the plasma ferritin is derived largely from the storage pool of body iron, its level is a good indicator of the adequacy of body iron stores.* In iron deficiency, serum ferritin is always below 12 μg/liter, whereas in iron overload, high values approaching 5000 μg/liter may be obtained. The physiologic importance of the storage iron pool is that it is readily mobilizable in the event of an increase in body iron requirements, as may occur after loss of blood.

Iron is transported in the plasma by an iron-binding glycoprotein called transferrin (Fig. 14–23), which is synthesized in the liver. In the normal individual, transferrin is about 33% saturated with iron, yielding serum levels that average 120 μg/dl in men and 100 mg/dl in women. Thus, the total iron-binding capacity of serum is in the range of 300 to 350 μg/dl. The major function of plasma transferrin is to deliver iron to the cells, including erythroid precursors, where iron is required for hemoglobin synthesis. Immature red cells possess high-affinity receptors for transferrin, and iron is transported into erythroblasts by receptor-mediated endocytosis.

The absorption of iron and its regulation are complex and poorly understood. The most active site of iron absorption is the duodenum, but the stomach, ileum, and colon may also participate to a small degree.

Mucosal uptake of iron occurs by two distinct pathways (Fig. 14–24). Approximately 25% of the heme iron derived from hemoglobin, myoglobin, and other animal proteins is absorbed. Released from its apoproteins by gastric acids, heme is taken up directly by the mucosal cells. Once inside the cells, heme is enzymatically degraded to release iron. In contrast, only 1% to 2% of nonheme iron is absorbed, by mechanisms that are complex and poorly understood. According to some investigators, three proteins are involved in the transfer of inorganic (nonheme) iron from the lumen of the gut to cytosol. At first, *luminal mucins* bind iron at the acid pH of the stomach. This complex keeps iron soluble and available for absorption in the more alkaline pH of the duodenum. At the surface of the duodenal mucosal cell, iron binds to an *integrin-like* molecule that somehow facilitates its passage across the cell membrane, possibly by an iron transporter. A cytosolic protein called *mobilferrin* accepts iron within the cell and delivers it to ferritin or transferrin[31] (Fig. 14–24). Recent studies have led to the identification of a candidate iron transporter protein that is required for the passage of iron across the enterocyte membrane. In mice, a mutation affecting this transport protein (called Nramp2) results in a hypochromic microcytic anemia that is similar to the anemia of iron deficiency in humans. In these mutant mice, iron cannot be transported into erythroid precursors as well, suggesting that Nramp2 protein is also needed for the delivery of transferrin-bound iron to the erythroblasts.[32, 33]

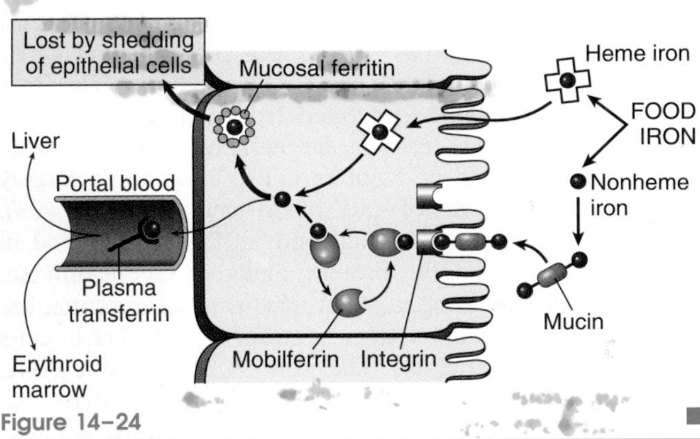

Figure 14–24

Diagrammatic representation of iron absorption. Mucosal uptake of heme and nonheme iron is depicted. Not illustrated is the iron transporter protein Nramp2 that is involved in the passage of iron across the mucosal cell membrane. When the storage sites of the body are replete with iron and erythropoietic activity is normal, most of the absorbed iron is lost into the gut by shedding of the epithelial cells. Conversely, when body iron needs to be increased or when erythropoiesis is stimulated, a greater fraction of the absorbed iron is transferred into plasma transferrin, with a concomitant decrease in iron loss through mucosal ferritin.

After absorption, both heme and nonheme iron appear to enter a common pool in the mucosal cell. Normally, a fraction of the iron that enters the cell is rapidly delivered to plasma transferrin. Most, however, is deposited as ferritin, some to be transferred more slowly to plasma transferrin, and some to be lost with exfoliation of mucosal cells. The extent to which the mucosal iron is distributed along these various pathways depends largely on the body's iron requirements. When the body is replete with iron, formation of ferritin within the mucosal cells is maximal, whereas transport into plasma is enhanced in iron deficiency.

Since body losses of iron are limited, iron balance is maintained largely by regulating the absorptive intake (mucosal block). The factors that regulate the absorption of available iron into the mucosal cell are largely unknown. It is known, however, that the rate and level of absorption are dependent on total body iron content as well as on erythropoietic activity, more specifically the iron needs of the erythroid precursors. As body stores rise, the percentage of iron absorbed falls, and vice versa. With ineffective erythropoiesis, as may occur in thalassemias, iron absorption is increased despite an excess of stored body iron. Some signal must be delivered to the mucosal cell, modifying its uptake and transfer of iron. The recently discovered *HFe* gene (also called *HLA-H)* is an attractive candidate for a regulator of iron absorption.[34] As discussed in Chapter 19, mutation in this gene leads to unregulated and excessive absorption of dietary iron, giving rise to hemochromatosis, a disease characterized by systemic iron overload.

Etiology. With this background of normal iron metabolism, we can discuss the causes and effects of iron deficiency.[35]

Iron requirements are best understood in the context of the fixed daily losses of iron, ranging between 1 and 1.5 mg. Thus, to maintain a normal iron balance, approximately 1 mg of iron must be absorbed from the diet every day. Because only 10% to 15% of the ingested iron is absorbed, the daily iron requirement is 5 to 10 mg for adult men and 7 to 20 mg for adult women. Since the average daily dietary intake of iron in the Western world is about 15 to 20 mg, most men ingest more than adequate iron, whereas many women consume just enough or marginally adequate amounts of iron.

The bioavailability of dietary iron is as important as the overall content. Heme iron is much more absorbable than inorganic iron. The absorption of the latter is influenced by other dietary contents. Ascorbic acid, citric acid, amino acids, and sugars in the diet enhance absorption of inorganic iron, but tannates (as in tea), carbonates, oxalates, and phosphates inhibit its absorption.

An iron deficiency may result from (1) dietary lack, (2) impaired absorption, (3) increased requirement, or (4) chronic blood loss.

Dietary lack is a rare cause of iron deficiency in industrialized countries having abundant food supplies (including meat) and where about two thirds of the dietary iron is in the readily assimilable heme form. The situation is different in developing countries, where food is less abundant and diets are predominantly vegetarian, containing poorly absorbable inorganic iron. Despite the availability of iron, dietary inadequacy is still encountered in privileged societies under the following circumstances:

- *The elderly* often have restricted diets with little meat for economic reasons or because of poor dentition.
- *The very poor,* often minority group individuals, are at risk for obvious reasons.
- *Infants* are also at high risk because the diet, predominantly milk, contains very small amounts of iron. Human breast milk, for example, provides only about 0.3 mg/liter of iron, which, however, has better bioavailability than cow's milk, which contains about twice as much iron but has poor bioavailability.
- *Children,* especially during the early years of life, have a critical need for dietary iron to accommodate growth and expansion of the blood volume.

Impaired absorption is encountered in sprue, other causes of intestinal steatorrhea, and chronic diarrhea. Gastrectomy impairs iron absorption by decreasing hydrochloric acid and transit time through the duodenum. Specific items in the diet, as is evident from the preceding discussion, may also affect absorption.

Increased requirement is an important potential cause of iron deficiency. Growing infants and children, adolescents, and premenopausal (particularly pregnant) women have a much greater requirement for iron than do nonmenstruating adults. Particularly at risk are economically deprived women having multiple, frequent pregnancies.

Chronic blood loss is the most important cause of iron deficiency in the Western world. Bleeding within the tissues or cavities of the body may be followed by total recovery and recycling of the iron. However, external hemorrhage depletes the reserves of iron. Such depletion may occur from the gastrointestinal tract (e.g., peptic ulcers, hemorrhagic gastritis, gastric carcinoma, colonic carcinoma, hemorrhoids, or hookworm or pinworm disease), from the urinary tract (e.g., renal, pelvic, or bladder tumors), or from the genital tract (e.g., menorrhagia, uterine cancer).

When all the potential causes of an iron deficiency are taken into consideration, *deficiency in adult men and postmenopausal women in the Western world should be considered to be caused by gastrointestinal blood loss until proven otherwise. To prematurely ascribe an iron lack in such individuals to any of the other possible origins is to run the risk of missing an occult gastrointestinal cancer or other bleeding lesion.*

Whatever the basis, iron deficiency induces a hypochromic microcytic anemia. Simultaneously, depletion of essential iron-containing enzymes in cells throughout the body may cause other changes, including koilonychia, alopecia, atrophic changes in the tongue and gastric mucosa, and intestinal malabsorption. These changes are seen in patients with severe and long-standing iron deficiency. Uncommonly, esophageal webs may appear, to complete the triad of major findings in the *Plummer-Vinson syndrome:* (1) microcytic hypochromic anemia, (2) atrophic glossitis, and (3) esophageal webs (Chapter 18).

At the outset of chronic blood loss or other states of negative iron balance, the reserves in the form of ferritin and hemosiderin may be adequate to maintain normal hemoglobin and hematocrit levels as well as normal serum iron and transferrin saturation. Progressive depletion of these reserves will eventually lower the serum iron and transferrin saturation levels but still may not give rise to anemia. Up to this stage of blood loss, there is increased erythroid activity in the bone marrow. Thereafter, anemia will appear when all iron stores are depleted, now accompanied by low levels of serum iron and transferrin saturation as well as low serum ferritin.

MORPHOLOGY. The bone marrow reveals a mild to moderate increase in erythropoietic activity, manifested by increased numbers of normoblasts. Specificity is lent to these changes by the disappearance of stainable iron from the mononuclear phagocytic cells in the bone marrow. In the peripheral blood smear, red cells appear smaller (microcytic) and much paler (hypochromic) than normal. In many cells, hemoglobin is seen only in the form of a narrow peripheral rim (Fig. 14–25).

The clinical manifestations related to the anemia are nonspecific and were detailed earlier. The dominating signs and symptoms frequently relate to the underlying cause of the anemia, for example, gastrointestinal or gynecologic disease, malnutrition, pregnancy, and malabsorption. Gastrointestinal disturbances may be present, associated with the disorder that led to the chronic blood loss (e.g., bleeding peptic ulcer or gastric carcinoma, diverticulitis, colonic cancer).

The diagnosis of iron deficiency anemia ultimately rests on laboratory studies. Both hemoglobin and hematocrit are depressed, usually to moderate levels, and are associated with hypochromia, microcytosis, and some poikilocytosis. *The serum iron and serum ferritin are low, and the total plasma iron-binding capacity (reflecting transferrin concentration) is high. Low serum iron with increased iron-binding capacity results in a reduction of transferrin saturation levels to below 15%.* As mentioned earlier, transferrin receptor, expressed on the surface of many cells, is required for the transport of iron into cells. The level of transferrin receptors is inversely related to available serum iron. With iron deficiency, the level of cell-bound transferrin receptors and their soluble forms that circulate in the blood is ele-

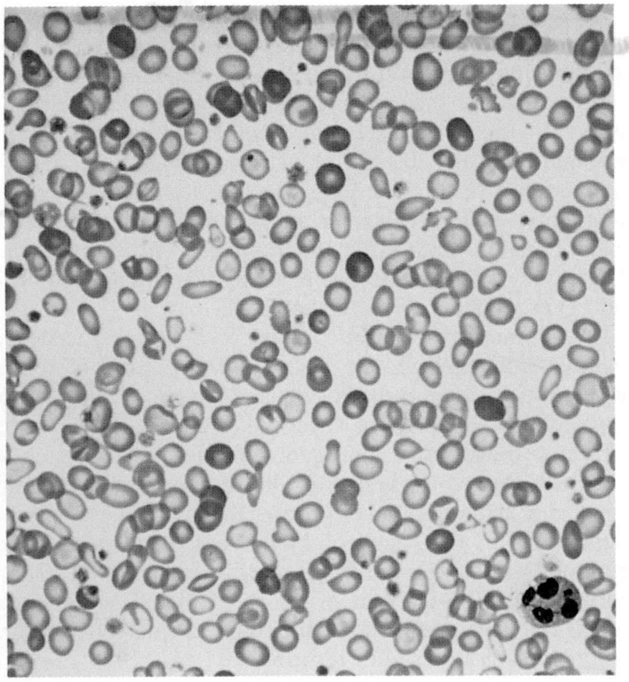

Figure 14–25

Hypochromic microcytic anemia of iron deficiency. Note the small red cells containing a narrow rim of hemoglobin at the periphery. Contrast with the scattered fully hemoglobinized cells derived from a recent blood transfusion given to the patient. (Courtesy of Dr. Robert W. McKenna, Department of Pathology, University of Texas Southwestern Medical School, Dallas, TX.)

vated. The level of transferrin receptors in the serum has been found to be an excellent test for the diagnosis of iron deficiency.[36] However, this test is not widely used. Reduced heme synthesis leads to elevation of free erythrocyte protoporphyrin. The alert clinician who investigates an unexplained iron deficiency anemia occasionally discovers an occult lesion or cancer and thereby saves a life.

ANEMIA OF CHRONIC DISEASE

Impaired red cell production associated with chronic diseases is perhaps the most common cause of anemia among hospitalized patients in the United States.[37] It is associated with reduced erythroid proliferation and impaired iron utilization and may therefore mimic iron deficiency. The chronic illnesses associated with this form of anemia can be grouped into three categories:

- Chronic microbial infections, such as osteomyelitis, bacterial endocarditis, and lung abscess
- Chronic immune disorders, such as rheumatoid arthritis and regional enteritis
- Neoplasms, such as Hodgkin disease and carcinomas of the lung and breast

The common features that characterize anemia in these diverse clinical settings are *low serum iron and reduced total iron-binding capacity in association with abundant stored iron in the mononuclear phagocytic cells.* This combination suggests a defect in the reuse of iron due to some block in the transfer of iron from the storage pool to the erythroid precursors. Although there is some impediment of iron reutilization, this form of anemia is caused largely by marrow hypoproliferation that results from an inappropriately low erythropoietin response for the degree of anemia. The reduction in renal erythropoietin generation is caused by the action of interleukin-1, tumor necrosis factor α (TNF-α), and interferon-γ. Secretion of these cytokines is triggered by the underlying chronic inflammatory or neoplastic disease. The anemia is usually mild, and the dominant symptoms are those of the underlying disease. The red blood cells may be normocytic and normochromic or may be hypochromic and microcytic as in anemia of iron deficiency. *The presence of increased storage iron in the marrow macrophages, a high serum ferritin level, and reduced total iron-binding capacity readily rule out iron deficiency as the cause of anemia.* In addition, the serum transferrin receptor level is within normal range. Treatment of the underlying condition corrects the anemia as does administration of recombinant erythropoietin.

APLASTIC ANEMIA

This somewhat misleading term is applied to pancytopenia characterized by (1) anemia, (2) neutropenia, and (3) thrombocytopenia. The basis for these changes is a failure or suppression of multipotent myeloid stem cells, with inadequate production or release of the differentiated cell lines.

Table 14–7. MAJOR CAUSES OF APLASTIC ANEMIA

Acquired
Idiopathic
  Primary stem cell defect
  Immune mediated
Chemical agents
  Dose related
    Alkylating agents
    Antimetabolites
    Benzene
    Chloramphenicol
    Inorganic arsenicals
  Idiosyncratic
    Chloramphenicol
    Phenylbutazone
    Organic arsenicals
    Methylphenylethylhydantoin
    Streptomycin
    Chlorpromazine
    Insecticides (e.g., DDT, parathion)
Physical agents (e.g., whole-body irradiation)
Viral infections
  Non-A, non-B hepatitis
  Cytomegalovirus infections
  Epstein-Barr virus infections
  Herpes varicella-zoster
Miscellaneous
  Infrequently, many other drugs and chemicals
Inherited
Fanconi anemia

Etiology. The major circumstances under which aplastic anemia may appear are listed in Table 14–7.

Most cases of aplastic anemia of so-called known etiology follow exposure to chemicals and drugs. With some agents, the marrow damage is predictable, dose related, and, in most instances, reversible when the use of the offending agent is stopped. Best documented as known myelotoxins are benzene, chloramphenicol, alkylating agents, and antimetabolites (e.g., 6-mercaptopurine, vincristine, and busulfan). In most cases, the pancytopenia appears as an apparent idiosyncratic reaction to very small doses of known myelotoxins (e.g., chloramphenicol) or after the use of such drugs as phenylbutazone, methylphenylethylhydantoin, streptomycin, and chlorpromazine, which are generally without effect in other individuals. In such idiosyncratic reactions, the aplasia may be severe and sometimes irreversible and fatal.

Whole-body *irradiation* is an obvious mechanism for destruction of hematopoietic stem cells. The effects of radiation are dose related. Persons at risk are those who receive therapeutic irradiation and individuals exposed to nuclear explosions or nuclear plant accidents.

Although aplastic anemia may appear after a variety of *infections* (including human immunodeficiency virus [HIV] infection), it most commonly follows viral hepatitis of the non-A, non-B, non-C, and non-G type.[38] Why certain individuals develop this hematologic complication in the course of their infection is not understood, but it is not related to the severity of infection.

Fanconi anemia is a rare autosomal recessive disorder characterized by defects in DNA repair (Chapter 8). In these patients, the marrow hypofunction becomes evident early in life and is accompanied by multiple congenital anomalies, such as hypoplasia of the kidney and spleen and hypoplastic anomalies of bone, particularly involving the thumbs or radii.

Despite all these possible causal influences, no provocative factor can be identified in fully 65% of the cases, and hence they are lumped into the *idiopathic* category.

Pathogenesis. The pathogenesis of aplastic anemia is not fully understood. Indeed, it is unlikely that a single mechanism underlies all cases of marrow aplasia. Two major mechanisms have been invoked: an immunologically mediated suppression and an intrinsic abnormality of stem cells. Each is considered next (Fig. 14–26).

Recent studies suggest that in a large proportion of cases, perhaps in as many as 70%, marrow failure results from inhibition of stem cell proliferation and differentiation by activated T cells.[39] It is postulated that at first the stem cells are antigenically altered by exposure to drugs, infectious agents, or other unidentified environmental insults. This then evokes a T cell–mediated immune response during which cytokines such as interferon-γ and TNF-α are produced by activated T cells. These cytokines are known to be potent inhibitors of stem cell function. This scenario is supported by the observation that immunosuppressive therapy with antithymocyte globulin combined with drugs such as cyclosporine has a salutary effect in 60% to 70% of patients.

The notion that aplastic anemia results from a fundamental stem cell abnormality is supported by studies that indicate that in many cases of aplastic anemia, cells in the peripheral blood are clonal descendants of a single stem cell.[40] Some forms of marrow insult presumably cause genetic damage that results in the generation of stem cells with poor proliferative and differentiative capacity. If one such altered stem cell dominates, the resultant picture is that of aplastic anemia. The occasional transformation of aplastic anemia into acute leukemia lends further credence to this hypothesis. These two mechanisms are not mutually exclusive. The genetically altered stem cells not only may have poor proliferative capacity but also may be antigenically altered, thus inducing a secondary T cell–mediated suppression.[41]

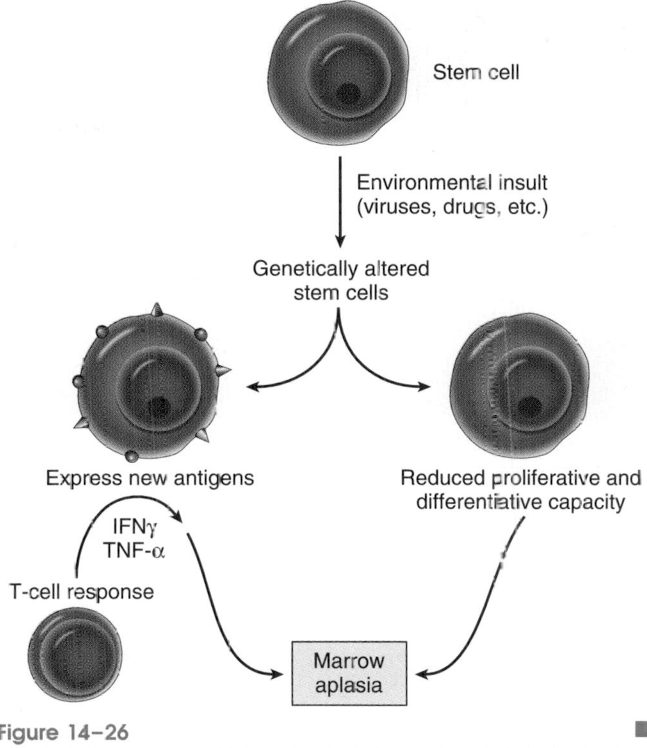

Figure 14–26

Pathophysiology of aplastic anemia. Insults to stem cells may produce progeny with new antigens and evoke an autoimmune reaction, or the altered stem cells may give rise to a clonal population with reduced proliferative capacity. Either pathway could lead to marrow aplasia.

MORPHOLOGY. The bone marrow is markedly hypocellular and is composed largely of empty marrow spaces populated by fat cells, fibrous stroma, and scattered or clustered foci of lymphocytes and plasma cells. Often, little material is aspirated ("dry tap"). Hence, compared with a smear, the marrow aplasia is better appreciated in a bone marrow biopsy (Fig. 14–27). A number of additional morphologic changes may accompany marrow failure. They are related to bacterial infections or hemorrhagic diatheses secondary to the granulocytopenia or thrombocytopenic, respectively. The toxic drug or agent may injure not

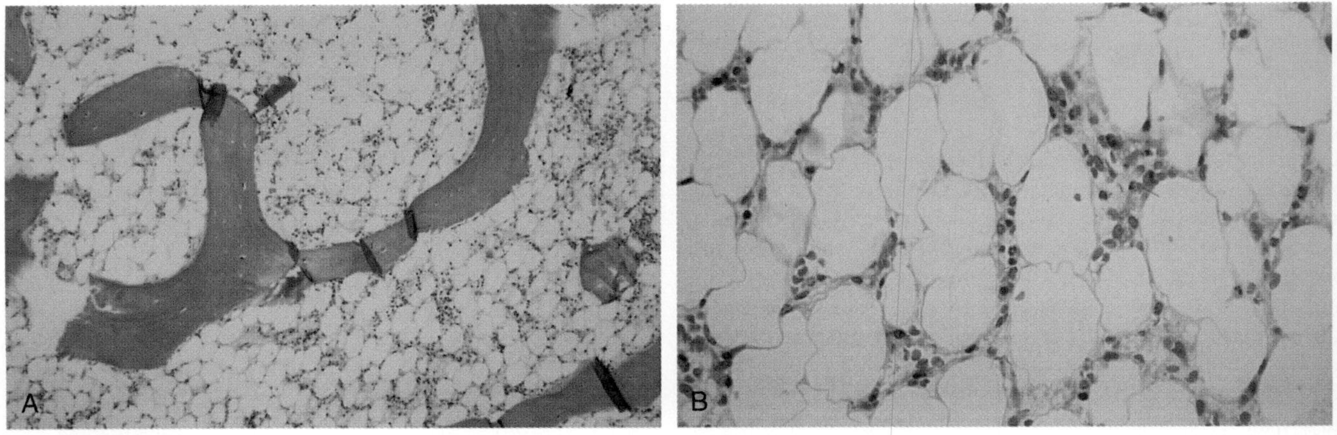

Figure 14–27

Aplastic anemia (bone marrow). The marrow is markedly hypocellular, composed largely of fat cells. *A*, Low power. *B*, High power. (Courtesy of Dr. Steven Kroft, Department of Pathology, University of Texas Southwestern Medical School, Dallas, TX.)

only the bone marrow but also the liver, the kidneys, and other structures. Benzene, for example, may cause fatty changes in the liver and kidneys. In some patients, especially those with multiple transfusions, systemic hemosiderosis is present.

Clinical Course. Aplastic anemia may occur at any age and in either sex. The onset is usually gradual, but in some cases the disorder strikes with suddenness and great severity. The initial manifestations vary somewhat, depending on the cell line predominantly affected. Anemia may cause the progressive onset of weakness, pallor, and dyspnea. Petechiae and ecchymoses may herald thrombocytopenia. Granulocytopenia may manifest itself only by frequent and persistent minor infections or by the sudden onset of chills, fever, and prostration. *Splenomegaly is characteristically absent, and if it is present, the diagnosis of aplastic anemia should be seriously questioned.* The red cells are typically normocytic and normochromic, although slight macrocytosis is occasionally present; *reticulocytosis is absent.*

The diagnosis rests on examination of bone marrow biopsy and peripheral blood. It is important to distinguish aplastic anemia from other causes of pancytopenia, such as "aleukemic" leukemia and myelodysplastic syndromes (Chapter 15). Since pancytopenia is common to all these conditions, their clinical manifestations are often indistinguishable. However, with aplastic anemia, the marrow is hypocellular owing to stem cell failure, whereas in leukemia and myelodysplasia, the marrow is populated by abnormal and immature myeloid cells. The prognosis of marrow aplasia is unpredictable. As mentioned earlier, withdrawal of toxic drugs may lead to recovery in some cases. The idiopathic form has a poor prognosis. Therapy consists of antithymocyte globulin along with cyclosporine to overcome the marrow suppressive effects of T cells. Alternatively, in selected patients, allogeneic bone marrow transplantation may be beneficial because it provides a new source of stem cells.[42]

PURE RED CELL APLASIA

Pure red cell aplasia is a rare form of marrow failure resulting from a specific aplasia of erythroid elements while granulopoiesis and thrombopoiesis remain normal.[43] Pure red cell aplasia may be primary, without any associated disease, or secondary to some neoplasm, particularly a thymic tumor (thymoma) and in some cases a leukemia of large granular lymphocytes (Chapter 15). The association with thymoma raises the question of some thymus-related immunologic mechanism, and indeed, in about half the patients, resection of the thymic tumor is followed by hematologic improvement. In all likelihood, the primary form is also related to autoimmunity against erythroid precursors, and immunosuppressive therapy may be beneficial in such patients. Plasmapheresis has also been used with success in refractory cases.

OTHER FORMS OF MARROW FAILURE

Space-occupying lesions that destroy significant amounts of bone marrow or perhaps disturb the marrow architecture depress its productive capacity. This form of marrow failure is referred to as *myelophthisic anemia.* As would be anticipated, all the formed elements of blood are concomitantly affected. However, characteristically immature forms of the red and white cells appear in the peripheral blood (leukoerythroblastosis). The infiltrative diseases of the marrow presumably destroy the normal marrow microenvironment, causing reactive fibrosis and thus allowing an inappropriate release of erythroid and myeloid precursors into the peripheral blood. The most common cause of myelophthisic anemia is metastatic cancer, arising most often from a primary lesion in the breast, lung, prostate, thyroid, or adrenals. Multiple myeloma, leukemia, osteosclerosis, and lymphomas are less commonly implicated. Myelophthisic anemia has also been observed with myelofibrosis, a diffuse fibrosis of the marrow. Such cases are variants of the myeloproliferative syndrome (Chapter 15).

Diffuse liver disease, whether it is toxic, infectious, or a form of cirrhosis, is for obscure reasons often associated with an anemia attributed to bone marrow failure. Other contributing factors include folate deficiency and iron deficiency due to gastrointestinal blood loss (varices, hemorrhoids). In most of these instances, there is a pure erythropoietic depression and the red cells are normocytic, but if folate deficiency is significant, they are macrocytic. Depression of the white cell count and platelets has been described but is infrequent.

Chronic renal failure, whatever its cause, is almost invariably associated with anemia that tends to be roughly proportional to the severity of the uremia. The basis of the anemia is multifactorial. There is evidence of an extracorpuscular defect inducing chronic hemolysis. Some patients have an iron deficiency secondary to the bleeding tendency often encountered in uremia. Concomitantly, there is reduced red cell production, related to advanced destruction of the kidneys, with inadequate formation of erythropoietin. This appears to be the dominant cause of anemia. Not surprisingly, therefore, administration of recombinant erythropoietin results in significant improvement of anemia in patients with renal failure.[44]

POLYCYTHEMIA

Polycythemia, or *erythrocytosis,* as it is sometimes referred to, denotes an increased concentration of red cells, usually with a corresponding increase in hemoglobin level. Such an increase may be *relative,* when there is hemoconcentration due to decreased plasma volume, or *absolute,* when there is an increase in total red cell mass. *Relative polycythemia* results from any cause of dehydration, such as deprivation of water, prolonged vomiting, diarrhea, or excessive use of diuretics. It is also associated with an obscure condition of unknown etiology called stress polycythemia, or Gaisböck syndrome. The affected individuals are usually hypertensive and obese and in a state of anxiety ("stress"). *Absolute polycythemia* is said to be *primary* when the increase in red cell mass results from an intrinsic abnormality of the myeloid stem cells and *secondary* when the red cell progenitors are normal but proliferate in response to increased levels of erythropoietin. Primary polycythemia (polycythemia vera) is one of several expressions of clonal, neoplastic proliferation of myeloid stem cells and is therefore best considered with other myeloproliferative disorders (Chapter 15). Another much less common form of "primary" polycythemia results from mutations in the erythropoietin receptor that cause the erythroid precursors to become exquisitely sensitive to erythropoietin. These individuals have congenital polycythemia. One such individual won an Olympic gold medal in cross-country skiing, having benefited from this natural form of blood doping! Secondary polycythemias may be caused by an increase in erythropoietin secretion that is physiologically appropriate or by an inappropriate (pathologic) secretion of erythropoietin (Table 14–8).

Table 14–8 PATHOPHYSIOLOGIC CLASSIFICATION OF POLYCYTHEMIA

Relative	Reduced plasma volume (hemoconcentration)
Absolute	
Primary	Abnormal proliferation of myeloid stem cells, normal or low erythropoietin levels (polycythemia vera)
Secondary	Increased erythropoietin levels
	Appropriate: lung disease, high-altitude living, cyanotic heart disease
	Inappropriate: erythropoietin-secreting tumors (e.g., renal cell carcinoma, hepatocellular carcinoma, cerebellar hemangioblastoma)

BLEEDING DISORDERS: HEMORRHAGIC DIATHESES

Excessive bleeding may result from (1) increased fragility of vessels, (2) platelet deficiency or dysfunction, (3) derangements in the coagulation mechanism, and (4) combinations of these.

Before these forms of bleeding disorders are discussed, it would be profitable to review normal hemostasis and the common laboratory tests used in the evaluation of a bleeding diathesis. It should be recalled from the discussion in Chapter 5 that the normal hemostatic response involves the blood vessel wall, the platelets, and the clotting cascade. The various tests used in the initial evaluation of patients with bleeding disorders are as follows:

- *Bleeding time.* This represents the time taken for a standardized skin puncture to stop bleeding. Measured in minutes, this procedure provides an in vivo assessment of platelet response to limited vascular injury. The reference range depends on the actual method employed and varies from 2 to 9 minutes. It is abnormal when there is a defect in platelet numbers or function.
- *Platelet counts.* These are obtained on anticoagulated blood by using an electronic particle counter. The reference range is 150 to 450 × $10^3/mm^3$. Counts outside this range must be confirmed by a visual inspection of a peripheral blood smear.
- *Prothrombin time (PT).* Measured in seconds, this procedure tests the adequacy of the extrinsic and common coagulation pathways. It represents the time needed for plasma to clot in the presence of an exogenously added source of tissue thromboplastin (e.g., brain extract) and Ca^{++} ions. A prolonged PT may result from a deficiency of factor V, factor VII, factor X, prothrombin, or fibrinogen.
- *Partial thromboplastin time (PTT).* This test is designed to assess the integrity of the intrinsic and common clotting pathways. In this test, the time (in seconds) needed for the plasma to clot in the presence of kaolin, cephalin, and calcium is measured. Kaolin serves to activate the contact-dependent factor XII, and cephalin substitutes for platelet phospholipids. Prolongation of PTT may be due to a deficiency of factor V, VIII, IX, X, XI, or XII or of prothrombin or fibrinogen.

In addition to these, more specialized tests include measurement of the levels of specific clotting factors, fibrinogen, and fibrin split products; determination of the presence of circulating anticoagulants; and platelet function tests. With this overview, we can turn to the various categories of bleeding disorders.

Bleeding Disorders Caused by Vessel Wall Abnormalities

Disorders within this category, sometimes called nonthrombocytopenic purpuras, are relatively common but do not usually cause serious bleeding problems. Most often, they induce small hemorrhages (petechiae and purpura) in the skin or mucous membranes, particularly the gingivae. On occasion, however, more significant hemorrhages may occur into joints, muscles, and subperiosteal locations or take the form of menorrhagia, nosebleeds, gastrointestinal bleeding, or hematuria. *The platelet count, bleeding time, and results of the tests of coagulation (PT, PTT) are usually normal.*

The varied clinical conditions in which hemorrhages can be related to abnormalities in the vessel wall include the following:

- Many *infections* induce petechial and purpuric hemorrhages, but especially implicated are meningococcemia, other forms of septicemia, infective endocarditis, and several of the rickettsioses. The involved mechanism is presumably microbiologic damage (vasculitis) to the microvasculature or disseminated intravascular coagulation (DIC).
- *Drug reactions* sometimes induce abnormal bleeding. In many instances, the vascular injury is mediated by the formation of drug-induced antibodies and the deposition of immune complexes in the vessel walls, with the production of a hypersensitivity (leukocytoclastic) vasculitis (Chapter 12).
- *Scurvy and the Ehlers-Danlos syndrome* represent examples of predisposition to hemorrhage related to impaired formation of the collagenous support of vessel walls. Essentially the same mechanism may be encountered in the very elderly, in whom atrophy of collagen is implicated. Similar is the predisposition to skin hemorrhages in *Cushing syndrome,* in which the protein-wasting effects of excessive corticosteroid production cause loss of perivascular supporting tissue.
- *Henoch-Schönlein purpura* is a systemic hypersensitivity disease of unknown cause characterized by a purpuric rash, colicky abdominal pain (presumably due to focal hemorrhages into the gastrointestinal tract), polyarthralgia, and acute glomerulonephritis (Chapter 21). All these changes are thought to result from the deposition of circulating immune complexes within vessels throughout the body and within the glomerular mesangial regions.
- *Hereditary hemorrhagic telangiectasia* is an autosomal dominant disorder characterized by dilated, tortuous blood vessels that have thin walls and hence bleed readily. Bleeding may occur anywhere in the body but is most common under the mucous membranes of the nose (epistaxis), tongue, mouth, and eyes.
- *Amyloid infiltration of blood vessels.* Systemic amyloidosis secondary to immunocyte dyscrasias may be associated with deposition of amyloid and consequent weakening of blood vessel wall. Patients may therefore present with mucocutaneous petechiae.

In most of these conditions, the hemorrhagic diathesis does not cause massive bleeding but more often calls attention to the underlying disorder.

Bleeding Related to Reduced Platelet Number: Thrombocytopenia

Reduction in platelet number constitutes an important cause of generalized bleeding. Platelet counts normally range between 150,000 and 300,000/mm^3, and a count below 100,000/mm^3 is generally considered to constitute thrombocytopenia. However, spontaneous bleeding does not become evident until the count falls below 20,000/mm^3. Platelet counts in the range of 20,000 to 50,000/mm^3 are associated with post-traumatic bleeding. Bleeding resulting from thrombocytopenia is associated with a prolonged bleeding time and normal PT and PTT.

The important role of platelets in hemostasis is discussed in Chapter 5. It hardly needs reiteration that they are vital to hemostasis in that they form temporary plugs and participate in the clotting reaction. Thus, thrombocytopenia is characterized principally by bleeding, most often from small vessels. The common sites of such hemorrhage are the skin and mucous membranes of the gastrointestinal and genitourinary tracts, where the bleeding is usually associated with the development of small petechiae. Intracranial bleeding is another danger in thrombocytopenic patients with markedly depressed platelet counts.

The many causes of thrombocytopenia can be classified into the four major categories cited in Table 14–9.

A few comments on each of these categories are offered before we turn to discussion of some common and clinically important causes of thrombocytopenia.

- *Decreased production of platelets.* This may accompany generalized diseases of bone marrow such as aplastic anemia and leukemias or result from diseases that affect the megakaryocytes somewhat selectively. In patients with vitamin B_{12} or folic acid deficiency, there is accelerated destruction of megakaryocytes within the bone marrow (ineffective megakaryopoiesis) because DNA synthesis is impaired.
- *Decreased platelet survival.* This is an important cause of thrombocytopenia and may be caused by immunologic or nonimmunologic mechanisms. In many cases, platelet destruction is caused by a circulating antiplatelet antibody or immune complexes. The antiplatelet antibodies may be directed against a self-antigen on the platelets (autoantibodies) or against platelet antigens that differ among different individuals (alloantibodies). The antigenic targets of both autoantibodies and alloantibodies are the platelet membrane glycoprotein complexes

Table 14–9. CAUSES OF THROMBOCYTOPENIA

Decreased Production of Platelets
Generalized diseases of bone marrow
Aplastic anemia: congenital and acquired (Table 14–7)
Marrow infiltration: leukemia, disseminated cancer
Selective impairment of platelet production
Drug-induced: alcohol, thiazides, cytotoxic drugs
Infections: measles, human immunodeficiency virus (HIV)
Ineffective megakaryopoiesis
Megaloblastic anemia
Paroxysmal nocturnal hemoglobinuria

Decreased Platelet Survival
Immunologic destruction
Autoimmune: idiopathic thrombocytopenic purpura, systemic lupus erythematosus
Isoimmune: post-transfusion and neonatal
Drug-associated: quinidine, heparin, sulfa compounds
Infections: infectious mononucleosis, HIV infection, cytomegalovirus
Nonimmunologic destruction
Disseminated intravascular coagulation
Thrombotic thrombocytopenic purpura
Giant hemangiomas
Microangiopathic hemolytic anemias

Sequestration
Hypersplenism

Dilutional

IIb-IIIa and Ib-IX. Autoimmune thrombocytopenias include idiopathic thrombocytopenic purpura (ITP), certain drug-induced thrombocytopenias, and HIV-associated thrombocytopenias. All of these are discussed later. Alloimmune thrombocytopenias arise when an individual is exposed to platelets of another person, as may occur after blood transfusion or during pregnancy. In the latter case, neonatal or even fetal thrombocytopenia occurs by a mechanism analogous to erythroblastosis fetalis.[45]

Nonimmunologic destruction of platelets may be caused by *mechanical injury*, in a manner analogous to red cell destruction in microangiopathic hemolytic anemia. The underlying conditions are also similar, including prosthetic heart valves and diffuse narrowing of the microvessels (e.g., malignant hypertension).

- *Sequestration.* Thrombocytopenia may appear unpredictably in any patient who has marked splenomegaly, or what has been referred to as *hypersplenism* (Chapter 15). The spleen normally sequesters 30% to 40% of the mass of circulating platelets; when enlarged, it sequesters as much as 90% of all platelets. Should the thrombocytopenia constitute an important part of the clinical problem, it can be cured by splenectomy.
- *Dilutional.* Massive *transfusions* may produce a dilutional thrombocytopenia. Blood stored for longer than 24 hours contains virtually no viable platelets; thus, plasma volume and red cell mass are reconstituted by transfusion, but the number of circulating platelets is relatively reduced.

IDIOPATHIC THROMBOCYTOPENIC PURPURA (ITP)

There are two clinical subtypes of ITP, acute and chronic; both are autoimmune disorders in which platelet destruction results from the formation of antiplatelet antibodies. We first discuss the more common chronic form of the disease; acute ITP, a self-limited disease of children, is discussed later.

Immunologically mediated destruction of platelets (immune thrombocytopenia) occurs in many different settings, including systemic lupus erythematosus, acquired immunodeficiency syndrome (AIDS), after viral infections, and as a complication of drug therapy. These *secondary forms of immune thrombocytopenia can sometimes mimic the idiopathic autoimmune variety*, and hence the diagnosis of this disorder should be made only after exclusion of other known causes of thrombocytopenia. Particularly important in this regard is systemic lupus erythematosus, a multisystem autoimmune disease (Chapter 7) that can present with thrombocytopenia.

Pathogenesis. It is well established that idiopathic autoimmune thrombocytopenia is caused by the formation of autoantibodies against platelet membrane glycoproteins, most often IIb-IIIa or Ib-IX.[46, 47] Antibodies reactive with these membrane glycoproteins can be demonstrated in the plasma as well as bound to the platelet surface (platelet-associated immunoglobulins) in approximately 80% of patients. In the overwhelming majority of cases, the antiplatelet antibodies are of the IgG class.

The mechanism of platelet destruction is similar to that seen in autoimmune hemolytic anemias. Opsonized platelets are rendered susceptible to phagocytosis by the cells of the mononuclear phagocyte system. About 75% to 80% of patients are remarkably improved after splenectomy, which suggests that the spleen is the major site of removal of sensitized platelets. Since it is also the major site of autoantibody synthesis, the beneficial effects of splenectomy may in part derive from removal of the source of autoantibodies. Although destruction of sensitized platelets is the major mechanism of thrombocytopenia, there is some evidence that megakaryocytes may be attacked as well, since some antiplatelet antibodies also react with megakaryocytes. In most cases, however, the megakaryocyte injury is not significant enough to deplete their numbers.

MORPHOLOGY. The principal morphologic lesions of thrombocytopenic purpura are found in the spleen and bone marrow. The secondary changes related to the bleeding diathesis may be found in any tissue or structure in the body.

The spleen is normal in size. On histologic examination, there is congestion of the sinusoids and hyperactivity and enlargement of the splenic follicles, manifested by the formation of prominent germinal centers. In many instances, megakaryocytes are found within the sinuses and sinusoidal walls. These splenic findings are not distinctive and cannot be considered pathognomonic of this disorder.

Bone marrow reveals an increased number of megakaryocytes. Some are apparently immature with large, nonlobulated, single nuclei. These findings are not characteristic of autoimmune thrombocytopenic purpura but merely represent accelerated thrombopoiesis. As such, they are seen in most forms of thrombocytopenia resulting from increased platelet destruction. The importance of the bone marrow examination is to rule out thrombocytopenias resulting from bone marrow failure. A decrease in the number of megakaryocytes virtually rules out the diagnosis of this condition.

The secondary changes relate to the hemorrhages that are dispersed throughout the body.

Clinical Features. Chronic ITP occurs most commonly in adult women younger than 40 years. The female to male ratio is 3:1. ITP is insidious in onset and is characterized by bleeding into the skin and mucosal surface. Cutaneous bleeding is seen in the form of *pinpoint hemorrhages* (petechiae), especially prominent in the dependent areas where the capillary pressure is higher. Petechial hemorrhages may become confluent and give rise to *ecchymoses*. Often there is a long history of easy bruising, nosebleeds, bleeding from the gums, and extensive hemorrhages into soft tissues from relatively minor trauma. Also, the disease may become manifest first by the appearance of melena, hematuria, or excessive menstrual flow. Subarachnoid hemorrhage and intracerebral hemorrhage are serious consequences of thrombocytopenic purpura but, fortunately, are rare in patients treated with steroids. Splenomegaly and lymphadenopathy are extremely uncommon in ITP, and their presence should lead one to consider other possible diagnoses.

The clinical signs and symptoms associated with ITP are not specific for this condition but rather are reflective of thrombocytopenia. Destruction of platelets as the cause of thrombocytopenia is supported by demonstration of low platelet counts with normal or increased megakaryocytes in the bone marrow. Accelerated thrombopoiesis also leads to the formation of abnormally large platelets (megathrombocytes), detected easily in a blood smear. The bleeding time is prolonged, but PT and PTT are normal. Tests for platelet autoantibodies are not widely available. *Therefore, a diagnosis of ITP should be made only after all the possible known causes for platelet deficiencies, such as those listed in Table 14–9, have been ruled out.*

Acute Idiopathic Thrombocytopenic Purpura

Although, like chronic ITP, this condition is caused by the formation of antiplatelet autoantibodies, its clinical features and course are distinct. Acute ITP is a disease of childhood occurring with equal frequency in both sexes. The onset of thrombocytopenia is usually abrupt, and in most cases it is preceded by a viral illness. The usual interval between the infection and onset of purpura is 2 weeks. Unlike the adult chronic form of ITP, the childhood disease is self-limited, and it usually resolves spontaneously within 6 months. Steroid therapy is indicated only if thrombocytopenia is severe. Approximately 20% of the children develop chronic ITP, defined by persistence of low platelet count beyond 6 months.

DRUG-INDUCED THROMBOCYTOPENIA

Like hemolytic anemia, thrombocytopenia may result from immunologically mediated destruction of platelets after drug ingestion. The drugs most commonly involved are quinine, quinidine, penicillins, thiazide diuretics, methyldopa, and heparin. Of particular importance is heparin-induced thrombocytopenia, because of the common use of this anticoagulant drug and because of the severity of the reaction.[48] Thrombocytopenia occurs in approximately 5% of patients receiving heparin.[46] Most patients develop the so-called type I thrombocytopenia that occurs rapidly after onset of therapy, is modest in severity, and is clinically insignificant. It results most likely from the platelet-aggregating effect of heparin.

Type II thrombocytopenia is more severe; it follows 5 to 14 days after commencement of therapy and is sometimes associated with life-threatening venous and arterial thrombosis. It is caused by an immune reaction directed against a complex of heparin and platelet factor 4. The antibodies, on the one hand, deplete platelets; on the other hand, they activate platelets, thus promoting thrombosis. Platelet activation, it seems, is caused by the cross-linking of Fc receptors on the platelet surface by IgG antibodies directed against the heparin–platelet factor 4 complex. Unless therapy is rapidly discontinued, patients with this complication may succumb to pulmonary thromboembolism.[49]

HIV-ASSOCIATED THROMBOCYTOPENIA

Thrombocytopenia is perhaps the most common hematologic manifestation of HIV infection. Both impaired platelet production and increased destruction are responsible. CD4, the receptor for HIV on T cells, has also been demonstrated on megakaryocytes, and it is believed that these cells can be infected by HIV. By destroying or otherwise impairing megakaryocyte function, HIV infection gives rise to reduced platelet generation. Antibodies directed against platelet membrane glycoprotein IIb-III complexes have also been detected in patients' sera. These autoantibodies cross-react with HIV-associated gp120, thus raising the possibility of molecular mimicry. Such cross-reactive antibodies are believed to opsonize platelets and favor their premature destruction in the spleen. Some studies have also implicated a nonspecific deposition of immune complexes on the platelet surface as being a factor in their removal by the mononuclear phagocyte system.

THROMBOTIC MICROANGIOPATHIES: THROMBOTIC THROMBOCYTOPENIC PURPURA (TTP) AND HEMOLYTIC-UREMIC SYNDROME (HUS)

The term "thrombotic microangiopathies" encompasses a spectrum of clinical syndromes that includes TTP and HUS. Traditionally, TTP has been characterized by its occurrence in adult women and the pentad of fever, thrombocytopenia, microangiopathic hemolytic anemia, transient neurologic deficits, and renal failure. HUS, like TTP, is also associated with microangiopathic hemolytic anemia and thrombocytopenia but is distinguished from it by the absence of neurologic symptoms, the dominance of acute renal failure, and onset in childhood. Recent studies have tended to blur these distinctions because many adult patients with TTP lack one or more of the five criteria and some patients with HUS have fever and neurologic dysfunction. Fundamental to both of these conditions is widespread formation of hyaline thrombi in the microcirculation, which are composed primarily of dense aggregates of platelets that are surrounded by fibrin. The development of myriad platelet aggregates induces *thrombocytopenia,* and the intravascular thrombi provide a rational explanation for *a microangiopathic form of hemolytic anemia* and widespread organ dysfunction. It is believed that the differences in the clinical manifestations of TTP and HUS are in all likelihood due to different distribution of microvascular lesions.[50]

Although these disorders may have diverse causes, endothelial injury and activation of intravascular thrombosis seem to be the initiating mechanisms (Chapter 21). Verotoxins produced by certain strains of *Escherichia coli* are the trigger for endothelial injury in HUS. Thus, HUS most commonly follows gastroenteritis caused by verotoxin-producing *E. coli* O157:H7. The affected children present with bloody diarrhea, and HUS makes its appearance a few days later. The inciting agent in TTP has not been identified, but prodromal symptoms resembling influenza are frequently reported, suggesting a viral illness. At one time these conditions were uniformly fatal, but with recent improvements in treatment, including plasma exchange, approximately 80% survival can be expected. Despite some similarities with disseminated intravascular coagulation (DIC), the two conditions are separate and distinct. Unlike in DIC, activation of the clotting system is not of primary importance, and hence results of laboratory tests of coagulation, such as PT and PTT, are usually normal.

Bleeding Disorders Related to Defective Platelet Functions

Qualitative defects of platelet function may be congenital or acquired. Several congenital disorders characterized by prolonged bleeding time and normal platelet count have been described. A brief discussion of these rare diseases is warranted by the fact that they provide excellent model systems for investigating the molecular mechanisms of platelet functions.[51]

Congenital disorders of platelet function may be classified into three groups on the basis of the predominant functional abnormality: (1) *defects of adhesion,* (2) *defects of aggregation,* and (3) *disorders of platelet secretion (release reaction).*

- Bleeding resulting from defective adhesion of platelets to the subendothelial collagen is best illustrated by the autosomal recessive *Bernard-Soulier syndrome.* In this disorder, there is an inherited deficiency of a platelet membrane glycoprotein complex (Ib-IX). This glycoprotein is a receptor for von Willebrand factor (vWF) and is essential for normal platelet adhesion to collagen (Chapter 5).
- Bleeding due to *defective platelet aggregation* is exemplified by *thrombasthenia,* which is also transmitted as an autosomal recessive trait. Thrombasthenic platelets fail to aggregate with adenosine diphosphate (ADP), collagen, epinephrine, or thrombin owing to a deficiency of glycoprotein IIb-IIIa, the fibrinogen receptor. In normal platelets, these glycoproteins favor aggregation by creating fibrinogen "bridges" between adjacent platelets (Chapter 5).
- *Disorders of platelet secretion* are characterized by normal initial aggregation with collagen or ADP, but the subsequent responses, such as secretion of prostaglandins and release of granule-bound ADP, are impaired. The underlying biochemical defects of the so-called *storage pool disease* are varied, complex, and beyond the scope of our discussion.

Among the *acquired defects* of platelet function, two are clinically significant.[52] The first is related to *ingestion of aspirin* and other nonsteroidal anti-inflammatory drugs, which may significantly prolong the bleeding time. Aspirin is a potent inhibitor of the enzyme cyclooxygenase and can suppress the synthesis of prostaglandins (Chapter 3), which are known to be involved in platelet aggregation and the subsequent platelet release reaction (Chapter 5). The antiplatelet effect of aspirin forms the basis of its use in the management of myocardial infarction (Chapter 13). *Uremia* (Chapter 21) is the other condition that exemplifies an acquired defect in platelet functions. Although the pathogenesis of bleeding in uremia is complex and poorly understood, several abnormalities of platelet function have been found.

Hemorrhagic Diatheses Related to Abnormalities in Clotting Factors

A deficiency of every one of the known clotting factors has been reported at one time or another as the cause of a bleeding disorder. The bleeding in these conditions differs somewhat from that encountered in platelet deficiencies. The apparent spontaneous appearance of petechiae or purpura is uncommon. More often, *the bleeding manifests as the development of large ecchymoses or hematomas after an injury, or as prolonged bleeding after a laceration or any form of surgical procedure.* Bleeding into the gastrointestinal and urinary tracts, and particularly into weight-bearing joints, is a common manifestation. Typical stories describe the patient who continues to ooze for days after a tooth extraction or who develops a hemarthrosis after a relatively trivial stress on a knee joint. History may well have been changed by the presence of a hereditary coagulation defect in the intermarried royal families of Great Britain and Europe. Clotting abnormalities may occur as acquired defects or, as mentioned, may be hereditary in origin.

Acquired disorders are usually characterized by multiple clotting abnormalities. Vitamin K deficiency (Chapter 10) results in depressed synthesis of factors II, VII, IX, and X and protein C. Since the liver makes virtually all the clotting factors, severe parenchymal liver disease may be associated with a hemorrhagic diathesis. Disseminated intravascular coagulation (DIC) produces a deficiency of multiple coagulation factors.

Hereditary deficiencies have been identified for each of the clotting factors. Deficiencies of factor VIII (hemophilia A) and of factor IX (Christmas disease, or hemophilia B) are transmitted as sex-linked recessive disorders. Most of the others follow autosomal patterns of transmission. *These hereditary disorders typically involve a single clotting factor.*

DEFICIENCIES OF FACTOR VIII–vWF COMPLEX

Hemophilia A and von Willebrand disease, two of the most common inherited disorders of bleeding, are caused by qualitative or quantitative defects involving the factor VIII–von Willebrand factor (vWF) complex. Before we can discuss these disorders, it is essential to review the structure and function of these proteins.[53, 54]

Plasma factor VIII–vWF is a complex made up of two separate proteins (factor VIII and vWF) *that can be distinguished by functional, biochemical, and immunologic criteria.* One component, which is required for the activation of factor X in the intrinsic coagulation pathway, is called *factor VIII procoagulant protein,* or *factor VIII* (Fig. 14–28; Chapter 5). Deficiency of factor VIII gives rise to hemophilia A. Through noncovalent bonds, factor VIII is linked to the much larger protein vWF that forms approximately 99% of the complex; vWF is not a discrete protein but exists in the form of a series of multimers that contain up to 100 subunits with molecular mass exceeding 20×10^6 daltons. vWF can also bind several other proteins that are involved in hemostasis, including collagen, heparin, and platelet membrane glycoproteins (Ib-IX and IIb-IIIa). Glycoprotein Ib-IX serves as the major receptor for vWF, and it is believed that it is through this receptor that vWF bridges collagen and platelets and also favors platelet aggregation (Fig. 14–28). Indeed, *the most important function of vWF in vivo is to facilitate the adhesion of platelets to subendothelial collagen.* vWF is crucial to the normal process of hemostasis (Chapter 5), and its absence in von Willebrand disease leads to a bleeding diathesis.

In addition to its function in platelet adhesion, vWF serves as a carrier for factor VIII and is important for its stability. The half-life of factor VIII in the circulation is 12 hours if vWF levels are normal but only 2.4 hours if it is deficient or abnormal (as in patients with von Willebrand disease).

vWF can be assayed by immunologic techniques or by the so-called *ristocetin aggregation test.* Ristocetin (once used as an antibiotic) binds to platelets in vitro and activates vWF receptors on their surface. This leads to platelet aggregation if vWF is available to "bridge" the platelets (Fig. 14–28). Thus, ristocetin-induced platelet aggregation can be used as a bioassay for vWF.

The two components of the factor VIII–vWF complex are coded by separate genes and are synthesized by different cells. vWF is produced by endothelial cells and megakaryocytes, and it can be demonstrated in platelet α-granules. *Endothelial cells are the major source of plasma vWF.* Factor VIII can be synthesized by several tissues, but in the absence of liver disease, hepatocytes are the major source of this protein. To summarize, *the two components of factor VIII–vWF complex, synthesized separately, come together and circulate in the plasma as a unit that serves to promote the clotting as well as the platelet–vessel wall interactions necessary to ensure hemostasis.* With this background, we can discuss the diseases resulting from deficiencies of factor VIII–vWF complex.

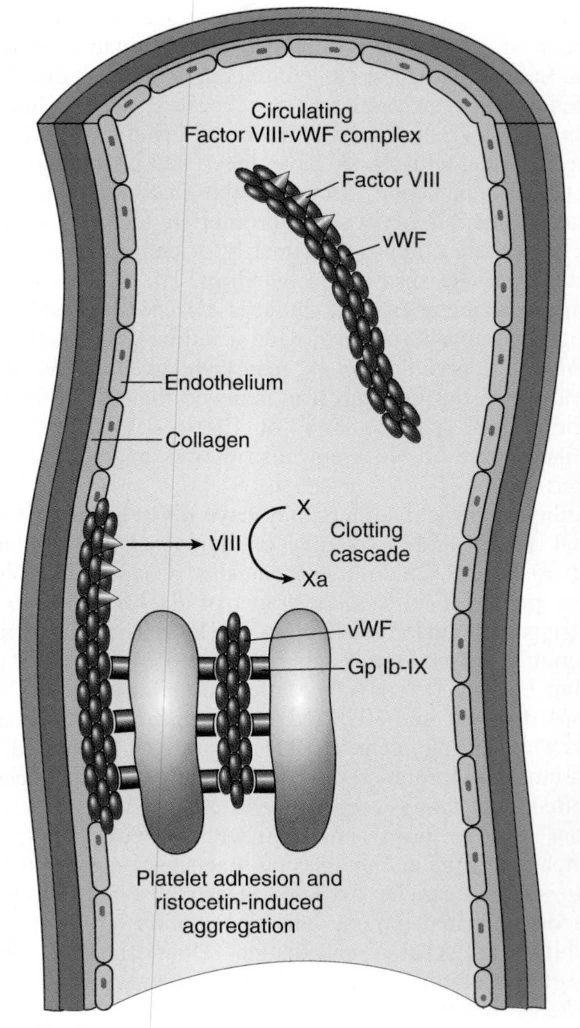

Figure 14–28

Structure and function of factor VIII–von Willebrand factor (vWF) complex. Factor VIII is synthesized by the liver and vWF in the endothelial cells. The two circulate as a complex in the circulation. Factor VIII takes part in the coagulation cascade by activating factor X. vWF causes adhesion of platelets to subendothelial collagen via the glycoprotein (Gp) Ib-IX platelet receptor. Ristocetin activates glycoprotein Ib-IX receptors in vitro and causes platelet aggregation if vWF is present.

VON WILLEBRAND DISEASE

With an estimated frequency of 1%, von Willebrand disease is believed to be one of the most common inherited disorders of bleeding in humans. According to some, it is even more common than hemophilia A. Clinically, it is characterized by spontaneous bleeding from mucous membranes, excessive bleeding from wounds, menorrhagia, and a prolonged bleeding time in the presence of a normal platelet count. In most cases, it is transmitted as an autosomal dominant disorder, but several rare autosomal recessive variants have been identified.[55]

More than 20 variants of von Willebrand disease have been described, and they can be grouped into two major categories:

- Type 1 and type 3 von Willebrand disease are associated with a *reduced quantity of circulating vWF*. Type 1, an autosomal dominant disorder, accounts for approximately 70% of all cases and is relatively mild. Reduced penetrance and variable expressivity characterize this type, and hence clinical manifestations are varied. Type 3 (an autosomal recessive disorder) is associated with extremely low levels of vWF, and the clinical manifestations are correspondingly severe. Fortunately, it is much less common than type 1. The molecular basis of reduced vWF levels in type 1 disease is virtually unknown; type 3 von Willebrand disease is associated with gene deletions and frameshift mutations.
- Type 2 von Willebrand disease is characterized by qualitative defects in vWF; there are several subtypes, of which type 2A is the most common. It is inherited as an autosomal dominant disorder. Because of missense mutations, the vWF that is formed is abnormal, and multimer assembly is defective. Large and intermediate multimers, representing the most active forms of vWF, are missing from plasma. Type 2 von Willebrand disease accounts for 25% of all cases and is associated with mild to moderate bleeding.

Patients with von Willebrand disease have *prolonged bleeding* time with *normal platelet count*. The plasma level of vWF, measured as the *ristocetin cofactor activity, is reduced.* Because vWF stabilizes factor VIII by binding to it, a deficiency of vWF gives rise to a secondary decrease in factor VIII levels. This may be reflected by a prolongation of PTT. *To summarize, patients with von Willebrand disease have a compound defect involving platelet function and the coagulation pathway.* However, except in the most severely affected patients, effects of factor VIII deficiency such as bleeding into the joints, which characterizes hemophilia, are uncommon.

HEMOPHILIA A (FACTOR VIII DEFICIENCY)

Hemophilia A is the most common *hereditary disease with serious bleeding.* It is caused by a reduction in the amount or activity of factor VIII. This protein serves as a cofactor for the activation of factor X in the coagulation cascade (Chapter 5). Hemophilia A is inherited as an X-linked recessive trait, and thus it occurs in males and in homozygous females. However, excessive bleeding has been described in heterozygous females, presumably caused by extremely "unfavorable lyonization" (inactivation of the normal X chromosome in most of the cells). Approximately 30% of the patients have no family history; their disease is presumably caused by new mutations.

Hemophilia A exhibits a wide range of clinical severity that correlates well with the level of factor VIII activity. Those with less than 1% of normal activity develop severe disease; levels between 2% and 5% of normal are associated with moderate disease; and patients with 6% to 50% of activity develop mild disease.[56] The variable degrees of deficiency in the level of factor VIII procoagulant are related to the type of mutation in the factor VIII gene.[57] As with β-thalassemias, several genetic lesions (deletions, nonsense mutations that create stop codons, splicing errors) have been documented. Most of the severely affected patients have an unusual mutation in which a large sequence of DNA becomes inverted, thus preventing any synthesis of factor VIII. In a minority of patients, the mutations do not affect the synthesis of factor VIII, but the functional domains are altered. In such cases, levels of factor VIII appear normal by immunoassay, but the protein is inactive.

In all symptomatic cases, there is a tendency toward easy bruising and massive hemorrhage after trauma or operative procedures. In addition, "spontaneous" hemorrhages are frequently encountered in regions of the body normally subject to trauma, particularly the joints, where they are known as hemarthroses. Recurrent bleeding into the joints leads to progressive deformities that may be crippling. *Petechiae are characteristically absent.*

Patients with hemophilia A typically have normal bleeding time and platelet counts, with prolonged PTT and normal PT. These tests point to an abnormality of the intrinsic coagulation pathway. Factor VIII assays are required for diagnosis.

Treatment of hemophilia A involves infusion of factor VIII, currently derived from human plasma. Approximately 15% of severely affected patients with low or absent factor VIII develop antibodies against factor VIII that can complicate replacement therapy. The basis of formation of these antibodies is not clear. There are other hazards of replacement therapy as well, the most serious of which is the risk of transmission of viral diseases. Until the mid-1980s, before routine screening of blood for HIV antibodies was instituted, thousands of hemophiliacs received factor VIII concentrates containing HIV, and many have developed AIDS (Chapter 7). With current blood banking practices, the risk of HIV transmission has been virtually eliminated, but the threat of other undetected infections remains. Ultimately, the only safe factor VIII will be one derived from the cloned factor VIII gene. Clinical trials of replacement therapy with recombinant factor VIII are now in progress. Efforts to develop somatic gene therapy for hemophilia are also under way.

HEMOPHILIA B (CHRISTMAS DISEASE, FACTOR IX DEFICIENCY)

Severe factor IX deficiency is a disorder that is clinically indistinguishable from hemophilia A. With the exception of DNA inversion, the spectrum of mutations found in hemophilia B is similar to that seen in hemophilia A. Moreover, it is also inherited as an X-linked recessive trait and may occur asymptomatically or with associated hemorrhage. In about 14% of these patients, factor IX is present but nonfunctional. As with hemophilia A, PTT is prolonged and PT is normal, as is bleeding time. Identification of Christmas disease (named after the first patient with this condition and not the holiday) is possible only by assay of the factor levels.

Disseminated Intravascular Coagulation (DIC)

DIC is an acute, subacute, or chronic thrombohemorrhagic disorder occurring as a secondary complication in a variety of diseases. It is characterized by activation of the coagulation sequence that leads to the formation of microthrombi throughout the microcirculation of the body, but often in a quixotically uneven distribution. Sometimes the coagulopathy is localized to a specific organ or tissue. *As a consequence of the thrombotic diathesis, there is consumption of platelets, fibrin, and coagulation factors and, secondarily, activation of fibrinolytic mechanisms.* Thus, DIC may present with signs and symptoms relating to tissue hypoxia, and infarction caused by the myriad microthrombi, or as a hemorrhagic disorder related to depletion of the elements required for hemostasis (hence, the term "consumption coagulopathy" is sometimes used to describe DIC). Activation of the fibrinolytic mechanism aggravates the hemorrhagic diathesis.

Etiology and Pathogenesis. At the outset, it must be emphasized that DIC is not a primary disease. It is a coagulopathy that occurs in the course of a variety of clinical conditions. In discussing the general mechanisms underlying DIC, it is useful to briefly review the normal process of blood coagulation and clot removal discussed in Chapter 5. It should be recalled that clotting may be initiated by either of two pathways: (1) the *extrinsic pathway,* which is triggered by the release of tissue factor ("tissue thromboplastin"); and (2) the *intrinsic pathway,* which involves the activation of factor XII by surface contact with collagen or other negatively charged substances. Both pathways, through a series of intermediate steps, result in the generation of thrombin, which in turn converts fibrinogen to fibrin. This process is regulated by *clot-inhibiting influences,* which include the activation of fibrinolysis involving generation of plasmin; the clearance of activated clotting factors by the mononuclear phagocyte system or by the liver; and the activation of endogenous anticoagulants such as protein C.

From this brief review, it can be concluded that DIC may result from pathologic activation of the extrinsic and/or intrinsic pathways of coagulation or impairment of clot-inhibiting influences. Since the latter rarely constitute primary mechanisms of DIC, we focus our attention on the abnormal initiation of clotting.[58]

Two major mechanisms trigger DIC: (1) release of tissue factor or thromboplastic substances into the circulation and (2) widespread injury to the endothelial cells. Tissue thromboplastic substances may be derived from a variety of sources, such as placenta in obstetric complications (Table 14–10) and the granules of leukemic cells in acute promyelocytic leukemia. Mucus released from certain adenocarcinomas can also act as a thromboplastic substance by directly activating factor X, independent of factor VII. In gram-negative sepsis (an important cause of DIC), bacterial endotoxins cause increased synthesis, membrane exposure, and release of tissue factor from monocytes. Furthermore, activated monocytes release interleukin-1 and TNF-α, both of which increase the expression of tissue factor on endothelial cell membranes and simultaneously decrease the expression of thrombomodulin.[59] The latter, you may recall, activates protein C, an anticoagulant. The result is both activation of the clotting system and inhibition of coagulation control. TNF-α is an extremely important mediator of DIC in septic shock. In addition to the effects previously mentioned, TNF-α up-regulates the expression of adhesion molecules on endothelial cells and thus favors adhesion of leukocytes, which in turn damage endothelial cells by releasing oxygen-derived free radicals and preformed proteases.[60]

Endothelial injury, the other major trigger, can initiate DIC by causing release of tissue factor, promoting platelet aggregation, and activating the intrinsic coagulation pathway. Even subtle endothelial injury can unleash procoagulant activity by enhancing membrane expression of tissue factor. Widespread endothelial injury may be produced by deposition of antigen-antibody complexes (e.g., systemic lupus erythematosus), temperature extremes (e.g., heat stroke, burns), or microorganisms (e.g., meningococci, rickettsiae).

Several disorders associated with DIC are listed in Table 14–10. Of these, DIC is most likely to follow *obstetric complications, malignant neoplasia, sepsis,* and *major*

Table 14–10. MAJOR DISORDERS ASSOCIATED WITH DISSEMINATED INTRAVASCULAR COAGULATION

Obstetric Complications
Abruptio placentae
Retained dead fetus
Septic abortion
Amniotic fluid embolism
Toxemia
Infections
Gram-negative sepsis
Meningococcemia
Rocky Mountain spotted fever
Histoplasmosis
Aspergillosis
Malaria
Neoplasms
Carcinomas of pancreas, prostate, lung, and stomach
Acute promyelocytic leukemia
Massive Tissue Injury
Traumatic
Burns
Extensive surgery
Miscellaneous
Acute intravascular hemolysis, snakebite, giant hemangioma, shock, heat stroke, vasculitis, aortic aneurysm, liver disease

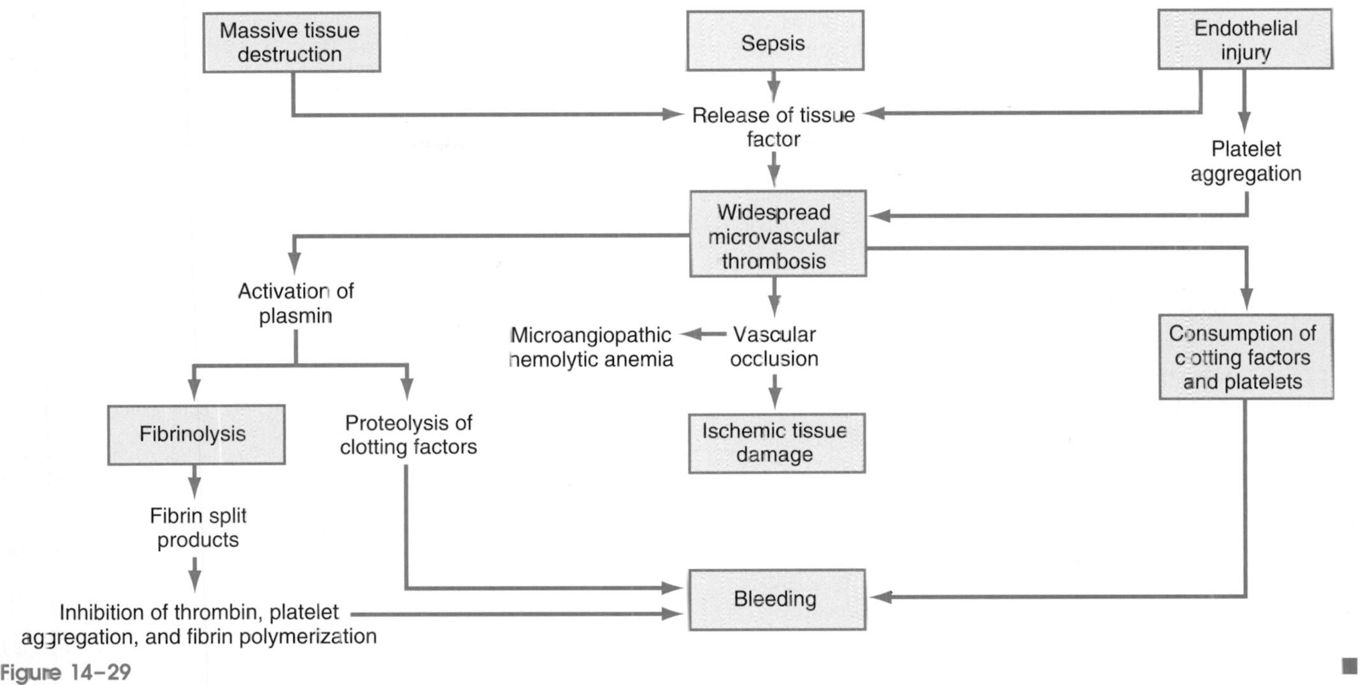

Figure 14–29

Pathophysiology of disseminated intravascular coagulation.

trauma. The initiating factors in these conditions are often multiple and interrelated. For example, in infections, particularly those caused by gram-negative bacteria, endotoxins released by the bacteria may activate both the intrinsic and the extrinsic pathways by producing endothelial cell injury and release of thromboplastins from inflammatory cells; furthermore, endotoxins inhibit the anticoagulant activity of protein C by suppressing thrombomodulin expression on endothelium. Endothelial cell damage may also be produced directly by meningococci, rickettsiae, and viruses. Antigen-antibody complexes formed during the infection can activate the classic complement pathway, and the complement fragments can secondarily activate both platelets and granulocytes. Endotoxins as well as other bacterial products are also capable of directly activating factor XII. In *massive trauma, extensive surgery,* and *severe burns,* the major mechanism of DIC is believed to be autoinfusion of tissue thromboplastins. In *obstetric* conditions, thromboplastins derived from the placenta, dead retained fetus, or amniotic fluid may enter the circulation. However, hypoxia, acidosis, and shock, which often coexist with the surgical and obstetric conditions, can also cause widespread endothelial injury. Supervening infection may complicate the problems further. Among cancers, acute promyelocytic leukemia and carcinomas of the lung, pancreas, colon, and stomach are most frequently associated with DIC. These tumors are associated with the release of a variety of thromboplastic substances, including tissue factors, proteolytic enzymes, mucin, and other undefined tumor products.

The consequences of DIC are twofold. First, there is *widespread deposition* of fibrin within the microcirculation. This may lead to ischemia of the more severely affected or more vulnerable organs and to a *hemolytic anemia* resulting from fragmentation of red cells as they squeeze through the narrowed microvasculature (microangiopathic hemolytic anemia). Second, a *hemorrhagic diathesis* may dominate the clinical picture. This results from consumption of platelets and clotting factors as well as activation of plasminogen. Plasmin not only can cleave fibrin but also can digest factors V and VIII, thereby reducing their concentration further. In addition, fibrinolysis leads to the formation of fibrin degradation products, which inhibit platelet aggregation and fibrin polymerization and have antithrombin activity. All of these influences lead to the hemostatic failure seen in DIC (Fig. 14–29).

MORPHOLOGY. In general, thrombi are found in the following sites in decreasing order of frequency: brain, heart, lungs, kidneys, adrenals, spleen, and liver. However, no tissue is spared, and thrombi are occasionally found in only one or several organs without affecting others. In giant hemangiomas, for example, they are localized to the neoplasm. In this condition, they are believed to result from local stasis and recurrent trauma to the poorly supported blood vessels. The affected kidneys may reveal small thrombi in the glomeruli that may evoke only a reactive swelling of endothelial cells; however, in severe cases, microinfarcts or even bilateral renal cortical necrosis may result. Numerous fibrin thrombi may be found in the alveolar capillaries, sometimes associated with pulmonary edema and exudation of fibrin, creating "hyaline membranes" reminiscent of adult respiratory distress syndrome (Chapter 16). In the central nervous system, microinfarcts may be caused by the fibrin thrombi, occasionally complicated by simultaneous fresh hemorrhage. Such changes are the basis for the bizarre neurologic signs and symptoms sometimes observed in this syndrome. The manifestations of DIC in the endocrine glands are of considerable interest. In meningococcemia, the massive adrenal hemorrhages of the Waterhouse-Friderichsen syndrome (Chapter 26) are probably related to fibrin thrombi within the microcirculation of the adrenal cortex. Similarly, Sheehan postpartum pituitary necrosis (Chapter 26) may be one of the expressions of DIC. In toxemia of pregnancy (Chapter 24), the placenta exhibits widespread microthrombi, providing a plausible explanation for the premature atrophy of the cytotrophoblast and syncytiotrophoblast encountered in this condition.

The bleeding manifestations of DIC are not dissimilar to those encountered in the hereditary and acquired disorders affecting the hemostatic mechanisms discussed earlier.

Clinical Course. The onset may be fulminant, as in endotoxic shock or amniotic fluid embolism, or it may be insidious and chronic, as in cases of carcinomatosis or retention of a dead fetus. Overall, about 50% of individuals with DIC are obstetric patients having complications of pregnancy. In this setting, the disorder tends to be reversible with delivery of the fetus. About 33% of the patients have carcinomatosis. The remaining cases are associated with the various entities previously listed.

It is almost impossible to detail all the potential clinical presentations, but a few common patterns may be cited. A microangiopathic hemolytic anemia may appear. Respiratory symptoms such as dyspnea, cyanosis, and extreme respiratory difficulty may predominate. Neurologic signs and symptoms including convulsions and coma represent another pattern. Renal changes such as oliguria and acute renal failure may dominate. Circulatory failure and shock may appear suddenly or develop progressively. In general, *acute DIC, associated with obstetric complications or major trauma, for example, is dominated by bleeding diathesis, whereas chronic DIC, such as may occur in a patient with cancer, tends to present initially with thrombotic complications.* Accurate clinical observation and laboratory studies are necessary for the diagnosis. It is usually necessary to monitor fibrinogen, platelets, PT, PTT, and fibrin degradation products.

The prognosis is highly variable and depends, to a considerable extent, on the underlying disorder. The management of these cases requires meticulous maneuvering between the Scylla of the thrombotic tendency and the Charybdis of the bleeding diathesis. Thus is posed the dilemma of whether to attempt to block coagulation or to control bleeding by the administration of coagulants. Each patient must be treated individually, and depending on the clinical picture, potent anticoagulants such as heparin or coagulants in the form of fresh-frozen plasma may be administered. Platelet transfusions may sometimes be necessary. DIC is another of the therapeutist's nightmares.

REFERENCES

1. Sieff CA, et al: The anatomy and physiology of hematopoiesis. In Nathan DG, Orkin SH (eds): Nathan and Oski's Hematology of Infancy and Childhood, 5th ed. Philadelphia, WB Saunders, 1998, p 161.
1a. Kondo M, et al: Identification of clonogenic common lymphoid progenitors in mouse bone marrow. Cell 91:661, 1997.
2. Gallagher PG, et al: Disorders of the erythrocyte membrane. In Nathan DG, Orkin SH (eds): Nathan and Oski's Hematology of Infancy and Childhood, 5th ed. Philadelphia, WB Saunders, 1998, p 544.
3. Eber SW: Ankyrin-1 mutations are the major cause of dominant and recessive hereditary spherocytosis. Nat Genet 13:214, 1996.
4. Jarolim P, et al: Characterization of 13 novel band 3 gene defects in hereditary spherocytosis with band 3 deficiency. Blood 88:4366, 1996.
5. Jandl JH, et al: Red cell filtration and the pathogenesis of certain hemolytic anemias. Blood 18:33, 1961.
6. Cynober T, et al: Red cell abnormalities in hereditary spherocytosis: relevance to diagnosis and understanding of the variable expression of clinical severity. J Lab Clin Med 128:259, 1996.
7. Beutler E: G6PD deficiency. Blood 84:3613, 1994.
8. Martini G, Ursini MV: A new lease of life for an old enzyme. Bioessays 18:631, 1996.
9. Mason PJ: New insights into G6PD deficiency. Br J Haematol 94: 585, 1996.
10. Bunn HF: Pathogenesis and treatment of sickle cell disease. N Engl J Med 337:762, 1997.
11. Ballas SK, Mohandas N: Pathophysiology of vaso-occlusion. Hematol Oncol Clin North Am 10:1221, 1996.
12. Hebbel RP, Vercellotti GM: The endothelial biology of sickle cell disease. J Lab Clin Med 129:288, 1997.
13. Lane PA: Sickle cell disease. Pediatr Clin North Am 43:639, 1996.
14. Smith JA: Bone disorders in sickle cell disease. Hematol Oncol Clin North Am 10:1345, 1996.
15. Charache S, et al: Effect of hydroxyurea on the frequency of painful crises in sickle cell anemia. N Engl J Med 332:1317, 1995.
16. Steinberg MH, et al: Fetal hemoglobin in sickle cell anemia: determinants of response to hydroxyurea. Multicenter study of hydroxyurea. Blood 89:1078, 1997.
17. Orkin SH, Nathan DG: The thalassemias. In Nathan DG, Orkin SH (eds): Nathan and Oski's Hematology of Infancy and Childhood, 5th ed. Philadelphia, WB Saunders, 1998, p 811.
18. Weatherall DJ: The thalassemias. In Beutler E, et al (eds): Williams Hematology, 5th ed. New York, McGraw-Hill, 1995, p 581.
19. Aljurf M, et al: Abnormal assembly of membrane protein in erythroid progenitors of patients with β-thalassemia major. Blood 87:2049, 1996.
20. Giardina PJ, Hilgartner MW: Update on thalassemia. Pediatr Rev 13: 55, 1992.
21. Rosse WF: Paroxysmal nocturnal hemoglobinuria as a molecular disease. Medicine (Baltimore) 76:63, 1997.
22. Engelfreit CP, et al: Autoimmune hemolytic anemia. Semin Hematol 29:3, 1992.
23. Petz LD: Drug-induced hemolysis. N Engl J Med 313:510, 1985.
24. Nydegger UE, et al: Immunopathologic and clinical features of hemolytic anemia due to cold agglutinins. Semin Hematol 28:66, 1991.
25. Hoffbrand A, Jackson BFA: Correction of the DNA synthesis defect in vitamin B_{12} deficiency by tetrahydrofolate: evidence in favour of the methyl-folate trap deficiency. Br J Haematol 83:643, 1993.
26. Chanarin I, et al: Cobalamin and folate: recent developments. J Clin Pathol 45:277, 1992.
27. Allen RH, et al: Metabolic abnormalities in cobalamin (vitamin B_{12}) and folate deficiency. FASEB J 7:1344, 1993.
28. Toh BA, Van Dreal IR, Gleeson PA: Pernicious anemia. N Engl J Med 337:1441, 1997.
29. Looker AC, et al: Prevalence of iron deficiency in the United States. JAMA 277:973, 1997.
30. Beard JL, et al: Iron metabolism: A comprehensive review. Nutr Rev 54:295, 1996.
31. Conrad ME, Umbreit JN: A concise review: iron absorption—the mucin-mobilferrin-integrin pathway: a competitive pathway for metal absorption. Am J Hematol 42:67, 1993.
32. Vulpe C, Gitscher J: Ironing out anemia. Nat Genet 16:319, 1997.

33. Fleming MD, et al: Microcytic anemia mice have a mutation in Nramp2, a candidate iron transporter gene. Nat Genet 16:383, 1997.
34. Fleet JC: Discovery of the hemochromatosis gene will require rethinking the regulation of iron metabolism. Nutr Rev 54:285, 1996.
35. Scrimshaw NS: Iron-deficiency and its functional consequences. Compr Ther 11:40, 1985.
36. Punnonen K, et al: Serum transferrin receptor and its ratio to serum ferritin in the diagnosis of iron deficiency. Blood 89:1052, 1997.
37. Sears DA: Anemia of chronic disease. Med Clin North Am 76:567, 1992.
38. Brown KE, et al: Hepatitis-associated aplastic anemia. N Engl J Med 336:1059, 1997.
39. Young NS, Maciejewski J: The pathophysiology of acquired aplastic anemia. N Engl J Med 336:1365, 1997.
40. Young NS: The problem of clonality in aplastic anemia: Dr. Dameshek's riddle, restated. Blood 29:1385, 1992.
41. Socie G: Could aplastic anemia be considered a pre-pre-leukemic disorder? Eur J Haematol 57(Suppl):60, 1996.
42. Fonseca R, Tefferi A: Practical aspects in the diagnosis and management of aplastic anemia. Am J Med Sci 313:160, 1997.
43. Freedman MH: Clinical annotation. Pure red cell aplasia in childhood and adolescence: pathogenesis and approaches to diagnosis. Br J Haematol 85:246, 1996.
44. Erslev AJ, Besarab A: Erythropoietin in the pathogenesis and treatment of the anemia of chronic renal failure. Kidney Int 51:662, 1997.
45. Bussell JB, et al: Fetal alloimmune thrombocytopenia. N Engl J Med 337:22, 1997.
46. Chang BH: Diagnosis, treatment and pathophysiology of autoimmune thrombocytopenias. Crit Rev Oncol Hematol 20:271, 1995.
47. Karpatkin S: Autoimmune (idiopathic) thrombocytopenic purpura. Lancet 349:1531, 1997.
48. Warkentin TE, et al: Heparin-induced thrombocytopenia in patients treated with low-molecular-weight heparin or unfractionated heparin. N Engl J Med 332:1330, 1995.
49. Warkentin TE, Kelton JG: A 14-year study of heparin-induced thrombocytopenia. Am J Med 101:502, 1996.
50. Ruggenenti P, et al: Pathogenesis and treatment of thrombotic microangiopathy. Kidney Int 51(Suppl 58):S-97, 1997.
51. Marcus AJ: Platelets and their disorders. In Ratnoff OD, Forbes CD (eds): Disorders of Hemostasis, 3d ed. Philadelphia, WB Saunders, 1996, p 79.
52. Bick RL: Acquired platelet function defects. Hematol Oncol Clin North Am 6:1203, 1992.
53. Nichols WC, Ginsburg D: von Willebrand disease. Medicine (Baltimore) 76:1, 1997.
54. Hoyer LW: Hemophilia-A. N Engl J Med 330:38, 1994.
55. Ewenstein BM: Von Willebrand disease. Annu Rev Med 48:525, 1997.
56. Cahill MR, Colvin BT: Hemophilia. Postgrad Med J 73:201, 1997.
57. Green PM, et al: The hemophilias. Adv Genet 32:99, 1995.
58. Moake JL: Hypercoagulable states. Adv Intern Med 35:235, 1990.
59. Thijs LG, et al: Coagulation disorders in septic shock. Intensive Care Med 19:S8, 1993.
60. Risberg B, et al: Disseminated intravascular coagulation. Acta Anaesthiol Scand 35(Suppl 95):60, 1991.

15

White Cells, Lymph Nodes, Spleen, and Thymus

Jon Aster and Vinay Kumar

White Cells and Lymph Nodes

NORMAL WHITE CELLS AND LYMPH NODES

LEUKOPENIA

NEUTROPENIA (AGRANULOCYTOSIS)

REACTIVE (INFLAMMATORY) PROLIFERATIONS OF WHITE CELLS AND NODES

LEUKOCYTOSIS

ACUTE NONSPECIFIC LYMPHADENITIS

CHRONIC NONSPECIFIC LYMPHADENITIS

NEOPLASTIC PROLIFERATIONS OF WHITE CELLS

LYMPHOID NEOPLASMS

Definitions and Classifications

Precursor B-Cell and T-Cell Neoplasms

Acute Lymphoblastic Leukemia/Lymphoma

Peripheral B-Cell Neoplasms

Chronic Lymphocytic Leukemia and Small Lymphocytic Lymphoma

Follicular Lymphoma

Diffuse Large B-Cell Lymphoma

Burkitt Lymphoma

Plasma Cell Neoplasms, Multiple Myeloma, and Related Entities

Lymphoplasmacytic Lymphoma (Waldenström Macroglobulinemia)

Mantle Cell Lymphoma

Marginal Zone Lymphoma (MALToma)

Hairy Cell Leukemia

Peripheral T-Cell and Natural Killer Cell Neoplasms

Peripheral T-Cell Lymphoma, Unspecified

Adult T-Cell Leukemia/Lymphoma

Mycosis Fungoides and Sézary Syndrome

Hodgkin Disease

MYELOID NEOPLASMS

Acute Myelogenous Leukemia

Myelodysplastic Syndromes

Chronic Myeloproliferative Disorders

Chronic Myelogenous Leukemia

Polycythemia Vera

Essential Thrombocytosis

Myelofibrosis with Myeloid Metaplasia

LANGERHANS CELL HISTIOCYTOSIS

ETIOLOGIC AND PATHOGENETIC FACTORS IN WHITE CELL NEOPLASIA: SUMMARY AND PERSPECTIVES

Spleen

NORMAL SPLEEN

SPLENOMEGALY

NONSPECIFIC ACUTE SPLENITIS

CONGESTIVE SPLENOMEGALY

SPLENIC INFARCTS

NEOPLASMS

CONGENITAL ANOMALIES

RUPTURE

Thymus

NORMAL THYMUS

DEVELOPMENTAL DISORDERS

THYMIC HYPERPLASIA

THYMOMAS

White Cells and Lymph Nodes

NORMAL WHITE CELLS AND LYMPH NODES

The origin and differentiation of white cells (granulocytes, monocytes, and lymphocytes) were briefly discussed in Chapter 14. Lymphocytes and monocytes not only circulate in the blood and lymph, but also accumulate in discrete, organized masses, the so-called lymphoreticular system. Components of this system include lymph nodes, thymus, spleen, tonsils, adenoids, and Peyer patches. Less discrete collections of lymphoid cells occur in the bone marrow, lungs, gastrointestinal tract, and other tissues. Lymph nodes are the most widely distributed and easily accessible component of the lymphoid tissue and are hence frequently examined for the diagnosis of lymphoreticular disorders. Therefore, it is advantageous to review the normal morphology of lymph nodes (shown schematically in Fig. 15–1).

Lymph nodes are discrete structures surrounded by a capsule composed of connective tissue and a few elastic

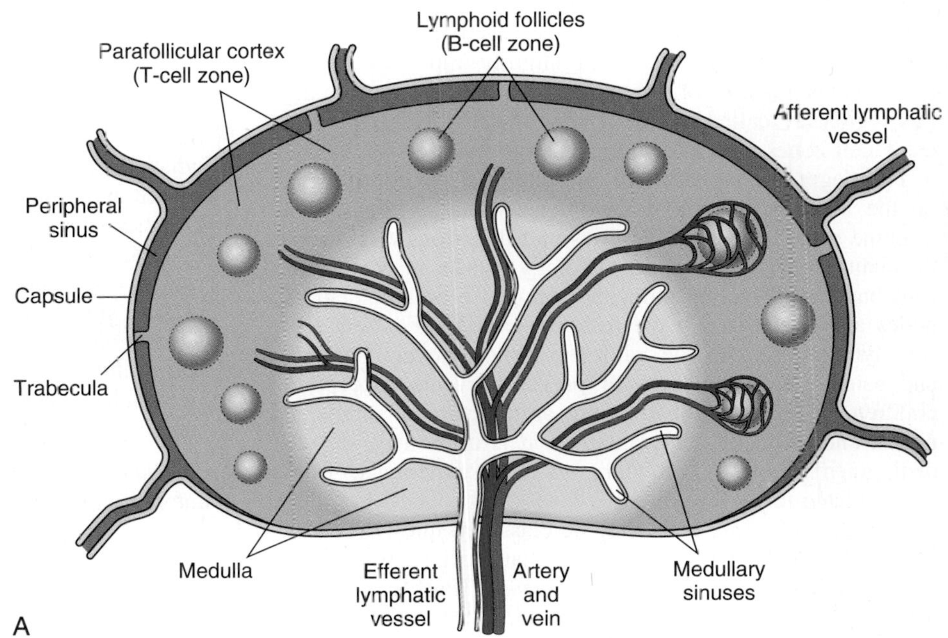

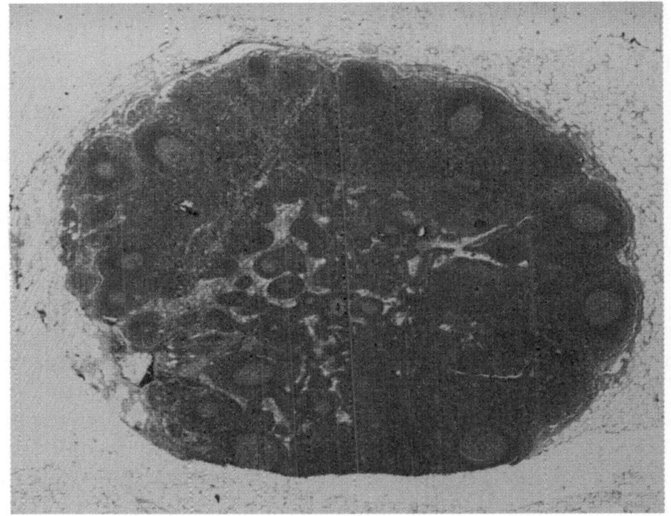

Figure 15–1

Normal lymph node architecture. *A*, Schematic diagram of a lymph node illustrating the blood and lymphatic supply and the distribution of B- and T-cell zones. *B*, Low-power view of a lymph node. (Modified from Abbas AK, et al [eds]: Cellular and Molecular Immunology, 3rd ed. Philadelphia, WB Saunders, 1997, p 30.)

fibrils. The capsule is perforated by multiple afferent lymphatics that empty into a fenestrated subcapsular peripheral sinus. Lymph extravasates from this sinus and slowly percolates through the node, eventually collecting in medullary sinusoids and exiting through a single efferent lymphatic vessel in the hilus, which also serves as the point of penetration by a single small artery and vein. Situated in the cortex subjacent to the peripheral sinus are spherical aggregates of lymphoid cells, the so-called primary follicles, that represent the B-lymphocyte areas. Between the primary follicles is the paracortex, a region rich in T lymphocytes. Deep to the cortex lies the medulla, a region containing numerous plasma cells and relatively few lymphocytes.

This morphologic description of the lymph node is highly idealized and falsely static. As secondary lines of defense, they are constantly responding to stimuli, even in the absence of clinical disease. Within several days of antigenic stimulation, the primary follicles enlarge and develop pale-staining germinal centers composed of follicular center cells that are surrounded by mantle zones containing small unchallenged B cells. In some reactive conditions, a rim of B lymphoid cells with slightly more cytoplasm accumulates outside of the mantle zone; cells occupying this region are called *marginal zone B cells*. The paracortical T-cell zones also frequently undergo hyperplasia.

The degree and pattern of morphologic change depend on the inciting factor and the intensity of the subsequent immune response. Trivial injuries and infections effect subtle changes in lymph node histology, while more significant bacterial infections inevitably produce enlargement of nodes and sometimes leave residual scarring. For this reason, lymph nodes in the adult are almost never "normal" and usually bear the scars of previous events. Except in children, it is difficult to find architecturally unaltered nodes, and in histologic evaluations it is often necessary to distinguish changes secondary to past experience from those related to present disease.

Disorders of white cells may be classified into two broad categories: *proliferative* and those characterized by a deficiency of leukocytes, that is, *leukopenias*. Proliferations of white cells may be *reactive* or *neoplastic*. Since their major function is host defense, reactive proliferation in response to an underlying primary, often microbial, disease is fairly common. Neoplastic disorders, although less frequent, are much more important. In the following discussion, we describe first the leukopenic states and summarize the common reactive disorders, then consider in some detail malignant proliferations of white cells.

LEUKOPENIA

The number of circulating white cells may be markedly decreased in a variety of disorders. An abnormally low white cell count (*leukopenia*) usually results from reduced numbers of neutrophils (*neutropenia, granulocytopenia*). *Lymphopenia* is less common, and in addition to the congenital immunodeficiency diseases (Chapter 7), it is most commonly observed in specific settings, such as advanced human immunodeficiency virus (HIV) infection, after therapy with glucocorticoids or cytotoxic drugs, autoimmune disorders, malnutrition, and certain acute viral infections. Only the more common leukopenias involving granulocytes are discussed further here.

Neutropenia (Agranulocytosis)

Reduction in the number of granulocytes in the peripheral blood (*neutropenia*) may be seen in a wide variety of circumstances. A marked reduction in neutrophil count has serious consequences by predisposing to infections. When of this magnitude, it is referred to as *agranulocytosis*.

Pathogenesis. A reduction in circulating granulocytes occurs if (1) there is reduced or ineffective production of neutrophils or (2) there is accelerated removal of neutrophils from the circulating blood. *Inadequate or ineffective granulopoiesis* is observed in the setting of

- Suppression of myeloid stem cells, as occurs in aplastic anemia (Chapter 14) and a variety of infiltrative marrow disorders (e.g., tumors, granulomatous disease)—in these conditions, granulocytopenia is accompanied by anemia and thrombocytopenia
- Suppression of the committed granulocytic precursors, which occurs after exposure to certain drugs, as discussed subsequently
- Disease states characterized by ineffective granulopoiesis, such as megaloblastic anemias caused by vitamin B_{12} or folate deficiency (Chapter 14) and myelodysplastic syndromes, in which defective precursors are susceptible to intramedullary death
- Rare inherited conditions (such as Kostmann syndrome) in which genetic defects in specific genes result in impaired granulocytic differentiation

Accelerated removal or destruction of neutrophils is encountered with

- Immunologically mediated injury to the neutrophils, which may be idiopathic, associated with a well-defined immunologic disorder (e.g., systemic lupus erythematosus), or produced by exposure to drugs
- Splenic sequestration, in which excessive destruction occurs secondary to enlargement of the spleen, usually also associated with increased destruction of red cells and platelets
- Increased peripheral use, as may occur in overwhelming bacterial, fungal, or rickettsial infections

Among the many associations mentioned, the *most significant neutropenias (agranulocyloses) are produced by drugs*. Certain drugs, such as alkylating agents and antimetabolites used in cancer treatment, produce agranulocytosis in a predictable, dose-related fashion. They cause a generalized suppression of the bone marrow, and therefore production of erythrocytes and platelets is also affected. Agranulocytosis may also be encountered as an idiosyncratic reaction to a large variety of agents. The roster of implicated drugs includes aminopyrine, chloramphenicol, sulfonamides, chlorpromazine, thiouracil, and phenylbutazone. The neutropenia induced by chlorpromazine and related phenothiazines is believed to result from a toxic effect on granulocytic precursors in the bone marrow. In contrast, agranulocytosis after administration of aminopyrine, thiouracil, and certain sulfonamides appears to stem from immunologically mediated destruction of mature neutrophils through mechanisms that are similar to those involved in drug-induced hemolytic anemias (Chapter 14).

In some patients with acquired neutropenia, no antecedent cause can be detected, but autoimmunity is suspected since serum antibodies directed against neutrophil-specific antigens can be detected.[1] Severe neutropenia may also occur in association with monoclonal proliferations of large granular lymphocytes (so-called LGL leukemia).[2] The mechanism of this neutropenia is not clear, but suppression of granulocytic progenitors in the bone marrow is considered most likely.

MORPHOLOGY. The anatomic alterations in the bone marrow depend on the underlying basis of the neutropenia. When it is caused by excessive destruction of the mature neutrophils, the marrow may be hypercellular with increased numbers of granulocytic precursors. Hypercellularity is also seen with ineffective granulopoiesis, as occurs in megaloblastic anemias and myelodysplastic syndromes. Agranulocytosis caused by agents that suppress the growth or lead to the destruction of granulocytic precursors is understandably associated with decreased numbers of maturing leukopoietic elements.

Infections are a characteristic feature of agranulocytosis. Ulcerating necrotizing lesions of the gingiva, floor of the mouth, buccal mucosa, pharynx, or anywhere within the oral cavity (agranulocytic angina) are quite characteristic of agranulocytosis. These ulcers are typically deep, undermined, and covered by gray to green-black necrotic membranes from which numerous bacteria or fungi can be isolated. Similar ulcerations may occur on the skin or in the vagina, anus, or gastrointestinal tract, but these sites are much less frequently involved. Severe necrotizing infections are also encountered, but less prominently, in the lungs, urinary tract, and kidneys. All these sites of infection are characterized by massive growth of bacteria (or other agents) with relatively poor leukocytic response. In many instances, the bacteria grow in colony formation (botryomycosis) as though they were cultured on nutrient media. The regional lymph nodes draining these infections are enlarged and inflamed.

Clinical Course. The symptoms and signs of neutropenias are those of bacterial or fungal infections. They include malaise, chills, and fever, followed in sequence by marked weakness and fatigability. In severe agranulocytosis with virtual absence of neutrophils, these infections may become so overwhelming as to cause death within a few days.

Characteristically the neutrophil count is reduced to less than 1000 cells/mm³ of blood, and when counts fall below 500/mm³, serious infections tend to occur. Because infections in this setting are often fulminant, neutropenic patients are commonly treated with broad-spectrum antibiotics at the first sign of infection. Additionally, after treatment with myelosuppressive chemotherapy, granulocyte colony-stimulating factor (G-CSF) may be used to decrease the duration and severity of the granulocytic nadir.

REACTIVE (INFLAMMATORY) PROLIFERATIONS OF WHITE CELLS AND NODES

Leukocytosis

Leukocytosis is a common reaction in a variety of inflammatory states.

Pathogenesis. The peripheral blood leukocyte count is influenced by several factors, including

- The size of the myeloid (for granulocytes and monocytes) and lymphoid (for lymphocytes) precursor and storage cell pools
- The rate of release of cells from the storage pool into the circulation
- The proportion of cells that are marginating at any one time (the marginating pool)
- The rate of extravasation of cells from the peripheral blood into tissues

As discussed in Chapters 3 and 14, leukocyte homeostasis is maintained by cytokines, growth factors, and adhesion molecules, which affect commitment, proliferation, differentiation, and extravasation of leukocytes and their progenitors in each of these compartments. The mechanisms of leukocytosis vary depending on the affected leukocyte pool and the particular factor. We have seen, for example, that interleukin 1 (IL-1)–induced and tumor necrosis factor (TNF)–induced release of cells from the bone marrow storage pool causes leukocytosis in acute infection (Chapter 3); in chronic infections, there is in addition enlargement of the pool of proliferating bone marrow progenitor cells caused by IL-1–driven and TNF-driven increases in CSFs. Figure 15–2 summarizes the major mechanisms of neutrophilic leukocytosis and their causes. Similar mechanisms underlie other types of leukocytosis. For example, IL-5 causes eosinophilic leukocytosis by stimulating the differentiation of eosinophilic precursor cells, while the c-*kit* ligand and IL-7 play a central role in lymphopoiesis and lymphocytosis. Such factors are differentially produced in response to various pathogenic stimuli, and as a result the five principal types of leukocytosis (neutrophilic, eosinophilic, and basophilic leukocytosis; monocytosis; and lymphocytosis) tend to be observed in particular clinical settings (Table 15–1).

In patients with sepsis or severe inflammatory disorders (such as Kawasaki disease), in addition to leukocytosis there may be morphologic changes in the neutrophils, such

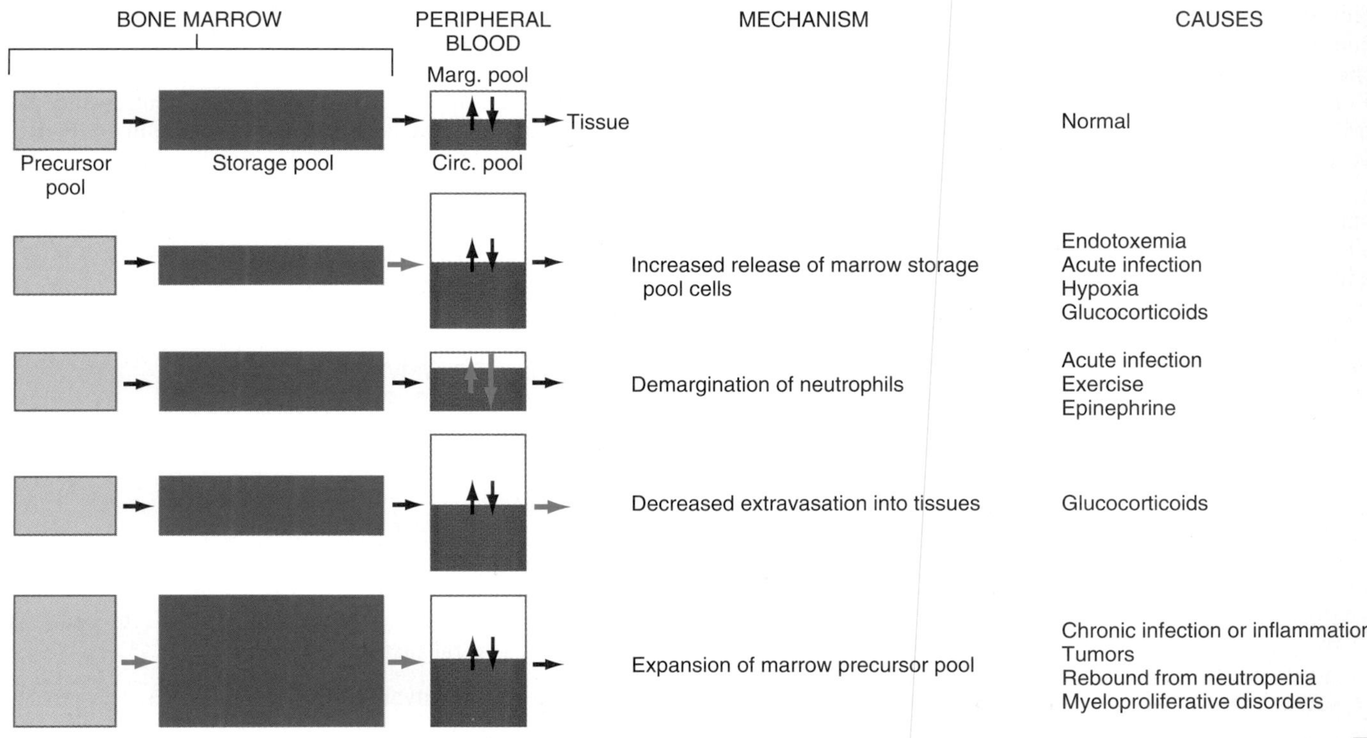

Figure 15–2

Mechanisms of neutrophilic leukocytosis. Neutrophils and their precursors are distributed in five pools: a bone marrow precursor pool, which includes progenitor cells and more committed, mitotically active precursors; a bone marrow storage pool, consisting of mitotically inactive mature and slightly immature neutrophils (band forms); a peripheral blood marginating pool (Marg. Pool); a peripheral blood circulating pool (Circ. Pool); and a tissue pool. The relative size of each pool is represented by the size of its corresponding box. The peripheral blood neutrophil count measures only the circulating peripheral blood pool, which can be enlarged by increased release of cells from the marrow storage pool, increased demargination, diminished extravasation into tissues, or expansion of the marrow precursor cell pool. (Modified from Finch SC: Hematology, 3rd ed. New York, McGraw-Hill, 1983, p 795.)

Table 15–1. CAUSES OF LEUKOCYTOSIS

Neutrophilic leukocytosis	Acute bacterial infections, especially those caused by pyogenic organisms; sterile inflammation caused by, for example, tissue necrosis (myocardial infarction, burns)
Eosinophilic leukocytosis (eosinophilia)	Allergic disorders such as asthma, hay fever, allergic skin diseases (e.g., pemphigus, dermatitis herpetiformis); parasitic infestations; drug reactions; certain malignancies (e.g., Hodgkin disease and some non-Hodgkin lymphomas); collagen vascular disorders and some vasculitides; atheroembolic disease (transient)
Basophilic leukocytosis (basophilia)	Rare, often indicative of a myeloproliferative disease (e.g., chronic myelogenous leukemia)
Monocytosis	Chronic infections (e.g., tuberculosis), bacterial endocarditis, rickettsiosis, and malaria; collagen vascular diseases (e.g., systemic lupus erythematosus); inflammatory bowel diseases (e.g., ulcerative colitis)

as toxic granulations, Döhle bodies, and cytoplasmic vacuoles (Fig. 15–3). *Toxic granules* are coarse and darker than the normal neutrophilic granules and are believed to represent abnormal azurophilic (primary) granules. *Döhle bodies* are patches of dilated endoplasmic reticulum that appear as cerulean blue cytoplasmic *puddles*.

In most instances, differentiation of reactive leukocytosis and leukocytosis caused by flooding of the peripheral blood by neoplastic white blood cells (leukemia) is not problematic, but difficulties may arise in two settings. Particularly in children, acute viral infections can produce the appearance of activated lymphocytes in the peripheral blood and marrow that resemble neoplastic lymphoblasts. Other times, particularly in inflammatory states, many immature granulocytes appear in the blood, simulating a picture of myelogenous leukemia (*leukemoid reaction*). In both settings, differentiation of reactive and neoplastic leukocytosis may require additional laboratory studies, as discussed later.

Infections and other inflammatory stimuli may not only cause leukocytosis, but also involve the lymph nodes, which act as defensive barriers. The infections that lead to lymphadenitis are numerous. Some that produce distinctive morphologic patterns are described in other chapters. In most instances, however, the lymphadenitis is entirely nonspecific, designated *acute* or *chronic nonspecific lymphadenitis*.

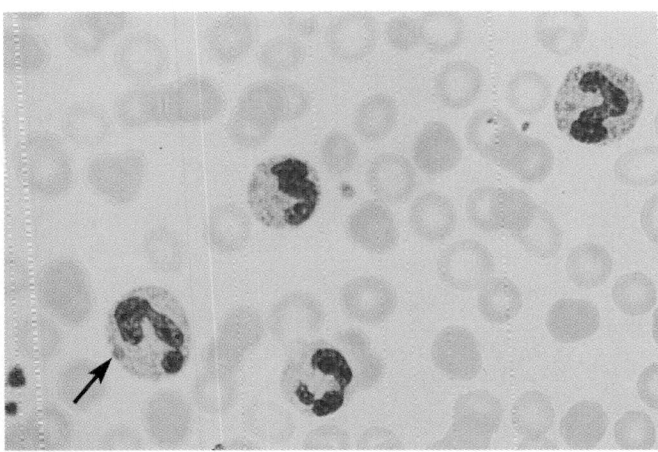

Figure 15–3

Reactive changes in neutrophils. Neutrophils containing coarse purple cytoplasmic granules (toxic granulations) and blue cytoplasmic patches of dilated endoplasmic reticulum (Döhle bodies) *(arrow)* are observed in this peripheral blood smear taken from a patient with bacterial sepsis.

Acute Nonspecific Lymphadenitis

Lymph nodes undergo reactive changes whenever challenged by microbiologic agents, cell debris, or foreign matter introduced into wounds or into the circulation. Acutely inflamed nodes are most commonly caused by direct microbiologic drainage and are seen most frequently in the cervical area in association with infections of the teeth or tonsils or in the axillary or inguinal regions secondary to infections in the extremities. Similarly, acute lymphadenitis is often found in mesenteric lymph nodes draining acute appendicitis. Other self-limited infections may also cause mesenteric adenitis and induce abdominal symptoms mimicking acute appendicitis, a differential diagnosis that plagues the surgeon. Systemic viral infections and bacteremia, particularly in children, often produce generalized lymphadenopathy.

MORPHOLOGY. Macroscopically the nodes become swollen, gray-red, and engorged. Histologically, there is prominence of the lymphoid follicles, with large germinal centers containing numerous mitotic figures. Histiocytes often contain particulate debris of bacterial origin or derived from necrotic cells. When pyogenic organisms are the cause of the reaction, the centers of the follicles may undergo necrosis; the entire node may sometimes be converted into a suppurative mass. With less severe reactions, there is sometimes a neutrophilic infiltrate about the follicles, and numerous neutrophils can be found within the lymphoid sinuses. The cells lining the sinuses become hypertrophied and cuboidal and may undergo hyperplasia.

Clinically, nodes with acute lymphadenitis are enlarged because of the cellular infiltration and edema. As a consequence of the distention of the capsule, they are tender to touch. When abscess formation is extensive, they become fluctuant. The overlying skin is frequently red, and sometimes penetration of the infection to the skin surface produces draining sinuses, particularly when the nodes have undergone suppurative necrosis. As might be expected, healing of such lesions is associated with scarring.

Chronic Nonspecific Lymphadenitis

Chronic reactions assume one of three patterns, depending on their cause.

MORPHOLOGY

- **Follicular hyperplasia:** Follicular hyperplasia is caused by inflammatory processes that activate B cells. It is distinguished by the prominence of large, round or oblong germinal centers (secondary follicles), which appear to bulge against a surrounding collar of small, resting B lymphocytes that constitute the mantle zone (Fig. 15–4). Within opposing poles of a reactive germinal center, two distinct regions are usually discernible: (1) a dark zone containing proliferating blastlike B cells (centroblasts) and (2) a light zone composed of B cells with irregular or cleaved nuclear contours (centrocytes). Also present throughout the follicle are phagocytic macrophages containing nuclear debris (tingible body macrophages) and a meshwork of inconspicuous dendritic cells that function in antigen presentation. Plasma cells, histiocytes, and occasionally neutrophils or eosinophils may be found in the parafollicular regions, and there generally is striking hyperplasia of the mononuclear phagocytic cells lining the lymphatic sinuses. Some specific causes of follicular hyperplasia include rheumatoid arthritis, toxoplasmosis, and early stages of HIV infection. This form of lymphadenitis may be confused morphologically with follicular lymphomas (see later discussion of lymphoid neoplasms). It is beyond the scope of this chapter to go into all the subtle morphologic features in this differential diagnosis, but several points may be noted. Favoring reactive follicular hyperplasia are (1) preservation of the lymph node architecture, including interfollicular T-cell zones and the sinusoids; (2) marked variation in the shape and size of lymphoid nodules; and (3) the presence of frequent mitotic figures, phagocytic macrophages, and recognizable light and dark zones, all of which tend to be absent from neo-

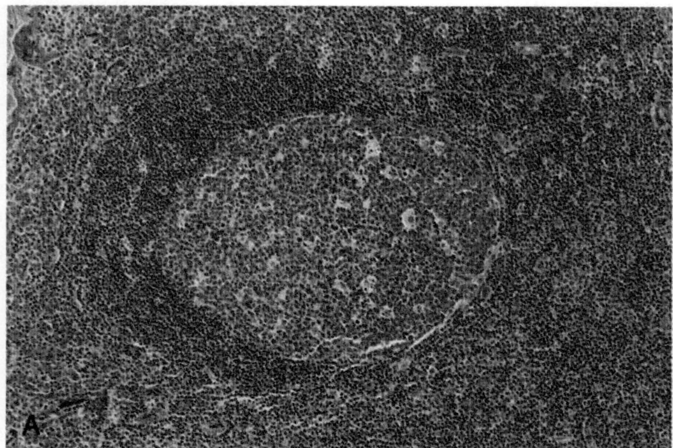

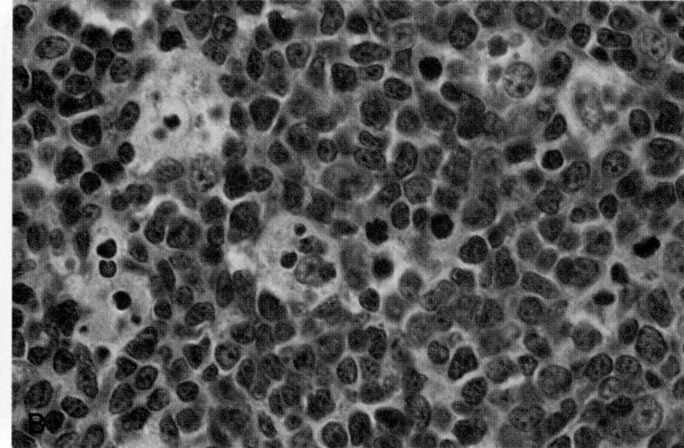

Figure 15–4

Follicular hyperplasia. *A*, Low-power view showing a reactive follicle and surrounding mantle zone. The dark-staining mantle zone is polarized, being much more prominent adjacent to the germinal center light zone in the left half of the follicle. The right half of the follicle consists of the dark zone. *B*, A high-power view of the dark zone shows several mitotic figures and numerous tingible body macrophages, indicative of ongoing apoptosis.

plastic follicles. Follicular hyperplasia is sometimes accompanied by **marginal zone B-cell hyperplasia.** In some immune reactions, particularly those caused by toxoplasmosis and early HIV infection, marginal zone B cells accumulate in a rim external to the mantle zone of germinal centers.

- **Paracortical lymphoid hyperplasia:** Paracortical lymphoid hyperplasia is characterized by reactive changes within the T-cell regions of the lymph node that encroach on and sometimes appear to efface the B-cell follicles. Within interfollicular regions, scattered activated T cells (immunoblasts) are often observed. These latter cells are three to four times the size of resting lymphocytes. In addition, there is hypertrophy of the sinusoidal and vascular endothelial cells and a mixed cellular infiltrate, principally of macrophages and sometimes of eosinophils. Such changes are encountered in immunologic reactions induced by drugs (especially phenytoin (Dilantin)); in acute viral infections, particularly infectious mononucleosis; and after vaccination against certain viral diseases.
- **Sinus histiocytosis (also called reticular hyperplasia):** Sinus histiocytosis refers to distention and prominence of the lymphatic sinusoids. Although nonspecific, this form of hyperplasia may be particularly prominent in lymph nodes draining cancers, such as carcinoma of the breast. The lining endothelial cells are markedly hypertrophied, and the sinuses may be virtually engorged with histiocytes. In the setting of cancer, this pattern of reaction has been thought to represent an immune response on the part of the host against the tumor or its products.

Characteristically, lymph nodes in chronic reactions are not tender because their capsules are not under increased pressure. Chronic lymphadenitis is particularly common in inguinal and axillary nodes, which drain relatively large areas of the body and so are frequently challenged.

NEOPLASTIC PROLIFERATIONS OF WHITE CELLS

Malignant proliferative diseases constitute the most important white cell disorders. The several categories of these diseases can be defined briefly as follows:

- *Lymphoid neoplasms* encompass a diverse group of entities. In many but not all instances, the phenotype of the neoplastic cell closely resembles that of a particular stage of normal lymphocyte differentiation, a feature that is used in the diagnosis and classification of these disorders.
- *Myeloid neoplasms* arise from hematopoietic stem cells that give rise to cells of the myeloid (i.e., erythroid, granulocytic, or thrombocytic) lineage. Three categories of myeloid neoplasia are recognized: *acute myelogenous leukemias*, in which immature progenitor cells accumulate in the bone marrow; *myelodysplastic syndromes*, associated with ineffective hematopoiesis and resultant

peripheral blood cytopenias; and *chronic myeloproliferative disorders*, in which increased production of one or more terminal differentiated myeloid elements (e.g, granulocytes) usually leads to an elevation of peripheral blood counts.

- The *histiocytoses* represent proliferative lesions of histiocytes, including rare neoplasms that present as malignant lymphomas. A special category of histiocytes referred to as *Langerhans cells* gives rise to a spectrum of neoplastic disorders, some of which behave as disseminated malignant tumors and others as localized benign proliferations. This group is called *Langerhans cell histiocytoses*.

As can be seen, the neoplastic disorders of white cells are extremely varied. In the following sections, each of the categories is treated separately.

Lymphoid Neoplasms

DEFINITIONS AND CLASSIFICATIONS

One of the confusing aspects of the lymphoid neoplasms concerns the use of the descriptive terms *lymphocytic leukemia* and *lymphoma*. *Leukemia* is used for lymphoid neoplasms that present with widespread involvement of the bone marrow, usually accompanied by the presence of large numbers of tumor cells in the peripheral blood. *Lymphoma* is used to describe proliferations arising as discrete tissue masses. Traditionally, these terms were attached to what were believed to be distinct entities The line between the *lymphocytic leukemias* and the *lymphomas*, however, often blurs. Many types of lymphoma occasionally present with a leukemic peripheral blood picture accompanied by extensive marrow involvement, and evolution to *leukemia* is not unusual with progression of incurable *lymphomas*. Conversely, tumors identical to leukemias sometimes arise as lymphomatous masses without evidence of bone marrow disease. Hence, when applied to particular neoplasms, the terms *leukemia* and *lymphoma* merely describe the usual tissue distribution of the disease.

Within the broad group of lymphomas, *Hodgkin disease* (HD) (Hodgkin lymphoma) is segregated from all other forms, which constitute the *non-Hodgkin lymphomas* (NHL). As seen subsequently, HD is clinically and histologically distinct from the NHLs. In addition, it is treated in a unique fashion, making the differentiation of HD and NHL of great practical importance.

The other important category of lymphoproliferative disease encompasses the *plasma cell neoplasms*, tumors composed of terminally differentiated B cells. Such tumors most commonly arise in the bone marrow, only rarely involving lymph nodes or producing a leukemic peripheral blood picture. In addition, as seen subsequently, certain features of their pathophysiology are related to the secretion of whole or partial immunoglobulin (Ig) fragments by the tumor cells.

The clinical presentation of the various lymphoid neoplasms is dictated by the anatomic distribution of disease. Two thirds of NHLs and virtually all cases of HD present with nontender nodal enlargement (often >2 cm) that may be localized or generalized. The remaining one third of NHLs arise at extranodal sites (e.g., skin, stomach, brain). In contrast, the leukemic forms (lymphocytic leukemia) most commonly come to clinical attention because of signs and symptoms related to suppression of normal hematopoiesis by tumor cells in the bone marrow. Lymphocytic leukemias also characteristically infiltrate and enlarge the spleen and liver. Finally, plasma cell neoplasms involving the skeleton cause local bony destruction and hence often present with pain owing to pathologic fractures.

Few areas of pathology have evoked as much controversy and confusion as the classification of NHL and related lymphoid neoplasms. In 1982, an international panel of hematopathologists attempted to stem the rising tide of classifications for NHL by proposing a Working Formulation for Clinical Usage,[3] which divided NHL on clinical grounds into three prognostic groups: low, intermediate, and high grade. Classification of NHL within each of these prognostic groups was based solely on morphologic criteria, particularly the pattern of tumor growth within lymph nodes (nodular or diffuse) and the size of the tumor cells (small, large, or mixed small and large). This approach to classification had the advantage of being simple and has been widely used, but further immunophenotypic and genotypic characterization of lymphoid neoplasms made it clear that a number of distinct entities had been lumped together or completely ignored in the Working Formulation. Of practical importance, some of the neoplasms not formally recognized in the Working Formulation (e.g., mantle cell lymphoma and marginal zone lymphoma) have proven to be fairly unique in their clinical behavior and response to therapy.

In an effort to correct the perceived deficiencies of the Working Formulation, a new classification emerged in 1994. Termed the *Revised European-American Classification of Lymphoid Neoplasms* (REAL),[4] it describes neoplasms that are believed to constitute distinct clinicopathologic entities based on clinical features, morphology, immunophenotype, and genotype; these entities are listed in Table 15–2, along with their Working Formulation equivalents. The REAL classification includes the lymphocytic leukemias, NHLs, and plasma cell neoplasms, thus eliminating the previous division between the various lymphoid neoplasms, which are now sorted into four broad categories, based on immunophenotype:

1. Precursor B-cell neoplasms (neoplasms of immature B cells)
2. Peripheral B-cell neoplasms (neoplasms of mature B cells)
3. Precursor T-cell neoplasms (neoplasms of immature T cells)
4. Peripheral T-cell and natural killer (NK) cell neoplasms (neoplasms of mature T cells and NK cells)

Diagnostic categories for HD were not modified by the REAL working group; the specific subtypes of HD are covered in a later section.

Table 15–2. *REAL* CLASSIFICATION OF THE LYMPHOID NEOPLASMS AND THEIR WORKING FORMULATION EQUIVALENTS

REAL Classification	Working Formulation Equivalent
I. Precursor B-Cell Neoplasms	
* Precursor B lymphoblastic leukemia/lymphoma	Leukemias not included; lymphomas classified as high-grade, lymphoblastic
II. Precursor T-Cell Neoplasms	
* Precursor T lymphoblastic leukemia/lymphoma	Leukemias not included; lymphomas classified as high-grade, lymphoblastic
III. Peripheral B-Cell Neoplasms	
● Chronic lymphocytic leukemia/small lymphocytic lymphoma	Low-grade, small lymphocytic
Lymphoplasmacytic lymphoma	Low-grade, small lymphocytic plasmacytoid
Mantle cell lymphoma	Most classified as intermediate-grade, diffuse small cleaved cell
● Follicular lymphoma	
Cytologic grade I	Low-grade, follicular, predominantly small cleaved cell
Cytologic grade II	Low-grade, follicular, mixed small and large cell
Cytologic grade III	Intermediate-grade, follicular, predominantly large cell
Marginal zone lymphoma	Most classified as low-grade, small lymphocytic
Hairy cell leukemia	Not included
● Plasmacytoma/plasma cell myeloma	Not included
● Diffuse large B-cell lymphoma	Intermediate-grade, diffuse large cell or high-grade, large cell immunoblastic
* Burkitt lymphoma	High-grade, small noncleaved cell
IV. Peripheral T-Cell and Natural Killer Cell Neoplasms	
T-cell chronic lymphocytic leukemia	Low-grade, small lymphocytic
Large granular lymphocytic leukemia	Low-grade, small lymphocytic
Mycosis fungoides and Sézary syndrome	Low-grade, mycosis fungoides
Peripheral T-cell lymphoma, unspecified	Variable; most often intermediate-grade, diffuse mixed small and large cell
Angioimmunoblastic T-cell lymphoma	Variable; most often intermediate-grade, diffuse mixed small and large cell
Angiocentric lymphoma (NK/T-cell lymphoma[4a])	Variable; most often intermediate-grade, diffuse mixed small and large cell
Intestinal T-cell lymphoma	Variable; most often high-grade, large cell immunoblastic
Adult T-cell leukemia/lymphoma	Variable; most often intermediate-grade, diffuse mixed small and large cell
Anaplastic large cell lymphoma	Variable; most often high-grade, large cell immunoblastic

● Most common tumors in adults.
* Most common tumors in children or adolescents.

Before discussing the specific entities described in the REAL classification, some important principles relevant to the lymphoid neoplasms need to be emphasized.

- The diagnosis of lymphoid neoplasia can be suspected from the clinical features, but *histologic examination of lymph nodes or other involved tissues is required for diagnosis.*
- *Although all lymphoid neoplasms have traditionally been considered to be malignant, a wide range of behavior from seemingly benign to rapidly fatal is observed.* It is perhaps more accurate to consider all clonal lymphoid proliferations as being potentially malignant because even the most indolent proliferations tend to transform over time into more aggressive, overtly malignant tumors.
- *The vast majority of lymphoid neoplasms (80 to 85%) are of B-cell origin, with most of the remainder being T-cell tumors; only rarely are tumors of NK or histiocytic origin observed.* Tumors of T and B cells may represent cells arrested at any stage along their differentiation pathways (Fig. 15–5). Figure 15–5 also illustrates the genotypic and phenotypic characteristics of differentiating T and B cells that are useful in subdividing this group of tumors. Some additional cell surface markers helpful in the study of lymphomas and leukemias are listed in Table 15–3.
- *As tumors of the immune system, lymphoid neoplasms tend to disrupt normal regulatory mechanisms, leading to frequent immune abnormalities.* Both a loss of vigilance (as evidenced by susceptibility to infection) and a breakdown of tolerance (manifested by autoimmunity) may be seen, sometimes in the same patient. In a further, ironic twist, patients with inherited or acquired immunodeficiency are themselves at high risk of developing certain lymphoid neoplasms.
- *All lymphoid neoplasms are derived from a single transformed cell and are therefore monoclonal.* Antigen receptor genes rearrange during normal B-cell and T-cell differentiation through a mechanism that ensures that each lymphocyte makes a single, unique antigen receptor (Chapter 7). *In most lymphoid neoplasms, antigen receptor gene rearrangement precedes transformation; as a result, the daughter cells derived from the malignant progenitor share the same antigen receptor gene configuration and sequence and synthesize identical antigen receptor proteins* (either Ig or T-cell receptors). For this reason, analysis of antigen receptor genes and their protein products is frequently used to differentiate monoclonal neoplasms from polyclonal reactive pro-

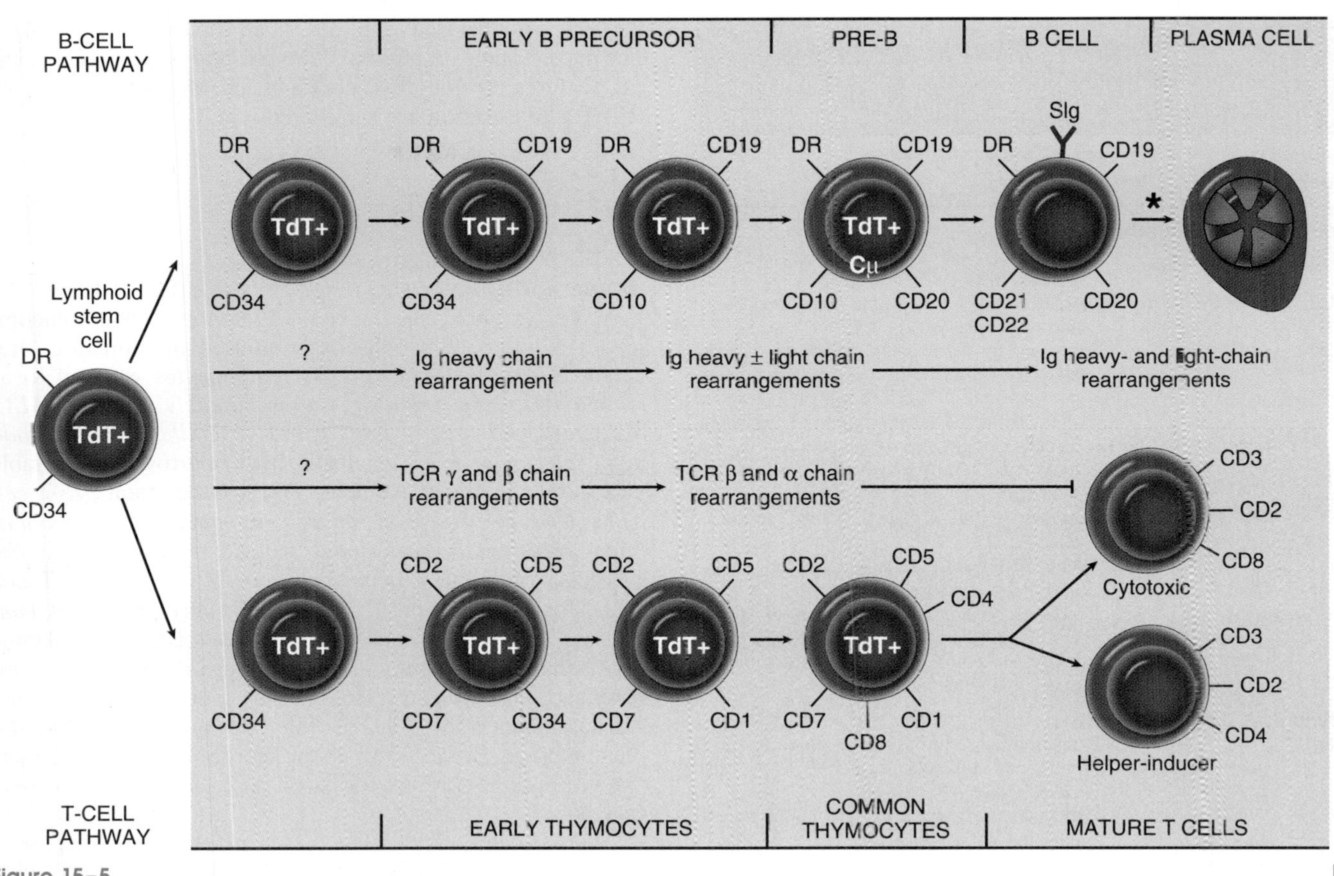

Figure 15-5

Schematic illustration of the phenotypic and genotypic changes associated with the differentiation of B cells and T cells. Not shown are some CD4+/CD8− cells (common thymocytes) that also express CD3. Stages between resting B cells and plasma cells are not depicted. CD, cluster designation; TdT, terminal deoxynucleotidyl transferase; Ig, immunoglobulin; TCR, T-cell receptor.

cesses. In addition, since a particular rearranged antigen receptor gene is unique to the neoplastic clone, it can be used as a highly specific marker that is useful for detecting minimal residual disease after treatment or recurrences before they become clinically apparent.[5]

- *Neoplastic B and T cells tend to home to and grow in areas where their normal counterparts reside.* This results in characteristic patterns of tissue involvement in certain lymphoid neoplasms. For example, follicular lymphomas proliferate in the B-cell areas of the lymph node, producing a nodular or follicular pattern of growth, whereas T-cell lymphomas typically grow in paracortical T-cell zones. It is thought that the tendency of particular lymphoid neoplasms to involve certain extranodal tissues also stems from a combination of homing and local trophic factors.
- *Given that normal B and T lymphoid cells recirculate through the lymphatics and peripheral blood to distant lymphoid tissues, it is not suprising that neoplastic lymphocytes show a similar wanderlust.* Using sensitive molecular techniques, most tumors appear to be widely disseminated at the time of diagnosis. This fits well with the clinical observation that cure is possible in most lymphoid neoplasms only with systemic therapy. The most notable exception to this rule is HD, which can be cured with local therapy.
- *HD spreads in an orderly fashion, and as a result staging is of great importance in determining therapy.* In contrast, the spread of NHL is less predictable, and, as noted previously, most patients are assumed to have systemic disease at the time of diagnosis. Hence, staging in particular NHLs provides useful prognostic information but is generally not as important in guiding therapy as in HD.

We now turn to the specific entities of the REAL classification. In the discussion that follows, we begin with neoplasms of immature lymphoid cells, then move on to tumors of mature B cells, T cells, and NK cells. We describe a relatively large variety of distinctive clinicopathologic entities. It is worth remembering, however, that *only four entities constitute the majority of lymphoid lymphomas and leukemias in adults: follicular lymphoma, large B-cell lymphoma, chronic lymphocytic leukemia/small lymphocytic lymphoma, and multiple myeloma. Similarly, two groups of neoplasms are most common (and therefore most important) in children and young adolescents: acute lymphoblastic leukemia/lymphoma and Burkitt lymphoma.* Thus,

Table 15-3. SOME IMMUNE CELL ANTIGENS DETECTED BY MONOCLONAL ANTIBODIES

Antigen Designation	Comments
Primarily T Cell Associated	
CD1	Expressed on cortical thymocytes and Langerhans histiocytes
CD2	Present on all T cells (thymic and peripheral) and NK cells
CD3	Expressed by thymocytes, peripheral T cells, and NK cells. Surface expression requires coexpression of T-cell receptor
CD4	Expressed on the helper subset of peripheral T cells, single positive medullary thymocytes, and CD4/CD8 double positive thymocytes
CD5	Expressed on all T cells and small subset of B cells
CD7	Expressed on all T cells and subset of myeloid cell precursors
CD8	Expressed on the cytotoxic subset of peripheral T cells, single positive medullary thymocytes, double positive cortical thymocytes, and some NK cells
Primarily B Cell Associated	
CD10	Expressed at high levels on marrow pre-B cells and follicular center B cells; also called CALLA
CD19	Present on marrow pre-B cells and mature B cells but not on plasma cells
CD20	Expressed on marrow pre-B cells after CD19 and mature B cells but not on plasma cells
CD21	EBV receptor; present on mature B cells and follicular dendritic cells
CD22	Present on mature B cells
CD23	Present on activated mature B cells
Primarily Monocyte or Macrophage Associated	
CD13	Expressed on immature and mature monocytes and granulocytes
CD14	Expressed on all monocytes
CD15	Expressed on all granulocytes; also expressed by Reed-Sternberg cells and variants in Hodgkin disease
CD33	Expressed on myeloid progenitors and monocytes
Primarily NK Cell Associated	
CD16	Present on all NK cells and granulocytes
CD56	Present on all NK cells and a subset of T cells
Primarily Stem Cell and Progenitor Cell Associated	
CD34	Expressed on pluripotent hematopoietic stem cells and progenitor cells of many lineages
Activation Markers	
CD30	Present on activated B cells, T cells, and monocytes
Present on All Leukocytes	
CD45	Also known as leukocyte common antigen (LCA)

CD, cluster designation; NK, natural killer; CALLA, common acute lymphoblastic leukemia antigen; EBV, Epstein-Barr virus.

they are emphasized and described first (Table 15–4A). The most salient immunophenotypic, karyotypic, and clinical features of the less common or rare entities of the REAL classification are summarized in Table 15–4B.

PRECURSOR B-CELL AND T-CELL NEOPLASMS

Acute Lymphoblastic Leukemia/Lymphoma

Acute lymphoblastic leukemia/lymphoma (ALL) encompasses a group of neoplasms composed of immature, precursor B (pre-B) or T (pre-T) lymphocytes referred to as *lymphoblasts. The majority (approximately 85%) of ALLs are pre-B cell tumors that typically manifest as childhood acute leukemias* with extensive bone marrow and variable peripheral blood involvement. The less common *pre-T cell ALLs tend to present in adolescent males as lymphomas, often with thymic involvement.* Considerable overlap is observed in the clinical behavior of pre-B cell and pre-T cell ALL; for example, pre-B cell tumors may present as *lymphomas*, and many pre-T cell tumors evolve to a leukemic peripheral blood picture. Malignant pre-B and pre-T lymphoblasts are also morphologically indistinguishable, and subclassification of ALL is thus dependent on immunophenotyping. Because of their morphologic and clinical similarities, the various forms of ALL are considered here together.

Approximately 2500 new cases of ALL are diagnosed each year in the United States, with most cases occurring in individuals younger than 15 years of age. It is almost twice as common in whites as in nonwhites and is slightly more frequent in boys than in girls. The peak incidence in children is at approximately 4 years of age. ALL also occurs in adults of all ages, but much less frequently.

MORPHOLOGY. Because of differing responses to chemotherapeutic agents, it is of great practical importance to differentiate ALL from acute myelogenous leukemia (AML), a neoplasm of immature myeloid cells that may cause identical signs and symptoms. Morphologic features that favor a lymphoid derivation for blasts include relatively condensed chromatin; the absence of conspicuous nucleoli; and the presence of scant, agranular cytoplasm (Fig. 15–6). Differentiation of AML and ALL on morphologic grounds alone is not possible in all cases, however, and for this reason leukemic blasts are typically analyzed for expression of myeloid and lymphoid surface markers (Fig. 15–7). Histochemical stains are also helpful, as lymphoblasts (in contrast to myeloblasts) lack peroxidase-positive granules and often contain cytoplasmic aggregates of periodic acid–Schiff (PAS)–positive material.

As noted, **ALLs with lymphomatous presentations are mostly of pre-T cell type, 50 to 70% of which are associated with mediastinal masses**

Table 15–4A. SUMMARY OF THE MOST COMMON LYMPHOID NEOPLASMS

Diagnosis	Immunophenotype	Genotype	Salient Clinical Features
Precursor B-cell acute lymphoblastic leukemia/lymphoma	Pre-B cells expressing TdT and lacking surface Ig; almost all positive for CD19, variable expression of CD10 and CD20	Diverse chromosomal translocations, many involving Ig loci. t(12;21) involving *TEL1* and *AML1* genes most common rearrangement	Predominantly children with symptoms relating to pancytopenia secondary to marrow involvement
Precursor T-cell acute lymphoblastic leukemia/lymphoma	Pre-T cells expressing CD1 and TdT; variable expression of other pan T-cell markers such as CD2, CD3, CD4, CD5, and CD8	Diverse chromosomal translocations, many involving T-cell receptor loci. Rearrangements of the *TAL1* gene are most common	Adolescent males with mediastinal masses. Variable splenic, hepatic, and bone marrow involvement
Small lymphocytic lymphoma/chronic lymphocytic leukemia	CD5-positive peripheral B-cell tumor; also expresses CD23, but negative for CD10. Expresses low levels of surface IgM	Trisomy 12, deletions of 11q23, abnormalities of 13q, t(14;19) (rare)	Older patients with bone marrow, lymph node, spleen, and liver disease. Most present with leukemic picture. Autoimmune hemolysis and thrombocytopenia in a minority
Follicular lymphoma	CD10-positive peripheral B-cell tumor; negative for CD5. Expresses high levels of surface Ig (usually IgG)	t(14;18) involving the *BCL2* gene; results in overexpression of BCL2 protein	Older patients with generalized lymphadenopathy and marrow involvement
Diffuse large B-cell lymphoma	Peripheral B-cell phenotype, with variable expression of CD5 and CD10. Usually surface Ig positive, negative for TdT	Diverse chromosomal aberrations. 30% contain the t(14;18); 20–30% have rearrangements of the *BCL6* gene on chromosome 3	All ages, but most common in adults. Often appears as a single rapidly growing mass. 30% extranodal
Burkitt lymphoma	Peripheral B cells expressing CD10 and surface IgM	Translocations involving c-*myc* and Ig loci; usually t(8;14), but also t(2;8) or t(8;22). African (endemic) cases latently infected with EBV	Adolescents or young adults with jaw or extranodal abdominal masses. Uncommonly presents similar to a leukemia (B-cell ALL)
Multiple myeloma/solitary plasmacytoma	Terminally differentiated B-cell tumor; expresses CD38 and cytoplasmic Ig	t(4;14)(p16.3;q32) (approximately 25% of cases), leading to increased expression of *FGFR3*	Myeloma; older patients with lytic bone lesions, pathologic fractures, hypercalcemia, renal failure, and primary amyloidosis. Plasmacytoma: isolated plasma cell masses in bone or soft tissue (e.g., oropharynx)

stemming from thymic involvement. Lymphadenopathy and splenomegaly are also more prevalent in pre-T cell ALL. Regardless of phenotype, the histologic appearance is similar, with normal tissue architecture completely effaced by lymphoblasts having scant cytoplasm and nuclei that are somewhat larger than those of small lymphocytes. **The nuclear chromatin is delicate and finely stippled, and nucleoli are either absent or inconspicuous.** In many cases, the nuclear membrane shows deep subdivision, imparting a convoluted (lobulated) appearance. In keeping with its aggressive growth, the tumor shows a high rate of mitosis, and as with other tumors having a high mitotic rate (e.g., Burkitt lymphomas), a **starry sky** pattern may be produced by interspersed benign macrophages.

Immunophenotype and Genetics. Immunostaining for terminal deoxytransferase (TdT), a specialized DNA polymerase that is expressed only by pre-B and pre-T lymphoblasts, is positive in greater than 95% of cases (Fig. 15–7). Subclassification of ALL is based on the origin of the lymphoblasts and their stage of differentiation and is summarized in Table 15–5. *Approximately 90% of patients with ALL have numerical or structural changes in the chromosomes of the leukemia cells,* most commonly hyperdiploidy (>50 chromosomes), but also pseudodiploidy; t(12;21); t(9;22) [Philadelphia chromosome]; and t(4;11). These alterations correlate with immunophenoytpe and sometimes affect prognosis. It is noteworthy that pre-B and pre-T ALL are associated with distinct sets of translocations, indicating that different molecular mechanisms underlie their pathogenesis.

Table 15–4B. SUMMARY OF THE LESS COMMON LYMPHOID NEOPLASMS

Diagnosis	Immunophenotype	Genotype	Salient Clinical Features
Lymphoplasmacytic lymphoma	Peripheral B-cell tumor; negative for CD5, CD10, and CD23. Expresses surface Ig (usually IgM) and cytoplasmic Ig in plasma cell component	t(9;14) in 50% of cases, apparently producing aberrant expression of PAX5, a transcription factor that is essential for normal B-cell differentiation	Older patients with marrow, lymph node, spleen, and liver disease. Often associated with a hyperviscosity syndrome (Waldenström macroglobulinemia). 10% have autoimmune hemolysis
Mantle cell lymphoma	CD5-positive peripheral B-cell tumor; negative for CD10 and CD23. Expresses surface IgM and IgD	t(11;14) involving the *BCL1* gene; results in overexpression of BCL1 protein (also known as cyclin D1)	Older male patients with lymphadenopathy and marrow involvement. May arise at extranodal sites or present as splenomegaly
Marginal zone lymphoma	Peripheral B-cell tumor; negative for CD5, CD10, and CD23. Expresses surface Ig and may have cytoplasmic Ig in plasma cell component	Trisomy 18, t(11;18)	Frequently arises at extranodal sites in adult patients with chronic inflammatory diseases. Tends to remain localized for long periods of time
Hairy cell leukemia	Peripheral B-cell tumor coexpressing CD11c, CD25, and surface Ig	No specific chromosomal rearrangements	Older males with pancytopenia and splenomegaly
Peripheral T-cell lymphoma, unspecified	Mature T-cell tumor; positive for pan T-cell markers and usually CD4 or CD8. Negative for TdT and CD1	Diverse chromosomal translocations. Clonal T-cell receptor rearrangements	Usually adult patients with generalized lymphadenopathy, sometimes accompanied by pruritus
Adult T-cell leukemia/lymphoma	CD4-positive mature T-cell tumor expressing CD25 (IL-2 receptor)	HTLV-1 provirus present in tumor cells	Adults with cutaneous lesions, marrow involvement, and hypercalcemia
Mycosis fungoides/Sézary syndrome	CD4-positive peripheral T-cell neoplasm expressing T-cell receptor α/β	No specific chromosomal abnormality described	Adult patients with cutaneous patches, plaques, nodules, or generalized erythema
Large granular lymphocytic leukemia[6–8]	Two types: (1) CD8-positive T cell expressing T-cell receptor α/β; and (2) true NK cell expressing CD2, CD16, and CD56	No specific chromosomal abnormality; NK tumors lack antigen receptor gene rearrangements	Adult patients with splenomegaly, neutropenia, and anemia, sometimes accompanied by autoimmune disease
Angiocentric lymphoma[9] (NK/T-cell lymphoma)	NK cell expressing CD2, cytoplasmic CD3, CD16, and CD56	No specific chromosomal abnormality. Clonal T-cell receptor rearrangements absent. Majority contain clonal EBV episomes	Adults with destructive sinonasal masses, often accompanied by hemophagocytic syndrome. Most common in China

TdT, terminal deoxytransferase; CD, cluster designation; Ig, immunoglobulin; EBV, Epstein-Barr virus; ALL, acute lymphoblastic leukemia/lymphoma; HTLV-1, human T-cell lymphotropic virus type 1; NK, natural killer.

Clinical Features. Although ALL and AML are immunophenotypically and genotypically distinct, they typically present with similar clinical features. This similarity stems from the fact that in both diseases there is an accumulation of neoplastic *blast* cells in the bone marrow that suppress normal hematopoiesis by physical crowding and other poorly understood mechanisms. The resultant failure of normal hematopoiesis is manifested by anemia, neutropenia, and thrombocytopenia, which underlie the major clinical features of both AML and ALL. These are listed, along with those features that are somewhat more characteristic of ALL, as follows:

- *Abrupt stormy onset*: Most patients present within days to a few weeks of the onset of symptoms.
- *Symptoms related to depression of normal marrow function*: Symptoms include fatigue mainly as a result of anemia; fever, reflecting an infection caused by absence of

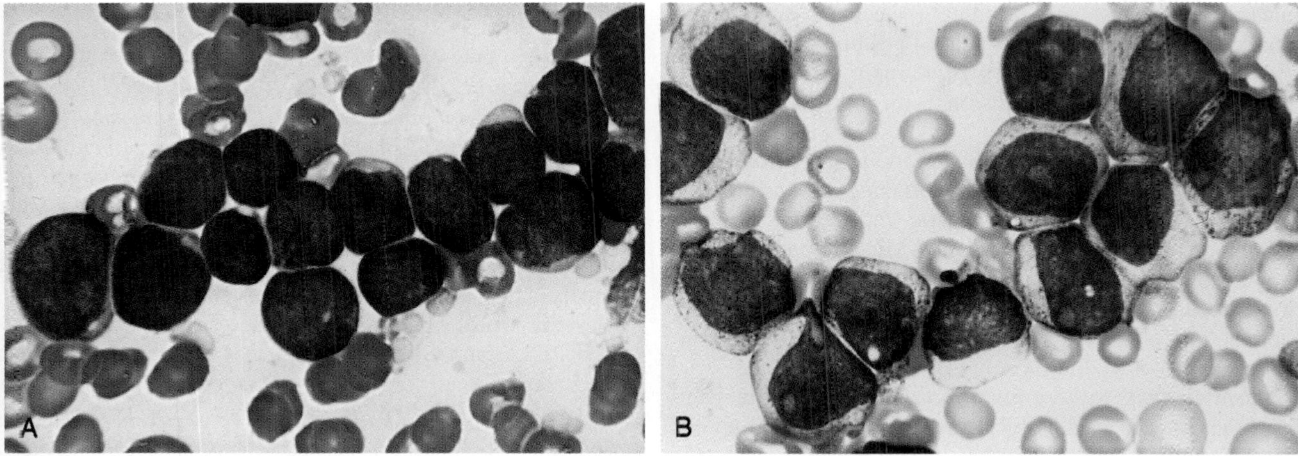

Figure 15–6

Morphologic comparison of lymphoblasts and myeloblasts. *A*, Acute lymphoblastic leukemia/lymphoma (ALL). Lymphoblasts have fewer nucleoli than do myeloblasts, and the nuclear chromatin is more condensed. Cytoplasmic granules are absent. *B*, Acute myeloblastic leukemia (AML, M1 subtype). Myeloblasts have delicate nuclear chromatin, prominent nucleoli, and fine azurophilic granules in the cytoplasm. (Courtesy of Dr. Robert W. McKenna, Department of Pathology, University of Texas Southwestern Medical School, Dallas, TX.)

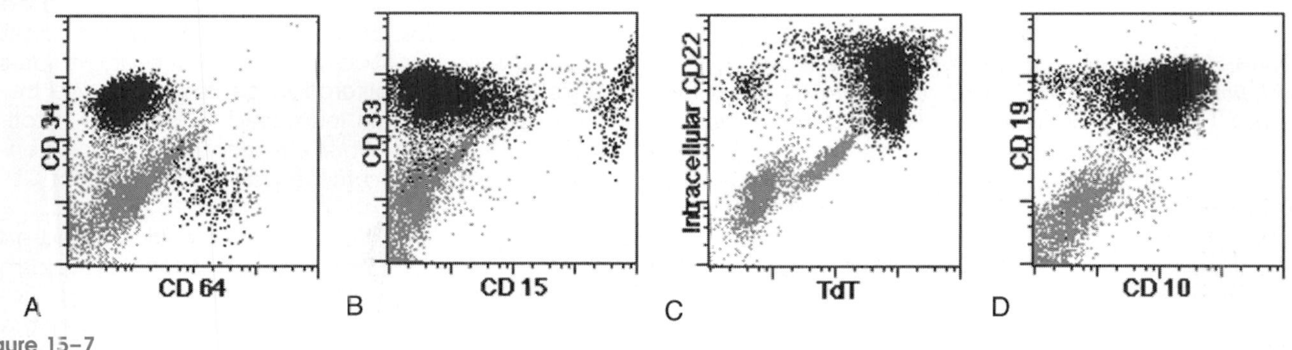

Figure 15–7

Immunophenotypic comparison of ALL and AML. *A* and *B* represent the phenotype of AML, M1 subtype (shown in 15–6*B*). The myeloid blasts, represented by the red dots, express CD34, a marker of multipotent stem cells, but do not express CD64, a marker of mature myeloid cells. In *B* the same myeloid blasts express CD33, a marker expressed by immature myeloid cells, and some cells also express CD15, a marker of more mature myeloid cells. Thus, these blasts are minimally differentiated myeloid cells. *C* and *D* represent the phenotype of a precursor B-cell ALL (shown in Fig. 15–6*A*). Note that the lymphoblasts represented by the red dots express TdT and the B-cell marker CD22 *(C)*. In *D* the same cells are seen to express two other B-cell markers, CD10 and CD19. Thus, these cells represent pre-B lymphoblasts. (Courtesy of Dr. Louis Picker, Department of Pathology, University of Texas Southwestern Medical School, Dallas, TX.)

Table 15–5. IMMUNOLOGIC CLASSIFICATION OF ACUTE LYMPHOBLASTIC LEUKEMIA/LYMPHOMA

	B Lineage Markers					T Lineage Markers			
Category	***TdT***	***CD19***	***CD10***	***Cμ***	***SIg***	***CD7***	***CD3***	***CD2***	**Frequency**
B lineage									
Very early pre-B	+	+	–	–	–	–	–	–	5–10%
Early pre-B	+	+	+	–	–	–	–	–	50–60%
Pre-B	+	+	+	+	–	–	–	–	20%
T lineage	+	–	–	–	–	+	+*	+	15%

TdT, terminal deoxytransferase; Cμ, cytoplasmic IgM heavy chain; SIg, surface immunoglobulin.
*CD3 staining may be cytoplasmic or membranous.

mature leukocytes; and bleeding (petechiae, ecchymoses, epistaxis, gum bleeding) secondary to thrombocytopenia.

- *Bone pain and tenderness*: Bone pain and tenderness result from marrow expansion with infiltration of the subperiosteum.
- *Generalized lymphadenopathy, splenomegaly, and hepatomegaly*: Lymphadenopathy, splenomegaly, and hepatomegaly are caused by neoplastic infiltration. Each is more common in ALL than in AML. In patients with pre-T cell ALL with a large mediastinal mass, symptoms related to invasion of large vessels or impending obstruction of airways may also be seen. Testicular involvement is also common in ALL.
- *Central nervous system manifestations*: Headache, vomiting, and nerve palsies resulting from meningeal spread are also more frequent in ALL than AML.

Truly dramatic advances have been made in the treatment of ALL. With aggressive chemotherapy (given together with prophylactic treatment of the central nervous system), more than 90% of children with ALL achieve complete remission, and at least two thirds can be considered cured. Children 2 to 10 years of age with early pre-B phenotype and hyperploidy, as well as those with a t(12;21) translocation, have an excellent prognosis. *Three factors have been consistently associated with a worse prognosis*: (1) *age under 2, possibly because of the strong association of infantile ALL with translocations involving the MLL gene on chromosome 11*[10]; (2) *presentation in adolescence or adulthood*; and (3) *the presence of the t(9;22) (the Philadelphia chromosome)*.[11] The t(9;22) is seen in only 3% of childhood ALL but is observed in up to 25% of adult cases, which may partially explain the poor outcome in adults.[12] Allogeneic bone marrow transplantation offers hope for those in poor prognostic categories.

PERIPHERAL B-CELL NEOPLASMS

Chronic Lymphocytic Leukemia and Small Lymphocytic Lymphoma

Chronic lymphocytic leukemia (CLL) and small lymphocytic lymphoma (SLL) are morphologically, phenotypically, and genotypically indistinguishable, differing only in the degree of peripheral blood lymphocytosis. Most patients have sufficient lymphocytosis to fullfill the diagnostic requirement for CLL (absolute lymphocyte count >4000/mm^3), which is the most common leukemia of adults in the Western world. In contrast, SLL constitutes only 4% of NHL. CLL and SLL are much less common in Japan and other Asian countries. *The tumor cells resemble a small subset of circulating B cells that express the surface marker CD5.*

MORPHOLOGY. Lymph node architecture is diffusely effaced by a predominant population of small lymphocytes of 6–12 μ containing round to slightly irregular nuclei with condensed chromatin and scant cytoplasm (Fig. 15–8). These cells are mixed with variable numbers of larger cells called **prolymphocytes.** In many cases, prolymphocytes gather together focally to form loose aggregates referred to as **proliferation centers,** so-called because they contain increased numbers of mitotically active cells. When present, proliferation centers are considered to be pathognomonic for CLL and SLL.[13]

In CLL, the peripheral blood contains increased small, round lymphocytes with scant cytoplasm (Fig. 15–9). These cells are fragile and are frequently disrupted in the process of making the

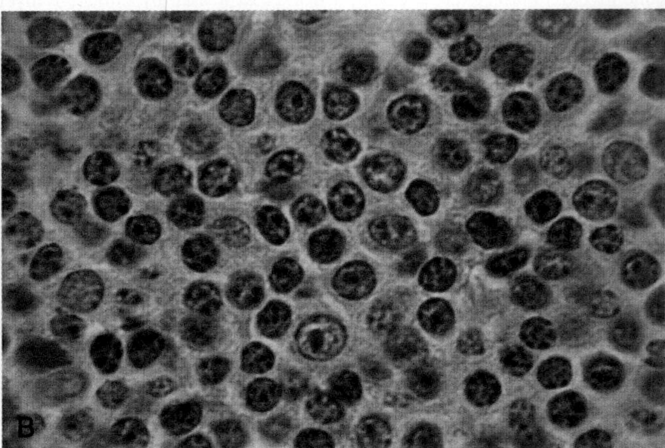

Figure 15–8

Nodal involvement by small lymphocytic lymphoma/chronic lymphocytic leukemia. *A*, Low-power view showing diffuse effacement of nodal architecture. At high power (*B*), most of the tumor cells have the appearance of small round lymphocytes. A single "prolymphocyte," a larger cell with a centrally-placed nucleolus, is also present in this field. (*A* courtesy of Dr. José Hernandez, Department of Pathology, University of Texas Southwestern Medical School, Dallas, TX.)

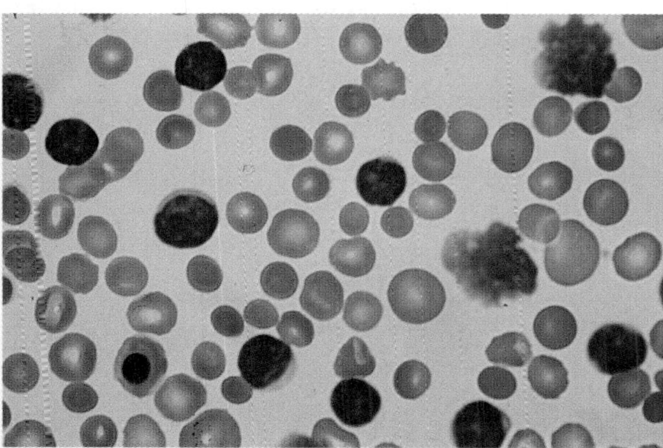

Figure 15–9

Chronic lymphocytic leukemia. This peripheral blood smear is flooded with small lymphocytes with condensed chromatin and scant cytoplasm. A characteristic finding is the presence of disrupted tumor cells (smudge cells). A coexistent autoimmune hemolytic anemia (see Chapter 14) has caused the appearance of spherocytes (hyperchromatic, round erythrocytes). In this case the severity of the anemia is such that immature erythroid forms are being released from the marrow; note the nucleated erythroid cell in the lower left-hand corner of the field. (Courtesy of Dr. Jacqueline Mitus.)

smear, producing so-called **smudge cells.** Involvement of the bone marrow is observed in all cases of CLL and most cases of SLL, taking the form of interstitial infiltrates or nonparatrabecular aggregates of small lymphocytes. Both the splenic white and red pulp and hepatic portal tracts (Fig. 15–10) are usually infiltrated by tumor cells, although the extent of involvement varies widely.

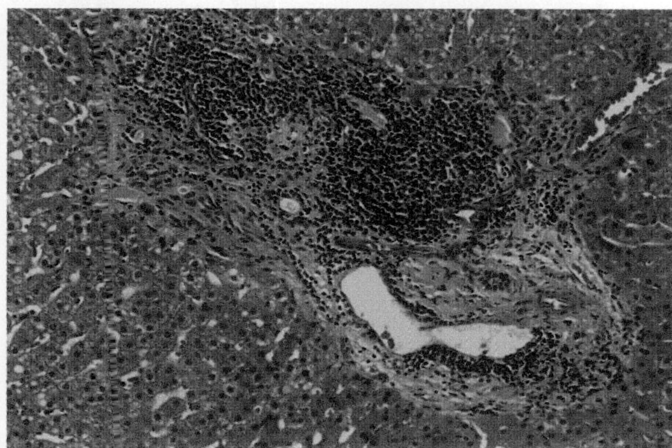

Figure 15–10

Small lymphocytic lymphoma/chronic lymphocytic leukemia in the liver. Low-power view of a typical periportal lymphocytic infiltrate. (Courtesy of Dr. Mark Fleming, Department of Pathology, Brigham and Women's Hospital, Boston, MA.)

Immunophenotype and Genetics. CLL and SLL have a distinctive immunophenotype. The tumor cells express the pan B-cell markers CD19 and CD20. In addition, CD5, a T-cell marker that is expressed only on a small subset of normal B cells, is present on the tumor cells. They typically also have low-level surface expression of Ig heavy chain (usually IgM or IgM and IgD) and either κ or λ light chain. The most common chromosomal anomalies are trisomy 12, deletions of 13q12-14, and deletions of 11q, each of which is seen in 20 to 30% of cases.[14,15]

Clinical Features. Most patients present at ages over 50 (median age, 60); a male predominance has been noted (2:1). *Patients with CLL and SLL are often asymptomatic.* When symptoms are present, they are nonspecific and include easy fatigability, weight loss, and anorexia. Generalized lymphadenopathy and hepatosplenomegaly are present in 50 to 60% of the cases. The total leukocyte count may be increased only slightly or may reach 200,000/mm^3. A small monoclonal Ig "spike" is present in the serum of some patients.

CLL and SLL disrupt normal immune function through uncertain mechanisms. Hypogammaglobulinemia is common and contributes to increased susceptibility to bacterial infections. Conversely, some 10 to 15% of patients develop autoantibodies directed against red blood cells or platelets that produce autoimmune hemolytic anemia or thrombocytopenia. These autoantibodies are polyclonal IgGs that are produced not by the tumor cells themselves, but by non-neoplastic, self-reactive B cells.[16]

The course and prognosis of CLL and SLL are extremely variable and depend primarily on the clinical stage. Overall the median survival is 4 to 6 years, but patients who present with minimal tumor burden may survive for 10 years or more. The presence of trisomy 12 and deletions of 11q correlate with higher-stage disease and portend a worse prognosis.[14,15]

An additional important factor in patient survival is the tendency of CLL and SLL to transform to more aggressive lymphoid neoplasms. Most commonly, this takes the form of *prolymphocytic transformation* (15 to 30% of patients) or transformation to diffuse large B-cell lymphoma (so-called *Richter syndrome*, seen in about 10% of patients). Prolymphocytic transformation is marked by appearance in the peripheral blood of large numbers of *prolymphocytes*, which are cells with a large nucleus containing a single, prominent, centrally placed nucleolus. In most cases, the transformed tumor is clonally related to the underlying CLL and SLL and retains a B-cell phenotype. Both prolymphocytic and large cell transformation are usually ominous events, with most patients surviving less than 1 year.[17]

Follicular Lymphoma

Follicular lymphoma is the most common form of NHL in the United States, comprising about 45% of adult lymphomas. It usually presents in middle age and afflicts men and women equally. It is less common in Europe and rare in Asian populations. *The neoplastic cells closely resemble normal germinal center B cells.*

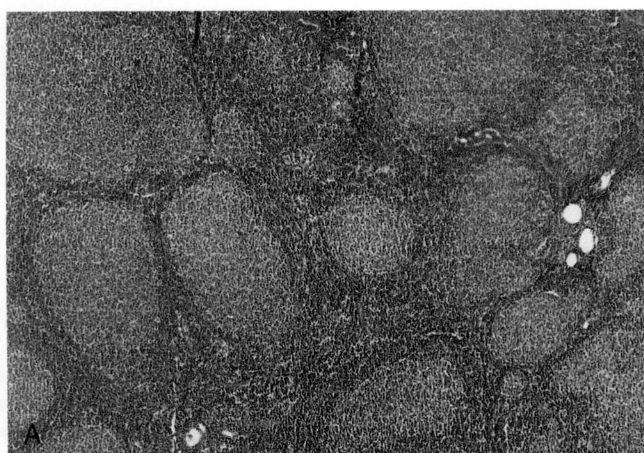

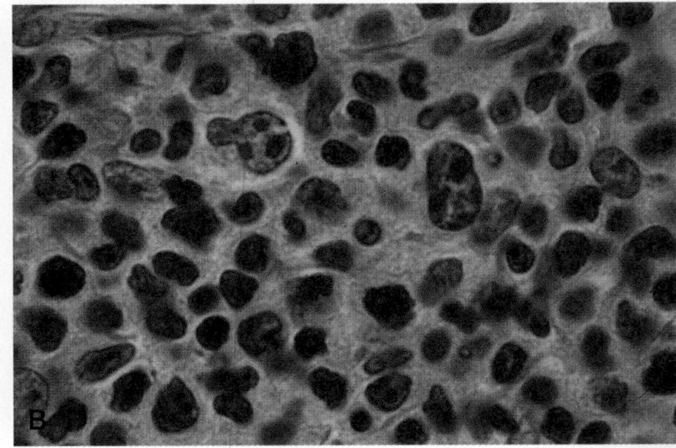

Figure 15–11

Non-Hodgkin lymphoma, follicular type, involving the lymph node. *A*, Nodular aggregates of lymphoma cells are present throughout the lymph node. At high magnification (*B*), small lymphoid cells with condensed chromatin and irregular or cleaved nuclear outlines (centrocytes) are mixed with a population of larger cells with nucleoli (centroblasts). (*A* courtesy of Dr. Robert W. McKenna, Department of Pathology, University of Texas Southwestern Medical School, Dallas, TX.)

MORPHOLOGY. In most cases, at low magnification, a predominantly nodular or nodular and diffuse growth pattern is observed in involved lymph nodes (Fig. 15–11). **Two principal cell types are observed in varying proportions: (1) small cells with irregular or cleaved nuclear contours and scant cytoplasm referred to as centrocytes (small cleaved cells)** and (2) **larger cells with open nuclear chromatin, several nucleoli, and modest amounts of cytoplasm referred to as centroblasts** (Fig. 15–11). In most follicular lymphomas, small cleaved cells compose the majority of the cellularity. Peripheral blood involvement sufficient to produce lymphocytosis (usually <20,000/mm^3) is seen in about 10% of patients. Bone marrow involvement occurs in 85% of patients and characteristically takes the form of paratrabecular lymphoid aggregates. Splenic white pulp (Fig. 15–12) and hepatic portal triads are also frequently involved.

Immunophenotype and Genetics. The neoplastic cells resemble normal follicular center B cells, expressing CD19, CD20, CD10 (common acute lymphoblastic leukemia antigen [CALLA]), and monotypic surface Ig. In contrast to CLL and SLL and mantle cell lymphoma, CD5 is not expressed. Follicular lymphoma cells also consistently express BCL2 protein, in distinction to normal follicular center B cells, which are BCL2 negative (Fig. 15–13).

The hallmark of follicular lymphoma is a (14;18) translocation, which leads to the juxtaposition of the IgH locus on chromosome 14 and the BCL2 locus on chromosome 18. This translocation is seen in most but not all follicular lymphomas[18] and leads to overexpression of BCL2 protein. BCL2, as seen in Chapters 1 and 7, is an antagonist of apoptotic cell death and appears to promote the survival of follicular lymphoma cells. Although reactive follicles contain numerous B cells undergoing apoptosis (as shown in Fig. 15–4), neoplastic follicles characteristically lack apoptotic cells.

Clinical Features. Follicular lymphomas tend to present with painless lymphadenopathy, which is frequently generalized. Involvement of extranodal sites, such as the gastrointestinal tract, central nervous system, or testis, is relatively uncommon. Although follicular lymphoma is incurable, it often follows an indolent waxing and waning course. The overall median survival is 7 to 9 years and is not improved

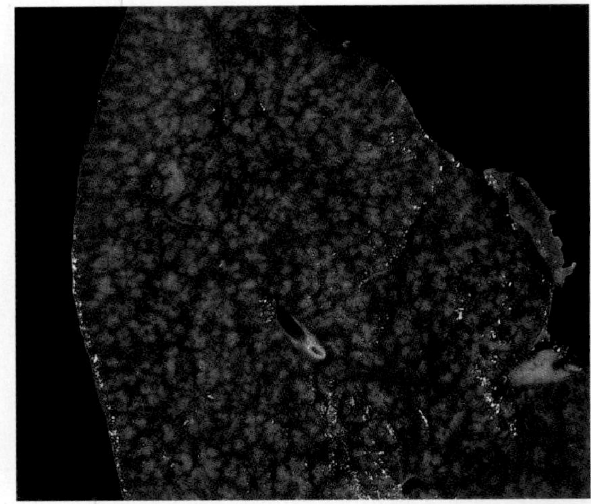

Figure 15–12

Non-Hodgkin lymphoma, follicular type, involving the spleen. Prominent nodules represent white pulp follicles expanded by follicular lymphoma cells. Other indolent B-cell lymphomas (small lymphocytic lymphoma, mantle cell lymphoma, marginal zone lymphoma) can produce an identical pattern of involvement. (Courtesy of Dr. Jeffrey Jorgenson, Department of Pathology, Brigham and Women's Hospital, Boston, MA.)

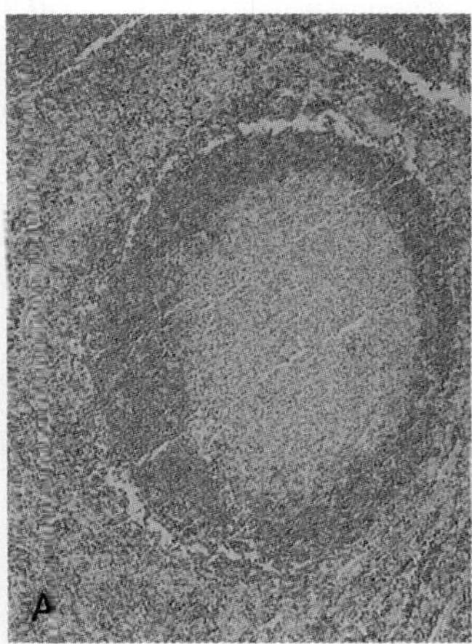
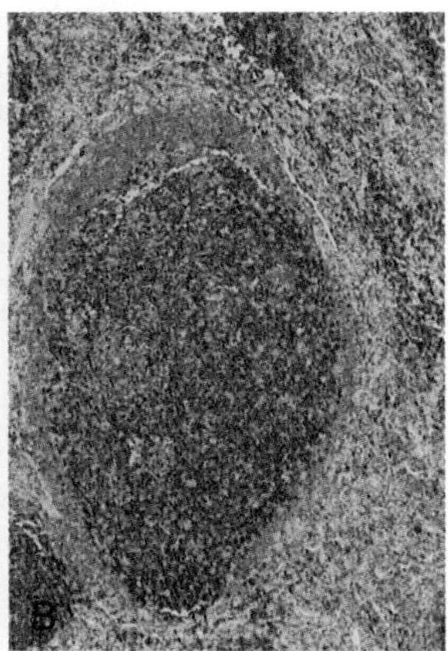

Figure 15–13 ■

BCL2 protein expression in reactive and neoplastic follicles. BCL2 protein was detected using an immunohistochemical technique that produces a brown stain. In reactive follicles (*A*), BCL2 is present in mantle zone cells but not follicular center B cells, whereas follicular lymphoma cells (*B*) exhibit strong BCL2 staining. (Courtesy of Dr. Jeffrey Jorgenson, Department of Pathology, Brigham and Women's Hospital, Boston, MA.)

by aggressive therapy; hence, the usual clinical approach is to palliate patients with low-dose chemotherapy or radiation when they become symptomatic.

Histologic transformation occurs in 30 to 50% of follicular lymphomas, most commonly to diffuse large B-cell lymphoma. Rarely, follicular lymphoma transforms to an aggressive tumor resembling lymphoblastic lymphoma or leukemia, an event usually associated with acquisition of a chromosomal translocation involving the c-*myc* locus. Median survival is less than 1 year after transformation.

Diffuse Large B-Cell Lymphoma

The diagnostic category of diffuse large B-cell lymphoma encompasses a heterogeneous group of tumors that together constitute about 20% of all NHL and 60 to 70% of aggressive lymphoid neoplasms. There is a slight male predominance, with a median age of about 60 years. The age range is wide, however, and diffuse large B-cell lymphoma constitutes about 5% of childhood lymphoma.

MORPHOLOGY. The common morphologic features that unite this group of neoplasms are a relatively large cell size (usually four to five times the diameter of a small lymphocyte) and a diffuse pattern of growth (Fig. 15–14). In other respects, there is a fair degree of morphologic variation. In most cases, the tumor cells have a round or oval nucleus that appears vesicular owing to margination of chromatin at the nuclear membrane, but large multilobated or cleaved nuclei predominate in some cases. Nucleoli may be two to three in number and located adjacent to the nuclear membrane or single and centrally placed. Cytoplasm is usually present in moderate abundance and may be pale or basophilic. Other more anaplastic tumors may contain multinucleated cells with large, inclusion-like nucleoli that closely resemble Reed-Sternberg (RS) cells (the tumor cell of HD), and in some difficult cases, phenotyping must be relied on to distinguish these two entities.

Immunophenotype and Genetics. These mature B-cell tumors express CD19 and CD20. Tumors of follicular center cell origin often express CD10. Most have surface Ig, and all are negative for TdT.

Within this group of tumors, about 30% contain the t(14;18), the characteristic chromosomal abnormality of follicular lymphoma.[18] Such tumors are considered to be of follicular center cell origin. An additional 20 to 30% of tumors contain various translocations that have in common a breakpoint involving the *BCL6* locus on chromosome 3.[19] The *BCL6* gene encodes a zinc-finger transcription factor that is normally expressed in germinal centers, consistent with a role in control of B-cell differentiation.[20] Tumors with *BCL6* rearrangements often arise at extranodal sites and uniformly lack *BCL2* rearrangements, suggesting the existence of at least two unique pathogenetic pathways for these neoplasms.

Special Subtypes. Two of several distinctive subtypes of large B-cell lymphoma, occuring in the setting of immunodeficiency states, including AIDS, are of sufficient pathogenetic interest to merit discussion.

- *Immunodeficiency-associated large B-cell lymphoma*: These tumors arise in the setting of severe T-cell immunodeficiency (e.g., end-stage HIV infection, severe combined immunodeficiency, allogeneic bone marrow transplantation, solid organ transplantation). *The neoplastic B cells are often latently infected with Epstein-Barr virus* (EBV), which is thought to play a critical pathogenic role. Restoration of T-cell immunity may lead to regression of such EBV-positive proliferations.

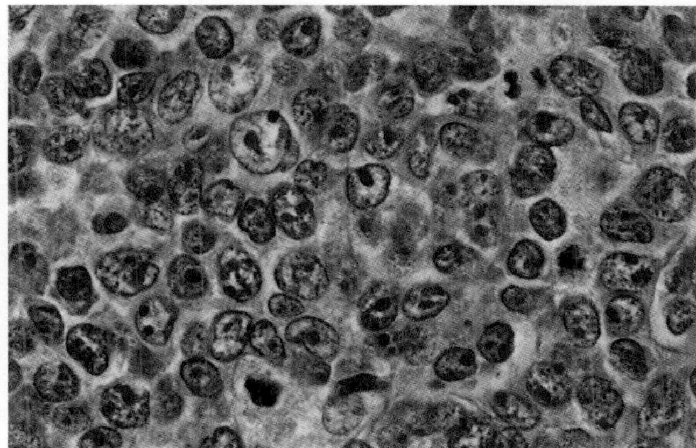

Figure 15–14 ■

Non-Hodgkin lymphoma, diffuse large B-cell type. Tumor cells have large nuclei, open chromatin, and prominent nucleoli. (Courtesy of Dr. Robert W. McKenna, Department of Pathology, University of Texas Southwestern Medical School, Dallas, TX.)

- *Body cavity large B-cell lymphoma*: These are large cell lymphomas that arise as malignant pleural or ascitic effusions. Most are seen in patients with advanced HIV infection, but a few cases have been observed in HIV-negative elderly adults.[21] The tumor cells often fail to express surface B-cell or T-cell markers but have clonal IgH gene rearrangements. *In all cases, the tumor cells are infected with human herpesvirus 8*, which may play a causal role in the development of this tumor.[22] Among the malignant lymphomas, human herpesvirus 8, which is also associated with Kaposi sarcoma (Chapter 7 and 12), has been observed only in this particular subtype.[23]

Clinical Course. *Patients with diffuse large B-cell lymphoma typically present with a rapidly enlarging, often symptomatic mass at a single nodal or extranodal site.* Involvement of the gastrointestinal tract, skin, bone, or brain may be the presenting feature. Waldeyer ring, the oropharyngeal lymphoid tissues that include the tonsils and adenoids, is also commonly involved. There may be large destructive masses in the liver and spleen (Fig. 15–15). Bone marrow involvement occurs late in the disease, and rarely a leukemic picture may emerge.

As a group, diffuse large B-cell lymphomas are aggressive tumors that are rapidly fatal if untreated. With intensive combination chemotherapy, however, complete remission can be achieved in 60 to 80% of the patients, and approximately 50% remain free from disease for several years and may be considered cured. Patients with limited disease fare better than patients with widespread disease or a large bulky tumor mass.[24] Tumors with *BCL6* rearrangements appear to have a better prognosis,[25] while the presence of *p53* mutations correlates with a worse outcome.[26]

Burkitt Lymphoma

Within the category of Burkitt lymphoma fall (1) African (endemic) Burkitt lymphoma, (2) sporadic (nonendemic) Burkitt lymphoma, and (3) a subset of aggressive lymphomas occurring in patients infected with HIV. Burkitt lymphomas occurring in these settings are histologically identical, but some clinical, genotypic, and virologic differences exist. The relationship of African Burkitt lymphoma to EBV is discussed in Chapter 7.

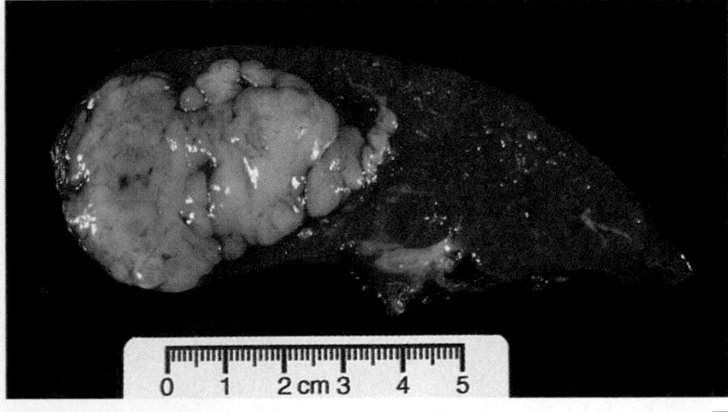

Figure 15–15

Non-Hodgkin lymphoma, large B-cell type, involving the spleen. The presence of an isolated large mass is typical. In contrast, indolent B-cell lymphomas usually produce multifocal expansion of white pulp (see Fig. 15–10). (Courtesy of Dr. Mark Fleming, Department of Pathology, Brigham and Women's Hospital, Boston, MA.)

MORPHOLOGY. Involved tissues are effaced by a diffuse infiltrate of intermediate-sized lymphoid cells, 10 to 25 μm in diameter, containing round or oval nuclei with coarse chromatin, several nucleoli, and a moderate amount of faintly basophilic or amphophilic cytoplasm (Fig. 15–16). The nuclear size approximates that of benign macrophages within the tumor. **A high mitotic index is typical, as is apoptotic tumor cell death,** accounting for the presence of numerous tissue macrophages with ingested nuclear debris. Because these benign macrophages, which are diffusely distributed among the tumor cells, are often surrounded by a clear space, they create a characteristic **starry sky pattern.** Occasionally, patients with Burkitt lymphoma present with a leukemic picture. In such cases, the tumor cells in marrow aspirates have slightly clumped nuclear chromatin, two to five distinct nucleoli, and royal blue cytoplasm containing multiple, clear cytoplasmic vacuoles.

Immunophenotype and Molecular Genetics. These are tumors of relatively mature B cells expressing surface IgM; monotypic κ or λ light chain; and CD19, CD20, and CD10.

*All forms of Burkitt lymphoma are highly associated with translocations of the c-*myc *gene on chromosome 8.* The partner is usually the IgH locus (t(8;14)), but may also be the κ (t(2;8)) or λ (t(8;22)) light-chain locus. There are subtle differences in the position of the chromosomal breakpoints in African and nonendemic Burkitt lymphoma that suggest that these two forms arise in different B-cell populations.[27] *Essentially all African tumors are latently infected with EBV*, which is also present in about 25% of HIV-associated tumors and in a minority of sporadic cases. Molecular analysis has shown that the configuration of the viral DNA is identical in all tumor cells within individual cases, indicating that infection precedes cellular transformation. While supporting a direct role for EBV in lymphomagenesis, this finding also raises interesting questions about the EBV negative tumors: Is another infectious agent involved in such cases, or can mutations in critical genes in the host genome mimic the effects of the transforming proteins of EBV on cell growth and differentiation?

Clinical Features. *Most tumors manifest at extranodal sites.* Endemic African Burkitt lymphoma often presents as a mass involving the mandible and shows an unusual predilection for involvement of abdominal viscera, particularly the kidneys, ovaries, and adrenal. In contrast, nonendemic Burkitt lymphoma most often presents as an abdominal mass involving the ileocecum and peritoneum. Both the African and the sporadic cases are found largely in children or young adults, accounting for approximately 30% of childhood NHLs in the United States. Evolution to a leuke-

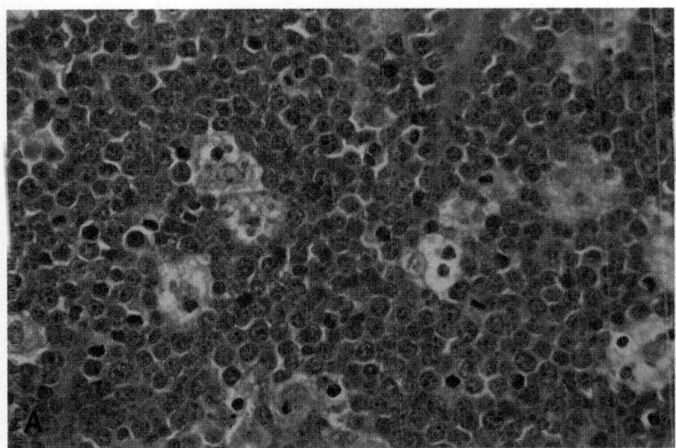
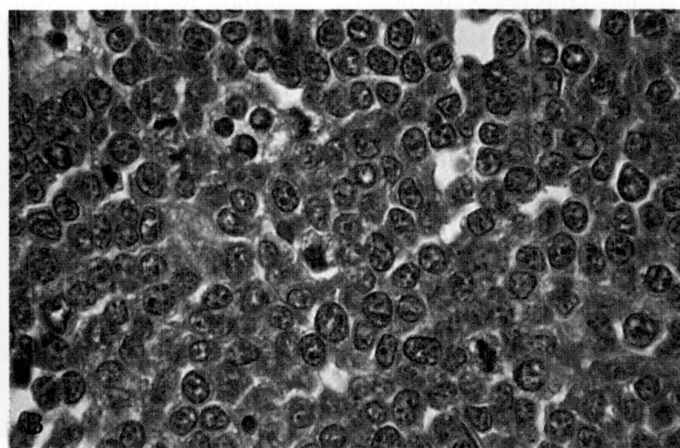

Figure 15–16

Burkitt lymphoma. At low power (*A*), numerous pale, tingible body macrophages are evident, producing a "starry sky" appearance. At high power (*B*), tumor cells have multiple small nucleoli and high mitotic index. The lack of significant variation in nuclear shape and size lends a monotonous appearance. (*B* courtesy of Dr. José Hernandez, Department of Pathology, University of Texas Southwestern Medical School, Dallas, TX.)

mic picture is uncommon, especially in African cases. Burkitt lymphoma is aggressive but responds well to short-term, high-dose chemotherapy, with many patients appearing to be cured.

Plasma Cell Neoplasms, Multiple Myeloma, and Related Entities

Plasma cell neoplasms and related entities are a group of lymphoid neoplasms of terminally differentiated B cells that have in common the expansion of a single clone of Ig-secreting plasma cells and a resultant increase in serum levels of a single homogeneous Ig or its fragments. In many but not all cases, these clonal proliferations (often referred to as *dyscrasias*) behave as malignant diseases. Collectively, these disorders account for about 15% of deaths from malignant white cell disease.

The monoclonal Ig identified in the blood is referred to as an M component in reference to *m*yeloma. Since complete M components have molecular weights of 160,000 or higher, they are restricted largely to circulating plasma and extracellular fluid. They may appear in the urine, however, when there is some form of glomerular damage with heavy proteinuria. *In normal plasma cells,* production and coupling of heavy and light chains is tightly balanced. *This balance is frequently lost in neoplastic plasma cells, leading to production of excess light or heavy chains along with complete Ig.* Occasionally, only light chains or heavy chains are produced, without complete Ig. The free light chains, known as *Bence Jones proteins*, are sufficiently small to be rapidly excreted in the urine and so are often totally cleared from the blood or present only at low levels. With renal failure or massive synthesis, however, they may appear in the blood in significant concentrations.

Designations applied to disorders associated with abnormal Ig include gammopathy, monoclonal gammopathy, dysproteinemia, and paraproteinemia. A variety of clinicopathologic entities are associated with monoclonal gammopathies, as follows:

- *Multiple myeloma* (*plasma cell myeloma*) is the most important and most common disorder. It is characterized by multiple tumorous masses of neoplastic plasma cells scattered throughout the skeletal system. *Solitary myeloma, or solitary plasmacytoma*, is an infrequent variant consisting of a solitary neoplastic mass of plasma cells found in bone or some soft tissue site.
- *Waldenström macroglobulinemia* is a syndrome stemming from serum hyperviscosity caused by high levels of IgM. It is most commonly seen in patients with lymphoplasmacytic lymphoma (and thus is discussed later in more detail under this entity) but may also be seen in association with tumors that morphologically resemble CLL and SLL and rare myelomas that secrete IgM. Although macroglobulinemia is unusual in myeloma, significant hyperviscosity is observed with some tumors, particularly those secreting large amounts of IgA or IgG_3.
- *Heavy-chain disease* is seen in a diverse group of disorders, including CLL and SLL, lymphoplasmacytic lymphoma, and an unusual small bowel lymphoma occurring in malnourished populations (so-called Mediterranean lymphoma). The common feature is synthesis and secretion of Ig heavy chain fragments.
- *Primary or immunocyte-associated amyloidosis* results from a monoclonal proliferation of plasma cells secreting free light chains (most commonly of λ isotype) that are subsequently processed and deposited as amyloid. While some patients with primary amyloidosis have overt multiple myeloma, others have only a minor clonal population of marrow plasma cells (Chapter 7).
- *Monoclonal gammopathy of undetermined significance* (*MGUS*) refers to instances in which M components are identified in the blood of patients having no symptoms or signs of any of the better-characterized monoclonal gammopathies.

Against this background, we can turn to some of the specific clinicopathologic entities. Primary amyloidosis was discussed along with other disorders of the immune system in Chapter 7.

Multiple Myeloma. *Multiple myeloma is a plasma cell neoplasm that is characterized by involvement of the skeleton at multiple sites.* Although bony disease dominates the clinical picture, it can also spread to lymph nodes and extranodal sites, such as the skin. Multiple myeloma causes 1% of all cancer deaths in Western countries. Its incidence is higher in men than in women, in people of African descent relative to the U.S. population at large, and in older adults as compared to the young.

Etiology and Pathogenesis. Although cells with mature plasma cell morphology and function accumulate within lesions, *phenotypic studies imply that the cell of origin is a less differentiated cell.* Small lymphoid cells within the peripheral blood have been shown to express Ig identical to that of neoplastic plasma cells, suggesting that they represent a progenitor cell population. Additionally, myeloma cells may express antigens typically associated with myelomonocytic cells (CD33), megakaryocytes (GpIIb/IIIa), and erythroid cells (glycophorin). Whether this is an example of neoplasia-induced *lineage infidelity* or an indication that the true cell of origin is a multipotent hematopoietic stem cell is unclear.

The proliferation and survival of myeloma cells seem to be dependent on several cytokines, most notably IL-6. Serum levels of this cytokine are increased in patients with active disease, and it appears that high serum IL-6 levels are associated with a poor prognosis.[28] IL-6 is produced by tumorous plasma cells and stromal cells in the marrow.[29] These observations have spurred therapeutic trials of antibodies directed against IL-6 in aggressive myeloma.[30] An interesting discovery is that marrow stromal cells of many myeloma patients are infected by human herpesvirus 8,[31] a virus implicated in other tumors (Kaposi sarcoma and certain large B-cell lymphomas), which carries a gene encoding a polypeptide structurally and functionally homologous to IL-6.

In addition to causing the growth of myeloma cells, *cytokines also mediate bone destruction—the major pathologic feature of multiple myeloma.* Loss of bone is in large part due to osteoclastic reabsorption induced by the tumor. A variety of cytokines produced by the tumor cells, particularly IL-1β and IL-6, serve as osteoclast-activating factors.[29]

The most frequent karyotypic abnormalities are deletions of 13q and rearrangements of 14q. Up to 30% of cases have a balanced translocation, t(4;14)(p16.3;q32), that places the *FGFR3* (fibroblast growth factor receptor 3) gene under the control of IgH promoter elements.[32] This results in increased expression of FGFR3, a member of a family of tyrosine kinase receptors implicated in control of cellular proliferation (Chapter 8).

MORPHOLOGY. Multiple myeloma presents most often as multifocal destructive bone lesions throughout the skeletal system. Although any bone may be affected, the following distribution was found in a large series of cases: vertebral column, 66%; ribs, 44%; skull, 41%; pelvis, 28%; femur, 24%; clavicle, 10%; and scapula, 10%. These focal lesions generally begin in the medullary cavity, erode the cancellous bone, and progressively destroy the cortical bone. Pathologic fractures are often produced by plasma cell lesions; they are most common in the vertebral column but may affect any of the numerous bones suffering erosion and destruction of their cortical substances. The bony defects are typically filled with soft, red tumor with a gelatinous consistency. **Most commonly, the lesions appear radiographically as punched-out defects, usually 1 to 4 cm in diameter** (Fig. 15–17), but in some of the cases only diffuse demineralization is evident.

Microscopic examination of the marrow reveals an increased number of plasma cells, which usually constitute greater than 30% of all cells. These cells may diffusely infiltrate the marrow or be present in sheetlike masses that completely replace normal elements. Similar to their normal counterparts, neoplastic plasma cells tend to have a perinuclear hof (owing to a prominent Golgi apparatus) and an eccentrically placed nucleus, features that allow their recognition (Fig. 15–18). Relatively normal-appearing plasma cells or a number of cytologic variants may predominate, including **plasmablasts,** having less condensed nuclear chromatin and prominent single nucleolus; **bizarre multinucleated cells,** which may

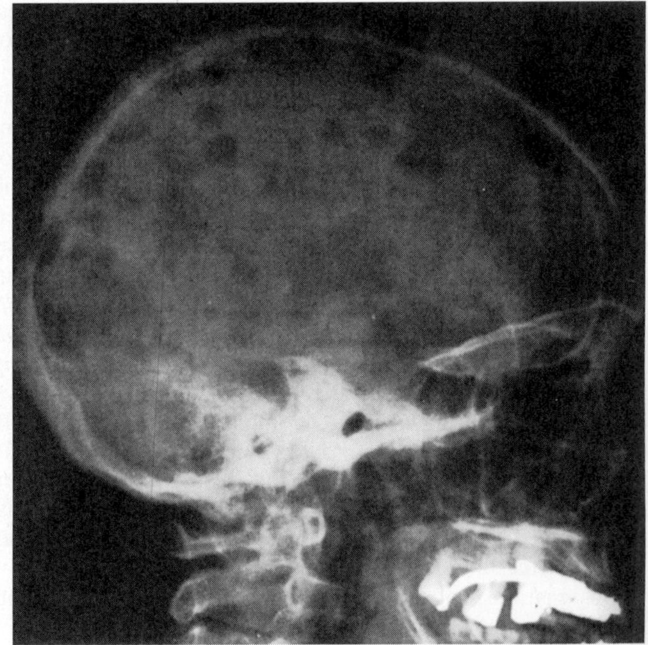

Figure 15–17

Multiple myeloma of the skull (radiograph, lateral view). The sharply punched-out bone lesions are most obvious in the calvarium.

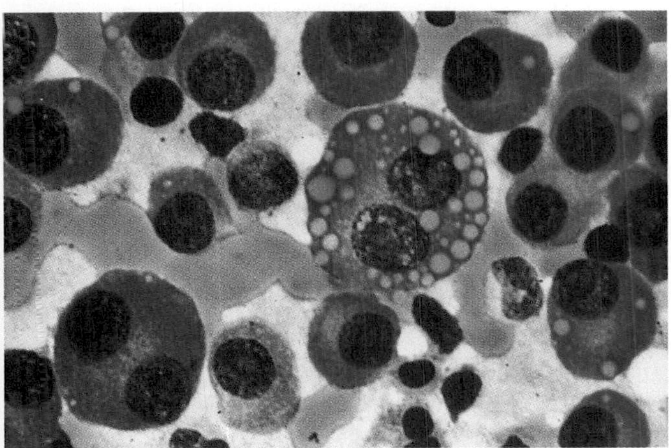

Figure 15–18

Multiple myeloma, bone marrow aspirate. Normal marrow cells are largely replaced by plasma cells, including atypical forms with multiple nuclei, prominent nucleoli, and cytoplasmic droplets containing immunoglobulin.

in some cases constitute most of the cellularity; **flame cells** with fiery red cytoplasm; **Mott cells,** having multiple blue, grapelike cytoplasmic droplets; and cells containing a variety of other cytoplasmic inclusions, including **fibrils, crystalline rods, Russell bodies, and their intranuclear counterpart, Dutcher bodies.** With progressive disease, plasma cell infiltrations of soft tissues may be encountered in the spleen, liver, kidneys, lungs, and lymph nodes or more widely.

Bence Jones proteins are excreted in the kidney and contribute to the renal involvement, generally called *myeloma kidney*, which is one of the more distinctive features of multiple myeloma. It is discussed in detail in Chapter 21.

Clinical Course. The peak age incidence of multiple myeloma is between 50 and 60 years. As previously stated, the *clinical features of myeloma stem from the effects of* (1) *infiltration of organs, particularly bones, by the neoplastic plasma cells*; (2) *the production of excessive Ig, which often has abnormal physicochemical properties*; and (3) *the suppression of normal humoral immunity.*

Infiltration of bones is manifested by pain and pathologic fractures. *Hypercalcemia* resulting from bone resorption may give rise to neurologic manifestations, such as confusion, weakness, lethargy, constipation, and polyuria, and also contributes to renal disease. Decreased production of normal Ig sets the stage for *recurrent infections* with bacteria such as *Streptococcus pneumoniae*, *Staphylococcus aureus*, and *Escherichia coli*. Cellular immunity is relatively unaffected. *Of great significance is renal insufficiency, which is second only to infections as a cause of death.* The pathogenesis of renal failure, which may occur in up to 50% of patients, is multifactorial and is discussed in Chapter 21. The most important factor appears to be Bence Jones proteinuria, since the excreted light chains are toxic to the tubular epithelial cells. *Amyloidosis* of the AL type occurs in some patients owing to excessive production of Ig light chains.

In 99% of patients with multiple myeloma, electrophoretic analysis reveals increased levels of Ig in the blood or light chains (Bence Jones proteins) in the urine, or both. The monoclonal Ig produces a high spike when serum or urine is subjected to electrophoresis. Immunoelectrophoresis or immunofixation is used to identify the nature of monoclonal Ig (Fig. 15–19). Quantitative analyses of monoclonal Ig usually reveal more than 3 gm of Ig per dl of serum and more than 6 mg of Bence Jones proteins per dl of urine. The most common serum monoclonal Ig (M protein) is IgG, which is found in 55% of patients. An

Normal serum

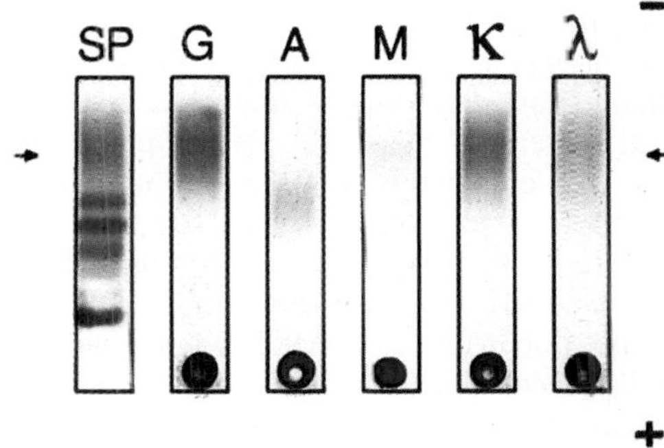

Patient serum

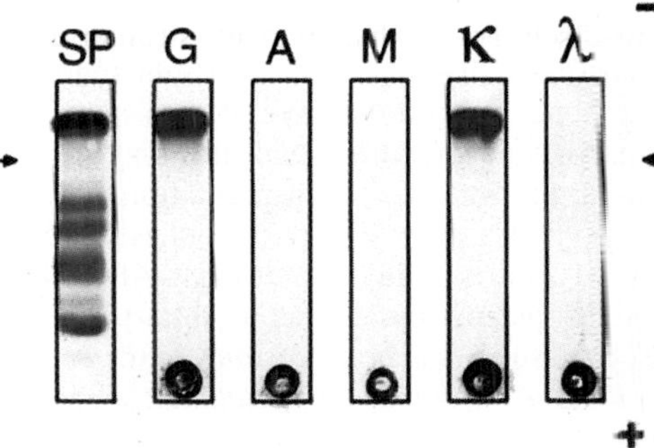

Figure 15–19

M-protein detection, multiple myeloma. Serum protein electrophoresis (SP) is used to screen for the presence of a monoclonal immunoglobulin (M protein). Polyclonal IgG in normal serum (denoted by the arrow) appears as a broad band; in contrast, serum from a patient with multiple myeloma contains a single sharp protein band in this region of the electropherogram. The suspected monoclonal immunoglobulin is then confirmed and characterized by immunofixation. In this procedure the electrophoresed proteins within the gel are reacted with specific antisera. After extensive washing, only proteins cross-linked by the antisera are retained in the gel, which is then stained for protein. Note that the sharp band in the immunoglobulin region of the patient's SP is recognized by antisera against IgG heavy chain (G) and kappa light chain (κ), indicating that this band is an IgGκ M protein. The levels of polyclonal IgG, IgA (A), and lambda light chain (λ) are also decreased in the patient serum relative to normal serum, a common finding in multiple myeloma. (Courtesy of Dr. David Sacks, Department of Pathology, Brigham and Women's Hospital, Boston, MA.)

additional 25% of cases are associated with an IgA M protein. Myelomas expressing IgM, IgD, or IgE occur but are rare. Excessive production and aggregation of M proteins leads to the hyperviscosity syndrome (described under lymphoplasmacytic lymphoma) in approximately 7% of patients, most of whom have tumors that secrete IgA or IgG_3.

Bence Jones proteinuria and a serum M protein are both observed in 60 to 70% of all myeloma patients. In approximately 20% of patients, however, Bence Jones proteinuria is present as a isolated finding. It should also be noted that about 1% of myelomas are nonsecretory and thus occur in the absence of detectable serum or urine M proteins. Hence, the absence of paraproteinemia and paraproteinuria does not exclude myeloma.

The clinicopathologic diagnosis of multiple myeloma rests on radiographic and laboratory findings. The radiographic changes are so distinctive that a reasonably certain diagnosis can usually be made. *Classically the individual lesions appear as sharply punched-out defects having a rounded soap-bubble appearance on x-ray film, but generalized osteoporosis may also be seen.* Marrow examination may reveal increased interstitial plasma cells or sheetlike aggregates that completely replace the normal elements. Extensive marrow involvement gives rise to a normocytic normochromic anemia, sometimes accompanied by moderate leukopenia and thrombocytopenia. Rarely, neoplastic plasma cells flood the peripheral blood, giving rise to *plasma cell leukemia.*

The prognosis for this condition is variable but generally poor. Patients with multiple bony lesions, if untreated, rarely survive for more than 6 to 12 months, whereas occasional patients with *indolent myeloma* can survive for many years. Chemotherapy in the form of alkylating agents induces remission in 50 to 70% of patients, but the median survival is still a dismal 3 years. Biphosphonates, drugs that inhibit bone resorption, have shown some promise in reducing pathologic fractures and limiting hypercalcemia. Autologous bone marrow transplantation after intensive chemotherapy may improve survival but is noncurative.[33]

Solitary Myeloma (Plasmacytoma). About 3 to 5% of plasma cell neoplasms present as a solitary lesion of either bone or soft tissue. *The bony lesions tend to occur in the same locations as in multiple myeloma. Extraosseous lesions are often located in the lungs, oronasopharynx, or nasal sinuses.* Modest elevations of M proteins in the blood or urine may be found in a minority of patients.

When patients with such localized disease are followed, *progression to classic multiple myeloma becomes manifest in most patients with osseous plasmacytoma, whereas extraosseous tumors disseminate in only a minor fraction of patients.* It appears that the solitary plasmacytoma involving the bones is an early stage of multiple myeloma, but in some individuals it may be present for 10 to 20 years without progression. Extraosseous plasmacytomas, particularly those involving the upper respiratory tract, represent limited disease that can often be cured by local resection.

Monoclonal Gammopathy of Uncertain Significance (MGUS). M proteins can be identified in the serum of 1% of asymptomatic healthy persons older than 50 years of age and in 3% older than 70 years of age. *This dysproteinemia without associated disease is considered MGUS,* which is the most common form of monoclonal gammopathy.

Approximately 20% of patients with MGUS develop an overt plasma cell dyscrasia (usually multiple myeloma) over a period of 10 to 15 years. The diagnosis of MGUS should be made with caution and after careful exclusion of other causes of monoclonal gammopathy, particularly indolent multiple myeloma. In general, patients with MGUS have less than 3 gm/dl of monoclonal protein in the serum and no Bence Jones proteinuria.

Whether a given patient with MGUS will follow a benign course, as most do, or develop a well-defined plasma cell neoplasm cannot be predicted, and hence periodic assessment of serum M component levels and Bence Jones proteinuria is warranted.

Lymphoplasmacytic Lymphoma (Waldenström Macroglobulinemia)

Lymphoplasmacytic lymphoma (LPL) is a B-cell neoplasm of older adults that usually presents in the sixth or seventh decade of life. It has gone by a variety of monikers, including *small lymphocytic lymphoma with plasmacytic differentiation* and *immunocytoma.* Although bearing a superficial resemblance to CLL and SLL, it differs in that a substantial fraction of the tumor cells undergo terminal differentiation to plasma cells. *Most commonly, the neoplastic plasma cells secrete monoclonal IgM, often in amounts sufficient to cause a hyperviscosity syndrome known as Waldenström macroglobulinemia.*

MORPHOLOGY. Typically, there is a diffuse, sparse-to-heavy infiltrate in the bone marrow of lymphocytes, plasma cells, and intermediate plasmacytoid lymphocytes (so-called **plymphocytes**), often accompanied by a reactive hyperplasia of mast cells (Fig. 15–20). PAS-positive inclusions containing Ig may be seen in the cytoplasm **(Russell bodies)** or nucleus **(Dutcher bodies)**. Tumorous masses causing bony erosions, a feature characteristic of multiple myeloma (described later), are not seen. A similar polymorphous infiltrate may be present in the lymph nodes, spleen, or liver in patients having disseminated disease. Infiltration of the nerve roots, meninges, and more rarely the brain may also occur.

Clinical Course. The dominant presenting complaints are weakness, fatigue, and weight loss—all nonspecific symptoms. Approximately half the patients have *lymphadenopathy, hepatomegaly,* and *splenomegaly.* Anemia caused by marrow infiltration is often present and may be exacerbated by *autoimmune hemolysis,* which is seen in about 10% of patients. Hemolysis is caused by *cold agglutinins,* IgM antibodies that bind to erythrocytes at temperatures of less than 37°C.

Patients with IgM-secreting tumors have additional complaints that stem from the physicochemical properties of macroglobulin.[34] Because of its large size and increased

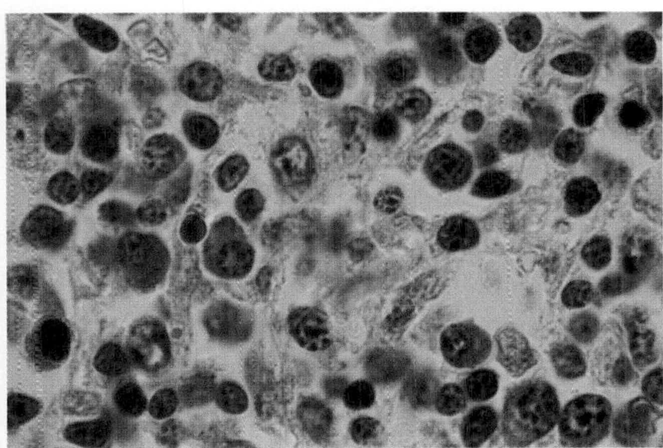

Figure 15-20

Lymphoplasmacytic lymphoma. Bone marrow biopsy shows a characteristic mixture of small lymphoid cells exhibiting various degrees of plasma cell differentiation. In addition, a mast cell with purplish-red cytoplasmic granules is present at the left-hand side of the field.

concentration in blood, IgM tends to increase the viscosity of the blood, giving rise to a *hyperviscosity syndrome*. This syndrome is characterized by the following features:

- *Visual impairment* resulting from the striking tortuosity and distention of retinal veins as well as retinal hemorrhages and exudates
- *Neurologic problems*, such as headaches, dizziness, deafness, and stupor, stemming from sluggish blood flow and sludging
- *Bleeding* related to the formation of complexes between macroglobulins and clotting factors as well as interference with platelet functions
- *Cryoglobulinemia* resulting from precipitation of macroglobulins at low temperatures, producing symptoms such as Raynaud phenomenon and cold urticaria

Lymphoplasmacytic lymphoma is an incurable progressive disease. Because IgM is mostly intravascular, symptoms caused by high levels of IgM (such as hyperviscosity and hemolysis) can be alleviated by plasmapheresis. Transformation to large cell lymphoma occurs uncommonly. Median survival is about 4 years.

Mantle Cell Lymphoma

Mantle cell lymphoma comstitutes about 3% of NHL in the United States and a somewhat higher fraction of NHL in Europe (7 to 9%). It usually presents in people in the forties to fifties and shows a male predominance. As the name implies, *the tumor cells closely resemble the normal mantle zone cells that surround follicular centers, and have distinctive cytogenetic and molecular abnormalities.*

MORPHOLOGY. Two patterns of lymph node involvement are observed: (1) a mantle zone pattern in which tumor cells surround or efface B-cell follicles, producing a vaguely nodular appearance at low power, and (2) a diffuse pattern. Regardless of the pattern, **in most cases, the proliferation consists of a homogeneous population of small lymphocytes with round to irregular to occasionally deeply clefted (cleaved) nuclear contours** (Fig. 15-21). Large cells resembling centroblasts are usually absent, as are proliferation centers, helping to distinguish mantle cell lymphoma from follicular lymphoma and CLL and SLL.[9] In most cases, the nuclear chromatin is condensed, nucleoli are inconspicuous, and cytoplasm is scant.

From 20 to 40% of patients have peripheral blood lymphocytosis, usually less than 20,000 mm³. The majority of patients present with bone marrow involvement, which usually takes the form of nonparatrabecular and paratrabecular lymphoid ag-

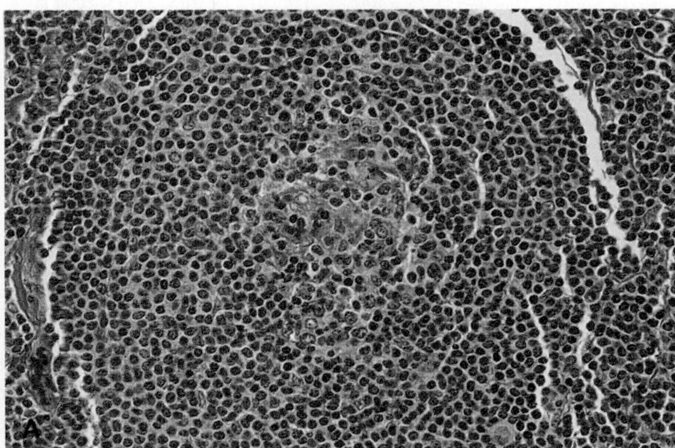

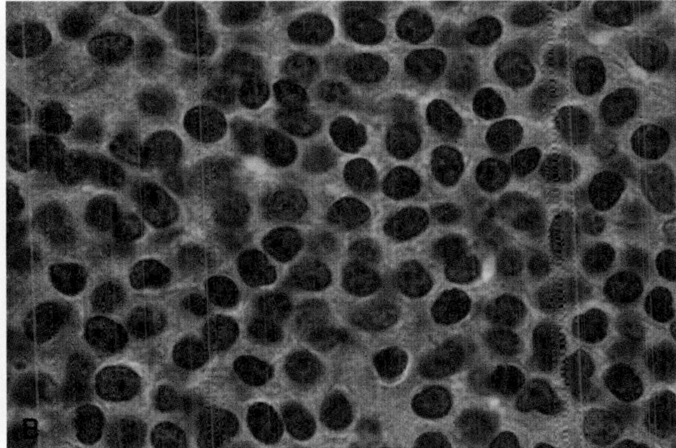

Figure 15-21

Non-Hodgkin lymphoma, mantle cell type. At low power (*A*), neoplastic lymphoid cells surround a small, atrophic germinal center, exhibiting a mantle zone pattern of growth. A high-power view (*B*) shows a homogeneous population of small lymphoid cells with somewhat irregular nuclear outlines, condensed chromatin, and scant cytoplasm. Large cells resembling "prolymphocytes" (seen in chronic lymphocytic leukemia) and centroblasts (seen in follicular lymphoma) are absent.

gregates. Splenic involvement is common, with tumor cells preferentially expanding white pulp zones, as is periportal infiltration of the liver. Extranodal disease is also relatively common in mantle cell lymphoma. Occasionally, multifocal mucosal involvement of the small bowel and colon produces **lymphomatoid polyposis**; of all forms of NHL, mantle cell lymphoma is most likely to spread in this fashion.

Immunophenotype and Genetics. Mantle cell lymphoma is a B-cell neoplasm that expresses CD19, CD20, moderately high levels of surface Ig heavy chain (usually IgM and IgD), and either κ or λ light chain. It is usually CD5 positive and CD23 negative, which can help to distinguish it from CLL and SLL. Expression of CD5 may be aberrant because normal mantle zone cells are CD5 negative.

Further distinctiveness is conferred to mantle cell lymphoma by the frequent occurrence of an (11;14) translocation involving the IgH locus on chromosome 14 and a locus on chromosome 11 variously known as BCL1 (not BCL2) or PRAD1. The t(11;14) is detected in about 70% of cases by cytogenetics and an even higher fraction of tumors analyzed by fluorescent in situ hybridization.[35] The *BCL1* locus encodes cyclin D1, a protein involved in the regulation of G_1 to S phase progression during the cell cycle. BCL1 rearrangements lead to increased expression of cyclin D1 protein,[36] which may contribute to tumorigenesis by causing loss of cell cycle control.

Clinical Features. Most patients present with generalized lymphadenopathy, bone marrow, and liver involvement. Splenomegaly is present in about 50% of patients. B symptoms (fever and weight loss) are observed in a minority of patients.

The prognosis for mantle cell lymphoma patients is poor, as the median survival is only 3 to 4 years. Mantle cell lymphoma is not curable with conventional chemotherapy, and most patients eventually succumb to organ dysfunction caused by tumor infiltration. For unclear reasons, histologic transformation occurs less frequently in mantle cell lymphoma than in CLL and SLL or follicular lymphoma.

Marginal Zone Lymphoma (MALToma)

The category of marginal zone lymphoma encompasses a heterogeneous group of B-cell tumors that may primarily arise within the lymph nodes, spleen, or within extranodal tissues. Although all marginal zone lymphomas share certain morphologic and immunophenotypic features, those arising at extranodal sites deserve special attention because of their unusual pathogenesis. These are predominantly tumors of middle-aged adults and are exceptional in three regards: (1) *they tend to arise within tissues involved by chronic inflammatory disorders of autoimmune (e.g., the salivary gland in Sjögren disease and the thyroid gland in Hashimoto thyroiditis) or infectious (e.g., the stomach in* Helicobacter *gastritis) origin*; (2) *they remain localized for prolonged periods at sites of origin, spreading systemically only late in their course*; and (3) *they are composed of cells at various stages of B lymphoid differentiation, often including terminally differentiated plasma cells.* Because these tumors were initially recognized at mucosal sites, they have been referred to as tumors of *m*ucosa-*a*ssociated *l*ymphoid *t*issues (or *MALT*oma). In most cases, the predominant tumor cell population bears a resemblance to normal marginal zone B cells, and under the REAL classification all are considered variants of marginal zone lymphoma.

The process begins as a reactive, polyclonal immune reaction.[37] Over time, a monoclonal B-cell neoplasm emerges, probably because of acquired genetic changes, that is still dependent on reactive T helper cells for growth and survival.[38] With further clonal evolution, spread to distant sites and transformation to diffuse large B-cell lymphoma may occur. This theme of polyclonal-to-monoclonal transition during lymphomagenesis is also applicable to the pathogenesis of human T-cell lymphotropic virus type 1 (HTLV-1)–induced and EBV–induced lymphoma and is more fully discussed in Chapter 8.

Hairy Cell Leukemia

Hairy cell leukemia is a rare but distinctive B-cell neoplasm of uncertain origin that constitutes about 2% of all leukemias. It is predominantly a disease of middle-aged white men (male-to-female ratio of 4:1).

MORPHOLOGY. Hairy cell leukemia derives its picturesque name from the appearance of the leukemic cells, which have fine hairlike projections that are best recognized under the phase-contrast microscope (Fig. 15–22). On routine peripheral blood smears, hairy cells have round, oblong, or reniform nuclei and modest amounts of pale blue cytoplasm, often with threadlike or bleblike extensions. The number of circulating cells is highly variable. The bone marrow is always involved by a diffuse interstitial infiltrate of cells with oblong or reniform nuclei, condensed chromatin, and abundant pale cytoplasm. Because these cells are usually entrapped in an extracellular matrix composed of reticulin fibrils, tumor cells are frequently absent from bone marrow aspirate smears. The red pulp of the spleen is preferentially infiltrated by hairy cells, leading to a beefy red, gross appearance and obliteration of white pulp. Hepatic portal triads are also frequently infiltrated.

Histochemistry and Immunophenotype. A cytochemical feature that is characteristic of hairy cell leukemia is the presence of tartrate-resistant acid phosphatase in the neoplastic B cells. The hairy cells also usually express the pan B-cell markers CD19 and CD20, surface IgH (usually IgG), and either κ or λ light chain, the monocyte-associated antigen CD11c, CD25 (the IL-2 receptor), and plasma cell-associated antigen-1 (PCA-1). The precise cell of origin is unknown.

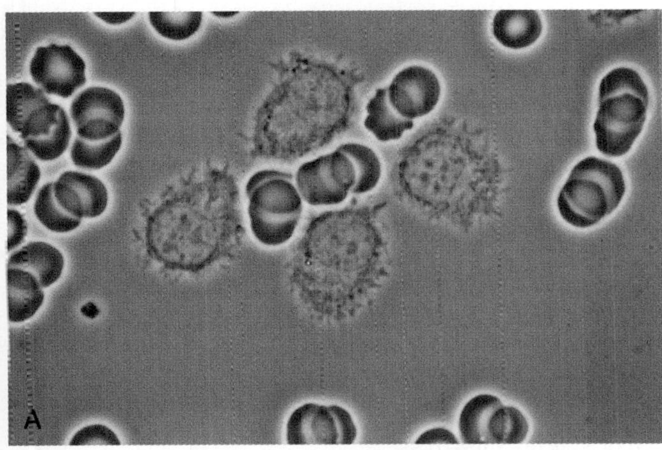

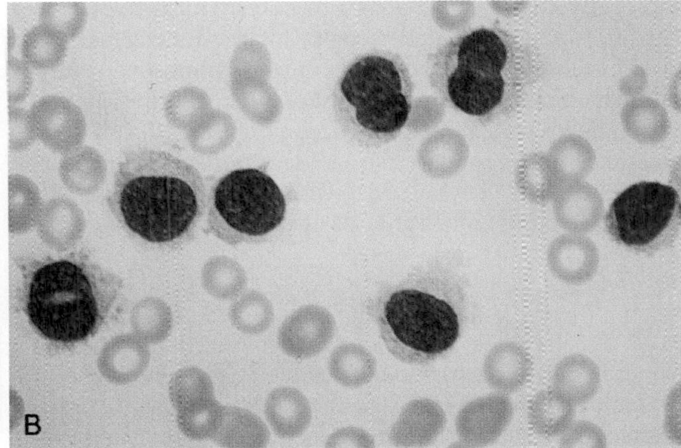

Figure 15–22

Hairy cell leukemia in peripheral blood. *A*, Phase contrast microscopy shows tumor cells with fine, hairlike cytoplasmic projections. In stained smears (*B*), these cells have round or folded nuclei and modest amounts of pale-blue, agranular cytoplasm. (Courtesy of Dr. David Weinberg, Department of Pathology, Brigham and Women's Hospital, Boston, MA.)

Clinical Features. Clinical manifestations largely result from infiltration of bone marrow, liver, and spleen. *Splenomegaly*, often massive, is the most common and sometimes the only abnormal physical finding. *Hepatomegaly* is less common and not as marked, and lymphadenopathy is distinctly rare. *Pancytopenia*, resulting from marrow failure and splenic sequestration, is seen in more than half the cases. About one third of patients present with *infections*. One unusual feature is a high incidence of atypical mycobacterial infection,[39] possibly related in part to frequent monocytopenia.

Hairy cell leukemia tends to follow an indolent course. For unclear reasons, the tumor cells are exceptionally sensitive to particular chemotherapeutic regimens, which produce long-lasting remissions in a majority of patients.[40] Whether such patients are truly cured is not yet known.

PERIPHERAL T-CELL AND NATURAL KILLER CELL NEOPLASMS

Peripheral T-cell and NK cell neoplasms include a heterogeneous group of neoplasms having phenotypes resembling mature T cells or NK cells. Peripheral T-cell tumors comprise about 15% of NHLs in the United States and Europe but are substantially more common in Asia. NK cell tumors are rare in the Westen hemisphere but also relatively common in the Far East.

Peripheral T-Cell Lymphoma, Unspecified

Although the REAL classification includes a number of distinct forms of peripheral T-cell neoplasia, peripheral T-cell lymphomas as a group are heterogeneous and not easily categorized. In recognition of this, a "wastebasket" diagnostic category, *peripheral T-cell lymphoma, unspecified*, has been created.

Although no morphologic feature is pathognomonic of peripheral T-cell lymphomas, certain findings are characteristic. The tumors diffusely efface the architecture of involved lymph nodes and are typically composed of a pleomorphic mixture of small, intermediate, and large-sized malignant T cells (Fig. 15–23). They may have a prominent infiltrate of reactive cells such as eosinophils and macrophages, probably attracted by T cell–derived cytokines. Prominent angiogenesis is also sometimes seen.

The diagnosis can be confirmed only by immunophenotyping. By definition, all peripheral T-cell lymphomas have a mature T-cell phenotype, lacking TdT and usually expressing CD2, CD5, surface CD3, and either T-cell $\alpha\beta$ or $\delta\gamma$ receptors. Many variations on this theme are possible, however, and some tumors have phenotypes that are considered aberrant for peripheral T cells, such as CD5 or

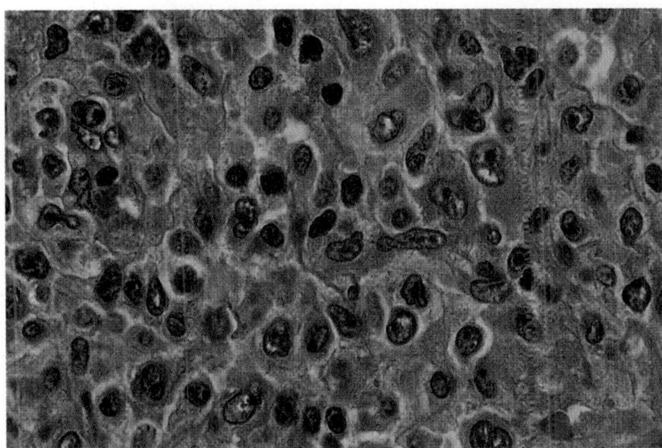

Figure 15–23

Peripheral T-cell lymphoma, unspecified, involving a lymph node. A spectrum of small, intermediate, and large lymphoid cells, many with irregular nuclear contours, is seen.

CD7 negative. In a high fraction of cases, clonal rearrangements of at least one T-cell receptor locus are detected.

Most patients present with generalized lymphadenopathy, sometimes accompanied by eosinophilia, pruritus, fever, and weight loss. Although cures of peripheral T-cell lymphoma have been reported, the incidence of relapse appears to be higher than that observed with aggressive mature B-cell neoplasms (e.g., diffuse large B-cell lymphoma).

Adult T-Cell Leukemia/Lymphoma

Adult T-cell leukemia/lymphoma is a neoplasm of CD4+ T cells observed in patients infected by *HTLV-1* (Chapter 7). It is most frequent in regions where HTLV-1 is endemic (southern Japan and the Caribbean basin) and is characterized by skin lesions, generalized lymphadenopathy, hepatosplenomegaly, peripheral blood lymphocytosis, and hypercalcemia. The appearance of the tumor cells varies widely, but frequently cells with multilobated nuclei, described as *cloverleaf* or *flower* cells, are found in involved tissues and peripheral blood. Less commonly, multinucleated giant cells resembling RS cells may be present. *The tumor cells contain clonal HTLV-1 provirus, compatible with direct pathogenic involvement of the virus in this neoplasm.*

Most patients present with rapidly progressive disease that is fatal within months to 1 year despite aggressive chemotherapy. Less commonly, the tumor primarily involves the skin and follows a much more indolent course resembling mycosis fungoides. It should be noted that in addition to causing lymphoid malignancies, HTLV-1 infection can also give rise to a progressive demyelinating disease that affects the central nervous system and the spinal cord (Chapter 30).

Mycosis Fungoides and Sézary Syndrome

Mycosis fungoides and Sézary syndrome appear to be different manifestations of a single neoplastic entity. It is an indolent disorder of peripheral CD4+ T cells that is characterized by the involvement of skin and therefore belongs to the group of *cutaneous T-cell lymphoid neoplasms.*

Clinically the cutaneous lesions of *mycosis fungoides* show three somewhat distinct stages (Chapter 27). Briefly, mycosis fungoides presents with an inflammatory *premycotic phase* and progresses through a *plaque phase* to a *tumor phase*. Histologically, there is infiltration of the epidermis and upper dermis by neoplastic T cells, which have an extremely unusual cerebriform nucleus, characterized by marked infolding of the nuclear membrane. Disease progression is characterized by extracutaneous spread, most commonly to lymph nodes and bone marrow.

Sézary syndrome is a variant in which skin involvement is characteristically manifested as a *generalized exfoliative erythroderma.* In contrast to mycosis fungoides, the skin lesions rarely proceed to tumefaction. In addition, *there is an associated leukemia of Sézary cells* that have the same cerebriform appearance noted in the tissue infiltrates of mycosis fungoides. Circulating tumor cells can also be identified in peripheral smears in up to 25% of cases of mycosis fungoides in the plaque or tumor phase, emphasizing the overlap between mycosis fungoides and Sézary syndrome.

Although cutaneous disease dominates the clinical picture in these disorders, sensitive molecular analyses have shown that tumor cells are present in the lymph nodes and bone marrow early in the course of all patients, indicating that tumor cells circulate widely. The basis for the striking epidermotropism is uncertain; tumor cells may preferentially home to skin or be dependent on skin-specific factors for growth or survival. *These are indolent tumors associated with a median survival of 8 to 9 years.* Transformation to large cell lymphoma of T-cell type occasionally occurs as a terminal event.

HODGKIN DISEASE

HD encompasses a group of disorders that differ from NHL in several respects. In contrast to NHLs, which frequently arise at extranodal sites and spread in an unpredictable fashion, HD arises in a single node or chain of nodes and spreads characteristically to the anatomically contiguous nodes. It is characterized morphologically by the presence of distinctive neoplastic giant cells, *RS cells*, which induce the accumulation of reactive lymphocytes, histiocytes, and granulocytes. In contrast to other lymphoid neoplasms, the neoplastic cells of HD typically make up a minor fraction (1 to 5%) of the total tumor cell mass. The origin of the neoplastic cell in the more common forms of HD has yet to be identified with certainty and has a phenotype unique from that observed in other lymphoid neoplasms.

HD accounts for 0.7% of all new cancers in the United States, with approximately 7400 new cases reported per year. Its importance stems from the fact that it is one of the most common forms of malignancy in young adults, with an average age at diagnosis of 32 years. Much progress has been made in the treatment of this disease in the last several decades, and it is now curable in most cases.

Classification. There are three major subtypes of HD:

- Nodular sclerosis
- Mixed cellularity
- Lymphocyte predominance

Additional variants, such as *lymphocyte depletion HD*, are rare and controversial entities[4a] and are not discussed here.

MORPHOLOGY.

The Reed-Sternberg Cell. A distinctive tumor giant cell known as the **RS cell** is considered to be the true neoplastic element in HD, and identification of RS cells and their variants is therefore essential for the histologic diagnosis (Fig. 15–24). **Classic RS cells are quite large (15 to 45 μ in diameter), binucleate or bilobed, with the two halves often appearing as mirror images of each other.** At other times, there are multiple nuclei, or the single nucleus is multilobate. The nucleus is enclosed

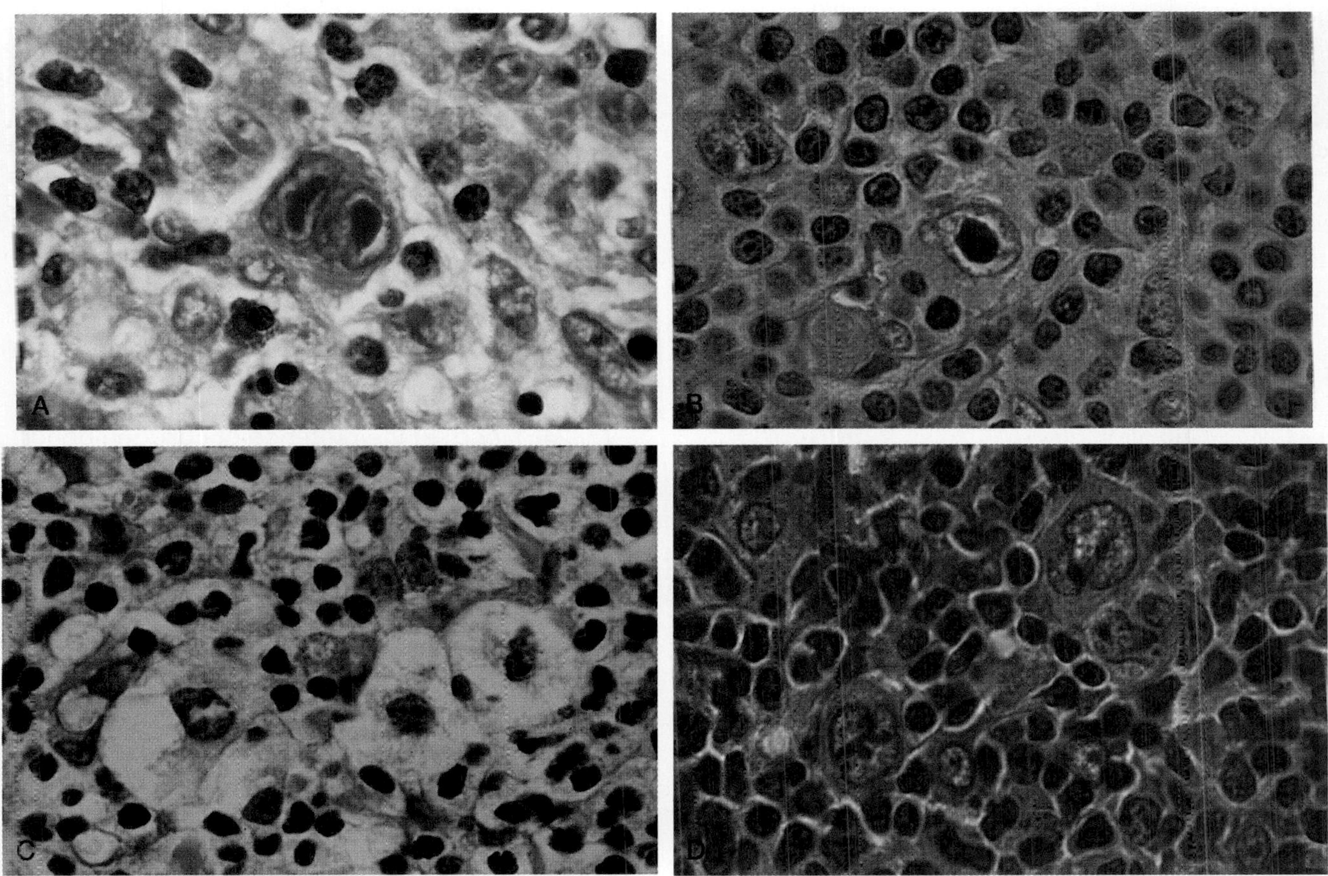

Figure 15–24

Reed-Sternberg cells and variants. *A*, Diagnostic Reed-Sternberg cell, with two nuclear lobes, large inclusion-like nucleoli, and abundant cytoplasm, surrounded by lymphocytes, macrophages, and an eosinophil. *B*, Reed-Sternberg cell, mononuclear variant. *C*, Reed-Sternberg cell, lacunar variant. This variant is usually seen in the nodular sclerosis subtype and has a folded nucleus or multilobate nucleus lying within a clear space created by retraction of its cytoplasm during processing of the tissue. *D*, Reed-Sternberg cell, lymphohistiocytic (L + H) variant. Several such variants with folded or multilobate nuclei, small nucleoli, fine chromatin, and abundant pale cytoplasm are present. (*A* courtesy of Dr. Robert W. McKenna, Department of Pathology, University of Texas Southwestern Medical School, Dallas, TX.)

within an abundant amphophilic cytoplasm and contains large, inclusion-like, **owl-eyed** nucleoli, generally surrounded by a clear halo, that are about the size of a small lymphocyte (5 to 7 μ in diameter).

Several variants of RS cells are also encountered. **Mononculear variants** contain only a single round or oblong nucleus with a large inclusion-like nucleolus. **Lacunar cells,** seen predominantly in the nodular sclerosis subtype, have more delicate folded or multilobate nuclei surrounded by abundant pale cytoplasm that is often disrupted during the cutting of sections, leaving the nucleus sitting in an empty hole (the lacune). **Lymphocytic and histiocytic variants (L + H cells)** with polypoid nuclei resembling popcorn kernels, inconspicuous nucleoli, and moderately abundant cytoplasm are specific to the lymphocyte predominance subtype.

The morphologic diagnosis of HD is complicated by the occasional presence of cells similar or identical in appearance to RS cells in other conditions, such as infectious mononucleosis, solid tissue cancers, and NHL. **Thus, although RS cells are requisite for the diagnosis, they must be present in an appropriate background of non-neoplastic inflammatory cells (lymphocytes, plasma cells, eosinophils).** In difficult cases, immunohistochemical markers and molecular genetic studies help in establishing the diagnosis.

Spread of HD and Staging. The spread of HD is remarkably predictable: Nodal disease precedes splenic disease, splenic disease usually precedes hepatic disease, and hepatic disease usually precedes marrow involvement and extranodal disease. Because of this uniform pattern of spread, patients with limited disease can be cured with local radiotherapy. For this reason, the **staging of**

Table 15–6. CLINICAL STAGING OF HODGKIN AND NON-HODGKIN LYMPHOMAS (ANN ARBOR CLASSIFICATION)

Stage*	Distribution of Disease
I	Involvement of a single lymph node region (I) or involvement of a single extralymphatic organ or site (I_E).
II	Involvement of two or more lymph node regions on the same side of the diaphragm alone (II) or with involvement of limited contiguous extralymphatic organ or tissue (II_E)
III	Involvement of lymph node regions on both sides of the diaphragm (III), which may include the spleen (III_S) and/or limited contiguous extralymphatic organ or site (III_E, III_{ES})
IV	Multiple or disseminated foci of involvement of one or more extralymphatic organs or tissues with or without lymphatic involvement

*All stages are further divided on the basis of the absence (A) or presence (B) of the following systemic symptoms: significant fever, night sweats, or unexplained weight loss of greater than 10% of normal body weight.

From Carbone PT, et al: Symposium (Ann Arbor): Staging in Hodgkin's disease. Cancer Res 31:1707, 1971.

HD (Table 15–6) is not only predictive of prognosis, but also guides the choice of therapy. Staging involves careful physical examination and several investigative procedures, including computed tomography of abdomen and pelvis, chest radiography, and biopsy of the bone marrow. These modalities still fail to detect splenic disease reliably, and staging laparotomy, which allows direct visualization of the intra-abdominal nodes, liver biopsy, and removal of the spleen, is still used in some patients being considered for radiotherapy. The presence of constitutional symptoms (fever, night sweats, and weight loss) are characteristic of HD but can also be seen in other lymphoid neoplasms.

With this background, we turn to the morphologic classification of HD into its subgroups and point out some of the salient immunophenotypic and clinical features of each (Table 15–7). Later the manifestations common to all are presented.

Hodgkin Disease, Nodular Sclerosis Type. The most common form of HD, constituting 65 to 75% of cases, the nodular sclerosis type is characterized by two features: (1) the presence of a particular variant of the RS cell, the **lacunar cell** (Fig. 15–24*C*), and (2) the presence of **collagen bands** that divide the lymphoid tissue into circumscribed nodules (Fig. 15–25). The fibrosis may be scant or abundant, and the neoplastic cells are found in a polymorphous background of small T lymphocytes, eosinophils, plasma cells, and macrophages. Classic RS cells are less frequent than in the mixed cellularity and lymphocyte depletion types. The tumor cells have a characteristic immunophenotype: positive for CD15 and CD30 and negative for CD45, B-cell, and T-cell markers. In early nodal disease, the tumor cells preferentially involve the paracortical T-cell zones. As in other forms of HD, involvement of the spleen, liver, bone marrow, and other organs and tissues may appear in due course and take the form of irregular, tumor-like nodules resembling that present in the nodes.

The nodular sclerosis type is the only form of HD that is more common in women and strikes adolescents or young adults. It has a propensity to involve the lower cervical, supraclavicular, and mediastinal lymph nodes. The prognosis is excellent.

Table 15–7. CLASSIFICATION OF HODGKIN DISEASE

Subtype	Morphology and Immunophenotype	Typical Clinical Features
Nodular sclerosis	Frequent lacunar cells and occasional diagnostic RS cells; background infiltrate composed of T lymphocytes, eosinophils, macrophages, and plasma cells; fibrous bands dividing cellular areas into nodules. RS cells CD15+, CD30+.	Stage 1 or 2 disease most common. Frequent mediastinal involvement. Females affected more than males, most patients young adults.
Mixed cellularity	Frequent mononuclear and diagnostic RS cells; background infiltrate rich in T lymphocytes, eosinophils, macrophages, plasma cells. RS cells CD15+, CD30+.	More than 50% present as stage 3 or 4 disease. Males affected more than females. Biphasic incidence, peaking in young adults and again in adults > 55.
Lymphocyte predominance	Frequent L + H (popcorn cell) variants in a background of follicular dendritic cells and reactive B cells. RS cells CD20+, CD15−, CD30−.	Young males with cervical or axillary lymphadenopathy. Mediastinal disease uncommon.
Lymphocyte depletion	Rare and somewhat controversial, with frequent RS or RS cells. Most cases prove to be large cell lymphoma. CD15+, CD30+.	Older male patients with disseminated disease. Also seen in HIV patients and developing countries.

RS, Reed-Sternberg; HIV, human immunodeficiency virus; L + H, lymphocytic-histiocytic.

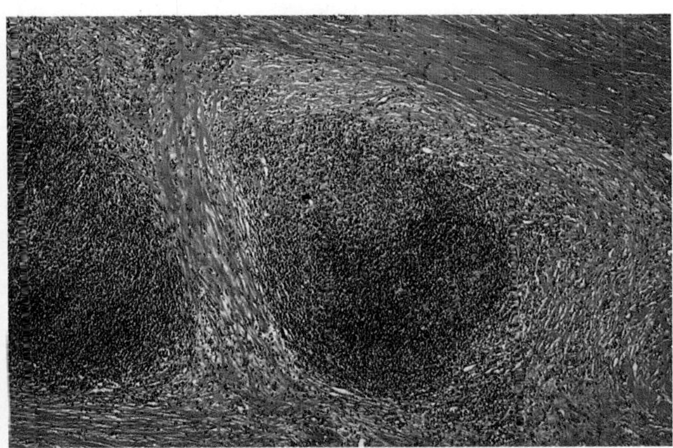

Figure 15–25

Hodgkin disease, nodular sclerosis type. A low-power view shows well-defined bands of pink, acellular collagen that have subdivided the tumor cells and associated reactive infiltrate into nodules. (Courtesy of Dr. Robert W. McKenna, Department of Pathology, University of Texas Southwestern Medical School, Dallas, TX.)

Hodgkin Disease, Mixed Cellularity Type. This form of HD constitutes about 25% of cases. The mixed cellularity type is rendered distinctive by **diffuse effacement** of lymph nodes by a heterogeneous cellular infiltrate, which includes small lymphocytes, eosinophils, plasma cells, and benign macrophages admixed with the neoplastic cells (Fig. 15–26). **Classic RS cells and mononculear variants are usually plentiful.** The immunophenotype is identical to that observed in the nodular sclerosis type. Small lymphocytes in the background are predominantly T cells, and early nodal disease preferentially involves paracortical T-cell zones. Uncommonly the background infiltrate is composed predominantly of a monotonous population of polyclonal small T lymphocytes with few admixed macrophages or other reactive elements. In such lymphocyte-rich cases, immunophenotyping may be needed to exclude the lymphocyte predominance type of HD or an unusual NHL.

The mixed cellularity form of HD is more common in men. Compared to the lymphocyte predominance and nodular sclerosis subtypes, it is more likely to be associated with older age, B symptoms, and advanced tumor stage. Nonetheless, the overall prognosis is good.

Hodgkin Disease, Lymphocyte Predominance Type. This uncommon variant, accounting for approximately 6% of all cases, is characterized by nodal effacement by a vaguely nodular infiltrate of small lymphocytes admixed with variable numbers of benign histiocytes (Fig. 15–27). Typical RS cells are extremely difficult to find. More common are so-called **lymphohistiocytic (L + H) variants** that have a delicate, multilobed nucleus that has been likened in appearance to popcorn (**popcorn cell**). Other cells, such as eosinophils, neutrophils, and plasma cells, are scanty or absent, and there is little evidence of necrosis or fibrosis.

Increasingly, **evidence is accruing that supports a follicular B-cell origin for the neoplastic cells of this subtype.** In contrast to other forms of HD, the tumor cells are positive for CD45 and CD20, a B-cell marker, and negative for CD15 and CD30.[41,42] The L + H cells within individual tumors share identical IgH gene rearrangments and have V_H segments that have undergone somatic hypermutation,[43,44] a modification that normally occurs only in follicular B cells. Finally, in contrast to other forms of HD, approximately 3 to 5% of tumors transform to diffuse large cell lymphomas, which are uniformly of B-cell type.

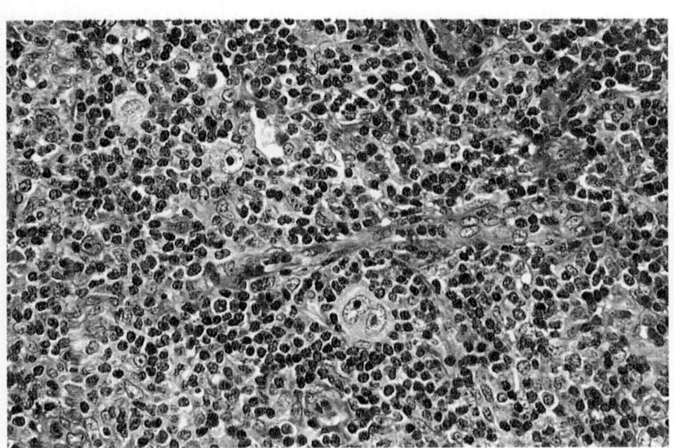

Figure 15–26

Hodgkin disease, mixed cellularity type. A diagnostic, binucleate Reed-Sternberg cell is surrounded by multiple cell types, including eosinophils (bright red cytoplasm), lymphocytes, and histiocytes. (Courtesy of Dr. Robert W. McKenna, Department of Pathology, University of Texas Southwestern Medical School, Dallas, TX.)

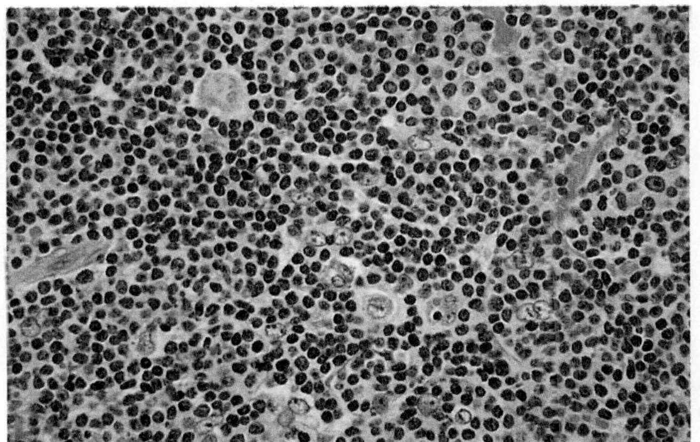

Figure 15–27

Hodgkin disease, lymphocyte predominance type. Numerous mature-looking lymphocytes surround scattered, large, pale-staining L + H variants ("popcorn" cells). (Courtesy of Dr. Robert W. McKenna, Department of Pathology, University of Texas Southwestern Medical School, Dallas, TX.)

A majority of patients are men, usually younger than 35 years of age, presenting with limited disease. Most patients have cervical or axillary lymphadenopathy. Mediastinal disease is rarely seen, and bone marrow involvement is rare. The overall prognosis is excellent.

Etiology and Pathogenesis. It is now widely accepted that HD is a clonal neoplastic disorder and that the RS cells and variants represent the transformed cells. In all likelihood, the characteristic accumulation of reactive cells occurs in response to *cytokines* secreted by the RS cells. Many cytokines, including IL-4, IL-5, TNF-α, GM-CSF, and transforming growth factor-β (TGF-β), have been detected in HD. Of these, IL-5 synthesis by RS cells correlates with eosinophil accumulation (a feature of mixed cellularity and nodular sclerosis subtypes).[45] TGF-β, a fibrogenic cytokine, is found almost exclusively in the nodular sclerosis variant, where it is produced by eosinophils.[46] Thus, the specific histologic pattern of HD may be determined by the unique combination of cytokines secreted by RS cells and the non-neoplastic cellular infiltrate.[47]

In the specific case of the lymphocyte predominance subtype, the evidence for a B-cell origin is fairly convincing. In the other subtypes of HD, the origin of these cells remains an enigma. The extensive studies on RS cell derivation in the nodular sclerosis and mixed cellularity subtypes can be summarized as follows:

- RS cells are aneuploid and contain clonal cytogenetic aberrations,[48] but no consistent abnormality has been detected.
- RS cells express surface markers, such as MHC class II antigens and B7, that are characteristic of antigen-presenting cells, such as macrophages or B lymphocytes.[49] Antigens specific for B cells or, in some cases, specific for T cells have been detected on RS cells and variants.[50] Certain markers specific for cells derived from the monocyte/macrophage series, however, are also expressed in a high fraction of cases.[51]
- Molecular analysis of Ig gene rearrangements has tended to support a B lymphoid origin. In one particularly well-studied case, a cell line derived from a patient with mixed cellularity HD was shown to have clonal rearrangements of the IgH and κ light chain loci.[52,53] Using single cell dissection, the identical rearrangements were then shown to be present in RS cells in the patient's tissues. Some, but not all, investigators have also detected clonal Ig rearrangements in the RS cells of nodular sclerosis and mixed cellularity HD.[54]

These studies indicate that RS cells in the mixed cellularity and nodular sclerosis subtypes often have molecular features of B lymphocytes, yet have some phenotypic attributes of monocyte/macrophages. It seems likely that cases with Ig rearrangements are most probably of B lymphoid origin, while the origin of tumors lacking Ig rearrangements remains uncertain.

Assuming that B lymphoid cells are the target of transformation in at least some cases of the mixed cellularity and nodular sclerosis subtypes, what causes the neoplastic change? For years, EBV has been suspected as an etiologic agent. Patients with a history of infectious mononucleosis or with elevated titers of antibodies against EBV antigens incur a slightly higher risk of HD. The seroepidemiologic evidence has been bolstered by molecular studies. EBV genomes and EBV-specific RNA transcripts can be identified in RS cells in 40% of cases of nodular sclerosis HD and 60 to 70% of cases of mixed cellularity HD[55–57] but is not seen in the lymphocyte predominance type. The configuration of the EBV DNA is the same in all tumor cells within a given case, indicating that infection occurred before cellular transformation.[58] Additionally, EBV-positive tumor cells express latent membrane protein-1,[59] a protein encoded by the EBV genome that has been shown to have transforming activity. Hence, EBV infection may be one of several steps involved in the pathogenesis of HD. It remains possible that other, as yet unknown, infectious agents could also be involved in HD, particularly in those cases that are EBV negative.

Clinical Course. HD, similar to NHL, usually presents with a painless enlargement of lymph nodes. Although distinction between HD and NHL can be made only by examination of a lymph node biopsy, several clinical features favor the diagnosis of the HD (Table 15–8). Younger patients with the more favorable histologic types tend to present in clinical stage I or II and are usually free from systemic manifestations. Patients with disseminated disease (stages III and IV) and the mixed cellularity or lymphocyte depletion subtypes are more likely to present with B symptoms. One curious paraneoplastic symptom that is rare but specific to HD is pain in involved lymph nodes that occurs only with consumption of alcohol.[60] Cutaneous energy resulting from depressed cell-mediated immunity is seen in most cases. The basis of this immune dysfunction is poorly understood, but it tends to persist even in sucessfully treated patients, possibly indicating that HD arises in the background of some underlying immune abnormality.

With modern treatment protocols, tumor burden (i.e., stage) rather than histologic type is the most important prognostic variable. Currently the 5-year survival rate of patients with stages I and IIA is close to 90%, and many appeared to be cured. Even with advanced disease (stages IVA and IVB), 60 to 70% 5-year disease-free survival can be achieved.

Table 15–8. CLINICAL DIFFERENCES BETWEEN HODGKIN AND NON-HODGKIN LYMPHOMAS

Hodgkin Disease	Non-Hodgkin Lymphoma
• More often localized to a single axial group of nodes (cervical, mediastinal, para-aortic)	• More frequent involvement of multiple peripheral nodes
• Orderly spread by contiguity	• Noncontiguous spread
• Mesenteric nodes and Waldeyer ring rarely involved	• Waldeyer ring and mesenteric nodes commonly involved
• Extranodal involvement uncommon	• Extranodal involvement common

Progress in the treatment of HD has created a new set of problems. Long-term survivors of chemotherapy and radiotherapy have an increased risk of developing second cancers. Myelodysplastic syndromes, AML, and lung cancer lead the list of second malignancies, but also included are NHL, breast cancer, gastric cancer, sarcoma, and malignant melanoma.[61] The risk of breast cancer is particularly high in women treated with radiation to the chest during adolescence,[62] and the risk of other solid tumors also seems to correlate with radiotherapy, whereas alkylating chemotherapeutic drugs appear to be responsible for the increased risk of AML and myelodysplasia. Non-neoplastic complications of radiotherapy have included pulmonary fibrosis and accelerated atherosclerosis. It appears that new combinations of chemotherapeutic drugs and more judicious use of radiotherapy may avoid these complications and yet be equally curative.

Myeloid Neoplasms

The common feature that unites this heterogeneous group of neoplasms is an origin in a progenitor cell that normally gives rise to terminally differentiated cells of the myeloid series (erythrocytes, granulocytes, monocytes, and platelets). As such, these diseases almost always primarily involve the bone marrow and to a lesser degree the secondary hematopoietic organs (spleen, liver, and lymph nodes) and present with altered hematopoiesis. Three broad categories of myeloid neoplasia exist:

1. AML, characterized by accumulation of immature myeloid cells in the bone marrow
2. Myelodysplastic syndromes (MDS) associated with ineffective hematopoiesis and associated cytopenias
3. Chronic myeloproliferative disorders (MPDs), usually associated with an increased production of terminally differentiated myeloid cells

The pathogenesis of myeloid neoplasms is best understood in the context of normal hematopoiesis, which involves a hierarchy of hematopoietic progenitor cells. At the top of the hierarchy sits the true pluripotent stem cell, which gives rise to multipotent progenitor cells that are committed to lymphoid or myeloid differentiation. The latter, in turn, produces more committed progenitors, which eventually give rise to terminally differentiated cells of a single type (e.g., erythrocyte, monocyte). In addition to giving birth to more committed daughter cells, hematopoietic progenitor cells must also be able to replicate themselves without differentiating (or else they would eventually disappear), a process known as *self-renewal.* Exactly how this balance between "stemness" and commitment to various cell fates is controlled is uncertain, but it appears to be disturbed in myeloid neoplasms. *The manifestations of myeloid neoplasms are likely influenced by three factors*: (1) *the position of the transformed cell within the hierarchy of progenitors*, (2) *the effect of transforming events on the capacity for self-renewal*, and (3) *the effect of the transforming events on differentiation.* We return to these themes as each type of myeloid neoplasia is discussed.

Given that all forms of myeloid neoplasia originate from a transformed hematopoietic progenitor cell, it should come as no surprise that the divisions between these neoplasms sometimes blur. Myeloid neoplasms, similar to other malignancies, tend to evolve over time to more aggressive forms of disease. In particular, both MDS and chronic MPDs often *transform* to AML. In the specific case of one of the MPDs, chronic myelogenous leukemia (CML), transformation to ALL may also be seen, probably because the tumor originates from a transformed pluripotent stem cell.

ACUTE MYELOGENOUS LEUKEMIA

AMLs affect primarily adults, peaking in incidence between the ages of 15 and 39 years, but are also observed in children and older adults. They constitute only 20% of childhood leukemias. AML is quite heterogeneous, reflecting the complexities of myeloid cell differentiation.

Pathophysiology. AML, similar to other forms of neoplasia, is associated with acquired (or, rarely, inherited) genetic alterations that result in the replacement of normal marrow elements by relatively undifferentiated blasts exhibiting one or more types of early myeloid differentiation. The replication rate of these blasts is actually lower than that of normal myeloid progenitors. Hence, the most important net effect of the genetic alterations is likely to be the inhibition of terminal differentiation (commitment).

As mentioned earlier in the discussion of ALL, neoplastic myeloid precursor cells accumulate in the marrow and suppress remaining normal hematopoietic progenitor cells by physical replacement as well as by other unknown mechanisms. Failure of normal hematopoiesis results in anemia, neutropenia, and thrombocytopenia, which are the basis for most of the major clinical complications seen in AML. Therapeutically the aim is to clear the bone marrow of the leukemic clone, thus permitting resumption of normal hematopoiesis. This can be accomplished by treatment with cytotoxic drugs or, in the specific case of acute promyelocytic leukemia, by overcoming the block in differentiation.

Classification. In the revised FAB classification (Table 15–9), AML is divided into eight (M0 to M7) categories.[63] This scheme takes into account both the degree of maturation (M0 to M3) and the lineage of the leukemic blasts (M4 to M7). Histochemical stains for peroxidase, specific esterase, and nonspecific esterase play an important role in classifying these tumors. Monoclonal antibodies that recognize common and lineage-specific determinants on myeloid cells are also useful in the diagnosis of AML (see Table 15–3), especially when morphologic and histochemical features are equivocal.

MORPHOLOGY. The diagnosis of AML is based on finding greater than 30% myeloid blasts in the bone marrow. In most cases, myeloid blasts can be distinguished from lymphoblasts in the usual Wright-Giemsa stain. Several types of myeloid blasts are recognized, but more than one type of blast, or blasts with hybrid features, can be seen

Table 15–9. REVISED FAB CLASSIFICATION OF ACUTE MYELOGENOUS LEUKEMIAS

Class	Incidence (% of AML)	Marrow Morphology and Comments
M0—Minimally differentiated AML	2–3%	Blasts lack definitive cytologic and cytochemical markers of myeloblasts (e.g., myeloperoxidase negative) but express myeloid lineage antigens and resemble myeloblasts ultrastructurally.
M1—AML without differentiation	20%	Very immature but ≥3% are peroxidase positive. Few granules or Auer rods and little maturation beyond the myeloblast stage.
M2—AML with maturation	30–40%	Full range of myeloid maturation through granulocytes. Auer rods present in most cases. Presence of t(8;21) defines a prognostically favorable subgroup.
M3—Acute promyelocytic leukemia	5–10%	Majority of cells are hypergranular promyelocytes, often with many Auer rods per cell. Patients are younger (median age 35–40 yr) and often develop DIC. The t(15;17) translocation is characteristic.
M4—Acute myelomonocytic leukemia	15–20%	Myelocytic and monocytic differentiation evident. Myeloid elements resemble M2 AML. Monoblasts are positive for nonspecific esterases. Presence of chromosome 16 abnormalities defines a subset (M4eo) with marrow eosinophilia and excellent prognosis.
M5—Acute monocytic leukemia	10%	In M5a subtype, monoblasts (peroxidase-negative, nonspecific esterase-positive) and promonocytes predominate in marrow and blood. In M5b subtype, mature monocytes predominate in the peripheral blood. M5a and M5b occur in older patients. Characterized by high incidence of organomegaly, lymphadenopathy, and tissue infiltration.
M6—Acute erythroleukemia	5%	Dysplastic erythroid precursors (some megaloblastoid, others with giant or multiple nuclei) predominate, and within the nonerythroid cells, >30% are myeloblasts; seen in advanced age; makes up 1% of de novo AML and 20% of therapy-related AML.
M7—Acute megakaryocytic leukemia	1%	Blasts of megakaryocytic lineage predominate. Blasts react with platelet-specific antibodies directed against GPIIb/IIIa or vWF. Myelofibrosis or increased marrow reticulin seen in most cases.

AML, acute myelogenous leukemia; DIC, disseminated intravascular coagulation; GP, glycoprotein; vWF, von Willebrand factor; FAB, French-American-British.

in individual patients. **Myeloblasts** have delicate nuclear chromatin, two to four nucleoli, and more voluminous cytoplasm than lymphoblasts (see Fig. 15–6). The cytoplasm often contains fine, azurophilic, **peroxidase-positive** granules. Distinctive red-staining rodlike structures called **Auer rods,** which represent abnormal azurophilic granules, are also present in many cases and are particularly numerous in the M3 type (acute promyelocytic leukemia) (Fig. 15–28). Histochemical stains may help to bring out the presence of rare Auer rods because they are intensely peroxidase positive. The presence of Auer rods is taken to be definitive evidence of myeloid differentiation. **Monoblasts** (Fig. 15–29) often have folded or lobulated nuclei, lack Auer rods, and usually do not express peroxidase but can be identified by staining for nonspecific esterase. M6 AML, so-called erythroleukemia, is somewhat of a misnomer. In this subtype, greater than 50% of the cells are erythroid progenitors, and among the nonerythroid nucleated cells, greater than 30% of the cellularity is composed of myeloblasts. M7 AML,

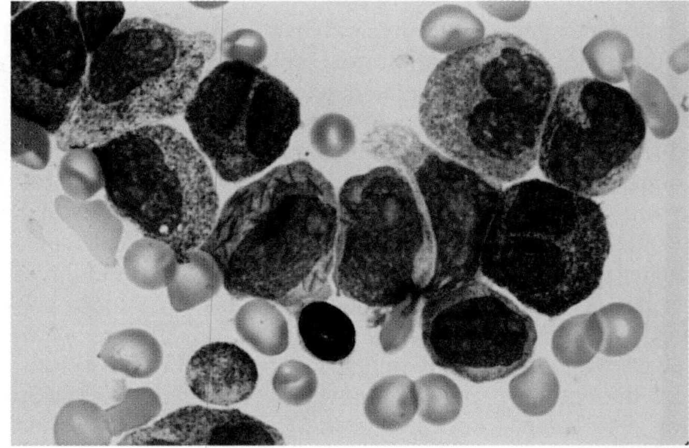

Figure 15–28

AML (acute promyelocytic leukemia [M3 subtype]). Bone marrow aspirate shows neoplastic promyelocytes with abnormally coarse and numerous azurophilic granules. Other characteristic findings include the presence of several cells with bilobed nuclei and a cell in the center of the field that contains multiple needle-like Auer rods. (Courtesy of Dr. Robert W. McKenna, Department of Pathology, University of Texas Southwestern Medical School, Dallas, TX.)

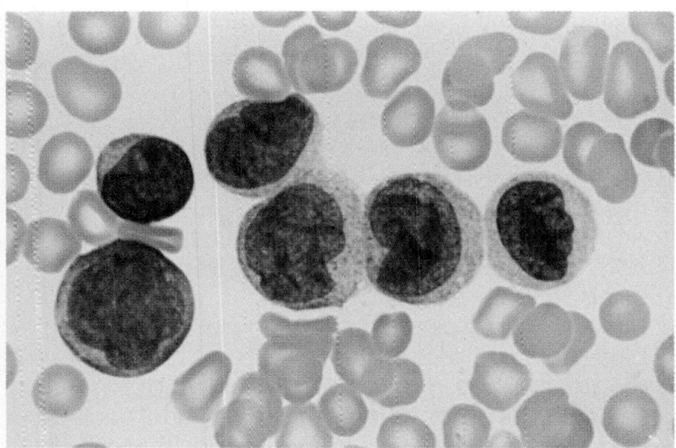

Figure 15–29

Acute monocytic leukemia (AML, M5a subtype). A peripheral smear shows one monoblast and five promonocytes with folded nuclear membranes. (Courtesy of Dr. Robert W. McKenna, Department of Pathology, University of Texas Southwestern Medical School, Dallas, TX.)

acute megakaryocytic leukemia, is often associated with marrow fibrosis, probably secondary to fibrogenic cytokines released from leukemic **megakaryoblasts.** Diagnosis of the M7 subtype usually requires the demonstration of platelet-specific markers on blast cells.[64]

The number of leukemic cells in the peripheral blood is highly variable, sometimes being more than 100,000 cells/μl, but being under 10,000 cells/μl in about 50% of the patients. **Occasionally the peripheral smear may not contain any blasts** (aleukemic leukemia). For this reason, bone marrow examination is essential to exclude acute leukemia in patients with pancytopenia.

Chromosomal Abnormalities. Special high-resolution banding techniques have revealed chromosomal abnormalities in approximately 90% of all AML patients. In 50 to 70% of the cases, the karyotypic changes can be detected by standard cytogenetic techniques. Many of the nonrandom chromosomal abnormalities have prognostic implications that are independent of other clinical prognostic factors.[65]

Particular chromosomal abnormalities correlate with the clinical setting in which the tumor occurs. AML arising de novo in patients with no risk factors are often associated with balanced chromosomal translocations. In contrast, AMLs that follow an MDS or that occur after exposure to DNA-damaging agents (such as chemotherapy or radiation therapy) are commonly associated with deletions or monosomies involving chromosomes 5 and 7 and usually lack chromosomal translocations. The exception to this rule is AMLs occurring after treatment with chemotherapeutic drugs that inhibit the enzyme topoisomerase II, which are often associated with translocations involving the *MLL* gene on chromosome 11 at band q23.[66]

The t(15;17) translocation characteristic of acute promyelocytic leukemia (M3) is of particular interest not only because of its pathogenetic importance, but also because of its effect on therapy. This translocation results in the fusion of a truncated retinoic acid receptor-α (*RAR-α*) gene on chromosome 17 to the *PML* (for promyelocytic leukemia) gene on chromosome 15.[67–69] Analogous to the *ABL-BCR* fusion in chronic myeloid leukemia, the *PML-RAR-α* rearrangement produces a hybrid mRNA that can be detected in most cases of M3 AML. The fusion gene encodes an abnormal retinoic acid receptor that blocks myeloid cell differentiation, probably by interfering with the function of other retinoid receptors.[70] Notably, pharmacologic doses of the vitamin A derivative *all-trans-retinoic acid* overcome this block in vitro and in vivo, causing neoplastic promyelocytes to differentiate into neutrophils.[71] Similar to normal neutrophils, neutrophils derived from the neoplastic clone are short-lived and rapidly die, thus clearing the marrow and allowing for resumption of normal hematopoiesis. Remarkably the same effect is also observed in patients treated with arsenic trioxide, which appears somehow to promote the degradation of the PML-RAR-α fusion protein.[72]

Although retinoic acid *differentiation therapy* induces remissions in a high fraction of patients with acute promyelocytic leukemia, all patients ultimately relapse, probably because retinoic acid fails to prevent continued self-renewal of the neoplastic progenitor cell. Nonetheless, this is the first example in which the molecular pathogenesis of a malignant tumor can be correlated with specific therapy.

Clinical Features. The clinical findings in AML are similar to ALL. *Most patients present within weeks or a few months of the onset of symptoms with findings related to anemia, neutropenia, and thrombocytopenia*, most notably fatigue, fever, and spontaneous mucosal and cutaneous bleeding. Many times, the bleeding diathesis caused by the thrombocytopenia is the most striking clinical and anatomic feature of the disease. Petechiae and ecchymoses are seen in the skin. Hemorrhages also occur into the serosal linings of the body cavities and into the serosal coverings of the viscera, particularly of the heart and lungs. Mucosal hemorrhages into the gingivae and urinary tract are common. Procoagulants released by leukemic cells, especially in acute promyelocytic leukemia (M3), may produce disseminated intravascular coagulation, further exacerbating the bleeding diathesis. Infections are common, particularly in the oral cavity, skin, lungs, kidneys, urinary bladder, and colon, and they are often caused by "opportunists" such as fungi, *Pseudomonas*, and commensals.

Signs and symptoms related to infiltration of tissues are usually less striking in AML than in ALL. Mild lymphadenopathy and organomegaly may be appreciated. In tumors with monocytic differentiation (M4 and M5), infiltration of the skin (leukemia cutis) and the gingiva may be observed, likely reflecting the normal tendency of non-neoplastic monocytes to extravasate into tissues. Central nervous system spread is less common than in ALL but is still seen. Quite uncommonly, patients present with localized masses composed of myeloblasts in the absence of marrow or peripheral blood involvement. Patients with these tumors, known variously as myeloblastomas, granulocytic sarcomas, or chloromas, almost inevitably progress to a typical AML picture over a period of up to several years.

Prognosis. AML is a difficult disease to treat. Approximately 60% of the patients achieve complete remission with chemotherapy, but only 15 to 30% of these remain free from disease for 5 years. As in ALL, prognosis is strongly influenced by particular chromosomal abnormalities. AMLs associated with an (8;21) chromosomal translocation or inversion of chromosome 16 have a relatively good prognosis, whereas those with the t(9;22) (Philadelphia chromosome) or translocations involving chromosome 11q23 have a poor outcome. The prognosis is especially dismal for those patients with AML arising out of a myelodysplastic syndrome or occuring after genotoxic therapy; such tumors often exhibit deletions or monosomies of chromosomes 5 or 7. Because of the generally poor outcome with standard therapy, an increasing number of patients with AML are being treated with allogeneic bone marrow transplantation.

MYELODYSPLASTIC SYNDROMES

Myelodysplastic syndrome (MDS) refers to a group of clonal stem cell disorders characterized by maturation defects resulting in ineffective hematopoiesis and an increased risk of transformation to AML. In patients with MDS, the bone marrow is partly or wholly replaced by the clonal progeny of a mutant multipotent stem cell that retains the capacity to differentiate into red cells, granulocytes, and platelets, but in a manner that is both ineffective and disordered. As a result, the bone marrow is usually *hypercellular* or *normocellular*, but the peripheral blood shows *pancytopenia*. MDS arises in two distinct settings:

- Idiopathic or primary MDS, occurring mainly in patients over age 50, often develops insidiously.
- Therapy-related MDS (t-MDS), a complication of previous myelosuppressive drug or radiation therapy, usually appears 2 to 8 years after exposure.

All forms of MDS can transform to AML, but transformation occurs most rapidly and with highest frequency in patients with t-MDS. Although characteristic morphologic changes are typically seen in the marrow and the peripheral blood, definitive diagnosis frequently requires correlation with other laboratory tests. Cytogenetic analysis is particularly helpful in confirming the diagnosis because certain chromosomal aberrations (discussed subsequently) are often observed.

Pathogenesis. The pathogenesis of MDS is unknown. Although the marrow is usually hypercellular at diagnosis, it may also be normocellular or, less commonly, hypocellular. Given this, the usual explanation for suppression of normal hematopoiesis (crowding out of normal elements) is difficult to apply, leading to the suggestion that MDS may arise out of a background of stem cell damage. Both primary MDS and t-MDS occurring after exposure to radiation or alkylating chemotherapeutic drugs are associated with similar clonal chromosomal abnormalities, including monosomy 5 and monosomy 7, deletions of 5q and 7q, trisomy 8, and deletions of 20q.[65]

MORPHOLOGY. The most characteristic finding is disordered (dysplastic) differentiation affecting all three lineages (erythroid, myeloid, and megakaryocytic) (Fig. 15–30). Within the erythroid series, common abnormalities include **ringed sideroblasts,** erythroblasts with iron-laden mitochondria that are visible as perinuclear granules in Prussian blue–stained aspirates or biopsy specimens; **megaloblastoid maturation** resembling that seen in vitamin B_{12} and folate deficiency; and **nuclear budding abnormalities,** recognized as nuclei with misshapen, often polypoid outlines. Neutrophils may contain decreased numbers of secondary granules or contain toxic granulations and Döhle bodies. **Pseudo-Pelger-Huët cells,** neutrophils with only two nuclear lobes, are frequently observed, and sometimes neutrophils appear that completely lack nuclear segmentation. Megakaryocytes with single nuclear lobes or multiple separate nuclei **(pawn ball megakaryocytes)** are also characteristic. **Myeloblasts** may be increased **but by definition constitute less than 30% of the overall marrow cellularity.** The peripheral blood often contains pseudo-Pelger-Huët cells, giant platelets, macrocytes, poikilocytes, and a relative or absolute monocytosis. Myeloblasts usually constitute less than 10% of the peripheral leukocytes.

Clinical Course. Primary MDS affects primarily individuals older than 60 years of age. As in acute leukemia, patients with this disorder present with weakness, infections, and hemorrhages, all owing to pancytopenia. Approximately half of the patients are asymptomatic, and the disease is discovered after incidental blood tests.

On the basis of specific morphologic features in the marrow and peripheral blood, primary MDS is divided into five categories, each with a somewhat different risk for transformation to overt AML.[73] In general, subtypes that are defined by having a higher proportion of blast cells in the marrow or peripheral blood are associated with a poorer prognosis. The presence of multiple clonal chromosomal abnormalities and the severity of peripheral blood cytopenias are independent risk factors that also portend a worse outcome.

The median survival in primary MDS varies from 9 to 29 months, but some individuals in good prognostic groups may live for 5 years or more. Overall, progression to AML occurs in 10 to 40% of individuals and is often accompanied by the appearance of additional clonal cytogenetic changes. Other patients succumb to complications of thrombocytopenia (bleeding) and neutropenia (infection). The outlook is even more grim in patients with t-MDS, who have an overall median survival of only 4 to 8 months. Cytopenias tend to be more severe than in primary MDS, and many patients progress rapidly to AML.

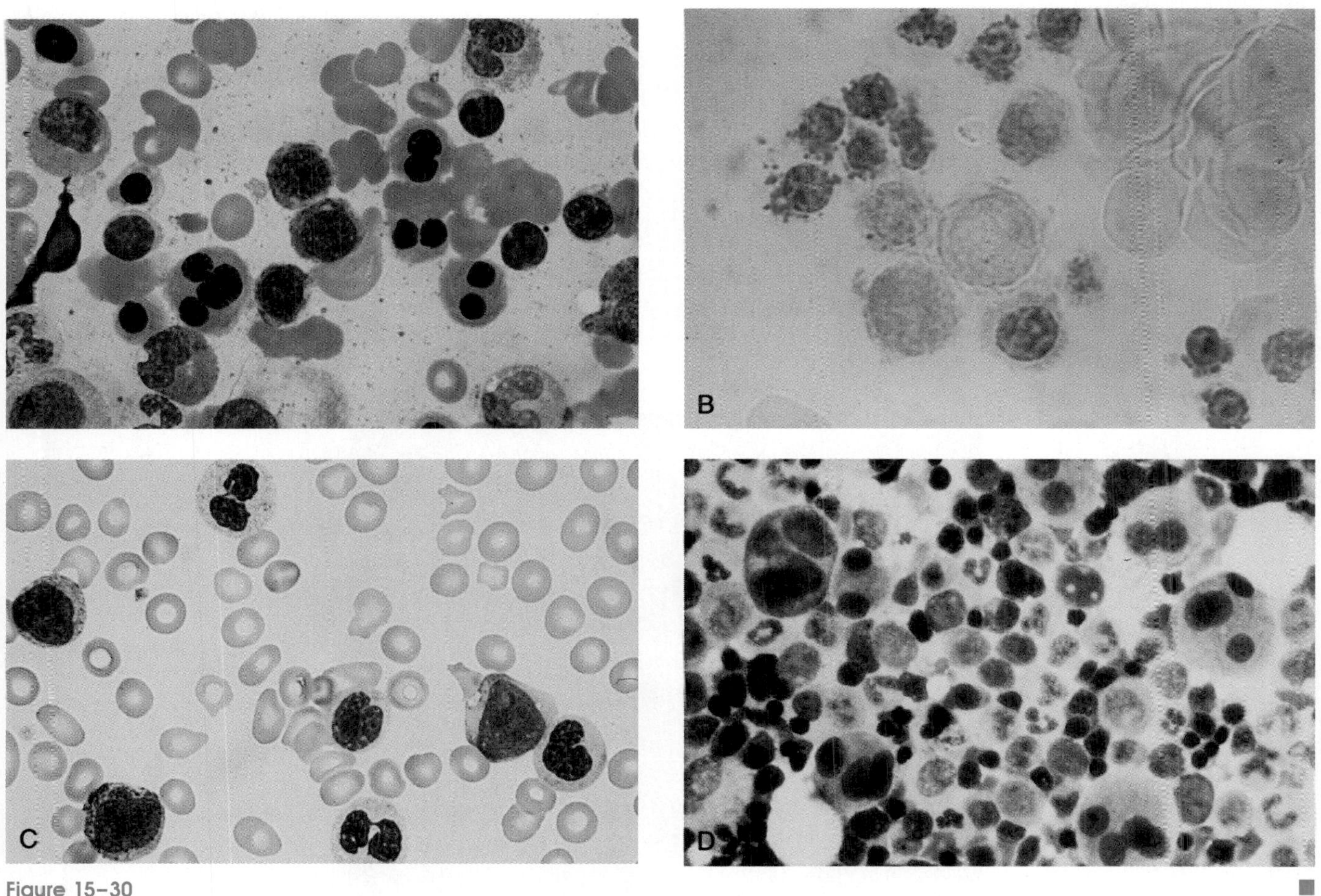

Figure 15-30

Myelodysplasia. Characteristic forms of dysplasia are shown. *A*, Nucleated red cell progenitors with multilobated or multiple nuclei. *B*, Ringed sideroblasts, erythroid progenitors with iron-laden mitochondria, seen as blue perinuclear granules (Prussian blue stain). *C*, Pseudo-Pelger-Huët cells, neutrophils with only two nuclear lobes instead of the normal three to four, are observed at the top and bottom of this field. *D*, Megakaryocytes with multiple nuclei, instead of the normal single multilobated nucleus. (*A*, *B*, and *D*, marrow aspirates; *C*, peripheral blood smear.)

Treatment options in MDS are limited. In younger patients, allogeneic bone marrow transplantation offers some hope for reconstitution of normal hematopoiesis and long-term survival. Older patients with MDS are treated supportively with antibiotics and blood product transfusions.

CHRONIC MYELOPROLIFERATIVE DISORDERS

In most chronic myeloproliferative disorders (MPDs), the target of neoplastic transformation is a multipotent progenitor cell capable of giving rise to mature erythrocytes, platelets, granulocytes, and monocytes. The singular exception is chronic myelogenous leukemia (CML), in which the pluripotent stem cell that can give rise to lymphoid and myeloid cells seems to be affected. Similar to AML, the neoplastic cells and their offspring flood the bone marrow and suppress residual normal progenitor cells; however, chronic MPDs differ in that terminal differentiation is initially unaffected. This combination leads to marrow hypercellularity and increased hematopoiesis, often accompanied by elevated peripheral blood counts.

Certain features are common to each of the four chronic MPDs: (1) CML, (2) polycythemia vera (PCV), (3) essential thrombocytosis, and (4) myelofibrosis with myeloid metaplasia. The neoplastic stem cells have the capacity to circulate and home to secondary hematopoietic organs, particularly the spleen, where they give rise to extramedullary hematopoiesis. As a result, all chronic MPDs cause varying degrees of splenomegaly. They also share the propensity to terminate in a spent phase characterized by marrow fibrosis and peripheral blood cytopenias. Further, all can progress over time to acute leukemia, but only CML does so invariably.

In contrast to the lymphoid neoplasms and AML, the pathologic findings in the chronic MPDs are not specific, having a considerable degree of overlap with one another and some reactive conditions that produce marrow hyperplasia. Diagnosis and classification depend on correlation of morphologic findings with other clinical and laboratory findings. Cytogenetic and molecular analyses also play an important role, as patients with CML uniformly possess the Philadelphia chromosome (Ph[1]) or variants thereof, whereas patients with other chronic MPDs lack the Ph[1].

Chronic Myelogenous Leukemia

CML is a disease primarily of adults between the ages of 25 and 60 years, with the peak incidence in the thirties and forties.

Genetics. *CML is distinguished from other chronic MPDs by the presence of a distinctive molecular abnormality—a translocation involving the BCR gene on chromosome 9 and the ABL gene on chromosome 22.* The resultant *BCR-ABL* fusion gene directs the synthesis of a 210-kD fusion protein with tyrosine kinase activity. In more than 90% of CML cases, karyotyping reveals the Ph[1], usually representing the reciprocal translocation t(9; 22)(q34;q11). In 5 to 10% of cases, however, the rearrangement can be complex or cytogenetically cryptic; in such cases, other methods such as *f*luorescent *in s*itu *hy*bridization (FISH) (Fig. 15–31), or the reverse transcriptase–polymerase chain reaction (RT-PCR) must be used to

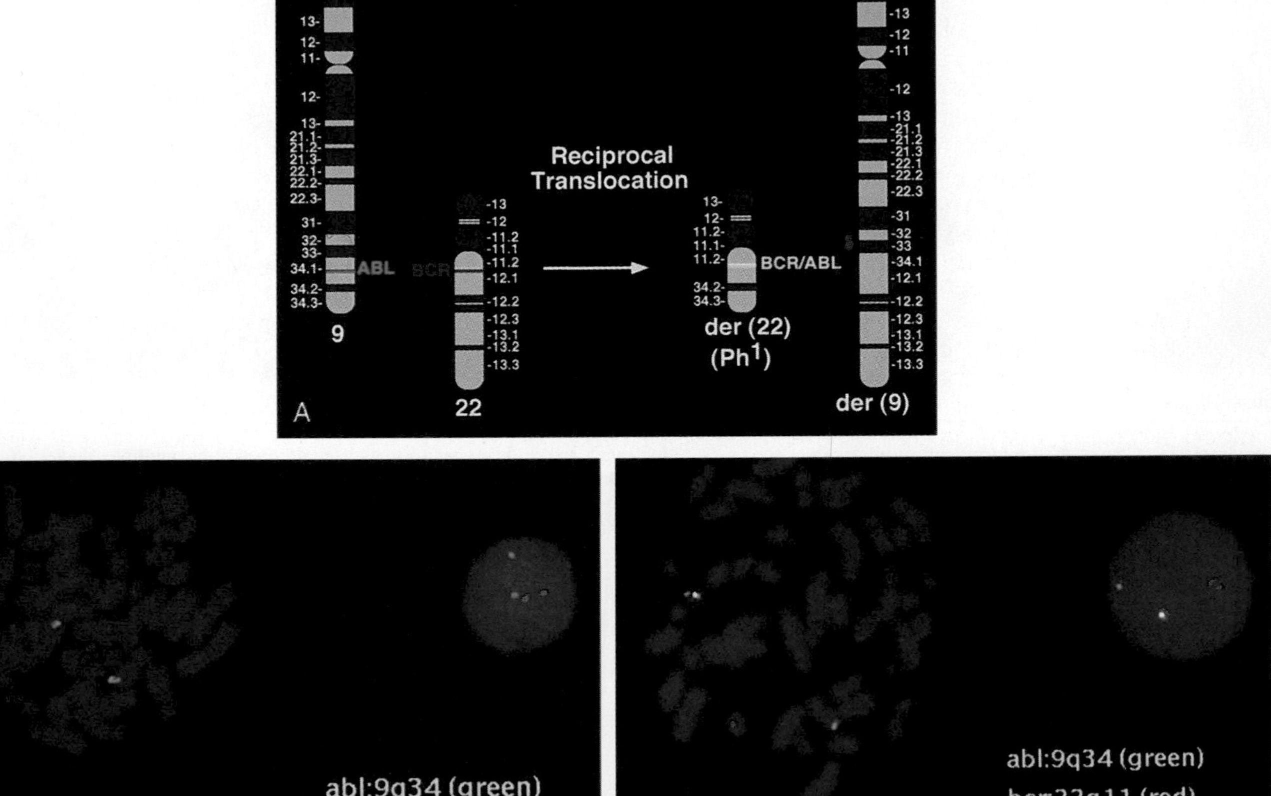

Figure 15–31

Detection of *BCR-ABL* fusion gene by fluorescent in situ hybridization (FISH). *A*, Idiogram depicting chromosomes 9 and 22 and the position of the *ABL* and *BCR* genes. The Philadelphia chromosome (Ph[1]) is created by a balanced chromosomal translocation that replaces the telomeric portion of 22q with the telomeric portion of 9q. At a molecular level, the breaking and rejoining of the DNA results in the formation of fusion gene on the Ph[1] derived from the 5′ end of *BCR* and the 3′ end of *ABL*, and hence brings *BCR* and *ABL* sequences that are normally far apart into close physical proximity. This abnormal colocalization of *BCR* and *ABL* can be detected by in situ hybridization with pairs of fluorescently tagged DNA probes complementary to genomic DNA sequences lying near *BCR* and *ABL* breakpoints. In *B* a green *ABL* probe and a red *BCR* probe have been hybridized to metaphase chromosomes and interphase nuclei prepared from the peripheral blood cells of a normal individual. Because of the pairing of sister chromatids during mitosis, signals on metaphase chromosomes may be seen as a single dot or a pair of closely spaced dots. Two pairs of red signals and two green signals are seen on the metaphase chromosomes, while two red and two green signals are present in the interphase nucleus, both indicating the presence of normal, spatially distant copies of *ABL* and *BCR*, respectively. *C*, In contrast, metaphase chromosomes and an interphase nucleus prepared from the bone marrow cells of a patient with CML show one normal *ABL* signal, one normal *BCR* signal, and an abnormal yellow signal created by superimposition of one *BCR* and one *ABL* signal, a finding indicative of the presence of a *BCR-ABL* fusion gene. (Courtesy of Dr. Cynthia Morton and Ms. Debbie Sandstrom, Department of Pathology, Brigham and Women's Hospital, Boston, MA.)

detect the *BCR-ABL* fusion gene or transcript. Introduction of the *BCR-ABL* fusion gene into murine bone marrow cells gives rise to a syndrome resembling human CML,[74] and hence its acquisition is considered to be a critical pathogenetic event.

There is a marked increase in neoplastic granulocytic precursors in the marrow, which coexist with a smaller number of *BCR-ABL* negative (normal) progenitor cells.[75] Although granulocytic proliferation dominates, genotypic studies have shown that other myeloid lineages, B lymphoid cells, and possibly T lymphoid cells also carry the Ph[1] or its molecular equivalent, indicating that the target of transformation is a pluripotent stem cell. Why there is preferential proliferation of granulocytic precursors is not known.

Figure 15–33

CML of the spleen showing an enlarged spleen (2630 gm; normal, 150–200 gm) with greatly expanded red pulp stemming from neoplastic hematopoiesis. (Courtesy of Dr. Daniel Jones, Department of Pathology, Brigham and Women's Hospital, Boston, MA.)

MORPHOLOGY. In contrast to normal bone marrow, which is usually about 50% cellular and 50% fat, CML marrows are usually 100% cellular, with most of the increased cellularity being composed of maturing granulocytic precursors. Increased numbers of megakaryocytes, often including small dysplastic forms, are frequently observed, whereas erythroid progenitors are usually present in normal or decreased numbers. A characteristic finding is the presence of scattered storage histiocytes with wrinkled, sea-blue cytoplasm (sea-blue histiocytes); similar cells may be seen in other disorders with increased marrow cell turnover. Increased deposition of reticulin fibers is typical, but overt marrow fibrosis is rare at presentation. Peripheral blood examination reveals a marked leukocytosis, often exceeding 100,000 cells/mm³ (Fig. 15–32). The circulating cells are predominantly neutrophils, metamyelocytes, and myelocytes, with less than 10% myeloblasts. Peripheral blood eosinophilia and basophilia are also common, and up to 50% of patients have thrombocytosis early in the course of their disease. Neoplastic extramedullary hematopoiesis within the splenic red pulp produces marked splenomegaly (Fig 15–33) that is often complicated by focal infarction. Extramedullary hematopoiesis may also lead to hepatomegaly and mild lymphadenopathy.

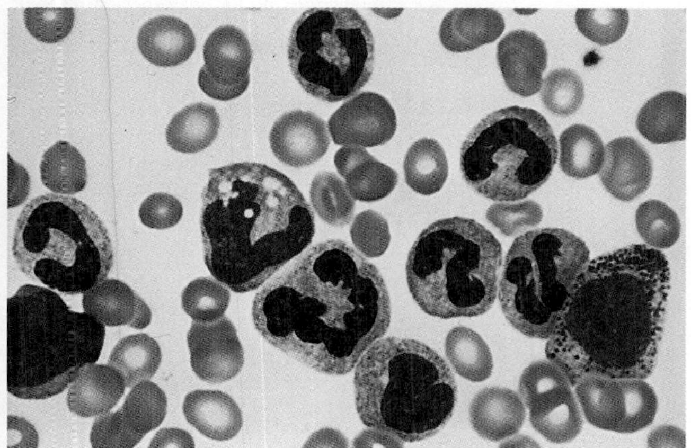

Figure 15–32

Chronic myelogenous leukemia (CML). A peripheral blood smear shows many mature neutrophils, some metamyelocytes, and a myelocyte. (Courtesy of Dr. Robert W. McKenna, Department of Pathology, University of Texas Southwestern Medical School, Dallas, TX.)

Clinical Features. The onset of CML is insidious, and the initial symptoms may be quite nonspecific. They are caused by mild to moderate anemia or by hypermetabolism owing to increased cell turnover and include easy fatigability, weakness, weight loss, and anorexia. Sometimes the first symptom is a dragging sensation in the abdomen caused by the extreme splenomegaly or acute onset of left-upper-quadrant pain caused by splenic infarction.

CML is best differentiated from other chronic MPDs by detection of the *BCR-cABL* fusion gene, either through chromosomal analysis or PCR-based molecular tests. Another informative laboratory finding in CML is the almost total lack of leukocyte alkaline phosphatase. In contrast, leukemoid reactions and other chronic MPDs are usually associated with an elevated leukocyte alkaline phosphatase. The only other hematologic disorder associated with low leukocyte alkaline phosphatase is paroxysmal nocturnal hemoglobinuria, which does not resemble CML in other respects and is therefore easily distinguished.

The course of CML is one of slow progression, and even without treatment a median survival of 3 years can be expected. After a variable period averaging 3 years, approximately 50% of patients enter an *accelerated phase*, during which there is a gradual failure of response to treatment accompanied by increasing anemia and thrombocytopenia and sometimes striking peripheral blood basophilia. Additional clonal cytogenetic abnormalities, such as trisomy 8, isochromosome 17q, or duplication of the Ph[1], may also appear. Within 6 to 12 months, the accelerated phase terminates in a picture resembling acute leukemia (*blast crisis*). In the remaining 50%, blast crises occur abruptly without an intermediate accelerated phase. In 70% of patients, the blasts have the morphologic and cytochemical features of myeloblasts, whereas in about 30% of patients the blasts contain the enzyme TdT and express early B lineage antigens such as CD10 and CD19. Rarely, the blasts resemble pre-T cells. These observations further support the notion that the target cell for transformation is a pluripotent stem cell.

CML can be controlled during the stable phase with low-dose chemotherapy, which, however, does not prevent progression to blast crisis. For this reason, the best hope for long-term survival is allogeneic bone marrow transplantation, which is most effective when performed in the stable phase. In patients with a suitable donor, the cure rate is about 75%. Other therapies include interferon-α, which suppresses CML progenitor cells through poorly understood mechanisms and allows the progeny of normal stem cells to reconstitute the bone marrow, or purification of residual normal stem cells ex vivo by using cell culture conditions that suppress the growth of CML progenitors. The hope is that these normal stem cells could then be used to reconstitute hematopoiesis after potentially curative high-dose cytotoxic therapy.

Polycythemia Vera

PCV is a neoplasm arising in a multipotent myeloid stem cell characterized by increased proliferation and production of erythroid, granulocytic, and megakaryocytic elements. Increased marrow production is reflected in the peripheral blood by erythrocytosis (polycythemia), granulocytosis, and thrombocytosis, but it is the absolute increase in red cell mass that is responsible for most of the clinical symptoms. PCV must be differentiated from relative polycythemia resulting from hemoconcentration (Chapter 14) and other causes of absolute polycythemia.

Pathophysiology. PCV progenitor cells require extremely small amounts of erythropoietin and other hematopoietic growth factors for proliferation and survival.[76] This accounts for the observation that PCV is associated with virtually undetectable levels of serum erythropoietin, whereas almost all other forms of absolute polycythemia are secondary to elevated erythropoietin. A thorough search for acquired erythropoietin receptor mutations in PCV has been unrevealing. The growth factor independence of PCV cells may be found to be caused by mutations in a factor or factors common to multiple hematopoietic growth factor signaling pathways.

MORPHOLOGY. The bone marrow is hypercellular, but some residual fat is often observed. The increase in erythroid progenitors can be quite subtle and is usually accompanied by increased numbers of maturing granulocytic precursors and megakaryocytes. At the time of diagnosis, a moderate to marked increased in marrow reticulin fibers is seen in approximately 10% of the patients. Mild organomegaly is common, being caused early in the course of PCV largely by congestion; at this stage, extramedullary hematopoiesis is minimal. The peripheral blood smear often shows increased basophils and abnormally large platelets.

Late in the course of some patients, the marrow may progress to a spent phase characterized by fibrosis that fills the intertrabecular space and displaces hematopoietic cells. At this time, extramedullary hematopoiesis increases in the spleen and liver, producing more prominent organomegaly (Fig. 15–34). Transformation to morphologically typical AML may also occur.

Clinical Course. PCV appears insidiously, usually in late middle age (median age at onset, 60 years). *Most symptoms are related to the increased red cell mass*, which is usually reflected by a markedly increased hematocrit. The elevation in hematocrit is usually accompanied by an increase in total blood volume, and together these two factors promote abnormal blood flow, vascular distention, and vascular stasis. Most of the excess blood is trapped in the venous circulation, which is greatly distended. Thus, patients are typically plethoric and somewhat cyanotic owing to stagnation and deoxygenation of blood in peripheral vessels. About 70% of patients are hypertensive. Headache, dizziness, and gastrointestinal symptoms are common. There is often intense pruritus and an increased tendency toward peptic ulceration, both possibly the result of an increased release of histamine from basophils. High cell turnover gives rise to hyperuricemia, and symptomatic gout is seen in 5 to 10% of cases.

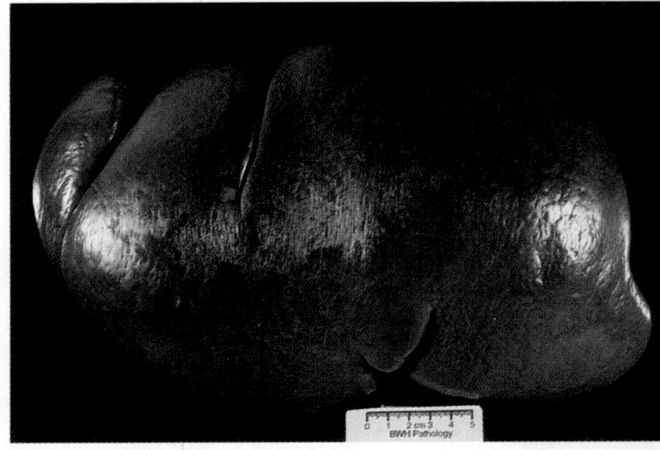

Figure 15–34

Polycythemia vera, spent phase. Massive splenomegaly (3020 gm; normal, 150–200 gm) largely due to extramedullary hematopoiesis occurred in the setting of advanced marrow myelofibrosis. (Courtesy of Dr. Mark Fleming, Department of Pathology, Brigham and Women's Hospital, Boston, MA.)

More ominously, *the abnormal blood flow (and possibly the abnormal platelet function) leads to increased risk of both major bleeding and thrombotic episodes.* About 25% of patients first come to clinical attention with thrombotic episodes, often manifesting as deep venous thrombosis, myocardial infarction, and stroke. Other common sites for thromboses include the hepatic veins (producing Budd-Chiari syndrome), the portal and mesenteric veins (leading to bowel infarction), and the venous sinuses of the brain (leading to hemorrhagic strokes). Minor hemorrhages (epistaxis, bleeding gums) are also common, while life-threatening hemorrhages occur in 5 to 10% of cases.

The hemoglobin concentration ranges from 14 to 28 gm/dl with hematocrit values of 60% or more. Occasionally, chronic bleeding may lead to iron deficiency. In some cases, the deficiency of iron may inhibit erythropoiesis sufficiently to lower the hematocrit into the normal range, a rare example of two defects counteracting one another to *correct* a laboratory abnormality. The white cell count is typically elevated, ranging between 12,000 and 50,000 cells/mm^3, and the platelet count is often greater than 500,000 cells/mm^3. In contrast to CML, leukocyte alkaline phosphatase levels are above normal and the Ph^1 is absent. The platelets usually exhibit morphologic abnormalities manifested as giant forms and megakaryocytic fragments and show defects in functional aggregation studies.

In patients who receive no treatment, death resulting from bleeding or thrombosis occurs within months after diagnosis. If the red cell mass is maintained at nearly normal levels by phlebotomies, however, median survival of 10 years can be achieved.

Extended survival with treatment has revealed that *the natural history of PCV involves a gradual transition to a spent phase, during which clinical and anatomic features of myelofibrosis with myeloid metaplasia develop.* Approximately 15 to 20% of patients undergo such a transformation after an average period of 10 years. This transition is brought about by obliterative fibrosis in the bone marrow (myelofibrosis) and marked by the appearance of extensive extramedullary hematopoiesis, principally in the spleen, which enlarges greatly. The pathogenetic basis for this transformation is not known.

Some patients with PCV develop a terminal AML, but at much lower frequency than in CML. AML occurs in 2% of patients treated with phlebotomy alone[77] but has been seen in up to 15% of those receiving myelosuppressive treatment with alkylating drugs or marrow irradiation with radioactive phosphorus, both of which are mutagenic. Because it is safe and effective, the current treatment of choice is phlebotomy. In contrast to CML, transformation to ALL is rarely observed, possibly indicating that the target of neoplastic transformation is a progenitor cell committed to myeloid differentiation.

Essential Thrombocytosis

In this hematopoietic stem cell disorder, the least common form of MPD, increased proliferation and production is largely confined to the megakaryocytic elements, with most patients having platelet counts exceeding 600,000 mm^3 (Fig. 15–35). Because all of the chronic MPDs can be associated with thrombocytosis, essential thrombocytosis is a diagnosis of exclusion. By definition, features characteristic of other chronic MPDs are absent. It must also be distinguished from reactive causes of thrombocytosis, including inflammatory disorders, asplenism, and iron deficiency. The pathogenetic basis for essential thrombocytosis is unknown.

Bone marrow examination is most helpful in excluding other chronic MPDs. Cellularity is usually mildly to moderately increased. Megakaryocytes are often markedly increased in number and include abnormally large forms. Deposition of delicate reticulin fibrils may be seen, but the overt fibrosis characteristic of myelofibrosis with myeloid metaplasia is absent. *Peripheral smears usually reveal abnormally large platelets* (Fig. 15–35), often accompanied by mild leukocytosis.

The major clinical manifestations are thrombosis and hemorrhage, probably reflecting both qualitative and quantitative abnormalities in platelets. Essential thrombocytosis is an indolent disorder with long asymptomatic periods punctuated by occasional thrombotic or hemorrhagic crises. Median survival times are 12 to 15 years.

Myelofibrosis with Myeloid Metaplasia

Myelofibrosis with myeloid metaplasia, similar to other chronic MPDs, is caused by neoplastic transformation of a multipotent myeloid stem cell. In contrast to other chronic MPDs, however, the hallmark of myelofibrosis with myeloid metaplasia is early progression to marrow fibrosis (myelofibrosis) that is histologically identical to the spent phase of the other chronic MPDs. Myelofibrosis suppresses bone marrow hematopoiesis, leading to peripheral blood cytopenias and extensive neoplastic extramedullary hematopoiesis in the spleen, liver, and lymph nodes.

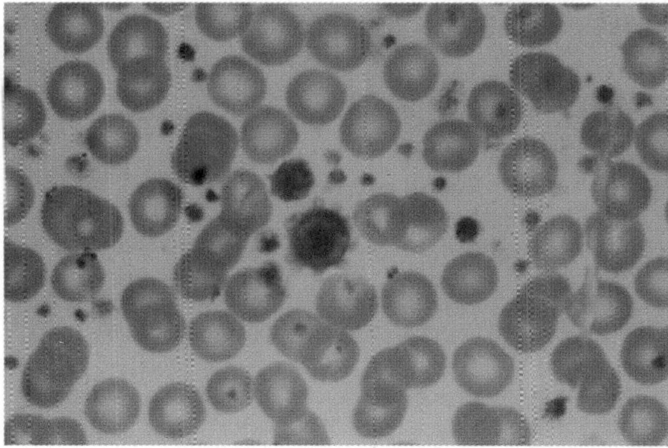

Figure 15–35 ■

Essential thrombocytosis (ET). A peripheral blood smear shows marked thrombocytosis, including giant platelets approximating the size of surrounding red cells. (Courtesy of Dr. Jacqueline Mitus.)

Pathophysiology. The pathologic features of myelofibrosis with myeloid metaplasia stem from extensive collagen deposition by non-neoplastic fibroblasts in the marrow. This fibrosis inexorably displaces hematopoietic elements, including stem cells, from the marrow, leading to extensive extramedullary hematopoiesis in the spleen, liver, and sometimes lymph nodes. The marrow fibrosis appears to be caused by the inappropriate release of fibrogenic factors from neoplastic megakaryocytes.[78,79] Two factors have been implicated: platelet-derived growth factor (PDGF) and TGF-β. Both are synthesized by megakaryocytes and released into the surrounding tissues either by leakage from the abnormal (neoplastic) cells or after intramedullary death. As you recall, PDGF and TGF-β are fibroblast mitogens. In addition, TGF-β promotes fibrosis and causes angiogenesis, both of which are observed in myelofibrosis. As marrow fibrosis progresses, circulating hematopoietic stem cells seed the spleen and liver, leading to extramedullary hematopoiesis.

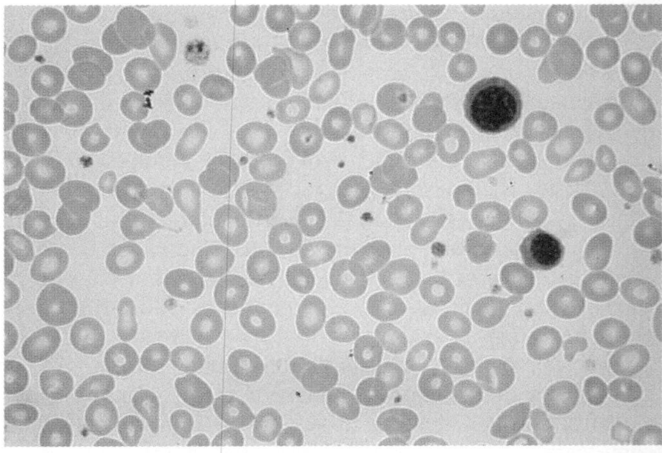

Figure 15–36

Myelofibrosis with myeloid metaplasia (MMM), peripheral blood smear. Two nucleated erythroid precursors and several teardrop-shaped red cells (dacryocytes) are evident. Immature myeloid cells were present in other fields. An identical picture can be seen in other diseases producing marrow distortion and fibrosis.

MORPHOLOGY. Early in the course, the marrow is often hypercellular with maturing cells of all lineages being increased. Morphologically the erythroid and granulocytic precursors appear normal, but megakaryocytes are large, dysplastic, and abnormally clustered. During this cellular phase, fibrosis is minimal. With progression, the marrow becomes hypocellular and diffusely fibrotic. Even at this stage, clusters of atypical megakaryocytes may be found in the sea of fibrosis. Late in the disease course, the fibrotic marrow space may be largely converted to bone, a development that is termed **osteosclerosis.**

Myelofibrotic obliteration of the marrow space leads to extensive extramedullary hematopoiesis, principally in the spleen, which is usually markedly enlarged, sometimes up to 4000 gm (see Fig. 15–39). On section, such spleens are firm and diffusely red to gray, with obliterated white pulp. As with CML, multiple subcapsular infarcts may be present. Histologically, there is trilineage hematopoietic proliferation, often with a predominance of **large, clustered megakaryocytes.** Initially, extramedullary hematopoiesis is confined to the sinusoids, but later it may extend to involve the cords. The **liver** may be moderately enlarged, with sinusoidal foci of extramedullary hematopoiesis. Hematopoiesis may also spread to lymph nodes, but significant lymphadenopathy is uncommon.

The peripheral blood reveals a number of characteristic findings in patients with full-blown myelofibrosis (Fig. 15–36). Fibrotic distortion of the marrow microenvironment leads to inappropriate release of nucleated erythroid progenitors and early granulocytes. Release of immature cells from sites of extramedullary hematopoiesis also contributes to the peripheral blood picture. **The presence of erythroid and granulocytic precursors in the peripheral blood is termed leukoerythroblastosis.** In addition, numerous teardrop erythrocytes (dacryocytes) are observed. Although characteristic of myelofibrosis with myeloid metaplasia, leukoerythroblastosis and dacryocytes can be observed in many infiltrative disorders of the bone marrow, including granulomatous diseases and metastatic tumors. Other common, albeit nonspecific, peripheral blood findings include abnormally large platelets and basophilia.

Clinical Course. Myelofibrosis with myeloid metaplasia is uncommon in individuals younger than 60 years of age. Except when preceded by PCV or CML, it usually comes to clinical attention because of either progressive anemia or marked splenic enlargement, producing a sensation of fullness in the left upper quadrant. Nonspecific symptoms such as fatigue, weight loss, and night sweats result from increased metabolism associated with the expanded mass of hematopoietic cells. Owing to a high rate of cell turnover, hyperuricemia and secondary gout may complicate the picture.

The laboratory findings are striking. There is usually a moderate to severe normochromic normocytic anemia accompanied by leukoerythroblastosis. The white cell count is usually normal or reduced but may be markedly elevated (80,000 to 100,000 cells/mm^3) during the early cellular phase. The platelet count is usually normal or elevated at the time of diagnosis, but thrombocytopenia supervenes as the disease progresses. Biopsy of the marrow to detect the early deposition of reticulin or the more advanced fibrosis is essential for diagnosis.

The course of this disease is difficult to predict. In different series, median survival time has varied from 1 to 5 years.[80] Threats to life are intercurrent infections, thrombotic episodes, bleeding related to platelet abnormalities, and, in 5 to 20% of cases, transformation to AML. In patients with extensive marrow fibrosis, AML may arise at unusual extramedullary sites, including lymph nodes and soft tissues.

Langerhans Cell Histiocytosis

The term *histiocytosis* is an umbrella designation for a variety of proliferative disorders of histiocytes or macrophages. Some, such as the rare histiocytic lymphomas, are clearly malignant, whereas others, such as the reactive histiocytic proliferations in lymph nodes, are clearly benign. Between these two extremes is a small cluster of conditions characterized by proliferation of a special type of histiocyte called the Langerhans cell (Chapter 6). The Langerhans cell histiocytoses represent clonal proliferations of these antigen-presenting dendritic cells,[81] which are normally readily seen in the skin but also found in other organs.

In the past, these disorders were referred to as histiocytosis X and subdivided into three categories: *Letterer-Siwe disease*, *Hand-Schüller-Christian disease*, and *eosinophilic granuloma*. These three conditions are now believed to represent different expressions of the same basic disorder. The tumor cells in each are dendritic and antigen presenting and express HLA-DR and CD1a.[82] They have abundant often vacuolated cytoplasm, with vesicular oval or indented nuclei. *Characteristic is the presence of HX bodies (Birbeck granules) in the cytoplasm. Under the electron microscope, these are seen to have a pentalaminar, rodlike, tubular structure, with characteristic periodicity and sometimes a dilated terminal end (tennis-racket appearance)* (Fig. 15–37). Because Birbeck granules are not seen in all tumor cells by electron microscopy, the detection of CD1a expression by immunohistochemical techniques aids in the diagnosis.

Langerhans cell histiocytosis presents as three clinicopathologic entities. Acute disseminated Langerhans cell histiocytosis (*Letterer-Siwe disease*) occurs most frequently before 2 years of age but occasionally may affect adults. The dominant clinical feature is the development of cutaneous lesions that resemble a seborrheic eruption secondary to infiltrations of Langerhans histiocytes over the front and back of the trunk and on the scalp. Most of those affected have concurrent hepatosplenomegaly, lymphadenopathy, pulmonary lesions, and eventually destructive osteolytic bone lesions. Extensive infiltration of the marrow often leads to anemia, thrombocytopenia, and predisposition to recurrent infections such as otitis media and mastoiditis. The course of untreated disease is rapidly fatal. With intensive chemotherapy, 50% of patients survive 5 years.

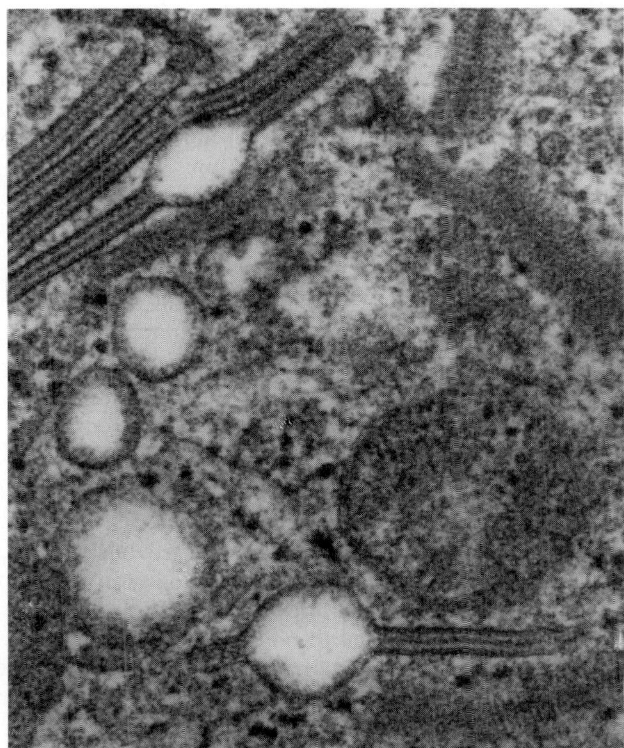

Figure 15–37

Langerhans cell histiocytosis. An electron micrograph shows rodlike Birbeck granules with characteristic periodicity and a dilated terminal end. (Courtesy of Dr. George Murphy, University of Pennsylvania School of Medicine, Philadelphia.)

Unifocal and multifocal Langerhans cell histiocytosis (*unifocal and multifocal eosinophilic granuloma*) are characterized by expanding, erosive accumulations of Langerhans cells, usually within the medullary cavities of bones. Histiocytes are variably admixed with eosinophils, lymphocytes, plasma cells, and neutrophils. The eosinophilic component ranges from scattered mature cells to sheetlike masses of cells. Virtually any bone in the skeletal system may be involved, most commonly the calvaria, ribs, and femur. Similar lesions may be found in the skin, lungs, or stomach, either as unifocal lesions or as components of the multifocal disease.

Unifocal lesions usually affect the skeletal system. They may be asymptomatic or may cause pain and tenderness and, in some instances, pathologic fractures. This is an indolent disorder that may heal spontaneously or be cured by local excision or irradiation.

Multifocal Langerhans cell histiocytosis usually affects children, who present with fever; diffuse eruptions, particularly on the scalp and in the ear canals; and frequent bouts of otitis media, mastoiditis, and upper respiratory tract infections. An infiltrate of Langerhans cells may lead to mild lymphadenopathy, hepatomegaly, and splenomegaly. In about

50% of patients, involvement of the posterior pituitary stalk of the hypothalamus leads to diabetes insipidus. The combination of calvarial defects, diabetes insipidus, and exophthalmos is referred to as the *Hand-Schüller-Christian triad.* Many patients experience spontaneous regression; others can be treated with chemotherapy.

ETIOLOGIC AND PATHOGENETIC FACTORS IN WHITE CELL NEOPLASIA: SUMMARY AND PERSPECTIVES

Having described the many types of white cell neoplasms, it is worth reviewing common themes pertaining to their cause and pathogenetic mechanisms.

- *Chromosomal translocations and oncogenes*
  - First we have seen that nonrandom karyotypic abnormalities, most commonly translocations, are present in the majority of white cell neoplasms. At a molecular level, translocations typically result in the fusion of elements from two genes. In some translocations, the DNA breaks fall within the coding sequence of both involved genes, leading to formation of a fusion gene encoding a novel chimeric protein. In other translocations, the coding sequence of one gene is juxtaposed to the noncoding regulatory elements of the second gene (often an Ig or T-cell receptor locus), resulting in inappropriate expression.
  - Certain chromosomal rearrangements involving protooncogenes are specifically associated with particular hematolymphoid tumors. For example, rearrangements of *TAL-1* are seen only in pre-T cell ALL, whereas *CBFβ* rearrangements are observed only in AML.
  - In contrast, other oncogenes are dysregulated in histogenetically heterogeneous forms of white cell neoplasia. For example, the Ph^1 may be found in AML, ALL, or CML. Such broad-spectrum oncogenes may have more general effects on the proliferation or differentiation of hematolymphoid progenitors.
  - In some instances, dysregulation of specific oncogenes produces hematolymphoid tumors in experimental models closely resembling their human counterparts, demonstrating that these genetic lesions constitute a critical step in tumorigenesis. For example, the expression of the *PML-RARα* gene in the bone marrow progenitors of mice results in the development of an AML that is responsive to treatment with retinoic acid,[83,84] as occurs in human M3 AML.
- *Inherited genetic factors*
  - As was discussed in Chapter 8, individuals with genetic diseases that promote genomic instability, such as Bloom syndrome, Fanconi anemia, and ataxia-telangiectasia, are at increased risk for development of acute leukemia.[85] In addition, Down syndrome (trisomy 21) and neurofibromatosis type I are both associated with an increased incidence of childhood leukemia.
- *Viruses and environmental agents*
  - Three viruses, HTLV-1, EBV, and human herpesvirus 8, have been implicated as causative agents. The possible mechanisms of transformation by viral agents were discussed earlier (Chapters 7 and 8).
  - Several environmental agents that lead to chronic immune stimulation predispose to lymphoid neoplasia. The most clear-cut associations are *Helicobacter pylori* infection and gastric marginal zone lymphoma,[37] and gluten-sensitive enteropathy and intestinal T-cell lymphoma.[86]
- *Iatrogenic factors*
  - Ironically, radiotherapy and certain forms of chemotherapy used to treat cancer increase the risk of subsequent hematolymphoid neoplasms, including MDS, AML, and NHL. This association is believed to stem from mutagenic effects of ionizing radiation and chemotherapeutic drugs on hematolymphoid progenitor cells.

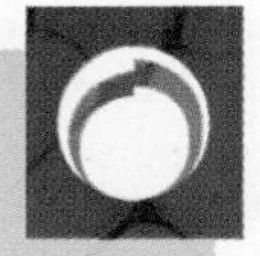

Spleen

NORMAL SPLEEN

The spleen is to the circulatory system as the lymph nodes are to the lymphatic system. Among its functions are filtration from the bloodstream of all *foreign* matter, including obsolescent and damaged blood cells, and participation in the immune response to all blood-borne antigens. Designed ingeniously for these functions, the spleen is a major repository of mononuclear phagocytic cells in the red pulp and of lymphoid cells in the white pulp. Normally in the adult, the spleen weighs about 150 gm and measures 12 cm in length, 7 cm in width, and 3 cm in thickness. It is enclosed within a thin, glistening connective tissue capsule that appears slate gray and through which the dusky red, friable parenchyma of the splenic substance can be seen. The cut surface of the spleen is dotted with gray specks, the splenic, or malpighian, follicles that constitute the white pulp. In three dimensions, this white pulp forms periarterial sheaths of lymphoid cells around the arteries, most abundant about the larger branches and progressively more attenuated as the arterial supply penetrates the splenic substance. A cross-section of such an arrangement reveals a central artery surrounded eccentrically by a collar of T lymphocytes, the so-called periarteriolar lymphatic sheath. At intervals, the lymphatic sheaths expand, usually on one side of the artery, to form lymphoid nodules composed principally of B lymphocytes (Fig. 15–38). On antigenic stimulation, typical germinal centers form within these B-cell areas. Eventually the arterial system terminates in fine penicilliary arterioles, which at first are enclosed within a thin mantle of lymphocytes, but which then enter the red pulp, leaving behind their "fellow-travelers."

The red pulp of the spleen is traversed by numerous thin-walled vascular sinusoids, separated by the splenic cords, or *cords of Billroth*. The endothelial lining of the sinusoid is of the open or discontinuous type, providing passage of blood cells between the sinusoids and cords. The splenic cords are spongelike and consist of a labyrinth of macrophages loosely connected through long dendritic processes to create both a physical and a functional filter through which the blood can slowly seep.

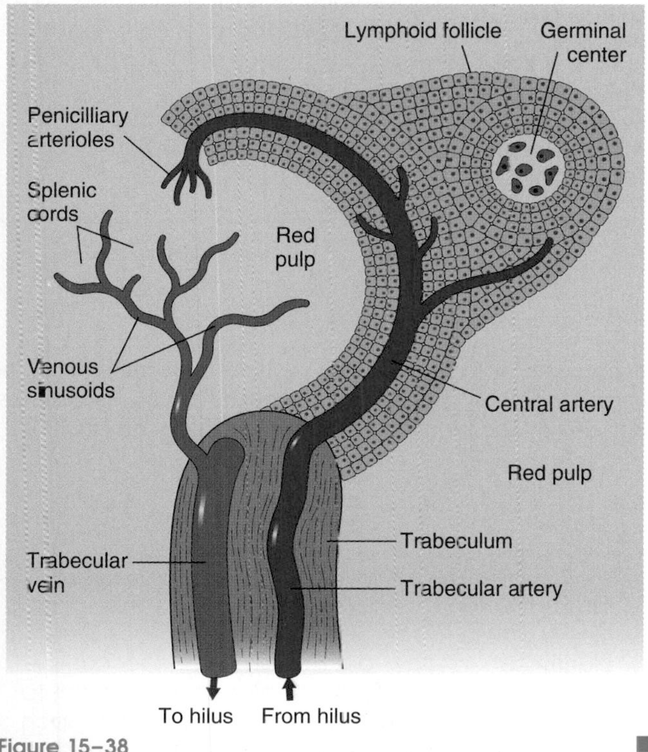

Figure 15–38

Schematic illustration of the normal splenic architecture. (Modified from Faller DV: Diseases of the spleen. In Wyngaarden JB, Smith LH [eds]: Cecil Textbook of Medicine, 18th ed. Philadelphia, WB Saunders, 1988, p 1036.)

It is widely believed that the blood, as it traverses the red pulp, takes two routes to reach the splenic veins.[87] Some of the capillary flow is into the splenic cords and is then gradually filtered out into the surrounding splenic sinusoids to reach the veins; this is the so-called open circulation, which is functionally the slow compartment. The other pathway involves direct passage from the capillaries to the splenic veins without the intervening stage of passage through the cords. This, the *closed circuit*, is understandably the more rapid compartment. According to current views, only a small fraction of the blood entering the spleen at any given time pursues the *open* route. Nevertheless, during the course of a day the total volume of blood passes through the filtration beds of the splenic cords, where it is exposed to the remarkably sensitive and effective phagocytic macrophages, which are able to screen the blood.

Most anatomic disorders of the spleen are secondary to some systemic disorder and thus are the consequence of normal splenic function. These can be segregated into four categories:

1. *Filtration of unwanted elements from the blood* by phagocytosis in the splenic cords is a major function of the spleen.[88] About 1/120 of all red cells are destroyed daily by phagocytosis in the reticuloendothelial system. This amounts to removal of approximately 2×10^{11} red cells/day in a 70-kg adult, about 50% of which are engulfed by splenic macrophages. The splenic phagocytes are also remarkably efficient in "culling" damaged red cells and leukocytes and red cells rendered foreign by antibody coating as well as the abnormal red cells encountered in several of the anemias (e.g., hereditary spherocytosis, sickle cell anemia). As discussed earlier (Chapter 14), the red cells have to undergo extreme deformation during passage from the cords into the sinusoids. In several hemolytic anemias, the reduced plasticity of the red cell membrane leads to trapping of the abnormal red cells within the cords and subsequent phagocytosis by the cordal macrophages. In addition to removal of the red cells, splenic macrophages are also involved in *pitting* of red cells, by which inclusions such as Heinz bodies are neatly excised without destruction of the erythrocytes. The phagocytes are also active in removal of other particulate matter from the blood, such as bacteria, cell debris, and abnormal macromolecules produced in some of the inborn errors of metabolism (e.g., Gaucher disease, Niemann-Pick disease).
2. The spleen is a *major secondary organ in the immune system.* The reticular network in the periarterial lymphatic sheaths traps antigen, permitting it to come into contact with effector lymphocytes.
3. The spleen is a *source of lymphoreticular cells and sometimes hematopoietic cells.* Splenic hematopoiesis normally ceases before birth, but in severe anemia,

extramedullary splenic hematopoiesis may be reactivated.

4. Because of its rich vascularization and phagocytic function, the spleen also constitutes a *reserve pool and storage site*. In humans, the normal spleen harbors only about 30 to 40 ml of erythrocytes, but with splenomegaly this reservoir is greatly increased. The normal spleen also stores approximately 30 to 40% of the total platelet mass in the body. With splenomegaly, this platelet storage may markedly increase, sometimes to up to 80 to 90% of the total platelet mass. Similarly, the enlarged spleen may trap a sufficient number of white cells to induce leukopenia.

In view of all these functions, it is no wonder that the spleen becomes secondarily involved in a wide variety of systemic disorders. As the largest unit of the mononuclear phagocyte system, the spleen is involved in all systemic inflammations and generalized hematopoietic disorders and many metabolic disturbances. It is rarely the primary site of disease. When the spleen is involved in systemic disease, splenic enlargement usually develops, and therefore splenomegaly is a major manifestation of disorders of this organ.

SPLENOMEGALY

Splenic enlargement may be an important diagnostic clue to the existence of an underlying disorder, but the condition itself may cause problems. When sufficiently enlarged, the spleen may cause a dragging sensation in the left upper quadrant and, through pressure on the stomach, cause discomfort after eating. In addition, its storage function may lead to the sequestration of significant numbers of blood elements, giving rise to a syndrome known as *hypersplenism*, which is characterized by the triad of (1) splenomegaly; (2) a reduction of one or more of the cellular elements of the blood, leading to anemia, leukopenia, thrombocytopenia, or any combination of these, in association with hyperplasia of the marrow precursors of the deficient cell type; and (3) correction of the blood cytopenia(s) by splenectomy. The precise cause of this syndrome is still uncertain, but increased sequestration of the cells and the consequent enhanced lysis by the splenic macrophages seem to be the likely explanation for the cytopenias.

Table 15–10 lists disorders associated with splenomegaly. The splenomegaly in virtually all the conditions mentioned has been discussed elsewhere. There remain only a few disorders that require consideration.

Table 15–10. DISORDERS ASSOCIATED WITH SPLENOMEGALY

Infections
Nonspecific splenitis
Infectious mononucleosis
Tuberculosis
Typhoid fever
Brucellosis
Cytomegalovirus
Syphilis
Malaria
Histoplasmosis
Toxoplasmosis
Kala-azar
Trypanosomiasis
Schistosomiasis
Leishmaniasis
Echinococcosis

Congestive States Related to Portal Hypertension
Cirrhosis of the liver
Portal or splenic vein thrombosis
Cardiac failure

Lymphohematogenous Disorders
Hodgkin disease
Non-Hodgkin lymphomas/leukemia
Multiple myeloma
Myeloproliferative disorders
Hemolytic anemias
Thrombocytopenic purpura

Immunologic-Inflammatory Conditions
Rheumatoid arthritis
Systemic lupus erythematosus

Storage Diseases
Gaucher disease
Niemann-Pick disease
Mucopolysaccharidoses

Miscellaneous
Amyloidosis
Primary neoplasms and cysts
Secondary neoplasms

Nonspecific Acute Splenitis

Enlargement of the spleen, sometimes also called *acute splenic tumor*, occurs in any blood-borne infection. The nonspecific splenic reaction in these infections may be caused not only by the microbiologic agents themselves, but also by the products of the inflammatory disease.

MORPHOLOGY. The spleen is enlarged (up to 200 to 400 gm) and soft. The splenic substance is sufficiently soft to flow out literally from the cut surface. Microscopically the major change is acute congestion of the red pulp, which may encroach on and sometimes virtually efface the lymphoid follicles. An infiltrate of neutrophils, plasma cells, and occasionally eosinophils is sometimes present throughout the white and red pulp. At times, there is acute necrosis of the centers of the splenic follicles, particularly when the causative agent is a hemolytic streptococcus. Rarely, abscess formation occurs.

Congestive Splenomegaly

Persistent or chronic venous congestion may cause enlargement of the spleen, referred to as *congestive splenomegaly*. The venous congestion may be systemic in origin, may be caused by intrahepatic derangement of portal venous drainage, or may be due to obstructive venous disorders in the portal or splenic veins. All these disorders ultimately lead to portal or splenic vein hypertension. *Systemic, or central venous, congestion* is encountered in cardiac decompensation involving the right side of the heart, as may occur in tricuspid or pulmonic valvular disease or chronic cor pulmonale or after left-sided heart failure. Such systemic passive congestion produces only moderate enlargement of the spleen, so that it rarely exceeds 500 gm in weight.

The only common causes of striking congestive splenomegaly are the various forms of cirrhosis of the liver. The diffuse fibrous scarring of alcoholic cirrhosis and pigment cirrhosis evokes the most extreme enlargements. Other forms of cirrhosis are less commonly implicated.

Congestive splenomegaly is also caused by obstruction of the extrahepatic portal vein or splenic vein. The venous obstruction may be due to *spontaneous portal vein thrombosis*, which is usually associated with some intrahepatic obstructive disease or may be initiated by inflammatory involvement of the portal vein (*pyelophlebitis*), such as follows intraperitoneal infections. Thrombosis of the splenic vein itself may be initiated by the pressure of tumors in neighboring organs, for example, carcinoma of the stomach or pancreas.

MORPHOLOGY. Long-standing congestive splenomegaly produces marked enlargement of the spleen (1000 gm or more); the organ is firm and becomes increasingly so the longer the congestion lasts. The weight may reach 5000 gm. The capsule may be thickened and fibrous but is otherwise uninvolved. The cut surface has a meaty appearance and varies from gray-red to deep red, depending on the amount of fibrosis. Often the malpighian corpuscles are indistinct. Microscopically, the pulp is suffused with red cells during the early phases but becomes increasingly more fibrous and cellular with time. The increased portal venous pressure causes deposition of collagen in the basement membrane of the sinusoids, which appear dilated owing to the rigidity of their walls. The resulting impairment of blood flow from the cords to the sinusoids prolongs the exposure of the blood cells to the cordal macrophages, resulting in excessive destruction (hypersplenism).[89] Foci of recent or old hemorrhage may be present with deposition of hemosiderin in histiocytes. Organization of these focal hemorrhages gives rise to Gandy-Gamna nodules—foci of fibrosis containing deposits of iron and calcium salts encrusted on connective tissue and elastic fibers.

Splenic Infarcts

Splenic infarcts are comparatively common lesions. Caused by occlusion of the major splenic artery or any of its branches, they are almost always due to emboli that arise in the heart. The spleen, along with kidneys and brain, ranks as one of the most frequent sites of localization of systemic emboli. The infarcts may be small or large, multiple or single, and sometimes involve the entire organ. They are usually of the bland, anemic type. Septic infarcts are found in infective endocarditis of the valves of the left side of the heart.

MORPHOLOGY. Infarcts are characteristically pale and wedge-shaped, with their bases at the periphery where the capsule is often covered with fibrin (Fig. 15–39). Septic infarction modifies this appearance as frank suppurative necrosis devel-

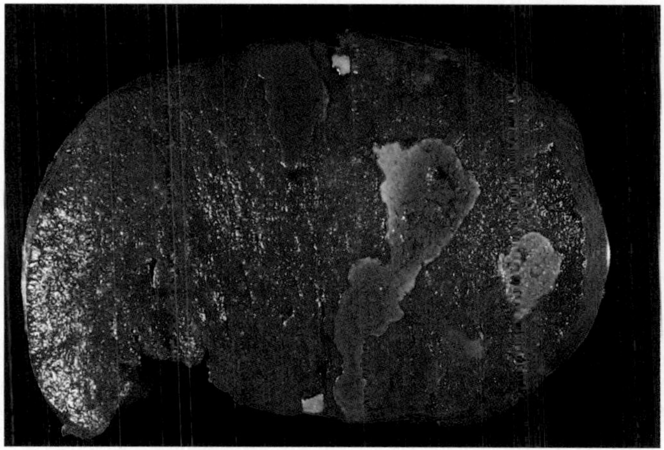

Figure 15–39

Splenic infarcts. Multiple well-circumscribed infarcts are present in this spleen (2820 gm; normal, 150–200 gm) that is massively enlarged by extramedullary hematopoiesis secondary to bone marrow myelofibrosis. Recent infarcts are hemorrhagic, whereas older, more fibrotic infarcts are pale yellow-gray.

ops. In the course of healing of these splenic infacts, large, depressed scars may develop.

NEOPLASMS

Neoplastic involvement of the spleen is rare except in tumors of the lymphohematopoietic system. When present, they induce splenomegaly. The following types of benign tumors may arise in the spleen: fibromas, osteomas, chondromas, lymphangiomas, and hemangiomas. The two last-named are the most common and are often cavernous in type. Some of the hemangiomas are better classified as hamartomas than as neoplasms. Splenic involvement occurs in a variety of leukemias and lymphomas, as already discussed.

CONGENITAL ANOMALIES

Complete absence of the spleen is rare and is usually associated with other congenital abnormalities, such as situs inversus and cardiac malformations. *Hypoplasia* is a more common finding.

Accessory spleens (spleniculi) are common and have been encountered singly or multiply in one fifth to one third of all postmortem examinations. They are usually small spherical structures that are histologically and functionally identical with the normal spleen, reacting to various stimuli in the same manner. They are generally situated in the gastrosplenic ligament or the tail of the pancreas but are sometimes located in the omentum or mesenteries of the small or large intestine. Accessory spleens may have great clinical importance. In some hematologic disorders, such as hereditary spherocytosis, thrombocytopenic purpura, and hypersplenism, splenectomy is a standard method of treatment. If a large accessory spleen is overlooked, the benefit from the removal of the definitive spleen may be lost.

RUPTURE

Rupture of the spleen is usually caused by a crushing injury or severe blow. Much less often, it is encountered in the apparent absence of trauma; this event is designated as spontaneous rupture. It is a clinical maxim that the normal spleen never ruptures spontaneously. In all instances of apparent nontraumatic rupture, some underlying condition should be suspected as the basis for the enlargement or weakening of this organ. Spontaneous rupture is encountered most often in infectious mononucleosis, malaria, typhoid fever, leukemia, and the other types of acute splenitis. Rupture is usually followed by extensive, sometimes massive, intraperitoneal hemorrhage. The condition usually must be treated by prompt surgical removal of the spleen to prevent death from loss of blood and shock.

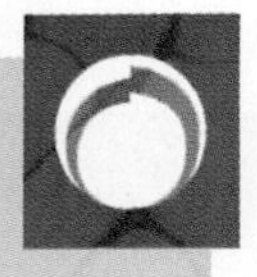

Thymus

NORMAL THYMUS

Once an organ buried in obscurity within the mediastinum, the thymus has risen to a star role in cell-mediated immunity, as detailed in Chapter 7. Here, interest centers on the disorders of the gland itself.

The thymus is embryologically derived from the third and, inconstantly, the fourth pair of pharyngeal pouches along with the lower pair of parathyroid glands. Not surprisingly, one or two parathyroids occasionally become enclosed within the thymic capsule, an aberrance that may plague the parathyroid surgeon. The thymus, or a portion of it, may be found in ectopic locations in the neck or on the pleural surface. At birth, the thymus weighs 10 to 35 gm and continues to grow in size until puberty, when it achieves a maximal weight of 20 to 50 gm. Thereafter, it undergoes progressive atrophy to little more than 5 to 15 gm in the elderly. This age-related involution is accompanied by replacement of the thymic parenchyma by fibrofatty tissue. The rate of thymic growth in the child and involution in the adult is extremely variable, and so it is difficult to determine weight appropriate for age. The thymus may also involute in children and young adults in response to episodes of severe stress, including HIV infection.

The fully developed thymus is pyramid shaped, well encapsulated, and composed of two fused lobes. Fibrous extensions of the capsule divide each lobe into numerous lobules, each of which has an outer cortical layer enclosing the central medulla. A diversity of cell types populate the thymus, but thymic epithelial cells and lymphocytes of T-cell lineage predominate (Chapter 7). Directly beneath the capsule, the epithelial cells are closely packed, but deeper in the cortex and medulla, they create a structural lattice containing lymphocytes. In the cortex, they have an abundant cytoplasm and pale vesicular nuclei with finely divided chromatin and only small nucleoli; cytoplasmic extensions interconnect with adjacent cells. In contrast, the epithelial cells in the medulla have only scant cytoplasm devoid of interconnecting processes; are more oval in shape; and may be *spindled* with oval, darkly staining nuclei. Whorls of these cells create the well-known *Hassall corpuscles* having keratinized cores.

As you know from the earlier consideration of the thymus in relation to immunity (Chapter 7), progenitor cells of marrow origin migrate to the thymus and there give rise to T cells. Peripherally, in the superficial cortex, there is a thin layer of relatively large prothymocytes that express early T-cell markers (such as CD2). These cells give rise to the more mature thymocytes found in the deeper cortex and the medulla. Most of the cortical thymocytes are small, compact cells bearing CD1a, CD2, and CD3 markers as well as both CD4 and CD8. The medullary thymocytes are fewer in number and slightly larger than the cortical thymocytes, and mostly express either CD4 or CD8.

In addition to thymocytes and epithelial cells, macrophages, dendritic cells, and rare neutrophils, eosinophils, B lymphocytes, and scattered myoid (muscle-like) cells may be found within the thymus. The myoid cells are of particular interest because, as seen subsequently, the thymus in some obscure manner is related to myasthenia gravis, a musculoskeletal disorder of apparent immune origin.

Morphologic lesions in the thymus are associated with a variety of systemic conditions ranging from immunologic to hematologic to neoplastic. The changes within the thymus itself are of relatively limited nature and can be adequately considered under the following headings: (1) developmental disorders, (2) thymic hyperplasia, and (3) thymomas. The changes associated with myasthenia gravis are considered in Chapter 28.

DEVELOPMENTAL DISORDERS

Thymic hypoplasia or *aplasia* is seen in DiGeorge syndrome accompanied by parathyroid developmental failures. As detailed in Chapter 7, this condition is marked by a total absence or severe lack of cell-mediated immunity and often hypoparathyroidism. Developmental defects may also involve the heart and great vessels as well as other sites.

Thymic cysts are uncommon lesions that are usually discovered incidentally at postmortem or at surgery. They are probably developmental in origin, rarely exceed 4 cm in diameter, may be spherical or arborizing, and are lined by stratified to columnar epithelium. The fluid contents may be serous to mucinous and are often modified by hemorrhage, recent or old. Cysts rarely distort the contour of the thymus itself and are without clinical significance.

THYMIC HYPERPLASIA

The term *thymic hyperplasia* in reality applies to the appearance of lymphoid follicles within the thymus, creating what is referred to as *thymic follicular hyperplasia.* The lymphoid follicles are not different from those encountered in lymph nodes, have germinal centers, and contain both follicular dendritic cells and B lymphocytes, which are present in scant numbers in the normal thymus. Although follicular hyperplasia may occur in chronic inflammatory and immunologic states, it is most frequently encountered in myasthenia gravis and is present in about 65 to 75% of these cases (Chapter 28). Similar thymic changes are sometimes encountered in Graves disease, systemic lupus erythematosus, scleroderma, and rheumatoid arthritis as well as other autoimmune disorders.

THYMOMAS

A diversity of neoplasms may arise in the thymus—germ cell tumors, lymphomas, Hodgkin disease, and carcinoids as well as others—but the *designation thymoma should be restricted to tumors of thymic epithelial cells.* Such tumors typically have in addition a scant or rich background of immature T cells (thymocytes), but this population of cells is secondary, not monoclonal, not tumorous, and therefore does not contribute to the biology or clinical behavior of these neoplasms.

Thymomas have been classified and reclassified in an effort to create subsets of clinical and prognostic usefulness. No effort is made here to present these varied classifications; we resort to one that has the virtues of simplicity and clinical usefulness. According to this approach, thymomas can be divided into the following categories:

- Benign or encapsulated thymoma: cytologically and biologically benign
- Malignant thymoma
  - Type I, also called *invasive thymoma*: cytologically benign but biologically aggressive and capable of local invasion and, rarely, distant spread
  - Type II, also called *thymic carcinoma*: cytologically malignant with all of the features of cancer and comparable behavior

All categories, benign and malignant, are tumors of adults, usually older than 40 years of age, and are rare in children. Males and females are affected equally. Most arise in the anterosuperior mediastinum but sometimes in the neck, thyroid, pulmonary hilus, or elsewhere. They are uncommon in the posterior mediastinum. They account for only 20 to 30% of tumors in the anterosuperior mediastinum because this is also a common location for the nodular sclerosis type of HD and certain forms of NHL.

MORPHOLOGY. Macroscopically, thymomas are lobulated, firm, gray-white masses up to 15 to 20 cm in longest dimension. They sometimes have areas of cystic necrosis and calcification even in tumors that later prove to be biologically benign. The majority appear encapsulated, but in about 20 to 25%, there is apparent penetration of the capsule and infiltration of perithymic tissues and structures.

Thymomas typically consist of jigsaw puzzle–type lobules that are separated by fibrous bands. Microscopically, virtually all thymomas are made up of a mixture of epithelial cells and a variable infiltrate of non-neoplastic thymocytes. The relative proportions of the epithelial and thymocytic components are of little significance.[90] In **benign thymomas,** the epithelial cells most often resemble those of the medulla and are often elongated or spindle-shaped, producing what is called a spindle cell or medullary thymoma (Fig. 15–40*A*). This pattern of thymoma often has few thymocytes. Frequently, there is an admixture of the plumper, rounder, cortical-type epithelial cells, producing a mixed pattern. The medullary and mixed patterns account for about 50% of all thymomas. Tumors that have a significant proportion of medullary-type epithelial cells are usually benign. Hassall corpuscles are rarely present with either pattern and, when found, often appear as poorly formed suggestive whorls. They are of no diagnostic significance because they may represent residual normal thymic tissue.

The designation **malignant thymoma type I** as used here implies a cytologically benign tumor, which is locally invasive and sometimes has the capacity for widespread metastasis (Fig. 15–40*B*). These tumors account for about 20 to 25% of all thymomas. They are composed of varying proportions of epithelial cells and thymocytes; the epithelial cells, however, tend to be of the cortical variety with abundant cytoplasm and rounded vesicular nuclei. Palisading of these cells about blood vessels is sometimes seen. Some spindled epithelial cells may be present as well. Typically, in a subset of these tumors, the neoplastic cells exhibit cytologic atypia, which correlates with a propensity for more aggressive behavior. **The critical distinguishing feature of these neoplasms is penetration of the capsule with invasion into surrounding structures.** The extent of invasion has been subdivided into various stages, which are somewhat beyond our scope, but it suffices that with minimal invasion, complete excision yields a

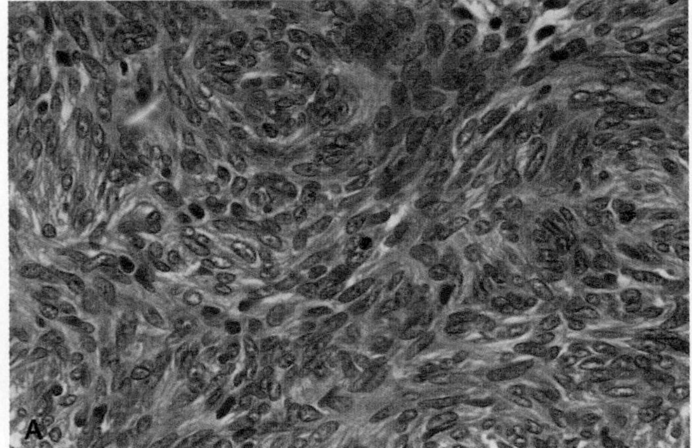

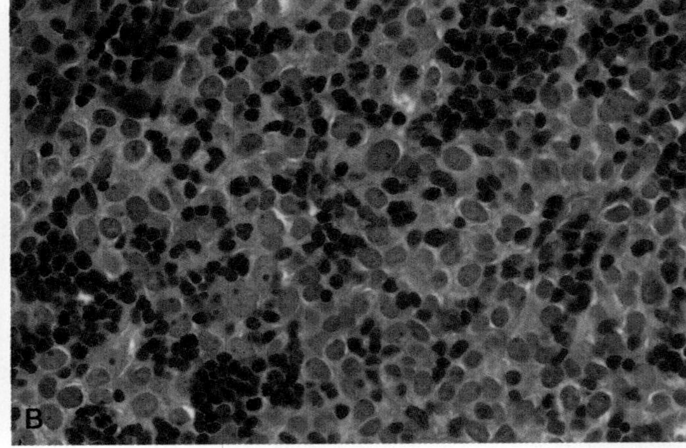

Figure 15–40

Benign and malignant thymoma. *A*, Benign thymoma (medullary type). The neoplastic epithelial cells are arranged in a swirling pattern and have bland, oval to elongated nuclei with inconspicuous nucleoli. Only a few small, reactive lymphoid cells are interspersed. *B*, Malignant thymoma type I. The neoplastic epithelial cells are polygonal and have round to oval, bland nuclei with inconspicuous nucleoli. Numerous small, reactive lymphoid cells are interspersed. The morphologic appearance of this tumor is identical to that of benign thymomas of the cortical type. In this case, however, the tumor was locally aggressive, invading adjacent lung and pericardium. (Courtesy of Dr. David Dorfman, Department of Pathology, Brigham and Women's Hospital, Boston, MA.)

greater than 90% 5-year survival. Extensive invasion is often accompanied by metastasis and is associated with a less than 50% 5-year survival.[91] These tumors tend to occur in younger patients.

Malignant thymoma type II is better designated **thymic carcinoma.** They represent about 5% of thymomas. In contrast to the type I malignant thymomas, these are cytologically malignant, having all of the features of anaplasia seen in most forms of cancer. Macroscopically, they are usually fleshy, obviously invasive masses sometimes accompanied by metastases to such sites as the lungs. The majority are **squamous cell carcinomas, either well or poorly differentiated.** The next most common malignant pattern is the so-called **lymphepithelioma** composed of cytologically anaplastic cortical-type epithelial cells scattered against a dense background of non-neoplastic thymocytes. Some lymphepitheliomas, particularly those occurring in Asian patients, contain clonal EBV genomes, suggesting a role for EBV in their pathogenesis. A variety of other histologic patterns of thymic carcinoma have been described, including sarcomatoid variants, basaloid carcinoma, and clear cell carcinoma. Thymic carcinoma cells, but not those of thymomas and nonthymic carcinomas, express CD5, a receptor molecule that signals cell growth in T cells.[92]

Clinical Course. Many thymomas are discovered incidentally during the course of some form of cardiac surgery. Of those that come to clinical attention, about 40% present as thymic masses either on imaging studies or because of local pressure symptoms and 30 to 45% because of their association with myasthenia gravis. Thymomas may be associated with other paraneoplastic syndromes, such as acquired hypogammaglobulinemia, pure red cell aplasia, Graves disease, pernicious anemia, dermatomyositis-polymyositis, and Cushing syndrome. The basis for these associations is still obscure.

REFERENCES

1. Dale DC: Immune and idiopathic neutropenia. Current Opin Hematol 5:33, 1998.
2. Loughran TP: Clonal diseases of large granular lymphocytes. Blood 82:1, 1993.
3. National Cancer Institute: Sponsored study of classification of non-Hodgkin's lymphomas: summary and description of Working Formulation for Clinical Usage. Cancer 49:2112, 1982.
4. Harris NL, et al: A revised European-American classification of lymphoid neoplasms: a proposal from the International Lymphoma Study Group. Blood 84:1361, 1994.

4a. Jaffe ES, et al: Society for Hematopathology Program—WHO classification of lymphomas and leukemia. Am J Surg Pathol 21:114, 1997.

5. Sklar J: Polymerase chain reaction: the molecular microscope of residual disease. J Clin Oncol 9:1521, 1991.
6. Semenzato G, et al: The lymphoproliferative disease of granular lymphocytes: updated criteria for diagnosis. Blood 89:256, 1997.
7. Lacy MQ, et al: Pure red cell aplasia: association with large granular lymphocyte leukemia and the prognostic value of cytogenetic abnormalities. Blood 87:3000, 1996.
8. Starkebaum G, et al: Immunogenetic similarities between patients with Felty's syndrome and those with clonal expansions of large granular lymphocytes in rheumatoid arthritis. Arthritis Rheum 40:624, 1997.
9. Jaffe ES, et al: Report of the Workshop on Nasal and Related Extranodal Angiocentric T/Natural Killer Cell Lymphomas: definitions, differential diagnosis, and epidemiology. Am J Surg Pathol 20:103, 1996.
10. Rubnitz JE, Look AT: Molecular genetics of childhood leukemias. J Pediatr Hematol Oncol 20:1, 1998.
11. Fletcher JA, et al: Extremely poor prognosis of pediatric acute lymphoblastic leukemia with translocation (9;22): updated experience. Leuk Lymphoma 8:75, 1992.
12. Rambaldi A, et al: Molecular diagnosis and clinical relevance of t(9; 22), t(4;11) and t(1;19) chromosome abnormalities in a consecutive group of 141 adult patients with acute lymphoblastic leukemia. Leuk Lymphoma 21:457, 1996.
13. Banks P, et al: Mantle cell lymphoma: a proposal for unification of morphologic, immunologic, and molecular data. Am J Surg Pathol 16: 637, 1992.
14. Dohner H, et al: 11q deletions identify a new subset of B-cell chronic lymphocytic leukemia characterized by extensive nodal involvement and inferior prognosis. Blood 89:2516, 1997.
15. Garcia-Marco JA, et al: Interphase cytogenetics in chronic lymphocytic leukemia. Cancer Genet Cytogenet 94:52, 1997.
16. Caligaris-Cappio F: B-chronic lymphocytic leukemia: a malignancy of anti-self B cells. Blood 87:2615, 1996.
17. O'Brien A, et al: Advances in the biology and treatment of B-cell chronic lymphocytic leukemia. Blood 85:307, 1995.
18. Weiss LM, et al: Molecular analysis of the t(14;18) chromosomal translocation in malignant lymphomas. N Engl J Med 317:1185, 1987.
19. Lo Coco F, et al: Rearrangements of the BCL6 gene in diffuse large cell non-Hodgkin's lymphoma. Blood 83:1757, 1994.
20. Cattoretti G, et al: BCL-6 protein is expressed in germinal-center B cells. Blood 86:45, 1995.
21. Nador RG, et al: Herpes-like DNA sequences in a body-cavity-based lymphoma in an HIV-negative patient. N Engl J Med 333:943, 1995.
22. Otsuki T, et al: Detection of HHV-8/KSHV DNA sequences in AIDS-associated extranodal lymphoid malignancies. Leukemia 10: 1358, 1996.
23. Gessain A, et al: Human herpes virus 8 (Kaposi's sarcoma herpes virus) and malignant lymphoproliferations in France: a molecular study of 250 cases including two AIDS-associated body cavity based lymphomas. Leukemia 11:266, 1997.
24. Shipp MA: Prognostic factors in aggressive non-Hodgkin's lymphoma: who has "high-risk" disease? Blood 83:1165, 1994.
25. Offit K, et al: Rearrangement of the bcl-6 gene as a prognostic marker in diffuse large-cell lymphoma. N Engl J Med 331:74, 1994.
26. Ichikawa A, et al: Mutations of the p53 gene as a prognostic factor in aggressive B-cell lymphoma. N Engl J Med 337:529, 1997.
27. Pelicci P, et al: Different regions of the immunoglobulin heavy-chain locus are involved in chromosomal translocations in distinct pathogenetic forms of Burkitt lymphoma. Proc Natl Acad Sci U S A 83: 2984, 1986.
28. Klein B, Bataille R: Cytokine network in human myeloma. Hematol Oncol Clin North Am 6:285, 1992.
29. Bataille R, Harousseau JL: Multiple myeloma. N Engl J Med 336: 1657, 1997.
30. Bataille R, et al: Biologic effects of anti-interleukin-6 murine monoclonal antibody in advanced multiple myeloma. Blood 86:685, 1995.
31. Rettig MB, et al: Kaposi's sarcoma-associated herpesvirus infection of bone marrow dendritic cells from multiple myeloma patients. Science 276:1851, 1997.
32. Chesi M, et al: Frequent translocation t(4;14)(p16.3;q32.3) in multiple

myeloma is associated with increased expression and activating mutations of fibroblast growth factor receptor 3. Nat Genet 16:260, 1997.
33. Kovacsovics TJ, Delaly A: Intensive treatment strategies in multiple myeloma. Semin Hematol 34:49, 1997.
34. Dimopoulos MA, Alexanian R: Waldenstrom's macroglobulinemia. Blood 83:1452, 1994.
35. Bigoni R, et al: Characterization of t(11;14) translocation in mantle cell lymphoma by fluorescent in situ hybridization. Oncogene 13:797, 1996.
36. Swerdlow SH, et al: Expression of cyclin D1 protein in centrocytic/mantle cell lymphomas with and without rearrangement of the BCL1/cyclin D1 gene. Hum Pathol 26:999, 1995.
37. Wetherspoon AC: Gastric lymphoma of mucosa-associated lymphoid tissue and *Helicobacter pylori.* Annu Rev Med 49:289, 1998.
38. Koulis A, et al: Characterization of tumor-infiltrating T lymphocytes in B-cell lymphomas of mucosa-associated lymphoid tissue. Am J Pathol 151:1353, 1997.
39. Bennett C, et al: Disseminated atypical mycobacterial infection in patients with hairy cell leukemia. Am J Med 80:891, 1986.
40. Piro L, et al: Lasting remissions in hairy cell leukemia induced by a single infusion of 2′-chlorodeoxyadenosine. Cancer 332:657, 1990.
41. Pinkus GS, Said JW: Hodgkin's disease, lymphocyte predominance type, nodular—a distinct entity? Unique staining profile for L&H variants of Reed-Sternberg cells defined by monoclonal antibodies to leukocyte common antigen, granulocyte-specific antigen, and B-cell-specific antigen. Am J Pathol 118:1, 1985.
42. Poppema S: Lymphocyte-predominance Hodgkin's disease. Semin Diagn Pathol 9:257, 1992.
43. Marafioti T, et al: Origin of nodular lymphocyte-predominant Hodgkin's disease from a clonal expansion of highly mutated germinal-center B cells. N Engl J Med 337:453,1997.
44. Ohno T, et al: Clonality in nodular lymphocyte-predominant Hodgkin's disease. N Engl J Med 337:459, 1997.
45. Samoszuk M, Nansen L: Detection of interleukin-5 messenger RNA in Reed-Sternberg cells of Hodgkin's disease with eosinophilia. Blood 75:13, 1990.
46. Kadin ME, et al: Immunohistochemical evidence of a role for transforming growth factor beta in the pathogenesis of nodular sclerosing Hodgkin's disease. Am J Pathol 136:1209, 1990.
47. Pinto A, et al: Human eosinophils express functional CD30 ligand and stimulate proliferation of a Hodgkin's disease cell line. Blood 88: 3299, 1996.
48. Inghirami G, et al: The Reed-Sternberg cells of Hodgkin's disease are clonal. Proc Natl Acad Sci USA 91:9842, 1994.
49. Delabie J, et al: The antigen-presenting cell function of Reed-Sternberg cells. Leuk Lymphoma 18:35, 1995.
50. Agnarsson BA, Kadin ME: The immunophenotype of Reed-Sternberg cells. A study of 50 cases of Hodgkin's disease using fixed frozen tissues. Cancer 63:2083, 1989.
51. Pinkus GS, et al: Fascin, a sensitive new marker for Reed-Sternberg cells of Hodgkin's disease. Evidence for a dendritic or B cell derivation? Am J Pathol 150:543, 1997.
52. Wolf J, et al: Peripheral blood mononuclear cells of a patient with advanced Hodgkin's lymphoma give rise to permanently growing Reed-Sternberg cells. Blood 87:3418, 1996.
53. Kanzler H, et al: Molecular single cell analysis demonstrates the derivation of a peripheral blood-derived cell line (L1236) from the Hodgkin/Reed-Sternberg cells of a Hodgkin's lymphoma patient. Blood 87:3429, 1996.
54. Wolf J, et al: Report on the workshop biology of the Third International Symposium on Hodgkin's Lymphoma in Cologne 1995. Ann Oncol 7:45, 1996.
55. Weiss LM, et al: Detection of Epstein-Barr viral genomes in Reed-Sternberg cells of Hodgkin's disease. N Engl J Med 320:502, 1989.
56. Haluska FG, et al: The cellular biology of the Reed-Sternberg cell. Blood 84:1005, 1994.
57. Niedobitek G: The role of Epstein-Barr virus in the pathogenesis of Hodgkin's disease. Ann Oncol 7:11, 1996.
58. Weiss LM, et al: Clonal antigen receptor gene rearrangements and Epstein-Barr viral DNA in tissues of Hodgkin's disease. Hematol Oncol 6:233, 1988.
59. Herbst H, et al: Epstein-Barr virus latent membrane protein expression in Hodgkin and Reed-Sternberg cells. Proc Natl Acad Sci USA 88:4766, 1991.
60. Atkinson K, et al: Alcohol pain in Hodgkin's disease. Cancer 37:895, 1976.
61. Tucker MA, et al: Risk of second cancers after treatment for Hodgkin's disease. N Engl J Med 318:76, 1988.
62. Hancock SL, et al: Breast cancer after treatment of Hodgkin's disease. J Natl Cancer Inst 85:25, 1993.
63. Bennett JM, et al: Proposal for the recognition of minimally differentiated acute myeloid leukaemia (AML-MO). Br J Haematol 78:325, 1991.
64. Bennett JM, et al: Criteria for the diagnosis of acute leukemia of megakaryocyte lineage (M7). A report of the French-American-British Cooperative Group. Ann Intern Med 103:460, 1985.
65. Scheinberg DA, et al: Acute leukemias. In DeVita VT, et al (eds): Cancer: Principles and Practice of Oncology, 5th ed. Philadelphia, Lippincott-Raven, 1997, p 2291.
66. Pui CH, et al: Epipodophyllotoxin-related acute myeloid leukemia: a study of 35 cases. Leukemia 9:1990, 1995.
67. de The H, et al: The t(15;17) translocation of acute promyelocytic leukaemia fuses the retinoic acid receptor alpha gene to a novel transcribed locus. Nature 347:558, 1990.
68. Kakizuka A, et al: Chromosomal translocation t(15;17) in human acute promyelocytic leukemia fuses RAR alpha with a novel putative transcription factor, PML. Cell 66:653, 1991.
69. de The H, et al: The PML-RAR alpha fusion mRNA generated by the t(15;17) translocatoin in acute promyelocytic leukemia encodes a functionally altered RAR. Cell 66:675, 1991.
70. Grignani F, et al: The acute promyelocytic leukemia-specific PML-RAR alpha fusion protein inhibits differentiation and promotes survival of myeloid precursor cells. Cell 74:423, 1993.
71. Warrell RP Jr, et al: Differentiation therapy of acute promyelocytic leukemia with tretinoin (all-trans-retinoic acid). N Engl J Med 324: 1385, 1991.
72. Shao W, et al: Arsenic trioxide as an inducer of apoptosis and loss of PML/RAR alpha protein in acute promyelocytic leukemia cells. J Natl Cancer Inst 90:124, 1998.
73. Varela BL, et al: Modifications in the classification of primary myelodysplastic syndromes: the addition of a scoring system. Hematol Oncol 3:55, 1985.
74. Daley GQ, et al: Induction of chronic myelogenous leukemia in mice by the P210bcr/abl gene of the Philadelphia chromosome. Science 247:824, 1990.
75. Leemhuis T, et al: Identification of BCR/ABL-negative primitive hematopoietic progenitor cells within chronic myeloid leukemia marrow. Blood 81:801, 1993.
76. Weinberg RS: In vitro erythropoiesis in polycythemia vera and other myeloproliferative disorders. Semin Hematol 34:64, 1997.
77. Ellis JT, et al: Studies of the bone marrow in polycythemia vera and the evolution of myelofibrosis and second hematologic malignancies. Semin Hematol 23:144, 1986.
78. Reilly JT: Idiopathic myelofibrosis: Pathogenesis, natural history, and management. Blood Rev 11:233, 1997.
79. Martyre MC: TGF-beta and megakaryocytes in the pathogenesis of myelofibrosis in myeloproliferative disorders. Leuk Lymphoma 20:39, 1995.
80. Tefferi A, Silverstein MN: Current perspective in agnogenic myeloid metaplasia. Leuk Lymphoma 22:169, 1996.
81. Willman CL, et al: Langerhans'-cell histiocytosis (histiocytosis X)—a clonal proliferative disease. N Engl J Med 331:154, 1994.
82. Pritchard J, et al: The proceedings of the Nikolas symposia on the histiocytoses. Br J Cancer 70:S1, 1994.
83. Brown D, et al: A PML-RARalpha transgene initiates murine acute promyelocytic leukemia. Proc Natl Acad Sci U S A 94:2551, 1997.
84. He LZ, et al: Acute leukemia with promyelocytic features in PML/RARalpha transgenic mice. Proc Natl Acad Sci U S A 94:5302, 1997.
85. Pui C-H: Childhood leukemias. N Engl J Med 332:1618, 1995.
86. Isaacson PG: Intestinal lymphoma and enteropathy. J Pathol 177:115, 1995.

87. Weiss L: The red pulp of the spleen: structural basis of blood flow. Clin Haematol 12:375, 1983.
88. Rosse WF: The spleen as a filter. N Engl J Med 317:704, 1987.
89. Bishop MB, Lansing LS: The spleen: a correlative overview of normal and pathologic anatomy. Hum Pathol 13:334, 1982.
90. Pan C-C, et al: The clinicopathological correlation of epithelial subtyping in thymoma: a study of 112 consecutive cases. Hum Pathol 25:893, 1994.
91. Masaoka A, et al: Follow-up study of thymomas with special reference to their clinical stages. Cancer 48:2485, 1981.
92. Hishima T, et al: CD5 expression in thymic carcinoma. Am J Pathol 145:268, 1994.

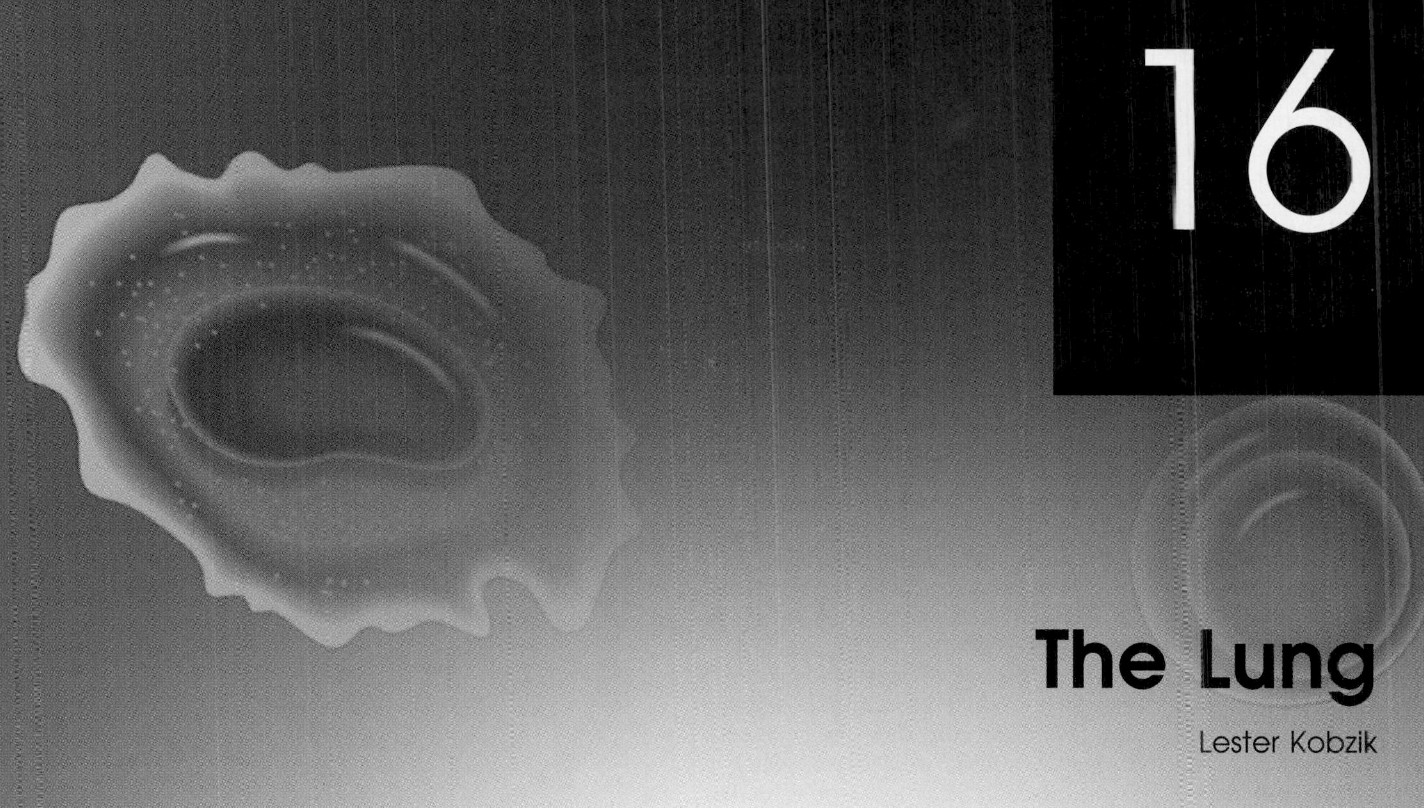

16 The Lung

Lester Kobzik

NORMAL LUNG

PATHOLOGY

CONGENITAL ANOMALIES

ATELECTASIS

DISEASES OF VASCULAR ORIGIN

- Pulmonary Congestion and Edema
  - *Hemodynamic Pulmonary Edema*
  - *Edema Caused by Microvascular Injury*
- Adult Respiratory Distress Syndrome (Diffuse Alveolar Damage)
- Pulmonary Embolism, Hemorrhage, and Infarction
- Pulmonary Hypertension and Vascular Sclerosis

OBSTRUCTIVE VERSUS RESTRICTIVE PULMONARY DISEASE

CHRONIC OBSTRUCTIVE PULMONARY DISEASE

- Emphysema
- Chronic Bronchitis
- Bronchial Asthma
- Bronchiectasis

PULMONARY INFECTIONS

- Bacterial Pneumonia
- Viral and Mycoplasmal Pneumonia (Primary Atypical Pneumonia)
- Lung Abscess
- Pulmonary Tuberculosis
  - *Primary Pulmonary Tuberculosis*
  - *Secondary (Reactivation) Pulmonary Tuberculosis*
  - *Progressive Pulmonary Tuberculosis*
- Pneumonia in the Immunocompromised Host

DIFFUSE INTERSTITIAL (INFILTRATIVE, RESTRICTIVE) DISEASES

- Pneumoconioses
  - *Coal Workers' Pneumoconiosis—Simple and Complicated (Progressive Massive Fibrosis)*
  - *Silicosis*
  - *Asbestos-Related Diseases*
  - *Beryiliosis*
- Sarcoidosis
- Idiopathic Pulmonary Fibrosis
- Desquamative Interstitial Pneumonitis
- Hypersensitivity Pneumonitis
- Pulmonary Eosinophilia (Pulmonary Infiltration With Eosinophilia)
- Bronchiolitis Obliterans-Organizing Pneumonia
- Diffuse Pulmonary Hemorrhage Syndromes
  - *Goodpasture Syndrome*
  - *Idiopathic Pulmonary Hemosiderosis*
  - *Other Hemorrhagic Syndromes*
- Pulmonary Involvement in Collagen Vascular Disorders
- Pulmonary Alveolar Proteinosis

COMPLICATIONS OF THERAPIES

- Drug-Induced Lung Disease
- Radiation-Induced Lung Disease
- Lung Transplantation

TUMORS

- Bronchogenic Carcinoma
  - *Paraneoplastic Syndromes*
- Bronchioloalveolar Carcinoma
- Neuroendocrine Tumors
  - *Bronchial Carcinoid*
- Miscellaneous Tumors
- Metastatic Tumors

PLEURA

- Inflammatory Pleural Effusions
- Noninflammatory Pleural Effusions
- Pneumothorax
- Pleural Tumors
  - *Solitary Fibrous Tumors (Pleural Fibroma)*
  - *Malignant Mesothelioma*

NORMAL LUNG

The lungs are ingeniously constructed to carry out their cardinal function, the exchange of gases between inspired air and the blood. The right lung is divided into three lobes; the left lung has only two lobes, its middle lobe equivalent being the *lingula*. The lung airways—the main right and left bronchi—arise from the trachea then branch dichotomously, giving rise to progressively smaller airways. The right main stem bronchus is more vertical and more directly in line with the trachea than is the left. As a consequence, aspirated foreign material, such as vomitus, blood, and foreign bodies, tends to enter the right lung rather than the left. Accompanying the branching airways is the double arterial supply to the lungs, that is, the pulmonary and bronchial arteries. In the absence of significant cardiac failure, the bronchial arteries of aortic origin can often sustain the vitality of the pulmonary parenchyma when pulmonary arterial supply is shut off, as by emboli.

Progressive branching of the bronchi forms *bronchioles,* which are distinguished from bronchi by the lack of cartilage and submucosal glands within their walls. Further branching of bronchioles leads to the *terminal bronchioles,* which are less than 2 mm in diameter. The part of the lung distal to the terminal bronchiole is called the *acinus*, or the *terminal respiratory unit*; it is approximately spherical in shape, with a diameter of about 7 mm. Acini contain alveoli and are thus the site of gas exchange. As illustrated in Figure 16–8*A*, an acinus is composed of *respiratory bronchioles* (emanating from the terminal bronchiole), which give off from their sides several alveoli; these bronchioles then proceed into the *alveolar ducts*, which immediately branch and empty into the *alveolar sacs*—the blind ends of the respiratory passages whose walls are formed entirely of alveoli. The alveoli open into the ducts through large mouths. In the correct plane of section, therefore, all alveoli are open and have incomplete walls. A cluster of three to five terminal bronchioles, each with its appended acini, is usually referred to as the pulmonary *lobule*. As seen subsequently, this lobular architecture assumes importance in distinguishing the major forms of emphysema.

From the microscopic standpoint, except for the vocal cords, which are covered by stratified squamous epithelium, nearly the entire respiratory tree, including the larynx, trachea, and bronchioles, is lined by pseudostratified, tall, columnar, ciliated epithelial cells, heavily admixed in the cartilaginous airways with mucus-secreting goblet cells. The bronchial mucosa also contains neuroendocrine cells that exhibit neurosecretory-type granules and contain serotonin, calcitonin, and gastrin-releasing peptide (bombesin). Numerous submucosal, mucus-secreting glands are dispersed throughout the walls of the trachea and bronchi (but not the bronchioles).

The microscopic structure of the alveolar walls (or alveolar septa) consists, from blood to air, of the following (Fig. 16–1):

- The *capillary endothelium* lining the intertwining network of anastomosing capillaries.
- A *basement membrane and surrounding interstitial tissue* separating the endothelial cells from the alveolar lining epithelial cells. In thin portions of the alveolar septum, the basement membranes of epithelium and endothelium are fused, whereas in thicker portions, they are separated by an interstitial space (*pulmonary interstitium*) containing fine elastic fibers, small bundles of collagen, a few fibroblast-like interstitial cells, smooth muscle cells, mast cells, and rarely lymphocytes and monocytes.

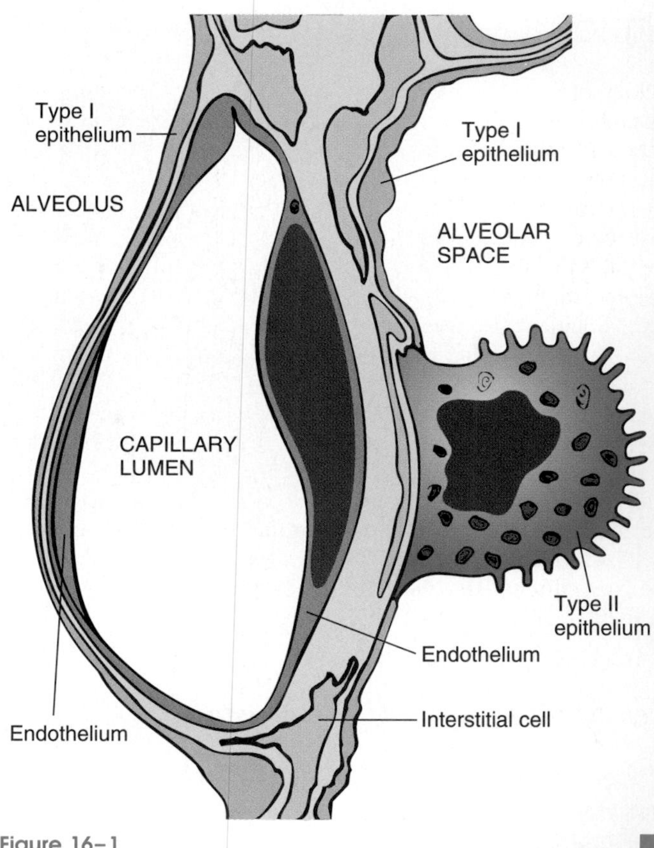

Figure 16–1

Microscopic structure of the alveolar wall. Note that the basement membrane *(yellow)* is thin on one side and widened where it is continuous with the interstitial space. Portions of interstitial cells are shown.

- *Alveolar epithelium,* comprising a continuous layer of two principal cell types: flattened, platelike pavement *type I pneumocytes* (or membranous pneumocytes) covering 95% of the alveolar surface and rounded *type II pneumocytes*. Type II cells are important for at least two reasons: (1) They are the source of *pulmonary surfactant*, contained in osmiophilic *lamellar bodies* seen with electron microscopy, and (2) they are the main cell type involved in the repair of alveolar epithelium after destruction of type I cells.
- *Alveolar macrophages,* loosely attached to the epithelial cells or lying free within the alveolar spaces, derived from blood monocytes and belonging to the mononuclear phagocyte system. Often, they are filled with carbon particles and other phagocytosed materials.

The alveolar walls are not solid but are perforated by numerous *pores of Kohn,* which permit the passage of bacteria and exudate between adjacent alveoli (see Fig. 16–20*B*). Adjacent to the alveolar cell membrane is the pulmonary surfactant layer (discussed in Chapter 11 in the section on respiratory distress syndrome in newborns).

PATHOLOGY

The importance of lung disease in the overall perspective of pathology and clinical medicine cannot be overemphasized. Primary respiratory infections, such as bronchitis, bronchopneumonia, and other forms of pneumonia, are commonplace in clinical and pathologic practice. In these days of cigarette smoking, air pollution, and other environmental inhalants, chronic bronchitis and emphysema have become rampant. Malignancy of the lungs has risen steadily in incidence, particularly in women, until it is now the most common lethal visceral malignancy in both men and women, surpassing even breast cancer in women. Moreover, the lungs are secondarily involved in almost all forms of terminal disease, so that some degree of pulmonary edema, atelectasis, or bronchopneumonia is present in virtually every dying patient. In the present consideration of the lung, emphasis is placed on primary diseases that affect this important organ. For detailed descriptions of less common conditions, the reader is referred to current comprehensive books of pulmonary disease.

Congenital Anomalies

Developmental defects of the lung[1] include the following:

- Agenesis or hypoplasia of both lungs, one lung, or single lobes
- Tracheal and bronchial anomalies
- Vascular anomalies
- Congenital lobar overinflation (emphysema)
- Congenital cysts
- Intralobar and extrapulmonary lobar sequestrations

The last two anomalies are seen more frequently and are discussed here. *Congenital cysts* represent an abnormal detachment of a fragment of primitive foregut, and most consist of *bronchogenic cysts.* Bronchogenic cysts may occur anywhere in the lungs as single or, on occasion, multiple cystic spaces from microscopic size to more than 5 cm in diameter. They are usually found adjacent to bronchi or bronchioles but may or may not have demonstrable connections with the airways. They are lined by bronchial-type epithelium and are usually filled with mucinous secretions or with air. Complications include infection of the secretions, with suppuration, lung abscess, or rupture into bronchi, causing hemorrhage and hemoptysis, or rupture into the pleural cavity, with pneumothorax or interstitial emphysema.

Bronchopulmonary sequestration refers to the presence of lobes or segments of lung tissue *without a normal connection to the airway system.* Blood supply to the sequestered area arises not from the pulmonary arteries but from the aorta or its branches. *Extralobar sequestrations* are external to the lung and may be found anywhere in the thorax or mediastinum. Found most commonly in infants as abnormal mass lesions, they may be associated with other congenital anomalies. *Intralobar sequestrations* are found within the lung substance and are usually associated with recurrent localized infection or bronchiectasis.

Atelectasis

Atelectasis refers either to incomplete expansion of the lungs or to the collapse of previously inflated lung substance, producing areas of relatively airless pulmonary parenchyma. Significant atelectasis reduces oxygenation and predisposes to infection. Acquired atelectasis, encountered principally in adults, may be divided into *obstruction* (or *resorption*), *compression*, and *contraction atelectasis* (Fig. 16–2).

Resorption atelectasis is the consequence of complete obstruction of an airway, which in time leads to *resorption* of the oxygen trapped in the dependent alveoli, without impairment of blood flow through the affected alveolar walls. Since lung volume is diminished, the mediastinum may shift *toward* the atelectatic lung. Resorption atelectasis is caused principally by excessive secretions (e.g., mucous plugs) or exudates within smaller bronchi and is therefore most often found in bronchial asthma, chronic bronchitis, bronchiectasis, and postoperative states and with aspiration

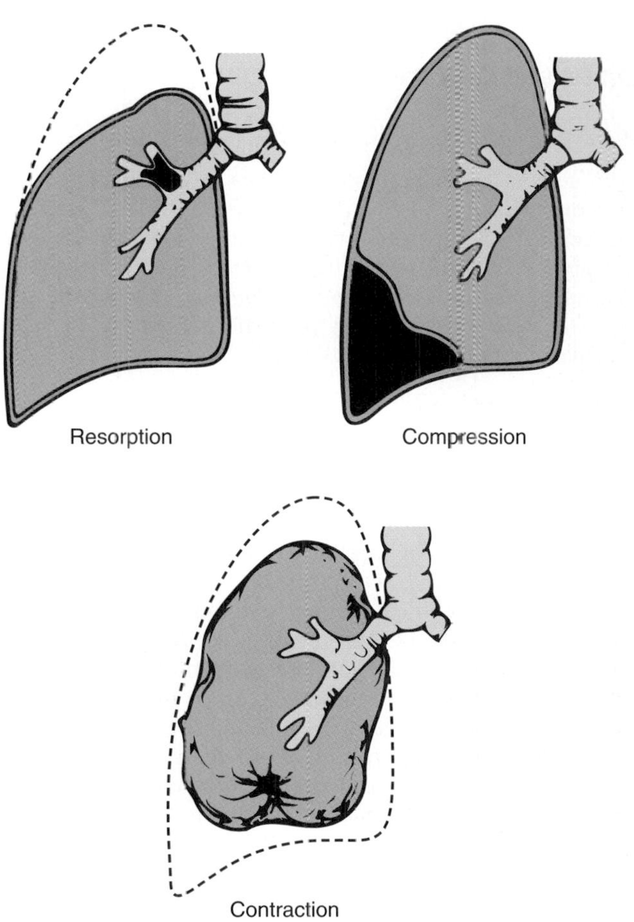

Figure 16–2 ■

Various forms of atelectasis in adults.

of foreign bodies. Although bronchial neoplasms can cause atelectasis, in most instances they cause subtotal obstruction and produce localized emphysema.

Compression atelectasis results whenever the pleural cavity is partially or completely filled by fluid exudate, tumor, blood, or air (the last-mentioned constituting *pneumothorax*) or, with *tension pneumothorax*, when air pressure impinges on and threatens the function of the lung and mediastinum, especially the major vessels. Compressive atelectasis is most commonly encountered in patients in cardiac failure who develop pleural fluid and in patients with neoplastic effusions within the pleural cavities. Similarly, abnormal elevation of the diaphragm, such as that which follows peritonitis or subdiaphragmatic abscesses or which occurs in seriously ill postoperative patients, induces basal atelectasis. With compressive atelectasis, the mediastinum shifts *away* from the affected lung. *Patchy atelectasis* develops when there is loss of pulmonary surfactant, as in neonatal and adult respiratory distress syndrome (ARDS). *Contraction atelectasis* occurs when local or generalized fibrotic changes in the lung or pleura prevent full expansion.

Because the collapsed lung parenchyma can be reexpanded, *atelectasis is a reversible disorder* (except that caused by contraction). Atelectatic parenchyma, however, is prone to developing superimposed infections.

Table 16–1. CLASSIFICATION AND CAUSES OF PULMONARY EDEMA

Hemodynamic Edema
Increased hydrostatic pressure
Left-sided heart failure
Mitral stenosis
Volume overload
Pulmonary vein obstruction
Decreased oncotic pressure
Hypoalbuminemia
Nephrotic syndrome
Liver disease
Protein-losing enteropathies
Lymphatic obstruction

Edema Due to Microvascular Injury
Infectious agents: viruses, *Mycoplasma,* other
Inhaled gases: oxygen, sulfur dioxide, cyanates, smoke
Liquid aspiration: gastric contents, near-drowning
Drugs and chemicals
  Chemotherapeutic agents: bleomycin, other
  Other medications: amphotericin B, colchicine, gold
  Other: heroin, kerosene, paraquat
Shock, trauma, and sepsis
Radiation
Miscellaneous

Edema of Undetermined Origin
High altitude
Neurogenic

Diseases of Vascular Origin

PULMONARY CONGESTION AND EDEMA

A general consideration of edema is in Chapter 5, and pulmonary congestion and edema are described briefly in the context of congestive heart failure (Chapter 13). Pulmonary edema can result from *hemodynamic* disturbances (*hydrodynamic* or *cardiogenic pulmonary edema*) or from direct *increases in capillary permeability*, owing to microvascular injury (Table 16–1).

Hemodynamic Pulmonary Edema

The most common *hemodynamic* mechanism of pulmonary edema is that attributable to *increased hydrostatic pressure*, as occurs in left-sided congestive heart failure. Accumulation of fluid in this setting can be accounted for by Starling's law of capillary interstitial fluid exchange (Chapter 5).

Whatever the clinical setting, pulmonary congestion and edema are characterized by heavy, wet lungs. Fluid accumulates initially in the basal regions of the lower lobes because hydrostatic pressure is greater in these sites. Histologically the alveolar capillaries are engorged, and an intra-alveolar granular pink precipitate is seen. Alveolar microhemorrhages and hemosiderin-laden macrophages ("heart failure" cells) may be present. In long-standing cases of pulmonary congestion, such as those seen in mitral stenosis, hemosiderin-laden macrophages are abundant, and fibrosis and thickening of the alveolar walls cause the soggy lungs to become firm and brown (*brown induration*). These changes not only impair normal respiratory function, but also predispose to infection.

Edema Caused by Microvascular Injury

The second mechanism leading to pulmonary edema is *injury to the capillaries of the alveolar septa.* Here the pulmonary capillary hydrostatic pressure is usually not elevated, and hemodynamic factors play a secondary role. The edema results from primary injury to the vascular endothelium or damage to alveolar epithelial cells (with secondary microvascular injury). This results in leakage of fluids and proteins first into the interstitial space and, in more severe cases, into the alveoli. When the edema remains localized, as it does in most forms of pneumonia, it is overshadowed by the manifestations of infection. When diffuse, however, alveolar edema is an important contributor to a serious and often fatal condition, *ARDS*, which is discussed in the following section.

ADULT RESPIRATORY DISTRESS SYNDROME (DIFFUSE ALVEOLAR DAMAGE)

ARDS and its many synonyms (including adult respiratory failure, shock lung, diffuse alveolar damage, acute alveolar injury, and traumatic wet lungs) are descriptive terms for a syndrome caused by diffuse alveolar capillary damage. It is characterized clinically by the rapid onset of severe life-threatening respiratory insufficiency, cyanosis, and severe arterial hypoxemia that is refractory to oxygen therapy and that may progress to extrapulmonary multisystem organ failure. In most patients, there is evidence of severe pulmonary edema (often called *noncardiogenic*, *low-pressure*, or *high-permeability pulmonary edema*), with chest radiographs showing a diffuse alveolar infiltration. Although hyaline membranes are a characteristic histologic feature of both ARDS and the respiratory distress syndrome of newborns (Chapter 11), the pathogenetic mechanisms are different.

ARDS is a well-recognized complication of numerous and diverse conditions, including both direct injuries to the lungs and systemic disorders (Table 16–2). Direct lung injuries causing ARDS include *diffuse* pulmonary and other viral infections, oxygen toxicity, inhalation of toxins and other irritants, and aspiration of gastric contents. Systemic conditions causing ARDS include septic shock, shock associated with trauma, hemorrhagic pancreatitis, burns, complicated abdominal surgery, narcotic overdose and other drug reactions, hypersensitivity reactions to organic solvents, hemodialysis, and cardiac surgery involving extracorporeal pumps. In many cases, a combination of the foregoing conditions is present (e.g., shock, oxygen therapy, and sepsis).

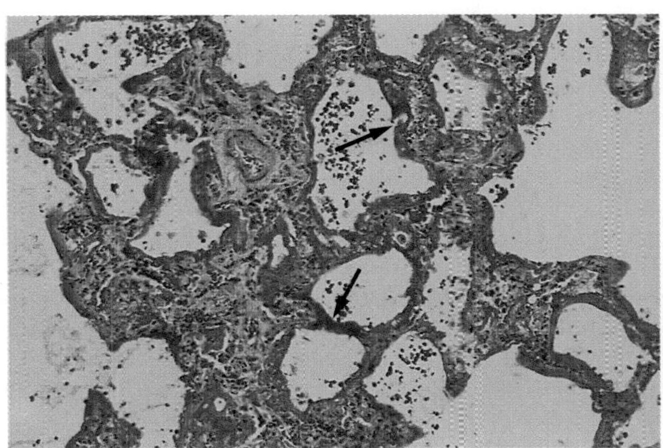

Figure 16–3 ■

Diffuse alveolar damage (adult respiratory distress syndrome) shown in a photomicrograph. Some of the alveoli are collapsed, others distended. Many contain dense proteinaceous debris, desquamated cells, and hyaline membranes *(arrows)*.

MORPHOLOGY. In the acute edematous stage, the lungs are heavy, firm, red, and boggy. They exhibit congestion, interstitial and intra-alveolar edema, and inflammation. In addition to the congestion and edema, there is fibrin deposition. The alveolar walls become lined with waxy **hyaline membranes** (Fig. 16–3) that are similar to those seen in hyaline membrane disease of neonates (Chapter 5). Alveolar hyaline membranes consist of fibrin-rich edema fluid mixed with the cytoplasmic and lipid remnants of necrotic epithelial cells. Subsequently, type II epithelial cells undergo proliferation in an attempt to regenerate the alveolar lining. Resolution is unusual; more commonly, there is organization of the fibrin exudate, with resultant intra-alveolar fibrosis. Marked thickening of the alveolar septa ensues, caused by proliferation of interstitial cells and deposition of collagen. Fatal cases often have superimposed bronchopneumonia.

Table 16–2. CONDITIONS ASSOCIATED WITH DEVELOPMENT OF ADULT RESPIRATORY DISTRESS SYNDROME

Infection
- Sepsis*
- Diffuse pulmonary infections*
  - Viral, *Mycoplasma,* and *Pneumocystis* pneumonia; miliary tuberculosis
- Gastric aspiration*

Physical/Injury
- Mechanical trauma, including head injuries*
- Pulmonary contusions
- Near-drowning
- Fractures with fat embolism
- Burns
- Ionizing radiation

Inhaled Irritants
- Oxygen toxicity
- Smoke
- Irritant gases and chemicals

Chemical Injury
- Heroin or methadone overdose
- Acetylsalicylic acid
- Barbiturate overdose
- Paraquat

Hematologic Conditions
- Multiple transfusions
- Disseminated intravascular coagulation

Pancreatitis

Uremia

Cardiopulmonary Bypass

* >50% of cases of adult respiratory distress syndrome are associated with these four conditions.

Pathogenesis. ARDS is best viewed as the clinical and pathologic end result of acute alveolar injury caused by a variety of insults and probably initiated by different mechanisms.[2] The final common pathway is *diffuse damage to the alveolar capillary walls*; this is followed by a relatively nonspecific, often predictable series of morphologic and physiologic alterations leading to respiratory failure. *In contrast, the mechanism of the respiratory distress syndrome of newborns is a deficiency in pulmonary surfactant* (Chapter 11). In ARDS, the initial injury is to either capillary endothelium (most frequently) or alveolar epithelium (occasionally), but eventually both are clearly affected. Damage to these cells leads to increased capillary permeability, interstitial and then intra-alveolar edema, fibrin exudation, and formation of hyaline membranes. Importantly the exudate and diffuse tissue destruction that occur with ARDS cannot be easily resolved, and the result is generally organization with scarring, producing severe chronic changes, in contrast to the transudate of cardiogenic pulmonary edema, which usually resolves.

The capillary defect in ARDS is believed to be produced by an interaction of leukocytes and mediators, including cytokines, oxygen radicals, complement, and eicosanoids, that damages the endothelium and allows fluid and proteins to leak across it.

Endotoxemia is important in initiating these cellular events in many patients. Endotoxin induces the release of proinflammatory cytokines from macrophages and increases endothelial expression of adhesion molecules for leukocytes (Fig. 16–4*A*). Endotoxin also amplifies complement-mediated responses of neutrophils, especially intrapulmonary leukocyte accumulation and subsequent damage to endothelial cells. In the absence of clear-cut endotoxemia, the initiating factors are unclear.

Neutrophils aggregate in the lung microvessels and have the capacity to injure pulmonary endothelial cells through release of toxic oxygen metabolites and destructive enzymes (Fig. 16–4*B*). In some situations, such as hemodialysis and cardiopulmonary bypass, neutrophil accumulation in the lung is induced by extrapulmonary activation of complement via the alternative pathway, as a result of blood contact with the membranes of these devices. Sepsis also causes nonspecific activation of complement. ARDS, however, can also develop in the face of systemic neutropenia and without pulmonary neutrophilic aggregates.

Macrophages are an alternative source of injury in patients with ARDS. Macrophages can generate toxic oxygen products, proteases, arachidonic acid metabolites, platelet-activating factor (PAF), and cytokines that regulate inflammation (Chapter 3). To some extent, neutrophilic inflammation in ARDS may be driven by macrophage-derived chemokines, for example, interleukin-8 (IL-8). Additional physiologic effects of these mediators include vasoconstriction and platelet aggregation, both of

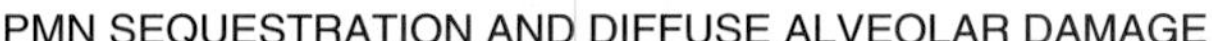

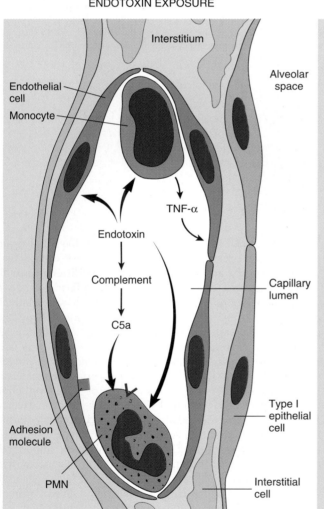

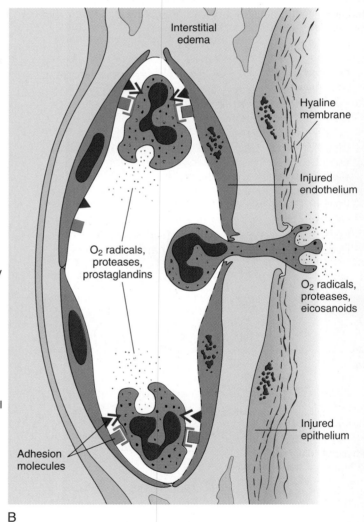

Figure 16–4

Simplified model for diffuse alveolar damage in endotoxemia. Endotoxin associated with gram-negative organisms acts on multiple targets. It induces monocytes and lung macrophages to release mediators, including tumor necrosis factor α (TNF-α) and chemotactic peptides (e.g., leukotriene B_4, interleukin 8). Endotoxin-induced activation of complement releases C5a, which together with bacterial lipopolysaccharide and TNF-α activates polymorphonuclear neutrophil leukocytes (PMNs) and up-regulates binding avidity of adhesion molecules. Endotoxin also activates endothelial cells to up-regulate adhesion molecules that facilitate binding of neutrophils. Activation of PMNs results in the release of oxidants, proteases, and prostaglandins. The net result is the sequestration (and extravasation) of PMNs in pulmonary capillaries, damage to endothelial and epithelial cells, and the development of interstitial edema and alveolar hyaline membranes.

which may decrease blood flow to aerated regions of the lungs.

Clinical Course. Patients who develop ARDS are usually hospitalized for one of the predisposing conditions listed earlier, and initially they may have no pulmonary symptoms. ARDS is heralded by profound dyspnea and tachypnea, but the chest radiograph is initially normal. Subsequently, there is increasing cyanosis and hypoxemia, respiratory failure, and the appearance of diffuse bilateral infiltrates on x-ray examination. Hypoxemia can then become unresponsive to oxygen therapy, and respiratory acidosis can develop.

The functional abnormalities in ARDS are not homogeneously distributed throughout the lungs. The lungs are focally stiff and have a decrease in functional volume. In essence, patients' lungs can be divided into areas that are infiltrated, consolidated, or collapsed (and thus poorly aerated and poorly compliant) and regions that have nearly normal levels of compliance and ventilation. Although blood is diverted away from poorly aerated regions in healthy lungs, lungs with ARDS continue to have perfusion of poorly aerated regions, contributing to ventilation-perfusion mismatching and hypoxemia. These patients can be helped by inhalation of nitric oxide, a potent vasodilator (Chapter 4), which decreases pulmonary artery pressure and pulmonary vascular resistance (usually elevated in ARDS), while not changing systemic arterial pressure and systemic vascular resistance.[3]

Therapy of ARDS is difficult, and this disorder is frequently fatal. The high concentrations of oxygen that are required to treat ARDS can themselves contribute to perpetuation of the damage (oxygen toxicity). Progression from one phase to the next can be rapid (a few hours), but some patients recover with resorption of the edema fluid and reexpansion of atelectatic areas. Despite improvements in supportive respiratory, however, the mortality rate among the 150,000 ARDS cases seen yearly in the United States is still about 60%.

PULMONARY EMBOLISM, HEMORRHAGE, AND INFARCTION

Occlusions of the pulmonary arteries by blood clot are almost always embolic in origin. Large-vessel in situ thromboses are rare and develop only in the presence of pulmonary hypertension, pulmonary atherosclerosis, and heart failure. The usual source of pulmonary emboli—thrombi in the deep veins of the leg in more than 95% of cases—and the magnitude of the clinical problem were discussed in Chapter 5, in which the disturbing frequency of pulmonary embolism and infarction was emphasized. Pulmonary embolism causes more than 50,000 deaths in the United States each year. Its incidence at autopsy has varied from 1% in the general population of hospital patients to 30% in patients dying after severe burns, trauma, or fractures to 65% of hospitalized patients in one study in which special techniques were applied to discover emboli at autopsy. It is the sole or a major contributing cause of death in about 10% of adults dying acutely in hospitals.

MORPHOLOGY. The morphologic consequences of embolic occlusion of the pulmonary arteries depend on the size of the embolic mass and the general state of the circulation. Large emboli may impact in the main pulmonary artery or its major branches or lodge at the bifurcation as a saddle embolus (Fig. 16–5). Sudden death often ensues, owing largely to the blockage of blood flow through the lungs. Death may also be caused by acute dilation of the right side of the heart (**acute cor pulmonale**). Smaller emboli can travel out into the more peripheral vessels, where they may or may not cause infarction. In patients with adequate cardiovascular function, the bronchial artery supply can often sustain the lung parenchyma despite obstruction to the pulmonary arterial system. Under these circumstances, hemorrhages may occur, but there is no infarction of the underlying lung parenchyma. Only about 10% of emboli actually cause infarction. Although the underlying pulmonary architecture may be obscured by the suffusion of blood, hemorrhages are distinguished by the preservation of the pulmonary alveolar architecture; in such cases, resorption of the blood permits reconstitution of the preexisting architecture.

Pulmonary embolism usually causes infarction only when the circulation is already inadequate, as in patients with heart or lung disease. For this reason, pulmonary infarcts tend to be uncommon in the young. About three fourths of all infarcts affect the lower lobes, and in more than half multiple lesions occur. They vary in size from lesions barely visible to the naked eye to massive involvement of large parts of an entire lobe. Characteristically, they extend to the periphery of the lung substance as a wedge with the apex pointing toward the hilus of the lung. In many cases,

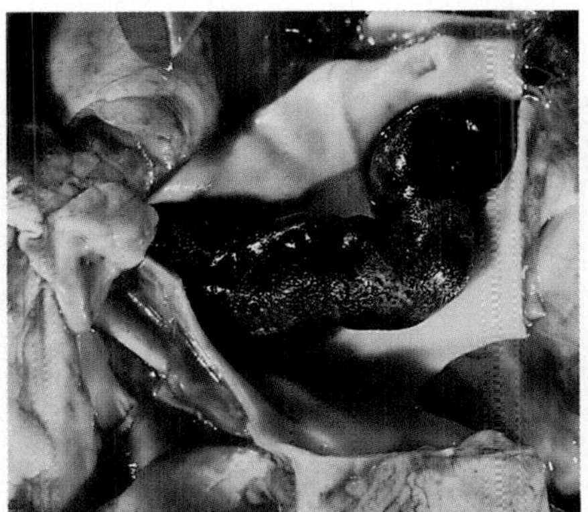

Figure 16–5

Large saddle embolus from the femoral vein lying astride the main left and right pulmonary arteries. (From the teaching collection of the Department of Pathology, University of Texas Southwestern Medical School, Dallas, TX.)

an occluded vessel can be identified near the apex of the infarct.

The pulmonary infarct is classically hemorrhagic and appears as a raised, red-blue area in the early stages (Fig. 16–6). Often the apposed pleural surface is covered by a fibrinous exudate. The red cells begin to lyse within 48 hours, and the infarct becomes paler and eventually red-brown as hemosiderin is produced. With the passage of time, fibrous replacement begins at the margins as a gray-white peripheral zone and eventually converts the infarct into a contracted scar. Histologically the diagnostic feature of acute pulmonary infarction is the ischemic necrosis of the lung substance within the area of hemorrhage, affecting the alveolar walls, bronchioles, and vessels. If the infarct is caused by an infected embolus, the infarct is modified by a more intense neutrophilic exudation and more intense inflammatory reaction. Such lesions are referred to as **septic infarcts,** and some convert to abscesses.

Clinical Course. Pulmonary embolism is a complication principally in patients already suffering from some underlying disorder, such as cardiac disease or cancer, or who are immobilized for long periods. Hypercoagulable states, either *primary* (e.g., antithrombin III or protein C deficiencies, defective fibrinolysis, and, paradoxically, the presence of lupus anticoagulant) or *secondary* (e.g., obesity, recent surgery, cancer, oral contraceptive use, pregnancy), frequently contribute to the original deep vein thrombus. Indwelling central venous lines can be a nidus for right atrial thrombus, which can be a source of pulmonary embolism.

The pathophysiologic response and clinical significance of pulmonary embolism depend on the extent to which the pulmonary artery blood flow is obstructed, size of the occluded vessel(s), number of emboli, overall status of the cardiovascular system, and release of vasoactive factors from platelets that accumulate at the site of thrombus, for example, thromboxane A_2. Emboli result in two main pathophysiologic consequences: *respiratory compromise* owing to the nonperfused, although ventilated segment and *hemodynamic compromise* owing to increased resistance to pulmonary blood flow engendered by the embolic obstruction. The latter leads to pulmonary hypertension and can cause acute failure of the right ventricle.

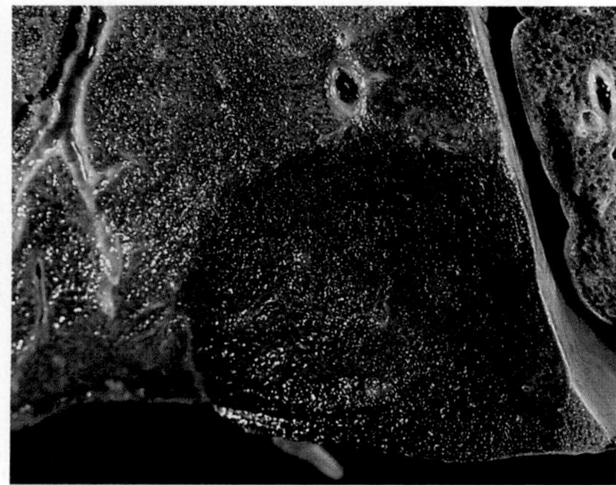

Figure 16–6

Recent, small, roughly wedge-shaped hemorrhagic pulmonary infarct.

A large pulmonary embolus is one of the few causes of virtually instantaneous death. During cardiopulmonary resuscitation in such instances, the patient frequently is said to have *electromechanical dissociation*, in which the electrocardiogram has a rhythm but no pulses are palpated because of the massive blockage of blood in the systemic venous circulation. If survival occurs after a sizable pulmonary embolus, however, the clinical syndrome may mimic myocardial infarction, with severe chest pain, dyspnea, shock, elevation of temperature, and increased levels of serum lactic dehydrogenase. Usually, however, *small emboli* induce only transient chest pain and cough or possibly pulmonary hemorrhages without infarction in persons with a normal cardiovascular system. Only in the predisposed in whom the bronchial circulation itself is inadequate do small emboli cause small infarcts. Such patients manifest dyspnea, tachypnea, fever, chest pain, cough, and hemoptysis. An overlying fibrinous pleuritis may produce a pleural friction rub.

The chest radiograph may disclose a pulmonary infarct, usually 12 to 36 hours after it has occurred, as a wedge-shaped infiltrate. Emboli can also be detected by pulmonary perfusion lung scanning after parenteral injection of macroaggregates of albumin labeled with radionuclides, such as technetium-99m. Pulmonary angiography is the most definitive diagnostic technique but entails more risk to the patient than do perfusion scans.

After the initial acute insult, emboli often resolve via contraction and fibrinolysis, particularly in the relatively young. Unresolved, multiple small emboli over the course of time may lead to pulmonary hypertension, pulmonary vascular sclerosis, and chronic cor pulmonale. Perhaps most important is the fact that a small embolus may presage a larger one. In the presence of an underlying predisposing factor, patients with a pulmonary embolus have a 30% chance of developing a second embolus.

Prevention of pulmonary embolism constitutes a major clinical problem for which there is no easy solution. Prophylactic therapy includes early ambulation in postoperative and postpartum patients, elastic stockings and isometric leg exercises for bedridden patients, and preventive anticoagulation in high-risk individuals. It is sometimes necessary to resort to insertion of a filter ("umbrella") into the inferior vena cava or to ligation of this vein, not minor procedures in an already serious ill patient. Treatment of existing pulmonary embolism often includes anticoagulation, preceded by thrombolysis in some cases.

PULMONARY HYPERTENSION AND VASCULAR SCLEROSIS

The pulmonary circulation is normally one of low resistance, and pulmonary blood pressure is only about one eighth of systemic blood pressure. Pulmonary hypertension (when mean pulmonary pressure reaches one fourth of systemic levels) is most frequently *secondary* to structural cardiopulmonary conditions that increase pulmonary blood flow or pressure (or both), pulmonary vascular resistance, or left heart resistance to blood flow. These include the following:

- *Chronic obstructive or interstitial lung diseases*: Patients with emphysema have hypoxia as well as destruction of lung parenchyma and hence have fewer alveolar capillaries. This causes increased pulmonary arterial resistance and, secondarily, pressure.
- *Antecedent congenital or acquired heart disease*: Pulmonary hypertension occurs in patients with mitral stenosis, for example, because of an increase in left atrial pressure that leads to an increase in pulmonary venous pressure and, consequently, to an increase in pulmonary artery pressure.
- *Recurrent thromboemboli*: Patients with recurrent pulmonary emboli may have pulmonary hypertension primarily owing to a reduction in the functional cross-sectional area of the pulmonary vascular bed brought about by the obstructing emboli, which, in turn, leads to an increase in pulmonary vascular resistance.

Uncommonly, pulmonary hypertension is encountered in patients in whom all known causes of increased pulmonary pressure are excluded, and this is referred to as *primary*, or *idiopathic, pulmonary hypertension*.

Pathogenesis. The endothelial cells in the lungs contribute in important ways to the dynamic regulation of pulmonary blood flow and pulmonary vascular resistance. Dysfunction of pulmonary vascular endothelial cells plays a central part in the vascular responses of both idiopathic (primary) and secondary pulmonary hypertension.[4, 5]

In *secondary forms of pulmonary hypertension*, endothelial cell dysfunction is produced by the process initiating the disorder, such as the increased shear and mechanical injury associated with left-to-right shunts or the biochemical injury produced by fibrin in thromboembolism. In *primary pulmonary hypertension*, endothelial dysfunction is idiopathic in most cases but is sometimes associated with autoimmune disorders, toxic substances, and perhaps specific genetic determinants. Decreased elaboration of prostacyclin, decreased production of nitric oxide, and increased release of endothelin all promote pulmonary vasoconstriction. Also, decreased elaboration of prostacyclin and nitric oxide promotes platelet adhesion and activation. Moreover, endothelial activation, as detailed in Chapters 3 and 12, makes endothelial cells thrombogenic and promotes the persistence of fibrin. Finally, production and release of growth factors and cytokines induce the migration and replication of vascular smooth muscle cells and elaboration of extracellular matrix.

Some patients with pulmonary hypertension have a vasospastic component; in such patients, pulmonary vascular resistance can be rapidly decreased with vasodilators. Pulmonary hypertension has also been reported after ingestion of certain plants or medicines, including the leguminous plant *Crotalaria spectabilis*, indigenous to the tropics and used medicinally in *bush tea*; the appetite depressant agent *aminorex*; adulterated olive oil; and most recently the antiobesity drugs fenfluramine and phentermine.[6] It has been suggested that such substances may act through endothelial dysfunction, by enhancing pulmonary vasoconstriction as described earlier.

MORPHOLOGY. A variety of vascular lesions occur in pulmonary hypertension.[7] Although they are not always specific and frequently overlap between primary and secondary forms, specific histologic appearances have diagnostic and prognostic implications.[8] The presence of many organizing or recanalized thrombi favors recurrent pulmonary emboli as the cause, and the coexistence of diffuse pulmonary fibrosis, or severe emphysema and chronic bronchitis, points to chronic hypoxia as the initiating event. The vessel changes can involve the entire arterial tree, from the main pulmonary arteries down to the arterioles (Fig. 16–7). In the most severe cases, atheromatous deposits form in the pulmonary artery and its major branches, resembling (but being lesser in degree than) systemic atherosclerosis. The arterioles and small arteries (40 to 300 mm in diameter) are most prominently affected, with striking increases in the muscular thickness of the media (medial hypertrophy) and intimal fibrosis, sometimes narrowing the lumina to pinpoint channels. These changes are present in all forms of pulmonary hypertension but are best developed in the primary form. One extreme in the spectrum of pathologic changes, present most prominently in primary pulmonary hypertension or congenital heart disease with left-to-right shunts, is **plexogenic pulmonary arteriopathy,** so-called because a tuft of capillary formations is present, producing a network, or web, that spans the lumens of dilated thin-walled arteries. Biopsy of the lung may be done in some cases to grade the degree of pulmonary hypertensive vascular abnormalities and thereby aid therapeutic decision making, especially in congenital heart disease, in which severe secondary pulmonary vascular changes may preclude surgical repair of the underlying cardiac anomaly (Chapter 13).

Clinical Course. Although secondary forms can occur at any age, primary pulmonary hypertension is most common in women who are 20 to 40 years of age and is also seen occasionally in young children. Clinical signs and symptoms of both the primary and the secondary forms of vascular sclerosis become evident only with advanced arterial disease. In cases of primary disease, the presenting features are usually dyspnea and fatigue, but some patients have chest pain of the anginal type. In the course of time, severe respiratory distress, cyanosis, and right ventricular hypertrophy occur, and death from decompensated cor pulmonale, often with superimposed thromboembolism and pneumonia, usually ensues within 2 to 5 years in 80% of patients.[9] Continuous therapy with vasodilators (e.g., cal-

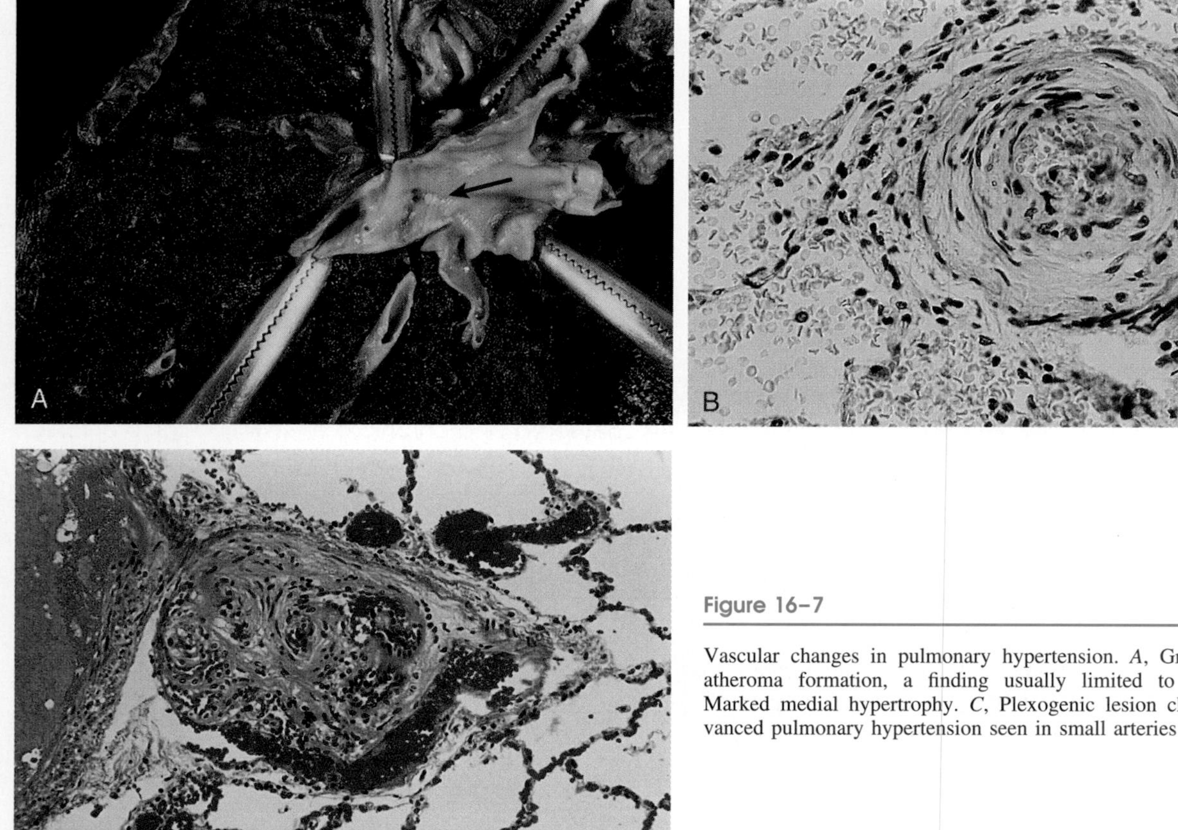

Figure 16–7

Vascular changes in pulmonary hypertension. *A*, Gross photograph of atheroma formation, a finding usually limited to large vessels. *B*, Marked medial hypertrophy. *C*, Plexogenic lesion characteristic of advanced pulmonary hypertension seen in small arteries and arterioles.

cium channel blockers or inhaled nitric oxide) and antithrombotic medications (e.g., warfarin, prostacyclin, and thromboxane receptor blockers), however, appears to improve the outcome in certain patients.

Obstructive Versus Restrictive Pulmonary Disease

Pulmonary physiologists have popularized the classification of *diffuse* pulmonary diseases into two categories: (1) *obstructive disease* (or *airway disease*), characterized by an increase in resistance to airflow owing to partial or complete obstruction at any level, from the trachea and larger bronchi to the terminal and respiratory bronchioles, and (2) *restrictive disease*, characterized by reduced expansion of lung parenchyma, with decreased total lung capacity. Although many conditions have both obstructive and restrictive components, distinction between the two patterns of pulmonary dysfunction is useful in correlating the results of pulmonary function tests with the radiologic and histologic findings in individual patients.

The major obstructive disorders (excluding tumor or inhalation of a foreign body) are *emphysema*, *chronic bronchitis*, *bronchiectasis*, and *asthma*. In patients with these diseases, pulmonary function tests show limitation of maximal airflow rates during forced expiration, usually measured by forced expiratory volume at 1 second (FEV_1). Expiratory airflow obstruction may result either from *anatomic airway narrowing*, such as is classically observed in asthma, or from *loss of elastic recoil of the lung*, which characteristically occurs in emphysema.

In contrast, restrictive diseases are identified by a reduced total lung capacity, while the expiratory flow rate is normal or reduced proportionately. The restrictive defect occurs in two general conditions: (1) *chest wall disorders in the presence of normal lungs* (e.g., neuromuscular diseases such as poliomyelitis, severe obesity, pleural diseases, and kyphoscoliosis) and (2) *acute or chronic interstitial and infiltrative diseases*. The classic acute restrictive disease is ARDS (see earlier). Chronic restrictive diseases include the dust diseases, or pneumoconioses, and most of the infiltrative conditions, discussed later.

Chronic Obstructive Pulmonary Disease

The term *chronic obstructive pulmonary disease* (COPD) refers to a group of conditions that share a major symptom—dyspnea—and are accompanied by chronic or recurrent obstruction to airflow within the lung. Because of the increase in cigarette smoking, environmental pollutants, and other noxious exposures, the incidence of COPD has in-

Table 16–3. DISORDERS ASSOCIATED WITH AIRFLOW OBSTRUCTION: THE SPECTRUM OF CHRONIC OBSTRUCTIVE PULMONARY DISEASE

Clinical Term	Anatomic Site	Major Pathologic Changes	Etiology	Signs/Symptoms
Chronic bronchitis	Bronchus	Mucous gland hyperplasia, hypersecretion	Tobacco smoke, air pollutants	Cough, sputum production
Bronchiectasis	Bronchus	Airway dilation and scarring	Persistent or severe infections	Cough; purulent sputum; fever
Asthma	Bronchus	Smooth muscle hyperplasia, excess mucus, inflammation	Immunologic or undefined causes	Episodic wheezing, cough, dyspnea
Emphysema	Acinus	Airspace enlargement; wall destruction	Tobacco smoke	Dyspnea
Small airway disease,* bronchiolitis	Bronchiole	Inflammatory scarring/obliteration	Tobacco smoke, air pollutants, miscellaneous	Cough, dyspnea

* A feature of chronic bronchitis (see text).

creased dramatically in the past few decades and now ranks as a major cause of activity-restricting or bed-confining disability in the United States.

In their prototypical forms, these individual disorders—chronic bronchitis, bronchiectasis, asthma, and emphysema—have distinct anatomic and clinical characteristics (Table 16–3). For example, patients with predominant emphysema and those with predominant bronchitis form distinct clinical categories (Table 16–4). Many patients, however, have overlapping features of damage at both the acinar (emphysema) and the bronchial (bronchitis) levels, almost certainly because one pathogenic mechanism—cigarette smoking—is common to both, as we shall see. Add the frequent component of reversible airway hyperreactivity (asthma) in these patients, and one can understand the utility and popularity of the broad umbrella term COPD.

EMPHYSEMA

Emphysema is a condition of the lung characterized by *abnormal permanent enlargement of the airspaces distal to the terminal bronchiole, accompanied by destruction of their walls,* and *without obvious fibrosis.*[10] In contrast, the enlargement of airspaces unaccompanied by destruction is termed *overinflation,* for example, the distention of airspaces in the opposite lung after unilateral pneumonectomy.

Types of Emphysema. Emphysema is defined in terms of the *anatomic nature* of the lesion, and it can be further classified according to its *anatomic distribution* within the lobule. Recall that the lobule is a cluster of acini, the alveolated terminal respiratory units. Although the term *emphysema* is sometimes loosely applied to diverse conditions, there are four major types: (1) *centriacinar,* (2) *panacinar,* (3) *paraseptal,* and (4) *irregular.* Of these, only the first two cause clinically significant airflow obstruction (Fig. 16–8). Centriacinar emphysema is far more common than the panacinar form (see later), constituting greater than 95% of cases. Clinical management does not rely on precise anatomic diagnosis and classification (thankfully, since this can be done only on postmortem specimens). The anatomic subtypes of emphysema, however, provide important clues to pathogenesis.

Centriacinar (Centrilobular Emphysema). The distinctive feature of this type of emphysema is the pattern of involvement of the lobules; *the central or proximal parts of the acini, formed by respiratory bronchioles, are af-*

Table 16–4. EMPHYSEMA AND CHRONIC BRONCHITIS

	Predominant Bronchitis	Predominant Emphysema
Age (yr)	40–45	50–75
Dyspnea	Mild; late	Severe; early
Cough	Early; copious sputum	Late; scanty sputum
Infections	Common	Occasional
Respiratory insufficiency	Repeated	Terminal
Cor pulmonale	Common	Rare; terminal
Airway resistance	Increased	Normal or slightly increased
Elastic recoil	Normal	Low
Chest radiograph	Prominent vessels; large heart	Hyperinflation; small heart
Appearance	*Blue bloater*	*Pink puffer*

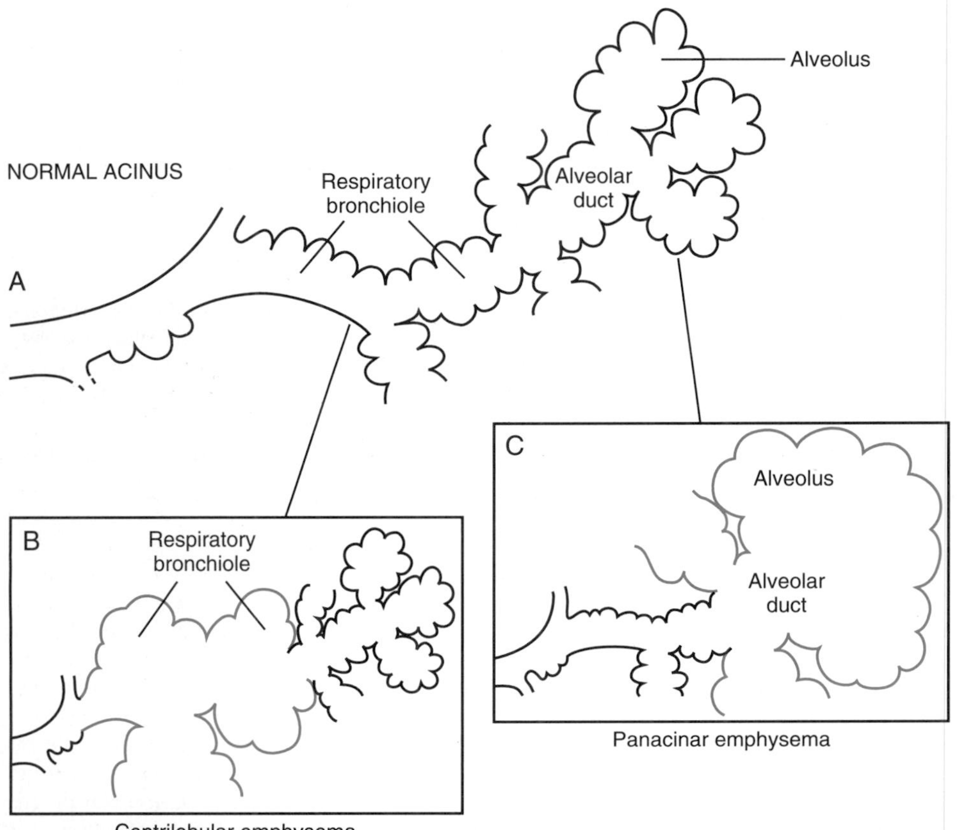

Figure 16–8

A, Diagram of normal structures within the acinus, the fundamental unit of the lung. A terminal bronchiole *(not shown)* is immediately proximal to the respiratory bronchiole. *B*, Centrilobular emphysema with dilation that initially affects the respiratory bronchioles. *C*, Panacinar emphysema with initial distention of the peripheral structures (i.e., the alveolus and alveolar duct); the disease later extends to affect the respiratory bronchioles.

fected, whereas distal alveoli are spared (Fig. 16–9*A*). Thus, both emphysematous and normal airspaces exist within the same acinus and lobule. The lesions are more common and usually more severe in the upper lobes, particularly in the apical segments. The walls of the emphysematous spaces often contain large amounts of black pigment. Inflammation around bronchi and bronchioles and in the septa is common. In severe centriacinar emphysema, the distal acinus may be involved, and differentiation from panacinar emphysema becomes difficult. Centriacinar emphysema occurs predominantly in heavy smokers, often in association with chronic bronchitis. In addition, some lesions of so-called coal workers' pneumoconiosis (see later in this chapter) bear a striking resemblance to centriacinar

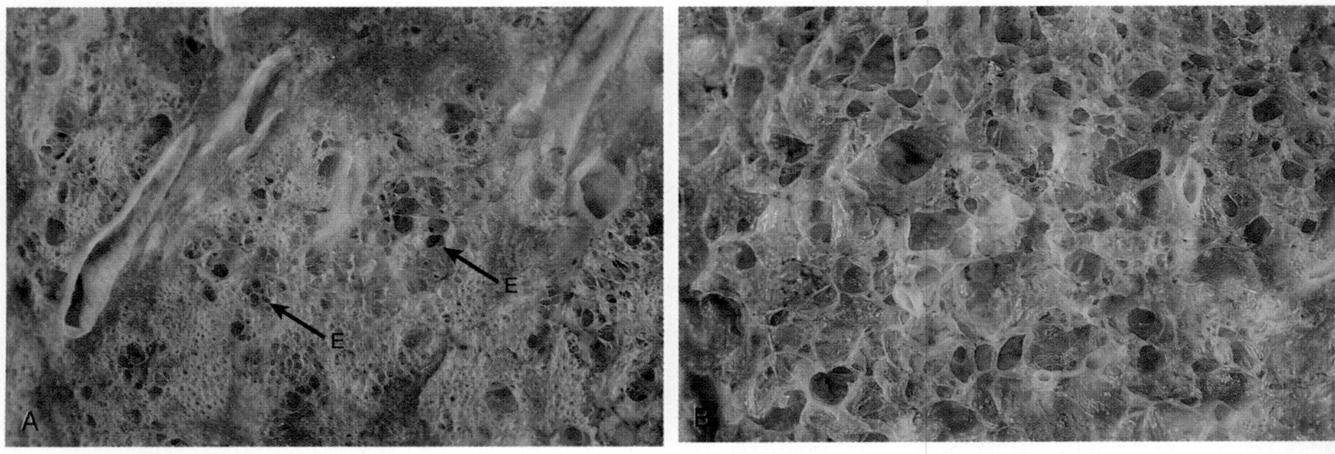

Figure 16–9

A, Centrilobular emphysema. Central areas show marked emphysematous damage (E), surrounded by relatively spared alveolar spaces. *B*, Panacinar emphysema involving the entire pulmonary architecture.

emphysema. These points suggest an important role for tobacco products and coal dust in the genesis of this type of emphysema.

Panacinar (Panlobular) Emphysema. In this type, the *acini are uniformly enlarged from the level of the respiratory bronchiole to the terminal blind alveoli* (Fig. 16–9*B*). The prefix *pan-* refers to the entire acinus but not to the entire lung. In contrast to centriacinar emphysema, panacinar emphysema tends to occur more commonly in the lower zones and in the anterior margins of the lung, and it is usually most severe at the bases. This type of emphysema is associated with *α_1-antitrypsin* (α_1-AT) *deficiency* (Chapter 19).

Paraseptal (Distal Acinar) Emphysema. In this type, the *proximal portion of the acinus is normal, but the distal part is dominantly involved.* The emphysema is more striking adjacent to the pleura, along the lobular connective tissue septa, and at the margins of the lobules. It occurs adjacent to areas of fibrosis, scarring, or atelectasis and is usually more severe in the upper half of the lungs. The characteristic findings are of multiple, continuous, enlarged airspaces from less than 0.5 mm to more than 2.0 cm in diameter, sometimes forming cystlike structures. This type of emphysema probably underlies many of the cases of spontaneous pneumothorax in young adults.

Irregular Emphysema. *Irregular emphysema, so named because the acinus is irregularly involved, is almost invariably associated with scarring.* Thus, it may be the most common form of emphysema because careful search of most lungs at autopsy shows one or more scars from a healed inflammatory process. In most instances, these foci of irregular emphysema are asymptomatic.

Incidence. Emphysema is a common disease. In one study, there was a 50% combined incidence of panacinar and centriacinar emphysema at autopsy, and the pulmonary disease was considered to be responsible for death in 6.5% of these patients.[11] *There is a clear-cut association between heavy cigarette smoking and emphysema,* and the most severe type occurs in men who smoke heavily. Although the emphysema does not become disabling until the forties to seventies, it is well known clinically that ventilatory deficits may make their first appearance decades earlier in those destined to develop the full-blown disease.

Pathogenesis. Although details of the genesis of the two common forms of emphysema—centriacinar and panacinar—remain unsettled, *the most plausible hypothesis to account for the destruction of alveolar walls is the protease-antiprotease mechanism.* This hypothesis is based on two important observations, one clinical and one experimental. The first is that homozygous patients with a genetic deficiency of the protease inhibitor α_1-AT have a markedly enhanced tendency to develop pulmonary emphysema, which is compounded by smoking.[12] α_1-AT deficiency is described in Chapter 19. α_1-AT (which is present in serum, tissue fluids, and macrophages) is a major inhibitor of proteases, particularly elastase, secreted by neutrophils during inflammation (Chapter 3). The normal α_1-AT phenotype, called *PiMM,*[75] is present in 90% of the population. Of the several phenotypes associated with α_1-AT deficiency, PiZZ is the most common. More than 80% of PiZZ phenotypes develop symptomatic emphysema that occurs at an earlier age and with greater severity if the individual smokes. Therefore, the most important therapeutic intervention in α_1-AT deficiency is cessation of smoking. The second observation bearing on the protease-antiprotease hypothesis is experimental, in that intratracheal instillation of the proteolytic enzyme papain, which degrades elastin, causes emphysema in experimental animals.[13]

The *protease-antiprotease theory* holds that alveolar wall destruction results from an imbalance between proteases (mainly elastase) and antiproteases in the lung (Fig. 16–10). The principal antielastase activity in serum and interstitial tissue is α_1-AT (others are *secretory leukoprotease inhibitor* in bronchial mucus and serum *α_2-macroglobulin*), and the principal cellular elastase activity is derived from neutrophils (other elastases are formed by macrophages, mast cells, pancreas, and bacteria). Neutrophil elastase is capable of digesting human lung, and this digestion can be inhibited by α_1-AT. Such elastase induces emphysema when instilled into the trachea of experimental animals.[14] Thus, the following sequence is postulated to explain the effect of α_1-AT deficiency on the lung: Neutrophils are normally sequestered in the lung (more in the lower zones than in the upper), and a few gain access to the alveolar space. Any stimulus that increases either the number of leukocytes (neutrophils and macrophages) in the lung or the release of their elastase-containing granules increases elastolytic activity. Stimulated neutrophils also release oxygen free radicals, which, as previously noted, inhibit α_1-AT activity. With low levels of serum α_1-AT, the process of elastic tissue destruction is unchecked, with consequent emphysema. *Thus, emphysema is seen to result from the destructive effect of high protease activity in subjects with low antiprotease activity.* The primacy of the neutrophil is accepted for patients with α_1-AT deficiency, but in the more common smoking-related emphysema, both neutrophil and macrophage proteases play a role.[15]

The protease-antiprotease hypothesis also explains the deleterious effect of cigarette smoking because both in-

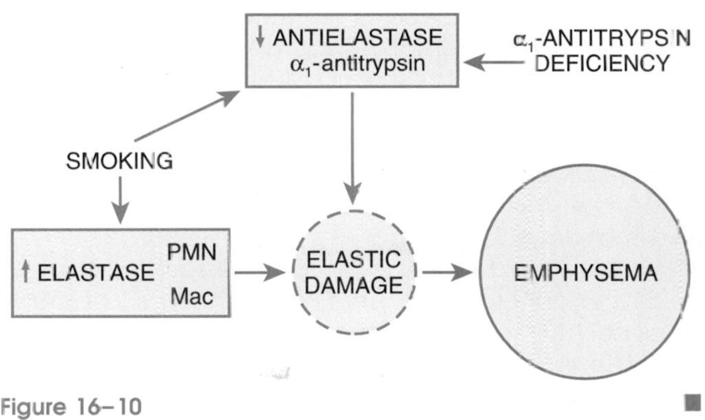

Figure 16–10

Protease-antiprotease mechanism of emphysema. Smoking inhibits antielastase and favors the recruitment of leukocytes and release of elastase. PMN, polymorphonuclear leukocytes; Mac, alveolar macrophages.

creased elastase availability and decreased antielastase activity occur in smokers, as follows (Fig. 16–10):

- *Smokers have greater numbers of neutrophils and macrophages in their alveoli.* The increased recruitment of neutrophils into the lung is likely to result, in part, from the release by activated alveolar macrophages of *neutrophil chemotactic factors* (*e.g.*, *IL-8*), this release being stimulated by smoking. In addition, nicotine is chemotactic for neutrophils, and cigarette smoke activates the alternative complement pathway.
- *Smoking stimulates release of elastase from neutrophils.*
- *Smoking enhances elastolytic protease(s) activity in macrophages.* Macrophage elastase is not inhibited by α_1-AT and can proteolytically digest this enzyme.
- *Oxidants in cigarette smoke and oxygen free radicals secreted by neutrophils inhibit α_1-AT* and thus decrease net antielastase activity in smokers.

It is thus postulated that impaction of smoke particles in the small bronchi and bronchioles, with the resultant influx of neutrophils and macrophages and increased elastase and decreased α_1-AT activity, causes the centriacinar emphysema seen in smokers. In contrast, it is postulated that the panacinar emphysema of α_1-AT-deficient individuals reflects total lack of antiprotease throughout the acinus and susceptibility to chronic low-level proteolysis from neutrophils in transit through the lung circulation. The predominantly lower lung distribution (where perfusion and neutrophil numbers are greatest) of panacinar emphysema is also consistent with this postulate. Finally, some speculate that the upper lobe distribution of centriacinar emphysema (see later) also reflects a relative lack of serum α_1-AT delivery to this less perfused region.

MORPHOLOGY. The diagnosis and classification of the emphysemas are based on naked eye (or hand lens) examination of lungs fixed in a state of inflation. Panacinar emphysema, when well developed, produces voluminous lungs, often overlapping the heart and hiding it when the anterior chest wall is removed. The macroscopic features of centriacinar emphysema are less impressive. The lungs may not appear particularly pale or voluminous unless the disease is well advanced. Generally the upper two thirds of the lungs are more severely affected. Large apical blebs or bullae are more characteristic of irregular emphysema secondary to scarring.

Microscopic examination is necessary to visualize the abnormal fenestrations in the walls of the alveoli, the complete destruction of septal walls, and the distribution of damage within the pulmonary lobule. With advance of the disease, adjacent alveoli fuse, producing even larger abnormal airspaces and possibly blebs or bullae. Often the respiratory bronchioles and vasculature of the lung are deformed and compressed by the emphysematous distortion of the airspaces, and, as mentioned, there may or may not be evidence of bronchitis or bronchiolitis.

Clinical Course. The clinical manifestations of emphysema do not appear until at least one third of the functioning pulmonary parenchyma is incapacitated. Dyspnea is usually the first symptom; it begins insidiously but is steadily progressive. In some patients, cough or wheezing is the chief complaint, easily confused with asthma. Cough and expectoration are extremely variable and depend on the extent of the associated bronchitis. Weight loss is common and may be so severe as to suggest a hidden malignant tumor. Classically the patient is barrel-chested and dyspneic, with obviously prolonged expiration, and sits forward in a hunched-over position, attempting to squeeze the air out of the lungs with each expiratory effort. Patients have a pinched face and breathe through pursed lips. *The only reliable and consistently present finding on physical examination is slowing of forced expiration.*

In patients with severe emphysema, cough is often slight, overdistention is severe, diffusing capacity is low, and blood gas values are relatively normal. Such patients may overventilate and remain well oxygenated and therefore are euphoniously if somewhat ingloriously designated as *pink puffers* (see Table 16–4). Patients with chronic bronchitis more often have a history of recurrent infection, abundant purulent sputum, hypercapnia, and severe hypoxemia, prompting the equally inglorious designation of *blue bloaters.* A hazard in severe bronchitis, in addition to the respiratory difficulties, is the development of cor pulmonale and eventual congestive heart failure, related to secondary pulmonary vascular hypertension. Death in most patients with COPD is due to (1) respiratory acidosis and coma, (2) right-sided heart failure, and (3) massive collapse of the lungs secondary to pneumothorax.

Other Types of Emphysema. Now we come to some conditions in which the term *emphysema* is applied less stringently and to some closely related conditions.

Compensatory Emphysema (Compensatory Hyperinflation). The term *compensatory emphysema* is sometimes used to designate dilation of alveoli but not destruction of septal walls in response to loss of lung substance elsewhere. It is best exemplified by the hyperexpansion of the residual lung parenchyma that follows surgical removal of a diseased lung or lobe.

Senile Emphysema. *Senile emphysema* refers to the overdistended, sometimes voluminous lungs found in the aged. These changes result from age-related alterations of the internal geometry of the lung—*larger alveolar ducts* and *smaller alveoli*—that occur without loss of elastic tissue or destruction of lung substance.

Obstructive Overinflation. *Obstructive overinflation refers to the condition in which the lung expands because air is trapped within it.* A common cause is subtotal obstruction by a tumor or foreign object. A classic example is *congenital lobar overinflation* in infants, probably resulting from hypoplasia of bronchial cartilage and sometimes associated with other congenital cardiac and lung abnormalities.

Overinflation in obstructive lesions occurs either (1) because of a ball-valve action of the obstructive agent, so that air enters on inspiration but cannot leave on expiration, or (2) because the bronchus may be totally obstructed, but ventilation through *collaterals* may bring in air from behind the obstruction. These collaterals are the *pores of Kohn* and other direct accessory *bronchioloalveolar connections* (the canals of Lambert). Obstructive overinflation can be a life-threatening emergency because the affected portion extends sufficiently to compress the remaining normal lung.

Bullous Emphysema. *Bullous emphysema* refers merely to any form of emphysema that produces large subpleural blebs or bullae (spaces >1 cm in diameter in the distended state) (Fig. 16–11). They represent localized accentuations of one of the four forms of emphysema, are most often subpleural, and occur near the apex, sometimes in relation to old tuberculous scarring. On occasion, rupture of the bullae may give rise to pneumothorax.

Interstitial Emphysema. *The entrance of air into the connective tissue stroma of the lung, mediastinum, or subcutaneous tissue is designated interstitial emphysema.* In most instances, alveolar tears in pulmonary emphysema provide the avenue of entrance of air into the stroma of the lung, but rarely a wound of the chest that allows air to be sucked in or a fractured rib that punctures the lung substance may underlie this disorder. Alveolar tears usually occur when there is a combination of coughing plus some bronchiolar obstruction, producing sharply increased pressures within the alveolar sacs. Children with whooping cough and bronchitis, patients with obstruction to the airways (by blood clots, tissue, or foreign bodies) or being artificially ventilated, and individuals who suddenly inhale irritant gases provide classic examples.

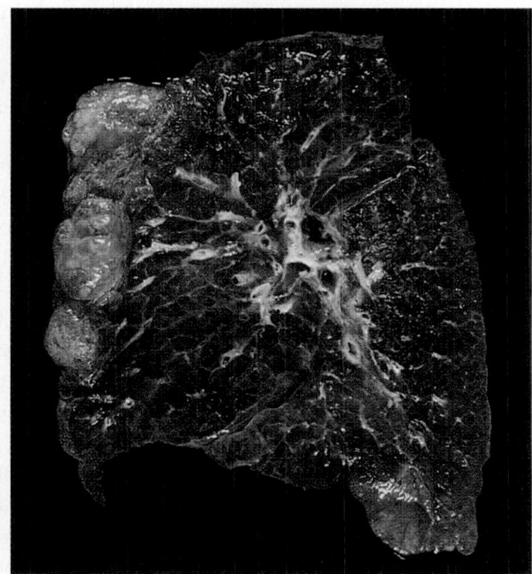

Figure 16–11

Bullous emphysema with large subpleural bullae *(upper left).*

CHRONIC BRONCHITIS

Chronic bronchitis, so common among habitual smokers and inhabitants of smog-laden cities, is not nearly so trivial as was once thought. When persistent for years, it may (1) be associated with chronic obstructive airway disease, as discussed earlier; (2) lead to cor pulmonale and heart failure; and (3) cause atypical metaplasia and dysplasia of the respiratory epithelium, providing a possible soil for cancerous transformation. Important definitions in bronchitis include the following:

- *Chronic bronchitis per se is defined clinically*: It is present in any patient who has persistent cough with sputum production for at least 3 months in at least 2 consecutive years.
- In *simple chronic bronchitis*, patients have a productive cough but no physiologic evidence of airflow obstruction.
- Some individuals may demonstrate hyperreactive airways with intermittent bronchospasm and wheezing. This condition is called *chronic asthmatic bronchitis*.
- Finally, some patients, especially heavy smokers, develop chronic airflow obstruction, usually with evidence of associated emphysema, and are classified as showing *obstructive chronic bronchitis*.

Pathogenesis. Two sets of factors are important in the genesis of chronic bronchitis: (1) chronic irritation by inhaled substances and (2) microbiologic infections. Both sexes and all ages may be affected, but chronic bronchitis is most frequent in middle-aged men. Cigarette smoking remains the paramount influence. Chronic bronchitis is 4 to 10 times more common in heavy smokers regardless of age, sex, occupation, and place of dwelling.

The hallmark and earliest feature of chronic bronchitis is *hypersecretion of mucus* in the large airways, and it is associated with hypertrophy of the submucosal glands in the trachea and bronchi.[16] As chronic bronchitis persists, there is also *a marked increase in goblet cells of small airways—small bronchi and bronchioles*—leading to excessive mucus production that contributes to airway obstruction. It is thought that both the submucosal gland hypertrophy and the increase in goblet cells are caused by tobacco smoke or other pollutants (e.g., sulfur dioxide, nitrogen dioxide).

Although mucus hypersecretion in large airways is the cause of sputum overproduction, it is now thought that accompanying *alterations in the small airways of the lung* (small bronchi and bronchioles, <2 to 3 mm in diameter) *can result in physiologically important and early manifestations of chronic airway obstruction.*[17, 18] Histologic studies of the small airways in young smokers disclose (1) goblet cell metaplasia with mucous plugging of the lumen, (2) clustering of pigmented alveolar macrophages, (3) inflammatory infiltration, and (4) fibrosis of the bronchiolar wall (in a somewhat older group of patients).[19, 20] It is postulated that smoking and other irritants, which cause the hypertrophy of mucous glands, also result in *bronchiolitis*,[21] or *small airway disease.* Certain physiologic studies suggest that this respiratory bronchiolitis is an important component in early and relatively mild airflow obstruction. *When bronchitis is accompanied by moderate to severe airflow obstruction, however, coexistent emphysema is the dominant lesion.*[18]

The role of *infection* appears to be secondary. It is not responsible for the initiation of chronic bronchitis but is probably significant in maintaining it and may be critical in producing acute exacerbations. Cigarette smoke predisposes to infection in more than one way: It interferes with ciliary action of the respiratory epithelium, may cause direct damage to airway epithelium, and inhibits the ability of bronchial and alveolar leukocytes to clear bacteria. Viral infections can also cause exacerbations of chronic bronchitis.

Following this review of the pathogenesis of both emphysema and chronic bronchitis, the reader is referred to Figure 16–12, which follows the evolution of both conditions into chronic obstructive airway disease.

MORPHOLOGY. Grossly, there may be hyperemia, swelling, and bogginess of the mucous membranes, frequently accompanied by excessive mucinous to mucopurulent secretions layering the epithelial surfaces. Sometimes, heavy casts of secretions and pus fill the bronchi and bronchioles. The characteristic histologic feature of chronic bronchitis is enlargement of the mucus-secreting glands of the trachea and bronchi. Although the numbers of goblet cells increase slightly, the **major increase is in the size of the mucous glands.** This increase can be assessed by the ratio of the thickness of the mucous gland layer to the thickness of the wall between the epithelium and the cartilage (**Reid index**). The Reid index (normally 0.4) is increased in chronic bronchitis, usually in proportion to the severity and duration of the disease. The bronchial epithelium may exhibit squamous metaplasia and dysplasia. There is marked narrowing of bronchioles caused by goblet cell metaplasia, mucous plugging, inflammation, and fibrosis. In the most severe cases, there may be obliteration of lumens (**bronchiolitis obliterans**). As discussed earlier, these bronchiolar changes probably contribute to the obstructive features in bronchitis patients.

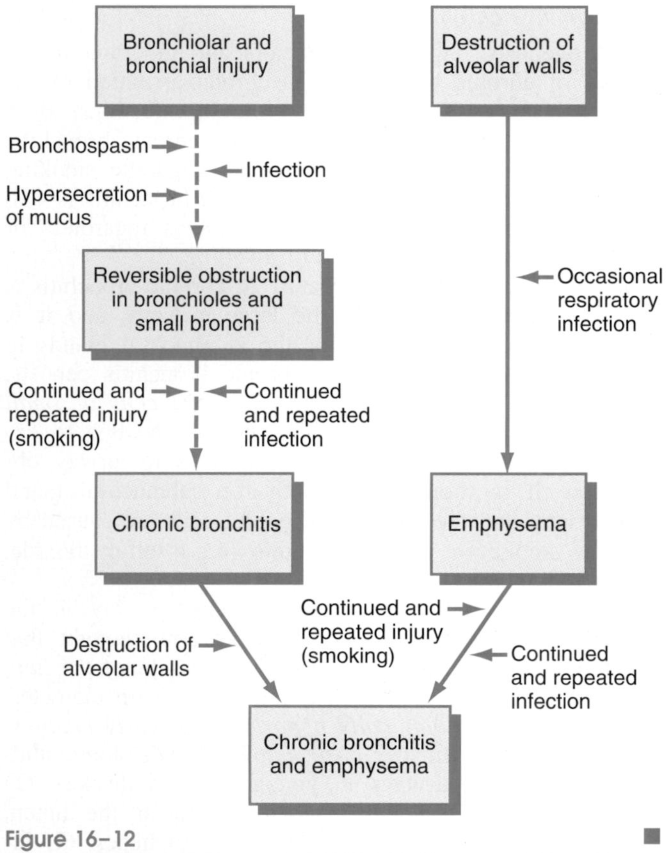

Figure 16–12

Schematic representation of evolution of chronic bronchitis *(left)* and emphysema *(right)*. Although both can culminate in chronic bronchitis and emphysema, the pathways are different, and either one may predominate. The dashed arrows on the left indicate that, in the natural history of chronic bronchitis, it is not known whether there is a predictable progression from obstruction in small airways to chronic (obstructive) bronchitis. (Redrawn from Fishman AP: The spectrum of chronic obstructive disease of the airways. In Fishman AP (ed): Pulmonary Diseases and Disorders, 2nd ed. New York, McGraw-Hill, 1988, p 1164.)

Clinical Features. The clinical sine qua non of chronic bronchitis is a persistent cough productive of copious sputum. For many years, no other respiratory functional impairment is present, but eventually dyspnea on exertion develops. With the passage of time, and usually with continued smoking, other elements of COPD may appear, including hypercapnia, hypoxemia, and mild cyanosis. Differentiation of pure chronic bronchitis from that associated with emphysema can be made in the classic case (see Table 16–3), but, as mentioned, many patients with COPD have both conditions. Long-standing severe chronic bronchitis commonly leads to cor pulmonale with cardiac failure. Death may also result from further impairment of respiratory function incident to acute intercurrent bacterial infections.

BRONCHIAL ASTHMA

Asthma is a chronic relapsing inflammatory disorder characterized by hyperreactive airways, leading to episodic, reversible bronchoconstriction, owing to increased responsiveness of the tracheobronchial tree to various stimuli.[22] Some of these stimuli would have little or no effect on nonasthmatics with normal airways. Most asthma is associated with atopy, which represents increased susceptibility to generate immunoglobulin E (IgE) in response to external allergens (Chapter 7).[22a]

Those afflicted experience unpredictable disabling attacks of severe dyspnea, coughing, and wheezing triggered by sudden episodes of bronchospasm. Between the attacks, patients may be virtually asymptomatic, but in some persons chronic bronchitis or cor pulmonale supervenes. Rarely a state of unremitting attacks (*status asthmaticus*) proves fatal; usually such patients have had a long history of asthma. In some cases, the attacks are triggered by exposure to an allergen to which the patient has previously been sensitized, but often no allergic trigger can be identified. There has been a significant increase in the incidence of asthma in the Western world in the past three decades.

Asthma has traditionally been divided into two basic types—extrinsic and intrinsic (idiosyncratic). *Extrinsic asthma* is initiated by a type I hypersensitivity reaction induced by exposure to an extrinsic antigen. Subtypes include *atopic (allergic) asthma*, occupational asthma, and *allergic bronchopulmonary aspergillosis*. The last-mentioned describes colonization of asthmatic airways with *Aspergillus* organisms, followed by development of additional IgE antibodies. In contrast, *intrinsic asthma* is initiated by diverse, nonimmune mechanisms, including ingestion of aspirin; pulmonary infections, especially viral; cold; inhaled irritants; stress; and exercise. As with other classification schemes, patients often ignore categories and manifest overlapping characteristics. For example, the patient with extrinsic asthma and increased airway hyperreactivity is also more likely to manifest bronchospasm after exposure to one of the agents associated with intrinsic asthma.

Pathogenesis. The two major components of asthma are chronic airway inflammation and bronchial hyperresponsiveness. *The inflammation involves many cell types and numerous inflammatory mediators,*[23] but the precise relationship of specific inflammatory cells and the mediators to airway hyperreactivity is not fully understood. The mechanisms have been best studied in atopic asthma, so this is presented first.

Atopic Asthma. This most common type of asthma usually begins in childhood. The disease is triggered by environmental antigens, such as dusts, pollens, animal dander, and foods, but potentially any antigen is implicated. A positive family history of atopy is common, and asthmatic attacks are often preceded by allergic rhinitis, urticaria, or eczema.

Candidate genes for predisposition to atopy and airway hyperresponsiveness are currently subjects of intensive search and include genes involved in antigen presentation (the HLA complex), T-cell activation (T-cell receptor complex, γ-interferon), regulation of cytokine production or function of relevant cytokines (IL-4, IL-5), and receptors for bronchodilators (β_2-adrenergic receptors).[22a] In any case, a skin test with the offending antigen in these patients results in an immediate wheal-and-flare reaction, a *classic example of type I IgE-mediated hypersensitivity reaction*, discussed in detail in Chapter 7. In the airways, the scene for the reaction is set in large part by initial sensitization to inhaled antigens (allergens), which stimulate induction of *Th2-type T cells*, which release cytokines such as IL-4 and IL-5 (Fig. 16–13*A*). These cytokines, in turn, promote IgE production by B cells, growth of mast cells (IL-4), and growth and activation of eosinophils (IL-5). Subsequent IgE-mediated reaction to inhaled allergens elicits an *acute response and a late-phase reaction.*

Recall that exposure of presensitized IgE-coated mast cells to the same or a cross-reacting antigen stimulates cross-linking of IgE and the release of chemical mediators. In the case of airborne antigens, the reaction occurs first on sensitized mast cells *on the mucosal surface* (Fig. 16–13*B*); the resultant mediator release opens the mucosal intercellular tight junctions and enhances penetration of antigen to the more numerous submucosal mast cells. In addition, direct stimulation of *subepithelial vagal* (parasympathetic) *receptors* provokes bronchoconstriction through both central and local reflexes (including those mediated by unmyelinated sensory C fibers). This occurs within minutes after stimulation and is called the *acute*, or *immediate*, response, which consists of bronchoconstriction, edema (owing to increased vascular permeability), mucus secretion, and, in extreme instances, hypotension. Mast cells also release cytokines that cause the influx of other leukocytes, including neutrophils and monocytes, lymphocytes, basophils, and particularly eosinophils (IL-5). These inflammatory cells set the stage for the *late-phase reaction*, which starts 4 to 8 hours later and may persist for 12 to 24 hours or more (Fig. 16–13*C*).

The *late-phase reaction,* as noted earlier, is mediated by the swarm of leukocytes recruited by the chemotactic factors and cytokines derived from mast cells[25] during the acute-phase response. However, mediators can also be produced by other cells in the affected bronchi, including inflammatory cells *already present* in asthmatics suffering a recurrent attack, or *vascular endothelium,* or *airway epithelial cells.* Epithelial cells are now known to produce a large variety of cytokines in response to infectious agents, drugs, and gases as well as to inflammatory mediators.[27] This second wave of mediators stimulates the late reaction. For example, *eotaxin*, produced by airway epithelial cells, is a potent chemoattractant and activator of eosinophils.[26] *The major basic protein of eosinophils, in turn, causes epithelial damage*[27] *and airway constriction.*[28] The presence of both immediate and delayed reactions in IgE-mediated events helps explain the prolonged manifestations of asthma.

Many mediators have been implicated in the asthmatic response, but the relative importance of each putative mediator in actual human asthma has been difficult to establish. The long list of "suspects" in acute asthma can be subclassified by the clinical efficacy of pharmacologic intervention with inhibitors or antagonists of the mediators.

- The first (disappointingly small) group includes putative mediators whose role in bronchospasm is clearly supported by efficacy of pharmacologic intervention: (1) *leukotrienes* C_4, D_4, and E_4, extremely potent mediators that cause prolonged bronchoconstriction as well as increased vascular permeability and increased mucus secretion, and (2) *acetylcholine*, released from intrapulmonary motor nerves, which can cause airway smooth muscle constriction by directly stimulating muscarinic receptors.
- A second group includes agents present at the *scene of the crime* and with potent asthma-like effects but whose actual clinical role in acute allergic asthma appears relatively minor based on lack of efficacy of potent antagonists or synthesis inhibitors: (1) *histamine*, a potent bronchoconstrictor; (2) *prostaglandin* D_2 (*PGD*$_2$), which elicits bronchoconstriction and vasodilation; and (3) *PAF*, which causes aggregation of platelets and release of histamine and serotonin from their granules. These mediators may yet prove important in other types of chronic or nonallergic asthma.

A. SENSITIZATION TO ALLERGEN

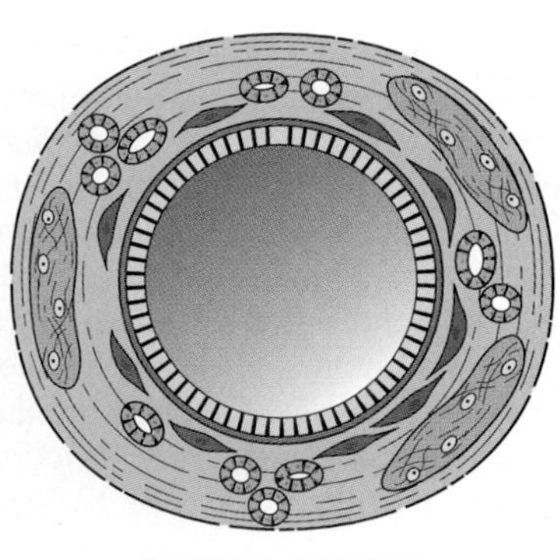

Pollen
Antigen
Mucosal lining
APC
IgE Fc receptor
TCR
IL-4
IL-5
IgE antibody
IgE B cell
IL-5
Mast cell
T_H2 cell
IL-5
Eosinophil recruitment

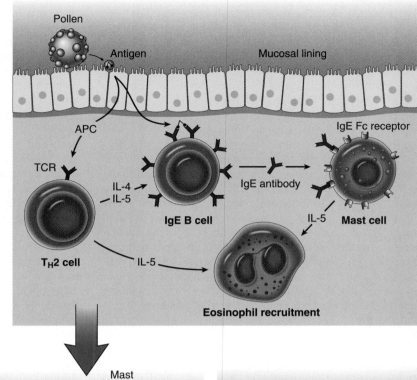

B. ALLERGEN-TRIGGERED ASTHMA

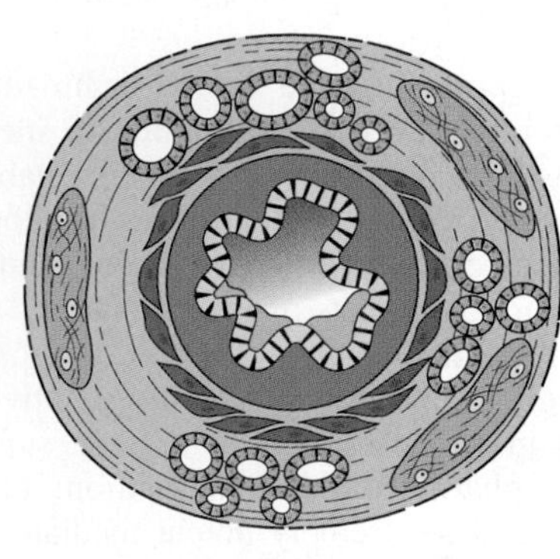

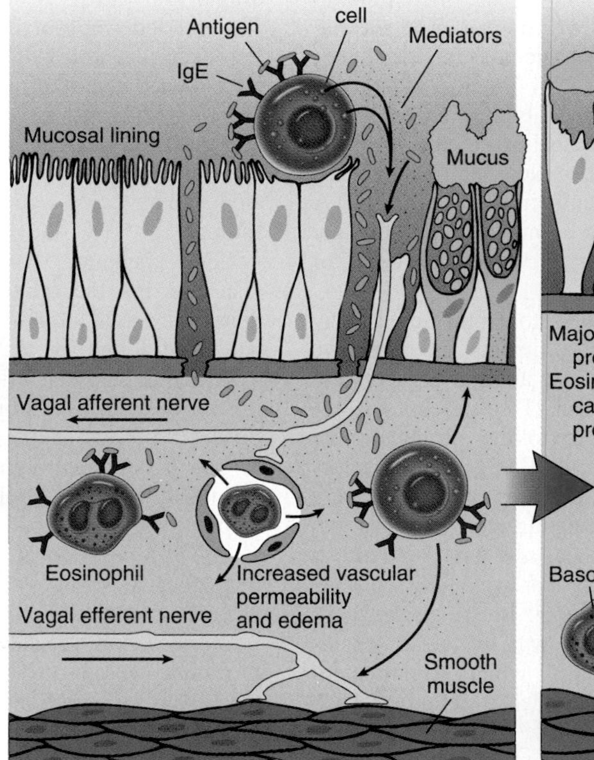

Mucus
Major basic
protein
Eosinophil
cationic
protein
Basophil
Eosinophil
Neutrophil

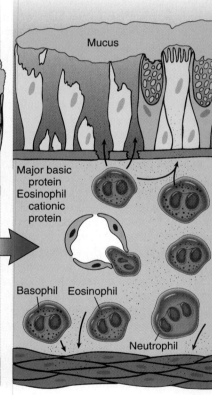

C. LATE PHASE (HOURS)

Figure 16–13

A model for allergic asthma. *A*, Inhaled allergens (antigen) elicit a Th2-dominated response favoring IgE production and eosinophil recruitment (priming or sensitization). *B*, On reexposure to antigen (Ag), the immediate reaction is triggered by Ag-induced cross-linking of IgE bound to IgE receptors on mast cells in the airways. These cells release preformed mediators that open tight junctions between epithelial cells. Antigen can then enter the mucosa to activate mucosal mast cells and eosinophils, which in turn release additional mediators. Collectively, either directly or via neuronal reflexes, the mediators induce bronchospasm, increased vascular permeability, and mucus production and recruit additional mediator-releasing cells from the blood. *C*, The arrival of recruited leukocytes (neutrophils, eosinophils, and basophils; also lymphocytes and monocytes [*not shown*]) signals the initiation of the late phase of asthma and a fresh round of mediator release from leukocytes, endothelium, and epithelial cells. Factors, particularly from eosinophils (e.g., major basic protein, eosinophil cationic protein), also cause damage to the epithelium.

■ Finally, a large third group comprises the *suspects* for whom specific antagonists or inhibitors are not available or insufficiently studied as of yet. These include numerous cytokines, such as IL-1, TNF, and IL-6 (some of which exist in a preformed state within the mast cell granules[24]), chemokines (e.g., eotaxin), neuropeptides, nitric oxide, bradykinin, and endothelins.

It is thus clear that multiple mediators contribute to the acute asthmatic response. Moreover, the composition of this mediator *soup* may differ among different individuals or types of asthma. The appreciation of the importance of inflammatory cells and mediators in asthma has led to greater emphasis on anti-inflammatory therapeutics in clinical practice.

Nonatopic Asthma. The second large group is the *nonatopic*, or *nonreaginic*, variety of asthma, which is most frequently triggered by respiratory tract infection. Viruses (e.g., rhinovirus, parainfluenza virus) rather than bacteria are the most common provokers.[29] A positive family history is uncommon, serum IgE levels are normal, and there are no other associated allergies. In these patients, skin test results are usually negative, and although hypersensitivity to microbial antigens may play a role, present theories place more stress on hyperirritability of the bronchial tree. *It is thought that virus-induced inflammation of the respiratory mucosa lowers the threshold of the subepithelial vagal receptors to irritants.* Inhaled air pollutants, such as sulfur dioxide, ozone, and nitrogen dioxide, may also contribute to the chronic airway inflammation and hyperreactivity present in some cases.

Drug-Induced Asthma. Several pharmacologic agents provoke asthma. *Aspirin-sensitive asthma* is an uncommon, yet fascinating type, occurring in patients with recurrent rhinitis and nasal polyps. These individuals are exquisitely sensitive to small doses of aspirin, and they experience not only asthmatic attacks, but also urticaria. It is probable that aspirin triggers asthma in these patients by inhibiting the cyclooxygenase pathway of arachidonic acid metabolism without affecting the lipoxygenase route, thus tipping the balance toward elaboration of the bronchoconstrictor leukotrienes.

Occupational Asthma. This form of asthma is stimulated by fumes (epoxy resins, plastics), organic and chemical dusts (wood, cotton, platinum), gases (toluene), and other chemicals (formaldehyde, penicillin products). Minute quantities of chemicals are required to induce the attack, which usually occurs after repeated exposure. The underlying mechanisms vary according to stimulus and include type I IgG-mediated reactions, direct liberation of bronchoconstrictor substances, and hypersensitivity responses of unknown origin.

MORPHOLOGY OF ASTHMA. The morphologic changes in asthma have been described principally in patients dying of status asthmaticus, but it appears that the pathology in nonfatal cases is similar. Grossly the lungs are overdistended because of overinflation, and there may be small areas of atelectasis. The most striking macroscopic finding is occlusion of bronchi and bronchioles by thick, tenacious **mucous plugs.** Histologically the mucous plugs contain whorls of shed epithelium, which give rise to the well-known **Curschmann spirals.** Numerous eosinophils and Charcot-Leyden crystals are present; the latter are collections of crystalloid made up of eosinophil membrane protein. The other characteristic histologic findings of asthma (Fig. 16–14) include

- Thickening of the basement membrane of the bronchial epithelium
- Edema and an inflammatory infiltrate in the bronchial walls, with a prominence of eosinophils, which form 5 to 50% of the cellular infiltrate
- An increase in size of the submucosal glands
- Hypertrophy of the bronchial wall muscle, a reflection of prolonged bronchoconstriction

While airflow obstruction is primarily attributed to muscular bronchoconstriction, the airway wall edema and inflammatory thickening may contribute as well. Emphysematous changes sometimes occur, and if chronic bacterial infection has supervened, bronchitis (described earlier) may appear.

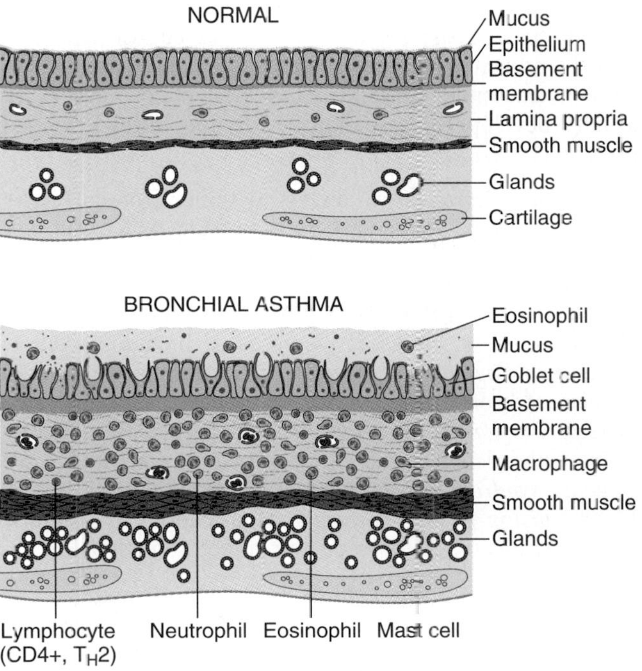

Figure 16–14

Comparison of a normal bronchiole with that in a patient with asthma. Note the accumulation of mucus in the bronchial lumen resulting from an increase in the number of mucus-secreting goblet cells in the mucosa and hypertrophy of submucosal mucous glands. In addition, there is intense chronic inflammation due to recruitment of eosinophils, macrophages, and other inflammatory cells. Basement membrane underlying the mucosal epithelium is thickened, and there is hypertrophy and hyperplasia of smooth muscle cells.

Clinical Course. The classic asthmatic attack lasts up to several hours and is followed by prolonged coughing; the raising of copious mucous secretions provides considerable relief of the respiratory difficulty. In some patients, these symptoms persist at a low level all the time. In its most severe form, *status asthmaticus*, the severe acute paroxysm persists for days and even weeks, and, under these circumstances, ventilatory function may be so impaired as to cause severe cyanosis and even death. The clinical diagnosis is aided by the demonstration of an elevated eosinophil count in the peripheral blood and the finding of eosinophils, Curschmann spirals, and Charcot-Leyden crystals in the sputum. In the usual case, with intervals of freedom from respiratory difficulty, the disease is more discouraging and disabling than lethal. With appropriate therapy to relieve the attacks, patients with asthma are able to maintain a productive life. Occasionally the disease disappears spontaneously. In the more severe forms, the progressive hyperinflation may eventually produce emphysema. Superimposed bacterial infections may lead to chronic persistent bronchitis, bronchiectasis, or pneumonia. In some cases, cor pulmonale and heart failure eventually develop.

BRONCHIECTASIS

Bronchiectasis is a chronic necrotizing infection of the bronchi and bronchioles leading to or associated with abnormal dilation of these airways. It is manifested clinically by cough, fever, and expectoration of copious amounts of foul-smelling, purulent sputum. To be considered bronchiectasis, the dilation should be permanent; reversible bronchial dilation often accompanies viral and bacterial pneumonia. Bronchiectasis has many origins and usually develops in association with the following conditions:[30]

- *Bronchial obstruction*, owing to tumor, foreign bodies, and occasionally mucous impaction, in which the bronchiectasis is localized to the obstructed lung segment, or owing to diffuse obstructive airway diseases, most commonly atopic asthma and chronic bronchitis
- *Congenital* or *hereditary conditions*, including *congenital bronchiectasis* (caused by a defect in the development of bronchi), *cystic fibrosis* (Chapter 11), *intralobar sequestration of the lung* (see earlier in this chapter), *immunodeficiency states,* and *immotile cilia* and *Kartagener syndromes* (see later)
- *Necrotizing pneumonia*, most often caused by the tubercle bacillus or staphylococci or mixed infections

Etiology and Pathogenesis. *Obstruction* and *infection* are the major influences associated with bronchiectasis, and it is likely that both are necessary for the development of full-fledged lesions. After bronchial obstruction (e.g., by tumors or foreign bodies), air is resorbed from the airways distal to the obstruction, with resultant atelectasis. Often accompanying atelectasis are early bronchial wall inflammation and the presence of intraluminal secretions that result in dilation of the walls of those airways that are patent. These changes are reversible. The changes, however, become irreversible (1) *if the obstruction persists*, especially during periods of growth, because the airways will not be able to develop normally, and (2) *if there is added infection.* Infection plays a role in the pathogenesis of bronchiectasis in two ways: (1) It produces bronchial wall inflammation, with weakening, and further dilation, and (2) the extensive bronchial and bronchiolar damage causes endobronchial obliteration, with atelectasis distal to the obliteration and subsequent bronchiectasis around atelectatic areas, as described earlier.

These mechanisms—infection and obstruction—are most readily apparent in the severe form of bronchiectasis associated with cystic fibrosis (Chapter 11). In this disorder, there is squamous metaplasia of the normal respiratory epithelium with impairment of normal mucociliary action, infection, necrosis of the bronchial and bronchiolar walls, and subsequent bronchiectasis. In younger children, the changes take the form of bronchiolitis (occlusion of the bronchioles by granulation tissue), but older children tend to develop full-blown bronchiectasis.

In *Kartagener syndrome*, characterized by bronchiectasis, sinusitis, and situs inversus, there is a *defect in ciliary motility, associated with structural abnormalities of cilia, most commonly absent or irregular dynein arms*—the structures on the microtubular doublets of cilia that are responsible for the generation of ciliary movement. The lack of ciliary activity interferes with bacterial clearance, predisposes the sinuses and bronchi to infection, and affects cell motility during embryogenesis, resulting in the situs inversus. Males with this condition tend to be infertile, owing to ineffective mobility of the sperm tail. The syndrome is inherited as an autosomal recessive trait and is variable, as about half the patients with defective cilia have no situs inversus for uncertain reasons. In some groups of patients, the cilia are not immobile but have abnormal movement (ciliary dyskinesia). More may be involved in the genesis of this syndrome than ciliary abnormalities, since some abnormal cilia may be found in otherwise normal individuals or in patients with viral illnesses and bronchial inflammation.[31]

MORPHOLOGY. Bronchiectasis usually affects the lower lobes bilaterally, particularly air passages that are most vertical, and is most severe in the more distal bronchi and bronchioles. When tumors or aspiration of foreign bodies leads to bronchiectasis, the involvement may be sharply localized to a single segment of the lungs. **The airways are dilated, sometimes up to four times normal size.** These dilations may produce long, tubelike enlargements (**cylindroid bronchiectasis**) or, in other cases, may cause **fusiform** or even sharply saccular distention (**saccular bronchiectasis**).

Characteristically the bronchi and bronchioles are sufficiently dilated that they can be followed, on gross examination, directly out to the pleural surfaces and may produce an almost cystic pattern to the cut surface of the lung (Fig. 16–15). By contrast, in the normal lung, the bronchioles cannot be followed by ordinary gross dissection beyond a point 2 to 3 cm removed from the pleural surfaces.

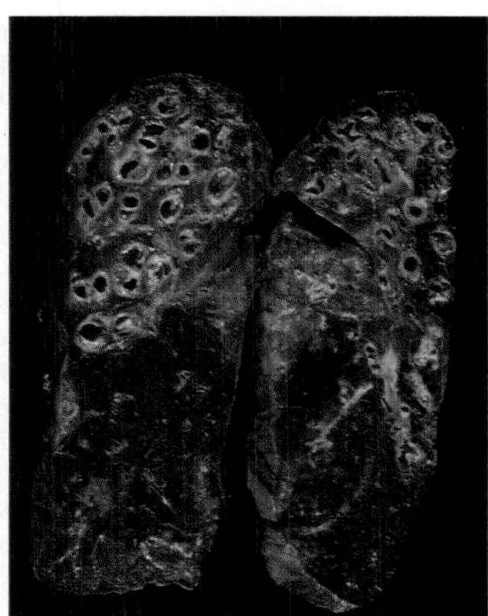

Figure 16–15

Bronchiectasis. Cut surface of lung showing transected, markedly distended peripheral bronchi, in this case predominantly in the upper lobes—an unusual localization.

The histologic findings vary with the activity and chronicity of the disease. In the full-blown, active case, there is an intense acute and chronic inflammatory exudation within the walls of the bronchi and bronchioles, associated with desquamation of the lining epithelium and extensive areas of necrotizing ulceration. There may be pseudostratification of the columnar cells or squamous metaplasia of the remaining epithelium. In some instances, the necrosis completely destroys the bronchial or bronchiolar walls and forms a lung abscess. Fibrosis of the bronchial and bronchiolar walls and peribronchiolar fibrosis develop in the more chronic cases.

Clinical Course. Bronchiectasis causes severe, persistent cough; expectoration of foul-smelling, sometimes bloody sputum; and dyspnea and orthopnea in severe cases. A systemic febrile reaction may occur when powerful pathogens are present. These symptoms are often episodic and are precipitated by upper respiratory tract infections or the introduction of new pathogenic agents. In the full-blown case, the cough is paroxysmal in nature. Such paroxysms are particularly frequent when the patient rises in the morning, and the changes in position lead to drainage into the bronchi of the collected pools of pus. Obstructive ventilatory insufficiency can lead to marked dyspnea and cyanosis. Cor pulmonale, *metastatic* brain abscesses, and amyloidosis are less frequent complications of bronchiectasis.

Pulmonary Infections

Respiratory tract infections are more frequent than infections of any other organ and account for the largest number of workdays lost in the general population. The vast majority are upper respiratory tract infections caused by viruses, but viral, mycoplasmal, bacterial, and fungal infections of the lung (pneumonia, bronchopneumonias, lung abscesses, and tuberculosis) still account for an enormous amount of morbidity and rank among the major immediate causes of death.[32] Many of these infections have been described in detail in Chapter 10. Here we review only those aspects of the pathology of pulmonary infections that need further discussion.

BACTERIAL PNEUMONIA

Bacterial invasion of the lung parenchyma evokes exudative solidification (*consolidation*) of the pulmonary tissue known as *bacterial pneumonia.* Many variables, such as the specific etiologic agent, the host reaction, and the extent of involvement, determine the precise form of pneumonia. Thus, classification may be made according to etiologic agent (e.g., pneumococcal or staphylococcal pneumonia), the nature of the host reaction (e.g., suppurative, fibrinous), or the gross anatomic distribution of the disease (lobular bronchopneumonia versus lobar pneumonia) (Fig. 16–16).

Patchy consolidation of the lung is the dominant characteristic of bronchopneumonia (Fig. 16–17). This parenchymal infection usually represents an extension of a preexisting bronchitis or bronchiolitis. It is an extremely common disease that tends to occur in the more vulnerable two extremes of life—infancy and old age. In the young, there is little previous experience with pathogenic organisms, rendering these patients susceptible to organisms of even low virulence. Resistance likewise falls in the aged, particularly in those already suffering from some serious disorder. Bronchopneumonia, a common finding on postmortem examinations, frequently terminates a long course of progressive heart failure or disseminated tumor.

Lobar pneumonia is an acute bacterial infection of a large portion of a lobe or of an entire lobe (Fig. 16–18). Classic lobar pneumonia is now infrequent, owing to the

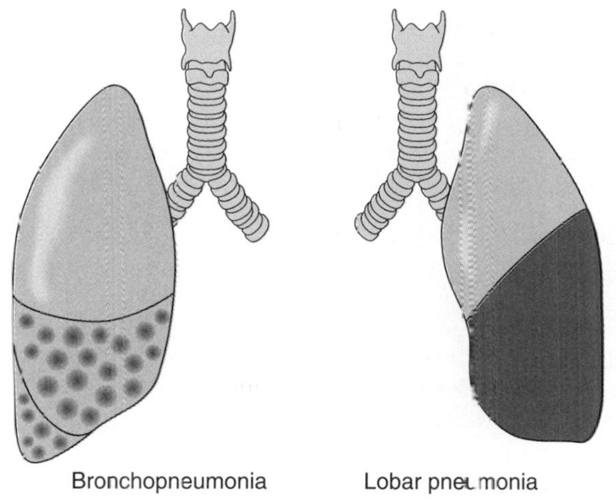

Figure 16–16

Comparison of bronchopneumonia and lobar pneumonia.

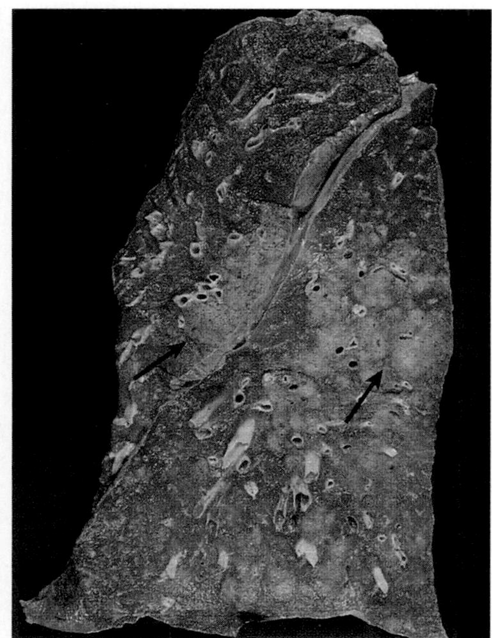

Figure 16–17

Bronchopneumonia. Gross section of lung showing patches of consolidation *(arrows)*.

effectiveness with which antibiotics abort these infections and prevent the development of full-blown lobar consolidation.

These anatomic but still classic categorizations are often difficult to apply in the individual case because patterns overlap. The lobular involvement may become confluent, producing virtually total lobar consolidation; in contrast, effective antibiotic therapy for any form of pneumonia may limit involvement to a subtotal consolidation. Moreover, the same organisms may produce lobular pneumonia in one patient, whereas in the more vulnerable individual a full-blown lobar involvement develops. *Most important, from the clinical standpoint, are identification of the causative agent and determination of the extent of disease.*

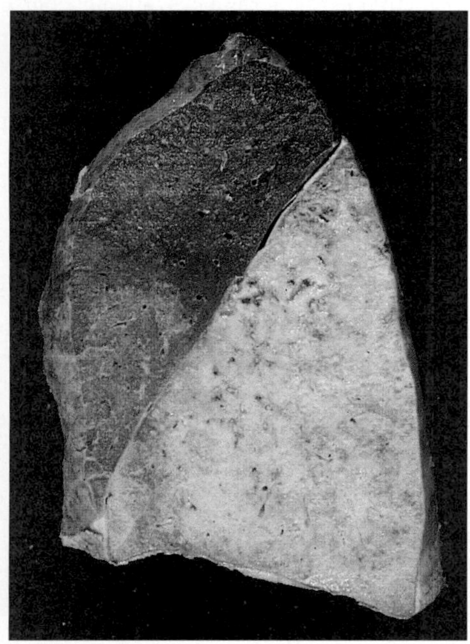

Figure 16–18

Lobar pneumonia—gray hepatization, gross photograph. The lower lobe is uniformly consolidated.

Pathogenesis. Each day, the respiratory airways and alveoli are exposed to more than 10,000 liters of air containing hazardous dusts, chemicals, and microorganisms. The fates of inhaled particles depend on their sizes. Thus, particles larger than 10 μm are deposited largely in the turbulent airflow of the nose and upper airways; particles of 3 to 10 μm lodge in the trachea and bronchi by impaction; and smaller particles, about the size of most bacteria, 1 to 5 μm, are deposited in the terminal airways and alveoli. Smaller particles (<1 μm) may remain suspended in the inspired air and can be exhaled.

The normal lung is free from bacteria. A number of potent defense mechanisms clear or destroy any bacteria inhaled with air or fortuitously deposited in the airway passages as follows (Fig. 16–19):

- *Nasal clearance*: Particles, including aerosolized droplets carrying microorganisms deposited near the front of the airway on the nonciliated epithelium, are normally removed by sneezing and blowing, whereas those deposited posteriorly are swept over the mucus-lined ciliated epithelium to the nasopharynx, where they are swallowed.
- *Tracheobronchial clearance*: This is accomplished by mucociliary action: The beating motion of cilia moves a film of mucus continuously from the lung toward the oropharynx; particles deposited on this film are eventually either swallowed or expectorated.
- *Alveolar clearance*: Bacteria or solid particles deposited in the alveoli are phagocytosed by *alveolar macrophages*. A particle is either digested or carried to the ciliated bronchioles. From here, the macrophage is propelled to the oropharynx and then swallowed. Alternatively the particle-laden macrophage may move through the interstitial space and either reenter the bronchioles or enter lymphatic capillaries. If the particle load is heavy and macrophage transport to the surface and alveolar pathways is overwhelmed, some particles may eventually reach the regional lymph nodes and, via the bloodstream, be carried elsewhere in the body.

Pneumonia can result whenever these defense mechanisms are impaired or whenever the resistance of the host in general is lowered. Factors that affect resistance in general include chronic diseases, immunologic deficiency, treatment with immunosuppressive agents, leukopenia, and unusually virulent infections. The clearing mechanisms can be interfered with by many factors, such as the following:

- *Loss or suppression of the cough reflex*, as a result of coma, anesthesia, neuromuscular disorders, drugs, or chest pain (this may lead to *aspiration* of gastric contents)

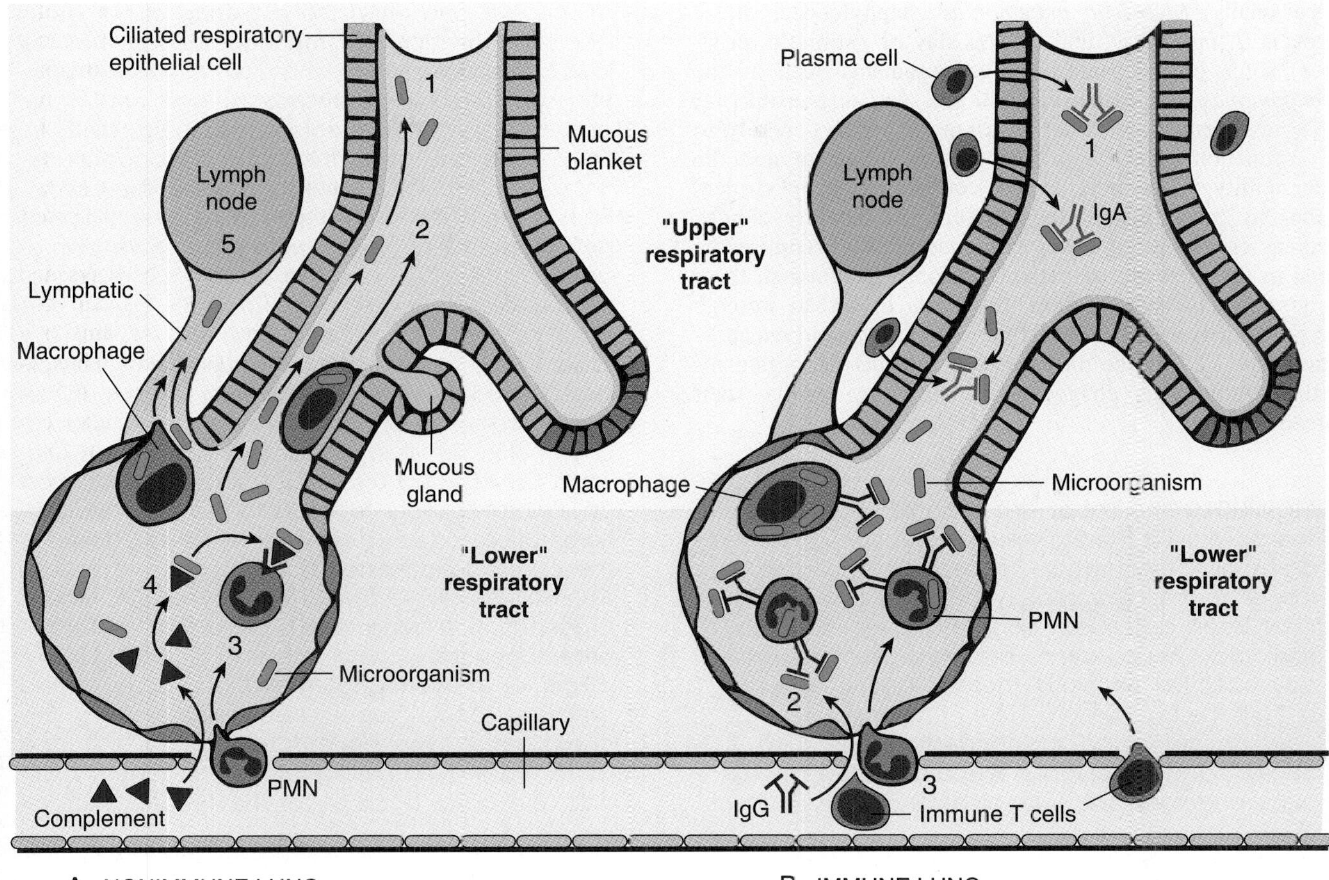

Figure 16–19

Lung defense mechanisms. *A*, In the nonimmune lung, removal of microbial organisms depends on ① entrapment in the mucous blanket (green) and removal via the mucociliary elevator, ② phagocytosis by alveolar macrophages that can kill and degrade organisms and remove them from the airspaces by migrating onto the mucociliary elevator, or ③ phagocytosis and killing by neutrophils recruited by macrophage factors. ④ Serum complement may enter the alveoli and be activated by the alternate pathway to provide the opsonin C3b that enhances phagocytosis. ⑤ Organisms, including those ingested by phagocytes, may reach the draining lymph nodes to initiate immune responses. *B*, Additional mechanisms operate in the immune lung. ① Secreted IgA can block attachment of the microorganism to epithelium in the upper respiratory tract. ② In the lower respiratory tract, serum antibodies (IgM, IgG) are present in the alveolar lining fluid. They activate complement more efficiently by the classic pathway, yielding C3b *(not shown)*. In addition, IgG is opsonic. ③ The accumulation of immune T cells is important for controlling infections by viruses and other intracellular microorganisms.

- *Injury to the mucociliary apparatus*, by either impairment of ciliary function or destruction of ciliated epithelium, owing to cigarette smoke, inhalation of hot or corrosive gases, viral diseases, or genetic disturbances (e.g., the immotile cilia syndrome)
- *Interference with the phagocytic or bactericidal action of alveolar macrophages*, by alcohol, tobacco smoke, anoxia, or oxygen intoxication
- *Pulmonary congestion and edema*
- *Accumulation of secretions* in conditions such as cystic fibrosis and bronchial obstruction

Several other points need to be emphasized. First, one type of pneumonia sometimes predisposes to another, especially in debilitated patients. For example, the most common cause of death in viral influenza epidemics is bacterial pneumonia. Second, although the portal of entry for most pneumonias is the respiratory tract, hematogenous spread from one focus to other foci can occur, and secondary seeding of the lungs may be difficult to distinguish from primary pneumonia. Finally, many patients with chronic diseases acquire terminal pneumonias while hospitalized (*nosocomial infection*). Bacteria common to the hospital environment may have acquired resistance to antibiotics; opportunities for spread are increased; invasive procedures, such as intubations and injections, are common; and bacteria may contaminate equipment used in respiratory care units.

Etiology. For bronchopneumonia, the common agents are staphylococci, streptococci, pneumococci, *Haemophilus influenzae*, *Pseudomonas aeruginosa*, and the coliform bacteria, although virtually any lung pathogen may also produce this pattern. In the case of lobar pneumonia, 90 to 95% are caused by pneumococci (*Streptococcus pneumoniae*). Most common are types 1, 3, 7, and 2. Type 3 causes a particularly virulent form of lobar pneumonia.

Occasionally, *Klebsiella pneumoniae*, staphylococci, streptococci, *H. influenzae*, and (in this day of antibiotic resistance) some of the gram-negative organisms such as the *Pseudomonas* and *Proteus* bacilli are also responsible for lobar involvement. A lobar distribution appears merely to be a function of the virulence of the organism and the vulnerability of the host. Heavy contamination by virulent pathogens may evoke this pattern in healthy adults, whereas organisms of lower virulence may accomplish the same in the predisposed patient. In lobar pneumonia, there is more extensive exudation that leads to spread through the pores of Kohn. Moreover, the copious mucoid encapsulation produced by the pneumococci protects the organisms against immediate phagocytosis and thus favors their spread.

MORPHOLOGY. Lobar pneumonia is a widespread fibrinosuppurative consolidation of large areas and even whole lobes of the lung. Four stages of the inflammatory response have classically been described: congestion, red hepatization, gray hepatization, and resolution. Present-day effective antibiotic therapy frequently slows or halts the progression.

In the first stage of **congestion,** the lung is heavy, boggy, and red. It is characterized by vascular engorgement, intra-alveolar fluid with few neutrophils, and often the presence of numerous bacteria. The stage of **red hepatization** that follows is characterized by massive confluent exudation with red cells (congestion) and neutrophils and fibrin filling the alveolar spaces (Fig. 16–20*A*). On gross examination, the lobe now appears distinctly red, firm, and airless with a liver-like consistency, hence the term **hepatization.** The stage of **gray hepatization** follows with progressive disintegration of red cells and the persistence of fibrinosuppurative exudate (Fig. 16–20*B*), giving the gross appearance of a grayish brown, dry surface. In the final stage of **resolution,** the consolidated exudate within the alveolar spaces undergoes progressive enzymatic digestion to produce a granular, semifluid debris that is resorbed (Fig. 16–20*C*), ingested by macrophages, or coughed up. Pleural fibrinous reaction to the underlying inflammation, often present in the early stages if the consolidation extends to the surface (**pleuritis**), may similarly resolve. More often, it undergoes organization, leaving fibrous thickening or permanent adhesions.

Foci of **bronchopneumonia** are consolidated areas of acute suppurative inflammation. The consolidation may be patchy through one lobe but is more often multilobar and frequently bilateral and basal because of the tendency of se-

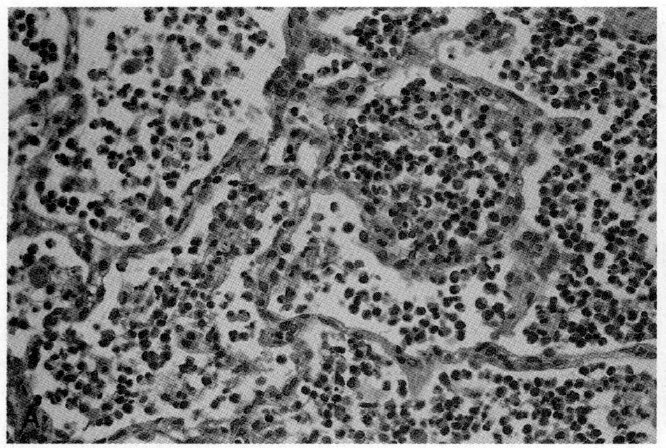

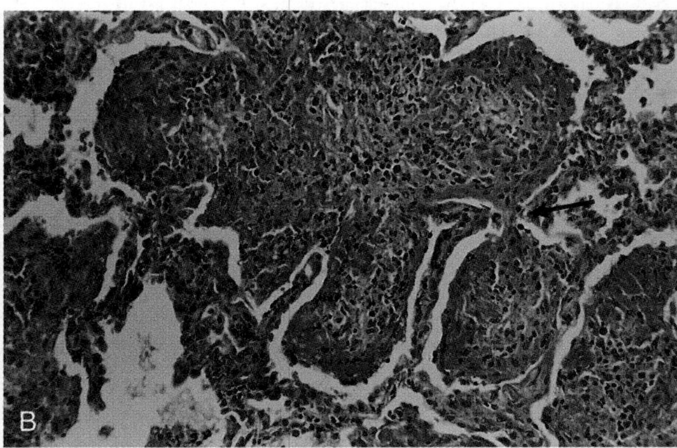

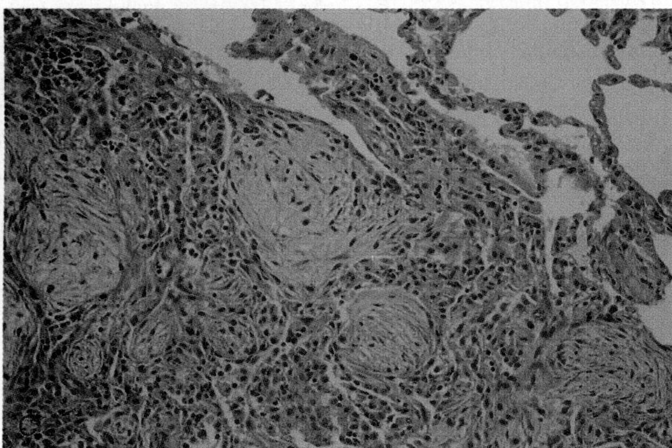

Figure 16–20

A, Acute pneumonia. The congested septal capillaries and extensive neutrophil exudation into alveoli corresponds to early red hepatization. Fibrin nets have not yet formed. *B*, Early organization of intra-alveolar exudate, seen in areas to be streaming through the pores of Kohn (*arrow*). *C*, Advanced organizing pneumonia (corresponding to gray hepatization), featuring transformation of exudates to fibromyxoid masses richly infiltrated by macrophages and fibroblasts.

cretions to gravitate into the lower lobes. Well-developed lesions are usually 3 to 4 cm in diameter, slightly elevated, dry, granular, gray-red to yellow, and poorly delimited at their margins (see Fig. 16–17). Histologically the reaction usually comprises a suppurative, neutrophil-rich exudate that fills the bronchi, bronchioles, and adjacent alveolar spaces (see Fig. 16–20*A*). Occasionally, consolidation of lung secondary to obstructive lesions (or, rarely, aspiration of mineral oils) causes a predominance of **lipid-laden foamy macrophages** and is designated **lipid pneumonia.**

Complications of pneumonia include (1) tissue destruction and necrosis, causing **abscess formation** (particularly common with type 3 pneumococci or *Klebsiella* infections); (2) spread of infection to the pleural cavity, causing the intrapleural fibrinosuppurative reaction known as **empyema;** (3) **organization** of the exudate, which may convert a portion of the lung into solid tissue (Fig. 16–20); and (4) **bacteremic dissemination** to the heart valves, pericardium, brain, kidneys, spleen, or joints, causing metastatic abscesses, endocarditis, meningitis, or suppurative arthritis.

Clinical Course. The major symptoms of pneumonia are malaise, fever, and cough productive of sputum. When fibrinosuppurative pleuritis is present, it is accompanied by pleuritic pain and pleural friction rub. The characteristic radiologic appearance of lobar pneumonia is that of a radiopaque, usually well-circumscribed lobe, whereas bronchopneumonia shows focal opacities.

The clinical picture is dramatically modified by the administration of antibiotics. Treated patients may be relatively afebrile with few clinical signs 48 to 72 hours after the initiation of antibiotics. The identification of the organism and the determination of its antibiotic sensitivity are the keystones to appropriate therapy. Fewer than 10% of patients with pneumonia severe enough to merit hospitalization now succumb, and in most such instances, death may be attributed either to a complication, such as empyema, meningitis, endocarditis, or pericarditis, or to some predisposing influence, such as debility or chronic alcoholism.

VIRAL AND MYCOPLASMAL PNEUMONIA (PRIMARY ATYPICAL PNEUMONIA)

The term *primary atypical pneumonia* was initially applied to an acute febrile respiratory disease characterized by patchy inflammatory changes in the lungs, largely confined to the alveolar septa and pulmonary interstitium. The term *atypical* denotes the lack of alveolar exudate, but a much more accurate designation is *interstitial pneumonitis.* The pneumonitis is caused by a variety of organisms, the most common being *Mycoplasma pneumoniae*. Other etiologic agents are viruses, including influenza virus types A and B, the respiratory syncytial viruses, adenovirus, rhinoviruses, rubeola, and varicella viruses; *Chlamydia* (psittacosis); and *Coxiella burnetti* (Q fever).[33] In some cases, the cause cannot be determined. Any one of these agents may cause merely an upper respiratory tract infection, recognized as the common cold, or a more severe lower respiratory tract infection. The circumstances that favor such extension of the infection are often mysterious but include malnutrition, alcoholism, and underlying debilitating illnesses.

MORPHOLOGY. All causal agents produce essentially similar morphologic patterns. The pneumonic involvement may be quite patchy or may involve whole lobes bilaterally or unilaterally. The affected areas are red-blue, congested, and subcrepitant. The pleura is smooth, and pleuritis or pleural effusions are infrequent.

The histologic pattern depends on the severity of the disease. **Predominant is the interstitial nature of the inflammatory reaction, virtually localized within the walls of the alveoli.** The alveolar septa are widened and edematous and usually have a mononuclear inflammatory infiltrate of lymphocytes, histiocytes, and occasionally plasma cells. In acute cases, neutrophils may also be present. The alveoli may be free from exudate, but in many patients there are intra-alveolar proteinaceous material, a cellular exudate, and characteristically pink hyaline membranes lining the alveolar walls, similar to those seen in hyaline membrane disease of infants. These changes reflect **alveolar damage** similar to that seen diffusely in ARDS (see Fig. 16–3). Subsidence of the disease is followed by reconstitution of the native architecture.

Superimposed bacterial infection modifies the histologic picture by causing ulcerative bronchitis and bronchiolitis and may yield the anatomic changes already described in the section on bacterial pneumonia. Some viruses, such as herpes simplex, varicella, and adenovirus, may be associated with necrosis of bronchial and alveolar epithelium and acute inflammation. Epithelial giant cells with intranuclear or intracytoplasmic inclusions may be present in cytomegalic inclusion disease. Other viruses produce cytopathic changes, as described in Chapter 9.

Clinical Course. The clinical course is extremely varied. Many cases masquerade as severe upper respiratory tract infections or as *chest colds.* Even patients with well-developed atypical pneumonia have few localizing symptoms. Cough may well be absent, and the major manifestations may consist only of fever, headache, muscle aches, and pains in the legs. The edema and exudation are both strategically located to cause an alveolocapillary block and thus evoke symptoms out of proportion to the scanty physical findings. One of the useful laboratory aids in differentiating viral atypical pneumonia from the *M. pneumoniae* form is detection of elevated cold agglutinin titers in the serum.

These are present in about half of patients with *Mycoplasma* and in 20% of adenovirus infections and are absent in other viral pneumonias.

The ordinary sporadic form of the disease is usually mild with a low mortality rate, below 1%. Interstitial pneumonia, however, may assume epidemic proportions with intensified severity and greater mortality, as documented in the highly fatal influenzal pandemics of 1915 and 1918 and the many smaller epidemics since then. Secondary bacterial infection by staphylococci or streptococci is common in such circumstances.

LUNG ABSCESS

The term pulmonary abscess describes a local suppurative process within the lung characterized by necrosis of lung tissue. Oropharyngeal surgical procedures, sinobronchial infections, dental sepsis, and bronchiectasis play important roles in their development.

Etiology and Pathogenesis. Although under appropriate circumstances any pathogen may produce an abscess, the commonly isolated organisms include aerobic and anaerobic streptococci, *Staphylococcus aureus*, and a host of gram-negative organisms. Mixed infections occur often because of the important causal role that inhalation of foreign material plays.[34] *Anaerobic organisms* normally found in the oral cavity, including members of the *Bacteroides*, *Fusobacterium*, and *Peptococcus* species, are the exclusive isolates in about 60% of cases. The causative organisms are introduced by the following mechanisms:

- *Aspiration of infective material* (the most frequent cause): This is particularly common in acute alcoholism, coma, anesthesia, sinusitis, gingivodental sepsis, and debilitation in which the cough reflexes are depressed. Aspiration of gastric contents is serious because the gastric acidity adds to the irritant role of the food particles, and in the course of aspiration mouth organisms are inevitably introduced.
- *Antecedent primary bacterial infection*: Postpneumonic abscess formations are usually associated with *S. aureus*, *K. pneumoniae*, and the type 3 pneumococcus. Fungal infections and bronchiectasis are additional antecedents to lung abscess formation. Post-transplant or otherwise immunosuppressed individuals are at special risk for this complication.
- *Septic embolism*: Infected emboli from thrombophlebitis in any portion of the systemic venous circulation or from the vegetations of infective bacterial endocarditis on the right side of the heart are trapped in the lung.
- *Neoplasia*: Secondary infection is particularly common in the bronchopulmonary segment obstructed by a primary or secondary malignancy (*postobstructive pneumonia*).
- *Miscellaneous*: Direct traumatic penetrations of the lungs; spread of infections from a neighboring organ, such as suppuration in the esophagus, spine, subphrenic space, or pleural cavity; and hematogenous seeding of the lung by pyogenic organisms all may lead to lung abscess formation.

When all these causes are excluded, there are still cases in which no reasonable basis for the abscess formation can be identified. These are referred to as *primary cryptogenic lung abscesses.*

MORPHOLOGY. Abscesses vary in diameter from lesions of a few millimeters to large cavities of 5 to 6 cm. They may affect any part of the lung and may be single or multiple. Pulmonary abscesses owing to aspiration are more common on the right (the more vertical main bronchus) and are most often single. Abscesses that develop in the course of pneumonia or bronchiectasis are usually multiple, basal, and diffusely scattered. Septic emboli and pyemic abscesses, by the haphazard nature of their genesis, are multiple and may affect any region of the lungs.

The cavity may or may not be filled with suppurative debris, depending on the presence or absence of a communication with one of the air passages. When such communications exist, the contained exudate may be partially drained to create an air-containing cavity. Superimposed saprophytic infections are prone to flourishing within the already necrotic debris of the abscess cavity. Continued infection leads to large, fetid, green-black, multilocular cavities with poor demarcation of their margins, designated **gangrene of the lung.** The **cardinal histologic change in all abscesses is suppurative destruction of the lung parenchyma within the central area of cavitation** (Fig. 16–21). In chronic cases, considerable fibroblastic proliferation produces a fibrous wall.

Clinical Course. The manifestations of pulmonary abscesses are much like those of bronchiectasis and are characterized principally by cough, fever, and copious amounts of foul-smelling purulent or sanguineous sputum. Fever, chest pain, and weight loss are common. Clubbing of the fingers and toes may appear within a few weeks after onset of an abscess. Diagnosis of this condition can be only suspected from the clinical findings and must be confirmed by roentgenography and bronchoscopy. Whenever an abscess is discovered, it is important to rule out an underlying carcinoma because this is present in 10 to 15% of cases.

The course of abscesses is variable. With antimicrobial therapy, most resolve with no major sequelae. Complications include extension of the infection into the pleural cavity, hemorrhage, the development of *brain abscesses* or *meningitis* from septic emboli, and (rarely) reactive secondary amyloidosis (type AA).

PULMONARY TUBERCULOSIS

A general discussion of tuberculosis appears in Chapter 9. Here we only briefly describe the effects of this infection on the lungs. As indicated earlier, the overwhelming

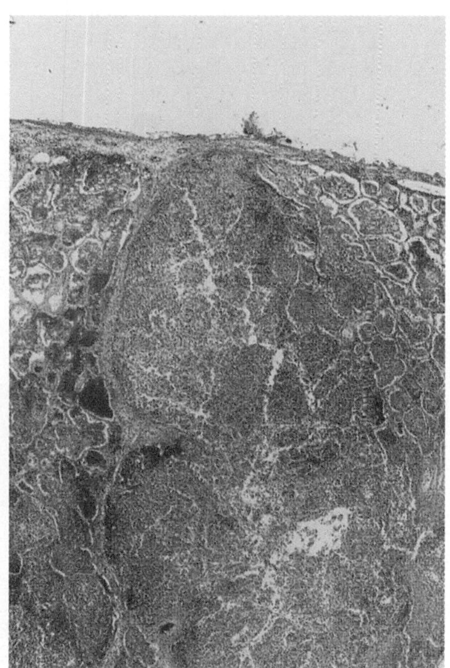

Figure 16–21 ■

Pyemic lung abscess in the center of section with complete destruction of underlying parenchyma within the focus of involvement.

preponderance of tuberculous infections affect the lungs and begin there. Pulmonary involvement is still the major cause of tuberculosis morbidity and mortality. The prevention and control of these pulmonary infections account for tuberculosis being a relatively uncommon cause of death today in the United States. The incidence of this infection in the United States began to increase again in the past decade, however, primarily reflecting infections in patients with acquired immunodeficiency syndrome (AIDS).[35] A further grim aspect of the resurgence of tuberculosis is the emergence of highly drug-resistant strains.[36] Moreover, in many parts of the world, underprivileged populations still suffer from death rates 20 times those of industrialized nations, and high-incidence pockets of infection are found among the poor in the most affluent countries.

Primary Pulmonary Tuberculosis

Except for the rare intestinal (bovine) tuberculosis and the even more uncommon skin, oropharyngeal, and lymphoidal primary sites, the lungs are the usual location of primary infections.[37] As detailed earlier (Chapter 9), the initial focus of primary infection is the *Ghon complex*, which consists of (1) a parenchymal subpleural lesion, often just above or just below the interlobar fissure between the upper and the lower lobes, and (2) enlarged caseous lymph nodes draining the parenchymal focus (Fig. 16–22).

The course and fate of this initial infection are variable, but in most cases patients are asymptomatic, and the lesions undergo fibrosis and calcification. Exceptionally, particularly in infants and children or immunodeficient adults, *progressive spread with cavitation, tuberculous pneumonia, or miliary tuberculosis* may follow a primary infection.

Secondary (Reactivation) Pulmonary Tuberculosis

Most cases of secondary pulmonary tuberculosis represent reactivation of an old, possibly subclinical infection. During primary infection, bacilli may disseminate, without producing symptoms, and establish themselves in sites with high oxygen tension, particularly the lung apices. Reactivation in such sites occurs in no more than 5 to 10% of the cases of primary infection. Secondary tuberculosis, however, tends to produce more damage to the lungs than does primary tuberculosis.

MORPHOLOGY. The **secondary pulmonary tuberculous lesion** is located in the apex of one or both lungs (Fig. 16–23). It begins as a **small focus of consolidation, usually less than 3 cm in diameter.** Less commonly, initial lesions may be located in other regions of the lung, particularly about the hilus. In almost every case of reinfection, the regional nodes develop foci of similar tuberculous activity. In the favorable case, the initial paren-

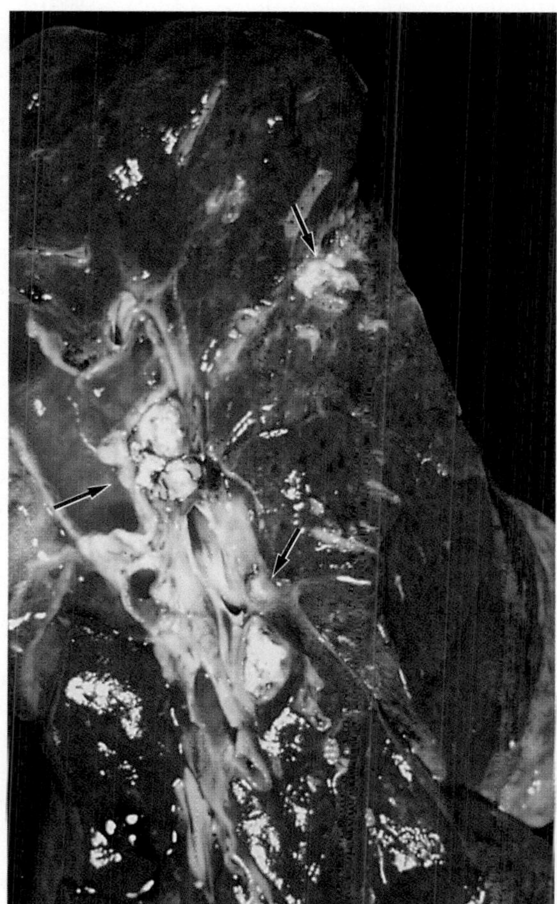

Figure 16–22 ■

Primary pulmonary tuberculosis, Ghon complex. The gray-white parenchymal focus is under the pleura in the lower part of the upper lobe *(topmost arrow)*. Hilar lymph nodes with caseation are seen *(lowermost arrows)*.

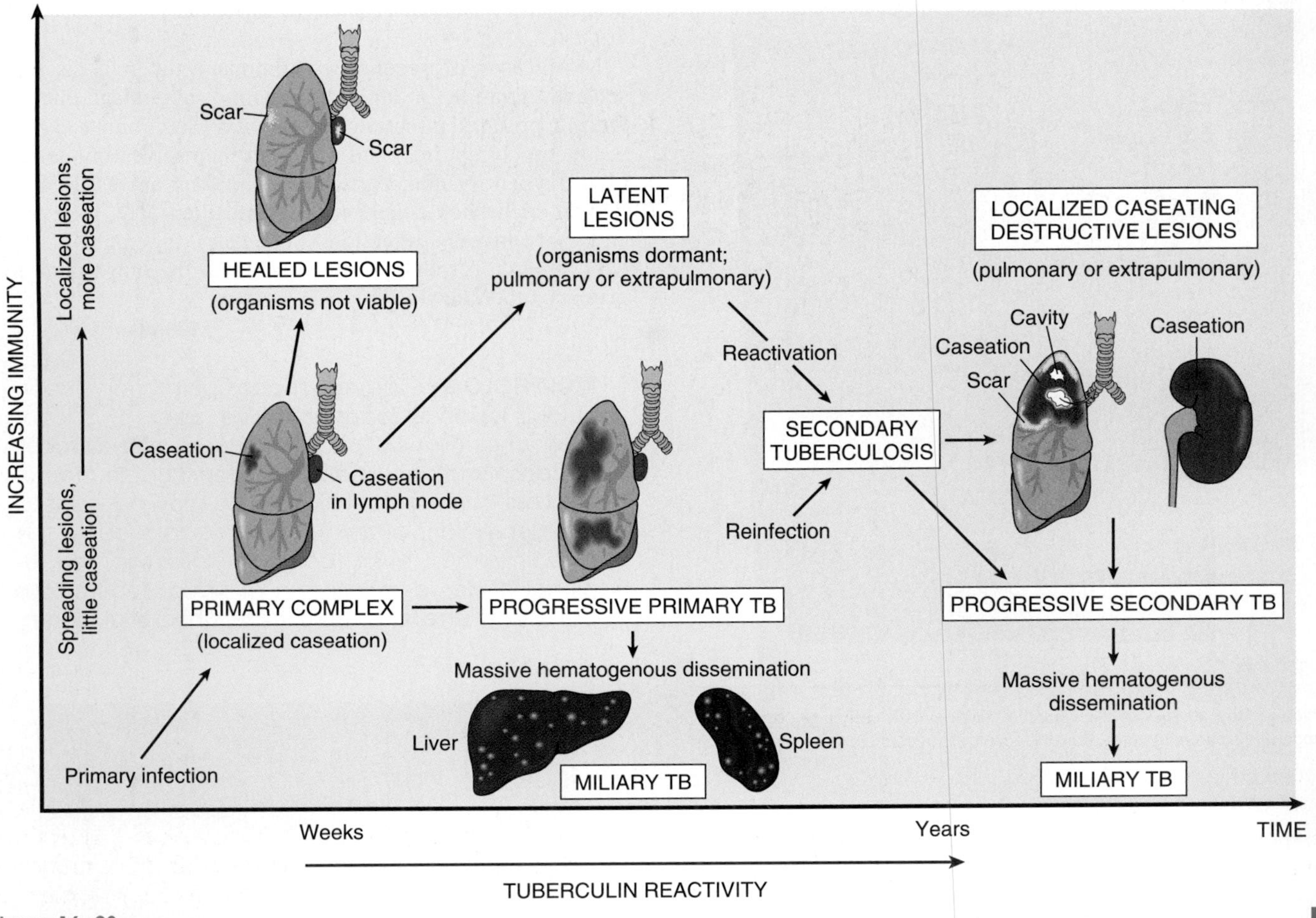

Figure 16–23

Natural history and spectrum of tuberculosis (TB). (Adapted from a sketch provided by Dr. R. K. Kumar, The University of New South Wales, School of Pathology, Sydney, Australia.)

chymal focus develops a small area of caseation necrosis that does not cavitate because it fails to communicate with a bronchus or bronchiole. The usual course is one of progressive fibrous encapsulation, leaving only fibrocalcific scars that depress and pucker the pleural surface and cause focal pleural adhesions. Sometimes, these fibrocalcific scars become secondarily blackened by anthracotic pigment.

Histologically, **coalescent granulomas are present, composed of epithelioid cells surrounded by a zone of fibroblasts and lymphocytes that usually contains Langhans giant cells. Some necrosis (caseation) is usually present in the centers of these tubercles,** the amount being entirely dependent on the sensitization of the patient and the virulence of the organisms (Fig. 16–24).

As the lesions progress, more tubercles coalesce to create a confluent area of consolidation. In the favorable case, either the entire area is eventually converted to a fibrocalcific scar, or the residual caseous debris becomes totally and heavily walled off by hyaline collagenous connective tissue. In these late lesions, the multinucleate giant cells tend to disappear.

In cases of suspected tuberculous tissue changes, the diagnosis is confirmed by histologic staining, smears, and cultures of acid-fast organisms. Tubercle bacilli can be demonstrated in the early exudative and caseous phases, but it is usually impossible to find them in the late fibrocalcific stages. Lesions with sparse organisms can be highly infective; one can estimate that finding a single acid-fast bacillus in a routine histologic sample from a 1-cm^3 granuloma indicates that a total of at least 2000 organisms are present within the granuloma. Hence, it cannot be assumed that their absence in histologic sections is tantamount to their total destruction because in many of these instances culture of the lesions or inoculation of this material into guinea pigs yields the organisms.

The subsequent course of the secondary lesions is variable. They either may heal spontaneously or with therapy, resulting in a fibrocalcific nodule, or may progress along the many pathways, discussed next.

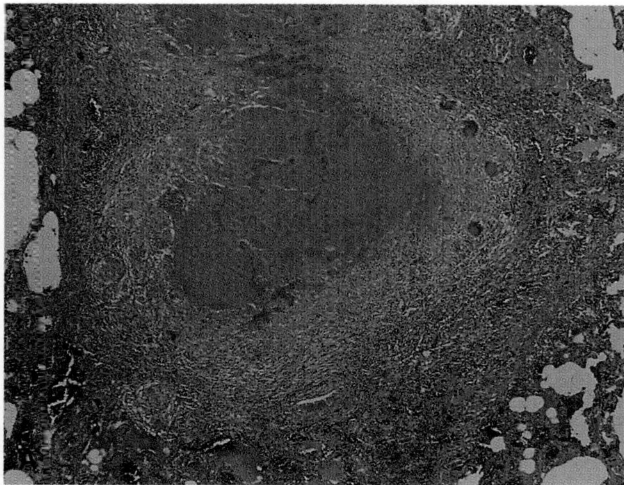

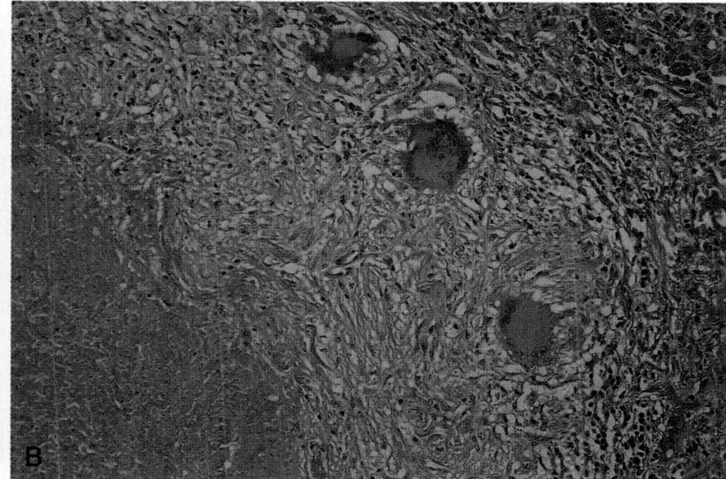

Figure 16–24

Characteristic tubercle at low magnification (*A*) and in detail (*B*), to illustrate central granular caseation and epithelioid and multinucleated giant cells.

Progressive Pulmonary Tuberculosis

A variable number of active lesions continue to progress over a period of months or years, causing further pulmonary and even distant organ involvement. The resultant clinicopathologic consequences include cavitary fibrocaseous tuberculosis (apical and advanced), miliary tuberculosis, and tuberculous bronchopneumonia (see Fig. 16–23).

CAVITARY FIBROCASEOUS TUBERCULOSIS. The name fairly well describes this stage of disease. By erosion into a bronchiole, drainage of the caseous focus transforms it into a cavity. Growth and multiplication of the tubercle bacilli under these conditions are favored by the increased oxygen tension.

In most cases, the cavity remains localized to the apex (apical cavitary fibrocaseous tuberculosis). The cavity is lined by a yellow-gray caseous material and is more or less walled off by fibrous tissue. Not uncommonly, thrombosed arteries may traverse these cavities to produce apparent fibrous bridging bands. When such cavitation occurs in the apices, the pathways for further dissemination of the tuberculous infection are prepared. The infective material may now disseminate through the airways to other sites in the lung or upper respiratory tract. Spread may also occur to the lymph nodes via the lymphatics, then retrogressively through other lymphatics to other areas of the lung or other organs. Miliary dissemination through the blood is a further hazard. Cavitary fibrocaseous tuberculosis may affect one, many, or all lobes of both lungs in the form of isolated minute tubercles, confluent caseous foci, or large areas of caseation necrosis (**advanced fibrocaseous tuberculosis**).

In the progress of this disease, the pleura is inevitably involved, and, depending on the chronicity of the disease, serous pleural effusions, frank tuberculous empyema, or massive obliterative fibrous pleuritis may be found. In the course of extensive fibrocaseous tuberculosis, it is almost inevitable that tubercle bacilli become implanted on the mucosal linings of the air passages to produce **endobronchial and endotracheal tuberculosis**. These lesions may later become ulcerated and produce irregular, ragged, necrotic, mucosal ulcers. Accompanying the endobronchial tuberculosis, **laryngeal seeding and intestinal tuberculosis** may occur. Fortunately, these complications of tuberculosis are now uncommon.

MILIARY TUBERCULOSIS. Lymphohematogenous dissemination may give rise to miliary tuberculosis, confined only to the lungs or involving other organs also. The distribution of miliary lesions depends on the pathways of dissemination. Tuberculous infection may drain via the lymphatics through the major lymphatic ducts into the right side of the heart, then spread into a diffuse, blood-borne pattern throughout the lungs **alone**. Despite their small size, most of the bacilli are usually filtered out by the alveolar capillary bed. Therefore, the infective material may not reach the arterial systemic circulation. Such limitation to the lungs usually is not complete, however, and some bacilli pass through the capillaries or through lymphatic-vascular anastomoses to enter the systemic circulation and produce distant organ seedings. Favored targets for miliary seeding are the bone marrow, liver, spleen, and retina, providing sites for biopsy or direct visualization of disease (retina). Occasionally, isolated organ involvement is found (e.g., kidneys, adrenals, testes).

In the miliary type of distribution, individual le-

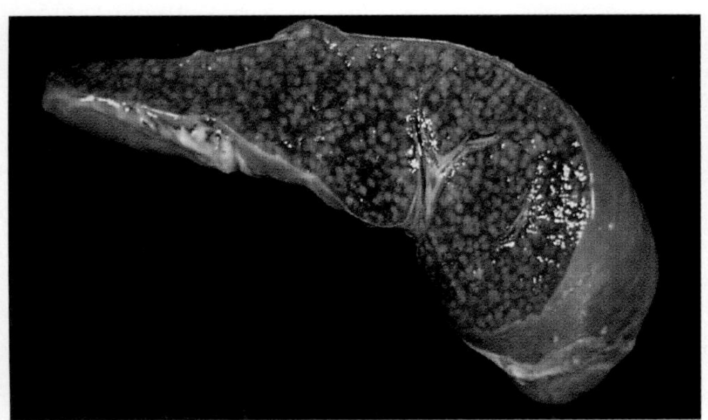

Figure 16–25

Miliary tuberculosis of the spleen. The cut surface shows numerous gray-white granulomas.

sions vary from one to several millimeters in diameter and are distinct, yellow-white, firm areas of consolidation that usually do not have grossly visible central caseation necrosis or cavitation at the time of examination (Fig. 16–25). Histologically, however, these present the characteristic pattern of individual or multiple confluent tubercles having microscopic central caseation.

TUBERCULOUS BRONCHOPNEUMONIA. In the highly susceptible, highly sensitized individual, the tuberculous infection may spread rapidly throughout large areas of lung parenchyma and produce a diffuse bronchopneumonia, or lobar exudative consolidation, at one time descriptively referred to as "galloping consumption." Sometimes, with such overwhelming disease, well-developed tubercles do not form, and it may be difficult to establish on histologic grounds the tuberculous nature of the pneumonic process. Numerous bacilli, however, are usually present in such exudates.

Clinical Course. The clinical course of pulmonary tuberculosis is extremely variable and depends entirely on the activity, extent, and pattern of distribution of the tuberculous pulmonary infection (Chapter 9). The great majority of cases respond to present-day chemotherapeutic measures unless the disease is advanced, the organisms are resistant to conventional therapies, or intercurrent problems such as diabetes mellitus, AIDS, or reactive amyloidosis complicate the outlook.

PNEUMONIA IN THE IMMUNOCOMPROMISED HOST

The appearance of a pulmonary infiltrate and signs of infection (e.g., fever) is one of the most common and serious complications in patients whose immune and defense systems are suppressed by disease, immunosuppression for organ transplants and tumors, or irradiation.[38] A wide variety of so-called opportunistic infectious agents, many of which rarely cause infection in normal hosts, can cause these pneumonias, and often more than one agent is involved. Mortality from these opportunistic infections is high. In the case of AIDS, nearly 100% of patients suffer from an opportunistic infection, most commonly caused by *P. carinii*.[39] Table 16–5 lists some of the opportunistic agents according to their prevalence and to whether they cause local or diffuse pulmonary infiltrates. Such infiltrates may also be due to drug reactions or to involvement of the lung by tumor. The specific infections are discussed in Chapter 9.

Diffuse Interstitial (Infiltrative, Restrictive) Diseases

Diffuse interstitial diseases are a heterogeneous group of diseases characterized predominantly by diffuse and usually chronic involvement of the pulmonary connective tissue, principally the most peripheral and delicate interstitium in the alveolar walls. The interstitium consists of the basement membrane of the endothelial and epithelial cells (fused in the thinnest portions), collagen fibers, elastic tissue, proteoglycans, fibroblasts, mast cells, and occasionally lymphocytes and monocytes.

There is no uniformity regarding terminology and classification of these disorders. Many of the entities are of unknown cause and pathogenesis, some have an intra-alveolar as well as an interstitial component, and there is frequent overlap in histologic features among the different conditions. Nevertheless, their similar clinical signs, symptoms, radiologic alterations, and pathophysiologic changes justify their consideration as a group. These disorders account for about 15% of noninfectious diseases seen by pulmonary physicians.

In general, the clinical and pulmonary functional changes are those of *restrictive rather than obstructive lung disease* (see the previous section on obstructive versus restrictive pulmonary disease). Patients have dyspnea, tachypnea, and

Table 16–5. CAUSES OF PULMONARY INFILTRATES IN IMMUNOCOMPROMISED HOSTS

Diffuse Infiltrate	Focal Infiltrate
Common	***Common***
Cytomegalovirus	Gram-negative rods
Pneumocystis carinii	*Staphylococcus aureus*
Drug reaction	*Aspergillus*
	Candida
	Malignancy
Uncommon	***Uncommon***
Bacteria	*Cryptococcus*
Aspergillus	*Mucor*
Cryptococcus	*Pneumocystis carinii*
Malignancy	*Legionella pneumophila*

eventual cyanosis, without wheezing or other evidence of airway obstruction. The classic physiologic features are reductions in oxygen-diffusing capacity, lung volumes, and compliance. *Chest radiographs show diffuse infiltration by small nodules, irregular lines, or ground-glass shadows*, hence the term *infiltrative*. Eventually, secondary pulmonary hypertension and right-sided heart failure with cor pulmonale may result. Although the entities can often be distinguished in the early stages, the advanced forms are hard to differentiate because they result in scarring and gross destruction of the lung, often referred to as *end-stage lung* or *honeycomb lung*.

Diffuse infiltrative diseases are categorized into those with known causes and those of unknown cause (Table 16–6), some of which can be defined either as clinicopathologic syndromes or as having characteristic histology.[40] Many of these entities are discussed in other sections of this book. Here we briefly review current concepts of pathogenesis that may be common to all and discuss those in which lung involvement is the primary or a major problem. In terms of frequency, the most common associations are environmental diseases (approximately 25%), sarcoidosis (approximately 20%), idiopathic pulmonary fibrosis (approximately 15%), and the collagen vascular diseases (approximately 10%). The remainder have more than 100 different causes and associations.

Pathogenesis. It is now thought that regardless of the type of interstitial disease or specific cause, the earliest common manifestation of most of the interstitial diseases is *alveolitis*,[41, 42] that is, an accumulation of inflammatory and immune effector cells within the alveolar walls and spaces (Fig. 16–26). Under normal conditions, these cells account for no more than 7% of the total lung cell population and consist of macrophages (93%), lymphocytes (7%), and neutrophils and eosinophils (<1%). In alveolitis, there is a marked increase in the number of these cells and a change in their relative proportions. The accumulation of leukocytes has two consequences: It distorts the normal alveolar structures and results in the release of mediators that can injure parenchymal cells and stimulate fibrosis. The final result is an end-stage fibrotic lung in which the alveoli are replaced by cystic spaces separated by thick bands of connective tissue interspersed with inflammatory cells.

The initial stimuli for alveolitis are as heterogeneous as the causes outlined in Table 16–6. Some of these stimuli, such as oxygen-derived free radicals and some chemicals, are directly toxic to endothelial cells, epithelial cells, or both. Beyond direct toxicity, a critical event is the *recruitment and activation of inflammatory and immune effector cells*. Neutrophil recruitment can be caused by complement activation in some disorders,[43] but in addition the alveolar macrophages, which increase in number in all interstitial diseases, release *chemotactic factors* for neutrophils (e.g., IL-8,[44] leukotriene B_4[45]). Some chemotactic agents also *activate* the neutrophils, causing them to secrete proteases and toxic oxygen free radicals, which contribute further to tissue damage and provide a mechanism for maintenance of the alveolitis. In diseases such as sarcoidosis, *cell-mediated immune reactions* result in the accumulation of monocytes and T lymphocytes and in the formation of granulomas (Chapter 7). It is thought that interactions among lymphocytes and macrophages and the release of lymphokines and monokines are responsible for the slowly progressive pulmonary fibrosis that ensues. The alveolar macrophage, in particular, plays a central role in the development of fibrosis, as reviewed in the discussion of chronic inflammation (Chapter 3).

Table 16–6. MAJOR CATEGORIES OF CHRONIC INTERSTITIAL LUNG DISEASE WITH SELECTED EXAMPLES

Known Etiology	Unknown Etiology
Lung Response: Alveolitis, Interstitial Inflammation, and Diffuse Fibrosis	
Environmental agents*	Collagen vascular diseases*
Asbestos, silica, fumes, gases	Scleroderma, rheumatoid arthritis, systemic lupus erythematosus, dermatomyositis, mixed connective tissue disease
Ionizing radiation	Idiopathic pulmonary fibrosis*
Following ARDS	Goodpasture syndrome
Drugs: busulfan, bleomycin	Idiopathic pulmonary hemosiderosis
Lung Response: As Above but With Granulomas	
Berylliosis	Sarcoidosis*
Hypersensitivity pneumonitis	Wegener granulomatosis

* Most common causes.
ARDS, adult respiratory distress syndrome.
Adapted from Reynolds HY: Interstitial lung diseases. In Isselbacher KJ, et al (eds): Harrison's Principles of Internal Medicine, 13th ed. New York, McGraw-Hill, 1994, p 1206.

PNEUMOCONIOSES

The term *pneumoconiosis* was originally coined to describe the non-neoplastic lung reaction to inhalation of mineral dusts (e.g., coal dust *anthracosis*, silica *silicosis*, asbestos *asbestosis*, and beryllium *berylliosis*) commonly encountered in the workplace. Less common mineral dust pneumoconioses include siderosis (iron dust), stannosis (tin dust), and baritosis (barium dust). The use of the term *pneumoconiosis* has been broadened to include diseases induced by organic as well as inorganic particulates and chemical fumes and vapors. A simplified classification is presented in Table 16–7. For all pneumoconioses, regulations limiting worker exposure have resulted in a decreased incidence of dust-associated diseases.

Although the pneumoconioses result from well-defined occupational exposure to specific airborne agents, there are also deleterious effects of particulate air pollution for the general population, especially in urban areas. Studies have found increased morbidity (e.g., asthma incidence) and mortality rates in populations exposed to increased ambient air particulate levels,[46, 47] leading to calls for greater efforts to reduce the levels of particulates in urban air.

General Pathogenesis. The specific changes caused by the more important dusts are presented in succeeding sections; however, certain pathogenetic principles apply to all. The development of a pneumoconiosis depends on (1) the

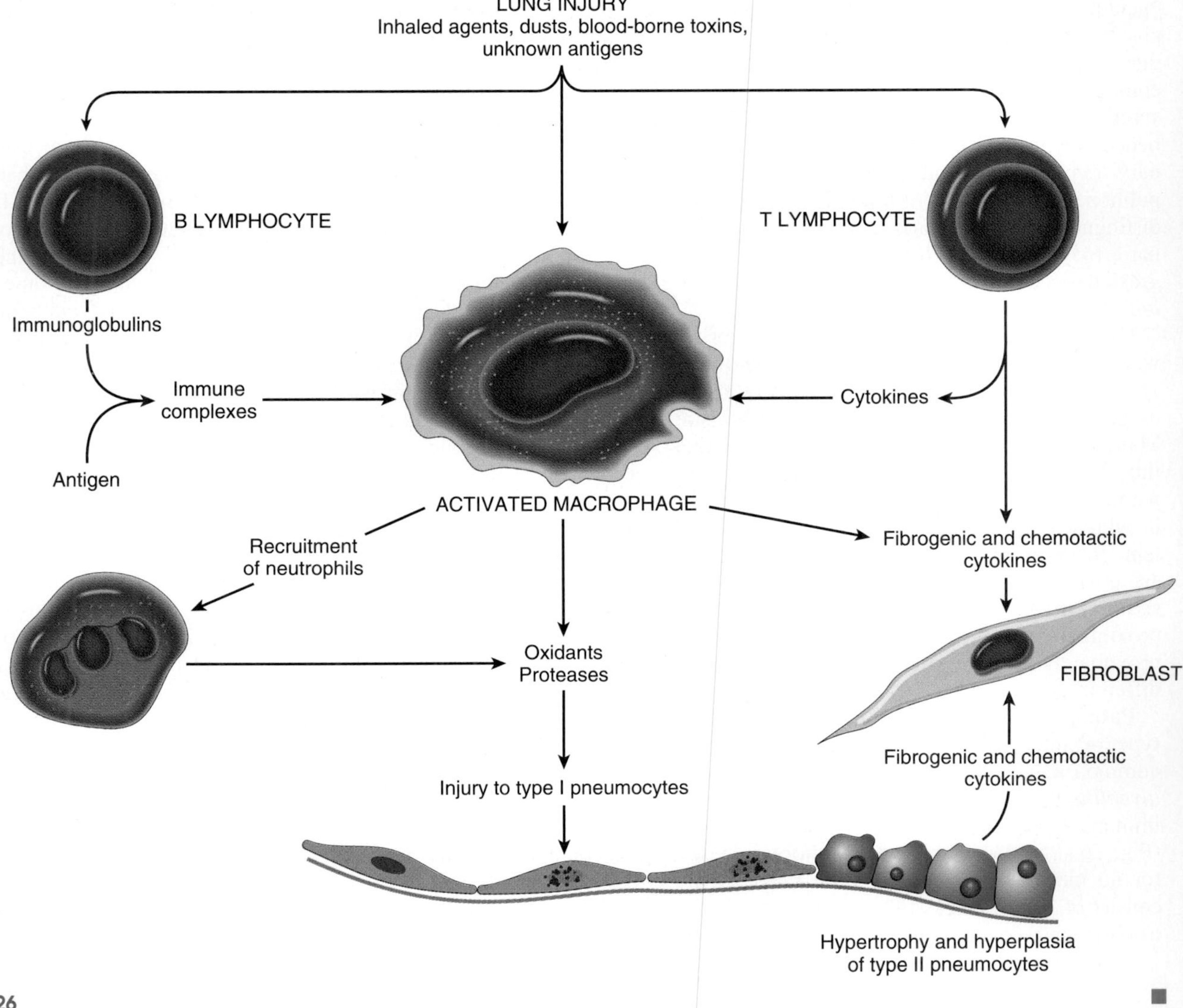

Figure 16–26

A possible schema of the pathogenesis of idiopathic pulmonary fibrosis.

amount of dust retained in the lung and airways; (2) the size, shape, and therefore buoyancy of the particles; (3) particle solubility and physiochemical reactivity; and (4) the possible additional effects of other irritants (e.g., concomitant tobacco smoking).

The amount of dust retained in the lungs is determined by the dust concentration in the ambient air, the duration of the exposure, and the effectiveness of clearance mechanisms. Recall (from the discussion of bacterial pneumonia in this chapter) that (1) any influence, such as cigarette smoking, that affects the integrity of the mucociliary apparatus significantly predisposes to the accumulation of dust, and (2) *the most dangerous particles range from 1 to 5 mm in diameter because they may reach the terminal small airways and air sacs and settle in their linings*. Under normal conditions, there is always a small pool of intra-alveolar macrophages that is expanded by recruitment of more macrophages when dust reaches the alveolar spaces. The protection provided by phagocytosis of particles, however, can be overwhelmed by the large dust burden deposited in occupational exposures and by specific chemical interactions of the particles with cells.

The *solubility and cytotoxicity of particles*, influenced to a considerable extent by their size, modify the nature of the pulmonary response. In general, the smaller the particle, the higher the surface area-to-mass ratio, and the more likely and more rapidly toxic levels will appear in the pulmonary fluids, depending, of course, on the solubility of the agent. Larger particles resist dissolution and so may persist within the lung parenchyma for years. These tend to evoke fibrosing collagenous pneumoconioses, such as is characteristic of silicosis. The reaction to crystalline silica illustrates how the *physiochemical reactivity* of particles contributes to pathogenesis. Quartz (a form of crystalline

Table 16–7. AIR POLLUTANT LUNG DISEASES

Agent	Disease	Exposure
Mineral Dusts		
Coal dust	Anthracosis Macules Progressive massive fibrosis Caplan syndrome	Coal mining (particularly hard coal)
Silica	Silicosis Caplan syndrome	Foundry work, sandblasting, hardrock mining, stone cutting, others
Asbestos	Asbestosis Pleural plaques Caplan syndrome Mesothelioma Carcinoma of the lung, larynx, stomach, colon	Mining, milling, and fabrication; installation and removal of insulation
Beryllium	Acute berylliosis Beryllium granulomatosis Bronchogenic carcinoma (?)	Mining, fabrication
Iron oxide	Siderosis	Welding
Barium sulfate	Baritosis	Mining
Tin oxide	Stannosis	Mining
Organic Dusts That Induce Hypersensitivity Pneumonitis		
Moldy hay Bagasse Bird droppings	Farmer's lung Bagassosis Bird-breeder's lung	Farming Manufacturing wallboard, paper Bird handling
Organic Dusts That Induce Asthma		
Cotton, flax, hemp Red cedar dust	Byssinosis Asthma	Textile manufacturing Lumbering, carpentry
Chemical Fumes and Vapors		
Nitrous oxide, sulfur dioxide, ammonia, benzene, insecticides	Bronchitis, asthma Pulmonary edema ARDS Mucosal injury Fulminant poisoning	Occupational and accidental exposure

silica) can cause direct injury to tissue and cell membranes by interaction with free radicals and other chemical groups on the particle surface. The resulting membrane damage may ultimately cause cell death. Of more importance, however, is the ability of silica to trigger macrophages to release a number of products that mediate an inflammatory response and initiate fibroblast proliferation and collagen deposition.[48, 49] Proinflammatory and fibrosing mediators are also critical in the pathogenesis of the pulmonary reaction to asbestos.[50] Many of the same mediators and cytokines discussed earlier in the pathogenesis of diffuse interstitial fibrosis are likely to play a role in the pathogenic response to inhaled particulates (details later).

Some of the particles may be taken up by epithelial cells or may cross the epithelial cell lining and interact directly with fibroblasts and interstitial macrophages. Some may reach the lymphatics either by direct drainage or within migrating macrophages and thereby initiate an immune response to components of the particulates or to self-proteins (or both), modified by the particles. This response leads to an amplification and extension of the local reaction. Although tobacco smoking worsens the effects of all inhaled mineral dusts, the effects of asbestos are particularly magnified by smoking.

Coal Workers' Pneumoconiosis—Simple and Complicated (Progressive Massive Fibrosis)

Coal, a form of combustible carbon, has long been mined for fuel. The spectrum of lung findings in coal workers is wide, varying from (1) asymptomatic anthracosis, in which pigment accumulates without a perceptible cellular reaction; to (2) simple coal workers' pneumoconiosis (CWP), in which accumulations of macrophages occur with little to no pulmonary dysfunction; to (3) complicated CWP, or progressive massive fibrosis (PMF), in which fibrosis is extensive and lung function is compromised.[51] Dust reduction measures in the coal mines around the globe have drastically reduced the incidence of coal dust–induced disease. Although statistics vary, it appears that fewer than 10% of cases of simple CWP progress to PMF. *PMF is a generic term that applies to a confluent, fibrosing reaction in the lung that can be a complication of any pneumoconiosis, although it is most common in CWP and silicosis.*

The pathogenesis of complicated CWP, and particularly what causes the lesions of simple CWP to progress to PMF, is incompletely understood. Contaminating silica in the coal dust can favor progressive disease. Evidence suggests, however, that in most cases carbon dust itself is the major culprit, and studies have shown that complicated lesions contain considerably more dust than simple lesions.

MORPHOLOGY. Anthracosis is the most innocuous coal-induced pulmonary lesion in coal miners and is also commonly seen in all urban dwellers and tobacco smokers. Inhaled carbon pigment is engulfed by alveolar or interstitial macrophages, which then accumulate in the connective tissue along the lymphatics, including the pleural lymphatics, or in organized lymphoid tissue along the bronchi or in the lung hilus. At autopsy, linear streaks and aggregates of anthracotic pigment readily identify pulmonary lymphatics and mark the pulmonary lymph nodes.

Simple CWP is characterized by **coal macules** (1 to 2 mm in diameter) and the somewhat larger **coal nodules.** The coal macule consists of carbon-laden macrophages; the nodule also contains small amounts of a delicate network of collagen fibers. Although these lesions are scattered throughout the lung, the upper lobes and upper zones of the lower lobes are more heavily involved. They are located primarily adjacent to respiratory bronchioles, the site of initial dust accumulation. In due course, dilation of adjacent alveoli occurs, a condition sometimes referred to as **centrilobular emphysema.** By definition, emphysema is associated with destruction of alveolar septa, and whether this occurs in primary CWP is not yet certain.

Complicated CWP (PMF) occurs on a background of simple CWP and generally requires many years to develop. It is characterized by intensely blackened scars larger than 2 cm, sometimes up to 10 cm in greatest diameter. They are usually multiple (Fig. 16–27). Microscopically the lesions consist of dense collagen and pigment. The center of the lesion is often necrotic, resulting most likely from local ischemia.

Caplan syndrome is defined as the coexistence of rheumatoid arthritis with a pneumoconiosis, leading to the development of distinctive nodular pulmonary lesions that develop fairly rapidly. Similar to rheumatoid nodules (Chapter 12), the nodular lesions in Caplan syndrome have central necrosis surrounded by fibroblasts, macrophages, and collagen. This syndrome can also occur in asbestosis and silicosis.

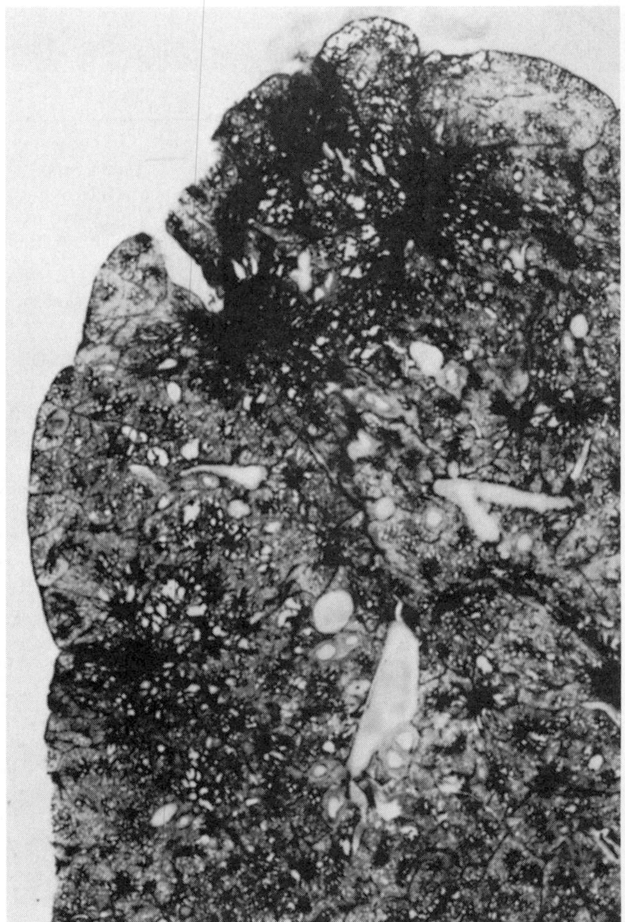

Figure 16–27

Progressive massive fibrosis superimposed on coal workers' pneumoconiosis. The large, blackened scars are located principally in the upper lobe. Note the extensions of scars into surrounding parenchyma and retraction of adjacent pleura. (Courtesy of Dr. Werner Laquer, Dr. Jerome Kleinerman, and the National Institute of Occupational Safety and Health, Morgantown, WV.)

Clinical Course. CWP is usually a benign disease that causes little decrement in lung function. Even mild forms of complicated CWP fail to demonstrate abnormalities of lung function. In a minority of cases, however, PMF develops, leading to increasing pulmonary dysfunction, pulmonary hypertension, and cor pulmonale. Once PMF develops, it may become progressive even if further exposure to dust is prevented. The incidence of clinical tuberculosis is increased in persons with CWP, but whether this reflects a greater vulnerability to infection or, instead, socioeconomic factors inherent in the life of miners is unclear. There is also some evidence that exposure to coal dust increases the incidence of chronic bronchitis and emphysema, independent of smoking, thus complicating the management of the patient with CWP. To date, however, there is no compelling evidence that CWP in the absence of smoking predisposes to cancer.

Silicosis

Silicosis is a lung disease caused by inhalation of crystalline silicon dioxide (silica).[52] *Currently the most preva-*

lent chronic occupational disease in the world, silicosis usually presents, after decades of exposure, as a slowly progressing, nodular, fibrosing pneumoconiosis. As shown in Table 16–7, workers in a large number of occupations are at risk, especially sandblasters and many mine workers. Less commonly, heavy exposure over months to a few years can result in acute silicosis, a lesion characterized by the generalized accumulation of a lipoproteinaceous material within alveoli (identical morphologically to alveolar proteinosis).

Pathogenesis. Silica occurs in both crystalline and amorphous forms, but crystalline forms (including quartz, crystobalite, and tridymite) are much more fibrogenic, revealing the importance of the physical form and surface properties in pathogenesis. Of these, quartz is most commonly implicated in silicosis. After inhalation, the particles interact with epithelial cells and macrophages to initiate injury and cause fibrosis. The mechanisms of tissue and cell injury by crystalline silica are thought to be based on the chemical reactivity of the particle surface. SiOH groups on the surface form bonds (hydrogen and electrostatic) with membrane proteins and phospholipids, which leads to denaturation of membrane proteins and damage to the lipid membranes. In addition, surface free radicals (which decay as a result of vigorous reactivity, with a half-life of 30 hours) are generated during the cleavage of silica (as occurs during crushing of stone in mining). This initially high surface chemical reactivity makes freshly ground silica substantially more cytotoxic in vitro than its aged counterpart.

Although lung macrophages that ingest the silica particles may ultimately succumb to the toxic effects described earlier, silica causes activation and release of mediators by viable macrophages. Mediators identified include IL-1, TNF, fibronectin, lipid mediators, oxygen-derived free radicals, and fibrogenic cytokines.[53] Especially compelling is evidence that anti-TNF monoclonal antibodies can block lung collagen accumulation in mice given silica intratracheally.[54] Animals exposed to silica demonstrate a steady recruitment of macrophages and lymphocytes to the alveolus and interstitium. These cells may further amplify the process.

As with CWP (discussed earlier), the initial lesions tend to localize in the upper lung zones, although the reasons for this distribution are obscure. In contrast with CWP, however, early lesions of silicosis are more fibrotic and less cellular. An interesting, perhaps related phenomenon is that quartz, when mixed with other minerals, has a reduced fibrogenic effect. This phenomenon is of practical importance because quartz in the workplace is rarely pure. Thus, miners of the iron-containing ore hematite may have more quartz in their lungs than some quartz-exposed workers and yet have relatively mild lung disease because the hematite provides a protective effect. This situation may reflect interaction of the other minerals with charged groups on the silica crystalline surface, dampening this component of the toxic interaction of silica and cell membranes. In the earth, much of the silicon combines with oxygen and other elements to form silicates. Although amorphous silicates are biologically less active than crystalline silica, heavy lung burdens of these minerals may also produce lesions. Talc, vermiculite, and mica are examples of noncrystalline silicates that are less common causes of pneumoconioses.

MORPHOLOGY. Silicosis is characterized grossly in its early stages by tiny, barely palpable, discrete pale to blackened (if coal dust is also present) nodules in the upper zones of the lungs. As the disease progresses, these nodules may coalesce into **hard collagenous scars** (Fig. 16–28). Some nodules may undergo central softening and cavitation. This change may be due to superimposed tuberculosis or to ischemia. The intervening lung parenchyma may be compressed or overexpanded, and a honeycomb pattern may develop. Fibrotic lesions may also occur in the hilar lymph nodes and pleura. Sometimes, thin sheets of calcification occur in the lymph nodes and are appreciated radiographically as **eggshell** calcification (i.e., calcium surrounding a zone lacking calcification). If the disease continues to progress, expansion and coalescence of lesions produce PMF. Histologically the nodular lesions consist of concentric layers of hyalinized collagen surrounded by a dense capsule of more condensed collagen (Fig. 16–29). Examination of the nodules by polarized microscopy reveals the birefringent silica particles.

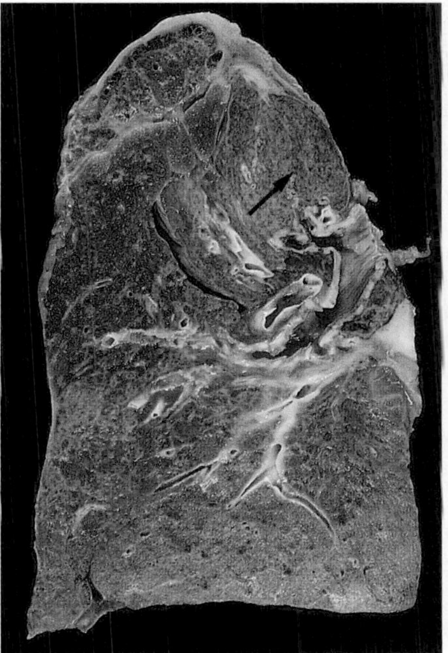

Figure 16–28 ■

Advanced silicosis seen on transection of lung. Scarring has contracted the upper lobe into a small dark mass *(arrow).* Note the dense pleural thickening. (Courtesy of Dr. John Godleski, Brigham and Women's Hospital, Boston, MA.)

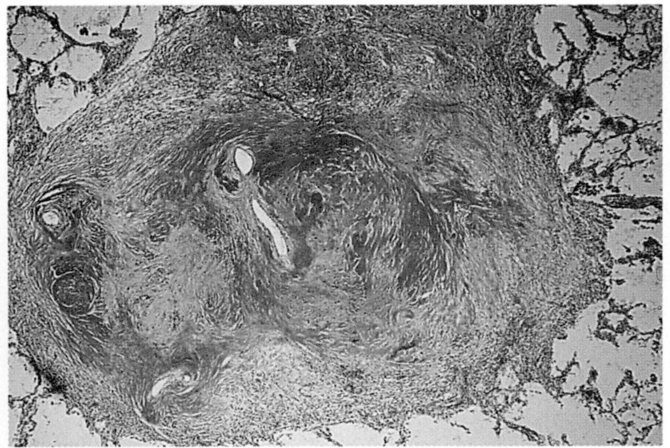

Figure 16–29

Several coalescent collagenous silicotic nodules. (Courtesy of Dr. John Godleski, Brigham and Women's Hospital, Boston, MA.)

Clinical Course. The disease is usually detected when routine chest radiography is performed on an asymptomatic worker. The radiographs typically show a fine nodularity in the upper zones of the lung, but pulmonary functions are either normal or only moderately affected. Most patients do not develop shortness of breath until late in the course, after PMF is present. At this time, the disease may be progressive, even if the patient is no longer exposed. The disease is slow to kill, but impaired pulmonary function may severely limit activity. Despite persistent controversy, there is no clear association of silica and the development of lung cancer in humans.[52]

Asbestos-Related Diseases

Asbestos is a family of crystalline hydrated silicates that form fibers. Based on epidemiologic studies, *occupational exposure* to asbestos is linked to

- Localized fibrous plaques or, rarely, diffuse pleural fibrosis
- Pleural effusions
- Parenchymal interstitial fibrosis (*asbestosis*)
- Bronchogenic carcinoma
- Mesotheliomas
- Laryngeal and perhaps other extrapulmonary neoplasms, including colon carcinomas[50, 55]

An increased incidence of asbestosis-related cancer in family members of asbestos workers has alerted the general public to the potential hazards of asbestos in the environment. The proper public health policy toward low-level exposures that might be encountered in old buildings or schools is controversial, with some experts questioning the wisdom of expensive asbestos abatement programs for environments with airborne fiber counts that are up to 100-fold lower than allowed by occupational standards.

Pathogenesis. Concentration, size, shape, and solubility of the different forms of asbestos dictate whether disease occurs. There are two distinct geometric forms of asbestos: *serpentine* (curly and flexible fibers) and *amphibole* (straight, stiff, and brittle fibers). The serpentine chrysotile chemical form accounts for most of the asbestos used in industry. Amphiboles include crocidolite, amosite, tremolite, anthophyllite, and actinolyte. This confusing array of terms is important because amphiboles, even though less prevalent, are more pathogenic than chrysotiles, particularly with respect to induction of malignant pleural tumors (mesotheliomas). Some studies of mesotheliomas have shown the link is almost always to amphibole exposure. The relatively few cases of mesotheliomas arising in chrysotile workers are in all likelihood due to contamination of chrysotile with the amphibole tremolite.

The greater pathogenicity of straight and stiff amphiboles is apparently related to their aerodynamic properties and solubility. Chrysotiles, with their more flexible, curled structure, are likely to become impacted in the upper respiratory passages and removed by the mucociliary elevator. Furthermore, once trapped in the lungs, chrysotiles are gradually leached from the tissues because they are more soluble than amphiboles. In contrast, the straight, stiff amphiboles may align themselves in the airstream and thus be delivered deeper into the lungs, where they can penetrate epithelial cells and reach the interstitium. The length of amphibole fibers also plays a role in pathogenicity, those longer than 8 mm and thinner than 0.5 mm being more injurious than shorter, thicker ones. Nevertheless, both amphiboles and serpentines are fibrogenic, and increasing doses are associated with a higher incidence of all asbestos-related disease except that only amphibole exposure correlates with mesothelioma. In contrast to other inorganic dusts, asbestos can also act as both a tumor initiator and a tumor promoter. Potentially toxic chemicals adsorbed onto the asbestos fibers, however, undoubtedly contribute to the oncogenicity of the fibers. For example, the adsorption of carcinogens in tobacco smoke onto asbestos fibers may well be important in the remarkable synergy between tobacco smoking and the development of bronchogenic carcinoma in asbestos workers. One study of asbestos workers found a 5-fold increase of bronchogenic carcinoma for asbestos exposure alone, while asbestos exposure and smoking together led to a 55-fold increase in the risk of lung cancer.[56]

Asbestosis, similar to the other pneumoconioses, depends on the interaction of inhaled fibers with lung macrophages and other parenchymal cells. The initial injury occurs at bifurcations of small airways and ducts, where the stiff fibers land and penetrate. Macrophages both alveolar and interstitial attempt to ingest and clear the fibers and are activated to release chemotactic factors and fibrogenic mediators that amplify the response. Chronic deposition of fibers and persistent release of mediators eventually leads to generalized interstitial pulmonary inflammation and interstitial fibrosis. It is not completely understood why silicosis is a nodular fibrosing disease and asbestosis a diffuse interstitial process. The more diffuse distribution may be related to the ability of asbestos to reach alveoli more consistently or its ability to penetrate epithelial cells, or to both.

MORPHOLOGY. Asbestosis is marked by **diffuse pulmonary interstitial fibrosis.** These changes are indistinguishable from those resulting from other causes of diffuse interstitial fibrosis except for the presence of **asbestos bodies.** Asbestos bodies appear as **golden brown, fusiform or beaded rods with a translucent center and consist of asbestos fibers coated with an iron-containing proteinaceous material** (Fig. 16–30). They arise when macrophages attempt to phagocytose asbestos fibers; the iron is presumably derived from phagocyte ferritin. Other inorganic particulates may become coated with similar iron protein complexes, and the term **ferruginous bodies** is better used where there is no evidence of an asbestos core. It should be noted that asbestos bodies can sometimes be found in the lungs of normal persons, but usually in much lower concentrations and without an accompanying interstitial fibrosis.

Asbestosis begins as fibrosis around respiratory bronchioles and alveolar ducts and extends to involve adjacent alveolar sacs and alveoli. The fibrous tissue distorts the native architecture, creating enlarged airspaces enclosed within thick fibrous walls; eventually the affected regions become honeycombed. In contrast to CWP and silicosis, asbestosis begins in the lower lobes and subpleurally, but the middle and upper lobes of the lungs become affected as fibrosis progresses. Simultaneously the visceral pleura undergoes fibrous thickening and sometimes binds the lungs to the chest wall. Large parenchymal nodules typical of Caplan syndrome may appear in a few patients who have concurrent rheumatoid arthritis. The scarring may trap and narrow pulmonary arteries and arterioles, causing pulmonary hypertension and cor pulmonale.

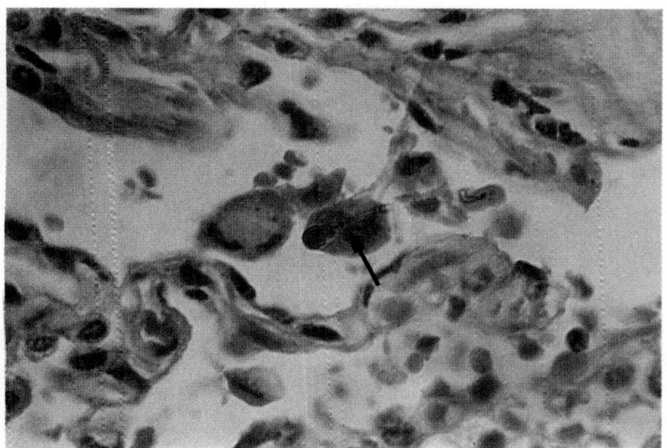

Figure 16–30 ■

High-power detail of an asbestos body, revealing the typical beading and knobbed ends (*arrow*).

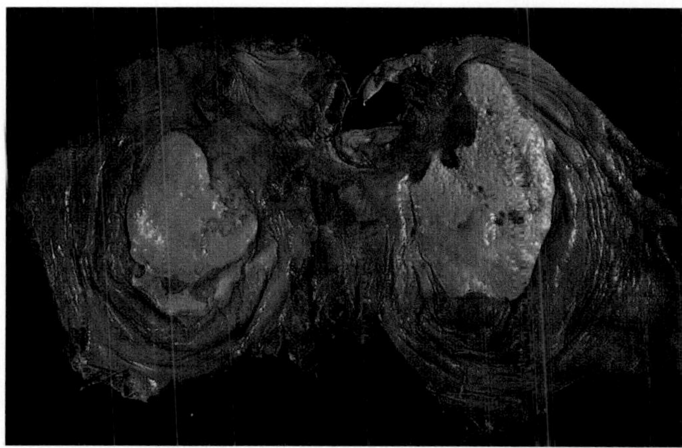

Figure 16–31 ■

Asbestos exposure evidenced by severe, discrete, characteristic fibrocalcific plaques on the pleural surface of the diaphragm. (Courtesy of Dr. John Godleski, Brigham and Women's Hospital, Boston, MA.)

Pleural plaques, the most common manifestation of asbestos exposure, are well-circumscribed plaques of dense collagen (Fig. 16–31), often containing calcium. They develop most frequently on the anterior and posterolateral aspects of the **parietal pleura** and over the domes of the diaphragm. They do not contain asbestos bodies, and only rarely do they occur in persons who have no history or evidence of asbestos exposure. Uncommonly, asbestos exposure induces pleural effusions, which are usually serous but may be bloody. Rarely, diffuse visceral pleural fibrosis may occur and, in advanced cases, bind the lung to the thoracic cavity wall.

Both bronchogenic carcinomas and mesotheliomas (pleural and peritoneal) develop in workers exposed to asbestos. The risk of bronchogenic carcinoma is increased about fivefold for asbestos workers; the relative risk of mesotheliomas, normally a rare tumor (2 to 17 cases per 1 million persons), is more than a 1000-fold greater. Concomitant cigarette smoking greatly increases the risk of bronchogenic carcinoma but not that of mesothelioma. These asbestos-related tumors are morphologically indistinguishable from cancers of other causes and are described later.

Clinical Course. The clinical findings in asbestosis are indistinguishable from those of any other diffuse interstitial lung disease (see earlier). Dyspnea is usually the first manifestation: at first, it is provoked by exertion, but later it is present even at rest. These manifestations rarely appear fewer than 10 years after first exposure and are more common after 20 years or more. The dyspnea is usually accompanied by a cough associated with production of sputum. The disease may remain static or progress to congestive heart failure, cor pulmonale, and death. Chest films reveal irregular linear densities, particularly in both lower lobes. With advancement of the pneumoconiosis, a honeycomb pattern develops. Pleural plaques are usually asymptomatic and are detected on radiographs as circumscribed densities. Asbestosis complicated by lung or pleural cancer is associated with a particularly grim prognosis.

Berylliosis

Heavy exposure to airborne dusts or to fumes of metallic beryllium or its oxides, alloys, or salts may induce acute pneumonitis; more protracted low-dose exposure may cause pulmonary and systemic granulomatous lesions that closely mimic sarcoidosis (see next section). Recognition of the hazards of beryllium exposure in the workplace and enactment in the late 1940s of standards for limiting worker exposure resulted in the disappearance of acute berylliosis. Currently, workers in the nuclear and aerospace industries working with beryllium alloys are at highest risk for exposure, but new cases of chronic berylliosis are reported only occasionally.

Chronic berylliosis is caused by induction of cell-mediated immunity.[57] Because only 2% of exposed workers develop disease, it appears that genetic susceptibility is necessary for the initiation of an immune response. The development of delayed hypersensitivity leads to the formation of noncaseating granulomas in the lungs and hilar nodes or, less commonly, in the spleen, liver, kidney, adrenals, and distant lymph nodes. The pulmonary granulomas become progressively fibrotic, giving rise to irregular, fine nodular densities detected on chest radiographs. Hilar adenopathy is present in about half the cases.

Chronic berylliosis often does not result in clinical manifestations until many years after exposure, when the patient presents with dyspnea, cough, weight loss, and arthralgias. Some cases stabilize, others remit and relapse, and still others progress to pulmonary failure. Epidemiologic evidence links heavy beryllium exposure to an increased incidence of lung cancer.

SARCOIDOSIS

Sarcoidosis is a systemic disease of unknown cause characterized by noncaseating granulomas in many tissues and organs. Sarcoidosis presents many clinical patterns, but bilateral hilar lymphadenopathy or lung involvement is visible on chest radiographs in 90% of cases. Eye and skin lesions are next in frequency. Since other diseases, including mycobacterial or fungal infections and berylliosis, can also produce noncaseating (*hard*) granulomas, the histologic diagnosis of sarcoidosis is made by exclusion.

The prevalence of sarcoidosis is higher in women than in men but varies widely in different countries and populations. In the United States, the rates are highest in the Southeast; they are ten times higher in American blacks than in whites. By contrast, among Chinese and Southeast Asians, the disease is almost unknown.

Etiology and Pathogenesis. The distinctive granulomatous tissue response seen in sarcoidosis suggests the presence of a persistent, poorly degradable antigen. Numerous intriguing immunologic abnormalities are present,[58] including increases in CD4+ lymphocytes within the lung and elevated levels of soluble IL-2 receptors in serum and lung lavage fluid. Alveolar macrophages also show an activated phenotype, with increased class II HLA expression and increased antigen-presenting capacity. The cytokines and factors secreted by these cells could well account for the influx of monocytes, alveolitis, and noncaseating granuloma formation in the lung and for the resulting progressive fibrosis, all characteristic features of pulmonary sarcoidosis. Similar to other T-cell responses to antigen, the T-cell proliferation in the sarcoid lung is oligoclonal, rather than a generalized, nonspecific response.[59] Nevertheless, numerous efforts at identifying bacterial or viral agents or other inciting agents have failed. Two developments have reawakened interest in a possible role for mycobacteria in sarcoidosis. First is the observation of elevated circulating $\gamma\delta$ T cells in some patients, a receptor subtype associated with response to mycobacterial antigens.[60] Second, polymerase chain reaction techniques are being applied to sarcoidal tissue in an attempt to detect minute amounts of mycobacterial DNA. True to its enigmatic self, sarcoid is providing conflicting results in these investigations[61] and must still be considered a disease of unknown etiology.

MORPHOLOGY. Histologically, all involved tissues show the classic **noncaseating granulomas** (Fig. 16–32), each composed of an aggregate of tightly clustered epithelioid cells, often with Langhans or foreign body–type giant cells. Central necrosis is unusual. In chronic disease, the granulomas may become enclosed within fibrous rims or may eventually be replaced by hyaline fibrous scars. Two other microscopic features are often present in the granulomas: (1) laminated concretions composed of calcium and proteins known as Schaumann bodies and (2) stellate inclusions known as asteroid bodies enclosed within giant cells found in approximately 60% of the granulomas. Although characteristic, these microscopic features are not pathognomonic of sarcoidosis because asteroid and Schaumann bodies may

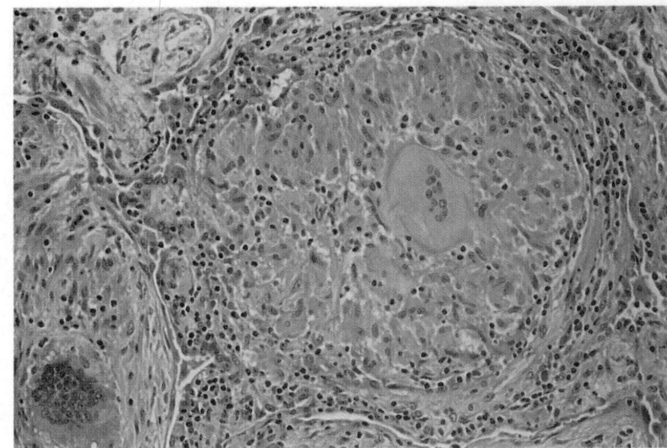

Figure 16–32

Characteristic sarcoid noncaseating granulomas in lung with many giant cells. (Courtesy of Dr. Ramon Blanco, Department of Pathology, Brigham and Women's Hospital, Boston, MA.)

be encountered in other granulomatous diseases (e.g., beryllliosis) (see preceding section on pneumoconiosis). Pathologic involvement of virtually every organ in the body has been cited at one time or another.

The **lungs** are common sites of involvement. Macroscopically, there is usually no demonstrable alteration, although at times the coalescence of granulomas may produce small nodules that are palpable or visible as 1- to 2-cm, noncaseating, noncavitated consolidations. Histologically the lesions are distributed primarily along the lymphatics around bronchi and blood vessels, although alveolar lesions are also seen. The relative frequency of granulomas in the bronchial submucosa accounts for the high diagnostic yield of bronchoscopic biopsies. There appears to be a strong tendency for lesions to heal in the lungs, so varying stages of fibrosis and hyalinization are often found, causing interstitial pulmonary fibrosis. The pleural surfaces are sometimes involved.

Lymph nodes are involved in almost all cases, specifically the hilar and mediastinal nodes, but any other node in the body may be involved. Nodes are characteristically enlarged, discrete, and sometimes calcified. The tonsils are affected in about one quarter to one third of cases.

The **spleen** is affected microscopically in about three quarters of the cases, but it is enlarged in only 18%. On occasion, granulomas may coalesce to form small nodules that are barely visible macroscopically. The capsule is not involved. The **liver** is affected slightly less often than the spleen. It may also be moderately enlarged and may contain scattered granulomas, more in portal triads than in the lobular parenchyma. Needle biopsy may permit the identification of these focal lesions. The **bone marrow** is an additional favored site of localization. Roentgenographic changes can be identified in about one fifth of cases of systemic involvement. The radiologically visible bone lesions have a particular tendency to involve phalangeal bones of the hands and feet, creating small circumscribed areas of bone resorption within the marrow cavity, a diffuse reticulated pattern throughout the cavity, with widening of the bony shafts or new bone formations on the outer surfaces.

Skin lesions are encountered in one third to one half of the cases. Sarcoidosis of the skin assumes a variety of macroscopic appearances (e.g. discrete subcutaneous nodules; focal, slightly elevated, erythematous plaques; or flat lesions that are slightly reddened and scaling and resemble those of lupus erythematosus). Lesions may also appear on the mucous membranes of the oral cavity, larynx, and upper respiratory tract. Involvement of the **eye, its associated glands, and the salivary glands** occurs in about one fifth to one half of the cases. The ocular involvement takes the form of iritis or iridocyclitis, either bilaterally or unilaterally. As a consequence, corneal opacities, glaucoma, and total loss of vision may occur. These ocular lesions are frequently accompanied by inflammations in the lacrimal glands, with suppression of lacrimation. Bilateral sarcoidosis of the parotid, submaxillary, and sublingual glands completes the **combined uveoparotid involvement designated as Mikulicz syndrome** (Chapter 17). Sarcoid granulomas occasionally occur in the heart, kidneys, central nervous system, and endocrine glands, particularly in the pituitary, as well as in other body tissues.

Clinical Course. Because of its varying severity and the inconstant distribution of the lesions, sarcoidosis is a protean clinical disease. Sarcoidosis may be discovered unexpectedly on routine chest films as bilateral hilar adenopathy or may have peripheral lymphadenopathy, cutaneous lesions, eye involvement, splenomegaly, or hepatomegaly as a presenting manifestation. In the great majority of cases, however, patients seek medical attention because of the insidious onset of respiratory abnormalities (shortness of breath, cough, chest pain, hemoptysis) or of constitutional signs and symptoms (fever, fatigue, weight loss, anorexia, night sweats).

Sarcoidosis follows a fairly unpredictable course characterized by either progressive chronicity or periods of activity interspersed with remissions, sometimes permanent, that may be spontaneous or initiated by steroid therapy. Overall, 65 to 70% of affected patients recover with minimal or no residual manifestations. Twenty per cent have permanent loss of some lung function or some permanent visual impairment. Of the remaining 10%, some die of cardiac or central nervous system damage, but most succumb to progressive pulmonary fibrosis and cor pulmonale. Patients presenting with hilar lymphadenopathy alone (stage I) have the best prognosis, followed by those with adenopathy and pulmonary infiltrates (stage II). Patients presenting with pulmonary disease and no adenopathy (stage III) have few spontaneous remissions and are most likely to develop chronic pulmonary fibrosis.

IDIOPATHIC PULMONARY FIBROSIS

The term *idiopathic pulmonary fibrosis* refers to a poorly understood pulmonary disorder characterized histologically by diffuse interstitial inflammation and fibrosis, which in the advanced case results in severe hypoxemia and cyanosis. There are at least 20 synonyms for this entity (e.g., chronic interstitial pneumonitis, Hamman-Rich syndrome), and in Britain it is known as *diffuse or cryptogenic* (*i.e., idiopathic*) *fibrosing alveolitis*. The term *usual interstitial pneumonitis* is employed by some to differentiate this condition from the desquamative type (*desquamative interstitial pneumonitis*), described later, and from other, rarer examples of so-called giant cell and lymphocytic interstitial pneumonitis.[62] Similar pathologic findings may occur as the result of well-defined entities, such as the pneumoconioses, hypersensitivity pneumonitis, oxygen toxicity pneumonitis, scleroderma, and irradiation injury. In about half the cases of interstitial fibrosis, however, there is no known underlying disease, and the term *idiopathic* is applied.

Pathogenesis. It is now thought that idiopathic pulmonary fibrosis represents a stereotyped inflammatory response of the alveolar wall to injuries of different types, durations, and intensities. The proposed sequence of events, described earlier, begins with some form of alveolar wall injury, which results in interstitial edema and accumulation of inflammatory cells (alveolitis). The type I membranous pneumocyte is particularly susceptible to injury. Subsequently, there is hyperplasia of type II pneumocytes in an attempt to regenerate the alveolar epithelial lining. Fibroblasts then proliferate, and progressive fibrosis of both the interalveolar septa and the intra-alveolar exudate results in obliteration of normal pulmonary architecture.

Immune mechanisms have been implicated in some cases. Granular deposits of IgG are sometimes seen in the alveolar walls, suggesting that immune complexes may play a pathogenetic role, but the nature of the antigens within the complexes is unknown. There are high levels of circulating immune complexes or cryoimmunoglobulins in the serum of some (but not all) patients with idiopathic interstitial pneumonia, but these can also be found in some individuals without lung disease, leaving the role of immune complexes, if any, unsettled.[63]

MORPHOLOGY. The morphologic changes vary according to the stage of the disease. In early cases, the lungs are firm in consistency and microscopically show pulmonary edema, intra-alveolar exudation, hyaline membranes, and infiltration of the alveolar septa with mononuclear cells. There is hyperplasia of type II pneumocytes, which appear as cuboidal or even columnar cells lining the alveolar spaces. With advancing disease, there is organization of the intra-alveolar exudate by fibrous tissue as well as thickening of the interstitial septa owing to fibrosis and variable amounts of inflammation. At this stage, the lungs become solid, with alternating areas of fibrosis and more normal-appearing lung. In the end stages of the disorder, the lung consists of spaces lined by cuboidal or columnar epithelium and separated by inflammatory fibrous tissue (Fig. 16–33). This gives the typical appearance of the **honeycomb lung**. Small cysts are often seen, and there is also intimal thickening of the pulmonary arteries and lymphoid hyperplasia. As mentioned earlier, this advanced picture can result from any of the disorders listed in Table 16–6. Thus, it is necessary to exclude the known causes of interstitial fibrosis by clinical, radiologic, or serologic means before the diagnosis of idiopathic fibrosis is made.

Clinical Course. As would be expected, patients exhibit varying degrees of respiratory difficulty and, in advanced cases, hypoxemia and cyanosis. The septal fibrosis constitutes a significant physiologic alveolocapillary block. Secondary pulmonary hypertension can be severe, and cor pulmonale and cardiac failure may result. The progression in an individual case is unpredictable, and in some patients the disease remits spontaneously. The process progresses in some rapidly, leading to fibrosis in a matter of weeks, whereas in others it develops over many years. The median survival is less than 5 years.

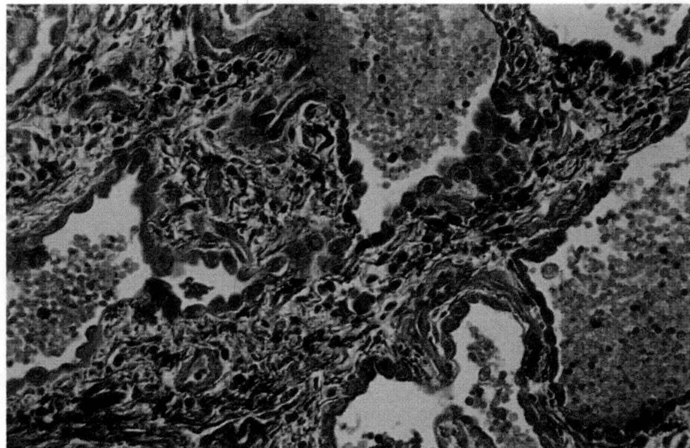

Figure 16–33

Diffuse interstitial fibrosis. Note the marked interstitial fibrosis (highlighted blue in this Masson trichrome stain), focal chronic inflammation, and dilated spaces lined by cuboidal type II epithelial cells.

DESQUAMATIVE INTERSTITIAL PNEUMONITIS

In some patients with interstitial pneumonitis, there is prominent aggregation of mononuclear cells (macrophages) within the alveoli, originally thought to be *desquamated* epithelial cells from the alveolar walls. These patients usually present with the slow development of cough and dyspnea, eventually leading to marked respiratory embarrassment, cyanosis, and clubbing of the fingers. Classically the radiologic picture is that of bilateral lower-lobe, ground-glass infiltrates.

MORPHOLOGY. The most striking histologic finding is the accumulation in the airspaces of a large number of macrophages containing lipid and periodic acid–Schiff (PAS)–positive granules. Some of the macrophages contain lamellar bodies (surfactant) within phagocytic vacuoles, presumably derived from necrotic type II pneumocytes. There is often an interstitial pneumonitis and an accompanying hyperplasia of the septal lining epithelial cells and desquamation of these cells into the airspaces (Fig. 16–34).

The cause is unknown. Patients benefit from steroid therapy, which often leads to clearing of the lungs. Some patients with desquamative interstitial pneumonitis have or subsequently develop significant interstitial fibrosis; for this reason, many authors object to the term *desquamative in-*

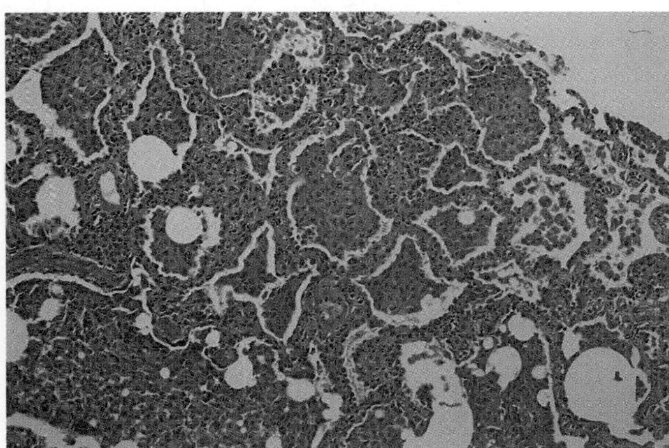

Figure 16–34 ■

Desquamative interstitial pneumonitis: medium-power detail of lung to demonstrate fibrous thickening of the alveolar walls and accumulation of large numbers of mononuclear cells within the alveolar spaces.

terstitial pneumonitis and consider the entity an early stage of usual idiopathic interstitial fibrosis (discussed earlier). Nevertheless, the presence of a prominent desquamative component has practical implications because such patients apparently have a better response to steroid therapy than those with the usual interstitial fibrotic pattern.[43]

HYPERSENSITIVITY PNEUMONITIS

The term *hypersensitivity pneumonitis* describes a spectrum of immunologically mediated, predominantly interstitial lung disorders caused by intense, often prolonged exposure to inhaled organic dusts and related occupational antigens.[64] Affected individuals have an abnormal sensitivity or heightened reactivity to the antigen, which, in contrast to that occurring in asthma, involves primarily the *alveoli. It is important to recognize these diseases early in their course because progression to serious chronic fibrotic lung disease can be prevented by removal of the environmental agent.*

Most commonly, hypersensitivity results from the inhalation of organic dust containing antigens made up of spores of thermophilic bacteria, true fungi, animal proteins, or bacterial products. Numerous specifically named syndromes are described, depending on the occupation or exposure of the individual. *Farmer's lung* results from exposure to dusts generated from harvested, humid, warm hay that permits the rapid proliferation of the spores of thermophilic actinomycetes. *Pigeon breeder's lung* (bird fancier's disease) is provoked by proteins from serum, excreta, or feathers of the birds. *Humidifier* or *air-conditioner lung* is caused by thermophilic bacteria in heated water reservoirs. There is also mushroom picker's lung, maple bark disease, and duck fever (from duck feathers). The evidence from experimental and human studies strongly suggests a type III immune complex pathogenesis for the early lesions, followed by a type IV delayed-hypersensitivity reaction for the granulomatous components.

MORPHOLOGY. Histologic information comes from biopsy specimens of patients with subacute and chronic forms, rather than from those with acute attacks. The alterations (Fig. 16–35) include (1) interstitial pneumonitis consisting primarily of lymphocytes, plasma cells, and macrophages (some of the last-mentioned having a foamy cytoplasm), (2) interstitial fibrosis, (3) obliterative bronchiolitis, and (4) outright granuloma formation. In more than half the patients, there is also evidence of an intra-alveolar infiltrate.

Clinical Features. The clinical manifestations are varied. Acute attacks, which follow inhalation of antigenic dust in sensitized patients, consist of recurring attacks of fever, dyspnea, cough, and leukocytosis. Diffuse and nodular infiltrates appear in the chest radiograph, and pulmonary function tests show an acute restrictive effect. Symptoms usually appear 4 to 6 hours after exposure. If exposure is continuous and protracted, a chronic form of the disease supervenes that no longer features the acute exacerbations on antigen re-exposure. Instead, there are signs of progressive respiratory failure, dyspnea, and cyanosis and a decrease in total lung capacity and compliance—a picture hard to differentiate from other forms of chronic interstitial disease.

Byssinosis is an occupational lung disease of textile workers that is apparently induced by the inhalation of airborne fibers of cotton, linen, and hemp. Acute effects include cough, wheezing, and airway obstruction, a picture that resembles bronchial asthma. Prolonged exposure leads to disabling chronic lung disease characterized by chronic bronchitis, emphysema, and interstitial granulomas. Evidence for an immunologic hypersensitivity in this disorder is not as clear as that in the other conditions described in this section.

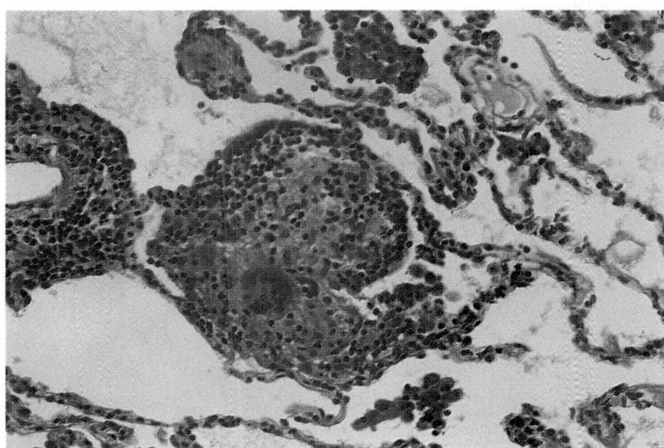

Figure 16–35 ■

Hypersensitivity pneumonitis, histologic appearance. Loosely formed interstitial granulomas and chronic inflammation are characteristic.

PULMONARY EOSINOPHILIA (PULMONARY INFILTRATION WITH EOSINOPHILIA)

A number of clinical and pathologic pulmonary entities are characterized by an infiltration of eosinophils, recruited in part by elevated alveolar levels of eosinophil attractants such as IL-5.[65] These diverse diseases are generally of immunologic but incompletely understood origins.[66] They have been divided into the following categories:

- *Simple pulmonary eosinophilia*, or Loffler syndrome
- *Tropical eosinophilia*, caused by infection with *microfilariae*
- *Secondary chronic pulmonary eosinophilia* (which occurs in a number of parasitic, fungal, and bacterial infections; in hypersensitivity pneumonitis; in drug allergies; and in association with asthma, allergic bronchopulmonary aspergillosis, or polyarteritis nodosa)
- So-called idiopathic *chronic eosophilic pneumonia*

Loffler syndrome is characterized by transient pulmonary lesions, eosinophilia in the blood, and a benign clinical course. Roentgenograms are often quite striking, with shadows of varying size and shape in any of the lobes, suggesting irregular intrapulmonary densities. The lungs show alveoli whose septa are thickened by an infiltrate composed of eosinophils and occasional interspersed giant cells, but there is no vasculitis, fibrosis, or necrosis. In some cases, eosinophils are found in a background of diffuse alveolar damage.[67]

Chronic eosinophilic pneumonia is characterized by focal areas of cellular consolidation of the lung substance distributed chiefly in the periphery of the lung fields. Prominent in these lesions are heavy aggregates of lymphocytes and eosinophils within both the septal walls and the alveolar spaces. Clinically, there is high fever, night sweats, and dyspnea, all of which respond to corticosteroid therapy. It is diagnosed when other causes of chronic pulmonary eosinophilia are excluded.

BRONCHIOLITIS OBLITERANS-ORGANIZING PNEUMONIA (BOOP)

Bronchiolitis obliterans-organizing pneumonia refers to what is now recognized to be a common response to infectious or inflammatory injury of the lungs.[68] Patients present with cough and dyspnea and often recall a recent respiratory tract infection. Patchy opacities or interstitial infiltrates are seen radiologically. The characteristic pathologic finding comprises polypoid plugs of loose, fibrous tissue filling both bronchioles (*bronchiolitis obliterans*) (Fig. 16–36) and alveoli (organizing pneumonia). A variable chronic inflammatory cell infiltrate usually accompanies what appears to be a prolonged effort to resolve or organize the pulmonary injury. Causes associated with bronchiolitis obliterans-organizing pneumonia include infections (viral, bacterial), inhaled toxins, drugs, collagen vascular disease, and graft-versus-host disease in bone marrow transplant recipients.[69] The bronchiolar injury and repair distinguish this process from routine pneumonias. In most cases, patients improve gradually or with steroid therapy.

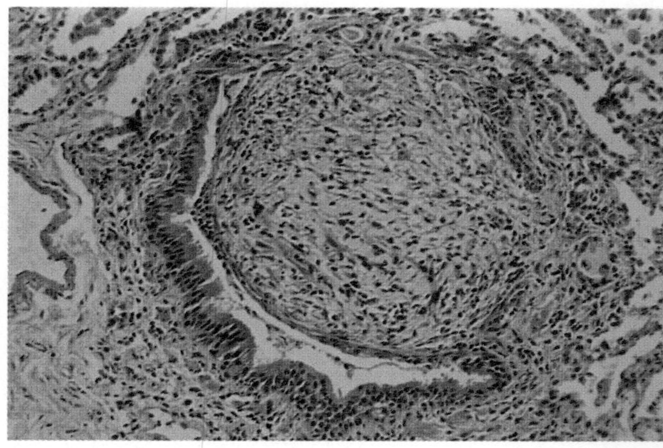

Figure 16–36

Bronchiolitis obliterans–organizing pneumonia (BOOP). The bronchiole shows a plug of organizing exudate.

DIFFUSE PULMONARY HEMORRHAGE SYNDROMES

Hemorrhage from the lung is a dramatic complication of some interstitial lung disorders.[70, 71] Among these so-called *pulmonary hemorrhage syndromes* (Fig. 16–37) are (1) Goodpasture syndrome; (2) idiopathic pulmonary hemosiderosis; and (3) vasculitis-associated hemorrhage, which is found in conditions such as hypersensitivity angiitis, Wegener granulomatosis, and lupus erythematosus (Chapter 12).

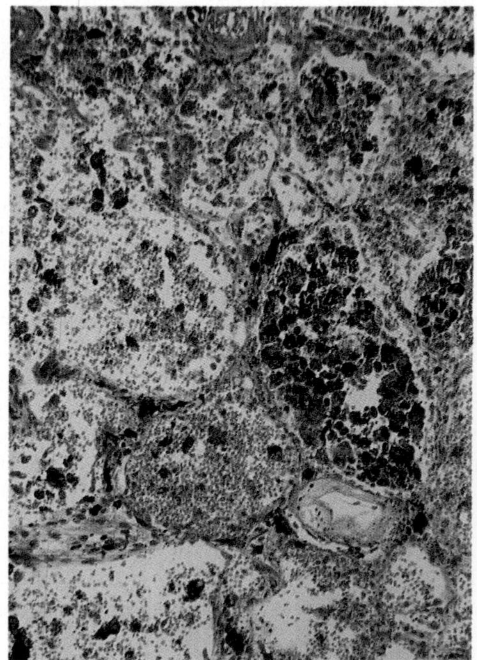

Figure 16–37

Acute intra-alveolar hemorrhage and hemosiderin-laden macrophages, reflecting previous hemorrhage, are common features of the diffuse pulmonary hemorrhage syndromes (Prussian blue stain for iron).

Goodpasture Syndrome

Goodpasture syndrome is an uncommon but intriguing condition characterized by the *simultaneous appearance of proliferative, usually rapidly progressive glomerulonephritis and a necrotizing hemorrhagic interstitial pneumonitis.* Most cases begin clinically with respiratory symptoms, principally hemoptysis, and radiographic evidence of focal pulmonary consolidations. Soon, manifestations of glomerulonephritis appear, leading to rapidly progressive renal failure. The common cause of death is uremia. Most cases occur in the teens or twenties, and there is a preponderance among men.

Pathogenesis. The evidence is quite substantial that the renal and pulmonary lesions are the consequence of antibodies evoked by antigens present in the glomerular and pulmonary basement membranes. The immunopathogenesis of the syndrome and the nature of the Goodpasture antigens are described in Chapter 21. The trigger initiating the anti–basement membrane antibodies is still unknown. In experimental animals, toxic pulmonary injury by toxic oxygen species or hydrocarbons increases fixation of antibodies onto basement membranes and induces pulmonary hemorrhage. In humans, virus infection, exposure to hydrocarbon solvents (used in the dry cleaning industry), and smoking have been implicated as cofactors in the causation of the syndrome and may act by a similar mechanism. As in other autoimmune disorders, a genetic predisposition is indicated by association with certain HLA subtypes (e.g., HLA-DR2).[70]

MORPHOLOGY. In the classic case, the lungs are heavy, with areas of red-brown consolidation. Histologically, there are acute focal necroses of alveolar walls associated with intra-alveolar hemorrhages, fibrous thickening of the septa, hypertrophy of lining septal cells, and (depending on the duration of the disease) organization of blood in the alveolar spaces. Often the alveoli contain hemosiderin-laden macrophages (Fig. 16–37). Immunofluorescence studies reveal linear deposits of immunoglobulins along the basement membranes of the septal walls. The kidneys reveal the characteristic findings of focal proliferative glomerulonephritis in the early cases, or crescentic glomerulonephritis in patients with rapidly progressive glomerulonephritis. Linear deposits of immunoglobulins and complement are also seen by immunofluorescence studies along the glomerular basement membranes, similar to those in the alveolar septa.

Clinical Features. The once dismal prognosis for this disease has been markedly improved by intensive *plasma exchange.* This procedure is thought to be beneficial by removing circulating anti–basement membrane antibodies as well as chemical mediators of immunologic injury. Simultaneous immunosuppressive therapy inhibits further antibody production. Both the lung hemorrhage and the glomerulonephritis improve with this form of therapy.

Idiopathic Pulmonary Hemosiderosis

Idiopathic pulmonary hemosiderosis is an uncommon pulmonary disease of obscure nature. It usually presents with an insidious onset of productive cough, hemoptysis, anemia, and weight loss associated with diffuse pulmonary infiltrations similar to Goodpasture syndrome. It tends to occur in younger adults and children, however.

MORPHOLOGY. The lungs are moderately increased in weight, with areas of consolidation that are usually red-brown to red. The cardinal histologic features of pulmonary hemosiderosis include prominent degeneration, shedding and hyperplasia of alveolar epithelial-cells, and marked alveolar capillary congestion. There are varying degrees of pulmonary interstitial fibrosis; hemorrhage into the alveolar spaces; and hemosiderosis, both within the alveolar septa and in macrophages lying free within the pulmonary alveoli.

The cause and pathogenesis are unknown, and no anti-basement membrane antibodies are detectable in serum or tissues.

PULMONARY INVOLVEMENT IN COLLAGEN VASCULAR DISORDERS

Diffuse interstitial fibrosis occurs classically in progressive systemic sclerosis (*scleroderma*), discussed in Chapter 7. Less commonly, patchy, transient parenchymal infiltrates are noted in *lupus erythematosus*, and occasionally severe lupus pneumonitis may occur and may be one of the major clinical problems in such patients. In *rheumatoid arthritis*, pulmonary involvement is common and may occur in one of five forms: (1) chronic pleuritis, with or without effusion; (2) diffuse interstitial pneumonitis and fibrosis; (3) intrapulmonary rheumatoid nodules; (4) rheumatoid nodules with pneumoconiosis (Caplan syndrome); and (5) pulmonary hypertension. Thirty per cent to 40% of patients with classic rheumatoid arthritis have abnormalities in pulmonary function. In certain patients, the disorder progresses to end-stage lung disease.

PULMONARY ALVEOLAR PROTEINOSIS

Pulmonary alveolar proteinosis is a disease of obscure cause that is characterized radiologically by diffuse pulmonary opacification and histologically by accumulation in the intra-alveolar spaces of a dense granular material that contains abundant lipid and PAS-positive (carbohydrate-containing) material.

Patients, for the most part, present with nonspecific respiratory difficulty of insidious onset, cough, and abundant sputum that often contains chunks of gelatinous material. Some have symptoms lasting for years, often with febrile illnesses. Progressive dyspnea, cyanosis, and respiratory insufficiency may occur, but some patients tend to have a benign course, with eventual resolution of the lesions. Pulmonary alveolar proteinosis does not usually progress to chronic fibrosis.

Pathogenesis. Pathogenesis remains unknown, but evidence points to a dysfunction of alveolar macrophages. For example, mice genetically deficient in granulocyte macrophage colony-stimulating factor (GM-CSF) receptors show an alveolar proteinosis that is prevented when normal macrophages repopulate the lungs after transplantation of wild-type bone marrow.[72] In addition, some patients with pulmonary alveolar proteinosis show a specific defect in GM-CSF receptor β-chain expression.[72a]

MORPHOLOGY. The disease is characterized by a peculiar, homogeneous, granular precipitate within the alveoli, causing focal-to-confluent consolidation of large areas of the lungs but without inflammatory reaction (Fig. 16–38). On section, turbid fluid exudes from these areas. As a consequence, there is a marked increase in the size and weight of the lung. The alveolar precipitate is PAS positive and also contains finely divided lipid. Biochemically the material is similar to surfactant but fails to show surfactant properties. By electron microscopy, the alveolar contents consist of necrotic alveolar macrophages and type II pneumocytes, amorphous precipitate, and considerable numbers of lamellar osmiophilic bodies morphologically resembling surfactant material. The involved alveoli are often lined with hyperplastic pneumocytes, and focal areas of necrosis of these cells are seen with the light microscope.

Some patients suffering from this disease may have occupational exposure to irritating dusts (including silica dust) and other chemicals. This disorder also occurs in immunosuppressed patients and in association with hematolymphoid malignancies and opportunistic infections.

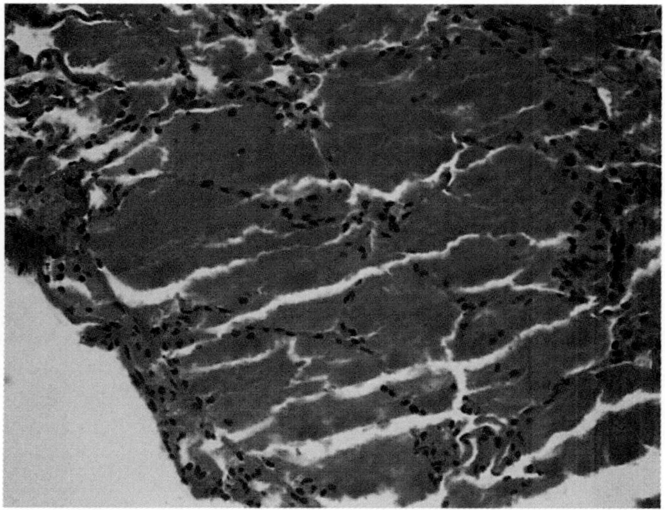

Figure 16–38 ■

Pulmonary alveolar proteinosis, histologic appearance. The alveoli are filled with a dense, amorphous, protein-lipid granular precipitate.

Table 16–8. EXAMPLES OF DRUG-INDUCED PULMONARY DISEASE

Drug	Pulmonary Disease
Cytotoxic drugs	
Bleomycin	Pneumonitis and fibrosis
Methotrexate	Hypersensitivity pneumonitis
Amiodarone	Pneumonitis and fibrosis
Nitrofurantoin	Hypersensitivity pneumonitis
Aspirin	Bronchospasm
β-antagonists	Bronchospasm

Complications of Therapies

DRUG-INDUCED LUNG DISEASE

Drugs can cause a variety of alterations in respiratory structure and function, including bronchospasm, pulmonary edema, chronic pneumonitis with fibrosis, and hypersensitivity pneumonitis (Table 16–8). For example, cytotoxic drugs used in cancer therapy (e.g., bleomycin) cause pneumonitis and pulmonary fibrosis as a result of direct toxicity of the drug and by stimulating the influx of inflammatory cells into the alveoli. Amiodarone, a drug that controls resistant cardiac arrhythmias, is preferentially concentrated in the lung and causes significant pneumonitis in 5 to 15% of patients receiving it.

RADIATION-INDUCED LUNG DISEASE

Radiation pneumonitis is a well-known complication of therapeutic radiation of pulmonary or other thoracic tumors (esophageal, breast, mediastinal).[73] *Acute radiation pneumonitis* occurs 1 to 6 months after therapy, manifested by fever, dyspnea, and radiologic infiltrates that correspond to an area of previous radiation. Morphologic changes are those of diffuse alveolar damage, including severe atypia of hyperplastic type II cells. Most patients respond to corticosteroid therapy. Some go on to manifest *chronic radiation pneumonitis*, with interstitial fibrosis in the affected area. Epithelial cell atypia and foam cells within vessel walls are also characteristic of radiation damage. The pathogenesis likely involves direct toxic injury to endothelial and epithelial cells from the radiation, with some blame going to additional injury from chemotherapeutic drugs or infections.

LUNG TRANSPLANTATION

Lung transplantation is the only effective treatment for a number of otherwise terminal lung diseases. These are generally bilateral, diffuse irreversible conditions, including severe idiopathic pulmonary fibrosis, primary pulmonary hypertension, emphysema, and cystic fibrosis. While double-lung and heart-lung transplants are possible, in many cases a single lung transplant is performed, offering sufficient improvement in pulmonary function for each of two recipients from a single (and all too scarce) donor. When chronic infection is present (cystic fibrosis, bronchiectasis), both lungs of the recipient are removed and replaced to minimize potential infectious complications related to immunosuppression.

MORPHOLOGY. The transplanted lung is subject to two major complications: infection and rejection.[74]

Pulmonary infections in lung transplant patients are essentially those of any immunocompromised host, discussed earlier. They include bacterial and viral (especially cytomegalovirus) bronchopneumonias, *Pneumocystis* pneumonia, and fungal infections. Moreover, despite routine immunosuppression postoperatively, rejection of the lung occurs to some degree in all patients.

Acute rejection occurs during the early weeks to months after surgery, presenting as fever, dyspnea, cough, and radiologic infiltrates. Since these are the exact same clinical features seen with infections, diagnosis often relies on transbronchial biopsy. The morphologic features of acute rejection are primarily those of mononuclear cell infiltrates, either around small vessels (Fig. 16–39) or in the submucosa of airways, or both.[75] Treatment with increased corticosteroids or other immunosuppressive drugs is usually successful in reversing the clinical decline and radiologic infiltrates.

Chronic rejection is a significant problem in 25 to 50% of all lung transplant patients. It is seen usually 6 to 12 months after surgery, manifested by cough and dyspnea. The major morphologic correlate of chronic rejection is **bronchiolitis obliterans,** the filling of small airways by an inflammatory-fibrous exudate. Evidence of ongoing cellular rejection around vessels is often also seen.

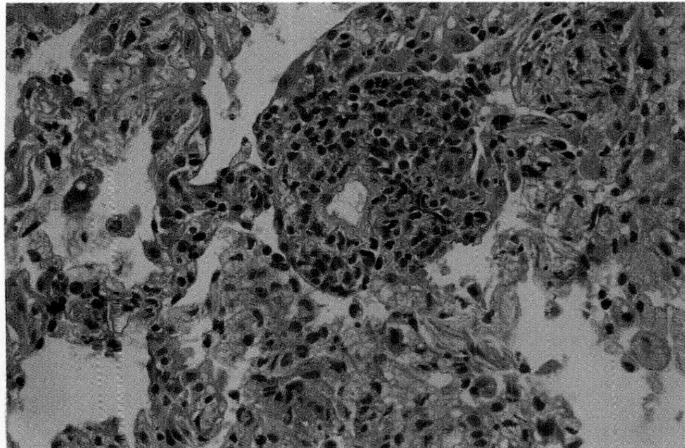

Figure 16–39

Acute rejection of a lung allograft is characterized by perivascular mononuclear cell infiltrates.

Although acute cellular airway rejection (the presumed forerunner of later, fibrous obliteration of these airways) is generally responsive to therapy, treatment of established bronchiolitis obliterans has been generally disappointing. Infrequent complications of lung transplantation include accelerated pulmonary arteriosclerosis in the graft and lymphoproliferative disease.

Tumors

A variety of benign and malignant tumors may arise in the lung,[76] but the vast majority (90 to 95%) are bronchogenic carcinomas. About 5% are bronchial carcinoids, and 2 to 5% are mesenchymal and other miscellaneous neoplasms. The term *bronchogenic* refers to the origin of these tumors in the bronchial (and sometimes bronchiolar) epithelium.

BRONCHOGENIC CARCINOMA

In industrialized nations, *public enemy number one* among cancers is bronchogenic carcinoma. It is the most common visceral malignancy in men; it alone accounts for approximately one third of all cancer deaths in men and more than 7% of all deaths in both sexes. The incidence is increasing dramatically in women, and lung cancer has passed breast carcinoma as a cause of cancer death in women. Overall, lung cancer is the most frequent fatal malignancy.

The annual number of deaths from lung cancer in the United States increased from 18,000 in 1950 to an estimated 158,000 in 1997.[77] In the same period, the age-adjusted death rate from cancer of the lung has more than trebled in men, rising from 19.9 to an outstanding 74 per 100,000 population. The death rate in women since 1950 has risen from 4.5 to 31 per 100,000, almost certainly the delayed consequence of increased cigarette smoking among women. Cancer of the lung now accounts for 13% of all cancers in both men and women. In 1996, an estimated 177,000 new cases of lung cancer occurred. Cancer of the lung occurs most often between ages 40 and 70 years, with a peak incidence in the fifties or sixties. Only 2% of all cases appear before the age of 40.

Etiology and Pathogenesis

Tobacco Smoking. The evidence provided by statistical and clinical observations establishing a positive relationship between tobacco smoking and lung cancer is incontrovertible.[78] Experimental data have also been pursued, but this approach is limited by species differences.

Statistical evidence is most compelling. In numerous retrospective studies of patients who died of bronchogenic carcinoma compared with control subjects, there was an invariable statistical association between the frequency of lung cancer and (1) the amount of daily smoking, (2) the tendency to inhale, and (3) the duration of the smoking habit. Compared with nonsmokers, average smokers of cigarettes have a 10-fold greater risk of developing lung cancer, and heavy smokers (more than 40 cigarettes per day for several years) have at least a 20-fold greater risk. Eighty per cent of lung cancers occur in smokers. Cessation of smoking for 10 years reduces risk to control levels. Epidemiologic studies also show an association between cigarette smoking and the following cancers: lip, tongue, floor of the mouth, pharynx, larynx, esophagus, urinary bladder, pancreas, and kidney.[79] Cigar and pipe smoking increase risk, although much more modestly than smoking of cigarettes.

Clinical evidence is obtained largely through observing histologic changes in the lining epithelium of the respiratory tract in smokers. A systematic study of the bronchial epithelium of smokers showed atypical and hyperplastic changes in about 10% of smokers, 1 to 2% of those smoking filter-tipped cigarettes, and 15% of patients who died of lung cancer. Nearly all (96.7%) of cigarette smokers showed some atypical cells in the bronchial tree, whereas 0.9% of control subjects had similar cells.[80, 81]

Experimental work has comprised mainly of attempts to induce cancer in experimental animals with extracts of tobacco smoke.[82] More than 1200 substances have been counted in cigarette smoke, and many of these are potential carcinogens. They include both initiators (polycyclic aromatic hydrocarbons such as benzo[*a*]pyrene) and promoters, such as phenol derivatives. Radioactive elements may also be found (polonium-210, carbon-14, potassium-40) as well as other contaminants, such as arsenic, nickel, molds, and additives. Protracted exposure of mice to these additives induces skin tumors. Efforts to produce lung cancer by exposing animals to tobacco smoke, however, have been unsuccessful. The few cancers that have been produced have been bronchioloalveolar carcinomas, a type of human tumor not strongly associated with smoking.

Industrial Hazards. Certain industrial exposures increase the risk of developing lung cancer. All types of *radiation* may be carcinogenic. There was an increased incidence of lung cancer among survivors of the Hiroshima and Nagasaki atomic bomb blasts. *Uranium* is weakly radioactive, but lung cancer rates among nonsmoking uranium miners are 4 times higher than those of the general population, and among smoking miners they are about 10 times higher.

The risk of lung cancer is increased with *asbestos*. Lung cancer is the most frequent malignancy in persons exposed to asbestos, which has become a universally recognized carcinogen, particularly when coupled with smoking.[56] Asbestos workers who do not smoke have a 5 times increased risk, and those who smoke have a 50 to 90 times greater risk of developing lung cancer than do nonsmoking control subjects. The latent period before the development of lung cancer is 10 to 30 years. Among asbestos workers, 1 death in 5 is due to bronchogenic carcinoma, 1 in 10 to pleural or peritoneal mesotheliomas (see later), and 1 in 10 to gastrointestinal carcinomas. There is also an increased risk of respiratory cancer among persons who work with *nickel*, *chromates*, *coal*, *mustard gas*, *arsenic*, *beryllium*, and *iron* and in newspaper workers, African gold miners, and haloether workers.

Air Pollution. Atmospheric pollutants may play some role in the increased incidence of bronchogenic carcinoma today. Attention has been drawn to the potential problem of *indoor* air pollution, especially by radon.[83, 84] Radon is a ubiquitous radioactive gas linked epidemiologically to increased lung cancer in miners exposed to relatively high concentrations. The pathogenetic mechanism is believed to be inhalation and bronchial deposition of radioactive decay products that become attached to environmental aerosols. These data have generated concern that low-level indoor exposure (e.g., in homes in areas of high radon in soil) may also lead to increased incidence of lung tumors, with some attributing the bulk of lung cancers in nonsmokers to this insidious carcinogen (Chapter 10). There remain substantial differences of opinion on the significance of the radon risk, with many skeptics awaiting more definitive studies.[85]

Molecular Genetics. Ultimately the exposures cited previously are thought to act by causing genetic alterations in lung cells, which accumulate and eventually lead to the neoplastic phenotype (Chapter 8). In lung cancers, it has been estimated that 10 to 20 genetic mutations have occurred by the time the tumor is clinically apparent.[86] As in other cancers, there is a role for dominant oncogenes and the frequent loss or inactivation of recessive tumor-suppressor genes in most lung cancer.[87, 88] The dominant oncogenes include c-*myc* in small cell carcinomas and K-*ras* in adenocarcinomas.[89] The commonly deleted or inactive recessive genes include *p53*, the retinoblastoma gene, and an unknown gene or genes on the short arm of chromosome 3. Noteworthy is the finding that in vitro exposure of human lung cells to the cigarette smoke carcinogen benzo[*a*]pyrene causes DNA damage (adduct formation) at the same codons of the *p53* gene that are the major mutational hotspots found in clinical lung cancers.[90] As established in colorectal and other cancers, multiple genetic changes are likely to accumulate during development of lung cancer. Although certain changes are known to be early (inactivation of chromosome 3p suppressor genes) or late (activation of *ras*), the temporal sequence is not as yet well defined. Occasional familial clustering has suggested a genetic predisposition, as has the variable risk even among heavy smokers. Attempts at defining markers of genetic susceptibility are ongoing and have, for example, identified a role for polymorphisms in the cytochrome P450 gene CYP1A1 (Chapter 8).

Scarring. Some lung cancers arise in the vicinity of pulmonary scars and are termed *scar cancers*. Histologically, these tumors are usually adenocarcinomas. In most cases, the scar is a desmoplastic response to the tumor,[91] but occasionally the scar has preceded the cancer. The scars incriminated are due to old infarcts, metallic foreign bodies, wounds, and granulomatous infections such as tuberculosis.

Classification. Numerous histologic classifications of bronchogenic carcinoma have been proposed, but the currently popular ones, based on classifications of the World Health Organization,[92] divide these tumors into four major categories (Table 16–9):

- Squamous cell carcinoma (25 to 40%)
- Adenocarcinoma (25 to 40%)
- Small cell carcinoma (20 to 25%)
- Large cell carcinoma (10 to 15%)

Table 16–9. HISTOLOGIC CLASSIFICATION OF BRONCHOGENIC CARCINOMA

- Squamous cell (epidermoid) carcinoma
- Adenocarcinoma
  - Bronchial derived
  - Acinar; papillary; solid
  - Bronchioloalveolar
- Small cell carcinoma
  - Oat cell (lymphocyte-like)
  - Intermediate cell (polygonal)
- Combined (usually with squamous)
- Large cell carcinoma
  - Undifferentiated; giant cell; clear cell
- Combined squamous cell carcinoma and adenocarcinoma

The incidence of adenocarcinoma has increased significantly in the last two decades, and it is now the most common form of lung cancer in women and, in many studies, men as well.[76, 93] The basis for this change is unclear. A possible factor is the increase in women smokers, but this only highlights our lack of knowledge about why women tend to show more adenocarcinomas. One interesting postulate is that changes in cigarette type (filter tips, lower tar and nicotine) have caused smokers to inhale more deeply and thereby expose more peripheral airways and cells (with a predilection to adenocarcinoma) to carcinogens.[94] There may be mixtures of histologic patterns, even in the same cancer. Thus, combined types of squamous cell carcinoma and adenocarcinoma or of small cell and squamous cell carcinoma are not infrequent. Another classification in common clinical use is based on response to available therapies: *small cell carcinomas* (high initial response to chemotherapy) versus *non–small cell carcinomas* (less responsive). The strongest relationship to smoking is with squamous cell and small cell carcinoma. From a histogenetic point of view, it seems most likely that all histologic variants of bronchogenic carcinoma, including small cell carcinoma as well as the bronchial carcinoid, to be described later, are derived from endoderm or a derivative—a view consistent with the frequency of tumors with mixed histologic patterns.

MORPHOLOGY. Bronchogenic carcinomas arise most often in and about the hilus of the lung. About three fourths of the lesions take origin from first-order, second-order, and third-order bronchi. A small number of primary carcinomas of the lung arise in the periphery of the lung substance from the alveolar septal cells or terminal bronchioles. These are predominantly adenocarcinomas, including those of the bronchioloalveolar type, to be discussed separately.

Carcinoma of the lung begins as an area of in situ cytologic atypia that, over an unknown interval of time, yields a small area of thickening or piling up of bronchial mucosa. With progression, this small focus, usually less than 1 cm² in area, assumes the appearance of an irregular, warty excrescence that elevates or erodes the lining epithelium (Fig. 16–40). The tumor may then follow a variety of paths. It may continue to fungate into the bronchial lumen to produce an intraluminal mass. It can also rapidly penetrate the wall of the bronchus to infiltrate along the peribronchial tissue (Fig. 16–40) into the adjacent region of the carina or mediastinum. In other instances, the tumor grows along a broad front to produce a cauliflower-like intraparenchymal mass that appears to push lung substance ahead of it. In almost all patterns, the neoplastic tissue is gray-white and firm to hard. Especially when the tumors are bulky, focal areas of hemorrhage or necrosis may appear to produce yellow-white mottling and softening. Sometimes these necrotic foci cavitate.

Extension may occur to the pleural surface and then within the pleural cavity or into the pericardium. Spread to the tracheal, bronchial, and mediastinal nodes can be found in most cases. The frequency of nodal involvement varies slightly with the histologic pattern but averages greater than 50%.

More distant spread of bronchogenic carcinoma occurs through both lymphatic and hematogenous pathways. These tumors have a distressing habit of spreading widely throughout the body and at an early stage in their evolution. Often the metastasis presents as the first manifestation of the underlying occult bronchogenic lesion. No organ or tissue is spared in the spread of these lesions, but the adrenals, for obscure reasons, are involved in more than half the cases. The liver (30 to 50%), brain (20%), and bone (20%) are additional favored sites of metastases.

Squamous Cell Carcinoma. Squamous cell carcinoma is most commonly found in men and is

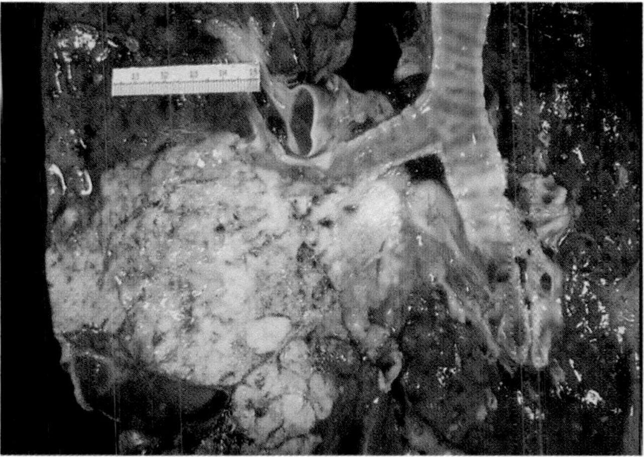

Figure 16–40

Bronchogenic carcinoma. The gray-white tumor tissue is seen infiltrating the lung substance. Histologically, this large tumor mass was identified as a squamous cell carcinoma.

closely correlated with a smoking history. The microscopic features are familiar in the form of production of keratin and intercellular bridges in the well-differentiated forms, but many less well-differentiated squamous cell tumors are encountered that begin to merge with the undifferentiated large cell pattern. This tumor arises in the larger, more central bronchi; tends to spread locally; and metastasizes somewhat later than the other patterns, but its rate of growth in its site of origin is usually more rapid than that of other types. Squamous metaplasia, epithelial dysplasia, and foci of frank carcinoma in situ are sometimes present in bronchial epithelium adjacent to the tumor mass.

Adenocarcinoma. Histologic classifications of adenocarcinomas include at least two forms: (1) the usual **bronchial-derived adenocarcinoma** and (2) a somewhat distinctive type termed **bronchioloalveolar carcinoma,** which probably arises from terminal bronchioles or alveolar walls. There may be overlap between these two forms, but the bronchioloalveolar carcinoma has sufficiently distinctive gross, microscopic, and epidemiologic features to be discussed later.

Adenocarcinoma is the most common type of lung cancer in women and nonsmokers. The lesions are usually more peripherally located, tend to be smaller, and vary histologically from well-differentiated tumors with obvious glandular elements to papillary lesions resembling other papillary carcinomas, to solid masses with only occasional mucin-producing glands and cells. About 80% contain mucin. Adenocarcinomas grow more slowly than squamous cell carcinomas. Peripheral adenocarcinomas are sometimes associated with areas of scarring (see earlier). Adenocarcinomas, including bronchioloalveolar carcinomas, are less frequently associated with a history of smoking (still, >75% found in smokers) than are squamous or small cell carcinomas (>98%).

Small Cell Carcinoma. This highly malignant tumor has a distinctive cell type. The epithelial cells are generally small, have little cytoplasm, and are round or oval and, occasionally, lymphocyte like (although they are about twice the size of a lym-

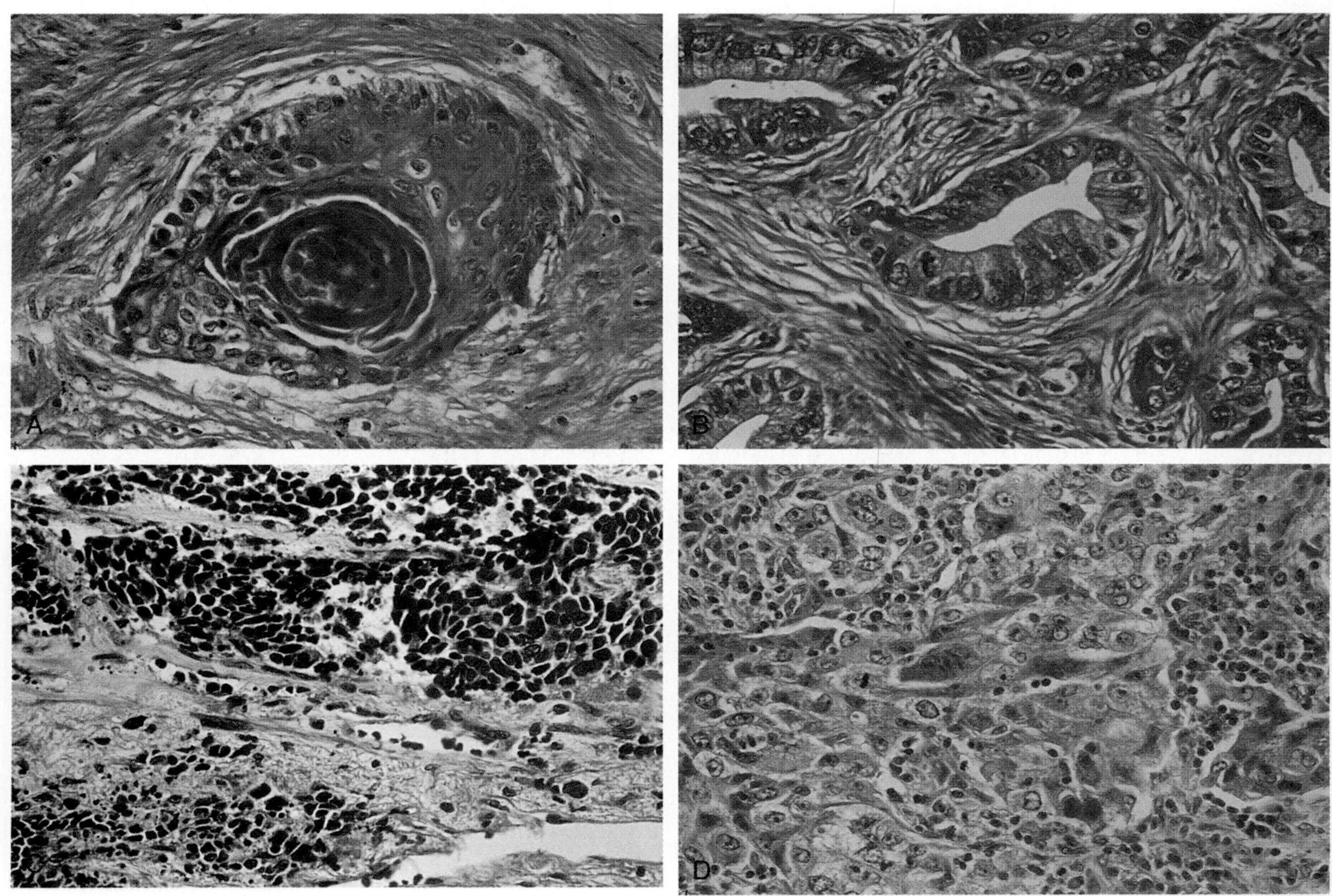

Figure 16–41

Histologic appearance of bronchogenic carcinoma: *A*, Well-differentiated squamous cell carcinoma showing keratinization. *B*, Gland-forming adenocarcinoma. *C*, Small cell carcinoma with islands of small deeply basophilic cells and areas of necrosis. *D*, Large cell carcinoma, featuring pleomorphic, anaplastic tumor cells and absence of squamous or glandular differentiation.

phocyte). This is the classic **oat cell** (Fig. 16-41*C*). Other small cell carcinomas have spindle-shaped or polygonal cells and may be thus classified (spindle or polygonal small cell carcinoma). The cells grow in clusters that exhibit neither glandular nor squamous organization.

Electron microscopic studies show dense-core neurosecretory granules in some of these tumor cells. The granules are similar to those found in the neuroendocrine argentaffin (Kulchitsky) cells present along the bronchial epithelium, particularly in the fetus and neonate. The occurrence of neurosecretory granules, the ability of some of these tumors to secrete polypeptide hormones, and the presence (ascertained by immunohistochemical stains) of neuroendocrine markers such as neuron-specific enolase and parathormone-like and other hormonally active products suggest derivation of this tumor from neuroendocrine cells of the lining bronchial epithelium.

Small cell carcinomas have a strong relationship to cigarette smoking; only about 1% occur in nonsmokers. Most often hilar or central, they are the most aggressive of lung tumors, metastasize widely, and are virtually incurable by surgical means. They are the most common pattern associated with ectopic hormone production (see later).

Large Cell Carcinoma. This anaplastic carcinoma has larger, more polygonal cells and vesicular nuclei. Large cell carcinomas probably represent squamous cell carcinomas and adenocarcinomas that are so undifferentiated that they can no longer be recognized. Some of these large cell carcinomas contain intracellular mucin, some exhibit larger numbers of multinucleate cells (**giant cell carcinoma**), some have cleared cells and are termed **clear cell carcinoma**, and some have a distinctly spindly histologic appearance (**spindle cell carcinoma**).

Secondary Pathology. Bronchogenic carcinomas cause related anatomic changes in the lung substance distal to the point of bronchial involvement. **Partial obstruction may cause marked focal emphysema; total obstruction may lead to atelectasis.** The impaired drainage of the airways is a common cause for **severe suppurative or ulcerative bronchitis or bronchiectasis. Pulmonary abscesses** sometimes call attention to a silent carcinoma that has initiated the chronic suppuration. Compression or invasion of the superior vena cava can cause venous congestion, dusky head and arm edema, and, ultimately, circulatory compromise—the **superior vena cava syndrome.** Extension to the pericardial or pleural sacs may cause **pericarditis** (Chapter 13) or **pleuritis** with significant effusions.

Staging. A uniform TNM system for staging cancer according to its anatomic extent at the time of diagnosis is extremely useful for many reasons, chiefly for comparing treatment results from different centers. The staging system in current use[95] is presented in Table 16–10.

Clinical Course. Lung cancer is one of the most insidious and aggressive neoplasms in the whole realm of oncology. In the usual case, it is discovered in patients in their fifties whose symptoms are of approximately 7 months' duration. The major presenting complaints are cough (75%), weight loss (40%), chest pain (40%), and dyspnea (20%). Increased sputum production is common and often contains diagnostic tumor cells when examined as cytologic specimens (Fig. 16–42*A*). Similarly, cytologic examination of a fine-needle aspirate of a tumor mass can often provide the diagnosis (Fig. 16–42*B*). Some of the more common local manifestations of tumor and their pathologic bases are listed in Table 16–11. Not infrequently, the tumor is discovered by its secondary spread during the course of investigation of an apparent primary neoplasm elsewhere.

The outlook is poor for most patients with bronchogenic carcinoma. Despite all efforts at early diagnosis by frequent radioscopic examination of the chest, cytologic examination of sputum and bronchial washings or brushings, and the many improvements in thoracic surgery, radiotherapy, and chemotherapy, the overall 5-year survival rate is on the order of 9%. In many large clinics, not more than 20 to

Table 16–10. NEW INTERNATIONAL STAGING SYSTEM FOR LUNG CANCER

T1	Tumor 3 cm without pleural or main stem bronchus involvement
T2	Tumor 3 cm or involvement of main stem bronchus 2 cm from carina, visceral, pleural, or lobar atelectasis
T3	Tumor with involvement of chest wall (including superior sulcus tumors), diaphragm, mediastinal pleura, pericardium, main stem bronchus 2 cm from carina, or entire lung atelectasis
T4	Tumor with invasion of mediastinum, heart, great vessels, trachea, esophagus, vertebral body, or carina or with a malignant pleural effusion
N0	No demonstrable metastasis to regional lymph nodes
N1	Ipsilateral hilar or peribronchial nodal involvement
N2	Metastasis to ipsilateral mediastinal or subcarinal lymph nodes
N3	Metastasis to contralateral mediastinal or hilar lymph nodes, ipsilateral or contralateral scalene, or supraclavicular lymph nodes
M0	No (known) distant metastasis
M1	Distant metastasis present

Stage Grouping

Stage Ia	T1	N0	M0
Stage Ib	T2	N0	M0
Stage IIa	T1	N1	M0
Stage IIb	T2	N1	M0
	T3	N0	M0
Stage IIIa	T1–3	N2	M0
	T3	N1	M0
Stage IIIb	Any T	N3	M0
	T3	N2	M0
	T4	Any N	M0
Stage IV	Any T	Any N	M1

Modified from Mountain C: Revisions in the International System for Staging Lung Cancer. Chest 111:1710, 1997.

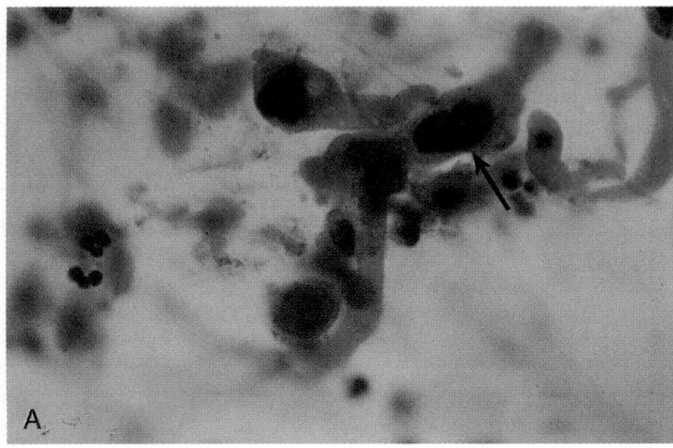

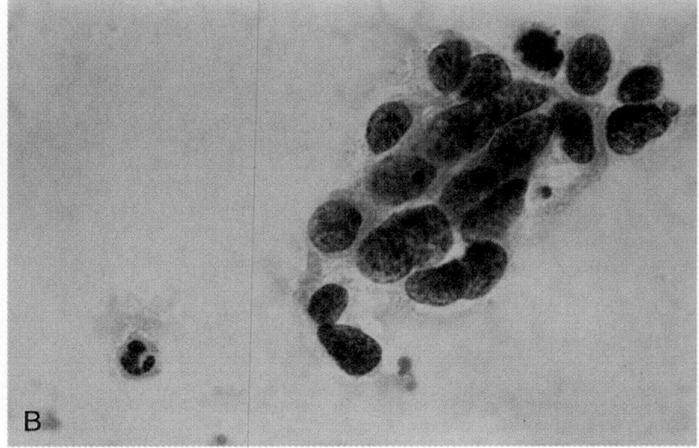

Figure 16–42

Cytologic diagnosis of lung cancer is often possible. *A*, A sputum specimen shows an organophilic, keratinized squamous carcinoma cell with a prominent hyperchromatic nucleus *(arrow)*. *B*, A fine-needle aspirate of an enlarged lymph node shows clusters of tumor cells from a small cell carcinoma, with molding and nuclear atypia characteristic of this tumor (see also Fig. 16–41*C*); note the size of the tumor cells compared with normal polymorphonuclear leukocytes in the left lower corner.

30% of lung cancer patients have lesions sufficiently localized to permit even an attempt at resection. In general, the adenocarcinoma and squamous cell patterns tend to remain localized longer and have a slightly better prognosis than do the undifferentiated cancers, which usually are advanced lesions by the time they are discovered. The overall 5-year survival rate of men is approximately 10% for squamous cell carcinoma and adenocarcinoma but only 3% for undifferentiated lesions. Surgical resection for *small cell carcinoma* is so ineffective that the diagnosis essentially precludes surgery. Untreated, the survival time for patients with small cell cancer is 6 to 17 weeks. This cancer is particularly sensitive to radiation and chemotherapy, and potential cure rates of 15 to 25% for limited disease have been reported in some centers. Most patients have distant metastases on diagnosis. Thus, even with treatment, the mean survival after diagnosis is about 1 year.

Table 16–11. LOCAL EFFECTS OF LUNG TUMOR SPREAD

Clinical Feature	Pathologic Basis
Pneumonia, abscess, lobar collapse	Tumor obstruction of airway
Lipid pneumonia	Tumor obstruction; accumulation of cellular lipid in foamy macrophages
Pleural effusion	Tumor spread into pleura
Hoarseness	Recurrent laryngeal nerve invasion
Dysphagia	Esophageal invasion
Diaphragm paralysis	Phrenic nerve invasion
Rib destruction	Chest wall invasion
SVC syndrome	SVC compression by tumor
Horner syndrome	Sympathetic ganglia invasion
Pericarditis, tamponade	Pericardial involvement

SVC, superior vena cava.

Despite this discouraging outlook, many patients have been cured by lobectomy or pneumonectomy, emphasizing the continued need for early diagnosis and adequate prompt therapy. Indeed, In the uncommon instance of *localized solitary tumors less than 4 cm in diameter, surgical resection results in up to 40% 5-year survival for patients with squamous cell carcinoma and 30% for patients with adenocarcinoma and large cell carcinoma.*

Paraneoplastic Syndromes

Bronchogenic carcinoma can be associated with a number of paraneoplastic syndromes[96] (Chapter 8), some of which may antedate the development of a gross pulmonary lesion. The hormones or hormone-like factors elaborated include

- *Antidiuretic hormone* (ADH), inducing hyponatremia owing to inappropriate ADH secretion
- *Adrenocorticotropic hormone* (ACTH), producing Cushing syndrome
- *Parathormone, parathyroid hormone–related peptide, prostaglandin E, and some cytokines*, all implicated in the hypercalcemia often seen with lung cancer
- *Calcitonin*, causing hypocalcemia
- *Gonadotropins*, causing gynecomastia
- *Serotonin*, associated with the carcinoid syndrome

The incidence of clinically significant syndromes related to these factors ranges from 1 to 10% of all lung cancer patients, although a much higher proportion of patients show elevated serum levels of these (and other) peptide hormones. Any one of the histologic types of tumors may occasionally produce any one of the hormones, but tumors producing ACTH and ADH are predominantly small cell carcinomas, whereas those producing hypercalcemia are mostly squamous cell tumors. The carcinoid syndrome is associated rarely with small cell carcinoma but is more common with the bronchial carcinoids, described later.

Other systemic manifestations of bronchogenic carcinoma include the *Lambert-Eaton myasthenic syndrome*, in which muscle weakness is caused by autoimmune antibodies (possibly elicited by tumor ionic channels) directed to the neuronal calcium channel;[94] *peripheral neuropathy*, usually purely sensory; dermatologic abnormalities, including *acanthosis nigricans* (Chapter 27); hematologic abnormalities, such as *leukemoid reactions*; and finally a peculiar abnormality of connective tissue called *hypertrophic pulmonary osteoarthropathy*, associated with clubbing of the fingers.

Apical lung cancers in the superior pulmonary sulcus tend to invade the neural structures around the trachea, including the cervical sympathetic plexus, and produce a group of clinical findings that includes severe pain in the distribution of the ulnar nerve and *Horner syndrome* (enophthalmos, ptosis, miosis, and anhidrosis) on the same side as the lesion. Such tumors are also referred to as *Pancoast tumors*.

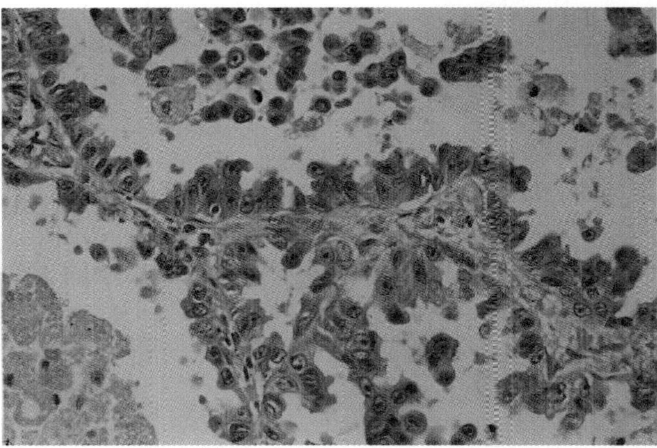

Figure 16–43

Terminal bronchioloalveolar carcinoma with characteristic tall, columnar cell papillary growth. Note the loose tumor cells in the alveoli, which may account for the "aerogenous" spread of tumor often observed.

BRONCHIOLOALVEOLAR CARCINOMA

As the name implies, bronchioloalveolar carcinoma occurs in the pulmonary parenchyma in the terminal bronchioloalveolar regions. It represents, in various series, 1 to 9% of all lung cancers. Changes are similar histologically to an apparently infectious disease of South African sheep known as *jagziekte*. Numerous efforts to identify an infectious agent in humans or to transmit the disease to sheep with cell-free extracts of human carcinoma, however, have been unavailing.

MORPHOLOGY. Macroscopically the tumor almost always occurs in the peripheral portions of the lung either as a single nodule or, more often, as multiple diffuse nodules that sometimes coalesce to produce a pneumonia-like consolidation. The parenchymal nodules have a mucinous, gray translucence when secretion is present and otherwise appear as solid, gray-white areas that can be confused with pneumonia on casual inspection.

Histologically, the tumor is characterized by distinctive, tall, columnar-to-cuboidal epithelial cells that line up along alveolar septa and project into the alveolar spaces in numerous branching papillary formations (Fig. 16–43). Tumor cells often contain abundant mucinous secretions. The degree of anaplasia is quite variable, but most tumors are well differentiated and tend to preserve the native septal wall architecture. Ultrastructurally, bronchioloalveolar carcinomas are a heterogeneous group, consisting of mucin-secreting bronchiolar cells, Clara cells, or, rarely, type II pneumocytes.

Clinical Course. These tumors occur in patients of all ages from the twenties to the advanced years of life. They are equally distributed among males and females. The symptoms, which usually appear late, are similar to those of bronchogenic carcinoma, with cough, hemoptysis, and pain the major presenting findings. Because the tumor does not involve major bronchi, atelectasis and emphysema are infrequent. Occasionally, they may produce a picture of diffuse interstitial pneumonitis. Solitary lesions are surgically resectable, resulting in a 50 to 75% 5-year survival rate, but the overall survival rate is about 25%. Metastases are not widely disseminated or large, and they do not occur early. Eventually, however, they appear in up to 45% of cases.

NEUROENDOCRINE TUMORS

Neuroendocrine tumors are pulmonary neoplasms that share morphologic and biochemical features with cells of the *dispersed neuroendocrine cell system* (Chapter 26).[97] The normal lung contains neuroendocrine cells within the epithelium as single cells or as clusters, the neuroepithelial bodies.[1, 95] Neoplasms of neuroendocrine cells in the lung include benign *tumorlets*, small, inconsequential hyperplastic neuroendocrine cells seen in areas of scarring or chronic inflammation; *carcinoids*; and the (already discussed) highly aggressive small cell carcinoma of the lung.

Bronchial Carcinoid

Bronchial carcinoids represent 1 to 5% of all lung tumors. They make up more than 90% of a group of bronchial tumors formerly classified as *bronchial adenoma* but now known to be often locally invasive or, occasionally, capable of metastasis. The remaining 10% of the group includes *adenoid cystic carcinoma* and *mucoepidermoid carcinoma*—tumors with histologic patterns reminiscent of similar tumors in salivary glands (Chapter 17). Most patients with carcinoid tumors are younger than 40 years of age, and the incidence is equal for both sexes There is no known relationship to cigarette smoking or other environmental factors. Bronchial carcinoids show the neuroendocrine differentiation of the Kulchitsky cells of bronchial mucosa and resemble intestinal carcinoids, described in detail in Chapter 18. They contain dense-core neurosecretory granules in their cytoplasm, secrete hormonally active polypeptides, and occasionally occur as part of multiple endocrine neoplasia.

MORPHOLOGY. On gross examination, the tumors grow as finger-like or spherical polypoid masses that commonly project into the lumen of the bronchus and are usually covered by an intact mucosa (Fig. 16–44*A*). They rarely exceed 3 to 4 cm in diameter. Most are confined to the main stem bronchi. Others, however, produce little intraluminal mass but instead penetrate the bronchial wall to fan out in the peribronchial tissue, producing the so-called collar-button lesion.

Histologically the tumor is composed of nests, cords, and masses of cells separated by a delicate fibrous stroma. In common with the lesions of the gastrointestinal tract, the individual cells are quite regular and have uniform round nuclei and infrequent mitoses (Fig. 16–44*B*). Occasional carcinoid adenomas display variation in the size and shape of cells and nuclei and, along with this pleomorphism, tend to demonstrate a more aggressive and more invasive behavior. On electron microscopy, the cells exhibit the dense-core granules characteristic of other neuroendocrine tumors and, by immunochemistry, are found to contain serotonin, neuron-specific enolase, bombesin, calcitonin, or other peptides.

Clinical Features. The clinical manifestations of bronchial carcinoids emanate from their intraluminal growth, their capacity to metastasize, and the ability of some of the lesions to elaborate vasoactive amines. Persistent cough, hemoptysis, impairment of drainage or respiratory passages with secondary infections, bronchiectasis, emphysema, and atelectasis all are byproducts of the intraluminal growth of these lesions.

Many carcinoids show infiltration or spread to local lymph nodes at the time of resection with apparently little ill effect on prognosis. Most interesting, albeit rare, are functioning lesions of the argentaffinoma pattern capable of producing the classic carcinoid syndrome, that is, intermittent attacks of diarrhea, flushing, and cyanosis. Overall, most bronchial carcinoids do not have secretory activity and do not metastasize to distant sites but follow a relatively benign course for long periods and are therefore amenable to resection. The reported 5- to 10-year survival rates for typical carcinoids are 50 to 95%. A minority (10%) of tumors show cytologic atypia, necrosis, and aggressive behavior (50% recurrence or metastasis after 2 years) and are designated *atypical carcinoids.*

MISCELLANEOUS TUMORS

Lesions of the complex category of benign and malignant mesenchymal tumors, such as fibroma, fibrosarcoma, leiomyoma, leiomyosarcoma, lipoma, hemangioma, hemangiopericytoma, and chondroma, may occur but are rare. Benign and malignant lymphoreticular tumors and tumor-like conditions, similar to those described in other organs, may also affect the lung, either as isolated lesions or, more commonly, as part of a generalized disorder. These include non-Hodgkin and Hodgkin lymphoma, lymphomatoid granulomatosis, pseudolymphoma, and plasma cell granuloma.

A lung *hamartoma* is a relatively common lesion usually discovered as an incidental, rounded focus of radiopacity (*coin lesion*) on a routine chest film. A new nodule in the lung requires clinical evaluation to determine whether a benign or malignant neoplasm has arisen. Pulmonary hamartomas are rarely greater than 3 to 4 cm in diameter and are composed principally of mature hyaline cartilage. Occasionally the cartilage contains cystic or cleftlike spaces, and

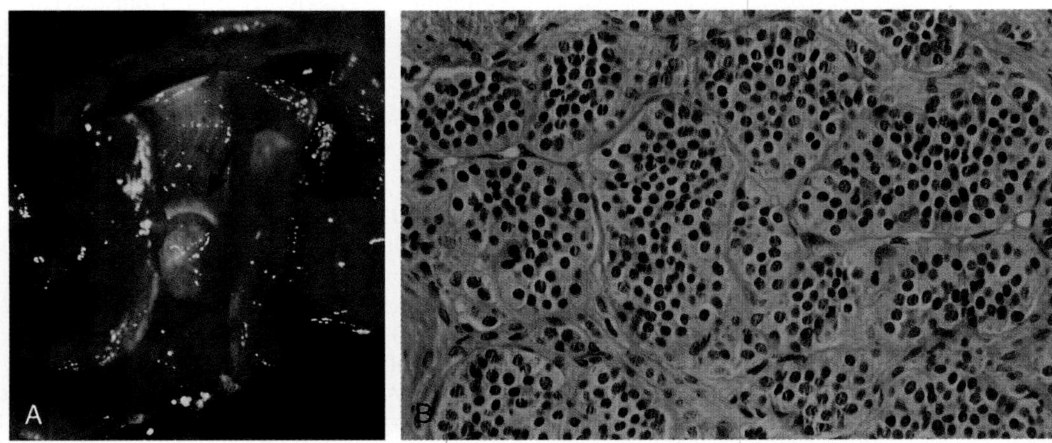

Figure 16–44

A, Bronchial carcinoid growing as a spherical, pale mass *(arrow)* protruding into the lumen of the bronchus. *B*, Histologic appearance of bronchial carcinoid, demonstrating small, rounded, uniform cells.

these may be lined by characteristic respiratory epithelium. At other times, there are admixtures of fibrous tissue, fat, and blood vessels. Recall that hamartomas are overgrowths of mature, normal tissues, in abnormal proportions (Chapter 8).

Tumors in the mediastinum either may arise in mediastinal structures or may be metastatic from the lung or other organs. They may also invade or compress the lungs. Table 16–12 lists the most common tumors in the various compartments of the mediastinum. Specific tumor types are discussed in appropriate sections of this book.

METASTATIC TUMORS

The lung is frequently the site of metastatic neoplasms. Both carcinomas and sarcomas arising anywhere in the body may spread to the lungs via the blood or lymphatics or by direct continuity. Growth of contiguous tumors into the lungs occurs most often with esophageal carcinomas and mediastinal lymphomas.

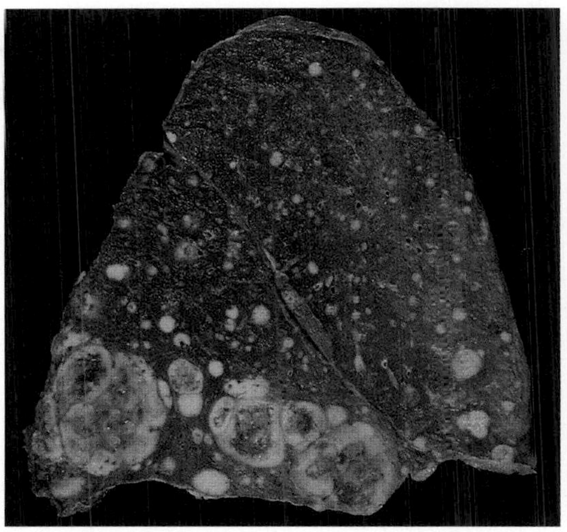

Figure 16–45 ■

Numerous metastases from a renal cell carcinoma. (Courtesy of Dr. Michelle Mantel, Brigham and Women's Hospital, Boston, MA.)

MORPHOLOGY. The pattern of metastatic growth within the lungs is quite variable. In the usual case, multiple discrete nodules are scattered throughout all lobes (Fig. 16–45). These discrete lesions tend to occur in the periphery of the lung parenchyma rather than in the central locations of the primary bronchogenic carcinoma.

As a second macroscopic variant, metastatic growth may be confined to peribronchiolar and perivascular tissue spaces, presumably when the tumor has extended to the lung through the lymphatics. Here the lung septa and connective tissue are diffusely infiltrated with the gray-white tumor. The subpleural lymphatics may be outlined by the contained tumor, producing a gross appearance referred to as *lymphangitis carcinomatosa.* Least commonly, the metastatic tumor is totally inapparent on gross examination and becomes evident only on histologic section as a diffuse intralymphatic dissemination dispersed throughout the peribronchial and perivascular channels. In certain instances, microscopic tumor emboli fill the small pulmonary vessels and may result in life-threatening pulmonary hypertension.

Table 16–12. MEDIASTINAL TUMORS AND OTHER MASSES

Superior Mediastinum
Lymphoma
Thymoma
Thyroid lesions
Metastatic carcinoma
Parathyroid tumors

Anterior Mediastinum
Thymoma
Teratoma
Lymphoma
Thyroid lesions
Parathyroid tumors

Posterior Mediastinum
Neurogenic tumors (schwannoma, neurofibroma)
Lymphoma
Gastroenteric hernia

Middle Mediastinum
Bronchogenic cyst
Pericardial cyst
Lymphoma

Pleura

Pathologic involvement of the pleura is, with rare exceptions, a secondary complication of some underlying disease. Secondary infections and pleural adhesions are particularly common findings at autopsy. Occasionally the secondary pleural disease assumes a dominant role in the clinical problem, as occurs in bacterial pneumonia with the development of empyema. Important primary disorders include (1) primary intrapleural bacterial infections that imply seeding of this space as an isolated focus in the course of a transient bacteremia and (2) a primary neoplasm of the pleura—mesothelioma (see later).

Pleural effusion is a common manifestation of both primary and secondary pleural involvements. Normally, no more than 15 ml of serous, relatively acellular, clear fluid lubricates the pleural surface. Increased accumulation of pleural fluid occurs in five setting as follows:

- Increased hydrostatic pressure, as in congestive heart failure
- Increased vascular permeability, as in pneumonia
- Decreased oncotic pressure, as in nephrotic syndrome
- Increased intrapleural negative pressure, as in atelectasis
- Decreased lymphatic drainage, as in mediastinal carcinomatosis

Table 16–13. PLEURAL SPACE FLUID ACCUMULATIONS

Condition	Type of Fluid	Common Associations
Inflammatory		
Serofibrinous pleuritis	Serofibrinous exudate	Inflammation in adjacent lung Collagen vascular disease
Suppurative pleuritis (empyema)	Pus	Suppurative infection in adjacent lung
Hemorrhagic pleuritis	Bloody exudate	Tumor
Noninflammatory		
Hydrothorax	Transudate	Congestive heart failure
Hemothorax	Blood	Ruptured aortic aneurysm, trauma
Chylothorax	Chyle (lymph)	Tumor obstruction of normal lymphatics

The character of the pleural effusion can be divided, for convenience, into inflammatory or noninflammatory, as summarized in Table 16–13.

INFLAMMATORY PLEURAL EFFUSIONS

Serous, *serofibrinous*, and fibrinous *pleuritis* all are caused by essentially the same processes. Fibrinous exudations generally reflect a later, more severe exudative reaction that, in an earlier developmental phase, might have presented as a serous or serofibrinous exudate.

The common causes of pleuritis are inflammatory diseases within the lungs, such as tuberculosis, pneumonia, lung infarcts, lung abscess, and bronchiectasis. Rheumatoid arthritis, disseminated lupus erythematosus, uremia, diffuse systemic infections, other systemic disorders, and metastatic involvement of the pleura can also cause serous or serofibrinous pleuritis. Radiation used in therapy for tumors in the lung or mediastinum often causes a serofibrinous pleuritis. In most instances, the serofibrinous reaction is only minimal, and the fluid exudate is resorbed with either resolution or organization of the fibrinous component. Accumulation of large amounts of fluid can sufficiently encroach on lung space to give rise to respiratory distress.

A purulent pleural exudate *(empyema)* usually results from bacterial or mycotic seeding of the pleural space. Most commonly, this seeding occurs by contiguous spread of organisms from intrapulmonary infection, but occasionally it occurs through lymphatic or hematogenous dissemination from a more distant source. Rarely, infections below the diaphragm, such as the subdiaphragmatic or liver abscess, may extend by continuity through the diaphragm into the pleural spaces, more often on the right side.

Empyema is characterized by yellow-green, creamy pus composed of masses of neutrophils admixed with other leukocytes. Although it may be difficult to visualize microorganisms on smears of the exudate, it should be possible to demonstrate them by culture. Although empyema may accumulate in large volumes (up to 500 to 1000 ml), usually the volume is small. Empyema may resolve, but this outcome is less common than organization of the exudate, with the formation of dense, tough fibrous adhesions that frequently obliterate the pleural space or envelop the lungs; either can seriously embarrass pulmonary expansion.

True *hemorrhagic pleuritis* manifested by sanguineous inflammatory exudates is infrequent and is found in hemorrhagic diatheses, rickettsial diseases, and neoplastic involvement of the pleural cavity. The sanguineous exudate must be differentiated from hemothorax (see later). When hemorrhagic pleuritis is encountered, careful search should be made for the presence of exfoliated tumor cells.

NONINFLAMMATORY PLEURAL EFFUSIONS

Noninflammatory collections of serous fluid within the pleural cavities are called *hydrothorax*. The fluid is clear and straw colored. Hydrothorax may be unilateral or bilateral, depending on the underlying cause. The most common cause of hydrothorax is cardiac failure, and for this reason it is usually accompanied by pulmonary congestion and edema. In cardiac failure, hydrothorax is usually, but not invariably, bilateral. Transudates may collect in any other systemic disease associated with generalized edema and are therefore found in renal failure and cirrhosis of the liver. Isolated right-sided hydrothorax occurs in Meig syndrome, an unusual combination of hydrothorax, ascites, and ovarian fibroma (Chapter 24).

In most instances, hydrothorax is not loculated, but in the presence of preexistent pleural adhesions, local collections may be found walled off by bridging fibrous tissue. Except for these localized collections, the fluid usually collects basally, when the patient is in an upright position, and causes compression and atelectasis of the regions of the lung surrounded by fluid. If the underlying cause is alleviated, hydrothorax may be resorbed, usually leaving behind no permanent alterations. Relief of respiratory distress is accomplished by the withdrawal of large pleural transudates.

The escape of blood into the pleural cavity is known as *hemothorax*. It is almost invariably a fatal complication of a ruptured aortic aneurysm or vascular trauma. Pure hemothorax is readily identifiable by the large clots that accompany the fluid component of the blood. Because this calamity often leads to death within minutes to hours, it is uncommon to find any inflammatory response within the pleural cavity. Rarely, nonfatal leakage of smaller amounts may provide a stimulus to organization and the development of pleural adhesions.

Chylothorax is an accumulation of milky fluid, usually of lymphatic origin, in the pleural cavity. Chyle is milky white because it contains finely emulsified fats. When it is allowed to stand, a creamy, fatty, supernatant layer separates. True chyle should be differentiated from turbid serous fluid, which does not contain fat and does not separate into an overlying layer of high fat content. Chylothorax may be bilateral but is more often confined to the left side. The volume of fluid is variable but rarely assumes the massive proportions of hydrothorax.

Chylothorax is most often caused by thoracic duct trauma or obstruction that secondarily causes rupture of major lymphatic ducts. This disorder is encountered in malignant conditions arising within the thoracic cavity that cause obstruction of the major lymphatic ducts. More distant cancers may metastasize via the lymphatics and grow within the right lymphatic or thoracic duct to produce obstruction.

PNEUMOTHORAX

Pneumothorax refers to air or gas in the pleural cavities and may be spontaneous, traumatic, or therapeutic. Spontaneous pneumothorax may complicate any form of pulmonary disease that causes rupture of an alveolus. An abscess cavity that communicates either directly with the pleural space or with the lung interstitial tissue may also lead to the escape of air. In the latter circumstance, the air may dissect through the lung substance or back through the mediastinum (interstitial emphysema), eventually entering the pleural cavity. Pneumothorax is most commonly associated with emphysema, asthma, and tuberculosis. Traumatic pneumothorax is usually caused by some perforating injury to the chest wall, but sometimes the trauma pierces the lung and thus provides two avenues for the accumulation of air within the pleural spaces. Resorption of the pleural space air occurs slowly in spontaneous and traumatic pneumothorax, provided that the original communication seals itself. Therapeutic pneumothorax was once a commonly practiced method of deflating the lung to favor the healing of tuberculous lesions.

Of the various forms of pneumothorax, the one that attracts greatest clinical attention is so-called *spontaneous idiopathic pneumothorax*. This entity is encountered in relatively young people; appears to be due to rupture of small, peripheral, usually apical subpleural blebs; and usually subsides spontaneously as the air is resorbed. Recurrent attacks are common and may be quite disabling.

Pneumothorax can be identified anatomically only by careful opening of the thoracic cavity under water to detect the escape of gas or air bubbles. Pneumothorax may have as much clinical significance as a fluid collection in the lungs because it also causes compression, collapse, and atelectasis of the lung and may be responsible for marked respiratory distress. Occasionally the lung collapse is marked. When the defect acts as a flap valve and permits the entrance of air during inspiration but fails to permit its escape during expiration, it effectively acts as a pump that creates the progressively increasing pressures of *tension pneumothorax*, which may be sufficient to compress the vital mediastinal structures and the contralateral lung.

PLEURAL TUMORS

The pleura may be involved in primary or secondary tumors. Secondary metastatic involvement is far more common than are primary tumors. The most frequent metastatic malignancies arise from primary neoplasms of the lung and breast. Advanced mammary carcinomas frequently penetrate the thoracic wall directly to involve the parietal and then the visceral pleura. They may also reach these cavities through the lymphatics and, more rarely, the blood. In addition to these cancers, malignancy from any organ of the body may spread to the pleural spaces. Ovarian carcinomas, for example, tend to cause widespread implants in both the abdominal and the thoracic cavities. In most metastatic involvements, a serous or serosanguineous effusion follows that may contain desquamated neoplastic cells. For this reason, careful cytologic examination of the sediment is of considerable diagnostic value.

Solitary Fibrous Tumors (Pleural Fibroma)

This benign pleural neoplasm, sometimes called *benign mesothelioma*, is a localized growth that is often attached to the pleural surface by a pedicle.[98] The tumor may be small (1 to 2 cm in diameter) or may reach an enormous size, but it always remains confined to the surface of the lung. These tumors do not usually produce a pleural effusion. Grossly, they consist of dense fibrous tissue with occasional cysts filled with viscid fluid; microscopically the tumors show whorls of reticulin and collagen fibers among which are interspersed spindle cells resembling fibroblasts. The tumor cells are CD34+, keratin-negative by immunostaining. This feature can be diagnostically useful in distinguishing these lesions from true malignant mesotheliomas (which show the opposite phenotype). The benign fibrous tumor has no relationship to asbestos exposure.

Malignant Mesothelioma

Malignant mesotheliomas in the thorax arise from either the visceral or the parietal pleura.[99,100] Although uncommon, they have assumed great importance in the past few years because of their increased incidence among persons with heavy exposure to asbestos (see the section on pneumoconioses earlier). In coastal areas with shipping industries in the United States and Great Britain and in Canadian and South African mining areas, up to 90% of reported mesotheliomas are asbestos-related. The lifetime risk of developing mesothelioma in heavily exposed individuals is as high as 7 to 10%. There is a long period of 25 to 45 years for the development of asbestos-related mesothelioma, and there seems to be no increased risk of mesothelioma in asbestos workers who smoke. *This is in contrast to the risk of asbestos-related bronchogenic carcinoma, already high, and is markedly magnified by smoking. Thus, for asbestos workers (particularly those who are also smokers), the risk of dying of lung carcinoma far exceeds that of developing mesothelioma.*

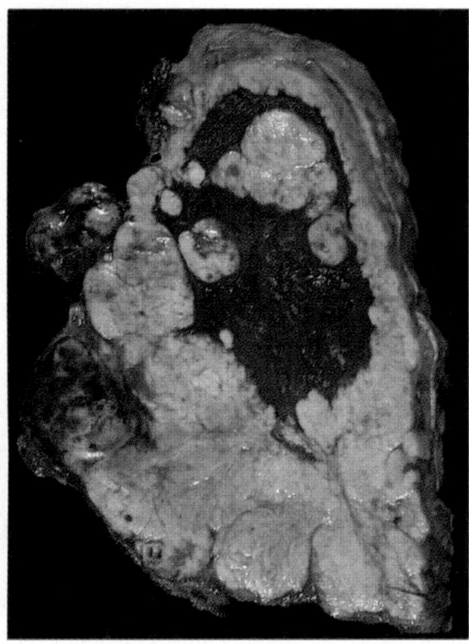

Figure 16–46

Malignant mesothelioma. Note the thick, firm, white, pleural tumor tissue that ensheathes this bisected lung.

Asbestos bodies (see Fig. 16–30) are found in increased numbers in the lungs of patients with mesothelioma, and mesotheliomas can be induced readily in experimental animals by intrapleural injections of asbestos.[101] Another marker of *asbestos exposure*, the *asbestos plaque*, has been previously discussed. There is little doubt about the carcinogenicity of asbestos; the mechanisms of cancer induction are discussed in Chapter 8.

MORPHOLOGY. Malignant mesothelioma is a diffuse lesion that spreads widely in the pleural space and is usually associated with extensive pleural effusion and direct invasion of thoracic structures. The affected lung is ensheathed by a thick layer of soft, gelatinous, grayish pink tumor tissue (Fig. 16–46).

Microscopically, malignant mesotheliomas consist of a mixture of two types of cells, either one of which might predominate in an individual case. Mesothelial cells have the potential to develop as either mesenchymal stromal cells or epithelium-like lining cells. The latter is the usual form of the mesothelium, an epithelium that lines the serous cavities of the body. The mesenchymal type of mesothelioma appears as a spindle cell sarcoma, resembling fibrosarcoma **(sarcomatoid type)**, whereas the papillary type consists of cuboidal, columnar, or flattened cells forming a tubular and papillary structure **(epithelial type)**, resembling adenocarcinoma (Fig. 16–47). Epithelial mesothelioma may at times be difficult to differentiate grossly and histologically from pulmonary adenocarcinoma. Special features that favor mesothelioma include the following[102]: (1) positive staining for acid mucopolysaccharide, which is inhibited by previous digestion by hyaluronidase; (2) lack of staining for carcinoembryonic antigen (CEA) and other epithelial glycoprotein antigens, markers generally expressed by adenocarcinoma; (3) strong staining for keratin proteins, with accentuation of perinuclear rather than peripheral staining (Fig. 16–48); and (4) on electron microscopy, the presence of long microvilli and abundant tonofilaments but absent microvillous rootlets and lamellar bodies (Fig. 16–48). The **mixed type** of mesothelioma contains both epithelial and sarcomatoid patterns. Cytogenetic abnormalities occur in mesotheliomas but not reactive mesothelial proliferations, a diagnostically useful feature.[99]

Clinical Course. The presenting complaints are chest pain, dyspnea, and, as noted, recurrent pleural effusions. Concurrent pulmonary asbestosis (fibrosis) is present in only 20% of patients with pleural mesothelioma. Fifty per cent of those with pleural disease die within 12 months of diagnosis, and few survive longer than 2 years. Aggressive therapy (extrapleural pneumonectomy, chemotherapy, radiation therapy) appears to improve this poor prognosis in some patients. The lung is invaded directly, and there is often metastatic spread to the hilar lymph nodes and, eventually, to the liver and other distant organs.

Mesotheliomas also arise in the peritoneum, pericardium, tunica vaginalis, and genital tract (benign adenomatoid tumor; Chapter 23). *Peritoneal mesotheliomas* are particularly related to heavy asbestos exposure; 50% of such patients also have pulmonary fibrosis. Although in about 50% of cases the disease remains confined to the abdominal cavity, intestinal involvement frequently leads to death from intestinal obstruction or inanition.

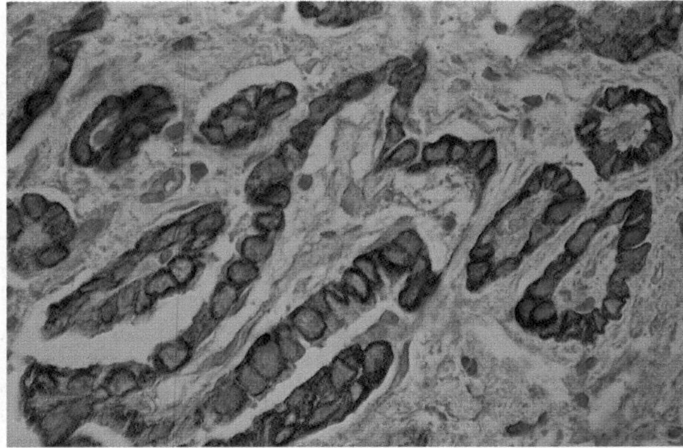

Figure 16–47

Malignant mesothelioma, epithelial type. The tumor cells are immunoperoxidase positive for keratin, as shown *(brown)*, but would be carcinoembryonic antigen negative.

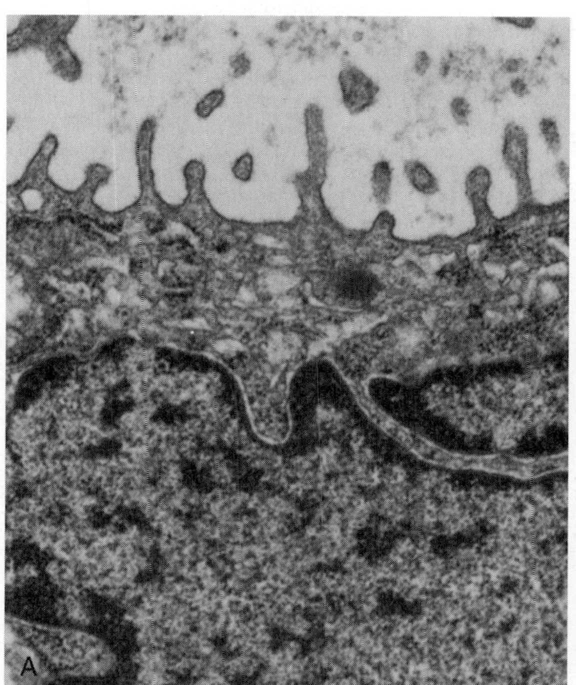

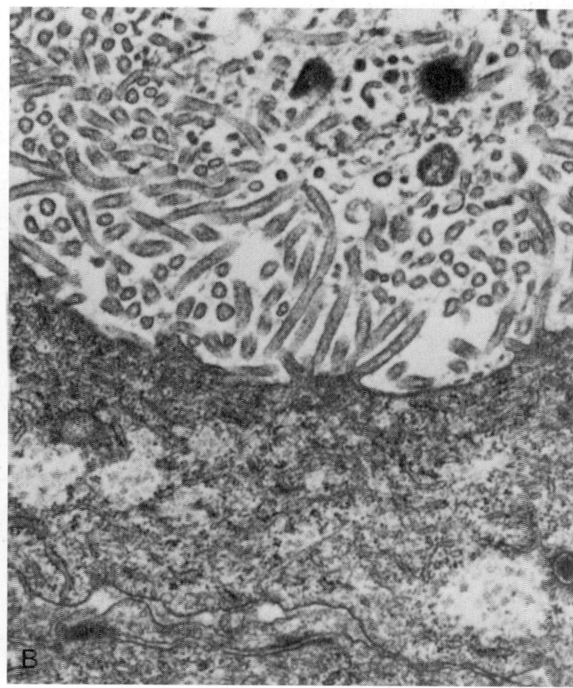

Figure 16–48

Ultrastructural features of pulmonary adenocarcinoma (*A*), characterized by short, plump microvilli, contrasted with those of mesothelioma (*B*), in which microvilli are numerous, long, and slender. (Courtesy of Dr. Noel Weidner, University of California, San Francisco, School of Medicine.)

REFERENCES

1. Gould S, Hasleton P: Congenital abnormalities. In Hasleton P (ed): Spencer's Pathology of the Lung. New York, McGraw-Hill, 1996, pp 57–114.
2. Bigatello LM, Zapol WM: New approaches to acute lung injury. Br J Anaesth 77:99, 1996.
3. Zapol W, Bloch K (eds): Nitric Oxide and the Lung. New York, Marcel Dekker, 1997.
4. Voelkel NF, Tuder RM: Cellular and molecular mechanisms in the pathogenesis of severe pulmonary hypertension. Eur Respir J 8: 2129, 1995.
5. Rubin LJ: Primary pulmonary hypertension. N Engl J Med 336:111, 1997.
6. Mark E, et al: Brief report: Fatal pulmonary hypertension associated with short-term use of fenfluramine and phentermine. N Engl J Med 337:602, 1997.
7. Burke A, et al: The pathology of primary pulmonary hypertension. Mod Pathol 4:269, 1991.
8. Pietra G, et al: Histopathology of primary pulmonary hypertension: A qualitative and quantitative study of pulmonary blood vessels from 58 patients in the National Heart, Lung, and Blood Institute primary pulmonary hypertension registry. Circulation 80:1198, 1989.
9. Fuster V, et al: Primary pulmonary hypertension: Natural history and the importance of thrombus. Circulation 70:580, 1984.
10. Snider GL, et al: The definition of emphysema. Report of the National Heart, Lung, and Blood Institute, Division of Lung Diseases Workshop. Am Rev Respir Dis 132:182, 1985.
11. Wright JL: Emphysema: concepts under change—a pathologist's perspective. Mod Pathol 8:873; 1995.
12. Lamb D: Chronic bronchitis, emphysema, and the pathological basis of chronic obstructive pulmonary disease. In Hasleton P (ed): Spencer's Pathology of the Lung. New York, McGraw-Hill, 1996, pp 597–630.
13. Gross P, et al: Enzymatically produced pulmonary emphysema: A preliminary report. J Occup Med 6:481, 1964.
14. Senior RM, et al: The induction of pulmonary emphysema with human leukocyte elastase. Am Rev Respir Dis 116:469, 1977.
15. Hautami R, et al: Requirement for macrophage elastase for cigarette smoke-induced emphysema in mice. Science 277:2002, 1997.
16. deMello D, Reid L: Chronic bronchitis. In Saldana M (ed): Pathology of Pulmonary Disease. Philadelphia, JB Lippincott, 1994, p 287.
17. Wright JL, et al: Diseases of the small airways. Am Rev Respir Dis 146:240, 1992.
18. Thurlbeck WM: Pathology of chronic airflow obstruction. In Cherniack NS (ed): Chronic Obstructive Pulmonary Disease. Philadelphia, WB Saunders, 1991, p 3.
19. Hogg JC, et al: Site and nature of airway obstruction in chronic obstruction lung disease. N Engl J Med 278:1355, 1968.
20. Cosio MG, et al: The relations between structural changes in small airways and pulmonary function tests. N Engl J Med 298:1277, 1978.
21. Colby TV: Bronchiolitis: pathologic considerations. Am J Clin Pathol 109:101, 1998.
22. Busse W, Holgate S: Asthma and Rhinitis. Boston, Blackwell Scientific, 1995.

22a. Holgate S: Asthma genetics: Waiting to exhale. Nat Genet 15:227, 1997.

23. Vogel G: New clues to asthma therapies. Science 276:1643, 1997.
24. Barnes P: Inflammatory mediators and neural mechanisms in severe asthma. In Szefler S, Leung D (ed): Severe Asthma: Pathogenesis and Clinical Management. New York, Marcel Dekker, 1996, p 129.
25. Galli SJ: The Paul Kallos Memorial Lecture: The mast cell: A versatile effector cell for a challenging world. Intl Arch Allergy Immunol 113:14, 1997.
26. Lilly CM, et al: Expression of eotaxin by human lung epithelial cells: Induction by cytokines and inhibition by glucocorticoids. J Clin Invest 99:1767, 1997.

27. Shelhamer J, et al: Airway inflammation. Ann Intern Med 123:288, 1995.
28. Costa JJ, et al: The cells of the allergic response: mast cells, basophils, and eosinophils. JAMA 278:1815, 1997.
29. Corne JM, Holgate ST: Mechanisms of virus induced exacerbations of asthma. Thorax 52:380, 1997.
30. Luce L: Bronchiectasis. In Murray J, Nadel J (eds): Textbook of Respiratory Medicine, Vol 2. Philadelphia, WB Saunders, 1994, pp 1398–1417.
31. Afzelius B: Ciliary dysfunction. In Crystal R, et al (eds): In The Lung: Scientific Foundations. Philadelphia, Lippincott-Raven, 1997, pp 2573–2578.
32. Pennington JE: Respiratory Infections: Diagnosis and Management, 3rd ed. New York, Raven Press, 1994.
33. Hasleton P: Atypical pneumonias. In Hasleton P (ed): Spencer's Pathology of the Lung. New York, McGraw-Hill, 1996, p 179.
34. Lomotan JR, et al: Aspiration pneumonia. Postgraduate Medicine 102:225, 229, 1997.
35. Barnes PF, et al: Tuberculosis in patients with human immunodeficiency virus infection. N Engl J Med 324:1644, 1991.
36. Bradford WZ, Daley CL: Multiple drug-resistant tuberculosis. Infect Dis Clin North Am 12:157, 1998.
37. Shinnick T (ed): Tuberculosis. Berlin, Springer, 1996.
38. Rosenow EC: Diffuse pulmonary infiltrates in the immunocompromised host. Clin Chest Med 11:55, 1990.
39. Nash G, et al: The pathology of AIDS. Mod Pathol 8:199, 1995.
40. Colby TV, Carrington CB: Interstitial lung disease. In Thurlbeck W, Churg A (eds): Pathology of the Lung. New York, Thieme Medical Publishers, 1995, p 589.
41. Chan-Yeung M, Muller NL: Cryptogenic fibrosing alveolitis. Lancet 350:651, 1997.
42. Kumar R, Lykke A: Messages and handshakes: Cellular interactions in pulmonary fibrosis. Pathology 27:18, 1995.
43. Vaillant P, et al: The role of cytokines in human lung fibrosis. Monaldi Arch Chest Dis 51:145, 1996.
44. Lynch JPI, et al: Neutrophilic alveolitis in idiopathic pulmonary fibrosis: The role of interleukin-8. Am Rev Respir Dis 145:1433, 1992.
45. Peters-Golden M: Lipid mediator synthesis by lung macrophages. In Lipscomb M, Russell S (eds): Lung Macrophages and Dendritic Cells in Health and Disease, Vol 102. New York, Marcel Dekker, 1997, pp 151–182.
46. Dockery D, et al: An association between air pollution and mortality in six U.S. cities. N Engl J Med 329:1753, 1993.
47. Pope C, et al: Health effects of particulate air pollution: Time for reassessment? Environ Health Perspect 103:472, 1995.
48. Vallyathan V, Shi X: The role of oxygen free radicals in occupational and environmental lung diseases. Environ Health Perspect 105(Suppl 1):165, 1997.
49. Vallyathan V, et al: Generation of free radicals from freshly fractured silica dust: Potential role in acute silica-induced lung injury. Am Rev Respir Dis 138:1213, 1988.
50. Kamp DW, Weitzman SA: Asbestosis: Clinical spectrum and pathogenic mechanisms. Proc Soc Exp Biol Med 214:12, 1997.
51. Green F, Vallyathan V: Coal workers' pneumoconiosis and pneumoconiosis due to other carbonaceous dusts. In Churg A, Green F (eds): Pathology of Occupational Lung Disease. Baltimore, Williams & Wilkins, 1998, p 129.
52. Godleski J: The pneumoconioses: Silicosis and silicatosis. In Saldana M (ed): Pathology of Pulmonary Disease. Philadelphia, JB Lippincott, 1994, p 387.
53. Vanhee D, et al: Cytokines and cytokine network in silicosis and coal workers' pneumoconiosis. Eur Respir J 8:834, 1995.
54. Piguet P, et al: Requirement of tumour necrosis factor for development of silica-induced pulmonary fibrosis. Nature 344:245, 1990.
55. Hammar S, Dodson R: Asbestos. In Hammar S, Dail D (eds): Pulmonary Pathology. New York, Springer-Verlag, 1996, pp 901–984.
56. Hammond E, et al: Asbestos exposure, cigarette smoking, and death rates. Ann N Y Acad Sci 330:473, 1979.
57. Tinkle SS, et al: Beryllium induces IL-2 and IFN-gamma in berylliosis. J Immunol 158:518, 1997.
58. Robinson B: Sarcoidosis. In Kradin R, Robinson B (eds): Immunopathology of Lung Disease. Boston, Butterworth-Heinemann, 1996, p 165.
59. Moller D, et al: Bias toward use of specific T cell receptor B-chain variable region in a subgroup of individuals with sarcoidosis. J Clin Invest 82:1183, 1988.
60. Balbi B, et al: Increased numbers of T lymphocytes with $\gamma\delta$-positive antigen receptors in a subgroup of individuals with pulmonary sarcoidosis. J Clin Invest 85:1353, 1990.
61. Mangiapan G, Hance AJ: Mycobacteria and sarcoidosis: An overview and summary of recent molecular biological data. Sarcoidosis 12:20, 1995.
62. Flint A, Colby TV: Surgical Pathology of Diffuse Infiltrative Lung Disease. Orlando, Grune & Stratton, 1987.
63. Richerson HB: Immune complexes and the lung: A skeptical review. Surv Synthesis Pathol Res 3:281, 1984.
64. Sharma OP, Fujimura N: Hypersensitivity pneumonitis: A noninfectious granulomatosis. Semin Respir Infect 10:96, 1995.
65. Kita H, et al: Cytokine production at the site of disease in chronic eosinophilic pneumonitis. Am J Respir Crit Care Med 153:1437, 1996.
66. Douglas N, Goetzl E: Pulmonary eosinophilia and eosinophilic granuloma. In Murray J, Nadel J (eds): Textbook of Respiratory Medicine. Philadelphia, WB Saunders, 1994, p 1913.
67. Tazelaar HD, et al: Acute eosinophilic pneumonia: Histopathologic findings in nine patients. Am J Respir Crit Care Med 155:296, 1997.
68. Katzenstein A-LA: Katzenstein and Askin's Surgical Pathology of Non-Neoplastic Lung Disease, 2nd ed. Philadelphia, WB Saunders, 1997.
69. Yousem SA: The histological spectrum of pulmonary graft-versus-host disease in bone marrow transplant recipients. Hum Pathol 26: 668, 1995.
70. Kelly PT, Haponik EF: Goodpasture syndrome: Molecular and clinical advances. Medicine 73:171, 1994.
71. Travis WD, Fleming MV: Vasculitis of the lung. Pathology 4:23, 1996.
72. Nishinakamura R, et al: The pulmonary alveolar proteinosis in granulocyte macrophage colony-stimulating factor/interleukins 3/5 beta c receptor-deficient mice is reversed by bone marrow transplantation. J Exp Med 183:2657, 1996.
72a. Dirksen V, Nishinakamura R, Groneck P, et al: Human pulmonary proteinosis associated with a defect in GM-CSF/IL-3/IL-5 receptor common β chain expression. J Clin Invest 100:2211, 1997.
73. Movsas B, et al: Pulmonary radiation injury. Chest 111:1061, 1997.
74. Hasleton P, Doran H: Pulmonary changes after transplantation. In Hasleton P (ed): Spencer's Pathology of the Lung. New York, McGraw-Hill, 1996, p 723.
75. Yousem SA, et al: Revision of the 1990 working formulation for the classification of pulmonary allograft rejection: lung rejection study group. J Heart Transplant 15:1, 1996.
76. Colby T, et al: Tumors of the Lower Respiratory Tract. Washington, DC, Armed Forces Institute of Pathology, 1995.
77. Landis SH, et al: Cancer statistics, 1998. CA Cancer J Clin 48:6, 1998.
78. Samet JM (ed): Epidemiology of Lung Cancer. New York, Marcel Dekker, 1994.
79. Smoking and Health: A National Status Report. A Report to Congress. Washington, DC, Department of Health and Human Services, 1987.
80. Auerbach O: Changes in bronchial epithelium in relationship to sex, age, residence, smoking and pneumonia. N Engl J Med 267:111, 1962.
81. Auerbach O: Changes in bronchial epithelium in relationship to cigarette smoking, 1955–1960 vs. 1970–1977. N Engl J Med 300: 285, 1979.
82. Marchevsky AM: Pathogenesis and experimental models of lung cancer. In Marchevsky AM (ed): Surgical Pathology of Lung Neoplasms. New York, Marcel Dekker, 1990, p 7.
83. Samet JM: Indoor radon and lung cancer: Estimating the risks. West J Med 156:25, 1992.
84. Pershagen G, et al: Residential radon exposure and lung cancer in Sweden [see comments]. N Engl J Med 330:159, 1994.
85. Abelson PH: Uncertainties about health effects of radon (editorial). Science 250:353, 1990.
86. Salgia R, Skarin AT: Molecular abnormalities in lung cancer. J Clin Oncol 16:1207, 1998.
87. Sundaresan V, Rabbits P: Genetics of lung tumors. In Hasleton P (ed): Spencer's Pathology of the Lung. New York, McGraw-Hill, 1996, p 987.

88. Gazdar A: The molecular and cellular basis of human lung cancer. Anticancer Res 13:261, 1994.
89. Cho JY, et al: Correlation between K-ras gene mutation and prognosis of patients with nonsmall cell lung carcinoma. Cancer 79:462, 1997.
90. Denissenko M, et al: Preferential formation of benzo[a]pyrene adducts at lung cancer mutational hotspots in p53. Science 274:430, 1996.
91. Barsky SH, et al: The extracellular matrix of pulmonary scar carcinomas is suggestive of a desmoplastic origin. Am J Pathol 124:412, 1986.
92. Yesner R, et al (eds): International Histological Classification of Tumors. Geneva, World Health Organization, 1982.
93. El-Torky M, et al: Significant changes in the distribution of histologic types of lung cancer. Cancer 65:2361, 1990.
94. Hoffman D, et al: The biological significance of tobacco-specific N-nitrosamines: Smoking and adenocarcinoma of the lung. Crit Rev Toxicol 26:199, 1996.
95. Mountain C: Revisions in the International System for Staging Lung Cancer. Chest 111:1710, 1997.
96. Patel A, et al: Paraneoplastic syndromes associated with lung cancer. Mayo Clin Proc 68:278, 1993.
97. Marchevsky AM: Neuroendocrine tumors of the lung. Pathology 4:103, 1996.
98. Steinetz C, et al: Localized fibrous tumor of the pleura: Correlation of histopathological, immunohistochemical and ultrastructural features. Pathol Res Pract 186:344, 1990.
99. Corson JM: Pathology of malignant mesothelioma. Semin Thorac Cardiovasc Surg 9:347, 1997.
100. Churg A: Neoplastic asbestos-induced diseases. In Churg A, Green F (eds): Pathology of Occupational Lung Disease. Baltimore, Williams & Wilkins, 1998, p 329.
101. Mossman BT, et al: Mechanisms of carcinogenesis and clinical features of asbestos-associated cancers. Cancer Invest 14:466, 1996.
102. Sheibani K, Stroup RM: Immunopathology of malignant mesothelioma. Pathology 4:191, 1996.

17

Head and Neck

ORAL CAVITY

INFLAMMATIONS

Herpes Simplex Virus Infections

Aphthous Ulcers (Canker Sores)

Oral Candidiasis (Thrush)

Glossitis

Xerostomia

REACTIVE LESIONS

ORAL MANIFESTATIONS OF SYSTEMIC DISEASE

Hairy Leukoplakia

TUMORS AND PRECANCEROUS LESIONS

Leukoplakia and Erythroplakia

Squamous Cell Carcinoma

ODONTOGENIC CYSTS AND TUMORS

UPPER AIRWAYS

NOSE

Inflammations

Necrotizing Lesions of the Nose and Upper Airways

NASOPHARYNX

Inflammations

TUMORS OF THE NOSE, SINUSES, AND NASOPHARYNX

LARYNX

Inflammations

Reactive Nodules (Vocal Cord Polyps)

Carcinoma of the Larynx

Squamous Papilloma and Papillomatosis

EAR

INFLAMMATORY LESIONS

OTOSCLEROSIS

TUMORS

NECK

BRANCHIAL CYST (LYMPHOEPITHELIAL CYST)

THYROGLOSSAL TRACT CYST

PARAGANGLIOMA (CAROTID BODY TUMOR)

SALIVARY GLANDS

INFLAMMATION (SIALADENITIS)

NEOPLASMS

Pleomorphic Adenoma

Warthin Tumor (Papillary Cystadenoma Lymphomatosum)

Mucoepidermoid Carcinoma

Other Salivary Gland Tumors

Diseases of the head and neck range from the common cold to the uncommon neoplasms of the nose. Those selected for discussion are assigned, sometimes arbitrarily, to one of the following anatomic sites: (1) oral cavity, particularly oral soft tissues, including the tongue; (2) upper airways, including the nose, pharynx, larynx, and nasal sinuses; (3) ears; (4) neck; and (5) salivary glands.

ORAL CAVITY

The oral cavity is a fearsome orifice guarded by ranks of upper and lower "horns" (lamentably, too subject to erosion), demanding constant gratification, and teeming with microorganisms, some of which are potentially harmful. Among the many disorders that affect its various parts, only the more important or frequent conditions involving the oral mucous membranes, lips, and tongue are considered. Disorders of the teeth and those limited to the gingiva are left for specialized dental texts, and those of the jaws for Chapter 28.

Inflammations

The oral mucosa is highly resistant to its indigenous flora, having many defenses, including the competitive suppression of potential pathogens by organisms of low virulence, the elaboration of secretory immunoglobulin A and other immunoglobulins by submucosal collections of lymphocytes and plasma cells, the antibacterial effects of saliva, and the diluting and irrigating effects of food and drink. Nonetheless, any lowering of these defenses, for example, with immunodeficiency or disruption of the microbiologic balance by antibacterial therapy, potentiates oral infection. Most of these infections are discussed in Chapter 9, and here we only briefly recapitulate the principal features.

HERPES SIMPLEX VIRUS INFECTIONS

Most orofacial herpetic infections (Chapter 9) are caused by herpes simplex virus type 1 (HSV-1) and are trivial "cold sores." Uncommonly, in children 2 to 4 years of age, they take the form of severe diffuse involvement of the oral and pharyngeal mucosa, the tongue, and the gingiva marked by fiery redness and swelling, soon followed by clusters of vesicles *(acute herpetic gingivostomatitis)*.

MORPHOLOGY. The vesicles range from lesions of a few millimeters to large bullae and, at first, are filled with a clear, serous fluid, but they often rupture to yield extremely painful, red-rimmed, shallow ulcerations. On microscopic examination, there is intracellular and intercellular edema (acantholysis), yielding clefts that may become transformed into macroscopic vesicles. Individual epidermal cells in the margins of the vesicle or lying free within the fluid sometimes develop eosinophilic **intranuclear viral inclusions,** or several cells fuse to produce giant cells **(multinucleate polykaryons),** changes that permit the diagnostic *Tzanck test* based on microscopic examination of the vesicle fluid. The vesicles and shallow ulcers usually spontaneously clear within 3 to 4 weeks, but the virus treks along the regional nerves and eventually becomes dormant in the local ganglia (e.g., the trigeminal).

The great preponderance of adults harbor latent HSV-1, but in some individuals, usually young adults, the virus becomes reactivated to produce the common but usually mild cold sore. The influences predisposing to activation are poorly understood but are thought to include upper respiratory tract infections; excessive exposure to cold, wind, or sunlight; and allergic reactions.

Recurrent herpetic stomatitis (in contrast to acute gingivostomatitis) takes the form of groups of small (1 to 3 mm) vesicles frequently on the lips, about the nasal orifices, or on the buccal mucosa. They resemble those already described in the primary infections but are much more limited in duration, are milder, usually dry up in 4 to 6 days, and heal within a week or 10 days.

APHTHOUS ULCERS (CANKER SORES)

These extremely common superficial ulcerations of the oral mucosa affect up to 40% of the population in the United States.[1] They are more common in the first two decades of life, are painful and often recurrent, and tend to be prevalent within certain families.

The lesions appear as single or multiple, shallow, hyperemic ulcerations covered by a thin exudate and rimmed by a narrow zone of erythema (Fig. 17–1). The underlying inflammatory infiltrate is at first largely mononuclear, but secondary bacterial infection introduces numerous neutrophils. The lesions may spontaneously clear within a week or be stubbornly persistent for weeks.

The causation of these lesions is obscure. Most ulcers are more painful than serious and require only symptomatic treatment.

ORAL CANDIDIASIS (THRUSH)

The many localizations of candidal infection are fully described in Chapter 9, and so it suffices here to merely emphasize that oral lesions typically take the form of a superficial, curdy, gray to white inflammatory membrane composed of matted organisms enmeshed in a fibrinosuppurative exudate that can be readily scraped off to reveal an underlying erythematous inflammatory base. As was pointed out, this fungus is a normal inhabitant of the oral cavity and causes mischief only in individuals who are diabetic, neutropenic, or immunoincompetent as in those with acquired immunodeficiency syndrome (AIDS); in those who have xerostomia or are otherwise debilitated; or when the normal flora of the oral cavity is perturbed by antibiotic therapy.

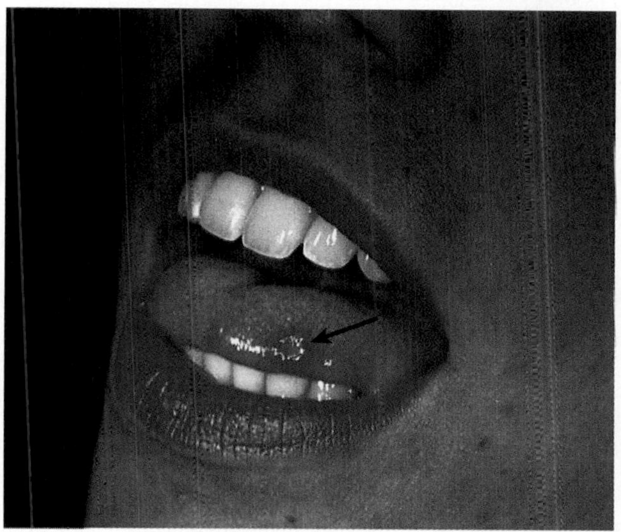

Figure 17–1

Aphthous ulcer of the tongue in a young woman. Doesn't it look painful? (Courtesy of Dr. John Sexton, Chief, Oral and Maxillofacial Surgery, Beth Israel Hospital, Boston, MA.)

GLOSSITIS

Although the designation glossitis implies inflammation of the tongue, it is sometimes applied to the beefy-red tongue encountered in certain deficiency states that results from atrophy of the papillae of the tongue and thinning of the mucosa, exposing the underlying vasculature. In some instances, the atrophic changes do indeed lead to inflammation and even shallow ulcerations. Such changes may be encountered in deficiencies of vitamin B_{12} (pernicious anemia), riboflavin, niacin, or pyridoxine. Similar alterations are sometimes encountered with sprue and iron deficiency anemia possibly complicated by one of the vitamin B deficiencies mentioned. *The combination of iron deficiency anemia, glossitis, and esophageal dysphagia usually related to webs is known as the Plummer-Vinson or Paterson-Kelly syndrome.* Glossitis, characterized by ulcerative lesions (sometimes along the lateral borders of the tongue), may also be seen with jagged carious teeth, ill-fitting dentures, and rarely syphilis, inhalation burns, or ingestion of corrosive chemicals.

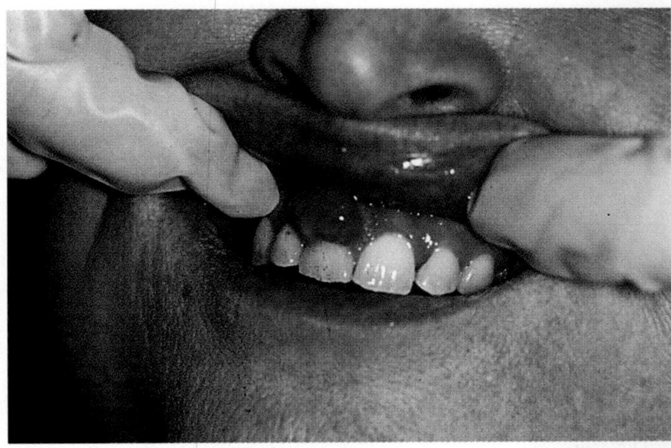

Figure 17–2 ■

"Pregnancy tumor" protruding from the margin of the upper gingiva. (Courtesy of Dr. John Sexton, Chief, Oral and Maxillofacial Surgery, Beth Israel Hospital, Boston, MA.)

XEROSTOMIA

Xerostomia refers to dry mouth; this manifestation is a major feature of the autoimmune disorder Sjögren syndrome in which it is usually accompanied by dry eyes (Chapter 7). A lack of salivary secretions may also be a residual of radiation therapy or may be drug induced by a wide variety of anticholinergic agents. The oral cavity may merely reveal dry mucosa or atrophy of the papillae of the tongue, with fissuring and ulcerations or, in Sjögren syndrome, concomitant inflammatory enlargement of the salivary glands.

Reactive Lesions

A number of soft tissue lesions of the oral cavity, which present as tumor masses, are indeed reactive in nature and represent inflammations and benign hyperplasias induced by irritation or by unknown mechanism. (All suspicious lesions, however, should be examined by biopsy.) Three deserve mention.

- The *irritation fibroma* mostly occurs in the buccal mucosa along the bite line or at the gingivodental margin. It consists of a nodular mass of fibrous tissue, with few inflammatory cells, covered by squamous mucosa.
- The *pyogenic granuloma* (Fig. 17–2) is a highly vascular, peduncular lesion usually occurring in the gingiva of children, young adults, and, commonly, pregnant women (pregnancy tumor). These lesions, which can also be considered a form of capillary hemangioma (Chapter 12), either regress, particularly after pregnancy, or undergo fibrous maturation and come to resemble a fibroma.
- The *peripheral giant cell granuloma (giant cell epulis)* is an unusual inflammatory lesion up to 1.5 cm in diameter that characteristically protrudes from the gingiva at some site of chronic inflammation. It is generally covered by intact gingival mucosa, but it may be ulcerated. On histologic evaluation, it is made up of a striking aggregation of multinucleate, foreign body–like giant cells separated by a fibroangiomatous stroma. Although not encapsulated, these lesions are usually well delimited and readily excised. They should be differentiated from central giant cell granulomas found within the maxilla or the mandible and from the histologically similar but frequently multiple reparative giant cell "brown tumors" seen in hyperparathyroidism (Chapter 28). The former may be locally aggressive, and some have a tendency to recur.

Oral Manifestations of Systemic Disease

As oral clinicians are at pains to emphasize, the mouth is a part of the body. Not surprisingly, then, many systemic diseases are associated with oral lesions. Some of the more common are cited in Table 17–1, with a few words about the associated oral changes. Only one—hairy leukoplakia—is characterized in more detail.

HAIRY LEUKOPLAKIA

Hairy leukoplakia is an uncommon oral lesion virtually restricted to patients with human immunodeficiency virus (HIV) infection.[2] Sometimes it calls attention to the existence of the infection. It takes the form of white, confluent patches of fluffy ("hairy") hyperkeratotic thickening situated anywhere on the oral mucosa. The distinctive microscopic appearance is attributable to piled up layers of keratotic squames based on underlying mucosal acanthosis. Sometimes there is koilocytosis of the superficial, nucleated epidermal cells, indicative of human papillomavirus (HPV) infection, and HIV transcripts have occasionally been

Table 17–1. ORAL MANIFESTATIONS OF SOME SYSTEMIC DISEASES

Infections	
Scarlet fever	Fiery red tongue with prominent papillae—raspberry tongue; white coated tongue through which hyperemic papillae project—strawberry tongue.
Measles	A spotty enanthema in the oral cavity often precedes the rash; ulcerations on the buccal mucosa about Stensen duct produce Koplik spots
Infectious mononucleosis	An acute pharyngitis and tonsillitis that may be coated with a gray-white exudative membrane; enlargement of lymph nodes in the neck
Diphtheria	A characteristic dirty white, fibrinosuppurative, tough, inflammatory membrane over the tonsils and retropharynx
Human immunodeficiency virus (HIV) infection–AIDS	Predisposition to opportunistic oral infections, particularly with herpesvirus, *Candida,* and other fungi; sometimes oral lesions of Kaposi sarcoma and hairy leukoplakia (described in text)
Dermatologic Conditions	
Lichen planus	Reticulate, lacelike, white keratotic lesions that rarely become bullous and ulcerated; seen in more than 50% of patients with cutaneous lichen planus and, rarely, is the sole manifestation
Pemphigus	Usually vulgaris; vesicles and bullae prone to rupture, leaving hyperemic erosions covered with exudate
Bullous pemphigoid	Oral lesions resemble macroscopically those of pemphigus but can be differentiated histologically (Chapter 27)
Erythema multiforme	A maculopapular, vesiculobullous eruption that sometimes follows an infection elsewhere, ingestion of drugs, development of cancer, or a collagen vascular disease; when it involves the lips and oral mucosa, it is referred to as *Stevens-Johnson syndrome*
Hematologic Disorders	
Pancytopenia (agranulocytosis, aplastic anemia)	Severe oral infections in the form of gingivitis, pharyngitis, tonsillitis; may extend to cellulitis of the neck *(Ludwig angina)*
Leukemia	With depletion of functioning neutrophils, oral lesions may appear like those in pancytopenia
Monocytic leukemia	Leukemic infiltration and enlargement of the gingivae, often with accompanying periodontitis
Miscellaneous	
Melanotic pigmentation	May appear in Addison disease, hemochromatosis, fibrous dysplasia of bone (Albright syndrome), and Peutz-Jegher syndrome (gastrointestinal polyposis)
Phenytoin (Dilantin) ingestion	Striking fibrous enlargement of the gingivae
Pregnancy	A friable, red, pyogenic granuloma protruding from the gingiva ("pregnancy tumor")
Rendu-Osler-Weber syndrome	Autosomal dominant disorder with multiple aneurysmal telangiectases from birth beneath the skin or mucosal surfaces of the oral cavity, lips, gastrointestinal tract, respiratory tract, and urinary tract as well as in internal viscera

found. However, Epstein-Barr virus (EBV) is present in most cases, and it is now accepted that EBV is the major cause of the condition.[3] Sometimes there is superimposed candidal infection on the surface of the lesions, adding to the "hairiness." When the hairy leukoplakia is a harbinger of HIV infection, manifestations of AIDS-related complex or AIDS generally appear within 2 or 3 years.

Tumors and Precancerous Lesions

Some common precancerous lesions and a variety of benign and malignant tumors occur in the oral soft tissues. Most of these tumors (e.g., hemangiomas, lymphomas) also occur elsewhere and are described adequately in other sections, and so only the precancerous leukoplakia, erythroplakia, papillomas, and squamous cell carcinoma are considered here.

LEUKOPLAKIA AND ERYTHROPLAKIA

The term leukoplakia means simply white plaque. It may be produced by several known conditions, such as lichen planus and candidiasis, as well as by other rarer lesions.[4] However, 85% to 90% of all white plaques are caused by epidermal proliferations, and so most experts recommend the following definition: *Leukoplakia is a white plaque on the oral mucous membranes that cannot be removed by scraping and cannot be classified clinically or microscopically as another disease entity.* All other white lesions are specified as to cause (e.g., lichen planus, candidal membrane). Thus defined, leukoplakic plaques range from benign epithelial thickenings to highly atypical lesions with dysplastic changes that merge with carcinoma in situ. Thus, *leukoplakia is a clinical term; until it is proved otherwise, it must be considered precancerous.*

Related to leukoplakia, but much less common and much more ominous, is *erythroplakia (dysplastic leukoplakia).* It represents a red, velvety, possibly eroded area within the oral cavity that usually remains level with or may be slightly depressed in relation to the surrounding mucosa. The epithelial changes in such lesions tend to be markedly atypical, incurring a much higher risk of malignant transformation than that with leukoplakia. Intermediate forms are occasionally encountered that have the characteristics of both leukoplakia and erythroplakia, termed *speckled leukoerythroplakia.*

Both leukoplakia and erythroplakia may be encountered in adults at any age, but they are usually found between the ages of 40 and 70 years, with a 2 to 1 male preponderance. *Although these lesions have multifactorial origins, the use of tobacco (cigarettes, pipes, cigars, and particularly chewing tobacco and buccal pouches) is the most common antecedent.* Other potentiating influences are alcohol, ill-fitting dentures, and chronic exposure to persistent irritants (lovers of hot pizza take note). HPV (human papillomavirus) sequences, particularly serotype 16, have been identified in tobacco-related lesions.[3]

MORPHOLOGY. Leukoplakias may occur anywhere in the oral cavity (favored locations are buccal mucosa, floor of the mouth, ventral surface of the tongue, hard palate). They appear as solitary or multiple, white patches or plaques with indistinct or sharply demarcated borders (Fig. 17–3*A*). They may be slightly thickened and smooth or wrinkled and indurated, or they may appear as raised, sometimes corrugated, verrucous plaques. On histologic examination, they present an epithelial spectrum ranging from hyperkeratosis overlying a thickened, acanthotic but orderly mucosal epithelium (Fig. 17–3*B*) to lesions with markedly dysplastic changes sometimes merging into carcinoma in situ. The more dysplastic or anaplastic the lesion, the more likely a subjacent inflammatory infiltrate of lymphocytes and macrophages.

The histologic changes in **erythroplakia** only rarely consist of orderly epidermal thickening; virtually all disclose superficial erosions with dysplasia, carcinoma in situ, or already developed carcinoma in the surrounding margins. An intense subepithelial inflammatory reaction with vascular dilation accounts for the red appearance of the lesion.

The frequency of carcinoma in situ or overt cancerous changes in leukoplakia varies among reports from 1% to 16%, but a reasonable average is 5% to 6%.[5] Ominous features are a speckled appearance, warty or verrucous thickening, and occurrence in "high-risk sites" (e.g., floor of the mouth and ventral surface of the tongue); hence the need for biopsy of persistent lesions that fail to respond to such simple measures as avoidance of tobacco and alcohol. In the case of erythroplakia, the malignant transformation rate is about 50% (some would say higher).

SQUAMOUS CELL CARCINOMA

At least 95% of cancers of the oral cavity (including the tongue) are squamous cell carcinomas. The small residual includes adenocarcinomas (of mucous gland origin), melanomas, various carcinomas, and other rarities. They represent about 3% of all cancers in the United States, and so they are by no means uncommon. Although most are readily accessible to discovery and biopsy, it is disheartening that many are detected late, and 50% of these lesions prove fatal. Squamous cell carcinomas are most frequently diagnosed in persons between the ages of 50 and 70 years.

Pathogenesis. The genesis of these cancers is linked to the use of tobacco and alcohol. Nondrinking smokers have a 2-fold to 4-fold greater risk of developing these cancers than matched control subjects do, which increases to 6-fold to 15-fold with both drinking and smoking. Particularly implicated are chewing tobacco and buccal pouches. The use of marijuana also increases risk. A major regional predisposing influence is the chewing of betel nuts and pan in India and parts of Asia. On the more pleasant side of the equation, several studies have reported that consumption of fruit and vegetables significantly reduces the risk.[6] Protracted irritation, as from ill-fitting dentures, jagged teeth, or chronic infections, is no longer thought to be an important direct antecedent to oral cancer, but it may contribute to leukoplakia, which, as has already been noted, is a subsoil for the development of oral cancer. HPV serotypes 6, 16, and 18 have been identified in half of the oral carcinomas arising in the Waldeyer tonsillar ring and in 10% to 15% of those in the tongue and other parts of the oral cavity.[7] Actinic radiation (sunlight) and, particularly, pipe smoking are known predisposing influences to cancer of the lower lip.

All these environmental influences presumably act on a fertile genetic soil, and indeed a number of chromosomal and molecular changes have been described in some but not all head and neck cancers.[8] These include deletions of chromosome regions 18q, 10p, 8p, and 3p; mutations in *p53*; and amplification of the *INT2* and *BCL1* oncogenes.[9, 10]

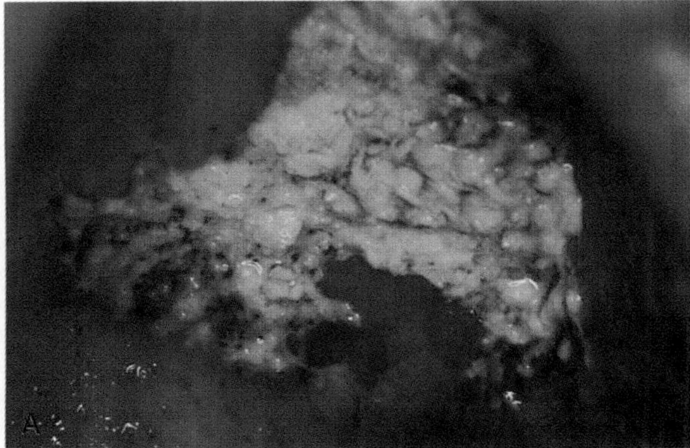

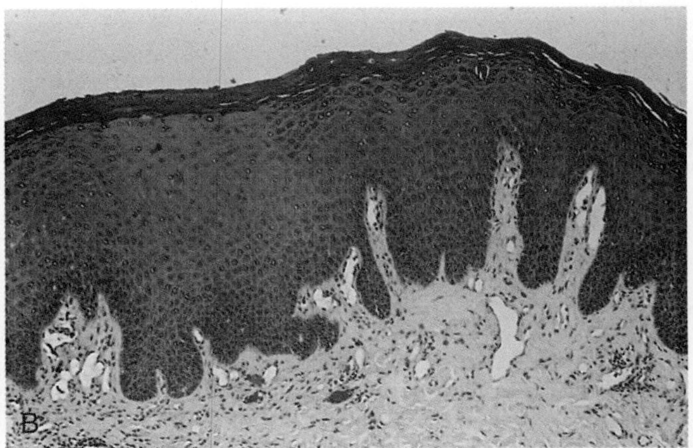

Figure 17–3

A, Leukoplakia of the hard palate. The numerous lesions have become virtually confluent. (Courtesy of Drs. E.E. Vokes, S. Lippman, et al, Department of Thoracic/Head and Neck Oncology, Texas Medical Center, Houston, TX. Reprinted with permission from The New England Journal of Medicine 328: 184, 1993.) *B*, Leukoplakia caused by marked epithelial thickening and hyperkeratosis.

MORPHOLOGY. Squamous cell carcinoma may arise anywhere in the oral cavity, but in large series, the favored locations are the floor of the mouth, tongue, hard palate, and base of tongue (Fig. 17–4). In the early stages, cancers of the oral cavity appear either as raised, firm, pearly plaques or as irregular, roughened, or verrucous areas of mucosal thickening, possibly mistaken for leukoplakia. Either pattern may be superimposed on a background of apparent leukoplakia or erythroplakia. As these lesions enlarge, they create protruding masses (Fig. 17–5) or undergo central necrosis, forming an irregular, shaggy ulcer rimmed by elevated, firm, rolled borders.

On histologic examination, these cancers begin as in situ lesions, sometimes with surrounding areas of epithelial atypicality or dysplasia. They range from well-differentiated keratinizing neoplasms to anaplastic, sometimes sarcomatoid tumors, and from slowly to rapidly growing lesions. As a group, they tend, in time, to infiltrate locally before they metastasize to other sites. The routes of extension depend on the primary site. Favored sites of metastasis are mediastinal lymph nodes, lungs, liver, and bones. Unfortunately, such distant metastases are often occult at the time of discovery of the primary lesion.[11]

As with all cancers, early diagnosis is the paramount prognostic factor. The prognosis is best with lip lesions, the 5-year recurrence-free rate approximating 90%, and poorest with tumors in the floor of the mouth and at the base of the tongue, yielding only 20% to 30% 5-year recurrence-free rates. All squamous cell carcinomas of the oral cavity take months to years to progress from carcinoma in situ to invasive cancer, and so every death they cause must be viewed as a preventable tragedy.

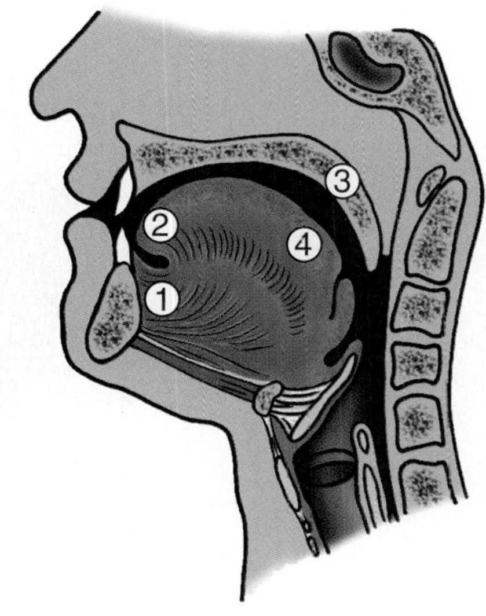

Figure 17–4

Schematic representation of the sites of origin of squamous cell carcinoma of the oral cavity, in numerical order of frequency.

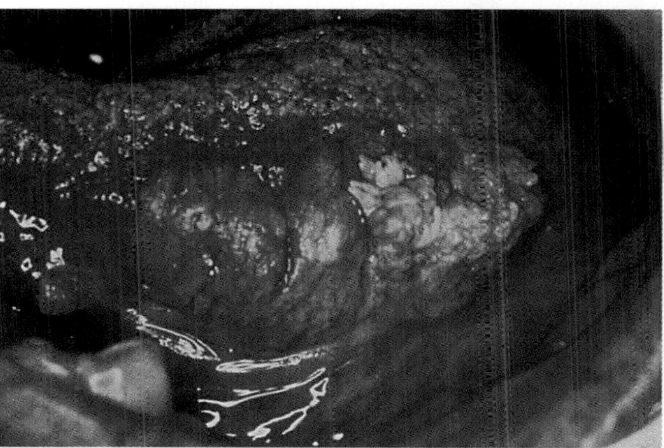

Figure 17–5

Carcinoma of the tongue. The tumor of the base of the tongue appears as a bulbous protruding mass. (Courtesy of Drs. E.E. Vokes, S. Lippman, et al, Department of Thoracic/Head and Neck Oncology, Texas Medical Center, Houston, TX. Reprinted with permission from The New England Journal of Medicine 328:184, 1993.)

Odontogenic Cysts and Tumors

These are specialized lesions that frequently affect dental structures and are beyond the scope of this discussion. However, some of them are associated with other systemic syndromes, and others present as soft tissue lesions in the oral cavity. For example, odontogenic cysts in the jaw, lined with keratinizing epithelium, are a component of the nevoid basal cell carcinoma syndrome (Gorlin syndrome), which as we shall see is related to mutations in the tumor-suppressor gene PATCHED (Chapter 27).

Odontogenic tumors are a complex group of lesions with diverse histology and clinical behavior.[3] Some are true neoplasms with malignant potential, and others are hamartomas. The two most common clinically significant tumors are

- *Ameloblastoma,* which arises from odontogenic epithelium and shows *no* ectomesenchymal differentiation. It is commonly cystic, slow forming, and locally invasive but has a benign course in most cases.
- *Odontoma,* the most common type of odontogenic tumor, which arises from epithelium but shows extensive depositions of enamel and dentin. Odontomas are probably hamartomas rather than true neoplasms and are cured by local excision.

UPPER AIRWAYS

The term upper airways is used here to include the nose, pharynx, and larynx and their related parts. Disorders of these structures are among the most common afflictions of humans, but fortunately the overwhelming majority are more nuisances than threats.

Nose

Inflammatory diseases, mostly in the form of the common cold, as everyone knows, are the most common disorders of the nose and accessory air sinuses. Most of these inflammatory conditions are viral in origin, but they are often complicated by superimposed bacterial infections having considerably greater significance. Much less common are a few destructive inflammatory nasal diseases and tumors primary in the nasal cavity or paranasal sinuses.

INFLAMMATIONS

Infectious Rhinitis. Infectious rhinitis, the more elegant way of saying "common cold," is in most instances caused by one or more viruses. Major offenders are adenoviruses, echoviruses, and rhinoviruses (Chapter 9). They evoke a profuse catarrhal discharge that is familiar to all and the bane of the kindergarten teacher. During the initial acute stages, the nasal mucosa is thickened, edematous, and red; the nasal cavities are narrowed; and the turbinates are enlarged. These changes may extend, producing a concomitant pharyngotonsillitis. Secondary bacterial infection enhances the inflammatory reaction and produces an essentially mucopurulent or sometimes frankly suppurative exudate. But as everyone knows, these infections soon clear up, usually in a week if appropriately treated but only after 7 days if ignored.

Allergic Rhinitis. Allergic rhinitis (hay fever) is initiated by sensitivity reactions to one of a large group of allergens, most commonly the plant pollens, fungi, animal allergens, and dust mites.[12] It affects 20% of the U.S. population. As is the case with asthma, allergic rhinitis is an immunoglobulin E–mediated immune reaction with an early- and late-phase response (see section on type I hypersensitivity in Chapter 7). The allergic reaction is characterized by marked mucosal edema, redness, and mucous secretion, accompanied by a leukocytic infiltration in which eosinophils are prominent.

Nasal Polyps. Recurrent attacks of rhinitis eventually lead to focal protrusions of the mucosa, producing so-called *nasal polyps,* which may reach 3 to 4 cm in length. On histologic examination, these polyps consist of edematous mucosa having a loose stroma, often harboring hyperplastic or cystic mucous glands and infiltrated with a variety of inflammatory cells, including prominently neutrophils, eosinophils, and plasma cells with occasional clusters of lymphocytes (Fig. 17–6). In the absence of bacterial infection, the mucosal covering of these polyps is intact, but with chronicity, it may become ulcerated or infected. When multiple or large, they may encroach on the airway and impair sinus drainage. Although the features of nasal polyps point to an allergic etiology, most patients with nasal polyps are not atopic, and only 0.5% of atopic patients develop polyps.[13]

Chronic Rhinitis. Chronic rhinitis is a sequel to repeated attacks of acute rhinitis, whether microbial or allergic in origin, with the eventual development of superimposed bacterial infection. A deviated nasal septum or nasal polyps with impaired drainage of secretions contribute to the microbial invasion. Frequently, there is superficial desquamation or ulceration of the mucosal epithelium and a variable inflammatory infiltrate of neutrophils, lymphocytes, and plasma cells subjacent to the epithelium. These suppurative infections sometimes extend into the air sinuses.

Sinusitis. Acute sinusitis is most commonly preceded by acute or chronic rhinitis, but maxillary sinusitis occasionally arises by extension of a periapical infection through the bony floor of the sinus. The offending agents are usually inhabitants of the oral cavity, and the inflammatory reaction is entirely nonspecific. Impairment of drainage of the sinus by inflammatory edema of the mucosa is an important contributor to the process and, when complete, may impound the suppurative exudate, producing *empyema* of the sinus. Obstruction of the outflow, most often of the

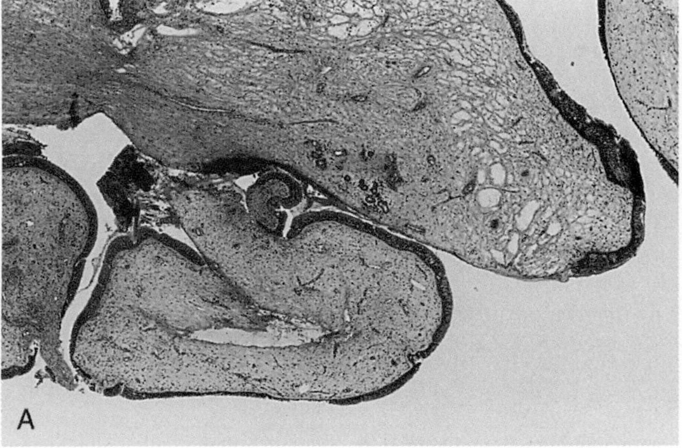

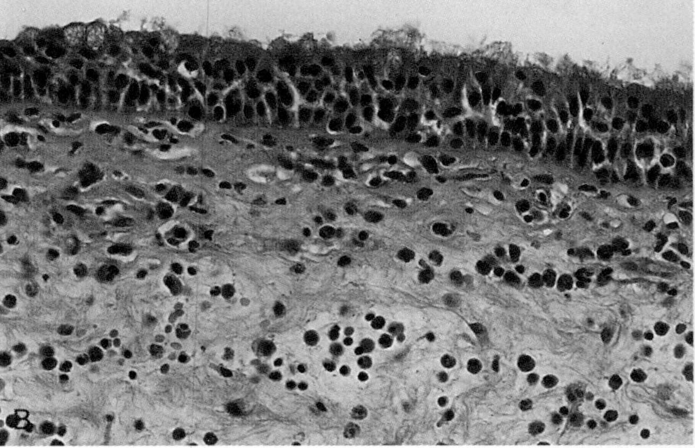

Figure 17–6

A, Nasal polyps. Low-power magnification showing edematous masses lined by epithelium. *B*, High-power views showing edema and eosinophil-rich inflammatory infiltrate.

frontal and next most often of the anterior ethmoid sinuses, occasionally leads to an accumulation of mucous secretions in the absence of direct bacterial invasion, producing a so-called *mucocele.* Acute sinusitis may, in time, give rise to *chronic sinusitis,* particularly when there is interference with drainage. There is usually a mixed microbial flora, largely of normal inhabitants of the oral cavity. Particularly severe forms of chronic sinusitis are caused by fungi (e.g., mucormycosis), especially in diabetics. Uncommonly, sinusitis is a component of *Kartagener syndrome,* which also includes bronchiectasis and situs inversus (Chapter 16). All these features are secondary to defective ciliary action. Although most instances of chronic sinusitis are more uncomfortable than disabling or serious, the infections have the potential of spreading into the orbit or of penetrating into the enclosing bone and producing osteomyelitis or, even, into the cranial vault, causing septic thrombophlebitis of a dural venous sinus.

NECROTIZING LESIONS OF THE NOSE AND UPPER AIRWAYS

Necrotizing ulcerating lesions of the nose and upper respiratory tract may be produced by

- Spreading fungal infections (principally mucormycosis [Chapter 9]), particularly in the diabetic
- Wegener granulomatosis (discussed in Chapter 12)
- A condition once called *lethal midline granuloma* or *polymorphic reticulosis* and now thought to represent, in most cases, angiocentric non-Hodgkin lymphoma, a neoplasm of natural killer cells[14] (Chapter 15). Ulceration and superimposed bacterial infection frequently complicate the process, confusing the histologic changes by producing tumor-related granulomatous inflammation. Concomitant lymphomatous lesions may be found in other organs and sites. At one time, these lesions were highly fatal owing to uncontrolled growth of the lymphoma, possibly with penetration into the cranial vault, or because of tumor necrosis with secondary bacterial infection and blood-borne dissemination of the infection. Currently, the treatment of the lymphoma with the usual modalities has proved to be effective, in many cases, in bringing the destructive process under control.

Nasopharynx

Although the nasopharyngeal mucosa, related lymphoid structures, and glands may be involved in a wide variety of specific infections (e.g., diphtheria, infectious mononucleosis discussed elsewhere) as well as by neoplasms, the only disorders mentioned here are nonspecific inflammations; tumors are discussed separately later.

INFLAMMATIONS

Pharyngitis and tonsillitis are frequent concomitants of the usual viral upper respiratory infections. Most often implicated are the multitudinous rhinoviruses, echoviruses, and adenoviruses, and less frequently respiratory syncytial viruses and the various influenzal strains. In the usual case, there is reddening and slight edema of the nasopharyngeal mucosa, with reactive enlargement of the related lymphoid structures. Bacterial infections may be superimposed on these viral involvements, or the bacteria may be primary invaders. The most common offenders are the β-hemolytic streptococci, but sometimes *Staphylococcus aureus* or other pathogens may be implicated. Particularly severe forms of pharyngitis and tonsillitis are seen in infants and children who have not yet developed any protective immunity to such agents and in adults rendered susceptible by neutropenia, some form of immunodeficiency, uncontrolled diabetes, or disruption of the normal oral flora by antibiotics. In these circumstances, microbial opportunists may be involved. The inflamed nasopharyngeal mucosa may be covered by an exudative membrane (pseudomembrane), and the nasopalatine and palatine tonsils may be enlarged and covered by exudate. A typical appearance is of enlarged, reddened tonsils (due to reactive lymphoid hyperplasia) dotted by pinpoints of exudate emanating from the tonsillar crypts, so-called *follicular tonsillitis.*

The major importance of streptococcal "sore throats" lies in the possible development of poststreptococcal complications, for example, rheumatic fever (Chapter 13) and glomerulonephritis (Chapter 21). Whether recurrent episodes of acute tonsillitis favor the development of chronic tonsillitis (true chronic tonsillitis is extremely rare) is open to debate, but they may leave residual enlargement of the lymphoid tissue, inviting the tender mercies of the otolaryngologist.

Tumors of the Nose, Sinuses, and Nasopharynx

Tumors in these locations are infrequent but include the entire category of mesenchymal and epithelial neoplasms.[14, 15] Brief mention may be made of somewhat distinctive types.

Nasopharyngeal Angiofibroma. This is a highly vascular tumor that occurs almost exclusively in adolescent males. Despite its benign nature, it may cause serious clinical problems because of its tendency to bleed profusely during surgery.

Inverted Papilloma. These are benign but locally aggressive neoplasms occurring in both the nose and the paranasal sinuses. As the name implies, the papillomatous proliferation of squamous epithelium, instead of producing an exophytic growth, extends into the mucosa, that is, is inverted (Fig. 17–7). If not adequately excised, it has a high rate of recurrence, with the potentially serious complication of invasion of the orbit or cranial vault; rarely, frank carcinoma may also develop. HPV DNA sequences have been identified in some patients.

Isolated Plasmacytomas. These extramedullary plasmacytomas (Chapter 15) arise in the lymphoid structures adjacent to the nose and sinuses. These may protrude within these cavities as polypoid growths, varying from 1 cm to several centimeters in diameter, covered usually by an in-

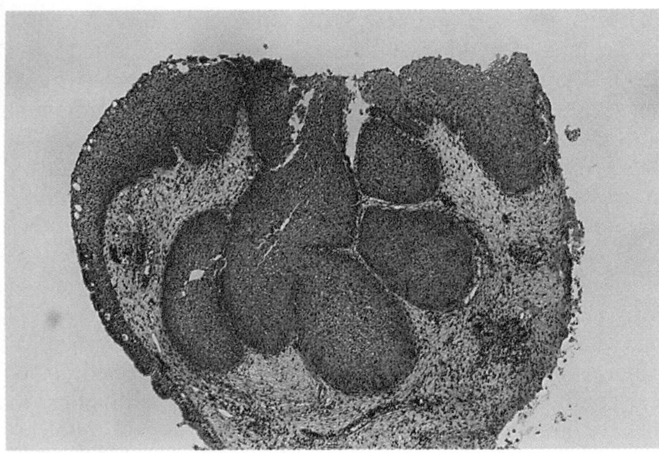

Figure 17–7

Inverted papilloma. The masses of squamous epithelium are growing inward; hence, the term *inverted.* (Courtesy of Dr. James Gulizia, Brigham and Women's Hospital, Boston, MA.)

tact overlying mucosa. The histology is that of a malignant plasma cell tumor and is identical to that described in Chapter 15. Only rarely do these lesions progress to multiple myeloma.

Olfactory Neuroblastomas (Esthesioneuroblastomas). These are uncommon, highly malignant tumors composed of small round cells resembling neuroblasts proliferating into lobular nests encircled by vascularized connective tissue. They arise most often superiorly and laterally in the nose from the neuroendocrine cells dispersed in the olfactory mucosa. The differential diagnosis of these neoplasms includes all other small cell tumors (Chapter 11), such as lymphoma, Ewing sarcoma, and embryonal rhabdomyosarcoma.[16] The cells are of neuroendocrine origin and thus exhibit membrane-bound secretory granules on electron microscopy and stain immunohistochemically for neuron-specific enolase, S-100 protein, and chromogranin. Although they are thus classifiable as primitive neuroectodermal tumors, many do not share the 11;22 translocation or fuscin-gene products typical of Ewing sarcoma of bone (Chapter 28) and other primitive neuroectodermal tumors.[16] Some of these tumors also reveal trisomy 8. Olfactory neuroblastomas tend to metastasize widely. Combinations of surgery, radiation, and chemotherapy yield a 5-year survival rate of 50% to 70%.[17]

Nasopharyngeal Carcinomas. This tumor is characterized by a distinctive geographic distribution, a close anatomic relationship to lymphoid tissue, and an association with EBV infection. It takes one of three patterns: (1) keratinizing squamous cell carcinomas, (2) nonkeratinizing squamous cell carcinomas, and (3) undifferentiated carcinomas that have an abundant non-neoplastic, lymphocytic infiltrate. The last pattern has often been called, erroneously, *lymphoepithelioma.*

Three sets of influences apparently affect the origins of these neoplasms: (1) heredity, (2) age, and (3) infection with EBV. Nasopharyngeal carcinomas are particularly common in parts of Africa, where they are the most frequent childhood cancer. In contrast, in southern China, they are the most common cancer in adults but rarely occur in children. In the United States, they are rare in both adults and children. Environment must play some role in this distribution, because migration from a high-incidence locale to a low-incidence locale is followed in the generations by a progressive decline in incidence. The EBV genome has been identified in the tumor epithelial cells (not the lymphocytes) of most undifferentiated and nonkeratinizing squamous cell nasopharyngeal carcinomas.[18] Its role in the pathogenesis of this tumor is discussed in Chapter 8.

MORPHOLOGY. On histologic examination, the keratinizing and nonkeratinizing squamous cell lesions more or less resemble usual well-differentiated and poorly differentiated squamous cell carcinomas arising in other locations. The undifferentiated variant is composed of large epithelial cells with oval or round vesicular nuclei, prominent nucleoli, and indistinct cell borders disposed in a syncytium-like array (Fig. 17–8). Admixed with the epithelial cells are abundant, mature, normal-appearing lymphocytes. The three histologic variants present as masses in the nasopharynx or sometimes in other locations, such as the tonsils, posterior tongue, or upper airways.

Nasopharyngeal carcinomas tend to grow silently until they have become unresectable and have often spread to cervical nodes or distant sites. Radiotherapy is the standard modality of treatment, yielding in most studies about a 50% to 70% 3-year survival rate. The undifferentiated carcinoma is the most radiosensitive, and the keratinizing the least radiosensitive.

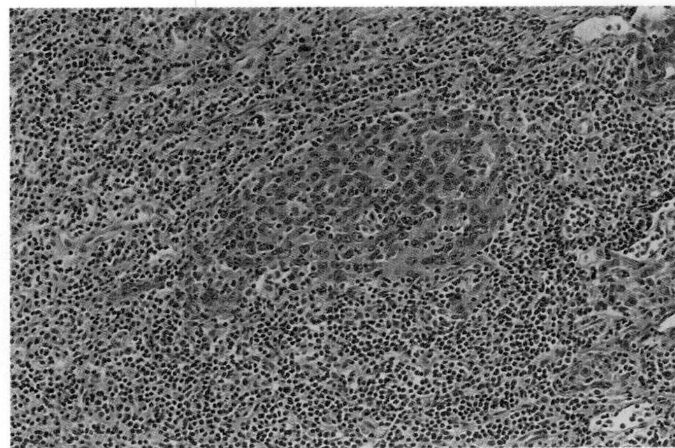

Figure 17–8

Nasopharyngeal carcinoma, lymphoepithelioma-type. The syncytium-like nests of epithelium are surrounded by lymphocytes. (Courtesy of Dr. James Gulizia, Brigham and Women's Hospital, Boston, MA.)

Larynx

The most common disorders that affect the larynx are inflammations. Tumors are uncommon but are amenable to resection, although often at the price of loss of natural voice.

INFLAMMATIONS

Laryngitis may occur as the sole manifestation of allergic, viral, bacterial, or chemical insult, but it is more commonly part of a generalized upper respiratory tract infection or the result of heavy exposure to tobacco smoke. The larynx may also be affected in many systemic infectious diseases, such as tuberculosis and diphtheria. Although most nonspecific microbiologic involvements are self-limited, they may at times be serious, especially in infancy or childhood, when mucosal congestion, exudation, or edema may cause laryngeal obstruction. In particular, laryngoepiglottitis, caused by *Haemophilus influenzae* or β-hemolytic streptococci in infants and young children with their small airways, may induce such sudden swelling of the epiglottis and vocal cords that a potentially lethal medical emergency is created. This form of disease is uncommon in adults owing to the larger size of the larynx and the stronger accessory muscles of respiration. *Croup* is the name given to laryngotracheobronchitis in children, in which the inflammatory narrowing of the airway produces the inspiratory stridor so frightening to parents. The most common form of laryngitis, encountered in heavy smokers, constitutes an important predisposition to the development of squamous epithelial changes in the larynx and sometimes overt carcinoma.

REACTIVE NODULES (VOCAL CORD POLYPS)

Reactive nodules, also called polyps, sometimes develop on the vocal cords, most often in heavy smokers or in individuals who impose great strain on their vocal cords *(singers' nodules).* Adults, predominantly men, are most often affected. These nodules constitute smooth, rounded, sessile or pedunculated excrescences, generally only a few millimeters in greatest dimension, located usually on the true vocal cords. They are usually covered by squamous epithelium that may become keratotic, hyperplastic, or even slightly dysplastic. The core of the nodule is a loose myxoid connective tissue that may be variably fibrotic or punctuated by numerous vascular channels. When nodules on opposing vocal cords impinge on each other, the mucosa may undergo ulceration.

Because of their strategic location, with corresponding greater inflammatory infiltration of the core of the lesion, they characteristically change the character of the voice and often cause progressive hoarseness. They virtually never give rise to cancers.

CARCINOMA OF THE LARYNX

Sequence of Hyperplasia, Dysplasia, Carcinoma. A spectrum of epithelial alterations is seen in the larynx. These are termed, from one end to the other, hyperplasia, atypical hyperplasia, dysplasia, carcinoma in situ, and invasive carcinoma.[19] Macroscopically, the epithelial changes range from smooth, white or reddened focal thickenings, sometimes roughened by keratosis, to irregular verrucous or ulcerated, white-pink lesions looking like cancer.

When first seen, the orderly thickenings have almost no potential for malignant transformation, but the risk rises to 1% to 2% during the span of 5 to 10 years with mild dysplasia and 5% to 10% with severe dysplasia. In essence, *there are all gradations of epithelial hyperplasia of the true vocal cords, and the likelihood of the development of an overt carcinoma is directly proportional to the level of atypia when the lesion is first seen.* Only histologic evaluation can determine the gravity of the changes.

The various changes described are most often related to tobacco smoke, the risk being proportional to the level of exposure. Indeed, up to the point of frank cancer, the changes often regress after cessation of smoking. However, alcohol is also clearly a risk factor and other factors may contribute to increased risk, including nutritional factors, exposure to asbestos, and irradiation.[20, 21] HPV sequences are present in about 5% of cases.[7]

MORPHOLOGY. About 95% of laryngeal carcinomas are typical squamous cell lesions. Rarely, adenocarcinomas are seen, presumably arising from mucous glands. The tumor usually develops directly on the vocal cords, but it may arise above or below the cords, on the epiglottis or aryepiglottic folds, or in the pyriform sinuses. Those confined within the larynx proper are termed **intrinsic,** whereas those that arise or extend outside the larynx are called **extrinsic.** Squamous cell carcinomas of the larynx follow the growth pattern of all squamous cell carcinomas. They begin as in situ lesions that later appear as pearly gray, wrinkled plaques on the mucosal surface, ultimately ulcerating and fungating (Fig. 17–9). The degree of anaplasia of the laryngeal tumors is highly variable. Sometimes massive tumor giant cells and multiple bizarre mitotic figures are seen. As expected with lesions arising from recurrent exposure to environmental carcinogens, adjacent mucosa may demonstrate squamous cell hyperplasia with foci of dysplasia, or even carcinoma in situ.

Carcinoma of the larynx manifests itself clinically by persistent hoarseness. At presentation, about 60% of these cancers are confined to the larynx; as a result, the prognosis is better than for those that have spread into adjacent structures. Later, laryngeal tumors may produce pain, dysphagia, and hemoptysis. Patients with this condition are extremely vulnerable to secondary infection of the ulcerating lesion. With surgery, radiation, or combined therapeutic treatments, many patients can be cured, but about one third die of the disease. The usual cause of death is infection of the distal respiratory passages or widespread metastases and cachexia.

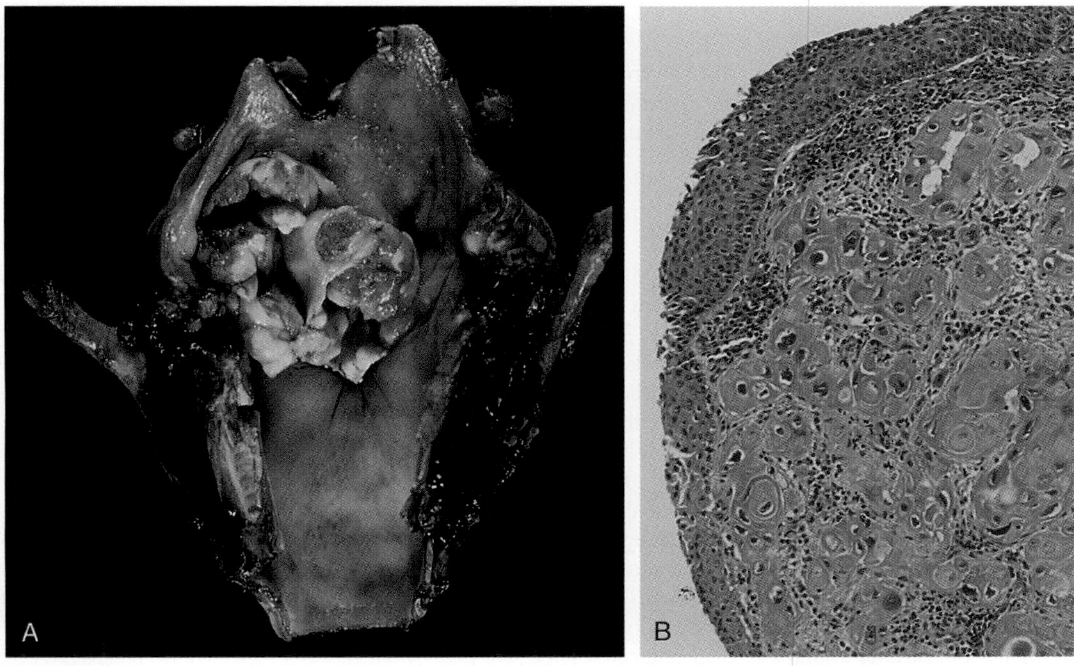

Figure 17–9

A, Laryngeal carcinoma. Note the large, ulcerated, fungating lesion involving the vocal cord and pyriform sinus. *B*, Histologic appearance of laryngeal squamous cell carcinoma. Note the atypical lining epithelium and invasive keratinizing cancer cells in the submucosa.

SQUAMOUS PAPILLOMA AND PAPILLOMATOSIS

Laryngeal squamous papillomas are benign neoplasms, usually on the true vocal cords, that form soft, raspberry-like excrescences rarely more than 1 cm in diameter (Fig. 17–10). On histologic examination, the papilloma consists of multiple, slender, finger-like projections supported by central fibrovascular cores and covered by an orderly, typical, stratified squamous epithelium. When the papilloma is on the free edge of the vocal cord, trauma may lead to ulceration that can be accompanied by hemoptysis.

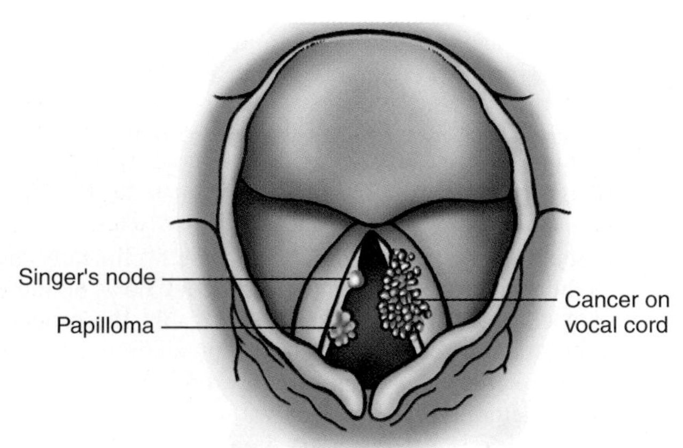

Figure 17–10

Diagrammatic comparison of a benign papilloma and an exophytic carcinoma of the larynx to highlight their quite different appearances.

Papillomas are usually single in adults but are often multiple in children, in whom they are referred to as *juvenile laryngeal papillomatosis.*[22] However, multiple recurring papillomas also occur in adults. *The lesions are caused by HPV types 6 and 11*, do not become malignant, but frequently recur. They often spontaneously regress at puberty, but some affected patients endure numerous surgeries before this occurs. Cancerous transformation is rare.

EAR

Although disorders of the ear rarely shorten the quantity of life, many impair its quality. The most common aural disorders, in descending order of frequency, are (1) acute and chronic otitis (most often involving the middle ear and mastoid), sometimes leading to a cholesteatoma; (2) symptomatic otosclerosis; (3) aural polyps; (4) labyrinthitis; (5) carcinomas, largely of the external ear; and (6) paragangliomas, found mostly in the middle ear. Only those conditions that have distinctive morphologic features are described. Paragangliomas are discussed later. All these entities are characterized here, save for labyrinthitis, which has few distinctive morphologic changes.

Inflammatory Lesions

Inflammations of the ear, *otitis media, acute or chronic,* occur mostly in infants and children. They usually produce a serous exudate (when viral in origin) but may become suppurative when bacterial infection becomes superimposed. The most common offenders are *Streptococcus pneumoniae, H. influenzae,* and β-hemolytic streptococci.

Repeated bouts of acute otitis media with failure of resolution lead to chronic disease. The causative agents of chronic disease are usually *Pseudomonas aeruginosa, Staphylococcus aureus,* or a fungus and, sometimes, a broadly mixed flora. Chronic infection has the potential to perforate the eardrum, encroaching on the ossicles or labyrinth, spreading into the mastoid spaces, and even penetrating into the cranial vault to produce there a temporal cerebritis or abscess. Otitis media in the diabetic person, when caused by *P. aeruginosa,* is especially aggressive and spreads widely (destructive necrotizing otitis media).

Cholesteatomas associated with chronic otitis media are not neoplasms, nor do they always contain cholesterol. Rather, they are cystic lesions 1 to 4 cm in diameter, lined by keratinizing squamous epithelium or metaplastic mucus-secreting epithelium, and filled with amorphous debris (derived largely from desquamated squames). Sometimes they contain spicules of cholesterol. The precise events involved in their development are not clear, but it is proposed that chronic inflammation and perforation of the eardrum with ingrowth of the squamous epithelium or metaplasia of the secretory epithelial lining of the middle ear are responsible for the formation of a squamous cell nest that becomes cystic. A chronic inflammatory reaction surrounds the keratinous cyst. Sometimes rupture not only enhances the inflammatory reaction but also induces the formation of giant cells that enclose partially necrotic squames and other particulate debris. These lesions, by progressive enlargement, can erode into the ossicles, the labyrinth, the adjacent bone, or the surrounding soft tissue and sometimes produce visible neck masses.

Otosclerosis

As the name implies, this condition refers to abnormal bone deposition in the middle ear about the rim of the oval window into which the footplate of the stapes fits. Both ears are usually affected. At first there is fibrous ankylosis of the footplate, followed in time by bony overgrowth anchoring it into the oval window. The degree of immobilization governs the severity of the hearing loss. This condition usually begins in the early decades of life; minimal degrees of this derangement are exceedingly common in the United States in young to middle-aged adults, but fortunately more severe symptomatic otosclerosis is relatively uncommon. In most instances it is familial, following autosomal dominant transmission with variable penetrance. The basis for the osseous overgrowth is completely obscure, but it appears to represent uncoupling of normal bone resorption and bone formation. Thus, it begins with bone resorption, followed by fibrosis and vascularization of the temporal bone in the immediate vicinity of the oval window, in time replaced by dense new bone anchoring the footplate of the stapes. In most instances, the process is slowly progressive during the span of decades, leading eventually to marked hearing loss.

Tumors

The large variety of epithelial and mesenchymal tumors that arise in the ear—external, medial, internal—are rare save for basal cell or squamous cell carcinomas of the pinna (external ear). These carcinomas tend to occur in elderly men and are thought to be associated with actinic radiation. By contrast, those within the canal tend to be squamous cell carcinomas, which occur in middle-aged to elderly women and are not associated with sun exposure. Wherever they arise, they morphologically resemble their counterparts in other skin locations, beginning as papules that extend and eventually erode and invade locally. Neither the basal cell nor the squamous cell lesions of the pinna often extend beyond local invasion, but squamous cell carcinomas arising in the external canal may invade the cranial cavity or metastasize to regional nodes and, indeed, account for a 5-year mortality of about 50%.

NECK

Most of the conditions that involve the neck have been described elsewhere (e.g., squamous cell and basal cell carcinomas of the skin, melanocarcinomas, lymphomas), or they are only a component of a systemic disorder (e.g., generalized rashes, the lymphadenopathy of infectious mononucleosis or tonsillitis). What remains for consideration here are a few uncommon lesions unique to the neck.

Branchial Cyst (Lymphoepithelial Cyst)

These benign cysts, usually appearing on the anterolateral aspect of the neck, arise either from remnants of the branchial arches or, as many believe, from developmental salivary gland inclusions within cervical lymph nodes.[23] Whatever their origin, they are circumscribed cysts, 2 to 5 cm in diameter, with fibrous walls usually lined by stratified squamous or pseudostratified columnar epithelium underlaid by an intense lymphocytic infiltrate or, more often, well-developed lymphoid tissue with reactive follicles. The cystic contents may be clear, watery to mucinous fluid or may contain desquamated, granular cellular debris. The cysts enlarge only slowly during the years, are rarely the site of cancerous transformation, and generally are readily excised. Similar lesions sometimes appear in the parotid gland or the oral cavity, beneath the tongue.

Thyroglossal Tract Cyst

Embryologically, the thyroid anlage begins in the region of the foramen caecum at the base of the tongue; as the gland develops, it descends to its definitive location in the anterior neck. Remnants of this developmental tract may persist, producing cysts, 1 to 4 cm in diameter, that may be lined by stratified squamous epithelium when the cyst is near the base of the tongue or by pseudostratified columnar epithelium in lower locations. Obviously, transitional patterns are also encountered. The connective tissue wall of the cyst may harbor lymphoid aggregates or remnants of recognizable thyroid tissue. If the excision is not complete, stubborn recurrence can be expected. Malignant transformation within the lining epithelium has been reported but is rare.

Paraganglioma (Carotid Body Tumor)

Paraganglia are clusters of neuroendocrine cells dispersed throughout the body, some connected with the sympathetic nervous system and others with the parasympathetic nervous system. The largest collection of these cells is found in the adrenal medulla, where they give rise to *pheochromocytomas* (Chapter 26). Tumors arising in extra-adrenal paraganglia are not surprisingly referred to as *paragangliomas*.[24] Paragangliomas develop in two general locations:

- Paravertebral paraganglia (e.g., organs of Zuckerkandl and rarely bladder). Such tumors have sympathetic connections and are chromaffin positive; about half elaborate catecholamines, as do pheochromocytomas.
- Paraganglia related to the great vessels of the head and neck, the so-called aorticopulmonary chain, including the *carotid bodies*; aortic bodies; jugulotympanic ganglia; ganglion nodosum of the vagus nerve; and clusters located about the oral cavity, nose, nasopharynx, larynx, and orbit. These are innervated by the parasympathetic nervous system, and their tumors are referred to as *nonchromaffin paragangliomas*. These tumors infrequently release catecholamines, but because the neuroendocrine cells that make up these lesions sense oxygen and carbon dioxide tensions within adjacent vessels, the tumors are also sometimes referred to as *chemodectomas*.

MORPHOLOGY. The **carotid body tumor** is a prototype of a parasympathetic paraganglioma. It rarely exceeds 6 cm in diameter and arises close to or envelops the bifurcation of the common carotid artery. The tumor tissue is red-pink to brown. The microscopic features of all paragangliomas, wherever they arise, are remarkably uniform. They are composed of nests **(zellballen)** of polygonal chief cells enclosed by trabeculae of fibrous and sustentacular elongated cells.[16] The tumor cells have abundant, clear or granular, eosinophilic cytoplasm and uniform, round to ovoid, sometimes vesicular nuclei (Fig. 17–11). In most tumors, there is little cell pleomorphism, and mitoses are scant. Electron microscopy often discloses well-demarcated neuroendocrine granules in paravertebral tumors, but they tend to be scant in nonfunctioning tumors. However, the cells in most tumors are argyrophilic and stain positively for neuroendocrine markers by immunohistochemistry (nonspecific enolase; S-100; chromogranin) as well as possibly other bioactive products (e.g., serotonin, gastrin, somatostatin, bombesin).

Carotid body tumors (and paragangliomas in general) are rare. They usually arise in the sixth decade of life. They commonly occur singly and sporadically but may be familial, with autosomal dominant transmission in the multiple endocrine neoplasia II syndrome (Chapter 26), and in this case, they are frequently multiple and sometimes bilaterally symmetric. Carotid body tumors frequently recur after incomplete resection, and despite their benign appearance, many metastasize to local and distant sites. About 50%

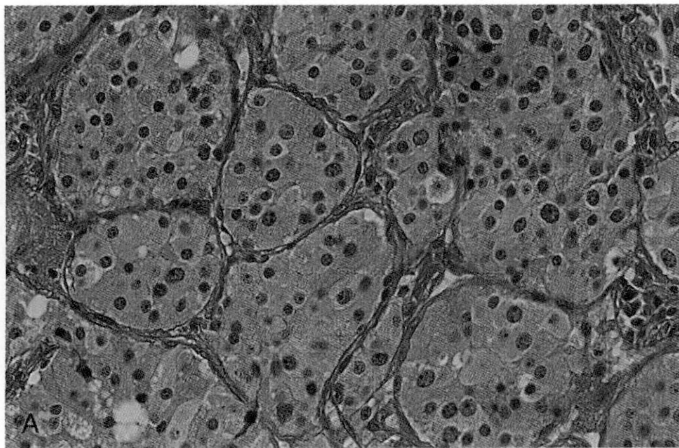

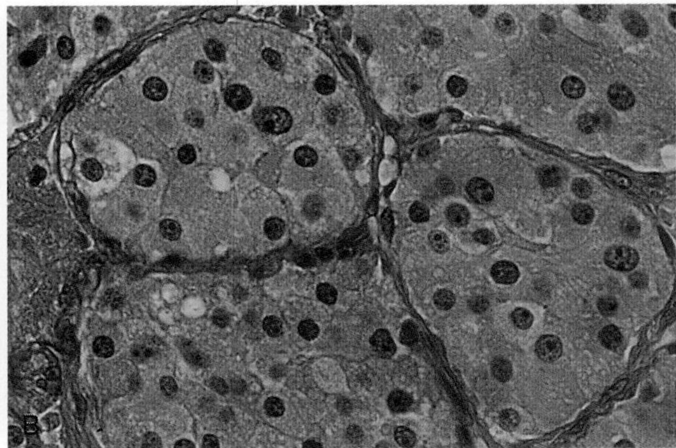

Figure 17–11

Carotid body tumor. *A*, Low-power view showing tumor clusters separated by septa (zellballen). *B*, High-power view of large, eosinophilic, slightly vacuolated tumor cells with elongated sustentacular cells in the septa.

ultimately prove fatal largely because of infiltrative growth. Unfortunately, it is almost impossible histologically to judge the clinical course of a carotid body tumor—mitoses, pleomorphism, and even vascular invasion are unreliable.[25]

SALIVARY GLANDS

There are three major salivary glands—parotid, submandibular, and sublingual—as well as innumerable minor salivary glands distributed throughout the mucosa of the oral cavity. All these glands, particularly the major ones, are subject to inflammation or to the development of neoplasms.

Inflammation (Sialadenitis)

Sialadenitis may be of viral, bacterial, or autoimmune origin. The most common form of viral sialadenitis is mumps, in which usually the major salivary glands, particularly the parotids, are affected (epidemic parotitis). Other glands (e.g., the pancreas and testes) may also be involved. Autoimmune disease underlies the inflammatory salivary changes of Sjögren syndrome, discussed in Chapter 7. In this condition, the widespread involvement of the salivary glands and the mucus-secreting glands of the nasal mucosa induces *xerostomia*—dry mouth; associated involvement of the lacrimal glands produces dry eyes—*keratoconjunctivitis sicca.* The combination of salivary and lacrimal gland inflammatory enlargement with xerostomia is sometimes called *Mikulicz syndrome,* a noncommittal term that includes all forms of involvement of these glands, including sarcoidosis, leukemia, lymphoma, and other tumors, that are sometimes accompanied by xerostomia. Xerostomia may also be secondary to radiation-induced salivary gland atrophy or to drugs (e.g., antihistamines, phenothiazines).

Sialolithiasis and Nonspecific Sialadenitis. Nonspecific bacterial sialadenitis most often involving the major salivary glands, particularly the submandibular glands, is an uncommon condition, usually secondary to ductal obstruction produced by stones *(sialolithiasis).* The common offenders are *Staphylococcus aureus* and *Streptococcus viridans.* The stone formation is sometimes related to obstruction of the orifices of the salivary glands by impacted food debris or by edema about the orifice after some injury. Frequently, the stones are of obscure origin. Dehydration with decreased secretory function may also predispose to secondary bacterial invasion, as sometimes occurs in patients receiving long-term phenothiazines that suppress salivary secretion. Perhaps dehydration with decreased secretion explains the development of bacterial suppurative parotitis in elderly patients with a recent history of major thoracic or abdominal surgery.

Whatever the origin, the obstructive process and bacterial invasion lead to a nonspecific inflammation of the affected glands that may be largely interstitial or, when induced by staphylococcal or other pyogens, may be associated with overt suppurative necrosis and abscess formation. Unilateral involvement of a single gland is the rule. The inflammatory involvement causes painful enlargement and sometimes a purulent ductal discharge.

Neoplasms

In view of their relatively undistinguished normal morphology, the salivary glands give rise to a surprising variety of benign and malignant tumors.[26–29] A classification and the relative incidence of benign and malignant tumors are shown in Table 17–2; not included are the rare benign and malignant mesenchymal tumors.

As indicated in Table 17–2, only a relatively few epithelial neoplasms make up more than 90% of salivary gland tumors, and so our consideration can be restricted to them. Overall, these neoplasms are relatively uncommon and represent less than 2% of tumors in humans. About 65% to 80% arise within the parotid, 10% in the submandibular gland, and the remainder in the minor salivary glands, including the sublingual glands. Fifteen per cent to 30% of tumors in the parotid glands are malignant, in contrast to about 40% in the submandibular glands, 50% in the minor salivary glands, and 70% to 90% of sublingual tumors.[18] *The likelihood then of a salivary gland tumor being malignant is more or less inversely proportional to the size of the gland.*

These tumors usually occur in adults, with a slight female predominance, but about 5% occur in children younger than 16 years. For unknown reasons, Warthin tumors occur much more often in males. The benign tumors most often appear in the fifth to seventh decades of life. The malignant ones tend, on average, to appear somewhat later. Whatever the histologic pattern, neoplasms in the parotid glands produce distinctive swellings in front of and below the ear. In general, when they are first diagnosed, both benign and malignant lesions range from 4 to 6 cm in diameter and are mobile on palpation except in the case of neglected malignant tumors. Although benign tumors are known to have been present usually for many months to

Table 17–2. HISTOLOGIC CLASSIFICATION AND APPROXIMATE INCIDENCE OF BENIGN AND MALIGNANT TUMORS OF THE SALIVARY GLANDS

Benign	Malignant
Pleomorphic adenoma (50%) (mixed tumor)	Mucoepidermoid carcinoma (15%)
Warthin tumor (5%–10%)	Adenocarcinoma (NOS) (10%)
Oncocytoma (1%)	Acinic cell carcinoma (5%)
Other adenomas (5%–10%)	Adenoid cystic carcinoma (5%)
Basal cell adenoma	Malignant mixed tumor (3%–5%)
Canalicular adenoma	Squamous cell carcinoma (1%)
Ductal papillomas	Other carcinomas (2%)

NOS, not otherwise specified. Data from Ellis GL, Auclair PL: Tumors of the Salivary Glands. Atlas of Tumor Pathology, Third Series. Washington, DC, Armed Forces Institute of Pathology, 1996.

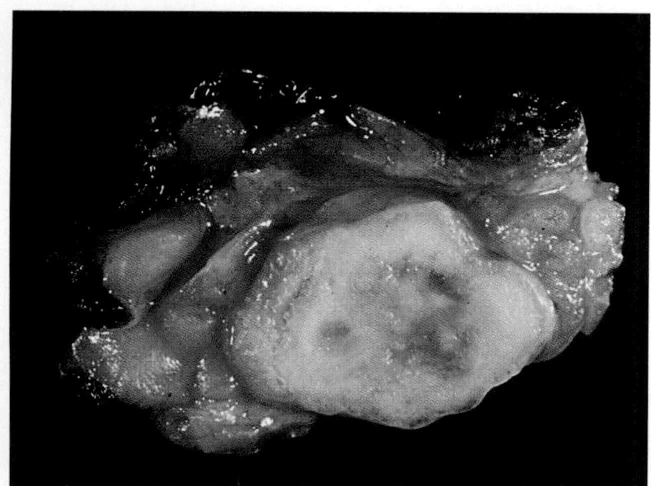

Figure 17–12

Pleomorphic adenoma of the parotid. The transected, sharply circumscribed, yellow-white tumor protrudes above the level of the surrounding glandular substance.

several years before coming to clinical attention, cancers seem to demand attention more promptly, probably because of their more rapid growth. Ultimately, however, there are no reliable criteria to differentiate, on clinical grounds, the benign from the malignant lesions, and morphologic evaluation is necessary.

PLEOMORPHIC ADENOMA

Because of their remarkable histologic diversity, these neoplasms have also been called *mixed tumors.* They represent about 60% of tumors in the parotid, are less common in the submandibular glands, and are relatively rare in the minor salivary glands. In essence, they are epithelium-derived benign tumors that show both epithelial and mesenchymal differentiation. They are thus composed of epithelial elements dispersed throughout a matrix showing varying degrees of myxoid, hyaline, chondroid (cartilaginous), and even osseous tissue. In some tumors, the epithelial elements predominate; in others, they are present only in widely dispersed foci.

Little is known about the origins of these neoplasms save that radiation exposure increases the risk.[27] Equally uncertain is the histogenesis of the various components, but favored today is the view that all neoplastic elements, including those that appear mesenchymal, are of either myoepithelial or ductal reserve cell origin (hence the designation *pleomorphic adenoma).*

MORPHOLOGY. Most pleomorphic adenomas present as basically rounded, well-demarcated masses rarely exceeding 6 cm in greatest dimension (Fig. 17–12). Although they are encapsulated, in some instances the capsule is not fully developed, and expansile growth produces tongue-like protrusions into the surrounding gland, rendering enucleation of the tumor (in contrast with limited parotidectomy) hazardous. The cut surface is gray-white with variegated myxoid and blue translucent areas of chondroid.

The dominant histologic feature is the great heterogeneity mentioned. The epithelial elements resembling ductal cells or myoepithelial cells are disposed in duct formations, acini, irregular tubules, strands, or sheets of cells. These elements

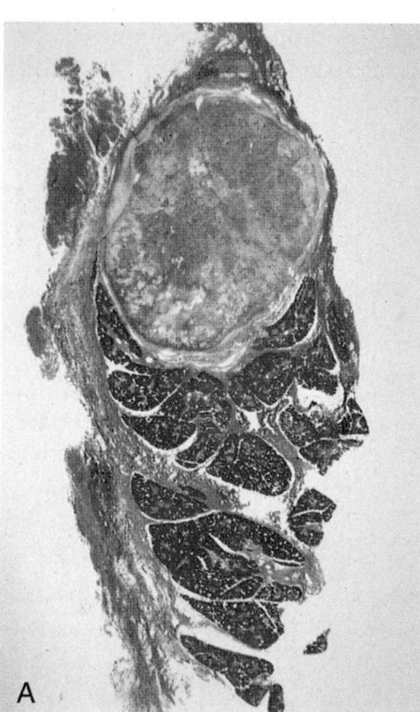

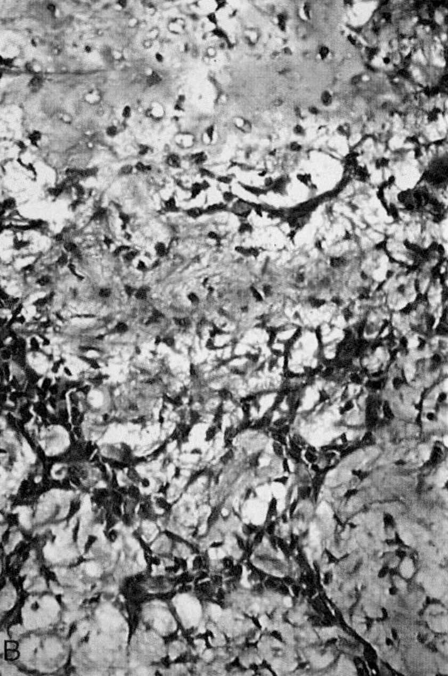

Figure 17–13

Pleomorphic adenoma. *A*, Low-power view showing a well-demarcated tumor with normal parotid acini below. *B*, High-power view showing amorphous myxoid stroma resembling cartilage, with interspersed islands and strands of myoepithelial cells. (Courtesy of Dr. E. Lee, Department of Pathology, University of Texas Southwestern Medical Center, Dallas, TX.)

are typically dispersed within a mesenchyme-like background of loose myxoid tissue containing islands of chondroid and, rarely, foci of bone (Fig. 17–13). Sometimes the epithelial cells form well-developed apparent ducts lined by cuboidal to columnar cells with an underlying layer of deeply chromatic, small myoepithelial cells. In other instances, there may be strands or sheets of myoepithelial cells. Islands of well-differentiated squamous epithelium may also occur. In most cases, there is no epithelial dysplasia or evident mitotic activity. There is no difference in biologic behavior between the tumors composed largely of epithelial elements and those composed only of seemingly mesenchymal elements.

Clinical Features. These tumors present as painless, slow-growing, mobile discrete masses within the parotid or submandibular areas or in the buccal cavity. The recurrence rate (perhaps months to years later) with adequate parotidectomy is about 4% but, with attempted enucleation, approaches 25% because of failure to recognize at surgery minute protrusions from the main mass.

A carcinoma infrequently arises in a pleomorphic adenoma, referred to variously as a *carcinoma ex pleomorphic adenoma* or a *malignant mixed tumor*. The incidence of malignant transformation increases with the duration of the tumor, being about 2% for tumors present less than 5 years and almost 10% for those of more than 15 years' duration. The cancer usually takes the form of an adenocarcinoma or undifferentiated carcinoma, and often it virtually completely overgrows the last vestiges of the preexisting pleomorphic adenoma; but to substantiate the diagnosis of carcinoma ex pleomorphic adenoma, recognizable traces of the latter must be found. Regrettably, these cancers, when they appear, are among the most aggressive of all salivary gland malignant neoplasms, accounting for a 30% to 50% mortality in 5 years.

WARTHIN TUMOR (PAPILLARY CYSTADENOMA LYMPHOMATOSUM)

This curious benign neoplasm with its intimidating histologic name is the second most common salivary gland neoplasm. It arises almost always in the parotid gland (the only tumor virtually restricted to the parotid) and occurs more commonly in males than in females, usually in the fifth to seventh decades of life. About 10% are multifocal and 10% bilateral. Smokers have eight times the risk of nonsmokers for developing tumors.

MORPHOLOGY. Most Warthin tumors (sometimes also called adenolymphomas) are round to oval, encapsulated masses, 2 to 5 cm in diameter, arising in most cases in the superficial parotid gland, where they are readily palpable. Transection reveals a pale gray surface punctuated by narrow cystic or cleft-like spaces filled with a mucinous or serous secretion. On microscopic examination, these spaces are lined by a double layer of epithelial cells resting on a dense lymphoid stroma sometimes bearing germinal centers (Fig. 17–14). The spaces are frequently narrowed by polypoid projections of the lymphoepithelial elements. The double layer of lining cells is distinctive, with a surface palisade of columnar cells having an abundant, finely granular, eosinophilic cytoplasm,

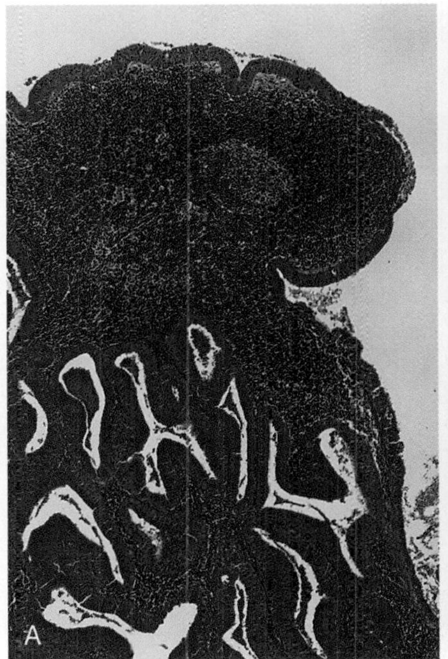

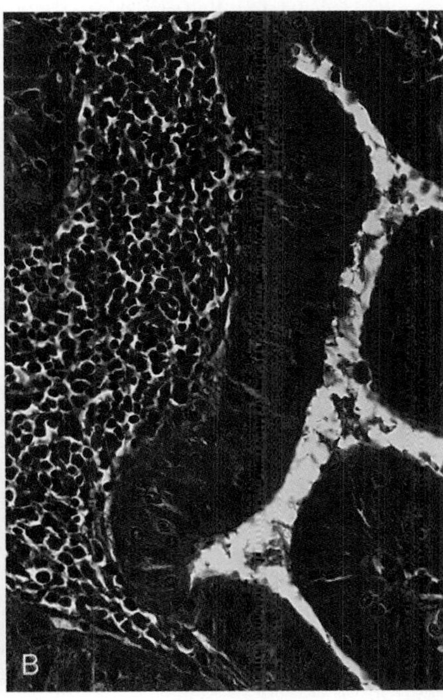

Figure 17–14

Warthin tumor. *A*, Lower-power view showing epithelial and lymphoid elements. Note the follicular germinal center beneath the epithelium. *B*, Cleftlike spaces separate the lobules of tumor covered by a regular double layer of eosinophilic epithelial cells based on a lymphoid stroma. (Courtesy of Dr. James Gulizia, Brigham and Women's Hospital, Boston, MA.)

imparting an oncocytic appearance, resting on a layer of cuboidal to polygonal cells. Oncocytes are epithelial cells stuffed with mitochondria that impart the granular appearance to the cytoplasm. Secretory cells are dispersed in the columnar cell layer, accounting for the secretion within the lumens. On occasion, there are foci of squamous metaplasia.

The histogenesis of these tumors has long been disputed. The occasional finding of small salivary gland rests in lymph nodes in the neck suggests that these tumors arise from the aberrant incorporation of similar inclusion-bearing lymphoid tissue in the parotids. Indeed, rarely, Warthin tumors have arisen within cervical lymph nodes, a finding that should not be misconstrued to imply a metastasis. These neoplasms are usually benign, with recurrence rates of only 2% after resection.

MUCOEPIDERMOID CARCINOMA

These neoplasms are composed of variable mixtures of squamous cells, mucus-secreting cells, and intermediate hybrids. They represent about 15% of all salivary gland tumors, and while they occur preponderantly (60% to 70%) in the parotids, they account for a large fraction of salivary gland neoplasms in the other glands, particularly the minor salivary glands. Overall, they are the most common form of *malignant* tumor primary in the salivary glands and are the most common radiation-induced neoplasm.

MORPHOLOGY. Mucoepidermoid carcinomas range up to 8 cm in diameter and, while apparently circumscribed, lack well-defined capsules and are often infiltrative at the margins. Pale gray-white on transection, they frequently reveal small, mucin-containing cysts. The basic histologic pattern is that of cords, sheets, or cystic configurations of squamous, mucous, or intermediate cells. The hybrid cell types often have squamous features, with small to large mucus-filled vacuoles, best seen when highlighted with mucin stains (Fig. 17–15*A*, *B*). The tumor cells may be regular and benign-appearing on one end of the spectrum or, alternatively, highly anaplastic and unmistakably malignant. Accordingly, mucoepidermoid carcinomas are subclassified into low, intermediate, or high grades. Low-grade lesions tend to be composed largely of mucus-secreting cells, often forming glandular spaces. On the other hand, high-grade tumors are composed largely of squamous cells with only a scattering of mucus-secreting cells.

The clinical course and prognosis depend on the grade of the neoplasm. Low-grade tumors may invade locally and recur in about 15% of cases, but only rarely do they metastasize and so yield a 5-year survival rate of more than 90%. By contrast, high-grade neoplasms and, to a somewhat lesser extent, intermediate-grade tumors are invasive and difficult to excise and so recur in about 25% to 30% of cases and, in 30% of cases, disseminate to distant sites. The 5-year survival rate of these tumors is only 50%.

OTHER SALIVARY GLAND TUMORS

Two less common neoplasms merit brief description, adenoid cystic carcinoma and acinic cell tumor.

Adenoid cystic carcinoma is a relatively uncommon tumor in the parotids but is the most common neoplasm in the other salivary glands, particularly the minor salivary glands about the mouth. Similar neoplasms have been reported in the nose, sinuses, and upper airways and elsewhere.

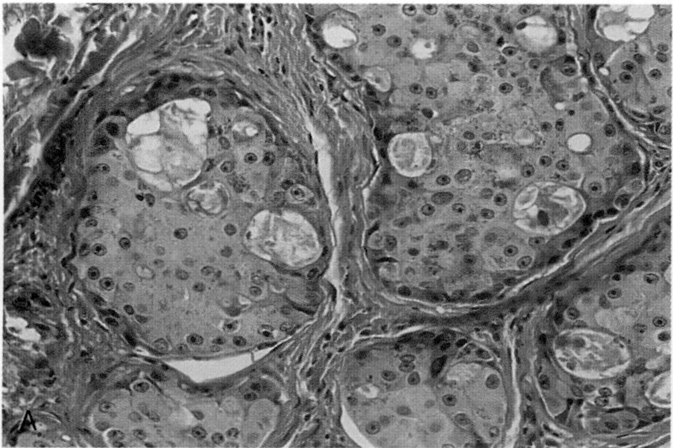

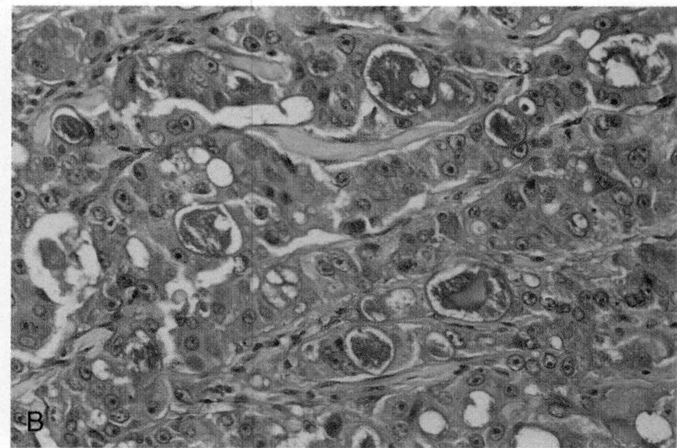

Figure 17–15

A, Mucoepidermoid carcinoma showing islands having squamous cells as well as clear cells containing mucin. *B*, Mucicarmine stains the mucin reddish-pink. (Courtesy of Dr. James Gulizia, Brigham and Women's Hospital, Boston, MA.)

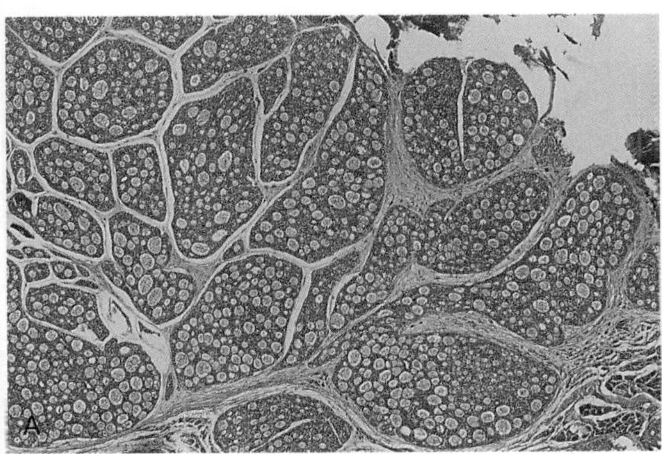

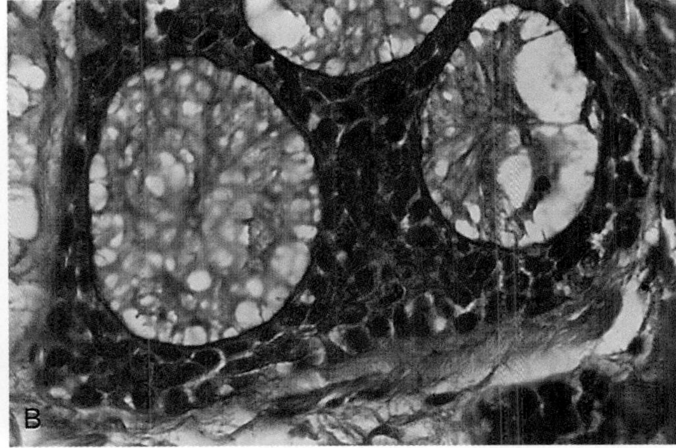

Figure 17–16

Adenoid cystic carcinoma in a salivary gland. *A*, Low-power view. The tumor cells have created a cribriform pattern enclosing secretions. *B*, High-power view showing polygonal tumor cells surrounding the cystic space filled with secretions.

MORPHOLOGY. In gross appearance, they are generally small, poorly encapsulated, infiltrative, gray-pink lesions. On histologic evaluation, they are composed of small cells having dark, compact nuclei and scant cytoplasm. These cells tend to be disposed in tubular, solid, or cribriform patterns reminiscent of cylindromas arising in the adnexa of the skin. The spaces between the tumor cells are often filled with a hyaline material thought to represent excess basement membrane (Fig. 17–16).

Although slowly growing, these are "sneaky," unpredictable tumors with a tendency to invade perineural spaces (making them the most painful salivary gland neoplasm), and they are stubbornly recurrent. Eventually, 50% or more disseminate widely to distant sites such as bone, liver, and brain, sometimes decades after attempted removal. Thus, although the 5-year survival rate is about 60% to 70%, it drops to about 30% at 10 years and 15% at 15 years. Neoplasms arising in the minor salivary glands have, on average, a poorer prognosis than those primary in the parotids.

The *acinic cell tumor* is composed of cells resembling the normal serous cells of salivary glands. They are relatively uncommon, representing only 2% to 3% of salivary gland tumors. Most arise in the parotids, the small remainder in the submandibular glands. They rarely involve the minor glands, which normally have only a scant number of serous cells. Like Warthin tumor, they are sometimes bilateral or multicentric. They are generally small, discrete lesions that may appear encapsulated. On histologic examination, they reveal a variable architecture and cell morphology. Most characteristically, the cells have apparent cleared cytoplasm, but the cells are sometimes solid or at other times vacuolated. The cells are disposed in sheets or microcystic, glandular, follicular, or papillary patterns. There is usually little anaplasia and few mitoses, but some tumors are occasionally slightly more pleomorphic.

The clinical course of these neoplasms is somewhat dependent on the level of pleomorphism. Overall, recurrence after resection is uncommon, but about 10% to 15% of these neoplasms metastasize to lymph nodes. The survival rate is in the range of 90% at 5 years and 60% at 20 years.

REFERENCES

1. Hutton KP, Rogers RS III: Recurrent aphthous stomatitis. Dermatol Clin 5:761, 1987.
2. Neville BW, et al (eds): Oral and Maxillofacial Pathology. Philadelphia, WB Saunders, 1995.
3. Sciubba JJ: Opportunistic oral infections in the immunosuppressed patient: oral hairy leukoplakia and oral candidiasis. Adv Dent Res 10: 69, 1996.
4. van der Waal I, et al: Oral leukoplakia: a clinicopathological review. Oral Oncol 33:291, 1997.
5. Hogewind WFC, et al: Oral leukoplakia with emphasis on malignant transformation: a follow-up study of 46 patients. J Craniomaxillofac Surg 17:128, 1989.
6. Boyle P, et al: Recent advances in the etiology and epidemiology of head and neck cancer. Curr Opin Oncol 2:529, 1990.
7. Paz IB, et al: Human papillomavirus (HPV) in head and neck cancer. An association of HPV 16 with squamous cell carcinoma of Waldeyer's tonsillar ring. Cancer 79:595, 1997.
8. Steinberg BM, DiLorenzo TP: A possible role for human papillomavirus in head and neck cancer. Cancer Metastasis Rev 15:91, 1996.
9. Jordan RC, Daley T: Oral squamous cell carcinoma: new insights. J Can Dent Assoc 63:517, 1997.
10. Cowan JM, et al: Cytogenetic evidence of the multistep origin of head and neck squamous cell carcinoma. J Natl Cancer Inst 84:793, 1992.
11. Carter RL: Patterns and mechanisms of spread of squamous carcinomas of the oral cavity. Clin Otolaryngol 15:185, 1990.
12. Naclerio R, Solomon W: Rhinitis and inhaled allergens. JAMA 278: 1842, 1997.
13. Slavin RG: Nasal polyps and sinusitis. JAMA 278:1845, 1997.
14. Hyams VJ, et al: Tumors of the Upper Respiratory Tract and Ear. Atlas of Tumor Pathology, Second Series. Washington, DC, Armed Forces Institute of Pathology, 1988.
15. Goodman ML, Pilch BZ: Tumors of the upper respiratory tract. In Fletcher DM (ed): Diagnostic Histopathology of Tumors. London, Churchill Livingstone, 1995, pp 79–126.

16. Argani P, et al: Olfactory neuroblastoma is not related to the Ewing family of tumors. Am J. Surg Pathol 22:391, 1998.
17. Broich G, et al: Esthesioneuroblastoma: a general review of the cases published since the discovery of the tumour in 1924. Anticancer Res 17:2683, 1997.
18. Hawkins EP, et al: Nasopharyngeal carcinoma in children—a retrospective review and demonstration of Epstein-Barr viral genomes in tumor cell cytoplasm: a report of the Pediatric Oncology Group. Hum Pathol 21:805, 1990.
19. Crissman JD, Zarbo RJ: Dysplasia, in situ carcinoma, and progression to invasive carcinoma of the upper aerodigestive tract. Am J Surg Pathol 13:5, 1989.
20. Cattaruzza MS, et al: Epidemiology of laryngeal cancer. Eur J Cancer B Oral Oncol 32B:293, 1996.
21. Koufman JA, Burke AJ: The etiology and pathogenesis of laryngeal carcinoma. Otolaryngol Clin North Am 30:1, 1997.
22. Bauman NM, Smith RJ: Recurrent respiratory papillomatosis. Pediatr Clin North Am 43:1385, 1996.
23. Regauer S, et al: Lateral neck cysts—the branchial theory revisited. A critical review and clinicopathological study of 97 cases with special emphasis on cytokeratin expression. APMIS 105:623, 1997.
24. Capella C, et al: Histopathology, cytology, and cytochemistry of pheochromocytomas and paragangliomas including chemodectomas. Pathol Res Pract 186:176, 1988.
25. Wick MR, Rosai JR: Neuroendocrine tumors of the mediastinum. Semin Diagn Pathol 8:35, 1991.
26. Ellis GL, Auclair PL: Tumors of the Salivary Glands. Atlas of Tumor Pathology, Third Series, Fascicle 17. Washington, DC, Armed Forces Institute of Pathology, 1996.
27. Simpson RH: Classification of salivary gland tumors—a brief histopathological review. Histol Histopathol 10:737, 1995.
28. Shrestha P, et al: Primary epithelial tumors of salivary glands—histogenesis, histomorphological and immunohistochemical implications—diagnosis and clinical management. Crit Rev Oncol Hematol 23:239, 1996.
29. Nagler RM, Laufer D: Tumors of the major and minor salivary glands: review of 25 years of experience. Anticancer Res 17:701, 1997.

18

The Gastrointestinal Tract

James M. Crawford

Esophagus

NORMAL ESOPHAGUS

PATHOLOGY

CONGENITAL ANOMALIES

LESIONS ASSOCIATED WITH MOTOR DYSFUNCTION

ESOPHAGITIS

- Reflux Esophagitis
- Barrett Esophagus
- Infectious and Chemical Esophagitis

ESOPHAGEAL VARICES

TUMORS

- Benign Tumors
- Malignant Tumors
  - *Squamous Cell Carcinoma*
  - *Adenocarcinoma*

Stomach

NORMAL STOMACH

GASTRIC MUCOSAL PHYSIOLOGY

PATHOLOGY

CONGENITAL ANOMALIES

- Pyloric Stenosis

GASTRITIS

- Acute Gastritis
- Chronic Gastritis (Including *Helicobacter* Infections)
  - *Special Forms of Gastritis*

PEPTIC ULCER DISEASE

- Peptic Ulcers
- Acute Gastric Ulceration

MISCELLANEOUS CONDITIONS

TUMORS

- Benign Tumors
- Gastric Carcinoma

Small and Large Intestines

NORMAL SMALL AND LARGE INTESTINES

PATHOLOGY

CONGENITAL ANOMALIES

- Atresia and Stenosis
- Meckel Diverticulum
- Congenital Aganglionic Megacolon—Hirschsprung Disease

ENTEROCOLITIS

- Diarrhea and Dysentery
- Infectious Enterocolitis
  - *Viral Gastroenteritis*
  - *Bacterial Enterocolitis*
  - *Necrotizing Enterocolitis*
  - *Antibiotic-Associated Colitis (Pseudomembranous Colitis)*
  - *Collagenous and Lymphocytic Colitis*
- Miscellaneous Intestinal Inflammatory Disorders
  - *Parasites and Protozoa*
  - *Acquired Immunodeficiency Syndrome*
  - *Transplantation*
  - *Drug-Induced Intestinal Injury*
  - *Radiation Enterocolitis*
  - *Neutropenic Colitis (Typhlitis)*
  - *Diversion Colitis*

MALABSORPTION SYNDROMES

- Celiac Sprue
- Tropical Sprue (Postinfectious Sprue)
- Whipple Disease
- Disaccharidase (Lactase) Deficiency
- Abetalipoproteinemia

IDIOPATHIC INFLAMMATORY BOWEL DISEASE

- Crohn Disease
- Ulcerative Colitis

VASCULAR DISORDERS

- Ischemic Bowel Disease
- Angiodysplasia
- Hemorrhoids

DIVERTICULAR DISEASE

INTESTINAL OBSTRUCTION

TUMORS OF THE SMALL AND LARGE INTESTINES

- Tumors of the Small Intestine
  - *Adenomas*
  - *Adenocarcinoma*
- Tumors of the Colon and Rectum
  - *Non-neoplastic Polyps*
  - *Adenomas*
  - *Familial Syndromes*
  - *Colorectal Carcinogenesis*
  - *Colorectal Carcinoma*
  - *Carcinoid Tumors*
- Gastrointestinal Lymphoma
- Mesenchymal Tumors

Appendix

NORMAL APPENDIX

PATHOLOGY

ACUTE APPENDICITIS

TUMORS OF THE APPENDIX

- Mucocele and Pseudomyxoma Peritonei

Peritoneum

INFLAMMATION

PERITONEAL INFECTION

MISCELLANEOUS CONDITIONS

TUMORS

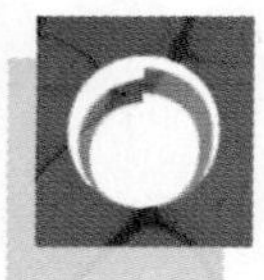

Esophagus

NORMAL ESOPHAGUS

The normal esophagus is a hollow, highly distensible muscular tube that extends from the pharynx to the gastroesophageal junction at the level of the T11 or T12 vertebra. Measuring between 10 and 11 cm in the newborn, it grows to a length of about 23 to 25 cm in the adult. Several points of luminal narrowing can be identified along its course—proximally at the cricoid cartilage, midway in its course alongside the aortic arch and at the anterior crossing of the left main bronchus and left atrium, and distally where it pierces the diaphragm. Manometric recordings of intraluminal pressures in the esophagus have identified two higher-pressure areas that remain relatively contracted in the resting phase. A 3-cm segment in the proximal esophagus at the level of the cricopharyngeus muscle is referred to as the *upper esophageal sphincter*. The 2- to 4-cm segment just proximal to the anatomic esophagogastric junction, at the level of the diaphragm, is referred to as the *lower esophageal sphincter* (LES).

The wall of the esophagus consists of a mucosa, submucosa, muscularis propria, and adventitia, reflecting the general structural organization of the gastrointestinal tract.[1] The *mucosa* is composed of a nonkeratinizing stratified squamous epithelial layer that overlies a lamina propria. A small number of specialized cell types, such as melanocytes, endocrine cells, and Langerhans cells (Chapter 27), are present in the deeper portion of the epithelial layer. The lamina propria is the nonepithelial portion of the mucosa, above the muscularis mucosae. It consists of areolar connective tissue and contains vascular structures and scattered leukocytes.

The *submucosa* consists of loose connective tissue containing blood vessels, a rich network of lymphatics, a sprinkling of leukocytes with occasional lymphoid follicles, nerve fibers (including the ganglia of Meissner plexus), and submucosal glands. The submucosal glands are considered to be continuations of the minor salivary glands of the oropharynx and are scattered along the entire esophagus but are more concentrated in the upper and lower portions. The muscularis propria of the proximal 6 to 8 cm of the esophagus also contains striated muscle fibers from the cricopharyngeus; this feature explains why skeletal muscle disorders can cause esophageal dysfunction.

In sharp contrast to the rest of the gastrointestinal tract, the esophagus is mostly devoid of a serosal coat. In the mediastinum, the intimate anatomic proximity to important thoracic viscera is of significance in permitting the ready and widespread dissemination of infections and tumors of the esophagus into the posterior mediastinum. Spread is further facilitated by the rich network of mucosal and submucosal lymphatics that run longitudinally along the esophagus.

The functions of the esophagus are to conduct food and fluids from the pharynx to the stomach and to prevent reflux of gastric contents into the esophagus. These functions require motor activity coordinated with swallowing—a wave of peristaltic contraction, relaxation of the LES in anticipation of the peristaltic wave, and closure of the LES after the swallowing reflex. The mechanisms governing this motor function are strikingly complex, involving both extrinsic and intrinsic innervation, humoral regulation, and properties of the muscle wall itself.

The control of the LES function is poorly understood. Both active inhibition of the muscle by inhibitory neurons and cessation of tonic neural excitation to the sphincter play a role. Disruption of the vagal fibers by truncal or selective vagotomy, however, has virtually no effect on LES tone or relaxation. Maintenance of sphincteric tone is necessary to prevent reflux of gastric contents, which are under positive pressure relative to the esophagus. Many chemical agents (e.g., gastrin, acetylcholine, serotonin, prostaglandin $F_{2\alpha}$, motilin, substance P, histamine, and pancreatic polypeptide) increase LES tone, but their precise roles in normal physiologic function remain unclear.

PATHOLOGY

Lesions of the esophagus run the gamut from highly lethal cancers to the merely annoying *heartburn* (which has affected many a partaker of a large, spicy meal). Esophageal varices, the result of cirrhosis and portal hypertension, are of major importance, since their rupture is frequently followed by massive hematemesis (vomiting of blood) and exsanguination. Esophagitis and hiatal hernias are far more frequent and rarely life-threatening. Distressing to the physician is that all disorders of the esophagus tend to produce similar symptoms.

Dysphagia (subjective difficulty in swallowing) is encountered both with deranged esophageal motor function and with diseases that narrow or obstruct the lumen. *Heartburn* (retrosternal burning pain) usually reflects regurgitation of gastric contents into the lower esophagus. *Pain* and *hematemesis* are sometimes evoked by esophageal disease, particularly by lesions associated with inflammation or ulceration of the esophageal mucosa. The clinical diagnosis of esophageal disorders often requires specialized procedures, such as esophagoscopy, radiographic barium studies, and manometry.

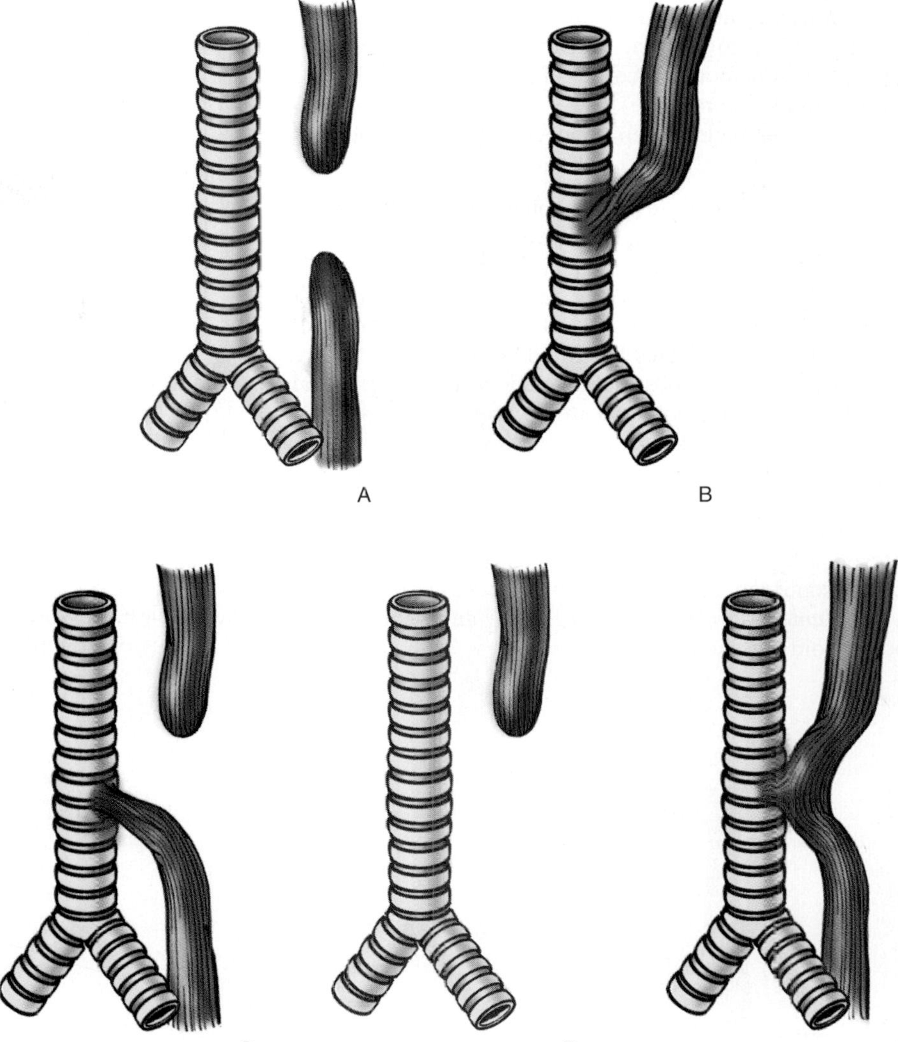

Figure 18–1 ■

Esophageal atresia and tracheoesophageal fistula. *A*, Blind upper and lower esophageal segments. *B*, Fistula between blind upper segment and trachea. *C*, Blind upper segment, fistula between blind lower segment and trachea. *D*, Blind upper segment only. *E*, Fistula between patent esophagus and trachea. Type C, in which the proximal esophagus ends in a blind pouch while the distal segment communicates with the trachea or a main stem bronchus, is the most common variety. (Adapted from Morson BC, Dawson IMP (eds): Gastrointestinal Pathology. Oxford, Blackwell Scientific Publications, 1972, p 8.)

Congenital Anomalies

ATRESIA AND FISTULAS

Although developmental defects in the esophagus are uncommon, they must be corrected early, since they are incompatible with life. Because they cause immediate regurgitation when feeding is attempted, they are usually discovered soon after birth. *Absence* (agenesis) of the esophagus is extremely rare; much more common are *atresia* and *fistula formation* (Fig. 18–1). In atresia, a segment of the esophagus is represented by only a thin, noncanalized cord, with a proximal blind pouch connected to the pharynx and a lower pouch leading to the stomach. Atresia is most commonly located at or near the tracheal bifurcation. Atresia rarely occurs alone but is usually associated with a fistula connecting the lower or upper pouch with a bronchus or the trachea. Often associated anomalies are congenital heart disease and other gastrointestinal malformations. Aspiration and paroxysmal suffocation from food are obvious hazards; pneumonia and severe fluid and electrolyte imbalances may also occur.

STENOSIS, WEBS, AND RINGS

Non-neoplastic constrictions of the esophagus are most often acquired conditions.

- *Stenosis* consists of fibrous thickening of the esophageal wall, particularly the submucosa, with atrophy of the muscularis propria. The lining epithelium is usually thin and sometimes ulcerated.
- *Mucosal webs* are uncommon ledgelike semicircumferential protrusions of the mucosa into the esophageal lumen. Those in the upper esophagus are often designated *webs*; those in the lower esophagus are designated *Schatzki rings*, located at or just above the esophagogas-

tric squamocolumnar junction. Well-developed webs rarely protrude more than 5 mm into the lumen, with a thickness of 2 to 4 mm. Upper esophageal webs are covered by squamous mucosa and contain a vascularized fibrous tissue core; the lower esophageal Schatzki rings have on their undersurface columnar gastric epithelium.

Stenosis is the result of severe esophageal injury with inflammatory scarring, as from gastroesophageal reflux, radiation, scleroderma, or caustic injury. Stenosis usually develops in adulthood and becomes manifest by progressive dysphagia, at first to solid foods only but eventually to all foods. Dysphagia constitutes the major symptom. In severe stenoses, virtually total obstruction may result. Esophageal webs and rings are encountered most frequently in women over age 40 and are of uncertain etiology. Episodic dysphagia is the main symptom associated with webs and rings, usually provoked when an individual bolts solid food. Pain is infrequent. When an upper esophageal web is accompanied by iron deficiency anemia, glossitis, and cheilosis, the condition is referred to as the *Paterson-Brown-Kelly* or *Plummer-Vinson syndrome*, with an attendant risk for postcricoid carcinoma.

Lesions Associated With Motor Dysfunction

Gravity alone is not sufficient to move food from the pharynx to the stomach or to prevent reflux of gastric contents. Coordinated motor function is critical to proper function of the esophagus; witness the blissful suckling of the supine infant. The four major entities that are caused by or induce motor dysfunction of the esophagus are diagrammed in Figure 18–2.

ACHALASIA

Achalasia is characterized by three major abnormalities: (1) aperistalsis, (2) partial or incomplete relaxation of the LES with swallowing, and (3) increased resting tone of the LES. The pathogenesis of primary achalasia is poorly understood but is thought to involve degenerative changes in neural innervation, either intrinsic to the esophagus[2] or in the extraesophageal vagus nerves and the dorsal motor nucleus of the vagus. Secondary achalasia may arise in Chagas disease, in which *Trypanosoma cruzi* causes destruction of the myenteric plexus of the esophagus, duodenum, co-

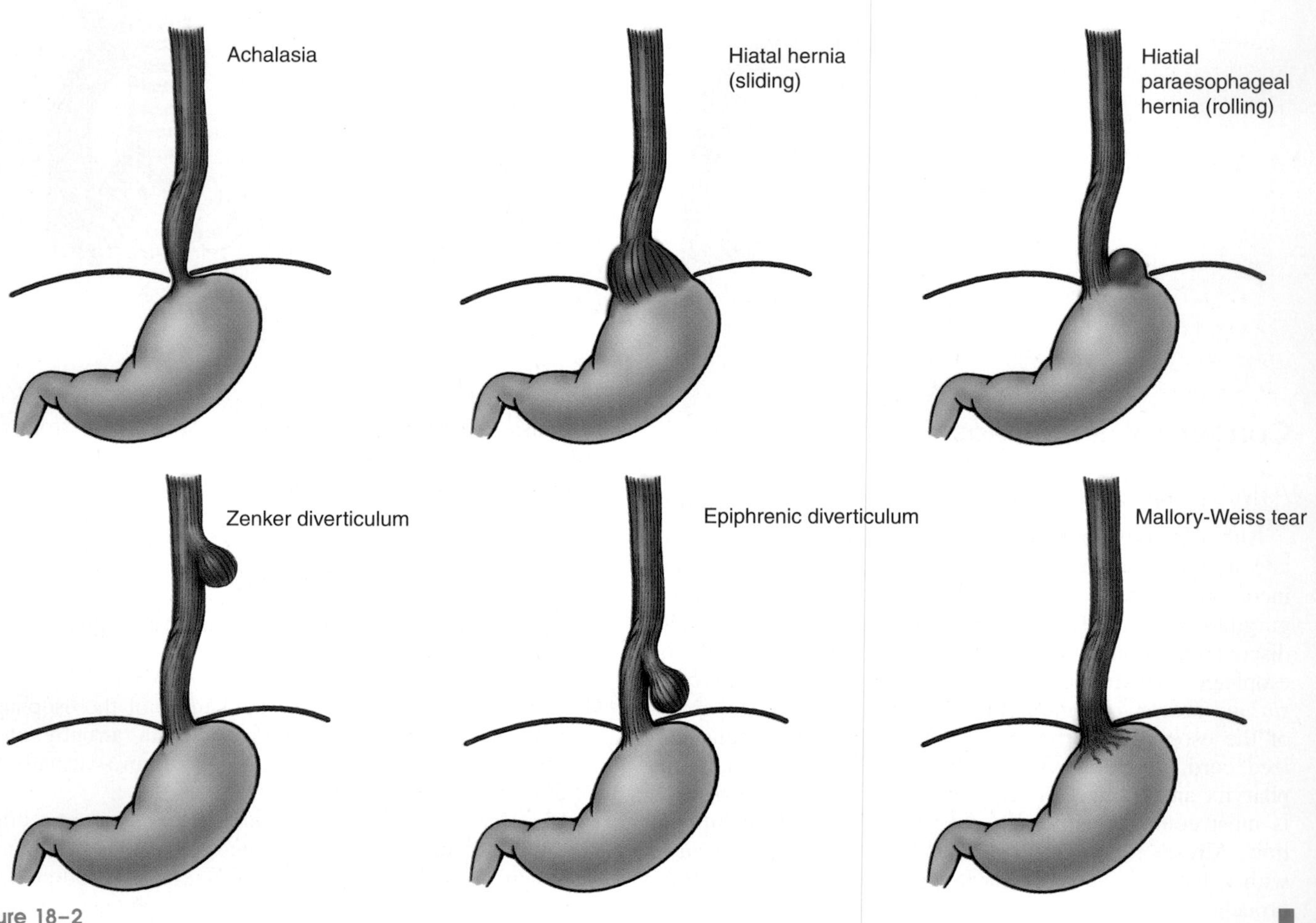

Figure 18–2

Major conditions associated with esophageal motor dysfunction (see text).

lon, and ureter, with resultant dilation of these viscera. Diseases of the dorsal motor nuclei, particularly polio or surgical ablation, can cause an achalasia-like illness, as can diabetic autonomic neuropathy, and infiltrative disorders, such as malignancy, amyloidosis, and sarcoidosis. *In most instances, however, achalasia occurs as a primary disorder of uncertain cause.*

MORPHOLOGY. In primary achalasia, there is progressive dilation of the esophagus above the level of the LES. The wall of the esophagus may be of normal thickness, thicker than normal owing to hypertrophy of the muscularis, or markedly thinned out by dilation. The myenteric ganglia are usually absent from the body of the esophagus but may or may not be reduced in number in the region of the lower sphincter. The mucosal lining may be unaffected, but sometimes inflammation, ulceration, or fibrotic thickening may be evident just above the lower sphincter.

Clinical Features. Achalasia usually becomes manifest in young adulthood but may appear in infancy or childhood. The classic clinical symptom of achalasia is progressive dysphagia. Nocturnal regurgitation and aspiration of undigested food may occur. The most serious aspect of this condition is the hazard of developing esophageal squamous cell carcinoma, said to occur in about 5% of patients, typically at an earlier age than those without this disease. Other complications include *Candida* esophagitis, lower esophageal diverticula (see later), and aspiration with pneumonia or airway obstruction.

HIATAL HERNIA

Hiatal hernia is characterized by separation of the diaphragmatic crura and widening of the space between the muscular crura and the esophageal wall. Two anatomic patterns are recognized (Fig. 18–2): the axial, or *sliding hernia*, and the nonaxial, or *paraesophageal hiatal hernia.* The sliding hernia constitutes 95% of cases; protrusion of the stomach above the diaphragm creates a bell-shaped dilation, bounded below by the diaphragmatic narrowing. In paraesophageal hernias, a separate portion of the stomach, usually along the greater curvature, enters the thorax through the widened foramen.

The cause of hiatal hernia is unknown. Reflux esophagitis (discussed later) is frequently seen in association with sliding hernias, but compromise of the LES with regurgitation of peptic juices into the esophagus is probably the result of, rather than the cause of, a sliding hernia. The uncommon paraesophageal hernias may be caused by previous surgery, including operations for sliding hernia.

Based on barographic studies, hiatal hernias are reported in 1 to 20% of adult subjects, increasing in incidence with age. Hiatal hernias, however, are well recognized in infants and children. Only about 9% of adults with a sliding hernia suffer from heartburn or regurgitation of gastric juices into the mouth. These symptoms are attributed to incompetence of the LES and are accentuated by positions favoring reflux (bending forward, lying supine) and obesity. Complications of hiatal hernias are numerous. Both types may ulcerate, causing bleeding and perforation. Paraesophageal hernias can become strangulated or obstructed, and early surgical repair has been advocated.

DIVERTICULA

A *diverticulum* is an outpouching of the alimentary tract that contains all visceral layers; a false diverticulum denotes an outpouching of mucosa and submucosa only. True diverticula are usually discovered in later life and may develop in three regions of the esophagus:

- *Zenker diverticulum* immediately above the upper esophageal sphincter
- *Traction diverticulum* near the midpoint of the esophagus
- *Epiphrenic diverticulum* immediately above the LES

Disordered cricopharyngeal motor dysfunction is implicated in the genesis of Zenker diverticulum. Scarring resulting from mediastinal lymphadenitis (as from tuberculosis) was a presumed cause of traction on the esophagus, giving rise to midesophageal diverticula. Arguments, however, have been advanced in favor of traction diverticula actually arising from motor dysfunction or being a congenital lesion. Dyscoordination of peristalsis and LES relaxation are the proposed cause of epiphrenic diverticula.

Zenker diverticula may reach several centimeters in size and accumulate significant amounts of food. Typical symptoms are food regurgitation in the absence of dysphagia and a mass in the neck; aspiration with resultant pneumonia is a significant risk. While midesophageal diverticula are generally asymptomatic, epiphrenic diverticula can give rise to nocturnal regurgitation of massive amounts of fluid.

LACERATIONS (MALLORY-WEISS SYNDROME)

Longitudinal tears in the esophagus at the esophagogastric junction are termed *Mallory-Weiss tears* and are believed to be the consequence of severe retching. They are encountered most commonly in alcoholics, attributed to episodes of excessive vomiting and refluxing of gastric contents in the setting of an alcoholic stupor.[3] Since these tears may occur in persons who have no history of vomiting or alcoholism, other mechanisms must exist; underlying inapparent hiatal hernias have been implicated.

MORPHOLOGY. The linear irregular lacerations are oriented in the axis of the esophageal lumen and are several millimeters to several centimeters in length. **They are usually found astride the esophagogastric junction or in the proximal gastric mucosa** (Fig. 18–3). The tears may involve only the mucosa or may penetrate deeply enough to perforate the wall. The histology is not distinctive and reflects trauma accompanied by fresh hemor-

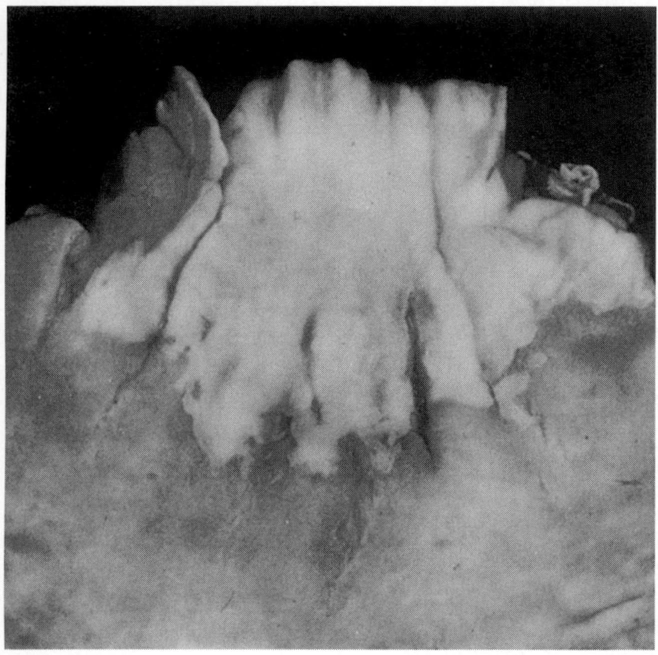

Figure 18–3

Esophageal laceration (Mallory-Weiss tears). Gross view demonstrating longitudinal lacerations extending from esophageal mucosa into stomach mucosa.

rhage and a nonspecific inflammatory response. Infection of the mucosal defect may lead to an inflammatory ulcer or to mediastinitis.

Clinical Features. Esophageal lacerations account for 5 to 10% of upper gastrointestinal bleeding episodes. Most often, bleeding is not profuse and ceases without surgical intervention, although massive hematemesis may occur. Supportive therapy, such as vasoconstrictive medications and transfusions and sometimes balloon tamponade, is usually all that is required. Healing tends to be prompt, with minimal to no residua. The rare instance of esophageal rupture is known as *Boerhaave syndrome* and may be a catastrophic event.

Esophagitis

Injury to the esophageal mucosa with subsequent inflammation is common worldwide. In the United States and other Western countries, esophagitis is present in about 5% of the adult population; much higher prevalence is encountered in selected regions, such as northern Iran and portions of China.

REFLUX ESOPHAGITIS

Reflux of gastric contents into the lower esophagus is the first and foremost cause of esophagitis. Many causative factors are involved, less well characterized than the name implies:[4]

- Decreased efficacy of esophageal antireflux mechanisms, particularly LES tone. Central nervous system depressants, hypothyroidism, pregnancy, systemic sclerosing disorders, alcohol or tobacco exposure, or the presence of a nasogastric tube may be contributing causes. In most instances, no antecedent cause is identified.
- Presence of a sliding hiatal hernia.
- Inadequate or slowed esophageal clearance of refluxed material.
- Delayed gastric emptying and increased gastric volume, contributing to the volume of refluxed material.
- Reduction in the reparative capacity of the esophageal mucosa by protracted exposure to gastric juices.

Any one of the aforementioned influences may assume primacy in an individual case, but more than one is likely to be involved in most instances. *The acid-peptic action of gastric juices is critical to the development of esophageal mucosal injury*; in severe cases, refluxed bile from the duodenum also may contribute to the mucosal disruption.

MORPHOLOGY. The anatomic changes depend on the causative agent and on the duration and severity of the exposure. Simple hyperemia (**redness**) may be the only alteration. In uncomplicated reflux esophagitis, three histologic features are characteristic (Fig. 18–4):[5]

1. The presence of inflammatory cells, including eosinophils, neutrophils, and excessive numbers of lymphocytes, in the epithelial layer
2. Basal zone hyperplasia exceeding 20% of the epithelial thickness
3. Elongation of lamina propria papillae with congestion, extending into the top third of the epithelial layer

Infiltrates of intraepithelial eosinophils are believed to be an early histologic abnormality, since they

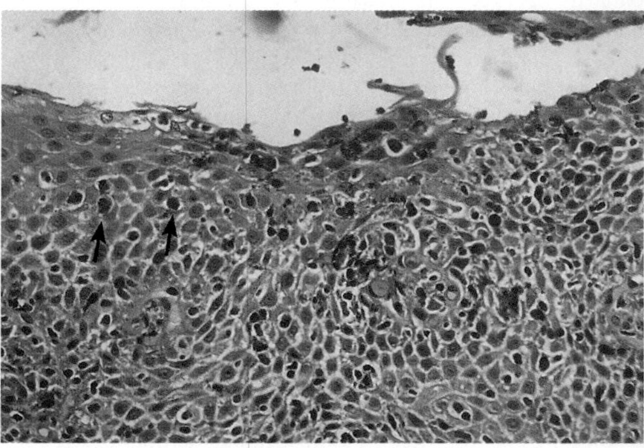

Figure 18–4

Reflux esophagitis showing the superficial portion of the mucosa. Numerous eosinophils *(arrows)* are present within the mucosa, and the stratified squamous epithelium has not undergone complete maturation owing to ongoing inflammatory damage.

occur even in the absence of basal zone hyperplasia. Intraepithelial neutrophils are markers of more severe injury, such as ulceration, rather than reflux esophagitis per se.

Clinical Features. Although largely limited to adults over age 40, reflux esophagitis is occasionally seen in infants and children. The clinical manifestations consist principally of dysphagia; heartburn; and sometimes regurgitation of a sour brash, hematemesis, or melena. *The severity of symptoms is not related closely to the presence or degree of histologic esophagitis*; most people experience reflux symptoms without damage to the distal esophageal mucosa, owing to the short duration of the reflux. Anatomic damage appears best correlated with prolonged exposure of the lower esophagus to refluxed material. Rarely, chronic symptoms are punctuated by attacks of severe chest pain that may be mistaken for a heart attack. The potential consequences of severe reflux esophagitis are bleeding, development of stricture, *and a tendency to develop Barrett esophagus,* with its attendant risks.

BARRETT ESOPHAGUS

Barrett esophagus is a complication of long-standing gastroesophageal reflux, occurring over time in up to 11% of patients with symptomatic reflux disease. *In Barrett esophagus, the distal squamous mucosa is replaced by metaplastic columnar epithelium, as a response to prolonged injury.* Barrett esophagus patients tend to have a long history of heartburn and other reflux symptoms and appear to have more massive reflux with more and longer reflux episodes than most reflux patients. It is unknown why the columnar epithelium develops in some patients with reflux and not in others.

The pathogenesis of Barrett esophagus is not clear.[6] Inflammation and ulceration followed by ingrowth of pluripotent stem cells had been proposed; these cells would then differentiate into a columnar epithelium that is more resistant to acid peptic injury. More recent studies suggest that true metaplasia of the esophageal mucosa occurs because the columnar cells of Barrett esophagus can exhibit ultrastructural and cytochemical features of both a squamous and a columnar epithelial phenotype.

MORPHOLOGY. Barrett esophagus seen grossly (Fig. 18–5*A*), or better still on endoscopy (Fig. 18–5*B*), is apparent as a red, velvety mucosa located between the smooth, pale esophageal squamous mucosa and the more lush light brown-pink gastric mucosa. It may exist as tongues or patches (islands) extending up from the gastroesophageal junction or as a broad circumferential band displacing the squamocolumnar junction cephalad. A small zone of metaplastic mucosa may be present only at the esophagogastric junction **(short-segment Barrett mucosa).** Microscopically the esophageal squamous epithelium is replaced by metaplastic columnar epithelium, complete with mucosal glands. The metaplastic mucosa

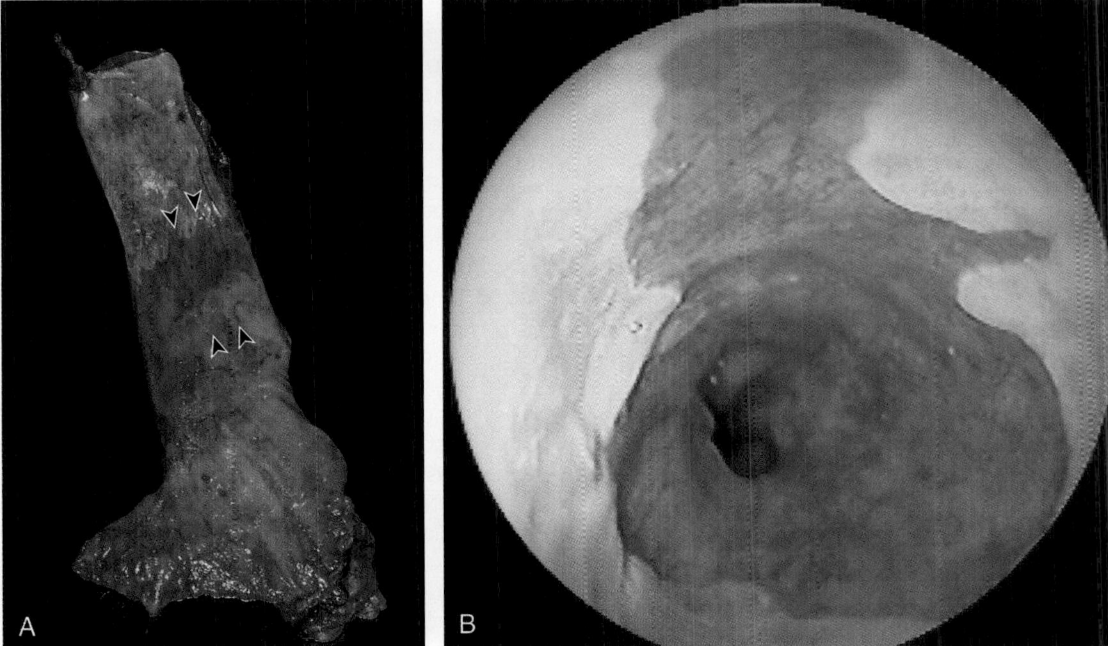

Figure 18–5

A, Gross view of the distal esophagus *(top)* and proximal stomach *(bottom)* showing the granular zone of Barrett esophagus *(arrowheads)*. *B*, Endoscopic view of Barrett esophagus showing red velvety gastrointestinal type mucosa extending from the gastroesophageal orifice. Note paler squamous esophageal mucosa. (*B*, courtesy of Dr. F. Farraye, Brigham and Women's Hospital, Boston, MA.)

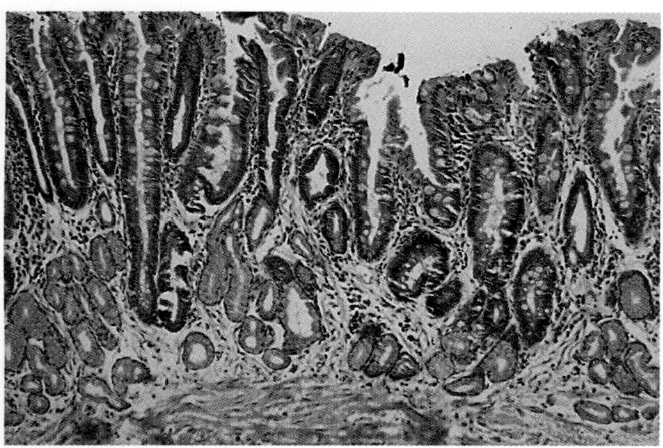

Figure 18–6

Barrett esophagus. Microscopic view showing mixed gastric and intestine-type columnar-epithelial cells in glandular mucosa.

may contain only gastric surface and glandular mucus-secreting cells, making clinical distinction from a hiatal hernia difficult. Diagnosis is more readily made when the columnar mucosa contains intestinal goblet cells (Fig. 18–6).

Critical to the pathologic evaluation of patients with Barrett mucosa is the search for dysplasia, the presumed precursor of malignancy, in columnar epithelium with intestinal metaplasia. Dysplasia is recognized by the presence of cytologic and architectural abnormalities extending to the luminal surface of the columnar epithelium. These abnormalities consist of enlarged, crowded, and stratified hyperchromatic nuclei and loss of intervening stroma between adjacent glandular structures.[7] Dysplasia is classified as **low grade** or **high grade**, with the predominant distinction being a basal epithelial orientation of all nuclei in low-grade dysplasia versus nuclei consistently reaching the apex of epithelial cells in high-grade dysplasia. Persistent high-grade dysplasia demands clinical intervention.

Clinical Features. In addition to the symptoms of reflux esophagitis, the clinical significance of Barrett esophagus relates to the secondary complications of local ulceration with bleeding and stricture. *Of greatest importance is the development of adenocarcinoma,* which, in patients with greater than 2 cm of Barrett mucosa, *occurs at an estimated 30-fold to 40-fold increased rate over the general population.* The presence of short-segment Barrett esophagus also appears to impart risk for adenocarcinoma but at what rate is not known. (See discussion under Carcinoma.)

INFECTIOUS AND CHEMICAL ESOPHAGITIS

In addition to gastroesophageal reflux (which is, in fact, a chemical injury), esophageal inflammation may have many origins, as follows:

- Ingestion of mucosal irritants, such as alcohol, corrosive acids or alkalis (in suicide attempts), and excessively hot fluids (e.g., hot tea in Iran), as well as heavy smoking.
- Cytotoxic anticancer therapy, with or without superimposed infection.
- Infection after bacteremia or viremia. Herpes simplex viruses and cytomegalovirus are the more common offenders in the immunosuppressed.
- Fungal infection in debilitated or immunosuppressed patients or during broad-spectrum antimicrobial therapy. Candidiasis is by far the most common; mucormycosis and aspergillosis may occur.
- Uremia in the setting of renal failure.

Esophageal inflammation may also arise after radiation treatment as well as in association with graft-versus-host disease or the desquamative dermatologic conditions of pemphigoid and epidermolysis bullosa.

MORPHOLOGY. Infectious and chemical causes of esophagitis exhibit their own characteristic features; the final common pathway for all is severe acute inflammation, superficial necrosis and ulceration with the formation of granulation tissue, and eventual fibrosis.

- In candidiasis, patches or all of the esophagus become covered by adherent gray-white pseudomembranes teeming with densely matted fungal hyphae.
- Herpes and cytomegalovirus cause punched-out ulcers of the esophageal mucosa; the nuclear inclusions of herpesvirus are found in a narrow rim of degenerating epithelial cells at the margin of the ulcer, whereas cytomegalic change tends to be found in capillary endothelium and stromal cells in the base of the ulcer.
- Pathogenic bacteria account for 10 to 15% of cases of infective esophagitis and exhibit bacterial invasion of the lamina propria with necrosis of the squamous epithelium.
- Chemically induced injury (lye, acids, detergents) may produce only mild erythema and edema, sloughing of the mucosa, or outright necrosis of the entire esophageal wall. Localized esophageal ulceration may result from pharmaceutical tablets or capsules **sticking** in the esophagus.
- After irradiation of the esophagus, submucosal and mural blood vessels exhibit marked intimal proliferation with luminal narrowing. The submucosa becomes severely fibrotic, and the mucosa exhibits atrophy, with flattening of the papillae and thinning of the epithelium.
- Graft-versus-host disease shares features with the skin manifestations, e.g., karyorrhexis of basal epithelial cells, atrophy, and fibrosis of the lamina propria with minimal inflammation.

Clinical Features. Infections of the esophagus may occur in otherwise healthy individuals but most often are in the debilitated or immunosuppressed. Chemical injury in children is usually accidental, as opposed to attempted suicide, which is an adult phenomenon.

Esophageal Varices

Regardless of cause, portal hypertension, when sufficiently prolonged or severe, induces the formation of collateral bypass channels wherever the portal and caval systems communicate. The pathogenesis of portal hypertension and the locations of these bypasses are considered in Chapter 19. Here we are concerned with the collaterals that develop in the region of the lower esophagus when portal blood flow is diverted through the coronary veins of the stomach into the plexus of esophageal mucosal and submucosal veins, thence into the azygos veins, and eventually into the systemic circulation. The increased pressure in the esophageal plexus produces dilated tortuous vessels called *varices* (Fig. 18–7*C*). *Varices develop in 90% of cirrhotic patients and are most often associated with alcoholic cirrhosis.* Worldwide, hepatic schistosomiasis is the second most common cause of variceal bleeding.

MORPHOLOGY. Varices appear as tortuous dilated veins lying primarily within the submucosa of the distal esophagus and proximal stomach; mucosal venous channels directly beneath the esophageal epithelium may also become massively dilated. The net effect is irregular protrusion of the overlying mucosa into the lumen, although varices are collapsed in surgical or postmortem specimens (Fig. 18–7*A*). When the varix is unruptured, the mucosa may be normal, but often it is eroded and inflamed because of its exposed position. **Variceal rupture produces massive hemorrhage into the lumen as well as suffusion of the esophageal wall with blood.** In this instance, the overlying mucosa appears ulcerated and necrotic (Fig. 18–7*B*). If rupture has occurred in the past, venous thrombosis and superimposed inflammation may be present.

Clinical Features. Varices produce no symptoms until they rupture, when massive hematemesis ensues. Among patients with advanced cirrhosis of the liver, half the deaths result from rupture of a varix. Some patients die as a direct consequence of the hemorrhage, and others die of hepatic coma triggered by the hemorrhage. Even when varices are present, they account for less than half of all episodes of hematemesis. Collectively, concomitant gastritis, esophageal laceration, and peptic ulcer are more common causes. Factors leading to rupture of a varix are unclear: Silent inflammatory erosion of overlying thinned mucosa, increased tension in progressively dilated veins, and vomiting with increased vascular hydrostatic pressure are likely to play roles. Once begun, the hemorrhage rarely subsides spontaneously, and endoscopic injection of thrombotic agents (*sclerotherapy*) or balloon tamponade is usually required. When varices bleed, 40% of patients die in the first episode. Among those who survive, rebleeding occurs in more than half within 1 year, with a similar rate of mortality for each episode.

Tumors

BENIGN TUMORS

Benign tumors of the esophagus are mostly mesenchymal in origin and lie within the esophageal wall. Most common are benign tumors of smooth muscle origin, traditionally called *leiomyomas* and considered the benign end of a spectrum of gastrointestinal stromal tumors. Fibromas, lipomas, hemangiomas, neurofibromas, and lymphangiomas also may arise. Mucosal polyps are usually composed of a combination of fibrous, vascular, or adipose tissue covered by an intact mucosa, descriptively titled *fibrovascular polyps* or *pedunculated lipomas* depending on their composition. *Squamous papillomas* are sessile lesions with a central core of connective tissue and a hyperplastic papilliform squamous mucosa. In rare instances, a mesenchymal mass of inflamed granulation tissue, called an *inflammatory polyp*, may resemble a malignant lesion, hence its alternative name *inflammatory pseudotumor*.

MALIGNANT TUMORS

In the United States, carcinomas of the esophagus represent about 6% of all cancers of the gastrointestinal tract but cause a disproportionate number of cancer deaths.[8] They remain asymptomatic during much of their development and are often discovered too late to permit cure. With rare exception, malignant esophageal tumors arise from the epithelial layer. For many years, most esophageal cancers were of squamous cell origin, but there has been a declining incidence of these tumors coupled with a steadily increasing incidence of adenocarcinomas. Worldwide, squamous cell cancers constitute 90% of esophageal cancers, but in the United States squamous cell carcinoma and adenocarcinoma exhibit comparable incidence rates. Rare cancers (undifferentiated, carcinoid, malignant melanoma, and adenocarcinomas arising from the submucosal glands) are not discussed.

Squamous Cell Carcinoma

Most squamous cell carcinomas occur in adults over age 50. The male-to-female ratio falls in the range of 2 : 1 to as high as 20 : 1. While squamous cell carcinoma of the esophagus occurs throughout the world, its incidence varies widely among countries and within regions of the same country. The region extending from Northern Iran across Central Asia to Northern China exhibits annual incidence rates exceeding 100 per 100,000, with deaths from cancer of the esophagus constituting more than 20% of all cancer deaths. Other areas of high incidence include Puerto Rico, South Africa, and Eastern Europe. In the United States, squamous cell carcinoma of the esophagus affects 2 to 8

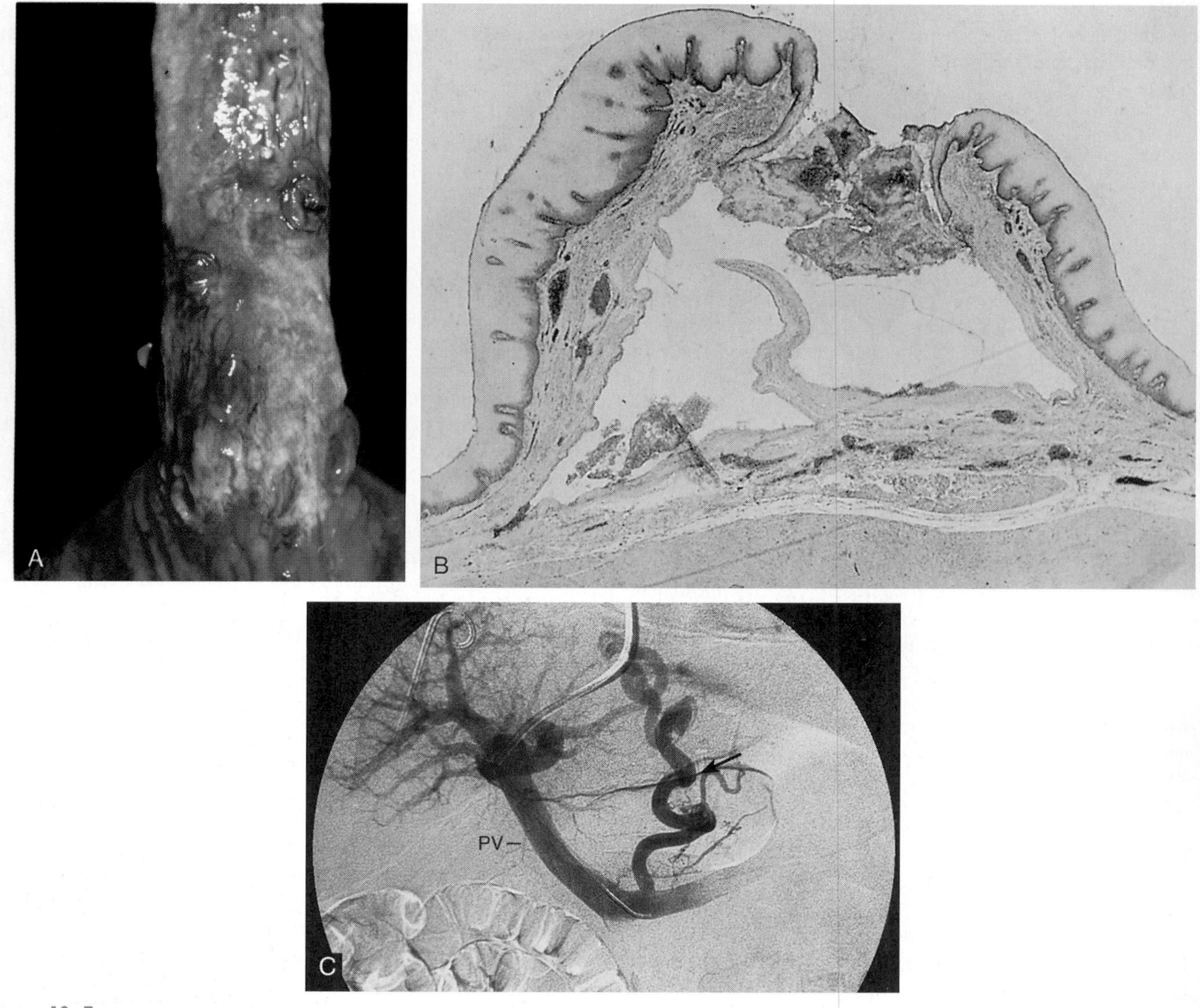

Figure 18–7

Esophageal varices. *A*, View of the everted esophagus and gastroesophageal junction showing dilated submucosal veins (varices). The blue-colored varices have collapsed in this postmortem specimen. *B*, Low-power cross-section of a dilated submucosal varix that has ruptured through the mucosa. *C*, Hepatic venogram after injection of dye into portal veins (PV) to show a large tortuous gastroesophageal varix (*arrow*) extending superiorly from the patent main portal vein. (*C*, courtesy of Dr. Emily Sedgwick, Brigham and Women's Hospital, Boston, MA.)

persons per 100,000 yearly and is predominantly a disease of men (male-to-female ratio, 4 : 1). Blacks throughout the world are at higher risk than are whites, reaching a fourfold higher incidence in the United States.

Etiology and Pathogenesis. The marked differences in epidemiology strongly implicate dietary and environmental factors (Table 18–1), with an ill-defined contribution from genetic predisposition.[9] The majority of cancers in Europe and the United States are attributable to alcohol and tobacco usage. Some alcoholic drinks contain significant amounts of such carcinogens as polycyclic hydrocarbons, fusel oils, and nitrosamines along with other mutagenic compounds. Nutritional deficiencies associated with alcoholism may contribute to the process of carcinogenesis.

Alcohol and tobacco cannot be invoked as risk factors in many high-incidence regions of the world. The presence of carcinogens, such as fungus-contaminated and nitrosamine-containing foodstuffs in China, may play a significant role in the extraordinary incidence of carcinoma in this region. Dietary deficiencies in vitamins and essential metals have been documented in China and South Africa. Human papillomavirus DNA is found frequently in esophageal squamous cell carcinomas from high-incidence regions. Its presence is infrequent, however, in cancer-bearing patients of North America.[10]

Based on the aforementioned considerations, dietary and environmental factors have been proposed to increase risk, with nutritional deficiencies acting as promoters or poten-

Table 18–1. FACTORS ASSOCIATED WITH THE DEVELOPMENT OF SQUAMOUS CELL CARCINOMA OF THE ESOPHAGUS

Dietary
Deficiency of vitamins (A, C, riboflavin, thiamine, pyridoxine)
Deficiency of trace metals (zinc, molybdenum)
Fungal contamination of foodstuffs
High content of nitrites/nitrosamines
Betel chewing

Lifestyle
Alcohol consumption
Tobacco use
Urban environment

Esophageal Disorders
Long-standing esophagitis
Achalasia
Plummer-Vinson syndrome

Genetic Predisposition
Long-standing celiac disease
Ectodermal dysplasia, epidermolysis bullosa
Tylosis palmaris et plantaris
Racial disposition

tiators of the tumorigenic effects of environmental carcinogens. For example, methylating nitroso compounds in the diet and in tobacco smoke may be the reason for the broad spectrum of *p53* point mutations, which are present in more than half of esophageal cancers. Mutations in *p16* and allelic loss (loss of heterogeneity) involving other chromosomes are prevalent in these cancers as well, in keeping with the concept that stepwise acquisition and accumulation of genetic alterations ultimately gives rise to cancer.[11] Notably absent from esophageal squamous cell carcinomas are K-*ras* and adenomatous polyposis coli (APC) gene mutations.

Finally, the chronic esophagitis so commonly observed in persons living in areas of high incidence may itself be the result of chronic exposure to such carcinogens. This esophagitis results in an increased epithelial cell turnover, which, over a length of time in a continuously carcinogenic environment, progresses to dysplasia and eventually to carcinoma.

MORPHOLOGY. Similar to squamous cell carcinomas arising in other locations, those of the esophagus begin as apparent in situ lesions. When they become overt, about 20% of these tumors are located in the upper third, 50% in the middle third, and 30% in the lower third of the esophagus. Early lesions appear as small, gray-white, plaquelike thickenings or elevations of the mucosa. In months to years, these lesions become tumorous masses and may eventually encircle the lumen. Three morphologic patterns are described: (1) **protruded (60%)—a polypoid exophytic** lesion that protrudes into the lumen (Fig. 18–8); (2) **flat (15%)—a diffuse, infiltrative form that tends to spread within the wall of the esophagus, causing thickening, rigidity, and narrowing of the lumen;** and (3) **excavated (25%)—a necrotic cancerous ulceration that excavates deeply into surrounding structures** and may erode into the respiratory tree (with resultant fistula and pneumonia) or aorta (with catastrophic exsanguination) or permeate the mediastinum and pericardium. The fortunate patient is found at the stage of **superficial esophageal carcinoma**, in which the malignant lesion is confined to the epithelial layer (in situ) or is superficially invading the lamina propria or submucosa (Fig. 18–9).

Most squamous cell carcinomas are moderately to well differentiated. Regardless of their degree of differentiation, most symptomatic tumors are quite large by the time they are diagnosed and have already invaded the wall or beyond. The

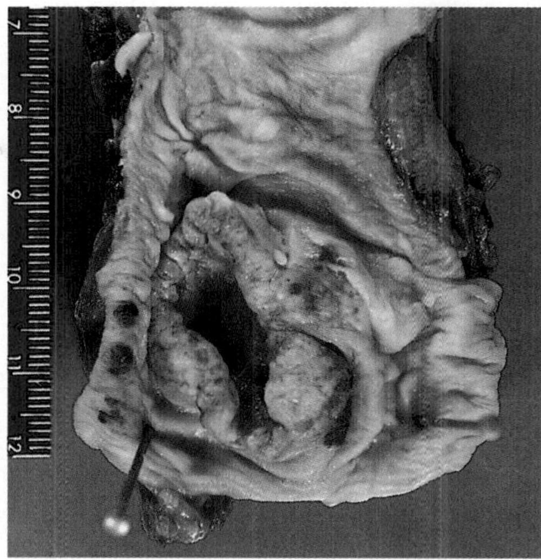

Figure 18–8

Large ulcerated squamous cell carcinoma of the esophagus.

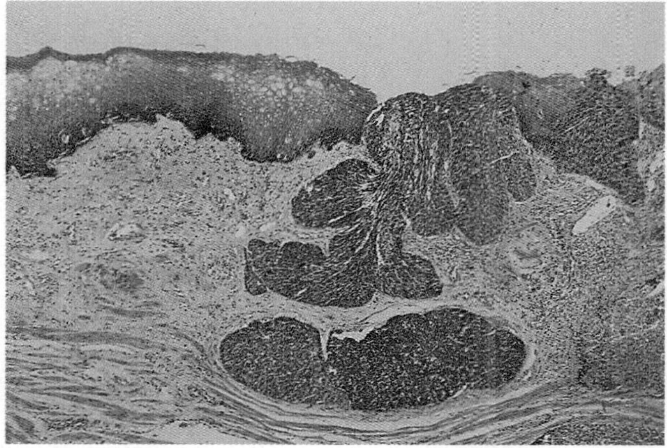

Figure 18–9

Squamous cell carcinoma of the esophagus. Low-power microscopic view showing invasion into the submucosa.

rich lymphatic network in the submucosa promotes extensive circumferential and longitudinal spread, and intramural tumor cell clusters may often be seen several centimeters away from the main mass. Local extension into adjacent mediastinal structures occurs early and often in this disease. Tumors located in the upper third of the esophagus also metastasize to cervical lymph nodes; those in the middle third to the mediastinal, paratracheal, and tracheobronchial nodes; and those in the lower third most often to the gastric and celiac groups of nodes.

Clinical Features. Esophageal carcinoma is insidious in onset and produces dysphagia and obstruction gradually and late. Patients subconsciously adjust to their increasing difficulty in swallowing by progressively altering their diet from solid to liquid foods. Extreme weight loss and debilitation result from both the impaired nutrition and the effects of the tumor itself. Hemorrhage and sepsis may accompany ulceration of the tumor. Occasionally the first alarming symptom is aspiration of food via a cancerous tracheoesophageal fistula. Although the insidious growth of these neoplasms often leads to large lesions by the time a diagnosis is established, resectability rates have improved modestly (from $<50\%$ to $>80\%$) with the advent of endoscopic screening in patient populations at risk. Five-year survival rates in patients with superficial esophageal carcinoma are about 75%, compared with 25% in patients undergoing *curative* surgery for more advanced disease and 5% for all patients with esophageal carcinoma. Local and distant recurrence after surgery is common. The presence of lymph node metastases at the time of resection significantly reduces the 5-year survival.

Adenocarcinoma

Because of confusion with gastric cancers arising at the gastroesophageal junction, true esophageal adenocarcinomas were thought to be unusual. With increasing recognition of Barrett mucosa, it is apparent that most adenocarcinomas in the lower third of the esophagus are true esophageal cancers, rather than gastric cancers straddling the esophagogastric junction.[12] Accordingly, adenocarcinoma now represents up to half of all esophageal cancers reported in the United States.

Etiology and Pathogenesis. Although the pathogenesis of Barrett esophagus is unclear, genetic alterations in this disease are well documented.[7] Overexpression of *p53* protein and increased proportions of cells with a G1/S DNA content are occasionally observed in metaplastic Barrett epithelium, presumably the result of chronic cell and DNA damage induced by gastric reflux. Allelic losses in *17p* or point mutations in *p53* are evident only in dysplastic foci, resulting in functional inactivation of the *p53* gene and abrogation of cell cycle control at the G1/S transition. Clonal progression of dysplastic foci to frank adenocarcinoma then occurs, with accumulation of further chromosomal abnormalities.

MORPHOLOGY. Adenocarcinomas arising in the setting of Barrett esophagus are usually located in the distal esophagus and may invade the adjacent gastric cardia. Initially appearing as flat or raised patches of an otherwise intact mucosa, they may develop into large nodular masses up to 5 cm in diameter or may exhibit diffusely infiltrative or deeply ulcerative features (Fig. 18–10*A*). Microscopically, most tumors are mucin-produc-

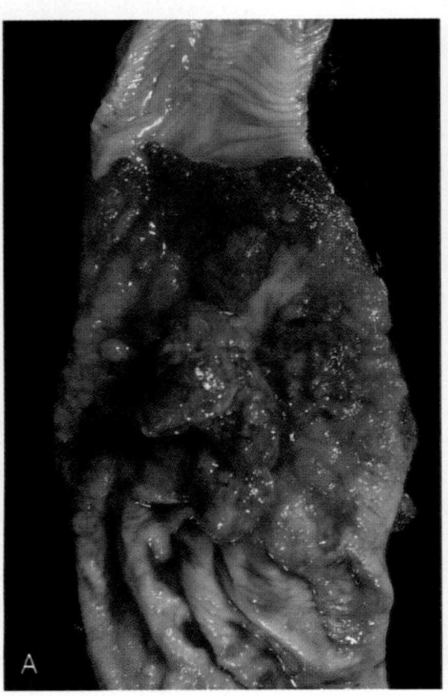

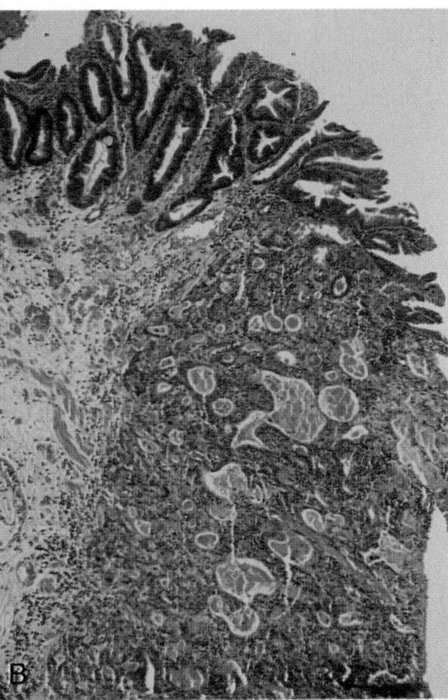

Figure 18–10

A, Gross view of an ulcerated, exophytic adenocarcinoma at the gastroesophageal junction, arising from mucosa of Barrett esophagus. The gray-white esophageal squamous mucosa is on top, and the folds of gastric mucosa below. A small patch of white squamous epithelium remains in center of tumor. (*A*, courtesy of Dr. James Gulizia, Brigham and Women's Hospital, Boston, MA.) *B*, Microscopic view of malignant intestinal-type glands in adenocarcinoma arising from Barrett esophagus.

ing glandular tumors exhibiting intestinal-type features (Fig. 18–10*B*) or, less often, are made up of diffusely infiltrative signet-ring cells of a gastric type.

Clinical Features. Adenocarcinomas arising in Barrett esophagus chiefly occur in patients over 40 years of age, with a median age in the fifties. In keeping with Barrett esophagus, adenocarcinoma is more common in men than women, and whites are affected more frequently than blacks, in contrast to squamous cell carcinomas. As in other forms of esophageal carcinoma, patients usually present because of dysphagia. Progressive weight loss, bleeding, chest pain, and vomiting may occur.

The prognosis of esophageal adenocarcinoma is as poor as that for other forms of esophageal cancer, with less than 30% 5-year survival. Identification and resection of early cancers with invasion limited to the mucosa or submucosa improves 5-year survival to greater than 80%. Although dysplasia appears to be a precursor for the development of adenocarcinoma, patients with low-grade dysplasia may not progress to cancer over long periods of follow-up, and apparent regression may occur.

Stomach

NORMAL STOMACH

The stomach is a saccular organ with a volume of 1200 to 1500 ml but a capacity of greater than 3000 ml. It extends from just left of the midline superiorly, where it is joined to the esophagus, to just right of the midline inferiorly, where it connects to the duodenum. The concavity of the right, inner curve is called the *lesser curvature*, and the convexity of the left, outer curve is the *greater curvature*. An angle along the lesser curvature, the *incisura angularis*, marks the approximate point at which the stomach narrows before its junction with the duodenum.

The stomach is divided into five anatomic regions (Fig. 18–11). The *cardia* is the narrow conical portion of the stomach immediately distal to the gastroesophageal junction. The *fundus* is the dome-shaped portion of the proximal stomach that extends superolaterally to the gastroesophageal junction. The *body*, or *corpus*, comprises the remainder of the stomach proximal to the incisura angularis. The stomach distal to this angle is the *antrum*, demarcated from the duodenum by the muscular *pyloric sphincter*.

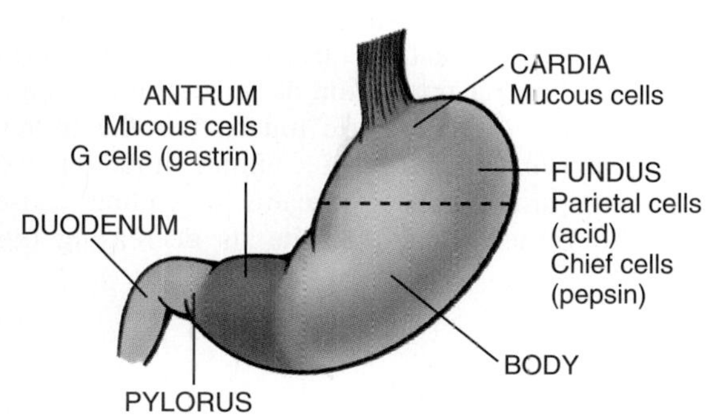

Figure 18–11

Anatomy of the stomach.

The gastric wall consists of mucosa, submucosa, muscularis propria, and serosa. The interior surface of the stomach exhibits coarse *rugae*. These infoldings of mucosa and submucosa extend longitudinally and are most prominent in the proximal stomach, flattening out when the stomach is distended. A finer mosaic-like pattern is delineated by small furrows in the mucosa. Finally, the delicate texture of the mucosa is punctuated by millions of gastric foveolae, or *pits*, leading to the mucosal glands.

The entire mucosal surface as well as the lining of the gastric pits is composed of surface foveolar cells. These tall, columnar mucin-secreting cells have basal nuclei and crowded, small, relatively clear mucin-containing granules in the supranuclear region. Deeper in the gastric pits are so-called *mucous neck cells*, which have a lower content of mucin granules and are thought to be the progenitors of both the surface epithelium and the cells of the gastric glands. Mitoses are extremely common in this region, as the entire gastric mucosal surface is totally replaced every 2 to 6 days.

The gastric glands vary between anatomic regions, as follows:

- *Cardia glands* contain mucus-secreting cells.
- *Gastric* or *oxyntic glands* are found in the fundus and body and contain parietal cells, chief cells, and scattered endocrine cells.
- *Antral* or *pyloric glands* contain mucus-secreting cells and endocrine cells.

The key cell types in the gastric glands are the following:

- *Mucous cells* populate the glands of the cardia and antral regions and secrete mucus and pepsinogen II. The mucous neck cells in the glands of the body and fundus secrete mucus as well as group I and II pepsinogens.
- *Parietal cells* line predominantly the upper half of gastric glands in the fundus and body. They are recognizable by their bright eosinophilia on hematoxylin and eosin preparations, attributable to their abundant mitochondria. The apical membrane of the parietal cell is invaginated, forming an extensive intracellular canalicu-

lar system complete with microvilli. In the resting state, vesicles lie in close approximation to the canalicular system. These vesicles contain the hydrogen ion pump, a unique H^+,K^+-ATPase that pumps hydrogen across membranes in exchange for potassium ions. Within minutes of parietal cell stimulation, the vesicles fuse with the canalicular system, thereby creating an apically directed, acid-secreting membrane of enormous surface area. Parietal cells also secrete *intrinsic factor*, which binds luminal vitamin B_{12} and permits its absorption in the ileum.

- *Chief cells* are concentrated more at the base of gastric fundus and body glands and are responsible for the secretion of the proteolytic proenzymes *pepsinogen I and II*. Chief cells are notable for their basophilic cytoplasm and ultrastructurally are classic protein-synthesizing cells, having an extensive subnuclear rough endoplasmic reticulum, a prominent supranuclear Golgi apparatus, and numerous apical secretory granules. On stimulation of chief cells, the pepsinogens contained in the granules are released by exocytosis. The pepsinogens are activated to *pepsin* by the low luminal pH and inactivated above pH 6 on entry into the duodenum.
- *Endocrine, or enteroendocrine, cells* are scattered among the epithelial cells of fundus, body, and antral glands. The cytoplasm of these triangular cells contains small, brightly eosinophilic granules that are concentrated on the basal aspect of the cell. These cells can act in an endocrine mode, releasing their products into the circulation, or a paracrine mode, via secretion into the local tissue.

Gastric Mucosal Physiology

ACID SECRETION

The hallmark of gastric physiology is secretion of hydrochloric acid, divided into three phases, as follows:

- The *cephalic phase*, initiated by the sight, taste, smell, chewing, and swallowing of palatable food, is mediated by vagal activity.
- The *gastric phase* involves stimulation of mechanical receptors by gastric distention and is mediated by vagal impulses and gastrin release from endocrine cells in the antral glands, designated *G cells*. Gastrin release also is promoted by luminal amino acids and peptides.
- The *intestinal phase*, initiated when food containing digested protein enters the proximal small intestine, involves a polypeptide distinct from gastrin.

All signals converge on the gastric parietal cell, as follows:[13]

- Cephalic-vagal or gastric-vagal afferents directly stimulate the parietal cell via the muscarinic type of cholinergic receptors for acetylcholine.
- Gastrin presumably activates a gastrin receptor.
- *An oxyntic gland endocrine cell designated the enterochromaffin-like cell plays a central role*: Gastrin and vagal afferents induce the release of histamine from the enterochromaffin-like cell, thereby stimulating the histamine$_2$ receptor on parietal cells.

MUCOSAL PROTECTION

At maximal secretory rates, the intraluminal concentration of hydrogen ion is *3 million times* greater than that of the blood and tissues. The *mucosal barrier* protects the gastric mucosa from autodigestion and is created by the following:[14]

- *Mucus secretion*: The thin layer of surface mucus in the stomach and duodenum exhibits a diffusion coefficient for H^+ that is one fourth that of water. Acid-containing and pepsin-containing fluid exits the gastric glands as *jets* passing through the surface mucous layer, entering the lumen directly without contacting surface epithelial cells.
- *Bicarbonate secretion*: Surface epithelial cells in both the stomach and the duodenum secrete bicarbonate into the boundary zone of adherent mucus, creating an essentially pH-neutral microenvironment immediately adjacent to the cell surface.
- *Epithelial barrier*: Intercellular tight junctions provide a barrier to the back-diffusion of hydrogen ions. Epithelial disruption is followed rapidly by *restitution*, in which existing cells migrate along the exposed basement membrane to fill in the defects and restore epithelial barrier integrity.
- *Mucosal blood flow*: The rich mucosal blood supply provides oxygen, bicarbonate, and nutrients to epithelial cells and removes back-diffused acid.

When the mucosal barrier is breached, the muscularis mucosa limits injury. Superficial damage, limited to the mucosa, can heal within hours to days. When damage extends into the submucosa, weeks are required for complete healing. Imperfect as our understanding of these defensive mechanisms may be, they are clearly a physiologic marvel, or gastric walls would suffer the same fate as a piece of swallowed meat.

PATHOLOGY

Gastric lesions are frequent causes of clinical disease. In Western industrialized nations, peptic ulcers develop in up to 10% of the general population at some point during life. Chronic infection of the gastric mucosa by the bacterium *Helicobacter pylori* is the most common infection worldwide. Lastly, gastric cancer remains a leading cause of death in the United States, despite its decreasing overall incidence.

Congenital Anomalies

Heterotopic rests of normal tissue may be present at any site in the gastrointestinal tract and are usually asymptomatic. With *pancreatic heterotopia*, nodules of essentially normal pancreatic tissue up to 1 cm in diameter may be present in the gastric or intestinal submucosa, in the muscle wall, or in a subserosal position. When in the pylorus, localized inflammation may lead to pyloric obstruction. With *gastric heterotopia*, small patches of ectopic gastric mucosa in the duodenum or in more distal sites may present as perplexing sources of bleeding, owing to peptic ulceration of adjacent mucosa.

Defective closure of the diaphragmatic anlage leads to weakness or partial-to-total absence of a region of the diaphragm, usually on the left. Resultant herniation of abdominal contents into the thorax in utero produces a *diaphragmatic hernia*. Usually the stomach or a portion of it insinuates into the pouch, but occasionally small bowel and even a portion of the liver accompany it. The herniation may be asymptomatic or may engender potentially lethal respiratory embarassment in the newborn.

PYLORIC STENOSIS

Congenital hypertrophic pyloric stenosis is encountered in infants as a disorder that affects boys three to four times more often than girls, occurring in 1 in 300 to 900 live births. Familial occurrence implicates a multifactorial pattern of inheritance; monozygotic twins have a high rate of concordance of the condition. Pyloric stenosis also may occur in association with Turner syndrome, trisomy 18, and esophageal atresia. Regurgitation and persistent, projectile, nonbilious vomiting usually appear in the second or third week of life. Physical examination reveals visible peristalsis and a firm, ovoid palpable mass in the region of the pylorus or distal stomach, the result of hypertrophy, and possibly hyperplasia, of the muscularis propria of the pylorus. Edema and inflammatory changes in the mucosa and submucosa may aggravate the narrowing. Surgical muscle splitting is curative.

Acquired pyloric stenosis in adults is one of the long-term risks of antral gastritis or peptic ulcers close to the pylorus. Carcinomas of the pyloric region, lymphomas, or adjacent carcinomas of the pancreas are more sinister causes. In these cases, inflammatory fibrosis or malignant infiltration narrows the pyloric channel, producing pyloric outlet obstruction. In rare instances, hypertrophic pyloric stenosis is the result of prolonged pyloric spasm or delayed appearance of the childhood pattern.

Gastritis

The diagnosis of gastritis is both overused and often missed—overused when it is applied loosely to any transient upper abdominal complaint in the absence of validating evidence, and missed because most patients with chronic gastritis are asymptomatic. *Gastritis is simply defined as inflammation of the gastric mucosa.* Inflammation may be predominantly *acute*, with neutrophilic infiltration, or *chronic*, with lymphocytes, plasma cells, or both predominating and associated intestinal metaplasia and atrophy.

ACUTE GASTRITIS

Acute gastritis is an acute mucosal inflammatory process, usually of a transient nature. The inflammation may be accompanied by hemorrhage into the mucosa and, in more severe circumstances, by sloughing of the superficial mucosa. This severe erosive form of the disease is an important cause of acute gastrointestinal bleeding.

Pathogenesis. The pathogenesis is poorly understood, in part because normal mechanisms for gastric mucosal protection are not clear. Acute gastritis is frequently associated with the following:

- Heavy use of nonsteroidal anti-inflammatory drugs (NSAIDs), particularly aspirin
- Excessive alcohol consumption
- Heavy smoking
- Treatment with cancer chemotherapeutic drugs
- Uremia
- Systemic infections (e.g., salmonellosis)
- Severe stress (e.g., trauma, burns, surgery)
- Ischemia and shock
- Suicidal attempts, as with acids and alkali
- Gastric irradiation or freezing
- Mechanical trauma (e.g., nasogastric intubation)
- After distal gastrectomy

One or more of the following influences are thought to be operative in these varied settings: increased acid secretion with back-diffusion, decreased production of bicarbonate buffer, reduced blood flow, disruption of the adherent mucus layer, and direct damage to the epithelium. Not surprisingly, mucosal insults can act synergistically. Thus, ischemic injury would worsen the effects of back-diffusion of hydrogen ions. Other mucosal insults have been identified, such as regurgitation of detergent bile acids and lysolecithins from the proximal duodenum and inadequate mucosal synthesis of prostaglandins. A substantial portion of patients have idiopathic gastritis, with no associated disorders.

MORPHOLOGY. In its mildest form, the lamina propria exhibits only moderate edema and slight vascular congestion. The surface epithelium is intact, and scattered neutrophils are present among the surface epithelial cells or within the epithelial layer and lumen of mucosal glands. **The presence of neutrophils above the basement membrane (within the epithelial space) is abnormal and signifies active inflammation (activity).** With more severe mucosal damage, erosion and hemorrhage develop. **Erosion denotes loss of the superficial epithelium, generating a defect in the mucosa that does not cross the muscularis mucosa. It is accompanied by a robust acute inflammatory infiltrate and extrusion of a fibrin-containing purulent exudate into the lumen.** Hemorrhage may occur independently, generating punctate dark spots in an otherwise hyperemic mucosa, or in association with erosion. Concurrent erosion and hemorrhage is termed **acute erosive gastritis** (Fig. 18–12*A*). Large areas of the gastric mucosa may

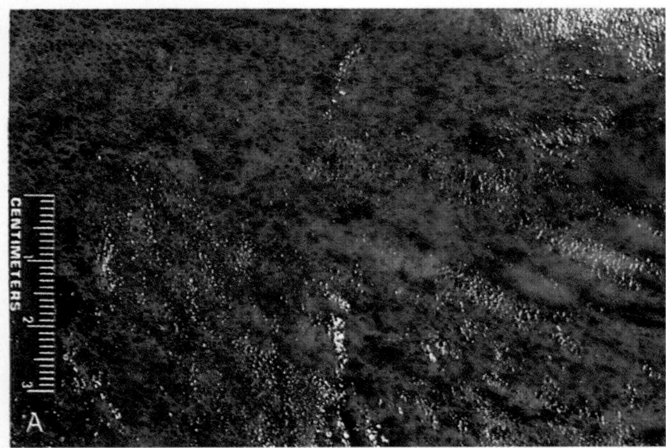

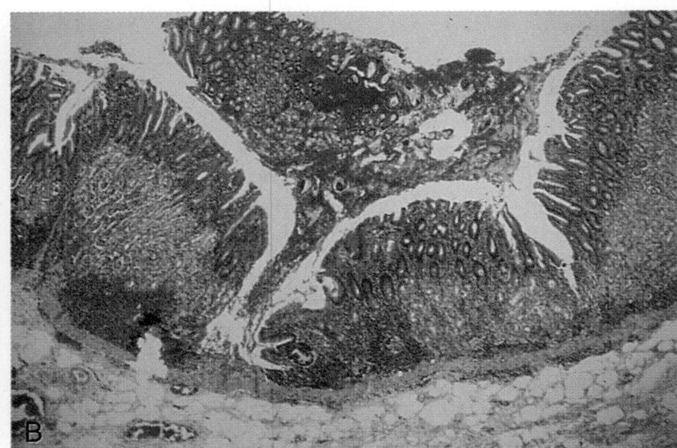

Figure 18–12

Acute gastritis. *A*, Gross view showing punctate erosions in an otherwise unremarkable mucosa; adherent blood is dark owing to exposure to gastric acid. *B*, Low-power microscopic view of focal mucosal disruption with hemorrhage; the adjacent mucosa is normal.

be denuded, but the involvement is superficial and rarely affects the entire depth of the mucosa (Fig. 18–12*B*). These lesions are but one step removed from stress ulcers, to be described later.

Clinical Features. Depending on the severity of the anatomic changes, acute gastritis may be entirely asymptomatic; may cause variable epigastric pain, nausea, and vomiting; or may present with overt hemorrhage, massive hematemesis, melena, and potentially fatal blood loss. Overall, it is one of the major causes of massive hematemesis, as in alcoholics. In particular settings, the condition is quite common. As many as 25% of persons who take daily aspirin for rheumatoid arthritis develop acute gastritis at some time, many with bleeding.

CHRONIC GASTRITIS (INCLUDING *HELICOBACTER* INFECTION)

Chronic gastritis is defined as the presence of chronic mucosal inflammatory changes leading eventually to mucosal atrophy and epithelial metaplasia, usually in the absence of erosions. The epithelial changes may become dysplastic and constitute a background for the development of carcinoma. Chronic gastritis is notable for distinct causal subgroups and for patterns of histologic alterations that vary in different parts of the world. In the Western world, the prevalence of histologic changes indicative of chronic gastritis exceeds 50% in the later decades of life.

Pathogenesis. The major etiologic associations of chronic gastritis are as follows:

- Chronic infection by *H. pylori* (Chapter 9)
- Immunologic (*autoimmune*), in association with pernicious anemia
- Toxic, as with alcohol ingestion and cigarette smoking
- Postsurgical, especially after antrectomy with gastroenterostomy with reflux of bilious duodenal secretions
- Motor and mechanical, including obstruction, bezoars (luminal concretions), and gastric atony
- Radiation
- Granulomatous conditions
- Miscellaneous—amyloidosis, graft-versus-host disease

Helicobacter pylori. By far the most important etiologic association is chronic infection by the bacillus *H. pylori.* As evident in this and later discussions, this organism plays a critical role in several major gastric diseases (Table 18–2). *H. pylori* is present in 90% of patients with chronic gastritis affecting the antrum. Colonization rates increase with age, reaching 50% in asymptomatic American adults over 50 years of age. Prevalence of infection among adults in Puerto Rico exceeds 80%. In this and other areas where infection is endemic, the organism seems to be acquired in childhood and persists for decades. *Most infected persons also have the associated gastritis but are asymptomatic.* Nevertheless, infected persons are at increased risk for the development of peptic ulcer disease and possibly gastric cancer.

H. pylori is a nonsporing, curvilinear gram-negative rod measuring approximately 3.5 × 0.5 μm.[15] *H. pylori* is part of a genus of bacteria that have adapted to the ecologic niche provided by gastric mucus. The specialized traits that allow *H. pylori* to flourish include the following:

- Motility (via flagella), allowing it to swim through viscous mucus
- Elaboration of a *urease*, which produces ammonia from

Table 18–2. DISEASES ASSOCIATED WITH *HELICOBACTER PYLORI* INFECTION

Chronic gastritis	Strong causal association
Peptic ulcer disease	Strong causal association
Gastric carcinoma	Postulated etiologic role
Gastric lymphoma	Postulated etiologic role

endogenous urea, thereby buffering gastric acid in the immediate vicinity of the organism

- Binding of *H. pylori* organisms to gastric epithelial cells via a bacterial *adhesin*; binding is enhanced with epithelial cells that bear the blood group O antigen

H. pylori strains that express the *cag*A gene are strongly associated with duodenal ulcer; the function of the 120- to 140-kD protein product is unknown. Such strains frequently express the *vac*A gene also, which codes for an 87-kD vacuolating cytotoxin. These two proteins, along with bacterial lipopolysaccharide (endotoxin) and other protein products, appear to act as proinflammatory substances. *H. pylori* appears to be capable of initiating and perpetuating a chronic state of gastric mucosal injury (Fig. 18–13). Patients with chronic gastritis and *H. pylori* usually improve when treated with antimicrobial agents, and relapses are associated with reappearance of this organism.

Autoimmune Gastritis. This form of gastritis accounts for less than 10% of cases of chronic gastritis. It results from the presence of autoantibodies to the gastric gland parietal cells and intrinsic factor, including one against the acid-producing enzyme, H^+,K^+-ATPase.[16] Gland destruction and mucosal atrophy lead to loss of acid production. In the most severe cases, production of intrinsic factor is lost, leading to pernicious anemia (Chapter 14). This uncommon form of gastritis is seen in association with other autoimmune disorders, such as Hashimoto thyroiditis and Addison disease.

MORPHOLOGY. Chronic gastritis may affect different regions of the stomach and exhibit varying degrees of mucosal damage.[17] **Autoimmune gastritis is characterized by diffuse mucosal damage of the body-fundic mucosa, with less intense-to-absent antral damage. Gastritis in the setting of environmental causes (including infection by *H. pylori*) tends to affect antral mucosa or both antral and body-fundic mucosa.** By visual inspection, the mucosa is usually reddened and has a coarser texture than normal. The inflammatory infiltrate may create a boggy-appearing mucosa with thickened rugal folds, mimicking early infiltrative lesions. Alternatively, with long-standing atrophic disease, the mucosa may become thinned and flattened. Regardless of cause or location, the histologic changes are similar. An inflammatory infiltrate of lymphocytes and plasma cells is present within the lamina propria (Fig. 18–14). **Active inflammation is signified by the presence of neutrophils within the glandular and surface epithelial layer.** Active inflammation may be prominent or absent. Lymphoid aggregates, some with germinal centers, are frequently observed within the mucosa. Several additional histologic features are characteristic.

Regenerative Change. A proliferative response to

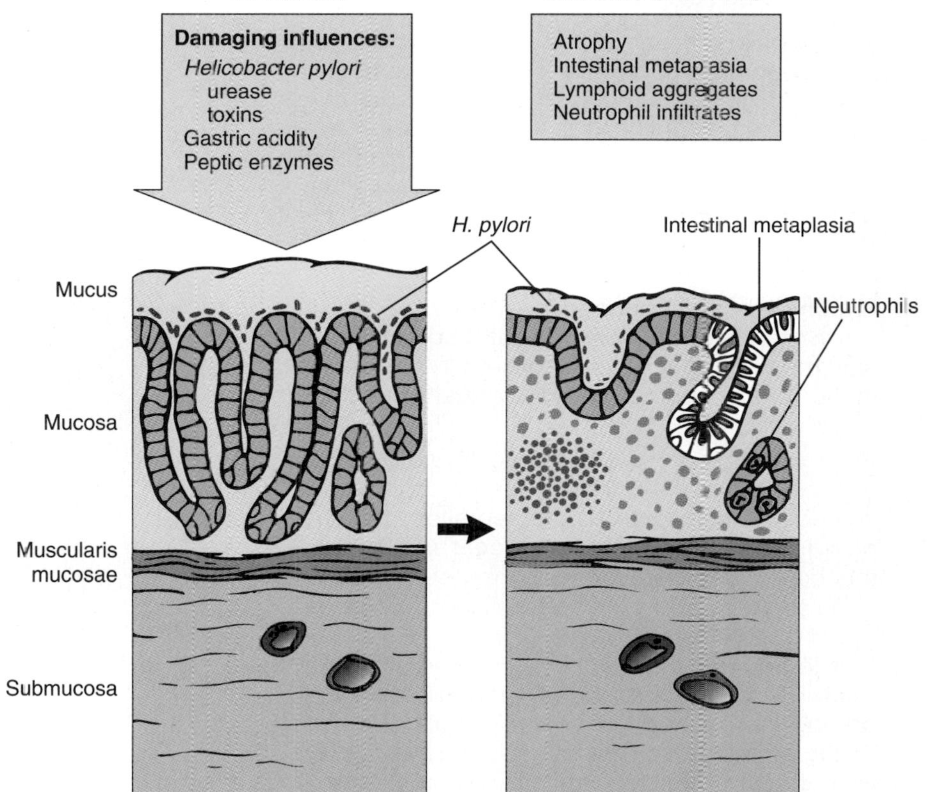

Figure 18–13

Schematic presentation of the presumed action of *Helicobacter pylori* in the development of chronic gastritis. *H. pylori* infection leads to exposure of the gastric mucosa to bacteria-derived urease and toxins, including lipopolysaccharide, *cag*A, and *vac*A. These, in concert with host-derived gastric acidity and peptic enzymes, produce a chronic state of gastric mucosal injury leading to chronic gastritis as depicted. Note that *H. pylori* do not colonize regions of intestinal metaplasia.

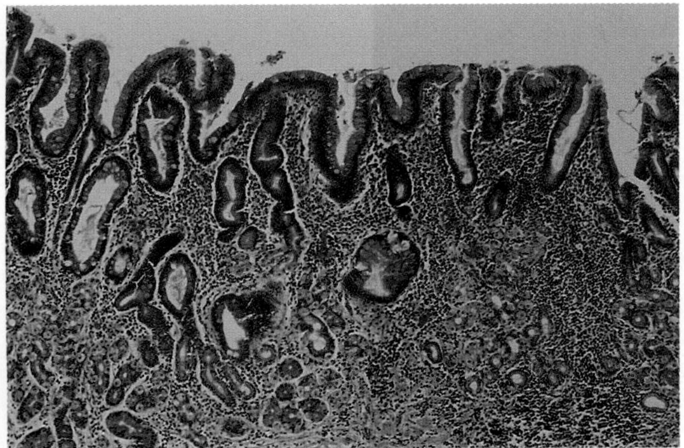

Figure 18–14

Chronic gastritis showing partial replacement of the gastric mucosal epithelium by intestinal metaplasia *(upper left)* and with inflammation of the lamina propria involving *(right)* lymphocytes and plasma cells.

the epithelial injury is a constant feature of chronic gastritis. In the neck region of the gastric glands, mitotic figures are increased. Epithelial cells of the surface mucosa, and to a lesser extent the glands, exhibit enlarged, hyperchromatic nuclei and a higher nuclear-to-cytoplasmic ratio. Mucus vacuoles are diminished or absent in the superficial cells. When regenerative changes are severe, particularly with ongoing active inflammation, distinguishing regenerative change from frank dysplasia may be difficult.

Metaplasia. Both antral and body-fundic mucosa may become partially replaced by metaplastic columnar absorptive cells and goblet cells of intestinal morphology (**intestinal metaplasia**), both along the surface epithelium and in rudimentary glands. Occasionally, villus-like projections may appear. Although small intestinal features predominate, in some instances features of colonic epithelium may be present.

Atrophy. Atrophic change is evident by marked loss in glandular structures. Parietal cells, in particular, may be conspicuously absent in the autoimmune form. Persisting glands frequently undergo cystic dilation.

Hyperplasia. **A particular feature of atrophic gastritis of autoimmune origin, or chronic gastritis treated by inhibitors of acid secretion, is hyperplasia of gastrin-producing G cells in the antral mucosa.** This hyperplasia is attributed to the hypochlorhydria or achlorhydria arising from severe loss of parietal cell acid secretion.

In individuals infected by *H. pylori*, the organism lies in the superficial mucous layer and among the microvilli of epithelial cells. The distribution of organisms can be patchy and irregular, with areas of heavy colonization adjacent to those with no organisms. In extreme cases, the organisms carpet the luminal surfaces of surface epithelial cells, the mucous neck cells, and the epithelial cells lining the gastric pits; they do not invade the mucosa. The organisms are most easily demonstrated with silver stains (Fig. 18–15), although organisms can be seen on Giemsa-stained and routine hematoxylin and eosin-stained tissue. Even in heavily colonized stomachs, **the organisms are absent from areas with intestinal metaplasia.** Conversely, organisms may be present in foci of pyloric metaplasia in an inflamed duodenum, and in gastric-type mucosa of Barrett esophagus.

Dysplasia. With long-standing chronic gastritis, the epithelium develops cytologic alterations, including variation in size, shape, and orientation of epithelial cells and nuclear enlargement and atypia. The cellular atypia tends to be most marked in long-standing autoimmune gastritis associated with pernicious anemia. **Dysplastic alterations may become so severe as to constitute in situ carcinoma.** As such, they probably account for the increased incidence of gastric cancer in atrophic forms of gastritis, particularly in association with pernicious anemia.

Clinical Features. Chronic gastritis usually causes few symptoms. Nausea, vomiting, and upper abdominal discomfort may occur. Individuals with advanced gastritis from *H. pylori* or other environmental causes are often hypochlorhydric, owing to parietal cell damage and atrophy of body-fundic mucosa. Because parietal cells are never completely destroyed, however, these patients do not develop achlorhydria or pernicious anemia. Serum gastrin levels are usually within the normal range or only modestly elevated.

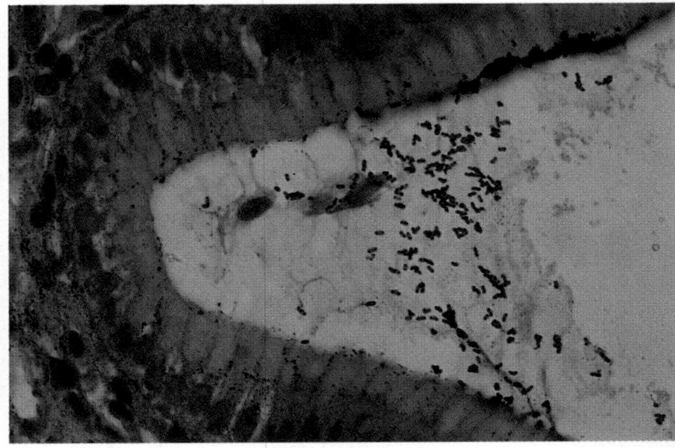

Figure 18–15

H. pylori. A Steiner silver stain demonstrates the numerous darkly stained *Helicobacter* organisms along the luminal surface of the gastric epithelial cells and within adherent mucus. Note that there is no tissue invasion by bacteria.

When severe parietal cell loss occurs in the setting of autoimmune gastritis, hypochlorhydria or achlorhydria and hypergastrinemia are characteristically present. Circulating autoantibodies to a diverse array of parietal cell antigens may be detected. A small subset of these patients (10%) may develop overt pernicious anemia after a period of years. The familial occurrence of pernicious anemia is well established; a high prevalence of gastric autoantibodies is also found in asymptomatic relatives of patients with pernicious anemia. The distribution suggests that the inheritance of autoimmune gastritis is autosomal dominant.

Most important is the relationship of chronic gastritis to the development of peptic ulcer and gastric carcinoma (see later). Most patients with a peptic ulcer, whether duodenal or gastric, have *H. pylori* infection. The long-term risk of gastric cancer in persons with autoimmune gastritis is 2 to 4%, which is considerably greater than the normal population. *H. pylori* has been implicated as contributing to the pathogenesis of both gastric carcinoma and lymphoma.

Special Forms of Gastritis

Several diseases merit separate mention. *Eosinophilic gastritis* is an idiopathic condition that features a prominent eosinophilic infiltrate of the mucosa, muscle wall, or all layers of the stomach, usually in the antral or pyloric region. Typically affecting middle-aged women, the primary symptom is abdominal pain, although swelling of the pylorus may produce gastric outlet obstruction. This disease may occur in association with *eosinophilic enteritis* and often is accompanied by a peripheral eosinophilia. Steroid therapy is usually effective. *Allergic gastroenteropathy* is a disorder of children that may produce symptoms of diarrhea, vomiting, and growth failure. An infiltrate of eosinophils limited to the mucosa can usually be demonstrated in antral biopsy specimens.

Lymphocytic gastritis is a condition in which lymphocytes densely populate the epithelial layer of the mucosal surface and pits. The intraepithelial lymphocytes are exclusively T lymphocytes, mostly CD8+ suppressor cells. This condition produces indistinct symptoms, such as abdominal pain, nausea, and vomiting. Although idiopathic in nature, it is increasingly associated with celiac sprue (see later).

The presence of intramucosal epithelioid granulomas can usually be attributed to Crohn disease, sarcoidosis, infection (tuberculosis, histoplasmosis, anisakiasis), a systemic vasculitis, or a reaction to foreign materials. *Granulomatous gastritis* is the term reserved for patients with no such conditions. This idiopathic disorder is clinically benign.

Peptic Ulcer Disease

An ulcer is defined as a breach in the mucosa of the alimentary tract, which extends through the muscularis mucosae into the submucosa or deeper. Although ulcers may occur anywhere in the alimentary tract, none are as prevalent as the peptic ulcers that occur in the duodenum and stomach. Acute gastric ulcers may also appear under conditions of severe systemic stress.

PEPTIC ULCERS

Peptic ulcers are chronic, most often solitary, lesions that occur in any portion of the gastrointestinal tract exposed to the aggressive action of acid-peptic juices. Peptic ulcers are usually solitary lesions less than 4 cm in diameter, located in the following sites, in order of decreasing frequency:

- Duodenum, first portion
- Stomach, usually antrum
- At the gastroesophageal junction, in the setting of gastroesophageal reflux
- Within the margins of a gastrojejunostomy
- In the duodenum, stomach, or jejunum of patients with Zollinger-Ellison syndrome
- Within or adjacent to a Meckel diverticulum that contains ectopic gastric mucosa

Epidemiology. In the United States, approximately 4 million people have peptic ulcers (duodenal and gastric), and 350,000 new cases are diagnosed each year. Around 100,000 patients are hospitalized yearly, and about 3000 people die each year as a result of peptic ulcer disease. The lifetime likelihood of developing a peptic ulcer is about 10% for American men and 4% for women.

Peptic ulcers are remitting, relapsing lesions that are most often diagnosed in middle-aged to older adults, but they may first become evident in young adult life. They often appear without obvious precipitating influences and may then, after a period of weeks to months of active disease, heal with or without therapy. *Even with healing, however, the propensity to develop peptic ulcers remains, in part because of the propensity for recurrent infections with H. pylori.* The male-to-female ratio for duodenal ulcers is about 3 : 1 and for gastric ulcers about 1.5 to 2 : 1. Women are most often affected at, or after, menopause. For unknown reasons, there has been a significant decrease in the prevalence of duodenal ulcers over the past decades but little change in the prevalence of gastric ulcers.

Pathogenesis. *Peptic ulcers appear to be produced by an imbalance between the gastroduodenal mucosal defense mechanisms and the damaging forces* (Fig. 18–16). *Gastric acid and pepsin are requisite for all peptic ulcerations.*[18] Hyperacidity is not a prerequisite because only a minority of patients with duodenal ulcers have hyperacidity, and it is even less common in those with gastric ulcers. Gastric ulceration can readily occur when mucosal defenses fall, however, as when mucosal blood flow drops, gastric emptying is delayed, or epithelial restitution is impaired.

The apparent role of H. pylori in peptic ulceration cannot be overemphasized. H. pylori infection is present in virtually all patients with duodenal ulcers and about 70% of those with gastric ulcers. Furthermore, antibiotic treatment of *H. pylori* infection promotes healing of ulcers and tends to prevent their recurrence. Hence, much interest is focused on the possible mechanisms by which this tiny spiral organism tips the balance of mucosal defenses. Some likely possibilities include the following:

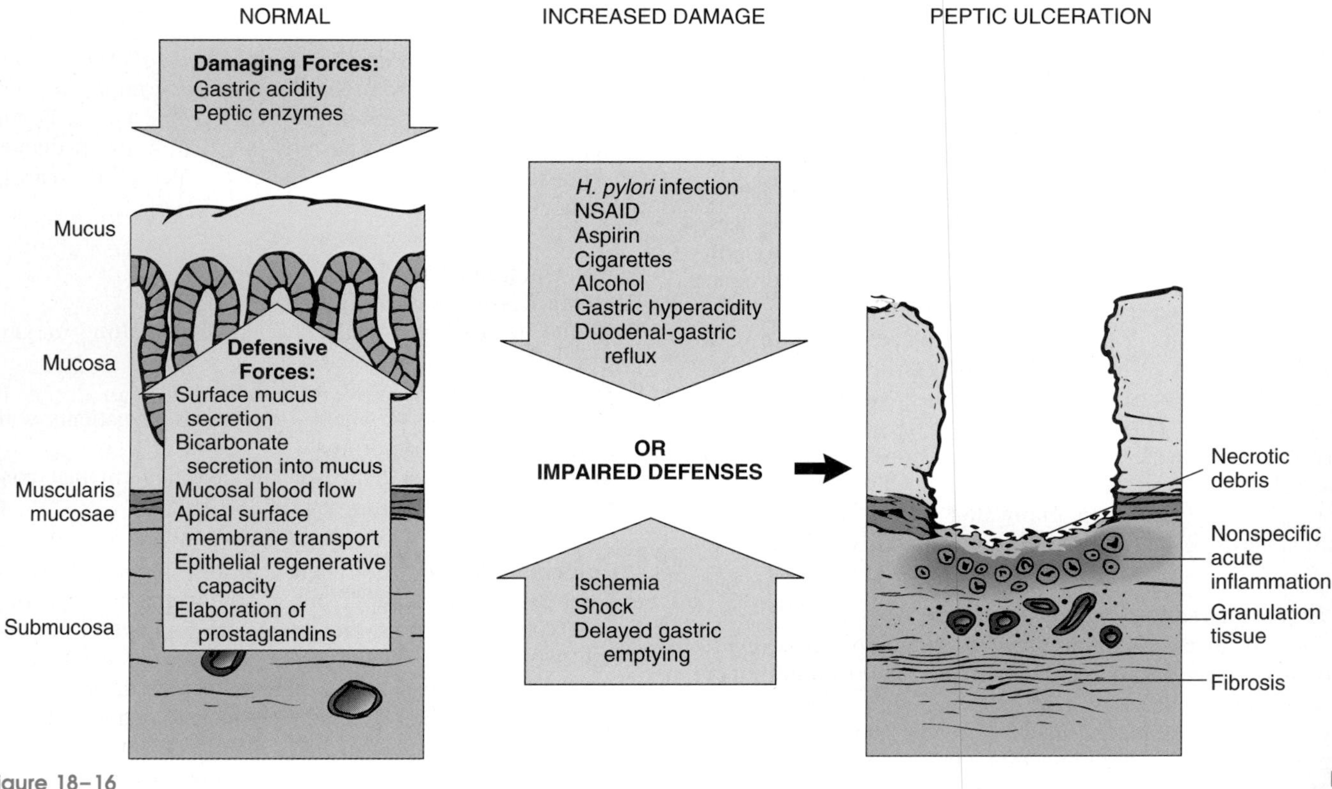

Figure 18–16

Diagram of aggravating causes of, and defense mechanisms against, peptic ulceration.

- *H. pylori* secretes a *urease*, which generates free ammonia, and a *protease*, which breaks down glycoproteins in the gastric mucus. The organisms also elaborate *phospholipases*, which damage surface epithelial cells and may release bioactive leukotrienes and eicosanoids.
- Neutrophils attracted by *H. pylori* release myeloperoxidase, which produces hypochlorous acid, yielding, in turn, monochloramine in the presence of ammonia. Both hypochlorous acid and monochloramine can destroy mammalian cells.
- Both mucosal epithelial cells and lamina propria endothelial cells are prime targets for the destructive actions of *H. pylori* colonization. Thrombotic occlusion of surface capillaries also is promoted by a bacterial platelet-activating factor.
- In addition to *H. pylori* elaboration of enzymes, other antigens (including lipopolysaccharide) recruit inflammatory cells to the mucosa. The chronically inflamed mucosa is more susceptible to acid injury.
- Finally, *damage to the mucosa is thought to permit leakage of tissue nutrients into the surface microenvironment, thereby sustaining the bacillus.*

Only 10 to 20% of individuals worldwide infected with *H. pylori* actually develop peptic ulcer. Hence, a key enigma is why most are spared and some are susceptible. Another perplexing observation is that in patients with duodenal ulcer, the actual infection by *H. pylori* is limited to the stomach. Some studies suggest that *H. pylori* ammonia elaboration stimulates gastrin release, thereby paradoxically increasing acid production. While the link between *H. pylori* infection and gastric and duodenal ulcers is established, the interactions leading to ulceration remain to be elucidated.

Other events may act alone or in concert with *H. pylori* to promote peptic ulceration. Gastric hyperacidity, when present, may be strongly ulcerogenic. Hyperacidity may arise from increased parietal cell mass, increased sensitivity to secretory stimuli, increased basal acid secretory drive, or impaired inhibition of stimulatory mechanisms such as gastrin release. *The Zollinger-Ellison syndrome* (Chapter 20) *exhibits multiple peptic ulcerations in the stomach, duodenum, and even jejunum, owing to excess gastrin secretion by a tumor and hence excess gastric acid production.*

Chronic use of nonsteroidal anti-inflammatory drugs (NSAIDs) suppresses mucosal prostaglandin synthesis; aspirin also is a direct irritant. *Cigarette smoking* impairs mucosal blood flow and healing. *Alcohol* has not been proved to cause peptic ulceration directly, but alcoholic cirrhosis is associated with an increased incidence of peptic ulcers. *Corticosteroids* in high dose and with repeated use promote ulcer formation. *In some patients with duodenal ulcers, there is too rapid gastric emptying, exposing the duodenal mucosa to an excessive acid load.* Duodenal ulcer also is more frequent in patients with alcoholic cirrhosis, chronic obstructive pulmonary disease, chronic renal failure, and hyperparathyroidism. In the last two conditions, hypercalcemia, whatever its cause, stimulates gastrin production and therefore acid secretion. Genetic influences appear to play no role in peptic ulceration. Finally, there are compelling arguments that *personality* and *psychological stress* are important contributing factors, even though hard data on cause and effect are lacking.

MORPHOLOGY. At least 98% of peptic ulcers are located in the first portion of the duodenum or in the stomach, in a ratio of about 4:1. Most duodenal ulcers are generally within a few centimeters of the pyloric ring. The anterior wall of the duodenum is more often affected than the posterior wall. Gastric ulcers are predominantly located along the lesser curvature, in or around the border zone between the corpus and the antral mucosa. Less commonly, they may occur on the anterior or posterior walls or along the greater curvature. Although the great majority of individuals have a single ulcer, in 10 to 20% of patients with gastric ulceration there may be a coexistent duodenual ulcer.

Wherever they occur, chronic peptic ulcers have a fairly standard, virtually diagnostic gross appearance (Fig. 18–17). Small lesions (<0.3 cm) are most likely to be shallow erosions; those greater than 0.6 cm are likely to be bona fide ulcers. Although more than 50% of peptic ulcers have a diameter less than 2 cm, about 10% of benign ulcers are greater than 4 cm. Since carcinomatous ulcers may be less than 4 cm in diameter, **size does not differentiate a benign from a malignant ulcer**.

The classic peptic ulcer is a round-to-oval, sharply punched-out defect with relatively straight walls. The mucosal margin may overhang the base slightly, particularly on the upstream portion of the circumference. Heaping-up of these margins is rare in the benign ulcer but is characteristic of the malignant lesion. The depth of these ulcers varies from superficial lesions involving only the mucosa and muscularis mucosa, to deeply excavated ulcers having their bases on the muscularis propria. When the entire wall is penetrated, the base of the ulcer may be formed by adherent pancreas, omental fat, or liver. Free perforation into the peritoneal cavity may occur.

The base of a peptic ulcer is smooth and clean, owing to peptic digestion of any exudate. At times, thrombosed or even patent blood vessels (the source of life-threatening hemorrhage) are evident in the base of the ulcer. Scarring may involve the entire thickness of the stomach; puckering of the surrounding mucosa creates mucosal folds, which radiate from the crater in spokelike fashion. The gastric mucosa surrounding a gastric ulcer is somewhat edematous and reddened, owing to the almost invariable gastritis.

The histologic appearance varies from active necrosis, to chronic inflammation and scarring, to healing (see Fig. 3–33*D*). In active ulcers with ongoing necrosis, four zones are demonstrable: (1) The base and margins have a superficial thin layer of necrotic fibrinoid debris not visible to the naked eye; (2) beneath this layer is the zone of a nonspecific inflammatory infiltrate, with neutrophils predominating; (3) in the deeper layers, especially in the base of the ulcer, there is active granulation tissue infiltrated with mononuclear leukocytes; and (4) the granulation tissue rests on a more solid fibrous or collagenous scar. Vessel walls within the scarred area are typically thickened by the surrounding inflammation and are occasionally thrombosed.

Chronic gastritis is virtually universal among patients with peptic ulcer disease, occurring in 85 to 100% of patients with duodenal ulcers and 65% with gastric ulcers. *H. pylori* infection is almost always demonstrable in these patients with gastritis. Gastritis remains after the ulcer has healed; recurrence of the ulcer does not appear to be related to progression of the gastritis. This feature is helpful in distinguishing peptic ulcers from acute erosive gastritis or stress ulcers because the adjacent mucosa is generally normal in the latter two conditions.

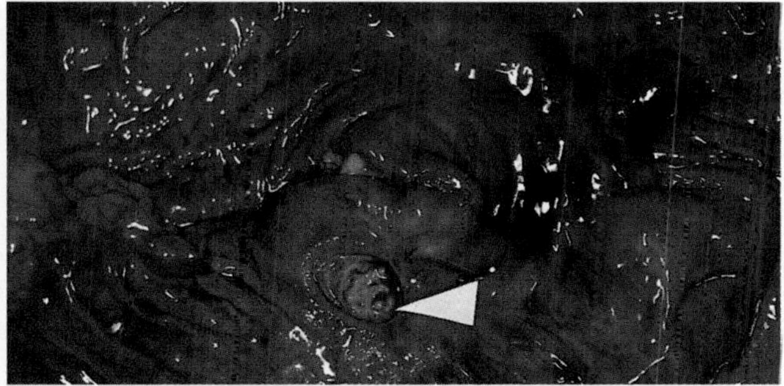

Figure 18–17

Perforating peptic ulcer of the duodenum (*arrowhead*). Note that the ulcer is small (2 cm) with a sharply punched-out appearance. Unlike cancerous ulcers, the margins are not elevated. The ulcer base shows a small amount of blood but is otherwise clean. Compare with the ulcerated carcinoma in Figure 18–23.

Clinical Features. The great majority of peptic ulcers cause epigastric gnawing, burning, or aching pain. A significant minority first come to light with complications such as anemia, frank hemorrhage, or perforation. The pain tends to be worse at night and occurs usually 1 to 3 hours after meals during the day. Classically the pain is relieved by alkalis or food, but there are many exceptions. Nausea, vomiting, bloating, belching, and significant weight loss (raising the fear of some hidden malignancy) are additional

Table 18–3. COMPLICATIONS OF PEPTIC ULCER DISEASE

Bleeding
- Occurs in 15–20% of patients
- Most frequent complication
- May be life-threatening
- Accounts for 25% of ulcer deaths
- May be first indication of an ulcer

Perforation
- Occurs in about 5% of patients
- Accounts for two thirds of ulcer deaths
- Rarely is first indication of an ulcer

Obstruction from edema or scarring
- Occurs in about 2% of patients
- Most often due to pyloric channel ulcers
- May also occur with duodenal ulcers
- Causes incapacitating, crampy abdominal pain
- Rarely may lead to total obstruction with intractable vomiting

Intractable pain

manifestations. Occasionally, with penetrating ulcers, the pain is referred to the back, the left upper quadrant, or chest. As with gastroesophageal reflux, the pain may be misinterpreted as being of cardiac origin.

Peptic ulcers are notoriously chronic, recurring lesions. They more often impair the quality of life than shorten it. When untreated, the average individual requires 15 years for healing of either a duodenal or gastric ulcer.[19] With present-day therapies aimed at neutralization of gastric acid, promotion of mucus secretion, and inhibition of acid secretion (H_2 receptor antagonists and parietal cell H^+,K^+-ATPase inhibitors), most ulcers heal within a few weeks, and patients avoid surgery.

The complications of peptic ulcer disease are shown in Table 18–3. Malignant transformation is unknown with duodenal ulcers and is extremely rare with gastric ulcers. When it occurs, the possibility exists that a seemingly benign lesion was from the outset a deceptive, ulcerative, gastric carcinoma. In addition, the underlying tendency toward dysplasia and carcinoma relates primarily to the associated chronic gastritis, rather than to the ulcer per se.

ACUTE GASTRIC ULCERATION

Focal, acutely developing gastric mucosal defects are a well-known complication of therapy with NSAIDs. Alternatively, they may appear after severe physiologic stress, whatever its nature—hence the term *stress ulcers*. Generally, there are multiple lesions located mainly in the stomach and occasionally in the duodenum. They range in depth from mere shedding of the superficial epithelium (*erosion*) to deeper lesions that involve the entire mucosal thickness (*ulceration*). The shallow erosions are, in essence, an extension of acute erosive gastritis (see earlier). The deeper lesions comprise well-defined ulcerations but are not precursors of chronic peptic ulcers, having a totally different pathobiology.

Stress erosions and ulcers are most commonly encountered in patients with shock, extensive burns, sepsis, or severe trauma; in any intracranial condition that raises intracranial pressure (e.g., trauma, brain surgery); and after intracranial surgery. Those occurring in the proximal duodenum and associated with severe burns or trauma are called *Curling ulcers*. Gastric, duodenal, and esophageal ulcers arising in patients with intracranial injury, operations, or tumors are designated *Cushing ulcers* and carry a high incidence of perforation.

The genesis of the acute mucosal defects in these varied clinical settings is poorly understood. No doubt, many factors are shared with the less severe acute gastritis, such as impaired oxygenation. In the case of cranial lesions, direct stimulation of vagal nuclei by increased intracranial pressure is proposed because hypersecretion of gastric acid is common in these patients. Systemic acidosis, a common finding in these clinical settings, may contribute to mucosal compromise, presumably by lowering the intracellular pH of mucosal cells already rendered hypoxic by stress-induced splanchnic vasoconstriction.

MORPHOLOGY. Acute stress ulcers are usually less than 1 cm in diameter and are circular and small. The ulcer base is frequently stained a dark brown by the acid digestion of extruded blood. In contrast to chronic peptic ulcers, acute stress ulcers are found anywhere in the stomach. They may occur singly or, more often, multiply throughout the stomach and duodenum (Fig. 18–18). The gastric rugal pattern is essentially normal, and the margins and base of the ulcer are not indurated. Microscopically, acute stress ulcers are abrupt lesions, with essentially unremarkable adjacent mucosa. Depending on the duration of the ulceration, there may be a suffusion of blood into the mucosa and submucosa and some inflammatory reaction. Conspicuously absent are scarring and thickening of blood vessels, as seen in chronic peptic ulcers. Healing with complete re-epitheliali-

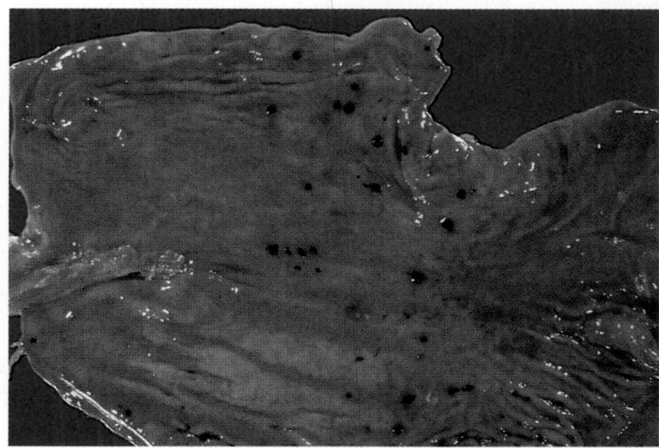

Figure 18–18 ■

Multiple stress ulcers of the stomach, highlighted by dark digested blood on their surface.

zation occurs after the causative factors are removed. The time required for complete healing varies from days to several weeks.

Clinical Features. About 5 to 10% of patients admitted to hospital intensive care units acutely develop superficial gastric erosions or ulcers. These may be asymptomatic or may create a hemodynamic emergency, as potentially lethal bleeding can occur. Although prophylactic antacid regimens and blood transfusions may blunt the impact of stress ulceration, *the most important determinant of clinical outcome is the ability to correct the underlying condition(s).* The gastric mucosa can recover completely if the patients do not succumb to their primary disease.

Miscellaneous Conditions

Gastric dilation may arise from gastric outlet obstruction (e.g., pyloric stenosis) or from the functional atony of the stomach and intestines (paralytic ileus) that may appear in patients with generalized peritonitis. The stomach may contain as much as 10 to 15 liters of fluid; on rare occasion, *gastric rupture* may occur. This is a calamitous event followed rapidly by shock or death if not treated immediately. Spontaneous gastric perforation may rarely occur in the newborn, during labor and delivery, severe vomiting, or cardiopulmonary rescuscitation, or after ingestion of extreme amounts of carbonated beverages.

The stomach is the major site for formation of luminal concretions of indigestible ingested material. *Phytobezoars* are derived from plant material, including fibers, leaves, roots, and skins of almost any plant matter. *Trichobezoars*, better known as *hairballs*, consist of ingested hair within a mucoid coat containing decaying foodstuff (Fig. 18–19). The dysmotility after partial gastrectomy or partial gastric outlet obstruction is conducive to bezoar formation from more conventional ingested food. Bizarre bezoars have developed among partakers of illicit pharmaceuticals, glue swallowers, and children or patients with neuropsychiatric disorders, who have been known to ingest pins, nails, razor blades, coins, gloves, and even leather wallets.

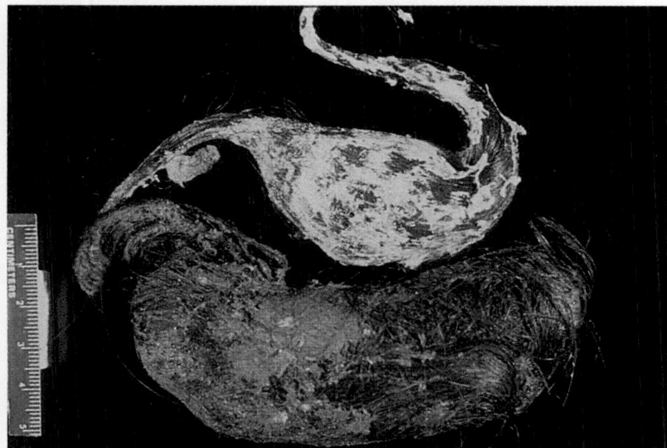

Figure 18–19 ■

Trichobezoar showing the agglomeration of hair, food, and mucus that occurred within the gastric lumen.

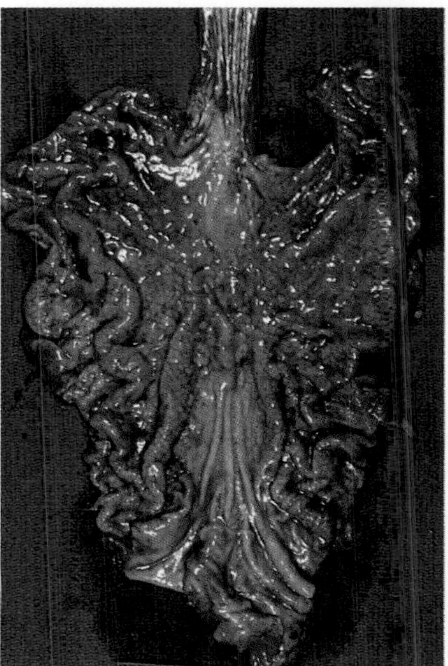

Figure 18–20 ■

Hypertrophic gastropathy showing markedly thickened gastric folds.

HYPERTROPHIC GASTROPATHY

Hypertrophic gastropathy encompasses a group of uncommon conditions, all characterized by giant cerebriform enlargement of the rugal folds of the gastric mucosa (Fig. 18–20). The rugal enlargement is caused not by inflammation but by hyperplasia of the mucosal epithelial cells. *Three variants are recognized:*[20]

1. *Ménétrier disease*, resulting from profound hyperplasia of the surface mucous cells with accompanying glandular atrophy
2. *Hypertrophic-hypersecretory gastropathy*, associated with hyperplasia of the parietal and chief cells within gastric glands
3. *Gastric gland hyperplasia secondary to excessive gastrin secretion*, in the setting of a gastrinoma (*Zollinger-Ellison syndrome*)

All three conditions are of clinical importance for two reasons: (1) *They may mimic infiltrative carcinoma or lymphoma of the stomach on radiographic examinations*, and (2) the enormous increase in acid secretions in the latter two conditions places patients at risk for peptic ulceration. A pure form of parietal cell hypertrophy, without hyperacidity, may occur in long-term takers of acid secretion inhibitors. Cessation of therapy invites transient rebound excess acid secretion.

Ménétrier disease, an idiopathic condition, is most often encountered in men (ratio 3 : 1) in their thirties to fifties but occasionally is encountered in children. Although the disorder may be asymptomatic, it often produces epigastric discomfort, diarrhea, weight loss, and sometimes bleeding related to superficial rugal erosions. The hypertrophic change may involve the body-fundus or antrum predominantly or may affect the entire stomach. The gastric secretions contain excessive mucus and, in many instances, little to no hydrochloric acid because of glandular atrophy. In some patients, there may be sufficient protein loss in the gastric secretions to produce hypoalbuminemia and peripheral edema, thus constituting a form of *protein-losing gastroenteropathy*. Infrequently the mucosal hyperplasia becomes metaplastic, providing a soil for the development of gastric carcinoma.

Tumors

As in the esophagus and intestines, tumors arising from the mucosa predominate over mesenchymal and stromal tumors. These can be classified as benign and malignant lesions.

BENIGN TUMORS

In the alimentary tract, the term polyp is applied to any nodule or mass that projects above the level of the surrounding mucosa. Use of the term is generally restricted to mass lesions arising in the mucosa, although occasionally a submucosal lipoma or leiomyoma may protrude, generating a polypoid lesion. Gastric polyps are uncommon, found in about 0.4% of adult autopsies and 3 to 5% of Japanese adults.[21] Although gastric polyps are usually found incidentally, dyspepsia or anemia resulting from blood loss may prompt the search for a gastrointestinal lesion.

MORPHOLOGY. The great majority of gastric polyps (>90%) are **non-neoplastic** and appear to be of a **hyperplastic** nature. These polyps are composed of a variable admixture of hyperplastic surface epithelium and cystically dilated glandular tissue, with a lamina propria containing increased inflammatory cells and smooth muscle. The surface epithelium may be regenerative in response to surface erosion and inflammation, but true dysplasia is not present. Most hyperplastic polyps are small and sessile; some may approach several centimeters in diameter and have an apparent stalk. Multiplicity, sometimes numbering by the score, is observed in about 20 to 25% of cases.

The adenoma of the stomach is a true neoplasm, representing 5 to 10% of the polypoid lesions in the stomach. **By definition, an adenoma contains proliferative dysplastic epithelium and thereby has malignant potential.** Adenomatous polyps are much more common in the colon (see later). Gastric adenomas may be **sessile** (without a stalk) or **pedunculated** (stalked). The most common location is the antrum. These lesions are usually single and may grow up to 3 to 4 cm in size before detection (Fig. 18–21). In contrast to the colon, adenomatous change may carpet a large region of flat gastric mucosa without forming a mass lesion.

Clinical Features. Hyperplastic polyps are seen most frequently in the setting of chronic gastritis. They are regarded as having no malignant potential as such but are nevertheless found in about 20% of stomachs resected for carcinoma. This occurrence is attributed to the tendency of chronically inflamed gastric mucosa both to form hyperplastic polyps and to degenerate into malignancy. As with the colonic counterpart, the incidence of gastric adenomas increases with age, particularly into and beyond the sixties. The male-to-female ratio is 2 : 1. Up to 40% of gastric adenomas contain a focus of carcinoma at the time of diagnosis, particularly the larger lesions.[22] The risk of cancer in the adjacent gastric mucosa may be as high as 30%. Autoimmune gastritis and colonic polyposis syndromes (see later) also have a propensity toward gastric adenoma formation.

Otherwise innocuous hyperplastic polyps may occasionally harbor foci of adenomatous epithelium. *Because hyperplastic and adenomatous polyps cannot reliably be distinguished endoscopically, histologic examination of gastric polyps is mandatory.*

GASTRIC CARCINOMA

Among the malignant tumors that occur in the stomach, carcinoma is overwhelmingly the most important and the most common (90 to 95%). Next in order of frequency are

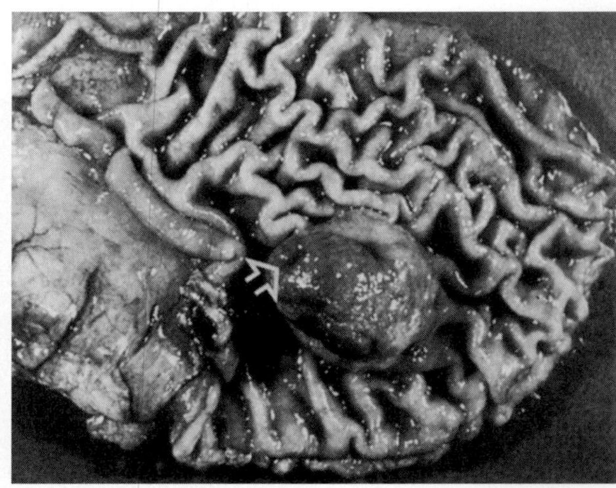

Figure 18–21

Adenomatous polyp of the stomach. Note the large size of the polyp and its lobulated configuration. A small ulceration (*arrow*) can be identified on its surface. (From Kasimer W, Dayal Y: Gastritis, gastric atrophy, and gastric neoplasia. In Chopra S, May RJ (eds): Pathophysiology of Gastrointestinal Disorders, Boston, Little, Brown, 1989.)

lymphomas (4%), carcinoids (3%), and malignant stromal cell tumors (2%).

Epidemiology. Gastric carcinoma is a worldwide disease. Its incidence, however, varies widely, being particularly high in countries such as Japan, Chile, China, Portugal, and Russia and fourfold to sixfold less common in the United States, United Kingdom, Canada, Australia, and France. It is more common in lower socioeconomic groups and exhibits a male-to-female ratio of about 2 : 1. In most countries, there has been a steady decline in both the incidence and the mortality of gastric cancer over the past six decades. In 1930, gastric cancer was the most common cause of cancer death in the United States. Since that time, the annual mortality rate in the United States has dropped from about 38 to 7 per 100,000 population for men and from 28 to 4 per 100,000 for women.[8] Yet it remains among the leading killer cancers, representing 2.5% of all cancer deaths in the United States and still exceeding lung cancer as the leading cause of cancer death worldwide.[23] Although 5-year survival rates have improved since the advent of endoscopy in the 1960, they remain poor at less than 20% overall.

Gastric carcinoma can be divided into two general histologic subtypes: (1) those exhibiting an *intestinal* morphology with the formation of bulky tumors composed of glandular structures and (2) those that are *diffuse* in the infiltrative growth of poorly differentiated discohesive malignant cells. The intestinal type exhibits a mean age of incidence of 55 years and a male-to-female ratio of 2 : 1. The diffuse type occurs in slightly younger patients (mean age, 48), with an approximately equal male-to-female ratio. The drop in incidence of gastric cancer has occurred only in the intestinal type. At the present time, the incidence is approximately the same for intestinal and diffuse cancer.

Pathogenesis. The major factors thought to affect the genesis of gastric cancer are summarized in Table 18–4. They apply more to the intestinal type, as the risk factors for diffuse gastric cancer are not well defined.

Environment. Environmental influences are thought to be the most important.[24] When families migrate from high-risk to low-risk areas (or the reverse), successive generations acquire the level of risk that prevails in the new locales. The *diet* is suspected to be a primary offender, and adherence to certain culinary practices is associated with a high risk of gastric carcinoma. The presence of carcinogens, such as *N*-nitroso compounds and benzopyrene, appears to be particularly important. Thus, lack of refrigeration; consumption of preserved, smoked, cured, and salted foods; water contamination with nitrates; and lack of fresh fruit and vegetables are common themes in high-risk areas. Conversely, intake of green, leafy vegetables and citrus fruits, which contain antioxidants such as ascorbate (vitamin C), α-tocopherol (vitamin E), and beta-carotene, is negatively correlated with gastric cancer.[23]

Alcohol intake has not been proven to increase risk. Cigarette smoking imparts a 1.5-fold to 3.0-fold increased risk, although there is no clear dose relationship. Despite initial concern, *to date there appears to be no increased risk of stomach cancer from the use of antacid drug therapies.* A role for occupational exposure has been difficult to establish.

Table 18–4. FACTORS ASSOCIATED WITH INCREASED INCIDENCE OF GASTRIC CARCINOMA

Environmental
Diet
Nitrites derived from nitrates (water, preserved food)
Smoked and salted foods, pickled vegetables
Lack of fresh fruit and vegetables
Low socioeconomic status
Cigarette smoking

Host Factors
Chronic gastritis
Hypochlorhydria: favors colonization with *Helicobacter pylori*
Intestinal metaplasia is a precursor lesion
Infection by *H. pylori*
Present in most cases of intestinal-type carcinoma
Partial gastrectomy
Favors reflux of bilious, alkaline intestinal fluid
Gastric adenomas
40% harbor cancer at time of diagnosis
30% have adjacent cancer at time of diagnosis
Barrett esophagus
Increased risk of gastroesophageal junction tumors

Genetic
Slightly increased risk with blood group A
Family history of gastric cancer
Hereditary nonpolyposis colon cancer syndrome

Host. *Host factors* are the second major area of scrutiny. Infection by *H. pylori* leading to chronic gastritis and intestinal metaplasia is thought to be a contributing, but not sufficient, factor for gastric carcinogenesis. *Autoimmune gastritis* also carries an increased risk, presumably owing to the same process of chronic inflammation and metaplasia. The relative risk for gastric cancer in both conditions is approximately threefold over the general population (recognizing that *H. pylori*–infected individuals represent more than 50% of the adult population in many locales). *Most persons infected with H. pylori never develop gastric cancer.* Chronic gastritis also appears to be the substratum from which diffuse gastric cancer arises.

Previous peptic ulcer disease per se does not impart increased risk. Only about 4% of patients with gastric cancer have a family history of this disease, and genetic factors are unlikely to be major influences.

Dysplasia of the gastric mucosa represents the final common pathway by which intestinal-type gastric cancers arise. Gastric adenomas are known to turn malignant, and these are simply raised lesions containing mucosal dysplasia. *The diffuse type of cancer appears to arise de novo, without evolution through dysplasia.* Molecular mechanisms underlying cancer promotion have not yet been defined, although many molecular events have been described. *In the intestinal type of gastric cancer,* the overall pattern of allelic losses shows similarities with colon cancer, with a cumulative series of gene alterations.[25] Abnormalities in several growth factor receptor systems, including c-*met*, K-*sam*, and *erb*, also occur, with markedly different frequencies between the two histologic types. In contrast to colon and pancreatic cancer, the *ras* oncogene is rarely mutated. Suffice it to say that the disparities in mutations implicate unique pathogenetic pathways, as yet unknown, for the development of intestinal and diffuse types of gastric cancer.

MORPHOLOGY. The location of gastric carcinomas within the stomach is as follows: pylorus and antrum, 50 to 60%; cardia, 25%; and the remainder in the body and fundus. The lesser curvature is involved in about 40% and the greater curvature in 12%. **Thus, a favored location is the lesser curvature of the antropyloric region.** Although less frequent, an ulcerative lesion on the greater curvature is more likely to be malignant.

Gastric carcinoma is classified on the basis of (1) depth of invasion, (2) macroscopic growth pattern, and (3) histologic subtype. The morphologic feature having the greatest impact on clinical outcome is the **depth of invasion. Early gastric carcinoma is defined as a lesion confined to the mucosa and submucosa, regardless of the presence or absence of perigastric lymph node metastases.** Some early tumors cover large areas of the gastric mucosa (up to 10 cm in diameter) and yet show no invasion into the muscular wall. **Early gastric carcinoma** is not synonymous with **carcinoma in situ**, as the latter is confined to the surface epithelial layer. **Advanced gastric carcinoma is a neoplasm that has extended below the submucosa into the muscular wall** and has perhaps spread more widely. All cancers presumably begin as **early** lesions, which develop over time into **advanced** lesions.

The three macroscopic growth patterns of gastric carcinoma, which may be evident at both the early and the advanced stages, are (1) **exophytic**, with protrusion of a tumor mass into the lumen; (2) **flat or depressed**, in which there is no obvious tumor mass within the mucosa; and (3) **excavated**, whereby a shallow or deeply erosive crater is present in the wall of the stomach (Fig. 18–22). Exophytic tumors are readily identified by radiographic techniques and at endoscopy and may contain portions of an adenoma. In contrast, **flat or depressed malignancy may be inapparent to even the experienced eye** except as regional effacement of the normal surface mucosal pattern. Excavated cancers may closely mimic, in size and appearance, chronic peptic ulcers. In advanced cases, cancerous craters can be identified by their heaped-up, beaded margins and shaggy, necrotic bases as well as the overt neoplastic tissue extending into the surrounding mucosa and wall (Fig. 18–23). Uncommonly a broad region of the gastric wall, or the entire stomach, is extensively infiltrated by malignancy, creating a rigid, thickened leather bottle-like stomach, termed **linitis plastica**. Metastatic

Early Gastric Carcinoma

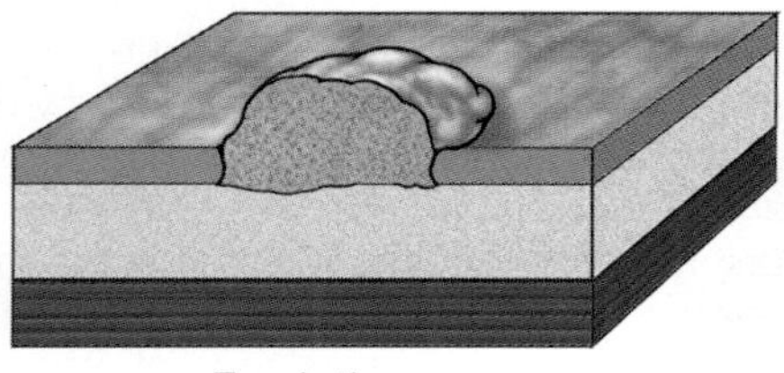
Exophytic

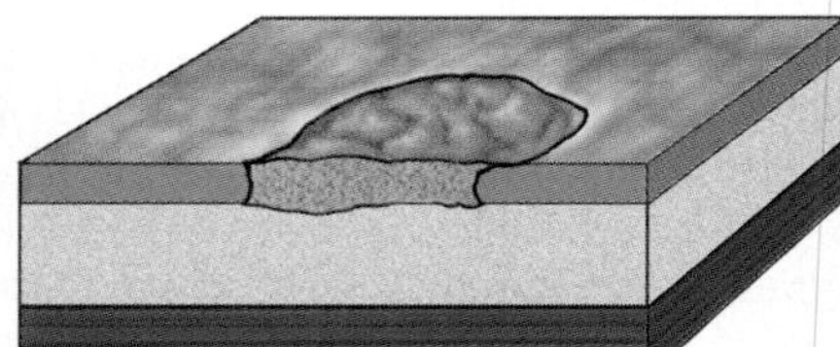
Flat or depressed

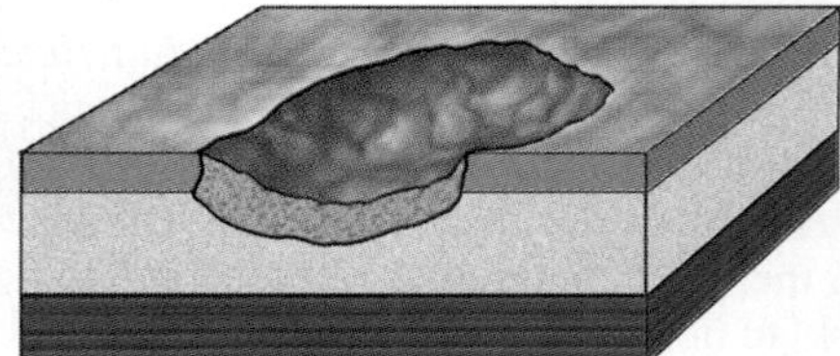
Excavated

Advanced Gastric Carcinoma

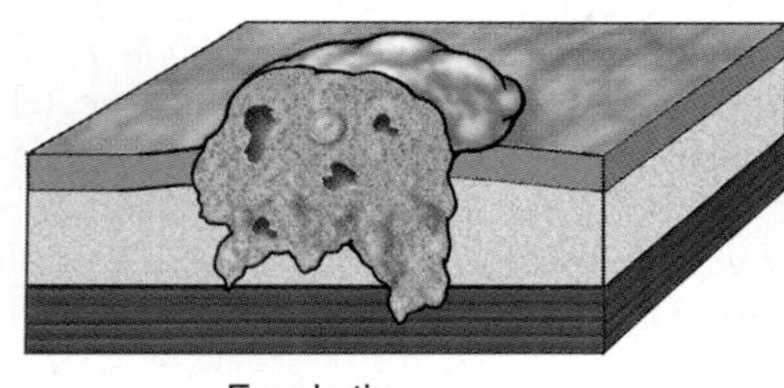
Exophytic

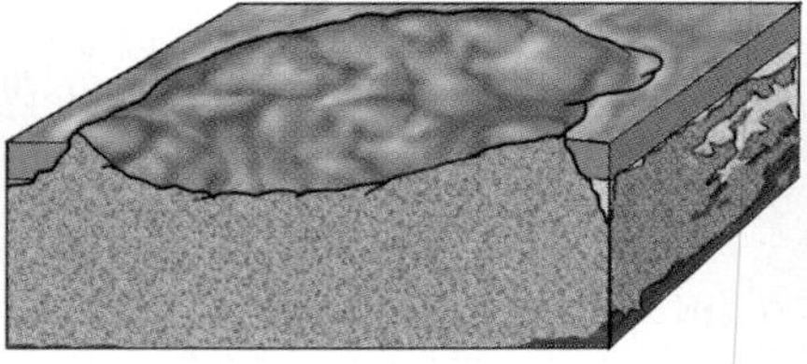
Linitis plastica

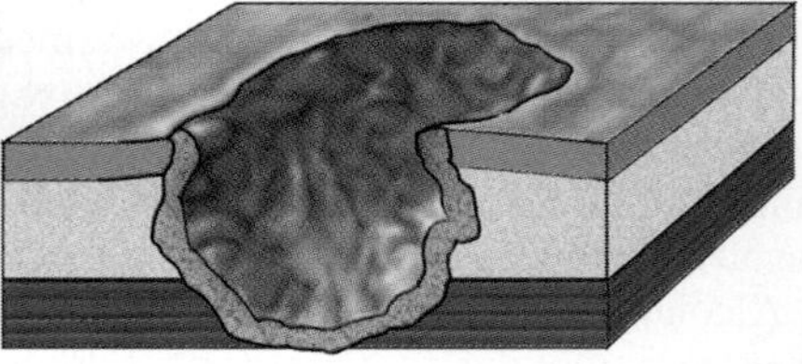
Excavated

Figure 18–22

Diagram of growth patterns and spread of gastric carcinoma. In early gastric carcinoma, tumor is confined to the mucosa and submucosa and may exhibit an exophytic, flat or depressed, or excavated conformation. Advanced gastric carcinoma extends into the muscularis propria and beyond. Linitis plastica is an extreme form of flat or depressed advanced gastric carcinoma.

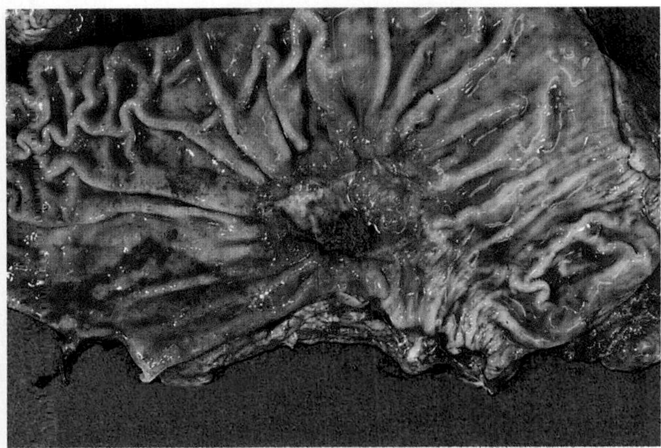

Figure 18–23

Ulcerative gastric carcinoma. The ulcer is large and irregular.

carcinoma, from the breast and lung, may generate a similar linitis plastica picture.

The histologic subtypes of gastric cancer have been variously subclassified, but **the two most important types, as noted earlier, are the intestinal type and diffuse type of the Lauren classification** (Fig. 18–24). **The intestinal variant is composed of neoplastic intestinal glands resembling those of colonic adenocarcinoma, which permeate the gastric wall but tend to grow along broad cohesive fronts in an expanding growth pattern**.[26] The neoplastic cells often contain apical mucin vacuoles, and abundant mucin may be present in gland lumens. **The diffuse variant is composed of gastric-type mucous cells, which generally do not form glands but rather permeate the mucosa and wall as scattered individual cells or small clusters in an infiltrative growth pattern.** These cells appear to arise from the middle layer of the mucosa, and the presence of intestinal metaplasia is not a prerequisite. In this variant, mucin formation expands the malignant cells and pushes the nucleus to periphery, creating a **signet ring** conformation (Fig. 18–24*B*). Regardless of cell type, the amount of mucin varies, and in poorly differentiated portions mucin may be absent.

Whatever the variant, all gastric carcinomas eventually penetrate the wall to involve the serosa and spread to regional and more distant lymph nodes. For obscure reasons, gastric carcinomas frequently metastasize to the supraclavicular sentinel (Virchow) node as the first clinical manifestation of an occult neoplasm. Local invasion into the duodenum, pancreas, and retroperitoneum is characteristic. At the time of death, widespread peritoneal seedings and metastases to the liver and lungs are common. A notable site of visceral metastasis is to one or both ovaries (**Krukenberg tumor**; Chapter 24).

Clinical Features. Gastric carcinoma is an insidious disease that is generally asymptomatic until late in its course. The symptoms include weight loss; abdominal pain; anorexia; vomiting; altered bowel habits; and, less frequently, dysphagia, anemic symptoms, and hemorrhage. Because these symptoms are essentially nonspecific, early detection of gastric cancer is difficult. In Japan, where mass endoscopy screening programs are in place, early gastric cancer constitutes about 35% of all newly diagnosed gastric cancers. In Europe and the United States, this figure has remained at 10 to 15% over several decades.

The prognosis for gastric carcinoma depends primarily on the depth of invasion and the extent of nodal and distant metastasis at the time of diagnosis; histologic type has minimal independent prognostic significance. The 5-year survival rate of surgically treated early gastric cancer is 90 to 95%, with only a small negative increment if lymph node metastases are present.[27] In contrast, the

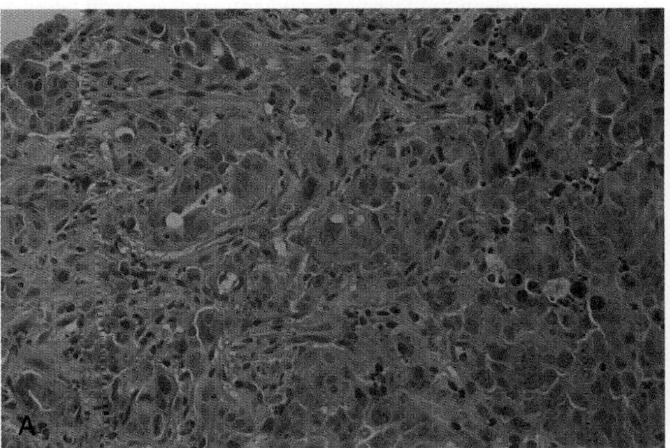

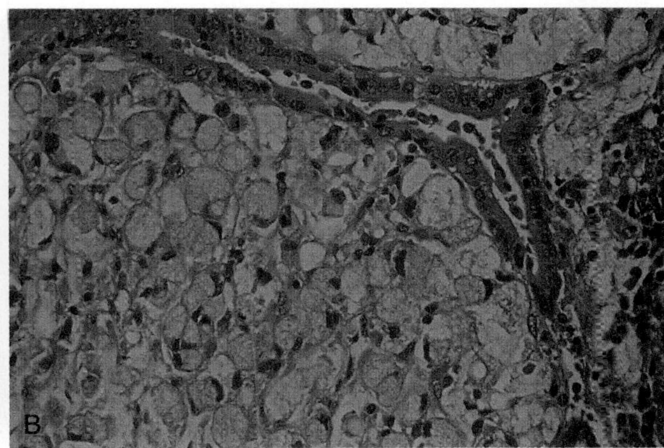

Figure 18–24

Gastric cancer. *A*, Poorly differentiated intestinal-type adenocarcinoma. Note small glands. *B*, Diffuse signet ring cell carcinoma of the stomach, surrounding a residual benign gastric gland in the mucosa. (Courtesy of Dr. Robert Odze, Brigham and Women's Hospital, Boston, MA.)

5-year survival rate for advanced gastric cancer remains below 15%.

LESS COMMON GASTRIC TUMORS

Gastric *lymphomas* represent 5% of all gastric malignancies and are similar to intestinal lymphomas; these are considered as a group later on. *Gastric neuroendocrine cell (carcinoid) tumors* are extremely rare and tend to be infiltrative tumors that metastasize in about one third of cases. These tumors are described in detail later. *Lipomas* are a benign neoplasm of adipose tissue, usually present in the submucosa.

A wide variety of mesenchymal neoplasms may arise in the stomach. They generally are of smooth muscle origin, hence the designations *leiomyoma* for the benign form and *leiomyosarcoma* for the malignant form. They may contain neural and fibroblastic elements, however, and as a class of tumors exhibit a spectrum of benign-to-malignant features, including a propensity to recurrence and metastasis. They are thus broadly classified under the term *gastrointestinal stromal tumors*. These lesions are discussed in the section on intestinal tumors.

The *inflammatory fibroid polyp* is a striking lesion, in that it is a bulky submucosal growth composed of inflamed vascularized fibromuscular tissue with a prominent eosinophilic infiltrate and a tenuous mucosa stretched over the surface. These polyps may occur anywhere in the alimentary tract but are found most frequently in the stomach. As they protrude into the lumen, they may occlude the pyloric channel and present abruptly as acute gastric outlet obstruction. Their origin is unknown, although it is postulated that they are a benign, polypoid growth of endothelium and smooth muscle.

Metastatic involvement of the stomach is unusual. The most common sources of gastric metastases are leukemia and generalized lymphoma. Metastases of malignant melanoma and carcinomas tend to be multiple and may develop central ulceration. Breast and lung carcinoma may mimic diffuse gastric carcinoma by diffusely infiltrating the gastric wall to generate *linitis plastica*, as described earlier.

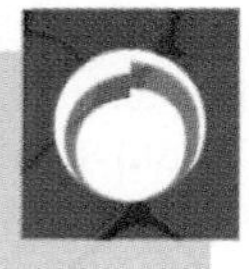

Small and Large Intestines

NORMAL SMALL AND LARGE INTESTINES

Anatomy

The *small intestine* in the human adult is approximately 6 meters in length and the *colon* (large intestine) approximately 1.5 meters. The first 25 cm of the small intestine, the duodenum, is retroperitoneal; the jejunum marks the entry of the small intestine into the peritoneal cavity, terminating where the ileum enters the colon at the ileocecal valve. The demarcation between jejunum and ileum is not clearly defined; the jejunum arbitrarily constitutes the proximal third of the intraperitoneal portion and the ileum the remainder. The colon is subdivided into the cecum and the ascending, transverse, descending, and sigmoid colon. The sigmoid colon begins at the pelvic brim and loops within the peritoneal cavity, becoming the rectum at about the level of the third sacral vertebra. Halfway along its 15-cm length, the rectum passes between the crura of the perineal muscles to become extraperitoneal. The reflection of the peritoneum from the rectum over the pelvic floor creates a cul-de-sac known as the *pouch of Douglas*.

Vasculature

The arterial supply of the intestine, from the proximal jejunum to the proximal transverse colon, is derived from the superior mesenteric artery. The inferior mesenteric artery feeds the remainder of the colon to the level of the rectum. Each artery progressively divides as it approaches the gut, with rich arterial interconnections via arching mesenteric arcades. Numerous collaterals connect the mesenteric circulation with the celiac arterial axis proximally and the pudendal circulation distally. The lymphatic drainage essentially parallels the vascular supply but does not have the intricate patterns of arcades.

The upper rectum is supplied by the superior hemorrhoidal branch of the inferior mesenteric artery. The lower portion receives its blood supply from the hemorrhoidal branches of the internal iliac or internal pudendal artery. The venous drainage follows essentially the same distribution and is connected by an anastomotic capillary bed between the superior and inferior hemorrhoidal veins, providing a connection between the portal and systemic venous systems. Since the colon is a retroperitoneal organ in the ascending and descending portions, it derives considerable accessory arterial blood supply and lymphatic drainage from a wide area of the posterior abdominal wall.

Small Intestinal Mucosa

The most distinctive feature of the small intestine is its mucosal lining, which is studded with innumerable *villi* (Fig. 18–25*A*). These extend into the lumen as finger-like projections covered by epithelial lining cells. The central core of lamina propria contains blood vessels; lymphatics; a minimal population of lymphocytes, eosinophils, and mast cells; and scattered fibroblasts and vertically oriented smooth muscle cells. Between the bases of the villi are the pitlike crypts, which extend down to the muscularis mucosae. The muscularis mucosae forms a smooth, continuous

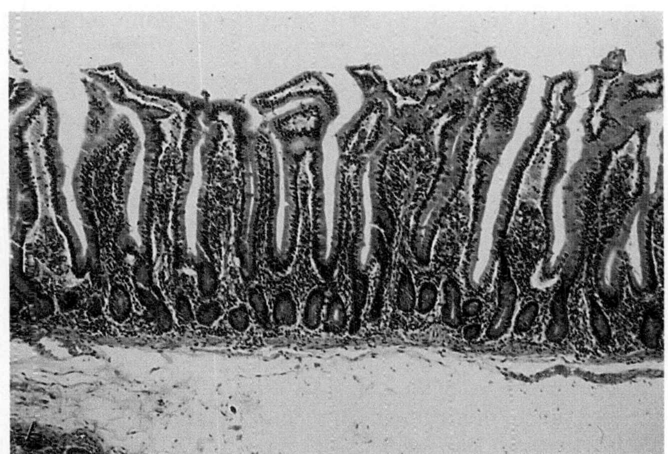

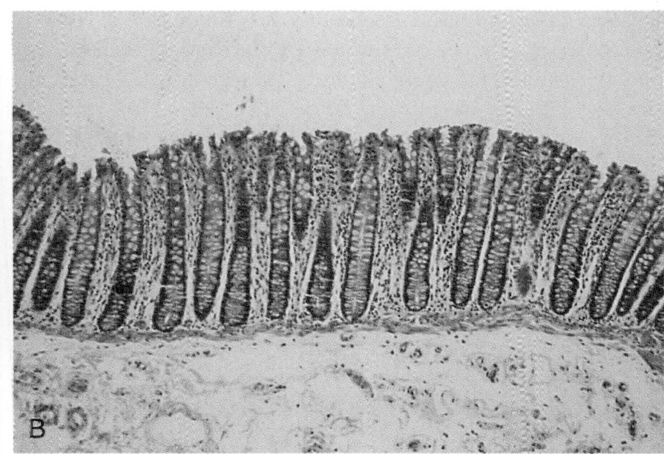

Figure 18–25

A, Normal small intestinal histology showing mucosal villi and crypts, lined by columnar cells. *B*, Normal colon histology showing a flat mucosal surface and abundant vertically oriented crypts.

sheet serving to anchor the configuration of villi and crypts alike. In normal individuals, the villus-to-crypt height ratio is about 4 to 5 : 1. Within the duodenum are abundant submucosal mucous glands, termed *Brunner glands*. These glands secrete bicarbonate ions, glycoproteins, and pepsinogen II and are virtually indistinguishable from the gastric pyloric mucous glands.

The surface epithelium of the villi contains three cell types. *Columnar absorptive cells* are recognized by the dense array of *microvilli* on their luminal surface (the *brush border*) and the underlying mat of microfilaments (the *terminal web*). Interspersed regularly between the absorptive cells are mucin-secreting *goblet cells* and a few *endocrine cells*, described subsequently. Within the crypts reside *undifferentiated crypt cells*, goblet cells, more abundant endocrine cells, and scattered *Paneth cells*. The last-mentioned cells have apically oriented bright eosinophilic granules containing a variety of antimicrobial proteins that play a role in mucosal immunity.[23]

The villi of the small intestinal mucosa are the site for terminal digestion and absorption of foodstuffs through the action of the columnar absorptive cells. The crypts secrete ions and water, deliver immunoglobulin A and antimicrobial peptides to the lumen, and serve as the site for cell division and renewal. The mucous cells of both crypts and villi generate an adherent mucous coat, which both protects the surface epithelium and provides an ideal local milieu for uptake of nutrients. Specific receptors for uptake of macromolecules also are present on the surface epithelial cells, such as those in the ileum for intrinsic factor–vitamin B_{12} complexes.

Colonic Mucosa

The small intestine accomplishes its absorptive function with a highly liquid luminal stream. The purpose of the colon is to reclaim luminal water and electrolytes. In contrast to the mucosa of the small intestine, the colonic mucosa has no villi and is flat. The mucosa is punctuated by numerous straight tubular crypts that extend down to the muscularis mucosa (Fig. 18–25*B*). The surface epithelium is composed of columnar absorptive cells, which have shorter, less abundant microvilli than found in the small intestine, and goblet mucous cells. The crypts contain abundant goblet cells, endocrine cells, and undifferentiated crypt cells. Paneth cells are occasionally present at the base of crypts in the cecum and ascending colon.

The regenerative capacity of the intestinal epithelium is remarkable. Cellular proliferation is confined to the crypts; differentiation and luminal migration serve to replenish superficial cells lost to senescence and surface abrasion. Within the small intestine, cells migrate out of the crypts and upward to the tips of the villi, where they are shed into the lumen. This journey normally takes between 96 and 144 hours, leading to normal renewal of the epithelial lining every 4 to 6 days. Turnover of the colonic surface epithelium takes 3 to 8 days. The rapid renewal of intestinal epithelium provides a remarkable capacity for repair but also renders the intestine particularly vulnerable to agents that interfere with cell replication, such as radiation and chemotherapy for cancer.

Endocrine Cells

A diverse population of *endocrine cells* is scattered among the epithelial cells lining the gastric glands, small intestinal villi, and small and large intestinal crypts. Comparable cells are present in the epithelia lining the pancreas, biliary tree, lung, thyroid, and urethra. As a population, gut endocrine cells exhibit characteristic morphologic features. In most cells, the cytoplasm contains abundant fine eosinophilic granules, which harbor secretory products. The cytoplasmic portion of the cell is at the base of the epithelium, and the nuclei reside on the luminal side of the cytoplasmic granules.

These cells exhibit a marked diversity of secretory peptides and distribution of cell subtypes. Secretory granules are released at the basal surface of the endocrine cell or along the basal part of its lateral surface; apical secretion (into the lumen) has never been observed. The various secretory products, some of which are present also in the mural autonomic neural plexus, act as chemical messengers and modulate normal digestive functions by a combination of endocrine, paracrine, and neurocrine mechanisms. Each endocrine cell type therefore exhibits a distribution tailored to meet the physiologic needs pertinent to a gut segment.

Intestinal Immune System

Throughout the small intestine and colon are nodules of *lymphoid tissue*, which either lie within the mucosa or span the mucosa and a portion of the submucosa. They distort the surface epithelium to produce broad domes rather than villi; within the ileum, confluent lymphoid tissue becomes macroscopically visible as *Peyer patches*. The surface epithelium over lymphoid nodules contains both columnar absorptive cells and *M (membranous) cells*, the latter found only in small and large intestinal lymphoid sites. M cells are able to transcytose antigenic macromolecules intact from the lumen to underlying lymphocytes, thus serving as an important afferent limb of the *intestinal immune system*. Throughout the intestines, T lymphocytes are scattered within the surface epithelium (*intraepithelial lymphocytes*), generally of cytotoxic phenotype (CD8+). The lamina propria contains helper T cells (CD4+) and educated B cells. The lymphoid nodules, mucosal lymphocytes, together with isolated lymphoid follicles in the appendix and mesenteric lymph nodes, constitute the *m*ucosa-*a*ssociated *l*ymphoid *t*issue (MALT).[29]

Neuromuscular Function

Small intestinal peristalsis, both *anterograde* and *retrograde*, mixes the food stream and promotes maximal contact of nutrients with the mucosa. Colonic peristalsis prolongs contact of the luminal contents with the mucosa. Although intestinal smooth muscle cells are capable of initiating contractions, *both small and large intestinal peristalsis are mediated by intrinsic (myenteric plexus) and extrinsic (autonomic innervation) neural control*. The myenteric plexus consists of two neural networks: *Meissner plexus* resides at the base of the submucosa, and *Auerbach plexus* lies between the inner circumferential and outer longitudinal muscle layers of the muscle wall; lesser neural twigs extend between smooth muscle cells and ramify within the submucosa.

PATHOLOGY

Many conditions, such as infections, inflammatory diseases, and tumors, affect both the small and large intestines. These two organs therefore are considered together. Collectively, disorders of the intestines account for a large portion of human disease.

Congenital Anomalies

Rare anomalies of gut formation may occur, as follows:

- *Duplication* of the small intestine or colon, usually in the form of saccular to long, cystic structures
- *Malrotation* of the entire bowel, resulting from improper embryologic rotation of the gut
- *Omphalocele*, in which the abdominal musculature fails to form, leading to birth of an infant with herniation of abdominal contents into a ventral membranous sac
- *Gastroschisis*, in which a portion of the abdominal wall fails to form altogether, with ensuing extrusion of the intestines

The above-listed lesions may be silent (malrotation) or catastrophic (gastroschisis). A far more common and innocuous lesion is *heterotopia*, usually of normal pancreatic tissue but occasionally gastric mucosa, appearing as small, 1- to 2-cm sized nodules in an aberrant gut location.

ATRESIA AND STENOSIS

Congenital intestinal obstruction is an uncommon but dramatic lesion that may affect any level of the intestines. Duodenal atresia is most common; the jejunum and ileum are equally involved and the colon virtually never. The obstruction may be complete (*atresia*) or incomplete (*stenosis*). Atresia may take the form of an imperforate mucosal diaphragm or a stringlike segment of bowel connecting intact proximal and distal intestine. Stenosis is less common and is due to a narrowed intestinal segment or a diaphragm with a narrow central opening. Single or multiple lesions appear to arise from developmental failure, intrauterine vascular accidents, or *intussusceptions* (telescoping of one intestinal segment within another) occurring after the intestine has developed. Failure of the cloacal diaphragm to rupture leads to an *imperforate anus*.

MECKEL DIVERTICULUM

Failure of involution of the vitelline duct, which connects the lumen of the developing gut to the yolk sac, produces a *Meckel diverticulum*. This solitary diverticulum lies on the antimesenteric side of the bowel, usually within 2 feet (85 cm) of the ileocecal valve (Fig. 18–26). *This is a true diverticulum, in that it contains all three layers of the normal bowel wall: mucosa, submucosa, and muscularis propria*. Meckel diverticula may take the form of only a small pouch or a blind segment having a lumen greater in diameter than that of the ileum and a length of up to 6 cm. Although the mucosal lining may be that of normal small intestine, *heterotopic rests of gastric mucosa (or pancreatic tissue) are found in about one half of these anomalies*. Meckel diverticula are present in an estimated 2% of the normal population, but most remain asymptomatic or are discovered incidentally. *When peptic ulceration occurs in the small intestinal mucosa adjacent to the gastric*

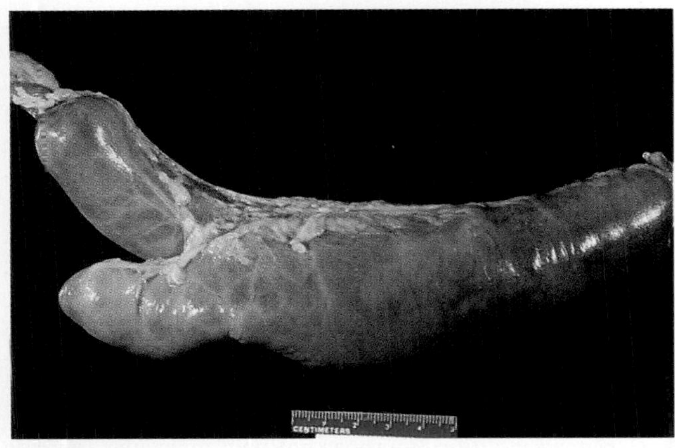

Figure 18–26

Meckel diverticulum. The blind pouch is on the antimesenteric side of the small bowel.

mucosa, mysterious intestinal bleeding or symptoms resembling those of an acute appendicitis may result. Alternatively, presenting symptoms may be related to intussusception, incarceration, or perforation.

CONGENITAL AGANGLIONIC MEGACOLON—HIRSCHSPRUNG DISEASE

This disorder is characterized by the absence of ganglion cells in the large bowel, leading to functional obstruction and colonic dilatation proximal to the affected segment. Most cases are sporadic, but familiar forms occur. It should be recalled that the intestinal neuronal plexus develops from neural crest cells that migrate into the bowel during development. Studies of familial forms and mouse models have traced the aganglionosis to heterogeneous defects in genes regulating migration and survival of neuroblasts (e.g., endothelin 3 and its receptor), neurogenesis (e.g., glial cell–derived growth factor, GDNF), and receptor tyrosine kinase activity.[30]

MORPHOLOGY. There is absence of ganglion cells in the muscle wall (Auerbach plexus) and submucosa (Meissner) of the affected segment. The rectum is always affected, with involvement of more proximal colon to variable extents. Most cases involve the rectum and sigmoid only, with longer segments in a fifth of cases and rarely the entire colon. This is sometimes accompanied by thickening and hypertrophy of nonmyelinated nerve fibers. **Proximal to the aganglionic segment, the colon undergoes progressive dilation and hypertrophy, beginning with the descending colon. With time, the proximal innervated colon may become massively distended, sometimes achieving a diameter of 15 to 20 cm (megacolon).** When distention outruns the hypertrophy, the colonic wall becomes markedly thinned and may rupture, usually near the cecum. Alternatively, mucosal inflammation or shallow, so-called **stercoral ulcers** may appear.

Clinical Features. Hirschsprung disease occurs in approximately 1 in 5000 to 8000 live births and is present with increased frequency (3.6%) in siblings of index cases. Males predominate 4 : 1. Short segment aganglionosis with megacolon is more common in boys, whereas long affected segments are more common in girls. Ten per cent of all cases of Hirschsprung disease occur in children with Down syndrome, and serious neurologic abnormalities are present in another 5%, raising the possibility that this disease is only one feature of more generalized abnormal development of the neural crest.

Hirschsprung disease usually manifests itself in the immediate neonatal period by failure to pass meconium, followed by obstructive constipation. In those instances when only a few centimeters of the rectum are affected, the build-up of pressure may permit occasional passage of stools or even intermittent bouts of diarrhea. Abdominal distention develops if a sufficiently large segment of colon is involved. The major threats to life in this disorder are superimposed enterocolitis with fluid and electrolyte disturbances and perforation of the colon or appendix with peritonitis.

Acquired megacolon is a condition of any age and may result from (1) *Chagas disease* (Chapter 8), in which the trypanosomes directly invade the bowel wall to destroy the enteric plexuses; (2) organic obstruction of the bowel as by a neoplasm or inflammatory stricture; (3) *toxic megacolon* complicating ulcerative colitis or Crohn disease (see later); or (4) a functional psychosomatic disorder. Except for Chagas disease, in which inflammatory involvement of the ganglia is evident, the remaining forms of megacolon are not associated with any deficiency of mural ganglia.

Enterocolitis

Diarrheal diseases of the bowel make up a veritable Augean stable of entities. Many are caused by microbiologic agents; others arise in the setting of malabsorptive disorders and idiopathic inflammatory bowel disease, discussed in subsequent sections. Consideration should first be given to the conditions known as *diarrhea* and *dysentery*.

DIARRHEA AND DYSENTERY

A typical adult in the United States imbibes 2 liters of fluid per day, to which is added 1 liter of saliva; 2 liters of gastric juice; 1 liter of bile; 2 liters of pancreatic juice, and 1 liter of intestinal secretions. Of these 9 liters of fluid presented to the intestine, less than 200 gm of stool are excreted per day, of which 65 to 85% is water. Jejunal absorption of water amounts to 3 to 5 liters/day; ileal absorption, 2 to 4 liters/day.[31] The colon normally absorbs 1 to 2 liters/day but is capable of absorbing almost 6 liters/day.

A precise definition of diarrhea is elusive, given the considerable variation in normal bowel habits. An increase in stool mass, stool frequency, or stool fluidity is perceived as diarrhea by most patients. For many individuals, this consists of daily stool production in excess of 250 gm, containing 70 to 95% water. More than 14 liters of fluid may be lost per day in severe cases of diarrhea (i.e., the equivalent of the circulating blood volume). Diarrhea is often accompanied by pain, urgency, perianal discomfort, and incontinence. Low-volume, painful, bloody diarrhea is known as *dysentery*. The major causes of diarrhea are presented in Table 18–5. The principal mechanisms of diarrhea, one or more of which may be operative in any one patient, are as follows:

- *Secretory diarrhea*: Net intestinal fluid secretion leads to the output of greater than 500 ml of fluid stool per day, which is isotonic with plasma and persists during fasting.
- *Osmotic diarrhea*: Excessive osmotic forces exerted by luminal solutes lead to output of greater than 500 ml of stool per day, which abates on fasting. Stool exhibits an osmotic gap (stool osmolality exceeds electrolyte concentration by ≥ 50 mOsm).
- *Exudative diseases*: Mucosal destruction leads to output of purulent, bloody stools, which persist on fasting; stools are frequent but may be small or large volume.
- *Malabsorption*: Improper absorption of gut nutrients produces voluminous, bulky stools with increased osmolarity combined with excess stool fat (steatorrhea). The diarrhea usually abates on fasting.
- *Deranged motility*: Improper gut neuromuscular function may produce highly variable patterns of increased stool volume; other forms of diarrhea must be excluded.

Table 18–5. MAJOR CAUSES OF DIARRHEAL ILLNESSES

Secretory Diarrhea
Infectious: viral damage to mucosal epithelium
- Rotavirus
- Norwalk virus
- Enteric adenoviruses

Infectious: enterotoxin mediated
- *Vibrio cholerae*
- *Escherichia coli*
- *Bacillus cereus*
- *Clostridium perfringens*

Neoplastic
- Tumor elaboration of peptides, serotonin, prostaglandins
- Villous adenoma in distal colon (non–hormone mediated)

Excess laxative use

Osmotic Diarrhea
Disaccharidase (lactase) deficiencies
Lactulose therapy (for hepatic encephalopathy, constipation)
Prescribed gut lavage for diagnostic procedures
Antacids ($MgSO_4$ and other magnesium salts)
Primary bile acid malabsorption

Exudative Diseases
Infectious: bacterial damage to mucosal epithelium
- *Shigella*
- *Salmonella*
- *Campylobacter*
- *Entamoeba histolytica*

Idiopathic inflammatory bowel disease
Typhlitis (neutropenic colitis in the immunosuppressed)

Malabsorption
Defective intraluminal digestion
Primary mucosal cell abnormalities
Reduced small intestinal surface area
Lymphatic obstruction
Infectious: impaired mucosal cell absorption
- *Giardia lamblia*

Deranged Motility
Decreased intestinal transit time
- Surgical reduction of gut length
- Neural dysfunction, including irritable bowel syndrome
- Hyperthyroidism
- Diabetic neuropathy
- Carcinoid syndrome

Decreased motility (increased intestinal transit time)
- Small intestinal diverticula
- Surgical creation of a *blind* intestinal loop
- Bacterial overgrowth in the small intestine

INFECTIOUS ENTEROCOLITIS

(see also Chapter 9)

Intestinal diseases of microbial origin are marked principally by diarrhea and sometimes ulceroinflammatory changes in the small or large intestine. *Infectious enterocolitis is a global problem of staggering proportions, causing more than 12,000 deaths per day from dehydration among children in developing countries and constituting one half of all deaths worldwide before age 5.*[32] *Although far less prevalent in industrialized nations, these infections still have attack rates of one to two illnesses per person per year, second only to the common cold in frequency.* This rate results in an estimated 99 million acute cases of either vomiting or diarrhea per year in the United States, equivalent to 40% of the population.[33]

Among the most common offenders are rotavirus and Norwalk virus and enterotoxigenic *Escherichia coli*. Many pathogens, however, can cause diarrhea; the major offenders vary with the age, nutrition, and immune status of the host; environment (living conditions, public health measures); and special predispositions, such as hospitalization, wartime dislocation, or foreign travel. In 40 to 50% of cases, the specific agent cannot be isolated.

The various organisms causing infectious enterocolitis have been discussed in Chapter 9, as have the major pathogenetic mechanisms. Here we consider clinical and pathologic features relevant to the gastrointestinal manifestations.

Viral Gastroenteritis

Symptomatic human infection is caused by several distinct groups of viruses (Table 18–6). *Rotavirus* is the most common and accounts for an estimated 140 million cases and 1 million deaths worldwide per year. The target population is children 6 to 24 months of age, but young infants and debilitated adults are susceptible to symptomatic infection. *The minimal infective inoculum is approximately 10 particles, whereas an individual with rotavirus gastroenteritis typically sheds up to 10^{12} particles/ml stool.* Thus, outbreaks among pediatric populations in hospitals and daycare centers are legion. The clinical syndrome consists of an incubation period of approximately 2 days followed by vomiting and watery diarrhea for several days.

Table 18–6. COMMON GASTROINTESTINAL VIRUSES

Virus	Genome	Size (nm)	% of US Childhood Hospitalizations	Host Age	Mode of Transmission	Prodrome/ Duration of Illness
Rotavirus (group A)	dsRNA	70	35–40	6–24 mo	Person-to-person, food, water	2 days/3–8 days
Enteric adenoviruses	dsDNA	80	5–20	Child <2 yr	Person-to-person	3–10 days/7+ days
Caliciviruses	ssRNA	35–40	3–5	Child	Person-to-person, water, cold foods, raw shellfish	1–3 days/4 days
Astroviruses	ssRNA	28	3–5	Child	Person-to-person, water, raw shellfish	24–36 hr/1–4 days
Norwalk virus/ small round structured viruses (SRSV)	ssRNA*	27	Not applicable	School age, adult	Person-to-person, water, cold foods, raw shellfish	1–2 days/12–60 hr

*Classified in the family *Caliciviridae*.
Adapted from Taterka JA, et al: Viral gastrointestinal infections. Gastroenterol Clin North Am 21:303–330, 1992.

Small round structured viruses, of which *Norwalk virus* is the prototype, are responsible for the majority of cases of nonbacterial food-borne epidemic gastroenteritis in older children and adults and are classified in the family *Caliciviridae*.[34] Infection in young children is unusual. Outbreaks occur after exposure of multiple individuals to a common source. The clinical syndrome consists of an incubation period of 1 to 2 days, followed by 12 to 60 hours of nausea, vomiting, watery diarrhea, and abdominal pain.

The morphologic changes consist of shortening and blunting of villi and infiltration of the lamina propria by lymphocytes. They are described in Chapter 9. In infants, rotavirus can produce a flat mucosa resembling celiac sprue (discussed later).

Bacterial Enterocolitis

Diarrheal illness induced by bacteria is caused by a variety of bacterial species (Table 18–7) and several pathogenic mechanisms, as follows:

- *Ingestion of preformed toxin*, present in contaminated food (major offenders are *Staphylococcus aureus*, *Vibrios*, and *Clostridium perfringens*)
- *Infection by toxigenic organisms*, which proliferate within the gut lumen and elaborate an enterotoxin
- *Infection by enteroinvasive organisms*, which proliferate, invade, and destroy mucosal epithelial cells

In the case of infection, key bacterial properties are (1) *the ability to adhere to the mucosal epithelial cells and replicate*, (2) *the ability to elaborate enterotoxins*, and (3) *the capacity to invade* (Chapter 9).

To produce disease, ingested organisms must adhere to the mucosa; otherwise, they are swept away by the fluid stream. Adherence of enterotoxigenic organisms such as *E. coli* and *Vibrio cholerae* is mediated by plasmid-coded adhesins. These proteins are expressed on the surface of the organism, sometimes in the form of fimbriae or *pili*. Adherence is also dependent on plasmid-coded proteins, but their form is not known. Adherence causes effacement of the apical enterocyte membrane, with destruction of the microvillus brush border and changes in the underlying cell cytoplasm.[35]

Bacterial enterotoxins are polypeptides that cause diarrhea. Some *enterotoxins* cause intestinal secretion of fluid and electrolytes without causing tissue damage; this is accomplished by binding of the toxin to the epithelial cell membrane, entry of a portion of the toxin into the cell, and massive activation of electrolyte secretion accompanied by water. *Cholera toxin, elaborated by V. cholerae, is the prototype secretagogue toxin*[36] (see Fig. 9–25). *Strains of* E. coli *that produce heat-labile and heat-stable secretagogue toxins are the major cause of traveler's diarrhea.* Leukocytes are absent from the stool in these patients. A second group of enterotoxins are *cytotoxins*, exemplified by Shiga toxin and toxins produced by enterohemorrhagic *E. coli*.

Bacterial Invasion. Both enteroinvasive *E. coli* and *Shigella* possess a large virulence plasmid that confers the capacity for epithelial cell invasion, apparently by microbe-stimulated endocytosis. Bacterial invasion is followed by intracellular proliferation, cell lysis, and cell-to-cell spread. *Salmonella* quickly pass through intestinal epithelial cells via transcytosis with minimal epithelial damage; entry into the lamina propria leads to a 5 to 10% incidence of bacteremia. *Yersinia enterocolitica* penetrates the ileal mucosa and multiplies within Peyer patches and regional lymph nodes.

MORPHOLOGY. Given the variety of bacterial pathogens, the pathologic manifestations of enteric bacterial disease are quite variable. Dramatic, even lethal, diarrhea may occur without a significant pathologic lesion, as in cholera resulting from *V. cholerae*. Alternatively, characteristic histology may enable diagnosis with reasonable

Table 18–7. MAJOR CAUSES OF BACTERIAL ENTEROCOLITIS

Organism	Pathogenic Mechanism	Source	Clinical Features
Escherichia coli			■ Traveler's diarrhea, including:
ETEC	Cholera-like toxin, no invasion	Food, water	Watery diarrhea
EHEC	Shiga-like toxin, no invasion	Undercooked beef products	Hemorrhagic colitis, HUS*
EPEC	Attachment, enterocyte effacement, no invasion	Weaning foods, water	Diarrhea, infants, and toddlers
EIEC	Invasion, local spread	Cheese, water, person-to-person	Fever, pain, diarrhea
Salmonella	Invasion, translocation, lymphoid inflammation, dissemination	Milk, beef, eggs, poultry	■ Fever, pain, diarrhea, dysentery, bacteremia, extraintestinal infection, common source outbreaks
Shigella	Invasion, local spread	Person-to-person, low inoculum	■ Fever, diarrhea, dysentery, epidemic spread
Campylobacter	Toxins, invasion	Milk, poultry, animal contact	■ Fever, pain, diarrhea, dysentery, food, animal reservoirs
Yersinia enterocolitica	Invasion, translocation, lymphoid inflammation, dissemination	Milk, pork	■ Fever, pain, diarrhea, adenitis, extraintestinal infection, food
Vibrio cholerae, other *Vibrio* species	Enterotoxin, no invasion	Water, shellfish, person-to-person spread	■ Watery diarrhea, cholera, pandemic spread
Clostridium difficile	Cytotoxin, local invasion	Nosocomial environmental spread	■ Fever, pain, bloody diarrhea, following antibiotics, nosocomial
Clostridium perfringens	Enterotoxin, no invasion	Meat, poultry, fish	■ Watery diarrhea, food sources, "pigbel" (enteritis necroticans)
Mycobacterium tuberculosis	Invasion, mural inflammatory foci with necrosis and scarring	Contaminated milk, swallowing of coughed-up organisms	■ Abdominal pain, malabsorption, stricture, perforation, fistulas, hemorrhage

* Hemolytic uremic syndrome; see Chapter 21.
ETEC, enterotoxigenic *E. coli;* EHEC, enterohemorrhagic *E. coli;* EPEC, enteropathogenic *E. coli;* EIEC, enteroinvasive *E. coli.*

certainty, as with *Clostridium difficile*–induced pseudomembranous colitis (discussed later). **Most bacterial infections exhibit a general nonspecific pattern of damage to the surface epithelium, decreased epithelial cell maturation, increased mitotic rate (regenerative change), hyperemia and edema of the lamina propria, and variable neutrophilic infiltration into the lamina propria and epithelial layer.** In the small intestine, modest villus blunting may occur; in the colon, mucosal architecture is usually preserved. With recovery, epithelial damage and neutrophilic inflammation subside, leaving the residua of regenerative change and lymphoplasmacytic infiltration of the lamina propria. Alternatively, progressive destruction of the mucosa leads to erosion, ulceration, and severe submucosal inflammation. Notable features of particular infections are summarized as follows:

- *Shigella*: Primarily distal colon; acute mucosal inflammation and erosion and purulent exudate (Fig. 18–27).
- *Campylobacter jejuni* and other species: Small intestine, appendix, and colon; villus blunting, multiple superficial ulcers, mucosal inflammation, and purulent exudate.
- *Y. enterocolitica* and *Y. pseudotuberculosis*: Ileum, appendix, and colon; mucosal hemorrhage and ulceration; bowel wall thickening; Peyer patch and mesenteric lymph node hypertrophy with necrotizing granulomas; systemic spread with peritonitis, pharyngitis, and pericarditis.
- *Salmonella* (multiple species, including *S. typhimurium* and *S. paratyphi*): Primarily ileum and colon; blunted villi, vascular congestion, mononuclear inflammation; Peyer patch involvement with swelling, congestion, and ulceration producing linear ulcers. With *S. typhimurium,* bacteremia, fever, and systemic dissemination constitute **typhoid fever**; this may result in chronic infection of biliary tree, joints, bones, meninges.
- *V. cholerae*: Small intestine, especially more proximal; essentially intact mucosa, with mucus-depleted crypts.
- *Clostridium perfringens*: Usually similar to *V. cholerae* but with some epithelial damage;

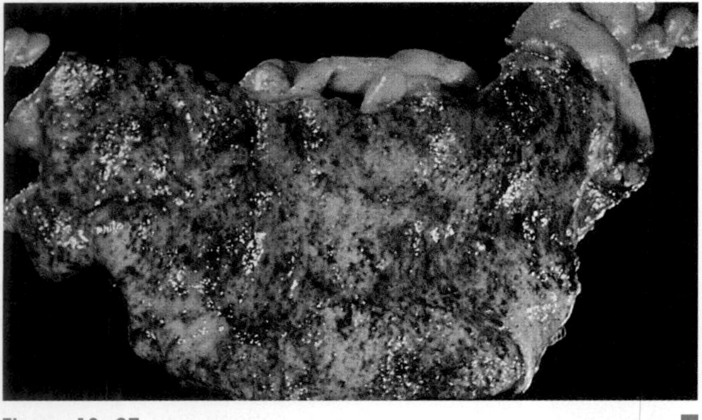

Figure 18–27

Infectious enterocolitis from *Shigella* infection. Segment of colon showing pale, granular, inflamed mucosa with patches of coagulated exudate.

some strains produce a severe necrotizing enterocolitis with perforation (**pigbel**).

Clinical Features. At the risk of oversimplification, bacterial enterocolitis takes the following forms:

- *Ingestion of preformed bacterial toxins*: Symptoms develop within a matter of hours; explosive diarrhea and acute abdominal distress herald an illness that passes within a day or so. Ingested systemic neurotoxins, as from *Clostridium botulinum*, may produce rapid, fatal respiratory failure.
- *Infection with enteric pathogens*: With ingestion of enteric pathogens, an incubation period of several hours to days is followed by *diarrhea and dehydration*, if the primary pathogenic mechanism is a secretory enterotoxin, or *dysentery*, if the primary mechanism is a cytotoxin or an enteroinvasive process. *Traveler's diarrhea* (Montezuma's revenge, turista) usually occurs after ingestion of fecally contaminated food or water; it begins abruptly and subsides within 2 to 3 days.
- *Insidious infection*: *Yersinia* and *Mycobacterium tuberculosis* may also present as subacute diarrheal illnesses. Tuberculosis is covered in detail in Chapter 9.

The complications of severe bacterial enterocolitis are the logical consequences of massive fluid loss or destruction of the intestinal mucosal barrier and include dehydration, sepsis, and perforation. Without quick intervention, death ensues rapidly, particularly in the very young. Alternatively an infection may produce extreme discomfort without being life-threatening. All enteroinvasive organisms can mimic acute onset of idiopathic inflammatory bowel disease (discussed later).

Necrotizing Enterocolitis

Necrotizing enterocolitis is an acute, necrotizing inflammation of the small and large intestine and is the most common acquired gastrointestinal emergency of neonates, particularly those who are premature or of low birth weight.[37] It may occur at any time in the first 3 months of life, but its peak incidence is around the time when infants are started on oral foods (2 to 4 days old). Necrotizing enterocolitis is believed to result from a combination of events, as follows:

- Immaturity of the gut immune system
- Initiation of oral feeding, which elicits release of a broad array of cytokines by the intestinal mucosa, including proinflammatory factors
- Gut colonization with bacteria on onset of oral feeding, with mucosal exposure to endotoxin and further release of proinflammatory cytokines
- Mucosal injury
- Deranged intestinal blood flow as a secondary event or, in some cases, as an initiating factor, further exacerbating intestinal mucosal injury

The net effect is a rapidly progressive spiral of injury affecting a major portion of the gut.

MORPHOLOGY. The disease primarily affects the terminal ileum and ascending colon, although in severe cases the entire small and large bowel may be involved. In early phases, the mucosa exhibits edema, hemorrhage, and necrosis. As the disease progresses, the full thickness of the bowel wall becomes hemorrhagic, inflamed, and gangrenous. Necrotic inflammatory debris may adhere to the mucosal surface, and frank intraluminal hemorrhage may be present. Bacterial overgrowth and mural gas formation are inconstant features. Reparative change (epithelial regeneration, granulation tissue formation, and fibrosis) may be prominent, suggesting evolution of the injury for several days before clinical presentation.

Clinical Features. The disease may present as a mild gastrointestinal disturbance or as a fulminant illness with intestinal gangrene, perforation, sepsis, and shock. The typical patient has abdominal distention, tenderness, ileus, and diarrhea with occult or frank blood. While treatment in early stages involves maintenance of fluid and electrolyte balance and blood pressure, onset of gangrene and perforation require prompt surgical intervention and usually massive resections. Long-term residua include a short bowel syndrome, malabsorption owing to ileal resection, strictures, and recurrence of disease.

Antibiotic-Associated Colitis (Pseudomembranous Colitis)

Antibiotic-associated colitis (pseudomembranous colitis) is *an acute colitis characterized by formation of an adherent inflammatory exudate (pseudomembrane) overlying sites of mucosal injury*. It is usually caused by two protein exotoxins (A and B) of *C. difficile*, a normal gut commensal.[38] This disease occurs most often in patients without a background of chronic enteric disease, after a course of

broad-spectrum antibiotic therapy. Nearly all antibacterial agents have been implicated. Presumably, toxin-forming strains flourish after alteration of the normal intestinal flora. Toxins bind to receptors on epithelial cells, inactivate the family of RhO cytoplasmic proteins, causing disaggregation of actin microfilaments and cell retraction. Toxin A also causes intestinal secretion and acute inflammation.[38a] The condition may rarely appear in the absence of antibiotic therapy, typically after surgery or superimposed on a chronic debilitating illness. Infrequently the small intestine is involved.

MORPHOLOGY. **Pseudomembranous colitis derives its name from the plaquelike adhesion of fibrinopurulent-necrotic debris and mucus to damaged colonic mucosa** (Fig. 18–28*A*)—**these are not true membranes because the coagulum is not an epithelial layer.** Pseudomembrane formation is not restricted to *C. difficile*–induced colitis: It also may occur after any severe mucosal injury, as in ischemic colitis or volvulus and with necrotizing infections (staphylococci, *Shigella, Candida,* necrotizing enterocolitis). What is striking about *C. difficile* toxin–induced colitis is the microscopic lesion (Fig. 18–28*B*). The surface epithelium is denuded, and the superficial lamina propria contains a dense infiltrate of neutrophils and occasional capillary fibrin thrombi. Superficially damaged crypts are distended by a mucopurulent exudate, which erupts out of the crypt to form a mushrooming cloud that adheres to the damaged surface—the coalescence of this cloud forms the pseudomembrane.

Clinical Features. Antibiotic-associated colitis occurs primarily in adults as an acute or chronic diarrheal illness, although it has been recorded as a spontaneous infection in young adults without predisposing influences. Diagnosis is confirmed by the detection of the *C. difficile* cytotoxin in stool. Response to treatment is usually prompt, but relapse occurs in up to 25% of patients.

Collagenous and Lymphocytic Colitis

Collagenous colitis is a distinctive disorder of the colon characterized by chronic watery diarrhea and patches of bandlike collagen deposits directly under the surface epithelium. *Lymphocytic colitis* is characterized by chronic watery diarrhea and a prominent intraepithelial infiltrate of lymphocytes. Collagenous colitis occurs primarily in middle-aged and older women; lymphocytic colitis affects men and women equally. Both sets of patients can have 3 to 20 nonbloody, watery bowel movements per day, accompanied by cramping abdominal pain. Radiographic studies are unremarkable, and endoscopy characteristically reveals normal mucosa. The pathogenesis of both these conditions remains unclear; they do appear to be separate conditions. Lymphocytic colitis shows a strong association with autoimmune diseases, including celiac sprue, thyroiditis, arthritis, and autoimmune gastritis. Both diseases are benign in nature, with neither debilitating weight loss nor malignancy as potential outcomes. Although collagenous colitis and lymphocytic colitis are uncommon, they must be considered in every adult patient who presents with a noninflammatory diarrhea.

MISCELLANEOUS INTESTINAL INFLAMMATORY DISORDERS

Parasites and Protozoa

Although viruses and bacteria are the predominant enteric pathogens in the United States, *parasitic disease and protozoal infection collectively affect more than half of the world population on a chronic or recurrent basis.* Infections covered in Chapter 9 include (1) *nematodes* (*roundworms*), such as *Strongyloides*, *Ascaris*, and hookworms; (2) *flatworms*, such as tapeworms and flukes; and (3) *pro-*

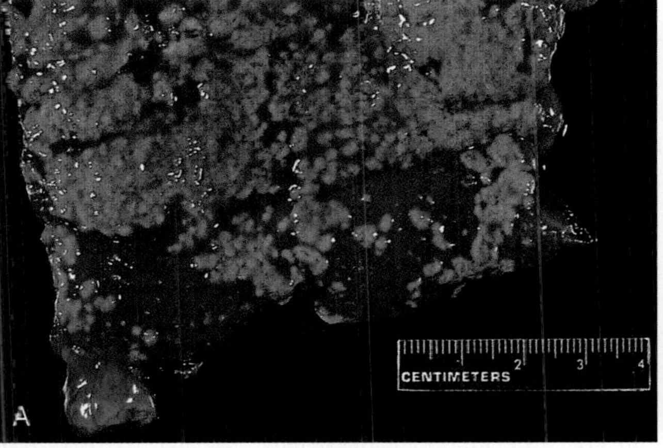

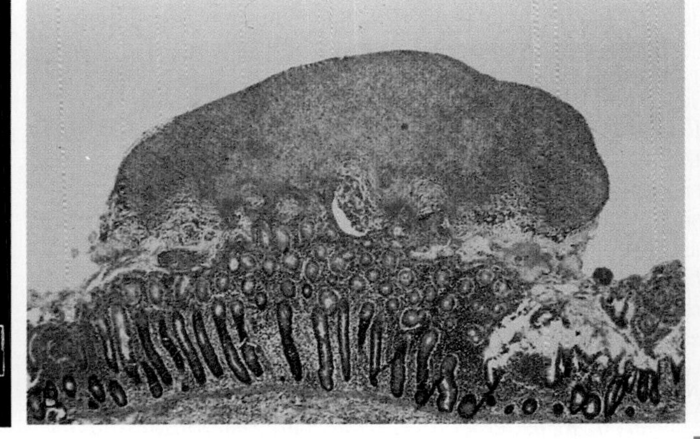

Figure 18–28

Pseudomembranous colitis from *Clostridium difficile* infection. *A*, Gross photograph. Close-up of mucosal surface showing plaques of yellow fibrin and inflammatory debris adherent to a reddened colonic mucosa. *B*, Low-power micrograph showing superficial erosion of the mucosa and an adherent "pseudomembrane" of fibrin, mucus, and inflammatory debris.

tozoa, such as microsporidia, cryptosporidia, and *Isospora belli*. Two protozoal agents merit specific comment.

Entamoeba histolytica is a dysentery-causing protozoan parasite spread by fecal-oral spread. Amebae invade the crypts of colonic glands and burrow into the lamina propria; the organisms then fan out laterally to create a flask-shaped ulcer with a narrow neck and broad base. In about 40% of patients with amebic dysentery, parasites penetrate portal vessels and embolize to the liver to produce solitary or, less often, multiple, discrete hepatic abscesses, some exceeding 10 cm in diameter. Occasional amebic abscesses are encountered in the lung, heart, kidneys and even brain. Such abscesses remain long after the acute intestinal illness has passed.

Giardia lamblia is an intestinal protozoan spread by fecal contaminated water. *Giardia* attaches to the small intestinal mucosa but does not appear to invade (Fig. 18–29). Small intestinal morphology may range from virtually normal to marked blunting of the villi with a mixed inflammatory infiltrate of the lamina propria. A malabsorptive diarrhea appears to arise from mucosal cell injury, by mechanisms that are not understood.

Acquired Immunodeficiency Syndrome

Diarrheal illness occurs in 30 to 60% of patients infected with *human immunodeficiency virus (HIV)*.[39] Some patients exhibit a malabsorptive syndrome with small intestinal villus atrophy or a colitic syndrome resembling ulcerative colitis (discussed later) in the absence of demonstrable pathogens. Although most cases are probably due to microorganisms that have been missed or have not yet been identified as pathogens, the concept of *acquired immunodeficiency syndrome (AIDS) enteropathy*, attributable to direct mucosal damage by HIV infection, is an attractive but as yet unproven pathogenic process. The spectrum of infections occurring in AIDS are discussed further in Chapter 7.

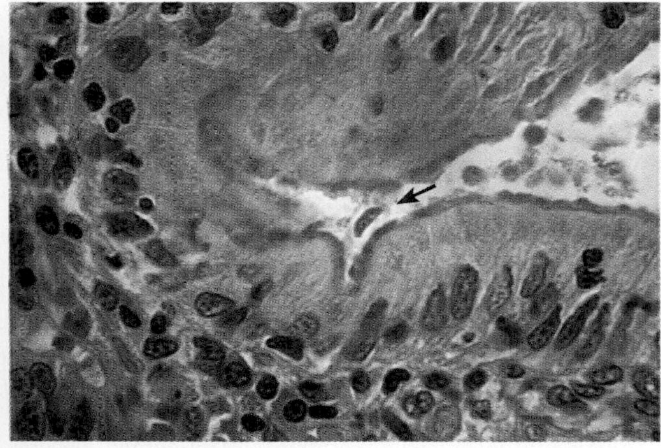

Figure 18–29

Giardia lamblia. Trophozoite *(arrow)* of the organism immediately adjacent to the duodenal surface of epithelium; note the double nuclei. The other luminal material is mucus *(bluish)* and an erythrocyte displaced by the biopsy procedure.

Complications of Transplantation

Diarrhea is a significant complication of *bone marrow transplantation*. Pretransplant conditioning may cause direct *toxic injury* to the small intestinal mucosa, evident as villus blunting, degeneration and flattening of crypt epithelial cells, decreased mitoses, and atypia of cell nuclei. Abrupt onset of severe watery diarrhea is a major feature of acute *graft-versus-host disease*. A distinctive histologic lesion is focal crypt cell necrosis, in which debris from apoptotic cells occupies lacunae within the epithelial layer, with minimal-to-absent inflammatory cell response in the lamina propria.[40] In more advanced graft-versus-host disease, necrosis may become so severe as to lead to total sloughing of the mucosa. In addition to fluid and electrolyte derangements, the life-threatening complications of sepsis and intestinal hemorrhage may ensue. Alimentary tract symptoms are less evident in chronic graft-versus-host disease but may include dysphagia, secondary to esophageal involvement, and occasionally malabsorption, secondary to chronic intestinal injury. *Small intestinal transplantation* also carries with it a spectrum of complications, including rejection and malabsorption.[41] Enteric cytomegalovirus infection may occur in any patient subjected to transplantation.

Drug-induced Intestinal Injury

When one considers the vast quantities of drugs ingested by humans, both licit and illicit, it is remarkable that the gastrointestinal tract escapes relatively unscathed. *Focal ulceration* can occur when a pill adheres to the mucosa and releases all of its contents locally, as may occur in the esophagus with *dry swallows*. Drug-induced acute erosive gastritis has been mentioned earlier. *The small intestine and colon are susceptible to drug-induced enterocolitis*, most commonly associated with the use of *NSAIDs*.[42] A nonspecific pattern of small intestinal inflammation may lead to malabsorption. Colonic inflammation may produce an acute or chronic diarrheal illness; ulceration and stricture formation also occur. *Drug-induced gastrointestinal injury must be considered whenever abdominal illness is encountered.* Considering this possibility may, on occasion, spare patients from erroneous assignment to other diagnostic categories.

Radiation Enterocolitis

Abdominal irradiation may severely impair the normal proliferative activity of the small intestinal and colonic mucosal epithelia. *Acute radiation enteritis* manifests as anorexia, abdominal cramps, and malabsorptive diarrhea, attributable to acute mucosal injury. *Chronic radiation enteritis* or *colitis* may exhibit more indolent symptoms than the acute form or may present as an inflammatory colitis. The mucosal damage may be perpetuated by radiation-induced vascular injury and accompanied by ischemic fibrosis and stricture.

Neutropenic Colitis (Typhlitis)

Typhlitis was a 19th century term for severe acute and chronic inflammation of the cecal and appendiceal region, which in retrospect was probably the outcome of untreated acute appendicitis. The term is now used to describe a life-threatening acute inflammatory destruction of the mucosa of the cecal region, occurring in neutropenic individuals. The presumed pathogenesis is impaired mucosal immunity in combination with compromised blood flow in the cecal region.

Diversion Colitis

Colonic enterocytes derive a significant portion of their caloric supply from short-chain fatty acids present in the luminal stream. Surgical diversion of the stream, as through an ileostomy, renders the colonic mucosa susceptible to nutritional deprivation. The changes may range from mild, with increased lamina propria lymphocytes, to a severe exudative diarrheal disease that resembles ulcerative colitis. Restoration of fecal flow through the colon or enemas containing short-chain fatty acids permit mucosal recovery.

Malabsorption Syndromes

Malabsorption is characterized by suboptimal absorption of fats, fat-soluble and other vitamins, proteins, carbohydrates, electrolytes and minerals, and water. At the most basic level, it is the result of disturbance of at least one of the following normal digestive functions:

1. *Intraluminal digestion*, in which proteins, carbohydrates, and fats are broken down into assimilable forms. The process begins in the mouth with saliva, receives a major boost from gastric peptic digestion, and continues in the small intestine, assisted by the detergent action of bile salts (Chapter 19).
2. *Terminal digestion*, which involves the hydrolysis of carbohydrates and peptides by disaccharidases and peptidases in the brush border of the small intestinal mucosa.
3. *Transepithelial transport*, in which nutrients, fluid, and electrolytes are transported across the epithelium of the small intestine for delivery to the intestinal vasculature. Absorbed fatty acids are converted to triglycerides and, with cholesterol, are assembled into chylomicrons for delivery to the intestinal lymphatic system.

The major diseases and disorders causing malabsorption are presented in Table 18–8. This classification is most helpful for diseases in which there is a single, clear-cut abnormality. In many malabsorptive disorders, a defect in one pathophysiologic process predominates, but others may contribute. Although many causes of malabsorption can be established clinically, diagnosis may require small intestinal mucosal biopsy to exclude celiac sprue satisfactorily.

Clinically the malabsorption syndromes resemble each other more than they differ. The consequences of malabsorption affect many organ systems, as follows:

- *Alimentary tract*: Diarrhea (both from nutrient malabsorption and from excessive intestinal secretions), flatus, abdominal pain, weight loss, and mucositis resulting from vitamin deficiencies
- *Hematopoietic system*: Anemia from iron, pyridoxine, folate, or vitamin B_{12} deficiency and bleeding from vitamin K deficiency

Table 18–8. MAJOR MALABSORPTION SYNDROMES

Defective Intraluminal Digestion
Digestion of fats and proteins
- Pancreatic insufficiency, owing to pancreatitis or cystic fibrosis
- Zollinger-Ellison syndrome, with inactivation of pancreatic enzymes by excess gastric acid secretion

Solubilization of fat, owing to defective bile secretion
- Ileal dysfunction or resection, with decreased bile salt uptake
- Cessation of bile flow from obstruction, hepatic dysfunction

Nutrient preabsorption or modification by bacterial overgrowth

Primary Mucosal Cell Abnormalities
Defective terminal digestion
- Disaccharidase deficiency (lactose intolerance)
- Bacterial overgrowth, with brush border damage

Defective epithelial transport
- Abetalipoproteinemia
- Primary bile acid malabsorption owing to mutations in the ileal bile acid transporter

Reduced Small Intestinal Surface Area
Gluten-sensitive enteropathy (celiac sprue)
Crohn disease

Lymphatic Obstruction
Lymphoma
Tuberculosis and tuberculous lymphadenitis

Infection
Acute infectious enteritis
Parasitic infestation
Tropical sprue
Whipple disease *(Tropheryma whippelii)*

Iatrogenic
Subtotal or total gastrectomy
Short-gut syndrome, following extensive surgical resection
Distal ileal resection or bypass

- *Musculoskeletal system*: Osteopenia and tetany from calcium, magnesium, vitamin D, and protein malabsorption
- *Endocrine system*: Amenorrhea, impotence, and infertility from generalized malnutrition and hyperparathyroidism from protracted calcium and vitamin D deficiency
- *Epidermis*: Purpura and petechiae from vitamin K deficiency; edema from protein deficiency; and dermatitis and hyperkeratosis from deficiencies of vitamin A, zinc, essential fatty acids, and niacin
- *Nervous system*: Peripheral neuropathy from vitamin A and vitamin B_{12} deficiencies

The passage of abnormally bulky, frothy, greasy, yellow or gray stools *(steatorrhea)* is a prominent feature of malabsorption, accompanied by weight loss, anorexia, abdominal distention, borborygmi, and muscle wasting. *The malabsorptive disorders most commonly encountered in the United States are celiac sprue, pancreatic insufficiency, and Crohn disease* (see later).

Pancreatic insufficiency, primarily from chronic pancreatitis or cystic fibrosis (Chapter 20), is a major cause of *defective intraluminal digestion*. Excessive growth of normal bacteria within the proximal small intestine (*bacterial overgrowth*) also impairs intraluminal digestion and can damage mucosal epithelial cells. Immunologic deficiencies, inadequate gastric acidity, and intestinal stasis, as from surgical alteration of small intestinal anatomy, predispose to bacterial overgrowth. Typical features of defective intraluminal digestion are an osmotic diarrhea from undigested nutrients and steatorrhea, which is excess output of undigested fat in stool. The intestinal mucosa in bacterial overgrowth either is normal or is minimally damaged.

CELIAC SPRUE

Celiac sprue is a relatively rare chronic disease, in which there is a characteristic mucosal lesion of the small intestine and impaired nutrient absorption, which improves on withdrawal of wheat gliadins and related grain proteins from the diet.[43] This condition is known by a variety of names—*gluten-sensitive enteropathy, nontropical sprue, celiac disease*. Celiac sprue occurs largely in whites and is rare or nonexistent among native Africans, Japanese, and Chinese.

Pathogenesis. *The fundamental disorder in celiac sprue is a sensitivity to gluten, which is the alcohol-soluble, water-insoluble protein component (gliadin) of wheat and closely related grains (oat, barley, and rye).*[44] Cell-mediated immunity appears to be important in the pathogenesis of this disease The small intestinal mucosa, when exposed to gluten, accumulates intraepithelial cytotoxic T cells and large numbers of lamina propria T helper cells that are sensitized to gliadin. Cytokine release by the T cells is thought to damage the intestinal enterocytes.

Although the genetic trends in this disease are variable, a specific HLA DQ α/β heterodimer appears to confer susceptibility through its interaction with gliadin. Ninety per cent to 95% of patients express the DQw2 histocompatibility antigen on chromosome 6, particularly a DQ α/β heterodimer, and familial clustering is well known in this disease. Because the DQ locus is linked with HLA B8, as many as 80% of patients express this latter antigen as well. An intriguing hypothesis invokes cross-reactivity of gliadin with a fragment of the E1b protein of type 12 adenovirus, raising the possibility that celiac disease results, in part, from environmental exposure to this virus.

MORPHOLOGY. The mucosa appears flat or scalloped or may be visually normal. Biopsy specimens demonstrate a **diffuse enteritis**, with marked atrophy or total loss of villi. The surface epithelium shows vacuolar degeneration, loss of the microvillus brush border, and an increased number of intraepithelial lymphocytes (Fig. 18–30). The crypts exhibit increased mitotic activity and are elongated, hyperplastic, and tortuous, so that the **overall mucosal thickness remains the same**. The lamina propria has an overall increase in plasma cells, lymphocytes, macrophages, eosinophils, and mast cells. All these structural changes are usually more marked in the proximal small intestine than in the distal because the duodenum and proximal jejunum are exposed to the highest concentration of dietary gluten. Although these changes are characteristic of celiac sprue, they can be mimicked by other diseases, most notably tropical sprue. Mucosal histology usually reverts to normal or near-normal after a period of gluten exclusion from the diet.

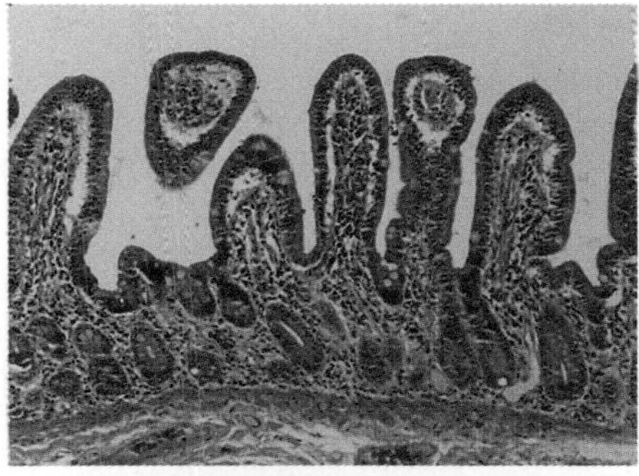

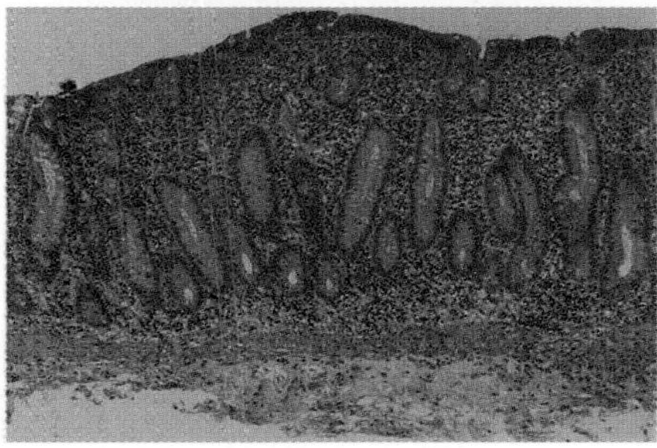

Figure 18–30

Celiac sprue (gluten-sensitive enteropathy) *(bottom)* compared with normal jejunum *(top)*. In sprue there is diffuse severe atrophy and blunting of villi, with a chronic inflammatory infiltrate of the lamina propria. (Courtesy of Dr. James Gulizia, Brigham and Women's Hospital, Boston, MA.)

Clinical Features. The symptoms of celiac sprue vary tremendously from patient to patient. Symptomatic diarrhea and failure to thrive may be evident during infancy, yet adults may seek attention only in their forties. The classic presentation includes diarrhea, flatulence, weight loss, and fatigue. Extraintestinal manifestations of malabsorption may overshadow the intestinal symptoms. Detection of circulating antigliadin or *antiendomesial* antibodies strongly favors the diagnosis. *Definitive diagnosis rests on* (1) *clinical documentation of malabsorption*, (2) *demonstration of the intestinal lesion by small bowel biopsy*, and (3) *unequivocal improvement in both symptoms and mucosal histology on gluten withdrawal from the diet.* If there is doubt about the diagnosis, gluten challenge followed by rebiopsy has been advocated.[45]

Most patients with celiac sprue who adhere to a gluten-free diet remain well indefinitely and ultimately die of unrelated causes. There is a long-term risk of malignant disease, although it may be less than a twofold increase over the usual rate. More than half of these malignancies are intestinal lymphomas, including a disproportionately high number of T-cell lymphomas. Other malignancies include gastrointestinal and breast carcinomas.

TROPICAL SPRUE (POSTINFECTIOUS SPRUE)

This condition is so named because this celiac-like disease occurs almost exclusively in people living in or visiting the tropics.[46] The distribution of the disease is curious: It is common in the Caribbean (but not in Jamaica), central and southern Africa, the Indian subcontinent and Southeast Asia, and portions of Central and South America. The disease may occur in endemic form, and epidemic outbreaks have occurred. No specific causal agent has been clearly associated with tropical sprue, but bacterial overgrowth by enterotoxigenic organisms (e.g., *E. coli* and *Haemophilus*) has been implicated.

MORPHOLOGY. Intestinal changes are extremely variable, ranging from near-normal to severe diffuse enteritis. In contrast to celiac sprue, injury is seen at all levels of the small intestine. Patients frequently have folate or vitamin B_{12} deficiency, leading to markedly atypical enlargement of the nuclei of epithelial cells (megaloblastic change), reminiscent of the changes seen in pernicious anemia.

Clinical Features. Malabsorption usually becomes apparent within days or a few weeks of an acute diarrheal enteric infection in visitors to endemic locales and may persist if untreated. The mainstay of treatment is broad-spectrum antibiotics, supporting an infectious cause. Intestinal lymphoma does not appear to be a hazard.

WHIPPLE DISEASE

Whipple disease is a rare, systemic condition, which may involve any organ of the body but principally affects the intestine, central nervous system, and joints. The causal organism is a gram-positive actinomycete, now named *Tropheryma whippelii,* on the basis of recent molecular phylogenetic analysis.[47]

MORPHOLOGY. The hallmark of Whipple disease is a small intestinal mucosa laden with distended macrophages in the lamina propria—the macrophages contain periodic acid–Schiff (PAS)–positive granules and rod-shaped bacilli by electron microscopy (Fig. 18–31). In untreated cases, bacilli can be seen in neutrophils, the extracellular space of the lamina propria, and even in epithelial cells. Expansion of the villi imparts a shaggy gross appearance to the intestinal mucosal surface; edema of the mucosa thickens the intestinal wall. Accompanying these changes is involvement of mesenteric lymph nodes by the same process and lymphatic dilation, suggesting lymphatic obstruction. Bacilli-laden macrophages also can be found in the synovial membranes of affected joints, the brain, cardiac valves, and elsewhere. **At each of these sites, inflammation is essentially absent.**

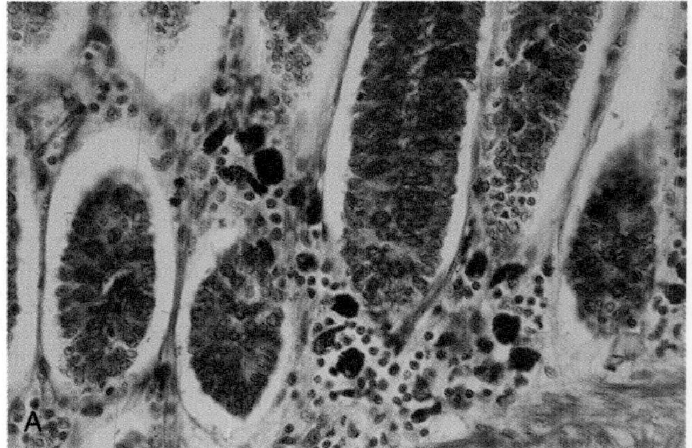

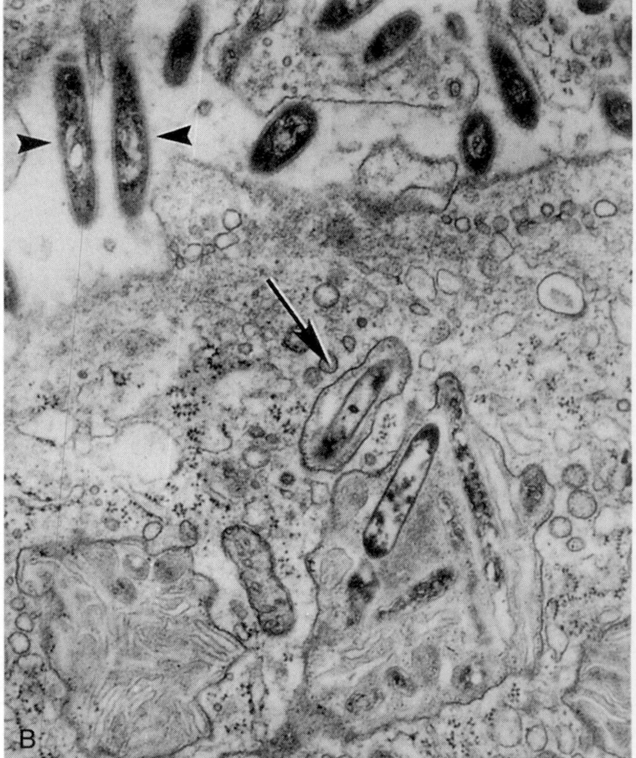

Figure 18–31

Whipple disease. *A*, PAS-positive strain showing large macrophages in lamina propria with PAS-positive material. *B*, Electron micrograph of a lamina propria macrophage and its adjacent extracellular space *(top)* from a jejunal biopsy specimen. Many bacilli are seen *(arrowheads)* and several disintegrating organisms are present within the macrophage *(arrow)*, contributing membranous material and intracellular granules. (*B*, From Trier JS, et al: Whipple's disease: light and electron microscope correlation of jejunal mucosal histology with antibiotic treatment and clinical status. Gastroenterology 48:684–707, 1965.)

Clinical Features. Whipple disease is principally encountered in whites in their thirties to forties, with a strong male predominance of 10:1. It usually presents as a form of malabsorption with diarrhea and weight loss, sometimes of years' duration. Atypical presentations, with polyarthritis, obscure central nervous system complaints, and other symptom complexes, are common. Lymphadenopathy and hyperpigmentation are present in more than half of patients. The diagnosis rests on light microscopic changes of PAS-positive macrophages, which contain rod-shaped organisms by electron microscopy. Response to antibiotic therapy is usually prompt, although some patients have a protracted, refractory course.

DISACCHARIDASE (LACTASE) DEFICIENCY

The disaccharidases, of which the most important is lactase, are located in the apical cell membrane of the villous absorptive epithelial cells. Congenital lactase deficiency is a rare condition, but acquired lactase deficiency is common, particularly among North American blacks. Incomplete breakdown of the disaccharide lactose into its monosaccharides, glucose and galactose, leads to osmotic diarrhea from the unabsorbed lactose. Bacterial fermentation of the unabsorbed sugars leads to increased hydrogen production, which is readily measured in exhaled air by gas chromatography.

When inherited as an enzyme deficiency, malabsorption becomes evident with the initiation of milk feeding. Infants develop explosive, watery, frothy stools and abdominal distention. Malabsorption is promptly corrected when exposure to milk and milk products is terminated. In the adult, lactase insufficiency apparently develops as an acquired disorder, sometimes in association with viral and bacterial enteric infections or other disorders of the gut. Neither light nor electron microscopy has disclosed abnormalities of the mucosal cells of the bowel in either the hereditary or the acquired form of the disease.

ABETALIPOPROTEINEMIA

Inability to synthesize apolipoprotein B is a rare inborn error of metabolism that is transmitted by autosomal recessive inheritance.[48] It is characterized by a defect in the synthesis and export of lipoproteins from intestinal mucosal cells. Free fatty acids and monoglycerides resulting from hydrolysis of dietary fat enter the absorptive epithelial cells and are re-esterified in the normal fashion but cannot be assembled into chylomicrons. As a consequence, triglycerides are stored within the cells, creating lipid vacuolation, which is readily evident under the light microscope, particularly with special fat stains. Concomitantly, there is complete absence in plasma of all lipoproteins containing apolipoprotein B (chylomicrons, very low-density lipoproteins, and low-density lipoproteins). The failure to absorb certain essential fatty acids leads to systemic abnormalities, including lipid membrane abnormalities, readily evident in the characteristic acanthocytic erythrocytes (*burr cells*). The disease becomes manifest in infancy and is dominated by failure to thrive, diarrhea, and steatorrhea.

Idiopathic Inflammatory Bowel Disease

Two inflammatory disorders of unknown cause affecting the intestinal tract are Crohn disease and ulcerative colitis. These diseases share many common features and are collectively known as *inflammatory bowel disease. Both Crohn disease and ulcerative colitis are chronic, relapsing inflammatory disorders of obscure origin. Crohn disease is a granulomatous disease that may affect any portion of the gastrointestinal tract from esophagus to anus but most often involves the small intestine and colon. Ulcerative colitis is a nongranulomatous disease limited to the colon. Both exhibit extraintestinal inflammatory manifestations.* Before considering these diseases separately, the pathogenesis of inflammatory bowel disease is considered.

ETIOLOGY AND PATHOGENESIS

The normal intestine is normally in a steady-state of physiologic inflammation, representing a dynamic balance between (1) factors that activate the host immune system (e.g., luminal microbes, dietary antigens, endogenous inflammatory stimuli) and (2) host defenses that maintain the integrity of the mucosa and down-regulate inflammation.[49] The search for the cause of loss of this balance in Crohn disease and ulcerative colitis has revealed many parallels, not the least of which is that *both diseases remain unexplained* and are thus best designated as *idiopathic.* While Crohn disease and ulcerative colitis share important pathophysiologic features, these two diseases may be partly or wholly distinct in their initial pathogenesis.

Genetic Predisposition. Familial aggregations in inflammatory bowel disease have been observed repeatedly, but a clear mendelian inheritance is not evident. Fifteen per cent of inflammatory bowel disease patients have affected first-degree relatives, and the lifetime risk if either a parent or sibling is affected is 9%. Dizygotic twins have the concordance rates expected for siblings; monozygotic twins exhibit a 30 to 50% concordance rate for Crohn disease. With the exception of monozygotic twins, familial occurrence can manifest either as Crohn disease or as ulcerative colitis. There is no increased risk for spouses of affected patients, pointing away from a pure environmental event.

Differential associations of Crohn disease and ulcerative colitis with the HLA class II locus on chromosome 6 suggest that these are genetically distinct disorders. An HLA-DR1/DQw5 allelic combination is observed in 27% of North American white patients with Crohn disease, whereas HLA-DR2 is increased in patients with ulcerative colitis.[50] HLA-B27 occurs with high frequency in patients with inflammatory bowel disease and ankylosing spondylitis. Although the HLA class II molecules are critical in antigen presentation during the immune response, it is possible that genetic predisposition is the result of linkage with other risk genes on chromosome 6, possibly the TNF-β gene.[51] A susceptibility locus on chromosome 16 in French families with multiple members affected by Crohn disease has been reported.[52]

Infectious Causes. The history of inflammatory bowel disease research is littered with candidate pathogens, including viruses, *Chlamydia*, atypical bacteria, and mycobacteria. Current attention is being given to *Mycobacterium paratuberculosis* and measles virus.[53] In the latter instance, persistent infection is purported to incite a chronic granulomatous vasculitis.[54] Given the success in explaining chronic gastritis on the basis of bacterial infection, the search also continues for a bacterial pathogen for inflammatory bowel disease. It is important to recognize that many bacteria (*Campylobacter, E. coli, Yersinia, Plesiomonas, Aeromonas, C. difficile*) cause diarrheal diseases that may be confused with inflammatory bowel disease.

Abnormal Host Immunoreactivity. *A fundamental emerging concept is that the host mucosal immunity is stimulated and then fails to down-regulate,* probably as a consequence of inappropriate exposure to luminal antigens, particularly ubiquitous bacterial cell wall products and secreted toxins. This view arises from observations in transgenic animals who develop inflammatory bowel disease as a result of deficiencies or overexpression of a number of immunoregulatory molecules. These models suggest that (1) defective immunoregulation is sufficient to produce chronic enterocolitis, (2) the chronic enterocolitis is mediated by immunoregulatory T lymphocytes, (3) genetic alterations in any of a number of immunoregulatory cytokines and signal-processing molecules can produce chronic intestinal inflammation, and (4) the host genetic background determines the incidence and aggressiveness of disease.[56] The fact that marked clinical improvement follows immunosuppressive therapy such as corticosteroids points toward an immune-mediated process. A satisfactory explanation for granuloma formation in Crohn disease is lacking.

Inflammation as the Final Common Pathway. *Both the clinical manifestations of inflammatory bowel disease and the diagnostic pathology are ultimately the result of activation of inflammatory cells whose products cause nonspecific tissue injury.* Neutrophils are among the most important cellular sources of these mediators, with lesser contributions from eosinophils, mast cells, and fibroblasts. Infiltrating mononuclear cells (lymphocytes and macrophages) also contribute their share of inflammatory cytokines.[49] Currently, most therapeutic agents act entirely or partly through nonspecific down-regulation of the immune system.

CROHN DISEASE

When first described in 1932, this idiopathic disorder was thought to be limited to the terminal ileum, hence the designation *terminal ileitis*. Recognition that sharply delineated bowel segments might be affected, with intervening unaffected (*skip*) areas, led to the alternate name *regional enteritis*. Predominant involvement of the colon gave rise to the term *granulomatous colitis*. It is now clear that any level of the alimentary tract may be involved and that there are systemic manifestations; thus the eponymic name *Crohn disease* is preferred. *When fully developed, Crohn disease is characterized pathologically by* (1) *sharply delimited and typically transmural involvement of the bowel by an inflammatory process with mucosal damage*, (2) *the presence of noncaseating granulomas*, and (3) *fissuring with formation of fistulas.*

Epidemiology. Crohn disease occurs throughout the world but primarily in Western developed populations. Its annual incidence in the United States is around 3 per 100,000.[57] It occurs at any age, from young childhood to advanced age, but peak ages of detection are the teens and twenties with a minor peak in the fifties and sixties. Females are affected slightly more often than males. Whites appear to develop the disease two to five times more often than do nonwhites. In the United States, Crohn disease occurs three to five times more often among Jews than among non-Jews. Smoking is a strong exogenous risk factor.

MORPHOLOGY. In Crohn disease, there is gross involvement of the small intestine alone in about 40% of cases, of small intestine and colon in 30%, and of the colon alone in about 30%. Crohn disease may involve the duodenum, stomach, esophagus, and even mouth, but these sites are distinctly uncommon. In diseased bowel segments, the serosa is granular and dull gray, and often the mesenteric fat wraps around the bowel surface (**creeping fat**). The mesentery of the involved segment is also thickened, edematous, and sometimes fibrotic. **The intestinal wall is rubbery and thick, the result of edema, inflammation, fibrosis, and hypertrophy of the muscularis propria.** As a result, the lumen is almost always narrowed; in the small intestine, this is evidenced on x-ray as the **string sign**, a thin stream of barium passing through the diseased segment. Strictures may occur in the colon but are usually less severe. **A classic feature of Crohn disease is the sharp demarcation of diseased bowel segments from adjacent uninvolved bowel. When multiple bowel segments are involved, the intervening bowel is essentially normal (skip lesions).**

A characteristic sign of early disease is focal mucosal ulcers resembling canker sores (**aphthous ulcers**), edema, and loss of the normal mucosal texture. With progressive disease, mucosal ulcers coalesce into long, serpentine **linear ulcers**, which tend to be oriented along the axis of the bowel (Fig. 18–32). As the intervening mucosa tends to be relatively spared, the mucosa acquires a coarsely textured, **cobblestone** appearance. **Narrow fissures develop between the folds of the mucosa,** often penetrating deeply through the bowel wall (Fig. 18–33) and leading to bowel adhesions. Further extension of fissures leads to **fistula or sinus tract formation**, to an adherent viscus, to the outside skin, or into a blind cavity. Free perforation or localized abscesses may also develop. The characteristic histologic features of Crohn disease are as follows.

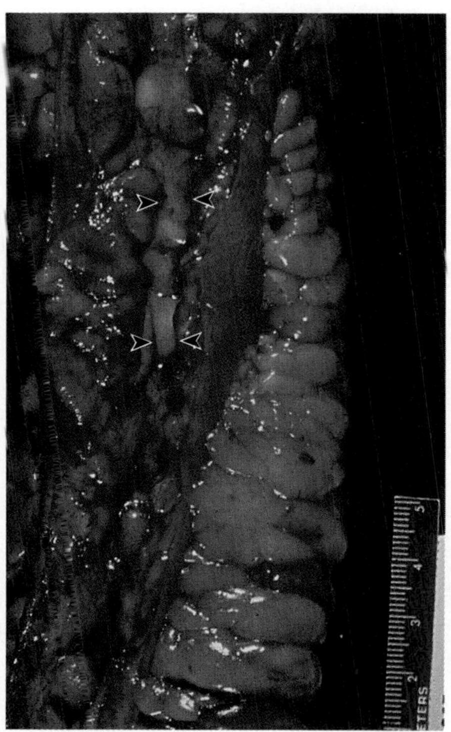

Figure 18–32

Crohn disease of the ileum showing narrowing of the lumen, bowel wall thickening, serosal extension of mesenteric fat ("creeping fat"), and linear ulceration of the mucosal surface *(arrowheads).*

Mucosal Inflammation. The earliest histologic lesion in Crohn disease appears to be focal neutrophilic infiltration into the epithelial layer, particularly overlying mucosal lymphoid aggregates. As the disease becomes more established, **neutrophils infiltrate isolated crypts; when a sufficient number of neutrophils have traversed the epithelium of a crypt (both in the small and large intestine), a crypt abscess is formed,** usually with ultimate destruction of the crypt.

Chronic Mucosal Damage. **The hallmark of inflammatory bowel disease, both Crohn disease and ulcerative colitis, is chronic mucosal damage. Architectural distortion** is manifest in the small intestine as variable villus blunting; in the colon, crypts exhibit irregularity and branching. Crypt destruction leads to progressive **atrophy,** particularly in the colon. The mucosa may undergo **metaplasia:** This may take the form of gastric antral-type glands **(pyloric metaplasia)** or as the development of Paneth cells in the distal colon, where they are normally absent **(Paneth cell metaplasia).**

Ulceration. Ulceration may be superficial, may undermine adjacent mucosa in a lateral fashion, or may penetrate deeply into underlying tissue layers. There is often an abrupt transition between ulcerated and adjacent normal mucosa.

Transmural Inflammation Affecting All Layers. Chronic inflammatory cells suffuse the affected mucosa and, to a lesser extent, all underlying tissue layers. **Lymphoid aggregates** are usually scattered throughout the bowel wall.

Noncaseating Granulomas. Present in about half of cases, sarcoid-like granulomas may be present in all tissue layers, both within areas of active disease and in uninvolved regions of the bowel (Fig. 18–34). **Granulomas have been documented throughout the alimentary tract, from mouth to rectum, in patients with Crohn disease limited to one bowel segment.** Conversely **the absence of granulomas does not preclude the diagnosis of Crohn disease.**

Other Mural Changes. In diseased segments, the muscularis mucosa usually exhibits reduplication, thickening, and irregularity. Fibrosis of the submucosa, muscularis propria, and mucosa eventually leads to stricture formation.

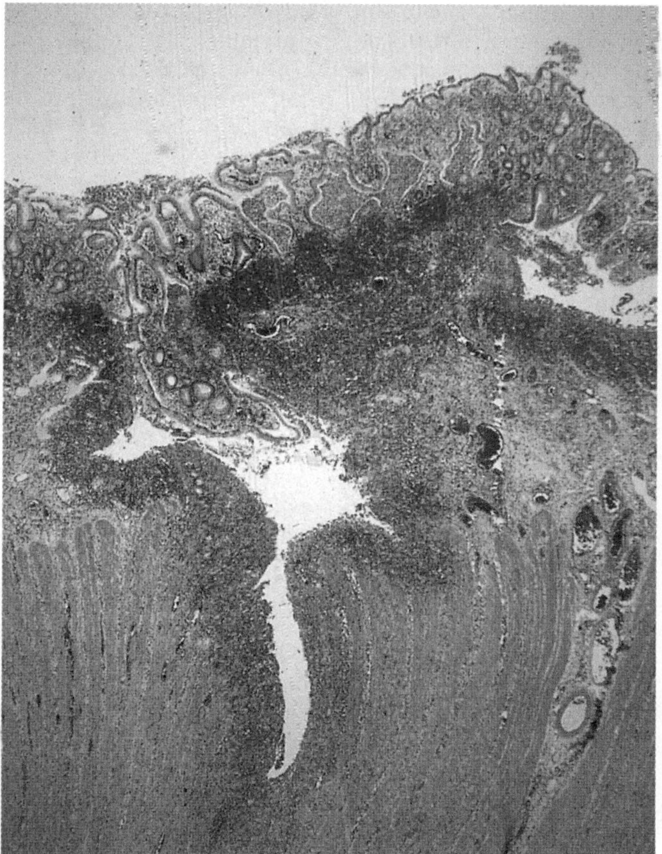

Figure 18–33

Crohn disease. Low power micrograph showing a deep fissure extending into the muscle wall *(center);* a second, shallow ulcer *(upper right);* and relative preservation of the intervening mucosa. Abundant lymphocyte aggregates are present, evident as dense blue patches of cells at the interface between mucosa and submucosa.

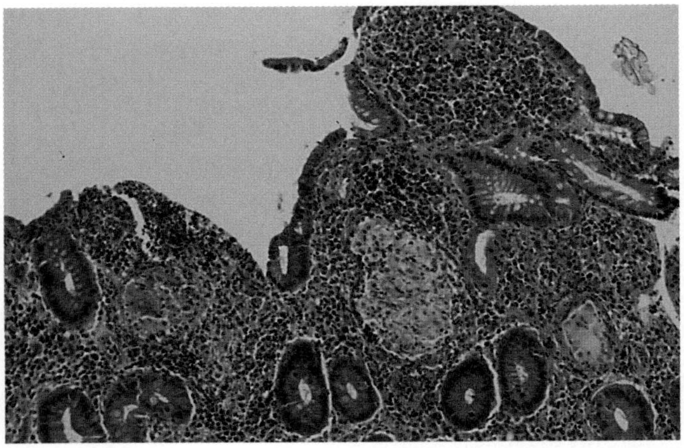

Figure 18–34

Crohn disease of the colon. Noncaseating granulomas are present in the lamina propria of a mildly inflamed region of colonic mucosa.

Clinical Features. The clinical manifestations of Crohn disease are extremely variable. The disease usually begins with intermittent attacks of relatively mild diarrhea, fever, and abdominal pain, spaced by asymptomatic periods lasting for weeks to many months. Often the attacks are precipitated by periods of physical or emotional stress. In those with colonic involvement, occult or overt fecal blood loss may lead to anemia over the span of time, but massive bleeding is uncommon. In about one fifth of patients, the onset is more abrupt, with acute right-lower-quadrant pain, fever, and diarrhea sometimes suggesting acute appendicitis or an acute bowel perforation.

During the lengthy, chronic disease, complications may arise from *fibrosing strictures*, particularly of the terminal ileum, and *fistulas* to other loops of bowel, the urinary bladder, vagina, or perianal skin or into a peritoneal abscess. Extensive involvement of the small bowel, including the terminal ileum, may cause *marked loss of albumin (protein-losing enteropathy), generalized malabsorption, specific malabsorption of vitamin B_{12}* (with consequential pernicious anemia), *or malabsorption of bile salts, leading to steatorrhea.*

Extraintestinal manifestations of this disease include migratory polyarthritis, sacroiliitis, ankylosing spondylitis, erythema nodosum, or clubbing of the fingertips. Hepatic primary sclerosing cholangitis (Chapter 19) occurs, but the association is not as strong as in ulcerative colitis. Any of these manifestations can develop before onset of intestinal symptoms. Deranged systemic immunity is thought to underly these related disorders. Uveitis, nonspecific mild hepatic pericholangitis, and renal disorders secondary to trapping of the ureters in the inflammatory process sometimes develop.

There is an increased incidence of cancer of the gastrointestinal tract in patients with long-standing progressive Crohn disease, representing a fivefold to sixfold increased risk over age-matched populations.[58] The risk of cancer in Crohn disease, however, appears to be considerably less than that in patients with chronic ulcerative colitis.

ULCERATIVE COLITIS

Ulcerative colitis is an ulceroinflammatory disease limited to the colon and affecting only the mucosa and submucosa except in the most severe cases. In contrast to Crohn disease, *ulcerative colitis extends in a continuous fashion proximally from the rectum. Well-formed granulomas are absent.* Similar to Crohn disease, ulcerative colitis is a systemic disorder associated in some patients with migratory polyarthritis, sacroiliitis, ankylosing spondylitis, uveitis, hepatic involvement (pericholangitis and primary sclerosing cholangitis; Chapter 19), and skin lesions.

Epidemiology. Ulcerative colitis is global in distribution and varies in incidence relative to Crohn disease, supporting the concept that they are separate diseases. In the United States, the incidence is about 4 to 12 per 100,000 population, slightly greater than Crohn disease. As with Crohn disease, the incidence of this condition has risen in recent decades. In the United States, it is more common among whites than among blacks, and women are affected more often than men. The onset of disease peaks between the ages of 20 and 25 years, but the condition may arise in both younger and considerably older individuals.

MORPHOLOGY. Ulcerative colitis involves the rectum and extends proximally in a retrograde fashion to involve the entire colon (pancolitis) in the more severe cases. It is a disease of continuity, and skip lesions such as occur in Crohn disease are not found (Fig. 18–35). In 10% of patients with severe pancolitis, the distal ileum may develop mild mucosal inflammation (**backwash ileitis**). The appendix may be involved with both Crohn disease and ulcerative colitis.

In the course of colonic involvement with ulcerative colitis, the mucosa may exhibit slight reddening and granularity with friability and easy bleeding. With fully developed severe, active inflammation, there may be extensive, broad-based ulceration of the mucosa in the distal colon or throughout its length (Fig. 18–36). Isolated islands of regenerating mucosa bulge upward to create **pseudopolyps**. As with Crohn disease, the ulcers of ulcerative colitis are frequently aligned along the axis of the colon, but rarely do they replicate the linear serpentine ulcers of Crohn disease. With indolent chronic disease or with healing of active disease, progressive mucosal atrophy leads to a flattened and attenuated mucosal surface. In contrast to Crohn disease, **mural thickening does not occur in ulcerative colitis, and the serosal surface is usually completely normal.** In the most severe cases, toxic damage to the muscularis propria and neural plexus lead to complete shutdown of neuromuscular function. In this instance, the colon progressively swells and becomes gangrenous (**toxic megacolon**) (Fig. 18–37).

The mucosal features of ulcerative colitis are similar to those of colonic Crohn disease, with mu-

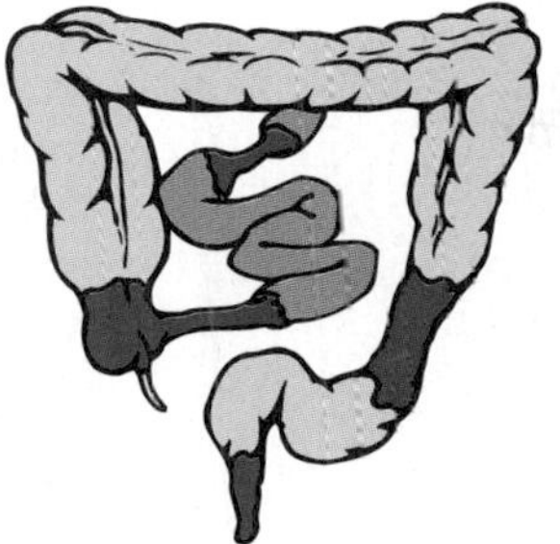

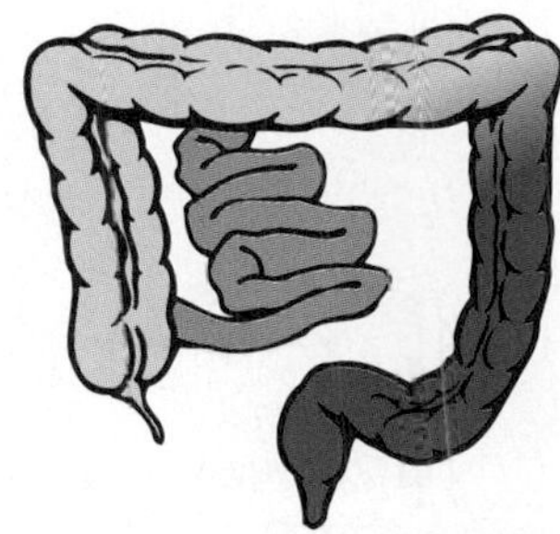

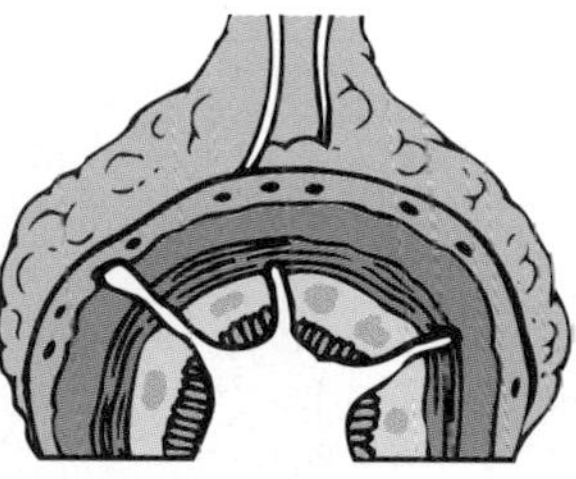

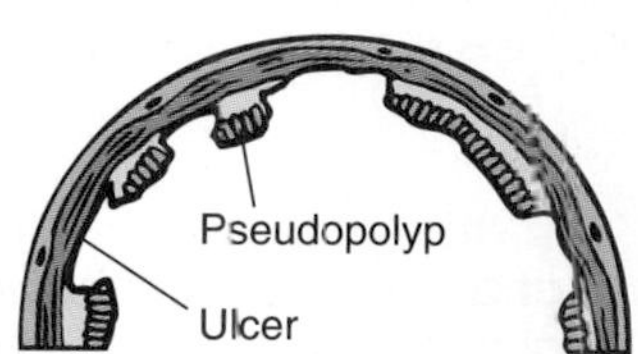

Figure 18–35

The distribution patterns of Crohn disease and ulcerative colitis are compared, as well as the different conformations of the ulcers and wall thickenings.

cosal inflammation, chronic mucosal damage, and ulceration (Figs. 18–38 and 18–39). First, **a diffuse, predominantly mononuclear inflammatory infiltrate in the lamina propria is almost universally present**, even at the time of clinical presentation. Neutrophilic infiltration of the epithelial layer may produce collections of neutrophils in crypt lumens (**crypt abscesses**) (Fig. 18–38). These are not specific for ulcerative colitis and may be observed in Crohn disease or any active inflammatory colitis. In contrast to Crohn disease, there are no granulomas. Second, **further destruction of the mucosa leads to outright ulceration, extending into the submucosa and sometimes leaving only the raw, exposed muscularis propria.** Third, with remission of active disease, granulation tissue fills in the ulcer craters, followed by regeneration

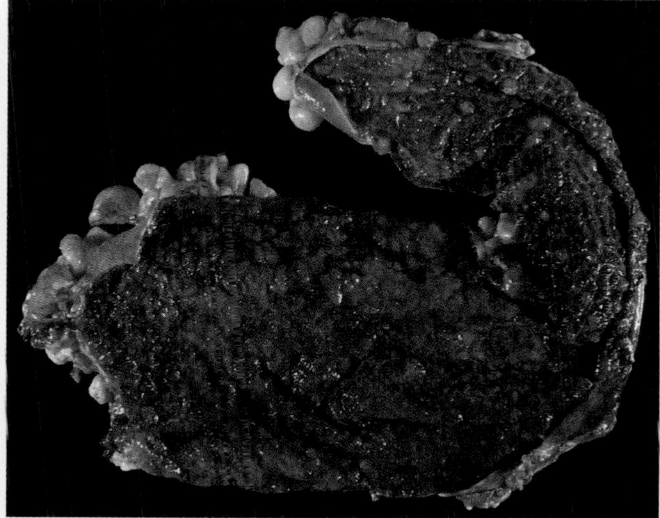

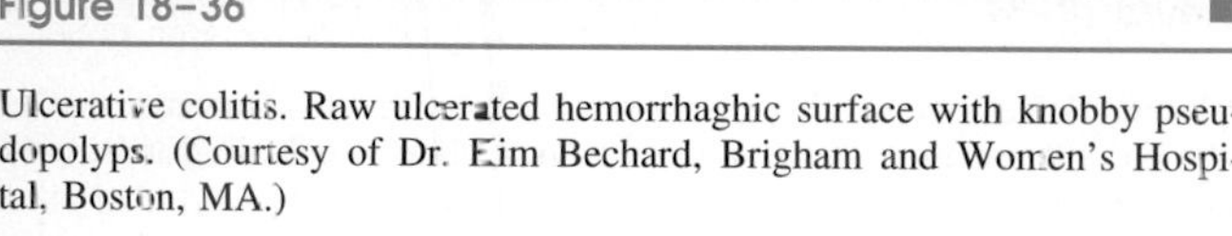

Figure 18–36

Ulcerative colitis. Raw ulcerated hemorrhaghic surface with knobby pseudopolyps. (Courtesy of Dr. Kim Bechard, Brigham and Women's Hospital, Boston, MA.)

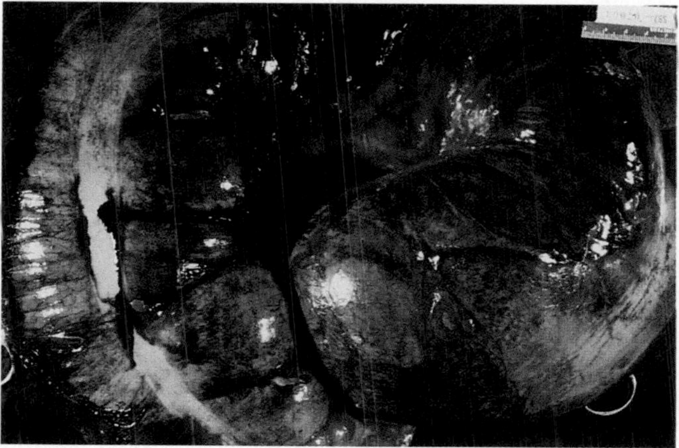

Figure 18–37

Toxic megacolon. Complete cessation of colon neuromuscular activity has led to massive dilation of the colon and black-green discoloration, signifying gangrene and impending rupture.

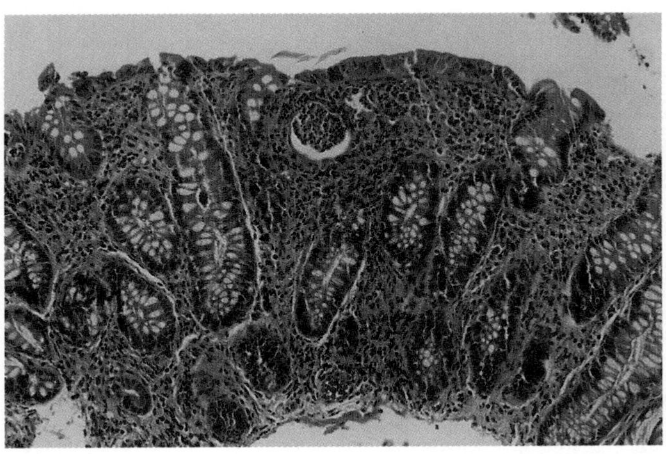

Figure 18–38

Ulcerative colitis with crypt abscess (middle of field, top). (Courtesy of Dr. James Gulizia, Brigham and Women's Hospital, Boston, MA.)

of the mucosal epithelium. **Submucosal fibrosis and mucosal architectural disarray and colonic gland atrophy may remain as residua of healed disease (Fig. 18–39).**

A key feature of ulcerative colitis is that the mucosal damage is continuous from the rectum and extending proximally. In Crohn disease, mucosal damage in the colon may be continuous but is just as likely to exhibit skip areas.

Particularly significant is the spectrum of epithelial changes signifying dysplasia and the progression to frank carcinoma. Nuclear atypia and loss of cytoplasmic differentiation may be present in inflamed or uninflamed colonic mucosa. Epithelial dysplasia is referred to as being **low grade** or **high grade.**[59] Plaquelike dysplastic lesions, overt polypoid dysplasia (adenomas), or invasive carcinoma are the ultimate lesions arising from flat dysplasia. Older patients with ulcerative colitis are also at risk for the banal sporadic adenoma.

Clinical Features. Ulcerative colitis typically presents as a relapsing disorder marked by attacks of bloody mucoid diarrhea that may persist for days, weeks, or months, then subside, only to recur after an asymptomatic interval of months to years or even decades. In the fortunate patient, the first attack is the last. At the other end of the spectrum, the explosive initial attack may lead to such serious bleeding and fluid and electrolyte imbalance as to constitute a medical emergency. In most patients, bloody diarrhea containing stringy mucus, accompanied by lower abdominal pain and cramps usually relieved by defecation, is the first manifestation of the disease. In a small number of patients, constipation may appear paradoxically, owing to disruption of normal peristalsis. Often the first attack is preceded by a stressful period in the patient's life. Spontaneously, or more often after appropriate therapy, these symptoms abate in the course of days to weeks. Flare-ups, when they do occur, may be precipitated by emotional or physical stress and rarely concurrent intraluminal growth of enterotoxin-forming *C. difficile*. Sudden cessation of bowel function with toxic dilation (toxic megacolon) rarely develops with severe acute attacks; perforation is a potentially lethal event.

About 60% of patients have clinically mild disease. In these individuals, the bleeding and diarrhea are not severe, and systemic signs and symptoms are absent. Almost all patients (97%), however, have at least one relapse during a 10-year period—about 30% of patients require colectomy within the first 3 years of onset because of uncontrollable disease.

The most feared long-term complication of ulcerative colitis is cancer. There is a tendency for dysplasia to arise in multiple sites, and the underlying inflammatory disease may mask the symptoms and signs of carcinoma. Historically the risk of cancer is highest in patients with pancolitis of 10 or more years' duration, in whom it exceeds by 20-fold to 30-fold that in a control population, equivalent to an absolute risk of colorectal cancer 35 years after diagnosis of 30%.[60] Screening programs of patients with ulcerative colitis, however, now indicate that *the rate of progression to dysplasia and carcinoma is, in fact, quite low, provided that initial examinations were negative for dysplasia.*[61, 62] Lastly, the features of Crohn disease and ulcerative colitis are compared in Table 18–9.

Vascular Disorders

ISCHEMIC BOWEL DISEASE

Ischemic lesions may be restricted to the small or large intestine or may affect both, depending on the particular vessel(s) affected. Acute occlusion of one of the three major supply trunks of the intestines—celiac, superior and inferior mesenteric arteries—may lead to infarction of several meters of intestine. *Insidious loss of one vessel may be without effect*, owing to the rich anastomotic interconnec-

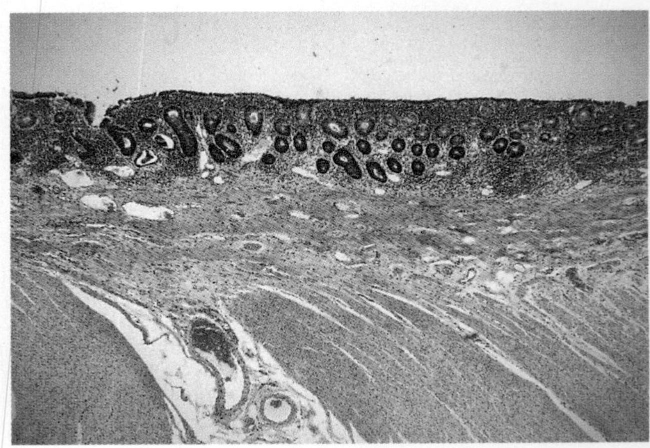

Figure 18–39

Chronic ulcerative colitis. Low-power micrograph showing marked chronic inflammation of the mucosa with atrophy of colonic glands, moderate submucosal fibrosis, and a normal muscle wall.

Table 18–9. DISTINCTIVE FEATURES OF CROHN DISEASE AND ULCERATIVE COLITIS*

Feature	Crohn Disease—SI	Crohn Disease—C	Ulcerative Colitis
Macroscopic			
Bowel region	Ileum ± colon	Colon ± ileum	Colon only
Distribution	Skip lesions	Skip lesions	Diffuse
Stricture	Early	Variable	Late/rare
Wall appearance	Thickened	Thin	Thin
Dilation	No	Yes	Yes
Microscopic			
Pseudopolyps	No to slight	Marked	Marked
Ulcers	Deep, linear	Deep, linear	Superficial
Lymphoid reaction	Marked	Marked	Mild
Fibrosis	Marked	Moderate	Mild
Serositis	Marked	Variable	Mild to none
Granulomas	Yes (50%)	Yes (50%)	No
Fistulas/sinuses	Yes	Yes	No
Clinical			
Fat/vitamin malabsorption	Yes	Yes, if ileum	No
Malignant potential	Yes	Yes	Yes
Response to surgery	Poor	Fair	Good

*Features not all present in a single case.
SI, Crohn disease of the small intestine; C, Crohn disease of the colon.

tions. Lesions within the end-arteries, which penetrate the gut wall, produce small, focal ischemic lesions. As depicted in Figure 18–40, the severity of injury ranges from (1) *transmural infarction* of the gut, involving all visceral layers; to (2) *mural infarction* of the mucosa and submucosa; to (3) *mucosal infarction*, if the lesion extends no deeper than the muscularis mucosae. *Almost always, transmural infarction implies mechanical compromise of the major mesenteric blood vessels. Mucosal or mural infarction more often results from hypoperfusion, either acute or chronic.* Mesenteric venous thrombosis is a less frequent cause of vascular compromise. The predisposing conditions for ischemia are as follows:

- *Arterial thrombosis*: Severe atherosclerosis (usually at the origin of the mesenteric vessel), systemic vasculitis (e.g., polyarteritis nodosa, Chapter 12), dissecting aneurysm, angiographic procedures, aortic reconstructive surgery, surgical accidents, hypercoagulable states, and oral contraceptives
- *Arterial embolism*: Cardiac vegetations, angiographic procedures, and aortic atheroembolism
- *Venous thrombosis*: Hypercoagulable states, oral contraceptives, antithrombin III deficiency, intraperitoneal sepsis, postoperative state, invasive neoplasms (particularly hepatocellular carcinoma), cirrhosis, and abdominal trauma
- *Nonocclusive ischemia*: Cardiac failure, shock, dehydration, vasoconstrictive drugs (e.g., digitalis, vasopressin, propranolol)
- *Miscellaneous*: Radiation injury, volvulus (see later), stricture, and internal or external herniation

Embolic arterial occlusion most often involves the branches of the superior mesenteric artery. The origin of the inferior mesenteric artery from the artery is more oblique, and this may contribute to the relative sparing of this arterial axis from embolism. Despite the multiplicity of possible causes, there remains a significant percentage of cases in which no well-defined basis for the vascular insufficiency can be identified. Mesenteric vascular spasm has been invoked in some cases, without definitive proof.

MORPHOLOGY. The severity of vascular compromise and the time frame during which it develops are major determinants of the morphology of ischemic bowel disease. The most severe, acute lesions are considered first.

Transmural Infarction. Small intestinal infarction af-

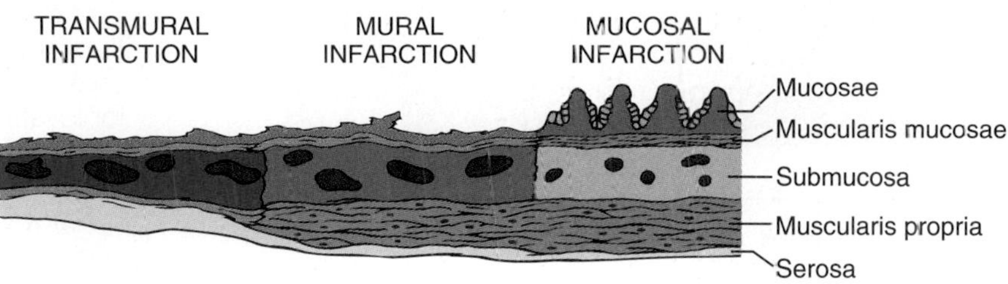

Figure 18–40 ■

Acute ischemic bowel disease. Schematic of the three levels of severity diagrammed for the small intestine (mucosal infarction, mural infarction, and transmural infarction).

ter sudden and total occlusion of mesenteric arterial blood flow may involve only a short segment but more often involves a substantial portion. Although the watershed between the distribution of the superior and inferior mesenteric arteries puts the splenic flexure of the colon at risk for ischemia, any portion of the colon may be affected. With mesenteric venous occlusion, anterograde and retrograde propagation of thrombus may lead to extensive involvement of the splanchnic bed. **Regardless of whether the arterial or venous side is occluded, the infarction appears hemorrhagic because of blood reflow into the damaged area.** In the early stages, the infarcted bowel appears intensely congested and dusky to purple-red (Fig. 18–41), with small and large foci of subserosal and submucosal ecchymotic discoloration. With time, the wall becomes edematous, thickened, rubbery, and hemorrhagic. The lumen commonly contains sanguineous mucus or frank blood. In arterial occlusions, the demarcation from normal bowel is usually sharply defined, but in venous occlusions the area of dusky cyanosis fades gradually into the adjacent normal bowel, having no clear-cut definition between viable and nonviable bowel. Histologically, there is obvious edema, interstitial hemorrhage, and sloughing necrosis of the mucosa. Normal features of the mural musculature, particularly cellular nuclei, become indistinct. **Within 1 to 4 days, intestinal bacteria produce outright gangrene and sometimes perforation of the bowel.** There may be little inflammatory response.

Mucosal and Mural Infarction. Mucosal and mural infarction may involve any level of the gut from the stomach to anus. The lesions may be multifocal or continuous and widely distributed. Affected areas of the bowel may appear dark red or purple owing to the accumulated luminal hemorrhage. **Hemorrhage and an inflammatory exudate are absent from the serosal surface.** On opening the bowel, there is hemorrhagic, edematous thickening of the mucosa, which may penetrate more deeply into the submucosa and muscle wall. Superficial ulceration may be present.

In the mildest form of ischemic injury, the superficial epithelium of the colon, or the tips of small intestinal villi, may be necrotic or sloughed. Inflammation is absent, and there may be only mild vascular dilation. With complete mucosal necrosis, epithelial sloughing leaves behind only the acellular scaffolding of the lamina propria (Fig. 18–42). When severe, there is extensive hemorrhage and necrosis of multiple tissue layers. Secondary acute and chronic inflammation is evident along the viable margins underlying and adjacent to the affected area. Bacterial superinfection and the formation of enterotoxic bacterial products (see earlier) may induce superimposed pseudomembrane inflammation, particularly in the colon. Thus, the mucosal changes may mimic enterocolitis of nonvascular origin.

Chronic Ischemia. With chronic vascular insufficiency to a region of intestine, mucosal inflammation and ulceration may develop, mimicking both acute enterocolitis from other causes and idiopathic inflammatory bowel disease (see earlier). **Submucosal chronic inflammation and fibrosis may lead to stricture** (Fig. 18–43). Although colonic strictures typically occur in the watershed area of the splenic flexure, **both acute and chronic mucosal ischemia are notoriously segmental and patchy, both on a microscopic and a macroscopic scale.**

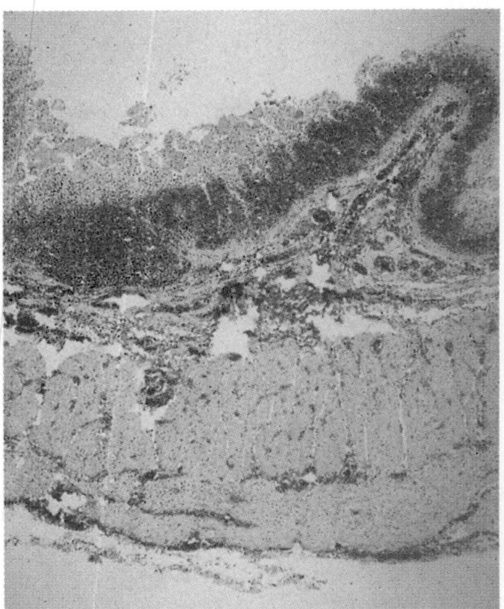

Figure 18–42

Mucosal infarction of the small bowel. The mucosa is hemorrhagic and there is no epithelial layer. The remaining layers of the bowel are intact.

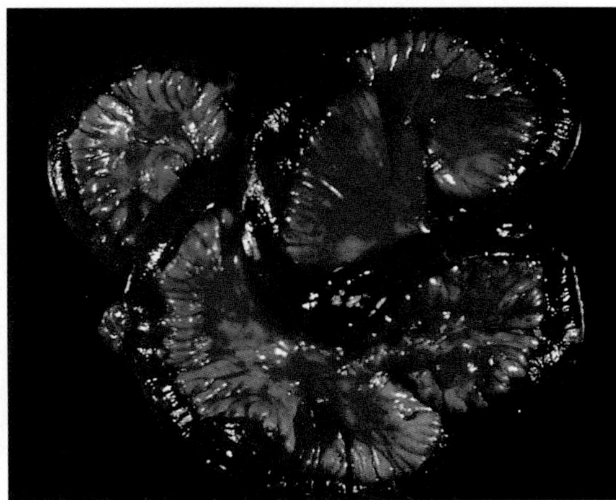

Figure 18–41

Infarcted small bowel secondary to acute thrombotic occlusion of the superior mesenteric artery.

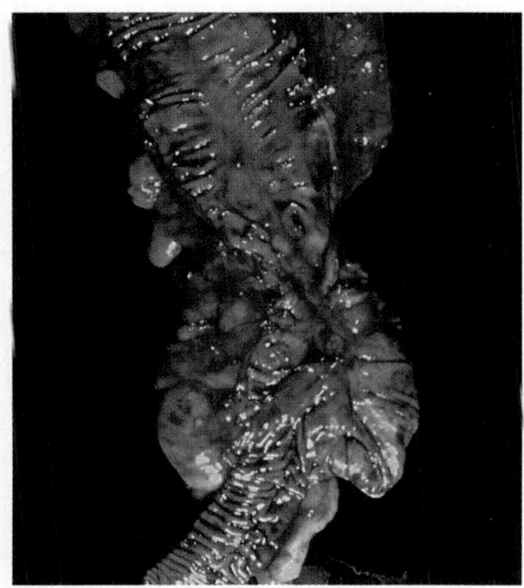

Figure 18-43

Chronic ischemia of the colon, resulting in chronic mucosal damage and a stricture of the ascending colon. The terminal ileum is in the lower portion of the photograph.

Clinical Features. Bowel infarction is an uncommon but grave disorder that imposes a 50 to 75% death rate, largely because the window of time between onset of symptoms and perforation is small. It tends to occur in older individuals, when cardiac and vascular diseases are most prevalent. Severe abdominal pain and tenderness develop suddenly in the setting of transmural infarction, sometimes accompanied by nausea, vomiting, and bloody diarrhea or grossly melanotic stool. Patients may progress to shock and vascular collapse within hours. Peristaltic sounds diminish or disappear, and spasm creates boardlike rigidity of the abdominal wall musculature.

Mucosal and mural infarction, by themselves, may not be fatal, particularly if the cause of vascular compromise is corrected. A confusing array of nonspecific abdominal complaints, combined with intermittent bloody diarrhea, may be the only indication of nonocclusive enteric ischemia. Nevertheless, bowel embarrassment may progress to more extensive infarction, and sepsis or serious blood loss may set in. Chronic ischemic colitis may present as an insidious inflammatory disease, with intermittent episodes of bloody diarrhea interspersed with periods of healing, mimicking inflammatory bowel disease (see earlier).

ANGIODYSPLASIA

Tortuous dilations of submucosal and mucosal blood vessels are seen most often in the cecum or right colon, usually only after the fifties.[63] Although the prevalence of these lesions is less than 1% in the adult population, *they account for 20% of significant lower intestinal bleeding; intestinal hemorrhage may be chronic and intermittent or acute and massive.* Most angiodysplasias span the mucosa and submucosa and contain a small amount of smooth muscle, suggesting that they are ectatic nests of preexisting veins, venules, and capillaries. The vascular channels may be separated from the intestinal lumen by only the vascular wall and a layer of attenuated epithelial cells, explaining the propensity toward bleeding.

The pathogenesis of angiodysplasia remains speculative but is attributed to mechanical factors operative in the colonic wall. Normal distention and contraction may intermittently occlude the submucosal veins that penetrate through the muscle wall. This occlusion then leads to focal dilation and tortuosity of overlying submucosal and mucosal vessels. According to LaPlace's law, tension in the wall of a cylinder is a function of intraluminal pressure and diameter. Because the cecum has the widest diameter of the colon, it develops the greatest wall tension, perhaps explaining the distribution of these lesions. Vascular degenerative changes related to aging may also play some role.

HEMORRHOIDS

Hemorrhoids are variceal dilations of the anal and perianal venous plexuses. These extremely common lesions affect about 5% of the general population and develop secondary to persistently elevated venous pressure within the hemorrhoidal plexus. The most frequent predisposing influences are constipation with straining at stool and the venous stasis of pregnancy. Except for pregnant women, they are rarely encountered in persons under the age of 30. More rarely but much more importantly, hemorrhoids may reflect collateral anastomotic channels that develop as a result of portal hypertension (Chapter 19).

MORPHOLOGY. The varicosities may develop in the inferior hemorrhoidal plexus and thus are located below the anorectal line (**external hemorrhoids**). Alternatively, they may develop from dilation of the superior hemorrhoidal plexus and produce **internal hemorrhoids**. Commonly, both plexuses are affected, and the varicosities are referred to as combined hemorrhoids. Histologically, these lesions consist only of thin-walled, dilated, submucosal varices that protrude beneath the anal or rectal mucosa. In their exposed, traumatized position, they tend to become thrombosed and, in the course of time, recanalized. Superficial ulceration, fissure formation, and infarction with strangulation may develop.

Diverticular Disease

A diverticulum is a blind pouch leading off the alimentary tract, lined by mucosa that communicates with the lumen of the gut. Congenital diverticula have all three layers of the bowel wall; the prototype is *Meckel diverticulum*, discussed earlier. Virtually all other diverticula are *acquired* and either lack or have an attenuated muscularis propria. Acquired diverticula may occur in the esophagus, stomach, and duodenum; duodenal diverticula occur in more than 1% of adults, possibly reflecting defects from healed peptic ulcer disease. Multiple diverticula of the jejunum and ileum are rare, occurring in the setting of abnormalities in the muscle wall or myenteric plexus.

Unless otherwise specified, however, diverticular disease refers to acquired outpouchings of the colonic mucosa and submucosa. *Colonic diverticula are rare in persons under age 30, but in Western adult populations over the age of 60 the prevalence approaches 50%. They generally occur multiply and are referred to as diverticulosis.* They are much less frequent in nonindustrialized tropical countries and in Japan.

MORPHOLOGY. Most colonic diverticula are **small flasklike or spherical outpouchings, usually 0.5 to 1 cm in diameter** and located in the sigmoid colon (Fig. 18–44*A*). The descending colon or entire colon, however, may be affected. They tend to occur alongside the taeniae coli and are elastic, compressible, and easily emptied of fecal contents. As these sacs dissect into the appendices epiploicae, they may be missed on casual inspection. Histologically, colonic diverticula have a thin wall composed of a flattened or atrophic mucosa, compressed submucosa, and attenuated or totally absent muscularis propria (Fig. 18–44*B*). Hypertrophy of the circular layer of the muscularis propria in the affected bowel segment is usually seen; the taeniae coli are also unusually prominent.

Obstruction or perforation of diverticula leads to inflammatory changes, producing peridiverticulitis and dissecting into the immediately adjacent pericolic fat. In time, the inflammation may lead to marked fibrotic thickening in and about the colonic wall, sometimes producing narrowing sufficient to resemble a colonic cancer. Extension of diverticular infection may lead to pericolic abscesses, sinus tracts, and sometimes pelvic or generalized peritonitis.

Pathogenesis. The morphology of colonic diverticula strongly suggests that *two factors are important in their genesis*: (1) *focal weakness in the colonic wall* and (2) *increased intraluminal pressure*.[64] The colon is unique in that the longitudinal muscle coat is not complete but is gathered into three equidistant bands (the taeniae coli). Where nerves and arterial vasa recta penetrate the inner circular muscle coat alongside the taeniae, focal defects in the muscle wall are created. The connective tissue sheaths accompanying these perforating vessels provide points of weakness for herniations. *Exaggerated peristaltic contractions, with spasmodic sequestration of bowel segments, are the putative cause of increased intraluminal pressure.* It has been proposed that diets low in fiber reduce stool bulk, which, in turn, leads to increased peristaltic activity, particularly in the sigmoid colon. Exaggerated contractions sequester segments of bowel (segmentation); this deranged motility can lead to symptoms in the absence of inflammation.

Clinical Features. Most individuals with diverticular disease remain asymptomatic throughout their lives—the lesions are most often discovered incidentally. Only about 20% of those affected ever develop manifestations: intermittent cramping or continuous lower abdominal discomfort, constipation, distention, and a sensation of never being able to empty the rectum completely. Patients sometimes experience alternating constipation and diarrhea. Occasionally, there may be minimal chronic or intermittent blood loss or, rarely, massive hemorrhages.

Longitudinal studies have shown that diverticula can regress early in their development or may become more numerous and prominent with time. Whether a high-fiber

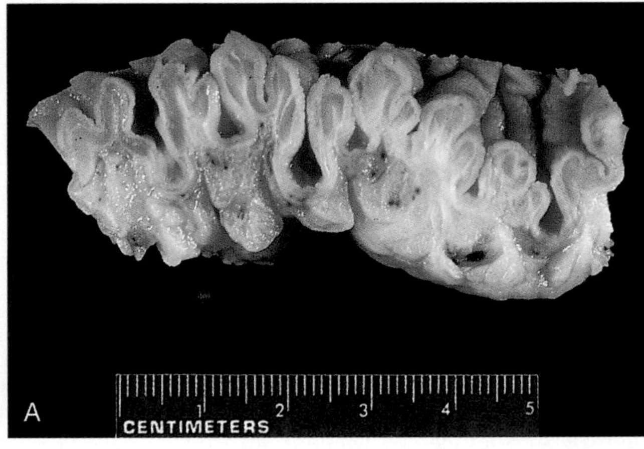

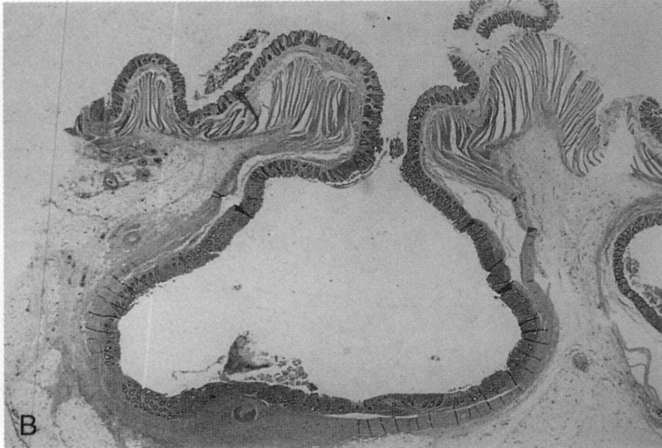

Figure 18–44

Diverticulosis. *A*, Section through the sigmoid colon showing multiple saclike diverticula protruding through the muscle wall into the mesentery. The muscularis propria in between the diverticular protrusions is markedly thickened. *B*, Low-power photomicrograph of diverticulum of the colon showing protrusion of mucosa and submucosa through the muscle wall. A dilated blood vessel at the base of the diverticulum was a source of bleeding; some blood clot is present within the diverticular lumen.

Table 18–10. MAJOR CAUSES OF INTESTINAL OBSTRUCTION

Mechanical Obstruction
Adhesions
Hernias, internal or external
Volvulus
Intussusception
Tumors
Inflammatory strictures
Obstructive gallstones, fecaliths, foreign bodies
Congenital strictures; atresias
Congenital bands
Meconium in mucoviscoidosis
Imperforate anus

Pseudo-obstruction
Paralytic ileus (e.g., postoperative)
Vascular—bowel infarction
Myopathies and neuropathies (e.g., Hirschsprung)

diet prevents such progression or protects against superimposed diverticulitis is still unclear. Relatively few patients require surgical intervention for obstructive or inflammatory complications.

Intestinal Obstruction

Obstruction of the gastrointestinal tract may occur at any level, but the small intestine is most often involved because of its narrow lumen. The causes of small and large intestinal obstruction are presented in Table 18–10. Tumors and infarction, although the most serious, account for only about 10 to 15% of small bowel obstructions. Four of the entities—hernias, intestinal adhesions, intussusception, and volvulus—collectively account for 80% (Fig. 18–45). The syndrome of intestinal obstruction features abdominal pain and distention, vomiting, obstipation, and failure to pass flatus. If the obstruction is mechanical or vascular in origin, immediate surgical intervention is usually required.

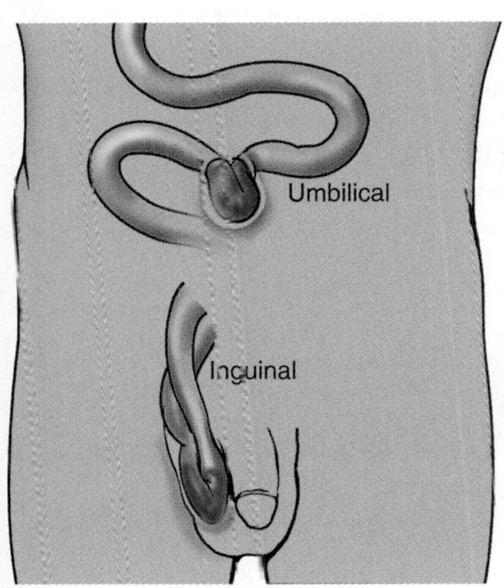

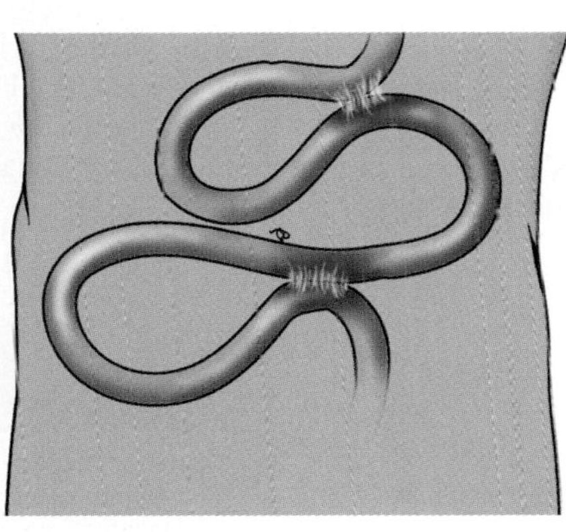

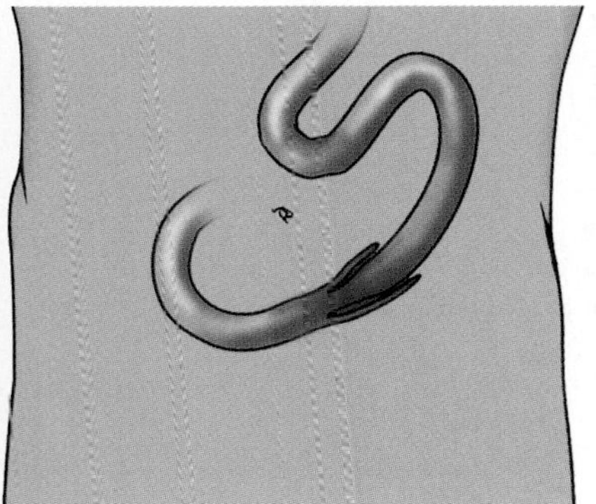

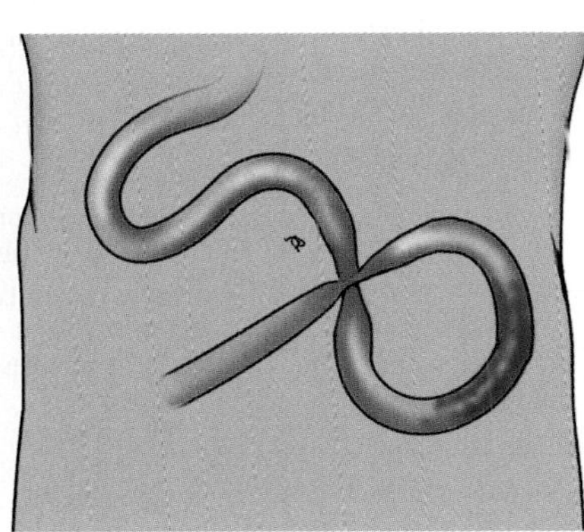

Figure 18–45

Schematic depicting the four major causes of intestinal obstruction: (1) herniation of a segment in the umbilical or inguinal regions; (2) adhesion between loops of intestine; (3) intussusception (see text); and (4) volvulus formation.

HERNIAS

A weakness or defect in the wall of the peritoneal cavity may permit protrusion of a pouchlike, serosa-lined sac of peritoneum, called a *hernial sac*. The usual sites of such weakness are anteriorly at the inguinal and femoral canals, at the umbilicus, and in surgical scars. Rarely, retroperitoneal hernias may occur, chiefly about the ligament of Trietz. *Hernias are of concern chiefly because segments of viscera frequently protrude and become trapped in them (external herniation).* This is particularly true with inguinal hernias because they tend to have narrow orifices and large sacs. The most frequent intruders are small bowel loops, but portions of omentum or large bowel also may become trapped. Pressure at the neck of the pouch may impair venous drainage of the trapped viscus. The resultant stasis and edema increase the bulk of the herniated loop, leading to permanent trapping, or *incarceration*. With time, compromise of arterial supply and venous drainage (*strangulation*) leads to infarction of the trapped segment.

ADHESIONS

Surgical procedures, infection, and even endometriosis often cause localized or more general peritoneal inflammation (*peritonitis*). As the peritonitis heals, adhesions may develop between bowel segments or the abdominal wall and operative site. These fibrous bridges can create closed loops through which other viscera may slide and eventually become trapped (*internal herniation*). The sequence of events after herniation—obstruction and strangulation—is much the same as with external hernias. Quite rarely, fibrous adhesions arise as congenital defects. Intestinal herniation must be considered then, even without a previous history of peritonitis or surgery.

INTUSSUSCEPTION

Intussusception occurs when one segment of the small intestine, constricted by a wave of peristalsis, suddenly becomes telescoped into the immediately distal segment of bowel. Once trapped, the invaginated segment is propelled by peristalsis farther into the distal segment, pulling its mesentery along behind it. When encountered in infants and children, there is usually no underlying anatomic lesion or defect in the bowel, and the patient is otherwise healthy. Intussusception in adults, however, signifies an intraluminal mass or tumor as the point of traction. In both settings, intestinal obstruction ensues, and trapping of mesenteric vessels leads to infarction.

VOLVULUS

Complete twisting of a loop of bowel about its mesenteric base of attachment also produces intestinal obstruction and infarction. This lesion occurs most often in large redundant loops of sigmoid, followed in frequency by the cecum, small bowel (all or portions), stomach, or (rarely) transverse colon. Recognition of this seldom encountered lesion demands constant awareness of its possible occurrence.

Tumors of the Small and Large Intestines

Epithelial tumors of the intestines are a major cause of morbidity and mortality worldwide. The colon (including the rectum) is host to more primary neoplasms than any other organ in the body. Colorectal cancer ranks second only to bronchogenic carcinoma among the cancer killers. Adenocarcinomas constitute the vast majority of colorectal cancers and represent 70% of all malignancies arising in the gastrointestinal tract. The small intestine is an uncommon site for benign or malignant tumors despite its great length and vast pool of dividing mucosal cells. The classification of intestinal tumors is the same for the small intestine and colon and is summarized in Table 18–11. Although small intestinal tumors are addressed first, the bulk of the discussion is devoted to colorectal neoplasia.

TUMORS OF THE SMALL INTESTINE

Although the small bowel represents 75% of the length of the alimentary tract, its tumors account for only 3 to 6% of gastrointestinal tumors, with a slight preponderance of benign tumors. The most frequent benign tumors in the small intestine are adenomas and smooth muscle tumors (see later discussion on gastrointestinal stromal tumors). Lipomas, angiomas, and rare hamartomatous mucosal lesions constitute the remainder. One of the enigmas of medicine is the rarity of malignant tumors of the small intestine—annual US death rate is under 1000, representing only about 1% of gastrointestinal malignancies. Small intestinal adenocarcinomas and carcinoids have roughly equal

Table 18–11. TUMORS OF THE SMALL INTESTINE AND COLON

Non-neoplastic (Benign) Polyps
- Hyperplastic polyps
- Hamartomatous polyps
  - Juvenile polyps
  - Peutz-Jeghers polyps
- Inflammatory polyps
- Lymphoid polyps

Neoplastic Epithelial Lesions
- Benign
  - Adenoma*
- Malignant
  - Adenocarcinoma*
  - Carcinoid tumor
  - Anal zone carcinoma

Mesenchymal Lesions
- Gastrointestinal stromal tumors (gradation from benign to malignant)
- Other benign lesions
  - Lipoma
  - Neuroma
  - Angioma
- Kaposi sarcoma

Lymphoma

*Benign and malignant counterparts of the most common neoplasms in the intestines; virtually all lesions are in the colon.

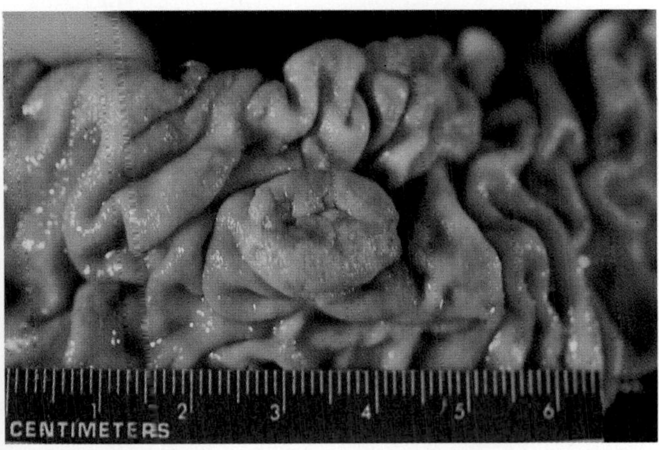

Figure 18–46 ■

Adenoma of the ampulla of Vater showing exophytic tumor at the ampullary orifice.

incidence, followed in order by lymphomas and sarcomas. Because the latter three exhibit a broader distribution than the small intestine, they are discussed later.

Adenomas

Adenomas account for approximately 25% of benign small intestinal tumors, with benign stromal tumors (leiomyomas), lipomas, and neuromatous lesions following in frequency. *Most adenomas occur in the region of the ampulla of Vater.* Patients usually present between the ages of 30 and 60 with occult blood loss and rarely with obstruction or intussusception; some are discovered incidentally during radiographic investigation. Patients with familial polyposis coli (discussed later) are particularly prone to developing periampullary adenomas. Macroscopically the ampulla of Vater is enlarged and exhibits a velvety surface (Fig. 18–46). Microscopically, these adenomas resemble their counterparts in the colon (discussed later). Frequently, there is extension of adenomatous tissue into the ampullary orifice, rendering surgical excision difficult, short of a pancreatoduodenectomy to remove the entire ampullary region.

Adenocarcinoma

The large majority of small intestinal adenocarcinomas occur in the duodenum and jejunum, with a presenting age usually between 40 and 70 years of age. These tumors grow in a napkin ring encircling pattern or as polypoid fungating masses, in a manner similar to colonic cancers. Tumors in the duodenum, particularly involving the ampulla of Vater, may present with obstructive jaundice early in their course. More typically, cramping pain, nausea, vomiting, and weight loss are the presenting signs and symptoms, resulting from intestinal obstruction. As with adenomas, fatigue from occult blood loss may be the only sign. Rarely the tumorous mass is a lead point for intussusception.

At the time of diagnosis, most tumors have already penetrated the bowel wall, invaded the mesentery or other segments of the gut, spread to regional nodes, and sometimes metastasized to the liver and more widely by the time of diagnosis. Despite these problems, wide *en bloc* excision of these cancers yields about a 70% 5-year survival rate.

TUMORS OF THE COLON AND RECTUM

Polyps of the colorectal mucosa are extraordinarily common in the older adult population. Before embarking on our discussion, several concepts pertaining to terminology must be emphasized (Fig. 18–47):

- A *polyp* is a tumorous mass that protrudes into the lumen of the gut. Presumably, all polyps start as small, *sessile* lesions without a definable stalk. In many instances, traction on the mass may create a stalked, or *pedunculated*, polyp.
- Polyps may be formed as the result of abnormal mucosal maturation, inflammation, or architecture. These polyps are *non-neoplastic* and do not have malignant potential per se. An example is the *hyperplastic polyp*.
- Epithelial polyps that arise as the result of proliferation and *dysplasia* are termed *adenomatous polyps*, or *adenomas. They are true neoplastic lesions (new growth) and are precursors of carcinoma.*
- Some polypoid lesions may be caused by submucosal or mural tumors. As with the stomach and small intestine, however, unless otherwise specified the term *polyp* refers to lesions arising from the epithelium of the mucosa.

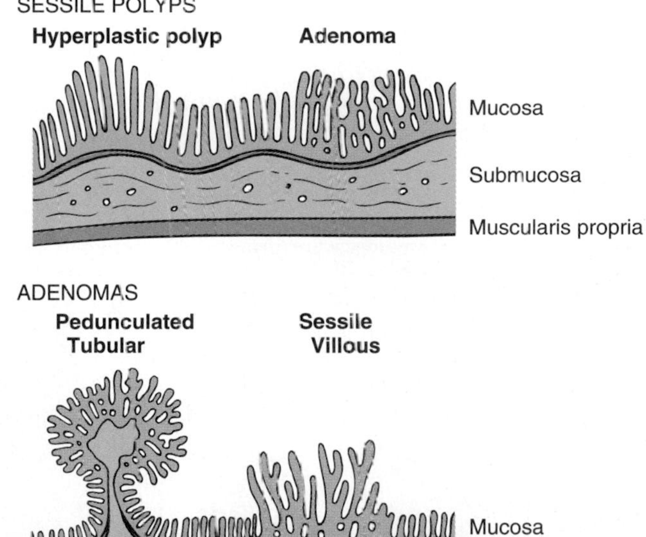

Figure 18–47 ■

Diagrammatic representation of two forms of sessile polyp (hyperplastic polyp and adenoma) and of two types of adenoma (pedunculated and sessile). There is only a loose association between the tubular architecture for pedunculated adenomas and the villous architecture for sessile adenomas.

Non-neoplastic Polyps

The overwhelming majority of intestinal polyps occur on a sporadic basis, particularly in the colon, and increase in frequency with age. Non-neoplastic polyps (mostly hyperplastic) represent about 90% of all epithelial polyps in the large intestine and are found in more than half of all persons age 60 years or older. Inflammatory (pseudo-) polyps, representing islands of inflamed regenerating mucosa surrounded by ulceration, are seen in patients with longstanding inflammatory bowel disease (i.e., ulcerative colitis or Crohn disease). Lymphoid polyps are an essentially normal variant of the mucosal bumps containing intramucosal lymphoid tissue. Three forms of non-neoplastic polyps deserve separate mention.

MORPHOLOGY. ***Hyperplastic Polyps.*** These are small (usually <5 mm in diameter) epithelial polyps, which may arise at any age but are usually discovered in patients in their fifties or sixties. They appear as nipple-like, hemispheric, smooth, moist protrusions of the mucosa. They often are multiple, and more than half are found in the rectosigmoid. Histologically, they are composed of well-formed glands and crypts lined by non-neoplastic epithelial cells, most of which show differentiation into mature goblet or absorptive cells. Delayed shedding of surface epithelial cells leads to infoldings of the crowded epithelial cells and fission of the crypts, creating a serrated epithelial profile and an irregular crypt architecture (Fig. 18–48*A*). Although large hyperplastic polyps may rarely coexist with foci of adenomatous change, **the usual small, hyperplastic polyp has virtually no malignant potential.**

Juvenile Polyps. These lesions represent focal hamartomatous malformations of the mucosal elements most frequently in the rectum. For the most part, they are sporadic lesions, with the vast majority occurring in children younger than age 5. Isolated hamartomatous polyps may be identified in the colon of adults; these incidental lesions are referred to as **retention polyps**. Juvenile polyps tend to be large (1 to 3 cm in diameter), rounded, smooth or slightly lobulated lesions with stalks up to 2 cm in length; retention polyps tend to be smaller (<1 cm in diameter). Histologically, lamina propria constitutes the bulk of the polyp, enclosing abundant cystically dilated glands. Inflammation is common, and the surface may be congested or eroded. In general, they occur singly and being hamartomatous lesions have no malignant potential. A rare autosomal dominant **juvenile polyposis syndrome** does carry a risk of adenomas and hence adenocarcinoma.

Peutz-Jeghers Polyps. These hamartomatous lesions may also occur singly or multiply in the **Peutz-Jeghers syndrome**. This rare autosomal dominant syndrome is characterized by multiple hamartomatous polyps scattered throughout the entire gastrointestinal tract and melanotic mucosal and cutaneous pigmentation around the lips, oral mucosa, face, genitalia, and palmar surfaces of the hands. Peutz-Jeghers polyps tend to be large and pedunculated with a firm lobulated contour. Histologically an arborizing network of connective tissue and well-developed smooth muscle extends into the polyp and surrounds normal abundant glands lined by normal intestinal epithelium rich in goblet cells (Fig. 18–48*B*). **While these hamartomatous polyps themselves do not have malignant potential, patients with the syndrome have an increased risk of developing carcinomas of the pancreas, breast, lung, ovary, and uterus.** When gastrointestinal adenocarcinoma occurs, it arises from concomitant adenomatous lesions.

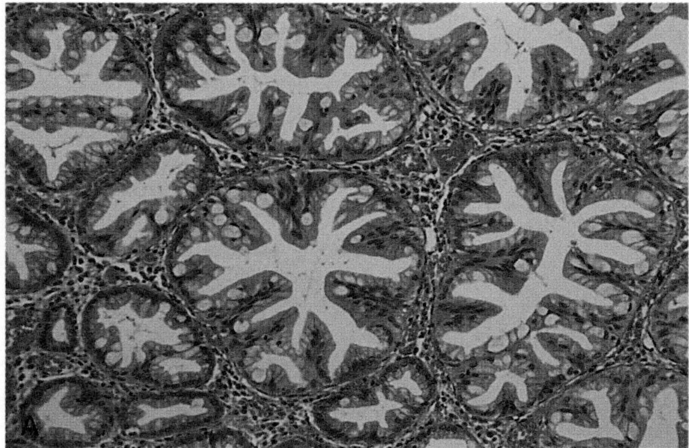

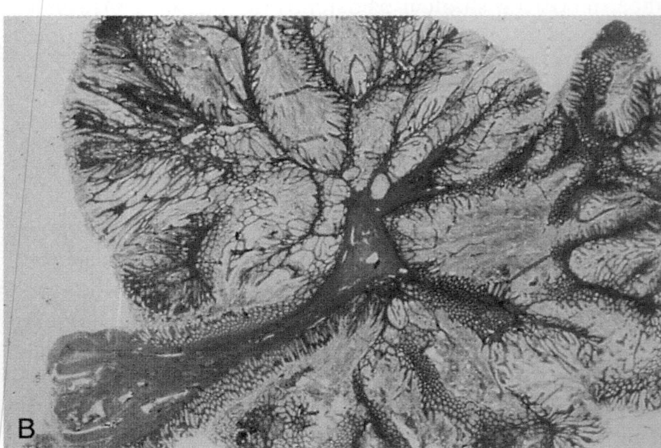

Figure 18–48

Non-neoplastic colonic polyps. *A*, Hyperplastic polyp, high-power view showing the serrated profile of the epithelial layer. *B*, Peutz-Jeghers polyp, low-power view showing the splaying of smooth muscle into the superficial portion of the pedunculated polyp.

Adenomas

Adenomatous polyps are neoplasms that range from small, often pedunculated lesions to large neoplasms that are usually sessile. The prevalence of colonic adenomas is about 20 to 30% before age 40, rising to 40 to 50% after age 60. Men and women are affected equally. There is a well-defined familial predisposition to sporadic adenomas, accounting for about a fourfold greater risk among first-degree relatives and also a fourfold greater risk of colorectal carcinoma.

Adenomatous polyps are segregated into three subtypes on the basis of the epithelial architecture:

- *Tubular adenomas*: Tubular glands
- *Villous adenomas*: Villous projections
- *Tubulovillous adenoma*: A mixture of the previous two

There is considerable overlap among these categories, so by convention, tubular adenomas exhibit greater than 75% tubular architecture, villous adenomas contain greater than 50% villous architecture, and tubulovillous adenomas contain 25 to 50% villous architecture. Tubular adenomas are by far the most common; about 5 to 10% of adenomas are tubulovillous, and only 1% are villous.

All adenomatous lesions arise as the result of epithelial proliferative dysplasia, which may range from mild to so severe as to constitute carcinoma in situ. Furthermore, there is strong evidence that adenomas are a precursor lesion for invasive colorectal adenocarcinomas (discussed subsequently). The period required for an adenoma to double in size is estimated at about 10 years. Thus, they are slow growing and must certainly have been present for many years before detection. The following concepts are pertinent:

- Most tubular adenomas are small and pedunculated; conversely, most pedunculated polyps are tubular.
- Villous adenomas tend to be large and sessile, and sessile polyps usually exhibit villous features.

The malignant risk with an adenomatous polyp is correlated with three interdependent features: polyp size, histologic architecture, and severity of epithelial dysplasia, as follows:[65]

- Cancer is rare in tubular adenomas smaller than 1 cm in diameter.
- The risk of cancer is high (approaching 40%) in sessile villous adenomas greater than 4 cm in diameter.
- Severe dysplasia, when present, is often found in villous areas.

Thus, the most worrisome lesions are villous adenomas greater than 4 cm in diameter. *Since all degrees of dysplasia (mild, moderate, and severe) and even invasive adenocarcinoma may be encountered in an adenoma of any subtype, however, it is impossible from gross inspection of a polyp to determine its clinical significance.*

MORPHOLOGY. *Tubular Adenomas.* Most (90%) are found in the colon, but they can occur in the stomach and small intestine. In about half of the instances, they occur singly; in the remainder, two or more lesions are distributed at random. The smallest tubular adenomas are smooth contoured and sessile; larger ones tend to be coarsely lobulated and have slender stalks (Fig. 18–49*A*). Un-

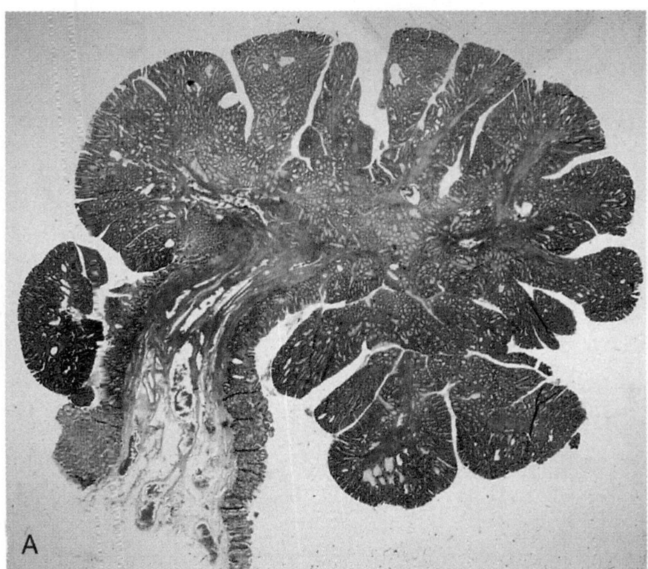

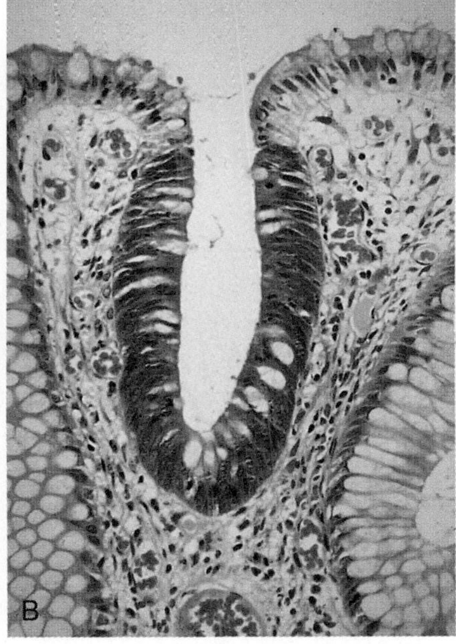

Figure 18–49

A, Pedunculated adenoma showing a fibrovascular stalk lined by normal colonic mucosa, and a head that contains abundant dysplastic epithelial glands. *B*, A small focus of adenomatous epithelium in an otherwise normal (mucin-secreting, clear) colonic mucosa, showing how the dysplastic columnar epithelium (deeply stained) can populate a colonic crypt and create a "tubular" architecture.

commonly, they exceed 2.5 cm in diameter. Histologically the stalk is composed of fibromuscular tissue and prominent blood vessels (derived from the submucosa), and it is usually covered by normal, non-neoplastic mucosa. Adenomatous epithelium, however, may extend down the stalk and into adjacent regions of the mucosa, particularly in the stomach. Whether small or large, adenomatous lesions are composed of neoplastic (dysplastic) epithelium, which lines glands as a tall, hyperchromatic, somewhat disordered epithelium, which may or may not show mucin vacuoles (Fig. 18–49*B*). In the clearly benign tubular adenoma, the branching glands are well separated by lamina propria, and the level of dysplasia is mild. All degrees of dysplasia may be encountered. **Severe dysplasia (carcinoma in situ) may merge with areas of overt malignant change confined to the mucosa (intramucosal carcinoma). Carcinomatous invasion into the submucosal stalk of the polyp constitutes invasive adenocarcinoma.**

Villous Adenomas. Villous adenomas are the larger and more ominous of the epithelial polyps. They tend to occur in older persons, most commonly in the rectum and rectosigmoid, but they may be located elsewhere. They generally are sessile, up to 10 cm in diameter, velvety or cauliflower-like masses projecting 1 to 3 cm above the surrounding normal mucosa. Their histology is that of frondlike villiform extensions of the mucosa (Fig. 18–50*A*), covered by dysplastic, somewhat disordered columnar epithelium (Fig. 18–50*B*). All degrees of dysplasia may be encountered. **When invasive carcinoma occurs, there is no stalk as a buffer zone, and invasion is directly into the wall of the colon (submucosa or deeper).**

Tubulovillous Adenomas. Tubulovillous adenomas are typically intermediate between the tubular and villous lesions in terms of their frequency of having a stalk or being sessile, their size, and the general level of dysplasia found in such lesions. The risk of harboring in situ or invasive carcinoma generally correlates with the proportion of the lesion that is villous.

Clinical Features. Colorectal tubular (and tubulovillous) adenomas may be asymptomatic, but many are discovered during evaluation of anemia or occult bleeding. Screening programs are intended to detect asymptomatic adenomas before they progress to malignancy.

The clinical impact of malignant change in an adenoma depends on the following:[66, 67]

- *Severe dysplasia (carcinoma in situ)* has not yet acquired the ability to metastasize and is still a benign lesion.
- Because lymphatic channels are largely absent in the colonic mucosa, *intramucosal carcinoma* also is regarded as having little to no metastatic potential.
- By crossing the muscularis mucosae into the submucosal space, *invasive adenocarcinoma* is a malignant lesion with metastatic potential. Nevertheless, *endoscopic removal of a pedunculated adenoma is regarded as an adequate excision, provided that three histologic conditions are met*: (1) The adenocarcinoma is superficial and does not approach the margin of excision across the

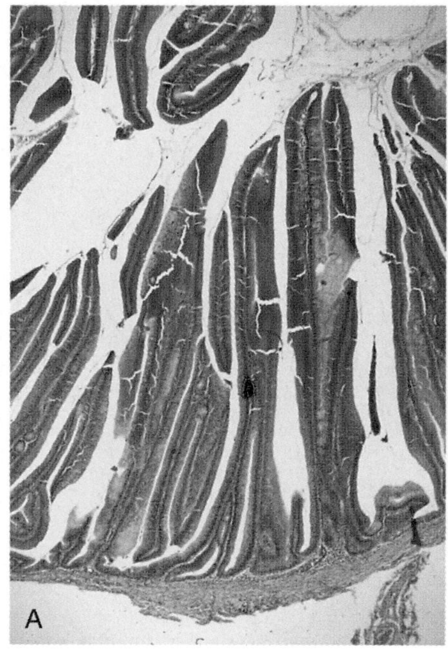

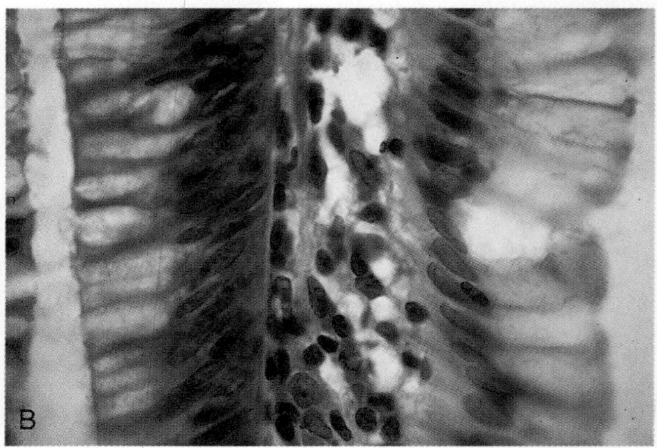

Figure 18–50

A, Sessile adenoma with villous architecture. Each frond is lined by dysplastic epithelium. *B*, Portion of a villous frond with dysplastic columnar epithelium on the left and normal colonic columnar epithelium on the right.

base of the stalk, (2) there is no vascular or lymphatic invasion, and (3) the carcinoma is not poorly differentiated.[67]

- *Invasive adenocarcinoma arising in a sessile polyp cannot be adequately resected by polypectomy*, and further surgery is required.
- Regardless of whether carcinoma is present, *the only adequate treatment for a pedunculated or sessile adenoma is complete resection.* If adenomatous epithelium remains behind in the patient, the patient still has a premalignant lesion or may even be harboring invasive carcinoma in the residual lesion.

Familial Syndromes

Familial polyposis syndromes are uncommon autosomal dominant disorders. Their importance lies in the propensity for malignant transformation and in the insights that such transformation has provided in unraveling the molecular basis of colorectal cancer. Peutz-Jeghers syndrome, described earlier, is characterized by hamartomatous polyps and a modestly increased risk of cancer, frequently in extragastrointestinal sites. *Familial adenomatous polyposis (FAP)* exhibits innumerable adenomatous polyps and has a frequency of progression to colon adenocarcinoma approaching 100%.

FAP is the archetype of the adenomatous polyposis syndromes. As discussed later, the genetic defect is in the APC gene on chromosome 5q21. Patients typically develop 500 to 2500 colonic adenomas that carpet the mucosal surface (Fig. 18–51). Occasionally, as few as 150 polyps are present; a minimum of 100 polyps is necessary for a diagnosis of FAP. Multiple adenomas may also be present elsewhere in the alimentary tract, including the region of the ampulla of Vater. Histologically the vast majority of polyps are tubular adenomas; occasional polyps may have villous features. Some patients already have cancer of the colon or rectum at the time of diagnosis. Cancer-preventive measures include a prophylactic colectomy as soon as possible and the early detection of the disease in siblings and first-degree relatives at risk.

Gardner syndrome is a variation of FAP, also autosomal dominant. Patients exhibit intestinal polyps identical to those in familial adenomatous polyposis combined with multiple osteomas (particularly of the mandible, skull, and long bones), epidermal cysts, and fibromatosis. Less frequent are abnormalities of dentition, such as unerupted and supernumerary teeth, and a higher frequency of duodenal and thyroid cancer. Most workers believe that both familial adenomatous polyposis and Gardner syndrome are variants of the same condition, with the wider spectrum of abnormalities seen in Gardner syndrome representing variable penetrance of a common genetic mutation. *Turcot syndrome* is a rare variant marked by the combination of adenomatous colonic polyposis and tumors of the central nervous system, mostly gliomas. The average age of onset of polyps in each of these adenomatous polyp syndromes is the teens to twenties, followed by cancer within 10 to 15 years unless surgical resections interrupt the natural progression.

Hereditary nonpolyposis colorectal cancer (HNPCC) is an autosomal dominant familial syndrome (extensively described by Henry Lynch, hence the alternative name of Lynch syndrome) characterized by an increased risk of colorectal cancer and extraintestinal cancer, particularly of the endometrium in women. Adenomas do occur in low numbers but considerably earlier than in the general adult population. The colonic malignancies often are multiple and are not always associated with preexisting adenomas. As described subsequently, the genetic defect involves DNA mismatch repair genes.

Colorectal Carcinogenesis

Adenoma-Carcinoma Sequence. The development of carcinoma from adenomatous lesions is referred to as the

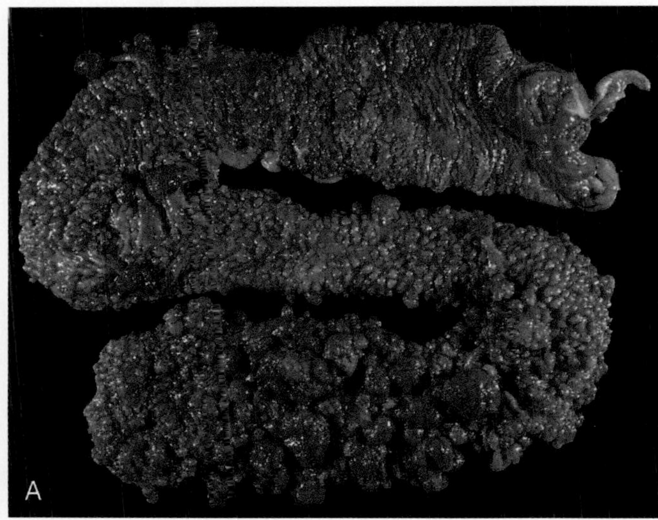

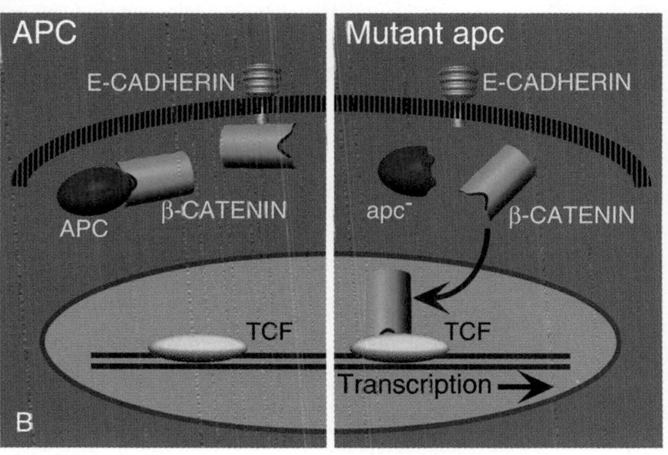

Figure 18–51

A, Familial adenomatous polyposis. The surface is carpeted by innumerable polypoid adenomas. (Courtesy of Dr. Tad Wieczorek, Brigham and Women's Hospital, Boston, MA.) *B*, Possible actions of the APC gene product (see text). (Courtesy of Dr. David Ferguson, Brigham and Women's Hospital, Boston, MA.)

adenoma-carcinoma sequence and is documented by the following observations:

- Populations that have a high prevalence of adenomas have a high prevalence of colorectal cancer, and vice versa.
- The distribution of adenomas within the colorectum is more or less comparable to that of colorectal cancer.
- The peak incidence of adenomatous polyps antedates by some years the peak for colorectal cancer.
- When invasive carcinoma is identified at an early stage, surrounding adenomatous tissue is often present.
- The risk of cancer is directly related to the number of adenomas and hence the virtual certainty of cancer in patients with familial polyposis syndromes.
- Programs that assiduously follow patients for the development of adenomas and remove all that are suspicious reduce the incidence of colorectal cancer.

The occurrence of colorectal carcinoma without evidence of adenomatous precursors suggests that some dysplastic lesions can degenerate into malignancy without passing through a polypoid stage.

Molecular Carcinogenesis. Virtually all colorectal carcinomas exhibit genetic alterations, the study of which has provided deep insights into the general mechanisms of carcinogenesis. Hence, this topic was covered in detail in Chapter 8; concepts specifically pertinent to colorectal carcinogenesis are illustrated in Figure 18–52. Key events involve the following genes.

Adenomatous Polyposis Coli (APC). The inherited defect underlying FAP and Gardner syndromes has been mapped to 5q21, site of the APC tumor-suppressor gene. The encoded protein binds to microtubule bundles and promotes cell migration and adhesion. APC protein also binds to the cytoskeletal protein *β-catenin* in a cellular adhesion molecular complex, which includes the intercellular adhesion molecule *E-cadherin* (Fig. 18–51*B*, *left*). β-Catenin can also act as an oncogene. When it is not bound to E-cadherin (thus participating in cell-cell adhesion), β-catenin binds to a family of protein partners called T cell factor–lymphoid enhancer factor (Tcf-Lef) proteins, which activate other genes. Genes activated by this β-catenin:Tcf complex are thought to include those stimulating cell proliferation and inhibiting apoptosis. APC binding to β-catenin directs β-catenin toward degradation, thereby inhibiting the β-catenin:Tcf signalling pathway. Mutations in the APC gene (Fig. 18–51*B*, *right*) reduce the affinity of APC protein for β-catenin, leading to loss of intercellular contact on the one hand and an increased cytoplasmic pool of β-catenin on the other. The resultant enhancement of Tcf-mediated cell proliferation initiates a sequence of events that predisposes to the development of carcinoma.[70] Hence, APC is regarded as a "gatekeeper" gene (Chapter 8). Mutations in APC underlie FAP, and are early events in the evolution of sporadic colon cancer; mutations can be found in 85% of colorectal carcinomas. *Notably, most of the tumors without mutations in APC show mutations in β-catenin.*

Hereditary Nonpolyposis Colon Carcinoma (HNPCC). Inherited mutations in any of four genes that are involved in DNA repair are putatively responsible for the familial syndrome of HNPCC. These human mismatch repair genes,

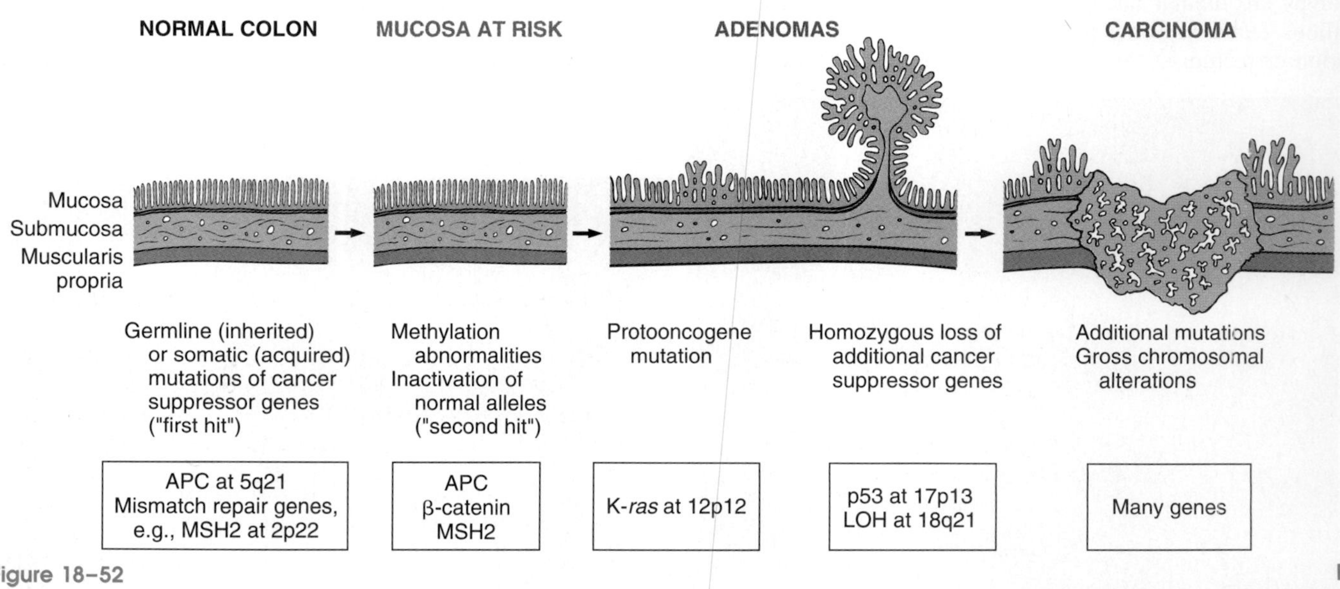

Figure 18–52

Schematic of the morphologic and molecular changes in the adenoma-carcinoma sequence. It is postulated that loss of one normal copy of the cancer suppressor "gatekeeper" gene APC and/or loss of DNA repair "caretaker" genes (e.g., MSH2) occurs early. Indeed, individuals may be born with one mutant allele of one of these genes, rendering them prone to develop colon cancer. The loss of the normal copy of the mismatch-repair gene or APC follows ("second hit"). Mutations of the oncogene K-*ras* seem to occur next. Additional mutations or losses of heterozygosity inactivate the tumor suppressor gene p53 and as yet unidentified loci on chromosome 18q, leading finally to the emergence of carcinoma, in which additional mutations occur. It is important to note that while there seems to be a temporal sequence of changes, as shown, the accumulation of mutations, rather than their occurrence in a specific order, is more important.

hMSH2 (chromosome 2p22), *hMLH1* (chromosome 3p21), *hPMS1* (chromosome 2q31-33), and *hPMS2* (chromosome 7p22), are involved in genetic "proofreading" during DNA replication, and *hence are referred to as "caretaker" genes.*[71] There are 50,000 to 100,000 dinucleotide repeat sequences in the human genome, and mutations in mismatch repair genes can be detected by the presence of widespread alterations in these repeats; this is referred to as *microsatellite instability*. Patients who inherit a mutant DNA repair gene have normal repair activity because of the remaining normal allele. However, cells in some organs (colon, stomach, endometrium) are susceptible to a second, somatic mutation that inactivates the wild-type allele. Mutation rates up to 1000 times normal ensue, such that most of the HNPCC tumors show microsatellite instability. About 10 to 15% sporadic colon cancers also have mutations in similar "caretaker" DNA repair genes, implicating somatic (acquired) mutations in these tumors as well. *Indeed, such mutations represent an alternative route for initiating the sequence leading to the development of colorectal cancer* (Chapter 8).

Methylation Abnormalities. A separate early recognizable change in colonic neoplasms is loss of methyl groups in DNA (hypomethylation).

K-ras. The K-*ras* gene (Chapter 6) is the most frequently observed activated oncogene in adenomas and colon cancers. K-*ras* (chromosome 12p12) plays a role in intracellular signal transduction and is mutated in fewer than 10% of adenomas less than 1 cm in size, in 50% of adenomas larger than 1 cm, and in 50% of carcinomas.

DCC. A common allelic loss in colon cancer is on 18q21, termed DCC (*d*eleted in *c*olon *c*ancer). The encoded protein, a cell adhesion molecule, normally is widely expressed on the colon mucosa. Its expression is reduced or absent in 70 to 75% of colon cancers, usually the result of loss of heterozygosity (LOH) of this region of 18q. Recently, the role of DCC in colorectal carcinogenesis has been questioned, since mutant mice lacking both alleles of DCC show no abnormalities of intestinal biology.[72] Whether a neighboring gene may in fact be the actual tumor suppressor gene on 18q remains to be determined.

p53. Losses at chromosome 17p have been found in 70 to 80% of colon cancers, yet comparable losses are infrequent in adenomas. These chromosomal deletions affect the *p53* gene, suggesting that mutations in *p53* occur late in colon carcinogenesis. The critical role of *p53* in cell cycle regulation was discussed in Chapter 6.

These considerations have led to the formulation of a multistage, *multihit* concept for colon cancer carcinogenesis. APC mutations are usually the earliest and possibly the initiating event in about 80% of sporadic colon cancers, with a less frequent contribution from mutations in mismatch repair genes. During the ensuing progression from adenoma to carcinoma, additional mutations ensue, such as late mutations or loss of heterozygosity (LOH) at p53 on chromosome 17p and the DCC region on chromosome 18q. *Cumulative alterations in the genome thus lead to progressive increases in size, level of dysplasia, and invasive potential of neoplastic lesions.*

Colorectal Carcinoma

Virtually 98% of all cancers in the large intestine are adenocarcinomas. They represent one of the prime challenges to the medical profession because they arise in polyps and produce symptoms relatively early and at a stage generally curable by resection. With an estimated 134,000 new cases per year and about 55,000 deaths, this disease accounts for 10% of all cancer-related deaths in the United States.[8]

Epidemiology, Etiology, and Pathogenesis. The peak incidence for colorectal carcinoma is 60 to 79 years; fewer than 20% of cases occur before the age of 50 years.[8] When colorectal carcinoma is found in a young person, preexisting ulcerative colitis or one of the polyposis syndromes must be suspected. Colorectal carcinoma has a worldwide distribution, with the highest death rates in the United States and Eastern European countries, up to tenfold lower rates in Mexico, South America, and Africa. Environmental factors, particularly dietary practices, are implicated in these striking geographic contrasts.[74, 75] In addition, dietary studies implicate obesity and physical inactivity as risk factors for colon cancer.[76]

The dietary factors receiving the most attention as predisposing to a higher incidence of cancer are[76] (1) excess energy intake relative to requirements, (2) a low content of unabsorbable vegetable fiber, (3) a corresponding high content of refined carbohydrates, (4) intake of red meat, and (5) decreased intake of protective micronutrients. It is theorized that reduced fiber content leads to decreased stool bulk, increased fecal transit time in the bowel, and an altered bacterial flora of the intestine. Potentially toxic oxidative byproducts of carbohydrate degradation by bacteria are therefore present in higher concentrations in the small stools and are held in contact with the colonic mucosa for longer periods of time. Moreover, high cholesterol intake in red meat enhances the synthesis of bile acids by the liver, which, in turn, may be converted into potential carcinogens by intestinal bacteria. Refined diets also contain less of vitamins A, C, and E, which may act as oxygen radical scavengers. Intriguing as these dietary speculations may be, the putative mechanisms remain unproven.

MORPHOLOGY. The distribution of the cancers in the colorectum is as follows: cecum and ascending colon, 38%; transverse colon, 18%; descending colon, 8%; sigmoid, 35%; and multiple sites at presentation, 1%.[77] As is evident, 99% of carcinomas occur singly, but when multiple carcinomas are present, they are often at widely disparate sites in the colon. While most cases occur sporadically, about 1 to 3% of colorectal carcinomas occur in patients with familial syndromes (i.e., familial adenomatous polyposis or HNPCC) or inflammatory bowel disease.

Although all colorectal carcinomas begin as in situ lesions, they evolve into different morphologic patterns. **Tumors in the proximal colon tend to grow as polypoid, exophytic masses** (Fig. 18–53), and obstruction is uncommon. **When carcinomas**

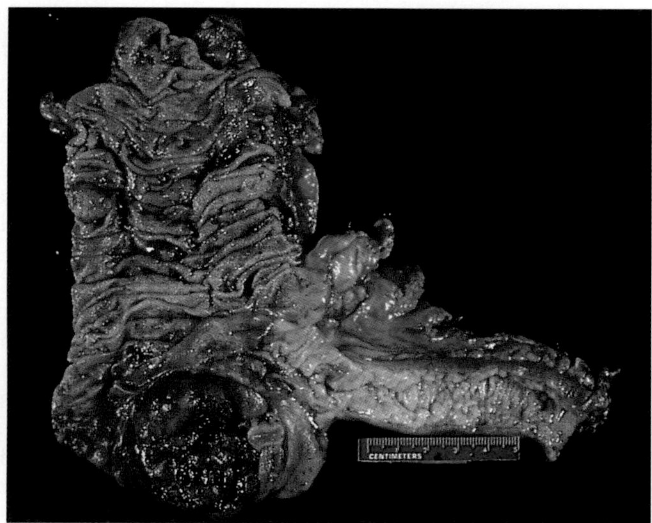

Figure 18–53

Carcinoma of the cecum. The exophytic carcinoma projects into the lumen but has not caused obstruction.

in the distal colon are discovered, they tend to be annular, encircling lesions that produce so-called napkin ring constrictions of the bowel (Fig. 18–54). The margins of the napkin ring are classically heaped up, beaded, and firm, and the mid-region is ulcerated. Both forms of neoplasm directly penetrate the bowel wall over the course of time and may appear as subserosal and serosal white, firm masses, frequently causing puckering of the serosal surface.

In contrast to the gross pathology, **the microscopic characteristics of right-sided and left-sided colonic adenocarcinomas are similar.** Differentiation may range from tall, columnar cells resembling their counterparts in adenomatous lesions (but are now invading the submucosa and muscularis propria) (Fig. 18–55), to undifferentiated, frankly anaplastic masses. Invasive tumor incites a strong desmoplastic stromal response, leading to the characteristic firm, hard consistency of most colonic carcinomas. Many tumors produce mucin, which is secreted into the gland lumens or into the interstitium of the gut wall. Because the mucinous secretion dissects through the gut wall, it aids the extension of the malignancy and worsens the prognosis.

Certain exceptions should be noted. Foci of endocrine differentiation may be found in about 10% of colorectal carcinomas. Alternatively, in some cancers, the cells take on a signet ring appearance. The small cell undifferentiated carcinoma appears to arise from endocrine cells per se and elaborates a variety of bioactive secretory products. Some cancers, particularly in the distal colon, have foci of squamous cell differentiation and are therefore referred to as **adenosquamous carcinomas**. In contrast, carcinomas arising in the anorectal canal constitute a distinct subgroup of tumors, dominated by squamous cell carcinoma.

Clinical Features. Colorectal cancers remain asymptomatic for years; symptoms develop insidiously and frequently have been present for months, sometimes years, before diagnosis. Cecal and right colonic cancers are most often called to clinical attention by the appearance of fatigue, weakness, and iron deficiency anemia. These bulky lesions bleed readily and may be discovered at an early stage, provided that the colon is examined thoroughly radiographically and during colonoscopy. Left-sided lesions come to attention by producing occult bleeding, changes in bowel habit, or crampy left-lower-quadrant discomfort. In theory, the chance for early discovery and successful removal should be greater with lesions on the left side because these patients usually have prominant disturbances in bowel function, such as melena, diarrhea, and constipation. Cancers of the rectum and sigmoid, however, tend to be more infiltrative at the time of diagnosis than proximal lesions and therefore have a somewhat poorer prognosis. *It is a clinical maxim that iron deficiency anemia in an older man means gastrointestinal cancer until proven otherwise.*

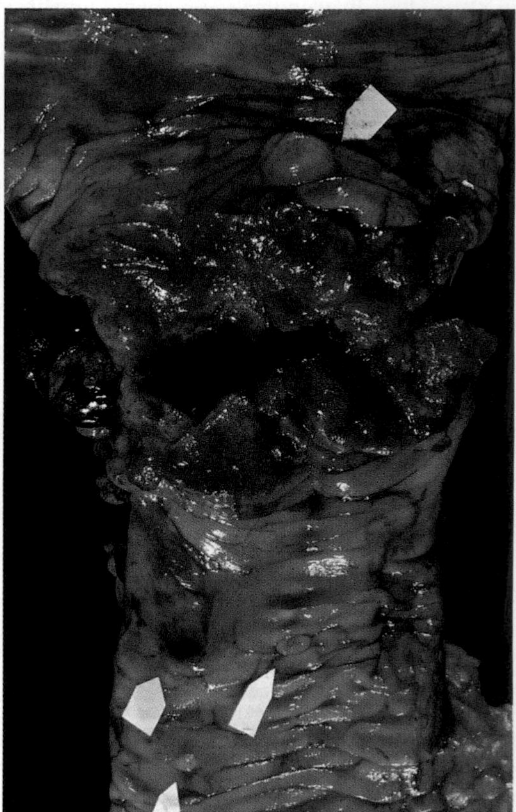

Figure 18–54

Carcinoma of the descending colon. This circumferential tumor has heaped-up edges and an ulcerated central portion. The arrows identify separate mucosal polyps.

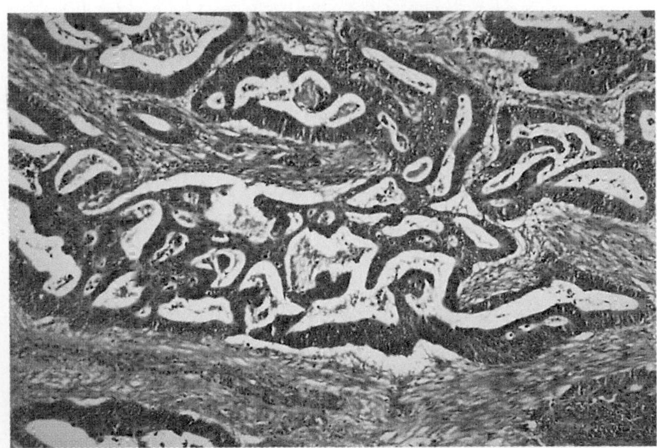

Figure 18–55

Invasive adenocarcinoma of the colon showing malignant glands infiltrating the muscle wall.

In women, the situation is less clear, since menstrual losses, multiple pregnancies, or abnormal uterine bleeding may underlie such an anemia. Systemic manifestations such as weakness, malaise, and weight loss are ominous, in that they usually signify more extensive disease.

All colorectal tumors spread by direct extension into adjacent structures and by metastasis through the lymphatics and blood vessels. In order of preference, the favored sites of metastatic spread are the regional lymph nodes, liver, lungs, and bones, followed by many other sites, including the serosal membrane of the peritoneal cavity, brain, and others. In general, the disease has spread beyond the range of curative surgery in 25 to 30% of patients. Anal region carcinomas are locally invasive and metastasize to regional lymph nodes and distant sites.

The most important prognostic indicator of colorectal carcinoma is the extent of the tumor at the time of diagnosis. A widely used staging system is that described by Astler and Coller in 1954 (Table 18–12 and Fig. 18–56), which represents a modification of classifications proposed by Dukes and Kirklin.[78] *Staging can be applied only after the neoplasm has been resected and the extent of spread determined by surgical exploration and anatomic examination.* A patient with an Astler-Coller A lesion has a virtual 100% chance for 5-year survival after resection, falling to 67% for a B1 lesion, 54% for a B2 lesion, 43% for a C1 lesion, and 23% for a C2 lesion.

Carcinoid Tumors

Cells generating bioactive compounds, particularly peptide and nonpeptide hormones, are normally dispersed along the length of the gastrointestinal tract mucosa and play a major role in coordinated gut function. Although they are derived from epithelial stem cells in the mucosal crypts, they are designated *endocrine* cells because of their endocrine and paracrine function and their resemblance to endocrine cells elsewhere, as in the pancreas. Mucosal en-

Table 18–12. ASTLER-COLLER CLASSIFICATION OF CARCINOMA OF THE COLON AND RECTUM*

Tumor Stage	Histologic Features of the Neoplasm
A	Limited to the mucosa
B1	Extending into the muscularis propria but not penetrating through it; uninvolved nodes
B2	Penetrating through the muscularis propria; uninvolved nodes
C1	Extending into the muscularis propria but not penetrating through it; involved nodes
C2	Penetrating through the muscularis propria; involved nodes
D	Distant metastatic spread

*Incorrectly assigned eponyms: Dukes; modified Dukes; Dukes Kirklin.

From Astler VB, Coller FA: The prognostic significance of direct extension of carcinoma of the colon and rectum. Ann Surg 139:846, 1954.

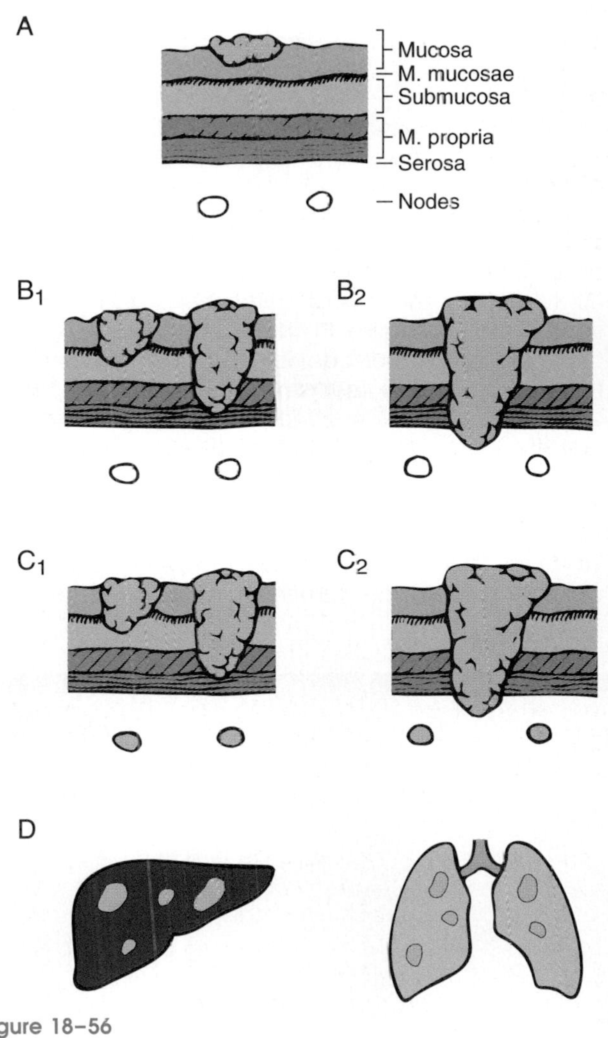

Figure 18–56

Pathologic staging of colorectal cancer according to the Astler-Coller system. Staging is based on the extent of local invasion and the presence of lymph node metastases (*A* to *C*) and distant visceral metastases (*D*).

docrine cells are abundant in other organs, including the lungs, but the great preponderance of tumors arising from these cells are in the gut. A scattering of tumors arises in the pancreas or peripancreatic tissue, lungs, biliary tree, and even liver. The peak incidence of these neoplasms is in the fifties, but they may appear at any age. They constitute less than 2% of colorectal malignancies but almost half of small intestinal malignant tumors.

Although all carcinoids are potentially malignant tumors, the tendency for aggressive behavior correlates with the site of origin, the depth of local penetration, and the size of the tumor. First, *appendiceal and rectal carcinoids infrequently metastasize, even though they may show extensive local spread.* By contrast, 90% of ileal, gastric, and colonic carcinoids that have penetrated halfway through the muscle wall have spread to lymph nodes and distant sites at the time of diagnosis, especially those tumors greater than 2 cm in diameter.

As with normal gut endocrine cells, the cells of carcinoid tumors can synthesize and secrete a variety of bioactive products and hormones. Although multiple factors may be synthesized by a single tumor, when a tumor secretes a predominant product to cause a clinical syndrome, it may be called by that name (e.g., gastrinoma, somatostatinoma, and insulinoma).

MORPHOLOGY. The appendix is the most common site of gut carcinoid tumors, followed by the small intestine (primarily ileum), rectum, stomach, and colon. The rectum, however, may represent up to half of those that come to clinical attention. Those that arise in the stomach and ileum are frequently multicentric, but the remainder tend to be solitary lesions. In the appendix, they appear as bulbous swellings of the tip, which frequently obliterate the lumen. Elsewhere in the gut, they appear as intramural or submucosal masses that create small, polypoid or plateau-like elevations rarely more than 3 cm in diameter (Fig. 18–57*A*). The overlying mucosa may be intact or ulcerated, and the tumors may permeate the bowel wall to invade the mesentery. **A characteristic feature is a solid, yellow-tan appearance on transection.** The tumors may cause angulation or kinking sufficient to cause obstruction. When present, visceral metastases are usually small, dispersed nodules and rarely achieve the size seen with the primary lesions. Notably, **rectal and appendiceal carcinoids almost never metastasize.**

Histologically the neoplastic cells may form discrete islands, trabeculae, strands, glands, or undifferentiated sheets. Whatever their organization, the tumor cells are monotonously similar, having a scant, pink granular cytoplasm and a round-to-oval stippled nucleus. In most tumors, there is minimal variation in cell and nuclear size, and mitoses are infrequent or absent (Fig. 18–57*B*). In unusual cases, there may be more significant anaplasia and sometimes mucin secretion within the cells and gland formations. By electron microscopy (Fig. 18–57*C*), the cells in most tumors contain cytoplasmic, well-formed, membrane-bound secretory granules with osmophilic centers (dense-core granules). Most carcinoids can be shown to contain chromogranin A, synaptophysin, and neuron-specific enolase. Specific hormonal peptides may occasionally be identified by immunocytochemical techniques.

Clinical Features. Gastrointestinal carcinoids may produce local symptoms owing to angulation or obstruction of the small intestine. Many (especially rectal and appendiceal) are asymptomatic and are found incidentally. The secretory products of some carcinoids may produce a variety of syndromes or endocrinopathies, depending on their anatomic site. Gastric, peripancreatic, and pancreatic carcinoids can release their products directly into the systemic circulation and can produce the *Zollinger-Ellison syndrome* related to excess elaboration of gastrin, Cushing syndrome associated with adrenocorticotropic hormone secretion, hyperinsulinism, and others. In some instances, these tumors may be less than 1.0 cm in size and extremely difficult to find, even during surgical exploration.

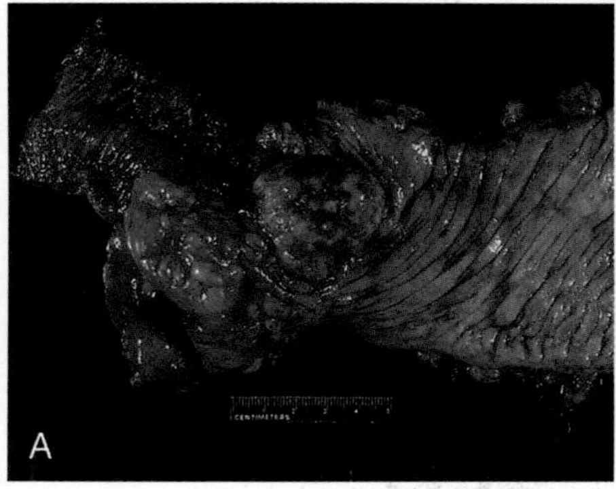

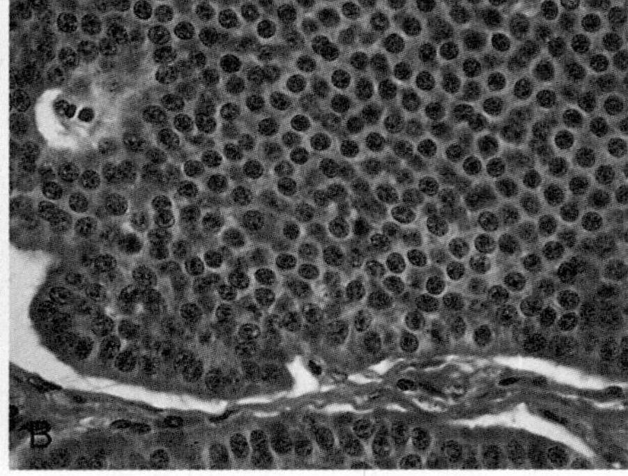

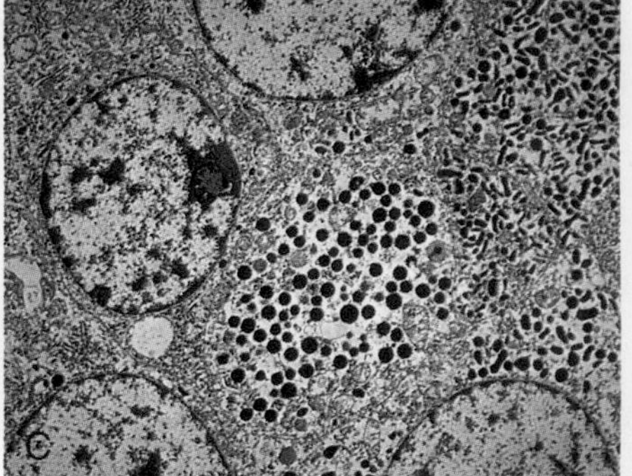

Figure 18–57

Carcinoid tumor. *A*, Multiple protruding tumors are present at the ileocecal junction. *B*, The tumor cells exhibit a monotonous morphology, with a delicate intervening fibrovascular stroma. *C*, Electron micrograph showing dense core bodies in the cytoplasm.

Table 18–13. CLINICAL FEATURES OF THE CARCINOID SYNDROME

- Vasomotor disturbances
  - Cutaneous flushes and apparent cyanosis (most patients)
- Intestinal hypermotility
  - Diarrhea, cramps, nausea, vomiting (most patients)
- Asthmatic bronchoconstrictive attacks
  - Cough, wheezing, dyspnea (about one third of patients)
- Hepatomegaly
  - Nodular liver owing to hepatic metastases (some patients)
- Systemic fibrosis (some patients)
  - Cardiac involvement
    - Pulmonic and tricuspid valve thickening and stenosis
    - Endocardial fibrosis, principally in the right ventricle
    - (Bronchial carcinoids affect the left side)
  - Retroperitoneal and pelvic fibrosis
  - Collagenous pleural and intimal aortic plaques

Some neoplasms are associated with a distinctive *carcinoid syndrome* (Table 18–13). The syndrome occurs in about 1% of all patients with carcinoids and in 20% of those with widespread metastases. Uncertainties remain in the precise origin of the carcinoid syndrome, but most manifestations are thought to arise from excess elaboration of serotonin (*5-hydroxytryptamine* [5-HT]). Elevated levels of 5-HT and its metabolite, *5-hydroxyindoleacetic acid* (5-HIAA), are present in the blood and urine of most patients with the classic syndrome. 5-HT is degraded in the liver to functionally inactive 5-HIAA. Thus, with gastrointestinal carcinoids, hepatic metastases must be present for the development of the syndrome. Not surprisingly, hepatic metastases are not required by extraintestinal carcinoids, such as those arising in the lungs or ovaries. Other secretory products of carcinoids, such as histamine, bradykinin, kallikrein, and prostaglandins, may contribute to the manifestations of the carcinoid syndrome.

The overall 5-year survival rate for carcinoids (excluding appendiceal) is approximately 90%. Even with small bowel tumors with hepatic metastases, it is better than 50%. Widespread disease, however, usually causes death.

GASTROINTESTINAL LYMPHOMA

Any segment of the gastrointestinal tract may be secondarily involved by systemic dissemination of non-Hodgkin lymphomas. Up to 40% of lymphomas arise in sites other than lymph nodes, and the gut is the most common location. Conversely, about 1 to 4% of all gastrointestinal malignancies are lymphomas. *By definition, primary gastrointestinal lymphomas exhibit no evidence of liver, spleen, or bone marrow involvement at the time of diagnosis*—regional lymph node involvement may be present. *Primary gastrointestinal lymphomas sometimes arise as sporadic neoplasms but occur more frequently in certain populations*: (1) *patients with* Helicobacter *gastritis*, (2) *natives of the Mediterranean region*, (3) *patients with congenital immunodeficiency states*, (4) *HIV-infected individuals*, (5) *individuals undergoing immunosuppresive therapy*, and (6) *patients with sprue*.

- *Sporadic lymphomas, also termed the Western type, are the most common form in the Western hemisphere.* These lymphomas appear to arise from the B cells of the gut mucosa-associated lymphoid tissue (MALT) (described earlier) and differ from node-based lymphomas in that (1) many behave as focal tumors in their early stages and are amenable to surgical resection; (2) relapse may occur exclusively in the gastrointestinal tract; (3) genotypic changes are different than those observed in nodal lymphomas: a unique (11;18) translocation has been found only in gut MALT lymphomas, whereas c-*myc* rearrangements may be unusually prevalent. This type of gastrointestinal lymphoma usually affects adults, lacks a sex predilection, and may arise anywhere in the gut: stomach (55 to 60% of cases), small intestine (25 to 30%), proximal colon (10 to 15%), and distal colon (up to 10%). The appendix and esophagus are only rarely involved. It is proposed that the random acquisition of genetic changes such as the t(11;18) leads to growth of a monoclonal β-cell population that is growth-dependent on cytokines produced by *H. pylori*–reactive T helper cells.[79] As a result, these tumors remain localized to the stomach for long periods of time, disseminating only late in their course. Successful treatment of the *Helicobacter* infection with antibiotics may lead to tumor regression, further highlighting its pathogenetic importance.[79]
- *Sprue-associated lymphoma* arises in some patients with a long-standing malabsorption syndrome that may or not be a true gluten-sensitive enteropathy. It occurs in relatively young individuals (30 to 40 years of age), often after a 10- to 20-year history of symptomatic malabsorption. Alternatively a diffuse enteropathy with malabsorption may accompany the development of a lymphoma. This form of lymphoma arises most often in the proximal small bowel. It is usually of T-cell origin, possibly in response to gluten-derived antigens, and its overall prognosis is poor.
- *Mediterranean lymphoma* refers to an unusual intestinal B-cell lymphoma arising in patients with Mediterranean ancestry, having a background of chronic diffuse mucosal plasmacytosis. The plasma cells synthesize abnormal IGA heavy chain, in which the variable portion has been deleted. A high proportion of patients have malabsorption preceding the development of the lymphoma. This condition is also referred to as *immunoproliferative small intestinal disease*. It sometimes regresses after antibiotic therapy, suggesting a role for bacterial infection in its pathogenesis.

MORPHOLOGY. Gastrointestinal lymphomas can assume a variety of gross appearances. Since all the gut lymphoid tissue is mucosal and submucosal, early lesions appear as plaquelike expansions of the mucosa and submucosa. Diffusely infiltrating lesions may produce full-thickness mural thickening, with effacement of the overlying mucosal folds and focal ulceration. Others may be polypoid, protruding into the lumen, or form large, fungating, ulcerated masses. Tumor infiltration into the muscularis propria splays the muscle fibers, gradually destroying them. Because of this feature, advanced lesions frequently cause motility problems with secondary obstruction. Large tumors sometimes perforate because of lack of stromal support; reduction in tumor bulk during chemotherapy also may lead to perforation.

The microscopic appearance varies according to subtype. In **MALT lymphomas** of the stomach, small lymphocytes with irregular nuclear contours expand the mucosa and infiltrate into epithelial glands, producing so-called lymphoepithelial lesions. Reactive-appearing germinal centers and variable numbers of neoplastic plasma cells are also commonly observed. **Mediterranean lymphoma** differs from gastric MALT lymphoma in that plasma cell infiltrates are more prominent, but it is otherwise similar. **Celiac sprue-associated lymphomas** tend to arise in the jejunum and form multifocal ulcerating plaques, masses, or strictures and are usually made up of large, pleomorphic cells. Overall, most gut lymphomas are of B-cell type (>95%). The rare T-cell tumors almost always occur in patients with preexistent celiac disease.

Clinical Features. Although gut lymphomas may occur as the result of obstruction or blood loss, their onset may be insidious with only vague symptoms of weakness and weight loss. Primary gastrointestinal lymphomas generally have a better prognosis than do those arising in other sites. Ten-year survival for patients with localized mucosal or submucosal disease approaches 85%. Early discovery is key to survival; thus gastric lymphomas generally have a better outcome than those of the small or large bowel. In general, the depth of local invasion, size of the tumor, histologic grade of the tumor, and extension into adjacent viscera are important determinants of prognosis.[80]

MESENCHYMAL TUMORS

Mesenchymal tumors may occur anywhere in the alimentary tract. Lipomas show a propensity for the submucosa of the small and large intestines, and lipomatous hypertrophy may occur in the ileocecal valve. A variety of spindle cell lesions may arise in the muscle wall of any gut segment. The great majority of these tumors are of smooth muscle origin and hence can be termed *leiomyomas* and *leiomyosarcomas*. Immunohistochemical methods, however, have shown some to possess features of neural, histiocytic, or dendritic origin. Since these tumors exhibit heterogeneity yet behave in a similar clinical fashion, they are grouped under the umbrella of *gastrointestinal stromal tumors*.[81] Both benign and malignant versions may occur at any age and in either sex. *Kaposi sarcomas* are considered elsewhere (Chapter 12).

MORPHOLOGY. Lipomas and benign stromal tumors are usually well-demarcated, firm nodules (almost always <4 cm in diameter) arising within the submucosa or muscularis propria. The overlying mucosa is stretched and attenuated. Rarely, they grow to larger size and produce hemispheric elevation of the mucosa with ulceration over the dome of the tumor. Malignant stromal tumors (primarily leiomyosarcoma) tend to produce large, bulky, intramural masses that eventually ulcerate into the lumen or project subserosally into the abdominal space. On cross-section, stromal tumors have a typical soft, fish-flesh appearance; are somewhat lobulated; and frequently have areas of hemorrhage, necrosis, or cystic softening. Histologically, lipomas, leiomyomas, and leiomyosarcomas resemble their counterparts encountered elsewhere (Chapter 8). In the case of the stromal tumors (e.g., leiomyomas and leiomyosarcomas), large size and a high mitotic rate are correlated with an aggressive course.

Clinical Features. Most mesenchymal tumors are asymptomatic. In the stomach, larger lesions (benign or malignant) may produce symptoms resembling those of peptic ulcer, particularly bleeding that is sometimes massive. Intestinal lesions may present with bleeding and for the small intestine, rare obstruction or intussusception. Benign lesions are easily resectable. Surgical removal is usually possible for the malignant lesions as well because they tend to grow as cohesive masses. Five-year survival rate for leiomyosarcoma, for example, is 50 to 60%. Metastases, however, are present in about one third of cases.

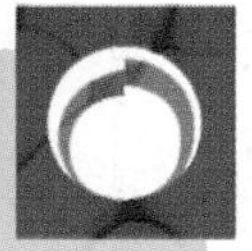

Appendix

NORMAL APPENDIX

Developmentally the appendix is an underdeveloped residuum of the otherwise voluminous cecum. The adult appendix averages 7 cm in length, is partially anchored by a mesenteric extension from the adjacent ileum, and has no known function. The appendix has the same four layers as the remainder of the gut and possesses a colonic-type mucosa. A distinguishing feature of this organ is the extremely rich lymphoid tissue of the mucosa and submucosa, which in young individuals forms an entire layer of germinal follicles and lymphoid pulp. This lymphoid tissue undergoes progressive atrophy during life to the point of complete disappearance in advanced age. In the elderly, the appendix, particularly the distal portion, sometimes undergoes fibrous obliteration.

PATHOLOGY

Diseases of the appendix loom large in surgical practice; appendicitis is the most common acute abdominal condition the surgeon is called on to treat. Appendicitis is one of the best-known medical entities and yet may be one of the most difficult diagnostic problems to confront the emergency physician. A differential diagnosis must include virtually every acute process that can occur within the abdominal cavity as well as some emergent conditions affecting organs of the thorax.

Acute Appendicitis

Inflammation in the right lower quadrant was considered a nonsurgical disease of the cecum (typhlitis or perityphlitis) until Fitz[82] recognized acute appendicitis as a distinct entity in 1886. Appendiceal inflammation is associated with obstruction in 50 to 80% of cases, usually in the form of a fecalith and, less commonly, a gallstone, tumor, or ball of worms (*Oxyuriasis vermicularis*). Continued secretion of mucinous fluid in the obstructed viscus presumably leads to a progressive increase in intraluminal pressure sufficient to cause eventual collapse of the draining veins. Ischemic injury then favors bacterial proliferation with additional inflammatory edema and exudation, further embarrassing the blood supply. Nevertheless, a significant minority of inflamed appendices have no demonstrable luminal obstruction, and the pathogenesis of the inflammation remains unknown.

MORPHOLOGY. At the earliest stages, only a scant neutrophilic exudate may be found throughout the mucosa, submucosa, and muscularis propria. Subserosal vessels are congested, and often there is a modest perivascular neutrophilic infiltrate. The inflammatory reaction transforms the normal glistening serosa into a dull, granular, red membrane; this transformation signifies **early acute appendicitis** for the operating surgeon. At a later stage, a prominent neutrophilic exudate generates a fibrinopurulent reaction over the serosa (Fig. 18–58). As the inflammatory process worsens, there is abscess formation within the wall, along with ulcerations and foci of suppurative necrosis in the mucosa. This state constitutes **acute suppurative appendicitis.** Further appendiceal compromise leads to large areas of hemorrhagic green ulceration of the mucosa, and green-black gangrenous necrosis through the wall extending to the serosa, creating **acute gangrenous appendicitis,** which is quickly followed by rupture and suppurative peritonitis.

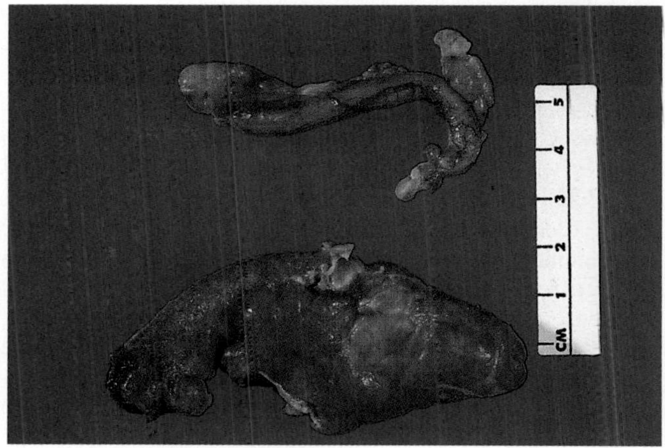

Figure 18–58 ■

Acute appendicitis. The inflamed appendix shown below is red, swollen, and covered with a fibrinous exudate. For comparison, a normal appendix is shown above.

The histologic criterion for the diagnosis of acute appendicitis is neutrophilic infiltration of the muscularis. Usually, neutrophils and ulcerations are also present within the mucosa. Since drainage of an exudate into the appendix from alimentary tract infection (e.g., *Campylobacter*) may also induce a mucosal neutrophilic infiltrate, evidence of muscular wall inflammation is requisite for the diagnosis.

Clinical Features. Acute appendicitis is mainly a disease of adolescents and young adults, but it may occur in any age group and affects males slightly more often than females. Classically, acute appendicitis produces the following manifestations, in the sequence given: (1) pain, at first periumbilical but then localizing to the right lower quadrant; (2) nausea, vomiting, or both; (3) abdominal tenderness, particularly in the region of the appendix; (4) mild fever; and (5) elevation of the peripheral white blood cell count up to 15,000 to 20,000 cell/mm^3. This classic presentation is more often absent than present. While pain, nausea, and vomiting usually develop, tenderness may be deceptively absent or maximal in atypical locations. In some cases, a retrocecal appendix may generate right flank or pelvic pain, while a malrotated colon may give rise to appendicitis in the left upper quadrant. The peripheral leukocytosis may be minimal or so high as to suggest alternative diagnoses. Nonclassic presentations are encountered more often in young children and in the very elderly, populations with a host of other plausible abdominal emergencies.

There is general agreement that highly competent surgeons make false-positive diagnoses of acute appendicitis and remove normal appendices about 20 to 25% of the time,[83] although newer imaging techniques may help reduce this false-positive rate.[84] *The discomfort and risks associated with an exploratory laparotomy and discovery of no disease are far outweighed by the morbidity and mortality (about 2%) associated with appendiceal perforation.* Besides perforation, uncommon complications of appendicitis include pylephlebitis with thrombosis of the portal venous drainage, liver abscess, and bacteremia. In instances when the appendix is normal, most often no disease of any kind is found during abdominal exploration. Definable conditions that mimic appendicitis are mesenteric lymphadenitis, usually secondary to an enterocolitis (often unrecognized) caused by *Yersinia* or a virus; systemic viral infection; acute salpingitis; ectopic pregnancy; *mittelschmerz* (pain caused by trivial pelvic bleeding at the time of ovulation); cystic fibrosis; and Meckel diverticulitis.

True *chronic inflammation* of the appendix is difficult to define as a pathologic entity, although occasionally granulation tissue and fibrosis associated with acute and chronic inflammation of the appendix suggest an organizing acute appendicitis. Much more frequently, recurrent acute attacks underlie a seemingly chronic condition. Since in some individuals the appendix is a mere fibrous cord from birth, it cannot be assumed that appendiceal fibrosis is the result of previous inflammation.

Tumors of the Appendix

The most common appendiceal tumor is the carcinoid, discussed earlier. It is usually discovered incidentally at the time of surgery or examination of a resected appendix. This neoplasm most frequently involves the distal tip of the appendix, where it produces a solid bulbous swelling up to 2 to 3 cm in diameter. Although intramural and transmural extension may be evident, nodal metastases are infrequent, and distant spread is rare.

Conventional adenomas or non–mucin-producing adenocarcinomas of the appendix may cause a typical neoplastic enlargement of this organ. Hyperplastic polyps as well may occur in this location. Benign and malignant mesenchymal growths resemble their counterparts in other areas.

MUCOCELE AND PSEUDOMYXOMA PERITONEI

Mucinous tumors of the appendix generally occur in adults and run the gamut from the innocuous mucocele to a mucin-secreting adenocarcinoma. In the latter instance, intraperitoneal spread may occur.

MORPHOLOGY. All mucinous lesions are associated with appendiceal dilation secondary to mucinous secretions. With **mucocele**, globular enlargement of the appendix by inspissated mucus occurs, usually the result of obstruction by a fecalith or other lesion such as an inflammatory stricture. Eventually the distention produces sufficient atrophy of the mucin-secreting mucosal cells and the secretions stop. Rarely a focus of mucin-secreting hyperplastic epithelium appears to be the culprit. This condition is usually asymptomatic; rarely a mucocele ruptures, spilling otherwise innocuous mucus into the peritoneal cavity.

The most common mucinous neoplasm is the benign **mucinous cystadenoma**, which replaces the appendiceal mucosa and distends the appendix with mucus. The luminal dilation is associated with appendiceal perforation in 20% of instances, producing localized collections of mucus attached to the serosa of the appendix or lying free within the peritoneal cavity. Histologic examination of the mucus, however, reveals no malignant cells.

Malignant *mucinous cystadenocarcinomas* are one fifth as common as cystadenomas. Macroscopically, they produce mucin-filled cystic dilation of the appendix indistinguishable from that seen with the benign cystadenomas. Penetration of the appendiceal wall by invasive cells and spread beyond the appendix in the form of localized or disseminated peritoneal implants, however, are frequently present (Fig. 18–59). In its fully developed state, continued cellular proliferation and mucin secretion fills the abdomen with tenacious, semisolid mucin—*pseudomyxoma peritonei.* Poorly differentiated adenocarcinomatous cells can be found, distinguishing this process from mucinous spillage. Instances in which pseudomyxoma peritonei is accompanied by both appendiceal and ovarian mucinous adenocarcinomas are usually ascribed to spread of an appendiceal primary lesion.[85]

Clinical Features. Mucoceles are generally encountered as an incidental lesion. Mucinous cystadenomas and adenocarcinomas may present with pain, attributable to distention of the viscus. Laparotomy for presumed acute appendicitis is a typical diagnostic setting. For lesions confined to the resected specimen (appendix or more radical excision), the outlook is excellent. Pseudomyxoma peritonei may be held in check for years by repeated debulking procedures but in most instances eventually runs its inexorable fatal course.

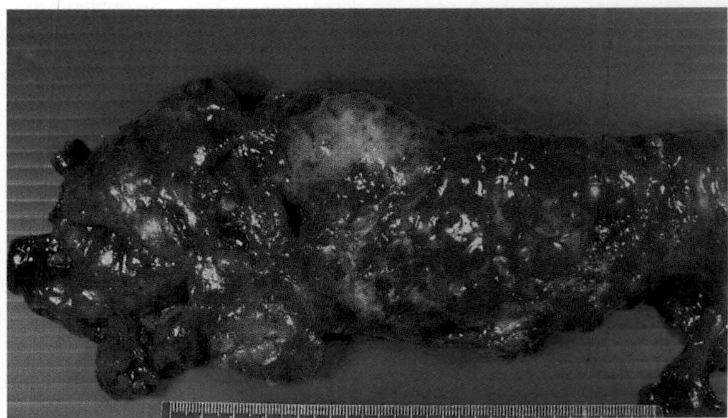

Figure 18–59

Mucinous cystadenocarcinoma of a markedly enlarged appendix.

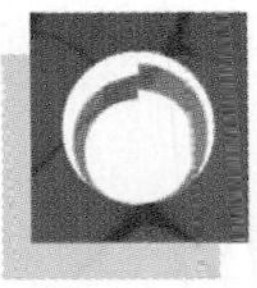

Peritoneum

INFLAMMATION

Peritonitis may result from bacterial invasion or chemical irritation. The most common causes of peritonitis are as follows:

- *Sterile peritonitis* from mild leakage of bile or pancreatic enzymes.
- *Perforation or rupture of the biliary system*, which evokes a highly irritating peritonitis, usually complicated by bacterial superinfection.
- *Acute hemorrhagic pancreatitis* (Chapter 20), with leakage of pancreatic enzymes and digestion of adipose tissue to produce fatty acids: These, in turn, precipitate with calcium to produce chalky white precipitates in areas of fat digestion and necrosis. Globules of free fat may be found floating in the peritoneal fluid; bacterial permeation of the bowel wall leads to a frank suppurative exudate after 24 to 48 hours.
- *Surgical procedures*: The reaction to surgically introduced foreign material such as talc is usually localized and minimal, leaving residual foreign body–type granulomas and fibrous tissue. Abrasion of serosal surfaces during abdominal surgery may lead to fibrous adhesions between visceral structures. Although usually asymptomatic, these occasionally are the points of internal herniation or intestinal obstruction.
- *Gynecologic conditions*: Endometriosis may introduce irritant blood into the peritoneal cavity, and ruptured dermoid cysts may invoke an intense peritoneal granulomatous reaction.

Peritoneal Infection

Bacterial peritonitis is almost invariably secondary to extension of bacteria through the wall of a hollow viscus or to rupture of a viscus. The more common disorders leading to such bacterial disseminations are *appendicitis, ruptured peptic ulcer, cholecystitis, diverticulitis, strangulation of bowel, acute salpingitis, abdominal trauma,* and *peritoneal dialysis*. Virtually every bacterial organism has been implicated, most commonly *E. coli*, α-hemolytic and β-hemolytic streptococci, *S. aureus*, enterococci, gram-negative rods, and *C. perfringens*. The last organism is a frequent inhabitant of the gut and contributor to peritonitis but rarely causes gas gangrene in the abdominal cavity. Gynecologic infections may introduce *gonococcus* and *Chlamydia*.

Spontaneous bacterial peritonitis may develop in the absence of an obvious source of contamination. It is an uncommon disorder seen most often in children, particularly those with the nephrotic syndrome. Among adults, 10% of cirrhotic patients with ascites develop spontaneous bacterial peritonitis during the course of their illness. The usual causal agents of the latter are *E. coli* and pneumococci, but the manner by which they invade the peritoneal cavity is unknown, possibly blood borne.

MORPHOLOGY. Depending on the duration of the peritonitis, the membranes show the following changes. Approximately 2 to 4 hours after initiation, there is loss of the gray, glistening quality of the peritoneal surface, and it becomes dull and lusterless. At this time, there is a small accumulation of essentially serous or slightly turbid fluid. Later the exudate becomes creamy and obviously suppurative. In some cases, it may be extremely thick and plastic and even inspissated, especially in dehydrated patients. The volume of exudates varies enormously. In many cases, it may be localized by the omentum and viscera to a small area of the abdominal cavity. In generalized peritonitis, an exudate may accumulate under and above the liver to form **subhepatic and subdiaphragmatic abscesses**. Collections in the lesser omental sac may likewise create residual persistent foci of infection.

The inflammatory process is typical of an acute bacterial infection anywhere and produces the characteristic neutrophilic infiltration with fibrinopurulent exudation. The reaction usually remains superficial and does not penetrate deeply into the visceral structures or abdominal wall. **Tuberculous peritonitis** tends to produce a plastic exudate studded with minute, pale granulomas.

These inflammatory processes can heal either spontaneously or with therapy. In the course of healing, the following may obtain: (1) **The exudate may be totally resolved, leaving no residual fibrosis;** (2) **residual, walled-off abscesses may persist, eventually to heal or serve as foci of new infection;** or (3) **organization of the exudate may occur, with the formation of fibrous adhesions that may be delicate or quite dense.**

Miscellaneous Conditions

Sclerosing Retroperitonitis. Dense fibromatous overgrowth of the retroperitoneal tissues may sometimes develop, designated *sclerosing retroperitonitis* or *retroperitoneal fibromatosis*. In some instances, the mesentery also is involved. The condition also causes ureteral obstruction and is discussed in Chapter 22.

Mesenteric Cysts. Large-to-small cystic masses are sometimes found within the mesenteries in the abdominal cavity or attached to the peritoneal lining of the abdominal wall. These cysts sometimes offer difficult clinical problems because they present on palpation as abdominal masses. Many classifications have been attempted; the most widely used is based on pathogenetic origins: (1) those arising from sequestered lymphatic channels; (2) those derived from pinched-off enteric diverticula of the developing foregut and hindgut; (3) those derived from the urogenital ridge or its derivatives (i.e., the urinary tract and male and female genital tracts); (4) those derived from walled-off infections or after pancreatitis, more properly called *pseudocysts* (see earlier); and (5) those of malignant origin, most often resulting from peritoneal involvement by intra-abdominal adenocarcinomas.

TUMORS

Virtually all tumors of the peritoneum are malignant and can be divided into primary and secondary forms. *Primary* tumors arising from the mesothelium of the peritoneum are extremely rare and are called *mesotheliomas*. These exactly duplicate mesotheliomas found in the pleura and the pericardium (Chapter 16). Similar to the supradiaphragmatic tumors, peritoneal mesotheliomas are associated with asbestos exposure in at least 80% of cases. How inhaled asbestos induces a peritoneal neoplasm remains a mystery.

Secondary tumors of the peritoneum are, in contrast, quite common. In any form of advanced cancer, penetration to the serosal membrane or metastatic seeding (peritoneal carcinomatosis) may occur. The most common tumors producing diffuse serosal implantation are ovarian and pancreatic. Appendiceal carcinomas, as noted earlier, may produce ensuing pseudomyxoma peritonei. Any type of intra-abdominal malignancy may be implicated in peritoneal seeding, however, and occasionally tumors from extra-abdominal locations.

Additional mention should be made of the uncommon tumors that may arise from retroperitoneal tissues (i.e., fat, fibrous tissue, blood vessels, lymphatics, nerves, and the lymph nodes alongside the aorta). These native structures may give rise to benign or malignant tumors derived from any of the indigenous mesenchymal cell types, resembling their counterparts arising elsewhere in the body.

ACKNOWLEDGMENT: Thanks are given to Drs. Yogeshwar Dayal and Ronald A. DeLellis for the use of material from their chapter "The Gastrointestinal Tract" in the fourth edition of this book.

REFERENCES

1. DeNardi FG, Riddell RH: The normal esophagus. Am J Surg Pathol 15:296, 1991.
2. Storch WB, et al: Autoantibodies to Auerbach plexus in achalasia. Cell Mol Biol 41:1033, 1995.
3. Weiss S, Mallory GK: Lesions of cardiac orifice of the stomach produced vomiting. JAMA 98:1353, 1932.
4. Galmiche J-P, Janssens J: The pathophysiology of gastro-oesophageal reflux disease: an overview. Scand J Gastroenterol 30(suppl 211):7, 1995.
5. Riddell RH: The biopsy diagnosis of gastroesophageal reflux disease, "carditis," and Barrett esophagus, and sequelae of therapy. Am J Surg Pathol 20(suppl 1):S31, 1996.
6. Spechler SJ, Goyal RK: The columnar-lined esophagus, intestinal metaplasia, and Norman Barrett. Gastroenterology 110:614, 1996.
7. Haggitt RC: Barrett esophagus, dysplasia, and adenocarcinoma. Hum Pathol 25:982, 1994.
8. Landis SH, et al: Cancer statistics, 1998. CA Cancer J Clin 48:6, 1998.
9. Riddell RH, Path FRC: Early detection of neoplasia of the esophagus and gastroesophageal junction. Am J Gastroenterol 91:853, 1996.
10. Turner JR, et al: Low prevalence of human papillomavirus infection in esophageal squamous cell carcinomas from North America: analysis by a highly sensitive and specific polymerase chain reaction-based approach. Hum Pathol 28:174, 1997.
11. Montesano R, et al: Genetic alterations in esophageal cancer and their relevance to etiology and pathogenesis: a review. Int J Cancer 69:225, 1996.
12. Pera M, et al: Increasing incidence of adenocarcinoma of the esophagus and esophagogastric junction. Gastroenterology 104:510, 1993.
13. Hersey SJ, Sachs G: Gastric acid secretion. Physiol Rev 75:155, 1995.
14. Allen A, et al: Gastroduodenal mucosal protection. Physiol Rev 73: 823, 1993.
15. Dekigai H, et al: Mechanism of *H. pylori*-associated gastric mucosal injury. Dig Dis Sci 40:1332, 1995.
16. Karlsson FA, et al: Major parietal cell antigen in autoimmune gastritis with pernicious anemia is the acid-producing H+,K+-adenosine triphosphatase of the stomach. J Clin Invest 81:475, 1988.
17. Dixon MF, et al: Classification and grading of gastritis—the updated Sydney System. Am J Surg Pathol 20:1161, 1996.
18. Soll AH: Pathogenesis of peptic ulcer and implications for therapy. N Engl J Med 322:909, 1990.
19. Fry J: Peptic ulcer: a profile. BMJ 2:809, 1964.
20. Komorowski RA, Caya JG: Hyperplastic gastropathy: clinicopathologic correlation. Am J Surg Pathol 15:577, 1991.
21. Ming S: Epithelial polyps of the stomach. In Ming S, Goldman H (eds): Pathology of the Gastrointestinal Tract. Philadelphia, WB Saunders, 1992, pp 547–569.
22. Dekker W, Op den Orth JO: Polyps of the stomach and duodenum: significance and management. Dig Dis 10:199, 1992.
23. Neuget AI, et al: Epidemiology of gastric cancer. Semin Oncol 23: 281, 1996.
24. Fuchs CS, Mayer RJ: Gastric carcinoma. N Engl J Med 333:32, 1995.
25. Tahara E: Molecular biology of gastric cancer. World J Surg 19:484, 1995.
26. Fenoglio-Preiser CM, et al: Pathologic and phenotypic features of gastric cancer. Semin Oncol 23:292, 1996.
27. Craanen ME, et al: Early gastric cancer: a clinicopathologic study. J Clin Gastroenterol 13:274, 1991.
28. Ouellette AJ, Selsted ME: Paneth cell defensins: endogenous peptide components of intestinal host defense. FASEB J 10:1280, 1996.
29. Gebert A, et al: M cells in Peyer patches of the intestine. Int Rev Cytol 167:91, 1996.
30. Wartiovaara K, et al: Hirschsprung's disease genes and the development of the enteric nervous system. Ann Med 30:66, 1998.
31. Chopra S, Trier JS: Diarrhea and malabsorption. In Chopra S, May RJ (eds): Pathophysiology of Gastrointestinal Diseases. Boston, Little, Brown, 1989, pp 125–169.
32. Guerrant RL, et al: Diarrhea in developed and developing countries: magnitude, special settings, and etiologies. Rev Infect Dis 12(suppl 1):S41–S50, 1990.
33. Garthright WE, et al: Estimates of incidence and costs of intestinal infectious diseases in the United States. Public Health Rep 103:107, 1988.
34. Cubitt WD, et al: Viral taxonomy: Classification and nomenclature. Sixth report of International Committee on the Taxonomy of Viruses. Arch Virol 10(suppl):359, 1995.
35. Knutton S, et al: Adhesion of enteropathogenic Escherichia coli to human intestinal enterocytes and cultured human intestinal mucosa. Infect Immun 55:69, 1987.

36. Lencer WI, et al: Signal transduction by cholera toxin: processing in vesicular compartments does not require acidification. Am J Physiol Gastrointest Liver Physiol 269:G548, 1995.
37. Neu J: Necrotizing enterocolitis—the search for a unifying pathogenic theory leading to prevention. Pediatr Clin North Am 43:409, 1996.
38. Gröschel DHM: *Clostridium difficile* infection. Crit Rev Clin Lab Sci 33:203, 1996.
38a. Castagliuolo I, et al: NK-1 receptor is required for *Clostridium difficile* enteritis. J Clin Invest 101:1547, 1998.
39. Orenstein JM, Kotler DP: Diarrheogenic bacterial enteritis in acquired immune deficiency syndrome: a light and electron microscopy study of 52 cases. Hum Pathol 26:481, 1995.
40. Snover DC, et al: A histopathologic study of gastric and small intestinal graft-versus-host disease following allogeneic bone marrow transplantation. Hum Pathol 16:387, 1985.
41. Lee RG, et al: Pathology of human intestinal transplantation. Gastroenterology 110:1820, 1996.
42. Lee FD: Drug-related pathological lesions of the intestinal tract. Histopathology 25:303, 1994.
43. Trier JS: Celiac sprue. N Engl J Med 325:1709, 1991.
44. Scott H, et al: Immunopathology of gluten-sensitive enteropathy. Semin Immunopathol 18:535, 1997.
45. Working Group of European Society of Paediatric Gastroenterology and Nutrition: Revised criteria for diagnosis of coeliac disease. Arch Dis Child 65:909, 1990.
46. Baker SJ, Mathan VI: Syndrome of tropical sprue in South India. Am J Clin Nutr 21:984, 1968.
47. Von Herbay A, et al: Whipple disease: staging and monitoring by cytology and polymerase chain reaction analysis of cerebrospinal fluid. Gastroenterology 113:434, 1997.
48. Isselbacher KJ, et al: Congenital B-lipoprotein deficiency: an hereditary disorder involving a defect in the absorption and transport of lipids. Medicine 43:347, 1964.
49. MacDermott RP: Alterations in the mucosal immune system in ulcerative colitis and Crohn disease. Med Clin North Am 78:1207, 1994.
50. Galperin C, Gershwin E: Immunopathogenesis of gastrointestinal and hepatobiliary diseases. JAMA 278:1946, 1997.
51. Plevy SE, et al: Tumor necrosis factor microsatellites define a Crohn disease-associated haplotype on chromosome 6. Gastroenterology 110: 1053, 1996.
52. Hugot JP, et al: Mapping of a susceptibility locus for Crohn disease on chromosome 16. Nature 379:821, 1996.
53. Thompson DE: The role of mycobacteria in Crohn disease. J Med Microbiol 41:74, 1994.
54. Wakefield AJ, et al: Crohn disease: pathogenesis and persistent measles virus infection. Gastroenterology 108:911, 1995.
55. Bjarnason I, et al: Intestinal permeability: an overview. Gastroenterology 108:1566, 1995.
56. Sartor RB: Insights into the pathogenesis of inflammatory bowel diseases provided by new rodent models of spontaneous colitis. Inflammatory Bowel Dis 1:64, 1995.
57. Russel MGVM, Stockbrügger RW: Epidemiology of inflammatory bowel disease: an update. Scand J Gastroenterol 31:417, 1996.
58. Ekbom A, et al: Increased risk of large-bowel cancer in Crohn disease with colonic involvement. Lancet 336:357, 1990.
59. Riddell RH, et al: Dysplasia in inflammatory bowel disease: standardized classification with provisional clinical applications. Hum Pathol 14:931, 1983.
60. Ekbom A, et al: Ulcerative colitis and colorectal cancer—a population-based study. N Engl J Med 323:1228, 1990.
61. Nugent FW, et al: Cancer surveillance in ulcerative colitis. Gastroenterology 100:1241, 1991.
62. Lashner BA, et al: Colon cancer surveillance in chronic ulcerative colitis: historical cohort study. Am J Gastroenterol 85:1083, 1990.
63. Mitsudo SM, et al: Vascular ectasia of the right colon in the elderly: a distinct pathologic entity. Hum Pathol 10:587, 1979.
64. Painter NS: The cause of diverticular disease of the colon, its symptoms and its complications. J R Coll Surg Edinb 30:118, 1985.
65. O'Brien MJ, et al: The National Polyp Study: Patient and polyp characteristics associated with high-grade dysplasia in colorectal adenomas. Gastroenterology 98:371, 1990.
66. Cranley JP, et al: When is endoscopic polypectomy adequate therapy for colonic polyps containing invasive carcinoma? Gastroenterology 91:419, 1986.
67. Haggitt RC, et al: Prognostic factors in colorectal carcinomas arising in adenomas: implications for lesions removed by endoscopic polypectomy. Gastroenterology 89:328, 1985.
68. Burt RW, et al: Genetics of colon cancer: impact of inheritance on colon cancer risk. Annu Rev Med 46:371, 1995.
69. Hermiston ML, Gordon JI: Inflammatory bowel disease and adenomas in mice expressing a dominant negative N-cadherin. Science 270: 1203, 1995.
70. Peifer M: Beta-catenin as oncogene: the smoking gun. Science 275: 1752, 1997.
71. Kinzler KW, Vogelstein B: Gatekeepers and caretakers. Nature 386: 761, 1997.
72. Fazeli A, et al: Phenotype of mice lacking functional deleted in colorectal cancer (DCC) gene. Nature 286:796, 1997.
73. Li ZH, et al: Telomerase activity is commonly detected in hereditary nonpolyposis colorectal cancers. Am J Pathol 148:1075, 1996.
74. Haenszel W, Kurihara M: Studies of Japanese migrants: 1. mortality from cancer and other diseases among Japanese in the United States. J Natl Cancer Inst 40:43, 1968.
75. Staszewski J, Haenszel W: Cancer mortality among the Polish born in the United States. J Natl Cancer Inst 35:291, 1965.
76. Giovannucci E, Willett WC: Dietary factors and risk of colon cancer. Ann Med 26:443, 1994.
77. Lawrence W Jr, et al: The National Cancer Data Base report on gastric cancer. Cancer 75:1734, 1995.
78. Kyriakos M: The President cancer, the Dukes classification, and confusion. Arch Pathol Lab Med 109:1063, 1985.
79. Qin Y, et al: Intraclonal offspring expansion of gastric low-grade MALT-type lymphoma: evidence for the role of antigen-driven high-affinity mutation in lymphomagenesis. Lab Invest 76:477, 1997.
80. Radaszkiewicz T, et al: Gastrointestinal malignant lymphomas of the mucosa-associated lymphoid tissue: factors relevant to prognosis. Gastroenterology 102:1628, 1992.
81. Franquemont DW: Differentiation and risk assessment of gastrointestinal stromal tumors. Am J Clin Pathol 103:41, 1995.
82. Fitz RH: Perforating inflammation of the vermiform appendix: with special references to its early diagnosis and treatment. Am J Med Sci 92:321, 1886.
83. Malt RA: The perforated appendix (editorial). N Engl J Med 315: 1546, 1986.
84. Rao PM, et al: Helical CT technique for the diagnosis of appendicitis: prospective evaluation of a focused appendix CT examination. Radiology 202:139, 1997.
85. Young RH, et al: Mucinous tumors of the appendix associated with mucinous tumors of the ovary and pseudomyxoma peritonei: a clinicopathological analysis of 22 cases supporting an origin in the appendix. Am J Surg Pathol 15:415, 1991.

19

The Liver and the Biliary Tract

James M. Crawford

The Liver

GENERAL MORPHOLOGIC AND FUNCTIONAL PATTERNS OF HEPATIC INJURY

HEPATIC INJURY

JAUNDICE AND CHOLESTASIS

- Bilirubin and Bile Formation
- Pathophysiology of Jaundice
- Cholestasis

HEPATIC FAILURE AND CIRRHOSIS

- Cirrhosis
- Portal Hypertension
  - *Ascites*
  - *Portosystemic Shunts*
  - *Splenomegaly*

INFECTIOUS DISORDERS

VIRAL HEPATITIS

- Hepatitis A Virus
- Hepatitis B Virus
- Hepatitis C Virus
- Hepatitis D Virus
- Hepatitis E Virus
- Other Hepatitis Viruses
- Clinicopathologic Syndromes
  - *The Carrier State*
  - *Asymptomatic Infection*
  - *Acute Viral Hepatitis*
  - *Chronic Viral Hepatitis*
  - *Fulminant Hepatitis*

BACTERIAL, PARASITIC, AND HELMINTHIC INFECTIONS

AUTOIMMUNE HEPATITIS

DRUG- AND TOXIN-INDUCED LIVER DISEASE

ALCOHOLIC LIVER DISEASE

INBORN ERRORS OF METABOLISM AND PEDIATRIC LIVER DISEASE

HEMOCHROMATOSIS

WILSON DISEASE

α_1-ANTITRYPSIN DEFICIENCY

NEONATAL HEPATITIS

INTRAHEPATIC BILIARY TRACT DISEASE

SECONDARY BILIARY CIRRHOSIS

PRIMARY BILIARY CIRRHOSIS

PRIMARY SCLEROSING CHOLANGITIS

ANOMALIES OF THE BILIARY TREE

CIRCULATORY DISORDERS

IMPAIRED BLOOD FLOW INTO THE LIVER

- Hepatic Artery Compromise
- Portal Vein Obstruction and Thrombosis

IMPAIRED BLOOD FLOW THROUGH THE LIVER

- Passive Congestion and Centrilobular Necrosis
- Peliosis Hepatis

HEPATIC VEIN OUTFLOW OBSTRUCTION

- Hepatic Vein Thrombosis (Budd-Chiari Syndrome)
- Veno-occlusive Disease

HEPATIC DISEASE ASSOCIATED WITH PREGNANCY

PREECLAMPSIA AND ECLAMPSIA

ACUTE FATTY LIVER OF PREGNANCY

INTRAHEPATIC CHOLESTASIS OF PREGNANCY

HEPATIC COMPLICATIONS OF ORGAN OR BONE MARROW TRANSPLANTATION

DRUG TOXICITY AFTER BONE MARROW TRANSPLANTATION

GRAFT-VERSUS-HOST DISEASE AND LIVER REJECTION

NONIMMUNOLOGIC DAMAGE TO LIVER ALLOGRAFTS

TUMORS AND TUMOROUS CONDITIONS

NODULAR HYPERPLASIAS

ADENOMAS

MALIGNANT TUMORS

- Primary Carcinoma of the Liver
- Metastatic Tumors

The Biliary Tract

CONGENITAL ANOMALIES

DISORDERS OF THE GALLBLADDER

CHOLELITHIASIS (GALLSTONES)

CHOLECYSTITIS

DISORDERS OF THE EXTRAHEPATIC BILE DUCTS

CHOLEDOCHOLITHIASIS AND ASCENDING CHOLANGITIS

BILIARY ATRESIA

CHOLEDOCHAL CYSTS

TUMORS

CARCINOMA OF THE GALLBLADDER

CARCINOMA OF THE EXTRAHEPATIC BILE DUCTS

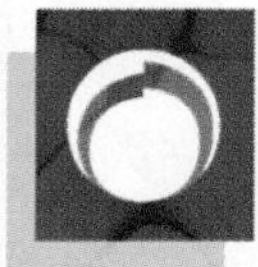

The Liver

NORMAL ANATOMY

The right upper quadrant of the abdomen is dominated by the liver and its companion biliary tree and gallbladder.

Residing at the crossroads between the digestive tract and the rest of the body, the liver has the enormous job of maintaining the body's metabolic homeostasis. This includes the processing of dietary amino acids, carbohydrates, lipids, and vitamins; synthesis of serum proteins; and detoxification and excretion into bile of endogenous waste products and pollutant xenobiotics. Hepatic disorders thus have far-reaching consequences.

The normal adult liver weighs 1400 to 1600 gm, representing 2.5% of body weight. Incoming blood arrives by the portal vein (60% to 70% of hepatic blood flow) and hepatic artery (30% to 40%) through the "gateway" of the liver, the *porta hepatis*; the common hepatic bile duct exits in this same region. The initial branches of artery, vein, and bile duct lie just outside the liver, but the remaining branches ramify roughly in parallel within the liver to form portal triads or *portal tracts*. The vast expanse of hepatic parenchyma is serviced by fenestrated terminal twigs of the portal vein and hepatic artery system, which enter the parenchyma at frequent intervals. Blood is collected into ramifications of the hepatic vein, which exits by the "back door" of the liver into the closely apposed inferior vena cava.

Microarchitecture. The liver has classically been divided into 1- to 2-mm-diameter hexagonal *lobules* oriented around the terminal tributaries of the hepatic vein (*terminal hepatic venules* or *"central" veins*). However, since hepatocytes near the central vein are most remote from the blood supply, it has been argued that they are at the periphery of "metabolic lobules," referred to as *acini*. Conceptualized as roughly triangular, the acini have the terminal twigs of hepatic artery and portal vein extending out from the portal tracts at their bases and the terminal hepatic venules at their apices[1] (Fig. 19–1). The parenchyma of the hepatic acinus is divided into three zones, zone 1 being closest to the vascular supply, zone 3 abutting the terminal hepatic venule, and zone 2 being intermediate. This zonation is of considerable metabolic consequence, since a lobular gradient of activity exists for many hepatic enzymes.[2] Moreover, many forms of hepatic injury exhibit a zonal distribution.

The hepatic parenchyma is organized into cribriform, anastomosing sheets or "plates" of hepatocytes, seen in microscopic sections as cords of cells (Fig. 19–2). Hepatocytes immediately abutting the portal tract are referred to as the *limiting plate*, forming a discontinuous rim around the mesenchyme of the portal tract. There is a radial orientation of the hepatocyte cords around the terminal hepatic vein. Hepatocytes exhibit minimal variation in overall size, but nuclei may vary in size, number, and ploidy, particularly with advancing age. Uninucleate, diploid cells tend to be the rule, but a significant fraction are binucleate, and the karyotype may range up to octaploidy.

Between the cords of hepatocytes are vascular sinusoids. Arterial and portal venous blood traverses the sinusoids and exits into the terminal hepatic vein through innumerable orifices in the vein wall. Hepatocytes are thus bathed on two sides by well-mixed portal venous and hepatic arterial blood, representing 25% of the cardiac output and placing hepatocytes among the most richly perfused cells in the body. The sinusoids are lined by fenestrated and discontinuous endothelial cells, which demarcate an extrasinusoidal *space of Disse*, into which protrude abundant mi-

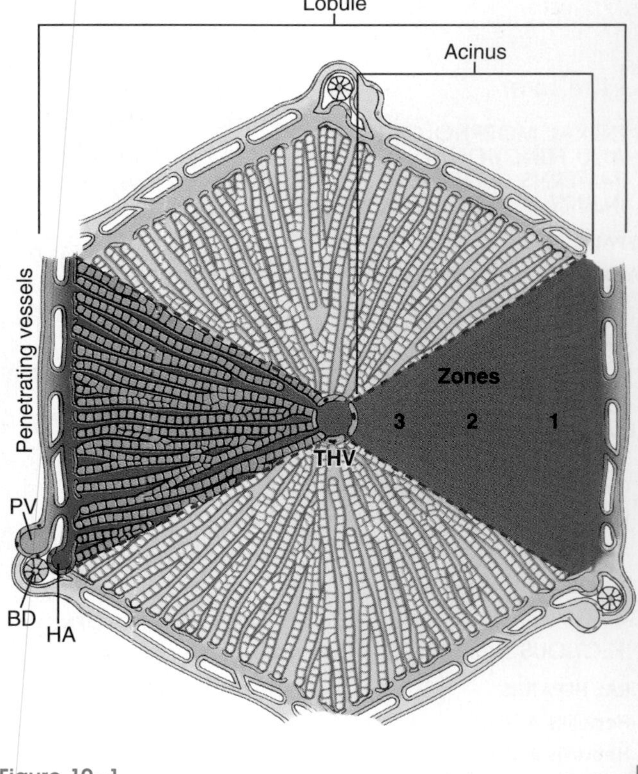

Figure 19–1

Microscopic liver architecture depicted schematically. The classic hexagonal lobule is centered around a central vein (terminal hepatic venule), with portal tracts at three of its apices. The triangular acinus has as its base the penetrating vessels, which extend from portal veins and hepatic arteries to penetrate the parenchyma. The apex is formed by the terminal hepatic vein. Zones 1, 2, and 3 represent metabolic regions increasingly distant from the blood supply.

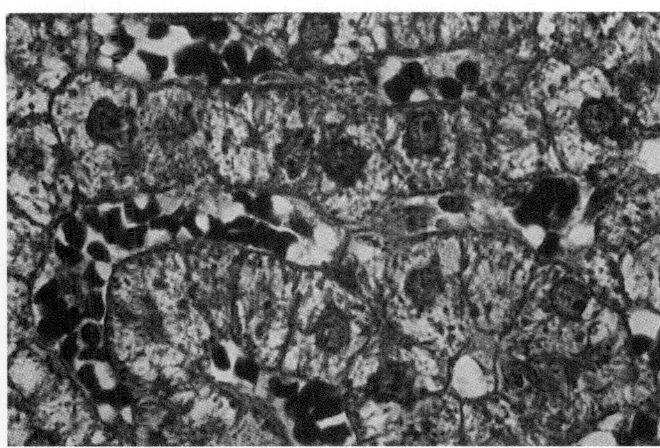

Figure 19–2 ■

Photomicrograph of liver. (Trichrome stain.) Note blood-filled sinusoids and cords of hepatocytes.

crovilli of hepatocytes. Scattered *Kupffer cells* of the monocyte-phagocyte system are attached to the luminal face of endothelial cells, and scattered fat-containing *hepatic stellate cells* (also called *Ito cells*) of mesenchymal origin are found in the space of Disse. These stellate cells play a role in the storage and metabolism of vitamin A and are transformed into collagen-producing myofibroblasts when there is inflammation and fibrosis of the liver, as we shall see.

Between abutting hepatocytes are *bile canaliculi*, which are channels 1 to 2 μm in diameter, formed by grooves in the plasma membranes of the facing cells and delineated from the vascular space by tight junctions. Numerous microvilli extend into these intercellular spaces, which constitute the outermost reaches of the biliary tree. Intracellular actin and myosin microfilaments surrounding the canaliculus help propel secreted biliary fluid along the canaliculi.[3] These channels begin in the centrilobular regions and progressively join to drain into the *canals of Hering*, the terminal parenchymal tributaries of the bile duct system. These canals are composed of a low cuboidal biliary epithelium. Biliary fluid is conveyed through their lumina to *interlobular bile ducts* within the portal tracts, which are lined by a more robust cuboidal epithelium.

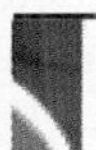

PATHOLOGY

GENERAL MORPHOLOGIC AND FUNCTIONAL PATTERNS OF HEPATIC INJURY

The liver is vulnerable to a wide variety of metabolic, toxic, microbial, circulatory, and neoplastic insults. In some instances, the disease is primary to the liver, as in viral hepatitis and hepatocellular carcinoma. More often the hepatic involvement is secondary, often to some of the most common diseases in humans, such as cardiac decompensation, disseminated cancer, alcoholism, and extrahepatic infections. The enormous functional reserve of the liver masks to some extent the clinical impact of early liver damage. However, with progression of diffuse disease or strategic disruption of bile flow, the consequences of deranged liver function become life threatening. Before specific disease processes are discussed, four general aspects of liver disease are reviewed: (1) general morphologic patterns of hepatic injury, (2) hepatic formation of bile, (3) hepatic failure, and (4) cirrhosis.

Hepatic Injury

From a morphologic standpoint, the liver is an inherently simple organ, with a limited repertoire of responses to injurious events. Regardless of cause, five general responses are seen.

DEGENERATION AND INTRACELLULAR ACCUMULATION. Damage from toxic or immunologic insult may cause hepatocytes to take on a swollen, edematous appearance **(ballooning degeneration)** with irregularly clumped cytoplasm and large clear spaces. Alternatively, retained biliary material may impart a diffuse foamy swollen appearance to the hepatocyte **(foamy degeneration)**. Substances may accumulate in viable hepatocytes, including iron and copper. Accumulation of fat droplets within hepatocytes is known as **steatosis.** Multiple tiny droplets that do not displace the nucleus are known as **microvesicular steatosis** and appear in such conditions as alcoholic liver disease and acute fatty liver of pregnancy. A single large droplet that displaces the nucleus, **macrovesicular steatosis,** may be seen in the alcoholic liver or in the livers of obese or diabetic individuals.

NECROSIS AND APOPTOSIS. Any significant insult to the liver may cause hepatocyte necrosis. In **ischemic coagulative necrosis,** the liver cells are poorly stained and "mummified" and often have lysed nuclei. With cell death that is toxic or immunologically mediated, isolated hepatocytes round up to form shrunken, pyknotic, and intensely eosinophilic **Councilman bodies** containing fragmented nuclei. This form of cell death is the consequence of **apoptosis** (Chapter 1). Alternatively, hepatocytes may osmotically swell and rupture, so-called **lytic necrosis.**

Necrosis frequently exhibits a zonal distribution. The most obvious is necrosis of hepatocytes immediately around the terminal hepatic vein **(centrilobular necrosis),** an injury that is characteristic of ischemic injury and a number of drug and toxic reactions. Pure **midzonal and periportal ne-**

crosis is rare; the latter may be seen in eclampsia. With most other causes of hepatic injury, a variable mixture of hepatocellular death and inflammation is encountered. The hepatocyte necrosis may be limited to scattered cells within hepatic lobules **(focal necrosis)** or to the interface between the periportal parenchyma and inflamed portal tracts **(interface hepatitis).** With more severe inflammatory injury, necrosis of contiguous hepatocytes may span adjacent lobules in a portal to portal, portal to central, or central to central fashion **(bridging necrosis).** Necrosis of entire lobules **(submassive necrosis)** or most of the liver **(massive necrosis)** is usually accompanied by hepatic failure. With disseminated candidal or bacterial infection, **macroscopic abscesses** may occur.

INFLAMMATION. Injury to the liver associated with an influx of acute or chronic inflammatory cells is termed hepatitis. Although hepatocyte necrosis may precede the onset of inflammation, the converse is also true. Attack on viable liver cells by sensitized T cells is a common cause of liver damage. Inflammation may be limited to the site of leukocyte entry (portal tracts) or spill over into the parenchyma. When hepatocytes undergo necrosis or apoptosis, scavenger macrophages engulf the dead cells within a few hours, generating clumps of inflammatory cells in an otherwise normal parenchyma. Foreign bodies, organisms, and a variety of drugs may incite a granulomatous reaction.

REGENERATION. The liver has enormous reserve, and regeneration occurs in all but the most fulminant diseases. Hepatocellular proliferation is signified by mitoses, thickening of the hepatocyte cords, and some disorganization of the parenchymal structure. Bile duct epithelial proliferation engenders an excess number of bile duct profiles within portal tracts. When hepatocellular necrosis occurs and leaves the connective tissue framework intact, almost perfect restitution of liver structure can occur, even when the necrosis is massive or submassive.

FIBROSIS. Fibrous tissue is formed in response to inflammation or direct toxic insult to the liver. Unlike all other responses, which are reversible, **fibrosis is generally an irreversible consequence of hepatic damage.** Deposition of collagen has lasting consequences on hepatic patterns of blood flow and perfusion of hepatocytes. In the initial stages, fibrosis may develop around portal tracts or the terminal hepatic vein, or it may be deposited directly within the space of Disse. **With continuing fibrosis, the liver is subdivided into nodules of regenerating hepatocytes surrounded by scar tissue, termed cirrhosis.** This end-stage form of liver disease is discussed later in this section.

The ebb and flow of hepatic injury may be imperceptible to the patient and detectable only by abnormal laboratory test results. Alternatively, hepatic function may be so impaired as to be life threatening. The major clinical consequences of liver disease are discussed next.

Jaundice and Cholestasis

Hepatic bile formation serves two major functions: (1) the promotion of dietary fat absorption in the lumen of the gut through the detergent action of bile salts and (2) the elimination of waste products. Bile constitutes the primary pathway for elimination of bilirubin, excess cholesterol, and xenobiotics that are insufficiently water soluble to be excreted into urine. Because bile formation is one of the most sophisticated functions of the liver, it is also one of the most readily disrupted. Such disruption becomes clinically evident as yellow discoloration of the skin and sclerae (*jaundice* or *icterus*, respectively), due to retention of pigmented bilirubin, and as *cholestasis*, characterized by systemic retention of not only bilirubin but also other solutes eliminated in bile.

BILIRUBIN AND BILE FORMATION

Bilirubin is the end product of heme degradation (Fig. 19–3). The majority of daily production (0.2 to 0.3 gm) is derived from breakdown of senescent erythrocytes by the mononuclear phagocyte system, especially in the spleen, liver, and bone marrow. Most of the remainder of bilirubin is derived from the turnover of hepatic hemoproteins (e.g., the P-450 cytochromes) and from premature destruction of newly formed erythrocytes in the bone marrow. The latter pathway is important in hematologic disorders associated with excessive intramedullary hemolysis of defective erythrocytes (ineffective erythropoiesis; Chapter 14).

Whatever the source, heme oxygenase oxidizes heme to biliverdin (step 1 in Figure 19–3), which is then reduced to bilirubin by biliverdin reductase. Bilirubin thus formed outside the liver is released and bound to serum albumin (step 2). Albumin binding is necessary since bilirubin is virtually insoluble in aqueous solutions at physiologic pH. The small fraction of unbound bilirubin in plasma may increase in severe hemolytic disease or when protein-binding drugs displace bilirubin from albumin.

Hepatic processing of bilirubin involves carrier-mediated uptake at the sinusoidal membrane (step 3), conjugation with one or two molecules of glucuronic acid by bilirubin uridine diphosphate–glucuronosyltransferase (UGT) in the endoplasmic reticulum (step 4), and excretion of the water-soluble, nontoxic bilirubin glucuronides into bile. Most bilirubin glucuronides are deconjugated by bacterial β-glucuronidases and degraded to colorless urobilinogens (step 5). The urobilinogens, and the residue of intact pigment, are largely excreted in feces. Approximately 20% of the urobilinogens formed are reabsorbed in the ileum and colon, returned to the liver, and promptly re-excreted into bile. The small amount that escapes this enterohepatic circulation is excreted in urine.

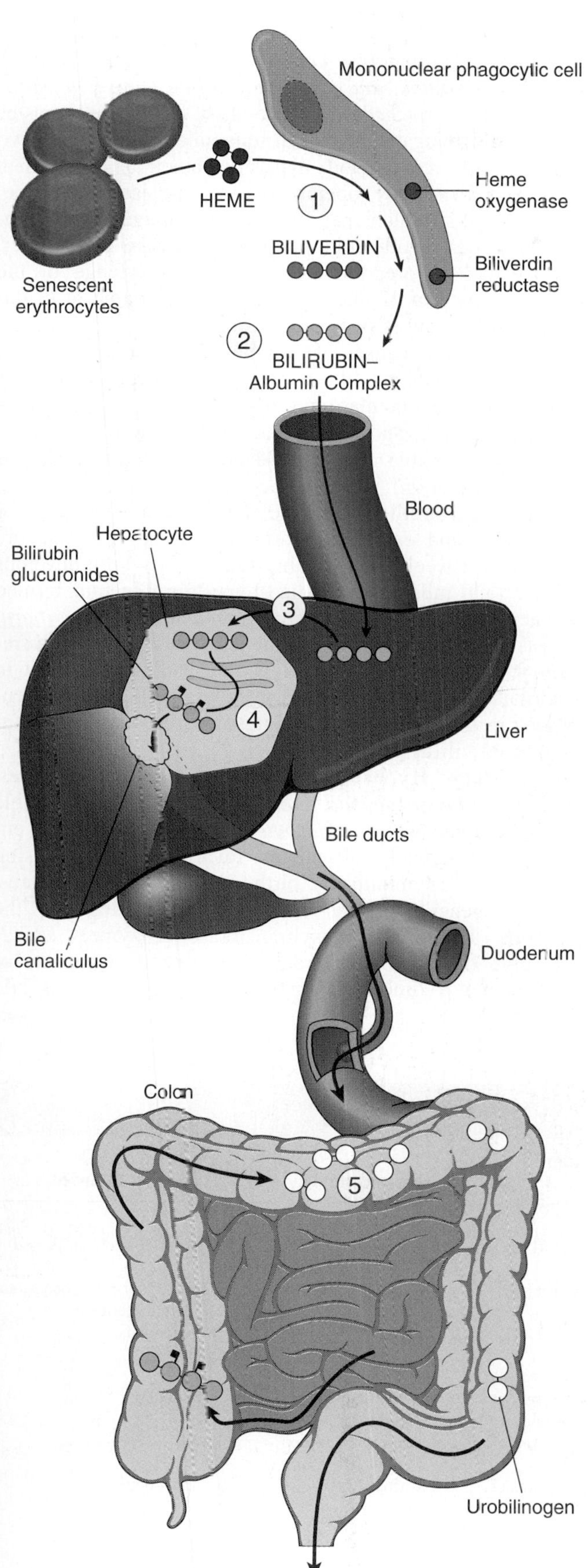

The brilliant yellow color of bilirubin makes it an easily identified component of hepatic bile formation. However, bilirubin metabolism and excretion is but a minor cog in the hepatic machinery that secretes 12 to 36 gm of bile acids into bile per day. Bile acids are carboxylated steroid molecules derived from cholesterol and are the detergent molecules primarily responsible for promoting bile flow and the secretion of phospholipid and cholesterol. The primary human bile acids are cholic acid and chenodeoxycholic acid, which are secreted as taurine and glycine conjugates. Ten per cent to 20% of excreted bile acids is deconjugated in the intestines by bacterial action. Virtually all conjugated and deconjugated bile acids are reabsorbed, primarily through the action of a sodium–bile acid cotransporter in the apical membrane of ileal enterocytes, and are returned to the liver for uptake, reconjugation, and resecretion. Fecal loss of bile acids (0.2 to 0.6 gm/day) is matched by de novo hepatic synthesis of bile acids from cholesterol. The *enterohepatic circulation* of bile acids provides an efficient mechanism for maintaining a large endogenous pool of bile acids for digestive and excretory purposes.

PATHOPHYSIOLOGY OF JAUNDICE

Both unconjugated bilirubin and bilirubin glucuronides may accumulate systemically and deposit in tissues, giving rise to the yellow discoloration of jaundice. This is particularly evident in the yellowing of the sclerae (icterus). There are two important pathophysiologic differences between the two forms of bilirubin. *Unconjugated bilirubin is virtually insoluble in water at physiologic pH and is tightly complexed to serum albumin. This form cannot be excreted in the urine even when blood levels are high.* A small amount of unconjugated bilirubin is normally present as an albumin-free anion in plasma. This fraction of unbound bilirubin may diffuse into tissues, particularly the brain in infants, and produce toxic injury. The unbound plasma fraction may increase in severe hemolytic disease or when protein-binding drugs displace bilirubin from albumin. Hence, *hemolytic disease of the newborn (erythroblastosis fetalis) may lead to accumulation of unconjugated bilirubin in the brain, which can cause severe neurologic damage, referred to as kernicterus*). In contrast, *conjugated bilirubin is water soluble, nontoxic, and only loosely bound to albumin. Because of its solubility and weak association with albumin, excess conjugated bilirubin in plasma can be ex-*

Figure 19–3

Bilirubin metabolism and elimination. 1, Normal bilirubin production from heme (0.2–0.3 gm/day) is derived primarily from the breakdown of senescent circulating erythrocytes, with a minor contribution from degradation of tissue heme-containing proteins. 2, Extrahepatic bilirubin is bound to serum albumin and delivered to the liver. 3, Hepatocellular uptake and (4) glucuronidation in the endoplasmic reticulum generate bilirubin mono- and diglucuronides, which are water soluble and readily excreted into bile. 5, Gut bacteria deconjugate the bilirubin and degrade it to colorless urobilinogens. The urobilinogens and the residue of intact pigments are excreted in the feces, with some reabsorption and excretion into urine.

Table 19–1. CAUSES OF JAUNDICE

Predominantly Unconjugated Hyperbilirubinemia

- Excess production of bilirubin
  - Hemolytic anemias
  - Resorption of blood from internal hemorrhage (e.g., alimentary tract bleeding, hematomas)
  - Ineffective erythropoiesis syndromes (e.g., pernicious anemia, thalassemia)
- Reduced hepatic uptake
  - Drug interference with membrane carrier systems
  - Some cases of Gilbert syndrome
- Impaired bilirubin conjugation
  - Physiologic jaundice of the newborn (decreased UGT activity, decreased excretion)
  - Breast milk jaundice (?inhibition of UGT activity)
  - Genetic deficiency of bilirubin UGT activity (Crigler-Najjar syndrome types I and II)
  - Gilbert syndrome (mixed etiologies)
  - Diffuse hepatocellular disease (e.g., viral or drug-induced hepatitis, cirrhosis)

Predominantly Conjugated Hyperbilirubinemia

- Decreased hepatic excretion of bilirubin glucuronides
- Deficiency in canalicular membrane transporters (Dubin-Johnson syndrome, Rotor syndrome)

UGT, uridine diphosphate–glucuronosyltransferase.

creted in urine. With prolonged conjugated hyperbilirubinemia, a portion of circulating pigment may become covalently bound to albumin (the *delta* fraction).

In the normal adult, total serum bilirubin levels vary between 0.3 and 1.2 mg/dl, and the rate of systemic bilirubin production is equal to the rates of hepatic uptake, conjugation, and biliary excretion. Jaundice becomes evident when the serum bilirubin levels rise above 2.0 to 2.5 mg/dl; levels as high as 30 to 40 mg/dl can occur with severe disease. Jaundice occurs when the equilibrium between bilirubin production and clearance is disturbed by one or more of the following mechanisms (Table 19–1): *(1) excessive production of bilirubin, (2) reduced hepatocyte uptake, (3) impaired conjugation, (4) decreased hepatocellular excretion, and (5) impaired bile flow (both intrahepatic and extrahepatic).* The first three mechanisms produce unconjugated hyperbilirubinemia, and the last two predominantly conjugated hyperbilirubinemia. More than one mechanism may operate to produce jaundice, especially hepatitis, which may produce unconjugated and conjugated hyperbilirubinemia. Generally speaking, however, one mechanism predominates, so that knowledge of the predominant form of plasma bilirubin is of value in evaluating possible causes of hyperbilirubinemia.

Of the various causes of jaundice listed in Table 19–1, the most common are due to bilirubin overproduction (as from hemolytic anemias and resorption of major hemorrhages), hepatitis, and obstruction to the flow of bile (considered later in this chapter). Several particular conditions merit consideration.

Neonatal Jaundice. Because the hepatic machinery for conjugating and excreting bilirubin does not fully mature until about 2 weeks of age, almost every newborn develops transient and mild unconjugated hyperbilirubinemia, termed neonatal jaundice or *physiologic jaundice of the newborn.* Breast-fed infants tend to exhibit jaundice with greater frequency, possibly the result of β-glucuronidases present in maternal milk. These enzymes deconjugate bilirubin glucuronides in the gut, increasing intestinal reabsorption of unconjugated bilirubin.

Hereditary Hyperbilirubinemias. *In rare instances, there may be a genetic lack of bilirubin UGT* (Table 19–2). *Crigler-Najjar syndrome type I,* in which the enzyme is completely absent, is invariably fatal, causing death within 18 months of birth secondary to kernicterus. Multiple genetic defects in the locus coding for the bilirubin UDP-glucuronosyltransferase enzyme, *UGT1,* may give rise to this disorder.[4] The liver is incapable of synthesizing a functional enzyme, and the colorless bile

Table 19–2. HEREDITARY HYPERBILIRUBINEMIAS

Disorder	Inheritance	Defects in Bilirubin Metabolism	Liver Pathology	Clinical Course
Unconjugated Hyperbilirubinemia				
Crigler-Najjar syndrome type I	Autosomal recessive	• Absent bilirubin UGT activity	Normal	Fatal in neonatal period
Crigler-Najjar syndrome type II	Autosomal dominant with variable penetrance	• Decreased bilirubin UGT activity	Normal	Generally mild, occasional kernicterus
Gilbert syndrome	?Autosomal dominant	• Decreased bilirubin UGT activity	Normal	Innocuous
Conjugated Hyperbilirubinemia				
Dubin-Johnson syndrome	Autosomal recessive	• Impaired biliary excretion of bilirubin glucuronides due to a canalicular membrane-carrier defect	Pigmented cytoplasmic globules; ?epinephrine metabolites	Innocuous
Rotor syndrome	Autosomal recessive	• ?Decreased hepatic uptake and storage ?Decreased biliary excretion	Normal	Innocuous

UGT, uridine diphosphate–glucuronosyltransferase.

contains only trace amounts of unconjugated bilirubin. The liver is morphologically normal by light and electron microscopy.

Crigler-Najjar syndrome type II is a less severe, nonfatal disorder exhibiting a partial defect in bilirubin conjugation; the major consequence is extraordinarily yellow skin. A mutation that disrupts the hydrophobic core of the signal peptide for bilirubin UGT has been reported for this syndrome.[5] Almost all patients develop normally, but there is a risk for some neurologic damage from kernicterus.

Gilbert syndrome is a relatively common, benign, somewhat heterogeneous inherited condition presenting with mild, fluctuating hyperbilirubinemia. The primary cause is reduction in hepatic bilirubin glucuronidating activity to about 30% of normal levels. Missense mutations and molecular anomalies in the promoter regions of the *UGT1* gene result in reduced expression of the enzyme.[6] Affecting some 6% of the population, the mild hyperbilirubinemia may go undiscovered for years and is not associated with functional derangements. When detected in adolescence or adult life, it is typically in association with stress, such as an intercurrent illness, strenuous exercise, or fasting. There is no clinical consequence of Gilbert syndrome except for the anxiety that a jaundiced sufferer might justifiably experience with this otherwise innocuous condition.

Dubin-Johnson syndrome results from a hereditary defect in hepatocellular excretion of bilirubin glucuronides across the canalicular membrane. The defect is attributable to an absence of the canalicular transport protein for bilirubin glucuronides and related organic anions.[7] The liver is darkly pigmented owing to coarse pigmented granules within the cytoplasm of hepatocytes (Fig. 19–4). Electron microscopy reveals coarse granules in hepatocellular lysosomes, which appear to be polymers of adrenaline (epinephrine) metabolites. The liver is otherwise normal. Apart from chronic or recurrent jaundice of fluctuating intensity, most patients are asymptomatic and have a normal life expectancy.

Rotor syndrome is a rare, separate form of asymptomatic conjugated hyperbilirubinemia with multiple defects in hepatocellular uptake and excretion of bilirubin pigments. The liver is not pigmented. As with Dubin-Johnson syndrome, patients with Rotor syndrome exhibit jaundice but otherwise live normal lives.

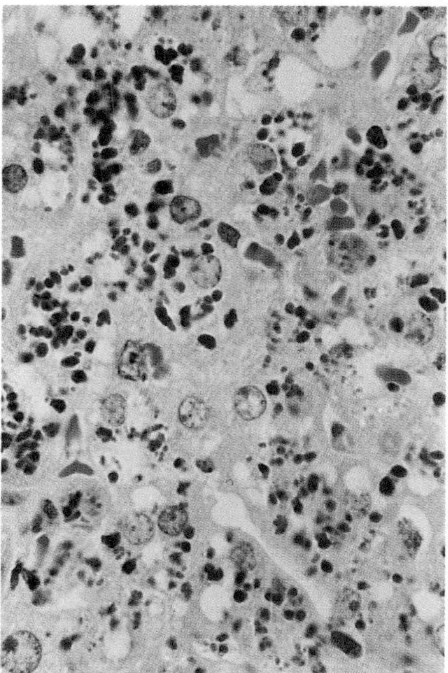

Figure 19–4

Dubin-Johnson syndrome, showing abundant pigment inclusions in otherwise normal hepatocytes. (H&E.)

CHOLESTASIS

Cholestatic conditions, which result from hepatocellular dysfunction or intrahepatic or extrahepatic biliary obstruction, may also present with jaundice. Alternatively, *pruritus* is a common presenting symptom, presumably related to the elevation in plasma bile acids and deposition in peripheral tissues, particularly skin. *Skin xanthomas* (focal accumulations of cholesterol) sometimes appear, the result of hyperlipidemia and impaired excretion of cholesterol. *A characteristic laboratory finding is elevated serum alkaline phosphatase*, an enzyme present in bile duct epithelium and in the canalicular membrane of hepatocytes. An isozyme is normally present in many other tissues such as bone, and so the increased levels must be verified as being hepatic in origin. Other manifestations of reduced bile flow relate to intestinal malabsorption, including nutritional deficiencies of the fat-soluble vitamins A, D, and K.

There is also a striking but heterogeneous group of autosomal recessively inherited conditions in which cholestasis results from impairment of bile salt or phospholipid secretion. One form causes progressive intrahepatic cholestasis *(Byler disease)*. The genetic defect appears to involve impaired biliary secretion of both bile acids and phosphatidylcholine.[8]

MORPHOLOGY. The morphologic features of cholestasis depend somewhat on its severity, duration, and underlying cause. **Common to both obstructive and hepatocellular cholestasis is the accumulation of bile pigment within the hepatic parenchyma** (Fig. 19–5). Elongated green-brown plugs of bile are visible in dilated bile canaliculi. Rupture of canaliculi leads to extravasation of bile, which is phagocytosed by Kupffer cells. Droplets of bile pigment also accumulate within hepatocytes, which can take on a wispy appearance (feathery or **foamy degeneration)**.

Obstruction to the biliary tree, either intrahepatic or extrahepatic, induces distention of upstream bile ducts by bile. The bile stasis and back-pressure induce proliferation of the duct epithelial cells and looping and reduplication of ducts, termed bile duct proliferation. The labyrinthine ducts further slow the flow of bile and favor the formation of concrements, which obstruct their lumens. Associated portal tract findings in-

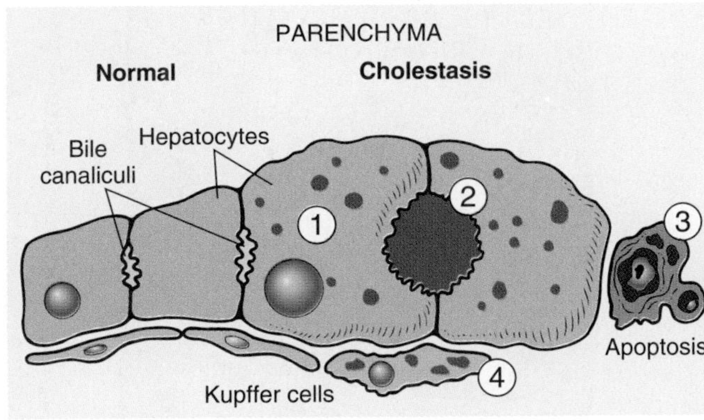

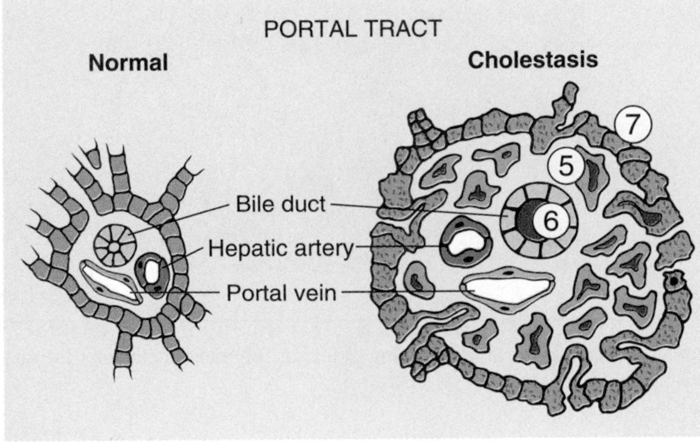

Figure 19–5

Illustration of the morphologic features of cholestasis (*right*) and comparison with normal liver (*left*). In the parenchyma (*upper panel*), cholestatic hepatocytes (1) are enlarged with dilated canalicular spaces (2). Apoptotic cells (3) may be seen, and Kupffer cells (4) frequently contain regurgitated bile pigments. In the portal tracts of obstructed livers (*lower panel*), there is also bile duct proliferation (5), edema, bile pigment retention (6), and eventually neutrophilic inflammation (not shown). Surrounding hepatocytes (7) are swollen and undergoing toxic degeneration.

clude edema and periductular infiltrates of neutrophils. Prolonged obstructive cholestasis leads not only to foamy change of hepatocytes but also to focal destruction of the parenchyma, giving rise to **bile lakes** filled with cellular debris and pigment. **Unrelieved obstruction leads to portal tract fibrosis,** which initially extends into and subdivides the parenchyma with relative preservation of hepatic architecture. Ultimately, an end-stage, bile-stained, cirrhotic liver is created (biliary cirrhosis, discussed later).

Extrahepatic biliary obstruction is frequently amenable to surgical alleviation; correct and prompt diagnosis is imperative. In contrast, cholestasis due to diseases of the intrahepatic biliary tree or hepatocellular secretory failure (collectively termed *intrahepatic cholestasis*) cannot be benefited by biliary surgery, and the patient's condition may be worsened by an operative procedure. *There is thus some urgency in making a correct diagnosis of the cause of jaundice and cholestasis.*

Hepatic Failure and Cirrhosis

The most severe clinical consequence of liver disease is hepatic failure. This may be the result of sudden and massive hepatic destruction. More often, it is the end point of progressive damage to the liver, either by insidious destruction of hepatocytes or by repetitive discrete waves of parenchymal damage. Whatever the sequence, 80% to 90% of hepatic functional capacity must be eroded before hepatic failure ensues. In many cases, the balance is tipped toward decompensation by intercurrent conditions that place demands on the liver. These include gastrointestinal bleeding, systemic infection, electrolyte disturbances, or severe stress such as major surgery or heart failure. In most cases of severe hepatic dysfunction, liver transplantation is the only hope for survival. The fortunate few can survive an acute event with conservative management until regeneration restores adequate hepatic function. Overall, mortality from hepatic failure is 70% to 95%.

The morphologic alterations that cause liver failure fall into three categories:

- *Massive hepatic necrosis*. This is most often due to fulminant viral hepatitis (hepatotropic viruses or nonhepatotropic). Drugs and chemicals may also induce massive necrosis, including acetaminophen, halothane, antituberculosis drugs (rifampin, isoniazid), antidepressant monoamine oxidase inhibitors, industrial chemicals such as carbon tetrachloride, and mushroom poisoning (*Amanita phalloides*). The mechanism may be direct toxic damage to hepatocytes (e.g., acetaminophen, carbon tetrachloride, mushroom toxins) but more often is a variable combination of toxicity and inflammation with immune-mediated hepatocyte destruction.
- *Chronic liver disease*. This is the most common route to hepatic failure and is the endpoint of relentless chronic hepatitis or alcoholic liver disease ending in cirrhosis.
- *Hepatic dysfunction without overt necrosis*. Less commonly, hepatocytes may be viable but unable to perform normal metabolic function, as with Reye syndrome, tetracycline toxicity, and acute fatty liver of pregnancy.

Clinical Features. Regardless of cause, the clinical signs of hepatic failure are much the same. Jaundice is an almost invariable finding. *Hypoalbuminemia*, which predisposes to peripheral edema, and *hyperammonemia*, which may play a role in cerebral compromise, are extremely worrisome developments. *Fetor hepaticus,* a characteristic body odor variously described as "musty" or "sweet and sour," occurs occasionally. It is related to the formation of mercaptans by the action of gastrointestinal bacteria on the sulfur-containing amino acid methionine and shunting of splanchnic blood from the portal into the systemic circulation (portosystemic shunting). Impaired estrogen metabolism and consequent hyperestrogenemia are the putative causes of *palmar erythema* (a reflection of local vasodilation) and *spider angiomas* of the skin. Each angioma is a central, pulsating, dilated arteriole from which small vessels radiate. In the male, hyperestrogenemia also leads to *hypogonadism* and *gynecomastia*.

Hepatic failure is life threatening, for a number of reasons. First, *with severely impaired liver function, patients are highly susceptible to failure of multiple organ systems.* Thus, respiratory failure with pneumonia and sepsis combine with renal failure to claim the lives of many patients with hepatic failure. A *coagulopathy* develops, attributable to impaired hepatic synthesis of blood clotting factors II, VII, IX, and X. The resultant bleeding tendency may lead to massive gastrointestinal bleeding as well as petechial bleeding elsewhere. Intestinal absorption of blood places a metabolic load on the liver, which worsens the extent of hepatic failure. The outlook of full-blown hepatic failure is grave: a rapid downhill course is usual, with death occurring within weeks to a few months in about 80%. A fortunate few can be tided over an acute episode until hepatocellular regeneration restores adequate hepatic function. Alternatively, liver transplantation may save the patient.

Two particular complications are important, since they herald the most grave stages of hepatic failure.

Hepatic encephalopathy is manifested by a spectrum of disturbances in consciousness, ranging from subtle behavioral abnormalities to marked confusion and stupor to deep coma and death. Associated fluctuating neurologic signs include rigidity, hyperreflexia, and particularly *asterixis*: nonrhythmic, rapid extension-flexion movements of the head and extremities, best seen when the arms are held in extension with dorsiflexed wrists. *Hepatic encephalopathy is caused by abnormal neurotransmission in the central nervous and neuromuscular systems*[9] and appears to be associated with elevated blood ammonia levels, which impair neuronal function and promote generalized brain edema.

Hepatorenal syndrome refers to *the appearance of acute renal failure in patients with severe liver disease, in whom there are no intrinsic morphologic or functional causes for the renal failure. Kidney function promptly improves if hepatic failure is reversed.* The pathogenesis of acute renal failure in this setting involves decreased renal perfusion as described in Chapter 21.[10]

Onset of this syndrome is typically heralded by a drop in urine output associated with rising blood urea nitrogen and creatinine concentrations. The prognosis is poor with a mortality of 80% to 95%. Alternatively, borderline renal insufficiency (serum creatinine concentration, 2 to 3 mg/dl) may persist for weeks to months, as in cirrhotic patients whose ascites is refractory to diuretic therapy.

CIRRHOSIS

Cirrhosis is among the top ten causes of death in the Western world. Although it is largely the result of alcohol abuse, other major contributors include chronic hepatitis, biliary disease, and iron overload. This end stage of chronic liver disease is defined by three characteristics:

- Bridging *fibrous septa* in the form of delicate bands or broad scars replacing multiple adjacent lobules
- *Parenchymal nodules* created by regeneration of encircled hepatocytes, varying from small (<3 mm in diameter, micronodules) to large (several centimeters in diameter, macronodules)
- *Disruption of the architecture of the entire liver*

Several features should be underscored:

- *The parenchymal injury and consequent fibrosis are diffuse*, extending throughout the liver; focal injury with scarring does not constitute cirrhosis.
- *Nodularity is requisite for the diagnosis* and reflects the balance between regenerative activity and constrictive scarring.
- *The fibrosis, once developed, is generally irreversible*, although regression is observed in rare instances of schistosomiasis and hemochromatosis.
- *Vascular architecture is reorganized* by the parenchymal damage and scarring, with the formation of abnormal interconnections between vascular inflow and hepatic vein outflow channels.

There is no satisfactory classification of cirrhosis save for specification of the presumed underlying cause. The terms micronodular and macronodular should not be used as a primary classification, although the size of the nodules may provide clues to etiology. Many forms of cirrhosis (particularly alcoholic) are initially micronodular, but there is a tendency for nodules to increase in size with time, counterbalanced by the constraints imposed by fibrous scarring.

The etiology of cirrhosis varies both geographically and socially. The following is the approximate frequency of etiologic categories in the Western world:

Alcoholic liver disease	60–70%
Viral hepatitis	10%
Biliary diseases	5–10%
Primary hemochromatosis	5%
Wilson disease	rare
α_1-Antitrypsin deficiency	rare
Cryptogenic cirrhosis	10–15%

Infrequent types of cirrhosis include (1) the cirrhosis developing in infants and children with galactosemia and tyrosinosis (Chapter 11); (2) liver destruction by a diffusely infiltrative cancer; (3) drug-induced cirrhosis (Chapter 10); and (4) syphilis (Chapter 9). Severe sclerosis can occur in the setting of cardiac disease (called cardiac cirrhosis, discussed later). After all the categories of cirrhosis of known causation have been excluded, a substantial number of cases remain. The magnitude of this "wastebasket" category, referred to as *cryptogenic cirrhosis*, speaks eloquently to the difficulties in discerning the many origins of cirrhosis. *Once cirrhosis is established, it is usually difficult to clearly distinguish an etiologic diagnosis on morphologic grounds alone.*

Pathogenesis. The central pathogenetic process in cirrhosis is progressive fibrosis. In the normal liver, interstitial collagens (types I and III) are concentrated in portal tracts and around central veins, with occasional bundles in the space of Disse. The collagen (reticulin) coursing alongside hepatocytes is composed of delicate strands of type IV collagen in the space of Disse. *In cirrhosis, types I and III collagen are deposited in the lobule, creating delicate or broad septal tracts.* New vascular channels in the septa connect the vascular structures in the portal region (hepatic arteries and portal veins) and terminal hepatic veins, shunting blood around the parenchyma. Continued deposition of collagen in the space of Disse within preserved parenchyma is accompanied by the loss of fenestrations in the sinusoidal endothelial cells. In the process, the sinusoidal space comes to resemble a capillary rather than a channel for exchange of solutes between hepatocytes and plasma. In particular, hepatocellular secretion of proteins (e.g., albumin, clotting factors, lipoproteins) is greatly impaired.

The major source of excess collagen in cirrhosis appears to be perisinusoidal *hepatic stellate cells* (Ito cells), which lie in the space of Disse. Although normally functioning as vitamin A fat-storing cells, they become activated during the development of cirrhosis, lose their retinyl ester stores, and transform into myofibroblast-like cells. As depicted in Figure 19–6, the stimuli for synthesis and deposition of collagen may come from several sources:

- Chronic inflammation, with production of inflammatory cytokines such as tumor necrosis factor (TNF)–α, transforming growth factor (TGF)–β, and interleukin-1
- Cytokine production by stimulated endogenous cells (Kupffer cells, endothelial cells, hepatocytes, and bile duct epithelial cells)
- Disruption of the extracellular matrix
- Direct stimulation of stellate cells by toxins

Acquisition of myofibers by perisinusoidal stellate cells and their transformation into myofibroblasts also increase vascular resistance within the liver parenchyma, since tonic contraction of these "myofibroblasts" constricts the sinusoidal vascular channels.

Throughout the process of liver damage and fibrosis, remaining hepatocytes are stimulated to regenerate, and they proliferate as spherical nodules within the confines of the fibrous septa. The net outcome is a fibrotic, nodular liver in which delivery of blood to hepatocytes is severely compromised, as is the ability of hepatocytes to secrete substances into plasma. Disruption of the interface between the parenchyma and portal tracts obliterates biliary channels as well. Thus, *the cirrhotic patient may develop jaundice and even hepatic failure, despite having a liver of normal mass.*

Clinical Features. All forms of cirrhosis may be clinically silent. When symptomatic, they lead to nonspecific clinical manifestations: anorexia, weight loss, weakness, osteoporosis, and, in advanced disease, frank debilitation. Incipient or overt hepatic failure may develop, usually precipitated by superimposition of a metabolic load on the liver, as from systemic infection or a gastrointestinal hem-

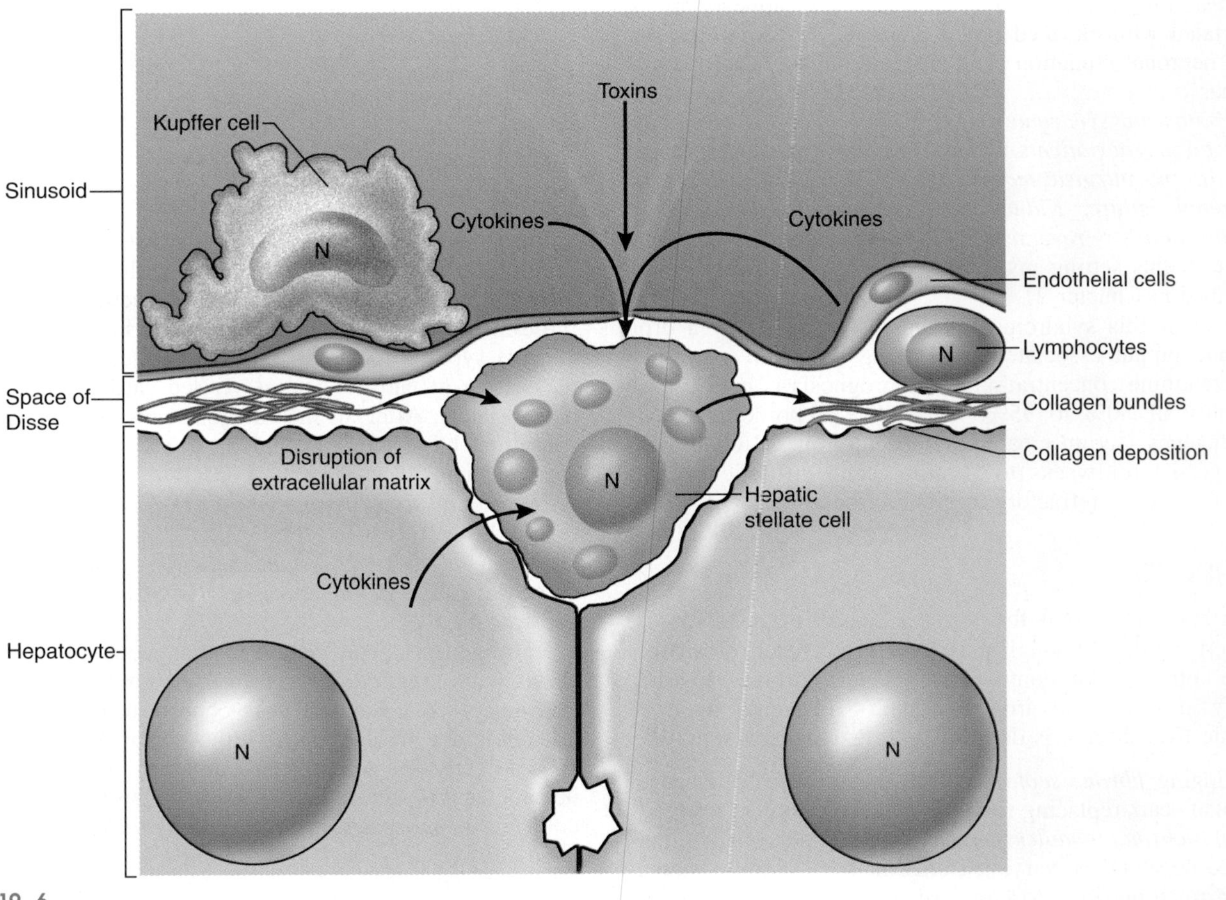

Figure 19–6

Proposed mechanisms for stimulation of collagen production by hepatic stellate cells in cirrhosis. Distortion of the extracellular matrix; secretion of cytokines from endothelial cells, Kupffer cells, hepatocytes, and inflammatory cells such as lymphocytes; and the direct action of toxins (or their metabolites) have all been proposed as possible stimuli for transforming hepatic stellate cells (lipocytes) into collagen-secreting myofibroblasts.

orrhage. Imbalances of pulmonary blood flow, which are poorly understood, may lead to severely impaired oxygenation (*hepatopulmonary syndrome*), further stressing the patient.[11] *The ultimate mechanism of most cirrhotic deaths is (1) progressive liver failure (discussed earlier), (2) a complication related to portal hypertension, or (3) the development of hepatocellular carcinoma.*

PORTAL HYPERTENSION

Increased resistance to portal blood flow may develop in a variety of circumstances, which can be divided into *prehepatic, intrahepatic, and posthepatic causes*. The major *prehepatic conditions* are obstructive thrombosis and narrowing of the portal vein before it ramifies within the liver. Massive splenomegaly may also shunt excessive blood into the splenic vein. The major *posthepatic causes* are severe right-sided heart failure, constrictive pericarditis, and hepatic vein outflow obstruction. These vascular disturbances are discussed later in this chapter. *The dominant intrahepatic cause is cirrhosis, accounting for most cases of portal hypertension.* Far less frequent are schistosomiasis, massive fatty change, diffuse fibrosing granulomatous disease such as sarcoidosis and miliary tuberculosis, and diseases affecting the portal microcirculation exemplified by nodular regenerative hyperplasia (also discussed later).

Portal hypertension in cirrhosis results from increased resistance to portal flow at the level of the sinusoids, and compression of central veins by perivenular fibrosis and expansile parenchymal nodules. Anastomoses between the arterial and portal systems in the fibrous bands also contribute to portal hypertension by imposing arterial pressure on the low-pressure portal venous system. *The four major clinical consequences are (1) ascites, (2) the formation of portosystemic venous shunts, (3) congestive splenomegaly, and (4) hepatic encephalopathy (discussed earlier).* These are illustrated in Figure 19–7.

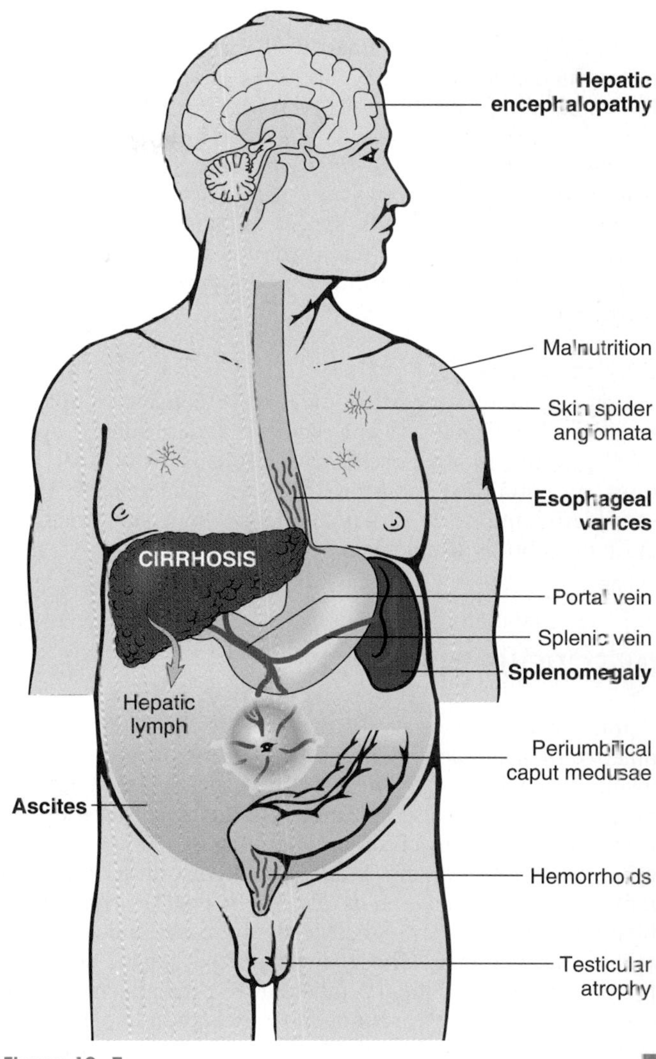

Figure 19–7

The major clinical consequences of portal hypertension in the setting of cirrhosis.

Ascites

Ascites refers to the collection of excess fluid in the peritoneal cavity. It usually becomes clinically detectable when at least 500 ml has accumulated, but many liters may collect and cause massive abdominal distention. It is generally a serous fluid having less than 3 gm/dl of protein (largely albumin) as well as the same concentrations as in the blood of solutes such as glucose, sodium, and potassium. Influx of neutrophils suggests secondary infection, whereas red cells point to possible disseminated intra-abdominal cancer. With long-standing ascites, seepage of peritoneal fluid through transdiaphragmatic lymphatics may produce hydrothorax, more often on the right side.

The *pathogenesis of ascites* is complex, involving the following mechanisms[12]:

- *Sinusoidal hypertension*, altering Starling forces and driving fluid into the space of Disse, which is then removed by hepatic lymphatics; this movement of fluid is also promoted by *hypoalbuminemia*.
- *Percolation of hepatic lymph into the peritoneal cavity.* Normal thoracic duct lymph flow approximates 800 to 1000 ml/day. With cirrhosis, hepatic lymphatic flow may approach 20 L/day, exceeding thoracic duct capacity. Hepatic lymph is rich in proteins and low in triglycerides, which is reflected in the protein-rich ascitic fluid.
- *Intestinal fluid leakage.* Portal hypertension also engenders increased perfusion pressure in intestinal capillaries. The osmotic action of the protein-rich ascitic fluid promotes movement of additional fluid out of intestinal capillaries into the abdomen.
- *Renal retention of sodium and water* due to secondary hyperaldosteronism (Chapter 26).

Portosystemic Shunts

With the rise in portal system pressure, bypasses develop wherever the systemic and portal circulation share common capillary beds. Principal sites are veins around and within the rectum (manifest as hemorrhoids); the cardioesophageal junction (producing esophagogastric varices); the retroperitoneum; and the falciform ligament of the liver (involving periumbilical and abdominal wall collaterals). Although hemorrhoidal bleeding may occur, it is rarely massive or life threatening. *Much more important are the esophagogastric varices that appear in about 65% of patients with advanced cirrhosis of the liver and cause massive hematemesis and death in about half of them* (see Fig. 18–7C). Abdominal wall collaterals appear as dilated subcutaneous veins extending from the umbilicus toward the rib margins (*caput medusae*) and constitute an important clinical hallmark of portal hypertension.

Splenomegaly

Long-standing congestion may cause congestive splenomegaly. The degree of enlargement varies widely up to 1000 gm and is not necessarily correlated with other features of portal hypertension. Massive splenomegaly may secondarily induce a variety of hematologic abnormalities attributable to hypersplenism.

INFECTIOUS DISORDERS

Inflammatory disorders of the liver dominate the clinical practice of hepatology. This is partly because virtually any insult to the liver can kill hepatocytes and recruit inflammatory cells[13] but also because inflammatory diseases are frequently long-term chronic conditions that must be managed medically. Among inflammatory disorders, infection ranks supreme. The liver is almost inevitably involved in blood-borne infections, whether they are systemic or arise within the abdomen. Those in which the hepatic lesion is prominent include miliary tuberculosis, malaria, staphylococcal bacteremia, the salmonelloses, candidiasis, and amebiasis. The foremost hepatic infections, however, are viral in origin.

Viral Hepatitis

Systemic viral infections that can involve the liver include (1) infectious mononucleosis (Epstein-Barr virus), which may cause a mild hepatitis during the acute phase; (2) cytomegalovirus infection, particularly in the newborn or immunosuppressed patient; and (3) yellow fever, which has been a major and serious cause of hepatitis in tropical countries. Infrequently in children and immunosuppressed patients, the liver is affected in the course of rubella virus, adenovirus, herpesvirus, or enterovirus infections.[14] However, *unless otherwise specified, the term "viral hepatitis" is reserved for infection of the liver caused by a group of viruses having a particular affinity for the liver* (Table 19–3). As these viruses cause overlapping patterns of disease, each virus is introduced before the pathology of viral hepatitis is discussed.

HEPATITIS A VIRUS

Hepatitis A, long known as infectious hepatitis and the scourge of military campaigns since antiquity, is a benign, self-limited disease with an incubation period of 2 to 6 weeks. *Hepatitis A virus (HAV) does not cause chronic hepatitis or a carrier state and only rarely causes fulminant hepatitis, and so the fatality rate associated with HAV is about 0.1%.* HAV occurs throughout the world and is endemic in countries with substandard hygiene and sanitation, so that most native populations have detectable anti-HAV by the age of 10 years. Clinical disease tends to be mild or asymptomatic and rare after childhood. In developed countries, the prevalence of seropositivity increases gradually with age, reaching 50% by age 50 years in the United States. In this population, acute HAV infection tends to be a sporadic overt febrile illness. Overall, HAV accounts for about 25% of clinically evident acute hepatitis worldwide.

Table 19–3. THE HEPATITIS VIRUSES

	Hepatitis A Virus	Hepatitis B Virus	Hepatitis C Virus	Hepatitis D Virus	Hepatitis E Virus	Hepatitis G Virus*
Agent	Icosahedral capsid, ssRNA	Enveloped dsDNA	Enveloped ssRNA	Enveloped ssRNA	Unenveloped ssRNA	ssRNA virus
Transmission	Fecal-oral	Parenteral; close contact	Parenteral; close contact	Parenteral; close contact	Water-borne	Parenteral
Incubation period	2–6 wk	4–26 wk	2–26 wk	4–7 wk	2–8 wk	Unknown
Carrier state	None	0.1%–1.0% of blood donors in U.S. and Western world	0.2%–1.0% of blood donors in U.S. and Western world	1%–10% in drug addicts and hemophiliacs	Unknown	1%–2% of blood donors in U.S.
Chronic hepatitis	None	5%–10% of acute infections	>50%	<5% coinfection, 80% superinfection	None	None
Hepatocellular carcinoma	No	Yes	Yes	No increase above HBV	Unknown, but unlikely	None

* At present, hepatitis G virus is not considered pathogenic.

HAV is a small, unenveloped, single-stranded RNA picornavirus that occupies its own genus, Hepatovirus. Ultrastructurally, HAV is an icosahedral capsid 27 nm in diameter. HAV is spread by ingestion of contaminated water and foods and is shed in the stool for 2 to 3 weeks before and 1 week after the onset of jaundice. Thus, close personal contact with an infected individual or fecal-oral contamination during this period accounts for most cases. This explains the outbreaks in institutional settings such as schools and nurseries and the water-borne epidemics under overcrowded, unsanitary conditions. HAV is not shed in any significant quantities in saliva, urine, or semen. Among developed countries, sporadic infections may be contracted by the consumption of raw or steamed shellfish (oysters, mussels, clams), which concentrate the virus from seawater contaminated with human sewage. *Because HAV viremia is transient, blood-borne transmission of HAV occurs only rarely, and therefore donated blood is not specifically screened for this virus.*

Serologic Diagnosis. Specific antibody against HAV of the immunoglobulin (Ig) M type appears in blood at the onset of symptoms, constituting a reliable marker of acute infection (Fig. 19–8). Fecal shedding of the virus ends as the IgM titer rises. The IgM response usually begins to decline in a few months and is followed by the appearance of IgG anti-HAV. The latter persists for years, perhaps for life, providing protective immunity against reinfection by all strains of HAV.

HEPATITIS B VIRUS

Hepatitis B virus (HBV), the cause of "serum hepatitis," can produce (1) acute hepatitis, (2) nonprogressive chronic hepatitis, (3) progressive chronic hepatitis ending in cirrhosis, (4) fulminant hepatitis with massive liver necrosis, (5) an asymptomatic carrier state, with or without progressive subclinical disease, and (6) the backdrop for hepatitis D virus (HDV). HBV also plays an important role in the development of hepatocellular carcinoma. The approximate clinical outcomes for HBV infection are depicted in Figure 19–9.

Liver disease due to HBV is an enormous problem globally, with an estimated worldwide carrier rate of 300 million; in the United States alone, there are 300,000 new infections per year. Unlike HAV, HBV remains in blood during the last stages of a prolonged incubation period (4 to 26 weeks) and during active episodes of acute and chronic hepatitis. It is also present in all physiologic and pathologic body fluids, with the exception of stool. HBV is a hardy virus and can withstand extremes of temperature and humidity. Thus, whereas blood and body fluids are the primary vehicles of transmission, virus may also be spread by contact with body secretions such as semen, saliva, sweat, tears, breast milk, and pathologic effusions. *Transfusion, blood products, dialysis, needle-stick accidents among health workers, intravenous drug abuse, and homosexual activity constitute the primary risk categories for HBV infection.* In one third of patients, the source of infection is unknown. In endemic regions such as Africa and Southeast Asia, spread from an infected mother to a neonate during birth (*vertical transmission*) is common. These neonatal infections often lead to the carrier state for life.

HBV is a member of the Hepadnaviridae, a family of DNA-containing viruses that cause hepatitis in multiple animal species. The mature HBV virion is a spherical double-layered "Dane particle" that has an outer surface envelope of protein, lipid, and carbohydrate enclosing a slightly hexagonal core. The genome of HBV is a partially double stranded circular DNA molecule (Fig. 19–10). The organization of the HBV genome is unique in that all regions of the viral genome encode protein sequences:

- A nucleocapsid "core" protein (HBcAg, hepatitis B core antigen) and a longer polypeptide transcript with a precore and core region, designated HBeAg (hepatitis B e antigen).
- Envelope glycoprotein (HBsAg, hepatitis B surface antigen). Infected hepatocytes are capable of synthesizing and secreting massive quantities of noninfective surface protein (HBsAg).
- A DNA polymerase that exhibits reverse transcriptase activity, and genomic replication occurs through an intermediate RNA template.
- A protein from the X region (HBX), which is necessary for virus replication and acts as a transcriptional transactivator of the viral genes and a wide variety of host gene promoters. HBX is also thought to play a key role in the causation of hepatocellular carcinoma.

HBV infections pass through two phases. During the *proliferative phase*, HBV DNA is present in episomal form, with formation of complete virions and all associated antigens. Cell surface expression of viral HBsAg and HBcAg in association with the major histocompatibility complex (MHC) class I molecules leads to activation of cytotoxic CD8+ T lymphocytes and hepatocyte destruc-

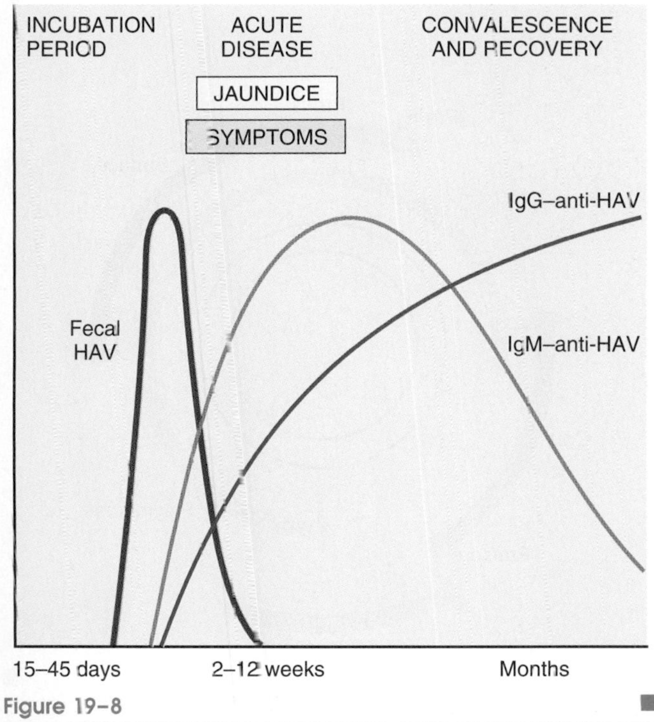

Figure 19–8

Sequence of serologic markers in acute hepatitis A viral hepatitis.

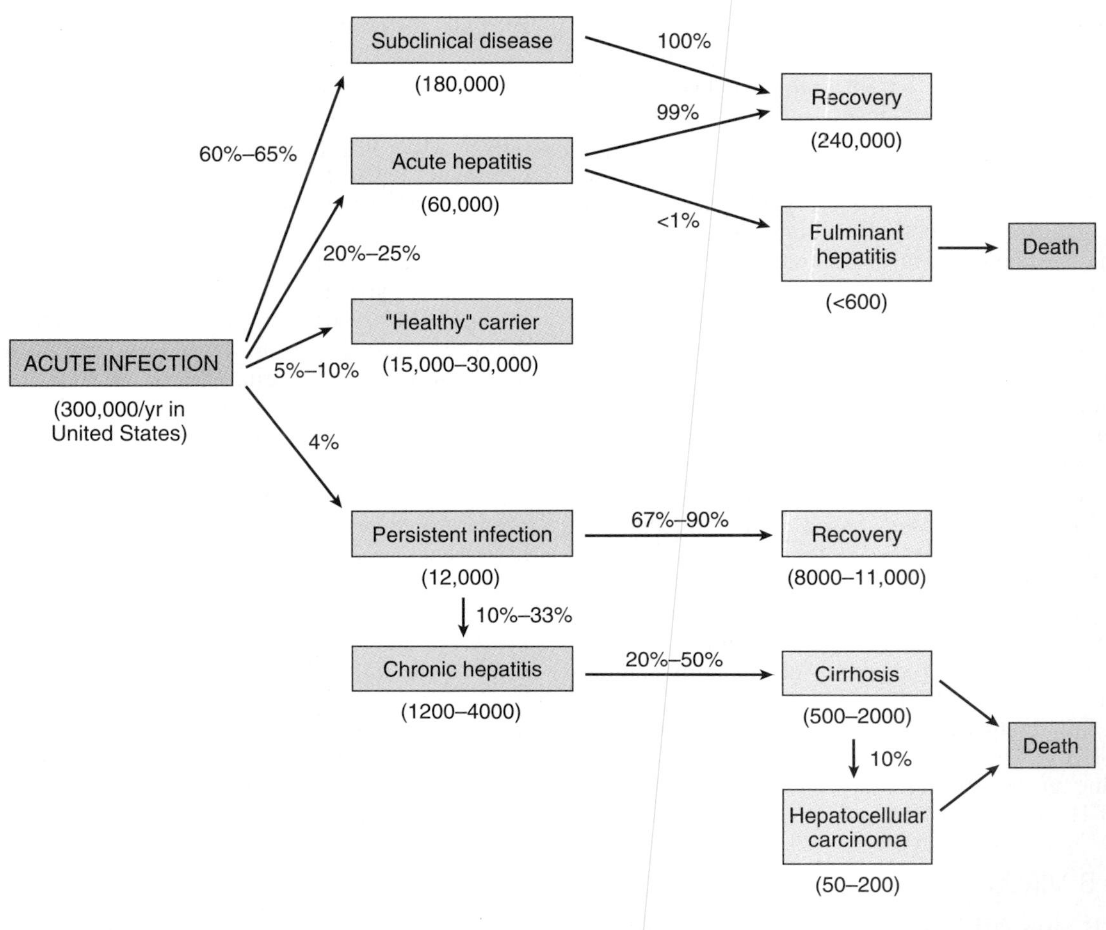

Figure 19–9

Schematic of the approximate outcomes of hepatitis B infection in adults, with their approximate annual frequencies in the United States. (Population estimates courtesy of John L. Gollan, MD, PhD, Brigham and Women's Hospital, Boston, MA.)

tion. An *integrative phase*, in which viral DNA is incorporated into the host genome, may occur in hepatocytes not destroyed by the immune response. With cessation of viral replication and the appearance of antiviral antibodies, infectivity ends and liver damage subsides. However, the risk of hepatocellular carcinoma persists.

On occasion, infectious mutant strains of HBV emerge during active replication of the wild type HBV strain, and some may have ominous consequences. First, some mutants replicate successfully but are incapable of HBeAg expression, despite continued HBcAg production. The loss of circulating HBeAg, and hence of anti-HBe antibody formation, is associated with fulminant hepatitis. Second, vaccine-induced escape mutants appear to replicate in the presence of vaccine-induced immunity.

Serologic Diagnosis. After exposure to HBV, the long asymptomatic 4- to 26-week incubation period (mean, 6 to 8 weeks) is followed by acute disease lasting many weeks to months (Fig. 19–11*A*). Most patients experience a self-limited illness:

- HBsAg appears before the onset of symptoms, peaks during overt disease, and then declines to undetectable levels in 3 to 6 months.

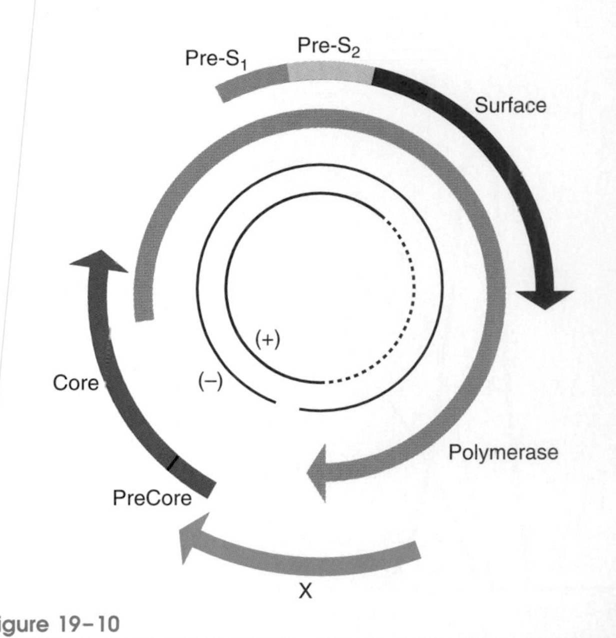

Figure 19–10

Diagrammatic representation of the structure and transcribed components of the hepatitis B virion.

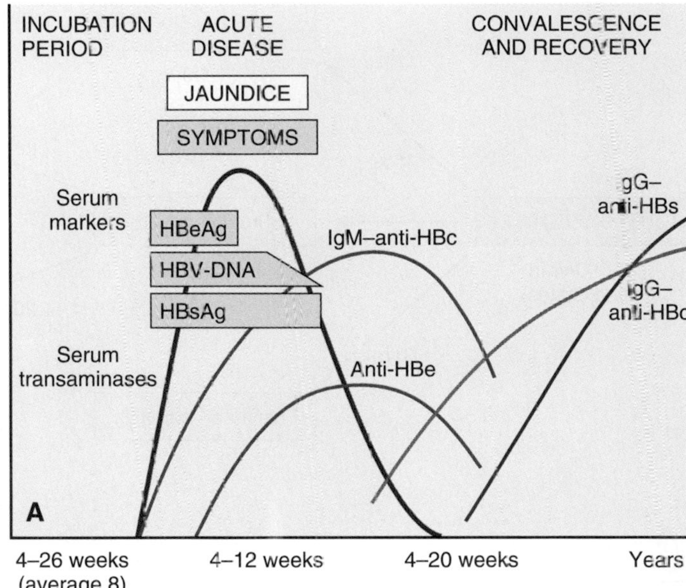

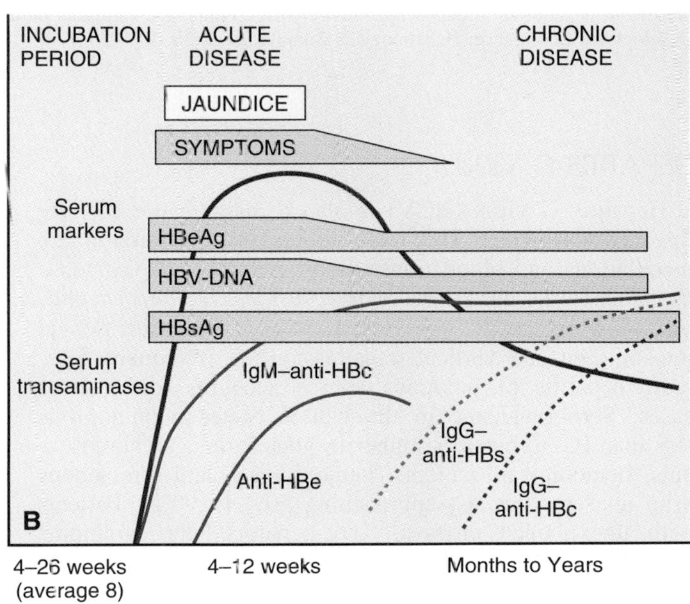

Figure 19–11

Sequence of serologic markers for hepatitis B viral hepatitis demonstrating *(A)* acute infection with resolution and *(B)* progression to chronic infection.

- HBeAg, HBV DNA, and DNA polymerase appear in the serum soon after HBsAg, and all signify active viral replication.
- IgM anti-HBc becomes detectable in serum shortly before the onset of symptoms, concurrent with the onset of elevated serum transaminase levels. During months, the IgM antibody is replaced by IgG anti-HBc.
- Anti-HBe is detectable shortly after the disappearance of HBeAg, implying that the acute infection has peaked and the disease is on the wane.
- IgG anti-HBs does not rise until the acute disease is over and is usually not detectable for a few weeks to several months after the disappearance of HBsAg. Anti-HBs may persist for life, conferring protection; this is the basis for current vaccination strategies using noninfectious HBsAg.

The carrier state is defined by the presence of HBsAg in serum for 6 months or longer after initial detection. The presence of HBsAg alone does not necessarily indicate replication of complete virions, and patients may be asymptomatic and without liver damage. In contrast, *chronic replication of HBV virions is characterized by persistence of circulating HBsAg, HBeAg, and HBV DNA, usually with anti-HBc and occasionally with anti-HBs* (Fig. 19–11*B*). In these patients, progressive liver damage may occur.

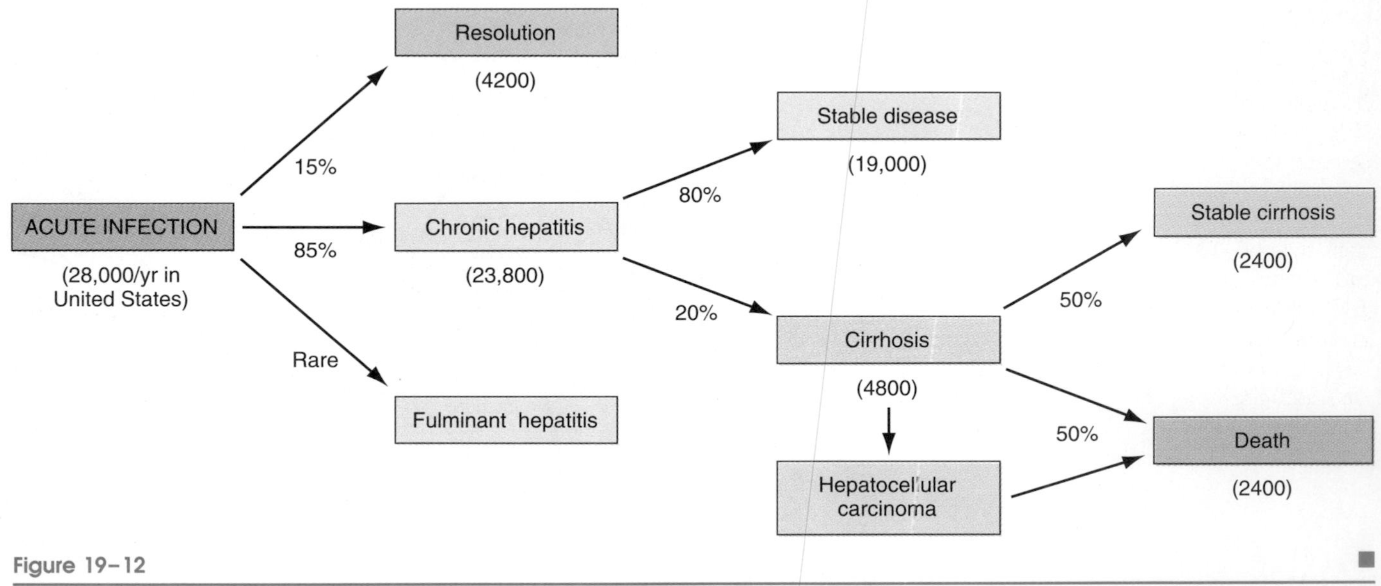

Figure 19–12

Schematic of the potential outcomes of hepatitis C infection in adults in the United States. The population estimates are for new infections. Including diagnoses of previously unsuspected cases of hepatitis C, the annual reported incidence of total cases actually exceeds 100,000, and total annual death rates from hepatitis C infection approach 10,000. (Population estimates based on the consensus report from the National Institutes of Health Consensus Development Conference. Hepatology 26:Suppl 1:1S–153S, 1997.)

HEPATITIS C VIRUS

Hepatitis C virus (HCV) is also a major cause of liver disease worldwide. The main routes of transmission are inoculations and blood transfusions. *HCV is believed to be the most important cause of transfusion-associated hepatitis, being responsible for 90% to 95% of all cases.* Sexual transmission and vertical transmission are infrequent. Sporadic hepatitis of unknown source accounts for 40% of cases. Seroprevalence in the United States population is less than 0.2%, but it is higher in house contacts, homosexuals, hemodialysis patients, hemophiliacs, and intravenous drug abusers (the last approaching 50% to 90%). Patients with unexplained cirrhosis and hepatocellular carcinoma have anti-HCV prevalence rates exceeding 50%. *In contrast to HBV, HCV has a high rate of progression to chronic disease or eventual cirrhosis, exceeding 50%* (Fig. 19–12). *Thus, HCV may in fact be the leading infectious cause of chronic liver disease in the Western world.*

HCV, and the closely related hepatitis G virus, occupy a genus in the Flaviviridae. HCV is a small, enveloped, single-stranded RNA virus with a genome that codes for a single polyprotein (Fig. 19–13). This peptide is subsequently processed into functional proteins. The HCV virus is inherently unstable, giving rise to multiple types and subtypes. This variability has seriously hampered efforts to develop an HCV vaccine. In particular, *elevated titers of anti-HCV IgG occurring after an active infection do not confer effective immunity.* A characteristic feature of HCV infection, therefore, is repeated bouts of hepatic damage, the result of reactivation of a preexisting infection or emergence of an endogenous, newly mutated strain. *Persistent infection and chronic hepatitis are the hallmarks of HCV infection*, despite the generally asymptomatic nature of the acute illness. *Cirrhosis can be present at the time of diagnosis or may develop during a period of 5 to 10 years.*

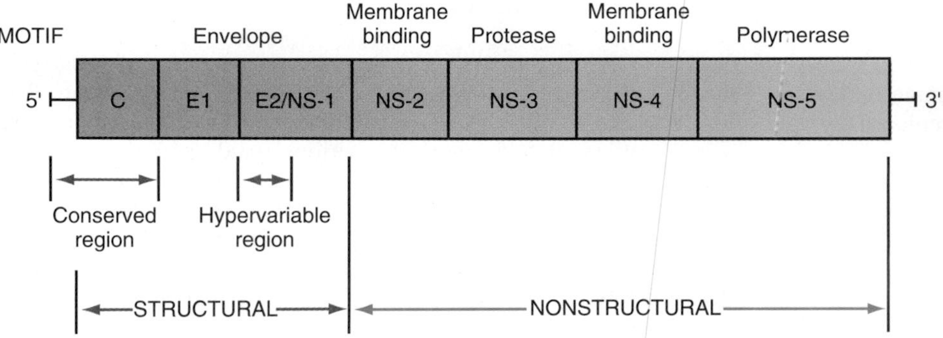

Figure 19–13

Diagrammatic representation of the genomic structure of hepatitis C virus. A single open reading frame codes for core (C) and envelope (E) proteins, as well as for a series of nonstructural (NS) proteins. Notably, most of the genome exhibits variability, with only the 5′ end being well-conserved among different genotypes.

Serologic Diagnosis. The incubation period for HCV hepatitis ranges from 2 to 26 weeks, with a mean between 6 and 12 weeks. HCV RNA is detectable in blood for 1 to 3 weeks, coincident with elevations in serum transaminases (Fig. 19–14*A*). Circulating RNA persists in many patients despite the presence of neutralizing antibodies, including more than 90% of patients with chronic disease. The clinical course of acute HCV hepatitis is likely to be milder than that of HBV, but individual cases may be severe and indistinguishable from HAV or HBV hepatitis. *In chronic HCV infection, a characteristic clinical feature is episodic elevations in serum transaminases, with intervening normal or near-normal periods* (Fig. 19–14*B*). Alternatively, transaminases may be persistently elevated or may remain normal.

HEPATITIS D VIRUS

Also called the delta agent and hepatitis delta virus, HDV is a unique RNA virus that is replication defective, causing infection only when it is encapsulated by HBsAg. Thus, *although taxonomically distinct from HBV, HDV is absolutely dependent on the genetic information provided by HBV for multiplication and causes hepatitis only in the presence of HBV.* Delta hepatitis thus arises in two settings[15] (Fig. 19–15):

- *Acute coinfection* occurs after exposure to serum containing both HDV and HBV. The HBV must become established first to provide the HBsAg necessary for development of complete HDV virions.
- *Superinfection* of a chronic carrier of HBV with a new

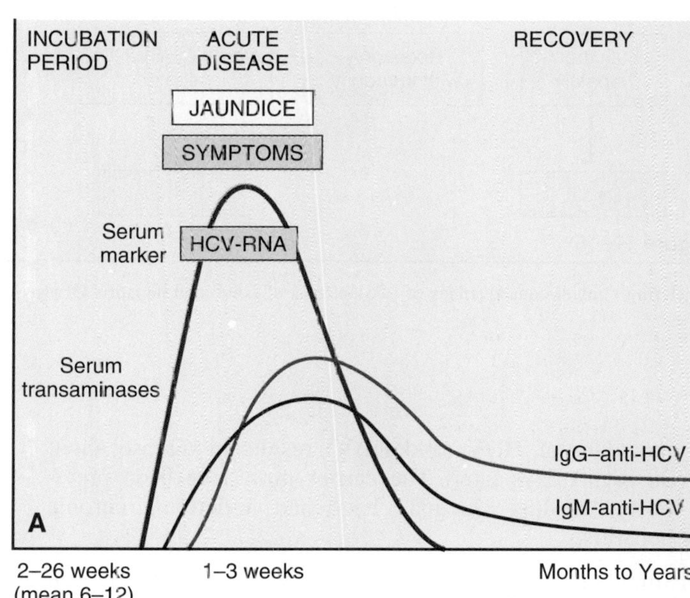

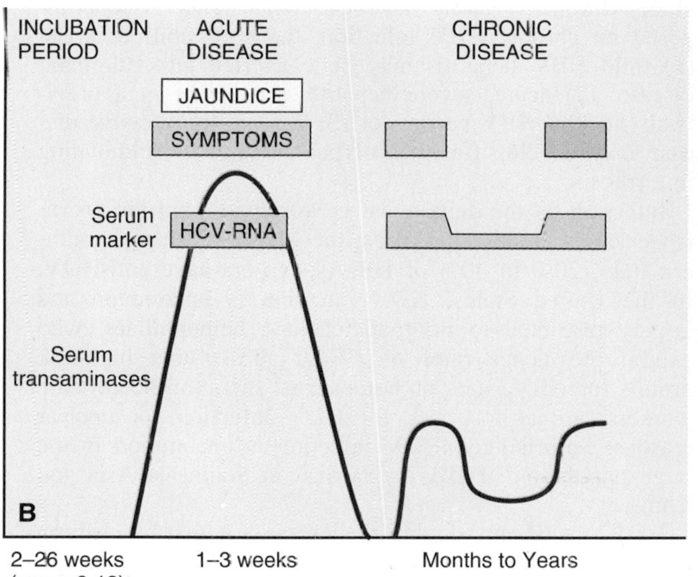

Figure 19–14

Sequence of serologic markers for hepatitis C viral hepatitis demonstrating *(A)* acute infection with resolution and *(B)* progression to chronic relapsing infection.

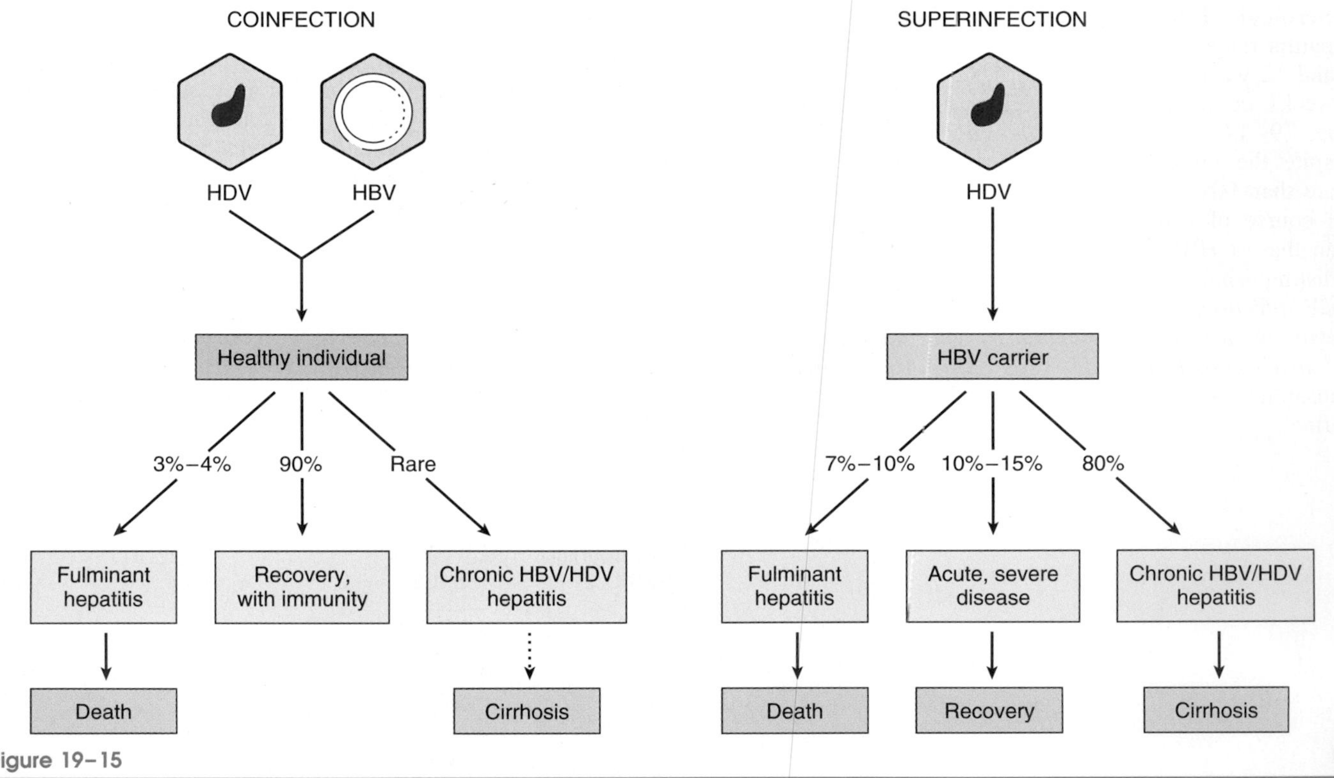

Figure 19–15

Differing clinical consequences of two patterns of combined hepatitis D virus and hepatitis B virus infection.

inoculum of HDV (and HBV) results in disease about 30 to 50 days later. The carrier may have been previously "healthy" or may have had underlying chronic hepatitis.

Simultaneous coinfection with HBV and HDV results in hepatitis ranging from mild to fulminant, with fulminant disease more likely (about 3% to 4%) than with HBV alone. Chronicity rarely develops. When HDV is superimposed on chronic HBV infection, three possibilities arise: (1) mild HBV hepatitis may be converted into fulminant disease; (2) acute, severe hepatitis may erupt in a previously healthy HBV carrier; or (3) chronic, progressive disease may develop (in 80% of patients), often culminating in cirrhosis.

Infection by the delta agent is worldwide, but the prevalence varies greatly. In Africa, the Middle East, and southern Italy, 20% to 40% of HBsAg carriers have anti-HDV. In the United States, HDV infection is uncommon and largely restricted to drug addicts and hemophiliacs, who exhibit prevalence rates of 1% to 10%. Other high-risk groups for HBV, such as homosexual men and health care workers, are at low risk for HDV infection for unclear reasons. Surprisingly, HDV infection is uncommon in the large population of HBsAg carriers in Southeast Asia and China.

HDV is a 35-nm, double-shelled particle that by electron microscopy resembles the Dane particle of HBV. The external coat antigen of HBsAg surrounds an internal polypeptide assembly, designated delta antigen (HDAg). Associated with HDAg is a circular molecule of single-stranded RNA, whose length is smaller than the genome of any known animal virus.[16] This RNA is considered "genomic," but HDAg is the only HDV-encoded protein product detected to date.

Serologic Diagnosis. HDV RNA is detectable in the blood and liver just before and in the early days of acute symptomatic disease (Fig. 19–16*A*). IgM anti-HDV is the most reliable indicator of recent HDV exposure, although its appearance is late and frequently short-lived. Nevertheless, acute coinfection by HDV and HBV is best indicated by detection of IgM against both HDAg and HBcAg (denoting new infection with hepatitis B). With chronic delta hepatitis arising from HDV superinfection (Fig. 19–16*B*), HBsAg is present in serum and IgM anti-HDV persists for months or longer.

HEPATITIS E VIRUS

Hepatitis E virus (HEV) hepatitis is an enterically transmitted, water-borne infection occurring primarily in young to middle-aged adults; sporadic infection and overt illness in children are rare.[17] Epidemics have been reported from Asia and the Indian subcontinent, sub-Saharan Africa, and Mexico. Sporadic infection seems to be uncommon and is seen mainly in travelers. *A characteristic feature of the infection is the high mortality rate among pregnant women,*

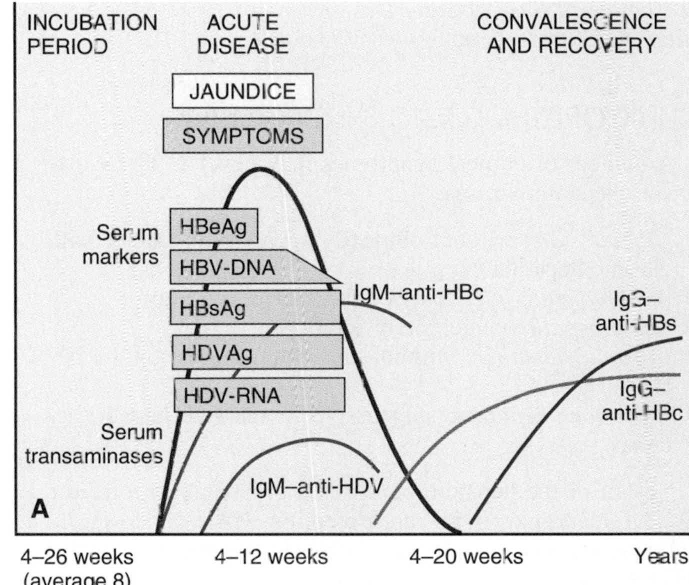

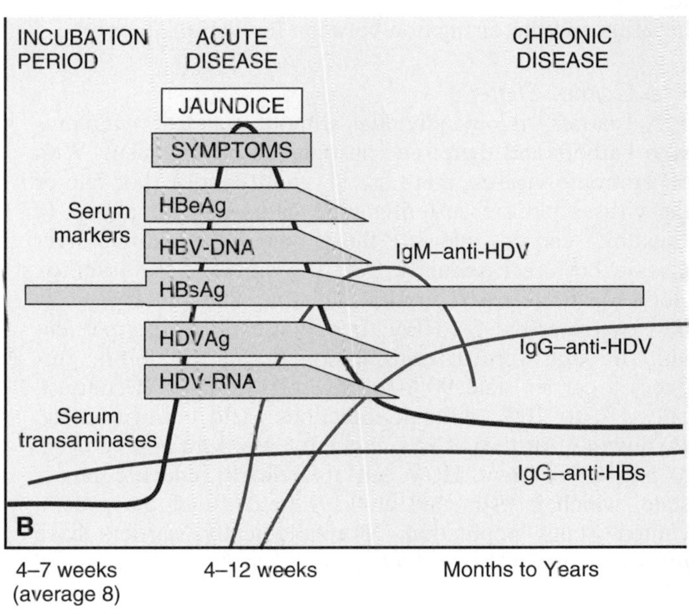

Figure 19–16 ■

Sequence of serologic markers for hepatitis D viral hepatitis depicting *(A)* coinfection with hepatitis B virus (HBV) and *(B)* superinfection of an HBV carrier.

approaching 20%. In most cases, the disease is self-limited; HEV is not associated with chronic liver disease or persistent viremia. The average incubation period after exposure is 6 weeks.

HEV is an unenveloped single-stranded RNA virus that is structurally similar to the Caliciviridae.[18] A specific antigen (HEV Ag) can be identified in the cytoplasm of hepatocytes during active infection, and virions are shed in stool during the acute illness.

Serologic Diagnosis. Before onset of clinical illness, HEV RNA and HEV virions can be detected in stool and liver. The onset of rising serum transaminases, clinical illness, and elevated IgM anti-HEV titers are virtually simultaneous. Symptoms resolve in 2 to 4 weeks, during which time the IgM is replaced with a persistent IgG anti-HEV titer.

OTHER HEPATITIS VIRUSES

Epidemiologic studies have established that some cases of hepatitis are caused by infectious agents other than those listed earlier. A viral agent bearing similarities to HCV has been cloned and designated hepatitis G virus (HGV). Transmission by transfusion has been documented, and evidence of HGV exposure has been found in 1% to 2% of blood donors in the United States. However, *HGV appears to be nonpathogenic, causing neither liver disease nor ex-*

acerbation of liver disease. Designation of HGV as a "hepatitis" virus may therefore be premature.

CLINICOPATHOLOGIC SYNDROMES

A number of clinical syndromes may develop after exposure to hepatitis viruses:

- *Carrier state*: without clinically apparent disease or with chronic hepatitis
- *Asymptomatic infection*: serologic evidence only
- *Acute hepatitis*: anicteric or icteric
- *Chronic hepatitis*: without or with progression to cirrhosis
- *Fulminant hepatitis*: submassive to massive hepatic necrosis

Not all of the hepatotropic viruses provoke each of these clinical syndromes; with rare exception, HAV and HEV do not generate a carrier state or cause chronic hepatitis. *Other infectious or noninfectious causes, particularly drugs and toxins, can lead to essentially identical syndromes.* Therefore, serologic studies are integral for the diagnosis of viral hepatitis and the distinction between the various types.

The Carrier State

A "carrier" is an individual without manifest symptoms who harbors and therefore can transmit an organism. With hepatotropic viruses, there are (1) those who harbor one of the viruses but are suffering little or no adverse effects (a "healthy" carrier) and (2) those who have chronic liver disease but are essentially free of symptoms or disability. Both constitute reservoirs of infection. The carrier state is best characterized for HBV. Infection early in life, particularly through vertical transmission during childbirth, produces a carrier state 90% to 95% of the time. In contrast, only 1% to 10% of adult infections yield a carrier state. *Individuals with impaired immunity are particularly likely to become carriers.* HCV can also clearly induce a carrier state, which is estimated at 0.2% to 0.6% of the general United States population. Morphologically, carriers have normal livers, a few ground-glass hepatocytes with sanded nuclei (HBV), or, in the case of HCV, evidence of chronic hepatitis.

Asymptomatic Infection

Not surprisingly, patients in this group are identified only incidentally on the basis of minimally elevated serum transaminases or after the fact by the presence of antiviral antibodies.

Acute Viral Hepatitis

Any one of the hepatotropic viruses can cause acute viral hepatitis. Whatever the agent, *the disease is more or less the same and can be divided into four phases: (1) an incubation period, (2) a symptomatic preicteric phase, (3) a symptomatic icteric phase, and (4) convalescence.* The *incubation period* for the different viruses is given in Table 19–5. Peak infectivity occurs during the last asymptomatic days of the incubation period and the early days of acute symptoms.

The *preicteric phase* is marked by nonspecific, constitutional symptoms. Malaise is followed in a few days by general fatigability, nausea, and loss of appetite. Weight loss, low-grade fever, headaches, muscle and joint aches, and pains and diarrhea are inconstant symptoms. About 10% of patients with acute hepatitis, most often those with hepatitis B, develop a serum sickness–like syndrome. This consists of fever, rash, and arthralgias attributable to circulating immune complexes. The true origin of all these symptoms is suggested by elevated serum aminotransferase levels. Physical examination reveals a mildly enlarged, tender liver.

In some patients, the nonspecific symptoms are more severe, with higher fever, shaking chills, and headache, sometimes accompanied by right upper quadrant pain and tender liver enlargement. Surprisingly, as jaundice appears and these patients enter the *icteric phase*, other symptoms begin to abate. The jaundice is caused predominantly by conjugated hyperbilirubinemia and hence is accompanied by dark-colored urine related to the presence of conjugated bilirubin. The stools may become light colored, and the retention of bile salts may cause distressing skin itching (pruritus). Laboratory findings include prolonged prothrombin time and hyperglobulinemia; the serum alkaline phosphatase is usually only mildly elevated. An icteric phase is usual in adults (but not children) with HAV but is absent in about half the cases of HBV and most cases of HCV. In a few weeks to perhaps several months, the jaundice and most of the other systemic symptoms clear as convalescence begins.

Chronic Viral Hepatitis

Chronic hepatitis is defined as symptomatic, biochemical, or serologic evidence of continuing or relapsing hepatic disease for more than 6 months, with histologically documented inflammation and necrosis. Although the hepatitis viruses are responsible for most cases of chronic hepatitis, there are many other causes of chronic hepatitis (described later). They include Wilson disease, α_1-antitrypsin deficiency, chronic alcoholism, drugs (isoniazid, methyldopa, methotrexate), and autoimmunity.

From 1968 to the early 1990s, chronic hepatitis was classified according to the histologic extent of inflammation. However, it is now apparent that *etiology rather than the histologic pattern is the single most important factor determining the probability of developing progressive chronic hepatitis.* In particular, HCV is notorious for causing a chronic hepatitis evolving to cirrhosis in a high percentage of patients (see Fig. 19–14), regardless of histologic features at the time of initial evaluation.

The clinical features of chronic hepatitis are extremely variable and are not predictive of outcome. In some patients, the only signs of chronic disease are persistent elevations of serum transaminases, hence the misleading designation "transaminitis." The most common symptom is fatigue; less commonly, there are malaise, loss of appetite, and occasional bouts of mild jaundice. Physical findings are few, the most common being spider angiomas, palmar erythema, mild hepatomegaly, hepatic tenderness, and mild splenomegaly. Laboratory studies may reveal prolongation

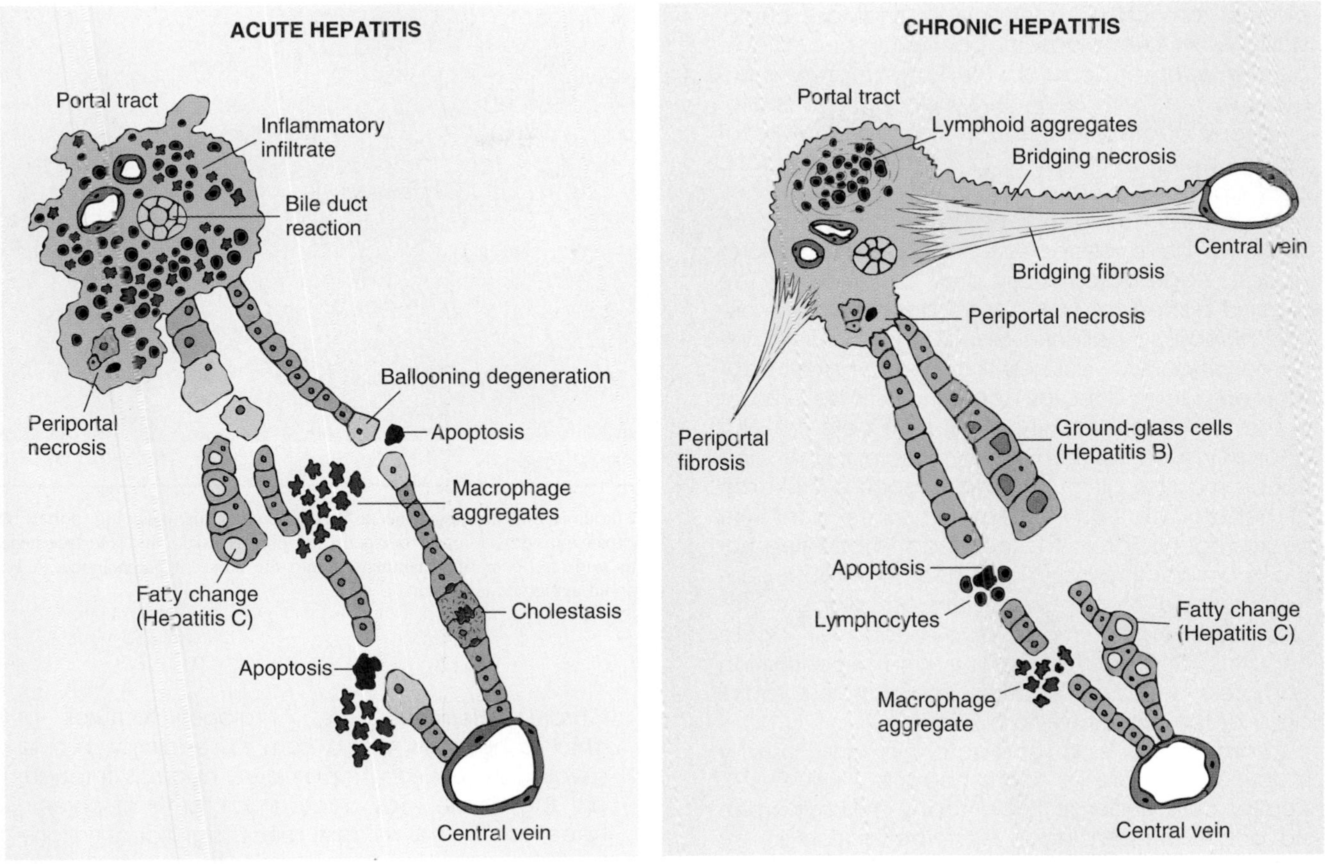

ACUTE HEPATITIS

Portal tract
Inflammatory infiltrate
Bile duct reaction
Ballooning degeneration
Apoptosis
Periportal necrosis
Macrophage aggregates
Fatty change (Hepatitis C)
Cholestasis
Apoptosis
Central vein

CHRONIC HEPATITIS

Portal tract
Lymphoid aggregates
Bridging necrosis
Central vein
Bridging fibrosis
Periportal necrosis
Periportal fibrosis
Ground-glass cells (Hepatitis B)
Apoptosis
Lymphocytes
Fatty change (Hepatitis C)
Macrophage aggregate
Central vein

Figure 19–17

Diagrammatic representation of the morphologic features of acute and chronic hepatitis.

of the prothrombin time and, in some instances, hyperglobulinemia, hyperbilirubinemia, and mild elevations in alkaline phosphatase levels. In cases of HBV and HCV infection, immune complex disease may occasionally develop secondary to the presence of circulating antibody-antigen complexes, taking the form of vasculitis (subcutaneous or visceral, Chapter 12) and glomerulonephritis (Chapter 22). Cryoglobulinemia is found in about 35% of patients with chronic HCV hepatitis.

MORPHOLOGY OF ACUTE AND CHRONIC HEPATITIS. The general morphologic features of viral hepatitis are depicted schematically in Figure 19–17. **The morphologic changes in acute and chronic viral hepatitis are shared among the hepatotropic viruses and can be mimicked by drug reactions.** Although most viruses do not impart specific cytopathic changes, **HBV infection may generate "ground-glass" hepatocytes** (Fig. 19–18): a finely granular, eosinophilic cytoplasm shown by electron microscopy to be spheres and tubules of HBsAg. Other HBV-infected hepatocytes may have **"sanded" nuclei** due to abundant HBcAg, indicating active viral replication.

Acute Hepatitis. With acute hepatitis, hepatocyte injury takes the form of diffuse swelling **(ballooning degeneration),** so that the cytoplasm looks empty and contains only scattered wisps of cyto-

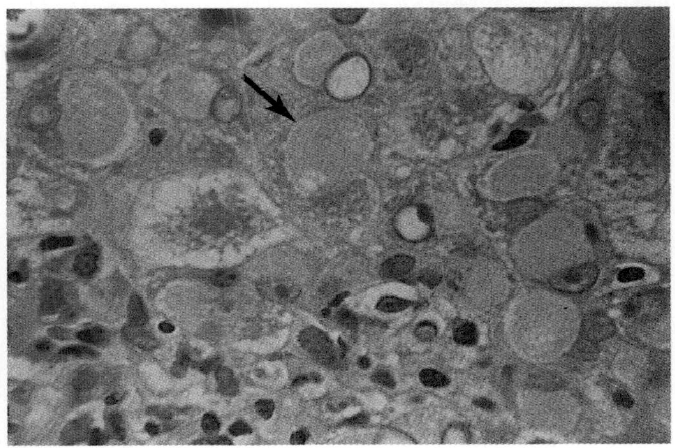

Figure 19–18

Ground-glass hepatocytes *(arrow)* in HBV infection (H & E.)

plasmic remnants. An inconstant finding is **cholestasis,** with bile plugs in canaliculi and brown pigmentation of hepatocytes. **Fatty change** is unusual except with HCV. Two patterns of hepatocyte cell death are seen. In the first, rupture of cell membranes leads to cytolysis. The necrotic cells appear to have "dropped out," with collapse of the collagen reticulin framework where the cells have disappeared; scavenger **macrophage aggregates** mark sites of dropout. The second pattern of cell death, **apoptosis,** is more conspicuous. Apoptotic hepatocytes shrink, become intensely eosinophilic, and have fragmented nuclei; effector T cells may still be present in the immediate vicinity. Apoptotic cells are also phagocytosed within hours by macrophages and hence may be difficult to find despite a brisk rate of hepatocyte injury. In severe cases, confluent necrosis of hepatocytes may lead to **bridging necrosis** connecting portal to portal, central to central, or portal to central regions of adjacent lobules, signifying a more severe form of acute hepatitis. Hepatocyte swelling and regeneration compress sinusoids, and the more or less radial array of the parenchyma is lost.

Inflammation is a characteristic and usually prominent feature of acute hepatitis (Fig. 19–19). **Kupffer cells undergo hypertrophy and hyperplasia** and are often laden with lipofuscin pigment because of phagocytosis of hepatocellular debris. **The portal tracts are usually infiltrated with a mixture of inflammatory cells.** The inflammatory infiltrate may spill over into the adjacent parenchyma to cause necrosis of periportal hepatocytes—this "interface hepatitis" can occur in both acute and chronic hepatitis. Finally, bile duct epithelia may become reactive and even proliferate to form poorly defined ductular structures, particularly in cases of HCV hepatitis.

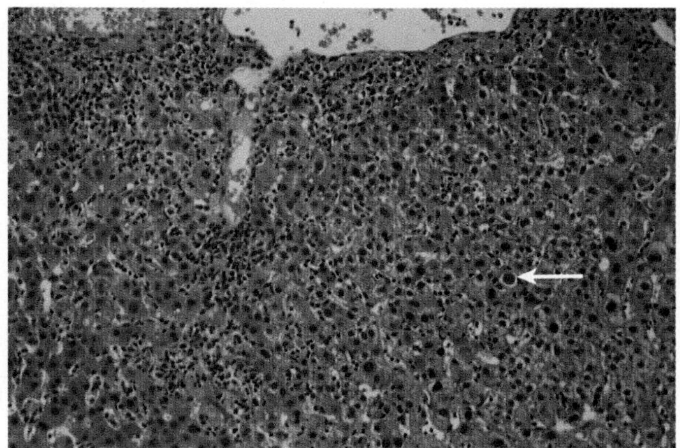

Figure 19–19

Acute viral hepatitis showing disruption of lobular architecture, inflammatory cells in the sinusoids, and hepatocellular apoptosis *(arrow).*

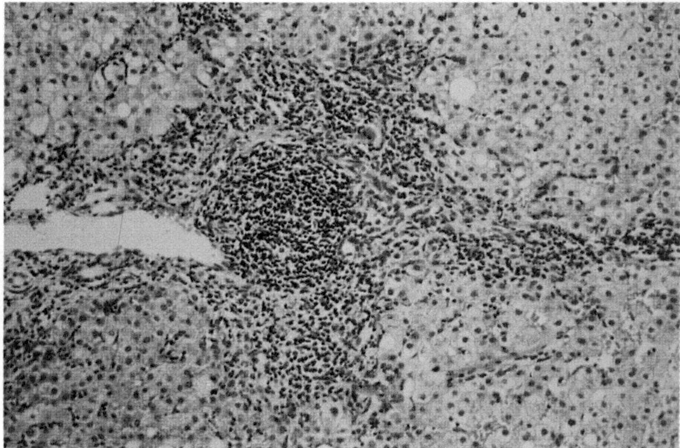

Figure 19–20

Chronic viral hepatitis due to hepatitis C virus, showing portal tract expansion with inflammatory cells and fibrous tissue, and interface hepatitis with spillover of inflammation into the adjacent parenchyma. A lymphoid aggregate is present.

Chronic Hepatitis. The histologic features of chronic hepatitis range from exceedingly mild to severe. Smoldering hepatocyte necrosis throughout the lobule may occur in all forms of chronic hepatitis. In the mildest forms, significant inflammation is limited to portal tracts and consists of lymphocytes, macrophages, occasional plasma cells, and rare neutrophils or eosinophils. **Lymphoid aggregates** in the portal tract are often seen in HCV infection (Fig. 19–20). Liver architecture is usually well preserved. Continued **interface hepatitis** and **bridging necrosis** are harbingers of progressive liver damage. **The hallmark of irreversible liver damage is the deposition of fibrous tissue.** At first, only portal tracts exhibit increased fibrosis, but **periportal fibrosis** occurs with time, followed by linking of fibrous septa between lobules **(bridging fibrosis).**

Continued loss of hepatocytes and fibrosis results in cirrhosis, with fibrous septa and hepatocyte regenerative nodules. This pattern of cirrhosis is characterized by irregularly sized nodules separated by variable but mostly broad scars (Fig. 19–21). Historically, this pattern of cirrhosis has been termed **postnecrotic cirrhosis,** but many other causes may give rise to a cirrhotic liver with large nodules, and the term is better avoided. In some cases that come to autopsy, the inciting cause of such broad scars cannot be determined at all ("cryptogenic cirrhosis").

The clinical course of viral hepatitis is unpredictable. Patients may experience spontaneous remission or may have indolent disease without progression for many years. Conversely, some patients have rapidly progressive disease and develop cirrhosis within a few years. The major causes

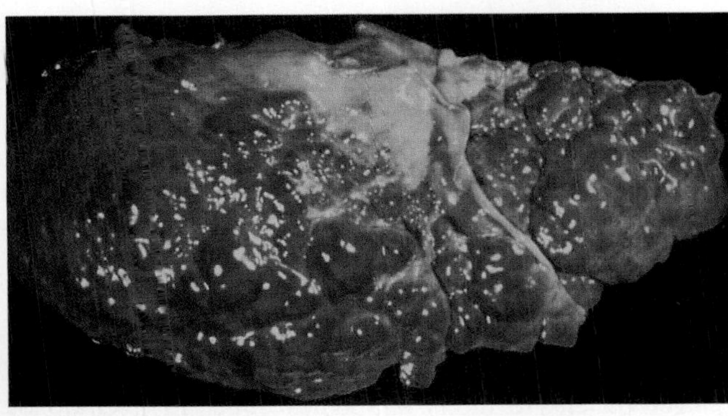

Figure 19–21

Cirrhosis resulting from chronic viral hepatitis. Note broad scar and coarse nodular surface.

of death are twofold: cirrhosis, with liver failure and hepatic encephalopathy or massive hematemesis from esophageal varices; and hepatocellular carcinoma in those with long-standing HBV (particularly neonatal) or HCV infection.

Fulminant Hepatitis

When hepatic insufficiency progresses from onset of symptoms to hepatic encephalopathy within 2 to 3 weeks, it is termed *fulminant hepatic failure*. A less rapid course, extending up to 3 months, is called *subfulminant failure*.

Fulminant viral hepatitis is the cause of 50% to 65% of cases of fulminant hepatic failure. It can be induced by hepatitis viruses A, B, C, D (either coinfection or superinfection with B virus), and E. Reactivation of chronic hepatitis B or acute herpesvirus infection is sometimes the cause.

Drug and chemical toxicity make up most of the remainder (25% to 30%), acting either as direct hepatotoxins or by idiosyncratic inflammatory reactions. Principally implicated are acetaminophen (in suicidal doses), isoniazid, antidepressants (particularly monoamine oxidase inhibitors), halothane, methyldopa, and the mycotoxins of the mushroom *Amanita phalloides*.

Much more rare, but just as life threatening, are ischemic hepatic necrosis, obstruction of the hepatic veins, massive malignant infiltration of the liver, Wilson disease, hyperthermia (heat stroke), and microvesicular steatosis syndromes, particularly acute fatty liver of pregnancy.

MORPHOLOGY. All causative agents produce essentially identical morphologic changes that vary with the severity of the necrotizing process. With all, the distribution of liver destruction is extremely capricious: **the entire liver may be involved, or only random areas.** With massive loss of substance, the liver may shrink to as little as 500 to 700 gm. In so doing, it is transformed into a limp, red organ covered by a wrinkled, too-large capsule. On transection, necrotic areas have a muddy red, mushy appearance with blotchy bile staining. On microscopic examination, complete destruction of hepatocytes in contiguous lobules leaves only a collapsed reticulin framework and preserved portal tracts. There may be surprisingly little inflammatory reaction. Alternatively, with survival for several days, there is a massive influx of inflammatory cells to begin the phagocytic cleanup process.

Survival of the patient for more than a week permits secondary regenerative activity of surviving hepatocytes. With zonal necrosis, the parenchymal framework is preserved, regeneration is orderly, and native liver architecture is restored in time. With more massive destruction of confluent lobules, regeneration is disorderly, yielding nodular masses of liver cells. Scarring may occur in patients with a protracted course of submassive or patchy necrosis, representing a route for developing so-called postnecrotic cirrhosis, as noted earlier.

Fulminant hepatic failure may present as jaundice, encephalopathy, and fetor hepaticus, as described previously. Notably absent on physical examination are stigmata of chronic liver disease (e.g., gynecomastia, spider angiomas). Life-threatening extrahepatic complications include coagulopathy and bleeding, cardiovascular instability, renal failure, adult respiratory distress syndrome, electrolyte and acid-base disturbances, and sepsis. Overall mortality ranges from 25% to 90% in the absence of liver transplantation.

Bacterial, Parasitic, and Helminthic Infections

Extrahepatic bacterial infections, particularly sepsis, can induce mild hepatic inflammation and varying degrees of hepatocellular cholestasis. The latter effect is attributable to the effects of proinflammatory cytokines, released by Kupffer cells and endothelial cells in response to circulating endotoxin. A number of bacteria can infect the liver directly, including *Staphylococcus aureus* in the setting of toxic shock syndrome, *Salmonella typhi* in the setting of typhoid fever, and secondary or tertiary syphilis. Alternatively, bacteria may proliferate in a biliary tree compromised by partial or complete obstruction. The bacterial composition reflects the gut flora, and the severe acute inflammatory response within the intrahepatic biliary tree is called *ascending cholangitis*.

Parasitic and helminthic infections are major causes of morbidity worldwide, and the liver is frequently involved. Diseases discussed in Chapter 9 include malaria, schistosomiasis, strongyloidiasis, cryptosporidiosis, leishmaniasis, and infections by the liver flukes *Fasciola hepatica, Clonorchis sinensis*, and *Opisthorchis viverrini*. A form of liver infection deserving special mention is the liver abscess.

In developing countries, liver abscesses are common; most represent parasitic infections, for example, amebic, echinococcal, and (less commonly) other protozoal and helminthic organisms. In developed countries, liver abscesses are uncommon; a low incidence of amebic diseases is encountered, usually in immigrants from endemic regions. Most abscesses are pyogenic, representing a complication of a bacterial infection elsewhere. The organisms reach the liver by (1) the portal vein, (2) arterial supply, (3) ascending infection in the biliary tract (ascending cholangitis), (4) direct invasion of the liver from a nearby source, or (5) a penetrating injury. The majority of hepatic abscesses used to result from portal spread of intra-abdominal infections (e.g., appendicitis, diverticulitis, colitis). With improved management of these conditions, spread now occurs primarily through the biliary tree or the arterial supply in patients suffering from some form of immune deficiency (e.g., old age with debilitating disease, immunosuppression, or cancer chemotherapy with marrow failure). In these settings, abscesses may develop without a primary focus elsewhere.

MORPHOLOGY. Pyogenic hepatic abscesses may occur as solitary or multiple lesions, ranging in size from millimeters to massive lesions many centimeters in diameter. Bacteremic spread through the arterial or portal system tends to produce multiple small abscesses, whereas direct extension and trauma usually cause solitary large abscesses. Biliary abscesses, which are usually multiple, may contain purulent material from adjacent bile ducts. Gross and microscopic features are those to be seen in any abscess. The causative organism can occasionally be identified in the case of fungal or parasitic abscesses. On rare occasion, abscesses located in the subdiaphragmatic region, particularly amebic, may burrow into the thoracic cavity to produce empyema or a lung abscess. Rupture of subcapsular liver abscesses has also led to peritonitis or localized peritoneal abscesses.

Liver abscesses are associated with fever and, in many instances, right upper quadrant pain and tender hepatomegaly. Jaundice may result from extrahepatic biliary obstruction. Although antibiotic therapy may control smaller lesions, surgical drainage is often necessary for the larger lesions. Because diagnosis is frequently delayed, and because patients are often elderly and have serious coexistent disease, the mortality rate with large liver abscesses ranges from 30% to 90%. With early recognition and management, up to 80% of patients may survive.[19]

AUTOIMMUNE HEPATITIS

Autoimmune hepatitis is a syndrome of chronic hepatitis in patients with a heterogeneous set of immunologic abnormalities. The histologic features are indistinguishable from chronic viral hepatitis. This disease may run an indolent or severe course and typically responds dramatically to immunosuppressive therapy. Salient features include

- Female predominance (70%), particularly young to perimenopausal women
- The absence of viral serologic markers
- Elevated serum IgG levels (>2.5 gm/dl)
- High serum titers of autoantibodies in 80% of cases, including antinuclear, anti–smooth muscle, and antimitochondrial antibodies
- An increased frequency of HLA-B8 or HLA-DRw3

Other forms of autoimmune disease are present in up to 60% of patients, including rheumatoid arthritis, thyroiditis, Sjögren syndrome, and ulcerative colitis. A subgroup of younger patients exhibits antibodies either to liver/kidney microsomes or "soluble liver antigen" (cytokeratins 8 and 18), suggesting that three types of autoimmune hepatitis exist.

Clinical presentation is similar to other forms of chronic hepatitis; these tend to be the more severely affected patients, for whom immunosuppressive therapy is indicated. Autoimmune hepatitis may present in an atypical fashion with associated disease involving other organ systems, hampering diagnostic efforts. Alternatively, clinical autoimmune hepatitis exhibiting destruction of bile ducts ("autoimmune cholangitis") may make distinction from primary biliary cirrhosis or primary sclerosing cholangitis (discussed later) difficult.[20]

DRUG- AND TOXIN-INDUCED LIVER DISEASE

As the major drug metabolizing and detoxifying organ in the body, the liver is subject to potential damage from an enormous array of pharmaceutical and environmental chemicals.[21] Injury may result (1) from direct toxicity, (2) by hepatic conversion of a xenobiotic to an active toxin, or (3) through immune mechanisms, usually by a drug or a metabolite acting as a hapten to convert a cellular protein into an immunogen.

Principles of drug and toxic injury are discussed in Chapter 10. Here it suffices to recall that drug reactions may be classified as *predictable (intrinsic)* reactions or *unpredictable (idiosyncratic)* ones. Predictable drug reactions may occur in anyone who accumulates a sufficient dose. Unpredictable reactions depend on idiosyncrasies of the host, particularly the host's propensity to mount an immune response to the antigenic stimulus and the rate at which the host metabolizes the agent. Major examples include chlorpromazine, an agent that causes cholestasis in those patients who are slow to metabolize it to an innocuous byproduct, and halothane, which can cause a fatal immune-mediated hepatitis in some patients exposed to this anesthetic on multiple occasions. A broad classification of offending agents is offered in Table 19–4. It should be noted that

- The injury may be immediate or take weeks to months to develop, presenting only after severe liver damage has developed.
- The injury may take the form of *hepatocyte necrosis*, *cholestasis*, or *insidious onset of liver dysfunction*.

■ *Drug-induced chronic hepatitis is clinically and histologically indistinguishable from chronic viral hepatitis, and hence serologic markers of viral infection are critical for making the distinction.*

Among the agents listed in Table 19–4, predictable drug reactions are ascribed to acetaminophen, tetracycline, antineoplastic agents, *Amanita phalloides* toxin, carbon tetrachloride, and, to a certain extent, alcohol. Many others, such as sulfonamides, methyldopa, and allopurinol, cause idiosyncratic reactions.

Reye syndrome, a potentially fatal syndrome of mitochondrial dysfunction in liver, brain, and elsewhere, occurs predominantly in children given acetylsalicylic acid (aspirin) for the relief of virus-induced fever. This disease, which features extensive accumulation of fat droplets within hepatocytes (microvesicular steatosis), is exceedingly rare. A causal relationship with use of salicylates was never established, but a national campaign in the 1970s and 1980s condemning the use of aspirin in children with febrile illness may have served to break the Reye syndrome epidemic.

Drug-induced liver disease is usually followed by recovery on removal of the drug. *Exposure to a toxin or therapeutic agent should always be included in the differential diagnosis of liver disease.*

Alcoholic Liver Disease

Excessive alcohol consumption is the leading cause of liver disease in most Western countries. These United States statistics attest to the magnitude of the problem[22]:

- More than 10 million Americans are alcoholics.
- Alcohol abuse causes 200,000 deaths annually, the fifth-leading cause of death, many related to automobile accidents.
- Twenty-five per cent to 30% of hospitalized patients have problems related to alcohol abuse.

Table 19–4. DRUG- AND TOXIN-INDUCED HEPATIC INJURY

Hepatocellular Damage	Examples
Microvesicular fatty change	• Tetracycline, salicylates, yellow phosphorus, ethanol
Macrovesicular fatty change	• Ethanol, methotrexate, amiodarone
Centrilobular necrosis	• Bromobenzene, CCl_4, acetaminophen, halothane, rifampin
Diffuse or massive necrosis	• Halothane, isoniazid, acetaminophen, methyldopa, trinitrotoluene, *Amanita phalloides* (mushroom) toxin
Hepatitis, acute and chronic	• Methyldopa, isoniazid, nitrofurantoin, phenytoin, oxyphenisatin
Fibrosis-cirrhosis	• Ethanol, methotrexate, amiodarone, most drugs that cause chronic hepatitis
Granuloma formation	• Sulfonamides, methyldopa, quinidine, phenylbutazone, hydralazine, allopurinol
Cholestasis (with or without hepatocellular injury)	• Chlorpromazine, anabolic steroids, erythromycin estolate, oral contraceptives, organic arsenicals

Chronic alcohol consumption has a variety of adverse effects, as pointed out in Chapter 10. Of greatest impact, however, are the three distinctive, albeit overlapping, forms of liver disease: (1) hepatic steatosis, (2) alcoholic hepatitis, and (3) cirrhosis, collectively referred to as alcoholic liver disease. Because the first two conditions may develop independently, they do not necessarily represent a continuum of changes. The morphology of the three forms of alcoholic liver disease is presented first, because this facilitates consideration of their pathogenesis. The various forms of alcoholic liver disease are depicted in Figure 19–22.

MORPHOLOGY. ***Hepatic Steatosis (Fatty Liver).*** After even moderate intake of alcohol, small **(microvesicular)** lipid droplets accumulate in hepatocytes. With chronic intake of alcohol, lipid accumulates to the point of creating large clear **macrovesicular** globules, compressing and displacing the nucleus to the periphery of the hepatocyte. This transformation is initially centrilobular, but it may involve the entire lobule in severe cases (Fig. 19–23). In macroscopic appearance, the fatty liver of chronic alcoholism is a large (up to 4 to 6 kg) soft organ that is yellow, greasy, and readily fractured. Although there is little or no fibrosis at the outset, fibrous tissue develops around the central veins and extends into the adjacent sinusoids with continued alcohol intake. **Up to the time that fibrosis appears, the fatty change is completely reversible if there is abstention from further intake of alcohol.**

Alcoholic Hepatitis. This is characterized by the following:

- **Hepatocyte swelling and necrosis.** Single or scattered foci of cells undergo swelling (ballooning) and necrosis. The swelling results from the accumulation of fat and water as well as proteins that normally are exported.
- **Mallory bodies.** Scattered hepatocytes accumulate tangled skeins of cytokeratin intermediate filaments and other proteins, visible as eosinophilic cytoplasmic inclusions in degenerating hepatocytes (Fig. 19–24). These inclusions are a characteristic but not specific feature of alcoholic liver disease, as they are also seen in primary biliary cirrhosis, Wilson disease, chronic cholestatic syndromes, and hepatocellular tumors.
- **Neutrophilic reaction.** Neutrophils permeate the lobule and accumulate around degenerating hepatocytes, particularly those having Mallory bodies. Lymphocytes and macrophages also enter portal tracts and spill into the parenchyma.

NORMAL LIVER
Exposure
Abstinence
Severe exposure
Abstinence
STEATOSIS
Fatty change
Perivenular fibrosis
Abstinence
Severe exposure
HEPATITIS
Liver cell necrosis
Inflammation
Mallory bodies
Fatty change
Repeated attacks
Continued exposure
CIRRHOSIS
Fibrosis
Hyperplastic nodules

Figure 19–22 ■

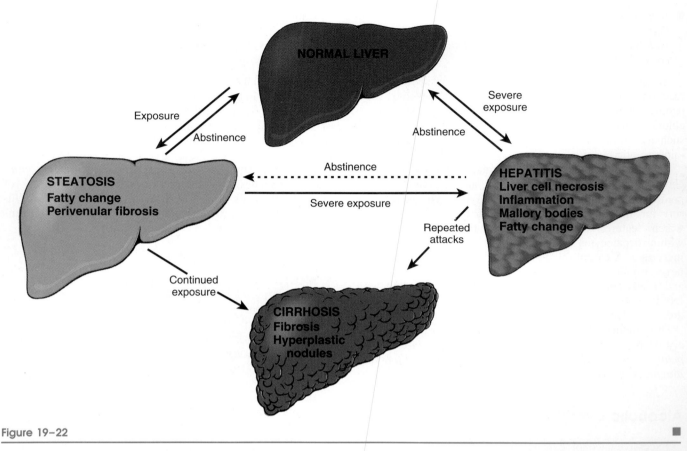

Alcoholic liver disease. The interrelationships among hepatic steatosis, hepatitis, and cirrhosis are shown, along with a depiction of key morphologic features at the morphologic level.

- **Fibrosis.** Alcoholic hepatitis is almost always accompanied by a brisk sinusoidal and perivenular fibrosis; periportal fibrosis may occasionally predominate, particularly with repeated bouts of heavy alcohol intake. In some cases, there is cholestasis and mild deposition of hemosiderin (iron) in hepatocytes and Kupffer cells.

In macroscopic appearance, the liver is mottled red with bile-stained areas. Although the liver may be of normal or increased size, it often contains visible nodules and fibrosis indicative of evolution to cirrhosis.

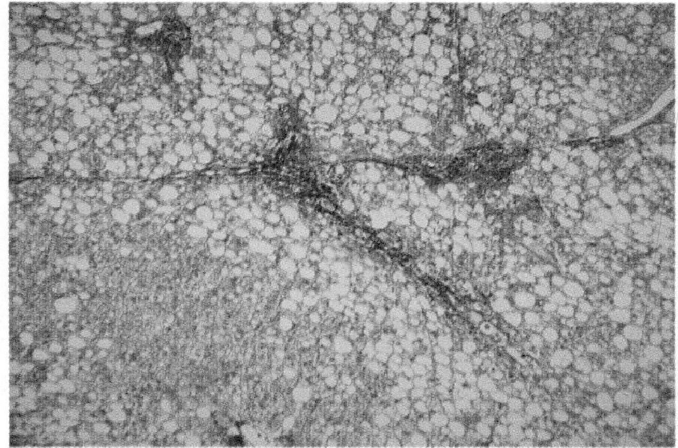

Figure 19–23 ■

Alcoholic liver disease: macrovesicular steatosis, involving most regions of the hepatic lobule. The intracytoplasmic fat is seen as clear vacuoles. Some early fibrosis *(stained blue)* is present. (Masson trichrome.)

Alcoholic Cirrhosis. The final and irreversible form of alcoholic liver disease usually evolves slowly and insidiously. At first the cirrhotic liver is yellow-tan, fatty, and enlarged, usually weighing more than 2 kg. During the span of years, it is transformed into a brown, shrunken, nonfatty organ, sometimes less than 1 kg in weight. Arguably, cirrhosis may develop more rapidly in the setting of alcoholic hepatitis, within 1 to 2 years. Initially, the developing fibrous septa are delicate and extend through sinusoids from central vein to portal regions as well as from portal tract to portal tract. Regenerative activity of entrapped parenchymal hepatocytes generates fairly uniformly sized "micronodules." With time, the nodularity becomes more prominent; scattered larger nodules create a "hobnail" appearance on the surface of the liver (Fig. 19–25*A*). As fibrous septa dissect and surround nodules, the liver becomes more fibrotic,

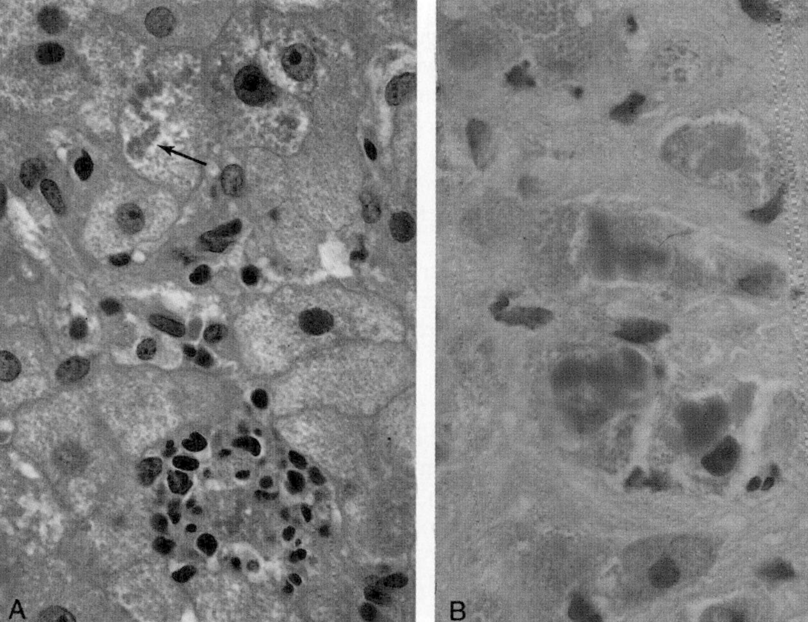

Figure 19–24

Alcoholic hepatitis. *A*, The cluster of inflammatory cells marks the site of a necrotic hepatocyte. A Mallory body is present in a second hepatocyte *(arrow)*. *B*, Eosinophilic Mallory bodies are seen in hepatocytes, which are surrounded by fibrous tissue. (H&E.)

loses fat, and shrinks progressively in size. Parenchymal islands are engulfed by ever wider bands of fibrous tissue, and the liver is converted into a mixed micronodular and macronodular pattern (Fig. 19–25*B*). Ischemic necrosis and fibrous obliteration of nodules eventually create broad expanses of tough, pale scar tissue (Laënnec cirrhosis). Bile stasis often develops; Mallory bodies are only rarely evident at this stage. Thus, **end-stage alcoholic cirrhosis comes to resemble, both macroscopically and microscopically, the cirrhosis developing from viral hepatitis and other causes.**

Pathogenesis. Short-term ingestion of up to 80 gm of ethanol (eight beers or 7 ounces of 80-proof liquor) generally produces mild, reversible hepatic changes, such as fatty liver. Daily intake of 80 gm or more of ethanol generates significant risk for severe hepatic injury, and daily ingestion of 160 gm or more for 10 to 20 years is associated more consistently with severe injury. *Only 10% to 15% of alcoholics, however, develop cirrhosis.* For reasons that may relate to decreased gastric metabolism of ethanol and differences in body composition, women appear to be more susceptible to hepatic injury than are men. Individual, possibly genetic susceptibility must exist, but no reliable genetic markers of susceptibility have been

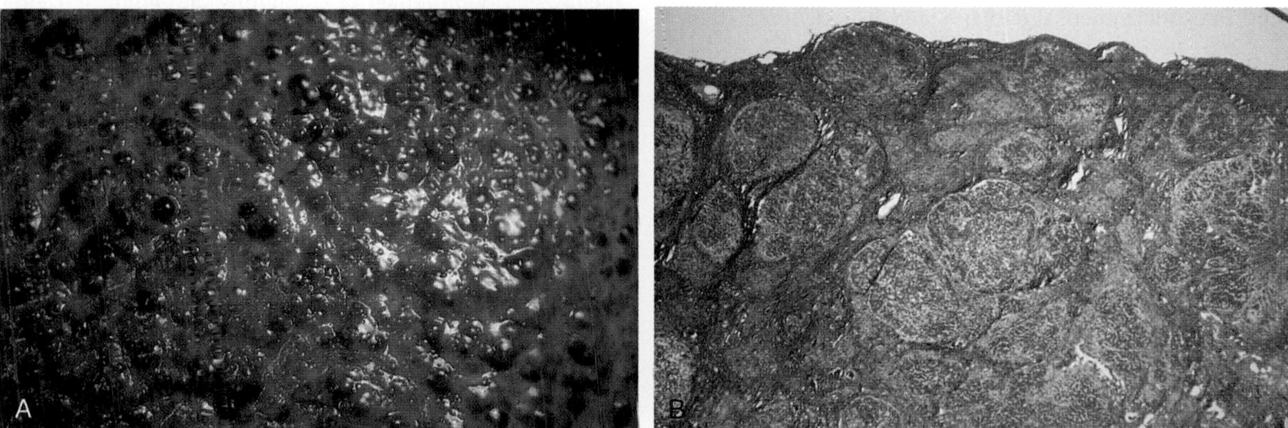

Figure 19–25

Alcoholic cirrhosis. *A*, The characteristic diffuse nodularity of the surface reflects the interplay between nodular regeneration and scarring. The average nodule size is 3 mm in this close-up view. The greenish tint of some nodules is due to bile stasis. *B*, The microscopic view shows nodules of varying sizes entrapped in blue-staining fibrous tissue. The liver capsule is at the top. (Masson trichrome.)

identified. In addition, the relationship between hepatic steatosis and alcoholic hepatitis as precursors to cirrhosis, both causally and temporally, is not yet clear. Cirrhosis may develop without antecedent evidence of steatosis or alcoholic hepatitis. *In the absence of a clear understanding of the pathogenetic factors influencing liver damage, no "safe" upper limit for alcohol consumption can be proposed* (despite the current popularity of red wines for amelioration of coronary vascular disease).

The pharmacokinetics and metabolism of alcohol are examined in Chapter 10. Pertinent to our discussion is the detrimental effect of alcohol and its byproducts on hepatocellular function:

- Hepatocellular steatosis results from (1) the shunting of normal substrates away from catabolism and toward lipid biosynthesis owing to generation of excess nicotinamide adenine dinucleotide (NADH) by the two major enzymes of alcohol metabolism, alcohol dehydrogenase and acetaldehyde dehydrogenase, (2) impaired assembly and secretion of lipoproteins, and (3) increased peripheral catabolism of fat.
- Induction of cytochrome P-450 leads to augmented transformation of other drugs to toxic metabolites.
- Free radicals, generated during microsomal ethanol-oxidizing system oxidation of alcohol, react with cellular membranes and proteins.
- Alcohol directly affects microtubular and mitochondrial function and membrane fluidity.
- Acetaldehyde (the major intermediate metabolite of alcohol en route to acetate production) induces lipid peroxidation and acetaldehyde-protein adduct formation, further disrupting cytoskeletal and membrane function.
- Alcohol induces immunologic attack on hepatic neoantigens, possibly the result of alcohol-induced or acetaldehyde-induced alteration in hepatic proteins.

In addition, alcohol is food and can become a major calorie source in the diet of an alcoholic, displacing other nutrients and leading to malnutrition and vitamin deficiencies (such as vitamin B_{12}). This is compounded by impaired digestive function, primarily related to chronic gastric and intestinal mucosal damage, and pancreatitis.

Collagen deposition by perisinusoidal hepatic stellate cells is a response to many converging events[23]:

- Kupffer cell activation, with release of proinflammatory cytokines (TNF-α, interleukins 1 and 6, transforming growth factor-β)
- Amplification of the cytokine stimuli by platelet-activating factor, a lecithin-related lipid released by endothelial cells and Kupffer cells
- Influx of neutrophils into the parenchyma in response to the proinflammatory cytokines, with release of their noxious substances

These events are set in motion by the local toxic effects of alcohol and by alcohol-induced release of bacterial endotoxin into the portal circulation from a compromised gut. Alcohol also induces release of vasoconstricting endothelins from sinusoidal endothelial cells. Endothelins induce the myofibroblast-like hepatic stellate cells to contract, decreasing sinusoidal perfusion and causing regional hypoxia.

The net effect is a chronic disorder featuring steatosis, hepatitis, progressive fibrosis, and marked derangement of vascular perfusion. In essence, alcoholic liver disease can be regarded as a maladaptive state in which cells in the liver respond in an increasingly pathologic manner to a stimulus (alcohol) that originally was only marginally harmful.

Clinical Course. *Hepatic steatosis* may become evident as hepatomegaly with mild elevation of serum bilirubin and alkaline phosphatase levels. Alternatively, there may be no clinical or biochemical evidence of liver disease. Severe hepatic compromise is unusual. Alcohol withdrawal and the provision of an adequate diet are sufficient treatment.

In contrast, *alcoholic hepatitis* tends to appear relatively acutely, usually after a bout of heavy drinking. Symptoms and laboratory manifestations may be minimal or those of fulminant hepatic failure. Between these two extremes are the nonspecific symptoms of malaise, anorexia, weight loss, upper abdominal discomfort, and tender hepatomegaly and the laboratory findings of hyperbilirubinemia, elevated alkaline phosphatase levels, and often a neutrophilic leukocytosis. An acute cholestatic syndrome may appear, resembling large bile duct obstruction. The outlook is unpredictable; each bout of hepatitis incurs about a 10% to 20% risk of death. With repeated bouts, cirrhosis appears in about one third of patients within a few years. Alcoholic hepatitis may also be superimposed on established cirrhosis. With proper nutrition and total cessation of alcohol consumption, the alcoholic hepatitis may clear slowly. However, in some patients, the hepatitis persists despite abstinence and progresses to cirrhosis.

The manifestations of *alcoholic cirrhosis* are similar to other forms of cirrhosis, presented earlier, and include those of portal hypertension (with life-threatening variceal hemorrhage), jaundice, ascites, and other stigmata (e.g., grossly distended abdomen, wasted extremities, caput medusae). Laboratory findings reflect the developing hepatic compromise, with elevated serum transaminase levels, hyperbilirubinemia, variable elevation of serum alkaline phosphatase, hypoproteinemia (globulins, albumin, and clotting factors), and anemia. In some instances, liver biopsy may be indicated, since experience teaches that in about 10% to 20% of cases of presumed alcoholic cirrhosis, another disease process is found on biopsy. Last, cirrhosis may be clinically silent, discovered only at autopsy or when stress such as infection or trauma tips the balance toward hepatic insufficiency.

The long-term outlook for alcoholics with liver disease is variable. Five-year survival approaches 90% in abstainers who are free of jaundice, ascites, or hematemesis; it drops to 50% to 60% in those who continue to imbibe. In the end-stage alcoholic, the proximate causes of death are (1) hepatic coma, (2) a massive gastrointestinal hemorrhage, (3) an intercurrent infection (to which these patients are predisposed), (4) hepatorenal syndrome after a bout of alcoholic hepatitis, and (5) hepatocellular carcinoma in 3% to 6% of cases.

Mention must be made of an uncommon condition resembling alcoholic hepatitis occurring in patients who do not drink alcohol. Entitled *nonalcoholic steatohepatitis*, this condition features liver biopsy findings of steatosis, a mixed inflammatory infiltrate of the parenchyma, Mallory hyaline, and sinusoidal fibrosis.[24] Patients are largely asymptomatic, with abnormalities in biochemical laboratory test results. Nonspecific constitutional symptoms of weakness, fatigue, and malaise may be present. Obesity is the most important risk factor; type II diabetes mellitus and hypertriglyceridemia are less common antecedent conditions. The chief risk is the development of cirrhosis, which occurs in a minority of patients.

INBORN ERRORS OF METABOLISM AND PEDIATRIC LIVER DISEASE

A distinct group of liver diseases are attributable to disorders of metabolism. Genetic hemochromatosis, Wilson disease, and α_1-antitrypsin deficiency are well-characterized inherited disorders. Reye syndrome is not an inherited disease but has metabolic features suggesting a predisposition to its development. We must also consider here neonatal hepatitis, a broad disease category encompassing rare inherited diseases and neonatal infections.

Hemochromatosis

Hemochromatosis is characterized by the excessive accumulation of body iron, most of which is deposited in parenchymal organs such as the liver and pancreas. Because humans do not have a major excretory pathway for iron, hemochromatosis results either from a genetic defect causing excessive iron absorption or as a consequence of parenteral administration of iron (usually in the form of transfusions). *Genetic hemochromatosis*, also called *hereditary hemochromatosis*, is a homozygous recessive heritable disorder. Acquired forms of hemochromatosis with known sources of excess iron are called *secondary hemochromatosis* (Table 19–5).

Table 19–5 CLASSIFICATION OF IRON OVERLOAD

I. Genetic Hemochromatosis

II. Secondary Hemochromatosis
- A. Parenteral iron overload
  - Transfusions
    - Long-term hemodialysis
    - Aplastic anemia
    - Sickle cell disease
    - Myelodysplastic syndromes
    - Leukemias
  - Iron-dextran injections
- B. Ineffective erythropoiesis with increased erythroid activity
  - β-Thalassemia
  - Sideroblastic anemia
  - Pyruvate kinase deficiency
- C. Increased oral intake of iron
  - African iron overload (Bantu siderosis)
- D. Congenital atransferrinemia
- E. Chronic liver disease
  - Chronic alcoholic liver disease
  - Porphyria cutanea tarda

As discussed in Chapter 14, the total body iron pool ranges from 2 to 6 gm in normal adults; about 0.5 gm is stored in the liver, 98% of which is in hepatocytes. In genetic hemochromatosis, total iron accumulation may exceed 50 gm, more than one third of which accumulates in the liver. The following features characterize this disease:

- Fully developed cases exhibit (1) *micronodular cirrhosis*—all patients; (2) *diabetes mellitus*—75% to 80%; and (3) *skin pigmentation*—75% to 80% of cases.
- Iron accumulation is lifelong; symptoms usually first appear in the fifth to sixth decades of life.
- The hemochromatosis gene is located on the short arm of chromosome 6, close to the HLA gene locus. This gene, called *HLA-H,* encodes a novel HLA class I–like molecule that in some uncharacterized manner influences iron absorption.[25] The most common mutation is a cysteine to tyrosine substitution at amino acid 282, which inactivates this 343–amino acid protein; other alleles have also been identified. HLA-H is in linkage disequilibrium with HLA-A3, thus accounting for the association of this haplotype with genetic hemochromatosis.
- Males predominate (5 to 7:1) with slightly earlier clinical presentation, partly because physiologic iron loss (menstruation, pregnancy) delays iron accumulation in women.

In white populations of northern European extraction, the gene frequency has been estimated at approximately 6%. The frequency for homozygosity is 0.45% (1 of every 220 persons) and 11% (1 of every 9 persons) for heterozygosity, making genetic hemochromatosis one of the most common inborn errors of metabolism.

Pathogenesis. It may be recalled that the total body content of iron is tightly regulated, whereby the limited daily losses of iron are matched by gastrointestinal absorption. *In genetic hemochromatosis, there is a primary defect in the intestinal absorption of dietary iron, leading to net iron accumulation of 0.5 to 1.0 gm/year.* The disease manifests itself typically after 20 gm of storage iron has accumulated. The exact mechanism by which a defect in *HLA-H* engenders excessive iron absorption is not yet known. Regulated transfer of iron from intestinal mucosal cells to plasma may be involved, since *HLA-H* is expressed on the mucosal cell surface and interacts with circulating β_2-microglobulin.[26] Mice defective in plasma β_2-microglobulin develop a syndrome resembling genetic hemochromatosis.[27]

Excessive iron appears to be directly toxic to host tissues by the following mechanisms: (1) lipid peroxidation through iron-catalyzed free radical reactions; (2) stimulation of collagen formation; and (3) direct interactions of iron with DNA, leading to lethal injury or predisposition to hepatocellular carcinoma. Whatever the deleterious effects of iron, they are reversible in cells not fatally injured, and removal of excess iron during therapy promotes recovery of tissue function.

The most common causes of secondary hemochromatosis

are the hemolytic anemias associated with ineffective erythropoiesis, discussed in Chapter 14. In these disorders, the excess iron may result not only from transfusions but also from increased intestinal absorption. Transfusions alone, as in aplastic anemias, lead to systemic hemosiderosis in which parenchymal organ injury tends to occur only in extreme cases. *Alcoholic cirrhosis* is often associated with a modest increase in stainable iron within liver cells. However, this represents alcohol-induced redistribution of iron, since total body iron is not significantly increased. A rather unusual form of iron overload resembling genetic hemochromatosis occurs in sub-Saharan Africa, the result of ingesting large quantities of alcoholic beverages fermented in iron utensils (Bantu siderosis). Home brewing in steel drums continues to this day, and a genetic susceptibility in this population has been implicated.[28]

MORPHOLOGY. The morphologic changes in genetic hemochromatosis are characterized principally by (1) the **deposition of hemosiderin** in the following organs (in decreasing order of severity): liver, pancreas, myocardium, pituitary, adrenal, thyroid and parathyroid glands, joints, and skin; (2) **cirrhosis**; (3) **pancreatic fibrosis**. In the liver, iron becomes evident first as golden yellow hemosiderin granules in the cytoplasm of periportal hepatocytes, which stain blue with the Prussian blue stain (Fig. 19–26). With increasing iron load, there is progressive involvement of the rest of the lobule, along with bile duct epithelium and Kupffer cell pigmentation. Iron is a direct hepatotoxin, and inflammation is characteristically absent. At this stage, the liver is typically slightly larger than normal, dense, and chocolate brown. Fibrous septa develop slowly, leading ultimately to a micronodular pattern of cirrhosis in an intensely pigmented liver.

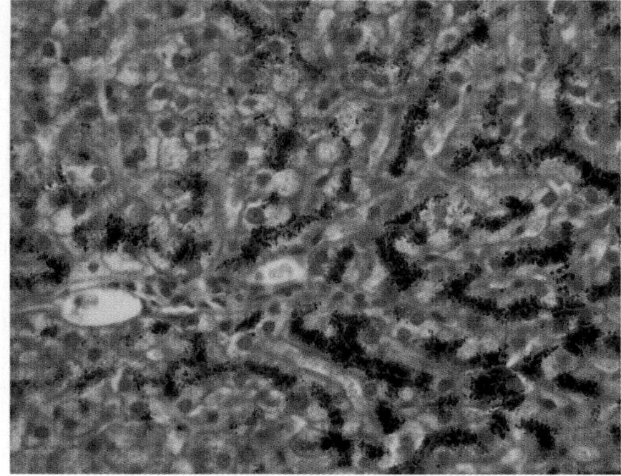

Figure 19–26 ■

Genetic hemochromatosis. Hepatocellular iron deposition is blue in this Prussian blue–stained section of an early stage of the disease, in which parenchymal architecture is normal.

Biochemical determination of hepatic iron concentration in unfixed tissue is the standard for quantitating hepatic iron content. In normal individuals, the iron content of unfixed liver tissue is less than 1000 μg per gram dry weight of liver. Adult patients with genetic hemochromatosis exhibit more than 10,000 μg iron per gram dry weight; hepatic iron concentrations in excess of 22,000 μg per gram dry weight are associated with the development of fibrosis and cirrhosis.

The **pancreas** becomes intensely pigmented, has diffuse interstitial fibrosis, and may exhibit some parenchymal atrophy. Hemosiderin is found in both the acinar and the islet cells and sometimes in the interstitial fibrous stroma. The **heart** is often enlarged and has hemosiderin granules within the myocardial fibers, inducing a striking brown coloration to the myocardium. A delicate interstitial fibrosis may appear. Although **skin** pigmentation is partially attributable to hemosiderin deposition in dermal macrophages and fibroblasts, most of the pigmentation results from increased epidermal melanin production. The combination of these pigments imparts a characteristic slate-gray color to the skin. With hemosiderin deposition in the **joint synovial linings**, an acute synovitis may develop. Excessive deposition of calcium pyrophosphate damages the articular cartilage, producing a disabling polyarthritis referred to as **pseudogout**. The **testes** may be small and atrophic but are not usually significantly pigmented. It is thought that the atrophy is secondary to a derangement in the hypothalamic-pituitary axis.

Clinical Features. Genetic hemochromatosis is more often a disease of males and rarely becomes evident before age 40 years. The principal manifestations include hepatomegaly, abdominal pain, skin pigmentation (particularly in sun-exposed areas), deranged glucose homeostasis or frank diabetes mellitus due to destruction of pancreatic islets, cardiac dysfunction (arrhythmias, cardiomyopathy), and atypical arthritis. In some patients, the presenting complaint is hypogonadism (e.g., amenorrhea in the female, and loss of libido and impotence in the male). The classic triad of pigment cirrhosis with hepatomegaly, skin pigmentation, and diabetes mellitus may not develop until late in the course of the disease. Death may result from cirrhosis or cardiac disease. A significant cause of death is hepatocellular carcinoma; the risk is 200-fold greater than in the general population, and treatment for iron overload does not remove the risk for this aggressive neoplasm.

Fortunately, genetic hemochromatosis can be diagnosed long before irreversible tissue damage has occurred. Screening involves demonstration of high levels of serum iron and ferritin, exclusion of secondary causes of iron overload, HLA gene molecular analysis, and liver biopsy if indicated. *Screening of family members of probands is important.* Heterozygotes for genetic hemochromatosis also accumulate excessive iron, but not to the degree required to cause significant tissue damage. Homozygotes may be identified before onset of clinical disease. Patients with genetic hemochromatosis diagnosed in the subclinical, precirrhotic stage and treated by regular phlebotomy have a normal life expectancy.

Wilson Disease

This autosomal recessive disorder is marked by *the accumulation of toxic levels of copper in many tissues and organs, principally the liver, brain, and eye.* Normally, 40% to 60% of daily ingested copper (2 to 5 mg) is absorbed in the stomach and duodenum and transported to the liver loosely complexed with albumin. Free copper dissociates and is transferred into hepatocytes, where it is incorporated into an α_2-globulin to form ceruloplasmin (a metallothionein) and resecreted into plasma. Ceruloplasmin accounts for 90% to 95% of plasma copper, although its biologic role is unknown since the contained six to seven atoms of copper per molecule are not readily exchangeable. Desialylated, senescent ceruloplasmin is endocytosed by the liver, degraded within lysosomes, and excreted into bile; this is the primary route for copper elimination. Estimated total body copper is only 50 to 150 mg.

The gene for Wilson disease, designated *ATP7B,* is on chromosome 13 and encodes a transmembrane copper-transporting ATPase, located on the hepatocyte canalicular membrane.[29] *The overwhelming majority of patients are compound heterozygotes containing different mutations of the Wilson disease gene on each allele.* The overall frequency of mutated alleles is 1:200, engendering an incidence of the disease of approximately 1:30,000. Defective biliary excretion leads to copper accumulation in the liver in excess of the metallothionein-binding capacity, causing toxic liver injury. Usually by 5 years of age, nonceruloplasmin-bound copper spills over into the circulation, causing hemolysis and pathologic changes at other sites such as brain, cornea, kidneys, bones, joints, and parathyroids. Concomitantly, urinary excretion of copper markedly increases from its normal minuscule levels.

MORPHOLOGY. The liver often bears the brunt of injury in Wilson disease; hepatic changes range from relatively minor to massive damage. **Fatty change** may be mild to moderate, with vacuolated nuclei (glycogen or water) and occasional hepatocyte focal necrosis. An **acute hepatitis** can exhibit features mimicking acute viral hepatitis, save possibly for the accompanying fatty change. A **chronic hepatitis** resembles chronic hepatitis of viral, drug, or alcoholic origin but may exhibit such distinguishing features as fatty change, vacuolated nuclei, and Mallory bodies. With progression of chronic hepatitis, **cirrhosis** will develop. **Massive liver necrosis** is a rare manifestation that is indistinguishable from that caused by viruses or drugs. Excess copper deposition can often be demonstrated by special stains (rhodanine stain for copper, orcein stain for copper-associated protein). Because copper also accumulates in chronic obstructive cholestasis, and because histology cannot reliably distinguish Wilson disease from viral and drug-induced hepatitis (and vice versa), demonstration of hepatic copper content in excess of 250 μg per gram dry weight is most helpful for making a diagnosis.

In the **brain**, toxic injury primarily affects the basal ganglia, particularly the putamen, which demonstrates atrophy and even cavitation. Nearly all patients with neurologic involvement develop **eye lesions** called **Kayser-Fleischer rings** (green to brown deposits of copper in Desçemet membrane in the limbus of the cornea)—hence the alternative designation of *hepatolenticular degeneration.*

Clinical Features. The age at onset and the clinical presentation of Wilson disease are extremely variable, but the disorder rarely manifests before age 6 years. The most common presentation is acute or chronic liver disease. Neuropsychiatric manifestations, including mild behavioral changes, frank psychosis, or a Parkinson disease–like syndrome, are the initial features in most of the remaining cases. The biochemical diagnosis of Wilson disease is based on *a decrease in serum ceruloplasmin, increase in hepatic copper content, and increased urinary excretion of copper.* Serum copper levels are of no diagnostic value, since they may be low, normal, or elevated, depending on the stage of evolution of the disease. Demonstration of Kayser-Fleischer rings further favors the diagnosis. Early recognition and long-term copper chelation therapy (as with D-penicillamine) have dramatically altered the usual progressive downhill course.

α_1-Antitrypsin Deficiency

α_1-Antitrypsin deficiency is an autosomal recessive disorder marked by abnormally low serum levels of this major protease inhibitor (Pi). The major function of this protein is the inhibition of proteases, particularly neutrophil elastase released at sites of inflammation. The deficiency leads to the development of *pulmonary emphysema,* because a relative lack of this protein permits tissue-destructive enzymes to run amok (discussed in Chapter 16).

α_1-Antitrypsin is a small, 394–amino acid plasma glycoprotein synthesized predominantly by hepatocytes. The gene, located on human chromosome 14, is polymorphic, and at least 75 α_1-antitrypsin forms have been identified, denoted alphabetically by their relative migration on an isoelectric gel. The most common genotype is PiMM, occurring in 90% of individuals. Most allelic variants exhibit conservative substitutions in the polypeptide chain and produce normal functioning levels of α_1-antitrypsin. Some *deficiency variants,* including the S variant, result in a reduction in serum concentrations of α_1-antitrypsin without clinical manifestations. However, homozygotes for the PiZZ protein have circulating α_1-antitrypsin levels that are

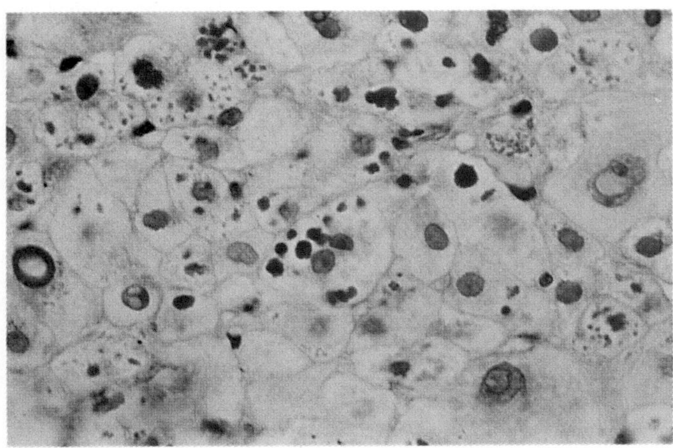

Figure 19–27

α_1-Antitrypsin deficiency. Periodic acid–Schiff stain of the liver, highlighting the characteristic red cytoplasmic granules. (Courtesy of Dr. I. Wanless, Toronto Hospital, Toronto, Ontario, Canada.)

only 10% of normal levels. These individuals are at high risk for developing clinical disease. Expression of alleles is autosomal codominant, and consequently PiMZ heterozygotes have intermediate plasma levels of α_1-antitrypsin. The gene frequency of PiZ is 0.0122 in the North American white population, yielding a PiZZ genotype frequency of approximately 1:7000. Rare variants termed Pi-null have no detectable serum α_1-antitrypsin.

Pathogenesis. With most allelic genes, the mRNA is translated and the protein is synthesized and secreted normally. Deficiency variants exhibit a selective defect in movement of this secretory protein from the endoplasmic reticulum to Golgi apparatus; this is most marked for the PiZ polypeptide, attributable to a single amino acid substitution of Glu_{342} to Lys_{342}. The mutant polypeptide (α_1-antitrypsin Z) is abnormally folded, blocking its movement along the remainder of the secretory pathway (Chapter 2). All individuals with the PiZZ genotype accumulate α_1-antitrypsin Z in the endoplasmic reticulum of hepatocytes; only 10% develop clinical liver disease. This subgroup of susceptible individuals also exhibit lags in the endoplasmic reticulum degradation pathway, a fundamental quality control apparatus of the normal cell designed to degrade abnormally folded or unassembled polypeptides. The mechanism by which endoplasmic reticulum retention of α_1-antitrypsin Z leads to liver injury is not known.

MORPHOLOGY. α_1-Antitrypsin deficiency is characterized by the presence of round to oval cytoplasmic globular inclusions in hepatocytes, which in routine hematoxylin and eosin stains are acidophilic and indistinctly demarcated from the surrounding cytoplasm. They are strongly periodic acid–Schiff (PAS) positive and diastase resistant (Fig. 19–27). The globules are also present in diminished size and number in intermediate deficiency states. The hepatic syndromes associated with PiZZ homozygosity are extremely varied, ranging from neonatal hepatitis without or with cholestasis and fibrosis (discussed shortly), to childhood cirrhosis, to a smoldering chronic inflammatory hepatitis or cirrhosis that becomes apparent only late in life. For the most part, the only distinctive feature of the hepatic disease is the PAS-positive globules; infrequently, fatty change and Mallory bodies are present.

Clinical Features. Neonatal hepatitis with cholestatic jaundice appears in 10% to 20% of newborns with the deficiency. In adolescence, presenting symptoms may be related to hepatitis or cirrhosis. Attacks of hepatitis may subside with apparent complete recovery, or they may become chronic and lead progressively to cirrhosis. Finally, the disease may remain silent until cirrhosis appears in middle to later life. Hepatocellular carcinoma develops in 2% to 3% of PiZZ adults, usually but not always in the setting of cirrhosis. The treatment, and cure, for severe hepatic disease is orthotopic liver transplantation. In patients with pulmonary disease, the single most important treatment is avoidance of cigarette smoking, since this behavior markedly accelerates the destructive lung disease associated with α_1-antitrypsin deficiency (Chapter 14).

Neonatal Hepatitis

Prolonged conjugated hyperbilirubinemia in the neonate, termed *neonatal cholestasis*, affects approximately 1 in 2500 live births. The major conditions causing it are (1) bile duct disease, primarily *extrahepatic biliary atresia* (see later), and (2) a variety of disorders causing conjugated hyperbilirubinemia in the neonate, collectively referred to as *neonatal hepatitis. Neonatal cholestasis and hepatitis are not specific entities, nor are the disorders necessarily inflammatory.* Instead, the finding of "neonatal cholestasis" should evoke a diligent search for recognizable toxic, metabolic, and infectious liver diseases[30] (Table 19–6). Once identifiable causes are excluded, one is left with the syndrome of "idiopathic" neonatal hepatitis, which shows considerable clinical overlap with extrahepatic biliary atresia.

Affected infants have jaundice, dark urine, light or acholic stools, and hepatomegaly. Variable degrees of hepatic synthetic dysfunction may be identified, such as hypoprothrombinemia. Liver biopsy is crucial in distinguishing neonatal hepatitis from an identifiable cholangiopathy.

MORPHOLOGY. The morphologic features of neonatal hepatitis are

1. Lobular disarray with focal liver cell necrosis
2. Panlobular giant cell transformation of hepatocytes
3. Prominent hepatocellular and canalicular cholestasis

Table 19–6 MAJOR CAUSES OF NEONATAL CHOLESTASIS

Bile duct obstruction
- Extrahepatic biliary atresia

Neonatal infection
- Cytomegalovirus
- Bacterial sepsis
- Urinary tract infection
- Syphilis

Toxic
- Drugs
- Parenteral nutrition

Metabolic disease
- Tyrosinemia
- Niemann-Pick disease
- Galactosemia
- Defective bile acid synthetic pathways
- α_1-Antitrypsin deficiency
- Cystic fibrosis

Miscellaneous
- Shock/hypoperfusion
- Indian childhood cirrhosis
- Alagille syndrome (paucity of bile ducts)

Idiopathic neonatal hepatitis

4. Mild mononuclear infiltration of the portal areas
5. Reactive changes in the Kupffer cells
6. Extramedullary hematopoiesis[31]

This predominantly parenchymal pattern of injury may blend imperceptibly into a ductal pattern of injury, with bile duct proliferation and fibrosis of portal tracts. Clear distinction from an obstructive cholangiopathy may thus be impossible. Specific features that permit diagnosis of a particular cause include the inclusions of α_1-antitrypsin or cytomegalovirus, and fatty change with cirrhosis in galactosemia and tyrosinemia. Electron microscopy may be helpful, for example, by showing phospholipid whorls in Niemann-Pick disease.

Despite the long list of disorders associated with neonatal cholestasis, most are rare. "Idiopathic" neonatal hepatitis represents 50% to 60% of cases; about 20% are due to extrahepatic biliary atresia and 15% to α_1-antitrypsin deficiency. Differentiation of the two most common causes assumes great importance, since definitive treatment of extrahepatic biliary atresia requires surgical intervention, whereas surgery may adversely affect the clinical course of a child with neonatal hepatitis. Fortunately, discrimination can be made with clinical data in conjunction with liver biopsy in about 90% of cases.

INTRAHEPATIC BILIARY TRACT DISEASE

In this section, we discuss three disorders of intrahepatic bile ducts that culminate in cirrhosis, as summarized in Table 19–7. It should be noted that biliary tract disorders cannot always be divided strictly into the two main types, intrahepatic or extrahepatic, because extrahepatic biliary disorders incite secondary changes within the liver. In addition, hepatic bile ducts are frequently damaged as part of more general liver disease, as in drug toxicity, viral hepatitis, and transplantation (both orthotopic liver transplantation and graft-versus-host disease after bone marrow transplantation).

Table 19–7. DISTINGUISHING FEATURES OF THE MAJOR INTRAHEPATIC BILE DUCT DISORDERS

	Secondary Biliary Cirrhosis	Primary Biliary Cirrhosis	Primary Sclerosing Cholangitis
Etiology	Extrahepatic bile duct obstruction: biliary atresia, gallstones, stricture, carcinoma of pancreatic head	Possibly autoimmune	Unknown, possibly autoimmune; 50%–70% associated with inflammatory bowel disease
Sex predilection	None	Female to male 6:1	Female to male 1:2
Symptoms and signs	Pruritus, jaundice, malaise, dark urine, light stools, hepatosplenomegaly	Same as secondary biliary cirrhosis; insidious onset	Same as secondary biliary cirrhosis; insidious onset
Laboratory findings	Conjugated hyperbilirubinemia, increased serum alkaline phosphatase, bile acids, cholesterol	Same as secondary biliary cirrhosis, plus elevated serum IgM autoantibodies (especially M2 form of antimitochondrial antibody)	Same as secondary biliary cirrhosis, plus elevated serum IgM, hypergammaglobulinemia
Important pathologic findings before cirrhosis develops	Prominent bile stasis in bile ducts, bile duct proliferation with surrounding neutrophils, portal tract edema	Dense lymphocytic infiltrate in portal tracts with granulomatous destruction of bile ducts	Periductal portal tract fibrosis, segmental stenosis of extra-hepatic and intrahepatic bile ducts

Secondary Biliary Cirrhosis

Prolonged obstruction to the extrahepatic biliary tree results in profound alteration of the liver itself. The most common cause of obstruction in adults is extrahepatic cholelithiasis (gallstones, described later), followed by malignant neoplasms of the biliary tree or head of the pancreas and strictures resulting from previous surgical procedures. Obstructive conditions in children include biliary atresia, choledochal cysts (a cystic anomaly of the extrahepatic biliary tree, see later), cystic fibrosis, and syndromes in which there are insufficient intrahepatic bile ducts (paucity of bile duct syndromes).[32] The initial morphologic features of *cholestasis,* described earlier, are entirely reversible with correction of the obstruction. However, secondary inflammation resulting from biliary obstruction initiates periportal fibrosis, which eventually leads to scarring and nodule formation, resulting in *secondary biliary cirrhosis.* Subtotal obstruction may promote secondary bacterial infection of the biliary tree (*ascending cholangitis*), which aggravates the inflammatory injury. Enteric organisms such as coliforms and enterococci are common culprits.

MORPHOLOGY. The end-stage obstructed liver exhibits extraordinary yellow-green pigmentation and is accompanied by marked icteric discoloration of body tissues and fluids. On cut surface, the liver is hard, with a finely granular appearance (Fig. 19–28). The histology is characterized by coarse fibrous septa that subdivide the liver in a jigsaw-like pattern. Embedded in the septa are distended small and large bile ducts, which frequently contain inspissated pigmented material. There is extensive proliferation of smaller bile ductules and edema, particularly at the interface between septa (formerly portal tracts) and the parenchyma. Cholestatic features in the parenchyma may be severe, with extensive feathery degeneration and formation of bile lakes. However, once regenerative nodules have formed, bile stasis may become less conspicuous. Onset of ascending bacterial infection incites a robust neutrophilic infiltration of bile ducts; severe pylephlebitis (inflammation of veins) and cholangitic abscesses may develop.

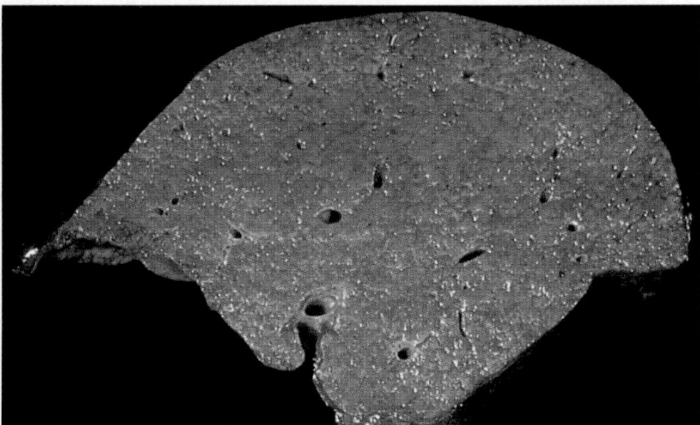

Figure 19–28

Biliary cirrhosis. Sagittal section through the liver demonstrates the fine nodularity and bile staining of end-stage biliary cirrhosis.

Primary Biliary Cirrhosis

Primary biliary cirrhosis is a chronic, progressive, and often fatal cholestatic liver disease characterized by the destruction of intrahepatic bile ducts, portal inflammation and scarring, and the eventual development of cirrhosis and liver failure. *The primary feature of this disease is a nonsuppurative, granulomatous destruction of medium-sized intrahepatic bile ducts.* Cirrhosis develops only after many years.

This is primarily a disease of middle-aged women, with a female to male predominance in excess of 6:1. Age at onset is between 20 and 80 years, with peak incidence between 40 and 50 years of age.

Serum alkaline phosphatase and cholesterol are almost always elevated; hyperbilirubinemia is a late development and usually signifies incipient hepatic decompensation. A striking feature of the disease is the presence of serum autoantibodies, especially antimitochondrial antibodies in more than 90% of patients. Particularly characteristic of primary biliary cirrhosis are circulating "antimitochondrial antibodies" against the E2 subunit of the pyruvate dehydrogenase complex, *dihydrolipoamide acetyltransferase,* located on the inner face of the inner mitochondrial membrane. However, 5% to 10% of patients with granulomatous destruction of bile ducts do not exhibit antimitochondrial antibodies.

Pathogenesis. Many lines of evidence indicate an autoimmune etiology for primary biliary cirrhosis, including aberrant neoexpression of MHC class II molecules on bile duct epithelial cells and accumulation of autoreactive T cells around bile ducts. The disease features a systemic polyclonal hypergammaglobulinemia, failure to convert IgM to IgG antibodies, and hypocomplementemia from complement activation and formation of immune complexes. Moreover, patients may develop extrahepatic autoimmune associations including Sjögren syndrome, scleroderma, thyroiditis, rheumatoid arthritis, Raynaud phenomenon, membranous glomerulonephritis, and celiac disease. However, the initiating events in primary biliary cirrhosis are not clear, nor is it understood how the antimitochondrial antibodies result in the formation of granulomas.

MORPHOLOGY. Primary biliary cirrhosis is the prototype of all conditions leading to small-duct biliary fibrosis and cirrhosis. **Primary biliary cirrhosis is a focal and variable disease, exhibiting different degrees of severity in different portions of the liver.** During the precirrhotic stage, interlobular

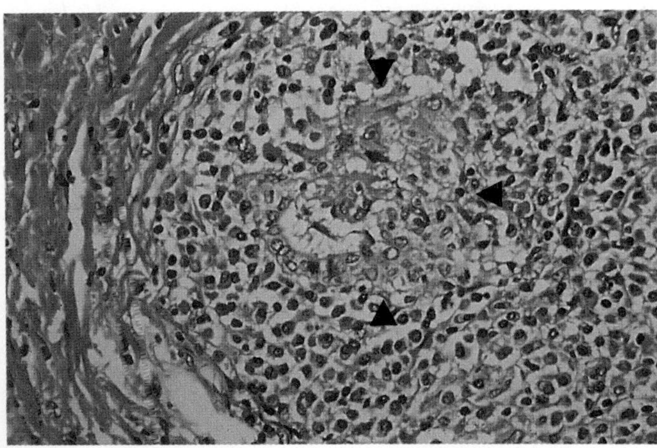

Figure 19–29

Primary biliary cirrhosis. A portal tract is markedly expanded by an infiltrate of lymphocytes and plasma cells. The granulomatous reaction to a bile duct undergoing destruction (florid duct lesion) is highlighted by the arrowheads.

bile ducts are destroyed by granulomatous inflammation (the **florid duct lesion),** accompanied by a dense portal tract infiltrate of lymphocytes, macrophages, plasma cells, and occasional eosinophils (Fig. 19–29). With time, the obstruction to intrahepatic bile flow leads to progressive hepatic damage. Portal tracts upstream from damaged bile ducts exhibit bile ductular proliferation, inflammation, and necrosis of the adjacent periportal hepatic parenchyma. The parenchyma develops generalized cholestasis. In years to decades, relentless portal tract scarring and bridging fibrosis lead to cirrhosis.

The liver does not at first appear abnormal macroscopically, but as the disease progresses, bile stasis stains the liver green. The capsule remains smooth and glistening until a fine granularity appears, culminating in a well-developed, uniform micronodularity. Liver weight is at first normal to increased (owing to inflammation); ultimately liver weight is slightly decreased. **In most cases, the end-stage picture is indistinguishable from secondary biliary cirrhosis or the cirrhosis that follows chronic active hepatitis.**

Clinical Features. The onset is insidious, usually presenting with pruritus. Jaundice develops late in the course. Hepatomegaly is typical. Xanthomas and xanthelasmas arise because of cholesterol retention. Stigmata of chronic liver disease are late features. During a period of two or more decades, patients develop hepatic decompensation, including portal hypertension with variceal bleeding, and hepatic encephalopathy. The major cause of death is liver failure, followed in order by massive variceal hemorrhage and intercurrent infection. Liver transplantation is the definitive treatment.

Primary Sclerosing Cholangitis

Primary sclerosing cholangitis is characterized by inflammation, obliterative fibrosis, and segmental constriction of the intrahepatic and extrahepatic bile ducts. Characteristic "beading" of a barium column in radiographs of the intrahepatic and extrahepatic biliary tree is attributable to the irregular strictures and secondary dilations of affected bile ducts. *Primary sclerosing cholangitis is commonly seen in association with inflammatory bowel disease* (Chapter 18), *particularly chronic ulcerative colitis, which coexists in approximately 70% of primary sclerosing cholangitis patients.* Conversely, the prevalence of primary sclerosing cholangitis in ulcerative colitis patients is about 4%. Primary sclerosing cholangitis tends to occur in the third through fifth decades of life, and males predominate 2:1 (Table 19–7).

Pathogenesis. The cause of primary sclerosing cholangitis is unknown, despite its clear association with inflammatory bowel disease. Hypothesized mechanisms include toxin release by the inflamed gut, immunologically mediated injury and ischemia, leading to bile duct loss.[34]

MORPHOLOGY. Primary sclerosing cholangitis is a fibrosing cholangitis of bile ducts, with a lymphocytic infiltrate, progressive atrophy of the bile duct epithelium, and obliteration of the lumen (Fig. 19–30). The concentric periductal fibrosis around affected ducts ("onion-skin fibrosis") is followed by their disappearance, leaving behind a solid, cordlike fibrous scar. In between areas of progressive stricture, bile ducts become ectatic and inflamed, presumably the result of downstream obstruction. As the disease progresses, the liver becomes markedly cholestatic, culminating in biliary cirrhosis much like that seen with primary and secondary biliary cirrhosis.

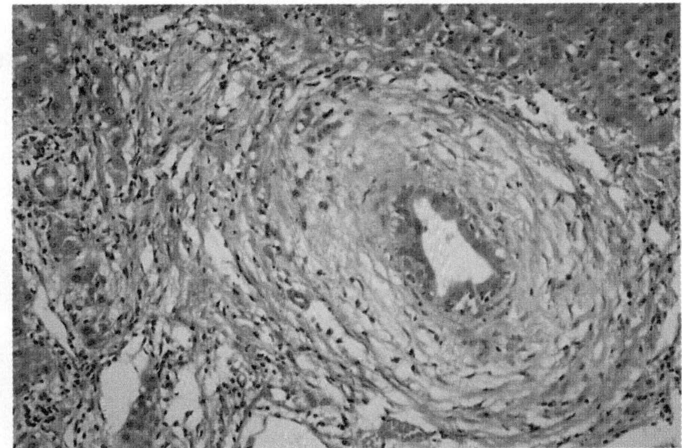

Figure 19–30

Primary sclerosing cholangitis. A bile duct undergoing degeneration is entrapped in a dense, "onion-skin" concentric scar.

Clinical Features. Asymptomatic patients may come to attention only on the basis of persistent elevation of serum alkaline phosphatase. Alternatively, progressive fatigue, pruritus, and jaundice may develop. Unlike in primary biliary cirrhosis, autoantibodies are present in less than 10% of patients. Severely afflicted patients exhibit symptoms associated with chronic liver disease, including weight loss, ascites, variceal bleeding, and encephalopathy. This disease also follows a protracted course for many years. There is an increased risk for the development of cholangiocarcinoma. As with primary biliary cirrhosis, liver transplantation is the definitive treatment.

Anomalies of the Biliary Tree (Including Liver Cysts)

A heterogeneous group of lesions exist in which the primary abnormality is altered architecture of the intrahepatic biliary tree. One form (von Meyenburg complexes) presumably arises as a result of incomplete involution of embryonic bile duct remnants.[35] Lesions may be found incidentally during radiographic studies or at autopsy. They may become manifest as hepatosplenomegaly and portal hypertension in the absence of hepatic dysfunction. Symptoms typically occur in late childhood, in adolescence, or during adult years. Histologic abnormalities are diagrammed in Figure 19–31. Some are associated with distinct cysts and fibrosis. Although one pattern usually predominates, it is not uncommon to find features of more than one pattern in the same liver.

MORPHOLOGY. ***Von Meyenburg Complexes.*** Close to or within portal tracts, these are small clusters of modestly dilated bile ducts embedded in a fibrous, sometimes hyalinized stroma. Although these "bile duct microhamartomas" may communicate with the biliary tree, they are generally free of pigmented material. A triangular bile duct hamartoma (misnamed bile duct adenoma) may occasionally lie just under the Glisson capsule.

Polycystic Liver Disease. The liver contains multiple diffuse cystic lesions numbering from a scattered few to hundreds. The cysts are lined by cuboidal or flattened biliary epithelium and contain straw-colored fluid. They do not contain pigmented material and appear to be detached from the biliary tree. Solitary liver cysts of biliary origin are occasionally identified, more commonly in women (4:1).

Congenital Hepatic Fibrosis. The portal tracts are enlarged by irregular and broad bands of collagenous tissue, forming septa and dividing the liver into irregular islands. Variable numbers of abnormally shaped bile ducts are embedded in the fibrous tissue, and bile duct remnants are distributed along the septal margins. Curved bile duct profiles are sometimes arranged in a concentric circle around portal tracts. The increased number of bile duct profiles is in continuity with the biliary tree.

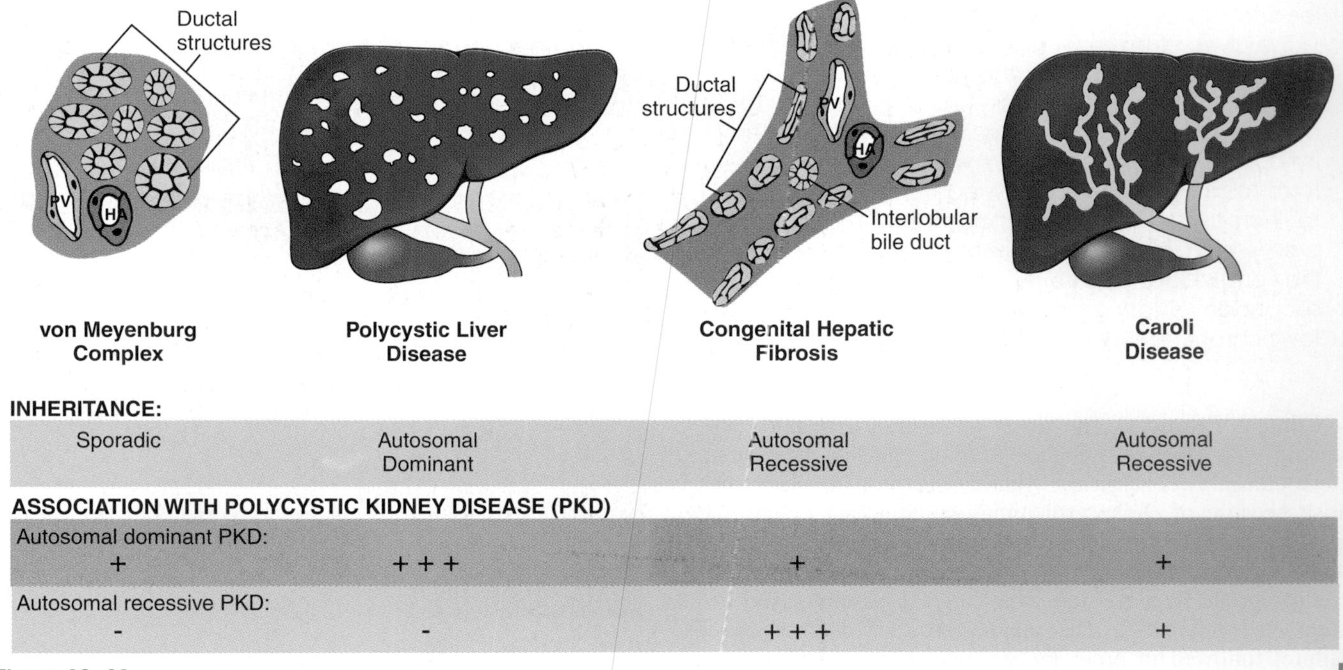

INHERITANCE:

	von Meyenburg Complex	Polycystic Liver Disease	Congenital Hepatic Fibrosis	Caroli Disease
	Sporadic	Autosomal Dominant	Autosomal Recessive	Autosomal Recessive
ASSOCIATION WITH POLYCYSTIC KIDNEY DISEASE (PKD)				
Autosomal dominant PKD:	+	+ + +	+	+
Autosomal recessive PKD:	-	-	+ + +	+

Figure 19–31

Bile duct anomalies. The morphologic features of the four major groups are diagrammed, along with apparent patterns of inheritance and associations with polycystic kidney disease.

Caroli Disease. The larger ducts of the intrahepatic biliary tree are segmentally dilated and may contain inspissated bile. Pure forms are rare; this disease is usually associated with portal tract fibrosis of the congenital hepatic fibrosis type.[36]

Clinical Features. Von Meyenburg complexes are common and usually without clinical significance, save to avoid being mistaken radiographically for metastatic carcinoma. Patients with *polycystic liver disease* may develop abdominal tenderness, or pain on stooping, occasionally requiring surgical intervention. There is a slight female predilection, with presentation common during pregnancy. Although patients with *congenital hepatic fibrosis* rarely develop cirrhosis, they may still face complications of portal hypertension, particularly bleeding varices. *Caroli disease* is frequently complicated by intrahepatic cholelithiasis (see later), cholangitis, and hepatic abscesses as well as by portal hypertension. There is an increased risk of cholangiocarcinoma (see later) with Caroli disease and congenital hepatic fibrosis.

As denoted in Figure 19–31, liver cysts represent the most frequent extrarenal manifestation of autosomal dominant polycystic kidney disease (Chapter 21), occurring in 15% to 40% of affected patients. Congenital hepatic fibrosis is strongly associated with the autosomal recessive form of polycystic kidney disease. In both situations, renal impairment dominates the clinical picture and outlook. It is presumed that a common pathogenesis underlies the renal and hepatic lesions.[37]

Alagille syndrome (syndromic paucity of bile ducts) is an uncommon autosomal dominant condition in which *the liver is almost normal, but portal tract bile ducts are completely absent.*[38] These patients exhibit a number of extrahepatic features including a peculiar facies, vertebral anomalies, and cardiovascular defects. Patients can survive into adulthood but are at risk for hepatic failure and hepatocellular carcinoma. Mutations in the gene *Jagged1* on chromosome 20p, which encodes a ligand for Notch1 and plays a role in epithelial-mesenchymal interactions, is proposed as the genetic event.[39]

CIRCULATORY DISORDERS

Given the enormous flow of blood through the liver, it is not surprising that circulatory disturbances have considerable impact on liver status. In most instances, clinically significant liver compromise does not develop, but hepatic morphology may be strikingly affected. These disorders can be grouped according to whether blood flow into, through, or from the liver is impaired (Fig. 19–32).

Impaired Blood Flow Into the Liver

HEPATIC ARTERY COMPROMISE

Liver infarcts are rare, thanks to the double blood supply to the liver. Nonetheless, thrombosis or compression of an intrahepatic branch of the hepatic artery by embolism, neo-

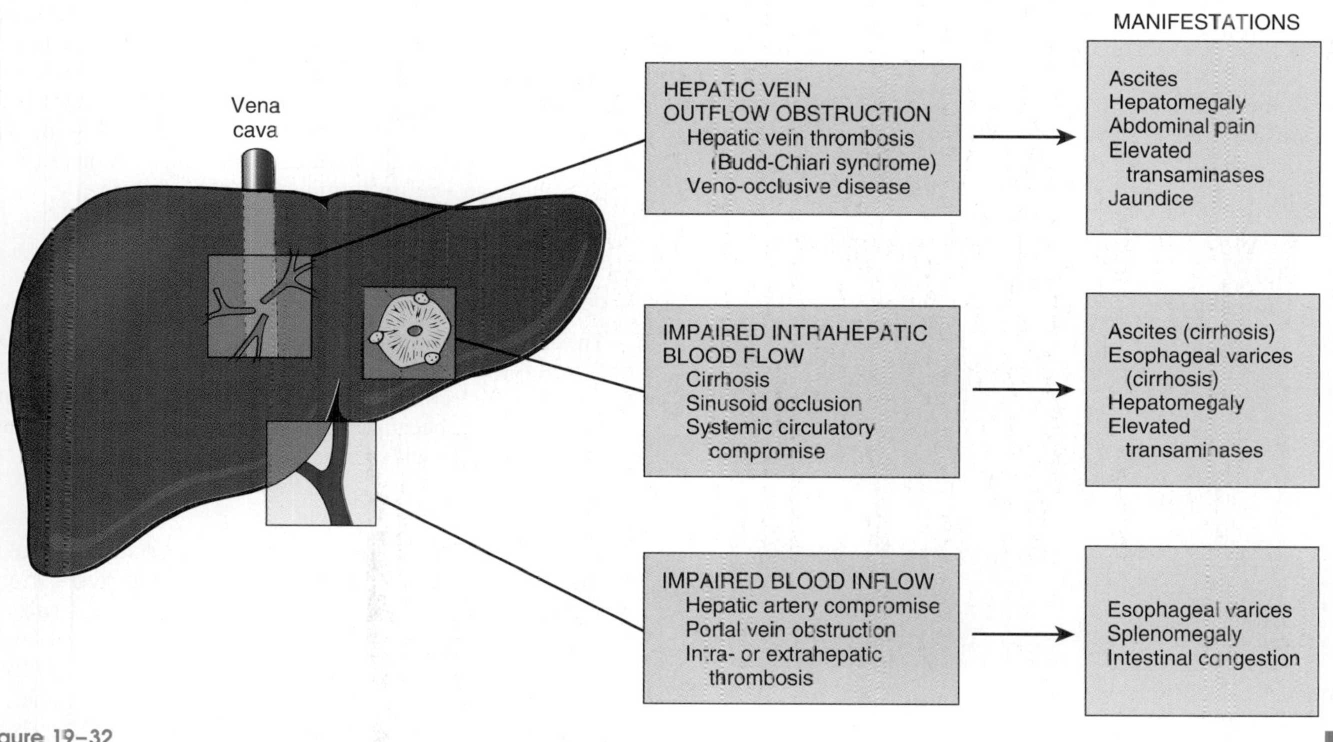

Figure 19–32

Hepatic circulatory disorders. The forms and clinical manifestations of compromised blood flow are contrasted.

plasia, polyarteritis nodosa (Chapter 12), or sepsis may result in a localized infarct that is usually anemic and pale tan or sometimes hemorrhagic owing to suffusion of portal blood (Fig. 19–33). Interruption of the main hepatic artery does not always produce ischemic necrosis of the organ, particularly if the liver is otherwise normal. Retrograde arterial flow through accessory vessels, when coupled with the portal venous supply, may be sufficient to sustain the liver parenchyma. The one exception is hepatic artery thrombosis in the transplanted liver, since the intrahepatic biliary tree is fed only by the hepatic artery. This generally leads to loss of the organ.

PORTAL VEIN OBSTRUCTION AND THROMBOSIS

Blockage of the main portal vein may be insidious and well tolerated, or it may be a catastrophic and potentially lethal event; most cases fall somewhere in between. Occlusive disease of the portal vein or its major radicles typically produces abdominal pain and, in most instances, ascites and other manifestations of portal hypertension, principally esophageal varices that are prone to rupture. The ascites, when present, is often massive and intractable. Acute impairment of visceral blood flow leads to profound congestion and bowel infarction.

Extrahepatic portal vein obstruction may arise from

- Peritoneal sepsis, for example, acute diverticulitis or appendicitis leading to *pylephlebitis* in the splanchnic circulation
- Lymphatic metastasis from abdominal cancers creating massive enlargement of hepatic hilar lymph nodes
- Pancreatitis that initiates splenic vein thrombosis that propagates into the portal vein
- Postsurgical thromboses after upper abdominal procedures
- Remote portal vein thrombosis, in which subclinical occlusion of the portal vein (as from neonatal omphalitis or umbilical vein catheterization) presents as variceal bleeding and ascites years after the occlusive event; the recanalization of an ectatic portal vein (cavernous transformation of the portal vein) and associated splenomegaly are sometimes called *Banti syndrome*

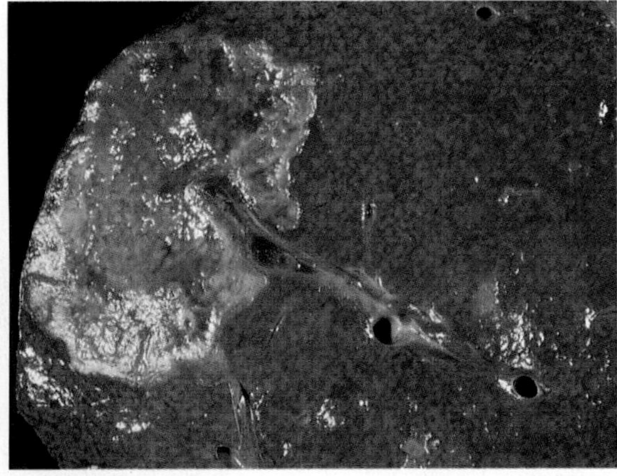

Figure 19–33

Liver infarct. A thrombus is lodged in a peripheral branch of the hepatic artery and compresses the adjacent portal vein; the distal hepatic tissue is pale, with a hemorrhagic margin.

Intrahepatic thrombosis of a portal vein radicle, when acute, does not cause ischemic infarction but instead results in a sharply demarcated area of red-blue discoloration (so-called *infarct of Zahn*). There is no necrosis, only hepatocellular atrophy and marked hemostasis in distended sinusoids. Vascular invasion by primary or secondary cancer in the liver can progressively occlude portal inflow to the liver; tongues of hepatocellular carcinoma can even occlude the main portal vein.

Idiopathic portal hypertension is a chronic, generally bland condition of progressive portal tract sclerosis leading to impaired portal vein inflow. In those instances in which a cause can be identified, it may be hypercoagulable myeloproliferative disorders, peritonitis, or chronic exposure to arsenicals.

Impaired Blood Flow Through the Liver

The most common *intrahepatic cause* of portal blood flow obstruction is *cirrhosis*, as described earlier.

Alternatively, physical occlusion of the *sinusoids* occurs in a small but striking group of diseases. In *sickle cell disease*, the hepatic sinusoids may become packed with sickled erythrocytes, both free within the vascular space and erythrophagocytosed by Kupffer cells, leading to panlobular parenchymal necrosis. *Disseminated intravascular coagulation* may occlude sinusoids. This is usually inconsequential except for the periportal sinusoidal occlusion and parenchymal necrosis that may arise in pregnancy as part of *eclampsia* (discussed shortly). Finally, metastatic tumor cells (e.g., breast carcinoma, lymphoma) may fill the hepatic sinusoids in the absence of a mass lesion. The attendant obstruction to blood flow and massive necrosis of hepatocytes can lead to fulminant hepatic failure.

PASSIVE CONGESTION AND CENTRILOBULAR NECROSIS

These hepatic manifestations of systemic circulatory compromise are considered together because they represent a morphologic continuum. Both changes are commonly seen at autopsy, because there is an element of preterminal circulatory failure with virtually every death.

MORPHOLOGY. Right-sided cardiac decompensation leads to **passive congestion of the liver.** The liver is slightly enlarged, tense, and cyanotic with rounded edges. On microscopic examination, there is congestion of centrilobular sinusoids. With time, centrilobular hepatocytes become atrophic, resulting in markedly attenuated liver cell cords. **Left-sided cardiac failure** or **shock** may lead to hepatic hypoperfusion and hypoxia. In this in-

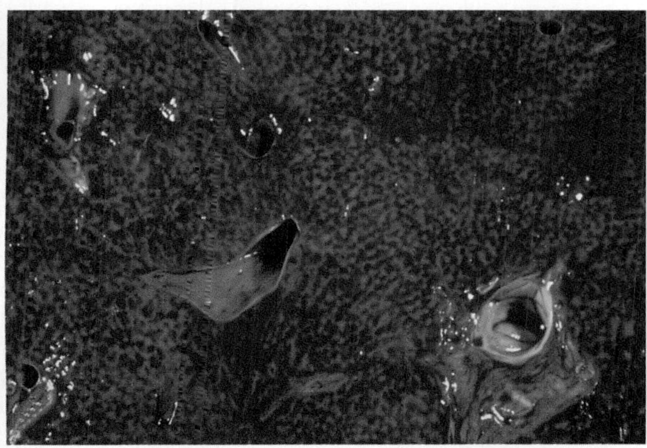

Figure 19–34 ■

Centrilobular hemorrhagic necrosis. The cut liver section, in which major blood vessels are visible, is notable for a variegated, mottled, red appearance (nutmeg liver).

stance, hepatocytes in the central region of the lobule undergo ischemic necrosis (centrilobular necrosis).

The combination of hypoperfusion and retrograde congestion acts synergistically to generate **centrilobular hemorrhagic necrosis.** The liver takes on a variegated mottled appearance reflecting hemorrhage and necrosis in the centrilobular regions, known traditionally as the **nutmeg liver** (Fig. 19–34). By microscopy, there is a sharp demarcation of viable periportal and necrotic pericentral hepatocytes, with suffusion of blood through the centrilobular region. An uncommon complication of sustained chronic severe congestive heart failure is so-called **cardiac sclerosis.** The pattern of liver fibrosis is distinctive, inasmuch as it is mostly centrilobular. The damage rarely fulfills the accepted criteria for the diagnosis of cirrhosis, but the historically sanctified term **cardiac cirrhosis** cannot easily be dislodged.

In most instances, the only clinical evidence of centrilobular necrosis is mild to moderate transient elevation of serum aminotransaminases. The parenchymal damage may be sufficient to induce mild to moderate jaundice.

PELIOSIS HEPATIS

Sinusoidal dilation occurs in any condition in which efflux of hepatic blood is impeded. *Peliosis hepatis* is a rare condition in which the dilation is primary. It is most commonly associated with exposure to anabolic steroids, and rarely oral contraceptives and danazol, although the pathogenesis is not known. In patients infected with human immunodeficiency virus, peliotic liver lesions can develop as a result of hepatic infection by *Bartonella henselae,* as a component of bacillary angiomatosis (Chapter 12). Although clinical signs are generally absent even in advanced peliosis, potentially fatal intra-abdominal hemorrhage or hepatic failure may occur. In the case of drug-induced peliosis, the lesions usually disappear after cessation of drug treatment.

Hepatic Vein Outflow Obstruction

HEPATIC VEIN THROMBOSIS (BUDD-CHIARI SYNDROME)

The Budd-Chiari syndrome was originally described for acute and usually fatal thrombotic occlusion of the hepatic veins. The definition has now been expanded to include subacute and chronic occlusive syndromes, characterized by hepatomegaly, weight gain, ascites, and abdominal pain. *Hepatic vein thrombosis is associated with (in order of frequency) polycythemia vera, pregnancy, the postpartum state, the use of oral contraceptives, paroxysmal nocturnal hemoglobinuria, and intra-abdominal cancers, particularly hepatocellular carcinoma.* All these conditions produce thrombotic tendencies or, in the case of liver cancers, sluggish blood flow. About 30% of cases are idiopathic in origin.

MORPHOLOGY. With acutely developing thrombosis of the major hepatic veins or inferior vena cava, the liver is swollen and red-purple and has a tense capsule (Fig. 19–35). On microscopic examination, the affected hepatic parenchyma reveals severe centrilobular congestion and necrosis. Centrilobular fibrosis develops in instances in which the thrombosis is more slowly developing. The major veins may contain totally occlusive fresh thrombi, subtotal occlusion, or in chronic cases, organized adherent thrombi.

The mortality of untreated acute Budd-Chiari syndrome is high. Prompt surgical creation of a portosystemic venous shunt permits reverse flow through the portal vein and considerably improves the prognosis; direct dilation of caval obstruction may be possible during angiography. The

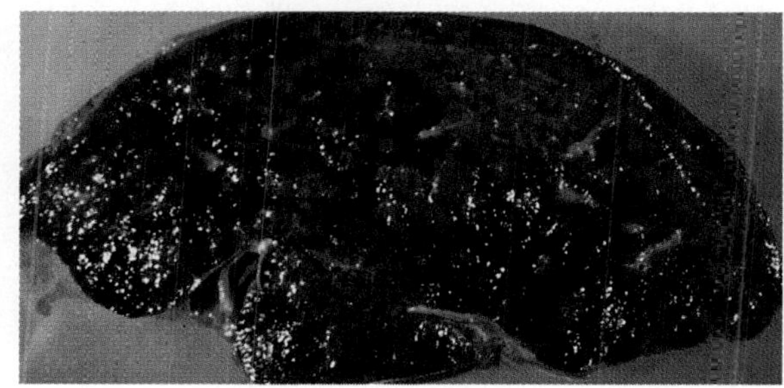

Figure 19–35 ■

Budd-Chiari syndrome. Thrombosis of the major hepatic veins has caused extreme blood retention in the liver.

chronic form of the syndrome is far less lethal, and about half the patients are alive after 5 years.

VENO-OCCLUSIVE DISEASE

Originally described in Jamaican drinkers of pyrrolizidine alkaloid–containing bush tea, veno-occlusive disease now occurs primarily in the weeks immediately after bone marrow transplantation. The incidence approaches 25% in recipients of allogeneic marrow transplants, with mortality rates of more than 30%. A diagnosis of veno-occlusive disease is frequently made on clinical grounds only (tender hepatomegaly, ascites, weight gain, and jaundice) because of the high risk of liver biopsy in these patients.

MORPHOLOGY. Veno-occlusive disease is characterized by obliteration of hepatic vein radicles by varying amounts of subendothelial swelling and fine reticulated collagen. In acute disease, there is striking centrilobular congestion with hepatocellular necrosis and accumulation of hemosiderin-laden macrophages. As the disease progresses, obliteration of the lumen of the venule is easily identified with use of special stains for connective tissue (Fig. 19–36). With chronic or healed veno-occlusive disease, dense perivenular fibrosis radiating out into the parenchyma may be present, frequently with total obliteration of the venule; hemosiderin deposition is evident in the scar tissue, and congestion is minimal.

The pathogenesis of veno-occlusive disease has been attributed (without rigorous proof) to toxic damage of the sinusoidal endothelium, allowing erythrocyte extravasation into the space of Disse, activation of the coagulation cascade, and downstream accumulation of debris in the central vein. Treatment of veno-occlusive disease has been largely supportive and has not significantly affected the mortality rates.

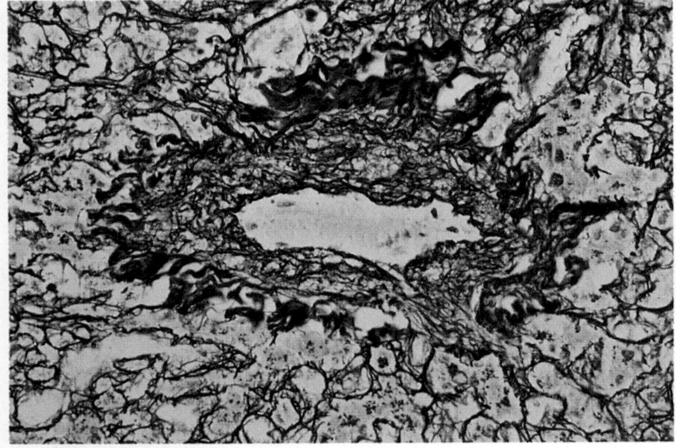

Figure 19–36

Veno-occlusive disease. A reticulin stain reveals the parenchyma framework of the lobule and the marked deposition of collagen within the lumen of the central vein.

HEPATIC DISEASE ASSOCIATED WITH PREGNANCY

Pregnancy can occur in patients with chronic liver disease, or liver diseases can become manifest during pregnancy. While these women require careful clinical management, their liver disease has no intrinsic differences from that of nonpregnant patients. However, a unique and small subgroup of pregnant patients (0.1%) develop hepatic complications directly attributable to pregnancy. In extreme cases, the outcome is fatal.

Preeclampsia and Eclampsia

Preeclampsia is a complication of pregnancy and is characterized by maternal hypertension, proteinuria, peripheral edema, coagulation abnormalities, and varying degrees of disseminated intravascular coagulation (Chapter 24). When hyperreflexia and convulsions occur, the condition is called *eclampsia*. Hepatic disease is distressingly common in preeclampsia, usually as part of a syndrome of *h*emolysis, *e*levated *l*iver enzymes, and *l*ow *p*latelets, dubbed the HELLP syndrome.[41]

MORPHOLOGY. The affected liver in preeclampsia is normal in size, firm, and pale with small red patches due to hemorrhage. Yellow or white patches of ischemic infarction can be seen occasionally. On microscopic examination, **the periportal sinusoids contain fibrin deposits with hemorrhage into the space of Disse,** leading to periportal hepatocellular coagulative necrosis. Blood under pressure may coalesce and expand to form a **hepatic hematoma; dissection of blood under the Glisson capsule may lead to catastrophic hepatic rupture** (Fig. 19–37).

Patients with hepatic involvement in preeclampsia may exhibit modest to severe elevation of serum transaminases and mild elevation of serum bilirubin. Development of a synthetic coagulopathy signifies far-advanced and potentially lethal disease. In mild cases, patients may be managed conservatively; *definitive treatment in severe cases requires termination of the pregnancy*. Patients who survive recover without sequelae.

Acute Fatty Liver of Pregnancy

This disease exhibits a spectrum ranging from modest or even subclinical hepatic dysfunction (evidenced by elevated transaminase serum levels) to hepatic failure, coma, and

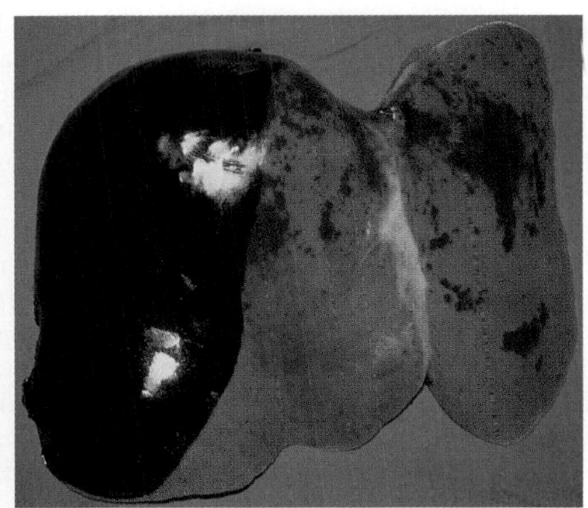

Figure 19–37

Eclampsia. Subcapsular hematoma dissecting under the Glisson capsule in a fatal case of eclampsia. (Courtesy of Dr. Brian Blackbourne, Los Angeles, CA.)

death. Affected women present in the latter half of pregnancy, usually in the third trimester. Symptoms are directly attributable to incipient hepatic failure, including bleeding, nausea and vomiting, jaundice, and coma. In 20% to 40% of cases, the presenting symptoms may be those of coexistent preeclampsia.

MORPHOLOGY. The diagnosis of acute fatty liver rests on biopsy confirmation of characteristic microvesicular fatty transformation of hepatocytes. In severe cases, there may be lobular disarray with hepatocyte dropout, reticulin collapse, and portal tract inflammation, making distinction from viral hepatitis difficult. **Diagnosis depends on (1) a high index of suspicion and (2) confirmation of microvesicular steatosis with use of special stains (oil red O or Sudan black).**

While this condition most commonly runs a mild course, patients with acute fatty liver of pregnancy can progress within days to hepatic failure and death. *The primary treatment of acute fatty liver of pregnancy is termination of the pregnancy.* A defect in intramitochondrial fatty acid oxidation has been identified: a substantial portion of mothers exhibit a heterozygous deficiency in long-chain 3-hydroxyacyl–coenzyme A dehydrogenase, and their fetuses are homozygously affected (with a heterozygous state in the father as well).[42]

Intrahepatic Cholestasis of Pregnancy

The onset of pruritus in the third trimester, followed by darkening of the urine and occasionally light stools and jaundice, heralds the development of this enigmatic syndrome. Serum bilirubin concentration (mostly conjugated) rarely exceeds 5 mg/dl; alkaline phosphatase may be slightly elevated. Liver biopsy reveals mild cholestasis without necrosis. Estrogenic hormones appear to play a causal role by inhibiting hepatocellular bile secretory function.[43] Although this is generally a benign condition, the mother is at risk for gallstones and malabsorption, and the incidence of fetal distress, stillbirths, and prematurity is modestly increased.

HEPATIC COMPLICATIONS OF ORGAN OR BONE MARROW TRANSPLANTATION

The increasing use of transplantation for bone marrow, renal, hepatic, and other organ disorders has generated a challenging group of hepatic complications. For patients undergoing bone marrow transplantation, the liver may be damaged by toxic drugs or graft-versus-host disease, whereas patients receiving a liver transplant may encounter graft failure or graft rejection. Although the clinical settings are obviously different for each population of patients, the common themes of toxic or immunologically mediated liver damage, infection of immunosuppressed hosts, recurrent disease, and post-transplant lymphoproliferative disorder are readily apparent. The following focuses on lesions peculiar to the liver.

Drug Toxicity After Bone Marrow Transplantation

"Liver toxicity" describes a syndrome of hepatic dysfunction that follows the cytoreductive therapy administered just before bone marrow transplantation. It affects up to half of all such patients and is heralded by weight gain, tender hepatomegaly, edema, ascites, hyperbilirubinemia, and a fall in urinary sodium excretion. The onset is typically on the days immediately after the donor marrow administration. A spectrum of centrilobular necroinflammatory changes is encountered, culminating in veno-occlusive disease (described earlier).[44] Clinical outcome is directly related to the severity of liver toxicity. Persistent severe liver dysfunction is a harbinger of a fatal outcome, with patients succumbing to septicemia, pneumonia, bleeding, or multiorgan failure. Another form of toxic liver damage evolving over weeks to several months, *nodular regenerative hyperplasia,* is discussed in the section on tumors.

Graft-Versus-Host Disease and Liver Rejection

The liver has the unenviable position of being attacked by graft-versus-host and host-versus-graft mechanisms in the setting of bone marrow transplantation and liver transplantation, respectively. Although these general processes are covered in detail in Chapter 7, morphologic features peculiar to the liver deserve comment.

MORPHOLOGY. Liver damage in acute graft-versus-host disease (10 to 50 days after bone marrow transplantation) is dominated by direct attack of donor lymphocytes on epithelial cells of the liver. This results in a hepatitis with necrosis of hepatocytes and bile duct epithelial cells, and inflammation of the parenchyma and portal tracts. In chronic hepatic graft-versus-host disease (usually more than 100 days after transplantation), portal tracts develop inflammation, selective **bile duct destruction,** and eventual fibrosis. Portal vein and hepatic vein radicles may exhibit **endotheliitis,** a process in which a subendothelial lymphocytic infiltrate lifts the endothelium from its basement membrane. Cholestasis may be observed in both acute and chronic graft-versus-host disease.

Acute cellular rejection of implanted livers exhibits features common to all solid organ transplants, including infiltration of a mixed population of inflammatory cells into portal tracts, bile duct and hepatocyte injury, and endotheliitis. With chronic rejection, a severe obliterative arteritis of small and larger arterial vessels will generate ischemic changes in the liver parenchyma. Alternatively, bile ducts are progressively obliterated owing to direct attack or obliteration of their arterial supply. Both may lead to loss of the graft.

Nonimmunologic Damage to Liver Allografts

Besides technical problems in the surgical procedure and the rare *hyperacute rejection*, revascularization and perfusion of the donor liver may result in *preservation injury*, attributable to the generation of oxygen radicals in a hypoxic organ with insufficient reserves of oxygen scavengers to prevent damage. *Sinusoidal endothelial injury is followed by Kupffer cell activation, neutrophil adhesion, platelet aggregation, and local cytokine release*. Hepatocyte ballooning and cholestasis follow, with variable degrees of centrilobular necrosis.[45] With severe injury, the portal tracts are also damaged, resulting in inflammation, bile duct proliferation, and fibrosis. These histologic features may take weeks to months to resolve.

In the days to weeks after transplantation, other complications may threaten the viability of the graft. Unlike in the native liver, *hepatic artery thrombosis* is a sufficiently severe vascular insult to cause severe hepatic compromise. Alternatively, *portal vein thrombosis* may be insidious and present only as variceal hemorrhage weeks to months later. *Bile duct obstruction*, particularly from stricture at the anastomosis with the native common bile duct, presents in the expected fashion.

TUMORS AND TUMOROUS CONDITIONS

Hepatic masses may come to attention for a variety of reasons. They may generate epigastric fullness and discomfort or be detected by routine physical examination or radiographic studies for other indications. The most common benign lesions are *cavernous hemangiomas*, identical to those occurring elsewhere (Chapter 12). They appear as discrete red-blue soft nodules, usually less than 2 cm in diameter, and often occur directly beneath the capsule. Their chief clinical significance is for them not to be mistaken for metastatic tumors in radiologic studies and for blind percutaneous biopsies not to be performed on them. *Cysts* have been addressed previously.

Nodular Hyperplasias

Solitary or multiple hyperplastic hepatocellular nodules may develop in the noncirrhotic liver. Two such conditions, having confusingly overlapping names, are *focal nodular hyperplasia* and *nodular regenerative hyperplasia.*

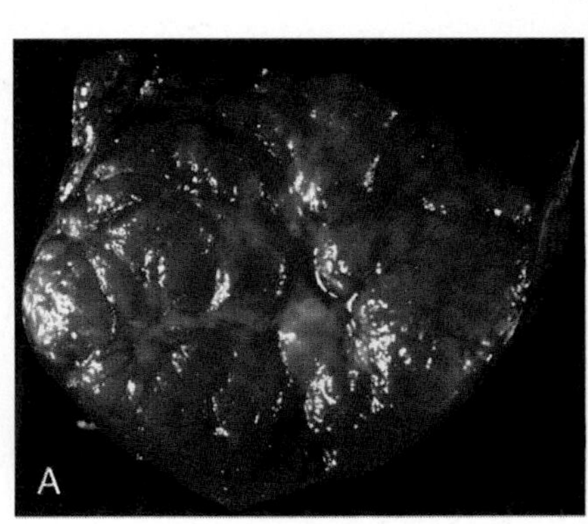

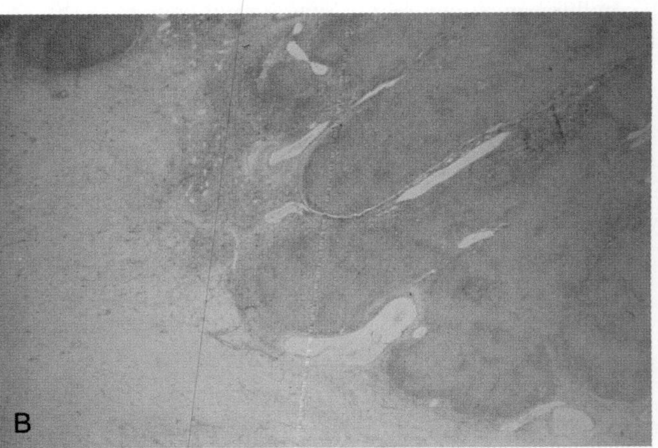

Figure 19–38

Focal nodular hyperplasia. *A*, Resected specimen showing lobulated contours and a central stellate scar. *B*, Microscopic view of the center of the lesion showing the stellate scar.

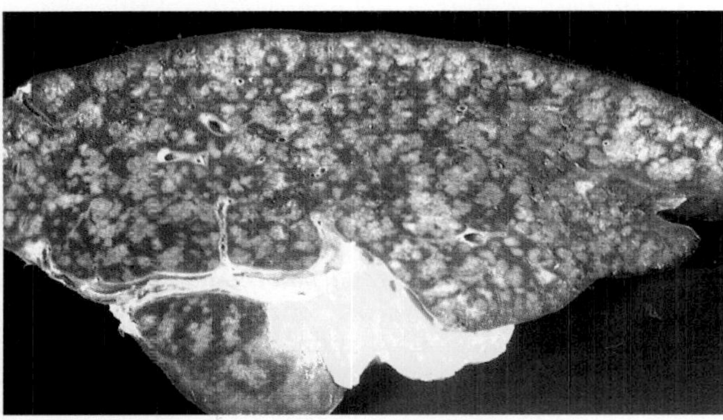

Figure 19–39

Nodular regenerative hyperplasia. Autopsied liver showing diffuse nodular transformation.

MORPHOLOGY. Focal nodular hyperplasia appears as a well-demarcated but poorly encapsulated nodule, ranging up to many centimeters in diameter (Fig. 19–38). The lesion is generally lighter in color than the surrounding liver and is sometimes yellow. There is typically a central gray-white, depressed stellate scar from which radiate fibrous septa to the periphery. The central scar contains large vessels, usually arterial, that typically exhibit fibromuscular hyperplasia with eccentric or concentric narrowing of the lumen. The radiating septa exhibit foci of intense lymphocytic infiltrates and exuberant bile duct proliferation along septal margins. The parenchyma between the septa is composed largely of normal hepatocytes.

Nodular regenerative hyperplasia, in contrast, affects the entire liver with roughly spherical nodules, in the absence of fibrosis (Fig. 19–39). On microscopic examination, plump hepatocytes are surrounded by rims of atrophic cells. The variation in parenchymal architecture may be missed on a hematoxylin and eosin stain, and reticulin staining is required to appreciate the changes in hepatocellular architecture.

Focal nodular hyperplasia presents as a spontaneous mass lesion, most frequently in young to middle-aged women, and has an excellent prognosis. Nodular regenerative hyperplasia, in contrast, is associated with the development of portal hypertension with its attendant complications. This lesion occurs in association with conditions affecting intrahepatic blood flow, including solid organ (particularly renal) transplantation, bone marrow transplantation, and vasculitic conditions. The common factor in both lesions appears to be heterogeneity in hepatic blood supply arising from focal obliteration of portal vein radicles with compensatory augmentation of arterial blood supply.[46]

Adenomas

Benign neoplasms developing from hepatocytes are called *liver cell adenomas*. These tend to occur in young women who have used oral contraceptives, and they regress on discontinuance of use. Liver cell adenomas have clinical significance for three reasons:

- When they present as an intrahepatic mass, they may be mistaken for the more ominous hepatocellular carcinoma.
- Subcapsular adenomas have a tendency to rupture, particularly during pregnancy (under estrogenic stimulation), causing severe intraperitoneal hemorrhage.
- Rarely, they may harbor hepatocellular carcinoma.

MORPHOLOGY. Liver cell adenomas are pale, yellow-tan, and frequently bile-stained nodules found anywhere in the hepatic substance but often beneath the capsule (Fig. 19–40). They may reach 30 cm in diameter. Although they are usu-

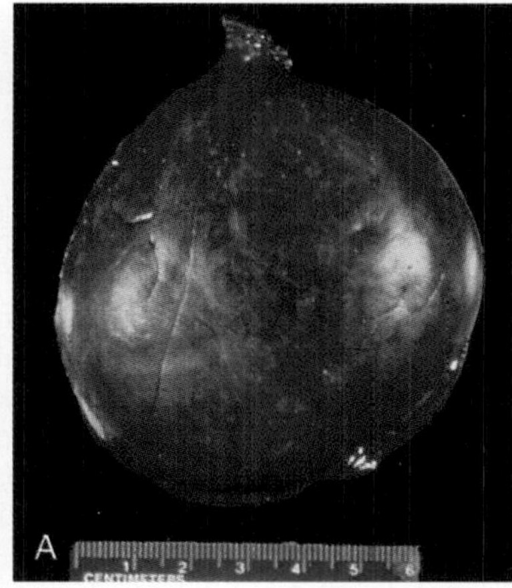

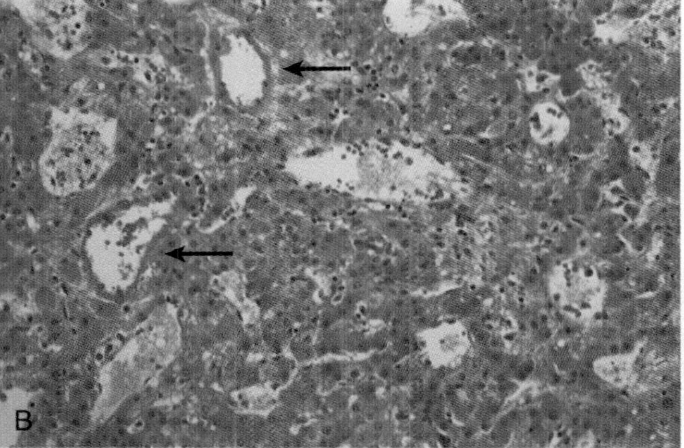

Figure 19–40

Adenoma. *A*, Resected specimen presenting as a pendulous mass arising from the liver. *B*, Microscopic view showing cords of hepatocytes, with an arterial vascular supply *(arrows)* and no portal tracts.

ally well demarcated, encapsulation may not be present. On histologic examination, liver cell adenomas are composed of sheets and cords of cells that may resemble normal hepatocytes or have some variation in cell and nuclear size. Abundant glycogen may generate a cleared cytoplasm. Portal tracts are absent; instead, prominent arterial vessels and draining veins are distributed through the substance of the tumor.

Malignant Tumors

The liver and lungs share the dubious distinction of being the visceral organs most often involved in the metastatic spread of cancers. Primary carcinomas of the liver are relatively uncommon in North America and Western Europe (0.5% to 2% of all cancers) but represent 20% to 40% of cancers in countries endemic for viral hepatitis. Before the major forms of malignant disease affecting the liver are discussed, two rare forms of primary liver cancer deserve brief mention.

The *hepatoblastoma,* a tumor of young childhood that is usually fatal within a few years if it is not resected, exhibits two anatomic variants:

- The *epithelial type*, composed of small, polygonal fetal cells or even smaller embryonal cells forming acini, tubules, or papillary structures vaguely recapitulating liver development
- The *mixed epithelial and mesenchymal type*, which contains foci of mesenchymal differentiation that may consist of primitive mesenchyme, osteoid, cartilage, or striated muscle

The *angiosarcoma* resembles those occurring elsewhere. The primary liver form is of interest because of its association with exposure to vinyl chloride, arsenic, or Thorotrast (Chapter 12). The latency period after exposure to the putative carcinogen may be several decades. These highly aggressive neoplasms metastasize widely and generally kill within a year.

PRIMARY CARCINOMA OF THE LIVER

There are two major types of primary carcinoma of the liver: *hepatocellular carcinoma* arising from hepatocytes, and *cholangiocarcinoma* arising from the bile duct epithelium. Hepatocellular carcinoma, grievously sometimes called a "hepatoma," accounts for more than 90% of all primary liver cancers. Virtually all the remainder are cholangiocarcinomas; the mixed pattern is uncommon.

Epidemiology. On a global basis, primary liver cancer constitutes the most common visceral malignant tumor (more than 350,000 cases per year) and in some populations is the most common cancer overall. Annual incidence rates for hepatocellular carcinoma of 2 to 4 cases per 100,000 population in North and South America, north and central Europe, and Australia compare with intermediate rates of up to 20 cases per 100,000 in countries bordering the Mediterranean. The highest annual incidence rates are found in Korea, Taiwan, Mozambique, and southeast China, approaching 150 per 100,000. Within each geographic area (low or high incidence), blacks have attack rates approximately fourfold higher than whites do. Worldwide, there is a clear predominance of males, ranging from 8:1 in countries with a high incidence of hepatocellular carcinoma to approximately 2:1 to 3:1 in populations with a low frequency.

The global distribution of hepatocellular carcinoma is strongly linked to the prevalence of HBV infection. In high-incidence regions, the HBV carrier state begins in infancy after vertical transmission of virus from infected mothers, conferring a 200-fold increased risk for hepatocellular carcinoma by adulthood.[47] In these regions, cirrhosis may be absent in up to half of hepatocellular carcinoma patients, and the cancer often occurs between 20 and 40 years of age. In the Western world, where HBV is not prevalent, cirrhosis is present in 85% to 90% of cases of hepatocellular carcinoma and the cancer rarely occurs before age 60 years. In these populations, the most common associations are chronic infection with HCV and alcohol.

None of the influences related to hepatocellular carcinoma has any bearing on the development of cholangiocarcinoma: the only recognized causal influences on this uncommon tumor are previous exposure to Thorotrast (formerly used in radiography of the biliary tract) and invasion of the biliary tract by the liver fluke *Opisthorchis sinensis* and its close relatives. Most cholangiocarcinomas arise without evidence of antecedent risk conditions.

Pathogenesis. The molecular origins of hepatocellular carcinoma remain unclear, but the following principles apply.[48]

- Repeated cycles of cell death and regeneration are important in the pathogenesis of HBV- and HCV-associated liver cancers. The accumulation of mutations during continuous cycles of cell division may eventually transform some hepatocytes.
- In virtually all cases of HBV-associated liver cancer, the viral DNA is integrated into the host cell genome, and the tumors are clonal with respect to these insertions. This indicates that the viral integration precedes or accompanies transformation.
- HBV DNA integration induces genomic instability, but the effects are widely distributed through the host genome rather than being limited to the integration site.
- The HBV genome contains only four open reading frames, so oncogenic candidates are few. *The HBV X protein is proposed to play a role in carcinogenesis, acting as a transactivator of cellular and viral promoters.* This protein is believed to disrupt normal growth control of infected cells by transcriptional activation of several host growth-promoting genes, such as insulin-like growth factor II and receptors for insulin-like growth factor I. HBV X protein also binds to the tumor suppressor gene *p53* and may interfere with its growth-suppressing activities.
- Aflatoxins, produced by food spoilage molds, are encountered in certain areas endemic for hepatocellular carcinoma. They are the most potent environmental factor implicated in hepatocellular carcinogenesis. Aflatox-

ins are activated in hepatocytes, and their products intercalate into DNA to form mutagenic adducts with guanosine. A particular susceptibility site for aflatoxin action is the guanosine base in codon 249 of the *p53* gene, leading to G to T transversion at this site. This specific *p53* mutation is found frequently in hepatocellular carcinomas from sub-Saharan Africa and China. It is these same world regions in which there are inherited susceptibilities to aflatoxin. Hepatocellular microsomal epoxide hydrolase and glutathione *S*-transferase are responsible for detoxifying aflatoxin, and in sub-Saharan Africa and China, patients with hepatocellular carcinoma exhibit mutant hepatic enzymes with little or no activity towards aflatoxin. *It appears that HBV infection, aflatoxin exposure, and genetic variation act synergistically in some world regions to increase risk for hepatocellular carcinoma.*

- In patients not infected with HBV, cirrhosis is the major risk factor for hepatocellular carcinoma. This includes patients with HCV infection, alcoholic cirrhosis, and primary hemochromatosis. Curiously, the highest incidence of hepatocellular carcinoma occurs in hereditary tyrosinemia, in which almost 40% of patients develop this tumor despite adequate dietary control. It would appear that stimulation of hepatocellular division in the midst of ongoing necrosis and inflammation is the fundamental theme common to hepatocellular carcinoma cases not associated with HBV infection.

Despite our incomplete understanding of hepatocellular carcinogenesis, one fact is clear: *universal vaccination of children against HBV in endemic areas may dramatically decrease the incidence of hepatocellular carcinoma.* Such a program was begun in Taiwan in 1984 and has reduced HBV infection rates from 10% to 1.3% in 10 years.[49] However, because of the latency period for hepatocellular carcinoma, three to four decades will be needed to fully determine the impact of HBV control on hepatocellular carcinoma incidence.

MORPHOLOGY. Hepatocellular carcinoma, cholangiocarcinoma, or the mixed pattern may appear grossly as (1) a **unifocal** (usually large) mass (Fig. 19–41*A*); (2) **multifocal,** widely distributed nodules of variable size; or (3) a **diffusely infiltrative** cancer, permeating widely and sometimes involving the entire liver. All three patterns may cause liver enlargement, particularly the unifocal massive and multifocal patterns. The diffusely infiltrative tumor may blend imperceptibly into a cirrhotic liver background.

Hepatocellular carcinomas are usually paler than the surrounding liver substance and sometimes take on a green hue when they are composed of well-differentiated hepatocytes capable of secreting bile. Cholangiocarcinomas are rarely bile stained, because differentiated bile duct epithelium does not synthesize bile. Infrequently with hepatocellular carcinoma but often with cholangiocarcinoma, the tumor substance is extremely firm and gritty, related to dense desmoplasia. **All patterns of hepatocellular carcinoma have a strong propensity for invasion of vascular channels.** Extensive intrahepatic metastases ensue, and occasionally long, snakelike masses of tumor invade the portal vein (with occlusion of the portal circulation) or inferior vena cava, extending even into the right side of the heart.

Hepatocellular carcinomas range from well-differentiated to highly anaplastic undifferentiated lesions. In well and moderately well differentiated tumors, cells recognizable as hepatocytic in origin are disposed either in a trabecular pattern (recapitulating liver cell plates) or in an acinar, pseudoglandular pattern (Fig. 19–41*B*). In poorly differentiated forms, tumor cells can take on a pleomorphic appearance with numerous ana-

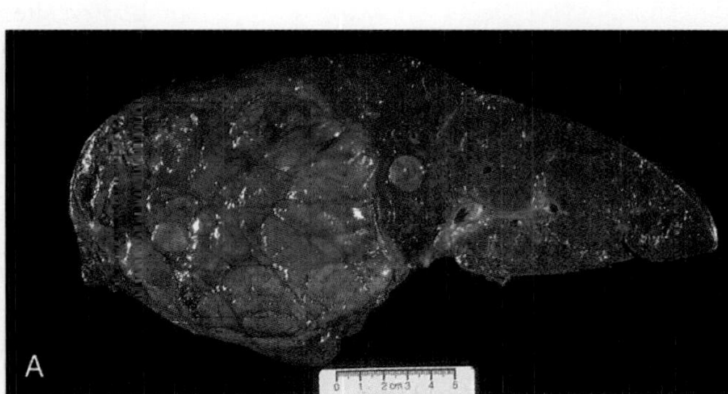

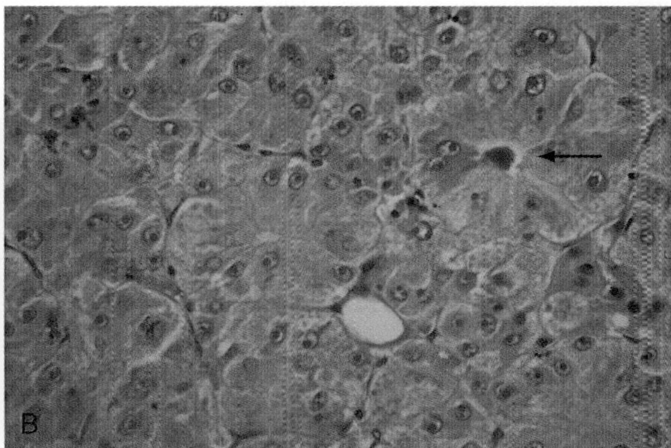

Figure 19–41

Hepatocellular carcinoma. *A*, Autopsied liver showing a unifocal, massive neoplasm replacing most of the right hepatic lobe in a noncirrhotic liver; a satellite tumor nodule is directly adjacent. *B*, In this microscopic view of a well-differentiated lesion, tumor cells are arranged in nests, sometimes with a central lumen, one of which contains bile *(arrow)*. Other tumor cells contain intracellular bile pigment.

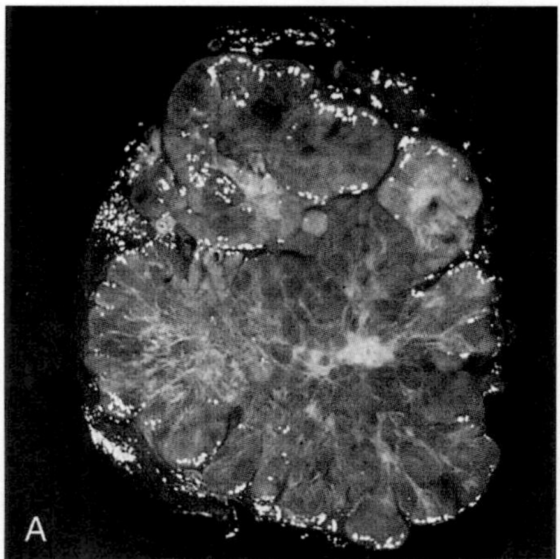
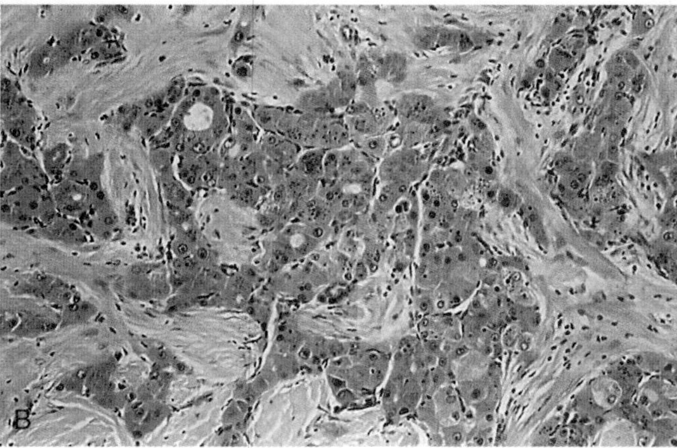

Figure 19–42

Fibrolamellar carcinoma. *A*, Resected specimen showing a demarcated nodule in an otherwise normal liver. *B*, Microscopic view showing nests and cords of malignant-appearing hepatocytes separated by dense bundles of collagen.

plastic giant cells, become small and completely undifferentiated cells, or even resemble a spindle cell sarcoma.

A distinctive variant of hepatocellular carcinoma is the **fibrolamellar carcinoma.** This tumor occurs in young male and female adults (20 to 40 years of age) with equal incidence, has no association with HBV or cirrhosis risk factors, and has a distinctly better prognosis. It usually constitutes a single large, hard "scirrhous" tumor with fibrous bands coursing through it. On histologic examination, it is composed of well-differentiated polygonal cells growing in nests or cords and separated by parallel lamellae of dense collagen bundles (Fig. 19–42).

Cholangiocarcinomas resemble adenocarcinomas arising in other parts of the body and may exhibit the full range of morphologic variation. However, most are moderately differentiated sclerosing adenocarcinomas with clearly defined glandular and tubular structures lined by somewhat anaplastic cuboidal to low columnar epithelial cells (Fig. 19–43). These neoplasms are often markedly desmoplastic, so that dense collagenous stroma separates the glandular elements.

The hepatocellular carcinoma and the cholangiocarcinoma differ somewhat in their patterns of spread. Hematogenous metastases to the lungs, bones (mainly vertebrae), adrenals, brain, or elsewhere are present at autopsy in about 50% of cases of cholangiocarcinoma. Hematogenous metastases are less frequent with hepatocellular carcinoma, despite obvious venous invasion, until late in the course of the disease, when the lungs are frequently involved. Lymph node metastases to the perihilar, peripancreatic, and para-aortic nodes above and below the diaphragm are

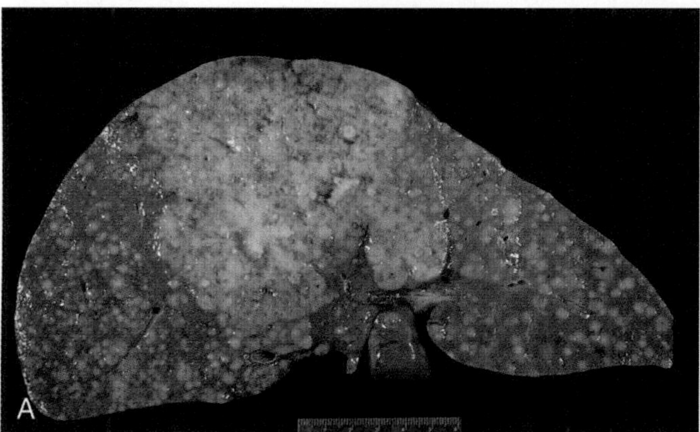
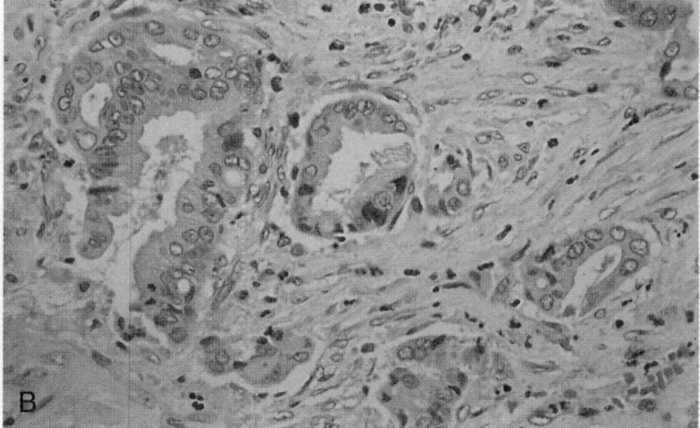

Figure 19–43

Cholangiocarcinoma. *A*, Autopsied liver showing a massive neoplasm in the right hepatic lobe and innumerable metastases permeating the entire liver. *B*, Microscopic view showing tubular glandular structures embedded in a dense sclerotic stroma.

found in about half of all cholangiocarcinomas and less frequently with hepatocellular carcinoma.

Clinical Features. The clinical manifestations of primary liver cancer are seldom characteristic and in the Western population are often masked by those related to the background cirrhosis or chronic hepatitis. In areas of high incidence such as tropical Africa, patients usually have no clinical history of liver disease, although cirrhosis may be detected at autopsy. In both populations, most patients have ill-defined upper abdominal pain, malaise, fatigue, weight loss, and sometimes awareness of an abdominal mass or abdominal fullness. In many cases, the enlarged liver can be felt on palpation, with sufficient irregularity or nodularity to permit differentiation from cirrhosis. Jaundice, fever, and gastrointestinal or esophageal variceal bleeding are inconstant findings.

Elevated levels of serum α-fetoprotein are found in 60% to 75% of patients with hepatocellular carcinoma. However, false-positive results are encountered with yolk sac tumors of the gonads and many non-neoplastic conditions including cirrhosis, massive liver necrosis, chronic hepatitis, normal pregnancy, fetal distress or death, and fetal neural tube defects such as anencephaly and spina bifida. This and other biochemical tests (such as elevated serum carcinoembryonic antigen levels) often fail to detect small lesions, when curative resection might be possible. Most valuable for small tumors are radiologic studies, ultrasonography, hepatic angiography, CT, and MRI.

The natural course of primary liver cancer is progressive enlargement of the primary mass until it encroaches on hepatic function or metastasizes, generally first to the lungs and then to other sites. Overall, death usually occurs within 10 months of diagnosis from (1) cachexia, (2) gastrointestinal or esophageal variceal bleeding, (3) liver failure with hepatic coma, or rarely (4) rupture of the tumor with fatal hemorrhage.[50]

The fibrolamellar variant of hepatocellular carcinoma is associated with a far more favorable outlook. It arises in otherwise healthy young adults and may be discovered while it is still amenable to surgical resection. About 60% of patients are alive at 5 years; the remainder succumb to progressive, unresectable disease. Cholangiocellular carcinoma is not usually detected until late in its course, and the clinical outlook is dismal; death characteristically comes within 6 months.

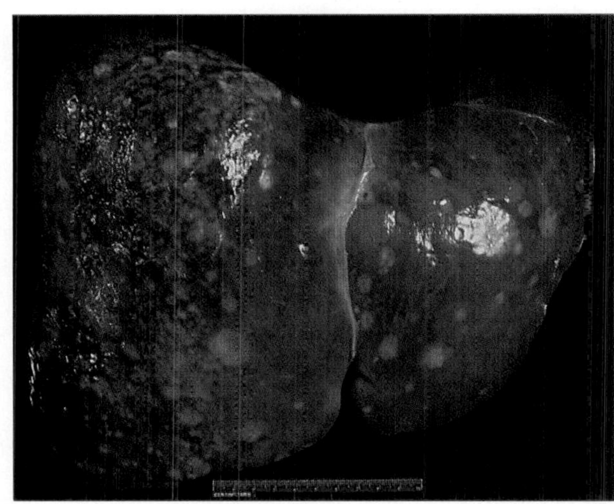

Figure 19–44

Multiple hepatic metastases from a primary colon adenocarcinoma.

METASTATIC TUMORS

Metastatic involvement of the liver is far more common than primary neoplasia. Although the most common primaries producing hepatic metastases are those of the breast, lung, and colon, any cancer in any site of the body may spread to the liver, including leukemias and lymphomas. Typically, multiple nodular implants are found that often cause striking hepatomegaly and may replace more than 80% of existent hepatic parenchyma (Fig. 19–44). The liver weight can exceed several kilograms. There is a tendency for metastatic nodules to outgrow their blood supply, producing central necrosis and umbilication when viewed from the surface of the liver. Always surprising is the amount of metastatic involvement that may be present in the absence of clinical or laboratory evidence of hepatic functional insufficiency. Often the only clinical telltale sign is hepatomegaly, sometimes with nodularity of the free edge. However, with massive or strategic involvement (obstruction of major ducts), jaundice and abnormal elevations of liver enzymes may appear.

The Biliary Tract

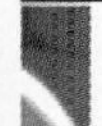

NORMAL

Disorders of the biliary tract affect a significant portion of the world's population. More than 95% of biliary tract disease is attributable to cholelithiasis (gallstones). In the United States, the annual cost of cholelithiasis and its complications is $6 to $8 billion, representing 1% of the national health care budget. Before further discussion, some comments about the normal structure and function of the biliary tree are in order.

Bile is the exocrine secretion of the liver, and humans secrete about 0.5 to 1.0 liter daily. Between meals, bile is stored in the gallbladder, which in the adult has a capacity of about 50 ml. Storage is facilitated by fivefold to tenfold concentration of bile through the active absorption of electrolytes, with passive movement of water. In response to cholecystokinin, the gallbladder contracts and releases stored bile into the gut. Although bile itself is critical for intestinal absorption of dietary fat, the gallbladder is not essential for biliary function; humans do not suffer from maldigestion or malabsorption of fat after cholecystectomy.

Anatomy. Unlike the rest of the gastrointestinal tract, the gallbladder lacks a muscularis mucosae and submucosa and consists only of (1) a mucosal lining with a single layer of columnar cells; (2) a fibromuscular layer; (3) a layer of subserosal fat with arteries, veins, lymphatics, nerves, and paraganglia; and (4) a peritoneal covering, save where the gallbladder lies adjacent to or is even embedded in the liver. The mucosal epithelium takes the form of numerous interlacing tiny folds, creating a honeycombed surface. In the neck of the gallbladder, these folds coalesce to form the *spiral valves of Heister*, which extend into the cystic duct. In combination with muscle action, these "valves" may assist in retaining bile between meals. The rapid taper of the gallbladder neck just proximal to the cystic duct is the site at which gallstones become impacted.

Small tubular channels (*ducts of Luschka*) are sometimes found buried within the gallbladder wall adjacent to the liver. The channels communicate with the intrahepatic biliary tree but only rarely form patent accessory bile ducts that directly enter the gallbladder lumen. Small outpouchings of the gallbladder mucosa may penetrate into and through the muscle wall (*Rokitansky-Aschoff sinuses*); their prominence in the settings of inflammation and gallstone formation suggests that they are acquired herniations.

The confluence of the biliary tree is the common bile duct, which courses through the head of the pancreas for about 2 cm before disgorging its contents through the *ampulla of Vater* into the duodenal lumen. In approximately 60% to 70% of individuals, the main pancreatic duct joins the common bile duct to drain through a common channel; in the remainder, the two ducts run in parallel without joining. Scattered along the length of both the intrahepatic and extrahepatic biliary tree are mucin-secreting accessory glands. These become prominent near the terminus of the common bile duct, appearing as microscopic outpouchings that interdigitate with the spiraling smooth muscle of the ampullary sphincter. To the unwary, these buried glands may be mistaken for invasive cancer.

Chemistry. Hepatic bile is a bicarbonate-rich fluid containing by weight about 3% organic solutes, of which two thirds are bile salts (Fig. 19–45). Bile salts are the major hepatic products of cholesterol metabolism and are a family of water-soluble sterols with carboxylated side chains. Bile salts act as highly effective detergents, solubilizing water-insoluble lipids secreted by the liver into the biliary tree and promoting dietary lipid absorption within the gut lumen. The principal secreted lipids (>95%) are *lecithins* (phosphatidylcholine), which are hydrophobic and have no appreciable aqueous solubility of their own, and *cholesterol*, which is a negligibly soluble steroid molecule with a single polar hydroxyl group. *Cholesterol solubility in bile is increased several million-fold by the presence of bile salts and lecithin.*[51]

About 95% of secreted bile salts is avidly reabsorbed in the intestines, primarily in the ileum, and returned to the liver by portal blood. *The enterohepatic circulation of bile salts constitutes a highly efficient mechanism for reuse of these essential physiologic molecules.*[52] Nevertheless, *the obligatory fecal loss of about half a gram of bile salts per day constitutes the major route for elimination of body cholesterol*, with a lesser contribution from free cholesterol secreted directly into bile.

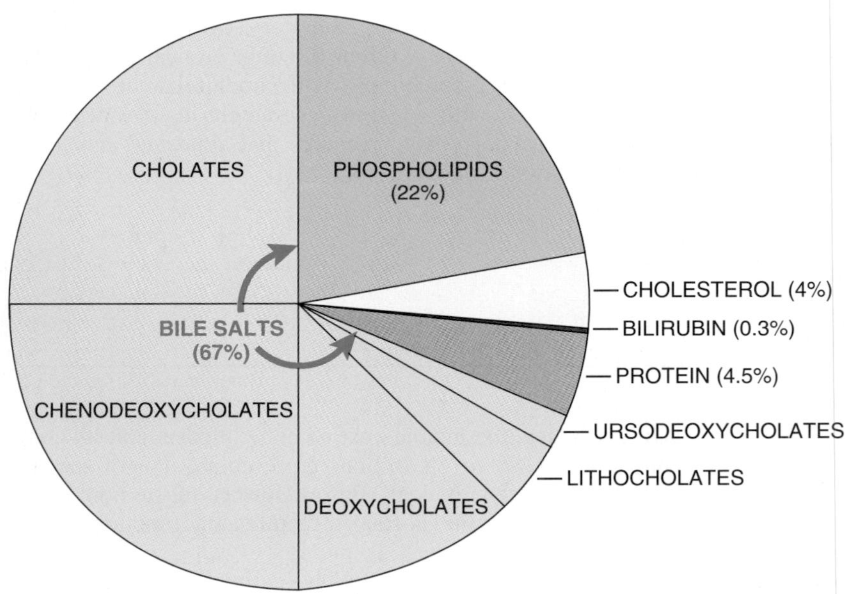

Figure 19–45

Typical solute composition of gallbladder and hepatic bile in health. (From Carey MC: Biliary lipids and gallstone formation. In Csomos G, Thaler H (eds): Clinical Hepatology. Berlin, Springer-Verlag, 1983, pp 52–69.)

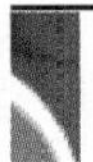

PATHOLOGY

CONGENITAL ANOMALIES

Although major developmental anomalies of the gallbladder and bile ducts are rare, anatomic variation is sufficiently common to present occasional surprises during surgery. The more distinctive variations, which may also be appreciated during ultrasonography, computed tomography, and magnetic resonance imaging scans, merit comment. The gallbladder may be *congenitally absent*, or there may be gallbladder *duplication* with conjoined or independent cystic ducts.[53] A longitudinal or transverse septum may create a *bilobed gallbladder. Aberrant locations* of the gallbladder occur in 5% to 10% of the population, most commonly partial or complete embedding in the liver substance. A *folded fundus* is the most common anomaly, creating the so-called *phrygian cap* (Fig. 19–46). *Agenesis* of all or any portion of the hepatic or common bile ducts and *hypoplastic* narrowing of biliary channels (true "biliary atresia") are rare malformations.

DISORDERS OF THE GALLBLADDER

Cholelithiasis (Gallstones)

Gallstones afflict 10% to 20% of adult populations in developed countries. It is estimated that more than 30,000,000 persons in the United States have gallstones, totaling some 25 to 50 tons in weight![54] About 1 million new patients annually are found to have gallstones, of whom half undergo surgery. Nevertheless, most gallstones (>80%) are "silent," and most individuals remain free of biliary pain or stone complications for decades. There are two main types of gallstones. In the West, *about 80% are cholesterol stones, containing more than 50% of crystalline cholesterol monohydrate. The remainder are composed predominantly of bilirubin calcium salts* and are designated *pigment stones.*

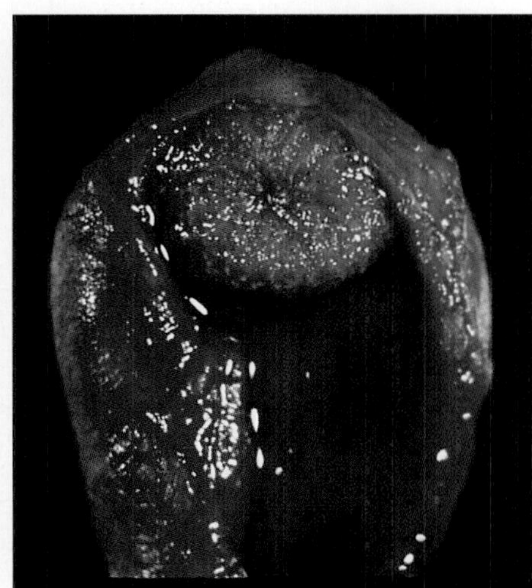

Figure 19–46 ■

Phrygian cap of the gallbladder; the fundus is folded inward.

Prevalence and Risk Factors. Certain populations are far more prone than others to develop gallstones. The following applies to cholesterol gallstones.[55]

Ethnic-Geographic. The prevalence rates of cholesterol gallstones approach 75% in Native Americans of the first migration from Asia, which includes the Pima, Hopi, and Navajo[56]—pigment stones are rare. Gallstones exhibit prevalence rates of around 25% in industrialized societies[57] but are uncommon in underdeveloped or developing societies.

Age and Sex. The prevalence of gallstones increases throughout life. In the United States, less than 5% of the population younger than 40 years has stones, in contrast to more than 30% of those older than 80 years. The prevalence in white women is about twice as high as in men (exceeding 50% by age 80 years). With both aging and gender, hypersecretion of biliary cholesterol appears to play the major role.

Environmental Factors. Estrogenic influences, including oral contraceptives and pregnancy, increase the expression of hepatic lipoprotein receptors and stimulate hepatic hydroxymethylglutaryl–coenzyme A (HMG CoA) reductase activity. Thus, both cholesterol uptake and biosynthesis, respectively, are increased. Clofibrate, used to lower blood cholesterol, increases hepatic HMG-CoA reductase and decreases conversion of cholesterol to bile acids by reducing cholesterol 7α-hydroxylase activity. The net result of these influences is excess biliary secretion of cholesterol. Obesity and rapid weight loss are also strongly associated with increased biliary cholesterol secretion.

Acquired Disorders. Although gastrointestinal conditions may severely impair intestinal resorption of bile salts, there is compensatory enhanced hepatic conversion of cholesterol to bile salts, leading to less cholesterol excretion, and no particular tendency to cholesterol stone formation. Gallbladder stasis, either neurogenic or hormonal, fosters a local environment favorable for both cholesterol and pigment gallstone formation.

Hereditary Factors. In addition to ethnicity, family history alone imparts increased risk, as do a variety of inborn errors of metabolism that (1) lead to impaired bile salt synthesis and secretion or (2) generate increased serum and biliary levels of cholesterol, such as defects in lipoprotein receptors (hyperlipidemia syndromes) that engender marked increases in cholesterol biosynthesis. Animal studies also implicate specific genetic susceptibilities from so-called lith genes to gallstone formation.[58]

Certain risk factors are well established for the development of pigment stones. Disorders that are associated with elevated levels of unconjugated bilirubin in bile include hemolytic syndromes, severe ileal dysfunction (or bypass), and bacterial contamination of the biliary tree. Pigment gallstones are the predominant type of gallstones in non-

Western populations, primarily arising in the biliary tree in the setting of infections and parasitic infestations.

Pathogenesis

Cholesterol Stones. Cholesterol is rendered soluble in bile by aggregation with water-soluble bile salts and water-insoluble lecithins, both of which act as detergents. *When cholesterol concentrations exceed the solubilizing capacity of bile (supersaturation), cholesterol can no longer remain dispersed and nucleates into solid cholesterol monohydrate crystals. Cholesterol gallstone formation involves a tetralogy of simultaneous defects* (Fig. 19–47).[58]

- Bile must be supersaturated with cholesterol.
- Gallbladder hypomotility promotes nucleation.
- Cholesterol nucleation in bile is accelerated.
- Mucus hypersecretion in the gallbladder traps the crystals, permitting their agglomeration into stones.

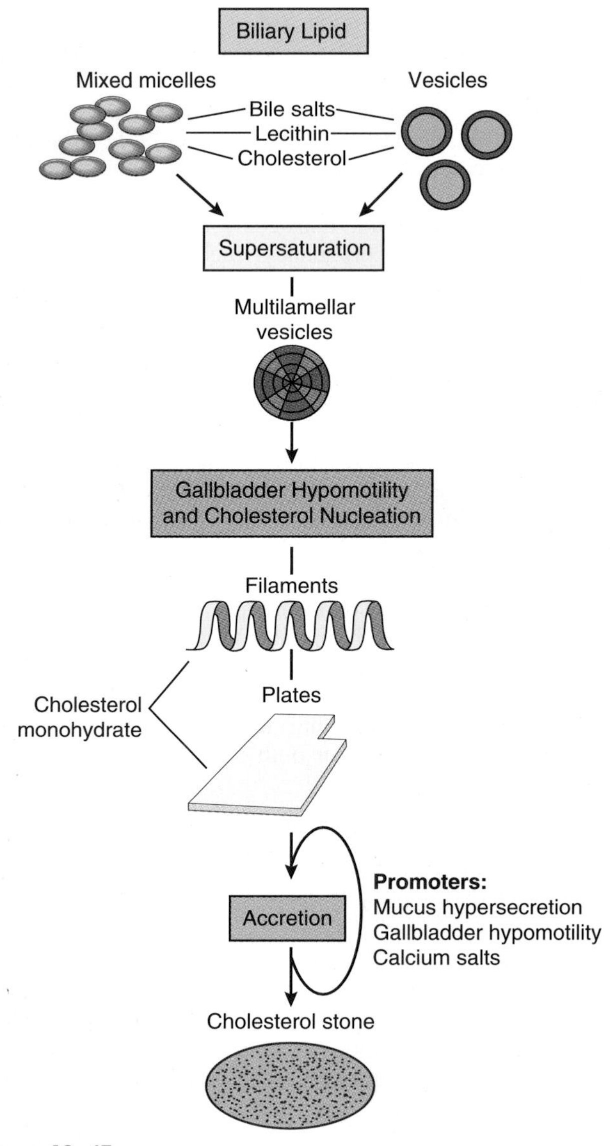

Figure 19–47

Schematic representation of the four contributing factors for cholelithiasis: supersaturation, gallbladder hypomotility, crystal nucleation, and accretion within the gallbladder mucous layer.

Biliary hypersecretion of cholesterol appears to be the primary defect, mediated possibly by enhanced delivery of plasma cholesterol in circulating lipoproteins to bile[59] and abnormal regulation of hepatic cholesterol biosynthetic pathways.[60] The abundant free cholesterol is toxic to the gallbladder, exceeding the ability of the mucosa to detoxify it by esterification. Hypomotility, mucin hypersecretion, and resultant sequestration of gallbladder bile promote nucleation and agglomeration. Superimposed environmental influences exacerbate defective gallbladder emptying: prolonged fasting, pregnancy, rapid weight loss, total parenteral nutrition, and spinal cord injury.

Pigment Stones. Pigment gallstones are mixtures of insoluble calcium salts of unconjugated bilirubin along with inorganic calcium salts.[61] Unconjugated bilirubin is normally a minor component of bile but increases when infection of the biliary tract leads to release of microbial β-glucuronidases, which hydrolyze bilirubin glucuronides. Thus, infection with *Escherichia coli*, *Ascaris lumbricoides*, or, in Asia, the liver fluke *Opisthorchis sinensis* increases the likelihood of pigment stone formation. Alternatively, intravascular hemolysis leads to increased biliary excretion of conjugated bilirubin. Since a low level (about 1%) of bilirubin glucuronides is deconjugated in the biliary tree even normally, the aqueous solubility of free bilirubin may easily be exceeded under hemolytic conditions.

MORPHOLOGY. Cholesterol stones arise exclusively in the gallbladder and contain cholesterol contents ranging from 100% down to around 50%. **Pure cholesterol stones** are pale yellow and round to ovoid and have a finely granular, hard external surface, which on transection reveals a glistening radiating crystalline palisade. With increasing proportions of calcium carbonate, phosphates, and bilirubin, the stones exhibit discoloration and may be lamellated and gray-white to black on transection (Fig. 19–48). Most often, multiple stones are present that range up to several centimeters in diameter. Rarely there is a single much larger stone that may virtually fill the fundus. Surfaces of multiple stones may be rounded or faceted owing to tight apposition. **Stones composed largely of cholesterol are radiolucent; sufficient calcium carbonate is found in 10% to 20% of cholesterol stones to render them radiopaque.**

Pigment gallstones are trivially classified as black and brown.[61] In general, black pigment stones are found in sterile gallbladder bile, and brown stones are found in infected intrahepatic or extrahepatic ducts. Black pigment stones are composed of oxidized polymers of the calcium salts of unconjugated bilirubin; lesser amounts of calcium carbonate, calcium phosphate, and mucin glycoprotein; and a modicum of cholesterol monohydrate crystals. Brown pigment stones contain pure calcium salts of unconjugated bilirubin,

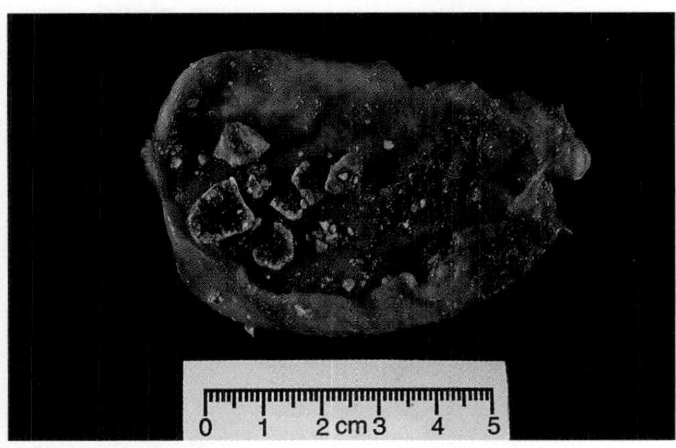

Figure 19–48 ■

Cholesterol gallstones. Mechanical manipulation during laparoscopic cholecystectomy has caused fragmentation of several cholesterol gallstones, revealing interiors that are pigmented because of entrapped bile pigments. The gallbladder mucosa is reddened and irregular as a result of coexistent chronic cholecystitis.

mucin glycoprotein, a substantial cholesterol fraction, and calcium salts of palmitate and stearate. The black stones are rarely greater than 1.5 cm in diameter, are almost invariably present in great number (Fig. 19–49), and may crumble to the touch. Their contours are usually spiculated and molded. Brown stones tend to be laminated and soft and may have a soaplike or greasy consistency. Because of calcium carbonates and phosphates, **approximately 50% to 75% of black stones are radiopaque.** Brown stones, which contain calcium soaps, are radiolucent. Mucin glycoproteins constitute the scaffolding and interparticle cement of all stones, whether pigment or cholesterol.

A incidental finding, pertinent to cholesterol biology but not directly related to gallstone formation, is **cholesterolosis.** Cholesterol normally entering the gallbladder mucosa by free exchange with the lumen may be esterified by acyl CoA: cholesterol acyltransferase. Cholesterol hypersecretion by the liver promotes excessive accumulation of cholesterol esters within the lamina propria of the gallbladder. The mucosal surface is studded with minute yellow flecks, producing the "strawberry gallbladder."

Clinical Features. Gallstones may be present for decades before symptoms develop, and 70% to 80% of patients remain asymptomatic throughout their lives. *It appears that asymptomatic patients convert to symptomatic ones at the rate of 1% to 3% per year, and the risk diminishes with time.*[62] Prominent among symptoms is biliary pain, which tends to be constant, or an excruciating "colicky" (spasmodic) pain due to the obstructive nature of gallstones in the gallbladder or biliary tree proper. Inflammation of the gallbladder (cholecystitis; see later), in association with stones, also generates pain. More severe complications include empyema, perforation, fistulas, inflammation of the biliary tree (cholangitis), and obstructive cholestasis or pancreatitis with ensuant problems. The larger the calculi, the less likely they are to enter the cystic or common ducts to produce obstruction—it is the very small stones, or "gravel," that are the more dangerous. A large stone may occasionally erode directly into an adjacent loop of small bowel, generating intestinal obstruction ("gallstone ileus"). On occasion, progressive mucosal removal of luminal lipids in obstructed, uninflamed gallbladders may leave clear mucinous secretions, so-called *hydrops* or *mucocele* of the gallbladder. Most notable is the increased risk for carcinoma of the gallbladder, discussed later.

Cholecystitis

Inflammation of the gallbladder may be acute, chronic, or acute superimposed on chronic. It almost always occurs in association with gallstones. In the United States, cholecystitis is one of the most common indications for abdominal surgery. Its epidemiologic distribution closely parallels that of gallstones.

ACUTE CHOLECYSTITIS

Acute calculous cholecystitis is an acute inflammation of the gallbladder, precipitated 90% of the time by gallstone obstruction of the neck or cystic duct. It is the primary complication of gallstones and the most common reason for emergency cholecystectomy. *Acute acalculous cholecystitis occurs in the absence of gallstones, generally in the severely ill patient.* Most of these cases occur in the following circumstances: (1) the postoperative state after major, nonbiliary surgery; (2) severe trauma (car accidents, war injuries); (3) severe burns; (4) multisystem organ fail-

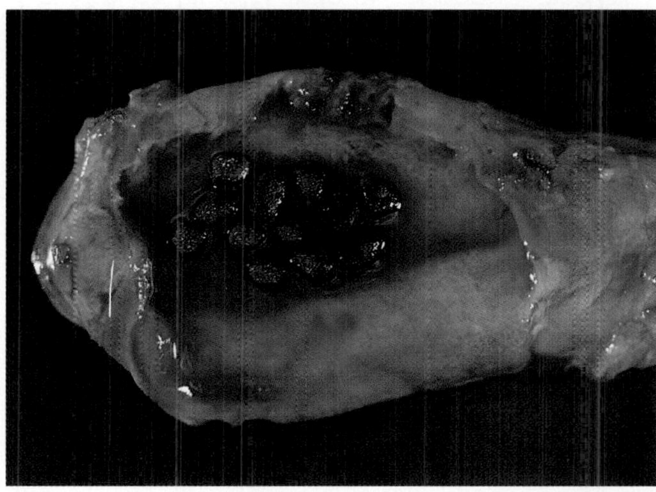

Figure 19–49 ■

Pigment gallstones. Several faceted black gallstones are present in this otherwise unremarkable gallbladder from a patient with a mechanical mitral valve prosthesis, leading to chronic intravascular hemolysis.

ure; (5) sepsis; (6) prolonged intravenous hyperalimentation; and (7) the postpartum state.

Pathogenesis. Acute calculous cholecystitis results from chemical irritation and inflammation of the obstructed gallbladder. The action of mucosal phospholipases hydrolyzes luminal lecithins to lysolecithins. The normally protective glycoprotein mucous layer is disrupted, exposing the mucosal epithelium to the direct detergent action of bile salts. Gallbladder dysmotility develops; distention and increased intraluminal pressure compromise blood flow to the mucosa. *These events occur in the absence of bacterial infection*; only later in the course may bacterial contamination develop.

Acute acalculous cholecystitis is thought to result from direct ischemic compromise. The cystic artery is an end-artery with essentially no collateral circulation. Contributing factors are thought to include[63]

- Dehydration and multiple blood transfusions, leading to a pigment load
- Gallbladder stasis, as may occur with hyperalimentation and assisted ventilation
- Accumulation of biliary sludge, viscous bile, and gallbladder mucus, causing cystic duct obstruction in the absence of frank stone formation
- Inflammation and edema of the wall, compromising blood flow
- Bacterial contamination and generation of lysolecithins

MORPHOLOGY. In **acute calculous cholecystitis,** the gallbladder is usually enlarged and tense; it may assume a bright red or blotchy, violaceous to green-black discoloration imparted by subserosal hemorrhages (Fig. 19–50). The serosal covering is frequently layered by fibrin and, in severe cases, by a definite suppurative, coagulated exudate. In most cases, an obstructing stone is present in the neck of the gallbladder or the cystic duct. In addition to other possible stones, the gallbladder lumen is filled with a cloudy or turbid bile that may contain large amounts of fibrin and frank pus as well as hemorrhage. When the contained exudate is virtually pure pus, the condition is referred to as **empyema of the gallbladder.** In mild cases, the gallbladder wall is thickened, edematous, and hyperemic. In more severe cases, it is transformed into a green-black necrotic organ, termed **gangrenous cholecystitis,** with small to large perforations. The inflammatory reactions are not histologically distinctive and consist of the usual patterns of acute inflammation, that is, edema, leukocytic infiltration, vascular congestion, frank abscess formation, or gangrenous necrosis.

There are no specific morphologic differences between acute calculous and acalculous cholecystitis, save for the absence of macroscopic stones. As a result of either delay in diagnosis or the disease itself, the incidence of gangrene and perforation is much higher than in calculous cholecystitis.[62] In rare instances, primary bacterial infection can give rise to acute acalculous cholecystitis, including agents such as *Salmonella typhi* and staphylococci. Acute emphysematous cholecystitis results from gas-forming organisms, notably clostridia and coliforms, typically in diabetics.

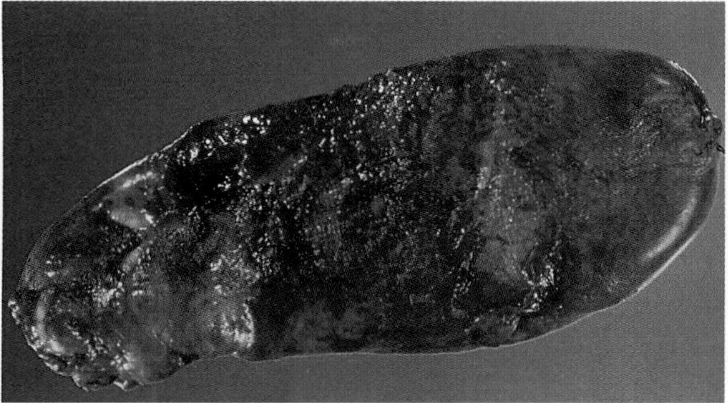

Figure 19–50

Acute calculous cholecystitis; the stone was not photographed.

Clinical Features. Patients with acute calculous cholecystitis usually but not always have experienced previous episodes of biliary pain. *Acute calculous cholecystitis may appear with remarkable suddenness and constitute an acute surgical emergency, or it may present with mild symptoms that resolve without medical intervention.* An attack of acute cholecystitis begins with progressive right upper quadrant or epigastric pain, frequently associated with mild fever, anorexia, tachycardia, diaphoresis, and nausea and vomiting. The upper abdomen is tender, but a distended tender gallbladder is not usually evident. Most patients are free of jaundice; the presence of hyperbilirubinemia suggests obstruction of the common bile duct. Mild to moderate leukocytosis may be accompanied by mild elevations in serum alkaline phosphatase values. In the absence of medical attention, the attack usually subsides in 7 to 10 days and frequently within 24 hours. However, up to 25% of patients develop progressively more severe symptoms, requiring immediate surgical intervention. In those patients who recover, recurrence is common.

Clinical symptoms of acute acalculous cholecystitis tend to be more insidious, since symptoms are obscured by the underlying conditions precipitating the attacks. A higher proportion of patients have no symptoms referable to the gallbladder; diagnosis therefore rests on a high index of suspicion. In the severely ill patient, early recognition of this condition is crucial, since failure to do so almost ensures a fatal outcome. A more indolent form of acute acalculous cholecystitis may occur in the outpatient population in the setting of systemic vasculitis, severe athero-sclerotic ischemic disease in the elderly, and acquired im-munodeficiency syndrome (with infection).[64]

CHRONIC CHOLECYSTITIS

Chronic cholecystitis may be a sequel to repeated bouts of mild to severe acute cholecystitis, but in many instances it develops in the apparent absence of antecedent attacks. Since it is associated with cholelithiasis in more than 90% of cases, the populations of patients are the same as for cholelithiasis. The evolution of chronic cholecystitis is ob-scure in that it is not clear that gallstones play a direct role in the initiation of inflammation or the development of pain. Microorganisms, usually *E. coli* and enterococci, can be cultured from the bile in about one third of cases. The symptoms for calculous chronic cholecystitis are similar to those of the acute form and range from biliary colic to indolent right upper quadrant pain and epigastric distress. Since most gallbladders removed at elective surgery for gallstones exhibit features of chronic cholecystitis, one must conclude that biliary symptoms often emerge after long-term coexistence of gallstones and low-grade inflam-mation.

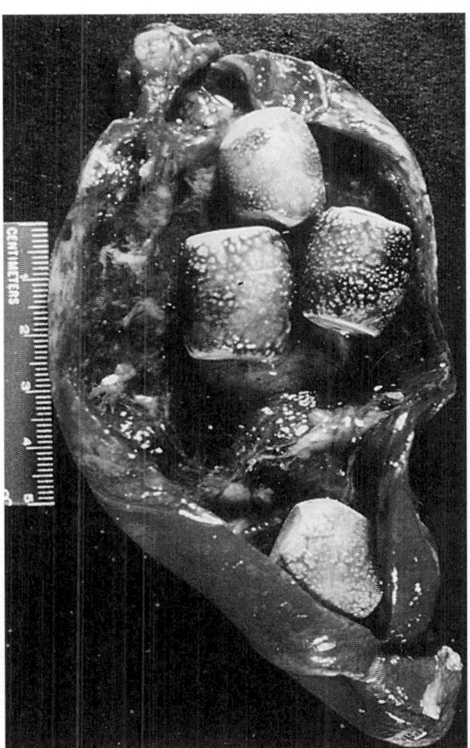

Figure 19–51

Chronic cholecystitis demonstrating a thickened gallbladder wall and lu-minal stones.

MORPHOLOGY. The morphologic changes in chronic cholecystitis are extremely variable and sometimes minimal. The serosa is usually smooth and glistening, but often it is dulled by subserosal fibrosis. Dense fibrous adhesions may remain as sequelae of preexistent acute inflammation. On sectioning, the wall is variably thickened, rarely to more than thrice normal. The wall has an opaque gray-white appearance and may be less flexible than normal. In the uncomplicated case, the lumen contains fairly clear, green-yellow, mucoid bile and usually stones (Fig. 19–51). The mucosa itself is generally preserved.

On histologic examination, the degree of in-flammatory reaction is variable. In more devel-oped cases, there is marked subepithelial and subserosal fibrosis, accompanied by mononuclear cell infiltration. Inflammatory proliferation of the mucosa and fusion of the mucosal folds may give rise to buried crypts of epithelium within the gall-bladder wall. Outpouchings of the mucosal epi-thelium through the wall **(Rokitansky-Aschoff si-nuses)** may be prominent. Superimposition of acute inflammatory changes implies acute exac-erbation of a previously chronically injured gall-bladder.

In rare instances, extensive dystrophic calcifi-cation within the gallbladder wall may yield a **porcelain gallbladder,** notable for a markedly increased incidence of associated cancer. In **xanthogranulomatous cholecystitis** the gallblad-der is shrunken and nodular and exhibits his-tiocytes packed with lipids admixed with an exuberant fibrous tissue response. Gallstones are usually present. This rare condition can be con-fused macroscopically with a malignant neo-plasm. Finally, an atrophic, chronically ob-structed gallbladder may contain only clear secretions, a condition known as **hydrops of the gallbladder.**

Clinical Features. Chronic cholecystitis does not have the striking manifestations of the acute forms and is usu-ally characterized by recurrent attacks of either steady or colicky epigastric or right upper quadrant pain. Nausea, vomiting, and intolerance for fatty foods are frequent ac-companiments.

Diagnosis of both acute and chronic cholecystitis is im-portant because of the following complications:

- Bacterial superinfection with cholangitis or sepsis
- Gallbladder perforation and local abscess formation
- Gallbladder rupture with diffuse peritonitis
- Biliary enteric (cholecystenteric) fistula, with drainage of bile into adjacent organs, entry of air and bacteria into the biliary tree, and potentially gallstone-induced intesti-nal obstruction (ileus)
- Aggravation of preexisting medical illness, with cardiac, pulmonary, renal, or liver decompensation

DISORDERS OF THE EXTRAHEPATIC BILE DUCTS

Choledocholithiasis and Ascending Cholangitis

These conditions are considered together, since they so frequently go hand-in-hand. *Choledocholithiasis is the presence of stones within the biliary tree*, occurring in about 10% of patients with cholelithiasis. In Western nations, almost all stones are derived from the gallbladder, although both cholesterol and pigmented stones can form de novo in the biliary tree. In the Orient, there is a much higher incidence of primary ductal and intrahepatic stone formation, usually pigmented. Choledocholithiasis may be asymptomatic or may cause symptoms from (1) obstruction, (2) pancreatitis, (3) cholangitis, (4) hepatic abscess, (5) secondary biliary cirrhosis, and (6) acute calculous cholecystitis.

Cholangitis is the term used for bacterial infection of the bile ducts. Cholangitis can result from any lesion creating obstruction to bile flow, most commonly choledocholithiasis. Uncommon causes include indwelling stents or catheters, tumors, acute pancreatitis, benign strictures, and rarely fungi, viruses, or parasites. Bacteria most likely enter the biliary tract through the sphincter of Oddi; infection of intrahepatic biliary radicles is termed *ascending cholangitis*. The bacteria are usually enteric gram-negative aerobes such as *E. coli, Klebsiella, Clostridium, Bacteroides,* or *Enterobacter* and group D streptococci. Cholangitis usually generates fever, chills, abdominal pain, and jaundice accompanied by acute inflammation of the wall of the bile ducts with entry of neutrophils into the luminal space. Intermittence of symptoms suggests bouts of partial obstruction. The most severe form of cholangitis is suppurative cholangitis, in which purulent bile fills and distends bile ducts, extending into the hepatic substance to cause liver abscesses. Because sepsis rather than cholestasis tends to dominate the picture, prompt diagnostic evaluation and intervention are imperative in these unstable patients.

Biliary Atresia

The infant presenting with neonatal cholestasis has been discussed previously in the context of intrahepatic disorders. A major contributor to neonatal cholestasis is *extrahepatic biliary atresia*, representing one third of infants with neonatal cholestasis and occurring in approximately 1:10,000 live births. *Extrahepatic biliary atresia is defined as a complete obstruction of bile flow due to destruction or absence of all or part of the extrahepatic bile ducts.*[65] It is the single most frequent cause of death from liver disease in early childhood and accounts for 50% to 60% of children referred for liver transplantation because of the rapidly progressing secondary biliary cirrhosis.

Pathogenesis. Most infants with extrahepatic biliary atresia are born with an intact biliary tree, which undergoes progressive inflammatory destruction in the weeks after birth. In rare cases, there is evidence of bile duct destruction before birth. The cause of extrahepatic biliary atresia remains unknown, despite efforts to ascribe the disease to

- Occult viral infection, particularly reovirus 3, cytomegalovirus, and rubella virus
- Exposure to environmental toxins
- Defective morphogenesis of bile ducts
- Disordered immunity with autoantibody formation to aberrant HLA class I or II antigen complexes
- Defects in the fetal and perinatal hilar blood flow

Arguably, biliary atresia should be viewed as a common phenotype of a heterogeneous group of disorders, since multiple pathogenetic mechanisms may be operative.

MORPHOLOGY. The salient features of extrahepatic biliary atresia include inflammation and fibrosing stricture of the hepatic or common bile ducts, periductular inflammation of intrahepatic bile ducts, and progressive destruction of the intrahepatic biliary tree (Fig. 19–52). On histologic examination of the liver, florid features of extrahepatic biliary obstruction are evident, that is, marked bile ductular proliferation, portal tract edema and fibrosis, and parenchymal cholestasis. When it is unrecognized or uncorrected, cirrhosis develops within 3 to 6 months of birth.

Clinical Features. Infants with extrahepatic biliary atresia present with neonatal cholestasis, discussed previously. These infants exhibit normal birth weight and postnatal weight gain, a slight female preponderance, and the progression of initially normal stools to acholic stools as the disease evolves. At the time of presentation, serum bilirubin values are usually in the 6 to 12 mg/dl range, with only moderately elevated transaminase and alkaline phosphatase levels.

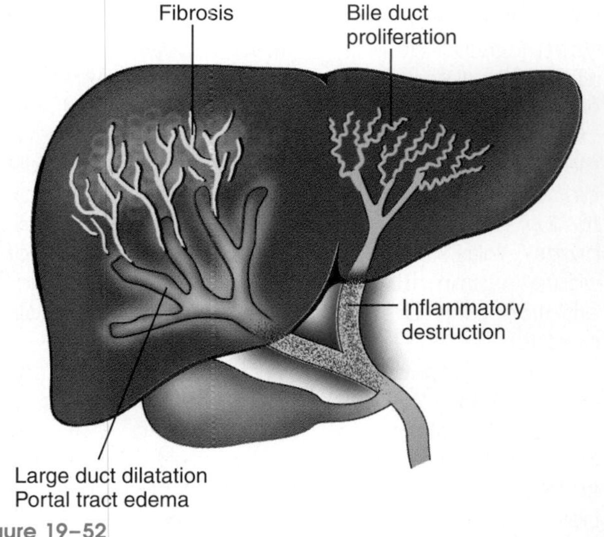

Figure 19–52

Biliary atresia, schematized to show the pattern of biliary tract injury.

There is considerable variability in extrahepatic biliary atresia. When the disease is limited to the common (type I) or hepatic bile ducts (type II) with patent proximal branches, the disease is surgically correctable. Unfortunately, 90% of patients have type III biliary atresia, in which there is also obstruction of bile ducts at or above the porta hepatis. These cases are noncorrectable, since there are no patent bile ducts amenable to surgical anastomosis. Moreover, in most patients, bile ducts within the liver are initially patent but are progressively destroyed. Liver transplantation with accompanying donor bile ducts remains the primary hope for these young patients. Without surgical intervention, death usually occurs within 2 years of birth.

Choledochal Cysts

Choledochal cysts are congenital dilations of the common bile duct, presenting most often in children before age 10 years with the nonspecific symptoms of jaundice or recurrent abdominal pain typical of biliary colic. Approximately 20% of cases become symptomatic only in adulthood; these sometimes occur in conjunction with cystic dilation of the intrahepatic biliary tree (Caroli disease, see earlier). The female to male ratio is 3 to 4:1.[66] These uncommon cysts may take the form of segmental or cylindrical dilation of the common bile duct; diverticula of the extrahepatic ducts; or choledochoceles, which are cystic lesions that protrude into the duodenal lumen. Choledochal cysts predispose to stone formation, stenosis and stricture, pancreatitis, and obstructive biliary complications within the liver. In the older patient, the risk of bile duct carcinoma is increased.

TUMORS

Although heterotopic tissues, carcinoids, hemangiomas, and stromal tumors have been described in the biliary tract, the neoplasms of primary clinical importance are those derived from the mucosa.[67] Adenomas are benign epithelial tumors representing localized neoplastic growth of the lining epithelium and are similar to adenomas found elsewhere in the alimentary tract. *Inflammatory polyps* are sessile mucosal projections with a surface of columnar epithelial cells covering a fibrous stroma infiltrated with chronic inflammatory cells and lipid-laden macrophages. These lesions may be difficult to differentiate from neoplasms on imaging studies. *Adenomyosis* of the gallbladder is characterized by hyperplasia of the muscularis, containing intramural hyperplastic glands.

Carcinoma of the Gallbladder

Carcinoma of the gallbladder is slightly more common in women and occurs most frequently in the seventh decade of life. Only rarely is it discovered at a resectable stage, and the mean 5-year survival has remained for many years at about 1%, despite surgical intervention. Gallstones are present in 60% to 90% of cases, but not 100%; in Asia, where pyogenic and parasitic disease of the biliary tree is common, the coexistence of gallstones is much lower. Presumably, gallbladders containing stones or infectious agents develop cancer as a result of irritative trauma and chronic inflammation. Carcinogenic derivatives of bile acids may also play a role.

MORPHOLOGY. Carcinomas of the gallbladder exhibit two patterns of growth, **infiltrating** or **exophytic.** The infiltrating pattern is more common and usually appears as a poorly defined area of diffuse thickening and induration of the gallbladder wall that may cover several square centimeters or may involve the entire gallbladder. Deep ulceration may cause direct penetration of the gallbladder wall or fistula formation to adjacent viscera into which the neoplasm has grown. These tumors are scirrhous and have a firm consistency. The exophytic pattern grows into the lumen as an irregular, cauliflower mass but at the same time invades the underlying wall. The luminal portion may be necrotic, hemorrhagic, and ulcerated (Fig. 19–53*A*). The most common sites of involvement are the fundus and neck; about 20% involve the lateral walls.

Most carcinomas of the gallbladder are adenocarcinomas. Some are papillary and others are infiltrative and poorly differentiated to undifferentiated (Fig. 19–53*B*). About 5% are squamous cell carcinomas or have adenosquamous differentiation. A minority may exhibit carcinoid or a variety of mesenchymal features. By the time these neoplasms are discovered, **most have invaded the liver centrifugally,** and many have extended to the cystic duct and adjacent bile ducts and porta hepatic lymph nodes. The peritoneum, gastrointestinal tract, and lungs are common sites of seeding.

Clinical Features. Preoperative diagnosis of carcinoma of the gallbladder is the exception rather than the rule, occurring in less than 20% of patients. Presenting symptoms are insidious and typically indistinguishable from those associated with cholelithiasis: abdominal pain, jaundice, anorexia, and nausea and vomiting. The fortunate patient will develop a palpable gallbladder and acute cholecystitis before extension of the tumor into adjacent structures or will have incidental carcinoma at the time of cholecystectomy for symptomatic gallstones.

Carcinoma of the Extrahepatic Bile Ducts

Carcinomas of the extrahepatic biliary tree, down to the level of the ampulla of Vater, are uncommon tumors. They are extremely insidious tumors and generally produce pain-

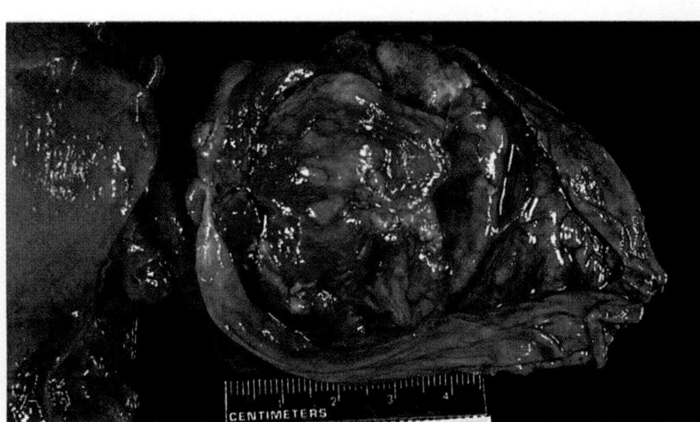

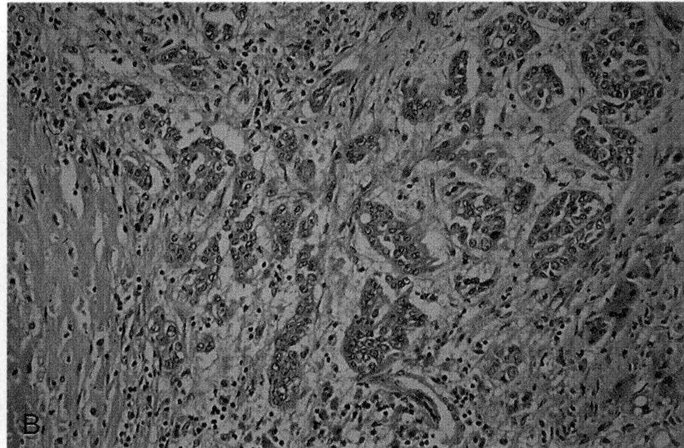

Figure 19–53

Gallbladder adenocarcinoma. *A*, The opened gallbladder contains a large, exophytic tumor that virtually fills the lumen. *B*, Malignant glandular structures are present within a densely fibrotic gallbladder wall.

less, progressively deepening jaundice. They occur in older individuals and, unlike cancers of the gallbladder, occur slightly more frequently in men. Gallstones are present in only about a third of cases. As with intrahepatic biliary tract carcinomas (cholangiocarcinomas), risk is increased in patients with biliary tree fluke infections (*Clonorchis sinensis*) in Asia or by preexisting primary sclerosing cholangitis, inflammatory bowel disease, or choledochal cysts.

A subgroup of biliary tree carcinomas are those arising in the immediate vicinity of the ampulla of Vater. Tumors of this region also include pancreatic carcinoma and adenomas of the duodenal mucosa (discussed in Chapters 20 and 18, respectively). Collectively, these tumors are referred to as periampullary carcinomas, and all are treated by surgical resection.

MORPHOLOGY. Because partial or complete obstruction of bile ducts rapidly leads to jaundice, these tumors tend to be relatively small at the time of diagnosis. Most tumors appear as firm, gray nodules within the bile duct wall; some may be diffusely infiltrative lesions creating ill-defined thickening of the wall; others are papillary, polypoid lesions. **Most bile duct tumors are adenocarcinomas** that may or may not be mucin secreting. Uncommonly, squamous features are present. For the most part, an abundant fibrous stroma accompanies the epithelial proliferation. Tumors arising at the confluence of the right and left hepatic ducts at the liver hilus are called **Klatskin tumors.**[68] These tumors are notable for their slow-growing behavior, marked sclerosing characteristics, and the infrequent occurrence of distal metastases.

Clinical Features. Jaundice generally arises because of obstruction, often accompanied by decoloration of the stools, nausea and vomiting, and weight loss. Hepatomegaly is present in about 50% and a palpable gallbladder in about 25% of cases. Associated changes are elevated levels of serum alkaline phosphatase and transaminases, bile-stained urine, and prolonged prothrombin time. Differentiation of obstructive jaundice due to calculous disease or other benign conditions from neoplasia is a major clinical problem, particularly because the presence of stones does not preclude the existence of concomitant malignant neoplasms. Despite their small size, most ductal cancers are not surgically resectable at the time of diagnosis. Mean survival times range from 6 to 18 months.

REFERENCES

1. Rapaport AM: The structural and functional units of the human liver (liver acinus). Microvasc Res 6:212, 1973.
2. Jungermann K, Kietzmann T: Zonation of parenchymal and nonparenchymal metabolism in liver. Annu Rev Nutr 16:179–203, 1996.
3. Tsukada N, et al: The structure and organization of the bile canalicular cytoskeleton with special reference to actin and actin-binding proteins. Hepatology 21:1106–1113, 1995.
4. Ciotti M, et al: Genetic defects at the *UGT1* locus associated with Crigler-Najjar type I disease, including a prenatal diagnosis. Am J Med Genet 68:173–178, 1997.
5. Seppen J, et al: A mutation which disrupts the hydrophobic core of the signal peptide of bilirubin UDP-glucuronosyltransferase, an endoplasmic reticulum membrane protein, causes Crigler-Najjar type II. FEBS Lett 390:294–298, 1996.
6. Bosma PJ, et al: The genetic basis of the reduced expression of bilirubin UDP-glucuronosyltransferase 1 in Gilbert's syndrome. N Engl J Med 333:1171–1175, 1995.
7. Kartenbeck J, et al: Absence of the canalicular isoform of the MRP gene-encoded conjugate export pump from the hepatocytes in Dubin-Johnson syndrome. Hepatology 23:1061–1066, 1996.
8. Bull LN, et al: A gene encoding a P-type ATPase mutated in two forms of hereditary cholestasis. Nat Genet 18:219–224, 1998.
9. Mousseau DD, Butterworth RF: Current theories on the pathogenesis of hepatic encephalopathy. Proc Soc Exp Biol Med 206:329–344, 1994.
10. Van Roey G, Moore K: The hepatorenal syndrome. Pediatr Nephrol 10:100–107, 1996.
11. Lange PA, Stoller JK: The hepatopulmonary syndrome. Ann Intern Med 122:521–529, 1995.

12. Henriksen JH: Cirrhosis: ascites and hepatorenal syndrome. Recent advances in pathogenesis. J Hepatol 23(Suppl 1):25–30, 1995.
13. Crawford JM: Cellular and molecular biology of the inflamed liver. Curr Opin Gastroenterol 13:175–185, 1997.
14. Soltis RD: New concepts in viral hepatitis. Geriatrics 36:62, 1981.
15. Hoofnagle JH: Type D (delta) hepatitis. JAMA 261:1321–1325, 1989.
16. Lai MMC: The molecular biology of hepatitis delta virus. Annu Rev Biochem 64:259–286, 1995.
17. Goldsmith R, et al: Enzyme-linked immunosorbent assay for diagnosis of acute sporadic hepatitis E in Egyptian children. Lancet 339: 328–331, 1992.
18. Mast EE, Krawczynski K: Hepatitis E: an overview. Annu Rev Med 47:257–266, 1996.
19. Bertel CK, et al: Treatment of pyogenic hepatic abscesses. Arch Surg 121:554–558, 1986.
20. Czaja AJ: The variant forms of autoimmune hepatitis. Ann Intern Med 125:588–598, 1996.
21. Lee WM: Medical progress—drug-induced hepatotoxicity. N Engl J Med 333:1118–1127, 1995.
22. Carithers RL Jr: Alcoholic hepatitis and cirrhosis. In Kaplowitz N (ed): Liver and Biliary Diseases. Baltimore, Williams & Wilkins, 1992, pp 334–346.
23. Lands WEM: Cellular signals in alcohol-induced liver injury: a review. Alcohol Clin Exp Res 19:928–938, 1995.
24. Neuschwander-Tetri BA, Bacon BR: Nonalcoholic steatohepatitis. Med Clin North Am 80:1147–1166, 1996.
25. Feder JN, et al: A novel MHC class I–like gene is mutated in patients with hereditary haemochromatosis. Nat Genet 13:399–408, 1996.
26. Feder JN, et al: The hemochromatosis founder mutation in HLA-H disrupts β_2-microglobulin interaction and cell surface expression. J Biol Chem 272:14025–14028, 1997.
27. Santos M, et al: Defective iron homeostasis in β_2-microglobulin knockout mice recapitulates hereditary hemochromatosis in man. J Exp Med 184:1975–1985, 1996.
28. Gordeuk V, et al: Iron overload in Africa: interaction between a gene and dietary iron content. N Engl J Med 326:95–100, 1992.
29. Schilsky ML: Wilson disease: genetic basis of copper toxicity and natural history. Semin Liver Dis 16:83–95, 1996.
30. Andres JM: Neonatal hepatobiliary disorders. Clin Perinatol 23:321–352, 1996.
31. Craig JM, Landing BH: Forms of hepatitis in neonatal period simulating biliary atresia. Arch Pathol Lab Med 54:321–333, 1952.
32. McEvoy CF, Suchy FJ: Biliary tract disease in children. Pediatr Clin North Am 43:75–98, 1996.
33. Berk PD: Primary biliary cirrhosis, Parts I and II. Semin Liver Dis 17:1–250, 1997.
34. Ludwig J, et al: Floxuridine-induced sclerosing cholangitis: an ischemic cholangiopathy? Hepatology 9:215–218, 1989.
35. Desmet VJ: Congenital diseases of intrahepatic bile ducts: variations on the theme "ductal plate malformation." Hepatology 16:1069–1083, 1992.
36. Caroli J: Diseases of the intrahepatic biliary tree. Clin Gastroenterol 2:147–161, 1973.
37. Gattone VH II, et al: Murine autosomal recessive polycystic kidney disease with multiorgan involvement induced by the *cpk* gene. Anat Rec 245:488–499, 1996.
38. Hoffenberg EJ, et al: Outcome of syndromic paucity of interlobular bile ducts (Alagille syndrome) with onset of cholestasis in infancy. J Pediatr 127:220–224, 1995.
39. Li LH, et al: Alagille syndrome is caused by mutations in human Jagged1, which encodes a ligand for Notch 1. Nat Genet 16:243–251, 1997.
40. European Polycystic Kidney Disease Consortium: The polycystic kidney disease 1 gene encodes a 14 kb transcript and lies within a duplicated region on chromosome 16. Cell 77:881–894, 1994.
41. Weinstein L: Syndrome of hemolysis, elevated liver enzymes, and low platelet count: a severe consequence of hypertension in pregnancy. Am J Obstet Gynecol 142:159–167, 1982.
42. Treem WR, et al: Acute fatty liver of pregnancy, hemolysis, elevated liver enzymes, and low platelets syndrome, and long chain 3-hydroxyacyl-coenzyme A dehydrogenase deficiency. Am J Gastroenterol 91: 2293–2300, 1996.
43. Green RM, Crawford JM: Hepatocellular cholestasis: pathobiology and histological outcome. Semin Liver Dis 15:372–389, 1995.
44. Shulman HM, et al: Venoocclusive disease of the liver after marrow transplantation: histological correlates of clinical signs and symptoms. Hepatology 19:1171–1181, 1994.
45. Ng IOL, et al: Hepatocellular ballooning after liver transplantation: a light and electronmicroscopic study with clinicopathological correlation. Histopathology 18:323–330, 1991.
46. Wanless IR: Micronodular transformation (nodular regenerative hyperplasia) of the liver: a report of 64 cases among 2,500 autopsies and a new classification of benign hepatocellular nodules. Hepatology 11:787–797, 1990.
47. Beasley RP: Hepatitis B virus, the major etiology of hepatocellular carcinoma. Cancer 61:1942–1956, 1988.
48. Geissler M, et al: Molecular mechanisms of hepatocarcinogenesis. In Okuda K, Tabor E (eds): Liver Cancer. New York, Churchill Livingstone, 1997, pp 59–88.
49. Chen HL, et al: Seroepidemiology of hepatitis B virus infection in children: ten years mass vaccination in Taiwan. JAMA 270 906–908, 1996.
50. Nagasue N, et al: The natural history of hepatocellular carcinoma. A study of 100 untreated cases. Cancer 54:1461–1465, 1984.
51. Carey MC, LaMont JT: Cholesterol gallstone formation. 1. Physical-chemistry of bile and biliary lipid secretion. Prog Liver Dis 10:139–163, 1992.
52. Carey MC, Cahalane MJ: The enterohepatic circulation. In Arias I, et al (eds): The Liver: Biology and Pathobiology, 2nd ed. New York, Raven Press, 1988, pp 573–616.
53. Janson JA, et al: Choledocholithiasis and a double gallbladder. Gastrointest Endosc 38:377–379, 1992.
54. Carey MC, O'Donovan MA: Gallstone disease: current concepts on the epidemiology, pathogenesis and management. In Harrison's Principles of Internal Medicine, Update V. New York, McGraw-Hill, 1984, pp 139–168.
55. LaMont JT, Carey MC: Cholesterol gallstone formation. 2. Pathobiology and pathomechanics. Prog Liver Dis 10:165–191, 1992.
56. Gibbons A: Geneticists trace the DNA trail of the first Americans. Science 259:312–313, 1993.
57. Jorgensen T, et al: Are autopsy studies reliable in assessing gallstone prevalence in the community? Int J Epidemiol 23:566–569, 1994.
58. Apstein MD, Carey MC: Pathogenesis of cholesterol gallstones: a parsimonious hypothesis. Eur J Clin Invest 26:343–352, 1996.
59. Kozarsky KF, et al: Overexpression of the HDL receptor SR-B1 alters plasma HDL and bile cholesterol levels. Nature 387:414–417, 1997.
60. Wang DQ-H, et al: Phenotypic characterizaton of Lith genes that determine susceptibility to cholesterol cholelithiasis in inbred mice: physical chemistry of gallbladder bile. J Lipid Res 38:1395–1411, 1997.
61. Cahalane MJ, et al: Physical-chemical pathogenesis of pigment gallstones. Semin Liver Dis 8:317–328, 1988.
62. Malet PF: Complications of cholelithiasis. In Kaplowitz N (ed): Liver and Biliary Diseases. Baltimore, Williams & Wilkins, 1992, pp 610–627.
63. Williamson RCN: Acalculous disease of the gallbladder. Gut 29:860–872, 1988.
64. Savoca PE, et al: The increasing prevalence of acalculous cholecystitis in outpatients. Ann Surg 211:433–437, 1990.
65. Balistreri WF, et al: Biliary atresia: current concepts and research directions—summary of a symposium. Hepatology 23:1682–1692, 1996.
66. Lipsett PA, et al: Biliary atresia and biliary cysts. Baillieres Clin Gastroenterol 11:619–641, 1997.
67. Albores-Saavedra J, et al: The WHO Histological Classification of Tumors of the Gallbladder and Extrahepatic Bile Ducts: a commentary on the second edition. Cancer 70:410–414, 1992.
68. Klatskin G: Adenocarcinoma of the hepatic duct at its bifurcation within the porta hepatis. Am J Med 38:241–256, 1965.

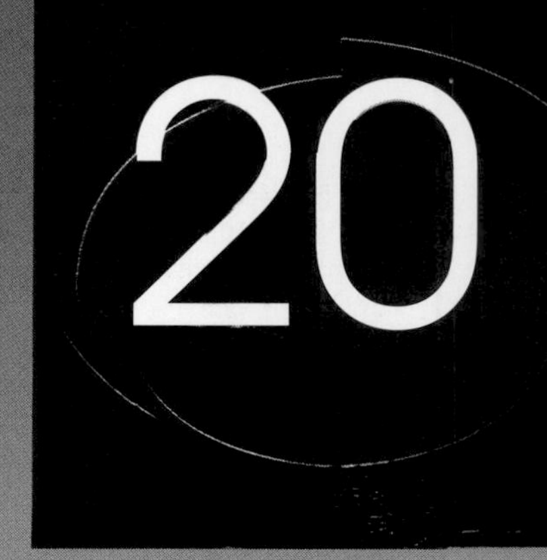

The Pancreas

James M. Crawford and Ramzi S. Cotran

The Exocrine Pancreas
CONGENITAL ANOMALIES
ECTOPIC PANCREAS
PANCREATITIS
ACUTE PANCREATITIS
CHRONIC PANCREATITIS
CYSTS
PSEUDOCYSTS
TUMORS
CYSTIC TUMORS
CARCINOMA OF THE PANCREAS
The Endocrine Pancreas
DIABETES MELLITUS
CLASSIFICATION AND INCIDENCE
PATHOGENESIS
MORPHOLOGY OF DIABETES AND ITS LATE COMPLICATIONS
CLINICAL FEATURES
ISLET CELL TUMORS
HYPERINSULINISM (INSULINOMA)
ZOLLINGER-ELLISON SYNDROME (GASTRINOMAS)
OTHER RARE ISLET CELL TUMORS

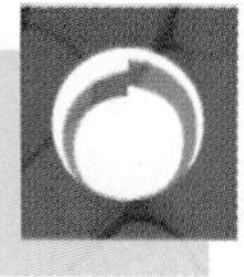

The Exocrine Pancreas

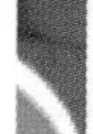

NORMAL

In its posterior location in the upper abdomen, the pancreas is one of the "hidden" organs in the body. It is virtually impossible to palpate clinically. Diseases that impair its function evoke signs or symptoms only when far advanced, because there is such a large reserve of both exocrine and endocrine function. Some life-threatening lesions are manifested only by encroachment on neighboring structures, particularly nerves that course through the retroperitoneal tissue. Thus, detection of pancreatic disease continues to be a source of frustration in modern medicine.

In adults the average pancreas is about 15 cm in length; weighs 60 to 140 gm; and consists of a head, body, and tail. The gross anatomic relationships of the pancreas include immediate proximity to the duodenum, ampulla of

Vater, superior mesenteric artery, portal vein, spleen and its vascular supply, stomach, transverse colon, left lobe of the liver, and lower recesses of the lesser omental cavity (Fig. 20–1). The pancreas is a pinkish tan organ with distinct coarse lobulations, the result of delicate collagen septa that subdivide the parenchyma into macroscopic lobules.

The pancreas arises from the duodenum in the form of a dorsal bud and a shorter ventral bud. Fusion of the two creates the composite head; the dorsal bud is the primary source of the tapering body and tail. Fusion of the ventral duct and distal portion of the dorsal duct creates the definitive pancreatic duct (*duct of Wirsung*). Occasionally, the proximal portion of the dorsal duct persists as the *accessory duct of Santorini.* Although there is much variability in the ductal system, *in two thirds of adults the major pancreatic duct does not empty directly into the duodenum but into the common bile duct just proximal to the ampulla of Vater, as the bile duct courses through the head of the pancreas.* Thus, in most individuals there is a common channel for pancreatic and biliary drainage.

Histologically, the pancreas has two separate components, the exocrine and endocrine glands. The endocrine pancreas is described later in this chapter. The exocrine portion, constituting 80% to 85% of the organ, is made up of numerous small glands (*acini*) containing columnar to pyramidal epithelial cells radially oriented about the gland circumference (Fig. 20–2). The acinar cells are deeply basophilic because of their abundant rough endoplasmic reticulum, located in the basal portion of the cell. The supranuclear Golgi complex is well developed and is part of an apically oriented secretory complex that forms abundant membrane-bound *zymogen granules* containing digestive enzymes. When acinar cells are stimulated, these zymogen-containing vesicles migrate to the apical plasma membrane and rupture at the point of attachment to release their contents into the acinar lumen. The extremely fine channels that drain each secretory acinus progressively anastomose to form the pancreatic ductal system. The lining epithelium is at first cuboidal but gradually becomes a tall, columnar, electrolyte- and mucus-secreting epithelium in the main ducts. About the larger ducts, there are numerous accessory mucous glands.

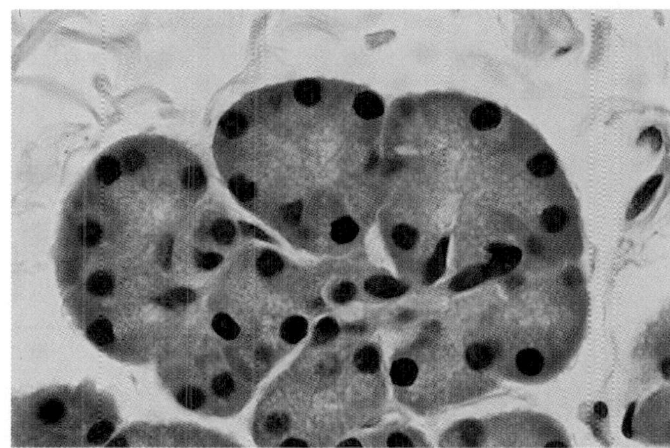

Figure 20–2

Pancreatic acini, showing the radial orientation of the pyramidal exocrine acinar cells. The cytoplasm is devoted to the synthesis and packaging of digestive enzymes for secretion into a central lumen.

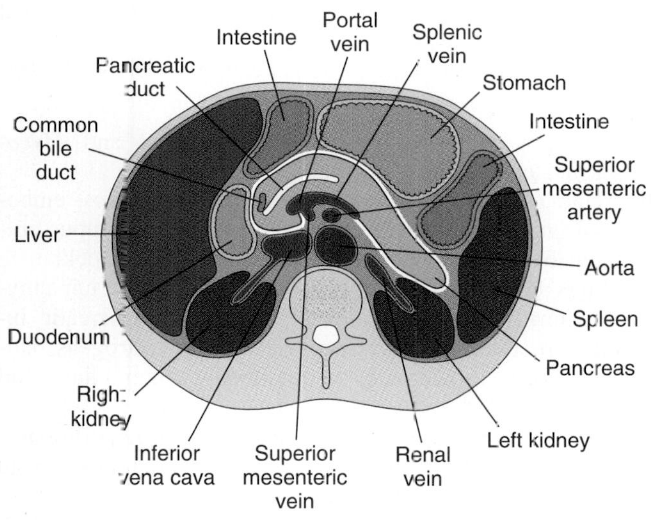

Figure 20–1

Anatomic relationships of the pancreas seen in a cross-section of the abdomen at the level of the upper lumbar vertebrae. (From Go VW, et al (eds): The Pancreas: Biology, Pathobiology, and Disease, 2nd ed. New York, Raven Press, 1993.)

The pancreas secretes 2 to 2.5 liters per day of a bicarbonate-rich fluid containing digestive enzymes and proenzymes. Regulation of this secretion involves both neural stimulation mediated by vagal nerves and humoral factors. The most important of the latter are the hormones *secretin* and *cholecystokinin*, produced in the duodenum. Secretin stimulates water and bicarbonate secretion by duct cells, and cholecystokinin promotes discharge of digestive enzymes by acinar cells. The primary stimulants of duodenal secretin production are an acid load from the gastric effluent and luminal fatty acids. Cholecystokinin is released from the duodenal mucosa predominantly in response to fatty acids and protein digestive products—peptides and amino acids.

The digestive enzymes consist of trypsin, chymotrypsin, aminopeptidases, elastase, amylases, lipase, phospholipases, and nucleases. Trypsin is a key enzyme, as it catalyzes activation of the other enzymes. Self-digestion of the pancreas is prevented by several means:

- The enzymes are synthesized as inactive proenzymes (with the exception of amylase and lipase).
- They are sequestered in membrane-bound zymogen granules in the acinar cells.
- Activation of proenzymes requires conversion of inactive trypsinogen to active trypsin by duodenal enteropeptidase (enterokinase).
- Trypsin inhibitors are present within acinar and ductal secretions.

- Intrapancreatic release of trypsin activates an enzyme or enzymes that degrade(s) other digestive enzymes to inert products.
- Lysosomal hydrolases are capable of degrading zymogen granules when normal acinar secretion is impaired or blocked.
- Acinar cells are remarkably resistant to the action of trypsin, chymotrypsin, and phospholipase A_2.

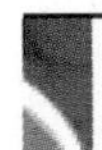

PATHOLOGY

The most significant disorders of the exocrine pancreas are cystic fibrosis (Chapter 11), acute and chronic pancreatitis, and tumors. From the standpoints of both morbidity and mortality, diabetes mellitus overshadows all other pancreatic disorders. This disorder of endocrine metabolism is considered in the second portion of this chapter. However, a knowledgeable alertness to exocrine pancreatic disease is very necessary. These disorders are difficult to diagnose because of the hidden position and large reserve function of this organ, and they may appear under such diverse guises as a catastrophic "acute abdomen" or the silent growth of a carcinoma.

CONGENITAL ANOMALIES

Variations in pancreatic anatomy are usually of little clinical import, with some notable exceptions. The pancreas may be totally absent (*agenesis*), a condition regularly associated with widespread severe malformations that are incompatible with life. Incomplete fusion of the two pancreatic anlagen creates *pancreas divisum* and predisposes to recurrent pancreatitis. The gland may exist as two separate structures if the dorsal and ventral pancreatic anlagen do not fuse at all. The head of the pancreas may encircle the duodenum as a collar (*annular pancreas*), sometimes causing subtotal duodenal obstruction. Variable ductal anatomy of the pancreas may present particular problems to the endoscopist and surgeon. For example, the ducts of Wirsung and of Santorini may persist as totally separate structures, with separate duodenal orifices. Failure to recognize aberrant ductal anatomy may lead to potential ligation or severance of ducts during surgery around the ampulla, causing serious sequelae.

Ectopic Pancreas

Aberrant, or *ectopic*, displaced pancreatic tissue is found in about 2% of careful routine postmortem examinations. The favored sites for ectopia are the stomach and duodenum, followed by the jejunum, Meckel diverticulum, and ileum. Usually, the embryologic rests are a few millimeters to centimeters in diameter, located in the submucosa. They are seen histologically to be composed of glands that appear completely normal, and not infrequently islets of Langerhans are present. Although usually incidental, such lesions may be visualized as sessile lesions, may cause pain from localized inflammation, or rarely may incite mucosal bleeding. About 2% of islet cell tumors arise in ectopic pancreatic tissue.

PANCREATITIS

Inflammation of the pancreas, almost always associated with acinar cell injury, is termed *pancreatitis*. Clinically and histologically, pancreatitis occurs as a spectrum, both in duration and severity. *Acute pancreatitis* includes a mild, self-limited form and a more serious type, *acute hemorrhagic pancreatitis*, which exhibits extensive hemorrhagic necrosis of the organ. *Chronic pancreatitis* is the process of continuous or relapsing inflammation of the pancreas, typically causing pain and leading to irreversible morphologic damage and permanent impairment of function.

Acute Pancreatitis

Acute pancreatitis is characterized by the acute onset of abdominal pain resulting from enzymatic necrosis and inflammation of the pancreas. It is a relatively common disorder, with an incidence rate in Western countries of 10 to 20 cases per 100,000. About 80% of cases are associated with two conditions: *biliary tract disease* and *alcoholism* (Table 20–1).[1] Gallstones are present in 35% to 60% of cases of pancreatitis, and *about 5% of patients with gallstones develop pancreatitis.* The proportion of cases of acute pancreatitis caused by alcoholism varies from 65% in the United States to 20% in Sweden and 5% or less in southern France and the United Kingdom.[2] The male-female ratio is 1:3 in the group with biliary tract disease and 6:1 in those with alcoholism.

The less common causes of pancreatitis include the following:

- Infections with mumps, coxsackieviruses, and *Mycoplasma pneumoniae.*
- Acute ischemia induced by vascular thrombosis, embolism, vasculitis (polyarteritis nodosa, systemic lupus erythematosus, Henoch-Schönlein purpura), and shock.
- Drugs cause abdominal pain and elevated serum amylase levels. Those implicated in causing pancreatic injury are thiazide diuretics, azathioprine, estrogens, sulfonamides, furosemide, methyldopa, pentamidine, and procainamide.[4]
- Pancreatitis is occasionally associated with hyperlipoproteinemia (types I and V) and with hyperparathyroidism and other hypercalcemia states.
- Occlusion of pancreatic ducts by *Ascaris lumbricoides* and *Clonorchis sinensis* organisms.

Of note, 10% to 20% of patients have no known associated processes, and their condition must be termed *idiopathic*.

Table 20-1. ETIOLOGIC FACTORS IN ACUTE PANCREATITIS

Metabolic
Alcoholism
Hyperlipoproteinemia
Hypercalcemia
Drugs (e.g., thiazide diuretics)
Genetic

Mechanical
Gallstones
Iatrogenic injury
  Perioperative injury
  Endoscopic procedures with dye injection

Vascular
Shock
Atheroembolism
Polyarteritis nodosa

Infectious
Mumps
Coxsackievirus
Mycoplasma pneumoniae

MORPHOLOGY. The morphology of acute pancreatitis stems directly from the action of activated pancreatic enzymes that are released into the pancreatic substance. The basic alterations are **(1) microvascular leakage, to cause edema, (2) necrosis of fat by lipolytic enzymes, (3) an acute inflammatory reaction, (4) proteolytic destruction of pancreatic substance, and (5) destruction of blood vessels with subsequent interstitial hemorrhage.** The extent and predominance of each of these alterations depend on the duration and severity of the process.

In the milder form, acute interstitial pancreatitis, histologic alterations are limited to interstitial edema and focal areas of fat necrosis in the pancreatic substance and peripancreatic fat (Fig. 20–3). Fat necrosis, as we have seen, results from enzymatic destruction of fat cells. The released fatty acids combine with calcium to form insoluble salts that precipitate in situ (Chapter 1).

In the more severe form, acute necrotizing pancreatitis, necrosis of pancreatic tissue affects acinar and ductal tissues as well as the islets of Langerhans. There may be sufficient damage to the vasculature to cause hemorrhage into the parenchyma of the pancreas. Macroscopically, the pancreatic substance exhibits areas of blue-black hemorrhage interspersed with foci of yellow-white, chalky fat necrosis (Fig. 20–4). Foci of fat necrosis may also be found in any of the fat depots, such as the omentum and the mesentery of the bowel, and even outside the abdominal cavity, such as in the subcutis. In most cases the peritoneal cavity contains a serous, slightly turbid, brown-tinged fluid in which globules of fat (derived from the action of enzymes on adipose tissue) can be identified.

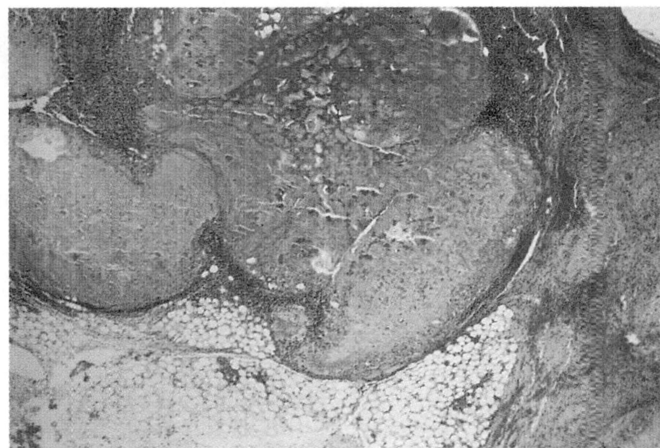

Figure 20–3

Acute pancreatitis. The microscopic field shows an advancing region of fat necrosis at the upper left, impinging upon preserved adipose tissue (*lower left*) and with accompanying local hemorrhage (*right*). (H&E.)

Pathogenesis. The anatomic changes of acute pancreatitis strongly suggest autodigestion of the pancreatic substance by inappropriately activated pancreatic enzymes. As is well known, pancreatic enzymes are present in the acini in the proenzyme form and have to be activated to fulfill their enzymatic potential. Among many possible activators, a major role is attributed to trypsin, which itself is synthesized as the proenzyme trypsinogen. Once trypsin is generated, it can in turn activate other proenzymes such as prophospholipase and proelastase, which then take part in the process of autodigestion. The activated enzymes so generated cause disintegration of fat cells and damage the

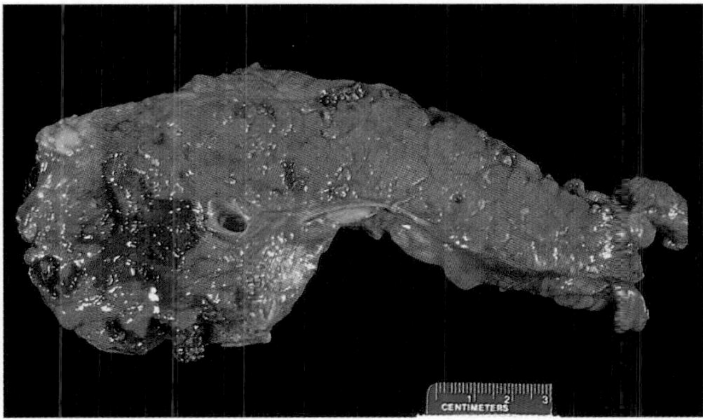

Figure 20–4

Acute pancreatitis. The pancreas has been sectioned across to reveal dark areas of hemorrhage in the head of the pancreas and a focal area of pale fat necrosis in the peripancreatic fat (*upper left*).

elastic fibers of blood vessels, respectively. Trypsin also converts prekallikrein to its activated form, thus bringing into play the kinin system—and by activation of Hageman factor the clotting and complement systems as well. In this way, the inflammation and small-vessel thromboses (which may lead to congestion and rupture of already weakened vessels) are amplified. Thus, activation of trypsinogen is an important triggering event in acute pancreatitis.

The mechanisms by which activation of pancreatic enzymes is initiated are not entirely clear, but there is evidence for three possible pathways (Fig. 20–5):

1. *Pancreatic duct obstruction.* Regardless of whether the common bile duct and pancreatic duct share a common channel or separate channels, impaction of a gallstone in the region of the ampulla of Vater raises intrapancreatic ductal pressure. Blockage to ductal flow favors the accumulation of an enzyme-rich interstitial fluid. This causes local fat necrosis, as lipase is already active. Resident tissue leukocytes are stimulated to release proinflammatory cytokines, initiating local inflammation and promoting the development of interstitial edema through a leaky microvasculature.[5] According to one hypothesis, *edema compromises local blood flow, causing vascular insufficiency and ischemic injury to acinar cells.*[6]
2. *Primary acinar cell injury.* This mechanism is most clearly involved in the pathogenesis of acute pancreatitis caused by certain viruses (e.g., mumps), drugs, and direct trauma to the pancreas, as well as that following the ischemia of shock. The mechanisms by which alcohol promotes acinar cell injury remain unclear.[7]
3. *Defective intracellular transport of proenzymes within acinar cells.* Aberrant acinar cell packaging of digestive enzymes has been shown to occur both when there is pancreatic duct obstruction or exposure to alcohol, and in experimental animal models of metabolic pancreatic injury.[8] In normal acinar cells, digestive enzymes and the lysosomal hydrolases are transported in separate pathways after being synthesized in the endoplasmic reticulum and packaged in the Golgi apparatus. The digestive enzymes make their way through zymogen granules to the apical cell surface, while lysosomal hydrolases are transported into the lysosomes. When acinar cells

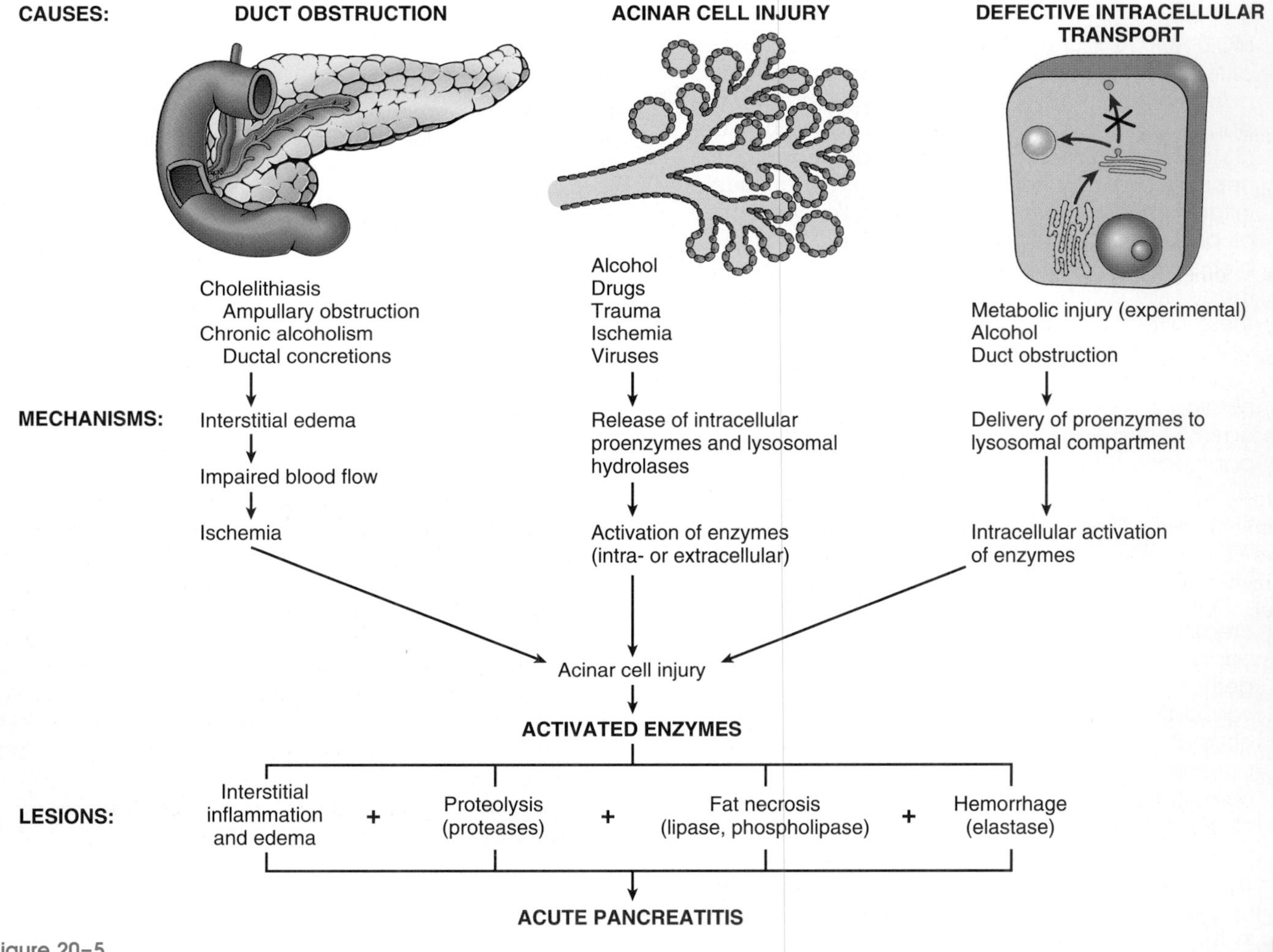

Figure 20–5

Three proposed pathways in the pathogenesis of acute pancreatitis.

are injured, the pancreatic proenzymes are delivered to an intracellular compartment containing lysosomal hydrolases, thereby permitting proenzyme activation, rupture of the lysosomes, and local release of activated enzymes.

The manner by which alcohol precipitates pancreatitis is unknown. Transient increases in pancreatic exocrine secretion, contraction of the sphincter of Oddi, and direct toxic effects on acinar cells have all been postulated from experimental studies. Many authorities now think that most cases of alcoholic pancreatitis are sudden exacerbations of chronic pancreatitis, presenting as apparent de novo acute pancreatitis.[7] According to this view, chronic alcohol ingestion causes secretion of protein-rich pancreatic fluid, leading to deposition of inspissated protein plugs and obstruction of small pancreatic ducts, followed by the train of events described above.

Clinical Features. Abdominal pain is the cardinal manifestation of acute pancreatitis. Its severity varies from mild and uncomfortable to severe and incapacitating. Suspected acute pancreatitis is primarily diagnosed by the presence of elevated plasma levels of amylase and lipase, and exclusion of other causes of abdominal pain.

Full-blown acute pancreatitis is a medical emergency of the first magnitude. These patients usually have the sudden calamitous onset of an "acute abdomen" that must be differentiated from diseases such as ruptured acute appendicitis, perforated peptic ulcer, acute cholecystitis with rupture, and occlusion of mesenteric vessels with infarction of the bowel. Characteristically, the pain is constant and intense and is often referred to the upper back.

Many of the systemic features of severe acute pancreatitis can be attributed to release of toxic enzymes, cytokines, and other mediators into the circulation and explosive activation of the systemic inflammatory response, resulting in *leukocytosis, hemolysis, disseminated intravascular coagulation, fluid sequestration, adult respiratory distress syndrome, and diffuse fat necrosis. Peripheral vascular collapse and shock with acute renal tubular necrosis may occur* (Fig. 20–6). Explanations for the rapid development of shock include loss of blood volume and electrolyte disturbances, endotoxemia, and release of cytokines and vasoactive agents such as bradykinin, prostaglandins, nitric oxide (NO), and platelet activating factor. Laboratory findings include marked elevation of serum amylase and lipase levels during the first 24 hours, followed within 72 to 96 hours by a rising serum lipase level. Glycosuria occurs in 10% of cases. Hypocalcemia may result from precipitation of calcium soaps in the fat necrosis; if persistent, it is a poor prognostic sign. Direct visualization of the enlarged inflamed pancreas by radiographic means is useful in the diagnosis of pancreatitis.

The key to management is "resting" the pancreas by total restriction of food and fluids and by supportive therapy. Although most patients with acute pancreatitis recover fully, about 5% die from shock during the first week of the clinical course. Acute adult respiratory distress syndrome and acute renal failure are ominous complications.[9] In surviving patients, sequelae may include a sterile *pancreatic abscess* and a *pancreatic pseudocyst* (discussed later). In

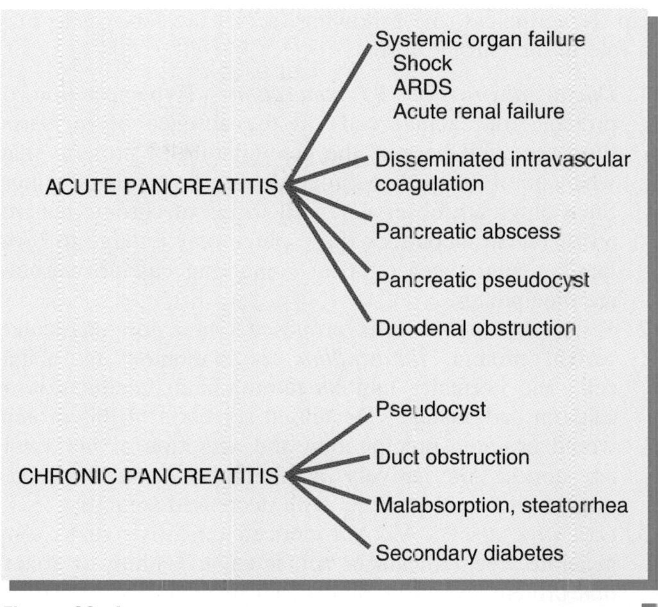

Figure 20–6

Comparison of the sequelae of acute and chronic pancreatitis.

40% to 70% of patients with acute necrotizing pancreatitis, the necrotic debris becomes infected, further complicating the clinical course.[10]

Chronic Pancreatitis

Chronic pancreatitis is a disease characterized by repeated bouts of mild to moderate pancreatic inflammation, with continued loss of pancreatic parenchyma and replacement by fibrous tissue.[11] The chief distinction between acute and chronic pancreatitis is whether the pancreas is normal before a symptomatic attack or already chronically damaged—this distinction may be impossible to apply in clinical settings. The disease is protean in its manifestations and most frequently affects middle-aged males, particularly alcoholics. Biliary tract disease plays a less important role in chronic pancreatitis than in the acute form of the disease; hypercalcemia and hyperlipoproteinemia also predispose to chronic pancreatitis. In up to 12% of patients, recurrent pancreatitis is associated with *pancreas divisum*, presumably because of the combination of an anomalous ductal system and stenosis of the duodenal papilla. There are relatively rare special forms of chronic pancreatitis, such as *nonalcoholic tropical pancreatitis* and *familial hereditary pancreatitis*. Hereditary pancreatitis begins in childhood and predisposes to the development of pancreatic carcinoma in later years. Up to 40% of patients with chronic pancreatitis have no recognizable predisposing factor.

Pathogenesis. As noted, the distinction between causes of acute and chronic pancreatitis remains blurred, and thus the pathogenetic mechanisms in these disorders may overlap. Nevertheless, the following factors are thought to play a role in the chronic forms:[7]

1. *Ductal obstruction by concretions.* Hypersecretion of protein from acinar cells in the absence of increased fluid secretion permits the precipitation of proteins that, when admixed with cellular debris, form ductal plugs. Such plugs are observed in all forms of chronic pancreatitis, but in alcoholics these plugs may enlarge to form laminar aggregates (stones) containing calcium carbonate precipitates.
2. *Secreted proteins.* It is proposed that a low-molecular-weight protein, *lithostathine,* is elaborated by acinar cells and normally inhibits intraluminal precipitation of calcium carbonates.[12] Decreased secretion of this protein would promote precipitation and accretion of intraluminal stones. Alternatively, alcohol may cause the secretion of abnormal proteins with decreased solubility.[13]
3. *Oxidative stress.* Alcohol-induced oxidative stress may generate free radicals in acinar cells, leading to abnormal protein secretion, acinar cell necrosis, inflammation, and fibrosis.
4. *Interstitial fibrosis.* It is proposed that acute pancreatitis initiates a sequence of perilobular fibrosis, duct distortion, and altered pancreatic secretion and ductal flow—the "necrosis-fibrosis" hypothesis.[14] Alternatively, abnormal intrapancreatic lipid metabolites may trigger the development of fibrosis.[15]

Protein-calorie malnutrition probably plays a role in the tropical pancreatitis seen in southeast Asia and parts of Africa, where alcohol consumption is extremely low. The rare *autosomal dominant hereditary pancreatitis* is associated with an arginine to histidine substitution at residue 117 of trypsinogen. This point mutation removes a proteolytic cleavage site in the activated enzyme, which would otherwise permit the enzyme's inactivation.[15]

MORPHOLOGY. Chronic pancreatitis is characterized by **irregularly distributed fibrosis, reduced number and size of acini with relative sparing of the islets of Langerhans, and variable obstruction of pancreatic ducts of all sizes** (Fig. 20–7*A*). The lesions have a macroscopic lobular distribution and may involve portions or all of the pancreas. A chronic inflammatory infiltrate around lobules and ducts is usually present. The interlobular and intralobular ducts are dilated and contain protein plugs in their lumens. The ductal epithelium may be atrophied or hyperplastic or may show squamous metaplasia, and ductal concretions may be evident (Fig. 20–7*B*). Remaining islets become embedded in sclerosed tissue or severely damaged lobules, before they too disappear. Grossly, the gland is hard, sometimes with extremely dilated ducts and grossly visible calcified concretions. Pseudocyst formation is common.

Clinical Features. Chronic pancreatitis has many faces. It may present as repeated attacks of moderately severe abdominal pain, recurrent attacks of mild pain, or persistent abdominal and back pain. Again, the local disease may be entirely silent until pancreatic insufficiency and diabetes develop, the latter from associated destruction of islets. In still other instances, recurrent attacks of jaundice or vague attacks of indigestion may hint at pancreatic disease. Attacks may be precipitated by alcohol abuse, overeating (which increases demand on the pancreas), or the use of opiates and other drugs.

The diagnosis of chronic pancreatitis requires a high degree of suspicion. During an attack of abdominal pain there may be mild fever and mild to moderate elevations

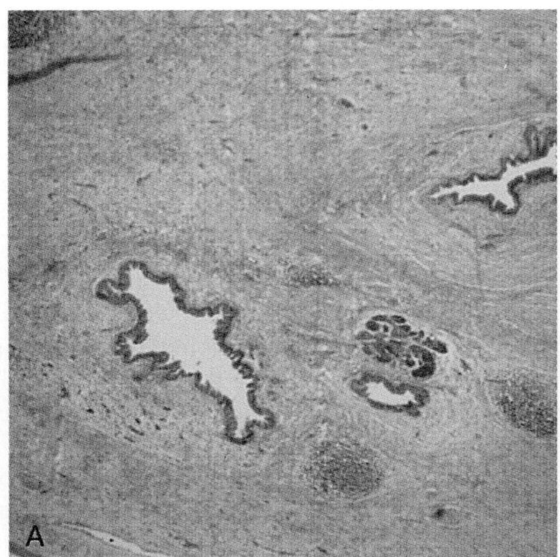

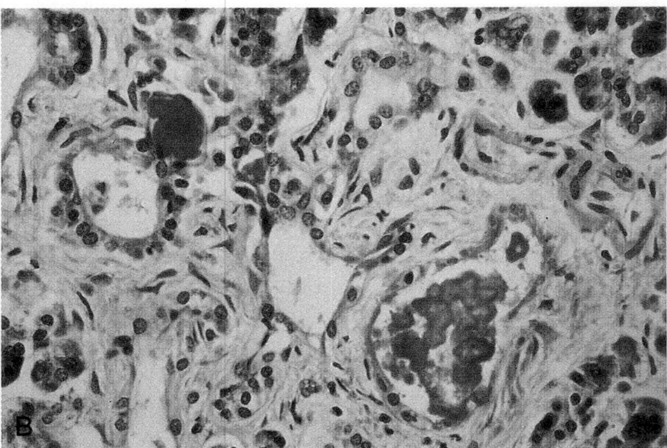

Figure 20–7

Chronic pancreatitis. *A*, Extensive fibrosis and atrophy has left only residual islets and ducts, with a sprinkling of chronic inflammatory cells and acinar tissue. *B*, A higher power demonstrating dilated ducts with inspissated eosinophilic ductal concretions.

of serum amylase. When the disease has been present for a long time, however, the destruction of acinar cells may preclude such diagnostic clues. Gallstone-induced obstruction may be evident as jaundice or elevations in serum levels of alkaline phosphatase. A very helpful finding is visualization of calcifications within the pancreas by computed tomography (CT) and ultrasonography. Weight loss and hypoalbuminemic edema may point toward pancreatic insufficiency.

For the most part, chronic pancreatitis is a disabling rather than life-threatening condition (Fig. 20–6). Severe pancreatic exocrine insufficiency and chronic malabsorption may develop, as can diabetes mellitus. Alternatively, severe chronic pain may become the dominant problem. Pancreatic pseudocysts develop in about 10% of patients. There is a modestly increased risk of pancreatic carcinoma, attributed to the risk imposed by smoking and alcohol consumption rather than a causal role of chronic pancreatitis per se.[16]

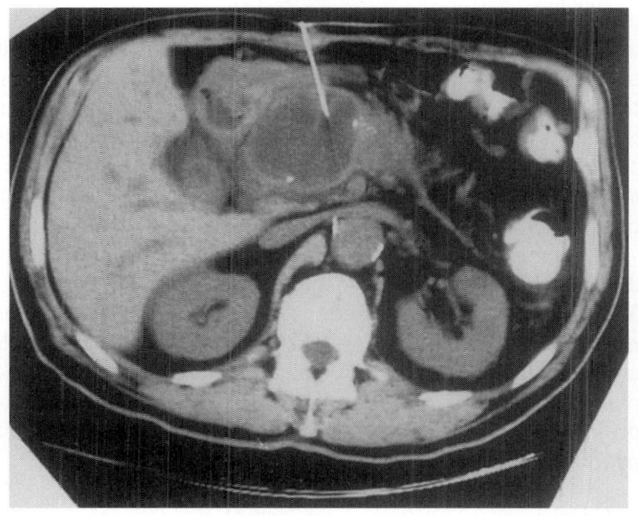

Figure 20–8 ■

Pancreatic pseudocyst. In this computed tomographic scan of the upper abdomen, a percutaneous needle has been placed into a large cystic lesion in the body of the pancreas. (Courtesy of Peter A. Banks, MD, Brigham and Women's Hospital, Boston, MA.)

CYSTS

A variety of cysts can arise in this organ. Most are non-neoplastic *pseudocysts* (see later), but neoplastic cystic tumors also occur and are discussed under "Tumors."

Congenital cysts are believed to result from anomalous development of the pancreatic ducts. Cysts in the kidney, liver, and pancreas frequently coexist in *polycystic disease* (discussed in Chapter 21). The pancreatic cysts range from microscopic lesions to cysts 3 to 5 cm in diameter. They are lined by a glistening, duct-type cuboidal epithelium or a completely attenuated cell layer, enclosed in a thin, fibrous capsule and filled with a clear to turbid mucoid or serous fluid. In *von Hippel-Lindau disease* (Chapter 21), angiomas are found in the retina and cerebellum or brain stem in association with cysts in the pancreas, liver, and kidney.

Pseudocysts

Pseudocysts are localized collections of pancreatic secretions that develop after inflammation of the pancreas. They are to be distinguished from sterile *pancreatic abscesses*, which involve liquefactive necrosis of severely damaged pancreatic parenchyma. Both entities lack a true epithelial lining, unlike congenital cysts. *Pseudocysts are by far the more common, and virtually all arise after acute or chronic pancreatitis*. Traumatic injury to the abdomen may also give rise to pseudocysts.

MORPHOLOGY. These cysts are usually solitary and may be situated within the pancreatic substance (Fig. 20–8) or immediately adjacent to the pancreas. They are formed by drainage of pancreatic secretions from damaged ducts into interstitial tissue, which becomes walled off by fibrous tissue to form a cystic space. Continued fluid drainage may lead to massive enlargement of the cyst to 5 to 10 cm in diameter.

Pseudocysts produce abdominal pain; hemorrhage and infection with generalized peritonitis are potential complications. However, their usual clinical significance lies in their being discovered as an abdominal mass in a location that strongly suggests a primary malignancy. They are usually unilocular, which assists in distinction from neoplastic cysts, which tend to be multiloculated.

TUMORS

A variety of benign and malignant tumors may arise in the exocrine and endocrine pancreas.[17] Endocrine tumors are described later. Most tumors of the exocrine pancreas are solid, malignant, glandular tumors, to which the common term *carcinoma of the pancreas* refers, and these are now common causes of cancer worldwide. Some, however, are cystic, and such tumors can be benign, borderline malignant, or malignant.

Cystic Tumors

Cystic tumors make up less than 5% of all pancreatic neoplasms and occur most often in elderly women. They are usually in the body or tail, and present as painless, slow-growing masses. Some are multiloculated, cystic neoplasms filled with mucinous secretions (*mucinous cystic tumors*), resembling their histologic counterpart in the ovary (Chapter 24). The only way to distinguish the entirely benign form (*cystadenoma*) from its malignant counterpart (*cystadenocarcinoma*, Fig. 20–9) is by pathologic assessment after complete surgical removal, usually by distal pancreatectomy. A rare cystic tumor with serous secretions (*microcystic adenoma*) is almost always benign.

The unusual *solid-cystic* (papillary-cystic) *tumor* is predominantly seen in adolescent girls and women under age 35.[18] It is a large, rounded, well-circumscribed mass that has solid and cystic zones. Histologically, the tumor cells are small and uniform and have a finely granular eosinophilic cytoplasm. They grow in solid sheets or papillary projections. The tumors cause abdominal discomfort and pain and are usually cured by resection.

Carcinoma of the Pancreas

Carcinoma of the pancreas is now the fifth most frequent cause of death from cancer in the United States, preceded only by lung, colon, breast, and prostate cancers.[19] Currently, 28,000 new patients are identified every year, of whom only 1000 are expected to survive 5 years.

Pathogenesis and Genetics. Unlike other cancers of the alimentary tract, little is known about the cause of pancreatic cancer. The strongest environmental influence is smoking, since incidence rates are several times higher in smokers than in nonsmokers.[20] Other environmental factors have been implicated, including chronic alcohol intake and consumption of a high-energy diet rich in fats, but these are not consistent risk factors. Pancreatic cancer arises with greater frequency in patients with chronic pancreatitis,[21] but a causal role for pancreatitis is not established, since smoking and alcohol usage in this patient population may underlie the association.[16] A similar argument applies to the association of diabetes with pancreatic cancer, since diabetes may develop as a consequence of chronic pancreatitis. Familial clustering of pancreatic cancer has been reported, but no genetic abnormality has been described. A rare form of pancreatitis, familial relapsing pancreatitis, is significantly associated with pancreatic cancer.

Point mutations at codon 12 of K-*ras* are found in over 90% of pancreatic cancers, and 60% to 80% exhibit mutations in *p53*.[22] K-*ras* mutations appear to be the early event, as they are detected frequently in patients with chronic pancreatitis. However, they do not seem to impart increased risk for pancreatic cancer in screening studies of patients with pancreatitis.[23, 24]

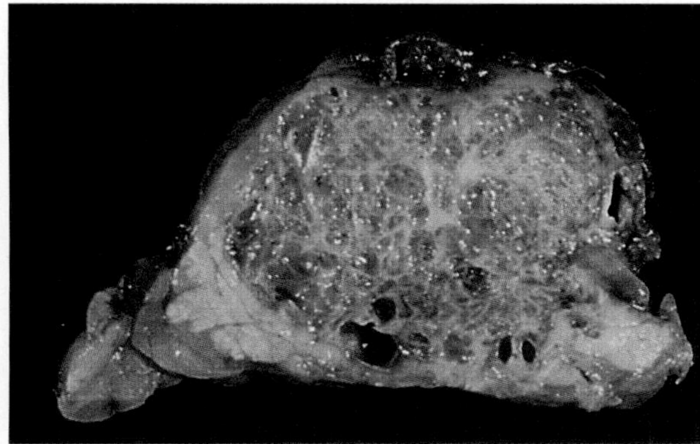

Figure 20–9

Pancreatic mucinous cystadenocarcinoma. Cross-section through a mucinous multiloculated cystic tumor in the body of the pancreas. The normal pancreatic tissue has been obliterated.

MORPHOLOGY. Approximately 60% of cancers of this organ arise in the head of the pancreas, 15% in the body, and 5% in the tail; in 20% the tumor diffusely involves the entire gland. Virtually all of these lesions are adenocarcinomas arising in the ductal epithelium. Some may secrete mucin, and many have an abundant fibrous stroma. These desmoplastic lesions therefore present as gritty, gray-white, hard masses. In its early stages, the tumor infiltrates locally and eventually extends into adjacent structures.

With carcinoma of the head of the pancreas, the ampullary region is invaded, obstructing the outflow of bile (Fig. 20–10*A*). Ulceration of the tumor into the duodenal mucosa may also occur. As a consequence of common bile duct obstruction, there is marked distention of the biliary tree in about 50% of patients with carcinoma of the head of the pancreas. In marked contrast, **carcinomas of the body and tail of the pancreas do not impinge on the biliary tract and hence remain silent for some time. They may be quite large and widely disseminated by the time they are discovered.** They extend through the retroperitoneal spaces; impinge on adjacent nerves, and occasionally invade the spleen, adrenals, vertebral column, transverse colon, and stomach. Peripancreatic, gastric, mesenteric, omental, and portahepatic nodes are frequently involved, and the liver is often enlarged owing to metastatic deposits. Distant metastases occur, principally to the lungs and bones.

Microscopically, there is no difference between carcinomas of the head of the pancreas and those of the body and tail of the pancreas. The appearance is usually that of a **moderately to poorly differentiated adenocarcinoma forming abortive tubular structures or cell clusters and exhibiting an aggressive, deeply infiltrative growth pattern** (Fig. 20–10*B*). Dense stromal fibrosis accompanies tumor invasion, and there is a proclivity for perineural invasion within and beyond the organ. The malignant glands are atypical, irregular, small, and bizarre and are usually lined by anaplastic cuboidal to columnar epithelial cells. Well-differentiated tumors are the exception. Careful examination may reveal regions of ductal dysplasia and intraductal tumor growth, in keep-

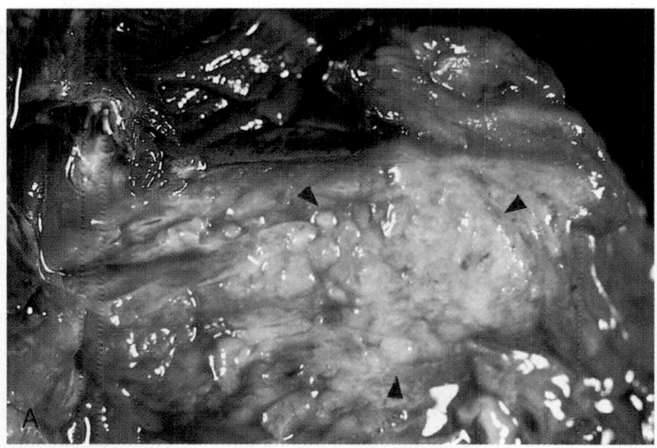

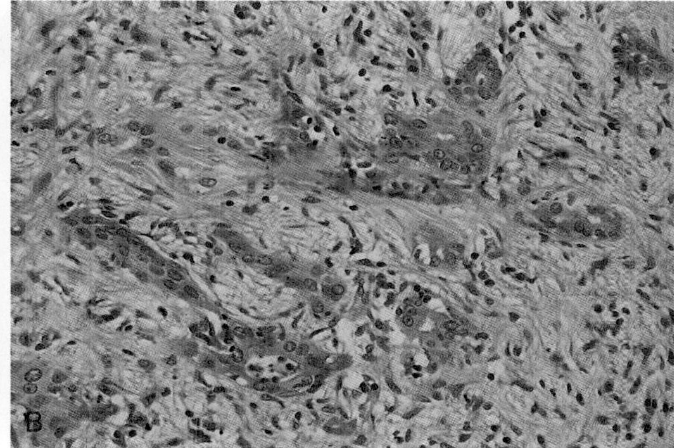

Figure 20–10

Carcinoma of the pancreas. *A*, A cross-section through the head of the pancreas and adjacent common bile duct shows both an ill-defined tumorous mass in the pancreatic substance (*arrowheads*) and the green discoloration of the duct resulting from total obstruction of bile flow. *B*, Poorly formed glands are present in densely fibrotic stroma within the pancreatic substance; there are some inflammatory cells. (H&E.)

ing with the ductal origin of most of these tumors. About 10% of tumors assume either an **adenosquamous pattern** or the uncommon pattern of extreme anaplasia with **giant cell formation** or a **sarcomatoid** histologic appearance. Rarely, carcinomas arise from acinar cells (**acinar cell carcinoma**) distinguished by the plump, polygonal eosinophilic appearance of the tumor cells.

Clinical Features. From the preceding discussion, it should be evident that carcinomas in the pancreas remain silent until their extension impinges on some other structure. It is when they erode to the posterior wall of the abdomen and affect nerve fibers that pain appears. Pain is usually the first symptom, but by the time pain appears, these cancers are usually beyond cure. Obstructive jaundice is associated with most cases of carcinoma of the head of the pancreas, but it rarely draws attention to the invasive cancer soon enough. Weight loss, anorexia, and generalized malaise and weakness tend to be signs of advanced disease. *Migratory thrombophlebitis*, known as the *Trousseau sign*, occurs in about 10% of patients, attributed to the elaboration of platelet-aggregating factors and procoagulants from the tumor or its necrotic products (Chapter 5). Ironically, Trousseau diagnosed his own fatal disease as cancer of the pancreas when he developed these spontaneously appearing and disappearing thromboses.

The symptomatic course of pancreatic carcinoma is typically brief and progressive. Despite the tendency of lesions of the head of the pancreas to obstruct the biliary system, less than 15% of pancreatic tumors overall are resectable at the time of diagnosis. There has long been a search for biochemical tests indicative of their presence.[26] As discussed earlier, the utility of screening tests for K-*ras* mutations remains unproven.[23, 25] Serum levels of many enzymes and antigens (e.g., carcinoembryonic antigen and CA19-9 antigen) have been found to be elevated, but these markers are unreliable. Several imaging techniques such as ultrasonography and CT have proved of great value in diagnosis; performance of percutaneous needle biopsy can obviate the need for exploratory laparotomy.

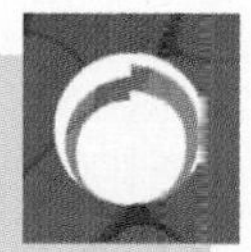

The Endocrine Pancreas

The endocrine pancreas consists of about 1 million microscopic clusters of cells, the islets of Langerhans. In the aggregate the islets in the adult human weigh only 1 to 1.5 gm. Embryologically, islet cells are of endodermal origin and form at many points along the pancreatic tubuloductal system. The first evidence of islet formation in the human fetus is seen at 9 to 11 weeks.[27]

In human adults, most islets measure 100 to 200 μm and consist of four major and two minor cell types. The four main types are β, α, δ, and PP (pancreatic polypeptide) cells. These make up about 68%, 20%, 10%, and 2%, respectively, of the adult islet cell population. They can be differentiated morphologically by their staining properties, by the ultrastructural structure of their granules, and by their hormone content (Fig. 20–11).

The β cell produces insulin, as detailed in the discussion of diabetes. The insulin-containing intracellular granules contain a crystalline matrix with a rectangular profiles, surrounded by a halo. *The α cell secretes glucagon*, inducing hyperglycemia by its glycogenolytic activity in the liver. α-

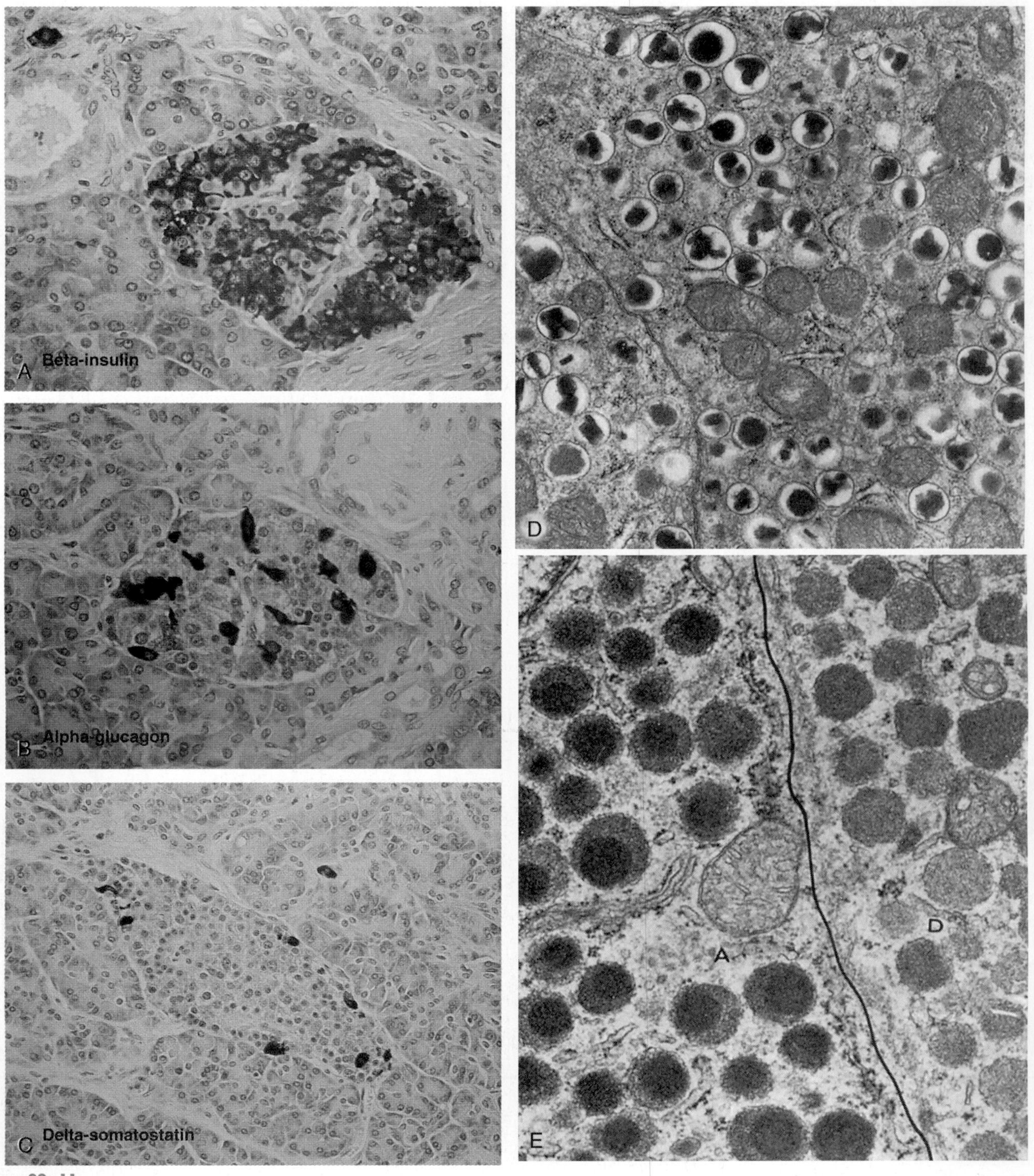

Figure 20–11

Immunoperoxidase staining shows a dark reaction product for insulin in ß cells (*A*), glucagon in α cells (*B*), and somatostatin in δ cells (*C*). *D*, Electron micrographs of β cells show the characteristic membrane-bound granules, each containing a dense, often rectangular core and distinct halo. *E*, Portions of an α cell (*left*) and δ cell (*right*) also exhibit granules, but with closely apportioned membranes. The α-cell granule exhibits a dense, round center. (Electron micrographs courtesy of Dr. A. Like, University of Massachusetts Medical School, Worcester, MA.)

Cell granules are round, with closely applied membranes and a dense center. *δ cells contain somatostatin,* which suppresses both insulin and glucagon release; they have large, pale granules with closely applied membranes. *PP cells contain a unique pancreatic polypeptide* that exerts a number of gastrointestinal effects, such as stimulation of secretion of gastric and intestinal enzymes and inhibition of intestinal motility. These cells have small, dark granules and are not only present in islets but also are scattered in the exocrine pancreas.

The two rare cell types are *D1 cells* and *enterochromaffin cells.* D1 cells elaborate *vasoactive intestinal polypeptide (VIP),* a hormone that induces glycogenolysis and hyperglycemia; it also stimulates gastrointestinal fluid secretion and causes secretory diarrhea. *Enterochromaffin cells synthesize serotonin* and are the source of pancreatic tumors that cause the carcinoid syndrome (Chapter 18).

We now turn to the two main disorders of islet cells: diabetes mellitus and islet cell tumors.

DIABETES MELLITUS

Diabetes mellitus is a chronic disorder of carbohydrate, fat, and protein metabolism. A defective or deficient insulin secretory response, which translates into impaired carbohydrate (glucose) use, is a characteristic feature of diabetes mellitus, as is the resultant hyperglycemia. About 3% of the world population, approximately 100 million people, suffer from diabetes, making this one of the most common noncommunicable diseases.

Classification and Incidence

Diabetes mellitus represents a heterogeneous group of disorders that have hyperglycemia as a common feature. It may occasionally arise secondarily from any disease causing extensive destruction of pancreatic islets, including pancreatitis, tumors, certain drugs, iron overload (hemochromatosis), certain acquired or genetic endocrinopathies, and surgical excision (Table 20–2).[28] However, *the most common and important forms of diabetes mellitus arise from primary disorders of the islet cell–insulin signaling system.* These can be divided into two common variants (type 1 and type 2) that differ in their patterns of inheritance, insulin responses, and origins, and less common specific genetic defects of β-cell functions (Table 20–3).

- *Type 1 diabetes,* also called insulin-dependent diabetes mellitus (IDDM) and previously referred to as juvenile-onset diabetes, accounts for about 10% of all cases of primary diabetes.
- Most of the remaining 80% to 90% of patients have the so-called *type 2 diabetes,* also called non–insulin-dependent diabetes mellitus (NIDDM) and previously referred to as adult-onset diabetes.
- The third group, commonly termed *maturity-onset diabetes of the young* (MODY), results from genetic defects of β-cell function. This group accounts for less than 5% of cases. MODY is manifested as a mild hyperglycemia and is transmitted as an autosomal dominant trait (see also under "Pathogenesis").

It should be stressed that while the major types of diabetes have different pathogenic mechanisms, *the long-term complications in blood vessels, kidneys, eyes, and nerves are the same and are the major causes of morbidity and death from diabetes.*

Diabetes affects an estimated 13 million people in the United States, although only about half of these are clinically diagnosed. With an annual mortality rate of about

Table 20–2. TYPES OF DIABETES MELLITUS

Primary Diabetes
- Type 1 (previously insulin-dependent diabetes mellitus, IDDM)
- Type 2 (previously non–insulin-dependent diabetes mellitus, NIDDM)
- Genetic defects of β-cell function (including maturity-onset diabetes of the young [MODY])
  - Chromosome 2, HNF 4α (MODY1)
  - Chromosome 7, glucokinase (MODY2)
  - Chromosome 12, HNF 1α (MODY3)
  - Mitochondrial DNA
  - Other genetic defects

Secondary Diabetes
- Infectious
  - Congenital rubella
  - Cytomegalovirus
- Endocrinopathies (e.g., adrenal, pituitary tumors)
- Drugs (corticosteroids, pentamidine, Vacor)
- Other genetic disorders (e.g., Down syndrome)
- Gestational diabetes mellitus

HNF, hepatocyte nuclear factor.
Modified from the Report of the Executive Committee on the Diagnosis and Classification of Diabetes Mellitus: Diabetic Care 20:1183–1197, 1997.

Table 20–3. TYPE 1 VS. TYPE 2 DIABETES MELLITUS

	Type 1 (IDDM)	Type 2 (NIDDM)
Clinical	Onset <20 yr Normal weight Decreased blood insulin Anti-islet cell antibodies Ketoacidosis common	Onset >30 yr Obese Normal or increased blood insulin No anti-islet cell antibodies Ketoacidosis rare
Genetics	50% concordance in twins HLA-D linked	90% to 100% concordance in twins No HLA association
Pathogenesis	Autoimmunity, immunopathologic mechanisms Severe insulin deficiency	Insulin resistance Relative insulin deficiency
Islet cells	Insulitis early Marked atrophy and fibrosis β-cell depletion	No insulitis Focal atrophy and amyloid deposits Mild β-cell depletion

54,000, diabetes is the seventh leading cause of death in the United States.[19] Diabetes increases in prevalence with age; about 50% of patients are over 55 years old. The lifetime risk of developing type 2 diabetes for the American adult population is estimated at 5% to 7%; for type 1 diabetes the lifetime risk is about 0.5%.

Pathogenesis

The pathogenesis of the two types is discussed separately, but first we briefly review normal insulin metabolism, since many aspects of insulin release and action are important in the consideration of pathogenesis.

NORMAL INSULIN PHYSIOLOGY

Normal glucose homeostasis is tightly regulated by three interrelated processes: *glucose production in the liver, uptake and utilization of glucose by peripheral tissues,* and *insulin secretion.* The insulin gene is expressed in the β cells of the pancreatic islets (Fig. 20–12). *Preproinsulin* is synthesized in the rough endoplasmic reticulum from insulin mRNA and delivered to the Golgi apparatus. There, a series of proteolytic cleavage steps by prohormone convertases generate the mature *insulin* and a cleavage peptide, *C peptide.*[29] Both C peptide and insulin are then stored in secretory granules and secreted together after physiologic stimulation.

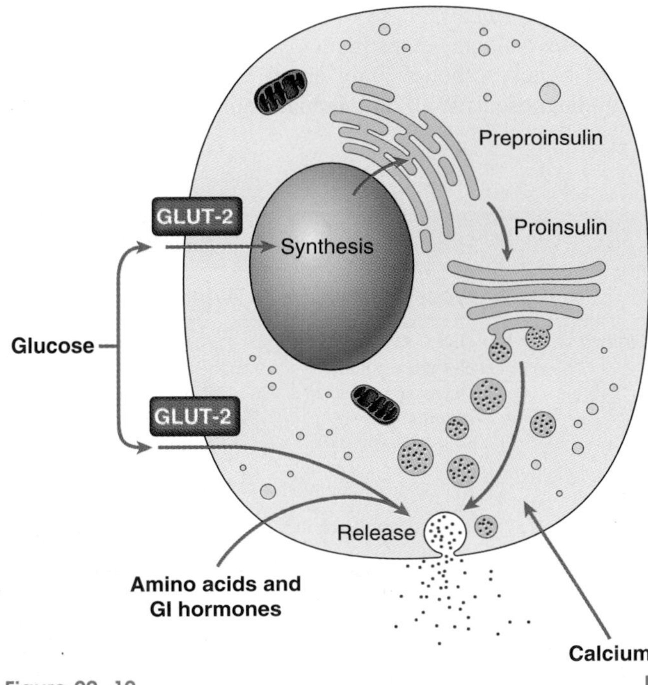

Figure 20–12

Insulin synthesis and secretion. Glucose stimulates both synthesis and calcium-dependent secretion of insulin, while other agents—amino acids and certain gastrointestinal hormones—induce only insulin secretion. GLUT-2 is an insulin-independent glucose transporter that facilitates entry of glucose into the cell.

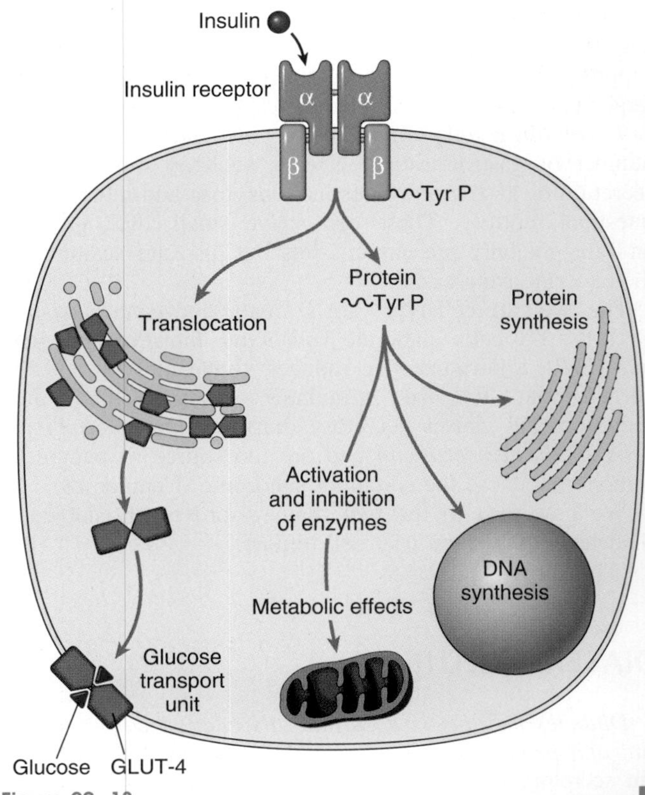

Figure 20–13

Insulin action on a target cell. Insulin binds to the α subunit of the insulin receptor and activates tyrosine-specific protein kinase autophosphorylation of the adjacent β subunit. This activates a cascade that stimulates DNA synthesis, protein synthesis (anabolism), and translocation of glucose transport units (GLUT proteins) from the Golgi apparatus to the plasma membrane.

The most important stimulus that triggers insulin release and synthesis is glucose. A rise in blood glucose levels results in glucose uptake into β cells, facilitated by an insulin-independent, glucose-transporting protein, GLUT-2. This calls forth an *immediate release of insulin,* presumably that stored in the β-cell granules. If the secretory stimulus persists, coupled with normal cholinergic input from the autonomic nervous system, a delayed and protracted response follows that involves *active synthesis of insulin.* Other agents, including intestinal hormones and certain amino acids (leucine and arginine), as well as the sulfonylureas, stimulate insulin release but not synthesis.

Insulin is a major anabolic hormone. It is necessary for (1) transmembrane transport of glucose and amino acids, (2) glycogen formation in the liver and skeletal muscles, (3) glucose conversion to triglycerides, (4) nucleic acid synthesis, and (5) protein synthesis. Its principal metabolic function is to increase the rate of glucose transport into certain cells in the body (Fig. 20–13).[30] These are the striated muscle cells (including myocardial cells), fibroblasts, and fat cells, *representing collectively about two thirds of the entire body weight.* In addition to these metabolic effects, *insulin and insulin-like growth factors initiate DNA synthesis in certain cells and stimulate their growth and differentiation.*

Insulin interacts with its target cells by first *binding to the insulin receptor*; hence, the number and function are important in regulating the action of insulin. The insulin receptor is composed of two glycoprotein subunits, α and β, possessing tyrosine kinase activity in the β-subunit cytosolic domain. Receptor-bound insulin triggers a cascade of intracellular responses, including activation of DNA and protein synthesis, and activation of anabolic metabolic pathways and inhibition of catabolic pathways (Fig. 20–13).[31] *One of the important early effects of insulin in target tissues involves translocation of glucose transport proteins (or units) (GLUTs) from the Golgi apparatus to the plasma membrane, thus facilitating cellular uptake of glucose.* There are several different forms of GLUTs, which differ in their tissue distribution, affinity for glucose, and sensitivity to insulin stimulation. GLUT-4, present in striated muscle and adipose tissue, is the major transporter regulated by insulin. On the other hand (as shown in Fig. 20–12), GLUT-2, present in liver hepatocytes and β cells of the pancreas, is insulin independent and serves to facilitate rapid equilibration of glucose between extracellular and intracellular compartments. Thus, whereas peripheral tissues utilize GLUT-4 to extract glucose from the blood, GLUT-2 serves primarily as a conduit for pancreatic and hepatic operation of the insulin-glucose feedback loop.

A singular feature of diabetes mellitus is impaired glucose tolerance. This is unmasked by a glucose challenge, such as an oral glucose tolerance test, in which blood glucose levels are sampled minutes to hours after an oral dose of glucose. In normal individuals, blood glucose levels rise only modestly, and a brisk pancreatic insulin response ensures a return to normoglycemic levels within an hour. *In diabetic individuals and in those in a preclinical stage, blood glucose rises to abnormally high levels for a sustained period.* As will become evident, this may result from an absolute lack of pancreatic insulin release, an impaired target tissue response to insulin, or both. Notably, screening programs using the glucose tolerance test indicate that *prevalence rates for preclinical diabetes (principally type 2) are the same as those for clinically diagnosed disease—about 3%.*

PATHOGENSIS OF TYPE 1 DIABETES MELLITUS

This form of diabetes results from a severe, absolute lack of insulin caused by a reduction in β-cell mass. Type 1 diabetes usually develops in childhood, becoming manifest and severe at puberty. Patients depend on insulin for survival; hence, the older term insulin-dependent diabetes mellitus (IDDM). Without insulin, they develop serious metabolic complications such as acute ketoacidosis and coma.

Three interlocking mechanisms are responsible for the islet cell destruction: genetic susceptibility, autoimmunity, and an environmental insult. A postulated sequence of events involving these three mechanisms is shown in Figure 20–14. It is thought that *genetic susceptibility* linked to specific alleles of the class II major histocompatibility complex (MHC) predisposes certain persons to the development of autoimmunity against β cells of the islets. The

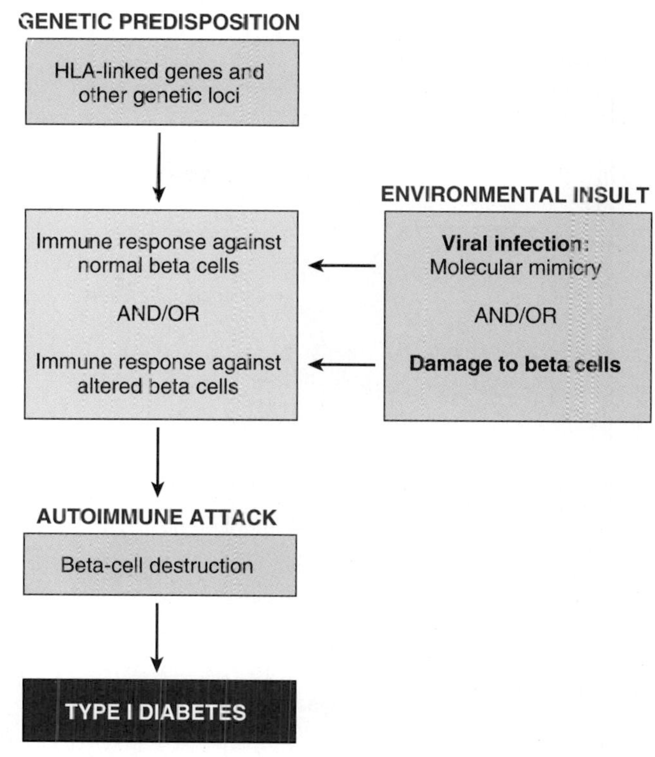

Figure 20–14

A simplified schema to show pathways of β-cell destruction leading to type 1 (insulin-dependent) diabetes mellitus. An environmental insult, possibly viral infection, is thought to provoke autoimmune attack of β cells in genetically susceptible individuals. Environmental insults may involve either molecular mimicry, in which a viral antigen evokes autoimmune attack of a similar β-cell antigen, or direct damage to β cells, causing abnormal expression of β-cell antigens.

autoimmune reaction either develops spontaneously or, more likely, is triggered by an *environmental event* that alters β cells, rendering them immunogenic. Overt diabetes appears after most of the β cells have been destroyed (Fig. 20–15). Let us now review the three mechanisms in the sequence.

Genetic Susceptibility. Type 1 diabetes mellitus occurs most frequently in persons of Northern European descent. The disease is much less common among other racial groups, including blacks, Native Americans, and Asians. Diabetes can aggregate in families; about 6% of children of first-order relatives with type 1 diabetes develop the disease. Among identical twins, the cumulative concordance risk (i.e., both twins affected) from birth to age 35 is 70%.[32] The fact that this number is not 100% implicates incomplete penetrance of genetic susceptibility traits or an additional role for environmental factors.

At least one of the susceptibility genes for type 1 diabetes resides in the region that encodes the class II antigens of the MHC on chromosome 6p21 (HLA-D).[33] You will recall (Chapter 7) that the HLA-D region contains three classes of genes (DP, DQ, and DR), that the class II molecules are highly polymorphic, and that each has numerous alleles. *About 95% of white patients with type 1 diabetes have either HLA-DR3 or HLA-DR4 alleles or both,*

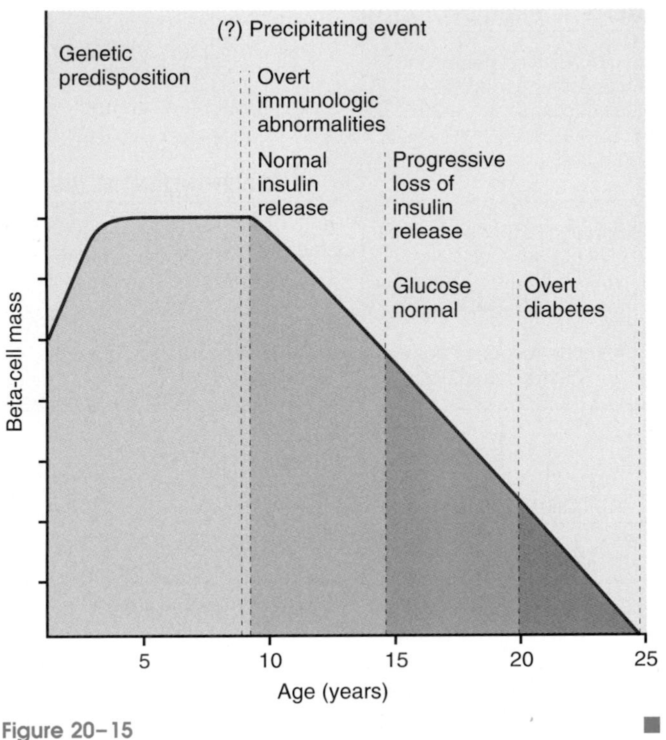

Figure 20–15

Stages in the development of type β-1 diabetes mellitus. The stages are listed from left to right, and hypothetical β-cell mass is plotted against age. (From Eisenbarth GE: Type 1 diabetes—a chronic autoimmune disease. N Engl J Med 314:1360, 1986. Copyright © 1986, Massachusetts Medical Society. All rights reserved.)

whereas in the general population the prevalence of these antigens is only 45%. There is an even stronger association with certain alleles (such as DQB1*0302), that are in linkage disequilibrium (i.e., coinherited) with HLA-DR genes. Notable is the finding that HLA-DQ β peptide chains with amino acid differences in the region close to the antigen-binding cleft of the molecule seem to affect the risk for type 1 diabetes in whites.

It is thought that genetic variations in the HLA class II molecule may alter recognition by the T-cell receptor, or may modify the presentation of the antigen because of variations in the antigen-binding cleft. Thus, *class II HLA genes may affect the degree of immune responsiveness to a pancreatic β-cell autoantigen, or a β-cell autoantigen may be presented in a manner that promotes an abnormal immunologic reaction.*

In addition to the established influence of HLA-linked genes, human genome analysis has revealed about 20 other chromosomal regions independently associated with predisposition to the disease. To date, these include 11p15 (the insulin gene region) and regions encoding loci of glucokinase and T-cell receptor peptides.[35] Collectively, these account for no more than 10% of the genetic risk.[36] Evaluation of these and other genes will be a major emphasis in coming years.

Autoimmunity. Although the clinical onset of type 1 diabetes is abrupt, this disease in fact results from a chronic autoimmune attack of β cells that usually exists for many years before the disease becomes evident.[37] The classic manifestations of the disease (hyperglycemia and ketosis) occur late in its course, after more than 90% of the β cells have been destroyed. Evidence for the importance of autoimmunity is as follows:

- *A lymphocyte-rich inflammatory infiltrate* ("insulitis") is observed in the islets of patients in early diabetes, and in animal models of autoimmune diabetes (see Fig. 20–19*A*). The infiltrate consists mostly of CD8 T lymphocytes, plus variable numbers of CD4 T cells and macrophages. CD4 T cells from animals with autoimmune diabetes can transfer diabetes to normal animals, thus establishing the primacy of T-cell autoimmunity in type 1 diabetes.[38]
- The insulitis is associated with *increased expression of class I MHC molecules and aberrant expression of class II MHC molecules on the β cells.* (However, aberrant MHC class II expression is not an absolute requisite for diabetes.[39]) This aberrant expression is mediated in part by *locally produced cytokines* (e.g., interferon-gamma [IFN-γ]) derived from activated T cells.[40] Genetic dysregulation of a cytokine that induces IFN-γ production promotes the development of diabetes in a mouse model.[41] Whether the abnormal expression of MHC genes is a cause or consequence of insulitis is unclear.
- About 70% to 80% of patients with type 1 diabetes have *islet cell autoantibodies* against intracellular islet cell antigens such as glutamic acid decarboxylase (GAD), "islet autoantigen 2" (IA-2, a tyrosine phosphatase), insulin, and gangliosides.[43] Whether these and other autoantibodies participate in causing damage to the β cells is unclear. Recent studies in an animal model strongly implicate GAD-reactive T cells in the pathogenesis of type 1 disease,[43] suggesting that GAD-reactive antibodies are formed *after* T-cell mediated injury to β cells. Regardless of their origin, *GAD autoantibodies can be detected long before the onset of clinical symptoms.*[44] Moreover, the simultaneous presence of GAD, IA-2, and insulin antibodies carries close to a 100% risk of the development of clinical diabetes within 5 years.[44] Asymptomatic relatives of patients with type 1 diabetes (who are therefore at increased risk) develop islet cell autoantibodies months to years before they manifest overt diabetes. Approximately 10% of persons with type 1 diabetes also have other organ-specific autoimmune disorders such as Graves disease, Addison disease, and thyroiditis.

To summarize, *overwhelming evidence implicates autoimmunity and immune-mediated injury as causes of β-cell loss in type 1 diabetes.* Indeed, immunosuppressive therapies have been shown to ameliorate type 1 diabetes in experimental animals and in children with new onset of the disease.

Environmental Factors. Assuming that a genetic susceptibility predisposes to autoimmune destruction of islet cells, what triggers the autoimmune reaction? Although the answer is unknown in most cases, there is compelling evidence that environmental factors are involved. Finnish children have a 60- to 70-fold greater risk of type 1 diabetes than Korean children. In the northeastern United States there has been a tripling of type 1 diabetes incidence in children under 15 years of age since the late 1960s. In three studies in Japan, Israel, and Canada, emigrants assume a risk of type 1 diabetes closer to that of their destination country than to that of their country of origin.

Viruses. Epidemiologic studies suggest the action of viruses. Seasonal trends that often correspond to the prevalence of common viral infections have long been noted in the diagnosis of new cases, as has the association between coxsackieviruses of group B and pancreatic diseases, including diabetes.[45] Other implicated viral infections include mumps, measles, cytomegalovirus, rubella, and infectious mononucleosis. Although many viruses are β-cell tropic, direct virus-induced injury is rarely severe enough to cause diabetes mellitus.

Several scenarios have been postulated for the role of viruses. *One is that viruses cause mild β-cell injury, which is followed by an autoimmune reaction against previously sequestered antigens in virally altered β cells in persons with HLA-linked susceptibility.* Type 1 diabetes would thus be a rare outcome of some relatively common viral infection, delayed by the long latency period necessary for progressive autoimmune loss of β cells to occur and dependent on the modifying effects of the genetic background, particular that of MHC class II molecules.

Another is that an immune response develops against a viral protein that shares amino acid sequences with a β cell protein ("molecular mimicry"). For example, a 6 amino acid sequence is shared between islet cell GAD and the P2-C replicative complex of Coxsackie B4 virus. The immunologic cross-over to self could occur from virus-induced activation of preexistent autoreactive lymphocytes, or from the mounting of an immune response to a viral neoantigen. Finally, an endogenous *retroviral* genome has recently been identified in diabetic islets that also serves as a superantigen (Chapter 7).[47] Whether the virus is a trigger, a precipitator, or simply a marker for diabetes is unknown.[48]

Others. Antigenic exposure may also come from other sources. Although the subject is controversial, it has been reported that children who ingest *cow's milk products* early in life (before age 4 months) have a 1.5-fold increased risk for type 1 diabetes relative to those who do not, raising the spectre of a cross-reacting antigen in cow's milk.[49] A number of *chemical toxins*, including streptozotocin, alloxan, and pentamidine, also induce islet cell destruction in animals. In humans, pentamidine, a drug used for the treatment of parasitic infections, has been occasionally associated with the development of abrupt-onset diabetes, and cases of diabetes have also been reported after accidental or suicidal ingestion of Vacor, a pharmacologic agent used as a rat exterminator. These chemicals act either directly on islet cells or indirectly by triggering a destructive autoimmune reaction.

PATHOGENESIS OF TYPE 2 DIABETES MELLITUS

While much has been learned in recent years, the pathogenesis of type 2 diabetes remains enigmatic. There is no evidence that autoimmune mechanisms are involved. Life style clearly plays a role, as will become evident when obesity is considered. Nevertheless, *genetic factors are even more important than in type 1 diabetes.* Among identical twins, the concordance rate is 60% to 80%. In first-degree relatives with type 2 diabetes (and in nonidentical twins) the risk of developing disease is 20% to 40%, versus 5% to 7% in the population at large.

Unlike type 1 diabetes, the disease is not linked to any HLA genes. Rather, *epidemiologic studies indicate that type 2 diabetes appears to result from a collection of multiple genetic defects or polymorphisms, each contributing its own predisposing risk and modified by environmental factors.*[50]

The two metabolic defects that characterize type 2 diabetes are (1) a derangement in β-cell secretion of insulin and (2) a decreased response of peripheral tissues to respond to insulin (insulin resistance) (Fig. 20–16). The primacy of the secretory defect versus insulin resistance is a matter of continuing debate.

Deranged β-Cell Secretion of Insulin. In populations at risk for developing type 2 diabetes (relatives of patients), a modest hyperinsulinemia may be observed, attributed to β-cell hyperresponsiveness to physiologic elevations in blood glucose. With the development of overt disease, the pattern of insulin secretion exhibits a subtle change. Early in the course of type 2 diabetes, insulin secretion appears to be normal and plasma insulin levels are not reduced. However, the normal pulsatile, oscillating pattern of insulin secretion is lost and the rapid first phase of insulin secretion triggered by glucose is obtunded. Collectively, these and

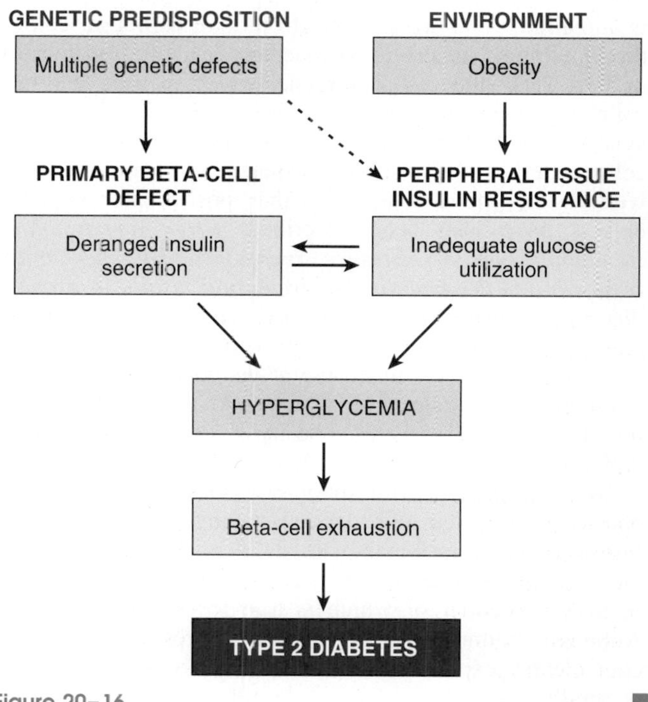

Figure 20–16

Pathogenesis of type 2 diabetes mellitus. Genetic predisposition and environmental influences converge to cause hyperglycemia and overt diabetes. The primacy of deranged β-cell insulin secretion and peripheral insulin resistance is not established; in patients with clinical disease, both defects can be demonstrated.

other observations suggest derangements in β-cell responses to hyperglycemia early in type 2 diabetes, rather than deficiencies in insulin synthesis per se.

Later in the course of type 2 diabetes, a mild to moderate deficiency of insulin develops, which is less severe than that of type 1. The cause of the insulin deficiency is not entirely clear, but irreversible β-cell damage does appear to be present. Unlike type 1 diabetes, there is no evidence of viral or immune-mediated injury to the islet cells. According to one view, all the somatic cells of predisposed individuals, including pancreatic β cells, are genetically vulnerable to injury, leading to accelerated cell turnover and premature aging, and ultimately to a modest reduction in β-cell mass. Chronic hyperglycemia may exhaust the ability of β cells to function (this is unfortunately called "glucose toxicity"), as a consequence of persistent β-cell stimulation.

Insulin Resistance. Although insulin deficiency is present late in the course of type 2 diabetes, it is not of sufficient magnitude to explain the metabolic disturbances. Rather, reduced responsiveness of peripheral tissues (insulin resistance) is a major factor in the development of type 2 diabetes. At the outset, it should be noted that insulin resistance is a complex phenomenon that is not restricted to the diabetes syndrome. In both obesity and pregnancy (gestational diabetes), insulin sensitivity of target tissues decreases (even in the absence of diabetes), and serum levels of insulin may be elevated to compensate for insulin resistance.

The molecular bases of insulin resistance are not clear. There may be a decrease in the number of insulin receptors, and more important, postreceptor signaling by insulin is impaired. You may recall from our earlier discussion that binding of insulin to its receptors leads to translocation of GLUTs to the cell membrane, which in turn facilitates cellular uptake of glucose. It is suspected that reduced synthesis and translocation of GLUTs in muscle and fat cells underlies the insulin resistance noted in obesity as well as in type 2 diabetes. Other postreceptor signaling defects have also been described. *From a physiologic standpoint, insulin resistance, regardless of its mechanism, results in (1) the inability of circulating insulin to properly direct the disposition of glucose (and other metabolic fuels), (2) a more persistent hyperglycemia, and therefore (3) more prolonged stimulation of the pancreatic β cell.*

Obesity. Regardless of which initiating event is proposed for type 2 diabetes, obesity is an extremely important environmental influence. Approximately 80% of type 2 diabetics are obese, with abdominal obesity (as opposed to obesity in subcutaneous depots) having a greater impact. Intra-abdominal fat catabolism delivers free fatty acids to the liver, yet is relatively resistant to the modulating effects of insulin (neither of which is true for subcutaneous fat). Although abdominal obesity and insulin resistance could be coincidental expressions of a third unknown factor, the possibility that they are causally related must be considered.[51]

Nondiabetic obese individuals can also exhibit insulin resistance and hyperinsulinemia, and a small proportion develop type 2 diabetes. However, when obese type 2 diabetics are compared with weight-matched nondiabetics, it appears that the insulin levels of obese diabetics are below those observed in obese nondiabetics, suggesting a relative insulin deficiency. Fortunately, for many obese diabetics, weight loss (and physical exercise) can reverse impaired glucose tolerance, especially early in the course of the disease.

Amylin. Current interest is also focused on the role of *amylin* in the pathogenesis of type 2 diabetes. This 37 amino acid peptide is normally produced by the β cells, copackaged with insulin and cosecreted with insulin in response to food ingestion. In patients with type 2 diabetes, amylin tends to accumulate in the sinusoidal space outside the β cells, in close contact with their cell membranes, eventually acquiring the tinctorial characteristics of amyloid.[52] It is unknown whether amylin deposition contributes to the disturbance in glucose sensing by the β cells, noted early in the course of type 2 diabetes, or is instead a result of disordered β-cell function.

To summarize, type 2 diabetes is a complex, multifactorial disorder involving both impaired insulin release leading to relative insulin deficiency and end-organ insensitivity. Insulin resistance, frequently associated with obesity, produces excessive stress on β cells, which may fail in the face of sustained need for a state of hyperinsulinism. Genetic factors are definitely involved, but how they fit into this puzzle remains mysterious.

GENETIC DEFECTS OF β-CELL FUNCTION

Maturity-Onset Diabetes of the Young (MODY). About 2% to 5% of diabetic patients do not fall clearly into either the type 1 or type 2 diabetes phenotype, yet may be confused clinically with either. However, because an insulin secretory defect occurs *without β-cell loss*, affected families have been intensively studied in the hope of gaining insights into type 2 diabetes. It now appears that MODY is the outcome of a heterogeneous group of genetic defects in β-cell function characterized by

- Autosomal dominant inheritance as a monogenic defect, with high penetrance.
- Early onset, usually before age 25, as opposed to after age 40 for most patients with type 2 diabetes.
- Impaired β-cell function, normal weight, lack of GAD antibodies, and lack of the insulin resistance syndrome.

Four distinct genetic defects have so far been identified. Some are characterized by severe β-cell insulin secretory defects (MODY1 and MODY3), while others (MODY2) feature mild chronic hyperglycemia due to reduced pancreatic β-cell responsiveness to glucose.

- *One form (MODY1) is caused by mutations in the gene for hepatocyte nuclear transcription factor-4a (HNF-4α) on chromosome 20*, a member of the steroid/thyroid hormone receptor superfamily and an upstream regulator of HNF-1α expression.[53]
- *MODY2 is caused by mutations in the glucokinase gene on chromosome 7.*
- *Mutations in the gene for hepatocyte nuclear factor-1α (HNF-1α) on chromosome 12q are associated with*

MODY3.[54] HNF-1α is a transcription factor that functions as a weak transactivator of the insulin-I gene.

- *Point mutations in mitochondrial DNA* have been found to be associated with diabetes mellitus and deafness.

The mechanisms by which mutations in these genes result in an autosomal dominant form of diabetes mellitus are not yet known but presumably involve abnormal insulin metabolism.

PATHOGENESIS OF THE COMPLICATIONS OF DIABETES

The morbidity associated with long-standing diabetes of either type results from a number of serious complications, namely *microangiopathy, retinopathy, nephropathy,* and *neuropathy.* Hence, the basis of these complications is the subject of a great deal of research.[55] *Most of the available experimental and clinical evidence suggests that the complications are a consequence of the metabolic derangements, mainly hyperglycemia.* For example, when kidneys are transplanted into diabetics from nondiabetic donors, the lesions of diabetic nephropathy develop within 3 to 5 years after transplantation. Conversely, kidneys with lesions of diabetic nephropathy demonstrate a reversal of the lesion when transplanted into normal recipients. Multicenter clinical trials clearly show delayed progression of microvasculature diabetic complications by strict control of the hyperglycemia.

Two metabolic events appear to be involved in the genesis of these complications (Fig. 20–17).[56]

Nonenzymatic Glycosylation. This refers to the process by which glucose chemically attaches to the amino group of proteins without the aid of enzymes. Glucose forms chemically reversible glycosylation products with protein (named Schiff bases) that may rearrange to form more stable Amadori-type early glycosylation products, which are also chemically reversible (Fig. 20–17*A*). The degree of enzymatic glycosylation is directly related to the level of blood glucose. Indeed, *the measurement of glycosylated hemoglobin (HbA_{1c}) levels in the blood is a useful adjunct in the management of diabetes mellitus.*

The early glycosylation products on collagen and other long-lived proteins in interstitial tissues and blood vessel walls, rather than dissociating, undergo a slow series of chemical rearrangements to form *irreversible advanced gly-*

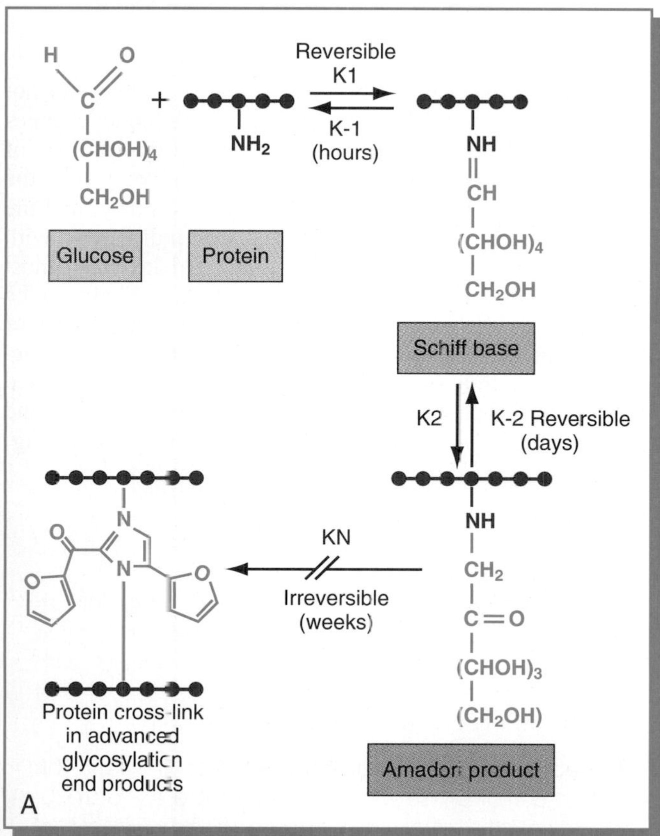

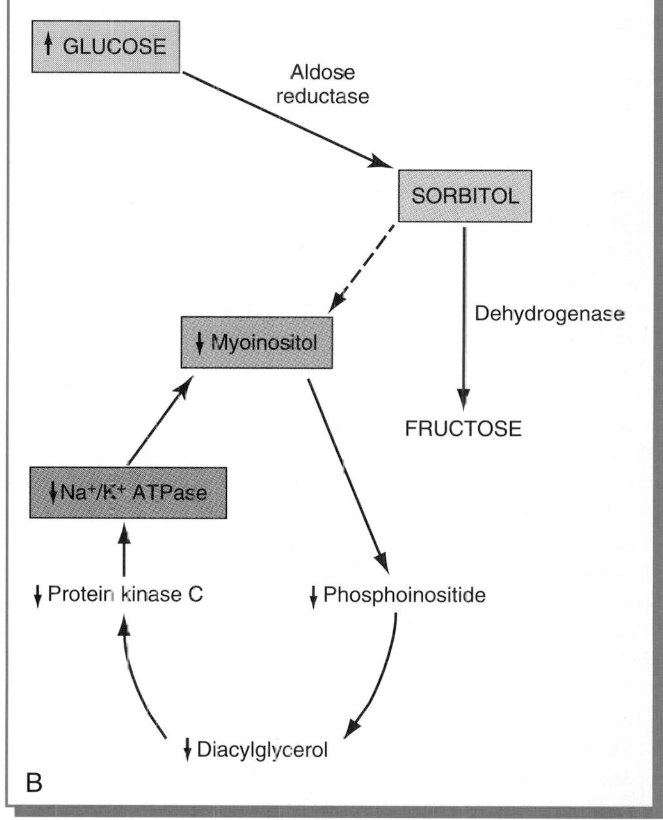

Figure 20–17

Chemical effects of diabetic hyperglycemia. *A*, Nonenzymatic glycosylation of proteins. The advanced glycosylation product involves protein-protein cross-linking. Note that whereas the early glycosylation products are reversible, advanced end products are irreversible. (Modified from Brownlee M, et al: Advanced glycosylation end products in tissue and the biochemical basis of diabetic complications. N Engl J Med 318:1315, 1988.) *B*, Intracellular hyperglycemia, the sorbitol pathway, and effects on *myo*-inositol. (Modified from Greene DA, et al: Sorbitol, phosphoinositides, and sodium potassium ATPase in the pathogenesis of diabetic complications. N Engl J Med 316:599, 1987.)

Table 20–4. RELEVANT CHEMICAL AND BIOLOGIC PROPERTIES OF ADVANCED GLYCOSYLATION END PRODUCTS

Chemical
Cross-link polypeptides of same protein (e.g., collagen)
Trap nonglycosylated proteins (e.g., LDL, Ig, complement)
Confer resistance to proteolytic digestion
Induce lipid oxidation
Inactivate nitric oxide
Bind nucleic acids

Biologic
Bind to AGE receptors on monocytes and mesenchymal cells
Induce: Monocyte emigration
Cytokines and growth factor secretion
Increased vascular permeability
Procoagulant activity
Enhanced cellular proliferation
Enhanced ECM production

ECM, extracellular matrix; LDL, low-density lipoprotein.
Adapted from Vlassara H, et al: Pathogenic effects of advanced glycosylation: biochemical, biological, and clinical indications. Lab Invest 70:138, 1994. ©United States and Canadian Academy of Pathology, Inc., 1994.

cosylation end products (AGE), which accumulate over the lifetime of the vessel wall. AGEs have a number of chemical and biologic properties that are potentially pathogenic (Table 20–4).[56a]

- *AGE* formation occurs on proteins, lipids, and nucleic acids. On proteins, such as collagen, they cause cross-links *between* polypeptides of the collagen molecule and also *trap* nonglycosylated plasma or interstitial proteins. In large vessels, trapping low-density lipoprotein (LDL), for example, retards its efflux from the vessel wall and enhances the deposition of cholesterol in the intima, thus accelerating atherogenesis (Chapter 12). In capillaries, including those of renal glomeruli, plasma proteins such as albumin bind to the glycosylated basement membrane, accounting in part for the increased basement membrane thickening characteristic of diabetic microangiopathy. *AGE cross-linked proteins are resistant to proteolytic digestion.* Thus, cross-linking decreases protein removal while enhancing protein deposition. AGE-induced cross-linking in collagen type IV in basement membrane may also impair the interaction of collagen with other matrix components (laminin, proteoglycans), resulting in structural and functional defects in the basement membranes.
- AGEs bind to receptors on many cell types—endothelium, monocytes, macrophages, lymphocytes, and mesangial cells. Binding induces a variety of biologic activities, including monocyte emigration; release of cytokines and growth factors from macrophages; increased endothelial permeability; increased procoagulant activity on endothelial cells and macrophages; and enhanced proliferation of and synthesis of extracellular matrix by fibroblasts and smooth muscle cells. All these effects can potentially contribute to diabetic complications.
- The importance of AGEs is supported by studies in which inhibition of their accumulation by pharmacologic agents abrogates the morphologic and functional defects in experimental models of diabetes.[56a]

Intracellular Hyperglycemia with Disturbances in Polyol Pathways. In some tissues that do not require insulin for glucose transport (e.g., nerves, lens, kidneys, blood vessels), hyperglycemia leads to an increase in intracellular glucose that is then metabolized by aldose reductase to *sorbitol,* a polyol, and eventually to fructose. These changes have several untoward effects. *The accumulated levels of sorbitol and fructose lead to increased intracellular osmolarity and influx of water, and eventually to osmotic cell injury.* In the lens, osmotically imbibed water causes swelling and opacity. *Sorbitol accumulation also impairs ion pumps and is believed to promote injury of Schwann cells and pericytes of retinal capillaries, with resultant peripheral neuropathy and retinal microaneurysms.* In keeping with this hypothesis, experimental inhibition of aldose reductase may ameliorate the development of cataracts and neuropathy. Finally, metabolic disposition of these polyols diverts the cellular machinery from processing of normal intermediary metabolites, thereby altering the complex balance between intracellular signaling networks and target enzymes.[57]

Morphology of Diabetes and its Late Complications

Pathologic findings in the pancreas are variable and not necessarily dramatic. The important morphologic changes are related to the many late systemic complications of diabetes. There is extreme variability among patients in the time of onset of these complications, their severity, and the particular organ or organs involved. In individuals with tight control of diabetes the onset may be delayed. In most patients, however, morphologic changes are likely to be found in arteries (*atherosclerosis*), basement membranes of small vessels (*microangiopathy*), kidneys (*diabetic nephropathy*), retina (*retinopathy*), nerves (*neuropathy*), and other tissues. These changes are seen in both type 1 and type 2 diabetes. A schematic overview is provided in Figure 20–18.

MORPHOLOGY

Pancreas. Lesions in the pancreas are inconstant and rarely of diagnostic value. Distinctive changes are more commonly associated with type 1 than with type 2 diabetes. One or more of the following alterations may be present.

- **Reduction in the number and size of islets.** This is most often seen in type 1 diabetes, particularly with rapidly advancing disease. Most of the islets are small, inconspicuous, and not easily detected.
- **Leukocytic infiltration of the islets** (insulitis) principally composed of T lymphocytes similar to that in models of autoimmune diabetes (Fig. 20–19*A*). This may be seen in type 1 diabetics

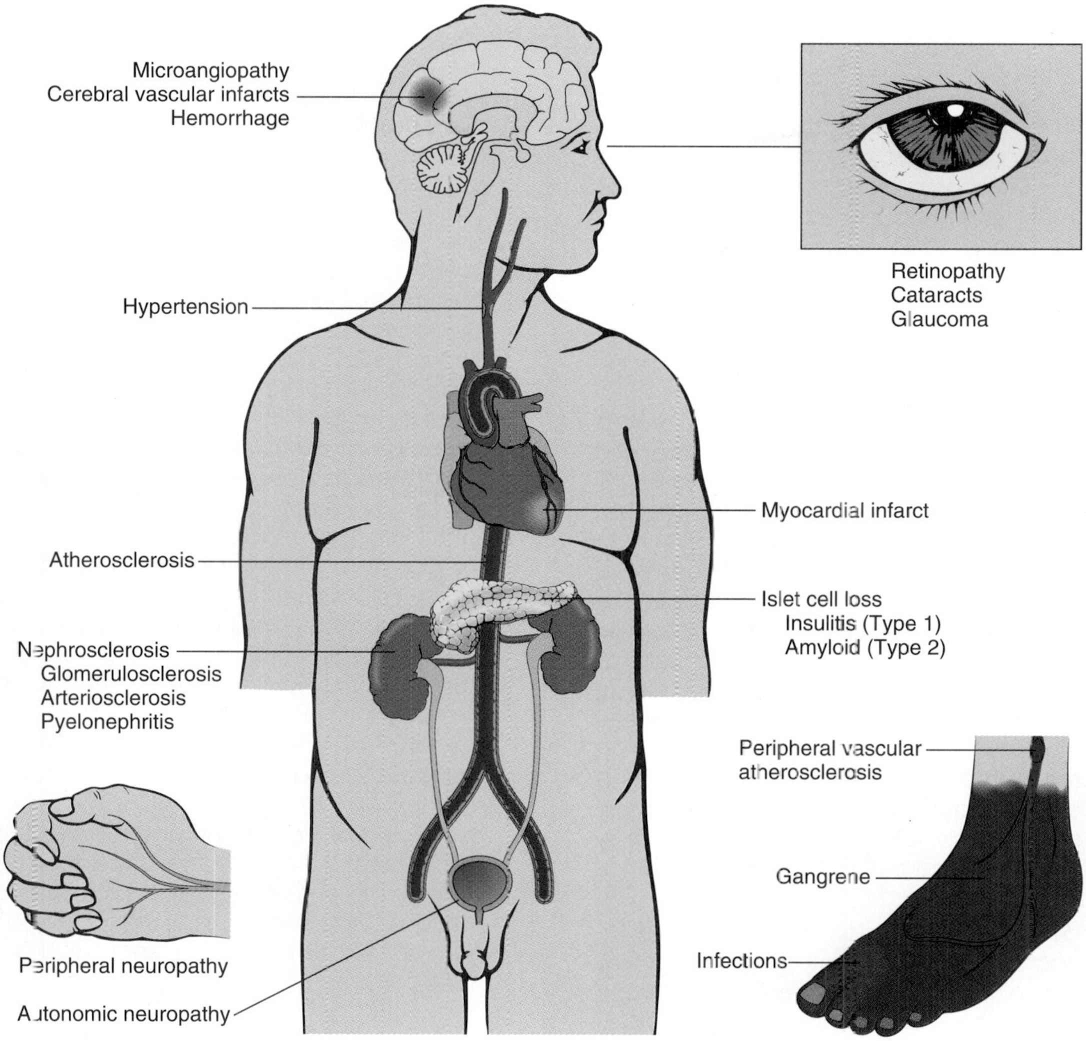

Microangiopathy
Cerebral vascular infarcts
Hemorrhage

Retinopathy
Cataracts
Glaucoma

Hypertension

Myocardial infarct

Atherosclerosis

Islet cell loss
Insulitis (Type 1)
Amyloid (Type 2)

Nephrosclerosis
Glomerulosclerosis
Arteriosclerosis
Pyelonephritis

Peripheral vascular atherosclerosis

Gangrene

Infections

Peripheral neuropathy

Autonomic neuropathy

Figure 20–18 ■

Long-term complications of diabetes.

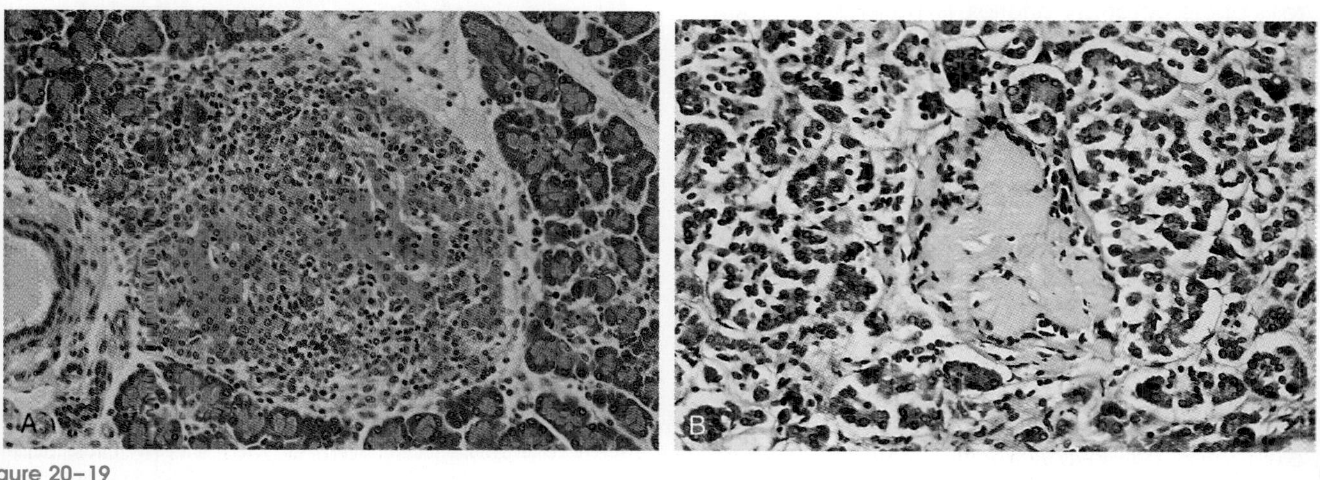

Figure 20–19 ■

A, Insulitis, shown here from a rat (BB) model of autoimmune diabetes, and seen in type 1 human diabetes. (Courtesy of Dr. Arthur Like, University of Massachusetts, Worchester, MA.) *B*, Amyloidosis of a pancreatic islet in type 2 diabetes.

at the time of clinical presentation. The distribution of insulitis may be strikingly uneven. Eosinophilic infiltrates may also be found, particularly in diabetic infants who fail to survive the immediate postnatal period.

- By electron microscopy, **β-cell degranulation** may be observed, reflecting depletion of stored insulin in already damaged β cells. This is more commonly seen in patients with newly-diagnosed type 1 disease, when some β cells are still present.
- **In type 2 diabetes, there may be a subtle reduction in islet cell mass**, demonstrated only by special morphometric studies.
- **Amyloid replacement of islets in type 2 diabetes** appears as deposition of pink, amorphous material beginning in and around capillaries and between cells. At advanced stages the islets may be virtually obliterated (Fig. 20–19*B*); fibrosis may also be observed. This change is often seen in long-standing cases of type 2 diabetes. As mentioned earlier, the amyloid is composed of amylin fibrils derived from the β cells. Similar lesions may be found in elderly nondiabetics, apparently as part of normal aging.
- **An increase in the number and size of islets is especially characteristic of nondiabetic newborns of diabetic mothers.** Presumably, fetal islets undergo hyperplasia in response to the maternal hyperglycemia.

Vascular System. **Accelerated atherosclerosis:** Diabetes exacts a heavy toll on the vascular system. Vessels of all sizes are affected, from the aorta down to the smallest arterioles and capillaries. **The aorta and large- and medium-sized arteries suffer from accelerated severe atherosclerosis.** Except for its greater severity and earlier age of onset, atherosclerosis in diabetics is indistinguishable from that in nondiabetics (Chapter 12). **Myocardial infarction, caused by atherosclerosis of the coronary arteries, is the most common cause of death in diabetics.** Significantly, it is almost as common in diabetic women as in diabetic men. In contrast, myocardial infarction is uncommon in nondiabetic women of reproductive age. **Gangrene of the lower extremities,** as a result of advanced vascular disease, is about 100 times more common in diabetics than in the general population. The larger renal arteries are also subject to severe atherosclerosis, but the most damaging effect of diabetes on the kidneys is exerted at the level of the glomeruli and the microcirculation. This is discussed later.

The pathogenesis of accelerated atherosclerosis is not well understood, and in all likelihood multiple factors are involved.[58, 59] About one third to one half of the patients have elevated blood lipid levels, known to predispose to atherosclerosis, but the remainder also have an increased predisposition to atherosclerosis. Qualitative changes in the lipoproteins brought about by excessive nonenzymatic glycosylation may affect their turnover and tissue deposition. Low levels of high-density lipoproteins (HDL) have been demonstrated in type 2 diabetes. Since HDL is a "protective molecule" against atherosclerosis (Chapter 12), this could contribute to increased susceptibility to atherosclerosis. Diabetics have increased platelet adhesiveness to the vessel wall, possibly owing to increased thromboxane A_2 synthesis and reduced prostacyclin. In addition to all these factors, diabetics tend to have an increased incidence of hypertension, which is a well-known risk factor for atherosclerosis.[60]

Hyaline arteriolosclerosis, the vascular lesion associated with hypertension (Chapters 12 and 21), is both more prevalent and more severe in diabetics than in nondiabetics, but it is not specific for diabetes and may be seen in elderly nondiabetics without hypertension. It takes the form of an amorphous, hyaline thickening of the wall of the arterioles, which causes narrowing of the lumen (Fig. 20–20). Not surprisingly, in diabetics it is related not only to the duration of the disease but also to the level of blood pressure.

Diabetic Microangiopathy. One of the most consistent morphologic features of diabetes is **diffuse thickening of basement membranes**. The thickening is most evident in the capillaries of the skin, skeletal muscle, retina, renal glomeruli, and renal medulla. However, it may also be seen in such nonvascular structures as renal tubules, the Bowman capsule, peripheral nerves, and placenta. By both light and electron microscopy, the basal lamina separating parenchymal or endothelial

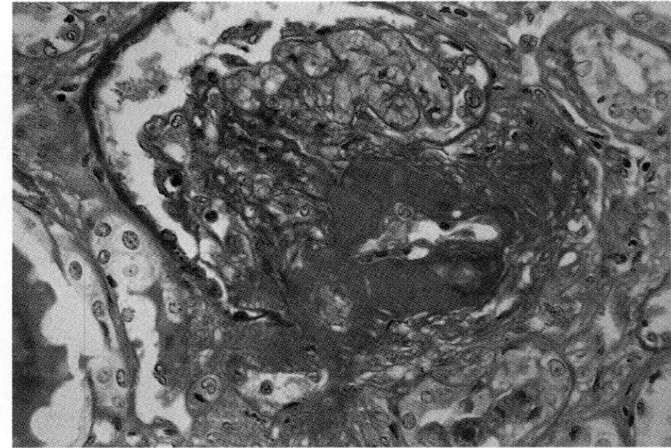

Figure 20–20

Severe renal hyaline arteriolosclerosis. Note a markedly thickened, tortuous afferent arteriole. The amorphous nature of the thickened vascular wall is evident. (Periodic acid–Schiff [PAS] stain; courtesy of M.A. Venkatachalam, MD, Department of Pathology, University of Texas Health Science Center at San Antonio, TX.)

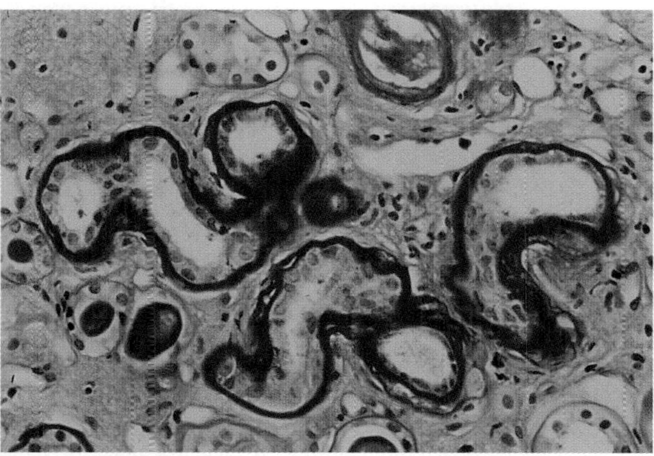

Figure 20–21

Renal cortex showing thickening of tubular basement membranes in a diabetic patient. (PAS stain.)

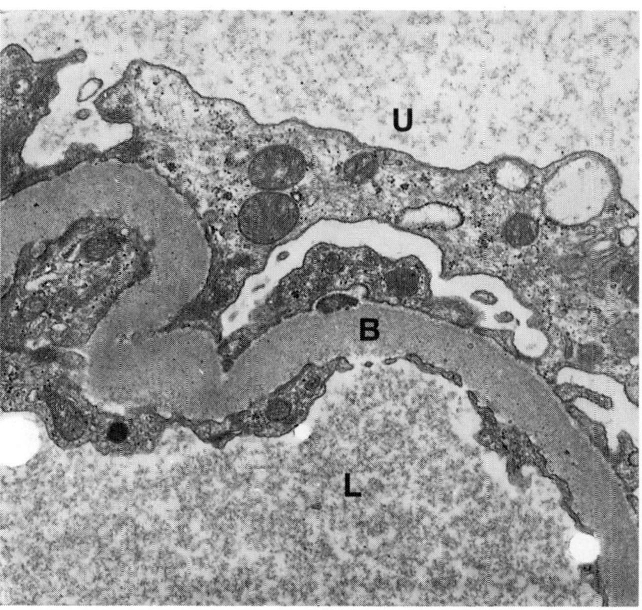

Figure 20–22

Renal glomerulus showing markedly thickened glomerular basement membrane (B) in a diabetic. L, glomerular capillary lumen; U, urinary space. (Courtesy of Michael Kashgarian, MD, Department of Pathology, Yale University School of Medicine.)

cells from the surrounding tissue is markedly thickened by concentric layers of hyaline material composed predominantly of type IV collagen (Fig. 20–21 and 20–22). It should be noted that **despite the increase in the thickness of basement membranes, diabetic capillaries are more leaky than normal to plasma proteins. The microangiopathy underlies the development of diabetic nephropathy and some forms of neuropathy.** An indistinguishable microangiopathy can be found in aged nondiabetic patients, but rarely to the extent seen in patients with long-standing diabetes. The microangiopathy is clearly related to the hyperglycemia.

Diabetic Nephropathy (See also Chapter 21). The kidneys are prime targets of diabetes.[61] Renal failure is second only to myocardial infarction as a cause of death from this disease. **Three lesions are encountered: (1) glomerular lesions; (2) renal vascular lesions, principally arteriolosclerosis; and (3) pyelonephritis, including necrotizing papillitis.**

The most important glomerular lesions are capillary basement membrane thickening, diffuse glomerulosclerosis, and nodular glomerulosclerosis. These are described in detail in Chapter 21. **The glomerular capillary basement membranes are thickened throughout their entire length.** This change can be detected by electron microscopy within a few years of the onset of diabetes, sometimes without any associated change in renal function.

Diffuse glomerulosclerosis consists of a diffuse increase in mesangial matrix along with mesangial cell proliferation and is always associated with basement membrane thickening. It is found in most patients with disease of more than 10 years' duration. When glomerulosclerosis becomes marked, patients manifest the nephrotic syndrome (Chapter 21), characterized by proteinuria, hypoalbuminemia, and edema.

Nodular glomerulosclerosis describes a glomerular lesion made distinctive by ball-like deposits of a laminated matrix within the mesangial core of the lobule (see Fig. 21–32). These nodules tend to develop in the periphery of the glomerulus, and since they arise within the mesangium, they push the glomerular capillary loops even more to the periphery. Often these capillary loops create halos about the nodule. This distinctive change has been called the **Kimmelstiel-Wilson lesion**, after the pioneers who described it. They usually contain trapped mesangial cells. Diffuse glomerulosclerosis is present in glomeruli not affected by nodular glomerulosclerosis.

Advanced glomerulosclerosis is associated with tubular ischemia and interstitial fibrosis. In addition, patients with uncontrolled glycosuria may reabsorb glucose and store it as glycogen in the tubular epithelium. This change does not affect tubular function.

Nodular glomerulosclerosis is encountered in perhaps 10% to 35% of diabetics and is a major cause of morbidity and mortality. Unlike the diffuse form, which may also be seen in association with old age and hypertension, the nodular form of glomerulosclerosis, for all practical purposes, implicates diabetes. Both the diffuse and the nodular forms of glomerulosclerosis induce sufficient ischemia to cause overall fine scarring of the kidneys, marked by a finely granular cortical surface (Fig. 20–23).

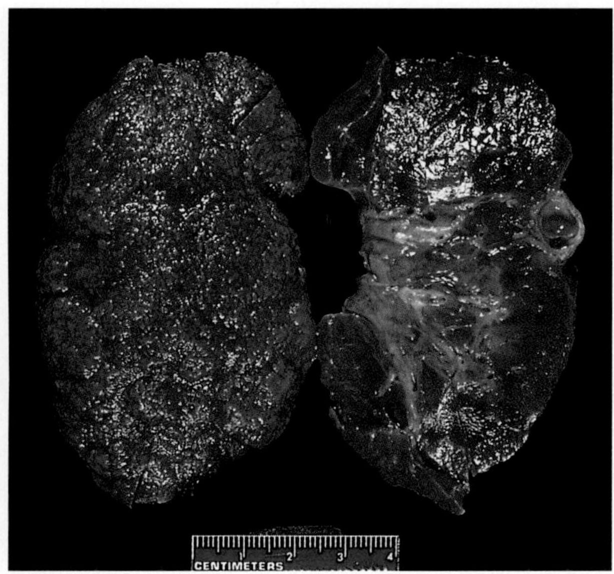

Figure 20–23

Nephrosclerosis in a patient with long-standing diabetes. The kidney has been bisected to demonstrate both diffuse granular transformation of the surface (*left*) and marked thinning of the cortical tissue (*right*). Additional features include some irregular depressions, the result of pyelonephritis, and an incidental cortical cyst (*far right*).

Renal atherosclerosis and arteriolosclerosis constitute part of the systemic involvement of blood vessels in diabetics. The kidney is one of the most frequently and severely affected organs; however, the changes in the arteries and arterioles are similar to those found throughout the body. **Hyaline arteriolosclerosis affects not only the afferent but also the efferent arteriole.** Such efferent arteriolosclerosis is rarely if ever encountered in persons who do not have diabetes.

Pyelonephritis is an acute or chronic inflammation of the kidneys that usually begins in the interstitial tissue and then spreads to affect the tubules. Both the acute and chronic forms of this disease occur in nondiabetics as well as in diabetics but are more common in diabetics than in the general population, and once affected, diabetics tend to have more severe involvement. One special pattern of acute pyelonephritis, **necrotizing papillitis** (or papillary necrosis), is much more prevalent in diabetics than in nondiabetics. These lesions are described more fully in Chapter 21.

Diabetic Ocular Complications. Visual impairment, sometimes even total blindness, is one of the more feared consequences of long-standing diabetes. This disease is currently the fourth leading cause of acquired blindness in the United States. **The ocular involvement may take the form of retinopathy, cataract formation, or glaucoma** and is discussed in Chapter 31.

Diabetic Neuropathy. The central and peripheral nervous systems are not spared by diabetes.[62] The neurologic manifestations are described in Chapters 29 and 30. The most frequent pattern of involvement is a peripheral, symmetric neuropathy of the lower extremities that affects both motor and sensory function but particularly the latter.

Clinical Features

It is difficult to sketch with brevity the diverse clinical presentations of diabetes mellitus. Only a few characteristic patterns will be presented.

Type 1 diabetes, which begins by age 20 years in most patients, is dominated by polyuria, polydipsia, polyphagia, and ketoacidosis—all resulting from metabolic derangements. As insulin is a major anabolic hormone in the body, *derangement of insulin function affects not only glucose metabolism but also fat and protein metabolism.* Unopposed secretion of counter-regulatory hormones (glucagon, growth hormone, epinephrine) also plays a role in these metabolic derangements. The assimilation of glucose into muscle and adipose tissue is sharply diminished or abolished. Not only does storage of glycogen in liver and muscle cease, but also reserves are depleted by glycogenolysis. Severe fasting hyperglycemia and glycosuria ensues. The glycosuria induces an osmotic diuresis and thus *polyuria*, causing a profound loss of water and electrolytes (Fig. 20–24).

The obligatory renal water loss combined with the hyperosmolarity resulting from the increased levels of glucose in the blood tends to deplete intracellular water, triggering the osmoreceptors of the thirst centers of the brain. In this manner, intense thirst (*polydipsia*) appears. With a deficiency of insulin, the scales swing from insulin-promoted anabolism to catabolism of proteins and fats. Proteolysis follows, and the gluconeogenic amino acids are removed by the liver and used as building blocks for glucose. The catabolism of proteins and fats tends to induce a negative energy balance, which in turn leads to increasing appetite (*polyphagia*), thus completing the classic triad of diabetes: *polyuria*, *polydipsia*, and *polyphagia*. Despite the increased appetite, catabolic effects prevail, resulting in weight loss and muscle weakness.

The combination of polyphagia and weight loss is paradoxical and should always raise the suspicion of diabetes. Plasma insulin is low or absent and the glucagon level is increased. Glucose intolerance is of the unstable or brittle type, in that blood glucose levels are quite sensitive to administered exogenous insulin, deviations from normal dietary intake, unusual physical activity, infection, or other forms of stress. Inadequate fluid intake or vomiting may rapidly lead to significant disturbances in fluid and electrolyte balance.

Thus, these patients are vulnerable, on the one hand, to *hypoglycemic episodes* (due to treatment with insulin), and on the other, to *ketoacidosis. This latter complication occurs almost exclusively in type 1 diabetes and is stimulated by severe insulin deficiency coupled with absolute or rela-*

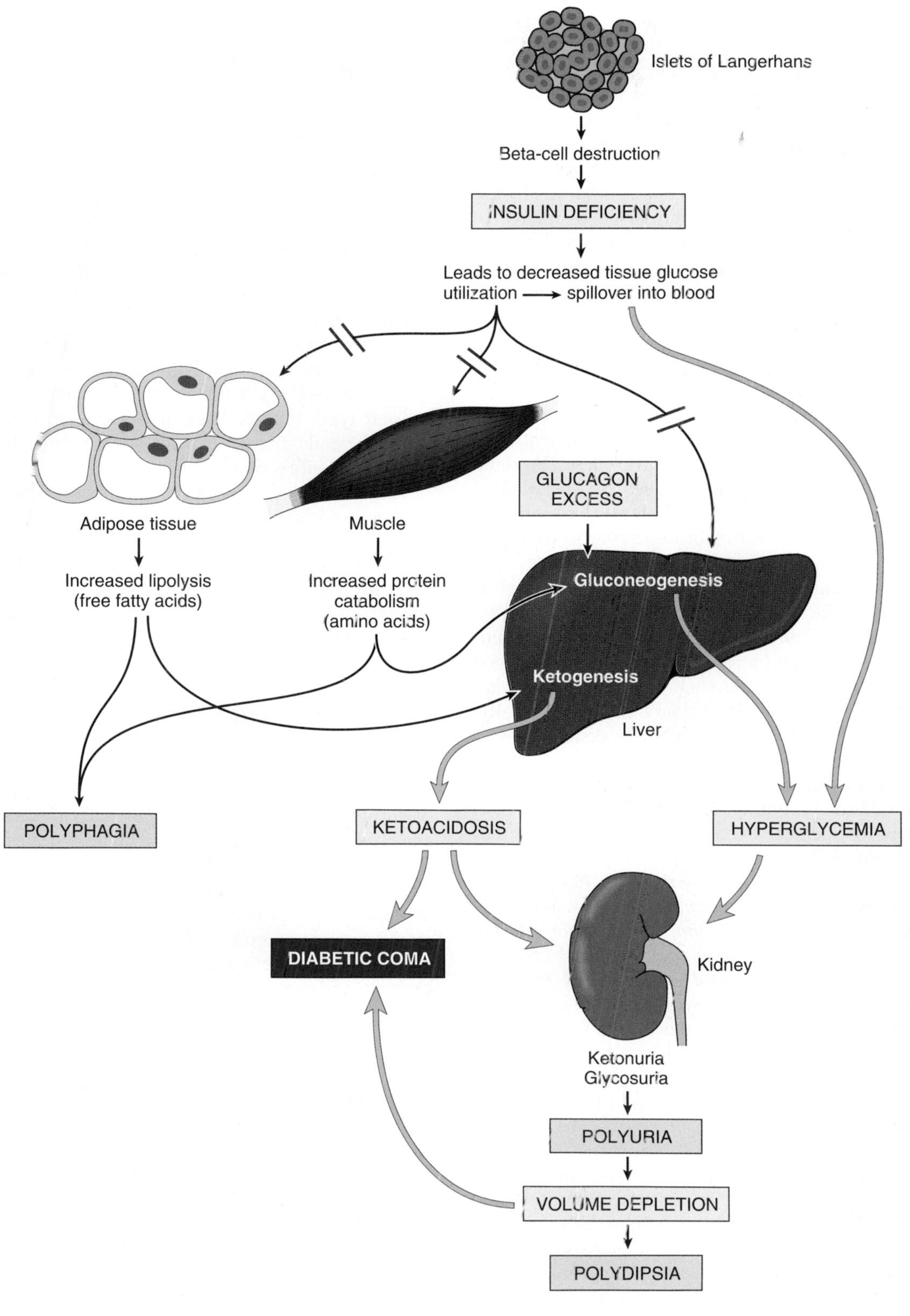

Figure 20–24

Sequence of metabolic derangements leading to diabetic coma in type 1 diabetes mellitus. An absolute insulin deficiency leads to a catabolic state, eventuating in ketoacidosis and severe volume depletion. These cause sufficient central nervous system compromise to cause coma, and eventual death if left untreated.

tive increases of glucagon (Fig. 20–24).[63] The insulin deficiency causes excessive breakdown of adipose stores, resulting in increased levels of free fatty acids. Oxidation of such free fatty acids within the liver through acetyl CoA produces ketone bodies (acetoacetic acid and β-hydroxybutyric acid). *Glucagon* is the hormone that accelerates such fatty acid oxidation. The rate at which ketone bodies are formed may exceed the rate at which acetoacetic acid and β-hydroxybutyric acid can be utilized by muscles and other tissues, thus leading to *ketonemia* and *ketonuria.* If the urinary excretion of ketones is compromised by dehydration, the plasma hydrogen ion concentration increases and systemic metabolic ketoacidosis results. Release of ketogenic amino acids by protein catabolism aggravates the ketotic state. Diabetics have increased susceptibility to infections. Because the stress of infection increases insulin requirements, infections often precipitate diabetic ketoacidosis.

Type 2 diabetes mellitus may also present with polyuria and polydipsia, but unlike type 1 diabetes, patients are often older (over 40 years) and frequently obese. In some cases medical attention is sought because of unexplained weakness or weight loss. Frequently, however, the diagnosis is made after routine blood or urine testing in asymptomatic persons. Although patients with type 2 diabetes also have metabolic derangements, these are easier to control and less severe. In the decompensated state, these patients develop *hyperosmolar nonketotic coma*, a syndrome engendered by the severe dehydration resulting from sustained hyperglycemic diuresis in patients who do not drink enough water to compensate for urinary losses. Typically, the patient is an elderly diabetic who is disabled by a stroke or an infection who is unable to maintain adequate water intake. Furthermore, the absence of ketoacidosis and its symptoms (nausea, vomiting, respiratory difficulties) delays the seeking of medical attention in these patients until severe dehydration and coma occur.

In both forms of long-standing diabetes, atherosclerotic events such as myocardial infarction, cerebrovascular accidents, gangrene of the leg, and renal insufficiency are the most threatening and most frequent concomitants.[64] *Diabetics are also plagued by enhanced susceptibility to infections of the skin and to tuberculosis, pneumonia, and pyelonephritis.* Such infections cause the deaths of about 5% of diabetic patients. A trivial infection in a toe may be the first event in a long succession of complications (gangrene, bacteremia, pneumonia) that ultimately lead to death.

Patients with type 1 diabetes are more likely to die from their disease than those with type 2. The causes of death, in descending order of importance, are myocardial infarction, renal failure, cerebrovascular disease, atherosclerotic heart disease, and infections, followed by a large number of other complications more common in diabetics than in nondiabetics (e.g., gangrene of an extremity). Fortunately, hypoglycemia and ketoacidosis are rare causes of death today.

As mentioned, this disease continues to be one of the top ten "killers" in the United States. It is hoped that islet cell transplantation, which is still in the experimental stage, or insights gained from new molecular studies will lead to a cure for diabetes mellitus. Until then, strict glycemic control offers the only hope for preventing the deadly complications of diabetes.

ISLET CELL TUMORS

Tumors of pancreatic islet cells are rare in comparison with tumors of the exocrine pancreas. They are most common in adults and can occur anywhere along the length of the pancreas, embedded in the substance of the pancreas or arising in the immediate peripancreatic tissues. They resemble in appearance their counterparts, carcinoid tumors, found elsewhere in the alimentary tract (Chapter 18).[65] Islet cell tumors may be single or multiple and benign or malignant, the latter metastasizing to lymph nodes and liver. When multiple, each tumor may be composed of a different cell type. Islet cell tumors have a propensity to elaborate pancreatic hormones, but some islet cell tumors may be totally nonfunctional.

The three most common and distinctive clinical syndromes associated with functional islet cell tumors are *(1) hyperinsulinism, (2) hypergastrinemia and the Zollinger-Ellison syndrome, and (3) multiple endocrine neoplasia.* The last of these is characterized by the occurrence of tumors in several endocrine glands, and so is described in Chapter 26.

Hyperinsulinism (Insulinoma)

β-Cell tumors (insulinomas) are the most common of islet cell tumors and may be responsible for the elaboration of sufficient insulin to induce clinically significant hypoglycemia. There is a characteristic clinical triad resulting from these pancreatic lesions: (1) attacks of hypglycemia occur with blood glucose levels below 50 mg/dl of serum; (2) the attacks consist principally of such central nervous system manifestations as confusion, stupor, and loss of consciousness; and (3) the attacks are precipitated by fasting or exercise and are promptly relieved by feeding or parenteral administration of glucose.

MORPHOLOGY. Insulinomas are most often found within the pancreas and are generally benign. Most are solitary lesions, although multiple tumors or tumors ectopic to the pancreas may be encountered. Bona fide carcinomas, making up only about 10% of cases, are diagnosed on the basis of local invasion and distant metastases. On rare occasions, an islet cell tumor may arise in ectopic pancreatic tissue.

Solitary tumors are usually small (often less than 2 cm in diameter) and are encapsulated, pale to red-brown nodules located anywhere in the pancreas. Histologically, these benign tumors look remarkably like giant islets, with preservation of the

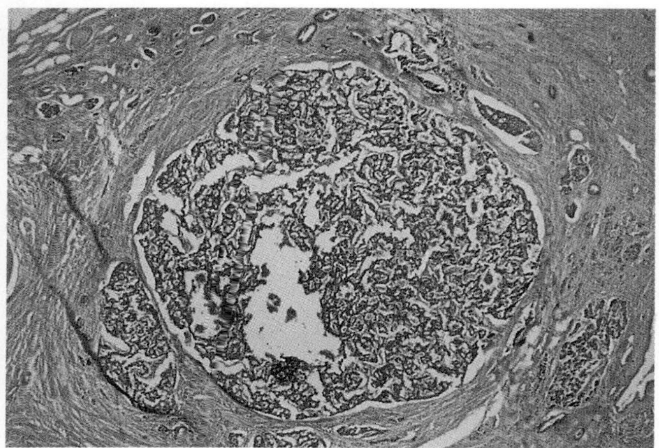

Figure 20–25

Pancreatic islet cell tumor less than 1 cm in diameter in a focal area of pancreatic fibrosis. Despite the small size of the tumor, clinical hypoglycemia was present.

regular cords of monotonous cells and their orientation to the vasculature (Fig. 20–25). Not even the malignant lesions present much evidence of anaplasia, and they may be deceptively encapsulated. By immunocytochemistry, insulin can be localized in the tumor cells. Under the electron microscope, neoplastic β cells, like their normal counterparts, display distinctive round granules that contain polygonal or rectangular dense crystals separated from the enclosing membrane by a distinct halo. It should be cautioned that granules may be present in the absence of clinically significant hormone activity.

Hyperinsulinism may also be caused by **diffuse hyperplasia of the islets.** This change is found occasionally in adults but is usually encountered in infants born of diabetic mothers. Long exposed to the hyperglycemia of maternal blood, the fetus responds by an increase in the size and number of its islets. In the postnatal period, these hyperactive islets may be responsible for serious episodes of hypoglycemia.

While up to 80% of islet cell tumors may demonstrate excessive insulin secretion, the hypoglycemia is mild in all but 20%, and many cases never become clinically symptomatic. The critical laboratory findings in insulinomas are high circulating levels of insulin and a high insulin-glucose ratio. Surgical removal of the tumor is usually followed by prompt reversal of the hypoglycemia.

It is important to note that *there are many other causes of hypoglycemia besides islet cell tumors.* The differential diagnosis of this frequently obscure metabolic abnormality includes such conditions as insulin sensitivity, diffuse liver disease, inherited glycogenoses, and ectopic formation of insulin by certain retroperitoneal fibromas and fibrosarcomas.

Zollinger-Ellison Syndrome (Gastrinomas)

Marked hypersecretion of gastrin usually has its origin in gastrin-producing tumors (*gastrinomas*), which are just as likely to arise in the duodenum and peripancreatic soft tissues as in the pancreas. There has been lack of agreement regarding the cell of origin for these tumors, save that endocrine cells of both the gut and pancreas can undergo dedifferentiation and express a broad array of gene products.[66] Zollinger and Ellison first called attention to the *association of pancreatic islet cell lesions with hypersecretion of gastric acid and severe peptic ulceration.* Ulcers are present in 90% to 95% of patients; the ratio of duodenal to gastric ulcers is 6:1 (Chapter 18).

MORPHOLOGY. Gastrinomas may arise in the pancreas, the peripancreatic region, or the wall of the duodenum. **Over half of gastrin-producing tumors are locally invasive or have already metastasized at the time of diagnosis.** In some instances, multiple gastrin-producing tumors are encountered in patients who have other endocrine tumors, thus conforming to multiple endocrine neoplasia type I (Chapter 26). As with insulin-secreting tumors of the pancreas, gastrin-producing tumors are histologically bland and rarely exhibit marked anaplasia.

In the classic case of the Zollinger-Ellison syndrome, hypergastrinemia from an islet cell tumor stimulates extreme gastric acid secretion, which in turn causes peptic ulceration. The duodenal and gastric ulcers, sometimes multiple, are identical to those found in the general population; they differ only in their intractability to usual modalities of therapy. In addition, ulcers may also occur in unusual locations such as the jejunum; when intractable jejunal ulcers are found, Zollinger-Ellison syndrome should be considered. More than 50% of the patients have diarrhea; in 30% it is the presenting symptom.

Treatment of the Zollinger-Ellison syndrome involves control of gastric acid secretion by use of histamine (H_2) receptor blockers and excision of the neoplasm. Total resection of the neoplasm, when possible, eliminates the syndrome. Patients with hepatic metastases have a significantly shortened life expectancy, with progressive tumor growth leading to liver failure usually within 10 years.

Other Rare Islet Cell Tumors

α-Cell tumors (glucagonomas) are associated with increased serum levels of glucagon and a syndrome consisting of mild diabetes mellitus; a characteristic migratory, necrotizing skin erythema; and anemia. They occur most frequently in peri- and postmenopausal women and are characterized by extremely high plasma glucagon levels.

δ-Cell tumors (somatostatinomas) are associated with diabetes mellitus, cholelithiasis, steatorrhea, and hypochlorhydria. They are exceedingly difficult to localize preoperatively. High plasma somatostatin levels are required for diagnosis.

VIPoma (diarrheogenic islet cell tumor) is an islet cell tumor that induces a characteristic syndrome of *watery diarrhea, hypokalemia*, and *achlorhydria*, caused by release of VIP from the tumor. Some of these tumors are locally invasive and metastatic. Neural crest tumors, such as ganglioneuroma, neuroblastoma, neurofibroma, and pheochromocytomas, can also be associated with the VIPoma syndrome.

Pancreatic carcinoid tumors producing serotonin and an atypical carcinoid syndrome are exceedingly rare. *Pancreatic polypeptide-secreting islet cell tumors* are endocrinologically asymptomatic, despite the presence of high levels of the hormone in plasma.

Some pancreatic and extrapancreatic tumors produce two or more hormones, usually simultaneously, and occasionally in sequence. In addition to insulin, glucagon, and gastrin, islet cell tumors may produce adrenocorticotropic hormone, melanocyte-stimulating hormone, vasopressin, serotonin, and norepinephrine. These *multihormonal tumors* are to be distinguished from the multiple endocrine neoplasias described in Chapter 26, in which a multiplicity of hormones are produced by tumors in several different glands.

REFERENCES

1. Beger HG, et al: Natural course of acute pancreatitis. World J Surg 21:130, 1997.
2. Ranson JHC: Risk factors in acute pancreatitis. Hosp Pract 20:69, 1985.
3. Steer ML: Etiology and pathophysiology of acute pancreatitis. In Go VLW, et al (eds): The Pancreas: Biology, Pathobiology, and Disease, 2nd ed. New York, Raven Press, 1993, pp 581–591.
4. Scarpelli DG: Toxicology of the pancreas. Toxicol Appl Pharmacol 101:543, 1989.
5. Norman J: Role of cytokines in the pathogenesis of acute pancreatitis. Am J Surg 175:76, 1998.
6. Blackstone MO: Hypothesis: vascular compromise is the central pathogenic mechanism for acute hemorrhagic pancreatitis. Perspect Biol Med 39:56, 1995.
7. Pitchumoni CS, Bordalo O: Evaluation of hypotheses on pathogenesis of alcoholic pancreatitis. Am Gastroenterol 91:637, 1996.
8. Steer ML: Pathogenesis of acute pancreatitis. Digestion 58 (suppl 1): 46, 1997.
9. Watanabe S: Acute pancreatitis: overview of medical aspects. Pancreas 16:307, 1998.
10. Friess H, et al: Acute pancreatitis: the role of infection. Dig Surg 13: 357, 1996.
11. Steer ML, et al: Chronic pancreatitis. N Engl J Med 332:1482, 1995.
12. Bertrand JA, et al: Crystal structure of human lithostathine, the pancreatic inhibitor of stone formation. EMBO J 15:2678, 1996.
13. Sarles H, et al: Pathogenesis and epidemiology of chronic pancreatitis. Annu Rev Med 40:453, 1989.
14. Amman RW, et al: Course of alcoholic chronic pancreatitis: a prospective clinicomorphologic long-term study. Gastroenterology 111: 224, 1996.
15. Adler G, Schmid RM: Chronic pancreatitis: still puzzling? Gastroenterology 112:1762, 1997.
16. Karlson B-M, et al: The risk of pancreatic cancer following pancreatitis: an association due to confounding? Gastroenterology 113:587, 1997.
17. Armed Forces Institute of Pathology: Atlas of Tumor Pathology; Tumors of the Pancreas. Bethesda, MD, Universities Associated for Research and Education in Pathology, 1997.
18. Nishihara K, et al: Papillary cystic tumors of the pancreas assessment of their malignant potential. Cancer 71:82, 1993.
19. Parker SL, et al: Cancer Statistics, 1997. Ca Cancer J Clin 47:5, 1997.
20. Ahlgren JD: Epidemiology and risk factors in pancreatic cancer. Semin Oncol 23:241, 1996.
21. Andren-Sandberg A, et al: Etiologic links between chronic pancreatitis and pancreatic cancer. Scand J Gastroenterol 32:97, 1997.
22. Weyrer K, et al: *p53*, Ki-*ras*, a DNA ploidy in human pancreatic ductal adenocarcinomas. Lab Invest 74:279, 1996.
23. Pinto M. M., et al: Ki-*ras* mutations and the carcinoembryonic antigen level in fine needle aspirates of the pancreas. Acta Cytol 41:427, 1997.
24. Furuya N, et al: Long-term follow-up of patients with chronic pancreatitis and *ras* gene mutations detected in pancreatic juice. Gastroenterology 113:593, 1997.
25. Schmielau J, et al: The role of cytokines in pancreatic cancer. Int J Pancreatol 19:157, 1996.
26. Urrutia R, DiMagno EP: Genetic markers: the key to early diagnosis and improved survival in pancreatic cancer? Gastroenterology 110: 306, 1996.
27. Falkmer S: Origin of the parenchymal cells of the endocrine pancreas: some phylogenic and ontogenetic aspects. Front Gastrointest Res 23:2, 1995.
28. American Diabetes Association, Alexandria, VA: Report of the expert committee on the diagnosis and classification of diabetes mellitus. Diabetes Care 20:1183, 1997.
29. Matthews DR, Clark A: Insulin secretion and the aetiology of non-insulin-dependent diabetes. Front Horm Res 22:179, 1997.
30. Kruszynska YT, Olefsky JM: Cellular and molecular mechanisms of non–insulin dependent diabetes mellitus. Invest Med 44:413, 1996.
31. Prentki M, et al: Signal transduction mechanisms in nutrient-induced insulin secretion. Diabetologia 40 suppl.2:S32, 1997.
32. Kyvik KO, et al: H. Concordance rates of insulin dependent diabetes mellitus: a population based study of young Danish twins. Br Med J 311:913, 1995.
33. Bain SC, et al: Genetic factors associated with insulin-dependent diabetes. Front Horm Res 22:23, 1997.
34. Reijonen H, Nepom GT: Role of HLA susceptibility in predisposing to insulin-dependent diabetes mellitus. Front Horm Res 22:46, 1997.
35. Reed P, et al: Evidence for a type 1 diabetes susceptibility locus (IDDM10) on human chromosome 10p11-q11. Hum Mol Genet 6: 1011, 1997.
36. Buhler J, et al: Linkage analyses in type 1 diabetes mellitus using CASPAR, a software and statistical program for conditional analysis of polygenic diseases. Hum Hered 47:211, 1997.
37. Bach J-F: Insulin-dependent diabetes mellitus as an autoimmune disease. Endocr Rev 15:516, 1994.
38. Grewal IS, Flavell RA: New insights into insulin dependent diabetes mellitus from studies with transgenic mouse models. Lab Invest 76:3, 1997.
39. Laufer TM, et al: Autoimmune diabetes can be induced in transgenic major histocompatibility complex class II–deficient mice. J Exp Med 178:589, 1993.
40. Rabinovitch A: Immunoregulatory and cytokine imbalances in the pathogenesis of IDDM: therapeutic intervention by immunostimulation? Diabetes 43:613, 1994.
41. Rothe H, et al: Active stage of autoimmune diabetes is associated with the expression of a novel cytokine IGIF, which is located near Idd2. J Clin Invest 99:469, 1997.
42. Sepe V, et al: Islet-related autoantigens and the pathogenesis of insulin-dependent diabetes mellitus. Front Horm Res 22:68, 1997.
43 Zekzer D, et al: GAD-reactive CD4+ Th 1 cells induce diabetes in NOD/SCJD mice. J Clin Invest 101:68, 1998.
44 Kulmala P, et al: Prediction of insulin-dependent diabetes mellitus in siblings of children with diabetes: a population-based study. J Clin Invest 101:327, 1998.
45. Verge CF, et al. Number of autoantibodies (against insulin, GAD or ICA512/IA) rather than particular autoantibody determines risk of type 1 diabetes. J Autoimmun 1997, 9:379, 1996.

46. Andreoletti L, et al: Detection of Coxsackie B virus RNA sequences in whole blood samples from adult patients at the onset of type 1 diabetes mellitus. J Med Virol 52:121, 1997.
46a. Atkinson MA: Molecular mimicry and the pathogenesis of insulin dependent diabetes mellitus—still just an attractive hypothesis. Ann Med 5:393, 1997.
47. Conrad B, et al: A human endogenous retroviral superantigen as candidate autoimmune gene in type I diabetes. Cell 90:303, 1997.
48. Benoist C, Mathis D: Retrovirus as trigger, precipitator or marker? Nature 388:833, 1997.
49. Gerstein H: Cow's milk exposure and type 1 diabetes. Diabetes Care 17:13, 1994.
50. Hattersley A: Genetic factors in the aetiology of non–insulin-dependent diabetes. Front Horm Res 22:157, 1997.
51. Groop LC: Etiology of non-insulin-dependent diabetes mellitus. Front Horm Res 22:131, 1997.
52. Sacks DB: Amylin—a glucoregulatory hormone involved in the pathogenesis of diabetes mellitus? Clin Chem 42:494, 1996.
53. Yamagata K, et al. Mutations in the hepatocyte nucleus factor-4α gene in maturity onset diabetes of the young (MODY1). Nature 384: 458, 1996.
54. Frayling TM, et al: Mutations in the hepatocyte nuclear factor-1α gene are a common cause of maturity-onset diabetes of the young in the U.K. Diabetes 46:720, 1997.
55. Semenkovich CF, Heinecke JW: The mystery of diabetes and atherosclerosis: time for a new plot. Diabetes 46:327, 1997.
56. Nathan DM: The pathophysiology of diabetic complications: how much does the glucose hypothesis explain? Ann Intern Med 124:86, 1996.
56a. Vlassara H: Recent progress in advanced glycation end products and diabetic complications. Diabetes 46(Suppl 2): S19, 1997.
57. Stehouwer CDA, et al: Endothelial dysfunction and pathogenesis of diabetic angiopathy. Cardiovasc Res 34:55, 1997.
58. Diabetes Control and Complications Trial Research Group: The effect of intensive treatment of diabetes on the development and progression of long-term complications in insulin-dependent diabetes mellitus. N Engl J Med 329:977, 1993.
59. Sowers JR, Epstein M: Diabetes mellitus and associated hypertension, vascular disease, and nephropathy: an update. Hypertension 26:869, 1995.
60. Epstein M: Diabetes and hypertension: the bad companions. J Hypertens 15 (suppl 2):S55, 1997.
61. Cooper ME, et al: Diabetic vascular complications. Clin Exp Pharmacol Physiol 24:770, 1997.
62. Mooradian AD: Central nervous system complications of diabetes mellitus—a perspective from the blood-brain barrier. Brain Res Rev 23:210, 1997.
63. Genuth SM: Diabetic ketoacidosis and hyperglycemic hyperosmolar coma. Curr Ther Endocrinol Metab 6:438, 1997.
64. Tooke JE: Microvasculature in diabetes. Cardiovasc Res 32:764, 1996.
65. Capella C, et al: Revised classification of neuroendocrine tumours of the lung, pancreas and gut. Virchows Arch 425:547, 1995.
66. Vassilopoulou-Sellin R, Ajani J: Islet cell tumors of the pancreas. Endocrinol Metab Clin North Am 23:53, 1994.

21

The Kidney

CLINICAL MANIFESTATIONS OF RENAL DISEASES

CONGENITAL ANOMALIES

CYSTIC DISEASES OF THE KIDNEY

Cystic Renal Dysplasia

Autosomal Dominant (Adult) Polycystic Kidney Disease

Autosomal Recessive (Childhood) Polycystic Kidney Disease

Cystic Diseases of Renal Medulla

Medullary Sponge Kidney

Nephronophthisis–Uremic Medullary Cystic Disease Complex

Acquired (Dialysis-Associated) Cystic Disease

Simple Cysts

GLOMERULAR DISEASES

CLINICAL MANIFESTATIONS

HISTOLOGIC ALTERATIONS

PATHOGENESIS OF GLOMERULAR INJURY

In Situ Immune Complex Deposition

Anti-GBM Nephritis

Heymann Nephritis

Antibodies Against Planted Antigens

Circulating Immune Complex Nephritis

Antibodies to Glomerular Cells

Cell-Mediated Immunity in Glomerulonephritis

Activation of Alternative Complement Pathway

Epithelial Cell Injury

Mediators of Glomerular Injury

Cells

Soluble Mediators

MECHANISMS OF PROGRESSION IN GLOMERULAR DISEASES

ACUTE GLOMERULONEPHRITIS

Acute Proliferative (Poststreptococcal, Postinfectious) Glomerulonephritis

Poststreptococcal Glomerulonephritis

Nonstreptococcal Acute Glomerulonephritis

RAPIDLY PROGRESSIVE (CRESCENTIC) GLOMERULONEPHRITIS

NEPHROTIC SYNDROME

MEMBRANOUS GLOMERULONEPHRITIS (MEMBRANOUS NEPHROPATHY)

MINIMAL CHANGE DISEASE (LIPOID NEPHROSIS)

FOCAL SEGMENTAL GLOMERULOSCLEROSIS

MEMBRANOPROLIFERATIVE GLOMERULONEPHRITIS

IgA NEPHROPATHY (BERGER DISEASE)

FOCAL PROLIFERATIVE AND NECROTIZING GLOMERULONEPHRITIS (FOCAL GLOMERULONEPHRITIS)

HEREDITARY NEPHRITIS

Alport Syndrome

Thin Membrane Disease (Benign Familial Hematuria)

CHRONIC GLOMERULONEPHRITIS

GLOMERULAR LESIONS ASSOCIATED WITH SYSTEMIC DISEASE

Systemic Lupus Erythematosus

Henoch-Schönlein Purpura

Bacterial Endocarditis

Diabetic Glomerulosclerosis

Amyloidosis

Fibrillary and Immunotactoid Glomerulonephritis

Other Systemic Disorders

DISEASES AFFECTING TUBULES AND INTERSTITIUM

ACUTE TUBULAR NECROSIS

TUBULOINTERSTITIAL NEPHRITIS

Pyelonephritis and Urinary Tract Infection

Acute Pyelonephritis

Chronic Pyelonephritis and Reflux Nephropathy

Tubulointerstitial Nephritis Induced by Drugs and Toxins

Acute Drug-Induced Interstitial Nephritis

Analgesic Abuse Nephropathy

Nephropathy Associated With Nonsteroidal Anti-Inflammatory Drugs

Other Tubulointerstitial Diseases

Urate Nephropathy

Hypercalcemia and Nephrocalcinosis

Multiple Myeloma

DISEASES OF BLOOD VESSELS

BENIGN NEPHROSCLEROSIS

MALIGNANT HYPERTENSION AND ACCELERATED NEPHROSCLEROSIS

RENAL ARTERY STENOSIS
THROMBOTIC MICROANGIOPATHIES
Classic (Childhood) Hemolytic-Uremic Syndrome
Adult Hemolytic-Uremic Syndrome/Thrombotic Thrombocytopenic Purpura
Idiopathic HUS/TTP
Other Vascular Disorders
Atherosclerotic Ischemic Renal Disease
Atheroembolic Renal Disease
Sickle Cell Disease Nephropathy
Diffuse Cortical Necrosis
Renal Infarcts
URINARY TRACT OBSTRUCTION (OBSTRUCTIVE UROPATHY)
UROLITHIASIS (RENAL CALCULI, STONES)
TUMORS OF THE KIDNEY
BENIGN TUMORS
Renal Papillary Adenoma
Renal Fibroma or Hamartoma (Renomedullary Interstitial Cell Tumor)
Angiomyolipoma
Oncocytoma
MALIGNANT TUMORS
Renal Cell Carcinoma (Hypernephroma, Adenocarcinoma of Kidney)
Classification of Renal Cell Carcinoma: Histology, Cytogenetics, and Genetics
Urothelial Carcinomas of Renal Pelvis

NORMAL

What is man but an ingenious machine designed to turn, with "infinite artfulness, the red wine of Shiraz into urine"? So said the storyteller in Isak Dinesen's *Seven Gothic Tales.*[1] More accurately but less poetically, human kidneys serve to convert more than 1700 liters of blood per day into about 1 liter of a highly specialized concentrated fluid called urine. In so doing, the kidney excretes the waste products of metabolism, precisely regulates the body's concentration of water and salt, maintains the appropriate acid balance of plasma, and serves as an endocrine organ, secreting such hormones as erythropoietin, renin, and prostaglandins. The physiologic mechanisms that the kidney has evolved to carry out these functions require a high degree of structural complexity.

Each human adult kidney weighs about 150 gm. As the ureter enters the kidney at the hilum, it dilates into a funnel-shaped cavity, the *pelvis,* from which derive two or three main branches, the *major calyces;* the latter subdivide again into about three or four *minor calyces.* There are about 12 minor calyces in the human kidney. On cut surface, the kidney is made up of a *cortex* and a *medulla,* the former 1.2 to 1.5 cm in thickness. The medulla consists of *renal pyramids,* the apices of which are called *papillae,* each related to a calyx. Cortical tissue extends into spaces between adjacent pyramids as the *renal columns of Bertin.* From the standpoint of its diseases, the kidney can be divided into four components: blood vessels, glomeruli, tubules, and interstitium.

Blood Vessels. The kidney is richly supplied by blood vessels, and although both kidneys make up only 0.5% of the total body weight, they receive about 25% of the cardiac output. Of this, the cortex is by far the more richly vascularized, receiving 90% of the total renal circulation. The main renal artery divides into anterior and posterior sections at the hilum. From these, *interlobar arteries* emerge, course between lobes, and give rise to the *arcuate arteries,* which arch between cortex and medulla, in turn giving rise to the *interlobular arteries.* From the interlobular arteries, *afferent arterioles* enter the glomerular tuft, where they progressively subdivide into 20 to 40 capillary loops arranged in several units or lobules. Capillary loops merge together to exit from the glomerulus as *efferent arterioles.* In general, efferent arterioles from superficial nephrons form a rich vascular network that encircles cortical tubules *(peritubular vascular network);* deeper juxtamedullary glomeruli give rise to the *vasa recta,* which descend as straight vessels to supply the outer and inner medulla. These descending arterial vasa recta then make several loops in the inner medulla and ascend as the *venous vasa recta.*

The anatomy of renal vessels has several important implications. First, because the arteries are largely end-arteries, *occlusion of any branch results in infarction of the specific area it supplies.* Glomerular disease that interferes with blood flow through the glomerular capillaries has profound effects on the tubules, within both the cortex and the medulla, because *all tubular capillary beds are derived from the efferent arterioles.* The peculiarities of the blood supply to the renal medulla render them especially vulnerable to ischemia; *the medulla is relatively avascular,* and the blood in the capillary loops in the medulla has a remarkably low hematocrit value. Thus, minor interference with the blood supply of the medulla may result in medullary necrosis.

Glomeruli. The glomerulus consists of an anastomosing network of capillaries lined by fenestrated epithelium invested by two layers of epithelium (Fig. 21–1). The visceral epithelium is incorporated into and becomes an intrinsic part of the capillary wall separated from endothelial cells by a basement membrane. The parietal epithelium lines Bowman space, the cavity in which plasma filtrate first collects.

The glomerular capillary wall is the filtering membrane and consists of the following structures[2] (Fig. 21–2):

- A thin layer of fenestrated *endothelial cells,* each fenestrum being about 70 to 100 nm in diameter.
- A *glomerular basement membrane* (GBM) with a thick electron-dense central layer, the *lamina densa,* and thinner electron-lucent peripheral layers, the *lamina rara interna* and *lamina rara externa.* The GBM consists of collagen (mostly type IV), laminin, polyanionic proteoglycans (mostly heparan sulfate), fibronectin, entactin, and several other glycoproteins. Type IV collagen forms a network suprastructure to which other glycoproteins attach. The building block (monomer) of this network is

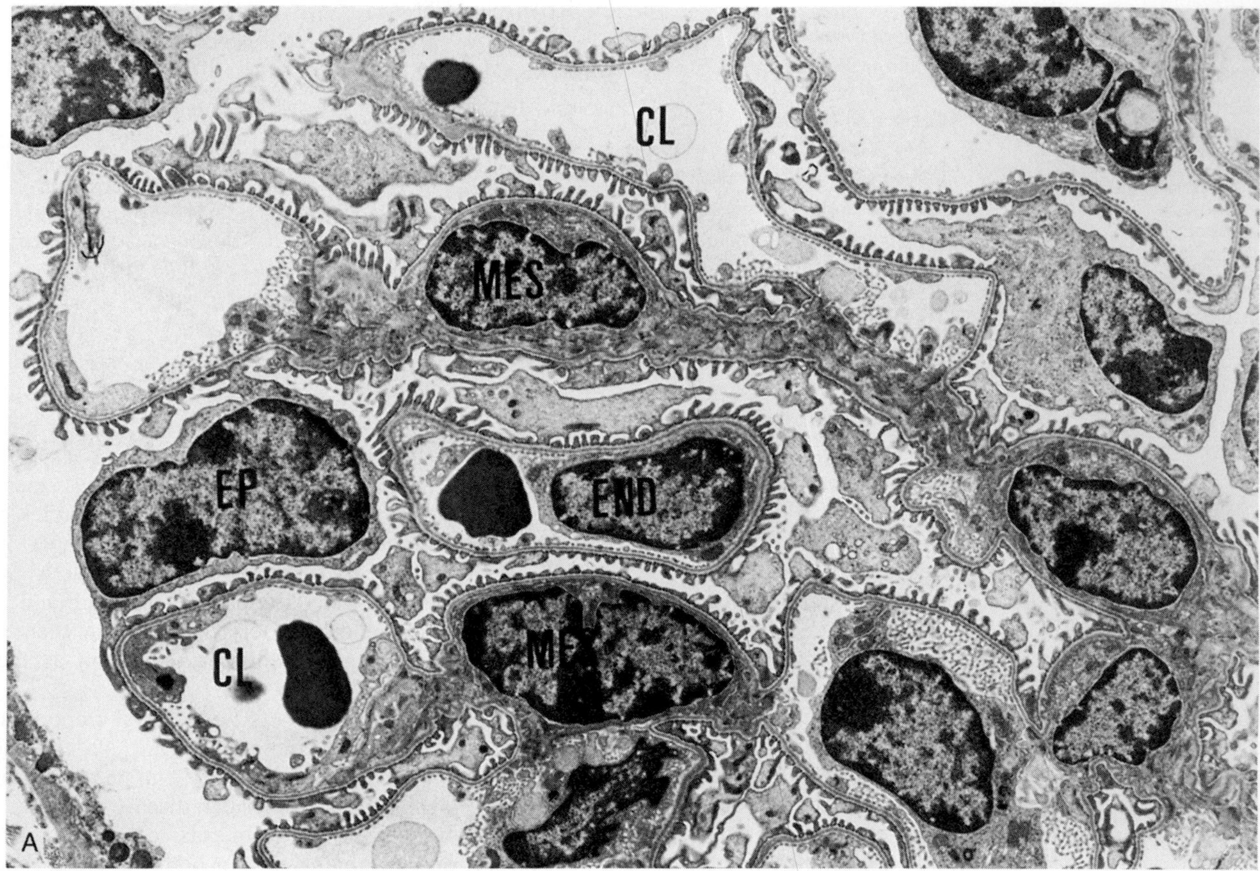

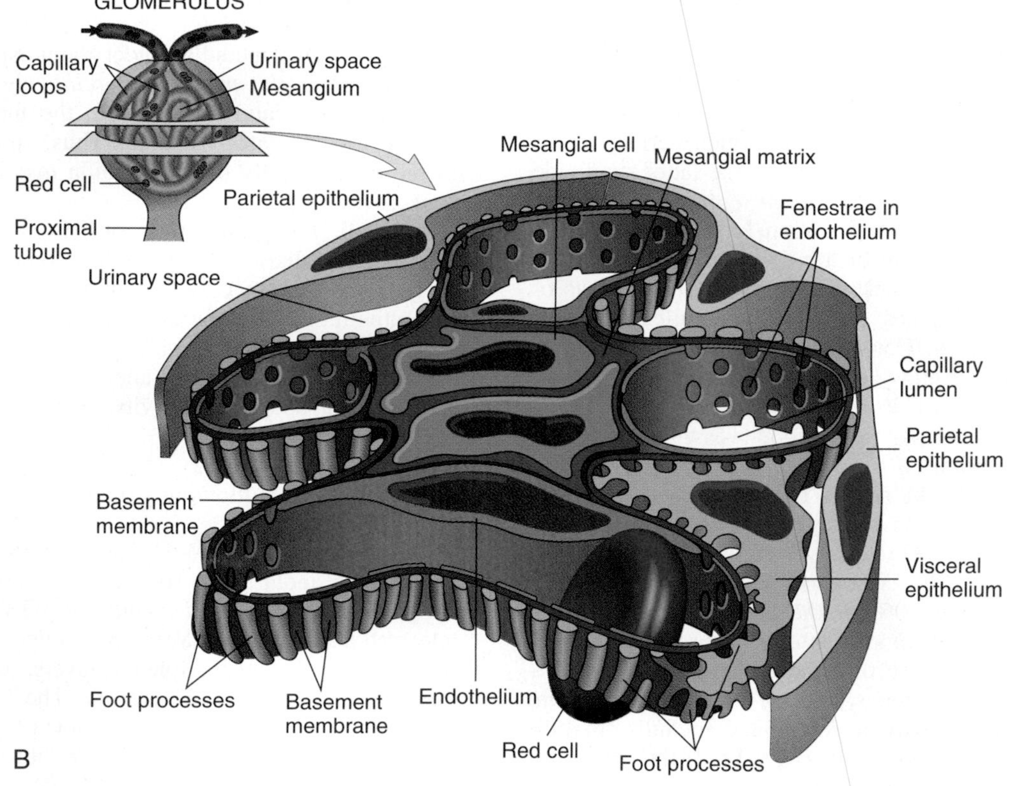

Figure 21–1

A, Low-power electron micrograph of renal glomerulus. CL, capillary lumen; MES, mesangium; END, endothelium; EP, visceral epithelial cells with foot processes. (Courtesy of Dr. Vicki Kelley, Brigham and Women's Hospital, Boston, MA.) *B*, Schematic representation of a glomerular lobe.

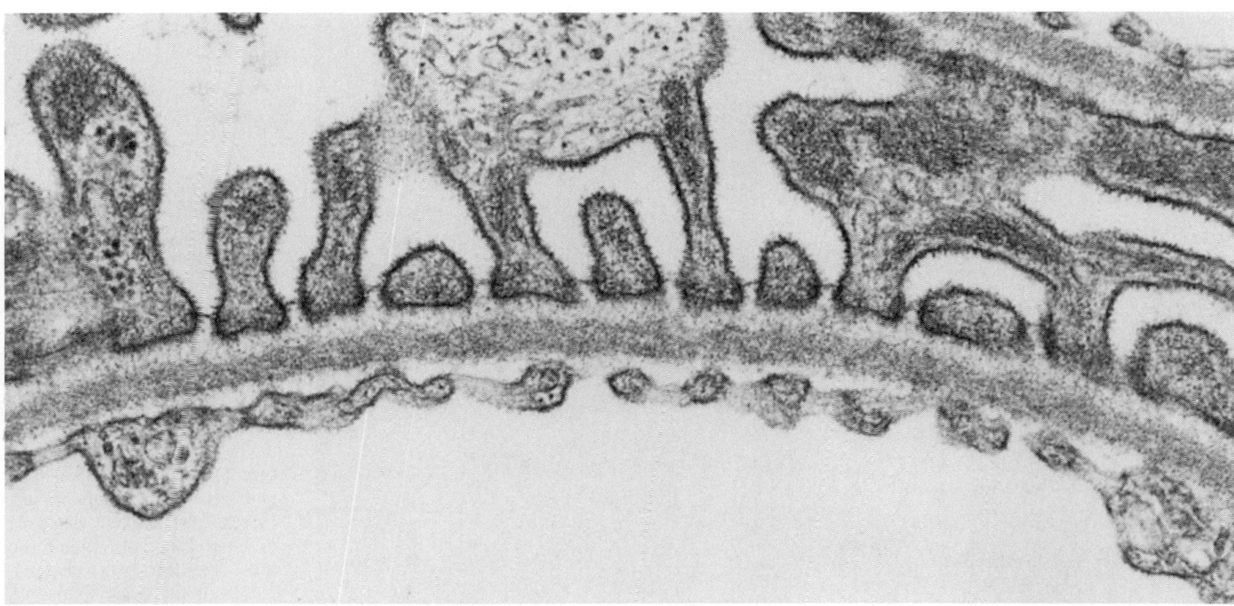

Figure 21–2

Glomerular filter consisting, from bottom to top, of fenestrated endothelium, basement membrane, and foot processes of epithelial cells. Note filtration slits and diaphragm. Note also that the basement membrane consists of a central lamina densa, sandwiched between two looser layers, the lamina rara interna and lamina rara externa. (Courtesy of Dr. Helmut Rennke, Brigham and Women's Hospital, Boston, MA.)

a triple-helical molecule made up of three α chains, composed of one or more of six types of α chains (α_1 to α_6 or COL4A1 to COL4A6), the most common consisting of α_1 α_2 α_1 (Fig. 21–3).[3] Each molecule consists of a 7S domain at the amino terminus, a triple-helical domain in the middle, and a globular noncollagenous domain (NC1) at the carboxyl terminus. The NC1 domain is important for helical formation and also for assembly of collagen monomers into dimers. The 7S domain, in turn, is involved in formation of tetramers, and thus a porous suprastructure evolves. Glycoproteins (laminin, entactin) and acidic proteoglycans (perlecan) attach to the collagenous suprastructure[4] (Fig. 21–4). *These biochemical determinants are critical to understanding glomerular diseases.* For example, as we shall see, the NC1 domain is the antigenic site in anti-GBM nephritis; genetic defects in the α chains underlie some forms of hereditary nephritis; and the acidic porous nature of the GBM determines its permeability characteristics.

- The *visceral epithelial cells* (podocytes), structurally complex cells that possess interdigitating processes embedded in and adherent to the lamina rara externa of the basement membrane. Adjacent *foot processes* (pedicels) are separated by 20- to 30-nm-wide *filtration slits,* which are bridged by a thin diaphragm. (see Fig. 21–2).
- The entire glomerular tuft is supported by *mesangial cells* lying between the capillaries. Basement membrane–like *mesangial matrix* forms a meshwork through which the mesangial cells are scattered. These cells, of mesenchymal origin, are contractile, phagocytic, and capable of proliferation, of laying down both matrix and

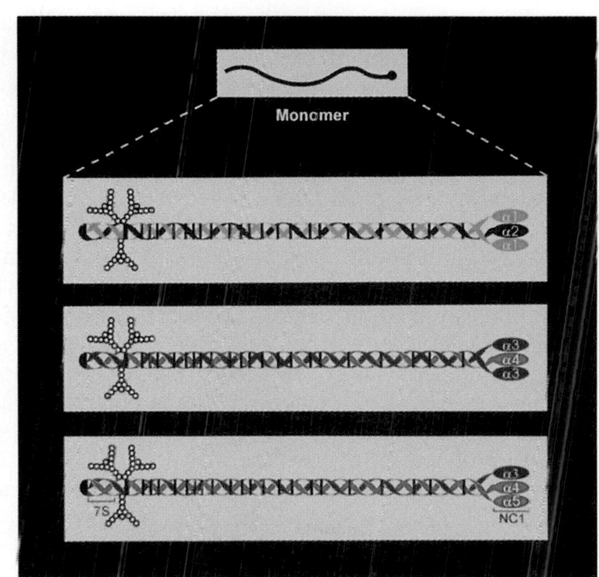

Figure 21–3

The structure of type IV collagen of the glomerular basement membrane (GBM), showing the building block of the collagen network: collagen type IV monomers composed of three α chains (of possible six α chain types, α_1 to α_6) arranged in a triple helix. The most common monomer is made up of α_1/α_2 chains, but α_3/α_4 and α_5/α_6 chains are also present in the kidney. Each monomer has an NC1 domain (carboxyl terminus), a triple-helical domain, and a 7S amino acid terminus domain. Monomers form dimers through their NC1 domains and tetramers at the 7S domain to develop a suprastructure to which other extracellular matrix components attach, as shown in Figure 21–4. (Courtesy of Dr. B. G. Hudson, University of Kansas.)

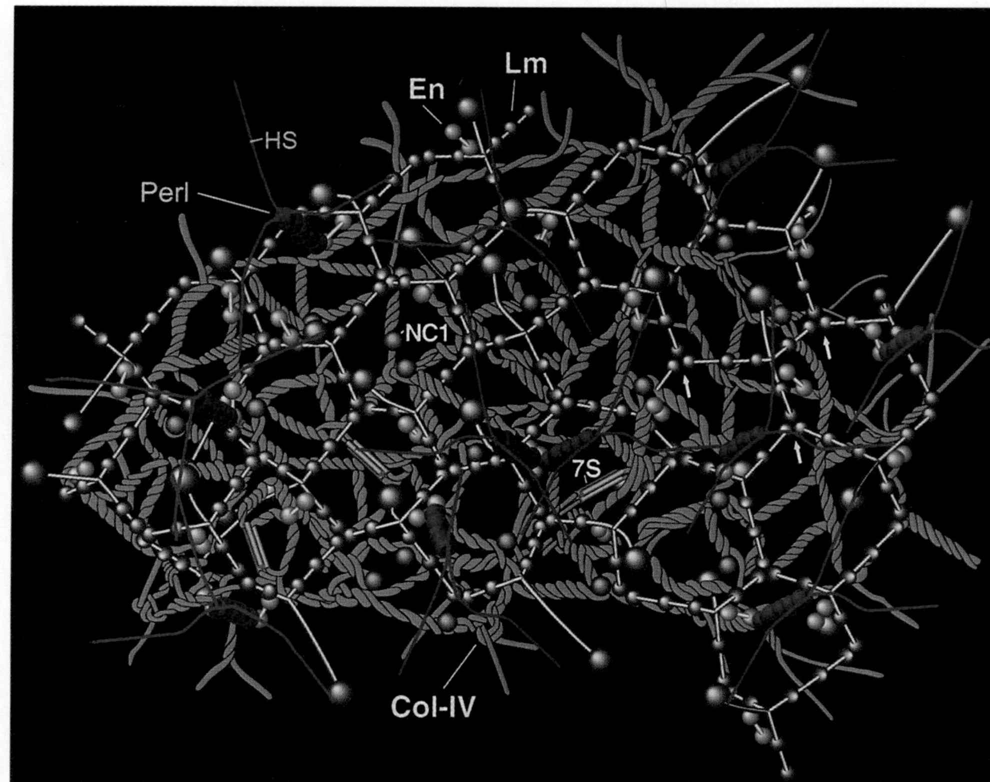

Figure 21–4

A proposed model of the GBM molecular architecture in which type IV collagen monomers (gray) form a stable network through their NC1 domains (dimeric interactions, gray spheres) and 7S domains (tetrameric interactions) and intertwine along the triple-helical domains. Laminin monomers (red) separately form a reversible meshwork. Entactin (green) connects laminin to the collagen network and binds to perlecan (blue), an anionic heparan sulfate proteoglycan. This anionic suprastructure determines the charged porous nature of the GBM. (Courtesy of Dr. Peter Yurchenco, Robert W. Johnson Medical School, Piscataway, NJ.)

collagen, and of secreting a number of biologically active mediators. They are, as we shall see, important players in many forms of human glomerulonephritis.

The major characteristics of glomerular filtration are an extraordinary high permeability to water and small solutes, accounted for by the highly fenestrated endothelium, and impermeability to proteins, such that molecules of the size of albumin (+3.6-nm radius; 70,000 MW). The latter property, called *glomerular barrier function,* discriminates among various protein molecules, depending on their size (the larger, the less permeable) and charge (the more cationic, the more permeable). This size- and charge-dependent barrier function is accounted for by the complex structure of the capillary wall, the collagenous porous charged suprastructure of the GBM, and the many anionic moieties present within the wall, including the acidic proteoglycans of the GBM (Fig. 21–4) and the sialoglycoproteins of epithelial and endothelial cell coats. The charge-dependent restriction is important in the virtually complete exclusion of albumin from the filtrate, because albumin is an anionic molecule of a pI 4.5. The *visceral epithelial cell* is important in the maintenance of glomerular barrier function: its slit diaphragm presents a distal diffusion barrier to the filtration of proteins, and it is the cell type that is largely responsible for synthesis of GBM components.

Tubules. The structure of renal tubular epithelial cells varies considerably at different levels of the nephron and, to a certain extent, correlates with function. For example, the highly developed structure of the *proximal tubular cells,* with their abundant long microvilli, numerous mitochondria, apical canaliculi, and extensive intercellular interdigitations, is correlated with their major functions: reabsorption of two thirds of filtered sodium and water as well as glucose, potassium, phosphate, amino acids, and proteins. The proximal tubule is particularly vulnerable to ischemic damage. Furthermore, toxins are frequently reabsorbed by the proximal tubule, rendering it also susceptible to chemical injury.

The *juxtaglomerular apparatus* snuggles closely against the glomerulus where the afferent arteriole enters it. The juxtaglomerular apparatus consists of (1) the *juxtaglomerular cells,* modified granulated smooth muscle cells in the media of the afferent arteriole that contain renin; (2) the *macula densa,* a specialized region of the distal tubule as it returns to the vascular pole of its parent glomerulus—here the tubular cells are more crowded and the cells are somewhat shorter and possess distinct patterns of interdigitation between adjacent membranes; and (3) the *lacis cells* or *nongranular cells,* which reside in the area bounded by the afferent arteriole, the macula densa, and the glomerulus. They resemble mesangial cells and appear to be continuous with them. The juxtaglomerular apparatus is a small endocrine organ, the juxtaglomerular cells being the principal sources of renin production in the kidney.

Interstitium. In the normal cortex, the interstitial space is compact, being occupied by the fenestrated peritubular capillaries and a small number of fibroblast-like cells. Any obvious expansion of the cortical interstitium is usually abnormal; this expansion can be due to edema or infiltration with acute inflammatory cells, as in acute interstitial diseases, or it may be caused by accumulation of chronic inflammatory cells and fibrous tissue, as in chronic interstitial diseases. The amounts of proteoglycans in the interstitial tissue of the medulla increase with age and in the presence of ischemia.

PATHOLOGY

Renal diseases are responsible for a great deal of morbidity but, fortunately, are not major causes of mortality. To place the problem in some perspective, approximately 35,000 deaths are attributed yearly to renal disease in the United States, in contrast to about 750,000 to heart disease, 400,000 to cancer, and 200,000 to stroke. Morbidity, however, is by no means insignificant. Millions of persons are affected annually by nonfatal kidney diseases, most notably infections of the kidney or lower urinary tract, kidney stones, and urinary obstruction. Twenty per cent of all women suffer from infection of the urinary tract or kidney at some time in their lives, and at least 1% of the United States population develop renal stones. Similarly, dialysis and transplantation keep many patients alive who would formerly have died of renal failure, adding to the pool of renal morbidity. The cost of such programs now exceeds several billion dollars annually. Renal disease also has special importance to the clinician because so many of the deaths occur in young people.

Diseases of the kidney are as complex as its structure, but their study is facilitated by dividing them into those that affect the four basic morphologic components: glomeruli, tubules, interstitium, and blood vessels. This traditional approach is useful, since the early manifestations of disease affecting each of these components tend to be distinct. Further, some components appear to be more vulnerable to specific forms of renal injury; for example, most *glomerular diseases are immunologically mediated, whereas tubular and interstitial disorders are frequently caused by toxic or infectious agents.* Nevertheless, some agents affect more than one structure. In addition, the anatomic interdependence of structure in the kidney implies that damage to one almost always secondarily affects the others. Disease primarily in the blood vessels, for example, inevitably affects all the structures dependent on this blood supply. Severe glomerular damage impairs the flow through the peritubular vascular system and also delivers potentially toxic products to tubules; conversely, tubular destruction, by increasing intraglomerular pressure, may induce glomerular atrophy. Thus, whatever the origin, there is a tendency for all forms of chronic renal disease ultimately to destroy all four components of the kidney, culminating in chronic renal failure and what has been called *end-stage kidneys.* The functional reserve of the kidney is large, and much damage may occur before there is evident functional impairment. For these reasons, the early signs and symptoms are particularly important clinically.

In this chapter, we briefly review the clinical manifestations, pathogenesis, and pathology of the major renal diseases. These are dealt with in great detail in two comprehensive texts of pathology[5, 6] and renal medicine[7, 8] and in electronic updates of nephrology.[9]

CLINICAL MANIFESTATIONS OF RENAL DISEASES

The clinical manifestations of renal disease can be grouped into reasonably well defined syndromes. Some are peculiar to glomerular diseases; others are present in diseases that affect any one of the components. Before we list the syndromes, a few terms must be clarified.

Azotemia is a biochemical abnormality that refers to an elevation of the blood urea nitrogen (BUN) and creatinine levels and is related largely to a decreased glomerular filtration rate (GFR). Azotemia is produced by many renal disorders, but it also arises from extrarenal disorders. *Prerenal azotemia* is encountered when there is hypoperfusion of the kidneys (e.g., in hemorrhage, shock, volume depletion, and congestive heart failure) that impairs renal function *in the absence of parenchymal damage.* Similarly, *postrenal azotemia* is seen whenever urine flow is obstructed below the level of the kidney. Relief of the obstruction is followed by correction of the azotemia.

When azotemia becomes associated with a constellation of clinical signs and symptoms and biochemical abnormalities, it is termed uremia. Uremia is characterized not only by failure of renal excretory function but also by a host of metabolic and endocrine alterations incident to renal damage. There is, in addition, secondary gastrointestinal (e.g., uremic gastroenteritis), neuromuscular (e.g., peripheral neuropathy), and cardiovascular (e.g., uremic fibrinous pericarditis) involvement, which is usually necessary for the diagnosis of uremia.

We can now turn to a brief description of the clinical presentations of renal disease, some of which cluster into relatively distinct syndromes.

- *Acute nephritic syndrome* is a glomerular syndrome dominated by the acute onset of usually grossly visible hematuria (red blood cells in urine), mild to moderate proteinuria, and hypertension; it is the classic presentation of acute poststreptococcal glomerulonephritis.
- The *nephrotic syndrome* is characterized by heavy proteinuria (more than 3.5 gm/day), hypoalbuminemia, severe edema, hyperlipidemia, and lipiduria (lipid in the urine).
- *Asymptomatic hematuria or proteinuria,* or a combination of these two, is usually a manifestation of subtle or mild glomerular abnormalities.
- *Acute renal failure* is dominated by oliguria or anuria (no urine flow), with recent onset of azotemia. It can result from glomerular (e.g., crescentic glomerulonephritis), interstitial, and vascular injury or acute tubular necrosis.
- *Chronic renal failure,* characterized by prolonged symptoms and signs of uremia, is the end result of all chronic renal diseases.
- *Renal tubular defects* are dominated by polyuria (excessive urine formation), nocturia, and electrolyte disorders

(e.g., metabolic acidosis). They are the result of either diseases directly affecting tubular structure (e.g., medullary cystic disease) or defects in specific tubular functions. The latter can be inherited (e.g., familial nephrogenic diabetes, cystinuria, renal tubular acidosis) or acquired (e.g., lead nephropathy).

- *Urinary tract infection* is characterized by bacteriuria and pyuria (bacteria and leukocytes in the urine). The infection may be *symptomatic* or *asymptomatic,* and it may affect the kidney *(pyelonephritis)* or the bladder *(cystitis)* only.
- *Nephrolithiasis* (renal stone) is manifested by renal colic, hematuria, and recurrent stone formation.
- *Urinary tract obstruction* and *renal tumors* represent specific anatomic lesions with often varied clinical manifestations.

Renal Failure. Acute renal failure implies a rapid and frequently reversible deterioration of renal function. As a characteristic syndrome with a complex pathogenesis, it is discussed separately. Here the discussion is limited to *chronic renal failure,* which is the end result of a variety of renal diseases and is the major cause of death from renal disease.

Although exceptions abound, the evolution from normal renal function to symptomatic chronic renal failure progresses through four stages that merge into one another.

Table 21–1. PRINCIPAL SYSTEMIC MANIFESTATIONS OF CHRONIC RENAL FAILURE AND UREMIA

Fluid and Electrolytes
Dehydration
Edema
Hyperkalemia
Metabolic acidosis
Calcium Phosphate and Bone
Hyperphosphatemia
Hypocalcemia
Secondary hyperparathyroidism
Renal osteodystrophy
Hematologic
Anemia
Bleeding diathesis
Cardiopulmonary
Hypertension
Congestive heart failure
Pulmonary edema
Uremic pericarditis
Gastrointestinal
Nausea and vomiting
Bleeding
Esophagitis, gastritis, colitis
Neuromuscular
Myopathy
Peripheral neuropathy
Encephalopathy
Dermatologic
Sallow color
Pruritus
Dermatitis

Diminished Renal Reserve. In this situation, the GFR is about 50% of normal. Serum BUN and creatinine values are normal, and the patients are asymptomatic. However, they are more susceptible to developing azotemia with an additional renal insult.

Renal Insufficiency. The GFR is 20% to 50% of normal. Azotemia appears, usually associated with anemia and hypertension. Polyuria and nocturia occur as a result of decreased concentrating ability. Sudden stress (e.g., with nephrotoxins) may precipitate uremia.

Renal Failure. The GFR is less than 20% to 25% of normal. The kidneys cannot regulate volume and solute composition, and patients develop edema, metabolic acidosis, and hypocalcemia. Overt uremia may ensue, with neurologic, gastrointestinal, and cardiovascular complications.

End-Stage Renal Disease. The GFR is less than 5% of normal; this is the terminal stage of uremia.

The details of the pathophysiology of chronic renal failure are beyond the scope of this book and are well covered in various nephrology texts.[8, 9] Table 21–1 lists the major systemic abnormalities in uremic renal failure.

CONGENITAL ANOMALIES

About 10% of all persons are born with potentially significant malformations of the urinary system. Renal dysplasias and hypoplasias account for 20% of chronic renal failure in children. Polycystic kidney disease (a congenital anomaly that becomes apparent in adults) is responsible for about 10% of chronic renal failure in humans.

Congenital renal disease can be hereditary but is most often the result of an acquired developmental defect that arises during gestation. As discussed in Chapter 11, defects in developmental genes, including the Wilms' tumor *(WT1)*–associated genes, cause urogenital anomalies. As a rule, developmental abnormalities involve structural components of the kidney and urinary tract. However, enzymatic or metabolic defects in tubular transport, such as cystinuria and renal tubular acidosis, also occur. Here we restrict the discussion to structural anomalies involving primarily the kidney. Anomalies of the lower urinary tract are discussed in Chapter 22.

Agenesis of the Kidney. Total bilateral agenesis, which is incompatible with life, is usually encountered in stillborn infants. It is often associated with many other congenital disorders (limb defects, hypoplastic lungs) and leads to early death. Unilateral agenesis is an uncommon anomaly that is compatible with normal life, if no other abnormalities exist. The opposite kidney is usually enlarged as a result of compensatory hypertrophy. Some patients eventually develop progressive glomerular sclerosis in the remaining kidney as a result of the adaptive changes in hypertrophied nephrons, discussed later in the chapter, and in time chronic renal failure.

Hypoplasia. Renal hypoplasia refers to failure of the kidneys to develop to a normal size. This anomaly may occur bilaterally, resulting in renal failure in early childhood, but it is more commonly encountered as a unilateral defect. True renal hypoplasia is extremely rare; most cases reported probably represent acquired scarring due to vascular, infectious, or other parenchymal diseases rather than an underlying developmental failure. Differentiation between congenital and acquired atrophic kidneys may be impossible, but *a truly hypoplastic kidney should show no scars and should possess a reduced number of renal lobes and pyramids:* six or fewer. In one form of hypoplastic kidney, *oligomeganephronia,* the kidney is small but the nephrons are markedly hypertrophied.

Ectopic Kidneys. The development of the definitive metanephros may occur in ectopic foci, usually at abnormally low levels. These kidneys lie either just above the pelvic brim or sometimes within the pelvis. They are usually normal or slightly smaller in size but otherwise are not remarkable. Because of their abnormal position, kinking or tortuosity of the ureters may cause some obstruction to urinary flow, which predisposes to bacterial infections.

Horseshoe Kidney. Fusion of the upper or lower poles of the kidneys produces a horseshoe-shaped structure continuous across the midline anterior to the great vessels. This anomaly is common and is found in about 1 in 500 to 1000 autopsies. Ninety per cent of such kidneys are fused at the lower pole, and 10% are fused at the upper pole.

Cystic Diseases of the Kidney

Although not all cysts of the kidney are congenital, all types of cysts are discussed here for convenience.

Cystic diseases of the kidney are a heterogeneous group comprising hereditary, developmental but nonhereditary, and acquired disorders. As a group, they are important for several reasons: (1) they are reasonably common and often represent diagnostic problems for clinicians, radiologists, and pathologists; (2) some forms, such as adult polycystic disease, are major causes of chronic renal failure; and (3) they can occasionally be confused with malignant tumors. A useful classification of renal cysts is as follows[10]:

1. Cystic renal dysplasia
2. Polycystic kidney disease
   a. Autosomal dominant (adult) polycystic disease
   b. Autosomal recessive (childhood) polycystic disease
3. Medullary cystic disease
   a. Medullary sponge kidney
   b. Nephronophthisis–uremic medullary cystic disease complex
4. Acquired (dialysis-associated) cystic disease
5. Localized (simple) renal cysts
6. Renal cysts in hereditary malformation syndromes (e.g., tuberous sclerosis)
7. Glomerulocystic disease
8. Extraparenchymal renal cysts (pyelocalyceal cysts, hilar lymphangitic cysts)

Only the more important of the cystic diseases are discussed.

CYSTIC RENAL DYSPLASIA

This disorder is due to an abnormality in metanephric differentiation *characterized histologically by the persistence in the kidney of abnormal structures—cartilage, undifferentiated mesenchyme, and immature collecting ductules—and by abnormal lobar organization.* Most cases are also associated with ureteropelvic obstruction, ureteral agenesis or atresia, and other anomalies of the lower urinary tract. Renal dysplasia occurs as a sporadic disorder, without familial clustering.

Dysplasia can be unilateral or bilateral and is almost always cystic. In gross appearance, the kidney is usually enlarged, extremely irregular, and multicystic (Fig. 21–5*A*). The cysts vary in size from small microscopic structures to some that are several centimeters in diameter. They are lined by flattened epithelium. On histologic examination, although normal nephrons are present, many have immature ducts. The characteristic feature is the *presence of islands of undifferentiated mesenchyme, often with cartilage, and immature collecting ducts* (Fig. 21–5*B*).

When unilateral, the dysplasia is discovered by the appearance of a flank mass that leads to surgical exploration and nephrectomy. Function in the opposite kidney is normal, and such patients have an excellent prognosis after surgical removal of the affected kidney. In bilateral renal dysplasia, renal failure may ultimately result.

AUTOSOMAL DOMINANT (ADULT) POLYCYSTIC KIDNEY DISEASE

Adult polycystic kidney disease is a hereditary disorder characterized by multiple expanding cysts of both kidneys that ultimately destroy the renal parenchyma and cause renal failure.[11, 12] It is a common condition affecting roughly 1 of every 400 to 1000 live births and accounting for about 10% of cases of chronic renal failure requiring transplantation or dialysis. The pattern of inheritance is *autosomal dominant,* with high penetrance. The disease is universally bilateral; reported unilateral cases probably represent multicystic dysplasia. The cysts initially involve only portions of the nephrons, so that renal function is retained until about the fourth or fifth decade of life. The likelihood of developing renal failure is less than 2% in affected individuals younger than 40 years but rises to 25% by age 50 years, 40% at age 60 years, and 75% by age 70 to 75 years. Although the major pathologic process is in the kidneys, adult polycystic kidney disease is a systemic disorder in which cysts and other anomalies also arise in other organs (see later).

Genetics and Pathogenesis. The disease is genetically heterogeneous, caused by mutations of three separate genes.

- The *PKD1* gene, located on chromosome 16p13.3, accounts for about 85% of cases and encodes a large (460 kD) protein named *polycystin 1.*[13] Polycystin is a complex cell membrane–associated protein with a long extracellular portion, a transmembrane domain, and a short cytoplasmic tail[13a] (Fig. 21–6). Although its precise

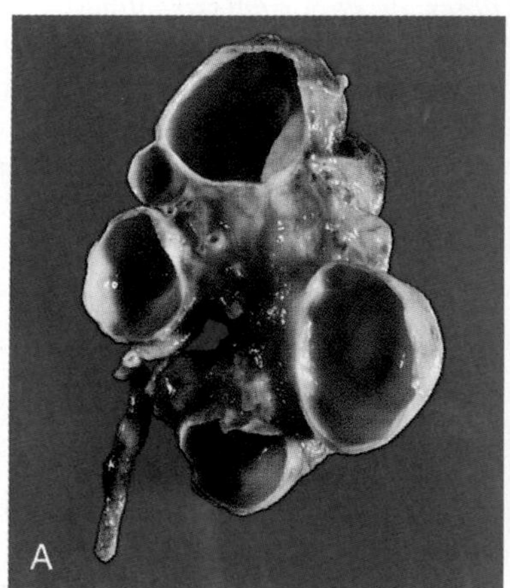

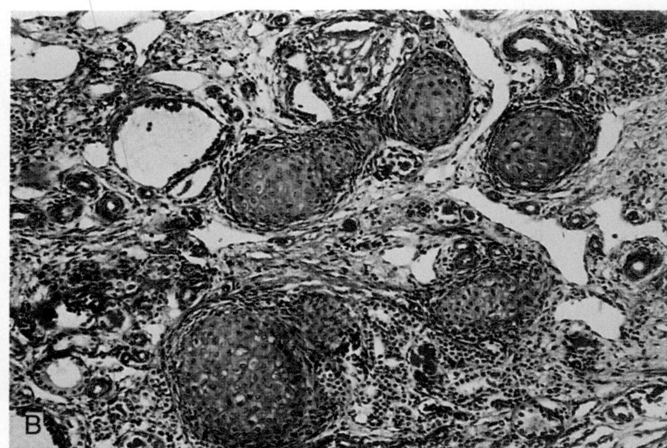

Figure 21–5

Renal dysplasia. *A*, Gross appearance, *B*, Histologic section showing disorganized architecture, dilated tubules, and islands of immature cartilage, PAS stain. (Courtesy of Dr. D. Schofield, Children's Hospital, Los Angeles, CA.)

function is unknown, it has domains with homology to proteins involved in cell-cell and cell-matrix interactions, as well as specific repeated so-called polycystic kidney disease (PKD) domains that may assume an immunoglobulin-like fold (Fig. 21–6).

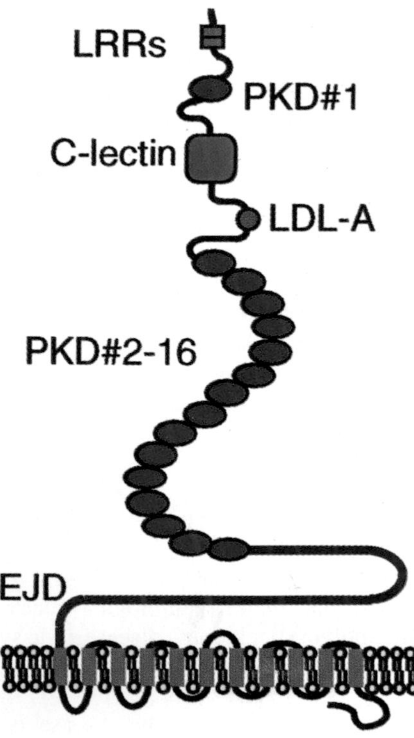

Figure 21–6

A schematic of human polycystin molecule, with various domains drawn approximately to scale. The long extracellular region consists primarily of the following domains: two leucine-rich repeats (LRRs); a C type lectin domain; a low-density lipoprotein (LDL-A) type module; 16 PKD repeats, each of which may assume an immunoglobulin-like fold; and an egg jelly type module (EJD). Eleven membrane-spanning segments are predicted, followed by a short cytoplasmic tail. (Courtesy of Dr. Amin Arnaout, Massachusetts General Hospital, Boston, MA.)

- The *PKD2* gene is on chromosome 4q13–23, and mutations in the gene are present in about 10% of families. The *PKD2* gene product, *polycystin 2,* is an integral membrane protein with homologies to certain calcium and sodium channel proteins as well as to a portion of polycystin 1.[14]
- A *PKD3* gene, responsible for a minority of cases, has yet to be mapped.

But how do defects in these proteins cause cyst formation, cyst expansion, and renal damage? Here speculations abound, since the normal function of the proteins is still unclear. Nevertheless, it is currently thought that the link may be in the role of the proteins in *cell-cell matrix interactions important in tubular epithelial cell growth and differentiation.*

It has long been known that epithelial cells lining cysts have a high proliferation rate, and that the nonproliferating cells in cysts exhibit abnormally simplified structure, with a relatively immature phenotype. Cysts are frequently detached from adjacent tubules and enlarge by active fluid *secretion* from the lining epithelial cells. In addition, the extracellular matrix (ECM) produced by cyst-lining cells is abnormal. These findings have led to the hypothetical scenario (Fig. 21–7) that cysts develop as a result of an abnormality in cell differentiation, associated with sustained cellular proliferation, transepithelial fluid secretion, remodeling of the ECM, and cyst formation.[12] In addition, cyst fluids have been shown to harbor mediators derived from epithelial cells that enhance fluid secretion and induce inflammation. This could potentially result in further enlargement of cysts and the interstitial fibrosis characteristic of progressive polycystic kidney disease.[15]

The distribution of polycystin 1 in developing renal tubules in fetal life and the structural homologies of some of its domains (see Fig. 21–6) are consistent with a role in the cell-cell and cell-matrix interactions critical to cell growth and differentiation. Indeed, targeted *PKD1* mutations in transgenic mice interfere with nephrogenesis and result in cyst formation.[16] Recent molecular analyses of *PKD* gene alleles in single cysts suggest that the *PKD1*

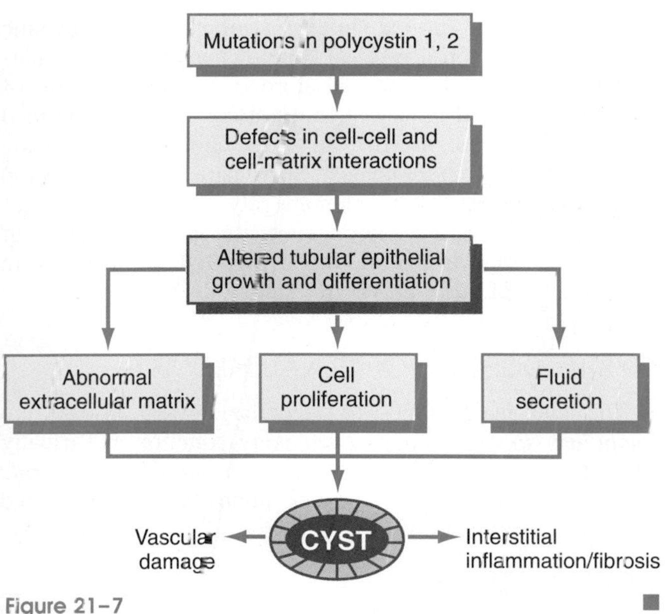

Figure 21–7

Possible mechanisms of cyst formation in polycystic kidney disease (see text).

gene serves a suppressor function—its loss leads to hyperplasia of epithelial cells.[17] Akin to tumor-suppressor genes (Chapter 8), a second somatic mutation is necessary for full expression of the defect. This intriguing speculation is thought to explain the variable phenotypic expression and focal nature of the initial cyst formation. There is also some evidence that normal *PKD1* and *PKD2* gene products interact (bind together) along some of their domains, thus influencing each other's function, probably accounting for the similar phenotype in the disease induced by two different genes.[18]

MORPHOLOGY. In gross appearance, the kidneys are usually bilaterally enlarged and may achieve enormous sizes; weights up to 4 kg for each kidney have been reported. The external surface appears to be composed solely of a mass of cysts, up to 3 to 4 cm in diameter, with no intervening parenchyma (Fig. 21–8). However, microscopic examination reveals functioning nephrons dispersed between the cysts. The cysts may be filled with a clear serous fluid or, more usually, with turbid, red to brown, sometimes hemorrhagic fluid. As these cysts enlarge, they may encroach on the calyces and pelvis to produce pressure defects. The cysts arise from the tubules throughout the nephron and therefore have variable lining epithelia. On occasion, papillary epithelial formations and polyps project into the lumen. Bowman capsules are occasionally involved in cyst formation, and glomerular tufts may be seen within the cystic space.

Clinical Features. Many of these patients remain asymptomatic until indications of renal insufficiency announce the presence of the underlying kidney disease. In others, hemorrhage or progressive dilation of cysts may produce pain. Excretion of blood clots causes renal colic. The larger masses usually apparent on abdominal palpation may induce a dragging sensation. The disease occasionally begins with the insidious onset of hematuria, followed by

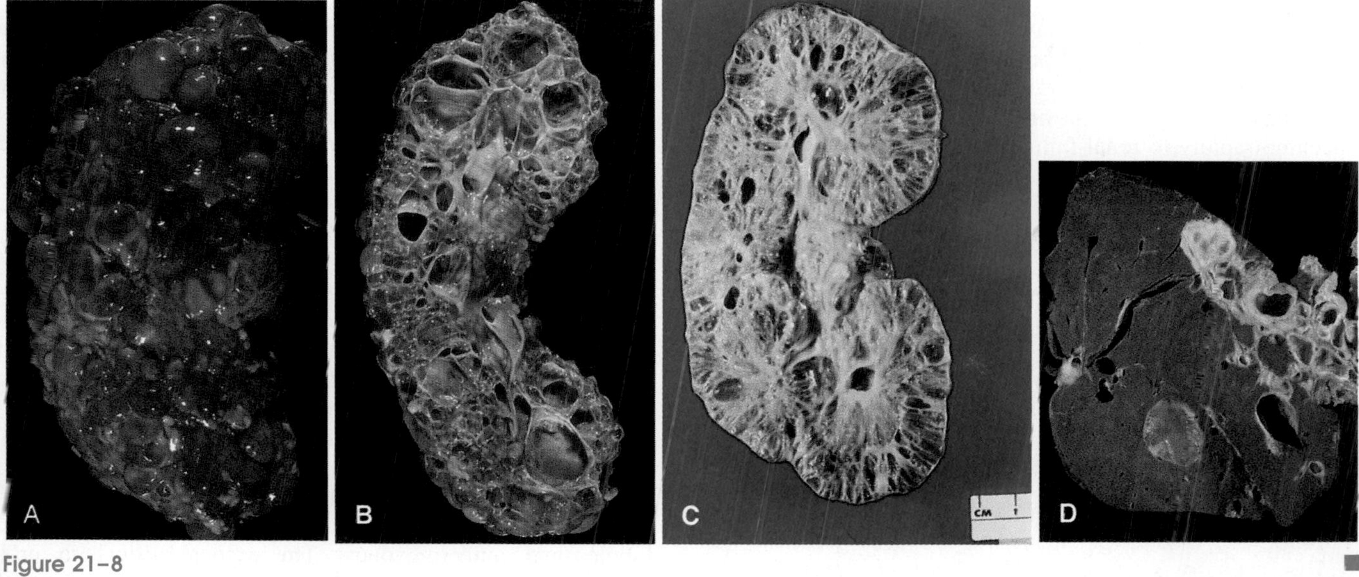

Figure 21–8

A and *B*, Autosomal dominant adult polycystic kidney, viewed from external surface and bisected. The kidney is markedly enlarged with numerous dilated cysts. *C*, Autosomal recessive childhood polycystic kidney disease, showing smaller cysts and dilated channels at right angles to the cortical surface. *D*, Liver with cysts in adult PKD.

other features of progressive chronic renal disease, such as proteinuria (rarely more than 2 gm/day), polyuria, and hypertension. Families with *PKD2* genotype tend to have an older age at onset and later development of renal failure. Progression is accelerated in blacks (largely correlated with sickle cell trait), in males compared with females, and in the presence of hypertension.

Patients with polycystic kidney disease also tend to have extrarenal congenital anomalies[19]: *about 40% have one to several cysts in the liver (polycystic liver disease) that are usually asymptomatic.* The cysts are derived from biliary epithelium. Cysts occur much less frequently in the spleen, pancreas, and lungs. *Intracranial berry aneurysms, presumably from altered expression of polycystin in vascular smooth muscle, arise in the circle of Willis,* and subarachnoid hemorrhages from these[20] account for death in about 4% to 10% of patients with polycystic kidney disease. *Mitral valve prolapse* and other valvular anomalies occur in 20% to 25% of patients, but most are asymptomatic. The clinical diagnosis is made by radiologic imaging techniques. Computed tomographic scanning is highly sensitive and can detect cysts a few millimeters in diameter. Ultrasound examination is the least invasive and can confirm the diagnosis.

This form of chronic renal failure is remarkable in that patients may survive for many years with azotemia slowly progressing to uremia. Dialysis prolongs life further. Ultimately, about 40% of adult patients die of coronary or hypertensive heart disease, 25% of infection, 15% of a ruptured berry aneurysm or hypertensive intracerebral hemorrhage, and the rest of other causes.

AUTOSOMAL RECESSIVE (CHILDHOOD) POLYCYSTIC KIDNEY DISEASE

This rare developmental anomaly is genetically distinct from adult polycystic kidney disease, having an *autosomal recessive* type of inheritance. *Perinatal, neonatal, infantile,* and *juvenile* subcategories have been defined, depending on time of presentation and presence of associated hepatic lesions. The first two are most common; serious manifestations are usually present at birth, and the young infant may succumb rapidly to renal failure.

MORPHOLOGY. Kidneys are enlarged and have a smooth external appearance. On cut section, numerous small cysts in the cortex and medulla give the kidney a spongelike appearance. Dilated elongated channels are present at right angles to the cortical surface, completely replacing the medulla and cortex (Fig. 21–8*C*). On microscopic examination, there is saccular or, more commonly, cylindrical dilation of all collecting tubules. The cysts have a uniform lining of cuboidal cells, reflecting their origin from the collecting tubules. The disease is invariably bilateral. **In almost all cases, there are multiple epithelium-lined cysts in the liver** (Fig. 21–8*D*) **as well as proliferation of portal bile ducts.**

Patients who survive infancy (infantile and juvenile form) may develop a peculiar type of hepatic fibrosis characterized by bland periportal fibrosis and proliferation of well-differentiated biliary ductules, a condition now termed *congenital hepatic fibrosis.* In older children, the hepatic picture in fact predominates. Such patients may develop portal hypertension with splenomegaly. Curiously, congenital hepatic fibrosis sometimes occurs in the absence of polycystic kidneys and has been reported occasionally in the presence of adult polycystic kidney disease.

CYSTIC DISEASES OF RENAL MEDULLA

The two major types of medullary cystic disease are *medullary sponge kidney,* a relatively common and usually innocuous structural change, and *nephronophthisis–uremic medullary cystic disease complex,* almost always associated with renal dysfunction.

Medullary Sponge Kidney

The term medullary sponge kidney should be restricted to lesions consisting of multiple cystic dilations of the collecting ducts in the medulla. The condition occurs in adults and is usually discovered radiographically, either as an incidental finding or sometimes in relation to secondary complications. The latter include calcifications within the dilated ducts, hematuria, infection, and urinary calculi. Renal function is usually normal. On gross inspection, the papillary ducts in the medulla are dilated, and small cysts may be present. The cysts are lined by cuboidal epithelium or occasionally by transitional epithelium. Unless there is superimposed pyelonephritis, cortical scarring is absent. The pathogenesis is unknown.

Nephronophthisis–Uremic Medullary Cystic Disease Complex

This is a group of progressive renal disorders that usually have their onset in childhood. The common characteristic is the presence of a variable number of *cysts in the medulla associated with significant cortical tubular atrophy and interstitial fibrosis.* Although the presence of medullary cysts is important, the *cortical tubulointerstitial damage is the cause of the eventual renal insufficiency,* and some prefer the term *hereditary tubulointerstitial nephritis for this group.*[10] Four variants are recognized: (1) *sporadic, nonfamilial* (20%); (2) *familial juvenile nephronophthisis,* (FJN), inherited as an autosomal recessive disease; (3) *renal-retinal dysplasia* (15%), recessively inherited and associated with retinitis pigmentosa; and (4) *adult-onset medullary cystic disease,* dominantly inherited (15%). As a group, this complex accounts for about 20% of cases of chronic renal failure in children and adolescents.

Affected children present first with polyuria and polydipsia, which reflect a marked tubular defect in concentrating ability. Sodium wasting and tubular acidosis are also prominent, findings consistent with initial injury to the distal tubules and collecting ducts. The expected course is progression to terminal renal failure during a period of 5 to 10 years.

Pathogenesis. The gene for many of the FJN pedigrees, on 2q13, encodes a protein with an SH3 domain, probably

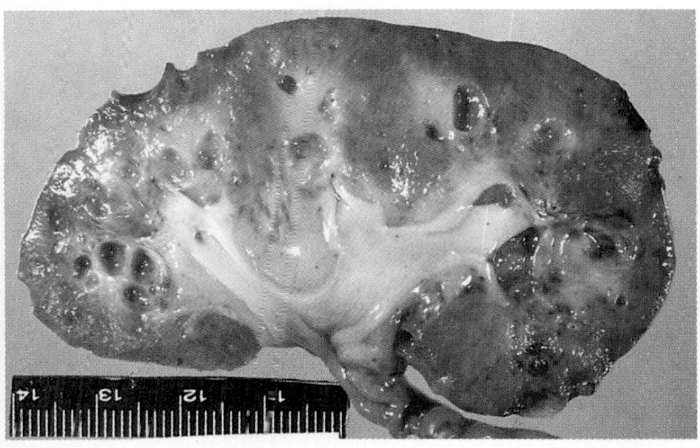

Figure 21–9

Uremic medullary cystic disease. Cut section of kidney showing cysts at the corticomedullary junction and in the medulla.

involved in protein–protein interactions and intracellular signaling.[21]

MORPHOLOGY. In gross appearance, the kidneys are small, have contracted granular surfaces, and show cysts in the medulla, most prominently at the corticomedullary junction (Fig. 21–9). Small cysts are also seen in the cortices. The cysts are lined by flattened or cuboidal epithelium and are usually surrounded by either inflammatory cells or fibrous tissue. In the cortex, there is widespread atrophy and thickening of the basement membranes of proximal and distal tubules together with interstitial fibrosis. Some glomeruli may be hyalinized, but in general, glomerular structure is preserved.

There are few specific clues to diagnosis, because the medullary cysts may be too small to be visualized radiographically. The disease should be strongly considered in children or adolescents with otherwise unexplained chronic renal failure, a positive family history, and chronic tubulointerstitial nephritis on biopsy.

ACQUIRED (DIALYSIS-ASSOCIATED) CYSTIC DISEASE

The kidneys from patients with end-stage renal disease who have undergone prolonged dialysis sometimes exhibit numerous cortical and medullary cysts. The cysts measure 0.5 to 2 cm in diameter, contain clear fluid, are lined by either hyperplastic or flattened tubular epithelium, and often contain calcium oxalate crystals. They probably form as a result of obstruction of tubules by interstitial fibrosis or by oxalate crystals.

Most are asymptomatic, but sometimes the cysts bleed, causing hematuria. The most ominous complication is the development of renal cell carcinoma in the walls of these cysts, occurring in 7% of dialyzed patients observed for 10 years.

Table 21–2. SUMMARY OF RENAL CYSTIC DISEASES

	Inheritance	Pathologic Features	Clinical Features or Complications	Typical Outcome	Diagrammatic Representation
Adult polycystic kidney disease	Autosomal dominant	Large multicystic kidneys, liver cysts, berry aneurysms	Hematuria, flank pain, urinary tract infection, renal stones, hypertension	Chronic renal failure beginning at age 40–60 yr	
Childhood polycystic kidney disease	Autosomal recessive	Enlarged, cystic kidneys at birth	Hepatic fibrosis	Variable, death in infancy or childhood	
Medullary sponge kidney	None	Medullary cysts on excretory urography	Hematuria, urinary tract infection, recurrent renal stones	Benign	
Familial juvenile nephronophthisis	Autosomal recessive	Corticomedullary cysts, shrunken kidneys	Salt wasting, polyuria, growth retardation, anemia	Progressive renal failure beginning in childhood	
Adult-onset medullary cystic disease	Autosomal dominant	Corticomedullary cysts, shrunken kidneys	Salt wasting, polyuria	Chronic renal failure beginning in adulthood	
Simple cysts	None	Single or multiple cysts in normal-sized kidneys	Microscopic hematuria	Benign	
Acquired renal cystic disease	None	Cystic degeneration in end-stage kidney disease	Hemorrhage, erythrocytosis, neoplasia	Dependence on dialysis	

SIMPLE CYSTS

These occur as multiple or single, usually cortical cystic spaces that vary in diameter over wide limits. They are commonly 1 to 5 cm but may reach 10 cm or more in size. They are translucent, lined by a gray, glistening, smooth membrane, and filled with clear fluid. On microscopic examination, these membranes are composed of a single layer of cuboidal or flattened cuboidal epithelium, which in many instances may be completely atrophic.

Simple cysts are common postmortem findings without clinical significance. On occasion, hemorrhage into them may cause sudden distention and pain, and calcification of the hemorrhage may give rise to bizarre radiographic shadows. The main importance of cysts lies in their differentiation from kidney tumors, when they are discovered either incidentally or because of hemorrhage and pain during life. Radiologic studies show that in contrast to renal tumors, renal cysts have smooth contours, are almost always avascular, and give fluid rather than solid signals on ultrasonography.

Table 21–2 summarizes the characteristic features of the principal renal cystic diseases.

Table 21–3. GLOMERULAR DISEASES

Primary Glomerulopathies
Acute diffuse proliferative glomerulonephritis
Poststreptococcal
Non-poststreptococcal
Rapidly progressive (crescentic) glomerulonephritis
Membranous glomerulopathy
Lipoid nephrosis (minimal change disease)
Focal segmental glomerulosclerosis
Membranoproliferative glomerulonephritis
IgA nephropathy
Focal proliferative glomerulonephritis
Chronic glomerulonephritis

Systemic Diseases
Systemic lupus erythematosus
Diabetes mellitus
Amyloidosis
Goodpasture syndrome
Polyarteritis nodosa
Wegener granulomatosis
Henoch-Schönlein purpura
Bacterial endocarditis

Hereditary Disorders
Alport syndrome
Thin membrane disease
Fabry disease

GLOMERULAR DISEASES

Glomerular diseases constitute some of the major problems in nephrology; indeed, chronic glomerulonephritis is one of the most common causes of chronic renal failure in humans. Glomeruli may be injured by a variety of factors and in the course of a number of systemic diseases. Immunologic diseases such as systemic lupus erythematosus (SLE), vascular disorders such as hypertension and polyarteritis nodosa, metabolic diseases such as diabetes mellitus, and some purely hereditary conditions such as Fabry disease often affect the glomerulus. These are termed *secondary glomerular diseases* to differentiate them from those in which the kidney is the only or predominant organ involved. The latter constitute the various types of *primary glomerulonephritis* or, because some do not have a cellular inflammatory component, *glomerulopathy. However, both the clinical manifestations and glomerular histologic changes in primary and secondary forms can be similar.*

Here we discuss the various types of primary glomerulonephritis and briefly review the secondary forms covered in other parts of this book.

Table 21–3 lists the most common forms of glomerulonephritis that have reasonably well defined morphologic and clinical characteristics. In reviewing the specific types of glomerulonephritis, it is useful to consider each in terms of (1) clinical presentation, (2) the morphology of the glomerular lesion, and (3) the cause and pathogenesis.

Clinical Manifestations

The clinical manifestations of glomerular disease are clustered into the five major glomerular syndromes described earlier and summarized in Table 21–4. Both the primary glomerulonephritides and the systemic diseases affecting the glomerulus can result in these syndromes. Thus, a critical point in the clinical differential diagnosis is first to exclude the major systemic disorders, of which the major four are *diabetes mellitus, SLE, vasculitis,* and *amyloidosis.*

Histologic Alterations

Various types of glomerulonephritis are characterized by one or more of four basic tissue reactions.

Hypercellularity. So-called *inflammatory diseases* of the glomerulus are associated with an increase in the number of cells in the glomerular tufts. This hypercellularity is associated with one or combinations of three of the following:

Table 21–4. THE GLOMERULAR SYNDROMES

Syndrome	Features
Acute nephritic syndrome	■ Hematuria, azotemia, variable proteinuria, oliguria, edema, and hypertension
Rapidly progressive glomerulonephritis	■ Acute nephritis, proteinuria, and acute renal failure
Nephrotic syndrome	■ >3.5 gm proteinuria, hypoalbuminemia, hyperlipidemia, lipiduria
Chronic renal failure	■ Azotemia → uremia progressing for years
Asymptomatic hematuria or proteinuria	■ Glomerular hematuria; subnephrotic proteinuria

- *Cellular proliferation* of mesangial, endothelial, or, in certain cases, parietal epithelial cells
- *Leukocytic infiltration,* consisting of neutrophils, monocytes, and, in some diseases, lymphocytes
- *Formation of crescents.* These are accumulations of cells composed of proliferating epithelial cells and infiltrating leukocytes.

Basement Membrane Thickening. By light microscopy, this change appears as thickening of the capillary walls, best seen in sections stained with periodic acid–Schiff (PAS). On electron microscopy, such thickening can be resolved as either (1) thickening of the basement membrane proper, as occurs in diabetic glomerulosclerosis, or more commonly (2) deposition of amorphous electron-dense material representing precipitated proteins on the endothelial or epithelial side of the basement membrane or within the GBM itself. *The most common type of thickening is due to extensive subepithelial deposition, as occurs in membranous glomerulonephritis,* discussed later. In most instances, the material is thought to be immune complexes, although fibrin, amyloid, cryoglobulins, and abnormal fibrillary proteins may also deposit in the GBM.

Hyalinization and Sclerosis. Hyalinization or hyalinosis, as applied to the glomerulus, denotes the accumulation of material that is homogeneous and eosinophilic by light microscopy. By electron microscopy, the hyalin is extracellular and consists of amorphous substance, made up of precipitated plasma protein as well as increased amounts of basement membrane or mesangial matrix. This change results in obliteration of structural detail of the glomerular tuft (sclerosis) and usually denotes the end result of various forms of glomerular damage.

Additional alterations include *intraglomerular thrombosis, fibrin deposition,* or *accumulation of lipid* and other metabolic materials. Because many of the primary glomerulonephritides are of unknown cause, they are often classified by their histology, as can be seen in Table 21–3. The histologic changes can be further subdivided into *diffuse,* involving all glomeruli; *global,* involving the entire glomerulus; *focal,* involving only a certain proportion of the glomeruli; *segmental,* affecting a part of each glomerulus; and *mesangial,* affecting predominantly the mesangial region. These terms are sometimes appended to the histologic classifications.

Pathogenesis of Glomerular Injury

Although we know little of etiologic agents or triggering events, it is clear that immune mechanisms underlie most cases of primary glomerulonephritis and many of the secondary glomerular involvements[22, 23] (Table 21–5). Glomerulonephritis can be readily induced experimentally by antigen-antibody reactions, and glomerular deposits of immunoglobulins, often with various components of complement, are found in more than 70% of patients with glomerulonephritis. Cell-mediated immune reactions also clearly play a role, usually in concert with antibody-mediated events. We therefore begin this discussion with a review of antibody-instigated injury.

Table 21–5. IMMUNE MECHANISMS OF GLOMERULAR INJURY

Antibody-Mediated Injury
- **In situ immune complex deposition**
  - Fixed intrinsic tissue antigens
    - Goodpasture antigen (anti-GBM nephritis)
    - Heymann antigen (membranous glomerulonephritis)
    - Mesangial antigens
    - Others
  - Planted antigens
    - Exogenous (infectious agents, drugs)
    - Endogenous (DNA, immunoglobulins, immune complexes, IgA)
- **Circulating immune complex deposition**
  - Endogenous antigens (e.g., DNA, tumor antigens)
  - Exogenous antigens (e.g., infectious products)
- **Cytotoxic antibodies**

Cell-Mediated Immune Injury

Activation of Alternative Complement Pathway

Two forms of antibody-associated injury have been established: (1) injury by *antibodies reacting in situ within the glomerulus, either with insoluble fixed (intrinsic) glomerular antigens or with molecules planted within the glomerulus,* and (2) injury resulting from deposition of *soluble circulating antigen-antibody complexes* in the glomerulus. In addition, there is experimental evidence that *cytotoxic antibodies* directed against glomerular cell components may cause glomerular injury. These pathways are not mutually exclusive, and in humans all may contribute to injury.

IN SITU IMMUNE COMPLEX DEPOSITION

In this form of injury, antibodies react directly with intrinsic tissue antigen, or antigens "planted" in the glomerulus from the circulation. There are two well-established experimental models for anti-tissue–mediated glomerular injury, for which there are counterparts in human disease: anti–glomerular basement membrane (anti-GBM) and Heymann nephritis.

Anti-GBM Nephritis

In this type of injury, *antibodies are directed against intrinsic fixed antigens that are normal components of the GBM proper.* It has its experimental counterpart in so-called Masugi or nephrotoxic nephritis, produced in rats by injections of anti–rat kidney antibodies prepared in rabbits by immunization with rat kidney tissue. The injected antibodies bind along the entire length of the GBM, *resulting in a homogeneous, diffuse linear pattern of staining for the antibodies by immunofluorescent techniques* (Fig. 21–10*B* and *E*). This is contrasted with the granular lumpy pattern seen in other in situ models or after deposition of circulating immune complexes.

In the Masugi model, the deposited immunoglobulin of the rabbit is foreign to the host and thus acts as an antigen eliciting antibodies in the rat. This rat antibody then reacts

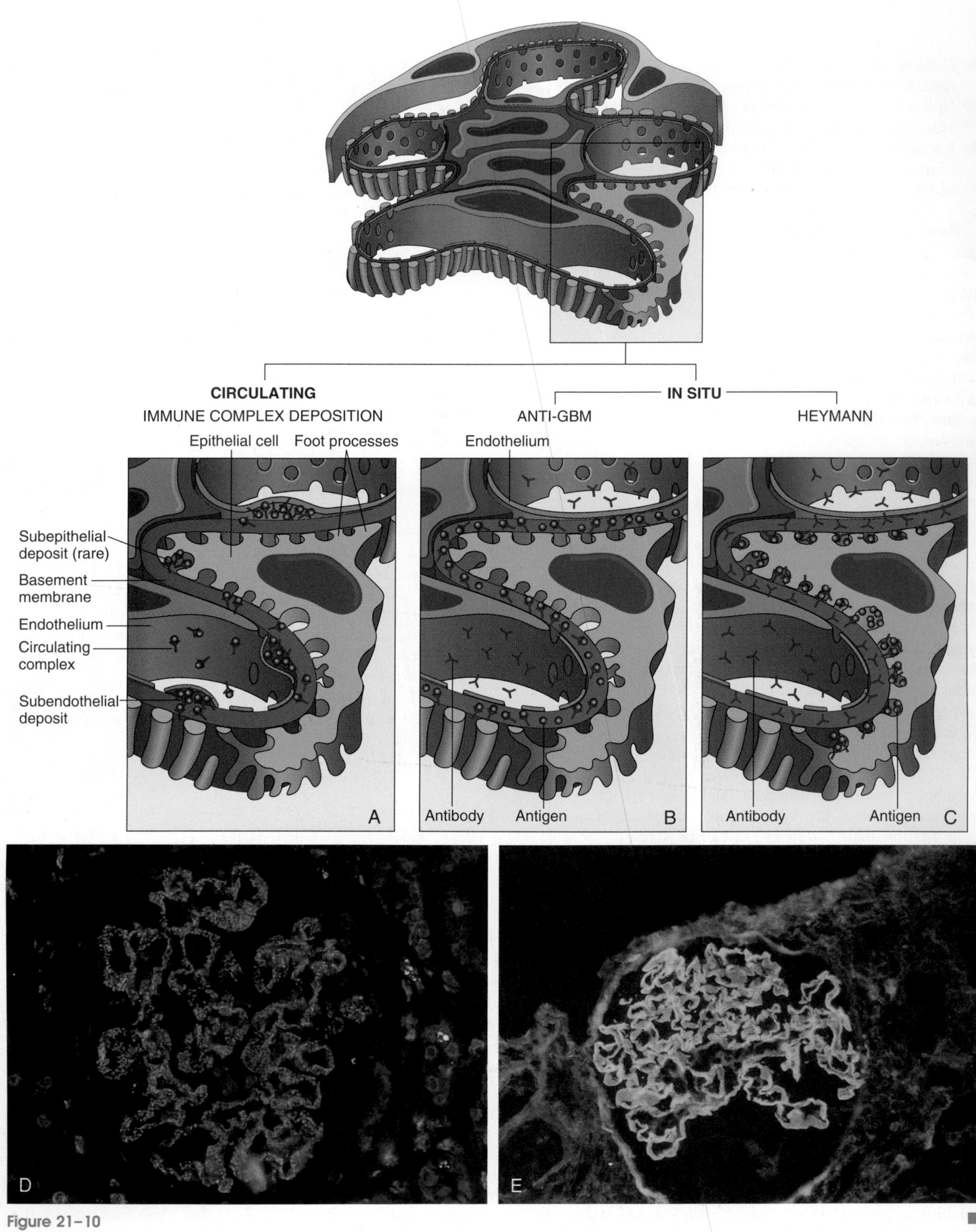

Figure 21–10

Antibody-mediated glomerular injury can result either from the deposition of circulating immune complexes (*A*) or more commonly from in situ formation of complexes exemplified by anti-GBM disease (*B*) or Heymann nephritis (*C*). *D* and *E*, Two patterns of deposition of immune complexes as seen by immunofluorescence microscopy: *D*, granular, characteristic of circulating and in situ immune complex nephritis; *E*, linear, characteristic of classic anti-GBM disease.

with the rabbit immunoglobulin within the basement membrane, leading to further glomerular injury. This is referred to as the *autologous phase* of nephrotoxic nephritis, to distinguish it from the initial *heterologous phase* caused by the anti-GBM antibody. Often the anti-GBM antibodies cross-react with other basement membranes, especially those in the lung alveoli, resulting in simultaneous lung and kidney lesions *(Goodpasture syndrome). The GBM antigen responsible for classic anti-GBM nephritis and Goodpasture syndrome is a component of the noncollagenous domain (NC1) of the α_3 chain of collagen type IV, which, as discussed earlier (see Fig. 21–3), is critical for maintenance of GBM superstructure.*[3] Anti-GBM nephritis accounts for less than 5% of cases of human glomerulonephritis. It is solidly established as the cause of injury in Goodpasture syndrome, discussed later. Most instances of anti-GBM nephritis are characterized by severe glomerular damage and the development of rapidly progressive renal failure.

Heymann Nephritis

The Heymann model of rat glomerulonephritis is induced by immunizing animals with an antigen originally made up of preparations of proximal tubular brush border (Fig. 21–10*C*). The rats develop antibodies to this antigen, and a membranous glomerulonephritis, resembling human membranous glomerulonephritis, develops (discussed later; see also Fig. 21–19). On electron microscopy, the nephritis is characterized by the presence of numerous electron-dense deposits (made up largely of immune reactants) along the *subepithelial aspect* of the basement membrane. The pattern of immune deposition by fluorescence microscopy is *granular* and *interrupted,* rather than linear (Fig. 21–10). It is now clear that this type of nephritis results largely from the reaction of antibody with an antigen complex located on the basal surface of visceral epithelial cells and cross-reacting with the brush border antigen used in the original experiments. This so-called Heymann antigen is a large 330-kD protein called *megalin,* having homology to the low-density lipoprotein receptor (Chapter 6), complexed to a smaller 44-kD protein, called *receptor-associated protein* (RAP). Antibody binding to cell membrane is followed by complement activation and then by patching, capping, and subsequent shedding of the immune aggregates from the cell surface to form the characteristic subepithelial deposits (Fig. 21–10*C*). Heymann nephritis most closely resembles human membranous glomerulonephritis, in which the epithelial cell antigen appears to be a homolog of the megalin complex.

It must be apparent that, in humans, anti-GBM disease and membranous glomerulonephritis are autoimmune diseases, caused by antibodies to endogenous tissue components. What triggers these autoantibodies is unclear, but any one of the several mechanisms responsible for autoimmunity, discussed in Chapter 7, may be involved. Several forms of autoimmune glomerulonephritis can be experimentally induced by drugs (e.g., mercuric chloride), infectious products (endotoxin), and the graft-versus-host reaction (Chapter 7). In such models, there is an induced alteration of immune regulation associated with *polyclonal B-cell activation* and the induction of an array of autoantibodies that react with renal antigens.

Antibodies Against Planted Antigens

Antibodies can react in situ with previously "planted" nonglomerular antigens. Such antigens may localize in the kidney by interacting with various intrinsic components of the glomerulus. There is increasing experimental support for such a mechanism. Planted antigens include cationic molecules that bind to glomerular capillary anionic sites; DNA, which has an affinity for GBM components; bacterial products; large aggregated proteins (e.g., aggregated immunoglobulin [Ig] G), which deposit in the mesangium because of their size; and immune complexes themselves, since they continue to have reactive sites for further interactions with free antibody, free antigen, or complement. There is no dearth of other possible planted antigens, including viral, bacterial, and parasitic products and drugs. Most of these planted antigens induce a granular or heterogeneous pattern of immunoglobulin deposition by fluorescence microscopy, the pattern found also in circulating immune complex nephritis, discussed next.

CIRCULATING IMMUNE COMPLEX NEPHRITIS

In this type of nephritis, glomerular injury is caused by the trapping of circulating antigen-antibody complexes within glomeruli. The antibodies have no immunologic specificity for glomerular constituents, and the complexes localize within the glomeruli because of their physicochemical properties and the hemodynamic factors peculiar to the glomerulus (Fig. 21–10*A*).

The pathogenesis of immune complex diseases (type III hypersensitivity reactions) is discussed in Chapter 7. Here we briefly review the salient features that relate to glomerular injury.

The evocative antigens may be of endogenous origin, as in the case of the glomerulopathy associated with SLE, or they may be exogenous, as is likely in the glomerulonephritis that follows certain infections. Antigens implicated include bacterial products (streptococci), the surface antigen of hepatitis B virus (HBsAg), hepatitis C virus antigen or RNA, various tumor antigens, *Treponema pallidum, Plasmodium falciparum,* and several viruses. The inciting antigen is frequently unknown.

Whatever the antigen may be, antigen-antibody complexes are formed in the circulation and then trapped in the glomeruli, where they produce injury, in large part through the binding of complement. The glomerular lesions usually consist of leukocytic infiltration in glomeruli and proliferation of mesangial and endothelial cells. Electron microscopy reveals the immune complexes as electron-dense deposits or clumps that lie *in the mesangium,* or between the endothelial cells and the GBM *(subendothelial deposits),* or rarely between the outer surface of the GBM and the podocytes *(subepithelial deposits).* Deposits may be located at more than one site in a given case. By immunofluorescence microscopy, *the immune complexes are seen as granular deposits either along the basement membrane or in the mesangium, or in both locations.* Once deposited in the kidney, immune complexes may eventually be degraded, mostly by phagocytic infiltrating monocytes and by mesangial cells, and the inflammatory changes may then subside. Such a course occurs when the exposure to the inciting antigen is short-lived and limited, as in most cases of poststreptococcal glomerulonephritis. However, if a continuous shower of antigens is provided, as may be seen in SLE or viral hepatitis B and C, repeated cycles of immune complex formation, deposition, and injury may occur, leading to a more chronic membranoproliferative type of glomerulonephritis.

Several factors affect glomerular localization of antigen, antibody, or complexes. The molecular charge and size of these reactants are clearly important. Highly cationic immunogens tend to cross the GBM, and the resultant complexes eventually achieve a subepithelial location. Highly anionic macromolecules are excluded from the GBM and either are trapped subendothelially or may, in fact, not be nephritogenic at all. Molecules with more neutral charge and their complexes tend to accumulate in the mesangium. Large circulating complexes are not usually nephritogenic because they are cleared by the mononuclear-phagocyte system and do not enter the GBM in sufficient quantities. The pattern of localization is also affected by changes in glomerular hemodynamics, mesangial function, and integrity of the charge-selective barrier in the glomerulus. These influences may underlie the variable pattern of immune reactant deposition and histologic change in various forms of glomerulonephritis, as shown in Figure 21–11.

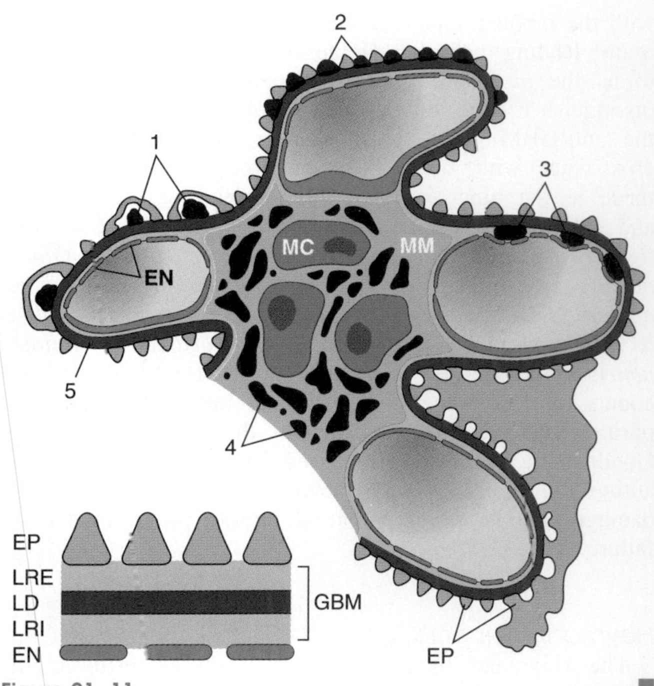

Figure 21–11

Localization of immune complexes in the glomerulus: (1) subepithelial humps, as in acute glomerulonephritis; (2) epimembranous deposits, as in membranous and Heymann glomerulonephritis; (3) subendothelial deposits, as in systemic lupus erythematosus and membranoproliferative glomerulonephritis; (4) mesangial deposits, as in IgA nephropathy; (5) basement membrane. LRE, lamina rara externa; LRI, lamina rara interna; LD, lamina densa; EP, epithelium; EN, endothelium; MC, mesangial cell; MM, mesangial matrix. (Modified from Couser WG: Mediation of immune glomerular injury. J Am Soc Nephrol 1:13, 1990.)

ANTIBODIES TO GLOMERULAR CELLS

In addition to causing immune deposits, antibodies directed to glomerular cell antigens may react with cellular components and cause injury by cytotoxic or other mechanisms. Antibodies to mesangial cell antigens, for example, cause mesangiolysis followed by mesangial cell proliferation; antibodies to endothelial cell antigens cause endothelial injury and intravascular thrombosis; and antibodies to certain visceral epithelial cell glycoproteins cause proteinuria in experimental animals. This mechanism may well play a role in certain human immune disorders not associated with demonstrable immune deposits.

To conclude the discussion of antibody-mediated injury, it must be stated that in the largest proportion of cases of human glomerulonephritis, the pattern of immune deposition is granular and along the basement membrane or in the mesangium. However, it may be difficult to determine whether the deposition has occurred in situ or by circulating complexes, or by both mechanisms—because, as discussed earlier, immune complex trapping can initiate in situ formation. Single etiologic agents, such as hepatitis B and C viruses, can cause either a membranous pattern of glomerulonephritis, suggesting in situ deposition, or a membranoproliferative pattern, more indicative of circulating complexes. It is best then to consider that *antigen-antibody deposition in the glomerulus is a major pathway of glomerular injury and that in situ immune reactions, trapping of circulating complexes, interactions between these two events, and local hemodynamic and structural determinants in the glomerulus all contribute to the diverse morphologic and functional alterations in glomerulonephritis.*

CELL-MEDIATED IMMUNITY IN GLOMERULONEPHRITIS

Although antibody-mediated mechanisms may initiate many forms of glomerulonephritis, there is now considerable evidence that sensitized nephritogenic T cells, as a reflection of cell-mediated immune reactions, cause some forms of glomerular injury and are involved in the progression of many glomerulonephritides.[25] Clues to its occurrence include the presence of activated macrophages and T cells and their products in the glomerulus in some forms of human and experimental glomerulonephritis; in vitro and in vivo evidence of lymphocyte activation on exposure to antigen in human and experimental glomerulonephritis; abrogation of glomerular injury by lymphocyte depletion; and successful attempts in which glomerular histologic alterations are transferred by T cells in experimental glomerulonephritis. The evidence is most compelling for certain types of experimental crescentic glomerulonephritis in which antibodies to GBM may initiate or facilitate glomerular injury by subsets of activated lymphocytes.[26]

ACTIVATION OF ALTERNATIVE COMPLEMENT PATHWAY

Alternative complement pathway activation occurs in the clinicopathologic entity called *membranoproliferative glomerulonephritis (MPGN type II),* sometimes independently of immune complex deposition, and also in some forms of proliferative glomerulonephritis. This mechanism is discussed later in the discussion of MPGN.

EPITHELIAL CELL INJURY

This can be induced by antibodies to visceral epithelial cell antigens; by toxins, as in an experimental model of proteinuria induced by puromycin aminonucleoside; conceivably by certain cytokines; or by still poorly characterized factors, as in the case of human lipoid nephrosis and focal glomerulosclerosis, discussed later. Such injury is reflected by morphologic changes in the visceral epithelial cells, which include loss of foot processes, vacuolization, retraction, and detachment of cells from the GBM, and functionally by proteinuria. It is hypothesized that the detachment of visceral epithelial cells is caused by loss of adhesive interactions with the basement membrane and that this detachment leads to protein leakage (Fig. 21–12).

MEDIATORS OF GLOMERULAR INJURY

Once immune reactants or sensitized T cells have localized in the glomerulus, how does the glomerular damage ensue? The mediators—both cells and molecules—are the usual suspects involved in acute and chronic inflammation, described in Chapter 3, and only a few are highlighted[27, 28] (Fig. 21–13).

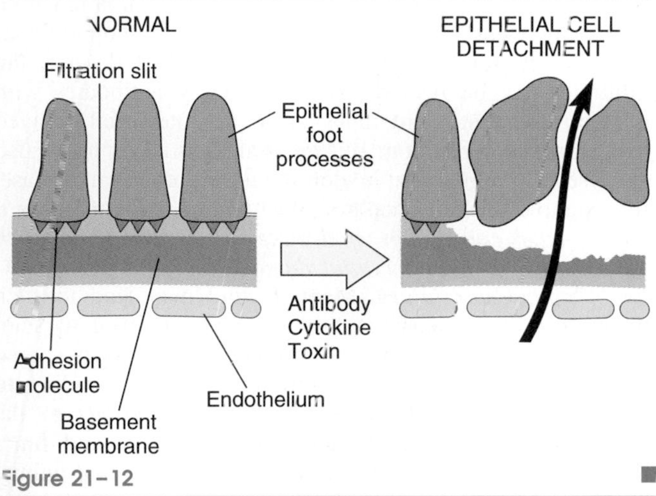

Figure 21–12

Epithelial cell injury. The postulated sequence is a consequence of antibodies against epithelial cell antigens, or toxins, or cytokines or other factors causing injury and detachment of epithelial cells, and protein leakage through defective GBM and filtration slits. (Adapted from Couser WG: Mediation of immune glomerular injury. Am Soc Nephrol 1:13, 1990.)

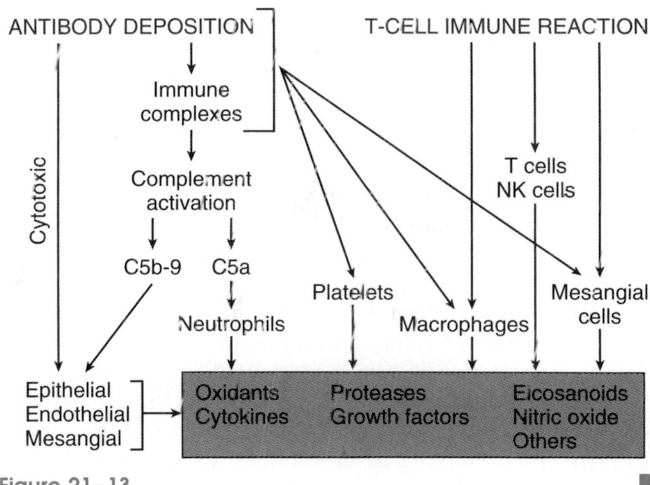

Figure 21–13

Mediators of immune glomerular injury including cells and soluble mediators (see text).

Cells

- *Neutrophils* infiltrate the glomerulus in certain types of glomerulonephritis, largely owing to activation of complement, resulting in generation of chemotactic agents (mainly C5a), but also by Fc-mediated immune adherence and by other mechanisms. Neutrophils release proteases, which cause GBM degradation; oxygen-derived free radicals, which cause cell damage; and arachidonic acid metabolites, which contribute to the reductions in GFR.
- *Macrophages, lymphocytes,* and *NK cells,* which infiltrate the glomerulus in antibody- and cell-mediated reactions, when activated release a vast number of biologically active molecules (described in Chapter 3).
- *Platelets* aggregate in the glomerulus during immune-mediated injury. Their release of eicosanoids and growth factors may contribute to the manifestations of glomerulonephritis. Antiplatelet agents have beneficial effects in both human and experimental glomerulonephritis.
- *Resident glomerular cells,* particularly mesangial cells, can be stimulated to produce several inflammatory mediators, including oxygen free radicals, cytokines, growth factors, eicosanoids, nitric oxide, and endothelin. In the absence of leukocytic infiltration, they may initiate inflammatory responses in the glomerulus.

Soluble Mediators

Virtually all the inflammatory chemical mediators have been implicated in glomerular injury.

- The *chemotactic complement components* induce leukocyte influx (complement-neutrophil–dependent injury) and C5b–C9, the lytic component. C5b–C9 causes cell lysis but in addition stimulates mesangial cells to produce oxidants, proteases, and other mediators. Thus, even in the absence of neutrophils, C5b–C9 can cause proteinuria, as has been postulated in membranous glomerulonephritis.

- *Eicosanoids, nitric oxide,* and *endothelin* are involved in the hemodynamic changes.
- *Cytokines,* particularly interleukin-1 and tumor necrosis factor, induce leukocyte adhesion and a variety of other effects.
- *Chemokines* such as monocyte chemoattractant protein 1 (MCP-1) and RANTES promote monocytes and lymphocyte influx. Of the *growth factors, platelet-derived growth factor* is involved in mesangial cell proliferation,[22] and *transforming growth factor (TGF)–β* appears to be critical in the ECM deposition and hyalinization leading to glomerulosclerosis in chronic injury.[29]
- The *coagulation system* is also a mediator of glomerular damage. Fibrin is frequently present in the glomeruli in glomerulonephritis, and fibrinogen may leak into Bowman space, serving as a stimulus to cell proliferation. Fibrin deposition is mediated largely by stimulation of macrophage procoagulant activity.

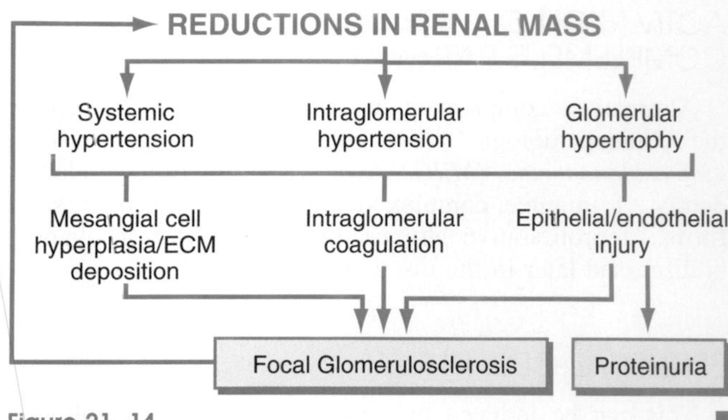

Figure 21–14

Renal ablation glomerulosclerosis. The adaptive changes in glomeruli (hypertrophy and glomerular capillary hypertension), as well as systemic hypertension, cause epithelial and endothelial injury and resultant proteinuria. The mesangial response, involving mesangial cell proliferation and extracellular matrix (ECM) production together with intraglomerular coagulation, causes the glomerulosclerosis. This results in further loss of functioning nephrons and a vicious circle of progressive glomerulosclerosis.

Mechanisms of Progression in Glomerular Diseases

Thus far we have discussed the immunologic mechanisms and mediators that *initiate* glomerular injury. The outcome of such injury depends on several factors, including the initial severity of renal damage, the nature and persistence of the antigens, the immune status of the host, and a variety of other factors.

But it has long been known that once any renal disease, glomerular or otherwise, destroys functioning nephrons and reduces the GFR to about 30% to 50% of normal, progression to end-stage renal failure proceeds at a relatively constant rate, independent of the original stimulus or activity of the underlying disease. The secondary factors that lead to progression are of great clinical interest since they can be targets of therapy that delays the inexorable journey to dialysis or transplantation.

The two major histologic characteristics of such progressive renal damage are *focal segmental glomerulosclerosis* and *tubulointerstitial inflammation and fibrosis,* and we discuss these separately.[30, 31]

Focal Segmental Glomerulosclerosis. Patients with this secondary change develop proteinuria, even if the primary disease was nonglomerular. The glomerulosclerosis appears to be initiated by the *adaptive change* that occurs in the relatively unaffected glomeruli of diseased kidneys.[32] Such a mechanism is suggested by experiments in rats subjected to ablation of renal mass by subtotal nephrectomy. *Compensatory hypertrophy* of the remaining glomeruli serves to maintain renal function in these animals, but proteinuria and glomerulosclerosis soon develop, leading eventually to total glomerular sclerosis and uremia. The glomerular hypertrophy is associated with *hemodynamic changes*, including increases in single-nephron GFR, blood flow, and transcapillary pressure (capillary hypertension), and often with systemic hypertension. The sequence of events (Fig. 21–14) thought to lead to sclerosis in this setting entails endothelial and epithelial cell injury, increased glomerular permeability to proteins, accumulation of proteins in the mesangial matrix, and fibrin deposition. This is followed by proliferation of mesangial cells, infiltration by leukocytes, increased deposition of ECM, and sclerosis of glomeruli. This results in further reductions in nephron mass and a vicious circle of continuing glomerulosclerosis. Most of the mediators of chronic inflammation and fibrosis, and particularly TGF-*β*, play a role in the induction of sclerosis. The role of this so-called *renal ablation glomerulosclerosis* in progression is supported by the protective effect of treatment with angiotensin-converting enzyme inhibitors, which reduces intraglomerular hypertension and actual progression in both animal and human studies.

Tubulointerstitial Damage. Tubulointerstitial injury, manifested by tubular damage and interstitial inflammation, is a component of many acute and chronic glomerulonephritides. In some instances, as in anti-GBM disease, the infiltrate may be related to cross-reacting antibodies with tubular basement membranes or to an interstitial delayed hypersensitivity reaction. But tubulointerstitial injury is also a cause of progression in nonimmune glomerular disease, for example, diabetic nephropathy. *Indeed, there is often a much better correlation of decline in renal function with the extent of tubulointerstitial damage than with the severity of glomerular injury.* Many factors may lead to such tubulointerstitial injury, including ischemia distal to sclerotic glomeruli, concomitant immune reactions to shared antigens, and phosphate or ammonia retention leading to interstitial fibrosis. However, current work points to the effects of *proteinuria* on tubular cell structure and function[30, 31] (Fig. 21–15). On the basis of in vitro and animal studies, proteinuria is thought to cause *direct injury to and activation of tubular cells*. Activated tubular cells in turn express adhesion molecules and elaborate proinflammatory cytokines and growth factors that contribute to interstitial fibrosis. Components of the filtered protein that produce these tubular effects include cytokines, complement prod-

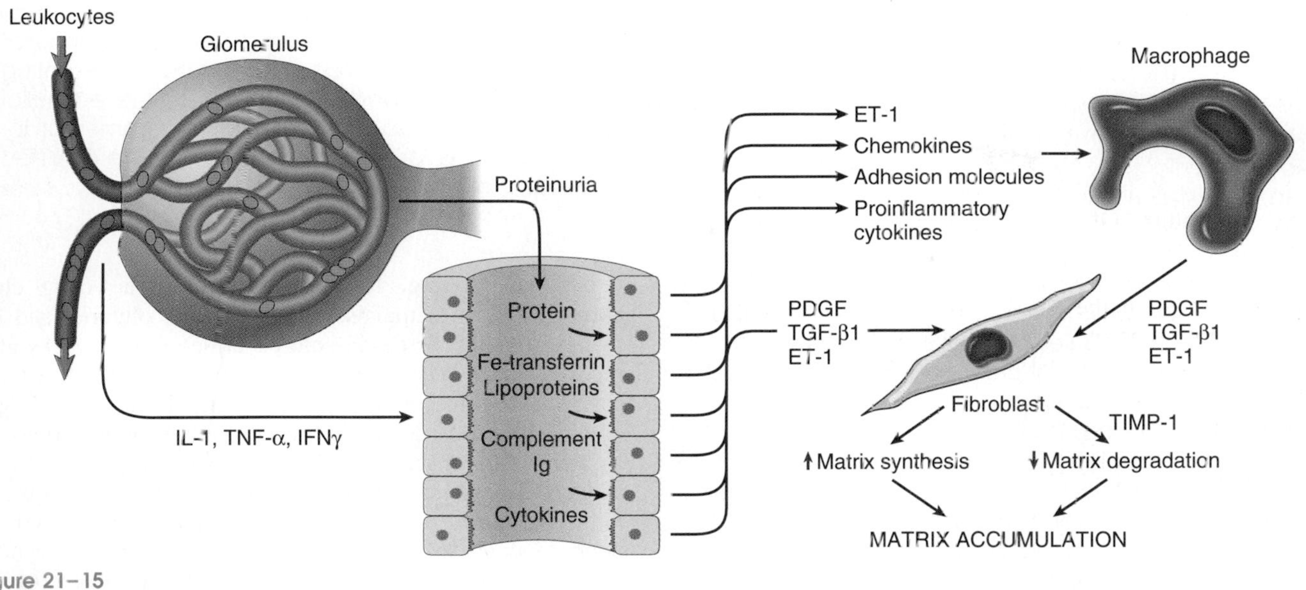

Figure 21–15

Mechanisms of chronic tubulointerstitial injury in glomerulonephritis (see text). Various components of the protein-rich filtrate and cytokines derived from leukocytes cause tubular cell activation and secretion of cytokines, growth factors, and other mediators. These, together with products of macrophages, incite interstitial inflammation and fibrosis. ET-1, endothelin-1; TIMP-1, tissue inhibitor of metalloproteinases. (Adapted and modified from references 30 and 31.)

ucts, the iron in transferrin, immunoglobulins, and lipid moieties.

Having discussed factors in the initiation and progression of glomerular injury, we now turn to a review of individual glomerular diseases.

Acute Glomerulonephritis

This group of glomerular diseases is *characterized anatomically by inflammatory alterations in the glomeruli and clinically by the syndrome of acute nephritis.* The nephritic patient usually presents with hematuria, red cell casts in the urine, azotemia, oliguria, and mild to moderate hypertension. The patient also commonly has proteinuria and edema, but these are not as severe as those encountered in the nephrotic syndrome, discussed later. The acute nephritic syndrome may occur in such multisystem diseases as SLE and polyarteritis nodosa. Typically, however, it is characteristic of acute proliferative glomerulonephritis and is an important component of crescentic glomerulonephritis, which is described later.

ACUTE PROLIFERATIVE (POSTSTREPTOCOCCAL, POSTINFECTIOUS) GLOMERULONEPHRITIS

As the name implies, this cluster of diseases is characterized histologically by diffuse proliferation of glomerular cells, associated with influx of leukocytes. These lesions are typically caused by immune complexes. The inciting antigen may be exogenous or endogenous. The prototype exogenous pattern is postinfectious glomerulonephritis, whereas that produced by an endogenous antigen is lupus erythematosus, described in Chapter 7. The most common infections are streptococcal, but the disorder has also been associated with other infections (see later).

Poststreptococcal Glomerulonephritis

This glomerular disease is decreasing in frequency in the United States but continues to be a fairly common disorder worldwide.[33] It usually appears 1 to 4 weeks after a streptococcal infection of the pharynx or skin (impetigo). It occurs most frequently in children 6 to 10 years of age, but adults of any age can be affected.

Etiology and Pathogenesis. Only certain strains of group A β-hemolytic streptococci are nephritogenic, more than 90% of cases being traced to types 12, 4, and 1, which can be identified by typing of M protein of the cell wall. Skin infections are commonly associated with overcrowding and poor hygiene.

Poststreptococcal glomerulonephritis is an immunologically mediated disease. The latent period between infection and onset of nephritis is compatible with the time required for the building up of antibodies. Elevated titers to one or more of the streptococcal products are present in a great majority of patients. Serum complement levels are low, compatible with involvement of the complement system. The presence of granular immune deposits in the glomeruli suggests an immune complex–mediated mechanism, and so does the finding of electron-dense deposits. The streptococcal antigenic component responsible for the immune reaction has eluded identification for years. A cytoplasmic antigen called *endostreptosin* and several *cationic antigens,* including a proteinase related to the streptococcal erythrogenic toxin, are present in affected glomeruli, but whether these represent planted antigens or part of circulating immune complexes, or both, is unknown. GBM and immunoglobulins altered by streptococcal enzymes have also been implicated as antigens at one time or another.

MORPHOLOGY. The classic diagnostic picture is one of enlarged, hypercellular glomeruli (Fig. 21–16). The hypercellularity is caused by (1) infiltration by leukocytes, both neutrophils and monocytes, and (2) proliferation of endothelial and mesangial cells and, in many cases, epithelial cells. The proliferation and leukocyte infiltration are diffuse, that is, involving all lobules of all glomeruli. There is also swelling of endothelial cells, and the combination of proliferation, swelling, and leukocyte infiltration obliterates the capillary lumens. Small deposits of fibrin within capillary lumens and mesangium can be demonstrated in most cases. There may be interstitial edema and inflammation, and the tubules often contain red cell casts.

By **immunofluorescence microscopy,** there are granular deposits of IgG, IgM, and C3 in the mesangium and along the basement membrane. Although universally present, they are often focal and sparse. The characteristic **electron microscopic findings** are the discrete, amorphous, electron-dense deposits on the epithelial side of the membrane, often having the appearance of "humps" (Fig. 21–16*B*), presumably representing the antigen-antibody complexes at the epithelial cell surface. Subendothelial and intramembranous deposits are also seen, and there is often swelling of endothelial and mesangial cells.

Clinical Course. In the classic case, a young child abruptly develops malaise, fever, nausea, oliguria, and hematuria (smoky or cocoa-colored urine) 1 to 2 weeks after recovery from a sore throat. The patients exhibit red cell casts in the urine, mild proteinuria (usually less than 1 gm/day), periorbital edema, and mild to moderate hypertension. In adults, the onset is more likely to be atypical, with the sudden appearance of hypertension or edema, frequently with elevation of BUN. During epidemics caused by nephritogenic streptococcal infections, glomerulonephritis may be asymptomatic, discovered only on screening for microscopic hematuria. Important laboratory findings include elevations of antistreptococcal antibody titers (anticationic proteinase and anti–DNase B), a decline in the serum concentration of C3, and the presence of cryoglobulins in the serum.

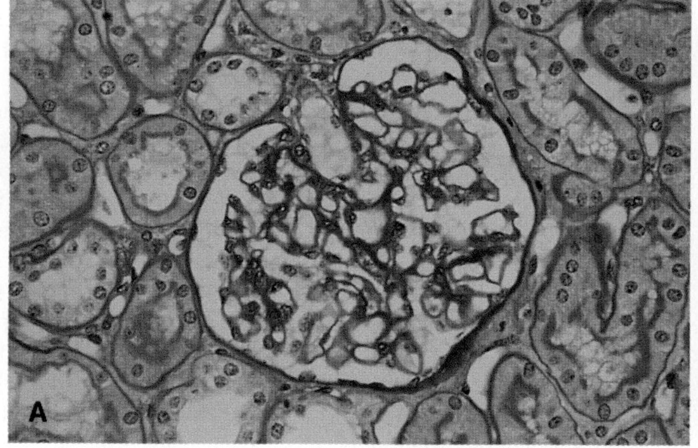

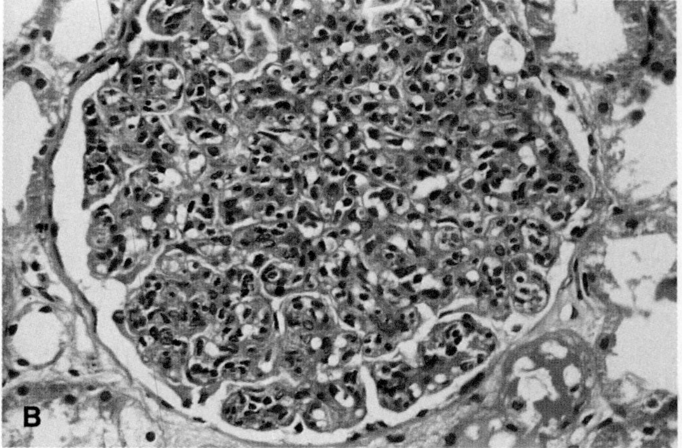

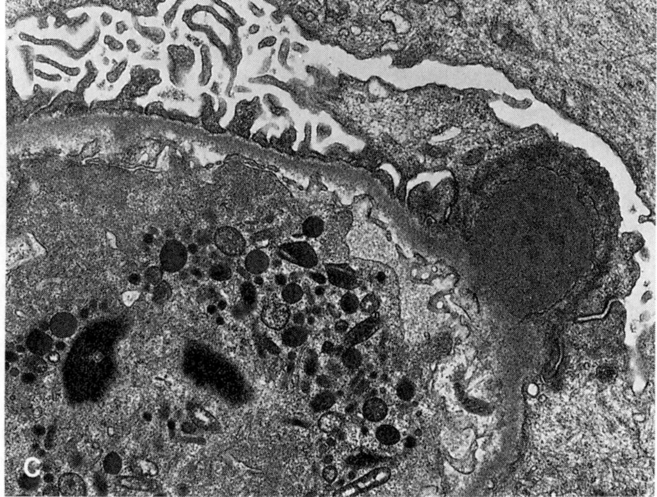

Figure 21–16

Acute proliferative glomerulonephritis. *A*, Normal glomerulus. *B*, Glomerular hypercellularity is due to intracapillary leukocytes and proliferation of intrinsic glomerular cells. *C*, Typical electron-dense subepithelial "hump" and a neutrophil in the lumen. (Courtesy of Dr. H. Rennke, Brigham and Women's Hospital, Boston, MA.)

More than 95% of affected children eventually recover totally with conservative therapy aimed at maintaining sodium and water balance. A small minority of children (perhaps less than 1%) do not improve, become severely oliguric, and develop a rapidly progressive form of glomerulonephritis (described later). Another 1% to 2% may undergo slow progression to chronic glomerulonephritis with or without recurrence of an active nephritic picture. Prolonged and persistent heavy proteinuria and abnormal GFR mark patients with an unfavorable prognosis.

In adults, the disease is less benign. Although the overall prognosis in epidemics is good, in only about 60% of *sporadic cases* do the patients recover promptly. Some patients develop rapidly progressive glomerulonephritis. In the remainder, the glomerular lesions fail to resolve quickly, as manifested by persistent proteinuria, hematuria, and hypertension. In some of these patients, the lesions eventually clear totally, but others develop chronic glomerulonephritis.

Nonstreptococcal Acute Glomerulonephritis

A similar form of glomerulonephritis occurs sporadically in association with other bacterial infections (e.g., staphylococcal endocarditis, pneumococcal pneumonia, and meningococcemia), viral disease (e.g., hepatitis B, hepatitis C, mumps, human immunodeficiency virus [HIV] infection, varicella, and infectious mononucleosis), and parasitic infections (malaria, toxoplasmosis). In all these, granular immunofluorescent deposits and subepithelial humps characteristic of immune complex nephritis are present.

Rapidly Progressive (Crescentic) Glomerulonephritis

Rapidly progressive glomerulonephritis (RPGN) is a syndrome associated with severe glomerular injury and does not denote a specific etiologic form of glomerulonephritis. It is characterized clinically by rapid and progressive loss of renal function associated with severe oliguria and (if untreated) death from renal failure within weeks to months. *Regardless of the cause, the histologic picture is characterized by the presence of crescents in most of the glomeruli* (crescentic glomerulonephritis). These are produced in part by proliferation of the parietal epithelial cells and Bowman capsule and in part by infiltration of monocytes and macrophages.

Classification and Pathogenesis. RPGN may be caused by a number of different diseases, some restricted to the kidney and others systemic.[34] Although no single mechanism can explain all cases, there is little doubt that in most cases the glomerular injury is immunologically mediated. Thus, a practical classification divides RPGN into three groups on the basis of immunologic findings (Table 21–6). In each group, the disease may be associated with a known disorder or it may be idiopathic.

Table 21–6. RAPIDLY PROGRESSIVE GLOMERULONEPHRITIS (RPGN)

- **TYPE I RPGN**
  - Idiopathic
  - Goodpasture syndrome
- **TYPE II RPGN** (immune complex)
  - Idiopathic
  - Postinfectious
  - Systemic lupus erythematosus
  - Henoch-Schönlein purpura (IgA)
  - Others
- **TYPE III RPGN** (pauci-immune) (ANCA associated)
  - Idiopathic
  - Wegener granulomatosis
  - Microscopic polyarteritis nodosa

Type I RPGN is best remembered as anti-GBM disease and hence is characterized by linear deposits of IgG and, in many cases, C3 in the GBM, as previously described. In some of these patients, the anti-GBM antibodies cross-react with pulmonary alveolar basement membranes to produce the clinical picture of pulmonary hemorrhages associated with renal failure (*Goodpasture syndrome*).

The Goodpasture antigen, as noted, resides in the noncollagenous portion of the α_3 chain of collagen type IV. What triggers the formation of these antibodies is unclear in most patients. Exposure to viruses or hydrocarbon solvents (found in paints and dyes) has been implicated in some patients, as have various drugs and cancers. Cigarette smoking appears to play a permissive role, since most patients who develop pulmonary hemorrhage are smokers. There is a high prevalence of certain HLA subtypes and haplotypes (e.g., HLA-DRB1), a finding consistent with the genetic predisposition to autoimmunity.[34]

Type II RPGN is an *immune complex–mediated disease.* It can be a complication of any of the immune complex nephritides, including postinfectious glomerulonephritis, SLE, IgA nephropathy, and Henoch-Schönlein purpura. In some cases, immune complexes can be demonstrated, but the underlying cause is undetermined. In all of these cases, immunofluorescence studies reveal the characteristic ("lumpy bumpy") granular pattern of staining. These patients cannot usually be helped by plasmapheresis, and they require treatment for the underlying disease.

Type III RPGN, also called *pauci-immune type,* is defined by the lack of anti-GBM antibodies or immune complexes by immunofluorescence and electron microscopy. Most of these patients have *antineutrophil cytoplasmic antibody* (ANCA) in the serum, which, as we have seen (Chapter 12), plays a role in some vasculitides. Hence, in some cases, type III RPGN is a component of a systemic vasculitis such as Wegener granulomatosis or microscopic polyarteritis. In many cases, however, pauci-immune crescentic glomerulonephritis is isolated and hence *idiopathic.* More than 90% of such idiopathic cases have C-ANCA or P-ANCA in the sera.

To summarize, all three types of RPGN may be associated with a well-defined renal or extrarenal disease, but in many cases (approximately 50%) the disorder is idiopathic. Of the idiopathic cases, about one fourth have anti-GBM disease (RPGN type I) without lung involvement; another one fourth have type II RPGN; and the remainder are pauci-immune or type III RPGN. *The common denominator in all types of RPGN is severe glomerular injury.*

MORPHOLOGY. The kidneys are enlarged and pale, often with petechial hemorrhages on the cortical surfaces. Depending on the underlying cause, the glomeruli may show focal necrosis, diffuse or focal endothelial proliferation, and mesangial proliferation. The histologic picture, however, is dominated by the formation of distinctive **crescents** (Fig. 21–17). Crescents are formed by proliferation of parietal cells and by migration of monocytes and macrophages into Bowman space. Neutrophils and lymphocytes may be present. The crescents eventually obliterate Bowman space and compress the glomerular tuft. **Fibrin strands are prominent between the cellular layers in the crescents,** and indeed the escape of fibrin into Bowman space is an important contributor to crescent formation. Electron microscopy may, as expected, disclose subepithelial deposits in some cases but in all cases shows distinct **ruptures in the GBM** (Fig. 21–18). In time, most crescents undergo sclerosis.

By immunofluorescence microscopy, postinfectious cases exhibit granular immune deposits; Goodpasture syndrome cases show linear fluorescence; and idiopathic cases may have granular, linear, or little deposition (pauci-immune).

Clinical Course. The renal manifestations of all forms include hematuria with red cell casts in the urine, moderate proteinuria occasionally reaching the nephrotic range, and variable hypertension and edema. In Goodpasture syndrome, the course may be dominated by recurrent hemoptysis or even life-threatening pulmonary hemorrhage. Serum analyses for anti-GBM, antinuclear antibodies, and ANCA are helpful in the diagnosis of specific subtypes. Although milder forms of glomerular injury may subside, the renal involvement is usually progressive during a matter of weeks, culminating in severe oliguria. Recovery of renal function may follow early intensive plasmapheresis (plasma exchange) combined with steroids and cytotoxic agents in Goodpasture syndrome. This therapy appears to reverse both pulmonary hemorrhage and renal failure. Other forms of RPGN also respond well to steroids and cytotoxic agents. Despite therapy, patients may eventually require chronic dialysis or transplantation.

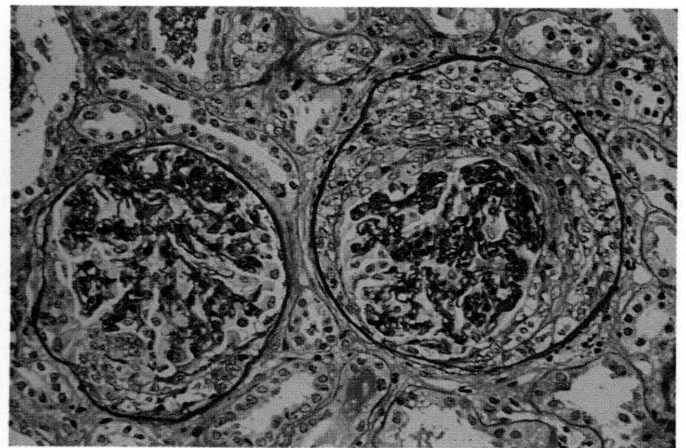

Figure 21–17

Crescentic glomerulonephritis (PAS stain). Note the collapsed glomerular tufts and the crescent-shaped mass of proliferating cells and leukocytes internal to Bowman capsule. (Courtesy of Dr. M.A. Venkatachalam, Department of Pathology, University of Texas Health Sciences Center, San Antonio, TX.)

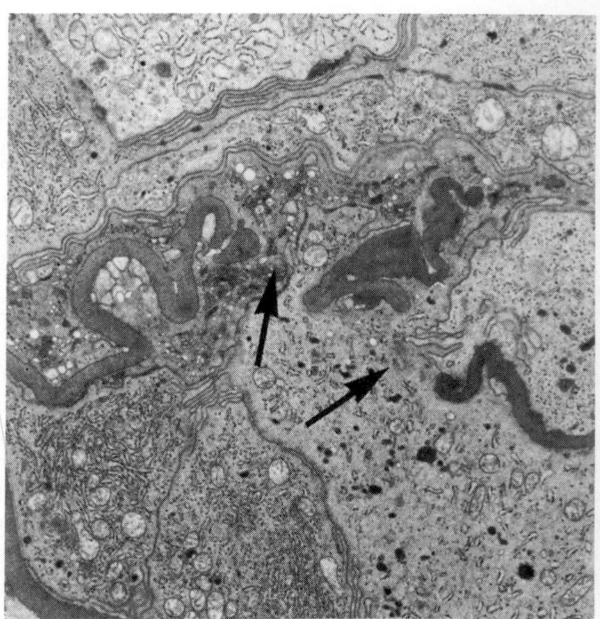

Figure 21–18

Rapidly progressive glomerulonephritis. Electron micrograph showing characteristic wrinkling of GBM with focal disruptions in its continuity (*arrows*).

Nephrotic Syndrome

Certain glomerular diseases virtually always produce the nephrotic syndrome. In addition, many other forms of primary and secondary glomerulonephritis discussed in this chapter may evoke it. Before the major diseases associated with nephrotic syndrome are presented, the pathophysiology of this clinical complex is briefly discussed and the causes are listed.[35]

Pathophysiology. The manifestations of the nephrotic syndrome include

1. *massive proteinuria*, with the daily loss of 3.5 gm or more of protein (less in children);
2. *hypoalbuminemia*, with plasma albumin levels less than 3 gm/dl;
3. *generalized edema*; and
4. *hyperlipidemia and lipiduria*.

The various components of nephrotic syndrome bear a logical relationship to one another. The initial event is a derangement in glomerular capillary walls resulting in *increased permeability to the plasma proteins.* It will be remembered that the glomerular capillary wall, with its endothelium, GBM, and visceral epithelial cells, acts as a size and charge barrier through which the glomerular filtrate must pass. Increased permeability resulting from either structural or physicochemical alterations allows protein to escape from the plasma into the glomerular filtrate. *Massive proteinuria results.*

The heavy proteinuria leads to depletion of serum albumin levels below the compensatory synthetic abilities of the liver, with consequent hypoalbuminemia and a reversed albumin-globulin ratio. Increased renal catabolism of filtered albumin also contributes to the hypoalbuminemia. The generalized edema is, in turn, the consequence of the loss of colloid osmotic pressure of the blood and the accumulation of fluid in the interstitial tissues. There is also *sodium and water retention,* which aggravates the edema (Chapter 5). This appears to be due to several factors, including compensatory secretion of aldosterone, mediated by the hypovolemia-enhanced antidiuretic hormone secretion; stimulation of the sympathetic system; and a reduction in the secretion of natriuretic factors, such as atrial peptides. Edema is characteristically soft and pitting, most marked in the periorbital regions and dependent portions of the body. It may be massive with pleural effusions and ascites.

The largest proportion of protein lost in the urine is albumin, but globulins are also excreted in some diseases. The ratio of low- to high-molecular-weight proteins in the urine in various cases of nephrotic syndrome determines the so-called *selectivity* of proteinuria. A *highly selective proteinuria* consists mostly of low-molecular-weight proteins (albumin 70,000; transferrin 76,000), whereas a *poorly selective proteinuria* consists of higher molecular weight globulins in addition to albumin.

The genesis of the *hyperlipidemia* is complex. Most patients have increased cholesterol, triglyceride, very-low-density lipoprotein, low-density lipoprotein, Lp(a) lipoprotein, and apoprotein concentrations, and there is a decrease in high-density lipoprotein concentration in some patients. These defects seem to be due, in part, to *increased synthesis of lipoproteins in the liver, abnormal transport of circulating lipid particles, and decreased catabolism. Lipiduria* follows the hyperlipidemia, because not only albumin molecules but also lipoproteins leak across the glomerular capillary wall. The lipid appears in the urine either as free fat or as *oval fat bodies,* representing lipoprotein resorbed by tubular epithelial cells and then shed along with the degenerated cells.

These patients are particularly vulnerable to *infection,* especially with staphylococci and pneumococci. The basis for this vulnerability could be related to loss of immunoglobulins or low-molecular-weight complement components (e.g., factor B) in the urine. *Thrombotic and thromboembolic complications* are also common in nephrotic syndrome, owing in part to loss of anticoagulant factors (e.g., antithrombin III) and antiplasmin activity through the leaky glomerulus. *Renal vein thrombosis,* once thought to be a cause of nephrotic syndrome, is most often a *consequence* of this hypercoagulable state.

Causes. The relative frequencies of the several causes of the nephrotic syndrome vary according to age. *In children younger than 15 years,* for example, the nephrotic syndrome is almost always caused by a lesion primary to the kidney; whereas among adults, it may often be associated with a systemic disease. Table 21–7 represents a composite derived from several studies of the causes of the nephrotic syndrome and is therefore only approximate. As Table 21–7 indicates, the most frequent *systemic causes* of the nephrotic syndrome are SLE, diabetes, and amyloidosis. The most important of the *primary glomerular lesions* are *lipoid nephrosis (minimal change disease), membranous glomerulonephritis,* and *focal segmental glomerulosclerosis.* The first is most common in children, the second in adults, and focal segmental glomerulosclerosis occurs at all ages.[35] These three lesions, as well as a fourth less common disorder, membranoproliferative glomerulonephritis, are discussed individually in the following sections. The fifth possible primary cause, diffuse proliferative glomerulonephritis, frequently presents with the nephritic syndrome and was discussed earlier.

Membranous Glomerulonephritis (Membranous Nephropathy)

Membranous glomerulonephritis is the most common cause of the nephrotic syndrome in adults. It is characterized by diffuse thickening of the glomerular capillary wall and the accumulation of electron-dense, immunoglobulin-containing deposits along the epithelial (subepithelial) side of the basement membrane.[36]

Membranous glomerulonephritis occurring in association with other systemic diseases and a variety of identifiable etiologic agents is referred to as *secondary membranous*

Table 21–7. CAUSES OF NEPHROTIC SYNDROME

	Prevalence (%) Children	Adults
Primary Glomerular Disease		
Membranous glomerulonephritis	5	40
Lipoid nephrosis	65	15
Focal segmental glomerulosclerosis	10	15
Membranoproliferative glomerulonephritis	10	7
Other proliferative glomerulonephritis (focal, "pure mesangial," IgA nephropathy)	10	23
Systemic Diseases		
Diabetes mellitus		
Amyloidosis		
Systemic lupus erythematosus		
Drugs (gold, penicillamine, "street heroin")		
Infections (malaria, syphilis, hepatitis B, acquired immunodeficiency syndrome)		
Malignant disease (carcinoma, melanoma)		
Miscellaneous (bee-sting allergy, hereditary nephritis)		

*Approximate prevalence of primary disease = 95% in children, 60% in adults. Approximate prevalence of systemic disease = 5% in children, 40% in adults.

glomerulonephritis. The most notable such associations are as follows:

- *Drugs* (penicillamine, captopril, gold, nonsteroidal anti-inflammatory drugs [NSAIDs]): 1% to 7% of patients with rheumatoid arthritis treated with penicillamine or gold develop membranous glomerulonephritis. In a recent report, membranous glomerulonephritis was attributable to NSAIDs in 10% of patients. NSAIDs, as we shall see, also cause minimal change disease.
- *Underlying malignant tumors,* particularly carcinoma of the lung and colon and melanoma. These are present in 5% to 10% of adults with membranous glomerulonephritis.
- *SLE.* About 15% of glomerulonephritis in SLE is of the membranous type.
- *Infections* (chronic hepatitis B, hepatitis C, syphilis, schistosomiasis, malaria)
- *Metabolic disorders* (diabetes mellitus, thyroiditis)

In about 85% of patients, no associated condition can be uncovered, and the disease is truly "idiopathic."

Etiology and Pathogenesis. Membranous glomerulonephritis is a form of chronic antigen-antibody–mediated disease. In secondary membranous glomerulonephritis, specific antigens can sometimes be implicated. For example, membranous glomerulonephritis in SLE is associated with deposition of autoantigen-antibody complexes. Exogenous (hepatitis B, *Treponema* antigens, insulin) or endogenous (thyroglobulin) antigens have been identified within deposits in some patients.

The lesions bear a striking resemblance to those of experimental Heymann nephritis, which, as you may recall, is induced by antibodies to a *megalin* antigenic complex, and a similar antigen is present in humans. Susceptibility to Heymann nephritis in rats and membranous glomerulonephritis in humans is linked to the HLA locus, which influences the ability to elaborate antibodies to the *nephritogenic* antigen. Thus, idiopathic membranous glomerulonephritis, like Heymann nephritis, is considered *an autoimmune disease linked to susceptibility genes and caused by antibodies to a renal autoantigen.*

How does the glomerular capillary wall become leaky in membranous glomerulonephritis? With the paucity of neutrophils, monocytes, or platelets in glomeruli and the virtually uniform presence of complement, experimental work suggests a direct action of C5b–C9, the membrane attack complex of complement. C5b–C9 causes activation of glomerular epithelial and mesangial cells, inducing them to liberate proteases and oxidants, which cause capillary wall injury and increased protein leakage.

MORPHOLOGY. By light microscopy, the glomeruli either appear normal in the early stages of the disease or exhibit **uniform, diffuse thickening of the glomerular capillary wall** (Fig. 21–19*A*). By electron microscopy, the apparent thickening is caused by irregular dense deposits between the basement membrane and the overlying epithelial cells, the latter having lost their foot processes (Fig. 21–19*B* and *D*). Basement membrane material is laid down between these deposits, appearing as irregular spikes protruding from the GBM. These spikes are best seen by silver stains, which color the basement membrane black. In time, these spikes thicken to produce domelike protrusions and eventually close over the immune deposits, burying them within a markedly thickened, irregular membrane. Immunofluorescence microscopy demonstrates that the granular deposits contain both immunoglobulins and various amounts of complement (Fig. 21–19*C*). As the disease advances, the membrane thickening progressively encroaches on the capillary lumens, and sclerosis of the mesangium may occur; in the course of time, glomeruli become totally hyalinized. The epithelial cells of the proximal tubules contain hyaline droplets, reflecting protein reabsorption, and there may be considerable mononuclear interstitial inflammation.

Clinical Course. In a previously healthy individual, this disorder usually begins with the insidious onset of the nephrotic syndrome or, in 15% of patients, with non-nephrotic proteinuria. Hematuria and mild hypertension are present in 15% to 35% of cases. It is necessary in any patient to first rule out the secondary causes described earlier, since treatment of the underlying condition (malignant neoplasm, infection, or SLE) or discontinuance of the offending drug may reverse progression.

The course is irregular but generally indolent. In contrast to minimal change disease, described later, the proteinuria is nonselective and does not usually respond well to corticosteroid therapy. Progression is associated with increasing sclerosis of glomeruli, rising BUN, relative reduction in the severity of proteinuria, and development of hypertension. Although proteinuria persists in more than 60% of patients, only about 10% die or progress to renal failure within 10 years, and no more than 40% eventually develop renal insufficiency. Spontaneous remissions and a relatively benign outcome occur more commonly in women and in those with non-nephrotic range proteinuria and mild glomerular changes on electron microscopy. Because of the notoriously variable course of the disease, it has been difficult to evaluate the overall effectiveness of corticosteroids or other immunosuppressive therapy in controlling the proteinuria or progression.

Minimal Change Disease (Lipoid Nephrosis)

This relatively benign disorder is the *most frequent cause of nephrotic syndrome in children. It is characterized by diffuse loss of foot processes of epithelial cells in glomeruli that appear virtually normal by light microscopy.* The peak incidence is between 2 and 6 years of age. The

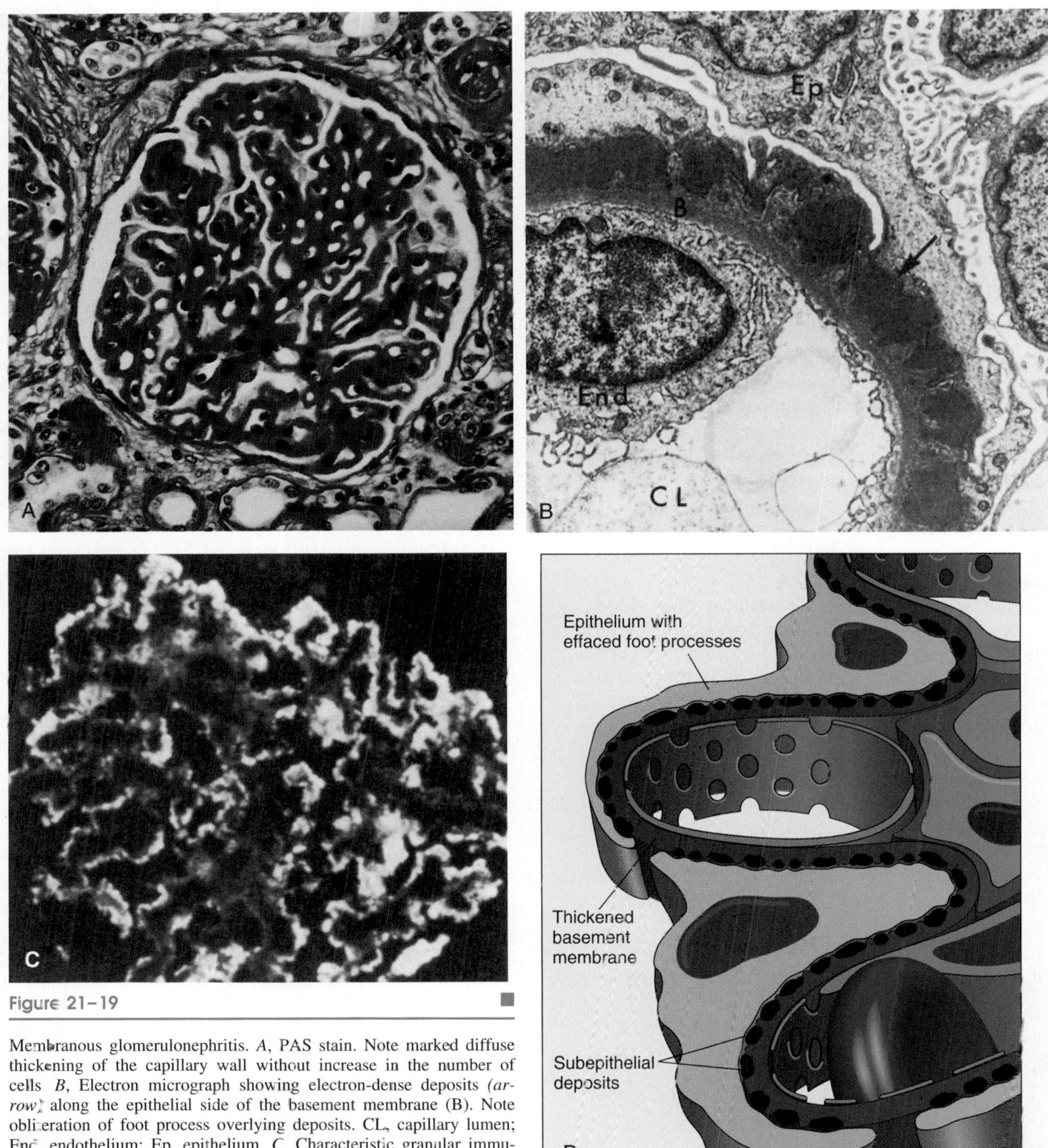

Figure 21–19

Membranous glomerulonephritis. *A*, PAS stain. Note marked diffuse thickening of the capillary wall without increase in the number of cells. *B*, Electron micrograph showing electron-dense deposits *(arrow)* along the epithelial side of the basement membrane (B). Note obliteration of foot process overlying deposits. CL, capillary lumen; End, endothelium; Ep, epithelium. *C*, Characteristic granular immunofluorescent deposits of IgG along GBM. *D*, Diagrammatic representation of membranous glomerulonephritis.

disease sometimes follows a respiratory infection or routine prophylactic immunization. *Its most characteristic feature is its usually dramatic response to corticosteroid therapy.*[37]

Etiology and Pathogenesis. Although the absence of immune deposits in the glomerulus excludes classic immune complex mechanisms, several features of the disease point to an immunologic basis,[38] including (1) the clinical association with respiratory infections and prophylactic immunization; (2) the response to corticosteroid and immunosuppressive therapy; (3) the association with other atopic disorders (e.g., eczema, rhinitis); (4) the increased prevalence of certain HLA haplotypes in patients with minimal change disease associated with atopy (suggesting a possible genetic predisposition); (5) the increased incidence of minimal change disease in patients with Hodgkin disease, in whom defects in T cell–mediated immunity are well recognized; (6) the recurrence of proteinuria after transplantation in patients with the related disorder focal segmental glomerulosclerosis, discussed later; and (7) reports of proteinuria-inducing factors in the plasma or lymphocyte supernatants of patients with lipoid nephrosis and focal glomerulosclerosis.

The current hypothesis is that lipoid nephrosis involves some immune dysfunction, eventually resulting in the elaboration of a cytokine-like circulating substance that affects visceral epithelial cells and causes proteinuria. The ultrastructural changes point to a primary *visceral epithelial cell injury,* and studies in animal models suggest the loss of glomerular polyanions; thus, defects in the charge barrier contribute to the proteinuria. Detachment of epithelial cells (see Fig. 21–12), a consequence of diminished adhesion to GBM, may also lead to protein loss. Recent clues might come from the discovery of mutations in a renal glomerular protein, termed *nephrin*, in a hereditary form of congenital nephrotic syndrome with minimal change morphology (Finnish type). This protein resembles immunoglobulin-like cell adhesion receptors that participate in cell-cell and cell-matrix interactions,[38a] thus supporting a role for epithelial adhesion defects in this disease.

MORPHOLOGY. The glomeruli are normal by light microscopy (Fig. 21–20). By **electron microscopy,** the basement membrane appears morphologically normal, and no electron-dense material is deposited. **The principal lesion is in the visceral epithelial cells, which show a uniform and diffuse effacement of foot processes,** these being replaced by a rim of cytoplasm often showing vacuolization, swelling, and villous hyperplasia (Fig. 21–21). This change, often incorrectly termed "fusion" of foot processes, actually represents simplification of the epithelial cell architecture with flattening, retraction, and swelling of foot processes. Such foot process loss is also present in other proteinuric states (e.g., membranous glomerulonephritis, diabetes). It is only when fusion is associated with normal glomeruli that the diagnosis of minimal change disease can be made. The visceral epithelial changes are completely reversible after corticosteroid therapy and remission of the proteinuria. The cells of the proximal tubules are often laden with lipid, reflecting tubular reabsorption of lipoproteins passing through diseased glomeruli (thus, the term **lipoid nephrosis**). Immunofluorescence studies show no immunoglobulin or complement deposits.

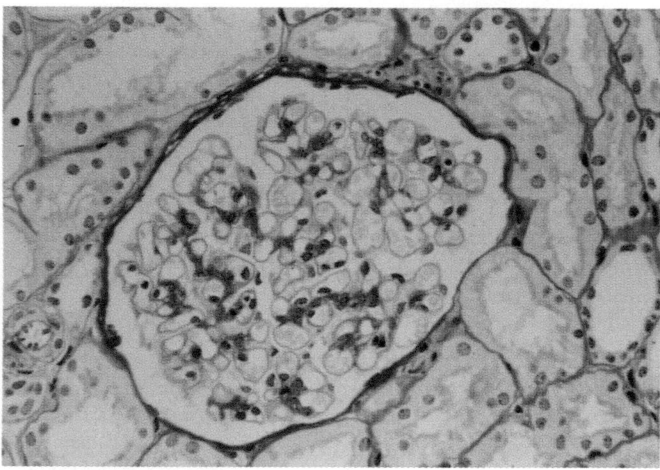

Figure 21–20

Minimal change disease. Thin section of glomerulus stained with PAS. Note thin basement membrane and absence of proliferation. Compare with membranous glomerulonephritis in Figure 21–19*A*.

Clinical Course. Despite massive proteinuria, renal function remains good, and there is commonly no hypertension or hematuria. The proteinuria usually is highly selective, most of the protein consisting of albumin. Most children (more than 90%) with minimal change disease respond rapidly to corticosteroid therapy. However, the nephrotic phase may recur, and some patients may become "steroid dependent or resistant." Nevertheless, the long-term prognosis for patients is excellent, and even steroid-dependent disease resolves when children reach puberty. Although adults are slower to respond, the long-term prognosis is also excellent.

As noted, minimal change disease in adults can be associated with Hodgkin disease and, less frequently, other lymphomas and leukemias. In addition, secondary minimal change disease may follow NSAID therapy, usually in association with acute interstitial nephritis, to be described later in this chapter.

Focal Segmental Glomerulosclerosis

As the name implies, *this lesion is characterized by sclerosis of some, but not all, glomeruli (thus, it is focal); and in the affected glomeruli, only a portion of the capillary tuft is involved (thus, it is segmental).* Focal segmental glomerulosclerosis is frequently accompanied clinically by the nephrotic syndrome or heavy proteinuria.

Classification and Types. Focal segmental glomerulosclerosis occurs in the following settings[39]:

1. in association with other known conditions, such as HIV infection and heroin addiction (HIV nephropathy, heroin addiction nephropathy), sickle cell disease, and massive obesity;
2. as a secondary event, reflecting glomerular scarring, in other forms of focal glomerulonephritis (e.g., IgA nephropathy);
3. as a component of the adaptive response in glomerular ablation nephropathy (described earlier) in advanced stages of other renal disorders such as reflux nephropathy, or with unilateral renal agenesis;
4. in certain inherited, congenital forms of nephrotic syndrome, where the disease, in certain pedigrees, has been linked to chromosome 19q13,[39] close to the locus of *nephrin*, described in the discussion of lipoid nephrosis; or

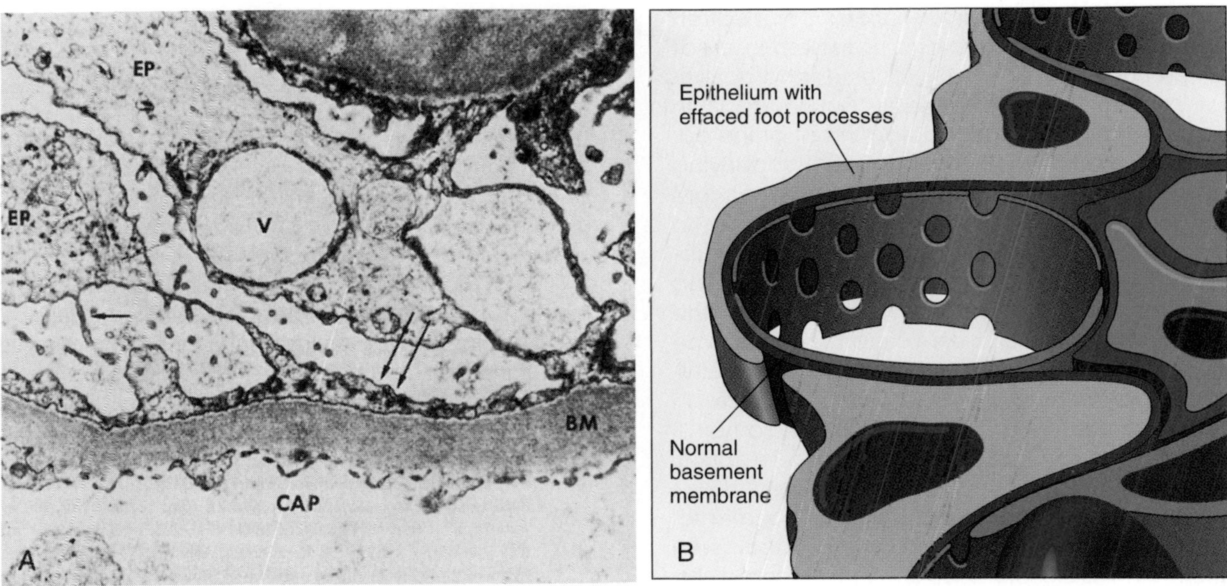

Figure 21–21

A, Ultrastructural characteristics of minimal change disease: loss of foot processes *(double arrows)*, absence of deposits, vacuoles (V), and microvilli in visceral epithelial cells *(single arrow)*. *B*, Schematic representation of minimal change disease, showing diffuse loss of foot processes.

5. as a primary disease (idiopathic focal segmental glomerulosclerosis).

Idiopathic focal segmental glomerulosclerosis accounts for 10% and 15% of cases of nephrotic syndrome in children and adults, respectively. Patients differ from the usual patients with minimal change disease in the following respects: (1) they have a higher incidence of hematuria, reduced GFR, and hypertension; (2) their proteinuria is more often nonselective; (3) they respond poorly to corticosteroid therapy; (4) many progress to chronic glomerulonephritis, and at least 50% develop end-stage renal disease within 10 years; and (5) immunofluorescence microscopy shows deposition of IgM and C3 in the sclerotic segment.

MORPHOLOGY. By light microscopy, the segmental lesions may involve only a minority of the glomeruli and may be missed if insufficient glomeruli are present in the biopsy specimen (Fig. 21–22*A*). The lesions initially tend to involve the juxtamedullary glomeruli, although they subsequently become more generalized. In the sclerotic segments, there is collapse of basement membranes, increase in matrix, and deposition of hyaline masses **(hyalinosis)**, often with lipoid droplets and foam cells (Fig. 21–22*B*). Glomeruli not exhibiting segmental lesions either appear normal on light microscopy or may show increased mesangial

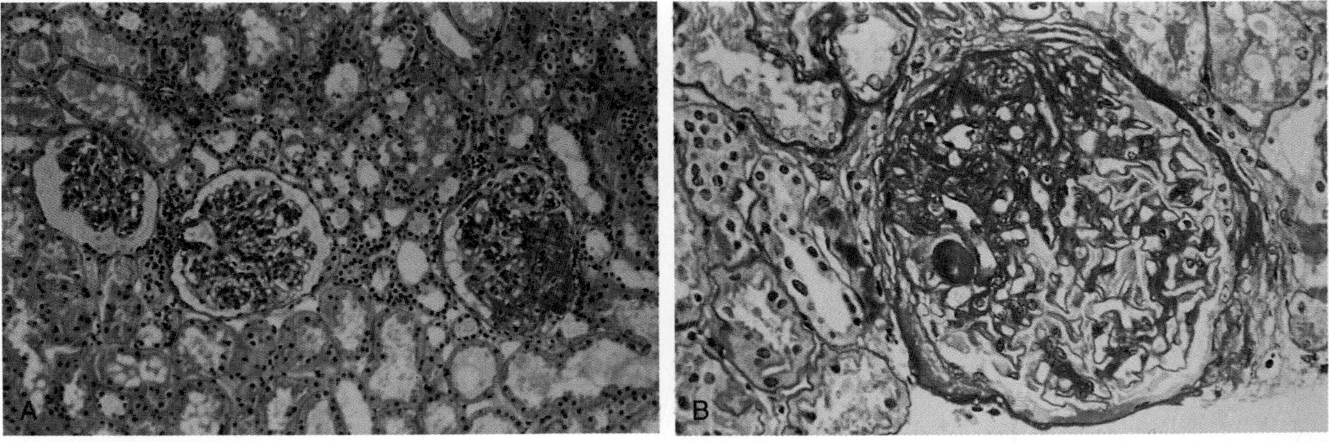

Figure 21–22

Focal segmental glomerulosclerosis. PAS stain. *A*, Low-power view showing segmental sclerosis in one of three glomeruli (at 3 o'clock). *B*, High-power view showing hyaline mass and lipid (small vacuoles) in sclerotic area.

matrix and mesangial proliferation. On electron microscopy, both sclerotic and nonsclerotic areas show the diffuse loss of foot processes characteristic of minimal change disease, but in addition there is **pronounced, focal detachment of the epithelial cells with denudation of the underlying GBM.** By immunofluorescence microscopy, IgM and C3 are present within the hyaline masses in the sclerotic areas. In addition to the focal sclerosis, there is often pronounced hyaline thickening of afferent arterioles. With the progression of the disease, increased numbers of glomeruli become involved, sclerosis spreads within each glomerulus, and there is an increase in mesangial matrix. In time this leads to total sclerosis of glomeruli, with pronounced tubular atrophy and interstitial fibrosis.

A morphologic variant of focal segmental glomerulosclerosis, called **collapsing focal segmental glomerulosclerosis,** is characterized by collapse and sclerosis of the entire glomerular tuft in addition to the usual focal segmental glomerulosclerosis lesions. Although it may be seen in idiopathic focal segmental glomerulosclerosis, it is more characteristic of the form associated with HIV infection. It has a particularly poor prognosis.[40]

Pathogenesis. Whether idiopathic focal segmental glomerulosclerosis represents a distinct disease or is simply a phase in the evolution of a subset of patients with minimal change disease is a matter of conjecture, most workers favoring the latter explanation. The characteristic degeneration and focal disruption of visceral epithelial cells are thought to represent an accentuation of the diffuse epithelial cell change typical of minimal change disease. *It is this epithelial damage that is the hallmark of focal segmental glomerulosclerosis.* The hyalinosis and sclerosis represent entrapment of plasma proteins in extremely hyperpermeable foci with increased ECM deposition. The recurrence of proteinuria, sometimes within 24 hours after transplantation, suggests a circulating factor, perhaps a cytokine, as the cause of the epithelial damage, and indeed a ±50-kD nonimmunoglobulin factor causing proteinuria has been isolated from sera of such patients.[41]

Renal ablation focal segmental glomerulosclerosis occurs as a complication of glomerular and nonglomerular diseases causing reduction in functioning renal tissue, particularly reflux nephropathy and unilateral agenesis. These may lead to progressive glomerulosclerosis and renal failure. The pathogenesis of focal segmental glomerulosclerosis in this setting has been detailed earlier in this chapter, under Pathogenesis.

Clinical Course. There is little tendency for spontaneous remission in idiopathic focal segmental glomerulosclerosis, and responses to corticosteroid therapy are variable. In general, children have a better prognosis than that of adults. Progression of renal failure occurs at variable rates. About 20% of patients follow an unusually rapid course *(malignant focal sclerosis),* with intractable massive proteinuria ending in renal failure within 2 years. Recurrences are seen in 25% to 50% of patients receiving allografts.

HIV-Associated Nephropathy. HIV infection can result in a number of renal complications, including acute renal failure induced by drugs, shock, and infection; postinfectious glomerulonephritis; membranous glomerulonephritis associated with hepatitis B infection; MPGN due to hepatitis C infection; and *most commonly a severe form of focal segmental glomerulosclerosis.*[42] The last occurs in 5% to 10% of HIV-infected patients, more frequently in blacks than in whites, and the nephrotic syndrome may precede the development of acquired immunodeficiency syndrome. The glomerular lesions resemble idiopathic focal segmental glomerulosclerosis, but with the following additional features:

- A high frequency of the *collapsing variant of focal segmental glomerulosclerosis,* with global involvement of the tuft
- A striking focal cystic dilation of tubule segments, filled with proteinaceous material, inflammation, and fibrosis
- The presence of large numbers of *tubuloreticular inclusions* in endothelial cells. Such inclusions, also present in SLE, have been shown to be induced by circulating interferon-α. They are not present in idiopathic focal segmental glomerulosclerosis and thus may have diagnostic value in a biopsy specimen.

The pathogenesis of HIV-related focal segmental glomerulosclerosis is unclear. It may be due to infection of glomerular cells by HIV, which has been shown in animal models, and the local release of cytokines.[43]

Membranoproliferative Glomerulonephritis

This group of disorders is characterized histologically by *alterations in the basement membrane, proliferation of glomerular cells, and leukocyte infiltration.*[44] Because the proliferation is predominantly in the mesangium, a frequently used synonym is *mesangiocapillary glomerulonephritis.* MPGN accounts for 5% to 10% of cases of idiopathic nephrotic syndrome in children and young adults. Some patients present only with hematuria or proteinuria in the non-nephrotic range, and others have a combined nephrotic-nephritic picture. Like many other glomerulonephritides, histologic MPGN either can be associated with other systemic disorders and known etiologic agents (secondary MPGN) or may be primary, without known cause (idiopathic) in the kidney.

Primary MPGN is divided into two major types on the basis of distinct ultrastructural, immunofluorescent, and pathogenic findings: type I and type II MPGN.

MORPHOLOGY. By light microscopy, both types are similar. The glomeruli are large and hypercellular. The hypercellularity is produced by proliferation of cells in the mesangium, although infiltrating leukocytes and parietal epithelial crescents are present in many cases The glomeruli have a "lobular" appearance accentuated by the proliferating mesangial cells and increased mesangial matrix (Fig. 21–23). The GBM is clearly thickened, often focally, most evident in the peripheral capillary loops. The glomerular capillary wall often shows a "double-contour" or "tram-track" appearance, especially evident in silver or PAS stains. This is caused by "duplication" of the basement membrane and the inclusion within the lamina rara interna of processes of cells extending into the peripheral capillary loops, so-called **mesangial and monocyte interposition.**

Types I and II have altogether different ultrastructural and immunofluorescent features (Fig. 21–24).

Type I MPGN (two thirds of cases) is characterized by the presence of **subendothelial electron-dense deposits.** Mesangial and occasional subepithelial deposits may also be present (Fig. 21–24*A*). By immunofluorescence, C3 is deposited in a granular pattern, and IgG and early complement components (C1q and C4) are often also present, suggesting an immune complex pathogenesis.

In type II lesions, the lamina densa of the GBM is transformed into an irregular, ribbon-like, extremely electron-dense structure because of the **deposition of dense material** of unknown composition in the GBM proper, giving rise to the term **dense-deposit disease.** In type II, C3 is present in irregular granular-linear foci in the basement membranes on either side, but not within the dense deposits. C3 is also present in the mesangium in characteristic circular aggregates (mesangial rings). **IgG is usually absent,** as are the early-acting complement components (C1q and C4).

Rare variants (type III) segregated because they exhibit both subendothelial and subepithelial deposits are associated with GBM disruption and reduplication.

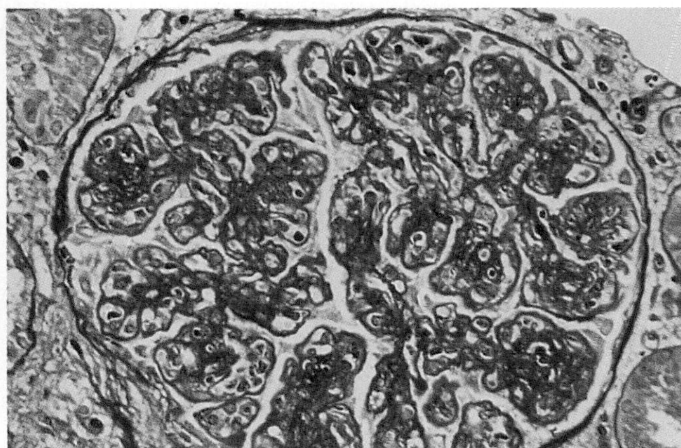

Figure 21–23

Membranoproliferative glomerulonephritis, showing mesangial cell proliferation, increased mesangial matrix, basement membrane thickening, and accentuation of lobular architecture. (Courtesy of Dr. H. Rennke, Brigham and Women's Hospital, Boston, MA.)

Pathogenesis. *Although there are exceptions, most cases of type I MPGN present evidence of immune complexes in the glomerulus and activation of both classic and alternative complement pathways. The antigens involved in idiopathic MPGN are unknown.*

Conversely, most patients with dense-deposit disease (type II) have abnormalities that suggest activation of the alternative complement pathway. These patients have a consistently *decreased serum C3,* but normal C1 and C4, the immune complex–activated early components of complement. They also have diminished serum levels of factor B and properdin, components of the alternative complement pathway. In the glomeruli, C3 and properdin are deposited, but not IgG. Recall that in the alternative complement pathway, C3 is directly cleaved to C3b (Fig. 21–25). The reaction depends on the initial interaction of C3 with such substances as bacterial polysaccharides, endotoxin, aggregates of IgA in the presence of factors B and D, and magnesium. This leads to the generation of C3b,Bb, the alternative pathway C3 convertase. The alternative C3 convertase is labile, being degraded by factors I and H, but it can be stabilized by properdin. More than 70% of patients with dense-deposit disease have a circulating antibody termed *C3 nephritic factor (C3NeF),* which is a conformational autoantibody that binds to the alternative C3 convertase (Fig. 21–25). Binding of the antibody stabilizes the convertase, protecting it from enzymatic degradation and thus favoring persistent C3 degradation and hypocomplementemia. There is also decreased C3 synthesis by the liver, further contributing to the profound hypocomplementemia.

Precisely how C3NeF is related to glomerular injury and the nature of the dense deposits are unknown. C3NeF activity also occurs in some patients with a genetically determined disease, *partial lipodystrophy,* some of whom develop type II MPGN.

Clinical Course. The principal mode of presentation is the nephrotic syndrome occurring in older children or young adults, but usually with nephritic component manifested by hematuria or, more insidiously, as mild proteinuria. Few remissions occur spontaneously in either type, and the disease follows a slowly progressive but unremitting course. Some patients develop numerous crescents and a clinical picture of RPGN. About 50% develop chronic renal failure within 10 years. Treatments with steroids, immunosuppressive agents, and antiplatelet drugs have not been proved to be materially effective. There is a high incidence of recurrence in transplant recipients, particularly in type II disease; dense deposits may recur in 90% of such patients, although renal failure in the allograft is much less common.

Secondary MPGN. Secondary MPGN arises in the following settings[45]:

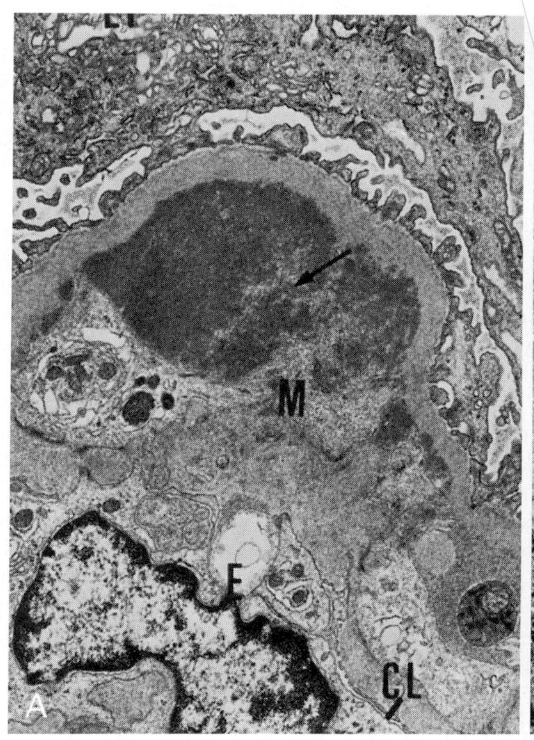

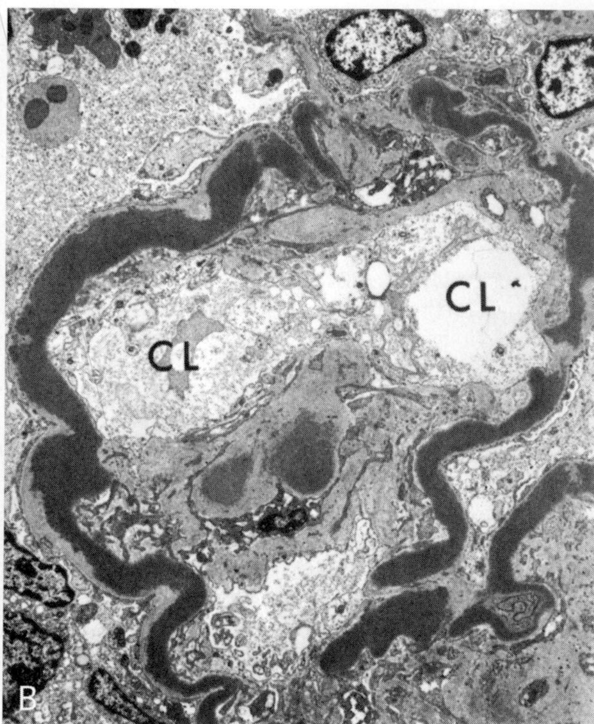

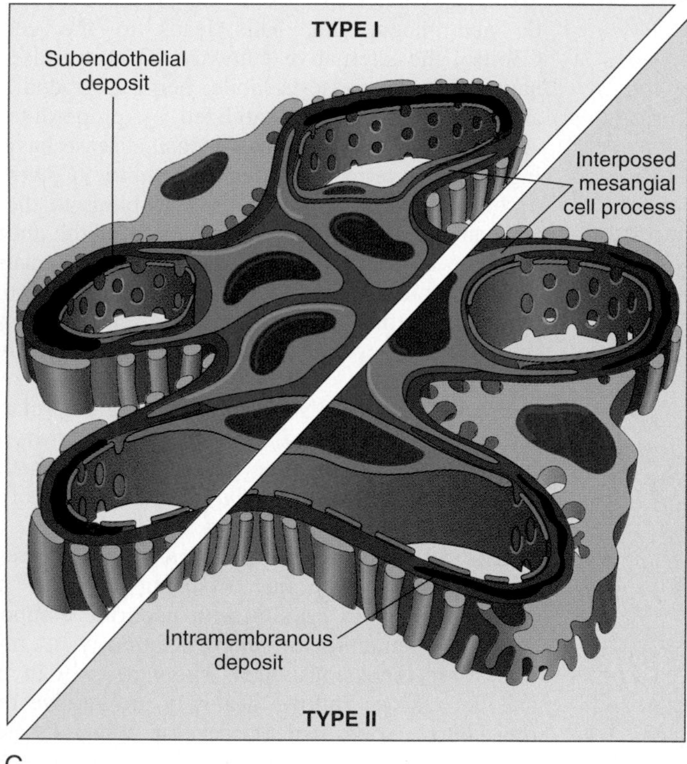

Figure 21–24

A, Membranoproliferative glomerulonephritis, type I. Note large subendothelial deposit *(arrow)* incorporated into mesangial matrix (M). E, endothelium; EP, epithelium; CL, capillary lumen. *B*, Type II membranoproliferative glomerulonephritis, dense-deposit disease. There are markedly dense homogeneous deposits within the basement membrane proper. CL, capillary lumen. *C*, Schematic representation of patterns in the two types of membranoproliferative GN. In type I there are subendothelial deposits; type II is characterized by intramembranous dense deposits (dense deposit disease). In both, mesangial interposition gives the appearance of split basement membranes when viewed in the light microscope.

- Chronic immune complex disorders, such as SLE; hepatitis B infection; hepatitis C infection, usually with cryoglobulinemia; endocarditis; infected ventriculoatrial shunts; chronic visceral abscesses; HIV infection; and schistosomiasis.
- Partial lipodystrophy associated with C3NeF (type 2)
- α_1-Antitrypsin deficiency
- Malignant diseases (chronic lymphocytic leukemia, lymphoma, melanoma)
- Hereditary complement deficiency states

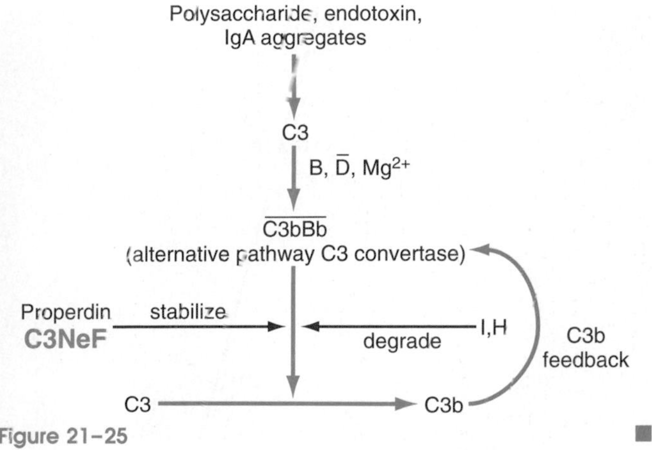

Figure 21–25

The alternative complement pathway. Note that C3NeF, present in the serum of patients with membranoproliferative glomerulonephritis, acts at the same step as properdin, serving to stabilize the alternative pathway C3 convertase, thus enhancing C3 breakdown and causing hypocomplementemia.

IgA Nephropathy (Berger Disease)

This form of glomerulonephritis is characterized by the presence of prominent IgA deposits in the mesangial regions, detected by immunofluorescence microscopy.[46] The disease can be suspected by light microscopic examination, but diagnosis is made only by immunocytochemical techniques (Fig. 21–26). *IgA nephropathy is a frequent cause of recurrent gross or microscopic hematuria* and is probably the most common type of glomerulonephritis worldwide. Mild proteinuria is usually present, and the nephrotic syndrome may occasionally develop. A patient may rarely present with rapidly progressive crescentic glomerulonephritis.

Whereas IgA nephropathy is an isolated renal disease, similar IgA deposits are present in a systemic disorder of children, *Henoch-Schönlein purpura,* to be discussed later, which has many overlapping features with IgA nephropathy. In addition, *secondary IgA nephropathy* occurs in patients with liver and intestinal diseases, as discussed under Pathogenesis.

Pathogenesis. IgA, the main immunoglobulin in mucosal secretions, is at low levels in normal serum, where it is present mostly in monomeric form, the polymeric forms being catabolized in the liver. In patients with IgA nephropathy, serum polymeric IgA is increased, and circulating IgA immune complexes are present in some patients. A genetic influence is suggested by the occurrence of this condition in families and in HLA-identical brothers and the increased frequency of certain HLA and complement phenotypes in some populations. The prominent mesangial deposition of IgA suggests entrapment of IgA immune complexes in the mesangium, and the absence of C1q and C4 in glomeruli points to activation of the alternative complement pathway.

Taken together, these clues suggest a genetic or acquired abnormality of immune regulation leading to increased mucosal IgA synthesis in response to respiratory or gastrointestinal exposure to environmental agents (e.g., viruses, bacteria, food proteins). IgA1 and IgA1-containing complexes are then entrapped in the mesangium, where they activate the alternative complement pathway and initiate glomerular injury. In support of this scenario, IgA nephropathy occurs with increased frequency in patients with *gluten enteropathy* (celiac disease), in whom intestinal mucosal defects are well defined, and in *liver disease,* in which there is defective hepatobiliary clearance of IgA complexes *(secondary IgA nephropathy).*

The nature of the antigens is unknown, and several infectious agents and food products have been implicated. The deposited IgA appears to be polyclonal, and it may be that a variety of antigens are involved in the course of the disease. Alternatively, it has been suggested that qualitative alterations in the IgA1 molecule itself make it more likely to bind to mesangial antigens, or that IgA antibodies react with mesangial cell autoantigens.

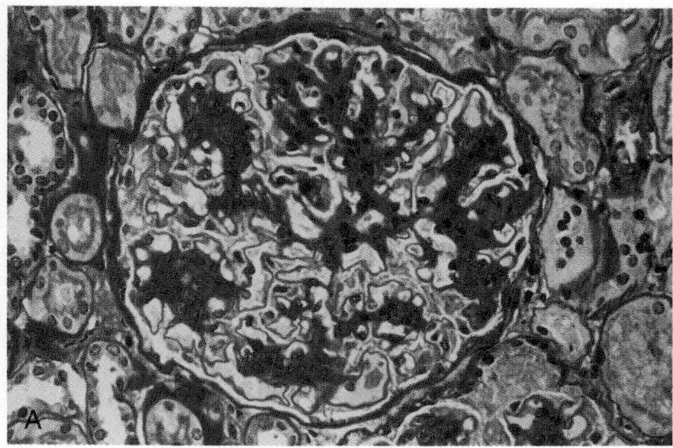

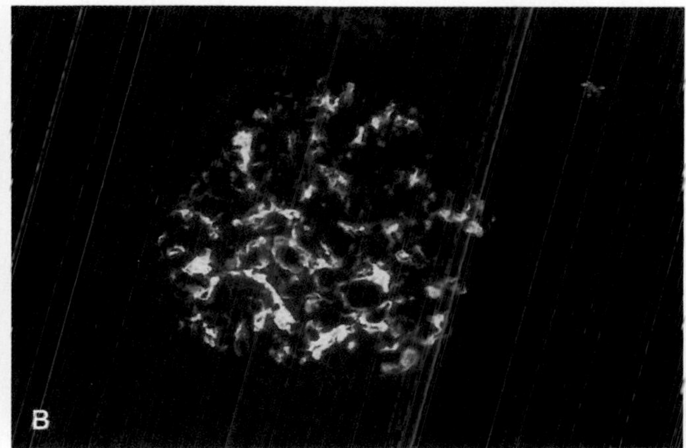

Figure 21–26

IgA nephropathy. *A,* Light microscopy showing mesangial proliferation and matrix increase. *B,* Characteristic immunofluorescence deposition of IgA, principally in mesangial regions.

MORPHOLOGY. On histologic examination, the lesions vary considerably. The glomeruli may be normal or may show mesangial widening and proliferation (mesangioproliferative), segmental proliferation confined to some glomeruli (focal proliferative glomerulonephritis), or rarely overt crescentic glomerulonephritis. Healing of the focal proliferative lesion may lead to focal segmental sclerosis. The characteristic immunofluorescent picture is of **mesangial deposition of IgA** (Fig. 21–26), often with C3 and properdin and lesser amounts of IgG or IgM. Early complement components are usually absent. Electron microscopy confirms the presence of electron-dense deposits in the mesangium in most cases. In some biopsy specimens, prominent hyaline thickening of arterioles is present, a feature associated with a greater likelihood of hypertension and progression to chronic renal failure.

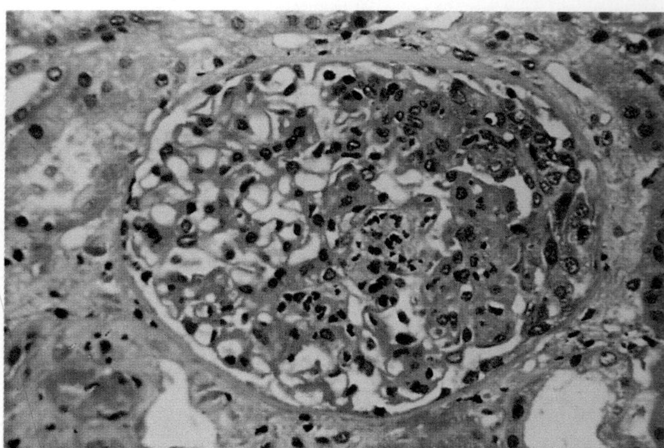

Figure 21–27

Focal glomerulonephritis in lupus erythematosus. There is segmental proliferation of cells and necrosis on the right. In the necrotic area, there are neutrophils and fragmented nuclei (nuclear dust). The remainder of the glomerulus is not involved.

Clinical Course. The disease affects children and young adults. More than half the patients present with gross hematuria after an infection of the respiratory or, less commonly, gastrointestinal or urinary tract; 30% to 40% have only microscopic hematuria, with or without proteinuria, and 5% to 10% develop a typical acute nephritic syndrome. The hematuria typically lasts for several days and then subsides, only to return every few months. The subsequent course is highly variable.[47] Many patients maintain normal renal function for decades. Slow progression to chronic renal failure occurs in 25% to 50% of cases during a period of 20 years. Onset in old age, heavy proteinuria, hypertension, and the extent of glomerulosclerosis on biopsy are clues to an increased risk of progression. Recurrence of IgA deposits in transplanted kidneys occurs in 20% to 60% of grafts; the resulting disease most frequently runs the same indolent, slowly progressive course as that of the primary IgA nephropathy.[47]

Focal Proliferative and Necrotizing Glomerulonephritis (Focal Glomerulonephritis)

Focal glomerulonephritis represents a histologic entity in which glomerular proliferation is restricted to segments of individual glomeruli and commonly involves only a certain proportion of glomeruli. The lesions are predominantly proliferative and should be differentiated from those of focal sclerosis. Focal necrosis and fibrin deposition within the lesions often occur (Fig. 21–27).

Focal glomerulonephritis occurs under three circumstances:

1. It may be an early or mild manifestation of a systemic disease that sometimes involves entire glomeruli; among these are SLE, polyarteritis nodosa, Henoch-Schönlein purpura, Goodpasture syndrome, subacute bacterial endocarditis, and Wegener granulomatosis.
2. It may be a component of a known glomerular disease, such as IgA nephropathy, as discussed earlier.
3. It can occur unrelated to any systemic or other renal disease and constitutes a form of *primary idiopathic focal glomerulonephritis.* It is necessary to exclude all other systemic disorders and IgA nephropathy by clinical and laboratory studies. The clinical manifestations may be mild, characterized by recurrent microscopic or gross hematuria or non-nephrotic proteinuria, but occasional cases present with a nephrotic syndrome.

Hereditary Nephritis

Hereditary nephritis refers to a group of heterogeneous hereditary-familial renal diseases associated primarily with glomerular injury. Two deserve discussion: *Alport syndrome,* because the lesions and genetic defects have been most well studied[48]; and *thin membrane disease*, the most common cause of *benign familial hematuria.*

ALPORT SYNDROME

Alport syndrome is the name usually given to the disease in which nephritis is accompanied by nerve deafness and various eye disorders, including lens dislocation, posterior cataracts, and corneal dystrophy.[49] Males tend to be affected more frequently and more severely than females and are more likely to progress to renal failure. Females, however, are not completely spared. The mode of inheritance is heterogeneous. Most patients have an X-linked dominant pattern, but autosomal recessive and autosomal dominant pedigrees also exist.

MORPHOLOGY. On histologic examination, the glomeruli are always involved. The most common early lesion is segmental proliferation or sclerosis, or both. There is an increase in mesangial matrix and, in some patients, the persistence of fetal-like glomeruli. In some kidneys, glomerular or tubular epithelial cells acquire a foamy appearance owing to accumulation of neutral fats and mucopolysaccharides **(foam cells).** As the disease progresses, there is increasing glomerulosclerosis, vascular narrowing, tubular atrophy, and interstitial fibrosis.

The characteristic findings are seen with the electron microscope and are found in some (but not all) patients with hereditary nephritis. The GBM shows irregular foci of thickening or attenuation (thinning), with pronounced splitting and lamination of the lamina densa (Fig. 21–28). Similar alterations are found in the tubular basement membranes. Although such basement membrane changes may be seen focally in diseases other than hereditary nephritis, they are most widespread and pronounced in patients with this disorder.

Immunohistochemistry is helpful in cases with absent or borderline basement membrane lesions, because antibodies to α_3, α_4, and α_5 collagen fail to stain both glomerular and tubular basement membranes. There is also absence of α_5 staining in skin biopsy specimens.

Pathogenesis. Defective GBM synthesis underlies the renal lesions. In patients with X-linked disease, the defect is caused by *mutations in the gene encoding the α_5 chain of collagen type IV (COL4A5),* a component of GBM[48] (see Fig. 21–3). The mutations are heterogeneous and affect all domains of the α_5 chain. This is thought to interfere with the structure and function of collagen type IV and thus the GBM suprastructure.[48] In addition, probably as a result of this defect, patients synthesize lesser amounts of other collagen components, including the α_3 chain, which as you recall includes the Goodpasture antigen and also the α_4 chain. Indeed, glomeruli lacking the α_3 chain fail to react with anti-GBM antibodies from patients with Goodpasture syndrome. Certain patients with the X-linked form associated with diffuse leiomyomatosis have additional mutations in the α_6 chain of collagen. In the autosomal recessive pedigrees, mutations in the α_3 and α_4 chains have been reported.

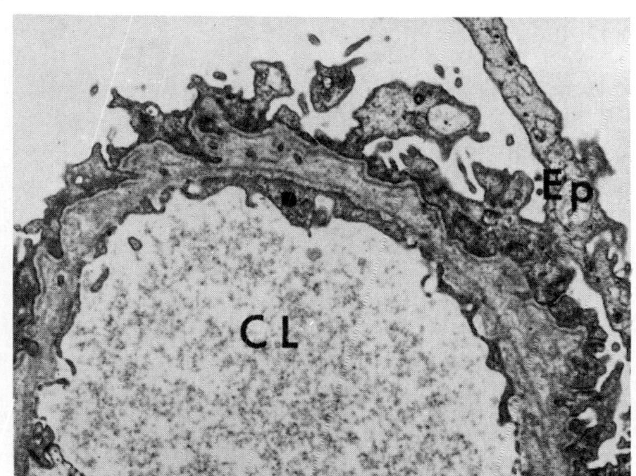

Figure 21–28 ■

Hereditary nephritis. Electron micrograph of glomerulus with irregular thickening of basement membrane, lamination of lamina densa, and foci of rarefaction. Such changes may be present in other diseases but are most pronounced and widespread in hereditary nephritis. CL, capillary lumen; Ep, epithelium.

Clinical Picture. The most common presenting sign is gross or microscopic hematuria, frequently accompanied by erythrocyte casts. Proteinuria may occur and, rarely, the nephrotic syndrome develops. Symptoms appear at ages 5 to 20 years, and the onset of overt renal failure is between ages 20 and 50 years in men. The auditory defects may be subtle, requiring sensitive testing.

THIN MEMBRANE DISEASE (BENIGN FAMILIAL HEMATURIA)

This is a recently appreciated and fairly common entity manifested *clinically by familial asymptomatic hematuria*—usually uncovered on routine urinalysis—*and morphologically by diffuse thinning of the GBM* to between 150 and 225 nm (compared with 300 to 400 nm in normal individuals). Although mild or moderate proteinuria may also be present, renal function is normal and prognosis is virtually uniformly excellent.

The disorder should be differentiated from IgA nephropathy, another common cause of hematuria, and X-linked classical Alport syndrome. Unlike Alport syndrome, hearing loss, ocular abnormalities, and a family history of renal failure are absent and skin biopsy specimens show presence of the α_5 chain of collagen type IV by immunohistochemistry.[48]

The anomaly in thin membrane disease has also been traced in some families to genes encoding α_3 and α_4 chains type IV collagen.[50] Most asymptomatic patients are heterozygous for the defective gene. The disorder in homozygotes resembles autosomal recessive Alport disease, and may progress to renal failure, even in women.

Chronic Glomerulonephritis

Chronic glomerulonephritis is best considered an end-stage pool of glomerular disease fed by a number of streams of specific types of glomerulonephritis, most of which have been described earlier in this chapter[51] (Fig. 21–29). Poststreptococcal glomerulonephritis is a rare antecedent of chronic glomerulonephritis, except in adults. Patients with RPGN, if they survive the acute episode, usually progress to chronic glomerulonephritis. Membranous glomerulonephritis, MPGN, and IgA nephropathy progress more slowly to chronic renal failure, whereas focal sclerosis often advances rapidly into chronic glomerulonephritis. *Nevertheless, in any series of patients with chronic glomerulonephritis, a variable percentage of cases arise mysteriously with no antecedent history of any of the well-recognized forms of early glomerulonephritis.* These cases must represent the end result of relatively asymptomatic

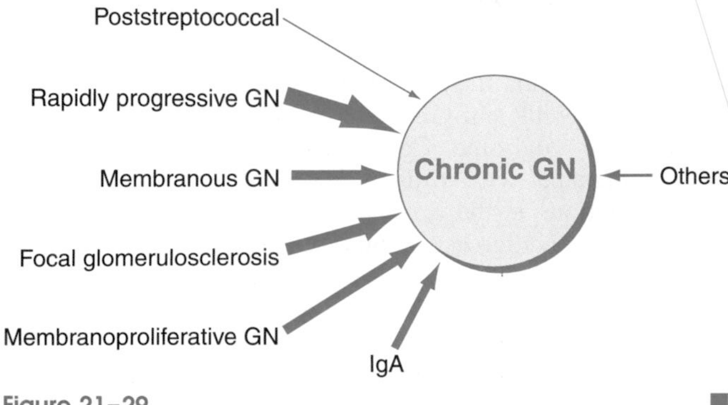

Figure 21–29

Primary glomerular diseases leading to chronic glomerulonephritis (GN). The thickness of the arrows reflects the approximate proportion of patients in each group who progress to chronic glomerulonephritis: poststreptococcal (1% to 2%); rapidly progressive (crescentic) (90%); membranous (50%); focal glomerulosclerosis (50% to 80%); membranoproliferative glomerulonephritis (50%); IgA nephropathy (30% to 50%).

forms of glomerulonephritis, either known or still unrecognized, that progress to uremia. Clearly, the proportion of such unexplained cases depends on the availability of renal biopsy material from patients early in their disease.

MORPHOLOGY. The kidneys are symmetrically contracted and have diffusely granular, cortical surfaces. On section, the cortex is thinned, and there is an increase in peripelvic fat. The glomerular histology depends on the stage of the disease. In early cases, the glomeruli may still show evidence of the primary disease (e.g., membranous glomerulonephritis or MPGN). However, there eventually ensues hyaline obliteration of glomeruli, transforming them into acellular eosinophilic masses. The hyaline represents a combination of trapped plasma proteins, increased mesangial matrix, basement membrane–like material, and collagen (Fig. 21–30). Because hypertension is an accompaniment of chronic glomerulonephritis, arterial and arteriolar sclerosis may be conspicuous. Marked atrophy of associated tubules, irregular interstitial fibrosis, and lymphocytic infiltration also occur.

Dialysis Changes. Kidneys from patients with end-stage disease on long-term dialysis exhibit a variety of changes that are unrelated to the primary disease. These include **arterial intimal thickening** caused by accumulation of smooth muscle–like cells and a loose, proteoglycan-rich stroma; calcification, most obvious in glomerular tufts and tubular basement membranes; **extensive deposition of calcium oxalate crystals** in tubules and interstitium; **acquired cystic disease,** discussed earlier; and increased numbers of renal **adenomas** and borderline **adenocarcinomas.**

Uremic Complications. Patients dying with chronic glomerulonephritis also exhibit pathologic changes **outside** the kidney that are related to the uremic state and are also present in other forms of chronic renal failure. Often clinically important, these include uremic **pericarditis,** uremic **gastroenteritis, secondary hyperparathyroidism** with nephrocalcinosis and renal osteodystrophy, **left ventricular hypertrophy** due to hypertension, and pulmonary changes of diffuse alveolar damage often ascribed to uremia **(uremic pneumonitis).**

Clinical Course. In most patients, chronic glomerulonephritis develops insidiously and slowly progresses to death in uremia during a span of years or possibly decades (see discussion of chronic renal failure). Not infrequently, patients present with such nonspecific complaints as loss of appetite, anemia, vomiting, or weakness. In some, the renal disease is suspected with the discovery of proteinuria, hypertension, or azotemia on routine medical examination. In others, the underlying renal disorder is discovered in the course of investigation of edema. *Most patients are hypertensive, and sometimes the dominant clinical manifestations are cerebral or cardiovascular.* In all, the disease is relentlessly progressive, although at widely varying rates. In nephrotic patients, as glomeruli become obliterated, the protein loss in the urine diminishes. If patients with chronic glomerulonephritis are not maintained with continued dialysis or if they do not receive a renal transplant, the outcome is invariably death.

Table 21–8 summarizes the main clinical and histologic features of the major forms of primary glomerulonephritis.

Glomerular Lesions Associated With Systemic Disease

Many immunologically mediated, metabolic, or hereditary systemic disorders are associated with glomerular injury; in some (e.g., SLE and diabetes mellitus), the glo-

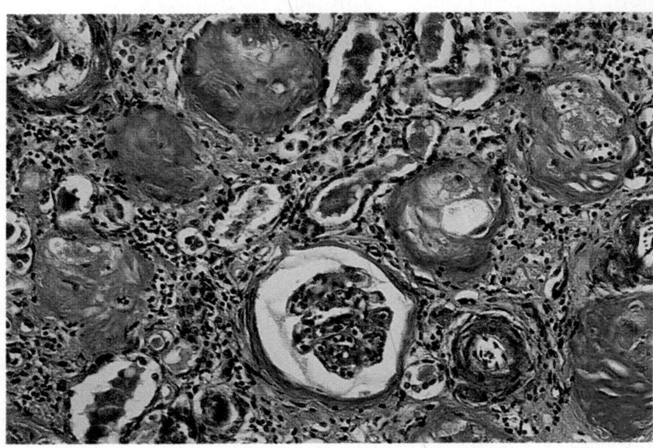

Figure 21–30

Chronic glomerulonephritis. A Masson trichrome preparation shows complete replacement of virtually all glomeruli by blue-staining collagen. (Courtesy of Dr. M.A. Venkatachalam, Department of Pathology, University of Texas Health Sciences Center, San Antonio, TX.)

Table 21–8. SUMMARY OF MAJOR PRIMARY GLOMERULONEPHRITIDES

Disease	Most Frequent Clinical Presentation	Pathogenesis	Glomerular Pathology: Light Microscopy	Glomerular Pathology: Fluorescence Microscopy	Glomerular Pathology: Electron Microscopy
Poststreptococcal glomerulonephritis	Acute nephritis	Antibody mediated; circulating or planted antigen	Diffuse proliferation; leukocytic infiltration	Granular IgG and C3 in GBM and mesangium	Subepithelial humps
Goodpasture syndrome	Rapidly progressive glomerulonephritis	Anti-GBM COL4-A3 antigen	Proliferation; crescents	Linear IgG and C3; fibrin in crescents	No deposits; GBM disruptions; fibrin
Idiopathic RPGN	Rapidly progressive glomerulonephritis	Anti-GBM Immune complex ANCA-associated	Proliferation; focal necrosis; crescents	Linear IgG and C3 Granular Negative or equivocal	No deposits Deposits may be present No deposits
Membranous glomerulonephritis	Nephrotic syndrome	In situ antibody-mediated antigen: megalin complex	Diffuse capillary wall thickening	Granular IgG and C3; diffuse	Subepithelial deposits
Lipoid nephrosis	Nephrotic syndrome	Unknown, loss of glomerular polyanion	Normal; lipid in tubules	Negative	Loss of foot processes; no deposits
Focal segmental glomerulosclerosis	Nephrotic syndrome; non-nephrotic proteinuria	Unknown Ablation nephropathy ?Plasma factor	Focal and segmental sclerosis and hyalinosis	Focal; IgM and C3	Loss of foot processes; epithelial denudation
Membranoproliferative glomerulonephritis Type I	Nephrotic syndrome	(I) Immune complex	Mesangial proliferation; basement membrane thickening; splitting	(I) IgG + C3; C1 + C4	(I) Subendothelial deposits
Type II	Hematuria Chronic renal failure	(II) Autoantibody: alternative complement pathway		(II) C3 ± IgG; no C1 or C4	(II) Dense-deposit disease
IgA nephropathy	Recurrent hematuria or proteinuria	Unknown; see text	Focal proliferative glomerulonephritis; mesangial widening	IgA + IgG, IgM, and C3 in mesangium	Mesangial and paramesangial dense deposits
Chronic glomerulonephritis	Chronic renal failure	Variable	Hyalinized glomeruli	Granular or negative	

ANCA, antineutrophil cytoplasmic antibody; GBM, glomerular basement membrane; RPGN, rapidly progressive glomerulonephritis.

merular involvement is a major clinical manifestation. Most of these diseases have been discussed elsewhere in this book. Here we briefly recall some of the lesions and discuss only those not considered in other sections.

SYSTEMIC LUPUS ERYTHEMATOSUS

The various types of lupus nephritis are described and illustrated in Chapter 7. As discussed, SLE gives rise to a heterogeneous group of lesions and clinical presentations. The clinical manifestations include recurrent microscopic or gross hematuria, acute nephritis, the nephrotic syndrome, chronic renal failure, and hypertension. Glomerular changes are classified histologically into *mesangial lupus nephritis, focal glomerulonephritis, diffuse proliferative glomerulonephritis, and diffuse membranous glomerulonephritis.*

HENOCH-SCHÖNLEIN PURPURA

This syndrome consists of *purpuric skin lesions characteristically involving the extensor surfaces of arms and legs as well as buttocks; abdominal manifestations including pain, vomiting, and intestinal bleeding; nonmigratory arthralgia; and renal abnormalities.* The renal manifestations occur in one third of patients and include gross or microscopic hematuria, proteinuria, and nephrotic syndrome. A small number of patients, mostly adults, develop a rapidly progressive form of glomerulonephritis with many crescents. Not all components of the syndrome need to be present, and individual patients may have purpura, abdominal pain, or urinary abnormalities as the dominant feature. The disease is most common in children 3 to 8 years old, but it also occurs in adults, in whom the renal manifestations are usually more severe.[51a] There is a strong background of atopy in about one third of patients, and onset often follows an upper respiratory infection. IgA is deposited in the glomerular mesangium in a distribution similar to that of IgA nephropathy. This has led to the notion that *IgA nephropathy and Henoch-Schönlein purpura are spectra of the same disease.*

MORPHOLOGY. On histologic examination, the renal lesions vary from mild focal mesangial proliferation to diffuse mesangial proliferation to relatively typical crescentic glomerulonephritis.

Whatever the histologic lesions, the prominent feature by fluorescence microscopy is the **deposition of IgA, sometimes with IgG and C3 in the mesangial region.** The skin lesions consist of subepidermal hemorrhages and a necrotizing vasculitis involving the small vessels of the dermis. IgA is also present in such vessels. Vasculitis can also occur in other organs, such as the gastrointestinal tract, but is rare in the kidney.

The course of the disease is variable, but recurrences of hematuria may persist for many years after onset. Most children have an excellent prognosis. Patients with the more diffuse lesions or with the nephrotic syndrome have a somewhat poorer prognosis, and renal failure occurs in those with the crescentic lesions.

BACTERIAL ENDOCARDITIS

Glomerular lesions occurring in the course of bacterial endocarditis represent a type of immune complex nephritis initiated by bacterial antigen-antibody complexes. Hematuria and proteinuria of various degrees characterize this entity clinically, but an acute nephritic presentation is not uncommon, and even RPGN may occur in rare instances. The histologic lesions, when present, generally reflect these clinical manifestations. Milder forms have a focal and segmental necrotizing glomerulonephritis, whereas more severe ones exhibit a diffuse proliferative glomerulonephritis, and the rapidly progressive forms show large numbers of crescents.

DIABETIC GLOMERULOSCLEROSIS (see also Chapter 20)

Diabetes mellitus is a major cause of renal morbidity and mortality, and diabetic nephropathy is one of the leading causes of chronic kidney failure in the United States. End-stage kidney disease occurs in as many as 30% of insulin-dependent type I diabetics and accounts for 20% of deaths in patients younger than 40 years. By far the most common lesions involve the glomeruli and are associated clinically with three glomerular syndromes, including non-nephrotic proteinuria, nephrotic syndrome, and chronic renal failure.[52] However, diabetes also affects the arterioles, causing *arteriolar sclerosis;* increases susceptibility to the development of pyelonephritis, and particularly *papillary necrosis;* and causes a variety of tubular lesions. The term *diabetic nephropathy* is applied to the conglomerate of lesions that often occur concurrently in the diabetic kidney.

Proteinuria, sometimes in the nephrotic range, occurs in about 50% of both type 1 and type 2 diabetics. It is usually discovered 12 to 22 years after the clinical appearance of diabetes and (particularly in type 1 diabetics) often heralds the progressive development of chronic renal failure ending in death or end-stage disease within a period of 4 to 5 years. The morphologic changes in the glomeruli include (1) capillary basement membrane thickening, (2) diffuse diabetic glomerulosclerosis, and (3) nodular glomerulosclerosis.

Pathogenesis. The pathogenesis of diabetic glomerulosclerosis is intimately linked with that of generalized diabetic microangiopathy, discussed in Chapter 20. The principal points are as follows.[53, 54]

1. The bulk of the evidence suggests that diabetic glomerulosclerosis *is caused by the metabolic defect,* that is, the insulin deficiency, or the resultant hyperglycemia, or some other aspects of glucose intolerance.
2. Biochemical alterations in diabetic GBM are significant and include increased amount and synthesis of collagen type IV and fibronectin and decreased synthesis of proteoglycan heparan sulfate.
3. *Nonenzymatic glycosylation* of proteins, known to occur in diabetics and giving rise to advanced glycosylation end products, may contribute to the glomerulopathy. The mechanisms by which advanced glycosylation end products cause their effects are discussed in Chapter 20 (see Table 20–6).
4. One hypothesis implicates *hemodynamic changes* in the initiation or progression of diabetic glomerulosclerosis. It is well known that early-onset type I diabetics have an increased GFR, increased glomerular filtration area, increased glomerular capillary pressure, and *glomerular hypertrophy.* Hemodynamic alterations and glomerular hypertrophy also occur in experimental streptozotocin-induced diabetes in rats, in which they are associated with proteinuria and can be reversed by diabetic control. It has been speculated that the subsequent morphologic alterations in the mesangium are somehow influenced by the glomerular hypertrophy and hemodynamic changes, akin to the adaptive responses to ablation of renal mass, discussed earlier.

To sum up, two processes seem to play a role in the fully developed diabetic glomerular lesions: a metabolic defect, possibly linked to advanced glycosylation end products, that accounts for the thickened GBM and increased mesangial matrix that occur in *all* patients; and hemodynamic effects, associated with glomerular hypertrophy, which leads to glomerulosclerosis in about 40% of patients.

MORPHOLOGY

Capillary Basement Membrane Thickening. Widespread thickening of the glomerular capillary basement membrane (GBM) occurs in virtually all diabetics, irrespective of the presence of proteinuria, and is part and parcel of the diabetic microangiopathy. Pure capillary basement membrane thickening can be detected only by electron microscopy. Careful morphometric studies demonstrate that this thickening begins as early as 2 years after the onset of type I diabetes and by 5 years amounts to about a 30% increase.[41] The thickening continues progressively and usually concurrently with mesangial widening (Fig. 21–31). Simultaneously there is thickening of the tubular basement membranes.

Diffuse Glomerulosclerosis. This consists of diffuse increase in mesangial matrix, with mild prolifera-

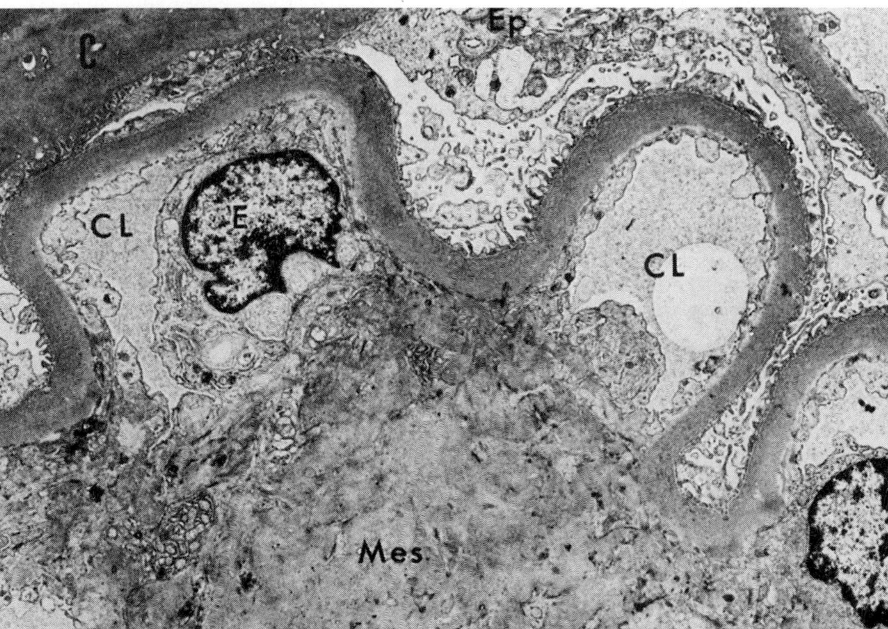

Figure 21–31

Electron micrograph of advanced diabetic glomerulosclerosis. Note massive increase in mesangial matrix (Mes) encroaching on glomerular capillary lumena (CL). GBM and Bowman capsule (C) are markedly thickened. Ep, epithelium; E, endothelium.

tion of mesangial cells, and is always associated with the overall thickening of the GBM. The increase in mesangial volume appears to lag slightly behind basement membrane widening but becomes pronounced after 10 to 20 years of diabetes. The matrix depositions are PAS positive. The changes almost always begin in the vascular stalk and sometimes seem continuous with the invariably present hyaline thickening of arterioles (Fig. 21–32). As the disease progresses, the mesangial areas expand further and obliterate the mesangial cells, gradually filling the entire glomerulus **(obliterative diabetic glomerulosclerosis).**

Nodular Glomerulosclerosis. This is also known as **intercapillary glomerulosclerosis or Kimmelstiel-Wilson disease.** The glomerular lesions take the form of ovoid or spherical, often laminated, hyaline masses situated in the periphery of the glomerulus. They lie within the mesangial core of the glomerular lobules and often are surrounded by peripheral patent capillary loops (Fig. 21–32). Usually, not all the lobules in the individual glomerulus are involved. **Uninvolved lobules and glomeruli all show striking diffuse glomerulosclerosis.** The nodules are PAS positive and contain lipids and fibrin. As the disease advances, the individual nodules enlarge and eventually compress and engulf capillaries, obliterating the glomerular tuft. As a consequence of the glomerular and arteriolar lesions, the kidney suffers from ischemia, develops tubular atrophy and interstitial fibrosis, and usually undergoes overall contraction in size.

Nodular glomerulosclerosis and the diffuse lesion are fundamentally similar lesions of the mesangium. The nodular lesion, however, is virtually pathognomonic of diabetes, so long as care is taken to exclude membranoproliferative (lobular) glomerulonephritis, the glomerulonephritis associated with light-chain disease, and amyloidosis. Approximately 15% to 30% of long-term patients with diabetes develop nodular glomerulosclerosis, and in most instances it is associated with renal failure.

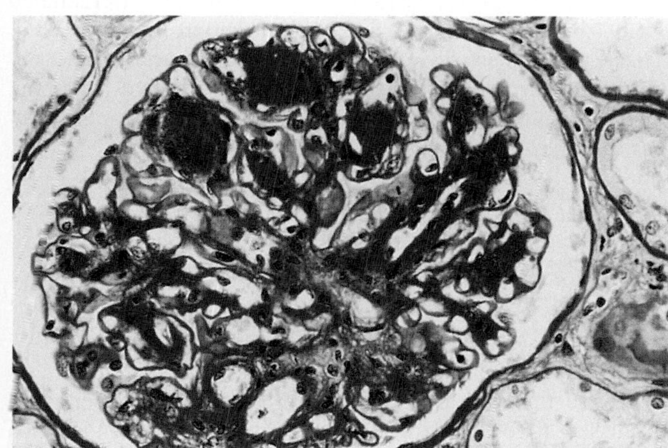

Figure 21–32

Diffuse and nodular diabetic glomerulosclerosis (PAS stain). Note diffuse increase in mesangial matrix and characteristic acellular PAS-positive nodules.

Clinical Course. The clinical manifestations of diabetic glomerulosclerosis are linked to those of diabetes. The increased GFR typical of early-onset type 1 diabetics is associated with *microalbuminuria,* defined as urinary albumin excretion of 30 to 300 mg/day of albumin. Microalbuminuria and increased GFR are important predictors of future overt diabetic nephropathy in these patients. Overt proteinuria then develops, which may be mild and asymptomatic initially but gradually increases to nephrotic levels in some patients. This is followed by progressive loss of GFR, leading to end-stage renal failure within a period of 5 years.

Systemic hypertension may precede the development of proteinuria and renal insufficiency. Indeed, the risk of renal disease in type 1 diabetics is associated with a genetic predisposition to hypertension, possibly related to polymorphisms in the genes encoding proteins of the renin-angiotensin system (Chapter 12). Hypertension in turn increases the susceptibility to developing diabetic nephropathy in the presence of poor hyperglycemic control.

Although the prevalence of proteinuria is comparable in type 1 and type 2 diabetics, the lesions are more heterogeneous and less predictable in type 2 diabetics.[55] Indeed, 20% to 50% of type 2 patients undergoing renal biopsy have other glomerular diseases (e.g., membranous glomerulonephritis). End-stage renal disease results in only 10% to 20% of patients with type 2 diabetes.

At present, most patients with end-stage diabetic nephropathy are maintained on long-term dialysis, and a few receive renal transplantation. Diabetic lesions may recur in the renal allografts. Precise control of the blood glucose level in diabetes has now been shown by several studies to delay or prevent the progression of glomerulopathy. Similarly, inhibition of angiotensin by converting enzyme inhibitors (captopril) has a beneficial effect on progression, possibly by reversing the increased intraglomerular capillary pressure.

AMYLOIDOSIS

The various forms of amyloidosis and their pathogenesis are discussed in Chapter 7. Most types of disseminated amyloidosis may be associated with deposits of amyloid within the glomeruli. The typical Congo red amyloid-positive fibrillary deposits are present within the mesangium and subendothelium and occasionally within the subepithelial space. Eventually, they obliterate the glomerulus completely. Recall that deposits of amyloid also appear in blood vessel walls and in the kidney interstitium. Patients with glomerular amyloid may present with heavy proteinuria or the nephrotic syndrome and later, owing to destruction of the glomeruli, die in uremia. Characteristically, kidney size tends to be either normal or slightly enlarged.

FIBRILLARY AND IMMUNOTACTOID GLOMERULONEPHRITIS

Fibrillary glomerulonephritis is a morphologic variant of glomerulonephritis associated with relatively characteristic fibrillar deposits in the mesangium and glomerular capillary that differ from amyloid fibrils both ultrastructurally and in that they do not stain with Congo red. The fibrils are 20 to 30 nm in diameter, rather than the 10 nm characteristic of amyloid. The glomerular lesions are membranoproliferative by light microscopy, and by immunofluorescence microscopy there is selective deposition of IgG4, with complement C3, and κ and λ light chains. Clinically, patients develop nephrotic syndrome, hematuria, and progressive renal insufficiency.

In *immunotactoid glomerulopathy*, a much rarer condition, the deposits are microtubular in structure and 30 to 50 nm in width. Patients often have circulating paraproteins and monoclonal immunoglobulin deposition in glomeruli.[56]

The precise nature and pathogenesis of both of these entities are unknown.

OTHER SYSTEMIC DISORDERS

Goodpasture syndrome (Chapter 16), *microscopic polyarteritis* and *Wegener granulomatosis* (Chapter 12) are commonly associated with glomerular lesions, as described in the discussion of these diseases. Suffice it to say here that the glomerular lesions in these three conditions can be similar. In the early or mild forms of involvement, there is focal and segmental, sometimes necrotizing, glomerulonephritis, and most of these patients will have hematuria with mild decline in GFR. In the more severe cases associated with RPGN, there is also extensive necrosis, fibrin deposition, and the formation of epithelial crescents.

Essential mixed cryoglobulinemia is another rare systemic condition in which deposits of cryoglobulins composed principally of IgG-IgM complexes induce cutaneous vasculitis, synovitis, and focal or diffuse proliferative glomerulonephritis. Cryoglobulinemia secondary to infection (e.g., hepatitis C) may be associated with glomerulonephritis, usually of the MPGN type.

Plasma cell dyscrasias may also induce glomerular lesions. *Multiple myeloma* is associated with (1) amyloidosis, (2) deposition of monoclonal cryoglobulins in glomeruli, and (3) peculiar nodular glomerular lesions, ascribed to the deposition of *nonfibrillar* light chains. This so-called *light-chain glomerulopathy* sometimes occurs in the absence of overt myeloma, usually associated with deposition of κ chains in glomeruli. The glomeruli show PAS-positive mesangial nodules, lobular accentuation, and mild mesangial hypercellularity, lesions that need to be differentiated from diabetic nodules and membranoproliferative GN. These patients usually present with proteinuria or the nephrotic syndrome, hypertension, and progressive azotemia. Other renal manifestations of multiple myeloma are discussed later.

DISEASES AFFECTING TUBULES AND INTERSTITIUM

Most forms of tubular injury involve the interstitium as well, and thus diseases affecting these two components are discussed together. Under this heading, we consider two major groups of processes: (1) ischemic or toxic tubular injury, leading to *acute tubular necrosis (ATN)* and acute renal failure, and (2) inflammatory reactions of the tubules and interstitium *(tubulointerstitial nephritis).*

Acute Tubular Necrosis

ATN is a clinicopathologic entity characterized morphologically by destruction of tubular epithelial cells and clinically by acute suppression of renal function. It is the most common cause of acute renal failure,[56a] which signifies acute suppression of renal function and urine flow, falling within 24 hours to less than 400 ml. It can be caused by a variety of conditions including:

1. *Organic vascular obstruction,* caused by diffuse involvement of the intrarenal vessels, such as in polyarteritis nodosa and malignant hypertension, and the hemolytic-uremic syndrome
2. *Severe glomerular disease,* such as RPGN
3. *Acute tubulointerstitial nephritis,* most commonly occurring as a hypersensitivity to drugs
4. *Massive infection* (pyelonephritis), especially when it is accompanied by papillary necrosis
5. *Disseminated intravascular coagulation*
6. *Urinary obstruction* by tumors, prostatic hypertrophy, or blood clots (so-called postrenal acute renal failure)
7. *Acute tubular necrosis* (ATN)

Here we discuss ATN, the major cause of acute renal failure, accounting for some 50% of cases in hospitalized patients. The other causes of acute renal failure are discussed elsewhere in this chapter.

ATN is a reversible renal lesion that arises in a variety of clinical settings. Most of these, ranging from severe trauma to acute pancreatitis, have in common a period of inadequate blood flow to the peripheral organs, usually accompanied by marked hypotension and shock. This pattern of ATN is called *ischemic ATN.* Mismatched blood transfusions and other hemolytic crises causing *hemoglobinuria,* and skeletal muscle injuries causing *myoglobinuria,* also produce a picture resembling ischemic ATN. The second pattern, called *nephrotoxic ATN,* is caused by a multitude of drugs, such as gentamicin and other antibiotics; radiographic contrast agents; poisons, including heavy metals (e.g., mercury); and organic solvents (e.g., carbon tetrachloride). In addition to its frequency, the potential reversibility of ATN adds to its clinical importance. Proper management means the difference between full recovery and death.

Pathogenesis. The critical events in both ischemic and nephrotoxic ATN are believed to be (1) tubular injury and (2) persistent and severe disturbances in blood flow[57] (Fig. 21–33).

- *Tubule cell injury:* Tubular epithelial cells are particularly sensitive to ischemia and are also vulnerable to toxins. Several factors predispose the tubules to toxic injury, including a vast electrically charged surface for tubular reabsorption, active transport systems for ions and organic acids, and the capability for effective concentration.

  Ischemia causes numerous structural and functional alterations in epithelial cells, as discussed in Chapter 1. The structural changes include those of reversible injury (such as cellular swelling, loss of brush border, blebbing, loss of polarity, and cell detachment) and those associated with lethal injury (necrosis and apoptosis). Biochemically, there is depletion of adenosine triphosphate; accumulation of intracellular calcium; activation of proteases (e.g., calpain), which cause cytoskeletal rearrangement, and phospholipases, which damage mem-

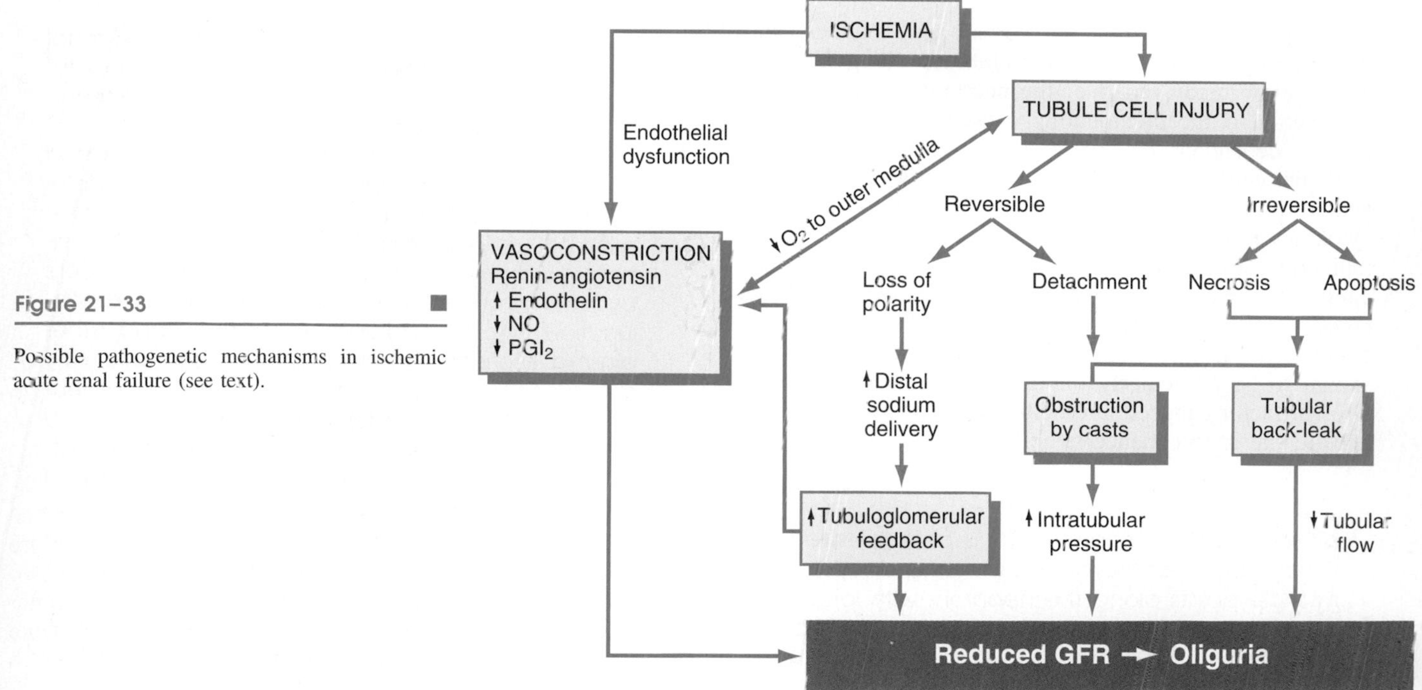

Figure 21–33 ■

Possible pathogenetic mechanisms in ischemic acute renal failure (see text).

branes; generation of reactive oxygen species; and activation of caspases, which induce apoptotic cell death. One early reversible result of ischemia is *loss of cell polarity* due to redistribution of membrane proteins (e.g., the enzyme Na^+,K^+-ATPase) from the basolateral to the luminal surface of the tubular cells, resulting in abnormal ion transport across the cells, and *increased sodium delivery to distal tubules.* The latter results in *tubuloglomerular feedback,* which, as will be described, incites vasoconstriction.[58] In addition, ischemic tubular cells express cytokines and adhesion molecules (such as ICAM-1), thus recruiting leukocytes that appear to participate in the subsequent injury.[59] In time, detached injured cells cause *luminal tubule obstruction,* increase intratubular pressure, and decrease the GFR. In addition, fluid from the damaged tubules could leak into the interstitium, resulting in increased interstitial pressure and collapse of the tubule. All these effects, as shown in Fig. 21–33 contribute to the decreased GFR.

- *Disturbances in blood flow:* Ischemic renal injury is also characterized by *hemodynamic alterations* that cause reduced GFR. The major one is *intrarenal vasoconstriction,* which results in both reduced glomerular plasma flow and reduced oxygen delivery to the functionally important tubules in the outer medulla (thick ascending limb and straight segment of the proximal tubule). A number of vasoconstrictor pathways have been implicated, including the renin-angiotensin mechanism, stimulated by increased distal sodium delivery (*glomerulotubular feedback*), and *sublethal endothelial injury,* leading to increased release of the endothelial vasoconstrictor *endothelin* and decreased production of the vasodilator *nitric oxide* and PGI_2. Finally, there is also some evidence of a direct effect of ischemia or toxins on the glomerulus, causing a reduced glomerular ultrafiltration coefficient, possibly due to mesangial contraction.

The patchiness of tubular necrosis and maintenance of the integrity of the basement membrane along many segments allow ready repair of the necrotic foci and recovery of function if the precipitating cause is removed. This repair is dependent on the capacity of *reversibly* injured epithelial cells to proliferate and differentiate. Re-epithelialization is mediated by a variety of growth factors and cytokines produced locally by the tubular cells themselves (autocrine stimulation) or by inflammatory cells in the vicinity of necrotic foci (paracrine stimulation).[60] Of these, epidermal growth factor (EGF), TGF-α, insulin-like growth factor type I, and hepatocyte growth factor have been shown to be particularly important in renal tubular repair. Growth factors, indeed, are being explored as possible therapeutic agents to enhance re-epithelialization in ATN.[60]

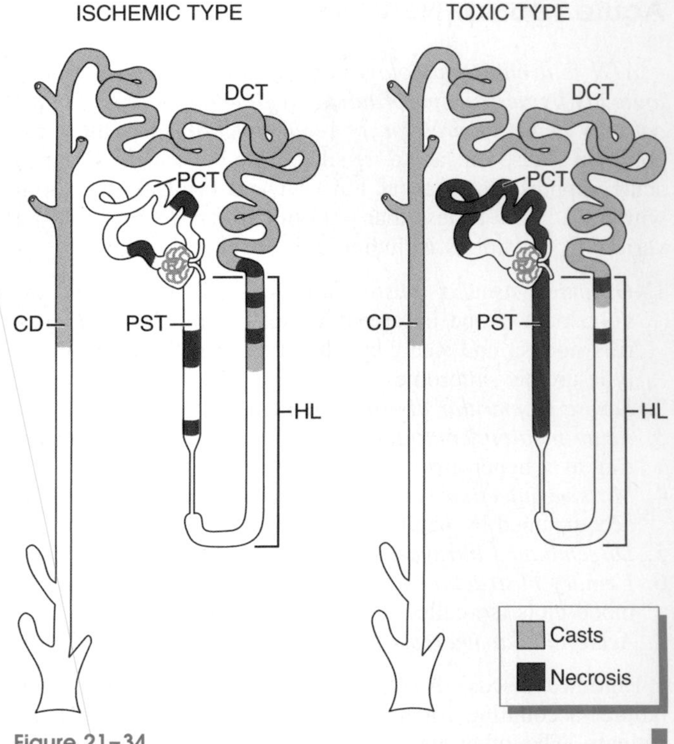

Figure 21–34

Patterns of tubular damage in ischemic and toxic acute tubular necrosis. In ischemic type, tubular necrosis is patchy, relatively short lengths of tubules are affected, and straight segments of proximal tubules (PST) and ascending limbs of Henle's loop (HL) are most vulnerable. In toxic acute tubular necrosis, extensive necrosis is present along proximal tubule segments (PCT) with many toxins (e.g., mercury), but necrosis of the distal tubule, particularly ascending Henle's loop, also occurs. In both types, lumens of distal convoluted tubules (DCT) and collecting ducts (CD) contain casts.

MORPHOLOGY. Ischemic ATN is characterized by focal tubular epithelial necrosis and apoptosis at multiple points along the nephron, with large skip areas in between, often accompanied by rupture of basement membranes (tubulorrhexis) and occlusion of tubular lumens by casts[61] (Figs. 21–34 and 21–35). The straight portion of the proximal tubule and the ascending thick limb in the renal medulla are especially vulnerable, but focal lesions may also occur in the distal tubule, often in conjunction with casts.

Eosinophilic hyaline casts, as well as pigmented granular casts, are common, particularly in distal tubules and collecting ducts. These casts consist principally of Tamm-Horsfall protein (a specific urinary glycoprotein normally secreted by the cells of ascending thick limb and distal tubules) in conjunction with hemoglobin, myoglobin, and other plasma proteins. Other findings in ischemic ATN are interstitial edema and accumulations of leukocytes within dilated vasa recta. There is also often evidence of epithelial regeneration: flattened epithelial cells with hyperchromatic nuclei and mitotic figures are often present. In the course of time, this regeneration repopulates the tubules so that if survival occurs, no residual evidence of damage can be seen.

Toxic ATN is manifested by acute tubular injury, most obvious in the proximal convoluted tubules (see Fig. 21–34). On histologic examination, the tubular necrosis may be entirely nonspecific but is

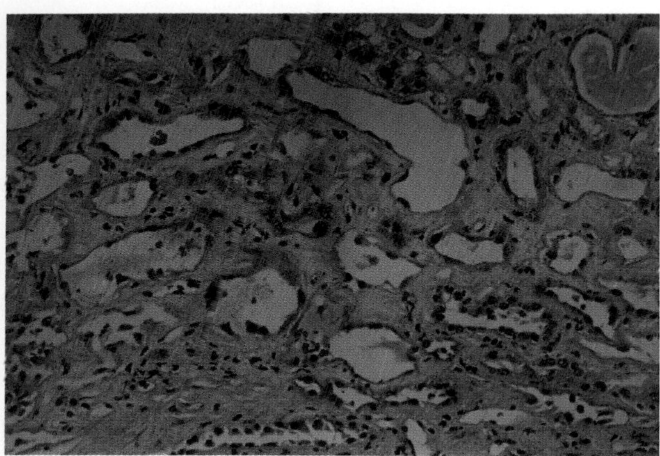

Figure 21–35 ■

Ischemic acute tubular necrosis. Some of the tubular epithelial cells in affected tubules are necrotic, whereas others are flattened, stretched out, and regenerating.

somewhat distinctive in poisoning with certain agents. With mercuric chloride, for example, severely injured cells not yet dead may contain large acidophilic inclusions. Later, these cells become totally necrotic, are desquamated into the lumen, and may undergo calcification. Carbon tetrachloride poisoning, in contrast, is characterized by the accumulation of neutral lipids in injured cells, but again, such fatty change is followed by necrosis. Ethylene glycol produces marked ballooning and hydropic or vacuolar degeneration of proximal convoluted tubules. Calcium oxalate crystals are often found in the tubular lumens in such poisoning.

Clinical Course. The clinical course of ATN is highly variable, but the classic case may be divided into *initiating, maintenance,* and *recovery* stages. The *initiating phase,* lasting for about 36 hours, is dominated by the inciting medical, surgical, or obstetric event in the ischemic form of ATN. The only indication of renal involvement is a slight decline in urine output with a rise in BUN. At this point, oliguria could be explained on the basis of a transient decrease in blood flow to the kidneys.

The *maintenance stage* is characterized by sustained decreases in urine output to between 40 and 400 ml/day (oliguria), with salt and water overload, rising BUN concentrations, hyperkalemia, metabolic acidosis, and other manifestations of uremia dominating this phase. With appropriate attention to the balance of water and blood electrolytes, including dialysis, the patient can be carried over this oliguric crisis.

The *recovery phase* is ushered in by a steady increase in urine volume that may reach up to 3 liters/day. The tubules are still damaged, so that large amounts of water, sodium, and potassium are lost in the urinary flood. *Hypokalemia, rather than hyperkalemia, becomes a clinical problem.* There is a peculiar increased vulnerability to infection at this stage. Eventually, renal tubular function is restored, with improvement in concentrating ability. At the same time, BUN and creatinine levels begin to return to normal. Subtle tubular functional impairment may persist for months, but most patients who reach this phase eventually recover completely.

The prognosis of ATN depends on the clinical setting surrounding its development. Recovery is expected with nephrotoxic ATN when the toxin has not caused serious damage to other organs, such as the liver or heart. With modern methods of care, 95% of those who do not succumb to the precipitating cause have a chance of recovery. Conversely, in shock related to sepsis or extensive burns, the mortality rate may rise to more than 50%.

Up to 50% of patients with ATN may not have oliguria and may in fact have increased urine volumes. This so-called *nonoliguric ATN* occurs particularly often with nephrotoxins, and generally it tends to follow a more benign clinical course.

Tubulointerstitial Nephritis

This group of renal diseases is characterized by histologic and functional alterations that involve predominantly the tubules and interstitium.[62, 62a] We have previously seen that chronic tubulointerstitial injury may occur in primarily glomerular diseases (see Fig. 21–15) and indeed that such injury may be an important cause of progression in these diseases. This *secondary tubulointerstitial nephritis* is also present in a variety of vascular, cystic (polycystic kidney disease), metabolic (diabetes), and renal disorders, in which it may also contribute to progressive damage. Here we discuss disorders in which tubulointerstitial injury appears to be a primary event. *These disorders have diverse causes and different pathogenetic mechanisms* (Table 21–9). Thus, the disorders are identified by cause or by associated disease (e.g., analgesic nephritis, irradiation nephritis). Glomerular and vascular abnormalities may also be present but either are mild or occur only in advanced stages of these diseases.

Tubulointerstitial nephritis can be acute or chronic. Acute tubulointerstitial nephritis has an acute clinical onset and is characterized histologically by interstitial edema, often accompanied by leukocytic infiltration and focal tubular necrosis. In *chronic interstitial nephritis,* there is infiltration with mononuclear cells, prominent interstitial fibrosis, and widespread tubular atrophy.

These conditions are clinically distinguished from the glomerular diseases by the absence, in early stages, of such hallmarks of glomerular injury as nephritic or nephrotic syndromes and by the presence of defects in tubular function. The latter may be subtle and include impaired ability to concentrate urine, evidenced clinically by polyuria or nocturia; salt wasting; diminished ability to excrete acids (metabolic acidosis); and isolated defects in tubular reabsorption or secretion. The advanced forms, however, may be difficult to distinguish clinically from other causes of renal insufficiency.

Some of the specific conditions listed in Table 21–9 are discussed elsewhere in this book. In this section, we deal

Table 21–9. TUBULOINTERSTITIAL NEPHRITIS

Infections
Acute bacterial pyelonephritis
Chronic pyelonephritis (including reflux nephropathy)
Other infections (e.g., viruses, parasites)

Toxins
Drugs
Acute hypersensitivity interstitial nephritis
Analgesic nephritis
Heavy metals
Lead, cadmium

Metabolic Diseases
Urate nephropathy
Nephrocalcinosis (hypercalcemic nephropathy)
Hypokalemic nephropathy
Oxalate nephropathy

Physical Factors
Chronic urinary tract obstruction
Radiation nephritis

Neoplasms
Multiple myeloma

Immunologic Reactions
Transplant rejection
Sjögren syndrome

Vascular Diseases

Miscellaneous
Balkan nephropathy
Nephronophthisis–medullary cystic disease complex
Other rare causes (sarcoidosis)
"Idiopathic" interstitial nephritis

principally with pyelonephritis and interstitial diseases induced by drugs.

PYELONEPHRITIS AND URINARY TRACT INFECTION

Pyelonephritis is a renal disorder affecting tubules, interstitium, and renal pelvis and is one of the most common diseases of the kidney. It occurs in two forms. *Acute pyelonephritis* is caused by bacterial infection and is the renal lesion associated with urinary tract infection. *Chronic pyelonephritis* is a more complex disorder: bacterial infection plays a dominant role, but other factors (vesicoureteral reflux, obstruction) are involved in its pathogenesis. Pyelonephritis is a serious complication of an extremely common clinical spectrum of *urinary tract infections* that affect the urinary bladder (cystitis) or the kidneys and their collecting systems (pyelonephritis), or both. Bacterial infection of the urinary tract may be completely asymptomatic (asymptomatic bacteriuria) and most often remains localized to the bladder without the development of renal infection. However, urinary tract infection always carries the potential of spread to the kidney.

Etiology and Pathogenesis.[63] The dominant etiologic agents, accounting for more than 85% of cases of urinary tract infection, are the gram-negative bacilli that are normal inhabitants of the intestinal tract. By far the most common is *Escherichia coli,* followed by *Proteus, Klebsiella,* and *Enterobacter. Streptococcus faecalis,* also of enteric origin, staphylococci, and virtually every other bacterial and fungal agent can also cause lower urinary tract and renal infection.

In most patients with urinary tract infection, the infecting organisms are derived from the patient's own fecal flora. This is thus a form of *endogenous infection.* There are two routes by which bacteria can reach the kidneys: (1) through the bloodstream (hematogenous infection) and (2) from the lower urinary tract (ascending infection) (Fig. 21–36). Although the hematogenous route is the less common of the two, acute pyelonephritis does result from seeding of the kidneys by bacteria from distant foci in the course of

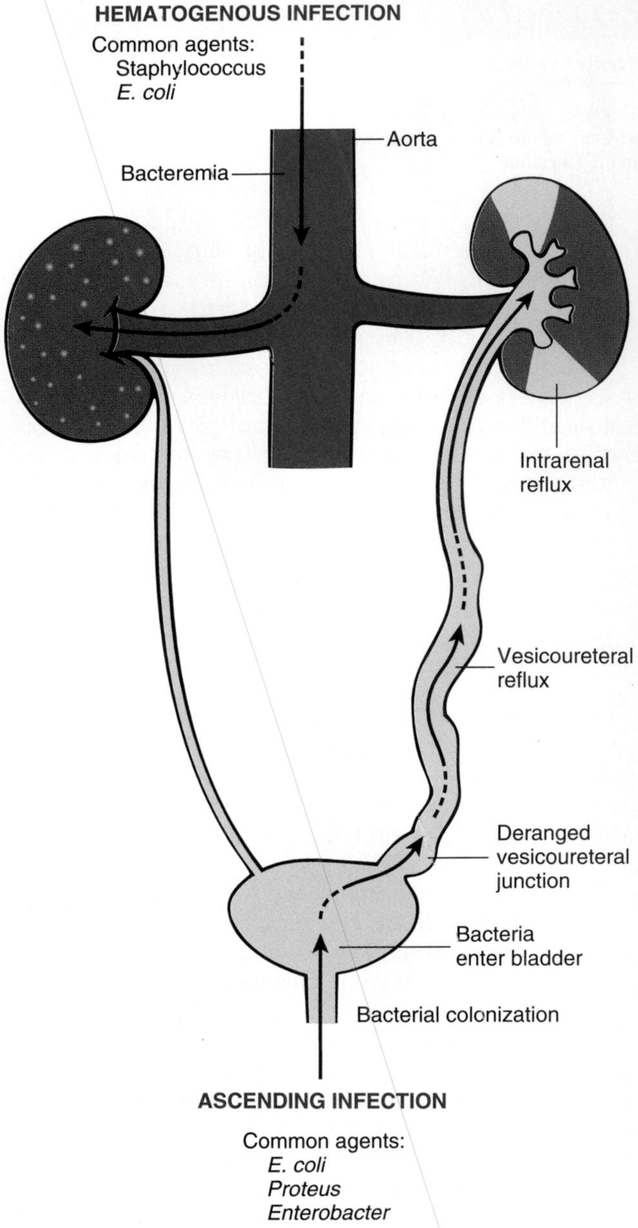

Figure 21–36

Schematic representation of pathways of renal infection. Hematogenous infection results from bacteremic spread. More common is ascending infection, which results from a combination of urinary bladder infection, vesicoureteral reflux, and intrarenal reflux.

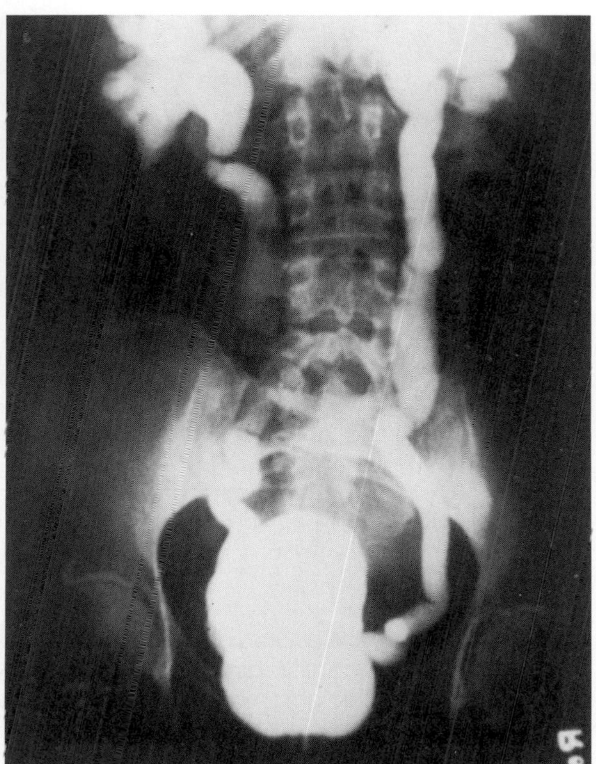

Figure 21–37

Vesicoureteral reflux demonstrated by a voiding cystourethrogram. Dye injected into the bladder refluxes into both dilated ureters, filling the pelvis and calcyes.

septicemia or infective endocarditis. Hematogenous infection is more likely to occur in the presence of ureteral obstruction, in debilitated patients, in patients receiving immunosuppressive therapy, and with nonenteric organisms, such as staphylococci and certain fungi.

Ascending infection is the most common cause of clinical pyelonephritis. Normal human bladder and bladder urine are sterile, and thus a number of steps must occur for renal infection to occur. The first step in the pathogenesis of ascending infection appears to be the *colonization of the distal urethra and introitus* (in the female) by coliform bacteria. This colonization is influenced by the ability of bacteria to adhere to urethral mucosal cells. Such bacterial adherence, as discussed in Chapter 9, involves adhesive molecules (adhesins) on the P-fimbriae (pili) of bacteria that interact with receptors on the surface of uroepithelial cells. Specific adhesins (e.g., the *pap* variant) are associated with infection. In addition, certain types of fimbriae promote renal tropism, or persistence of infection, or an enhanced inflammatory response to bacteria.[64]

- *From the urethra to the bladder,* organisms gain entrance during urethral catheterization or other instrumentation. Long-term catheterization, in particular, carries a risk of infection. In the absence of instrumentation, *urinary infections are much more common in females,* and this has been variously ascribed to the shorter urethra in females, the absence of antibacterial properties such as are found in prostatic fluid, hormonal changes affecting adherence of bacteria to the mucosa, and urethral trauma during sexual intercourse or a combination of these factors.[65]
- *Multiplication in the bladder.* Ordinarily, organisms introduced into the bladder are cleared by the continual flushing of voiding and by antibacterial mechanisms. However, outflow obstruction or bladder dysfunction results in incomplete emptying and increased residual volume of urine. In the presence of stasis, bacteria introduced into the bladder can multiply unhindered without being unceremoniously flushed or destroyed by the bladder wall. Accordingly, urinary tract infection is particularly frequent among patients with lower urinary tract obstruction, such as may occur with benign prostatic hypertrophy, tumors, or calculi.
- *Vesicoureteral reflux.* Although obstruction is an important predisposing factor in the pathogenesis of ascending infection, *it is incompetence of the vesicoureteral valve* that allows bacteria to ascend the ureter into the pelvis. The normal ureteral insertion into the bladder is a competent one-way valve that prevents retrograde flow of urine, especially during micturition, when the intravesical pressure rises. An incompetent vesicoureteral orifice allows the reflux of bladder urine into the ureters *(vesicoureteral reflux)*[65] (Fig. 21–37). Reflux is most often due to a congenital, inherited absence or shortening of the intravesical portion of the ureter (Fig. 21–38), such that the ureter is not compressed during micturition. In addition, bladder infection itself, probably as a result of the action of bacterial or inflammatory products on ureteral contractility, can cause or accentuate vesicoureteral reflux, particularly in children. *Acquired vesicoureteral reflux* in adults can result from persistent bladder atony caused by spinal cord injury. The effect of vesicoureteral reflux is similar to that of an obstruction in that after voiding there is residual urine in the urinary tract, which favors bacterial growth.

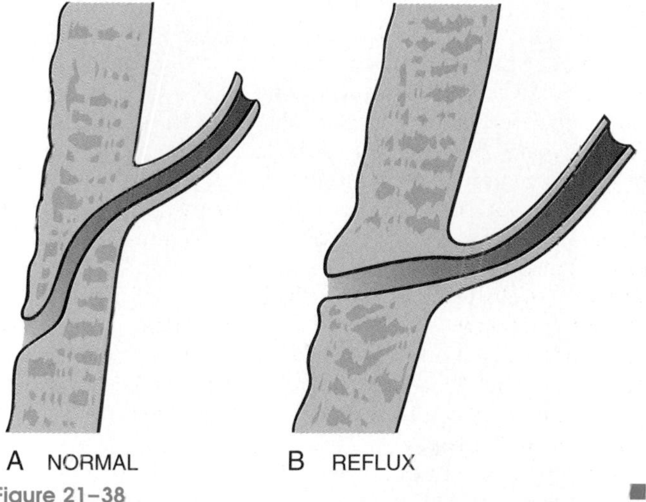

Figure 21–38

The vesicoureteric junction. In normal individuals (*A*), the intravesical portion of the ureter is oblique, such that the ureter is closed by muscle contraction during micturition. The most common cause of reflux is congenital complete or partial absence of the intravesical ureter (*B*).

- *Intrarenal reflux.* Vesicoureteral reflux also affords a ready mechanism by which the infected bladder urine can be propelled up to the renal pelvis and deep into the renal parenchyma through open ducts at the tips of the papillae (intrarenal reflux). Intrarenal reflux is most common in the upper and lower poles of the kidney, where papillae tend to have flattened or concave tips rather than the convex pointed type present in the midzones of the kidney (and depicted in most textbooks). Reflux can be demonstrated radiographically by a voiding cystourethrogram: the bladder is filled with a radiopaque dye, and films are taken during micturition. Vesicoureteral reflux can be demonstrated in about 50% of infants and children with urinary tract infection (see Fig. 21–37).

In the absence of vesicoureteral reflux, infection usually remains localized in the bladder. Thus, the majority of patients with repeated or persistent bacterial colonization of the urinary tract suffer from cystitis and urethritis *(lower urinary tract infection)* rather than pyelonephritis.

ACUTE PYELONEPHRITIS

Acute pyelonephritis is an acute suppurative inflammation of the kidney caused by bacterial infection—whether hematogenous and induced by septicemic spread or ascending and associated with vesicoureteral reflux.

MORPHOLOGY. The hallmarks of acute pyelonephritis are **patchy interstitial suppurative inflammation and tubular necrosis.** The suppuration may occur as discrete focal abscesses involving one or both kidneys or as large, wedge-shaped areas of coalescent suppuration (Fig. 21–39). The distribution of these lesions is unpredictable and haphazard, but in pyelonephritis associated with reflux, damage occurs most commonly in the lower and upper poles.

In the early stages, the neutrophilic infiltration is limited to the interstitial tissue. Soon, however, the reaction involves tubules and produces a characteristic abscess with the destruction of the engulfed tubules (Fig. 21–40). Since the tubular lumens present a ready pathway for the extension of the infection, large masses of neutrophils frequently extend along the involved nephron into the collecting tubules. Characteristically, the glomeruli appear to be resistant to the infection. Large areas of severe necrosis, however, eventually destroy the glomeruli, and fungal pyelonephritis (e.g., *Candida)* often affects glomeruli.

Three complications of acute pyelonephritis are encountered in special circumstances.

- **Papillary necrosis** is seen mainly in diabetics and in those with urinary tract obstruction. Papillary necrosis is usually bilateral but may be unilateral. One or all of the pyramids of the affected kidney may be involved. On cut section, the tips or distal two thirds of the pyramids have gray-white to yellow necrosis that resembles infarction (Fig. 21–41). On microscopic examination, the necrotic tissue shows characteristic coagulative infarct necrosis, with preservation of outlines of tubules. The leukocytic response is limited to the junctions between preserved and destroyed tissue.
- **Pyonephrosis** is seen when there is total or almost complete obstruction, particularly when it is high in the urinary tract. The suppurative exudate is unable to drain and thus fills the renal pelvis, calyces, and ureter, producing pyonephrosis.
- **Perinephric abscess** implies extension of suppu-

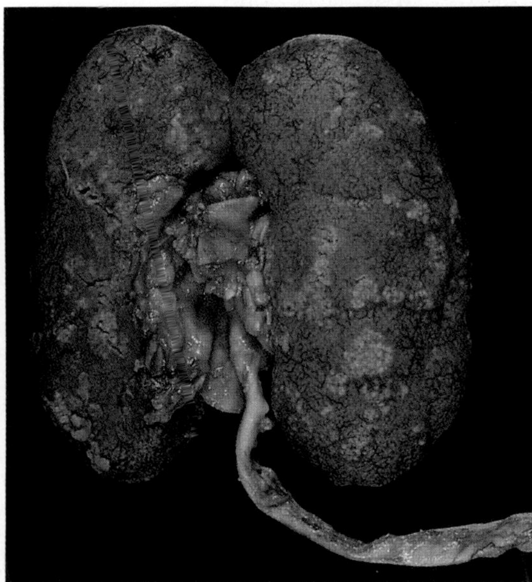

Figure 21–39

Acute pyelonephritis. Cortical surface exhibits grayish white areas of inflammation and abscess formation.

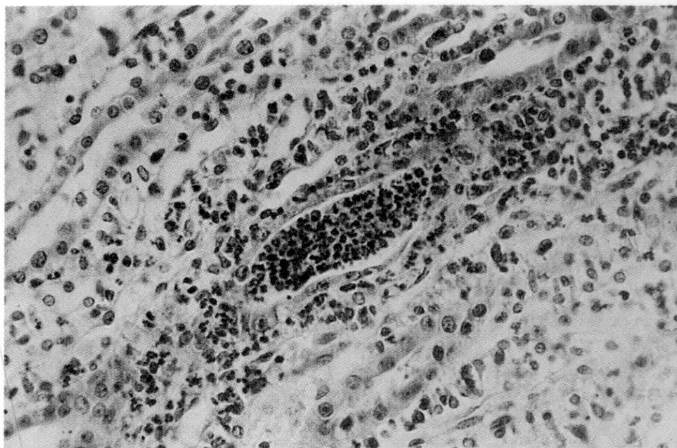

Figure 21–40

Acute pyelonephritis marked by an acute neutrophilic exudate within tubules and the renal substance.

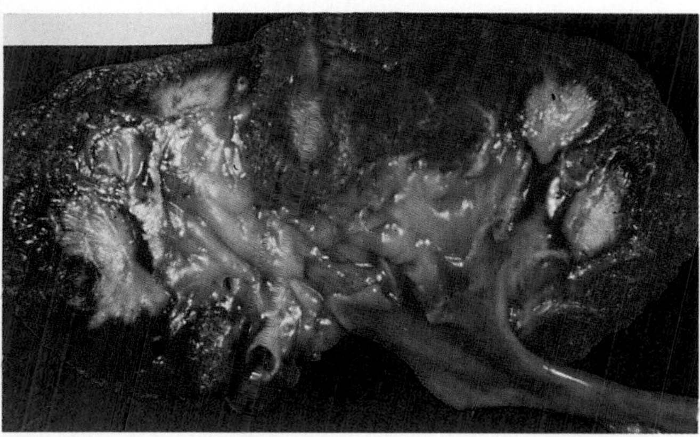

Figure 21–41

Papillary necrosis. Areas of pale gray necrosis are limited to the papillae.

rative inflammation through the renal capsule into the perinephric tissue.

After the acute phase of pyelonephritis, healing occurs. The neutrophilic infiltrate is replaced by one that is predominantly mononuclear with macrophages, plasma cells, and (later) lymphocytes. The inflammatory foci are eventually replaced by scars that can be seen on the cortical surface as fibrous depressions. Such scars are characterized microscopically by atrophy of tubules, interstitial fibrosis, and lymphocyte infiltrate and may resemble scars produced by ischemic or other types of injury to the kidney. **However, the pyelonephritic scar is almost always associated with inflammation, fibrosis, and deformation of the underlying calyx and pelvis**, reflecting the role of ascending infection and vesicoureteral reflux in the pathogenesis of the disease.

Clinical Course. Acute pyelonephritis is often associated with predisposing conditions, some of which were covered in the discussion of pathogenetic mechanisms. These include the following:

- *Urinary obstruction,* either congenital or acquired
- *Instrumentation* of the urinary tract, most commonly catheterization
- *Vesicoureteral reflux*
- *Pregnancy.* Four per cent to 6% of pregnant women develop bacteriuria sometime during pregnancy, and 20% to 40% of these eventually develop symptomatic urinary infection if not treated.
- *Patient's sex and age.* After the first year of life (when congenital anomalies in males commonly become evident) and up to around age 40 years, infections are much more frequent in females. With increasing age, the incidence in males rises owing to the development of prostatic hypertrophy and frequent instrumentation.
- *Preexisting renal lesions,* causing intrarenal scarring and obstruction
- *Diabetes mellitus,* in which acute pyelonephritis is caused by more frequent instrumentation, the general susceptibility to infection, and the neurogenic bladder dysfunction exhibited by patients
- *Immunosuppression and immunodeficiency*

When acute pyelonephritis is clinically apparent, the onset is usually sudden, with pain at the costovertebral angle and systemic evidence of infection, such as fever and malaise. There are usually indications of bladder and urethral irritation, such as dysuria, frequency, and urgency. The urine contains many leukocytes (pyuria) derived from the inflammatory infiltrate, but pyuria does not differentiate upper from lower urinary tract infection. The finding of leukocyte casts (pus casts) indicates renal involvement, because casts are formed only in tubules. The diagnosis of infection is established by quantitative urine culture.

Uncomplicated acute pyelonephritis usually follows a benign course, and the symptoms disappear within a few days after the institution of appropriate antibiotic therapy. Bacteria, however, may persist in the urine, or there may be recurrence of infection with new serologic types of *E. coli* or other organisms. Such bacteriuria then either disappears or may persist sometimes for years. In the presence of unrelieved urinary obstruction, diabetes mellitus, and immunocompromise, acute pyelonephritis may be more serious, leading to repeated septicemic episodes. The superimposition of *papillary necrosis* may lead to acute renal failure.

CHRONIC PYELONEPHRITIS AND REFLUX NEPHROPATHY

Chronic pyelonephritis is a chronic tubulointerstitial renal disorder in which *chronic tubulointerstitial inflammation and renal scarring are associated with pathologic involvement of the calyces and pelvis* (Fig. 21–42). Pelvocalyceal damage is important in that virtually all the diseases listed in Table 21–9 produce chronic tubulointerstitial alterations, but except for chronic pyelonephritis and analgesic nephropathy, none affects the calyces. Chronic pyelonephritis is an important cause of end-stage kidney disease, being found in 10% to 20% of patients in renal transplant or dialysis units.

Chronic pyelonephritis can be divided into two forms: chronic obstructive and chronic reflux-associated.

Chronic Obstructive Pyelonephritis. We have seen that obstruction predisposes the kidney to infection. Recurrent infections superimposed on diffuse or localized obstructive lesions lead to recurrent bouts of renal inflammation and scarring, resulting in a picture of chronic pyelonephritis. In this condition, the effects of obstruction contribute to the parenchymal atrophy, and indeed it is sometimes difficult to differentiate the effects of bacterial infection from those of obstruction alone. The disease can be bilateral, as with obstructive anomalies of the urinary tract (e.g., posterior urethral valves), resulting in renal insufficiency unless the anomaly is corrected; or unilateral, such as occurs with calculi and unilateral obstructive anomalies of the ureter.

Reflux Nephropathy. This is by far the more common form of chronic pyelonephritic scarring. Renal involvement in reflux nephropathy occurs early in childhood, as a result

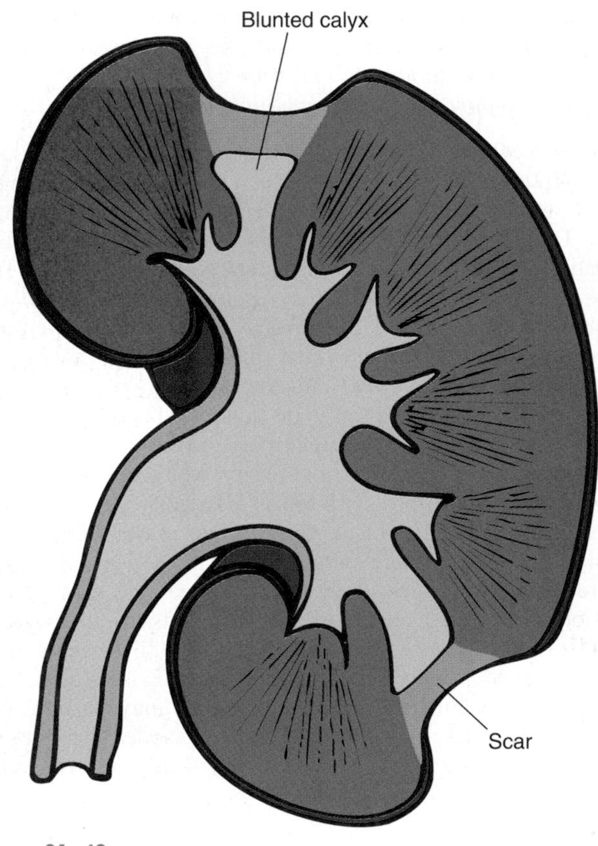

Figure 21–42

Typical coarse scars of chronic pyelonephritis associated with vesicoureteral reflux. The scars are usually polar and are associated with underlying blunted calyces.

of superimposition of a urinary infection on congenital vesicoureteral reflux and intrarenal reflux, the latter conditioned by the number of potentially refluxing papillae. Reflux may be unilateral or bilateral; thus, the resultant renal damage either may cause scarring and atrophy of one kidney or may involve both and lead to chronic renal insufficiency. Vesicoureteral reflux occasionally causes renal damage in the absence of infection (sterile reflux) but only in the presence of severe obstruction.

MORPHOLOGY. The characteristic morphologic changes of chronic pyelonephritis are seen on gross examination (Fig. 21–42). The kidneys usually are irregularly scarred; if bilateral, the involvement is asymmetric. This contrasts with chronic glomerulonephritis, in which the kidneys are diffusely and symmetrically scarred. The hallmark of chronic pyelonephritis is the coarse, discrete, corticomedullary scar overlying a dilated, blunted, or deformed calyx (Fig. 21–43). The scars can vary from one to several in number and may affect one or both kidneys. Most are in upper and lower poles, consistent with the frequency of reflux in these sites.

The microscopic changes involve predominantly tubules and interstitium. The tubules show atrophy in some areas and hypertrophy in others, or dilation. Dilated tubules may be filled with colloid casts **(thyroidization)**. There are varying degrees of chronic interstitial inflammation and fibrosis in the cortex and medulla. In the presence of active infection, there may be neutrophils in the interstitium and pus casts in the tubules. Arcuate and interlobular vessels disclose obliterative endarteritis in the scarred areas; and in the presence of hypertension, hyaline arteriosclerosis is seen in the entire kidney. There is often fibrosis around the calyceal mucosa as well as marked chronic inflammatory infiltrate. Glomeruli may appear normal except for periglomerular fibrosis, but a variety of glomerular changes may be present, including ischemic fibrous obliteration as well as proliferation and necrosis ascribed to hyperten-

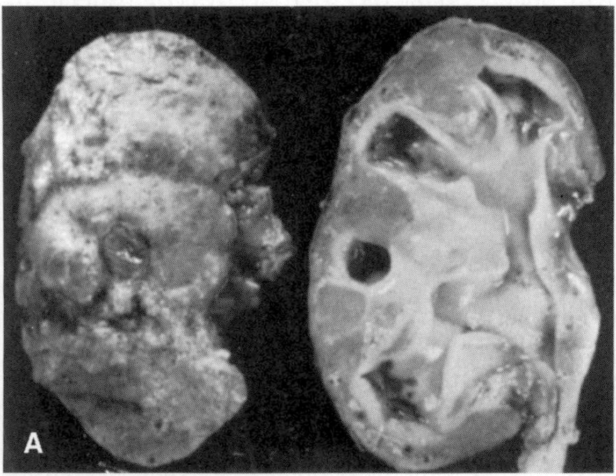

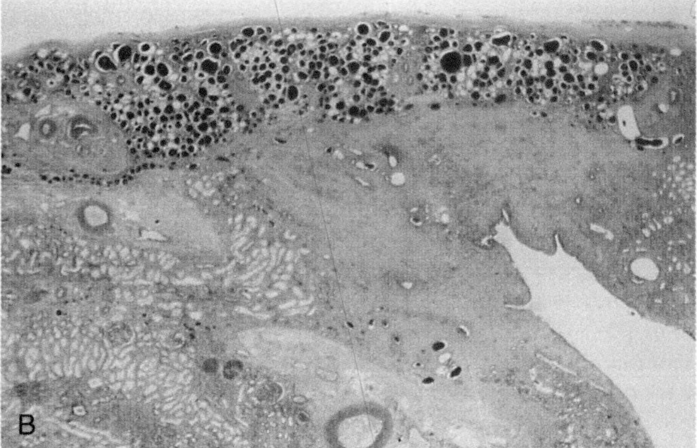

Figure 21–43

A, Chronic pyelonephritis. Surface *(left)* is irregularly scarred. Cut section *(right)* reveals characteristic dilation and blunting of calyces. Ureter is dilated and thickened—a finding consistent with chronic vesicoureteral reflux. *B*, Low-power view showing corticomedullary renal scar with an underlying dilated deformed calyx. Note thyroidization of tubules in the cortex.

sion. Patients with chronic pyelonephritis and reflux nephropathy who develop proteinuria in advanced stages exhibit secondary **focal segmental glomerulosclerosis**, as described later.

Xanthogranulomatous pyelonephritis is an unusual and relatively rare form of chronic pyelonephritis characterized by accumulation of foamy macrophages intermingled with plasma cells, lymphocytes, polymorphonuclear leukocytes, and occasional giant cells. Often associated with *Proteus* infections and obstruction, the lesions sometimes produce large, yellowish orange nodules that may be confused with renal cell carcinoma.

Clinical Course. Chronic obstructive pyelonephritis may be insidious in onset or may present the clinical manifestations of acute recurrent pyelonephritis with back pain, fever, frequent pyuria, and bacteriuria. Chronic pyelonephritis associated with reflux may have a silent onset. These patients come to medical attention relatively late in the course of their disease because of the gradual onset of renal insufficiency and hypertension or because of the discovery of pyuria or bacteriuria on routine examination. Reflux nephropathy is a common cause of hypertension in children. Loss of tubular function—in particular of concentrating ability—gives rise to polyuria and nocturia. Radiographic studies show asymmetrically contracted kidneys with characteristic coarse scars and blunting and deformity of the calyceal system. Significant bacteriuria may be present, but it is often absent in the late stages.

Although proteinuria is usually mild, some patients with pyelonephritic scars develop *focal segmental glomerulosclerosis* with significant proteinuria, even in the nephrotic range, usually several years after the scarring has occurred and often in the absence of continued infection or persistent vesicoureteral reflux. The appearance of proteinuria and focal segmental glomerulosclerosis is a poor prognostic sign, and such patients may proceed to chronic end-stage renal failure. The glomerulosclerosis, as we have discussed, may be attributable to the adaptive glomerular alterations secondary to loss of renal mass caused by pyelonephritic scarring (renal ablation nephropathy).

TUBULOINTERSTITIAL NEPHRITIS INDUCED BY DRUGS AND TOXINS

Toxins and drugs can produce renal injury in at least three ways: (1) they may trigger an interstitial immunologic reaction, exemplified by the acute hypersensitivity nephritis induced by such drugs as methicillin; (2) they may cause acute renal failure, as described earlier; and (3) they may cause subtle but cumulative injury to tubules that takes years to become manifest, resulting in chronic renal insufficiency. The last type of damage is especially treacherous because it may be clinically unrecognized until significant renal damage has occurred. Such is the case with analgesic abuse nephropathy, which is usually detected only after the onset of chronic renal insufficiency.

Acute Drug-Induced Interstitial Nephritis

This is a well-recognized adverse reaction to a constantly increasing number of drugs. First reported after the use of sulfonamides, acute tubulointerstitial nephritis most frequently occurs with synthetic penicillins (methicillin, ampicillin), other synthetic antibiotics (rifampin), diuretics (thiazides), NSAIDs (phenylbutazone), and miscellaneous drugs (phenindione, cimetidine).[66, 66a] The disease begins about 15 days (range, 2 to 40) after exposure to the drug and is characterized by *fever, eosinophilia* (which may be transient), *a rash* in about 25% of patients, and *renal abnormalities.* The last include hematuria, mild proteinuria, and leukocyturia (including eosinophils). A *rising serum creatinine level or acute renal failure with oliguria develops in about 50% of cases,* particularly in older patients.

MORPHOLOGY. On histologic examination, the abnormalities are in the interstitium, which shows pronounced edema and infiltration by mononuclear cells, principally lymphocytes and macrophages. Eosinophils and neutrophils may be present (Fig. 21–44), often in large numbers, and plasma cells and basophils are sometimes found in small numbers. With some drugs (e.g., methicillin, thiazides), interstitial **granulomas** with giant cells may be seen. Variable degrees of tubular necrosis and regeneration are present. The glomeruli are normal except in some cases caused by NSAIDs when minimal change disease and the nephrotic syndrome develop concurrently (see discussion under NSAIDs, later).

Pathogenesis. Many features of the disease suggest an immune mechanism. Clinical evidence of hypersensitivity includes the latent period, the eosinophilia and rash, the

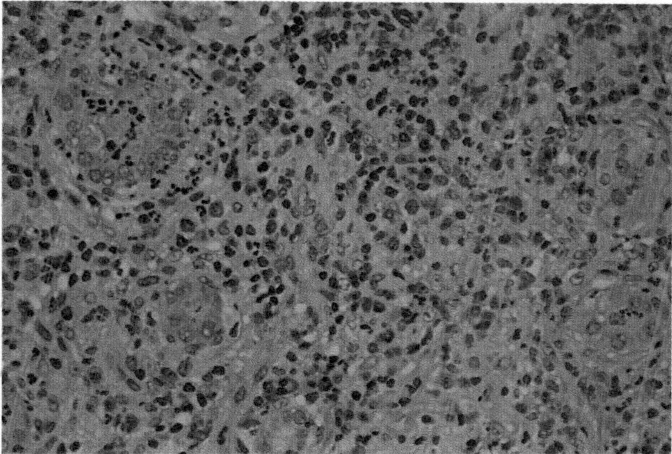

Figure 21–44

Drug-induced interstitial nephritis, with prominent eosinophilia and mononuclear infiltrate. (Courtesy of Dr. H. Rennke, Brigham and Women's Hospital, Boston, MA.)

fact that the onset of nephropathy is not dose related, and the recurrence of hypersensitivity after re-exposure to the same or a cross-reactive drug. IgE serum levels are increased in some patients, and IgE-containing plasma cells and basophils are sometimes present in the lesions, suggesting that an IgE-mediated *late-phase response* hypersensitivity may be involved in the pathogenesis (Chapter 7). The mononuclear or granulomatous infiltrate, together with positive results of skin tests to drug haptens, suggests a delayed hypersensitivity type reaction (type IV).

The most likely sequence of events is that the drugs act as haptens, which, during secretion by tubules, covalently bind to some cytoplasmic or extracellular component of tubular cells and become immunogenic. The resultant injury is then due to IgE and cell-mediated immune reactions to tubular cells or their basement membranes.

Clinical Features. It is important to recognize drug-induced renal failure because withdrawal of the offending drug is followed by recovery, although it may take several months for renal function to return to normal and irreversible damage may occur occasionally in older subjects.

Analgesic Abuse Nephropathy

This is a form of chronic renal disease caused by excessive intake of analgesic mixtures and characterized morphologically by chronic tubulointerstitial nephritis with renal papillary necrosis.[67, 68]

Analgesic nephropathy is of worldwide distribution. Its incidence reflects consumption of analgesics in various populations. In some parts of Australia, it ranks as one of the most common causes of chronic renal insufficiency. Its incidence in the United States is relatively low but varies between states, being highest in the Southeast. Overall it accounts for 9%, 3%, and 1% of patients undergoing dialysis in Australia, Europe, and the United States, respectively. The renal damage was first ascribed to phenacetin, but the analgesic mixtures consumed often contain, in addition, aspirin, caffeine, acetaminophen (a metabolite of phenacetin), and codeine. Patients who develop this disease usually ingest large quantities of mixtures of at least two antipyretic analgesics. In most countries, restriction of over-the-counter sale of phenacetin or analgesic mixtures has reduced the incidence of the disorder but has not eradicated it, presumably because non–phenacetin-containing mixtures are also available.

Pathogenesis. Papillary necrosis is readily induced experimentally by a mixture of aspirin and phenacetin, usually combined with water depletion. Most patients consume phenacetin-containing mixtures, and cases ascribed to ingestion of aspirin, phenacetin, or acetaminophen alone are uncommon. It is now clear that in the sequence of events leading to renal damage, *papillary necrosis occurs first, and cortical tubulointerstitial nephritis is a secondary phenomenon.* The phenacetin metabolite acetaminophen injures cells by both *covalent binding and oxidative damage.* Aspirin induces its potentiating effect by inhibiting the vasodilatory effects of prostaglandin, predisposing the papilla to ischemia. Thus, the papillary damage may be due to a combination of direct toxic effects of phenacetin metabolites and ischemic injury to both tubular cells and vessels.

MORPHOLOGY. In gross appearance, the kidneys are either normal or slightly reduced in size, and the cortex exhibits depressed and raised areas, the depressed areas representing cortical atrophy overlying necrotic papillae. The papillae show various stages of necrosis, calcification, fragmentation, and sloughing. **This gross appearance contrasts with the papillary necrosis seen in diabetic patients, in which all papillae are at the same stage of acute necrosis.** On microscopic examination, the papillary changes may take one of several forms: in early cases, there is patchy necrosis; but in the advanced form, the entire papilla is necrotic, often remaining in place as a structureless mass with ghosts of tubules and foci of dystrophic calcification (Fig. 21–45). Segments of entire portions of the papilla may then be sloughed and excreted in the urine.

The cortical changes consist of loss and atrophy of these tubules and interstitial fibrosis and inflammation. These changes are mainly due to obstructive atrophy caused by the tubular damage in the papilla, but superimposed pyelonephritic changes may be present. **The cortical columns of Bertin are characteristically spared from this atrophy.** The small vessels in the papilla and submucosa of the urinary tract exhibit characteristic PAS-positive basement membrane thickening (analgesic microangiopathy).

Clinical Course. Analgesic nephropathy is more common in women than in men and is particularly prevalent in individuals with recurrent headaches and muscle pain, in psychoneurotic patients, and in factory workers. Early renal findings include inability to concentrate the urine, as would be expected with lesions in the papilla. Acquired distal renal tubular acidosis contributes to the development of renal stones. Headache, anemia, gastrointestinal symptoms, and hypertension are common accompaniments of analgesic nephropathy. The anemia in particular is out of proportion to the renal insufficiency, owing to damage to red cells by the phenacetin metabolites. Urinary tract infection complicates about 50% of cases. On occasion, entire tips of necrotic papillae are excreted, and these may cause gross hematuria or renal colic due to obstruction of the ureter by necrotic fragments. Computed tomographic imaging is helpful in detecting papillary necrosis and calcifications. Progressive impairment of renal function may lead to chronic renal failure, but with *drug withdrawal and proper therapy for infection, renal function may either stabilize or actually improve.*

Unfortunately, a complication occurs in a small percentage of patients who have survived because of their discontinuance of the offending drugs—namely, the development of *transitional papillary carcinoma of the renal pelvis.* Whether the carcinogenic effect is due to a metabolite of phenacetin or to some other component of the analgesic compounds is unsettled.

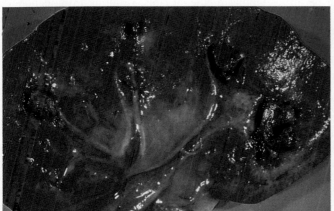

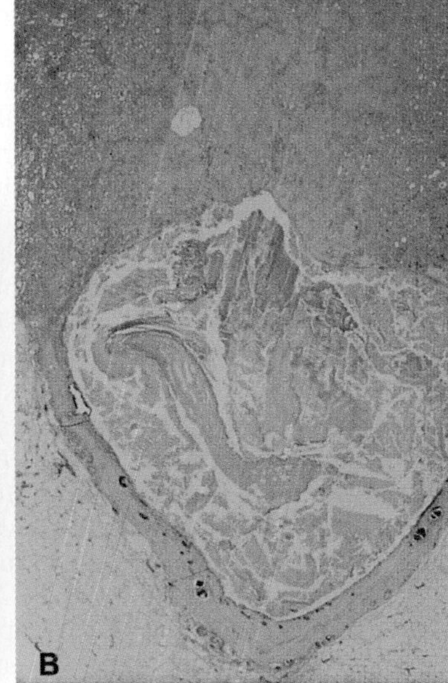

Figure 21–45

Analgesic nephropathy. *A*, The brownish necrotic papilla, transformed to a necrotic, structureless mass, fills the pelvis. *B*, Microscopic view. Note fibrosis in the medulla. (Courtesy of Dr. F. J. Gloor, Institut für Pathologie, Kantonsspital, St. Gallen, Switzerland.)

Papillary necrosis is not specific for analgesic nephropathy. In addition to diabetes mellitus, it can occur in urinary tract obstruction, sickle cell anemia or trait, and focally in renal tuberculosis. Table 21–10 lists certain features of papillary necrosis in these conditions.

Nephropathy Associated With Nonsteroidal Anti-Inflammatory Drugs

NSAIDs are one of the most common classes of drugs currently in use and produce several forms of renal injury. Although these complications are fortunately uncommon, they need to be kept in mind, since NSAIDs are frequently administered to patients with other potential causes of renal disease. NSAID-associated renal syndromes include

- Hemodynamically induced *acute renal failure*, due to the inhibition of vasodilatory prostaglandin synthesis by NSAIDs. This is particularly likely to occur in the setting of other renal diseases or conditions causing volume depletion.
- Acute hypersensitivity interstitial nephritis, resulting in acute renal failure, as described earlier.
- Acute interstitial nephritis and lipoid nephrosis. This curious association of two diverse renal conditions, one leading to renal failure and the other to nephrotic syndrome, remains unexplained.
- Membranous glomerulonephritis, with the nephrotic syndrome, is a recently appreciated association, also of unclear pathogenesis.[69]

Whether prolonged use of NSAIDs by decreasing prostaglandin synthesis causes papillary necrosis and chronic interstitial disease, such as occurs with analgesics, is currently unproven.[68]

OTHER TUBULOINTERSTITIAL DISEASES

Urate Nephropathy

- Three types of nephropathy can occur in patients with hyperuricemic disorders. *Acute uric acid nephropathy* is

Table 21–10. PAPILLARY NECROSIS

	Diabetes Mellitus	Analgesic Nephropathy	Sickle Cell Disease	Obstruction
Male-to-female ratio	1:3	1:5	1:1	9:1
Time course	10 years	7 years of abuse	Variable	Variable
Infection	80%	25%	±	90%
Calcification	Rare	Frequent	Rare	Frequent
Number of papillae affected	Several; all of same stage	Almost all; different stages of necrosis	Few	Variable

Modified from Seshan S, et al (eds): Classification and Atlas of Tubulointerstitial and Vascular Diseases. Baltimore, Williams & Wilkins (in press).

caused by the precipitation of uric acid crystals in the renal tubules, principally in collecting ducts, leading to obstruction of nephrons and the development of acute renal failure. This type is particularly likely to occur in patients with leukemias and lymphomas who are undergoing chemotherapy; the drugs increase the destruction of neoplastic nuclei and the elaboration of uric acid. Precipitation of uric acid is favored by the acidic pH in collecting tubules.

- *Chronic urate nephropathy,* or gouty nephropathy, occurs in patients with more protracted forms of hyperuricemia. The lesions are ascribed to the deposition of monosodium urate crystals in the acidic milieu of the distal tubules and collecting ducts as well as in the interstitium. *These deposits have a distinct histologic appearance, in the form of birefringent, needle-like crystals present either in the tubular lumina or in the interstitium* (Fig. 21–46). The urates induce a *tophus* often surrounded by foreign body giant cells, other mononuclear cells, and a fibrotic reaction (Chapter 28). Tubular obstruction by the urates causes cortical atrophy and scarring. Arterial and arteriolar thickening is common in these kidneys, owing to the relatively high frequency of hypertension in patients with gout. Clinically, urate nephropathy is a subtle disease associated with tubular defects that may progress slowly. Patients with gout who actually develop a chronic nephropathy commonly have evidence of increased exposure to lead, mostly by way of drinking "moonshine" whiskey contaminated with lead.
- The third renal syndrome in hyperuricemia is *nephrolithiasis;* uric acid stones are present in 22% of patients with gout and 42% of those with secondary hyperuricemia (see later discussion of renal stones).

Hypercalcemia and Nephrocalcinosis

Disorders characterized by hypercalcemia, such as hyperparathyroidism, multiple myeloma, vitamin D intoxication, metastatic bone disease, or excess calcium intake (milk-alkali syndrome), may induce the formation of calcium stones and deposition of calcium in the kidney (nephrocalcinosis). Extensive degrees of calcinosis, under certain conditions, may lead to a form of chronic tubulointerstitial disease and renal insufficiency. The first damage induced by the hypercalcemia is at the *intracellular level,* in the tubular epithelial cells, resulting in mitochondrial distortion and evidence of cell injury. Subsequently, calcium deposits can be demonstrated within the mitochondria, cytoplasm, and basement membrane. Calcified cellular debris then aids in obstruction of the tubular lumens and causes obstructive atrophy of nephrons with interstitial fibrosis and nonspecific chronic inflammation. Atrophy of entire cortical areas drained by calcified tubules may occur, and this accounts for the alternating areas of normal and scarred parenchyma seen in such kidneys.

The earliest functional defect is an inability to elaborate a concentrated urine. Other tubular defects, such as tubular acidosis and salt-losing nephritis, may also occur. With further damage, a slowly progressive renal insufficiency develops. This is usually due to nephrocalcinosis, but many of these patients also have calcium stones and secondary pyelonephritis.

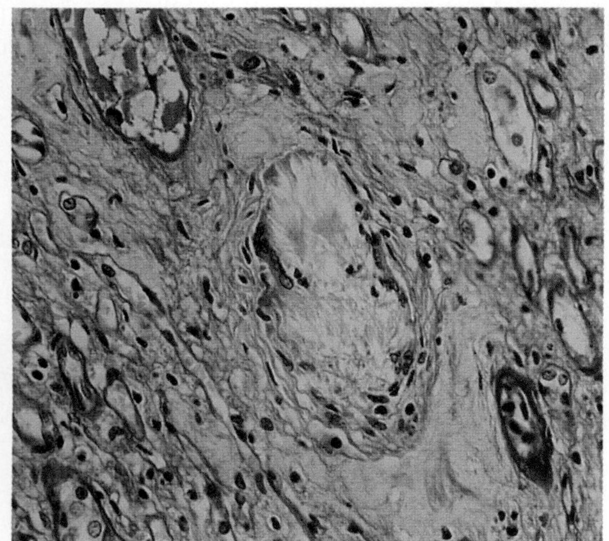

Figure 21–46 ■

Urate crystals in the renal medulla. Note giant cells and fibrosis around the crystals.

Multiple Myeloma

Nonrenal malignant tumors, particularly those of hematopoietic origin, affect the kidneys in a number of ways (Table 21–11). The most common involvements are tubulointerstitial, caused by complications of the tumor (hypercalcemia, hyperuricemia, obstruction of ureters) or therapy (irradiation, hyperuricemia, chemotherapy, infections in immunosuppressed patients). As the survival rate of patients with malignant neoplasms increases, so do these renal complications. We limit the discussion to the renal lesions in *multiple myeloma* that sometimes dominate the clinical picture in patients with this disease.

Renal involvement is a sometimes ominous manifestation of multiple myeloma; overt renal insufficiency occurs in half the patients with this disease. Several factors contribute to renal damage:

- *Bence Jones proteinuria and cast nephropathy.* The main cause of renal dysfunction is related to Bence Jones (light-chain) proteinuria, because renal failure correlates well with the presence and amount of such proteinuria and is extremely rare in its absence. Two mechanisms appear to account for the renal toxicity of Bence Jones proteins. First, some light chains are directly toxic to epithelial cells; different light chains have different nephrotoxic potential. Second, Bence Jones proteins combine with the urinary glycoprotein (Tamm-Horsfall protein) under acidic conditions to form large, histologically distinct tubular casts that obstruct the tubular lumina and also induce a peritubular inflammatory reaction (cast nephropathy).
- *Amyloidosis,* which occurs in 6% to 24% of patients with myeloma
- *Light-chain nephropathy.* In some patients, light chains deposit in glomeruli in nonfibrillar forms, causing a glo-

Table 21–11. RENAL INVOLVEMENT BY NONRENAL NEOPLASMS

Direct tumor invasion of renal parenchyma
  Ureters (obstruction)
  Artery (renovascular hypertension)
Hypercalcemia
Hyperuricemia
Amyloidosis
Excretion of abnormal proteins (multiple myeloma)
Radiotherapy
Chemotherapy
Infection
Glomerulopathy
  Immune complex glomerulonephritis (carcinomas)
  Lipoid nephrosis (Hodgkin disease)

merulopathy (described earlier), or around tubules, causing a tubulointerstitial nephritis.

- *Hypercalcemia and hyperuricemia*, which are often present in these patients
- *Vascular disease* in the usually elderly population affected with myeloma
- *Urinary tract obstruction* with secondary pyelonephritis

MORPHOLOGY. The tubulointerstitial changes in multiple myeloma are fairly characteristic. The Bence Jones tubular casts appear as pink to blue amorphous masses, sometimes concentrically laminated, filling and distending the tubular lumens. Some of the casts are surrounded by multinucleate giant cells, derived from either reactive tubular epithelium or mononuclear phagocytes (Fig. 21–47). The epithelium surrounding the cast is often necrotic, and the adjacent interstitial tissue usually shows a nonspecific inflammatory response. On occasion, the casts erode their way from the tubules into the interstitium and here evoke a granulomatous inflammatory reaction.

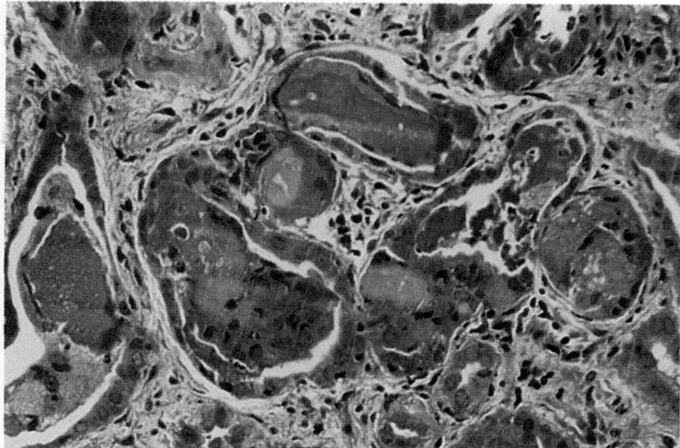

Figure 21–47 ■

Myeloma kidney. Note tubular casts with multinucleate cells around them. (Courtesy of Dr. C. Alpers, University of Washington, Seattle, WA.)

The histologic features of amyloidosis, light-chain nephropathy, and nephrocalcinosis and infection, described elsewhere, may also be present.

Clinically, the renal manifestations are of several types. In the most common form, *chronic renal failure* develops insidiously and usually progresses slowly during a period of several months to years. Another form occurs suddenly and is manifested by *acute renal failure* with oliguria. Precipitating factors in these patients include dehydration, hypercalcemia, acute infection, and treatment with nephrotoxic antibiotics. *Proteinuria* occurs in 70% of patients with myeloma; the presence of significant non–light-chain proteinuria (e.g., albumin) suggests secondary amyloidosis or light-chain glomerulopathy.

DISEASES OF BLOOD VESSELS

Nearly all diseases of the kidney involve the renal blood vessels secondarily. Systemic vascular diseases, such as various forms of vasculitis, also affect renal vessels, and often their effects on the kidney are clinically important. Hypertension, as we discussed in Chapter 12, is intimately linked with the kidney, because kidney disease can be both the cause and consequence of increased blood pressure.[70, 70a] In this chapter, we discuss benign and malignant nephrosclerosis and renal artery stenosis, lesions associated with hypertension, and sundry lesions involving mostly smaller vessels of the kidney.

Benign Nephrosclerosis

Benign nephrosclerosis is the term used for the kidney associated with sclerosis of renal arterioles and small arteries. The resultant effect is focal ischemia of parenchyma supplied by the thickened narrowed vessels. Some degree of nephrosclerosis is present at autopsy with increasing age, more in blacks than whites, preceding or in the absence of hypertension.[71] Hypertension and diabetes mellitus, however, increase the incidence and severity of the lesions.

Pathogenesis. Two processes participate in inducing the arterial lesions:

- Medial and intimal thickening, as a response to hemodynamic changes, genetic defects, or both
- Hyaline deposition in arterioles, caused partly by extravasation of plasma proteins through injured endothelium and partly by increased deposition of basement membrane matrix

MORPHOLOGY. In gross appearance, the kidneys are either normal in size or moderately reduced to average weights between 110 and 130 gm. The cortical surfaces have a fine, even granularity

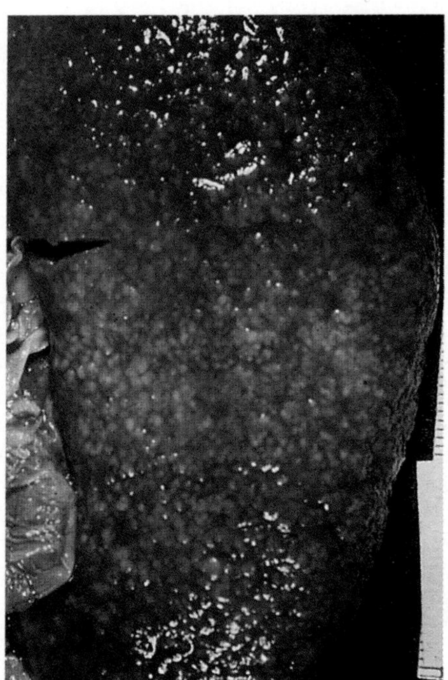

Figure 21–48

Close-up of gross appearance of the cortical surface in benign nephrosclerosis illustrating fine leathery granularity of the surface.

that resembles grain leather (Fig. 21–48). On section, the loss of mass is due mainly to cortical narrowing.

On histologic examination, there is narrowing of the lumens of arterioles and small arteries, caused by thickening and hyalinization of the walls (Fig. 21–49) **(hyaline arteriolosclerosis).**

In addition to arteriolar hyalinization, the interlobular and arcuate arteries exhibit a characteristic lesion that consists of medial hypertrophy, reduplication of the elastic lamina, and increased myofibroblastic tissue in the intima, with consequent narrowing of the lumen. This change, called **fibroelastic hyperplasia,** often accompanies hyaline arteriolosclerosis and increases in severity with age and in the presence of hypertension.

Consequent to the vascular narrowing, there is patchy ischemic atrophy, which consists of (1) foci of tubular atrophy and interstitial fibrosis and (2) a variety of glomerular alterations. The latter include collapse of GBMs, deposition of collagen within the Bowman space, periglomerular fibrosis, and total sclerosis of glomeruli.

Clinical Features. Uncomplicated benign nephrosclerosis alone unusually causes renal insufficiency or uremia. There are usually moderate reductions in renal plasma flow, but the GFR is normal or slightly reduced. On occasion, there is mild proteinuria. However, three groups of hypertensives with benign nephrosclerosis are at increased risk of developing renal failure: blacks; patients with more severe blood pressure elevations; and patients with a second underlying disease, especially diabetics. In these groups, renal insufficiency may supervene after prolonged benign hypertension, but more rapid renal failure results from the development of the malignant or accelerated phase of hypertension, discussed next.

Malignant Nephrosclerosis and Accelerated Hypertension

Malignant nephrosclerosis is the form of renal disease associated with the malignant or accelerated phase of hypertension.[71, 71a] This dramatic pattern of hypertension may occasionally develop in previously normotensive individuals but often is superimposed on preexisting essential benign hypertension, or secondary forms of hypertension, or an underlying chronic renal disease, particularly glomerulonephritis or reflux nephropathy (Table 21–12). It is also a frequent cause of death from uremia in patients with scleroderma. Malignant hypertension is relatively uncommon, occurring in 1% to 5% of all patients with elevated blood pressure. In its pure form, it usually affects younger individuals, with a high preponderance in men and in blacks.

Pathogenesis. The basis for this turn for the worse in hypertensive subjects is unclear, but the following sequence of events is suggested. The initial event appears to be some form of vascular damage to the kidneys. This most commonly results from long-standing benign hypertension, with eventual injury to the arteriolar walls, or it may spring from arteritis or a coagulopathy. In either case, the result is increased permeability of the small vessels to fibrinogen and other plasma proteins, endothelial injury, and platelet deposition. This leads to the appearance of *fibrinoid necro-*

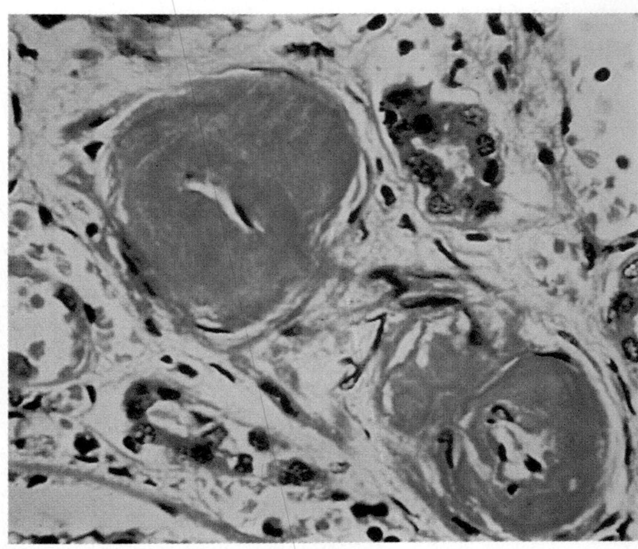

Figure 21–49

Hyaline arteriolosclerosis. High-power view of two arterioles with hyaline deposition, marked thickening of the walls, and a narrowed lumen. (Courtesy of Dr. M.A. Venkatachalam, Department of Pathology, University of Texas Health Sciences Center, San Antonio, TX.)

Table 21–12. TYPES OF HYPERTENSION

Primary or Essential Hypertension

Secondary Hypertension

- Renal
  - Acute glomerulonephritis
  - Chronic renal disease
  - Renal artery stenosis
  - Renal vasculitis
  - Renin-producing tumors
- Endocrine
  - Adrenocortical hyperfunction (Cushing syndrome)
  - Oral contraceptives
  - Pheochromocytoma
  - Acromegaly
  - Myxedema
  - Thyrotoxicosis (systolic)
- Vascular
  - Coarctation of aorta
  - Polyarteritis nodosa
  - Aortic insufficiency (systolic)
- Neurogenic
  - Psychogenic
  - Increased intracranial pressure
  - Polyneuritis, bulbar poliomyelitis, others

sis of arterioles and small arteries and intravascular thrombosis. Mitogenic factors from platelets (e.g., platelet-derived growth factor [PDGF]), plasma and other cells cause intimal smooth hyperplasia of vessels, resulting in the hyperplastic arteriolosclerosis typical of malignant hypertension and further narrowing of the lumens. The kidneys become markedly ischemic. With severe involvement of the renal afferent arterioles, the renin-angiotensin system receives a powerful stimulus, and indeed *patients with malignant hypertension have markedly elevated levels of plasma renin.* This then sets up a self-perpetuating cycle in which angiotensin II causes intrarenal vasoconstriction, and the attendant renal ischemia perpetuates renin secretion. Other vasoconstrictors (e.g., endothelin) and loss of vasodilators (nitric oxide) may also contribute to vasoconstriction. Aldosterone levels are also elevated, and salt retention undoubtedly contributes to the elevation of blood pressure. The consequences of the markedly elevated blood pressure on the blood vessels throughout the body are known as *malignant arteriosclerosis*, and the renal disorder is malignant nephrosclerosis.

MORPHOLOGY. On gross inspection, the kidney size is dependent on the duration and severity of the hypertensive disease. Small, pinpoint petechial hemorrhages may appear on the cortical surface from rupture of arterioles or glomerular capillaries, giving the kidney a peculiar "flea-bitten" appearance.

Two histologic alterations characterize blood vessels in malignant hypertension (Fig. 21–50):

- **Fibrinoid necrosis of arterioles.** This appears as an eosinophilic granular change in the blood vessel wall, which stains positively for fibrin by histochemical or immunofluorescence techniques. In addition, there is often an inflammatory infiltrate within the wall, giving rise to the term **necrotizing arteriolitis.**
- In the interlobular arteries and arterioles, there is intimal thickening caused by a proliferation of elongated, concentrically arranged cells, smooth muscle cells, together with fine concentric layering of collagen. This alteration is known as **hyperplastic arteriolitis,** also referred to as onion-skinning. The lesion correlates well with renal failure in malignant hypertension. Sometimes the glomeruli become necrotic and infiltrated with neutrophils, and the glomerular capillaries may thrombose **(necrotizing glomerulitis).** The arteriolar and arterial lesions result in considerable narrowing of all vascular lumens, with ischemic atrophy and infarction distal to the abnormal vessels.

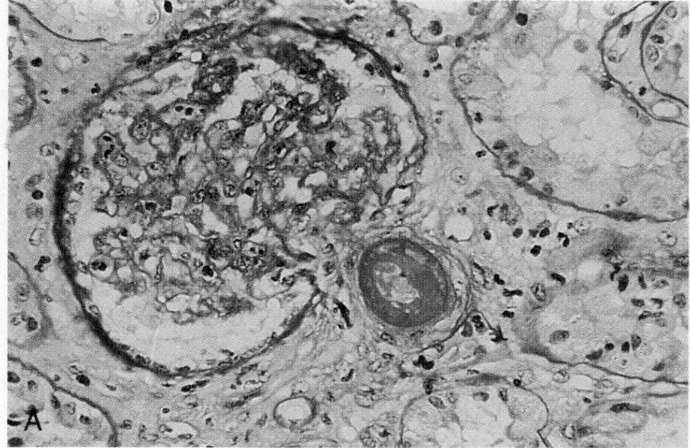

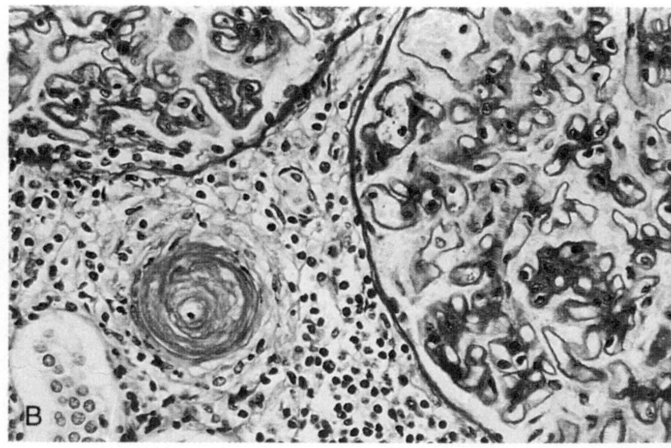

Figure 21–50

Malignant hypertension. *A*, Fibrinoid necrosis of afferent arteriole (PAS stain). *B*, Hyperplastic arteriolitis (onion-skin lesion). (Courtesy of Dr. H. Rennke, Brigham and Women's Hospital, Boston, MA.)

Clinical Course. The full-blown syndrome of malignant hypertension is characterized by diastolic pressures greater than 130 mm Hg, papilledema retinopathy, encephalopathy, cardiovascular abnormalities, and renal failure. Most often, the early symptoms are related to increased intracranial pressure and include headaches, nausea, vomiting, and visual impairments, particularly the development of scotomas or spots before the eyes. "Hypertensive crises" are sometimes encountered, characterized by episodes of loss of consciousness or even convulsions. At the onset of rapidly mounting blood pressure, there is marked proteinuria and microscopic or sometimes macroscopic hematuria but no significant alteration in renal function. Soon, however, renal failure makes its appearance. The syndrome is a true medical emergency requiring the institution of aggressive and prompt antihypertensive therapy before the development of irreversible renal lesions. Before introduction of the new antihypertensive drugs, malignant hypertension was associated with a 50% mortality rate within 3 months of onset, progressing to 90% within a year. At present, however, about 75% of patients will survive 5 years, and 50% survive with precrisis renal function.

Renal Artery Stenosis

Unilateral renal artery stenosis is a relatively uncommon cause of hypertension, responsible for 2% to 5% of cases, but it is of importance because it is a potentially curable form of hypertension, surgical treatment being successful in 70% to 80% of carefully selected cases in humans.[72] Furthermore, much early knowledge of renal mechanisms in hypertension has come from studies of experimental and human renal artery stenosis.

Pathogenesis. The classic experiments of Goldblatt[73] in 1934 showed that constriction of one renal artery in dogs results in hypertension and that the magnitude of the effect is roughly proportional to the amount of constriction. Later experiments in rats confirmed these results, and in time it was shown that the hypertensive effect, at least initially, is due to stimulation of renin secretion by cells of the juxtaglomerular apparatus and the subsequent production of the vasoconstrictor angiotensin II. A large proportion of patients with renovascular hypertension have elevated plasma or renal vein renin levels, and almost all show a reduction of blood pressure when given competitive antagonists of angiotensin II. Further, unilateral renal renin hypersecretion can be normalized after renal revascularization, in association with a decrease in blood pressure. Other factors, however, contribute to the maintenance of renovascular hypertension after the renin-angiotensin system has initiated it, including *sodium retention* and, possibly, endothelin and loss of nitric oxide.

MORPHOLOGY. The most common cause of renal artery stenosis (70% of cases) is occlusion by an atheromatous plaque at the origin of the renal artery. This lesion occurs more frequently in men, the incidence increasing with advancing age and diabetes mellitus. The plaque is usually concentrically placed, and superimposed thrombosis often occurs.

The second type of lesion leading to stenosis is so-called **fibromuscular dysplasia** of the renal artery. This is a heterogeneous group of lesions characterized by fibrous or fibromuscular thickening and may involve the intima, the media, or the adventitia of the artery. These lesions are thus subclassified into **intimal, medial,** and **adventitial hyperplasia**—the medial type being by far the most common (Fig. 21–51). The stenoses, as a whole, are more common in women and tend to occur in younger age groups (i.e., in the third and fourth decades). The lesions may consist of a single well-defined constriction or a series of narrowings, usually in the middle or distal portion of the renal artery. They may also involve the segmental branches and may be bilateral.

The ischemic kidney is usually reduced in size and shows signs of diffuse ischemic atrophy, with crowded glomeruli, atrophic tubules, interstitial fibrosis, and focal inflammatory infiltrate. The arterioles in the ischemic kidney are usually protected from the effects of high pressure, thus showing only mild arteriolosclerosis, in contrast to the contralateral nonischemic kidney, which may exhibit hyaline arteriolosclerosis, depending on the severity of the preceding hypertension.

Clinical Course. Few distinctive features suggest the presence of renal artery stenosis, and in general, these patients resemble those presenting with essential hypertension. On occasion, a bruit can be heard on auscultation of the kidneys. Elevated plasma or renal vein renin, response to angiotensin-converting enzyme inhibitor, renal scans,

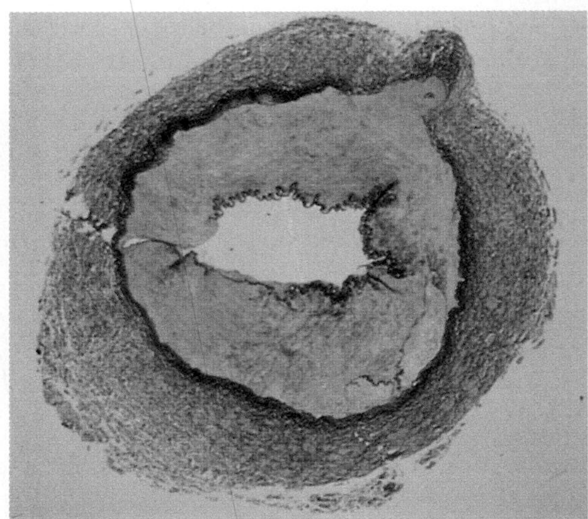

Figure 21–51

Fibromuscular dysplasia of the renal artery, medial type (elastic tissue stain). The medium shows marked fibrous thickening, and the lumen is stenotic. (Courtesy of Dr. Seymour Rosen, Beth Israel Hospital, Boston, MA.)

and intravenous pyelography may aid with diagnosis, but arteriography is required to localize the stenotic lesion. As noted, the cure rate after surgery is 70% to 80% in well-selected cases.

Thrombotic Microangiopathies

As described in Chapter 14, these represent a group of disorders with overlapping clinical manifestations that are *characterized morphologically by thrombosis in capillaries and arterioles throughout the body* (Fig. 21–52) *and clinically by microangiopathic hemolytic anemia, thrombocytopenia, and, in certain conditions, renal failure.*[74] The renal failure is associated with platelet or platelet-fibrin thrombi in the interlobular renal arteries and glomeruli, together with necrosis and thickening of the vessel walls (Fig. 21–52).

The classification of these diseases is somewhat muddied by the fact that two of the conditions, hemolytic-uremic syndrome (HUS) and thrombotic thrombocytopenic purpura (TTP), show considerable overlap; indeed, they are now termed the HUS/TTP syndrome.[74] A useful categorization by cause and condition is as follows:

1. Classic childhood HUS, most frequently associated with intestinal infection by verocytotoxin-releasing bacteria
2. Adult HUS, associated with
   a. Infection
   b. Antiphospholipid antibodies
   c. Complications of pregnancy and contraceptives
   d. Vascular renal diseases such as scleroderma and hypertension
   e. Chemotherapeutic and immunosuppressive drugs
3. Idiopathic HUS/TTP

The morphologic changes may be similar to those seen in malignant hypertension; but in these conditions, they may precede development of hypertension or may be seen in its absence.

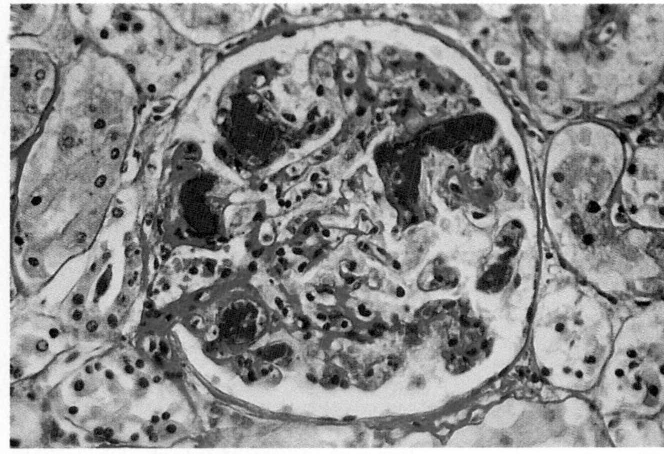

Figure 21–52 ■

Fibrin stain showing platelet-fibrin thrombi (red) in glomerular capillaries characteristic of microangiopathic disorders.

Pathogenesis. Although these disorders may have diverse causes, two processes dominate the pathogenetic sequence of events: (1) *endothelial injury and activation,* with subsequent intravascular thrombosis, and (2) *platelet aggregation.* Both of these events cause *vascular obstruction* and *vasoconstriction* and thus precipitate distal ischemia.[75]

Endothelial Injury. The triggers for endothelial injury and activation as described in Chapters 3 and 12 can be bacterial endotoxins and cytotoxins, cytokines, viruses, drugs, or possibly antiendothelial antibodies. In childhood HUS associated with diarrheal infections, *verocytotoxin,* as we shall see, is clearly the culprit.[76] Still uncharacterized factors in sera of patients with both idiopathic and secondary HUS have recently been shown to cause *apoptosis* of cultured endothelial cells.[76] But it must be admitted that in many cases, the proximate endothelial toxin is unknown.

Endothelial injury may mediate the microangiopathy in several ways.

- Endothelial denudation exposes a potentially thrombogenic subendothelial ECM.
- Reduced production of prostaglandin I_2 and nitric oxide (both of which normally cause vasodilation and inhibit platelet aggregation) enhances platelet aggregation and causes vasoconstriction. Vasoconstriction can also be induced by endothelial-derived endothelin. Endothelial cells may also be *activated,* increasing their adhesivity to leukocytes, which themselves contribute to thrombosis, as described in Chapter 5.
- Endothelial cells elaborate abnormal multimers of von Willebrand factor, which cause platelet aggregation (Chapter 14).

Platelet Aggregation. Because many thrombi in HUS/TTP are composed largely of aggregated platelets with scant fibrin, serum factors *causing* platelet aggregation, or decreased levels of factors that normally *inhibit* platelet aggregation, have been sought. These include unusually large von Willebrand factor multimers and certain proteases, including a cysteine protease called calpain, of uncertain origin. Some of these factors presumably induce aggregation by activating platelet surface glycoproteins (Chapter 5). It is not clear, however, whether the platelet defects are primary or secondary to endothelial dysfunction. As we noted, damaged endothelial cells elaborate abnormal von Willebrand factor multimers.

CLASSIC (CHILDHOOD) HEMOLYTIC-UREMIC SYNDROME

This is the most well characterized of the hemolytic-uremic syndromes, since as many as 75% of cases occur in children after intestinal infection with verocytotoxin-producing *E. coli* (e.g., type O157:H7).[77] Verocytotoxins (so called because they cause damage to *Vero* cells in culture) are similar to *Shiga* toxins produced by *Shigella* and described in Chapter 9. Some epidemics have been traced to ingestion of infected ground meat (hamburgers).

The disease is one of the main causes of acute renal failure in children. It is characterized by the *sudden onset, usually after a gastrointestinal or influenza-like prodromal episode, of bleeding manifestations* (especially hematemesis and melena), *severe oliguria, hematuria, a microangiopathic hemolytic anemia, and (in some patients) prominent neurologic changes.* Hypertension is present in about half the patients.

The *pathogenesis* of this syndrome is clearly related to the Shiga-like toxin. The toxin has a variety of effects on endothelium, causing increased adhesion of leukocytes; increased endothelin production and loss of endothelial nitric oxide (both favoring vasoconstriction); and in the presence of cytokines, such as TNF, endothelial lysis. The resultant endothelial effects enhance both thrombosis and vasoconstriction, resulting in the characteristic microangiopathy. Verocytotoxin also binds to erythrocytes, activates monocytes, and affects platelet function.

MORPHOLOGY. In gross appearance, the kidneys may show patchy or widespread renal cortical necrosis (described later). On microscopic examination, the glomeruli show thickening of capillary walls, due largely to endothelial and subendothelial swelling, and deposits of fibrin-related materials in the capillary lumens, subendothelially, and in the mesangium. Interlobular and afferent arterioles show fibrinoid necrosis and intimal hyperplasia and are often occluded by thrombi.

If the renal failure is managed properly with dialysis, most patients experience recovery in a matter of weeks. However, the long-term (15 to 25 years) prognosis is not uniformly favorable. In one study, only 10 of 25 patients had normal renal function, and 7 had chronic renal failure.[78]

ADULT HEMOLYTIC-UREMIC SYNDROME/ THROMBOTIC THROMBOCYTOPENIC PURPURA

HUS/TTP occurs in adults under a variety of settings:

1. *In association with infection,* such as typhoid fever, *E. coli* septicemia, viral infections, and shigellosis (postinfectious HUS). *Endotoxin,* or *Shiga toxin* (from *Shigella* species), plays a role in the pathogenesis of such cases.
2. In the *antiphospholipid syndrome*, either primary or secondary to SLE (lupus anticoagulant). The syndrome is described in detail in Chapter 5. The microangiopathic changes in the kidney tend to be more chronic—healing of the thrombotic changes in glomeruli results in changes mimicking membranoproliferative glomerulonephritis.
3. In women in relation to complications of pregnancy (placental hemorrhage) or the postpartum period. So-called *postpartum renal failure* usually occurs after an uneventful pregnancy, 1 day to several months after delivery, and is characterized by microangiopathic hemolytic anemia, oliguria, anuria, and initially mild hypertension. The condition has a grave prognosis, although recovery may occur in milder cases.
4. Associated with *vascular renal diseases,* such as scleroderma, and malignant hypertension.
5. In patients treated with chemotherapeutic and immunosuppressive drugs, such as mitomycin, cyclosporine, bleomycin, and cisplatin.

IDIOPATHIC HUS/TTP

Classic idiopathic TTP, discussed earlier (Chapter 14), is manifested by fever, neurologic symptoms, hemolytic anemia, thrombocytopenic purpura, and the presence of thrombi in glomerular capillaries and afferent arterioles. The disease is more common in women, and most patients are younger than 40 years. Idiopathic TTP and various forms of HUS overlap considerably both clinically and morphologically. In classic TTP, however, central nervous system involvement is the dominant feature, whereas renal involvement occurs in only about 50% of patients. In the kidney, eosinophilic granular thrombi are present predominantly in the terminal part of the interlobular arteries, afferent arterioles, and glomerular capillaries. The thrombi are composed largely of platelets and are found in arterioles of many organs throughout the body. Untreated, the disease was once highly fatal, but exchange transfusions and corticosteroid therapy have reduced mortality to less than 50%.

OTHER VASCULAR DISORDERS

Atherosclerotic Ischemic Renal Disease

We have seen that atherosclerotic unilateral artery stenosis can lead to hypertension. *Bilateral* disease, usually diagnosed definitively by arteriography, now appears to be a fairly common cause of chronic ischemia, with renal insufficiency, in older individuals sometimes in the absence of hypertension.[71, 79] The importance of recognizing this condition is that surgical revascularization is beneficial in reversing further decline in renal function.

Atheroembolic Renal Disease

Embolization of fragments of atheromatous plaques from the aorta or renal artery into intraparenchymal renal vessels occurs in elderly patients with severe atherosclerosis, especially after surgery on the abdominal aorta, aortography, or intra-aortic cannulization. These emboli can be recognized in the walls of arcuate and interlobular arteries by their content of cholesterol crystals, which appear as rhomboid clefts (Fig. 21–53). The clinical consequences of atheroemboli vary according to the number of emboli and the preexisting state of renal function. Frequently, they have no functional significance. However, acute renal failure may result in elderly patients in whom renal function is already compromised, principally after abdominal surgery on atherosclerotic aneurysms.

Sickle Cell Disease Nephropathy

Sickle cell disease in both the homozygous and the heterozygous forms may lead to a variety of alterations in renal morphology and function, some of which, fortunately uncommonly, produce clinically significant abnormalities. The various manifestations are termed sickle cell nephropathy.

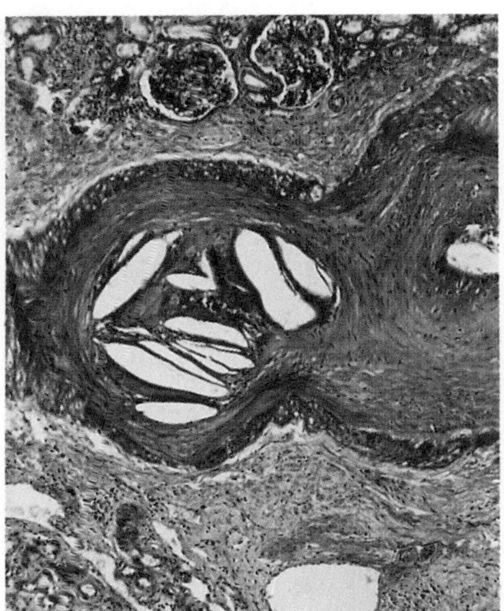

Figure 21–53

Atheroemboli with typical cholesterol clefts in the interlobar artery.

The most common clinical and functional abnormalities are *hematuria* and a *diminished concentrating ability.* These are thought to be largely due to accelerated sickling in the hypertonic hypoxic milieu of the renal medulla, which increases the viscosity of the blood during its passage through the vasa recta, leading to plugging of vessels and decreased flow. Patchy *papillary necrosis* may occur in both homozygotes and heterozygotes; this is sometimes associated with cortical scarring. *Proteinuria* is also common in sickle cell disease, occurring in about 30% of patients. It is usually mild to moderate, but on occasion the overt nephrotic syndrome arises, associated with a membranoproliferative glomerular lesion.

Diffuse Cortical Necrosis

This is an uncommon condition that occurs most frequently after an obstetric emergency, such as abruptio placentae (premature separation of the placenta), septic shock, or extensive surgery. When bilateral and symmetric, it is uniformly fatal, but patchy cortical necrosis may permit survival. The cortical destruction has all the earmarks of ischemic necrosis. Glomerular and arteriolar microthrombi are found in some but by no means all cases; if present, they clearly contribute to the necrosis and renal damage. It is thought that the disorder results from disseminated intravascular coagulation (Chapter 5) and vasoconstriction.

MORPHOLOGY. The gross alterations of the massive ischemic necrosis are sharply limited to the cortex (Fig. 21–54). The histologic appearance is that of acute ischemic infarction. The lesions may be patchy, with areas of apparently better preserved cortex. Intravascular and intraglomerular thromboses may be prominent but are usually focal, and acute necroses of small arterioles and capillaries may occasionally be present. Hemorrhages occur into the glomeruli, together with the precipitation of fibrin in the glomerular capillaries.

Massive acute cortical necrosis is of grave significance, since it gives rise to sudden anuria, terminating rapidly in uremic death. Instances of unilateral or patchy involvement are compatible with survival.

Renal Infarcts

The kidneys are favored sites for the development of infarcts, as one fourth of the cardiac output passes through these organs. Although thrombosis in advanced atherosclerosis and the acute vasculitis of polyarteritis nodosa may occlude arteries, most infarcts are due to embolism. The major source of such emboli is mural thrombosis in the left atrium and ventricle as a result of myocardial infarction. Vegetative endocarditis, thrombosis in aortic aneurysms, and aortic atherosclerosis are less frequent sites for the origin of emboli.

MORPHOLOGY. Because the arterial supply to the kidney is of the "end-organ" type, most infarcts are of the "white" anemic type. They may occur as solitary lesions or may be multiple and bilateral. Within 24 hours, infarcts become sharply demarcated, pale, yellow-white areas that may contain small irregular foci of hemorrhagic discoloration. They are usually ringed by a zone of intense hyperemia.

On section, they are wedge shaped, with the base against the cortical surface and the apex pointing toward the medulla. There may be a narrow rim of preserved subcortical tissue that has been spared by the collateral capsular circulation. In time, these acute areas of ischemic necrosis undergo progressive fibrous scarring, giving rise to depressed, **pale, gray-white scars** that

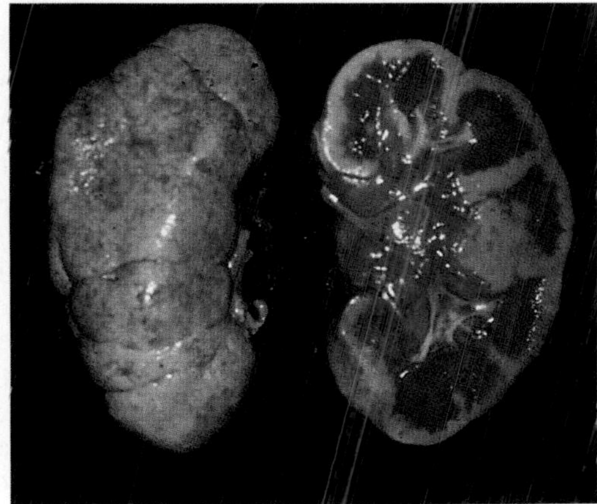

Figure 21–54

Diffuse cortical necrosis. Pale ischemic necrotic areas are confined to the cortex and columns of Bertin.

assume a V shape on section. The histologic changes in renal infarction are those of ischemic coagulation necrosis, described in Chapter 1.

Many renal infarcts are clinically silent. Sometimes, pain with tenderness localized to the costovertebral angle occurs, and this is associated with showers of red cells in the urine. Large infarcts of one kidney are a well-known basis for hypertension.

URINARY TRACT OBSTRUCTION (OBSTRUCTIVE UROPATHY)

Recognition of urinary obstruction is important *because obstruction increases susceptibility to infection and to stone formation, and unrelieved obstruction almost always leads to permanent renal atrophy,* termed *hydronephrosis or obstructive uropathy.* Fortunately, many causes of obstruction are surgically correctable or medically treatable.

Obstruction may be sudden or insidious, partial or complete, unilateral or bilateral; it may occur at any level of the urinary tract from the urethra to the renal pelvis. It can be caused by lesions that are *intrinsic* to the urinary tract or *extrinsic* lesions that compress the ureter. The common causes are as follows (Fig. 21–55):

1. *Congenital anomalies:* posterior urethral valves and urethral strictures, meatal stenosis, bladder neck obstruction; ureteropelvic junction narrowing or obstruction; severe vesicoureteral reflux
2. *Urinary calculi*
3. *Benign prostatic hypertrophy*
4. *Tumors:* carcinoma of the prostate, bladder tumors, contiguous malignant disease (retroperitoneal lymphoma), carcinoma of the cervix or uterus
5. *Inflammation:* prostatitis, ureteritis, urethritis, retroperitoneal fibrosis
6. *Sloughed papillae or blood clots*
7. *Normal pregnancy*
8. *Uterine prolapse and cystocele*
9. *Functional disorders:* neurogenic (spinal cord damage) and other functional abnormalities of the ureter or bladder (often termed *dysfunctional obstruction)*

Hydronephrosis is the term used to describe dilation of the renal pelvis and calyces associated with progressive atrophy of the kidney due to obstruction to the outflow of urine. Even with complete obstruction, glomerular filtration persists for some time because the filtrate subsequently diffuses back into the renal interstitium and perirenal spaces, where it ultimately returns to the lymphatic and venous systems. Because of this continued filtration, the affected calyces and pelvis become dilated, often markedly so. The high pressure in the pelvis is transmitted back through the collecting ducts into the cortex, causing renal atrophy, but it also compresses the renal vasculature of the medulla, causing a diminution in inner medullary plasma flow. The medullary vascular defects are reversible, but if protracted, obstruction will lead to medullary functional disturbances. Accordingly, the initial functional alterations are largely tubular, manifested primarily by impaired concentrating ability. Only later does the GFR begin to diminish. *Obstruction also triggers an interstitial inflammatory reaction, mediated by activated tubular cells and leukocytes, leading eventually to interstitial fibrosis,* by mechanisms similar to those discussed earlier (see Fig. 21–15).[80]

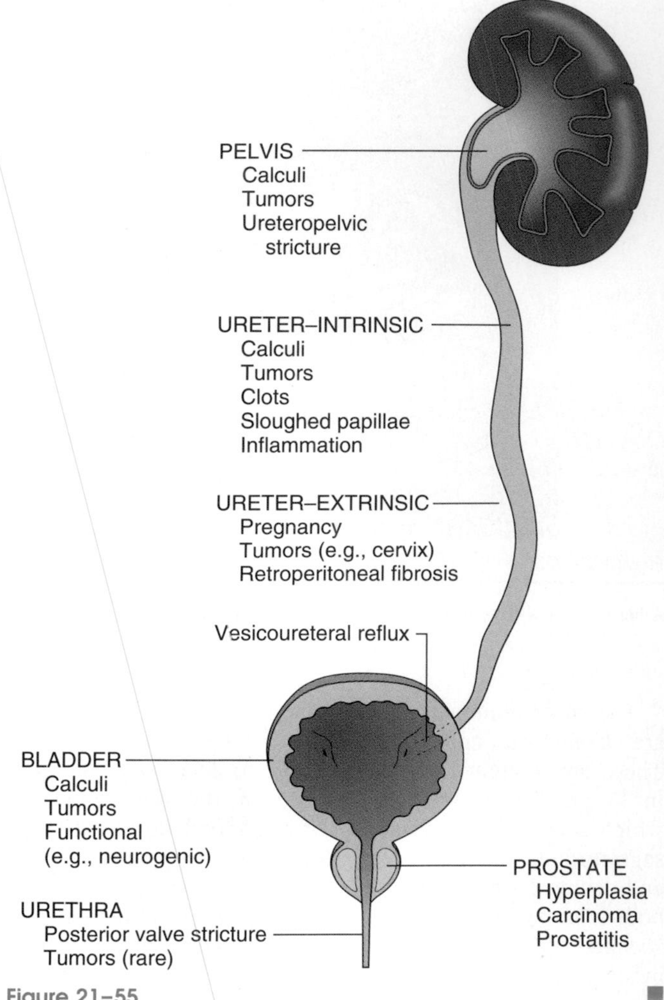

Figure 21–55

Obstructive lesions of the urinary tract.

MORPHOLOGY. When the obstruction is sudden and complete, the reduction of glomerular filtration usually leads to mild dilation of the pelvis and calyces but sometimes to atrophy of the renal parenchyma. When the obstruction is subtotal or intermittent, glomerular filtration is not suppressed, and progressive dilation ensues. Depending on the level of urinary block, the dilation may affect first the bladder or ureter and then the kidney.

In gross appearance, the kidney may have slight to massive enlargement. The earlier features are those of simple dilation of the pelvis and calyces, but in addition there is often significant interstitial inflammation, even in the absence of infection. In chronic cases, the picture is one of cortical tubular atrophy with marked diffuse interstitial fibrosis. Progressive blunting of the apices of the pyramids occurs, and eventually these become cupped. In far-advanced cases, the kidney may become transformed into a thin-walled cystic structure having a diameter of up to 15 to 20 cm (Fig. 21–56) with striking parenchymal atrophy, total obliteration of the pyramids, and thinning of the cortex.

Clinical Course. *Acute obstruction* may provoke pain attributed to distention of the collecting system or renal capsule. Most of the early symptoms are produced by the basic cause of the hydronephrosis. Thus, calculi lodged in the ureters may give rise to renal colic, and prostatic enlargements to bladder symptoms.

Unilateral, complete, or partial hydronephrosis may remain silent for long periods, since the unaffected kidney can maintain adequate renal function. Sometimes its existence first becomes apparent in the course of intravenous pyelography. It is regrettable that this disease tends to remain asymptomatic, because it has been shown that in its early stages, perhaps the first few weeks, relief of such obstruction is compatible with reversion to normal function. *Ultrasonography* is a useful noninvasive technique in the diagnosis of obstructive uropathy.

In *bilateral partial obstruction,* the earliest manifestation is that of inability to concentrate the urine, reflected by polyuria and nocturia. Some patients will have acquired distal tubular acidosis, renal salt wasting, secondary renal calculi, *and a typical picture of tubulointerstitial nephritis* with scarring and atrophy of the papilla and medulla. Hypertension is common in such patients.

Complete bilateral obstruction results in oliguria or anuria and is incompatible with long survival unless the obstruction is relieved. Curiously, after relief of complete urinary tract obstruction, postobstructive *diuresis* occurs. This can often be massive, with the kidney excreting large amounts of urine rich in sodium chloride.

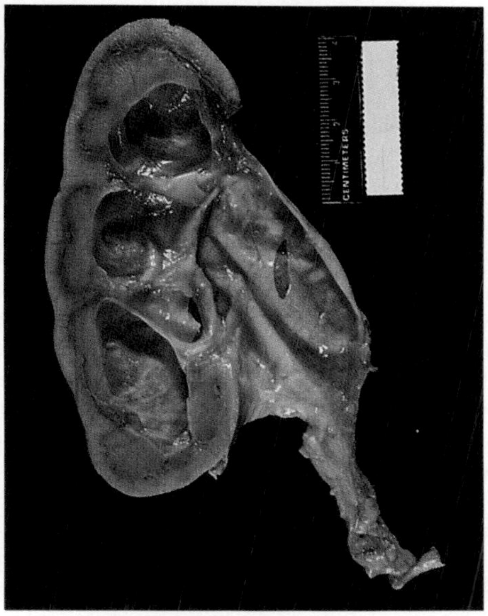

Figure 21–56 ■

Hydronephrosis of the kidney, with marked dilation of the pelvis and calyces and thinning of the renal parenchyma.

UROLITHIASIS (RENAL CALCULI, STONES)

Stones may form at any level in the urinary tract, but most arise in the kidney. Urolithiasis is a frequent clinical problem, affecting 5% to 10% of Americans in their lifetime.[81] Men are affected more often than women are, and the peak age at onset is between 20 and 30 years. Familial and hereditary predisposition to stone formation has long been known. Many of the inborn errors of metabolism, such as gout, cystinuria, and primary hyperoxaluria, provide good examples of hereditary disease characterized by excessive production and excretion of stone-forming substances.

Cause and Pathogenesis. There are four main types of calculi[81, 82] (Table 21–13): (1) *most stones (about 75%) are calcium containing,* composed largely of calcium oxalate, or calcium oxalate mixed with calcium phosphate; (2) another 15% are so-called *triple stones* or *struvite stones,* composed of magnesium ammonium phosphate; (3) *6% are uric acid stones;* and (4) *1% to 2% are made up of cystine.* An organic matrix of mucoprotein, making up 1% to 5% of the stone by weight, is present in all calculi. Al-

Table 21–13. PREVALENCE OF VARIOUS TYPES OF RENAL STONES

	Percentage of All Stones
Calcium Oxalate (Phosphate)	75
Idiopathic hypercalciuria (50%)	
Hypercalciuria and hypercalcemia (10%)	
Hyperoxaluria (5%)	
Enteric (4.5%)	
Primary (0.5%)	
Hyperuricosuria (20%)	
Hypocitraturia	
No known metabolic abnormality (15%–20%)	
Struvite (Magnesium Ammonium Phosphate)	10–15
Uric Acid	6
Associated with hyperuricemia	
Associated with hyperuricosuria	
Idiopathic (50% of uric stones)	
Cystine	1–2
Others or Unknown	±10

though there are many causes for the initiation and propagation of stones, *the most important determinant is an increased urinary concentration of the stones' constituents, such that it exceeds their solubility in urine (supersaturation). A low urine volume* in some metabolically normal patients may also favor supersaturation.

Calcium oxalate stones (Table 21–13) are associated in about 5% of patients with both *hypercalcemia* and *hypercalciuria,* occasioned by hyperparathyroidism, diffuse bone disease, sarcoidosis, and other hypercalcemic states. About 55% have *hypercalciuria without hypercalcemia.* This is caused by several factors, including hyperabsorption of calcium from the intestine *(absorptive hypercalciuria),* an intrinsic impairment in renal tubular reabsorption of calcium *(renal hypercalciuria),* or *idiopathic fasting hypercalciuria with normal parathyroid function.* As many as 20% are associated with increased uric acid secretion *(hyperuricosuric calcium nephrolithiasis),* with or without hypercalciuria. The mechanism of stone formation in this setting involves "nucleation" of calcium oxalate by uric acid crystals in the collecting ducts. Five per cent are associated with *hyperoxaluria,* either hereditary (primary oxaluria) or, more commonly, acquired by intestinal overabsorption in patients with enteric diseases. The latter, so-called *enteric hyperoxaluria,* also occurs in vegetarians, because much of their diet is rich in oxalates. *Hypocitraturia* associated with acidosis and chronic diarrhea of unknown cause may produce calcium stones. *In a variable proportion of patients with calcium stones,* no cause can be found (idiopathic calcium stone disease).

Magnesium ammonium phosphate stones are formed largely after infections by urea-splitting bacteria (e.g., *Proteus* and some staphylococci), which convert urea to ammonia. The resultant alkaline urine causes the precipitation of magnesium ammonium phosphate salts. These form some of the largest stones, as the amounts of urea excreted normally are huge. Indeed, so-called *staghorn calculi* are almost always associated with infection.

Uric acid stones are common in patients with hyperuricemia, such as gout, and diseases involving rapid cell turnover, such as the leukemias. However, *more than half of all patients with urate calculi have neither hyperuricemia nor increased urinary excretion of uric acid.* In this group, it is thought that an unexplained tendency to excrete urine of pH below 5.5 may predispose to uric acid stones, because uric acid is insoluble in relatively acidic urine. In contrast to the radiopaque calcium stones, uric acid stones are radiolucent.

Cystine stones are caused by genetic defects in the renal reabsorption of amino acids, including cystine, leading to cystinuria. Stones form at low urinary pH.

It can thus be appreciated that increased concentration of stone constituents, changes in urinary pH, decreased urine volume, and the presence of bacteria influence the formation of calculi. *However, many calculi occur in the absence of these factors, and conversely patients with hypercalciuria, hyperoxaluria, and hyperuricosuria often do not form stones.* It has, therefore, been postulated that stone formation is enhanced by a *deficiency in inhibitors of crystal formation in urine.* The list of such inhibitors is long, including pyrophosphate, diphosphonate, citrate, glycosaminoglycans, and a glycoprotein called *nephrocalcin.*

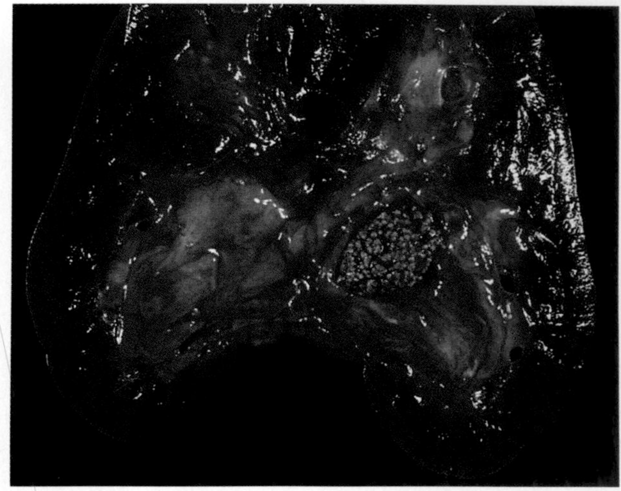

Figure 21–57

Nephrolithiasis. Large stone impacted in the renal pelvis. (Courtesy of Dr. E. Mosher, Brigham and Women's Hospital, Boston, MA.)

MORPHOLOGY. Stones are unilateral in about 80% of patients. The favored sites for their formation are within the renal calyces and pelves (Fig. 21–57) and in the bladder. If formed in the renal pelvis, they tend to remain small, having an average diameter of 2 to 3 mm. These may have smooth contours or may take the form of an irregular, jagged mass of spicules. Often, many stones are found within one kidney. On occasion, progressive accretion of salts leads to the development of branching structures known as staghorn stones, which create a cast of the pelvic and calyceal system.

Clinical Course. Stones are of importance when they obstruct urinary flow or produce ulceration and bleeding. They may be present without producing any symptoms or significant renal damage. In general, smaller stones are most hazardous, because they may pass into the ureters, producing pain referred to as colic (one of the most intense forms of pain) as well as ureteral obstruction. Larger stones cannot enter the ureters and are more likely to remain silent within the renal pelvis. Commonly, these larger stones first manifest themselves by hematuria. Stones also predispose to superimposed infection, both by their obstructive nature and by the trauma they produce.

TUMORS OF THE KIDNEY

Both benign and malignant tumors occur in the kidney.[83, 84] With the exception of oncocytoma, the benign tumors are incidental findings at autopsy and rarely have clinical significance. Malignant tumors, on the other hand, are of great importance clinically and deserve considerable emphasis. By far the most common of these malignant tumors is renal cell carcinoma, followed by Wilms' tumor, which is found in children and described in Chapter 11, and finally urothelial tumors of the calyces and pelves.

Benign Tumors

RENAL PAPILLARY ADENOMA

Small, discrete adenomas having origin in the renal tubules are found commonly (7% to 22%) at autopsy. They are most frequently papillary and are thus called *papillary adenomas* in the most recent international classifications.[85]

MORPHOLOGY. These are small tumors, usually less than 5 mm in diameter.[85] They are present invariably within the cortex and appear grossly as pale yellow-gray, discrete, seemingly encapsulated nodules. On microscopic examination, they are composed of complex, branching, papillomatous structures with numerous complex fronds that project into a cystic space. Cells may also grow as tubules, glands, cords, and totally undifferentiated masses of cells. The cell type for all these growth patterns is regular and free of atypia. The cells are cuboidal to polygonal in shape, have regular small central nuclei, and have a clear cytoplasm.

By histologic criteria, these tumors do not differ from low-grade papillary renal cell adenocarcinoma and indeed share some immunohistochemical and cytogenetic features (trisomies 7 and 17) with papillary cancers, to be discussed later, although less extensively. The size of the tumor was once used as a prognostic feature, with a cutoff of 3 cm separating those that metastasize from those that rarely do. However, because tumors of relatively small size, 1 to 3 cm in diameter, are increasingly being detected during x-ray procedures performed for non-renal symptoms, the current view is to consider and treat those as early cancers, until an unequivocal marker of benignity is discovered.

RENAL FIBROMA OR HAMARTOMA (RENOMEDULLARY INTERSTITIAL CELL TUMOR)

On occasion, at autopsy, small foci of gray-white firm tissue, usually less than 1 cm in diameter, are found within the pyramids of the kidneys. Microscopic examination of these discloses fibroblast-like cells and collagenous tissue. Ultrastructurally, the cells have features of renal interstitial cells. The tumors have no malignant propensities.

ANGIOMYOLIPOMA

This is a benign tumor consisting of vessels, smooth muscle, and fat. *Angiomyolipomas are present in 25% to 50% of patients with tuberous sclerosis,* a disease characterized by lesions of the cerebral cortex that produce epilepsy and mental retardation as well as a variety of skin abnormalities (Chapter 27).

ONCOCYTOMA

This is an epithelial tumor composed of large, eosinophilic cells having small, rounded, benign-appearing nuclei. It is thought to arise from the intercalated cells of collecting ducts. It is not an uncommon tumor, accounting for 5% of surgically resected neoplasms. *Ultrastructurally, the eosinophilic cells have numerous prominent mitochondria.* In gross appearance, the tumors are tan or mahogany brown, relatively homogeneous, and usually well encapsulated. However, they may achieve a large size (up to 12 cm in diameter). Although anecdotal cases with metastases have been reported, the tumor is considered benign.

Malignant Tumors

RENAL CELL CARCINOMA (HYPERNEPHROMA, ADENOCARCINOMA OF KIDNEY)

Renal cell carcinomas represent about 1% to 3% of all visceral cancers and account for 85% of renal cancers in adults. There are 30,000 new cases per year and 12,000 deaths from the disease.[86] The tumors occur most often in older individuals, usually in the sixth and seventh decades of life, showing a male preponderance in the ratio of 2 to 3:1. Because of their gross yellow color and the resemblance of the tumor cells to clear cells of the adrenal cortex, they were at one time called *hypernephroma.* It is now clear that all these tumors arise from tubular epithelium and are therefore renal adenocarcinomas.

Epidemiology. Tobacco is the most prominent risk factor. Cigarette smokers have double the incidence of renal cell carcinoma, and pipe and cigar smokers are also more susceptible. An international study has identified additional risk factors, including obesity (particularly in women); hypertension; unopposed estrogen therapy; and exposure to asbestos, petroleum products, and heavy metals.[87] There is also increased incidence in patients with chronic renal failure and acquired cystic disease (see earlier) and in tuberous sclerosis.

Most renal cancer is sporadic, but unusual forms of autosomal dominant familial cancers occur, usually in younger individuals. Although they account for only 4% of renal cancers, familial variants have been enormously instructive in studying renal carcinogenesis.

- *Von Hippel–Lindau (VHL) syndrome:* Half to two thirds of patients with VHL (Chapter 30)—characterized by hemangioblastomas of the cerebellum and retina—develop renal cysts and bilateral, often multiple renal cell carcinomas (nearly all, if they live long enough). As we shall see, *current studies implicate the VHL gene in carcinogenesis of both familial and sporadic clear cell tumors.*

- *Hereditary (familial) clear cell carcinoma*, confined to the kidney, without the other manifestations of VHL, but with abnormalities involving the same or a related gene.
- *Hereditary papillary carcinoma.* This autosomal dominant form is manifested by multiple bilateral tumors with papillary histology. These tumors exhibit a series of cytogenetic abnormalities and, as will be described, mutations in the *MET* protooncogene.

Classification of Renal Cell Carcinoma: Histology, Cytogenetics, and Genetics

The classification of renal cell carcinoma has recently undergone revision, based on correlative cytogenetic, genetic, and histologic studies of both familial and sporadic tumors.[85] The major types of tumor are as follows (Fig. 21–58):

1. *Clear cell (nonpapillary) carcinoma.* This is the most common type, accounting for 70% to 80% of renal cell cancers. On histologic examination, the tumors are made of cells with clear or granular cytoplasm and are *nonpapillary*. They can be familial, associated with VHL disease, or in most cases sporadic. In 98% of these tumors, *whether familial, sporadic, or associated with VHL,* there is a deletion or unbalanced chromosomal translocation (3;6, 3;8, 3;11) resulting in losses of the smallest overlapping region of chromosome 3—3p14 to 3p26. This region harbors the *VHL* gene (3p25.3).[88] A second nondeleted allele of the *VHL* gene shows somatic mutations, or hypermethylation-induced inactivation in about 80% of clear cell cancers, indicating that the *VHL* gene acts as a tumor-suppressor gene in both sporadic and familial forms. The *VHL* gene encodes a protein that inhibits the generation of a transcriptional elongation complex, called *elongin,* and presumably the rate of transcription of important distal genes.[89] How these defects contribute to renal cancer is still unclear.
2. *Papillary carcinoma* accounts for 10% to 15% of renal cancers.[90] It is characterized by a papillary growth pattern and also occurs in both familial and sporadic forms. These tumors are not associated with 3p deletions. The most common cytogenetic abnormalities are trisomies 7, 16, and 17 and loss of Y in male patients [t(X,1)] in the sporadic form, and trisomy 7 in the familial form. The gene for the familial form has been mapped to a locus on chromosome 7, encompassing the locus for *MET*, a protooncogene that serves as the tyrosine kinase receptor for *hepatocyte growth factor.* Described in Chapter 4, hepatocyte growth factor (also called scatter factor) mediates growth, cell mobility, invasion, and morphogenetic differentiation.[91] Both germ line and somatic mutations in the tyrosine kinase domain of the *MET* gene have been identified, making mutated *MET* a likely candidate oncogene in the cancers. A second gene called *PRCC* (for papillary renal cell carcinoma) on chromosome 1 has also been implicated in sporadic tumors, largely in children, exhibiting characteristic X;1 translocations.[92]
3. *Chromophobe renal carcinoma* represents 5% of renal cell cancers and is manifested by cells with prominent cell membranes and pale eosinophilic cytoplasm, usually with a halo around the nucleus. On cytogenetic examination, these tumors exhibit multiple chromosome losses and extreme hypodiploidy. They are, like the benign oncocytoma, thought to grow from intercalated cells of collecting ducts and have an excellent prognosis compared with that of the clear cell and papillary cancers.

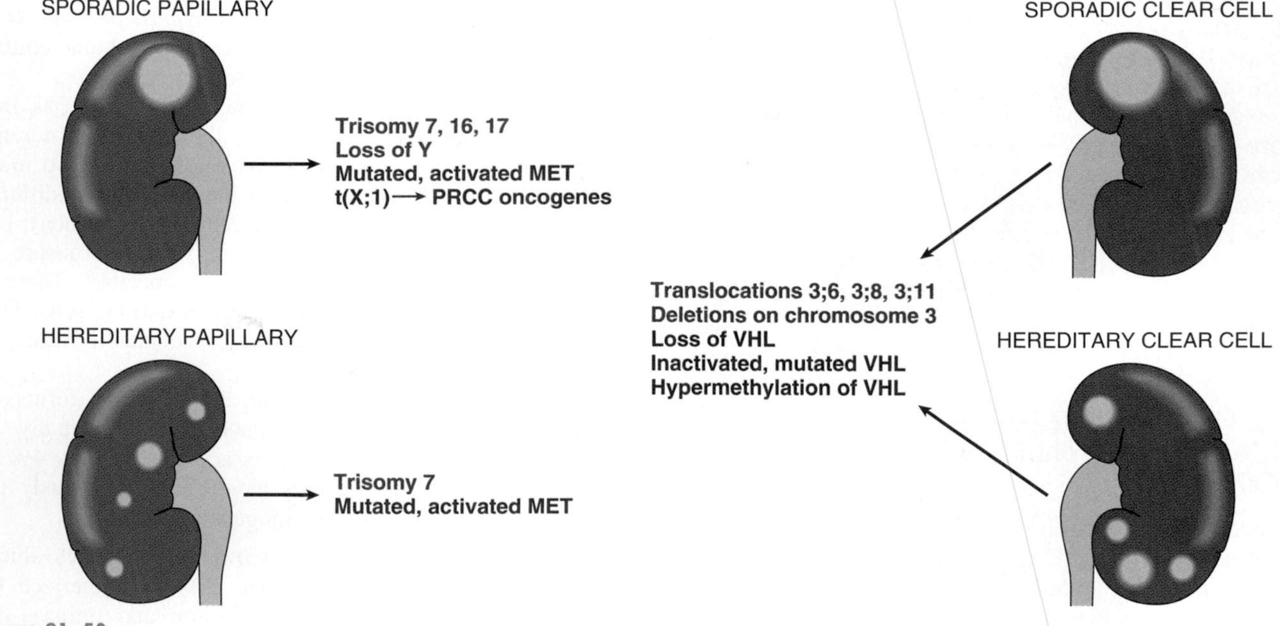

Figure 21–58

Cytogenetics (in blue) and genetics (in red) of clear cell versus papillary renal cell carcinoma. (Courtesy of Dr. Keith Ligon, Brigham and Women's Hospital, Boston, MA.)

MORPHOLOGY. In its macroscopic appearance, the renal cell carcinoma tumor is characteristic. It may arise in any portion of the kidney, but more commonly it affects the poles, particularly the upper one. Clear cell neoplasms occur as solitary unilateral lesions They are spherical masses, 3 to 15 cm in diameter, composed of bright yellow-gray-white tissue that distorts the renal outline. There are commonly large areas of ischemic, opaque, gray-white necrosis, foci of hemorrhagic discoloration, and areas of softening. The margins are usually sharply defined and confined within the renal capsule (Fig. 21–59). **Papillary tumors** can be multifocal and bilateral. They are typically hemorrhagic and cystic, especially when large. The papillae may be seen grossly as golden yellow flakes.

As tumors enlarge, they may bulge into the calyces and pelvis and eventually may fungate through the walls of the collecting system to extend even into the ureter. One of the striking characteristics of this tumor is its tendency to invade the renal vein (Fig. 21–59) and grow as a solid column of cells within this vessel. Further extension produces a continuous cord of tumor in the inferior vena cava and even in the right side of the heart.

In **clear cell carcinoma,** the growth pattern varies from solid to trabecular (cordlike) or tubular (resembling tubules). The tumor cells have a rounded or polygonal shape and abundant clear or granular cytoplasm; the latter on special stains contains glycogen and lipids (Fig. 21–60*A*). The tumors have delicate branching vasculature and may exhibit cystic as well as solid areas. Most tumors are well differentiated, but some show marked nuclear atypia with formation of bizarre nuclei and giant cells. **Papillary carcinoma** is composed of cuboidal or low columnar cells arranged in papillary formations. Interstitial foam cells are common in the papillary cores (Fig. 21–60*B*). **Psammoma** bodies may be present. The stroma is usually scanty but highly vascularized. **Chromophobe renal carcinoma** is made up of pale eosinophilic cells, often with a perinuclear halo, arranged in solid sheets with a concentration of the largest cells around blood vessels (Fig. 21–60*C*). **Collecting duct carcinoma** is a rare variant showing irregular channels lined by highly atypical epithelium with a hobnail pattern. **Sarcomatoid** changes arise infrequently in all types of renal cell carcinoma and are a decidedly ominous feature of these tumors.

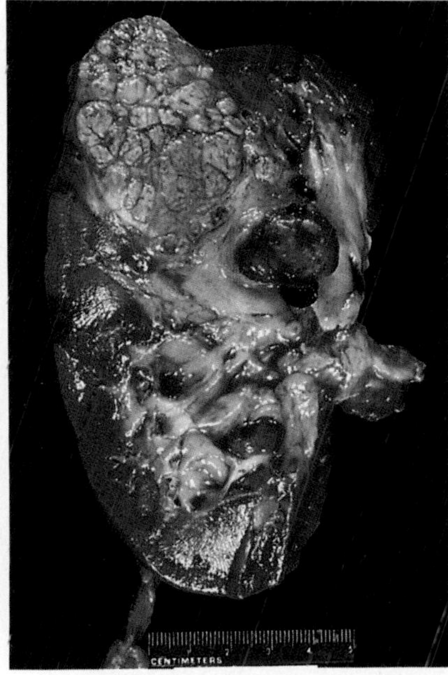

Figure 21–59 ■

Renal cell carcinoma. Typical cross-section of yellowish, spherical neoplasm in one pole of the kidney. Note tumor in the dilated thrombosed renal vein.

Clinical Course. The three classic diagnostic features of *costovertebral pain, palpable mass,* and *hematuria* unfortunately appear in only 10% of cases. The most reliable of the three is hematuria, but it is usually intermittent and may be microscopic; thus, the tumor may remain silent until it attains a large size. At this time, it gives rise to generalized constitutional symptoms, such as fever, malaise, weakness, and weight loss. This pattern of asymptomatic growth occurs in many patients, so that the tumor may have reached a diameter of more than 10 cm when it is discovered. In current times, however, many of these tumors are being discovered in the asymptomatic state by incidental radiologic studies (e.g., computed tomographic scan or magnetic resonance imaging) usually performed for non-renal indications.

Renal cell carcinoma is classified as one of the great "mimics" in medicine, because it tends to produce a diversity of systemic symptoms not related to the kidney. In addition to the fever and constitutional symptoms mentioned earlier, renal cell carcinomas produce a number of paraneoplastic syndromes (Chapter 8), ascribed to abnormal hormone production, including *polycythemia, hypercalcemia, hypertension, hepatic dysfunction, feminization or masculinization, Cushing syndrome, eosinophilia, leukemoid reactions, and amyloidosis.*

One of the common characteristics of this tumor is its *tendency to metastasize widely before giving rise to any local symptoms or signs.* In 25% of new patients with renal cell carcinoma, there is radiologic evidence of metastases at presentation. The most common locations of metastasis are the lungs (more than 50%) and bones (33%), followed in order by the regional lymph nodes, liver and adrenals, and brain.

The average 5-year survival of patients with renal cell carcinoma is about 45% and up to 70% in the absence of distant metastases. With renal vein invasion or extension into the perinephric fat, the figure is reduced to approximately 15% to 20%. Nephrectomy is the treatment of choice.

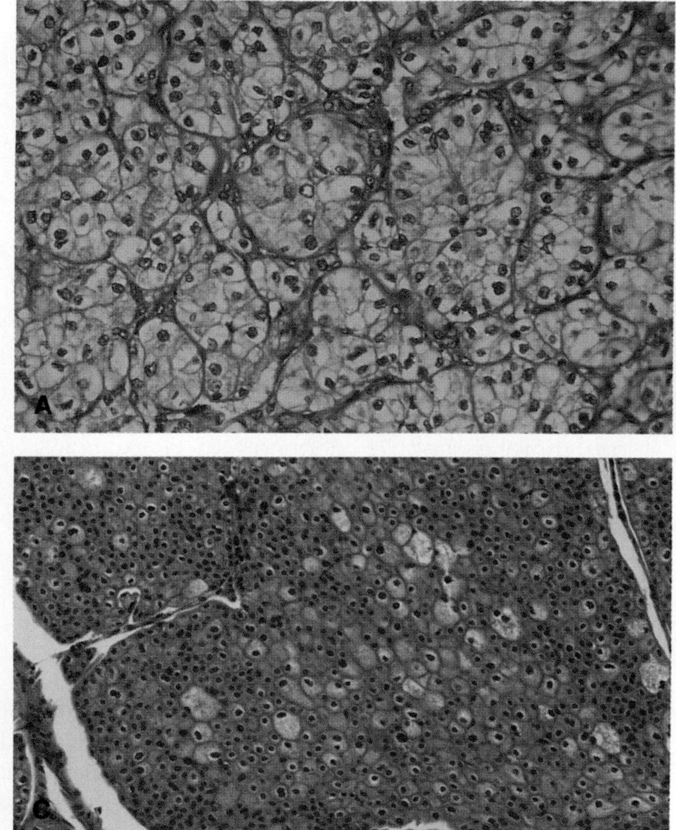

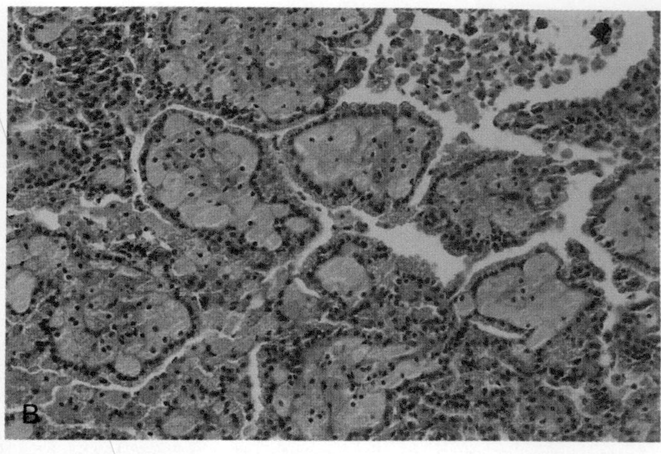

Figure 21–60

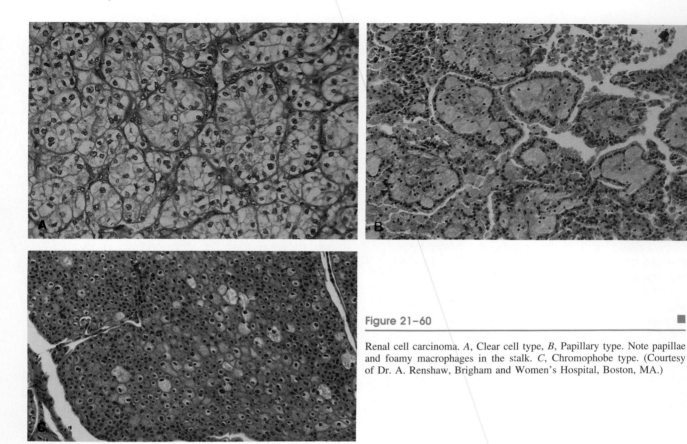

Renal cell carcinoma. *A*, Clear cell type, *B*, Papillary type. Note papillae and foamy macrophages in the stalk. *C*, Chromophobe type. (Courtesy of Dr. A. Renshaw, Brigham and Women's Hospital, Boston, MA.)

UROTHELIAL CARCINOMAS OF RENAL PELVIS

Approximately 5% to 10% of primary renal tumors occur in the renal pelvis (Fig. 21–61). These tumors span the range from apparently benign papillomas to frank papillary carcinomas, but as with bladder tumors, the benign papillomas are difficult to differentiate from the low-grade papillary cancers.

Renal pelvic tumors usually become clinically apparent within a relatively short time because they lie within the pelvis and, by fragmentation, produce noticeable hematuria. They are almost invariably small when discovered. These tumors are almost never palpable clinically; however, they may block the urinary outflow and lead to palpable hydronephrosis and flank pain. On histologic examination, pelvic tumors are the exact counterpart of those found in the urinary bladder; for further details, reference should be made to that section.

Urothelial tumors may occasionally be multiple, involving the pelvis, ureters, and bladder. In 50% of renal pelvic tumors, there is a preexisting or concomitant bladder urothelial tumor. On histologic examination, there are also foci of atypia or carcinoma in situ in grossly normal urothelium remote from the pelvic tumor. There is an increased incidence of urothelial carcinomas of the renal pelvis and bladder in patients with analgesic nephropathy.

Infiltration of the wall of the pelvis and calyces is common. For this reason, despite their apparently small, deceptively benign appearance, the prognosis for these tumors is not good. Five-year survival rates vary from 50% to 70% for low-grade superficial lesions to 10% with high-grade infiltrating tumors.

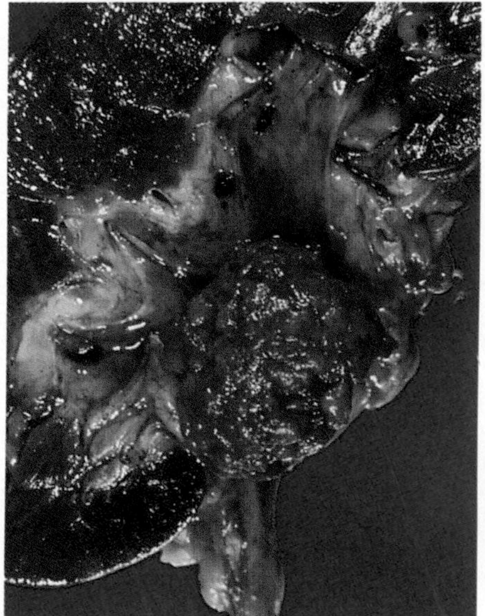

Figure 21–61

Urothelial carcinoma of the renal pelvis. Pelvis has been opened to expose the nodular irregular neoplasm, just proximal to the ureter.

REFERENCES

1. Dinesen I: Seven Gothic Tales. New York, Modern Library, 1939.
2. Kanwar YS, Venkatachalam MA: Morphology of the glomerulus and juxtaglomerular apparatus. In Handbook of Physiology, Section of Renal Physiology, 2nd ed. Washington, DC, American Physiological Society, 1990.
3. Hudson BG, et al: Structure, gene organization and role in human diseases of type IV collagen. J Biol Chem 268:1, 1993.
4. Timpl R, Brown JC: Supramolecular assembly of basement membranes. Bioassays 18:123, 1997.
5. Jennette JC, et al: Heptinstall's Pathology of the Kidney, 5th ed. Philadelphia, Lippincott-Raven, 1998.
6. Tisher C, Brenner BM: Renal Pathology, with Clinical and Pathological Correlations, 3rd ed. Philadelphia, JB Lippincott, 1999.
7. Schrier RW, Gottschalk CW (eds): Diseases of the Kidney, 6th ed. Boston, Little, Brown, 1997.
8. Brenner BM, Rector F (eds): The Kidney, 5th ed. Philadelphia, WB Saunders, 1996.
9. Rose's Up To Date in Medicine—Nephrology, Vol. 6, No. 1. Up To Date, Inc. Wellesley, MA, 1998.
10. Gardner KD Jr, Bernstein J: The Cystic Kidney. Dordrecht, Kluwer Academic Publishers, 1990.
11. Gabow PA: Autosomal dominant polycystic kidney disease. N Engl J Med 329:332, 1993.
12. Grantham JJ: The pathogenesis, etiology and treatment of autosomal dominant polycystic kidney disease. Am J Kidney Dis 28:788, 1996.
13. The International Polycystic Kidney Disease Consortium. Polycystic kidney disease: the complete structure of the *PKD1* gene and its protein. Cell 81:289, 1995.
13a. Hughes J, et al: The polycystic kidney disease 1 *(PKD1)* gene encodes a novel protein with multiple cell recognition domains. Nat Genet 10:151, 1995.
14. Mochizuki T, et al: *PKD2,* a gene for polycystic kidney disease that encodes an integral membrane protein. Science 272:1339, 1996.
15. Grantham JJ, et al: Evidence for inflammatory and secretagogue lipids in cyst fluids from patients with autosomal dominant polycystic kidney disease. Proc Assoc Am Physicians 109:397, 1997.
16. Lu W, et al: Perinatal lethality with kidney and pancreas defects in mice with a targeted *PKD-1* mutation. Nat Gen 17:179, 1997.
17. Qian F, et al: The molecular basis of focal cyst formation in human autosomal dominant polycystic kidney disease type I. Cell 87:979, 1996.
18. Qian F, et al: *PKD1* interacts with *PKD2* through a probable coiled-coil domain. Nat Genet 16:184, 1997.
19. Watson MC: Complications of APKD. Kidney Int 51:353, 1997.
20. Griffin MD, et al: Vascular expression of polycystin. J Am Soc Nephrol 8:616, 1997.
21. Hildebrandt F, et al: A novel gene encoding on SH-3 domain protein is mutated in juvenile nephronophthisis type 1. Nat Genet 17:149, 1997.
22. Nielsen EG, Couser WG: Immunologic Renal Diseases. New York, Lippincott-Raven, 1997.
23. Wilson CB: Renal response to immunological injury. In Brenner BM, Rector F (eds): The Kidney, 5th ed. Philadelphia, WB Saunders, 1996, pp 1253–1391.
24. Farquhar M, et al: The Heymann nephritis antigenic complex: megalin (gp330) and RAP. J Am Soc Nephrol 6:35, 1996.
25. Bolton WK, et al: New avian model of experimental glomerulonephritis consistent with mediation by cellular immunity. Nonhumorally mediated glomerulonephritis in chickens. J Clin Invest 73:1263, 1984.
26. Kalluri R, et al: Susceptibility to anti–glomerular basement membrane disease and Goodpasture syndrome is linked to MHC class II genes and emergence of T cell–mediated immunity in mice. J Clin Invest 100:2263, 1997.
27. Couser WG: Mediation of immune glomerular injury. J Am Soc Nephrol 1:13, 1990.
28. Johnson RJ: Cytokines, growth factors and renal injury. Kidney Int 52:S2, 1997.
29. Border WA, Noble NA: TGF-β in kidney fibrosis: a target for gene therapy. Kidney Int 51:1389, 1997.
30. Remuzzi G, Ruggenenti P, Benigni A: Understanding the nature of renal disease progression. Kidney Int 51:2, 1997.
31. Schena FP, et al: Progression of renal damage in human glomerulonephritis. Kidney Int 52:1439, 1997.
32. Rennke HG, et al: The progression of renal disease: structural and functional correlations. In Tisher CC, Brenner B (eds): Renal Pathology, 2nd ed. Philadelphia, JB Lippincott, 1994, pp 116–139.
33. Rodriguez-Iturbe J: Acute post-streptococcal glomerulonephritis. In Schrier RW, Gottschalk CW (eds): Diseases of the Kidney, 5th ed. Boston, Little, Brown, 1993, pp 1715–1730.
34. Fisher M, et al: Susceptibility to anti–glomerular basement membrane disease is strongly associated with HLA-DRB1 genes. Kidney Int 51: 222, 1997.
35. Haas M, et al: Changing etiologies of unexplained adult nephrotic syndrome. Am J Kidney Dis 30:621, 1997.
36. Wasserstein AG: Membranous glomerulonephritis. J Am Soc Nephrol 8:664, 1997.
37. A Report on the International Study of Kidney Disease in Children. The primary nephrotic syndrome in children: identification of patients with minimal change nephrotic syndrome from initial response to prednisone. J Pediatr 98:561, 1981.
38. D'Agati V: The many masks of focal segmental glomerulosclerosis. Kidney Int 46:1223, 1994.
38a. Kestila M, et al: Positionally cloned gene for a novel glomerular protein—nephrin—is mutated in congenital nephrotic syndrome. Mol Cell 1:575, 1998.
39. Mathis BJ: A locus for inherited focal segmental glomerulosclerosis maps to chromosome 19q13. Kidney Int 53:282, 1998.
40. Humphreys MH: HIV-associated glomerulonephritis. Kidney Int 48: 311, 1995.
41. Savin V, et al: Circulating factor associated with increased permeability to albumin in recurrent focal segmental glomerulosclerosis. N Engl J Med 334:878, 1996.
42. D'Agati V, Appel GB: HIV infection and the kidney. J Am Soc Nephrol 8:139, 1997.
43. Bruggerman LA, et al: Nephropathy in human HIV-1 transgenic mice is due to renal trans gene expression. J Clin Invest 46:759, 1997.
44. White RH: Mesangiocapillary glomerulonephritis. In Edelman CM Jr (ed): Pediatric Kidney. Boston, Little, Brown, 1992, pp 1307–1324.
45. Rennke HG: Secondary MPGN. Kidney Int 47:643, 1995.
46. Emancipator SN: Primary and secondary forms of IgA nephritis. In Jennette JC (ed): Heptinstall's Pathology of the Kidney, 5th ed. Boston, Little, Brown, 1998.
47. Donadio JV, Grande JP: Immunoglobulin A nephropathy: a clinical perspective. J Am Soc Nephrol 8:1324, 1997.
48. Kashtan CE, Michael AF: Perspectives in clinical nephrology: Alport syndrome. Kidney Int 50:1445, 1996.
49. Grunfeld JP: The clinical spectrum of hereditary nephritis. Kidney Int 27:83, 1985.
50. Hemmink HH, et al: Benign familial hematuria due to a mutation of the type IV collagen $\alpha 4$ gene. J Clin Invest 98:1114, 1996.
51. Cameron SJ: The long-term outcome of glomerular diseases. In Schrier RW, Gottschalk CW (eds): Diseases of the Kidney, 5th ed. Boston, Little, Brown, 1993, pp 1895–1958.
51a. Blanco R, et al: Henoch-Schönlein purpura in adulthood and childhood. Two different expressions of the same syndrome. Arthritis Rheum 40:859, 1997.
52. Mauer M, et al: Diabetic glomerulosclerosis. In Schrier RW, Gottschalk CW (eds): Diseases of the Kidney, 5th ed. Boston, Little, Brown, 1993, pp 2153–2189.
53. Ibrahim H, Hostetter TH: Diabetic nephropathy. Am Soc Nephrol 8: 487, 1997.
54. Vlassara H: Recent progress in advanced glycation end products and diabetic complications. Diabetes 46:519, 1997.
55. Gambara V, et al: Heterogeneous nature of renal lesions in type 2 diabetes. J Am Soc Nephrol 3:1458, 1993.
56. Fogo A, et al: Morphologic and clinical features of fibrillary versus immunotactoid glomerulonephropathy. Am J Kidney Dis 22:367, 1993.
56a. Liebenthal WL: Biology of acute renal failure. Kidney Int 52:1102, 1997.
57. Brezis M, Epstein FH: Cellular mechanisms of acute ischemic injury to the kidney. Annu Rev Med 44:27, 1993.
58. Edelstein CL, et al: The nature of renal cell injury. Kidney Int 51: 341, 1997.

59. Rabb H, et al: Leukocytes, cell adhesion molecules and ischemic renal failure. Kidney Int 51:1463, 1997.
60. Humes DH, et al: Acute renal failure: growth factors, cell therapy and gene therapy. Proc Am Assoc Physicians 109:547, 1997.
61. Oliver J, et al: The pathogenesis of acute renal failure associated with traumatic and toxic injury, renal ischemia, nephrotoxic damage, and the ischemic episode. J Clin Invest 30:1307, 1951.
62. Cavallo T: Tubulointerstitial nephritis. In Jennette JC, et al (eds): Heptinstall's Pathology of the Kidney, 5th ed. Philadelphia, Lippincott-Raven, 1998, p 667.
62a. Seshan S, et al (eds): Classification and Atlas of Tubulo-interstitial and Vascular Diseases. Baltimore, Williams & Wilkins, 1998.
63. Rubin RH, et al: Urinary tract infection, pyelonephritis, and reflux nephropathy. In Brenner BM (ed): Brenner and Rector's The Kidney, 5th ed. Philadelphia, WB Saunders, 1996, pp 1597–1654.
64. Langermann S, et al: Prevention of mucosal *Escherichia coli* infection by FimH-adhesin–based systemic vaccination. Science 276:607, 1997.
65. Kunin CM: Urinary Tract Infections: Detection, Prevention, and Management, 5th ed. Baltimore, Williams & Wilkins, 1997.
66. Appel GB: Acute interstitial nephritis. In Nielsen E, Couser WG (eds): Immunologic Renal Disease. Philadelphia, Lippincott-Raven, 1997.
66a. Michel D, Kelly CJ: Acute interstitial nephritis. J Am Soc Nephrol 9:506, 1998.
67. Kincaid Smith P, Nanra RS: Lithium-induced and analgesic-induced renal disease. In Schrier RW, Gottschalk CW (eds): Diseases of the Kidney, 5th ed. Boston, Little, Brown, 1993, pp 1099–1130.
68. De Broe ME, Elseveirs MM: Analgesic nephropathy. N Engl J Med 338:446, 1998.
69. Radford MG, et al: Reversible membranous nephropathy associated with the use of nonsteroidal antiinflammatory drugs. JAMA 276:466, 1996.
70. Kurokawa K, et al (eds): Hypertension: causes and consequences of renal injury. Kidney Int 49(Suppl 55):S1, 1997.
70a. Preston RA, et al: Renal parenchymal hypertension. Present concepts. Arch Intern Med 156:602, 1996.
71. Meyrier A, et al: Ischemic renal diseases: new insights into old entities. Kidney Int 54:2, 1998.
71a. Kitiyakara C, Guzman NJ: Malignant hypertension and hypertensive emergencies. J Am Soc Nephrol 9:128, 1998.
72. Working Group on Renovascular Hypertension: Detection, evaluation, and treatment. Ann Intern Med 147:820, 1987.
73. Goldblatt H, et al: Studies on experimental hypertension: I. Production of persistent elevation of systolic blood pressure by means of renal ischemia. J Exp Med 59:347, 1934.
74. Kwaan HC, et al (eds): Thrombotic thrombocytopenic purpura and the hemolytic uremic syndrome. Semin Hematol 34:81, 1997.
75. Remuzzi G, Ruggenenti P: The hemolytic uremic syndrome. Kidney Int 48:2, 1995.
76. Mitra D, et al: Thrombotic thrombocytopenic purpura and sporadic hemolytic-uremic syndrome plasmas induce apoptosis in restricted lineages of human microvascular endothelial cells. Blood 89:1224, 1997.
77. Boyce TG, et al: *Escherichia coli* O157:H7 and the hemolytic uremic syndrome. N Engl J Med 333:364, 1995.
78. Gagnuandou MF, et al: Long-term (15–25 years) prognosis of hemolytic-uremic syndrome. J Am Soc Nephrol 4:275, 1993.
79. Greco BA, Breyer JA: Atherosclerotic ischemic renal disease. Am J Kidney Dis 29:167, 1997.
80. Klahr S: Obstructive nephropathy. Kidney Int 54:286, 1998.
81. Pak CT: Urolithiasis. In Schrier RW, Gottschalk CW (eds): Diseases of the Kidney, 5th ed. Boston, Little, Brown, 1993, pp 729–743.
82. Coe FL, et al: The pathogenesis and treatment of kidney stones. N Engl J Med 327:1141, 1993.
83. Murphy WM, et al: Tumors of the urinary bladder, urethra, ureters, renal pelves, and kidneys. Atlas of Tumor Pathology, 3rd Series, Fascicle 11. Washington, DC, Armed Forces Institute of Pathology, 1994.
84. Eble JN (Ed.): Tumors of the kidney. Semin Diagn Pathol 15:1–81, 1998.
85. Storkel S, et al: Classification of renal cell carcinoma. Cancer 80:987, 1997.
86. Motzer RJ, et al: Medical progress: renal cell carcinoma. N Engl J Med 335:865, 1996.
87. Savage PD: Renal cell carcinoma. Curr Opin Oncol 8:247, 1996.
88. Neumann HPH, Zbar B: Renal cysts, renal cancer and von Hippel–Lindau disease. Kidney Int 51:16, 1997.
89. Iliopoulos O, Kaelin WG: The molecular basis of von Hippel Lindau disease. Mol Med 3:289, 1997.
90. Lager DJ, et al: Papillary renal tumors. Cancer 76:669, 1995.
91. Jeffers M, et al: Activating mutations for the Met tyrosine kinase receptor in human cancer. Proc Natl Acad Sci USA 94:11445, 1997.
92. Sidhar SK, et al: The t(X;1)(p11.2;q21.2) translocation in papillary renal cell carcinoma fuses a novel gene *PRCC* to the *TFE3* transcription factor gene. Hum Mol Genet 5:1333, 1996.

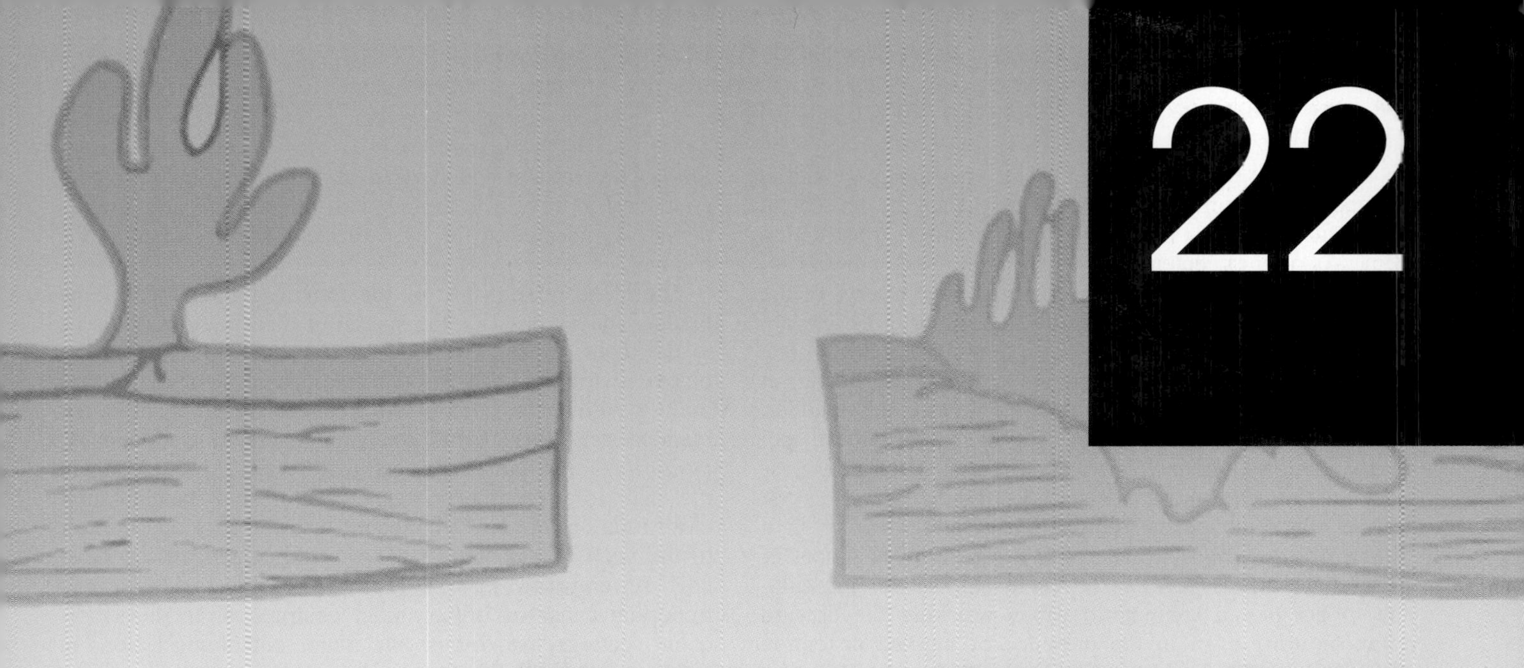

The Lower Urinary Tract

Ureters

CONGENITAL ANOMALIES
INFLAMMATIONS
TUMORS AND TUMOR-LIKE LESIONS
OBSTRUCTIVE LESIONS

Urinary Bladder

CONGENITAL ANOMALIES
INFLAMMATIONS
ACUTE AND CHRONIC CYSTITIS
SPECIAL FORMS OF CYSTITIS
NEOPLASMS
UROTHELIAL (TRANSITIONAL CELL) TUMORS
MESENCHYMAL TUMORS
SECONDARY TUMORS
OBSTRUCTION

Urethra

INFLAMMATIONS
TUMORS

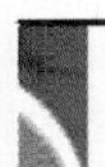

NORMAL

Despite differing embryonic origins, the various components of the lower urinary tract come to have many morphologic similarities. The renal pelves, ureters, bladder, and urethra (save for its terminal portion) are lined by a special form of transitional epithelium (urothelium) that is two to three cells thick in the pelvis, three to five cells thick in the ureters, and three to seven cells thick in the bladder. The surface layer consists of large, flattened "umbrella cells" that cover several underlying cells. The umbrella cells have a trilaminar asymmetric unit membrane and possess apical plaques composed of specific proteins called *uroplakins.* Toward the basal layer, the cells become smaller, or more cylindrical (particularly in contracted bladders), but are capable of some flattening when the underlying wall is stretched. This epithelium rests on a well-developed basement membrane, beneath which there is a lamina propria. The lamina propria in the urinary bladder may have wisps of smooth muscle, but a well-developed muscularis mucosae occurs in less than 5% of normal human bladders. It is important to differentiate the muscularis mucosae from the deeper well-defined rounded muscle fibers of the detrusor muscle, since bladder cancers are staged on the basis of invasion of the latter. The bladder musculature in the ureters and bladders is capable, with obstruction to the flow of urine, of great thickening. The normal epithelial cells express surface blood group antigens (A, B, H) and receptors for growth factors.

Several variants of the normal epithelial pattern may be encountered. Nests of urothelium or inbudding of the surface epithelium may be found occasionally in the mucosa lamina propria; these are sometimes referred to as *Brunn nests.* Similarly, small cystic inclusions lined by cuboidal or columnar epithelium are sometimes found in the lamina propria.

Several points about the gross anatomy of these structures may come to have clinical significance. The ureters lie throughout their course in a retroperitoneal position. Retroperitoneal tumors or fibrosis may trap the ureters in neoplastic or dense, fibrous tissue, sometimes obstructing them. As ureters enter the pelvis, they pass anterior to either the common iliac or the external iliac artery. In the female pelvis, they lie close to the uterine arteries and are therefore vulnerable to injury in operations on the female genital tract. There are three points of slight narrowing: at the ureteropelvic junction, where they enter the bladder, and where they cross the iliac vessels, all providing loci where renal calculi may become impacted when they pass from the kidney to the bladder. As the ureters enter the bladder, they pursue an oblique course, terminating in a slitlike orifice. The obliquity of this intramural segment of the ureteral orifice permits the enclosing bladder musculature to act like a sphincteric valve, blocking the upward reflux of urine even in the presence of marked distention of the urinary bladder. As discussed in Chapter 21, a defect in the intravesical portion of the ureter leads to vesicoureteral reflux. The orifices of the ureters and urethra demarcate an area at the base of the bladder known as the trigone.

The close relationship of the female genital tract to the bladder makes possible the spread of disease from one tract to the other. In middle-aged and elderly women, relaxation of pelvic support leads to prolapse (descent) of the uterus, pulling with it the floor of the bladder. In this fashion, the bladder is protruded into the vagina, creating a pouch—*cystocele*—that fails to empty readily with micturition. In the man, the seminal vesicles and prostate have similar close relationships, being situated just posterior and inferior to the neck of the bladder. Thus, enlargement of the prostate, so common in middle to later life, constitutes an important cause of urinary tract obstruction. In the subsequent sections, we discuss the major pathologic lesions in the ureters, urinary bladder, and urethra separately.[1, 2]

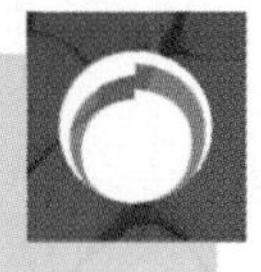

Ureters

CONGENITAL ANOMALIES

Congenital anomalies of the ureters occur in about 2% or 3% of all autopsies. Although most have little clinical significance, certain anomalies may contribute to obstruction to the flow of urine and thus cause clinical disease. Anomalies of the ureterovesical junction, potentiating reflux, are discussed with pyelonephritis in Chapter 21.

Double and bifid ureters. Double ureters (derived from a double or split ureteral bud) are almost invariably associated either with totally distinct double renal pelves or with the anomalous development of a large kidney having a partially bifid pelvis terminating in separate ureters. Double ureters may pursue separate courses to the bladder but commonly are joined within the bladder wall and drain through a single ureteral orifice.

Ureteropelvic junction obstruction, a congenital disorder, results in hydronephrosis. It usually presents in infants or children, much more commonly in boys, usually in the left ureter. However, it is bilateral in 20% of cases and may be associated with other congenital anomalies. In adults, ureteropelvic junction obstruction is more common in women and is most often unilateral. The condition has been ascribed to abnormal organization of smooth muscle bundles at the ureteropelvic junction, to excess stromal deposition of collagen between smooth muscle bundles, or in unusual cases to congenitally extrinsic compression by polar renal vessels. There is agenesis of the kidney on the opposite side in a significant number of cases, probably resulting from obstructive lesions in utero.[3]

Diverticula, saccular outpouchings of the ureteral wall, are uncommon lesions. They appear as congenital or acquired defects and are of importance as pockets of stasis and secondary infections. Dilation, elongation, and tortuosity of the ureters *(hydroureter)* may occur as congenital anomalies or as acquired defects. Congenital hydroureter is thought to reflect some neurogenic defect in the innervation of the ureteral musculature. Massive enlargement of the ureter is known as *megaloureter* and is probably due to a functional defect of ureteral muscle. These anomalies are sometimes associated with some congenital defect of the kidney.

INFLAMMATIONS

Ureteritis may develop as one component of urinary tract infections. The morphologic changes are entirely nonspecific. Only infrequently does such ureteritis make a significant contribution to the clinical problem. Persistence of infection or repeated acute exacerbations may give rise to chronic inflammatory changes within the ureters.

MORPHOLOGY. In certain cases of long-standing chronic ureteritis, specialized reaction patterns are sometimes observed. The accumulation or aggregation of lymphocytes in the subepithelial region may cause slight elevations of the mucosa and produce a fine granular mucosal surface **(ureteritis follicularis)**. At other times, the mucosa may become sprinkled with fine cysts varying in diameter from 1 to 5 mm **(ureteritis cystica)**. These changes are also found in the bladder (they receive fuller description later, in the section on urinary bladder). The cysts may aggregate to form

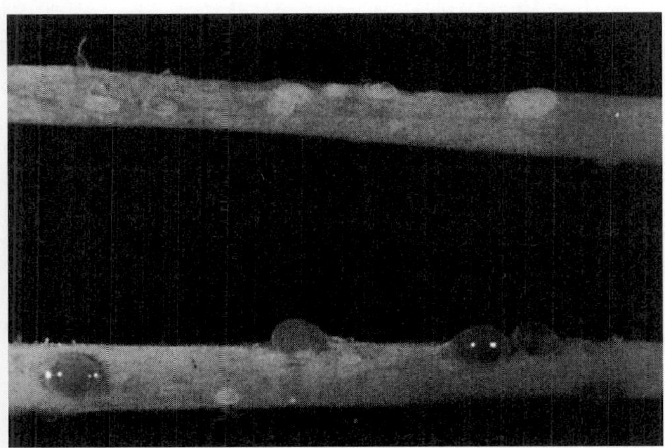

Figure 22–1

Opened ureters showing ureteritis cystica. Note smooth cysts projecting from the mucosa.

small, grapelike clusters (Fig. 22–1). Histologic sections through such cysts demonstrate a lining of modified transitional epithelium with some flattening of the superficial layer of cells.

TUMORS AND TUMOR-LIKE LESIONS

Primary neoplasia of the ureter is rare. Metastatic seeding from other primary lesions occurs much more often than primary growths.

Small *benign tumors* of the ureter are generally of mesenchymal origin. The two most common are fibroepithelial polyps and leiomyomas. The *fibroepithelial polyp* is a tumor-like lesion that grossly presents as a small mass projecting into the lumen. The lesion occurs more commonly in the ureters (left more often than right) but may also appear in the bladder, renal pelves, and urethra. The polyp presents as a loose, vascularized connective tissue mass lying beneath the mucosa.

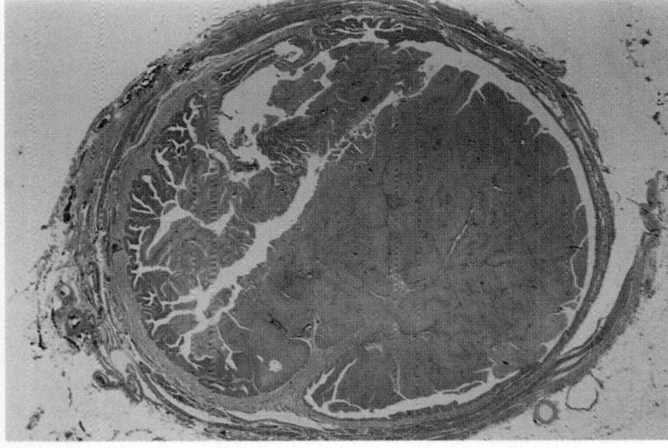

Figure 22–2

A papillary transitional cell carcinoma arising in the ureter and virtually filling the cross-section of the ureter. (Courtesy of Dr. Christopher Corless, University of Oregon, Eugene, OR.)

The primary *malignant tumors* of the ureter follow patterns similar to those arising in the renal pelvis, calyces, and bladder, and the majority are transitional cell carcinomas (Fig. 22–2). They cause obstruction of the ureteral lumen and are found most frequently during the sixth and seventh decades of life. They are sometimes multiple and occasionally occur concurrently with similar neoplasms in the bladder or renal pelvis.

OBSTRUCTIVE LESIONS

A great variety of pathologic lesions may obstruct the ureters and give rise to hydroureter, hydronephrosis, and sometimes pyelonephritis (Chapter 21). Obviously, it is not the ureteral dilation that is of significance in these cases, but the consequent involvement of the kidneys. The more important causes, divided into those of intrinsic and those of extrinsic origin, are cited in Table 22–1 (see also Fig. 21–55). Only sclerosing retroperitoneal fibrosis is discussed further.

Sclerosing Retroperitoneal Fibrosis. This refers to an uncommon cause of ureteral narrowing or obstruction characterized by a *fibrous proliferative inflammatory process*

Table 22–1. MAJOR CAUSES OF URETERAL OBSTRUCTION

Intrinsic	
Calculi	Of renal origin, rarely more than 5 mm in diameter Larger renal stones cannot enter ureters Impact at loci of ureteral narrowing—ureteropelvic junction, where ureters cross iliac vessels, and where they enter bladder—and cause excruciating "renal colic"
Strictures	Congenital or acquired (inflammations, sclerosing retroperitoneal fibrosis)
Tumorous masses	Transitional cell carcinomas arising in ureters Rarely, benign tumors or fibroepithelial polyps
Blood clots	Massive hematuria from renal calculi, tumors, or papillary necrosis
Neurogenic causes	Interruption of the neural pathways to the bladder
Extrinsic	
Pregnancy	Physiologic relaxation of smooth muscle or pressure on ureters at pelvic brim from enlarging fundus
Periureteral inflammation	Salpingitis, diverticulitis, peritonitis, sclerosing retroperitoneal fibrosis
Endometriosis	With pelvic lesions, followed by scarring
Tumors	Cancers of the rectum, bladder, prostate, ovaries, uterus, cervix, lymphomas, sarcomas. Ureteral obstruction is one of the major causes of death from cervical carcinoma

encasing the retroperitoneal structures and causing hydronephrosis. The disorder occurs in middle to late age. In some cases, specific causes can be identified, such as drugs (ergot derivatives, β-adrenergic β-blockers), adjacent inflammatory conditions (vasculitis, diverticulitis, Crohn disease), or malignant disease (lymphomas, urinary tract carcinomas). However, 70% of cases have no obvious cause and are considered primary, or idiopathic. Several cases have been reported with similar fibrotic changes in other sites (referred to as mediastinal fibrosis, sclerosing cholangitis, and Riedel fibrosing thyroiditis), suggesting that the disorder is systemic in distribution but preferentially involves the retroperitoneum. Thus, an autoimmune reaction, sometimes triggered by drugs, has been proposed.

On microscopic examination, the inflammatory fibrosis is marked by a prominent inflammatory infiltrate of lymphocytes, often with germinal centers, plasma cells, and eosinophils. Sometimes, foci of fat necrosis and granulomatous inflammation are seen in and about the fibrosis.

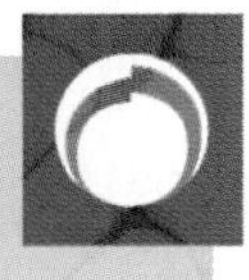

Urinary Bladder

Diseases of the bladder, particularly inflammation (cystitis), constitute an important source of clinical signs and symptoms. Usually, however, these disorders are more disabling than lethal. Cystitis is particularly common in young women of reproductive age and in older age groups of both sexes. Tumors of the bladder are an important source of both morbidity and mortality.

CONGENITAL ANOMALIES

Diverticula. A bladder or vesical diverticulum consists of a pouchlike eversion or evagination of the bladder wall. Diverticula may arise as congenital defects but more commonly are acquired lesions from persistent urethral obstruction.

The *congenital form* may be due to a focal failure of development of the normal musculature or to some urinary tract obstruction during fetal development. *Acquired diverticula* are most often seen with prostatic enlargement (hyperplasia or neoplasia), producing obstruction to urine outflow and marked muscle thickening of the bladder wall. The increased intravesical pressure causes outpouching of the bladder wall and the formation of diverticula. They are frequently multiple and have narrow necks located between the interweaving hypertrophied muscle bundles. In both the congenital and the acquired forms, the diverticulum usually consists of a round to ovoid, saclike pouch that varies from less than 1 cm to 5 to 10 cm in diameter (Fig. 22–3).

Diverticula are of clinical significance because they constitute sites of urinary stasis and predispose to infection and the formation of bladder calculi. They may also predispose to vesicoureterial reflux. Rarely, carcinomas may arise in bladder diverticuli.

Exstrophy. Exstrophy of the bladder implies the presence of a developmental failure in the anterior wall of the abdomen and the bladder, so that the bladder either communicates directly through a large defect with the surface of the body or lies as an opened sac (Fig. 22–4). The exposed bladder mucosa may undergo colonic glandular metaplasia and is subject to the development of infections that often spread to upper levels of the urinary system. In the course of persistent chronic infections, the mucosa often becomes converted into an ulcerated surface of granulation tissue, and the preserved marginal epithelium becomes transformed into a stratified squamous type. There is an increased tendency toward the development later in life of carcinoma, mostly adenocarcinoma. These lesions are amenable to surgical correction, and long-term survival is possible.

Miscellaneous Anomalies. *Vesicoureteral reflux* is the most common and serious anomaly. As a major contributor to renal infection and scarring, it was taken up earlier in Chapter 21 in the consideration of pyelonephritis. Abnormal connections between the bladder and the vagina, rectum, or uterus may create *congenital vesicouterine fistulas.*

Rarely, the *urachus* may remain patent in part or in whole (persistent urachus). When it is totally patent, a fistulous urinary tract is created that connects the bladder with the umbilicus. At times, the umbilical end or the bladder end remains patent, while the central region is obliterated. A sequestered umbilical epithelial rest or bladder diverticulum is formed that may provide a site for the

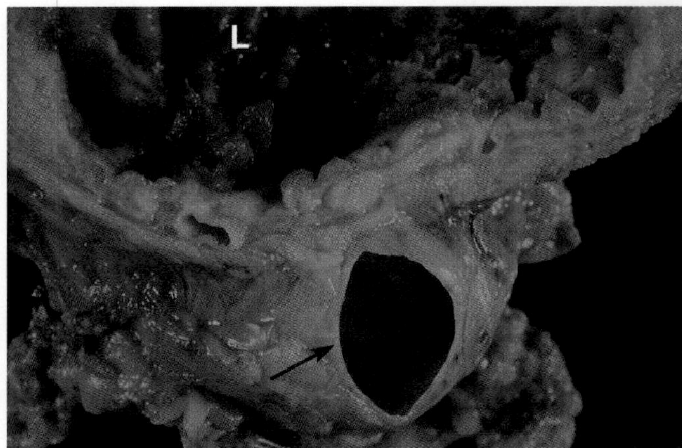

Figure 22–3

Bladder diverticulum *(arrow)* seen here in the bladder wall. Bladder lumen (L) lined by reddened mucosa is on the top. (Courtesy of Dr. Andrew Renshaw, Brigham and Women's Hospital, Boston, MA.)

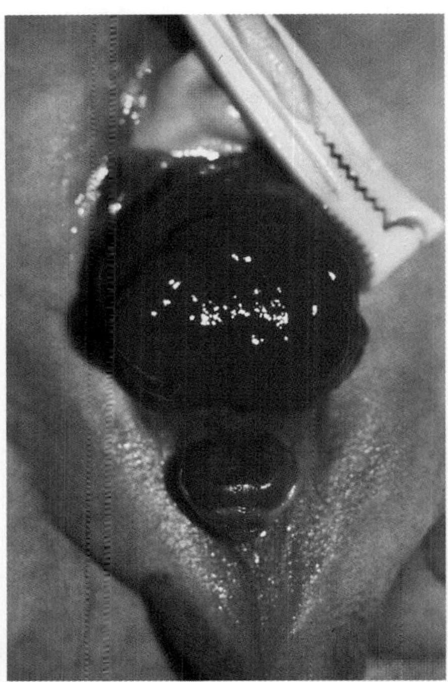

Figure 22-4

Exstrophy of the bladder in a newborn boy. The clamped umbilical cord is seen above the hyperemic mucosa of the everted bladder. Below is an incompletely formed penis with marked epispadias. (Courtesy of Dr. Hardy Hendren, Surgeon-in-Chief, Children's Hospital, Boston, MA.)

development of infection. At other times, only the central region of the urachus persists, giving rise to *urachal cysts,* lined by either transitional or metaplastic epithelium. *Carcinomas,* mostly glandular tumors resembling colonic adenocarcinomas, arise in such cysts. These account for only a minority of all bladder cancers (0.1% to 0.3%) but 20% to 40% of bladder adenocarcinomas.[2]

INFLAMMATIONS

Acute and Chronic Cystitis

The pathogenesis of cystitis and the common bacterial etiologic agents are discussed in Chapter 21 in the consideration of urinary tract infections. As emphasized earlier, bacterial pyelonephritis is frequently preceded by infection of the urinary bladder, with retrograde spread of microorganisms into the kidneys and their collecting systems. The common etiologic agents of cystitis are the coliforms—*Escherichia coli,* followed by *Proteus, Klebsiella,* and *Enterobacter. Tuberculous cystitis* is almost always a sequel to renal tuberculosis. *Candida albicans (Monilia)* and, much less often, cryptococcal agents cause cystitis, particularly in immunosuppressed patients or those receiving long-term antibiotics. Schistosomiasis *(Schistosoma haematobium)* is rare in the United States but is common in certain Middle Eastern countries, notably Egypt. Viruses (e.g., adenovirus), *Chlamydia,* and *Mycoplasma* may also be causes of cystitis. Patients receiving *cytotoxic antitumor drugs,* such as cyclophosphamide, sometimes develop hemorrhagic cystitis.[4] Finally, radiation of the bladder region gives rise to *radiation cystitis.*

MORPHOLOGY. Most cases of cystitis take the form of nonspecific acute or chronic inflammation of the bladder. In gross appearance, there is hyperemia of the mucosa, sometimes associated with exudate. When there is a hemorrhagic component, the cystitis is designated **hemorrhagic cystitis.** This form of cystitis sometimes follows radiation injury or antitumor chemotherapy and is often accompanied by epithelial atypia. Adenovirus infection also causes a hemorrhagic cystitis.

The accumulation of large amounts of suppurative exudate may merit the designation of **suppurative cystitis.** When there is ulceration of large areas of the mucosa, or sometimes the entire bladder mucosa, this is known as ulcerative cystitis.

Persistence of the infection leads to **chronic cystitis,** which differs from the acute form only in the character of the inflammatory infiltrate (Fig. 22-5). There is more extreme heaping up of the epithelium with the formation of a red, friable, granular, sometimes ulcerated surface. Chronicity of the infection gives rise to fibrous thickening in the tunica propria and consequent thickening and inelasticity of the bladder wall. Histologic variants include **follicular cystitis,** characterized by the aggregation of lymphocytes into lymphoid follicles within the bladder mucosa and underlying wall, and **eosinophilic cystitis,** manifested by infiltration with submucosal eosinophils together with fibrosis and occasionally giant cells.

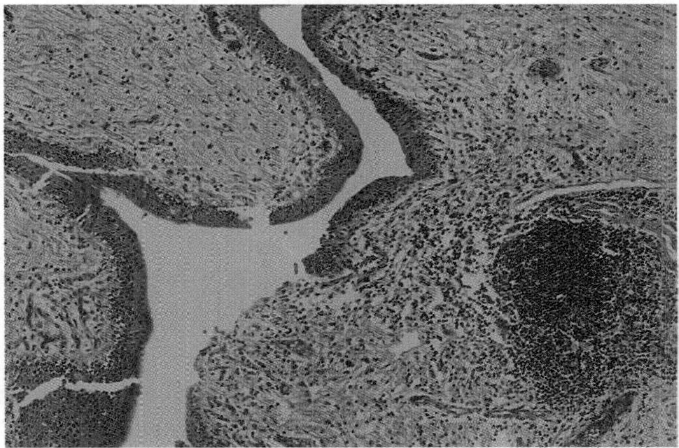

Figure 22-5

Chronic cystitis with subepithelial edema, inflammation, and a lymphoid aggretate in the lamina propria. (Courtesy of Dr. Andrew Renshaw, Brigham and Women's Hospital, Boston, MA.)

All forms of cystitis are characterized by a triad of symptoms: (1) frequency, which in acute cases may necessitate urination every 15 to 20 minutes; (2) lower abdominal pain localized over the bladder region or in the suprapubic region; and (3) dysuria—pain or burning on urination. Associated with these localized changes, there may be systemic signs of inflammation such as elevation of temperature, chills, and general malaise. In the usual case, the bladder infection does not give rise to such a constitutional reaction.

The local symptoms of cystitis may be disturbing, but these infections are also important as antecedents to pyelonephritis. Cystitis is sometimes a secondary complication of some underlying disorder such as prostatic enlargement, cystocele of the bladder, calculi, or tumors. These primary diseases must be corrected before the cystitis can be relieved.

Special Forms of Cystitis

Several special variants of cystitis are distinctive by either their morphologic appearance or their causation.

Interstitial Cystitis (Hunner Ulcer). This is a *persistent, painful form of chronic cystitis occurring most frequently in women and associated with inflammation and fibrosis of all layers of the bladder wall.* It is characterized clinically by intermittent, often severe suprapubic pain, urinary frequency, urgency, hematuria and dysuria without evidence of bacterial infection, and cystoscopic findings of fissures in the bladder mucosa after luminal distention. Some but not all patients exhibit morphologic features of chronic mucosal ulcers *(Hunner ulcers).* Inflammatory cells and granulation tissue may involve the mucosa, lamina propria, and muscularis, and *mast cells* may be particularly prominent. The condition is of unknown etiology but is thought by some to be of autoimmune origin, particularly because it is sometimes associated with lupus erythematosus and other autoimmune disorders.

Malacoplakia. This designation refers to *a peculiar pattern of vesical inflammatory reaction characterized macroscopically by soft, yellow, slightly raised mucosal plaques 3 to 4 cm in diameter* (Fig. 22–6), and *histologically by infiltration with large, foamy macrophages with occasional multinucleate giant cells and interspersed lymphocytes.* The macrophages have an abundant granular cytoplasm. The granularity is periodic acid–Schiff positive and due to phagosomes stuffed with particulate and membranous debris of bacterial origin. In addition, laminated mineralized concretions known as *Michaelis-Gutmann bodies* are typically present, both within the macrophages and between cells (Fig. 22–7). Similar lesions have been described in the colon, lungs, bones, kidneys, prostate, and epididymis.

Malacoplakia is clearly related to chronic bacterial infection, mostly by *E. coli* or occasionally *Proteus* species. It occurs with increased frequency in immunosuppressed transplant recipients. The unusual-appearing macrophages and giant phagosomes point to defects in phagocytic or degradative function of macrophages, such that phagosomes become overloaded with undigested bacterial products.

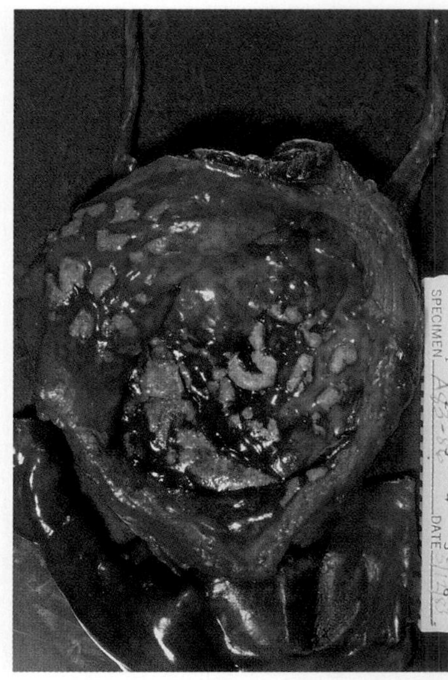

Figure 22–6 ■

Cystitis with malacoplakia of bladder showing inflammatory exudate and broad, flat plaques.

Cystitis Glandularis and Cystitis Cystica. These terms refer to common lesions of the urinary bladder in which nests of transitional epithelium (Brunn nests) grow downward into the lamina propria and undergo transformation of their central epithelial cells into cuboidal or columnar epithelium lining slitlike *(cystitis glandularis)* or cystic spaces *(cystitis cystica).* Typical goblet cells are sometimes present, and the epithelium resembles intestinal mucosa *(intestinal metaplasia).* Both variants are common microscopic incidental findings in relatively normal bladders, and

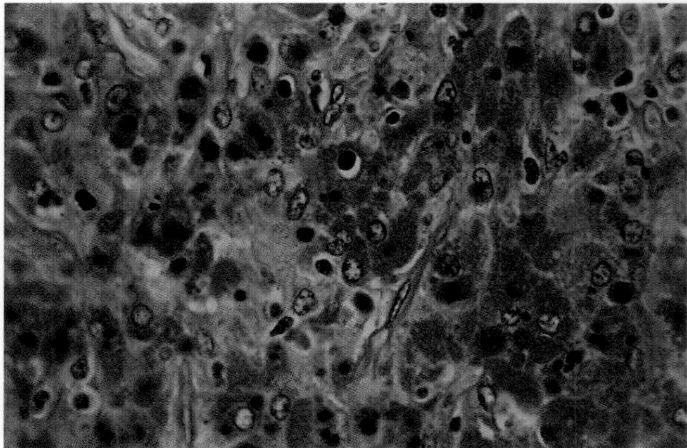

Figure 22–7 ■

Malacoplakia, PAS stain. Note the large macrophages with granular PAS-positive cytoplasm and several dense, round Michaelis-Gutmann bodies surrounded by artifactual cleared holes in the upper middle field.

Table 22–2. TUMORS OF THE URINARY BLADDER

Urothelial (transitional cell) tumors
- Inverted papilloma
- Papilloma (exophytic)
- Urothelial tumors of low malignant potential
- Urothelial carcinoma
- Carcinoma in situ

Squamous cell carcinoma
Mixed carcinoma
Adenocarcinoma
Small cell carcinoma
Sarcomas

thus some experts classify them as metaplasias rather than a form of cystitis. They are, however, more prominent in inflamed and chronically irritated bladders. *Lesions exhibiting extensive intestinal metaplasia are at increased risk for the development of adenocarcinoma.*

In *cystitis cystica,* the cysts are usually 0.1 to 1 cm in diameter, filled with clear fluid, and lined by cuboidal or urothelial cells. As noted, similar cysts occur in the pelvis and ureter (ureteritis and pyelitis cystica).

NEOPLASMS

Neoplasms of the bladder pose biologic and clinical challenges. Despite significant inroads into their origins and improved methods of diagnosis and treatment, they continue to exact a high toll in morbidity and mortality. The incidence of the epithelial tumors in the United States has been steadily increasing during the past years and is now more than 50,000 new cases annually.[5] Despite improvements in detection and management of these neoplasms, the death toll remains at about 10,000 annually, because the increased prevalence offsets such gains as have been made.

About 95% of bladder tumors are of epithelial origin, the remainder being mesenchymal tumors (Table 22–2). Most epithelial tumors are composed of urothelial (transitional cell) type and are thus interchangeably called urothelial or transitional tumors, but squamous and glandular carcinomas also occur. Here we discuss the transitional cell tumors in some detail and only touch on the others.

Urothelial (Transitional Cell) Tumors

These represent about 90% of all bladder tumors and run the gamut from small benign lesions that may never recur, to tumors of low or indeterminate malignant potential, to lesions that invade the bladder wall and metastasize frequently. Many of these tumors are multifocal at presentation. Histologic grading of these tumors, as a means to predict behavior, has been a subject of great debate, as there is poor interobserver reproducibility and no uniformly accepted grading system. There is, however, growing consensus that the majority of tumors can be segregated, *at the time of initial diagnosis,* into two major categories.[6]

- Low-grade urothelial tumors. These are always papillary, noninvasive lesions that recapitulate normal transitional epithelium and exhibit limited cellular and nuclear pleomorphism. They are usually DNA diploid, show limited chromosome and gene abnormalities, and retain blood group antigens. Patients with these tumors may develop new lesions after excision, commonly called *recurrences* (although many appear to be new primaries), but they have an excellent prognosis except for the relatively few patients (2% to 10%) in whom higher grade lesions develop as recurrences.
- High-grade urothelial carcinoma. These tumors may be papillary, nodular, or both and exhibit considerable cellular pleomorphism and anaplasia. The lesions are nearly always aneuploid, have a high frequency of chromosome and gene abnormalities, and usually lack blood group antigens. They have metastatic potential and are lethal in about 60% of cases within 10 years of diagnosis.

In Table 22–3, we have listed two of many systems of grading these tumors. The older (1972), commonly used World Health Organization (WHO) classification (currently being revised) grades tumors into a rare totally benign papilloma and three grades of transitional cell carcinoma (grades I, II, and III). A more recent classification, based on a consensus reached at a conference by the International Society of Urological Pathology (ISUP) in 1998, is currently being prepared.[7] It recognizes a rare benign papilloma, a group of papillary urothelial neoplasms of low malignant potential, and two grades of carcinoma (low and high grade).

MORPHOLOGY. The gross patterns of urothelial cell tumors vary from purely papillary to nodular or flat to mixed papillary and nodular. The tumors may also be invasive or noninvasive (Fig. 22–8). The papillary lesions appear as red elevated excrescences varying in size from less than 1 cm in diameter to large masses up to 5 cm in diameter. Multicentric origins may produce separate tumors. As noted, the histologic changes encompass a spectrum from benign papilloma to highly aggressive anaplastic cancers. Overall, about half of bladder cancers are high-grade lesions. Most

Table 22–3. GRADING OF UROTHELIAL (TRANSITIONAL CELL) TUMORS

WHO Grading	ISUP CONSENSUS*
Papilloma	Urothelial papilloma
TCC Grade I	Urothelial neoplasm of low malignant potential
TCC Grade II	Urothelial carcinoma, low grade
TCC Grade III	Urothelial carcinoma, high grade

WHO, World Health Organization; ISUP, International Society of Urological Pathology; TCC, transitional cell carcinoma.
* Tentative (*Grades in WHO classification do not strictly correspond to ISUP terminology*).

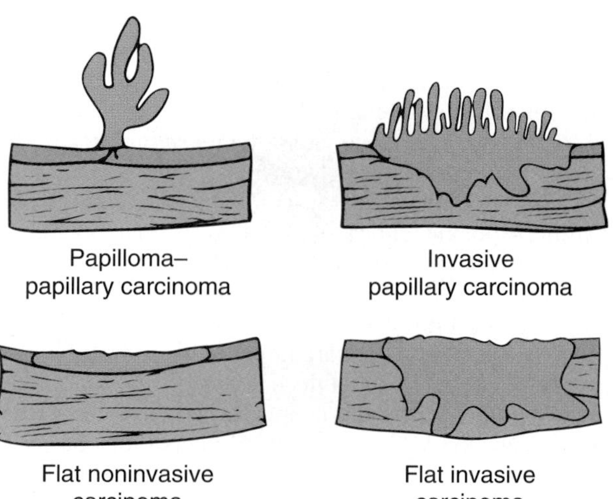

Figure 22–8

Four morphologic patterns of bladder tumors.

arise from the lateral or posterior walls at the bladder base.

- **Papilloma.** This term is used to describe a rare variant, representing 1% or less of bladder tumors, seen in younger patients. The tumors usually arise singly as small (0.5 to 2.0 cm), delicate, soft structures, superficially attached to the mucosa by a stalk. The individual finger-like papillae have a central core of loose fibrovascular tissue covered by transitional epithelial cells that are *histologically identical to normal urothelium* (Fig. 22–9). True recurrences rarely if ever occur.
- **Grade I** of the WHO classification corresponds more or less to the *urothelial neoplasms of low malignant potential* in the ISUP consensus terminology. The gross appearance is similar to that of papilloma (Fig. 22–10). The tumor cells display some cytologic and architectural atypia but are well differentiated and closely resemble normal transitional cells. Mitoses are rare. There may be a significant increase in the number of layers of cells but only slight loss of polarity (see Fig. 22–11). Most recurrences are benign, but sometimes (about 3% to 5% of cases) they are of higher grade. The line between the papilloma and grade I tumor is finely drawn, *but fortunately all such well-differentiated papillary neoplasms seldom become invasive and provide a 95% to 98% 10-year survival rate.*
- **Grade II.** The histologic criteria are difficult to pin down. Most of the tumors are papillary, but they may have contiguous flat regions. The tumor cells are still recognizable as of transitional origin. The number of layers of cells is increased, as is the number of mitoses, and there is greater loss of polarity. Greater variability in cell size, shape, and chromaticity is present.

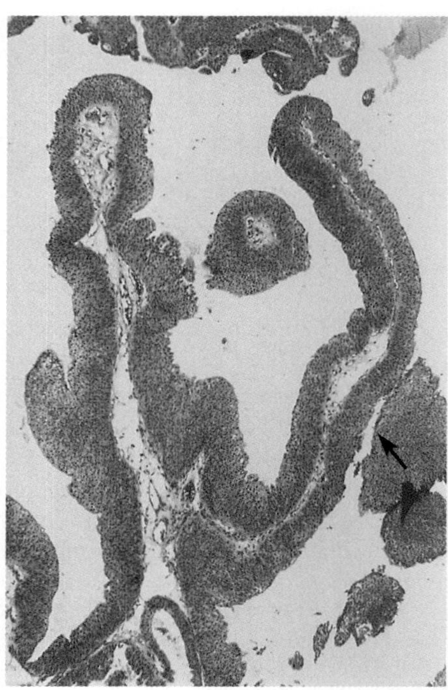

Figure 22–9

Low-power view of typical papillomatous growth of bladder. Note delicate axial stromal framework. (Courtesy of Dr. Christopher Corless, University of Oregon, Eugene, OR.)

The lower spectrum of grade II lesions of the WHO classification is included in the *low-grade urothelial carcinoma* of the ISUP consensus. These tumors may be associated with invasion at the time of diagnosis but have a low risk of progression.

- **Grade III.** These tumors are part of the *high-grade carcinomas* of the ISUP consensus

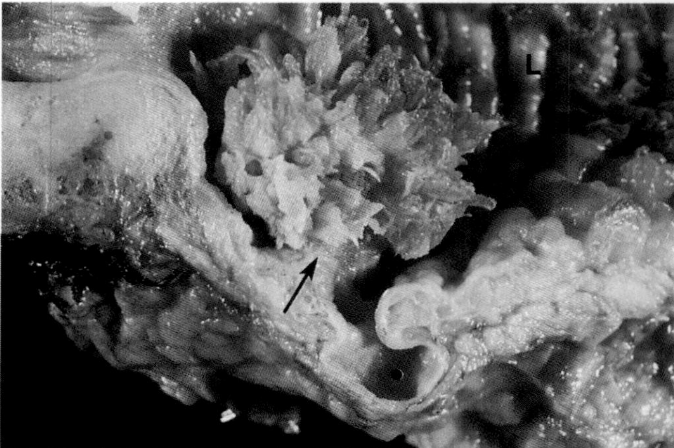

Figure 22–10

Sectioned bladder showing a papillary transitional cell carcinoma projecting into the lumen *(arrow).* Note delicate arborizing structure and small stalk. Note also the small diverticulum adjacent to the attachment site of the stalk. L, lumen, •, diverticulum.

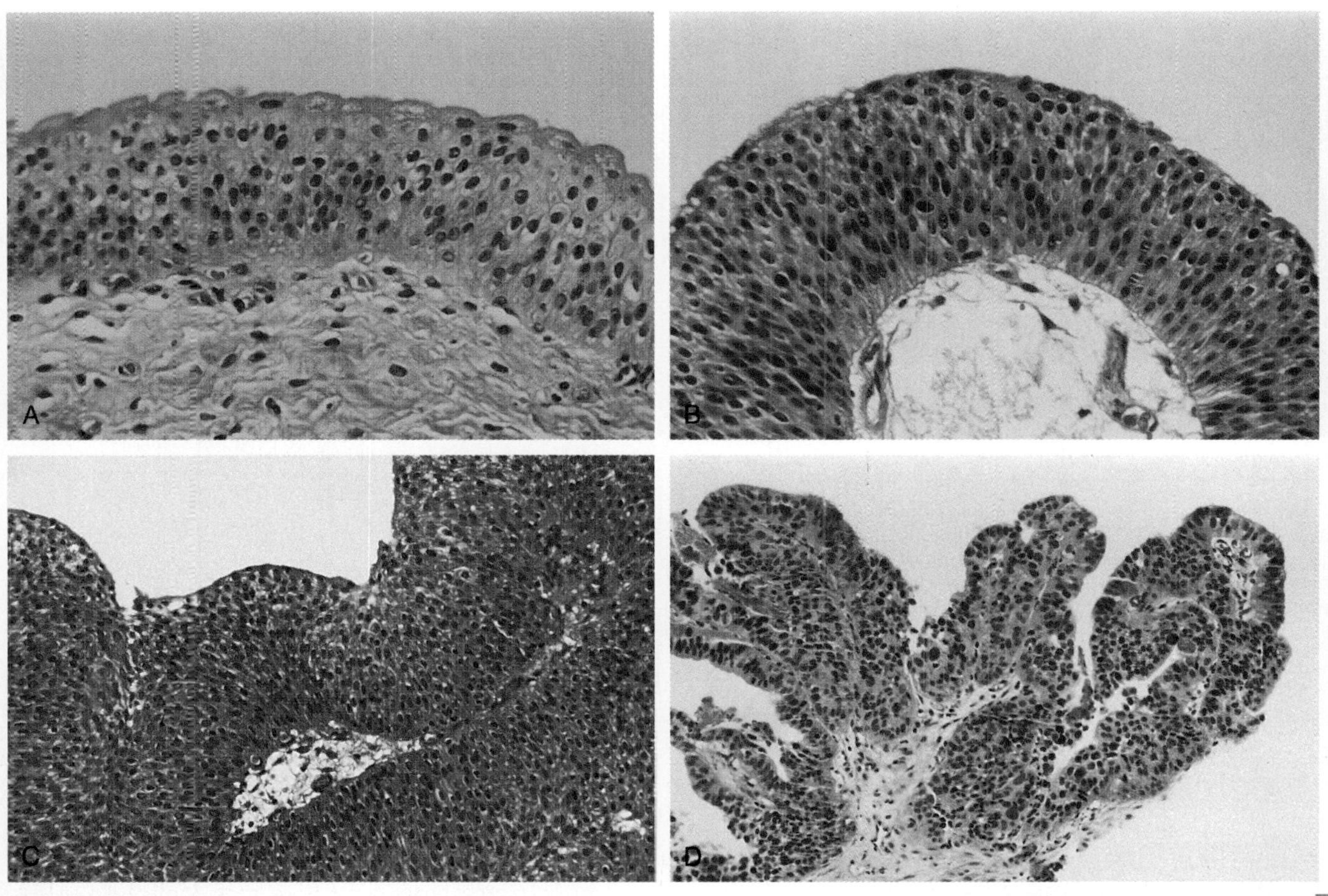

Figure 22–11

A, Normal bladder mucosa. *B–D*, Urothelial tumors. *B*, Grade I or low malignant potential; *C*, Grade II (low grade); *D*, Grade III (high grade). (*A, B, D*, Courtesy of Dr. Christopher Corless, University of Oregon, Eugene, OR. *C*, Courtesy of Dr. Donald Antonioli, Beth Israel Hospital, Boston, MA.)

(which also include the higher spectrum of the WHO grade II lesions). These tumors can be papillary, flat, or both. They tend to be larger, to be more extensive, and to show a high preponderance for invasion of the muscularis. Many of the tumor cells show anaplastic changes. In particular, there is evident disarray of cells with loosening and fragmentation of the superficial layers of cells (Fig. 22–11*D*). Occasional giant cells may be present. Sometimes the cells tend to flatten out, and the lesions come to resemble squamous cell carcinomas. Alternatively, foci of glandular differentiation may be present. The tumors have a much higher incidence of invasion into the muscular layer, a higher risk of progression than low-grade lesions, and significant metastatic potential.

Despite the heterogeneity of gross and microscopic appearance, a few points can be made. Papillomas and low-grade lesions are almost always papillary. Higher grades may be flat or papillary. Many high-grade III lesions may be fungating, necrotic, sometimes ulcerative tumors that have unmistakably invaded deeply (Fig. 22–12). With the higher grade neoplasms, in areas of the bladder devoid of tumor, there may frequently be areas of mucosal hyperplasia, dysplasia, or carcinoma in situ. In most analyses, less than 10% of low-grade cancers invade, but as many as 80% of high-grade transitional cell carcinomas are invasive. Aggressive tumors may extend only into the bladder wall, but the more advanced stages invade the adjacent prostate, seminal vesicles, ureters, and retroperitoneum, and some produce fistulous communications to the vagina or rectum. About 40% of these deeply invasive tumors metastasize to regional lymph nodes. Hematogenous dissemination, principally to the liver, lungs, and bone marrow, generally occurs late, and only with highly anaplastic tumors.

Carcinoma in situ is defined as a high-grade flat abnormality confined to the bladder mucosa (Fig. 22–13). It usually appears as an area of mucosal reddening, granularity, or thickening without producing an evident intraluminal mass. It is commonly multifocal and may involve most of the

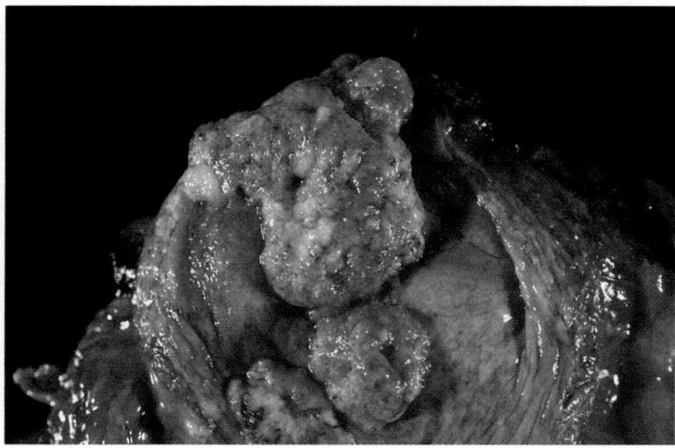

Figure 22–12

Opened bladder showing a high-grade invasive transitional cell carcinoma at an advanced stage. The aggressive multinodular neoplasm has fungated into the bladder lumen and spread over a wide area. Normal bladder mucosa. (Courtesy of Dr. Andrew Renshaw, Brigham and Women's Hospital, Boston, MA.)

Table 22–4. PATHOLOGIC STAGING OF BLADDER CARCINOMA

Depth of Invasion	AJCC/UICC
Noninvasive, papillary	Ta
Noninvasive, flat	TIS
Lamina propria	T1
Superficial muscularis propria	T2
Deep muscularis propria	T3a
Perivesical fat	T3b
Adjacent structures	T4
Lymph node metastases	N1–3*
Distant metastases	M1

* N1, regional lymph node <2 cm; N2, regional lymph nodes 2 to 5 cm; N3, regional lymph nodes >5 cm or other lymph nodes.

AJCC/UICC, American Joint Commission on Cancer/Union Internationale Contre le Cancer.

bladder surface and extend into the ureters and urethra. Although carcinoma in situ is most often found in bladders harboring well-defined transitional cell carcinoma, about 1% to 5% of cases occur in the absence of such tumors. In time, some of these lesions become invasive.

The extent of spread at the time of initial diagnosis is the most important factor in determining the outlook for a patient. Thus, **staging,** in addition to grade, is critical in the assessment of bladder neoplasms. The staging system most commonly used is given in Table 22–4.

Other Types of Carcinoma

Squamous cell carcinomas represent about 3% to 7% of bladder cancers in the United States, but in countries endemic for urinary schistosomiasis, they occur much more frequently. Pure squamous cell carcinomas are nearly always associated with chronic bladder irritation and infection. *Mixed transitional cell carcinomas with areas of squamous carcinoma* are more frequent than pure squamous cell carcinomas. Most are invasive, fungating tumors or infiltrative and ulcerative. True papillary patterns are almost never seen. The level

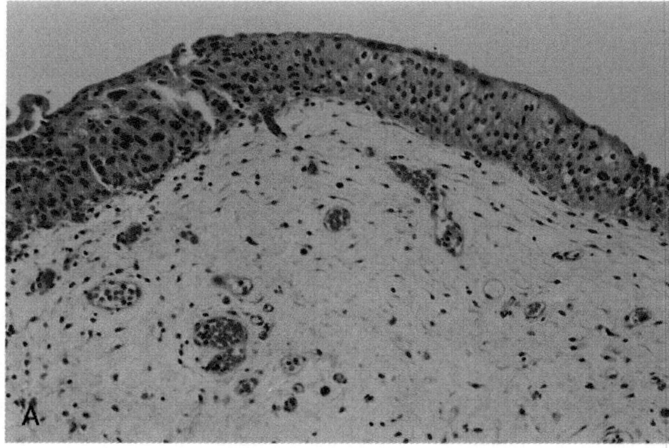

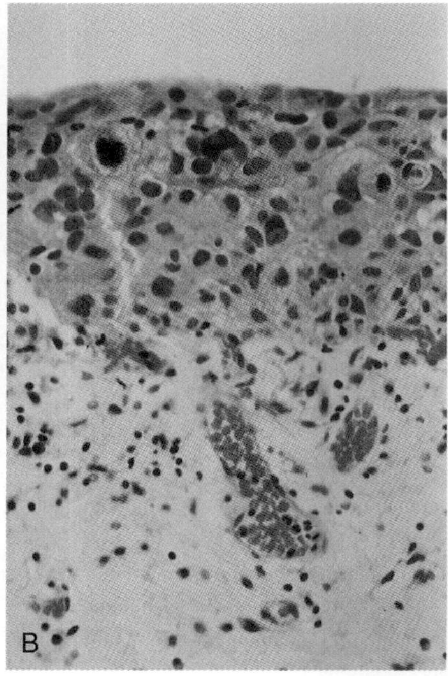

Figure 22–13

A, Low-power view of bladder with focus of carcinoma in situ on the left side of the illustration. *B,* High-power view of carcinoma confined to the epithelium. (Courtesy of Dr. Christopher Corless, University of Oregon, Eugene, OR.)

of cytologic differentiation varies widely, from the highly differentiated lesions producing abundant keratohyaline pearls to anaplastic giant cell tumors showing little evidence of squamous differentiation. They often cover large areas of the bladder and are deeply invasive by the time of discovery.

Adenocarcinomas of the bladder are rare. Some arise from urachal remnants or in association with extensive intestinal metaplasia (discussed earlier). Rare variants are **small cell carcinoma,** the highly malignant **signet-ring cell carcinoma,** and **mixed adenocarcinoma** and transitional cell carcinomas.

Epidemiology and Pathogenesis. The incidence of carcinoma of the bladder resembles that of bronchogenic carcinoma, being more common in men than in women, in industrialized than in developing nations, and in urban than in rural dwellers. The male to female ratio for transitional cell tumors is approximately 3:1. About 80% of patients are between the ages of 50 and 80 years.

A number of factors have been implicated in the causation of transitional cell carcinoma. Some of the more important contributors include the following:

- *Cigarette smoking* is clearly the most important influence, increasing the risk threefold to sevenfold, depending on the pack-years and smoking habits. Fifty per cent to 80% of all bladder cancers among men are associated with the use of cigarettes. Cigars, pipes, and smokeless tobacco invoke a much smaller risk.
- *Industrial exposure to arylamines,* particularly 2-naphthylamine as well as related compounds, as pointed out in the earlier discussion of chemical carcinogenesis (Chapter 8). The cancers appear 15 to 40 years after the first exposure.
- *Schistosoma haematobium* infections in areas where these are endemic (Egypt, Sudan) are an established risk. The ova are deposited in the bladder wall and incite a brisk chronic inflammatory response that induces progressive mucosal squamous metaplasia and dysplasia and, in some instances, neoplasia. Seventy per cent of the cancers are squamous, the remainder being transitional cell carcinoma.
- Long-term use of analgesics, implicated also in analgesic nephropathy (Chapter 21).
- Heavy long-term exposure to cyclophosphamide, an immunosuppressive agent, induces as noted hemorrhagic cystitis and increases the risk of bladder cancer.

How these influences induce cancer is unclear, but a number of genetic alterations have been observed in transitional cell carcinoma. The cytogenetic and molecular alterations are heterogeneous. Particularly common (occurring in 30% to 60% of tumors studied) are chromosome 9 monosomy or deletions of 9p and 9q as well as deletions of 17p, 13q, 11p, and 14q.[8] The *chromosome 9 deletions are the only genetic changes present frequently in superficial papillary tumors and occasionally in noninvasive flat tumors.* The 9p deletions (9p21) involve the tumor-suppressor gene *p16 (MTS1, INK4a),* which encodes an inhibitor of a cyclin-dependent kinase (Chapter 8), and also the related *p15.*[9, 10] The 9q deletion includes numerous potential tumor-suppressor foci, but the identity of this putative second tumor-suppressor locus is not yet known. On the other hand, many invasive transitional cell carcinomas show *deletions of 17p,* including the region of the *p53* gene, as well as mutations in the *p53* gene, suggesting that alterations in *p53* contribute to the progression of transitional cell carcinoma. Mutations in *p53* are also found in flat in situ cancer lesions. The *13q* deletion is that of the *retinoblastoma gene* and is also present in invasive tumors. Deletions of *14q* are seen exclusively in flat lesions or invasive tumors but not in papillary tumors, and a putative tumor-suppressor gene is being pursued. Increased expression of *ras,* c-*myc,* and epidermal growth factor receptors is also seen in some bladder cancers.

On the basis of these findings, two models for bladder carcinogenesis have been proposed. In the two-pathway model,[10] the first pathway is *initiated by deletions of tumor-suppressor genes* on 9p and 9q leading to superficial papillary or occasionally flat tumors, a few of which may then acquire *p53* mutations and progress to invasion; a second pathway, possibly *initiated by p53 mutations,* directly results in the induction of potentially invasive tumors. The second model is a linear model of progression,[11] beginning with inactivation of tumor-suppressor genes on chromosome 9 (or 14 for flat lesions), through loss of *p53* function and a variety of other genetic alterations, as has been proposed for colonic cancer[12] (Chapter 8).

Clinical Course of Bladder Cancer. Bladder tumors classically produce painless hematuria. This is their dominant and sometimes only clinical manifestation. Frequency, urgency, and dysuria occasionally accompany the hematuria. When the ureteral orifice is involved, pyelonephritis or hydronephrosis may follow. About 60% of neoplasms, when first discovered, are single, and 70% are localized to the bladder.

Patients with urothelial tumors, whatever their grade, have a tendency to develop new tumors after excision, and recurrences may exhibit a higher grade. Overall, about 50% of papillomas and low-grade carcinomas recur, in contrast to 80% to 90% of high grade tumors. In many instances, the recurrences seen at a different site, and the question of whether these represent new primaries or are true recurrences is difficult to ascertain.

The prognosis depends on the histologic grade of the tumor and on the stage when it is first diagnosed. Papillomas and grade I cancers (those of low malignant potential) yield a 98% 10-year survival rate regardless of the number of recurrences; only a few patients (< 10%) have progression of their disease to higher grade lesions. In contrast, only about 40% of individuals with a grade III cancer survive 10 years; the tumor is progressive in 65%. Approximately 70% of patients with squamous cell carcinomas are dead within the year. Other factors may influence the prognosis. The expression of blood group antigens by tumor cells correlates with tumor behavior. Patients whose tumor cells express A, B, H antigens have a better prognosis than those that do not or lose this capacity. Analogously, the detection of multiple chromosome and gene mutations (cited earlier) worsens the outlook.

The clinical challenge with these neoplasms is early detection and adequate follow-up. Although cystoscopy and biopsy are the mainstays of diagnosis, carcinoma in situ producing no or only subtle gross mucosal changes and early small papillary lesions may be difficult to detect. Of value in these circumstances are *cytologic examinations possibly augmented by flow cytometric analyses of urinary sediment.* The latter diagnostic approach for DNA content is effective in differentiating the high-grade tumors from the benign ones and detecting aneuploid high-grade lesions when there is uncertainty as to diagnosis.

Mesenchymal Tumors

Benign. A great variety of benign mesenchymal tumors may arise in the bladder. Collectively, they are rare. The most common is *leiomyoma.* They all tend to grow as isolated, intramural, encapsulated, oval to spherical masses, varying in diameter up to several centimeters. On occasion, they assume submucosal pedunculated positions. They have the histologic features of their counterparts elsewhere.

Sarcomas. True sarcomas are distinctly uncommon in the bladder. Inflammatory pseudotumors, postoperative spindle cell nodules, and various carcinomas may assume sarcomatoid growth patterns, all sometimes mistaken histologically for sarcomas.[13] As a group, sarcomas tend to produce large masses (varying up to 10 to 15 cm in diameter) that protrude into the vesical lumen. Their soft, fleshy, gray-white gross appearance suggests their sarcomatous nature. *Rhabdomyosarcoma* takes one of two forms. The "adult" form occurs mostly in adults older than 40 years and shows a range of histology similar to rhabdomyosarcomas of striated muscle (Chapter 28). The other variant is the *embryonal rhabdomyosarcoma,* or *sarcoma botryoides,* encountered chiefly in infancy or childhood, and similar to those that occur in the female genital tract (Chapter 24).

Secondary Tumors

Secondary malignant involvement of the bladder is most often by direct extension from primary lesions in nearby organs, cervix, uterus, prostate, and rectum, in the order given. They may, on casual inspection of the bladder, appear as primary carcinomas of this organ. Hemorrhage, ureteral obstruction, and vesicovaginal fistulas are the common sequelae. Distinction between primary adenocarcinoma of the bladder (urethral or otherwise) from local extension of colorectal cancer can be difficult.

OBSTRUCTION

Obstruction to the bladder neck is of major clinical importance, not only for the changes induced in the bladder but also because of its eventual effect on the kidney. A great variety of intrinsic and extrinsic diseases of the bladder may narrow the urethral orifice and cause partial or complete vesical obstruction. In the male patient, the most important lesion is enlargement of the prostate gland due either to nodular hyperplasia or to carcinoma (Fig. 22–14). Vesical obstruction is somewhat less common in the female patient and is most often caused by cystocele of the bladder. The more infrequent causes can be listed as (1) congenital narrowings or strictures of the urethra; (2) inflammatory strictures of the urethra; (3) inflammatory fibrosis and contraction of the bladder after varying types of cystitis; (4) bladder tumors, either benign or malignant, when strategically located; (5) secondary invasion of the bladder neck by growths arising in perivesical structures, such as the cervix, vagina, prostate, and rectum; (6) mechanical obstructions caused by foreign bodies and calculi; and (7) injury to the innervation of the bladder causing neurogenic or cord bladder.

MORPHOLOGY. In the early stages, there is only some thickening of the bladder wall, presumably due to hypertrophy of the smooth muscle. The mucosal surface at this time may be entirely normal. With progressive hypertrophy of the muscle coat, the individual muscle bundles greatly enlarge and produce trabeculation of the bladder wall. In the course of time, crypts form and may then become converted into true acquired diverticula.

In some cases of acute obstruction or in terminal disease when the patient's normal reflex mechanisms are depressed, the bladder may become extremely dilated. The enlarged bladder may reach the brim of the pelvis or even the level of the umbilicus. In these cases, the bladder wall is markedly thinned, and the trabeculation becomes totally inapparent.

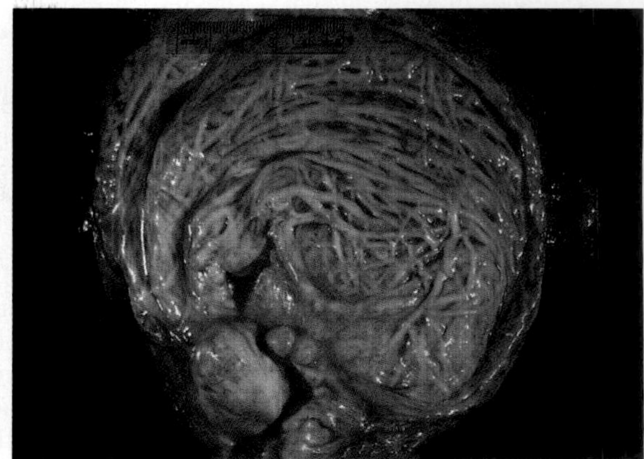

Figure 22–14

Hypertrophy and trabeculation of bladder wall secondary to polypoid hyperplasia of the prostate.

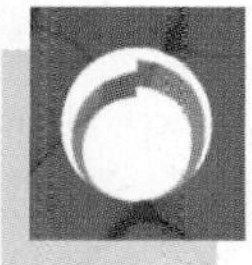

Urethra

INFLAMMATIONS

Urethritis is classically divided into gonococcal and nongonococcal urethritis. As noted earlier, gonococcal urethritis is one of the earliest manifestations of this venereal infection. Nongonococcal urethritis is common and can be caused by a variety of bacteria, among which *E. coli* and other enteric organisms predominate. Urethritis is often accompanied by cystitis in women and by prostatitis in men. In many instances, bacteria cannot be isolated. Various strains of *Chlamydia* (e.g., *C. trachomatis*) are the cause of 25% to 60% of nongonococcal urethritis in men and about 20% in women. *Mycoplasma (Ureaplasma urealyticum)* also accounts for the symptoms of urethritis in many cases. Urethritis is also one component of *Reiter syndrome,* which comprises the clinical triad of arthritis, conjunctivitis, and urethritis.

The morphologic changes are entirely typical of inflammation in other sites within the urinary tract. The urethral involvement is not itself a serious clinical problem but may cause considerable local pain, itching, and frequency and may represent a forerunner of more serious disease in higher levels of the urogenital tract.

TUMORS

Urethral caruncle is an inflammatory lesion presenting a small, red, painful mass about the external urethral meatus in the female patient. Caruncles may be found at any age but are more common in later life. The lesion consists of a hemispheric, friable, 1- to 2-cm nodule that occurs singly, either just outside or just within the external urethral meatus. It may be covered by an intact mucosa but is extremely friable, and the slightest trauma may cause ulceration of the surface and bleeding. On histologic examination, it is composed of a *highly vascularized, young, fibroblastic connective tissue, more or less heavily infiltrated with leukocytes.* The overlying epithelium, where present, is either transitional or squamous cell in type. Surgical excision affords prompt relief and cure.

Papillomas of the urethra occur usually just within or on the external meatus. They may be of viral origin, analogous to those affecting the vulva.

Carcinoma of the urethra is an uncommon lesion. It tends to occur in advanced age in women and, in most instances, begins about the external meatus or on the immediately surrounding structures, such as the glans penis or the introitus in the female patient. Some apparently begin just inside the external meatus or even at a higher level within the urethra. Those that occur at or protrude from the external meatus appear as warty, papillary growths that at first resemble the sessile papillary carcinomas described in the bladder. As they progress, they tend to become ulcerated on their surfaces and to assume the characteristics of a fungating, ulcerating lesion (Fig. 22–15).

Most of these malignant neoplasms are squamous cell carcinomas. The papillary lesions that protrude from the external meatus are likely to show a transitional cell growth that further heightens their similarity to bladder carcinoma. Uncommonly, an adenocarcinomatous growth pattern is found. Overall, they are more aggressive than bladder cancers, more often invasive, and more difficult to eradicate despite the fact that they seldom metastasize, probably because most lead to death within a few years.

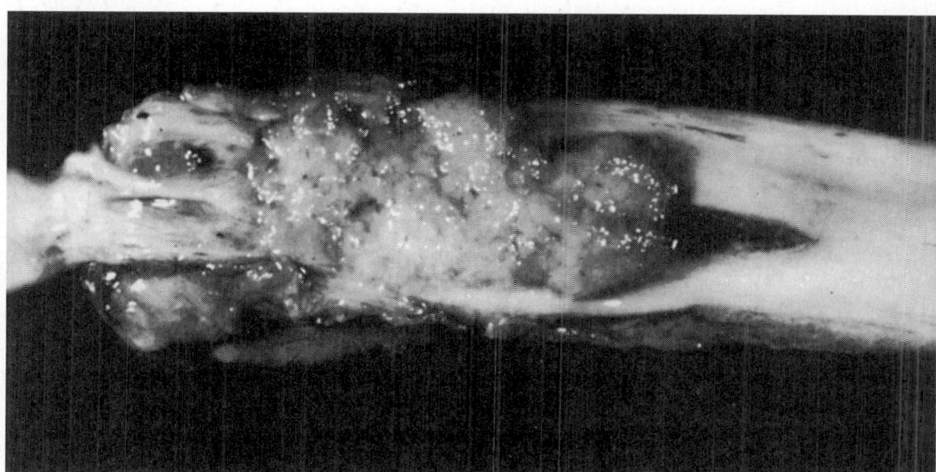

Figure 22–15 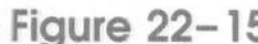

Carcinoma of urethra with typical fungating growth.

REFERENCES

1. Bostwick DG, Eble JN (eds): Urologic Surgical Pathology. St. Louis, Mosby, 1997.
2. Murphy WM (ed): Urologic Pathology, 2nd ed. Philadelphia, WB Saunders, 1997.
3. Benacerraf BR, et al: The prenatal evolution of renal cystic dysplasia in the setting of obstructive hydronephrosis seen sonographically. J Clin Ultrasound 19:446, 1991.
4. de Vries CR, Freiha FS: Hemorrhagic cystitis: a review. J Urol 143:1, 1990.
5. Landis SH, et al: Cancer statistics. CA Cancer J Clin 48:6, 1998.
6. Murphy WM et al: Tumors of the kidney, bladder, and related structures. Atlas of Tumor Pathology, 3rd Series, Fascicle 11. Washington, DC, Armed Forces Institute of Pathology, 1994.
7. Epstein JI, et al: International Society of Urological Pathology (ISUP) consensus classification of urothelial (transitional cell) lesions. Personal communication and consensus Conference Summary.
8. Gibas C, Gibas L: Cytogenetics of bladder cancer. Cancer Genet Cytogenet 95:108, 1997.
9. Orlow I, et al: Deletion of the *p16* and *p15* genes in human bladder tumors. J Natl Cancer Inst 87:1524, 1995.
10. Balazs M, et al: Frequent homozygous deletion of cyclin-dependent kinase inhibitor 2 (*MTS-1, p16*) in superficial bladder cancer. Genes Chromosomes Cancer 19:84, 1997.
11. Cairns P, Sidransky D: Bladder cancer. In Vogelstein B, Kinzler A (eds): Genetic Basis of Human Cancer. New York, McGraw-Hill, 1998, pp 639–645.
12. Spruck CH, et al: Two molecular pathways for transitional carcinoma of the bladder. Cancer Res 54:784, 1994.
13. Jones EC, et al: Inflammatory pseudotumor of the urinary bladder. Am J Surg Pathol 17:264, 1993.

23

The Male Genital Tract

PENIS

CONGENITAL ANOMALIES

- Hypospadias and Epispadias
- Phimosis

INFLAMMATIONS

TUMORS

- Benign Tumors
  - *Condyloma Acuminatum*
- Carcinoma in Situ
- Carcinoma

TESTIS AND EPIDIDYMIS

CONGENITAL ANOMALIES

- Cryptorchidism

REGRESSIVE CHANGES

- Atrophy

INFLAMMATIONS

- Nonspecific Epididymitis and Orchitis
- Granulomatous (Autoimmune) Orchitis
- Specific Inflammations
  - *Gonorrhea*
  - *Mumps*
  - *Tuberculosis*
  - *Syphilis*

VASCULAR DISTURBANCES

- Torsion

TESTICULAR TUMORS

- Germ Cell Tumors
  - *Seminoma*
  - *Spermatocytic Seminoma*
  - *Embryonal Carcinoma*
  - *Yolk Sac Tumor*
  - *Choriocarcinoma*
  - *Teratoma*
  - *Mixed Tumors*
- Tumors of Sex Cord–Gonadal Stroma
  - *Leydig (Interstitial) Cell Tumors*
  - *Sertoli Cell Tumors (Androblastoma)*
- Testicular Lymphoma

MISCELLANEOUS LESIONS OF TUNICA VAGINALIS

PROSTATE

INFLAMMATIONS

BENIGN ENLARGEMENT

- Nodular Hyperplasia (Benign Prostatic Hypertrophy or Hyperplasia)

TUMORS

- Carcinoma

PENIS

The penis can be affected by congenital anomalies, inflammations, and tumors, the most important of which are inflammations and tumors. The venereal infections (e.g., syphilis and gonorrhea) usually begin with penile lesions. Carcinoma of the penis, although not one of the more common neoplasms in North America, accounts for about 1% of cancers in men.

Congenital Anomalies

The penis is the site of many varied forms of congenital anomalies, only some of which have clinical significance. These range from congenital absence and hypoplasia to hyperplasia, duplication, and other aberrations in size and form. Most of these deviations are extremely uncommon and readily apparent on inspection. Certain other anomalies are more frequent and thus have greater clinical significance.

HYPOSPADIAS AND EPISPADIAS

Malformation of the urethral groove and urethral canal may create abnormal openings either on the *ventral surface of the penis (hypospadias)* or on the *dorsal surface (epispadias).*[1] Although more frequent with epispadias, either of these two anomalies may be associated with failure of normal descent of the testes and with malformations of the urinary tract. Hypospadias, the more common of the two, occurs in approximately 1 in 300 live male births.[2] Even when isolated, these urethral defects may have clinical significance because often the abnormal opening is constricted, resulting in urinary tract obstruction and an increased risk of ascending urinary tract infections. When the orifices are situated near the base of the penis, normal ejaculation and insemination are hampered or totally blocked. These lesions therefore are possible causes of sterility in men.

PHIMOSIS

When the orifice of the prepuce is too small to permit its normal retraction, the condition is designated *phimosis.* Such an abnormally small orifice may result from anomalous development but is more frequently the result of repeated attacks of infection that cause scarring of the preputial ring.[3] Phimosis is important because it interferes with cleanliness and permits the accumulation of secretions and detritus under the prepuce, favoring the development of secondary infections and possibly carcinoma. When a phimotic prepuce is forcibly retracted over the glans penis, marked constriction and subsequent swelling may block the replacement of the prepuce, creating what is known as *paraphimosis.* This condition is not only extremely painful, but also it may be a potential cause of urethral constriction and serious acute urinary retention.

Inflammations

Inflammations of the penis almost invariably involve the glans and prepuce and include a wide variety of specific and nonspecific infections. The specific infections—syphilis, gonorrhea, chancroid, granuloma inguinale, lymphopathia venerea, genital herpes—are sexually transmitted and are discussed in Chapter 9. Only the nonspecific infections causing so-called balanoposthitis need description here.

Balanoposthitis refers to infection of the glans and prepuce caused by a wide variety of organisms. Among the more common agents are *Candida albicans*, anaerobic bacteria, *Gardnerella*, and pyogenic bacteria.[4] Most cases occur as a consequence of poor local hygiene in uncircumcised males, with accumulation of desquamated epithelial cells, sweat, and debris, termed *smegma,* acting as local irritant. Persistence of such infections leads to inflammatory scarring and, as mentioned earlier, is a common cause of phimosis.

Tumors

Tumors of the penis are, on the whole, uncommon. The most frequent neoplasms are carcinomas and a benign epithelial tumor—condyloma acuminatum. In addition to the clearly defined benign and malignant categories, however, there are several forms of carcinoma in situ, exemplified by Bowen disease.

BENIGN TUMORS

Condyloma Acuminatum

Condyloma acuminatum is a benign tumor caused by human papillomavirus (HPV). It is related to the common wart (verruca vulgaris) and may occur on any moist mucocutaneous surface of the external genitals in either sex. There is ample evidence that HPV and associated diseases are sexually transmitted.[5] Of the various antigenically and genetically distinct types of HPV that have been identified, type 6, and less frequently type 11, have been clearly associated with condylomata acuminata.[6] The antigens and genome of these HPV types can be demonstrated in most lesions by immunoperoxidase and DNA hybridization techniques, respectively.

MORPHOLOGY. As mentioned, condylomata acuminata may occur on the external genitalia or perineal areas. On the penis, these lesions occur most often about the coronal sulcus and inner surface of the prepuce. They consist of single or multiple sessile or pedunculated, red papillary excrescences that vary from 1 mm to several millimeters in diameter (Fig. 23–1). Histologically a branching, villous, papillary connective tissue stroma is covered by a thickened hyperplastic epithelium that may have considerable superficial hyperkeratosis and thickening of the underlying

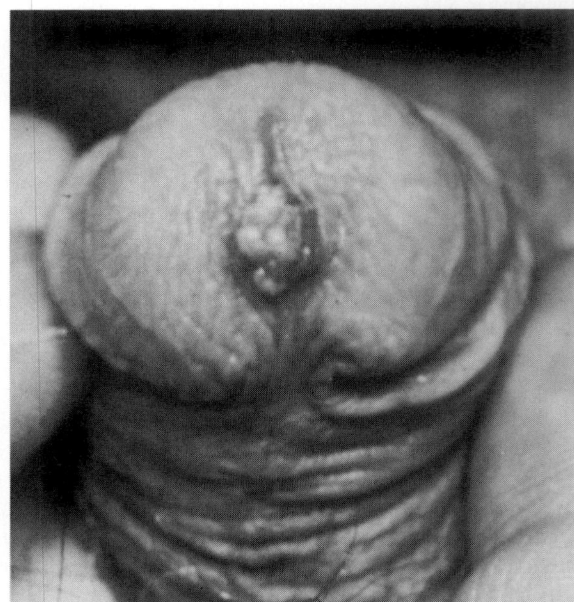

Figure 23–1

Condyloma acuminatum of the penis.

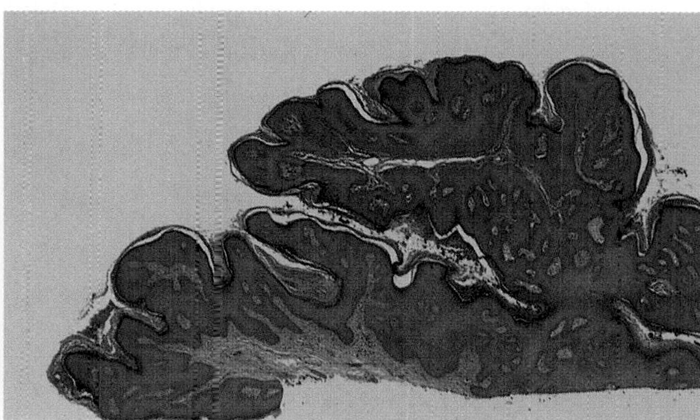

Figure 23–2

Condyloma acuminatum of the penis. Low magnification reveals the papillary (villous) architecture. (Courtesy of Dr. Jag Bhawan, Boston University School of Medicine, Boston, MA.)

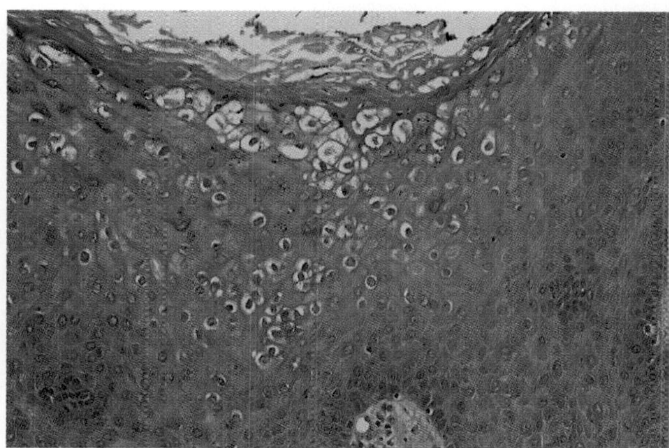

Figure 23–3

Condyloma acuminatum of the penis. The epithelium shows vacuolization (koilocytosis) characteristic of human papillomavirus (HPV) infection. (Courtesy of Dr. Jag Bhawan, Boston University School of Medicine, Boston, MA.)

epidermis (acanthosis) (Fig. 23–2). The normal orderly maturation of the epithelial cells is preserved. Clear vacuolization of the prickle cells (koilocytosis), characteristic of HPV infection, is noted in these lesions (Fig. 23–3). The basement membrane is intact, and there is no evidence of invasion of the underlying stroma. Condylomata acuminata tend to recur but do not evolve into invasive cancers.

CARCINOMA IN SITU

As discussed in Chapter 8, *carcinoma in situ* is a histologic term used to describe epithelial lesions having the cytologic changes of malignancy confined to the epithelium with no evidence of local invasion or distant metastases. It is considered a precancerous condition because of its potential to evolve into invasive cancer. In the external male genitalia, three lesions that display histologic features of carcinoma in situ have been described: *Bowen disease, erythroplasia of Queyrat,* and *bowenoid papulosis.*[7] Whether these are distinct clinical entities or instead are variants of a single underlying disorder is controversial, as is evident from the following brief descriptions. All these lesions have a strong association with infection by HPV. Data compiled from a large number of studies reveal that HPV DNA, most commonly type 16, is found in approximately 80% of cases.[8]

Bowen disease occurs in the genital region of both men and women, usually in those over the age of 35 years. In men, it is prone to involve the skin of the shaft of the penis and the scrotum. Grossly, it appears as a solitary, thickened, gray-white, opaque plaque with shallow ulceration and crusting. Histologically the epidermis shows proliferation with numerous mitoses, some atypical. The cells are markedly dysplastic with large hyperchromatic nuclei and lack of orderly maturation (Fig. 23–4). Nevertheless, *the dermal-epidermal border is sharply delineated by an intact basement membrane.* Over the span of years, Bowen disease may become invasive and transform into typical squamous cell carcinoma in approximately 10% of patients. Another feature said to be associated with Bowen disease is the occurrence of visceral cancer in approximately one third of the patients. This view has been challenged, however, and hence this issue remains unresolved.[7]

Erythroplasia of Queyrat generally appears on the glans and prepuce as single or multiple shiny red, sometimes velvety plaques. Histologically, it is indistinguishable from Bowen disease. Similar to Bowen disease, it has the potential to develop into invasive carcinoma. Hence, the distinction between Bowen disease and erythroplasia of Queyrat is tenuous. Most authorities use *Bowen disease* for carcinoma in situ involving the skin and *erythroplasia of*

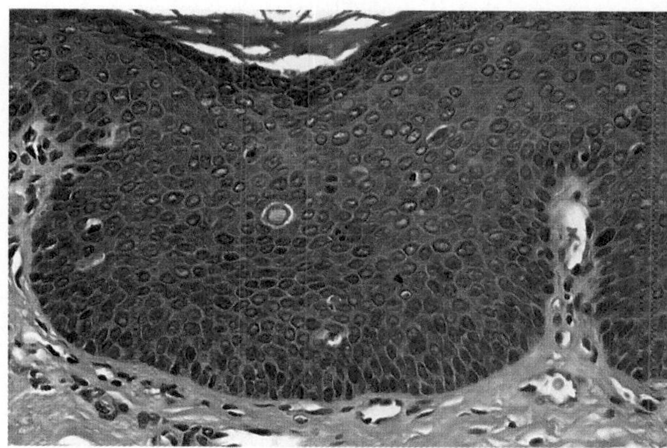

Figure 23–4

Bowen disease (carcinoma in situ) of the penis. Note the intact basement membrane and hyperchromatic, dysplastic epithelial cells with scattered mitoses above the basal layer. (Courtesy of Dr. Jag Bhawan, Boston University School of Medicine, Boston, MA.)

Queyrat for similar lesions that affect the mucosal surface such as glans penis.

Bowenoid papulosis, the third member of the carcinoma in situ family of lesions affecting the external genitalia, occurs in sexually active adults. Clinically, it differs from Bowen disease by the younger age of patients and the presence of multiple (rather than solitary), pigmented (reddish brown) papular lesions. In some cases, the lesions may be verrucoid and readily mistaken for condyloma acuminatum. Histologically, bowenoid papulosis is indistinguishable from Bowen disease. In contrast to the other two forms of carcinoma in situ, bowenoid papulosis virtually never develops into an invasive carcinoma.

CARCINOMA

Squamous cell carcinoma of the penis is an uncommon malignancy in the United States, accounting for less than 1% of cancers in males.[9] By contrast, the incidence of squamous cell carcinoma of the penis ranges from 10 to 20% of male malignancies in some parts of Asia, Africa, and South America. A striking correlation exists between the practice of circumcision and the occurrence of penile cancer. Circumcision confers protection, and hence this cancer is extremely rare among Jews and Moslems and is correspondingly more common in populations in which circumcision is not routinely practiced. It is postulated that circumcision is associated with better genital hygiene, which, in turn, reduces exposure to carcinogens that may be concentrated in smegma and decreases the likelihood of infection with potentially oncogenic human papillomavirus (HPV). This notion is supported by the observation that HPV DNA can be detected in the cancer cells in approximately 50% of patients.[8] HPV type 16 is the most frequent culprit, but as with other genitourinary malignancies, HPV 18 is also implicated. Carcinoma in situ (Bowen disease), the presumed precursor lesion of invasive squamous cell carcinoma of the penis, has a much stronger association with HPV, being detected in 80% of lesions. This disparity suggests that infection with HPV is not sufficient for transformation and that it probably acts in concert with other carcinogenic influences. These may include carcinogens in cigarette smoke; cigarette smoking elevates the risk of developing cancer of the penis.[10] Carcinomas are usually found in patients between the ages of 40 and 70.

MORPHOLOGY. Squamous cell carcinoma of the penis usually begins on the glans or inner surface of the prepuce near the coronal sulcus. Two macroscopic patterns are seen—papillary and flat. The papillary lesions simulate condylomata acuminata and may produce a cauliflower-like fungating mass. Flat lesions appear as areas of epithelial thickening accompanied by graying and fissuring of the mucosal surface. With progression, an ulcerated papule develops (Fig. 23–5). Histologically, both the papillary and the flat lesions are squamous cell carcinomas with varying degrees of differentiation. **Verrucous carcinoma,** also called **giant condyloma** or **Buschke-Löwenstein tumor,** is an uncommon, well-differentiated variant of squamous cell carcinoma that has low malignant potential. These tumors are locally invasive, but they rarely metastasize. As the name indicates, these tumors have a verrucous (papillary) appearance, similar to condylomata acuminata, but they are larger than the usual condylomata. Similar to condylomata acuminata, these lesions are believed to be caused by HPV types 6 and 11, and they also reveal the koilocytic change in the superficial layers. In contrast to condylomata acuminata, however, verrucous carcinomas penetrate the underlying tissues.

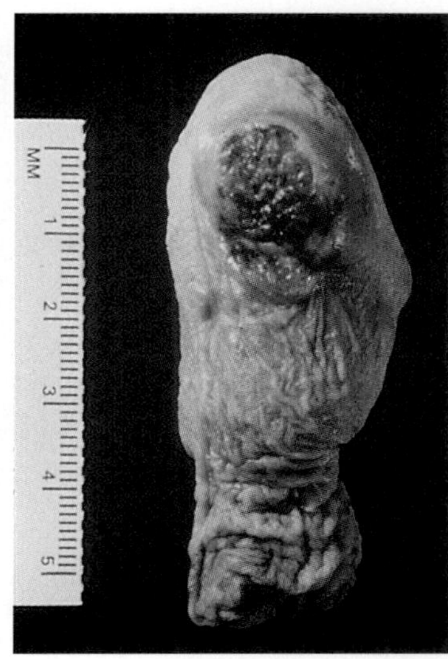

Figure 23–5

Carcinoma of the penis. The glans penis is deformed by a firm, ulcerated, infiltrative mass. (Courtesy of Dr. Kyle Molberg, Department of Pathology, University of Texas Southwestern Medical Center, Dallas, TX.)

Clinical Course. Invasive squamous cell carcinoma of the penis is a slowly growing, locally metastasizing lesion[11] that often has been present for a year or more before it is brought to medical attention. The lesions are nonpainful until they undergo secondary ulceration and infection. Frequently, they bleed. Metastases to inguinal and iliac lymph nodes characterize the early stage, but widespread dissemination is extremely uncommon until the lesion is far advanced. The prognosis is related to the stage of the tumor. In persons with limited lesions without invasion of the inguinal lymph nodes, there is a 66% 5-year survival rate, whereas metastasis to the lymph nodes carries a grim 27% 5-year survival.

TESTIS AND EPIDIDYMIS

The major pathologic involvements of the testis and epididymis are quite distinct. In the case of the epididymis, the most important and frequent involvements are inflammatory diseases, whereas in the testis, the major lesions are tumors. Their close anatomic relationship, however, permits the extension of any of these processes from one organ to the other.

Congenital Anomalies

With the exception of incomplete descent of the testes (cryptorchidism), congenital anomalies are extremely rare and include absence of one or both testes, fusion of the testes (so-called *synorchism*), and the formation of relatively insignificant cysts within the testis.

CRYPTORCHIDISM

Cryptorchidism is synonymous with undescended testes and is found in approximately 1% of 1-year-old boys.[12] This anomaly represents a complete or incomplete failure of the intra-abdominal testes to descend into the scrotal sac. It usually occurs as an isolated anomaly but may be accompanied by other malformations of the genitourinary tract, such as hypospadias.

Testicular descent occurs in two morphologically and hormonally distinct phases.[13] During the first, transabdominal, phase, the testis comes to lie within the lower abdomen or brim of the pelvis. This phase is believed to be controlled by a hormone called *müllerian-inhibiting substance*. In the second, or the inguinoscrotal, phase, the testes descend through the inguinal canal into the scrotal sac. This phase is androgen dependent and is possibly mediated by androgen-induced release of calcitonin gene–related peptide, from the genitofemoral nerve. Although testes may be arrested anywhere along their pathway of descent, defects in transabdominal descent are uncommon, accounting for approximately 5 to 10% of cases. In most patients, the undescended testis is palpable in the inguinal canal. The precise cause of cryptorchidism is still poorly understood. Despite the fact that testicular descent is controlled by hormonal factors, cryptorchidism is only rarely associated with hormonal disorders. It may be one of several congenital defects in chromosomal disorders, such as trisomy 13. The condition is completely asymptomatic, and it is found by the patient or the examining physician only when the scrotal sac is discovered not to contain the testis.

MORPHOLOGY. Cryptorchidism is unilateral in most cases, but it may be bilateral in 25% of patients. Histologic changes in the malpositioned testis begin as early as 2 years of age. They are characterized by an arrest in the development of germ cells associated with marked hyalinization and thickening of the basement membrane of the spermatic tubules (Fig. 23–6). Eventually the tubules appear as dense cords of hyaline connective tissue outlined by prominent basement membranes. There is concomitant increase in interstitial stroma. Because Leydig cells are spared, they appear to be prominent. As might be expected with progressive tubular atrophy, the cryptorchid testis is small in size and is firm in consistency owing to fibrotic changes. Histologic deterioration, leading to a paucity of germ cells, has also been noted in the contralateral (descended) testis in patients with unilateral cryptorchidism, supporting a hormonal basis for the development of this condition.

Cryptorchidism is of more than academic interest for many reasons. When the testis lies in the inguinal canal, it is particularly exposed to trauma and crushing against the ligaments and bones. A concomitant inguinal hernia ac-

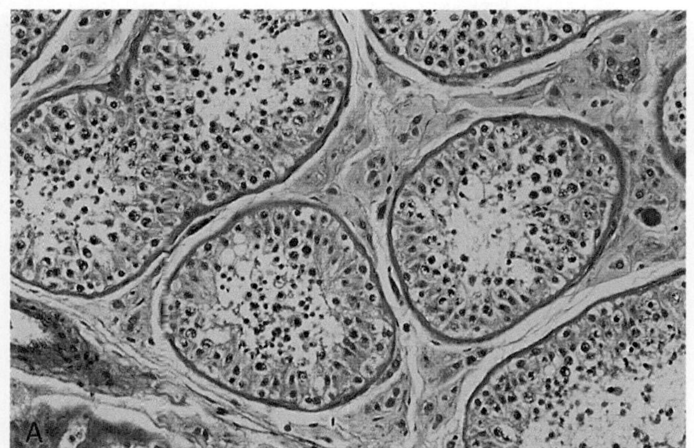

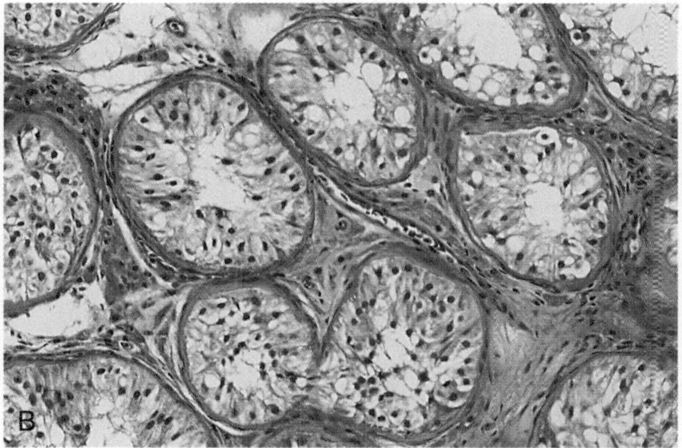

Figure 23–6

A, Normal testis shows tubules with active spermatogenesis. *B*, Testicular atrophy. The tubules show Sertoli cells but no spermatogenesis. There is thickening of basement membranes. (Courtesy of Dr. Arthur Weinberg, Department of Pathology, University of Texas Health Science Center, Dallas, TX.)

companies such malposition of the testis in about 10 to 20% of cases. From the morphologic changes, it is apparent that bilateral cryptorchidism may result in sterility. Infertility, however, is also noted in a significant number of cases with uncorrected unilateral cryptorchidism because, as mentioned earlier, the contralateral descended testis may also be deficient in germ cells. In addition, the undescended testis is at a greater risk of developing testicular cancer than is the descended testis. It is generally accepted that cryptorchid patients have a fivefold to tenfold increase in the chance of developing a testicular tumor.[14] The undescended testis requires surgical correction, preferably before histologic deterioration sets in at around 2 years of age.[12] Orchiopexy (placement in the scrotal sac) does not guarantee fertility; deficient spermatogenesis has been reported in 10 to 60% of patients in whom surgical repositioning was performed.[12,15] To what extent the risk of cancer is reduced after orchiopexy is also unclear. According to some studies, orchiopexy of unilateral cryptorchidism before 10 years of age protects against cancer development.[16] This is not universally accepted, however.[17] Malignant change may occur in the contralateral, normally descended testis. These observations suggest that cryptorchidism is associated with an intrinsic defect in testicular development and cellular differentiation that is unrelated to anatomic position.

Regressive Changes

ATROPHY

Atrophy is the only important regressive change that affects the scrotal testis, and it may have a number of causes, including (1) progressive atherosclerotic narrowing of the blood supply in old age; (2) the end stage of an inflammatory orchitis, whatever the etiologic agent; (3) cryptorchidism; (4) hypopituitarism; (5) generalized malnutrition or cachexia; (6) obstruction to the outflow of semen; (7) irradiation; (8) prolonged administration of female sex hormones, such as is used in treatment of patients with carcinoma of the prostate; and (9) exhaustion atrophy, which may follow the persistent stimulation produced by high levels of follicle-stimulating pituitary hormone. The gross and microscopic alterations follow the pattern already described for cryptorchidism. When the process is bilateral, as it frequently is, sterility results. Atrophy or sometimes improper development of the testes occasionally occurs as a primary failure of genetic origin. The resulting condition, called *Klinefelter syndrome*, represents a sex chromosomal disorder (discussed in detail in Chapter 6, along with other cytogenetic diseases).

Inflammations

Inflammations are distinctly more common in the epididymis than in the testis. It is classically taught that, of the three major specific inflammatory states, *gonorrhea and tuberculosis almost invariably arise in the epididymis, whereas syphilis affects first the testis.*

NONSPECIFIC EPIDIDYMITIS AND ORCHITIS

Epididymitis and possible subsequent orchitis are commonly related to infections in the urinary tract (cystitis, urethritis, genitoprostatitis), which presumably reach the epididymis and the testis through either the vas deferens or the lymphatics of the spermatic cord.

The cause of epididymitis varies with the age of the patient. Although uncommon in children, epididymitis in childhood is usually associated with a congenital genitourinary abnormality and infection with gram-negative rods. In sexually active men younger than age 35 years, the sexually transmitted pathogens *Chlamydia trachomatis* and *Neisseria gonorrhoeae* are the most frequent culprits. In men older than age 35, the common urinary tract pathogens, such as *Escherichia coli* and *Pseudomonas*, are responsible for most infections.

MORPHOLOGY. The bacterial invasion sets up a nonspecific acute inflammation characterized by congestion, edema, and infiltration by neutrophils, macrophages, and lymphocytes. Although the infection, in the early stage, is more or less limited to the interstitial connective tissue, it rapidly extends to involve the tubules and may progress to frank abscess formation or complete suppurative necrosis of the entire epididymis (Fig. 23–7). Usually, having involved the epididymis, the infection extends into the testis to evoke a similar inflammatory reaction. Such inflammatory involvement of the epididymis and testis is often followed by fibrous scarring, which, in many cases, leads to sterility. Usually the interstitial cells of Leydig are not totally destroyed, so sexual activity is not disturbed. Any such nonspecific infection may become chronic.

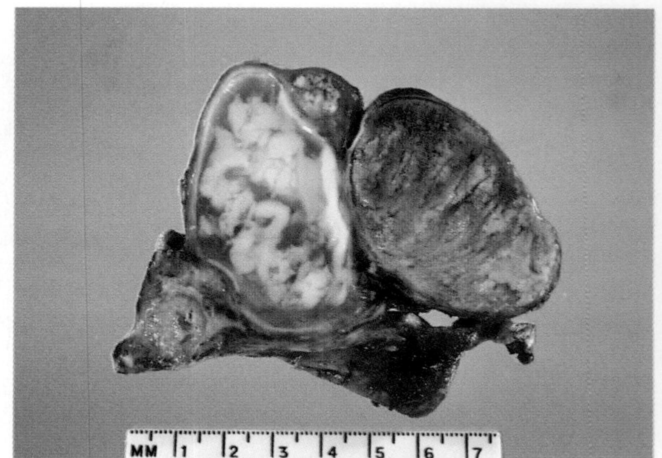

Figure 23–7

Acute epididymitis caused by gonococcal infection. The epididymis is replaced by an abscess. Normal testis is seen on the right.

GRANULOMATOUS (AUTOIMMUNE) ORCHITIS

Among middle-aged men, a rare cause of unilateral testicular enlargement is nontuberculous, granulomatous orchitis. It usually presents as a moderately tender testicular mass of sudden onset sometimes associated with fever. It may appear insidiously, however, as a painless testicular mass mimicking a testicular tumor, hence its importance.[18] Histologically the orchitis is distinguished by granulomas seen both within spermatic tubules and in the intertubular connective tissue. The lesions closely resemble tubercles but differ somewhat in having plasma cells and occasional neutrophils interspersed within the enclosing rim of fibroblasts and lymphocytes. Although an autoimmune basis is suspected, the cause of these lesions remains unknown.

SPECIFIC INFLAMMATIONS

Gonorrhea

Extension of infection from the posterior urethra to the prostate, seminal vesicles, and then to the epididymis is the usual course of a neglected gonococcal infection. Inflammatory changes similar to those described in the nonspecific infections occur, with the development of frank abscesses in the epididymis, resulting in extensive destruction of this organ. In the more neglected cases, the infection may then spread to the testis and produce a suppurative orchitis.

Mumps

Mumps is a systemic viral disease that most commonly affects school-aged children. Testicular involvement is extremely uncommon in this age group. In postpubertal males, however, orchitis may develop and has been reported in 20 to 30% of male patients. Most often, the acute interstitial orchitis develops about 1 week after onset of swelling of the parotid glands. Rarely, cases of orchitis precede the parotitis or may be unaccompanied by parotid gland involvement.

Tuberculosis

Tuberculosis almost invariably begins in the epididymis and may spread to the testis. In many of these cases, there is associated tuberculous prostatitis and seminal vesiculitis, and it is believed that epididymitis usually represents a secondary spread from these other involvements of the genital tract. The infection invokes the classic morphologic reactions of caseating granulomatous inflammation characteristic of tuberculosis elsewhere.

Syphilis

The testis and epididymis are affected in both acquired and congenital syphilis, but *almost invariably the testis is involved first by the infection.* In many cases, the orchitis is not accompanied by epididymitis. The morphologic pattern of the reaction takes two forms: the production of gummas or a diffuse interstitial inflammation characterized by edema and lymphocytic and plasma cell infiltration with the characteristic hallmark of all syphilitic infections (i.e., obliterative endarteritis with perivascular cuffing of lymphocytes and plasma cells).

Vascular Disturbances

TORSION

Twisting of the spermatic cord may cut off the venous drainage and the arterial supply to the testis. Usually, however, the thick-walled arteries remain patent so that intense vascular engorgement and venous infarction follow. The usual precipitating cause of such torsion is some violent movement or physical trauma. In most instances, however, there are predisposing causes, such as incomplete descent, absence of the scrotal ligaments or the gubernaculum testis, atrophy of the testis so it is abnormally mobile within the tunica vaginalis, abnormal attachment of the testis to the epididymis, or other abnormalities.

MORPHOLOGY. Depending on the duration of the process, the morphologic changes range from intense congestion to widespread extravasation of blood into the interstitial tissue of the testis and epididymis. Eventually hemorrhagic infarction of the entire testis occurs (Fig. 23–8). In these late stages, the testis is markedly enlarged and is converted virtually into a sac of soft, necrotic, hemorrhagic tissue.

Testicular Tumors

Testicular neoplasms span an amazing gamut of anatomic types. They are divided into two major categories: germ cell tumors and nongerminal tumors derived from stroma or sex cord. Approximately 95% arise from germ cells. Most of these germinal tumors are highly aggressive cancers capable of rapid, wide dissemination, although with current therapy most can be cured.[19] Nongerminal tumors,

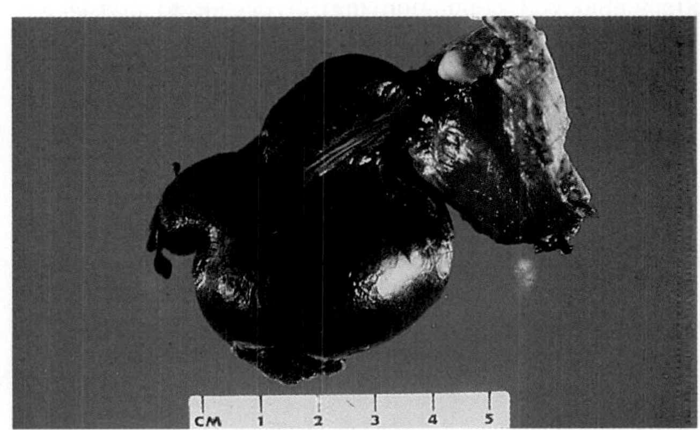

Figure 23–8

Torsion of testis.

in contrast, are generally benign, but some elaborate steroids leading to interesting endocrinologic syndromes.

GERM CELL TUMORS

The incidence of testicular tumors in the United States is approximately 6 per 100,000. For unexplained reasons, there is a worldwide increase in the incidence of these tumors. In the 15- to 34-year age group, when these neoplasms have a peak incidence, they constitute the most common tumor of men and cause approximately 10% of all cancer deaths. In the United States, these tumors are much more common in whites than in blacks (ratio 5 : 1).

Classification and Histogenesis. Classifications of the testicular germ cell tumors abound and, regrettably, vary widely. The major problems are the differing concepts of the histogenesis of these lesions and the endless variability in morphology among the various categories of neoplasms as well as within a single tumor. As one might guess, germ cells are multipotential, and once they become cancerous, they are not inhibited in their lines of differentiation. Table 23–1 shows the World Health Organization (WHO) classification, most widely used in the United States. The proposed histogenesis of germ cell tumors of the testis follows.

Table 23–1. WHO PATHOLOGIC CLASSIFICATION OF TESTICULAR TUMORS

GERM CELL TUMORS

Tumors of one histologic pattern

- Seminoma
- Spermatocytic seminoma
- Embryonal carcinoma
- Yolk sac tumor (embryonal carcinoma, infantile type)
- Polyembryoma
- Choriocarcinoma
- Teratomas
  - Mature
  - Immature
  - With malignant transformation

Tumors showing more than one histologic pattern

- Embryonal carcinoma plus teratoma (teratocarcinoma)
- Choriocarcinoma and any other types (specify types)
- Other combinations (specify)

SEX CORD—STROMAL TUMORS

Well-differentiated forms

- Leydig cell tumor
- Sertoli cell tumor
- Granulosa cell tumor

Mixed forms (specify)

Incompletely differentiated forms

Testicular germ cell tumors may be divided into two categories, on the basis of whether they are composed of a single histologic pattern or more than one. Tumors with a single histologic pattern constitute about 40% of all testicular neoplasms and are listed in Table 23–1. In approximately 60% of the tumors, there is a *mixture of two or more of the histologic patterns.* The most common mixture is that of teratoma, embryonal carcinoma, yolk sac tumor, and elements of choriocarcinoma.

The WHO classification is based on the view that most tumors in this group originate from intratubular testicular germ cells. *Indeed, a focus of carcinoma in situ is found in the vicinity of most testicular germ cell tumors.* It is from these intratubular, preinvasive lesions that most germ cell cancers are presumed to arise. Despite their common origin, the precise relationship between the various histologic subtypes of germ cell tumors is not clear. According to one view, the neoplastic germ cells may differentiate along gonadal lines to give rise to *seminoma* or transform into a totipotential cell population that gives rise to *nonseminomatous tumors.* Such totipotential cells may remain largely undifferentiated to form embryonal carcinoma or may differentiate along extraembryonic lines to form *yolk sac tumors* or *choriocarcinomas.* Teratoma results from differentiation of the embryonic carcinoma cells along the lines of all three germ cell layers. Some studies suggest that seminomas are not end-stage neoplasms. Similar to embryonal carcinomas, seminomas may also act as precursors from which other forms of testicular germ cell tumors originate.[20] This view is supported by the fact that cells that form intratubular germ cell tumors (the presumed precursors of all types of germ cell tumors) share morphologic and molecular characteristics with tumor cells in seminomas.[21] Despite the fascination of pathologists with the heterogeneity of testicular tumors, from a clinical standpoint there are only two important categories of germ cell tumors: seminomas and nonseminomatous tumors. As discussed later, this clinical distinction has important bearings on treatment and prognosis.

Pathogenesis. As with all neoplasms, little is known about the ultimate cause of germ cell tumors. Several predisposing influences, however, may be important: (1) cryptorchidism, (2) genetic factors, and (3) testicular dysgenesis, all of which may contribute to a common denominator—germ cell maldevelopment. Reference has already been made to the increased incidence of neoplasms in *undescended testes.* In most large series of testicular tumors, approximately 10% are associated with cryptorchidism.[18] The higher the location of the undescended testicle (intra-abdominal versus inguinal), the greater is the risk of developing cancer.

Genetic predisposition also seems to be important, although no well-defined pattern of inheritance has been identified. In support, striking racial differences in the incidence of testicular tumors can be cited. Blacks in Africa have an extremely low incidence of these neoplasms, which is unaffected by migration to the United States. Familial clustering has been reported, and according to one study, sibs of affected individuals have a tenfold higher risk of developing testicular cancer as compared with the general population.[17]

Patients with disorders of testicular development (testicular dysgenesis), including testicular feminization and Klinefelter syndrome, harbor an increased risk of developing germ cell tumors. The risk is highest in patients with testicular feminization. In cryptorchid and dysgenetic testes, foci of intratubular germ cell neoplasms can be detected at a high frequency, before the development of invasive tumors.

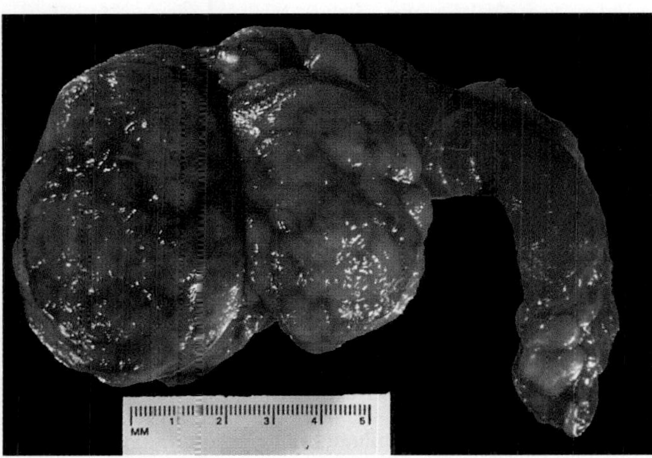

Figure 23–9

Seminoma of the testis appears as a fairly well circumscribed, pale, fleshy, homogeneous mass. (Courtesy of Dr. Kyle Molberg, Department of Pathology, University of Texas Southwestern Medical Center, Dallas, TX.)

As with all tumors, genomic changes are undoubtedly important in the pathogenesis of testicular cancers. An isochromosome of the short arm of chromosome 12, i(12p), is found in virtually all germ cell tumors, regardless of their histologic type.[19] In the approximately 10% of cases in which i(12p) is not detected, extra genetic material derived from 12p is found on other chromosomes. Obviously, dosage of genes located on 12p is critical for the pathogenesis of germ cell tumors, but no candidate genes have been identified. It is of interest that i(12p) is also noted in ovarian germ cell neoplasms, suggesting that the events leading to this alteration may be critical to the molecular pathogenesis of all germ cell neoplasms.

With this background of pathogenesis, we can discuss the morphologic patterns of germ cell tumors, followed by the clinical features common to most germinal tumors.[21] The student can take comfort in the fact that some of the tumors listed in Table 23–1 are sufficiently rare to justify exclusion from the following discussion.

Seminoma

Seminomas are the most common type of germinal tumor (50%) and the type most likely to produce a uniform population of cells. They almost never occur in infants; they peak in the thirties, somewhat later than the collective peak. A nearly identical tumor arises in the ovary, where it is called *dysgerminoma* (Chapter 24).

MORPHOLOGY. Three histologic variants of seminoma are described: typical (85%), anaplastic (5 to 10%), and spermatocytic (4 to 6%). The last-mentioned, despite its nosologic similarity, is actually a distinct tumor; it has been segregated into a separate category and is discussed later. All produce bulky masses, sometimes ten times the size of the normal testis.

The typical seminoma has a homogeneous, gray-white, lobulated cut surface, usually devoid of hemorrhage or necrosis (Fig. 23–9). In more than half the cases, the entire testis is replaced. Generally the tunica albuginea is not penetrated, but occasionally extension to the epididymis, spermatic cord, or scrotal sac occurs.

Microscopically the typical seminoma presents sheets of uniform, so-called seminoma cells divided into poorly demarcated lobules by delicate septa of fibrous tissue (Fig. 23–10*A*). **The classic seminoma cell is large and round-to-polyhedral and has a distinct cell membrane; a clear or watery-appearing cytoplasm; and a large, central nucleus with one or two prominent nucleoli** (Fig. 23–10*B*). Mitoses are infrequent. The cytoplasm contains varying amounts of glycogen and, rarely, lipid vacuoles. Classic seminoma cells do not contain α-fetoprotein (AFP) or human chori-

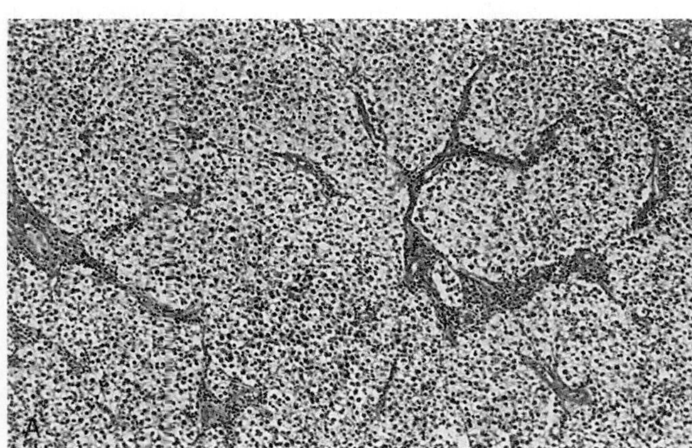

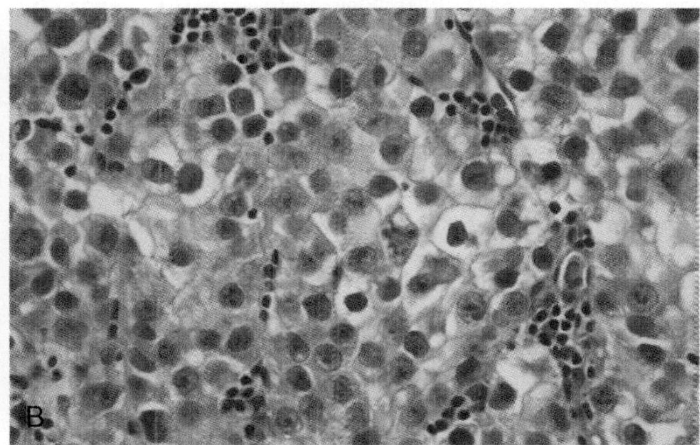

Figure 23–10

Seminoma. *A*, Low magnification shows clear seminoma cells divided into poorly demarcated lobules by delicate septa. *B*, Microscopic examination reveals large cells with distinct cell borders, pale nuclei, prominent nucleoli, and a sparse lymphocytic infiltrate.

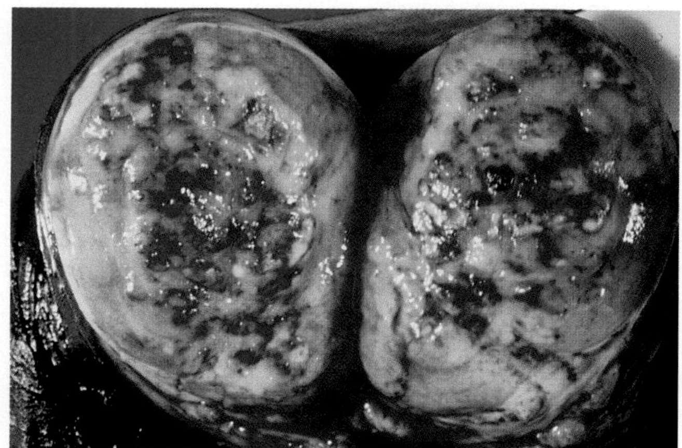

Figure 23–11

Embryonal carcinoma. In contrast to the seminoma illustrated in Figure 23–9, the embryonal carcinoma is a hemorrhagic mass. (Courtesy of Dr. Kyle Molberg, Department of Pathology, University of Texas Southwestern Medical Center, Dallas, TX.)

onic gonadotropin (HCG). The tumor cells stain positively for placental alkaline phosphatase.

Approximately 15% of seminomas contain syncytial giant cells that resemble the syncytiotrophoblast of the placenta both morphologically and in that they contain HCG. In this subset of patients, serum HCG levels are also elevated. The amount of stroma in typical seminomas varies greatly. Sometimes it is scant and at other times abundant. Usually, well-defined fibrous strands are present, creating lobules of neoplastic cells. The septa are usually infiltrated with T lymphocytes, and in some tumors they also bear prominent granulomas.

The anaplastic seminoma, as the name indicates, presents greater cellular and nuclear irregularity with more frequent tumor giant cells and many mitoses. Most critical to the identification of this pattern are the size of the cells and the presence of three or more mitoses per high-power field.

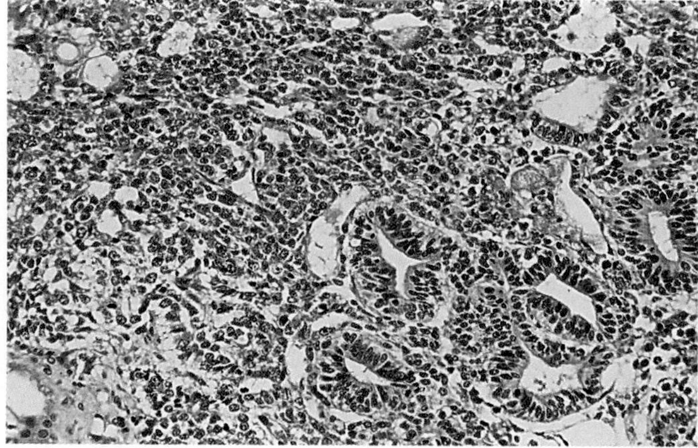

Figure 23–12

Embryonal carcinoma shows sheets of undifferentiated cells as well as glandular differentiation. The nuclei are large and hyperchromatic. (Courtesy of Dr. Trace Worrell, Department of Pathology, University of Texas Southwestern Medical Center, Dallas, TX.)

Spermatocytic Seminoma

Although related by name to seminoma, spermatocytic seminoma is a distinctive tumor both clinically and histologically. It is one of the two variants of germ cell tumors that do not arise from an intratubular germ cell neoplasm, the other being teratomas of children. Spermatocytic seminoma is an uncommon tumor, representing 1 to 2% of all testicular germ cell neoplasms. The age of involvement is much later than for most testicular tumors: Affected individuals are generally over the age of 65 years. In contrast to classic seminoma, it is a slow-growing tumor that rarely if ever produces metastases, and hence the prognosis is excellent.

MORPHOLOGY. Grossly, spermatocytic seminoma tends to be larger than classic seminoma and presents with a pale gray, soft, and friable cut surface. Spermatocytic seminomas have three cell populations, all intermixed: (1) medium-sized cells (15 to 18 μm), the most numerous, containing a round nucleus and eosinophilic cytoplasm; (2) smaller cells (6 to 8 μm), with a narrow rim of eosinophilic cytoplasm resembling secondary spermatocytes; and (3) scattered giant cells (50 to 100 μm), either uninucleate or multinucleate. With the electron microscope, tumor cells show nuclear and cytoplasmic features of spermatocytic maturation, thus justifying the term **spermatocytic seminoma**.

Embryonal Carcinoma

Embryonal carcinomas occur mostly in the 20- to 30-year age group. These tumors are more aggressive than seminomas.

MORPHOLOGY. Grossly, the tumor is smaller than seminoma and usually does not replace the entire testis. On cut surfaces, the mass is often variegated, poorly demarcated at the margins, and punctuated by foci of hemorrhage or necrosis (Fig. 23–11). Extension through the tunica albuginea into the epididymis or cord is not infrequent. **Histologically the cells grow in glandular, alveolar, or tubular patterns, sometimes with papillary convolutions** (Fig. 23–12). **More undifferentiated lesions may present sheets of cells.** The neoplastic cells have an epithelial appearance and are large and anaplastic, with angry-looking hyperchromatic nuclei having prominent nucleoli. In contrast to seminoma, the cell borders are usually indistinct, and there is considerable variation in cell and nuclear size and shape. Mitotic figures and tumor giant cells are frequent. **Within this background, syncytial cells containing HCG or cells containing AFP, or both, may be detected by immunoperoxidase techniques. Because HCG and AFP are products of trophoblastic and yolk sac cells, respectively, their presence is indicative of a mixed tumor.**

If tumors containing HCG or AFP, or both, are excluded, it is estimated that pure embryonal cell carcinomas constitute about 3% of testicular germ cell tumors. If one includes mixed tumors, however, embryonal carcinoma cells are present in about 45% of tumors.

Yolk Sac Tumor

Also known as *infantile embryonal carcinoma* or *endodermal sinus tumor*, the yolk sac tumor is of interest because it is the most common testicular tumor in infants and children up to 3 years of age, and in this age group it has a very good prognosis. In adults, the pure form of this tumor is rare; instead, yolk sac elements frequently occur in combination with embryonal carcinoma.

MORPHOLOGY. Grossly, the tumor is nonencapsulated, and on cross-section it presents a homogeneous, yellow-white, mucinous appearance. Characteristic on microscopic examination is a lacelike (reticular) network of medium-sized cuboidal or elongated cells. In addition, papillary structures or solid cords of cells may be found. In approximately 50% of tumors, the so-called endodermal sinuses may be seen; these consist of a mesodermal core with a central capillary and a visceral and parietal layer of cells resembling primitive glomeruli. Present within and outside the cytoplasm are eosinophilic, hyalin-like globules in which AFP and α_1-antitrypsin can be demonstrated by immunocytochemical staining. The presence of AFP in the tumor cells is highly characteristic, and it underscores their differentiation into yolk sac cells.

Choriocarcinoma

Choriocarcinoma is a highly malignant form of testicular tumor that is composed of both cytotrophoblast and syncytiotrophoblast. Identical tumors may arise in the placental tissue, ovary, or sequestered rests of totipotential cells (e.g., in the mediastinum or abdomen). In its "pure" form, choriocarcinoma is rare, constituting less than 1% of all germ cell tumors. As emphasized later, foci of choriocarcinoma are much more common in mixed patterns.

MORPHOLOGY. Despite their aggressive behavior, pure choriocarcinomas are usually small lesions. **Often, they cause no testicular enlargement and are detected only as a small palpable nodule.** Because they are rapidly growing, they may outgrow their blood supply, and sometimes the primary testicular focus is replaced by a small fibrous scar, leaving only widespread metastases. Typically, these tumors are small, rarely larger than 5 cm in diameter. Hemorrhage and necrosis are extremely common. Histologically the tumors contain two cell types (Fig. 23-13). The syncytiotrophoblastic cell is large and has many irregular or lobular hyperchromatic nuclei and an abundant eosinophilic vacuolated cytoplasm. As might be expected, HCG can be readily demonstrated in the cytoplasm of syncytiotrophoblastic cells. The cytotrophoblastic cells are more regular and tend to be polygonal with distinct cell borders and clear cytoplasm; they grow in cords or masses and have a single, fairly uniform nucleus. More anatomic details are available in the discussion of these neoplasms in the female genital tract (Chapter 24).

Teratoma

The designation *teratoma* refers to a group of complex tumors having various cellular or organoid components reminiscent of normal derivatives from more than one germ layer. They may occur at any age from infancy to adult life. Pure forms of teratoma are fairly common in infants and children, second only in frequency to yolk sac tumors. In adults, pure teratomas are rare, constituting 2 to 3% of germ cell tumors. As with embryonal carcinomas, their frequency in combination with other histologic types is about 45%.

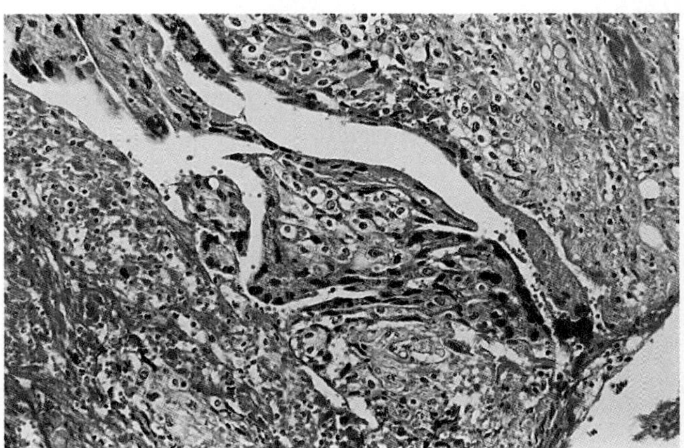

Figure 23-13

Choriocarcinoma shows clear cytotrophoblastic cells with central nuclei and syncytiotrophoblastic cells with multiple dark nuclei embedded in eosinophilic cytoplasm. Hemorrhage and necrosis are seen in the upper right field. (Courtesy of Dr. Trace Worrell, Department of Pathology, University of Texas Southwestern Medical School, Dallas, TX.)

MORPHOLOGY. Grossly, teratomas are usually large, ranging from 5 to 10 cm in diameter. Because they are composed of various tissues, the gross appearance is heterogeneous with solid, sometimes cartilaginous and cystic areas (Fig. 23–14). Hemorrhage and necrosis usually indicate admixture with embryonal carcinoma, choriocarcinoma, or both.

Histologically, three variants are recognized, based on the degree of differentiation. **Mature teratomas** are composed of a heterogeneous, helter-skelter collection of differentiated cells or organoid structures, such as neural tissue, muscle bundles, islands of cartilage, clusters of squamous epithelium, structures reminiscent of thyroid gland, bronchial or bronchiolar epithelium, and bits of intestinal wall or brain substance, all embedded in a fibrous or myxoid stroma. All the elements are differentiated. This mature variant occurs with relatively greater frequency in infancy and childhood. Similar tumors may occur in adults, but there is a far greater risk of small hidden foci of immature or malignant components that may escape detection despite rigorous sampling of the lesion. Thus, although teratomas may appear entirely mature and benign, such a diagnosis in an adult must be made with circumspection. Dermoid cysts, common in the ovary (Chapter 24), are rare in the testis. They represent a special form of mature teratoma.

Immature teratomas can be viewed as intermediate between mature teratoma and embryonal carcinoma. In contrast to the mature teratoma, elements of the three germ cell layers are incompletely differentiated and not arranged in organoid fashion. Even though the differentiation is incomplete, the nature of the embryonic tissue can be clearly identified; thus, poorly formed cartilage, neuroblasts, loose mesenchyme, and clusters of glandular structures may be seen lying helter-skelter. In some areas, more mature forms of these tissues may also be seen. Although these tumors are clearly malignant, they may not display clear-cut cytologic features of malignancy.

In contrast, the third variant—**teratoma with malignant transformation**—shows clear evidence of malignancy in derivatives of one or more germ cell layers. Thus, there may be a focus of squamous cell carcinoma, mucin-secreting adenocarcinoma, or a sarcoma. Immature and frankly malignant teratomas occur more commonly in adults.

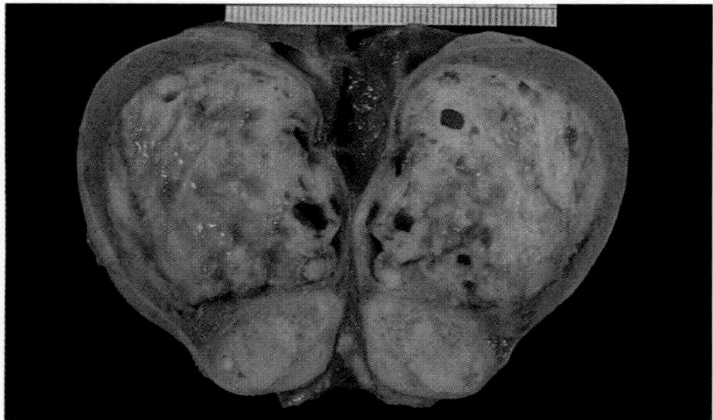

Figure 23–14 ■

Teratoma of testis. The variegated cut surface with cysts reflects the multiplicity of tissue found histologically.

In the child, differentiated mature teratomas may be expected to behave as benign tumors, and almost all these patients have a good prognosis. In the adult, it is difficult to be certain because, as pointed out, even apparently differentiated mature teratomas may harbor minute foci of cancer and should therefore be treated as malignant tumors.

Mixed Tumors

About 60% of testicular tumors are composed of more than one of the "pure" patterns. The most common mixture is that of teratoma, embryonal carcinoma, yolk sac tumor, and HCG-containing syncytiotrophoblast (Fig. 23–15). Tumors with such a combination constitute 14% of testicular germ cell tumors. Other combinations include seminoma with embryonal carcinoma and embryonal carcinoma with teratoma. The latter has been called *teratocarcinoma.* In most instances, the prognosis is worsened by the inclusion of more aggressive elements (e.g., the teratoma with a focus of choriocarcinoma has a poorer outlook than that of pure teratoma).

Clinical Features of Testicular Tumors. From a clinical standpoint, tumors of the testis are segregated into two broad categories: *seminoma* and *nonseminomatous* germ cell tumors (NSGCT). *NSGCT* is an umbrella designation that includes tumors of one histologic type such as embryonal cell carcinoma as well as those with more than one histologic pattern. As is evident from the later discussion, seminomas and NSGCT not only present with somewhat distinctive clinical features, but also they differ with respect to therapy and prognosis. First we offer some general comments on the clinical manifestations of testicular tumors as a group. Although *painless enlargement of the testis* is a characteristic feature of germ cell neoplasms, any testicular mass should be considered neoplastic unless proved otherwise. Many tumors present with swelling and diffuse testicular pain.[19] Clinical differentiation between various types of germ cell tumors, detailed subsequently, is at best imperfect because there are no specific clinical features to the testicular masses produced by tumors of different histologic types. Hence, biopsy is essential for diagnosis.

Testicular tumors have a characteristic mode of spread, the knowledge of which is helpful in treatment. Lymphatic spread is common to all forms of testicular tumors, and in general retroperitoneal para-aortic nodes are the first to be

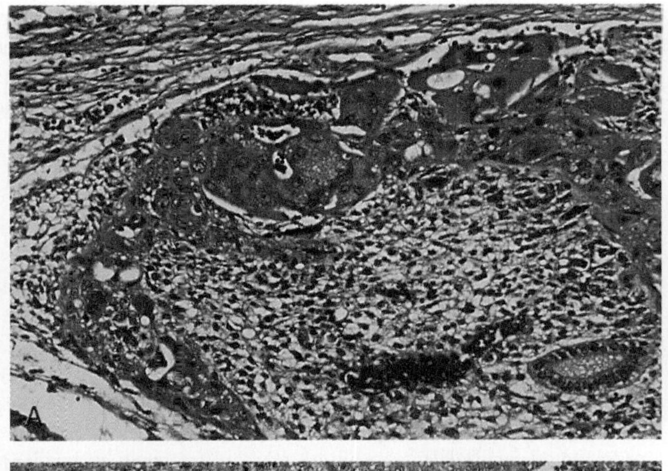

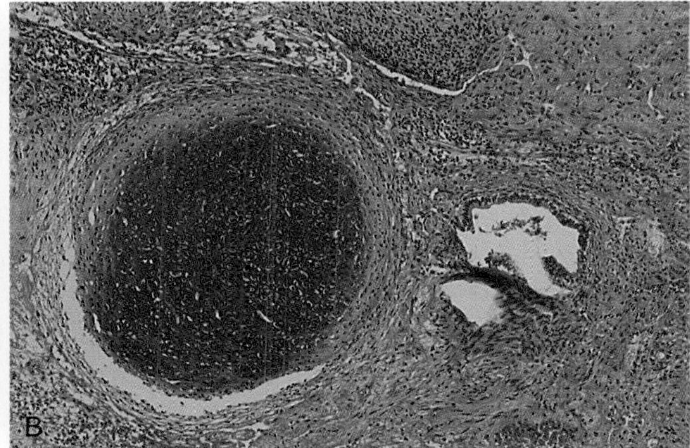

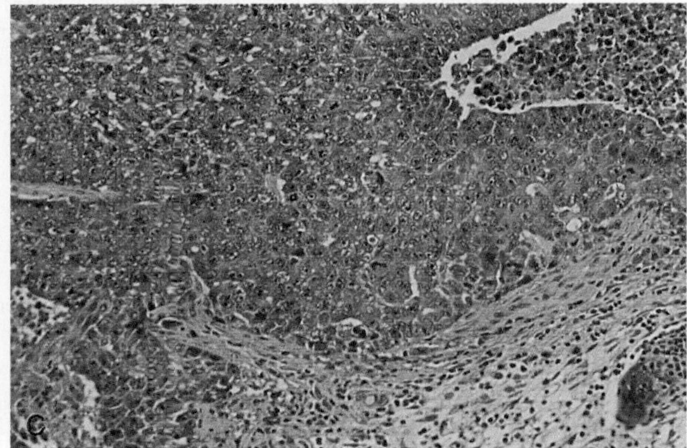

Figure 23–15

Mixed germ cell tumor. Three fields from the same tumor demonstrate a mixture of various cell types. *A*, An area with elements of choriocarcinoma: cytotrophoblasts (clear cells) surrounded by syncytiotrophoblast. *B*, Prominent collection of cartilage cells. *C*, Sheets of epithelial cells resembling liver cells. The areas *B* and *C* represent teratomatous elements. Other parts of the tumor revealed embryonal carcinoma and yolk sac tumor. (Courtesy of Dr. Kyle Molberg, Department of Pathology, University of Texas Southwestern Medical Center, Dallas, TX.)

involved. Subsequent spread may occur to mediastinal and supraclavicular nodes. Hematogenous spread is primarily to the lungs, but liver, brain, and bones may also be involved. Although most testicular tumors metastasize "true," the histology of metastases may sometimes be different from that of the testicular lesion. Thus, an embryonal carcinoma may present a teratomatous picture in the secondary deposits. Conversely, a teratoma may show foci of choriocarcinoma in the lymph nodes. As discussed earlier, because all these tumors are derived from totipotential germ cells, the apparent "forward" and "backward" differentiation seen in different locations is not entirely surprising.

With this background, we now highlight the differences between seminoma and NSGCT. Seminomas tend to remain localized to the testis for a long time, and hence approximately 70% present in clinical stage I (see later). In contrast, approximately 60% of patients with NSGCT present with advanced clinical disease (stages II and III). Metastases from seminomas typically involve lymph nodes. Hematogenous spread occurs later in the course of dissemination. NSGCT not only metastasize earlier, but also use the hematogenous route more frequently. The rare choriocarcinoma is the most aggressive of NSGCT. It may not cause any testicular enlargement but instead spreads predominantly and rapidly by the bloodstream. Therefore, lungs and liver are involved early in virtually every case. From a therapeutic viewpoint, seminomas are extremely radiosensitive, whereas NSGCT are relatively radioresistant. To summarize, as compared with seminomas, NSGCT are biologically more aggressive and in general have a poorer prognosis.

In the United States, three clinical stages of testicular tumors are defined:

- Stage I: Tumor confined to the testis, epididymis, or spermatic cord
- Stage II: Distant spread confined to retroperitoneal nodes below the diaphragm
- Stage III: Metastases outside the retroperitoneal nodes or above the diaphragm

Stages II and III are further subdivided ("early" or "advanced") on the basis of tumor burden in the secondary deposits.

Germ cell tumors of the testis often secrete polypeptide hormones and certain enzymes that can be detected in blood by sensitive assays. Such *biologic markers* include HCG, AFP, placental alkaline phosphatase, placental lactogen, and lactate dehydrogenase (LDH). HCG, AFP, and LDH are widely used clinically and have proved to be valuable in the diagnosis and management of testicular cancer.[22]

LDH is produced in many tissues, including skeletal and cardiac muscles, and hence elevations of this enzyme are not specific for testicular tumors. The degree of LDH elevation correlates with the mass of tumor cells, however, and the levels of this enzyme provide a tool to assess tumor burden.

AFP is the major serum protein of the early fetus and is synthesized by the fetal gut, liver cells, and yolk sac. One year after birth, the serum levels of AFP fall to less than 16 ng/ml, which is undetectable except by the most sensitive assays. HCG is a glycoprotein consisting of two dissimilar polypeptide units called α and β. It is normally synthesized and secreted by the placental syncytiotrophoblast. The β subunit of HCG has unique sequences not shared with other human glycoprotein hormones, and therefore the detection of HCG in the serum is based on a radioimmunoassay using antibodies to its β chain. As might be expected from the histogenesis and morphology, elevated levels of these markers are most often associated with nonseminomatous tumors. Yolk sac tumors produce AFP exclusively, and choriocarcinomas elaborate only HCG. Either or both of these markers are elevated in more than 80% of patients with NSGCT at the time of diagnosis. In passing, it might be noted that elevated serum levels of AFP are also encountered with liver cell carcinomas. In the context of testicular tumors, the value of serum markers is fourfold:

- In the evaluation of testicular masses
- In the staging of testicular germ cell tumors. For example, after orchiectomy, persistent elevation of HCG or AFP indicates stage II disease even if the lymph nodes appear of normal size by computed tomography scanning.
- In assessing tumor burden. The levels of LDH in particular are related to tumor mass and provide an independent prognostic marker in patients with these tumors.
- In monitoring the response to therapy. After eradication of tumors, there is a rapid fall in serum level of AFP and HCG. With serial measurements, it is often possible to predict recurrence before the patients become symptomatic or develop any other clinical signs of relapse.

As stated earlier, approximately 15% of seminomas have syncytiotrophoblast and an associated elevation of HCG levels. The prognosis of these tumors, however, is no different than those without HCG elevation.

The therapy and prognosis of testicular tumors depend largely on clinical stage and on the histologic type. Seminoma, which is extremely radiosensitive and tends to remain localized for long periods, has the best prognosis. More than 95% of patients with stage I and II disease can be cured. Among nonseminomatous tumors, the histologic subtype does not influence the prognosis significantly, and hence these are treated as a group. Although they do not share the excellent prognosis of seminoma, approximately 90% of patients with nonseminomatous tumors can achieve complete remission with aggressive chemotherapy, and most can be cured.

TUMORS OF SEX CORD–GONADAL STROMA

As indicated in Table 23–1, sex cord–gonadal stroma tumors are subclassified based on their presumed histogenesis and differentiation. The two most important members of this group—Leydig cell tumors (derived from the stroma) and Sertoli cell tumors (derived from the sex cord)—are described here. Details of these tumors and others not described may be found in a review.[23]

Leydig (Interstitial) Cell Tumors

Tumors of Leydig cells are particularly interesting because they may elaborate androgens or androgens and estrogens, and some have also elaborated corticosteroids. They arise at any age, although most of the reported cases have been noted between 20 and 60 years of age. As with other testicular tumors, the most common presenting feature is testicular swelling, but in some patients gynecomastia may be the first symptom. In children, hormonal effects, manifested primarily as sexual precocity, are the dominating features.

MORPHOLOGY. These neoplasms form circumscribed nodules, usually less than 5 cm in diameter. They have a distinctive golden brown, homogeneous cut surface. Histologically, tumorous Leydig cells usually are remarkably similar to their normal forebears in that they are large and round or polygonal, and they have an abundant granular eosinophilic cytoplasm with a round central nucleus. Cell boundaries are often indistinct. The cytoplasm frequently contains lipid granules, vacuoles, or lipofuscin pigment, but, most characteristically, rod-shaped crystalloids of Reinke occur in about 25% of the tumors. Approximately 10% of the tumors in adults are invasive and produce metastases; most are benign.

Sertoli Cell Tumors (Androblastoma)

These tumors may be composed entirely of Sertoli cells or may have a component of granulosa cells. Some induce endocrinologic changes. Either estrogens or androgens may be elaborated but only infrequently in sufficient quantity to cause precocious masculinization or feminization. Occasionally, as with Leydig cell tumors, gynecomastia appears.

MORPHOLOGY. These neoplasms appear as firm, small nodules with a homogeneous gray-white to yellow cut surface. Histologically the tumor cells are arranged in distinctive trabeculae with a tendency to form cordlike structures resembling immature seminiferous tubules. Most Sertoli cell tumors are benign, but occasional tumors (approximately 10%) are more anaplastic and pursue a malignant course.

TESTICULAR LYMPHOMA

Although not primarily a tumor of the testis, testicular lymphoma is included here because affected patients present with only a testicular mass. *Lymphomas account for 5% of testicular neoplasms and constitute the most common form of testicular cancer in men over the age of 60.* In most cases, disseminated disease is already present at the time of detection of the testicular mass; only rarely does it remain confined to the testis. The histologic type in almost all cases is the diffuse large cell lymphoma (see non-Hodgkin lymphomas, Chapter 15). The prognosis is extremely poor.

Miscellaneous Lesions of Tunica Vaginalis

Brief mention should be made of the tunica vaginalis. As a serosa-lined sac immediately proximal to the testis and epididymis, it may become involved by any lesion arising in these two structures. Clear serous fluid may accumulate from neighboring infections or tumors, often spontaneously and without apparent cause (*hydrocele*). Considerable enlargement of the scrotal sac is produced, which can be readily mistaken for testicular enlargement. By transillumination, however, it is usually possible to define the clear, translucent character of the contained substance, and many times the opaque testis can be outlined within this fluid-filled space.

Hematocele indicates the presence of blood in the tunica vaginalis. It is an uncommon condition usually encountered only when there has been either direct trauma to the testis or torsion of the testis with hemorrhagic suffusion into the surrounding tunica vaginalis or in hemorrhagic diseases associated with widespread bleeding diatheses.

Chylocele refers to the accumulation of lymph in the tunica and is almost always found in patients with elephantiasis who have widespread, severe lymphatic obstruction. For clarity's sake, mention should be made of the *spermatocele* and *varicocele*, which refer respectively to a small cystic accumulation of semen (spermatocele) or to a dilated vein in the spermatic cord (varicocele).

PROSTATE

In the normal adult, the prostate weighs approximately 20 gm. The prostate is a retroperitoneal organ encircling the neck of the bladder and urethra and is devoid of a distinct capsule. Classically, the prostate has been divided into five lobes, to which are attributed distinctive significance in the development of tumors and benign enlargements. These five lobes include a posterior, middle, and anterior lobe and two lateral lobes. These subdivisions, however, can be recognized only in the embryo. In the adult, prostatic parenchyma can be divided into four biologically and anatomically distinct zones or regions: the peripheral, central, transitional, and periuretheral zones (Fig. 23–16). The types of proliferative lesions are different in each region. For example, most hyperplasias arise in the transitional and periuretheral zones, whereas most carcinomas originate in the peripheral zone.

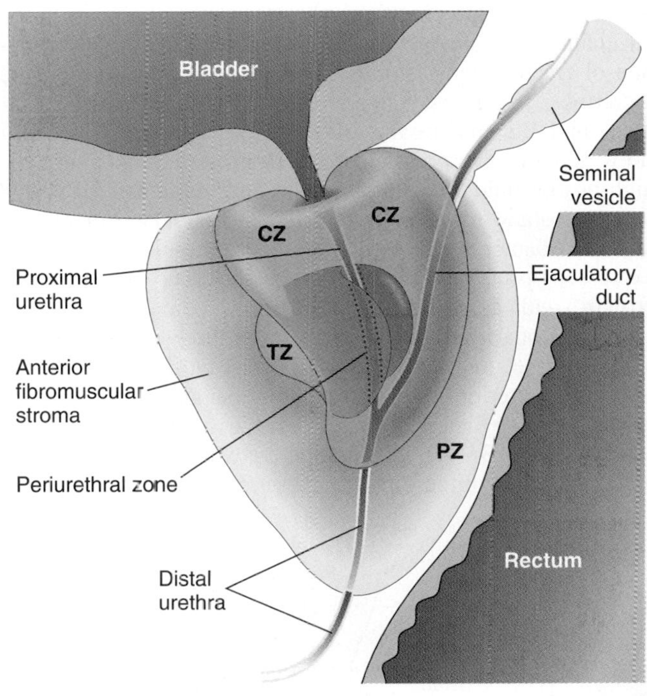

Figure 23–16

Adult prostate. The normal prostate contains several distinct regions, including a central zone (CZ), a peripheral zone (PZ), a transitional zone (TZ), and a periurethral zone. Most carcinomas arise from the peripheral glands of the organ and are often palpable during digital examination of the rectum. Nodular hyperplasia, in contrast, arises from more centrally situated glands and is more likely to produce urinary obstruction early on than is carcinoma.

Histologically, the prostate is a compound tubuloalveolar gland, which, in one plane of section, presents small to fairly large glandular spaces lined by epithelium. Characteristically, the glands are lined by two layers of cells: a basal layer of low cuboidal epithelium covered by a layer of columnar mucus-secreting cells. In many areas, there are small villous projections or papillary inbuddings of the epithelium. These glands all have a distinct basement membrane and are separated by an abundant fibromuscular stroma. Testicular androgens are clearly of prime importance in controlling prostatic growth because castration leads to atrophy of the prostate.

Only three pathologic processes affect the prostate gland with sufficient frequency to merit discussion: inflammation, benign nodular enlargement, and tumors. Of these three, the benign nodular enlargements are by far the most common and occur so often in advanced age that they can almost be construed as a "normal" aging process. Prostatic carcinoma is also an extremely common lesion in men and therefore merits careful consideration. The inflammatory processes are, for the most part, of less clinical significance and can be treated briefly.

Inflammations

Prostatitis may be divided into three categories: *acute* and *chronic bacterial prostatitis* and *chronic abacterial prostatitis.*[24] Differentiation among these entities is based on quantitative bacterial cultures and microscopic examination of fractionated urine specimens and expressed prostatic secretions. If the first voided 10 ml of urine (urethral specimen) and the midstream urine (bladder specimen) do not show pyuria, the presence of 10 or more leukocytes per high-power field in prostatic secretions obtained by transrectal prostatic massage is considered diagnostic of prostatitis.[25] In bacterial prostatitis (acute or chronic), cultures of expressed prostatic secretions are positive for bacterial growth, and the quantitative bacterial counts are significantly (1 logarithm) higher than in cultures of urethral and bladder urine. In chronic abacterial prostatitis, however, the prostatic secretions are consistently negative for bacterial growth despite unambiguous evidence of prostatic inflammation (Fig. 23–17). Distinction between the three forms of prostatitis is important because treatment differs. In the ensuing discussion, the three conditions are characterized first, then the morphologic features of all the forms are described together.

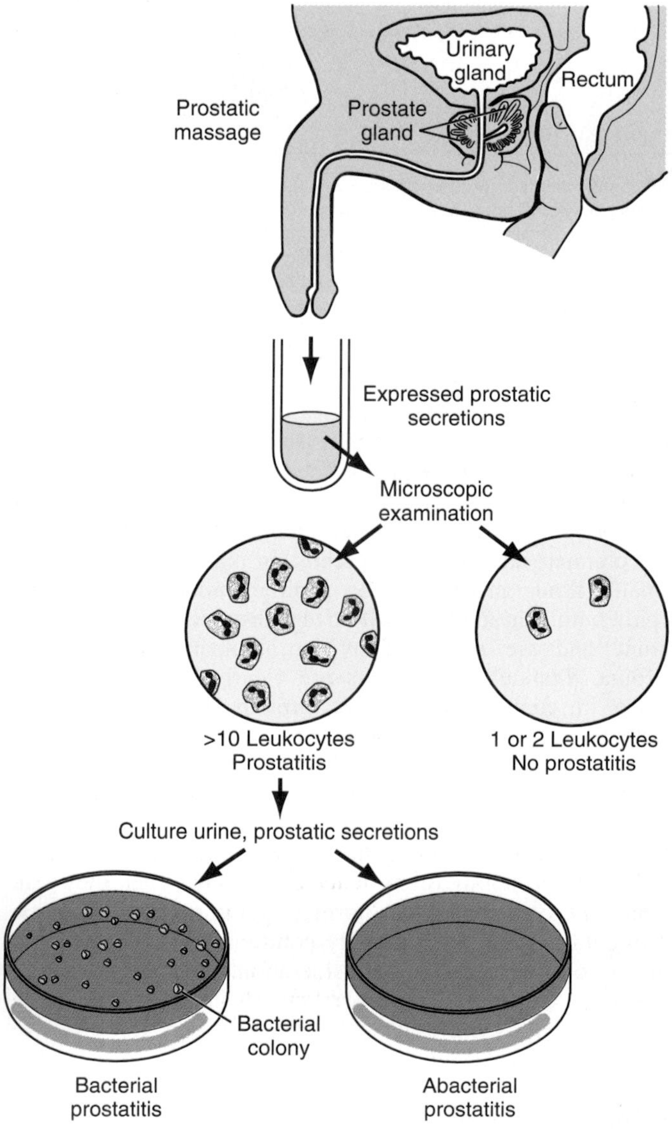

Acute bacterial prostatitis consists of an acute focal or diffuse suppurative inflammation in the prostatic substance. The bacteria responsible are similar in type and in incidence to those that cause urinary tract infections. Thus, most cases are caused by various strains of *E. coli*, other gram-negative rods, enterococci, and staphylococci. The organisms become implanted in the prostate usually by intraprostatic reflux of urine from the posterior urethra or from the urinary bladder, but occasionally they seed the prostate by the lymphohematogenous routes from distant foci of infection. Prostatitis sometimes follows some surgical manipulation on the urethra or prostate gland itself, such as catheterization, cystoscopy, urethral dilation, or resection procedures on the prostate. Clinically, acute bacterial prostatitis is associated with fever, chills, and dysuria. On rectal examination, the prostate is exquisitely tender and boggy. The diagnosis can be established by urine culture and clinical features.

Chronic bacterial prostatitis is difficult to diagnose and treat. It may present with low back pain, dysuria, and perineal and suprapubic discomfort. Alternatively, it may be virtually asymptomatic. *A common historical characteristic is recurrent urinary tract infections (cystitis, urethritis) caused by the same organism.* Because most antibiotics penetrate the prostate poorly, bacteria find safe haven in the parenchyma and constantly seed the urinary tract. Diagnosis of chronic bacterial prostatitis depends on the documentation of leukocytosis in the expressed prostatic secretions along with positive bacterial cultures in the prostatic secretions. In most cases, there is no antecedent acute attack, and the disease appears insidiously and without obvious provocation. The implicated organisms are the same as those cited as causes of acute prostatitis.

Chronic abacterial prostatitis is the most common form of prostatitis seen today. *Clinically, it is indistinguishable from chronic bacterial prostatitis. There is no history, however, of recurrent urinary tract infection.* Expressed prostatic secretions contain more than 10 leukocytes per high-power field, but bacterial cultures are uniformly negative. Because the affected patients are usually sexually active men, several sexually transmitted pathogens have been implicated. *C. trachomatis, Ureaplasma urealyticum*, and *Mycoplasma hominis* remain on trial as offending agents, but firm evidence is lacking.[25]

Figure 23–17

Prostatitis, bacterial and abacterial.

MORPHOLOGY. Acute prostatitis may appear as minute, disseminated abscesses; as large, coalescent focal areas of necrosis; or as a diffuse edema, congestion, and boggy suppuration of the entire gland. When these reactions are fairly diffuse, they cause an overall soft, spongy enlargement of the gland.

Histologically, depending on the duration and severity of the inflammation, there may be minimal stromal leukocytic infiltrate accompanied by increased elaboration of prostatic secretion or leukocytic infiltration within gland spaces. When abscess formation has occurred, focal or large areas of the prostatic substance may become necrotic. Such inflammatory reactions may totally subside and leave behind only some fibrous scarring and calcification. Alternatively, they may become chronic, particularly when the excretory ducts are plugged and the infection continues to smolder within walled-off minute abscesses in the prostatic substance.

Chronic prostatitis, both bacterial and abacterial, when correctly diagnosed, should be restricted to those cases of inflammatory reaction in the prostate characterized by the aggregation of numerous lymphocytes, plasma cells, and macrophages as well as neutrophils within the prostatic substance. It should be pointed out that, in the normal aging process, aggregations of lymphocytes are prone to appear in the fibromuscular stroma of this gland. All too often, such nonspecific aggregates are diagnosed as chronic prostatitis, even though the pathognomonic inflammatory cells, the macrophages and neutrophils, are not present.

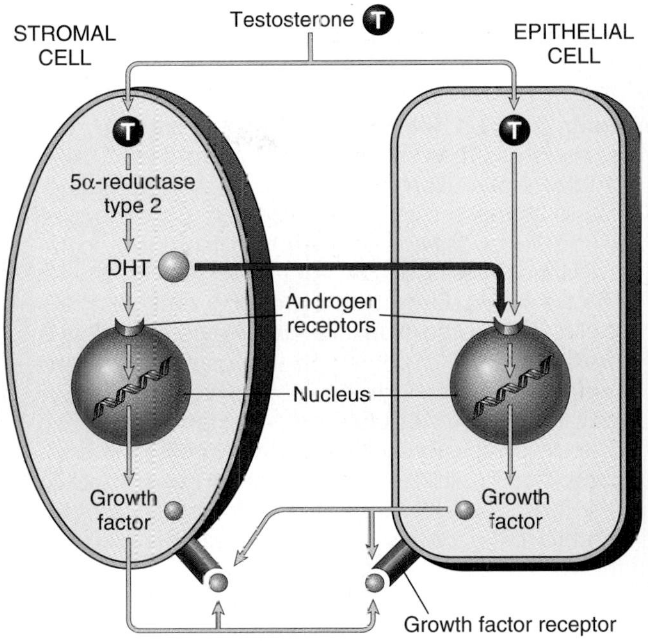

Figure 23–18

Simplified scheme of the pathogenesis of prostatic hyperplasia. The central role of the stromal cells in generating dihydrotestosterone should be noted.

Benign Enlargement

NODULAR HYPERPLASIA (BENIGN PROSTATIC HYPERTROPHY OR HYPERPLASIA)

Nodular hyperplasia, still referred to by the redundant term *benign prostatic hyperplasia* (all hyperplasias are benign), is an extremely common disorder in men over age 50. It is characterized by hyperplasia of prostatic stromal and epithelial cells, resulting in the formation of large, fairly discrete nodules in the periurethral region of the prostate. When sufficiently large, the nodules compress and narrow the urethral canal to cause partial, or sometimes virtually complete, obstruction of the urethra.[26]

Incidence. Histologic evidence of nodular hyperplasia can be seen in approximately 20% of men 40 years of age, a figure that increases to 70% by age 60 and to 90% by age 70.[27] There is no direct correlation, however, between histologic changes and clinical symptoms. Only 50% of those who have microscopic evidence of nodular hyperplasia have clinically detectable enlargement of the prostate, and of these individuals, only 50% develop clinical symptoms. Nodular hyperplasia of prostate is a problem of enormous magnitude. More than 400,000 transurethral resections of the prostate are performed every year in the United States. In men older than 65 years of age, this surgical procedure is second only to cataract extraction.

Etiology and Pathogenesis. Much has been learned about the origins of prostatic hyperplasia. There is little doubt that this form of prostatic enlargement is related to the action of androgens (Fig. 23–18).[28] Dihydrotestosterone (DHT), a metabolite of testosterone, is the ultimate mediator of prostatic growth. It is synthesized in the prostate from circulating testosterone by the action of the enzyme 5α-reductase, type 2. This enzyme is localized principally in the stromal cells, and hence these cells are the main site for the synthesis of DHT. Once synthesized, DHT can act in an autocrine fashion on the stromal cells or in paracrine fashion by diffusing into nearby epithelial cells. In both of these cell types, DHT binds to nuclear androgen receptors and signals the transcription of growth factors that are mitogenic to the epithelial and stromal cells. Although testosterone can also bind to the androgen receptors and cause growth stimulation, DHT is ten times more potent because it dissociates from the androgen receptor more slowly.

The importance of DHT in causing nodular hyperplasia is supported by clinical observations in which an inhibitor of 5α-reductase was given to men with this condition. Therapy with 5α-reductase inhibitor markedly reduces the DHT content of the prostate, and in a proportion of cases, there is a decrease in prostatic volume and urinary obstruction.[29] The fact that all patients do not benefit from androgen-depriving therapy suggests that prostatic hyperplasia may be etiologically heterogeneous, and in some cases, factors other than androgens may be more important. There is some experimental evidence that DHT-mediated prostatic hyperplasia is aided and abetted by estrogens. In castrated young dogs, prostatic hyperplasia can be induced by administration of androgens, an effect markedly enhanced by simultaneous administration of 17β-estradiol. In aging men, estradiol levels increase, and it is believed that estrogens induce an increase in androgen receptors, thus rendering cells more susceptible to the action of DHT.

MORPHOLOGY. In the usual case of prostatic enlargement, the nodules weigh between 60 and 100 gm. Not uncommonly, however, aggregate weights of up to 200 gm are encountered, and even larger masses have been recorded. Careful studies have demonstrated that nodular hyperplasia of the prostate originates almost exclusively in the inner aspect of the prostate gland, in the transitional and periurethral zones (see Fig. 23–16). The first nodules, composed almost entirely of epithelial cells, arise from the transitional zone; later, predominantly stromal nodules arise in the periurethral zone.[30] From their origin in this strategic location, the nodular enlargements may encroach on the lateral walls of the urethra to compress it to a slitlike orifice. In some cases, nodular enlargement may project up into the floor of the urethra as a hemispheric mass directly beneath the mucosa of the urethra.

On cross-section of the affected prostate, the nodules usually are fairly readily identified (Fig. 23–19). They vary in color and consistency. In nodules with primarily glandular proliferation, the tissue is yellow-pink with a soft consistency, and a milky white prostatic fluid oozes out of these areas. In those primarily due to fibromuscular involvement, each nodule is pale gray, is tough, does not exude fluid, and is less clearly demarcated from the surrounding prostatic capsule. Although the nodules do not have true capsules, the compressed surrounding prostatic tissue creates a plane of cleavage about them, used by the surgeon in the enucleation of prostatic masses in so-called suprapubic prostatectomies.

Microscopically the nodularity may be due to glandular proliferation or dilation or to fibrous or muscular proliferation of the stroma. Although all three elements are involved in almost every case, the stromal (fibroblastic) component predominates in most cases. Glandular proliferation takes the form of aggregations of small to large to cystically dilated glands, lined by two layers, an inner columnar and an outer cuboidal or flattened epithelium, based on an intact basement membrane (Fig. 23–20). The epithelium is characteristically thrown up into numerous papillary buds and infoldings, which are more prominent than in the normal prostate. Two other histologic changes are frequently found: (1) foci of squamous metaplasia and (2) small areas of infarction. The former tend to occur in the margins of the foci of infarction as nests of metaplastic, but orderly, squamous cells.

Clinical Course. Symptoms of nodular hyperplasia, when present, relate to two secondary effects: (1) compression of the urethra with difficulty in urination and (2) retention of urine in the bladder with subsequent distention and hypertrophy of the bladder, infection of the urine, and development of cystitis and renal infections. Patients experience frequency, nocturia, difficulty in starting and stopping the stream of urine, overflow dribbling, and dysuria (painful micturition). In many cases, sudden, acute urinary retention appears for unknown reasons and persists until the patient receives emergency catheterization. In addition to these difficulties in urination, prostatic enlargement results in the inability to empty the bladder completely. Presumably, this inability is due to the raised level of the urethral floor so that, at the conclusion of micturition, a considerable amount of residual urine is left. This residual urine provides a static fluid that is vulnerable to infection. On this basis, catheterization or surgical manipulation provides a real danger of the introduction of organisms and the development of pyelonephritis.

Many secondary changes occur in the bladder, such as hypertrophy, trabeculation, and diverticulum formation (Chapter 22). Hydronephrosis or acute retention, with sec-

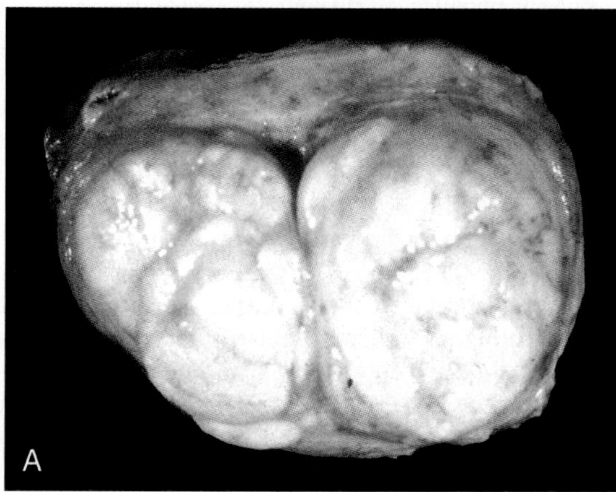

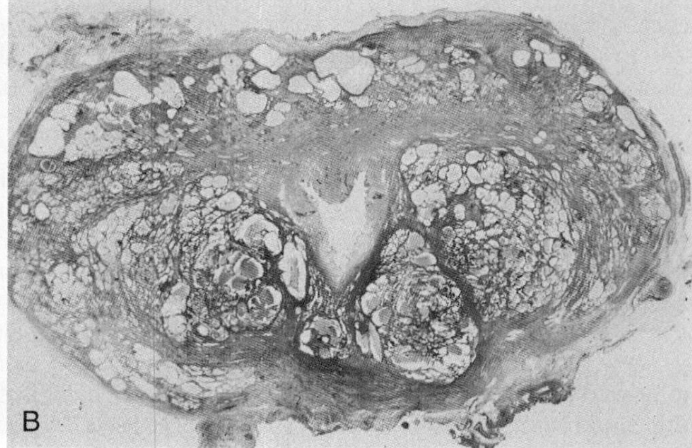

Figure 23–19

Nodular prostatic hyperplasia. *A*, Well-defined nodules bulge from the cut surface. The proximity of the nodules to the urethra accounts for the urinary obstruction associated with the lesion. *B*, A microscopic view of a whole mount of the prostate shows nodules of hyperplastic glands on both sides of the urethra. (*B* courtesy of Dr. Kyle Molberg, Department of Pathology, University of Texas Southwestern Medical Center, Dallas, TX.)

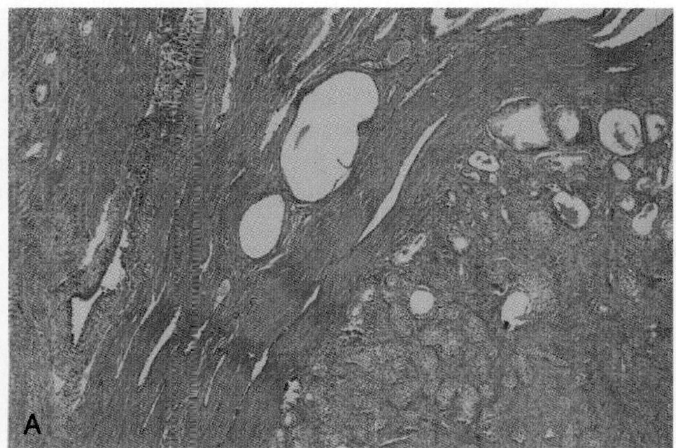

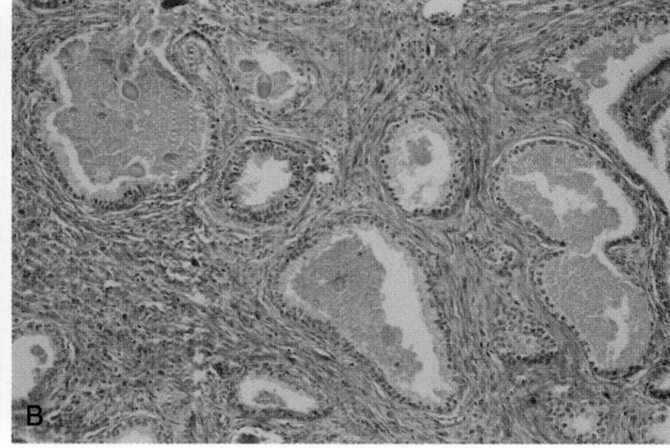

Figure 23–20

Nodular hyperplasia of prostate. *A*, A low-power view shows proliferation of glands, some cystically dilated within a well-defined nodule. *B*, A high-power view shows hyperplastic glands with two layers of cells: an inner columnar and an outer cuboidal or flattened. (Courtesy of Dr. Trace Worrell, Department of Pathology, University of Texas Southwestern Medical Center, Dallas, TX.)

ondary urinary tract infection and even azotemia or uremia, may develop. Finally, it should be noted that despite earlier claims that nodular hyperplasia predisposes to cancer of the prostate, most studies deny any association, and hence nodular hyperplasia is not considered to be a premalignant lesion.

Tumors

CARCINOMA

Carcinoma of the prostate is the most common form of cancer in men (followed closely by lung cancer) and the second leading cause of cancer death. It is estimated that more than 300,000 new cases are detected every year, of which approximately 41,000 prove to be lethal.[31] In addition to these lethal neoplasms, there is an even more frequent anatomic form of prostatic cancer in which a microscopic focus of cancer is discovered as an incidental finding, either at postmortem examination or in a surgical specimen removed for other reasons (e.g., nodular hyperplasia). Approximately 90% of these lesions do not cause trouble in the lifetime of the host; but which ones are the "bad apples"?[32]

Incidence. Cancer of the prostate is a disease of men over age 50. Only 1% of prostate cancers are diagnosed before 50 years of age. The age-adjusted incidence in the United States is 69 per 100,000.[33] The incidence of latent prostatic cancer is even higher. It increases from 20% in men in their fifties to approximately 70% in men between the ages of 70 and 80 years. There are some remarkable and puzzling national and racial differences in the incidence of this disease. Prostatic cancer is extremely rare in Asians. The age-adjusted incidence (per 100,000) among Japanese is in the range of 3 to 4 and for the Chinese in Hong Kong only 1, as compared with a rate of 50 to 60 among whites in the United States. The disease is even more prevalent among blacks, who have the highest rate among 24 countries having reasonably accurate mortality data.[34] Despite the greater than tenfold differences in the incidence of clinically evident cancers, the age-adjusted incidence of the so-called latent or histologic form of prostate cancer is virtually identical in Japanese and US white populations. Assuming that prostate cancer, similar to other cancers, arises from accumulation of multiple genetic events, these observations indicate that whereas the initial molecular events that give rise to latent cancers occur at the same rate in Japanese and American men, the probability of acquiring additional mutations, presumably environmentally induced, is lower in Japanese men. This notion is supported by the fact that in Japanese immigrants to the United States the incidence of the disease seems to have risen, but not nearly to the level of that of native-born Americans.

Etiology. Little is known about the causes of prostatic cancer. Several risk factors, such as age, race, family history, hormone levels, and environmental influences, are suspected of playing roles. The association of this form of cancer with advancing age and the enigmatic differences among races have already been mentioned. The tendency for the incidence of this disease to rise among those enjoying a low-incidence rate when they migrate to a high-incidence locale is consistent with a role for environmental influences. There are many candidate environmental factors, but none has been proven to be causative. For example, increased consumption of fats has been implicated. It has been proposed that dietary fat intake influences the levels of hormones such as testosterone, which, in turn, affect the growth of prostate. Other dietary factors, such as intake of vitamin A and beta-carotene, are also under scrutiny.[35]

As with nodular hyperplasia of prostate, androgens are believed to play a role in the pathogenesis of prostate cancer. Support for this general thesis lies in the inhibition of these tumors that can be achieved with orchiectomy. Neoplastic epithelial cells, similar to their normal counterparts, possess androgen receptors, which suggests that they

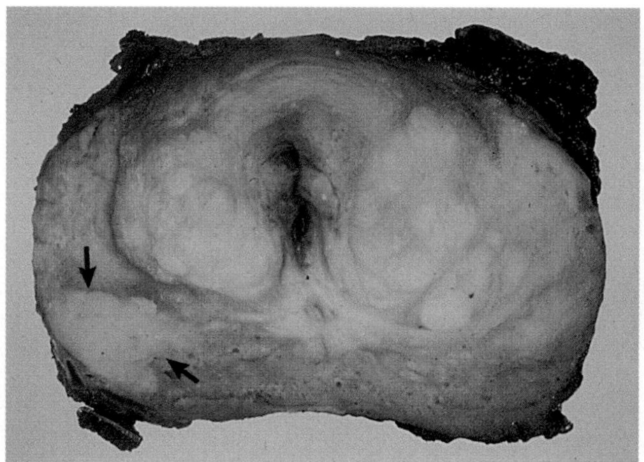

Figure 23–21

Nodular hyperplasia and carcinoma of the prostate. Carcinomatous tissue is seen on the posterior aspect (*arrows*). Compare the location of the cancer with that of the hyperplastic prostate on either side of the urethra. (Courtesy of Dr. Kyle Molberg, Department of Pathology, University of Texas Southwestern Medical Center, Dallas, TX.)

are responsive to these hormones. No significant or consistent alterations in the levels or metabolism of testosterone, however, have been disclosed in any studies. It seems more likely, therefore, that the role of hormones in this malignancy is essentially permissive because androgens are required for the maintenance of the prostatic epithelium.

Much interest has focused on the genetics and molecular pathogenesis of prostate cancer. In approximately 10% of white American men, the development of prostate cancer has been linked to germ line inheritance of prostate cancer susceptibility genes. In one third of these familial cases, a susceptibility gene has been mapped to chromosome 1q24-25.[36] The identification of the relevant gene at this locus is in progress. In addition, putative cancer-suppressor genes that are lost early in prostate carcinogenesis have been localized to chromosomes 8p, 10q, 12p, and 16q.[37] At some of these locations, putative cancer-suppressor genes have been mapped (e.g., E-cadherin at 16q22), but in most instances the identity of the relevant genes is unknown. The role of E-cadherin in tumorigenesis is discussed in Chapter 8.

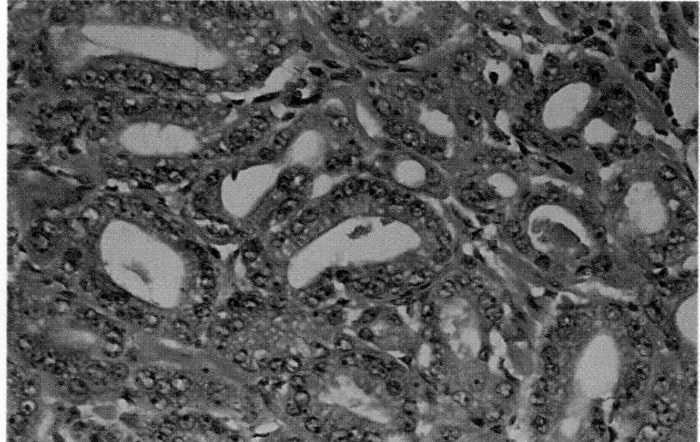

Figure 23–22

Photomicrograph of well-differentiated adenocarcinoma of the prostate demonstrating crowded, "back-to-back" glands lined by a single layer of cuboidal cells. Glandular differentiation is much less obvious in some higher-grade lesions. (Courtesy of Dr. Kyle Molberg, Department of Pathology, University of Texas Southwestern Medical Center, Dallas, TX.)

Morphology. In approximately 70% of cases, carcinoma of the prostate arises in the peripheral zone of the gland, classically in a posterior location, often rendering it palpable on rectal examination (Fig. 23–21). Characteristically, on cross-section of the prostate, **the neoplastic tissue is gritty and firm, but when embedded within the prostatic substance, it may be extremely difficult to visualize and be more readily apparent on palpation.** Spread of prostate cancer occurs by direct local invasion and through the bloodstream and lymph. Local extension most commonly involves the seminal vesicles and the base of the urinary bladder, which may result in ureteral obstruction. Hematogenous spread occurs chiefly to the bones, particularly the axial skeleton, but some lesions spread widely to viscera. Massive visceral dissemination is an exception rather than the rule. The bony metastases may be osteolytic, but osteoblastic lesions are frequent and in men point strongly to prostatic cancer. The bones commonly involved, in descending order of frequency, are lumbar spine, proximal femur, pelvis, thoracic spine, and ribs. Lymphatic spread occurs initially to the obturator nodes followed by perivesical, hypogastric, iliac, presacral, and para-aortic nodes. Lymph node spread occurs frequently and often precedes spread to the bones. As we discuss later, metastases to the lymph nodes in apparently localized prostatic cancer have a significant impact on the prognosis.

Histologically, most lesions are adenocarcinomas that produce well-defined, readily demonstrable gland patterns.[38] The glands are lined by a single uniform layer of cuboidal or low columnar epithelium. The outer basal layer of cells typical of normal and hyperplastic glands is often absent. Occasionally the glands are somewhat larger, with a papillary or cribriform pattern. The cytoplasm of the tumor cells is unremarkable, but the nuclei are large and vacuolated and contain one or more large nucleoli. There is some variation in nuclear size and shape, but in general pleomorphism is not marked. Mitotic figures are extremely uncommon. When such well-differentiated tumors occur in sharply delimited rounded masses, they have to be distinguished from nodular hyperplasia. In general, malignant acini are smaller and closely spaced, "back-to-back" with little intervening stroma and are lined by a single layer of cells (Fig. 23–22). Not all prostatic can-

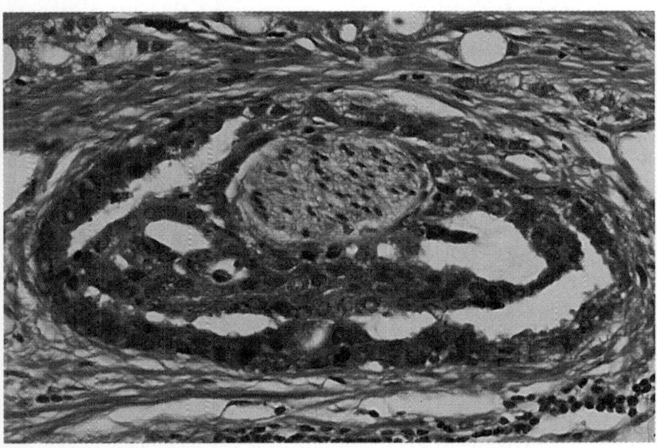

Figure 23–23

Carcinoma of prostate showing perineurial invasion by malignant glands. (Courtesy of Dr. Kyle Molberg, Department of Pathology, University of Texas Southwestern Medical Center, Dallas, TX.)

cers, however, are well differentiated. In less differentiated lesions, the tumor cells tend to grow in cords, nests, or sheets. Stromal production may be scant or quite extensive in certain lesions, producing a scirrhous-like consistency to the neoplasm.

The most reliable hallmarks of malignancy, especially in well-differentiated tumors, are clear evidence of invasion of the capsule with its lymphatic and vascular channels, perineurial invasion, or both (Fig. 23–23). The perineurial spaces, which are involved in most cases, are not lined by endothelium, and they do not represent lymphatics, as formerly believed.

In approximately 80% of cases, prostatic tissue removed for carcinoma also harbors presumptive precursor lesions, referred to as duct-acinar dysplasia, or simply **prostatic intraepithelial neoplasia (PIN)**.[39] These lesions consist of multiple, although sometimes single, foci of glands with intra-acinar proliferation of cells that demonstrate nuclear anaplasia. In contrast to frank cancer, however, there is no invasion, and the dysplastic cells are surrounded by a layer of basal cells and an intact basement membrane. Studies have revealed that many of the molecular changes seen in invasive cancers are also present in PIN. These include aneuploidy as well as loss of heterozygosity at several loci. At certain loci (e.g., 8p12), there is loss of heterozygosity in 64% of foci of PIN and 91% of cancers, compared with 0% in benign tissues. Such data strongly support the argument that PIN is an intermediate lesion between normal and frankly malignant tissue.[37] In keeping with this notion, follow-up studies reveal that in about one third of cases, PIN progresses to invasive cancer within a period of 10 years, presumably after additional genetic changes have accumulated.

Grading and Staging. Carcinomas of the prostate, similar to most other forms of cancer, are graded and staged. Several grading systems have been described, of which the Gleason system is the best known.[38,40] According to the Gleason system, prostate cancers are stratified into five grades on the basis of glandular patterns and degree of differentiation as seen under low magnification. Grade 1 represents the most well differentiated tumors, in which the neoplastic glands are uniform and round in appearance and are packed into well-circumscribed nodules. By contrast, grade 5 tumors show no glandular differentiation, and the tumor cells infiltrate the stroma in the form of cords, sheets, and nests. The other grades fall in between. Because most tumors contain more than one pattern, it is usual to assign a primary grade to the dominant pattern and a secondary grade to the subdominant pattern. The two numerical grades are then added to obtain a combined Gleason grade or score. Thus, for example, a tumor with a dominant grade 3 and a secondary grade 4 would achieve a Gleason score of 7. Tumors with only one pattern are treated as if their primary and secondary grades are the same, and, hence, the number is doubled. Thus, under this schema the most well differentiated tumors have a Gleason score of 2 (1 + 1) and the least-differentiated tumors merit a score of 10 (5 + 5). *Grading is of particular importance in prostatic cancer because there is in general fairly good correlation between the prognosis and the degree of differentiation.*

Staging of prostatic cancer is also important in the selection of the appropriate form of therapy and in establishing a prognosis. A staging system that is widely used in the United States is depicted in Figure 23–24.

Clinical Course. As discussed earlier, the incidence of stage A cancers increases with age and approaches 70% or more in men past the age of 80 years. These microscopic cancers are asymptomatic and are discovered incidentally at autopsy or in tissue removed for nodular hyperplasia of the prostate. The long-term significance of these lesions is still not entirely clear. It is generally accepted that most patients with stage A1 cancer do not show evidence of progressive disease when followed for 10 or more years. Five per cent to 25% of patients, however, do develop local or distant spread. This is more likely in younger patients (<60 years), who have a longer life expectancy. For patients in this age group, some authorities recommend careful follow-up studies so that if progression occurs, the cancer may be detected early, at a stage amenable to surgical cure.[41] Stage A2 lesions are more ominous. Approximately 30 to 50% can be expected to progress over a period of 5 years, with a mortality of 20% if left untreated.

Approximately 60% of patients with prostate cancer present with clinically localized disease (i.e., stage A or B). One third of these have micrometastases, and hence they truly belong to stage D. These patients do not have urinary symptoms, and the lesion is discovered by the finding of a suspicious nodule on rectal examination or elevated serum prostate-specific antigen level (discussed later). Most prostatic cancers arise in a subcapsular location removed from the urethra, and therefore urinary symptoms occur late. Most of the localized lesions are destined to progress unless eradicated by surgery or radiation.

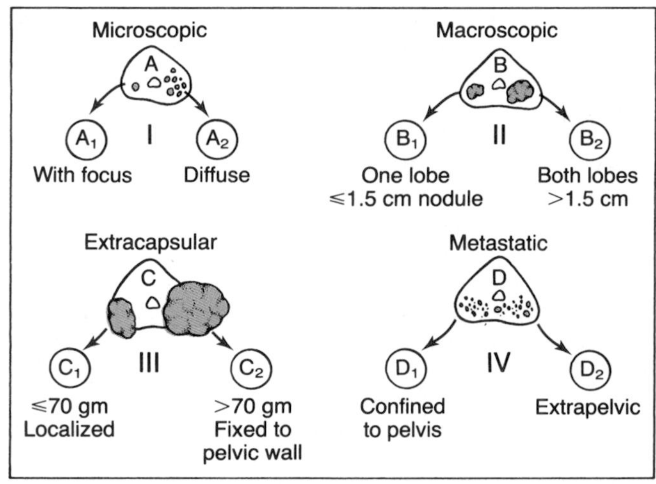

Figure 23–24

Staging of prostate cancer. Stage A: microscopic, not clinically palpable tumor (A_1, with focus in less than 5% of tissue examined, low grade; A_2, with multiple areas [more than 5%] or Gleason grade higher than 4). Stage B: palpable, macroscopic tumor (B_1, ≤1.5 cm in diameter, in only one lobe; B_2, >1.5 cm in diameter, or several nodules in both lobes). Stage C: tumor with extracapsular extension but still clinically localized (C_1, palpably extending into the seminal vesicle but not fixed to the pelvic wall; C_2, fixed to the pelvic wall). Stage D: demonstrated metastatic tumor (D_1, metastases limited to three pelvic nodes or fewer; D_2, more extensive nodal or extrapelvic metastases, e.g., to bone). The tumor, node, and metastasis (TNM) staging for local tumors is indicated by Roman numerals I to IV. (Redrawn from Gittes RF: Carcinoma of the prostate. N Engl J Med 324:240, 1991. Copyright © 1991 Massachusetts Medical Society. All rights reserved.)

With combined clinical and pathologic staging, more than 50% of patients with prostatic cancer present with stage C or D cancer. They come to clinical attention usually because of urinary symptoms, such as difficulty in starting or stopping the stream, dysuria, frequency, or hematuria. Pain is a late finding, reflecting involvement of capsular perineurial spaces. Some patients in stage D come to attention because of back pain caused by vertebral metastases. *The finding of osteoblastic metastases in bone is virtually diagnostic of this form of cancer in men* (Fig. 23–25). The outlook for these patients is poor.

Careful digital rectal examination is a useful, direct method for detection of early prostatic carcinoma because the posterior location of most tumors renders them easily palpable. Transrectal ultrasonography is an important adjunct for early detection as well as assessment of local spread. A transperineal or transrectal *biopsy is required to confirm the diagnosis.* Several procedures are used to determine the extent of disease. The involvement of lymph nodes may be detected by computed tomography scans or magnetic resonance imaging. Because microscopic metastases may be missed by either of these two procedures, many centers use pelvic lymphadenectomy as a staging procedure. If pelvic lymph nodes are involved, curative surgery (radical prostatectomy) is not warranted. Osseous metastases may be detected by skeletal surveys or the much more sensitive radionuclide bone scanning.

Two biochemical markers, prostatic acid phosphatase and prostate-specific antigen (PSA), have been used in the diagnosis and management of prostate cancer. Both are produced by normal as well as neoplastic prostatic epithelium. PSA has largely supplanted prostatic acid phosphatase in the management of prostate cancer.[42] PSA is a product of prostatic epithelium and is normally secreted in the semen. It is a serine protease whose function is to cleave and liquefy the seminal coagulum formed after ejaculation. In normal men, only minute amounts of PSA circulate in the serum. Elevated blood levels of PSA occur in association with localized as well as advanced cancer. In most laboratories, a serum level of 4 ng/ml is used as a cut-off point between normal and abnormal. *PSA is organ specific, however, and not cancer specific.* Thus, elevations in PSA levels occur not only in cancer, but also in non-neoplastic conditions, such as nodular hyperplasia of the prostate and prostatitis. Although serum levels of PSA are elevated to a lesser extent in benign nodular hyperplasia, there is considerable overlap. For instance, 25 to 30% of men with nodular hyperplasia and 80% with histologically documented cancer have serum PSA levels greater than 4.0 ng/ml.[43] Furthermore, 20 to 40% of patients with organ-confined prostate cancer have a PSA value of 4.0 ng/ml or less.

In view of such overlap, several refinements in the estimation and interpretation of PSA values have been proposed. These include the ratio between the serum PSA value and volume of prostate gland (PSA density), the rate of change in PSA value with time (PSA velocity), the use

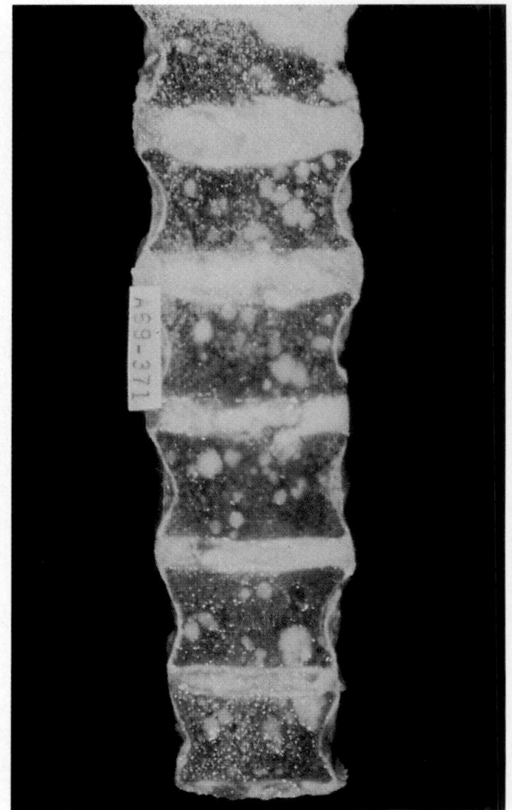

Figure 23–25

Metastatic osteoblastic prostatic carcinoma within vertebral bodies.

of age-specific reference ranges, and the ratio of free and bound PSA in the serum. While many of these parameters are still under investigation, there seems to be an emerging consensus that detection of percent free PSA is of particular value for distinguishing prostatic cancer from non-neoplastic conditions.[43,44] Studies have revealed that immunoreactive PSA (the form detected by the widely used antibody test) exists in two forms: a major fraction bound to α_1-antichymotrypsin and a minor free fraction. The percentage of free PSA (free PSA ÷ total PSA × 100) is lower in men with prostate cancer than in men with benign prostatic diseases. Furthermore, it appears that percent free PSA is most valuable in discriminating between benign and malignant disease when the total PSA level is in the "gray zone" of 4 to 10 ng/ml.[45] Until the value of these refinements in the estimation and interpretations of PSA levels is better established, serum PSA by itself cannot be used for detection of early cancer. When combined with rectal examination and transrectal ultrasonography, however, measurement of PSA antigen levels is considered useful in detection of early-stage cancers. Because many small cancers localized to the prostate may never progress to clinically significant invasive cancers, there is considerable uncertainty regarding the management of small lesions that are detected because of an elevated PSA level. Much effort is therefore focused in devising criteria by which those localized lesions most likely to advance can be distinguished from those that may remain innocuous.[46]

Although serum PSA levels are less than perfect for detection of early prostate cancer, there is little doubt that serial measurements of PSA are of great value in assessing the response to therapy. For example, an elevated PSA level after radical prostatectomy for localized disease is indicative of disseminated disease. Rising PSA levels after initial control of cancer herald recurrence or dissemination. Immunohistochemical localization of PSA is also helpful in determining whether a metastatic tumor originated in the prostate.

Cancer of the prostate is treated by surgery, radiotherapy, and hormonal manipulations. As might be expected, surgery and radiotherapy are most suited for treatment of patients with localized (stage A or B) disease. More than 90% of patients in this group can expect to live for 15 years. Endocrine therapy is the mainstay for treatment of advanced, metastatic carcinoma. Because prostatic cancer cells depend on androgens for their sustenance, the aim of endocrine manipulations is to deprive the tumor cells of testosterone. This can be achieved by orchiectomy or by administration of estrogens or synthetic agonists of luteinizing hormone–releasing hormone. Although estrogens can inhibit testicular androgen synthesis directly, their principal effect appears to be suppression of pituitary luteinizing hormone secretion, which, in turn, leads to reduced testicular output of testosterone. Synthetic analogues of luteinizing hormone–releasing hormone act similarly. Long-term administration of luteinizing hormone–releasing hormone agonists (after an initial transient increase in luteinizing hormone secretion) suppresses luteinizing hormone release, achieving in effect a pharmacologic orchiectomy. Although antiandrogen therapy does induce remissions, tumor progression leads to emergence of testosterone-insensitive clones, and hence despite all forms of treatment, patients with disseminated cancers have a poor prognosis.

REFERENCES

1. Diamond DA, Ransley PG: Male epispadias. J Urol 154:2150, 1995.
2. Belman AB: Hypospadias update. Urology 49:166, 1997.
3. Davenport M: ABC of general surgery in children: problems with penis and prepuce. BMJ 312:299, 1996.
4. Edwards S: Balanitis and balanoposthitis: a review. Genitourin Med 72:155, 1996.
5. Grossman HB: Premalignant and early carcinoma of the penis and scrotum. Urol Clin North Am 19:221, 1992.
6. Strohmeyer TG, Slamon D: Protooncogenes and tumor suppressor genes in human urologic malignancies. J Urol 151:1479, 1994.
7. Gerber GS: Carcinoma in situ of the penis. J Urol 151:829, 1994.
8. Cupp MR, et al: The detection of human papilloma virus deoxyribonucleic acid in intraepithelial, in situ, verrucous and invasive carcinoma of the penis. J Urol 154:1024, 1995.
9. Micalli G, et al: Squamous cell carcinoma of the penis. J Am Acad Dermatol 35:432, 1996.
10. Holly EA, Palefsky JM: Factors related to risk of penile cancer: new evidence from a study of Pacific Northwest. J Natl Cancer Inst 85:2, 1993.
11. Burgers JK, et al: Penile cancer: clinical presentation, diagnosis, and staging. Urol Clin North Am 19:267, 1992.
12. Rozanski TA, Bloom D: The undescended testis: theory and management. Urol Clin North Am 22:107, 1995.
13. Hutson J, et al: Normal testicular descent and the etiology of cryptorchidism. Adv Anat Embryol Cell Biol 132:1, 1996.
14. Swerdlow AJ, et al: Risk of testicular cancer in cohort of boys with cryptorchidism. BMJ 314:1507, 1997.
15. Davenport M: ABC of general pediatric surgery: inguinal hernia, hydrocele, and the undescended testis. BMJ 312:564, 1996.
16. Forman D, et al: Aetiology of testicular cancer: association with congenital abnormalities, age at puberty, infertility and exercise. BMJ 308:1393, 1994.
17. Beutow SA: Epidemiology of testicular cancer. Epidemiol Rev 17:433, 1995.
18. Klein FA, et al: Bilateral granulomatous orchitis: manifestation of idiopathic systemic granulomatosis. J Urol 134:762, 1985.
19. Bosl GJ, Motzer RJ: Testicular germ-cell cancer. N Engl J Med 337:242, 1997.
20. Czaja JT, Ulbright TM: Evidence for the transformation of seminoma to yolk sac tumor, with histogenetic considerations. Am J Clin Pathol 97:468, 1992.
21. Ulbright TM: Germ cell neoplasms of the testis. Am J Surg Pathol 17:1075, 1993.
22. Doherty AP, et al: The role of tumor markers in the diagnosis and treatment of testicular germ cell cancers. Br J Urol 79:247, 1997.
23. Dilworth JP, et al: Non-germ cell tumors of testis. Urology 37:399, 1991.
24. Meares EM: Prostatitis. Med Clin North Am 75:405, 1991.
25. Doble A: Chronic prostatitis. Br J Urol 74:537, 1994.
26. Steers WD, Zorn B: Benign prostatic hyperplasia. Dis Mon 41:437, 1995.
27. Arrighi HM, et al: Natural history of benign prostatic hyperplasia and risk of prostatectomy: The Baltimore Longitudinal Study of Aging. Urology 38(suppl):4, 1991.
28. Droller MJ: Medical approaches to the management of prostate disease. Br J Urol 79:42, 1997.
29. Walsh PC: Treatment of benign prostatic hyperplasia. N Engl J Med 335:586, 1996.
30. Oesterling JE: Benign prostatic hyperplasia: a review of histogenesis and natural history. Prostate 6(suppl):67, 1996.
31. Boring CC, et al: Cancer statistics, 1994. CA Cancer J Clin 44:7, 1994.
32. Isaacs JT: Molecular markers of prostate cancer metastases. Am J Pathol 150:1511, 1997.
33. Dijkman GA, Debrune FMJ: Epidemiology of prostate cancer. Eur Urol 30:281, 1996.
34. Meilke AW, Smith JA: Epidemiology of prostate cancer. Urol Clin North Am 17:709, 1990.

35. Ekman P, et al: Environmental and genetic factors: a possible link with prostate cancer. Br J Urol 79(suppl 2):35, 1997.
36. Smith JR, et al: Major susceptibility locus for prostate cancer on chromosome 1 suggested by genome-wide search. Science 274:1371, 1996.
37. Botswick DG, et al: Molecular biology of prostatic intraepithelial neoplasia. Prostate 29:117, 1996.
38. Mostofi FK, et al: Pathology of carcinoma of the prostate. Cancer 70(suppl):235, 1992.
39. Bostwick DG: Progression of prostatic intraepithelial neoplasia to eary invasive cancer. Eur Urol 30:145, 1996.
40. Foster CS, Deshmukh N: Grading prostate cancer. In Foster CS, Botswick DG (eds): Pathology of Prostate. Philadelphia, WB Saunders, 1998, p 191.
41. Whitmore W: Stage A prostate cancer. J Urol 136:883, 1986.
42. Arcangeli CG, et al: Prostate-specific antigen as a screening test for prostate cancer: the United States experience. Urol Clin North Am 24:299, 1997.
43. Catalona WJ: Clinical utility of measurements of free and total prostate-specific antigen (PSA): a review. Prostate 7(suppl):64, 1996.
44. Vashi AR, Oesterling JE: Percent free prostate-specific antigen: entering a new era in the detection of prostate cancer. Mayo Clin Proc 72: 337, 1997.
45. Catalona WJ, et al: Use of the percentage of free prostate-specific antigen to enhance differentiation of prostate cancer from benign prostatic disease. A prospective multicenter clinical trial. JAMA 279: 1542, 1998.
46. Partin AW, et al: Combination of prostate-specific antigen, clinical stage, and Gleason score to predict pathologic stage of localized prostate cancer: a multiinstitutional update. JAMA 277:1445, 1997.

24

The Female Genital Tract

Christopher P. Crum

EMBRYOLOGY

ANATOMY

FEMALE GENITAL INFECTIONS

- INFECTIONS CONFINED TO THE LOWER GENITAL TRACT
- INFECTIONS INVOLVING THE LOWER AND UPPER GENITAL TRACT

VULVA

BARTHOLIN CYST

VESTIBULAR ADENITIS

NON-NEOPLASTIC EPITHELIAL DISORDERS

- LICHEN SCLEROSUS
- SQUAMOUS HYPERPLASIA

TUMORS

- BENIGN TUMORS
- PREMALIGNANT AND MALIGNANT NEOPLASMS
  - Paget Disease

VAGINA

CONGENITAL ANOMALIES

PREMALIGNANT AND MALIGNANT NEOPLASMS

- VAGINAL INTRAEPITHELIAL NEOPLASIA AND SQUAMOUS CELL CARCINOMA
- ADENOCARCINOMA
- EMBRYONAL RHABDOMYOSARCOMA

CERVIX

INFLAMMATIONS

- ACUTE AND CHRONIC CERVICITIS
- ENDOCERVICAL POLYPS

INTRAEPITHELIAL AND INVASIVE SQUAMOUS NEOPLASIA

- CERVICAL INTRAEPITHELIAL NEOPLASIA
- SQUAMOUS CELL CARCINOMA

BODY OF UTERUS AND ENDOMETRIUM

ENDOMETRIAL HISTOLOGY IN THE MENSTRUAL CYCLE

FUNCTIONAL ENDOMETRIAL DISORDERS

- ANOVULATORY CYCLE
- INADEQUATE LUTEAL PHASE
- ORAL CONTRACEPTIVES AND INDUCED ENDOMETRIAL CHANGES
- MENOPAUSAL AND POSTMENOPAUSAL CHANGES

INFLAMMATIONS

- CHRONIC ENDOMETRITIS

ADENOMYOSIS

ENDOMETRIOSIS

ENDOMETRIAL POLYPS

ENDOMETRIAL HYPERPLASIA

MALIGNANT TUMORS

- CARCINOMA OF THE ENDOMETRIUM

MIXED MÜLLERIAN AND MESENCHYMAL TUMORS

- MALIGNANT MIXED MÜLLERIAN TUMORS

TUMORS OF THE MYOMETRIUM

- LEIOMYOMAS
- LEIOMYOSARCOMAS
- ENDOMETRIAL STROMAL TUMORS

FALLOPIAN TUBES

INFLAMMATIONS

TUMORS AND CYSTS

OVARIES

NON-NEOPLASTIC FUNCTIONAL CYSTS

- FOLLICULAR AND LUTEAL CYSTS
- POLYCYSTIC OVARIES AND STROMAL HYPERTHECOSIS

OVARIAN TUMORS

- TUMORS OF SURFACE (COELOMIC) EPITHELIUM
- GERM CELL TUMORS
- SEX CORD–STROMAL TUMORS

GESTATIONAL AND PLACENTAL DISORDERS

DISORDERS OF EARLY PREGNANCY

- SPONTANEOUS ABORTION
- ECTOPIC PREGNANCY

DISORDERS OF LATE PREGNANCY

- PLACENTAL ABNORMALITIES AND TWIN PLACENTAS
- PLACENTAL INFLAMMATIONS AND INFECTIONS
- TOXEMIA OF PREGNANCY (PREECLAMPSIA AND ECLAMPSIA)

GESTATIONAL TROPHOBLASTIC DISEASE

- HYDATIDIFORM MOLE (COMPLETE AND PARTIAL)
- INVASIVE MOLE
- CHORIOCARCINOMA
- PLACENTAL SITE TROPHOBLASTIC TUMOR

NORMAL

EMBRYOLOGY

The embryology of the female genital tract is relevant to both anomalies in this region and the histogenesis of various tumors. The primordial germ cells arise in the wall of the yolk sac by the fourth week of gestation; by the fifth or sixth week, they migrate into the urogenital ridge. The mesodermal epithelium of the urogenital ridge then proliferates eventually to produce the epithelium and stroma of the gonad, and the dividing germ cells—of endodermal origin—are incorporated into these proliferating epithelial cells to form the ovary.[1] Failure of germ cells to develop may result in either absence of ovaries or premature ovarian failure. Disruption of normal migration may account for extragonadal distribution of germ cell midline structures (retroperitoneum, mediastinum, and even pineal gland) and may rarely lead to tumors in these sites.

A second component of female genital development is the müllerian duct. At about the sixth week, invagination and subsequent fusion of the coelomic lining epithelium form the lateral müllerian (or paramesonephric) ducts. Müllerian ducts progressively grow caudally to enter the pelvis, where they swing medially to fuse. Further caudal growth brings these fused ducts into contact with the urogenital sinus, which eventually becomes the vestibule of the external genitalia. Normally, the unfused portions mature into the fallopian tubes, the fused caudal portion developing into the uterus and upper vagina and the urogenital sinus forming the lower vagina and vestibule (Fig. 24–1). Consequently, the entire lining of the uterus and tubes as well as the ovarian surface is derived from coelomic epithelium (mesothelium). The fact that these various surfaces are derived from a similar origin explains the histologic similarities in both benign and malignant tumors at these sites.

In males, müllerian inhibitory substance[2] from the developing testis causes regression of the müllerian ducts, and the paired wolffian (or mesonephric) ducts form the epididymis and the vas deferens. Normally, the mesonephric duct regresses in the female, but remnants may persist into adult life as epithelial inclusions adjacent to the ovaries, tubes, and uterus. In the cervix and vagina, these rests may be cystic and are termed Gartner duct cysts.

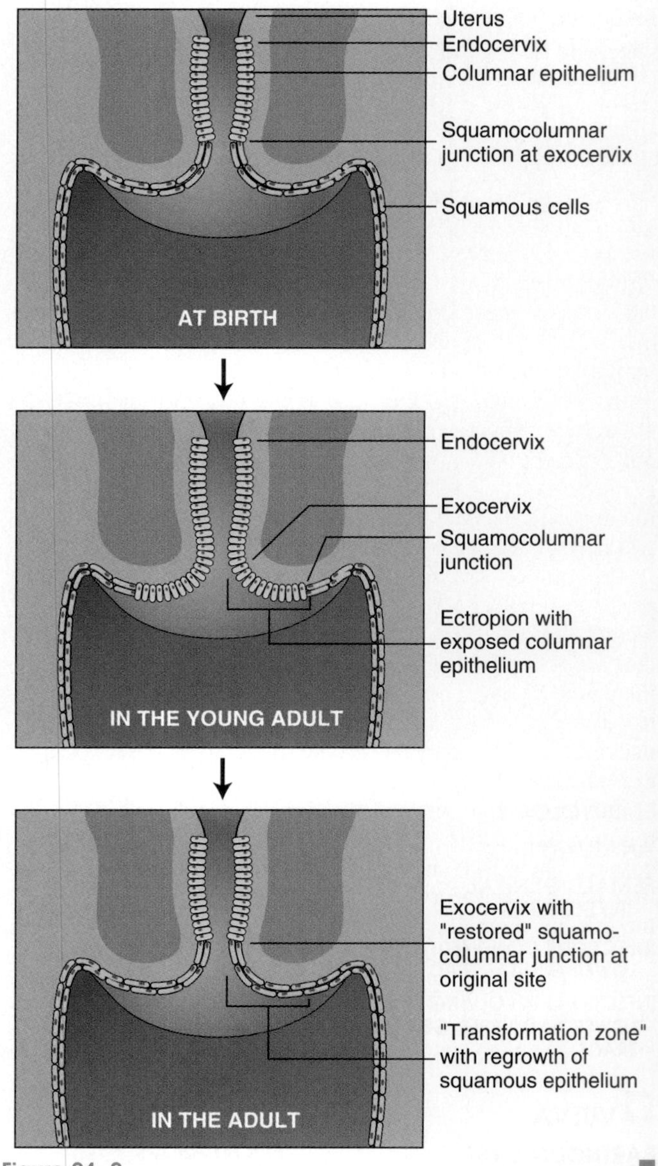

Figure 24–2

Schematic of the development of the cervical transformation zone.

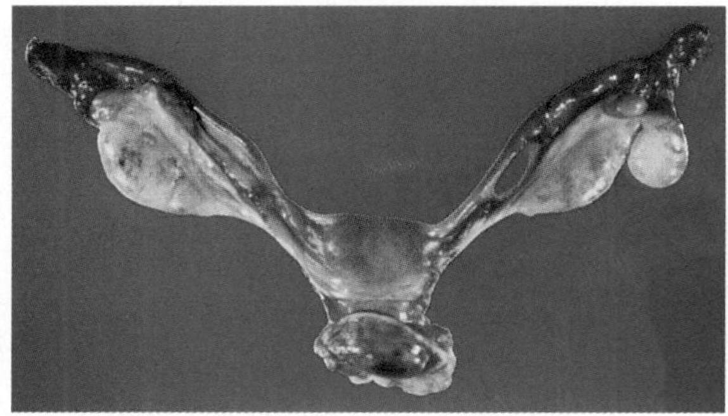

Figure 24–1

Anatomy of the female genital tract. This specimen depicts the normal cervix, uterus, fallopian tubes, and ovaries. A small paratubal cyst is present on the right.

ANATOMY

During active reproductive life, the ovaries measure about 4 × 2.5 × 1.5 cm in dimension. The ovary is divided into a cortex and a medulla. The cortex consists of a layer of closely packed spindle cells that resemble plump fibroblasts with scant intercellular ground substance and a thin outer layer of relatively acellular collagenous connective tissue. Follicles in varying stages of maturation are found within the outer cortex. With each menstrual cycle, one follicle develops into a graafian follicle en route to ovulation and after ovulation is transformed into a corpus luteum. Corpora lutea of varying ages as well as corpora albicantia are also present in the cortex of the adult.

The medulla of the ovary is made up of a more loosely arranged mesenchymal tissue and may contain small clusters of round to polygonal, epithelial-appearing cells around vessels and nerves. These "hilus" cells, presumed to be vestigial remains of the gonad from its primitive "ambisexual" phase, are steroid producing and thus resemble the interstitial cells of the testis. Rarely, these cells give rise to masculinizing tumors (hilar cell tumors).

In the fallopian tube, the mucosa is thrown up into numerous delicate folds (plica) that on cross-section produce a papillary appearance. The lining epithelium consists of three cell types: ciliated columnar cell; nonciliated, columnar secretory cells; and so-called intercalated cells, which may simply represent inactive secretory cells.

The uterus varies in size, depending on the age and parity of the individual. During active reproductive life, it weighs about 50 gm and measures about 8.0 × 6.0 × 3.0 cm in dimension. Pregnancies may leave small residual increases in these dimensions (up to 70 gm in weight) because the uterus rarely involutes completely to its original size. After menopause, the uterus undergoes atrophy, diminishing by up to half in dimension.

The uterus has three distinctive anatomic and functional regions: the cervix, the lower uterine segment, and the corpus. The cervix is further divided into the vaginal portion and the endocervix. The anatomic portion is visible to the eye on vaginal examination. It is covered by a stratified nonkeratinizing squamous epithelium continuous with the vaginal vault. The squamous epithelium converges centrally at a small opening termed the external os. In the normal cervix of nulliparous women, this os is virtually closed. Just cephalad to the os is the endocervix, which is lined by columnar, mucus-secreting epithelium that dips down into the underlying stroma to produce crypts (endocervical glands). The point at which the squamous and glandular epithelium meet is the squamocolumnar junction. The position of the junction is variable. Although its original position is at the cervical os (Fig. 24–2, top), in virtually all adult women who have borne children, the endocervix is everted, exposing the squamocolumnar junction to the naked eye (Fig. 24–2, middle). A combination of ingrowth of the squamous epithelium portion (epidermidalization) and intrinsic squamous differentiation of subcolumnar reserve cells (squamous metaplasia) transforms this area into squamous epithelium and produces the *transformation zone* (Fig. 24–2, bottom). During reproductive life, the squamocolumnar junction migrates cephalad on the leading edge of the transformation zone and may be invisible to the naked eye after menopause (Fig. 24–3). As we shall see, it is in this transformation zone, including the squamocolumnar junction, where squamous carcinomas or precancerous lesions develop. The lower uterine segment, or isthmus, is the portion between the endocervix and the endometrial cavity.

The endometrial changes that occur during the menstrual cycle are keyed to the rise and fall in the levels of ovarian hormones, and the student should be familiar with the complex but fascinating interactions among hypothalamic, pituitary, and ovarian factors underlying maturation of ovarian follicles, ovulation, and the menstrual cycle. Suffice it to say that under the influence of the pituitary follicle-stimulating hormone and luteinizing hormone, development and ripening of a single ovum occur, and estrogen production by the enlarging ovarian follicle progressively rises during the first 2 weeks of the usual 28-day menstrual cycle. It reaches a peak, presumably just before ovulation, and then falls. After ovulation, the estrogen lev-

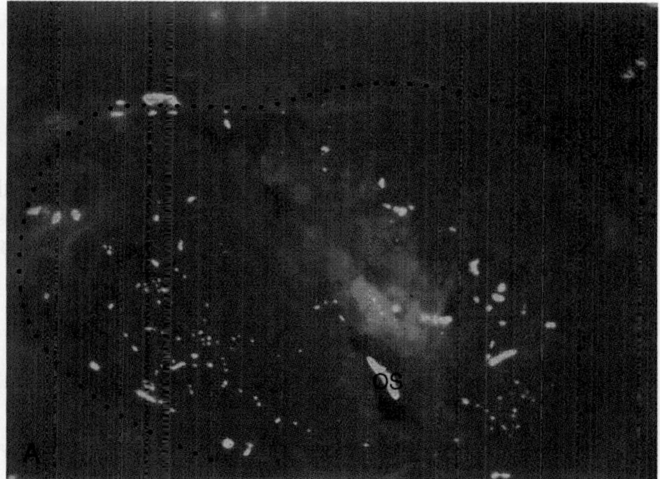

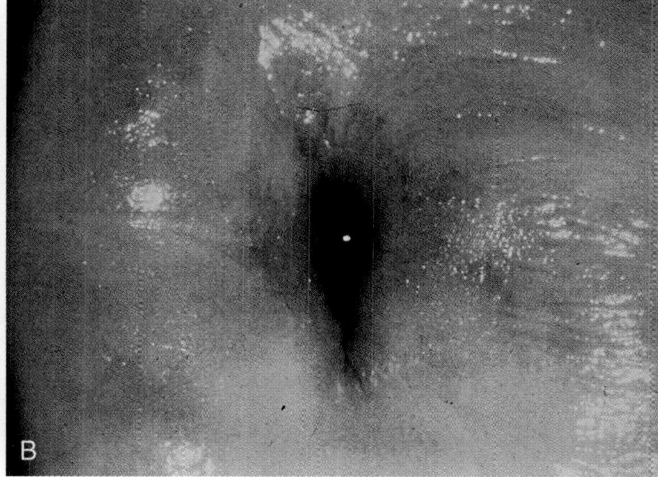

Figure 24–3

A, Colpophotograph of the cervix in a reproductive age woman. The portio epithelium (peripheral) merges with (at dotted boundary) and eventually replaces the endocervical columnar epithelium (red and grapelike) to form the transformation zone. The os is in the center. *B*, The postmenopausal cervix. The epithelial surface is smooth and completely covered by squamous epithelium. The squamocolumnar junction is not visible and is inside the endocervical canal. (*A* and *B* courtesy of Dr. Alex Ferenczy, McGill University, Montreal, Quebec.)

els again begin to rise to a plateau at about the end of the third week, but these levels are never as high as the preovulatory peak. The level of this hormone then progressively falls, beginning 3 to 4 days before the onset of menstruation. Progesterone, produced by the corpus luteum, rises throughout the last half of the menstrual cycle to fall to basal levels just before the onset of menstrual bleeding. The histology of the normal and abnormal endometrial cycle is discussed later in the section on the endometrium.

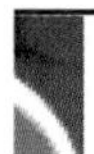

PATHOLOGY

Diseases of the female genital tract are extremely common in clinical and pathologic practice and include complications of pregnancy, inflammations, tumors, and hormonally induced effects. The following discussion presents the pathology of the majority of clinical problems. Details can be found in current books of obstetric and gynecologic pathology and medicine.[3–7] The pathologic conditions peculiar to each segment of the female genital tract are discussed separately, but first we briefly review pelvic inflammatory disease (PID) and other infections because they can affect many of the segments concomitantly.

FEMALE GENITAL INFECTIONS

A large variety of organisms can infect the female genital tract and, in total, account for considerable suffering and morbidity (Table 24–1). Some, such as *Candida* infections, trichomoniasis, and *Gardnerella* infections, are extremely common and may cause significant discomfort with no serious sequelae. Others, such as gonorrhea and *Chlamydia* infection, are major causes of female infertility, and others still, such as *Mycoplasma* infections, are implicated in spontaneous abortions. Viruses, principally the human papillomaviruses (HPV), appear to be involved in the pathogenesis of vulvar and cervical cancer.

Many of these infections are sexually transmitted, including trichomoniasis, gonorrhea, chancroid, granuloma inguinale, lymphogranuloma venereum, syphilis, mycoplasmal infection, chlamydial infection, herpes, and HPV infection.[8] Most of these conditions have been adequately considered in Chapter 9. Here we touch only on selected aspects relevant to the female genital tract, including pathogens confined to the lower genital tract (vulva, vagina, and cervix) and those that involve the entire genital tract and are implicated in PID. Papillomaviruses are discussed subsequently under tumors.

Infections Confined to the Lower Genital Tract

Herpes simplex infection is common and usually involves the vulva, vagina, and cervix.[8] In sexually transmitted disease clinics, approximately half of patients have current or prior evidence of infection versus less than 10% of unselected women.[9] The frequency of genital herpes has increased dramatically in the past two decades, particularly in teenagers and young women, and herpes simplex virus type 2 (HSV-2) infection is now one of the major sexually transmitted diseases. Of individuals infected, clinical symptoms are seen in about one third.[9] The lesions begin 3 to 7 days after sexual relations and consist of painful red papules in the vulva that progress to vesicles and then coalescent ulcers. Cervical or vaginal involvement causes severe leukorrhea (genital discharge), and the initial infection produces systemic symptoms, such as fever, malaise, and tender inguinal lymph nodes. The vesicles and ulcers contain numerous virus particles, accounting for the high transmission rate during active infection. The lesions heal spontaneously in 1 to 3 weeks, but as with herpetic infections elsewhere, latent infection of regional nerve ganglia persists. About two thirds of affected women suffer recurrences, which are less painful. Transmission may occur

Table 24–1. ANATOMIC DISTRIBUTION OF COMMON FEMALE GENITAL INFECTIONS

		Location and Manifestations of Infection				
Organism	**Source**	***Vulva***	***Vagina***	***Cervix***	***Corpus***	***Adnexa***
Herpesvirus	STD	Herpetic ulcers				
Molluscum contagiosum	STD	Molluscum lesions				
HPV	STD	Genital warts, intrapeithelial neoplasia, invasive carcinoma				
Chlamydia trachomatis	STD			Follicular cervicitis, endometritis, salpingo-oophoritis		
Neisseria gonorrhoeae	STD	Skene gland adenitis	Vaginitis in children	Acute cervicitis	Acute endometritis and salpingitis	
Candida	Endogenous	Vulvovaginitis				
Trichomonas	STD		Cervicovaginitis			

HPV, human papillomavirus; STD, sexually transmitted disease.

during active or inactive (latent) phases, although it is much less likely in asymptomatic carriers. The gravest consequence of HSV infection is transmission to the neonate during birth. This risk is highest if the infection is active during delivery and particularly if it is a primary (initial) infection in the mother.[10]

Mycotic and *yeast (Candida) infections* are common; about 10% of women are thought to be carriers of vulvovaginal fungi. Diabetes mellitus, oral contraceptives, and pregnancy may enhance the development of infection, which manifests as small white surface patches similar to monilial lesions elsewhere. It is accompanied by leukorrhea and pruritus. The diagnosis is made by finding the organism in wet mounts of the lesions.

Trichomonas vaginalis is a large, flagellated ovoid protozoan that can be readily identified in wet mounts of vaginal discharge in infected patients (see Fig. 9–32 in Chapter 9). Infections may occur at any age and are seen in about 15% of women in sexually transmitted disease clinics.[11] They are associated with a purulent vaginal discharge and discomfort; the underlying vaginal and cervical mucosa typically has a characteristic fiery red appearance, called strawberry cervix. On histologic examination, the inflammatory reaction is usually limited to the mucosa and immediately subjacent lamina propria.

Mycoplasma species account for some cases of vaginitis and cervicitis and have been implicated in spontaneous abortion and chorioamnionitis. *Gardnerella* is a gram-negative, small bacillus that is implicated in cases of vaginitis when other organisms *(Trichomonas,* fungi) cannot be found.

Infections Involving the Lower and Upper Genital Tract

PELVIC INFLAMMATORY DISEASE (PID)

PID is a common disorder characterized by pelvic pain, adnexal tenderness, fever, and vaginal discharge; it results from infection by one or more of the following groups of organisms: gonococcus, chlamydiae, and enteric bacteria. The gonococcus continues to be a common cause of PID, the most serious complication of gonorrhea in women (Chapter 9). *Chlamydia* infection is now another well-recognized cause of PID. Besides these two, infections after spontaneous or induced abortions and normal or abnormal deliveries (called puerperal infections) are important in the production of PID. Such PID is polymicrobial and is caused by staphylococci, streptococci, coliform bacteria, and *Clostridium perfringens.*

Gonococcal inflammation usually begins in Bartholin and other vestibular glands or periurethral glands; cervix involvement is common and frequently asymptomatic. From any of these loci, the organisms may spread upward to involve the tubes and tubo-ovarian region. The adult vagina is remarkably resistant to the gonococcus, but in the child, presumably because of a more delicate lining mucosa, vulvovaginitis may develop. The nongonococcal bacterial infections that follow induced abortion, dilation and curettage of the uterus, and other surgical procedures on the female genital tract are thought to spread from the uterus upward through the lymphatics or venous channels rather than on the mucosal surfaces. These infections therefore tend to produce less mucosal involvement but more reaction within the deeper layers.

MORPHOLOGY. With the gonococcus, approximately 2 to 7 days after inoculation of the organism, inflammatory changes appear in the affected glands. Wherever it occurs, gonococcal disease is characterized by an acute suppurative reaction with inflammation largely confined to the superficial mucosa and underlying submucosa. Smears of the inflammatory exudate should disclose the intracellular gram-negative diplococcus, but absolute confirmation requires culture. If spread occurs, the endometrium is usually spared, for obscure reasons. Once it is within the tubes, an **acute suppurative salpingitis** ensues. The tubal serosa becomes hyperemic and layered with fibrin, the tubal fimbriae are similarly involved, and the lumen fills with purulent exudate that may leak out of the fimbriated end. In days or weeks, the fimbriae may seal or become plastered against the ovary to create a **salpingo-oophoritis.** Collections of pus within the ovary and tube **(tubo-ovarian abscesses)** or tubal lumen **(pyosalpinx)** may occur. Adhesions of the tubal plica may produce glandlike spaces (follicular salpingitis) (Fig. 24–4). In the course of time, the infecting organisms may disappear, the pus undergoing proteolysis to a thin, serous fluid, to produce a **hydrosalpinx** or hydrosalpinx follicularis.

PID caused by staphylococci, streptococci, and the other puerperal invaders tends to have less exudation within the lumens of the tube and less

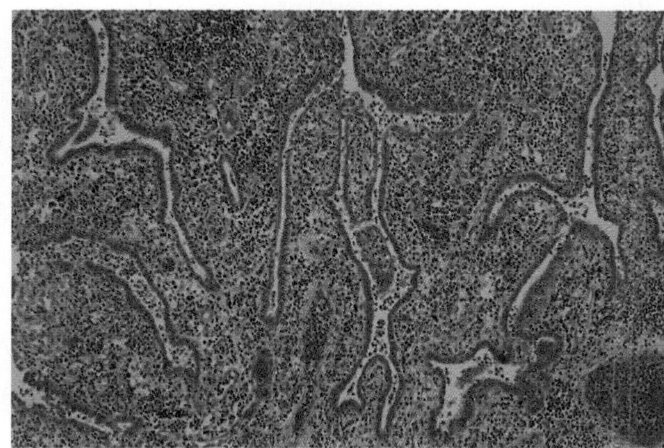

Figure 24–4 ■

A, Acute salpingo-oophoritis with tubo-ovarian abscess. The fallopian tubes and ovaries have coalesced into an inflammatory mass adherent to the uterus. Compare with Figure 24–1. *B,* Chronic salpingitis with fusion of the tubal plicae and inflammatory cell infiltrates.

involvement of the mucosa, with a greater inflammatory response within the deeper layers. The infection tends to spread throughout the wall to involve the serosa and may often track into the broad ligaments, pelvic structures, and peritoneum. Bacteremia is a more frequent complication of streptococcal or staphylococcal PID than of gonococcal infections.

The complications of PID include

- Peritonitis
- Intestinal obstruction due to adhesions between the small bowel and the pelvic organs
- Bacteremia, which may produce endocarditis, meningitis, and suppurative arthritis
- Infertility, one of the most commonly feared consequences of long-standing chronic PID

In the early stages, gonococcal infections are readily controlled with antibiotics, although penicillin-resistant strains have regrettably emerged. When the infection becomes walled off in suppurative tubes or tubo-ovarian abscesses, it is difficult to achieve a sufficient level of antibiotic within the centers of such suppuration to control these infections effectively. Postabortion and postpartum PIDs are also amenable to antibiotics but are far more difficult to control than the gonococcal infections. It sometimes becomes necessary to remove the organs surgically.

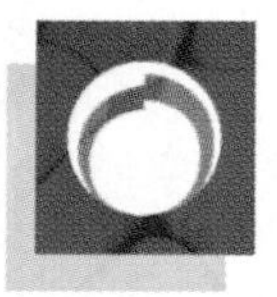

VULVA

Diseases of the vulva in the aggregate constitute only a small fraction of gynecologic practice. Many inflammatory dermatologic diseases that affect hair-bearing skin elsewhere on the body may also occur on the vulva, so vulvitis may be encountered in psoriasis, eczema, and allergic dermatitis. The vulva is prone to skin infections because it is constantly exposed to secretions and moisture. Nonspecific vulvitis is particularly likely to occur in blood dyscrasias, uremia, diabetes mellitus, malnutrition, and avitaminoses. Most skin cysts (epidermal inclusion cysts) and tumors can also occur in the vulva. Here we discuss disorders peculiar to the vulva, including Bartholin cyst, vestibular adenitis, vulvar dystrophies, and tumors of the vulva.

BARTHOLIN CYST

Acute infection of the Bartholin gland produces an acute inflammation of the gland (adenitis) and may result in a Bartholin abscess. Bartholin cysts are relatively common, occur at all ages, and result from obstruction of the Bartholin duct, usually by a preceding infection. These cysts may become large, up to 3 to 5 cm in diameter. The cyst is lined by either the transitional epithelium of the normal duct or squamous metaplasia. The cysts produce pain and local discomfort; the cysts are either excised or opened permanently (marsupialization).

VESTIBULAR ADENITIS

The vulvar vestibule is located in the posterior introitus at the entrance to the vagina and contains small glands in the submucosa (vestibular glands). Inflammation of these glands is associated with a chronic, recurrent, and exquisitely painful condition known as vestibular adenitis. The inflammatory condition, which involves the glands and mucosa, produces small ulcerations, which account for extreme point tenderness in the vestibule. The cause of the condition is unknown, and the condition is relieved, in some but not in all cases, by surgical removal of the inflamed mucosa.[12]

NON-NEOPLASTIC EPITHELIAL DISORDERS

A spectrum of inflammatory lesions of the vulva is characterized by opaque, white, scaly, plaquelike mucosal thickenings that produce vulvar discomfort and itching (pruritus). Because of their white appearance, these disorders have traditionally been termed leukoplakia by clinicians. This is a clinical descriptive term because *white plaques may indicate a variety of benign, premalignant, or malignant lesions.*[13] Hence, a biopsy of "leukoplakia" may reveal one of several conditions: (1) vitiligo (loss of pigment); (2) inflammatory dermatoses (e.g., psoriasis, chronic dermatitis [Chapter 27]); (3) carcinoma in situ, Paget disease, or even invasive carcinoma; and (4) a variety of alterations of unknown etiology that elude proper classification. To eliminate the confusion generated by using multiple terms to characterize white vulvar lesions (e.g., kraurosis vulvae, leukoplakia, atrophic vulvitis), clinical descriptive terminology has been separated from histologic diagnosis. Excluding neoplasms and specific disease entities, nonspecific inflammatory alterations of the vulva are now classified with use of accepted dermatologic diagnoses (such as lichen simplex chronicus) or placed within two additional categories: (1) *lichen sclerosus,* a characteristic disorder manifested by subepithelial fibrosis, and (2) *squamous hyperplasia,* manifested by epithelial hyperplasia and hyperkeratosis. The two forms may coexist in different areas of the same vulva, and the lesions are often multiple,

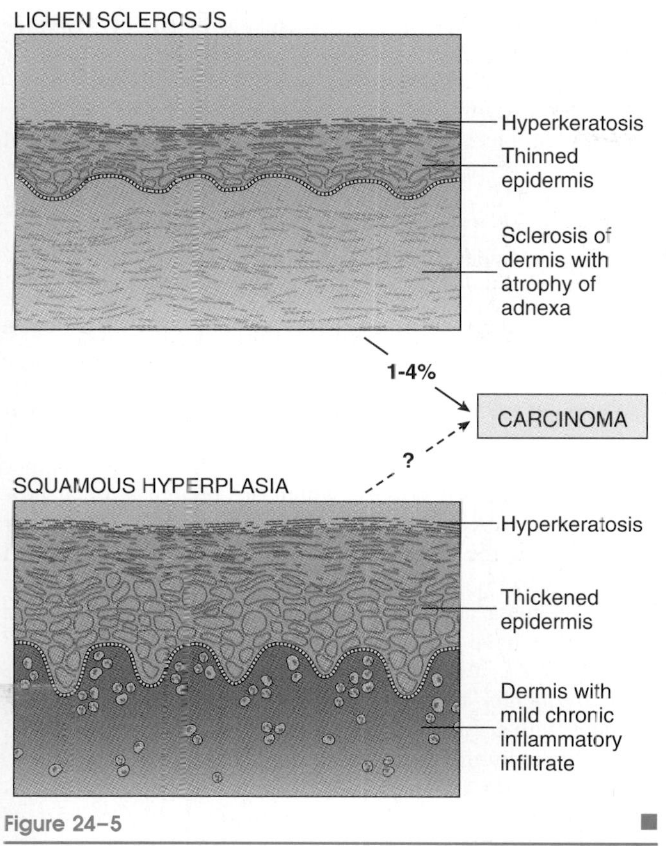

Figure 24–5

Schematic composition of lichen sclerosus (*top*) and squamous hyperplasia (*bottom*) of the vulvar mucosa.

making their clinical management particularly difficult[14] (Fig. 24–5).

Lichen Sclerosus

Lichen sclerosus leads to atrophy, fibrosis, and scarring, and is also called chronic atrophic vulvitis. The skin becomes pale gray and parchment-like, the labia are atrophied, and the introitus is narrowed (Fig. 24–6). On histologic examination, there is usually thinning of the epidermis, with disappearance of the rete pegs and replacement of the underlying dermis by dense collagenous fibrous tissue (Fig. 24–7). There is often marked hyperkeratosis and a mononuclear cell infiltrate about blood vessels. Lichen sclerosus occurs clinically in all age groups but is most common after menopause. The pathogenesis is unclear, but genetic predisposition, autoimmunity, and hormonal factors have been implicated.[14] At all ages, the disorder tends to be slow in developing, insidious, and progressive. It causes considerable discomfort and predisposes to acute infection but is usually of little systemic significance. Lichen sclerosus is not recognized as a precancerous condition, but it increases the risk of subsequent carcinoma. A small proportion of patients (about 1% to 4%) have been observed to develop carcinoma.[15]

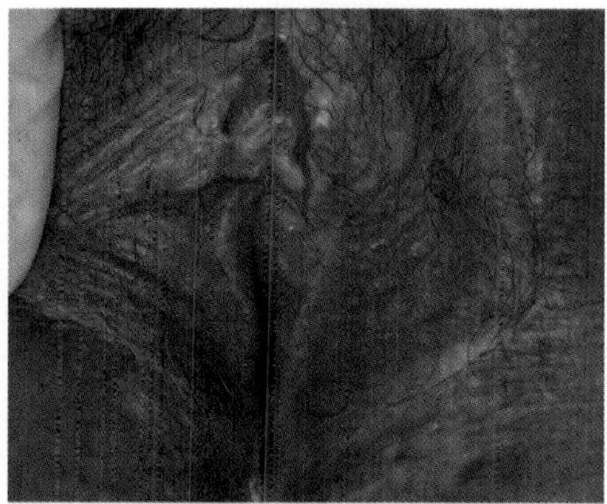

Figure 24–6

Lichen sclerosus. Note the white parchment-like patches of the skin of the vulva and labial atrophy.

Squamous Hyperplasia

Previously called hyperplastic dystrophy, this lesion denotes hyperplasia of the vulvar squamous epithelium, frequently with hyperkeratosis. The epithelium is thickened and may show increased mitotic activity in both the basal and prickle cell layers (Fig. 24–8) with variable leukocytic infiltration of the dermis. Similar to lichen sclerosus, squamous hyperplasia is sometimes associated with carcinoma. It is not, however, considered a significant cancer precursor unless there is coexisting epithelial atypia, in which case it

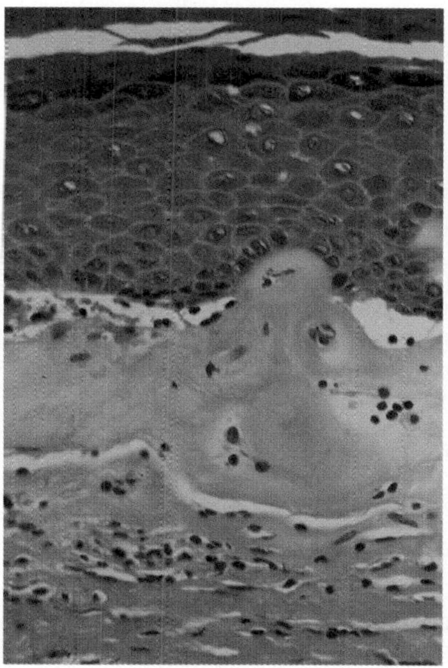

Figure 24–7

The histologic hallmark of lichen sclerosus is a dense band of hyaline collagen beneath the epithelium.

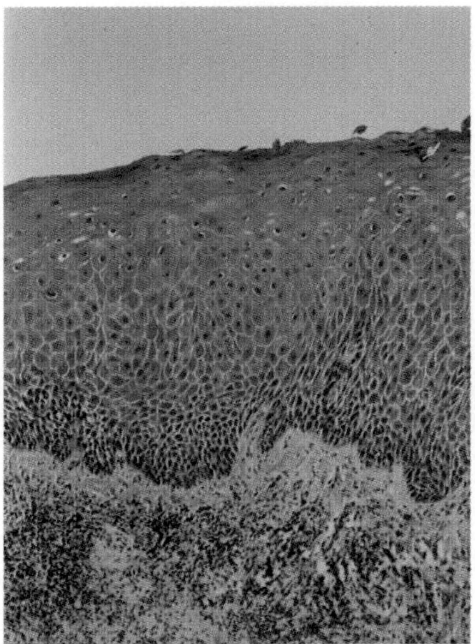

Figure 24–8

Squamous hyperplasia. Epithelial hyperplasia and dermal chronic inflammation.

is classified as a precancerous lesion (vulvar intraepithelial neoplasia).[16]

The pathogenesis of squamous hyperplasia is unknown. Because the lesions may present as white vulvar plaques, they may be indistinguishable clinically from more serious disorders. Thus, biopsy is indicated in all lesions, even those that are remotely suspicious.

TUMORS

Tumors of the vulva are the most important lesions to affect this region. Many types have been recorded, both benign and malignant, including fibromas, neurofibromas, angiomas, sweat gland tumors, carcinomas, malignant melanomas, and various types of sarcoma. All these forms are uncommon and moreover are histologically analogous to similar tumors occurring elsewhere in the body. Therefore, attention is focused on the more common tumors and other proliferative lesions distinctive of the vulva.

Benign Tumors

PAPILLARY HIDRADENOMA

Like the breast, the vulva contains modified apocrine sweat glands. In fact, the vulva may contain tissue closely resembling breast ("ectopic breast") and develop two tumors with counterparts in the breast. One of these, papillary hidradenoma, is identical in appearance to intraductal papillomas of the breast. The other, Paget disease, is discussed later. Hidradenoma presents as a sharply circumscribed nodule, most commonly on the labia majora or interlabial folds, and may be confused clinically with carcinoma because of its tendency to ulcerate. On histologic examination, hidradenomas consist of tubular ducts lined by a single or double layer of nonciliated columnar cells, with a layer of flattened "myoepithelial cells" underlying the epithelium. These myoepithelial elements are characteristic of sweat glands and sweat gland tumors.

CONDYLOMA ACUMINATUM

Benign raised or wartlike (verrucous) conditions of the vulva occur in three forms. (1) By far the most common is the condyloma acuminatum, a papillomavirus-induced squamous lesion also called venereal wart. (2) Another consists of mucosal polyps, which are benign stromal proliferations covered with squamous epithelium. (3) Another raised lesion, the syphilitic condyloma latum, is described in Chapter 9.

Condylomata acuminata are sexually transmitted, benign tumors that have a distinctly verrucous gross appearance[17] (Fig. 24–9*A*). Although they may be solitary, they are more frequently multiple and often coalesce; they involve perineal, vulvar, and perianal regions as well as the vagina and, less commonly, the cervix. The lesions are identical to those found on the penis and around the anus in males (Chapter 23). On histologic examination, they consist of branching, treelike proliferation of stratified squamous epithelium supported by a fibrous stroma (Fig. 24–9*B*). Acanthosis, parakeratosis, hyperkeratosis, and, most specifically, nuclear atypia in the surface cells with perinuclear vacuolization (called *koilocytosis)* are present. Condylomata are caused by HPV, principally types 6 and 11,[18] which are associated with benign genital lesions and replicate in the squamous epithelium. The virus life cycle is completed in the epithelium, specifically the mature superficial cells. This dependence of viral growth on squamous maturation is typical of HPV and produces a distinct cytologic change in the mature cells—*koilocytotic atypia* (nuclear atypia and perinuclear vacuolization)—that is considered a viral "cytopathic" effect. Except in immunosuppressed individuals, condylomata acuminata frequently regress spontaneously and are not considered to be precancerous lesions. They are, however, a marker for sexually transmitted disease.[18]

Premalignant and Malignant Neoplasms

CARCINOMA AND VULVAR INTRAEPITHELIAL NEOPLASIA

Carcinoma of the vulva is an uncommon malignant neoplasm (approximately one eighth as frequent as cervical cancer) representing about 3% of all genital cancers in the female; approximately two thirds occur in women older than 60 years.[19] Eighty-five per cent of these malignant tumors are squamous cell carcinomas, the remainder being basal cell carcinomas, melanomas, or adenocarcinomas. In

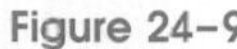

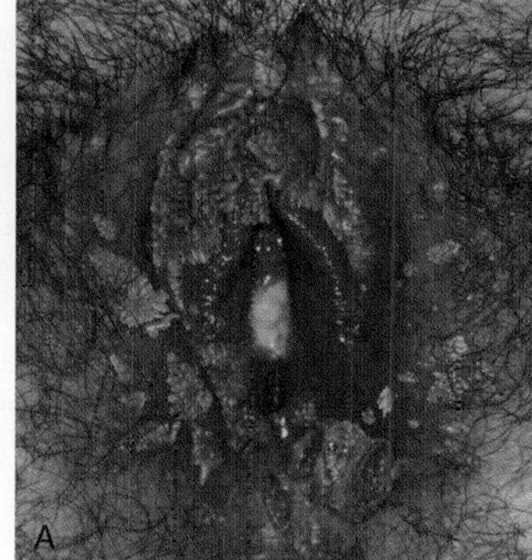

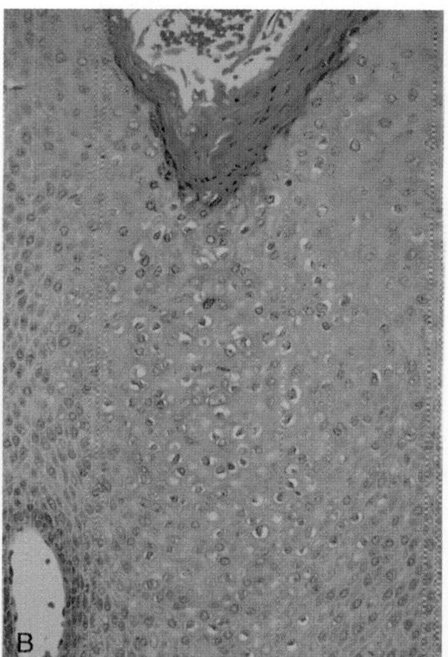

Figure 24–9

A, Numerous condylomas of the vulva encircling the introitus. (Courtesy of Dr. Alex Ferenczy, McGill University, Montreal, Quebec.) *B*, Histopathology of condyloma acuminatum showing acanthosis, hyperkeratosis, and cytoplasmic vacuolation (koilocytosis, *center*).

terms of etiology, pathogenesis, and clinical presentation, vulvar squamous cell carcinomas may be divided into two general groups.

The first group is associated with cancer-related (high-risk) HPV, may be multicentric, and frequently coexists with or is preceded by a classic and easily recognized precancerous change called vulvar intraepithelial neoplasia (VIN). This form of VIN is also termed carcinoma in situ or Bowen disease.[20] VIN is characterized by nuclear atypia in the epithelial cells, increased mitoses, and lack of surface differentiation (Fig. 24–10). It is analogous to high-grade squamous intraepithelial lesions of the cervix (see under cervix). These lesions usually present as white or pigmented plaques on the vulva; identical lesions are encountered in the male. VIN is appearing with increasing frequency in women younger than 40 years. With or without associated invasive carcinoma, VIN is frequently multicentric, and 10% to 30% are associated with another primary squamous neoplasm in the vagina or cervix. This association indicates a common etiologic agent. Indeed, 90% of cases of VIN and many associated cancers contain HPV DNA, specifically types 16, 18, and other cancer-associated (high-risk) types.[20] Spontaneous regression of VIN lesions has been reported; the risk of progression to invasive cancer increases in older (older than 45 years) or immunosuppressed women.[20]

The second group of squamous cell carcinomas are associated with squamous cell hyperplasia and lichen sclerosus. The etiology of this group of carcinomas is unclear, and they are infrequently associated with HPV. In one scenario, genetic alterations arise in lichen sclerosus or hyperplasia, leading directly to invasion, or by an intermediate step in which atypia develops within hyperplasia or lichen sclerosus (differentiated VIN).[21] These tumors have also been associated with mutations in *p53* and appear to have a significantly worse prognosis than HPV-positive tumors do.[22] A variety of chromosome abnormalities are linked to invasive vulvar cancer, some of which may be specific for HPV-positive tumors.[23]

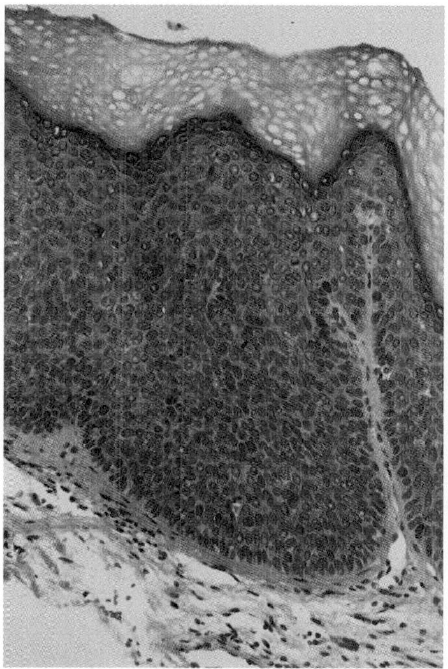

Figure 24–10

Histopathology of vulvar intraepithelial neoplasia with diffuse cellular atypia, nuclear crowding, and increased mitotic index.

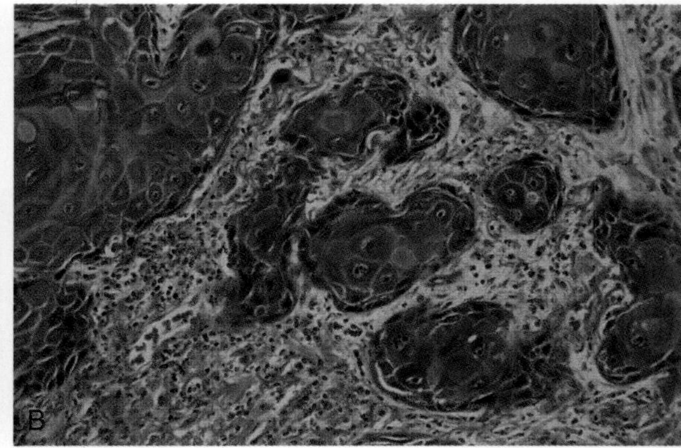

Figure 24–11

A, Poorly differentiated vulvar carcinoma associated with human papillomaviruses (HPV). *B*, Well-differentiated keratinizing vulvar carcinoma, typically HPV negative.

MORPHOLOGY. Vulvar squamous cell carcinomas begin as small areas of epithelial thickening that resemble leukoplakia but, in the course of time, progress to create firm, indurated, **exophytic** tumors or ulcerated, endophytic lesions. Although vulvar carcinomas are external tumors that are obviously apparent to the patient and the clinician, many are misinterpreted as dermatitis, eczema, or leukoplakia for long periods. The clinical manifestations evoked are chiefly those of pain, local discomfort, itching, and exudation because superficial secondary infection is common.

On histologic examination, tumors associated with HPV or VIN frequently exhibit cohesive invasive growth patterns that mimic intraepithelial neoplasia. These "intraepithelial-like" patterns may be well (warty) or poorly differentiated (basaloid)[20,24] (Fig. 24–11*A*). HPV-negative tumors, which at times arise from lichen sclerosus or squamous hyperplasia, typically exhibit an invasive pattern with prominent keratinization (Fig. 24–11*B*).

Risk of metastatic spread is linked to the size of tumor, depth of invasion, and involvement of lymphatic vessels. The inguinal, pelvic, iliac, and periaortic lymph nodes are most commonly involved. Ultimately, lymphohematogenous dissemination involves the lungs, liver, and other internal organs. Patients with lesions less than 2 cm in diameter have a 60% to 80% 5-year survival rate after treatment with one-stage vulvectomy and lymphadenectomy; larger lesions with lymph node involvement yield a less than 10% 5-year survival rate.

Rare variants of squamous cell carcinoma include **verrucous carcinoma,** which may resemble condyloma acuminatum and presents as a large fungating tumor. Local invasion confirms the malignant nature of the lesion, but it rarely metastasizes and can be cured by wide excision.

EXTRAMAMMARY PAGET DISEASE

This curious and rare lesion of the vulva, and sometimes the perianal region, is similar in its skin manifestations to Paget disease of the breast[15] (Chapter 25). As a vulvar neoplasm, it manifests as a pruritic red, crusted, sharply demarcated, maplike area, occurring usually on the labia majora. It may be accompanied by a palpable submucosal thickening or tumor. The diagnostic microscopic feature of this lesion is the presence of large tumor cells lying singly

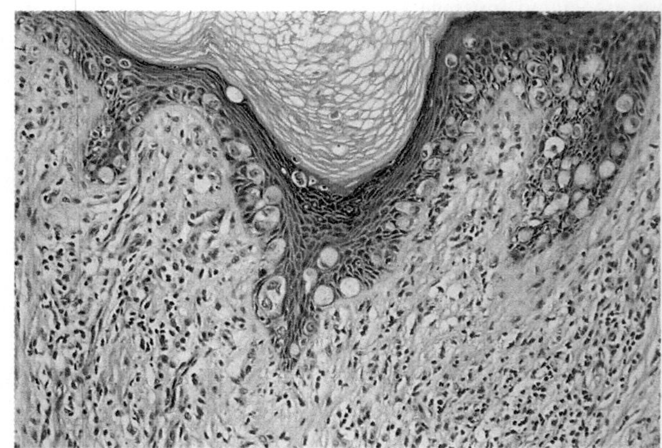

Figure 24–12

Paget disease of the vulva with a cluster of large clear tumor cells within the squamous epithelium.

or in small clusters within the epidermis and its appendages. These cells are distinguished by a clear separation ("halo") from the surrounding epithelial cells (Fig. 24–12) and a finely granular cytoplasm containing periodic acid–Schiff stain–, Alcian blue–, or mucicarmine-positive mucopolysaccharide. Ultrastructurally, Paget cells display apocrine, eccrine, and keratinocyte differentiation and presumably arise from primitive epithelial progenitor cells.

In contrast to Paget disease of the nipple, in which 100% of patients show an underlying ductal breast carcinoma, vulvar lesions are most frequently confined to the epidermis of the skin and adjacent hair follicles and sweat glands. The prognosis of Paget disease is poor in the uncommon cases with associated carcinoma, but intraepidermal Paget disease may persist for many years, even decades, without the development of invasion. However, because Paget cells often extend into skin appendages and may extend beyond the confines of the grossly visible lesion, they are prone to recurrence.

MALIGNANT MELANOMA

Melanomas of the vulva are rare, representing less than 5% of all vulvar cancers and 2% of all melanomas in women. Their peak incidence is in the sixth or seventh decade; they tend to have the same biologic and histologic characteristics as melanomas occurring elsewhere and are capable of widespread metastatic dissemination. The overall survival rate is less than 32%, presumably owing to delays in detection and a generally poor prognosis for mucosal melanomas. Prognosis is linked principally to depth of invasion, with greater than 60% mortality for lesions invading deeper than 1 mm.[25] Because it is initially confined to the epithelium, melanoma may resemble Paget disease, both grossly and histologically. It can usually be differentiated by its uniform reactivity, with immunoperoxidase techniques, with antibodies to S100 protein, absence of reactivity with antibodies to carcinoembryonic antigen, and lack of mucopolysaccharides.

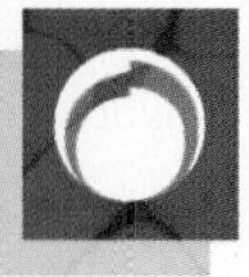

VAGINA

The vagina is a portion of the female genital tract that is remarkably free from primary disease. In the adult, inflammations often affect the vulva and perivulvar structures and spread to the cervix without significant involvement of the vagina. The major serious primary lesion of this structure is the uncommon primary carcinoma. The remaining entities can therefore be cited briefly.

CONGENITAL ANOMALIES

Atresia and total absence of the vagina are both extremely uncommon. The latter usually occurs only when there are severe malformations of the entire genital tract. Septate, or double, vagina is also an uncommon anomaly that arises from failure of total fusion of the müllerian ducts and accompanies double uterus (uterus didelphys).

Gartner duct cysts are relatively common lesions found along the lateral walls of the vagina and derived from wolffian duct rests. They are 1- to 2-cm fluid-filled cysts that occur submucosally. Other cysts include mucous cysts, which occur in the proximal vagina, are derived from müllerian epithelium, and often contain squamous metaplasia. Another müllerian-derived lesion (endometriosis, described later) may occur in the vagina and simulate a neoplasm.

PREMALIGNANT AND MALIGNANT NEOPLASMS

Most benign tumors of the vagina occur in reproductive-age women and consist of skeletal muscle (rhabdomyomas) or stromal (stromal polyps) tumors. The latter may contain cellular atypia but are benign, localized, and self-limited. Others include benign leiomyomas, hemangiomas, and rare mixed tumors. Clinically important malignant tumors in terms of frequency and biologic behavior are carcinoma and embryonal rhabdomyosarcoma (sarcoma botryoides).

Vaginal Intraepithelial Neoplasia and Squamous Cell Carcinoma

Primary carcinoma of the vagina is an extremely uncommon cancer (about 0.6 per 100,000 women yearly) accounting for about 1% of malignant neoplasms in the female genital tract, and of these, 95% are squamous cell carcinomas. Most are associated with HPV. The greatest risk factor is a previous carcinoma of the cervix or vulva; 1% to 2% of patients with an invasive cervical carcinoma eventually develop a vaginal squamous carcinoma.

MORPHOLOGY. Most often the tumor affects the upper posterior vagina, particularly along the posterior wall at the junction with the ectocervix. It begins as a focus of epithelial thickening, often in association with dysplastic changes, progressing to a plaquelike mass that extends centrifugally and invades, by direct continuity, the cervix and perivaginal structures. The lesions in the lower two thirds metastasize to the inguinal nodes, whereas upper lesions tend to involve the regional iliac nodes.

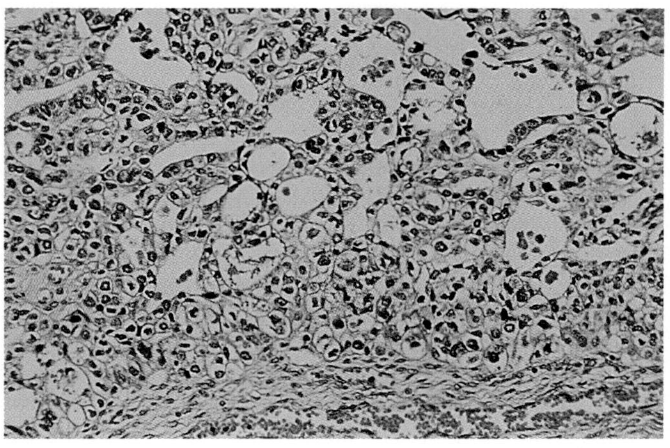

Figure 24–13

Clear cell adenocarcinoma showing vacuolated tumor cells in clusters and forming glands.

These tumors first come to the patient's attention by the appearance of irregular spotting or the development of a frank vaginal discharge (leukorrhea). At other times, they remain totally silent and become clinically manifest only with the onset of urinary or rectal fistulas.

Adenocarcinoma

Adenocarcinomas are rare but have received attention because of the increased frequency of clear cell adenocarcinomas in young women whose mothers had been treated with diethylstilbestrol (DES) during pregnancy (for a threatened abortion).[26] Fortunately, less than 0.14% of such DES-exposed young women develop adenocarcinoma. These tumors are usually discovered between the ages of 15 and 20 years and are often composed of vacuolated, glycogen-containing cells, hence the term clear cell carcinoma (Fig. 24–13).

MORPHOLOGY. The tumors are most often located on the anterior wall of the vagina, usually in the upper third, and vary in size from 0.2 to 10 cm in greatest diameter. These cancers can also arise in the cervix. A probable precursor of the tumor is *vaginal adenosis,* a condition in which glandular columnar epithelium of müllerian type either appears beneath the squamous epithelium or replaces it.[27] Adenosis presents clinically as red, granular foci contrasting with the normal pale pink, opaque vaginal mucosa. On microscopic examination, the glandular epithelium may be either mucus secreting, resembling endocervical mucosa, or so-called tuboendometrial, often containing cilia. Adenosis has been reported in 35% to 90% of the offspring of estrogen-treated mothers, but as mentioned earlier, malignant transformation is extremely rare.

Because of its insidious, invasive growth, vaginal cancer (squamous and adenocarcinomatous) is difficult to cure. Thus, early detection by careful follow-up is mandatory in DES-exposed women. Surgery and irradiation have successfully eradicated DES-related tumors in up to 80% of patients. Extension of cervical carcinoma to the vagina is much more common than are primary malignant neoplasms of the vagina. Accordingly, before a diagnosis of primary vaginal carcinoma can be made, a preexisting cervical lesion must be ruled out.

Embryonal Rhabdomyosarcoma

Also called *sarcoma botryoides,* this is an interesting but uncommon vaginal tumor most frequently found in infants and in children younger than 5 years. The tumor consists predominantly of malignant embryonal rhabdomyoblasts and is thus a type of rhabdomyosarcoma.[28]

MORPHOLOGY. These tumors tend to grow as polypoid, rounded, bulky masses that sometimes fill and project out of the vagina; they have the appearance and consistency of grapelike clusters (hence the designation botryoides, meaning grapelike) (Fig. 24–14). On histologic examination, the tumor cells are small and have oval nuclei, with small protrusions of cytoplasm from one end, so they resemble a tennis racket. Striations can

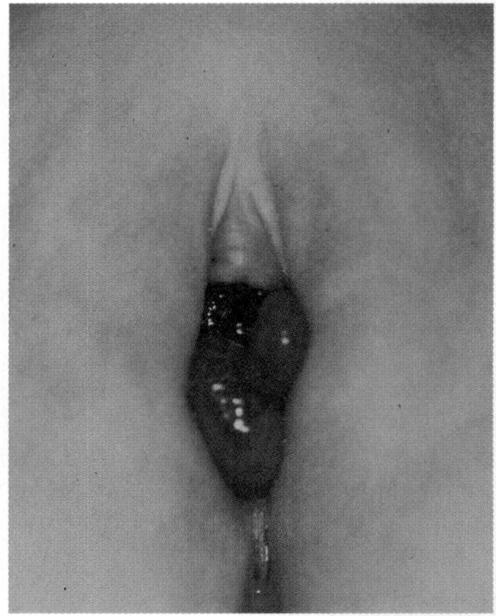

Figure 24–14

Sarcoma botryoides (embryonal rhabdomyosarcoma) of the vagina appearing as a polypoid mass protruding from the vagina. (Courtesy of Dr. Michael Donovan, Children's Hospital, Boston.)

rarely be seen within the cytoplasm. Beneath the vaginal epithelium, the tumor cells are crowded in a so-called cambium layer; but in the deep regions, they lie within a loose fibromyxomatous stroma that is edematous and may contain many inflammatory cells. For this reason, the lesions can be mistaken for benign inflammatory polyps, leading to unfortunate delays in diagnosis and treatment. These tumors tend to invade locally and cause death by penetration into the peritoneal cavity or by obstruction of the urinary tract.

Conservative surgery, coupled with chemotherapy, appears to offer the best results in cases diagnosed sufficiently early.[29]

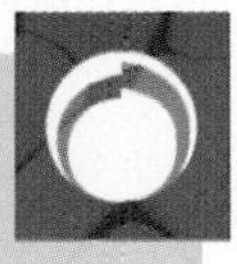

CERVIX

The cervix is both a sentinel for potentially serious upper genital tract infections and a target for viral and other carcinogens, which may lead to invasive carcinoma. Infection constitutes one of the most common clinical complaints in gynecologic practice and frequently vexes both patient and clinician. The potential threat of cancer, however, is central to Papanicolaou smear screening programs and histologic interpretation of biopsy specimens by the pathologist. Worldwide, cervical carcinoma alone is responsible for about 5% of all cancer deaths in women.

INFLAMMATIONS

Acute and Chronic Cervicitis

At the onset of menarche, the production of estrogens by the ovary stimulates maturation (glycogen uptake) of cervical and vaginal squamous mucosa. As these cells are shed, the glycogen provides a substrate for endogenous vaginal aerobes and anaerobes, streptococci, enterococci, *Escherichia coli,* and staphylococci. The bacterial growth produces a drop in vaginal pH. The exposed endocervix is sensitive to these changes in chemical environment and bacterial flora and responds by undergoing a transformation from columnar to squamous epithelium, as detailed previously. The process of transformation is also hastened by trauma and other infections occurring in the reproductive years. As the squamous epithelium overgrows and obliterates the surface columnar papillae, it covers and obstructs crypt openings, with the accumulation of mucus in deeper crypts (glands) to form mucous (nabothian) cysts. This process is invariably associated with an inflammatory infiltrate composed of a mixture of polymorphonuclear leukocytes and mononuclear cells, and if the inflammation is severe, it may be associated with loss of the epithelial lining (erosion or ulceration) and epithelial repair (reparative atypia or dysplasia of repair). All of these components characterize what is known as *chronic cervicitis* (Fig. 24–15).

Some degree of cervical inflammation may be found in virtually all multiparous and in many nulliparous adult women, and it is usually of little clinical consequence.

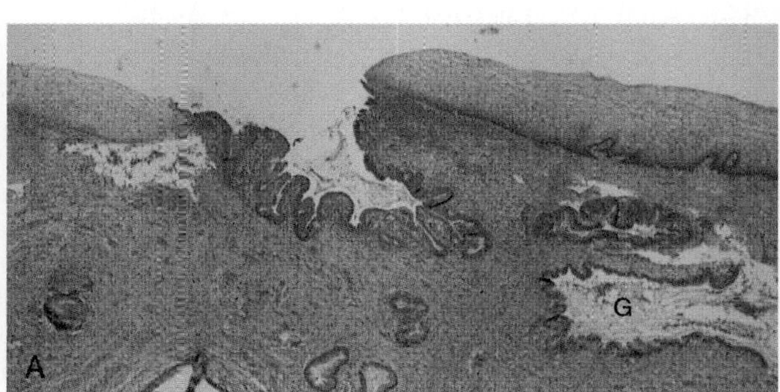

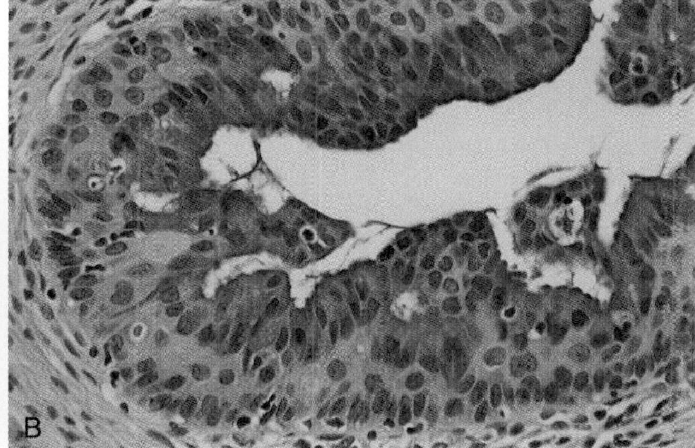

Figure 24–15

A, Low-power histology of chronic cervicitis and the cervical transformation zone. Mature squamous epithelium (epidermidalization) has replaced the columnar epithelium on the surface and covers the glands (G). An inflammatory infiltrate is present in the submucosa. *B*, Immature squamous metaplasia developing in an endocervical gland. Layers of immature squamous cells displace columnar cells toward the gland lumen.

Principal concerns include the potential presence of organisms, which may be clinically important. Specific infections by gonococci, chlamydiae, mycoplasmas, and herpesvirus (mostly type 2) may produce significant acute or chronic cervicitis and should be identified for their relevance to upper genital tract disease, pregnancy complications, or sexual transmission.

MORPHOLOGY. The pathologic correlates of acute and chronic cervicitis include epithelial spongiosis (intercellular edema), submucosal edema, and a combination of epithelial and stromal changes. Acute cervicitis includes acute inflammatory cells, erosion, and reactive or reparative epithelial change. Chronic cervicitis includes inflammation, usually mononuclear, with lymphocytes, macrophages, and plasma cells. Necrosis and granulation tissue may also be present. Although the inflammation alone is not specific, some patterns are associated with certain organisms. Herpesvirus is most strongly associated with epithelial ulcers (often with intranuclear inclusions in epithelial cells) and a lymphocytic infiltrate, and *C. trachomatis* with lymphoid germinal centers and a prominent plasmacytic infiltrate[30] (Fig. 24–16). Epithelial spongiosis is associated with *T. vaginalis* infection.[31]

All the aforementioned changes are more pronounced in patients with clinical symptoms (mucopurulent cervicitis) or in whom specific organisms can be identified. These changes, however, may be observed in culture-negative or asymptomatic women, underscoring the combined importance of culture, clinical evaluation, and Papanicolaou smear examination. Severe reparative changes may shed atypical-appearing squamous cells that mimic precancerous lesions because cells undergoing repair are depleted of their normal content of glycogen and may contain nuclear atypia.

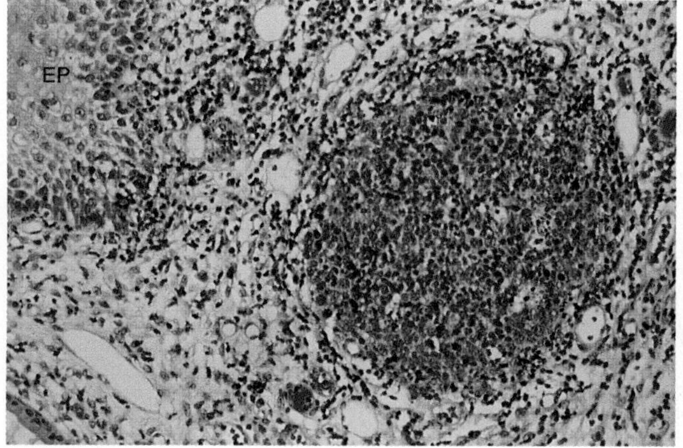

Figure 24–16

Severe chronic cervicitis with prominent lymphoid follicles (follicular cervicitis), typically associated with chlamydial infection. The epithelium (EP) is in the upper left.

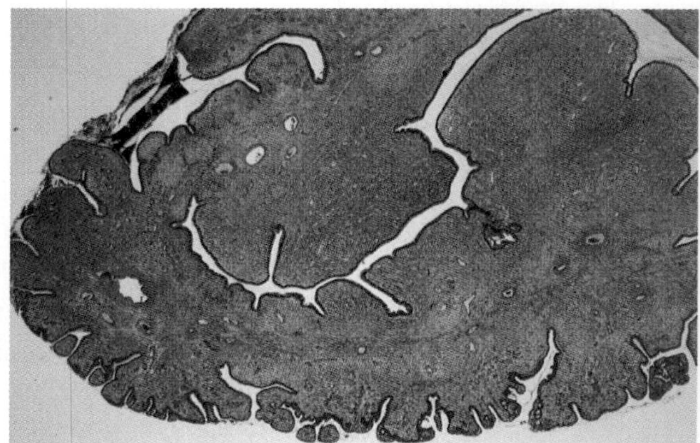

Figure 24–17

Endocervical polyp composed of a dense fibrous stroma covered with endocervical columnar epithelium.

Endocervical Polyps

Endocervical polyps are relatively innocuous, inflammatory tumors that occur in 2% to 5% of adult women. Perhaps the major significance of polyps lies in their production of irregular vaginal "spotting" or bleeding that arouses suspicion of some more ominous lesion. Most polyps arise within the endocervical canal and vary from small and sessile to large, 5-cm masses that may protrude through the cervical os. All are soft, almost mucoid, and are composed of a loose fibromyxomatous stroma harboring dilated, mucus-secreting endocervical glands often accompanied by inflammation and squamous metaplasia (Fig. 24–17). In almost all instances, simple curettage or surgical excision effects a cure.

INTRAEPITHELIAL AND INVASIVE SQUAMOUS NEOPLASIA

No form of cancer better documents the remarkable effects of prevention, early diagnosis, and curative therapy on the mortality rate than does cancer of the cervix. Fifty years ago, carcinoma of the cervix was the leading cause of cancer deaths in women in the United States, but the death rate has declined by two thirds to its present rank as the eighth source of cancer mortality, causing about 4500 deaths annually (behind lung, breast, colon, pancreas, ovary, lymph nodes, and blood). In sharp contrast to this reduced mortality, the detection frequency of early cancers and precancerous conditions is high. Much credit for these dramatic gains belongs to the effectiveness of the Papanicolaou cytologic test in detecting cervical precancers and to the accessibility of the cervix to colposcopy and biopsy.

There are an estimated 13,000 cases of new invasive cancer annually and nearly 1 million precancerous conditions (squamous intraepithelial lesions) of varying grade. Thus, it is evident that Papanicolaou smear screening has increased the detection of potential curable cancers and the detection and eradication of preinvasive lesions, some of which would progress to cancer if not discovered.

Pathogenesis. To understand the pathogenesis of cervical cancer, it is important to understand the components involved in its development, which have been identified from a series of clinical, epidemiologic, pathologic, and molecular studies. Epidemiologic data have long implicated a sexually transmitted agent specifically on the basis of the risk factors for cervical cancer, which include

- Early age at first intercourse
- Multiple sexual partners
- A male partner with multiple previous sexual partners

All other risk factors are subordinate to these three influences, primarily multiple sexual partners. Potential risk factors that remain poorly understood include oral contraceptive use, cigarette smoking, parity, family history, associated genital infections, and lack of circumcision in the male sexual partner.[32,33]

Concerning sexually transmitted agents, HPV is currently considered an important factor in cervical oncogenesis. As noted earlier, this virus is the known cause of the sexually transmitted vulvar condyloma acuminatum and has been isolated from vulvar and vaginal squamous cell carcinomas; it is also suspected of being an oncogenic agent in a variety of other squamous tumors or proliferative lesions of skin and mucous membranes, as detailed in Chapter 8.[34]

There is mounting evidence linking HPV to cancer in general and cervical cancer in particular. First, HPV DNA is detected by hybridization techniques in approximately 85% of cervical cancers and in approximately 90% of cervical condylomata and precancerous lesions.[34] Second, specific HPV types are associated with cervical cancer (high risk) versus condylomata (low risk); low-risk types include types 6, 11, 42, and 44, and high-risk types include 16, 18, 31, 33, and others (Fig. 24–18*A*).[35] Third, in vitro studies indicate that the high-risk HPV types have the capability to transform cells in culture (Chapter 8), and this ability is linked to specific viral oncogenes (*E6* and *E7* genes), which differ in sequence between the high-risk and low-risk HPV types. Introduction of these nucleic acids into cultured keratinocytes produces morphologic changes nearly identical to precancerous changes, and under certain circumstances, these cells may form squamous tumors when they are injected into mice. Fourth, the physical state of the virus differs in cancers, being covalently linked (integrated) with the host genomic DNA. This is in contrast to free (episomal) viral DNA in condylomata and most precancerous lesions.[34,36] Fifth, the E6 oncoprotein of HPV types 16 and 18 (but not low-risk type 11) binds to the tumor-suppressor gene *p53* and accelerates its proteolytic degradation; the E7 protein binds to the retinoblastoma gene (*RB*) and displaces transcription factors normally sequestered by *RB*. Both of these properties affect cell cycle regulation (Chapters 4 and 8). Sixth, certain chromosome abnormalities, including amplification of 3q, have been associated with cancers containing specific (HPV-16) papillomaviruses.[37]

The evidence does not implicate HPV as the only factor. A high percentage of young women are infected with one or more HPV types during their reproductive years, and only a few develop cancer. Other cocarcinogens, the immune status of the individual, nutrition, and many other factors influence whether the HPV infection remains subclinical (latent), turns into a precancer, or eventually progresses to cancer. In addition, some cervical cancers are associated with p53 mutations, implying other modes of cancer development, including host gene mutations.[38] Figure 24–18 presents one attempt to explain the role of HPV in cervical carcinogenesis and its impact on the population in the United States.

Cervical Intraepithelial Neoplasia

The reason that Papanicolaou smear screening is so effective in preventing cervical cancer is that the majority of cancers are preceded by a precancerous lesion. This lesion may exist in the noninvasive stage for as long as 20 years and shed abnormal cells that can be detected on cytologic examination.[39] These precancerous changes should be viewed with the following in mind: (1) they represent a continuum of morphologic change with relatively indistinct boundaries; (2) they will not invariably progress to cancer and may spontaneously regress, with the risk of persisting or progressing to cancer increasing with the severity of the precancerous change; (3) they are associated with papillomaviruses, and high-risk HPV types are found in increasing frequency in the higher grade precursors.[40,41]

Cervical precancers have been classified in a variety of ways. The oldest system is the dysplasia/carcinoma in situ system with mild dysplasia on one end and severe dysplasia/carcinoma in situ on the other. Another is the cervical intraepithelial neoplasia (CIN) classification, with mild dysplasias termed CIN grade I and carcinoma in situ lesions termed CIN III.[40] Still another reduces these entities to two, terming them low-grade and high-grade intraepithelial lesions.[40] Because these systems describe noninvasive lesions of indeterminate biology that are usually easily treated, none of these classifications is indispensable to clinical management or immune to revision. In this chapter, we refer to lesions by the CIN terminology.[40]

MORPHOLOGY. Figures 24–19 and 24–20 illustrate a spectrum of morphologic alterations that range from normal to the highest grade precancer.

On the extreme low end of the spectrum are lesions that are indistinguishable histologically from condylomata acuminata and may be either raised (acuminatum) or macular (flat condyloma) in appearance (Figs. 24–19*A* and 24–20). These lesions exhibit koilocytotic atypia (viral cytopathic effect) with few alterations in the other cells in the epithelium and fall within the range of CIN I. They often contain abundant papillomavirus nucleic

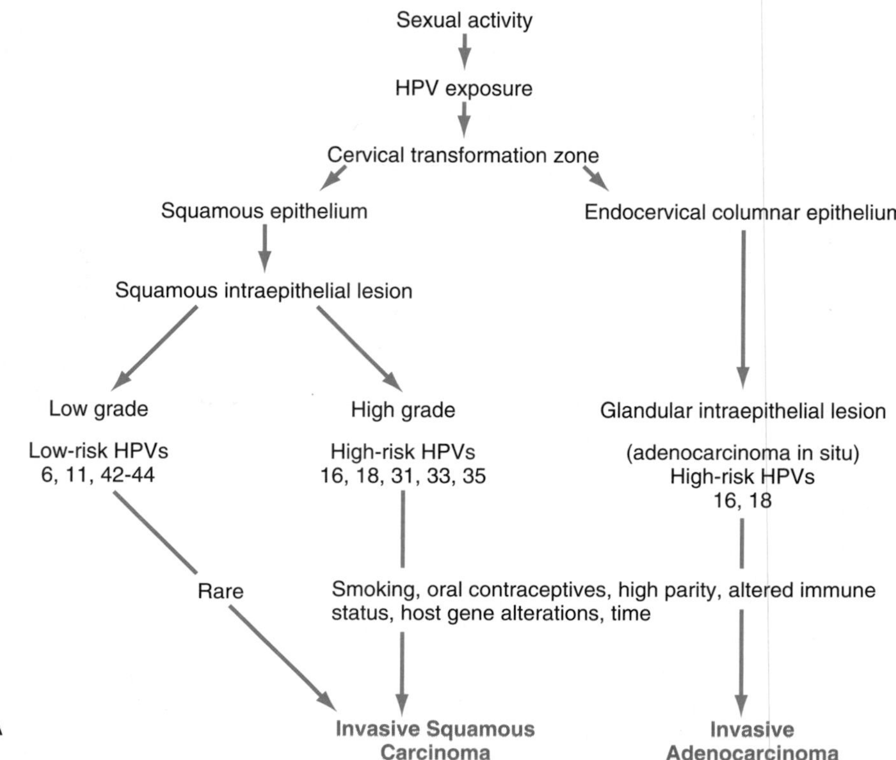

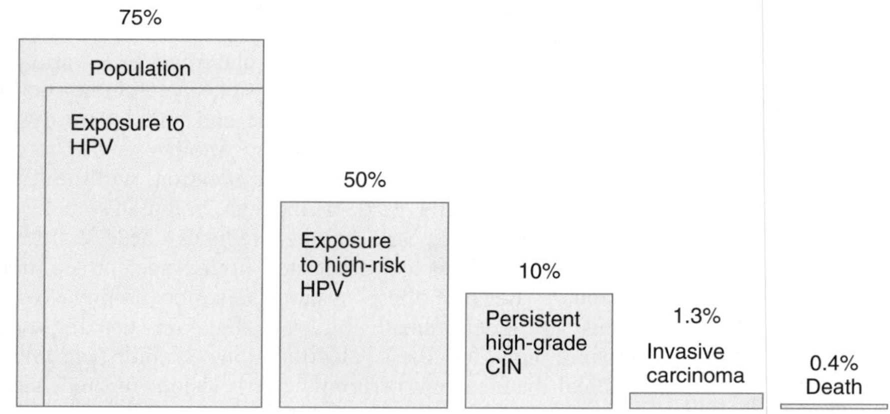

Figure 24–18 ■

A, Postulated steps in the pathogenesis of cervical neoplasia. Conditions influencing progression are listed at the lower center of the diagram. *B*, Approximate lifetime risks of acquiring HPV infection (*left*) and dying of cervical cancer (*right*). The intermediate steps include risks of infection with high-risk HPV types, development of advanced cervical intraepithelial neoplasia (CIN), and progression to invasive carcinoma.

acids (Fig. 24–19*B*). These changes correlate strongly (but not invariably) with low-risk HPV types and genetically diploid or polyploid cell populations.

The next change in the spectrum consists of the appearance of atypical cells in the lower layers of the squamous epithelium but nonetheless with persistent (but abnormal) differentiation toward the prickle and keratinizing cell layers. The atypical cells show changes in nucleocytoplasmic ratio; variation in nuclear size (anisokaryosis); loss of polarity; increased mitotic figures, including abnormal mitoses; and hyperchromasia—in other words, they take on some of the characteristics of malignant cells. These lesions fall within the range of CIN II (Fig. 24–20). These features have been associated with aneuploid cell populations and correlate strongly with high-risk HPV types, probably reflecting early changes associated with the viral oncogenes of these viruses. As the spectrum evolves, there is progressive loss of differentiation with involvement of more and more layers of the epithelium, until it is totally replaced by immature atypical cells, exhibiting no surface differentiation

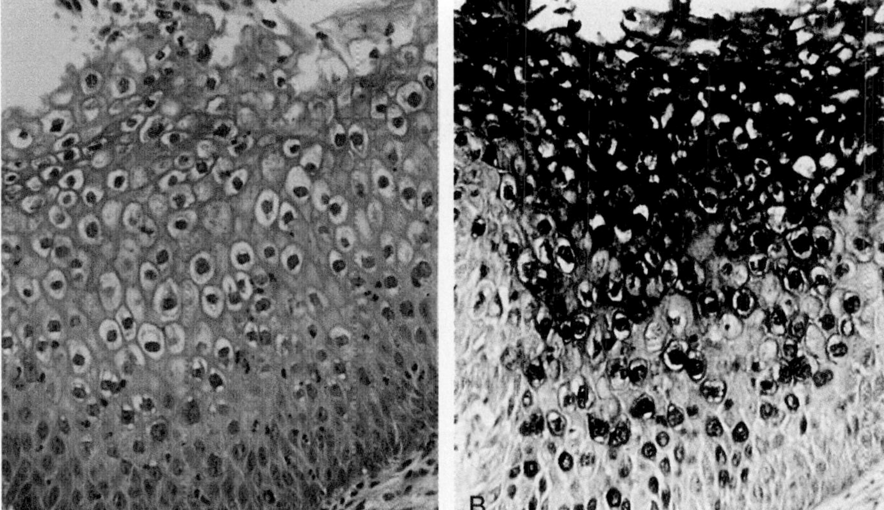

Figure 24–19

A, Histology of a cervical condyloma illustrating the prominent koilocytotic atypia in the upper epithelial cells, as evidenced by the prominent perinuclear halos. *B*, Nucleic acid in situ hybridization of the same lesion for HPV nucleic acids. The blue staining denotes HPV DNA, which is typically most abundant in the koilocytes.

(CIN III) (Fig. 24–20).[41,42] The cellular changes on Papanicolaou smear that correspond to this histologic spectrum are illustrated in Figure 24–21.

CIN almost always begins at the squamocolumnar junction, in the transformation zone. The lowest grade CIN lesions, including condylomata, most likely do not progress, whereas lesions containing greater degrees of cellular atypia are at greater risk. Not all lesions begin as condylomata or as CIN I, and they may enter at any point in the spectrum, depending on the associated HPV type and other host factors. The rates of progression are by no means uniform, and although HPV type is a potential predictor of lesion behavior it is difficult to predict the outcome in an individual patient. These findings underscore that risk of cancer is conferred only in part by HPV type and depends on other carcinogens or genetic alterations that bring about the evolution of a precancer. Predictably, lesions that have completely evolved (CIN III) constitute the greatest risk. CIN III is most frequently associated with invasive cancer when the latter is identified. Progression to invasive carcinoma, when it occurs, may develop in a few months to more than 20 years.[43]

Squamous Cell Carcinoma

Squamous cell carcinoma may occur at any age from the second decade of life to senility. The peak incidence is occurring at an increasingly younger age: 40 to 45 years for invasive cancer and about 30 years for high-grade pre-

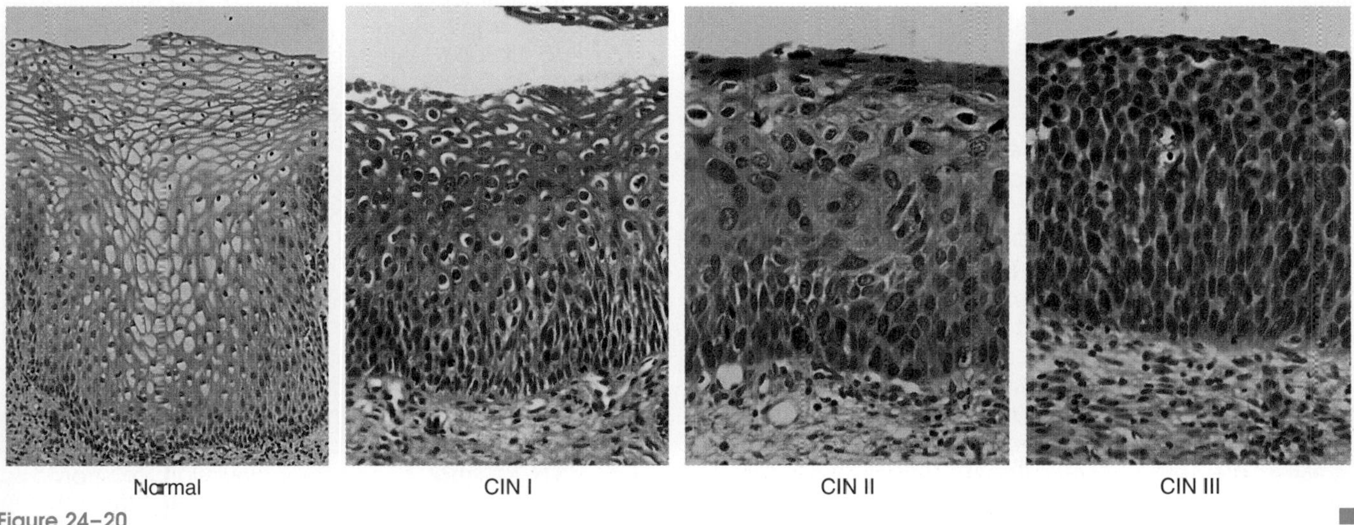

Figure 24–20

Spectrum of cervical intraepithelial neoplasia: normal squamous epithelium for comparison; CIN I with koilocytotic atypia; CIN II with progressive atypia in all layers of the epithelium; CIN III, (carcinoma in situ) with diffuse atypia and loss of maturation.

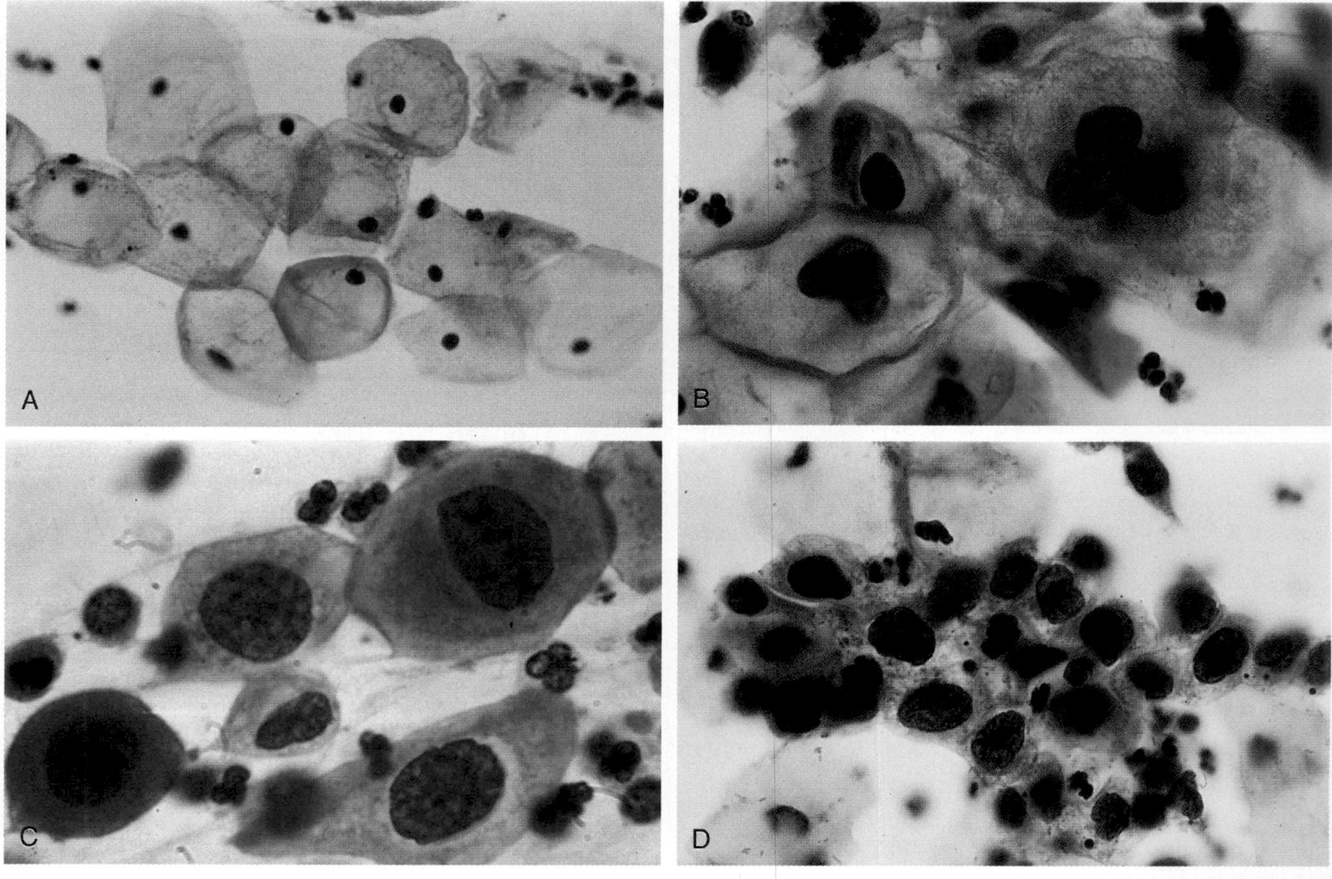

Figure 24–21

The cytology of cervical intraepithelial neoplasia as seen on the Papanicolaou smear. *A*, Normal exfoliated superficial squamous epithelial cells. *B*, CIN I. *C*, CIN II. *D*, CIN III. Note the reduction in cytoplasm and the increase in the nucleus to cytoplasm ratio, which occurs as the grade of the lesion increases. This reflects the progressive loss of cellular differentiation on the surface of the lesions from which these cells are exfoliated (see Figure 24–20). (Courtesy of Dr. Edmund S. Cibas, Department of Pathology, Brigham & Women's Hospital, Boston.)

cancers. This represents the combination of earlier onset of sexual activity (i.e., earlier acquisition of HPV infection) and active Papanicolaou smear screening programs in the United States, which detect either cancers or precancerous lesions at an earlier point in life.

MORPHOLOGY. Invasive cervical carcinoma manifests in three somewhat distinctive patterns: **fungating (or exophytic), ulcerating, and infiltrative cancer.** The most common variant is the fungating tumor, which produces an obviously neoplastic mass that projects above the surrounding mucosa (Fig. 24–22*A*). Advanced cervical carcinoma extends by direct continuity to involve every contiguous structure, including the peritoneum, urinary bladder, ureters, rectum, and vagina. Local and distant lymph nodes are also involved. Distant metastasis occurs to the liver, lungs, bone marrow, and other structures.

On histologic examination, about 95% of squamous carcinomas are composed of relatively **large cells,** either **keratinizing** (well-differentiated) or **nonkeratinizing** (moderately differentiated) patterns. A small subset of tumors (less than 5%) are poorly differentiated small cell squamous or, more rarely, small cell undifferentiated carcinomas **(neuroendocrine or oat cell carcinomas).** The latter closely resemble oat cell carcinomas of lung and have an unusually poor prognosis owing to early spread by lymphatics and systemic spread. These tumors are also frequently associated with a specific high-risk HPV, type 18.[44]

Cervical cancer is staged as follows:

Stage 0. Carcinoma in situ (CIN III)
Stage I. Carcinoma confined to the cervix
Ia. Preclinical carcinoma, that is, diagnosed only by microscopy but showing
Ia1. Minimal microscopic invasion of stroma (minimally invasive carcinoma) (Fig. 24–22*B*)
Ia2. Microscopic invasion of stroma of less than 5 mm in depth (microinvasive carcinoma)

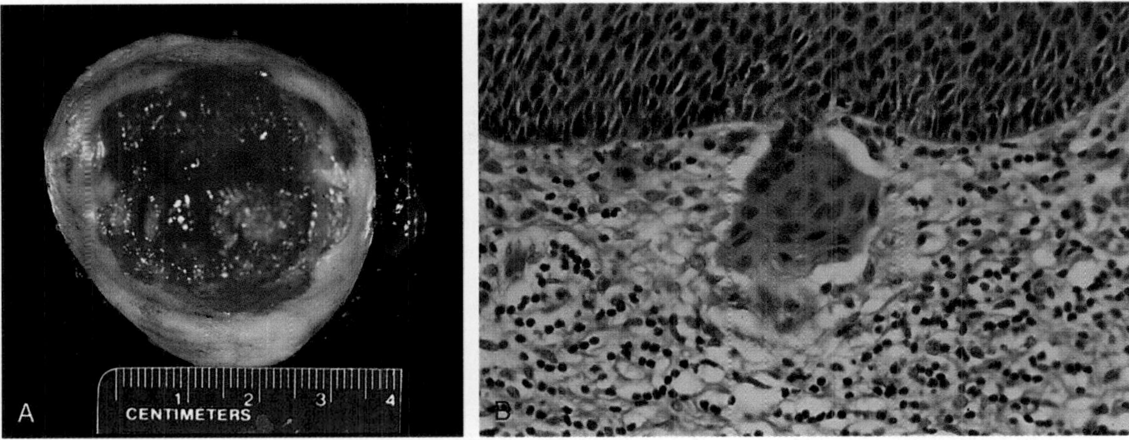

Figure 24–22

The spectrum of invasive cervical cancer. *A*, Carcinoma of the cervix, well advanced. *B*, Early stromal invasion occurring in a cervical intraepithelial neoplasm.

Ib. Histologically invasive carcinoma of the cervix that is greater than stage Ia2

Stage II. Carcinoma extends beyond the cervix but not onto the pelvic wall. Carcinoma involves the vagina but not the lower third.

Stage III. Carcinoma has extended onto pelvic wall. On rectal examination, there is no cancer-free space between the tumor and the pelvic wall. The tumor involves the lower third of the vagina.

Stage IV. Carcinoma has extended beyond the true pelvis or has involved the mucosa of the bladder or rectum. This stage obviously includes those with metastatic dissemination.

Ten per cent to 25% of cervical carcinomas constitute **adenocarcinomas, adenosquamous carcinomas, undifferentiated carcinomas,** or other rare histologic types. The adenocarcinomas presumably arise in the endocervical glands. They look grossly and behave like the squamous cell lesions and are frequently associated with HPV type 18 but arise in a slightly older age group.[45] The **adenosquamous carcinomas** have mixed glandular and squamous patterns and are thought to arise from the reserve cells in the basal layers of the endocervical epithelium. They tend to have a less favorable prognosis than does squamous cell carcinoma of similar stage. **Clear cell adenocarcinomas** of the cervix in DES-exposed women are similar to those occurring in the vagina, described earlier.

Clinical Course. It is apparent from the preceding discussion that cancer of the cervix and its precursors evolve slowly in the course of many years. During this interval, the only sign of disease may be the shedding of abnormal cells from the cervix. For these reasons, it is generally acknowledged that periodic Papanicolaou smears should be performed on all women after they become sexually active. Reduction in cervical cancer deaths would theoretically be greatest if all women were screened and if the accuracy of detecting Papanicolaou smear abnormalities was maximized.

Cytologic examination merely detects the possible presence of a cervical precancer or cancer; it does not make an absolute diagnosis, which requires histologic evaluation of appropriate biopsy specimens. Identification of abnormalities is facilitated by colposcopic examination of the cervix, in which CIN lesions are characterized by white patches on the cervix after the application of acetic acid.[39] In addition, distinct vascular mosaic or punctuation patterns can be appreciated. Highly abnormal vascular patterns regularly accompany invasive cervical cancer. Ultimately, when these cancers become clinically overt, they usually produce irregular vaginal bleeding, leukorrhea, bleeding or pain on coitus, and dysuria.

Modes of treatment of squamous neoplasia of the cervix depend on the stage of the neoplasm; treatment of precursors includes Papanicolaou smear follow-up (for mild lesions), cryotherapy, laser, wire loop excision, and cone biopsy. Invasive cancers usually result in hysterectomy and, for advanced lesions, radiation. Approximately 1 in 500 patients with a treated CIN III eventually develops an invasive cancer. The prognosis and survival for invasive carcinomas depend largely on the stage at which cancer is first discovered.

With current methods of treatment, there is a 5-year survival rate of about 80% to 90% with stage I, 75% with stage II, 35% with stage III, and 10% to 15% with stage IV disease. Most patients with stage IV cancer die as a consequence of local extension of the tumor (e.g., into and about the urinary bladder and ureters, leading to ureteral obstruction, pyelonephritis, and uremia) rather than distant metastases.

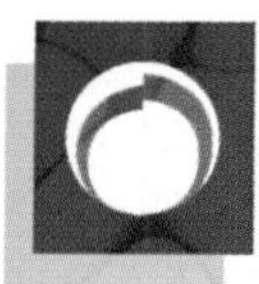

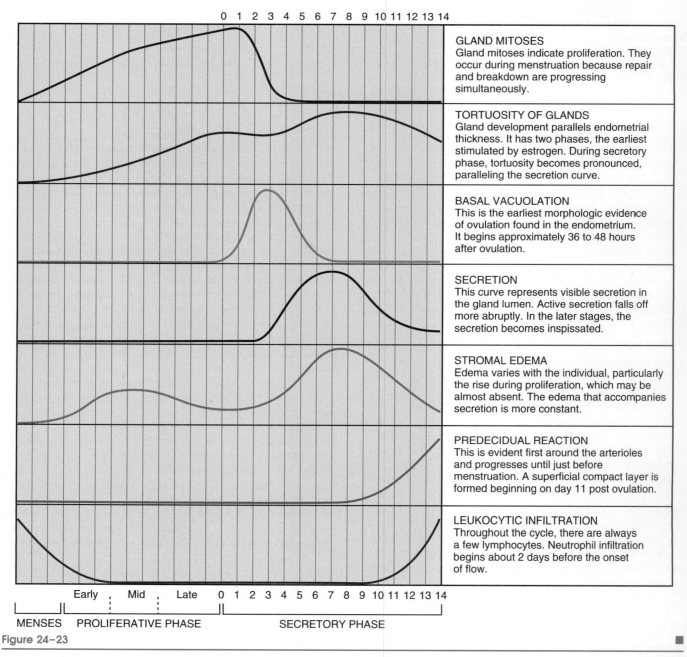

BODY OF UTERUS AND ENDOMETRIUM

The uterus, stimulated continually by hormones, denuded monthly of its endometrial mucosa, and inhabited periodically by fetuses, is subject to a variety of disorders, the most common of which result from endocrine imbalances, complications of pregnancy, and neoplastic proliferation. Together with the lesions that affect the cervix, the lesions of the corpus of the uterus and the endometrium account for the great preponderance of gynecologic practices.

0 1 2 3 4 5 6 7 8 9 10 11 12 13 14

GLAND MITOSES
Gland mitoses indicate proliferation. They occur during menstruation because repair and breakdown are progressing simultaneously.

TORTUOSITY OF GLANDS
Gland development parallels endometrial thickness. It has two phases, the earliest stimulated by estrogen. During secretory phase, tortuosity becomes pronounced, paralleling the secretion curve.

BASAL VACUOLATION
This is the earliest morphologic evidence of ovulation found in the endometrium. It begins approximately 36 to 48 hours after ovulation.

SECRETION
This curve represents visible secretion in the gland lumen. Active secretion falls off more abruptly. In the later stages, the secretion becomes inspissated.

STROMAL EDEMA
Edema varies with the individual, particularly the rise during proliferation, which may be almost absent. The edema that accompanies secretion is more constant.

PREDECIDUAL REACTION
This is evident first around the arterioles and progresses until just before menstruation. A superficial compact layer is formed beginning on day 11 post ovulation.

LEUKOCYTIC INFILTRATION
Throughout the cycle, there are always a few lymphocytes. Neutrophil infiltration begins about 2 days before the onset of flow.

Early | Mid | Late 0 1 2 3 4 5 6 7 8 9 10 11 12 13 14

MENSES PROLIFERATIVE PHASE SECRETORY PHASE

Figure 24–23

Approximate quantitative changes in seven morphologic criteria found to be most useful in dating human endometrium. (Modified from Noyes RW: Normal phases of the endometrium. In Norris HJ, et al (eds): The Uterus. Baltimore, Williams & Wilkins, 1973.)

ENDOMETRIAL HISTOLOGY IN THE MENSTRUAL CYCLE

"Dating" the endometrium by its histologic appearance is helpful clinically to assess hormonal status, document ovulation, and determine causes of endometrial bleeding and infertility. We can begin with the shedding of the upper one half to two thirds of the endometrium during the menstrual period (Fig. 24–23). The basal third does not respond to the ovarian steroids and is retained at the conclusion of the menstrual flow. From the basal third of this preovulatory proliferative phase of the cycle, there is extremely rapid growth of both glands and stroma (proliferative phase). The glands are straight, tubular structures lined by regular, tall, pseudostratified columnar cells. Mitotic figures are numerous, and there is no evidence of mucus secretion or vacuolation (Fig. 24–24*A*). The endometrial stroma is composed of thickly compacted spindle cells that have scant cytoplasm but abundant mitotic activity.

At the time of ovulation, the endometrium slows in its growth, and it ceases apparent mitotic activity within days immediately after ovulation. The postovulatory endometrium is initially marked by basal secretory vacuoles beneath the nuclei in the glandular epithelium (Fig. 24–24*B*). This secretory activity is most prominent during the third week of the menstrual cycle, when the basal vacuoles progressively push past the nuclei. By the fourth week, the secretions are discharged into the gland lumens. When secretion is maximal, between 18 and 24 days, the glands are dilated. By the fourth week, the glands are tortuous, producing a serrated appearance when they are cut in their long axis (Fig. 24–5). This serrated or "saw-toothed" appearance is accentuated by secretory exhaustion and shrinking of the glands.

The stromal changes in late secretory phase are important for dating the endometrium and consist of the development of prominent spiral arterioles by days 21 to 22. A considerable increase in ground substance and edema between the stromal cells occurs (Fig. 24–24*C*) and is followed in days 23 to 24 by stromal cell hypertrophy with accumulation of cytoplasmic eosinophilia (predecidual change) and resurgence of stromal mitoses (Fig. 24–24*D*). Predecidual changes spread throughout the functionalis (the hormonally responsive upper zone) during days 24 to 28 and are accompanied by scattered neutrophils and occasional lymphocytes (Fig. 24–24*E*), which here do not imply inflammation. This is followed by disintegration of the functionalis and escape of blood into the stroma, which marks the beginning of menstrual shedding (Fig. 24–24*F*).

The proliferative phase exhibits mitotic activity in glandular and stromal cells; ovulation is confirmed by prominent basal vacuolation of glandular epithelial cells, secretory exhaustion, or predecidual changes. Obviously, ovulation cannot be confirmed during the proliferative phase or in the late stages of endometrial shedding when only the basalis is present.

FUNCTIONAL ENDOMETRIAL DISORDERS (DYSFUNCTIONAL UTERINE BLEEDING)

During active reproductive life, the endometrium is constantly engaged in the dynamics of shedding and regrowth. It is controlled by the rise and fall of pituitary and ovarian hormones, and this control is executed by proper timing of hormonal release in both absolute and relative amounts. Alterations in this fine-tuning mechanism may result in a spectrum of disturbances, including atrophy, abnormal proliferative or secretory patterns, and hyperplasia.[46]

By far the most common problem is the occurrence of excessive bleeding during or between menstrual periods. The causes of abnormal bleeding from the uterus are many and vary among women of different age groups (Table 24–2). In some instances, bleeding is the result of a well-defined organic lesion, such as submucosal leiomyoma, endometrial polyp, or adenocarcinoma; however, the largest single group is so-called dysfunctional uterine bleeding. This is defined as abnormal bleeding in the presence of a functional disturbance rather than an organic lesion of the endometrium or uterus.[46]

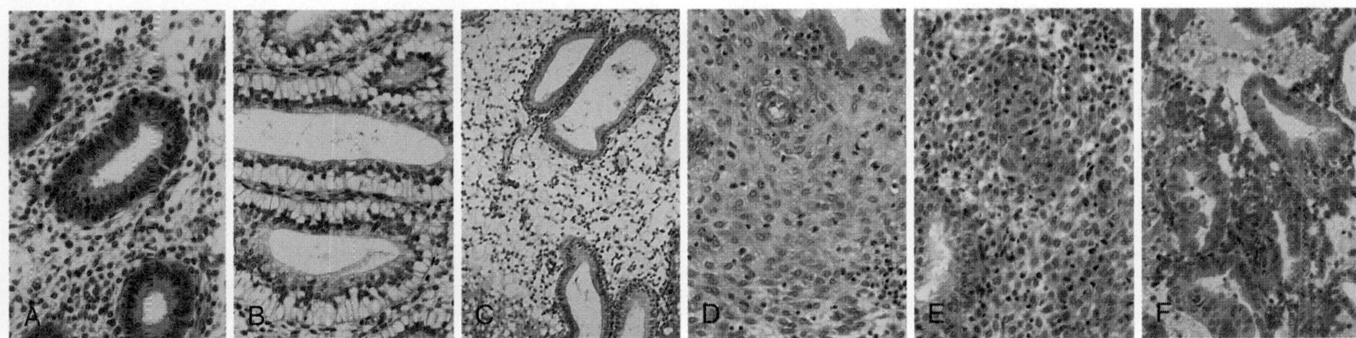

Figure 24–24

Histopathology of the menstrual cycle, including the proliferative phase with mitoses (*A*), the early secretory phase with subnuclear vacuoles (*B*) followed by secretory exhaustion (*C*), predecidual changes (*D*), stromal granulocytes (*E*), and stromal breakdown at the onset of menses (*F*) (see text).

Table 24–2. CAUSES OF ABNORMAL UTERINE BLEEDING BY AGE GROUP

Age Group	Causes
Prepuberty	Precocious puberty (hypothalamic, pituitary, or ovarian origin)
Adolescence	Anovulatory cycle
Reproductive age	Complications of pregnancy (abortion, trophoblastic disease, ectopic pregnancy) Organic lesions (leiomyoma, adenomyosis, polyps, endometrial hyperplasia, carcinoma) Anovulatory cycle Ovulatory dysfunctional bleeding (e.g., inadequate luteal phase)
Perimenopausal	Anovulatory cycle Irregular shedding Organic lesions (carcinoma, hyperplasia, polyps)
Postmenopausal	Organic lesions (carcinoma, hyperplasia, polyps) Endometrial atrophy

Anovulatory Cycle

In most instances, dysfunctional bleeding is due to the occurrence of an anovulatory cycle, which results in excessive and prolonged estrogenic stimulation without the development of the progestational phase that regularly follows ovulation. Less commonly, lack of ovulation is the result of (1) an endocrine disorder, such as thyroid disease, adrenal disease, or pituitary tumors; (2) a primary lesion of the ovary, such as a functioning ovarian tumor (granulosa-theca cell tumors) or polycystic ovaries (see section on ovaries); or (3) a generalized metabolic disturbance, such as marked obesity, severe malnutrition, or any chronic systemic disease. In most patients, however, anovulatory cycles are unexplainable, probably occurring because of subtle hormonal imbalances. Anovulatory cycles are most common at menarche and the perimenopausal period.

Failure of ovulation results in prolonged, excessive endometrial stimulation by estrogens. Under these circumstances, the endometrial glands undergo mild architectural changes, including cystic dilation (persistent proliferative endometrium). Unscheduled breakdown of the stroma may also occur ("anovulatory menstrual"), with no evidence of the endometrial secretory activity (Fig. 24–25). More severe consequences of anovulation are discussed under endometrial hyperplasia.

Inadequate Luteal Phase

This term refers to the occurrence of inadequate corpus luteum function and low progesterone output, with an irregular ovulatory cycle. The condition often manifests clinically as infertility, with either increased bleeding or amenorrhea. Endometrial biopsy performed at an estimated postovulatory date shows secretory endometrium, which, however, lags in its secretory characteristics with respect to the expected date.

Oral Contraceptives and Induced Endometrial Changes

As might be suspected, the use of oral contraceptives containing synthetic or derivative ovarian steroids induces a wide variety of endometrial changes, depending on the steroid used and the dose. A common response pattern is a discordant appearance between glands and stroma,[47] usually with inactive glands amidst a stroma showing large cells with abundant cytoplasm reminiscent of the decidua of pregnancy. When such therapy is discontinued, the endometrium reverts to normal. All these changes have been minimized with the newer low-dose contraceptives.

Menopausal and Postmenopausal Changes

Because the menopause is characterized by anovulatory cycles, architectural alterations in the endometrial glands may be present transiently, followed by ovarian failure and atrophy of the endometrium. As discussed next, a component of anovulatory cycles and uninterrupted estrogen production includes mild hyperplasias with cystic dilation of glands. If this is followed by complete ovarian atrophy and loss of stimulus, the cystic dilation may remain, while the ovarian stroma and gland epithelium undergo atrophy. In this case, so-called cystic atrophy results. Such cystic changes should not be confused with more active cystic hyperplasia, which exhibits evidence of glandular and stromal proliferation.

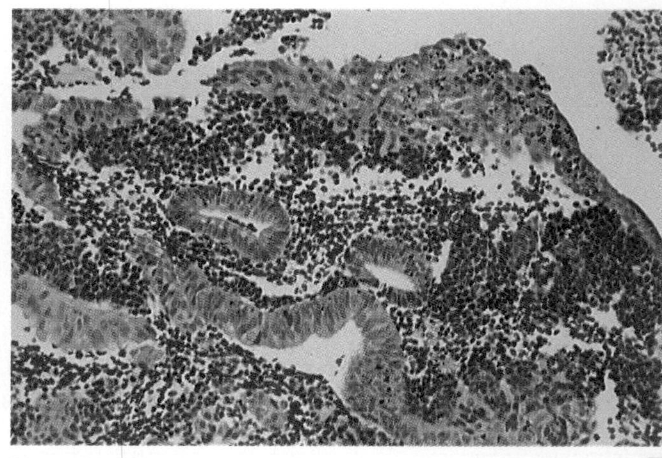

Figure 24–25 ■

Anovulatory endometrium with stromal breakdown. Note breakdown associated with proliferative glands.

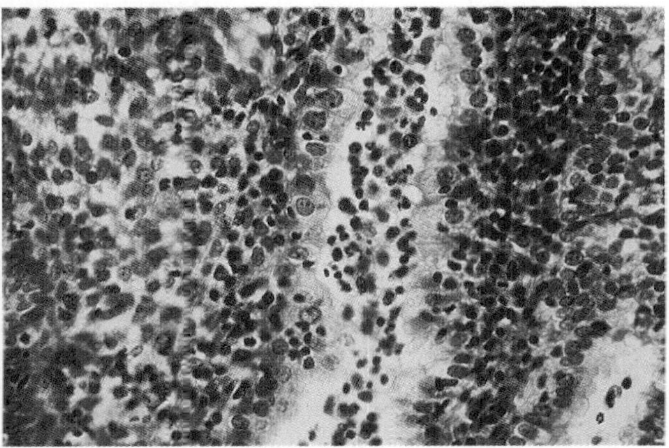

Figure 24–26

Chronic endometritis with inflammatory infiltrates and leukocytes in the gland lumen.

INFLAMMATIONS

The endometrium and myometrium are relatively resistant to infections, primarily because the endocervix normally forms a barrier to ascending infection. Thus, although chronic inflammation in the cervix is an expected and frequently insignificant finding, it is a concern in the endometrium, excluding the menstrual phase. Acute endometritis is uncommon and limited to bacterial infections that arise after delivery or miscarriage. Retained products of conception are the usual predisposing influence, causative agents including group A hemolytic streptococci, staphylococci, and other bacteria. The inflammatory response is chiefly limited to the interstitium and is entirely nonspecific. Removal of the retained gestational fragments by curettage is promptly followed by remission of the infection.

Chronic Endometritis

Chronic inflammation of the endometrium occurs in the following settings: (1) in patients suffering from chronic PID; (2) in patients with postpartal or postabortal endometrial cavities, usually due to retained gestational tissue; (3) in patients with intrauterine contraceptive devices; and (4) in patients with tuberculosis, either from miliary spread or more commonly from drainage of tuberculous salpingitis. The last is distinctly rare in Western countries. The chronic endometritis in all these cases represents a secondary disease, and under these circumstances there is a plausible cause.

In about 15% of cases, no such primary cause is obvious, yet plasma cells (which are not present in normal endometrium) are seen together with macrophages and lymphocytes (Fig. 24–26). Some women with this so-called nonspecific chronic endometritis have such gynecologic complaints as abnormal bleeding, pain, discharge, and infertility. *Chlamydia* may be involved and is commonly associated with both acute (polymorphonuclear leukocytes) and chronic (e.g., lymphocytes, plasma cells) inflammatory cell infiltrates. The organisms may or may not be successfully cultured.[30,31,48] Importantly, antibiotic therapy is indicated because it may prevent other sequelae (e.g., salpingitis).

ADENOMYOSIS

The endomyometrial interface is usually sharply demarcated. Some endometrial glands, however, may extend beneath this interface to form nests deep within the myometrium, producing a condition known as adenomyosis. The cause is unknown; it occurs in approximately 15% to 20% of uteri. Adenomyosis causes expansion (enlargement) of the uterine wall and may be visible on gross examination as numerous small cysts. On microscopic examination, irregular nests of endometrial stroma, with or without glands, are arranged within the myometrium, separated from the basalis by at least 2 to 3 mm. In some patients, the most important consequence of adenomyosis relates to shedding of the endometrium during the menstrual cycle (Fig. 24–27). Hemorrhage within these small adenomyotic nests results in menorrhagia, colicky dysmenorrhea, dyspareunia, and pelvic pain, particularly during the premenstrual period.

ENDOMETRIOSIS

Endometriosis is the term used to describe the presence of endometrial glands or stroma in abnormal locations outside the uterus. It occurs in the following sites, in descending order of frequency: (1) ovaries; (2) uterine ligaments; (3) rectovaginal septum; (4) pelvic peritoneum; (5) laparot-

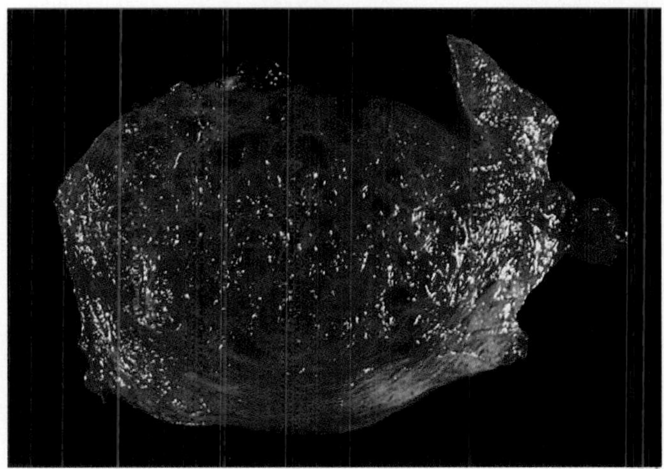

Figure 24–27

Adenomyosis. An unusual variant with functional endometrial nests producing foci of hemorrhagic cysts within the uterine wall.

omy scars; and (6) rarely in the umbilicus, vagina, vulva, or appendix.

Endometriosis is an important clinical condition; it often causes infertility, dysmenorrhea, pelvic pain, and other problems. The disorder is principally a disease of women in active reproductive life, most often in the third and fourth decades, and afflicts approximately 10% of women.

Three potential explanations exist to explain the origin of these dispersed lesions; they are not mutually exclusive (Fig. 24–28).

1. The regurgitation theory. Retrograde menstruation through the fallopian tubes occurs regularly even in normal women and could mediate spread of endometrial tissue to the peritoneal cavity.
2. The metaplastic theory. Endometrium could arise directly from coelomic epithelium, which in the last analysis is the origin of the endometrium itself.
3. The vascular or lymphatic dissemination theory. This theory would explain the presence of endometriotic lesions in the lungs or lymph nodes, a phenomenon not explainable by the first two theories.

Genetic, hormonal, and immune factors have also been postulated to increase susceptibility of some women to endometriosis. Based on the finding of aromatase cytochrome P450 in endometriotic tissue but not in normal endometrium, it has been suggested that the endometriotic tissue per se possesses the capacity to produce its own estrogens via this enzyme.[49] This and other studies suggest important biochemical differences between endometriotic tissue and normal uterine endometrium.

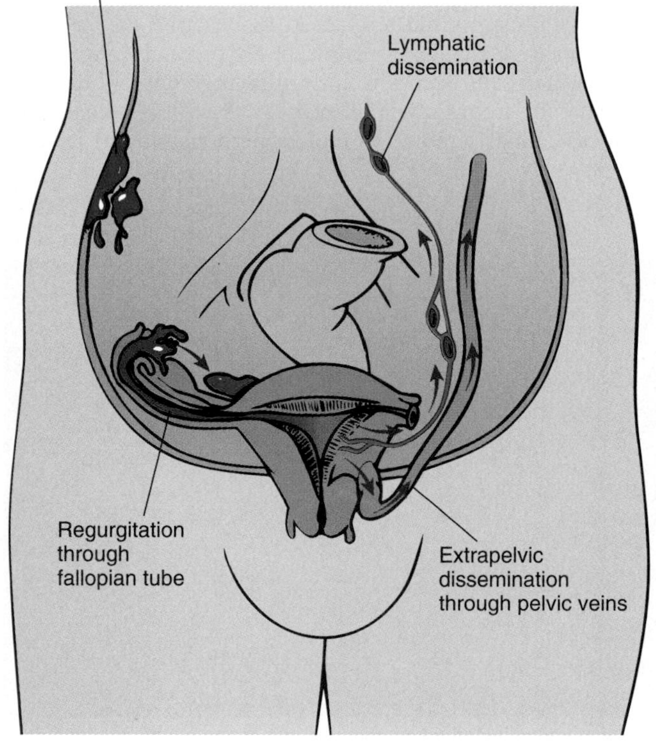

Figure 24–28

The potential origins of endometriosis implants.

MORPHOLOGY. The foci of endometrium are almost invariably under the influence of the ovarian hormones and therefore undergo the cyclic menstrual changes with periodic bleeding. This produces nodules with a red-blue to yellow-brown appearance on or just beneath the serosal surfaces in the site of involvement. When the disease is extensive, organizing hemorrhage causes extensive fibrous adhesions between tubes, ovaries, and other structures and obliteration of the pouch of Douglas. The ovaries may become markedly distorted by large cystic spaces (3 to 5 cm in diameter) filled with brown blood debris to form so-called chocolate cysts (Fig. 24–29*A*).

The histologic diagnosis of endometriosis is usually straightforward but may be difficult in long-standing cases in which the endometrial tissue is obscured by the fibro-obliterative response. A histologic diagnosis of endometriosis is satisfied if two of the three following features are identified: endometrial glands, stroma, and hemosiderin pigment (Fig. 24–29*B*).

Clinical Course. Clinical signs and symptoms usually consist of severe dysmenorrhea, dyspareunia, and pelvic pain due to the intrapelvic bleeding and periuterine adhesions. Pain on defecation reflects rectal wall involvement, and dysuria reflects involvement of the serosa of the bladder. Intestinal disturbances may appear when the small intestine is affected. Menstrual irregularities are common, and infertility is the presenting complaint in 30% to 40% of women. Rarely, malignancies may develop in endometriotic lesions.

ENDOMETRIAL POLYPS

Endometrial polyps are sessile masses of variable size that project into the endometrial cavity. They may be single or multiple and are usually 0.5 to 3.0 cm in diameter but occasionally large and pedunculated. Polyps may be asymptomatic or may cause abnormal bleeding if they ulcerate or undergo necrosis. They are generally of two histologic types made up of (1) functional endometrium, paralleling the adjacent cycling endometrium, or (2) more commonly hyperplastic endometrium, mostly of the cystic variety. Such polyps may develop in association with generalized endometrial hyperplasia and are responsive to the growth effect of estrogen but exhibit no progesterone response (Fig. 24–30). Rarely, adenocarcinomas may arise within endometrial polyps. Endometrial polyps have been observed in association with the administration of tamoxifen, an antiestrogen frequently used in the therapy of breast cancer.[50] Cytogenetic studies indicate that the stromal cells

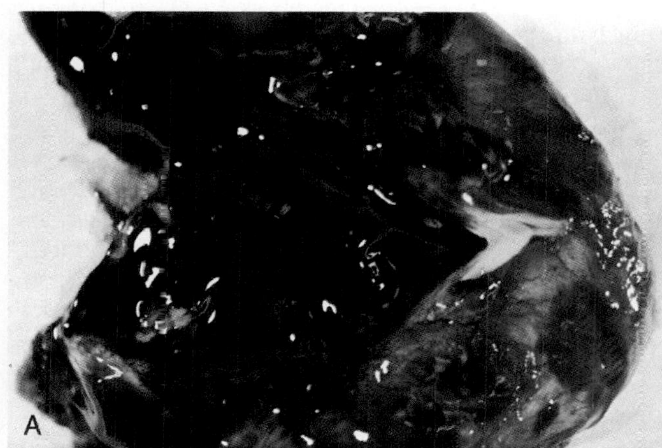

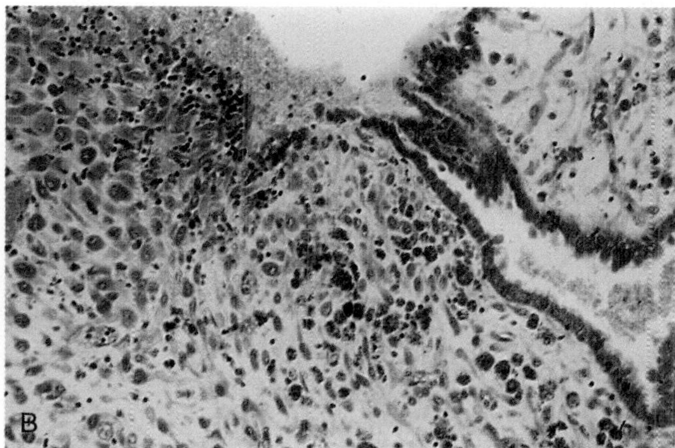

Figure 24–29

Endometriosis. *A*, This ovary has been sectioned to reveal a large endometriotic cyst containing necrotic brown material consisting of degenerated blood (chocolate cyst). *B* Lining of an endometriotic cyst from a pregnant patient. On the right is an endometrial gland; on the left is endometrial stroma with plump stromal cells characteristic of decidual changes. In the center are numerous macrophages containing hemosiderin.

in endometrial polyps are clonal with chromosome (6p21) rearrangements, indicating that genetic alterations may play a role in their development.[51]

ENDOMETRIAL HYPERPLASIA

Endometrial hyperplasia is another cause of abnormal bleeding that differs from typical anovulation by the degree of glandular epithelial alterations in the endometrium. Endometrial hyperplasia deserves special attention because of its relationship to endometrial carcinoma. More than 50 years ago, Hertig and Sommers[52] proposed a progression of endometrial changes from hyperplasia through a spectrum of atypical changes leading eventually, in some cases, to endometrial carcinoma. Numerous studies have since largely confirmed the malignant potential of certain endometrial hyperplasias and the concept of a continuum of glandular atypia culminating, in some cases, in carcinoma.[53]

As mentioned previously, endometrial hyperplasia is related to an abnormally high, prolonged level of estrogenic stimulation with diminution or absence of progestational activity. Thus, hyperplasia occurs most commonly around menopause or in association with persistent anovulation in younger women. Conditions leading to hyperplasia include polycystic ovarian disease (including Stein-Leventhal syndrome), functioning granulosa cell tumors of the ovary, excessive cortical function (cortical stroma hyperplasia), and prolonged administration of estrogenic substances (estrogen replacement therapy). These are the same influences postulated to be of pathogenetic significance in a portion of endometrial carcinomas, discussed later.

MORPHOLOGY. Endometrial hyperplasia exhibits a continuum of alterations in gland architecture, epithelial growth pattern, and cytology, and the grade increases as a function of the severity of these changes.

Lower grade hyperplasias include simple hyperplasia and complex hyperplasia. **Simple hyperplasia,** also known as cystic or mild hyperplasia, is characterized by the presence of architectural alterations in glands of various sizes, producing irregularity in gland shape with cystic alterations.

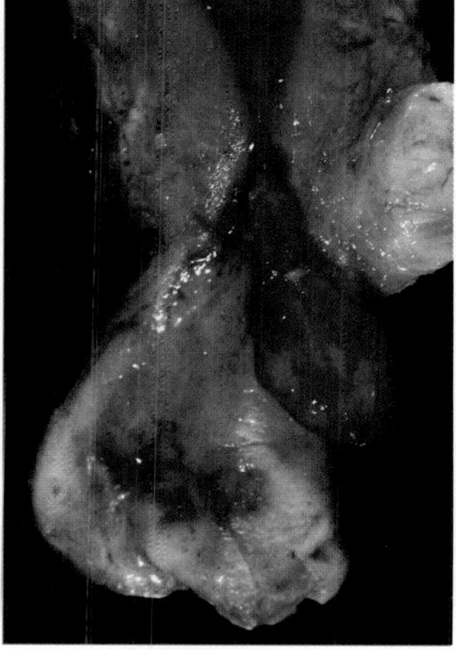

Figure 24–30

Endometrial polyp projecting from a think stalk at the junction of the endometrium (*left*) and endocervix (*right*).

The epithelial growth pattern and cytology are similar to proliferative endometrium, although mitoses are not as prominent (Fig. 24–31*A*). The stroma between glands is also frequently increased. These lesions uncommonly progress to adenocarcinoma; cystic hyperplasia frequently evolves into cystic atrophy in which the epithelium and stroma become atrophic. **Complex hyperplasia,** also known as adenomatous hyperplasia without atypia, exhibits an increase in the number and size of endometrial glands, with gland crowding and a disparity in their size and irregularity in their shape. The glands undergo "budding" with finger-like outpouchings into the adjacent endometrial stroma. The lining epithelium may appear more stratified than simple hyperplasia but is regular in contour and devoid of conspicuous cytologic atypia (Fig. 24–31*B*). In the absence of cytologic atypia, less than 5% of these lesions evolve into carcinoma.

Higher grade hyperplasias are usually termed **atypical hyperplasia,** or adenomatous hyperplasia with atypia. In addition to glandular crowding and complexity, epithelial lining is irregular, characterized by stratification, scalloping, and tufting. Importantly, there is cellular atypia with cytomegaly, loss of polarity, hyperchromatism, prominence of nucleoli, and altered nuclear cytoplasmic ratio (Fig. 24–31*C*). Mitotic figures are common. Predictably, in the most severe forms, cytologic and architectural atypia may resemble frank adenocarcinoma, and an accurate distinction between atypical hyperplasia and cancer may not be made without hysterectomy. In one study, 23% of patients with atypical hyperplasias eventually developed adenocarcinoma.[53] In another study in which atypical hyperplasias were treated with progestin therapy alone, 50% persisted despite therapy, 25% recurred, and 25% progressed to carcinoma.[54]

Many endometrial hyperplasias exhibit altered cellular differentiation (metaplasia), including the presence of squamous, ciliated cell and mucinous metaplasia (Fig. 24–31*D*). Interpretation of endometrial hyperplasia may be highly subjective, and thus precise classification is elusive. Therefore, in any assessment of a hyperplastic lesion, it is

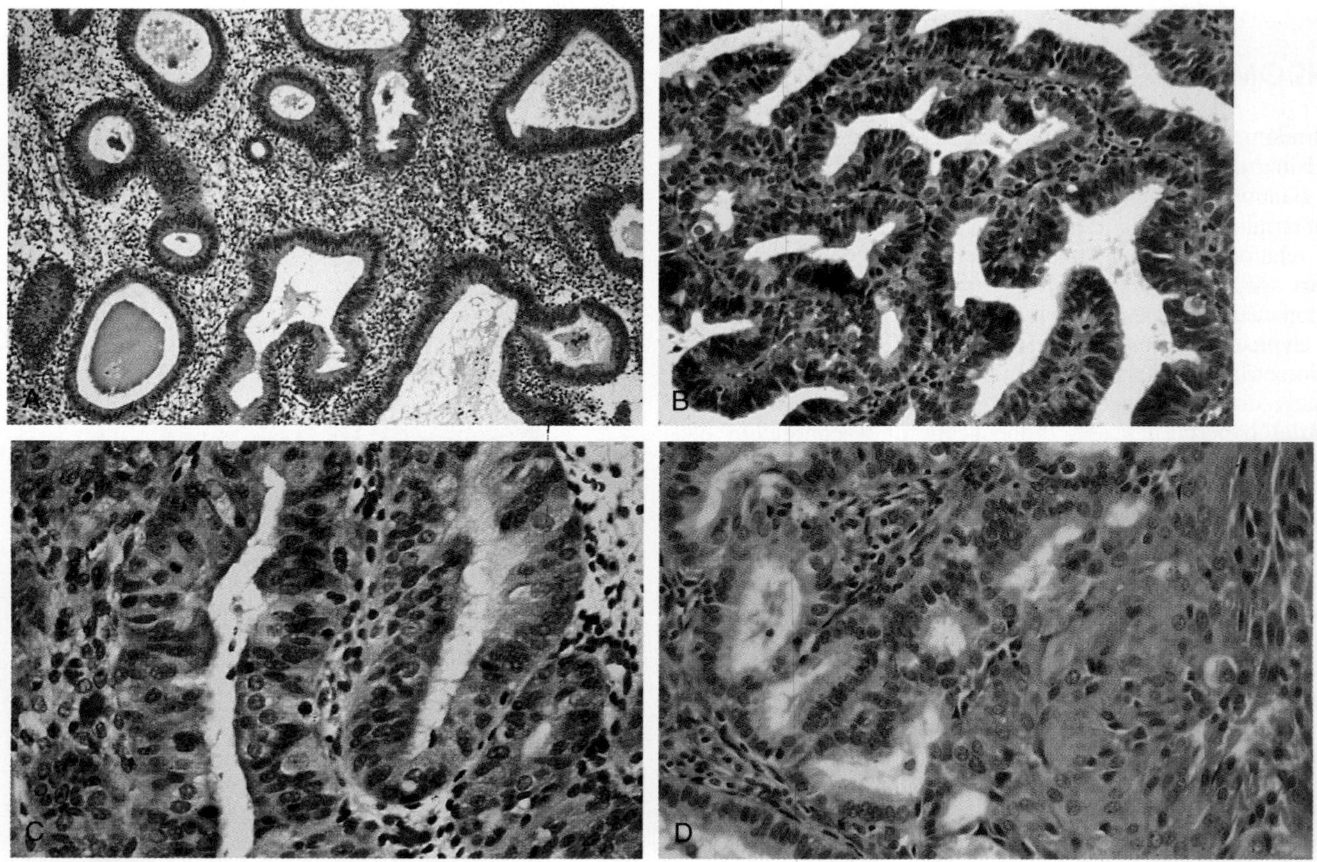

Figure 24–31

Low-grade hyperplasias of the endometrium: *A*, simple (cystic); *B*, complex. Both lesions contain minimal epithelial stratification or atypia. *C*, High-grade (atypical) hyperplasia with epithelial stratification and cellular atypia. *D*, Endometrial hyperplasia with squamous metaplasia.

important for the pathologist to indicate the degree of atypia in a manner clearly understandable by the clinician. The selection of diagnostic terminology may mean the difference between cyclic progestin therapy on one hand and continuous high-dose progestin therapy or hysterectomy (or both) on the other.

MALIGNANT TUMORS OF THE ENDOMETRIUM

Carcinoma of the Endometrium

Endometrial carcinoma is the most common invasive cancer of the female genital tract and accounts for 7% of all invasive cancer in women, excluding skin cancer. At one time, it was far less common than cancer of the cervix, but earlier detection and eradication of CIN and an increase in endometrial carcinomas in younger age groups have reversed this ratio. There are now 34,000 new endometrial cancers per year, compared with 13,000 new invasive cervical cancers. Despite their high frequency, endometrial cancers arise mainly in postmenopausal women, causing abnormal (postmenopausal) bleeding. This permits early detection and cure at an early stage.

Incidence and Pathogenesis. Carcinoma of the endometrium is uncommon in women younger than 40 years. The peak incidence is in the 55- to 65-year-old woman. A higher frequency of this form of neoplasia is seen with (1) obesity, (2) diabetes (abnormal glucose tolerance is found in more than 60%), (3) hypertension, and (4) infertility (women who develop cancer of the endometrium tend to be single and nulliparous and to give a history of functional menstrual irregularities consistent with anovulatory cycles). Infrequently, both endometrial and breast carcinomas arise in the same patient.[55]

In terms of potential pathogenesis, two general groups of endometrial cancer can be identified. The first develops on a background of prolonged estrogen stimulation and *endometrial hyperplasia.*[56] Both conditions, hyperplasia and cancer, appear closely related. Support for this conclusion includes the following. First, both are also linked with obesity and anovulatory cycles. Second, women with ovarian estrogen-secreting tumors have a higher risk of endometrial cancer. Third, endometrial cancer is extremely rare in women with ovarian agenesis and in those castrated early in life. Fourth, estrogen replacement therapy is associated with increased risk in women, and prolonged administration of DES to laboratory animals may produce endometrial polyps, hyperplasia, and carcinoma. Fifth, in postmenopausal women, there is greater synthesis of estrogens in body fats from adrenal and ovarian androgen precursors, a finding that may partly explain why there is increased risk of endometrial cancer with age and obesity. Endometrial carcinomas that are associated with hyperplasia and the aforementioned risk factors tend to be well differentiated and mimic normal endometrial glands *(endometrioid)* in histologic appearance. This group of tumors is associated with a more favorable prognosis.[56]

A second subset of patients with endometrial cancer less commonly exhibits the stigmata of hyperestrinism or preexisting hyperplasia and acquires the disease at a somewhat older average age. In this group, tumors are generally more poorly differentiated, including tumors that resemble subtypes of ovarian carcinomas *(serous carcinomas).* Overall, these tumors have a poorer prognosis than estrogen-related cancers do. Some endometrioid tumors have been associated with microsatellite instability, and serous subtypes are linked to overexpression of *p53.*[57,58]

MORPHOLOGY. In gross appearance, endometrial carcinoma presents either as a localized polypoid tumor or as a diffuse tumor involving the entire endometrial surface (Fig. 24–32*A*). Spread generally occurs by direct myometrial invasion with eventual spread to the periuterine structures by direct continuity. Spread into the broad ligaments may create a clinically palpable mass. Dissemination to the regional lymph nodes eventually occurs, and in the late stages, the tumor may be hematogenously borne to the lungs, liver, bones, and other organs. In certain types, specifically papillary serous carcinoma, relatively superficial endometrial involvement may be associated with extensive peritoneal disease, suggesting spread by routes (i.e., tubal or lymphatic transmission) other than direct invasion.

On histologic examination, most endometrial carcinomas (about 85%) are **adenocarcinomas** characterized by more or less well defined gland patterns lined by malignant stratified columnar epithelial cells (Fig. 24–32*B*). They are classically defined as well differentiated (grade 1), with easily recognizable glandular patterns; moderately differentiated (grade 2), showing well-formed glands mixed with solid sheets of malignant cells; or poorly differentiated (grade 3), characterized by solid sheets of cells with barely recognizable glands and a greater degree of nuclear atypia and mitotic activity.

The more well differentiated tumors tend to be those of endometrioid differentiation. Two per cent to 20% of endometrioid carcinomas contain foci of squamous differentiation. Squamous elements most commonly are histologically benign in appearance (called **adenocarcinoma with squamous metaplasia** or, more traditionally, **adenoacanthoma)** when they are associated with well-differentiated adenocarcinomas. Less commonly, moderate or poorly differentiated endometrioid carcinomas contain squamous elements that appear frankly malignant. Such tumors have also been termed **adenosquamous carcinomas** if more than 10% of the tumor is squamous.[59]

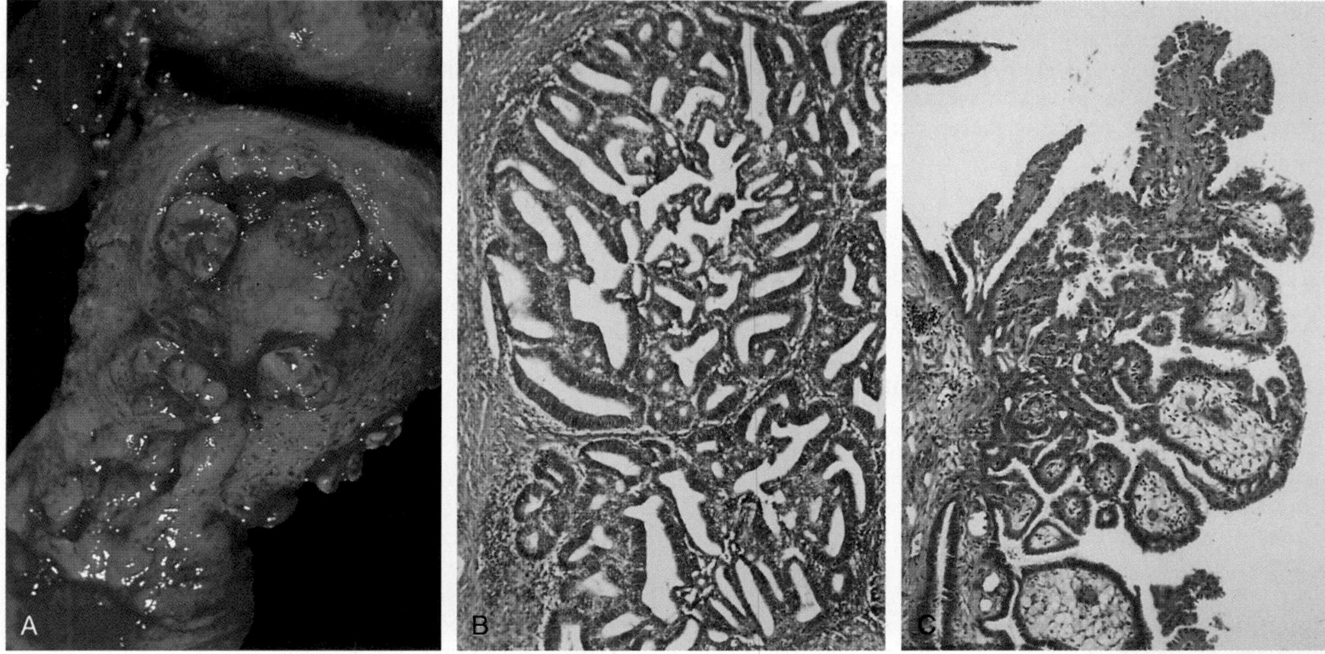

Figure 24–32

A, Endometrial adenocarcinoma presenting as a fungating mass in the fundus of the uterus. *B*, Well-differentiated endometrial adenocarcinoma. Discrete glands are less easily identified because the epithelium is arranged in a confluent pattern without intervening stroma. *C*, Papillary serous carcinoma of the endometrium.

Although classification as a poorly differentiated adenocarcinoma typically requires a loss of glandular differentiation and the presence of solid growth, two histologic patterns behave as poorly differentiated regardless of their degree of differentiation and include **papillary serous carcinomas** and **clear cell carcinomas** (Fig. 24–32*C*). Serous carcinomas in particular are a highly aggressive form of uterine cancer.[60]

Staging of endometrial adenocarcinoma is as follows[61]:

Stage I. Carcinoma is confined to the corpus uteri itself.

Stage II. Carcinoma has involved the corpus and the cervix.

Stage III. Carcinoma has extended outside the uterus but not outside the true pelvis.

Stage IV. Carcinoma has extended outside the true pelvis or has obviously involved the mucosa of the bladder or the rectum.

Cases in various stages can also be subgrouped with reference to histologic type of adenocarcinoma as follows:

G1. Well-differentiated adenocarcinoma

G2. Differentiated adenocarcinoma with partly solid areas

G3. Predominantly solid or entirely undifferentiated carcinoma, including all serous and clear cell carcinomas

Clinical Course. Carcinoma of the endometrium may be asymptomatic for periods of time but usually produces irregular vaginal bleeding with excessive leukorrhea. Uterine enlargement in the early stages may be deceptively absent. Cytologic detection on Papanicolaou smears is variable and most likely with serous carcinomas, which shed discohesive clusters of cells. The diagnosis must ultimately be established by curettage and histologic examination of the tissue.

As would be anticipated, the prognosis depends heavily on the clinical stage of the disease when it is discovered and its histologic grade and type. In the United States, most women (about 80%) have stage I disease clinically and have well-differentiated or moderately well differentiated lesions histologically. Surgery, alone or in combination with irradiation, yields close to 90% 5-year survival in stage I disease. This rate drops to 30% to 50% in stage II and to less than 20% in any of the other more advanced stages of the disease.

MIXED MÜLLERIAN AND MESENCHYMAL TUMORS

Sarcomas collectively make up 5% or less of uterine tumors; mixed mesodermal tumors, leiomyosarcomas, and endometrial stromal sarcomas are the most common variants.

Malignant Mixed Müllerian Tumors (Carcinosarcomas)

Malignant mixed müllerian tumors consist of endometrial adenocarcinomas in which malignant mesenchymal (stromal) differentiation takes place.[62] They are called carcinosarcomas because they consist of malignant glandular and stromal (sarcomatous) elements, and the latter tend to differentiate into a variety of malignant mesodermal components, including muscle, cartilage, and even osteoid. Both components are presumably derived originally from the same cell, a concept supported by the fact that the stromal cells often stain positive with epithelial cell markers. Carcinosarcomas occur in postmenopausal women and manifest similarly to adenocarcinoma, with postmenopausal bleeding. Many affected patients give a history of previous radiation therapy.

MORPHOLOGY. In gross appearance, such tumors are somewhat more fleshy than adenocarcinomas, may be bulky and polypoid, and sometimes protrude through the cervical os. On histology, the tumors consist of adenocarcinoma admixed with the stromal (sarcoma) elements; alternatively, the tumor may comprise two distinct and separate epithelial and mesenchymal components. Sarcomatous components may mimic extrauterine tissues (i.e., striated muscle cells, cartilage, adipose tissue, and bone).

Outcome is determined primarily by depth of invasion and stage. Similar to that of endometrial carcinoma, the prognosis may be influenced in addition by the grade and type of the adenocarcinoma, being poorest with serous differentiation. It is noteworthy that carcinosarcomas usually metastasize as adenocarcinomas. The tumors are highly malignant, and patients have a 5-year survival rate of 25% to 30%.[62]

TUMORS OF THE MYOMETRIUM

Leiomyomas

Leiomyomas are the most common tumors in women and are referred to in colloquial usage as fibroids. The tumors are found in at least 25% of women in active reproductive life and are more common in blacks. These tumors are estrogen responsive; they regress or even calcify after castration or menopause and may undergo rapid increase in size during pregnancy. Their cause is unknown, although, similar to the pathogenesis of endometrial polyps, chromosome aberrations may play a role.[63]

MORPHOLOGY. Leiomyomas are sharply circumscribed, discrete, round, firm, gray-white tumors varying in size from small, barely visible nodules to massive tumors that fill the pelvis. Except in rare instances, they are found within the myometrium of the corpus. Only infrequently do they involve the uterine ligaments, lower uterine segment, or cervix. They can occur within the myometrium **(intramural)**, just beneath the endometrium **(submucosal)** (Fig. 24–33*A*), or beneath the serosa **(subserosal)**.

Whatever their size, the characteristic whorled pattern of smooth muscle bundles on cut section usually makes these lesions readily identifiable on gross inspection. Large tumors may develop areas of yellow-brown to red softening (red degeneration).

On histologic examination, the leiomyoma is composed of whorled bundles of smooth muscle cells that resemble the architecture of the uninvolved myometrium (Fig. 24–33*B*). Usually, the individual muscle cells are uniform in size and shape and have the characteristic oval nucleus and long, slender bipolar cytoplasmic processes. Mitotic figures are scarce. Benign variants of

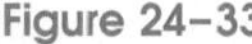

Figure 24–33

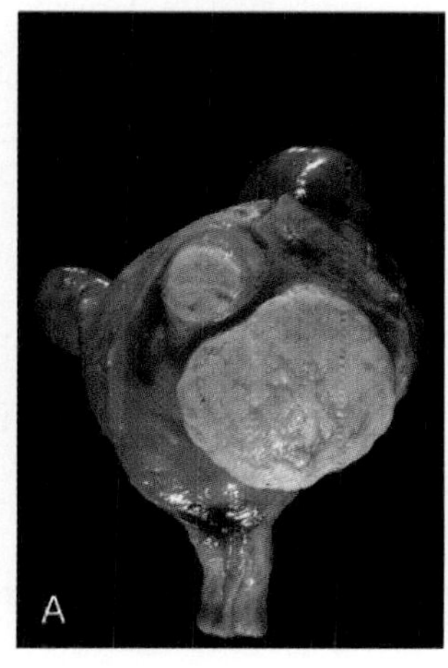

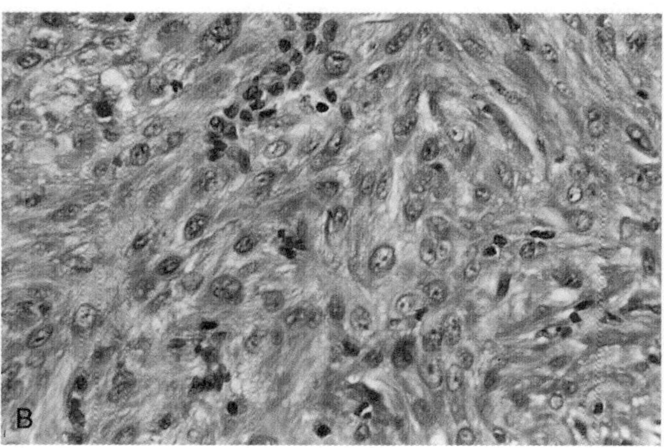

A, Leiomyomas of the myometrium. The uterus is opened to reveal the tumors bulging into the endometrial cavity and displaying a firm white appearance on sectioning. *B*, Leiomyoma showing well-differentiated, regular, spindle-shaped smooth muscle cells.

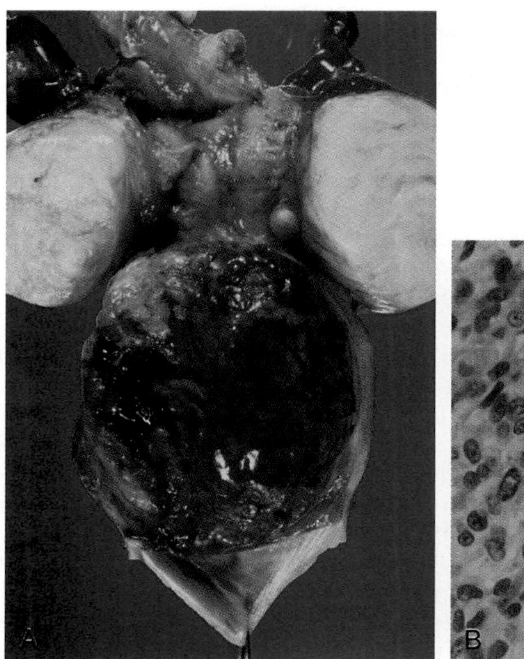

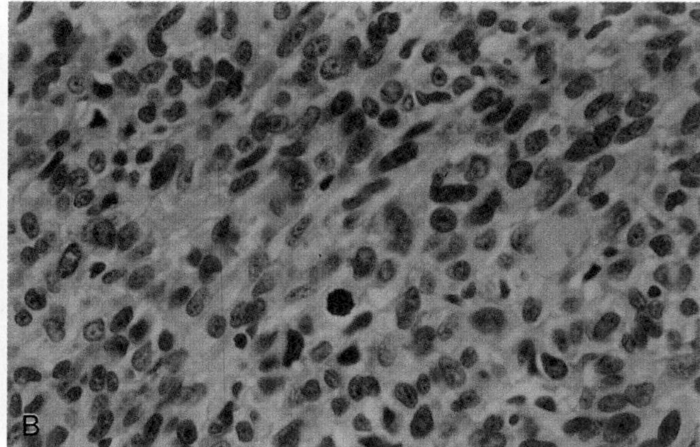

Figure 24–34

Leiomyosarcoma. *A*, A large hemorrhagic tumor mass distends the lower corpus and is flanked by two leiomyomas. *B*, The tumor cells are irregular in size and have hyperchromatic nuclei.

leiomyoma include atypical or bizarre (symplastic) tumors with nuclear atypia and giant cells and cellular leiomyomas. Importantly, both contain a low mitotic index. An extremely rare variant, **benign metastasizing leiomyoma,** consists of a uterine tumor that extends into vessels and migrates to other sites, most commonly the lung.

Leiomyomas of the uterus, even when they are extensive, may be asymptomatic. The most important symptoms are produced by submucosal leiomyomas (abnormal bleeding), compression of the bladder (urinary frequency), sudden pain if disruption of blood supply occurs, and impaired fertility. Myomas in pregnant women increase the frequency of spontaneous abortion, fetal malpresentation, uterine inertia, and postpartum hemorrhage. Malignant transformation (leiomyosarcoma) within a leiomyoma is extremely rare.

Leiomyosarcomas

These uncommon malignant neoplasms arise de novo directly from the myometrium or endometrial stroma, which undergoes smooth muscle differentiation. Their origin from a preexisting leiomyoma is a controversial issue, and most believe that such occurrences are extremely rare.

MORPHOLOGY. Leiomyosarcomas grow within the uterus in two somewhat distinctive patterns: bulky, fleshy masses that invade the uterine wall, or polypoid masses that project into the uterine lumen (Fig. 24–34*A*). On histologic examination, they contain a wide range of atypia, from those that are extremely well differentiated to anaplastic lesions that have the cytologic abnormalities of wildly growing sarcomas (Fig. 24–34*B*). The distinction of leiomyosarcomas from leiomyomas is based on the combination of degree of nuclear atypia, mitotic index, and zonal necrosis. With few exceptions, the presence of ten or more mitoses per ten high-power (×400) fields indicates malignancy, with or without cellular atypism. If the tumor contains nuclear atypia or large (epithelioid) cells, five mitoses per ten high-power fields are sufficient to justify a diagnosis of malignancy.[64,65] Rare exceptions include mitotically active leiomyomas in young or pregnant women, and caution should be exercised in interpreting such neoplasms as malignant. A proportion of smooth muscle neoplasms may be impossible to classify and are termed smooth muscle tumors of "uncertain malignant potential."[65]

Leiomyosarcomas are equally common before and after menopause, with a peak incidence at 40 to 60 years of age.

These tumors have a striking tendency to recur after removal, and more than half the cases eventually metastasize through the bloodstream to distant organs, such as lungs, bone, and brain. Dissemination throughout the abdominal cavity is also encountered. The 5-year survival rate averages about 40%. The well-differentiated lesions have a better prognosis than the anaplastic lesions, which have a low 5-year survival rate of about 10% to 15%.

Endometrial Stromal Tumors

The endometrial stroma occasionally gives rise to neoplasms involving the myometrium that may closely or remotely resemble normal stromal cells. Similar to most neoplasms, they may be well or poorly differentiated. Stromal neoplasms are divided into three categories: (1) benign stromal nodules; (2) low-grade stromal sarcoma, or endolymphatic stromal myosis; and (3) endometrial stromal sarcoma.

Stromal nodule is a well-circumscribed aggregate of endometrial stromal cells in the myometrium and is of little consequence. *Low-grade stromal sarcoma* consists of well-differentiated endometrial stroma lying between muscle bundles of the myometrium and is distinguished from stromal nodules by the penetration of lymphatic channels, hence the term *endolymphatic stromal myosis.* About half of these tumors recur, sometimes after 10 to 15 years; distant metastases and death from metastatic tumor occur in about 15% of cases. *Endometrial stromal sarcoma* is the overtly malignant subset of stromal tumors. These tumors infiltrate the stroma with indistinct margins and contain cells with a wide range of atypia, with numerous mitoses. Like all sarcomas, these cancers invade vessels and are capable of widespread metastasis. Five-year survival rates average 50%.

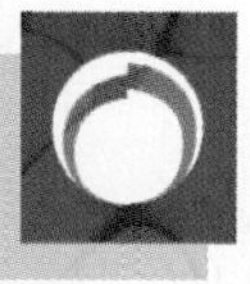

FALLOPIAN TUBES

The most common disorders in these structures are inflammations, followed in frequency by ectopic (tubal) pregnancy (see discussion later in this chapter) and endometriosis.

INFLAMMATIONS

Suppurative salpingitis may be caused by any of the pyogenic organisms, and often more than one is involved. The gonococcus still accounts for more than 60% of cases of suppurative salpingitis, with chlamydiae less often a factor. These tubal infections are a part of PID described earlier in this chapter.

Tuberculous salpingitis is extremely uncommon in the United States and accounts for probably not more than 1% to 2% of all forms of salpingitis. It is more common, however, in parts of the world where tuberculosis is prevalent and is an important cause of infertility in these areas.

TUMORS AND CYSTS

The most common primary lesions of the fallopian tube (excluding endometriosis) are minute, 0.1- to 2-cm translucent cysts filled with clear serous fluid, called paratubal cysts. Larger varieties are found near the fimbriated end of the tube or in the broad ligaments and are referred to as *hydatids of Morgagni.* These cysts are presumed to arise in remnants of the müllerian duct and are of little more than academic significance.

Tumors of the fallopian tube are uncommon. Benign tumors include *adenomatoid tumors* (mesotheliomas), which occur subserosally on the tube or sometimes in the mesosalpinx. These small nodules are the exact counterparts of those already described in relation to the testes or epididymides (Chapter 23) and are benign. *Adenocarcinoma* of the fallopian tubes is rare and has a papillary architecture with tubal (papillary serous) differentiation. Because these tumors commonly are undiagnosed when they are confined to the tube, they have a poor prognosis. For adenocarcinoma to be distinguished as a primary tubal cancer versus a metastasis of ovarian or endometrial origin, the bulk of the tumor must be in the tube, involve the lumen, and arise from the mucosa.

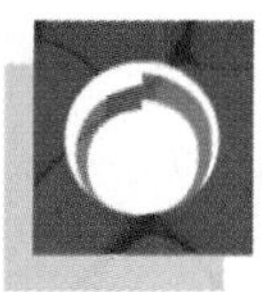

OVARIES

The most common types of lesions encountered in the ovary include functional or benign cysts and tumors. Intrinsic inflammations of the ovary (oophoritis) are uncommon, usually accompanying tubal inflammation. Rarely, a primary inflammatory disorder involving ovarian follicles (autoimmune oophoritis) occurs and is associated with infertility.

NON-NEOPLASTIC AND FUNCTIONAL CYSTS

Follicular and Luteal Cysts

Cystic follicles in the ovary are so common as to be virtually physiologic. They originate in unruptured graafian follicles or in follicles that have ruptured and immediately sealed.

MORPHOLOGY. These cysts are usually multiple. They range in size up to 2 cm in diameter, are filled with a clear serous fluid, and are lined by a gray, glistening membrane. On occasion, larger cysts exceeding 2 cm (follicular cysts) may be diagnosed by palpation or ultrasonography and cause pelvic pain. Granulosa lining cells can be identified histologically if the intraluminal pressure has not been too great. The outer theca cells may be conspicuous with increased cytoplasm and a pale appearance (luteinized). As discussed subsequently, when this alteration is pronounced (hyperthecosis), it may ultimately result in increased estrogen production and endometrial abnormalities. An impressive physiologic condition accompanying pregnancy is theca-lutein hyperplasia of pregnancy, in which the theca interna proliferates and may form small nodules in the ovarian cortex.

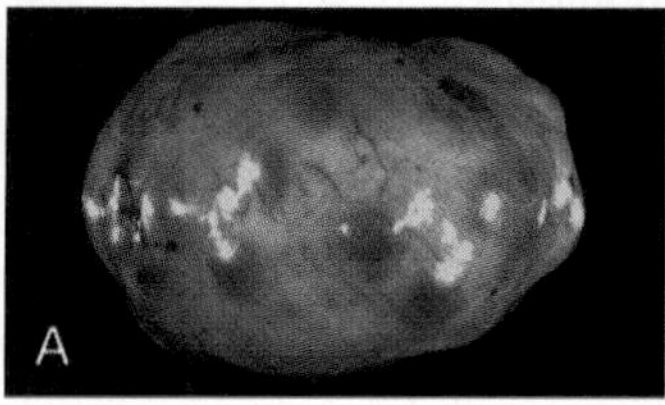

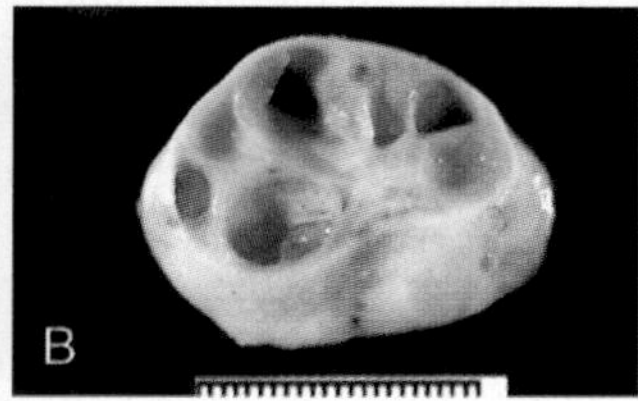

Figure 24–35

Polycystic ovarian disease. *A*, The ovarian cortex reveals numerous clear cysts. *B*, A section of the cortex reveals several subcortical cystic follicles.

Granulosa **luteal cysts** (cystic corpora lutea) are normally present in the ovary. These cysts are lined by a rim of bright yellow luteal tissue containing luteinized granulosa cells. They occasionally rupture and cause a peritoneal reaction. When advanced, the combination of old hemorrhage and fibrosis may make their distinction from endometriotic cysts difficult.

Polycystic Ovaries and Stromal Hyperthecosis

In polycystic ovarian disease, the central pathologic abnormality is numerous cystic follicles or follicle cysts. When it is associated with oligomenorrhea, the clinical term *Stein-Leventhal syndrome* has been applied. These patients have persistent anovulation, obesity (40%), hirsutism (50%), and, rarely, virilism.[66]

MORPHOLOGY. The ovaries are usually twice normal size, are gray-white with a smooth outer cortex, and are studded with subcortical cysts 0.5 to 1.5 cm in diameter. On histologic examination, there is a thickened superficial cortex beneath which are innumerable follicle cysts with hyperplasia of the theca interna (follicular hyperthecosis) (Fig. 24–35). Corpora lutea are frequently but not invariably absent.

The initiating event in polycystic ovarian disease is not clear, but increased secretion of luteinizing hormone theoretically stimulates the theca-lutein cells of the follicles, with excessive production of androgen (androstenedione), which is converted to estrone. For years, these endocrine abnormalities were attributed to primary ovarian dysfunction because large wedge resections of the ovaries sometimes restored fertility. It is now believed that a variety of enzymes involved in androgen biosynthesis are poorly regulated in polycystic ovarian disease, including insulin, growth factors, and luteinizing hormones. Genetic defects have also been proposed.[67]

Stromal hyperthecosis, also called cortical stromal hyperplasia, is a disorder of ovarian stroma most commonly seen in postmenopausal women but may blend with polycystic ovarian disease in younger women. The disorder is characterized by uniform enlargement of the ovary (up to 7 cm) with a white to tan appearance on sectioning. The involvement is usually bilateral and microscopically consists of hypercellular stroma with luteinization of the stromal cells, which are visible as discrete nests with vacuolated cytoplasm. The clinical presentation and effects on the endometrium are similar to those of polycystic ovarian disease, although virilization may be striking.[66]

OVARIAN TUMORS

Tumors of the ovary are common forms of neoplasia in women.[68,69] Among cancers of the female genital tract, the incidence of ovarian cancer ranks below only carcinoma of the cervix and the endometrium. Ovarian cancer accounts for 6% of all cancers in the female and is the fifth most common form of cancer in women in the United States (excluding skin cancer). In addition, because many of these ovarian neoplasms cannot be detected early in their development, they account for a disproportionate number of fatal cancers, being responsible for almost half of the deaths from cancer of the female genital tract. There are numerous types of ovarian tumors, both benign and malignant. About 80% are benign, and these occur mostly in young women between the ages of 20 and 45 years. The malignant tumors are more common in older women between the ages of 40 and 65 years.

Risk factors for ovarian cancer are much less clear than for other genital tumors[70] with general agreement on two: nulliparity and family history. There is a higher frequency of carcinoma in unmarried women and in married women with low parity. Gonadal dysgenesis in children is associated with a higher risk of ovarian cancer. The risk of developing ovarian cancer in women 40 to 59 years of age who have taken oral contraceptives is reduced.[71] The most intriguing risk factor is genetic and candidate host genes, which may be altered in susceptible families (i.e., ovarian cancer genes). Several are being considered, and as discussed in Chapter 25, mutations in both *BRCA1*[72] and *BRCA2*[73] increase susceptibility to ovarian cancer. *BRCA1* mutations occur in about 5% of patients younger than 70 years with ovarian cancer. The estimated risk of ovarian cancer in women bearing *BRCA1* or *BRCA2* is 16% by the age of 70 years.[73] Most of these cancers are serous cystadenocarcinomas. Approximately 30% of ovarian adenocarcinomas express high levels of *HER2/neu* oncogene, which correlates with a poor prognosis. Mutations in a host tumor-suppressor gene *p53* are found in 50% of ovarian carcinomas.[74]

The classification of ovarian tumors given in Table 24–3 and Figure 24–36 is a simplified version of the World Health Organization Histological Classification, which separates ovarian neoplasms according to the most probable tissue of origin. It is now believed that tumors of the ovary arise ultimately from one of three ovarian components: (1) the surface coelomic epithelium, which embryologically gives rise to the müllerian epithelium, that is, the fallopian tubes (ciliated columnar serous cells), the endometrial lining (nonciliated, columnar cells), or the endocervical glands (mucinous nonciliated cells); (2) the germ cells, which migrate to the ovary from the yolk sac and are totipotential; and (3) the stroma of the ovary, which includes the sex cords, forerunners of the endocrine apparatus of the postnatal ovary. There is, as usual, a group of tumors that defy classification, and finally there are secondary or metastatic tumors, the ovary being a common site of metastases from a variety of other cancers.

Although some of the specific tumors have distinctive features and are hormonally active, most are nonfunctional and tend to produce relatively mild symptoms until they have reached a large size. Malignant tumors have usually spread outside the ovary by the time a definitive diagnosis is made. Some of these tumors, principally epithelial tumors, tend to be bilateral. Table 24–4 lists these tumors and their subtypes and shows the frequency of bilateral occurrence. Abdominal pain and distention, urinary and

Table 24–3. OVARIAN NEOPLASMS (1993 WHO CLASSIFICATION)

Surface epithelial-stromal tumors
- Serous tumors
  - Benign (cystadenoma)
  - Of borderline malignancy
  - Malignant (serous cystadenocarcinoma)
- Mucinous tumors, endocervical-like and intestinal type
  - Benign
  - Of borderline malignancy
  - Malignant
- Endometrioid tumors
  - Benign
  - Of borderline malignancy
  - Malignant
  - Epithelial-stromal
    - Adenosarcoma
    - Mesodermal (müllerian) mixed tumor
  - Clear cell tumors
    - Benign
    - Of borderline malignancy
    - Malignant
  - Transitional cell tumors
    - Brenner tumor
    - Brenner tumor of borderline malignancy
    - Malignant Brenner tumor
    - Transitional cell carcinoma (non-Brenner type)

Sex cord–stromal tumors
- Granulosa-stromal cell tumors
  - Granulosa cell tumors
  - Tumors of the thecoma-fibroma group
- Sertoli-stromal cell tumors; androblastomas
- Sex cord tumor with annular tubules
- Gynandroblastoma
- Steroid (lipid) cell tumors

Germ cell tumors
- Teratoma
  - Immature
  - Mature (adult)
    - Solid
    - Cystic (dermoid cyst)
  - Monodermal (e.g., struma ovarii, carcinoid)
- Dysgerminoma
- Yolk sac tumor (endodermal sinus tumor)
- Mixed germ cell tumors

Malignant, not otherwise specified

Metastatic nonovarian cancer (from nonovarian primary)

Modified from the WHO Classification. (Courtesy Dr. Robert Scully, Massachusetts General Hospital, Boston, MA.)

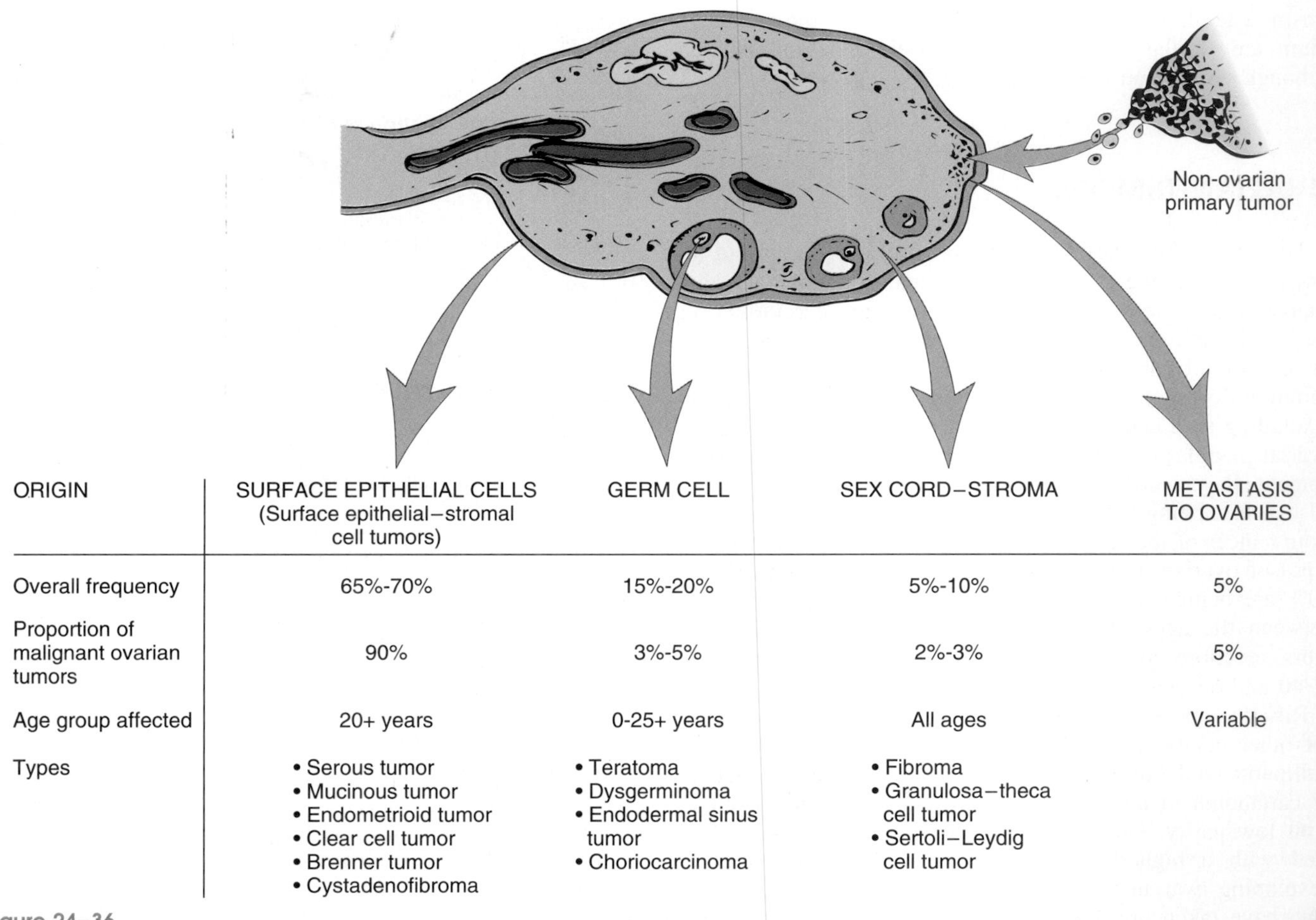

ORIGIN	SURFACE EPITHELIAL CELLS (Surface epithelial–stromal cell tumors)	GERM CELL	SEX CORD–STROMA	METASTASIS TO OVARIES
Overall frequency	65%-70%	15%-20%	5%-10%	5%
Proportion of malignant ovarian tumors	90%	3%-5%	2%-3%	5%
Age group affected	20+ years	0-25+ years	All ages	Variable
Types	• Serous tumor • Mucinous tumor • Endometrioid tumor • Clear cell tumor • Brenner tumor • Cystadenofibroma	• Teratoma • Dysgerminoma • Endodermal sinus tumor • Choriocarcinoma	• Fibroma • Granulosa–theca cell tumor • Sertoli–Leydig cell tumor	

Figure 24–36

Derivation of various ovarian neoplasms and some data on their frequency and age distribution.

Table 24–4. CERTAIN FREQUENCY DATA FOR MAJOR OVARIAN TUMORS

Type	Percentage of Malignant Ovarian Tumors	Percentage That Are Bilateral
Serous	40	
Benign (60%)		25
Borderline (15%)		30
Malignant (25%)		65
Mucinous	10	
Benign (80%)		5
Borderline (10%)		10
Malignant (10%)		20
Endometrioid carcinoma	20	40
Undifferentiated carcinoma	10	—
Clear cell carcinoma	6	40
Granulosa cell tumor	5	5
Teratoma		15
Benign (96%)		
Malignant (4%)	1	Rare
Metastatic	5	>50
Others	3	—

gastrointestinal tract symptoms due to compression by tumor or cancer invasion, and abdominal and vaginal bleeding are the most common symptoms. The benign forms may be entirely asymptomatic and occasionally are unexpected findings on abdominal or pelvic examination or during surgery.

Tumors of Surface (Coelomic) Epithelium

Most primary neoplasms in the ovary fall within this category. There are three major types of such tumors: serous, mucinous, and endometrioid. Mixtures of these epithelia frequently occur in the same tumor. Neoplasms composed of these three cell types range from clearly benign, to tumors of borderline malignancy, to malignant tumors.[69] These neoplasms range in size and composition. Tumors may be small and grossly imperceptible or massive, filling the pelvis and even the abdominal cavity. Components of the tumors may include cystic areas (cystadenomas), cystic and fibrous areas (cystadenofibromas), and predominantly

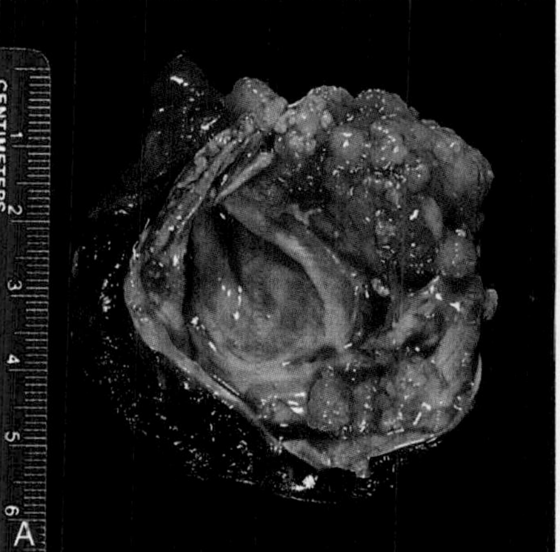

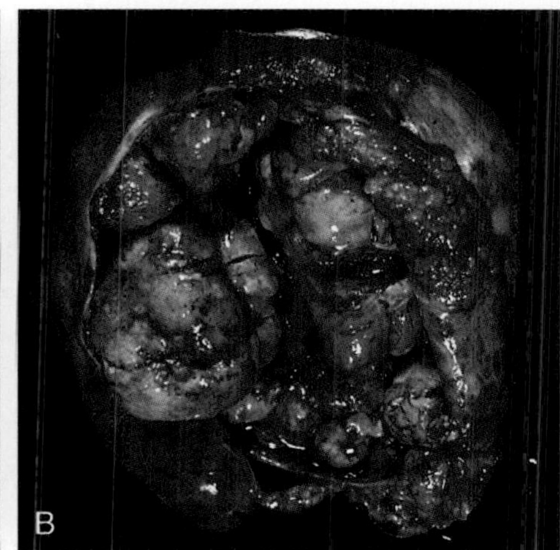

Figure 24–37

A, Borderline serous cystadenoma opened to display a cyst cavity lined by delicate papillary tumor growths. *B*, Cystadenocarcinoma. The cyst is opened to reveal a large, bulky tumor mass.

fibrous areas (adenofibromas). On gross examination, the risk of malignancy increases as a function of the amount of discernible solid epithelial growth, including papillary projections of soft tumor, thickened tumor lining the cyst spaces, or solid necrotic friable tissue depicting necrosis.

Although epithelial in differentiation, these tumors are derived from coelomic mesothelium and are graphic reminders of this tissue's ability to evolve into serous (tubal), endometrioid (endometrium), and mucinous (cervix) epithelia present in the normal female genital tract. Why these tumors predominate in the ovary is a mystery but appears linked to the incorporation of coelomic epithelium into the ovarian cortex to form mesothelial inclusion cysts. This incorporation occurs by the formation of surface adhesions, atrophy with epithelial infolding, and repair of ovulation sites. The close association of ovarian carcinomas with either the ovarian surface mesothelium or inclusion cysts may explain the development of extraovarian carcinomas of similar histology from similar coelomic epithelial rests (so-called endosalpingiosis) in the mesentery.

SEROUS TUMORS

These common cystic neoplasms are lined by tall, columnar, ciliated epithelial cells and are filled with clear serous fluid. Although the term serous appropriately describes the cyst fluid, it has become synonymous with the tubal-like epithelium in these tumors. Together the benign, borderline, and malignant types account for about 30% of all ovarian tumors. About 75% are benign or of borderline malignancy, and 25% are malignant. Serous cystadenocarcinomas account for approximately 40% of all cancers of the ovary and are the most common malignant ovarian tumors. Benign and borderline tumors are most common between the ages of 20 and 50 years. Cystadenocarcinomas occur later in life on average, although somewhat earlier in familial cases.

MORPHOLOGY. In gross appearance, the characteristic serous tumor has one or a few fibrous walled cysts averaging 10 to 15 cm in diameter and occasionally up to 40 cm. Benign tumors contain a smooth glistening cyst wall with no epithelial thickening or small papillary projections (i.e., papillary cystadenoma). Borderline tumors contain an increasing amount of papillary projections (Fig. 24–37*A*). Larger amounts of solid or papillary tumor mass, irregularity in the tumor mass, and fixation or nodularity of the capsule are all important indicators of probable malignancy (Fig. 24–37*B*). Bilaterality is common, occurring in 20% of benign cystadenomas, 30% of borderline tumors, and approximately 66% of cystadenocarcinomas. On histologic examination, the lining epithelium is composed of columnar epithelium with abundant cilia in benign tumors (Fig. 24–38). Microscopic papillae may be found. Tumors of borderline malignancy contain increased complexity of the stromal papillae with stratification of the epithelium and nuclear atypia, but destructive infiltrative growth into the stroma is not seen (Fig. 24–39). Cystadenocarcinomas exhibit even more

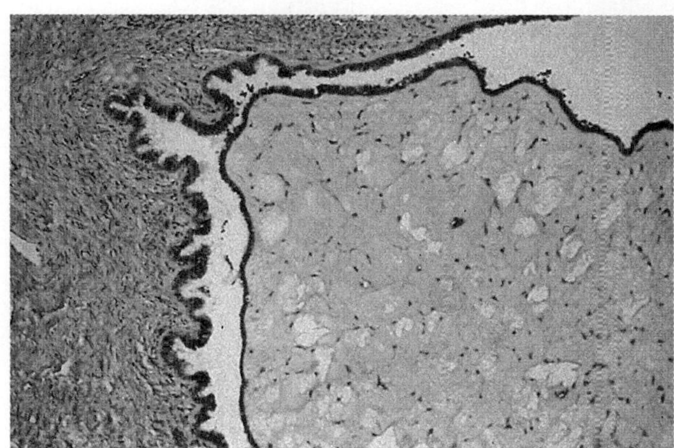

Figure 24–38

Histopathology of papillary serous cystadenoma revealing stromal papillae with a columnar epithelium.

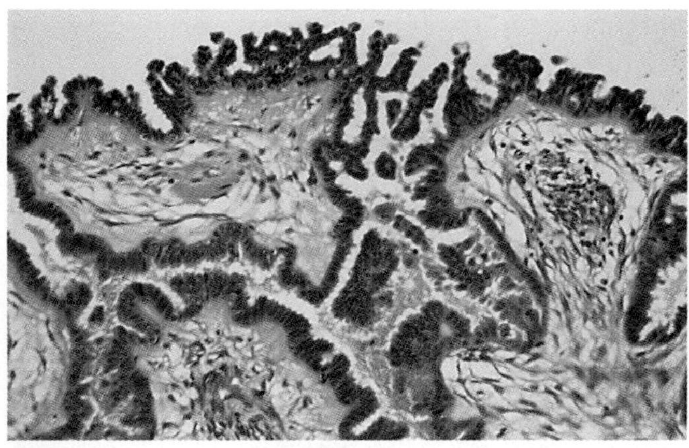

Figure 24–39

Borderline serous cystadenoma exhibiting increased architectural complexity and epithelial cell stratification.

complex growth with infiltration or frank effacement of the underlying stroma by solid growth (Fig. 24–40). The individual tumor cells in the carcinomatous lesions display the usual features of all malignant neoplasia, and with the more extreme degrees of atypia, the cells may become undifferentiated. Concentric calcifications (psammoma bodies) characterize serous tumors, although they are not specific for neoplasia when they are found alone.

The biologic behavior of serous tumors depends on both degree of differentiation and distribution. Importantly, serous tumors may occur on the surface of the ovaries and, rarely, as primary tumors of the peritoneal surface (Fig. 24–41). Predictably, unencapsulated serous tumors of the ovarian surface are more likely to extend to the peritoneal surfaces, and prognosis is closely related to the histologic

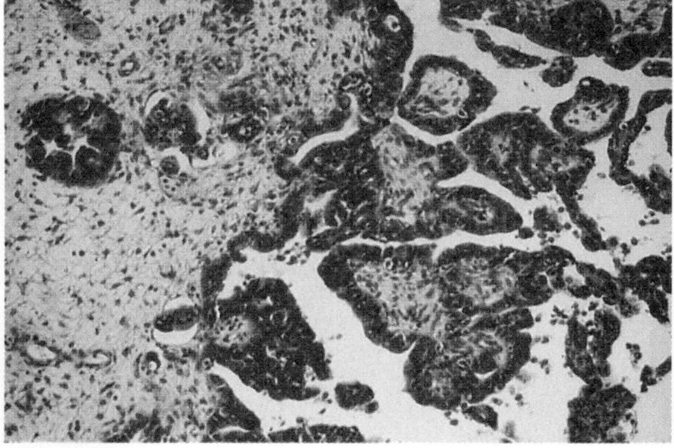

Figure 24–40

Papillary serous cystadenocarcinoma of the ovary with invasion of underlying stroma.

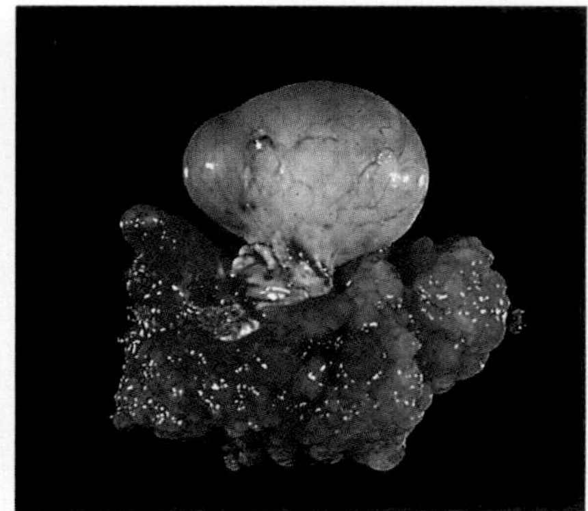

Figure 24–41

Serous epithelial tumor growth from the surface of the ovary (*above*).

appearance of the tumor and its growth pattern on the peritoneum. Borderline tumors can also originate from or extend to the peritoneal surfaces and may remain localized, causing no symptoms, or slowly spread, producing intestinal obstruction or other complications after many years. Frank carcinomas infiltrate the soft tissue and form large intra-abdominal masses and rapid deterioration. For this reason, careful pathologic classification of the tumor, even if it has extended to the peritoneum, is relevant to both prognosis and selection of therapy.[75] The 5-year survival rate for borderline and malignant tumors confined within the ovarian mass is 100% and 70%, whereas the 5-year survival rate for the same tumors involving the peritoneum is about 90% and 25%, respectively. Because of their protracted course, borderline tumors may recur after many years, and 5-year survival is not synonymous with cure.

MUCINOUS TUMORS

These tumors closely resemble their serous counterparts. They are somewhat less common, accounting for about 25% of all ovarian neoplasms. They occur principally in middle adult life and are rare before puberty and after menopause. Eighty per cent are benign or borderline, and about 15% are malignant. Mucinous cystadenocarcinomas are relatively uncommon and account for only 10% of all ovarian cancers.

MORPHOLOGY. In gross appearance, the mucinous tumors differ from the serous variety in several ways. They are characterized by more cysts of variable size and a rarity of surface involvement and are less frequently bilateral. Approximately 5% of mucinous cystadenomas and 20% of mucinous cystadenocarcinomas are bilateral. Mucinous tumors tend to produce larger cystic masses, and some have been recorded with weights of more than 25 kg. They appear grossly as multiloculated tumors filled with sticky, gelatinous fluid rich in glycoproteins (Fig. 24–42*A*).

On histologic examination, benign mucinous tu-

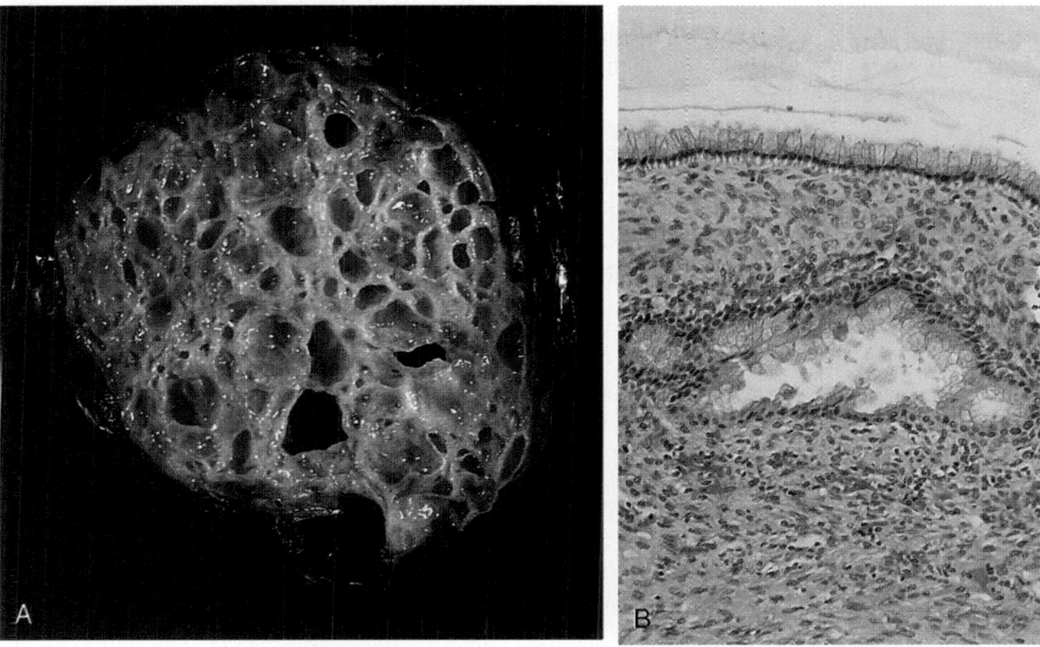

Figure 24–42

A, A mucinous cystadenoma with its multicystic appearance and delicate septa. Note the presence of glistening mucin within the cysts. *B*, Columnar cell lining of mucinous cystadenoma.

mors are characterized by a lining of tall columnar epithelial cells with apical mucin and the absence of cilia, akin to benign cervical or intestinal epithelia (Fig. 24–42*B*). Borderline tumors exhibit abundant glandlike or papillary growth with nuclear atypia and stratification and are strikingly similar to tubular adenomas or villous adenomas of the intestine. Cystadenocarcinomas contain more solid growth with conspicuous epithelial cell atypia and stratification, loss of gland architecture, and necrosis and are similar to colonic cancer in appearance. Because both borderline and malignant mucinous cystadenomas form complex glands in the stroma, the documentation of clear-cut stromal invasion, which is uncomplicated in serous tumors, is subjective, and some authors describe a category of "noninvasive" mucinous carcinomas for those tumors with marked epithelial atypia without obvious stromal alterations. Approximate 10-year survival rates for stage I borderline, noninvasive malignant, and frankly invasive malignant tumors are greater than 95%, 90%, and 66%, respectively.[76]

A condition associated with mucinous ovarian neoplasms is *pseudomyxoma peritonei.* This disorder combines the presence of an ovarian tumor with extensive mucinous ascites, cystic epithelial implants on the peritoneal surfaces, and adhesions (Fig. 24–43). Pseudomyxoma peritonei, if extensive, may result in intestinal obstruction and death. Recent evidence strongly supports an extraovarian (usually appendiceal) primary mucinous tumor in many cases, with secondary ovarian and peritoneal spread[77] (Chapter 18).

ENDOMETRIOID TUMORS

These neoplasms account for approximately 20% of all ovarian cancers, excluding endometriosis, which is considered non-neoplastic. Most endometrioid tumors are carcinomas. Less commonly, benign forms—usually cystadenofi-

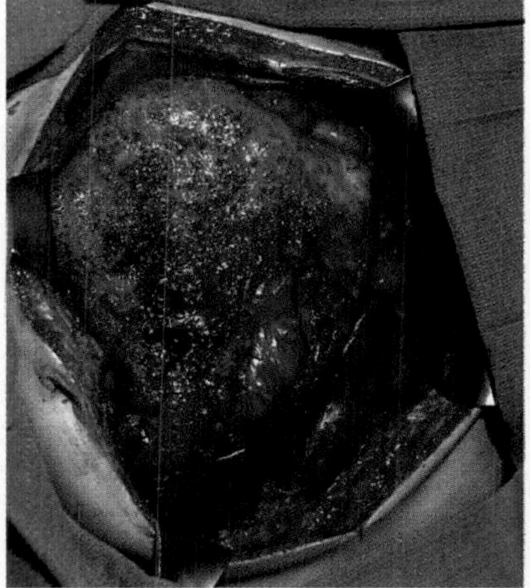

Figure 24–43

Pseudomyxoma peritonei viewed at laparotomy revealing massive overgrowth of a gelatinous metastatic tumor originating from the appendix. (Courtesy of Dr. Paul H. Sugarbaker, Washington Hospital Cancer Center, Washington, DC.)

bromas—are encountered.[78] They are distinguished from serous and mucinous tumors by the presence of tubular glands bearing a close resemblance to benign or malignant endometrium. For obscure reasons, 15% to 30% of endometrioid carcinomas are accompanied by a carcinoma of the endometrium, and the relatively good prognosis in such cases suggests that the two may arise independently rather than by metastatic spread from one another.[79] About 15% of cases with endometrioid carcinoma coexist with endometriosis, although an origin directly from ovarian coelomic epithelium is also possible.

MORPHOLOGY. In gross appearance, endometrioid carcinomas present as a combination of solid and cystic areas, similar to other cystadenocarcinomas. Forty per cent involve both ovaries, and such bilaterality usually, although not always, implies extension of the neoplasm beyond the female genital tract. On histologic examination, glandular patterns bearing a strong resemblance to those of endometrial origin are seen. The overall 5-year survival rate is 40% to 50%.

CLEAR CELL ADENOCARCINOMA

This uncommon pattern of surface epithelial tumor of the ovary is characterized by large epithelial cells with abundant clear cytoplasm. Because these tumors sometimes occur in association with endometriosis or endometrioid carcinoma of the ovary and resemble clear cell carcinoma of the endometrium, they are now thought to be of müllerian duct origin and variants of endometrioid adenocarcinoma.[69] The clear cell tumors of the ovary can be predominantly solid or cystic. In the solid neoplasm, the clear cells are arranged in sheets or tubules. In the cystic variety, the neoplastic cells line the spaces. The 5-year survival rate is approximately 50% when the tumors are confined to the ovaries; however, these tumors tend to be aggressive, and with spread beyond the ovary, a survival of 5 years is exceptional.

CYSTADENOFIBROMA

Cystadenofibromas are variants in which there is more pronounced proliferation of the fibrous stroma that underlies the columnar lining epithelium. These benign tumors are usually small and multilocular and have simple papillary processes that do not become so complicated and branching as those found in the ordinary cystadenoma. They may be composed of mucinous, serous, endometrioid, and transitional (Brenner tumors) epithelium. Borderline lesions with cellular atypia and, rarely, tumors with focal carcinoma occur, but metastatic spread of either is extremely uncommon.

BRENNER TUMOR

Brenner tumors are uncommon adenofibromas in which the epithelial component consists of nests of transitional cells resembling those lining the urinary bladder. Less frequently, the nests contain microcysts or glandular spaces lined by columnar, mucin-secreting cells. For reasons not clear, Brenner tumors are occasionally encountered in mucinous cystadenomas.

MORPHOLOGY. These neoplasms may be solid or cystic, are usually unilateral (approximately 90%), and vary in size from small lesions less than 1 cm in diameter to massive tumors up to 20 and 30 cm (Fig 24–44*A*). The fibrous stroma, resembling that of the normal ovary, is marked by sharply demarcated nests of epithelial cells resembling the epithelium of the urinary tract, often with mucinous glands in their center (Fig. 24–44*B*). Infrequently, the stroma is composed of somewhat plump fibroblasts resembling theca cells, and

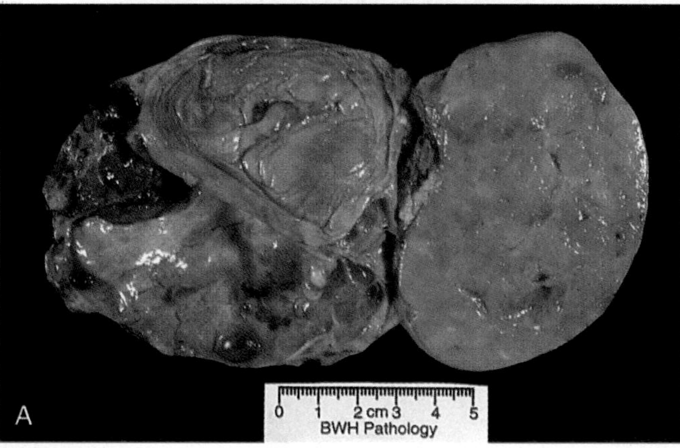

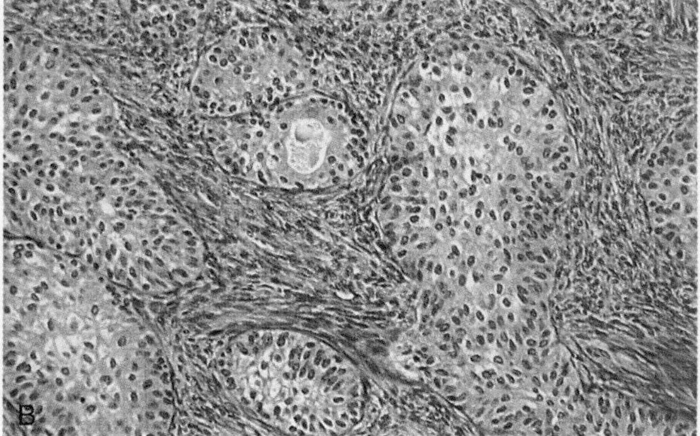

Figure 24–44

A, Brenner tumor (*right*) associated with a benign cystic teratoma (*left*). *B*, Histologic detail of characteristic epithelial nests within the ovarian stroma.

such neoplasms may have hormonal activity. Most Brenner tumors are benign, but borderline (proliferative Brenner tumor) and malignant counterparts have been reported.

Several reports have emphasized the occurrence of ovarian tumors that are composed in part or all of neoplastic epithelium similar to transitional carcinoma of the bladder but without a coexisting Brenner component. Referred to as *transitional cell carcinoma,* these tumors arise from coelomic epithelium or from selective differentiation of existing carcinomas. This form of differentiation is of interest because of speculation, albeit controversial, that transitional cell tumors are susceptible to chemotherapy, with correspondingly more favorable prognosis.[80]

CLINICAL COURSE OF SURFACE EPITHELIAL TUMORS

All ovarian epithelial carcinomas produce similar clinical manifestations, most commonly lower abdominal pain and abdominal enlargement. Gastrointestinal complaints, urinary frequency, dysuria, pelvic pressure, and many other symptoms may appear. Benign lesions are easily resected with cure. The malignant forms, however, tend to cause the progressive weakness, weight loss, and cachexia characteristic of all malignant neoplasms. If the carcinomas extend through the capsule of the tumor to seed the peritoneal cavity, massive ascites is common. Characteristically, the ascitic fluid is filled with diagnostic exfoliated tumor cells. The peritoneal seeding that these malignant neoplasms produce is distinctive: they tend to seed all serosal surfaces diffusely with 0.1- to 0.5-cm nodules of tumor. These surface implants rarely invade deeply into the underlying parenchyma of the organ. The regional nodes are often involved, and metastases may be found in the liver, lungs, gastrointestinal tract, and elsewhere. Metastasis across the midline to the opposite ovary is discovered in about half the cases by the time of laparotomy and heralds a progressive downhill course to death within a few months or years.

Because ovarian carcinomas often remain undiagnosed until they are large, or originate on the ovarian surface from where they readily spread to the pelvis, many patients are first seen with lesions that are no longer confined to the ovary. This is perhaps the primary reason for the relatively poor 5- and 10-year survival rates for these patients, compared with rates in cervical and endometrial carcinoma. For these reasons, specific biochemical markers for tumor antigens or tumor products in the plasma of these patients are being sought vigorously. One such marker is a high-molecular-weight glycoprotein present in more than 80% of serous and endometrioid carcinomas, known as CA-125, but whether its use will influence outcome is unproven.[81]

Germ Cell Tumors

Germ cell tumors constitute 15% to 20% of all ovarian tumors.[69] Most are benign cystic teratomas, but the remainder, which are found principally in children and young adults, have a higher incidence of malignant behavior and pose problems in histologic diagnosis and in therapy. They bear a remarkable homology to germ tumors in the male testis (Chapter 23) and arise from germ cell differentiation in a similar manner (Fig. 24–45).

TERATOMAS

Teratomas are divided into three categories: (1) mature (benign), (2) immature (malignant), and (3) monodermal or highly specialized.

Mature (Benign) Teratomas. Most benign teratomas are cystic and are better known in clinical parlance as dermoid cysts. These neoplasms are invariably benign and

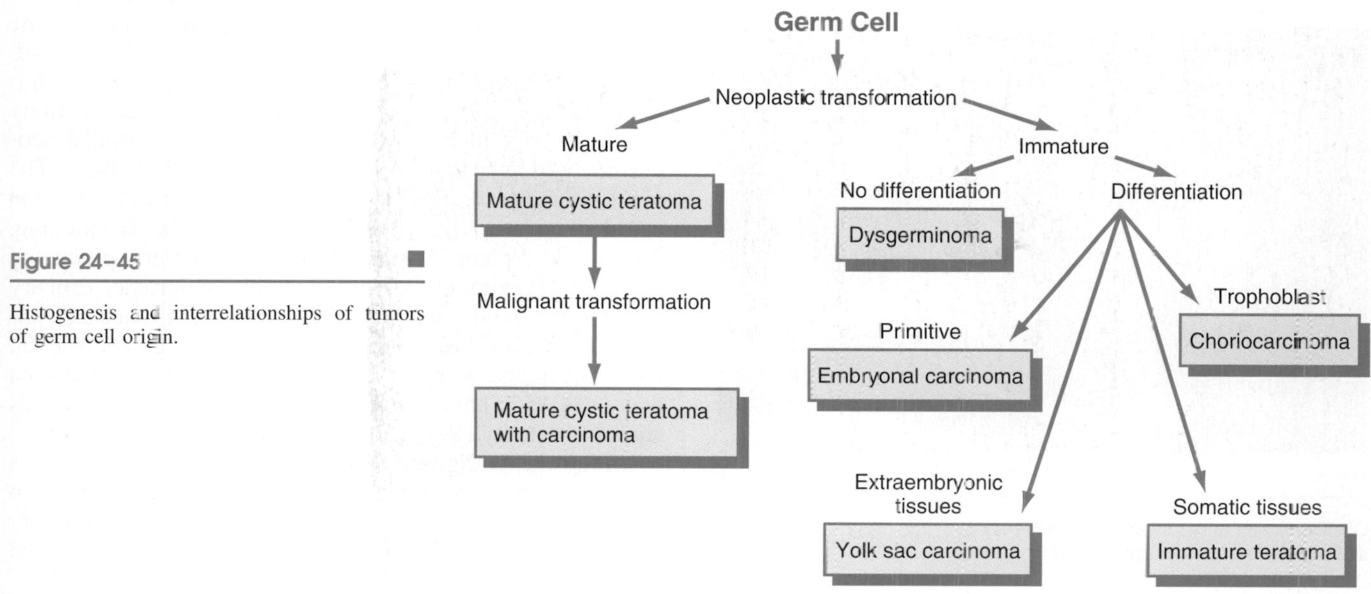

Figure 24–45

Histogenesis and interrelationships of tumors of germ cell origin.

are presumably derived from the ectodermal differentiation of totipotential cells. Cystic teratomas are usually found in young women during the active reproductive years.[69]

MORPHOLOGY. Benign teratomas are bilateral in 10% to 15% of cases. Characteristically, they are unilocular cysts containing hair and cheesy sebaceous material (Fig. 24–46). On section, they reveal a thin wall lined by an opaque, gray-white, wrinkled, apparent epidermis. From this epidermis, hair shafts frequently protrude. Within the wall, it is common to find tooth structures and areas of calcification.

On histologic examination, the cyst wall is composed of stratified squamous epithelium with underlying sebaceous glands, hair shafts, and other skin adnexal structures (Fig. 24–47). In most cases, structures from other germ layers can be identified, such as cartilage, bone, thyroid tissue, and other organoid formations. Dermoid cysts are sometimes incorporated within the wall of a mucinous cystadenoma. **About 1% of the dermoids undergo malignant transformation of any one of the component elements (e.g., thyroid carcinoma, melanoma, but most commonly squamous cell carcinoma).**

In rare instances, a teratoma is solid but is composed entirely of benign-looking heterogeneous collections of tissues and organized structures derived from all three germ layers. These tumors presumably have the same histogenetic origin as dermoid cysts but lack preponderant differentiation into ectodermal derivatives. **These neoplasms may be initially difficult to differentiate from the malignant, immature teratomas, which almost always are largely solid.**

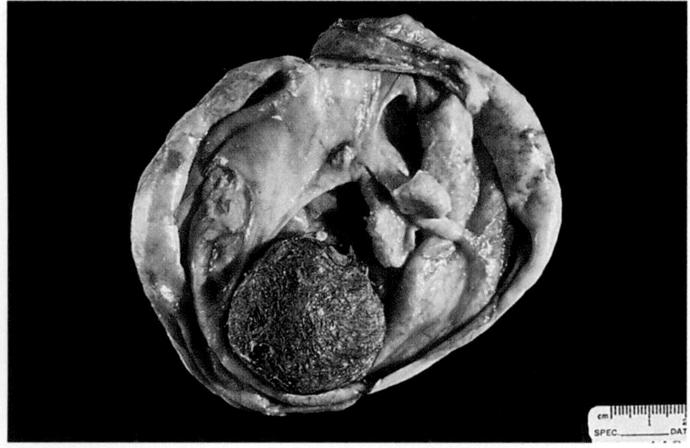

Figure 24–46

Opened mature cystic teratoma (dermoid cyst) of the ovary. Hair (bottom) and a mixture of tissues are evident.

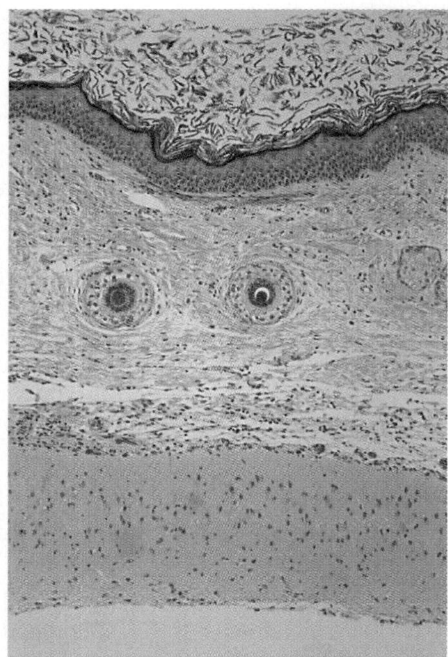

Figure 24–47

Benign cystic teratoma. Low-power view of skin (*top*), beneath which there is brain tissue (*bottom*).

The origin of teratomas has been a matter of fascination for centuries. Some common beliefs blamed witches, nightmares, or adultery with the devil. The current parthenogenetic theory suggests origin from a meiotic germ cell. The karyotype of all benign ovarian teratomas is 46,XX. From the results of chromosome banding techniques and the distribution of electrophoretic variants of enzymes in the normal and teratoma cells, Linder and coworkers[82] suggested that tumors arise from an ovum after the first meiotic division. Other derivations have been proposed.[83]

Monodermal or Specialized Teratomas. The specialized teratomas are a remarkable, rare group of tumors, the most common of which are struma ovarii and carcinoid. They are always unilateral, although a contralateral teratoma may be present. Struma ovarii is composed entirely of mature thyroid tissue. Interestingly, these thyroidal neoplasms may hyperfunction, producing hyperthyroidism. The ovarian carcinoid, which presumably rises from intestinal epithelium in a teratoma, might in fact be functioning, particularly in large (greater than 7 cm) tumors, producing 5-hydroxytryptamine and the carcinoid syndrome. Primary ovarian carcinoid can be distinguished from metastatic intestinal carcinoid, the latter virtually always bilateral. Even more rare is the strumal carcinoid, a combination of struma ovarii and carcinoid in the same ovary. Primary carcinoids are uncommonly (less than 2%) malignant.

Immature Malignant Teratomas. These are rare tumors that differ from benign teratomas in that the component tissue resembles that observed in the fetus or embryo rather than the adult. The tumor is found chiefly in prepubertal

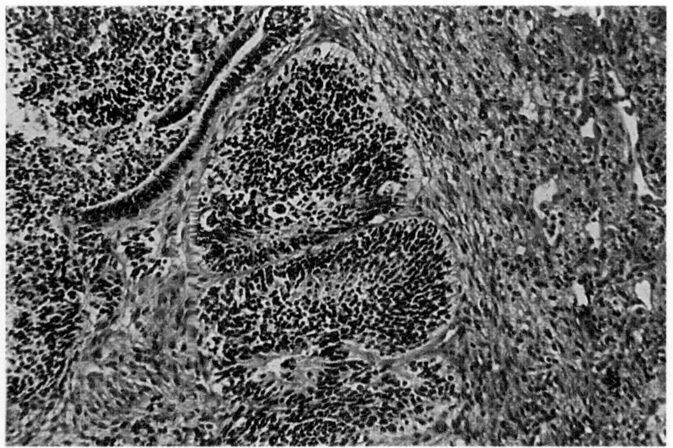

Figure 24–48 ■

Immature teratoma of the ovary illustrating primitive neuroepithelium.

adolescents and young women, the mean age being 18 years.[84]

MORPHOLOGY. The tumors are bulky and have a smooth external surface. On section, they have a solid or predominantly solid structure. There are areas of necrosis and hemorrhage. Hair, grumous material, cartilage, bone, and calcification may be present. On microscopic examination, there are varying amounts of immature tissue differentiating toward cartilage, glands, bone, muscle, nerve, and others. An important risk for subsequent extraovarian spread is the histologic grade of tumor (I through III), which is based on the proportion of tissue (in histologic sections) containing immature neuroepithelium (Fig. 24–48).

Immature teratomas grow rapidly and frequently penetrate the capsule with spread or metastases. Stage I tumors, however, particularly those with low-grade (grade I) histology, have an excellent prognosis. Higher grade tumors confined to the ovary are generally treated with prophylactic chemotherapy. Most recurrences develop in the first 2 years, and absence of disease beyond this period carries an excellent chance of cure.

DYSGERMINOMA

The dysgerminoma[85] is best remembered as the ovarian counterpart of the seminoma of the testis. Similar to the seminoma, it is composed of large vesicular cells having a cleared cytoplasm, well-defined cell boundaries, and centrally placed regular nuclei. Relatively uncommon tumors, the dysgerminomas account for about 2% of all ovarian cancers yet form about half of malignant germ cell tumors. They may occur in childhood, but 75% occur in the second and third decades. Some occur in patients with gonadal dysgenesis, including pseudohermaphroditism. Most of these tumors have no endocrine function. A few produce elevated levels of chorionic gonadotropin and may have syncytiotrophoblastic giant cells on histologic examination.

MORPHOLOGY. Usually unilateral (80% to 90%), they most frequently are solid tumors ranging in size from barely visible nodules to masses that virtually fill the entire abdomen. On cut surface, they have a yellow-white to gray-pink appearance and are often soft and fleshy. On histologic examination, the dysgerminoma cells are dispersed in sheets or cords separated by scant fibrous stroma (Fig. 24–49). As in the seminoma, the fibrous stroma is infiltrated with mature lymphocytes and occasional granulomas. On occasion, small nodules of dysgerminoma are encountered in the wall of an otherwise benign cystic teratoma; conversely, a predominantly dysgerminomatous tumor may contain a small cystic teratoma.

All dysgerminomas are malignant, but the degree of histologic atypia is variable, and only about one third are aggressive. Thus, a unilateral tumor that has not broken through the capsule and has not spread has an excellent prognosis (up to 96% cure rate) after simple salpingo-oophorectomy. These neoplasms are extremely radiosensitive, and even those that have extended beyond the ovary can generally be controlled by radiotherapy. Overall survival exceeds 80%.

ENDODERMAL SINUS (YOLK SAC) TUMOR

This tumor is rare but is the second most common malignant tumor of germ cell origin. It is thought to be

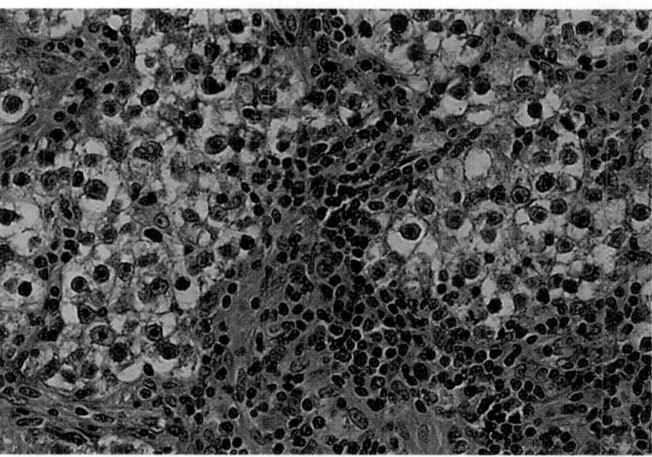

Figure 24–49 ■

Histopathology of dysgerminoma showing polyhedral tumor cells with round nuclei and adjacent inflammation.

derived from a multipotential embryonal carcinoma by selection and differentiation toward yolk sac structure (Fig. 24–45). Similar to the yolk sac, the tumor is rich in α-fetoprotein and α_1-antitrypsin. Its characteristic histologic feature is a glomerulus-like structure composed of a central blood vessel enveloped by germ cells within a space similarly lined by germ cells (Schiller-Duval body) (Fig. 24–50). Similar structures are observed in the yolk sac of the rat placenta. Conspicuous intracellular and extracellular hyaline droplets are present in all tumors, and some of these can be stained for α-fetoprotein by immunoperoxidase techniques.

Most patients are children or young women presenting with abdominal pain and a rapidly developing pelvic mass. The tumors usually appear to involve a single ovary but grow rapidly and aggressively. These tumors were once almost uniformly fatal within 2 years of diagnosis, but combination chemotherapy has measurably improved the outcome.

CHORIOCARCINOMA

More commonly of placental origin, the choriocarcinoma, similar to the endodermal sinus tumor, is an example of extraembryonic differentiation of malignant germ cells. It is generally held that a germ cell origin can be certified only in the prepubertal girl because after this age, an origin from an ovarian ectopic pregnancy cannot be excluded.

Most ovarian choriocarcinomas exist in combination with other germ cell tumors, and pure choriocarcinomas are extremely rare. They are histologically identical with the more common placental lesions, described later. These ovarian primaries are ugly tumors that generally have metastasized widely through the bloodstream to the lungs, liver, bone, and other viscera by the time of diagnosis. Like all choriocarcinomas, they elaborate high levels of chorionic gonadotropins that are sometimes helpful in establishing the diagnosis or highlighting recurrences. In contrast to choriocarcinomas arising in placental tissue, those arising in the ovary are generally unresponsive to chemotherapy and are highly fatal.

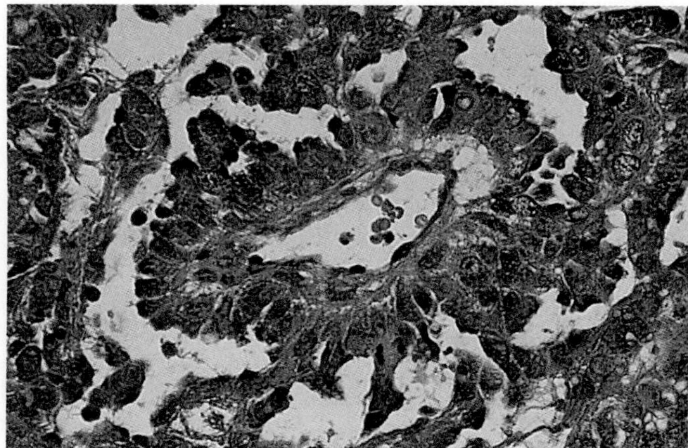

Figure 24–50

A Schiller-Duval body in yolk sac carcinoma.

OTHER GERM CELL TUMORS

These include (1) embryonal carcinoma, another highly malignant tumor of primitive embryonal elements, histologically similar to tumors arising in the testes (Chapter 23); (2) polyembryoma, a malignant tumor containing so-called embryoid bodies; and (3) mixed germ cell tumors containing various combinations of dysgerminoma, teratoma, endodermal sinus tumor, and choriocarcinoma.

Sex Cord–Stromal Tumors

These ovarian neoplasms are derived from the ovarian stroma, which in turn is derived from the sex cords of the embryonic gonad. Because the undifferentiated gonadal mesenchyme eventually produces structures of specific cell type in both male (Sertoli and Leydig) and female (granulosa and theca) gonads, tumors emulating all of these cell types can be identified in the ovary.[86] Moreover, because some of these cells normally secrete estrogens (theca cells) or androgens (Leydig cells), their corresponding tumors may be either feminizing (granulosa-theca cell tumors) or masculinizing (Leydig cell tumors).

GRANULOSA-THECA CELL TUMORS

This designation embraces ovarian neoplasms composed of varying proportions of granulosa and theca cell differentiation. These tumors are composed almost entirely of granulosa cells or a mixture of granulosa and theca cells. Collectively, these neoplasms account for about 5% of all ovarian tumors. Although they may be discovered at any age, approximately two thirds occur in postmenopausal women.

MORPHOLOGY. Granulosa cell tumors are usually unilateral and vary from microscopic foci to large, solid, and cystic encapsulated masses. Tumors that are endocrinologically active have a yellow coloration to their cut surfaces, produced by contained lipids. The pure thecomas are solid, firm tumors.

The granulosa cell component of these tumors takes one of many histologic patterns. The small, cuboidal to polygonal cells may grow in anastomosing cords, sheets, or strands (Fig. 24–51). In occasional cases, small, distinctive, glandlike structures filled with an acidophilic material recall immature follicles (Call-Exner bodies). When these structures are evident, the diagnosis is rendered considerably more simple. The thecoma component consists of clusters or sheets of cuboidal to polygonal cells. In some tumors, the granulosa or theca cells may appear more plump with ample

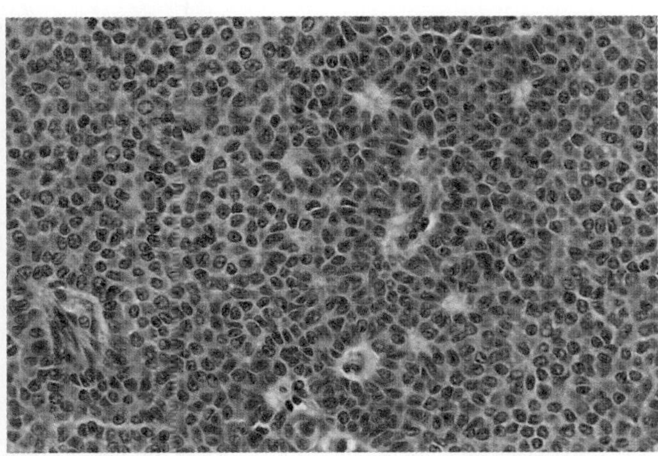

Figure 24–51

Granulosa cell tumor. The tumor cells are arranged in sheets punctuated by small follicle-like structures (Call-Exner bodies).

cytoplasm characteristic of luteinization (i.e., luteinized granulosa-theca cell tumors).

Granulosa-theca cell tumors have clinical importance for two reasons: (1) their potential elaboration of large amounts of estrogen and (2) the small but distinct hazard of malignancy in the granulosa cell forms. Functionally active tumors in young girls (juvenile granulosa cell tumors) may produce precocious sexual development in prepubertal girls. In adult women, they may be associated with endometrial hyperplasia, cystic disease of the breast, and endometrial carcinoma. About 10% to 15% of patients with steroid-producing tumors eventually develop an endometrial carcinoma. Occasional granulosa cell tumors produce androgens, masculinizing the patient.

The additional clinical significance of these tumors lies in the fact that all are potentially malignant. It is difficult, from the histologic evaluation of granulosa cell tumors, to predict their biologic behavior.[84] The estimates of clinical malignancy (recurrence, extension) range from 5% to 25%. In general, malignant tumors pursue an indolent course in which local recurrences may be amenable to surgical therapy. Recurrences within the pelvis and abdomen may appear many years (10 to 20) after removal of the original tumor. The 10-year survival rate is approximately 85%. Tumors composed predominantly of theca cells are almost never malignant.

THECOMA-FIBROMAS

Tumors arising in the ovarian stroma that are composed of either fibroblasts (fibromas) or more plump spindle cells with lipid droplets (thecomas) are relatively common and account for about 4% of all ovarian tumor types (Fig. 24–52*A*). Because many tumors contain a mixture of these cells, they are termed fibroma-thecomas. Pure thecomas are rare, but tumors in which these cells predominate may be hormonally active. Most are composed principally of fibroblasts and are for practical purposes hormonally inactive.

Fibroma-thecomas of the ovary are unilateral in about 90% of cases and are usually solid, spherical or slightly lobulated, encapsulated, hard, gray-white masses covered by glistening, intact ovarian serosa (Fig. 24–52*B*). On histologic examination, they are composed of well-differentiated fibroblasts with a more or less scant collagenous connective tissue interspersed between the cells. Areas of thecal differentiation may be identified and can be confirmed by fat stains. This exercise, however, is considered unnecessary on clinical grounds.

In addition to the relatively nonspecific findings of pain and pelvic mass, the tumors may be accompanied by two curious associations. The first is ascites, found in about 40% of cases, in which the tumors measure more than 6 cm in diameter. Uncommonly, there is also hydrothorax,

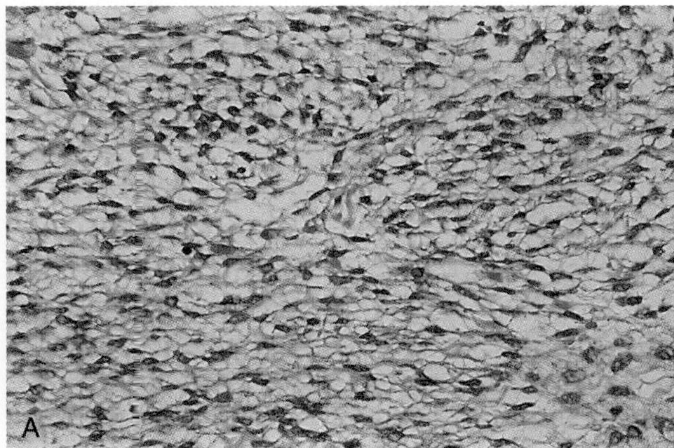

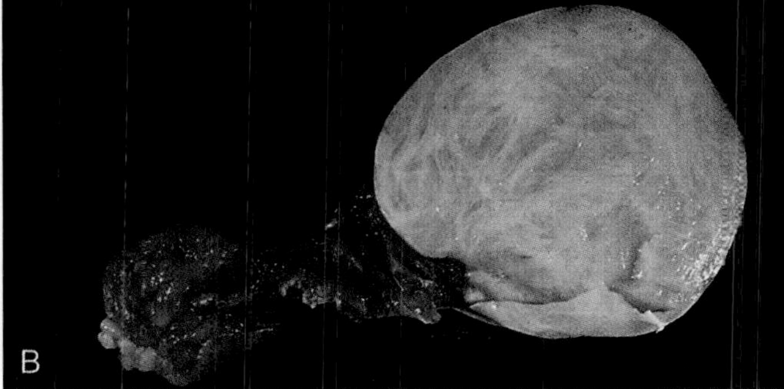

Figure 24–52

A, Thecoma-fibroma composed of plump, differentiated stromal cells with thecal appearance. *B*, Large bisected fibroma of the ovary apparent as a white, firm mass (*right*). The fallopian tube is attached.

usually only of the right side. This combination of findings (i.e., ovarian tumor, hydrothorax, and ascites) is designated Meigs syndrome. The genesis is unknown. The second association is with the basal cell nevus syndrome, described in Chapter 27. Rarely, cellular tumors with mitotic activity and increased nuclear cytoplasmic ratio are identified; because they may pursue a malignant course, they are termed fibrosarcomas.[87]

SERTOLI-LEYDIG CELL TUMORS (ANDROBLASTOMAS)

These tumors recapitulate, to a certain extent, the cells of the testis at various stages of development.[88] They commonly produce masculinization or at least defeminization, but a few have estrogenic effects. They occur in women of all ages, although the peak incidence is in the second and third decades. The embryogenesis of such male-directed stromal cells remains a puzzle. These tumors are unilateral and resemble granulosa-theca cell neoplasms.

The cut surface is usually solid and varies from gray to golden brown in appearance (Fig. 24–53*A*). On histologic examination, the well-differentiated tumors exhibit tubules composed of Sertoli cells or Leydig cells interspersed with stroma (Fig. 24–53*B*). The intermediate forms show only outlines of immature tubules and large eosinophilic Leydig cells. The poorly differentiated tumors have a sarcomatous pattern with a disorderly disposition of epithelial cell cords. Leydig cells may be absent. Heterologous elements, such as mucinous glands, bone, and cartilage, may be present in some tumors.

The incidence of recurrence or metastasis by Sertoli-Leydig cell tumors is less than 5%. These neoplasms may block normal female sexual development in children and may cause defeminization of women, manifested by atrophy of the breasts, amenorrhea, sterility, and loss of hair. The syndrome may progress to striking virilization, that is, hirsutism, male distribution of hair, hypertrophy of the clitoris, and voice changes.

OTHER SEX CORD–STROMAL TUMORS

The ovarian hilum normally contains clusters of polygonal cells arranged around vessels (hilar cells). *Hilus cell tumors (pure Leydig cell tumor)* are derived from these cells and are rare, unilateral, and characterized histologically by large lipid-laden cells with distinct borders. A typical cytoplasmic structure characteristic of Leydig cells (Reinke crystalloids) is usually present. Typically, the patients present clinically with evidence of masculinization, hirsutism, voice changes, and clitoral enlargement. The tumors are unilateral. The most consistent laboratory finding is an elevated 17-ketosteroid excretion level unresponsive to cortisone suppression. Treatment is surgical excision. True hilus cell tumors are almost always benign. On occasion, histologically identical tumors occur in the cortical stroma *(nonhilar Leydig cell tumors).*

In addition to Leydig cell tumors, the stroma rarely may give rise to tumors composed of pure luteinized cells, producing small benign tumors rarely more than 3 cm in diameter. The tumor may produce the clinical effects of androgen, estrogen, or progestogen stimulation.

As mentioned previously, the ovary in pregnancy may exhibit microscopic nodular proliferations of theca cells in response to gonadotropins. A frank tumor may rarely develop (termed *pregnancy luteoma)* that closely resembles a corpus luteum of pregnancy. These tumors have been associated with virilization in pregnant patients and in their respective female infants.

Gonadoblastoma is an uncommon tumor thought to be composed of germ cells and sex cord–stroma derivatives. It occurs in individuals with abnormal sexual development and in gonads of indeterminate nature. Eighty per cent are phenotypic females, and 20% are phenotypic males with undescended testicles and female internal secondary organs. On microscopic examination, the tumor consists of nests of a mixture of germ cells and sex cord derivatives resembling immature Sertoli and granulosa cells. A coexistent dysgerminoma occurs in 50% of the cases. The prognosis is excellent if the tumor is completely excised.[89]

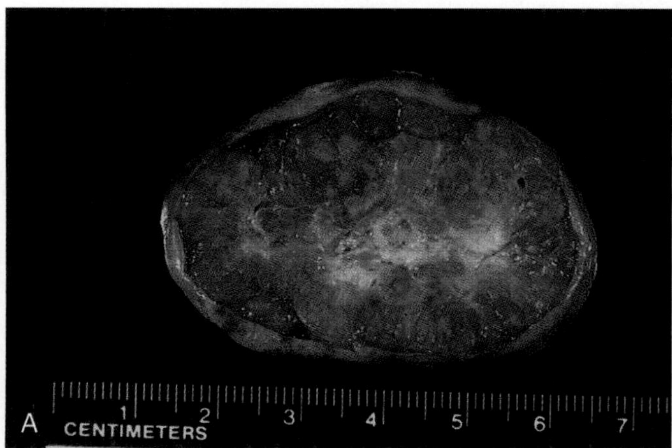

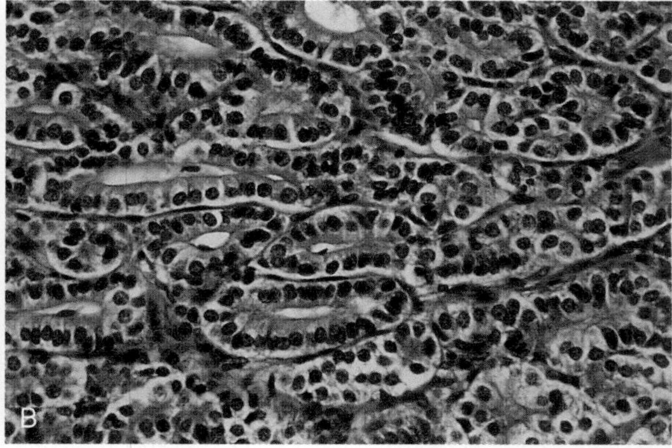

Figure 24–53

Sertoli cell tumor. *A*, Gross photograph illustrating characteristic golden yellow appearance of the tumor. *B*, Photomicrograph showing well-differentiated Sertoli cell tubules. (Courtesy of Dr. William Welch, Brigham and Women's Hospital, Boston, MA.)

Another tumor of possible stromal origin is small cell carcinoma of the ovary. These malignant tumors occur predominantly in young women and may be associated with hypercalcemia.[90]

METASTATIC TUMORS

The most common "metastatic" tumors of the ovary are probably derived from tumors of müllerian origin: the uterus, fallopian tube, contralateral ovary, or pelvic peritoneum. Although technically metastases, they are accepted as part of the "field effect" of müllerian neoplasia. The most common extramüllerian primaries are the breast and gastrointestinal tract, including stomach, biliary tract, and pancreas. A classic example of metastatic gastrointestinal neoplasia to the ovaries is termed Krukenberg tumor, characterized by bilateral metastases composed of mucin-producing, signet-ring cancer cells, most often of gastric origin.[91]

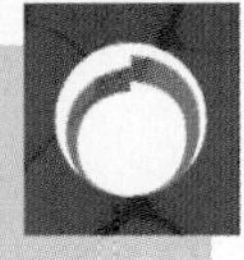

Gestational and Placental Disorders

Diseases of pregnancy and pathologic conditions of the placenta are important causes of intrauterine or perinatal death, congenital malformations, intrauterine growth retardation, maternal death, and a great deal of morbidity for both mother and child.[5, 92] Here we discuss only a limited number of disorders in which knowledge of the morphologic lesions contributes to an understanding of the clinical problem. This discussion is confined to selected disorders of early pregnancy, complications of late pregnancy, and trophoblastic neoplasia.

DISORDERS OF EARLY PREGNANCY

Spontaneous Abortion

Ten per cent to 15% of recognized pregnancies terminate in spontaneous abortion. However, studies using highly sensitive immunoassay of chorionic gonadotropin to detect pregnancy identified an additional 22% loss of presumably fertilized and implanted ova in otherwise healthy women.[93] The causes for this early loss of pregnancy are still mysterious.

The causes of recognized spontaneous abortion are both fetal and maternal. Defective implantation inadequate to support fetal development and death of the ovum or fetus in utero because of some genetic or acquired abnormality constitute the major origins of spontaneous abortion. Numerous studies have indicated chromosome abnormalities in more than half of spontaneous abortuses.[94]

Maternal influences, which are less well understood, include inflammatory diseases, both localized to the placenta and systemic; uterine abnormalities; and possibly trauma. The role of trauma is generally overemphasized and must be considered a rare to exceptional trigger of spontaneous abortion. *Toxoplasma, Mycoplasma, Listeria,* and viral infections have also been implicated as causes of abortion.

The morphologic changes usually seen in endometrial curettage specimens depend, of course, on the interval between fetal death and passage of the products of conception.[95] In general, there are focal areas of decidual necrosis with intense neutrophilic infiltrations, thrombi within decidual blood vessels, and considerable amounts of hemorrhage, both recent and old, within the necrotic decidua. Placental villi may be markedly edematous and devoid of blood vessels. The changes encountered in the ovum or fetus are highly variable. In many spontaneous abortions, no fetal products can be identified, but when they are present, they should be carefully examined for anomalies that would suggest specific genetic or karyotypic defects. Chromosomal studies are recommended in (1) habitual or recurrent abortion and (2) when there is a malformed fetus.

Ectopic Pregnancy

Ectopic pregnancy is the term applied to implantation of the fetus in any site other than a normal uterine location. The most common site is within the tubes (approximately 90%).[96] The other sites are the ovary, the abdominal cavity, and the intrauterine portion of the fallopian tube (cornual pregnancy). Ectopic pregnancies occur about once in every 150 pregnancies. The most important predisposing condition in 35% to 50% of patients is PID with chronic salpingitis. Other factors are peritubal adhesions due to appendicitis or endometriosis, leiomyomas, and previous surgery. Fifty per cent, however, occur in tubes that are apparently normal. Intrauterine devices may also increase risk.

Ovarian pregnancy is presumed to result from the rare fertilization and trapping of the ovum within the follicle just at the time of its rupture. Abdominal pregnancies may develop when the fertilized ovum drops out of the fimbriated end of the tube. In all these abnormal locations, the fertilized ovum undergoes its usual development with the formation of placental tissue, amniotic sac, and fetus, and the host implantation site develops decidual changes.

MORPHOLOGY. In tubal pregnancy, the placenta is poorly attached to the wall of the tube. Intratubal hemorrhage may thus occur from partial placental separation without tubal rupture (Fig. 24–54). Tubal pregnancy is the most common cause of hematosalpinx and should always be sus-

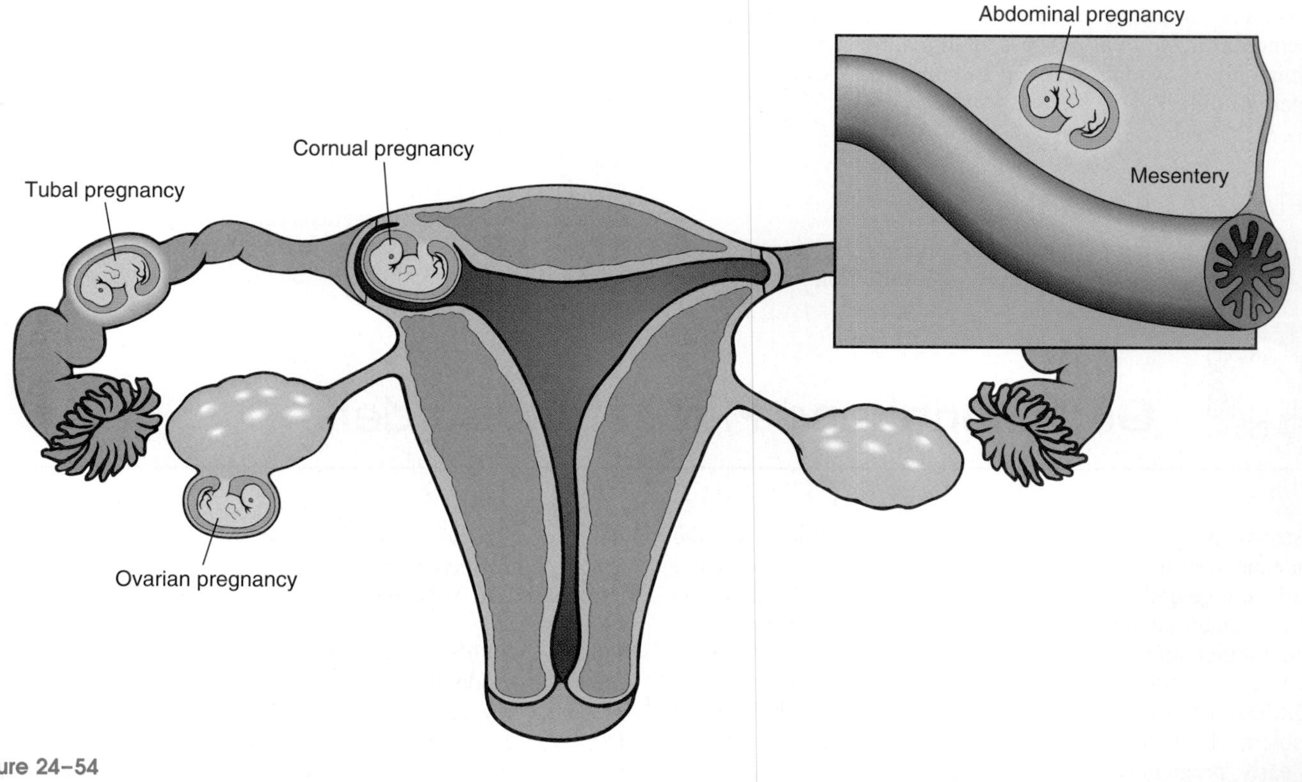

Figure 24–54

Potential sites for ectopic pregnancy, including the fallopian tube, ovary, cornu, and abdominal viscera.

pected when a tubal hematoma is present. More often, the placental tissue invades the tubal wall and causes tubal rupture and intraperitoneal hemorrhage. Less commonly, the tubal pregnancy may undergo spontaneous regression and resorption of the entire gestation. Still less commonly, the tubal pregnancy is extruded through the fimbriated end into the abdominal cavity (tubal abortion).

The clinical course of ectopic pregnancy is punctuated by the onset of severe abdominal pain about 6 weeks after a previous normal menstrual period, when rupture of the tube leads to a pelvic hemorrhage. In such cases, the patient may rapidly develop a shocklike state with signs of an acute abdomen, and early diagnosis becomes critical. Chorionic gonadotropin assays, ultrasound studies, and laparoscopy may be helpful. Endometrial biopsy specimens may or may not disclose decidual changes but, excluding the extremely rare dual pregnancy, do not exhibit chorionic villi. Rupture of a tubal pregnancy constitutes a medical emergency.

DISORDERS OF LATE PREGNANCY

The multitude of disorders that may occur in the third trimester reflect the complex anatomy of the maturing placenta (Fig. 24–55). Any interruption of blood flow through the umbilical cord (such as constricting knots or compression) will be lethal to the fetus. Ascending infections involving the chorioamnionic membranes may lead to premature rupture and delivery. Retroplacental hemorrhage at the interface of placenta and myometrium (abruptio placentae) will threaten both mother and fetus. Rupture of the fetal vessels in terminal villi (intervillous hemorrhage) may produce a sudden drop in fetal blood volume, with fetal stress or death. Uteroplacental insufficiency can be precipitated by abnormal placentation, altered placental development, or maternal vascular thrombosis, and the effects may range from mild intrauterine growth retardation to severe uteroplacental ischemia and maternal toxemia. The more common of these conditions are discussed.

Placental Abnormalities and Twin Placentas

Abnormalities in placental shape, structure, and implantation are not uncommon. Accessory placental lobes, bipartite placenta (placenta made up of two equal segments), and circumvallate placenta (having an extrachorial part) are examples of abnormalities that have limited clinical significance.

Placenta accreta is caused by partial or complete absence of the decidua with adherence of the placenta di-

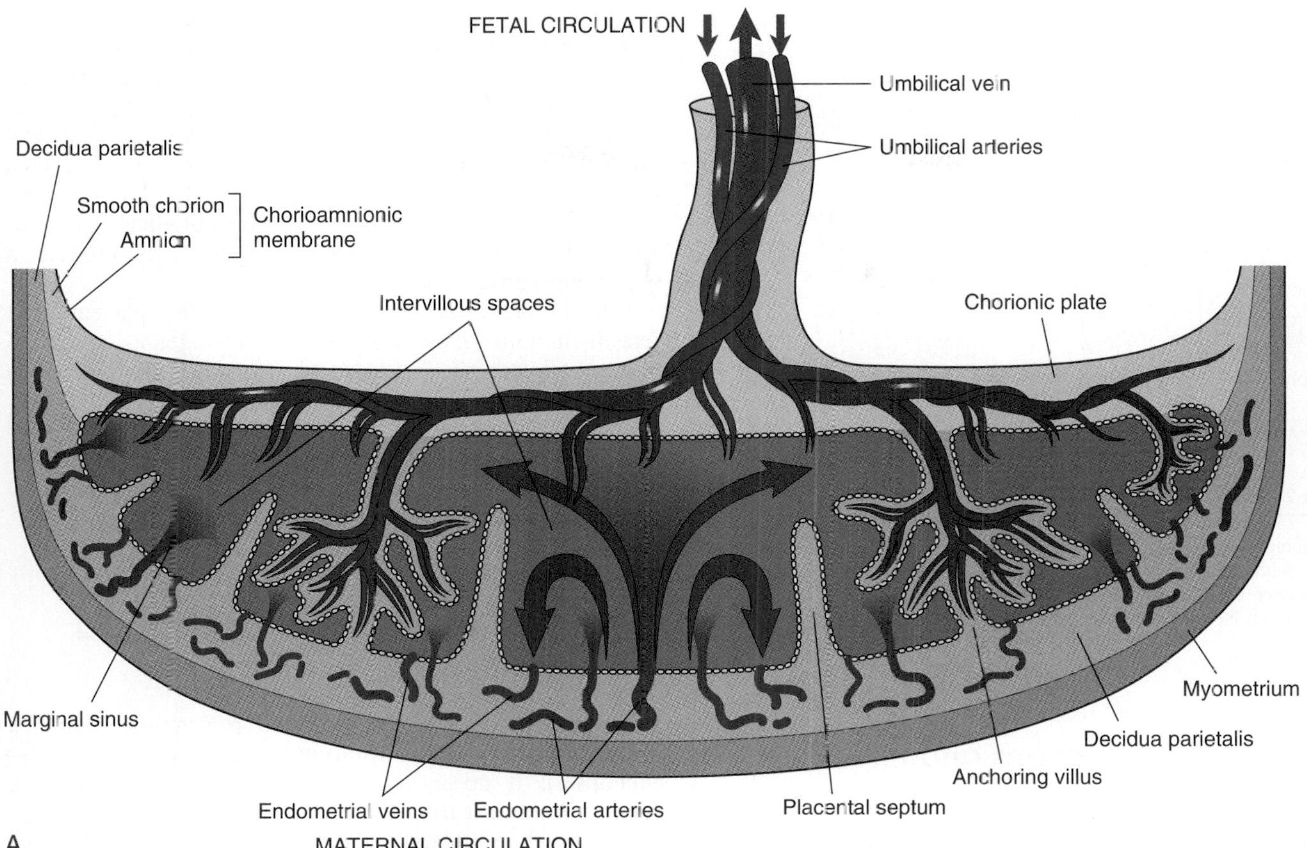

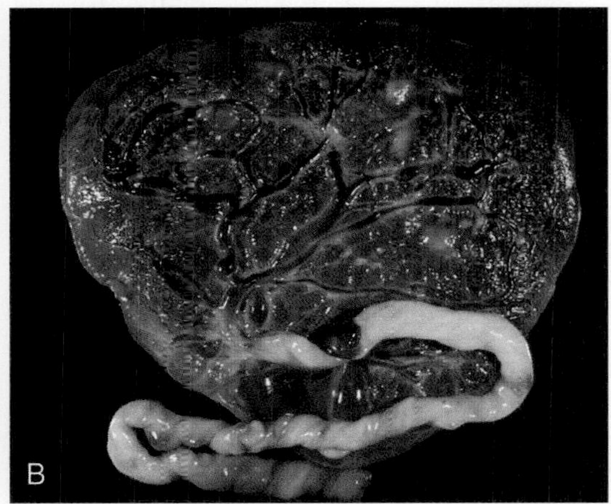

Figure 24–55

A, Diagram of placental anatomy. *B*, Normal term placenta with umbilical cord.

rectly to the myometrium. It is important for two reasons: (1) postpartum bleeding, often life-threatening, occurs because of failure of placental separation; (2) in up to 60% of cases, it is associated with placenta previa, a condition in which the placenta implants in the lower uterine segment or cervix, often with serious antepartum bleeding and premature labor. Many cases of placenta previa–associated accreta occur in patients with cesarean section scars.

Twin pregnancies arise from fertilization of two ova (dizygotic) or from division of one fertilized ovum (monozygotic). There are three basic types of twin placentas[97] (Fig. 24–56) dichorionic diamnionic (which may be fused), monochorionic diamnionic, and monochorionic monoamnionic. Monochorionic placentas imply monozygotic (identical) twins, and the time at which splitting occurs determines whether one or two amnions are present. Dichorionic gestation may occur with either monozygotic or dizygotic twins and is not specific.

One complication of twin pregnancy is twin-twin transfusion, in which placental vascular anastomoses (connections) create an abnormal sharing of fetal circulations through shunting. If an imbalance in blood flow occurs, a marked disparity in fetal blood volumes may result in the death of one or both fetuses (Fig. 24–57).

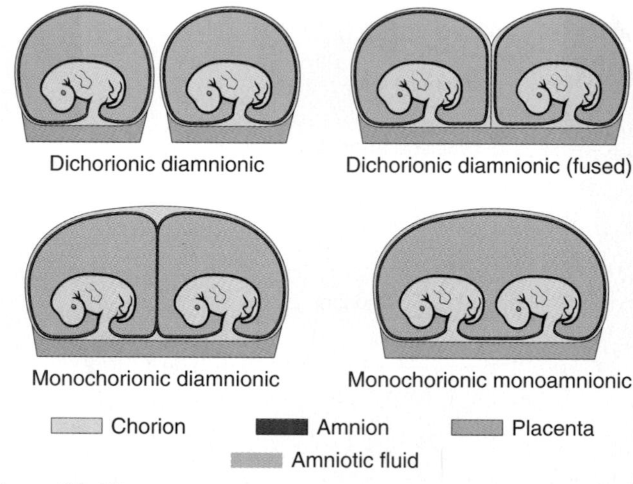

Figure 24–56

Diagrammatic representation of the various types of twin placentation and their membrane relationships. (Adapted from Gersell D, et al: Diseases of the placenta. In Kurman, R (ed): Blaustein's Pathology of the Female Genital Tract. New York, Springer-Verlag, 1994.)

Placental Inflammations and Infections

Infections may occur in the placenta (placentitis, villitis), in the fetal membranes (chorioamnionitis), and in the umbilical cord (funisitis).[98] They reach the placenta by two pathways: (1) ascending infection through the birth canal and (2) hematogenous (transplacental) infection. Ascending infections are by far the most common and are most often bacterial; in many such instances, localized infection of the membranes by an organism produces premature rupture of membranes and entry for the organisms. Sexual intercourse has been implicated in enhancing ascending infections.[98] The amniotic fluid may be cloudy with purulent exudate, and the chorion-amnion histologically contains a leukocytic polymorphonuclear infiltration with accompanying edema and congestion of the vessels (Fig. 24–58). The infection frequently elicits a fetal response with umbilical cord vasculitis. Extension into the villous space may produce a septic intervillous thrombus.

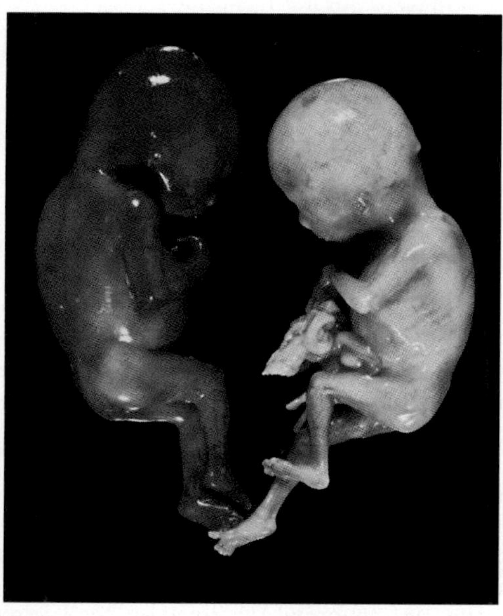

Figure 24–57

Twin-twin transfusion syndrome resulting in the death of both fetuses because of excessive (*left*) or deficient (*right*) blood volume.

Uncommonly, bacterial infections of the placenta and fetal membranes may arise by the hematogenous spread of bacteria directly to the placenta. The villi are most often affected histologically (villitis). Classically, TORCH (toxoplasmosis and others [syphilis, tuberculosis, listeriosis], rubella, cytomegalovirus, herpes simplex) should be considered, although the cause is usually obscure and may involve immunologic phenomena.[5] (See also Chapter 11.)

Toxemia of Pregnancy (Preeclampsia and Eclampsia)

Toxemia of pregnancy refers to a symptom complex characterized by hypertension, proteinuria, and edema (preeclampsia). It occurs in about 6% of pregnant women, usually in the last trimester and more commonly in primiparas than in multiparas. Certain of these patients become more seriously ill, developing convulsions; this more severe form is termed eclampsia. Patients with eclampsia develop disseminated intravascular coagulation (DIC) with lesions in the liver, kidneys, heart, placenta, and sometimes the brain. There is no absolute correlation between the severity of eclampsia and the magnitude of the anatomic changes.

Pathogenesis. The many theories on the nature of toxemia of pregnancy[99] are beyond our scope, but three events that seem to be of prime importance in this disorder are addressed: placental ischemia, hypertension, and DIC (Fig. 24–59).

The causes of the initial events of toxemia are unknown, but evidence points to an abnormality of placentation, leading to *placental ischemia*. This may involve an abnormality in both trophoblast invasion and the development of the physiologic alterations in the placental vessels required to perfuse the placental bed adequately. Immunologic, genetic, and other factors have been postulated as causes of these abnormalities. The net effect is a shallow implantation with incomplete conversion of decidual vessels to vessels adequate for the pregnancy state.[100] Investigators have hypothesized that an intrinsic defect in the invading trophoblast may contribute to altered vascular flow. This abnormality is manifest by the inability of the invading cytotrophoblast to assume the phenotype of normal endothelial cells, which normally includes the expression of adhesion receptors. These defects in trophoblastic conversion may further influence remodeling of uterine vasculature, reducing blood flow and leading to *placental ischemia, the basis for the toxemic placenta.*[101, 102] It is thought that this decreased uteroplacental perfusion induces stimulation of vasocon-

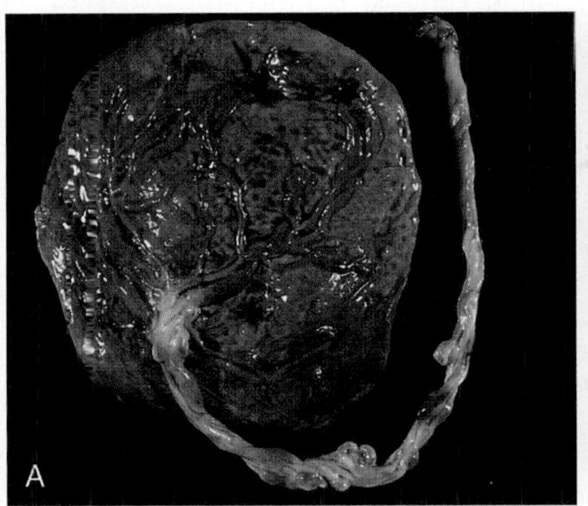

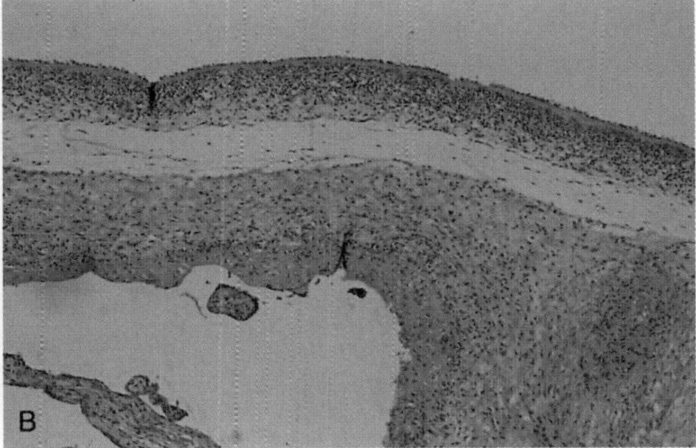

Figure 24–58

Acute chorioamnionitis. *A*, On gross examination, the placenta contains greenish opaque membranes. Compare with Figure 24–55*B*. *B*, A photomicrograph illustrates a dense bandlike inflammatory exudate on the amniotic surface (*top*).

strictor substances (thromboxane, angiotensin, endothelin) and the inhibition of vasodilator influences (prostaglandin I_2, prostaglandin E_2, nitric oxide) from the ischemic placenta. The resultant DIC, hypertension, and organ damage ensue (Fig. 24–59).

As to the pathogenesis of DIC in toxemia, endothelial damage, abnormalities in the level and activities of coagulation factors, and primary platelet alteration may play a role.[103] For example, during toxemia, the placental ischemia leads to a higher output of thromboplastic substances, and antithrombin III levels are reduced. The characteristic lesions in eclampsia are in large part due to thrombosis of arterioles and capillaries throughout the body, particularly in the liver, kidneys, brain, pituitary, and placenta.

The mechanism of toxemic hypertension appears to involve the renin-angiotensin mechanism and prostaglandins.[104] Normal pregnant women develop a resistance to the vasoconstrictive and hypertensive effects of angiotensin, but women with toxemia lose such resistance, developing a tendency to hypertension. Prostaglandins of the E series, produced in the uteroplacental vascular bed during pregnancy, are thought to mediate the normal resistance of pregnant women to angiotensin, and prostaglandin production is indeed decreased in the placenta of toxemic women. Thus, the increase in angiotensin hypersensitivity, characteristic of toxemia, may be due to decreased synthesis of prostaglandin by the toxemic placenta. There is also evidence that renin production by the toxemic placenta is increased, another potentially vasoconstrictive event. Figure 24–59 presents a hypothetical schema for the pathogenesis of eclampsia.

MORPHOLOGY. The **liver** lesions, when present, take the form of irregular, focal, subcapsular, and intraparenchymal hemorrhages. On histologic examination, there are fibrin thrombi in the portal capillaries with foci of characteristic peripheral hemorrhagic necrosis.

The **kidney** lesions are variable. Glomerular lesions are diffuse, at least when they are assessed by electron microscopy. They consist of striking swelling of endothelial cells, the deposition of fibrinogen-derived amorphous dense deposits on the endothelial side of the basement membrane, and mesangial cell hyperplasia. Immunofluorescent studies confirm the abundance of fibrin in glomeruli. In the more well defined cases, fibrin thrombi are present in the glomeruli and capillaries of the cortex. When the lesion is far advanced, it may produce complete destruction of the cortex in the pattern referred to as bilateral renal cortical necrosis (Chapter 21).

The **brain** may have gross or microscopic foci of hemorrhage along with small-vessel thromboses. Similar changes are often found in the **heart** and the **anterior pituitary**. The **placenta** is the site of variable changes, most of which reflect ischemia and vessel injury. (1) Placental infarcts, which occur in normal full-term placentas, are larger and more numerous. (2) There is increased frequency of retroplacental hematomas. (3) There is evidence of increased villous ischemia: formation of prominent syncytial knots, thickening of trophoblastic basement membrane, and villous hypovascularity. (4) A characteristic finding in the walls of uterine vessels is striking fibrinoid necrosis and intramural lipid deposition (acute atherosis) (Fig. 24–60).

Clinical Course. Preeclampsia usually starts after the 32nd week of pregnancy but begins earlier in patients with hydatidiform mole or preexisting kidney disease or hypertension. The onset is usually insidious, characterized by hypertension and edema, with proteinuria following within several days. Headaches and visual disturbances are common. Eclampsia is heralded by central nervous system in-

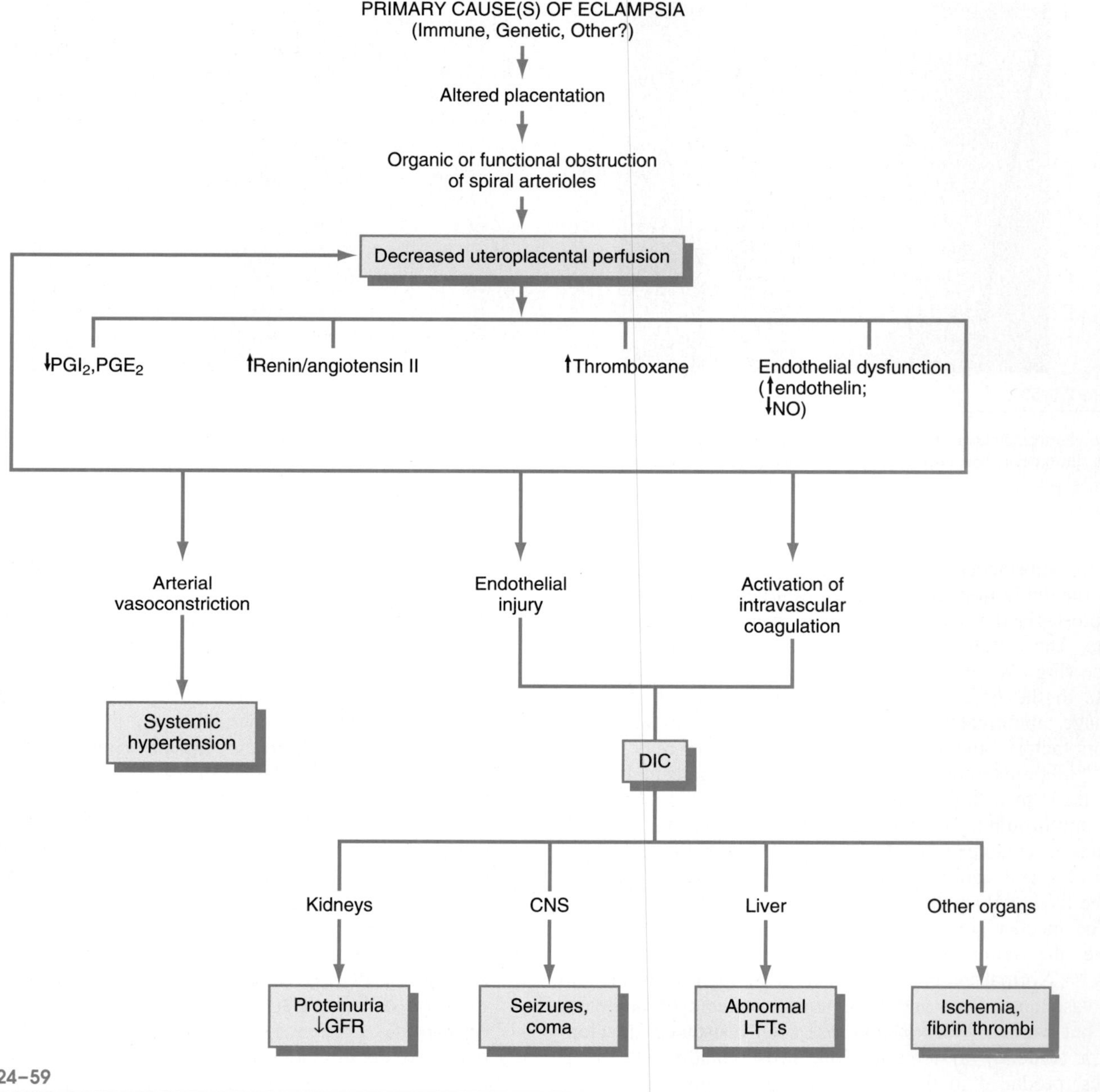

Figure 24–59

Proposed sequence of events in the pathogenesis of toxemia of pregnancy. The main features are (1) decreased uteroplacental perfusion; (2) increased vasoconstrictors and decreased vasodilators, resulting in local and systemic vasoconstriction; and (3) disseminated intravascular coagulation (DIC). (Adapted from Friedman SA: Pre-eclampsia: a review of the role of prostaglandins. Obstet Gynecol 71:122, 1988. Reprinted by permission of the American College of Obstetricians and Gynecologists; and Khong TY, et al: Inadequate maternal vascular response to placentation in pregnancies complicated by pre-eclampsia and by small for gestational age infants. Br J Obstet Gynecol 93:1049, 1986.)

volvement, including convulsions and eventual coma. Mild and moderate forms of toxemia can be controlled by bed rest, a balanced diet, and antihypertensive agents, but induction of delivery is the only definitive treatment of established preeclampsia and eclampsia. Proteinuria and hypertension usually disappear within 1 or 2 weeks after delivery except in patients in whom these findings predated the pregnancy.

GESTATIONAL TROPHOBLASTIC DISEASE

Gestational trophoblastic disease constitutes a spectrum of tumors and tumor-like conditions characterized by proliferation of pregnancy-associated trophoblastic tissue of progressive malignant potential. The lesions include the hydatidiform mole (complete and partial), the invasive

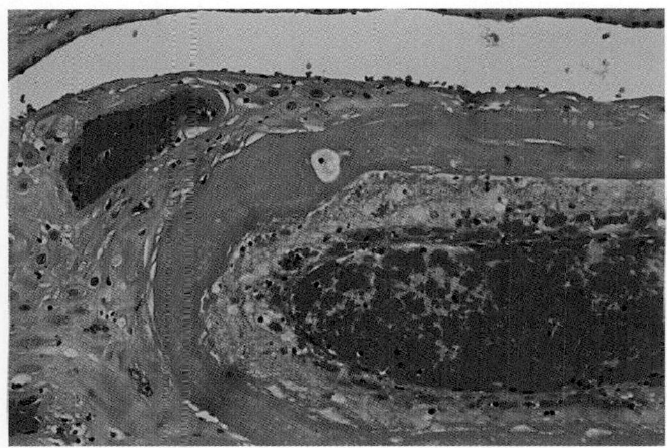

Figure 24–60

Acute atherosis of uterine vessels in eclampsia. Note fibrinoid necrosis of the vessel walls, subendothelial macrophages and perivascular lymphocytic infiltrate. (Courtesy of Dr. Drucilla J. Roberts, Massachusetts General Hospital, Boston.)

mole, and the frankly malignant choriocarcinoma.[105] Gestational trophoblastic disease is important for the following reasons:

- The hydatidiform mole is a common complication of gestation, occurring about once in every 1000 to 2000 pregnancies in the United States and, curiously, far more commonly in the Far East.
- It has become possible, by monitoring the circulating levels of human chorionic gonadotropin, to determine the early development of persistent trophoblastic disease.
- Choriocarcinoma, once a dreaded and uniformly fatal complication, is now highly responsive to chemotherapy.[106]

Hydatidiform Mole (Complete and Partial)

Hydatidiform mole is characterized by cystic swelling of the chorionic villi, accompanied by variable trophoblastic proliferation. The most important reason for the correct recognition of true moles is that they may precede choriocarcinoma.[105] Most patients present in the fourth or fifth month of pregnancy with vaginal bleeding and with a uterus that is usually, but not always, larger than expected for the duration of pregnancy. These moles can occur at any age during active reproductive life, but the risk is higher in pregnant women in their teens or between the ages of 40 and 50 years. For poorly explained reasons, the incidence varies considerably in different regions of the world: 1 in 1000 pregnancies in the United States but 10 in 1000 in Indonesia.[107]

Types and Pathogenesis. Two types of benign, noninvasive moles—complete and partial—can be differentiated by histologic, cytogenetic, and flow cytometric studies[108] (Table 24–5). In complete (or classic mole), all or most of

Table 24–5. FEATURES OF COMPLETE VERSUS PARTIAL HYDATIDIFORM MOLE

Feature	Complete Mole	Partial Mole
Karyotype	46,XX (46,XY)	Triploid
Villous edema	All villi	Some villi
Trophoblast proliferation	Diffuse; circumferential	Focal; slight
Atypia	Often present	Absent
Serum hCG	Elevated	Less elevated
hCG in tissue	++++	+
Behavior	2% choriocarcinoma	Rare choriocarcinoma

hCG, human chorionic gonadotropin.

the villi are edematous, and there is diffuse trophoblast hyperplasia. Cytogenetic studies of these moles show that more than 90% have a 46,XX diploid pattern, all derived from the sperm (a phenomenon called androgenesis). They are presumed to be derived from fertilization by a single sperm of an egg that has lost its chromosomes (Fig. 24–61). The remaining 10% are from the fertilization of such an empty egg by two sperm (46,XX and 46,XY). In both circumstances, embryonic development does not occur, and thus complete moles show no fetal parts.

In partial moles, some of the villi are edematous, and other villi show only minor changes; the trophoblastic proliferation is focal. In these moles, the karyotype is triploid (e.g., 69,XXY) or even occasionally tetraploid (92,XXXY). The moles result from fertilization of an egg with one or two sperm (Fig. 24–61). The embryo is viable for weeks, and thus fetal parts may be present when the resultant mole is aborted. In contrast to complete moles, partial moles are rarely followed by choriocarcinoma.

MORPHOLOGY. In most instances, moles develop within the uterus, but they may occur in any ectopic site of pregnancy. When discovered, usually in the fourth or fifth month of gestation, the uterus is usually larger (but may be of normal size, or even smaller) than anticipated for the duration of the pregnancy. The uterine cavity is filled with a delicate, friable mass of thin-walled, translucent, cystic, grapelike structures (Fig. 24–62). Careful dissection may disclose a small, usually collapsed amniotic sac. Fetal parts are frequently seen in partial moles but are never found in complete moles (unless there is a twin pregnancy).

In **partial moles** (Fig. 24–63*A*), the villous edema involves only a proportion of villi, and the trophoblastic proliferation is focal and slight.

On microscopic examination, the **complete mole** shows hydropic swelling of most chorionic villi and virtual absence or inadequate development of vascularization of villi. The central substance of the villi is a loose, myxomatous, edematous stroma, and they may be covered by a layer of chorionic epithelium, both cytotrophoblast and

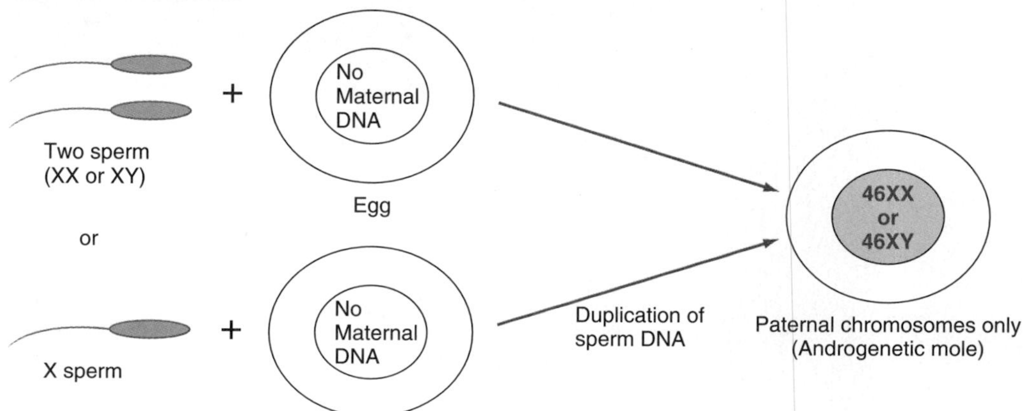

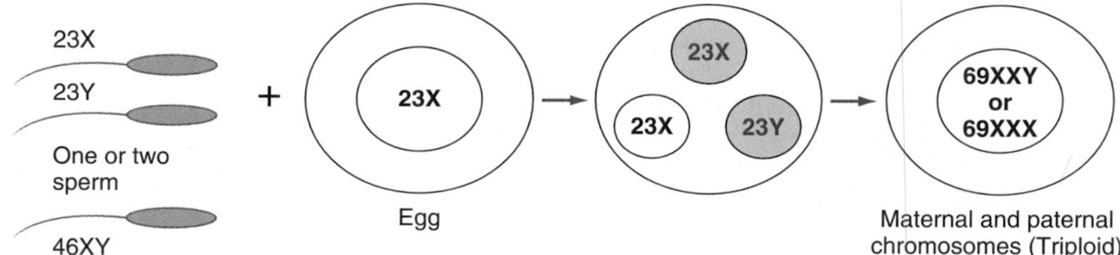

Figure 24–61 ■

Patterns of fertilization to account for chromosomal origin of complete (46,XX) and triploid partial moles (XXY). In a complete mole, one or two sperm fertilize an egg that has lost its chromosomes. Partial moles are due to fertilization of an egg by one diploid, or two haploid sperm, depicted in this example as one 23,X and one 23,Y.

syncytiotrophoblast (Fig. 24–63*B*). At the opposite end of the spectrum are moles having similar cystic dilation of villi, accompanied, however, by circumferential and striking proliferation of the chorionic epithelium to produce sheets and masses of both cytotrophoblast and syncytiotrophoblast. Histologic grading does not predict the outcome[109]; therefore, all moles should be carefully observed by monitoring of the human chorionic gonadotropin levels.

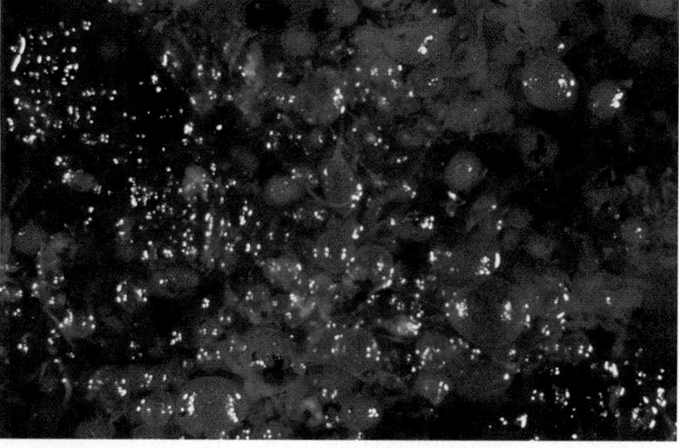

Figure 24–62 ■

Complete hydatidiform mole suspended in saline showing numerous swollen (hydropic) villi.

Clinical Course. Most patients have abnormal uterine bleeding that usually begins early in the course of the pregnancy and is accompanied by the passage of a thin, watery fluid and bits of tissue seen as small, grapelike masses. The uterine enlargement is more rapid than anticipated. Ultrasound examination permits a definitive diagnosis in most cases.

In the classic case, quantitative analysis of human chorionic gonadotropin shows levels of hormone greatly exceeding those produced by a normal pregnancy of similar age. Serial hormone determination indicates a rapidly mounting level that climbs faster than the usual normal single or even multiple pregnancy.

Once the diagnosis is made, the mole must be removed by thorough curettage. In patients not desirous of further childbearing, hysterectomy may be performed. The course after curettage alone depends on the malignant potential of the removed uterine contents. From many studies, it is clear that 80% to 90% of these moles remain benign and give no further difficulty. Ten per cent develop into invasive moles and 2.5% into choriocarcinoma.[110]

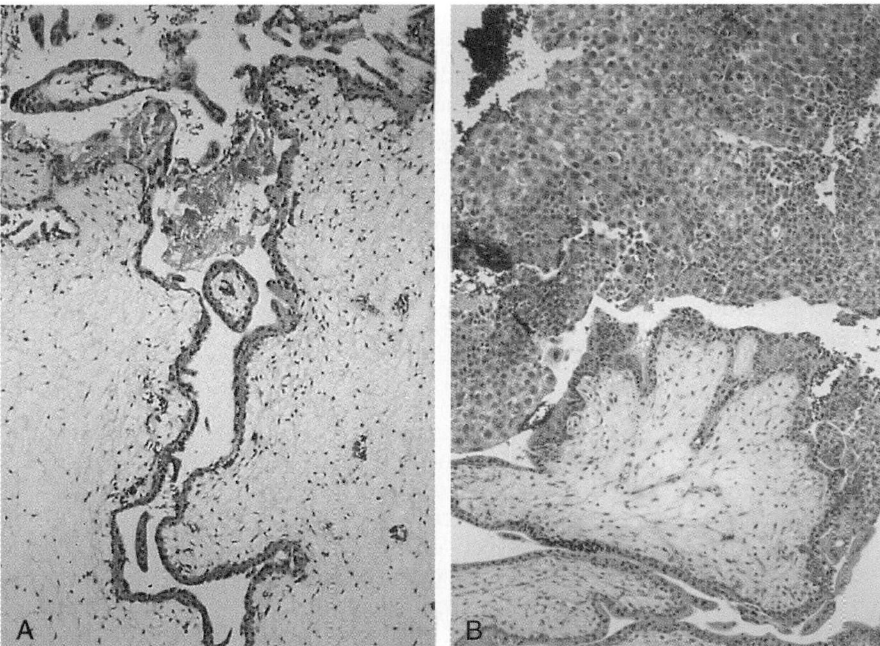

Figure 24–63

A, Photomicrograph of partial hydatidiform mole revealing swollen villi and slight hyperplasia of the surface trophoblast. *B*, Complete hydatidiform mole with extensive cytotrophoblastic hyperplasia (*lower field*).

Invasive Mole

This is defined as a mole that penetrates and may even perforate the uterine wall. There is invasion of the myometrium by hydropic chorionic villi, accompanied by proliferation of both cytotrophoblast and syncytiotrophoblast (Fig. 24–64). The tumor is locally destructive and may invade parametrial tissue and blood vessels. Hydropic villi may embolize to distant sites, such as lungs and brain, but do not grow in these organs as true metastases, and even before the advent of chemotherapy, they eventually regressed unless fatal hemorrhage occurred. The tumor is manifested clinically by vaginal bleeding and irregular uterine enlargement. It is always associated with a persistent elevated human chorionic gonadotropin level and varying degrees of luteinization of the ovaries. The tumor responds well to chemotherapy. Although invasive mole is biologically benign, rupture of the uterus may lead to hemorrhage.

Choriocarcinoma

Gestational choriocarcinoma is an epithelial malignant neoplasm of trophoblastic cells derived from any form of previously normal or abnormal pregnancy.[105] Although most cases arise in the uterus, ectopic pregnancies provide extrauterine sites of origin. Choriocarcinoma is a rapidly

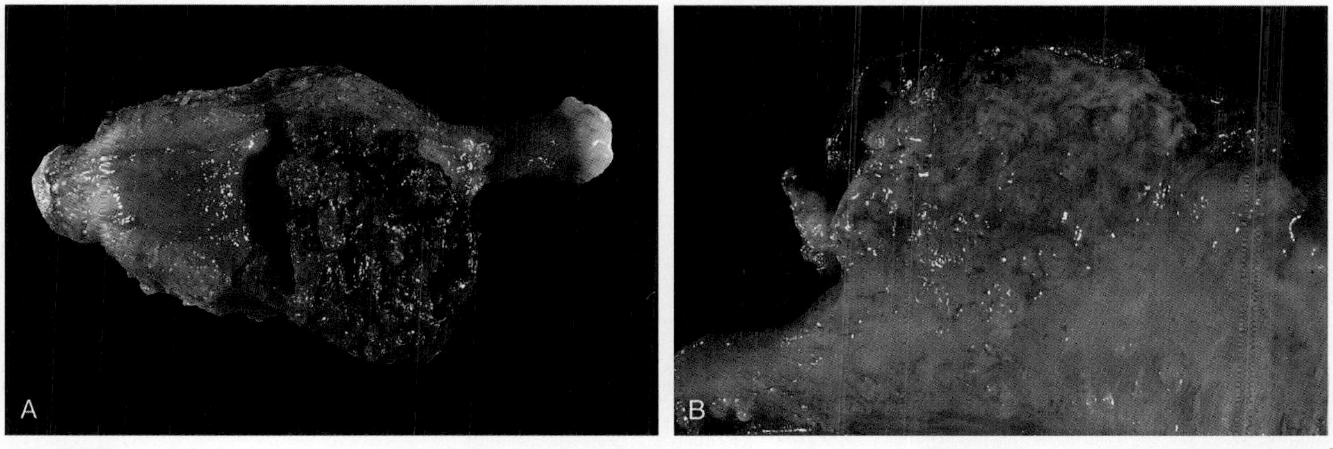

Figure 24–64

A, Invasive mole presenting as a hemorrhagic mass adherent to the uterine wall. *B*, On cross-section, the tumor invades into the myometrium. (Courtesy of Dr. David R. Genest, Brigham and Women's Hospital, Boston, MA.)

invasive, widely metastasizing malignant neoplasm, but once it is identified, it responds well to chemotherapy.

Incidence. This is an uncommon condition that arises in 1 in 20,000 to 30,000 pregnancies in the United States. It is much more common in some African countries; for example, it occurs in 1 in 2500 pregnancies in Ibadan, Nigeria. It is preceded by several conditions: 50% arise in hydatidiform moles, 25% in previous abortions, approximately 22% in normal pregnancies, and the rest in ectopic pregnancies and genital and extragenital teratomas. About 1 in 40 hydatidiform moles may be expected to give rise to a choriocarcinoma, in contrast to 1 in approximately 150,000 normal pregnancies.

MORPHOLOGY. The choriocarcinoma is classically a soft, fleshy, yellow-white tumor with a marked tendency to form large pale areas of ischemic necrosis, foci of cystic softening, and extensive hemorrhage (Fig. 24–65*A*). On histologic examination, it is a purely epithelial cellular malignancy that does not produce chorionic villi and that grows, as do other cancers, by the abnormal proliferation of both cytotrophoblast and syncytiotrophoblast (Fig. 24–65*B*).

It is sometimes possible to identify anaplasia within such abnormal proliferation replete with abnormal mitoses. The tumor invades the underlying myometrium, frequently penetrates blood vessels and lymphatics, and in some cases extends out onto the uterine serosa and adjacent structures. In its rapid growth, it is subject to hemorrhage, ischemic necrosis, and secondary inflammatory infiltration.

In fatal cases, metastases are found in the lungs, brain, bone marrow, liver, and other organs. On occasion, metastatic choriocarcinoma is discovered without a detectable primary in the uterus (or ovary), presumably because the primary has undergone total necrosis.

Clinical Course. The uterine choriocarcinoma does not classically produce a large, bulky mass. It becomes manifest only by irregular spotting of a bloody, brown, sometimes foul-smelling fluid. This discharge may appear in the course of an apparently normal pregnancy, after a miscarriage, or after a curettage.

Sometimes the tumor does not appear until months later. Usually, by the time the tumor is discovered locally, radiographs of the chest and bones already disclose the presence of metastatic lesions. The human chorionic gonadotropin titers are elevated to levels above those encountered in hydatidiform moles. Occasional tumors, however, produce little hormone, and some tumors have become so necrotic as to become functionally inactive.

Widespread metastases are characteristic of these tumors. Favored sites of involvement are the lungs (50%) and vagina (30% to 40%), followed in descending order of frequency by the brain, liver, and kidney.

The treatment of trophoblastic neoplasms depends on the type and stage of tumor and includes evacuation of the contents of the uterus, surgery, and chemotherapy. The results of chemotherapy for gestational choriocarcinoma are spectacular and have resulted in up to 100% cure or remission in all patients except some who had high-risk metastatic trophoblastic disease. Many of the cured patients have had normal subsequent pregnancies and deliveries. By

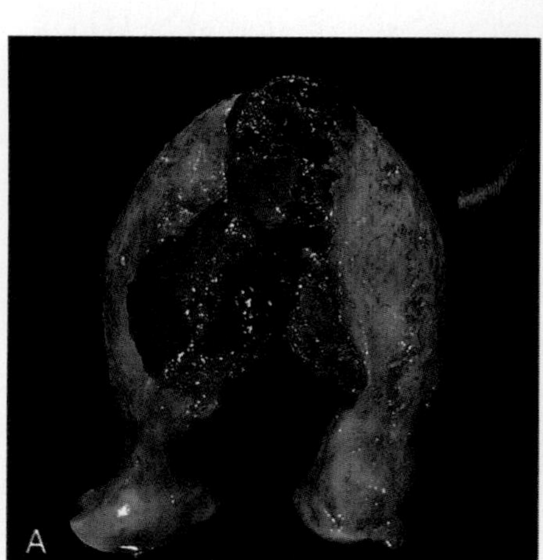

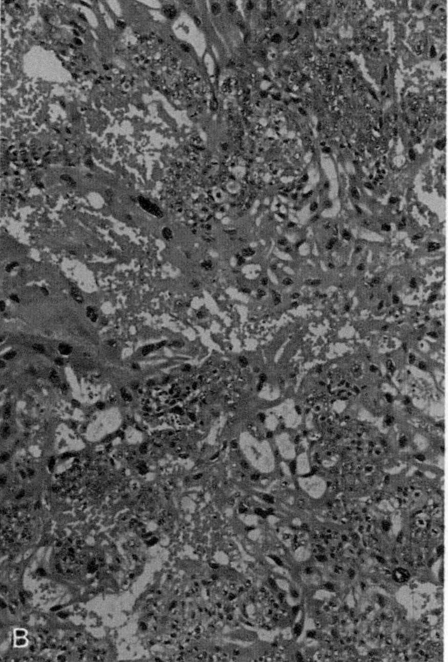

Figure 24–65

A, Choriocarcinoma presenting as a bulky hemorrhagic mass invading the uterine wall. *B*, Photomicrograph of choriocarcinoma illustrating both neoplastic cytotrophoblast and syncytiotrophoblast. (Courtesy of Dr. David R. Genest, Brigham and Women's Hospital, Boston, MA.)

contrast, nongestational choriocarcinomas are much more resistant to therapy.

Placental Site Trophoblastic Tumor

This rare tumor is characterized by the presence of proliferating trophoblastic tissue deeply invading the myometrium and is composed largely of an *intermediate trophoblast.* These cells are usually mononuclear, rather than syncytial, but are larger and have more abundant cytoplasm than the regular cytotrophoblast; in contrast to syncytiotrophoblast (which produces human chorionic gonadotropin), intermediate trophoblast cells are immunoreactive for human placental lactogen. This lesion differs from choriocarcinoma in the absence of cytotrophoblastic elements and in the low level of human chorionic gonadotropin production. The tumors are locally invasive, but many are self-limited and subject to cure by curettage. Malignant variants, however, have been reported; they are distinguished by a high mitotic index, extreme cellularity, extensive necrosis, local spread, or even widespread metastases. About 10% result in disseminated metastases and death.[105,111]

REFERENCES

1. Robboy SJ, et al: Embryology of the female genital tract. In Kurman R (ed): Blaustein's Pathology of the Female Genital Tract, 4th ed. New York, Springer-Verlag, 1994, pp 3–31.
2. Malasanos TH: Sexual development of the fetus and pubertal child. Clin Obstet Gynecol 40:153, 1997.
3. Kurman R (ed): Blaustein's Pathology of the Female Genital Tract, 4th ed. New York, Springer-Verlag, 1994.
4. Fox H (ed): Haines and Taylor's Obstetrical and Gynaecologic Pathology, 4th ed. Edinburgh, Churchill Livingstone, 1987.
5. Benirschke K, Kaufmann P: Pathology of the Human Placenta, 3rd ed. New York, Springer-Verlag, 1995.
6. Scott JR (ed): Danforth's Obstetrics and Gynecology, 7th ed. Philadelphia, JB Lippincott, 1994.
7. Knapp RC, Berkowitz RS (eds): Gynecologic Oncology, 2nd ed. New York, McGraw-Hill, 1993.
8. Holmes KK, et al (eds): Sexually Transmitted Diseases, 2nd ed. New York, McGraw-Hill, 1990.
9. Brugha R, et al: Genital herpes infection: a review. Int J Epidemiol 26:698, 1997.
10. Prober CG: Herpetic vaginitis in 1993. Clin Obstet Gynecol 36:177, 1993.
11. Heine P, McGregor JA: Trichomonas vaginalis: a reemerging pathogen. Clin Obstet Gynecol 36:137, 1993.
12. Mann MS, et al: Vulvar vestibulitis: significant clinical variables and treatment outcome. Obstet Gynecol 79:1, 1992.
13. Wilkinson EJ: Normal histology, and nomenclature of the vulva and malignant neoplasms, including VIN. Dermatol Clin 10:283, 1992.
14. Wilkinson EJ, Stone KI: Atlas of Vulvar Disease. Baltimore, Williams & Wilkins, 1995.
15. Wilkinson EJ: Premalignant and malignant diseases of the vulva. In Kurman R (ed): Blaustein's Pathology of the Female Genital Tract, 4th ed. New York, Springer-Verlag, 1994, pp p 87.
16. Crum CP: Vulvar intraepithelial neoplasia: histology and associated viral changes. Contemp Issues Surg Pathol 9:119, 1987.
17. Sykes NL: Condyloma Acuminatum. Int J Dermatol 34:297, 1995.
18. zur Hausen H: Papillomavirus infections—a major cause of human cancers. Biochim Biophys Acta 1288:F55, 1996.
19. Kurman RJ, et al: Tumors of the Cervix, Vagina, and Vulva. Atlas of Tumor Pathology, Third Series, Fascicle 4. Washington, DC, Armed Forces Institute of Pathology, 1992, p 191.
20. Crum CP: Carcinoma of the vulva: epidemiology and pathogenesis. Obstet Gynecol 79:3, 1992.
21. Leibowitch M, et al: The epithelial changes associated with squamous cell carcinoma of the vulva: a review of the clinical, histological and viral findings in 78 women. Br J Obstet Gynaecol 97:1135, 1990.
22. Monk BJ, et al: Prognostic significance of human papillomavirus DNA in vulvar carcinoma. Obstet Gynecol 85:709, 1995.
23. Worsham MJ, et al: Consistent chromosome abnormalities in squamous cell carcinoma of the vulva. Genes Chromosomes Cancer 3:420, 1991.
24. Kurman RJ, et al: Basaloid and warty carcinomas of the vulva. Distinctive types of squamous cell carcinoma frequently associated with human papillomaviruses [published erratum appears in Am J Surg Pathol 17:536, 1993]. Am J Surg Pathol 17:133, 1993.
25. Duntion CJ: Malignant melanoma of the vulva: a review. Obstet Gynecol Surv 50:739, 1995.
26. Mittendof R, Herbst AL: DES exposure: an update. Contemp Pediatr 11:59, 1994.
27. Scully RE, Welch WR: Pathology of the female genital tract after prenatal exposure to diethylstilbestrol. In Herbst AL, Bern HA (eds): Developmental Effects of Diethylstilbestrol in Pregnancy. New York, Thieme-Stratton, 1981, pp 26–45.
28. Copeland LJ, et al: Sarcoma botryoides of the female genital tract. Obstet Gynecol 66:262, 1985.
29. Andrassy RJ, et al: Conservative surgical management of vaginal and vulvar pediatric rhabdomyosarcoma: a report from the Intergroup Rhabdomyosarcoma Study III. J Pediatr Surg 30:1034, 1995.
30. Winkler B, Crum CP: *Chlamydia trachomatis* infection of the female genital tract. Pathogenetic and clinicopathologic correlations. Pathol Annu 5:193, 1984.
31. Kiviat NB, et al: Histopathology of endocervical infection by *Chlamydia trachomatis,* herpes simplex virus, *Trichomonas vaginalis,* and *Neisseria gonorrhoeae.* Hum Pathol 21:831, 1990.
32. Koutsky LA, et al: A cohort study of the risk of cervical intraepithelial neoplasia grade 2 or 3 in relation to papillomavirus infection. N Engl J Med 327:1272, 1992.
33. Herrero R, et al: Sexual behavior, venereal diseases, hygiene practices and invasive cervical cancer in a high-risk population. Cancer 65:380, 1990.
34. Alani RM, Munger K: Human papillomaviruses and associated malignancies. J Clin Oncol 16:330, 1997.
35. Lorincz AT, et al: Human papillomavirus infection of the cervix: relative risk associations of 15 common anogenital types. Obstet Gynecol 79:328, 1992.
36. Crum CP, Nuovo GJ: Genital Papillomaviruses and Related Neoplasms. New York, Raven Press, 1991.
37. Heselmeyer K, et al: Gain in chromosome 3q defines the transition from severe dysplasia to invasive carcinoma of the uterine cervix. Proc Natl Acad Sci USA 93:479, 1996.
38. Benjamin I, et al: Expression and mutational analysis of p53 in stage IB and IIA cervical cancers. Am J Obstet Gynecol 175:1266, 1996.
39. Wright T, et al: Precancerous lesions of the cervix. In Kurman R (ed): Blaustein's Pathology of the Female Genital Tract, 4th ed. New York, Springer-Verlag, 1994, pp 229.
40. Crum CP, et al: Pathology of Early Cervical Neoplasia. New York, Churchill Livingstone, 1996.
41. Crum CP, et al: Cervical papillomaviruses segregate within morphologically distinct precancerous lesions. J Virol 54:675, 1985.
42. The Bethesda System for reporting cervical/vaginal cytologic diagnoses. Report of the 1991 Bethesda Workshop. Am J Surg Pathol 16:914, 1992.
43. Ostor AG: Natural history of cervical intraepithelial neoplasia: a critical review. Int J Gynaecol Pathol 12:186, 1993.
44. Stoler MH, et al: Small-cell neuroendocrine carcinoma of the cervix. A human papillomavirus type-18 associated tumor. Am J Surg Pathol 15:28, 1991.
45. Smotkin D, et al: Human papillomavirus DNA in adenocarcinoma and adenosquamous carcinoma of the uterine cervix. Obstet Gynecol 68:241, 1986.
46. Dahlenbach-Hellweg G: Histopathology of the Endometrium. 4th ed. New York, Springer-Verlag, 1993.

47. Deligdisch L: Effects of hormone therapy on the endometrium. Mod Pathol 6:94, 1993.
48. Kiviat NB, et al: Endometrial histopathology in patients with culture-proved upper genital tract infection and laparoscopically diagnosed acute salpingitis. Am J Surg Pathol 14:167, 1990.
49. Noble LS, et al: Prostaglandin E2 stimulates aromatase expression in endometriosis-derived stromal cells. J Clin Endocrinol Metab 82: 600, 1997.
50. Corley D, et al: Postmenopausal bleeding from unusual endometrial polyps in women on chronic tomoxifen therapy. Obstet Gynecol 79: 111, 1992.
51. Fletcher JA, et al: Clonal 6p21 rearrangement is restricted to the mesenchymal component of an endometrial polyp. Genes Chromosomes Cancer 5:260, 1992.
52. Hertig AT, Sommers SC: Genesis of endometrial carcinoma. 1. Study of prior biopsies. Cancer 2:964, 1949.
53. Kurman RJ, et al: The behavior of endometrial hyperplasia. A long-term study of untreated hyperplasia in 170 patients. Cancer 56:403, 1985.
54. Ferenczy A, Gelfand M: The biologic significance of cytologic atypia in progestogen-treated endometrial hyperplasia. Am J Obstet Gynecol 160:126, 1989.
55. Brinton LA, et al: Reproductive, menstrual, and medical risk factors for endometrial cancer: results from a case-control study. Am J Obstet Gynecol 167:1317, 1992.
56. Silverberg SG, Kurman RJ: Tumors of the Uterine Corpus and Gestational Trophoblastic Disease. Atlas of Tumor Pathology, Third Series, Fascicle 3. Washington, DC, Armed Forces Institute of Pathology, 1991, pp 219–287.
57. Mutter GL, et al: Allelotype mapping of unstable microsatellites establishes direct lineage continuity between endometrial precancers and cancer. Cancer Res 56:4483, 1996.
58. Tashiro H, et al: *p53* gene mutations are common in uterine serous carcinoma and occur early in their pathogenesis. Am J Pathol 150: 177, 1997.
59. Rose PG: Endometrial carcinoma. N Engl J Med 335:640, 1997.
60. Nicklin JL, Copeland LJ: Endometrial papillary serous carcinoma: patterns of spread and treatment. Clin Obstet Gynecol 39:686, 1996.
61. Creasman WT, Eddy GL: Recent advances in endometrial cancer. Semin Surg Oncol 6:339, 1990.
62. Silverberg SG, et al: Carcinosarcoma (malignant mixed mesodermal tumor of the uterus). Int J Gynaecol Pathol 9:1, 1990.
63. Quade BJ: Pathology, cytogenetics, and molecular biology of uterine leiomyomas and other smooth muscle lesions. Curr Opin Obstet Gynecol 7:35, 1995.
64. Buscema J, et al: Epithelioid leiomyosarcoma. Cancer 47:1192, 1986.
65. Bell SW, et al: Problematic uterine smooth muscle neoplasms. A clinicopathologic study of 213 cases. Am J Surg Pathol 18:535, 1994.
66. Young RH, Scully RE: Ovarian pathology in infertility. In Kraus FT (ed): Pathology of Reproductive Failure. Baltimore, Williams & Wilkins, 1991, pp 104–139.
67. Homburg R: Polycystic ovary syndrome—from gynaecological curiosity to multisystem endocrinopathy. Hum Reprod 11:29, 1996.
68. Russel P, Bannatyne P: Surgical Pathology of the Ovaries. Edinburgh, Churchill Livingstone, 1989.
69. Young RH, et al: The ovary. In Sternberg S, et al (eds): Diagnostic Surgical Pathology. New York, Raven Press, 1994, p 2195.
70. Baker TR, Piver MS: Etiology, biology, and epidemiology of ovarian cancer. Semin Surg Oncol 10:224, 1994.
71. Schlesseljan JJ: Net effect of oral contraceptive use on the risk of cancer in women in the United States. Obstet Gynecol 85(pt 1):793, 1995.
72. Stratton JF, et al: Contribution of *BRCA1* mutations to ovarian cancer. N Engl J Med 336:1125, 1997.
73. Streuwing JP, et al: The risk of cancer associated with specific mutations of *BRCA1* and *BRCA2* among Ashkenazi Jews. N Engl J Med 336:1401, 1997.
74. Bast RC, et al: Malignant transformation of ovarian epithelium. J Natl Cancer Inst 84:557, 1992.
75. Bell DA, et al: Peritoneal implants of ovarian serous borderline tumors. Cancer 62:2212, 1988.
76. Watkin W, et al: Mucinous carcinoma of the ovary. Cancer 69:208, 1992.
77. Young RH, et al: Mucinous tumors of the appendix associated with mucinous tumors of the ovary and pseudomyxoma peritonei. A clinicopathologic analysis of 22 cases supporting an origin in the appendix. Am J Surg Pathol 15:415, 1991.
78. Snyder RR, et al: Endometrial proliferative and low malignant potential tumors of the ovary. Am J Surg Pathol 12:661, 1988.
79. Eifel P, et al: Simultaneous presentation of carcinoma involving the ovary and uterine corpus. Cancer 50:163, 1982.
80. Silva EG, et al: Ovarian carcinomas with transitional cell carcinoma pattern. Cancer 93:457, 1990.
81. Berek JS, Bast RC Jr: Ovarian cancer screening. The use of serial complementary tumor markers to improve sensitivity and specificity for early detection. Cancer 76(Suppl):2092, 1995.
82. Linder D, et al: Pathogenetic origin of benign ovarian teratomas. N Engl J Med 292:63, 1975.
83. Mutter GL: Teratoma genetics and stem cells: a review. Obstet Gynecol Surv 42:661, 1987.
84. O'Connor DM, Norris HJ: The influence of grade on the outcome of stage I ovarian immature (malignant) teratomas. The reproducibility of grading. Int J Gynecol Pathol 13:283, 1994.
85. Gordon T, et al: Dysgerminoma. A review of 158 cases from the Emil Novak ovarian tumor registry. Obstet Gynecol 58:497, 1981.
86. Young RH, Scully R: Ovarian sex cord–stromal tumors. Recent progress. Int J Gynaecol Pathol 1:101, 1982.
87. Prat J, Scully RE: Cellular fibromas and fibrosarcomas of the ovary. Cancer 47:2663, 1981.
88. Roth LM, et al: Sertoli-Leydig cell tumors: a clinicopathologic study of 34 cases. Cancer 48:187, 1981.
89. Hart WR, Burkons DM: Germ all neoplasms arising in gonadoblastomas. Cancer 43:669, 1979.
90. Eichhorn JH, et al: DNA content and proliferative activity in ovarian small cell carcinomas of the hypercalcemic type. Implications for diagnosis, prognosis and histogenesis. Am J Clin Pathol 98:579, 1992.
91. Young RH, Scully RE: Metastatic tumors of the ovary. In Kurman RJ (ed): Blaustein's Pathology of the Female Genital Tract, 4th ed. New York, Springer-Verlag, 1994, pp 939–974.
92. Kaplan C: Placental pathology for the nineties. Pathol Annu 28:15, 1993.
93. Wilcox AJ: Incidence of early loss of pregnancy. N Engl J Med 319:189, 1988.
94. Kalousek DK, Lau AE: Pathology of spontaneous abortion. In Dimmick JE, Kalousek DK (eds): Developmental Pathology of the Embryo and Fetus. Philadelphia, JB Lippincott, 1992, p 62.
95. Rushton DI: Examination of products of conception from previable human pregnancies. J Clin Pathol 34:819, 1981.
96. Saxon D, et al: A study of ruptured tubal ectopic pregnancy. Obstet Gynecol 90:46, 1997.
97. Gersell DJ, Kraus FT: Diseases of the placenta. In Kurman RJ (ed): Blaustein's Pathology of the Female Genital Tract. New York, Springer-Verlag, 1994, p 975.
98. Grossman JH: Infections affecting the placenta. In Lavery JP (ed): The Placenta. Rockville, MD, Aspen Publishing, 1987, pp 131–134.
99. Weiner GP: The clinical spectrum of preeclampsia. Am J Kidney Dis 9:312, 1987.
100. Khong TY, et al: Inadequate maternal vascular response to placentation in pregnancies complicated by preeclampsia and by small for gestational age infants. BMJ 93:1049, 1986.
101. Zhou Y, et al: Human cytotrophoblasts adopt a vascular phenotype as they differentiate. A strategy for succesful endovascular invasion? J Clin Invest 99:2139, 1997.
102. Zhou Y, et al: Preeclampsia is associated with failure of human cytotrophoblasts to mimic a vascular adhesion phenotype. One cause of defective endovascular invasion in this syndrome? J Clin Invest 99:2152, 1997.
103. Ferris TF: Pregnancy, preeclampsia and the endothelial cell. N Engl J Med 325:1439, 1991.
104. Friedman SA: Pre-clampsia: a review of the role of prostaglandins. Obstet Gynecol 71:122, 1988.

105. Redline RW, Abdul-Karim FW: Pathology of gestational trophoblastic disease. Semin Oncol 22:96, 1995.
106. Berkowitz RS, Goldstein DP: Management of molar pregnancy and gestational trophoblastic tumors. In Knapp RC, Berkowitz RS (eds): Gynecologic Oncology. New York, McGraw-Hill, 1993, pp 328–340.
107. Bracken MB, et al: Epidemiology of hydatidiform mole and choriocarcinoma. Epidemiol Rev 6:52, 1984.
108. Lage JM: Gestational trophoblastic tumors: refining histologic diagnosis by using DNA flow and image cytometry. Curr Opin Obstet Gynecol 6:359, 1994.
109. Genest DR, et al: A clinico-pathologic study of 153 cases of complete hydatidiform mole (1980–1990): histologic grade lacks prognostic significance. Obstet Gynecol 78:402, 1991.
110. Lurain JR, et al: Natural history of hydatidiform mole after primary evacuation. Am J Obstet Gynecol 145:591, 1983.
111. Finkler NJ, et al: Clinical experience with placental site trophoblastic tumors at the New England Trophoblastic Disease Center. Obstet Gynecol 71:854, 1988.

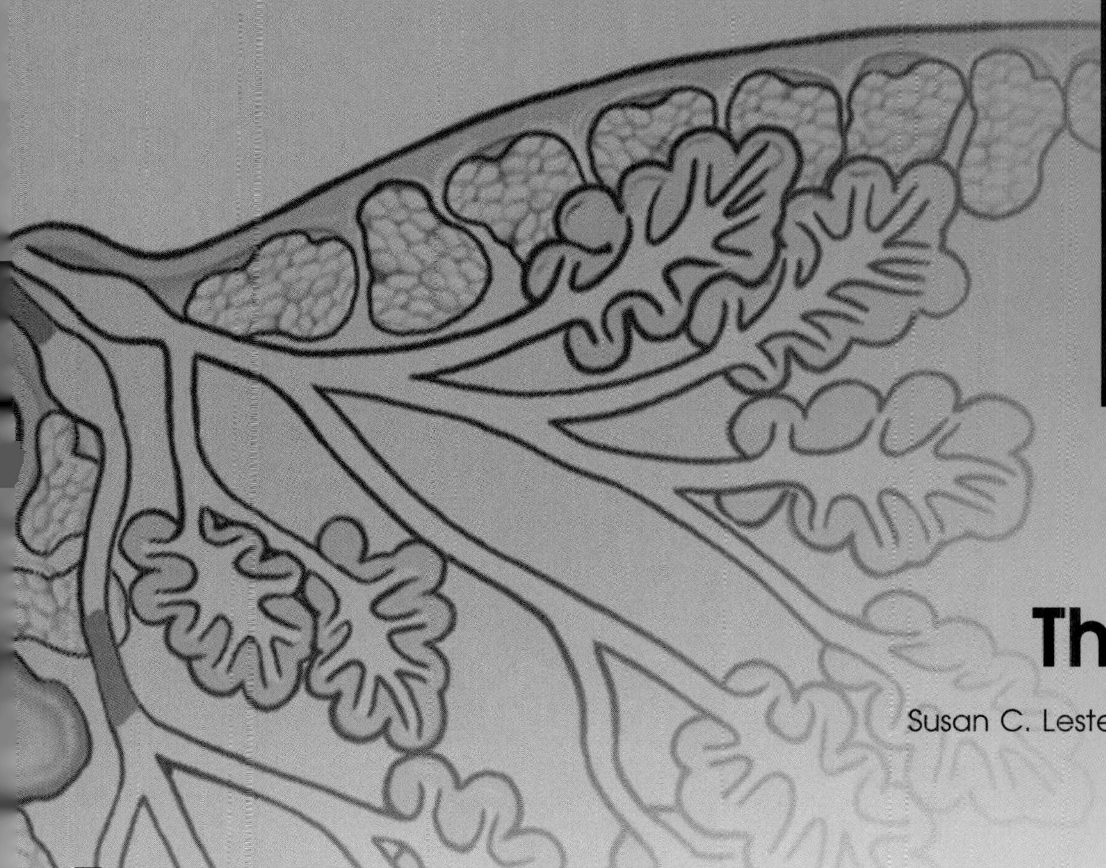

25

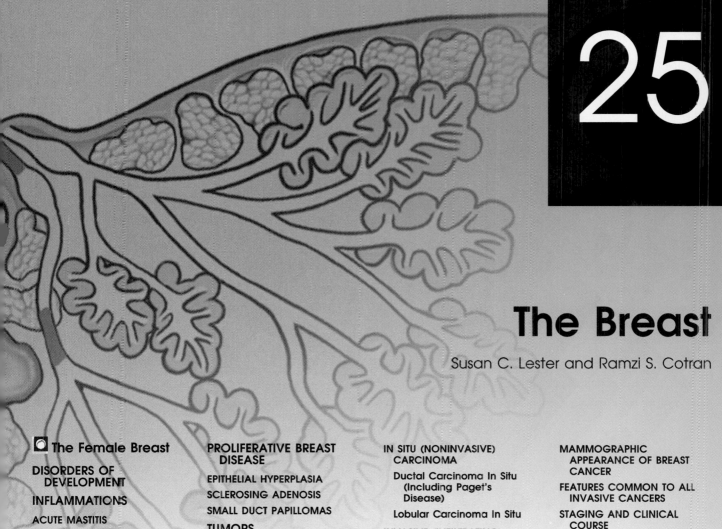

The Breast

Susan C. Lester and Ramzi S. Cotran

The Female Breast

DISORDERS OF DEVELOPMENT

INFLAMMATIONS

ACUTE MASTITIS

PERIDUCTAL MASTITIS (RECURRENT SUBAREOLAR ABSCESS, SQUAMOUS METAPLASIA OF LACTIFEROUS DUCTS)

MAMMARY DUCT ECTASIA

FAT NECROSIS

GRANULOMATOUS MASTITIS

SILICONE BREAST IMPLANTS

FIBROCYSTIC CHANGES

PROLIFERATIVE BREAST DISEASE

EPITHELIAL HYPERPLASIA

SCLEROSING ADENOSIS

SMALL DUCT PAPILLOMAS

TUMORS

STROMAL TUMORS

Fibroadenoma

Phyllodes Tumor

Sarcomas

EPITHELIAL TUMORS

Large Duct Papilloma

CARCINOMA OF THE BREAST

IN SITU (NONINVASIVE) CARCINOMA

Ductal Carcinoma In Situ (Including Paget's Disease)

Lobular Carcinoma In Situ

INVASIVE (INFILTRATING) CARCINOMA

Invasive Ductal Carcinoma, No Special Type

Invasive Lobular Carcinoma

Medullary Carcinoma

Colloid (Mucinous) Carcinoma

Tubular Carcinoma

Invasive Papillary Carcinoma

MAMMOGRAPHIC APPEARANCE OF BREAST CANCER

FEATURES COMMON TO ALL INVASIVE CANCERS

STAGING AND CLINICAL COURSE

MISCELLANEOUS MALIGNANT NEOPLASMS

The Male Breast

GYNECOMASTIA

CARCINOMA

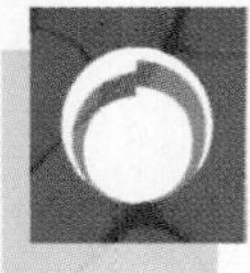

The Female Breast

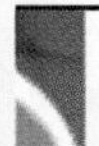

NORMAL

Anatomy and Histology. The resting mammary gland consists of six to ten major duct systems, each of which is subdivided into lobules, the functional units of the mammary parenchyma. Each ductal system drains through a separate main excretory duct or *lactiferous sinus.* Successive branching of the large ducts distally eventually leads to the terminal ducts. Before puberty, the complex system of branching ducts ends blindly, but at the beginning of menarche, it proliferates distally, giving rise to lobules consisting of a cluster of epithelium-lined *ductules* or *acini.*[1] Each terminal duct and its ductules compose the *terminal duct lobular unit* (Figs. 25–1 and 25–2*A*).

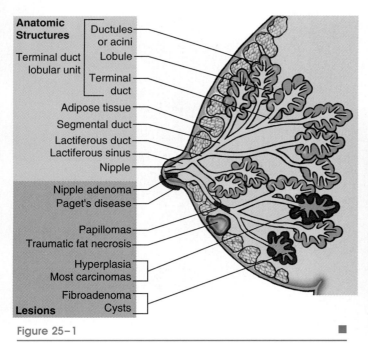

Anatomic Structures
Terminal duct lobular unit
Ductules or acini
Lobule
Terminal duct
Adipose tissue
Segmental duct
Lactiferous duct
Lactiferous sinus
Nipple
Nipple adenoma
Paget's disease
Papillomas
Traumatic fat necrosis
Hyperplasia
Most carcinomas
Fibroadenoma
Cysts
Lesions

Figure 25–1

Anatomy of the breast and major lesions at each site within the various units.

The nipple and areola are covered by stratified squamous epithelium. The areolar skin is pigmented and supported by smooth muscle. Numerous areolar glands (of Montgomery) become more prominent during pregnancy and function in nipple lubrication. The major lactiferous ducts open onto the skin surface at the nipple. The squamous epithelium continues into the duct orifice and then abruptly changes to a double-layered cuboidal epithelium. A basement membrane faithfully follows the contour of skin, ducts, and ductules.[1] A low, flattened layer of contractile cells containing myofilaments *(myoepithelial cells)* can be identified beneath the more prominent lining epithelium. The majority of breast stroma consists of dense fibroconnective tissue admixed with adipose tissue *(interlobular stroma)* containing elastic fibers supporting the large ducts. Lobules are enclosed by a breast-specific hormonally responsive loose, delicate, myxomatous stroma that contains a scattering of lymphocytes *(intralobular stroma).*

Just as the endometrium rises and ebbs with each menstrual cycle, so does the breast.[2] In the first half or follicular phase of the menstrual cycle, the lobules are relatively quiescent. After ovulation, under the influence of estrogen and rising progesterone levels, cell proliferation increases as does the number of acini per lobule, and there is vacuolization of basal epithelial cells. Lobular stromal edema becomes marked. This combined stimulatory effect of estrogen and progesterone on the intralobular breast elements accounts for the sense of fullness commonly experienced by women during the premenstrual phase of the cycle. When menstruation occurs, the fall in estrogen and progesterone levels is followed by epithelial cell death (apoptosis), disappearance of the stromal edema, lymphocytic infiltration, and overall regression in the size of the lobules.

It is only with the onset of pregnancy that the breast assumes its complete morphologic maturation and func-

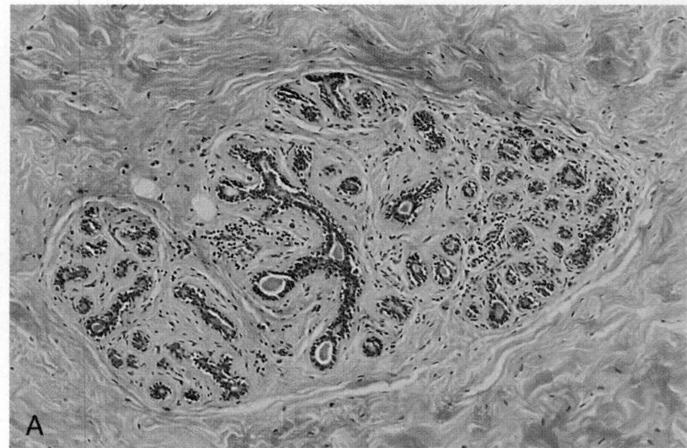

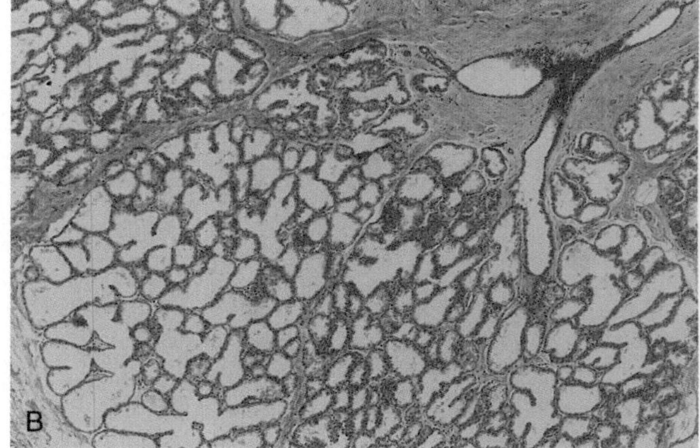

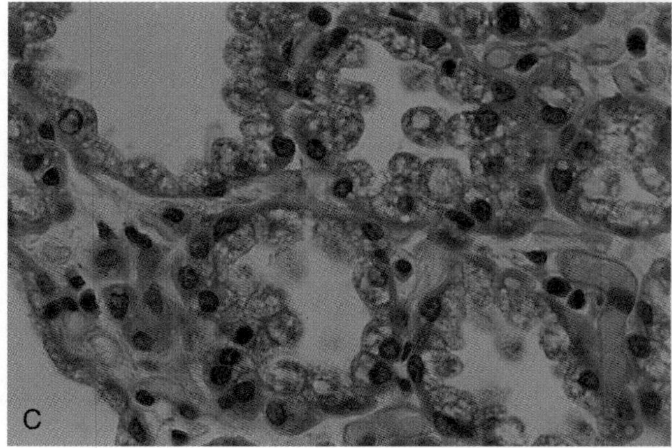

Figure 25–2

A, Terminal duct lobular unit demonstrating myoepithelial and epithelial cells lining the duct and the acini. The loose cellular intralobular stroma invests the lobule, whereas the less cellular and denser interlobular stroma is found between lobules. *B,* Enlarged lobule of pregnancy and lactation showing increased numbers of dilated acini per lobule. *C,* The milk producing epithelial cells of the lactating breast are filled with secretory vacuoles. Note that the cells of the large duct system (seen in the upper right-hand corner in *B*) do not undergo lactational change.

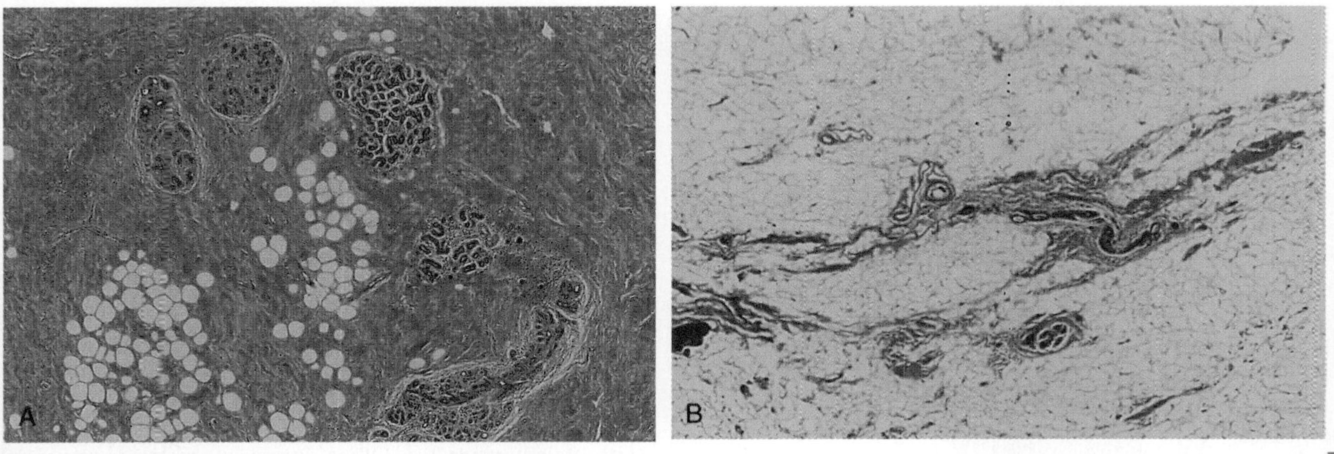

Figure 25–3

A, Premenopausal normal breast. The breast consists of ducts and lobules surrounded by dense interlobular stroma interspersed with small islands of adipose tissue. *B*, Postmenopausal normal breast. Lobules and specialized stroma gradually regress leaving only ducts. The interlobular stroma consists predominantly of adipose tissue.

tional activity. From each terminal duct, numerous true secretory glands pouch out to form grapelike clusters. As a consequence, there is a reversal of the usual stromal-epithelial relationship so that, by the end of the pregnancy, the breast is composed almost entirely of lobules separated by a relatively scant amount of stroma (Fig. 25–2*B*). The lobules are lined by cuboidal cells, and in the third trimester, secretory vacuoles of lipid material are found within the cells (Fig. 25–2*C*). Immediately after birth, the secretion of milk begins. Breast lesions excised during pregnancy may exhibit similar secretory changes (e.g., lactating adenoma or fibroadenoma).

After cessation of lactation, the lobules regress and atrophy, and the total breast size diminishes remarkably. However, complete regression to the stage of the normal nulliparous breast usually does not occur, and some increase in the size and number of lobules remains as a permanent residual.

After the third decade, the ducts and lobules further atrophy with more shrinkage of the intralobular and interlobular stroma. The lobular acini and stroma may almost totally disappear in the very aged, leaving only ducts to create a morphologic pattern that comes close to that of the male breast. However, in most women, there is sufficient persistent estrogenic stimulation, possibly of adrenal origin or from stores of body fat, to maintain the vestigial remnants of lobules that differentiate even the very aged female breast from the male breast. The radiodense interlobular stroma of the young female breast (Fig. 25–3*A*) is progressively replaced by radiolucent adipose tissue (Fig. 25–3*B*). Most breast neoplasms do not contain adipose tissue and appear mammographically as denser masses in contrast to the surrounding breast stroma. Thus, mammography is less sensitive in young women in whom such masses may be obscured by surrounding dense tissue.

PATHOLOGY

Lesions of the breast are preponderantly confined to the female. In the male, the breast is a rudimentary structure relatively insensitive to endocrine influences and apparently resistant to neoplastic growth. In the female, on the other hand, the more complex breast structure, the greater breast volume, and the extreme sensitivity to endocrine influences all predispose this organ to a number of pathologic conditions.

Most diseases of the breast present as palpable masses, inflammatory lesions, nipple secretion, or mammographic abnormalities. Although fortunately most are benign, cancer of the breast is the second most common cause of cancer deaths and one of the most dreaded diseases of women. In this chapter, therefore, the conditions described should be considered in terms of their possible confusion clinically with cancer.[3, 4]

An overall perspective of the frequency of various breast problems can be gained from an analysis of a large series of patients with breast complaints who were seen in a surgical outpatient department.[5] About 30% of the women were considered, after careful evaluation, to have no breast disease. Almost 40% were diagnosed as having fibrocystic changes. Slightly more than 10% had biopsy-proven cancer, and about 7% had a benign tumor (fibroadenoma). The remainder were suffering from a miscellany of benign lesions (Fig. 25–4). Three features of this study deserve particular note. First, *a significant proportion of women having no recognizable breast disease have sufficient irregularity of the "normal" breast tissue to cause concern and to necessitate clinical evaluation.* Second, *fibrocystic changes are the dominant breast problem.* Third, *cancer, unhappily, is all too frequent.*

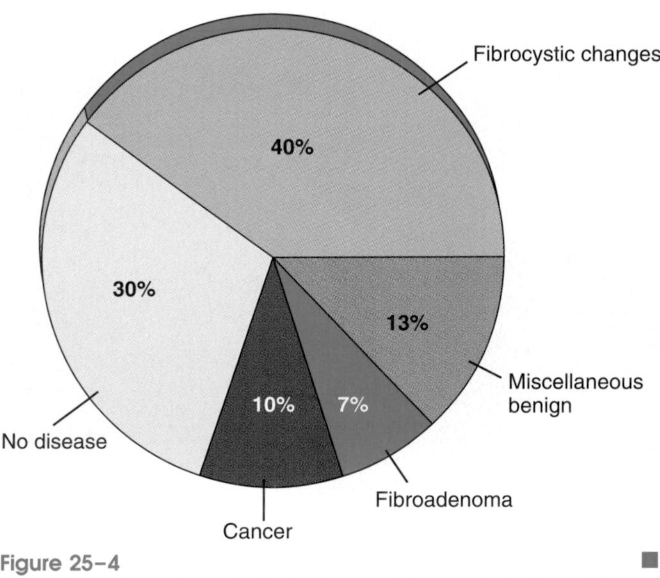

Figure 25–4

Representation of the findings in a series of women seeking evaluation of apparent breast "lumps."

DISORDERS OF DEVELOPMENT

Congenital anomalies run the gamut from congenital absence to abnormal numbers of breasts, but as a group, these entities are of limited clinical significance.

Supernumerary Nipples or Breasts. These result from the persistence of epidermal thickenings along the milk line, extending from the axilla to the perineum, both below the adult breast and above it in the anterior axillary fold. The disorders that affect the normally situated breast may rarely arise in these heterotopic foci, and occasionally the cyclic changes of the menstrual cycle cause painful premenstrual enlargements.

Accessory Axillary Breast Tissue. The normal ductal system can extend over the entire anterolateral chest wall and into the axillary fossa. Mastectomies may not remove all breast epithelium. Thus, prophylactic mastectomies reduce but do not completely eliminate the risk of developing breast cancer. Such tissue may undergo lactational changes or give rise to tumors that appear to be outside the breast and, therefore, may be misidentified as lesions of the axillary lymph nodes or metastases from an occult breast cancer.

Congenital Inversion of Nipples. This occurs in many women, particularly those who have large or pendulous breasts. This inversion is commonly corrected during the growth activity of pregnancy, or it may sometimes be corrected by simple traction on the nipples. Nipple inversion is of clinical significance, since it may frustrate attempts at nursing and may also be confused with acquired retraction of the nipple, sometimes observed in mammary cancer and in inflammation of the breasts.

Macromastia. The appropriate breast size is subjective and influenced by cultural norms. However, some women develop severe back pain and disability because of very large breasts. The large size may be due to variations in body habitus or to an unusual tissue response to hormonal changes during puberty resulting in massive rapid breast growth (juvenile hypertrophy). Reduction mammaplasty removes breast tissue but preserves the nipple.

INFLAMMATIONS

Inflammations of the breast are, on the whole, uncommon and consist of only a relatively few forms of acute and chronic disease. Of these, the most important is acute mastitis, virtually confined to the lactating period. Women with pituitary prolactinomas may present occasionally with symptoms of acute mastitis or duct ectasia, often associated with galactorrhea.[6, 7] Other forms of mastitis are nipple related (periductal mastitis and duct ectasia), post-traumatic lesions (fat necrosis), and granulomatous mastitis. "Inflammatory breast cancer" mimics inflammation by obstructing dermal vasculature with tumor emboli resulting in an enlarged erythematous breast and should always be suspected in a nonlactating woman with the clinical appearance of mastitis.

Acute Mastitis

During the early weeks of nursing, the breast is rendered vulnerable to bacterial infection by the development of cracks and fissures in the nipples. From this portal of entry, *Staphylococcus aureus* usually, or streptococci less commonly, invade the breast substance. Mastitis is rare outside the postpartum state and is often related to periductal mastitis (see later) with secondary bacterial infection.

MORPHOLOGY. The disease is usually unilateral. The staphylococcus tends to produce a localized area of acute inflammation that may progress to the formation of single or multiple abscesses. The streptococcus tends to cause, as it does in all tissues, a diffuse spreading infection that eventually involves the entire organ. Surgical drainage and antibiotic therapy may limit the spread of the infection, but when extensive necrosis occurs, the destroyed breast substance is replaced by fibrous scar as a permanent residual of the inflammatory process. Such scarring may create a localized area of increased consistency sometimes accompanied by retraction of the skin or the nipple, changes that may later be mistaken for a neoplasm.

Periductal Mastitis (Recurrent Subareolar Abscess, Squamous Metaplasia of Lactiferous Ducts)

In this condition, known by a variety of names descriptive of the histologic changes, women present with a painful erythematous subareolar mass, usually clinically thought to be an infectious process. Recurrences are common if it is treated with incision and drainage alone. In recurrent cases, a fistula tract often tunnels under the smooth muscle of the nipple and opens onto the skin at the edge of the areola. Fibrosis and scarring usually occur, followed by nipple inversion.

MORPHOLOGY. The main histologic feature is keratinizing squamous epithelium extending to an abnormal depth into the orifices of the nipple ducts. Keratin is trapped within the ductal system and causes dilation and eventually rupture of the duct (Fig. 25–5). An intense chronic and granulomatous inflammatory response develops to keratin spilled into periductal tissue. Incision and drainage may remove the abscess cavity but usually do not remove the causative keratinizing epithelium. Appropriate clinical management requires removing the involved duct and fistula tract in continuity.[8] However, multiple ducts may be involved, leading to further recurrences. Secondary infections with skin bacteria or with mixed anaerobes are common.

More than 90% of women with periductal mastitis are smokers, suggesting that tobacco use alters the epithelium of the lactiferous sinuses.[8] This condition is not associated with lactation, a specific reproductive history, or age.

Mammary Duct Ectasia

This disorder tends to occur in the fifth or sixth decade of life, usually in multiparous women, and, unlike periductal mastitis, is not associated with cigarette smoking. Patients present with a poorly defined palpable periareolar mass, sometimes with skin retraction, often accompanied by a thick cheesy nipple secretion. Pain and erythema are uncommon.

MORPHOLOGY. This lesion is characterized chiefly by dilation of ducts, inspissation of breast secretions, and a marked periductal and interstitial chronic granulomatous inflammatory reaction.[4] The dilated ducts are filled by granular, necrotic, acidophilic debris that contains principally lipid-laden macrophages. The lining epithelial cells of the ducts may persist in small foci but for the most part are necrotic and atrophic. The periductal and interductal inflammation is manifested by heavy infiltrates of lymphocytes and histiocytes, with a striking predominance of plasma cells in some cases. On occasion, there is a granulomatous inflammation around cholesterol deposits. Fibrosis may eventually produce skin retraction that can be confused with carcinoma. Squamous metaplasia of nipple ducts is not a feature of this disorder.

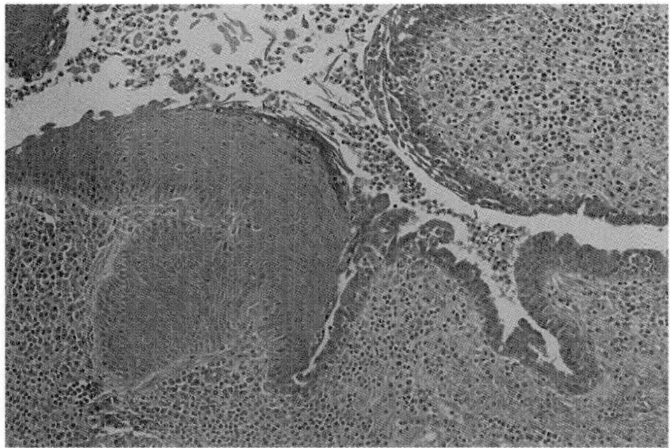

Figure 25–5

Periductal mastitis. Squamous metaplasia is present in a lactiferous duct, and keratin debris is within the lumen. The duct is surrounded by an inflammatory response.

This lesion is of clinical significance because it can be mistaken for a carcinoma clinically, grossly, and by mammographic examination.

Fat Necrosis

Focal necrosis of fat tissues in the breast, followed by an inflammatory reaction, is an uncommon lesion that tends to occur as an isolated, sharply localized process in one breast. If strict criteria are used to differentiate this entity from mammary duct ectasia, many patients give a history of trauma, prior surgical intervention, or radiation therapy.[4]

MORPHOLOGY. Grossly, the lesion may consist of hemorrhage in the early stages and, later, central liquefactive necrosis of fat. Still later, it may be an ill-defined nodule of gray-white, firm tissue containing small foci of chalky white or hemorrhagic debris.

On histologic examination, the central focus of necrotic fat cells is surrounded by lipid-filled macrophages and an intense neutrophilic infiltration. Then, during the next few days, progressive fibroblastic proliferation, increased vascularization, and lymphocytic and histiocytic infiltration wall off the focus. By this time, the central necrotic fat cells have disappeared and may be represented only by foamy, lipid-laden macrophages and spicules of crystalline lipids. Subsequently, foreign body giant cells, calcium salts, and blood pigments make their appearance, and eventually the focus is replaced by scar tissue or is encysted and walled off by collagenous tissue (Fig. 25–6). On mammography, fat necrosis often has the characteristic appearance of a calcified cyst.

The major clinical significance of the condition is its possible confusion with a tumor, when fibrosis has created a clinically palpable mass or focal calcification is seen on mammography.

Granulomatous Mastitis

Granulomas in the breast are caused by a wide variety of diseases, all of them rare, and account for less than 1% of all breast biopsy results. Systemic granulomatous diseases (e.g., Wegener granulomatosis, sarcoidosis) may involve the breast, and on occasion the breast may be the presenting site of involvement. Infections (mycobacterial, fungal) occur, most commonly in immunocompromised patients or in the setting of a breast prosthesis. Granulomatous lobular mastitis is an uncommon breast-limited disease distinguished by granulomas involving lobular epithelium. Only parous women are affected, and it is possible the disease represents a hypersensitivity reaction mediated by prior alterations in lobular epithelium during lactation.

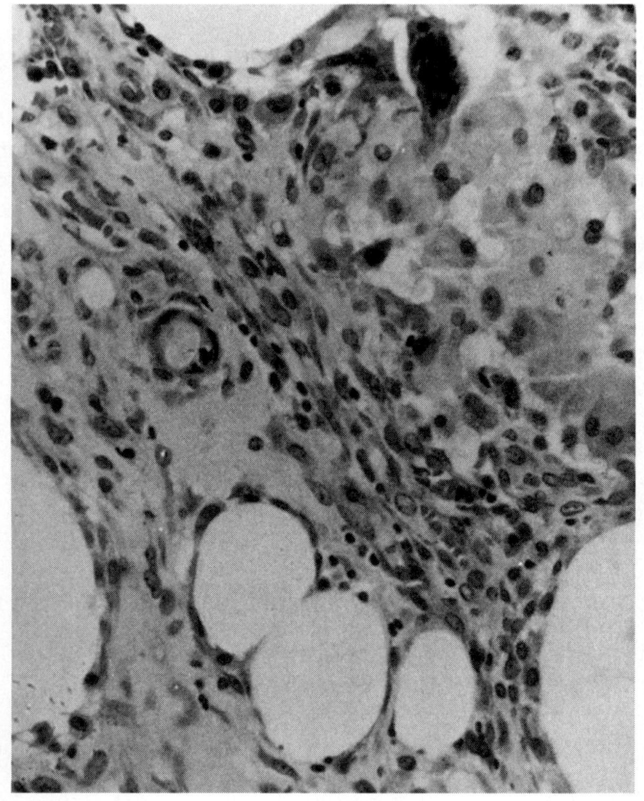

Figure 25–6

Fat necrosis. Note foamy macrophages and giant cell *(top right),* inflammation, and beginning fibrosis.

Silicone Breast Implants

Breast implants were developed in the early 1960s to replace breast tissue after mastectomy or for cosmetic augmentation. Silicone, a polymer of silica, oxygen, and hydrogen, can be produced in liquid, gel, and solid forms by varying the length of the polymer. Silicone implants consist of a solid silicone shell filled with either silicone gel or saline.

MORPHOLOGY. The typical histologic response to silicone implants is a chronic inflammatory infiltrate of lymphocytes, macrophages, and giant cells with associated fibrosis. In some cases, the lining cells take on a papillary villous appearance resembling joint synovium.[9] Silicone gel seeps ("bleeds") through intact shells and is frequently seen in the surrounding tissue. A fibrous capsule usually forms and may contract, causing cosmetic deformity. This capsule can limit the spread of silicone after implant rupture. However, if the capsule is also ruptured, silicone gel can escape into surrounding tissues and be transported into axillary lymph nodes. Migration to more distant sites from implants has been shown in animals but not definitively in humans.[10] After long periods of implantation, the outer shell can weaken and rupture in the absence of trauma. Some implants become heavily calcified.

Case reports have suggested linkage of implants to "human adjuvant disease," an autoimmune-like illness in response to foreign material. However, multiple large epidemiologic studies failed to show a connection between implants and objective evidence of rheumatologic disease.[11, 12] Nevertheless, the long-term consequences of implants are unknown. There are approximately 2 million women in the United States with implants, and the number of women with implantation more than 20 years ago will rapidly increase in the next three decades.

FIBROCYSTIC CHANGES

There is a miscellany of morphologic alterations in the female breast often grouped under the term fibrocystic changes. Despite the many "good-byes to fibrocystic disease,"[13] the term, although unsatisfactory, seems to be ingrained in clinical use. The term "fibrocystic changes" is more appropriate, since the alterations are present in most women and are often of no clinical significance. Alterations conferring an increased risk of carcinoma are termed proliferative disease and are discussed separately in the following section.

Incidence and Pathogenesis. Fibrocystic changes represent the single most common disorder of the breast and

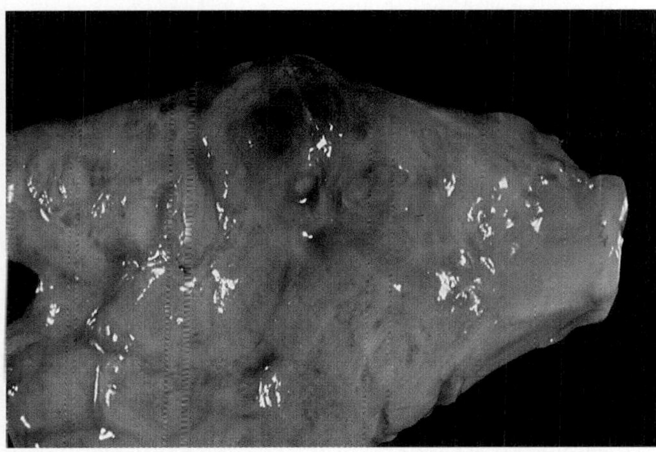

Figure 25–7

Cystic change of breast, showing a "blue-dome cyst."

account for more than half of all surgical operations on the female breast. In a study of the so-called normal breast, that is, in unselected forensic postmortem cases, grossly evident cystic changes and fibrosis were found in 20% but histologic changes were present in 59% of women.[14] The condition is unusual before adolescence, is diagnosed frequently between the ages of 20 and 40 years, peaks at or just before the menopause, and rarely develops after the menopause. However, premenopausal lesions may persist into the more advanced years.

Hormonal imbalances are considered to be basic to the development of this multipatterned disorder. The excess of estrogens may represent an absolute increase, as in the rarely associated functioning ovarian tumors, or may be related to a deficiency of progesterone, as seen in anovulatory women. There is also some evidence of abnormal end-organ metabolism of hormones in the pathogenesis of cystic disease. Oral contraceptive use decreases the risk of fibrocystic changes, presumably because it supplies a balanced source of progesterone and estrogen.

MORPHOLOGY. There are three principal patterns of morphologic change: (1) **cyst formation, often with apocrine metaplasia**; (2) **fibrosis**; and (3) **adenosis.**

Cysts. A large, grossly evident cyst may be formed within one breast, but the disorder is usually multifocal and often bilateral. As a result of cystic dilation of ducts and lobules, the involved areas, by palpation, have an ill-defined diffuse increase in consistency as well as discrete nodularities. Closely aggregated, small cysts produce a shotty texture. Larger, particularly solitary, cysts evoke the greatest alarm as isolated firm masses that are deceptively unyielding. Secretory products within cysts calcify, resulting in microcalcifications detected by mammography. Unopened, these cysts are brown to blue **(blue-dome cysts)** due to the contained semitranslucent, turbid fluid (Fig. 25–7). Frequently, cysts are lined by large polygonal cells having an abundant granular, eosinophilic cytoplasm, with small, round, deeply chromatic nuclei resembling the apocrine epithelium of sweat glands **(apocrine metaplasia)** (Fig. 25–8). Such apocrine metaplasia is found not uncommonly in the normal breast and is virtually always benign. Epithelial overgrowth and papillary projections are common in cysts lined by apocrine epithelium. In larger cysts, lining cells may be flattened or may be totally atrophic.

Fibrosis. Cysts frequently rupture with release of secretory material into the adjacent stroma. The resulting chronic inflammation and scarring fibrosis contribute to the palpable firmness of the breast.

Adenosis. Adenosis is recognized as an increase in the number of acinar units per lobule. A physiologic adenosis occurs during pregnancy, but this change can also be seen in nonpregnant women. The gland lumens are often enlarged (blunt duct adenosis) and are not distorted as is seen in the distinctly proliferative lesion, described later, termed sclerosing adenosis. Calcifications are occasionally present within lumens.

Clinical Significance. In the absence of proliferative breast disease (described later), fibrocystic changes do not elevate the risk of developing cancer. However, these changes may come to clinical attention when they mimic carcinoma by producing palpable lumps, mammographic densities or calcifications, or nipple discharge. Cysts and fibrosis produce the "lumpy bumpy" findings on physical examination that may make detection of other breast masses more difficult. Solitary enlarged cysts may form

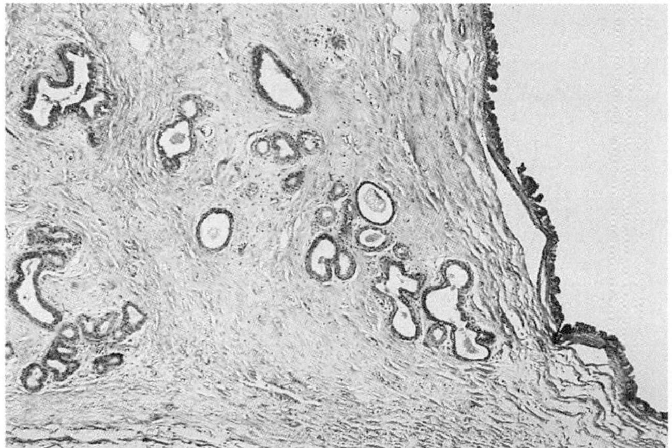

Figure 25–8

Microscopic detail of fibrocystic change of the breast revealing dilation of ducts producing microcysts and, at right, the wall of a large cyst with visible lining epithelial cells. (Courtesy of Dr. Kyle Molberg, Department of Pathology, University of Texas Southwestern Medical School, Dallas, TX.)

mammographic densities or palpable masses but can usually be diagnosed by disappearance of the mass after fine-needle aspiration of cyst contents. Cysts containing solid debris or clusters of small cysts are more difficult to diagnose and may require surgical excision. Calcifications are commonly found in cysts and adenosis and often form mammographically suspicious clusters. Cystic changes are also rarely associated with spontaneous unilateral nipple discharge.

PROLIFERATIVE BREAST DISEASE

Changes in the breast conferring an increased risk of developing carcinoma have been identified by large epidemiologic reviews of "benign" breast biopsy specimens from women who later developed breast cancer.[15, 16] Increased risk is associated with (1) moderate or florid epithelial hyperplasia with or without atypia, (2) sclerosing adenosis, and (3) small duct papillomas. These lesions are often accompanied by the fibrocystic changes described earlier.

Epithelial Hyperplasia

In normal breast, only a double layer of myoepithelial and epithelial cells is present above the basement membrane. Epithelial hyperplasia is defined by an increase in the layers of cells and may be due to increased proliferation or, more likely, failure of cells to undergo apoptosis. If more than four cell layers are present, there is an increased risk of developing carcinoma. This is not to say that all foci of epithelial hyperplasia (termed *epitheliosis* by British pathologists) are premalignant, leading inevitably to carcinoma; indeed, only a small proportion apparently are. But it is this pattern of alteration that should concern the pathologist, who is called to differentiate among benign hyperplasia, atypical but still noncancerous hyperplasia, and carcinoma.

MORPHOLOGY. Epithelial hyperplasia is usually not grossly evident. The proliferating epithelium takes the form of solid masses extending and encroaching into the duct lumen, partially obliterating it, but irregular lumens **(fenestrations)** can usually be discerned at the periphery of the cellular masses (Fig. 25–9*A*). Various degrees of cellular and architectural atypia may be present **(atypical hyperplasia).** The differentiation of the latter from carcinoma in situ, discussed later, may be difficult. In general, greater cellular homogeneity with nuclear hyperchromasia, architectural uniformity, and more extensive distribution favor carcinoma in situ.

Atypical ductal hyperplasia is recognized by its histologic resemblance to ductal carcinoma in situ. However, the lesions are characteristically limited in extent, and the cells are not completely monomorphic in type or fail to completely fill ductal spaces (Fig. 25–9*B*). At least 40% of atypical ductal hyperplasias are clonal and show microsatellite DNA instability.[17] In breasts with invasive cancer, multiple independent atypical hyperplastic clones may be present, suggesting that this is a multicentric process and that only a minority of these lesions progress to malignancy.[18]

Atypical lobular hyperplasia refers to proliferation of a population of cells that resemble those of lobular carcinoma in situ (described later) but do not fill or distend more than 50% of the acini within a lobule.[19] Atypical lobular hyperplasia can also extend to ducts (rather than only acini), and this finding is associated with an increased risk of developing invasive carcinoma.[19]

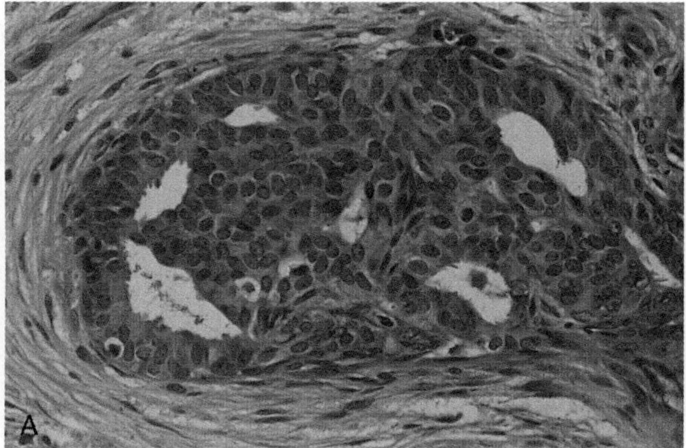

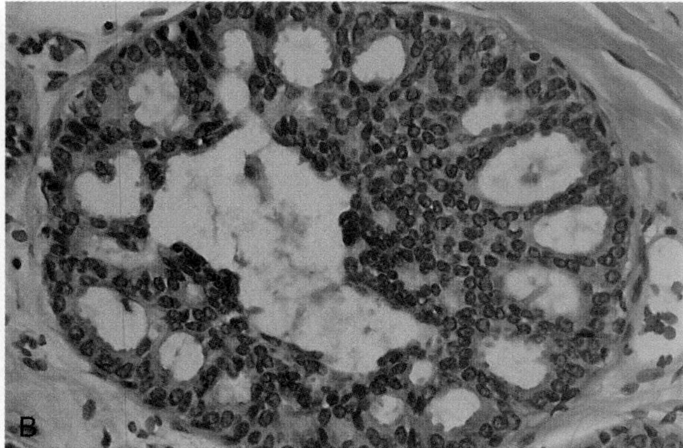

Figure 25–9

A, Hyperplasia. The lumen is filled with a heterogeneous population of round and spindle cells. The fenestrations are slitlike and peripherally located. *B*, Atypical ductal hyperplasia. The cell population is homogeneous and the spaces are more regular in shape and evenly spaced. (Courtesy of Dr. Stuart Schnitt, Beth Israel Hospital, Boston.)

Sclerosing Adenosis

This lesion is characterized histologically by increased numbers of distorted and compressed acini. Small lesions commonly present as mammographic calcifications, and larger lesions may form mammographic densities or, rarely, palpable masses.

MORPHOLOGY. On gross inspection, areas of sclerosing adenosis sometimes have a hard cartilaginous consistency that begins to approximate that found in breast cancer. On section, the involved area is not well localized and does not have the chalky yellow-white foci and streaks that identify breast carcinoma, an important gross differential feature.

The number of acini per terminal duct is increased to at least twofold the number found in uninvolved lobules. The lobular arrangement is maintained. The acini are compressed and distorted in the central portions of the lesion but characteristically dilated at the periphery. Myoepithelial cells are often prominent. On occasion, stromal fibrosis may totally compress the lumens to create the appearance of solid cords or double strands of cells lying within dense stroma, a histologic pattern that at times verges on the appearance of carcinoma (Fig. 25–10).

Other less common sclerosing lesions of the breast include **complex sclerosing lesions (radial scars)** and **sclerosing papillomas.** Complex sclerosing lesions exhibit abundant central fibrosis and elastosis. Sclerosing papillomas contain papillary projections. Both often have a component of sclerosing adenosis. These lesions at times may be difficult to distinguish from carcinomas both radiologically and histologically.

Although long thought to be a completely innocuous lesion, sclerosing adenosis has been shown to confer a slightly increased risk of subsequent cancer.[20]

Small Duct Papillomas

Small papillomas occur deep within the breast and are often associated with the other changes of proliferative breast disease. These small papillomas are usually clinically silent and are probably etiologically distinct from the large duct papillomas associated with nipple discharge discussed later.

MORPHOLOGY. Fibrovascular cores extend into small duct lumens and are lined by a normal two-cell layer (Fig. 25–11). However, epithelial hyperplasia may also be present in papillomas. The distinction between a benign but atypical small duct papilloma and an intraductal papillary carcinoma may be difficult in some cases. In general, a monomorphic cell population, the absence of myoepithelial cells, delicate vascular connective tissue cores, the presence of cribriform or micropapillary areas, and the absence of hyalinization or apocrine metaplasia favor a malignant rather than benign papillary tumor.

Clinical Significance of Proliferative Disease. The number of women diagnosed with proliferative breast disease has increased because of the association of some of the changes with mammographic abnormalities (calcifications and densities) and because they are present in the large number of breast biopsies performed to evaluate

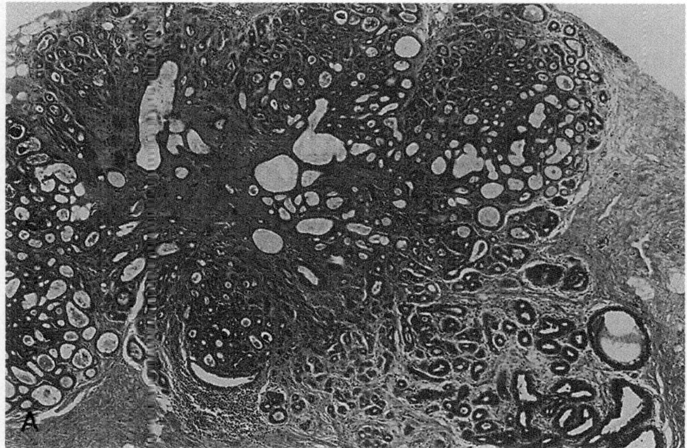

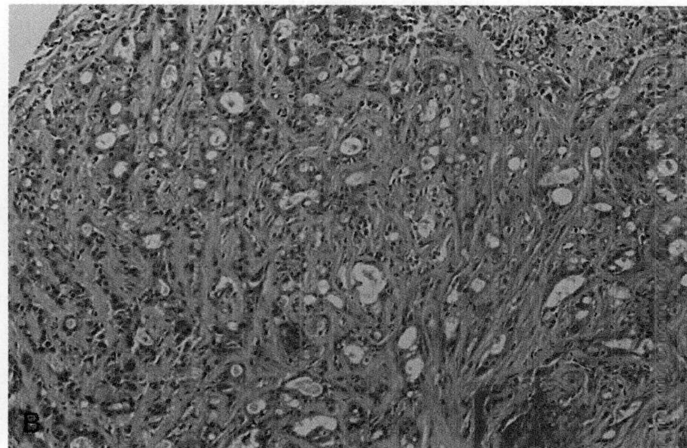

Figure 25–10

A, Sclerosing adenosis. The number of acini exceeds that seen in a normal lobule. Central dilated terminal ducts are present as well as characteristic dilated acini at the periphery. *B*, The acini are compressed and distorted by the surrounding fibrotic stroma and can appear to be solid nests or cords of cells.

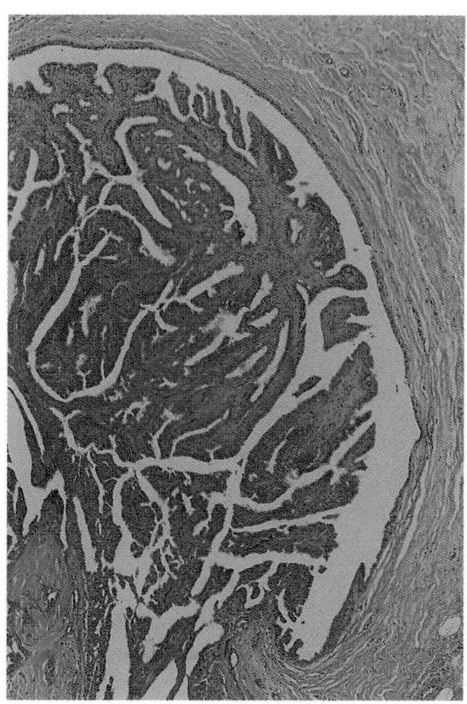

Figure 25–11 ■

Small duct papilloma with a fibrovascular central core lined by a normal two-cell epithelium.

palpable masses. Current evidence suggests that the increased risk of cancer is proportional to the type of proliferative breast disease and to the presence of atypia. The increased risk for the various types of changes is as follows:

- *No increased risk of breast carcinoma:* adenosis, cystic changes, apocrine metaplasia, mild epithelial hyperplasia
- *Slightly increased risk, 1.5 to 2 times:* sclerosing adenosis, epithelial hyperplasia (moderate to florid), papillomas
- *Moderately increased risk, 4 to 5 times:* atypical epithelial hyperplasia, ductal or lobular
- *A family history of breast cancer increases the risk in all categories,* for example, to about tenfold with atypical hyperplasia

Fortunately, among women undergoing breast biopsies for benign disease, about 50% will have no proliferative disease, and of the 50% with proliferative changes, only 5% to 10% will have atypical hyperplasia.[16] Of the latter, less than 15% will develop cancer. Atypical lobular hyperplasia is associated with a higher risk of cancer in premenopausal women, whereas risk associated with atypical ductal hyperplasia is equivalent for both premenopausal and postmenopausal women.[21] When cancer develops, both breasts are at equal risk, even if the initial lesion was unilateral.

TUMORS

Neoplasms constitute the most important, albeit not the most common, lesions of the female breast. A great variety of tumors may occur in the female breast, made up as it is of a covering integument, adult fat, mesenchymal connective tissue, and epithelial structures. These tumors run the gamut of the neoplasms that may arise from squamous epithelium, glandular structures, and connective tissue. Only the more common tumors of the breast are described, and the main discussion focuses on breast cancer.

Stromal Tumors

The two types of stroma in the breast, intralobular and interlobular (see under Normal), give rise to distinct types of neoplasms. Breast-specific intralobular stroma is the progenitor of the breast-specific biphasic tumors fibroadenoma and phyllodes tumor. The specialized stroma may elaborate growth factors for epithelial cells resulting in the associated proliferation of the non-neoplastic epithelial component of these tumors. Interlobular stroma is the source of the same types of tumors found in connective tissue in other sites of the body (e.g., lipomas, angiosarcomas).

FIBROADENOMA

This is the most common benign tumor of the female breast. As the name implies, it is *a new growth composed of both fibrous and glandular tissue.* Some fibroadenomas represent hyperplasias and are polyclonal in origin.[22] For example, almost half of women receiving cyclosporin A after renal transplantation develop fibroadenomas.[23] The tumors are frequently multiple and bilateral and are likely to be due to drug-related growth stimulation. On the other hand, there is a subset of fibroadenomas that are benign neoplasms of stromal cells. Multiple studies have shown that in some tumors, the fibrous (stromal) component is clonal and may have cytogenetic aberrations, but the epithelial component is polyclonal.[4, 24] Occurring at any age within the reproductive period of life, fibroadenomas are somewhat more common before age 30 years. Young women usually present with a palpable mass and older women with a mammographic density (Fig. 25–12*B*). Fibroadenomas are associated with a mild increase in the risk of subsequent breast cancer, especially when they are associated with fibrocystic changes, proliferative breast disease, or a family history of breast cancer.[25]

MORPHOLOGY. The fibroadenoma grows as a spherical nodule that is usually sharply circumscribed and freely movable from the surrounding breast substance. These tumors frequently occur in the upper outer quadrant of the breast. They vary in size from less than 1 cm to giant forms 10 to 15 cm in diameter **(giant fibroadenoma)**, but most are surgically removed when they are 2 to 4

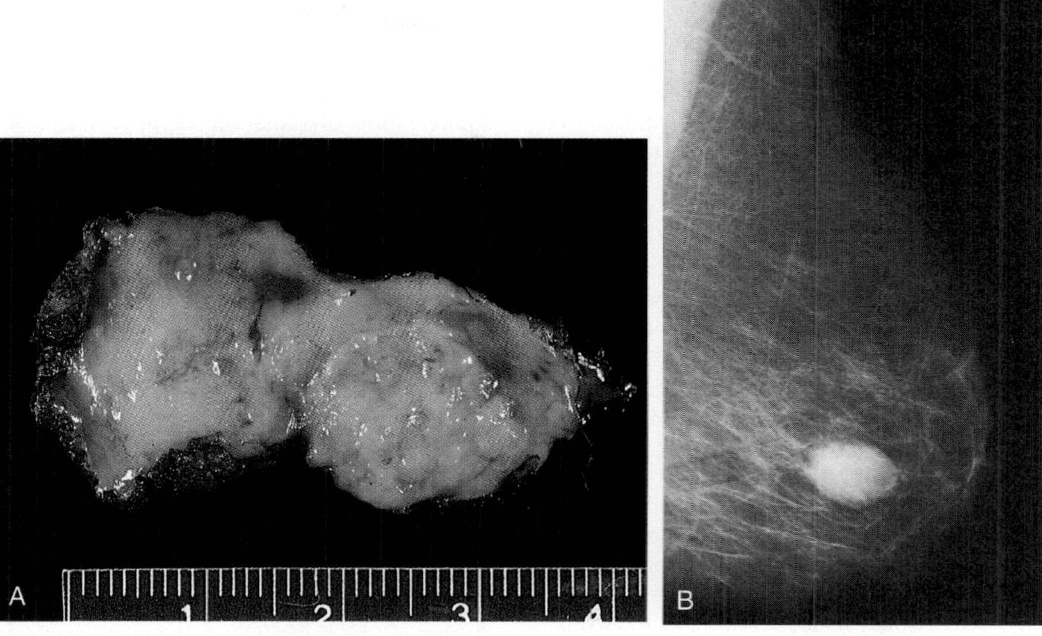

Figure 25–12 ■

A, Fibroadenoma. The white well-circumscribed mass is clearly demarcated from the surrounding yellow adipose tissue. *B*, A well-circumscribed mammographic density most commonly corresponding to a fibroadenoma. (Courtesy of Dr. Jack G. Meyer, Brigham and Women's Hospital, Boston, MA.)

cm in diameter (Fig. 25–12*A*). On section, they are grayish white and often contain slit-like spaces.

The histologic pattern is essentially one of delicate, cellular, fibroblastic stroma resembling intralobular stroma, enclosing glandular and cystic spaces lined by epithelium. The epithelium may be surrounded by stroma or compressed and distorted by it (Fig. 25–13).

The epithelium of the fibroadenoma is hormonally responsive, and a slight increase in size may occur during the late phases of each menstrual cycle. An increase in size due to lactational changes, or not uncommonly infarction and inflammation, may lead to a fibroadenoma mimicking carcinoma during pregnancy. Regression usually occurs postmenopausally. The stroma often becomes densely hyalinized and may calcify. Large ("popcorn") calcifications have a characteristic mammographic appearance, but small calcifications may appear clustered and require surgical excision to exclude carcinoma.

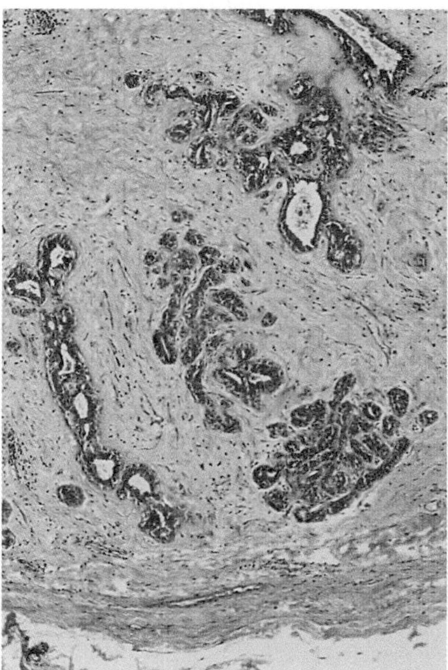

Figure 25–13 ■

Microscopic view of fibroadenoma of the breast. The fibrous capsule *(below)* sharply delimits the tumor from the surrounding tissue. (Courtesy of Dr. Trace Worrell, Department of Pathology, University of Texas Southwestern Medical School, Dallas, TX.)

PHYLLODES TUMOR

Phyllodes tumors, like fibroadenomas, arise from intralobular stroma. Although they can occur at any age, most present in the sixth decade, 10 to 20 years later than the average presentation of a fibroadenoma. Most are low-grade tumors that may recur locally but only rarely metastasize. Rare high-grade lesions behave aggressively, exhibiting local recurrences commonly and distant hematogenous metastases in about one third of cases.[26] As is true of other stromal malignant neoplasms, lymph node metastases are rare. The term *cystosarcoma phyllodes* is sometimes used for these lesions; however, the majority of the tumors behave in a relatively benign fashion.

MORPHOLOGY. The tumors vary in size from a few centimeters to massive lesions involving the entire breast. The larger lesions often have bulbous protrusions (phyllodes is Greek for leaflike) due to the presence of nodules of proliferating stroma covered by epithelium (Fig. 25–14). This growth pattern can also occasionally be seen in larger fibroadenomas and is not an indicator of malignancy. Phyllodes tumors are distinguished from the more common fibroadenomas on the basis of cellularity, mitotic rate, nuclear pleomorphism, stromal overgrowth, and infiltrative borders. On histologic evaluation, lower grade lesions resemble fibroadenomas but with increased cellularity and mitotic figures. High-grade lesions may be difficult to distinguish from other types of soft tissue sarcomas and may have foci of heterologous mesenchymal differentiation (e.g., rhabdomyosarcoma).

SARCOMAS

Tumors of the extrinsic connective tissue of the breast include the same types of benign and malignant lesions seen elsewhere in the body. Malignant lesions include angiosarcoma, rhabdomyosarcoma, liposarcoma, leiomyosarcoma, chondrosarcoma, and osteosarcoma. Sarcomatous differentiation also occurs in phyllodes tumors and in carcinomas ("metaplastic carcinomas"). Sarcomas usually present as bulky palpable masses. Lymph node metastases are rare; hematogenous spread to the lung is commonly seen.

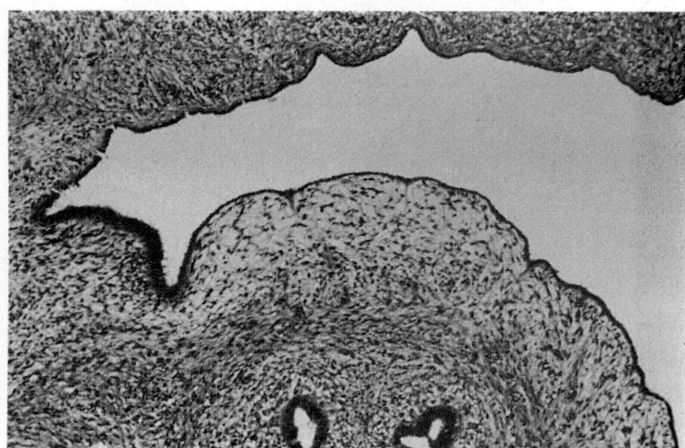

Figure 25–14 ■

Phyllodes tumor. Note the increased stromal cellularity and a typical stromal nodule projecting into a slitlike space, resulting in the gross phyllode (leaflike) pattern.

Angiosarcomas of the breast arise spontaneously or as a complication of radiation therapy. There is a 0.3% to 4% risk of angiosarcoma after radiation therapy for breast cancer, with most cases arising 5 to 10 years after treatment.[4] Angiosarcomas can also arise in the skin of a chronically edematous arm after mastectomy (Stewart-Treves syndrome), but this complication has become much less common with greater attention to surgical techniques.

Epithelial Tumors

Large Duct Papilloma

Most of these lesions are solitary and are found within the principal lactiferous ducts or sinuses. They represent papillary clonal proliferations of duct epithelial cells and are thus classified as true neoplasms.[27] More than 80% present as spontaneous unilateral serous or bloody nipple discharge, the remainder as small palpable masses or mammographic densities. Although nipple discharge is most commonly due to such benign papillomas, it is associated with carcinoma in 7% of women younger than 60 years and in 30% of women older than 60 years.

MORPHOLOGY. The tumors are rarely more than 1 cm in diameter and are composed of multiple branching papillae, each having a connective tissue axis covered by epithelial and myoepithelial cells (Fig. 25–15). Growth occurs within a dilated duct or lactiferous sinus close to the nipple. Apocrine metaplasia is common. The papilloma can spontaneously infarct, possibly because of torsion on the stalk, resulting in hemorrhagic discharge.

The present consensus is that most solitary intraductal papillomas are benign and are **not** the precursors of papillary carcinoma. However, **multiple small duct papillomas** should be distinguished from the group, since they are associated with an increased risk of development of carcinoma.

Nipple adenoma and **florid papillomatosis of the nipple** are terms used to describe tumors of the nipple exhibiting adenosis of the duct epithelium sometimes associated with papillary areas. They should be differentiated from intraductal papilloma, as they are associated with concomitant or subsequent carcinoma in 16% of cases, often found elsewhere in the breast.[4]

CARCINOMA OF THE BREAST

One of nine women in the United States will develop breast cancer in her lifetime; a third of these women will succumb to the disease, resulting in more than 44,000

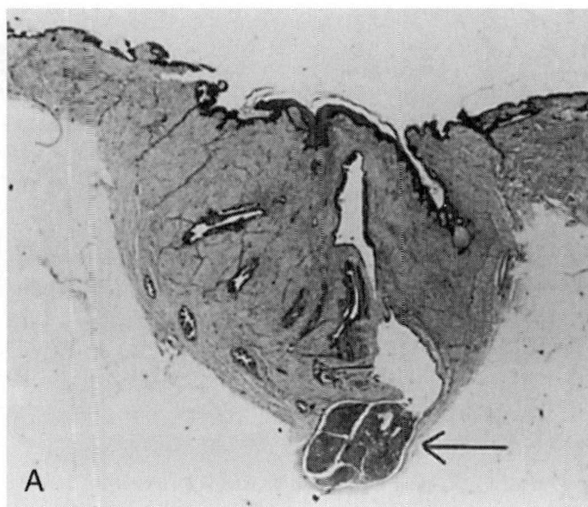

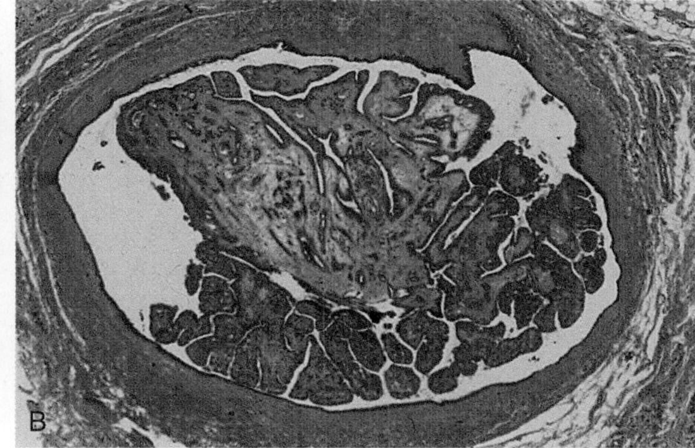

Figure 25–15

Intraductal papilloma. *A*, Low-power view of the nipple showing tumor in the lactiferous duct *(arrow)*. *B*, Large duct papilloma. The lesion has a thick fibrovascular core.

deaths each year. Understandably, then, breast cancer has received a great deal of appropriate publicity and has been the focus of intensive study relative to its origins, diagnostic methods, and treatment. Much has been gained, particularly in early diagnosis, and after remaining stable for many decades, the mortality rate from breast cancer in white women in the United States decreased slightly between 1989 and 1992. Unfortunately, the mortality rate for black women increased during the same period. It is both ironic and tragic that a neoplasm arising in an exposed organ, readily accessible to self-examination and clinical diagnosis, continues to exact such a heavy toll, second only to lung cancer among women.

Incidence and Epidemiology. Cancer of the female breast is rarely found before the age of 25 years except in certain familial cases. The incidence then increases with age from 1 in 232 in the fourth decade to 1 in 29 in the seventh decade. The overall incidence of breast cancer in the population increased steadily up to 1988 but has been stable since that time.

Few cancers have been subjected to more intensive epidemiologic study. Observations bearing on the incidence of this disease can be summarized as follows.

Genetic Predisposition. A family history is a risk factor for the development of breast cancer, and 5% to 10% of breast cancer is attributable to inheritance of an autosomal dominant gene.[28] The probability of genetic inheritance increases if there are multiple affected relatives and the cancers occur at young ages. Two genes, *BRCA1* and *BRCA2* (Table 25–1), account for the majority of hereditary breast cancers.[29, 30] However, less than 20% of women with a family history of breast cancer will carry these genes.[31, 32] Genetic susceptibility due to other genes is much less common. Breast cancer affects the majority of women with the Li-Fraumeni syndrome (multiple sarcomas and carcinomas), which, as described in Chapter 8, is associated with germ line mutations of the tumor-suppressor gene *p53*. Women with Cowden disease ("multiple hamartoma syndrome" due to a mutation of a gene on chromosome 10q) have a 30% to 50% risk of breast cancer by age 50 years, and heterozygous carriers for ataxia-telangiectasia *(ATM* gene) have an 11% risk at the same age.

Although the overall incidence of breast cancer is lower in black women, women in this group present at a more advanced stage and have an increased mortality rate compared with white women. Social factors such as decreased access to health care and lower use of mammography account for some of the difference, but genetic factors may also play a role. A greater number of breast cancers are diagnosed in young black women than in white women younger than 40 years, and breast carcinomas in black women have a higher nuclear grade, more frequently lack hormone receptors, and have different types of sporadic *p53* mutations.

Increasing Age. Breast cancer is uncommon before age 25 years, but then there is a steady rise to the time of menopause, followed by a slower rise throughout life. The average age at diagnosis is 64 years.

Proliferative Breast Disease. Proliferative breast disease is associated with an increased risk, as noted in the earlier discussion of this condition.

Carcinoma of the Contralateral Breast or Endometrium. Increased risk is associated with carcinoma of the contralateral breast or endometrium.

Radiation Exposure. Women exposed to therapeutic radiation or after atom bomb exposure have a higher rate of breast cancer. Risk increases with younger age and higher radiation doses.

Geographic Influences. The incidence of breast cancer varies fourfold to sevenfold when Asian and other countries are compared, with the United States and northern European countries having the highest rates. The specific factors have not been identified but probably include many of those listed in the following.

Length of Reproductive Life. Risk increases with early menarche and late menopause.

Parity. Breast cancer is more frequent in nulliparous than in multiparous women.

Table 25–1. PROPERTIES AND ROLES OF *BRCA1* AND *BRCA2*

	BRCA1	*BRCA2*
Chromosome	17q21	13q12
Gene	100 kb	70 kb
Protein	1863 amino acids Component of RNA polymerase holoenzyme	3418 amino acids
Function	Tumor suppressor Interacts with nuclear proteins Possible role in DNA repair	Tumor suppressor Interacts with nuclear proteins Possible role in DNA repair
Mutations	>500 identified	>200 identified
Risk of breast cancer	More than 70% by age 80 years	More than 60% by age 70 years
Age at onset	Younger age (40s to 50s)	50 years; older than *BRCA1*
Risk of other tumors	30%–60% risk of ovarian cancer by age 70 years Prostate, colon	Male breast cancer, ovary, bladder, prostate, pancreas
Mutations in nonfamilial breast cancer	Very rare (<5%)	<5%
Epidemiology	Specific mutations more common in some ethnic groups (e.g., one mutation present in 20% to 30% of breast cancers in Ashkenazi Jews)	Specific mutations more common in some ethnic groups
Pathology of breast cancers	Greater incidence (13%) of medullary carcinomas and higher grade tumors Ductal carcinoma in situ less frequent	Variable types, may depend on specific mutations

Age at First Child. Risk is increased in women older than 30 years at the time of their first child.

Obesity. There is decreased risk in obese women younger than 40 years owing to the association with anovulatory cycles and lower progesterone levels late in the cycle. There is increased risk in postmenopausal obese women attributed to synthesis of estrogens in fat depots.

Exogenous Estrogens. The role of postmenopausal hormone replacement therapy or oral contraceptives as risk factors for developing breast cancer remains controversial.[33] Any risk, if present, is small.

Etiology and Pathogenesis. The epidemiologic data cited and studies of mammary tumors in vitro and in experimental animals point to three sets of important influences in breast cancer: (1) genetic factors, (2) hormonal influences, and (3) environmental factors.

Genetic Factors. Genetic predisposition clearly exists. As noted, germ line mutations in *BRCA1, BRCA2, p53,* a locus on 10q in Cowden syndrome, and the *ATM* gene (ataxia-telangiectasia) account for the majority of rare cases of autosomally inherited familial cancer. These genes probably act as tumor-suppressor genes (limiting cell growth) or in DNA repair (Chapter 8), and the features of *BRCA1* and *BRCA2* that are salient to breast cancer are shown in Table 25–1.

Hormonal Influences. *Endogenous estrogen excess,* or more accurately, hormonal imbalance, clearly plays a significant role. Many of the risk factors mentioned—long duration of reproductive life, nulliparity, and late age at first child—imply increased exposure to estrogen peaks during the menstrual cycle. Functioning ovarian tumors that elaborate estrogens are associated with breast cancer in postmenopausal women. Mildly increased breast cancer risk has been documented in postmenopausal women with high-normal levels of circulating estrogens.[34] There are also hints of how the estrogens may act. Normal breast epithelium possesses estrogen and progesterone receptors. These have been identified in some but not all breast cancers. A variety of growth promoters (transforming growth factor-α/epidermal growth factor, platelet-derived growth factor, and fibroblast growth factor) and growth inhibitors (transforming growth factor-β) are secreted by human breast cancer cells, and many studies suggest that they are involved in an autocrine mechanism of tumor progression. Production of these growth factors is dependent on estrogen, and it is thought that interactions between circulating hormones, hormone receptors on cancer cells, and autocrine growth factors induced by tumor cells are involved in breast cancer progression (Chapter 8).[35]

Environmental Factors. Environmental influences are suggested by the variable incidence of breast cancer in genetically homogeneous groups and the geographic differences in prevalence. Historically, breast cancer incidence rates in the United States and other Western countries have been four to seven times higher than in non-Western countries. However, the risk of breast cancer in immigrants to the United States increases during several generations, suggesting that much of the increased risk is due to modifiable factors. Indeed, as Japan and Taiwan have adopted a more Western life style, breast cancer incidence in these countries has also increased.

Women in their teens and 20s (but not at older ages) undergoing mantle radiation for Hodgkin disease have a 20% to 30% risk of developing breast cancer 10 to 30 years after treatment.[36] "Windows of susceptibility" for other exogenous factors may exist but have been difficult to establish because critical exposure may have occurred decades before development of the disease. Mammographic screening uses low doses of radiation and is unlikely to increase risk unless there is an underlying predisposition to radiation sensitivity, such as heterozygosity for ataxia-telangiectasia.

Various items in diet, in particular dietary fat, have been implicated, but specific foods that can modify risk have not been identified.[37] Coffee addicts will be pleased to know that there is no substantial evidence that caffeine consumption increases the risk, but studies do suggest that moderate or heavy alcohol consumption is associated with an increased risk of breast cancer. Cigarette smoking is not associated with breast cancer. The role of *viruses* has been pursued since Bittner's brilliant discovery in 1936 that a filterable agent, transmitted through the mother's milk, causes breast cancer in suckling mice.[38] The virus, called mouse mammary tumor virus, was later identified as a retrovirus. Subsequently, there have been many hints of the existence of an analogous virus in breast cancer of humans, but a direct link has not been established.[39] There is also concern that environmental contaminants such as organochlorine pesticides may have estrogenic effects on humans. The possible effect of environmental toxins on breast cancer risk is being intensively investigated.[40]

Cellular Changes in Breast Cancer Progression. Much has been learned of the specific cellular changes that occur in the progression to breast cancer and indeed forms the basis of some of our current views on cancer progression (Chapter 8).[41, 42] One of the earliest detectable changes is loss of normal regulation of cell number, resulting in epithelial hyperplasia or sclerosing adenosis. Next, genetic instability occurs in multiple small clonal populations of cells recognizable histologically as atypical hyperplasia. After progression to carcinoma, numerous cellular alterations can be identified, including increased expression of oncogenes (e.g., c-*erb-B2*, *Her2/neu*, *INT2*, c-*ras*, c-*myc*), decreased expression or function of tumor-suppressor genes (e.g., *NM23*, *p53*, *RB*), alterations in cell structure (e.g., increased expression of vimentin, decreased expression of fodrin), loss of cell adhesion (e.g., loss of E-cadherin in lobular carcinomas, loss of integrins in poorly differentiated carcinomas), increased expression of cell cycle proteins (e.g., cyclins, Ki-67, proliferating cell nuclear antigen), increased expression of angiogenic factors (e.g., vascular endothelial growth factor, fibroblast growth factor), and increased expression of proteases (e.g., cathepsin-D, stromelysins). All of these changes occur in some but not all cancers, suggesting that the malignant phenotype is due to an accumulation of multiple changes rather than an orderly progression. In addition, many of these changes can also be found in in situ carcinomas, and the specific factors necessary for stromal invasion and metastasis remain to be established.

Classification and Distribution. Curiously, carcinoma is more common in the left breast than in the right, in a ratio of 110:100. The cancers are bilateral or sequential in the same breast in 4% or more of cases.

Among breast carcinomas small enough for their general areas of origin to be identified, approximately 50% arise in the upper outer quadrant; 10% in each of the remaining quadrants; and about 20% in the central or subareolar region. As will be seen, the site of origin influences the pattern of nodal metastasis to a considerable degree.

Carcinoma is divided into noninvasive or in situ carcinomas and invasive carcinomas. Carcinoma in situ was originally classified as ductal or lobular on the basis of resemblance of the involved spaces to ducts and lobules. Although these descriptive terms are still used, all carcinomas are thought to arise from the terminal duct lobular unit, and "ductal" and "lobular" no longer imply a site or cell type of origin.[43] The most common histologic types of invasive breast carcinoma are listed in Table 25–2. Other less common types (apocrine carcinomas, carcinomas with neuroendocrine differentiation, clear cell carcinomas) are clinically similar to carcinomas of no special type in behavior and prognosis and are not listed. Inflammatory carcinoma refers to the clinical presentation of a carcinoma extensively involving dermal lymphatics resulting in an enlarged erythematous breast and is not a specific histologic type.

Table 25–2. DISTRIBUTION OF HISTOLOGIC TYPES OF BREAST CANCER

	Total Cancers*	
In Situ Carcinoma	15%–30%	
Ductal carcinoma in situ		80%
Lobular carcinoma in situ		20%
Invasive Carcinoma	70%–85%	
Ductal carcinoma (no special type)		79%
Lobular carcinoma		10%
Tubular/cribriform carcinoma		6%
Colloid (mucinous) carcinoma		2%
Medullary carcinoma		2%
Papillary carcinoma		1%

*The proportion of in situ carcinomas detected is dependent on the number of women undergoing mammographic screening and ranges from less than 5% in unscreened populations to almost 50% in patients with screen-detected cancers. Current observed numbers are between these two extremes.

The data on invasive carcinomas are modified from Dixon JM, et al: Long-term survivors after breast cancer. Br J Surg 72:445, 1985.

In Situ (Noninvasive) Carcinoma

DUCTAL CARCINOMA IN SITU (INCLUDING PAGET'S DISEASE)

The number of cases of ductal carcinoma in situ (DCIS) has rapidly increased in the past two decades from less than 5% of all carcinomas before mammographic screening to 15% to 30% of carcinomas in well-screened populations (Table 25–2). Among mammographically detected cancers, almost half are DCIS. The lesion consists of a malignant population of cells that lack the capacity to invade through the basement membrane and, therefore, are incapable of distant metastasis. However, these cells can spread throughout a ductal system and produce extensive lesions involving an entire sector of a breast. When DCIS involves

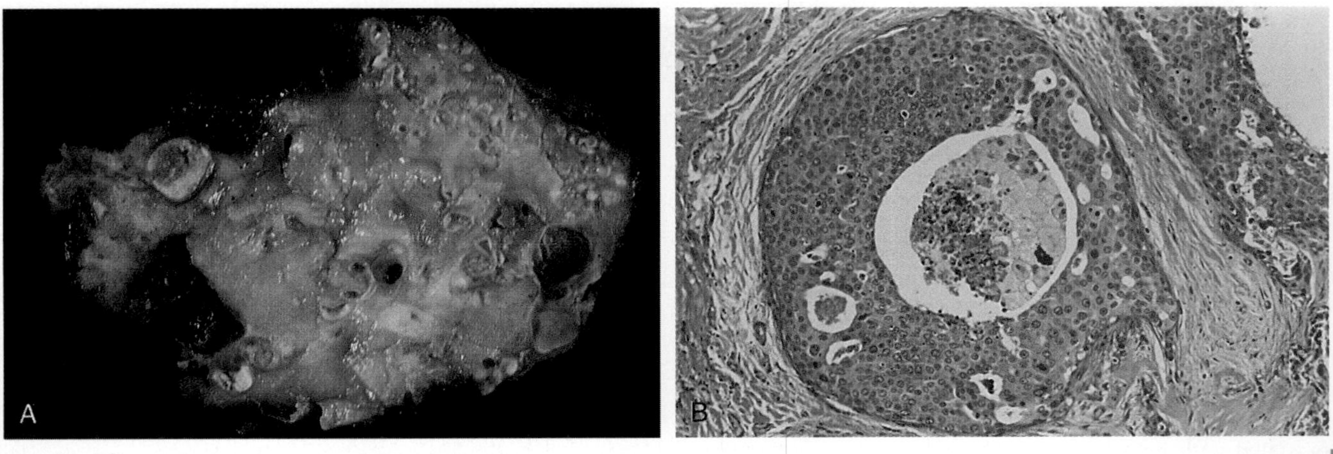

Figure 25–16

A, Gross appearance of comedocarcinoma showing typical white necrotic centers. *B*, Comedocarcinoma showing intraductal proliferation of malignant cells with central necrosis and calcifications.

lobules, the acini are often distorted and unfolded and take on the appearance of small ducts.

Historically, DCIS has been divided into five architectural subtypes: *comedocarcinoma, solid, cribriform, papillary,* and *micropapillary*. Some cases of DCIS will have a single growth pattern, but the majority demonstrate a mixture of patterns.

Comedocarcinoma is characterized by solid sheets of high-grade malignant cells and central necrosis (Fig. 25–16*B*). The necrosis commonly calcifies and is detected on mammography as clusters or linear and branching microcalcifications. Punctate areas of necrotic material ("comedone"-like) can be seen grossly (Fig. 25–16*A*). Periductal concentric fibrosis and chronic inflammation occur commonly, and extensive lesions are sometimes palpable as an area of vague nodularity.

Noncomedo DCIS can have nuclear grades ranging from low to high. Calcifications are seen associated with central necrosis, but more commonly when there are intraluminal secretions (Fig. 25–17*A*). The cells appear monomorphic. In **cribriform DCIS**, intraepithelial spaces are evenly distributed and regular in shape. **Papillary DCIS** typically lacks the normal myoepithelial cell layer (Fig. 25–17*B*). **Micropapillary DCIS** is recognized by bulbous protrusions without a fibrovascular core, often forming complex intraductal patterns.

Paget's disease of the nipple is a form of DCIS that extends from nipple ducts into the contiguous skin of the nipple and areola. The most striking gross characteristics of this lesion involve the skin

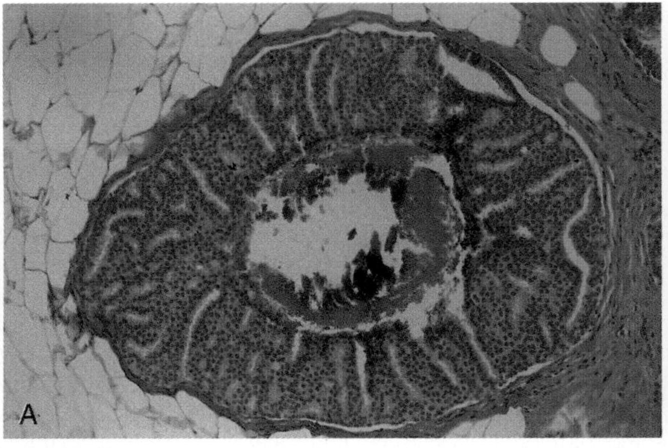

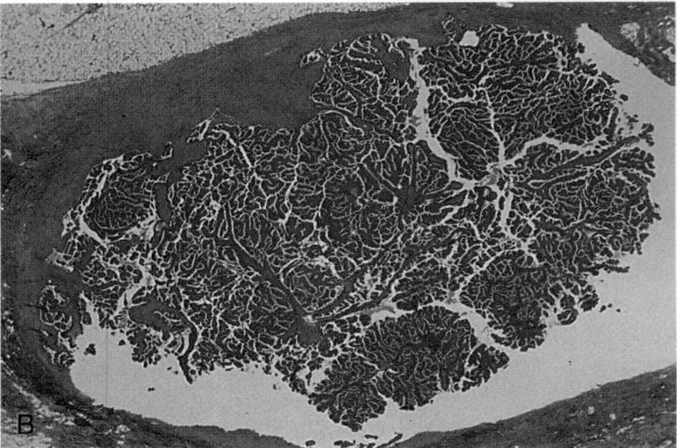

Figure 25–17

Noncomedo DCIS. *A*, Cribriform DCIS with-low grade nuclei and central necrosis with calcifications. *B*, Papillary DCIS growing within a dilated space. Delicate fibrovascular cores are present.

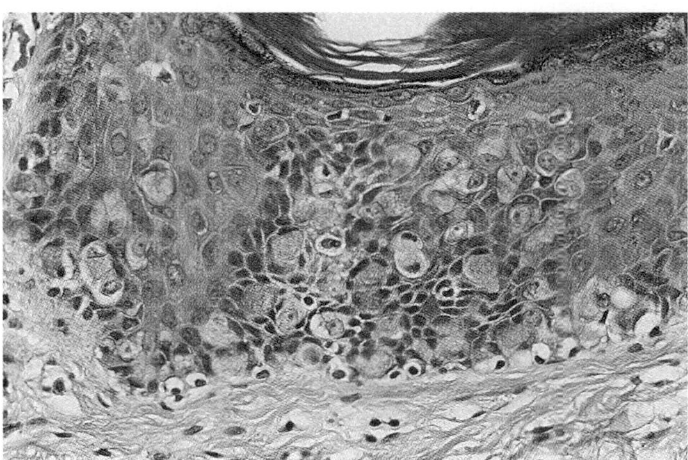

Figure 25–18

Paget's disease of the breast. Paget cells with abundant clear cytoplasm and pleomorphic nuclei dot the epithelium.

of the nipple and areola, which is frequently fissured, ulcerated, and oozing. There is surrounding inflammatory hyperemia and edema and, occasionally, total nipple ulceration. An underlying palpable mass is present in 50% to 60% of cases and usually indicates the presence of invasive carcinoma. **The histologic hallmark of this entity is the involvement of the epidermis by malignant cells,** referred to as Paget cells. These cells are large and have abundant clear or lightly staining cytoplasm and nuclei with prominent nucleoli (Fig. 25–18). The cells often contain mucin and are immunoreactive for epithelial membrane antigens, *c-erb-B2 (Her2/neu),* and low-molecular-weight keratins. In addition to the Paget cells, the other histologic criteria of ductal carcinoma are present. Prognosis is dependent on the extent of the underlying carcinoma.

DCIS with microinvasion is recognized by the coexistence of foci of tumor cells less than 0.1 cm in size invading the stroma. Microinvasion is most commonly seen in association with comedocarcinoma. Rare cases of DCIS with lymph node metastases are probably due to small invasive foci that may go undetected, particularly when the area involved by DCIS is large (e.g., more than 5 cm). However, in general, the prognosis of DCIS with microinvasion is similar to that of DCIS alone.

The natural history of DCIS has been difficult to examine since in the past all women were treated with mastectomy, and the current practice of surgical excision usually followed by radiation is largely curative. In a small cohort of 28 women with small noncomedo largely low-grade DCIS initially misdiagnosed as benign disease and treated with biopsy alone, 32% developed invasive carcinoma in the same area when they were observed for almost 30 years.[4-] It is thus now thought that many cases of low-grade DCIS, and probably most cases of high-grade DCIS, may progress to invasive carcinoma, emphasizing the importance of proper diagnosis and appropriate therapy in this condition.

LOBULAR CARCINOMA IN SITU

Lobular carcinoma in situ (LCIS) is manifested by proliferation, in one or more terminal ducts or ductules (acini), of a monomorphic population of cells that are loosely cohesive, are somewhat larger than normal, and have oval or round nuclei with small nucleoli (Fig. 25–19). Signet-ring cells containing mucin are commonly present. LCIS rarely distorts the underlying architecture, and the involved lobules remain recognizable. LCIS is an incidental finding in biopsies performed for other reasons because it is only rarely associated with calcifications and never forms a mass.

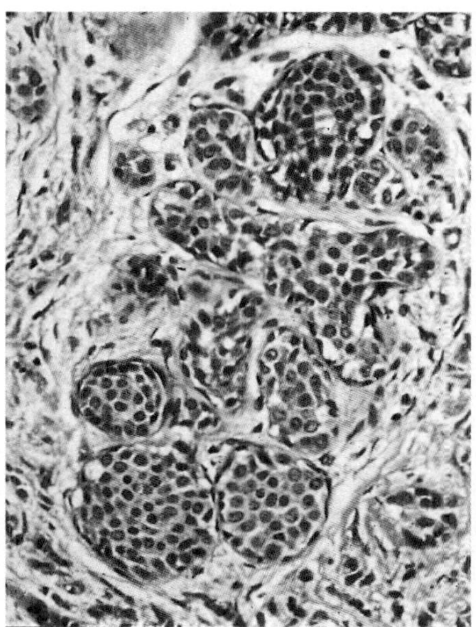

Figure 25–19

Lobular carcinoma in situ. Note the monomorphic population of cells that expands and distorts the terminal duct and lobule. (Courtesy of Dr. Kyle Molberg, Department of Pathology, University of Texas Southwestern Medical School, Dallas, TX.)

Thus, it remains infrequent (1% to 6% of all carcinomas) in mammographically screened populations (Table 25–2). LCIS is bilateral in 50% to 70% of women when both breasts are examined, compared with 10% to 20% in cases of DCIS. However, most incidentally detected lesions do not progress to clinically recognized disease.

Women diagnosed with LCIS by biopsy develop invasive carcinomas at a frequency similar to that of women with untreated DCIS. In patients observed for more than 20 years, invasive carcinoma develops in 25% to 35%.[4] However, unlike in DCIS, both breasts are at equal risk. Invasive carcinomas developing in women after a diagnosis of LCIS are threefold more likely to be of lobular type compared with carcinomas overall, but the majority do not show specific lobular differentiation.

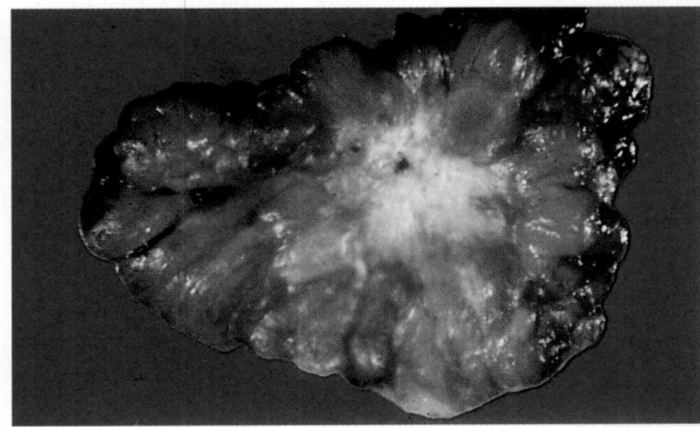

Figure 25–20

Cut section of invasive ductal carcinoma of the breast. The lesion is retracted, infiltrating the surrounding breast substance, and would be stony hard on palpation.

Invasive (Infiltrating) Carcinoma

INVASIVE DUCTAL CARCINOMA, NO SPECIAL TYPE (NST)

Invasive ductal carcinoma NST includes the majority of carcinomas (70% to 80%) that cannot be classified as any other subtype.

Most of these cancers exhibit a marked increase in dense, fibrous tissue stroma, giving the tumor a hard consistency **(scirrhous carcinoma).** These growths occur as fairly sharply delimited nodules of stony-hard consistency that average 1 to 2 cm in diameter and rarely exceed 4 to 5 cm. On palpation, they may have an infiltrative attachment to the surrounding structures with fixation to the underlying chest wall, dimpling of the skin, and retraction of the nipple. The mass is characteristic on cut section. It is retracted below the cut surface, has a hard cartilaginous consistency, and produces a grating sound when scraped. Within the central focus, there are small pinpoint foci or streaks of chalky white elastotic stroma and occasionally small foci of calcification (Fig. 25–20).

On histologic examination, the tumor consists of malignant cells disposed in cords, solid cell nests, tubules, anastomosing masses, and mixtures of all these invading into stroma (Fig. 25–21). The cytologic detail of tumor cells varies from small cells with moderately hyperchromatic regular nuclei to huge cells with large irregular and hyperchromatic nuclei. Frequently, invasion of lymphatic and perineural spaces is readily evident.

Aneuploidy and absence of hormone receptors vary with grade, being found in more than half of poorly differentiated tumors and in less than half of well-differentiated tumors.

INVASIVE LOBULAR CARCINOMA

Although making up only 5% to 10% of breast carcinomas, *invasive lobular carcinomas* are of particular interest for the following reasons:

- They tend to be bilateral far more frequently than other subtypes, the likelihood of cancer in the contralateral breast being on the order of 20%.
- They tend to be multicentric within the same breast.
- They often have a diffusely invasive pattern that can make both primary tumors and metastases difficult to

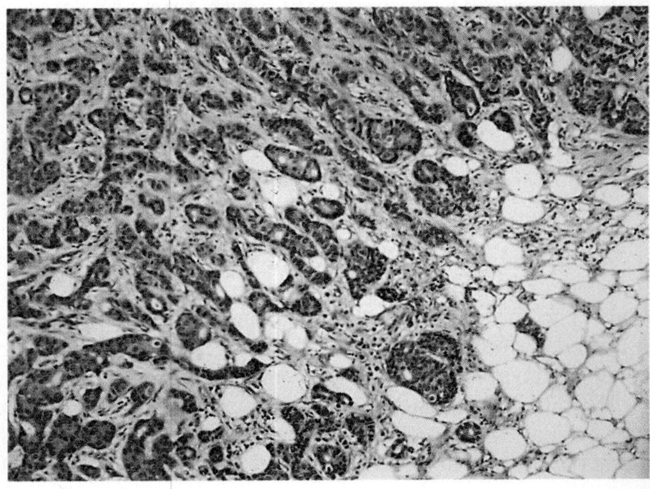

Figure 25–21

Invasive ductal carcinoma (no special type) infiltrating into, and replacing, adjacent adipose tissue.

detect either by physical examination or by radiologic studies.

- They more frequently metastasize to cerebrospinal fluid, serosal surfaces, ovary and uterus, and bone marrow compared with other subtypes.

On gross inspection, the tumor is rubbery and poorly circumscribed but sometimes appears as a typical scirrhous type. On histologic examination, strands of infiltrating tumor cells, often only one cell in width (in the form of a single file), are loosely dispersed throughout the fibrous matrix (Fig. 25–22). The cells have the same cytologic features of LCIS and lack cohesion without formation of tubules or papillae. In the classic type, the cells are small with relatively little nuclear pleomorphism. Signet-ring cells are common. Irregularly shaped, solid nests may also occur in continuity with the single-file pattern. Tumor cells are frequently arranged in concentric rings about normal ducts.

Classic well-differentiated invasive lobular carcinomas are usually diploid, exhibit hormone receptors, are associated with LCIS in more than 90% of cases, and have a better prognosis than carcinomas of no special type. Virtually all invasive lobular carcinomas, as well as LCIS, lack the cell-cell adhesion molecule E-cadherin compared with only 52% of invasive ductal carcinomas.[45]

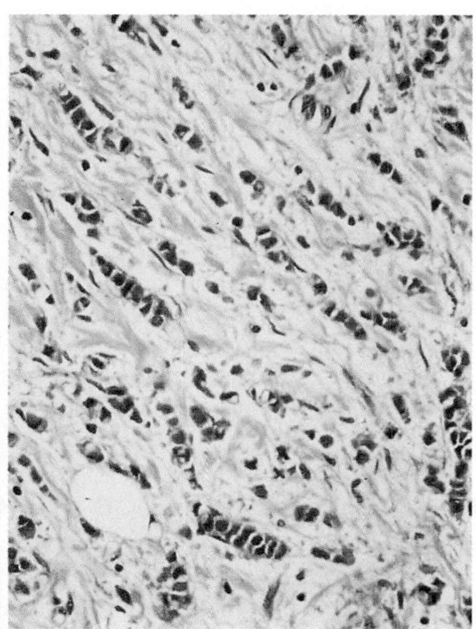

Figure 25–22

Invasive lobular carcinoma. Parallel arrays of single files of small, poorly cohesive cells are embedded within a dense fibrous stroma.

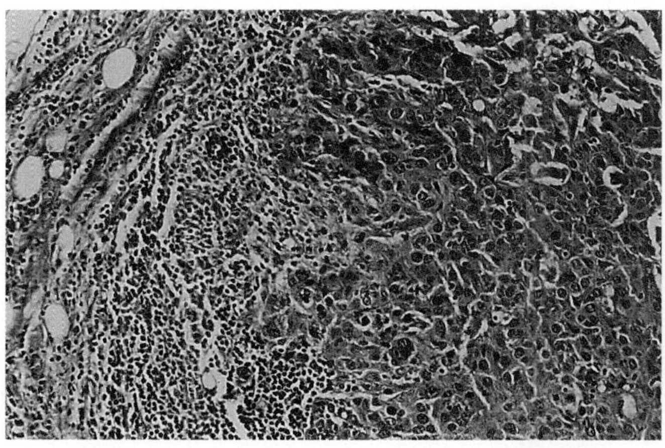

Figure 25–23

Medullary carcinoma with lymphoid infiltrate. Note the lymphocytes infiltrating sheets of high-grade tumor cells.

MEDULLARY CARCINOMA

Medullary carcinoma accounts for 1% to 5% of all mammary carcinomas and occurs in younger than average women. They are, however, disproportionately reported in women carrying the *BRCA1* gene, in which group they account for 13% of cancers.

The typical size is 2 to 3 cm, but some produce large, fleshy tumor masses up to 5 cm in diameter or greater. These tumors do not have the striking desmoplasia of the usual carcinoma and, therefore, are distinctly more yielding on external palpation and on cut section. The tumor has a soft, fleshy consistency (medulla is Latin for marrow, referring to a soft structure) and is well circumscribed. The carcinoma is characterized histologically by (1) solid, syncytium-like sheets (occupying more than 75% of the tumor) of large cells with vesicular, often pleomorphic nuclei, containing prominent nucleoli and frequent mitoses; (2) a moderate to marked lymphoplasmacytic infiltrate surrounding and within the tumor; and (3) a pushing (noninfiltrative) border (Fig. 25–23).

Medullary carcinomas have a slightly better prognosis than do carcinomas of no special type, despite the almost universal presence of poor prognostic factors including high nuclear grade, aneuploidy, absence of hormone receptors, *p53* expression, and high proliferative rates. The syncytial growth pattern and pushing borders may reflect retention or overexpression of adhesion molecules that could potentially limit metastatic potential. Tumor cells have been reported to strongly express HLA-DR.[4]

COLLOID (MUCINOUS) CARCINOMA

This unusual variant (1% to 6% of all carcinomas) tends to occur in older women and grows slowly during the course of many years.

The tumor is extremely soft and has the consistency and appearance of pale gray-blue gelatin. Colloid carcinomas are usually well circumscribed and may mimic benign lesions on physical examination and mammographically.

On histologic examination, there are large lakes of lightly staining, amorphous mucin that dissect and extend into contiguous tissue spaces and planes of cleavage. Floating within this mucin are small islands and isolated neoplastic cells, sometimes forming glands (Fig. 25–24). Neuroendocrine differentiation in the form of argyrophilic granules is present in 14% to 50%.

Colloid carcinomas are usually diploid, and the majority exhibit hormone receptors. The survival rate is appreciably greater in colloid carcinoma than in carcinomas of no special type, and lymph node metastases are present in less than 20% of patients.

TUBULAR CARCINOMA

Tubular carcinomas accounted for only 2% of all breast carcinomas before mammographic screening but have increased in frequency and represent up to 10% of carcinomas less than 1 cm in size. Tubular carcinomas are usually detected as mammographic spiculated (irregular) masses. Women tend to be younger than average and usually present in their late 40s. Tumors are multifocal within one breast in 10% to 56% of cases or bilateral in 9% to 38%.

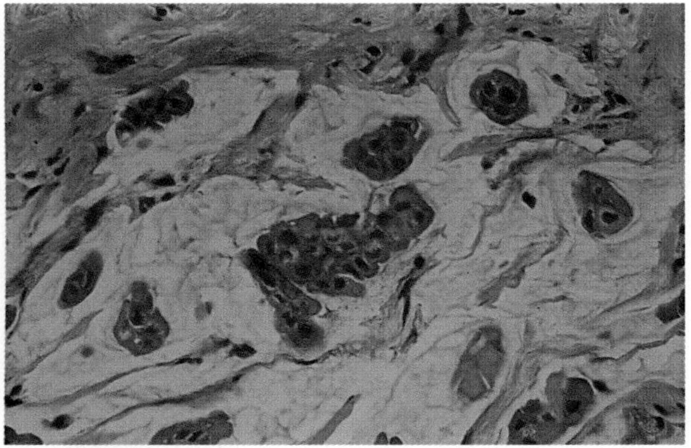

Figure 25–24

Colloid carcinoma. Note the lakes of lightly staining mucin with small islands of tumor cells.

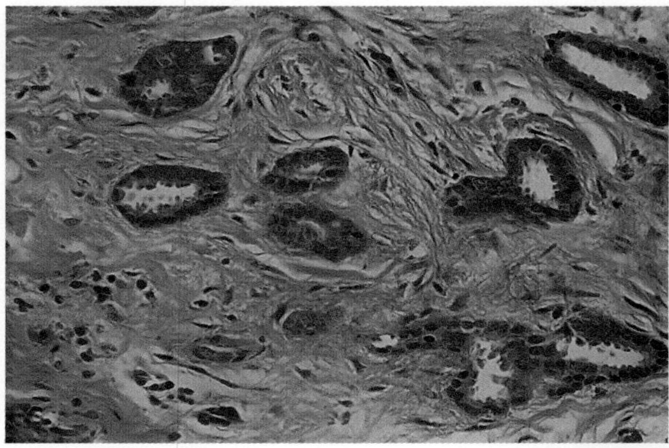

Figure 25–25

Tubular carcinoma. Note the well-formed tubules lined by a single layer of cells with apocrine snouts.

These tumors consist exclusively of well-formed tubules and are sometimes mistaken for a benign sclerosing lesion (Fig. 25–25). However, a myoepithelial cell layer is absent, and tumor cells are in direct contact with stroma. Cribriform spaces may also be present. Apocrine snouts are typical, and calcifications may be present within the lumens. DCIS is present in 40% and LCIS in 10% of cases.

More than 95% of all tubular carcinomas are diploid and exhibit hormone receptors. By definition, all are well differentiated. Axillary metastases occur in less than 10% of cases except in cases of multifocal disease. This subtype is important to recognize because of its excellent prognosis with only rare deaths reported in women with stage I disease.

INVASIVE PAPILLARY CARCINOMA

Invasive carcinomas with a papillary architecture are rare and represent less than 1% of all invasive cancers. Papillary architecture is more commonly seen in DCIS. The clinical presentation is similar to that of carcinomas of no special type, but the overall prognosis is better.

Mammographic Appearance of Breast Cancer

The use of mammography has increased the detection of DCIS and small invasive tumors before they reach palpable size (Table 25–3). Nonpalpable lesions detected by mammography can be sampled either by mammographically guided large-core needle biopsy or by placement of a local-

Table 25–3. INVASIVE AND IN SITU CARCINOMA IN BIOPSIES FOR PALPABLE AND MAMMOGRAPHIC LESIONS

	Invasive Carcinoma (%)*	Average Size of Invasive Carcinoma (cm)	DCIS (%)*	LCIS (%)*
Pre-mammography data		3.5	<5	<5
Palpable masses	20	2.0	2	0.4
Mammographic density	28	1.1	3	3
Calcifications	7	0.6	22	3

* Percentage of biopsies with carcinoma.
DCIS, ductal carcinoma in situ; LCIS, lobular carcinoma in situ.
S. Lester, unpublished data.

izing wire within the lesion to guide surgical excision. The principal radiologic signs of breast carcinoma are (1) densities, (2) architectural distortion, (3) calcifications, and (4) changes over time.

Densities. Most neoplasms grow as solid masses and are radiologically denser than the intermingled connective and adipose tissue of the normal breast. Invasive carcinomas most commonly present as a mammographic density (Table 25–3). The most common presentation of an invasive carcinoma is as a spiculated density with irregular infiltration of the surrounding tissue (Fig. 25–26). Postinflammatory changes, for example prior surgical sites, or complex sclerosing lesions rarely present in this way. DCIS may rarely form a dense mass. Well-circumscribed densities with smooth borders are most often benign lesions such as cysts or fibroadenomas (Fig. 25–12*B*). However, invasive carcinomas, most typically medullary and mucinous carcinomas, can also be well circumscribed.

Architectural Distortion. Architectural distortion is a rarely seen alteration in the normal parenchymal pattern. Although patchy involutional changes can underlie this finding, diffusely invasive carcinomas that infiltrate in and around adipose tissue without replacing it, most commonly lobular carcinomas, may produce distortion without the presence of a discrete density.

Calcifications. Calcifications are due to either calcified secretory material or necrotic debris. Calcifications associated with malignancy are more commonly small, irregular, numerous, and clustered or linear and branching. DCIS is the most common malignant neoplasm associated with calcifications (Table 25–3). Benign calcifications are usually associated with clusters of apocrine cysts, sclerosing adenosis, fat necrosis, or hyalinized fibroadenomas.

Changes Over Time. The examination of serial mammograms may reveal subtle changes of malignancy. Developing densities, architectural distortion, or increasing numbers of calcifications may indicate the inexorable growth of an underlying malignant neoplasm.

Some carcinomas, even if they are palpable, are not detectable by mammography. The principal reasons are surrounding dense tissue (especially in younger women), absence of calcifications, small size, or location close to the chest wall or in the periphery of the breast.

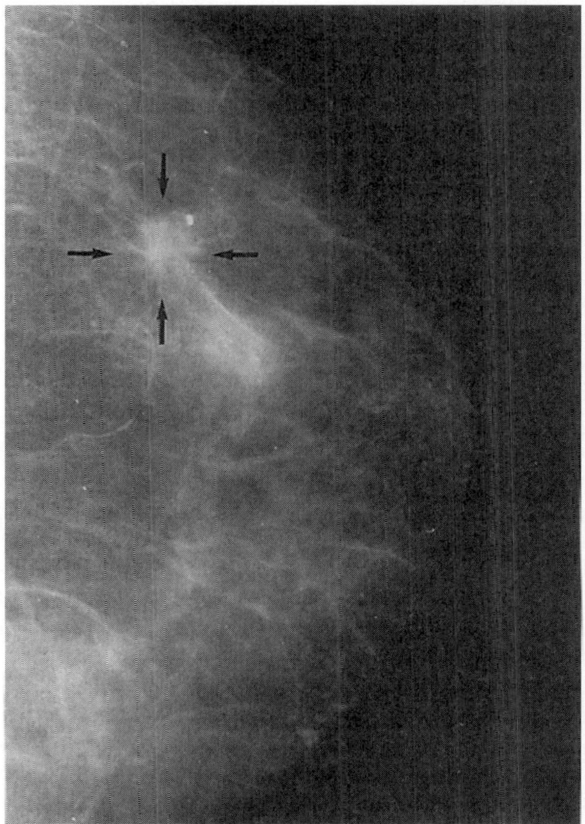

Figure 25–26

Cranial caudal-view mammogram. Invasive carcinoma with a spiculated border *(arrows)*. There is a small, superimposed, incidental calcification. (Courtesy of Dr. Jack E. Meyer, Brigham and Women's Hospital, Boston, MA.)

Other imaging modalities are useful adjuncts for mammography. Ultrasonography can distinguish solid and cystic lesions and can define more precisely the borders of solid lesions. Magnetic resonance imaging detects cancers by the rapid uptake of contrast agents due to increased tumor vascularity. It has been most useful in determining the extent of chest wall invasion in locally advanced cancers and for the evaluation of breast implant rupture.

Features Common to All Invasive Cancers

There are additional morphologic features common to all invasive breast carcinomas, whatever the histologic type. As focal lesions, they extend progressively in all directions. In the course of time, they may become adherent to the deep fascia of the chest wall and thus become fixed in position. Extension to the skin may cause not only fixation but also retraction and dimpling of the skin, an important characteristic of malignant growth. At the same time, the lymphatics may become so involved as to block the local area of skin drainage and cause lymphedema and thickening of the skin, a change that has for years been referred to as *peau d'orange*. Tethering of the skin to the breast by Cooper ligaments creates the appearance of an orange peel. When the tumor involves the central portion of the breast, retraction of the nipple may develop. Certain carcinomas tend to infiltrate widely through the breast substance, involve the majority of dermal lymphatics, and produce acute swelling and redness with tenderness of the breast, referred to clinically as *inflammatory carcinoma*. There is a high incidence of systemic metastases.

Spread of the tumor eventually occurs through the lymphohematogenous routes. The pathways of lymphatic dissemination are in all possible directions: lateral to the axilla, superior to the nodes above the clavicle and the neck, medial to the other breast, inferior to the abdominal viscera and lymph nodes, and deep to the nodes within the chest, particularly along the internal mammary arteries. The two most favored directions of drainage are the axillary nodes and the nodes along the internal mammary artery.

Overall, about one third of all patients have metastases to lymph nodes at the time of initial diagnosis of breast cancer. The pattern of nodal spread is heavily influenced by the location of the cancer in the breast. Larger tumors arising in the outer quadrants involve the axillary nodes alone in about 50% of cases and have both internal mammary and axillary involvement in an additional 15% of cases. In contrast, cancers arising in the inner quadrants and center of the breast affect the axilla alone in about 25% of cases. In an additional 40%, internal mammary nodes are affected, along with axillary involvement. The supraclavicular nodes are the third most favored site of nodal spread. Distant metastases through the bloodstream may affect virtually any organ of the body. Favored sites for dissemination are the lungs, bones, liver, adrenals, brain, and meninges. In these locations, cancer cells can be detected in pleural, peritoneal cavity, or cerebrospinal fluid by cytologic examination (Fig. 25–27).

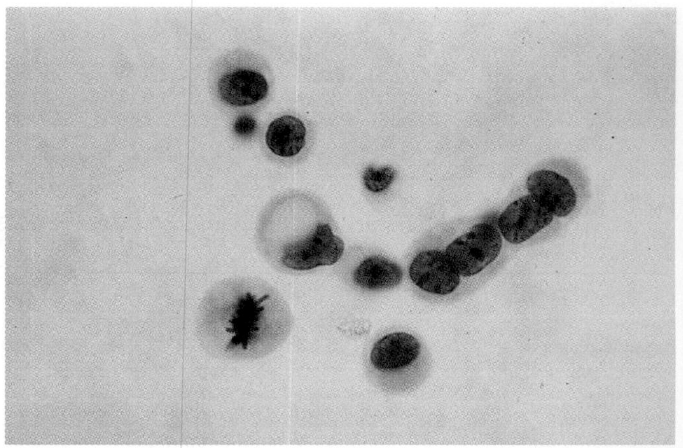

Figure 25–27

Cerebrospinal fluid showing metastatic breast cancer cells. Note the duct-like structure; a signet-ring, mucus-containing cell; and a mitotic figure. (Courtesy of Dr. Edmund Cibas, Brigham and Women's Hospital, Boston, MA.)

Staging and Clinical Course

Breast cancer has been divided into smaller groups to standardize comparisons of results of various therapeutic modalities among clinics and guide treatment.

The American Joint Committee on Cancer Staging[46] divides the clinical stages as follows:

Stage 0. DCIS or LCIS (5-year survival rate 92%)

Stage I. Invasive carcinoma 2 cm or less in size (including carcinoma in situ with microinvasion) without nodal involvement and no distant metastases (5-year survival rate 87%)

Stage II. Invasive carcinoma 5 cm or less in size with involved but movable axillary nodes and no distant metastases, or a tumor greater than 5 cm without nodal involvement or distant metastases (5-year survival rate 75%)

Stage III. Breast cancers greater than 5 cm in size with nodal involvement; or any breast cancer with fixed axillary nodes; or any breast cancer with involvement of the ipsilateral internal mammary lymph nodes; or any breast cancer with skin involvement, pectoral and chest wall fixation, edema, or clinical inflammatory carcinoma, if distant metastases are absent (5-year survival rate 46%)

Stage IV. Any form of breast cancer with distant metastases (including ipsilateral supraclavicular lymph nodes) (5-year survival rate 13%)

Stage II and stage III cancers are also subdivided according to the number of involved axillary lymph nodes for therapeutic decision making and enrollment in clinical trials. If no axillary metastases are present, some patients may not receive systemic therapy, depending on other characteristics of the tumor. Almost all women with one to three positive axillary nodes receive some form of standard systemic treatment, either hormonal therapy or chemotherapy. Women with four to nine positive axillary nodes are eligible for clinical trials using high-dose chemotherapy. If ten or more nodes are positive, women are eligible for other experimental treatments such as autologous bone marrow transplantation.

Clinical Course. Cancers of the breast are usually first discovered by a woman or her physician as a solitary, painless mass in the breast or because of mammographic abnormalities during screening. The older the patient with a single breast lesion, the more likely it is to be cancer. On average, palpable invasive carcinomas are 2 to 3 cm in size when they are first found, and approximately one third have already spread to axillary or other nodes. In contrast, mammographically detected invasive carcinomas average 1 cm in size, and less than one fifth will have axillary metastases. DCIS is most commonly detected as mammographic calcifications and only rarely as a palpable or radiographic mass or nipple discharge (Table 25–3). DCIS is important to detect because it is limited to the breast and most cases can be cured by local treatment.

Once distant metastases are present, cure is unlikely, although long-term remissions and palliation can be achieved, especially for women with hormonally responsive tumors. A number of factors influence the prognosis of women with breast cancer without distant metastases.[4]

1. *Lymph node metastases.* Axillary lymph node status is the most important prognostic factor. With no involvement, the 10-year disease-free survival rate is close to 70% to 80%, which falls to 35% to 40% with one to three positive nodes and 10% to 15% in the presence of more than ten positive nodes. The size of the metastatic deposit (macrometastases versus only micrometastases less than 0.2 cm) and the presence of invasion through the capsule are also indicators of poorer prognosis.
2. *Locally advanced disease.* Tumors invading into skin or skeletal muscle are frequently associated with concurrent or subsequent distant disease. With increased awareness of breast cancer detection, such cases have happily decreased in frequency and are now rare at initial presentation.
3. *Tumor size.* More than 98% of women with tumors less than 1 cm survive for 5 years. More than 96% of women with node-negative tumors less than 2 cm in size survive for the same period. However, very small tumors are capable, although rarely, of distant metastasis.
4. *Histologic subtypes.* The 30-year survival of women with special types of invasive carcinomas (tubular, colloid, medullary, lobular, and papillary) is more than 60%, compared with less than 20% for women with cancers of no special type ("ductal carcinomas").[47] As discussed earlier, tubular and colloid carcinomas have an exceptionally good prognosis.[48] However, if the tumor is not "pure" in type, or poor prognostic factors are present such as large tumor size, poor nuclear grade, or lymph node involvement, the favorable prognosis may be diminished or eliminated.
5. *Tumor grade.* The most commonly used grading system (modified Bloom and Richardson grading system) combines nuclear grade, tubule formation, and mitotic rate. More than 80% of women with grade I tumors survive 16 years, whereas less than 60% of women with grade II and grade III tumors survive for the same period. Certain large-scale studies suggest that mitotic rate alone can be as predictive as the grading system.
6. *Estrogen and progesterone receptors.* Fifty per cent to 85% of tumors exhibit estrogen receptors, and such tumors are more commonly found in postmenopausal women. Seventy per cent of tumors with estrogen receptors regress after hormonal manipulation, whereas only 5% of those that are negative respond. The highest response rates are in patients with tumors exhibiting both estrogen and progesterone receptors. Cancers with high levels of hormone receptors have a slightly better prognosis than those without receptors.
7. *Lymphovascular invasion.* Tumor cells are sometimes seen within vascular spaces (either lymphatics or small capillaries) surrounding tumors. This finding is strongly associated with the presence of lymph node metastases and is a poor prognostic factor in women without lymph node metastases. The presence of tumor cells in lymphatics of the dermis is strongly associated with the clinical appearance of inflammatory cancer and bodes a very poor prognosis with 3-year survival only 3% to 10%.
8. *Proliferative rate.* Proliferation can be measured by flow cytometry (as the S-phase fraction [Fig. 25–28]), by thymidine labeling index, by mitotic counts, or by immunohistochemical detection of cellular proteins (e.g., cyclins, Ki-67) produced during the cell cycle. Tumors with high proliferation rates have a worse prognosis, but the most reliable method to assess proliferation has not yet been established.[49]
9. *DNA content.* The amount of DNA per tumor cell can be determined by flow cytometric analysis or by image analysis of tissue sections. Tumors with a DNA index of 1 have the same amount of DNA as normal diploid cells, although marked karyotypic changes may be present. Aneuploid tumors are those with abnormal DNA indices and have a slightly worse prognosis (Fig. 25–28).
10. *Expression of oncogenes or loss of expression of tumor-suppressor genes.* Changes in expression of c-*erb-B2* (*Her2/neu*), c-*myc, ras* p21, and *INT2, p53,* and *NM23* are associated with a poorer prognosis and are commonly found in cancers with other poor prognostic factors.
11. *Angiogenesis.* Most studies have shown a correlation between vessel density (reflecting angiogenesis; Chapter 8) and the subsequent development of metastases[50] (Fig. 25–29).
12. *Proteases.* Stromal proteases may be involved in tumor invasion by degrading extracellular matrix (Chapter 8), and some studies have shown that estimation of tumor protease content correlates with poorer prognosis.

Although axillary node status is the single most important prognostic factor, 20% to 30% of patients with histologically negative lymph nodes suffer recurrences and die of their disease within 10 years. Despite the prognostic indicators listed, it is impossible in an individual case to predict the outcome. Sadly, only time tells this story! For these reasons, there are continued searches for better or refined biologic markers of prognosis and more effective treatment modalities.

Current therapeutic approaches include local and regional control, using combinations of surgery (mastectomy or breast conservation) and postoperative irradiation, and systemic control, using hormonal treatment or chemotherapy or both. Axillary node dissection is performed for prognostic purposes, but the axilla can also be adequately treated with radiation alone. Newer therapeutic strategies include inhibition (by pharmacologic agents or specific antibodies) of membrane-bound growth factor receptors (e.g., *Her 2/neu*), stromal proteases, and angiogenesis.[51]

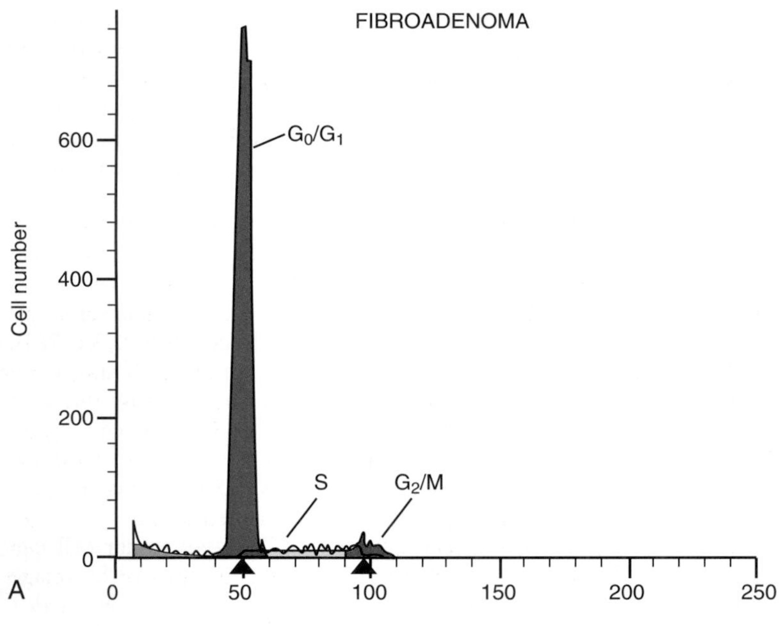

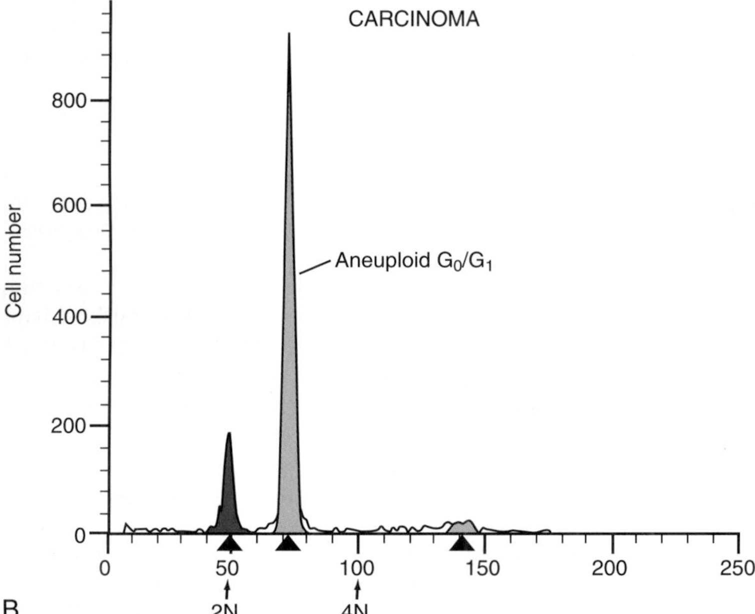

Figure 25–28

Flow cytometric histograms of a fibroadenoma *(top)* and an invasive carcinoma *(bottom)* plotted using ModFit LT cell cycle analysis software (Verity, Topsham, ME). The histogram of the fibroadenoma contains a single peak, representing G_0/G_1 phase euploid nuclei having a normal 2N DNA content (colored red). The histogram of the carcinoma shows, in addition, an aneuploid population having near-triploid G_0/G_1 phase DNA content (colored yellow). The smaller peaks to the right represent the G_2/M cell population and are used to calculate the S-phase fraction. (Courtesy of Dr. David Dorfman, Brigham and Women's Hospital, Boston, MA.)

Such therapies are based on models of breast cancer spread that have evolved as our understanding of its biology has changed. Earlier models proposed that breast cancer spreads in a contiguous fashion by direct extension from breast to nodes and could thus be cured by en bloc surgical resection. However, radical surgery, including mastectomies with removal of pectoralis muscles, internal mammary nodes, and even supraclavicular nodes, failed to decrease mortality. A subsequent model, based on studies demonstrating that *lumpectomy* (removal of the breast mass) and radiation were equivalent to mastectomy, postulated that all cancers had spread systemically by the time of diagnosis, and that local or regional treatment was unimportant for overall survival. In the current era of increased detection of in situ lesions and small invasive carcinomas by mammography, a third model that combines the first two is thought to be more appropriate to guide therapy[52]: while many women already have systemic involvement at first presentation and cannot be cured by local and regional control, in situ and early carcinomas can be limited to the breast, and local and regional treatment with intent to cure must be the goal for such cancers.[51]

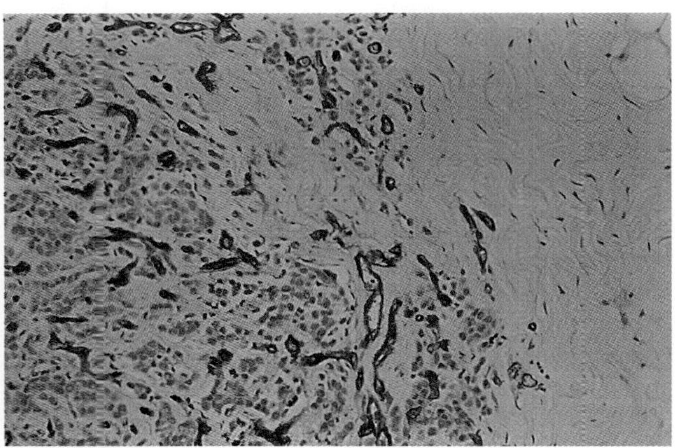

Figure 25–29

Invasive carcinoma *(left)* showing immunoreactivity in endothelial cells for factor VIII (brown color). Note the markedly increased density of blood vessels (angiogenesis) in the tumor compared with the surrounding stroma *(right)*. (Courtesy of Dr. Noel Weidner, University of California at San Francisco.)

Thus, this discussion of breast cancer ends virtually where it began. The clinical problem is monumental despite great efforts to solve it, and there is much yet to be learned.

Miscellaneous Malignant Neoplasms

Malignant neoplasia may arise from the skin of the breast, sweat glands, sebaceous glands, and hair shafts and is identical to its counterparts found in other sites of the body. Lymphomas may arise primarily in the breast, or the breasts may be secondarily involved by a systemic lymphoma. Most are of large cell type of B-cell origin. Young women with Burkitt lymphoma may present with massive bilateral breast involvement and are often pregnant or lactating. Metastases to the breast are rare and most commonly arise from a contralateral breast carcinoma. The most frequent nonmammary metastases are from melanomas and lung cancers.

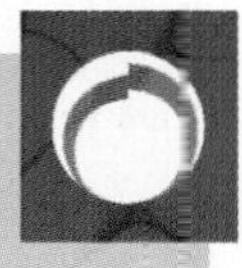

The Male Breast

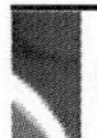

PATHOLOGY

The rudimentary male breast is relatively free from pathologic involvement. Only two processes occur with sufficient frequency to merit consideration.

GYNECOMASTIA

Like the female breast, the male breast is subject to hormonal influences, and gynecomastia (enlargement of the male breast) may occur as a result of an imbalance between estrogens, which stimulate breast tissue, and androgens, which counteract these effects. It is encountered under a variety of normal and abnormal circumstances. It may be found at the time of puberty or in the very aged, in the latter presumably owing to a relative increase in adrenal estrogens as the androgenic function of the testis fails. It is one of the manifestations of Klinefelter syndrome and may occur in those with functioning testicular neoplasms, such as Leydig cell and, rarely, Sertoli cell tumors. It may occur at any time during adult life when there is cause for hyperestrinism. The most important cause of hyperestrinism in the male is cirrhosis of the liver, since the liver is responsible for metabolizing estrogen. Drugs such as alcohol, marijuana, heroin, anabolic steroids used by some athletes and body builders, and some psychoactive agents have also been associated with gynecomastia.[53]

MORPHOLOGY. The lesion may be unilateral or bilateral. A button-like, subareolar enlargement develops. In farther advanced cases, the swelling may simulate the adolescent female breast.

On microscopic examination, there is proliferation of a dense, periductal hyaline, collagenous connective tissue, but more striking are the changes in the epithelium of the ducts. There is marked micropapillary hyperplasia of the ductal linings (Fig. 25–30). The individual cells are fairly regular, columnar to cuboidal with regular nuclei. Lobule formation is rare.

The lesion is readily apparent on clinical examination and must be differentiated only from the seldom-occurring carcinoma of the male breast. Gynecomastia is chiefly of importance as an indicator of hyperestrinism, suggesting the possible existence of a functioning testicular tumor or the possible presence of cirrhosis of the liver.

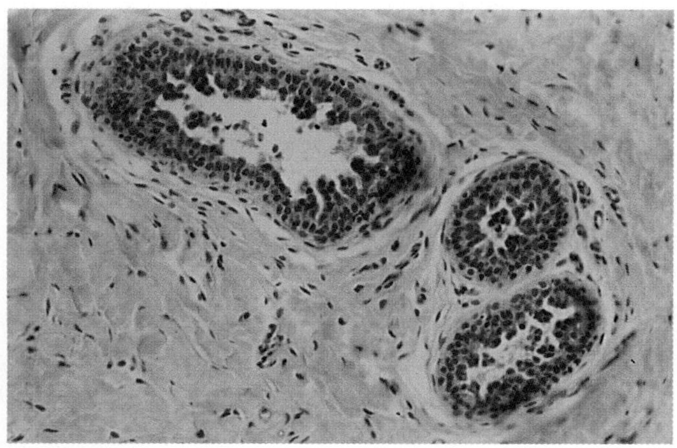

Figure 25–30

Gynecomastia. Note the ducts with hyperplastic multilayered epithelium and periductal hyalinization and fibrosis.

CARCINOMA

Carcinoma arising in the male breast is a rare occurrence, with a frequency ratio to breast cancer in the female of less than 1:100. Risk factors are similar to those in women and include residency in Western countries, first-degree relatives with breast cancer, increasing age, infertility, obesity, exposure to exogenous estrogens, prior benign breast disease, and exposure to ionizing radiation.[54] Decreased testicular function (e.g., Klinefelter syndrome) is also a risk factor. Prognostic factors are also similar in men and women. Male breast cancer is strongly associated with *BRCA2* in some families but is not associated with *BRCA1*.

DCIS and LCIS are rare in men. The same histologic subtypes of invasive cancer are present, and specialized types also have a better prognosis. However, male breast cancers are more likely to have estrogen receptors.

Because of the scant amount of breast substance in the man, the malignant neoplasm rapidly infiltrates to become attached to the overlying skin and underlying thoracic wall. Ulceration through the skin is perhaps more common than in women. Dissemination follows the same pattern as in women, and axillary lymph node involvement is present in about half of cases at the time of discovery of the lesion. Distant metastases to the lungs, brain, bone, and liver are common. Although men present at higher stages, when they are matched by stage, prognosis is similar in men and women.

REFERENCES

1. Ellis H, et al: Surgical embryology and anatomy of the breast and its related anatomic structures. Surg Clin North Am 73:611, 1993.
2. Longacre TA, Bartow SA: A correlative morphologic study of human breast and endometrium in the menstrual cycle. Am J Surg Pathol 10: 382, 1986.
3. Donegan WL, Spratt JS: Cancer of the Breast. Philadelphia, WB Saunders, 1995.
4. Rosen PP, Oberman HA: Tumors of the Mammary Gland. Atlas of Tumor Pathology, Third Series, Fascicle 7. Washington, DC, Armed Forces Institute of Pathology, 1993.
5. Ellis H, Cox PJ: Breast problems in 1,000 consecutive referrals to surgical out-patients. Postgrad Med J 60:653, 1984.
6. Peters F, Schuth W: Hyperprolactinemia and nonpuerperal mastitis (duct ectasia). JAMA 261:1618, 1989.
7. Shousha S, et al: Mammary duct ectasia and pituitary adenoma. Am J Surg Pathol 12:180, 1988.
8. Meguid M, et al: Pathogenesis-based treatment of recurring subareolar breast abscesses. Surgery 118:775, 1995.
9. Hameed MR, et al: Capsular synovial-like hyperplasia around mammary implants similar to detritic synovitis, a morphologic and immunohistochemical study of 15 cases. Am J Surg Pathol 19:433, 1995.
10. Barnard JJ, et al: Distribution of organosilicon polymers in augmentation mammaplasties at autopsy. Plast Reconstr Surg 100:197, 1997.
11. Noone RB: A review of the possible health implications of silicone breast implants. Cancer 79:1747, 1997.
12. Yoshida SH, et al: Silicon and silicone: theoretical and clinical implications of breast implants. Regul Toxicol Pharmacol 17:3, 1993.
13. Hutter RVP: Good-by to "fibrocystic disease." N Engl J Med 312: 179, 1985.
14. Bartow SA, et al: Fibrocystic disease: a continuing enigma. Pathol Annu 17:93, 1982.
15. Page DL, Dupont WD: Premalignant conditions and markers of elevated risk in the breast and their management. Surg Clin North Am 70:831, 1990.
16. London SJ, et al: A prospective study of benign breast disease and the risk of breast cancer. JAMA 267:941, 1992.
17. Rosenberg CL, et al: Detection of monoclonal microsatellite alterations in atypical breast hyperplasia. J Clin Invest 98:1095, 1996.
18. Rosenberg CL, et al: Microsatellite alterations indicating monoclonality in atypical hyperplasias associated with breast cancer. Hum Pathol 28:214, 1997.
19. Page DL, et al: Ductal involvement by cells of atypical lobular hyperplasia in the breast. Hum Pathol 19:201, 1988.
20. Jensen RA, et al: Invasive breast cancer risk in women with sclerosing adenosis. Cancer 64:1977, 1989.
21. Marshall LM, et al: Risk of breast cancer associated with atypical hyperplasia of lobular and ductal types. Cancer Epidemiol Biomarkers Prev 6:297, 1997.
22. Noguchi S, et al: Clonal analysis of fibroadenoma and phyllodes tumor of the breast. Cancer Res 53:4071, 1993.
23. Baildam AD, et al: Cyclosporin A and multiple fibroadenomas of the breast. Br J Surg 83:1755, 1996.
24. Koerner FC, O'Connell JX: Fibroadenoma: morphological observations and a theory of pathogenesis. Pathol Annu 29(pt 1):1, 1994.
25. Dupont WD, et al: Long-term risk of breast cancer in women with fibroadenoma. N Engl J Med 331:10, 1994.
26. Cohn-Cedermark G, et al: Prognostic factors in cystosarcoma phyllodes. Cancer 68:2017, 1991.
27. Noguchi S, et al: Clonal analysis of solitary intraductal papilloma of the breast by means of polymerase chain reaction. Am J Pathol 144: 1320, 1994.
28. Radford DM, Zehnbauer BA: Inherited breast cancer. Surg Clin North Am 76:205, 1996.
29. Miki Y, et al: A strong candidate for the breast and ovarian cancer susceptibility gene *BRCA1*. Science 266:66, 1994.

29a. Zhang H, et al: BRCA 1, BRCA 2, and DNA damage response: collision or collusion? Cell 92:433, 1998.

30. Wooster R, et al: Identification of the breast cancer susceptibility gene *BRCA2*. Nature 378:789, 1995.

30a. Bertwistle D, Ashworth A: Functions of the BRCA 1 and BRC 2 genes. Curr Opin Genet Dev 8:14, 1998.

31. Newman B, et al: Frequency of breast cancer attributable to *BRCA1* in a population-based series of American women. JAMA 279:915, 1996.
32. Malone KE, et al: *BRCA1* mutations and breast cancer in the general population. Analyses in women before age 35 years and in women before age 45 years with first-degree family history. JAMA 279:922, 1998.
33. Helzlsouer KJ, Couzi R: Hormones and breast cancer. Cancer 76(Suppl):2059, 1995.
34. Toniolo PG, et al: A prospective study of endogenous estrogens and

breast cancer in postmenopausal women. J Natl Cancer Inst 87:190, 1995.
35. Dickson RB, Lippman ME: Molecular determinants of growth, angiogenesis, and metastases in breast cancer. Semin Oncol 19:286, 1992.
36. Aisenberg AC, et al: High risk of breast carcinoma after irradiation of young women with Hodgkin's disease. Cancer 79:1203, 1997.
37. Kohlmeier L, Mendez M: Controversies surrounding diet and breast cancer. Proc Nutr Soc 56:369, 1997.
38. Bittner JJ: Some possible effects of nursing on mammary gland tumor incidence in mice. Science 84:162, 1936.
39. Ziegler J: An unlikely link? Researchers probe viral role in breast cancer [news]. J Natl Cancer Inst 89:608, 1997.
40. Ahlborg UG, et al: Organochlorine compounds in relation to breast cancer, endometrial cancer, and endometriosis: an assessment of the biological and epidemiological evidence. Crit Rev Toxicol 25:463, 1995.
41. Shay JW, et al: Toward a molecular understanding of human breast cancer: a hypothesis. Breast Cancer Res Treat 25:83, 1993.
42. Leslie KO, Howard P: Oncogenes and antioncogenes in human breast carcinoma. Pathol Annu 27(pt 1):321, 1992.
43. Wellings SR: A hypothesis of the origin of human breast cancer from the terminal ductal lobular unit. Pathol Res Pract 166:515, 1980.
44. Page DL, et al: Continued local recurrence of carcinoma 15–25 years after a diagnosis of low grade ductal carcinoma in situ of the breast treated only by biopsy. Cancer 76:1197, 1995.
45. Siitonen SM, et al: Reduced E-cadherin expression is associated with invasiveness and unfavorable prognosis in breast cancer. Am J Clin Pathol 105:394, 1996.
46. AJCC Cancer Staging Manual. Philadelphia, Lippincott-Raven, 1997, pp 171–180.
47. Simpson JF, Page DL: Prognostic value of histopathology in the breast. Semin Oncol 19:254, 1992.
48. Fisher ER, et al: Pathologic findings from the National Surgical Adjuvant Breast and Bowel Projects (NSABP): prognostic discriminants for 8-year survival for node-negative invasive breast cancer patients. Cancer 65:2121, 1990.
49. Weinberg DS: Proliferation indices in solid tumors. Adv Pathol Lab Med 5:163, 1992.
50. Folkman J: The influence of angiogenesis research on management of patients with breast cancer. Breast Cancer Res Treat 36:109, 1995.
51. Sledge GW Jr: Implications of the new biology for therapy in breast cancer. Semin Oncol 23(Suppl 2):76, 1996.
52. Hellman S: Natural history of small breast cancers. J Clin Oncol 12: 2229, 1994.
53. Braunstein GD: Gynecomastia. N Engl J Med 328:490, 1993.
54. Donegan WL, Redlich PN: Breast cancer in men. Surg Clin North Am 76:343, 1996.

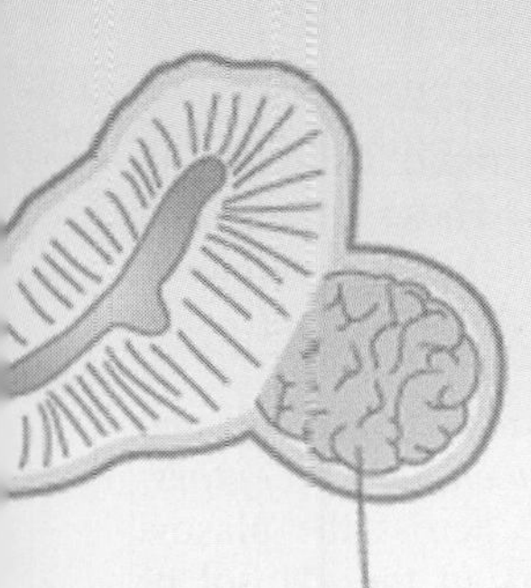
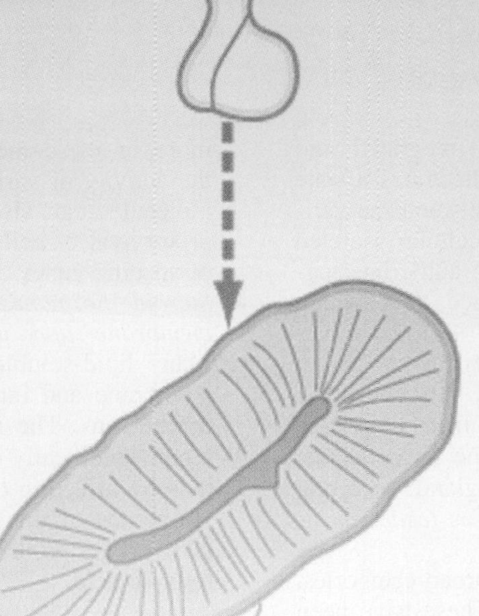

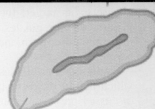

26

The Endocrine System

Pituitary

PITUITARY GLAND

HYPERPITUITARISM AND PITUITARY ADENOMAS

PROLACTINOMAS

GROWTH HORMONE (SOMATOTROPH CELL) ADENOMAS

CORTICOTROPH CELL ADENOMAS

OTHER ANTERIOR PITUITARY ADENOMAS

HYPOPITUITARISM

POSTERIOR PITUITARY SYNDROMES

HYPOTHALAMIC SUPRASELLAR TUMORS

Thyroid

THYROID GLAND

HYPERTHYROIDISM

HYPOTHYROIDISM

CRETINISM

MYXEDEMA

THYROIDITIS

HASHIMOTO THYROIDITIS

SUBACUTE (GRANULOMATOUS) THYROIDITIS

SUBACUTE LYMPHOCYTIC (PAINLESS) THYROIDITIS

GRAVES DISEASE

DIFFUSE AND MULTINODULAR GOITER

DIFFUSE NONTOXIC (SIMPLE) GOITER

MULTINODULAR GOITER

NEOPLASMS OF THE THYROID

ADENOMAS

OTHER BENIGN TUMORS

CARCINOMAS

Papillary Carcinoma

Follicular Carcinoma

Medullary Carcinoma

Anaplastic Carcinoma

CONGENITAL ANOMALIES

Parathyroid

PARATHYROID GLANDS

HYPERPARATHYROIDISM

PRIMARY HYPERPARATHYROIDISM

SECONDARY HYPERPARATHYROIDISM

HYPOPARATHYROIDISM

PSEUDOHYPOPARA-THYROIDISM

Adrenal Cortex

ADRENOCORTICAL HYPERFUNCTION (HYPERADRENALISM)

HYPERCORTISOLISM (CUSHING SYNDROME)

PRIMARY HYPERALDOSTERONISM

ADRENOGENITAL SYNDROMES

21-Hydroxylase Deficiency

ADRENAL INSUFFICIENCY

PRIMARY ACUTE ADRENOCORTICAL INSUFFICIENCY

WATERHOUSE-FRIDERICHSEN SYNDROME

PRIMARY CHRONIC ADRENOCORTICAL INSUFFICIENCY (ADDISON DISEASE)

SECONDARY ADRENOCORTICAL INSUFFICIENCY

ADRENOCORTICAL NEOPLASMS

OTHER LESIONS OF THE ADRENAL

Adrenal Medulla

PHEOCHROMOCYTOMA

TUMORS OF EXTRA-ADRENAL PARAGANGLIA

NEUROBLASTOMA

MULTIPLE ENDOCRINE NEOPLASIA SYNDROMES

Pineal

PINEAL GLAND

PINEALOMAS

The endocrine system contains a highly integrated and widely distributed group of organs that orchestrates a state of metabolic equilibrium, or homeostasis, between the various organs of the body. Signaling by extracellular secreted molecules can be classified into three types: autocrine, paracrine, or endocrine, based on the distance over which the signal acts. In endocrine signaling, the secreted molecules, which are frequently called *hormones,* act on target cells distant from their site of synthesis. An endocrine hormone is frequently carried by the blood from its site of release to its target. Increased activity of the target tissue, in turn, down-regulates the activity of the gland, secreting the stimulating hormone, a process known as *feedback inhibition.*

Hormones can be classified into several broad categories, which act on different types of receptors. These have been discussed previously, and only a few comments about each class follow:

- *Signaling molecules, which interact with cell-surface receptors:* This large class of compounds is composed of two groups: (1) peptide hormones, such as growth hormone and insulin, and (2) small molecules, such as epinephrine and histamine, that are derived from amino acids and function as hormones. Binding of these hormones to cell surface receptors leads to an increase in intracellular signaling molecules, termed *second messengers,* such as cyclic adenosine monophosphate (AMP); an increase in membrane phospholipids (e.g., inositol 1,4,5-trisphosphate or IP_3); and shifts in the intracellular levels of ionized calcium. The elevated levels of one or more of these messengers trigger a rapid alteration in the activity of various target proteins. These intracellular molecules can also control proliferation, differentiation, or survival of cells, in part, by regulating the expression of specific genes.
- *Steroid hormones, which diffuse across the plasma membrane and interact with intracellular receptors:* Many lipid-soluble hormones diffuse across the plasma membrane and interact with receptors in the cytosol or the nucleus. The resulting hormone receptor complexes bind specifically to recognition elements in DNA, thereby affecting the expression of specific target genes. Hormones of this type include the steroids (e.g., estrogen, progesterone, and glucocorticoids), thyroxine, and retinoic acid.

A number of processes may disturb the normal activity of the endocrine system, including impaired synthesis or release of hormones, abnormal interactions between hormones and their target tissues, and abnormal responses of target organs to their hormones. Endocrine diseases can be generally classified as (1) diseases of *underproduction or overproduction* of hormones and their resulting biochemical and clinical consequences and (2) diseases associated with the development of *mass lesions.* Such lesions may be nonfunctional, or they may be associated with overproduction or underproduction of hormones. A complete understanding of endocrine diseases requires a careful integration of morphologic findings with biochemical measurements of the levels of hormones, their regulators, and other metabolites.

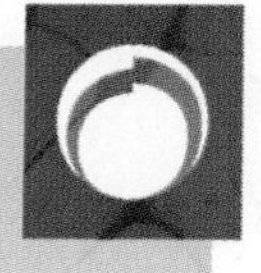

Pituitary

PITUITARY GLAND

Few organs in the body are smaller or more important than the pituitary gland. It is located at the base of the brain, where it lies nestled within the confines of the sella turcica in close proximity to the optic chiasm and the cavernous sinuses. The pituitary is a small bean-shaped organ that measures about 1 cm in greatest diameter and weighs about 0.5 gm, although it enlarges during pregnancy. The pituitary is attached to the hypothalamus by the pituitary stalk, which passes out of the sella through an opening in the dura mater surrounding the brain. Along with the hypothalamus, the pituitary gland plays a critical role in the regulation of most of the other endocrine glands. The pituitary is composed of two morphologically and functionally distinct components: the anterior lobe (adenohypophysis) and the posterior lobe (neurohypophysis).

The *anterior pituitary,* or adenohypophysis, constitutes about 80% of the gland. It is derived embryologically from Rathke pouch, which is an extension of the developing oral cavity. It is eventually cut off from its origins by the growth of the sphenoid bone, which creates a saddle-like depression, the sella turcica. Along its tract, squamous epithelial rests may be left. The anterior pituitary has a portal vascular system that is the conduit for the transport of hypothalamic releasing hormones from the hypothalamus to the anterior pituitary. Hypothalamic neurons have terminals in the median eminence where the hormones are released into the portal system, which traverse the pituitary stalk and enter the anterior pituitary gland. Most pituitary hormones are controlled predominantly by positive-acting releasing factors from the hypothalamus. Prolactin is the major exception, since its primary hypothalamic control is inhibitory through the action of dopamine. In routine histologic sections of the anterior pituitary, a colorful array of cells is present containing eosinophilic cytoplasm (acidophils), basophilic cytoplasm (basophils), or poorly staining cytoplasm *(chromophobic)* cells (Fig. 26–1). Specific antibodies against the pituitary hormones identify five cell types:

1. *Somatotrophs,* producing growth hormone (GH): These acidophilic cells constitute half of all the hormone-producing cells in the anterior pituitary.

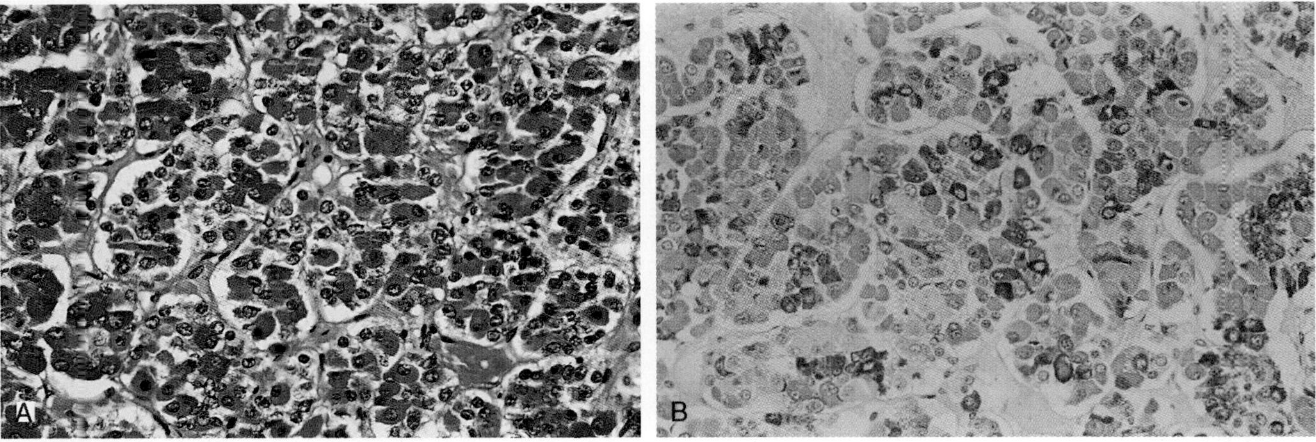

Figure 26–1

Photomicrograph of normal pituitary (*A*) and immunostain for human growth hormone (*B*).

2. *Lactotrophs* (mammotrophs), producing prolactin: These acidophilic cells secrete prolactin, which is essential for lactation.
3. *Corticotrophs:* These basophilic cells produce adrenocorticotropic hormone (ACTH), pro-opiomelanocortin, melanocyte-stimulating hormone (MSH), endorphins, and lipotropin.
4. *Thyrotrophs:* These pale basophilic cells produce thyroid-stimulating hormone (TSH).
5. *Gonadotrophs:* These basophilic cells produce both follicle-stimulating hormone (FSH) and luteinizing hormone (LH). FSH stimulates the formation of graafian follicles in the ovary, and LH induces ovulation and the formation of corpora lutea in the ovary.

The *posterior pituitary,* or neurohypophysis, consists of modified glial cells (termed *pituicytes*) and axonal processes extending from nerve cell bodies in the supraoptic and paraventricular nuclei of the hypothalamus, through the pituitary stalk to the posterior lobe, where the two posterior lobe hormones, *oxytocin* and *vasopressin,* are stored. The posterior pituitary is derived embryologically from an outpouching of the floor of the third ventricle, which grows downward alongside the anterior lobe. In contrast to the anterior lobe, the posterior lobe of the pituitary is supplied by an artery and drains into a vein, where its hormones are released directly into the systemic circulation. Thus, the pituitary has a dual circulation, composed of arteries and veins and a portal venous system linking the hypothalamus and the anterior lobe.

Diseases of the pituitary can be divided into those that primarily affect the anterior lobe and those that predominantly affect the posterior lobe. Diseases of the anterior pituitary may come to clinical attention because of increased or decreased secretion of hormones, designated *hyperpituitarism* or *hypopituitarism.* In most cases, *hyperpituitarism* is caused by a functional adenoma within the anterior lobe. *Hypopituitarism* may be caused by a variety of destructive processes, including ischemic injury, radiation, inflammatory reactions, and nonfunctioning neoplasms. In addition to endocrine abnormalities, diseases of the anterior pituitary may also be manifested by *local mass effects,* including radiographic enlargement of the sella turcica, visual field abnormalities caused by encroachment of mass lesions on the visual pathways, and evidence of increased intracranial pressure. Diseases of the posterior pituitary may come to clinical attention because of increased or decreased secretion of one of its products, *antidiuretic hormone* (ADH).

HYPERPITUITARISM AND PITUITARY ADENOMAS

In many instances, excess production of anterior pituitary hormones is caused by the presence of an adenoma arising in the anterior lobe.[1] Other less common causes include hyperplasias and carcinomas of the anterior pituitary, secretion of hormones by some pituitary tumors, and certain hypothalamic disorders. As we shall see, pituitary adenomas may be nonfunctional and may also cause hypopituitarism as they encroach on and destroy adjacent native anterior pituitary parenchyma. Functional pituitary adenomas are usually composed of a single cell type and produce a single predominant hormone, although exceptions are known to occur. Some pituitary adenomas are composed of a single cell type but secrete more than one hormone (e.g., GH and prolactin), and occasionally adenomas contain more than one cell population.

Pituitary adenomas are responsible for about 10% of intracranial neoplasms and are discovered incidentally in up to 25% of routine autopsies. They are usually found in adults, with a peak incidence from the thirties to the fifties.[2] Most pituitary adenomas occur as isolated lesions. In about 3% of cases, however, adenomas are associated with *multiple endocrine neoplasia (MEN) type I* (discussed later). Pituitary adenomas are designated, somewhat arbitrarily, *microadenomas* if less than 1 cm in diameter and *macroademomas,* if they exceed 1 cm in diameter. Nonfunctional adenomas are likely to come to clinical attention

Table 26–1. PITUITARY ADENOMAS

Type	Frequency (%)
Prolactin cell adenoma	20–30
Growth hormone cell adenomas	5
Mixed growth hormone–prolactin adenomas	5
ACTH cell adenomas	10–15
Gonadotroph cell adenomas	10–15
Null cell adenomas	20
Thyroid-stimulating hormone cell adenomas	1
Other pleurihormonal adenomas	15

ACTH, adrenocorticotropic hormone.
Modified from Burger PC, Scheithaurer BW, Vogel FS: Pituitary neoplasia. In Surgical Pathology of the Nervous System and its Coverings, 3rd ed. New York, Churchill Livingstone, 1991.

at a later stage than those associated with endocrine abnormalities and are therefore more likely to be macroadenomas.

The great majority of pituitary adenomas are monoclonal in origin, even those that are plurihormonal, suggesting that most arise from a single somatic cell.[3] Some plurihormonal tumors may arise from clonal expansion of primitive stem cells, which then differentiate in several directions simultaneously. Molecular studies have revealed mutations constitutively activating guanosine triphosphate (GTP)–binding proteins in subsets of pituitary adenomas.[4] About 40% of GH-secreting tumors harbor single base pair missense mutations within the α subunit of Gs, converting it into an oncogene termed *gsp*. These mutations stabilize the G protein in its active conformation by inhibiting its GTPase activity, thus mimicking the effect of specific extracellular growth factors. Other molecular alterations have been identified but are rare and sporadic, and the pathogenesis of the other pituitary adenomas remains largely unknown. The various types of anterior pituitary adenomas and their relative frequencies are listed in Table 26–1.

MORPHOLOGY. The common pituitary adenoma is a soft, well-circumscribed lesion that may be confined to the sella turcica. Larger lesions typically extend superiorly through the diaphragm sella into the suprasellar region, where they often compress the optic chiasm and adjacent structures, such as some of the cranial nerves (Fig. 26–2). As these adenomas expand, they frequently erode the sella turcica and anterior clinoid processes. They may also extend locally into the cavernous and sphenoid sinuses. In up to 30% of cases, the adenomas are grossly nonencapsulated and infiltrate adjacent bone, dura, and (rarely) brain. Such lesions are designated invasive adenomas. Foci of hemorrhage and necrosis are common in larger adenomas. On occasion, acute hemorrhage into an adenoma is associated with clinical evidence of a rapidly enlarging mass, a situation sometimes designated **pituitary apoplexy.**

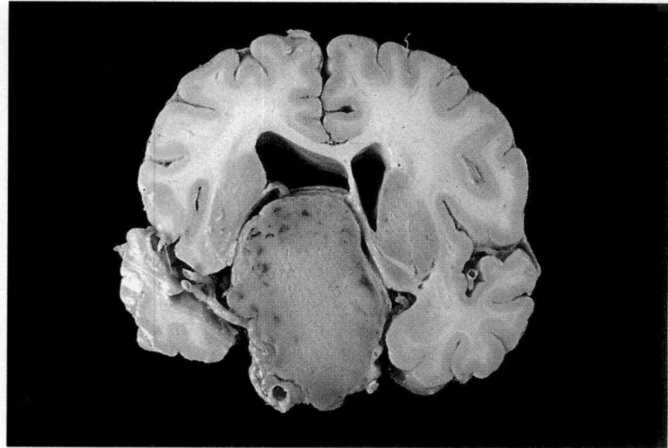

Figure 26–2 ■

Gross view of a pituitary adenoma. This massive, nonfunctional adenoma has grown far beyond the confines of the sella turcica and has distorted the overlying brain. Nonfunctional adenomas tend to be larger at the time of diagnosis than those that secrete a hormone.

Histologically, pituitary adenomas are composed of relatively uniform, polygonal cells arrayed in sheets or cords. Supporting connective tissue, or reticulin, is sparse, accounting for the soft, gelatinous consistency of many of these lesions. The nuclei of the neoplastic cells may be uniform or pleomorphic. Mitotic activity is usually modest. The cytoplasm of the constituent cells may be acidophilic, basophilic, or chromophobic, depending on the type and amount of secretory product within the cells, but it is generally uniform throughout the cytoplasm. This cellular monomorphism and the absence of a significant reticulin network distinguish pituitary adenomas from nonneoplastic anterior pituitary parenchyma (Fig. 26–3). The functional status of the adenoma cannot

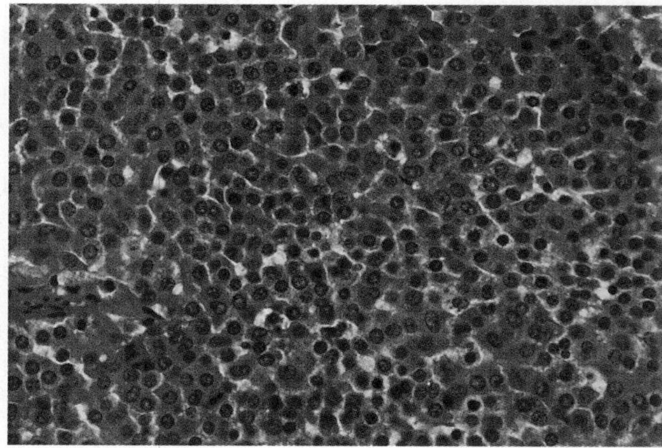

Figure 26–3 ■

Photomicrograph of pituitary adenoma. The monomorphism of these cells contrasts markedly with the mixture of cells seen in the normal anterior pituitary. Note also the absence of reticulin network.

be reliably predicted from its histologic appearance.

Clinical Course. The signs and symptoms of pituitary adenomas include endocrine abnormalities and mass effects. The abnormalities associated with the secretion of excessive quantities of anterior pituitary hormones are outlined with the specific types of pituitary adenoma. Local mass effects may be encountered in any type of pituitary tumor. Among the earliest changes resulting from such an effect are *radiographic abnormalities of the sella turcica,* including sellar expansion, bony erosion, and disruption of the diaphragm sellae. Because of the close proximity of the optic nerves and chiasm to the sella, expanding pituitary lesions often compress the nerve fibers in the optic chiasm. This gives rise to *visual field abnormalities,* classically in the form of defects in the lateral (temporal) visual fields—a so-called *bitemporal hemianopsia.* In addition, a variety of other visual field abnormalities may be caused by asymmetric growth of many tumors. As in the case of any expanding intracranial mass, pituitary adenomas may produce signs and symptoms of elevated *intracranial pressure,* including headache, nausea, and vomiting. Finally, expanding pituitary adenomas may compress the adjacent non-neoplastic anterior pituitary or the pituitary stalk sufficiently to compromise their functions, resulting in *hypopituitarism.* Acute hemorrhage into an adenoma is sometimes associated with a rapid increase in local mass effects, as noted previously.

Prolactinomas

Prolactinomas (lactotroph adenoma) are the most frequent type of hyperfunctioning pituitary adenoma, accounting for about 30% of all clinically recognized pituitary adenomas. These lesions range from small microadenomas to large, expansile tumors associated with substantial mass effect.[5] Microscopically, most prolactinomas are composed of weakly acidophilic or chromophobic cells. Prolactin can be demonstrated within the cytoplasm of the cells using immunohistochemical approaches and is contained within secretory granules (Fig. 26–4). Prolactin secretion by these adenomas is characterized by its *efficiency*—even microadenomas secrete sufficient prolactin to cause hyperprolacti-

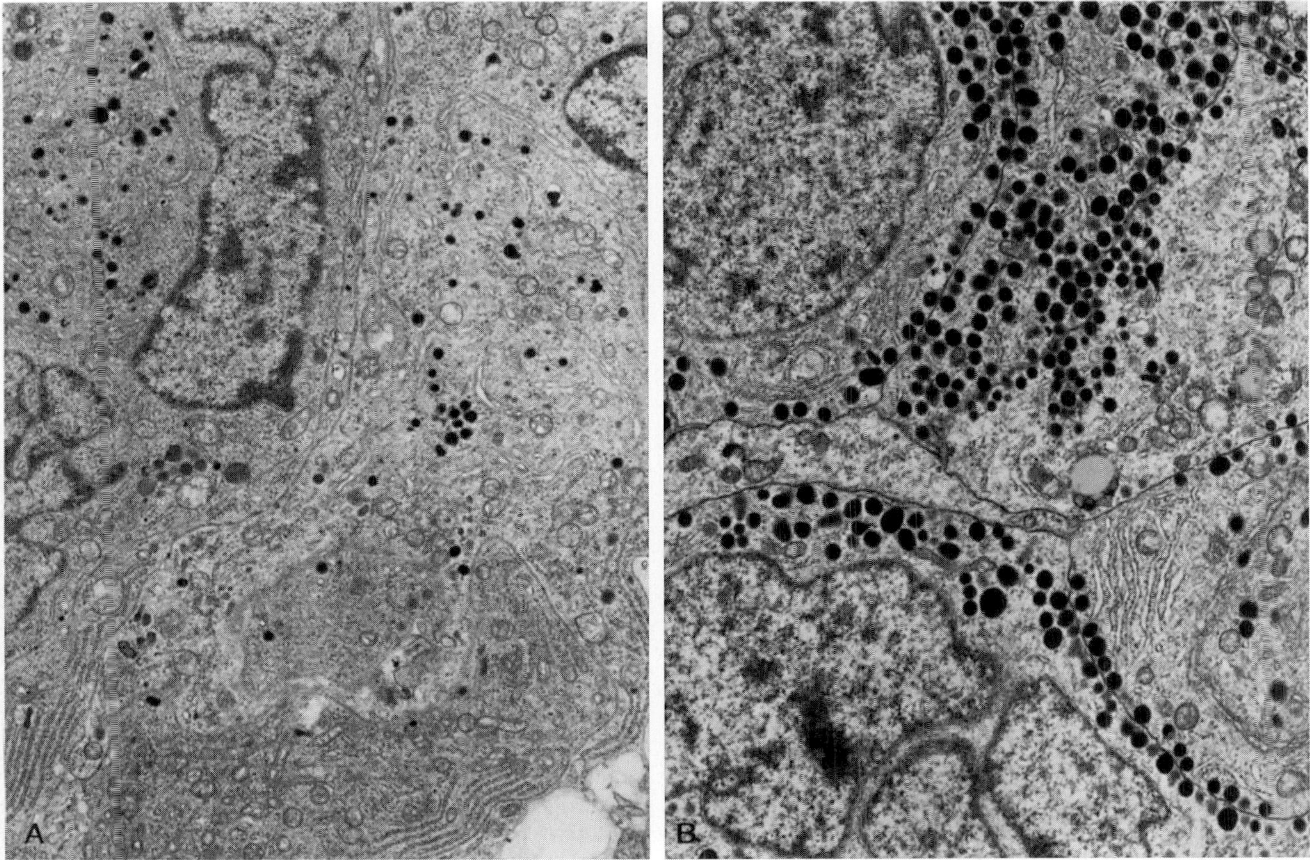

Figure 26–4

A, Electron micrograph of a sparsely granulated prolactinoma. The tumor cells contain abundant granular endoplasmic reticulum (indicative of active protein synthesis) and small numbers of secretory granules (6000×). *B,* Electron micrograph of densely granulated growth hormone–secreting adenoma. The tumor cells are filled with large membrane-bound secretory granules (6000×). (Courtesy of Dr. Eva Horvath, St. Michael's Hospital, Toronto, Ontario, Canada.)

nemia—and by its *proportionality,* in that serum prolactin concentrations tend to correlate with the size of the adenoma.

Increased serum levels of prolactin, or *prolactinemia,* cause amenorrhea, galactorrhea, loss of libido, and infertility. The diagnosis of an adenoma is made more readily in women than in men, especially between the ages of 20 and 40 years, presumably because of the sensitivity of menses to disruption by hyperprolactinemia. This tumor underlies almost a quarter of cases of amenorrhea. In contrast, in men and older women, the hormonal manifestations may be subtle, allowing the tumors to reach considerable size before being detected clinically.

Hyperprolactinemia may result from causes other than prolactin-secreting pituitary adenomas. Physiologic hyperprolactinemia occurs in pregnancy, where serum prolactin levels increase throughout pregnancy, reaching a peak at delivery. Prolactin levels are also elevated by nipple stimulation, as occurs during suckling in lactating women, and as a response to many types of stress. Pathologic hyperprolactinemia can also result from *lactotroph hyperplasia,* such as when there is interference with normal dopamine inhibition of prolactin secretion. This may occur as a result of damage to the dopaminergic neurons of the hypothalamus, pituitary stalk section (e.g., owing to head trauma), or drugs that block dopamine receptors on lactotroph cells. *Any mass in the suprasellar compartment may disturb the normal inhibitory influence of the hypothalamus on prolactin secretion, resulting in hyperprolactinemia—a phenomenon called the stalk effect. Therefore a mild elevation in serum prolactin in a patient with a pituitary adenoma does not necessarily indicate a prolactin-secreting tumor.* Several classes of drugs can cause hyperprolactinemia, including dopamine receptor antagonists such as the neuroleptic drugs (phenothiazines, haloperidol), and older antihypertensive drugs, such as reserpine, which inhibit dopamine storage. Other causes of hyperprolactinemia include estrogens, renal failure, and hypothyroidism. Prolactinomas are treated with bromocriptine, a dopamine receptor agonist, which causes the lesions to diminish in size.

Growth Hormone (Somatotroph Cell) Adenomas

GH-secreting tumors are the second most common type of functioning pituitary adenoma. These tumors, similar to other pituitary adenomas, arise from a monoclonal expansion of a single cell that has undergone somatic mutation. As we have mentioned, 40% of somatotroph cell adenomas express an oncogene *(gsp)*, which is a mutant GTPase-deficient α subunit of the G protein, Gs. Somatotroph cell adenomas may be quite large by the time they come to clinical attention because the manifestations of excessive GH may be subtle. Histologically, GH-containing adenomas are composed of granulated cells, which appear acidophilic or chromophobic in routine sections. Immunocytochemical stains demonstrate GH within the cytoplasm of the neoplastic cells. In addition, small amounts of immunoreactive prolactin are often present.

Persistent hypersecretion of GH stimulates the hepatic secretion of insulin-like growth factor-I (IGF-I), which causes many of the clinical manifestations.[6] If a somatotrophic adenoma appears in children before the epiphyses have closed, the elevated levels of GH result in *gigantism.* This is characterized by a generalized increase in body size, with disproportionately long arms and legs. If the increased levels of GH are present after closure of the epiphyses, patients develop *acromegaly.* In this condition, growth is most conspicuous in skin and soft tissues; viscera (thyroid, heart, liver, and adrenals); and bones of the face, hands, and feet. Bone density may be increased (hyperostosis) in both the spine and the hips. Enlargement of the jaw results in its protrusion (prognathism), with broadening of the lower face. The hands and feet are enlarged with broad, sausage-like fingers. In most instances, gigantism is also accompanied by evidence of acromegaly. These changes develop for decades before being recognized, hence the opportunity for the adenomas to reach substantial size. GH excess is also correlated with a variety of other disturbances, including gonadal dysfunction, diabetes mellitus, generalized muscle weakness, hypertension, arthritis, congestive heart failure, and an increased risk of gastrointestinal cancers. Prolactin can be demonstrated in a substantial fraction of GH-producing adenomas and in some cases may be released in sufficient quantities to produce hyperprolactinemia.

The goals of treatment are to restore GH levels to normal and to decrease symptoms referable to a pituitary mass lesion, while not causing hypopituitarism. To achieve these goals, the tumor can be removed surgically by a transsphenoidal approach or destroyed by radiation therapy, or GH secretion can be reduced by drug therapy. When effective control of GH hypersecretion is achieved, the characteristic tissue overgrowth and related symptoms gradually recede, and the metabolic abnormalities improve.

Corticotroph Cell Adenomas

Corticotroph adenomas are usually small microadenomas at the time of diagnosis. These tumors are basophilic or chromophobic and stain positively with periodic acid–Schiff (PAS) stains because of the presence of carbohydrate in the ACTH precursor molecule.

Excess production of ACTH by the corticotroph adenoma leads to adrenal hypersecretion of cortisol and the development of *hypercortisolism* (also known as *Cushing syndrome*). This syndrome is discussed in more detail later with the diseases of the adrenal gland. It can be caused by a wide variety of conditions in addition to ACTH-producing pituitary tumors. When the hypercortisolism is due to excessive production of ACTH by the pituitary, the process is designated *Cushing disease.* Large destructive adenomas can develop in patients after surgical removal of the adrenal glands for treatment of Cushing syndrome. This condition, known as *Nelson syndrome,* occurs in most cases because of a loss of the inhibitory effect of adrenal corticosteroids on a preexisting corticotroph microadenoma. Because the adrenals are absent in patients with this disorder, hypercortisolism does not develop. In contrast, patients present with mass effects of the pituitary tumor. In addition, there can be hyperpigmentation because of the stimulatory effect of other products of the ACTH precursor molecule on melanocytes.

Other Anterior Pituitary Adenomas

Pituitary adenomas may elaborate more than one hormone. As described earlier, somatotroph adenomas commonly contain immunoreactive prolactin. In some tumors, designated *mixed adenomas,* more than one cell population is present. In other cases, a single cell type is apparently capable of synthesizing more than one hormone. A few comments are made about several of the less frequent functioning tumors.

Gonadotroph (LH-producing and FSH-producing) adenomas constitute 10 to 15% of pituitary adenomas. These tumors can be difficult to recognize because they secrete hormones inefficiently and variably, and the secretory products usually do not cause a recognizable clinical syndrome. Gonadotroph adenomas are most frequently found in middle-aged men and women when they become large enough to cause neurologic symptoms, such as impaired vision, headaches, diplopia, or pituitary apoplexy.[7] Pituitary hormone deficiencies can also be found, most commonly impaired secretion of LH. This causes decreased energy and libido in men (due to reduced testosterone) and amenorrhea in premenopausal women. The neoplasms are basophilic or chromophobic and can reach substantial size before they are detected.

Thyrotroph (TSH-producing) adenomas are rare, accounting for approximately 1% of all pituitary adenomas.[8] Thyrotroph adenomas are chromophobic or basophilic and are a rare cause of hyperthyroidism.

A substantial number of pituitary adenomas generate no detectable hormonal product and are designated *null cell adenomas.* These nonfunctional tumors account for approximately 20% of all pituitary adenomas. These tumors are either chromophobic or contain cells with granular, eosinophilic cytoplasm. In contrast to the hormonally active tumors, the granular cytoplasm in such tumors is due largely to the presence of numerous mitochondria, whereas secretory granules are infrequent. Patients with null cell adenomas typically present with mass effects. These lesions may also compromise the residual anterior pituitary sufficiently to produce hypopituitarism. This may occur as a result of gradual enlargement of the adenoma or after abrupt enlargement of the tumor because of acute hemorrhage (pituitary apoplexy).

Pituitary carcinomas are quite rare, and most are not functional. These malignant tumors range from well differentiated, resembling somewhat atypical adenomas, to poorly differentiated, with variable degrees of pleomorphism and the features characteristic of carcinomas in other locations. The diagnosis of carcinoma requires the demonstration of metastases, usually to lymph nodes, bone, liver, and sometimes elsewhere.

HYPOPITUITARISM

Hypopituitarism refers to decreased secretion of pituitary hormones, which can result from diseases of the hypothalamus or of the pituitary. Hypofunction of the anterior pituitary occurs when approximately 75% of the parenchyma is lost or absent. This may be congenital or the result of a variety of acquired abnormalities that are intrinsic to the pituitary. Most cases of hypofunction arise from destructive processes directly involving the anterior pituitary, such as tumors, ischemic necrosis of the pituitary, and the empty sella syndrome, although other mechanisms have been identified.

- *Tumors and other mass lesions:* Pituitary adenomas, other benign tumors arising within the sella, primary and metastatic malignancies, and cysts can induce hypopituitarism. Any mass lesion in the sellae can cause damage by exerting pressure on adjacent pituitary cells.
- *Pituitary surgery or radiation:* Surgical excision of a pituitary adenoma may inadvertently extend to nonadenomatous pituitary. If sufficient normal tissue is removed, hypopituitarism may ensue. Radiation of the pituitary, used to prevent regrowth of residual tumor after surgery, exposes the nonadenomatous pituitary to the same radiation.
- *Rathke cleft cyst:* These cysts, lined by ciliated cuboidal epithelium with occasional goblet cells and anterior pituitary cells, can accumulate proteinaceous fluid and expand causing symptoms.
- *Pituitary apoplexy:* As has been mentioned, this is a sudden hemorrhage into the pituitary gland, often occurring into a pituitary adenoma. In its most dramatic presentation, apoplexy causes the sudden onset of excruciating headache, diplopia owing to pressure on the oculomotor nerves, and hypopituitarism.
- *Ischemic necrosis of the pituitary and Sheehan syndrome:* Ischemic necrosis of the anterior pituitary is an important cause of pituitary insufficiency. In general, the anterior pituitary tolerates ischemia reasonably well; loss of as much as half to the anterior parenchyma can occur without clinical consequence. With damage to 75% or more, however, evidence of hypopituitarism develops. *Sheehan syndrome,* or postpartum necrosis of the anterior pituitary, is the most common form of clinically significant ischemic necrosis of the anterior pituitary.[9] During pregnancy, the anterior pituitary enlarges to almost twice its normal size. This physiologic expansion of the gland is not accompanied by an increase in blood supply from the low-pressure venous system, and hence there is relative anoxia of the pituitary. Thus, sudden infarction of the anterior lobe precipitated by obstetric hemorrhage or shock may occur. Sudden systemic hypotension precipitates vasospasm of the vessels and thus ischemic necrosis of much of the anterior lobe. The posterior pituitary, because it receives its blood directly from arterial branches, is much less susceptible to ischemic injury in this setting and is therefore usually not affected. Pituitary necrosis may also be encountered in other conditions, such as disseminated intravascular coagulation and (more rarely) sickle cell anemia, elevated

intracranial pressure, traumatic injury, and shock of any origin. Whatever the pathogenesis, the infarcted adenohypophysis at the outset appears soft, pale, and ischemic or hemorrhagic. Over time, the ischemic area is resorbed and replaced by fibrous tissue. In some long-standing cases, the gland scars down to a fibrous nubbin weighing less than 0.1 gm, attached to the wall of an empty sella (Fig. 26–5).

- *Empty sella syndrome:* Any condition that destroys part or all of the pituitary gland, such as ablation of the pituitary by surgery or radiation, can result in an *empty sella.* The *empty sella syndrome* refers to the presence of an enlarged, empty sella turcica that is not filled with pituitary tissue.[10] There are two types: (1) In a *primary* empty sella, there is a defect in the diaphragma sellae that allows the arachnoidea mater and cerebrospinal fluid to herniate into the sella, resulting in expansion of the sella and compression of the pituitary. Classically the affected patients are obese women with a history of multiple pregnancies. The empty sella syndrome may be associated with visual field defects and occasionally with endocrine anomalies, such as hyperprolactinemia owing to interruption of inhibitory hypothalamic effects. Only rarely is it associated with hypopituitarism because sufficient functioning parenchyma is maintained. (2) In a *secondary* empty sella, a mass, such as a pituitary adenoma, enlarges the sella but then is removed by surgery or radiation. Hypopituitarism can result from the treatment or spontaneous infarction.
- *Genetic defects:* Rare congenital deficiencies of one or more pituitary hormones have been recognized in children. A defect has been identified in a gene that encodes *pit-1,* a transcription factor that is important in the expression of pituitary-specific genes, such as GH, prolactin, and TSH. The defective form of the protein can bind to the DNA response element but does not activate the target genes. Consequently, children born with this deficiency cannot synthesize these hormones.[11]

Less frequently, disorders that interfere with the delivery of pituitary hormone–releasing factors from the *hypothalamus,* such as hypothalamic tumors, may also cause hypofunction of the anterior pituitary. Any disease involving the hypothalamus can alter secretion of one or more of the hypothalamic hormones that influence secretion of the corresponding pituitary hormones. In contrast to diseases that involve the pituitary directly, any of these conditions can also diminish the secretion of ADH, resulting in diabetes insipidus (discussed later). Such hypothalamic lesions are

- *Tumors* include benign lesions that arise in the hypothalamus, such as craniopharyngiomas, and malignant tumors that metastasize to that site, such as breast and lung carcinomas. Hypothalamic hormone deficiency can ensue when brain or nasopharyngeal tumors are treated with radiation.
- *Infiltrative disorders and infections,* such as sarcoidosis or tuberculous meningitis, can cause deficiencies of anterior pituitary hormones and diabetes insipidus.

The clinical manifestations of anterior pituitary hypo-

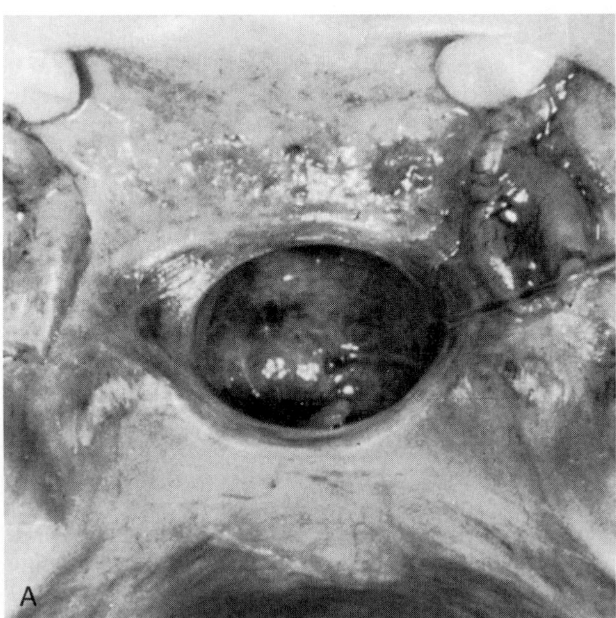

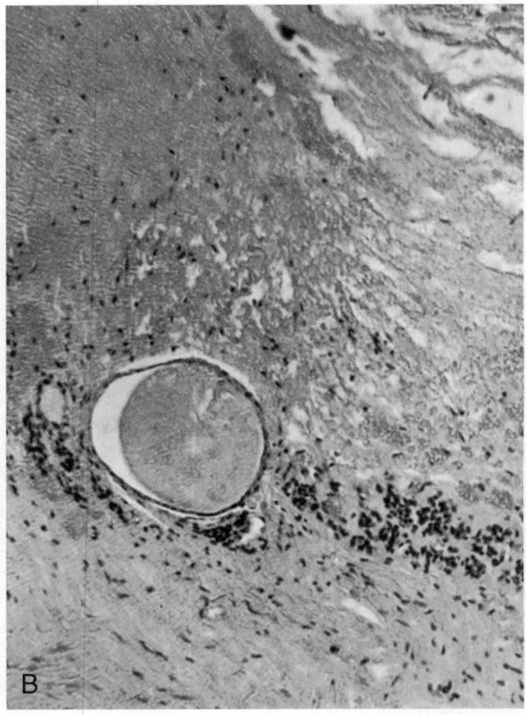

Figure 26–5

A, View of sella turcica in a patient dying with chronic pituitary insufficiency. A tiny nubbin of residual pituitary can be seen protruding from the posterior wall of the sella *(below). B,* Photomicrograph of residual anterior pituitary illustrated in *A.* Most of the gland has been replaced by dense fibrous tissue except for a few residual cells in the pars intermedia.

function depend on the nature and extent of the causative process as well as the type and degree of hormonal insufficiency. These changes are related to decreased function of the adrenal cortex, thyroid, and gonads. Specific manifestations of hypothyroidism and hypoadrenalism are discussed later. Additional alterations of hypopituitarism include pallor, as a result of loss of melanocyte-stimulating hormone (MSH) atrophy of the genitalia with resultant amenorrhea, impotence, and loss of libido; and loss of pubic and axillary hair.

POSTERIOR PITUITARY SYNDROMES

The posterior pituitary is composed of modified glial cells (designated *pituicytes*) and axonal processes extending from nerve cell bodies in the supraoptic and paraventricular nuclei of the hypothalamus. These neurons produce two peptides: *ADH* and *oxytocin*. The hormones are stored in axon terminals in the posterior pituitary and are released into the circulation in response to appropriate stimuli. Oxytocin stimulates contraction of the uterine smooth muscle cells in the gravid uterus and cells surrounding the lactiferous ducts of the mammary glands. Inappropriate oxytocin secretion has not been associated with clinical abnormalities. ADH is a nonapeptide hormone synthesized predominantly in the supraoptic nucleus. In response to a number of different stimuli, including increased plasma oncotic pressure, left atrial distention, exercise, and certain emotional states, ADH is released from the axon terminals in the neurohypophysis into the general circulation. The clinically relevant posterior pituitary syndromes involve ADH and include *diabetes insipidus and secretion of inappropriately high levels of ADH.* Glial tumors can also arise, rarely, from the pituicytes.

- *Diabetes insipidus:* ADH deficiency causes diabetes insipidus, a condition characterized by excessive urination (polyuria) owing to an inability of the kidney to resorb water properly from the urine. It can result from a variety of processes, including head trauma, tumors, and inflammatory disorders of the hypothalamus and pituitary as well as surgical procedures involving these organs. The condition can arise spontaneously, in the absence of an underlying disorder. The clinical manifestations include the excretion of large volumes of dilute urine with an inappropriately low specific gravity. Serum sodium and osmolality are increased owing to excessive renal loss of free water, resulting in thirst and polydipsia. Patients who can drink water can generally compensate for urinary losses; patients who are obtunded, bedridden, or otherwise limited in their ability to obtain water may develop life-threatening dehydration.
- *Syndrome of inappropriate ADH (SIADH) secretion:* ADH excess causes resorption of excessive amounts of free water, resulting in *hyponatremia.* The most frequent causes of SIADH include the secretion of ectopic ADH by malignant neoplasms (particularly small cell carcinomas of the lung), non-neoplastic diseases of the lung, and local injury to the hypothalamus or posterior pituitary (or both).[12] The clinical manifestations of SIADH are dominated by hyponatremia, cerebral edema, and resultant neurologic dysfunction. Although total body water is increased, blood volume remains normal, and peripheral edema does not develop.

HYPOTHALAMIC SUPRASELLAR TUMORS

Neoplasms in this location may induce hypofunction or hyperfunction of the anterior pituitary, diabetes insipidus, or combinations of these manifestations. The most commonly implicated lesions are *gliomas* (sometimes arising in the chiasm, Chapter 30) and *craniopharyngiomas.*[13] The craniopharyngioma is thought to be derived from vestigial remnants of Rathke pouch. These slow-growing tumors account for 1% to 5% of intracranial tumors; some of these lesions arise within the sella, but most are suprasellar. Although they occur most commonly during childhood and adolescence, about 50% present clinically after age 20. Children usually come to clinical attention because of endocrine deficiencies such as growth retardation, whereas adults usually present with visual disturbances. Pituitary hormonal deficiencies, including diabetes insipidus, are common.

MORPHOLOGY. Craniopharyngiomas average 3 to 4 cm in diameter; they may be encapsulated and solid but more commonly are cystic and sometimes multiloculated. More than three fourths of these tumors contain sufficient calcification to be visualized radiographically. In their strategic location, they often encroach on the optic chiasm or cranial nerves and not infrequently bulge into the floor of the third ventricle and base of the brain. Two histologic forms can be distinguished—adamantinomatous and papillary.

The **adamantinomatous craniopharyngioma** consists of nests or cords of stratified squamous or columnar epithelium embedded in a spongy reticulum. Often the nests of squamous cells gradually merge into a peripheral layer of columnar cells. Keratin formation is seen, and this form of the tumor is frequently calcified. Additional features typical of adamantinomatous craniopharyngioma include cholesterol-rich cyst contents, fibrosis, and chronic inflammatory reaction. These tumors extend fingerlets of epithelium into adjacent brain, where they elicit a brisk glial reaction.

The *papillary craniopharyngioma* usually lacks the keratin, calcification, and cyst content. The squamous cells of the solid sections of the tumor do not have the columnar sheet at the periphery and do not typically generate a spongy reticulum in the internal layers.

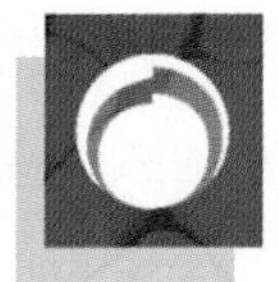

Thyroid

THYROID GLAND

The thyroid gland is unique among the organs of the endocrine system because of its size and superficial location. It consists of two bulky lateral lobes connected by a relatively thin isthmus, usually located below and anterior to the larynx. Normal variants in the structure of the thyroid gland include the presence of a pyramidal lobe above the isthmus.

The thyroid gland develops embryologically from an evagination of the developing pharyngeal epithelium that descends to its normal position in the anterior neck. This pattern of descent explains the occasional presence of thyroid tissue in atypical locations. Incomplete descent may lead to the formation of the thyroid at loci abnormally high in the neck, producing a lingual or aberrant subhyoid thyroid. Excessive descent leads to substernal thyroid glands. Malformations of branchial pouch differentiation may result in intrathyroidal sites of the thymus or parathyroid glands. The implication of these deviations becomes evident in the patient who has a total thyroidectomy and subsequently develops hypoparathyroidism.

The weight of the normal adult thyroid is approximately 15 to 20 gm. The thyroid has a rich intraglandular capillary network that is supplied by the superior and inferior thyroidal arteries. Nerve fibers from the cervical sympathetic ganglia indirectly influence thyroid secretion by acting on the blood vessels. The thyroid is divided into lobules composed of about 20 to 40 evenly dispersed follicles. The follicles range from uniform to variable in size and are lined by cuboidal-to-low columnar epithelium, which is filled with thyroglobulin. In response to trophic factors from the hypothalamus, TSH is released by thyrotrophs in the anterior pituitary into the circulation. TSH acts on the thyroid, causing the follicular epithelial cells of the thyroid to pinocytize colloid and ultimately convert thyroglobulin into *thyroxine* (T_4) and lesser amounts of *triiodothyronine* (T_3) (Fig. 26–6). T_4 and T_3 are released into the systemic circulation, where most of these peptides are reversibly bound to circulating plasma proteins, such as thyroxine-binding globulin (TBG), for transport to peripheral tissues.[14] The binding proteins serve to maintain the serum free T_3 and T_4 concentrations within narrow limits, yet ensure that the hormones are readily available to the tissues. The unbound T_3 and T_4 enter cells and interact with nuclear receptors, which change gene expression and ultimately up-regulate carbohydrate and lipid catabolism and stimulate protein synthesis in a wide range of cells. The net effect of these processes is an increase in the *basal metabolic rate.*

The thyroid gland is one of the most responsive organs in the body. The gland responds to many stimuli and is in a constant state of adaptation. During puberty, pregnancy, and physiologic stress from any source, the gland increases in size and becomes more active. This functional lability is reflected in transient hyperplasia of the thyroidal epithelium. At this time, thyroglobulin is resorbed, and the follicular cells become tall and columnar, sometimes forming small infolded buds or papillae. When the stress abates, involution occurs; that is, the height of the epithelium falls, colloid accumulates, and the follicular cells resume their normal size and architecture. Failure of this normal balance between hyperplasia and involution may produce major or minor deviations from the usual histologic pattern.

The function of the thyroid gland can be inhibited by a variety of chemical agents, collectively referred to as *goi-*

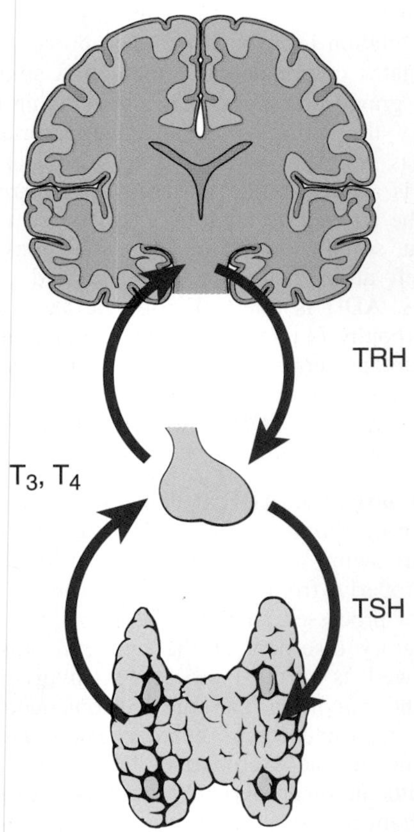

Figure 26–6

Diagram of relationship between the hypothalamus, anterior pituitary, and a peripheral endocrine gland, exemplified here by the thyroid gland. Secretion of thyroid hormones (T_3 and T_4) is controlled by trophic factors secreted by both the hypothalamus and the anterior pituitary. Decreased levels of T_3 and T_4 stimulate the release of thyrotropin-releasing hormone (TRH) from the hypothalamus and thyroid-stimulating hormone (TSH) from the anterior pituitary, causing T_3 and T_4 levels to rise. Elevated T_3 and T_4 levels, in turn, suppress the secretion of both TRH and TSH. This relationship is termed a *negative-feedback loop.* (Modified from Dr. Ronald A. DeLellis, New England Medical Center, Boston.)

trogens. Because they suppress T_3 and T_4 synthesis, the level of TSH increases, and subsequent hyperplastic enlargement of the gland (goiter) follows. The antithyroid agent propylthiouracil inhibits the oxidation of iodide and blocks production of the thyroid hormones. Iodide, when given to patients with thyroid hyperfunction, also blocks the release of thyroid hormones but through different mechanisms. Iodides in large doses inhibit proteolysis of thyroglobulin. Thus, thyroid hormone is synthesized and incorporated within increasing amounts of colloid, but it is not released into the blood.

In the interfollicular stroma, the thyroid gland also contains a population of *parafollicular cells,* or C cells, which synthesize and secrete the hormone *calcitonin.* This hormone promotes the absorption of calcium by the skeletal system and inhibits the resorption of bone by osteoclasts.

Diseases of the thyroid are of great importance because most are amenable to medical or surgical management. They include conditions associated with excessive release of thyroid hormones (hyperthyroidism), those associated with thyroid hormone deficiency (hypothyroidism), and mass lesions of the thyroid. We first consider the clinical consequences of disturbed thyroid function, then focus on the disorders that generate these problems.

Table 26–2. DISORDERS ASSOCIATED WITH HYPERTHYROIDISM

Common
Diffuse toxic hyperplasia (Graves disease)
Toxic multinodular goiter
Toxic adenoma

Uncommon
Acute or subacute thyroiditis
Hyperfunctioning thyroid carcinoma
Choriocarcinoma or hydatidiform mole
Thyroid-stimulating hormone–secreting pituitary adenoma
Neonatal thyrotoxicosis associated with maternal Graves disease
Struma ovarii (ovarian teratomatous thyroid)
Iodide-induced hyperthyroidism
Iatrogenic (exogenous) hyperthyroidism

HYPERTHYROIDISM

Thyrotoxicosis is a hypermetabolic state caused by elevated levels of free T_3 and T_4.[15] It is often referred to as *hyperthyroidism* because it is caused most commonly by hyperfunction of the thyroid gland. When these elevated levels arise from hyperfunction of the thyroid, as occurs in Graves disease, the thyrotoxicosis may correctly be called *hyperthyroidism.* When the increased hormone levels reflect excessive leakage of hormone out of a nonhyperactive gland, however, it is properly referred to as *thyrotoxicosis.* Long usage often equates these terms. By either name, the syndrome is manifested by nervousness, palpitations, rapid pulse, fatigability, muscular weakness, weight loss with good appetite, diarrhea, heat intolerance, warm skin, excessive perspiration, emotional lability, menstrual changes, a fine tremor of the hand (particularly when outstretched), eye changes, and variable enlargement of the thyroid gland. Thyrotoxicosis can be caused by a variety of disorders (Table 26–2):

- *Diffuse hyperplasia* of the thyroid associated with Graves disease (accounts for 85% of cases)
- Ingestion of *exogenous thyroid hormone* (administered for hypothyroidism)
- Hyperfunctional *multinodular goiter*
- Hyperfunctional *adenoma* of the thyroid
- Thyroiditis

The terms *primary* and *secondary hyperthyroidism* are sometimes used to designate hyperthyroidism arising from an intrinsic thyroid abnormality and that arising from processes outside of the thyroid, such as a TSH-secreting pituitary tumor. Less common causes of secondary hyperthyroidism include secretion of excessive amounts of thyroid hormone by ectopic thyroid arising in ovarian teratomas *(struma ovarii).*

Clinical Course. The clinical manifestations of hyperthyroidism include changes referable to the *hypermetabolic state* induced by excess thyroid hormone as well as those related to overactivity of the *sympathetic nervous system.* Excessive levels of thyroid hormone result in an increase in the basal metabolic rate. *Cardiac manifestations are among the earliest and most consistent features of hyperthyroidism.*[16] Patients with hyperthyroidism can have an increase in cardiac output, owing to both increased cardiac contractility and increased peripheral oxygen requirements. Tachycardia, palpitations, and cardiomegaly are common. Arrhythmias, particularly atrial fibrillation, occur frequently and are more common in older patients. The basis for these arrhythmias is not clear. Congestive heart failure may develop, particularly in elderly patients with preexisting cardiac disease. Myocardial changes, such as foci of lymphocytic and eosinophilic infiltration, mild fibrosis in the interstitium, fatty changes in myofibers, and an increase in size and number of mitochondria, have been described. These changes are not frequent, and other possible concomitant pathogeneses have not been rigorously ruled out, so debate continues about so-called *thyrotoxic cardiomyopathy.*

Other findings throughout the body include atrophy and fatty infiltration of skeletal muscle, sometimes with focal interstitial lymphocytic infiltrates; minimal fatty changes in the liver, sometimes accompanied by mild periportal fibrosis and a mild lymphocytic infiltrate; osteoporosis; and generalized lymphoid hyperplasia with lymphadenopathy.

Ocular changes often call attention to hyperthyroidism. A wide, staring gaze and lid lag are present because of sympathetic overstimulation of the levator palpebrae superioris (Fig. 26–7). Only patients with Graves disease have ophthalmopathy (see later).

In the *neuromuscular system,* overactivity of the sympathetic nervous system produces tremor, hyperactivity, emotional lability, anxiety, inability to concentrate, and insom-

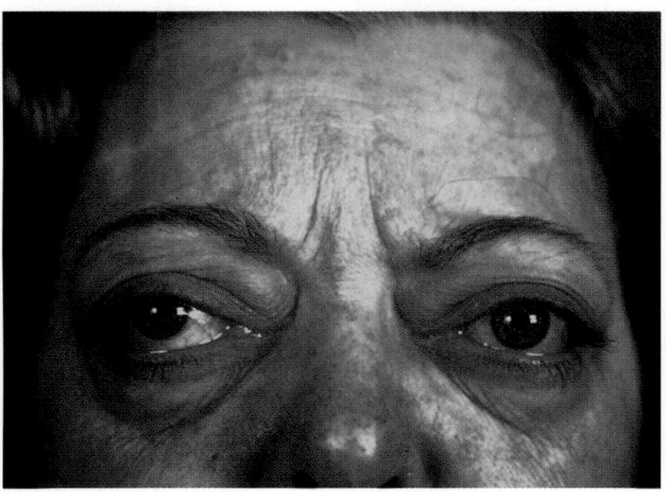

Figure 26–7

Photograph of a patient with hyperthyroidism. A wide-eyed, staring gaze, caused by overactivity of the sympathetic nervous system, is one of the features of this disorder. In Graves disease, one of the most important causes of hyperthyroidism, accumulation of loose connective tissue behind the eyeballs also adds to the protuberant appearance of the eyes.

nia. Proximal muscle weakness is common with decreased muscle mass.

The *skin* of thyrotoxic patients tends to be warm, moist, and flushed because of increased blood flow and peripheral vasodilation to increase heat loss. Sweating is increased because of higher levels of calorigenesis. Infiltrative dermopathy is seen only in Graves hyperthyroidism and is discussed later.

In the *gastrointestinal system,* increased gut motility results from increased sympathetic activity. There is an increase in appetite and hyperphagia. Despite the increase in appetite, weight loss occurs primarily as a result of increased energy expenditure but also increased bowel motility.

The *skeletal system* is also affected in hyperthyroidism. Thyroid hormone stimulates bone resorption, resulting in increased porosity of cortical bone and reduced volume of trabecular bone. The net effect is osteoporosis and an increased risk of fractures in patients with chronic hyperthyroidism.

A diagnosis of hyperthyroidism is made using both clinical and laboratory findings. *Determining the serum TSH concentration, in conjunction with a measurement of unbound (free) T_4, provides the best initial screen for cases of suspected hyperthyroidism. Free T_4 levels* are usually increased. *TSH levels* are extremely sensitive to free T_4 levels and are thus decreased to low levels in patients with primary hyperthyroidism (i.e., hyperthyroidism owing to intrinsic thyroid disease). TSH levels, however, are not a reliable indicator of thyroid function in patients with thyrotoxicosis caused by hypothalamic or primary pituitary disease (e.g., TSH-secreting pituitary adenomas). Determining TSH levels after the injection of TRH *(TRH stimulation test)* is used in the evaluation of cases of suspected hyperthyroidism with equivocal changes in the baseline serum TSH level. A normal rise in TSH after administration of TRH excludes secondary hyperthyroidism. Measurement of *radioactive iodine uptake* provides an additional direct indication of the level of activity within the thyroid gland. An unusual variant of hyperthyroidism is *T_3-hyperthyroidism*, or T_3-thyrotoxicosis, in which serum TSH is low and circulating levels of free T_3 are high, but free T_4 is normal. This results from an increase in thyroidal T_3 secretion and increased extrathyroidal conversion of T_4 to T_3 and can be seen in Graves disease or any form of primary hyperthyroidism. The therapeutic options for hyperthyroidism include multiple medications, each of which has a different mechanism of action. Typically, these include a β-blocker, to control symptoms induced by increased adrenergic tone; a thionamide, to block new hormone synthesis; an iodine solution, to block the release of thyroid hormone; and agents that inhibit peripheral conversion of T_4 to T_3. Radioiodine, which is incorporated into thyroid tissues, resulting in ablation of thyroid function over a period of 6 to 18 weeks, may also be used.

HYPOTHYROIDISM

Hypothyroidism is caused by any structural or functional derangement that interferes with the production of adequate levels of thyroid hormone. It can result from a defect anywhere in the hypothalamic-pituitary-thyroid axis. As in the case of hyperthyroidism, this disorder is divided into primary and secondary categories, depending on whether the hypothyroidism arises from an intrinsic abnormality in the thyroid or occurs as a result of hypothalamic or pituitary disease. The causes of hypothyroidism can be divided into several categories (Table 26–3).

Primary hypothyroidism accounts for the vast majority of cases of hypothyroidism. The most common cause of

Table 26–3. CAUSES OF HYPOTHYROIDISM

Insufficient thyroid parenchyma
Developmental
Radiation injury (radioiodine, external radiation)
Surgical ablation
Hashimoto thyroiditis
Interference with thyroid hormone synthesis
Idiopathic primary hypothyroidism (possible immune blockade of TSH receptors)
Heritable biosynthetic defects
Iodine deficiency
Drugs (lithium, iodides, *p*-aminosalicylic acid, others)
Hashimoto thyroiditis
Suprathyroidal
Pituitary lesions reducing TSH secretion
Hypothalamic lesions that reduce thyrotropin-releasing hormone delivery

TSH, thyroid-stimulating hormone.

hypothyroidism in iodine-sufficient areas of the world is *chronic autoimmune thyroiditis,* or Hashimoto thyroiditis.[17] This condition is variously reported to cause 15 to 60% of cases of hypothyroidism. Both cellular and humoral factors contribute to the thyroid injury and hypothyroidism in chronic autoimmune thyroiditis.

Hypothyroidism can follow thyroid surgery or radiation, be drug induced, or occur as a result of an infiltrative disorder. A large resection of the gland (total thyroidectomy) for the treatment of hyperthyroidism or excision of a primary neoplasm is a common cause of hypothyroidism. The gland may also be ablated by radiation, whether in the form of radioiodine administered for the treatment of hyperthyroidism, or exogenous irradiation, such as external radiation therapy to the neck. Drugs given intentionally to decrease thyroid secretion (e.g., methimazole and propylthiouracil) can cause hypothyroidism, as can agents used to treat nonthyroid conditions (e.g., lithium). Finally, infiltrative diseases such as hemochromatosis, amyloid, and sarcoid are rare causes of hypothyroidism.

Secondary hypothyroidism is that caused by TSH deficiency, and tertiary (central) hypothyroidism is caused by TRH deficiency. Secondary hypothyroidism can result from any of the causes of hypopituitarism, frequently a pituitary tumor; other causes include postpartum pituitary necrosis, trauma, and nonpituitary tumors, as previously discussed. Tertiary (central) hypothyroidism can be caused by any disorder that damages the hypothalamus or interferes with hypothalamic-pituitary portal blood flow, thereby preventing delivery of TRH to the pituitary. This can result from hypothalamic damage from tumors, trauma, radiation therapy, or infiltrative diseases. Classic clinical manifestations of hypothyroidism include cretinism and myxedema.

Cretinism

Cretinism refers to hypothyroidism developing in infancy or early childhood. The term *cretin* was derived from the French *chrétien,* meaning Christian or Christ-like, and was applied to these unfortunates because they were considered to be so mentally retarded as to be incapable of sinning. In the past, this disorder occurred fairly commonly in areas of the world where dietary iodine deficiency is endemic, such as the Himalayas, inland China, and Africa and other mountainous areas. It has become much less frequent in recent years, owing to the widespread supplementation of foods with iodine. On rare occasions, cretinism may also result from inborn errors in metabolism (e.g., enzyme deficiencies) that interfere with the biosynthesis of normal levels of thyroid hormone (*sporadic* cretinism).

Clinical features of cretinism include impaired development of the skeletal system and central nervous system, manifested by severe mental retardation, short stature, coarse facial features, a protruding tongue, and umbilical hernia. The severity of the mental impairment in cretinism appears to be directly influenced by the time at which thyroid deficiency occurs in utero. Normally, maternal hormones, including T_3 and T_4, cross the placenta and are critical to fetal brain development. If there is maternal thyroid deficiency before the development of the fetal thyroid gland, mental retardation is severe. In contrast, reduction in maternal thyroid hormones later in pregnancy, after fetal thyroid has developed, allows normal brain development.

Myxedema

The term *myxedema* is applied to hypothyroidism developing in the older child or adult. The clinical manifestations vary with the age of onset of the deficiency. The older child shows signs and symptoms intermediate between those of the cretin and those of the adult with hypothyroidism. In the adult, the condition appears insidiously and may take years to reach the level of clinical suspicion.

Clinical features of myxedema are characterized by a slowing of physical and mental activity. The initial symptoms include generalized fatigue; apathy, and mental sluggishness, which may mimic depression in the early stages of the disease. Speech and intellectual functions become slowed. Patients with myxedema are *listless, cold intolerant,* and frequently overweight. Reduced cardiac output probably contributes to shortness of breath and decreased exercise capacity, two frequent complaints in patients with hypothyroidism. Decreased sympathetic activity results in constipation and decreased sweating. The skin in these patients is cool and pale because of decreased blood flow. Histologically, there is an accumulation of matrix substances, such as glycosaminoglycans and hyaluronic acid in skin; subcutaneous tissue; and a number of visceral sites. This results in edema, a broadening and coarsening of facial features, enlargement of the tongue, and deepening of the voice.

Laboratory studies play an important role in the diagnosis of suspected hypothyroidism. As with hyperthyroidism, estimations of free T_4 and TSH levels are used as screening tests for hypothyroidism. In patients with overt hypothyroidism caused by disease of the thyroid gland, decreased serum concentrations of T_4 and T_3 result in a loss of feedback inhibition on TSH production by the pituitary. The TSH level is not increased in patients with hypothyroidism because of primary hypothalamic or pituitary disease. *T_4 levels are decreased* in patients with hypothyroidism of any origin.

THYROIDITIS

Thyroiditis, or inflammation of the thyroid gland, encompasses a diverse group of disorders characterized by some form of thyroid inflammation. These diseases include conditions that result in acute illness with severe thyroid pain (e.g., infectious thyroiditis, subacute granulomatous thyroiditis) and disorders in which there is relatively little inflammation and the illness is manifested primarily by thyroid dysfunction (subacute lymphocytic [painless] thyroiditis and fibrous [Reidel] thyroiditis).

Infectious thyroiditis may be either acute or chronic. Acute infections, may reach the thyroid via hematogenous spread or through direct seeding of the gland; such as via a fistula from the piriform sinus adjacent to the larynx. Other infections of the thyroid, including mycobacterial, fungal, and *Pneumocystis* infections, are more chronic and frequently occur in immunocompromised patients. Whatever the cause, the inflammatory involvement may cause sudden onset of neck pain and tenderness in the area of the gland and is accompanied by fever, chills, and other signs of infection. Infectious thyroiditis can be self-limited or can be controlled with appropriate therapy. Thyroid function is usually not significantly affected, and there are few residual effects except for possible small foci of scarring. This section focuses on the more common and clinically significant types of thyroiditis: (1) Hashimoto thyroiditis, (2) subacute granulomatous thyroiditis, and (3) subacute lymphocytic thyroiditis.

Hashimoto Thyroiditis

Hashimoto thyroiditis is the most common cause of hypothyroidism in areas of the world where iodine levels are sufficient. It is characterized by gradual thyroid failure because of autoimmune destruction of the thyroid gland: The name Hashimoto thyroiditis is derived from the 1912 report by Hashimoto describing patients with goiter and intense lymphocytic infiltration of the thyroid (e.g., *struma lymphomatosa*). This disorder is most prevalent between 45 and 65 years of age and is more common in women than in men, with a female predominance of 10:1 to 20:1. Although it is primarily a disease of older women, it can occur in children and is a major cause of nonendemic goiter in children. The disease clusters in families, and the concordance rate in monozygotic twins is 30% to 60%. Some cases of Hashimoto thyroiditis are associated with HLA-DR5; a minority are characterized by severe thyroid atrophy and are linked to HLA-DR3. This suggests that two different pathogenic mechanisms may play a role in the development of the disorder. The usual course of Hashimoto thyroiditis is gradual loss of thyroid function; although the inflammatory process early in the disorder may be sufficiently severe to cause thyroid follicular disruption and transient hyperthyroidism. The frequency of other autoimmune disorders, such as systemic lupus erythematosus and rheumatoid arthritis, is increased in patients with Hashimoto disease, as it is in individuals with Graves disease.

Pathogenesis. Although both cellular and humoral factors contribute to thyroid injury and hypothyroidism in Hashimoto thyroiditis, this disease is believed to be caused primarily by a defect in T cells. One model for this disorder proposes that T cells from patients with this disorder recognize processed thyroid antigens in association with specific types of major histocompatibility complex (MHC) antigens. Diminished suppressor T cells may also play a role in the emergence of thyroid-specific helper T cells. These activated T cells have two roles in the disease: (1) They interact with B cells and stimulate the secretion of a variety of antithyroid antibodies, which may activate antibody-dependent cytotoxicity mechanisms, and (2) the helper T cells may induce the formation of CD8+ cells, which can be cytotoxic to thyroid cells.

B lymphocytes from thyroid tissue of patients with Hashimoto thyroiditis are activated and secrete a number of *autoantibodies* directed against thyroid antigens:

- *Thyroglobulin and thyroid peroxidase:* Thyroglobulin is synthesized by follicular cells and secreted into the lumen of the thyroid follicle, where it is stored as colloid. Thyroid peroxidase is located on the luminal surface of the microvilli of thyroid epithelial cells and catalyzes both tyrosine iodination and coupling of iodotyrosyl residues to form T_3 and T_4. Nearly all patients with Hashimoto thyroiditis have antibodies to both thyroglobulin and thyroid peroxidase, although these autoantibodies are not specific for the disorder. The induction of experimental autoimmune thyroiditis using either thyroglobulin or thyroid peroxidase as antigens provides support for their potential role in Hashimoto thyroiditis.[18]
- *TSH receptor:* This is a G protein–coupled transmembrane receptor. TSH receptor antibodies are specific for Hashimoto and Graves diseases, in contrast to the antibodies to thyroglobulin and thyroid peroxidase, which are found in patients with many other thyroid diseases. In Hashimoto disease, the anti-TSH receptor antibodies block the action of TSH, thus accounting for the hypothyroidism, whereas in Graves disease the antibody can have a thyroid-stimulating activity.
- *Iodine transporter:* Iodine transporter mediates the transport of iodide into the thyroid as the first step in thyroid hormone synthesis. Antibodies to the iodine transporter occur in a few patients and may have a role in hypothyroidism.

Many thyroid autoantibodies can fix complement. As a result, complement-dependent, antibody-mediated cytotoxicity may contribute to destruction of thyroid tissue in patients with Hashimoto thyroiditis. The importance of this action, however, in comparison with the T cell–mediated effects is uncertain.

Apoptosis mediated by the Fas-FasL system[19] has also been implicated in the pathogenesis of Hashimoto thyroiditis. FasL is constitutively expressed by both normal and Hashimoto thyroid epithelial cells. Interleukin IL-1β is abundant in Hashimoto glands and induces the expression of Fas on the cells: This triggers Fas-FasL interactions among the thyroid epithelial cells and activates the apoptotic cell death program.

MORPHOLOGY. The thyroid is diffusely enlarged, although more localized enlargement may be seen in some cases. The capsule is intact, and the gland is well demarcated from adjacent structures. The cut surface is pale, gray-tan, firm, and somewhat nodular: Microscopic examination reveals extensive infiltration of the parenchyma by a **mononuclear inflammatory infiltrate** containing small lymphocytes, plasma cells, and well-developed **germinal centers** (Fig. 26–8). The thyroid follicles are small and are lined in many areas by

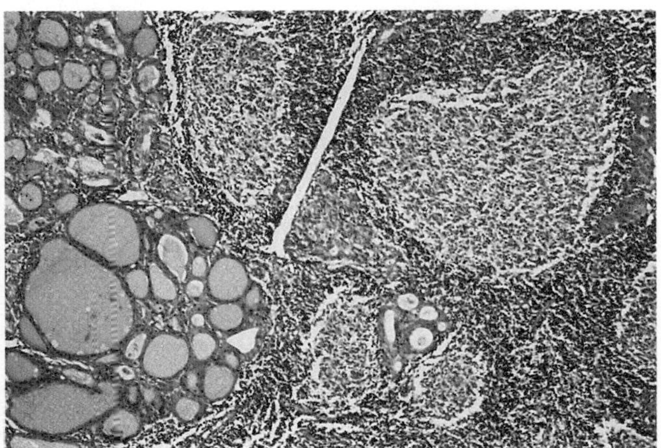

Figure 26–8

Photomicrograph of Hashimoto thyroiditis. The thyroid parenchyma contains a dense lymphocytic infiltrate with germinal centers. Residual thyroid follicles lined by deeply eosinophilic *Hürthle* cells are also seen.

epithelial cells with abundant eosinophilic, granular cytoplasm, termed **Hürthle** cells. Interstitial connective tissue is increased and may be abundant. The fibrosis does not extend beyond the capsule of the gland. A less common variant reveals a thyroid that is small and atrophic owing to more extensive fibrosis.

Clinical Course. Hashimoto thyroiditis comes to clinical attention as painless enlargement of the thyroid, *usually associated with some degree of hypothyroidism,* in a middle-aged woman. The enlargement of the gland is usually symmetric and diffuse, but in some cases it may be sufficiently localized to raise a suspicion of neoplasm. In the usual clinical course, hypothyroidism develops gradually. In some cases, however, it *may be preceded by transient thyrotoxicosis* caused by disruption of thyroid follicles, with secondary release of thyroid hormones. During this phase, free T_4 and T_3 levels are elevated, TSH is diminished, and radioactive iodine uptake is decreased. As hypothyroidism supervenes, T_4 and T_3 levels progressively fall, accompanied by a compensatory increase in TSH. Patients with Hashimoto disease are at increased risk for the development of B-cell lymphomas.

Subacute (Granulomatous) Thyroiditis

Subacute thyroiditis, which is also referred to as *granulomatous thyroiditis* or *DeQuervain thyroiditis,* occurs much less frequently than does Hashimoto disease. The disorder is most common between the ages of 30 and 50 and, similar to other forms of thyroiditis, affects women considerably more often than men (3 to 5 : 1).[20]

Pathogenesis. Subacute thyroiditis is believed to be caused by a *viral infection* or a postviral inflammatory process. The majority of patients have a history of an upper respiratory infection just before the onset of thyroiditis. The disease has a seasonal incidence with occurrences peaking in the summer, and clusters of cases have been reported in association with coxsackievirus, mumps, measles, adenovirus, and other viral illnesses. There is a fairly strong association with HLA-B35 in some ethnic groups.

One unifying pathogenic model suggests that the disorder results from a viral infection that provides an antigen, either viral or resulting from virus-induced host tissue damage. This antigen is presented by macrophages in the context of HLA-B35 and stimulates the formation of cytotoxic T lymphocytes, which then damage thyroid follicular cells. In contrast to autoimmune thyroid disease, the immune response is not self-perpetuating, so the process is limited.

MORPHOLOGY. The gland may be unilaterally or bilaterally enlarged and firm, with an intact capsule. It may be slightly adherent to surrounding structures. On cut section, the involved areas are firm and yellow-white and stand out from the more rubbery, normal brown thyroid substance. Histologically the changes are patchy and depend on the stage of the disease. Early in the active inflammatory phase, scattered follicles may be entirely disrupted and replaced by neutrophils forming microabscesses. Later the more characteristic features appear in the form of aggregations of lymphocytes, histiocytes, and plasma cells about collapsed and damaged thyroid follicles. **Multinucleate giant cells** enclose naked pools or fragments of colloid (Fig. 26–9), hence the designation *granulomatous thyroiditis.* In later stages of the disease, a chronic inflammatory infiltrate and fibrosis may replace the foci of injury. Different histologic stages are sometimes found in the same gland, suggesting waves of destruction over a period of time.[21]

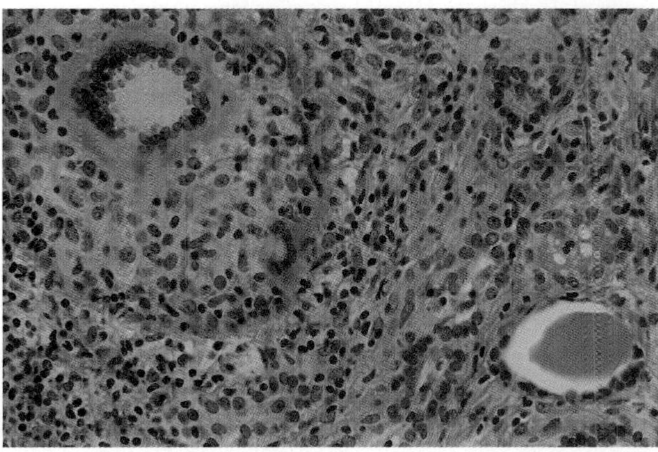

Figure 26–9

Subacute thyroiditis. The thyroid parenchyma contains a chronic inflammatory infiltrate with a multinucleate giant cell *(above left)* and a colloid follicle *(bottom right).*

Clinical Course. The presentation of subacute thyroiditis may be sudden or gradual. It is characterized by pain in the neck, which may radiate to the upper neck, jaw, throat, or ears, particularly when swallowing. Fever, fatigue, malaise, anorexia, and myalgia accompany a variable enlargement of the thyroid. The resultant thyroid inflammation and hyperthyroidism are transient, usually diminishing in 2 to 6 weeks, even if the patient is not treated. It may be followed by a period of transient, usually asymptomatic hypothyroidism lasting from 2 to 8 weeks, but recovery is virtually always complete.

The transient hyperthyroidism, as in other cases of thyroiditis, is due to disruption of thyroid follicles and release of excessive thyroid hormone. Nearly all patients have high serum T_4 and T_3 and low serum TSH levels. Radioactive iodine uptake is low because of suppression of TSH. The serum T_4 and T_3 levels are only modestly elevated. However, unlike in hyperthyroid states, radioactive iodine uptake is diminished. After recovery, generally in 6 to 8 weeks, normal thyroid function returns.

Subacute Lymphocytic (Painless) Thyroiditis

Subacute thyroiditis, which is also referred to as *painless thyroiditis, silent thyroiditis,* or *lymphocytic thyroiditis,* is an uncommon cause of hyperthyroidism. It usually comes to clinical attention because of mild hyperthyroidism or goitrous enlargement of the gland, or both. Although it may occur at any age, it is most often seen in middle-aged adults and is more common in women, especially during the postpartum period, than in men. The frequency of this form of thyroiditis varies considerably, from 1% to about 10% of cases of hyperthyroid patients.

The origin of this form of thyroiditis and its place in the spectrum of thyroiditis is not resolved. Subacute lymphocytic thyroiditis is associated with specific HLA haplotypes, notably HLA-DR3 and -DR5, suggesting an inherited susceptibility. It is considered by some as a variant form of Hashimoto thyroiditis, suggesting that it is part of the spectrum of thyroid autoimmune disease. The two disorders have elevated levels of antibodies to thyroglobulin and thyroid peroxidase, many patients have a family history of thyroid autoimmune disease, and some subsequently develop overt chronic autoimmune thyroiditis several years later. There is no evidence that points toward a particular viral or other agent.

MORPHOLOGY. Except for possible mild symmetric enlargement, the thyroid appears normal on gross inspection. Microscopic examination of the gland reveals a multifocal inflammatory infiltrate composed predominantly of small lymphocytes and patchy disruption and collapse of thyroid follicles. Plasma cells and germinal centers are not conspicuous and, when present, suggest the possibility of Hashimoto disease.

Clinical Course. The principal clinical manifestation of painless thyroiditis is hyperthyroidism. Symptoms usually develop over 1 to 2 weeks and last from 2 to 8 weeks before subsiding. The patient may have any of the common findings in hyperthyroidism (e.g., palpitations, tachycardia, tremor, weakness, and fatigue). The thyroid gland is not usually tender but is minimally and diffusely enlarged. Infiltrative ophthalmopathy and other manifestations of Graves disease (see later) are not present. Some patients have no signs or symptoms, and the disorder is incidentally detected during routine thyroid testing.

Laboratory findings during periods of thyrotoxicosis include *elevated levels of T_4 and T_3* and *depressed levels of TSH.* In contrast to Graves disease, in which radioactive iodine uptake is increased, the radioactive iodine uptake is *consistently decreased in thyrotoxicosis associated with thyroiditis.*

Other, less common forms of thyroiditis include *Reidel thyroiditis,* a rare disorder of unknown cause, characterized by extensive fibrosis involving the thyroid and contiguous neck structures. It may be associated with idiopathic fibrosis in other sites in the body, such as the retroperitoneum.

GRAVES DISEASE

Graves reported in 1835 on his observations of a disease characterized by "violent and long continued palpitations in females" associated with enlargement of the thyroid gland.[22] *Graves disease is the most common cause of endogenous hyperthyroidism.* It is characterized by a *triad* of clinical findings:

1. *Hyperthyroidism* owing to hyperfunctional, diffuse enlargement of the thyroid
2. Infiltrative *ophthalmopathy* with resultant exophthalmos
3. Localized, infiltrative *dermopathy* sometimes called *pretibial myxedema,* which is present in a minority of patients

Graves disease has a peak incidence between the ages of 20 and 40, with *women being affected up to seven times more commonly than men.* This is a very common disorder that is said to be present in 1.5 to 2.0% of women in the United States. Genetic factors are important in the causation of Graves disease. An increased incidence of Graves disease occurs among family members of affected patients, and the concordance rate in monozygotic twins is as high as 60%. The occurrence of this disorder is strongly associated with the presence of major histocompatibility haplotypes HLA-B8 and -DR3, although how these associations increase disease susceptibility is not clear.

Pathogenesis. Graves disease is an autoimmune disorder produced by autoantibodies to the TSH receptor. At least some of these autoantibodies appear to play a direct role in the pathogenesis of Graves disease:

- *Autoantibodies to the TSH receptor* or thyroid-stimulating immunoglobulin (TSI): Almost 50 years ago, serum from patients with Graves disease was found to contain a long-acting thyroid stimulator (LATS), so named because it stimulated thyroid function slower than TSH. LATS proved to be an IgG immunoglobulin that binds to the TSH receptor and stimulates adenylate cyclase activity, with resultant increased release of thyroid hormones. Almost all patients with Graves disease have detectable autoantibodies to the TSH receptor. As noted previously, this antibody is relatively specific for Graves disease, in contrast to thyroglobulin and thyroid peroxidase antibodies.

- *Thyroid growth-stimulating immunoglobulins:* Also directed against the TSH receptor, thyroid growth-stimulating immunoglobulins have been implicated in the proliferation of thyroid follicular epithelium.[23]
- *TSH-binding inhibitor immunoglobulins:* These anti-TSH receptor antibodies prevent TSH from binding normally to its receptor on thyroid epithelial cells. In so doing, some forms of TSH-binding inhibitor immunoglobulins mimic the action of TSH, resulting in the stimulation of thyroid epithelial cell activity, whereas other forms may actually *inhibit* thyroid cell function.

The trigger for the initiation of the autoimmune reaction in Graves disease remains uncertain, although two themes have emerged in the development of the disorder.

- *Molecular mimicry:* Molecular mimicry implies structural similarity between some infectious or other exogenous agent and human cell proteins, such that antibodies formed in response to the exogenous agent react with one or more of the thyroid proteins (Chapter 7). To date, however, there is no compelling evidence that infections or other exposures lead directly to autoimmune thyroid disease.[24]
- *Primary T-cell autoimmunity:* Thyroid epithelial cells can express specific types of MHC proteins, notably some related to the HLA-DR gene products. T cells recognize these MHC proteins, in association with processed peptides derived from thyroid antigens, and become activated. These activated T cells then cooperate with B cells, enhancing formation of a range of thyroid-specific autoantibodies from B cells, including antibodies against the TSH receptor. A causative role for T cells in Graves hyperthyroidism is supported by reports in which the antigen receptors of T cells isolated from thyroid tissue have been noted to be the products of a limited number of variable (V) gene families.[25] This finding suggests that the thyroid tissue of these patients attracts and expands T cells with particular types of antigen receptors, rather than nonspecifically. The limited T cell heterogeneity in Graves disease is similar to that seen in synovial tissue from patients with rheumatoid arthritis.

An autoimmune response also seems to play a role in the development of the infiltrative ophthalmopathy characteristic of Graves disease.[26] In Graves ophthalmopathy, the volume of both the retro-orbital connective tissue and the extraocular muscles is increased, owing to inflammation and the accumulation of extracellular matrix components, including proteoglycans and hyaluronic acid. These changes displace the eyeball forward and can interfere with the function of the extraocular muscles.

Both T cells and autoantibodies probably play a role in the ophthalmopathy. T cells (CD4+ or CD8+) are abundant in the inflammatory infiltrate, and these T cells react with the extraocular eye muscles. There are also reports of autoantibodies to retro-orbital tissues, particularly to extraocular muscle. The expression of the TSH receptor by extraocular muscle has stimulated speculation that this receptor may be the antigen involved in the pathogenesis of the ophthalmopathy.

In concluding this discussion of the role of autoimmunity in Graves disease, it must be emphasized that autoimmune disorders of the thyroid span a broad spectrum. In this spectrum, Graves disease, characterized by hyperfunction of the thyroid, lies at one extreme and Hashimoto disease, manifesting as hypothyroidism, occupies the other end. Antibodies against thyroidal antigens are common to both, but their specific epitopes are different, and hence their functional consequences differ. Sometimes the hyperthyroidism supervenes on preexisting Hashimoto thyroiditis, referred to as *hashitoxicosis.* As might be expected, other autoimmune diseases, such as systemic lupus erythematosus, pernicious anemia, type I diabetes, and Addison disease, occur with greater than chance frequency in patients with Graves disease.

MORPHOLOGY. The thyroid gland is usually symmetrically enlarged because of the presence of **diffuse hypertrophy and hyperplasia** of thyroid follicular epithelial cells. Increases in weight to over 80 gm are not uncommon. The gland is usually smooth and soft, and its capsule is intact. On cut section, the parenchyma has a soft, meaty appearance resembling normal muscle. Histologically the dominant feature is **too many cells.** The follicular epithelial cells in untreated cases are tall and more crowded than usual. This crowding often results in the formation of small papillae, which project into the follicular lumen and encroach on the colloid (Fig. 26–10). The colloid within the follicular lumen is pale, with scalloped margins. Such papillae lack fibrovascular cores, in contrast to those of papillary carcinoma (discussed later). On occasion, the papillae are sufficiently large to expand out and virtually fill the follicles. There is a striking increase in the amount of lymphoid tissue in the interfollicular stroma, and in some areas, large lymphoid aggregates consisting of autoreactive B cells are present.

Preoperative therapy alters the morphology of the thyroid in Graves disease. Preoperative administration of iodine causes involution of the epithelium and the accumulation of colloid by blocking thyroglobulin secretion. Alternatively, treatment with the antithyroid drug propylthiouracil, for example, exaggerates the epithelial hypertrophy and hyperplasia by stimulating TSH secretion. Thus, it is impossible from histologic examination to evaluate the functional activity of pretreated surgical specimens.

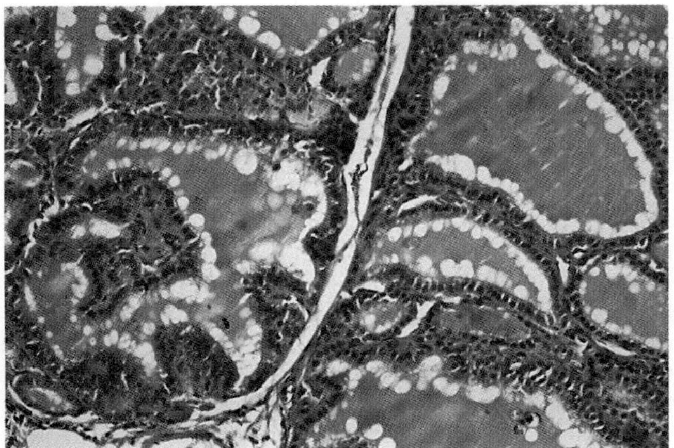

Figure 26–10

Photomicrograph of a diffusely hyperplastic gland in a case of Graves disease. The follicles are lined by tall, columnar epithelium. The crowded, enlarged epithelial cells project into the lumens of the follicles. These cells actively resorb the colloid in the centers of the follicles; resulting in the scalloped appearance of the edges of the colloid.

Changes in extrathyroidal tissue include generalized lymphoid hyperplasia. The heart may be hypertrophied, and ischemic changes may be present, particularly in patients with preexisting coronary artery disease. In patients with ophthalmopathy, the tissues of the orbit are edematous because of the presence of hydrophilic mucopolysaccharides. In addition, there is infiltration by lymphocytes and fibrosis. Orbital muscles are edematous initially but may undergo fibrosis late in the course of the disease.

Clinical Course. The clinical findings in Graves disease include changes referable to *thyrotoxicosis* as well as those associated uniquely with Graves disease—*diffuse hyperplasia of the thyroid, ophthalmopathy,* and *dermopathy.* The degree of thyrotoxicosis varies from case to case and may sometimes be less conspicuous than other manifestations of the disease. Diffuse enlargement of the thyroid is present in all cases of Graves disease. The *thyroid enlargement* may be accompanied by increased flow of blood through the hyperactive gland, often producing an audible bruit. The *ophthalmopathy* in the disorder is caused by a combination of the sympathetic overactivity that accompanies thyrotoxicosis and the deposition of matrix components behind the eyeball. These produce a characteristic wide, staring gaze and lid lag, and the eyes protrude abnormally. The extraocular muscles are often weak. The proptosis may persist or progress despite successful treatment of the thyrotoxicosis, sometimes resulting in corneal injury. The infiltrative dermopathy, or *pretibial myxedema,* is most common in the skin overlying the shins, where it presents as scaly thickening and induration of the skin. However, it is present only in a minority of patients. The skin lesions may be slightly pigmented papules or nodules and often have an orange-peel texture.

Laboratory findings in Graves disease include *elevated free T_4 and T_3* levels and *depressed TSH* levels. Because of ongoing stimulation of the thyroid follicles by thyroid-stimulating immunoglobulins, *radioactive iodine uptake is increased, and radioiodine scans show a diffuse uptake of iodine.*

Treatment of Graves disease consists of decreasing the symptoms of hyperthyroidism that are induced by increased β-adrenergic tone (e.g., tachycardia, palpitations, tremulousness, and anxiety), and measures aimed at decreasing thyroid hormone synthesis, such as the administration of thionamides (e.g., propylthiouracil), radioiodine ablation, and surgical intervention.[27]

DIFFUSE AND MULTINODULAR GOITER

Enlargement of the thyroid, or *goiter,* is the most common manifestation of thyroid disease. *Diffuse and multinodular goiters reflect impaired synthesis of thyroid hormone,* most often caused by dietary iodine deficiency. Impairment of thyroid hormone synthesis leads to a compensatory rise in the serum TSH level, which, in turn, causes hypertrophy and hyperplasia of thyroid follicular cells and, ultimately, gross enlargement of the thyroid gland. The degree of thyroid enlargement is proportional to the level and duration of thyroid hormone deficiency.

Diffuse Nontoxic (Simple) Goiter

Diffuse nontoxic (simple) goiter specifies a form of goiter that diffusely involves the entire gland without producing nodularity. Because the enlarged follicles are filled with colloid, the term *colloid goiter* has been applied to this condition. This disorder occurs in both an endemic and a sporadic distribution.

Endemic goiter occurs in geographical areas where the soil, water, and food supply contain only low levels of iodine. The term *endemic* is used when goiters are present in more than 10% of the population in a given region. Such conditions are particularly common in mountainous areas of the world, including the Alps, Andes, and Himalayas. The lack of iodine leads to decreased synthesis of thyroid hormone and a compensatory increase in TSH, leading to follicular cell hypertrophy and hyperplasia and goitrous enlargement. With increasing dietary iodine supplementation, the frequency and severity of endemic goiter have declined significantly.

Variations in the prevalence of endemic goiter in regions with similar levels of iodine deficiency point to the existence of other causative influences, particularly dietary substances, referred to as *goitrogens.* The ingestion of substances that interfere with thyroid hormone synthesis at some level, such as excessive calcium and vegetables belonging to the Brassica and Cruciferae families (e.g., cabbage, cauliflower, Brussels sprouts, turnips, and cassava), has been documented to be goitrogenic. Native populations subsisting on cassava root are particularly at risk. Cassava contains a thiocyanate that inhibits iodide transport within the thyroid, worsening any possible concurrent iodine deficiency.

Sporadic goiter occurs less frequently than does endemic goiter. There is a striking female preponderance and a peak incidence at puberty or in young adult life. Sporadic goiter can be caused by a number of conditions, including the ingestion of substances that interfere with thyroid hormone synthesis. In other instances, goiter may result from hereditary enzymatic defects that interfere with thyroid hormone synthesis, all transmitted as autosomal recessive conditions. The four major ones are (1) iodide transport defect, (2) organification defect, (3) dehalogenase defect, and (4) iodotyrosine coupling defect.[28] In most cases, however, the cause of sporadic goiter is not apparent.

MORPHOLOGY. Two stages can be identified in the evolution of diffuse nontoxic goiter, the **hyperplastic stage** and **colloid involution.** In the hyperplastic stage, the thyroid gland is diffuse and symmetrically enlarged, although the increase is modest, and the gland rarely exceeds 100 to 150 gm. The follicles are lined by crowded columnar cells, which may pile up and form projections similar to those seen in Graves disease. The accumulation is not uniform throughout the gland, and some follicles are hugely distended, whereas others remain small. If dietary iodine subsequently increases or if the demand for thyroid hormone decreases, the stimulated follicular epithelium involutes to form an enlarged, colloid-rich gland **(colloid goiter).**[29] In these cases, the cut surface of the thyroid is usually brown, somewhat glassy, and translucent. Histologically the follicular epithelium is flattened and cuboidal, and colloid is abundant during periods of involution.

Clinical Course. In children, sporadic goiter caused by a congenital biosynthetic defect may induce cretinism (see section on hypothyroidism and cretinism). By contrast, the clinical significance of nontoxic diffuse goiter in adults depends largely on its ability to achieve a state of euthyroidism, which is generally the rule. Rare patients are hyperthyroid, and the TSH level is almost invariably elevated, as it may be to a lesser extent in marginally euthyroid individuals. The goitrous enlargement may be plainly evident or nonvisible, even with the head raised.

Multinodular Goiter

With time, recurrent episodes of hyperplasia and involution combine to produce a more irregular enlargement of the thyroid, termed *multinodular goiter.* Virtually all long-standing simple goiters convert into multinodular goiters. They may be nontoxic or may induce thyrotoxicosis (toxic multinodular goiter). *Multinodular goiters produce the most extreme thyroid enlargements and are more frequently mistaken for neoplastic involvement than any other form of thyroid disease.* Because they derive from simple goiter, they occur in both sporadic and endemic forms, having the same female-to-male distribution and presumably the same origins but affecting older individuals because they are late complications.

The pathogenesis of nodules in multinodular goiters has many similarities to the molecular events involved in the formation of benign neoplasm of the thyroid.[30] Because normal thyroid cells are heterogeneous with respect to response to TSH and ability to replicate, the development of nodules may reflect clonal proliferation of cells having differing proliferative potentials. Thyroid cells with high intrinsic growth potential may be affected by the activation of oncogenes, generating autonomously growing cells that expand and form a nodule. Consistent with this model, somatic mutations have been identified in a subset of thyroid nodules, and many thyroid nodules, such as thyroid adenomas (see later), are clonal in origin. Both clonal and polyclonal nodules, however, coexist within the same nodular goiter.[31] The coexistence of both types of nodules suggests that different pathogenetic mechanisms may occur simultaneously or that monoclonal nodules may emerge secondarily from a polyclonal population because of a growth advantage. With such uneven follicular hyperplasia, generation of new follicles and uneven accumulation of colloid, tensions, and stresses are produced that lead to rupture of follicles and vessels followed by hemorrhages, scarring, and sometimes calcifications. The scarring adds to the tensions, and in this cyclical manner nodularity appears. Moreover, the preexistent stromal framework of the gland may more or less enclose areas of expanded parenchyma, contributing to the nodularity.[32]

MORPHOLOGY. Multinodular goiters are multilobulated, asymmetrically enlarged glands, which may achieve a weight of more than 2000 gm (Fig. 26–11). The pattern of enlargement is quite unpredictable and may involve one lobe far more than the other, producing lateral pressure on midline structures, such as the trachea and esophagus. In other instances, the goiter grows behind the sternum and clavicles to produce the so-called **intrathoracic** or **plunging goiter.** Occasionally, most of it is hidden behind the trachea and esophagus, yet in other instances, one nodule may so stand out as to impart the clinical appearance of a solitary nodule. On cut section, irregular nodules containing variable amounts of brown, gelatinous colloid are present. Regressive changes occur frequently, particularly in older lesions, and include areas of hemorrhage, fibrosis, calcification, and cystic change. The microscopic appearance includes colloid-rich follicles lined by flattened, inactive epithelium and areas of follicular epithelial hypertrophy and hyperplasia, accompanied by the degenerative changes noted previously.

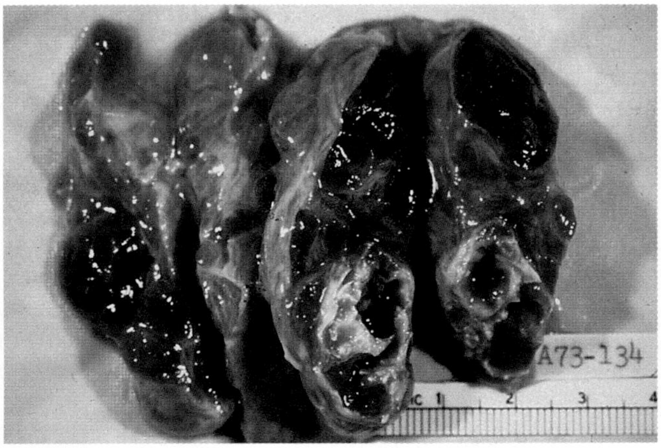

Figure 26–11

Gross photograph of nodular goiter. The gland is coarsely nodular and contains areas of fibrosis and cystic change.

Clinical Course. The dominant clinical features of goiter are those caused by the *mass effects* of the enlarged gland. In addition to the obvious cosmetic effects of a large neck mass, goiters may also cause airway obstruction, dysphagia, and compression of large vessels in the neck and upper thorax. Most patients are euthyroid, but in a substantial minority of patients, a hyperfunctioning nodule may develop within the goiter, resulting in *hyperthyroidism*—toxic multinodular goiter. This condition, known as *Plummer syndrome,* is not accompanied by the infiltrative ophthalmopathy and dermopathy of Graves disease. Less commonly, goiter may be associated with clinical evidence of *hypothyroidism.* Radioiodine uptake is uneven, reflecting varied levels of activity in different regions. Hyperfunctioning nodules concentrate radioiodine and appear "hot." Goiters are also of clinical significance because of their ability to mask or to mimic neoplastic diseases arising in the thyroid.

NEOPLASMS OF THE THYROID

The solitary thyroid nodule is a palpably discrete swelling within an otherwise apparently normal thyroid gland. The estimated incidence of solitary palpable nodules in the adult population of the United States is about 2 to 4%, although it is significantly higher in endemic goitrous regions. Single nodules are about four times more common in women than in men. The incidence of thyroid nodules increases throughout life.

From a clinical standpoint, the possibility of neoplastic disease is of major concern in patients who present with thyroid nodules. Fortunately the overwhelming majority of solitary nodules of the thyroid prove to be benign lesions, either follicular adenomas or localized, non-neoplastic conditions (e.g., nodular hyperplasia, simple cysts, or foci of thyroiditis). When such nodules prove to be neoplastic, in well over 90% of instances, they are adenomas. Carcinomas of the thyroid, in contrast, are uncommon, accounting for well under 1% of solitary thyroid nodules and representing about 15,000 new cancer cases each year. Moreover, as seen subsequently, most are indolent, permitting a 90% survival at 20 years. Several clinical criteria may provide a clue to the nature of a given thyroid nodule:

- *Solitary nodules,* in general, are more likely to be neoplastic than are multiple nodules.
- *Nodules in younger patients* are more likely to be neoplastic than are those in older patients.
- *Nodules in males* are more likely to be neoplastic than are those in females.
- A history of *radiation* treatment to the head and neck region is associated with an increased incidence of thyroid malignancy.
- Nodules that take up radioactive iodine in imaging studies (*hot* nodules) are more likely to be benign than malignant.

Such general trends and statistics, however, are of little significance in the evaluation of a given patient, in whom the timely recognition of a malignancy, however uncommon, can be life-saving. Ultimately, it is the morphologic evaluation of a given thyroid nodule, in the form of fine-needle aspiration biopsy and histologic study of surgically resected thyroid parenchyma, that provides the most definitive information about its nature. Using this diagnostic modality, false-positive results are uncommon.[33] In the following sections, we consider the major thyroid neoplasms, including adenoma and carcinoma in its various forms.

Adenomas

Adenomas of the thyroid are discrete, solitary masses. With rare exception, they all are derived from follicular epithelium and so might all be called *follicular adenomas.* They can be classified according to the size or presence of follicles and the type and degree of cellularity. Simple colloid (macrofollicular) adenomas, the most common form, closely resemble normal thyroid tissue. The others recapitulate stages in the embryogenesis of the normal thyroid and share architectural features with follicular carcinoma. There is little virtue in these classifications because mixed patterns are common, and ultimately all have the same clinical and biologic significance. Clinically, they may be difficult to distinguish, on one hand, from foci of follicular hyperplasia or, on the other hand, from the less common follicular carcinomas. Numerous studies have made it clear that adenomas are not forerunners of cancer except in the exceptional instance.

Pathogenesis. Important in the pathogenesis of thyroid adenomas is the function of the *TSH receptor,* which is a member of the seven transmembrane family of G protein–coupled receptors.[34] The TSH receptor preferentially couples to the α subunit of the stimulating guanine nucleotide binding protein Gs, which, in turn, activates adenylate cyclase. Increases in the intracellular levels of cAMP, a second messenger, activate genes that control the production of thyroid hormone and the proliferation of thyroid epithelial cells.

Somatic mutations in some of the components of this signaling system cause chronic stimulation of the cAMP pathway, generating cells that acquire a growth advantage. This results in clonal expansion of specific epithelial cells, leading to the formation of autonomously functioning monoclonal thyroid adenomas. Somatic mutations have been identified in Gsα in 12 to 38% of thyroid adenomas. These mutations result in constitutive activation of the cAMP cascade by mimicking an exaggerated TSH stimulation of thyroid follicular cells. Recall that mutations in this signal transduction component were first noted in pituitary somatotroph adenomas, discussed earlier. A series of constitutively activating mutations have also been identified in the thyrotropin receptor. These structural changes also increase thyrotropin-independent cAMP production. Overall, mutations leading to constitutive activation of the cAMP cascade appear to be the cause of a large proportion (50 to 75%) of autonomously functioning thyroid adenomas.

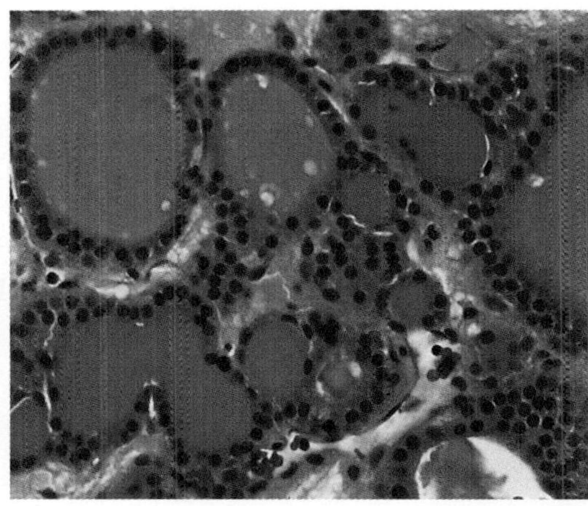

Figure 26–13

Photomicrograph of a follicular adenoma. Well-differentiated follicles resemble normal thyroid parenchyma.

MORPHOLOGY. The typical thyroid adenoma is a solitary, spherical, encapsulated lesion that is well demarcated from the surrounding thyroid parenchyma (Fig. 26–12). Follicular adenomas average about 3 cm in diameter, but some are smaller and others are much larger (up to 10 cm in diameter). In freshly resected specimens, the adenoma bulges from the cut surface and compresses the adjacent thyroid. The color ranges from gray-white to red-brown, depending on the cellularity of the adenoma and its colloid content. Areas of hemorrhage, fibrosis, calcification, and cystic change similar to those encountered in multinodular goiters are common, particularly within larger lesions. The neoplastic cells are demarcated from the adjacent parenchyma by a well-defined, intact capsule. Careful evaluation of the integrity of the capsule is important in the distinction of follicular adenomas from well-differentiated follicular carcinomas.

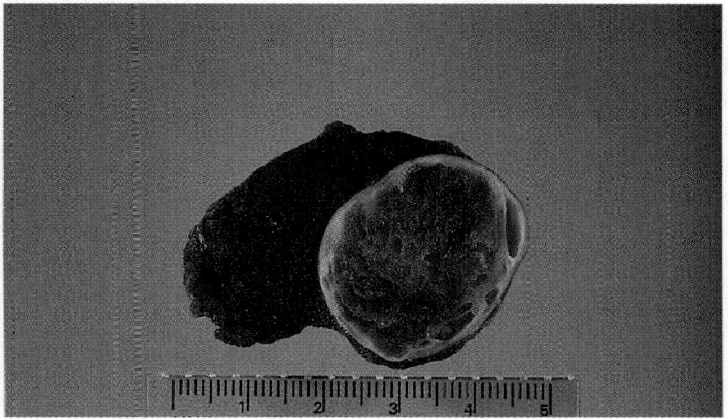

Figure 26–12

Follicular adenoma of the thyroid. A solitary, well-circumscribed nodule is seen.

Microscopically the constituent cells often form uniform-appearing follicles that contain colloid (Fig. 26–13). Various histologic subtypes of adenomas are recognized, based on the degree of follicle formation and the colloid content of the follicles: macrofollicular (simple colloid), microfollicular (fetal), embryonal (trabecular), Hürthle cell (oxyphil, oncocytic) adenomas, atypical adenomas, and adenomas with papillae. **Colloid adenomas** are lesions with large colloid-filled follicles lined by flattened epithelial cells. **Fetal adenomas** have numerous small, well-developed follicles lined by flattened epithelial cells widely separated by an abundant loose myxoid stroma. Others have follicles of normal size lined by cuboidal cells with scant interfollicular connective tissue. **Trabecular adenomas** are composed of closely packed cells forming cords or trabeculae of cells with only here and there small abortive follicles. Cytologically the epithelial cells in all reveal little variation in cell and nuclear morphology. Infrequently, adenomas are composed of tightly packed spindle cells with some significant variation in cellular size and nuclear morphology. These have been variously called spindle cell adenomas or **atypical adenomas.** The term **atypical,** however, is generally reserved for follicular adenomas revealing some pleomorphism and variability in cell and nuclear size. This pleomorphism can be so marked that it verges on that seen in follicular carcinoma, to be described, and in all likelihood many atypical lesions represent well-differentiated follicular carcinomas. Another rare variant is the **Hürthle cell adenoma,** composed of large, eosinophilic, granular cells identical to those encountered in various non-neoplastic thyroidal lesions (e.g., Hashimoto thyroiditis) (Fig. 26–14). A final variation is the so-called **papillary adenoma** distinguished by papillary excrescences within large follicular or cystic spaces. The

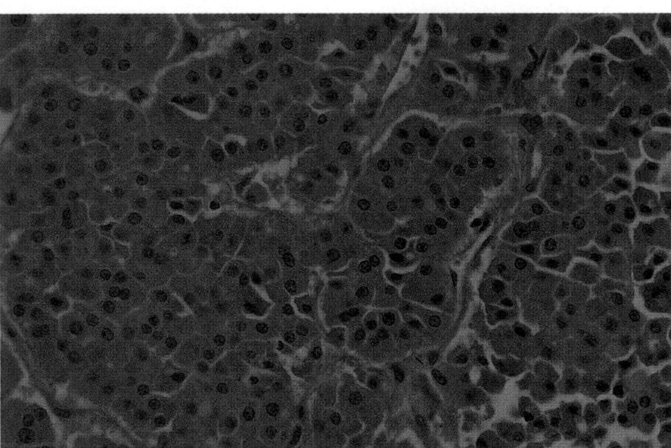

Figure 26–14

Photomicrograph of a Hürthle cell tumor. A high-power view showing that the tumor is composed of cells with abundant eosinophilic cytoplasm and small regular nuclei. (Courtesy of Dr. Mary Sunday, Brigham and Women's Hospital, Boston, MA.)

papillae may be large and branched and show some variation in cytologic morphology. Papillary change is not a typical feature of adenomas and, if present, should raise suspicion about the possibility of encapsulated papillary carcinoma (discussed later).

Clinical Features. Many thyroid adenomas present as a painless mass, often discovered during a routine physical examination. Larger masses may produce local symptoms, such as difficulty in swallowing.

Most adenomas take up less radioactive iodine less avidly than does normal thyroid parenchyma. On radionuclide scanning, therefore, adenomas appear as *cold* nodules relative to the adjacent thyroid when scanned. Up to 10% of cold nodules eventually prove to be malignant. By contrast, malignancy is rare in *hot* nodules. In a minority of cases, adenomas may be hyperfunctional, producing signs and symptoms of hyperthyroidism. In these adenomas, thyroid hormone is secreted autonomously, thereby suppressing thyrotropin secretion, so that the extranodular tissue becomes quiescent. On radionucleotide imaging of the hyperfunctioning adenoma, it appears hot, as compared with the paranodular thyroid tissue, which is deprived of thyrotropin stimulation. Although theoretically autonomous, an adenoma occasionally has some dependence on TSH and can be induced to regress by the administration of thyroid hormones, which suppress TSH secretion.

Additional techniques used in the preoperative evaluation of suspected adenomas are ultrasonography and fine needle aspiration biopsy. Suspected adenomas of the thyroid are usually removed surgically, with the definitive diagnosis of adenoma based on careful histologic examination of the resected specimen. Current evidence suggests that thyroid carcinomas arise de novo and that malignant transformation of adenomas does not occur.

Other Benign Tumors

Solitary nodules of the thyroid gland may also prove to be cysts.[33] The great preponderance of these lesions represent cystic degeneration of a follicular adenoma; the remainder probably arise in multinodular goiters. They are often filled with a brown, turbid fluid containing blood, hemosiderin pigment, and cell debris. Additional benign rarities include dermoid cysts, lipomas, hemangiomas, and teratomas (seen mainly in infants).

Carcinomas

Carcinomas of the thyroid are relatively uncommon in the United States, accounting for about 1.5% of all cancers. Most cases occur in adults, although some forms, particularly papillary carcinomas, may present in childhood.[35] A female predominance has been noted among patients developing thyroid carcinoma in the early and middle adult years, likely related to the expression of estrogen receptors on neoplastic thyroid epithelium. In contrast, cases presenting in childhood and late adult life are distributed equally among males and females. Most thyroid carcinomas are well-differentiated lesions. The major subtypes of thyroid carcinoma and their relative frequencies include

- Papillary carcinoma (75 to 85% of cases)
- Follicular carcinoma (10 to 20% of cases)
- Medullary carcinoma (5% of cases)
- Anaplastic carcinoma (<5% of cases)

Because of the unique clinical and biologic features associated with each variant of thyroid carcinoma, these subtypes are described separately.

Pathogenesis. The major risk factor predisposing to thyroid cancer is exposure to *ionizing radiation,* particularly during the first two decades of life.[36] In the past, radiation therapy was liberally employed in the treatment of a number of head and neck lesions in infants and children, including reactive tonsillar enlargement, acne, and tinea capitis. Up to 9% of people receiving such treatment during childhood have subsequently developed thyroid malignancies, usually several decades after exposure. The importance of radiation as a risk factor for thyroid carcinoma was demonstrated by the increased incidence of papillary thyroid carcinomas in children in the Marshall Islands after atomic bomb testing and, more recently, by the dramatic rise in the incidence of pediatric thyroid carcinoma among children exposed to ionizing radiation after the Chernobyl nuclear disaster in the Ukraine in 1986. More than 100 cases of pediatric thyroid carcinoma were observed in this region of Belorussia between the time of the incident and the present, a number far in excess of the usual incidence for this area.

Certain thyroid diseases such as nodular goiter and autoimmune thyroid disease (Hashimoto thyroiditis) have been implicated as predisposing factors.[35] As noted previously, there is little evidence that follicular adenomas progress to carcinoma.

The activation or mutation of certain *oncogenes* is important in the development of some thyroid carcinomas. Perhaps the most notable is the *RET protooncogene, which plays a role in both papillary and medullary thyroid carcinomas* (Chapter 8).[37] The RET protooncogene encodes a tyrosine kinase receptor that is not normally expressed by thyroid follicular cells. Two different mutational mechanisms have been implicated in the genesis of these tumors. In many papillary thyroid carcinomas, especially those occurring after irradiation, *rearrangements* of chromosome 10 place the tyrosine kinase portion of the RET protooncogene under the transcriptional control of a regulatory region (promoter) of a gene that is constitutively expressed by thyroid epithelial cells. In these alterations, the normal control sequences for RET and the sequences encoding the extracellular domain are lost. This results in a gene, which has been designated the *papillary thyroid carcinoma oncogene* (RET/PTC), that expresses the tyrosine kinase portion of receptor at a high level in the affected cells. This constitutively activated gene provides the thyroid cells with an unregulated growth signal.

The RET protooncogene also plays a role in the genesis of *medullary thyroid carcinomas.* This tumor arises in the thyroid parafollicular cells and is discussed in more detail later. Structural analysis of the RET gene in patients with hereditary medullary thyroid carcinoma reveals *germline point mutations* that affect residues in the cysteine-rich extracellular and in the intracellular tyrosine kinase domains. These mutations thus constitutively activate the receptor and, because the RET gene is normally expressed in the parafollicular cells, they undergo neoplastic transformation. The RET gene is mutated in 95% of families with *MEN-2,* a heritable disorder that involves a triad of medullary thyroid carcinoma, pheochromocytoma, and hyperparathyroidism (see later).

Activating point mutations in RAS genes are found with a similar frequency in thyroid adenomas and carcinomas, suggesting that these alterations represent an early event in thyroid tumorigenesis.[38] In contrast, inactivating point mutations in the *p53* tumor-suppressor gene are rare in well-differentiated thyroid carcinomas but common in those with anaplastic (undifferentiated) tumors.[39]

PAPILLARY CARCINOMA

Papillary carcinomas are the most common form of thyroid cancer. They occur at any age but occur most often in the twenties to forties and account for the vast majority of thyroid carcinomas associated with previous exposure to ionizing radiation.[36] A high incidence of papillary carcinomas has been found in patients with Gardner syndrome (familial adenomatous polyposis coli) and Cowden disease (familial goiter and skin hamartomas).

MORPHOLOGY. Papillary carcinomas are solitary or multifocal lesions within the thyroid. Some tumors may be well circumscribed and even encapsulated, whereas others may infiltrate the adjacent parenchyma with ill-defined margins. The lesions may contain areas of fibrosis and calcification and are often cystic. On the cut surface, they may appear granular and may sometimes contain grossly discernible papillary foci. The definitive diagnosis of papillary carcinoma can be made only after microscopic examination. The characteristic hallmarks of papillary neoplasms include the following:

- Papillary carcinomas can reveal branching **papillae** having a fibrovascular stalk covered by a single to multiple layers of cuboidal epithelial cells. In most neoplasms, the epithelium covering the papillae comprises well-differentiated, uniform, orderly, cuboidal cells, but at the other extreme are those with fairly anaplastic epithelium showing considerable variation in cell and nuclear morphology. When present, the papillae of papillary carcinoma differ from those seen in areas of hyperplasia. In contrast to hyperplastic papillary lesions, the neoplastic papillae have dense fibrovascular cores.
- The nuclei of papillary carcinoma cells contain finely dispersed chromatin, which imparts an **optically clear** or **empty** appearance, giving rise to the designation **ground-glass** or **Orphan Annie** nuclei (Fig. 26–15). As currently used, the diagnosis of **papillary carcinoma** is based on nuclear features rather than a papillary architecture.
- Eosinophilic intranuclear inclusions or grooves representing invaginations of cytoplasm are present.
- Concentrically calcified structures termed **psammoma bodies** are often present within

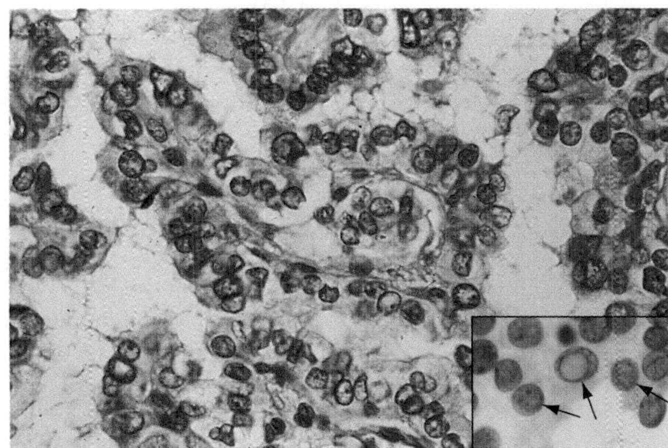

Figure 26–15 ■

Papillary carcinoma of the thyroid. This particular example contains well-formed papillae lined by cells with characteristic empty-appearing nuclei, sometimes termed *Orphan Annie eye* nuclei. *Inset* shows cells obtained by fine-needle aspiration of a papillary carcinoma. Characteristic intranuclear *inclusions* (*arrows*) are visible in cytologic preparations. (Courtesy of Dr. Edmund Cibas, Brigham & Women's Hospital, Boston.)

the lesion, usually within the cores of papillae. These structures are almost never found in follicular and medullary carcinomas and so, when present, are diagnostic of a papillary carcinoma. It is said that whenever a psammoma body is found within a lymph node or perithyroidal tissues, a **hidden** papillary carcinoma must be suspected.

There are variant forms of papillary carcinoma that are important to recognize because, despite their differences, they behave like the more common lesions.[40] The **encapsulated variant** constitutes about 10% of all papillary neoplasms. It is usually confined to the thyroid gland, is well encapsulated, rarely presents with vascular or lymph node dissemination, and so in most cases has an excellent prognosis. Such lesions in the past have been called **papillary adenoma.**

The **follicular variant** has the characteristic nuclei of the papillary carcinoma but has an almost totally follicular architecture. Similar to most papillary cancers, they are unencapsulated and infiltrative. The true follicular carcinoma is usually encapsulated, frequently shows vascular or focal capsular invasion, and has a less favorable prognosis.

A **tall cell variant** is marked by tall columnar cells with intensely eosinophilic cytoplasm covering the papillary structures and lining the follicular patterns. These tumors tend to be large with prominent vascular invasion and often are associated with local and distant metastases. They tend to occur in older individuals and have the poorest prognosis of all forms of papillary carcinoma. Because of their eosinophilic cytoplasm, they may be misdiagnosed as Hürthle cell tumors.

Foci of lymphatic invasion by tumor are often present, but involvement of blood vessels is relatively uncommon, particularly in smaller lesions. Metastases to adjacent cervical lymph nodes are estimated to occur in about half of cases.

Clinical Course. Most papillary carcinomas present as asymptomatic thyroid nodules, but the first manifestation may be a mass in a cervical lymph node. The carcinoma, which is usually a single nodule, moves freely during swallowing and is not distinguishable from a benign nodule. Hoarseness, dysphagia, cough, or dyspnea suggests advanced disease.

A variety of diagnostic tests have been employed to separate benign from malignant thyroid nodules, including radionuclide scanning and fine-needle aspiration. Most papillary lesions are *cold* masses on scintiscans. Improvements in cytologic analysis have made fine-needle aspiration cytology the best test for distinguishing between benign and malignant nodules.

The prognosis of a patient with thyroid cancer is related to the type of tumor. The overall 10-year survival rates are 98% for papillary and 92% for follicular carcinomas. Five per cent to 20% of patients have local or regional occurrences, and 10 to 15% have distant metastases. In general, the prognosis is less favorable among elderly patients, patients with invasion of extrathyroidal tissues, and patients with distant metastases.

FOLLICULAR CARCINOMA

Follicular carcinomas are the second most common form of thyroid cancer, accounting for 10 to 20% of all thyroid cancers. As a general rule, they tend to present in women at an older age than do papillary carcinomas, with a peak incidence in the forties and fifties. The incidence of follicular carcinoma is increased in areas of dietary iodine deficiency, suggesting that, in some cases, nodular goiter may predispose to the development of the neoplasm. There is no compelling evidence that follicular carcinomas arise from preexisting adenomas.[35,36]

MORPHOLOGY. Follicular carcinomas are single nodules that may be well circumscribed or infiltrative (Fig. 26–16) Sharply demarcated lesions may be exceedingly difficult to distinguish from follicular adenomas by gross examination. Larger lesions may penetrate the capsule and infiltrate well beyond the thyroid capsule into the adjacent neck.

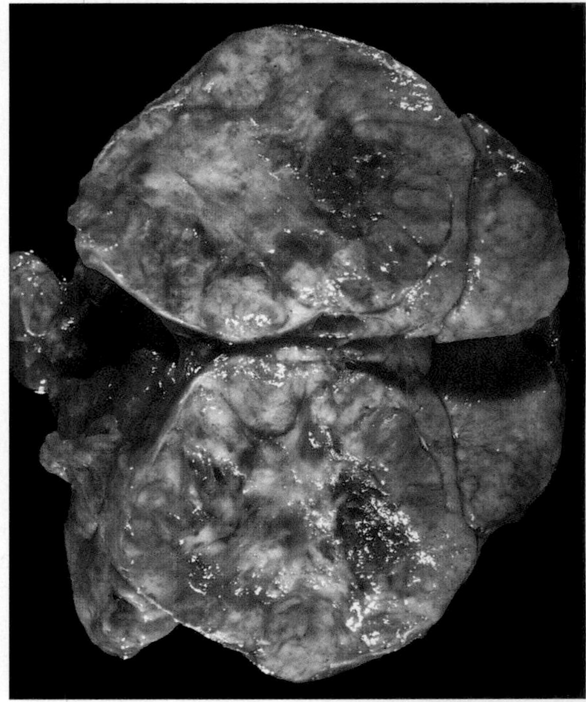

Figure 26–16

Follicular carcinoma. Cut surface of a follicular carcinoma with substantial replacement of the lobe of the thyroid. The tumor has a light-tan appearance and contains small foci of hemorrhage.

They are gray to tan to pink on cut section and, on occasion, are somewhat translucent when large, colloid-filled follicles are present. Degenerative changes, such as central fibrosis and foci of calcification, are often found.

Microscopically, most follicular carcinomas are composed of fairly uniform cells forming small follicles containing colloid, quite reminiscent of normal thyroid (Fig. 26–17). In other cases, follicular differentiation may be less apparent. Occasional tumors are dominated by cells with abundant granular, eosinophilic cytoplasm (Hürthle cells). Whatever the pattern, the nuclei lack the features typical of papillary carcinoma, and psammoma bodies are not present. It is important to note the absence of these details because some papillary carcinomas may appear almost entirely follicular. Follicular lesions in which the nuclear features are typical of papillary carcinomas should be treated as papillary cancers. Extensive invasion of adjacent thyroid parenchyma makes the diagnosis of carcinoma obvious. In other cases, however, invasion may be limited to microscopic foci of capsular or vascular invasion. Such lesions may require extensive histologic sampling before they can be distinguished from follicular adenomas. When both capsule and blood vessels are invaded, distant metastases are present in about half of the cases. With more evident extension through and beyond the capsule as well as vascular invasion, the rate of metastases approaches 75%.

Less commonly, follicular carcinomas present trabecular architecture or solid sheets of polygonal to spindled cells, but abortive follicles can generally be found. The cells in these variants may be somewhat more variable in size and shape, but marked anaplasia is unusual. An additional variant is composed mostly or entirely of eosinophilic oxyphilic cells, which have abundant cytoplasm and relatively uniform, round-to-oval nuclei, closely simulating Hürthle cells. Despite the cytologic variability, all patterns of follicular carcinoma have the same biologic behavior.

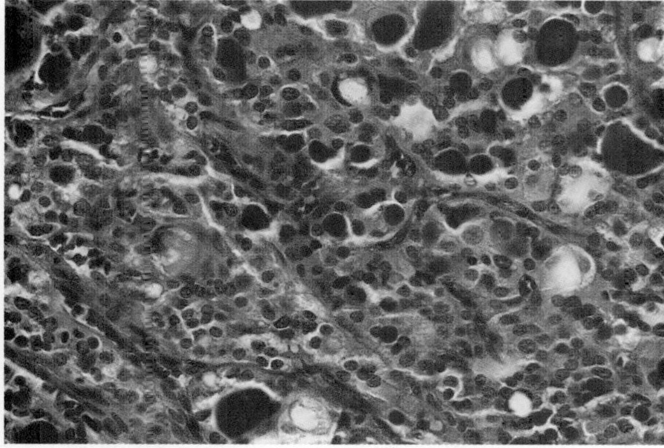

Figure 26–17

Follicular carcinoma of the thyroid. A few of the glandular lumens contain recognizable colloid.

Clinical Course. Follicular carcinomas present as slowly enlarging painless nodules. Most frequently, they are *cold* nodules on scintigrams, although in rare cases, the better-differentiated lesions may be hyperfunctional, take up radioactive iodine, and appear *warm* on scintiscan. Follicular carcinomas have little propensity for invading lymphatics, and therefore regional lymph nodes are rarely involved, but vascular invasion is common, with spread to bone, lungs, liver, and elsewhere. The prognosis depends on the size of the primary, the presence or absence of capsular and vascular invasion, and to some extent the level of anaplasia in the lesion. Follicular carcinomas are treated with lobectomy or subtotal thyroidectomy. Because better-differentiated lesions may be stimulated by TSH, patients are usually treated with thyroid hormone after surgery to suppress endogenous TSH. Widely invasive tumors are treated with total thyroidectomy followed by the administration of radioactive iodine. Well-differentiated metastases may take up radioactive iodine, which can be used to identify and ablate such lesions.

MEDULLARY CARCINOMA

Medullary carcinomas of the thyroid are *neuroendocrine* neoplasms derived from the parafollicular cells, or C cells, of the thyroid. The cells of medullary carcinomas, similar to normal C cells, secrete *calcitonin,* the measurement of which plays an important role in the diagnosis and postoperative follow-up of patients.[42] In some instances, the tumor cells elaborate other polypeptide hormones, such as carcinoembryonic antigen (CEA), somatostatin, serotonin, and vasoactive intestinal peptide (VIP). The tumors arise sporadically in about 80% of cases. The remainder occur in the setting of MEN syndrome IIA or IIB (see later) or as familial tumors without an associated MEN syndrome. Germ line mutations in the *RET protooncogene* play an important role in the development of medullary carcinomas associated with the MEN IIA syndrome. More recently, RET protooncogene mutations have been identified in some sporadic cases as well. This oncogene is also involved in the origin of papillary thyroid carcinoma. Cases associated with MEN II occur in younger patients and may even arise during childhood. In contrast, sporadic medullary carcinomas as well as some familial tumors are lesions of adulthood, with a peak incidence in the forties and fifties.

MORPHOLOGY. Medullary carcinomas can arise as a solitary nodule or may present as multiple lesions involving both lobes of the thyroid. The sporadic neoplasms tend to originate in one lobe

(Fig. 26–18). In contrast, bilaterality and **multicentricity** are particularly common in familial cases. Larger lesions often contain areas of necrosis and hemorrhage and may extend through the capsule of the thyroid. The tumor tissue in both types of lesions is firm, pale gray-to-tan, and infiltrative. There may be foci of hemorrhage and necrosis in the larger lesions.

Microscopically, medullary carcinomas are composed of polygonal to spindle-shaped cells, which may form nests, trabeculae, and even follicles.[43] Small, more anaplastic cells are present in some tumors and may be the predominant cell type. Acellular **amyloid deposits,** derived from altered calcitonin molecules, are present in the adjacent stroma in many cases (Fig. 26–19). Calcitonin is readily demonstrable within the cytoplasm of the tumor cells by immunohistochemical methods. Electron microscopy reveals variable numbers of membrane-bound electron-dense granules within the cytoplasm of the neoplastic cells (Fig. 26–20). Multiple foci of **C cell hyperplasia** are present in the surrounding thyroid parenchyma in many familial cases but are usually absent in sporadic lesions.

Clinical Course. Sporadic cases of medullary carcinoma come to medical attention most often as a mass in the neck, sometimes associated with local effects such as dysphagia or hoarseness. In some instances, the initial manifestations are those of a paraneoplastic syndrome, caused by the secretion of a peptide hormone (e.g., diarrhea owing

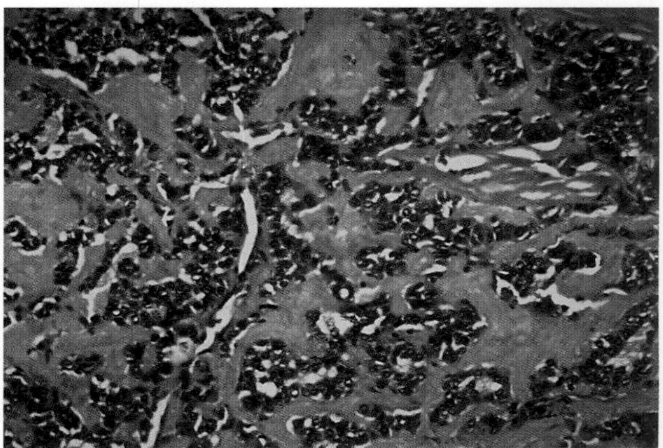

Figure 26–19

Medullary carcinoma of the thyroid. These tumors typically contain amyloid, visible here as homogeneous extracellular material, derived from calcitonin molecules secreted by the neoplastic cells.

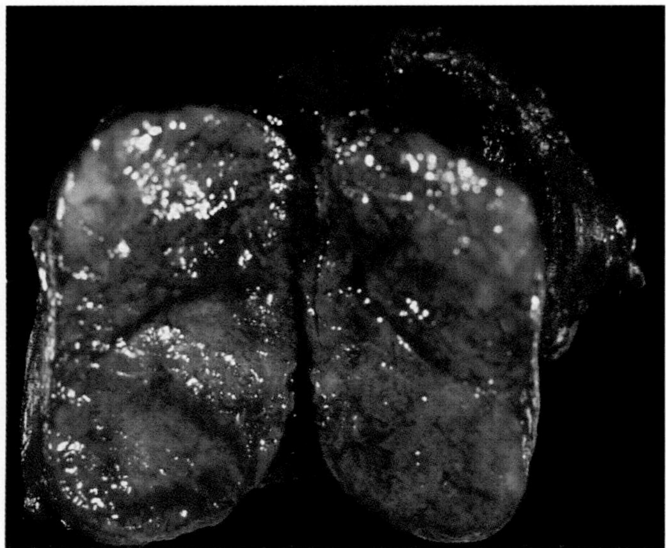

Figure 26–18

Medullary carcinoma of thyroid. These tumors typically show a solid pattern of growth and do not have connective tissue capsules. (Courtesy of Dr. Joseph Corson, Brigham and Women's Hospital, Boston, MA.)

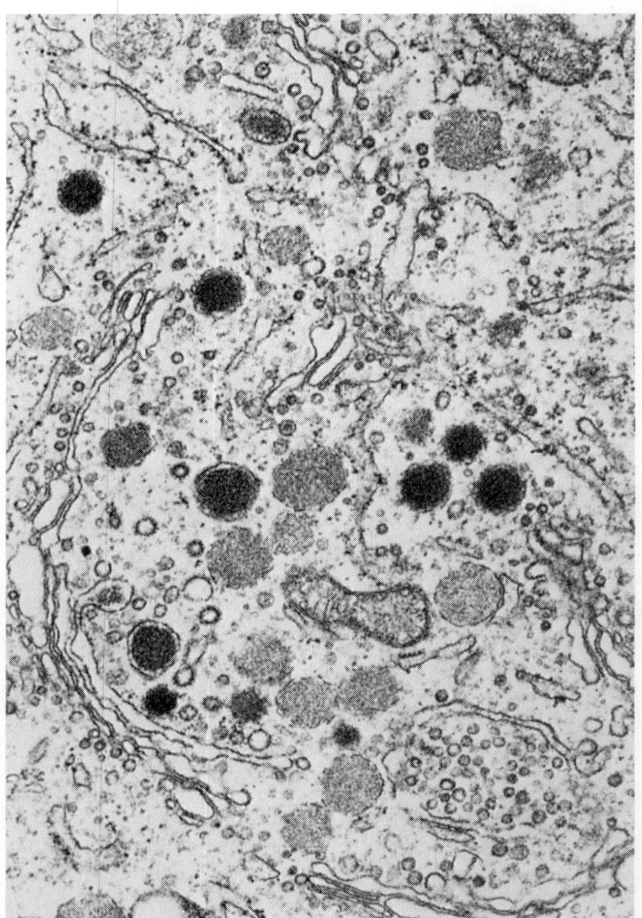

Figure 26–20

Electron micrograph of medullary thyroid carcinoma. These cells contain membrane-bound secretory granules that are the sites of storage of calcitonin and other peptides (30,000×).

to the secretion of VIP). In contrast, in the familial setting, medullary carcinoma is usually asymptomatic and is discovered by screening of relatives of patients with medullary carcinoma for elevated calcitonin levels. Sporadic medullary carcinomas and those arising in patients with MEN IIB are aggressive lesions, with a propensity to metastasize via the bloodstream and 5-year survival rates of about 50%. Familial medullary carcinomas not associated with MEN, in contrast, are often fairly indolent lesions.

ANAPLASTIC CARCINOMA

Anaplastic carcinomas of the thyroid are undifferentiated tumors of the thyroid follicular epithelium. In striking contrast to the differentiated thyroid carcinomas, anaplastic carcinomas are aggressive tumors, with a mortality approaching 100%.[44] These tumors account for less than 5% of all thyroid cancers. Patients with anaplastic carcinoma are older than those with other types of thyroid cancer, with a mean age of 65 years. About half of the patients have a history of multinodular goiter, whereas 20% of the patients with these tumors have a history of differentiated carcinoma; another 20 to 30% have a concurrent differentiated thyroid tumor, frequently a papillary carcinoma. These findings have led to speculation that anaplastic carcinoma develops from more differentiated tumors as a result of one or more genetic changes, possibly the loss of the *p53* tumor-suppressor gene.[45]

MORPHOLOGY. Microscopically, these neoplasms are composed of highly anaplastic cells, which may take one of three histologic patterns: (1) large, pleomorphic giant cells; (2) spindle cells with a sarcomatous appearance; and (3) small anaplastic cells resembling those seen in small cell carcinomas arising in other sites. A significant number of such small cell tumors ultimately prove to be medullary carcinomas (discussed previously). Small cell carcinomas must also be distinguished from malignant lymphomas, which may also occur in the thyroid but have a much better prognosis. Foci of papillary or follicular differentiation may be present in some tumors, suggesting origin from a better-differentiated carcinoma.

Clinical Course. Anaplastic carcinomas present as a rapidly enlarging bulky neck mass. In most cases, the disease has already spread beyond the thyroid capsule into adjacent neck structures or metastasized to the lungs at the time of presentation. Compression and invasion symptoms, such as dyspnea, dysphagia, hoarseness, and cough, are common. There is no effective therapy for anaplastic thyroid carcinoma, and the disease is uniformly fatal. Although metastases to distant sites are common, in most cases death occurs in less than 1 year as a result of aggressive growth and compromise of vital structures in the neck.

CONGENITAL ANOMALIES

Thyroglossal duct or *cyst* is the most common clinically significant congenital anomaly. A persistent sinus tract may remain as a vestigial remnant of the tubular development of the thyroid gland. Parts of this tube may be obliterated, leaving small segments to form cysts. These occur at any age and may not become evident until adult life. Mucinous, clear secretions may collect within these cysts to form either spherical masses or fusiform swellings, rarely over 2 to 3 cm in diameter. These are present in the midline of the neck anterior to the trachea. Segments of the duct and cysts that occur high in the neck are lined by stratified squamous epithelium, which is essentially identical with that covering the posterior portion of the tongue in the region of the foramen cecum. Those anomalies that occur in the lower neck more proximal to the thyroid gland are lined by epithelium resembling the thyroidal acinar epithelium. Characteristically, subjacent to the lining epithelium, there is an intense lymphocytic infiltrate. Superimposed infection may convert these lesions into abscess cavities, and rarely they give rise to cancers.

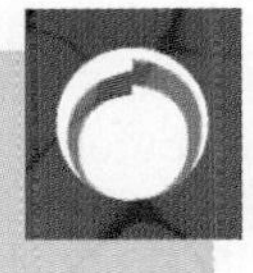

Parathyroid

PARATHYROID GLANDS

The *parathyroid glands* are derived from the developing pharyngeal pouches that also give rise to the thymus. The four glands normally lie in close proximity to the upper and lower poles of each thyroid lobe but may also be found anywhere along the pathway of descent of the pharyngeal pouches, including the carotid sheath, the thymus, and elsewhere in the anterior mediastinum. Of note, 10% of individuals have only two or three glands.

In the adult, the parathyroid is a yellow-brown, ovoid encapsulated nodule weighing approximately 35 to 40 mg. Most of the gland is composed of *chief cells*. The chief cells vary from light to dark pink with hematoxylin and eosin stains, depending on their glycogen content. They are polygonal; are 12 to 20 mm in diameter; and have central, round, uniform nuclei. In addition, they contain secretory granules of *parathyroid hormone (PTH)*. Sometimes, these cells have a *water clear* appearance owing to lakes of glycogen. *Oxyphil cells* and transitional oxyphils are found throughout the normal parathyroid either singly or in small clusters. They are slightly larger than the chief cells, have acidophilic cytoplasm, and are tightly packed with mitochondria. Glycogen granules are also present in these cells, but secretory granules are sparse or absent. In early infancy and childhood, the parathyroids are composed almost entirely of solid sheets of chief cells. The amount of stromal fat increases up to age 25, to reach a maximum of approximately 30% of the gland, and then it plateaus. The precise proportion of fat is determined largely by constitutional factors; fat individuals have fat glands, and vice versa.

The activity of the parathyroid glands is controlled by the level of free (ionized) calcium in the bloodstream, rather than by trophic hormones secreted by the hypothalamus and pituitary. Normally, decreased levels of free calcium stimulate the synthesis and secretion of *PTH.* Circulating PTH is an 84–amino acid linear polypeptide derived by sequential cleavage in the chief cell of a larger *pre-pro* form. Its biologic activity resides within the 34 residues at the amino terminus. Smaller nonfunctional fragments of the hormone, apparently lacking the critical amino-terminal domain, also circulate. These assume importance because, although they are biologically inert, they contain epitopes that react in certain radioimmunoassays for PTH.

The hormone binds specifically to a seven transmembrane receptor, which interacts with G proteins leading to the stimulation of adenylate cyclase and the generation of cAMP as well as to the activation of phospholipase C and the conversion of phosphatidylinositol diphosphate (PIP_2) to inositol trisphosphate (IP_3) and diacylglycerol (DAG).[46] The metabolic functions of PTH in supporting serum calcium level can be summarized as follows:

- PTH activates osteoclasts, thereby mobilizing calcium from bone.
- It increases the renal tubular reabsorption of calcium, thereby conserving free calcium.
- It increases the conversion of vitamin D to its active dihydroxy form in the kidneys.
- It increases urinary phosphate excretion, thereby lowering serum phosphate level.
- It augments gastrointestinal calcium absorption.

The net result of these activities is an increase in the level of free calcium, which, in turn, inhibits further PTH secretion in a classic feedback loop.

Hypercalcemia is one of a number of changes induced by elevated levels of PTH. As discussed in Chapter 8, hypercalcemia is a relatively common complication of malignancy, occurring with both solid tumors and hematologic malignancies, notably breast and lung cancers and multiple myeloma. Hypercalcemia of malignancy is due to increased bone resorption and subsequent release of calcium. It suffices here that there are two major mechanisms by which this can occur: (1) *osteolytic metastases and local release of cytokines,* and (2) *release of PTH-related protein (PTHrP).*[47]

- *Osteolytic metastases:* Tumor cells and infiltrating inflammatory cells release cytokines, which induce local osteolysis. TNF-α and IL-1 appear to be important in stimulating the differentiation of committed osteoclast precursors into mature cells. IL-6 is often produced by tumors and directly stimulates osteoblast production. Additionally, IL-6 enhances bone resorption mediated by PTHrP.
- *PTH-related protein:* The most frequent cause of hypercalcemia with nometastatic solid tumors is the release of PTHrP. This protein is immunologically distinct from PTH, yet is similar enough in structure to permit binding to identical receptors and simulation of second messengers. This accounts for the ability of PTHrP to induce most of the actions of PTH, including increases in bone resorption and inhibition of proximal tubule phosphate transport. In general, patients with PTHrP-induced hypercalcemia have advanced cancer and a poor prognosis.

Similar to the other endocrine organs, abnormalities of the parathyroids include both hyperfunction and hypofunction. *Tumors of the parathyroid glands, in contrast to thyroid tumors, usually come to attention because of excessive secretion of PTH, rather than because of mass effects.*

HYPERPARATHYROIDISM

Hyperparathyroidism occurs in two major forms, *primary* and *secondary,* and, less commonly, *tertiary* hyperparathyroidism. The first condition represents an autonomous, spontaneous overproduction of PTH, whereas the latter two conditions typically occur as secondary phenomena in patients with chronic renal insufficiency.

Primary Hyperparathyroidism

Primary hyperparathyroidism is one of the most common endocrine disorders, and it is an important cause of *hypercalcemia.* The frequency of the various parathyroid lesions underlying the hyperfunction is as follows:

- Adenoma—75 to 80%
- Primary hyperplasia (diffuse or nodular)—10 to 15%
- Parathyroid carcinoma—less than 5%

Primary hyperparathyroidism is usually a disease of adults and is more common in women than in men. The annual incidence is now estimated to be about 25 cases per 100,000 population in the United States and Europe.[48] Most cases occur in the fifties or later in life. A history of irradiation to the head and neck, on average 30 to 40 years before the development of hyperparathyroidism, can be obtained in some patients.

Studies have begun to provide a molecular understanding of the pathogenesis of primary hyperparathyroidism. In more than 95% of cases, the disorder is caused by sporadic parathyroid adenomas or sporadic hyperplasia. Some cases are caused by inherited syndromes, such as MEN I. The cells in the abnormal parathyroid tissue are usually monoclonal, including both adenomas and hyperplasias, suggesting that one important step in tumor development, i.e., mutation in a progenitor cell, has occurred in these lesions. Among the *sporadic adeno-*

mas, there are two notable tumor-specific (i.e., not germ line) chromosome defects that appear related to the clonal origin in some of these tumors.

- *Parathyroid adenoma 1 (PRAD 1):* PRAD 1 encodes cyclin D1, a major regulator of the cell cycle. An inversion on chromosome 11 results in relocation of the PRAD 1 protooncogene so that it is positioned adjacent to the 5′-PTH gene-regulatory sequences.[49] As a consequence of these changes, a regulatory element from the 5′-PTH gene directs overexpression of cyclin D1, forcing the cells to proliferate. Ten percent to 20% of adenomas have this defect.
- *Multiple endocrine neoplasia 1 (MEN 1):* Homozygous loss of a putative suppressor gene on chromosome 11q13 can be demonstrated in most familial cases of parathyroid adenoma. The *MEN 1 gene* was localized to this region of chromosome 11, and mutations in the gene were found in 14 of 15 kindreds with familial MEN I.[50] Significantly, about 20% of sporadic parathyroid tumors had a mutation in the MEN1 gene, suggesting that somatic mutation of the MEN1 gene contributes to parathyroid tumors not associated with the MEN I syndrome.[51]

Many of the parathyroid tumors examined to date do not have these defects. Furthermore, mutations similar to those in MEN IIA or IIB are not found in sporadic hyperparathyroidism, suggesting that other tumor suppressors may be involved.

MORPHOLOGY. The morphologic changes seen in primary hyperparathyroidism include those in the parathyroid glands as well as those in other organs affected by elevated levels of calcium. Parathyroid **adenomas** are almost always solitary and, similar to the normal parathyroids, may lie in close proximity to the thyroid gland, or in an ectopic site (e.g., the mediastinum). The typical parathyroid adenoma averages 0.5 to 5.0 gm; is a well-circumscribed, soft, tan nodule; and is invested by a delicate capsule (Fig. 26–21). In contrast to primary hyperplasia, the remaining glands are usually normal in size or somewhat shrunken because of feedback inhibition by elevations in serum calcium. Microscopically, parathyroid adenomas are often composed predominantly of fairly uniform, polygonal **chief** cells with small, centrally placed nuclei (Fig. 26–21). In most cases, at least a few nests of larger cells containing oxyphil cells or cells with more abundant clear cytoplasm are present as well. Follicles reminiscent of those seen in the thyroid are present in some cases. Mitotic figures are rare. A rim of compressed, non-neoplastic parathyroid tissue is often visible at the edge of the adenoma. In contrast to the normal parathyroid parenchyma, adipose tissue is inconspicuous within the adenoma.

Primary hyperplasia may occur sporadically or as a component of MEN syndrome I or IIA. Although classically all four glands are involved, frequently there is asymmetry with apparent sparing of one or two glands, making the distinction between hyperplasia and adenoma difficult. The combined weight of all glands rarely exceeds 1.0 gm and is often less. Microscopically the most common pattern seen is that of chief cell hyperplasia, which may involve the glands in a diffuse or multinodular pattern. Less commonly the constituent cells contain abundant water-clear cells. In many instances, there are islands of oxyphils and poorly developed, delicate fibrous strands may envelop the nodules. As in the case of adenomas, stromal fat is inconspicuous within the foci of hyperplasia.

Parathyroid carcinomas may be fairly circumscribed lesions that are difficult to distinguish from adenomas or from clearly invasive neoplasms. These tumors enlarge one parathyroid gland and

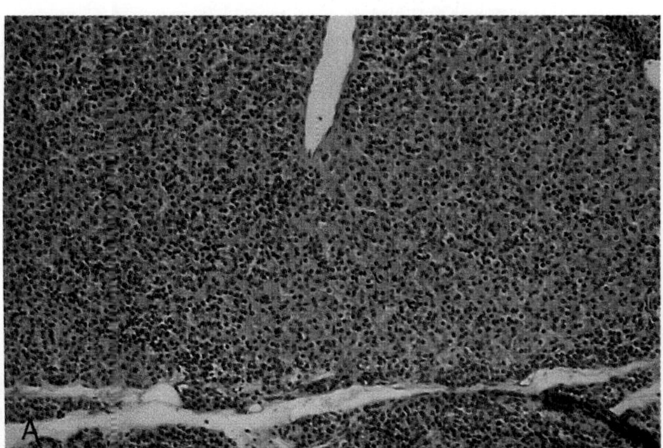

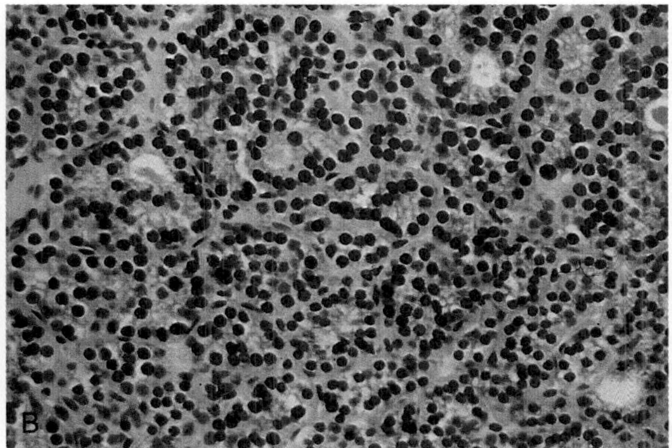

Figure 26–21

A, Solitary chief cell parathyroid adenoma (low-power view) revealing clear delineation from the residual gland below. *B,* High-power detail of a chief cell parathyroid adenoma. There is some slight variation in nuclear size but no anaplasia and some slight tendency to follicular formation.

consist of gray-white, irregular masses that sometimes exceed 10 gm in weight. The cells of parathyroid carcinomas are usually uniform and not too dissimilar from normal parathyroid cells. They are arrayed in nodular or trabecular patterns with a dense fibrous capsule enclosing the mass. There is general agreement that a **diagnosis of carcinoma based on cytologic detail is unreliable, and local invasion and metastasis are the only reliable criteria of malignancy.** Local recurrence occurs in one third of the cases and more distant dissemination in another third.

Morphologic changes in other organs deserving special mention include skeletal and renal lesions. **Skeletal changes** include prominence of osteoclasts, which, in turn, erode bone matrix and mobilize calcium salts, particularly in the metaphyses of long tubular bones. Bone resorption is accompanied by increased osteoblastic activity and the formation of new bone trabeculae. In many cases, the resultant bone contains widely spaced, delicate trabeculae reminiscent of those seen in osteoporosis. In more severe cases, the cortex is grossly thinned, and the marrow contains increased amounts of fibrous tissue accompanied by foci of hemorrhage and cyst formation (osteitis fibrosa cystica). Aggregates of osteoclasts, reactive giant cells, and hemorrhagic debris occasionally form masses that may be mistaken for neoplasms (**brown tumors** of hyperparathyroidism). PTH-induced hypercalcemia favors formation of **urinary tract stones** (nephrolithiasis) as well as calcification of the renal interstitium and tubules (nephrocalcinosis). Metastatic calcification secondary to hypercalcemia may also be seen in other sites, including the stomach, lungs, myocardium, and blood vessels.

Clinical Course. Primary hyperparathyroidism presents in one of two general ways: (1) It may be asymptomatic and be identified after a routine chemistry profile, or (2) patients may have the classic clinical manifestations of primary hyperparathyroidism.

Asymptomatic Hyperparathyroidism. Because serum calcium levels are routinely assessed in the work-up of most patients who need blood tests for unrelated conditions, clinically silent hyperparathyroidism is detected early. Hence many of the classic clinical manifestations, particularly those referable to bone and renal disease, are seen much less frequently in clinical practice. The *most common manifestation of primary hyperparathyroidism is an increase in the level of serum ionized calcium.* Patients with asymptomatic primary hyperparathyroidism do not have symptoms of hyperparathyroidism or hypercalcemia. It should be recalled that other conditions produce hypercalcemia. Malignancy, in particular, is the most common cause of clinically significant hypercalcemia in adults and must be excluded by appropriate clinical and laboratory investigations in patients with suspected hyperparathyroidism. *In patients with primary hyperparathyroidism, serum PTH levels are inappropriately elevated for the level of serum calcium, whereas PTH levels are low to undetectable in hypercalcemia because of nonparathyroid diseases.* In patients with hypercalcemia caused by secretion of PTHrP by certain nonparathyroid tumors, radioimmunoassays specific for PTH and PTHrP can distinguish between the two molecules. Other laboratory alterations referable to PTH excess include hypophosphatemia and increased urinary excretion of both calcium and phosphate. Secondary renal disease may lead to phosphate retention with normalization of serum phosphates.

Symptomatic Primary Hyperparathyroidism. The signs and symptoms of hyperparathyroidism reflect the combined effects of increased PTH secretion and hypercalcemia. Primary hyperparathyroidism has been traditionally associated with a constellation of symptoms that included "painful bones, renal stones, abdominal groans, and psychic moans." The symptomatic presentation involves a diversity of clinical manifestations[52]:

- *Bone disease* includes bone pain secondary to fractures of bones weakened by osteoporosis or osteitis fibrosa cystica.
- *Nephrolithiasis* (renal stones) occurs in 20% of newly diagnosed patients, with attendant pain and obstructive uropathy. Chronic renal insufficiency and a variety of abnormalities in renal function are found, including polyuria and secondary polydipsia.
- Gastrointestinal disturbances include constipation, nausea, peptic ulcers, pancreatitis, and gallstones.
- Central nervous system alterations, include depression, lethargy, and eventually seizures.
- Neuromuscular abnormalities include complaints of weakness and fatigue.
- Cardiac manifestations include aortic or mitral valve calcifications (or both).

The abnormalities most directly related to hyperparathyroidism are nephrolithiasis and bone disease, whereas those attributable to hypercalcemia include fatigue, weakness, and constipation. The pathogenesis of many of the other manifestations of the disorder remain poorly understood.

Secondary Hyperparathyroidism

Secondary hyperparathyroidism is caused by any condition associated with a chronic depression in the serum calcium level because low serum calcium leads to compensatory overactivity of the parathyroid glands. *Renal failure is, by far, the most common cause of secondary hyperparathyroidism,* although a number of other diseases, including inadequate dietary intake of calcium, steatorrhea, and vitamin D deficiency, may also cause this disorder. Chronic renal insufficiency is associated with decreased phosphate excretion, which results, in turn, in hyperphosphatemia. The elevated serum phosphate levels directly depress serum calcium levels and thereby stimulate parathyroid gland activity.

MORPHOLOGY. The **parathyroid glands in secondary hyperparathyroidism are hyperplastic.** As in the case of primary hyperplasia, the degree of glandular enlargement is not necessarily symmetric. Microscopically the hyperplastic glands contain an increased number of chief cells, or cells with more abundant, clear cytoplasm (so-called transition water-clear cells) in a diffuse or multinodular distribution. Fat cells are decreased in number. **Bone changes** similar to those seen in primary hyperparathyroidism may also be present. **Metastatic calcification** may be seen in many tissues, including lungs, heart, stomach, and blood vessels

Clinical Course. The clinical features of secondary hyperparathyroidism are usually dominated by those associated with chronic renal failure. Bone abnormalities (renal osteodystrophy) and other changes associated with PTH excess are, in general, less severe than are those seen in primary hyperparathyroidism. The vascular calcification associated with secondary hyperparathyroidism may occasionally result in significant ischemic damage to skin and other organs, a process sometimes referred to as *calciphylaxis.* In a minority of patients, parathyroid activity may become autonomous and excessive, with resultant hypercalcemia, a process sometimes termed *tertiary hyperparathyroidism.* Parathyroidectomy may be necessary to control the hyperparathyroidism in such patients.

HYPOPARATHYROIDISM

Hypoparathyroidism is far less common than is hyperparathyroidism. There are a substantial number of possible causes of deficient PTH secretion resulting in hypoparathyroidism:

- *Surgically induced* hypoparathyroidism occurs with inadvertent removal of all the parathyroid glands during thyroidectomy, excision of the parathyroid glands in the mistaken belief that they are lymph nodes during radical neck dissection for some form of malignant disease, or removal of too large a proportion of parathyroid tissue in the treatment of primary hyperparathyroidism.
- *Congenital absence* of all glands, as in certain developmental abnormalities, such as thymic aplasia (DiGeorge syndrome).
- *Primary (idiopathic)* atrophy of the glands most likely represents an autoimmune disease. Sixty percent of the patients with this disorder have autoantibodies directed against the calcium-sensing receptor in the parathyroid gland. Antibody binding to the receptor may prevent the release of PTH.
- *Familial hypoparathyroidism* is often associated with chronic mucocutaneous candidiasis and primary adrenal insufficiency. The syndrome typically presents in childhood with the onset of candidiasis, followed several years later by hypoparathyroidism, then adrenal insufficiency during adolescence.

The major clinical manifestations of hypoparathyroidism are referable to hypocalcemia and are related to the severity and chronicity of the hypocalcemia.

- The hallmark of hypocalcemia is *tetany,* which is characterized by *neuromuscular irritability,* resulting from decreased serum ionized calcium concentration. These findings can range from circumoral numbness or paresthesias (tingling) of the distal extremities and carpopedal spasm, to life-threatening laryngospasm and generalized seizures. The classic findings on physical examination of patients with neuromuscular irritability are *Chvostek sign* and *Trousseau sign.* Chvostek sign is elicited with subclinical disease by tapping along the course of the facial nerve, which induces contractions of the muscles of the eye, mouth, or nose. Occluding the circulation to the forearm and hand by inflating a blood pressure cuff about the arm for several minutes induces carpal spasm, which disappears as soon as the cuff is deflated (Trousseau sign).
- *Mental status changes* can include emotional instability, anxiety and depression, confusional states, hallucinations, and frank psychosis.
- *Intracranial manifestations* include parkinsonian-like movement disorders and papilledema.
- *Ocular disease* results in calcification of the lens leading to cataract formation.
- *Cardiovascular manifestations* include a conduction defect, which produces a characteristic prolongation of the QT interval in the electrocardiogram.
- *Dental abnormalities* occur when hypocalcemia is present during early development. These findings are highly characteristic of hypoparathyroidism and include dental hypoplasia, failure of eruption, defective enamel and root formation, and abraded carious teeth.

PSEUDOHYPOPARATHYROIDISM

Resistance of the organs to normal or elevated levels of PTH occurs with various forms of pseudohypoparathyroidism. The actions of PTH on bone and kidney are mediated by an interaction of the hormone receptor complex with GTP binding proteins and the generation of cyclic AMP. Two types of defects have been identified in pseudohypoparathyroidism:

1. *Pseudohypoparathyroidism type 1* is associated with diminished cyclic AMP response to PTH and is caused by a deficiency of the $Gs\alpha$ protein or by abnormalities in the level of the hormone receptor complex.[53] Patients with this disorder often have round facies, short stature, and short metacarpal and metatarsal bones (Albright hereditary osteodystrophy).
2. *Pseudohypoparathyroidism type 2* is characterized by normal PTH-induced cyclic AMP, with a blunted response to the second messenger.

Hypocalcemia results, leading to secondary parathyroid hyperfunction, unanticipated elevated serum PTH levels, and a constellation of skeletal and other developmental abnormalities.

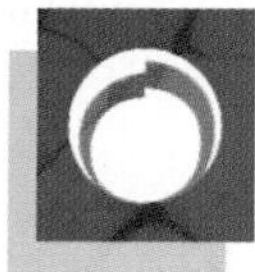

Adrenal Cortex

The *adrenal glands* are paired endocrine organs consisting of both cortex and medulla, which differ in their development, structure, and function. In the adult, the normal adrenal gland weighs about 4 gm, but with acute stress, lipid depletion may reduce the weight or, with prolonged stress, such as dying after a long chronic illness, may induce hypertrophy and hyperplasia of the cortical cells and more than double the weight of the normal gland. Beneath the capsule of the adrenal is the narrow layer of zona glomerulosa. An equally narrow zona reticularis abuts the medulla. Intervening is the broad zona fasciculata, which makes up about 75% of the total cortex. The *adrenal cortex* synthesizes three different types of steroids (Fig. 26–22): (1) *glucocorticoids* (principally cortisol), which are synthesized primarily in the zona fasciculata with a small contribution from the zona reticularis; (2) *mineralocorticoids,* the most important being aldosterone, which is generated in the zona glomerulosa; and (3) *sex steroids* (estrogens and androgens), which are produced largely in the zona reticularis. The *adrenal medulla* is composed of chromaffin cells, which synthesize and secrete *catecholamines,* mainly epinephrine. Catecholamines have many effects that allow rapid adaptations to changes in the environment. This section deals only with disorders of the adrenal cortex. Later, those of the medulla are considered. Diseases of the adrenal cortex can be conveniently divided into those associated with cortical hyperfunction and those characterized by cortical hypofunction.

ADRENOCORTICAL HYPERFUNCTION (HYPERADRENALISM)

Just as there are three basic types of corticosteroids elaborated by the adrenal cortex (glucocorticoids, mineralocorticoids, and sex steroids), so there are three distinctive hyperadrenal clinical syndromes: (1) *Cushing syndrome,* characterized by an excess of cortisol; (2) *hyperaldosteronism;* and (3) *adrenogenital* or virilizing syndromes with an excess of androgens. The clinical features of some of these syndromes overlap somewhat because of the overlapping functions of some of the adrenal steroids.

Hypercortisolism (Cushing Syndrome)

Pathogenesis. This disorder is caused by any condition that produces an elevation in glucocorticoid levels. There are four possible sources of excess cortisol (Fig. 26–23).[54]

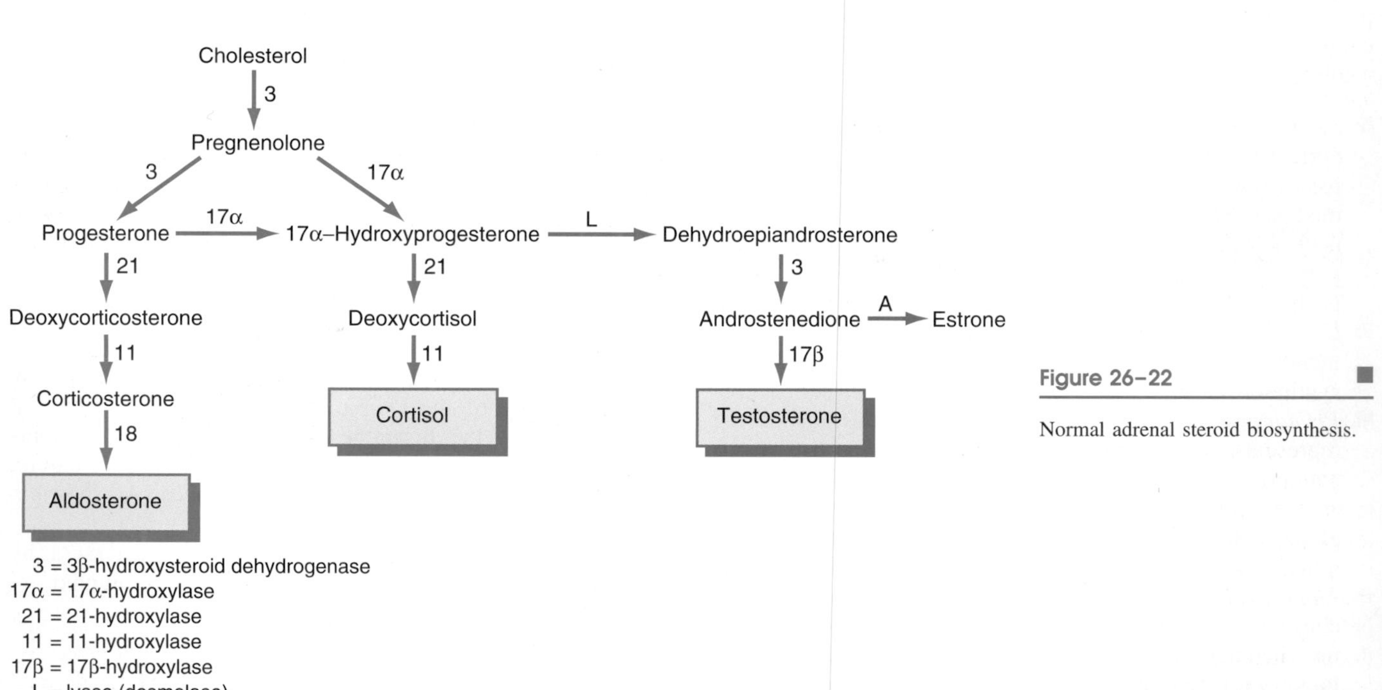

Figure 26–22

Normal adrenal steroid biosynthesis.

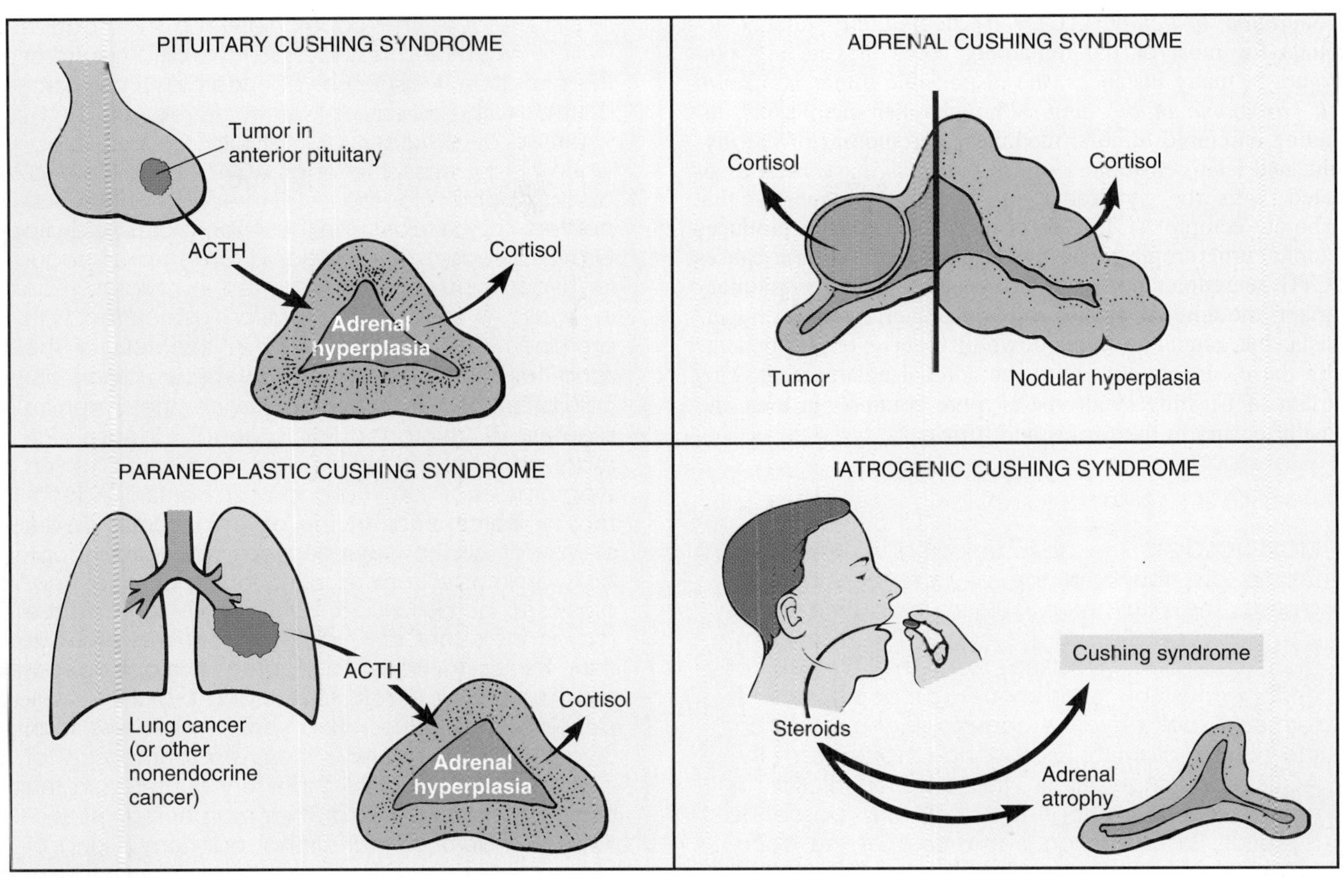

Figure 26–23

A schematic representation of the various forms of Cushing syndrome, illustrating the three endogenous forms as well as the more common exogenous (iatrogenic) form. ACTH, adrenocorticotropic hormone.

In clinical practice, *most causes of Cushing syndrome are the result of the administration of exogenous glucocorticoids.* The other three sources of the hypercortisolism can be categorized as *endogenous* Cushing syndrome:

- Primary hypothalamic-pituitary diseases associated with hypersecretion of ACTH
- Hypersecretion of cortisol by an adrenal adenoma, carcinoma, or nodular hyperplasia
- The secretion of ectopic ACTH by a nonendocrine neoplasm

Primary hypersecretion of ACTH accounts for more than half of cases of endogenous hypercortisolism. Out of deference to the neurosurgeon who first published the full description of this syndrome and related it to a pituitary lesion, this pituitary form of Cushing syndrome is referred to as *Cushing disease.* The disorder affects women about five times more frequently than men, and it occurs most frequently during the twenties to thirties. In most of these patients, the pituitary gland contains a small ACTH-producing adenoma that does not produce mass effects in the brain. The responsible adenoma may be composed of either basophilic or chromophobe cells. In most of the remaining cases, the anterior pituitary contains areas of corticotroph cell hyperplasia without a discrete adenoma. In at least some patients, the pituitary abnormality appears to result from excessive stimulation of ACTH release by the hypothalamus. The adrenal glands in patients with Cushing disease are characterized by variable degrees of nodular cortical hyperplasia (discussed later), caused by elevated levels of ACTH. The cortical hyperplasia, in turn, is responsible for hypercortisolism.

Primary adrenal neoplasms, such as adrenal adenoma, carcinoma, and cortical hyperplasia, are responsible for about 15 to 30% of cases of endogenous Cushing syndrome. This form of Cushing syndrome is also designated *ACTH-independent Cushing syndrome* or adrenal Cushing syndrome because the adrenals function autonomously. Adenomas and carcinomas are about equally common in adults; in children, carcinomas predominate. Autonomous hyperplasia is uncommon, as detailed later. The cortical carcinomas tend to produce more marked hypercortisolism than the adenomas or hyperplastic processes. In those instances with a unilateral neoplasm, the uninvolved adrenal cortex and that in the opposite gland undergo atrophy because of suppression of ACTH secretion. Thus, adrenal Cushing syndrome is marked by elevated levels of cortisol but low serum levels of ACTH.

Secretion of ectopic ACTH by nonpituitary tumors accounts for most of the remaining cases of Cushing syndrome. In many instances, the responsible tumor is a *small cell carcinoma of the lung,* although other neoplasms, including carcinoid tumors, medullary carcinomas of the thyroid, and islet cell tumors of the pancreas, have been associated with the syndrome. In addition to tumors that elaborate ectopic ACTH, an occasional neoplasm produces ectopic corticotropin-releasing factor, which, in turn, causes ACTH secretion and hypercortisolism. As in the pituitary variant, the adrenal glands undergo bilateral cortical hyperplasia, but often the rapid downhill course of the patients with these cancers cuts short the adrenal enlargement. This variant of Cushing syndrome is more common in men and usually occurs in the forties and fifties.

MORPHOLOGY. The basic lesions of Cushing syndrome are found in the pituitary and adrenal glands. The **pituitary** in Cushing syndrome shows changes regardless of the cause. The most common alteration, resulting from high levels of endogenous or exogenous glucocorticoids, is termed **Crooke hyaline change.** In this condition, the normal granular, basophilic cytoplasm of the ACTH-producing cells in the anterior pituitary is replaced by homogeneous, lightly basophilic material. This alteration is the result of the accumulation of intermediate keratin filaments in their cytoplasm.

The morphology of the **adrenal glands** depends on the cause of the hypercortisolism. The adrenals have one of the following abnormalities: (1) cortical atrophy; (2) diffuse hyperplasia; (3) nodular hyperplasia; and (4) an adenoma, rarely a carcinoma. In patients in whom the syndrome results from exogenous glucocorticoids, suppression of endogenous ACTH results in bilateral **cortical atrophy,** owing to lack of stimulation of the zonae fasciculata and reticularis by ACTH. In cases of endogenous hypercortisolism, in contrast, the adrenals either are hyperplastic or contain a cortical neoplasm. **Diffuse hyperplasia** is found in 60 to 70% of cases of Cushing syndrome. Both glands are enlarged, either subtly or markedly, weighing up to 25 to 40 gm. The adrenal cortex is diffusely thickened and yellow, owing to an increase in the size and number of lipid-rich cells in the zonae fasciculata and reticularis. Some degree of nodularity is common but is pronounced in **nodular hyperplasia.** This takes the form of bilateral, 0.5- to 2.0-cm, yellow nodules scattered throughout the cortex, separated by intervening areas of widened cortex. The uninvolved cortex and nodules are composed of a mixture of lipid-laden and lipid-poor compact cells showing some variability in cell and nuclear size with occasional binucleate forms. The combined adrenals may weigh up to 30 to 50 gm. This macronodularity appears to be an extension of the diffuse hyperplasia because the cortex between the nodules exactly resembles that found in the diffuse form of this condition. Most cases of hyperplasia are associated with elevated serum levels of ACTH whether of pituitary or ectopic origin. Rarely, when no increased level of ACTH can be found, autoantibodies to the ACTH receptors are suspected as the basis for the hyperplasia (as with Graves disease). An additional rare form of nodular hyperplasia, seen more often in children than in adults, is a familial condition associated with prominent lipofuscin deposits in the cells of the zona fasciculata and resultant brown-black discoloration of the adrenals, hence the synonym **pigmented micronodular adrenal disease. Primary adrenocortical neoplasms** causing Cushing syndrome may be malignant or benign. Adenomas or carcinomas of the adrenal cortex as the source of cortisol secretion are not macroscopically distinctive from nonfunctioning adrenal neoplasms to be described. Both the benign and the malignant lesions are more common in women in their thirties to fifties. The adrenocortical **adenomas** are yellow tumors surrounded by thin or well-developed capsules, and most weigh less than 30 gm. Microscopically, they are composed of cells that are similar to those encountered in the normal zona fasciculata. Their morphology is identical to that of nonfunctional adenomas and of adenomas associated with hyperaldosteronism (discussed later). The **carcinomas** associated with Cushing syndrome, by contrast, tend to be larger than the adenomas. These tumors are unencapsulated masses frequently exceeding 200 to 300 gm in weight, having all of the anaplastic characteristics of cancer, as detailed later. With both functioning benign and malignant tumors, the adjacent adrenal cortex and that of the contralateral adrenal gland are atrophic owing to suppression of endogenous ACTH by high cortisol levels.

Clinical Course. Developing slowly over time, Cushing syndrome, similar to many other endocrine abnormalities, can be quite subtle in its early manifestations.[55] Early stages of the disorder include hypertension and weight gain (Table 26–4). With time, the more characteristic central pattern of adipose tissue deposition becomes apparent, with resultant truncal obesity, moon facies, and accumulation of fat in the posterior neck and back *(buffalo hump).* Hypercortisolism causes selective atrophy of fast-twitch (type II) myofibers, resulting in decreased muscle mass and proximal limb weakness. Glucocorticoids induce gluconeogenesis and inhibit the uptake of glucose by cells with resultant *hyperglycemia, glucosuria, and polydipsia.* The catabolic effects on proteins cause loss of collagen and resorption of bones. Consequently the *skin is thin, fragile, and easily bruised;* wound healing is poor; cutaneous striae are particularly common in the abdominal area. Bone resorption re-

Table 26–4. MAJOR FEATURES OF CUSHING SYNDROME WITH APPROXIMATE FREQUENCY

Clinical Features	Percentages
Central obesity (about trunk and upper back)	85–90
Moon facies	85
Weakness and fatigability	85
Hirsutism	75
Hypertension	75
Plethora	75
Glucose intolerance/diabetes	75/20
Osteoporosis	75
Neuropsychiatric abnormalities	75–80
Menstrual abnormalities	70
Skin striae (sides of lower abdomen)	50

sults in the development of *osteoporosis,* with consequent backache and increased susceptibility to fractures. Patients with Cushing syndrome are at increased risk for a variety of infections because glucocorticoids suppress the immune response. Additional manifestations include a number of *mental disturbances,* including mood swings, depression, and frank psychosis, as well as *hirsutism* and *menstrual abnormalities.*

Cushing syndrome is diagnosed in the laboratory with the following: (1) the 24-hour urine free cortisol level, which is increased, and (2) loss of normal diurnal pattern of cortisol secretion. Determining the cause of Cushing syndrome depends on the level of serum ACTH and measurement of urinary steroid excretion after administration of dexamethasone. Three general patterns can be obtained:

1. In pituitary Cushing syndrome, the most common form, ACTH levels are elevated and cannot be suppressed by the administration of a low dose of dexamethasone. Hence there is no reduction in urinary excretion of 17-hydroxycorticosteroids. After higher doses of injected dexamethasone, however, the pituitary responds by reducing ACTH secretion, which is reflected by suppression of urinary steroid secretion.
2. Ectopic ACTH secretion results in an elevated level of ACTH, but its secretion is completely insensitive to low or high doses of exogenous dexamethasone.
3. When Cushing syndrome is caused by an adrenal tumor, the ACTH level is quite low because of feedback inhibition of the pituitary. As with ectopic ACTH secretion, both low-dose and high-dose dexamethasone fail to suppress cortisol excretion.

Primary Hyperaldosteronism

Primary hyperaldosteronism is the generic term for a small group of closely related, uncommon syndromes, all characterized by chronic excess aldosterone secretion. *Excessive levels of aldosterone cause sodium retention and potassium excretion, with resultant hypertension and hypokalemia.* Hyperaldosteronism may be primary, or it may be a secondary event resulting from an extra-adrenal cause.[56]

Primary hyperaldosteronism indicates an autonomous overproduction of aldosterone, with resultant suppression of the renin-angiotensin system and decreased plasma renin activity. Primary hyperaldosteronism is caused either by an aldosterone-producing adrenocortical neoplasm, usually an adenoma, or by primary adrenocortical hyperplasia (Fig. 26–24). In approximately 80% of cases, primary hyperaldosteronism is caused by an aldosterone-secreting adenoma in one adrenal gland, a condition referred to as *Conn syndrome.* This syndrome occurs most frequently in adult middle life and is more common in women than in men (2:1).

In *secondary hyperaldosteronism,* in contrast, aldosterone release occurs in response to activation of the renin-angiotensin system. It is characterized by increased levels of plasma renin and is encountered in conditions such as congestive heart failure, decreased renal perfusion (e.g., arteriolar nephrosclerosis, renal arterial stenosis), hypoalbuminemia, and pregnancy (owing to estrogen-induced increases in plasma renin substrate).

MORPHOLOGY. Aldosterone-producing adenomas are almost always solitary, small (<2 cm in diameter), encapsulated lesions, more often found on the left than on the right (Fig. 26–25). They tend to occur in women more often than men in the thirties and forties. They are often sufficiently buried within the gland not to produce visible enlargement, a point to be remembered when interpreting sonographic or scanning images. They are bright yellow on cut section and, surprisingly, are composed of lipid-laden cortical cells more closely resembling fasciculata cells than glomerulosa cells (the normal source of aldosterone). In general, the cells tend to be uniform in size and shape and resemble mature cortical cells, but occasionally there is some nuclear and cellular pleomorphism but no evidence of anaplasia.

Bilateral idiopathic hyperplasia (Fig. 26–26) is marked by diffuse and focal hyperplasia of cells resembling those of the normal zona glomerulosa interspersed with small adrenocortical nodules composed of lipid-laden cells having the electron microscopic features of normal zona fasciculata. These changes are highly reminiscent of those found in the nodular hyperplasia of Cushing syndrome, suggesting prolonged exposure to an abnormal secretagogue of as yet unknown nature. Several potential candidates have been described, most of the evidence favoring a non-ACTH pituitary glycoprotein.

Glucocorticoid-suppressible hyperaldosteronism is an uncommon cause of primary hyperaldosteronism that runs in families and appears to be the result of a mutation leading to some developmental derangement in the zonation of the adrenal cortex (which normally progresses from the capsule inward). As a result, hybrid cells appear in

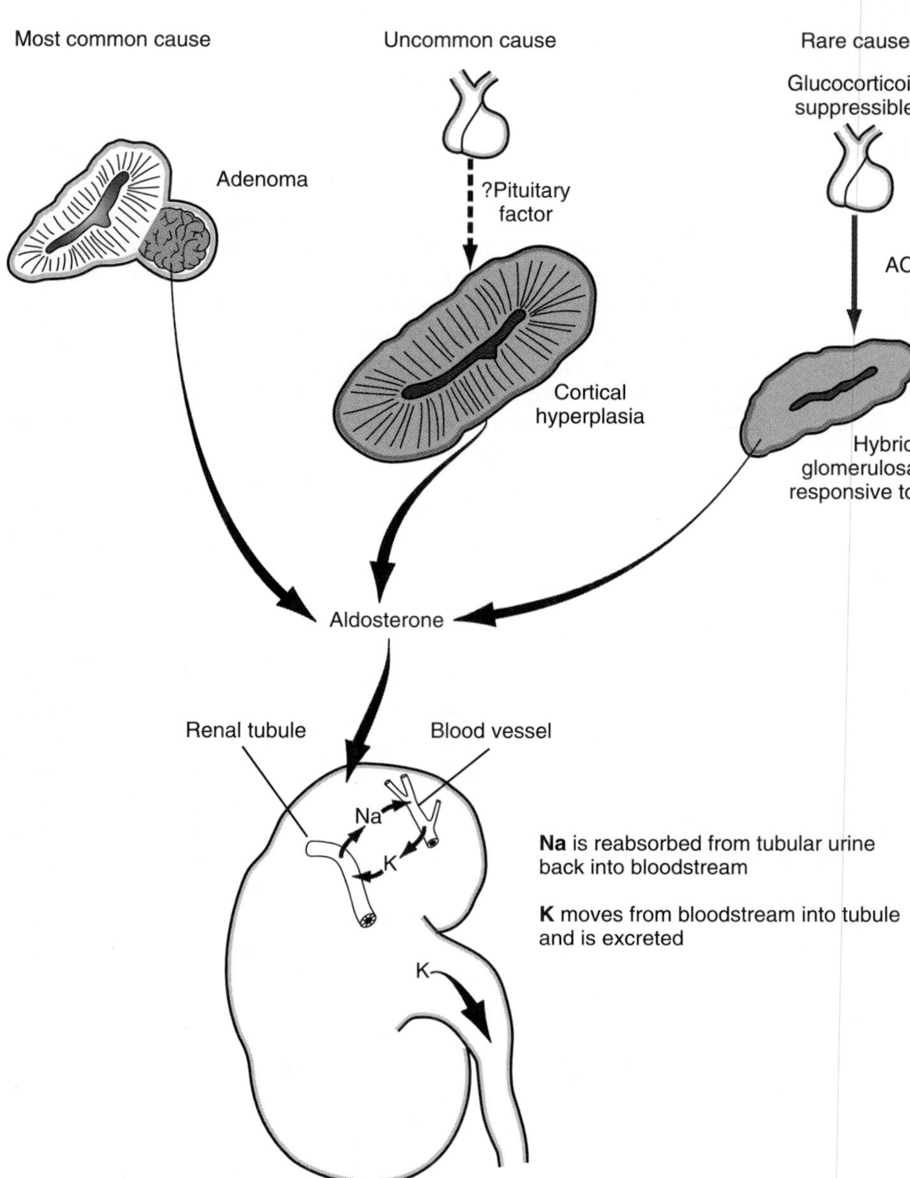

Figure 26–24 ■

The major causes of primary hyperaldosteronism and its principal effects on the kidney.

the interface between the zona glomerulosa and the zona fasciculata, which elaborate hybrid steroids in addition to both cortisol and aldosterone. The prolonged activation of aldosterone secretion appears to be under the continuous influence of ACTH and hence is suppressible by exogenous administration of dexamethasone.

Clinical Course. The clinical manifestations of primary hyperaldosteronism are hypertension and hypokalemia. Serum renin, as mentioned previously, is low. Hypokalemia results from renal potassium wasting and can cause a variety of neuromuscular manifestations, including weakness, paresthesias, visual disturbances, and occasionally frank tetany. Sodium retention increases the total body sodium and expands the extracellular fluid volume, leading to elevation of the serum sodium concentration and an increase in intracellular sodium with increased vascular reactivity. The hypertension is, in some part, a result of the sodium retention. The expanded extracellular fluid volume and hypokalemia both impose a burden on the heart, sometimes causing electrocardiographic changes and cardiac decompensation. The diagnosis of primary hyperaldosteronism is confirmed by the elevated levels of aldosterone and depressed levels of renin in the circulation. Even when the diagnosis of primary hyperaldosteronism is made, it is necessary to distinguish among the various causes, particularly the differentiation of an adenoma, which is amenable to surgical excision, and bilateral idiopathic hyperplasia, calling for medical therapy. Uncommon as primary hyperaldosteronism may be, it should not be overlooked clinically

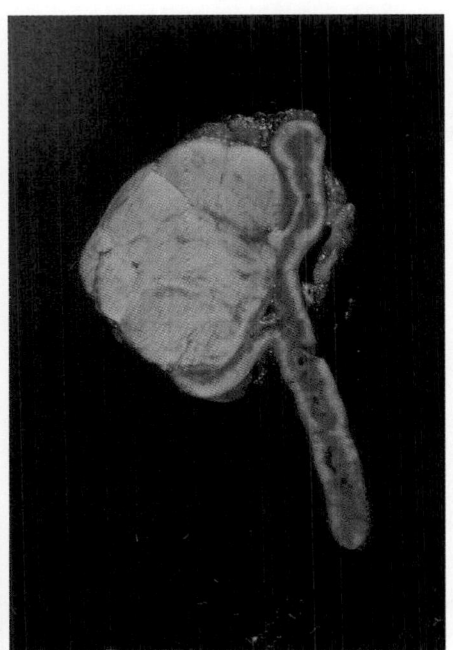

Figure 26–25 ■

Adrenal cortical adenoma. The adenoma is distinguished from nodular hyperplasia by its solitary, circumscribed nature. The functional status of an adrenal cortical adenoma cannot be predicted from its gross or microscopic appearance.

because it provides an opportunity to cure a form of hypertension.

Adrenogenital Syndromes

Disorders of sexual differentiation, such as virilization, may be caused by primary gonadal disorders and several primary adrenal disorders. The latter group of disorders include *adrenocortical neoplasms* and a group of disorders that have been designated *congenital adrenal hyperplasia.*

Adrenocortical neoplasms associated with virilization are more likely to be caused by an androgen-secreting adrenal carcinoma than adenomas. These tumors are morphologically identical to other cortical neoplasms and are discussed later.

Congenital adrenal hyperplasias represent a group of autosomal recessive, inherited metabolic errors, each characterized by a deficiency or total lack of a particular enzyme involved in the biosynthesis of cortical steroids, particularly cortisol. Steroidogenesis is then channeled into other pathways leading to increased production of androgens, which accounts for virilization. Simultaneously the deficiency of cortisol results in increased secretion of ACTH, resulting in adrenal hyperplasia. Certain enzyme defects may also impair aldosterone secretion, adding *salt wasting* to the virilizing syndrome. Other enzyme deficiencies may be incompatible with life or, in a rare instance, may involve only the aldosterone pathway without involving cortisol synthesis. Thus, there is a spectrum of these syndromes, and with each one there may be a total lack of a particular enzyme or a mutation that only mildly impairs the effectiveness of the enzyme. The following remarks focus on the most common of these disorders.

21-HYDROXYLASE DEFICIENCY

Defective conversion of progesterone to 11-deoxycorticosterone by 21-hydroxylase (CYP21A2) accounts for approximately 90% of cases of congenital adrenal hyperplasia.[57] Figure 26–27 illustrates normal adrenal steroidogenesis and the consequences of 21-hydroxylase deficiency. 21-Hydroxylase deficiency may range from a total lack to a mild loss, depending on the nature of the mutation. Three distinctive syndromes have been segregated: (1) salt-wasting adrenogenitalism, (2) simple virilizing adrenogenitalism, and (3) nonclassic adrenogenitalism, which implies mild disease that may be entirely asymptomatic or associated only with symptoms of androgen excess during childhood or puberty.

The *salt-wasting syndrome* results from an inability to convert progesterone into deoxycorticosterone because of a total lack of the hydroxylase. Thus, there is virtually no synthesis of mineralocorticoids and concomitantly a block in the conversion of hydroxyprogesterone into deoxycortisol with deficient cortisol synthesis. This pattern usually comes to light soon after birth because in utero the electrolytes and fluids can be maintained by the maternal kidneys. There is *salt wasting, hyponatremia,* and *hyperkalemia,* which induce acidosis, *hypotension,* cardiovascular collapse, and possibly death. The concomitant block in cortisol synthesis and excess production of androgens, however, lead to virilization, which is easily recognized in the female at birth or in utero but is difficult to recognize in the

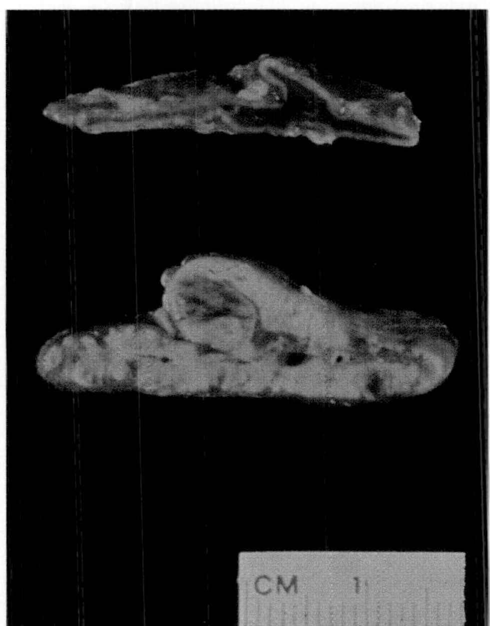

Figure 26–26 ■

Cross-section of nodular hyperplasia contrasted with normal adrenal.

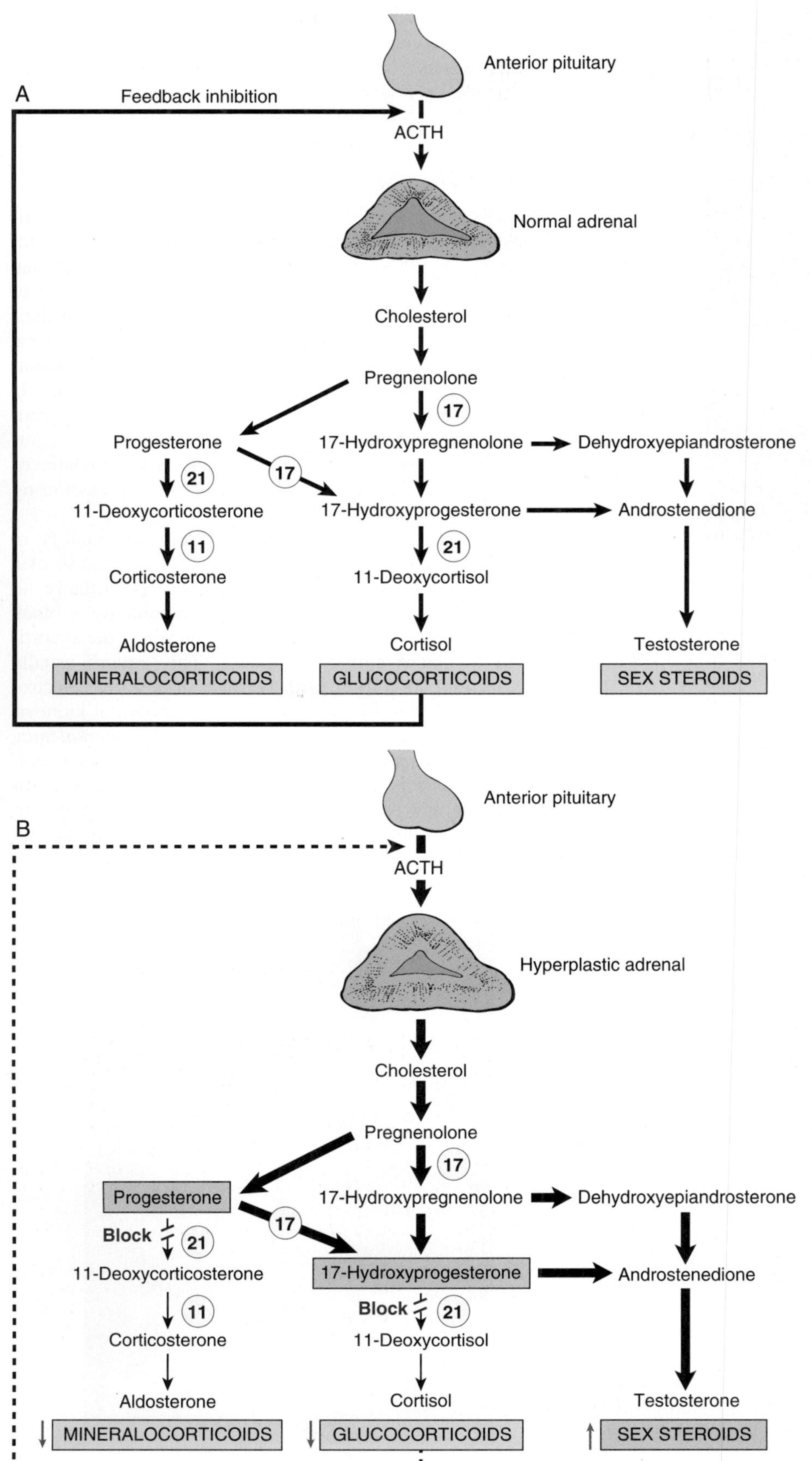

Figure 26–27

Simplified flow chart demonstrating normal adrenal steroidogenesis (*A*) and consequences of C-21 hydroxylase deficiency (*B*). 21-Hydroxylase deficiency impairs the synthesis of both cortisol and aldosterone. The resultant decrease in feedback inhibition *(dashed line)* causes increased secretion of adrenocorticotropic hormone, resulting ultimately in adrenal hyperplasia and increased synthesis of testosterone.

male. Various degrees of virilization are encountered, ranging from mild clitoral enlargement to complete labioscrotal fusion to marked clitoral enlargement enclosing the urethra, thus producing a phalloid organ. Males with this disorder are generally unrecognized at birth but come to clinical attention 5 to 15 days later because of some salt-losing crisis.

Simple virilizing adrenogenital syndrome without salt wasting (presenting as genital ambiguity) may appear with a less than total 21-hydroxylase defect because with less severe deficiencies the level of mineralocorticoid, although reduced, is sufficient for salt reabsorption, but the lowered glucocorticoid level fails to cause feedback inhibition of ACTH secretion. Thus, the level of aldosterone is mildly reduced, testosterone is increased, and ACTH is elevated, with resultant adrenal hyperplasia.

Nonclassic or late-onset adrenal virilism is much more common than the classic patterns already described. These patients may be virtually asymptomatic or have mild manifestations, such as hirsutism. The diagnosis can be made only by demonstration of biosynthetic defects in steroidogenesis and by genetic studies, as will become evident subsequently.

MORPHOLOGY. In all cases of congenital adrenal hyperplasia, the adrenals are hyperplastic bilaterally, sometimes expanding to 10 to 15 times their normal weights because of the sustained elevation in ACTH. The adrenal cortex is thickened and nodular, and on cut section, the widened cortex appears brown owing to total depletion of all lipid. The adrenal cells are identical to those seen in other forms of cortical hyperplasia and appear relatively normal in size and shape. Hyperplasia of corticotroph (ACTH-producing) cells is present in the anterior pituitary.

Clinical Course. The clinical features of these disorders are determined by the specific enzyme deficiency and include abnormalities related to androgen excess, sodium deficiency, and, in severe cases, glucocorticoid deficiency. Depending on the nature and severity of the enzymatic defect, the onset of clinical symptoms may occur in the perinatal period, later childhood, or less commonly in adulthood. For example, in 21-hydroxylase deficiency, excessive androgenic activity causes signs of masculinization in females, ranging from clitoral hypertrophy and pseudohermaphroditism in infants, to oligomenorrhea, hirsutism, and acne in postpubertal females. In males, androgen excess is associated with enlargement of the external genitalia and other evidence of precocious puberty in prepubertal patients and oligospermia in older males.

Patients with congenital adrenal hyperplasia are treated with exogenous glucocorticoids, which, in addition to providing adequate levels of glucocorticoids, suppress ACTH levels and thus decrease the excessive synthesis of the steroid hormones responsible for many of the clinical abnormalities.

ADRENAL INSUFFICIENCY

Adrenocortical insufficiency, or hypofunction, may be caused by either primary adrenal disease (primary hypoadrenalism) or decreased stimulation of the adrenals owing to a deficiency of ACTH (secondary hypoadrenalism) (Table 26–5). The patterns of adrenocortical insufficiency can be considered under the following headings: (1) primary acute adrenocortical insufficiency (adrenal crisis), (2) primary chronic adrenocortical insufficiency (Addison disease), and (3) secondary adrenocortical insufficiency.[58]

Primary Acute Adrenocortical Insufficiency

Acute adrenal cortical insufficiency occurs in a variety of clinical settings (Table 26–5), as follows:

- As a *crisis* in patients with chronic adrenocortical insufficiency precipitated by any form of stress that requires an immediate increase in steroid output from glands incapable of responding
- In patients maintained on exogenous corticosteroids, in whom rapid withdrawal of steroids, or failure to increase steroid doses in response to an acute stress, may precipitate an adrenal crisis, owing to the inability of the atrophic adrenals to produce glucocorticoid hormones
- As a result of massive adrenal hemorrhage, which destroys the adrenal cortex sufficiently to cause acute adrenocortical insufficiency. This occurs
  - In newborns, following prolonged and difficult delivery, with considerable trauma and hypoxia, leading to extensive adrenal hemorrhages beginning in the medulla and extending into the cortex. Newborns are particularly vulnerable because they are often deficient in prothrombin for at least several days after birth.
  - In some patients maintained on anticoagulant therapy

Table 26–5. ADRENOCORTICAL INSUFFICIENCY

Primary Insufficiency	Secondary Insufficiency
Loss of cortex	Hypothalamic pituitary disease
Idiopathic (autoimmune)	Neoplasm, inflammation (sarcoidosis, tuberculosis, pyogens, fungi)
Infection (mycobacteria, fungi)	Hypothalamic pituitary suppression
AIDS, opportunistic microbes	Long-term steroid administration
Acute hemorrhagic necrosis (Waterhouse-Friderichsen syndrome)	Steroid-producing neoplasms
Amyloidosis	
Sarcoidosis, hemochromatosis	
Metastatic carcinoma	
Metabolic failure in hormone production	
Congenital adrenal hypoplasia	
Drug- and steroid-induced inhibition of adrenocorticotropic hormone or cortical cell function	

- In postsurgical patients who develop disseminated intravascular coagulation with consequent hemorrhagic infarction of the adrenals.
- When massive adrenal hemorrhage complicates a bacteremic infection, in this setting called the *Waterhouse-Friderichsen* syndrome

Waterhouse-Friderichsen Syndrome

This uncommon but catastrophic syndrome is characterized by the following:

- An overwhelming bacterial infection, which is classically associated with *Neisseria meningitidis* septicemia but occasionally is caused by other highly virulent organisms, such as *Pseudomonas* species, pneumococci, *Haemophilus influenzae,* or staphylococci
- Rapidly progressive hypotension leading to shock
- Disseminated intravascular coagulation with widespread purpura, particularly of the skin
- Rapidly developing adrenocortical insufficiency associated with massive bilateral adrenal hemorrhage

The Waterhouse-Friderichsen syndrome may occur at any age but is somewhat more common in children. The basis for the adrenal hemorrhage is uncertain but could be attributable to direct bacterial seeding of small vessels in the adrenal, the development of disseminated intravascular coagulation, endotoxin-induced vasculitis, or some form of hypersensitivity vasculitis. *Whatever the basis, the adrenals are converted to sacs of clotted blood virtually obscuring all underlying detail* (Fig. 26–28). Histologic examination reveals that the hemorrhage starts within the medulla in relationship to thin-walled venous sinusoids, then suffuses peripherally into the cortex, often leaving islands of recognizable cortical cells. When recognized promptly and treated effectively with antibiotics, recovery is possible, but the clinical course is usually devastatingly abrupt, and prompt recognition and appropriate therapy must be instituted immediately or death follows within hours to a few days.

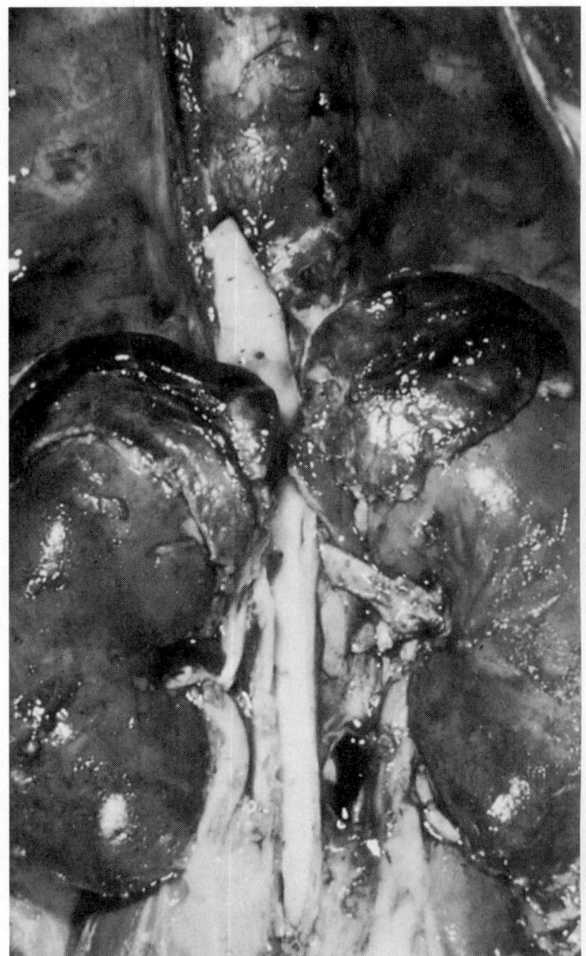

Figure 26–28 ■

Waterhouse-Friderichsen syndrome in a child. The dark, hemorrhagic adrenal glands are distended with blood.

Primary Chronic Adrenocortical Insufficiency (Addison Disease)

Addison disease, or chronic adrenocortical insufficiency, is an uncommon disorder resulting from progressive destruction of the adrenal cortex. In general, clinical manifestations of adrenocortical insufficiency do not appear until at least 90% of the adrenal cortex has been compromised. The causes of chronic adrenocortical insufficiency are listed in Table 26–5. Although all races and both sexes may be affected, certain causes of Addison disease (such as autoimmune adrenalitis) are much more common in whites, particularly in women.

Pathogenesis. A large number of diseases may attack the adrenal cortex, including lymphomas, amyloidosis, sarcoidosis, hemochromatosis, fungal infections, and adrenal hemorrhages, but more than 90% of all cases are attributable to *autoimmune adrenalitis, tuberculosis, or metastatic cancers.*[58]

Autoimmune adrenalitis accounts for 60 to 70% of cases. It may occur as a sporadic or familial disorder. In about half of these cases, the adrenal is the sole target of an autoimmune reaction, but in the remainder, other autoimmune disease, such as Hashimoto disease, pernicious anemia, type I diabetes mellitus, and idiopathic hypoparathyroidism, coexist. The term *polyglandular syndromes* has been used to designate the various combinations of organ involvement that may be encountered. Circulating antiadrenal antibodies are present in about half of the cases of autoimmune adrenalitis as well as other types of antibodies related to involvement of other organs or tissues. The frequency of autoimmune adrenalitis is increased in association with certain histocompatibility antigens, particularly HLA-B8 and DR-3, suggesting some genetic predisposition. As with other autoimmune endocrine disorders, the factors that initiate autoimmunity remain obscure.

Infections, particularly tuberculosis and those produced by fungi, may also cause primary chronic adrenocortical insufficiency. Tuberculous adrenalitis, which once accounted for as much as 90% of Addison disease, has become less common with the development of antituberculous agents. With the resurgence of tuberculosis in most urban centers and the persistence of the disease in developing countries, however, this cause of adrenal insufficiency must be kept in mind. When present, tuberculous adrenalitis is usually associated with active infection in other sites, particularly in the lungs and genitourinary tract. Among the fungi, disseminated infections caused by *Histoplasma capsulatum* and *Coccidioides immitis* may also result in chronic adrenocortical insufficiency.

Metastatic neoplasms involving the adrenals are another potential cause of adrenal insufficiency. The adrenals are a fairly common site for metastases in patients with disseminated carcinomas. Although adrenal function is preserved in most such patients, the metastatic tumors occasionally destroy enough adrenal cortex to produce a degree of adrenal insufficiency. Carcinomas of the lung and breast are the source of a majority of metastases in the adrenals, although many other neoplasms, including gastrointestinal carcinomas, malignant melanoma, and hematopoietic neoplasms, may also metastasize to this organ.

MORPHOLOGY. The anatomic changes in the adrenal glands of course depend on the underlying disease. **Primary autoimmune adrenalitis** is characterized by irregularly shrunken glands, which may be difficult to identify within the suprarenal adipose tissue. Histologically the cortex contains only scattered residual cortical cells in a collapsed network of connective tissue. A variable lymphoid infiltrate is present in the cortex and may extend into the subjacent medulla, although the medulla is otherwise preserved (Fig. 26–29). In cases of **tuberculous and fungal disease,** the adrenal architecture is effaced by a granulomatous inflammatory reaction identical to that encountered in other sites of infection. When hypoadrenalism is caused by **metastatic carcinoma,** the adrenals are enlarged, and their normal architecture is obscured by the infiltrating neoplasm.

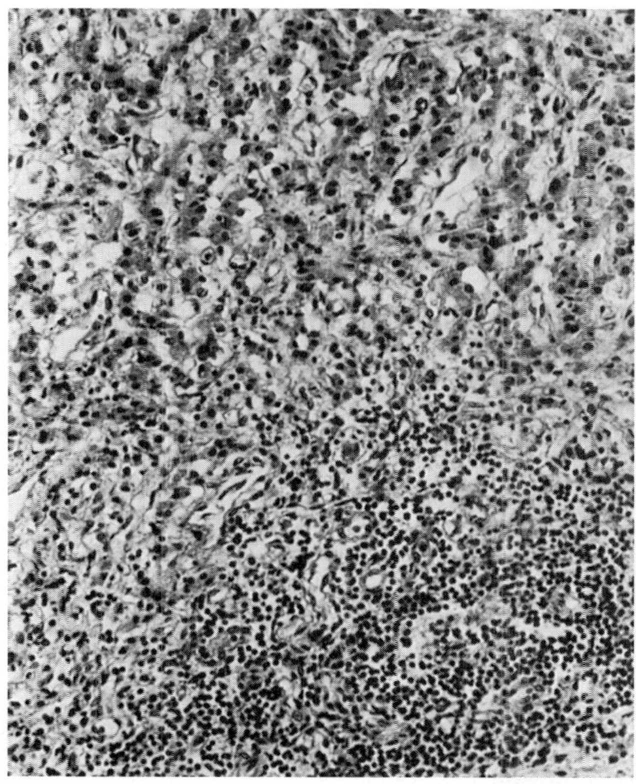

Figure 26–29

Autoimmune adrenalitis. In addition to loss of all but a subcapsular rim of cortical cells, there is an extensive mononuclear cell infiltrate.

Clinical Course. Addison disease begins insidiously and does not come to attention until at least 90% of the cortex of both glands is destroyed, and the levels of circulating glucocorticoids and mineralocorticoids are significantly decreased. The initial manifestations include progressive weakness and easy fatigability, which may be dismissed as nonspecific complaints. *Gastrointestinal* disturbances are common and include anorexia, nausea, vomiting, weight loss, and diarrhea. In patients with primary adrenal disease, increased circulating levels of ACTH precursor hormone stimulate melanocytes, with resultant *hyperpigmentation* of the skin, particularly of sun-exposed areas and at pressure points, such as the neck, elbows, knees, and knuckles. By contrast, hyperpigmentation is not seen in patients with adrenocortical insufficiency caused by primary pituitary or hypothalamic disease. Decreased mineralocorticoid activity in patients with primary adrenal insufficiency results in potassium and sodium loss, with consequent *hyperkalemia, hyponatremia, volume depletion, and hypotension.* The heart is frequently smaller than normal, probably because of chronic hypovolemia. Hypoglycemia may occasionally occur as a result of glucocorticoid deficiency and impaired glucogenesis. Stresses such as infections, trauma, or surgical procedures in such patients may precipitate an acute adrenal crisis, manifested by intractable vomiting, abdominal pain, hypotension, coma, and vascular collapse. Death occurs rapidly unless corticosteroid therapy begins immediately.

Secondary Adrenocortical Insufficiency

Any disorder of the hypothalamus and pituitary, such as metastatic cancer, infection, infarction, or irradiation, that reduces the output of ACTH leads to a syndrome of hypoadrenalism having many similarities to Addison disease. Analogously, prolonged administration of exogenous glucocorticoids suppresses the output of ACTH and adrenal function. *With secondary disease, the hyperpigmentation of primary Addison disease is lacking because melanotropic hormone levels are low.* The manifestations also differ inasmuch as secondary hypoadrenalism is characterized by deficient cortisol and androgen output but normal or near-normal aldosterone synthesis. Thus, in adrenal insufficiency secondary to pituitary malfunction, there is no marked hyponatremia and hyperkalemia, although a liberal intake of water may induce dilutional lowering of the serum sodium level.

ACTH deficiency may occur alone, but in some instances, it is only one part of panhypopituitarism, associated with multiple primary tropic hormone deficiencies. The differentiation of secondary disease from Addison disease can be confirmed with demonstration of low levels of plasma ACTH in the former. In patients with primary disease, the destruction of the adrenal cortex does not permit a response to exogenously administered ACTH in the form of increased plasma levels of cortisol, whereas in those with secondary hypofunction, there is a prompt rise in plasma cortisol levels.

MORPHOLOGY. In cases of hypoadrenalism secondary to hypothalamic or pituitary disease (**secondary hypoadrenalism**), depending on the extent of ACTH lack, the adrenals may be moderately to markedly reduced in size. They are reduced to small, flattened structures that usually retain their yellow color owing to a small amount of residual lipid. They may come to have a leaf-like appearance and be extremely difficult to find in the periadrenal fat. The cortex may be reduced to a thin ribbon having an unusually heavy fibrous capsule and scattered subcapsular cortical cells composed largely of zona glomerulosa. The medulla is unaffected.

ADRENOCORTICAL NEOPLASMS

It should be evident from preceding sections that functional adrenal neoplasms may be responsible for any of the various forms of hyperadrenalism. Not all adrenocortical neoplasms elaborate steroid hormones, however. The functional and nonfunctional adrenocortical neoplasms cannot be distinguished on the basis of morphologic features.[59] Determining whether a cortical neoplasm is functional or not is based on clinical assessment and measurement of the hormone in the laboratory.

MORPHOLOGY. Most **adrenocortical adenomas** are nonfunctional tumors and are usually encountered as incidental lesions at the time of autopsy. Whether functional or nonfunctional, the typical cortical adenoma is a well-circumscribed, nodular lesion up to 2.5 cm that expands the adrenal. Some nestle within the adrenal cortex, others appear to be within the medulla, and others protrude under the capsule. Some may achieve a larger size and exhibit areas of hemorrhage, cystic degeneration, and calcification. The encapsulation may be poorly defined and may appear at places to be deficient. In contrast to functional adenomas, which are associated with atrophy of the adjacent cortex, the cortex adjacent to nonfunctional adenomas is of normal thickness. On cut surface, adenomas are usually yellow to yellow-brown because of the presence of lipid within the tumor cells. Microscopically, adenomas are composed of cells similar to those populating the normal adrenal cortex. The nuclei are small, although some degree of pleomorphism may be seen even in benign lesions, even though mitotic activity is generally inconspicuous.

Adrenocortical carcinomas are rare neoplasms that may occur at any age, including childhood. They are more likely to be functional than adeno-

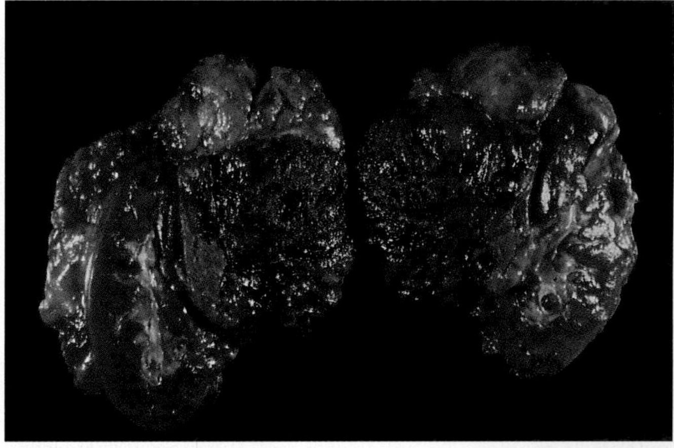

Figure 26–30

Adrenal carcinoma. The bright yellow tumor dwarfs the kidney and compresses the upper pole. It is largely hemorrhagic and necrotic.

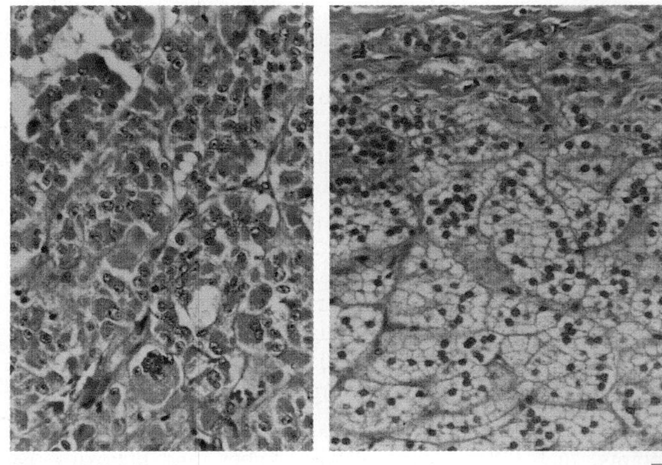

Figure 26–31

Adrenal carcinoma *(left)* revealing marked anaplasia, contrasted with normal cortical cells *(right)*.

mas and are therefore often associated with virilism or other clinical manifestations of hyperadrenalism. These tumors are highly malignant and usually large when discovered, many exceeding 20 cm in diameter. On cut section, they are predominantly yellow but frequently have hemorrhagic, cystic, and necrotic areas (Fig. 26–30). Many appear to be more or less encapsulated. Histologically, they range from lesions showing mild degrees of atypia to wildly anaplastic neoplasms composed of monstrous giant cells (Fig. 26–31). Between these extremes are found cancers with moderate degrees of anaplasia, some predominantly composed of spindle cells. Carcinomas, particularly those of bronchogenic origin, may metastasize to the adrenals, and they may be extremely difficult to differentiate from primary cortical carcinomas.

Adrenal cancers have a strong tendency to invade the adrenal vein, vena cava, and lymphatics. Metastases to regional and periaortic nodes are common as well as distant hematogenous spread to the lungs and other viscera. Bone metastases are unusual.

OTHER LESIONS OF THE ADRENAL

Adrenal cysts are relatively uncommon lesions; however, with the use of sophisticated abdominal imaging techniques, the frequency of these lesions appears to be increasing. The larger cysts may produce an abdominal mass and flank pain. Both cortical and medullary neoplasms may undergo necrosis and cystic degeneration and may present as "nonfunctional" cysts.

The adrenal myelolipoma is an unusual lesion composed of mature fat and hematopoietic cells. Although most of these lesions represent incidental findings, occasional myelolipomas may reach massive proportions. Foci of myelolipomatous change may be seen in cortical tumors and in adrenals with cortical hyperplasia.

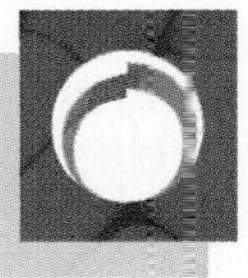

Adrenal Medulla

The adrenal medulla is developmentally, functionally, and structurally distinct from the adrenal cortex. It is composed of specialized neural crest (neuroendocrine) cells, termed *chromaffin* cells, and their supporting (sustentacular) cells. The chromaffin cells are round-to-oval, have prominent cytoplasmic membrane-bound granules of stored catecholamines, and are supported by a richly vascularized scant stroma of spindled and sustentacular cells. These cells, so named because of their brown-black color after exposure to potassium dichromate (e.g., Zenker), synthesize and secrete catecholamines in response to signals from preganglionic nerve fibers in the sympathetic nervous system. The adrenal medulla is the major source of catecholamines—epinephrine, norepinephrine—in the body. Norepinephrine functions as a local neurotransmitter, chiefly of sympathetic postganglionic neurons. Only small amounts reach the circulation. Epinephrine (adrenaline) is secreted into the vascular system. It interacts with α-adrenergic and β-adrenergic receptors in various cells, which then activate second messengers and a cascade of enzymatic reactions mediating the systemic actions of epinephrine, for example, increasing the force and rate of myocardial contractions and causing vasoconstriction of most vascular beds. Because the secretory cells are a part of the neuroendocrine system, they are also capable of synthesizing a variety of bioactive amines and peptides, such as histamine, serotonin, renin, chromogranin A, and neuropeptide hormones.

Neuroendocrine cells similar to chromaffin cells are widely dispersed in an extra-adrenal system of clusters and nodules, which together with the adrenal medulla make up the paraganglion system. These extra-adrenal paraganglia are closely associated with the autonomic nervous system and can be divided into three groups based on their anatomic distribution: (1) branchiomeric, (2) intravagal, and (3) aorticosympathetic (Fig. 26–32). The branchiomeric and intravagal paraganglia associated with the parasympathetic system are located close to the major arteries and cranial nerves of the head and neck and include the carotid bodies (Chapter 17). The intravagal paraganglia, as the term implies, are distributed along the vagus nerve. The aorticosympathetic chain is found in association with segmental ganglia of the sympathetic system and therefore is distributed mainly alongside of the abdominal aorta. The notorious organs of Zuckerkandl, close to the aortic bifurcation, belong to this group. The visceral paraganglia, as the term implies, are located within organs such as the urinary bladder. Histologically, all of the paraganglia are composed of cells closely resembling those of the adrenal medulla. Although many are functional, some are nonfunctional, and there is poor correspondence between the chromaffin reaction and the level of catecholamine release. Certain of the branchiomeric paraganglia, the carotid bodies in particular, are chemoreceptors capable of monitoring the oxygen and carbon dioxide levels in the blood. The most important diseases of the adrenal medulla are neoplasms, which include neoplasms of chromaffin cells (pheochromocytomas) and neuronal neoplasms (including neuroblastomas and more mature ganglion cell tumors).

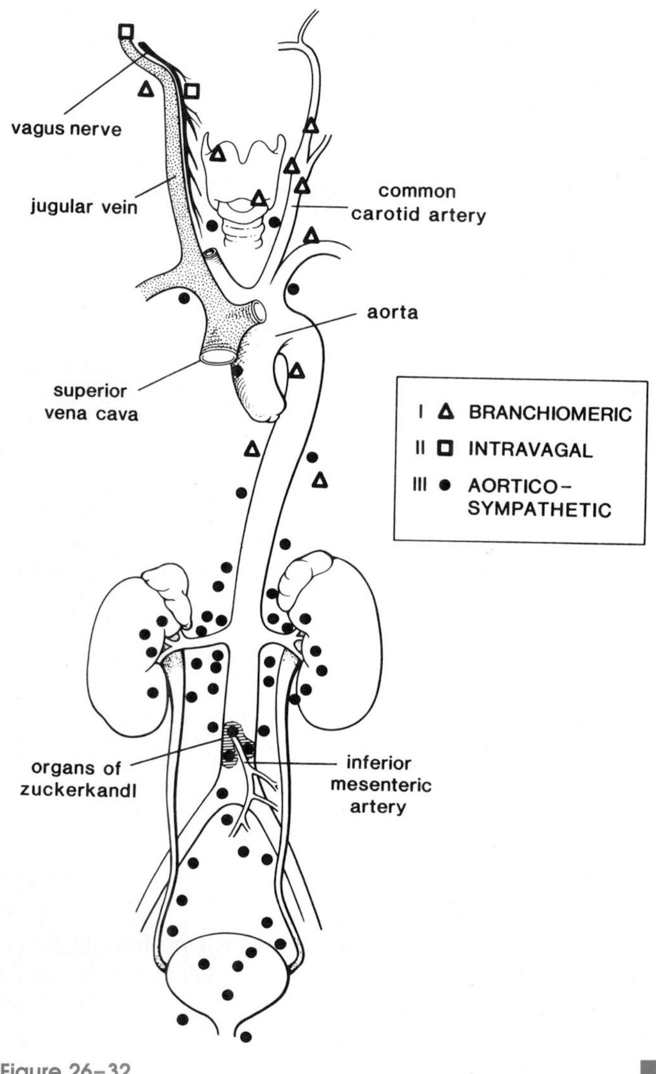

Figure 26–32

Schematic representation of paraganglion system demonstrates sites of paraganglion cell nests, in which neoplasms may form. Extra-adrenal portion of paraganglion system is grouped into three families based on anatomic distribution, innervation, and microscopic structure: (1) branchiomeric, (2) intravagal, and (3) aorticosympathetic. (From Whalen RK, et al: Extra-adrenal pheochromocytoma. J Urol 147:1–10, 1992; copyright Williams & Wilkins, 1992.)

PHEOCHROMOCYTOMA

Pheochromocytomas are uncommon neoplasms composed of chromaffin cells, which synthesize and release catecholamines and in some instances peptide hormones.[60] These tumors are important because they (similar to aldosterone-secreting adenomas) give rise to surgically correctable forms of hypertension. Although only about 0.1 to 0.3% of hypertensive patients have an underlying pheochromocytoma, the hypertension can be fatal when the pheochromocytoma goes unrecognized. Occasionally, one of these tumors produces other steroids or peptides and so may be associated with Cushing syndrome or some other endocrinopathy. About 85% of pheochromocytomas arise in the medulla of the adrenals, the remainder in any of the extra-adrenal paraganglia, more often below the diaphragm. Extra-adrenal tumors that are chromaffin negative are sometimes called *paragangliomas* to differentiate them from functioning pheochromocytomas. Although 90% of pheochromocytomas occur sporadically, about 10% occur in one of the several, mostly autosomal dominant, familial syndromes listed in Table 26–6. These include the MEN syndromes described later in this chapter, type I neurofibromatosis (Chapter 6), von Hippel–Lindau disease (Chapter 30), and Sturge-Weber syndrome (Chapter 12).[61] Although the nonfamilial pheochromocytomas most often occur in adults between 40 and 60 years of age, with a slight female preponderance, in the familial syndromes many arise in childhood, with a strong male preponderance. Most tumors in the familial syndromes are bilateral (70%), but in the nonfamilial setting only 10 to 15% are bilateral. Another highly significant difference is that frank malignancy is more common in tumors arising in extra-adrenal sites (20 to 40%) than it is in adrenal pheochromocytomas (10%).

MORPHOLOGY. Pheochromocytomas range from small, circumscribed lesions confined to the adrenal (Fig. 26–33) to large hemorrhagic masses

Table 26–6. FAMILIAL SYNDROMES WITH PHEOCHROMOCYTOMA

Syndrome	Components
MEN, type II or IIA	Medullary thyroid carcinomas and C cell hyperplasia Pheochromocytomas and adrenal medullary hyperplasia Parathyroid hyperplasia
MEN, type III or IIB	Medullary thyroid carcinomas and C cell hyperplasia Pheochromocytomas and adrenal medullary hyperplasia Mucosal neuromas Marfanoid features
von Hippel–Lindau	Renal, hepatic, pancreatic, and epididymal cysts Renal cell carcinomas Pheochromocytomas Angiomatosis Cerebellar hemangioblastomas
von Recklinghausen	Neurofibromatosis Café au lait skin spots Schwannomas, meningiomas, gliomas Pheochromocytomas
Sturge-Weber	Cavernous hemangiomas of fifth cranial nerve distribution Pheochromocytomas

MEN, multiple endocrine neoplasia.
Modified from Silverman ML, Lee AK: Anatomy and pathology of the adrenal glands. Urol Clin North Am *16*:417, 1989.

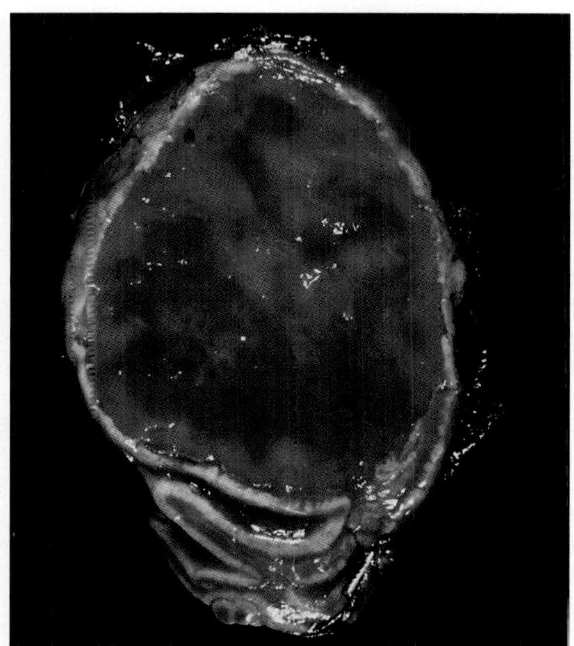

Figure 26–33

The gray-pink pheochromocytoma with areas of hemorrhage is enclosed within an attenuated cortex. The comma-shaped residual adrenal is seen below.

weighing kilograms. The average weight of a pheochromocytoma is 100 gm, but variations from just over 1 gm to almost 4000 gm have been reported. The larger tumors are well demarcated by either connective tissue or compressed cortical or medullary tissue. Fibrous trabeculae, richly vascularized, pass into the tumor and produce a lobular pattern. In many tumors, remnants of the adrenal gland can be seen, stretched over the surface or attached at one pole. On section, the cut surfaces of smaller pheochromocytomas are yellow-tan. Larger lesions tend to be hemorrhagic, necrotic, and cystic and typically efface the adrenal gland. Incubation of fresh tissue with a potassium dichromate solution turns the tumor a dark brown color owing to oxidation of stored catecholamines, thus the term *chromaffin.*

The histologic pattern in pheochromocytoma is quite variable. The tumors are composed of polygonal to spindle-shaped chromaffin cells, clustered with their supporting cells into small nests or alveoli **(zellballen),** by a rich vascular network. Uncommonly the dominant cell type is a spindle or small cell. Various patterns can be found in any one tumor. The cytoplasm has a finely granular appearance, best demonstrated with silver stains, owing to the appearance of granules containing catecholamines. Electron microscopy reveals variable numbers of membrane-bound, electron dense granules, representing catecholamines and sometimes other peptides (Fig. 26–34). Cellular and nuclear pleomorphism is often present, especially in the alveolar group of lesions, and giant and bizarre cells are commonly seen. Mitotic figures are rare and do not imply malignancy. Both capsular and vascular invasion may be encountered in benign lesions. Therefore the diagnosis of malignancy in pheochromocytomas is based exclusively on the presence of metastases.[62] These may involve regional lymph nodes as well as more distant sites, including liver, lung, and bone.

Clinical Course. The dominant clinical feature in patients with pheochromocytoma is *hypertension.* Classically this is described as an abrupt, precipitous elevation in blood pressure, associated with tachycardia, palpitations, headache, sweating, tremor, and a sense of apprehension. These episodes may also be associated wtih pain in the

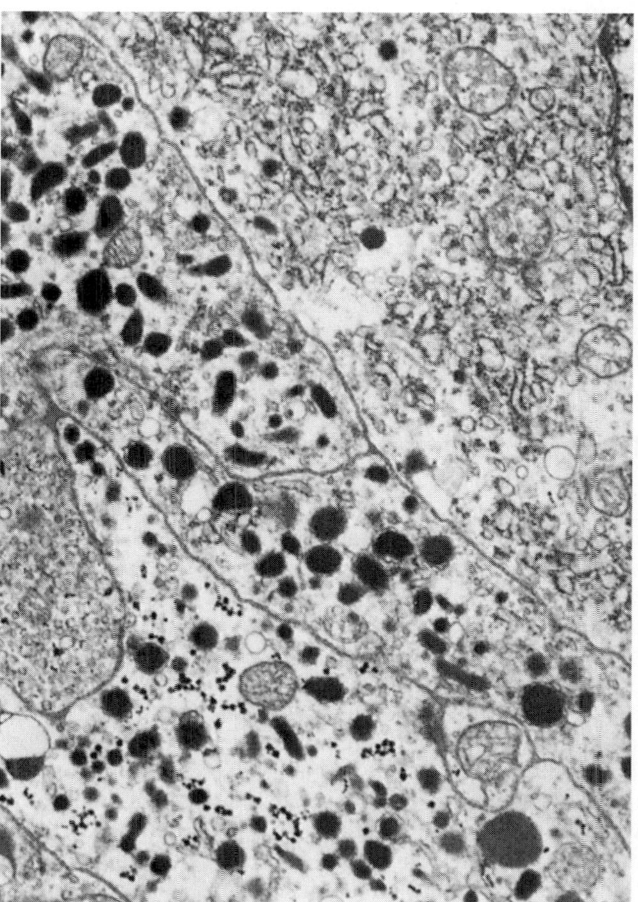

Figure 26–34

Electron micrograph of pheochromocytoma. This tumor contains membrane-bound secretory granules in which catecholamines are stored (30,000×).

abdomen or chest, nausea, and vomiting. In practice, isolated paroxysmal episodes of hypertension occur in less than half of patients. In about two thirds of patients, the hypertension occurs in the form of chronic, sustained elevation in blood pressure, although an element of labile hypertension is also present. The paroxysms may be precipitated by emotional stress, exercise, changes in posture, and palpation in the region of the tumor. The elevations of pressure are induced by the sudden release of catecholamines that may acutely precipitate congestive heart failure, pulmonary edema, myocardial infarction, ventricular fibrillation, and cerebrovascular accidents. The cardiac complications have been attributed to what has been called *catecholamine cardiomyopathy,* or catecholamine-induced myocardial instability and ventricular arrhythmias. The myocardial changes have been attributed to ischemic damage secondary to the catecholamine-induced vasomotor constriction of the myocardial circulation or to direct toxicity. Histologically, there are focal areas of myocytolysis and occasionally myofiber necrosis and interstitial fibrosis, sometimes with mononuclear inflammatory infiltrates. These cardiac lesions are often superimposed on hypertensive changes or alterations incident to coronary artery disease, and so, not surprisingly, patients may have anginal chest pain. In some cases, pheochromocytomas secrete other hormones, such as ACTH and somatostatin, and may therefore be associated with clinical features related to the secretion of these or other peptide hormones.

The laboratory diagnosis of pheochromocytoma is based on the demonstration of increased urinary excretion of free catecholamines and their metabolites, such as vanillylmandelic acid (VMA) and metanephrines. Isolated benign tumors are treated with surgical excision, after pre-operative and intraoperative medication of patients with adrenergic-blocking agents. Multifocal lesions require long-term medical treatment for hypertension.

Tumors of Extra-Adrenal Paraganglia

Pheochromocytomas that develop in paraganglia other than the adrenal medulla are often designated *paragangliomas,* although some restrict the term to the nonfunctioning tumors. Paragangliomas may arise in any organ that contains paraganglionic tissue. Tumors arising in the carotid body are designated carotid body tumors, whereas those originating in the jugulotympanic body are sometimes referred to as *chemodectomas* because these paraganglia sense the oxygen and carbon dioxide levels of the blood. The *carotid body tumor* is a typical paraganglioma, forming a palpable mass in the neck enveloping the carotid vessels. Paragangliomas are uncommon and occur about one tenth as frequently as adrenal pheochromocytomas. Most are discovered in the teens and twenties, with no significant sex predisposition. They are, however, much more often multicentric (15 to 25% of cases) than adrenal tumors. Despite the infrequency and small size of paragangliomas, they are of great clinical importance because from 10 to 40% are malignant and recur after resection, and overall about 10% metastasize widely, causing death.

MORPHOLOGY. Typically, these lesions range from 1 to 6 cm in diameter and are firm and tan-red. Despite encapsulation, well developed or scant, they are often densely adherent to adjacent vessels and difficult to excise. Histologically, they are composed of well-differentiated neuroendocrine cells with indistinct outlines, so they may give the appearance of syncytia. The cells are arranged typically in small clusters (zellballen) or cords separated by prominent fibrovascular stroma. Some tumors completely mimic the appearance of adrenal pheochromocytomas. Distinctive within the cells in most tumors are dark neurosecretory granules that contain catecholamines. Sometimes the cells are spindle shaped. Mitoses are usually infrequent, but occasional tumors are overtly anaplastic and pleomorphic and contain numerous mitoses. The malignancy rates (up to 40%) for paraganglion tumors are significantly higher than those for adrenal pheochromocytomas. The more anaplastic lesions may disseminate widely and cause death.

NEUROBLASTOMA

Neuroblastoma is the most common extracranial solid tumor of childhood. It originates in the adrenal medulla or anywhere in the sympathetic nervous system. Most neuroblastomas are sporadic, although familial cases occur. These tumors are discussed along with the other pediatric neoplasms in Chapter 11.

MULTIPLE ENDOCRINE NEOPLASIA SYNDROMES

The MEN syndromes are a group of familial diseases associated with hyperplasias or neoplasms (or both) of several endocrine organs. The disorders are inherited as autosomal dominant traits. The principal features of these syndromes are summarized in Table 26–7.

MEN I, or *Wermer syndrome,* is characterized by abnormalities involving the *parathyroids, pancreas,* and *pituitary glands;* thus the mnemonic device, the *3Ps.* It is a rare heritable disorder with a prevalence of about 2 per 100,000. *Primary hyperparathyroidism* is the most common manifestation of MEN I and is the initial manifestation of the disorder in most patients, appearing in almost all patients by age 40 to 50.[63] Parathyroid abnormalities include both hyperplasia and adenomas. The pancreatic le-

Table 26-7. MULTIPLE ENDOCRINE NEOPLASIA (MEN) SYNDROMES

	MEN I (Wermer Syndrome)	MEN II or IIA (Sipple Syndrome)	MEN IIB or III
Pituitary	Adenomas		
Parathyroid	Hyperplasia+++ Adenomas+	Hyperplasia+ Adenomas	Hyperplasia
Pancreatic islets	Hyperplasia+ Adenomas+++ Carcinoma++		
Adrenal	Cortical hyperplasia++	Pheochromocytoma++	Pheochromocytoma+++
Thyroid	C-cell hyperplasia	Medullary carcinoma+++	Medullary carcinoma++
Extraendocrine changes			Mucocutaneous ganglioneuromas Marfanoid habitus
Mutant gene locus	MEN I	RET	RET

Relative frequency: +, uncommon; +++, common.

sions include islet cell tumors, which may secrete a wide range of peptide hormones, including insulin, glucagon, gastrin, somatostatin, and vasoactive intestinal peptide (VIP). The most common type of anterior pituitary tumor in MEN I is prolactinoma, although other types of tumors can occur. The spectrum of this disease has been expanded beyond the *3Ps.* The duodenum is a common site of gastrinomas in these patients, and carcinoid tumors, thyroid and adrenocortical adenomas, and lipomas are more frequent than in the general population. The genetic defect in MEN I has been linked to a novel gene on chromosome 11 (11q13) that has been shown to be mutated in 14 of 15 families with MEN I.[50] The MEN I gene product shows no significant homology to known proteins, and the biochemical and cellular functions of the protein are not known. As noted previously, mutations in this gene have also been found in 16% of sporadic nonfamilial parathyroid adenomas, further supporting the relationship between the mutations and tumorigenesis.[51]

The dominant clinical manifestations of MEN I are usually defined by the peptide hormones and include such abnormalities as recurrent hypoglycemia in insulinomas and recurrent peptic ulcers in patients with gastrin-secreting neoplasms (Zollinger-Ellison syndrome). The pancreatic islet cell tumors are often multiple and may either be malignant or benign. Pituitary adenomas of any type may be encountered but are usually a less prominent feature than are abnormalities referable to the parathyroid or pancreas.

MEN II is subclassified into three distinct syndromes: MEN IIA, MEN IIB, and familial medullary thyroid cancer.[63] *MEN IIA,* or *Sipple syndrome,* is characterized by *pheochromocytoma, medullary carcinoma,* and *parathyroid hyperplasias.* Medullary carcinomas of the thyroid occur in almost 100% of patients. They are usually multifocal and virtually always associated with foci of C cell hyperplasia. The medullary carcinomas may elaborate calcitonin and other active products and are usually clinically aggressive. Forty percent to 50% of patients with MEN IIA have pheochromocytomas, which are often bilateral and may arise in extra-adrenal sites. As in the case of pheochromocytomas in general, they may be benign or malignant. Ten percent to 20% of patients have parathyroid hyperplasia and evidence of hypercalcemia or renal stones. MEN II is clinically and genetically distinct from MEN I and has been linked to germ line mutations in the *RET protooncogene* on chromosome 10.[37] As noted earlier, the RET protooncogene is a receptor tyrosine kinase that binds *glial-derived neurotrophic factor* and transmits growth and differentiation signals (Chapter 8). These germ line mutations *constitutively activate* the receptor, resulting in gain of function. This is different from most other inherited predispositions to neoplasia, which are due to heritable loss of function mutations that inactivate tumor-suppressor proteins (Chapter 8). In contrast to MEN I, in which the long-term benefit of early diagnosis via genetic screening is not well established, diagnosis via screening of at-risk family members in MEN IIA kindreds is important because medullary thyroid carcinoma is a life-threatening disease that can be prevented by early thyroidectomy.

MEN IIB, also known as MEN III, is clinically similar to MEN IIA. It is genetically distinct and involves a mutation in the RET protooncogene that is different from those associated with MEN IIA. A single amino acid change appears to be responsible for virtually all cases of MEN IIB and affects a critical region of the tyrosine kinase catalytic core. In addition to medullary carcinomas and pheochromocytomas, MEN IIB is also accompanied by *neuromas* or ganglioneuromas involving the skin, oral mucosa, eyes, respiratory tract, and gastrointestinal tract. These additional features distinguish MEN IIB from MEN IIA.

Familial medullary thyroid cancer is a variant of MEN IIA, in which there is a strong predisposition to medullary thyroid cancer but not the other clinical manifestations of MEN IIA (or IIB). A substantial majority of cases of medullary thyroid cancer are sporadic, but as many as 25% may be familial. As noted, germ line mutations of RET are responsible for this heritable disease.

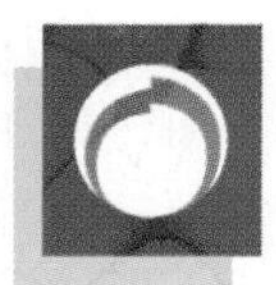

Pineal

PINEAL GLAND

The rarity of clinically significant lesions (virtually only tumors) justifies brevity in the consideration of the pineal gland. It is a minute, pine cone–shaped organ (hence its name), weighing 100 to 180 mg and lying between the superior colliculi at the base of the brain. It is composed of a loose, neuroglial stroma enclosing nests of epithelial-appearing pineocytes containing well-defined neurosecretory granules (melatonin). Silver impregnations reveal that these cells have long, slender processes reminiscent of primitive neuronal precursors intermixed with the processes of astrocytic cells.

All tumors involving the pineal are rare; most (50 to 70%) arise from sequestered embryonic germ cells. They most commonly take the form of so-called *germinomas* replicating testicular seminoma (Chapter 23) or ovarian dysgerminoma (Chapter 24). Other lines of germ cell differentiation include embryonal carcinomas; choriocarcinomas; mixtures of germinoma, embryonal carcinoma, and choriocarcinoma; and, uncommonly, typical teratomas (usually benign). Whether to characterize these germ cell neoplasms as pinealomas is still a subject of debate, but most "pinealophiles" favor restricting the term *pinealoma* to neoplasms arising from the pineocytes.

PINEALOMAS

These neoplasms are divided into two categories, pineoblastomas and pineocytomas, based on their level of differentiation, which, in turn, correlates with their neoplastic aggressiveness.[64]

MORPHOLOGY. Pineoblastomas are encountered mostly in young people and appear as soft, friable, gray masses punctuated with areas of hemorrhage and necrosis. They typically invade surrounding structures, that is, hypothalamus, midbrain, and lumen of the third ventricle. Histologically, they are composed of masses of pleomorphic cells two to four times the diameter of an erythrocyte. Large hyperchromatic nuclei appear to occupy almost the entire cell, and mitoses are frequent. The cytology is that of medulloblastoma-neuroblastoma of the brain. Large, poorly formed rosettes are sometimes present in the pineoblastoma, reminiscent of those seen in their "first cousins" in the brain. A further similarity is the tendency of pineoblastomas to spread via the cerebrospinal fluid. As might be expected, the enlarging mass may compress the aqueduct of Sylvius, giving rise to internal hydrocephalus and all its consequences. Survival beyond 1 or 2 years is rare.

In contrast, **pineocytomas** occur mostly in adults and are much slower growing than pineoblastomas. They tend to be well-circumscribed, gray, or hemorrhagic masses that compress but do not infiltrate surrounding structures. **Histologically, they exhibit divergent glial and neuronal differentiation.** On one hand, the neoplasm may be largely astrocytomatous. These areas stain positively for glial fibrillary acidic protein. On the other hand, it may be composed largely of pineocytes having darkly staining, round-to-oval, fairly regular nuclei that stain for neuron-specific enolase. Particularly distinctive of the pineocytoma are the pseudorosettes rimmed by rows of pineocytes. The centers of these rosettes are filled with eosinophilic cytoplasmic material representing tumor cell processes. These cells are set against a background of thin, fibrovascular, anastomosing septa that divide the tumor into lobular masses.

In addition to the monomorphic pineocytomas, there are many instances in which mixed patterns are encountered, in part astrocytic, in part pineocytomatous, sometimes having neuronal-type cells.

The clinical course of patients with pineocytomas is prolonged, averaging 7 years. The manifestations are the consequence of their pressure effects and consist of visual disturbances, headache, mental deterioration, and sometimes dementia-like behavior. The lesions being located where they are, it is understandable that successful excision is at best difficult.

REFERENCES

1. Yeh PJ, Chen JW: Pituitary tumors: surgical and medical management. Surg Oncol 6:67, 1997.
2. Mindermann T, Wilson CB: Age-related and gender-related occurrences of pituitary adenomas. Clin Endocrinol 41:359, 1994.
3. Alexander JM: Clinically nonfunctioning pituitary tumors are monoclonal in origin. J Clin Invest 86:336, 1990.
4. Lyons J, et al: Two G protein oncogenes in human endocrine tumors. Science 249:655, 1990.
5. Schlechte J, et al: The natural history of untreated hyperprolactinemia. J Clin Endocrinol Metab 68:412, 1989.
6. Melmed S, et al: Recent advances in pathogenesis diagnosis and management of acromegaly. J Clin Endocrinol Metab 80:3395, 1995.
7. Ho DM, et al: The clinicopathological characteristics of gonadotroph cell adenomas. Hum Pathol 28:905, 1997.
8. Beck-Peccoz P, et al: Thyrotropin-secreting pituitary tumors. Endocr Rev 17:610, 1997.

9. Sheehan HL: Postpartum necrosis of the anterior pituitary. J Pathol Bacteriol 45:189, 1987.
10. Barkan A Pituitary atrophy in patients with Sheehan's syndrome. Am J Med Sci 298:39, 1989.
11. Pfaffle RW, et al: Mutation of the POU-specific domain of pit-1 and hypopituitarism without pituitary hypoplasia. Science 257:1118, 1992.
12. Maesaka JK: An expanded view of SIADH. Clin Nephrol 46:79, 1996.
13. DeVile CJ, et al: Growth and endocrine sequelae of craniopharyngioma. Arch Dis Child 75:108, 1996.
14. Brent GA The molecular basis of thyroid hormone action. N Engl J Med 331:847, 1994.
15. Trzepacz PT, et al: Graves' disease: an analysis of thyroid hormone levels and hyperthyroid signs and symptoms. Am J Med 87:558, 1989.
16. Klein I, Levey GS: The cardiovascular system in thyrotoxicosis. In Braverman L, Utiger R (eds): Werner and Ingbar's The Thyroid, 7th ed. Philadelphia, Lippincott-Raven, 1996, p 607.
17. Dayan CM, Daniels GH: Chronic autoimmune thyroiditis. N Engl J Med 335:99, 1996.
18. Hutchings PR, et al: A thyroxine-containing peptide can induce murine experimental autoimmune thyroiditis. J Exp Med 175:869, 1992.
19. Giordano C, et al: Potential involvement of Fas and its ligand in the pathogenesis of Hashimoto's thyroiditis. Science 275:960, 1997.
20. Lazarus JH: Silent thyroiditis and subacute thyroiditis. In Braverman L, Utiger R (eds): Werner and Ingbar's The Thyroid, 7th ed. Philadelphia, Lippincott-Raven, 1996, p 577.
21. Harach HR, Williams ED: The pathology of granulomatous diseases of the thyroid. Sarcoidosis 7:19, 1990.
22. Graves RJ: Newly observed affection of the thyroid. London Medical and Surgical Journal 7:515, 1835.
23. Brown RS: Immunoglobulins affecting thyroid growth: a continuing controversy. J Clin Endocrinol Metab 80:1506, 1995.
24. Tomer Y, Davies TF: Infection, thyroid disease and autoimmunity. Endocr Rev 14:107, 1993.
25. Davies TF, et al: Evidence of limited variability of antigen receptors on intrathyroidal T cells in autoimmune thyroid disease. N Engl J Med 325:238, 1991.
26. Bahn RS, Heufelder AE: Pathogenesis of Graves' ophthalmopathy. N Engl J Med 329:1468, 1993.
27. Singer PA, et al: Treatment guidelines for patients with hyperthyroidism and hypothyroidism. JAMA 273:808, 1995.
28. Leonard JL, Koehrle J: Intracellular pathways of iodothyronine metabolism. In Braverman L, Utiger R (eds): Werner and Ingbar's The Thyroid, 7th ed. Philadelphia, Lippincott-Raven, 1996, p 125.
29. Studer H, Ramelli F: Simple goiter and its variants: euthyroid and hyperthyroid multinodular goiters. Endocr Rev 3:40, 1982.
30. Derwahl M: Molecular aspects of the pathogenesis of nodular goiters, thyroid nodules and adenomas. Exp Clin Endocrinol Diabetes 4:32, 1996.
31. Kopp P, et al: Polyclonal and monoclonal thyroid nodules coexist within human multinodular goiters. J Clin Endocrinol Metab 79:134, 1994.
32. Ramelli F, et al: Pathogenesis of thyroid nodules in multinodular goiter. Am J Pathol 109:215, 1982.
33. Mazzaferri EL: Management of a solitary thyroid nodule. N Engl J Med 328:553, 1993.
34. Paschke R, Ludgate M: The thyrotropin receptor in thyroid disease. N Engl J Med 337:1675, 1997.
35. Gagel RF, et al: Changing concepts in the pathogenesis and management of thyroid carcinoma. CA Cancer J Clin 46:261, 1996.
36. Schlumberger MJ: Papillary and follicular thyroid cancer. N Engl J Med 338:297, 1998.
37. Eng C: The RET proto-oncogene in multiple endocrine neoplasia type 2 and Hirschsprung's disease. N Engl J Med 335:943, 1996.
38. Challeton C, et al: Pattern of ras and gsp oncogene mutations in radiation-associated human thyroid tumors. Oncogene 11:601, 1995.
39. Fagin JA, et al: High prevalence of mutations of the p53 gene in poorly differentiated human thyroid carcinomas. J Clin Invest 91:179, 1993.
40. Rosai J, et al: Tumors of the thyroid gland. In: Atlas of Tumor Pathology, Washington, DC, Armed Forces Institute of Pathology, 1990, p 49.
41. Gillialan FD, et al: Prognostic factors for thyroid carcinoma. Cancer 79:564, 1997.
42. Ball DW, et al: Medullary thyroid carcinoma. In Braverman LE, Utiger RD (eds): Werner and Ingbar's The Thyroid, 7th ed. Philadelphia, Lippincott-Raven, 1996, p 946.
43. LiVolsi VA: Surgical pathology of the thyroid. In Bennington JL (ed): Major Problems in Pathology, vol 22. Philadelphia, WB Saunders, 1990.
44. Tan RK: Anaplastic carcinoma of the thyroid. Head Neck 17:41, 1995.
45. Ito T, et al: Unique association of p53 mutations with undifferentiated but not with differentiated carcinomas of the thyroid gland Cancer Res 52:1369, 1992.
46. Brown EM, et al: The extracellular calcium-sensing receptor: its role in health and disease. Annu Rev Med 49:15, 1998.
47. Ikeda K, Ogata E: Humoral hypercalcemia of malignancy: Some enigmas on the clinical features. J Cell Biochem 57:384, 1995.
48. Wermers RA, et al: The rise and fall of primary hyperparathyroidism: a population based study. Ann Intern Med 126:433, 1997.
49. Hsi ED, et al: Cyclin D1/PRAD1 expression in parathyroid adenomas. J Clin Endocrinol Metab 81:1736, 1996.
50. Chandrasekharappa SC, et al: Positional cloning of the gene for multiple endocrine neoplasia-type 1. Science 276:404, 1997.
51. Heppner C, et al: Somatic mutation of the MEN1 gene in parathyroid tumors. Nat Genet 16:375, 1997.
52. Silverberg SJ, Bilezikian JP: Evaluation and management of primary hyperparathyroidism. J Clin Endocrinol Metab 81:2036, 1996.
53. Shapira H, et al: Pseudohypoparathyroidism type 1a: two new heterozygous frameshift mutations in the Gs alpha gene. Hum Genet 97:73, 1996.
54. Tsigos C, Chrousos GP: Differential diagnosis and management of Cushing's syndrome. Annu Rev Med 47:443, 1996.
55. Orth DN: Medical progress: Cushing's syndrome. N Engl J Med 332:791, 1995.
56. Blumenfeld JD, et al: Diagnosis and treatment of primary hyperaldosteronism. Ann Intern Med 121:877, 1994.
57. Newfield RS, New MI: 21-hydroxylase deficiency. Ann N Y Acad Sci 816:219, 1997.
58. Oelkers W: Adrenal insufficiency. N Engl J Med 335:1206, 1996.
59. Lack EE: Tumors of the adrenal gland and extra-adrenal paraganglia. In: Atlas of Tumor Pathology. Washington, DC, Armed Forces Institute of Pathology, 1997.
60. Bravo EL: Evolving concepts in the pathophysiology, diagnosis, and treatment of pheochromocytoma. Endocr Rev 15:356, 1994.
61. Neumann HP, et al: Pheochromocytomas, multiple endocrine neoplasia type 2 and von Hippel-Lindau disease. N Engl J Med 329:1531, 1993.
62. Pattarino F, Bouloux P-M: The diagnosis of malignancy in pheochromocytoma. Clin Endocrinol 44:239, 1996.
63. Trump D, et al: Clinical studies of multiple endocrine neoplasia type 1 (MEN1). QJM 89:653, 1996.
64. Disclafani A, et al: Pineocytomas. Cancer 63:302, 1989.

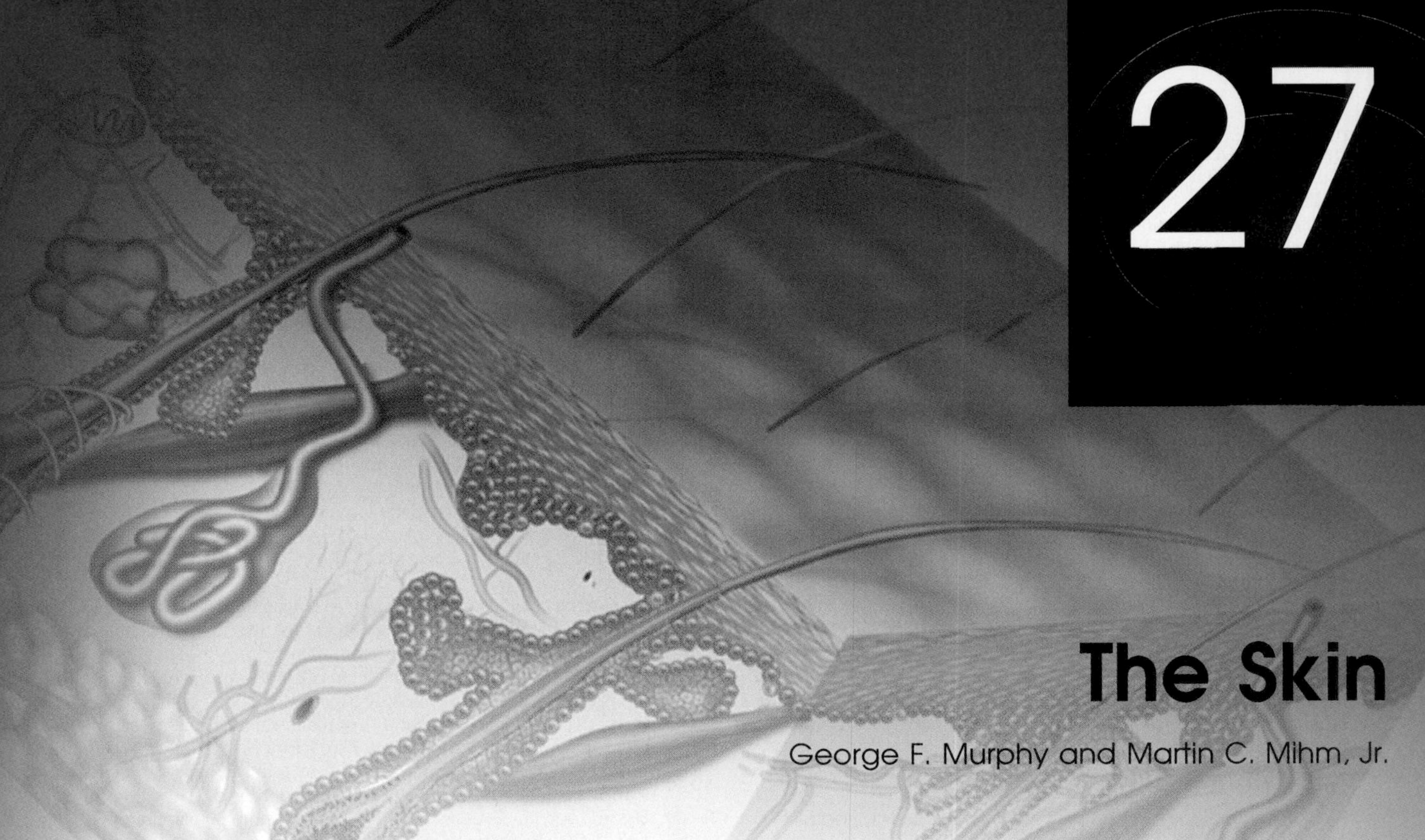

27

The Skin

George F. Murphy and Martin C. Mihm, Jr.

THE SKIN AS A PROTECTIVE ORGAN

DISORDERS OF PIGMENTATION AND MELANOCYTES

VITILIGO

FRECKLE (EPHELIS)

MELASMA

LENTIGO

NEVOCELLULAR NEVUS (PIGMENTED NEVUS, MOLE)

DYSPLASTIC NEVI

MALIGNANT MELANOMA

BENIGN EPITHELIAL TUMORS

SEBORRHEIC KERATOSES

ACANTHOSIS NIGRICANS

FIBROEPITHELIAL POLYP

EPITHELIAL CYST (WEN)

KERATOACANTHOMA

ADNEXAL (APPENDAGE) TUMORS

PREMALIGNANT AND MALIGNANT EPIDERMAL TUMORS

ACTINIC KERATOSIS

SQUAMOUS CELL CARCINOMA

BASAL CELL CARCINOMA

MERKEL CELL CARCINOMA

TUMORS OF THE DERMIS

BENIGN FIBROUS HISTIOCYTOMA

DERMATOFIBROSARCOMA PROTUBERANS

XANTHOMAS

DERMAL VASCULAR TUMORS

TUMORS OF CELLULAR IMMIGRANTS TO THE SKIN

HISTIOCYTOSIS X

MYCOSIS FUNGOIDES (CUTANEOUS T-CELL LYMPHOMA)

MASTOCYTOSIS

DISORDERS OF EPIDERMAL MATURATION

ICHTHYOSIS

ACUTE INFLAMMATORY DERMATOSES

URTICARIA

ACUTE ECZEMATOUS DERMATITIS

ERYTHEMA MULTIFORME

CHRONIC INFLAMMATORY DERMATOSES

PSORIASIS

LICHEN PLANUS

LUPUS ERYTHEMATOSUS

BLISTERING (BULLOUS) DISEASES

PEMPHIGUS

BULLOUS PEMPHIGOID

DERMATITIS HERPETIFORMIS

NONINFLAMMATORY BLISTERING DISEASES: EPIDERMOLYSIS BULLOSA, PORPHYRIA

DISORDERS OF EPIDERMAL APPENDAGES

ACNE VULGARIS

PANNICULITIS

ERYTHEMA NODOSUM AND ERYTHEMA INDURATUM

INFECTION AND INFESTATION

VERRUCAE (WARTS)

MOLLUSCUM CONTAGIOSUM

IMPETIGO

SUPERFICIAL FUNGAL INFECTIONS

ARTHROPOD BITES, STINGS, AND INFESTATIONS

THE SKIN AS A PROTECTIVE ORGAN

More than 100 years ago, Virchow portrayed the skin as a protective covering for more delicate and functionally sophisticated internal viscera.[1] At that time, the skin was appreciated primarily as a passive barrier to fluid loss and mechanical injury. During the past three decades, however, enormously productive avenues of scientific inquiry have demonstrated skin to be a complex organ in which precisely regulated cellular and molecular interactions govern many crucial responses to our environment.

We now know that skin is composed of a number of interdependent cell types and structures that work toward a common protective goal (Fig. 27–1). *Melanocytes* within the epidermis are cells responsible for the production of a brown pigment (melanin) that represents an important endogenous screen against harmful ultraviolet rays in sunlight. *Langerhans cells* are epidermal dendritic cells that take up and process antigenic signals and communicate this information to lymphoid cells. *Squamous epithelial cells (keratinocytes)* are major sites for the biosynthesis of soluble molecules (cytokines) which are important in the regulation of adjacent epidermal cells as well as cells in the dermis, as illustrated in Figure 27–2.[2] *Neural end-organs and axonal processes* warn of potentially damaging physical factors in the environment and have recently been found to assist in regulation of immunocompetent cells.[3] *Sweat glands* guard against deleterious variations in body temperature, and *hair follicles* contain protected repositories of epithelial stem cells[4] capable of regenerating superficial skin layers that have been disrupted by a variety of hostile external and internal agents. Specialized dermal cells *(dendrocytes)* are probably engineered for antigen presentation as well as for production of molecules (e.g., factor XIIIa) capable of coordinating the assembly of macromolecular complexes important in the early stages of wounds affecting the deeper cutaneous layers.[5] Although the human integument may be superficially drab compared with the skin and pelage of certain other members of the animal kingdom, it is indeed extraordinarily vibrant with regard to the diversity and complexity of protective functions that it serves.

Factors affecting the delicate homeostasis that exists among skin cells may result in conditions as diverse as wrinkles and hair loss, blisters and rashes, and even life-threatening cancers and disorders of immune regulation. For example, chronic exposure to sunlight fosters premature cutaneous aging, blunting of immunologic responses to environmental antigens, and the development of a variety of premalignant and malignant cutaneous neoplasms. Ingested agents, such as therapeutic drugs, can cause an enormous number of rashes or exanthems. Internal disorders, such as diabetes mellitus, amyloidosis, and lupus erythematosus, may also have important manifestations in the skin.

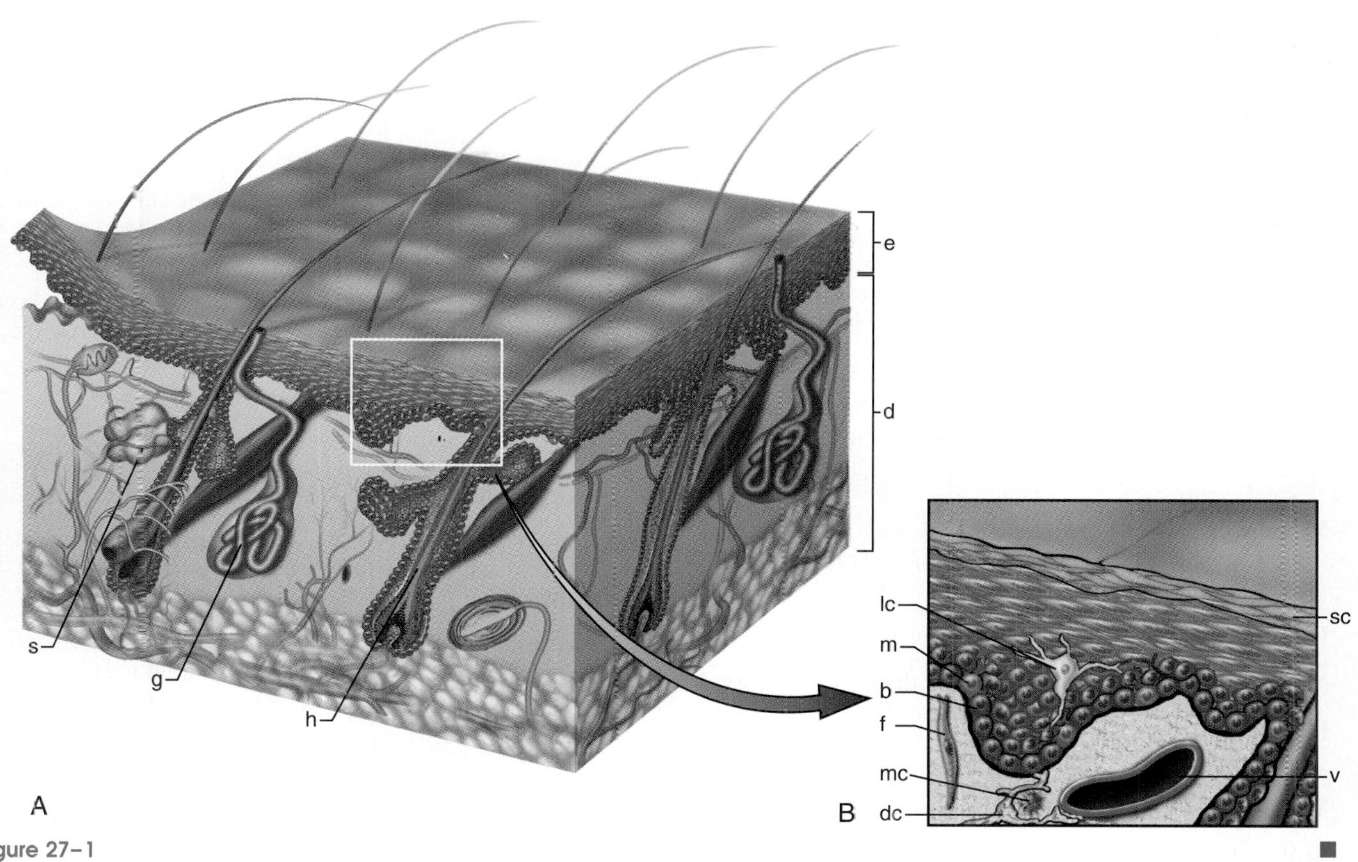

Figure 27–1

A, The skin is composed of an epidermal layer (e) from which specialized adnexa (hair follicles, h; sweat glands, g; and sebaceous glands, s) descend into the underlying dermis (d). *B*, This projection of the epidermal layer (e) and underlying superficial dermis demonstrates the progressive upward maturation of basal cells (b) into cornified squamous epithelial cells of the stratum corneum (sc). Melanin-containing dendritic melanocytes (m) and midepidermal dendritic Langerhans cells (Lc) are also present. The underlying dermis contains small vessels (v), fibroblasts (f), perivascular mast cells (mc), and dendrocytes (dc), potentially important in dermal immunity and repair.

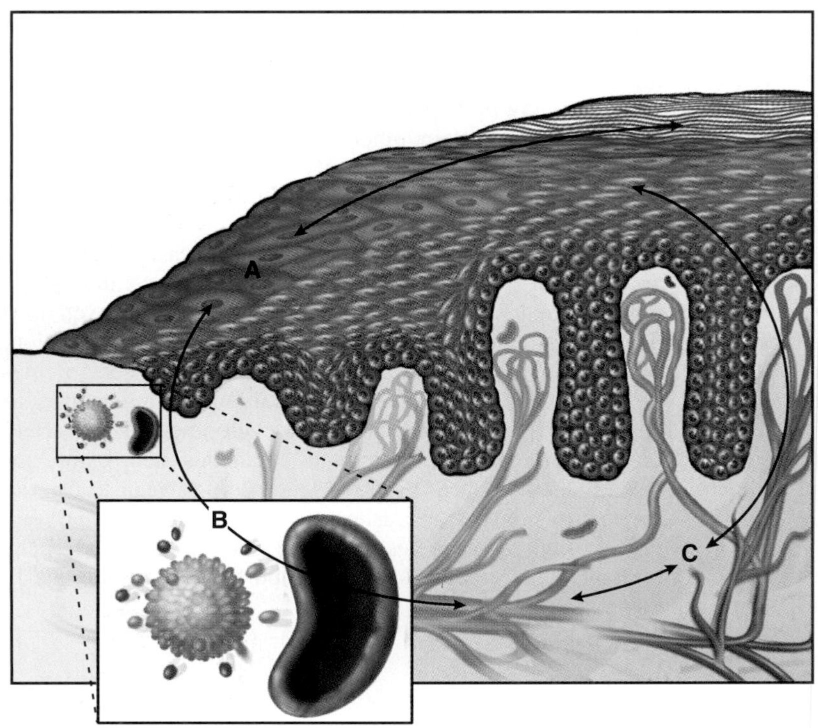

Figure 27–2

Schematic representation of dynamic interaction between the epidermal layer and the dermal layer. Keratinocytes at the edge of an ulcer (A) produce cytokines and factors that influence both keratinization and the function of underlying dermal cells (B). In turn, dermal cells (B), such as mast cells, also release cytokines (green granules) and proteases (red granules), which may regulate both endothelial cells and overlying keratinocytes. Perturbations in these interactions between epidermal cells and dermal cells may contribute to pathologic processes, such as psoriasis (C), in which both compartments become morphologically abnormal. (See discussion on psoriasis.)

Definition of Terms

Accurate description of the clinical appearance of the skin at a macroscopic level is critical, since lesions before biopsy are, in effect, the gross pathology. Correlation between the gross and histologic appearances is often critical in formulating diagnoses and in understanding pathogenesis. Accordingly, efforts are made in the following pages to depict and describe clinical lesions whenever possible and to relate these findings to the microscopic appearance of lesions.

MACROSCOPIC TERMS

Macule Circumscribed area of any size characterized by its flatness and usually distinguished from surrounding skin by its coloration

Papule Elevated solid area 5 mm or less across

Nodule Elevated solid area greater than 5 mm across

Plaque Elevated flat-topped area, usually greater than 5 mm across

Vesicle Fluid-filled raised area 5 mm or less across

Bulla Fluid-filled raised area greater than 5 mm across

Blister Common term used for vesicle or bulla

Pustule Discrete, pus-filled, raised area

Wheal Itchy, transient, elevated area with variable blanching and erythema formed as the result of dermal edema

Scale Dry, horny, platelike excrescence; usually the result of imperfect cornification

Lichenification Thickened and rough skin characterized by prominent skin markings; usually the result of repeated rubbing in susceptible persons

Excoriation A traumatic lesion characterized by breakage of the epidermis, causing a raw linear area (i.e., a deep scratch). Such lesions are often self-induced.

Onycholysis Loss of integrity of the nail substance

MICROSCOPIC TERMS

Hyperkeratosis Hyperplasia of the stratum corneum often associated with a qualitative abnormality of the keratin

Parakeratosis Modes of keratinization characterized by the retention of the nuclei in the stratum corneum. On mucous membranes, parakeratosis is normal.

Acanthosis Epidermal hyperplasia

Dyskeratosis Abnormal keratinization occurring prematurely within individual cells or groups of cells below the stratum granulosum

Acantholysis Loss of intercellular connections resulting in loss of cohesion between keratinocytes

Papillomatosis Hyperplasia of the papillary dermis with elongation or widening of the dermal papillae

Lentiginous Referring to a linear pattern of melanocyte proliferation within the epidermal basal cell layer. Lentiginous melanocytic hyperplasia can occur as a reactive change or as part of a neoplasm of melanocytes

Spongiosis Intercellular edema of the epidermis

Exocytosis Infiltration of the epidermis by inflammatory or circulating blood cells

Erosion Discontinuity of the skin exhibiting incomplete loss of the epidermis

Ulceration Discontinuity of the skin exhibiting complete loss of the epidermis and often of portions of the dermis and even subcutaneous fat

Vacuolization Formation of vacuoles within or adjacent to cells; often refers to basal cell–basement membrane zone area

DISORDERS OF PIGMENTATION AND MELANOCYTES

Skin pigmentation has historically had major societal implications. Cosmetic desire for increased pigmentation (tanning) has resulted in many deleterious alterations that are described in the pages that follow. Focal or widespread loss of normal protective pigmentation not only renders individuals extraordinarily vulnerable to the harmful effects of sunlight (as in albinism) but also has resulted in severe emotional stresses and, in some cultures, profound social and economic discrimination (as in vitiligo). Change in preexisting skin pigmentation may signify important primary events in the skin (e.g., malignant transformation of a mole) or disorders of internal viscera (e.g., in Addison disease).

Vitiligo

Vitiligo is a common disorder characterized by partial or complete loss of pigment-producing melanocytes within the epidermis. All ages and races are affected, but lesions are most noticeable in darkly pigmented individuals. Lesions may be entirely inapparent in lightly pigmented skin until tanning occurs in the surrounding normal skin.

Clinical lesions are asymptomatic, flat, well-demarcated zones (macules) of pigment loss (Fig. 27–3*A*); their size varies from few to many centimeters. Vitiligo often involves the hands and wrists; axillae; and perioral, periorbital, and anogenital skin.

MORPHOLOGY. On histologic examination, vitiligo is characterized by loss of melanocytes, as defined by electron microscopy (Fig. 27–3*B*). This is in contrast to some forms of **albinism,** in which melanocytes are present but no melanin pigment is produced because of a lack of or defect in the tyrosinase enzyme. Both conditions may be differentiated from other forms of hypopigmentation (unrelated to the absence of melanocytes or tyrosinase enzyme) by demonstrating diminished or absent activity of melanocyte tyrosinase on the melanin pigment precursor dopa (dihydroxyphenylalanine). This histochemical stain is useful because melanocytes or their melanogenic potential cannot be reliably quantified in routine hematoxylin and eosin (H&E) sections.

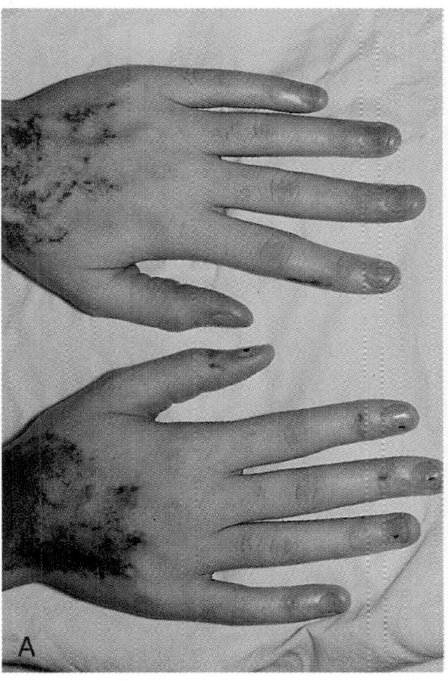

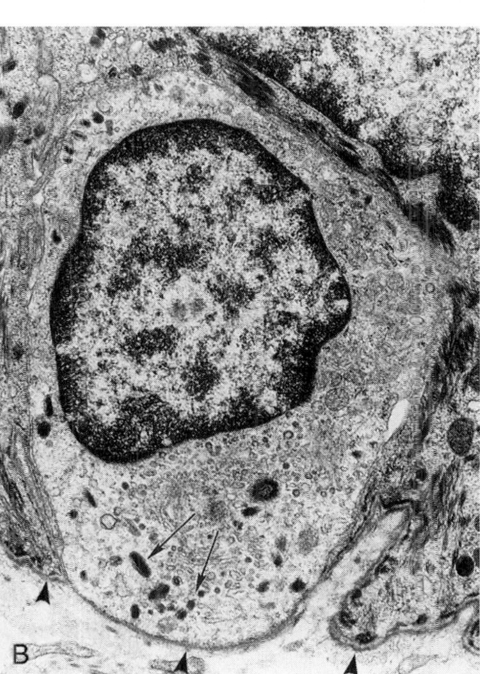

Figure 27–3

A, Clinical appearance of vitiligo. Well-demarcated zones of pigment loss result from depletion of melanocytes that produce small melanin granules. In the hands of this darkly pigmented patient, areas of melanin loss predominate. *B*, Electron microscopy of the melanocyte. These cells are difficult to identify by routine light microscopy, contain characteristic melanosomes *(arrows)* by electron microscopy, and are lost in lesions of vitiligo. (Arrowheads indicate basement membrane zone separating epidermis and dermis.)

Why are melanocytes progressively lost or destroyed in vitiligo? Theories of pathogenesis include (1) autoimmunity, (2) neurohumoral factors, and (3) self-destruction of melanocytes by toxic intermediates of melanin synthesis. Most evidence supports autoimmune causation, focusing on the presence of circulating antibodies against melanocytes[6] and the association of vitiligo with other autoimmune disorders, such as pernicious anemia, Addison disease, and autoimmune thyroiditis. Abnormalities in macrophages,[7] in T lymphocytes in skin,[8] and in the peripheral blood have been described recently, suggesting that aberrations in cell-mediated immunity may also be operative in the pathogenesis of vitiligo.

Freckle (Ephelis)

Freckles are the most common pigmented lesions of childhood in lightly pigmented individuals. They are small (1 to 10 mm in diameter), tan-red or light brown macules that first appear in early childhood after sun exposure. Once present, freckles will fade and reappear in a cyclic fashion with winter and summer, respectively.

MORPHOLOGY. The observed hyperpigmentation of the freckle is the result of increased amounts of melanin pigment within basal keratinocytes; melanocytes are relatively normal in number, although they may be slightly enlarged. It is unclear whether the freckle represents a focal abnormality in pigment production by a discrete field of melanocytes, enhanced pigment donation to adjacent basal keratinocytes, or both.

Melasma

Melasma is a masklike zone of facial hyperpigmentation commonly seen in association with pregnancy—hence its designation as the "mask of pregnancy." It presents as poorly defined, blotchy macules involving the cheeks, temples, and forehead bilaterally. Sunlight may accentuate this pigmentation, which often resolves spontaneously, particularly after the end of pregnancy.

MORPHOLOGY. Two histologic patterns have been recognized: an **epidermal type,** in which there is increased melanin deposition in the basal layers, and a **dermal type,** characterized by macrophages in the superficial (papillary) dermis that have phagocytosed melanin from the adjacent epidermal layer (a process referred to as **melanin pigment incontinence**). These two types may be distinguished by the use of a Wood's light. This is important because melasma of the epidermal type may respond to the topical bleaching agent hydroquinone.

The pathogenesis of melasma appears to relate to functional alterations in melanocytes resulting in enhanced pigment transfer to basal keratinocytes or to dermal macrophages. Apart from its association with pregnancy, melasma may occur during the administration of oral contraceptives or hydantoins, or it may be idiopathic.

Lentigo

Until now, we have been addressing disorders of pigmentation that do not involve proliferation of melanocytes. The term lentigo (plural, lentigines) refers to a common benign localized hyperplasia of melanocytes occurring at all ages but often in infancy and childhood. There is no sex or racial predilection, and the cause and pathogenesis are unknown. These lesions may involve mucous membranes as well as the skin, and they appear as small (5 to 10 mm across), oval, tan-brown macules. Unlike freckles, lentigines do not darken when they are exposed to sunlight.

MORPHOLOGY. The essential histologic feature of the lentigo is linear melanocytic hyperplasia (hyperplasia restricted to the cell layer immediately above the basement membrane) that produces a hyperpigmented basal cell layer. So characteristic is this linear melanocytic hyperplasia that the term **lentiginous** is often used to describe similar patterns of growth in unrelated melanocytic tumors, such as in lentiginous nevi and acral lentiginous melanomas. Elongation and thinning of the rete ridges are also commonly seen in a lentigo.

Nevocellular Nevus (Pigmented Nevus, Mole)

Most of us have at least a few moles and probably regard them as mundane and uninteresting. It may be surprising to learn, then, that moles or nevi represent one of the most diverse, dynamic, and biologically interesting tumors of the skin! Strictly speaking, the term nevus denotes any congenital lesion of the skin. Nevocellular nevus, however, refers to any congenital or acquired neoplasm of melanocytes.

In clinical appearance, common acquired nevocellular nevi are tan to brown, uniformly pigmented, small (usually less than 6 mm across), solid regions of relatively flat (macules) to elevated skin (papules) with well-defined, rounded borders (Figs. 27–4*A* and 27–5*A*). There are numerous clinical and histologic types of nevocellular nevi, and the clinical appearance may be variable. Table 27–1 provides a comparative summary of salient clinical and histologic features of the more commonly encountered forms of melanocytic nevi.

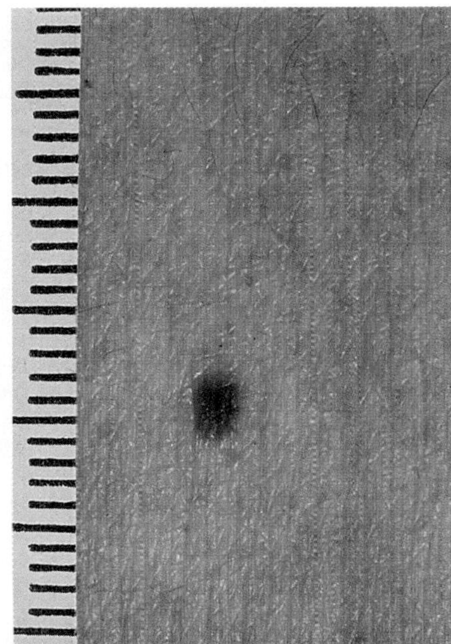

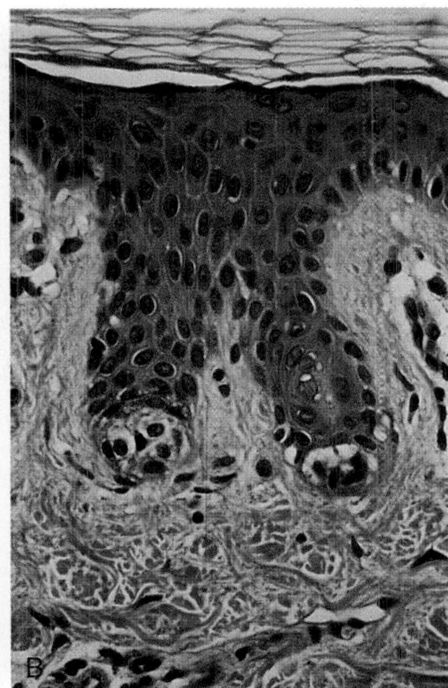

Figure 27–4 ■

Nevocellular nevus, junctional type. *A*, In clinical appearance, lesions are small, relatively flat, symmetric, and uniform. *B*, On histologic examination, junctional nevi are characterized by rounded nests of nevus cells originating at the tips of rete ridges along the dermoepidermal junction. (From Murphy GF, Herzberg AJ: Atlas of Dermatopathology. Philadelphia, WB Saunders, 1996, p 177.)

MORPHOLOGY. Nevocellular nevi are initially formed by melanocytes that have been transformed from highly dendritic single cells normally interspersed among basal keratinocytes to round to oval cells that grow in aggregates, or "nests," along the dermal-epidermal junction (Fig. 27–4*B*). Nuclei of nevus cells are uniform and rounded in contour, contain inconspicuous nucleoli, and show little or no mitotic activity. Such lesions are believed to represent an early developmental stage in nevocellular nevi and are called **junctional nevi.** Eventually, most junctional nevi grow into the underlying dermis as nests or cords of cells (Fig. 27–5*B*) **(compound nevi),** and in older lesions, the epidermal nests may be lost entirely to form pure **dermal nevi.** Clinically, compound and dermal nevi are often more elevated than junctional nevi.

Progressive growth of nevus cells from the dermoepidermal junction into the underlying dermis is accompanied by a process termed maturation. Whereas less mature, more superficial nevus cells are larger, tend to produce melanin pigment, and grow in nests, more mature, deeper nevus cells are smaller, produce little or no pigment,

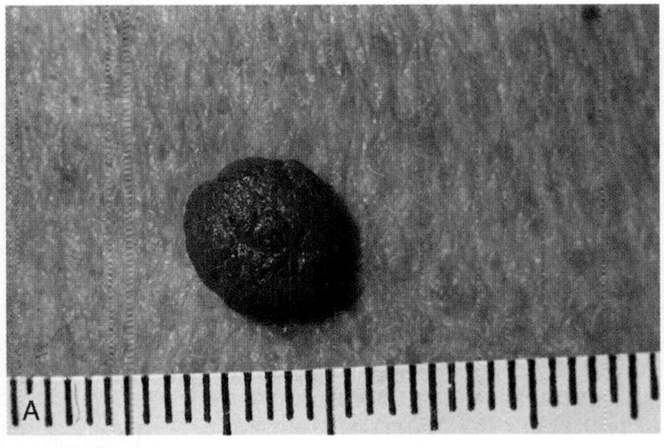

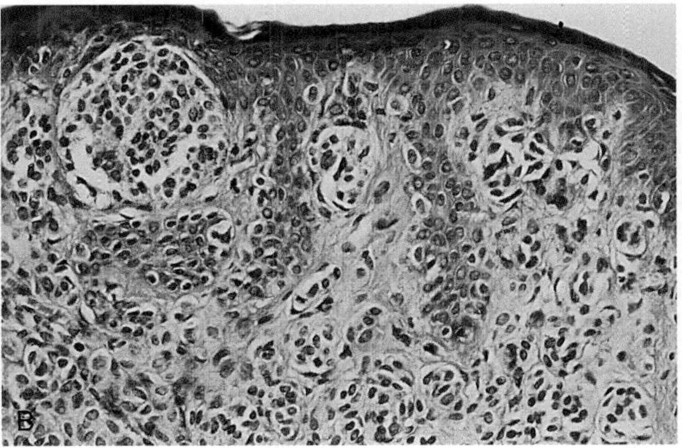

Figure 27–5 ■

Nevocellular nevus, compound type. In contrast to the junctional nevus, the compound nevus *(A)* is more raised and dome shaped. The symmetry and uniform pigment distribution suggest a benign process. Histologically *(B)*, compound nevi combine the features of junctional nevi (intraepidermal nevus cell nests) with nests and cords of nevus cells in the underlying dermis. (From Murphy GF, Herzberg AJ: Atlas of Dermatopathology. Philadelphia, WB Saunders, 1996, pp 177 and 178.)

Table 27–1. VARIANT FORMS OF NEVOCELLULAR NEVI

Nevus Variant	Diagnostic Architectural Features	Diagnostic Cytologic Features	Clinical Significance
Congenital nevus	Deep dermal and sometimes subcutaneous growth around adnexa, neurovascular bundles, and blood vessel walls	Identical to ordinary acquired nevi	Present at birth; large variants have increased melanoma risk
Blue nevus	Nonnested dermal infiltration, often with associated fibrosis	Highly dendritic, heavily pigmented nevus cells	Black-blue nodule; often confused with melanoma clinically
Spindle and epithelioid cell nevus (Spitz nevus)	Fascicular growth	Large, plump cells with pink-blue cytoplasm; fusiform cells	Common in children; red-pink nodule; often confused with hemangioma clinically
Halo nevus	Lymphocytic infiltration surrounding nevus cells	Identical to ordinary acquired nevi	Host immune response against nevus cells and surrounding normal melanocytes
Dysplastic nevus	Large, coalescent intraepidermal nests	Cytologic atypia	Potential precursor of malignant melanoma

and grow in cords. The most mature nevus cells may be found at the deepest extent of lesions, where they often acquire fusiform contours and grow in fascicles resembling neural tissue. This striking metamorphosis correlates with enzymatic changes (progressive loss of tyrosinase activity and acquisition of cholinesterase activity in deeper, nonpigmented, nervelike nevus cells). **This sequence of maturation of individual nevus cells is of diagnostic importance in distinguishing some benign nevi from melanomas, which usually show little or no maturation.**

Although nevocellular nevi are common, their clinical and histologic diversity necessitates thorough knowledge of their appearance and natural evolution, lest they become confused with other skin conditions, notably malignant melanoma. The biologic importance of some nevi, however, resides in their recent recognition as an important model of tumor progression (dysplastic nevi and the heritable melanoma syndrome).

Dysplastic Nevi

The association of nevocellular nevi with malignant melanoma was made more than 175 years ago,[9] although it was not until 1978 that a true precursor of malignant melanoma was described in detail. In 1978, Clark and colleagues[10] detailed the characteristics of lesions they termed BK moles (a name derived from the first letters of the last names of the initial two families studied).

Clinically, BK moles—or dysplastic nevi, as they are frequently called—are larger than most acquired nevi (often greater than 5 mm across) and may occur as hundreds of lesions on the body surface (Fig. 27–6*A*, inset). They are flat macules, slightly raised plaques with a "pebbly" surface, or target-like lesions with a darker raised center and irregular flat periphery. They usually show variability in pigmentation (variegation) and borders that are irregular in contour. Unlike ordinary moles, dysplastic nevi have a tendency to occur on non–sun-exposed as well as on sun-exposed body surfaces. Dysplastic nevi have been documented in multiple members of families prone to the development of malignant melanoma *(the heritable melanoma syndrome)*.[11] In these cases, genetic analyses have demonstrated the trait to be inherited as an autosomal dominant, possibly involving genes located on 1p36, 9p21, 12g14, and others. (See discussion under Malignant Melanoma.)[12,13] Transitions from these lesions to early melanoma have actually been documented clinically and histologically within a period as short as several weeks. However, most dysplastic nevi are clinically stable lesions. Dysplastic nevi may also occur as isolated lesions not associated with the heritable melanoma syndrome, in which case the risk of malignant change appears to be low.

MORPHOLOGY. On histologic examination (Fig. 27–6*A* and *B*), dysplastic nevi consist of compound nevi with both architectural and cytologic evidence of abnormal growth. **Nevus cell nests within the epidermis may be enlarged and exhibit abnormal fusion or coalescence with adjacent nests. As part of this process, single nevus cells begin to replace the normal basal cell layer along the dermoepidermal junction, producing so-called lentiginous hyperplasia** (recall the definition of this term earlier). Cytologic atypia consisting of irregular, often angulated, nuclear contours and hyperchromasia is frequently observed (Fig. 27–6*B*). Associated alterations also occur in the superficial dermis. These consist of a usually sparse lymphocytic infiltrate, loss of melanin pig-

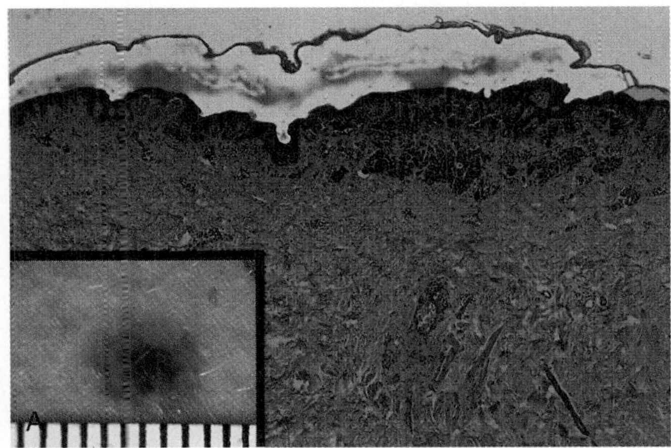

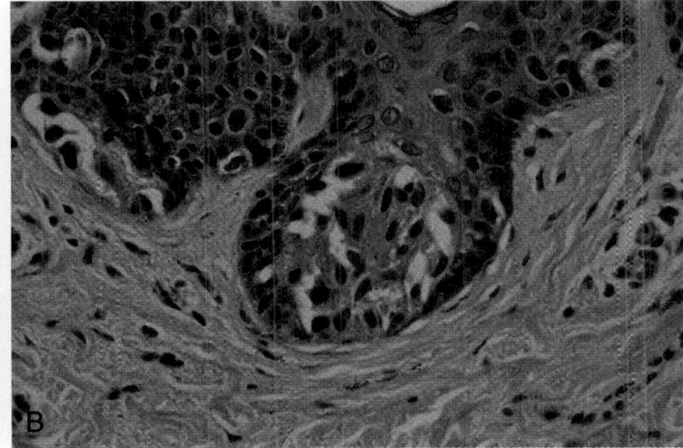

Figure 27–6

Dysplastic nevus. *A*, The lesion often has a compound nevus component (right side of scanning field) and an asymmetric "shoulder" composed of a junctional nevus component (left side of scanning field). The former correlates clinically with the more pigmented and raised central zone, and the latter with the less pigmented, flat peripheral rim *(inset)*. *B*, An important feature is the presence of cytologic atypia (irregularly shaped, dark-staining nuclei) at high magnification. The dermis underlying the atypical cells characteristically shows linear, or lamellar, fibrosis.

ment from presumably destroyed nevus cells, phagocytosis of this pigment by dermal macrophages (melanin pigment incontinence), and a peculiar linear fibrosis surrounding the epidermal rete ridges that are involved by the nevus. All of these features assist in the histologic recognition of a dysplastic nevus.

Several lines of evidence support the concept that some *dysplastic nevi are precursors of malignant melanoma*. In one study,[14] it was shown that in a large number of families prone to the development of melanoma, more than 5% of family members developed melanoma during an 8-year follow-up period, and new melanomas occurred only in individuals with dysplastic nevi. From this database, it was concluded that the actuarial probability of persons with the dysplastic nevus syndrome developing melanoma is 56% at age 59 years. Dysplastic nevi also demonstrate expression of some abnormal cell surface antigens,[15] karyotypic abnormalities,[16] and in vitro vulnerability to mutagenic effects of ultraviolet light.[17]

Clark and associates[18] have proposed steps whereby benign nevi may undergo aberrant differentiation to become dysplastic and eventually metastasizing malignant tumors (Fig. 27–7). Parallels may be found in neoplasia involving other organ systems, and thus dysplastic nevi are regarded by some as a general model of tumor progression.

Malignant Melanoma

Malignant melanoma is a relatively common neoplasm that not long ago was considered almost uniformly deadly. Although the great preponderance of melanomas arise in the skin, other sites of origin include the oral and anogenital mucosal surfaces, esophagus, meninges, and notably the eye. The following comments apply to cutaneous melanomas. Intraocular melanomas are discussed in Chapter 31.

Today as a result of increased public awareness of the earliest signs of skin melanomas, most are cured surgically.[19] Nonetheless, the incidence of these lesions is on the rise, necessitating vigorous surveillance for their development.

As with epithelial malignant neoplasms of the skin (see later), sunlight appears to play an important role in the development of skin malignant melanoma. For example, men commonly develop this tumor on the upper back, whereas women have a relatively high incidence on both the back and the legs. Lightly pigmented individuals are at higher risk for the development of melanoma than are darkly pigmented individuals. Sunlight, however, does not seem to be the only predisposing factor, and the presence of a preexisting nevus (e.g., a dysplastic nevus), hereditary factors, or even exposure to certain carcinogens (as in the case of experimental melanomas in rodent models) may play a role in lesion development and evolution.[20]

Molecular Genetics. The molecular basis for nonheritable forms of melanoma is incompletely understood, and much of our current knowledge is based upon evaluation of the approximately 10% of melanomas that tend to run in families. As stated before, these melanomas are often (but not invariably) associated with multiple dysplastic nevi. Some of the suspected melanoma-associated genes in this setting include[12]: (1) the CMM1 gene, on chromosome 1p36; (2) the tumor suppressor gene p16, mapped to chromosome 9p21 (Genetic analyses have revealed germline mutations in this gene in certain melanoma patients and their family members.[13] It may be recalled that this tumor suppressor gene is an inhibitor of cyclin-dependent kinase 4 [CDK 4] and as such negatively regulates the cell cycle [Chapter 8]); and (3) the cyclin-dependent kinase gene CDK4, on chromosome 12q14.[12] Transgenic mice with melanocyte-specific expression of activated *ras* on a ge-

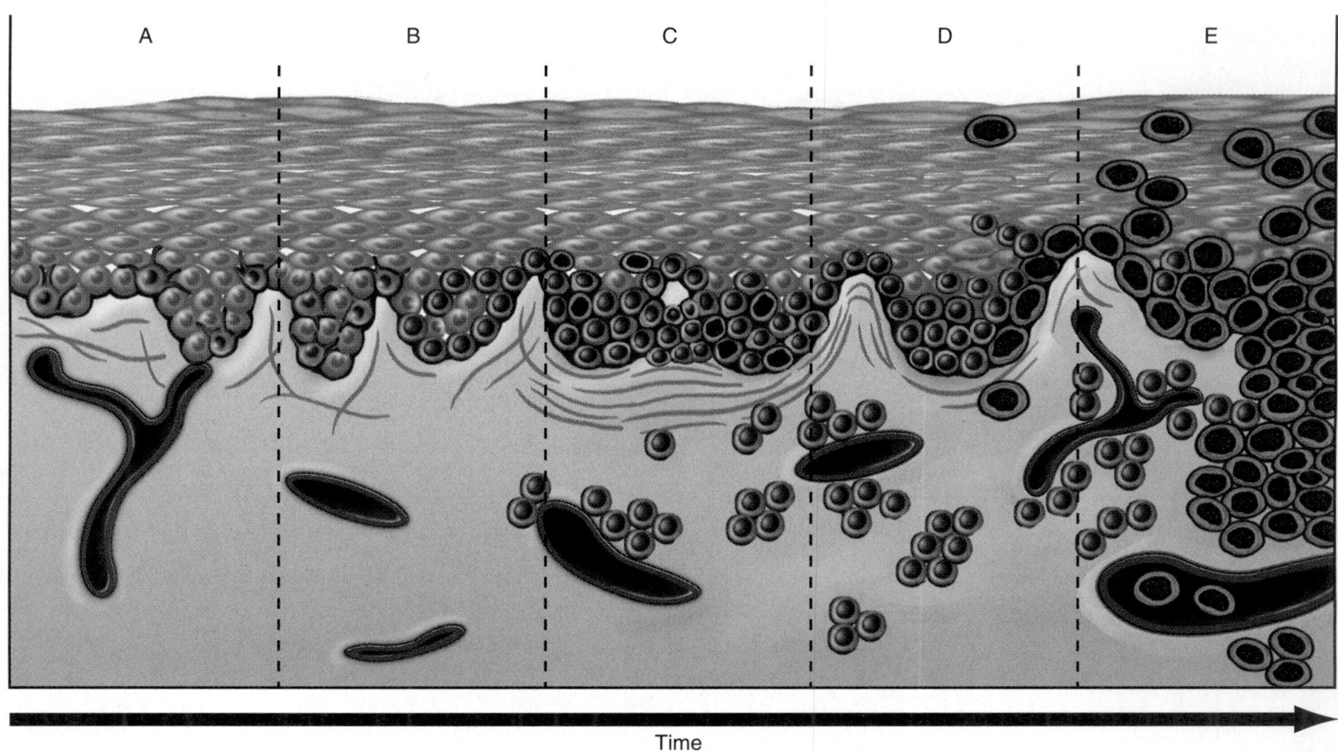

Figure 27–7

Steps of tumor progression in dysplastic nevi: *A*, Lentiginous melanocytic hyperplasia. *B*, Lentiginous junctional nevus. *C*, Lentiginous compound nevus with abnormal architectural and cytologic features (dysplastic nevus). *D*, Early melanoma, or radial growth phase melanoma (large dark cells in epidermis). *E*, Advanced melanoma (vertical growth phase) with malignant spread into the dermis and vessels.

netic background deficient for alleles of p16 exhibit accelerated development of melanoma, thus confirming the role of this tumor suppressor in the pathogenesis of melanomas.[20a]

Clinical Features. Malignant melanoma of the skin is usually asymptomatic, although itching may be an early manifestation. *The most important clinical sign of the disease is change in color in a pigmented lesion.* Unlike benign (nondysplastic) nevi, melanomas exhibit striking variations in pigmentation, appearing in shades of black, brown, red, dark blue, and gray (Fig. 27–8*A*). On occasion, zones of white or flesh-colored hypopigmentation are also present. The borders of melanomas are not smooth, round, and uniform, as in nevocellular nevi, but irregular and often "notched." In summary, the clinical warning signs of melanoma are (1) enlargement of a preexisting mole, (2) itching or pain in a preexisting mole, (3) development of a new pigmented lesion during adult life, (4) irregularity of the borders of a pigmented lesion, and (5) variegation of color within a pigmented lesion.

GROWTH PATTERNS AND MORPHOLOGY. Central to understanding the complicated histology of malignant melanoma is the concept of **radial and vertical growth.** Simply stated, radial growth indicates the tendency of a melanoma to grow horizontally within the epidermal and superficial dermal layers, often for a prolonged time (Fig. 27–8*B*). During this stage of growth, melanoma cells do not have the capacity to metastasize. Specific types of radial growth phase melanoma include lentigo maligna, superficial spreading, and acral/mucosal lentiginous. These are defined on the basis of architectural and cytologic features of growth within the epidermal layer as well as biologic behavior. For example, lentigo maligna type of radial growth typically occurs on sun-damaged facial skin of the elderly and may continue for as long as several decades before the tumor develops the capacity to metastasize. With time, the pattern of growth assumes a vertical component, and the melanoma now grows downward into the deeper dermal layers as an expansile mass lacking cellular maturation, without a tendency for the cells to become smaller as they descend into the reticular dermis (Fig. 27–8*C*). **This event is heralded clinically by the development of a nodule in the relatively flat radial growth phase and correlates with the emergence of a clone of cells with true metastatic potential.** Interestingly, the probability of metastasis in such lesions may be predicted by simply measuring in millimeters the depth of invasion of this vertical growth phase nodule below the granular cell layer of the overly-

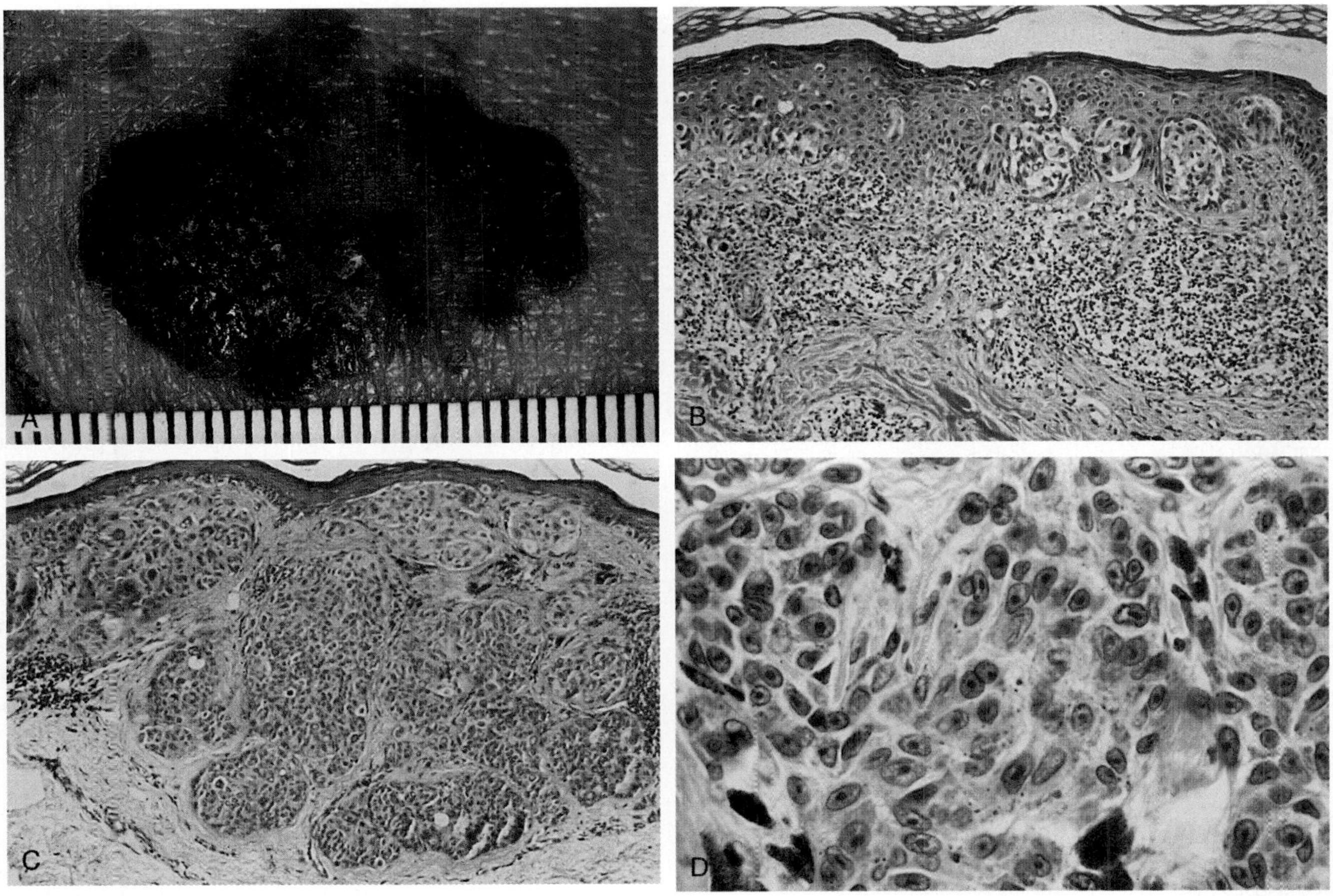

Figure 27–8

Malignant melanoma. *A*, In clinical appearance, lesions are irregular in contour and pigmentation. Macular areas correlate with the radial growth phase, while raised areas usually correspond to nodular aggregates of malignant cells in the vertical phase of growth. *B*, Radial growth phase of malignant melanoma, showing irregular nested and single-cell growth of melanoma cells within the epidermis, and an underlying inflammatory response within the dermis. *C*, Photomicrograph of lesion in the vertical phase of growth demonstrating nodular aggregates of infiltrating cells. *D*, High-power view of malignant melanoma cells.

ing epidermis.[21] Prediction of clinical outcome has recently been refined further by taking into account factors such as number of mitoses and degree of infiltrative lymphocytic response within the tumor nodule.[22]

Individual melanoma cells are usually considerably larger than nevus cells. They contain large nuclei with irregular contours, having chromatin characteristically clumped at the periphery of the nuclear membrane and prominent red (eosinophilic) nucleoli (Fig. 27–8*D*). These cells proliferate as poorly formed nests or as individual cells at all levels of the epidermis (Fig. 27–8*B*) in the radial phase of growth and, in the dermis, as expansile, balloon-like nodules in the vertical phase of growth (Fig. 27–8*C*). **The nature and extent of the vertical growth phase determine the biologic behavior of malignant melanoma,** and thus it is important to observe and record vertical growth phase parameters in a pathology report.

BENIGN EPITHELIAL TUMORS

Benign epithelial neoplasms are common and usually biologically inconsequential, although they may represent significant sources of psychologic discomfort for the patient. These tumors, derived from the keratinizing stratified squamous epithelium of the epidermis and hair follicles (keratinocytes) and the ductular epithelium of cutaneous glands, may recapitulate the cell layers from which they arise. They are often confused clinically with malignancy, particularly when they are pigmented or inflamed, and histologic examination of a biopsy specimen is frequently required to establish a definitive diagnosis.

Seborrheic Keratoses

These common epidermal tumors occur most frequently in middle-aged or older individuals. They arise spontaneously and may become particularly numerous on the trunk, although the extremities, head, and neck may also be involved. In people of color, multiple small lesions on the face are termed *dermatosis papulosa nigra.*

Seborrheic keratoses have characteristic clinical features. They appear as round, flat, coinlike plaques that vary in diameter from millimeters to several centimeters (Fig. 27–9*A*). They are uniformly tan to dark brown and usually show a velvety to granular surface. Lesions may give the impression that they are "stuck on" and may be easily peeled off. Inspection with a hand lens will usually reveal small, round, porelike ostia impacted with keratin, a feature helpful in differentiating these pigmented lesions from melanomas.

MORPHOLOGY. On histologic examination, these neoplasms are exophytic and demarcated sharply from the adjacent epidermis. They are composed of sheets of small cells that most resemble basal cells of the normal epidermis (Fig. 27–9*B*). Variable melanin pigmentation is present within these basaloid cells, accounting for the brown coloration clinically. Exuberant keratin production (hyperkeratosis) occurs at the surface of seborrheic keratoses, and small keratin-filled cysts (horn cysts) and downgrowths of keratin into the main tumor mass (pseudo–horn cysts) are characteristic features. Interestingly, when seborrheic keratoses become irritated and inflamed, they undergo squamous differentiation[23] and are characterized by foci of "whirling" squamous cells resembling eddy currents in a stream. A biologic explanation for this intriguing phenomenon awaits discovery. When seborrheic keratoses involve the epithelium of hair follicles, they may grow in an endophytic (downward) fashion, and they generally also show the effects of inflammation; such lesions are termed **inverted follicular keratoses.**

Seborrheic keratoses may occur explosively in large numbers, as part of a paraneoplastic syndrome *(sign of Leser-Trélat).* TGF-α produced by tumor cells is thought to contribute to the development of such lesions.[24]

Acanthosis Nigricans

Acanthosis nigricans is used to describe thickened (acanthosis = hyperplasia of the stratum spinosum of the epidermis), hyperpigmented zones of skin involving most commonly the flexural areas (axillae, skin folds of the neck, groin, and anogenital regions). It is an important cutaneous marker for associated benign and malignant conditions and, accordingly, is divided into two types.[25] The *benign type,* which constitutes about 80% of all cases, develops gradually and usually occurs in childhood or during puberty. It may occur (1) as an autosomal dominant trait with variable penetrance, (2) in association with obesity or endocrine abnormalities (particularly with pituitary and pineal tumors and with diabetes), and (3) as part of a number of rare congenital syndromes. As with seborrheic keratoses, acanthosis nigricans may result from abnormal production of epidermal growth-promoting factors by a variety of tumors. This occurrence may account for many instances of the *malignant type,* in which lesions arise in middle-aged and older individuals, often in association with an underlying adenocarcinoma.

MORPHOLOGY. All forms of acanthosis nigricans have similar histologic features. The epidermis undulates sharply to form numerous repeating peaks and valleys. Variable hyperplasia may be seen, along with hyperkeratosis and slight basal cell layer hyperpigmentation (but no melanocytic hyperplasia).

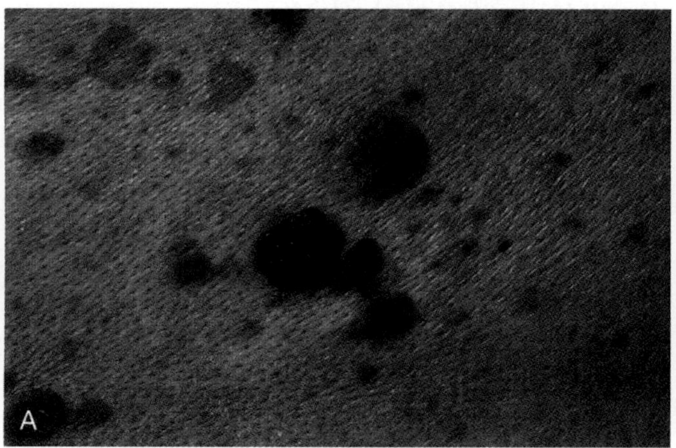

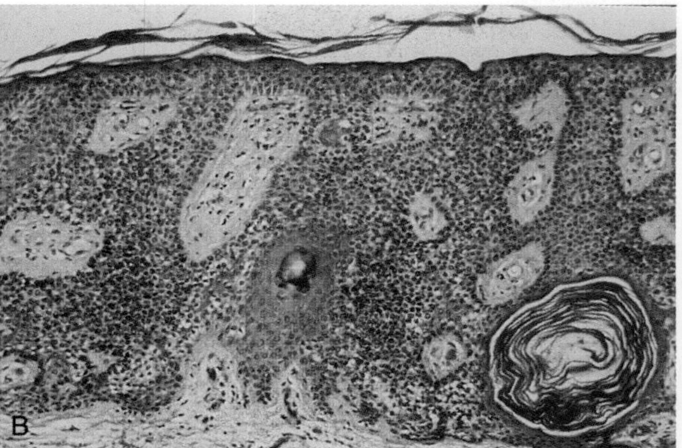

Figure 27–9

Seborrheic keratoses. Multiple coinlike pigmented lesions on the back *(A)* are composed of well-demarcated, orderly proliferations of basaloid cells forming small, keratin-filled cysts *(B).*

Because the occurrence of acanthosis nigricans may *precede* the overt clinical symptoms and signs of the underlying process, knowledge and recognition of this entity are of great diagnostic importance.

Fibroepithelial Polyp

The fibroepithelial polyp has many names (acrochordon, squamous papilloma, skin tag) and is one of the most common cutaneous lesions. It is generally detected as an incidental finding in middle-aged and older individuals on the neck, trunk, face, and intertriginous areas as a soft, flesh-colored, baglike tumor attached to the skin surface by a small, often slender stalk.

MORPHOLOGY. On histologic examination, these tumors are merely fibrovascular cores covered by benign squamous epithelium. It is not uncommon to discover ischemic necrosis in histologic sections (the result of torsion that produced the pain and swelling that may precipitate their removal).

Fibroepithelial polyps are usually biologically inconsequential, although they have been associated with diabetes and intestinal polyposis. It is of interest that along with nevocellular nevi (discussed earlier) and hemangiomas (see later), they often become more numerous or prominent during pregnancy.

Epithelial Cyst (Wen)

Epithelial cysts are common lesions formed by the downgrowth and cystic expansion of the epidermis or of the epithelium forming the hair follicle. The lay term, wen, derives from the Anglo-Saxon *wenn,* meaning a lump or tumor. These cysts are filled with keratin and variable amounts of admixed, lipid-containing debris derived from sebaceous secretions. Clinically, they are dermal or subcutaneous, well-circumscribed, firm, and often moveable nodules. When large, they may be dome shaped and flesh colored and often become painful on traumatic rupture.

MORPHOLOGY. Epithelial cysts are divided into several histologic types according to the structural components of their walls. The **epidermal inclusion cyst** has a wall nearly identical to the epidermis and is filled with laminated strands of keratin. **Pilar** or **trichilemmal cysts** have a wall that resembles follicular epithelium, without a granular cell layer and filled by a more homogeneous mixture of keratin and lipid. The **dermoid cyst** is similar to the epidermal inclusion cyst, but it also shows multiple appendages (such as small hair follicles) budding outward from its wall. Finally, **steatocystoma multiplex** constitutes a curious cyst with a wall resembling the sebaceous gland duct from which numerous compressed sebaceous lobules originate. The importance of recognition of this cyst derives from the often dominantly heritable nature of the lesion.

Keratoacanthoma

Keratoacanthoma is a rapidly developing neoplasm that clinically and histologically may mimic well-differentiated squamous cell carcinoma (see later discussion), but it may heal spontaneously, without treatment! Men are more often affected than women are, and lesions most frequently affect sun-exposed skin of whites older than 50 years.[26]

Keratoacanthomas appear clinically as flesh-colored, dome-shaped nodules with a central, keratin-filled plug, imparting a crater-like topography (Fig. 27–10*A*). Lesions range in size from 1 cm to several centimeters across and have a predilection for facial skin including the cheeks, nose, and ears and the dorsa of the hands.

MORPHOLOGY. Keratoacanthomas are characterized histologically by a central, keratin-filled crater surrounded by proliferating epithelial cells that extend upward in a liplike fashion over the sides of the crater and downward into the dermis as irregular tongues (Fig. 27–10*B*). This epithelium is composed of enlarged cells showing evidence of reactive cytologic atypia. These cells have a characteristically "glassy" eosinophilic cytoplasm (Fig. 27–10*C*) and produce keratin abruptly (without the development of an intervening granular cell layer). This mode of keratinization is analogous to that of the normal hair follicle and similar to that seen in the pilar cyst described earlier, giving rise to speculation that the keratoacanthoma is a neoplasm of follicular epithelium. The early tumor infiltrates into the collagen and elastic fibers and entraps them (note that Figure 27–10*B* shows an elastic stain originally performed for this purpose). Little if any host inflammatory response is present during this rapidly proliferative phase, but as the lesion evolves, there is some stromal response that is fibrotic and contains numerous inflammatory cells.

There is growing belief that keratoacanthomas may represent a form of squamous cell carcinoma (see later) that regresses as a consequence of interactions with host tissue that fail to support inexorable growth. The majority of keratoacanthomas have detectable p53 oncoprotein, and occasional tumors show a point mutation in the *p53* gene.[27]

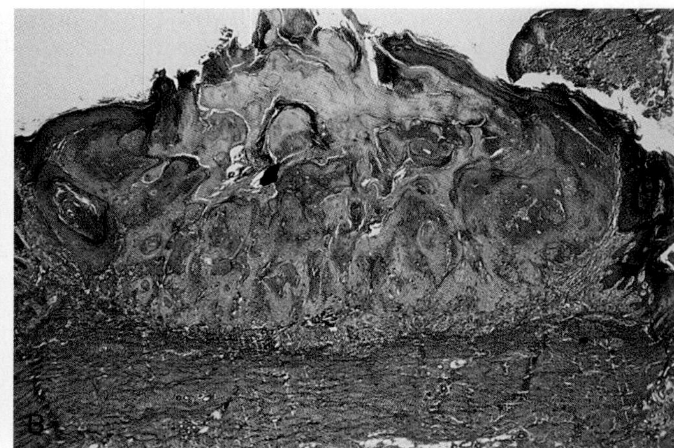

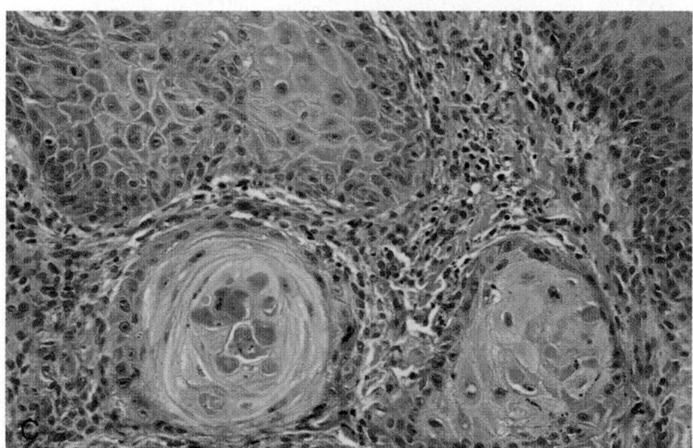

Figure 27–10

Keratoacanthoma. *A*, This symmetric crater-like nodule has a prominent central keratin plug. *B*, At low power, the crater-like architecture may be appreciated with an elastic tissue stain where the dermis is red, epithelial elements are gray, and the central keratin plug is yellow. *C*, Higher power view shows keratoacanthoma to be composed of large, glassy squamous cells and central islands of eosinophliic keratin. (*A* and *B* from Murphy GF, Herzberg AJ: Atlas of Dermatopathology. Philadelphia, WB Saunders, 1996, pp 143 and 144.)

Adnexal (Appendage) Tumors

There are literally hundreds of benign neoplasms arising from cutaneous appendages.[28] Although some show no aggressive behavior and remain localized, they may be confused with certain types of cutaneous cancers (e.g., basal cell carcinoma; see later discussion). Certain appendage tumors are associated with mendelian patterns of inheritance and occur as multiple disfiguring lesions. In some instances, these lesions serve as markers for internal malignancy, as in the case of multiple trichilemmomas and breast carcinoma of Cowden syndrome.[29] Selected examples are provided here to illustrate neoplasms of hair follicles, eccrine glands, and apocrine glands.

Appendage tumors are often clinically nondescript, solitary or multiple papules and nodules. Some have a predisposition for occurrence on specific body surfaces. For example, the *eccrine poroma* occurs predominantly on the palms and soles. The *cylindroma,* an appendage tumor with apocrine differentiation, usually occurs on the forehead and scalp (Fig. 27–11*A*), where coalescence of nodules with time may produce a hatlike growth, hence the name *turban tumor.* These lesions may be dominantly inherited and first appear early in life. *Syringomas,* lesions of eccrine differentiation, in comparison, usually occur as multiple, small, tan papules in the vicinity of the lower eyelids. *Trichoepitheliomas,* showing follicular differentiation, are dominantly inherited when they are seen as multiple, semitransparent, dome-shaped papules that involve the face, scalp, neck, and upper trunk (Fig. 27–11*C*).

MORPHOLOGY. The **cylindroma** is composed of islands of basaloid cells that seem to fit together like pieces of a jigsaw puzzle within a fibrous dermal matrix (Fig. 27–11*B*). The **trichoepithelioma** is a proliferation of basaloid cells that forms primitive hair follicle–germ structures (Fig. 27–11*D*). **Mixed tumor (chondroid syringoma)** is composed of variably dilated sweat gland–like ducts surrounded by a blue-gray matrix with features of true cartilage (Fig. 27–12*A*). The **trichilemmoma** is a localized proliferation of pale pink, glassy cells that resembles the uppermost portion of the hair follicle (infundibulum) (Fig. 27–12*B*). **Hidradenoma papilliferum** is composed of ducts lined by apocrine type cells that show characteristic decapitation secretion and a fibrous stroma (Fig. 27–12*C*). Table 27–2 summarizes common adnexal tumors according to histologic features that recapitulate mature adnexal counterparts.

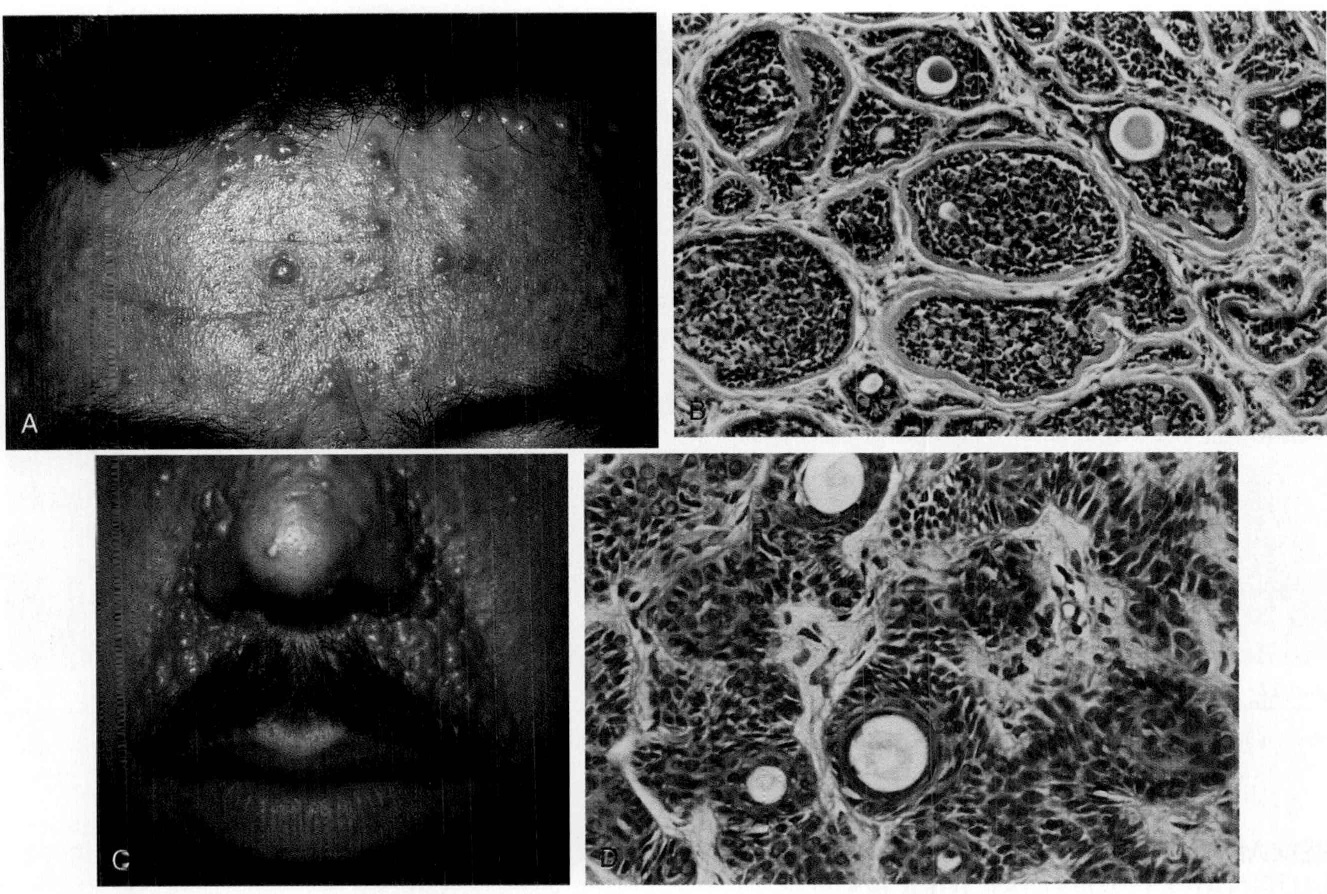

Figure 27–11

Adnexal tumors. The clinical appearance is often nondescript (*A* shows multiple cylindromas and *C* shows multiple trichoepitheliomas). *B*, on histologic examination, the cylindroma is composed of islands of basaloid cells containing occasional ducts and seemingly fitting together like pieces of a jigsaw puzzle. *D*, Trichoepithelioma is composed of buds of basaloid cells that resemble primitive hair follicles. Here the small ductlike structures are actually keratin-filled microcysts. (*B*, *C*, and *D* from Murphy GF, Herzberg AJ: Atlas of Dermatopathology. Philadelphia, WB Saunders, 1996, pp 162 and 165.)

Although most appendage tumors are benign, malignant variants do exist. *Sebaceous carcinoma,* for example, arises from the meibomian glands of the eyelid and may follow an aggressive biologic course with systemic metastases. *Eccrine* and *apocrine carcinomas* are often confused with metastatic adenocarcinomas to the skin because of their tendency for abortive gland formation.

Table 27–2. COMMON ADNEXAL TUMORS AND MATURE COUNTERPARTS

Adnexal Tumors	Mature Counterpart	Histologic Features	Clinical Significance
Trichoepithelioma Trichofolliculoma	Hair follicle	Hair matrix, outer root sheath differentiation	Multiple trichoepitheliomas, dominant inheritance
Sebaceous adenoma Sebaceous epithelioma	Sebaceous gland	Cytoplasmic lipid vacuoles	Association with internal malignancy
Syringocystadenoma papilliferum	Apocrine gland	Apocrine type ("decapitation") secretion	May develop in mixed epidermal-adnexal hamartomas of face and scalp termed nevus sebaceus
Syringoma	Eccrine gland	Eccrine ducts lined by membranous eosinophilic cuticles; tadpole-like epithelial structures	May be confused with basal cell carcinoma clinically

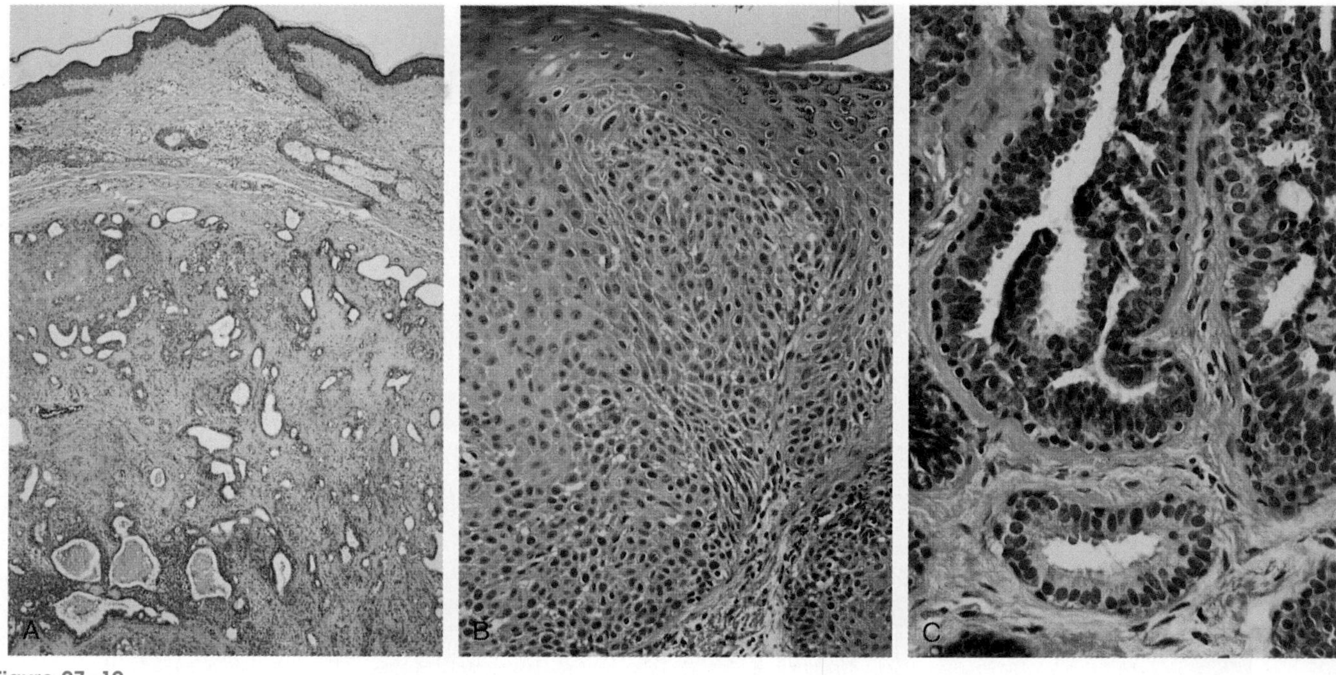

Figure 27–12

Adnexal tumors. *A*, Mixed tumor (chondroid syringoma). *B*, Trichilemmoma. *C*, Hidradenoma papilliferum.

PREMALIGNANT AND MALIGNANT EPIDERMAL TUMORS

Actinic Keratosis

Before the development of overt malignancy of the epidermis, a series of progressively dysplastic changes occur, a phenomenon analogous to the atypia that precedes carcinoma of the squamous mucosa of the uterine cervix (Chapter 24). Because this dysplasia is usually the result of chronic exposure to sunlight and is associated with build-up of excess keratin, these lesions are called actinic keratoses. As would be expected, they occur in a particularly high incidence in lightly pigmented individuals. Exposure to ionizing radiation, hydrocarbons, and arsenicals may induce similar lesions.

Actinic keratoses are usually less than 1 cm in diameter; are tan-brown, red, or skin colored; and have a rough, sandpaper-like consistency. Some lesions may produce so much keratin that a "cutaneous horn" develops (Fig. 27–13*A*). Such horns may become so prominent that they actually resemble the horns of animals! Skin sites commonly involved by sun exposure (face, arms, dorsum of hands) are most frequently affected. The lips may also develop similar lesions (actinic cheilitis).

MORPHOLOGY. Cytologic atypia is seen in the lowermost layers of the epidermis and may be associated with hyperplasia of basal cells (Fig. 27–13*B*) or, alternatively, with early atrophy that results in diffuse thinning of the epidermal surface of the lesion. The atypical basal cells usually have evidence of dyskeratosis with pink or reddish cytoplasm. Also, intercellular bridges are present, in contrast to basal cell carcinoma (see later discussion), in which the cytoplasm is usually basophilic and the cells lack intercellular bridges identifiable by light microscopy. The dermis contains thickened, blue-gray elastic fibers (elastosis), a probable result of abnormal dermal elastic fiber synthesis by sun-damaged fibroblasts[30] within the superficial dermis. The stratum corneum is thickened, and unlike in normal skin, nuclei in the cells in this layer are often retained (a pattern termed parakeratosis).

Whether all actinic keratoses would eventuate in skin cancer (usually squamous cell carcinoma), if given enough time, is conjectural. Many believe that certain lesions may regress or remain stable during a normal life span. However, enough do become malignant to warrant local eradication of these potential precursor lesions. This can usually be accomplished by gentle curettage, freezing, or topical application of chemotherapeutic agents.

Squamous Cell Carcinoma

Squamous cell carcinoma is the most common tumor arising on sun-exposed sites in older people. Except for lesions on the lower legs, these tumors have a higher incidence in men than in women. Implicated as predisposing factors, in addition to sunlight, are industrial carcino-

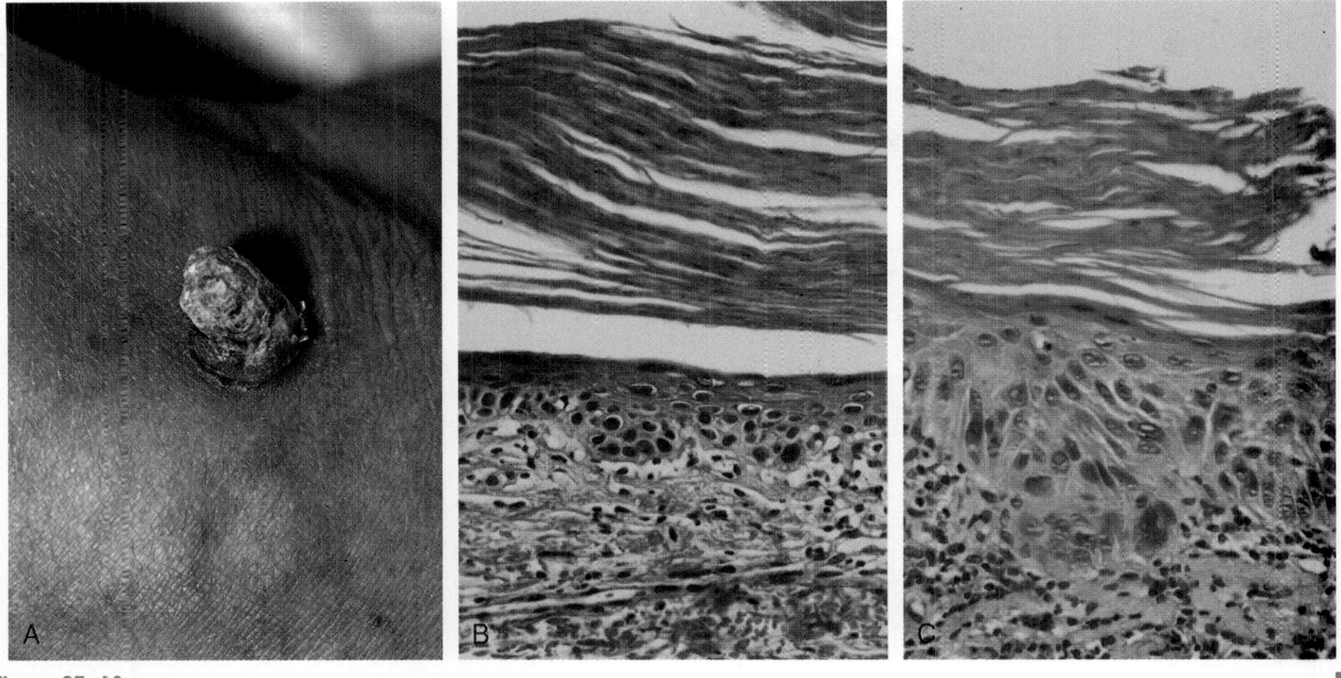

Figure 27–13

Actinic keratosis. *A*, Excessive scale formation in this lesion has produced a "cutaneous horn." *B*, Basal cell layer atypia is associated with marked hyperkeratosis and parakeratosis. *C*, Progression to full-thickness nuclear atypia, with or without the presence of superficial epidermal maturation, heralds the development of early squamous cell carcinoma in situ.

gens (tars and oils), chronic ulcers and draining osteomyelitis, old burn scars, ingestion of arsenicals, ionizing radiation, and (in the oral cavity) tobacco and betel nut chewing.

The most commonly accepted exogenous cause of squamous cell carcinoma is exposure to ultraviolet light with subsequent DNA damage and associated mutagenicity. Individuals who are immunosuppressed as a result of chemotherapy or organ transplantation, or who have xeroderma pigmentosum, are at increased risk for developing neoplasms.[31] A considerable proportion of these are squamous cell carcinomas, implicating aberrations in local immune networks in the skin in the production of an atmosphere permissive to neoplasia. Sunlight, in addition to its effect on DNA, also seems to have a direct and at least a transient immunosuppressive effect on skin by affecting the normal surveillance function of antigen-presenting Langerhans cells in the epidermis.[32] In experimental animals, it now appears that although Langerhans cells responsible for T-lymphocyte activation are injured by ultraviolet light, similar cells responsible for the selective induction of suppressor lymphocyte pathways are resistant to ultraviolet damage.[33] Such a phenomenon could result in local imbalances in T-cell function that would favor tumorigenesis and progression. DNA sequences of certain viruses (e.g., human papillomavirus type 36) have been detected in DNA extracted from potential precursors of squamous cell carcinoma,[34] suggesting a role for these agents in the evolution of certain cutaneous epithelial neoplasms. Finally, certain chemical agents appear to have direct mutagenic effects by producing DNA adducts with subsequent oncogene activation.[35]

MORPHOLOGY. Squamous cell carcinomas that have not invaded through the basement membrane of the dermoepidermal junction (**in situ carcinoma**) appear as sharply defined, red scaling plaques. More advanced, invasive lesions are nodular, show variable keratin production appreciated clinically as hyperkeratosis, and may ulcerate (Fig. 27–14*A*). Well-differentiated lesions may be indistinguishable from keratoacanthoma (see previous section). When the oral mucosa is involved, a zone of white thickening is seen, an appearance caused by a variety of disorders and referred to clinically as *leukoplakia.*

Unlike actinic keratoses, squamous cell carcinoma in situ is characterized by cells with atypical (enlarged and hyperchromatic) nuclei at **all levels** of the epidermis (see Fig. 27–13*C*). When these cells break through the basement membrane, the process has become invasive. Invasive squamous cell carcinoma (Fig. 27–14*B* and *C*) exhibits variable differentiation, ranging from tumors formed by polygonal squamous cells, arranged in orderly lobules and exhibiting numerous large zones of keratinization, to neoplasms formed by highly anaplastic, rounded cells with foci of necrosis and only abortive, single-cell keratinization

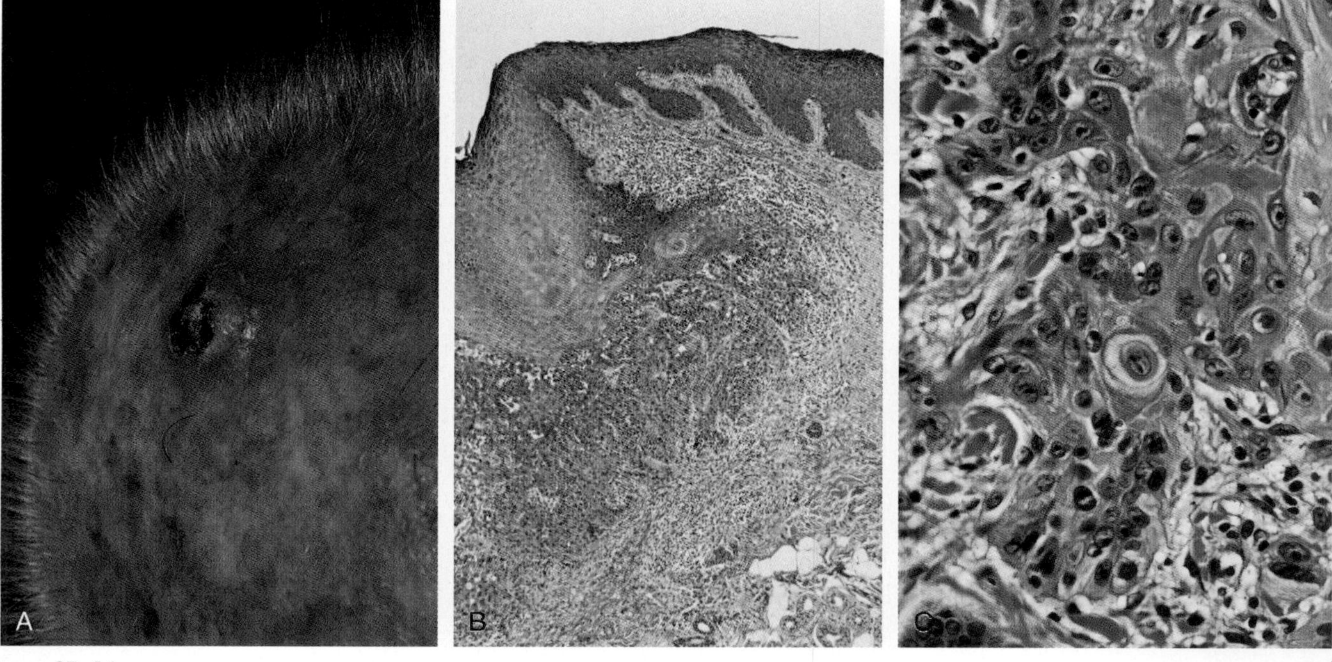

Figure 27–14

Invasive squamous cell carcinoma. *A*, Lesions are often nodular and ulcerated. *B*, Tongues of atypical squamous epithelium have transgressed the basement membrane, invading deeply into the dermis. *C*, Invasive tumor cells exhibit enlarged nuclei with angulated contours and prominent nucleoli.

(dyskeratosis). These latter tumors may be so poorly differentiated that electron microscopy for the detection of keratinocyte intercellular attachment sites (desmosomes) or reaction of tissue with antibodies to keratin or epithelial membrane–associated antigens may be necessary to definitively establish cell lineage.

Invasive squamous cell carcinomas are usually discovered while they are small and resectable; less than 5% have metastases to regional nodes.

Basal Cell Carcinoma

Basal cell carcinomas are common, slow-growing tumors that rarely metastasize. They have a tendency to occur at sites subject to chronic sun exposure and in lightly pigmented people. As with squamous cell carcinoma, the incidence of basal cell carcinoma rises sharply with immunosuppression and in patients with inherited defects in DNA replication or repair (xeroderma pigmentosum; Chapter 8).

These tumors present clinically as pearly papules often containing prominent, dilated subepidermal blood vessels (telangiectasias) (Fig. 27–15*A*). Some tumors contain melanin pigment and, thus, appear similar to nevocellular nevi or melanomas. Advanced lesions may ulcerate, and extensive local invasion of bone or facial sinuses may occur after many years of neglect or in unusually aggressive tumors, justifying the past designation "rodent ulcers."

MORPHOLOGY. On histologic examination, tumor cells resemble those in the normal basal cell layer of the epidermis. They arise from the epidermis or follicular epithelium and do not occur on mucosal surfaces. Two patterns are seen: **multifocal growths** originating from the epidermis and extending over several square centimeters or more of skin surface (multifocal superficial type); and **nodular lesions** growing downward deeply into the dermis as cords and islands of variably basophilic cells with hyperchromatic nuclei, embedded in a mucinous matrix, and often surrounded by many fibroblasts and lymphocytes (Fig. 27–15*B*). The cells forming the periphery of the tumor cell islands tend to be arranged radially with their long axes in approximately parallel alignment (palisading). The stroma shrinks away from the epithelial tumor nests (Fig. 27–15*C*), creating clefts or separation artifacts that assist in differentiating basal cell carcinomas from certain appendage tumors also characterized by proliferation of basaloid cells (e.g., trichoepithelioma).

Basal Cell Nevus Syndrome. This rare, dominantly inherited basal cell nevus syndrome[36] is associated with the development of numerous basal cell carcinomas in early life and with abnormalities of bone, nervous system, eyes, and reproductive organs.

Mutations in the tumor-suppressor gene PATCHED

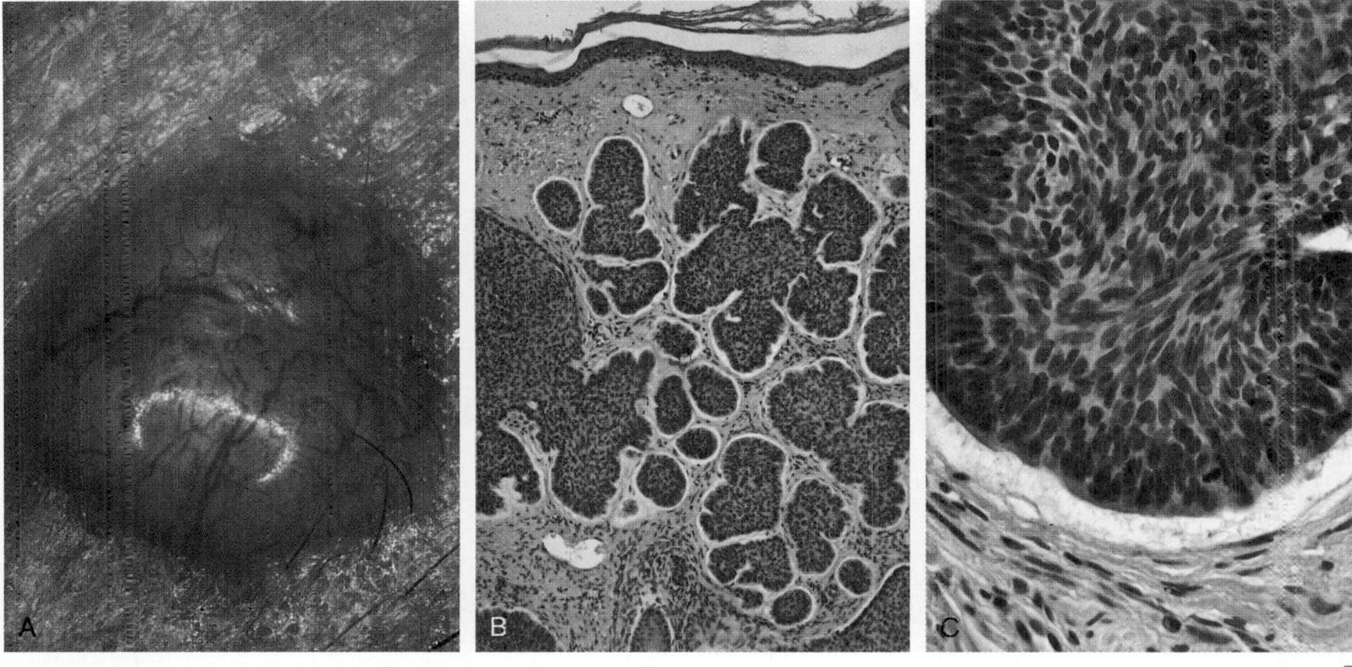

Figure 27–15

Basal cell carcinoma. Pearly, telangiectatic nodules *(A)* are composed of nests of basaloid cells within the dermis *(B)* that are often separated from the adjacent stroma by thin clefts *(C)*.

(PTC) are found in these patients. Mice genetically engineered to overexpress the ligand for *PTC,* the patterning gene "Sonic hedgehog" (or SHH), mimic the loss of *PTC* function, which is sufficient to induce basal cell carcinomas in these mice.[37] Thus, defects in PTC–SHH interactions may play a role in human skin carcinogenesis.

Merkel Cell Carcinoma

This rare neoplasm is derived from the infrequent and functionally obscure *Merkel cell* of the epidermis, a neural crest–derived cell putatively important for tactile sensation in lower animals.[38] These potentially lethal tumors are composed of small, round malignant cells containing neurosecretory type cytoplasmic granules. Pathologists must be aware of this rare primary skin tumor since it may closely resemble metastatic small cell carcinoma from lung or certain lymphomas that spread to the dermis.

TUMORS OF THE DERMIS

The dermis is composed of a variety of different elements, including smooth muscle, pericytes, fibroblasts, neural tissue, and endothelium. All of these components can give rise to neoplasia within the skin, but many of these tumors also arise in soft tissue and viscera unrelated to skin (e.g., leiomyosarcoma) or occur as part of a syndrome primarily affecting another organ system (e.g., as with cutaneous neurofibromas in neurofibromatosis). In this section, therefore, only representative dermal neoplasms that arise primarily in the skin, that have unique characteristics in the skin, or that have not been detailed in other chapters are considered.

Benign Fibrous Histiocytoma

Benign fibrous histiocytoma refers to a heterogeneous family of morphologically and histogenetically related benign dermal neoplasms of fibroblasts and histiocytes. (They are also discussed with the soft tissue tumors in Chapter 28.) These tumors are usually seen in adults and often occur on the legs of young to middle-aged women. Their biologic behavior is indolent, and they should not be confused with the unrelated malignant fibrous histiocytoma, which arises de novo in skin and in extracutaneous sites and often has an aggressive clinical course.

On gross inspection, these neoplasms are tan to brown, firm papules (Fig. 27–16*A*). Lesions are asymptomatic to slightly tender, and their size may increase and decrease slightly over time. Actively growing lesions may reach several centimeters in diameter, and with time, they often become flattened. The tendency for fibrous histiocytomas to dimple inward on lateral compression is helpful in distinguishing them from nodular melanomas, which protrude when they are similarly manipulated.

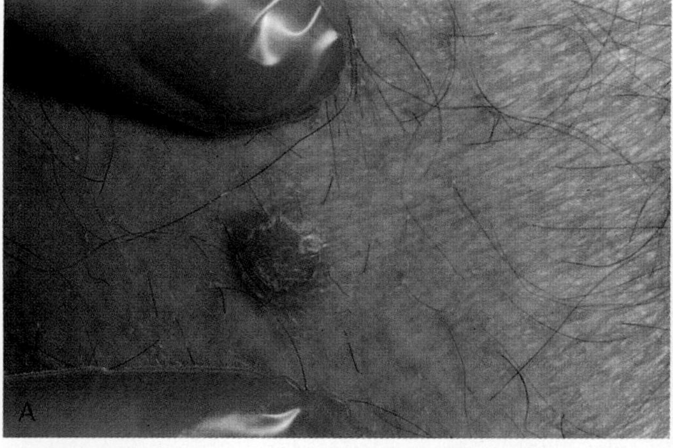

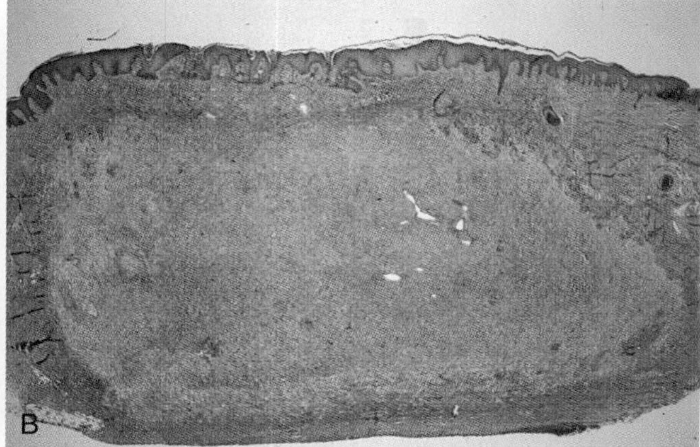

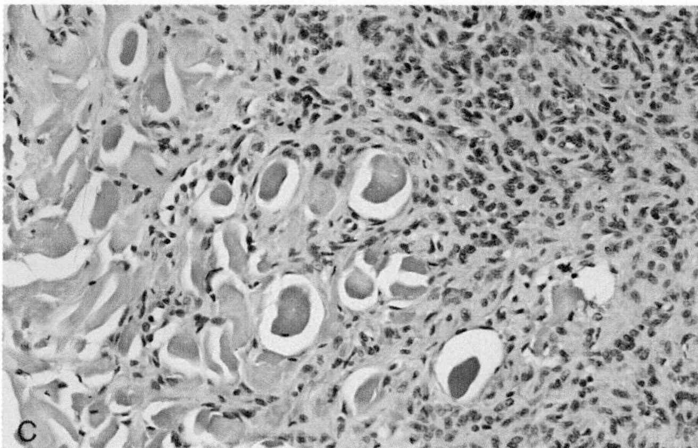

Figure 27–16

A, Benign fibrous histiocytoma (dermatofibroma). *B* and *C*, On excision, this firm, tan papule on the leg shows a localized nodular proliferation of benign-appearing fibroblasts within the dermis. Note the characteristic overlying epidermal hyperplasia and the tendency of fibroblasts to surround individual collagen bundles.

MORPHOLOGY. The most common form of fibrous histiocytoma is referred to as a **dermatofibroma.** These tumors are formed by benign, spindle-shaped fibroblasts arranged in a well-defined, nonencapsulated mass within the mid-dermis (Fig. 27–16*B* and *C*). Extension of these cells into the subcutaneous fat is frequently observed. The majority of cases demonstrate a peculiar form of overlying epidermal hyperplasia, characterized by downward elongation of hyperpigmented rete ridges ("dirty fingers" pattern). Although foamy histiocytes may be seen in dermatofibromas, they are generally not conspicuous. Certain variants are composed predominantly of these foamy histiocytes admixed with a paucity of fibroblasts. Finally, variants containing numerous blood vessels and deposits of hemosiderin may be encountered **(sclerosing hemangiomas).**

The histogenesis of fibrous histiocytomas remains a mystery. Many cases have a history of antecedent trauma, suggesting an abnormal response to injury, perhaps analogous to the deposition of increased amounts of altered collagen in a hypertrophic scar or keloid.

Dermatofibrosarcoma Protuberans

Dermatofibrosarcoma protuberans is best regarded as a well-differentiated, primary fibrosarcoma of the skin. These tumors are slow growing, and although they are locally aggressive, they rarely metastasize.

Clinically, they are firm, solid nodules that arise most frequently on the trunk. They often develop as aggregated "protuberant" tumors within a firm (indurated) plaque that may ulcerate.

MORPHOLOGY. On microscopic examination, these neoplasms are cellular, composed of fibroblasts arranged radially, reminiscent of blades of a pinwheel, a pattern referred to as storiform. Mitoses are usually present but are not as numerous as in a moderately or poorly differentiated fibrosarcoma (see section on soft tissue tumors in Chapter 28). In contrast to that in dermatofibroma, the overlying epidermis is generally thinned. Deep extension from the dermis into subcutaneous fat producing a characteristic "honeycomb" pattern is frequently present, hindering attempts at complete surgical removal.

Xanthomas

Xanthomas are tumor-like collections of foamy histiocytes within the dermis. They may be associated with familial (Chapter 6) or acquired disorders resulting in hyperlipidemia, with lymphoproliferative malignant neoplasms, or with no underlying disorder.

On the basis of clinical appearance, xanthomas are divided into five types. Because identification of these types may provide important clinical markers of the underlying hyperlipoproteinemia (Chapter 12), the classes of lipid abnormality (types I to V) are specified for each kind of clinical lesion.[39] *Eruptive xanthomas* (types I, IIB, III, IV, V) occur as sudden showers of yellow papules that wax and wane according to variations in plasma triglyceride and lipid content. They occur on the buttocks, posterior thighs, knees, and elbows. *Tuberous* (types IIA, III; rarely IIB, IV) and *tendinous* (types IIA, III; rarely IIIB) *xanthomas* occur as yellow nodules; the latter frequently are found on the Achilles tendon and the extensor tendons of the fingers. *Plane xanthomas* (type III; IIA associated with primary biliary cirrhosis) are linear yellow lesions in the skinfolds, especially the palmar creases. *Xanthelasma* (types IIA, III; also without lipid abnormality) refers to soft yellow plaques on the eyelids.

MORPHOLOGY. All types are characterized histologically by dermal accumulation of benign-appearing histiocytes with abundant, finely vacuolated (foamy) cytoplasm. Cholesterol (free and esterified), phospholipids, and triglycerides are present within cells. The cellularity of the infiltrate is variable, and with the exception of xanthelasma, lesions may also be surrounded by inflammatory cells and fibrosis about the central zone of lipid-laden cells.

Dermal Vascular Tumors

Benign vascular neoplasms (capillary and cavernous hemangiomas), malformations (nevus flammeus or "port-wine stain"), multifocal angioproliferative lesions (Kaposi sarcoma, bacillary angiomatosis), vascularized variants of other tumors (e.g., the sclerosing hemangioma variant of benign fibrous histiocytoma), and malignant vascular tumors (angiosarcomas) are frequently encountered in the skin. Most are discussed in depth in Chapter 12. The capillary hemangioma is by far the most commonly encountered form of cutaneous hemangioma. It appears clinically either in childhood ("strawberry hemangioma") or with advancing age as discrete deeply erythematous papules. In adults, lesions may slowly enlarge and occasionally thrombose, whereas in young children, they usually regress by fibrosis.

MORPHOLOGY. Cutaneous hemangiomas must be differentiated from dermal vascular hyperplasias (as may occur in venous stasis), reactive vascular proliferations (as in pyogenic granulomas), unregulated multifocal vascular proliferations (as seen in Kaposi sarcoma), and vascular malignant tumors (angiosarcoma). Typically, hemangiomas are represented histologically by well-formed, blood-filled vascular spaces lined by benign endothelial cells within the superficial and sometimes deep dermis.

TUMORS OF CELLULAR IMMIGRANTS TO THE SKIN

Aside from tumors that arise directly from epidermal and dermal cells, several proliferative disorders of the skin involve primarily cells whose progenitors have arisen elsewhere but that exhibit a peculiar homing to the cutaneous microenvironment. Examples of such cells are epidermal Langerhans cells, which arise from precursors in the bone marrow and, in their mature form, traffic freely from skin to regional lymph nodes by way of dermal lymphatics; T lymphocytes that are normally in residence in low numbers in the dermis and epidermis; and dermal mast cells derived from marrow precursors. The proliferative lesions discussed in this section—namely, histiocytosis X, cutaneous T-cell lymphoma (CTCL), and mastocytosis—are primary cutaneous disorders that arise from these three cell types, respectively.

Histiocytosis X

Histiocytosis X, also called Langerhans cell histiocytosis, is described in detail in Chapter 15. In the skin, this condition presents in multiple forms, including solitary or multiple lesions ranging from papules to nodules to scaling erythematous plaques that in infants may resemble seborrheic dermatitis (Fig. 27–17*A*).

MORPHOLOGY OF SKIN LESIONS. Histiocytosis X involving the skin has several histologic patterns, all of which may show marked infiltration of the skin. The first is that of a diffuse dermal infiltrate of large, round to ovoid cells with pale pink cytoplasms containing indented, often bland nuclei (Fig. 27–17*B*). A second pattern consists of a clustering of similar cells into small aggregates that resemble granulomas. The third is characterized by a dermal infiltrate of cells with foamy, xanthoma-like cytoplasm. Variable numbers of eosinophils may also be observed, particularly with the first pattern. Because these patterns are not specific, special immunohistochemical methods to identify cell surface markers common to Langerhans cells and histiocytosis X cells (CD1a antigen)[40] may be necessary to establish a definitive

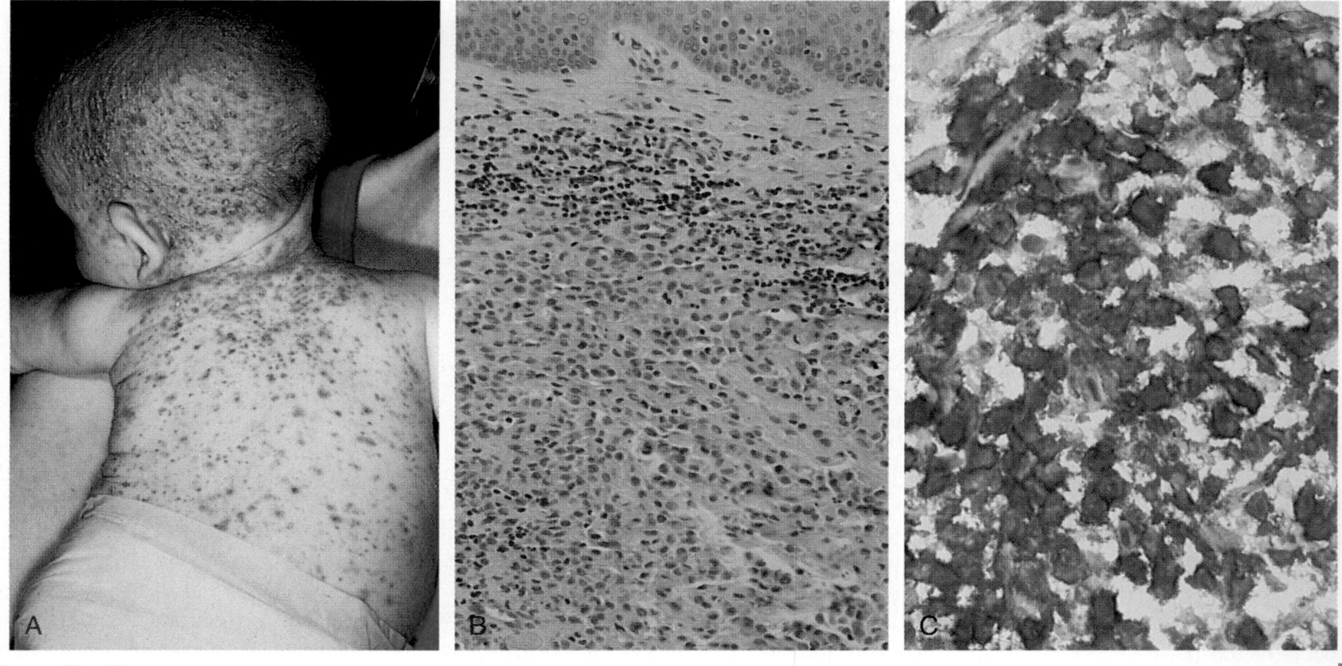

Figure 27–17

Histiocytosis X. *A*, Lesions may appear clinically as papules and nodules or, in this case, as erythematous scaling plaques mimicking the infantile form of seborrheic dermatitis. *B*, Dermal infiltration by bland mononuclear cells with infolded nuclei presents a nonspecific histologic pattern. *C*, Immunohistochemical demonstration of CD1a antigen confirms their origin from Langerhans cells. (*A* from Murphy GF, Herzberg AJ: Atlas of Dermatopathology. Philadelphia, WB Saunders, 1996, p 205.)

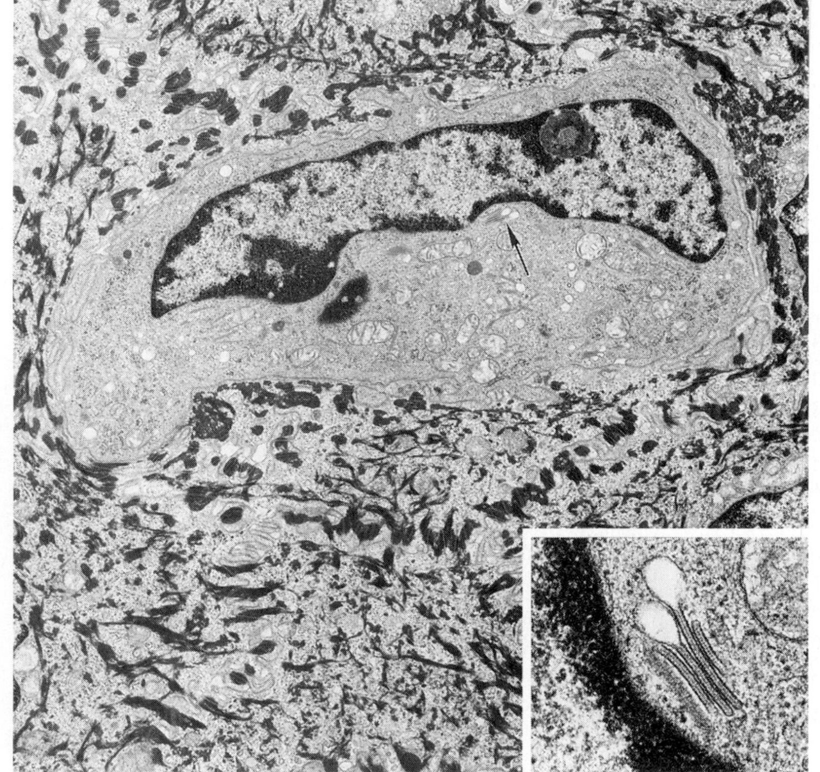

Figure 27–18

Histiocytosis X. Ultrastructural detection of Birbeck granules, as seen in normal Langerhans cells (*arrow* and *inset*), permitted accurate diagnosis in this case.

histologic diagnosis (Fig. 27–17*C*). In addition, ultrastructural identification of specific organelles (Birbeck granules) characteristic of the epidermal Langerhans cells from which histiocytosis X cells are believed to originate (Fig. 27–18) is also helpful.

Mycosis Fungoides (Cutaneous T-cell Lymphoma)

CTCL represents a spectrum of lymphoproliferative disorders affecting the skin (see also Chapter 15). Two types of malignant T-cell disorders were originally recognized: mycosis fungoides, a chronic proliferative process; and a nodular eruptive variant, *mycosis fungoides d'emblée.* It is now known that a variety of presentations of T-cell lymphoma occur, including mycosis fungoides, the eruptive nodular type, and an adult T-cell leukemia or lymphoma type. The latter disorder may have a rapid progressive downhill course.

Mycosis fungoides is the T-cell lymphoproliferative disorder that arises primarily in the skin and that may evolve into generalized lymphoma.[41] Most affected individuals have disease that remains localized to the skin for many years; a minority have rapid systemic dissemination. This condition may occur at any age, but most commonly it afflicts persons older than 40 years.

Clinically, lesions of the mycosis fungoides type of CTCL include scaly, red-brown patches; raised, scaling plaques that may even be confused with psoriasis; and fungating nodules. Eczema-like lesions typify early stages of disease when obvious visceral or nodal spread has not occurred. Raised, indurated, irregularly outlined, erythematous plaques may then supervene. Development of multiple, large (up to 10 cm or more in diameter), red-brown nodules correlates with systemic spreading. Sometimes plaques and nodules ulcerate, as depicted in Figure 27–19*A*. Lesions may affect numerous body surfaces, including the trunk, extremities, face, and scalp. In some individuals, seeding of the blood by malignant T cells is accompanied by diffuse erythema and scaling of the entire body surface (erythroderma), a condition known as *Sézary syndrome* (Chapter 15).

MORPHOLOGY. The hallmark of CTCL of the mycosis fungoides type histologically is the identification of the **Sézary-Lutzner** cells. These are T-helper cells (CD4 antigen-positive) that characteristically form bandlike aggregates within the superficial dermis (Fig. 27–19*B*) and invade the epidermis as single cells and small clusters **(Pautrier microabscesses).** These cells have markedly infolded nuclear membranes, imparting a "hyperconvoluted" or "cerebriform" contour. Although patches and plaques show pronounced epidermal infiltration by Sézary-Lutzner cells (epidermotropism), in more advanced nodular lesions the malignant T cells often lose this epidermotropic tendency, grow deeply into the dermis, and eventually seed lymphatics and the peripheral circulation.

As described in Chapters 8 and 15, HTLV-I has been implicated in certain forms of T-cell lymphoma,[41] and CTCL may also have an infectious causation. The proliferating cells in CTCL are clonal populations of lymphocytes of the CD4 subset.[42] These cells often express aberrant cell surface antigens as well as clonal T-cell receptor gene rearrangements, and detection of these features may be of diagnostic assistance in difficult cases.[43]

Topical therapy with steroids or ultraviolet light is often employed for early lesions of CTCL, whereas more aggressive systemic chemotherapy is indicated for advanced disease.

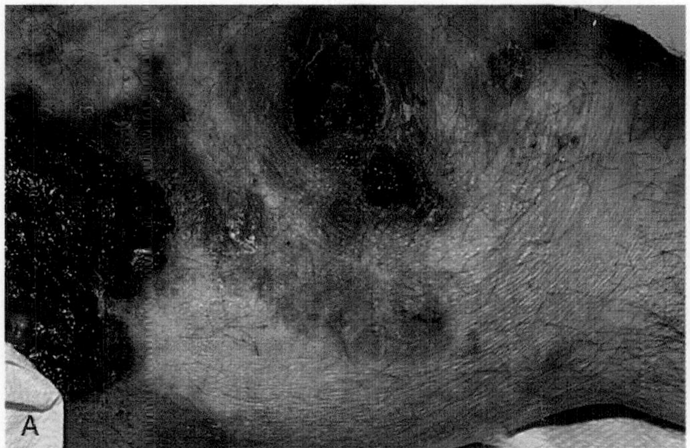

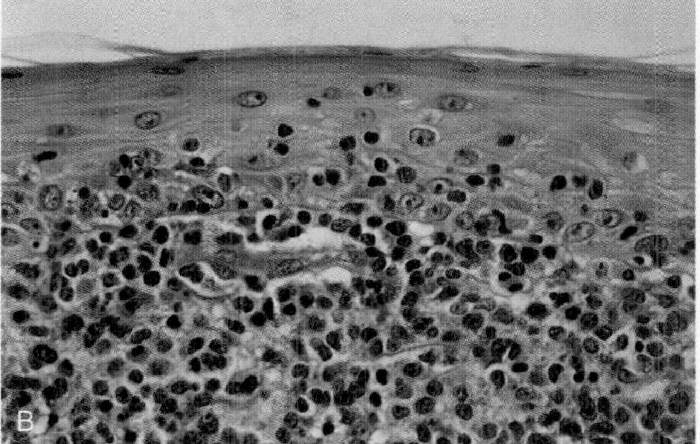

Figure 27–19

Cutaneous T-cell lymphoma. The histologic correlate of ill-defined, erythematous, often scaling, and occasionally ulcerated plaques *(A)* is an infiltrate of atypical lymphocytes that show a tendency to accumulate beneath the epidermal layer *(B)* and to invade the epidermis as small microabscesses.

Mastocytosis

The term mastocytosis refers to a spectrum of rare disorders characterized by increased numbers of mast cells in the skin and, in some instances, in other organs. A localized cutaneous form of the disease that affects predominantly children and accounts for more than 50% of all cases is termed *urticaria pigmentosa.* These lesions are multiple, although solitary mastocytomas may also occur, usually shortly after birth. About 10% of patients with mast cell disease have overt systemic mastocytosis, with mast cell infiltration of many organs. These individuals are often adults, and unlike the case with localized cutaneous disease, the prognosis may be poor.

The clinical picture of mastocytosis is highly variable. In urticaria pigmentosa, lesions are multiple and widely distributed, consisting of round to oval, red-brown, nonscaling papules and small plaques. Solitary mastocytomas present as one or several pink to tan-brown nodules that may be pruritic or exhibit blister formation (Fig. 27–20*A*). In systemic mastocytosis, skin lesions similar to those of urticaria pigmentosa are accompanied by mast cell infiltration of bone marrow, liver, spleen, and lymph nodes. Many of the signs and symptoms of mastocytosis are due to the effects of histamine, heparin, and other substances released as a result of degranulation. *Darier sign* refers to a localized area of dermal edema and erythema (wheal) that occurs when lesional skin is rubbed. *Dermatographism* refers to an area of dermal edema resembling a hive that occurs in normal skin as a result of localized stroking with a pointed instrument. In systemic disease, all of the following may be seen: pruritus and flushing triggered by certain foods, temperature changes, alcohol, and certain drugs (morphine, codeine, aspirin); watery nasal discharge (rhinorrhea); rarely, gastrointestinal or nasal bleeding, possibly due to the anticoagulant effects of heparin; and bone pain as a result of osteoblastic and osteoclastic involvement.

MORPHOLOGY. The histologic picture varies from a subtle increase in the numbers of spindle-shaped and stellate mast cells about superficial dermal blood vessels to large numbers of tightly packed, round to oval mast cells in the upper to mid-dermis (Fig. 27–20*B*) in urticaria pigmentosa or solitary mastocytoma. Variable fibrosis, edema, and small numbers of eosinophils may also be present. Mast cells may be difficult to differentiate from lymphocytes in routine, H&E-stained sections, and special "metachromatic" stains (toluidine blue or Giemsa) must be used to visualize their granules (Fig. 27–20*C*). Even with these stains, extensive degranulation may result in failure to detect these cells by light microscopy, and ultrastructural analysis must then be performed.

The pathogenesis of at least some cases of mastocytosis now appears to involve a clonal proliferation of mast cells

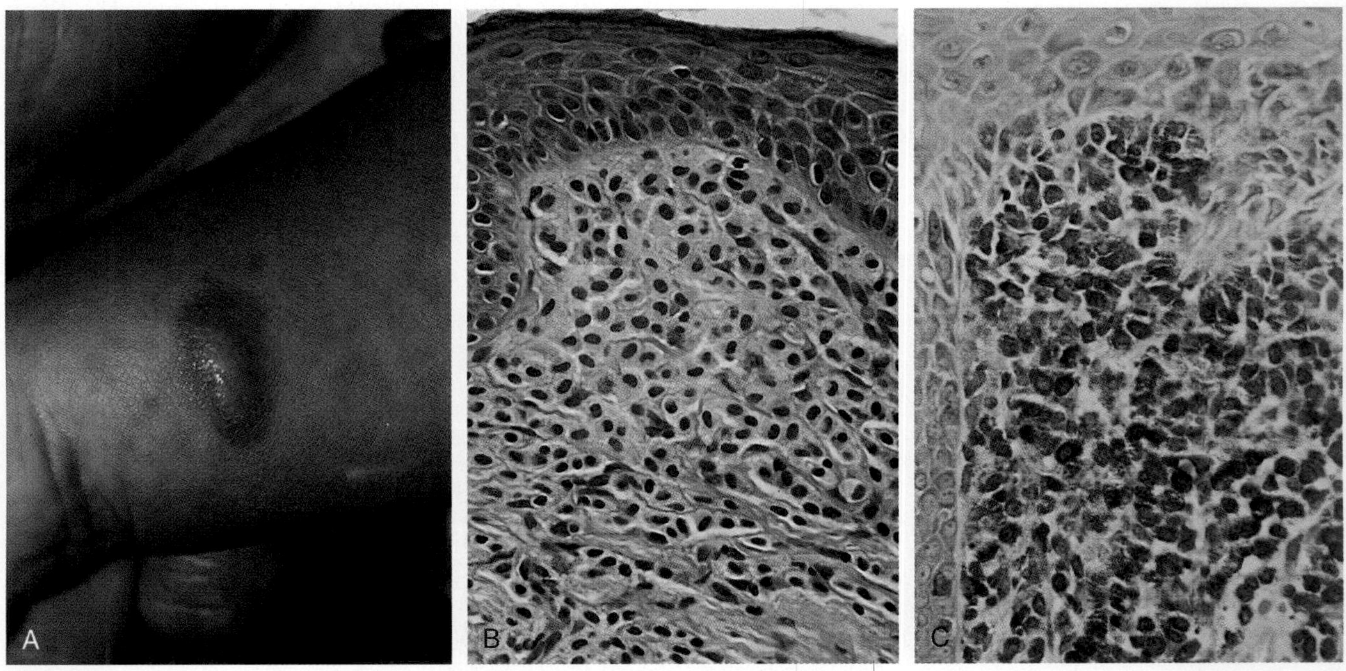

Figure 27–20

Mastocytosis. *A*, Solitary mastocytoma in a 1-year-old child. *B*, By routine histology, numerous ovoid cells with uniform, centrally located nuclei are observed in the dermis. *C*, Giemsa staining reveals purple, "metachromatic" granules within the cytoplasm of the cells. (*A* from Murphy GF, Herzberg AJ: Atlas of Dermatopathology. Philadelphia, WB Saunders, 1996, p 207.)

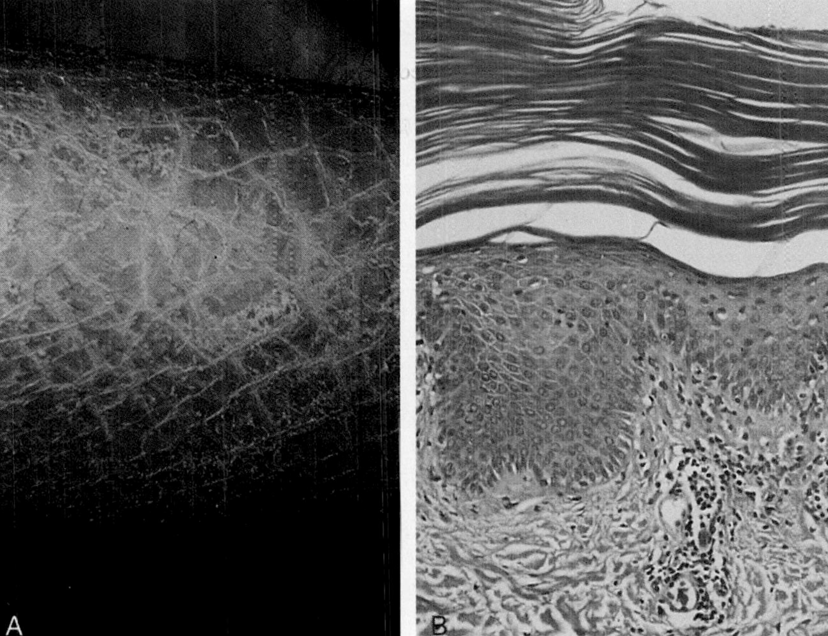

Figure 27–21

Ichthyosis. Note prominent fish-like scales *(A)* and compacted hyperorthokeratosis *(B)*.

containing a point mutation of the c-*kit* proto-oncogene that is known to cause activation of a type III receptor tyrosine kinase expressed by mast cells and involved in their growth and differentiation.[44] Although some clonal proliferations of mast cells thus have features of true neoplasia, the cells remain subject to certain phenotypic modifications in differing tissue microenvironments.[45] Such heterogeneity has resulted in the previous misconception that the disorder is exclusively a hyperplasia of mast cells.

DISORDERS OF EPIDERMAL MATURATION

Ichthyosis

Of the numerous disorders that impair epidermal maturation, ichthyosis is perhaps one of the most striking. The term is derived from the Greek root *ichthy-*, meaning fishy, and accordingly this group of genetically inherited disorders is associated with excessive keratin build-up (hyperkeratosis) that results clinically in fishlike scales (Fig. 27–21*A*). Most ichthyoses become apparent either at or around the time of birth. Acquired (noninherited) variants exist, and in the acquired vulgaris type in adults, there is an association with lymphoid and visceral malignant neoplasms. The various clinical types of ichthyosis vary according to the mode of inheritance, histology, and clinical features; the primary categories include ichthyosis vulgaris (autosomal dominant or acquired), congenital ichthyosiform erythroderma (autosomal recessive), lamellar ichthyosis (autosomal recessive), and X-linked ichthyosis.

MORPHOLOGY. The general histology of all forms of ichthyosis is often subtle build-up of compacted stratum corneum, with loss of the normal basket-weave pattern seen in this layer when it involves nonpalmar and plantar surfaces (Fig. 27–21*B*). There is generally little or no inflammation, and subtle associated variations in the thickness of the epidermis and the stratum granulosum, along with the clinical picture, assist in assigning the correct diagnostic subclassification.

The primary abnormality in some forms of ichthyosis may reside in defective mechanisms of desquamation, leading to retention of abnormally formed scale. For example, in X-linked ichthyosis, affected homozygotes demonstrate a deficiency in steroid sulfatase, an enzyme important to the removal of proadhesive cholesterol sulfate secreted into the intercellular spaces along with adhesive organelles called Odland bodies, or membrane-coating granules. Accumulation of this nondegraded cholesterol sulfate results in persistent cell-cell adhesion within the stratum corneum, hindering the desquamation process. Compare this with pemphigus vulgaris (see later), in which dramatically different lesions form as a consequence of decreased cell-cell adhesion!

ACUTE INFLAMMATORY DERMATOSES

Inflammatory dermatoses are usually mediated by local or systemic immunologic factors, although the causes for many remain a mystery. Literally thousands of specific

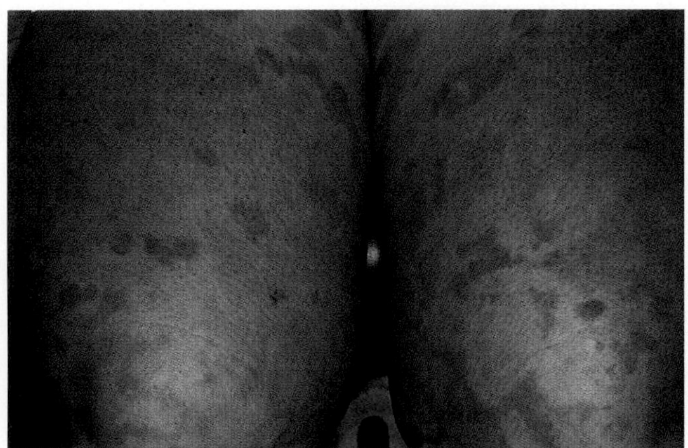

Figure 27-22

Urticaria. Clinically, there are erythematous, edematous, often circular plaques covered by a normal epidermal surface. (From Murphy GF, Herzberg AJ: Atlas of Dermatopathology. Philadelphia, WB Saunders, 1996, p 83.)

inflammatory dermatoses exist. In general, acute lesions last from days to weeks and are characterized by inflammation (often marked by mononuclear cells, not neutrophils), edema, and, in some, epidermal, vascular, or subcutaneous injury. Chronic lesions, on the other hand, persist for months to years and often show significant components of altered epidermal growth (atrophy or hyperplasia) or dermal fibrosis. The lesions discussed here are selected as examples of the more commonly encountered dermatoses within the acute category.

Urticaria

Urticaria (hives) is a common disorder of the skin characterized by localized mast cell degranulation and resultant dermal microvascular hyperpermeability, culminating in pruritic edematous plaques called wheals. Angioedema is closely related to urticaria and is characterized by deeper edema of both the dermis and the subcutaneous fat.

Urticaria most often occurs between the ages of 20 and 40 years, although all age groups are susceptible. Individual lesions develop and fade within hours (usually less than 24 hours), and episodes may last for days or persist for months. Lesions vary from small, pruritic papules to large edematous plaques (Fig. 27-22). Individual lesions may coalesce to form annular, linear, or arciform configurations. Sites of predilection for urticarial eruptions include any area exposed to pressure, such as the trunk, distal extremities, and ears. Persistent urticaria may simply be the result of inability to eliminate the causative antigen or may herald underlying disease (e.g., collagen vascular disorders, Hodgkin disease).

MORPHOLOGY. The histologic features of urticaria may be so subtle that many biopsy specimens at first resemble normal skin. There is usually a sparse superficial perivenular infiltrate consisting of mononuclear cells and rare neutrophils. Eosinophils may also be present. Collagen bundles are more widely spaced than in normal skin, a result of superficial dermal edema fluid that does not stain in routinely prepared tissue (Fig. 27-23). Superficial lymphatic channels are dilated in an attempt to accommodate this transudated edema fluid.

In most cases, urticaria results from antigen-induced release of vasoactive mediators from mast cell granules through sensitization with specific immunoglobulin E (IgE) antibodies. This *IgE-dependent* degranulation can follow exposure to a number of antigens (pollens, foods, drugs, insect venom) and specifically results from bridging between mast cell-bound IgE molecules by multivalent ligand, as discussed in Chapter 7. *IgE-independent* urticaria may result from substances that in certain individuals directly incite the degranulation of mast cells, such as opiates, certain antibiotics, curare, and radiographic contrast media. Another cause of IgE-independent urticaria is exposure to chemicals, such as aspirin, that suppress prostaglandin synthesis from arachidonic acid. Hereditary angioneurotic edema (Chapter 7) is the result of an inherited deficiency of C1 activator (C1 esterase inhibitor) that results in uncontrolled activation of the early components of the complement system (so-called complement-mediated urticaria).[46]

Acute Eczematous Dermatitis

Eczema is a clinical term that embraces a number of pathogenetically different conditions. All are characterized by red, papulovesicular, oozing, and crusted lesions early on that, with persistence, eventuate into raised, scaling plaques. In time, acute spongiotic dermatitis may evolve to a more chronic form in which epidermal hyperplasia and excessive scale, rather than blistering, dominate the clinical and histologic picture (Fig. 27-24). Clinical differences

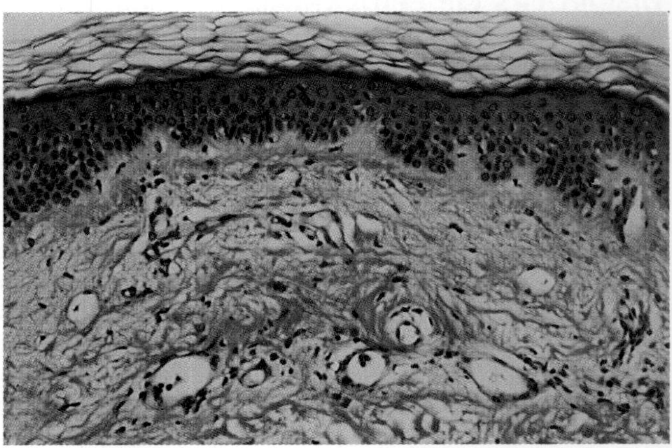

Figure 27-23

Urticaria. Histologically, there is superficial dermal edema and dilated lymphatic and blood-filled vascular spaces. The edema is manifested by widening of spaces that separate the collagen bundles. (From Murphy GF, Herzberg AJ: Atlas of Dermatopathology. Philadelphia, WB Saunders, 1996, p 83.)

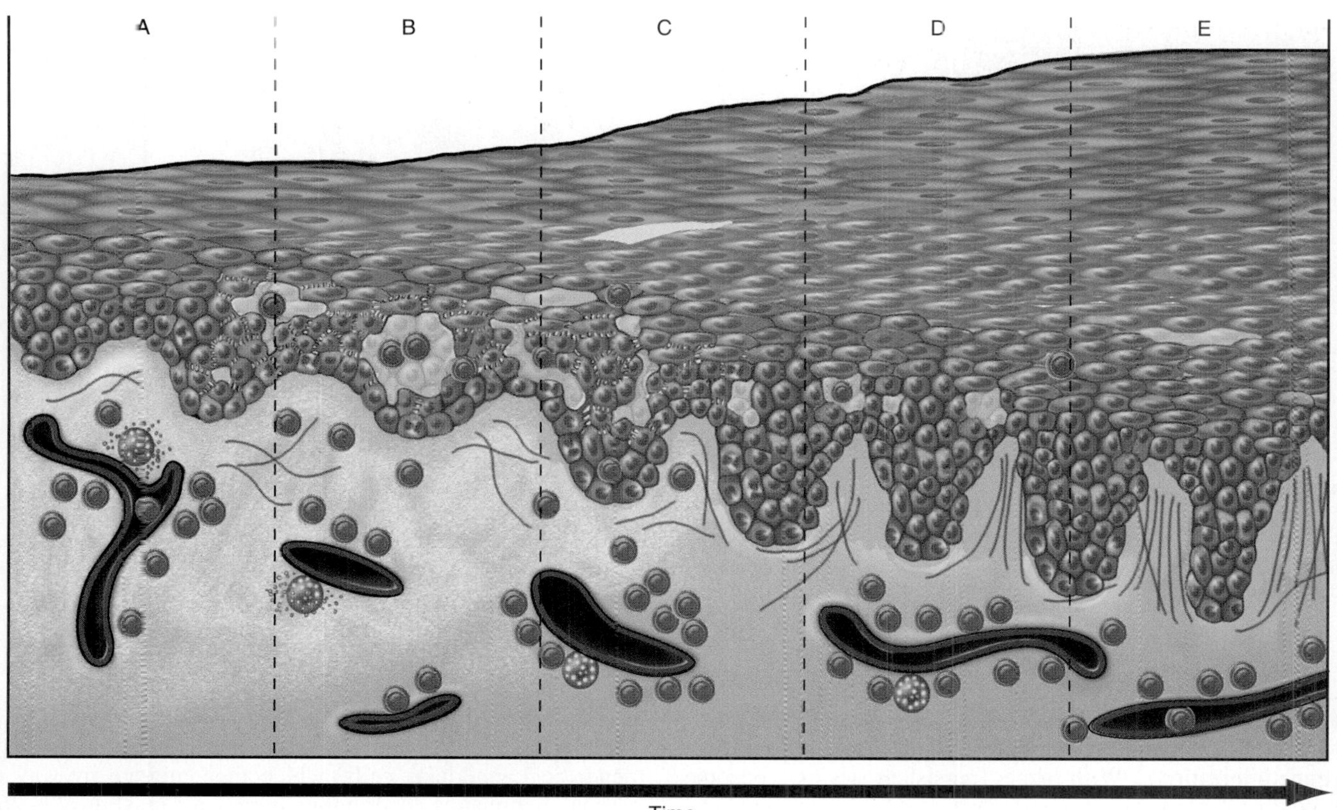

Figure 27–24

Evolutionary stages of spongiotic dermatitis. *A*, Initial dermal edema and perivascular infiltration by inflammatory cells is followed within 24 to 48 hours by epidermal spongiosis and microvesicle formation *(B)*. *C*, Abnormal scale, including parakeratosis, follows, along with progressive epidermal hyperplasia *(D)* and hyperkeratosis *(E)* as the lesion enters into a more chronic stage.

permit classification of eczematous dermatitis into the following categories: (1) allergic contact dermatitis, (2) atopic dermatitis, (3) drug-related eczematous dermatitis, (4) photoeczematous dermatitis, and (5) primary irritant dermatitis (Table 27–3).

The Greek word *eczema,* meaning "to boil over," vividly describes the clinical appearance of acute eczematous dermatitis. The most obvious example is an acute contact reaction to poison ivy, characterized by pruritic, edematous, oozing plaques, often containing small and large blisters

Table 27–3. CLASSIFICATION OF ECZEMATOUS DERMATITIS

Type	Cause or Pathogenesis	Histology*	Clinical Features
Contact dermatitis	Topically applied antigens Pathogenesis: delayed hypersensitivity	Spongiotic dermatitis	Marked itching or burning or both; requires antecedent exposure
Atopic dermatitis	Unknown, may be heritable	Spongiotic dermatitis	Erythematous plaques in flexural areas; family history of eczema, hay fever, or asthma
Drug-related eczematous dermatitis	Systemically administered antigens or haptens (e.g., penicillin)	Spongiotic dermatitis; eosinophils often present in infiltrate; deeper infiltrate	Eruption occurs with administration of drug; remits when drug is discontinued
Photoeczematous eruption	Ultraviolet light	Spongiotic dermatitis; deeper infiltrate	Occurs on sun-exposed skin; phototesting may help in diagnosis
Primary irritant dermatitis	Repeated trauma (rubbing)	Spongiotic dermatitis in early stages; epidermal hyperplasia in late stages	Localized to site of trauma

*All types, with time, may develop chronic changes.

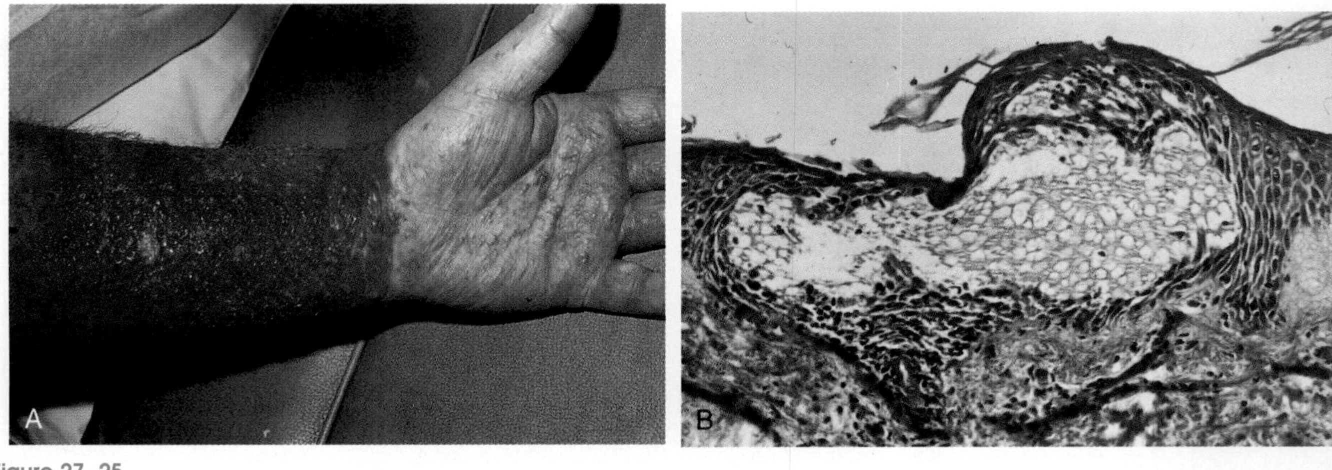

Figure 27–25

Eczematous dermatitis. *A*, In an acute allergic contact dermatitis, numerous vesicles appear at the site of antigen exposure (in this case, laundry detergent that persisted in clothing). *B*, Histologically, intercellular edema produces widened intercellular spaces within the epidermis, eventually resulting in small, fluid-filled intraepidermal vesicles.

(vesicles and bullae) (Fig. 27–25*A*). Such lesions are prone to bacterial superinfection, which produces a yellow crust (impetiginization). With time, persistent lesions become less "wet" (fail to ooze or form vesicles) and become progressively scaly (hyperkeratotic) as the epidermis thickens (acanthosis).

Pathogenesis: This has been well studied in dermatitis due to contact hypersensitivity (e.g., poison ivy dermatitis). Initially, antigens at the epidermal surface are taken up by dendritic Langerhans cells, which then migrate by way of dermal lymphatics to draining lymph nodes (Fig. 27–26). Here, antigens now processed by the Langerhans cell are presented to naive CD4 T cells, which subsequently develop immunologic memory. On antigen re-exposure, these

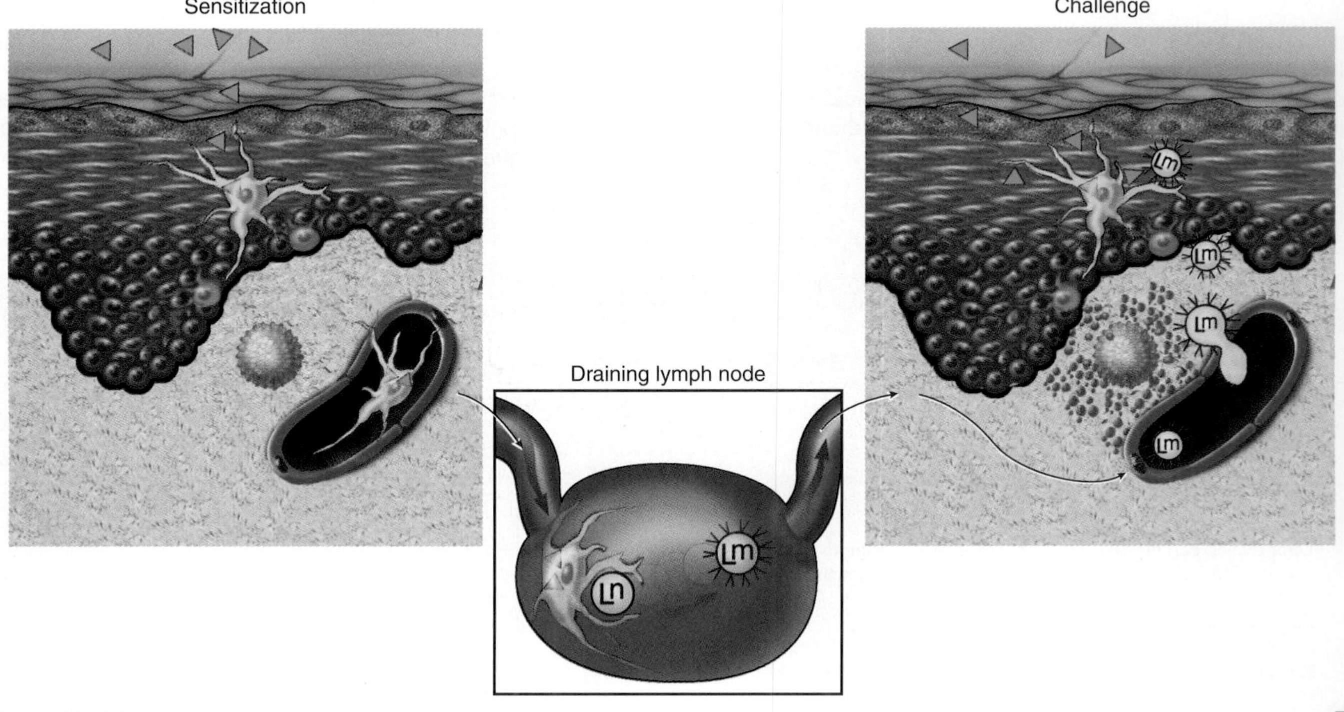

Figure 27–26

Schematic diagram of mechanisms of allergic contact dermatitis. ▲, antigen; Ln, naive T cell; Lm, memory T cell.

memory T cells migrate to affected skin sites where they release cytokines and factors that recruit the numerous inflammatory cells responsible for the clinical lesion of spongiotic dermatitis.

An early event in the genesis of T-cell recruitment to the challenge site is local cytokine release in the vicinity of dermal postcapillary venules.[48, 49] This results in "endothelial activation" whereby endothelial cells express molecules on their plasma membranes that promote adhesion of circulating T lymphocytes with immunologic memory for the sensitizing antigen or hapten. Once these memory T cells enter the site of antigen challenge through activated microvessels, they elaborate a potent array of lymphokines that signal recruitment of large numbers of inflammatory cells to the site of antigen contact. This process occurs within 24 hours and accounts for the initial erythema and pruritus that characterize cutaneous delayed hypersensitivity in the acute, spongiotic phase.

MORPHOLOGY. Spongiosis—the accumulation of edema fluid within the intercellular spaces of the epidermis—characterizes acute eczematous dermatitis, hence the synonym spongiotic dermatitis. Whereas edema is localized to the perivascular spaces of the superficial dermis in urticaria, edema seeps into the intercellular spaces of the epidermis in spongiotic dermatitis, splaying apart keratinocytes located primarily in the stratum spinosum. Intercellular bridges appear prominent, giving a "spongy" appearance to the epidermis. Mechanical shearing of intercellular attachment sites (desmosomes) and cell membranes by progressive accumulation of intercellular fluid may result in the formation of intraepidermal vesicles (Fig. 27–25*B*).

During the earliest stages of the evolution of spongiotic dermatitis, there is a superficial, perivascular, lymphocytic infiltrate associated with papillary dermal edema and mast cell degranulation. The pattern and composition of this infiltrate may provide clues to the underlying cause.[47] For example, spongiotic dermatitis resulting from certain drugs will show a lymphocytic infiltrate, **often containing eosinophils,** and extending around deep as well as superficial dermal vessels.

Erythema Multiforme

Erythema multiforme is an uncommon, self-limited disorder that appears to be a hypersensitivity response to certain infections and drugs. Erythema multiforme is a prototype of a cytotoxic reaction pattern (one typified by extensive epithelial cell degeneration and death). This disorder affects individuals of any age and is associated with the following conditions: (1) infections such as herpes simplex, mycoplasmal infections, histoplasmosis, coccidioidomycosis, typhoid, and leprosy, among others; (2) administration of certain drugs (sulfonamides, penicillin, barbiturates, salicylates, hydantoins, and antimalarials); (3) malignant disease (carcinomas and lymphomas); and (4) collagen vascular diseases (lupus erythematosus, dermatomyositis, and periarteritis nodosa).

Patients present clinically with an array of "multiform" lesions including macules, papules, vesicles, and bullae as well as the characteristic target lesion consisting of a red macule or papule with a pale, vesicular, or eroded center (Fig. 27–27*A*). Although lesions may be widely distributed, symmetric involvement of the extremities frequently occurs. An extensive and symptomatic febrile form of the disease, which is more common in children, is called the *Stevens-Johnson syndrome*. Typically, erosions and hemorrhagic crusts involve the lips and oral mucosa, although the

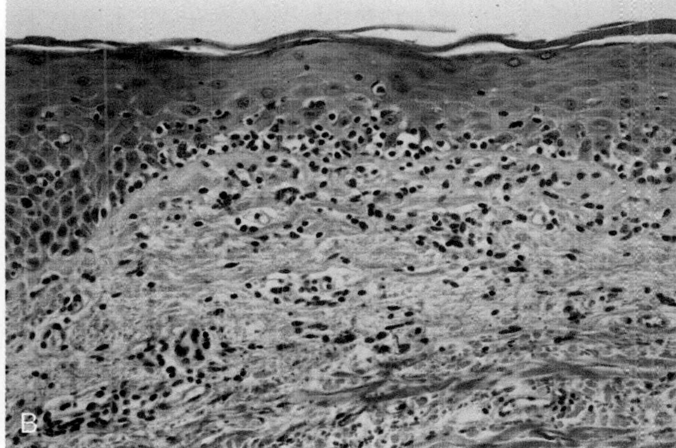

Figure 27–27

Erythema multiforme. *A*, The target-like clinical lesions consist of a central blister or zone of epidermal necrosis surrounded by macular erythema. *B*, Early lesions show lymphocytes collecting along the dermal epidermal junction where basal keratinocytes have begun to become vacuolated. (From Murphy GF, Herzberg AJ: Atlas of Dermatopathology. Philadelphia, WB Saunders, 1996, p 71.)

conjunctiva, urethra, and genital and perianal areas may also be affected. Infection of involved areas may result in life-threatening sepsis. Another variant, termed *toxic epidermal necrolysis,* results in diffuse necrosis and sloughing of cutaneous and mucosal epithelial surfaces, producing a clinical situation analogous to an extensive burn.

MORPHOLOGY. On histologic examination, early lesions show a superficial perivascular, lymphocytic infiltrate associated with dermal edema and margination of lymphocytes along the dermoepidermal junction, where they are intimately associated with degenerating and necrotic keratinocytes (Fig. 27–27*B*). With time, there is upward migration of lymphocytes into the epidermis. Discrete and confluent zones of epidermal necrosis occur with concomitant blister formation. Epidermal sloughing leads to shallow erosions. The **target lesion** exhibits central necrosis surrounded by a rim of perivenular inflammation.

Erythema multiforme has potential immunologic similarities to other conditions characterized by cytotoxic epidermal cell injury (e.g., acute graft-versus-host disease,[50] skin allograft rejection,[51] and fixed drug eruptions[52]). Many of the lymphocytes responsible for the cytotoxic response are of the cytotoxic phenotype, expressing CD8 molecules on their surfaces.

CHRONIC INFLAMMATORY DERMATOSES

This category focuses on those persistent inflammatory dermatoses that exhibit their most characteristic clinical and histologic features for many months to years. Unlike the normal cutaneous surface, the skin surface in some chronic inflammatory dermatoses is roughened as a result of excessive or abnormal scale formation and shedding. However, not all scaling lesions are inflammatory. Witness the hereditary ichthyoses with fishlike scales as the result of some defect in the adhesive properties of cells in the stratum corneum (see earlier).

Psoriasis

Psoriasis is a common chronic inflammatory dermatosis affecting as many as 1% to 2% of people in the United States. Persons of all ages may develop the disease. Psoriasis is sometimes associated with arthritis, myopathy, enteropathy, spondylitic heart disease, or the acquired immunodeficiency syndrome. Psoriatic arthritis may be mild or may produce severe deformities resembling the joint changes seen in rheumatoid arthritis.

Clinically, psoriasis most frequently affects the skin of the elbows, knees, scalp, lumbosacral areas, intergluteal cleft, and glans penis. The most typical lesion is a well-demarcated, pink to salmon-colored plaque covered by loosely adherent scales that are characteristically silver-white in color (Fig. 27–28). Variations exist, with some lesions occurring in annular, linear, gyrate, or serpiginous configurations. Psoriasis can be one cause of total body erythema and scaling known as *erythroderma.* Nail changes[53] occur in 30% of cases of psoriasis and consist of yellow-brown discoloration (often likened to an oil slick), with pitting, dimpling, separation of the nail plate from the underlying bed (onycholysis), thickening, and crumbling. In the rare variant called *pustular psoriasis,* multiple small pustules form on erythematous plaques. This type of psoriasis is either benign and localized (hands and feet) or generalized and life-threatening, with associated fever, leukocytosis, arthralgias, diffuse cutaneous and mucosal pustules, secondary infection, and electrolyte disturbances.

MORPHOLOGY. Established lesions of psoriasis have a characteristic histologic picture. Increased epidermal cell turnover results in marked epidermal thickening (acanthosis), with regular downward elongation of the rete ridges (Fig. 27–29). Mitotic figures are easily identified well above the basal cell layer, where mitotic activity is confined in normal skin. **The stratum granulosum is thinned or absent, and extensive overlying parakeratotic scale is seen.** Typical of psoriatic plaques is thinning of the portion of the epidermal cell layer that overlies the tips of dermal papillae (suprapapillary plates) and dilated, tortuous blood vessels within these papillae. This constellation of changes results in abnormal proximity of dermal vessels within the dermal papillae to the overlying

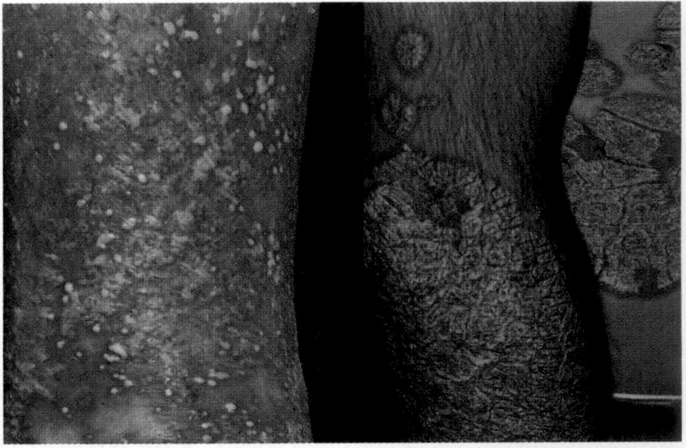

Figure 27–28

Clinical evolution of psoriasis. Early and eruptive lesions may be dominated by signs of inflammation and erythema *(left).* Established, chronic lesions demonstrate erythema surmounted by characteristic silver-white scale *(right).* Rarely, the early inflammatory phase predominates throughout the course of the disease (pustular psoriasis).

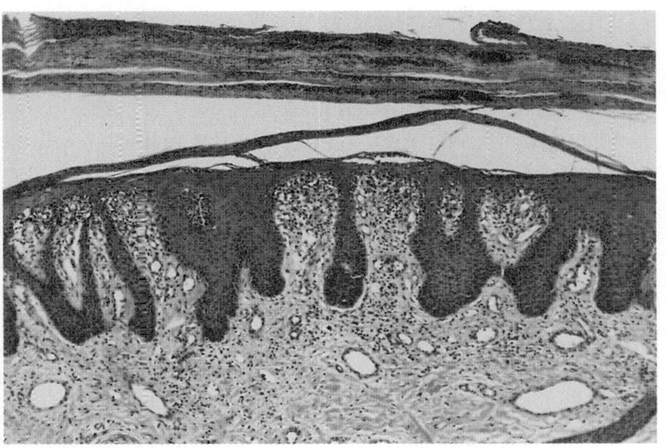

Figure 27–29

Psoriasis. Histologically, established lesions demonstrate marked epidermal hyperplasia, parakeratotic scale, and, importantly, minute microabscesses of neutrophils within the superficial epidermal layers.

parakeratotic scale, and it accounts for the characteristic clinical phenomenon of multiple, minute, bleeding points when the scale is lifted from the plaque **(Auspitz sign)**. Neutrophils form small aggregates within slightly spongiotic foci of the superficial epidermis **(spongiform pustules)** and within the parakeratotic stratum corneum **(Munro microabscesses)**. In pustular psoriasis, larger abscess-like accumulations of neutrophils are present directly beneath the stratum corneum.

Determination of the pathogenesis of psoriasis is one of the most important challenges in dermatopathologic research. An increased incidence of disease in association with certain HLA types suggests that genetic factors participate in the predisposition for disease development. The genesis of new lesions at sites of trauma (the *Koebner phenomenon*) provides certain clues. Numerous theories exist, including those that suggest that lesions may result from unmasking of stratum corneum antigens with related antibody and complement deposition, or that lesions evolve at sites containing abnormally reactive endothelial cells. Recent data suggest that lymphocytes from patients with psoriasis are capable of inducing abnormal growth of keratinocytes and dermal blood vessels.[54] If these results hold, then psoriasis is a systemic disorder of the immune system capable of provoking activation and disordered growth of certain skin cells.

Lichen Planus

"Pruritic, purple, polygonal papules" are the presenting signs of this disorder of skin and mucous membranes. Lichen planus is self-limiting and generally resolves spontaneously 1 to 2 years after onset, often leaving zones of postinflammatory hyperpigmentation (see later). Oral lesions may persist for years. Malignant degeneration has been noted to occur in chronic mucosal and paramucosal lesions of lichen planus, although the direct pathogenetic relationship has not been shown.[55]

Cutaneous lesions consist of itchy, violaceous, flat-topped papules that may coalesce focally to form plaques (Fig. 27–30*A*). These papules are often highlighted by white dots or lines called *Wickham striae*. In darkly pigmented individuals, lesions may acquire a dark brown color due to loss of melanin pigmentation into the dermis as the basal cell layer is destroyed. Multiple lesions are characteristic and are symmetrically distributed, particularly on the extremities, often about the wrists and elbows, and on the glans penis. In 70% of cases, oral lesions are present as white, reticulated, or netlike areas involving the mucosa. As in psoriasis, the Koebner phenomenon (see earlier) may be seen in lichen planus.

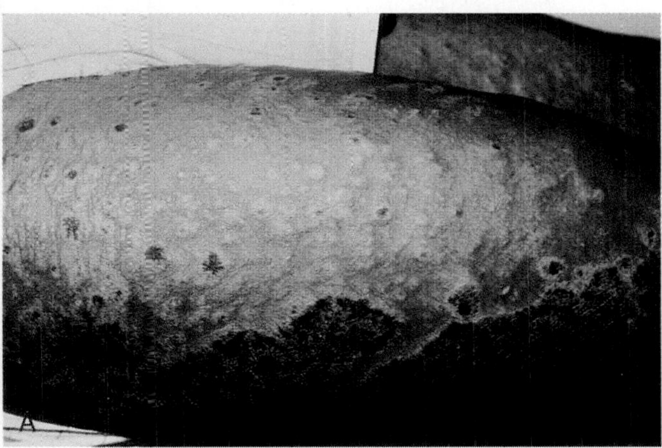

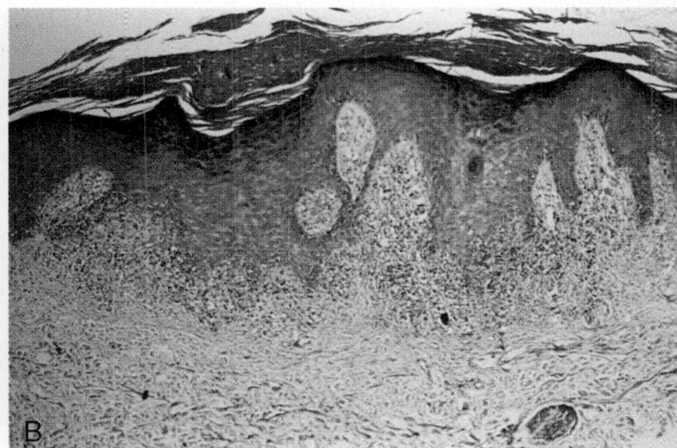

Figure 27–30

Lichen planus. *A*, An erythematous and hyperpigmented plaque has resulted from coalescence of multiple small papules. *B*, Biopsy of one of the lesions demonstrates the bandlike infiltrate of lymphocytes at the dermoepidermal junction and pointed rete ridges ("saw-toothing"; compare with Figure 27–1). (From Murphy GF, Herzberg AJ: Atlas of Dermatopathology. Philadelphia, WB Saunders, 1996, p 75.)

MORPHOLOGY. Lichen planus is characterized histologically by a dense, continuous infiltrate of lymphocytes along the dermoepidermal junction (Fig. 27–30*B*). The lymphocytes are intimately associated with basal keratinocytes, which show degeneration, necrosis, and a resemblance in size and contour to more mature cells of the stratum spinosum (squamatization). A consequence of this destructive infiltration of lymphocytes is a redefinition of the normal, smoothly undulating configuration of the dermoepidermal interface to a more angulated zigzag contour ("saw-toothing"). Anucleate, necrotic basal cells may become incorporated into the inflamed papillary dermis, where they are referred to as **colloid** or **Civatte bodies.** Although this destructive relationship between lymphocytes and epidermal cells bears some similarities to that in erythema multiforme (discussed previously), lichen planus shows changes of chronicity, namely, epidermal hyperplasia (or rarely atrophy) and thickening of the granular cell layer and stratum corneum (hypergranulosis and hyperkeratosis, respectively). Lichen planus preferentially affecting the epithelium of hair follicles is referred to as **lichen planopilaris.**

The precise pathogenesis of lichen planus is not known. It is plausible that release of antigens at the levels of the basal cell layer and the dermoepidermal junction may elicit a cell-mediated immune response in lichen planus. Supporting this notion are data indicating that infiltrates of primarily T lymphocytes associated with hyperplasia of Langerhans cells are fundamental to lesion formation and evolution.[56]

Lupus Erythematosus

The manifestations of systemic lupus erythematosus (SLE) are described in detail in Chapter 7. However, a localized, cutaneous form of lupus erythematosus, with no associated systemic manifestations, occurs and is called *discoid lupus erythematosus (DLE).* Patients who present with DLE usually do not go on to develop systemic disease. However, more than one third of patients with SLE may exhibit, during their course, lesions that are clinically and histologically indistinguishable from those of the discoid type. Thus, it is often impossible to distinguish patients with SLE from those with DLE on the basis of clinical and histologic inspection of skin lesions alone.

Cutaneous lesions usually consist of either poorly defined malar erythema (usually seen in systemic disease) or large, sharply demarcated erythematous scaling plaques (Fig. 27–31*A*). These "discoid" plaques may occur in either pure cutaneous lupus erythematosus or SLE. Cutaneous manifestations of lupus erythematosus may develop or worsen with sun exposure. The epidermal surface of lesions is shiny or scaly, and lateral compression often produces wrinkling, a sign of epidermal atrophy. Through this thinned epidermis, dilated and tortuous blood vessels (telangiectasia) and small zones of hypopigmentation and hyperpigmentation may be seen. Small, keratotic plugs in follicular ostia may be appreciated with a hand lens.

MORPHOLOGY. Lesions of DLE are characterized histologically by an infiltrate of lymphocytes along the dermoepidermal or the dermal-follicular epithelial junction, or both (Fig. 27–31*B*). Deep perivascular and periappendageal (e.g., around sweat glands) infiltrates are also observed, and

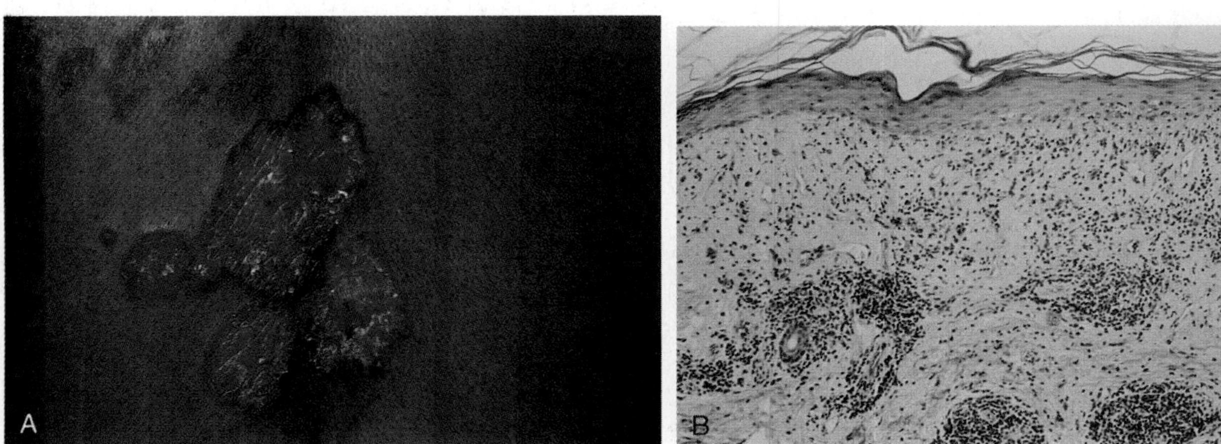

Figure 27–31

Lupus erythematosus. *A,* Discoid plaques show erythema and excessive scale. The histology of a biopsy specimen taken from the center of such a plaque is depicted in *B. B,* There is an infiltrate of lymphocytes within the superficial and deep dermis, marked thinning of the epidermis with loss of normal rete ridges, and hyperkeratosis. (From Murphy GF, Herzberg AJ: Atlas of Dermatopathology. Philadelphia, WB Saunders, 1996, pp 74 and 75.)

Figure 27–32

Granular deposits of immunoglobulin (here IgG) and complement at the dermoepidermal junction constitute a positive "band test" in lupus erythematosus. (From Murphy GF, Herzberg AJ: Atlas of Dermatopathology. Philadelphia, WB Saunders, 1996, p 27.)

preferential infiltration of subcutaneous fat is called **lupus profundus.** The basal cell layer generally shows diffuse vacuolization. The epidermal layer is markedly thinned or atrophied, with loss of the normal rete ridge pattern. Variable hyperkeratosis is present on the epidermal surface. Involved hair follicles may also show epithelial atrophy, and their infundibula are frequently dilated and plugged with keratin. Periodic acid–Schiff (PAS) stain of established lesions reveals marked thickening of the epidermal basement membrane zone, and **direct immunofluorescence shows a characteristic granular band of immunoglobulin and complement along the dermoepidermal and dermal-follicular junctions (so-called lupus band test**[57]) (Fig. 27–32). Such bands are typically seen in lesional skin but not normal skin in DLE and in both lesional and normal skin in many cases of SLE.

The immunopathogenesis of lupus erythematosus is discussed in Chapter 7. In the skin, it is believed that both humoral and cell-mediated mechanisms collaborate to result in destruction of pigment-containing basal cells. Humoral mechanisms of injury may involve both formation and deposition of immune complexes and components C5b to C9 ("membrane attack complex")[58] at the dermoepithelial junction.

BLISTERING (BULLOUS) DISEASES

Although vesicles and bullae (blisters) occur as a secondary phenomenon in a number of unrelated conditions (e.g., herpesvirus infection, spongiotic dermatitis, erythema multiforme, and thermal burns), there exists a group of disorders in which blisters are the primary and most distinctive features. These bullous diseases, as they are called, produce visually dramatic clinical lesions and in some instances (e.g., pemphigus vulgaris) are uniformly fatal if untreated. Blisters can occur at multiple levels within the skin (Fig. 27–33), and assessment of these levels is essential to formulating an accurate histologic diagnosis.

Pemphigus

Pemphigus is an autoimmune blistering disorder resulting from loss of the integrity of normal intercellular attachments within the epidermis and mucosal epithelium.[59] Although rare, its clinical consequences without treatment

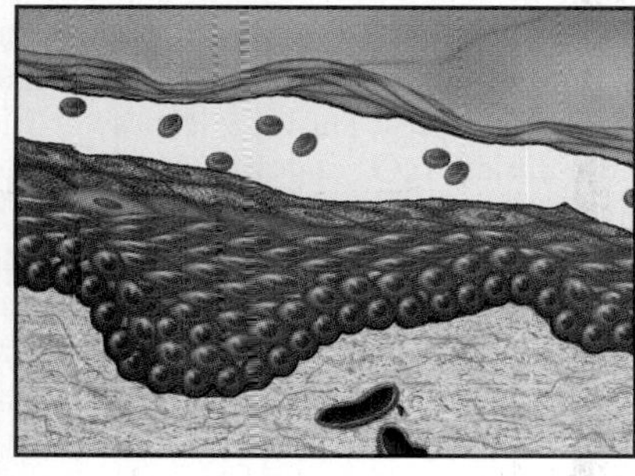

A Subcorneal

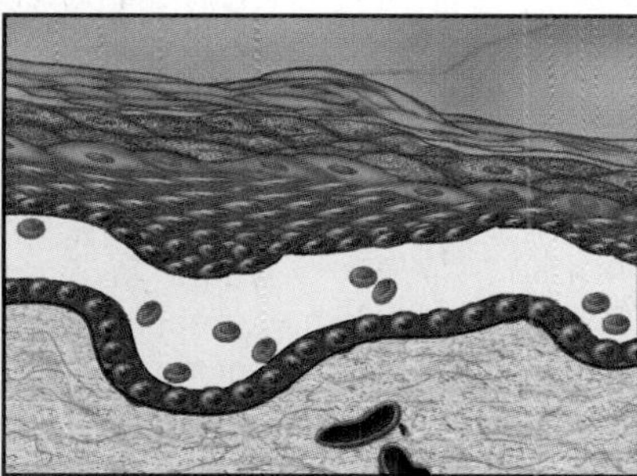

B Suprabasal

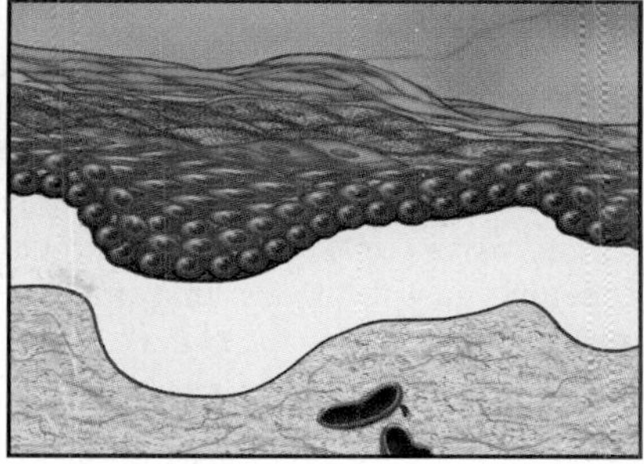

C Subepidermal

Figure 27–33

Schematic representation of sites of blister formation. *A*, In a subcorneal blister, the stratum corneum forms the roof of the bulla (as in impetigo or pemphigus foliaceus). *B*, In a suprabasal blister, a portion of the epidermis including the stratum corneum forms the roof (as in pemphigus vulgaris). *C*, In a subepidermal blister, the entire epidermis separates from the dermis (as in bullous pemphigoid and dermatitis herpetiformis).

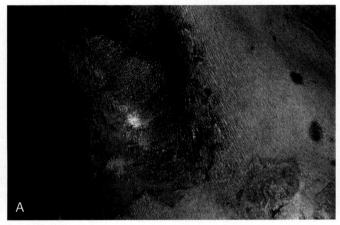

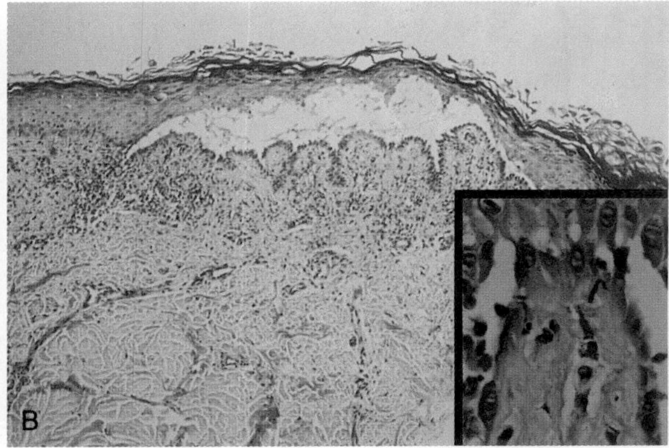

Figure 27–34

Pemphigus vulgaris. *A*, Eroded plaques are formed on rupture of confluent, thin-roofed bullae, here affecting axillary skin. *B*, Suprabasal acantholysis results in an intraepidermal blister in which rounded (acantholytic) epidermal cells are identified *(inset)*. (*A* from Murphy GF, Herzberg AJ: Atlas of Dermatopathology. Philadelphia, WB Saunders, 1996, p 63.)

may be life-threatening, and its pathobiology provides important insight into molecular mechanisms of keratinocyte adhesion. The majority of individuals who develop pemphigus are in the fourth to sixth decades of life, and men and women are affected equally. There are four clinical and pathologic variants: (1) pemphigus vulgaris, (2) pemphigus vegetans, (3) pemphigus foliaceus, and (4) pemphigus erythematosus.

Pemphigus vulgaris, by far the most common type (accounting for more than 80% of cases worldwide), involves mucosa and skin, especially on the scalp, face, axilla, groin, trunk, and points of pressure. It may present as oral ulcers that persist sometimes for months before skin involvement appears. Primary lesions are superficial vesicles and bullae that rupture easily, leaving shallow erosions covered with dried serum and crust (Fig. 27–34*A*). *Pemphigus vegetans* is a rare form that usually presents not with blisters but with large, moist, verrucous (wartlike), vegetating plaques studded with pustules on the groin, axilla, and flexural surfaces. *Pemphigus foliaceus* is a more benign form of pemphigus that occurs in an epidemic form in South America as well as in isolated cases in other countries. Sites of predilection are the scalp, face, chest, and back, and the mucous membranes are only rarely affected. Bullae are so superficial that only zones of erythema and crusting, sites of previous blister rupture, are usually present on physical examination. *Pemphigus erythematosus* is considered to be a localized, less severe form of pemphigus foliaceus that may selectively involve the malar area of the face in a lupus erythematosus–like fashion.

MORPHOLOGY. The common denominator, histologically, in all forms of pemphigus is **acantholysis.** This term implies dissolution, or lysis, of the intercellular adhesion sites within a squamous epithelial surface. Acantholytic cells that are no longer attached to other epithelial cells lose their polyhedral shape and characteristically become rounded. In pemphigus vulgaris and pemphigus vegetans, acantholysis selectively involves the layer of cells immediately above the basal cell layer. (The vegetans variant has considerable overlying epidermal hyperplasia.) The **suprabasal acantholytic blister** that forms is characteristic of pemphigus vulgaris (Fig. 27–34*B*). The single layer of intact basal cells that forms the blister base has been likened to a row of "tombstones." In pemphigus foliaceus, a blister forms by similar mechanisms but, unlike the case with pemphigus vulgaris, selectively involves the superficial epidermis at the level of the stratum granulosum. Variable superficial dermal infiltration by lymphocytes, histiocytes, and eosinophils accompanies all forms of pemphigus.

Sera from patients with pemphigus contain antibodies (IgG) to intercellular cement substance of skin and mucous membranes.[60] This phenomenon is the basis for direct and indirect diagnostic immunofluorescence testing of skin and serum, respectively. Lesional sites show a characteristic netlike pattern of intercellular IgG deposits localized to sites of developed or incipient acantholysis (Fig. 27–35). It is now known that the pemphigus antibody reacts with the desmoglein 3 molecules, a component of the desmosomes that appear to bind keratinocytes together. When the gene for desmoglein 3 is disrupted in genetically engineered mice, suprabasal blisters akin to pemphigus develop owing to lack of desmosome adhesion (Fig. 27–36). This suggests a direct role for pemphigus autoantibodies in interfering with the function of this protein.[61] Some of the acantholytic process may also be the consequence of synthesis and liberation of a serine protease, plasminogen activator, by epidermal cells, an event that is triggered by the pemphigus antibody.[62,63]

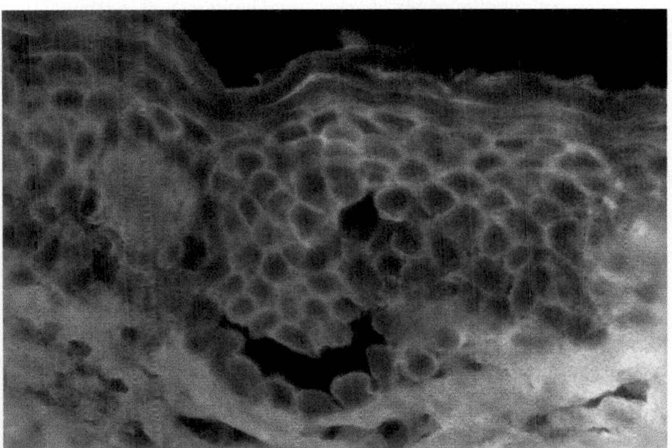

Figure 27–35 ■

Direct immunofluorescence of pemphigus vulgaris. There is deposition of immunoglobulin along the plasma membranes of epidermal keratinocytes in a fishnet-like pattern. Also note the early suprabasal separation due to loss of cell-cell adhesion (acantholysis).

Bullous Pemphigoid

Originally considered to be a form of pemphigus, bullous pemphigoid has been recognized for almost the last four decades as a distinct and relatively common autoimmune, vesiculobullous disease. Generally affecting elderly individuals, bullous pemphigoid shows a wide range of clinical presentations, with localized to generalized cutaneous lesions and involvement of mucosal surfaces.

Clinically, lesions are tense bullae, filled with clear fluid, on normal or erythematous skin (Fig. 27–37*A*). The size may reach 4 to 8 cm in diameter. The bullae do not rupture as easily as do the blisters seen in pemphigus and, if uncomplicated by infection, heal without scarring. Sites of occurrence include the inner aspects of the thighs, flexor surfaces of the forearms, axillae, groin, and lower abdomen. Oral involvement is present in up to one third of patients, usually after the development of cutaneous lesions. Some patients may present with urticarial plaques, with extreme associated pruritus.

MORPHOLOGY. The separation of bullous pemphigoid from pemphigus, establishing the former as a distinctive entity, was based on the seminal observation that pemphigoid resulted from a **subepidermal, nonacantholytic** blister.[64] Early lesions show a superficial and sometimes deep perivascular infiltrate of lymphocytes and variable numbers of eosinophils, occasional neutrophils, superficial dermal edema, and associated basal cell layer vacuolization (Fig. 27–37*B*). The vacuolated basal cell layer eventually gives rise to a fluid-filled blister.

In bullous pemphigoid[65] there is *linear* basement membrane zone deposition of immunoglobulin and complement (Fig. 27–38*A*) (recall that the pattern for lupus erythematosus is similar, but granular in character). Ultrastructural studies have shown that circulating antibody reacts with antigen present in the basal cell–basement membrane attachment plaques (hemidesmosomes) (Fig. 27–38*B*). The actual blister develops at the level of a narrow clear zone (lamina lucida) of the epidermal basement membrane that separates the underlying lamina densa from the plasma membrane of the basal cells. The antigens present at these sites have been named bullous pemphigoid antigens 1 and 2, and they are now recognized as normal constituents of the hemidesmosomes that bind basal cells at the dermoepidermal junction. In bullous pemphigoid, it is likely that the generation of autoantibodies to these basement membrane components results in the fixation of complement and sub-

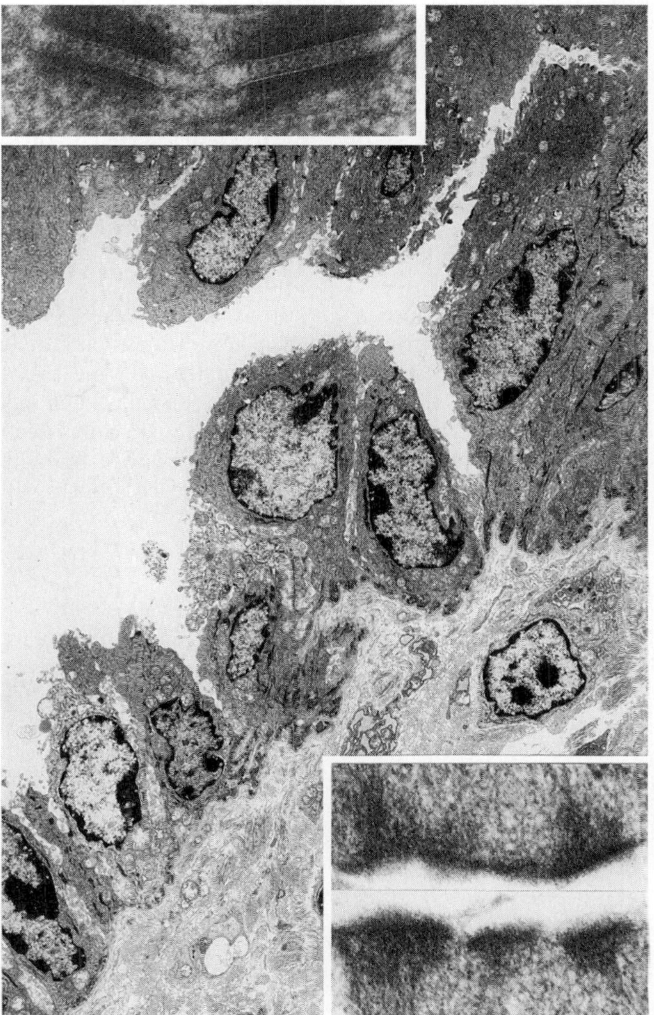

Figure 27–36 ■

Electron microscopy of pemphigus vulgaris–like acantholysis in a mouse with targeted disruption of desmoglein 3 gene. There is a blister forming directly above an intact basal cell layer. Unlike normal desmosomes that bind together plasma membranes of adjacent keratinocytes *(inset, upper left)*, desmosomes in the region of the forming blister in the desmoglein 3–deficient mouse are separated *(inset, lower right)*.

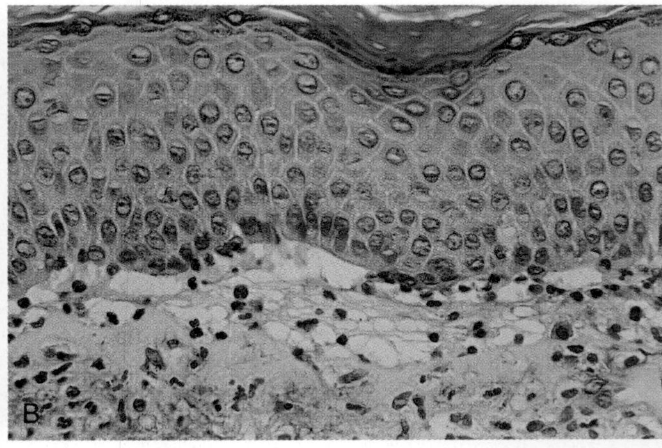

Figure 27–37

Bullous pemphigoid. Clinical bullae *(A)* result from basal cell layer vacuolization, producing a subepidermal blister *(B)*. Eosinophils, as well as lymphocytes and occasional neutrophils, may be intimately associated with basal cell layer destruction, creating a subepidermal cleft.

sequent tissue injury at this site through locally recruited neutrophils[66] and eosinophils.

Dermatitis Herpetiformis

Dermatitis herpetiformis[67] is a rare and fascinating entity characterized by urticaria and vesicles. Males tend to be affected more frequently than are females, and the age at onset is often in the third and fourth decades, although disease has been known to develop at any age after weaning. A major association is with celiac disease (Chapter 18); both the vesicular dermatosis and the enteropathy respond to a diet free of gluten (see later).

The urticarial plaques and vesicles of dermatitis herpetiformis are extremely pruritic. They characteristically occur bilaterally and symmetrically, involving preferentially the extensor surfaces, elbows, knees, upper back, and buttocks. Vesicles are frequently grouped, as are those of true herpesvirus, and hence the name herpetiform (Fig. 27–39*A*).

MORPHOLOGY. The early lesions of dermatitis herpetiformis are histologically characteristic. Fibrin and neutrophils accumulate selectively at the **tips of dermal papillae,** forming small "microabscesses" (Fig. 27–39*B*). The basal cells overlying these microabscesses show vacuolization, and minute zones of dermoepidermal separation (microscopic blisters) may occur at the tips of in-

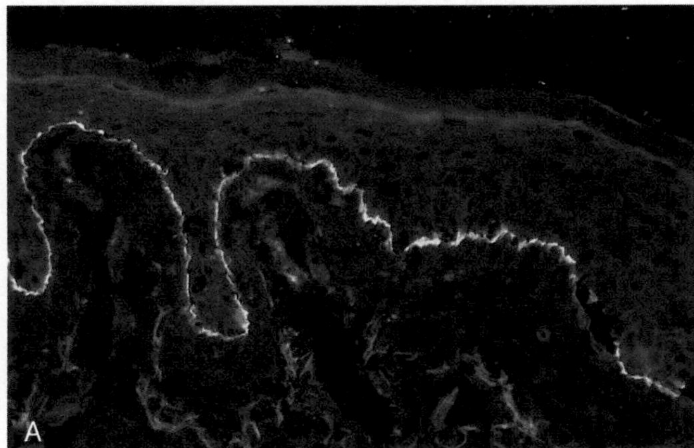

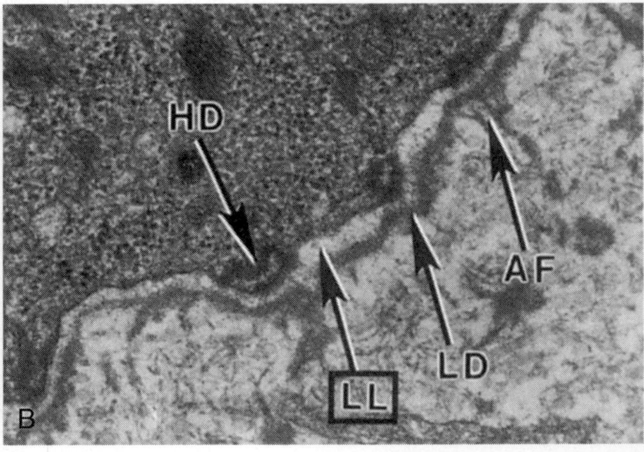

Figure 27–38

A, Linear deposition of complement along the dermal-epidermal junction in bullous pemphigoid; the pattern has been likened to "ribbon candy." *B*, Bullous pemphigoid antigen is located in the lowermost portion of the basal cell cytoplasm in association with hemidesmosomes (HD), with blister formation affecting the lamina lucida (LL) of the basement membrane zone. LD, lamina densa; AF, anchoring fibrils.

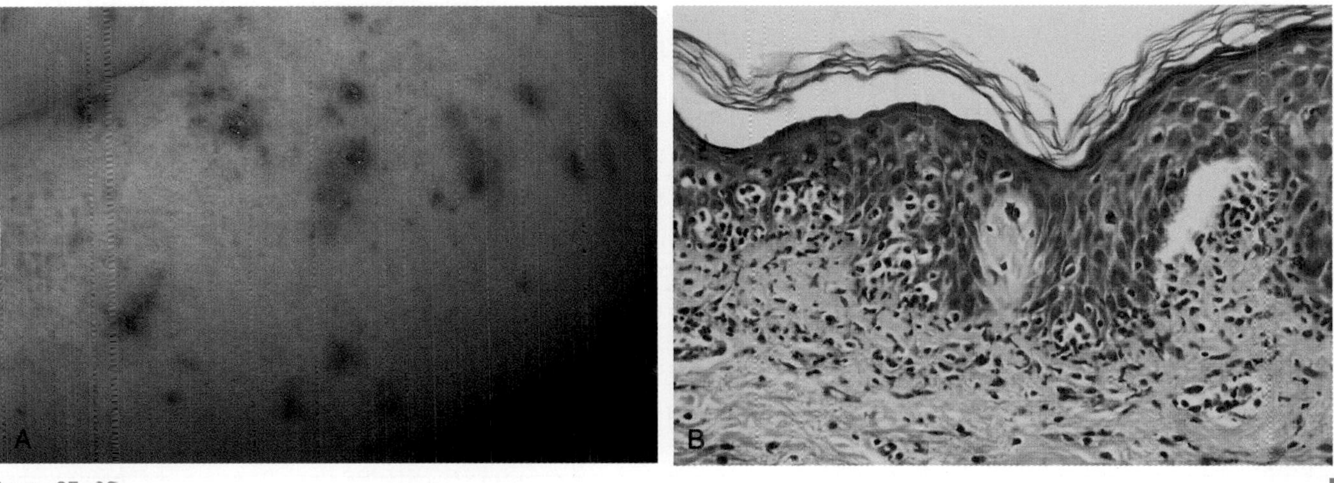

Figure 27–39

Dermatitis herpetiformis. *A*, Clinical lesions consist of intact and eroded erythematous blisters that are often grouped together. *B*, Histologically, neutrophilic microabscesses selectively involve the dermal papilla.

volved papillae (Fig. 27–40*A*). In time, these zones coalesce to form a true subepidermal blister. Eosinophils may occur in the infiltrates of older lesions, creating confusion with the histologic picture of bullous pemphigoid. Attention to the early alterations at the blister edge, however, usually allows separation of these two disorders. By direct immunofluorescence, dermatitis herpetiformis shows granular deposits of **IgA** selectively localized in the tips of dermal papillae, where they are deposited on anchoring fibrils (Fig. 27–40*B*).

Gluten is the protein moiety that persists subsequent to the removal of water and starch from defatted flour. Gliadin is a class of protein found in the gluten fraction of flour. Patients with dermatitis herpetiformis may develop antibodies of the IgA and IgG classes to gliadin and reticulin, a component of the anchoring fibrils that tether the epidermal basement membrane to the superficial dermis. In addition, individuals with certain histocompatibility types (HLA-B8 and HLA-DRw3) are particularly prone to this disease. It is thus thought that genetically predisposed persons may develop IgA antibodies in the gut to components of dietary gluten and that these antibodies (or immune complexes) then cross-react or are deposited in the dermal papillae of the skin, resulting in clinical disease. Some individuals with dermatitis herpetiformis and enteropathy respond to a gluten-free diet (as with celiac disease).[68]

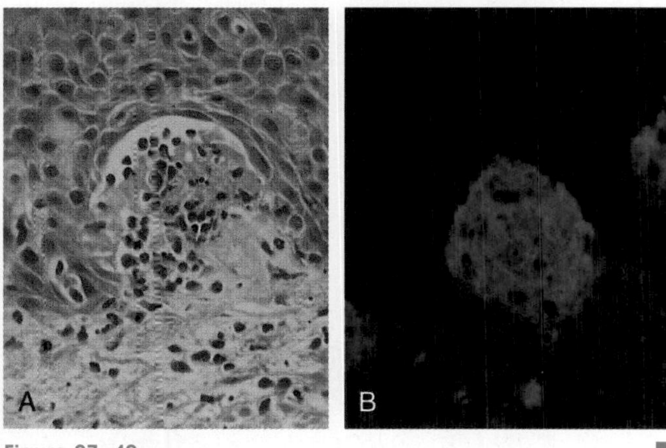

Figure 27–40

Dermatitis herpetiformis. *A*, Papillary dermal microabscesses are associated with zones of dermal-epidermal cleavage that eventually coalesce to form a clinical blister. *B*, By direct immunofluorescence, these abscesses are rich in IgA and fibrin deposits.

Noninflammatory Blistering Diseases: Epidermolysis Bullosa, Porphyria

To this point, we have discussed inflammatory blistering diseases. However, some primary disorders characterized by vesicles and bullae are not mediated by inflammatory mechanisms. Two such diseases are *epidermolysis bullosa* and *porphyria.*

Epidermolysis bullosa constitutes a group of disorders unified by the common link of blisters that develop at sites of pressure, rubbing, or trauma, at or soon after birth. The different types of epidermolysis bullosa, however, are likely to be unrelated with regard to pathogenesis. In the *simplex type,* for example, degeneration of the basal cell layer of the epidermis results in clinical bullae. In the *junctional type,* blisters occur in otherwise histologically normal skin at precisely the level of the lamina lucida (Fig. 27–41). In the scarring *dystrophic types,* blisters develop beneath the lamina densa, presumably in association with rudimentary or defective anchoring fibrils. The histologic changes are so subtle that electron microscopy may be required to differentiate among these types in clinically ambiguous settings.

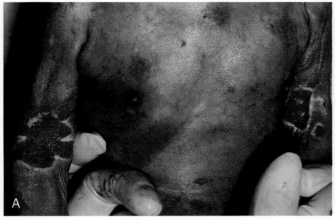

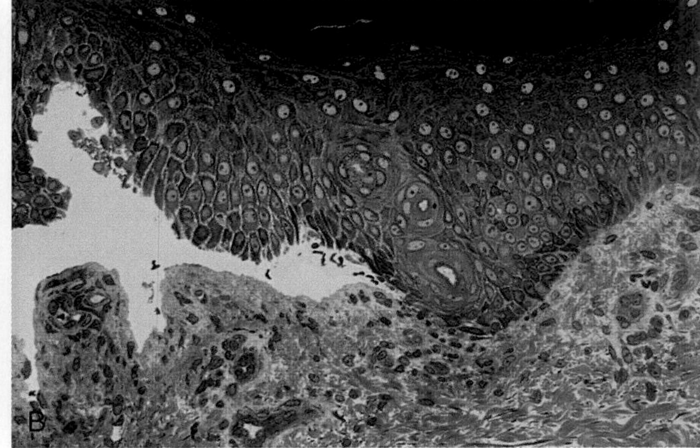

Figure 27–41

Epidermolysis bullosa. *A*, Junctional epidermolysis bullosa showing typical erosions in flexural creases. *B*, A noninflammatory subepidermal blister in this case has formed at the level of the lamina lucida. (*A* from Murphy GF, Herzberg AJ: Atlas of Dermatopathology. Philadelphia, WB Saunders, 1996, p 67.)

Porphyria refers to a group of uncommon inborn or acquired disturbances of porphyrin metabolism. Porphyrins are pigments normally present in hemoglobin, myoglobin, and cytochromes. The classification of porphyrias is based on both clinical and biochemical features. The five major types are (1) congenital erythropoietic porphyria, (2) erythrohepatic protoporphyria, (3) acute intermittent porphyria, (4) porphyria cutanea tarda, and (5) mixed porphyria. Cutaneous manifestations consist of urticaria and vesicles that heal with scarring and that are exacerbated by exposure to sunlight. The primary alterations by light microscopy are a *subepidermal vesicle* (Fig. 27–42A) *with associated marked thickening of superficial dermal vessels.* The pathogenesis of these alterations is not well understood, although serum proteins, including immunoglobulins, typically form glassy deposits in the walls of superficial dermal microvessels.

DISORDERS OF EPIDERMAL APPENDAGES

Acne Vulgaris

Virtually universal in the middle to late teenage years, acne vulgaris affects both males and females, although males tend to have more severe disease. Acne is seen in all races, but it is said to be milder in people of Asian descent. Acne vulgaris in adolescents is believed to occur as a result of physiologic hormonal variations and alterations in hair follicle maturation. The clinical features of acne may be induced or exacerbated by drugs (corticosteroids, adrenocorticotropic hormone, testosterone, gonadotropins, contraceptives, trimethadione, iodides, and bromides), occupational contactants (cutting oils, chlorinated hydrocarbons, and coal tars), and occlusive conditions such as heavy clothing and tropical climates. Some families seem to be particularly affected by acne, suggesting a heritable factor.

Acne is divided into noninflammatory and inflammatory types, although both may coexist. The former consists of open and closed comedones. *Open comedones* consist of small follicular papules containing a central black keratin plug. This color is the result of oxidation of melanin pigment (not dirt). *Closed comedones* are follicular papules without a visible central plug. Because the keratin plug is trapped beneath the epidermal surface, these lesions are potential sources of follicular rupture and inflammation. Inflammatory acne is characterized by erythematous pap-

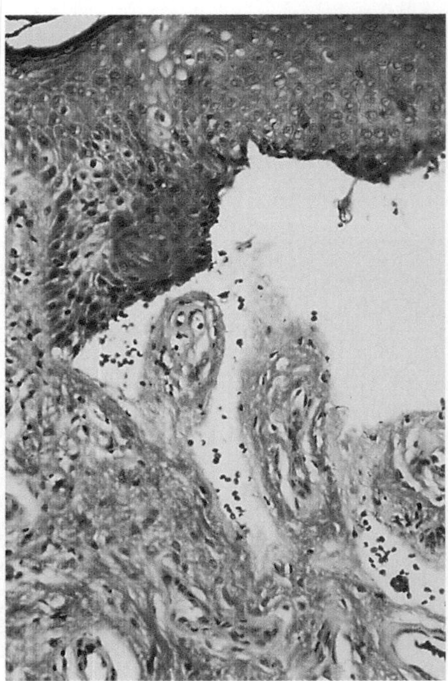

Figure 27–42

Porphyria. A noninflammatory blister is forming at the dermal-epidermal junction; note the seemingly rigid dermal papillae at the base that contain the altered superficial vessels.

ules, nodules, and pustules (Fig. 27–43*A*). Severe variants (e.g., acne conglobata) result in sinus tract formation and physical scarring, in addition to the emotional scars.

MORPHOLOGY. On histologic examination, comedones form as an expanding mass of lipid (sebum) and keratin within the midportion of the hair follicle. With gradual expansion, the follicle becomes dilated and the follicular epithelium and sebaceous glands atrophy. Resultant open comedones have large, patulous orifices, whereas those of closed comedones are identifiable only microscopically. Variable lymphohistiocytic infiltrates are present in and around affected follicles, and extensive acute and chronic inflammation accompanies follicular rupture. Dermal abscesses may form in association with rupture (Figs. 27–43*B*), and gradual resolution, often with scarring, ensues.

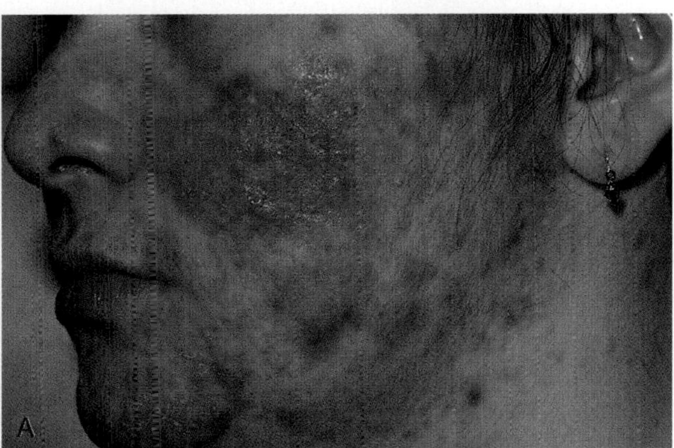

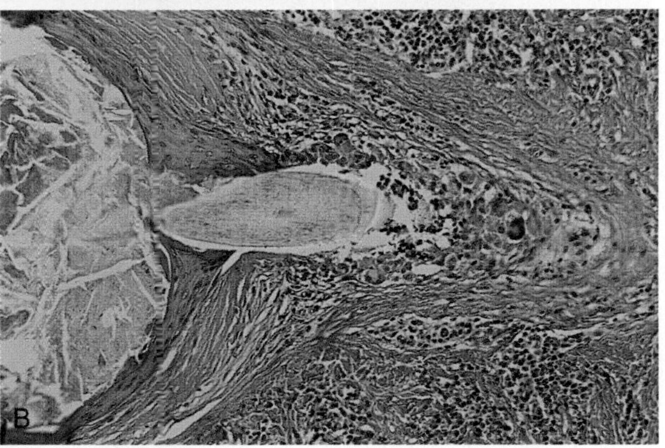

Figure 27–43 ■

Acne. *A*, Inflammatory acne is characterized clinically by erythematous papules and pustules, with the possibility of eventual scarring. *B*, A portion of a hair shaft piercing the follicular epithelium and eliciting an inflammatory response and fibrosis.

The pathogenesis of acne is incompletely understood. Endocrine factors have been implicated (especially androgens) because castrated persons never develop the condition. However, these do not appear to be the sole or primary cause.[69] It has been postulated that bacterial lipases of *Propionibacterium acnes* break down sebaceous oils, liberating highly irritating fatty acids resulting in the earliest inflammatory phases of acne.[70] Inhibition of lipase production is a rationale for administration of antibiotics to patients with inflammatory acne.[71] The synthetic vitamin A derivative 13-*cis*-retinoic acid (isotretinoin) has brought about remarkable clinical improvement in some cases of severe acne.[72]

PANNICULITIS

Erythema Nodosum and Erythema Induratum

Panniculitis is an inflammatory reaction in the subcutaneous fat that may affect (1) principally the connective tissue septa separating lobules of fat or (2) predominantly the lobules of fat themselves. *Erythema nodosum* is the most common form of panniculitis and usually has an acute presentation. Its occurrence is often associated with infections (β-hemolytic streptococcal infection, tuberculosis, and, less commonly, coccidioidomycosis, histoplasmosis, and leprosy), drug administration (sulfonamides, oral contraceptives), sarcoidosis, inflammatory bowel disease, and certain malignant neoplasms, but many times a cause cannot be elicited. Many types of panniculitis have a subacute to chronic course.

Panniculitis often involves the lower legs. Erythema nodosum presents as poorly defined, exquisitely tender, erythematous nodules that may be better felt than seen. Fever and malaise may accompany the cutaneous signs. During the course of weeks, lesions usually flatten and become bruiselike, leaving no residual clinical scars, while new lesions develop. Biopsy of a deep wedge of tissue is usually required to establish a definitive diagnosis.

Erythema induratum is an uncommon type of panniculitis that affects primarily adolescents and menopausal women. Although the cause is not known, most observers today regard this disorder as the result of a primary vasculitis affecting deep vessels supplying lobules of the subcutis, with subsequent necrosis and inflammation within the fat. Erythema induratum presents as an erythematous, slightly tender nodule that usually goes on to ulcerate. Originally considered a hypersensitivity response to tuberculosis, erythema induratum today most commonly occurs without an associated underlying disease.

MORPHOLOGY. The histopathology of erythema nodosum is distinctive. In early lesions, widening of the connective tissue **septa** is due to edema, fibrin exudation, and neutrophilic infiltration. Later, infiltration by lymphocytes, histiocytes, multinucleated giant cells, and occasional eosinophils is associated with septal fibrosis. Vasculitis is not present. In erythema induratum, on the other hand, the fat **lobule** is involved by granulomatous inflammation and zones of caseous necrosis. Early lesions show necrotizing vasculitis affecting small to medium-sized arteries and veins in the deep dermis and subcutis.

Erythema nodosum and erythema induratum are but two examples of many types of panniculitis. *Weber-Christian disease (relapsing febrile nodular panniculitis)* is a rare form of lobular, nonvasculitic panniculitis seen in children and adults. It is marked by crops of erythematous plaques or nodules, predominantly on the lower extremities, created by deep-seated foci of inflammation with aggregates of foamy histiocytes admixed with lymphocytes, neutrophils, and giant cells. *Factitial panniculitis,* as a result of self-inflicted trauma or injection of foreign or toxic substances, is a form of secondary panniculitis that often poses profound problems in definitive clinical and pathologic diagnosis and may present a distinct set of therapeutic challenges. Deep mycotic infections in immunocompromised individuals may produce histologic changes that mimic primary panniculitis. Finally, disorders such as lupus erythematosus (see earlier) may occasionally have deep inflammatory components with associated panniculitis.

INFECTION AND INFESTATION

Although the skin is a protective organ, it frequently succumbs to the attack of microorganisms, parasites, and insects. We have already discussed the possible role of bacteria in the pathogenesis of common acne, and the dermatoses resulting from viruses are too numerous to list. In the setting of the immunocompromised patient, ordinarily trivial cutaneous infections may be life-threatening.

Many disorders, such as herpes simplex and herpes zoster, the viral exanthems, and deep fungal infections, are discussed in Chapter 9. In addition, immune reactions in skin provoked by infectious agents, such as the annular erythema termed erythema chronicum migrans, a harbinger of Lyme disease, are also discussed in Chapter 9. Here we address a representative sampling of common infections and infestations whose primary clinical manifestations are in the skin.

Verrucae (Warts)

Verrucae are common lesions of children and adolescents, although they may be encountered at any age. They are caused by human papillomaviruses. Transmission of disease usually involves direct contact between individuals or autoinoculation. Verrucae are generally self-limited, regressing spontaneously within 6 months to 2 years.

The classification of verrucae is based largely on clinical morphology and location. *Verruca vulgaris* is the most common type of wart. These lesions occur anywhere but most frequently on the hands, particularly on the dorsal surfaces and periungual areas, where they appear as gray-

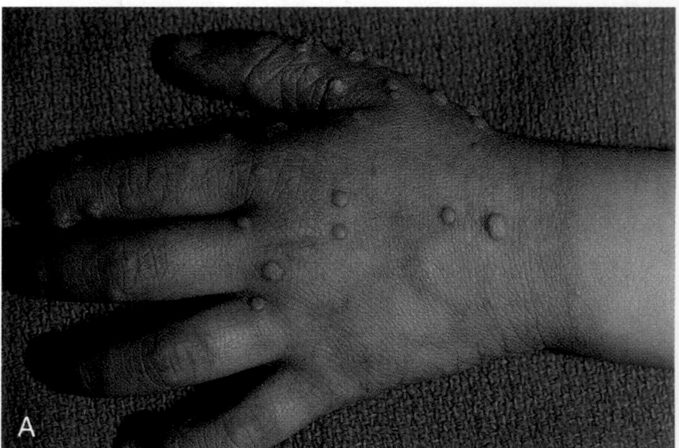

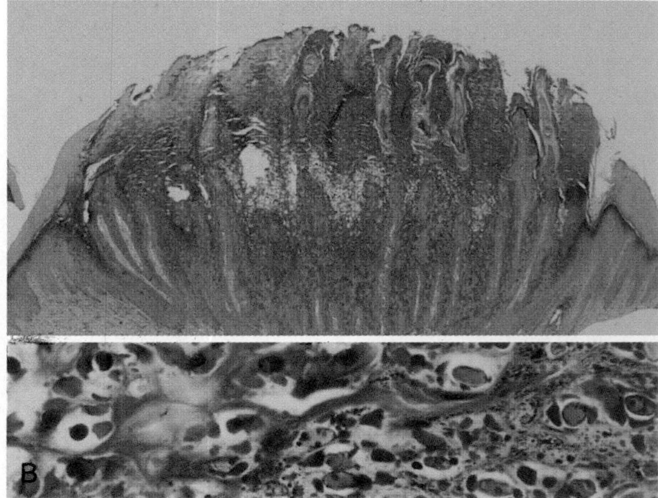

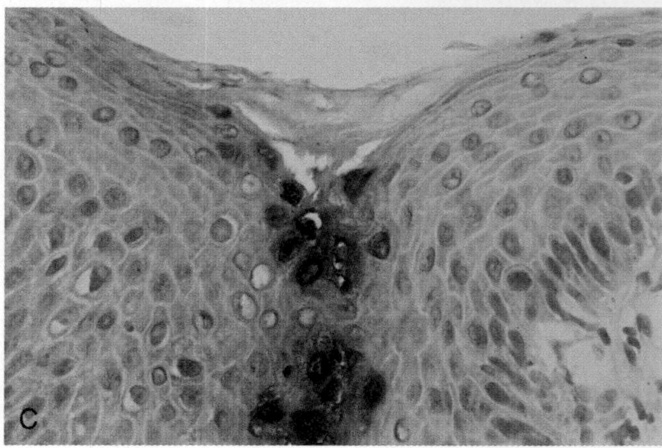

Figure 27–44

Verruca vulgaris. *A*, Multiple papules with rough, pebble-like surfaces are present. *B*, Histologically, such lesions show papillomatous epidermal hyperplasia and cytopathic alterations that include nuclear pallor and prominent keratohyaline granules *(inset panel at bottom)*. *C*, In situ hybridization reveals sites of viral DNA within infected epidermal cells.

white to tan, flat to convex, 0.1- to 1-cm papules with a rough, pebble-like surface (Fig. 27–44*A*). *Verruca plana,* or *flat wart,* is common on the face or the dorsal surfaces of the hands. These warts are slightly elevated, flat, smooth, tan papules that are generally smaller than verruca vulgaris. *Verruca plantaris* and *verruca palmaris* occur on the soles and palms, respectively. Rough, scaly lesions may reach 1 to 2 cm in diameter, coalesce, and be confused with ordinary calluses. *Condyloma acuminatum (venereal wart)* occurs on the penis, female genitalia, urethra, perianal areas, and rectum. These lesions appear as soft, tan, cauliflower-like masses that in occasional cases reach many centimeters in diameter.

MORPHOLOGY. Histologic features common to verrucae include epidermal hyperplasia that is often undulant in character (so-called verrucous or papillomatous epidermal hyperplasia; Fig. 27–44*B*) and cytoplasmic vacuolization (koilocytosis) that preferentially involves the more superficial epidermal layers, producing halos of pallor surrounding infected nuclei. Electron microscopy of these zones reveals numerous viral particles within nuclei. Infected cells may also demonstrate prominent and apparently condensed keratohyaline granules and jagged eosinophilic intracytoplasmic keratin aggregates as a result of viral cytopathic effects. These cellular alterations are not as prominent in condylomas; hence, their diagnosis is based primarily on hyperplastic papillary architecture containing wedge-shaped zones of koilocytosis.

It is now recognized that the clinically different types of warts just described result not solely because of the anatomically different sites in which they arise but also as a consequence of distinct types of human papillomavirus. More than 49 types of papillomavirus that can produce warts in humans have been identified in studies using molecular hybridization (Fig. 27–44*C*) and restriction enzyme analyses. For example, anogenital warts are caused predominantly by papillomavirus types 6 and 11. In contrast, there is a tendency for lesions induced by type 16 to show some degree of associated dysplasia.[73] Moreover, type 16 has also been associated with in situ squamous cell carcinoma of the genitalia and with *bowenoid papulosis* (genital lesions of young adults with the histology of in situ carcinoma but with a biologic course of spontaneous regression).[74] These findings are consonant with previous observations of the association of types 16 and 18 with carcinomas of the uterine cervix[75] (Chapter 24). The potential relationship of papillomavirus to carcinoma is reinforced by the rare heritable condition termed *epidermodysplasia verruciformis.* In this disorder, patients develop multiple flat warts, some of which evolve to become invasive squamous cell carcinomas. The genomes of papillomavirus types 5 and 8 have been detected in some of these cutaneous tumors.[76] Thus, the types of papillomavirus differ not only in the morphology of the lesions they produce but also in their oncogenic potential (Chapter 8).

Molluscum Contagiosum

Molluscum contagiosum is a common, self-limited viral disease of the skin caused by a poxvirus. The virus is characteristically brick shaped, has a dumbbell-shaped DNA core, and measures 300 nm in maximal dimension. Infection is usually spread by direct contact, particularly among children and young adults.

Clinically, multiple lesions may occur on the skin and mucous membranes, with a predilection for the trunk and anogenital areas. Individual lesions are firm, often pruritic, pink to skin-colored umbilicated papules generally ranging in diameter from 0.2 to 0.4 cm. Rarely, "giant" forms occur measuring up to 2.0 cm in diameter. A curdlike material can be expressed from the central umbilication. Smearing this material onto a glass slide and staining with Giemsa reagent often shows diagnostic "molluscum bodies."

MORPHOLOGY. On microscopic examination, lesions show cuplike verrucous epidermal hyperplasia. The diagnostically-specific structure is the **molluscum body,** which occurs as a large (up to 35 μm), ellipsoid, homogeneous, cytoplasmic inclusion in cells of the stratum granulosum and the stratum corneum (Fig. 27–45). These inclusions are

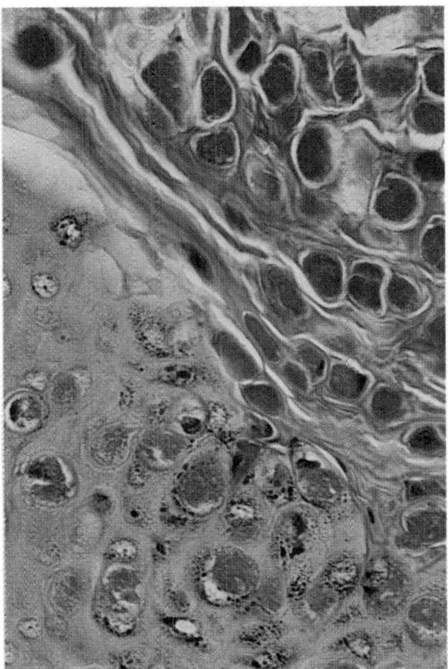

Figure 27–45

Molluscum contagiosum. A focus of verrucous epidermal hyperplasia contains numerous cells with ellipsoid cytoplasmic inclusions (molluscum bodies) within the stratum granulosum and stratum corneum.

eosinophilic in the blue-purple (on H&E stain) stratum granulosum and acquire a pale blue hue in the red stratum corneum. Numerous virions are present within molluscum bodies.

Impetigo

This common superficial infection of the skin usually caused by staphylococci or streptococci is discussed in Chapter 9. Impetigo is frequently seen in normal children as well as in adults in poor health. Cultures most frequently grow coagulase-positive staphylococci or group A β-hemolytic streptococci, or both. Nephritogenic strains of *Streptococcus* cause impetigo, particularly in tropical areas and in the southern United States.[77]

The condition usually involves exposed skin, particularly that of the face and hands. Initially it is an erythematous macule, but multiple small pustules rapidly supervene. As pustules break, shallow erosions form, covered with drying serum, giving the characteristic clinical appearance of *honey-colored crust.* If the crust is not removed, new lesions form about the periphery and extensive epidermal damage may ensue. A bullous form of impetigo occurs in children.

MORPHOLOGY. The characteristic microscopic feature of impetigo is accumulation of neutrophils beneath the stratum corneum, often with the formation of a subcorneal pustule. Special stains reveal the presence of bacteria in these foci. Nonspecific, reactive epidermal alterations and superficial dermal inflammation accompany these findings. Rupture of pustules results in superficial layering of serum, neutrophils, and cellular debris to form the characteristic crust.

Superficial Fungal Infections

As opposed to deep fungal infections, superficial fungal infections of the skin are confined to the stratum corneum, where they are caused primarily by dermatophytes. These organisms grow in the soil and on animals and produce a number of diverse and characteristic clinical lesions.

Tinea capitis usually occurs in children and is only rarely seen in infants and adults. It is a dermatophytosis of the scalp characterized by asymptomatic, often hairless patches of skin associated with mild erythema, crust formation, and scale. *Tinea barbae* is a dermatophyte infection of the beard area that affects adult men; it is a relatively uncommon disorder. *Tinea corporis,* on the other hand, is a common superficial fungal infection of the body surface that affects persons of all ages, but particularly children. Predisposing factors include excessive heat and humidity, exposure to infected animals, and chronic dermatophytosis of the feet or nails. The most common type of tinea corporis is an expanding, round, slightly erythematous plaque with an elevated scaling border (Fig. 27–46*A*). *Tinea cruris* occurs most frequently in the inguinal areas of obese men during warm weather. Heat, friction, and maceration all predispose to its development. The infection usually first appears on the upper inner thighs, with gradual extension of moist, red patches that have raised, scaling borders. *Tinea pedis (athlete's foot)* affects 30% to 40% of the population at some time in their lives. There is diffuse erythema and scaling, often initially localized to the web spaces. Most of the inflammatory tissue reaction, however, has recently been shown to be the result of bacterial superinfection and not directly related to the primary dermatophytosis.[78] Spread to or primary infection of the nails is referred to as *onychomycosis.* This produces discoloration, thickening, and deformity of the nail plate. *Tinea versicolor* usually occurs on the upper trunk and is highly distinctive in appearance. Caused by *Malassezia furfur,* the lesions consist of groups of macules of all sizes, lighter or darker than surrounding skin, with a fine peripheral scale.

MORPHOLOGY. The histologic features of all dermatophytoses are variable, depending on the antigenic properties of the organism, the corresponding host response, and the degree of bacterial superinfection that occurs. It may take the form of a mild eczematous dermatitis (Fig. 27–46*B*). Fungal cell walls, rich in mucopolysaccharides, stain bright pink to red with PAS stain. They are present in the anucleate cornified layer of lesional skin, hair, or nails (Fig. 27–46*C*), and scraping of these areas and subsequent culture of organisms will usually produce colonial growth that permits definitive classification of the offending species.

Arthropod Bites, Stings, and Infestations

Arthropods are ubiquitous, and we all are susceptible to the bites, stings, and other discomforts they cause. The arthropods include Arachnida (spiders, scorpions, ticks, and mites); Insecta (lice, bedbugs, bees, wasps, fleas, flies, and mosquitoes); and Chilopoda (centipedes). All can cause skin lesions, but there is a wide variability in clinical patterns of reaction. Some persons suffer minimal symptoms, others considerable discomfort, and some may die as a consequence of a bite or sting. Arthropods can produce lesions in several ways: (1) by direct irritant effects of insect parts or secretions; (2) by immediate or delayed hypersensitivity responses (including an anaphylactic reaction) to retained or injected body parts or secretions; (3) by specific effects of venoms (e.g., the black widow spider venom produces severe cramps and excruciating pain; the brown recluse spider venom contains potent enzymes that produce tissue necrosis); and (4) by serving as vectors for secondary invaders, such as bacteria, rickettsiae, and parasites.

Macroscopically, arthropod bites may be urticarial or in-

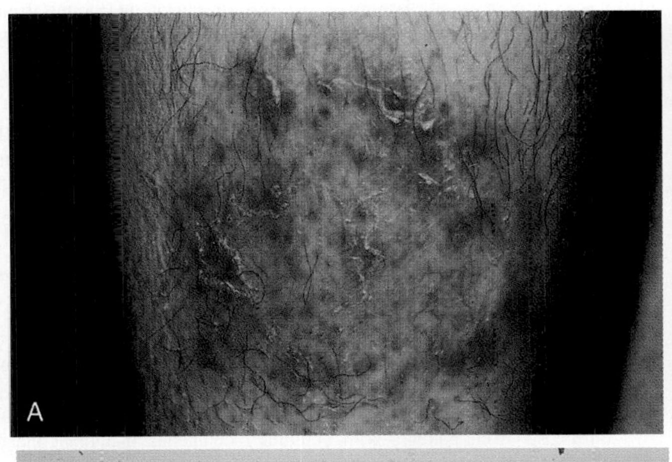

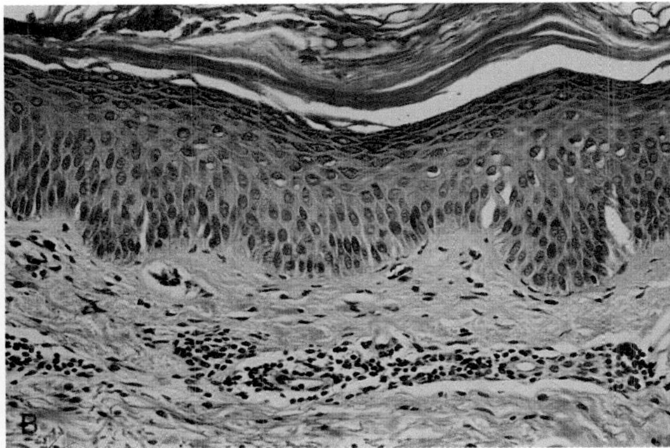

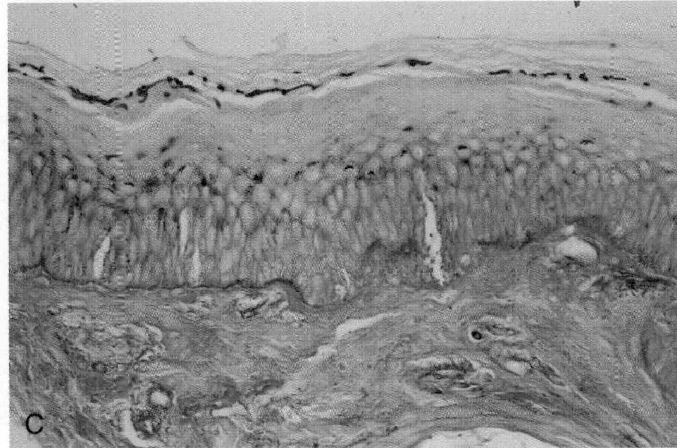

Figure 27–46

Tinea. *A*, Characteristic plaque of tinea corporis. Routine histology *(B)* shows the picture of mild eczematous (spongiotic) dermatitis, and periodic acid–Schiff stain reveals deep red hyphae and yeast forms *(C)* within the stratum corneum. (From Murphy GF, Herzberg AJ: Atlas of Dermatopathology. Philadelphia, WB Saunders, 1996, p 46.)

flamed papules and nodules, sometimes with ulceration. Individual lesions may last for several weeks. In the case of the tick bite caused by *Ixodes dammini,* the vector for the spirochete that causes Lyme disease (Chapter 9), a characteristic expanding, erythematous plaque (erythema chronicum migrans) develops. Such extensive necrosis may result from the bite of the brown recluse spider that radical surgical excision of the involved area is often necessary. *Pediculosis* is caused by the head louse, crab louse, and body louse. The disease is pruritic, and the louse, or its eggs, attached to hair shafts can usually be seen with the unaided eye (Fig. 27–47*A*). In pediculosis of the scalp, impetigo and enlarged cervical lymph nodes may be frequent complications, especially in children. The pubic

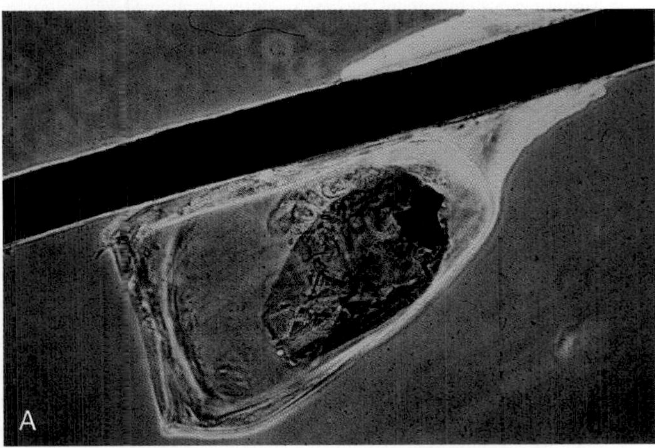

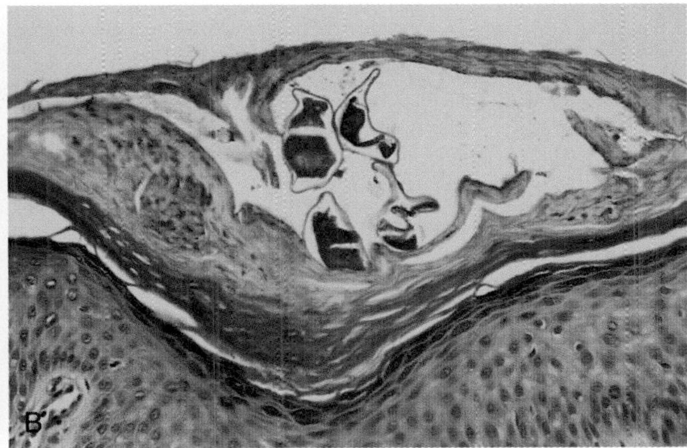

Figure 27–47

A, Pediculosis. Egg case (nit) of head louse attached to hair shaft. *B*, Portions of a scabies mite within a burrow involving the stratum corneum.

louse may be transmitted through sexual contact. Infection with the body louse ("vagabond's disease") is usually characterized by areas of hyperpigmentation and scratch marks (excoriations). *Scabies* is a contagious, pruritic dermatosis caused by the mite *Sarcoptes scabiei.* The female mite burrows under the stratum corneum (Fig. 27–47*B*), producing burrows (linear, poorly defined streaks, 0.2 to 0.6 cm in length) on the interdigital skin, palms, wrists, periareolar skin of women, and genital skin of men.

MORPHOLOGY. The histologic picture of arthropod bites is highly varied. The classic lesion shows a wedge-shaped perivascular infiltrate of lymphocytes, histiocytes, and eosinophils within the dermis. There may be a central zone of exceedingly focal epidermal necrosis, directly under which birefringent insect mouthparts may be found (the site of the bite is called the punctum). In some bites, a primarily urticarial reaction is seen histologically, whereas in others the inflammatory infiltrate is so florid and dense that it may superficially resemble a cutaneous lymphoma. Spongiosis, resulting in intraepidermal blisters, is present in some biopsy specimens, and in certain settings, insect bites even resemble bullous pemphigoid.

Careful correlation with a clinical history of exposure to insects and the clinical finding of clustered or linear lesions facilitate the clinicopathologic diagnosis.

ACKNOWLEDGMENTS: Dr. Gerald Lazarus graciously provided many of the clinical photographs. Dr. Michael Ioffreda provided original illustrations from which final versions were adapted and conceptualized. Dr. Arlene Herzberg was of invaluable assistance in obtaining many of the photomicrographs. Dr. Marcia Monteiro provided editorial input that greatly facilitated the updating of the material in this chapter.

REFERENCES

1. Virchow R: Cellular Pathology. London, John Churchill, 1860, p 33.
2. Williams IR, Kupper TS: Immunity at the surface: homeostatic mechanisms of the skin immune system. Life Sci 58:1485, 1996.
3. Murphy GF: The secret of "NIN," a novel neural immunological network potentially integral to immunologic function in human skin. In Nickoloff BJ (ed): Mast Cells, Macrophages and Dendritic Cells in Skin Disease. Boca Raton, FL, CRC Press, 1993, pp 227–244.
4. Cotsarellis G, et al: Label-retaining cells reside in the bulge area of the pilo-sebaceous unit: implications for follicular stem cells, hair cycle, and skin carcinogenesis. Cell 61:1329, 1990.
5. Sueki H, et al: Novel interactions between dermal dendrocytes and mast cells in human skin: implications for hemostasis and matrix repair. Lab Invest 69:160, 1993.
6. Fishman P, et al: Autoantibodies to tyrosinase: the bridge between melanoma and vitiligo. Cancer 79:1461, 1997.
7. Le Poole IC, et al: Presence of T cells and macrophages in inflammatory vitiligo skin parallels melanocyte disappearance. Am J Pathol 148:1219, 1996.
8. Badri AM, et al: An immunohistological study of cutaneous lymphocytes in vitiligo. J Pathol 170:149, 1993.
9. Norris W: A case of fungoid disease. Edinburgh Med Surg J 16:562, 1820.
10. Clark WH Jr, et al: Origin of familial malignant melanomas from heritable melanotic lesions: the BK mole syndrome. Arch Dermatol 114:732, 1978.
11. Reimer RR, et al: Precursor lesions in familial melanoma: a new genetic preneoplastic syndrome. JAMA 239:744, 1978.
12. Greene MH: Genetics of cutaneous melanoma and nevi [review]. Mayo Clin Proc 72:467, 1997.
13. Monzon J, et al: CDKN2A mutations in multiple primary melanomas. New Engl J Med 338:879, 1998.
14. Greene MH, et al: The high risk of melanoma in melanoma prone families with dysplastic nevi. Ann Intern Med 102:458, 1985.
15. van Duinen CM, et al: The distribution of cellular adhesion molecules in pigmented skin lesions. Cancer 73:2131, 1994.
16. Caporaso N, et al: Cytogenetics in hereditary malignant melanoma and dysplastic nevus syndrome: is dysplastic nevus syndrome a chromosome instability disorder? Cancer Genet Cytogenet 24:299, 1987.
17. Smith PJ, et al: Abnormal sensitivity to UV-radiation in cultured skin fibroblasts from patients with hereditary cutaneous malignant melanoma and dysplastic nevus syndrome. Int J Cancer 30:39, 1987.
18. Clark WH, et al: A study of tumor progression: the precursor lesions of superficial spreading and nodular melanoma. Hum Pathol 15:1147, 1985.
19. Mihm MC: The clinical diagnosis, classification and histogenetic concepts of the early stages of cutaneous malignant melanomas. N Engl J Med 284:1078, 1971.
20. Barnhill RL, et al: Neoplasms: malignant melanoma. In Fitzpatrick TB, et al (eds): Dermatology in General Medicine. New York, McGraw-Hill, 1993, chapter 82.

20a. Chin L, et al: Cooperative effects of ONK4a and ras in melanoma susceptibility in vivo. Genes Dev 11:2822, 1997.

21. Breslow A: Thickness, cross-sectional areas and depth of invasion in the prognosis of cutaneous melanoma. Ann Surg 182:572, 1970.
22. Clark WH Jr, et al: Model predicting survival in stage I melanoma based on tumor progression. J Natl Cancer Inst 81:1893, 1989.
23. Chen M, et al: Acantholytic variant of seborrheic keratosis. J Cutan Pathol 17:27, 1990.
24. Ellis DL, et al: Melanoma, growth factors, acanthosis nigricans, the sign of Leser-Trélat, and multiple acrochordons. A possible role for alpha-transforming growth factor in cutaneous paraneoplastic syndromes. N Engl J Med 317:1582, 1987.
25. Matsuoka LY, et al: Acanthosis nigricans. Clin Dermatol 11:21, 1993.
26. Schwartz RA: Keratoacanthoma. J Am Acad Dermatol 30:1, 1994.
27. Perez MI, et al: *P53* oncoprotein expression and gene mutations in some keratoacanthomas. Arch Dermatol 133:189, 1997.
28. Murphy GF, Elder D: Non-Melanocytic Tumors of the Skin. Atlas of Tumor Pathology, Third Series, Fascicle 1. Washington, DC, Armed Forces Institute of Pathology, 1991, pp 61–154.
29. Starink TM, et al: The cutaneous pathology of Cowden's disease: new findings. J Cutan Pathol 12:83, 1985.
30. Thielmann HW, et al: DNA repair synthesis in fibroblast strains from patients with actinic keratosis, squamous cell carcinoma, basal cell carcinoma, or malignant melanoma after treatment with ultraviolet light, *N*-acetoxy-2-acetyl-aminofluorene methyl methanesulfonate, and *N*-methyl-*N*-nitrosourea. J Cancer Res Clin Oncol 113:171, 1987.
31. Penn I: Neoplastic consequences of transplantation and chemotherapy. Cancer Detect Prev 1(Suppl):149, 1987.
32. Cooper KD, et al: Effects of ultraviolet radiation on human epidermal cell alloantigen presentation: initial depression of Langerhans cell–dependent function is followed by the appearance of T6 Dr$^+$ cells that enhance epidermal alloantigen presentation. J Immunol 134:129, 1985.
33. Granstein RD, et al: Epidermal cells in activation of suppressor lymphocytes: further characterization. J Immunol 138:4055, 1987.
34. Kawashima M, et al: Characterization of a new type of human papillomavirus (HPV) related to HPV5 from a case of actinic keratosis. Virology 154:389, 1986.
35. Hochwalt AE, et al: Mechanism of H-*ras* oncogene activation in mouse squamous carcinoma induced by an alkylating agent. Cancer Res 48:556, 1988.
36. Bale AE: The nevoid basal cell carcinoma syndrome: genetics and mechanism of carcinogenesis. Cancer Invest 15:180, 1997.
37. Oro AE, et al: Basal cell carcinoma in mice overexpressing sonic hedgehog. Science 276:817, 1997.

38. Al-Ghazal SK, et al: Merkel cell carcinoma of the skin. Br J Plast Surg 49:49_, 1996.
39. Lever WF, Schaumburg-Lever G: Histopathology of the Skin. Philadelphia, JB Lippincott, 1997, p 593.
40. Murphy GF, et al: Distribution of T cell antigens in histiocytosis X cells. Quantitative immunoelectron microscopy using monoclonal antibodies. Lab Invest 48:90, 1983.
41. Murphy GF: Cutaneous T cell lymphoma. In Fenoglio-Preiser CM (ed): Advances in Pathology. Chicago, Year Book Medical Publishers, 1988, pp 131–156.
42. Uchiyama T: Human T cell leukemia virus type I (HTLV-1) and human disease. Ann Rev Immunol 15:15, 1997.
43. Bakels V, et al: Immunophenotyping and gene rearrangement analysis provide additional criteria to differentiate between cutaneous T-cell lymphomas and pseudo-T-cell lymphomas. Am J Pathol 150:1941, 1997.
44. Longley BJ, et al: Somatic c-KIT activating mutation in urticaria pigmentosa and aggressive mastocytosis: establishment of clonality in a human mast cell neoplasm. Nat Genet 12:312, 1996.
45. Longley BJ, et al: Chronically KIT-stimulated clonally-derived human mast cells show heterogeneity in different tissue microenvironments. J Invest Dermatol 108:792, 1997.
46. Venencie PY: Classification of urticaria and genetic angioedema. Allerg Immunol 25:327, 1993.
47. Murphy GF, et al: Reaction patterns in the skin and special dermatologic techniques. In Moschella S (ed): Dermatology. Philadelphia, WB Saunders, 1984, p 104.
48. Waldorf HA, et al: Early cellular events in evolving cutaneous delayed hypersensitivity in humans. Am J Pathol 131:477, 1991.
49. Walsh LJ, et al: Human dermal mast cells contain and release tumor necrosis factor alpha, which induces leukocyte adhesion molecule 1. Proc Natl Acad Sci USA 88:4220, 1991.
50. Guillen FJ, et al: Acute cutaneous graft-versus-host disease to minor histocompatibility antigens in a murine model: evidence that large granular lymphocytes are the effector cells in the immune response. Lab Invest 137:1874, 1986.
51. Guillen FJ, et al: Inhibition of rat skin allograft rejection by cyclosporin. In situ characterization of the impaired local immune response. Transplantation 41:734, 1986.
52. Murphy GF, et al: Cytotoxic T lymphocytes and phenotypically abnormal epidermal dendritic cells in fixed cutaneous eruptions. Hum Pathol 16:1264, 1985.
53. de Jong EM: Psoriasis of the nails associated with disability in a large number of patients: results of a recent interview with 1,728 patients. Dermatology 193:300, 1996.
54. Wrone-Smith T, Nickoloff BJ. Dermal injection of immunocytes induces psoriasis. J Clin Invest 98:1878, 1996.
55. Franck JM, Young AW Jr: Squamous cell carcinoma in situ arising within lichen planus of the vulva. Dermatol Surg 21:890, 1995.
56. Bhan AK, et al: T cell subset populations in lichen planus: in situ characterization using monoclonal anti–T cell antibodies. Br J Dermatol 105:617, 1981.
57. Harrist TJ, Mihm MC: The specificity and usefulness of the lupus band test. Arthritis Rheum 23:479, 1980.
58. Boumpas DT, et al: Systemic lupus erythematosus: emerging concepts. Part 2: Dermatologic and joint disease, the antiphospholipid antibody syndrome, pregnancy. Ann Intern Med 123:42, 1995.
59. Becker BA, Gaspari AA: Pemphigus vulgaris and vegetans. Dermatol Clin 11:429, 1993.
60. Beutner EH, Jordan RE: Demonstration of skin antibodies in sera of pemphigus vulgaris patients by indirect immunofluorescent staining. Proc Soc Exp Biol Med 117:505, 1964.
61. Koch PJ, et al: Targeted disruption of the pemphigus vulgaris antigen (desmoglein 3) gene in mice causes loss of keratinocyte cell adhesion with a phenotype similar to pemphigus vulgaris. J Cell Biol 137: 1091, 1997.
62. Hashimoto K, et al: Anti–cell surface pemphigus autoantibody stimulates plasminogen activator activity of human epidermal cells. J Exp Med 157:259, 1983.
63. Seishima M, et al: Pemphigus IgG induces expression of urokinase plasminogen activator receptor on the cell surface of cultured keratinocytes. J Invest Dermatol 10:650, 1997.
64. Lever WF: Pemphigus. Medicine (Baltimore) 32:1, 1953.
65. Imber MJ, et al: The immunopathology of bullous pemphigoid. In Ahmed AR (ed): Clinics in Dermatology—Bullous Pemphigoid. Philadelphia, JB Lippincott, 1987, p 81.
66. Liu Z, et al: A major role for neutrophils in experimental bullous pemphigoid J Clin Invest 100:1256, 1997.
67. Duhring L: Dermatitis herpetiformis. JAMA 3:225, 1884.
68. Ahmed AR, Hameed A: Bullous pemphigoid and dermatitis herpetiformis. Clin Dermatol 11:47, 1993.
69. Walton S, et al: Clinical, ultrasound and hormonal markers of androgenicity in acne vulgaris. Br J Dermatol 133:249, 1995.
70. Leyden JJ: New understandings of the pathogenesis of acne. J Am Acad Dermatol 32(pt 3):S15, 1995.
71. Webster GF, et al: Inhibition of lipase production in *Propionibacterium acnes* by sub-minimal inhibitory concentrations of tetracycline and erythromycin. Br J Dermatol 104:453, 1981.
72. Berson DS, Shalita AR: The treatment of acne: the role of combination therapies. J Am Acad Dermatol 32(pt 3):S31, 1995.
73. de Villiers EM: Papillomavirus and HPV typing. Clin Dermatol 15:199, 1997.
74. Fang BS, et al: Human papillomavirus type 16 variants isolated from vulvar Bowenoid papulosis. J Med Virol 41:49, 1993.
75. Majewski S, Jablonska S: Human papillomavirus–associated tumors of the skin and mucosa. J Am Acad Dermatol 36(pt 1):659, 1997.
76. Harris AJ, et al: A novel human papillomavirus identified in epidermodysplasia verruciformis. Br J Dermatol 136:587, 1997.
77. Sadick NS: Current aspects of bacterial infections of the skin. Dermatol Clin 15:341, 1997.
78. Leyden JJ, Aly R: Tinea pedis. Semin Dermatol 12:280, 1993.

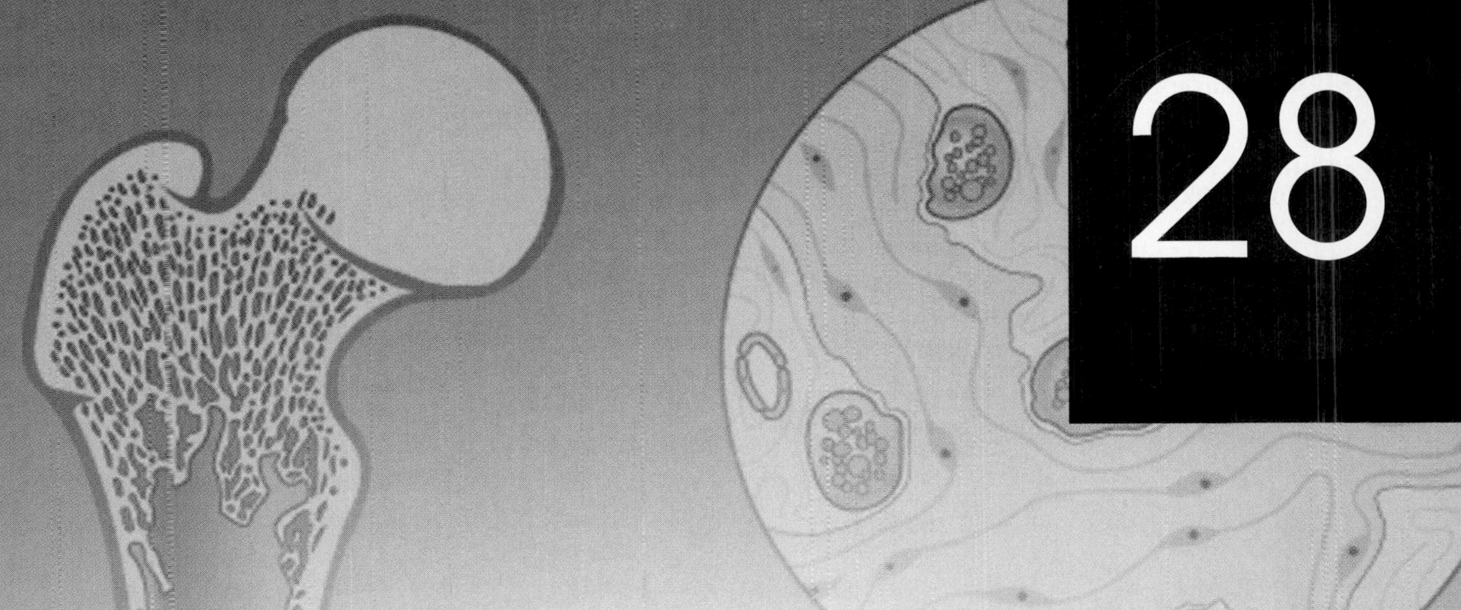

Bones, Joints, and Soft Tissue Tumors

Andrew Rosenberg

Bones

NORMAL SKELETAL SYSTEM

BONE MODELING AND REMODELING

BONE GROWTH AND DEVELOPMENT

PATHOLOGY

DEVELOPMENTAL ABNORMALITIES

Malformations

Achondroplasia and Thanatophoric Dwarfism

DISEASES ASSOCIATED WITH ABNORMAL MATRIX

Diseases Associated With Abnormal Metabolism of Collagen

Type 1 Collagen Diseases (Osteogenesis Imperfecta)

Diseases Associated With Abnormal Metabolism of Types 2, 10, and 11 Collagen

Mucopolysaccharidoses

Osteoporosis

DISEASES CAUSED BY OSTEOCLAST DYSFUNCTION

Osteopetrosis

Paget Disease (Osteitis Deformans)

DISEASES ASSOCIATED WITH ABNORMAL MINERAL HOMEOSTASIS

Rickets and Osteomalacia

Hyperparathyroidism

Renal Osteodystrophy

FRACTURES

OSTEONECROSIS (AVASCULAR NECROSIS)

INFECTIONS—OSTEOMYELITIS

Pyogenic Osteomyelitis

Tuberculous Osteomyelitis

Skeletal Syphilis

BONE TUMORS AND TUMOR-LIKE LESIONS

Bone-Forming Tumors

Osteoma

Osteoid Osteoma and Osteoblastoma

Osteosarcoma (Osteogenic Sarcoma)

Cartilage-Forming Tumors

Osteochondroma

Chondromas

Chondroblastoma

Chondromyxoid Fibroma

Chondrosarcoma

Fibrous and Fibro-osseous Tumors

Fibrous Cortical Defect and Nonossifying Fibroma

Fibrous Dysplasia

Fibrosarcoma and Malignant Fibrous Histiocytoma

MISCELLANEOUS TUMORS

Ewing Sarcoma and Primitive Neuroectodermal Tumor

Giant Cell Tumor

Metastatic Disease

Joints

NORMAL JOINTS

PATHOLOGY

ARTHRITIS

Osteoarthritis

Rheumatoid Arthritis

Juvenile Rheumatoid Arthritis

Seronegative Spondyloarthropathies

Ankylosing Spondyloarthritis

Reiter Syndrome

Enteropathic Arthritis

Psoriatic Arthritis

Infectious Arthritis

Suppurative Arthritis

Tuberculous Arthritis

Lyme Arthritis

Viral Arthritis

Gout and Gouty Arthritis

Calcium Pyrophosphate Crystal Deposition Disease (Pseudogout)

TUMORS AND TUMOR-LIKE LESIONS

Ganglion and Synovial Cyst

Giant Cell Tumor of Tendon Sheath and Pigmented Villonodular Synovitis

Soft Tissue Tumors and Tumor-like Lesions

PATHOGENESIS AND GENERAL FEATURES

FATTY TUMORS

LIPOMAS

LIPOSARCOMA

FIBROUS TUMORS AND TUMOR-LIKE LESIONS

REACTIVE PSEUDOSARCOMATOUS PROLIFERATIONS

Nodular Fasciitis

Myositis Ossificans

FIBROMATOSES

Superficial Fibromatosis (Palmar, Plantar, and Penile Fibromatoses)

Deep-seated Fibromatosis (Desmoid Tumors)

FIBROSARCOMA

FIBROHISTIOCYTIC TUMORS

BENIGN FIBROUS HISTIOCYTOMA (DERMATOFIBROMA AND SCLEROSING HEMANGIOMA)

MALIGNANT FIBROUS HISTIOCYTOMA

TUMORS OF SKELETAL MUSCLE

RHABDOMYOSARCOMA

TUMORS OF SMOOTH MUSCLE

LEIOMYOMAS

LEIOMYOSARCOMA

SYNOVIAL SARCOMA

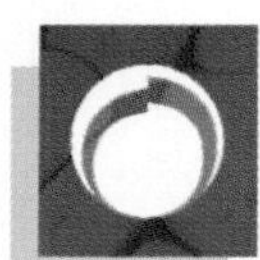

Bones

NORMAL SKELETAL SYSTEM

The skeletal system is as vital to life as any organ system because it plays an essential role in mineral homeostasis, houses the hematopoietic elements, provides mechanical support for movement, and protects and determines the attributes of body size and shape. The skeletal system is composed of 206 bones that vary in size and shape (tubular, flat, cuboid), and this diversity is an example of how form reflects function. The bones are interconnected by a variety of joints that allow for a wide range of movement while maintaining stability.

Bone is a type of connective tissue and is unique because it is one of the few tissues that normally mineralizes. Biochemically, it is defined by its special blend of organic matrix (35%) and inorganic elements (65%). The inorganic component, calcium hydroxyapatite [$Ca_{10}(PO_4)_6(OH)_2$], is the mineral that gives bone strength and hardness and is the storehouse for 99% of the body's calcium, 85% of the body's phosphorus, and 65% of the body's sodium and magnesium. The formation of hydroxyapatite crystal in bone is a phase transformation from liquid to solid analogous to the conversion of water to ice. The process involves the initiation and induction of mineralization by the organic matrix and is tightly regulated by numerous factors many of which are still unknown.[1] The rate of mineralization can vary, but normally there is a 12- to 15-day lag time between the formation of the matrix and its mineralization. Bone that is unmineralized is known as *osteoid.*

The organic component includes the cells of bone and the proteins of the matrix. The bone-forming cells include the osteoprogenitor cells, osteoblasts and osteocytes. The generation and stimulation of these cells are regulated by cytokines and growth factors such as fibroblast growth factor (FGF), platelet-derived growth factor (PDGF), insulin-like growth factor, and transforming growth factor-β (TGF-β).[2]

- *Osteoprogenitor* cells are pluripotential mesenchymal stem cells that are located in the vicinity of all bony surfaces; when appropriately stimulated, they have the capacity to undergo cell division and produce offspring that differentiate into osteoblasts. The transcription factor CBFA1 has been identified as being essential and specific for osteoblastic differentiation and stimulating osteoblast-specific gene expression (Chapter 2).[3] The generation of osteoblasts from osteoprogenitor cells is vital to growth, remodeling, and repair of bone.
- *Osteoblasts* are located on the surface of bone and synthesize, transport, and arrange the many proteins of matrix detailed later (Fig. 28–1). They also initiate the process of mineralization. Osteoblasts exhibit cell surface receptors, which bind many hormones (parathyroid

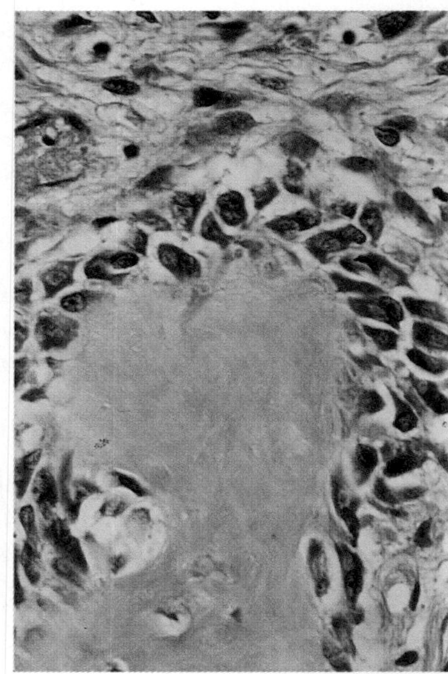

Figure 28–1

Active osteoblasts synthesizing bone matrix. The surrounding spindle cells represent osteoprogenitor cells.

hormone, vitamin D, and estrogen), cytokines and growth factors, and extracellular matrix proteins. Once osteoblasts become surrounded by matrix, they are known as *osteocytes*.

- *Osteocytes* are more numerous than any other bone-forming cell, and although encased by bone, they communicate with each other and surface cells via an intricate network of tunnels through the matrix known as *canaliculi*. The osteocytic cell processes traverse the canaliculi, and their contacts along gap junctions allow the transfer of surface membrane potentials and substrates. The large number of osteocytic processes and their distribution throughout bone tissue enable them to be the prime cell in several biologic processes. Studies have shown that this network may be important in controlling the second-to-second fluctuations in serum calcium and phosphorus levels by altering the concentration of these minerals in the local extracellular fluid compartment. Osteocytes also have the capability to detect mechanical forces and translate them into biologic activity, including the release of chemical mediators by signal transduction pathways involving cyclic adenosine monophosphate (AMP)[4] (Chapter 4).
- The *osteoclast* is the cell responsible for bone resorption and is derived from hematopoietic progenitor cells that also give rise to monocytes and macrophages. Cytokines crucial for osteoclast differentiation and maturation include interleukin (IL)-1, IL-3, IL-6, IL-11, tumor necrosis factor (TNF), granulocyte-macrophage colony-stimulating factor (GM-CSF), and macrophage colony-stimulating factor (M-CSF).[5] The mature multinucleated osteoclast (containing 6 to 12 nuclei) forms from fusion of circulating mononuclear precursors and is intimately related to the bone surface (Fig. 28–2). Osteoclast activity is initiated by binding to matrix adhesion proteins. The scalloped *resorption pits* they produce, and frequently reside in, are known as *Howship lacunae*. The portion of the osteoclast cell membrane overlying the resorption surface is modified by numerous villous extensions, known as the *ruffled border*, which serve to increase the membrane surface area. The plasmalemma bordering this region is specialized and forms a seal with the underlying bone preventing leakage of digestion products. This self-contained extracellular space is analogous to a secondary lysosome, and the osteoclast acidifies it with a hydrogen pump system that solubilizes the mineral. The osteoclast also releases into this space a multitude of enzymes that help disassemble the matrix proteins into amino acids and liberate and activate growth factors and enzymes (such as collagenase), which have been previously deposited and bound to the matrix by osteoblasts. *Thus, as bone is broken down to its elemental units, substances are released that initiate its renewal.*

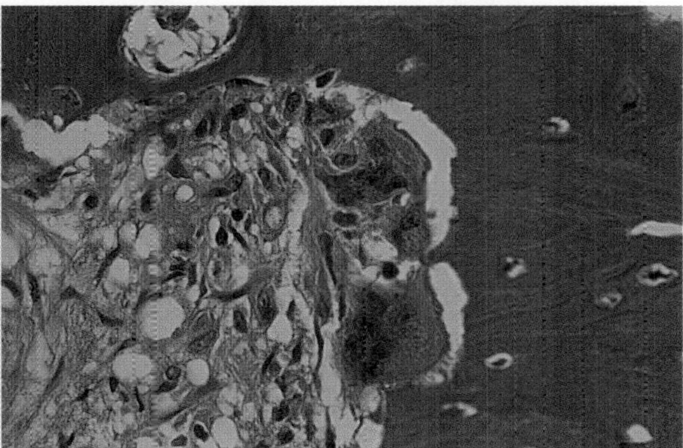

Figure 28–2

Two osteoclasts resorbing bone.

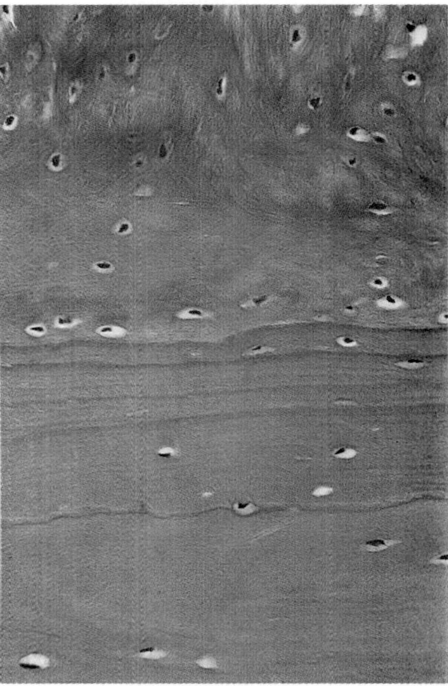

Figure 28–3

Woven bone (*top*) deposited on the surface of preexisting lamellar bone (*bottom*).

- The *proteins of bone* include type 1 collagen and a family of noncollagenous proteins that are derived mainly from osteoblasts. Type 1 collagen forms the backbone of matrix and accounts for 90% of the organic component. Osteoblasts deposit collagen either in a random weave known as *woven bone* or in an orderly layered manner designated *lamellar bone* (Fig. 28–3). Normally, woven bone is seen in the fetal skeleton and is formed at growth plates. Its advantages are that it is produced quickly, and it resists forces equally from all directions. The presence of woven bone in the adult is always indicative of a pathologic state; however, it is not diagnostic of a particular disease. For instance, in circumstances requiring rapid reparative stability, such as a fracture, woven bone is produced. It is also formed around sites of infection and composes the matrix of bone-forming tumors. *Lamellar bone, which gradually replaces woven bone during growth, is deposited much more slowly and is stronger than woven bone.* There are

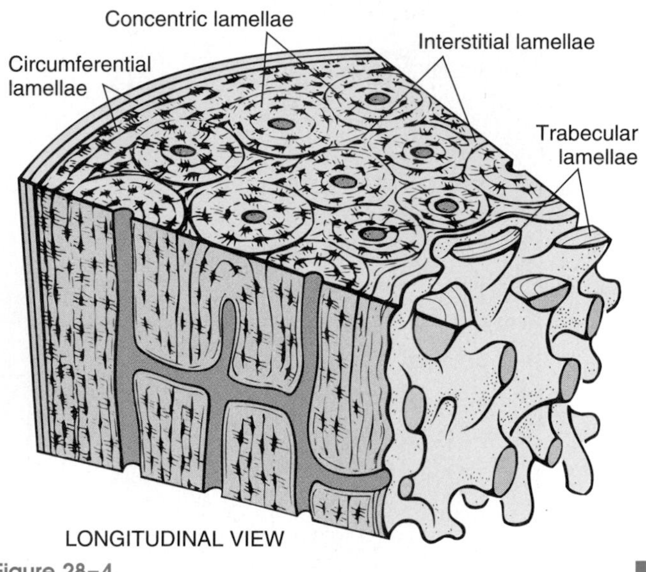

Figure 28–4

The schematic of normal bone structure reveals the subperiosteal and endosteal circumferential lamellae, concentric lamellae about vascular cores creating haversian systems, and the interstitial lamellae that fill the spaces in between the haversian systems. The trabecular lamellae extend from the endosteal surface. The individual lamellae are punctuated by osteocytic lacunae with their finely ramifying and interconnecting canals, which contain cell processes.

four different types of lamellar bone. Three are present only in the cortex—circumferential, concentric, and interstitial (Fig. 28–4). The fourth type, *trabecular lamellae*, composes the bone trabeculae in which the lamellae are oriented parallel to the long axis of the trabeculum.

The noncollagenous proteins of bone are bound to the matrix and grouped according to their function as adhesion proteins, calcium-binding proteins, mineralization proteins, enzymes, cytokines, and growth factors (Table 28–1).[6] Of these, only osteocalcin is unique to bone. It is measurable in the serum and used as a sensitive and specific marker for osteoblast activity. The cytokines and growth factors control bone cell proliferation, maturation, and metabolism.[7] They serve an important messenger function in translating mechanical and metabolic signals into local bone cell activity and eventual skeletal adaptation. The skeleton is uniquely able to adapt to new physical forces; witness the repositioning of teeth by the forces of braces.

Table 28–1. PROTEINS OF BONE MATRIX

Proteins of Bone Matrix
Osteoblast-Derived Proteins
Type 1 collagen
Cell adhesion proteins
Osteopontin, fibronectin, thrombospondin
Calcium-binding proteins
Osteonectin, bone sialoprotein
Proteins involved in mineralization
Osteocalcin
Enzymes
Collagenase, alkaline phosphatase
Growth factors
IGF-1, TGF-β, PDGF
Cytokines
Prostaglandins, IL-1, IL-6
Proteins Concentrated From Serum
β_2-microglobulin
Albumin

IGF, insulin-like growth factor; TGF, transforming growth factor; PDGF, platelet-derived growth factor; IL, interleukin.

Bone Modeling and Remodeling

Osteoblasts and osteoclasts act in coordination and are considered the functional unit of bone known as the *basic multicellular unit*. The processes of bone formation and resorption are tightly coupled, and their balance determines skeletal mass at any point in time.[8] As the skeleton grows and enlarges (modeling), bone formation predominates. Once the skeleton has reached maturity, the breakdown and renewal of bone that constitutes skeletal maintenance is called *remodeling*. Peak bone mass is determined by a variety of factors, including the type of vitamin D receptor inherited, state of nutrition, level of physical activity, age, and hormonal status. Peak bone mass is achieved in early adulthood, and at this stage, approximately 5% to 10% of the skeleton is turned over or remodeled yearly and the amount of bone formed and resorbed by the basic multicellular units is in equilibrium. Beginning in the fourth decade, however, the amount of bone resorbed exceeds that which has been formed so that there is a steady decrement in skeletal mass.

In the formation and maintenance of the skeletal system, the *osteoblast provides much of the local control because it not only produces bone matrix, but also plays an important role in mediating osteoclast activity*. Many of the primary stimulators of bone resorption, such as parathyroid hormone, parathyroid hormone–related protein (PHRP) (Chapter 26), IL-1, and TNF have minimal or no direct effect on osteoclasts. The osteoblast has receptors for these substances, and evidence suggests that once the osteoblast receives the appropriate signal, it releases a soluble mediator that induces osteoclast bone resorption. The cytokines and growth factors, especially TGF-β, released from the matrix during its digestion act as a feedback loop and trigger the formation and activation of osteoblasts to synthesize and deposit an equivalent amount of new bone in the resorption pit (Fig. 28–5). In this fashion, bone formation and resorption are temporally and spatially related and can be controlled by systemic and local factors.

Bone Growth and Development

The patterning and architectural arrangement of the skeleton are regulated by the *homeobox genes*. Their expression results in the production of localized cellular condensations of primitive mesenchyme in the sites of future bones, and these are the earliest precursors of the skeleton.

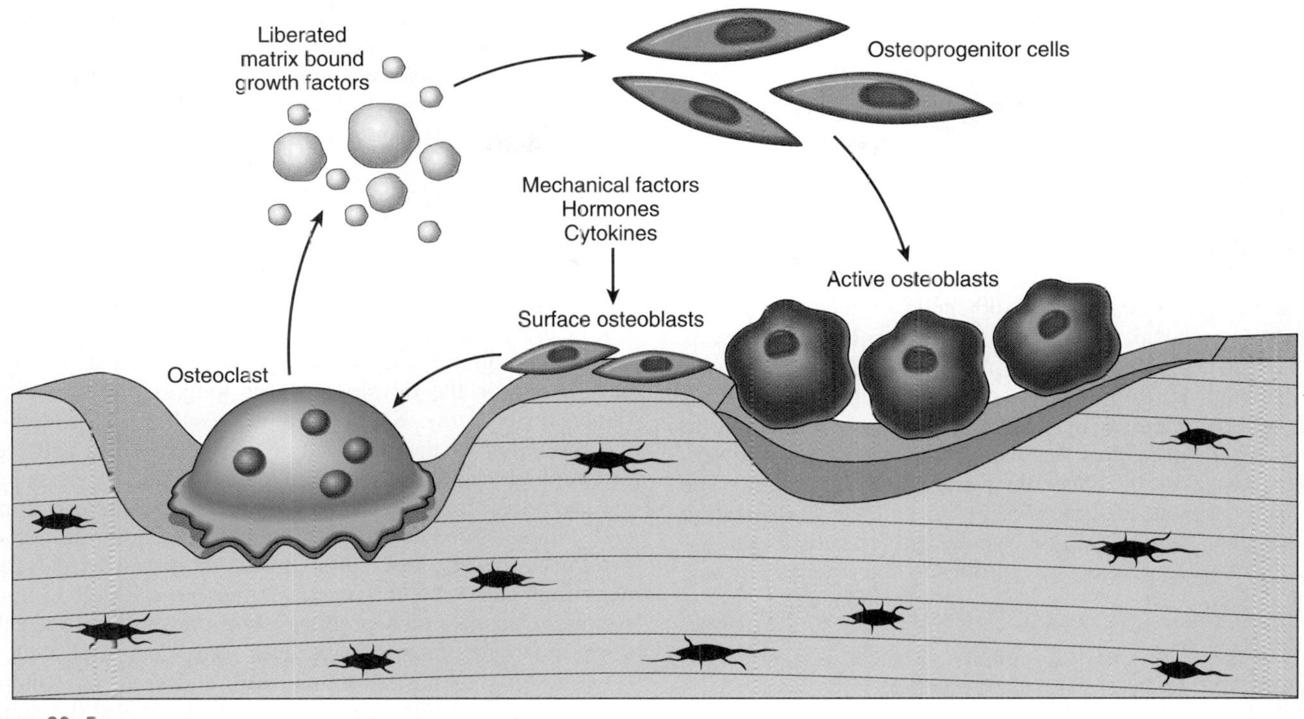

Figure 28–5

Bone resorption and formation are coupled processes that are controlled by systemic factors and local cytokines, some of which are deposited in the bone matrix. Cytokines are key in the communication between osteoblasts and osteoclasts.

In the process of *enchondral bone formation*, the mesenchyme first differentiates into a cartilaginous model, or anlage, of the future bone. Subsequently, around the eighth week of gestation, the cartilage in the center of the anlage undergoes degradative changes, mineralizes, and is removed by osteoclast-type cells. This process, which progresses up and down the length of the bone, allows for the ingrowth of blood vessels and osteoprogenitor cells that provide the bone-forming cells. Concurrently the periosteum in the midshaft of the anlage produces osteoblasts that deposit the beginnings of the cortex, and this region is known as the *primary center of ossification*. In the epiphyses, a similar sequence of events leading to the removal of cartilage occurs (*secondary center of ossification*) such that a plate of the cartilage model becomes entrapped between the expanding centers of ossification, and this structure is known as the *physis* or *growth plate*. The chondrocytes within the growth plate undergo a series of events, including proliferation, growth, maturation, and necrosis, and the matrix eventually mineralizes (Fig. 28–6). PHRP is important in regulating this sequence. Cartilage mineralization is a signal for its resorption, and remnant struts act as scaffolding for the deposition of bone on its surfaces. These structures form the primary spongiosa. The process of enchondral ossification also occurs at the base of articular cartilage, and by these mechanisms bones increase in length, and articular surfaces increase in diameter. In contrast, bones derived from *intramembranous formation*, such as the cranium and portions of the clavicles, are formed by osteoblasts directly from a fibrous layer of tissue that was derived from the mesenchyme.

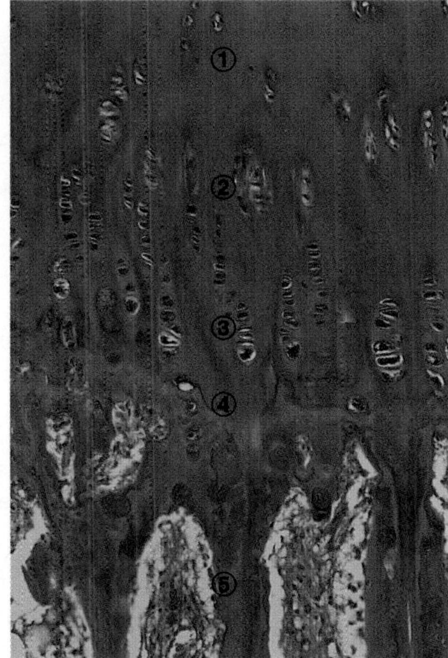

Figure 28–6

Active growth plate with ongoing enchondral ossification. 1, Reserve zone. 2, Zone of proliferation. 3, Zone of hypertrophy. 4, Zone of mineralization. 5, Primary spongiosa.

Bone tissue is made only by osteoblasts. After its formation, further increase in size is achieved only by the deposition of new bone on a preexisting surface. This mechanism of *appositional growth* is key to understanding the facets of bone growth and modeling.

PATHOLOGY

The skeletal system is as subject to circulatory, inflammatory, neoplastic, metabolic, and congenital disorders as are the other organ systems of the body. The complexity of its growth, development, maintenance, and relationships with other organ systems makes it unusually vulnerable to adverse influences. Not surprisingly, then, primary and secondary diseases of bone are varied and numerous. The spectrum of bone disorders is broad and the classification system not standardized, and so we prefer here to categorize the various disorders according to their perceived biologic defect.

Developmental Abnormalities

Developmental abnormalities of the skeleton vary from a simple loss of phalanx to widespread fatal deformities. These diseases are complex because they may have an impact on the skeleton during any of its stages of development. They thus have variable manifestations and may involve one, multiple, or all bones of the body. Many are heritable, and much has been learned about their genetic bases. The mutations responsible for these disorders have been shown to affect transcription factors (e.g., homeobox genes), cellular signaling mechanisms (e.g., growth factors), and matrix components (e.g., types 1 and 2 collagen) (Table 28–2)[9, 10] (Chapter 11).

Table 28–2. MOLECULAR GENETICS OF DISEASES OF THE SKELETON

Human Disorder	Gene Mutation
Defects in Mesenchymal Condensation and Related Cell Differentiation	
Synpolydactyly	HOXD-13
Waardenburg syndrome	PAX-3
Greig syndrome	GL13
Campomelic dysplasia	SOX9
Abnormal Proliferation or Maturation of Chondrocytes and Osteoblasts	
Achondroplasia	FGFR3
Hypochondroplasia	FGFR3
Thanatophoric dwarfism	FGFR3
Crouzon syndrome	FGFR2
Abnormal Metabolism of Collagen and Noncollagenous Proteins	
Osteogenesis imperfecta types 1–4	COL1A1, COL1A2
Achondrogenesis II	COl2A1
Hypochondrogenesis	COl2A1
Stickler syndrome	COL2A1, COL11A1,2
Diatrophic dysplasia	DTDST

Modified from Mundlos S, Olsen BR: Heritable diseases of the skeleton: Part I. Molecular insights into skeletal development-transcription factors and signaling pathways. FASEB J 11:125, 1997; and Mundlos S, Olsen BR: Heritable diseases of the skeleton: Part II. Molecular insights into skeletal development-matrix components and their homeostasis. FASEB J 11:227, 1997.

MALFORMATIONS

Congenital malformations of bone are relatively uncommon. The more simple anomalies include failure of development of a bone (e.g., congenital absence of a phalanx, rib, or clavicle); the formation of extra bones (supernumerary ribs or digits); the fusion of two adjacent digits (syndactylism); or the development of long, spider-like digits (arachnodactylism). Some of these result from defects in the formation of the mesenchymal condensations and their differentiation into the cartilage anlage. They are caused by genetic alterations that affect transcription factors, especially those coded for by the homeobox genes, and certain cytokines. An example of a defect in mesenchymal condensation is a mutation in the homeobox HOXD-13 transcription factor, which produces an extra digit between the third and fourth fingers as well as some degree of syndactyly.[9] Anomalies that affect the skull and vertebral column, such as *craniorachischisis* (failure of closure of the spinal column and skull), are frequently of great clinical importance. This defect produces a persistent opening through which the meninges and central nervous system herniate to produce a meningomyelocele or meningoencephalocele (Chapters 11 and 30).

ACHONDROPLASIA AND THANATOPHORIC DWARFISM

Achondroplasia is the most common disease of the growth plate and is a major cause of dwarfism. Achondroplasia is an example of a disease that is caused by a defect in cell signaling, and it manifests as a reduction in the proliferation of the chondrocytes in the growth plate. Patients with this disorder have a point mutation (usually Arg for Gly[375]) in the gene that codes for FGF receptor 3 (FGFR3).[9] In the normal growth plate, activation of FGFR3 *inhibits* cartilage proliferation, and in achondroplasia the mutation causes the receptor to be in the state of constant activation.

Achondroplasia is an autosomal dominant disorder, with approximately 80% of the cases representing new mutations. The affected infant has shortened proximal extremities, a trunk of relative normal length, and an enlarged head with bulging forehead and conspicuous depression of the root of the nose. The skeletal abnormalities are usually not associated with changes in longevity, intelligence, or reproductive status.

MORPHOLOGY. The histologic abnormalities in achondroplasia can be found in the growth plates. The zones of proliferation and hypertrophy are narrowed and disorganized and contain clusters of large chondrocytes instead of well-formed columns. At the base of the growth plate, there is premature deposition of horizontal struts of bone that seals the plate and prevents further growth. Appositional intramembranous bone formation is not disrupted; therefore the cortices form normally and appear thickened in relation to the short length of the bone.

Thanatophoric dwarfism is the most common lethal form of dwarfism and affects about 1 in every 20,000 live births. It is also caused by a mutation in FGFR3 that is either a missense mutation or a point mutation that is different than that in achondroplasia.[9] The affected patients have micromelic shortening of the limbs, frontal bossing with relative macrocephaly, a small chest cavity, and a bell-shaped abdomen. The underdeveloped thoracic cavity leads to respiratory insufficiency, and the patients frequently die at birth or soon after. The histologic changes in the growth plate show diminished proliferation of chondrocytes and poor columnation in the zone of proliferation.

Diseases Associated With Abnormal Matrix

Many of the organic bone matrix components have been only recently identified, and their interactions are far more complex than originally imagined. Therefore, this field of skeletal pathology is still in its early stages of discovery. Examples of the potential importance of abnormalities in bone matrix are the diseases associated with deranged metabolism of collagen, various mucopolysaccharide disorders, and decreased bone mass.

DISEASES ASSOCIATED WITH ABNORMAL METABOLISM OF COLLAGEN

The skeletal diseases associated with abnormal collagen metabolism (Table 28–2) result from mutations in those genes that code for the collagens that are important in bone and cartilage, including types 1, 2, 10, and 11 (Chapter 4). Their clinical manifestations are variable and range from lethal disease to premature osteoarthritis.

Type 1 Collagen Diseases (Osteogenesis Imperfecta)

Osteogenesis imperfecta is a group of phenotypically related disorders that are caused by deficiencies in the synthesis of type 1 collagen. Although osteogenesis imperfecta, or brittle bone disease, has prominent skeletal manifestations, other anatomic structures rich in type 1 collagen, such as joints, eyes, ears, skin, and teeth, are affected as well. The genetic defects in osteogenesis imperfecta reside in mutations in the genes that code for the α_1 and α_2 chains of the collagen molecule,[11] common ones inherited in an autosomal dominant fashion. Mutations resulting in the production of qualitatively normal collagen that is synthesized in decreased amounts are associated with mild skeletal abnormalities. More severe or lethal phenotypes result from genetic defects producing abnormal polypeptide chains that cannot form the triple helix of collagen.

The clinical expression of osteogenesis imperfecta constitutes a spectrum of disorders all marked by extreme skeletal fragility. Four major subtypes have been segregated (Table 28–3). New and less well characterized variants are still being identified. The recognition of particular variants and their modes of inheritance is of importance in genetic counseling.

The type II variant is at one end of the spectrum and is uniformly fatal in utero or during the perinatal period. It is characterized by extraordinary bone fragility with multiple fractures occurring when the fetus is still within the womb (Fig. 28–7). In contrast, the *type I form*, which is more often due to an acquired rather than a hereditary mutation, permits a normal life span but with an increased number of fractures during childhood. These decrease in frequency after puberty. Other findings include *blue sclerae* caused by a decrease in collagen content, making the sclera translucent and allowing partial visualization of the underlying choroid; *hearing loss* related to both a sensorineural deficit and impeded conduction owing to abnormalities in the

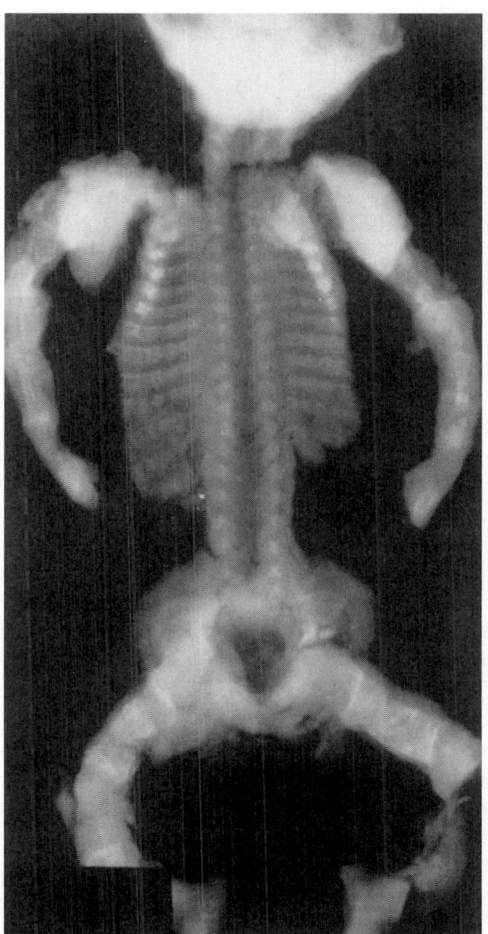

Figure 28–7 ■

Skeletal radiograph of a fetus with lethal type II osteogenesis imperfecta. Note the numerous fractures of virtually all bones, resulting in accordion-like shortening of the limbs.

Table 28–3. OSTEOGENESIS IMPERFECTA

	Subtype	Inheritance	Collagen Defect	Major Clinical Features
OI I	Postnatal fractures, blue sclerae	Autosomal dominant	Decreased synthesis pro-a1(1) chain Abnormal pro-a1(1) or pro-a2(1) chains	Compatible with survival Normal stature Skeletal fragility Dentinogenesis imperfecta Hearing impairment Joint laxity Blue sclerae
OI II	Perinatal lethal	Most autosomal recessive Some autosomal dominant ?New mutations	Abnormally short pro-a1(1) chain Unstable triple helix Abnormal or insufficient pro-a2(1)	Death in utero or within days of birth Skeletal deformity with excessive fragility and multiple fractures Blue sclerae
OI III	Progressive deforming	Autosomal dominant (75%) Autosomal recessive (25%)	Altered structure of propeptides of pro-a2(1) Impaired formation of triple helix	Compatible with survival Growth retardation Multiple fractures Progressive kyphoscoliosis Blue sclerae at birth that become white Hearing impairment Dentinogenesis imperfecta
OI IV	Postnatal fractures, normal sclerae	Autosomal dominant	Short pro-a2(1) chain Unstable triple helix	Compatible with survival Moderate skeletal fragility Short stature Sometimes dentinogenesis imperfecta

OI, osteogenesis imperfecta.

bones of the middle and inner ear; and *dental imperfections* (small, misshapen, and blue-yellow teeth) secondary to a deficiency in dentin. Morphologically *the basic abnormality in all forms of osteogenesis imperfecta is too little bone,* thus constituting a type of osteoporosis with marked cortical thinning and attenuation of trabeculae. In some variants, the skeleton fails to model properly, and there are persistent foci of hypercellular woven bone.[12]

Diseases Associated With Abnormal Metabolism of Types 2, 10, and 11 Collagen

Types 2, 10, and 11 collagen are important structural components of hyaline cartilage. Mutations that result in their abnormal metabolism, although uncommon, produce a spectrum of disorders ranging from those that are fatal to those compatible with life but associated with early destruction of joints (see Table 28–2). Greater than 30 mutations have been discovered in the type 2 collagen gene, and all have affected the triple helical component of the molecule. In the severe disorders, the type 2 collagen molecules are not secreted by the chondrocytes, and insufficient bone formation occurs. In the milder phenotypes, a nonfunctioning or *null* collagen gene allele is formed leading to a reduced content of type 2 collagen in the cartilage.[10]

MUCOPOLYSACCHARIDOSES

The mucopolysaccharidoses, as discussed earlier (Chapter 6) are a group of lysosomal storage diseases that are caused by deficiencies in the enzymes that degrade dermatan sulfate, heparan sulfate, and keratan sulfate. The implicated enzymes are mainly acid hydrolases. Mesenchymal cells, especially chondrocytes, play an important role in the metabolism of extracellular matrix mucopolysaccharides and therefore are most severely affected. Consequently, many of the skeletal manifestations of the mucopolysaccharidoses result from abnormalities in hyaline cartilage, including the cartilage anlage, growth plates, costal cartilages, and articular surfaces. It is not surprising therefore that these patients are frequently of short stature and have chest wall abnormalities and malformed bones.

OSTEOPOROSIS

Osteoporosis is a term that denotes increased porosity of the skeleton resulting from a reduction in bone mass. The associated structural changes predispose the bone to fracture. The disorder may be localized to a certain bone or region, as in *disuse osteoporosis of a limb*, or may involve the entire skeleton, as a manifestation of a *metabolic bone disease*. Generalized osteoporosis, in turn, may be primary or secondary to a large variety of conditions (Table 28–4).[13]

When the term osteoporosis is used in an unqualified manner, it usually refers to the most common forms, senile and postmenopausal osteoporosis, in which the critical loss of bone mass makes the skeleton vulnerable to fractures. About 15 million individuals suffer from primary osteoporosis in the United States, and their medical care costs close to $1 billion annually. Effective treatment and prevention are imperative. The following discussion relates largely to this dominant form of osteoporosis.

Pathogenesis. Peak bone mass is achieved during young adulthood. Its magnitude is determined largely by heredi-

Table 28–4. CATEGORIES OF GENERALIZED OSTEOPOROSIS

Primary	
Postmenopausal	Idiopathic
Senile	
Secondary	
Endocrine disorders	**Rheumatologic disease**
Hyperparathyroidism	**Drugs**
Hypo-hyperthyroidism	Anticoagulants
Hypogonadism	Chemotherapy
Pituitary tumors	Corticosteroids
Diabetes, type 1	Anticonvulsants
Addison disease	Alcohol
Neoplasia	**Miscellaneous**
Multiple myeloma	Osteogenesis imperfecta
Carcinomatosis	Immobilization
Gastrointestinal	Pulmonary disease
Malnutrition	Homocystinuria
Malabsorption	Anemia
Hepatic insufficiency	
Vitamin C, D deficiencies	

tary factors, especially the allele for the vitamin D receptor molecule. Physical activity, muscle strength, diet, and hormonal state, however, all contribute.[14] Once maximal skeletal mass is attained, a small deficit in bone formation accrues with every resorption and formation cycle of each basic multicellular unit. This is because the remodeling sequence is not completely effective. Accordingly, age-related bone loss—which may average 0.7% per year—is a normal and predictable biologic phenomenon, similar to the graying of hair. Both sexes are affected equally and whites more so than blacks. Differences in the peak skeletal mass in men versus women and in blacks versus whites may partially explain why certain populations are prone to develop this disorder.

Although much remains unknown, discoveries in the molecular biology of bone have provided intriguing new hypotheses in the pathogenesis of osteoporosis (Fig. 28–8):

- *Age-related changes* in bone cells and matrix have a strong impact on bone metabolism. Osteoblasts from elderly individuals have reduced reproductive and biosynthetic potential when compared with osteoblasts from younger individuals.[15] Also, proteins bound to the extracellular matrix (such as growth factors, which both are mitogenic to osteoprogenitor cells and stimulate osteoblastic synthetic activity) lose their biologic punch over time. The end result is a skeleton populated by bone-forming cells that have a diminished capacity to make bone. This form of osteoporosis, also known as *senile osteoporosis*, is categorized as a *low turnover variant.*
- *Reduced physical activity* increases the rate of bone loss in experimental animals and humans because mechanical forces are important stimuli for normal bone remodeling. The bone loss seen in an immobilized or paralyzed extremity, the reduction of skeletal mass observed in astronauts subjected to a gravity-free environment for prolonged periods, and the higher bone density in athletes as compared with nonathletes all support a role for physical activity in preventing bone loss. The type of exercise is important because load magnitude influences bone density more than the number of load cycles. Because muscle contraction is the dominant source of skeletal loading, it is logical that resistance exercises such as weight training are more effective stimuli for increasing bone mass than repetitive endurance activities such as jogging. Certainly the decreased physical activity that is associated with aging contributes to senile osteoporosis.
- *Genetic factors are also important*, as noted previously. The type of vitamin D receptor molecule that is inherited accounts for approximately 75% of the maximal peak mass achieved. Polymorphism in the vitamin D receptor molecule is associated with either a higher or lower maximal bone mass. However, increased parathyroid hormone levels or insufficient intake of vitamin D cannot be ascribed significant roles in the development of senile and postmenopausal osteoporosis.
- The body's calcium *nutritional state* is important. It has been shown that adolescent girls (but not boys) have insufficient calcium intake levels in the diet. This calcium deficiency occurs during a period of rapid bone growth, stunting the peak bone mass ultimately achieved; thus, these individuals are at greater risk of developing osteoporosis.
- *Hormonal influences.* In the decade after menopause, yearly reductions in bone mass may reach up to 2% of cortical bone and 9% of cancellous bone. Women may lose as much as 35% of their cortical bone and 50% of their trabecular bone within the 30 to 40 years after menopause. It is thus no surprise that 1 out of every 2 women suffers an osteoporotic fracture, in contrast to 1 in 40 men. *Postmenopausal* osteoporosis is characterized by a hormone-dependent acceleration of bone loss that occurs during the decade after menopause. *Estrogen deficiency plays the major role in this phenomenon, and estrogen replacement at the menopause is protective against bone loss.* The effects of estrogen on bone mass

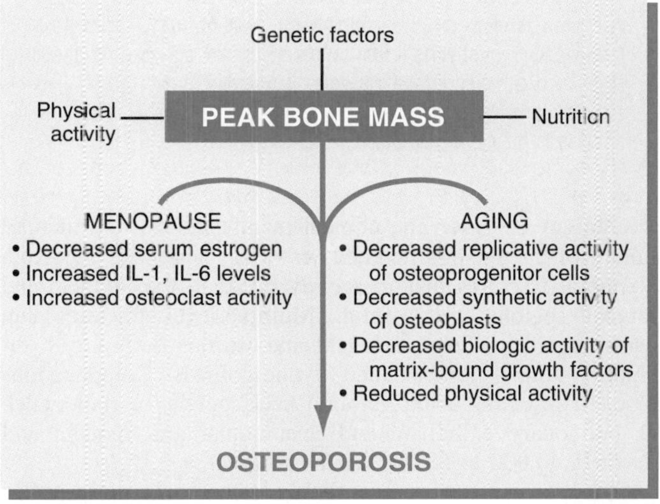

Figure 28–8

Pathophysiology of postmenopausal and senile osteoporosis (see text).

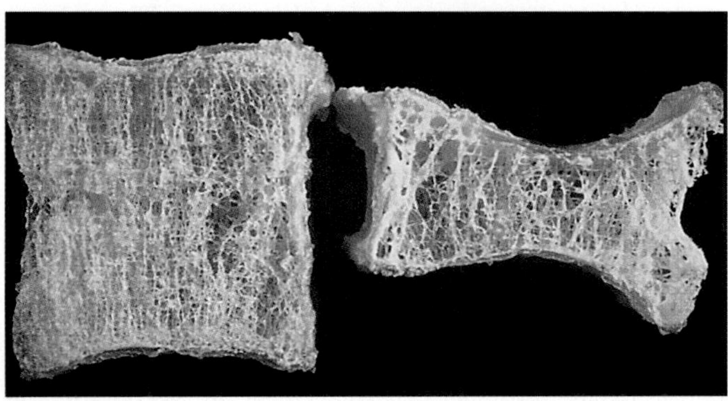

Figure 28–9

Osteoporotic vertebral body *(right)* shortened by compression fractures compared with a normal vertebral body. Note that the osteoporotic vertebra has a characteristic loss of horizontal trabeculae and thickened vertical trabeculae.

are mediated by cytokines. Decreased estrogen levels result in increased secretion of IL-1, IL-6, and TNF-α by blood monocytes and bone marrow cells.[16, 17] These cytokines are potent stimulators of osteoclast recruitment and activity. Compensatory osteoblastic activity occurs, but it does not keep pace, leading to what is classified as a high turnover form of osteoporosis.

MORPHOLOGY. The entire skeleton is affected in postmenopausal and senile osteoporosis (Fig. 28–9), but certain regions tend to be more severely involved than others. In **postmenopausal** osteoporosis, the increase in osteoclast activity affects mainly bones or portions of bones that have increased surface area, such as the cancellous compartment of vertebral bodies. The osteoporotic trabeculae are thinned and lose their interconnections, leading to progressive microfractures and eventual vertebral collapse. In senile osteoporosis, the osteoporotic cortex is thinned by subperiosteal and endosteal resorption, and the haversian systems are widened. In severe cases, the haversian systems are so enlarged that the cortex mimics cancellous bone. The bone that remains is of normal composition.

Clinical Course. The clinical manifestations of structural failure of the skeleton depend on which bones are involved. Vertebral fractures that frequently occur in the thoracic and lumbar regions are painful. Multiple-level fractures can cause significant loss of height and various deformities, including lumbar lordosis and kyphoscoliosis. Complications of overt fractures of the femoral neck, pelvis, or spine, such as pulmonary embolism and pneumonia, are frequent and result in 40,000 to 50,000 deaths per year.

Osteoporosis cannot be reliably detected in plain radiographs until 30% to 40% of the bone mass is lost, and measurement of blood levels of calcium, phosphorus, and alkaline phosphatase are not diagnostic. Osteoporosis is thus a difficult condition to diagnose accurately since it remains asymptomatic until skeletal fragility is well advanced. Currently the best procedures that accurately estimate the amount of bone loss, aside from biopsy, are specialized radiographic imaging techniques, such as single-energy photon absorptiometry, dual-energy absorptiometry, and quantitative computed tomography, which measure bone density.

Diseases Caused by Osteoclast Dysfunction

OSTEOPETROSIS

Osteopetrosis refers to a group of rare hereditary diseases that are characterized by osteoclast dysfunction, resulting in diffuse symmetric skeletal sclerosis (Fig. 28–10). The term *osteopetrosis* was coined because of the stonelike quality of the bones; however, the bones are abnormally brittle and fracture like a piece of chalk. Osteopetrosis, which is also known as *marble bone disease* and *Albers-Schönberg disease*, is classified into variants based on both the mode of inheritance and the clinical findings. The autosomal recessive malignant type and the autosomal dominant benign type are the most common variants.

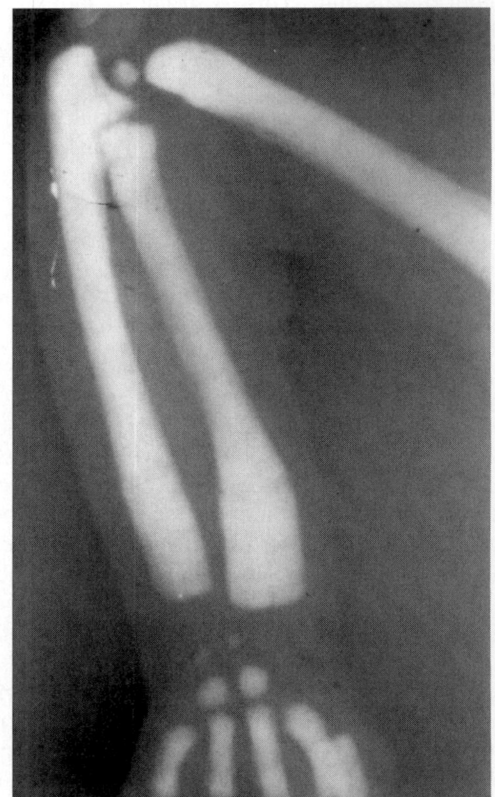

Figure 28–10

Radiograph of the upper extremity in a patient with osteopetrosis. The bones are diffusely sclerotic, and the distal metaphyses of the ulna and radius are poorly formed (Erlenmeyer flask deformity).

Pathogenesis. The precise nature of the osteoclast dysfunction in most cases is unknown. One exception is the variant associated with *carbonic anhydrase II* deficiency. Carbonic anhydrase II is required by osteoclasts and renal tubular cells to excrete hydrogen ions and acidify their environment. The absence of this enzyme prevents osteoclasts from solubilizing and resorbing matrix and blocks the acidification of urine by the renal tubular cells. In another form of the disease, it has been suggested that osteoclasts cannot generate superoxide; these patients have received some benefit from the administration of interferon-γ. In animals, osteopetrosis can also be caused by a retrovirus infection, a targeted mutation in the gene coding for M-CSF, and mutations in the *c-src* gene.[18] It is likely that some of these mechanisms will be linked to the human disorders.

MORPHOLOGY. The morphologic changes of osteopetrosis are explained by deficient osteoclast activity. Grossly the bones lack a medullary canal, and the ends of long bones are bulbous (Erlenmyer flask deformity) and misshapen. The neural foramina are small and compress exiting nerves. The primary spongiosa, which is normally removed during growth, persists and fills the medullary cavity leaving no room for the hematopoietic marrow and prevents the formation of mature trabeculae (Fig. 28–11). Bone that forms is not remodeled and tends to be woven in architecture. In the end, these intrinsic abnormalities cause the bone to be brittle. Histologically, there are no consistent changes in osteoclast number; they have been reported to be increased, normal, or decreased in number.

Clinical Features. The malignant autosomal recessive pattern usually becomes evident in utero or soon after birth. Fractures, anemia, and hydrocephaly are often seen resulting in postpartum mortality. Patients who survive into their infancy have cranial nerve problems (optic atrophy, deafness, facial paralysis) and repeated, often fatal infections because of inadequacies of the marrow produced in extramedullary sites. The extramedullary hematopoiesis also causes prominent hepatosplenomegaly. The autosomal dominant benign form may not be detected until adolescence or adulthood, when it is discovered on x-rays performed because of repeated fractures. These patients may also have milder cranial nerve deficits and anemia.

Because osteoclasts are derived from marrow monocyte stem cells, bone marrow transplants provide affected patients with progenitor cells that can produce normal functioning osteoclasts. Follow-up studies in transplanted patients have shown reversal of many of the skeletal abnormalities.

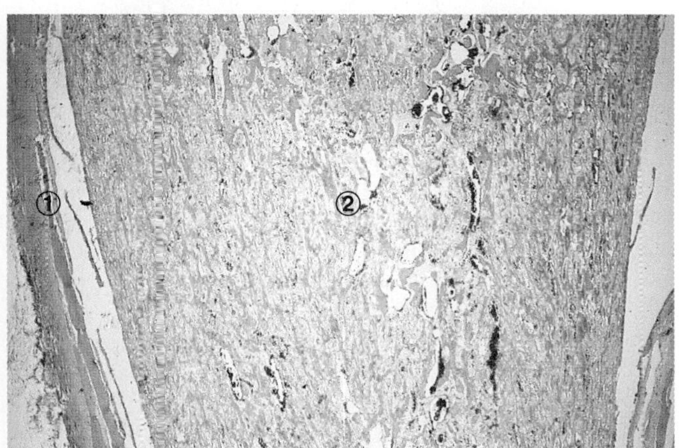

Figure 28–11

Section of proximal tibial diaphysis from a fetus with osteopetrosis. The cortex (1) is being formed and the medullary cavity (2) is abnormally filled with primary spongiosa replacing the hematopoietic elements.

PAGET DISEASE (OSTEITIS DEFORMANS)

This unique skeletal disease can be characterized as a *collage of matrix madness*. At the outset, Paget disease is marked by regions of furious osteoclastic bone resorption, which is followed by a period of hectic bone formation. The net effect, as the bone cell activity quiets down, is a *gain in bone mass*. The newly formed bone is disordered and architecturally unsound. *This repetitive and overlapping sequence forms the basis of dividing Paget disease into (1) an initial osteolytic stage, followed by (2) a mixed osteoclastic-osteoblastic stage, which ends with a predominance of osteoblastic activity and evolves ultimately into (3) a burnt-out quiescent osteosclerotic stage* (Fig. 28–12).

Paget disease usually begins during mid adulthood and becomes progressively more common thereafter. An intriguing aspect is the striking variation in prevalence both within certain countries and throughout the world. Paget disease is relatively common in whites in England, France, Austria, regions of Germany, Australia, New Zealand, and the United States. The exact incidence is hard to determine because most affected individuals are asymptomatic, but it is estimated to affect 5% to 11% of the adult populations in these countries. In contrast, Paget disease is rare in the native populations of Scandinavia, China, Japan, and Africa.

Pathogenesis. When Sir James Paget first described this condition in 1876, he attributed the skeletal changes to an inflammatory process, hence the term *osteitis deformans*. It is ironic that after numerous subsequent hypotheses were proposed, Paget may be finally proven correct. Current evidence suggests a slow virus infection by a *paramyxovirus* as the cause of Paget disease. This likens it to other slow virus diseases, such as subacute sclerosing leukoencephalitis, produced by the same family of viruses (Chapter 30). Viral particles resembling the nucleocapsids of paramyxovirus have been seen in the cytoplasm and nuclei of osteoclasts, and immunologic analyses have identified antigens associated with both the measles and respiratory syncytial viruses (both paramyxoviruses) in osteoclasts from affected sites. Additionally, measles virus transcripts were

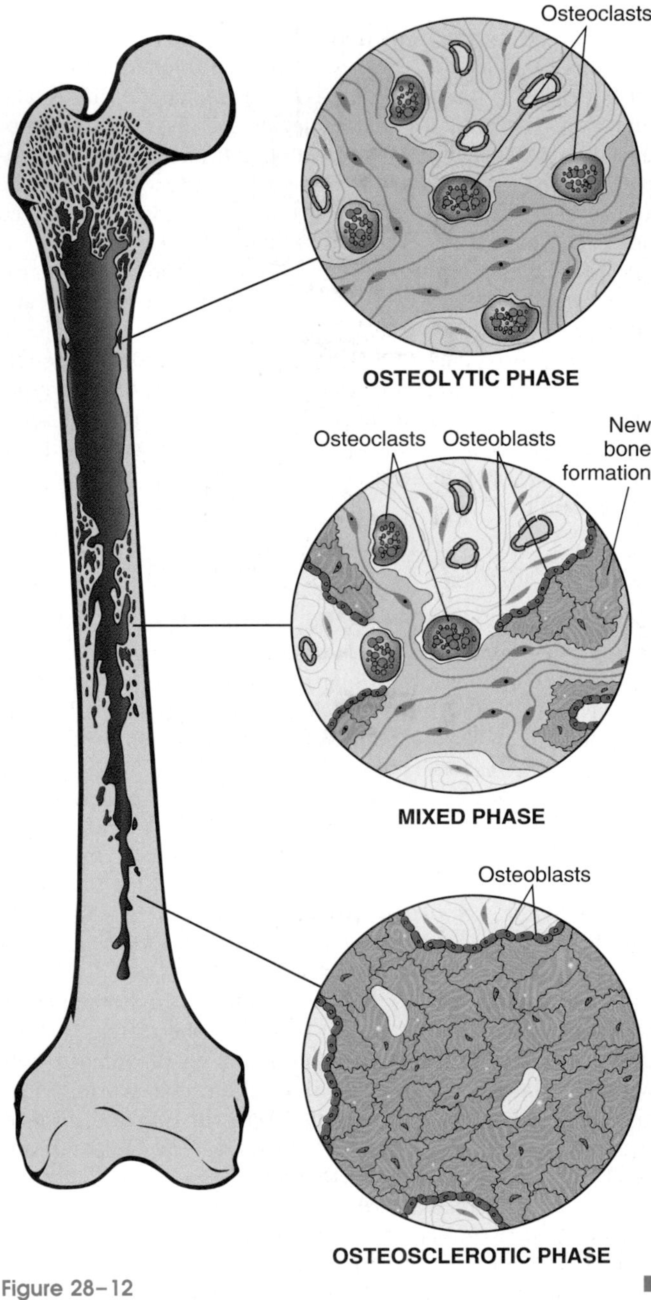

Figure 28–12

Diagrammatic representation of Paget disease of bone demonstrating the three phases in the evolution of the disease.

identified in the granulocyte-monocyte-colony forming unit cells, preosteoclasts, and peripheral blood mononuclear cells in patients with Paget disease.[19] One hypothesis suggests that the target of the virus is the osteoblast with permissive transmission to the osteoclast. The viral particles, however, have been identified only in the osteoclasts. Retroviruses such as the paramyxovirus can also induce the secretion of IL-6 from infected cells, and this cytokine is produced in large amounts by osteoblasts and is a potent stimulator of osteoclast recruitment and resorptive activity.[20] Intriguing as these observations may be, to date no virus has been isolated from affected tissue.

MORPHOLOGY. Paget disease is a focal process with remarkable variation in its stage of development in separate sites. The histologic hallmark is the **mosaic pattern** of lamellar bone. This pattern, which is likened to a jigsaw puzzle, is produced by prominent cement lines that anneal haphazardly oriented units of lamellar bone (Fig. 28–13*A*). In the initial lytic phase, there are the waves of osteoclastic activity and numerous resorption pits. The osteoclasts are abnormally large and have many more than the normal 10 to 12 nuclei; sometimes 100 nuclei are present. Osteoclasts persist in the mixed phase, but now many of the bone surfaces are lined by prominent osteoblasts. The marrow adjacent to the bone-forming surface is replaced by loose connective tissue that contains osteoprogenitor cells and numerous blood vessels, which transport nutrients and catabolites to and from these metabolically active sites. The newly formed bone may be woven or lamellar, but eventually all of it is remodeled into lamellar bone. As the mosaic pattern unfolds and the cell activity decreases, the fibrovascular lining tissue recedes and is replaced by normal marrow. In the end, the bone becomes a caricature of itself: larger than normal and composed of coarsely thickened trabeculae (Fig. 28–13*B*) and cortices that are soft and porous and lack structural stability. These aspects make the bone vulnerable to deformation under stress and to fracture.

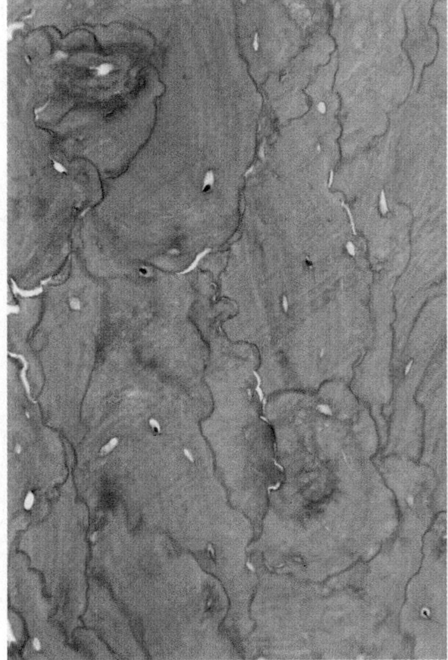

Figure 28–13

Mosaic pattern of lamellar bone pathognomonic of Paget disease.

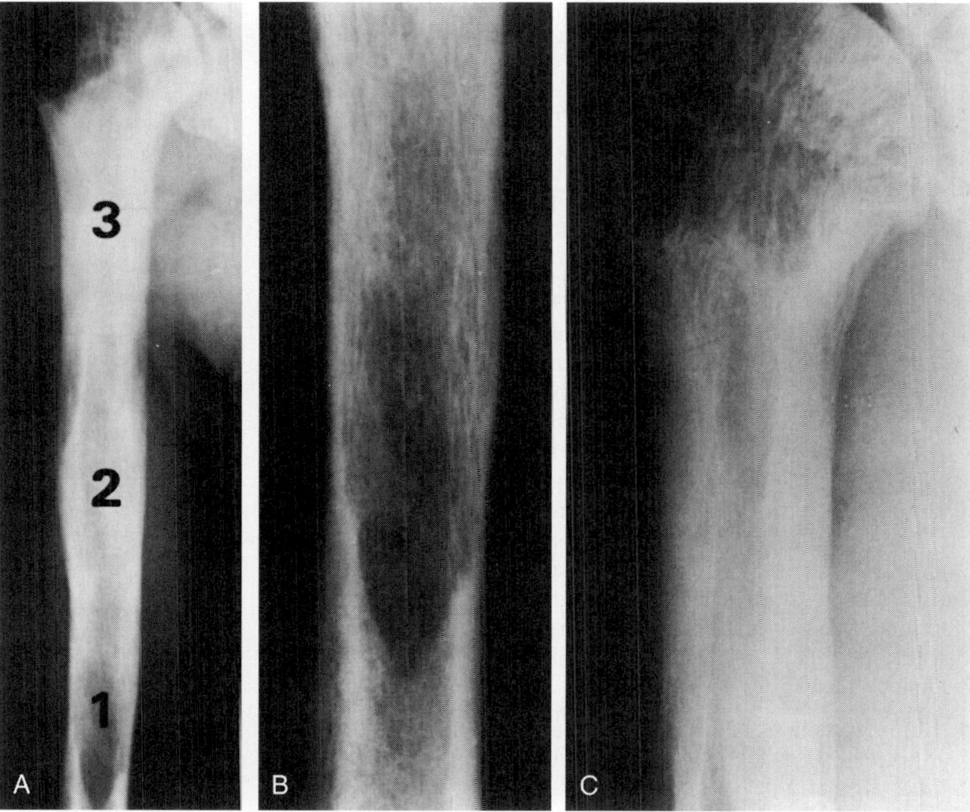

Figure 28–14

Paget disease of the humerus. *A*, The three sequential stages: (1) lytic, (2) mixed, and (3) sclerotic. *B*, Area 1, the lytic stage, is seen in close-up. Area 2, the mixed stage (*upper portion of B*) reveals central and endosteal cortical resorption and replacement by less compact new bone. *C*, Area 3, the sclerotic stage, with irregular thickening of both cortical and trabecular bone. (From Maldague B, Malghem J: Dynamic radiologic pattern of Paget's disease of bone. Clin Orthop 217:127, 1987.)

Clinical Course. Paget disease occurs in one or more bones. It is monostotic (tibia, ilium, femur, skull, vertebra, humerus) in about 15% of cases and polyostotic (pelvis, spine, skull) in the remainder. The axial skeleton or proximal femur is involved in up to 80% of cases. Even though no bone is immune, involvement of the ribs, fibula, and small bones of the hands and feet is unusual.

The diagnosis can frequently be made from the radiographic findings. Pagetic bone is typically enlarged with thick, coarsened cortices and cancellous bone (Fig. 28–14). Many patients exhibit an elevated serum level of alkaline phosphatase and increased urinary excretion of hydroxyproline. Clinical findings are extremely variable and depend on the extent and site of the disease. Most cases are mild and are discovered as an incidental radiographic finding. Paget disease can, however, produce a variety of skeletal, neuromuscular, and cardiovascular complications.

Pain is the most common problem and is localized to the affected bone. It is caused by a combination of microfractures and bone overgrowth that compresses spinal and cranial nerve roots. Bone overgrowth in the craniofacial skeleton may produce *leontiasis ossea* and a cranium so heavy that it becomes difficult for the patient to hold the head erect. The weakened pagetic bone may lead to invagination of the base of the skull (*platybasia*) and compression of the posterior fossa structures. Weight bearing causes anterior bowing of the femora and tibiae and distorts the femoral heads, resulting in the development of *severe secondary osteoarthritis*. *Chalkstick-type* fractures are the next most common complication and usually occur in the long bones of the lower extremities. Compression fractures of the spine result in spinal cord injury and the development of kyphoses. The hypervascularity of pagetic bone warms the overlying skin, and in severe polyostotic disease the increased blood flow behaves as an arteriovenous shunt leading to high-output heart failure or exacerbation of underlying cardiac disease.

A variety of tumor and tumor-like conditions develop in pagetic bone. The benign lesions include giant cell tumor, giant cell reparative granuloma, and extraosseous masses of hematopoiesis. The most dreaded complication is the development of sarcoma, which occurs in 5% to 10% of patients with severe polyostotic disease. The sarcomas are usually osteosarcoma, malignant fibrous histiocytoma, or chondrosarcoma,[21] and they arise in the long bones, pelvis, skull, and spine. In the absence of malignant transformation, Paget disease is usually not a serious or life-threatening disease. Most patients have mild symptoms that are readily suppressed by calcitonin and diphosphonates.

Diseases Associated With Abnormal Mineral Homeostasis

RICKETS AND OSTEOMALACIA

Rickets and osteomalacia represent a group of diseases of divergent causes that are characterized by a defect in matrix mineralization, most often related to a lack of vitamin D or some disturbance in its metabolism. The term *rickets* refers to the disorder in children in which deranged bone growth produces distinctive skeletal deformities. In the adult, the disorder is called *osteomalacia* because the bone that forms during the remodeling process is undermineralized. This results in osteopenia and predisposition to insufficiency fractures. Both rickets and osteomalacia are discussed in Chapter 10.

HYPERPARATHYROIDISM

Hyperparathyroidism is classified into primary and secondary types as discussed in Chapter 26. Primary hyperparathyroidism results from autonomous hyperplasia or a tumor, usually an adenoma, of the parathyroid gland, whereas secondary hyperparathyroidism is commonly caused by prolonged states of hypocalcemia resulting in compensatory hypersecretion of parathyroid hormone. Whatever the basis, the increased parathyroid hormone levels are detected by receptors on osteoblasts, which then initiate the release of mediators that stimulate osteoclast activity. Thus, through a chain of signals, the skeletal manifestations of hyperparathyroidism are caused by unabated osteoclastic bone resorption. The following points should be noted:

- Similar to all metabolic bone disease, the entire skeleton is affected in hyperparathyroidism, even though some sites are more severely affected than others.
- The anatomic changes of severe hyperparathyroidism, known as *osteitis fibrosa cystica*, are now rarely encountered because hyperparathyroidism is currently being diagnosed and treated at an early stage for reasons previously discussed.
- Secondary hyperparathyroidism is usually not as severe or as prolonged as primary hyperparathyroidism, hence the skeletal abnormalities tend to be milder.

MORPHOLOGY. For reasons unknown, the increased osteoclast activity in hyperparathyroidism affects cortical bone (subperiosteal, osteonal, and endosteal surfaces) more severely than cancellous bone. Subperiosteal resorption produces thinned cortices and the loss of the lamina dura around the teeth. The x-ray pattern, which is virtually diagnostic of hyperparathyroidism, is most frequently identified along the radial aspect of the middle phalanges of the index and middle fingers. Intracortical bone resorption is caused by a spearhead arrangement of osteoclasts that bore along and enlarge haversian and Volkmann canals. These cortical cutting cones are characteristic of hyperparathyroidism. In cancellous bone, osteoclasts tunnel into and dissect centrally along the length of the trabeculae creating the appearance of railroad tracks and producing what is known as **dissecting osteitis** (Fig. 28–15). The correlative radiographic finding is a decrease in bone density or osteopenia. Since bone resorption and formation are coupled processes, it is not surprising that osteoblast activity is also increased in hyperparathyroidism. In the regions of bone cell activity, the marrow spaces around the affected surfaces are replaced by fibrovascular tissue.

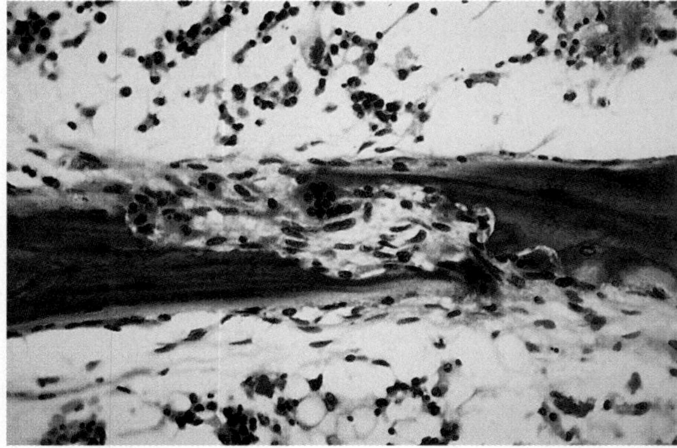

Figure 28–15

Hyperparathyroidism with osteoclasts boring into the center of the trabeculum (dissecting osteitis).

Microfractures and secondary hemorrhages occur that elicit an influx of multinucleated macrophages and an ingrowth of reactive fibrous tissue to create an apparent mass known as a brown tumor (Fig. 28–16). The brown color of this reactive lesion is the result of the vascularity, hemorrhage, and hemosiderin deposition. Frequently, these lesions undergo cystic degeneration. The combined picture of increased bone cell activity, peritrabecular fibrosis, and cystic brown tumors is the hallmark of severe hyperparathyroidism and is known as **generalized osteitis fibrosa cystica (von Recklinghausen disease of bone).**

The decrease in bone mass predisposes to fractures, deformities caused by the stress of weight bearing, and joint

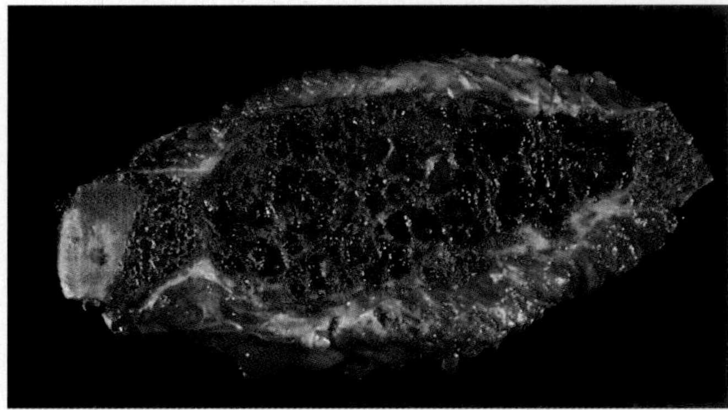

Figure 28–16

Resected rib, harboring an expansile brown tumor adjacent to the costal cartilage.

pain and dysfunction as the lines of normal weight bearing are altered. Control of the hyperparathyroidism allows the bony changes to regress significantly or disappear completely.

RENAL OSTEODYSTROPHY

The term *renal osteodystrophy* is used to describe collectively all of the skeletal changes of chronic renal disease, including (1) increased osteoclastic bone resorption mimicking osteitis fibrosa cystica, (2) delayed matrix mineralization (osteomalacia), (3) osteosclerosis, (4) growth retardation, and (5) osteoporosis. The interrelation between renal failure, secondary hyperparathyroidism, and altered vitamin D metabolism is well recognized, and as advances in medical technology have prolonged the lives of patients with renal diseases, their impact on skeletal homeostasis has assumed greater clinical importance.

The various changes are divided into two major types of bone disorders in patients with end-stage renal failure.[22] *High-turnover osteodystrophy* is characterized by increased bone resorption and formation with the former predominating. In contrast, *low-turnover or aplastic disease* is manifested by a marked reduction in the rate of bone mineralization, formation, and resorption. Many patients have a mixed pattern of disease.

Pathogenesis. The pathogenesis of the mix of skeletal lesions can be summarized as follows:

- Chronic renal failure results in *phosphate retention* and hyperphosphatemia.
- Hyperphosphatemia, in turn, induces *secondary hyperparathyroidism* because phosphate appears to regulate parathyroid hormone secretion directly.
- Hypocalcemia develops as the levels of vitamin D 1,25-dihydroxyvitamin D_3 (1,25-$[OH]_2D_3$) fall because of decreased conversion from the vitamin D metabolite 25-$(OH)D_3$ by damaged kidneys; inhibition of the renal hydroxylase involved in the conversion of 25-$(OH)D_3$ to the more active metabolite 1,25-$(OH)D_3$ by the high levels of phosphorus; and reduced intestinal absorption of calcium because of low levels of 1,25-$(OH)_2D_3$.
- Parathyroid hormone secretion markedly increases at all levels of serum calcium. 1,25-$(OH)_2D_3$ suppresses parathyroid hormone gene expression and secretion; in renal failure, there is a decrease in the binding of 1,25-$(OH)_2D_3$ to parathyroid cells; and there is decreased degradation and excretion of parathyroid hormone because of compromised renal function.
- The resultant *secondary hyperparathyroidism* produces increased osteoclast activity.
- *Metabolic acidosis* associated with renal failure stimulates bone resorption and the release of calcium hydroxyapatite from the matrix.
- Other factors that are important in the genesis of renal osteodystrophy are iron accumulation in bone and aluminum deposition at the site of mineralization. *Aluminum deposition,* in particular, has received a great deal of attention because of its iatrogenic origin. The sources of the aluminum include dialysis solutions prepared from water with a high aluminum content and oral aluminum-containing phosphate binders. The aluminum interferes with the deposition of calcium hydroxyapatite and hence results in osteomalacia. Aluminum is not only toxic to bone, but also has been implicated as the cause of dialysis encephalopathy and microcytic anemia in patients with chronic renal failure.
- Another complication seen in association with renal osteodystrophy is the deposition of masses of *amyloid* in bone and periarticular structures. The amyloid is formed from β_2-microglobulin, which is increased in the serum of patients who undergo long-term hemodialysis (Chapter 7).

Fractures

Traumatic and nontraumatic fractures are some of the most common pathologic conditions affecting bone. Fractures are classified as *complete* or *incomplete*; *closed (simple)*, when the overlying tissue is intact; *compound*, when the fracture site *communicates* with the skin surface; *comminuted*, when the bone is splintered; or *displaced*, when the ends of the bone at the fracture site are not aligned. If the break occurs in bone already altered by a disease process, it is described as a *pathologic fracture*. A *stress fracture* is a slowly developing fracture that follows a period of increased physical activity in which the bone is subjected to new repetitive loads—as in sports training or marching in military boot camp.

Bone is unique in its ability to repair itself; it can completely reconstitute itself by reactivating processes that normally occur during embryogenesis. This process is a highly regulated cascade that can be separated into overlapping histologic, biochemical, and biomechanical stages. The completion of each stage initiates the successive stage, and this is accomplished by a series of interactions and communications among the various cellular and acellular constituents of the healing zone.

- Immediately after fracture, rupture of blood vessels results in a hematoma, which fills the fracture gap and surrounds the area of bone injury. This also provides a fibrin mesh, which helps seal off the fracture site and at the same time serves as a framework for the influx of inflammatory cells and ingrowth of fibroblasts and new capillary vessels. Simultaneously, degranulated platelets and migrating inflammatory cells release PDGF, TGF-β, FGF, and ILs, which activate the osteoprogenitor cells in the periosteum, medullary cavity, and surrounding soft tissues and stimulate the production of osteoclastic and osteoblastic activity.[23] Thus, by the end of the first week, the hematoma is organizing, the adjacent tissue is being modulated for future matrix production, and the fractured ends of the bones are being remodeled. This fusiform and predominantly uncalcified tissue—called *soft tissue callus or procallus*—provides some anchorage between the ends of the fractured bones but offers no structural rigidity for weight bearing.
- Subsequently the activated osteoprogenitor cells deposit subperiosteal trabeculae of woven bone that are oriented

perpendicular to the cortical axis and within the medullary cavity. The activated mesenchymal cells in the soft tissues surrounding the fracture line may also differentiate into chondroblasts that make fibrocartilage and hyaline cartilage enveloping the fracture site. However, not all fractures contain cartilage as a component of the callus. In an uncomplicated fracture, the repair tissue reaches its maximal girth at the end of the second or third week, which helps stabilize the fracture site, but it is not yet strong enough for weight bearing. As the intramedullary and subperiosteal reactive woven bone approaches the newly formed cartilage along the fracture line, the cartilage undergoes enchondral ossification, such as normally occurs at the growth plate. In this fashion, the fractured ends are bridged by a *bony callus*, and as it mineralizes, the stiffness and strength of the callus increases to the point that controlled weight bearing can be tolerated (Fig. 28–17).

■ In the early stages of callus formation, an excess of fibrous tissue, cartilage, and bone is produced. If the bones are not perfectly aligned, the volume of callus is greatest in the concave portion of the fracture site. As the callus matures and transmits weight-bearing forces, the portions that are not physically stressed are resorbed, and in this manner the callus is reduced in size until the shape and outline of the fractured bone has been reestablished. The medullary cavity is also restored, and after this has been completed it may be impossible to demonstrate the site of previous injury.

The sequence of events in the healing of a fracture can be easily impeded or even blocked. Displaced and comminuted fractures frequently result in some deformity. The devitalized fragments of splintered bone require resorption, and this delays healing, enlarges the callus, and requires extremely long periods of remodeling so that in essence there is a permanent abnormality. Inadequate immobilization permits constant movement at the fracture site so that the normal constituents of callus do not form. Consequently the callus may be composed mainly of fibrous tissue and cartilage, perpetuating the instability and resulting in delayed union and nonunion. If a nonunion allows for too much motion along the fracture gap, the central portion of the callus undergoes cystic degeneration, and the

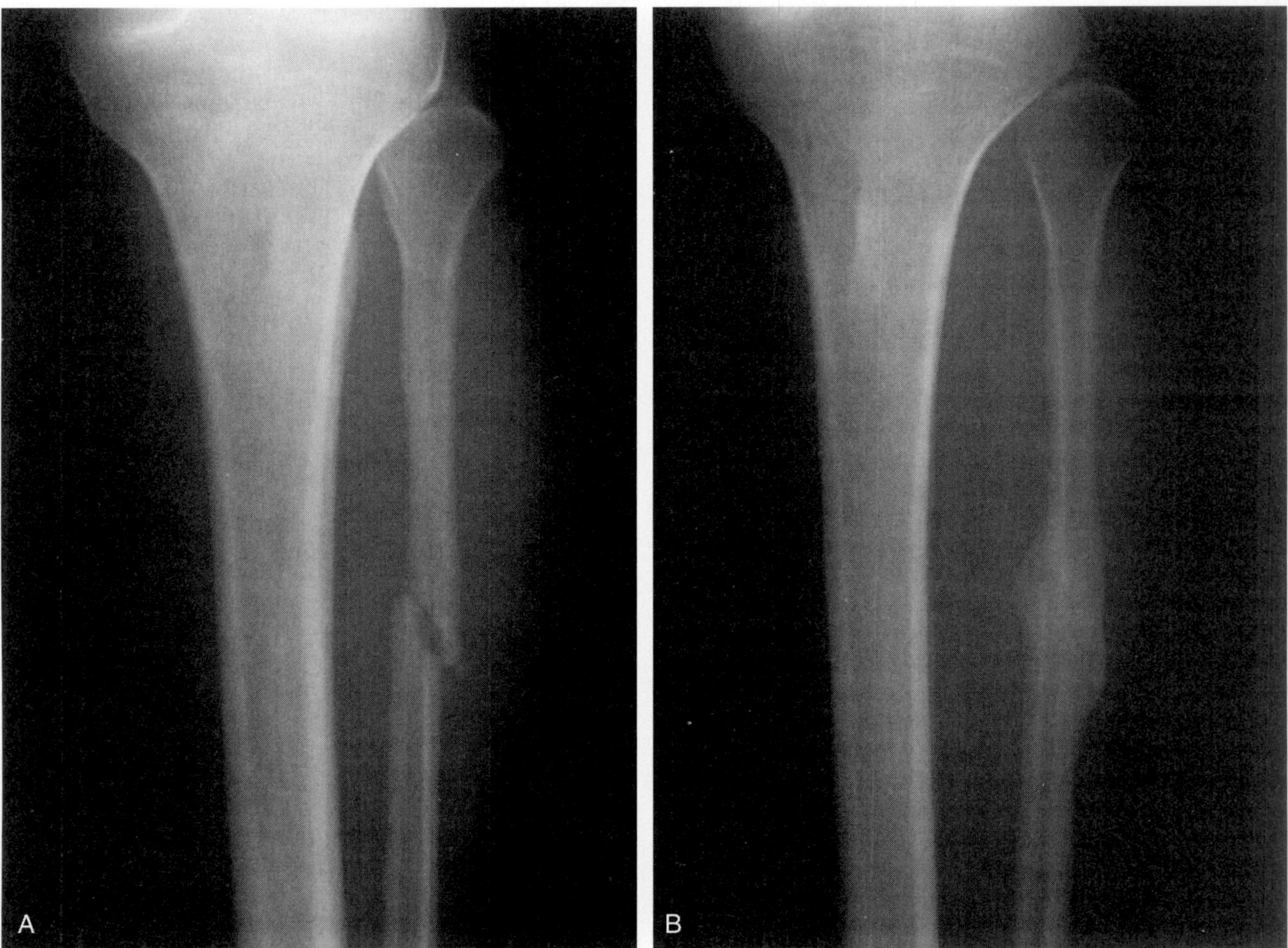

Figure 28–17

A, Recent fracture of the fibula. *B*, Marked callus formation 6 weeks later. (Courtesy of Dr. Barbara Weissman, Brigham and Women's Hospital, Boston, MA.)

Table 28-5. DISORDERS ASSOCIATED WITH OSTEONECROSIS

Idiopathic
Trauma
Corticosteroid administration
Infection
Dysbarism
Radiation therapy
Connective tissue disorders
Pregnancy
Gaucher disease
Sickle cell and other anemias
Alcohol abuse
Chronic pancreatitis
Tumors
Epiphyseal disorders

luminal surface can actually become lined by synovial-like cells creating a false joint or *pseudoarthrosis*. In the setting of a nonunion or pseudoarthrosis, the normal healing process can be reinstituted if the interposed soft tissues are removed and the fracture site stabilized. A serious obstacle to healing is *infection* of the fracture site, which is a risk in comminuted and open fractures. The infection must be eradicated before bony union can also be achieved. Bone repair can also be derailed by inadequate levels of calcium or phosphorus, vitamin deficiencies, systemic infection, diabetes, and vascular insufficiency.

Generally, with children and young adults, in whom most uncomplicated fractures are found, practically perfect reconstitution can be anticipated. In older age groups in whom fractures tend to occur on a background of some other disease (e.g., osteoporosis, osteomalacia), repair is less optimal and often requires mechanical methods of immobilization to facilitate healing.

Osteonecrosis (Avascular Necrosis)

Infarction of bone and marrow is a relatively common event and can occur in the medullary cavity of the metaphysis or diaphysis and the subchondral region of the epiphysis. All forms of bone necrosis result from ischemia. The mechanisms that produce ischemia are varied, however, and include (1) mechanical vascular interruption (fracture), (2) corticosteroids, (3) thrombosis and embolism (nitrogen bubbles in dysbarism) (Chapter 10), (4) vessel injury (vasculitis, radiation therapy), (5) increased intraosseous pressure with vascular compression, and (6) venous hypertension.[24] Nevertheless, although the disease states associated with bone infarcts are diverse (Table 28–5), in many the cause of the necrosis is uncertain. Aside from fracture, most cases of bone necrosis are either idiopathic or follow corticosteroid administration. The pathophysiology underlying steroid-induced bone infarcts is obscure. They follow high-dose steroid therapy for short periods, long-term administration of smaller doses, and even intra-articular injections.

MORPHOLOGY. The pathologic features of bone necrosis are the same regardless of the cause. In medullary infarcts, the necrosis is spotty and involves the cancellous bone and marrow. The cortex is usually not affected because of its collateral blood flow. In subchondral infarcts, a triangular or wedge-shaped segment of tissue that has the subchondral bone plate as its base and the center of the epiphysis as its apex undergoes necrosis. The overlying articular cartilage remains viable because it receives nutrition from the synovial fluid. The dead bone, recognized by its empty lacunae, is surrounded by necrotic adipocytes that frequently rupture, releasing their fatty acids, which bind calcium and form insoluble calcium soaps that may remain for life. In the healing response, osteoclasts resorb the necrotic trabeculae; however, those that remain act as scaffolding for the deposition of new living bone in a process known as **creeping substitution**. In subchondral infarcts, the pace of creeping substitution is too slow to be effective so there is eventual collapse of the necrotic cancellous bone and distortion of the articular cartilage (Fig. 28–18).

Clinical Course. The symptoms depend on the location and extent of infarction. Typically, subchondral infarcts cause chronic pain that is initially associated only with activity but then becomes progressively more constant until finally it is present at rest. In contrast, medullary infarcts are clinically silent except for large ones occurring in Gaucher disease, dysbarism, and hemoglobinopathies. Medullary infarcts usually remain stable over time and rarely are the site of malignant transformation. Subchondral infarcts, however, often collapse and may predispose to severe, secondary osteoarthritis. More than 10% of the 500,000 joint replacements performed annually in the United States are for treatment of the complications of osteonecrosis.

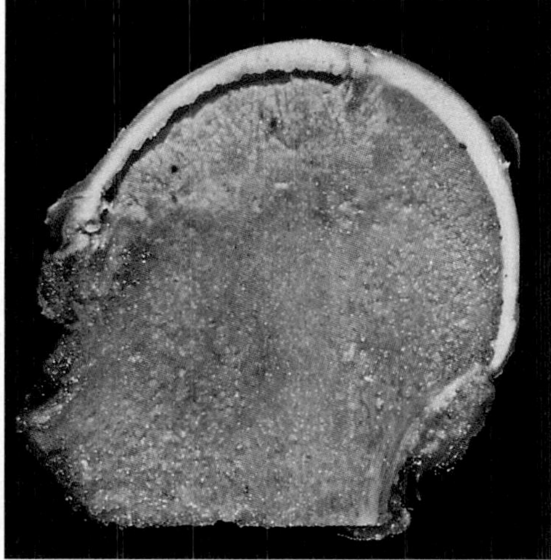

Figure 28–18

Femoral head with a subchondral, wedge-shaped pale yellow area of osteonecrosis. The space between the overlying articular cartilage and bone is caused by trabecular compression fractures without repair.

Infections—Osteomyelitis

Osteomyelitis denotes inflammation of bone and marrow, and the common use of the term virtually always implies infection. Osteomyelitis may be a complication of any systemic infection, but frequently manifests as a primary solitary focus of disease. All types of organisms, including viruses, parasites, fungi, and bacteria, can produce osteomyelitis, but infections caused by certain pyogenic bacteria and mycobacteria are the most common. Currently in the United States, exotic infections in third world immigrants and opportunistic infections in immunosuppressed patients have made the diagnosis and treatment of osteomyelitis ever more challenging.

PYOGENIC OSTEOMYELITIS

Pyogenic osteomyelitis is almost always caused by bacteria. Organisms may reach the bone by (1) hematogenous spread, (2) extension from a contiguous site, and (3) direct implantation. Most cases of osteomyelitis are hematogenous in origin and develop in the long bones or vertebral bodies in otherwise healthy individuals.[25] The initiating bacteremia may follow trivial occurrences, such as occult injury to the intestinal mucosa during defecation, vigorous chewing of hard foods, or minor infections of the skin.

Staphylococcus aureus is responsible for 80% to 90% of the cases of pyogenic osteomyelitis in which an organism is recovered. Its propensity to infect bone may be related to the fact that it expresses receptors to bone matrix components, thereby facilitating its adherence to bone tissue. *Escherichia coli*, *Pseudomonas*, and *Klebsiella* are more frequently isolated from patients with genitourinary tract infections or who are intravenous drug abusers. Mixed bacterial infections are seen in the setting of direct spread or inoculation of organisms during surgery or open fractures. In the neonatal period, *Haemophilus influenzae* and group B streptococci are frequent pathogens, and patients with sickle cell disease, for unknown reasons, are predisposed to *Salmonella* infection. In almost 50% of cases, no organisms can be isolated.

The location of the lesions within specific bones is influenced by the vascular circulation, which varies with age. In the neonate, the metaphyseal vessels penetrate the growth plate, resulting in frequent infection of the metaphysis, epiphysis, or both. In children, localization of microorganisms in the metaphysis is typical. After growth plate closure, the metaphyseal vessels reunite with their epiphyseal counterparts and provide a route for the bacteria to seed the epiphyses and subchondral regions in the adult.

MORPHOLOGY. The morphologic changes in osteomyelitis depend on the stage (acute, subacute, or chronic) and location of the infection. Once localized in bone, the bacteria proliferate and induce an acute inflammatory reaction and cause cell death. The entrapped bone undergoes necrosis within the first 48 hours, and the bacteria and inflammation spread within the shaft of the bone and may percolate throughout the haversian systems to reach the periosteum. In children, the periosteum is loosely attached to the cortex; therefore sizable **subperiosteal** abscesses may form, which can trek for long distances along the bone surface. Lifting of the periosteum further impairs the blood supply to the affected region, and both the suppurative and the ischemic injury may cause segmental bone necrosis; the dead piece of bone is known as the **sequestrum**. Rupture of the periosteum leads to a soft tissue abscess and the eventual formation of a **draining sinus**. Sometimes the sequestrum crumbles and forms free foreign bodies that pass through the sinus tract.

In infants but uncommonly in adults, epiphyseal infection spreads through the articular surface or along capsular and tendoligamentous insertions into a joint, to produce septic or suppurative arthritis, sometimes causing extensive destruction of the articular cartilage and permanent disability. An analogous process involves the vertebrae in which the infection destroys the hyaline cartilage end plate and intervertebral discs and spreads into adjacent vertebrae.

Over time, the host response evolves, and after the first week of infection chronic inflammatory cells become more numerous and their release of cytokines stimulates osteoclastic bone resorption, ingrowth of fibrous tissue, and the deposition of reactive bone in the periphery. In the presence of a sequestrum, the reactive woven or lamellar bone may be deposited as a sleeve of living tissue known as the *involucrum*, around the segment of devitalized bone (Fig. 28–19). Several

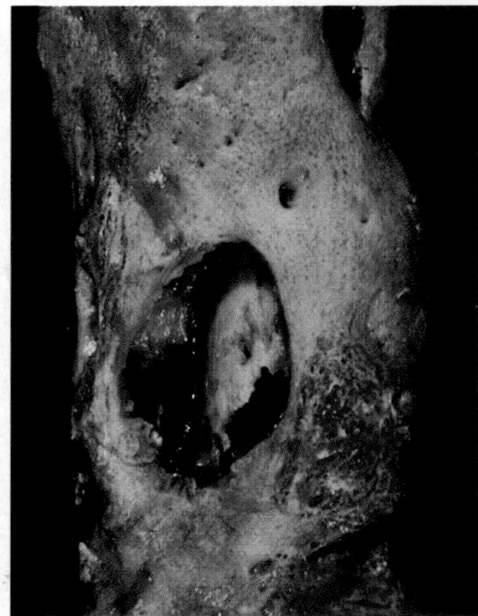

Figure 28–19 ■

Resected femur in a patient with draining osteomyelitis. The drainage tract in the subperiosteal shell of viable new bone (involucrum) reveals the inner native necrotic cortex (sequestrum).

morphologic variants of osteomyelitis have been given eponyms because of their distinguishing features: *Brodie abscess* is a small intraosseous abscess that frequently involves the cortex and is walled off by reactive bone; *sclerosing osteomyelitis of Garré* typically develops in the jaw and is associated with extensive new bone formation that obscures much of the underlying osseous structure.

Clinical Course. Clinically, hematogenous osteomyelitis may manifest as an acute systemic illness with malaise, fever, chills, leukocytosis, and marked-to-intense throbbing pain over the affected region. The presentation may be more subtle with only unexplained fever, particularly in infants, or only localized pain in the absence of fever in the adult. The diagnosis can be strongly suggested by the characteristic x-ray findings of a lytic focus of bone destruction surrounded by a zone of sclerosis. In many untreated cases, blood cultures are positive, but biopsy and bone cultures are required to identify the pathogen in most instances. The combination of antibiotics and surgical drainage is usually curative. In 5% to 25% of cases, acute osteomyelitis fails to resolve and persists as chronic infection. Chronicity may develop when there is delay in diagnosis, extensive bone necrosis, abbreviated antibiotic therapy, inadequate surgical debridement, and weakened host defenses. Acute flare-ups may mark the clinical course of chronic infection. They can occur after years of dormancy, are usually spontaneous, and have no obvious cause. Other complications of chronic osteomyelitis include pathologic fracture, secondary amyloidosis, endocarditis, sepsis, development of squamous cell carcinoma in the sinus tract, and rarely sarcoma in the infected bone.

TUBERCULOUS OSTEOMYELITIS

A resurgence of tuberculous osteomyelitis is occurring in industrialized nations, attributed to the influx of immigrants from third world countries and the greater numbers of immunosuppressed people. In developing countries, the affected individuals are usually adolescents or young adults, whereas in the indigenous population of the United States, the victims tend to be older except for those who are immunosuppressed. One per cent to 3% of patients with pulmonary or extrapulmonary tuberculosis have osseous infection.

MORPHOLOGY. The organisms are usually blood borne and originate from a focus of active visceral disease. Direct extension (e.g., from a pulmonary focus into a rib or from tracheobronchial nodes into adjacent vertebrae) or spread via draining lymphatics may also occur. The bony infection is usually solitary and in some cases may be the only manifestation of tuberculosis. Similar to the more common pulmonary form, it may fester for years before being recognized. In patients with acquired immunodeficiency syndrome (AIDS), the bone infection is frequently multifocal.

The spine (especially the thoracic and lumbar vertebrae) followed by the knees and hips are the most common sites of skeletal involvement. Tuberculous osteomyelitis tends to be more destructive and resistant to control than pyogenic osteomyelitis. The infection spreads through large areas of the medullary cavity and causes extensive necrosis. In the spine (**Pott disease**), the infection breaks through intervertebral discs to involve multiple vertebrae and extends into the soft tissues forming abscesses.

Typically, patients present with pain on motion, localized tenderness, low-grade fevers, chills, and weight loss. In remarkable cases, the patients may complain of an inguinal mass, which represents a cold fluctuant psoas abscess. Severe destruction of vertebrae frequently results in permanent compression fractures that produce significant scoliotic or kyphotic deformities and neurologic deficits secondary to spinal cord and nerve compression. Other complications of tuberculous osteomyelitis include tuberculous arthritis, sinus tract formation, and amyloidosis.

SKELETAL SYPHILIS

Syphilis (*Treponema pallidum*) and yaws (*Treponema pertenue*) both can involve bone. Currently, syphilis is experiencing a resurgence; however, bone involvement remains infrequent because the disease is readily diagnosed and treated before this stage develops.

In congenital syphilis, the bone lesions begin to appear about the fifth month of gestation and are fully developed at birth. The spirochetes tend to localize in areas of active enchondral ossification (osteochondritis) and in the periostium (periostitis). In acquired syphilis, bone disease may begin early in the tertiary stage, which is usually 2 to 5 years after the initial infection. The bones most frequently involved are those of the nose, palate, skull, and extremities, especially the long tubular bones such as the tibia. The syphilitic *saber shin* is produced by massive reactive periosteal bone deposition on the medial and anterior surfaces of the tibia.

MORPHOLOGY. The histology of congenital syphilitic bone infection is characterized by edematous granulation tissue containing numerous plasma cells and necrotic bone. This type of response is also seen in acquired syphilis. Gummata also occur in the acquired disease. The spirochetes can be demonstrated in the inflammatory tissue with special silver stains.

Bone Tumors and Tumor-like Lesions

Bone tumors are diverse in size and gross and histologic features and range in their biologic potential from the innocuous to the rapidly fatal. This diversity makes it critical to diagnose tumors correctly, stage them accurately, and treat them appropriately, so that the patients can not only survive, but also maintain optimal function of the affected body parts.

Most bone tumors are classified according to the normal cell or tissue type they recapitulate. Lesions that do not have normal tissue counterparts are grouped according to their distinct clinicopathologic features (Table 28–6). Overall, matrix-producing and fibrous tumors are the most common, and among the benign tumors, osteochondroma and fibrous cortical defect are most frequent. Excluding malignant neoplasms of marrow origin (myeloma, lymphoma, and leukemia), osteosarcoma is the most common primary cancer of bone, followed by chondrosarcoma and Ewing sarcoma.

The precise incidence of specific bone tumors is not known because many benign lesions are not biopsied. Benign tumors outnumber their malignant counterparts, however, by at least several hundred fold. Benign tumors have their greatest frequency within the first three decades of life, whereas in the elderly a bone tumor is likely to be malignant. In the United States, about 2100 new cases of bone sarcoma are diagnosed annually, and approximately 1300 deaths from bone sarcoma occur per year.

Although as a group these neoplasms affect all ages and arise in virtually every bone, specific types of tumors target certain age groups and anatomic sites.[26] For instance, most osteosarcomas occur during adolescence, and about half arise around the knee either in the distal femoral or proximal tibial metaphysis. These are the sites of greatest skeletal growth activity. In contrast, chondrosarcomas tend to develop in mid to late adulthood and to involve the trunk, limb girdles, and proximal long bones. Chondroblastomas and giant cell tumors almost always arise in the epiphysis of long bones, and in comparison, Ewing sarcoma, osteofibrous dysplasia, and adamantinoma most often arise in the diaphysis. Thus, the location of a tumor provides important diagnostic information.

Although the cause of most bone tumors is unknown, genetic alterations similar to those that occur in other tumors clearly play a role. For instance, bone sarcomas occur in the Li-Fraumeni and hereditary retinoblastoma cancer syndromes, which are linked to mutations in chromosomes *p53* and *Rb* (Chapter 8). Bone infarcts, chronic osteomyelitis, Paget disease, radiation, and metal prostheses are also associated with an increased incidence of bone neoplasia. Such secondary neoplasms, however, account for only a small fraction of all skeletal tumors.

Clinically, bone tumors present in various ways. The more common benign lesions are frequently asymptomatic and are detected as incidental findings. Many tumors, however, produce pain or are noticed as a slow-growing mass. In some circumstances, the first hint of a tumor's presence is a sudden pathologic fracture. Radiographic analysis plays an important role in diagnosing these lesions. In addition to providing the exact location and extent of the tumor, imaging studies can detect features that help limit diagnostic possibilities and give clues to the aggressiveness of the tumor. Ultimately in most instances, biopsy and histologic study are necessary. In addition to classifying the tumor, histologic *grade* must also be determined. This has been shown to be the most important prognostic feature of a bone sarcoma and has been incorporated into the major staging systems of bone neoplasms.

BONE-FORMING TUMORS

Common to all these neoplasms is the production of bone by the neoplastic cells. Except in osteoma, the tumor bone is usually deposited as woven trabeculae and is variably mineralized.

Table 28–6. CLASSIFICATIONS OF PRIMARY TUMORS INVOLVING BONES

Histologic Type	Benign	Malignant
Hematopoietic (40%)		■ Myeloma Malignant lymphoma
Chondrogenic (22%)	■ Osteochondroma Chondroma Chondroblastoma Chondromyxoid fibroma	■ Chondrosarcoma Dedifferentiated chondrosarcoma Mesenchymal chondrosarcoma
Osteogenic (19%)	■ Osteoid osteoma Osteoblastoma	■ Osteosarcoma
Unknown origin (10%)	■ Giant cell tumor	■ Ewing tumor Giant cell tumor Adamantinoma
Histiocytic origin	■ Fibrous histiocytoma	■ Malignant fibrous histiocytoma
Fibrogenic	■ Metaphyseal fibrous defect (fibroma)	■ Desmoplastic fibroma Fibrosarcoma
Notochordal		■ Chordoma
Vascular	■ Hemangioma	■ Hemangioendothelioma Hemangiopericytoma
Lipogenic	■ Lipoma	■ Liposarcoma
Neurogenic	■ Neurilemmoma	

Data on percentage of each type from Unni KK: Dahlin's Bone Tumors, 5th ed. Philadelphia, Lippincott-Raven, 1996, p 4; by permission of Mayo Foundation.

Osteoma

Osteomas are bosselated, round-to-oval sessile tumors that project from the subperiosteal or endosteal surfaces of the cortex. Subperiosteal osteomas most often arise on or inside the skull and facial bones. They are usually solitary and detected in middle-aged adults. Multiple osteomas are seen in the setting of *Gardner syndrome* (Chapter 18). They are composed of a composite of woven and lamellar bone that is frequently deposited in a cortical pattern with haversian-like systems. Some variants contain a component of trabecular bone in which the intertrabecular spaces are filled with hematopoietic marrow. Histologically the reactive bone induced by infection, trauma, or hemangiomas may simulate an osteoma and should be considered in the differential diagnosis.

Osteomas are generally slow-growing tumors of little clinical significance except when they cause obstruction of a sinus cavity, impinge on the brain or eye, interfere with function of the oral cavity, or produce cosmetic problems. Osteomas do not transform into osteosarcoma.

Osteoid Osteoma and Osteoblastoma

Osteoid osteoma and *osteoblastoma* are terms used to describe benign bone tumors that have identical histologic features but that differ in size, sites of origin, and symptoms. *Osteoid osteomas* are by definition less than 2 cm in greatest dimension and usually occur in the teens and twenties. Seventy-five per cent of patients are less than 25 years old, and men outnumber women 2 : 1. They can arise in any bone but have a predilection for the appendicular skeleton. Fifty per cent of cases involve the femur or tibia, where they commonly arise in the cortex and less frequently within the medullary cavity. Osteoid osteomas are painful lesions. The pain, which is caused by excess prostaglandin E_2 production, is severe in relation to the small size of the lesion and is characteristically nocturnal and dramatically relieved by aspirin.[28] *Osteoblastoma* differs from osteoid osteoma in that it involves the spine more frequently, the pain is dull, achy, and not responsive to salicylates, and it is not associated with a marked bony reaction.

MORPHOLOGY. Grossly, both osteoid osteoma and osteoblastoma are round-to-oval masses of hemorrhagic gritty tan tissue. Histologically, they are well circumscribed and composed of a morass of randomly interconnecting trabeculae of woven bone that are prominently rimmed by osteoblasts (Fig. 28–20). The stroma surrounding the tumor bone consists of loose connective tissue that contains many dilated and congested capillaries. The relative small size and well-defined margins of these tumors in combination with the benign cytologic features of the neoplastic osteoblasts helps distinguish them from osteosarcoma. Osteoid osteomas, especially those that arise beneath the periostium, usually elicit a tremendous amount of reactive bone formation that encircles the lesion. The actual tumor, known as the **nidus**, manifests radiographically as a small round lucency that is variably mineralized (Fig. 28–21).[27]

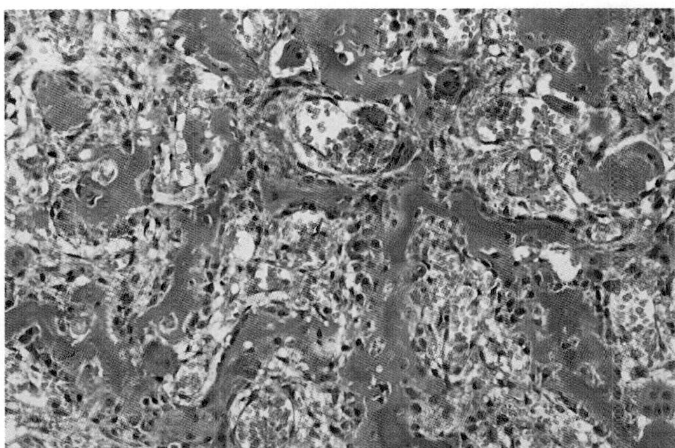

Figure 28–20

Osteoid osteoma composed of haphazardly interconnecting trabeculae of woven bone that are rimmed by prominent osteoblasts. The intertrabecular spaces are filled by vascular loose connective tissue.

Osteoid osteoma and osteoblastoma are readily treated by conservative surgery; if not entirely excised, they can recur. The possibility of malignant transformation is remote

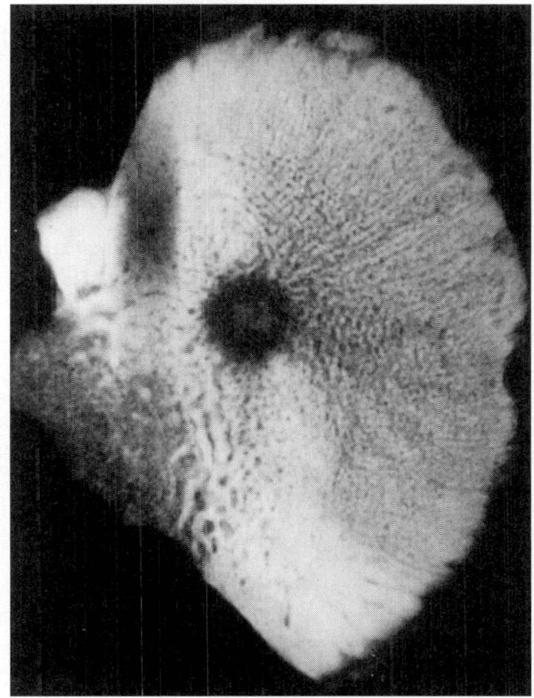

Figure 28–21

Specimen radiograph of intracortical osteoid osteoma. The round radiolucency with central mineralization represents the lesion and is surrounded by abundant reactive bone that has massively thickened the cortex.

except when treated with radiation, which promotes this dreaded complication.

Osteosarcoma (Osteogenic Sarcoma)

Osteosarcoma is defined as a malignant mesenchymal tumor in which the cancerous cells produce bone matrix. It is the most common primary malignant tumor of bone, exclusive of myeloma and lymphoma, and accounts for approximately 20% of primary bone cancers. Osteosarcoma occurs in all age groups but has a bimodal age distribution; 75% occur in patients younger than 20 years of age.[28] The smaller second peak occurs in the elderly, who frequently suffer from conditions known to be associated with the development of osteosarcoma—Paget disease, bone infarcts, and prior irradiation. Overall, men are more commonly affected than women (1.6 : 1). The tumors usually arise in the metaphyseal region of the long bones of the extremities, and almost 50% occur about the knee (Fig. 28–22). Any bone may be involved, however, and in persons beyond the age of 25, the incidence in flat bones and long bones is almost equal.

Pathogenesis. Genetic mutations are fundamental to the development of osteosarcoma. Patients with hereditary retinoblastomas have several hundred–fold greater risk of subsequently developing osteosarcoma, attributed to mutations in the *Rb* gene. Mutations in the *Rb* gene are uncommon in sporadic osteosarcoma. Mutations in *p53* are frequently present, however. Overexpression of MDM2 has been implicated in the genesis of nonhereditary osteosarcoma because it binds *p53* and inactivates its growth arrest and apoptotic functions[29] (Chapter 8). It is also noteworthy that many osteosarcomas develop at sites of greatest bone growth, where bone cell mitotic activity is at its peak. Large dog breeds such as St. Bernards and Great Danes have a high incidence of this type of tumor.

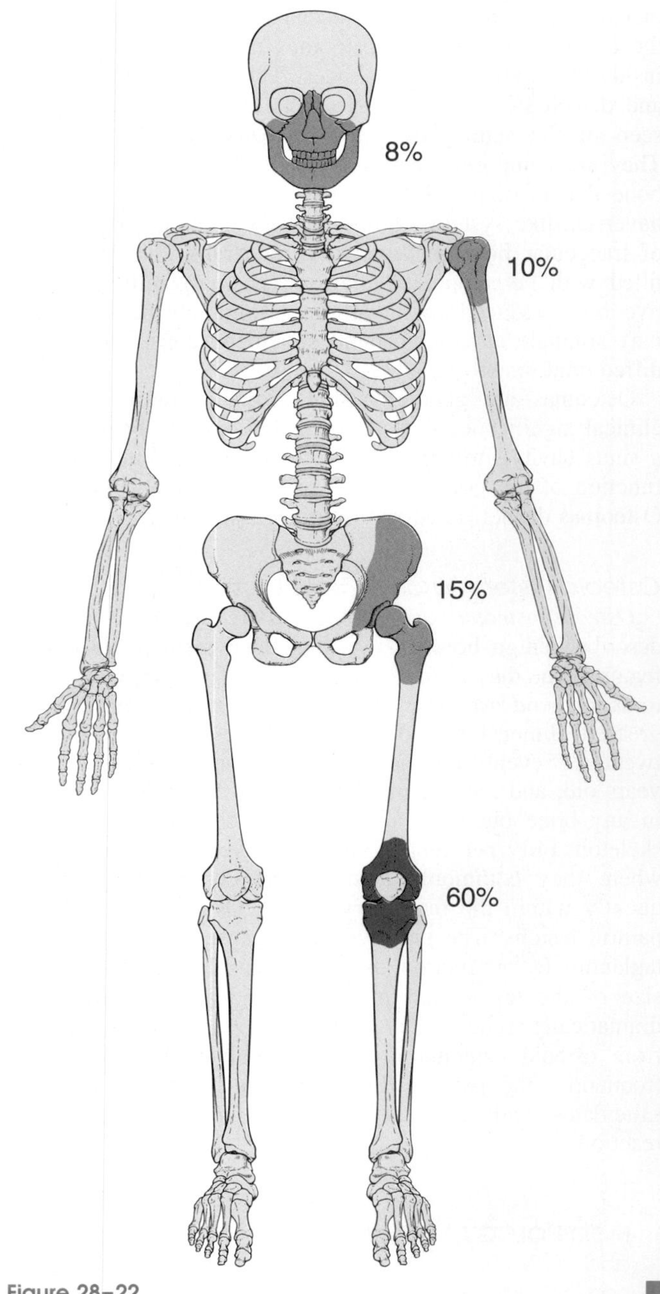

Figure 28–22

Major sites of origin of osteosarcomas. The numbers in parentheses are approximate percentages.

MORPHOLOGY. Several subtypes of osteosarcoma are described. They are grouped according to

- The anatomic portion of the bone from which they arise (intramedullary, intracortical, or surface)
- Degree of differentiation
- Multicentricity (synchronous, metachronous)
- Primary or secondary (e.g., osteosarcoma associated with preexisting disorders such as benign tumors, Paget disease, bone infarcts, previous radiation)
- Histologic variants (osteoblastic, chondroblastic, fibroblastic, telangiectatic, small cell, and giant cell)[30]

The most common subtype is osteosarcoma that arises in the metaphysis of long bones and is primary, solitary, intramedullary, and poorly differentiated and produces a predominantly bony matrix.

Grossly, osteosarcomas are big bulky tumors that are gritty, are gray-white, and often contain areas of hemorrhage and cystic degeneration (Fig. 28–23). The tumors frequently destroy the overlying cortex and produce a soft tissue mass. They spread widely in the medullary canal, infiltrating and replacing the marrow surrounding the preexisting bone trabeculae. Infrequently, they penetrate the epiphyseal plate or enter the joint. When joint invasion occurs, the tumor grows into it along tendinoligamentous structures or through the insertion site of the joint capsule. The tumor cells vary in size and shape and frequently have

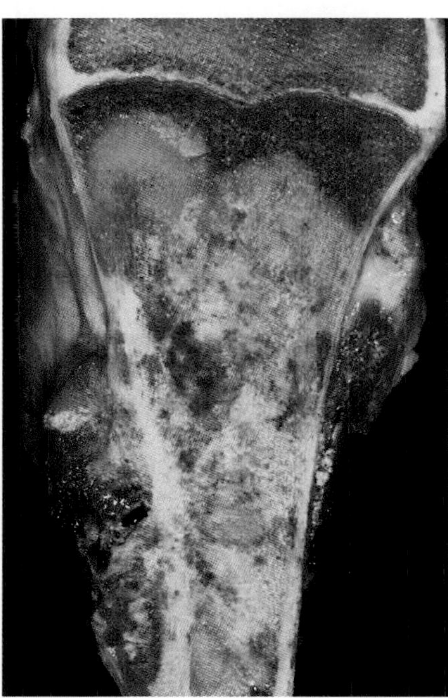

Figure 28–23

Osteosarcoma of the upper end of the tibia. The tan-white tumor fills most of the medullary cavity of the metaphysis and proximal diaphysis. It has infiltrated through the cortex, lifted the periosteum, and formed soft tissue masses on both sides of the bone.

large hyperchromatic nuclei. Bizarre tumor giant cells are common, as are mitoses. **The formation of bone by the tumor cells is most characteristic of osteosarcoma** (Fig. 28–24). The neoplastic bone has a coarse, lacelike architecture but is also deposited in broad sheets or as primitive trabeculae. Other matrices, including cartilage or fibrous tissue, may be present in varying amounts. When malignant cartilage is abundant, the tumor is called **chondroblastic osteosarcoma**. Vascular invasion is usually conspicuous, and up to 50% to 60% of an individual tumor may demonstrate spontaneous necrosis.

Clinical Course. Osteosarcomas typically present as painful and progressively enlarging masses. Sometimes a sudden fracture of the bone is the first symptom. These aggressive neoplasms spread through the bloodstream, and at the time of diagnosis, approximately 20% of patients have demonstrable pulmonary metastases. In those who die of the neoplasm, 90% have metastases to the lungs, bones, brain, and elsewhere. Radiographs of the primary tumor usually show a large destructive, mixed lytic and blastic mass that has permeative margins (Fig. 28–25). The tumor frequently breaks through the cortex and lifts the periosteum resulting in reactive periosteal bone formation. The triangular shadow between the cortex and raised ends of periostium is known radiographically as *Codman triangle* and is characteristic but not diagnostic of this tumor.

Advances in treatment have substantially improved the prognosis of osteosarcoma. Long-term survival is 60%, compared with previous rates of 25%.[31] Standard treatment now includes chemotherapy and limb-salvage therapy. An important factor determining chemosensitivity of the tumor cells is their expression of the *MDR1 gene product p-glycoprotein*, which mediates multidrug resistance. The expression of p-glycoprotein by tumor cells correlates with effectiveness of the chemotherapeutic drugs and prognosis (Chapter 8).

CARTILAGE-FORMING TUMORS

Cartilage tumors are characterized by the formation of hyaline or myxoid cartilage; fibrocartilage and elastic cartilage are rare components. As in most types of bone tumors, benign cartilage tumors are much more common than malignant ones.

Osteochondroma

Osteochondroma, also known as an *exostosis*, is a benign cartilage-capped outgrowth that is attached to the underlying skeleton by a bony stalk. It is a relatively common lesion and can be solitary or multiple. Multiple osteochondromas occur in *multiple hereditary exostosis*, which is an autosomal dominant hereditary disease that is genetically heterogeneous. Involvement of chromosomes 8, 11, and 19 has been implicated in its genesis. Osteochondromas develop only in bones of endochondral origin and are believed to result from displacement of the lateral portion of the growth plate, which then proliferates in a direction diagonal to the long axis of the bone and away from the

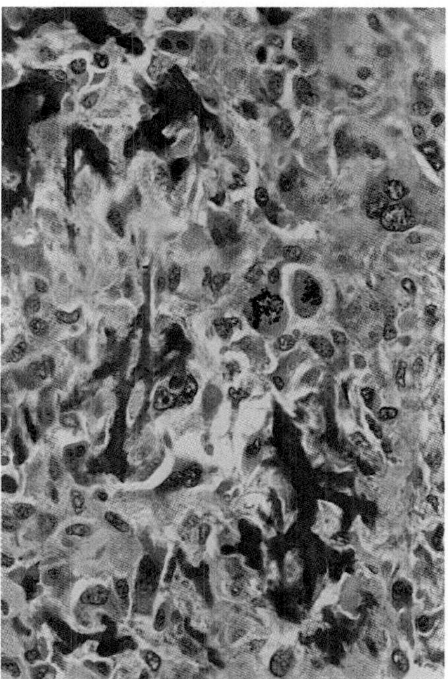

Figure 28–24

Coarse, lacelike pattern of neoplastic bone produced by anaplastic malignant tumor cells. Note the mitotic figures.

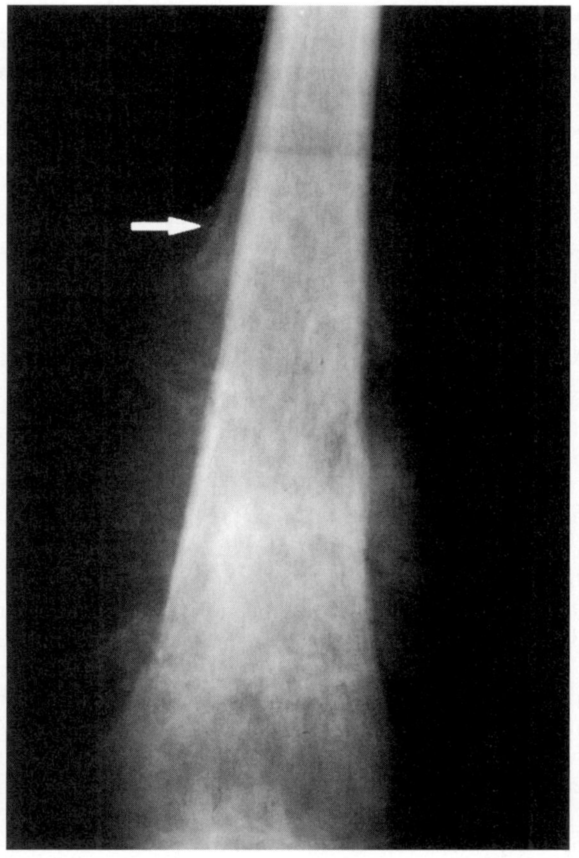

Figure 28–25

Distal femoral osteosarcoma with prominent bone formation extending into the soft tissues. The periosteum, which has been lifted, has laid down a proximal triangular shell of reactive bone known as a Codman triangle (*arrow*).

nearby joint (Fig. 28–26). Solitary osteochondromas are usually first diagnosed in late adolescence and early adulthood, but multiple osteochondromas become apparent during childhood. For unknown reasons, men are affected three times more often than women. Osteochondromas usually arise from the metaphysis near the growth plate of long tubular bones, especially about the knee. Occasionally, they develop from bones of the pelvis, scapula, and ribs, and in these sites they are frequently sessile and have short stalks. Rarely, these benign lesions involve the short tubular bones of the hands and feet.

MORPHOLOGY. Osteochondromas are mushroom shaped and range in size from 1 to 20 cm. The outer layer of the head of the osteochondroma is composed of benign hyaline cartilage varying in thickness and is delineated peripherally by perichondrium. The cartilage has the appearance of disorganized growth plate and undergoes enchondral ossification with the newly made bone forming the inner portion of the head and stalk. The cortex of the stalk merges with the cortex of the host bone so that the medullary cavity of the osteochondroma and bone are in continuity.

Clinically, osteochondromas present as slow-growing masses, which can be painful if they impinge on a nerve or if the stalk is fractured. In many cases, they are detected as an incidental finding. In multiple hereditary exostosis, the underlying bones may be bowed and shortened, reflecting an associated disturbance in epiphyseal growth. Osteochondromas usually stop growing at the time of growth plate closure. Rarely (less than 1% of cases), they give rise to a chondrosarcoma or some other type of sarcoma. The risk of this complication is substantially higher in patients with the hereditary syndrome.

Chondromas

Chondromas are benign tumors of hyaline cartilage. They may arise within the medullary cavity, where they are known as *enchondromas*, or on the surface of bone, where they are called *subperiosteal* or *juxtacortical chondromas*. Enchondromas are the most common of the intraosseous cartilage tumors. They are most frequent in the twenties to forties.

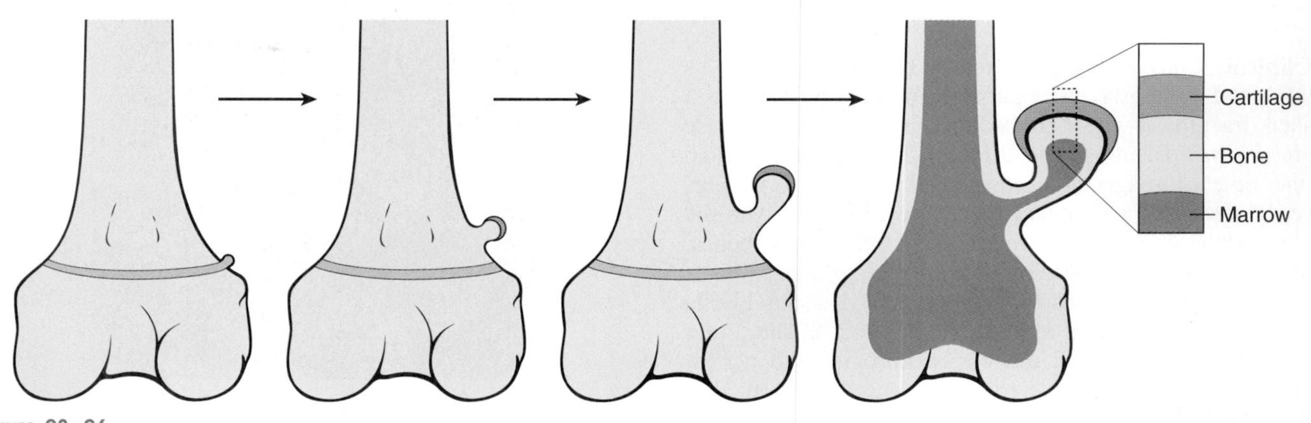

Figure 28–26

Schematic of the development over time of an osteochondroma, beginning with an outgrowth from the epiphyseal cartilage.

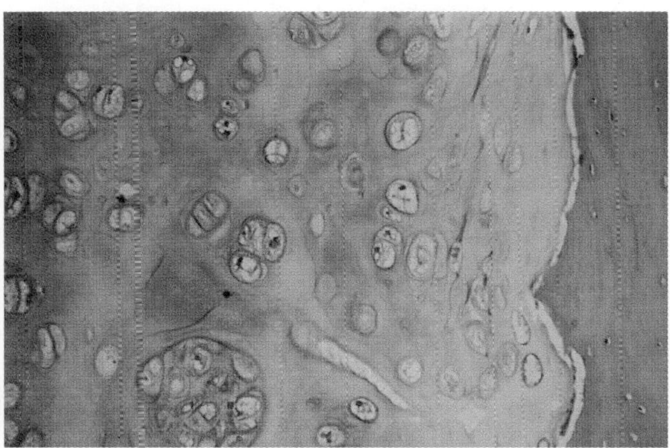

Figure 28–27

Enchondroma with a nodule of hyaline cartilage encased by a thin layer of reactive bone.

Enchondromas are usually solitary, located in the metaphyseal region of tubular bones, and the favored sites are the short tubular bones of the hands and feet.[32] *The syndrome of multiple enchondromas or enchondromatosis is known as Ollier disease. If the enchondromatosis is associated with soft tissue hemangiomas, the disorder is called Maffucci syndrome.* Chondromas are thought to develop from rests of growth plate cartilage that subsequently proliferate and slowly enlarge. Based on this theory, it is not surprising that these tumors arise mainly in bones that develop from enchondral ossification.

MORPHOLOGY. Enchondromas are usually smaller than 3 cm and grossly are gray-blue and translucent and have a nodular configuration. Microscopically the nodules of cartilage are well circumscribed, the nodules have a hyaline matrix, and the neoplastic chondrocytes that reside in lacunae are cytologically benign (Fig. 28–27). At the periphery of the nodules, the cartilage undergoes enchondral ossification, and the center frequently calcifies and dies. The chondromas in Ollier disease and Maffucci syndrome may demonstrate a greater degree of cellularity and cytologic atypia and may be difficult to distinguish from chondrosarcoma.

Most enchondromas are asymptomatic and are detected as incidental findings. Occasionally, they are painful and cause pathologic fracture. The cartilage tumors in enchondromatosis may be numerous and large, producing severe deformities. The radiographic features are characteristic, as the unmineralized nodules of cartilage produce well-circumscribed oval lucencies that are surrounded by a thin rim of radiodense bone (*O ring sign*).[31] If the matrix calcifies, it is detected as irregular opacities. The nodules scallop the endosteum, and in long bones they do not result in complete cortical destruction (Fig. 28–28). The growth potential of chondromas is limited, and most remain stable. They may recur if incompletely excised surgically. Solitary chondromas rarely undergo sarcomatous transformation, but those associated with enchondromatoses do so more frequently. Patients with Maffucci syndrome are at risk of developing other types of malignancies, including ovarian carcinomas and brain gliomas.

Chondroblastoma

Chondroblastoma is a rare benign tumor that accounts for less than 1% of primary bone tumors. It usually occurs in young patients in their teens with a male-to-female ratio of 2 : 1. Most arise about the knee. Less common sites such as the pelvis and ribs are affected in older patients. Chondroblastoma has a striking predilection for epiphyses and apophyses (epiphyseal equivalents, i.e., iliac crest).[33]

MORPHOLOGY. The tumor is cellular and is composed of sheets of compact polyhedral chondroblasts that have well-defined cytoplasmic borders, moderate amounts of pink cytoplasm, and nuclei that are hyperlobulated with longitudinal grooves (Fig. 28–29). Mitotic activity and necrosis are frequently present. The tumor cells are surrounded by hyaline matrix in a lacelike fashion; nodules of well-formed hyaline cartilage are distinctly uncommon. When the matrix calcifies, it produces a characteristic chicken-wire pattern of minerali-

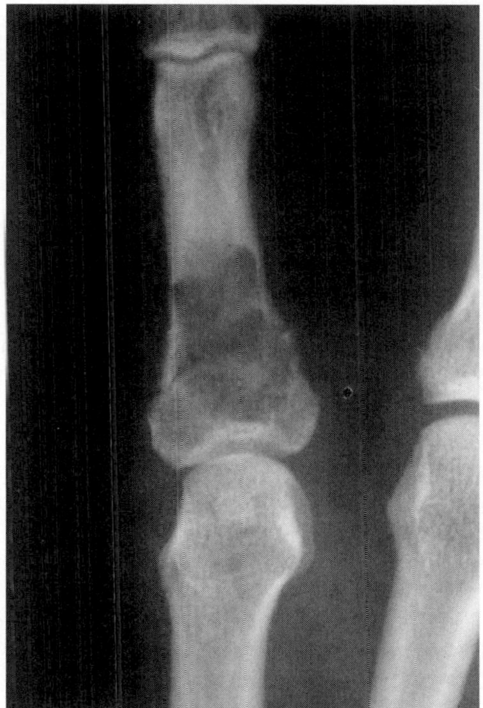

Figure 28–28

Enchondroma of the phalanx with a pathologic fracture. The radiolucent nodules of hyaline cartilage scallop the endosteal surface.

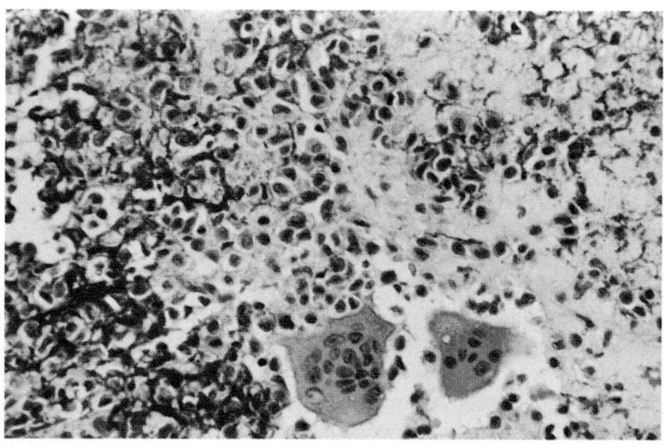

Figure 28–29

Chondroblastoma with scant mineralized matrix surrounding chondroblasts in a chicken wire–like fashion.

zation (Fig. 28–29). Scattered through the lesion are non-neoplastic osteoclast-type giant cells. Occasionally the tumors undergo prominent hemorrhagic cystic degeneration.

Chondroblastomas are usually painful, and because of their location near a joint they also cause effusions and restrict joint mobility. Radiographically, they produce a well-defined geographic lucency that commonly has spotty calcifications. Recurrences are not uncommon after surgical excision or curettage. Pulmonary metastases occur rarely in lesions that have undergone prior pathologic fracture or repeated curettage. Apparently, in these circumstances, the tumor cells are pushed into ruptured vessels, giving them access to the systemic circulation.

Chondromyxoid Fibroma

Chondromyxoid fibroma is the rarest of cartilage tumors and because of its varied morphology can be mistaken for sarcoma. It affects patients in their teens and twenties with a definite male preponderance. The tumors most frequently arise in the metaphysis of long tubular bones; however, they may involve virtually any bone of the body.

MORPHOLOGY. The tumors range from 3 to 8 cm in greatest dimension and are well circumscribed, solid, and glistening tan-gray. Microscopically, there are nodules of poorly formed hyaline cartilage and myxoid tissue delineated by fibrous septae. The cellularity varies; the areas of greatest cellularity are at the periphery of the nodules. In the cartilaginous regions, the tumor cells are situated in lacunae; however, in the myxoid areas, the cells are stellate, and their delicate cell processes extend through the mucinous ground substance and approach or contact neighboring cells (Fig. 28–30). In contrast to other benign cartilage tumors, the neoplastic cells in chondromyxoid fibroma show varying degrees of cytologic atypia, including the presence of large hyperchromatic nuclei. Other findings include small foci of calcification of the cartilaginous matrix and scattered non-neoplastic, osteoclast-type giant cells.[34]

Patients with chondromyxoid fibroma usually complain of localized dull, achy pain. In most instances, x-rays demonstrate an eccentric geographic lucency that is well delineated from the adjacent bone by a rim of sclerosis. Occasionally the tumor expands the overlying cortex. The treatment of choice is simple curettage, and even though they may recur, they do not pose a threat for malignant transformation or metastasis.

Chondrosarcoma

Chondrosarcomas comprise a group of tumors that have a broad spectrum of clinical and pathologic findings. The feature common to them all is the production of neoplastic cartilage. Chondrosarcoma is subclassified according to site as *intramedullary* and *juxtacortical* and histologically as *conventional (hyaline and/or myxoid), clear cell, dedifferentiated*, and *mesenchymal* variants.

Chondrosarcoma of the skeleton is about half as frequent as osteosarcoma and is the second most common malignant matrix-producing tumor of bone. Patients with chondrosarcoma are usually in their forties or older. The clear cell and especially the mesenchymal variants occur in younger patients, in their teens or twenties. The tumor affects men twice as frequently as women and has no race predilection. Although a significant number of conventional chondrosarcomas arise in association with a preexisting enchondroma, few develop within an osteochondroma, chondroblastoma, or fibrous dysplasia or in the setting of Paget disease.

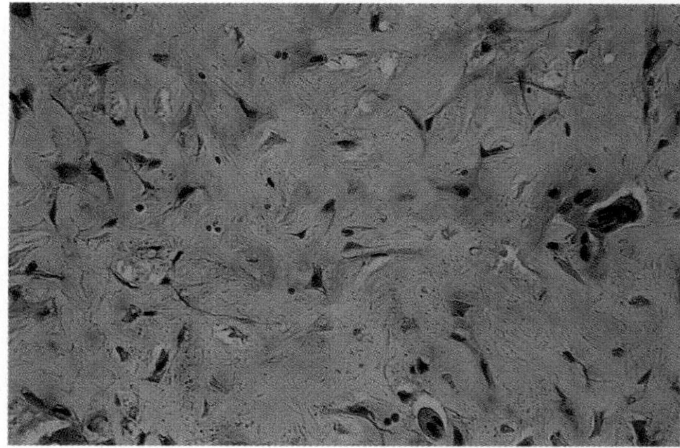

Figure 28–30

Chondromyxoid fibroma with prominent stellate and spindle cells surrounded by myxoid matrix. Occasional osteoclast-type giant cells are also present.

MORPHOLOGY. Conventional chondrosarcoma is composed of malignant hyaline and myxoid cartilage. The large bulky tumors are made up of nodules of gray-white, somewhat translucent glistening tissue (Fig. 28–31). In predominantly myxoid variants, the tumors are viscous and gelatinous and ooze from the cut surface. Spotty calcifications are typically present, and central necrosis may create cystic spaces. The adjacent cortex is thickened or eroded, and the tumor grows with broad pushing fronts into the surrounding soft tissue. The malignant cartilage infiltrates the marrow space and surrounds preexisting bony trabeculae. The tumors vary in degree of cellularity, cytologic atypia, and mitotic activity (Fig. 28–32). Low-grade or grade 1 lesions demonstrate mild hypercellularity, and the chondrocytes have plump vesicular nuclei with small nucleoli. Binucleate cells are sparse, and mitotic figures are difficult to find. Portions of the matrix frequently mineralize, and the cartilage may undergo enchondral ossification. By contrast, grade 3 chondrosarcomas are characterized by marked hypercellularity and extreme pleomorphism with bizarre tumor giant cells and mitoses. Pure grade 3 chondrosarcomas are uncommon. Such malignant cartilage is more frequently a component of **chondroblastic osteosarcoma** (see earlier).

Approximately 10% of conventional low-grade chondrosarcomas have a second high-grade component that has the morphology of a poorly differentiated sarcoma, such as malignant fibrous histiocytoma, fibrosarcoma, or osteosarcoma (dedifferentiated chondrosarcomas). The hallmark of **clear cell chondrosarcoma** is sheets of large malignant chondrocytes that have abundant clear cytoplasm, numerous osteoclast-type giant cells, and intralesional reactive bone formation. The last-mentioned aspect often causes confusion with osteosarcoma. **Mesenchymal chondrosarcoma** is composed of islands of well-differentiated hyaline cartilage surrounded by sheets of small round cells.

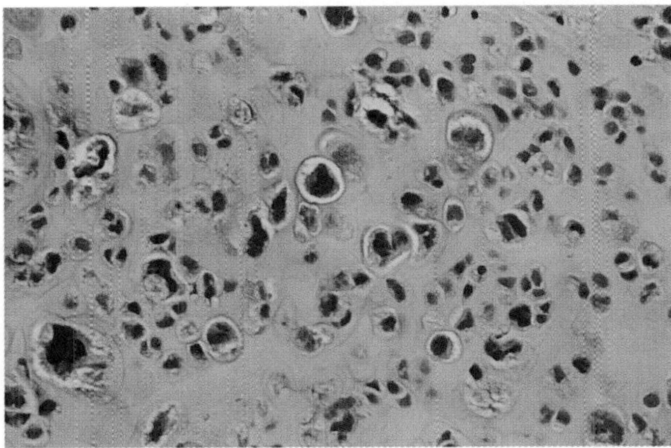

Figure 28–32

Anaplastic chondrocytes within a chondrosarcoma.

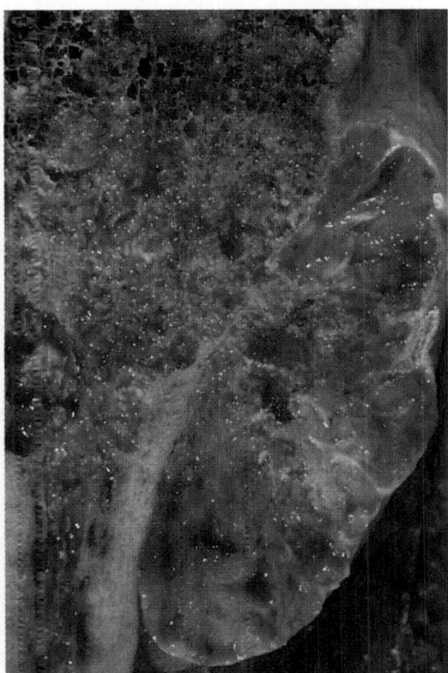

Figure 28–31

Chondrosarcoma with lobules of hyaline and myxoid cartilage permeating throughout the medullary cavity, growing through the cortex, and forming a relatively well circumscribed soft tissue mass.

Chondrosarcomas commonly arise in the central portions of the skeleton, including the pelvis, shoulder, and ribs. The clear cell variant is unique in that it originates in the epiphyses of long tubular bones. *In contrast to enchondroma, chondrosarcoma rarely involves the distal extremities.* These tumors usually present as painful, progressively enlarging masses. The nodular growth pattern of the cartilage produces prominent endosteal scalloping radiographically. The calcified matrix appears as foci of flocculent density. The more radiolucent the tumor, the greater the likelihood it is high grade. A slow-growing, low-grade tumor causes reactive thickening of the cortex, whereas a more aggressive high-grade neoplasm destroys the cortex and forms a soft tissue mass.[35] There is a direct correlation between the grade and the biologic behavior of the tumor. Fortunately, most conventional chondrosarcomas are indolent and fall into the range of grade 1 and grade 2. In one analysis, the 5-year survival rates were 90%, 81%, and 43% in grades 1 through 3. None of the grade 1 tumors metastasized, whereas 70% of the grade 3 tumors disseminated. Another prognostic feature is size. Tumors greater than 10 cm behave significantly more aggressively than smaller tumors. When chondrosarcomas metastasize, they spread preferentially to the lungs and skeleton. The treatment of conventional chondrosarcoma is wide surgical excision. The mesenchymal and dedifferentiated tumors are treated with chemotherapy in addition, because of their aggressive clinical course.

FIBROUS AND FIBRO-OSSEOUS TUMORS

Tumors composed solely or predominantly of fibrous elements are diverse and include some of the most common lesions of the skeleton.

Fibrous Cortical Defect and Nonossifying Fibroma

Fibrous cortical defects are extremely common, found in 30% to 50% of all children older than 2 years. They are believed to be developmental defects rather than neoplasms. The vast majority arise eccentrically in the metaphysis of the distal femur and proximal tibia, and almost one half are bilateral or multiple. Often, they are small, about 0.5 cm in diameter. Those that grow to 5 or 6 cm in size develop into *nonossifying fibromas* and are usually not detected until adolescence.

MORPHOLOGY. Both fibrous cortical defects and nonossifying fibromas produce elongated, sharply demarcated radiolucencies that are surrounded by a thin zone of sclerosis (Fig. 28–33). They consist of gray and yellow-brown tissue and are cellular lesions composed of fibroblasts and histiocytes.

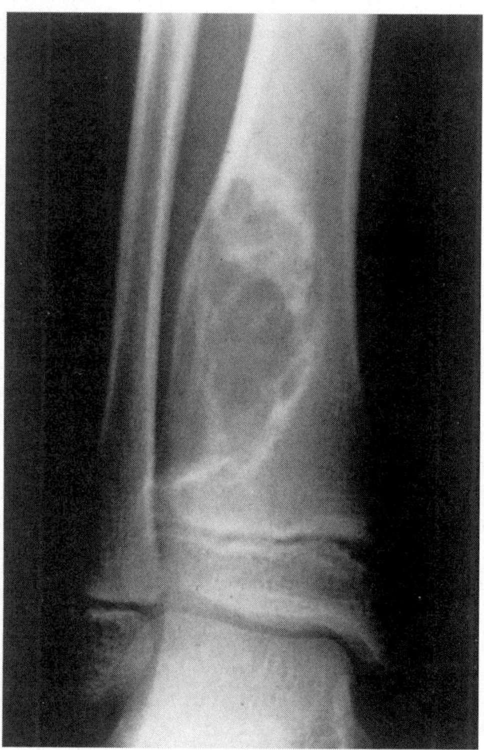

Figure 28–33

Nonossifying fibroma of the distal tibial metaphysis producing an eccentric lobulated radiolucency surrounded by a sclerotic margin.

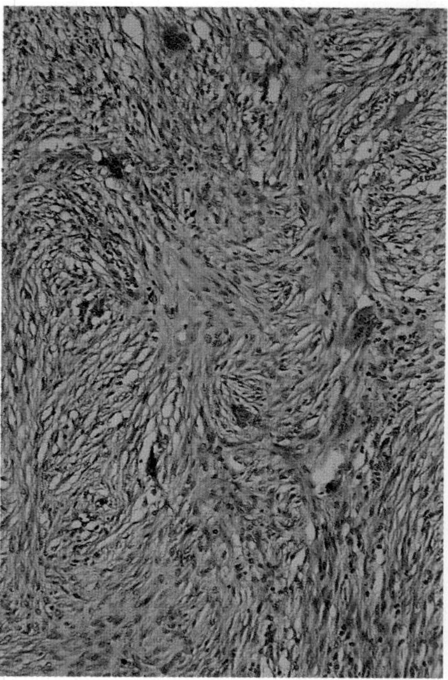

Figure 28–34

Storiform pattern created by benign spindle cells with scattered osteoclast-type giant cells characteristic of a fibrous cortical defect and nonossifying fibroma.

The cytologically benign fibroblasts are frequently arranged in a storiform (pinwheel) pattern, and the histiocytes are either multinucleated giant cells or clusters of foamy macrophages (Fig. 28–34).

Fibrous cortical defects are asymptomatic and are usually detected on x-ray as an incidental finding. The vast majority have limited growth potential and undergo spontaneous resolution within several years, being replaced by normal cortical bone. The few that progressively enlarge into nonossifying fibromas may present with pathologic fracture or require biopsy and curettage to exclude other types of tumors.

Fibrous Dysplasia

Fibrous dysplasia is a benign tumor-like lesion of bone that is best characterized as a localized developmental arrest; all of the components of normal bone are present, but they do not differentiate into their mature structures. The lesions appear in three distinctive but sometimes overlapping clinical patterns: (1) involvement of a single bone (monostotic); (2) involvement of multiple, but never all, bones (polyostotic); and (3) polyostotic disease, associated with café-au-lait skin pigmentations and endocrine abnormalities, especially precocious puberty.

Monostotic fibrous dysplasia accounts for 70% of all cases. It occurs equally in boys and girls, usually in early adolescence, and often stops growing at the time of growth plate closure. The ribs, femur, tibia, jaw bones, calvaria, and humerus are most commonly affected in descending order of frequency. The lesion is asymptomatic and usually discovered incidentally. Fibrous dysplasia can cause marked enlargement and distortion of bone, so that if the craniofacial skeleton is involved, disfigurement occurs. Monostotic disease does not evolve into the polyostotic form.

Polyostotic fibrous dysplasia without endocrine dysfunction accounts for 27% of all cases. It appears at a slightly earlier age than the monostotic type and may continue to cause problems into adulthood. The bones affected in descending order of frequency are the femur, skull, tibia, humerus, ribs, fibula, radius, ulna, mandible, and vertebrae. Craniofacial involvement is present in 50% of patients who have a moderate number of bones affected and in 100% of patients with extensive skeletal disease. All forms of polyostotic disease have a propensity to involve the shoulder and pelvic girdles resulting in severe, sometimes crippling deformities (e.g., shepherd-crook deformity of the proximal femur) and spontaneous and often recurrent fractures.

Polyostotic fibrous dysplasia associated with café-au-lait skin pigmentation and endocrinopathies is known as the McCune-Albright syndrome and accounts for 3% of all cases. The endocrinopathies and skeletal lesions result from a somatic (not hereditary) mutation occurring during embryogenesis and include sexual precocity, hyperthyroidism, pituitary adenomas that secrete growth hormone, and primary adrenal hyperplasia. The mutation involves the gene that codes for a guanine nucleotide–binding protein, and it results in the excess production of cyclic AMP leading to endocrine gland hyperfunction.[36] It has also been identified in the osseous lesions from patients without McCune-Albright syndrome but who have either the monostotic or polyostotic forms of the disease. The severity of manifestations in McCune-Albright syndrome depends on the number and cell types that harbor the mutation. The most common clinical presentation is precocious sexual development, and in this setting girls are affected more often than boys. The bone lesions are often unilateral, and the skin pigmentation is usually limited to the same side of the body. The cutaneous macules are classically large; are dark to café-au-lait; have irregular serpiginous borders (coastline of Maine); and are found primarily on the neck, chest, back, shoulder, and pelvic region.

MORPHOLOGY. Grossly the lesions of fibrous dysplasia are well circumscribed, are intramedullary, and vary greatly in size. Larger lesions expand and distort the bone. The lesional tissue is tan-white and gritty and is composed of curvilinear trabeculae of woven bone surrounded by a moderately cellular fibroblastic proliferation. The shapes of the trabeculae mimic Chinese letters, and the bone lacks osteoblastic rimming (Fig. 28–35). Nodules of hyaline cartilage with the appearance of disorganized growth plate are also present in approximately 20% of cases. Cystic degeneration, hemorrhage, and foamy macrophages are other common findings.

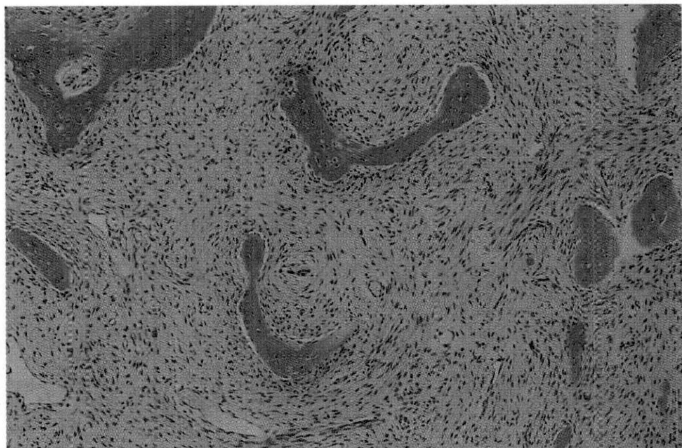

Figure 28–35

Fibrous dysplasia composed of curvilinear trabeculae of woven bone that lack conspicuous osteoblastic rimming and arise in a background of fibrous tissue.

Clinical Course. The natural history of fibrous dysplasia is variable and depends on the extent of skeletal involvement. Patients with monostotic disease usually have minimal symptoms. The lesion is readily diagnosed by x-ray because of its typical ground-glass appearance and well-defined margination. Lesions that fracture or cause significant symptoms are readily cured by conservative surgery. Polyostotic involvement is frequently associated with progressive disease, and the earlier the age at diagnosis, the more likely the skeletal complications are severe, such as recurring fractures, long bone deformities, and distorting involvement of the craniofacial bones. A rare complication usually in polyostotic involvement is malignant transformation of a lesion into a sarcoma, such as osteosarcoma, or malignant fibrous histiocytoma. The risk of this occurrence is increased if the lesion has been irradiated.

Fibrosarcoma and Malignant Fibrous Histiocytoma

Fibrosarcoma and malignant fibrous histiocytoma are fibroblastic collagen-producing sarcomas of bone. They have overlapping clinical, radiographic, and pathologic features, and their distinction is based on somewhat arbitrary morphologic criteria. They occur at any age, but most affect the middle-aged and elderly. Fibrosarcoma has a nearly equal sex distribution, whereas malignant fibrous histiocytoma occurs more frequently in men. Both sarcomas usually arise de novo; however, a minority are secondary tumors and develop in preexisting benign tumors, bone infarcts, pagetic bone, and previously radiated tissue.

MORPHOLOGY. Grossly, these tumors are large, hemorrhagic, tan-white masses that destroy the underlying bone and frequently extend into the soft tissues. Fibrosarcoma is composed of malignant fibroblasts arranged in a herringbone pattern. The level of differentiation determines the amount of collagen produced and degree of cytologic atypia. Bizarre multinucleated cells are not common, and most fibrosarcomas have the appearance of a low-to-intermediate-grade malignancy. Malignant fibrous histiocytoma consists of a background of spindled fibroblasts admixed with large, ovoid, bizarre multinucleated tumor giant cells. Morphologically, some tumor cells resemble neoplastic histiocytes; however, the evidence shows they are actually fibroblasts. Malignant fibrous histiocytoma of bone is generally a high-grade pleomorphic tumor.[37]

Fibrosarcoma and malignant fibrous histiocytoma present as enlarging painful masses that usually arise in the metaphyses of long bones and pelvic flat bones. Pathologic fracture is a frequent complication. Radiographically, they are permeative and lytic and often extend into the adjacent soft tissue. The prognosis of these two sarcomas depends on their grade; high-grade tumors have a poor prognosis.

Miscellaneous Tumors

EWING SARCOMA AND PRIMITIVE NEUROECTODERMAL TUMOR

Ewing sarcoma is a primary malignant *small round cell tumor* of bone (Chapter 11). It has long posed a difficult diagnostic problem because the tumors resemble those of lymphoma, rhabdomyosarcoma, neuroblastoma, and oat cell carcinoma.[38] Current evidence indicates that Ewing sarcoma tumor cells exhibit a neural phenotype. The expression of the oncogene c-*myc* and the identification of a specific chromosome translocation in both Ewing sarcoma and similar tumors of soft tissue, called *primitive neuroectodermal tumors* (*PNET*), further support this contention. Thus, Ewing sarcoma and PNET of bone are closely related tumors that differ in their degree of differentiation. Tumors that demonstrate neural differentiation by light microscopy, immunohistochemistry, or electron microscopy are labeled PNETs, and those that are undifferentiated by these analyses are diagnosed as Ewing sarcoma.

Ewing sarcoma and PNET account for approximately 6% to 10% of primary malignant bone tumors and follow osteosarcoma as the second most common group of bone sarcomas in children. Of all bone sarcomas, Ewing sarcoma has the youngest average age at presentation as most patients are 10 to 15 years old, and approximately 80% are younger than 20 years. Boys are affected slightly more frequently than girls, and there is a striking predilection for whites; blacks are rarely afflicted. In approximately 85% of Ewing sarcomas and PNETs, there is a t(11;22)(q24;q12) translocation; in 5% to 10% of cases, the translocation is t(21;21)(q21;q12); and in less than 1% of tumors, a t(7;22)(q22;12) translocation is present. Evidence suggests that the fusion genes (EWS-FLI1) generated from these translocations act as dominant oncogenes, and the chimeric proteins are transcription factors playing roles in tumor cell proliferation.[39]

MORPHOLOGY. Arising in the medullary cavity, Ewing sarcoma usually invades the cortex and periosteum producing a soft tissue mass. The tumor is tan-white and frequently contains areas of hemorrhage and necrosis. It is composed of sheets of uniform small, round cells that are slightly larger than lymphocytes (Fig. 28–36). They have scant cytoplasm, which may appear clear because it is rich in glycogen. The presence of Homer-Wright rosettes (where the tumor cells are arranged in a circle about a central fibrillary space) is indicative of neural differentiation. Although the tumor contains fibrous septae, there is generally little stroma. Necrosis may be prominent, and there are relatively few mitotic figures in relation to the dense cellularity of the tumor.

Ewing sarcoma usually arises in the diaphysis of long tubular bones, especially the femur and the flat bones of the pelvis. It presents as a painful enlarging mass, and the affected site is frequently tender, warm, and swollen. Some patients have systemic findings, including fever, elevated sedimentation rate, anemia, and leukocytosis, which mimic infection. Plain x-rays show a destructive lytic tumor that has permeative margins. The characteristic periosteal reaction produces layers of reactive bone deposited in an *onion-skin* fashion.

The treatment of Ewing sarcoma includes chemotherapy and surgery with or without radiation. The advent of effective chemotherapy has dramatically improved the prognosis from a dismal 5% to 15% to a 75% 5-year survival; at least 50% are long-term cures.

GIANT CELL TUMOR

Giant cell tumor is so named because it contains a profusion of multinucleated osteoclast type giant cells, giving rise to the synonym *osteoclastoma*. Giant cell tumor is a

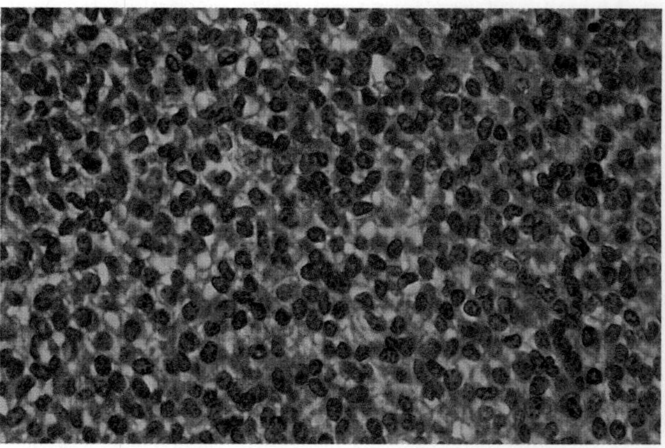

Figure 28–36 ■

Ewing sarcoma composed of sheets of small round cells with small amounts of clear cytoplasm.

relatively uncommon benign but locally aggressive neoplasm. It usually arises during the twenties to forties. Giant cell tumors are postulated to have a monocyte-macrophage lineage,[40] and the giant cells are believed to form via fusion of mononuclear cells.

MORPHOLOGY. These tumors are large and red-brown and frequently undergo cystic degeneration. They are composed of uniform oval mononuclear cells that have indistinct cell membranes and appear to grow in a syncytium. The mononuclear cells are the proliferating component of the tumor, and mitoses are frequent. Scattered within this background are numerous osteoclast-type giant cells having 100 or more nuclei that are identical to those of the mononuclear cells (Fig. 28–37). Necrosis, hemorrhage, hemosiderin deposition, and reactive bone formation are common secondary features. The histologic differential diagnosis includes other giant cell lesions, such as the brown tumor seen in hyperparathyroidism, giant cell reparative granuloma, chondroblastoma, and pigmented villonodular synovitis. The morphologic identity between the nuclei of the stromal cells and those of the giant cells helps distinguish giant cell tumor from these other lesions.

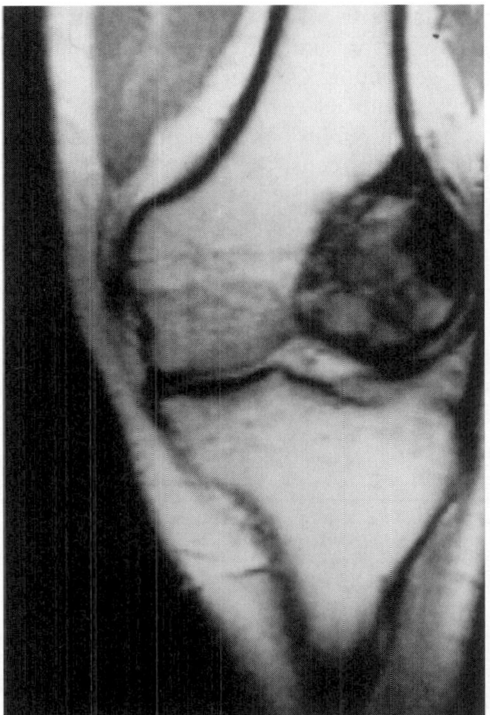

Figure 28–38

Magnetic resonance image of a giant cell tumor that replaces most of the femoral condyle and extends to the subchondral bone plate.

Clinical Course. Giant cell tumors in adults involve both the epiphyses and the metaphyses, but in adolescents they are confined proximally by the growth plate and are limited to the metaphysis. The majority of giant cell tumors arise around the knee (distal femur and proximal tibia), but virtually any bone may be involved. The location of these tumors in the ends of bones near joints frequently causes patients to complain of arthritic symptoms. Occasionally, they present as pathologic fractures. Most are solitary; however, multiple or multicentric tumors do occur, especially in the distal extremities. Radiographically, giant cell tumors are large, purely lytic, and eccentric and erode into the subchondral bone plate (Fig. 28–38). The overlying cortex is frequently destroyed producing a bulging soft tissue mass delineated by a thin shell of reactive bone. The margins with the adjacent bone are fairly circumscribed but seldom sclerotic. The biologic unpredictability of these neoplasms complicates their management. Conservative surgery such as curettage is associated with a 40% to 60% recurrence rate. Up to 4% metastasize to the lungs. The metastatic deposits have the same morphology as the primary tumor. Sarcomatous transformation of a giant cell tumor, either de novo or after previous treatment, is a rare event.

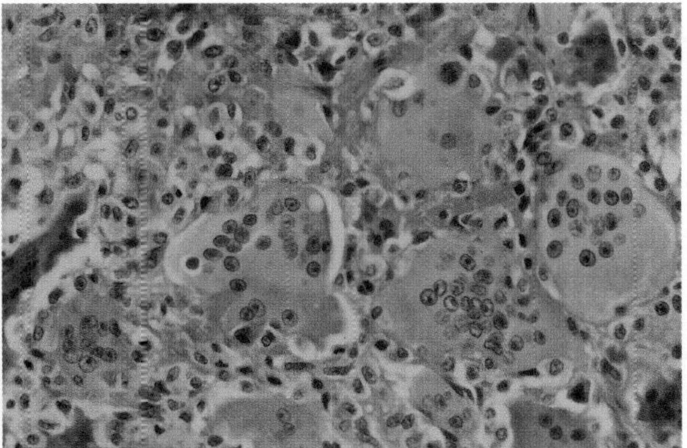

Figure 28–37

Benign giant cell tumor illustrating an abundance of multinucleated giant cells with background mononuclear stromal cells.

METASTATIC DISEASE

Metastatic tumors are the most common form of skeletal malignancy. The pathways of spread include (1) direct extension, (2) lymphatic or vascular dissemination, and (3) intraspinal seeding (Batson plexus of veins). Any cancer can spread to bone, but in adults, more than 75% of skeletal metastases originate from cancers of the prostate, breast, kidney, and lung. In children, metastases to bone originate from neuroblastoma, Wilms' tumor, osteosarcoma, Ewing sarcoma, and rhabdomyosarcoma.

Skeletal metastases are typically multifocal; however, carcinomas of the kidney and thyroid are notorious for producing solitary lesions. The metastases may occur in any bone, but most involve the axial skeleton (vertebral column, pelvis, ribs, skull, sternum), proximal femur, and humerus in descending order of frequency. The red marrow in these areas with its rich capillary network, slow blood flow, and nutrient environment facilitates implantation and growth of the tumor cells. Metastases to the small bones of the hands and feet are uncommon and usually originate in cancers of the lung, kidney, or colon.

The radiographic manifestations of metastases may be purely lytic, purely blastic, or mixed lytic and blastic. In lytic lesions, the metastatic cells secrete substances such as prostaglandins, ILs, and parathyroid hormone–related protein that stimulate osteoclastic bone resorption; the tumor cells themselves do not directly resorb bone. Carcinomas of the kidney, lung, and gastrointestinal tract and malignant melanoma produce this type of bone destruction. Similarly, metastases that elicit a sclerotic response, particularly prostate adenocarcinoma, do so by stimulating osteoblastic bone formation. Most metastases induce a mixed lytic and blastic reaction.

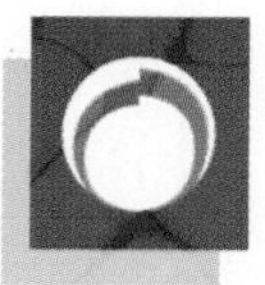

Joints

NORMAL JOINTS

Joints are constructed to provide both movement and mechanical support. Their anatomy is directly related to their function, and they are classified as solid (nonsynovial) and cavitated (synovial). The solid joints, known as *synarthroses*, provide structural integrity and allow for minimal movement. They lack a joint space and are grouped according to the type of connective tissue (fibrous tissue or cartilage) that bridges the ends of the bones; fibrous synarthroses include the cranial sutures and the bonds between roots of teeth and the jaw bones; cartilaginous synarthroses (synchondroses) are represented by the symphyses (manubriosternalis and pubic). *Synovial joints*, in contrast, have a joint space that allows for a wide range of motion. Situated between the ends of bones formed via enchondral ossification, they are strengthened by a dense fibrous capsule reinforced by ligaments and muscles. The boundary of the joint space is formed by the synovial membrane, which is firmly anchored to the underlying capsule. Its contour is smooth except near the osseous insertion, where it is thrown into numerous villous folds. The surface lining of cuboidal cells or synoviocytes is arranged one to four cell layers deep. They are not present over the cartilage surfaces. Traditionally, they are segregated into type A cells (macrophage-like), which are phagocytic and synthesize hyaluronic acid, and type B cells (fibroblast-like), which produce various proteins. The type A and B cells are now best considered one cell population that alters its phenotype according to the functional demands. The synovial lining lacks a basement membrane and merges with the underlying loose connective tissue stroma that is generally very vascular. The absence of a basement membrane allows for quick exchange between blood and synovial fluid. The clear, viscous synovial fluid is a filtrate of plasma containing hyaluronic acid that acts as a lubricant and provides nutrition for the articular hyaline cartilage.

Hyaline cartilage is a unique connective tissue ideally suited to serve as an elastic shock absorber and wear-resistant surface. It lacks a blood supply and does not have lymphatic drainage or innervation. Adult articular cartilage varies in thickness from 2 to 4 mm and is thickest both at the periphery of concave surfaces and in the central portions of convex surfaces. Hyaline cartilage is composed of type 2 collagen, water, proteoglycans, and chondrocytes, each of which have specific functions. The collagen fibers are arranged in arches so that near the surface they are horizontal in orientation—this allows the cartilage to resist tensile stresses and transmit vertical loads. The water and proteoglycans give hyaline cartilage its turgor and elasticity and play an important role in limiting friction. The chondrocytes synthesize the matrix as well as enzymatically digest it, with the half-life of the different components ranging from weeks (proteoglycans) to years (type 2 collagen). Matrix turnover is carefully controlled as chondrocytes secrete the degradative enzymes in an inactive form and enrich the matrix with enzyme inhibitors. Diseases that destroy articular cartilage do so by activating the catabolic enzymes and decreasing the production of inhibitors, thereby accelerating the rate of matrix breakdown. The chondrocytes react by increasing matrix production; however, the response is usually inadequate. Cytokines such as IL-1 and TNF trigger the degradative process, and their sources include chondrocytes, synoviocytes, fibroblasts, and inflammatory cells. Destruction of articular cartilage by indigenous cells is an important mechanism in many joint diseases.

PATHOLOGY

Arthritis

OSTEOARTHRITIS

Osteoarthritis, also called *degenerative joint disease*, is the most common type of joint disease. *It is characterized by the progressive erosion of articular cartilage.* Billions of dollars are spent annually for its treatment and for lost days of work. The term *osteoarthritis* implies an inflammatory disease. Although inflammatory cells may be present, osteoarthritis is considered to be an intrinsic disease of cartilage in which biochemical and metabolic alterations result in its breakdown.

In the great majority of instances, osteoarthritis appears insidiously, without apparent initiating cause, as an aging phenomenon (idiopathic or primary osteoarthritis). In these cases, the disease is usually oligoarticular (affects few joints) but may be generalized. In about 5% of cases, osteoarthritis may appear in younger individuals having some predisposing condition, such as previous macrotraumatic or repeated microtraumatic injuries to a joint; a congenital developmental deformity of a joint(s); or some underlying systemic disease such as diabetes, ochronosis, hemochromatosis, or marked obesity. In these settings, the disease is called *secondary osteoarthritis* and often involves one or several predisposed joints—witness the shoulder or elbow involvements in baseball players and knees in basketball players. Gender has some influence on distribution. The knees and hands are more commonly affected in women and the hips in men.

Pathogenesis. The association between osteoarthritis and aging is nonlinear; the prevalence increases exponentially beyond the age of 50. About 80% to 90% of individuals, of both sexes, have evidence of osteoarthritis by the time they reach age 65. Thus, osteoarthritis joins heart disease and cancer as one of the dividends of growing older. The age-related changes in cartilage include alterations in proteoglycans and collagen, which decrease tensile strength and shorten fatigue life. Despite this relationship, it is an oversimplification to consider osteoarthritis as merely a disease of cartilage wear and tear. Chondrocytes play a primary role in the process and constitute the cellular basis of the disease.[41] For example, chondrocytes in osteoarthritic cartilage produce IL-1 and TNF-α, which are known to stimulate the production of catabolic metalloproteinases, and inhibit the synthesis of both type 2 collagen and proteoglycans. The effects of these cytokines are potentiated because their receptors show increased sensitivity. Other mediators, such as prostaglandin derivatives and IL-6, also have a role in this cascade of matrix degradation.[42] Most of these cytokines also have proinflammatory properties, and inflammatory cells are present in many osteoarthritic joints. The precise events that lead to the secretion of cytokines, however, are not clear.

MORPHOLOGY. In the early stages of osteoarthritis, the chondrocytes proliferate forming clones. This process is accompanied by biochemical changes as the water content of the matrix increases and the concentration of proteoglycans decreases. Subsequently, vertical and horizontal fibrillation and cracking of the matrix occur as the superficial layers of the cartilage are degraded. Gross examination at this stage reveals a granular articular surface that is softer than normal. Eventually, full-thickness portions of the cartilage are sloughed, and the exposed subchondral bone plate becomes the new articular surface. Friction smoothes and burnishes the exposed bone giving it the appearance of polished ivory (**bone eburnation**) (Fig. 28–39). Concurrently, there is rebuttressing and sclerosis of the underlying cancellous bone. Small fractures through the articulating bone are common, and the dislodged pieces of cartilage and subchondral bone tumble into the joint forming loose bodies (**joint mice**). The fracture gaps allow synovial fluid to be forced into the subchondral regions in a one-way, ball-valve-like mechanism. The loculated fluid collection increases in size forming fibrous walled cysts. Mushroom-shaped osteophytes (bony outgrowths) develop at the margins of the articular surface and are capped by fibrocartilage and hyaline cartilage that gradually ossify. The synovium shows minor alterations in comparison to the destruction of the articular surface and is congested and fibrotic and may have scattered chronic inflammatory cells. In severe disease, a fibrous synovial pannus covers the peripheral portions of the articular surface.

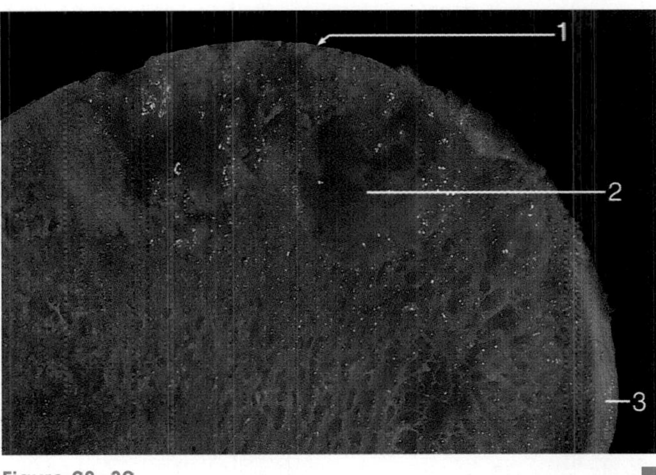

Figure 28–39

Severe osteoarthritis with small islands of residual articular cartilage next to exposed subchondral bone. *1,* Eburnated articular surface. *2,* Subchondral cyst. *3,* Residual articular cartilage.

Clinical Course. Osteoarthritis is an insidious disease. Patients with primary disease are usually asymptomatic until they are in their fifties. If a young patient has significant manifestations of osteoarthritis, a search for some underlying cause should be made. Characteristic symptoms include deep, achy pain that worsens with use, morning stiffness, crepitus, and limitation of range of movement. Impingement on spinal foramina by osteophytes results in cervical and lumbar nerve root compression with radicular pain, muscle spasms, muscle atrophy, and neurologic deficits. Typically, only one or a few joints are involved except in the uncommon generalized variant. The joints commonly involved include the hips, knees, lower lumbar and cervical vertebrae, proximal and distal interphangeal joints of the fingers, first carpometacarpal joints, and first tarsometatarsal joints of the feet (Fig. 28–40). Characteristic in women, but not in men, are *Heberden nodes* in the fingers representing prominent osteophytes at the distal interphalangeal joints. The wrists, elbows, and shoulders are usu-

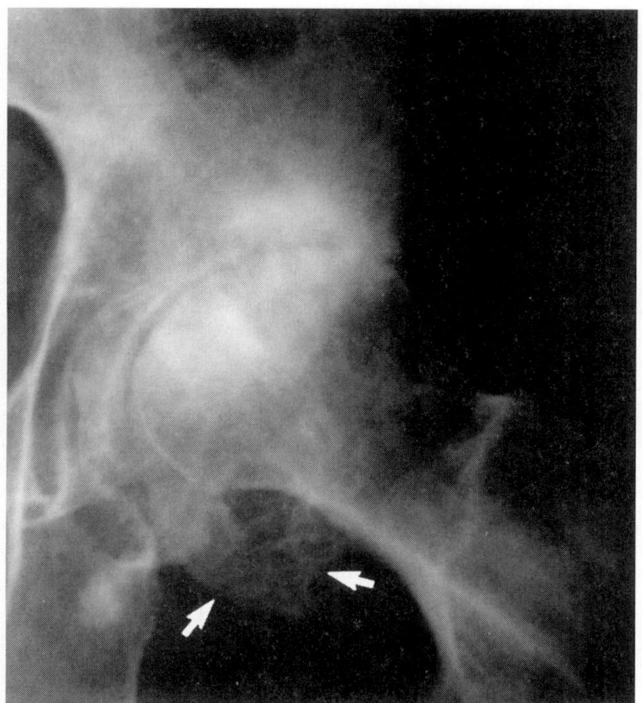

Figure 28–40

Severe osteoarthritis of the hip. The joint space is narrowed, and there is subchondral sclerosis with scattered oval radiolucent cysts and peripheral osteophyte lipping *(arrows)*.

ally spared. There are still no satisfactory means of preventing primary osteoarthritis, and there are no methods of halting its progression. The disease may stabilize for years at any stage but more often is slowly progressive over the remaining years of life and is second only to cardiovascular diseases in causing long-term disability.

RHEUMATOID ARTHRITIS

Rheumatoid arthritis (RA) is a chronic systemic inflammatory disorder that may affect many tissues and organs—skin, blood vessels, heart, lungs, and muscles—but principally attacks the joints, producing a nonsuppurative proliferative synovitis that often progresses to destruction of the articular cartilage and ankylosis of the joints. Although the cause of RA remains unknown, autoimmunity plays a pivotal role in its chronicity and progression.

About 1% of the world's population is afflicted by RA, women three to five times more often than men. The peak incidence is in the twenties and forties, but no age is immune. We first consider the morphology as a background to discuss pathogenesis.

MORPHOLOGY

Joints. RA causes a broad spectrum of morphologic alterations; the most severe are manifested in the joints. Initially the synovium becomes grossly edematous, thickened, and hyperplastic, transforming its smooth contour to one covered by delicate and bulbous fronds (Fig. 28–41). The characteristic histologic features include (1) infiltration of synovial stroma by a dense **perivascular inflammatory infiltrate** composed of lymphoid follicles (mostly CD4+ helper T cells), plasma cells, and macrophages filling the synovial stroma; (2) **increased vascularity** owing to vasodilation and angiogenesis, with superficial hemosiderin deposits; (3) aggregation of **organizing fibrin** covering

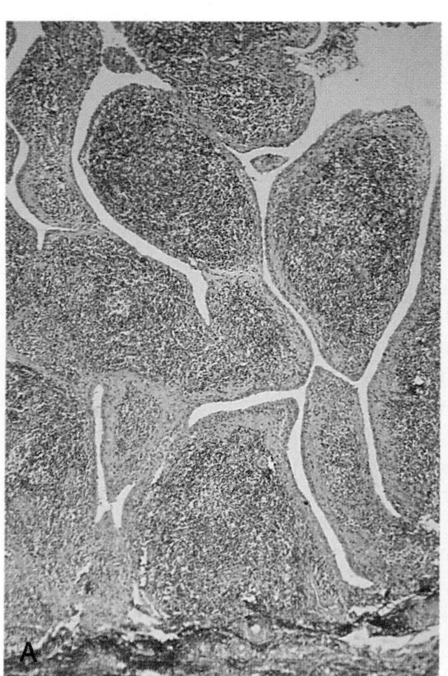

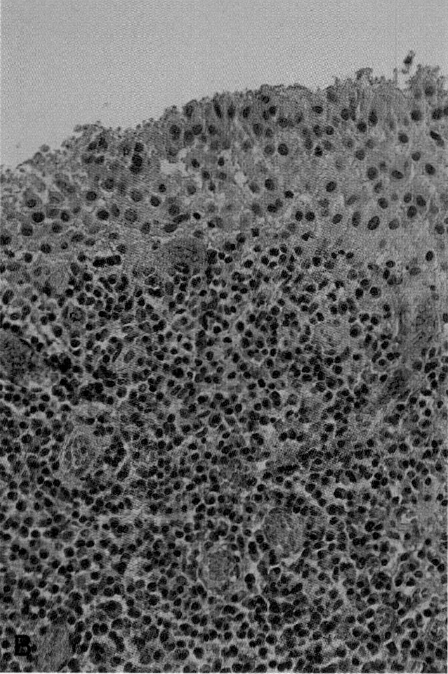

Figure 28–41

Rheumatoid arthritis. *A*, Low magnification reveals marked synovial hypertrophy with formation of villi. *B*, At higher magnification, subsynovial tissue containing a dense lymphoid aggregate is seen.

portions of the synovium and floating in the joint space as rice bodies; (4) **accumulation of neutrophils** in the synovial fluid and along the surface of synovium but usually not deep in the synovial stroma; (5) osteoclastic activity in underlying bone, allowing the synovium to penetrate into the bone forming **juxta-articular erosions, subchondral cysts,** and **osteoporosis;** and (6) **pannus** formation—the pannus is a fibrocellular mass of synovium and synovial stroma consisting of inflammatory cells, granulomatous tissue, and fibroblasts, which causes erosion of the underlying cartilage. In time, after the cartilage has been destroyed, the pannus bridges the apposing bones forming a **fibrous ankylosis**, which eventually ossifies ultimately resulting in **bony ankylosis**. Inflammation in the tendons, ligaments, and occasionally the adjacent skeletal muscle frequently accompanies the arthritis.

Skin. **Rheumatoid nodules** are the most common cutaneous lesion. They occur in approximately 25% of patients, usually those with severe disease, and arise in regions of the skin that are subjected to pressure, including the ulnar aspect of the forearm, elbows, occiput, and lumbosacral area. Less commonly, they form in the lungs, spleen, pericardium, myocardium, heart valves, aorta, and other viscera. Rheumatoid nodules are firm, nontender, and round to oval and in the skin arise in the subcutaneous tissue. Microscopically, they have a central zone of fibrinoid necrosis surrounded by a prominent rim of epithelioid histiocytes and numerous lymphocytes and plasma cells (Fig. 28–42).

Blood Vessels. Patients with severe erosive disease, rheumatoid nodules, and high titers of rheumatoid factor are at risk of developing vasculitic syndromes (Chapter 12). Rheumatoid vasculitis is a potentially catastrophic complication of RA, particularly when it affects vital organs. The involvement of medium-to-small size arteries is similar to that occurring in polyarteritis nodosa except that in RA the kidneys are not involved. Frequently, segments of small arteries such as **vasa nervorum** and **digital arteries** are obstructed by an obliterating endarteritis resulting in peripheral neuropathy, ulcers, and gangrene. Leukocytoclastic venulitis produces purpura, cutaneous ulcers, and nail bed infarction.

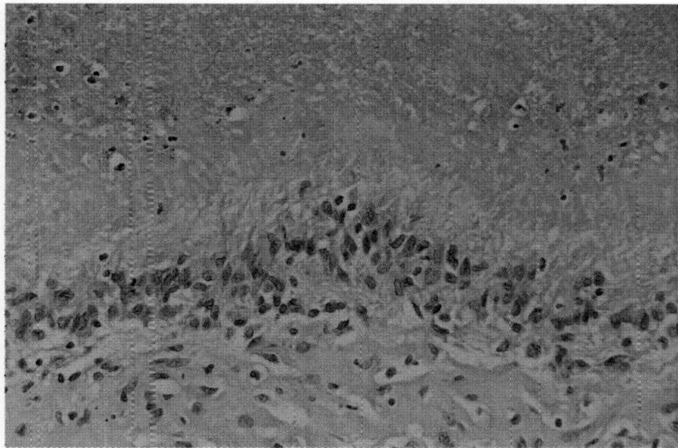

Figure 28–42 ■

Subcutaneous rheumatoid nodule with an area of necrosis (*top*) surrounded by a palisade of macrophages and scattered chronic inflammatory cells.

Pathogenesis. Although much remains uncertain, it is currently believed that *RA is triggered by exposure of an immunogenetically susceptible host to an arthritogenic microbial antigen.* In this manner, an acute arthritis is initiated, but it is the continuing *autoimmune reaction*, the activation of CD4+ helper T cells, and the local release of inflammatory mediators and cytokines that ultimately destroys the joint (Fig. 28–43). Involved therefore in the pathogenesis are (1) genetic susceptibility, (2) a primary exogenous arthritogen, (3) an autoimmune reaction to joint components, and (4) mediators of the joint damage.

- *Genetic susceptibility* is clearly a major determinant of susceptibility to RA. There is a high rate of concordance between monozygotic twins and a well-defined familial predisposition. More importantly, the majority (65% to 80%) of individuals who develop RA are HLA-DR4 or -DR1 or both, and 75% of patients with RA in the United States and Europe have the motif Q(K/R)RA in the antigen-binding DRB1-HV3 region of the T-cell antigen receptor. All the DR alleles associated with susceptibility to RA share a common region of four amino acids located in the antigen-binding cleft of the DR molecule adjacent to the T-cell receptor. This location is presumably the specific binding site of the arthritogen(s) that initiates the inflammatory synovitis.
- *Microbial agents*: It is thought that the *initiator of the disease* is a microbial agent, but its identity continues to be elusive. Epstein-Barr virus is a current suspect, but closely following are retroviruses, parvoviruses, mycobacteria, *Borrelia*, and *Mycoplasma* as well as numerous others.[43] For each, tentative support is offered, but the evidence implicating Epstein-Barr virus is particularly intriguing. Autoimmunity to type 2 collagen can be demonstrated in most patients with RA. The Epstein-Barr virus and type 2 collagen have some homologous HLA-DRβ chain epitopes, and conceivably an immunologic reaction against the Epstein-Barr virus might cross over to affect joint cartilage rich in type 2 collagen.
- *Autoimmunity*: Once an inflammatory synovitis has been initiated by an exogenous agent, an *autoimmune reaction*—in which T cells play the pivotal role—is responsible for the chronic destructive nature of RA. The antigen inducing this reaction has not been identified with certainty. The possible role of type 2 collagen was mentioned earlier, but there is additional evidence suggesting that human cartilage glycoprotein-39 is an autoantigen. This protein is a product of hyaline cartilage chondrocytes and has been shown to bind to DR4 peptides,

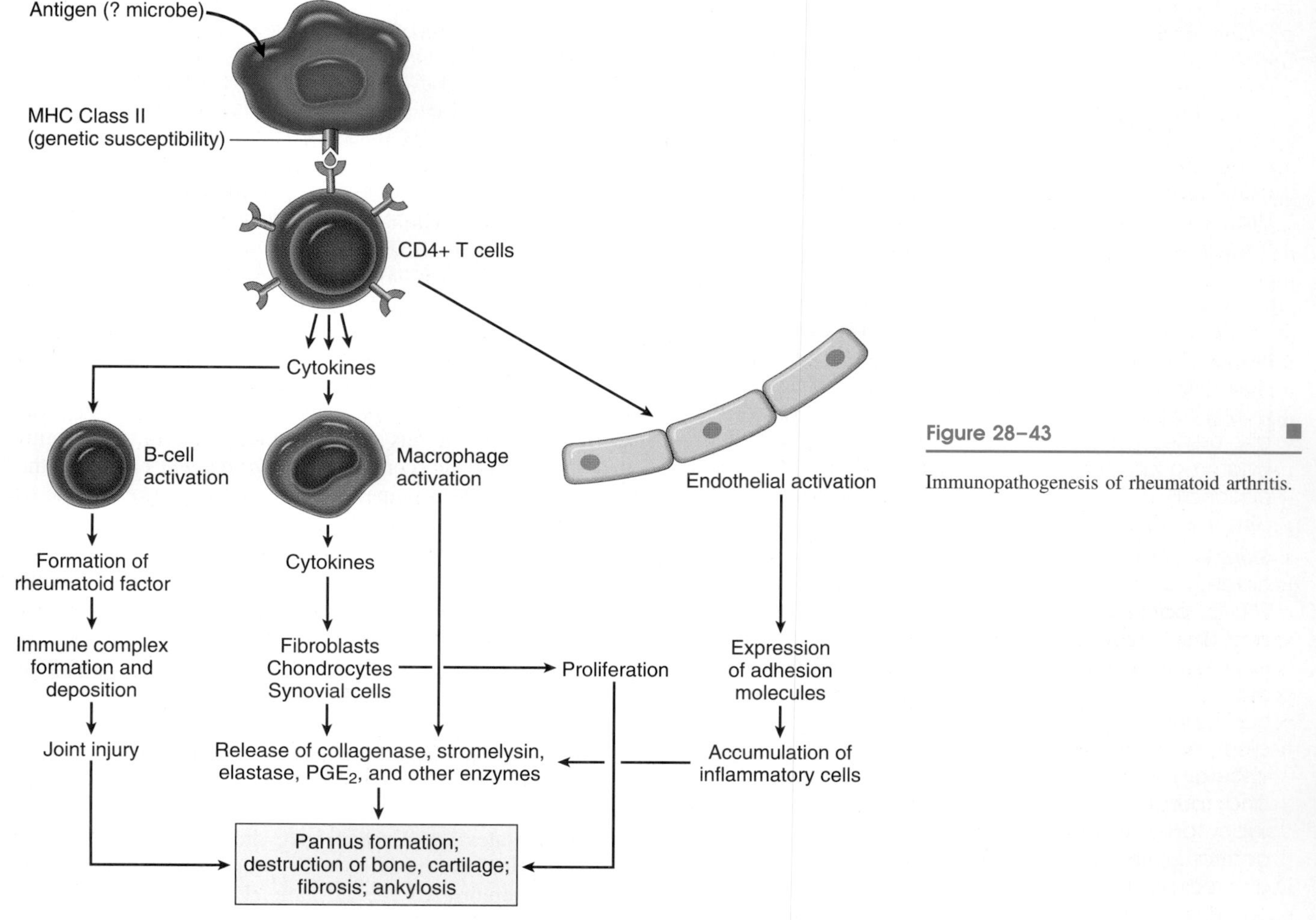

Figure 28–43

Immunopathogenesis of rheumatoid arthritis.

thereby making it a potential target of the T cell–regulated immune reaction.[44] Regardless, T cells, mainly CD4+ memory cells, appear within the affected joints early in the development of RA. Soon the endothelial cells of synovial capillaries are activated, with the expression of intercellular adhesion molecule-1 (ICAM-1) leading to further attachment and transmigration of other inflammatory cells, including CD4 and T cells. This sequence is further enhanced by release of cytokines by inflammatory cells and the sequence of cell/cytokine loops described in Chapter 3, leading to chronic immunologic injury. In RA, a role for IL-15, secreted by activated T cells and macrophages, seems prominent.[45]

Activated CD4+ cells simultaneously activate B cells resulting in antibody production in affected joints. *About 80% of individuals with RA have autoantibodies to the Fc portion of autologous IgG (rheumatoid factors).* These are mostly IgM antibodies, perhaps generated within joints, but may be of other classes. These self-associate (RA-IgG) to form immune complexes in the sera, synovial fluid, and synovial membranes. The circulating immune complexes underlie many of the extra-articular manifestations of RA. They are localized within the inflamed cartilage, activating complement, augmenting the synovial inflammatory reaction, and contributing to the degradation of cartilage. Rheumatoid factor, however, is not present in some patients with the disease (seronegative), is sometimes found in other disease states and even in otherwise healthy people, and is probably not critical to the causation of RA.

What *mediators* then bring about the destructive-proliferative synovitis? These represent the "usual suspects," including cytokines, TNF, IL-1, IL-6, IL-15, interferon-γ, and growth factors (GM-CSF, TFG-β) as well as proteases and elastases released by leukocytes and synoviocytes. TNF-α and IL-1 produced locally by macrophages play an early role. As discussed in Chapter 3, TNF-α and IL-1 up-regulate expression of adhesion molecules by endothelial cells, resulting in the accumulation of white cells in the inflamed synovium. Some of these adhesion molecules (VCAM-1) are also up-regulated in synoviocytes. The pannus then becomes lined by VCAM-1 expressing activated synoviocytes, which more easily adhere to the cartilage matrix, facilitating the destruction of the articular surface by enzymes produced by synoviocytes. Cartilage destruction, both at the interface with the pannus and distant from it, is further enhanced by IL-1 and TNF-α as these cytokines also stimulate the chondrocytes to produce more degradative enzymes and inhibit their synthesis of reparative proteoglycans.[46] *In the end, there is sustained, irreversible cartilage destruction.* Significantly, antibodies to TNF-α or IL-1 have a protective effect on a collagen-induced arthritis in mice.

Clinical Course. The clinical course of RA is extremely variable. The disease begins slowly and insidiously in more than half of patients. Initially, there is malaise, fatigue, and generalized musculoskeletal pain, and only after several weeks to months do the joints become involved. The pattern of joint involvement varies, but generally the small joints are affected before the larger ones. Symptoms usually develop in the small bones of the hands (metacarpophalangeal and proximal interphalangeal joints) and feet followed by the wrists, ankles, elbows, and knees. Uncommonly the upper spine is involved, but the lumbosacral region and hips are usually spared.

The involved joints are swollen, warm, painful, and particularly stiff on arising or following inactivity. Approximately 10% of patients have an acute onset with severe symptoms and polyarticular involvement developing within a few days. In the typical patient, progressive joint involvement occurs over a period of months to years, with initial minimal limitation of motion that in time becomes more severe. The disease course may be slow or rapid and fluctuate over a period of years, with the greatest damage occurring during the first 4 or 5 years. Approximately 20% of patients enjoy periods of partial or complete remission, but the symptoms inevitably return and involve previously unaffected joints.

The radiographic hallmarks are joint effusions and juxta-articular osteopenia with erosions and narrowing of the joint space with loss of articular cartilage (Fig. 28–44). Destruction of tendons, ligaments, and joint capsules produces characteristic deformities, including radial deviation of the wrist, ulnar deviation of the fingers, and flexion-hyperextension abnormalities of the fingers (swan neck, boutonnière). The end result is deformed joints that have no stability and minimal or no range of motion. Large synovial cysts, such as the Baker cyst in the posterior knee, may develop as the increased intra-articular pressure causes outpouchings of the synovium.

No specific laboratory tests are diagnostic of RA. As pointed out, rheumatoid factor may not be present and also appears in many other conditions. Analysis of synovial fluid confirms an inflammatory arthritis with neutrophils, high protein content, and low mucin content but is nonspecific. The diagnosis is made primarily on the clinical features and includes the presence of four of the following criteria: (1) morning stiffness, (2) arthritis in three or more joint areas, (3) arthritis of hand joints, (4) symmetric arthritis, (5) rheumatoid nodules, (6) serum rheumatoid factor, and (7) typical radiographic changes.

It is difficult to predict the natural history of the disease for individuals. Fortunate patients have a mild onset and relatively short-term symptoms with no sequelae. Most, however, have progressive disease for life. Overall, life expectancy is reduced by a mean of 3 to 7 years. The fatalities are usually due to the complications of RA, such as systemic amyloidosis and vasculitis, or to iatrogenic effects of therapy—in particular, gastrointestinal bleeding related to long-term use of anti-inflammatory drugs (aspirin, nonsteroidal anti-inflammatory drugs) and infections associated with chronic steroid use.

JUVENILE RHEUMATOID ARTHRITIS

Juvenile rheumatoid arthritis (JRA) is one of the more common connective tissue diseases of children and is a

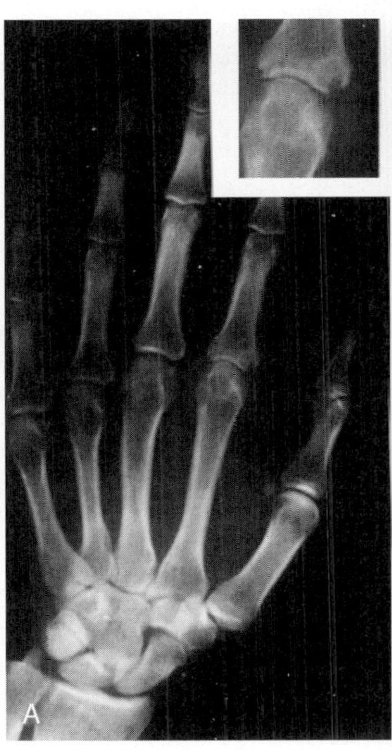

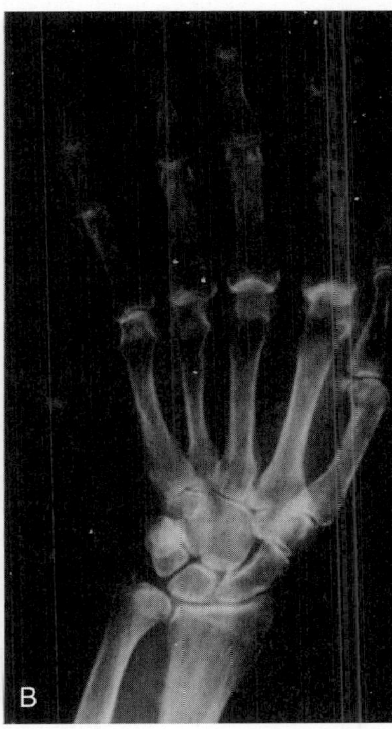

Figure 28–44

Rheumatoid arthritis. *A*, Early disease, most marked in the second metacarpophalangeal joint, where there is narrowing of joint space and marginal erosions on both radial and ulnar aspects of the proximal phalanx (*see inset*). *B*, More advanced disease with loss of articular cartilage, narrowing of joint spaces of virtually all the small joints, and ulnar deviation of the fingers. There is dislocation of the second, third, and fourth proximal phalanges produced by advanced articular disease. (Courtesy of Dr. John O'Connor, Boston University Medical Center, Boston, MA.)

major cause of functional disability in children.[47] By definition, it begins before the age of 16, and most patients are diagnosed during early childhood. There is a 2 : 1 female predominance except in the subgroup that has systemic onset, in which the sexes are equally affected. JRA is classified into oligoarticular (<5 joints involved), polyarticular (≥5 joints involved), and systemic variants.

JRA differs from RA in adults in the following points: (1) Oligoarthritis is more common, (2) systemic onset is more frequent, (3) large joints are affected more often than small joints, (4) rheumatoid nodules and rheumatoid factor are usually absent, and (5) antinuclear antibody seropositivity is common. Pathogenetic factors, similar to those in RA, include genetic association with particular HLA haplotypes (DRB1); mycobacterial, bacterial, or viral infection; abnormal immunoregulation with the prevalence of activated CD4+ T cells within involved joints; and cytokine production.[48] The morphologic changes in joint pathology are similar to those seen in adult RA.

Commonly targeted joints are the knees, wrists, elbows, and ankles. They become warm and swollen and are often involved symmetrically. Pericarditis, myocarditis, pulmonary fibrosis, glomerulonephritis, uveitis, and growth retardation are potential extra-articular manifestations. A systemic onset may begin rather abruptly, associated with high spiking fevers, migratory and transient skin rash, hepatosplenomegaly, and serositis. Satisfactory recovery occurs in 70% to 90% of patients, and in only 10% do severe joint deformities persist.

SERONEGATIVE SPONDYLOARTHROPATHIES

The seronegative spondyloarthropathies are a group of diseases characterized by inflammatory peripheral or axial arthritis and associated with other, usually infectious, disorders. They include *ankylosing spondylitis, reactive arthritis (Reiter syndrome and enteropathic arthritis), psoriatic arthritis, and arthritis associated with inflammatory bowel disease* (ulerative colitis, Crohn disease). They share overlapping clinical features, and many are associated with HLA B-27 and a triggering infection.

Ankylosing Spondyloarthritis

Also known as *rheumatoid spondylitis* and *Marie-Strümpell disease*, ankylosing spondyloarthritis is a chronic inflammatory joint disease of axial joints, especially the sacroiliac joints. It usually occurs in boys and begins in adolescence. Approximately 90% of affected individuals are HLA-B27 positive; however, certain HLA-B27 subtypes are not associated with disease susceptibility.[49] Analogous to RA, this immunogenetic phenotype may predispose to the development of autoantibodies directed at joint elements after infection. Histologically a chronic synovitis causes destruction of articular cartilage and bony ankylosis, especially in the sacroiliac and apophyseal joints (between tuberosities and processes). Inflammation of tendinoligamentous insertion sites eventuates in bony outgrowths, which compound the fibrous and bony ankylosis producing severe spinal immobility. The patients characteristically present with low back pain, which frequently follows a chronic progressive course. Involvement of peripheral joints, such as the hips, knees, and shoulders, occurs in at least one third of patients. Uveitis, aortitis, and amyloidosis are other recognized complications.

Reiter Syndrome

Reiter syndrome is defined by a triad of arthritis, nongonococcal urethritis or cervicitis, and conjunctivitis. Most affected individuals are men in their twenties or thirties, and more than 80% are positive for HLA-B27. The evidence suggests that the disease is caused by an autoimmune reaction initiated by prior infection. The implicated infections are gastrointestinal—*Shigella, Salmonella, Yersinia, Campylobacter*—and genitourinary—*Chlamydia*. Arthritic symptoms usually develop within several weeks of the inciting bout of urethritis or diarrhea. Joint stiffness and low back pain are common early symptoms. The ankles, knees, and feet are affected most often, frequently in an asymmetric pattern. Synovitis of digital tendon sheath produces the *sausage* finger or toe and leads to calcaneal spurs and bony outgrowths from tendons. Patients with severe chronic disease have involvement of the spine that is indistinguishable from ankylosing spondylitis. Extra-articular involvement manifests as inflammatory balanitis conjunctivitis, cardiac conduction abnormalities, and aortic regurgitation. The natural behavior of Reiter syndrome is extremely variable. The episodes of arthritis usually wax and wane over a period of several weeks to 6 months. Almost 50% of patients have recurrent arthritis, tendinitis, fasciitis, and lumbosacral back pain that can cause significant functional disability.

Enteropathic Arthritis

Enteropathic arthritis is induced by bowel infection with a variety of microorganisms, including *Yersinia, Salmonella, Shigella*, and *Campylobacter*. These organisms all have lipopolysaccharide as a major component in their outer cell membrane, and their derived antigens stimulate an array of immunologic responses.[50] The affected individuals are usually HLA-B27 positive. The arthritis appears abruptly and tends to involve the knees and ankles but sometimes the wrists, fingers, and toes. The arthritis lasts for about a year then generally clears and only rarely is accompanied by ankylosing spondylitis. Microbial components and not live organisms are found in the affected joints.

Psoriatic Arthritis

Psoriatic arthritis affects 5% of the psoriatic population. The disease manifests itself between the ages of 35 and 45. The joint symptoms develop slowly but are acute in onset in one third of patients. The patterns of joint involvement are diverse. The distal interphalangeal joints of the hands and feet are first affected in an asymmetric distribution in more than 50% of patients. The large joints such as the ankles, knees, hips, and wrists may be involved as well.[54] Inflammation of the digital tendon sheaths produces the sausage finger. Sacroiliac and spinal disease occurs in 20% to 40% of patients. Aside from conjunctivitis and iritis, extra-articular manifestations are uncommon and are similar in scope to those in the other seronegative spondyloarthropathies. Histologically, psoriatic arthritis is similar to

RA. Psoriatic arthritis, however, is usually not as severe, remissions are more frequent, and joint destruction is less frequent.

INFECTIOUS ARTHRITIS

Microorganisms of all types can seed joints during hematogenous dissemination. Articular structures can also become infected by direct inoculation or from contiguous spread from a soft tissue abscess or focus of osteomyelitis. Infectious arthritis is potentially serious because it can cause rapid destruction of the joint and produce permanent deformities.

Suppurative Arthritis

Bacterial infections almost always cause an acute suppurative arthritis. The bacteria usually seed the joint during an episode of bacteremia; however, in neonates, there is an increased incidence of contiguous spread from underlying epiphyseal osteomyelitis. The most common organisms are gonococcus, *Staphylococcus*, *Streptococcus*, *Haemophilus influenzae*, and gram-negative bacilli (*E. coli*, *Salmonella*, *Pseudomonas*, and others). *H. influenzae* arthritis predominates in children under 2 years of age, *S. aureus* is the main causative agent in older children and adults, and gonococcus is prevalent during late adolescence and young adulthood. Individuals with sickle cell disease are prone to infection with *Salmonella* at any age. These joint infections affect the sexes equally except for gonococcal arthritis, which is seen mainly in sexually active women. Predisposing conditions include immune deficiencies (congenital and acquired), debilitating illness, joint trauma, chronic arthritis of any cause, and intravenous drug abuse.

The classic presentation is the sudden development of an acutely painful and swollen infected joint that has a restricted range of motion. Systemic findings of fever, leukocytosis, and elevated sedimentation rate are common. In disseminated gonococcal infection, the symptoms are more subacute. In 90% of nongonococcal cases, the arthritis involves only a single joint, usually the knee followed in frequency by the hip, shoulder, elbow, wrist, and sternoclavicular joints. Axial articulations are more commonly involved in drug addicts. Prompt recognition and effective therapy prevent rapid joint destruction.

Tuberculous Arthritis

Tuberculous arthritis (Chapter 9) is a chronic progressive monarticular disease that occurs in all age groups, especially adults. It usually develops as a complication of adjoining osteomyelitis or after hematogenous dissemination from a visceral (usually pulmonary) site of infection. Onset is insidious and causes gradual progressive pain. Systemic symptoms may or may not be present. Mycobacterial seeding of the joint induces the formation of confluent granulomas with central caseous necrosis. The affected synovium may grow as a pannus over the articular cartilage and erode into bone along the joint margins. Chronic disease results in severe destruction with fibrous ankylosis and obliteration of the joint space. The weight-bearing joints are usually affected, especially the hips, knees, and ankles in descending order of frequency.

Lyme Arthritis

As previously discussed (Chapter 9), Lyme arthritis is caused by infection with the spirochete *Borrelia burgdorferi*. The initial infection of the skin is followed within several days or weeks by dissemination of the organism to other sites, especially the joints.

Approximately 80% of patients with Lyme disease develop joint symptoms within a few weeks to 2 years after the onset of the disease. The arthritis is the dominant feature of late disease and tends to be remitting and migratory and primarily involves large joints, especially the knees, shoulders, elbows, and ankles in descending order of frequency. Usually one or two joints are affected at a time, and the attacks last for a few weeks to months with periods of remission. Infected synovium takes the form of a chronic papillary synovitis with synoviocyte hyperplasia, fibrin deposition, mononuclear cell infiltrates (especially helper/inducer T cells), and onion-skin thickening of arterial walls. The morphology in severe cases can closely resemble that of RA. Silver stains may reveal small numbers of organisms in the vicinity of blood vessels in approximately 25% of cases. Chronic arthritis with pannus formation resulting in permanent deformities develops in approximately 10% of patients, and it is unclear whether this form of arthritis is caused by persistent joint infection or the initiation of an immune reaction.[51]

Viral Arthritis

Arthritis can occur in the setting of a variety of viral infections, including parvovirus B19, rubella, and hepatitis C virus. The clinical manifestations of the arthritis are variable and range from acute to subacute symptoms. It is unclear whether the joint symptoms are caused by direct infection of the joint by the virus or whether the viral infection generates an autoimmune reaction as seen in other forms of reactive arthritides.[52] The possible role of viruses in the generation of chronic joint diseases such as RA has been previously discussed. A variety of different rheumatic conditions, including reactive arthritis, psoriatic arthritis, and septic arthritis, have developed in patients infected with human immunodeficiency virus (HIV). Its role in causing chronic arthritis similar to RA is suspect, however.

GOUT AND GOUTY ARTHRITIS

Articular crystal deposits are associated with a variety of acute and chronic joint disorders. Endogenous crystals shown to be pathogenic include monosodium urate (gout), calcium pyrophosphate dihydrate, and basic calcium phosphate (hydroxyapatite). Exogenous crystals, such as corticosteroid ester crystals, talcum, polyethylene, and methyl methacrylate, may also induce joint disease. Silicone, polyethylene, and methyl methacrylate are used in prosthetic joints, and their debris that accumulates with long use and wear may result in local arthritis and failure of the prosthesis. Endogenous and exogenous crystals produce disease by triggering the cascade that results in cytokine-mediated cartilage destruction. Here we discuss the two most important crystal arthropathies: gout, caused by urates, and pseudogout, associated with calcium pyrophosphate.

Gout is the common end point of a group of disorders that produce hyperuricemia. It is marked by transient attacks of *acute arthritis* initiated by crystallization of urates within and about joints leading eventually to *chronic gouty arthritis* and the deposition of masses of urates in joints and other sites creating *tophi*. Tophi represent large aggregates of urate crystals and the surrounding inflammatory reaction (see later). Most, but not all, patients with chronic gout also develop urate nephropathy. Although hyperuricemia is a sine qua non for the development of gout, it is not the sole determinant. More than 10% of the population of the Western hemisphere have hyperuricemia, but gout develops in less than 0.5% of the population. A plasma urate level above 7 mg/dl is considered elevated because it exceeds the saturation value for urate at normal body temperature and blood pH. The various conditions producing hyperuricemia and gout (Table 28–7) are divided into those that produce primary gout, in which the basic metabolic defect is unknown or gout is the main manifestation of a known defect, and secondary gout, in which the cause of the hyperuricemia is known or gout is not the main clinical dysfunction.

Table 28–7. CLASSIFICATION OF GOUT

Clinical Category	Metabolic Defect
Primary Gout (90% of cases)	
Enzyme defects unknown (85 to 90% of primary gout)	■ Overproduction of uric acid Normal excretion (majority) Increased excretion (minority) Underexcretion of uric acid with normal production
Known enzyme defects—e.g., partial HGPRT deficiency (rare)	■ Overproduction of uric acid
Secondary Gout (10% of cases)	
Associated with increased nucleic acid turnover—e.g., leukemias	■ Overproduction of uric acid with increased urinary excretion
Chronic renal disease	■ Reduced excretion of uric acid with normal production
Inborn errors of metabolism—e.g., complete HGPRT deficiency (Lesch-Nyhan syndrome)	■ Overproduction of uric acid with increased urinary excretion

HGPRT, hypoxanthine guanine phosphoribosyl transferase.

Pathogenesis. Uric acid is the end product of purine metabolism. Two pathways are involved in purine synthesis[53]: (1) a de novo pathway in which purines are synthesized from nonpurine precursors and (2) a salvage pathway in which free purine bases derived from the breakdown of nucleic acids of endogenous or exogenous origin are recaptured (salvaged) (Fig. 28–45). The enzyme hypoxanthine guanine phosphoribosyl transferase (HGPRT) is involved in the salvage pathway. A deficiency of this enzyme leads to increased synthesis of purine nucleotides through the de novo pathway and hence increased production of uric acid. A complete lack of HGPRT occurs in the uncommon X-linked *Lesch-Nyhan syndrome*, seen only in males and characterized by hyperuricemia, severe neurologic deficits with mental retardation, self-mutilation, and in some cases

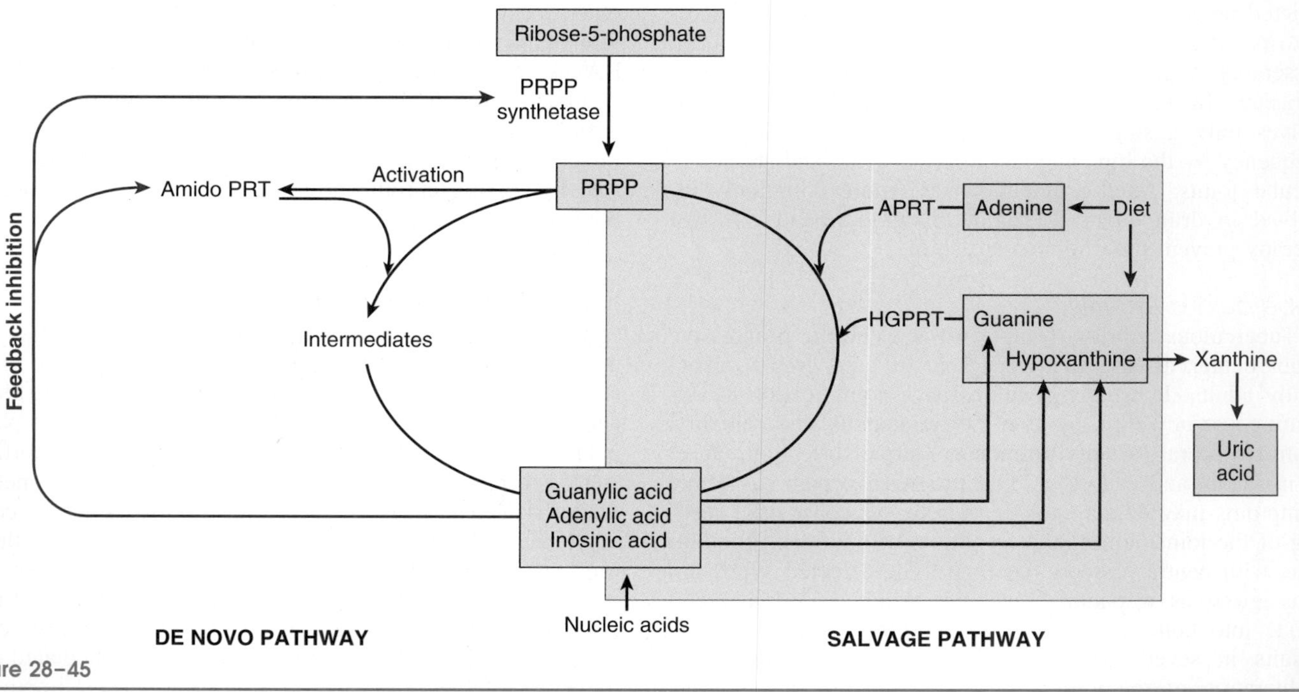

Figure 28–45

Purine metabolism. The conversion of PRPP to purine nucleotides is catalyzed by amido PRT in the de novo pathway and by APRT and HGPRT in the salvage pathway.

gouty arthritis. Less severe deficiencies of the enzyme may also induce hyperuricemia and gouty arthritis with only mild neurologic deficits, but together these causes of gout are uncommon. The great majority of cases of gout are primary in which the metabolic defect underlying the increased levels of uric acid is unknown.

As stated earlier, hyperuricemia does not necessarily lead to gouty arthritis. Many factors contribute to the conversion of asymptomatic hyperuricemia into primary gout, including the following:

- *Age* of the individual and duration of the hyperuricemia are factors. Gout rarely appears before 20 to 30 years of hyperuricemia.
- *Genetic predisposition* is another factor. In addition to the well-defined X-linked abnormalities of HGPRT, primary gout follows multifactorial inheritance and runs in families.
- Heavy *alcohol* consumption predisposes to attacks of gouty arthritis.
- *Obesity* increases the risk of asymptomatic gout.
- Certain *drugs* (e.g., thiazides) predispose to the development of gout.
- *Lead toxicity* increases the tendency to develop saturnine gout (Chapter 10).

Central to the pathogenesis of the arthritis is precipitation of monosodium urate crystals into the joints (Fig. 28–46). Synovial fluid is a poorer solvent for monosodium urate than plasma, and so with hyperuricemia the urates in the joint fluid become supersaturated, particularly in the peripheral joints (ankle), which may have temperatures as low as 20°C. With prolonged hyperuricemia, crystals and microtophi of urates develop in the synovial lining cells and in the joint cartilage. Inorganic crystals, including monosodium urate, can stimulate the formation of specific antibodies, which then can rapidly accelerate the formation of new crystals.[54] Some unknown event, possibly trauma, then initiates release of crystals into the synovial fluid followed by a cascade of events. The released crystals are chemotactic to leukocytes and also activate complement, with the generation of C3a and C5a leading to the accumulation of neutrophils and macrophages in the joints and synovial membranes. Phagocytosis of crystals induces release of toxic free radicals and leukotrienes (LTB_4). Activated neutrophils release destructive lysosomal enzymes,

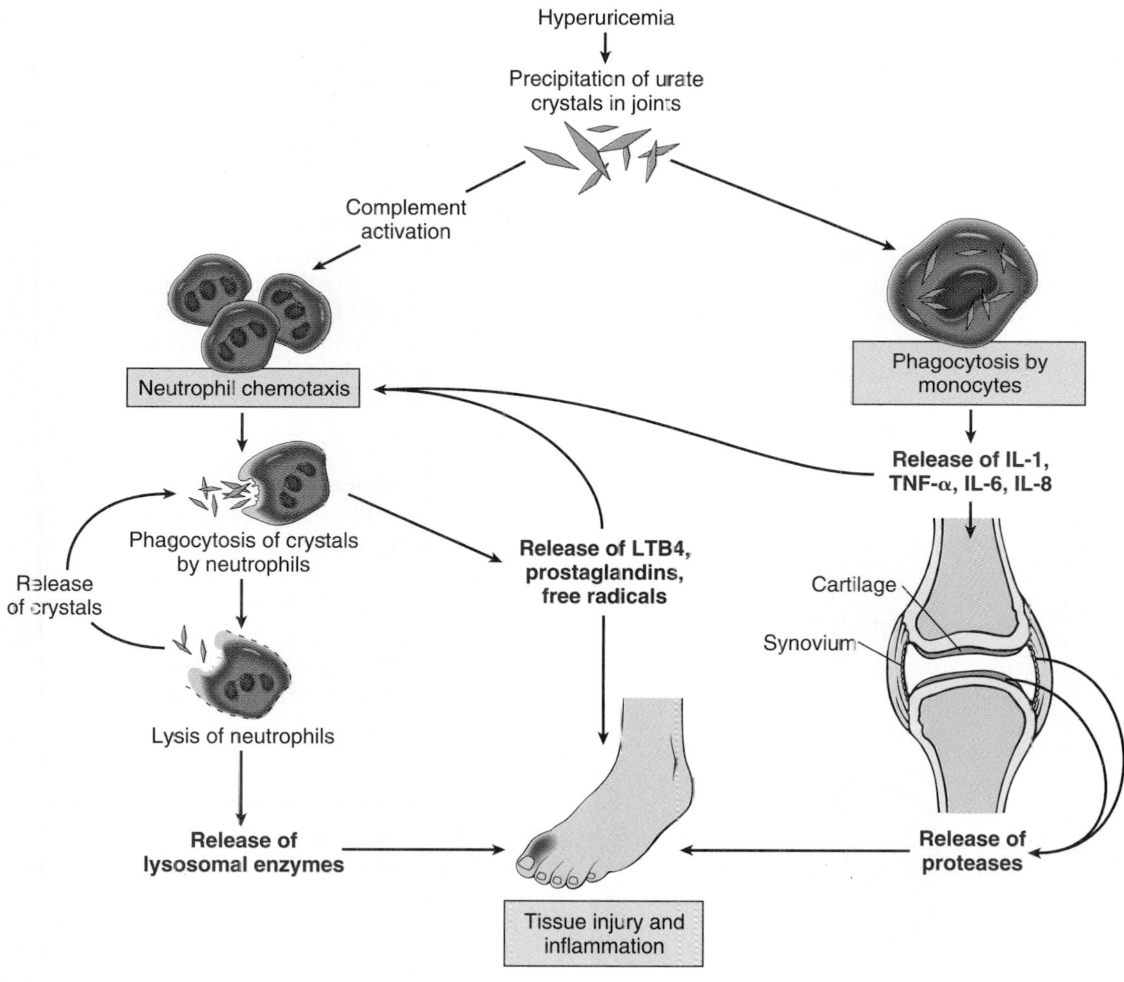

Figure 28–46

Pathogenesis of acute gouty arthritis.

and the macrophages and synoviocytes secrete a variety of mediators, which further intensify the inflammatory reaction and augment the injury to the articular structures.[55] Activation of Hageman factor pours fuel onto the fire. Thus comes about an acute arthritis, which typically remits (days to weeks) even untreated. A scheme of these events is shown in Figure 28–46.

Repeated attacks of acute arthritis lead eventually to chronic arthritis and the formation of tophi in the inflamed synovial membranes and periarticular tissue as well as elsewhere. In time, severe damage to the cartilage and the function of the joints develops. Unknown is why the chronic arthritis is asymptomatic for intervals of days to months, even though synovial crystals are undoubtedly present in abundance in the joints.

MORPHOLOGY. The distinctive morphologic changes in gout are (1) acute arthritis, (2) chronic tophaceous arthritis, (3) tophi in various sites, and sometimes (4) gouty nephropathy. **Acute arthritis** is characterized by a dense neutrophilic infiltrate that permeates the synovium and synovial fluid. The monosodium urate crystals are frequently found in the cytoplasm of the neutrophils and are arranged in small clusters in the synovium. They are long, slender, and needle shaped and are negatively birefringent. The synovium is edematous and congested and also contains scattered lymphocytes, plasma cells, and macrophages. When the episode of crystallization abates and the crystals are resolubilized, the acute attack remits.

Chronic tophaceous arthritis evolves from the repetitive precipitation of urate crystals during acute attacks. The urates may heavily encrust the articular surfaces and form visible deposits in the synovium (Fig. 28–47). The synovium becomes hyperplastic, fibrotic, and thickened by inflammatory cells and forms a pannus that destroys the underlying cartilage leading to juxta-articular bone erosions. In severe cases, fibrous or bony ankylosis ensues resulting in partial to complete loss of joint function.

Tophi are the pathognomonic hallmark of gout. They are formed by large aggregations of urate crystals surrounded by an intense inflammatory reaction of macrophages, lymphocytes, and large foreign body giant cells, which may have completely or partially engulfed masses of crystals (Fig. 28–48). Tophi may appear in the articular cartilage of joints and in the periarticular ligaments, tendons, and soft tissues, including the olecranon and patellar bursae, Achilles tendons, and ear lobes. Less frequently, they may appear in the kidneys, nasal cartilages, skin of the fingertips, palms, or soles as well as elsewhere. Superficial tophi can lead to large ulcerations of the overlying skin.

Gouty nephropathy (Chapter 21) refers to the renal disorder associated with the deposition of monosodium urate crystals in the renal medullary interstitium, sometimes forming tophi, intratubular precipitations, or free uric acid crystals, and the production of uric acid renal stones. Secondary complications, such as pyelonephritis, may ensue, particularly when the urates induce some urinary obstruction.

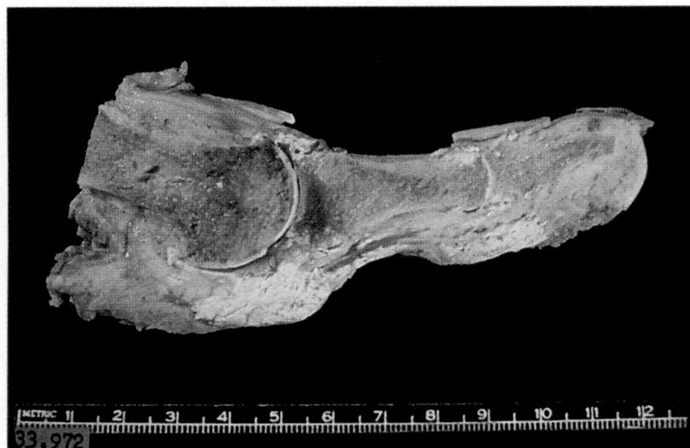

Figure 28–47 ■

Amputated great toe with white tophi involving the joint and soft tissues.

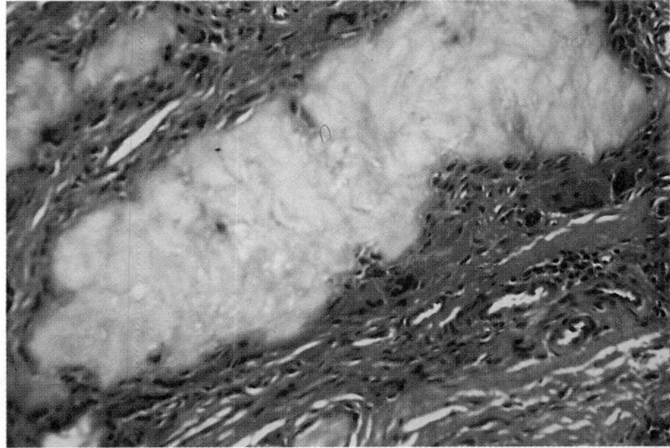

Figure 28–48 ■

Photomicrograph of a gouty tophus. An aggregate of dissolved urate crystals is surrounded by reactive fibroblasts, mononuclear inflammatory cells, and giant cells.

Clinical Course. The natural history of gout is said to pass through four stages: (1) asymptomatic hyperuricemia, (2) acute gouty arthritis, (3) intercritical gout, and (4) chronic tophaceous gout. *Asymptomatic hyperuricemia* appears around puberty in males and after the menopause in females. After a long interval of years, *acute arthritis* appears in the form of the sudden onset of excruciating joint pain associated with localized hyperemia, warmth, and exquisite tenderness. Yet constitutional symptoms are uncommon except possibly mild fever. The vast majority of first attacks are monarticular; 50% occur in the first metatarsophalangeal joint. Eventually, about 90% of patients experience acute attacks in the following locations (in descending order of frequency): insteps, ankles, heels, knees, wrists, fingers, and elbows. Untreated, acute gouty arthritis may last for hours to weeks, but gradually there is complete resolution and the patient enters an *asymptomatic intercritical period.* Although some patients never have another attack, most experience a second acute episode within months to a few years. In the absence of appropriate therapy, the attacks recur at shorter intervals and frequently become polyarticular. Eventually, over the span of years, symptoms fail to resolve completely with the development of disabling *chronic tophaceous gout.* On average, it takes about 12 years between the initial acute attack and the development of chronic tophaceous arthritis. At this stage, x-rays show characteristic juxta-articular bone erosion caused by the crystal deposits and loss of the joint space. Progression leads to severe crippling disease.

Hypertension is common in patients with gout. Renal manifestations sometimes appear in the form of renal colic associated with the passage of gravel and stones and may proceed to chronic gouty nephropathy. About 20% of those with chronic gout die of renal failure. The diagnosis of gout should not be delayed because numerous drugs are available to abort or prevent acute attacks of arthritis and mobilize tophaceous deposits. Their use is important because many aspects of the disease are related to the duration and severity of the hyperuricemia. Generally, gout does not materially shorten the life span, but it may impair quality of life.

CALCIUM PYROPHOSPHATE CRYSTAL DEPOSITION DISEASE (PSEUDOGOUT)

Calcium pyrophosphate crystal deposition disease (CPPD), also known as *pseudogout* and *chondrocalcinosis*, is one of the more common disorders associated with intra-articular crystal formation. It usually occurs in individuals over 50 years of age and becomes more common with increasing age, rising to a prevalence of 30% to 60% in those 85 years or older. The sexes and races are equally affected. CPPD is divided into sporadic (idiopathic), hereditary, and secondary types. In the hereditary variant, the crystals develop relatively early in life and are associated with severe osteoarthritis. One family with this disorder showed linkage of the disease with chromosome 8q. The secondary form is associated with various disorders, including previous joint damage, hyperparathyroidism, hemochromatosis, hypomagnesemia, hypothyroidism, ochronosis, and diabetes. The conditions leading to crystal formation are not entirely known but include altered activity of the matrix enzymes that produce and degrade pyrophosphate, resulting in its accumulation and eventual crystallization with calcium.

The crystals first develop in the articular matrix, menisci, and intervertebral discs, and as the deposits enlarge, they may rupture and seed the joint. Once released into the joint, they elicit an inflammatory infiltrate rich in neutrophils. Neutrophils are thought to produce damage through the release of oxygen metabolites and cytokines, calling forth the more chronic reactions associated with macrophages and fibrosis.[56] The crystals form chalky white friable deposits, which are seen histologically in stained preparations as oval blue-purple aggregates. Individual crystals are generally 0.5 to 5 μ in greatest dimension and weakly birefringent (Fig. 28–49). Rarely the crystals are deposited in masslike aggregates simulating tophi.

CPPD is frequently asymptomatic; however, it is a great simulator because it produces acute, subacute, or chronic arthritis that may mimic other disorders, such as osteoarthritis or RA. The joint involvement may last from several days to weeks and may be monarticular or polyarticular; the knees, followed by the wrists, elbows, shoulders, and ankles, are most commonly affected. Ultimately, approximately 50% of patients experience significant joint damage. Therapy is supportive. There is no known treatment that prevents or retards crystal formation.

Tumors and Tumor-like Lesions

Reactive tumor-like lesions, such as ganglions, synovial cysts, and osteochondral loose bodies, commonly involve

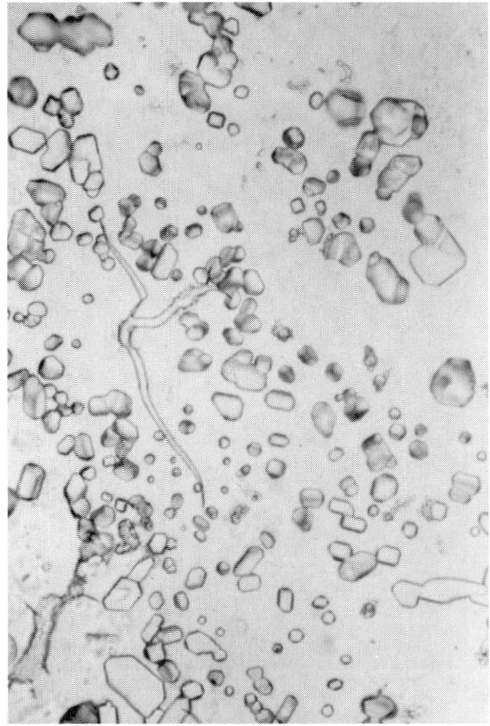

Figure 28–49 ■

Smear preparation of calcium pyrophosphate crystals.

joints and tendon sheaths. They usually result from trauma or degenerative processes and are much more common than neoplasms. Primary neoplasms are unusual and tend to recapitulate the cells and tissue types (synovial membrane, fat, blood vessels, fibrous tissue, and cartilage) native to joints and related structures. Benign tumors are much more frequent than their malignant counterparts, which are rare and discussed with the soft tissue tumors.

GANGLION AND SYNOVIAL CYST

A *ganglion* is a small (1 to 1.5 cm) cyst that is almost always located near a joint capsule or tendon sheath. A common location is around the joints of the wrist, where it appears as a firm, fluctuant, pea-sized translucent nodule. It arises as a result of cystic or myxoid degeneration of connective tissue, hence the cyst wall lacks a true cell lining. The lesion may be multilocular and enlarges through coalescence of adjacent areas of myxoid change. The fluid that fills the cyst is similar to synovial fluid; however, there is no communication with the joint space.

Herniation of synovium through a joint capsule or massive enlargement of a bursa may produce a *synovial cyst.* A well-recognized example is the synovial cyst that forms in the popliteal space in the setting of RA (Baker cyst). The synovial lining may be hyperplastic and contain inflammatory cells and fibrin but is otherwise unremarkable.

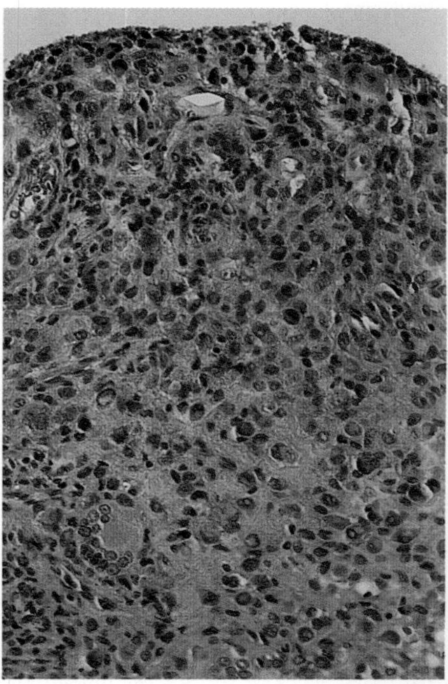

Figure 28–51

Sheets of proliferating cells in PVNS bulging the synovial lining.

GIANT CELL TUMOR OF TENDON SHEATH AND PIGMENTED VILLONODULAR SYNOVITIS

Villonodular synovitis is the term for several closely related benign neoplasms that develop in the synovial lining of joints, tendon sheaths, and bursae. They were previously considered reactive synovial proliferations (hence the designation *synovitis*); however, cytogenetic studies have demonstrated consistent chromosomal aberrations in these lesions indicating that they arise from a clonal proliferation of cells and are neoplastic.[57] The prototypes of these tumors are pigmented villonodular synovitis (PVNS), also known as *diffuse-type giant cell tumor of tendon sheath* (GCT). GCT is also known as *localized nodular tenosynovitis.* Whereas PVNS tends to involve one or more joints diffusely, GCT usually occurs as a discrete nodule on a tendon sheath. Both PVNS and GCT usually arise in the twenties to forties and affect the sexes equally.

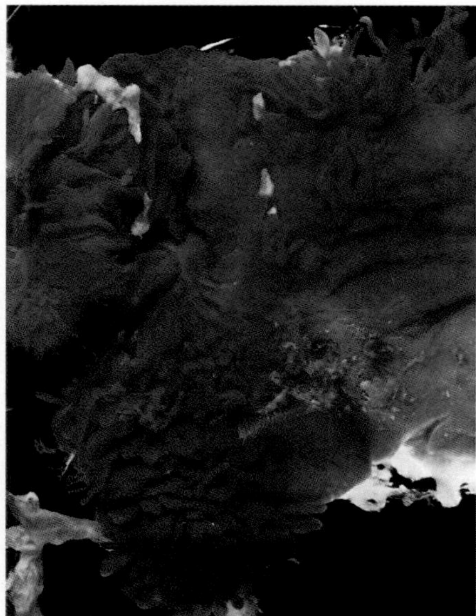

Figure 28–50

Excised synovium with fronds and nodules typical of pigmented villonodular synovitis (PVNS), best seen at 6 o'clock.

Grossly the lesions of PVNS and GCT are both red-brown to mottled orange-yellow. In PVNS, the normally smooth synovium in a joint, most often the knee, is converted into a tangled mat by red-brown folds and finger-like projections (Fig. 28–50). In contrast, GCT is localized and well circumscribed and resembles a small walnut. The tumor cells in both lesions are polyhedral, are moderately sized, and resemble synoviocytes (Fig. 28–51). In PVNS, they spread along the surface and infiltrate the subsynovial compartment. In GCT, the cells grow in a solid nodular aggregate that may be attached to the synovium by a pedicle. Other frequent findings in both lesions include hemosiderin deposits, foamy macrophages, multinucleated giant cells, and zones of sclerosis.

PVNS usually presents as a monarticular arthritis that affects the knee in 80% of cases, followed in frequency by the hip, ankle, and calcaneocuboid joints. Patients typically complain of pain, locking, and recurrent swelling. Tumor progression limits the range of movement of the joint and causes it to become stiff and firm. Sometimes a palpable mass can be appreciated. Aggressive tumors erode into adjacent bones and soft tissues, causing confusion with other types of neoplasia. In contrast, GCT manifests as a solitary, slow-growing, painless mass that frequently involves the tendon sheaths along the wrists and fingers; it is the most common mesenchymal neoplasm of the hand. Cortical erosion of adjacent bone occurs in approximately 15% of cases. Surgery is the recommended treatment for both lesions; PVNS has a significant recurrence rate because it is difficult to excise, and GCT often recurs locally.

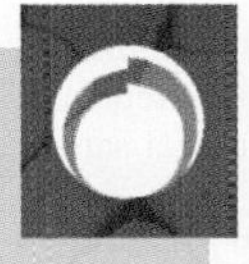

Soft Tissue Tumors and Tumor-like Lesions

Traditionally, soft tissue tumors are defined as mesenchymal proliferations that occur in the extraskeletal, nonepithelial tissues of the body, excluding the viscera, coverings of the brain, and lymphoreticular system. They are classified according to the tissue they *recapitulate* (muscle, fat, fibrous tissue, vessels, and nerves) (Table 28–8), although there is little evidence that they actually arise from the normal differentiated counterpart. Some have no normal tissue counterpart but have constant clinicopathologic features warranting their designation as distinct entities. The true frequency of soft tissue tumors is difficult to estimate because most benign lesions are not removed. A conservative estimate is that benign tumors outnumber their malignant counterparts by a ratio of at least 100:1. In the United States, only 7200 sarcomas are diagnosed annually (0.8% of invasive malignancies), yet they are responsible for 2% of all cancer deaths, reflecting their lethal nature.

Table 28–8. SOFT TISSUE TUMORS

- **Tumors of adipose tissue**
  - Lipomas
  - Liposarcoma
- **Tumors and tumor-like lesions of fibrous tissue**
  - Nodular fasciitis
  - Fibromatoses
    - Superficial fibromatoses
    - Deep fibromatoses
  - Fibrosarcoma
- **Fibrohistiocytic tumors**
  - Fibrous histiocytoma
  - Dermatofibrosarcoma protuberans
  - Malignant fibrous histiocytoma
- **Tumors of skeletal muscle**
  - Rhabdomyoma
  - Rhabdomyosarcoma
- **Tumors of smooth muscle**
  - Leiomyoma
  - Leiomyosarcoma
  - Smooth muscle tumors of uncertain malignant potential
- **Vascular tumors**
  - Hemangioma
  - Lymphangioma
  - Hemangioendothelioma
  - Hemangiopericytoma
  - Angiosarcoma
- **Peripheral nerve tumors**
  - Neurofibroma
  - Schwannoma
  - Malignant peripheral nerve sheath tumors
- **Tumors of uncertain histogenesis**
  - Granular cell tumor
  - Synovial sarcoma
  - Alveolar soft part sarcoma
  - Epithelioid sarcoma

PATHOGENESIS AND GENERAL FEATURES

The cause of most soft tissue tumors is unknown. There are documented associations, however, between radiation therapy and rare instances in which chemical burns, heat burns, or trauma were associated with subsequent development of a sarcoma. Exposure to phenoxyherbicides and chlorophenols has also been implicated in some cases. Kaposi sarcoma in patients with AIDS and in immunosuppressed patients is related to viruses and defective immunocompetence (Chapters 7 and 12). Most soft tissue tumors occur sporadically, but a small minority are associated with genetic syndromes, the most notable of which are neurofibromatosis type 1 (neurofibroma, malignant schwannoma), Gardner syndrome (fibromatosis), Li-Fraumeni syndrome (soft tissue sarcoma), and Osler-Weber-Rendu syndrome (telangiectasia). Cytogenetic and molecular analyses of soft tissue tumors have provided significant insight into their biology. Specific chromosomal abnormalities and genetic derangements can not only be used as diagnostic markers, but also provide important clues about the genesis of the neoplasms.[58] For example, many of the mutations target oncogenes that regulate transcription factors or cell cycle proteins, and their dysfunction results in uncontrolled cell proliferation (Table 28–9).

Soft tissue tumors may arise in any location, although approximately 40% occur in the lower extremity, especially the thigh, 20% in the upper extremities, 10% in the head and neck, and 30% in the trunk and retroperitoneum. Regarding sarcomas, males are affected more frequently than females (1.4 : 1), and the incidence generally increases with

Table 28–9. CHROMOSOMAL AND GENETIC ABNORMALITIES IN SOFT TISSUE SARCOMAS

Tumor	Cytogenetic Abnormality	Genetic Abnormality
Extraosseous Ewing sarcoma	t(11:22)(q24;q12)	FLI-1-EWS fusion gene
Primitive neuroectodermal tumor	t(21:22)(q22;q12)	ERG-EWS fusion gene
	t(7;22)(q22;q12)	ETV1-EWS fusion gene
Liposarcoma-myxoid and round cell type	t(12:16)(q13;p11)	CHOP/TLS fusion gene
Synovial sarcoma	t(x;18)(p11;q11)	SYT-SSX fusion gene
Rhabdomyosarcoma-alveolar type	t(2;13)(q35;q14)	PAX3-FKHR fusion gene
	t(1;13)(p36;q14)	PAX7-FKHR fusion gene
Extraskeletal myxoid chondrosarcoma	t(9;22)(q22;q12)	CHN-EWS fusion gene
Desmoplastic small round cell tumor	t(11;22)(p13;q12)	EWS-WT1 fusion gene
Clear cell sarcoma	t(12;22)(q13;q12)	EWS-ATF1 fusion gene

age. Fifteen per cent arise in children and constitute the fourth most common malignancy in this age group, following brain tumors, hematopoietic cancers, and Wilms' tumor in frequency. Specific sarcomas tend to appear in certain age groups (e.g., rhabdomyosarcoma in children, synovial sarcoma in young adulthood, and liposarcoma and malignant fibrous histiocytoma in mid to late adult life).

Some features of soft tissue tumors influence the prognosis:

- Accurate histologic classification contributes significantly to establishing the prognosis of a sarcoma. Important diagnostic features are cell morphology and architectural arrangement (Tables 28–10 and 28–11). Often these features are not sufficient to distinguish one sarcoma from another, particularly with poorly differentiated aggressive tumors. Great reliance must often be placed on immunohistochemistry, electron microscopy, cytogenetics, and molecular genetics.
- Whatever the type, the *grade* of a soft tissue sarcoma is of great importance. Grading, usually I to III, is based largely on the degree of differentiation, the average number of mitoses per high-power field, cellularity, pleomorphism, and an estimate of the extent of necrosis (presumably a reflection of rate of growth). Mitotic activity and extent of necrosis are thought to be particularly significant. The size, depth, and stage of the tumor also provide important diagnostic information.[59]
- Staging determines the prognosis and chances of successful excision of a tumor. Several staging systems have been proposed for these sarcomas.
- In general, tumors arising in superficial locations (e.g., skin and subcutis) have a better prognosis than deep-seated lesions. In patients with deep-seated, high-grade sarcomas, metastatic disease develops in 80% of those with a tumor larger than 20 cm and 30% of those with a tumor larger than 5 cm. Overall the 10-year survival rate for sarcomas is approximately 40%.

Table 28–10. MORPHOLOGY OF CELLS IN SOFT TISSUE TUMORS

Cell Type	Features	Tumor Type
Spindle cell	Rod-shaped, long axis twice as great as short axis	Fibrous, fibrohistiocytic, smooth muscle, Schwann cell
Small round cell	Size of a lymphocyte with little cytoplasm	Rhabdomyosarcoma, primitive neuroectodermal tumor
Epithelioid	Polyhedral with abundant cytoplasm, nucleus is centrally located	Smooth muscle, Schwann cell endothelial, epithelioid sarcoma

Table 28–11. ARCHITECTURAL PATTERNS IN SOFT TISSUE TUMORS

Pattern	Tumor Type
Fascicles of eosinophilic spindle cells intersecting at right angles	Smooth muscle
Short fascicles of spindle cells radiating from a central point (like spokes on a wheel)—storiform	Fibrohistiocytic
Nuclei arranged in columns—palisading	Schwann cell
Herringbone	Fibrosarcoma
Mixture of fascicles of spindle cells and groups of epithelioid cells—biphasic	Synovial sarcoma

With this brief background, we now turn to the individual tumors and tumor-like lesions. Some of the soft tissue tumors are presented elsewhere—tumors of peripheral nerve (Chapter 30); tumors of vascular origin, including Kaposi sarcoma (Chapter 12); and tumors of smooth muscle origin (Chapter 23).

FATTY TUMORS

Lipomas

Benign tumors of fat, known as lipomas, are the most common soft tissue tumor of adulthood. They are subclassified according to particular morphologic features as conventional lipoma, fibrolipoma, angiolipoma, spindle cell lipoma, myelolipoma, and pleomorphic lipoma. Some of the variants have characteristic chromosomal abnormalities;

for example, conventional lipomas often show rearrangements of 12q14-15, 6p, and 13q, and spindle cell and pleomorphic lipomas have rearrangements of 16q and 13q.

MORPHOLOGY. The conventional lipoma, the most common subtype, is a well-encapsulated mass of mature adipocytes that varies considerably in size. It arises in the subcutis of the proximal extremities and trunk, most frequently during mid-adulthood. Infrequently, lipomas are large, intramuscular, and poorly circumscribed. Histologically, they consist of mature fat cells with no evidence of pleomorphism or abnormal growth.

Lipomas are soft, mobile, and painless (except angiolipoma) and are usually cured by simple excision.

Liposarcoma

Liposarcomas are one of the most common sarcomas of adulthood and appear in the forties to sixties; they are uncommon in children. They usually arise in the deep soft tissues of the proximal extremities and retroperitoneum and are notorious for developing into large tumors.

MORPHOLOGY. Histologically, liposarcomas can be divided into well-differentiated, myxoid, round cell, and pleomorphic variants. The cells in well-differentiated liposarcomas are readily recognized as lipocytes. In the other variants, most of the tumor cells are not obviously adipogenic, but some cells indicative of fatty differentiation are almost always present. They are known as **lipoblasts**, which mimic fetal fat cells (Fig. 28–52). They contain round cytoplasmic vacuoles of lipid that scallop the nucleus. The myxoid and round cell variant of liposarcoma has a t(12;16) chromosomal abnormality in most cases.

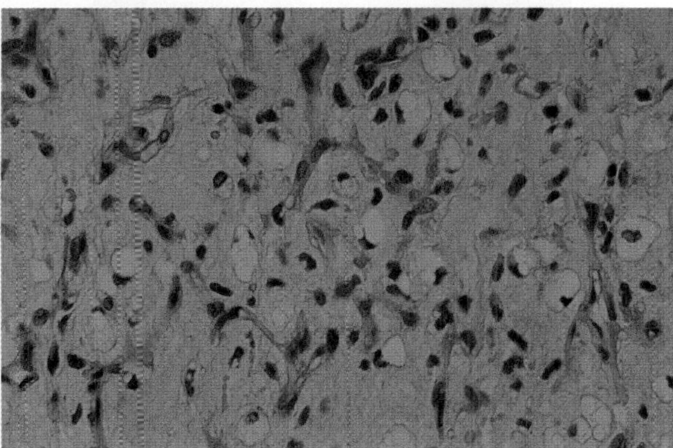

Figure 28–52

Myxoid liposarcoma with abundant ground substance in which are scattered adult-appearing fat cells and more primitive cells, some containing small lipid vacuoles (lipoblasts).

The well-differentiated variant is relatively indolent, the myxoid type is intermediate in its malignant behavior, and the round cell and pleomorphic variants usually are aggressive and frequently metastasize. All types of liposarcoma recur locally and often repeatedly unless adequately excised.

FIBROUS TUMORS AND TUMOR-LIKE LESIONS

Reactive Pseudosarcomatous Proliferations

Reactive pseudosarcomatous proliferations are non-neoplastic lesions that either develop in response to some form of local trauma (physical or ischemic) or are idiopathic. They are composed of plump reactive fibroblasts or related mesenchymal cells. Clinically, they are alarming because they develop suddenly and grow rapidly, and histologically, they cause concern because they mimic sarcomas owing to their hypercellularity, mitotic activity, and a primitive appearance. Representative of this family of lesions are *nodular fasciitis* and *myositis ossificans*.

NODULAR FASCIITIS

Nodular fasciitis, also known as *infiltrative* or *pseudosarcomatous fasciitis*, is the most common of the reactive pseudosarcomas. It most often occurs in adults on the volar aspect of the forearm, followed in order of frequency by the chest and back. Patients typically present with a several-week history of a solitary, rapidly growing, and sometimes painful mass. Preceding trauma is noted in only 10% to 15% of cases.

MORPHOLOGY. Nodular fasciitis lesions arise in the deep dermis, subcutis, or muscle. Grossly the lesion is several centimeters in greatest dimension, is nodular in configuration, and has poorly defined margins. By light microscopy, nodular fasciitis is richly cellular and consists of plump, immature-appearing fibroblasts arranged randomly (simulating cells growing in tissue culture) or in irregular short fascicles (Fig. 28–53). The cells vary in size and shape (spindle to stellate) and have conspicuous nucleoli and abundant mitotic figures. Frequently the stroma is myxoid and contains lymphocytes and extravasated red blood cells. The histologic differential is extensive, but important lesions that should be excluded are fibromatosis

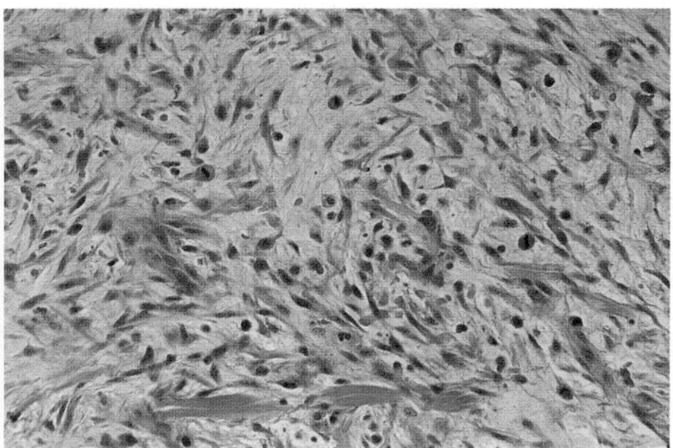

Figure 28–53

Nodular fasciitis with plump, randomly oriented spindle cells surrounded by myxoid stroma. Note the mitotic activity and extravasated red blood cells.

and spindle cell sarcomas. Because nodular fasciitis is reactive, the lesion rarely recurs after excision.

Other pseudosarcomas related to nodular fasciitis are *proliferative fasciitis* and *proliferative myositis.* These lesions occur in slightly older patients and develop in the trunk or proximal extremities. The proliferating fibroblasts are often large and round, have prominent nucleoli, and resemble ganglion cells.

MYOSITIS OSSIFICANS

Myositis ossificans is distinguished from the other fibroblastic proliferations by the presence of *metaplastic bone.* It usually develops in athletic adolescents and young adults and follows an episode of trauma in more than 50% of cases. The lesion arises in the subcutis and musculature of the proximal extremities. The clinical findings are related to its stage of development; in the early phase, the involved area is swollen and painful, and within the subsequent several weeks, it becomes more circumscribed and firm. Eventually, it evolves into a painless, hard, well-demarcated mass.

MORPHOLOGY. Grossly the usual lesion is 3 to 6 cm in greatest dimension. Most are well delineated and have soft, glistening centers and a firm, gritty periphery. The microscopic findings vary according to the age of the lesion; in the earliest phase, the lesion is the most cellular and consists of plump, elongated fibroblast-like cells simulating nodular fasciitis (see earlier). Morphologic zonation begins within 3 weeks; the center retains its population of fibroblasts; however, it merges with an adjacent intermediate zone that contains osteoblasts, which deposit ill-defined trabeculae of woven bone. The most peripheral zone contains well-formed, mineralized trabeculae that closely resemble cancellous bone. Frequently, skeletal muscle fibers and regenerating muscle giant cells are trapped within the margins. Eventually the entire lesion ossifies, and the intertrabecular spaces become filled with bone marrow. The mature lesion is completely ossified.

The radiographic findings parallel the morphologic progression. Initially the x-rays may show only soft tissue fullness, but at about 3 weeks, patchy flocculent radiodensities form in the periphery. The radiodensities become more extensive with time and slowly encroach on the radiolucent center (Fig. 28–54). Myositis ossificans must be distinguished from extraskeletal osteosarcoma. The latter usually occurs in elderly patients, the proliferating cells are cytologically malignant, and the tumor lacks the zonation of myositis ossificans. To be noted, the most peripheral regions of osteosarcoma are the most cellular and primitive, which is the reverse of myositis ossificans. Simple excision of myositis ossificans is usually curative.

Fibromatoses

SUPERFICIAL FIBROMATOSIS (PALMAR, PLANTAR, AND PENILE FIBROMATOSES)

Palmar, plantar, and penile fibromatoses, more bothersome than serious lesions, constitute a small group of su-

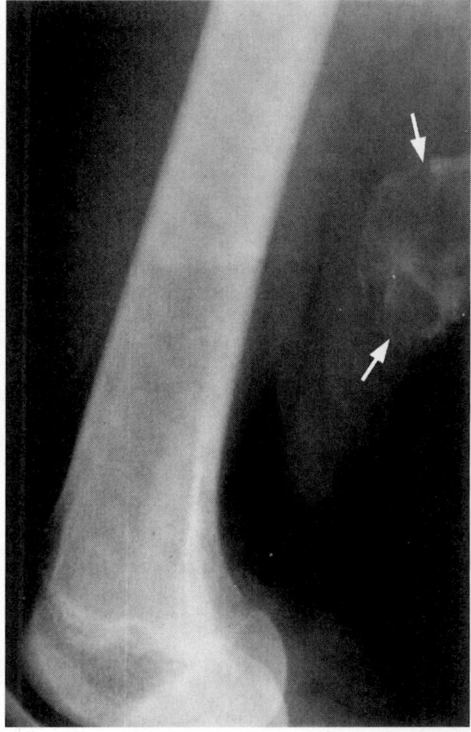

Figure 28–54

Peripherally mineralized myositis ossificans involving the posterior thigh.

perficial fibromatoses. They are characterized by nodular or poorly defined fascicles of mature-appearing fibroblasts surrounded by abundant dense collagen. Immunohistochemical and ultrastructural studies indicate that many of these cells are *myofibroblasts* (Chapter 4). Several nonrandom karyotypic abnormalities have been described in these tumors (e.g., trisomy 3 and 8), but their significance is still unclear.[60]

In the palmar variant (*Dupuytren contracture*), there is irregular or nodular thickening of the palmar fascia either unilaterally or bilaterally (50%). Over a span of years, attachment to the overlying skin causes puckering and dimpling. At the same time, a slowly progressive flexion contracture develops mainly of the fourth and fifth fingers of the hand. Essentially similar changes are seen with *plantar fibromatosis* except that flexion contractures are uncommon and bilateral involvement is infrequent. In *penile fibromatosis* (*Peyronie disease*), a palpable induration or mass appears usually on the dorsolateral aspect of the penis. It may cause eventually abnormal curvature of the shaft or constriction of the urethra, or both.

Although not surprisingly, males are affected more frequently than females in Peyronie disease, male predominance is true of the other patterns as well. In about 20% to 25% of cases, the palmar and plantar fibromatoses stabilize and do not progress, in some instances resolving spontaneously. Some recur after excision, particularly the plantar lesion.

DEEP-SEATED FIBROMATOSIS (DESMOID TUMORS)

Biologically, deep-seated fibromatoses lie in the interface between exuberant fibrous proliferations and low-grade fibrosarcomas. On the one hand, they present frequently as large, infiltrative masses that may recur after incomplete excision, and on the other, they are composed of banal well-differentiated fibroblasts that do not metastasize. They may occur at any age but are most frequent in the teens to thirties. Desmoids are divided into *extra-abdominal*, *abdominal*, and *intra-abdominal*, but all have essentially similar gross and microscopic features. Extra-abdominal desmoids occur in men and women with equal frequency and arise principally in the musculature of the shoulder, chest wall, back, and thigh. Abdominal desmoids generally arise in the musculoaponeurotic structures of the anterior abdominal wall in women during or after pregnancy. Intra-abdominal desmoids tend to occur in the mesentery or pelvic walls, often in patients having familial adenomatous polyposis (Gardner syndrome) (Chapter 18).

MORPHOLOGY. These lesions occur as unicentric, gray-white, firm, poorly demarcated masses varying from 1 to 15 cm in greatest diameter. They are rubbery and tough and infiltrate surrounding structures. Histologically the central region, presumably the oldest part of the growth, is often largely densely collagenous, whereas the periphery is made up of plump fibroblasts having minimal variation in cell and nuclear size (Fig. 28–55). Mitoses are infrequent. Regenerative muscle cells when trapped within these lesions may take on the appearance of multinucleated giant cells.

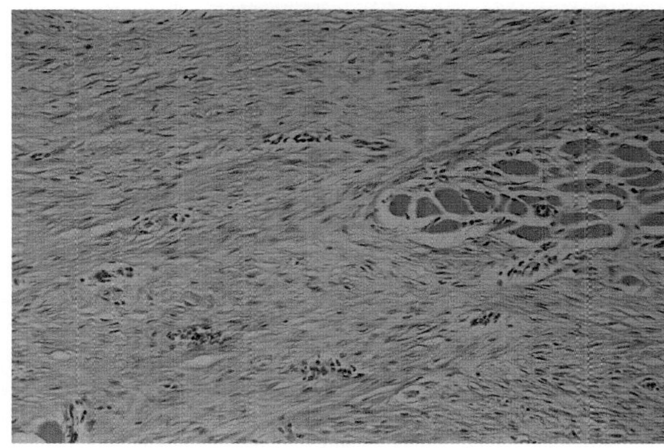

Figure 28–55

Fibromatosis infiltrating between skeletal muscle cells.

In addition to their possibly being disfiguring or disabling, desmoids are occasionally painful. Although curable by adequate excision, they frequently recur locally and persistently when incompletely removed. Some tumors have responded to treatment with tamoxifen, and in other cases chemotherapy or irradiation has been effective. The rare reports of metastasis of a desmoid must be interpreted as misdiagnosis of fibrosarcoma.

Fibrosarcoma

Fibrosarcomas are rare but may occur anywhere in the body, most commonly in the retroperitoneum, the thigh, the knee, and the distal extremities. Many tumors previously considered fibrosarcoma have been reclassified as aggressive fibromatosis (desmoid), malignant fibrous histiocytoma, malignant peripheral nerve sheath tumors, or synovial sarcomas.

MORPHOLOGY. Typically, these neoplasms are unencapsulated, infiltrative, soft, fish-flesh masses often having areas of hemorrhage and necrosis. Better-differentiated lesions may appear deceptively encapsulated. Histologic examination discloses all degrees of differentiation, from slowly growing tumors that closely resemble cellular fibromas sometimes having spindled cells growing in a herringbone fashion (Fig. 28–56) to highly cellular neoplasms dominated by architectural disarray, pleomorphism, frequent mitoses, and areas of necrosis.

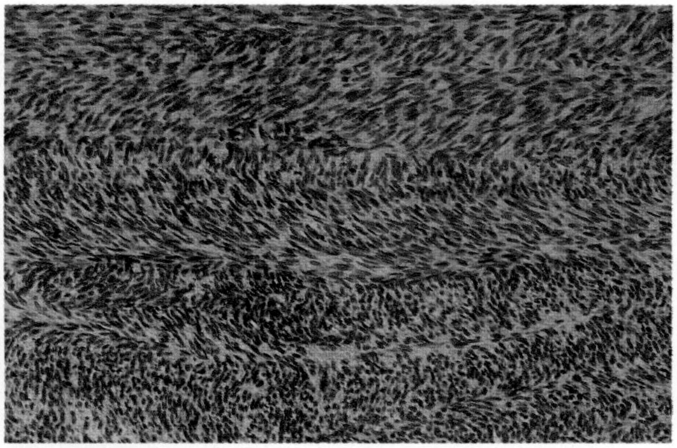

Figure 28–56

Fibrosarcoma composed of malignant spindle cells arranged in a herringbone pattern.

Because true fibrosarcomas are often difficult to diagnose, data on their properties are variable. They are aggressive tumors, however, recurring in more than 50% of the cases and metastasizing in more than 25%.

FIBROHISTIOCYTIC TUMORS

Fibrohistiocytic tumors contain cellular elements that resemble both fibroblasts and histiocytes. Originally, they were believed to be neoplasms of histiocytes, but studies suggest that the fundamental phenotype of the neoplastic cells most closely resembles fibroblasts. Thus, the term *fibrohistiocytic* should be viewed as descriptive in nature and not one that connotes histogenetic origin.

Benign Fibrous Histiocytoma (Dermatofibroma and Sclerosing Hemangioma)

Benign fibrous histiocytoma is a relatively common lesion that usually occurs in the dermis and subcutis. It is painless and slow growing and most often presents in mid-adult life as a firm, small (up to 1 cm) mobile nodule.

MORPHOLOGY. Most benign fibrous histiocytomas consist of a proliferation of bland spindle cells arranged in a storiform pattern. These are often referred to as **dermatofibromas**. Other variants may contain numerous blood vessels and hemosiderin deposition giving rise to the designation **sclerosing hemangioma**. Still others may be richly punctuated with foamy histiocytes and are called **histiocytomas**. All are variations on a common theme, and in all the margins are infiltrative, but the tumor does not invade the overlying epidermis, which is frequently hyperplastic. Adequate treatment is simple excision.

Malignant Fibrous Histiocytoma

Once considered the most common sarcoma of adults, *malignant fibrous histiocytoma* refers to a heterogeneous group of aggressive soft tissue tumors characterized by considerable cytologic pleomorphism, the presence of bizarre multinucleate cells, a storiform architecture, and a background of inflamed collagenous stroma, often with foamy macrophages. The cell of origin is uncertain but is clearly not histiocytic. Immunochemical and ultrastructural studies have shown many of these tumors to be pleomorphic variants of liposarcoma, leiomyosarcoma, rhabdomyosarcoma, and myxofibrosarcoma. Thus, some authors question categorization of malignant fibrous histiocytoma as a distinct entity. Nevertheless, some cases with the histologic features described show no distinct differentiation and can be thus classified. Malignant fibrous histiocytoma usually arises in the musculature of the proximal extremities and the retroperitoneum. Cutaneous variants are also known as *atypical fibroxanthomas*.

MORPHOLOGY. These tumors are usually gray-white unencapsulated masses but often appear deceptively circumscribed. They are frequently large (5 to 20 cm). Malignant fibrous histiocytomas have been categorized into **storiform-pleomorphic, myxoid, inflammatory, giant cell,** and **angiomatoid** variants based on their histologic features. The storiform-pleomorphic type is the most common and as the name indicates is composed of malignant spindle cells oriented in a storiform pattern with scattered, large round pleo-

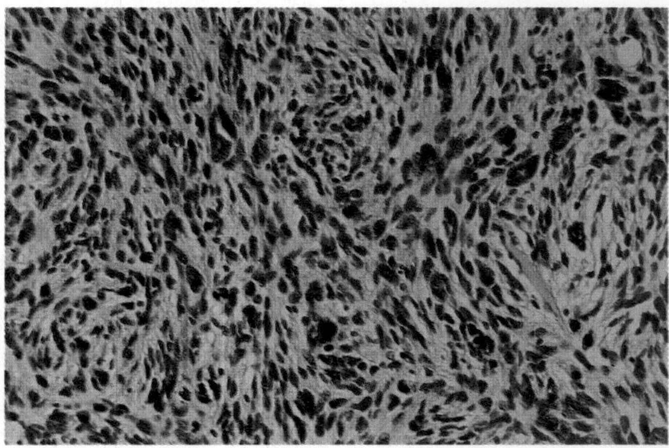

Figure 28–57

Malignant fibrous histiocytoma revealing fascicles of plump spindled cells in a swirling (storiform) pattern, typical but not pathognomonic of this neoplasm. (Courtesy of Dr. J. Corson, Brigham and Women's Hospital, Boston, MA.)

morphic cells (Fig. 28–57). As noted earlier, some of these tumors show differentiation toward well-recognized lipoid, fibrous, muscle, or myxoid tumors and in these instances should be thus designated.

Most variants of malignant fibrous histiocytoma are aggressive, recur unless widely excised, and have a metastatic rate of 30% to 50% except for the cutaneous tumors, which rarely disseminate. The angiomatoid variant is also indolent and in contrast to the other types occurs in adolescents and young adults.

TUMORS OF SKELETAL MUSCLE

Skeletal muscle neoplasms, in contrast to other groups of tumors, are almost all malignant. The benign variant, rhabdomyoma, is distinctly rare. The so-called cardiac rhabdomyoma is probably hamartomatous in origin and is discussed in Chapter 13.

Rhabdomyosarcoma

Rhabdomyosarcomas, the most common soft tissue sarcomas of childhood and adolescence, usually appear before age 20. They may arise in any anatomic location, but most occur in the head and neck or genitourinary tract, where there is little if any skeletal muscle as a normal constituent.[61] Only in the extremities do they appear in relation to skeletal muscle.

MORPHOLOGY. Rhabdomyosarcoma is histologically subclassified into the **embryonal, alveolar**, and **pleomorphic** variants. The rhabdomyoblast—the diagnostic cell in all types—contains eccentric eosinophilic granular cytoplasm rich in thick and thin filaments. The rhabdomyoblasts may be round or elongate; the latter are known as tadpole or strap cells (Fig. 28–58). Ultrastructurally, rhabdomyoblasts contain sarcomeres, and immunohistochemically they stain with antibodies to vimentin, actin, desmin, and myoglobin.

Embryonal rhabdomyosarcoma is the most common type, accounting for 66% of rhabdomyosarcomas. It includes the **sarcoma botryoides** described in Chapter 24 and spindle cell variants. The tumor occurs in children under the age of 10 years and typically arises in the nasal cavity, orbit, middle ear, prostate, and paratesticular region. The sarcoma botryoides subtype develops in the walls of hollow, mucosal-lined structures, such as the nasopharynx, common bile duct, bladder, and vagina.

The tumor presents as a soft gray infiltrative mass. The tumor cells mimic skeletal muscle cells at various stages of embryogenesis and consist of sheets of both malignant round and spindled cells in a variably myxoid stroma. Sarcoma botryoides grows in a polypoid fashion producing the appearance of a cluster of grapes protruding into a hollow structure such as the bladder or vagina. Where the tumor abuts the mucosa of an organ, they form a submucosal zone of hypercellularity known as the **cambium layer**. Rhabdomyoblasts with visible cross-striations may be present.

Alveolar rhabdomyosarcoma is most common in early to mid adolescence and commonly arises in the deep musculature of the extremities. Histologically the tumor is traversed by a network of fibrous septae that divide the cells into clusters or aggregates; as the central cells degenerate and drop out, a crude resemblance to pulmonary alveolce is created (Fig. 28–59). The tumor cells are discohesive and moderate in size, and many

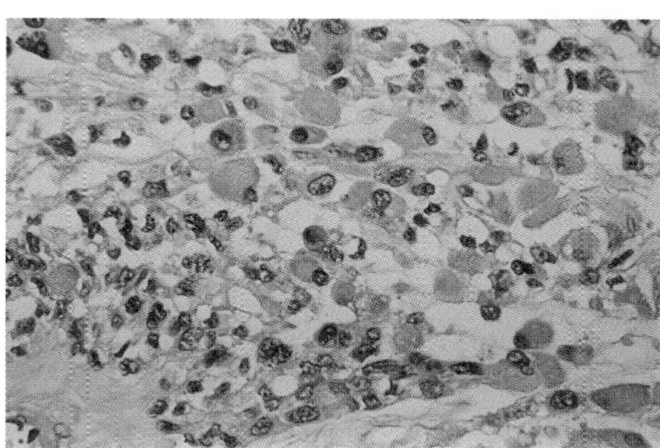

Figure 28–58

Rhabdomyosarcoma composed of malignant small round cells. The rhabdomyoblasts are large and round and have abundant eosinophilic cytoplasm; no cross-striations are evident.

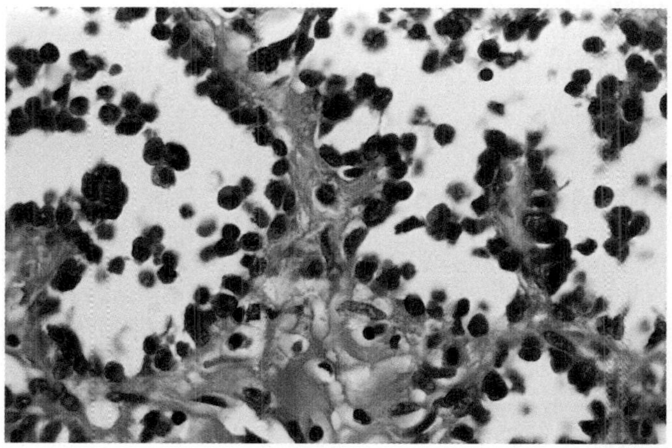

Figure 28–59

Alveolar rhabdomyosarcoma with numerous spaces lined by tumor cells.

have little cytoplasm. Cells with cross-striations are identified in about 25% of cases. Cytogenetic studies have shown that this variant of rhabdomyosarcoma has a t(2,13) or t(1;13) chromosomal aberration.

Pleomorphic rhabdomyosarcoma is characterized by numerous large, sometimes multinucleated, bizarre eosinophilic tumor cells. This variant is uncommon, has a tendency to arise in the deep soft tissue of adults, and, as noted earlier, can resemble malignant fibrous histiocytoma histologically.

Rhabdomyosarcomas are aggressive neoplasms and are usually treated with a combination of surgery and chemotherapy with or without radiation. The histologic variant and location of the tumor influence survival. The botryoid subtype has the best prognosis followed by the embryonal, pleomorphic, and alveolar variants. Overall, approximately 65% of children are cured of their disease,[62] but adults fare less well.

TUMORS OF SMOOTH MUSCLE

Leiomyomas

Leiomyomas, the benign smooth muscle tumors, often arise in the uterus where they represent the most common neoplasm in women (Chapter 24). Leiomyomas may also arise in the skin and subcutis from the arrector pili muscles found in the skin, nipples, scrotum, and labia (genital leiomyomas) and less frequently develop in the deep soft tissues. Those arising in the arrector muscles (*pilar leiomyomas*) are frequently multiple and painful. The tendency to develop multiple lesions is thought to be hereditary and transmitted as an autosomal dominant trait. In whatever setting, these lesions tend to occur in adolescence and early adult life.

They are usually not larger than 1 to 2 cm in greatest dimension and are composed of fascicles of spindle cells that tend to intersect each other at right angles. The tumor cells have blunt-ended elongated nuclei and show minimal atypia and few mitotic figures. Solitary lesions are easily cured; however, they may be so numerous that complete surgical removal is impractical.

Leiomyosarcoma

Leiomyosarcomas account for 10% to 20% of soft tissue sarcomas. They occur in adults and afflict women more frequently than men. Most develop in the skin and deep soft tissues of the extremities and retroperitoneum.

MORPHOLOGY. Leiomyosarcomas present as painless firm masses. Retroperitoneal tumors may be large and bulky and cause abdominal symptoms. Histologically, they are characterized by malignant spindle cells that have cigar-shaped nuclei arranged in interweaving fascicles. Morphologic variants include tumors with a prominent myxoid stroma and others with epithelioid cells. Ultrastructurally, malignant smooth muscle cells contain bundles of thin filaments with dense bodies and pinocytotic vesicles, and individual cells are surrounded by basal lamina. Immunohistochemically, they stain with antibodies to vimentin, actin, and desmin.

Treatment depends on the size, location, and grade of the tumor. Superficial or cutaneous leiomyosarcomas are usually small and have a good prognosis, whereas those of retroperitoneum are large, cannot be entirely excised, and cause death by both local extension and metastatic spread.

SYNOVIAL SARCOMA

Synovial sarcoma is so named because it was once believed to recapitulate synovium, but the cell of origin is still unclear. In addition, although the term *synovial sarcoma* implies an origin from the joint linings, less than 10% are intra-articular. Synovial sarcomas account for approximately 10% of all soft tissue sarcomas and rank as the fourth most common sarcoma. Most occur in the twenties to forties. The majority develop in the vicinity of the large joints of the extremities, and about 60% to 70% involve the lower extremity, especially around the knee and thigh. Patients usually present with a deep-seated mass that has been noted for several years. Uncommonly, these tumors occur in the parapharyngeal region or in the abdominal wall.

MORPHOLOGY. The histologic hallmark of synovial sarcoma is the biphasic morphology of the tumor cells (i.e., epithelial-like and spindle cells). Despite the mimicry of synovium, the tumor cells do not have the features of synoviocytes. The epithelial cells are cuboidal to columnar and form glands or grow in solid cords. The spindle cells are arranged in densely cellular fascicles that surround the epithelial cells (Fig. 28–60). Most synovial sarcomas are *monophasic* in that they are composed of only spindled or epithelial cells. Lesions composed solely of spindled cells are easily mistaken for fibrosarcomas. A characteristic feature when present are calcified concretions that can sometimes be detected radiographically. Immunohistochemistry is helpful in identifying these tumors, since the epithelioid and spindle cell portions yield positive reactions for keratin and epithelial membrane antigen, differentiating these tumors from most other sarcomas. In addition, most synovial sarcomas show a characteristic chromosomal translocation t(x;18)[63] and fused gene (SYT-SSX).[64]

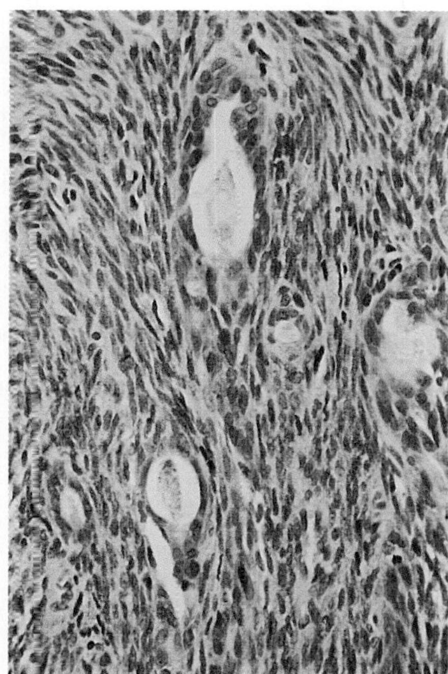

Figure 28–60 ■

Synovial sarcoma revealing the classic biphasic spindle cell and glandular-like histologic appearance.

Synovial sarcomas are treated aggressively with limb-sparing therapy. The 5-year survival rate varies from 25% to 62%, and only 11% to 30% live for 10 years or longer. Common sites of metastases are the regional lymph nodes, lung, and skeleton.

REFERENCES

1. Glimcher MJ: The nature of the mineral component of bone and the mechanism of calcification. In Avioli LV, Krane SM (eds): Metabolic Bone Disease and Clinical Related Disorders, 2nd ed. Philadelphia, WB Saunders, 1990.
2. Mundy GR: Local control of bone formation by osteoblasts. Clin Orthop Rel Res 313:19, 1995.
3. Rodan GA, Harada S: The missing bone. Cell 89:677, 1997.
4. Duncan RL, Turner CH: Mechanotransduction and the functional response of bone to mechanical strain. Calcif Tissue Int 57:344, 1995.
5. Athanasou NA: Cellular biology of bone-resorbing cells. J Bone Joint Surg 78(A):1096, 1996
6. Young MF, et al: Structure, expression and reglation of the major non-collagenous matrix proteins of bone. Clin Orthop Rel Res 281: 275, 1992.
7. MacDonald BR, Gowen M: Cytokines and bone. Br J Rheumatol 31: 149, 1992.
8. Marcus R: Normal and abnormal bone remodeling in man. Ann Rev Med 38:129, 1987.
9. Mundlos S, Olsen BR: Heritable diseases of the skeleton: Part I. Molecular insights into skeletal development—transcription factors and signaling pathways. FASEB J 11:125, 1997.
10. Mundlos S, Olsen BR: Heritable diseases of the skeleton: Part II. Molecular insights into skeletal development—matrix components and their homeostasis. FASEB J 11:227, 1997.
11. Byers PH, Steiner RD: Osteogenesis imperfecta. Annu Rev Med 43: 269, 1992.
12. Bullough PG, et al: The morbid anatomy of the skeleton in osteogenesis imperfecta. Clin Orthop Rel Res 159:42, 1981.
13. Gallager JC: Pathophysiology of osteoporosis. Semin Nephrol 12:109, 1992.
14. Chestnut CH: Theoretical overview: bone development, peak bone loss, bone loss, and fracture risk. Am J Med 91(suppl 5B):25, 1991.
15. Rubin CT, et al: Suppression of the osteogenic response in the aging skeleton. Calcif Tissue Int 50:306, 1992.
16. Pacifici R: Estrogens, cytokines and pathogenesis of postmenopausal osteoporosis. J Bone Miner Res 11:1043, 1996.
17. Manolagas SC, et al: Sex steroids, cytokines and the bone marrow: new concepts on the pathogenesis of osteoporosis. Ciba Res Found Symp 191:187, 1995
18. Felix R, et al: Recent developments in understanding of the pathophysiology of osteopetrosis. Eur J Endocrinology 134:143, 1996.
19. Fraser WD: Paget disease of bone. Curr Opin Rheumatol 9:347, 1997.
20. Ooi CG, Fraser WD: Paget disease of bone. Postgrad Med 73:69, 1996.
21. Hadjipavlou A, et al: Malignant transformation in Paget disease of bone. Cancer 70:2802, 1992.
22. Bushinsky DA: Bone disease in moderate renal failure: cause, nature and prevention. Ann Rev Med 48:167, 1997.
23. Bolander M: Regulation of fracture repair by growth factors. Proc Soc Exp Biol Med 200:165, 1992.
24. Mankin H: Nontraumatic necrosis of bone (osetonecrosis). N Engl J Med 326:1473, 1992.
25. Lew SP, Waldvogel FA: Osteomyelitis. N Engl J Med 336:999, 1997.
26. Senac MO, et al: Primary lesions of bone in the first decade of life: retrospective survey of biopsy results. Radiology 160:491, 1986.
27. Klein MH, Shankman S: Osteoid osteoma: radiologic and pathologic correlation. Skeletal Radiol 21:23, 1992.
28. Klein MJ, et al: Osteosarcoma: clinical and pathological considerations. Orthop Clin North Am 20:327, 1989.
29. Lonardo F, et al: P53 and MDM2 alterations in osteosarcoma: correlation with clinicopathologic features and proliferation rates. Cancer 79:1541, 1997.
30. Unni KK, Dahlin DC: Osteosarcoma: pathology and classification. Semin Roentgenol 24:143, 1989.
31. Hahn M, Dorman JP: Primary bone malignancies in children. Curr Opin Pediatr 8:71, 1996.
32. Ragsdale BD, et al: Radiology as gross pathology in evaluating chondroid lesions. Hum Pathol 20:930, 1989.
33. Turcotte RE, et al: Chondroblastoma. Hum Pathol 24:944, 1993.
34. Zillmer DA, Dorfman HD: Chondromyoid fibroma of bone: thirty-six cases with clinicopathologic correlation. Hum Pathol 20:952, 1989.
35. Brien EW, et al: Benign and malignant cartilage tumors of bone and joint: Their anatomic and theoretical basis with an emphasis on radiology, pathology and clinical biology. Skeletal Radiol 26:325, 1997.
36. Ringle MD, et al: Clinical implications of genetic defects in G proteins: the molecular basis of McCune-Albright syndrome and Albright hereditary osteodystrophy. Medicine 75:171, 1996.
37. Huvos AG, et al: Malignant fibrous histiocytoma of bone: a clinicopathologic study of 81 patients. Cancer 79:482, 1997.
38. Vlasak R, Sim FH: Ewing sarcoma. Orthop Clin North Am 27:591, 1996.
39. May WA, Denny CT: Biology of EWS/FL1 and related fusion genes in Ewing sarcoma and primitive neuroectodermal tumor. Curr Top Microbiol Immunol 220:143, 1997.
40. Meideiros LJ, et al: Giant cells and mononuclear cells of giant cell tumor of bone resemble histiocytes. Appl Immunohistochem 1:115, 1993.
41. Kraus VB: Pathogenesis and treatment of osteoarthritis. Med Clin North Am 81:85, 1997.
42. Westacott CI, Shariff M: Cytokines in osteoarthritis: Mediators or markers of joint destruction. Semin Arthritis Rheum 25:254, 1996.
43. Krause A, et al: Potential infectious agents in the induction of arthritides. Curr Opin Rheumatol 8:203, 1996.
44. Breedveld FC, Verweij CL: T-cells in rheumatoid arthritis. Br J Rheumatol 36:617, 1997.
45. Panayi GS: T-cell-dependent pathways in rheumatoid arthritis. Curr Opin Rheumatol 9:236, 1997.
46. Muller-Ladner U: Molecular and cellular interactions in rheumatoid synovium. Curr Opin Rheumatol 8:210, 1996.
47. Cassidy JT, et al: The development of classification criteria for children with juvenile rheumatoid arthritis. Bull Rheum Dis 38:1, 1989.

48. Sakkas LI, Platsoucas CD: Immunopathogenesis of juvenile rheumatoid arthritis: role of T cells and MHC. Immunol Res 14:218, 1995.
49. Brown M, Wordsworth P: Predisposing factors to spondyloarthropathies. Curr Opin Rheumatol 9:308, 1997.
50. Granfors K: Host-microbe interaction in HLA-B27-associated diseases. Ann Med 29:153, 1997.
51. Sigal LH: Lyme disease: a review of aspects of its immunology and immunopathogenesis. Ann Rev Immunol 15:63, 1997.
52. Phillips PE: Viral arthritis. Curr Opin Rheumatol 9:337, 1997.
53. German DC, Holmes EW: Hyperuricemia and gout. Med Clin North Am 70:419, 1986.
54. Gross M: Crystallographic antibodies. Nature 373:105, 1995.
55. DiGiovine FS, et al: Interleukin 1 (IL-1) as a mediator of crystal arthritis: stimulation of T cell and synovial fibroblast mitogenesis by urate crystal–induced IL-1. J Immunol 138:3213, 1987.
56. Rull M: Calcium-crystal diseases and miscellaneous crystals. Curr Opin Rheumatol 9:274, 1997.
57. Fletcher JA, et al: Trisomy 5 and trisomy 7 are nonrandom aberrations in pigmented villonodular synovitis: confirmation of trisomy 7 in unclutured cells. Genes Chrom Cancer 4:264, 1992.
58. Choong PF, et al: Musculoskeletal oncology—advances in cytogenetics and molecular genetics and their clinical implications. Acta Oncol 36:245, 1997.
59. Guillou L, et al: Comparative study of the National Cancer Institute and French Federation of Cancer Centers Sarcoma Group grading systems in a population of 420 adult patients with soft tissue sarcoma. J Clin Oncol 15:350, 1997.
60. Hasegawa S, Fletcher C. Fibromatosis in the adult. Adv Pathol 9:259, 1996.
61. Malogolowkin M, Ortega JA: Rhabdomyosarcoma of childhood. Pediatr Ann 17:253, 1992.
62. Pappo AS, et al: Rhabdomyosarcoma: biology and treatment. Pediatr Clin North Am 44:953, 1997.
63. Dal Cin P, Van den Berghe H: Ten years of the cytogenetics of soft tissue tumors. Cancer Genet Cytogenet 95:59, 1997.
64. Kawai A, et al: SYT-SSX fusion as a determinant of morphology and prognosis in synovial sarcoma. New Eng J Med 338:153, 1998.

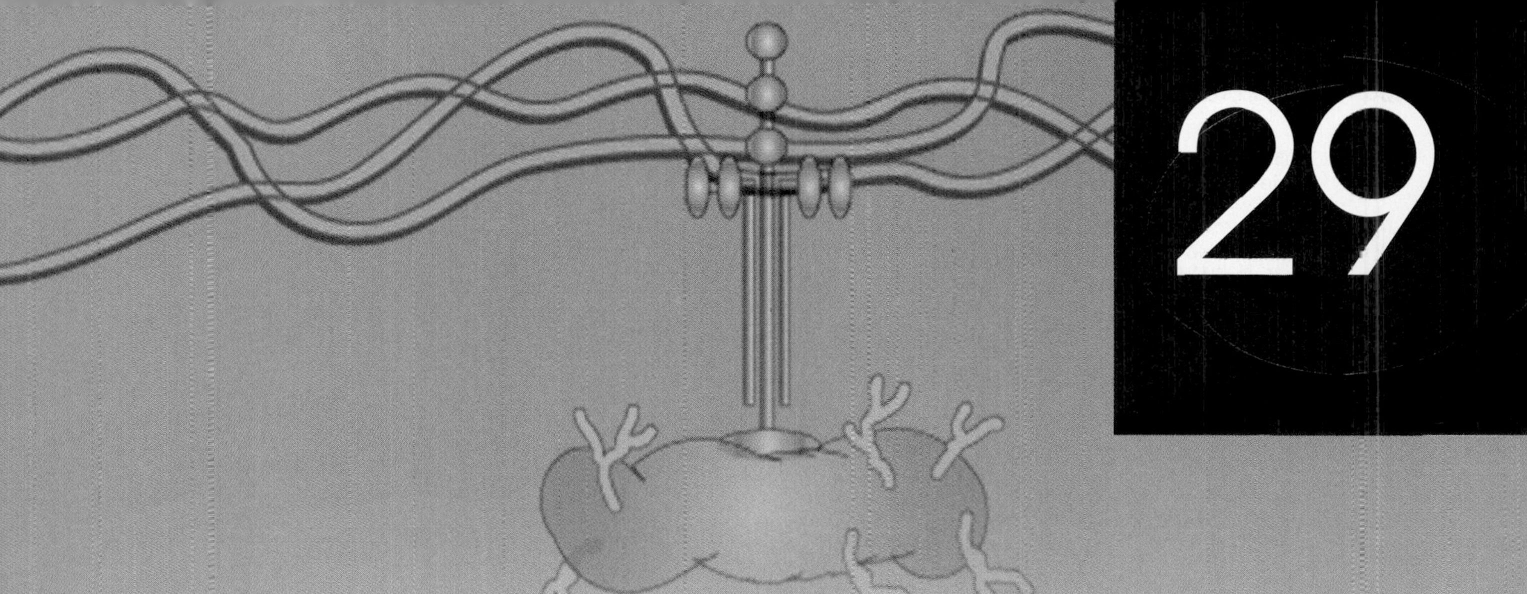

29

Peripheral Nerve and Skeletal Muscle

Umberto De Girolami, Douglas C. Anthony, and Matthew P. Frosch

NORMAL STRUCTURE

NORMAL PERIPHERAL NERVE

NORMAL SKELETAL MUSCLE

GENERAL REACTIONS OF THE MOTOR UNIT

SEGMENTAL DEMYELINATION

AXONAL DEGENERATION AND MUSCLE FIBER ATROPHY

NERVE REGENERATION AND REINNERVATION OF MUSCLE

REACTIONS OF THE MUSCLE FIBER

DISEASES OF PERIPHERAL NERVE

INFLAMMATORY NEUROPATHIES

Immune-Mediated Neuropathies

Guillain-Barré Syndrome (Acute Inflammatory Demyelinating Polyradiculoneuropathy)

Chronic Inflammatory Demyelinating Polyradiculoneuropathy

INFECTIOUS POLYNEUROPATHIES

Leprosy

Diphtheria

Varicella-Zoster Virus

HEREDITARY NEUROPATHIES

Hereditary Motor and Sensory Neuropathy I (HMSN I, CMT1)

Other Hereditary Motor and Sensory Neuropathies

HMSN II

Dejerine-Sottas Disease (HMSN III)

ACQUIRED METABOLIC AND TOXIC NEUROPATHIES

Peripheral Neuropathy in Adult-Onset Diabetes Mellitus

Metabolic and Nutritional Peripheral Neuropathies

Neuropathies Associated With Malignancy

Toxic Neuropathies

TRAUMATIC NEUROPATHIES

TUMORS OF PERIPHERAL NERVE

DISEASES OF SKELETAL MUSCLE

DENERVATION ATROPHY

Spinal Muscular Atrophy (Infantile Motor Neuron Disease)

MUSCULAR DYSTROPHIES

X-Linked Muscular Dystrophy (Duchenne Muscular Dystrophy and Becker Muscular Dystrophy)

Autosomal Muscular Dystrophies

Myotonic Dystrophy

ION CHANNEL MYOPATHIES (CHANNELOPATHIES)

CONGENITAL MYOPATHIES

MYOPATHIES ASSOCIATED WITH INBORN ERRORS OF METABOLISM

Lipid Myopathies

Mitochondrial Myopathies (Oxidative Phosphorylation Diseases)

INFLAMMATORY MYOPATHIES

TOXIC MYOPATHIES

Thyrotoxic Myopathy

Ethanol Myopathy

Drug-Induced Myopathies

DISEASES OF THE NEUROMUSCULAR JUNCTION

Myasthenia Gravis

Lambert-Eaton Myasthenic Syndrome

TUMORS OF SKELETAL MUSCLE

NORMAL STRUCTURE

The functional unit of the neuromuscular system is the *motor unit,* which consists of (1) a *lower motor neuron* in the anterior horn of the spinal cord or cranial nerve motor nucleus in the brain stem, (2) the *axon* of that neuron, and (3) the multiple *muscle fibers* it innervates (Fig. 29–1). Lower motor neurons distributed in the anterior horns in columns or groups are arranged somatotopically so that cells lying medially innervate proximal muscles, and those

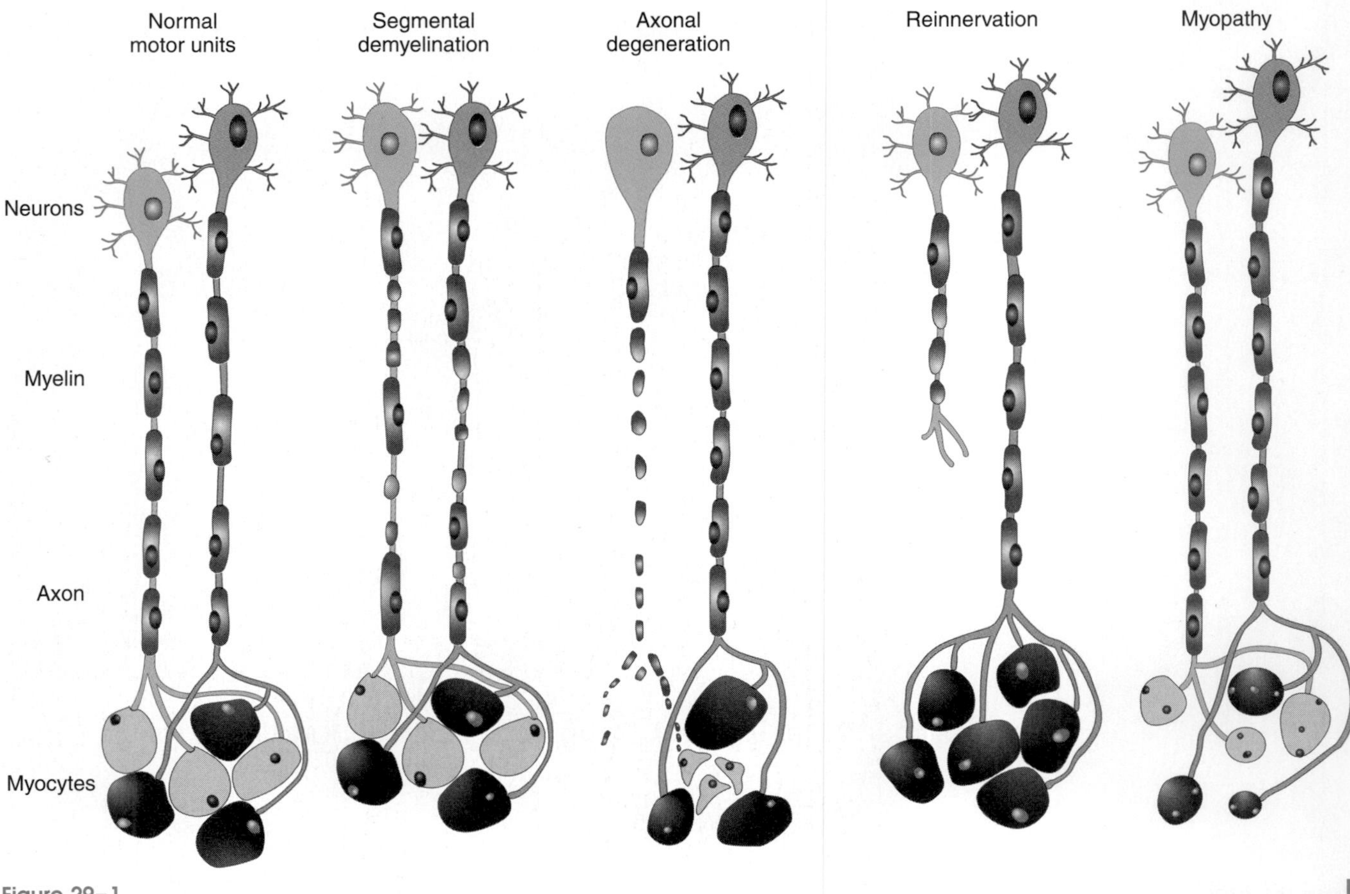

Figure 29–1

Normal and abnormal motor units. Two adjacent units are shown. *Segmental demyelination:* Random internodes of myelin are injured and are remyelinated by multiple Schwann cells, while the axon and myocytes remain intact. *Axonal degeneration:* The axon and its myelin sheath undergo anterograde degeneration (shown for the green neuron), with resulting denervation atrophy of the myocytes within its motor unit. *Reinnervation of muscle:* Sprouting of adjacent (red) uninjured motor axons leads to fiber type grouping of myocytes, while the injured axon attempts axonal sprouting. *Myopathy:* Scattered myocytes of adjacent motor units are small (degenerated or regenerated), whereas the neurons and nerve fibers are normal.

lying laterally supply the distal musculature. The number of muscle fibers within each unit varies considerably. Muscles with highly refined movements, like the extrinsic muscles of the eye, have a high neuron to muscle-fiber ratio (1 : 10); those with relatively coarse and stereotyped movements, like calf muscles, have a much lower ratio (1 : 2000).[1]

Normal Peripheral Nerve

The principal structural component of peripheral nerve is the *nerve fiber* (an axon with its Schwann cells and myelin sheath). A nerve consists of numerous fibers that are grouped into fascicles by connective tissue sheaths. *Myelinated* and *unmyelinated* nerve fibers are intermingled within the fascicle (Fig. 29–2). In the sural nerve, the nerve most commonly examined by biopsy and a relatively pure sensory nerve, myelinated fibers range between 2 and 16 μm in diameter and have a bimodal distribution; the smaller axons, which average 4 μm, are about twice as numerous as the larger axons, which average 11 μm.[2] Axons are myelinated in segments (*internodes*) separated by *nodes of Ranvier.* A single Schwann cell supplies the myelin sheath for each internode. The thickness of the myelin sheath is directly proportional to the diameter of the axon,[3] and the larger the axon diameter, the longer the internodal distance. Myelin in the peripheral nervous system is similar in overall lipid and protein composition to central nervous system myelin; however, peripheral nervous system myelin contains a higher proportion of sphingomyelins and glycoproteins. Some myelin proteins are specific to peripheral nervous system myelin, whereas others are shared with central nervous system myelin. Myelin protein zero (MPZ) is the major protein, comprising nearly 50% of peripheral nervous system myelin protein. In the compacted lipid bilayers, MPZ is a transmembrane protein, the external portion of which may function in the compaction of apposing layers of myelin. Myelin basic protein is the second most abundant protein; it is located topographically on the internal surface of bilayers at the major dense line of myelin. Peripheral myelin protein 22 (PMP22) is a 22-kD transmembrane protein located in compacted myelin.[4]

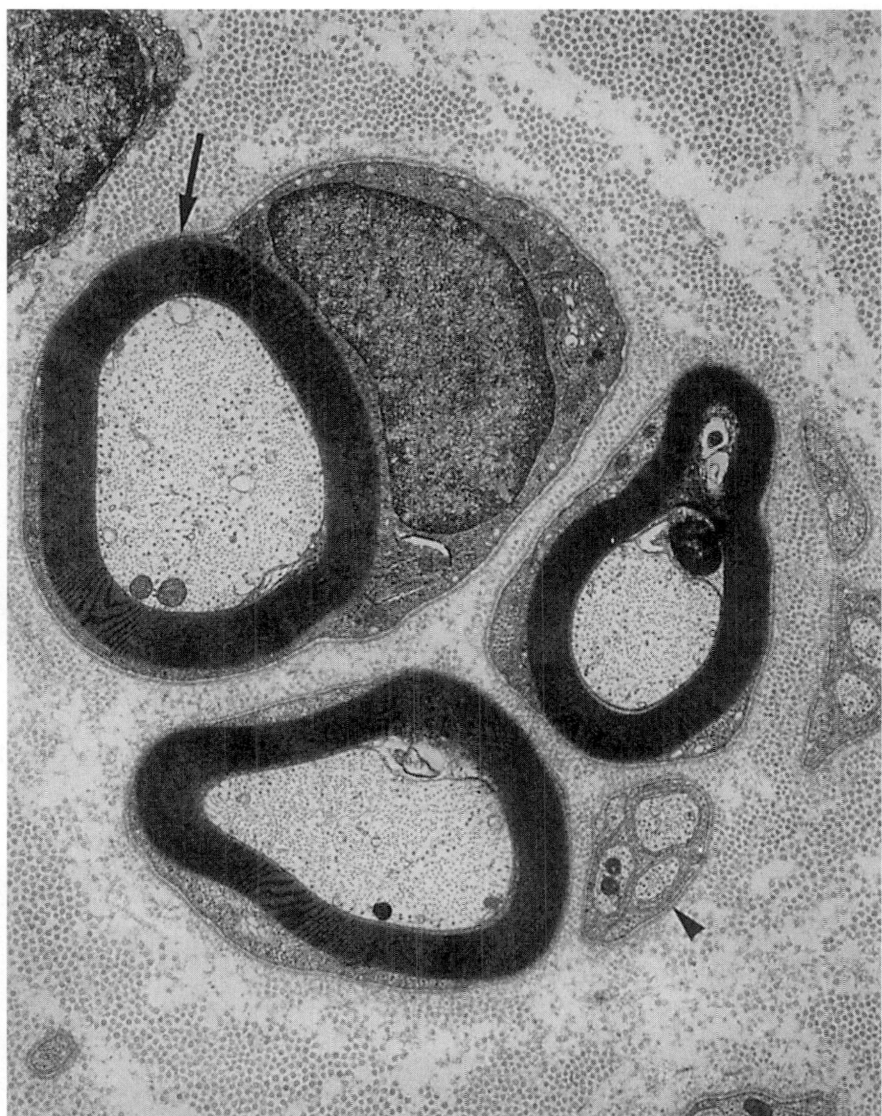

Figure 29–2 ■

Electron micrograph of myelinated *(arrow)* and unmyelinated *(arrowhead)* fibers in human sural nerve. One Schwann cell nucleus is present.

Unmyelinated axons are more numerous than myelinated axons. They range in size from 0.2 to 3 μm. The cytoplasm of one Schwann cell envelops, and isolates from each other, a variable number of unmyelinated fibers (5 to 20). The Schwann cells associated with either myelinated or unmyelinated fibers have pale oval nuclei with an even chromatin distribution and an elongated bipolar cell body. By electron microscopy, Schwann cells, unlike endoneurial fibroblasts and histiocytes, have a basement membrane.

Peripheral axons contain organelles and cytoskeletal structures, including microfilaments, neurofilaments, microtubules, mitochondria, vesicles, smooth endoplasmic reticulum, and lysosomes. Dense-core granules and coated vesicles are located in the nerve terminals. Protein synthesis does not occur in the axon, and axoplasmic flow delivers proteins and other substances synthesized in the perikaryon down the axon.[5,6] A retrograde transport system serves as a feedback system for the cell body.

There are three major connective tissue components of peripheral nerve: the *epineurium*, which encloses the entire nerve; the *perineurium*, a multilayered concentric connective tissue sheath that encloses each fascicle; and the *endoneurium*, which surrounds individual nerve fibers. The nerve microenvironment is regulated by the *perineurial barrier* (formed by the tight junctions between perineurial cells), the *blood-nerve barrier*, and the *nerve–cerebrospinal fluid* (CSF) barrier.[7] Endoneurial capillaries derive from the vasa nervorum, and their endothelial cells form tight junctions to establish the blood-nerve barrier. This barrier has been found to be relatively less competent within nerve roots, dorsal root ganglia, and autonomic ganglia than along the rest of the nerve. The nerve-CSF barrier is formed by the tight junctions between the cells that form the outer layer of the arachnoid membrane. These cells fuse with the perineurium of the roots and cranial nerves as they leave the subarachnoid space. The motor and sensory fibers, which are separated within anterior and posterior roots, intermingle within the mixed sensorimotor nerves that exit the spinal canal.

Normal Skeletal Muscle

Skeletal muscle fibers (*muscle fibers, myocytes*) form syncytia derived from the fusion of a contiguous series of individual embryonic cells and are therefore characterized by multinucleation. The multiple nuclei are located normally just beneath the plasma membrane (*sarcolemma*) of the myocyte. Transverse sections of muscle also demonstrate the subsarcolemmal position of the nucleus in most fibers. Under normal circumstances, the nucleus in 3% to 5% of muscle fibers is located within the interior of the muscle fiber[8]; internalized nuclei occur more often in some pathologic conditions. *Satellite cells*, a reserve cell population, are located adjacent to the sarcolemma and are covered by basement membrane, which encircles the entire muscle fiber.

Most of the cytoplasm of muscle fibers is filled with *myofilaments*, which form the contractile apparatus of *myofibrils* (Fig. 29–3). A myofibril consists of identical repeating units (*sarcomeres*) composed of interlaced, longitudinally directed thin filaments (actin) and thick filaments (myosin) and perpendicularly disposed *Z bands* (primarily α-actinin). The T-tubule system, involved in calcium release during excitation, is an invagination of the sarcolemmal membrane into the interior of the cell. The T system runs parallel to the Z bands, accompanied on each side by sarcoplasmic reticulum. Between the myofibrils is the myocyte cytoplasm (sarcoplasm), which accounts for 40% of the volume of the fiber and contains myoglobin, glycogen, mitochondria, lysosomes, and lipid vacuoles.

The adult muscle fiber on transverse section is polygonal; in infancy, fibers tend to be round, as are those of the extrinsic eye muscles and some facial muscles in adults. The cross-sectional diameter of individual fibers varies, depending on the specific muscle and its functional status. In humans, two major types of fibers, *type 1* and *type 2*, have been defined on the basis of histochemistry and physiology (Table 29–1). Type 1 fibers are high in myoglobin and oxidative enzymes and have many mitochondria, in keeping with their ability to perform tonic contraction; operationally, they are most often defined by their dark staining for adenosine triphosphatase (ATPase) at pH 4.2 but light staining at pH 9.4. Type 2 fibers are rich in glycolytic enzymes and are involved in rapid phasic contractions; they stain dark for ATPase at pH 9.4 but light at pH 4.2. *Since the motor neuron determines fiber types, all fibers of a single unit are of the same type.* These fibers are distributed randomly across the muscle, giving rise to the checkerboard pattern of alternating light and dark fibers as demonstrated especially well with ATPase (Fig. 29–4*A*). Normally, there is some variability in the relative abundance of type 1 and type 2 fibers among different mus-

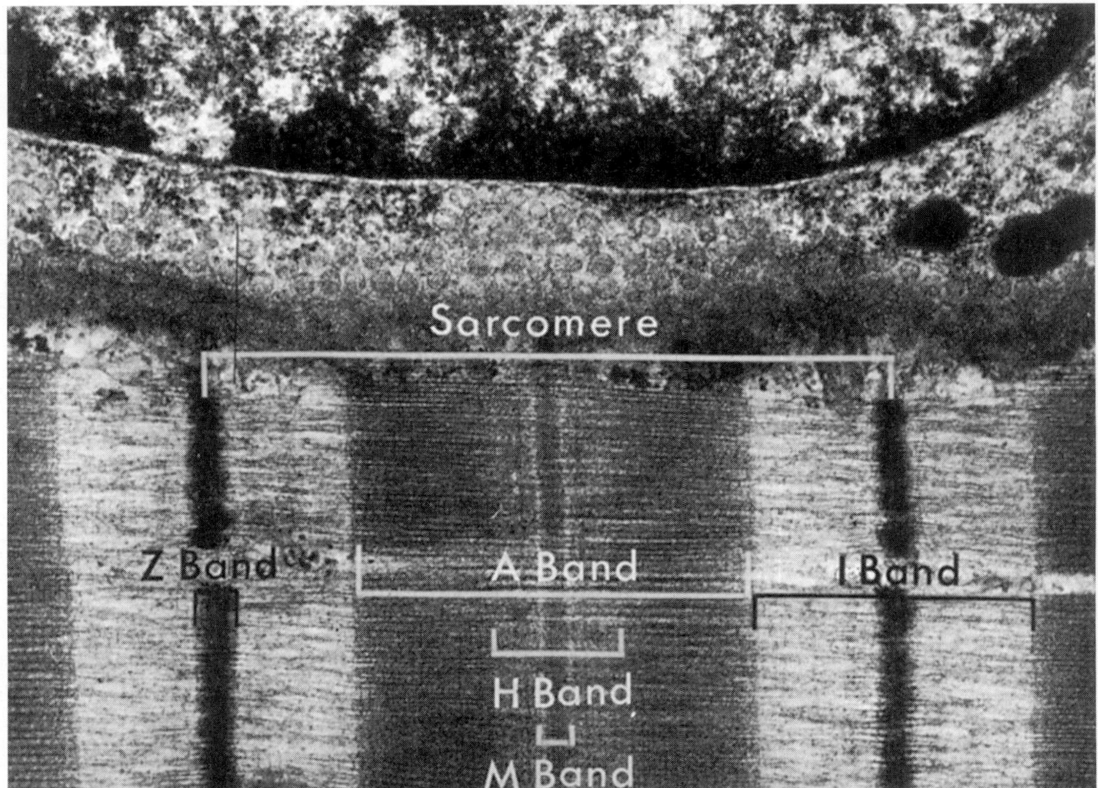

Figure 29–3

Electron micrograph of parts of two cells with the nucleus of one above and the most superficial myofibrils of a muscle cell below. Principal features of the pattern of cross-striations are identified on the illustration (×34,000). (Courtesy of Bloom W, Fawcett DW: A Textbook of Histology, 11th ed. Philadelphia, WB Saunders, 1986.)

Table 29–1. MUSCLE FIBER TYPES

	Type 1	Type 2
Action	Sustained force Weight-bearing	Sudden movements Purposeful motion
Enzyme content	NADH dark staining ATPase pH 4.2 dark staining ATPase pH 9.4 light staining	NADH light staining ATPase pH 4.2 light staining ATPase pH 9.4 dark staining
Lipids	Abundant	Scant
Glycogen	Scant	Abundant
Ultrastructure	Many mitochondria Wide Z band	Few mitochondria Narrow Z band
Physiology	Slow-twitch	Fast-twitch
Color	Red	White
Prototype	Soleus (pigeon)	Pectoral (pigeon)

cles.[8] The mnemonic "*one* (type 1 fiber) *slow* (twitch) *fat* (lipid-rich) *red* (appearance) *ox* (oxidative)" is useful to keep the physiology-morphology of the fiber types in mind.

Muscle spindles are fusiform structures that respond to stretch in muscles and have a role in maintaining tone. They consist of specialized muscle and nerve fibers, delimited by a connective tissue capsule.

The connective tissue sheath of muscles includes the *endomysium*, which surrounds individual muscle fibers; the *perimysium*, which groups muscle fibers into primary and secondary bundles (fasciculi); and the *epimysium*, which envelops single muscles or large groups of fibers.

GENERAL REACTIONS OF THE MOTOR UNIT

The two main responses of peripheral nerve to injury are based on the target of the insult: either the Schwann cell or the axon. Diseases that affect primarily the Schwann cell lead to a loss of myelin, referred to as *segmental demyelination.* In contrast, primary involvement of the neuron and its axon leads to axonal degeneration. In some diseases, axonal degeneration may be followed by *axonal regeneration* and *reinnervation* of muscle. The two principal pathologic processes seen in skeletal muscle are denervation

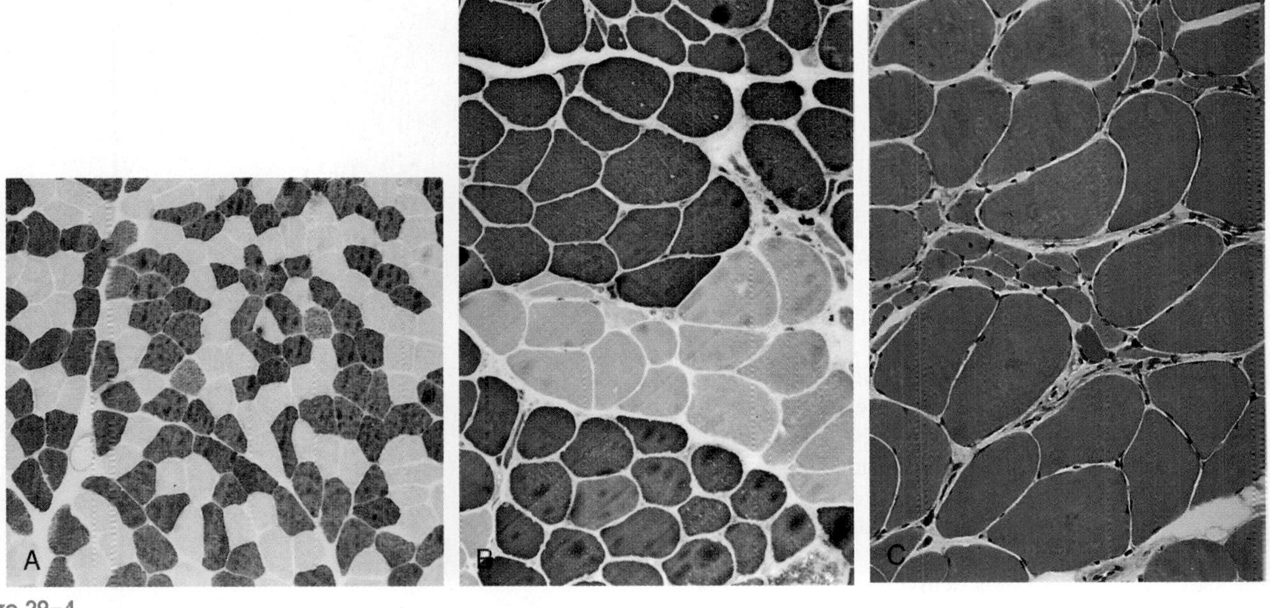

Figure 29–4

A, ATPase histochemical staining, at pH 9.4, of normal muscle showing checkerboard distribution of intermingled type 1 (light) and type 2 (dark) fibers. *B,* In contrast, fibers of either histochemical type are grouped together after reinnervation of muscle. *C,* A cluster of atrophic fibers (group atrophy) in the center.

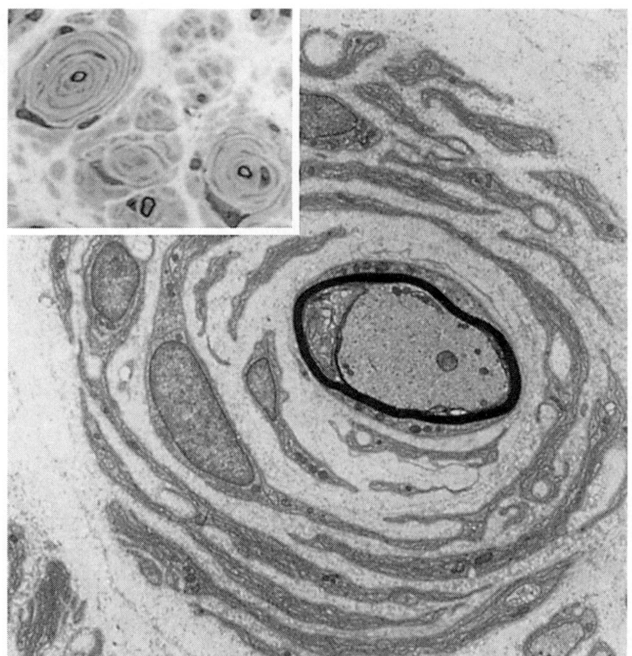

Figure 29–5

Electron micrograph of a single, thinly myelinated axon surrounded by concentrically arranged proliferating Schwann cells, forming an onion bulb. (Courtesy of G. Richard Dickersin, MD, from Diagnostic Electron Microscopy: A Text-Atlas. New York, Igaku-Shoin Medical Publishers, 1988, p 600.) *Inset,* Light microscopic appearance of an onion bulb neuropathy.

atrophy, which follows loss of axons, and those due to a primary abnormality of the muscle fiber itself, referred to as *myopathy*. We now consider the general features of these processes.

Segmental Demyelination

Segmental demyelination occurs when there is dysfunction of the Schwann cell or damage to the myelin sheath; there is no primary abnormality of the axon. The process affects some Schwann cells and their corresponding internodes while sparing others (see Fig. 29–1). The disintegrating myelin is engulfed initially by Schwann cells and later by macrophages. The denuded axon provides a stimulus for remyelination. A population of cells within the endoneurium has the capacity to replace injured Schwann cells. These cells proliferate and encircle the axon and, in time, remyelinate the denuded portion.[9] Newly formed myelinated internodes are shorter than normal, however, and several are required to bridge the demyelinated region (see Fig. 29–1). The new myelin sheath is also thin in proportion to the diameter of the axon.

With sequential episodes of demyelination and remyelination, there is an accumulation of tiers of Schwann cell processes that on transverse section appear as concentric layers of Schwann cell cytoplasm and redundant basement membrane that surround a thinly myelinated axon (*onion bulbs*) (Fig. 29–5). In time, many chronic demyelinating neuropathies give way to axonal injury.

Axonal Degeneration and Muscle Fiber Atrophy

Axonal degeneration is the result of primary destruction of the axon, with secondary disintegration of its myelin sheath. Damage to the axon may be due either to a focal event occurring at some point along the length of the nerve (such as trauma or ischemia) or to a more generalized abnormality affecting the neuron cell body (*neuronopathy*) or its axon (*axonopathy*). When axonal injury occurs as the result of a focal lesion, such as traumatic transection of a nerve, the distal portion of the fiber undergoes *wallerian degeneration* (Fig. 29–6). Within a day, the axon breaks down, and the affected Schwann cells begin to catabolize myelin and later engulf axon fragments, forming small oval compartments (*myelin ovoids*). Macrophages are recruited into the area and participate in the phagocytosis of axonal and myelin-derived debris.[10, 11] The stump of the proximal portion of the severed nerve shows degenerative changes involving only the most distal two or three internodes and then undergoes regenerative activity. In the slowly evolving neuronopathies or axonopathies, evidence of myelin breakdown is scant because only a few fibers are degenerating at any given time.

When axonal degeneration occurs, the muscle fibers within the affected motor unit lose their neural input and undergo *denervation atrophy*. Denervation of muscle leads to down-regulation of myosin and actin synthesis, with a

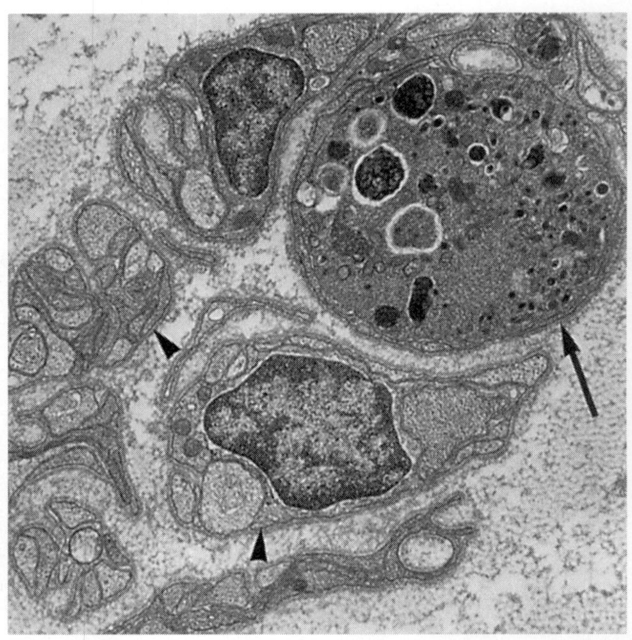

Figure 29–6

Electron micrograph of a degenerating axon *(arrow)* adjacent to several intact unmyelinated fibers *(arrowheads).* The axon is markedly distended and contains numerous degenerating organelles and dense bodies.

decrease in cell size and resorption of myofibrils, but cells remain viable.[12] In cross-section, the atrophic fibers are smaller than normal and have a roughly triangular shape ("angulated"). There is also cytoskeletal reorganization of some muscle cells, which results in a rounded zone of disorganized filaments (*target fiber*).

Type-specific atrophy is characteristic of some disease states. Type 2 fiber atrophy is a relatively common finding and is associated with inactivity or disuse. This type of "disuse atrophy" may occur after fracture of a limb and application of a plaster cast, in pyramidal tract degeneration, or in neurodegenerative diseases.

Nerve Regeneration and Reinnervation of Muscle

The proximal stumps of degenerated axons can develop new growth cones as the axon regrows. These growth cones will use the Schwann cells vacated by the degenerated axons to guide them. The presence of multiple, closely aggregated, thinly myelinated small-caliber axons is evidence of regeneration (*regenerating cluster*). This regrowth of axons is a slow process, apparently limited by the rate of the slow component of axonal transport, the movement of tubulin, actin, and intermediate filaments, on the order of 2 mm/day.[13] In spite of its slow pace, axonal regeneration accounts for some of the potential for functional recovery after peripheral axonal injury.

Reinnervation of the atrophic muscle fibers within an injured motor unit occurs when the normal neighboring axons belonging to an unaffected unit extend sprouts to reinnervate the denervated myocytes and incorporate them into the healthy motor unit. The number of muscle fibers within the healthy reinnervating motor unit will thus be increased. Furthermore, since muscle fiber typing is imparted by the innervating neuron, the newly adopted reinnervated fibers assume the fiber type of their neighboring new siblings. The result of reinnervation is the loss of the checkerboard pattern and the occurrence of a patch of contiguous myocytes having the same histochemical type (*type grouping*) (see Fig. 29–4*B*). *Group atrophy* ensues when a type group, in turn, becomes denervated because it is affected in the course of progression of the disease (see Fig. 29–4*C*).

Reactions of the Muscle Fiber

Although a wide spectrum of diseases may affect muscle, there is a relatively limited number of pathologic reactions of myocytes. The following pathologic changes may be seen in myopathies as well as in diseases in which the pathogenesis involves factors outside of the muscle and only secondarily involves the muscle cells. The most common forms of reaction include the following:

- *Segmental necrosis*, destruction of only a portion of the length of a myocyte, may be followed by *myophagocytosis* as macrophages infiltrate the region. Whatever the cause, the loss of muscle fibers in time leads to extensive deposition of collagen and fatty infiltration.
- *Vacuolation, alterations in structural proteins or organelles, and accumulation of intracytoplasmic deposits* may be seen in a wide variety of diseases.
- *Regeneration* occurs when peripherally located satellite cells proliferate and reconstitute the destroyed portion of the fiber. The regenerating muscle fiber has large internalized nuclei and prominent nucleoli, and the cytoplasm, laden with RNA, becomes basophilic.
- Fiber *hypertrophy* occurs in response to increased load, either in the setting of exercise or in pathologic conditions in which muscle fibers are injured. Large fibers may divide along a segment (*muscle fiber splitting*) so that, in cross-section, a single large fiber contains a cell membrane traversing its diameter, often with adjacent nuclei.

DISEASES OF PERIPHERAL NERVE

Peripheral nerve is subject to the same wide range of categories of disease (inflammatory, traumatic, metabolic, toxic, genetic, neoplastic) as other tissues. The pattern of disease, however, reflects the unique structure and function of nerves.

Inflammatory Neuropathies

These diseases are characterized by inflammatory cell infiltrates into peripheral nerves, roots, and sensory and autonomic ganglia. In some, an infectious agent elicits the inflammatory responses; in others, an autoimmune mechanism is presumed to underlie the inflammation.

IMMUNE-MEDIATED NEUROPATHIES

Guillain-Barré Syndrome (Acute Inflammatory Demyelinating Polyradiculoneuropathy)

Guillain-Barré syndrome is one of the most common life-threatening diseases of the peripheral nervous system, with an overall annual incidence of 1 to 3 cases per 100,000 persons in the United States.[14, 15] The disease is characterized clinically by weakness beginning in the distal limbs but rapidly advancing to affect more proximal muscle functions (ascending paralysis) and histologically by inflammation and demyelination of peripheral nerves and spinal nerve roots (radiculoneuropathy).

Pathogenesis. Approximately two thirds of cases are preceded by an acute, influenza-like illness, usually viral, from which the patient has recovered by the time the neuropathy becomes symptomatic. There has been no consistent demonstration of any infectious agent in peripheral nerves in these patients, and an immunologically mediated disorder is now generally favored.[16, 17] A similar inflammatory disease of peripheral nerves can be induced in experimental animals by sensitization to peripheral nerve myelin or its components. A T cell–mediated immune response ensues, accompanied by segmental demyelination effected by macrophages. Transfer of these T cells to a naive animal results in comparable lesions.[18] Moreover, lymphocytes from patients with Guillain-Barré syndrome have been shown to produce demyelination in tissue cultures of myelinated nerve fibers. Circulating antibodies may also play a part,[19] and plasmapheresis has been reported to be an effective treatment.

MORPHOLOGY. The dominant histopathologic finding is **inflammation of peripheral nerve,** manifested as perivenular and endoneurial infiltration by lymphocytes, macrophages, and a few plasma cells. The invading inflammatory cells vary in number from a sparse seeding of the perivenous spaces to large collections of mononuclear cells disseminated throughout the entire nerve. Segmental demyelination affecting peripheral nerves is the primary lesion,[16] but damage to axons is also characteristic, particularly when the disease is severe. Electron microscopy has identified an early effect on myelin sheaths. The cytoplasmic processes of macrophages penetrate the basement membrane of Schwann cells, particularly in the vicinity of the nodes of Ranvier, and extend between the myelin lamellae, stripping away the myelin sheath from the axon. Ultimately, the remnants of the myelin sheath are engulfed by the macrophages. Remyelination follows the demyelination.

Inflammatory foci and demyelination are widely distributed throughout the peripheral nervous system, although their intensity is so variable that they may be difficult to identify in an individual case. The most intense inflammatory reaction is often localized in spinal and cranial motor roots and the adjacent parts of the spinal and cranial nerves.

Clinical Course. The clinical picture is dominated by the ascending paralysis. Deep tendon reflexes disappear early in the process; although sensory involvement can often be detected, it is less troublesome than the weakness. The nerve conduction velocity is slowed because of the multifocal destruction of myelin segments involving many axons within a nerve; there is elevation of the CSF protein due to inflammation and altered permeability of the microcirculation within the spinal roots as they traverse the subarachnoid space. Inflammatory cells are contained within the roots, however, and there is little to no CSF pleocytosis. Many patients spend weeks in hospital intensive care units before recovering normal function. With improved respiratory care and support, the mortality rate has fallen from 25% in the past but is still considerable, with some 2% to 5% dying of respiratory paralysis, autonomic instability, and the complications of tracheostomy.[14]

Chronic Inflammatory Demyelinating Polyradiculoneuropathy

In some patients, inflammatory demyelinating polyradiculoneuropathy, instead of occurring as an acute illness as in Guillain-Barré syndrome, follows a subacute or chronic course usually with relapses and remissions over the course of several years.[17] There is often a symmetric, mixed sensorimotor polyneuropathy, although some patients have predominantly sensory or motor impairment. Clinical remissions may occur with steroid treatment and plasmapheresis. Biopsies of sural nerves show evidence of recurrent demyelination and remyelination with well-developed onion bulb structures.[20]

Infectious Polyneuropathies

Many infectious processes may affect peripheral nerve. Here we briefly review the changes in leprosy, diphtheria, and varicella-zoster because they cause unique and specific pathologic changes in nerves. They are discussed further in Chapter 9.

LEPROSY

There is peripheral nerve involvement in both lepromatous and tuberculoid leprosy (Chapter 9). In lepromatous leprosy, Schwann cells are often invaded by *Mycobacterium leprae*, which proliferate and eventually infect other cells. There is evidence of segmental demyelination and remyelination and loss of both myelinated and unmyelinated axons. As the infection advances, endoneurial fibrosis and multilayered thickening of the perineurial sheaths occur. Clinically, these patients develop a symmetric polyneuropathy that prominently involves pain fibers; the loss of sensation that results contributes to the tissue injury of the disease. Tuberculoid leprosy shows evidence of active cell-mediated immune response to *M. leprae*, with nodular granulomatous inflammation situated in the dermis. The inflammation injures cutaneous nerves in the vicinity; axons, Schwann cells, and myelin are lost, and there is fibrosis of the perineurium and endoneurium. With this form of leprosy, patients have much more localized nerve involvement but do develop areas of abnormal sensation from the injury.

DIPHTHERIA

Peripheral nerve involvement results from the effects of the diphtheria exotoxin and begins with paresthesias and weakness; early loss of proprioception and vibratory sensation is common. The earliest changes are seen in the sensory ganglia, where the incomplete blood-nerve barrier allows entry of the toxin.[21] There is selective demyelination of axons that extends into adjacent anterior and posterior roots as well as into the mixed sensorimotor nerve.

VARICELLA-ZOSTER VIRUS

This virus is one of the few that produce lesions in the peripheral nervous system. Latent infection of neurons in the sensory ganglia of the spinal cord and brain stem follows chickenpox, and reactivation leads to a painful, vesicular skin eruption in the distribution of sensory dermatomes *(shingles),* most frequently thoracic or trigeminal.

The virus may be transported along the sensory nerves to the skin, where it establishes an active infection of epidermal cells. In a small proportion of patients, weakness is also apparent in the same distribution. Although the factors giving rise to reactivation are not fully understood, decreased cell-mediated immunity is of major importance in many cases.[22]

Affected ganglia show neuronal destruction and loss, usually accompanied by abundant mononuclear inflammatory infiltrates. Regional necrosis with hemorrhage may also be found. Peripheral nerve shows axonal degeneration after the death of the sensory neurons. Focal destruction of the large motor neurons of the anterior horns or cranial nerve motor nuclei may be seen at the corresponding levels. Intranuclear inclusions generally are not found in the peripheral nervous system.

Hereditary Neuropathies

This is a group of heterogeneous, typically progressive, and often disabling syndromes that affect peripheral nerves. The genetic and molecular basis of many of the hereditary peripheral neuropathies is just now becoming clear, and as they are further defined, adjustments in the current classification scheme can be anticipated.[23] They can be divided into several groups:

- Most hereditary neuropathies affect both strength and sensation and have been termed *hereditary motor and sensory neuropathies* (HMSN).
- In others, symptoms are usually limited to numbness, pain, and autonomic dysfunction such as orthostatic hypotension, and these are called *hereditary sensory and autonomic neuropathies* (HSAN) (Table 29–2).
- Some are notable for the deposition of amyloid within the nerve. These *familial amyloid polyneuropathies* have a clinical presentation similar to HSAN, but most kindreds exhibit mutations of the *transthyretin* gene, located on chromosome 18q11.2–q12.1, with deposition within nerve of amyloid fibrils composed of transthyretin protein, a protein involved in serum binding and transport of thyroid hormone.
- Various other inherited disorders may cause neuropathies; the characteristics of some of these associated with known biochemical abnormalities are presented in Table 29–3.[24]

The pathologic findings of many of the hereditary neuropathies are those of an axonal neuropathy. Fiber loss is the most prominent finding.

HEREDITARY MOTOR AND SENSORY NEUROPATHY I (HMSN I, CMT1)

The most common hereditary peripheral neuropathy, *Charcot-Marie-Tooth (CMT) disease, hypertrophic form (HMSN I)*, usually presents in childhood or early adulthood. A characteristic progressive muscular atrophy of the calf seen in these patients gives rise to the common clinical term *peroneal muscular atrophy*. Patients may be asymptomatic, but when they present, it is often with symptoms such as distal muscle weakness, atrophy of the calf, or secondary orthopedic problems of the foot (such as *pes cavus*).

Molecular Genetics. The disease is genetically heterogeneous. In most pedigrees (known as HMSN IA or CMT1A), there is a duplication of a large region of chromosome 17p11.2–p12 resulting in "segmental trisomy" of the duplicated region. The duplicated segment includes the gene for peripheral myelin protein 22 (PMP22), but whether the disease is caused by overexpression of PMP22, through a gene dosage effect,[25, 26] or by other adjacent duplicated genes is not clear. A separate genetic locus with the same clinical phenotype (HMSN IB) on chromosome 1 involves myelin protein zero (MPZ).[27] A third set of pedigrees shows no linkage to either of these sites (type IC). In addition, some pedigrees have a genetic locus on the X chromosome, with mutations in the gene for the gap junction protein connexin-32.[28]

MORPHOLOGY. CMT1 is a demyelinating neuropathy, both by nerve conduction velocity studies and pathologically. Histologic examination shows the consequences of repetitive demyelination and remyelination, with multiple onion bulbs, more pronounced in distal than in proximal nerves (see Fig. 29–5). The axon is often present in the center of the onion bulb, and the myelin sheath is usually thin or absent. The redundant layers of Schwann cell hyperplasia surrounding individual axons are associated with enlargement of individual peripheral nerves that may be individually palpable, which has led to the term "hypertrophic" neuropathy. In the longitudinal plane, individual segments of the axon may show evidence of segmental demyelination. Autopsy studies of affected individuals have shown degeneration of the posterior columns of the spinal cord.

Table 29–2 HEREDITARY SENSORY AND AUTONOMIC NEUROPATHIES

Disease	Clinical and Pathologic Findings
HSAN I; autosomal dominant	Predominantly sensory neuropathy, presenting in young adults Axonal degeneration (mostly myelinated fibers)
HSAN II; autosomal recessive (some cases are sporadic)	Predominantly sensory neuropathy, presenting in infancy Axonal degeneration (mostly myelinated fibers)
HSAN III (Riley-Day syndrome: familial dysautonomia); autosomal recessive (most often in Jewish children; locus on chromosome 9q31–q33)	Predominantly autonomic neuropathy, presenting in infancy Axonal degeneration (mostly unmyelinated fibers); atrophy and loss of sensory and autonomic ganglion cells

Table 29–3. HEREDITARY NEUROPATHIES WITH KNOWN METABOLIC CAUSE

Disease	Metabolic Defect	Inheritance	Clinical Findings	Pathologic Findings
Adrenoleukodystrophy	Peroxisomal transporter enzyme; *ALD* gene	X-linked; 4% of female carriers are symptomatic	Mixed motor and sensory neuropathy, adrenal insufficiency, spastic paraplegia Onset between 10 and 20 years for males (leukodystrophy), between 20 and 40 years for females (myeloneuropathy)	Axonal degeneration (myelinated and unmyelinated) Segmental demyelination, with onion bulbs Electron microscopy: linear inclusions in Schwann cells
Familial amyloid polyneuropathies	Point mutations in transthyretin, rarely other molecules	Autosomal dominant	Sensory and autonomic dysfunction Age at onset varies with site of mutation	Amyloid deposits in vessel walls and connective tissue with axonal degeneration
Porphyria, acute intermittent or variegate coproporphyria	Enzymes involved in heme synthesis (acute intermittent porphobilinogen deaminase deficiency)	Autosomal dominant	Acute episodes of neurologic dysfunction, psychiatric disturbances, abdominal pain, seizures, proximal weakness, autonomic dysfunction Attacks may be precipitated by drugs	Acute and chronic axonal degeneration Regenerating clusters
Refsum disease	Phytanoyl CoA α-hydroxylase (peroxisomal enzyme)	Autosomal recessive	Mixed motor and sensory neuropathy with palpable nerves Ataxia, night blindness, retinitis pigmentosa, ichthyosis Age at onset before 20 years (a genetically distinct infantile form also exists)	Severe onion bulb formation

Clinical Course. The disorder is usually autosomal dominant, and although it is slowly progressive, the disability of sensorimotor deficits and associated orthopedic problems such as pes cavus are usually limited in severity and a normal life span is typical. The relationship between the molecular abnormalities and the observed peripheral nerve pathology is not well understood.

OTHER HEREDITARY MOTOR AND SENSORY NEUROPATHIES

HMSN II

This is a neuronal form of autosomal dominant Charcot-Marie-Tooth disease that presents with signs and symptoms similar to those of HMSN I, although nerve enlargement is not seen and the disease presents at a slightly later age. This form is less common than HMSN I and in some families (designated CMT2A) is linked to chromosome 1p35–p36.[29] Nerve biopsy specimens in this disorder show loss of myelinated axons as the predominant finding. Segmental demyelination of internodes is infrequent. These findings suggest that the site of primary cellular dysfunction is the axon or neuron.

Dejerine-Sottas Disease (HMSN III)

Dejerine-Sottas disease is a slowly progressive, autosomal recessive disorder beginning in early childhood, manifested by delay in the developmental milestones, such as the acquisition of motor skills. In contrast to HMSN I and HMSN II, in which the atrophy is limited to the leg musculature, both trunk and limb muscles are involved. On physical examination, *enlarged peripheral nerves* can be detected by inspection and palpation. The deep tendon reflexes are depressed or absent, and nerve conduction velocity is slowed. Several families have been identified with mutations of the same genes, *PMP22* and *MPZ,* that are affected in the hypertrophic forms of Charcot-Marie-Tooth disease (HMSN I).[30] Morphologically, the size of individual peripheral nerve fascicles is increased, often dramatically, with abundant onion bulb formation as well as segmental demyelination. There is usually evidence of axonal loss, and those axons that remain are often of diminished caliber. These findings are most severe in the distal portions of the peripheral nervous system; however, autopsy studies have shown that similar findings may be present in spinal roots.

Other less common forms of HMSN are characterized by

additional neurologic and ophthalmologic abnormalities, such as retinitis pigmentosa and deafness.

Acquired Metabolic and Toxic Neuropathies

Functional and structural changes in peripheral nerve develop in response to various metabolic alterations—either from endogenous disorders or from exogenous agents. The most common of these processes are discussed here.

PERIPHERAL NEUROPATHY IN ADULT-ONSET DIABETES MELLITUS

Several distinct patterns of diabetes-related peripheral nerve abnormalities have been recognized (Chapter 20). They are categorized as *distal symmetric sensory or sensorimotor neuropathy, autonomic neuropathy,* and *focal or multifocal asymmetric neuropathy.* Individuals may develop any combination of these lesions, and in fact the first two (sensorimotor and autonomic) are often found together. The most common of these patterns of injury is the symmetric neuropathy that involves distal sensory and motor nerves. These patients develop decreased sensation in the distal extremities with comparably less evident motor abnormalities. The loss of pain sensation can result in the development of ulcers that heal poorly because of the diffuse vascular injury in diabetes and are a major cause of morbidity.

MORPHOLOGY. The predominant pathologic finding is an axonal neuropathy; as with other chronic axonal neuropathies, there is also some segmental demyelination. There is a relative loss of small myelinated fibers and of unmyelinated fibers, but large fibers are also affected. Endoneurial arterioles show thickening, hyalinization, and intense periodic acid–Schiff (PAS) positivity in their walls and extensive reduplication of the basement membrane[31, 32] (Fig. 29–7). Whether the lesions are due to ischemia[33] or a metabolic dysfunction is unclear.

Clinical Course. The prevalence of peripheral neuropathy in patients with diabetes mellitus depends on the duration of the disease, with up to 50% of diabetic patients having peripheral neuropathy clinically after 25 years of diabetes and up to 100% having conduction abnormalities electrophysiologically. Another manifestation of diabetic neuropathy is *dysfunction of the autonomic nervous system;* this affects 20% to 40% of diabetics, nearly always in association with a distal sensorimotor neuropathy.[34] The basis of autonomic dysfunction is unknown. In some patients, especially elderly adults with a long history of diabetes, neuropathy manifests itself as a disorder of single individual peripheral or cranial (oculomotor nerve) nerves *(mononeuropathy)* or of several individual nerves in an asymmetric distribution *(multiple mononeuropathy or mononeuropathy multiplex).*

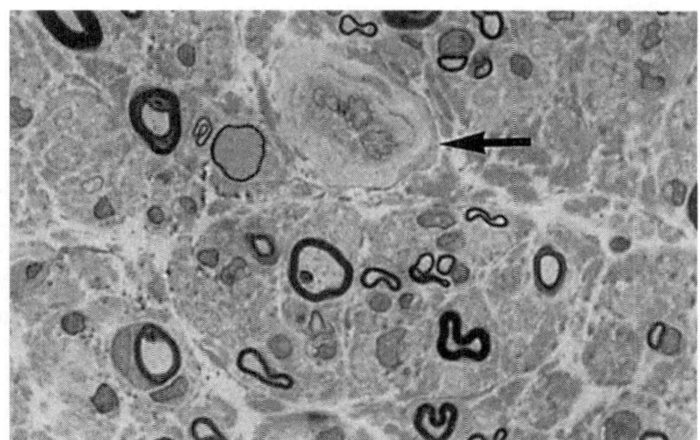

Figure 29–7 ■

Diabetic neuropathy with marked loss of myelinated fibers, a thinly myelinated fiber, and thickening of endoneurial vessel wall *(arrow).*

METABOLIC AND NUTRITIONAL PERIPHERAL NEUROPATHIES

As many as 65% of patients with renal failure have clinical evidence of peripheral neuropathy before dialysis *(uremic neuropathy).*[35] This is typically a distal, symmetric neuropathy that may be asymptomatic or may be associated with muscle cramps, distal dysesthesias, and diminished deep tendon reflexes. In these patients, axonal degeneration is the primary event, with degenerating fibers and fiber loss; occasionally there is secondary demyelination. Regeneration and recovery are common after dialysis.

Peripheral neuropathy can also develop in patients with chronic liver disease, chronic respiratory insufficiency,[35] and thyroid dysfunction. *Thiamine deficiency* is characterized by axonal neuropathy, a clinical condition termed neuropathic *beriberi.* Axonal neuropathies also occur with deficiencies of vitamins B_{12} (cobalamin), B_6 (pyridoxine), and E (α-tocopherol).

NEUROPATHIES ASSOCIATED WITH MALIGNANCY

Direct infiltration or compression of peripheral nerves by tumor is a common cause of mononeuropathy and may be the presenting symptom of cancer. These neuropathies include *brachial plexopathy* from neoplasms of the apex of the lung, *obturator palsy* from pelvic malignant neoplasms, and *cranial nerve palsies* from intracranial tumors and tumors of the base of the skull. A *polyradiculopathy* involving the lower extremity may develop when the cauda equina is involved by meningeal carcinomatosis.

A diffuse, symmetric peripheral neuropathy may occur in patients with a distant carcinoma and is considered a remote, or *paraneoplastic,* effect (Chapters 8 and 30). The most common manifestation is a sensorimotor neuropathy characterized by weakness and sensory deficits that are often more pronounced in the lower extremities and that progress during months to years. The neuropathy is most frequently associated with small cell carcinoma of the lung; as many as 2% to 5% of patients with lung cancer may have clinical evidence of peripheral neuropathy. Patients with the less frequent pure sensory neuropathy present with numbness and paresthesias, symptoms that may precede the identification of the malignant neoplasm by 6 to 15 months.[36] An immunologic mechanism for the neuropathy has been suggested on the basis of the presence of inflammatory infiltrates within the dorsal root ganglia and the identification of a circulating polyclonal immunoglobulin G antibody (anti-Hu) in such patients that binds to a 35- to 38-kD RNA-binding protein expressed by neurons and the tumor.[37]

Paraneoplastic neuropathy may also develop in patients with plasma cell dyscrasias in one of two ways. The first is through the deposition of light-chain amyloid in peripheral nerves, particularly AL type amyloid (Chapter 6). The second is independent of the presence or deposition of amyloid and may be related to the binding of monoclonal immunoglobulin M to myelin-associated glycoprotein.[38]

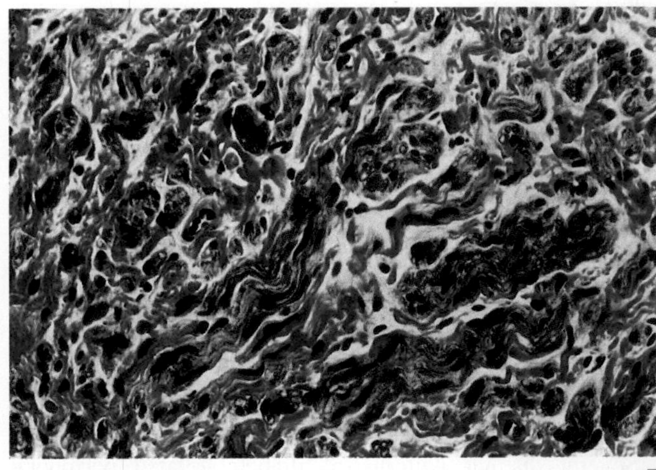

Figure 29–8 ■

Traumatic neuroma showing disordered orientation of nerve fiber bundles (purple) intermixed with connective tissue (blue).

TOXIC NEUROPATHIES

Peripheral neuropathies can occur after exposure to industrial or environmental chemicals, biologic toxins, or therapeutic drugs.[39] Prominent among the environmental chemicals are heavy metals, including lead and arsenic (Chapter 10). In addition, many organic compounds are known to be neurotoxic.

Traumatic Neuropathies

Peripheral nerves are commonly injured in the course of trauma. *Lacerations* result from cutting injuries and can complicate fractures when a sharp fragment of bone lacerates the nerve. *Avulsions* occur when tension is applied to a peripheral nerve, often as the result of a force applied to one of the limbs. The direct severance of nerves is associated with hemorrhage, and there is transection of the connective tissue planes. Regeneration of peripheral nerve axons does occur, albeit slowly. Regrowth may be complicated by discontinuity between the proximal and distal portions of the nerve sheath as well as by the misalignment of individual fascicles. Axons, even in the absence of correctly positioned distal segments, may continue to grow, resulting in a mass of tangled axonal processes known as a *traumatic neuroma (pseudoneuroma or amputation neuroma).* Within this mass, small bundles of axons appear randomly oriented; each, however, is surrounded by organized layers containing Schwann cells, fibroblasts, and perineurial cells (Fig. 29–8).

Compression neuropathy (entrapment neuropathy) occurs when a peripheral nerve is compressed, often within an anatomic compartment. *Carpal tunnel syndrome* is the most common entrapment neuropathy and results from compression of the median nerve at the level of the wrist within the compartment delimited by the transverse carpal ligament. Women are more commonly affected than men are, and the problem is frequently bilateral. The disorder may be observed with any condition that can cause decreased available space within the carpal tunnel, such as tissue edema, but predisposing factors include pregnancy, degenerative joint disease, hypothyroidism, amyloidosis (especially that related to β_2-microglobulin deposition in renal dialysis patients), and excessive usage of the wrist.[40, 41] Symptoms are limited to dysfunction of the median nerve, including numbness and paresthesias of the tips of the thumb and first two digits. Additional compression neuropathies include involvement of the ulnar nerve at the level of the elbow, the peroneal nerve at the level of the knee, and the radial nerve in the upper arm as seen after sleeping with the arm improperly positioned ("Saturday night palsy"). Another form of compression neuropathy is found in the foot, affecting the interdigital nerve at intermetatarsal sites. This problem, which occurs more often in women than in men, leads to foot pain (metatarsalgia). The histologic findings of the lesion (*Morton neuroma*) include evidence of chronic compressive injury.

Tumors of Peripheral Nerve

Both benign and malignant tumors can be derived from elements of the nerve sheath. These are discussed in association with tumors of the central nervous system (Chapter 30).

DISEASES OF SKELETAL MUSCLE

Denervation Atrophy

Neurogenic atrophy of muscle is caused by any process that affects the anterior horn cell or its axon in the peripheral nervous system. The tissue response denervation and the histologic changes attending reinnervation are described earlier.

SPINAL MUSCULAR ATROPHY (INFANTILE MOTOR NEURON DISEASE)

Motor neuron diseases are progressive neurologic illnesses that include, within the spectrum of neuronal degeneration throughout the central nervous system, an abnormality of the anterior horn cells in the spinal cord that results in their destruction. Motor neuron diseases in adults are discussed in Chapter 30. Spinal muscular atrophy (SMA) is a distinctive group of autosomal recessive motor neuron diseases beginning in childhood or adolescence that are discussed here because the weakness in children is commonly considered with the childhood myopathies and because the pathologic findings in skeletal muscle are so characteristic.

Genetics. All forms of SMA are syngeneic and associated with a locus on chromosome 5, which harbors the survival motor neuron gene *(SMN)* and is strongly linked with the disease phenotype. Deletion of *SMN* occurs in 98% of patients with the SMA phenotype, and contiguous deletion of the nearby neuronal apoptosis inhibitory protein gene *(NAIP)* is associated with the most severe clinical phenotype (Chapter 1).[42]

MORPHOLOGY. The typical histologic finding in muscle is large numbers of atrophic fibers, often only a few micrometers in diameter (Fig. 29–9). This is unlike the groups of angulated atrophic fibers seen in denervation atrophy of muscle in adults. These atrophic fibers often involve an entire fascicle—**panfasciular atrophy**. There are also scattered large fibers that are two to four times normal size.

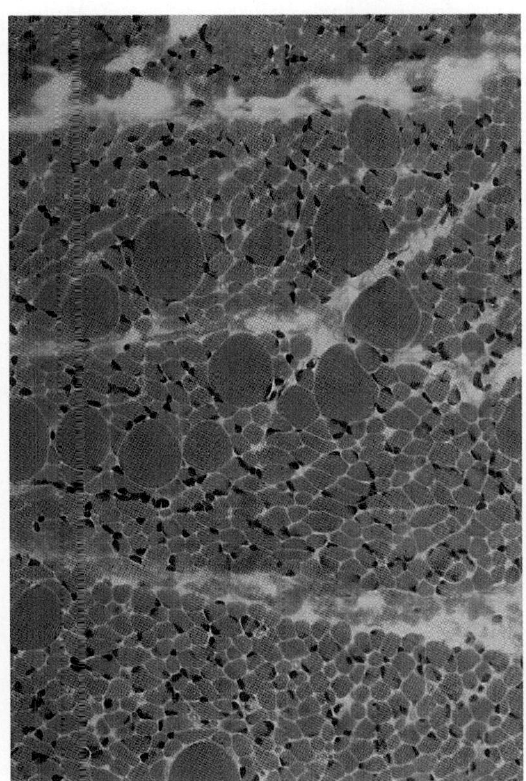

Figure 29–9 ■

Spinal muscular atrophy with groups of atrophic muscle fibers resulting from denervation atrophy of muscle in early childhood.

Clinical Course. The most common form of spinal muscular atrophy, Werdnig-Hoffmann disease (SMA type 1), has onset at birth or within the first 4 months of life and usually leads to death within the first 3 years of life. The other two forms (SMA 2 and SMA 3) present at later ages, either in early childhood (between 3 and 15 months in SMA 2) or later childhood (after 2 years in SMA 3). The clinical progression is related to the subtype, with shorter survival (more than 4 years) in the earlier onset form (SMA 2) than in patients with SMA 3, who often survive into adulthood.

Muscular Dystrophies

The muscular dystrophies are a heterogeneous group of inherited disorders, often beginning in childhood, characterized clinically by progressive muscle weakness and wasting.

X-LINKED MUSCULAR DYSTROPHY (DUCHENNE MUSCULAR DYSTROPHY AND BECKER MUSCULAR DYSTROPHY)

The two most common forms of muscular dystrophy are X-linked: *Duchenne muscular dystrophy* (DMD) and *Becker muscular dystrophy* (BMD). DMD is the most severe and the most common form of muscular dystrophy, with an incidence of about 1 per 10,000 males.[43]

Clinical Course. DMD becomes clinically manifest by the age of 5 years with weakness leading to wheelchair dependence by 10 to 12 years of age and progresses relentlessly until death by the early 20s. Boys with DMD are normal at birth, and early motor milestones are met on time. Walking, however, is often delayed, and the first indications of muscle weakness are clumsiness and inability to keep up with peers. Weakness begins in the pelvic girdle muscles and then extends to the shoulder girdle. Enlargement of the calf muscles associated with weakness, a phenomenon termed *pseudohypertrophy*, is an important clinical finding. The increased muscle bulk is caused initially by an increase in the size of the muscle fibers and then, as the muscle atrophies, by an increase in fat and connective tissue. Pathologic changes are also found in the heart, and patients may develop heart failure or arrhythmias. Although there are no well-established structural abnormalities of the central nervous system, cognitive impairment appears to be a component of the disease and is severe enough in some patients to be considered mental retardation.[44] Serum creatine kinase is elevated during the first decade of life but returns to normal in the later stages of the disease. Death results from respiratory insufficiency, pulmonary infection, and cardiac decompensation.

Although BMD involves the same genetic locus, it is less common and much less severe than DMD. The onset occurs later in childhood or in adolescence and is accompanied by a slower and more variable rate of progression, although there is considerable variation between pedigrees. Many patients have a nearly normal life span. Cardiac disease is much rarer in these patients.

Pathogenesis and Genetics. The gene for DMD and BMD is located in the Xp21 region and encodes a 427-kD protein termed *dystrophin*.[45] Deletions appear to represent a large proportion of mutations, with frameshift and point mutations accounting for the rest. Approximately one third of cases of DMD represent new mutations[43]; in the remaining families, obligate female carriers are usually clinically asymptomatic but often have elevated serum creatine kinase and show minimal myopathic histologic abnormalities on muscle biopsy.

Dystrophin is normally located adjacent to the sarcolemmal membrane in myocytes. Muscle biopsy specimens from patients with DMD show minimal evidence of dystrophin by both staining and direct measurements (Western blot).[46] BMD patients, who also have mutations in the dystrophin gene, have diminished amounts of dystrophin, usually of an abnormal molecular weight, reflecting mutations that allow synthesis of the protein (Fig. 29–10*B*). The molecule has been further localized to sites of I and M bands and has been suggested to play a role in maintaining the integrity of the myocyte membrane during the shape changes associated with contraction. Various other proteins that interact with dystrophin have been found to underlie other muscle disease (see later).

MORPHOLOGY. Histopathologic abnormalities common to DMD and BMD include (1) **variation in fiber size** (diameter) due to the presence of both small and giant fibers, sometimes with fiber splitting; (2) **increased numbers of internalized nuclei** (beyond the normal range of 3% to 5%); (3) **degeneration, necrosis, and phagocytosis of muscle fibers**; (4) **regeneration of muscle fibers**; and (5) **proliferation of endomysial connective tissue** (Fig. 29–10*A*). DMD cases also often show enlarged, rounded, hyaline fibers that have lost their normal cross-striations, believed to be hypercontracted fibers; this finding is rare in BMD. Both type 1 and type 2 fibers are involved, and no alterations in the proportion or distribution of fiber types are evident. Histochemical reactions sometimes fail to identify distinct fiber types in DMD. In later stages, the muscles eventually become almost totally replaced by fat and connective tissue, an appearance indistinguishable from the end stage of other severe muscle diseases. Cardiac involvement, when present, consists of interstitial fibrosis, more prominent in the subendocardial layers. Despite the clinical evidence of central nervous system dysfunction in DMD, no consistent neuropathologic abnormalities have been described.

AUTOSOMAL MUSCULAR DYSTROPHIES

Other forms of muscular dystrophy share many of the histologic features of DMD and BMD but have distinct clinical and pathologic features. Some of these muscular dystrophies affect specific muscle groups and the specific diagnosis is based largely on the pattern of clinical muscle weakness (Table 29–4). A group of the autosomal muscular dystrophies, however, affect the proximal musculature of the trunk and limbs similar to the X-linked muscular dystrophies and are termed *limb girdle muscular dystrophies*.

Limb girdle muscular dystrophies are inherited in either an autosomal dominant (type 1) or recessive (type 2) pat-

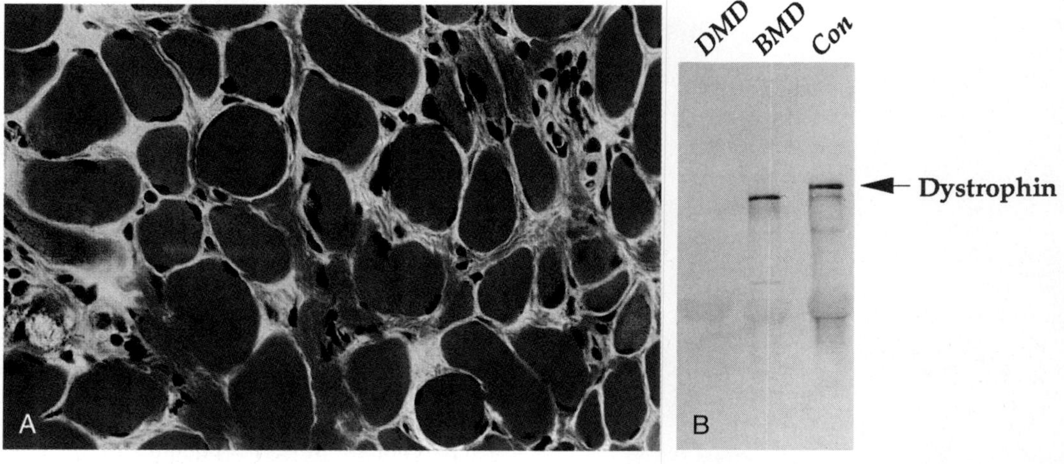

Figure 29–10

A, Duchenne muscular dystrophy (DMD) showing variation in muscle fiber size, increased endomysial connective tissue, and regenerating fibers (blue hue). *B*, Western blot showing absence of dystrophin in DMD and altered dystrophin size in Becker muscular dystrophy (BMD) compared with control (Con). (Courtesy of Dr. L. Kunkel, Children's Hospital, Boston, MA.)

Table 29–4. OTHER MUSCULAR DYSTROPHIES

Disease	Inheritance	Clinical Findings	Pathologic Findings
Facioscapulohumeral muscular dystrophy	Autosomal dominant (Type 1A—gene localized to 4q35-qter)	Variable age at onset (most commonly 10–30 years) Weakness of muscles of face, neck, and shoulder girdle	Dystrophic myopathy, but also often including inflammatory infiltrates of muscle.
Oculopharyngeal muscular dystrophy	Autosomal dominant (gene localized to 14q11–q13)	Onset in midadult life Ptosis and weakness of extraocular muscles Difficulty in swallowing	Dystrophic myopathy, but often including rimmed vacuoles in type 1 fibers
Emery-Dreifuss muscular dystrophy	X-linked (Xq28 EMD gene)	Variable onset (most commonly 10–20 years) Prominent contractures, especially of elbows and ankles	Mild myopathic changes Absent emerin by immunohistochemistry
Congenital muscular dystrophy	Autosomal recessive Two subtypes: merosin-negative (mutations in merosin/laminin αII gene), and merosin-positive	Neonatal hypotonia, respiratory insufficiency, delayed motor milestones	Variable fiber size and extensive endomysial fibrosis

tern. Three subtypes of the dominant dystrophies (1A, 1B, 1C) and seven subtypes of the recessive limb girdle dystrophies (2A to 2G) have been identified. Mutations of the *sarcoglycan complex of proteins* have been identified in four of the limb girdle muscular dystrophies (2C, 2D, 2E, and 2F) (Table 29–5). These membrane proteins interact with dystrophin through another transmembrane protein, β-dystroglycan (Fig. 29–11).

MYOTONIC DYSTROPHY

Myotonia, the sustained involuntary contraction of a group of muscles, is the cardinal neuromuscular symptom in this disease.[47] Patients often complain of "stiffness" and have difficulty in releasing their grip, like after a handshake. Myotonia can often be elicited by percussion of the thenar eminence.

Pathogenesis. Inherited as an autosomal dominant trait, the disease tends to increase in severity and appear at a younger age in succeeding generations, a phenomenon termed *anticipation.* The gene for myotonic dystrophy, localized to 19q13.2–13.3, encodes a protein kinase termed *myotonin protein kinase.*[48] Located in the 3′ untranslated region of the gene, it is a trinucleotide repeat, consisting of $(CTG)_n$. (See also Chapter 6.) The disease phenotype is associated with expansion of this region: in normal subjects, fewer than 30 repeats are present; in severely affected individuals, several thousand may be present.[49] The mutation is not stable within a pedigree; with each generation, more repeats accumulate, and this appears to correspond to the clinical feature of anticipation. Expansion of the trinucleotide repeat influences the eventual level of protein product.

MORPHOLOGY. Skeletal muscle may show pathologic features of a dystrophy similar to DMD. In addition, there is a striking increase in the number of internal nuclei, which on longitudinal section may form conspicuous chains. Another well-recognized abnormality is the **ring fiber**, with a subsarcolemmal band of cytoplasm that appears distinct from the center of the fiber. The rim contains myofibrils that are oriented circumferentially around the longitudinally oriented fibrils in the rest of the fiber. The ring fiber may be associated with an irregular mass of sarcoplasm **(sarcoplasmic mass)** extending outward from the ring. These stain blue with hematoxylin and eosin, red with Gomori trichrome, and intensely blue with the nicotinamide adenine dinucleotide–tetrazolium reductase (NADH-TR) histochemical reaction. The relation of the ring fiber to clinical myotonia is not understood. Histochemical techniques have demonstrated a relative atrophy of type 1 fibers early in the course of the disease in some cases. Of all the dystrophies, only myotonic dystrophy shows pathologic changes in the intrafusal fibers of muscle spindles, with fiber splitting, necrosis, and regeneration.

Clinical Course. The disease often presents in late childhood with abnormalities in gait secondary to weakness of foot dorsiflexors and subsequently progresses to weakness of the hand intrinsic muscles and wrist extensors. Atrophy of muscles of the face and ptosis ensue, leading to the typical facial appearance. Cataracts, which are present in virtually every patient, may be detected early in the course of the disease with slit-lamp examination. Other associated abnormalities include frontal balding, gonadal atrophy, cardiomyopathy, smooth muscle involvement, decreased plasma immunoglobulin G, and an abnormal glucose tolerance test response. Dementia has been reported in some cases. The disease may present as congenital weak-

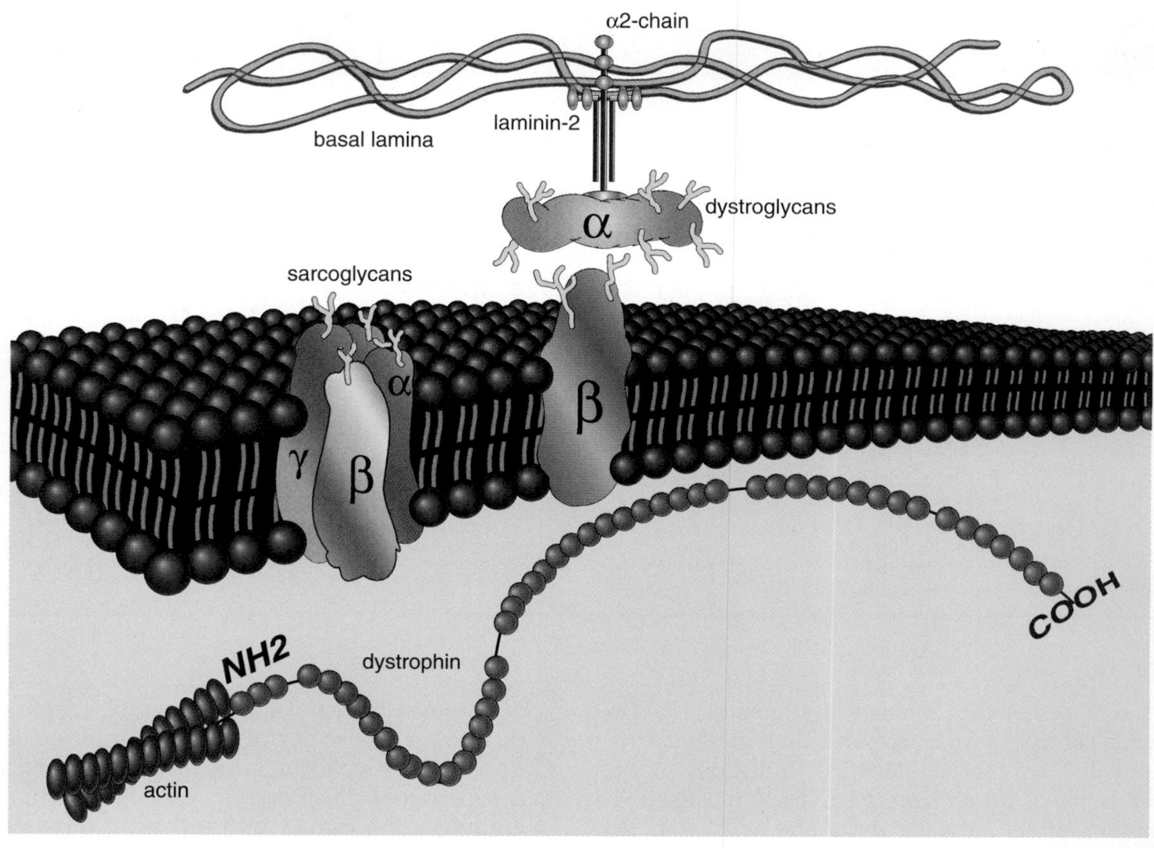

Figure 29–11

Diagram showing the relationship between the cell membrane (sarcolemma) and the sarcolemmal-associated proteins. Dystrophin, an intracellular protein, forms an interface between the cytoskeletal proteins and groups of transmembrane proteins, the dystroglycans and the sarcoglycans. These transmembrane proteins have interactions with the extracellular matrix, including the laminin proteins. Mutations in dystrophin are associated with the X-linked muscular dystrophies, mutations in the sarcoglycan proteins with the autosomal limb girdle muscular dystrophies, and mutations in α2-laminin (merosin) with a form of congenital muscular dystrophy.

Table 29–5. LIMB GIRDLE MUSCULAR DYSTROPHIES

Type	Inheritance	Locus Site	Gene	Clinicopathologic Features
1A	Autosomal dominant	5q22.3–q31.3	Unknown	■ Onset in adult life with slow progression of limb weakness, but sparing of facial muscles
1B	Autosomal dominant	1q11–q21	Unknown	■ Onset before the age of 20 years in lower limbs, progression during many years with cardiac involvement
1C	Autosomal dominant	3p25	Caveolin-3	■ Onset before the age of 20, clinically similar to type 1B
2A	Autosomal recessive	15q15.1–21.1	Calpain 3	■ Onset in late childhood to middle age; slow progression during 20 to 30 years
2B	Autosomal recessive	2p13	Unknown	■ Mild clinical course with onset in early adulthood
2C	Autosomal recessive	13q12	γ-Sarcoglycan	■ Severe weakness during childhood, rapid progression; dystrophic myopathy on muscle biopsy
2D	Autosomal recessive	17q21	α-Sarcoglycan	■ Severe weakness during childhood, rapid progression; dystrophic myopathy on muscle biopsy
2E	Autosomal recessive	4q12	β-Sarcoglycan	■ Onset in early childhood, with Duchenne-like clinical course
2F	Autosomal recessive	5q33–34	δ-Sarcoglycan	■ Early onset and severe myopathy; dystrophic myopathy on muscle biopsy
2G	Autosomal recessive	17q11–q12	Unknown	■ Distal weakness with limb-girdle weakness in late childhood to adulthood; rimmed vacuoles in muscle cells

ness and is then associated with maternal inheritance. In these cases, symptoms are severe, with facial muscle weakness (diplegia), feeding difficulties, and respiratory insufficiency.

Ion Channel Myopathies (Channelopathies)

The *ion channel myopathies* or channelopathies are a group of autosomal dominant familial diseases characterized clinically by myotonia, relapsing episodes of hypotonic paralysis (induced by vigorous exercise, cold, or a high-carbohydrate meal), or both. Hypotonia variants are recognized that are associated with elevated, depressed, or normal serum potassium levels at the time of the attack—*hyperkalemic, hypokalemic, and normokalemic periodic paralysis.* Conditions characterized by myotonia include either an autosomal dominant form, *myotonia congenita* (Thomsen disease), or a rare recessive variant (Becker myotonia). *Paramyotonia congenita* is a disorder of childhood wherein myotonia and periods of hypotonia appear during exercise and increase with continued exercise, especially with exposure to cold.

Pathogenesis. Different defects on the same gene on chromosome 17 cause hyperkalemic periodic paralysis and paramyotonia congenita. The gene controls the production of a sodium channel protein, which regulates the entry of sodium in muscle during contraction. The gene for hypokalemic periodic paralysis encodes a voltage-gated calcium channel.[50] Both the dominant and recessive forms of myotonia congenita are channelopathies linked to the human skeletal muscle chloride channel on chromosome 7.[50]

MORPHOLOGY. The principal histologic finding in the periodic paralyses, especially the hyperkalemic form, is the presence of PAS-positive intermyofibril vacuoles, especially evident during episodes of acute weakness. Ultrastructural examination demonstrates dilation of the sarcoplasmic reticulum. Also characteristic are tubular aggregates, faintly basophilic deposits found in both the interior and periphery of muscle fibers that can be well demonstrated with the NADH-TR but not with succinic dehydrogenase; ultrastructurally, they appear as fascicular arrays of parallel double-walled 60- to 90-nm tubules that have a distinctive hexagonal array in transverse section.

Malignant hyperpyrexia (malignant hyperthermia) is a rare clinical syndrome characterized by a dramatic hypermetabolic state (tachycardia, tachypnea, muscle spasms, and later hyperpyrexia) triggered by the induction of anesthesia, ordinarily halogenated inhalational agents and succinylcholine. The clinical syndrome may also occur in predisposed individuals with hereditary muscle diseases including congenital myopathies, dystrophinopathies, and metabolic myopathies. The only reliable method of diagnosis is the muscle biopsy and in vitro demonstration of contracture on exposure to anesthetic. Different genes have been identified in families with susceptibility to malignant hyperthermia, including genes encoding a voltage-gated calcium channel (lq32), an L-type voltage-dependent calcium channel (7q21–q22), and a ryanodine receptor (19q13).

Congenital Myopathies

The congenital myopathies are a group of disorders defined largely on the basis of the pathologic findings within muscle. Most of these conditions share common clinical features, including onset in early life, nonprogressive or slowly progressive course, proximal or generalized muscle weakness, and hypotonia. Those affected at birth or in

Table 29–6. CONGENITAL MYOPATHIES

Disease	Inheritance	Clinical Findings	Pathologic Findings
Central core disease	Autosomal dominant (ryanodine receptor-1 gene; 19q13.1) Sporadic	Early-onset hypotonia and nonprogressive weakness Associated skeletal deformities May develop malignant hyperthermia	Cytoplasmic cores are lightly eosinophilic and distinct from surrounding sarcoplasm; found only in type 1 fibers, which usually predominate
Nemaline myopathy	Autosomal recessive (unknown gene) Autosomal dominant (tropomyosin 3)	Weakness, hypotonia, and delayed motor development in childhood; may also be seen in adults Usually nonprogressive Involves proximal limb muscles most severely Skeletal abnormalities may be present	Aggregates of subsarcolemmal spindle-shaped particles *(nemaline rods)*; occur predominantly in type 1 fibers; derived from Z-band material (α-actinin)
Centronuclear myopathy	Autosomal recessive (unknown gene) X-linked (Xq28) Sporadic	Presents in infancy or early childhood with prominent involvement of extraocular and facial muscles, hypotonia, and slowly progressive limb muscle weakness	Abundance of centrally located nuclei involving the majority of muscle fibers Central nuclei are usually confined to type 1 fibers, which are small in diameter, but can occur in both fiber types

early infancy may present as "floppy babies" because of hypotonia or may have severe joint contractures *(arthrogryposis);* however, both hypotonia and arthrogryposis may also be caused by other neuromuscular dysfunction.

The best characterized congenital myopathies are listed in Table 29–6. Figure 29–12 shows the structural characteristics of nemaline myopathy, one of the most distinctive types.

Myopathies Associated With Inborn Errors of Metabolism

Many of the myopathies associated with metabolic disease are found in the setting of disorders of glycogen synthesis and degradation (Chapter 6). Myopathies can also result from disorders of mitochondrial function.

LIPID MYOPATHIES

To undergo β-oxidation, cytoplasmic fatty acyl coenzyme A (acyl-CoA) esters are conjugated with carnitine through the action of carnitine palmitoyltransferase (CPT), transported across the inner mitochondrial membrane, and then re-esterified to acyl-CoA esters that are then catabolized to acetyl-CoA units by the acyl-CoA dehydrogenases. Deficiencies affecting the carnitine transport system or deficiencies of the mitochondrial dehydrogenase enzyme systems can lead to the accumulation of lipid droplets within muscle (lipid myopathies) and can result from a deficiency of carnitine, acyl-CoA dehydrogenase, or CPT.[51]

Carnitine deficiency may be limited to muscle (myopathic carnitine deficiency) or may be secondary to diminished systemic levels (systemic carnitine deficiency). The cardinal symptom of the so-called myopathic form of disease is weakness; the age at onset is variable. Systemic

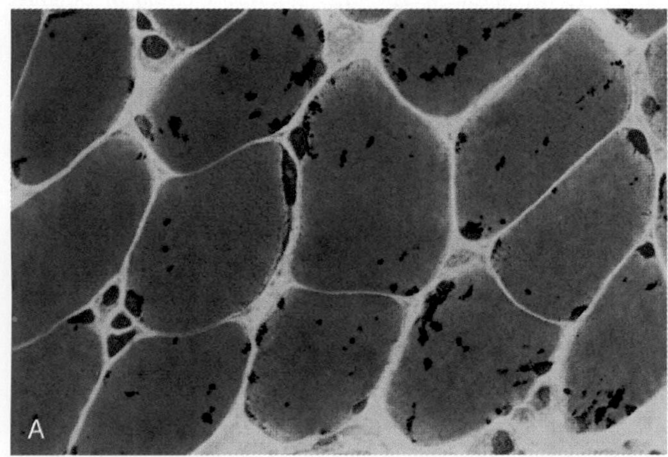

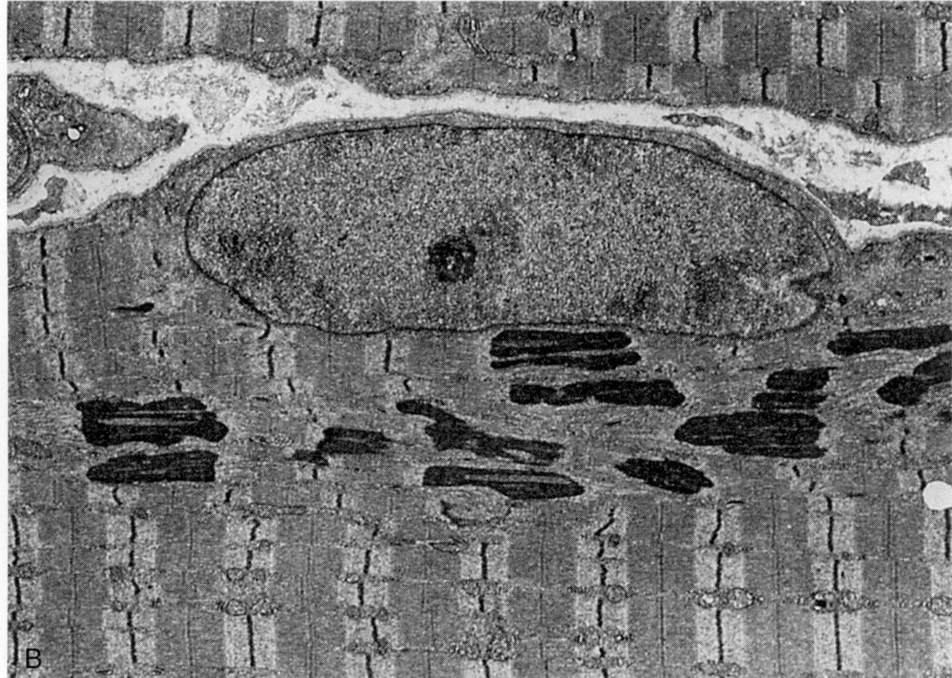

Figure 29–12 ■

A, Nemaline myopathy with numerous rod-shaped, intracytoplasmic inclusions (dark purple structures). *B*, Electron micrograph of subsarcolemmal nemaline bodies, showing material of Z-band density.

carnitine deficiency may result from impaired renal reabsorption of carnitine but more often is only secondary to the disorders of β-oxidation of fatty acids, most commonly medium-chain acyl-CoA dehydrogenase deficiency.[51]

In contrast, CPT deficiency often presents as recurrent myoglobinuria.[52] The most common form (CPT II deficiency) presents in teenagers and young adults with episodic acute myonecrosis (rhabdomyolysis) after prolonged exercise and leads to the release of myoglobin into plasma, which gives the urine an alarmingly dark color (myoglobinuria) when it is excreted. Renal failure can occur after massive episodes of rhabdomyolysis and is a serious complication of CPT II deficiency. A more severe infantile form of CPT deficiency (CPT I deficiency) is related to a separate gene product.[51]

In all of the lipid myopathies, the principal morphologic characteristic is accumulation of lipid within myocytes. The myofibrils are separated by vacuoles that stain with oil red O or Sudan black and have the typical appearance of lipid by electron microscopy. The vacuoles occur predominantly in type 1 fibers, and they are dispersed diffusely throughout the fiber.

MITOCHONDRIAL MYOPATHIES (OXIDATIVE PHOSPHORYLATION DISEASES)

Approximately one fifth of the proteins involved in mitochondrial oxidative phosphorylation are encoded by the mitochondrial genome (mtDNA); additionally, this circular genome codes for mitochondrial-specific tRNA and rRNA species.[53] The remainder of the mitochondrial enzyme complexes are encoded in the nuclear genome. Mutations in both nuclear and mitochondrial genes cause the so-called *mitochondrial myopathies.* Diseases that involve the mtDNA show maternal inheritance, since the oocyte contributes the mitochondria to the embryo. There is a high mutation rate for mtDNA compared with nuclear DNA. Mitochondrial metabolic defects identified so far include defects in respiratory chain protein complexes I, III, and IV.[54] The mitochondrial diseases may present in young adulthood and manifest with proximal muscle weakness, sometimes with severe involvement of the muscles that move the eyes (external ophthalmoplegia). The weakness may be accompanied by other neurologic symptoms, lactic acidosis, and cardiomyopathy, so that this group of disorders is sometimes classified as mitochondrial encephalomyopathies (Chapter 30).

MORPHOLOGY. The most consistent pathologic finding is aggregates of abnormal mitochondria that are demonstrable only by special techniques. These occur subsarcolemmally in early stages, but with severe involvement, they may extend throughout the fiber. The abnormal mitochondria impart a blotchy red appearance to the muscle fiber on the modified Gomori trichrome stain. Since they are also associated with distortion of the myofibrils, the muscle fiber contour becomes irregular on cross-section, and the descriptive term **ragged red fibers** has been applied to them (Fig. 29–13*A*).[55] The electron microscopic appearance is often distinctive: there are increased numbers of, and abnormalities in the shape and size of, mitochondria, some of which contain paracrystalline **parking lot inclusions** or alterations in the structure of cristae[56] (Fig. 29–13*B*).

Clinical Course and Genetics. The relationship between clinical course in the mitochondrial disorders and the genetic alterations is not entirely clear; however, three general categories have been defined.[57] *Class I mutations* involve the genes encoded by nuclear DNA and show autosomal dominant or recessive inheritance. Some cases of subacute necrotizing encephalopathy (Leigh syndrome), exertional myoglobinuria, and infantile X-linked cardioskeletal myopathy (Barth syndrome) are due to mutations in nuclear DNA. *Class II mutations* involve point mutations in mtDNA, and some examples include myoclonic epilepsy with ragged red fibers (MERFF), Leber hereditary optic neuropathy (LHON), and mitochondrial encephalomyopathy with lactic acidosis and stroke-like episodes (MELAS).[58, 59] *Class III mutations* have deletions or duplications of mtDNA. *Chronic progressive external ophthalmoplegia (CPEO)* is characterized by a myopathy with prominent weakness of external ocular movements. *Kearns-Sayre syndrome (KSS)* ("ophthalmoplegia plus") is also characterized by ophthalmoplegia but in addition includes pigmentary degeneration of the retina and complete heart block. Other findings include short stature and cerebellar ataxia.[60] Both CPEO and KSS are associated with Class III deletions.

Inflammatory Myopathies

There are three subgroups of inflammatory muscle diseases and the entities within these have been discussed elsewhere in this text: infectious myositis (Chapter 9), noninfectious inflammatory muscle disease (polymyositis, dermatomyositis, and inclusion body myositis; Chapter 7), and systemic inflammatory diseases that involve muscle along with other organs (Chapter 7).

Toxic Myopathies

THYROTOXIC MYOPATHY

Thyrotoxic myopathy presents most commonly as an acute or a chronic proximal muscle weakness that may precede the onset of other signs of thyroid dysfunction. *Exophthalmic ophthalmoplegia* is characterized by swelling of the eyelids, edema of the conjunctiva, and diplopia. In *hypothyroidism*, there may be cramping or aching of muscles, and movements and reflexes are slowed. Findings include fiber atrophy, an increased number of internal nuclei, glycogen aggregates, and occasionally deposition of mucopolysaccharides in the connective tissue.

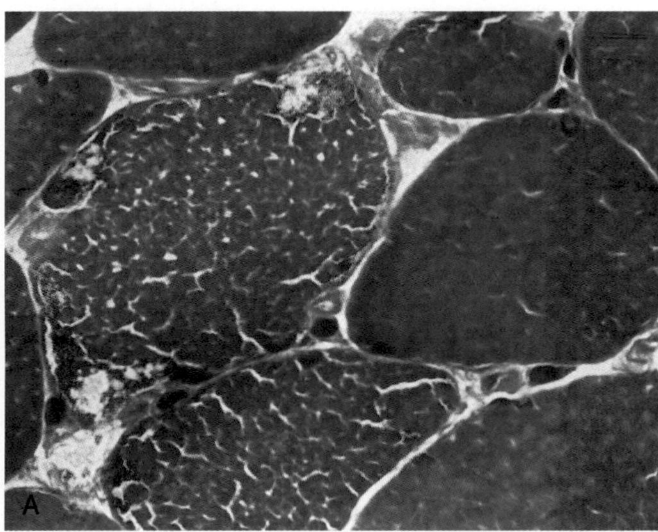

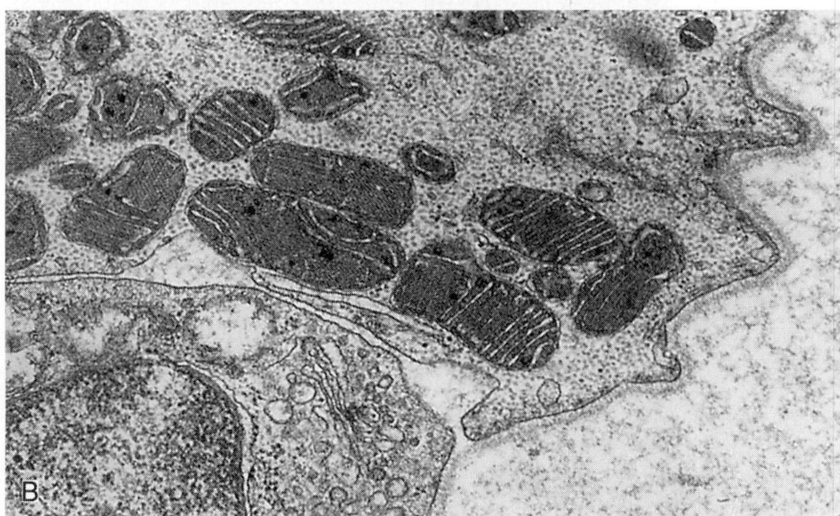

Figure 29–13

A, Mitochondrial myopathy showing an irregular fiber with subsarcolemmal collections of mitochondria that stain red with the modified Gomori trichrome stain (ragged red fiber). *B*, Electron micrograph of mitochondria from biopsy specimen in *A* showing "parking lot" inclusions.

Another muscle disease associated with thyroid dysfunction is *thyrotoxic periodic paralysis*, which is characterized by episodic weakness that is often accompanied by hypokalemia. Males are affected four times more often than are females, with a high incidence in individuals of Japanese descent. In thyrotoxic myopathy, there is myofiber necrosis, regeneration, and interstitial lymphocytosis. In chronic thyrotoxic myopathy, there may be only slight variability of muscle fiber size, mitochondrial hypertrophy, and focal myofibril degeneration; fatty infiltration of muscle is seen in severe cases. Exophthalmic ophthalmoplegia is limited to the extraocular muscles, which may be edematous and enlarged.

ETHANOL MYOPATHY

"Binge" drinking of alcohol is known to produce an acute toxic syndrome of rhabdomyolysis with accompanying myoglobinuria, which may lead to renal failure. Clinically, the patient may acutely develop pain that is either generalized or confined to a single muscle group. Some patients have a complicated clinicopathologic syndrome consisting of proximal muscle weakness with electrophysiologic evidence of myopathy superimposed on alcoholic neuropathy. On histologic examination, there is swelling of myocytes, with fiber necrosis, myophagocytosis, and regeneration. There may also be evidence of denervation.

DRUG-INDUCED MYOPATHIES

Proximal muscle weakness and atrophy can occur as a result of the deleterious effects of steroids on muscle, whether in Cushing syndrome or during therapeutic administration of steroids, a condition known as *steroid myopathy*. The severity of clinical disability is variable and not directly related to the steroid level or the therapeutic regimen. It is characterized by muscle fiber atrophy, predominantly affecting type 2 fibers.[8] When the myopathy is severe, there may be a bimodal distribution of fiber sizes, with type 1 fibers of nearly normal caliber and markedly atrophic type 2 fibers. Electron microscopy has shown dilation of the sarcoplasmic reticulum and thickening of the basal laminae.

Chloroquine, originally used in treatment of malaria but

subsequently used in other clinical settings, can produce a proximal myopathy in humans. The most prominent finding in chloroquine myopathy is the presence of vacuoles within myocytes.[61] Two types of vacuoles have been described: autophagic membrane-bound vacuoles containing membranous debris and curvilinear bodies with short curved membranous structures with alternating light and dark zones. Vacuoles can be seen in as many as 50% of the myocytes, most commonly type 1 fibers, and with progression, myocyte necrosis may develop.

Diseases of the Neuromuscular Junction

MYASTHENIA GRAVIS

Now recognized as one of the most well defined forms of autoimmune disease, *myasthenia gravis is a muscle disease caused by immune-mediated loss of acetylcholine receptors and having characteristic temporal and anatomic patterns as well as drug responses.* The disease has a prevalence of about 3 in 100,000 persons.[62] When arising before age 40 years, it is most commonly seen in women, but there is equal occurrence between the sexes in older patients. Thymic hyperplasia is found in 65% and thymoma in 15% of patients. Analysis of neuromuscular transmission in myasthenia gravis shows a decrease in the number of muscle acetylcholine receptors (AChRs), and circulating antibodies to the AChR are present in nearly all patients with myasthenia gravis.[63] The disease can be passively transferred to animals with serum from affected patients.

MORPHOLOGY. By light microscopic examination, muscle biopsy specimens from patients with myasthenia are usually unrevealing. In severe cases, disuse changes with type 2 fiber atrophy may be found. The postsynaptic membrane is simplified, with loss of AChRs from the region of the synapse. Immune complexes as well as the membrane attack complex of the complement cascade (C5–Cq) can be found along the postsynaptic membrane as well.

Pathogenesis. Electrophysiologic studies are notable for decrement in motor responses with repeated stimulation; nerve conduction study findings are normal. Sensory as well as autonomic functions are not affected. The circulating anti-AChR antibodies apparently increase the degradation rate of the AChR,[64] leading to a decreased receptor number, and also appear to fix complement and lead to direct injury to the postsynaptic membrane. Despite the evidence that these antibodies play a critical pathogenic role in the disease, there is not always a correlation between antibody levels and neurologic deficit. Interestingly, in light of the immune-mediated etiology of the disease, thymic abnormalities are common in these patients, but the precise link for autoimmunity to AChRs is uncertain. Regardless of the pattern of thymic pathology, most patients show improvement after thymectomy.

Clinical Course. Typically, weakness begins with extraocular muscles; drooping eyelids (ptosis) and double vision (diplopia) cause the patient to seek medical attention. However, the initial symptoms may include generalized weakness. The weakness fluctuates, with alterations occurring during days, hours, or even minutes, and intercurrent medical conditions can lead to exacerbations of the weakness. Patients show improvement in strength in response to administration of anticholinesterase agents. This remains a most useful test on clinical examination.[63] Respiratory compromise was a major cause of mortality in the past; 95% of patients survive after 5 years because of improved methods of treatment and better ventilatory support. Effective forms of treatment include anticholinesterase drugs, prednisone, plasmapheresis, and resection of thymoma if it is present.

LAMBERT-EATON MYASTHENIC SYNDROME

Lambert-Eaton myasthenic syndrome is a disease of the neuromuscular junction that is distinct from myasthenia gravis. It usually develops as a paraneoplastic process, most commonly with small cell carcinoma of the lung (60% of cases), although it can occur in the absence of underlying malignant disease.[65] Patients develop proximal muscle weakness along with autonomic dysfunction. No clinical improvement is found with the Tensilon test, and electrophysiologic studies show evidence of enhanced neurotransmission with repetitive stimulation. These clinical features allow this disorder to be distinguished from myasthenia gravis.

The content of anticholinesterase is normal in neuromuscular junction synaptic vesicles, and the postsynaptic membrane is normally responsive to anticholinesterase, but fewer vesicles are released in response to each presynaptic action potential. Some patients have antibodies that recognize presynaptic calcium channels, and a similar disease can be transferred to animals with these antibodies.[56] This suggests that autoimmunity to the calcium channel causes the disease.

Tumors of Skeletal Muscle

Skeletal muscle tumors are discussed with other soft tissue tumors (Chapter 28).

REFERENCES

1. Adams RD, et al: Principles of Neurology, 6th ed. New York, McGraw-Hill, 1997, p 1387.
2. Dyck PJ, et al: The morphometric composition of myelinated fibers by nerve, level, and species related to nerve micro-environment and ischaemia. Electroencephalogr Clin Neurophysiol Suppl 36:39–55, 1982.
3. Smith KJ, et al: Internodal myelin volume and axon surface area. J Neurol Sci 55:231–246, 1982.
4. Trapp BD, et al: Molecular pathogenesis of peripheral neuropathy. Rev Neurol 152:314–319, 1996.

5. Walker RA, Sheetz MP: Cytoplasmic microtubule associated motors. Annu Rev Biochem 62:429–451, 1993.
6. Grafstein B, Forman DS: Intracellular transport in neurons. Physiol Rev 60:1167–1283, 1980.
7. Rechthand E, Rapoport SI: Regulation of the microenvironment of peripheral nerve: role of the blood-nerve barrier. Prog Neurobiol 28: 303–343, 1987.
8. Dubowitz V: Muscle Biopsy: A Practical Approach, 2nd ed. London, Baillière Tindal, 1985, p 720.
9. DeVries GH: Schwann cell proliferation. In Dyck PJ, et al (eds): Peripheral Neuropathy. Philadelphia, WB Saunders, 1993, pp 290–298.
10. Brück W, et al: Mechanisms of macrophage recruitment in Wallerian degeneration. Acta Neuropathol 89:363–367, 1995.
11. Stoll G, et al: Wallerian degeneration in the peripheral nervous system: participation of both Schwann cells and macrophages in myelin degradation. J Neurocytol 18:671–683, 1989.
12. Tischler ME, et al: Different mechanisms of increased proteolysis in atrophy induced by denervation or unweighting of rat soleus muscle. Metabolism 39:756–763, 1990.
13. Wujek JR, Lasek RJ: Correlation of axonal regeneration and slow component B in two branches of a single axon. J Neurosci 3:243–251, 1983.
14. Rees JH, et al: Epidemiological study of Guillain-Barré syndrome in southeast England. J Neurol Neurosurg Psychiatr 64:74–77, 1998.
15. Prevots DR, Sutter RW: Assessment of Guillain-Barré syndrome mortality and morbidity in the United States: implications for acute flaccid paralysis surveillance. J Infect Dis 175(Suppl 1):S151–155, 1997.
16. Hartung HP, Toyka KV: T-cell and macrophage activation in experimental autoimmune neuritis and Guillain-Barré syndrome. Ann Neurol 27:S57–S63, 1990.
17. van der Meche FG, van Doorn PA: Guillain-Barré syndrome and chronic inflammatory demyelinating polyneuropathy: immune mechanisms and update on current therapies. Ann Neurol 37(Suppl)1:S14–S31, 1995.
18. Linington C, et al: Cell adhesion molecules of the immunoglobulin supergene family as tissue-specific autoantigens: induction of experimental allergic neuritis (EAN) by P0 protein-specific T cell lines. Eur J Immunol 22:1813–1817, 1992.
19. Ilyas AA, et al: Anti-GM1 IgA antibodies in Guillain-Barré syndrome. J Neuroimmunol 36:69–76, 1992.
20. Barohn RJ, et al: Chronic inflammatory demyelinating polyradiculoneuropathy. Clinical characteristics, course, and recommendations for diagnostic criteria. Arch Neurol 46:878–884, 1989.
21. Waksman BH: Experimental study of diphtheritic polyneuritis in the rabbit and guinea pig. III. The blood-nerve barrier in the rabbit. J Neuropathol Exp Neurol 20:35–77, 1961.
22. Wilson A, et al: Subclinical varicella-zoster virus viremia, herpes zoster, and T lymphocyte immunity to varicella-zoster viral antigens after bone marrow transplantation. J Infect Dis 165:119–126, 1992.
23. Suter U, Snipes GJ: Biology and genetics of hereditary motor and sensory neuropathies. Ann Rev Neurosci 18:45–75, 1995.
24. Yamamoto K, et al: Familial amyloid polyneuropathy in Taiwan: identification of transthyretin variant (Leu55–>Pro). Muscle Nerve 17:637–641, 1994.
25. Lupski JR, et al: Gene dosage is a mechanism for Charcot-Marie-Tooth disease type 1A. Nat Genet 1:29–33, 1992.
26. Chance PF, et al: Trisomy 17p associated with Charcot-Marie-Tooth neuropathy type 1A phenotype: evidence for gene dosage as a mechanism in CMT1A. Neurology 42:2295–2299, 1992.
27. Hayasaka K, et al: Charcot-Marie-Tooth neuropathy type 1B is associated with mutations of the myelin P0 gene. Nat Genet 5:31–34, 1993.
28. Bergoffen J, et al: Connexin mutations in X-linked Charcot-Marie-Tooth disease. Science 262:2039–2042, 1993.
29. Ben Othmane K, et al: Localization of a gene *(CMT2A)* for autosomal dominant Charcot-Marie-Tooth disease type 2 to chromosome 1p and evidence of genetic heterogeneity. Genomics 17:370–375, 1993.
30. Roa BB, et al: Dejerine-Sottas syndrome associated with point mutation in the peripheral myelin protein 22 *(PMP22)* gene. Nat Genet 5: 269–273, 1993.
31. Behse F, et al: Nerve biopsy and conduction studies in diabetic neuropathy. J Neurol Neurosurg Psychiatry 40:1072–1082, 1977.
32. Beggs J, et al: Innervation of the vasa nervorum: changes in human diabetics. J Neuropathol Exp Neurol 51:612–629, 1992.
33. Dyck PJ, Giannini C: Pathologic alterations in the diabetic neuropathies of humans: a review. J Neuropathol Exp Neurol 55:1181–1193, 1996.
34. Llewelyn JG, et al: Sural nerve morphometry in diabetic autonomic and painful sensory neuropathy. A clinicopathological study. Brain 114:867–892, 1991.
35. Asbury AK: Neuropathies with renal failure, hepatic disorders, chronic respiratory insufficiency, and critical illness. In Dyck PJ, et al (eds): Peripheral Neuropathy. Philadelphia, WB Saunders, 1993, pp 1251–1265.
36. Dayan AD, et al: Association of carcinomatous neuromyopathy with different histological types of carcinoma of the lung. Brain 88:435–448, 1965.
37. Hughes R, et al: Carcinoma and the peripheral nervous system. J Neurol 243:371–376, 1996.
38. Latov N, et al: Peripheral neuropathy and anti-MAG antibodies. Crit Rev Neurobiol 3:301–332, 1988.
39. Spencer PS, Schaumburg HH: Experimental and Clinical Neurotoxicology. Baltimore, Williams & Wilkins, 1980, p 929.
40. Fuchs PC, et al: Synovial histology in carpal tunnel syndrome. J Hand Surg Am 16:753–758, 1991.
41. Ullian ME, et al: Beta-2-microglobulin–associated amyloidosis in chronic hemodialysis patients with carpal tunnel syndrome. Medicine (Baltimore) 68:107–115, 1989.
42. Somerville MJ, et al: Clinical application of the molecular diagnosis of spinal muscular atrophy: deletions of neuronal apoptosis inhibitory protein and survival motor neuron genes. Am J Med Genet 69:159–165, 1997.
43. van Essen AJ, et al: Birth and population prevalence of Duchenne muscular dystrophy in The Netherlands. Hum Genet 88:258–266, 1992.
44. Hodgson SV, et al: Correlation of clinical and deletion data in Duchenne and Becker muscular dystrophy, with special reference to mental ability. Neuromuscul Disord 2:269–276, 1992.
45. Hoffman EP, et al: Dystrophin: the protein product of the Duchenne muscular dystrophy locus. Cell 51:919–928, 1987.
46. Gold R, et al: The use of monoclonal antibodies in diagnostic tests for Becker and Duchenne muscular dystrophy. J Neurol 240:21–24, 1993.
47. Ptacek LJ, et al: Genetics and physiology of the myotonic muscle diseases. N Engl J Med 328:482–489, 1993.
48. Shelbourne P, et al: Direct diagnosis of myotonic dystrophy with a disease-specific DNA marker. N Engl J Med 328:471–475, 1993.
49. Brook JD, et al: Molecular basis of myotonic dystrophy: expansion of a trinucleotide (CTG) repeat at the 3′ end of a transcript encoding a protein kinase family member. Cell 68:799–808, 1992.
50. Ptacek LJ. Channelopathies: ion channel disorders as a paradigm for paroxysmal disorders of the nervous system. Neuromuscul Disord 7: 250–255, 1997.
51. Roe CR, Coates PM: Mitochondrial fatty acid oxidation disorders. In Scriver CR, et al (eds): The Metabolic and Molecular Bases of Inherited Diseases. New York, McGraw-Hill, 1995, pp 1501–1533.
52. Tonin P, et al: Metabolic causes of myoglobinuria. Ann Neurol 27: 181–185, 1990.
53. Clayton DA: Structure and function of the mitochondrial genome. J Inherit Metab Dis 15:439–447, 1992.
54. Hammans SR, et al: A molecular genetic study of focal histochemical defects in mitochondrial encephalomyopathies. Brain 115:343–365, 1992.
55. Rowland LP, et al: Clinical syndromes associated with ragged red fibers. Rev Neurol (Paris) 147:467–473, 1991.
56. Lindal S, et al: Mitochondrial diseases and myopathies: a series of muscle biopsy specimens with ultrastructural changes in the mitochondria. Ultrastruct Pathol 16:263–275, 1992.
57. Shoffner JM, Wallace DC: Oxidative phosphorylation diseases. In Scriver CR, et al (eds). The Metabolic and Molecular Bases of Inherited Diseases. New York, McGraw-Hill, 1995, pp 1535–1609.
58. Moraes CT, et al: The mitochondrial tRNA(Leu(UUR)) mutation in mitochondrial encephalomyopathy, lactic acidosis, and strokelike epi-

sodes (MELAS): genetic, biochemical, and morphological correlations in skeletal muscle. Am J Hum Genet 50:934–949, 1992.
59. Ciafaloni E, et al: MELAS: clinical features, biochemistry, and molecular genetics. Ann Neurol 31:391–398, 1992.
60. Sparaco M, et al: Neuropathology of mitochondrial encephalomyopathies due to mitochondrial DNA defects. J Neuropathol Exp Neurol 52:1–10, 1993.
61. Kumamoto T, et al: Experimental chloroquine myopathy: morphological and biochemical studies. Eur Neurol 29:202–207, 1989.
62. Phillips LH Jr, et al: The epidemiology of myasthenia gravis in central and western Virginia. Neurology 42:1888–1893, 1992.
63. Phillips LH Jr, Melnick PA: Diagnosis of myasthenia gravis in the 1990s. Semin Neurol 10:62–69, 1990.
64. Tzartos SJ, et al: The main immunogenic region (MIR) of the nicotinic acetylcholine receptor and the anti-MIR antibodies. Mol Neurobiol 5:1–29, 1991.
65. Gutmann L, et al: Trends in the association of Lambert-Eaton myasthenic syndrome with carcinoma. Neurology 42:848–850, 1992.
66. Kim YI, Neher E: IgG from patients with Lambert-Eaton syndrome blocks voltage-dependent calcium channels. Science 239:405–408, 1988.

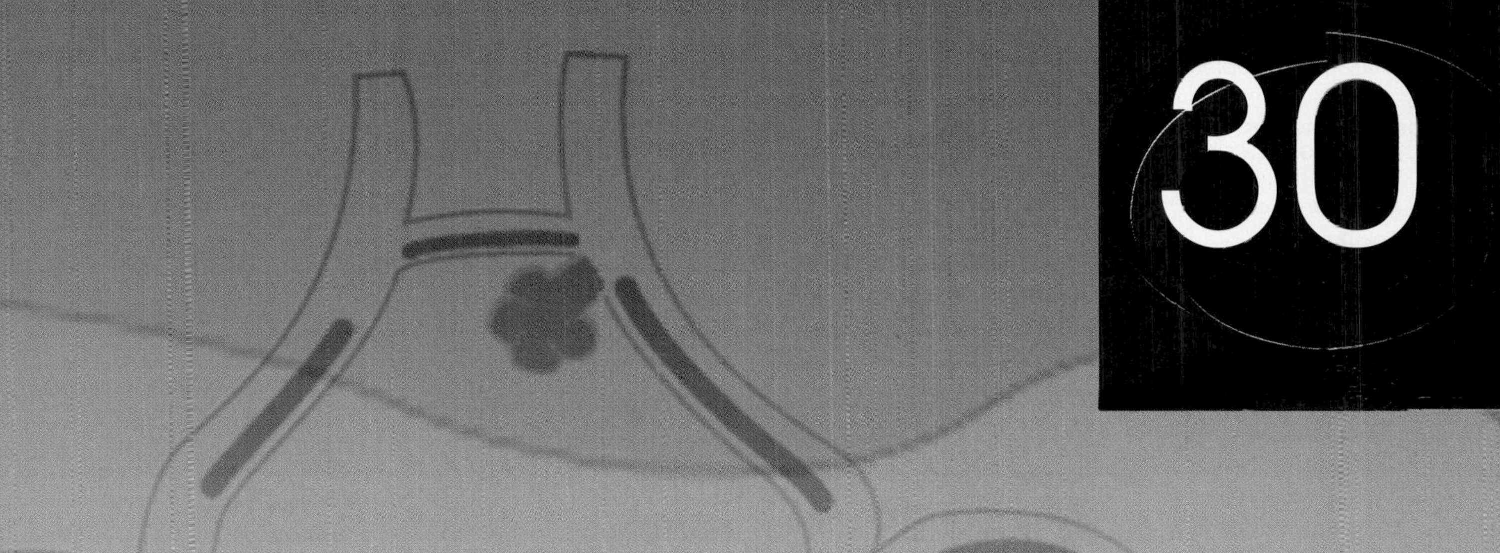

The Central Nervous System

Umberto De Girolami, Douglas C. Anthony, and Matthew P. Frosch

NORMAL CELLS AND CELLULAR PATHOLOGY
NEURONS
GLIA
Astrocytes
Oligodendrocytes
Ependymal Cells
Microglia
CEREBRAL EDEMA, RAISED INTRACRANIAL PRESSURE AND HERNIATION, AND HYDROCEPHALUS
CEREBRAL EDEMA
RAISED INTRACRANIAL PRESSURE AND HERNIATION
HYDROCEPHALUS
MALFORMATIONS AND DEVELOPMENTAL DISEASES
NEURAL TUBE DEFECTS
FOREBRAIN ANOMALIES
POSTERIOR FOSSA ANOMALIES
SYRINGOMYELIA AND HYDROMYELIA
PERINATAL BRAIN INJURY
TRAUMA
SKULL FRACTURES
PARENCHYMAL INJURIES
Concussion
Direct Parenchymal Injury
Axonal Injury
TRAUMATIC VASCULAR INJURY
Epidural Hematoma
Subdural Hematoma
SEQUELAE OF BRAIN TRAUMA
SPINAL CORD TRAUMA
CEREBROVASCULAR DISEASES
PATHOPHYSIOLOGIC CONSIDERATIONS: HYPOXIA, ISCHEMIA, AND INFARCTION
Hypotension, Hypoperfusion, and Low-Flow States—Global Cerebral Ischemia
Focal Cerebral Ischemia—Infarction From Obstruction of Local Blood Supply
INTRACRANIAL HEMORRHAGE
Intracerebral (Intraparenchymal) Hemorrhage
Subarachnoid Hemorrhage and Ruptured Berry Aneurysms
Vascular Malformations
HYPERTENSIVE CEREBROVASCULAR DISEASE
Lacunar Infarcts
Slit Hemorrhages
Hypertensive Encephalopathy
INFECTIONS
ACUTE MENINGITIS
Acute Pyogenic (Bacterial) Meningitis
Acute Aseptic (Viral) Meningitis
ACUTE FOCAL SUPPURATIVE INFECTIONS
Brain Abscess
Subdural Empyema
Extradural Abscess
CHRONIC BACTERIAL MENINGOENCEPHALITIS
Tuberculosis and Mycobacterioses
Neurosyphilis
Neuroborreliosis (Lyme Disease)
VIRAL MENINGOENCEPHALITIS
Arthropod-Borne (Arbo) Viral Encephalitis
Herpes Simplex Virus Type 1
Herpes Simplex Virus Type 2
Varicella-Zoster Virus (Herpes Zoster)
Cytomegalovirus
Poliomyelitis
Rabies
Human Immunodeficiency Virus 1
HIV-1 Meningoencephalitis (Subacute Encephalitis)
Vacuolar Myelopathy
AIDS-Associated Myopathy, Peripheral Neuropathy
AIDS in Children
Progressive Multifocal Leukoencephalopathy
Subacute Sclerosing Panencephalitis
FUNGAL MENINGOENCEPHALITIS
OTHER INFECTIOUS DISEASES OF THE NERVOUS SYSTEM
TRANSMISSIBLE SPONGIFORM ENCEPHALOPATHIES (PRION DISEASES)
DEMYELINATING DISEASES
MULTIPLE SCLEROSIS
MULTIPLE SCLEROSIS VARIANTS
ACUTE DISSEMINATED ENCEPHALOMYELITIS AND ACUTE NECROTIZING HEMORRHAGIC ENCEPHALOMYELITIS
OTHER DISEASES WITH DEMYELINATION
DEGENERATIVE DISEASES

DEGENERATIVE DISEASES AFFECTING THE CEREBRAL CORTEX
Alzheimer Disease
Pick Disease
DEGENERATIVE DISEASES OF BASAL GANGLIA AND BRAIN STEM
Parkinsonism
Idiopathic Parkinson Disease (Paralysis Agitans)
Progressive Supranuclear Palsy
Corticobasal Degeneration
Multiple System Atrophy
Striatonigral Degeneration
Shy-Drager Syndrome
Olivopontocerebellar Atrophy
Huntington Disease
SPINOCEREBELLAR DEGENERATIONS
Spinocerebellar Ataxias
Friedreich Ataxia
Ataxia-Telangiectasia
DEGENERATIVE DISEASES AFFECTING MOTOR NEURONS
Amyotrophic Lateral Sclerosis (Motor Neuron Disease)
Bulbospinal Atrophy (Kennedy Syndrome)
Spinal Muscular Atrophy
INBORN ERRORS OF METABOLISM
LEUKODYSTROPHIES
Krabbe Disease
Metachromatic Leukodystrophy
Adrenoleukodystrophy
Pelizaeus-Merzbacher Disease
Canavan Disease
MITOCHONDRIAL ENCEPHALOMYOPATHIES
Leigh Disease
Other Mitochondrial Encephalomyopathies
TOXIC AND ACQUIRED METABOLIC DISEASES
VITAMIN DEFICIENCIES
Thiamine (Vitamin B_1) Deficiency
Vitamin B_{12} Deficiency
NEUROLOGIC SEQUELAE OF METABOLIC DISTURBANCES
Hypoglycemia
Hyperglycemia
Hepatic Encephalopathy
TOXIC DISORDERS
Carbon Monoxide
Methanol
Ethanol
Radiation
Combined Methotrexate and Radiation-Induced Injury
TUMORS
GLIOMAS
Astrocytoma
Fibrillary (Diffuse) Astrocytoma and Glioblastoma Multiforme
Pilocytic Astrocytoma
Pleomorphic Xanthoastrocytoma
Brain Stem Glioma
Oligodendroglioma
Ependymoma and Related Paraventricular Mass Lesions
NEURONAL TUMORS
POORLY DIFFERENTIATED NEOPLASMS
Medulloblastoma
OTHER PARENCHYMAL TUMORS
Primary Brain Lymphoma
Germ Cell Tumors
Pineal Parenchymal Tumors
MENINGIOMAS
METASTATIC TUMORS
PARANEOPLASTIC SYNDROMES
PERIPHERAL NERVE SHEATH TUMORS
Schwannoma
Neurofibroma
Malignant Peripheral Nerve Sheath Tumor (Malignant Schwannoma)
NEUROCUTANEOUS SYNDROMES (PHAKOMATOSES)
Neurofibromatosis
TYPE 1 Neurofibromatosis (NF1)
TYPE 2 Neurofibromatosis (NF2)
Tuberous Sclerosis
Von Hippel–Lindau Disease

The human central nervous system (CNS) is an enormously complex tissue serving the organism as a processing center linking information between the body and the outside world. It is estimated that 50% or more of the human genome codes for genes that are nervous system specific. The principal functional unit of the CNS is the neuron; the best estimates are that there are about 10^{11} neurons in the human brain.[1] Neurons, although similar in many ways to other cells in the body, are unique in their ability to receive, store, and transmit information. Neurons differ greatly from one another in many important properties—their functional roles (such as sensory, motor, autonomic), the distribution of their interconnections, the neurotransmitters they use for synaptic transmission, their metabolic requirements, and their levels of electrical activity at a given moment. A set of neurons, not necessarily clustered together in a given brain region, may thus be singled out for destruction—*selective vulnerability*—because they share one or more of these properties. Furthermore, and of particular importance in medicine, beyond embryonic development, neurons are postmitotic cells incapable of cell division, so that destruction of even a relatively small number of neurons responsible for a specific function may leave the patient with a severe clinical neurologic deficit. In comparison to other organ systems of the body, the nervous system has several unique anatomic and physiologic characteristics: the protective bony enclosure of the skull and spinal column that contains it, a specialized system of *autoregulation* of cerebral blood flow, metabolic substrate requirements, the absence of a conventional lymphatic system, a special cerebrospinal fluid (CSF) circulation, limited immunologic surveillance, and distinctive responses to injury and wound healing. As a result of these special characteristics, the CNS is vulnerable to unique pathologic processes, and the reactions of CNS tissue to injury may differ considerably from those encountered elsewhere.[2,3]

NORMAL CELLS AND CELLULAR PATHOLOGY

The principal cells of the CNS are neurons, glia, and the cells that compose the meninges and blood vessels.

Neurons

In the CNS, neurons are topographically organized either as aggregates (nuclei, ganglia) or as elongated columns or layers (such as the intermediolateral gray column of the spinal cord or the six-layered cerebral cortex).[4] Functional domains have been assigned to many of these anatomically defined regions (such as the hypoglossal nucleus of the medulla: motor fibers of the 12th cranial nerve; calcarine cortex of the occipital lobe: visual cortex). In addition, as a further dimension of anatomic-functional specificity, some cortical and subcortical neurons and their projections are arranged somatotopically (such as motor neurons supplying the leg: interhemispheric medial aspect of precentral gyrus of isocortex).[5] Neurons vary considerably in structure and size throughout the nervous system and within a given brain region. With conventional histologic preparations, an anterior horn cell neuron in the spinal cord has a cell body (perikaryon) that is about 50 μm wide, a large and somewhat eccentrically placed nucleus, a prominent nucleolus, and abundant Nissl substance; the nucleus of a granule cell neuron of the cerebellar cortex is about 10 μm across, and its perikaryon and nucleolus are not readily visible. Electron microscopic study reveals further variability among neurons in cytoplasmic content and the shape of the cells and their processes.[6] Characteristic ultrastructural features common to many neurons include neurotubules, neurofilaments, a prominent Golgi apparatus and rough endoplasmic reticulum, and synaptic specializations. Immunohistochemical markers for neurons and their processes commonly used in diagnostic work include neurofilament protein, neuron-specific enolase, and synaptophysin.[7]

There are several well-characterized basic histopathologic *neuronal reactions to injury;* these include those related to neuronal degeneration and cell death and those associated with reparative events. Neuronal degeneration either occurs in the context of programmed cell death (apoptosis), as when there is elimination of sets of neurons during the course of fetal brain development, or is the result of acute or slowly progressive cell injury.

- *Acute neuronal injury (red neuron)* refers to a spectrum of changes that accompany acute CNS hypoxia/ischemia or infectious and toxic insults that ultimately lead to death of the cell. Red neurons are evident with hematoxylin and eosin (H&E) preparations at about 12 to 24 hours after an irreversible hypoxic/ischemic insult. The morphologic features consist of shrinkage of the cell body, pyknosis of the nucleus, disappearance of the nucleolus, and loss of Nissl substance, with intense eosinophilia of the cytoplasm. Often, the nucleus assumes the angulated shape of the shrunken perikaryon. Experimental studies have defined even earlier (4 to 8 hours) structural changes that attend irreversible neuronal injury consisting of small vacuoles within the cell body[8]; these are difficult to detect in human tissue examined post mortem.
- *"Simple" neuronal atrophy ("degeneration")* refers to situations of neuronal death occurring as a result of a progressive disease process of long duration, as is seen in certain slowly evolving neurologic diseases (such as amyotrophic lateral sclerosis). The characteristic histologic feature is cell loss, often selectively involving functionally related systems of neurons, and reactive gliosis. When the process is at an early stage, this cell loss is difficult to detect; the associated glial changes are often the best indicator of the pathologic process at this stage. Neuronal *transsynaptic degeneration* is seen when there is a destructive process that interrupts the majority of the afferent input to a group of neurons, such as in the degeneration of sets of lateral geniculate neurons after eye enucleation.
- *Axonal reaction.* This refers to the reaction within the cell body that attends regeneration of the axon; it has been extensively studied in motor neurons in experimental animals.[9] In the anterior horn cells of the spinal cord, axonal reaction occurs when motor axons are cut or seriously damaged. This reparative process is associated with up-regulation of protein synthesis, and its most important effect is axonal sprouting. Morphologic changes that at first are visible in the perikaryon consist of enlargement and rounding up of the cell body, peripheral displacement of the nucleus, enlargement of the nucleolus, and dispersion of Nissl substance, particularly in the center of the cell *(central chromatolysis).* The regenerative and degenerative changes that occur over the course of time at the site of axotomy (proximal and distal ends, respectively) are discussed in Chapter 29.
- A wide range of subcellular alterations in the neuronal organelles and cytoskeleton are recognized. *Neuronal inclusions* may occur as a manifestation of aging when there are intracytoplasmic accumulations of complex lipids, proteins, and carbohydrates *(lipofuscin),* believed to be residual bodies derived from lysosomes. Abnormal intracytoplasmic deposition of complex lipids and other substances also occurs in genetically determined disorders of metabolism in which substrate or other intermediates accumulate (Chapter 6). In these conditions, the neuronal cell body at first becomes greatly swollen because of the intracytoplasmic accumulation of the abnormal metabolite that, as time evolves, causes death of the cell. Viral diseases can lead to abnormal intranuclear inclusions, as seen in herpetic infection (Cowdry body), intracytoplasmic inclusions, as seen in rabies (Negri body), or both (cytomegalovirus [CMV]).
- Some diseases of the CNS are associated with neuronal intracytoplasmic deposits, such as *neurofibrillary tangles* of Alzheimer disease and *Lewy bodies* of Parkinson disease; others cause abnormal vacuolization of the perikaryon and neuronal cell processes in the neuropil (Creutzfeldt-Jakob disease). A number of neurodegenerative diseases (discussed later) are associated with intracellular or extracellular depositions of aggregated or fibrillar proteins that are characteristic histologic features of the disease (Table 30–1). These aggregates are highly resistant to degradation, contain proteins with altered conformation, and result from mutations in proteins that affect protein folding, ubiquitization, and intracellular trafficking (see discussion of protein folding in Chapter 2). They are sometimes referred to as *proteinopathies.*

Glia

Glia are derived from neuroectoderm (macroglia: astrocytes, oligodendrocytes, ependyma) or from bone marrow (microglia). Glial cells act as a supporting system for the neurons and their dendritic and axonal processes; they also have a primary role in a wide range of normal functions and reactions to injury, including inflammation, repair, fluid balance, and energy metabolism. The size and shape of the nucleus generally serve to distinguish one glial cell type

Table 30–1. NEURODEGENERATIVE DISEASES ASSOCIATED WITH AGGREGATED PROTEINS

Disease	Protein	Normal Structure	Aggregate/Inclusion	Location
Transmissible spongiform encephalopathies (Prion disease)	Prion protein (PrP)	α-Helix and random coil	β-pleated sheet, protein-ase K–resistant	Extracellular (see Fig. 30–35*D*)
Alzheimer disease	Amyloid precursor protein (APP)	α-Helix and random coil	β-pleated sheet, amyloid (fragment of APP)	Extracellular (see Fig. 30–29*C*)
Parkinson disease	α-Synuclein	Random coil, repeats	Aggregated, Lewy bodies	Intracytoplasmic (see Fig. 30–31*C*)
Huntington disease	Huntingtin	Trinucleotide repeats	Insoluble aggregates	Nuclear
Spinocerebellar ataxias	Ataxins	Trinucleotide repeats	Insoluble aggregates	Nuclear

Modified from Welch WJ, Gambetti P: Chaperoning brain diseases. Nature 392:23–24, 1998.

from another, as their cytoplasmic processes are not apparent on H&E preparations and can be demonstrated only with the use of metallic impregnation, immunohistochemical, or electron microscopic methods. *Astrocytes* have round to oval nuclei (10 μm wide) with evenly dispersed, pale chromatin; *oligodendrocytes* have a denser, more homogeneous chromatin in a rounder and smaller nucleus (8 μm); and *microglia* have an elongated, irregularly shaped nucleus (5 to 10 μm) with clumped chromatin. *Ependymal cells,* on the other hand, do have visible cytoplasm; seen with H&E, they are columnar epithelial-like cells with a ciliated/microvillous border facing the ventricular surface and with a pale, vesiculated nucleus, about 8 μm, at the abluminal end of the cell.

ASTROCYTES

This glial cell is found throughout the CNS in both gray and white matter. *Protoplasmic* astrocytes occur mainly in the gray matter, *fibrous* astrocytes in white and gray matter. The cell derives its name from its star-shaped appearance imparted by the multipolar, branching cytoplasmic processes that emanate from the cell body; these are well seen in tissue sections only with metallic impregnation techniques (e.g., Golgi method) (Fig. 30–1*A*) or immunohistochemical preparations (e.g., glial fibrillary acidic protein [GFAP]) (Fig. 30–1*B*). Intracytoplasmic intermediate filaments are characteristic of astrocytes on ultrastructural examination, either aggregated in fascicles (protoplasmic astrocyte) or dispersed diffusely throughout the cytoplasm (fibrous astrocyte). Some astrocytic processes are directed toward neurons and their processes and synapses, where they are believed to act as metabolic buffers or detoxifiers, suppliers of nutrients, and electrical insulators. Others surround capillaries or extend to the subpial and subependymal zones, where they contribute to barrier functions controlling the flow of macromolecules between the blood, the CSF, and the brain. Finally, astrocytes are the principal cells responsible for repair and scar formation in the brain.

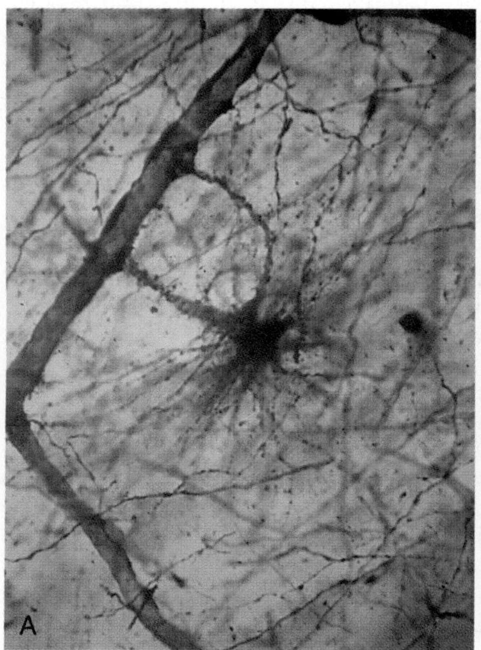

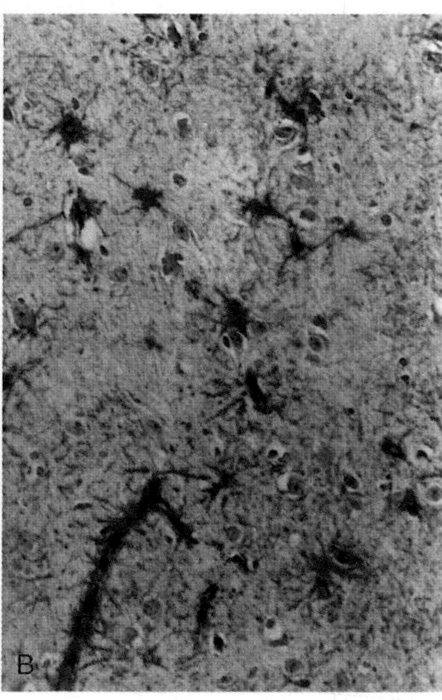

Figure 30–1

A, Astrocytes and their processes. Some processes extend toward blood vessels (Golgi). *B,* Immunoperoxidase staining for glial fibrillary acidic protein shows astrocytic perinuclear cytoplasm and well-developed processes (*red*).

Fibroblasts, which have a major role in wound healing elsewhere, are located mainly around large CNS blood vessels and in the subarachnoid space; they participate in wound healing only to a limited extent.

The cellular pathology of astrocytes may be subdivided into those reactive responses that accompany the cell's proliferation *(gliosis)* and the sets of reactions to injury that lead to death or degeneration.

- *Gliosis* is the most important histopathologic indicator of CNS injury, regardless of etiology. Astrocytes participate in this process by undergoing both hypertrophy and hyperplasia. The nucleus enlarges and becomes vesicular, and the nucleolus is prominent. The previously scant cytoplasm expands to a bright pink, somewhat irregular swath around an eccentric nucleus, from which emerge numerous stout, ramifying processes *(gemistocytic astrocyte)*. Immunohistochemistry for GFAP splendidly demonstrates the extraordinary metamorphosis. In long-standing lesions, the nuclei become small and dark and lie in a dense net of processes. These processes, *glial "fibrils,"* are not true extracellular fibers. Proliferation of astrocytes between the molecular and granule cell layers of the cerebellum—*Bergmann gliosis*—is a regular accompaniment of anoxic injury associated with death of Purkinje cells.
- *Rosenthal fibers* are thick, elongated, brightly eosinophilic structures that are somewhat irregular in contour and occur within astrocytic processes. They have a dense core that consists of an osmiophilic mass containing two heat-shock proteins, αB-crystallin and hsp27. Rosenthal fibers are typically found in regions of long-standing gliosis; they are also characteristic of cerebellar pilocytic astrocytoma (see later). In *Alexander disease,* a leukodystrophy, they are present in abundance in periventricular, perivascular, and subpial locations.
- *Corpora amylacea,* or polyglucosan bodies, are round, faintly basophilic, periodic acid–Schiff (PAS)–positive, concentrically lamellated structures ranging between 5 and 50 μm and located wherever there are astrocytic end processes, especially in the subpial and perivascular zones. Although consisting primarily of glucose polymers, they also contain heat-shock proteins and ubiquitin. They represent a degenerative change in the astrocyte, and they occur in increasing numbers with advancing age and in a rare condition called *adult polyglucosan body disease.* The *Lafora bodies* seen in the cytoplasm of neurons (as well as hepatocytes, myocytes, and other cells) in myoclonic epilepsy (Lafora body myoclonus with epilepsy) are of similar structure and biochemical composition.
- Glial cytoplasmic inclusions consisting of silver-positive meshes of 20- to 40-nm intermediate filaments are characteristic of a number of CNS degenerative diseases, including multiple system atrophy.[10]
- The *Alzheimer type II astrocyte* is a gray matter astrocyte with a large (two to three times normal) nucleus, pale-staining central chromatin, an intranuclear glycogen droplet, and a prominent nuclear membrane and nucleolus. Despite its name, it is unrelated to Alzheimer disease; rather, it occurs especially in patients with hyperammonemia due to chronic liver disease, Wilson disease, or hereditary metabolic disorders of the urea cycle.
- *Cellular swelling.* Swelling of the astrocyte cytoplasm occurs regularly in acute insults when there is a failure of the cell's pump systems, as occurs in hypoxia, in hypoglycemia, and in toxic injuries; it is also seen in Creutzfeldt-Jakob disease.[11]

OLIGODENDROCYTES

Oligodendroglial cytoplasmic processes wrap around the axons of neurons to form myelin in a manner analogous to the Schwann cells of the peripheral nervous system. In routine sections, oligodendroglia are recognizable by their small, rounded, lymphocyte-like nuclei, often arranged in linear arrays. Injury to oligodendroglial cells is a feature of acquired demyelinating disorders (e.g., multiple sclerosis) and is also seen in the leukodystrophies. Oligodendroglial nuclei may harbor viral inclusions in certain conditions such as progressive multifocal leukoencephalopathy.

EPENDYMAL CELLS

Ependymal cells line the ventricular system. They are closely related to the cuboidal cells lining the choroid plexus. Disruption of ependymal cells is often associated with a local proliferation of subependymal astrocytes to produce small irregularities on the ventricular surfaces termed *ependymal granulations.* Certain infectious agents, particularly CMV, may produce extensive ependymal injury, and viral inclusions may be seen in ependymal cells.

MICROGLIA

Microglia are mesoderm-derived cells whose primary function is to serve as a fixed macrophage system. They express many marker antigens in common with peripheral monocytes/macrophages (such as CR3 and CD4). They respond to injury by (1) proliferation; (2) developing elongated nuclei *(rod cells),* as in neurosyphilis; (3) forming aggregates about small foci of tissue necrosis *(microglial nodules);* or (4) congregating around portions of dying neurons *(neuronophagia).* In addition to microglia, blood-derived macrophages are the principal phagocytic cells present in inflammatory foci.[12–14]

CEREBRAL EDEMA, RAISED INTRACRANIAL PRESSURE AND HERNIATION, AND HYDROCEPHALUS

The brain and spinal cord exist within a rigid compartment defined by the skull, vertebral bodies, and dura mater. The advantage of housing as vital and delicate a structure as the CNS in a protective environment is obvious. On the other hand, such rigid confines provide little room for brain parenchymal expansion. A number of disorders may upset the delicate balance between brain parenchymal volume and the fixed boundaries of the intracranial vault. These include generalized brain edema, hydrocephalus, and more localized expanding mass lesions.

Cerebral Edema

Cerebral edema or, more appropriately, brain parenchymal edema may arise in the setting of a number of diseases. Broadly speaking, it may be categorized as vasogenic edema and cytotoxic edema.

Vasogenic edema occurs when the integrity of the normal blood-brain barrier is disrupted, allowing fluid to escape from the vasculature into the intercellular space of the brain. The paucity of lymphatics in the brain greatly impairs the resorption of excess intercellular fluid. Vasogenic edema may be either localized, (when it results from abnormally permeable vessels adjacent to abscesses and neoplasms) or generalized.

Cytotoxic edema, in contrast, implies an increase in intracellular fluid secondary to cellular injury, as might be encountered in a patient with a generalized hypoxic/ischemic insult.

In practice, conditions associated with generalized edema have elements of both vasogenic and cytotoxic edema.

Interstitial edema (hydrocephalic edema) occurs especially around the lateral ventricles when there is an abnormal flow of fluid from the intraventricular CSF to the periventricular white matter in a setting of hydrocephalus.

MORPHOLOGY. The edematous brain is softer than normal and often appears to "overfill" the cranial vault. In generalized edema, the gyri are flattened, the intervening sulci are narrowed, and the ventricular cavities are compressed. As the brain expands, herniation may occur.

Raised Intracranial Pressure and Herniation

Raised intracranial pressure is an increase in mean CSF pressure above 200 mm water with the patient recumbent. It occurs when the intracranial volume increases beyond the leeway permitted by compression of veins and displacement of CSF. Most cases are associated with a mass effect, either diffuse, as in generalized brain edema, or focal, as with tumors, abscesses, or hemorrhages. Because the cranial vault is subdivided by rigid dural folds (falx and tentorium), a focal expansion of the brain causes it to be displaced in relation to these partitions. If the expansion is sufficiently severe, a *herniation* of the brain will occur (Fig. 30–2).

1. *Subfalcine (cingulate gyrus) herniation* occurs when unilateral or asymmetric expansion of the cerebral hemisphere displaces the cingulate gyrus under the falx cerebri. This is often associated with compression of branches of the anterior cerebral artery.

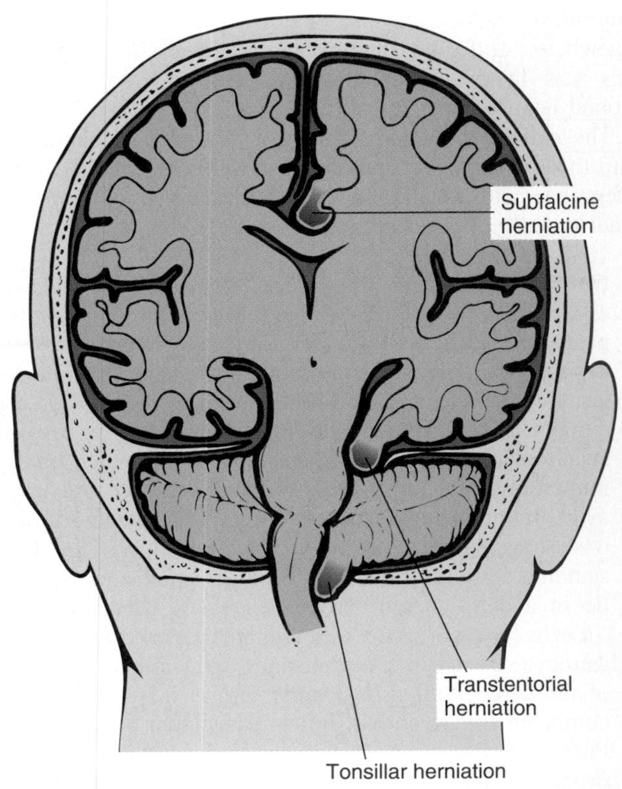

Figure 30–2

Herniations of the brain: (1) subfalcine, (2) transtentorial, and (3) tonsillar. (Adapted from Fishman RA: Brain edema. N Engl J Med 293:706, 1975. Copyright © 1975, Massachusetts Medical Society. All rights reserved.)

2. *Transtentorial (uncal, mesial temporal) herniation* occurs when the medial aspect of the temporal lobe is compressed against the free margin of the tentorium cerebelli. As displacement of the temporal lobe extends, the third cranial nerve is compressed, resulting in pupillary dilation and impairment of ocular movements on the side of the lesion. The posterior cerebral artery is also often compressed, resulting in ischemic injury to the territory supplied by that vessel, including the primary visual cortex. Progression of transtentorial herniation is often accompanied by hemorrhagic lesions in the midbrain and pons, termed *secondary brain stem,* or *Duret, hemorrhages* (Fig. 30–3). These linear or flame-shaped lesions usually occur in the midline and paramedian regions.
3. *Tonsillar herniation* refers to displacement of the cerebellar tonsils through the foramen magnum. This pattern of herniation is life-threatening because it causes brain stem compression and compromises vital respiratory centers in the medulla oblongata.

Hydrocephalus

In the normal brain, CSF is produced by the choroid plexus within the lateral and fourth ventricles. The CSF normally circulates through the ventricular system and en-

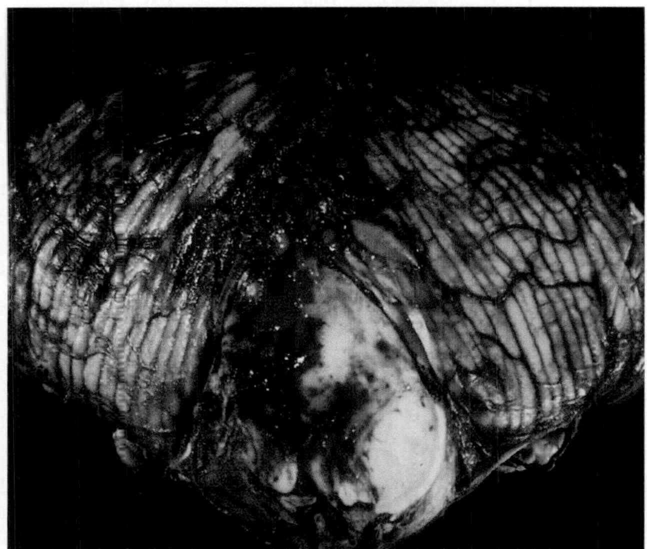

Figure 30–3

Duret hemorrhage involving the midline at the junction of the pons and midbrain.

ters the cisterna magna at the base of the brain stem through the foramina of Luschka and Magendie. Subarachnoid CSF bathes the superior cerebral convexities and is absorbed by the arachnoid granulations.[15] *Hydrocephalus* refers to the accumulation of excessive CSF within the ventricular system of the brain. Most such cases occur as a consequence of decreased resorption of CSF, although in rare instances (e.g., tumors of the choroid plexus), overproduction of CSF may be responsible. Whatever its origin, an increase in CSF within the ventricles expands them and causes an elevation in intracranial pressure.

If hydrocephalus develops before closure of the cranial sutures, there is enlargement of the head, manifested by an increase in head circumference. Hydrocephalus developing after fusion of the sutures, in contrast, is associated with expansion of the ventricles and increased intracranial pressure, without a change in head circumference (Fig. 30–4).

The term *hydrocephalus ex vacuo* refers to dilation of the ventricular system with a compensatory increase in CSF volume secondary to a loss of brain parenchyma.

MALFORMATIONS AND DEVELOPMENTAL DISEASES

The importance of human developmental neuropathology is emphasized by recent estimates suggesting that as many as 17% of youngsters have some form of developmental disability.[16] Prenatal or perinatal insults may either cause failure of normal CNS development or result in tissue destruction. The anatomic pattern of the malformation reflects the stage of formation of the brain at the time of injury.[17,18] Although the pathogenesis and etiology of CNS malformations are largely unknown, both genetic and environmental factors clearly play a role and have been the topic of intensive research in recent years, as detailed in Chapter 11. Signaling molecules and homeotic and other genes control body patterning, and such genes are expressed in a regulated fashion during the segmental development of the CNS.[19–21] Finally, many toxic compounds and infectious agents are known to have teratogenic effects in humans and experimental animals (Chapter 10).

Neural Tube Defects

Failure of a portion of the neural tube to close, or reopening of a region of the tube after successful closure,

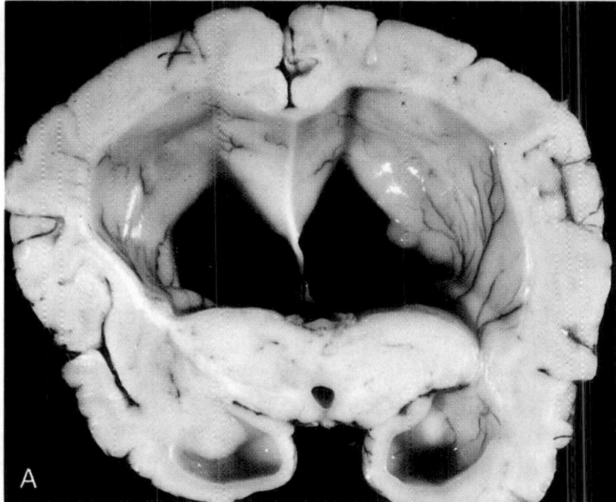

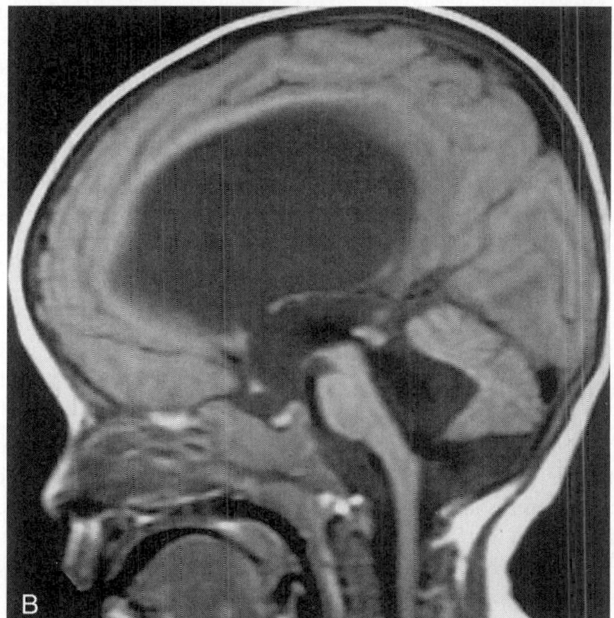

Figure 30–4

A, Hydrocephalus. Dilated lateral ventricles seen in a coronal section through the midthalamus. *B*, Midsagittal plane T1-weighted magnetic resonance image of a child with communicating hydrocephalus, involving all ventricles. (*B*, Courtesy of Dr. P. Barnes, Children's Hospital, Boston, MA.)

may lead to one of several malformations. All are characterized by abnormalities involving both neural tissue and overlying bone or soft tissues. Collectively, these are the most common CNS malformations.

Anencephaly is a malformation of the anterior end of the neural tube, with absence of the brain and calvarium. It occurs in 1 to 5 per 1000 live births, more commonly in females, and is thought to develop at approximately 28 days of gestation. Forebrain development is disrupted, and all that remains in its place is the *area cerebrovasculosa*, a flattened remnant of disorganized brain tissue with admixed ependyma, choroid plexus, and meningothelial cells. The posterior fossa structures are often spared.

An *encephalocele* is a diverticulum of malformed CNS tissue extending through a defect in the cranium. It most often occurs in the occipital region or in the posterior fossa.

The most common forms of neural tube defects in newborns involve the spinal cord and are caused by a failure of closure or reopening of the caudal portions of the neural tube. *Spinal dysraphism* or *spina bifida* may be an asymptomatic bony defect (spina bifida occulta) or a severe malformation with a flattened, disorganized segment of spinal cord, associated with an overlying meningeal outpouching. *Myelomeningocele* (or meningomyelocele) refers to extension of CNS tissue through a defect in the vertebral column; the term *meningocele* applies when there is only a meningeal extrusion. Clinical neurologic dysfunction is most often related to the structural abnormality of the cord itself and to superimposed infection that extends from the thin, overlying skin. Myelomeningoceles occur most commonly in the lumbosacral region, and the patient manifests clinical deficits referable to motor and sensory function in the lower extremities as well as disturbances of bowel and bladder control.

The etiology of neural tube defects is unknown; their frequency varies widely among ethnic groups. Antenatal diagnosis has been facilitated by new imaging methods and the screening of maternal blood samples for evidence of elevated α-fetoprotein. The overall recurrence rate for a neural tube defect in subsequent pregnancies has been estimated at 4% to 5%. Folate deficiency during the initial weeks of gestation has been implicated as a risk factor.[22]

Forebrain Anomalies

Polymicrogyria is characterized by a loss of the normal external contour of the convolutions, which on macroscopic examination appear small, unusually numerous, and irregularly formed. The gray matter is composed of four layers (or fewer), with entrapment of apparent meningeal tissue at points of fusion of what would otherwise be the cortical surface. Animal studies suggest that polymicrogyria can be induced by localized tissue injury during the time of neuronal migration.[20] More than 25 human genetic syndromes have been recognized to be associated with malformations of cortical development, including polymicrogyria.[23]

The volume of brain may be abnormally large *(megalencephaly)* or small *(microencephaly)*. Microencephaly, by far the more common of the two, can occur in a wide range of clinical settings, including chromosome abnormalities, fetal alcohol syndrome, and human immunodeficiency virus 1 (HIV-1) infection acquired in utero. A reduction in the number of neurons that reach the neocortex is postulated, and this leads to a simplification of the gyral folding. This can range from a noticeable decrease in the number of gyri to total absence, leaving a smooth-surfaced brain, *lissencephaly (agyria)*. In the Miller-Dieker syndrome (seizures, mental retardation, and lissencephaly) about 90% of patients have a deletion in chromosome 17p13.3; the cloned deleted gene has been termed *LIS1*—it is normally localized in the CNS but absent in the disorder.[23,24] Abnormal gyral patterns are also found in chondrodysplasias; *thanatophoric dwarfism* is a lethal form characterized by abnormally large and hyperconvoluted temporal lobes and skeletal anomalies (micromelia, chest and skull deformities).

The migration of neurons from the germinal matrix (the periventricular region of neuronal and glial proliferation), through the deeper structures to reach their final destinations in the cerebral cortex, is a complicated process that can go awry.[5] Stranded clusters of neurons *(neuronal heterotopias)* may then be found strewn along the path of migration, either as large conglomerates or as small clusters within the white matter.

Holoprosencephaly is a spectrum of malformations characterized by incomplete separation of the cerebral hemispheres across the midline (Fig. 30–5). Extreme forms manifest midline facial abnormalities, including cyclopia; less severe variants (arrhinencephaly) show absence of the olfactory cranial nerves and related structures. Intrauterine diagnosis of severe forms by ultrasound examination is now possible. Holoprosencephaly is associated with trisomy 13 (rarely, with trisomy 18), and there is an increased incidence in the offspring of maternal diabetics. Comparable malformations have been induced in animals with a plant alkaloid. Mutations in the human Sonic hedgehog gene (a member of a family of secreted proteins synthesized by the notochord and neural plate during induction) have been shown in some cases of holoprosencephaly.[25]

In *agenesis of the corpus callosum,* a relatively common malformation, there is an absence of the white matter bundles that carry cortical projections from one hemisphere to the other (Fig. 30–6). Radiologic imaging studies show misshapen lateral ventricles ("bat-wing" deformity); on coronal whole-mount sections of the brain, bundles of anteroposteriorly oriented white matter can be demonstrated. Agenesis of the corpus callosum can be found in patients with mental retardation or in clinically normal individuals. Unlike patients with surgically induced callosal section who show clinical evidence of hemispheric disconnection, patients with this malformation can be shown to have only minimal deficits even with neuropsychologic testing. The malformation may be complete or partial; in the latter case, the caudal portion of the callosum is absent, and a lipoma sometimes occupies the defect.

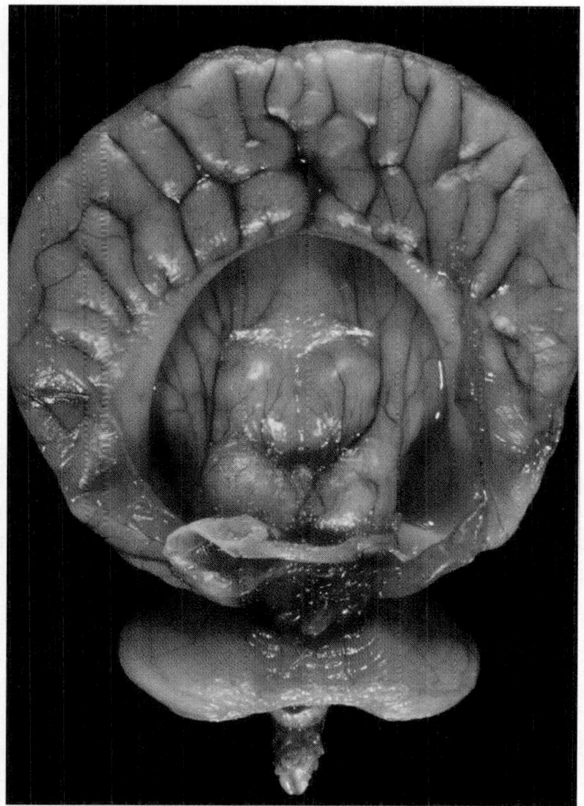

Figure 30–5

Holoprosencephaly. View of the dorsal surface showing a lack of separation of cerebral hemispheres, a single ventricle, and fused basal ganglia.

Posterior Fossa Anomalies

The *Arnold-Chiari malformation* (Chiari type II malformation) consists of a small posterior fossa, a misshapen midline cerebellum with downward extension of *vermis* through the foramen magnum (Fig. 30–7), and, almost invariably, hydrocephalus and a lumbar myelomeningocele. Other associated changes include caudal displacement of the medulla, malformation of the tectum, aqueductal stenosis, cerebral heterotopias, and hydromyelia (see later). In the Chiari I malformation, low-lying cerebellar *tonsils* extend down the vertebral canal and may cause symptoms referable to obstruction of CSF flow and medullary compression that are amenable to neurosurgical intervention.

In contrast, the *Dandy-Walker malformation* is characterized by an *enlarged* posterior fossa. The cerebellar vermis is absent or present only in rudimentary form in its anterior portion. In its place is a large midline cyst that is lined by ependyma and is contiguous with leptomeninges on its outer surface. This cyst represents the expanded, roofless fourth ventricle in the absence of a normally formed vermis. Dysplasias of brain stem nuclei are commonly found in association with Dandy-Walker malformation.

Syringomyelia and Hydromyelia

These are disorders characterized by a discontinuous multisegmental or confluent expansion of the ependyma-lined central canal of the cord *(hydromyelia)* or by the formation of a fluid-filled cleftlike cavity in the inner portion of the cord *(syringomyelia, syrinx)*. These lesions are associated with destruction of the adjacent gray and white matter and are surrounded by a dense feltwork of reactive gliosis. The cervical spinal cord is most often affected, and the slitlike cavity may extend into the brain stem *(syringo-*

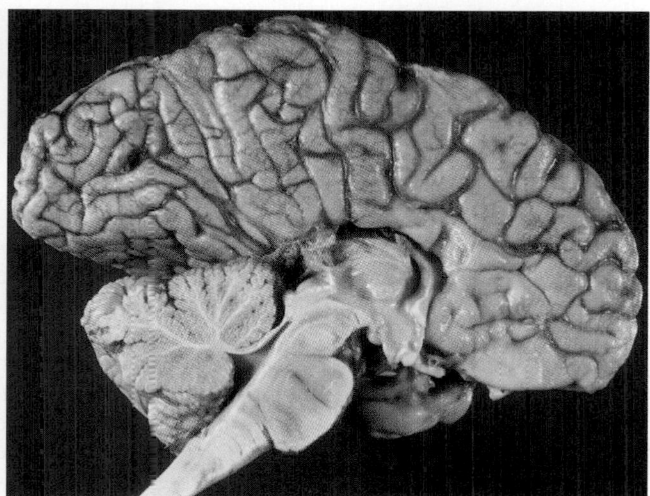

Figure 30–6

Agenesis of the corpus callosum. The sagittal section shows the lack of a corpus callosum above the third ventricle.

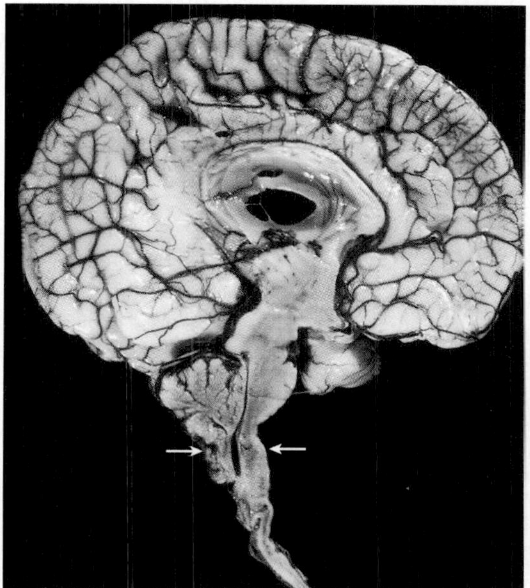

Figure 30–7

Arnold-Chiari malformation. Midsagittal section showing small posterior fossa contents, downward displacement of the cerebellar vermis, and deformity of the medulla (arrows indicate the approximate level of the foramen magnum).

bulbia). Associated anomalies of the spinal column are common (vertebral fusions, scoliosis, platybasia).

As many as 90% of cases of syringomyelia have the Chiari I malformation; a minority are associated with intraspinal tumors or follow traumatic injury. In general, the histologic appearance of the lesions is comparable. The disease generally becomes manifest in the second or third decade of life. The distinctive initial clinical symptoms and signs of a syrinx are progressive evolution of dissociated sensory loss of pain and temperature sensation in the upper extremities, retention of position sense, and absence of motor deficits due to early involvement of the crossing anterior spinal commissural fibers.

PERINATAL BRAIN INJURY

A variety of exogenous factors may injure the developing brain. Injuries that occur early in gestation may destroy brain without evoking the usual "reactive" changes in the parenchyma and may be difficult to distinguish from malformations. Brain injury occurring in the perinatal period is an important cause of childhood neurologic disability.

The broad clinical term *cerebral palsy* refers to a nonprogressive neurologic motor deficit characterized by spasticity, dystonia, ataxia/athetosis, and paresis attributable to insults occurring during the prenatal and perinatal periods.[2,26] Signs and symptoms may be inapparent at birth and only later declare themselves as development occurs. Postmortem examination of children with this syndrome has shown a wide range of neuropathologic findings, including hemorrhages and infarctions.[27]

In premature infants, there is an increased risk of *intraparenchymal hemorrhage* within the germinal matrix, near the junction between the thalamus and the caudate nucleus. Hemorrhages may remain localized or extend into the ventricular system and thence to the subarachnoid space, sometimes leading to hydrocephalus.

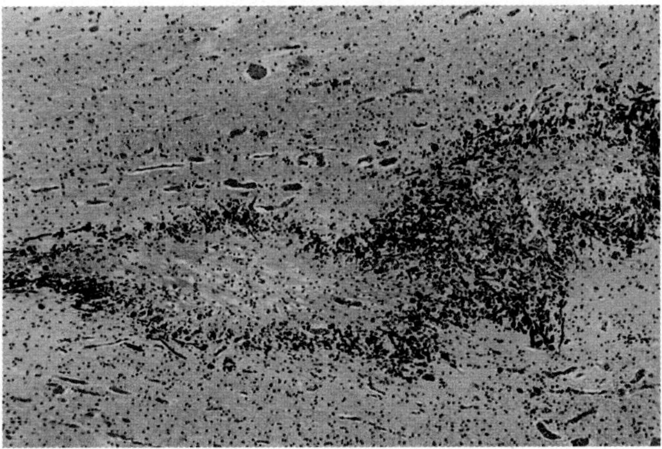

Figure 30–8

Periventricular leukomalacia. Central focus of white matter necrosis with a peripheral rim of mineralized axonal processes (staining blue).

Infarcts may occur in the supratentorial periventricular white matter *(periventricular leukomalacia),* especially in premature babies. These are chalky yellow plaques consisting of discrete regions of white matter necrosis and mineralization (Fig. 30–8). Cyst formation may follow in cases in which there has been extensive ischemic damage; when both gray and white matter are involved, large destructive lesions develop through the hemispheres; this condition is termed *multicystic encephalopathy.*

In perinatal ischemic lesions of the cerebral cortex, the depths of sulci bear the brunt of injury and result in thinned-out, gliotic gyri *(ulegyria).* The basal ganglia and thalamus may also suffer ischemic injury, with patchy neuronal loss and reactive gliosis. Later, with the advent of myelination at about 6 months of age, aberrant and irregular myelin formation gives rise to a marble-like appearance of the deep nuclei—*status marmoratus.* Clinically, because the lesions are in the caudate, putamen, and thalamus, choreoathetosis and related movement disorders are important sequelae.

TRAUMA

The anatomic location of the lesion and the limited capacity of the brain for functional repair are two factors of great significance in CNS trauma. Necrosis of several cubic centimeters of brain parenchyma may be clinically silent (frontal lobe), severely disabling (spinal cord), or fatal (brain stem).

The magnitude and distribution of a traumatic brain lesion depend on the shape of the object causing the trauma, the force of impact, and whether the head is in motion at the time of injury. A blow to the head may be *penetrating* or *blunt;* it may cause either an *open* or a *closed injury.* Severe brain damage can occur in the absence of external signs of head injury, and conversely, severe lacerations and even skull fractures do not necessarily indicate damage to the underlying brain. Physical forces cause their effects by inducing three types of injury: *skull fractures, parenchymal injury,* and *vascular injury;* all three are often present in combination.[28–30]

Skull Fractures

In general, the kinetic energy that causes a fracture is dissipated at a fused suture; fractures that cross sutures are termed *diastatic.* With multiple points of impact or repeated blows to the head, the fracture lines of subsequent injuries do not extend across fracture lines of prior injury. A fracture in which bone is displaced into the cranial cavity by a distance greater than the thickness of the bone is called a *displaced skull fracture.* The thickness of the cranial bones varies, and therefore their resistance to fracture differs greatly. Also, the relative incidence of fractures among skull bones is related to the pattern of falls. When an individual falls while awake, such as might occur when stepping off a ladder, the site of impact is often in the occipital portion of the skull; in contrast, a fall that follows loss of consciousness, as might follow a syncopal attack, commonly results in a frontal impact. Basal skull fractures typically follow an impact to the occiput or sides of the head rather than a blow to the vertex; these fractures are difficult to detect at postmortem examination and require careful removal of the dura, which normally is tightly adherent to the base of the skull. Symptoms referable to the lower cranial nerves or the cervicomedullary region, and the presence of orbital or mastoid hematomas distant from the point of impact, raise the clinical suspicion of a basal skull fracture; CSF discharge from the nose or ear and infection (meningitis) may follow.

Parenchymal Injuries

CONCUSSION

Concussion is a *clinical* syndrome of alteration of consciousness secondary to head injury typically brought about by a change in the momentum of the head (movement of the head arrested by a rigid surface). The characteristic neurologic picture includes instantaneous onset of transient neurologic dysfunction, including loss of consciousness, temporary respiratory arrest, and loss of reflexes.[1] Although neurologic recovery is complete, amnesia for the event persists, and many postconcussive neuropsychiatric syndromes have been described. The pathogenesis of the sudden disruption of nervous activity is unknown; but biochemical and physiologic abnormalities occur, such as depolarization due to excitatory amino acid–mediated ionic fluxes across cell membranes, depletion of mitochondrial adenosine triphosphate (ATP), and alterations in vascular permeability. Some patients who die after a postconcussive syndrome may show evidence of direct parenchymal injury, but in others there is no evidence of damage.

DIRECT PARENCHYMAL INJURY

Contusion and *laceration* are conditions in which direct parenchymal injury of the brain has occurred, either through transmission of kinetic energy to the brain and bruising analogous to what is seen in soft tissues (contusion) or by penetration of an object and tearing of tissue (laceration). As with any other organ, a blow to the surface of the brain, transmitted through the skull, leads to rapid tissue displacement, disruption of vascular channels, and subsequent hemorrhage, tissue injury, and edema (Figs. 30–9 and 30–10). The crests of gyri are most susceptible, whereas cerebral cortex along the sulci is less vulnerable. The most common locations where contusions occur correspond to the most frequent sites of direct impact and to regions of the brain that overlie a rough and irregular calvarial surface, such as the frontal lobes, along the orbital gyri, and the temporal lobes. They are less frequent over the occipital lobes, brain stem, and cerebellum, unless these points are adjacent to a skull fracture *(fracture contusions).*

A patient who suffers a blow to the head may develop a cerebral injury at the point of contact (a *coup* injury) or damage to the brain surface diametrically opposite to it (a *contrecoup* injury). Both coup and contrecoup lesions are contusions. Since their macroscopic and microscopic appearance is indistinguishable, the distinction between them is based on forensic identification of the point of impact and the circumstances attending the incident. In general, if the head is immobile at the time of trauma, only a fracture contusion is found. When the head is mobile, there may be

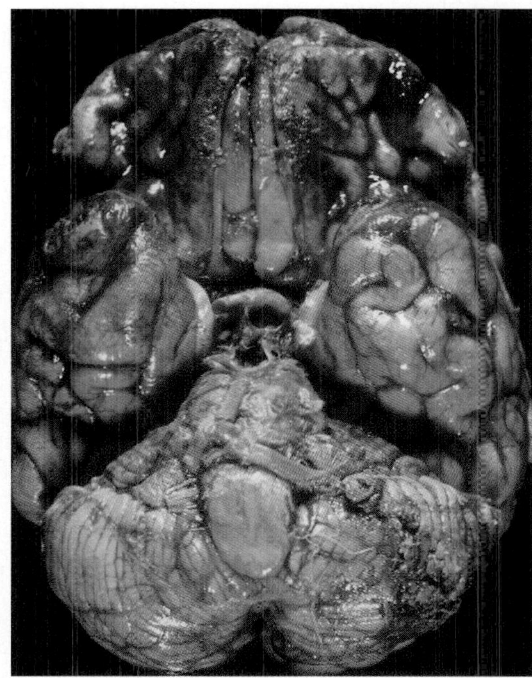

Figure 30–9 ■

Multiple contusions involving the cerebellum, inferior surfaces of frontal lobes, and temporal tips.

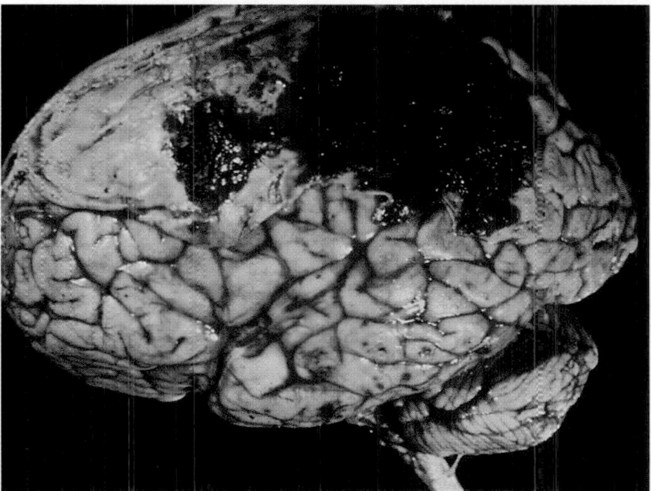

Figure 30–10 ■

Epidural hematoma covering a portion of the dura. Multiple small contusions are seen in the temporal lobe. (Courtesy of Dr. Raymond D. Adams, Massachusetts General Hospital, Boston, MA).

coup lesions beneath the site of impact and also contrecoup lesions. Whereas the coup lesion is caused by the force of direct impact between the brain and skull at the site of impact, the contrecoup contusion is thought to develop when the brain strikes the opposite inner surface of the skull after sudden deceleration.

MORPHOLOGY. Contusions, when seen on cross-section, are wedge shaped, with the broad base spanning the surface and centered on the point of impact. The histologic appearance of contusions is independent of the type of trauma. In the earliest stages, there is evidence of edema and hemorrhage, which is pericapillary. During the next few hours, the extravasation of blood extends throughout the involved tissue, across the width of the cerebral cortex, and into the white matter and subarachnoid spaces. Morphologic evidence of injury in the neuronal cell body (pyknosis of nucleus, eosinophilia of the cytoplasm, disintegration of cell) takes about 24 hours to appear, although functional brain injury occurs earlier. Axonal swellings develop in the vicinity of damaged neurons or at great distances away. The inflammatory response to the injured tissue follows its usual course, with neutrophils preceding the appearance of macrophages. Old traumatic lesions on the surface of the brain have a characteristic macroscopic appearance: they are depressed, retracted, yellowish brown patches involving the crests of gyri most commonly located at the sites of contrecoup lesions (inferior frontal cortex, temporal and occipital poles). The term **plaque jaune** is applied to these lesions; they can be foci of clinical seizure discharges. More extensive hemorrhagic regions of brain trauma give rise to larger cavitated lesions, which can resemble remote infarcts. In sites of old contusions, gliosis and residual hemosiderin-laden macrophages predominate.

Sudden impacts that result in violent posterior or lateral hyperextension of the neck (as occurs when a pedestrian is struck from the rear by a vehicle) may actually avulse the pons from the medulla, or the medulla from the cervical cord, causing instantaneous death.

DIFFUSE AXONAL INJURY

The surface of the brain is not the only region of damage in traumatic injury, although it is often the most striking. The deep centroaxial white matter regions—in the supratentorial compartment, particularly the corpus callosum, paraventricular and hippocampal areas; the brain stem, along the cerebral peduncles, brachium conjunctivum, superior colliculi, and deep reticular formation—may also be involved. The microscopic findings include axonal swellings, indicative of *diffuse axonal injury* and of focal hemorrhagic lesions. Angular acceleration alone, in the absence of impact, can cause diffuse axonal injury as well as hemorrhage. As many as 50% of patients who develop coma shortly after trauma, even without cerebral contusions, are believed to have white matter damage and diffuse axonal injury. The most widely accepted explanation for diffuse axonal injury is that mechanical forces damage the integrity of the axon at the node of Ranvier, with subsequent alterations in axoplasmic flow.[31]

MORPHOLOGY. The histopathology of diffuse axonal injury is characterized by the wide but often asymmetric distribution of axonal swellings that appear within hours of the injury and may persist for much longer. These are best demonstrated with silver impregnation techniques or with immunoperoxidase methods for axons. Later, there are increased numbers of microglia in related areas of cerebral cortex and, subsequently, degeneration of the involved fiber tracts.

Traumatic Vascular Injury

Vascular injury is a frequent component of CNS trauma and results from direct trauma and disruption of the vessel wall, leading to hemorrhage. Depending on the anatomic position of the ruptured vessel, hemorrhage will occur in any of several compartments (sometimes in combination): *epidural, subdural, subarachnoid,* and *intraparenchymal* (Fig. 30–11). In the cavernous sinus, a traumatic tear of the carotid artery leads to the formation of an arteriovenous fistula.

EPIDURAL HEMATOMA

The epidural space is a potential space—the dura is closely applied to the internal surface of the skull and is fused with the periosteum. Vessels that course within the dura, most importantly the middle meningeal artery, are vulnerable to injury, particularly with skull fractures. Trauma to the skull, especially in the region of the temporal bone, can lead to laceration of this artery if the fracture lines cross the course of the vessel. In children, in whom the skull is deformable, a temporary displacement of the skull bones leading to laceration of a vessel can occur in the absence of a skull fracture.

Once a vessel has been torn, the accumulation of blood under arterial pressure can cause separation of the dura off the inner surface of the skull. The expanding hematoma has a smooth inner contour that compresses the brain surface. Clinically, patients can be lucid for several hours between the moment of trauma and the development of neurologic signs. An epidural hematoma may expand rapidly and is a neurosurgical emergency requiring prompt drainage.

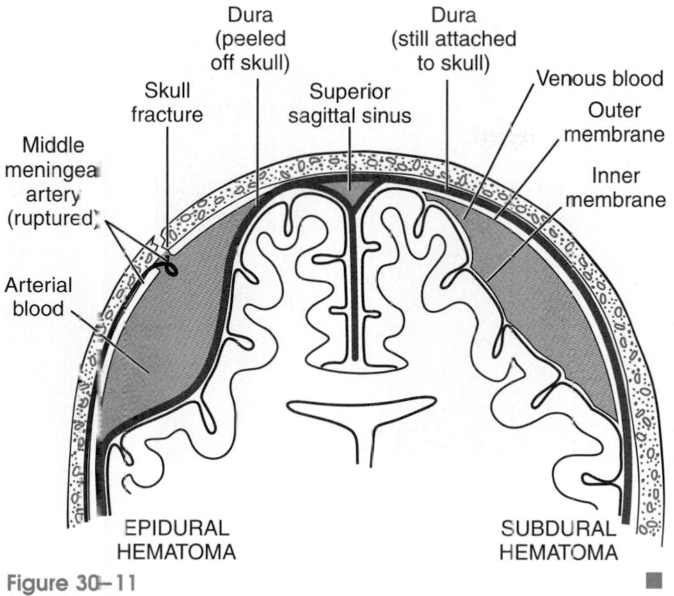

Figure 30–11

Epidural hematoma (*left*) in which rupture of a meningeal artery, usually associated with a skull fracture, leads to accumulation of arterial blood between the dura and the skull. In a subdural hematoma (*right*), damage to bridging veins between the brain and the superior sagittal sinus leads to the accumulation of blood between the dura and the arachnoid.

SUBDURAL HEMATOMA

The space beneath the inner surface of the dura mater and the outer arachnoid layer of the leptomeninges is also a potential space. *Bridging veins* traverse from the surface of the convexities of the cerebral hemispheres through the subarachnoid space and the subdural space to empty with dural vessels into the superior sagittal sinus. Similar anatomic relationships exist with other dural sinuses. These vessels are particularly prone to tearing along their course through the subdural space; they are the source of bleeding in most cases of subdural hematoma. The most commonly accepted mechanism of damage postulates that the brain, floating freely in its bath of CSF, can move within the skull, but the venous sinuses are fixed. The displacement of the brain that occurs in trauma can tear the veins at the point where they penetrate the dura. In elderly patients with brain atrophy, the bridging veins are stretched out and the brain has additional space for movement, hence the increased rate of subdural hematomas in these patients, even after relatively minor head trauma.

Subdural hematomas most often become clinically manifest within the first 48 hours after injury. They are most common over the lateral aspects of the cerebral hemispheres and are bilateral in about 10% of cases. Neurologic signs commonly observed are attributable to the pressure exerted on the adjacent brain. There may be focal signs, but often the clinical manifestations are nonlocalizing and include headache or confusion. In time, there may be slowly progressive neurologic deterioration, but rarely, acute decompensation occurs.

MORPHOLOGY. On macroscopic examination, the acute subdural hematoma appears as a collection of freshly clotted blood apposed along the contour of the brain surface, without extension into the depths of sulci (Fig. 30–12). The underlying brain is flattened, and the subarachnoid space is often clear. Typically, venous bleeding is self-limited; breakdown and organization of the hematoma take place in time. The course of organization of subdural hematomas may be approximated as follows, but it is extremely difficult to date subdural hematomas with the precision required in cases of criminal litigation.

- Lysis of the clot (about 1 week)
- Growth of fibroblasts from the dural surface into the hematoma (2 weeks)
- Early development of hyalinized connective tissue (1 to 3 months)

A remarkable macroscopic characteristic of an organized hematoma is that the lesion is firmly attached by fibrous tissue only to the inner surface of the dura and is not at all adherent to the underlying smooth arachnoid, which does not contribute to its formation. The lesion can eventually retract as the granulation tissue matures. Lesions that evolve to this stage of healing are referred to as **chronic subdural hematomas.** A common finding in subdural hematomas, however, is the occurrence of multiple episodes of rebleeding, presumably from the thin-walled vessels of the granulation tissue. The risk of rebleeding is greatest in the first few months after the initial hemorrhage. The treatment of subdural hematomas is to remove the organized blood and surrounding reactive connective tissue ("subdural membranes").

Subarachnoid and intraparenchymal hemorrhages most often occur concomitantly in the setting of brain trauma with superficial contusions and lacerations. **Spät-apoplexie** (delayed post-traumatic hemorrhage) is a syndrome of sudden, deep intracerebral hemorrhage that follows even minor head trauma by an interval of 1 to 2 weeks.

Sequelae of Brain Trauma

The broad range of neurologic syndromes that become manifest months or years after brain trauma of any cause have gained increasing importance in the context of legal medicine and litigation involving issues of compensation of victims in the work force and the military services. *Post-traumatic hydrocephalus* is largely due to obstruction of CSF resorption from hemorrhage into the subarachnoid spaces. *Post-traumatic dementia* and the *punch-drunk syndrome* (dementia pugilistica) follow repeated head trauma during a protracted period; the neuropathologic findings include hydrocephalus, thinning of the corpus callosum,

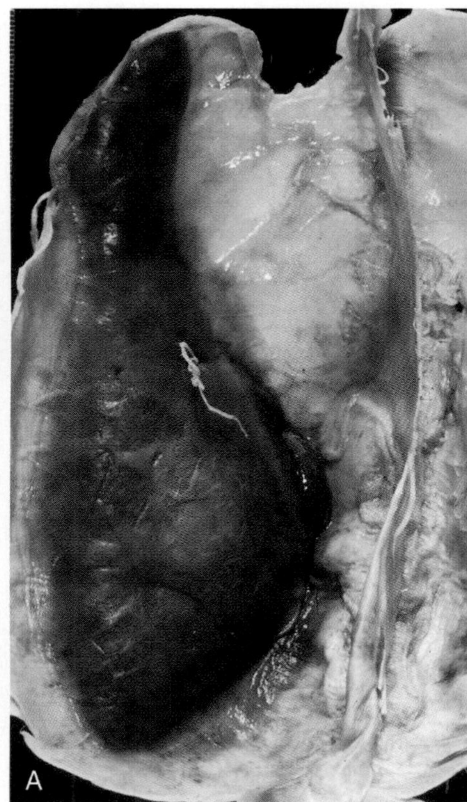

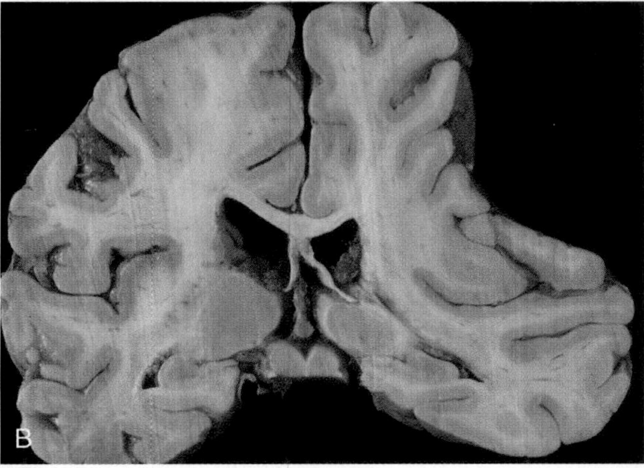

Figure 30–12

A, Large organizing subdural hematoma attached to the dura. *B*, Coronal section of the brain showing compression of the hemisphere underlying the hematoma.

diffuse axonal injury, neurofibrillary tangles (mainly in the medial temporal areas), and diffuse Aβ-positive plaques (see section on Alzheimer disease). Other important sequelae of brain trauma include post-traumatic epilepsy, brain tumors (meningioma), infectious diseases, and psychiatric disorders.[2]

Spinal Cord Trauma

The spinal cord, normally protected within the bony vertebral canal, is vulnerable to trauma from its skeletal encasement. Most injuries that damage the cord are associated with displacement of the spinal column, either rapid and temporary or persistent. The level of cord injury determines the extent of neurologic manifestations: lesions involving the thoracic vertebrae or below can lead to paraplegia; cervical lesions result in quadriplegia; and those above C-4 can, in addition, lead to respiratory compromise from paralysis of the diaphragm. Segmental damage to the descending and ascending white matter tracts isolates the distal spinal cord from its cortical connections to the cerebrum and brain stem; this interruption, rather than the segmental gray matter damage that may occur at the level of the impact, causes the principal clinical deficits. Besides traumatic tissue disruption, progression and extension of the lesion occur secondary to vascular injury/ischemia and excitotoxicity.[32,33]

MORPHOLOGY. The histologic changes of traumatic injury of the spinal cord are similar to those found at other sites in the CNS. At the level of injury, the acute phase consists of hemorrhage, necrosis, and axonal swellings in the surrounding white matter. The lesion tapers above and below the injured level. In time, the central necrotic lesion becomes cystic and gliotic; cord sections above and below the lesion show, respectively, secondary ascending and descending wallerian degeneration involving the long white matter tracts affected at the site of trauma.

CEREBROVASCULAR DISEASES

Cerebrovascular disease is the third leading cause of death (after heart disease and cancer) in the United States; it is also the most prevalent neurologic disorder in terms of both morbidity and mortality. The term cerebrovascular disease denotes any abnormality of brain caused by a pathologic process of blood vessels; "stroke" is the clinical designation that applies to these conditions, particularly when symptoms begin acutely.[2,34] Cerebrovascular diseases, from the clinical point of view, include three major categories: thrombosis, embolism, and hemorrhage; this operational division is useful especially because the management of patients differs greatly in each group. From the standpoint of pathophysiology and pathologic anatomy, it is convenient to consider cerebrovascular disease as two processes:

- Hypoxia, ischemia, and infarction resulting from impairment of blood supply and oxygenation of CNS tissue
- Hemorrhage resulting from rupture of CNS vessels

Some forms of hypertensive cerebrovascular disease combine aspects of both and are discussed separately.

Pathophysiologic Considerations: Hypoxia, Ischemia, and Infarction

The brain requires a constant supply of glucose and oxygen, which is delivered by the circulation and accounts for 15% of the resting cardiac output and 20% of the total body oxygen consumption. Cerebral blood flow, normally about 50 ml per minute for each 100 gm of tissue (with considerable regional variations between white and gray matter and among different portions of the gray matter), remains constant over a wide range of blood pressure and intracranial pressure because of autoregulation of vascular resistance. The brain is a highly aerobic tissue, with oxygen rather than metabolic substrate serving as the limiting substance. The brain may be deprived of oxygen by any of several mechanisms: *functional hypoxia* in a setting of a low inspired partial pressure of oxygen (Po_2), impaired oxygen-carrying capacity, or inhibition of oxygen use by tissue; or *ischemia*, either *transient* or *permanent*, after interruption of the normal circulatory flow. Cessation of blood flow can result from a reduction in perfusion pressure, as in hypotension, or be secondary to small- or large-vessel obstruction.

When blood flow to a portion of the brain is reduced, the survival of the tissue at risk depends on a number of *modifying factors:* the availability of collateral circulation, the duration of ischemia, and the magnitude and rapidity of the reduction of flow. These factors will determine, in turn, the precise anatomic site and size of the lesion and, consequently, the clinical deficit. Two principal types of acute ischemic injury are recognized:

- *Global cerebral ischemia* (ischemic/hypoxic encephalopathy) occurs when there is a generalized reduction of cerebral perfusion, such as in cardiac arrest, shock, and severe hypotension.
- *Focal cerebral ischemia* follows reduction or cessation of blood flow to a localized area of the brain due to large-vessel disease (such as embolic or thrombotic arterial occlusion) or to small-vessel disease (such as vasculitis).

HYPOTENSION, HYPOPERFUSION, AND LOW-FLOW STATES—GLOBAL CEREBRAL ISCHEMIA

The outcome of a severe hypotensive episode that produces *global cerebral ischemia (diffuse hypoxic/ischemic encephalopathy)* varies with the severity of the insult. In mild cases, there may be only a transient postischemic confusional state, with eventual complete recovery and no irreversible tissue damage. On the other hand, irreversible damage of CNS tissue does occur in some patients who suffer mild or transient global ischemic insults. There is a hierarchy of CNS cells that show preferential susceptibility *(selective vulnerability).* Neurons are the most sensitive cells, although glial cells (oligodendrocytes and astrocytes) are also vulnerable. There is also great variability in the susceptibility of different populations of neurons in different regions of the CNS; this is based in part on differences in regional cerebral blood flow and cellular metabolic requirements. In severe global cerebral ischemia, widespread brain infarction, irrespective of regional vulnerability, occurs. Patients who survive in this state often remain severely impaired neurologically and deeply comatose—persistent vegetative state. Other patients meet the current clinical criteria for "brain death," including persistent evidence of diffuse cortical injury (isoelectric—"flat"—electroencephalogram) as well as brain stem damage, including absent reflexes and respiratory drive, and absent perfusion. When patients with this pervasive form of injury are maintained on mechanical ventilation, the brain gradually undergoes an autolytic process, leading to soft disintegrated tissue that does not fix well in formalin and stains poorly with dyes.

MORPHOLOGY. On macroscopic examination, the brain is swollen, the gyri are widened, and the sulci are narrowed. The cut surface shows poor demarcation between gray and white matter. The histopathologic changes that attend irreversible ischemic injury (infarction) are grouped into three categories. **Early changes,** occurring 12 to 24 hours after the insult, include the acute neuronal cell change (red neurons) characterized at first by microvacuolization, then eosinophilia of the neuronal cytoplasm, and later nuclear pyknosis and karyorrhexis. Similar acute changes occur somewhat later in astrocytes and oligodendroglia. Pyramidal cells of the Sommer sector (CA1) of the hippocampus, Purkinje cells of the cerebellum, and pyramidal neurons in the neocortex are the most susceptible to irreversible injury. **Subacute changes,** occurring at 24 hours to 2 weeks, include necrosis of tissue, influx of macrophages, vascular proliferation, and reactive gliosis. **Repair,** seen after 2 weeks, is characterized by removal of all necrotic tissue, loss of normally organized CNS structure, and gliosis. In the cerebral cortex, the neuronal loss and gliosis produce an uneven destruction of the neocortex, with preservation of some layers and involvement of others—a pattern termed pseudolaminar necrosis.

Border zone infarcts ("watershed") are wedge-shaped areas of infarction that occur in those regions of the brain and spinal cord that lie at the most distal fields of arterial irrigation. In the cerebral hemispheres, the border zone between the anterior and the middle cerebral artery distributions is at greatest risk. Damage to this region produces a sickle-shaped band of necrosis over the cerebral convexity a few centimeters lateral to the interhemispheric fissure. Border zone infarcts are usually seen after hypotensive episodes.

FOCAL CEREBRAL ISCHEMIA—INFARCTION FROM OBSTRUCTION OF LOCAL BLOOD SUPPLY

Cerebral arterial occlusion may lead to focal ischemia and ultimately, if it is sustained, to infarction of a specific region of CNS tissue within the territory of distribution of the compromised vessel. The area of the brain affected determines whether the patient remains asymptomatic or develops a hemiplegia, a sensory deficit, blindness, aphasia, or some other deficit. The deficit evolves over time, and the outcome either is fatal or is characterized by some degree of slow improvement during a period of months.

The size, location, and shape of the infarct and the extent of tissue damage that results from focal cerebral ischemia brought about by occlusion of a blood vessel are determined by the *modifying factors* mentioned before, most importantly the adequacy of collateral flow. The major source of collateral flow is the circle of Willis (supplemented by the external carotid–ophthalmic pathway). Partial and inconstant reinforcement is available over the surface of the brain for the distal branches of the anterior, middle, and posterior cerebral arteries through cortical-leptomeningeal anastomoses. In contrast, there is little if any collateral flow for the deep penetrating vessels supplying structures such as the thalamus, basal ganglia, and deep white matter.

Occlusive vascular disease of severity sufficient to lead to cerebral infarction may be due to *in situ thrombosis* or *embolization* from a distant source; the pathology of these conditions is discussed in Chapters 5 and 12.

The majority of thrombotic occlusions are due to *atherosclerosis;* the most common sites of involvement are the carotid bifurcation, the origin of the middle cerebral artery, and at either end of the basilar artery.[35] The evolution of arterial stenosis varies from progressive narrowing of the lumen and thrombosis, which may be accompanied by anterograde extension, to fragmentation and distal embolization. Another important aspect of occlusive cerebrovascular disease is its frequent association with systemic diseases such as hypertension and diabetes.

Arteritis of small and large vessels, in association with syphilis and tuberculosis, formerly accounted for cerebral infarcts; infectious vasculitis in now more commonly seen in the setting of immunosuppression and opportunistic infection (such as toxoplasmosis, aspergillosis, and CMV encephalitis). Polyarteritis nodosa and other collagen-vascular diseases may involve cerebral vessels and cause single or multiple infarcts throughout the brain. *Granulomatous angiitis of the nervous system* (GANS) is an inflammatory disorder that involves multiple small to medium-sized parenchymal and subarachnoid vessels characterized by chronic inflammation, multinucleated giant cells, and destruction of the vessel wall. Affected individuals manifest a diffuse encephalopathic or multifocal clinical picture, often with cognitive dysfunction; patients improve with steroid and immunosuppressive treatment. Other conditions that may cause thrombosis and infarction (and intracranial hemorrhage) include hematologic disease with hypercoagulable states, dissecting aneurysm of extracranial arteries in the neck vessels supplying the brain, and drug abuse (amphetamines, heroin, cocaine).

Cerebral autosomal dominant arteriopathy with subcortical infarcts and leukoencephalopathy (CADASIL) is a rare hereditary cause of stroke first described in Sweden and France; the gene has now been mapped to chromosome 19q12 and may involve the *Notch3* gene.[36,37] The disease is characterized clinically by recurrent strokes (usually infarcts, less often hemorrhages) and dementia. Histopathologic study has shown abnormalities of white matter and subarachnoid arteries (also involving non-CNS vessels) consisting of concentric thickening of the media and adventitia. Basophilic, PAS-positive granules, which appear as osmiophilic compact granules by electron microscopy, have been consistently detected in the smooth muscle cells of affected vessels.

Embolism to the brain occurs from a wide range of origins. Cardiac mural thrombi are the most common sources; myocardial infarct, valvular disease, and atrial fibrillation are important predisposing factors. Next in importance are thromboemboli arising in arteries, most often originating over atheromatous plaques within the carotid arteries. Other sources of emboli include paradoxical emboli, particularly in children with cardiac anomalies; emboli associated with cardiac surgery; and emboli of other material (tumor, fat, or air). The territory of distribution of the middle cerebral artery is the brain region most frequently affected by embolic infarction; the incidence is about equal in the hemispheres. Emboli tend to lodge where blood vessels branch or in areas of preexisting luminal stenosis. In many cases, the site of occlusion cannot be identified at postmortem examination, perhaps because the embolus has lysed by the time the tissue is examined. "Shower embolization," as in fat embolism, may occur after fractures; affected patients manifest generalized cerebral dysfunction with disturbances of higher cortical function and consciousness, often without localizing signs.

Infarcts are subdivided into two broad groups based on their macroscopic and corresponding radiologic appearance (Fig. 30–13). *Hemorrhagic (red) infarction*, characterized macroscopically by multiple, sometimes confluent, petechial hemorrhages, is typically associated with embolic events. The hemorrhage is presumed to be secondary to reperfusion of damaged vessels and tissue, either through collaterals or directly after dissolution of intravascular occlusive material. In contrast, *nonhemorrhagic (pale, bland,*

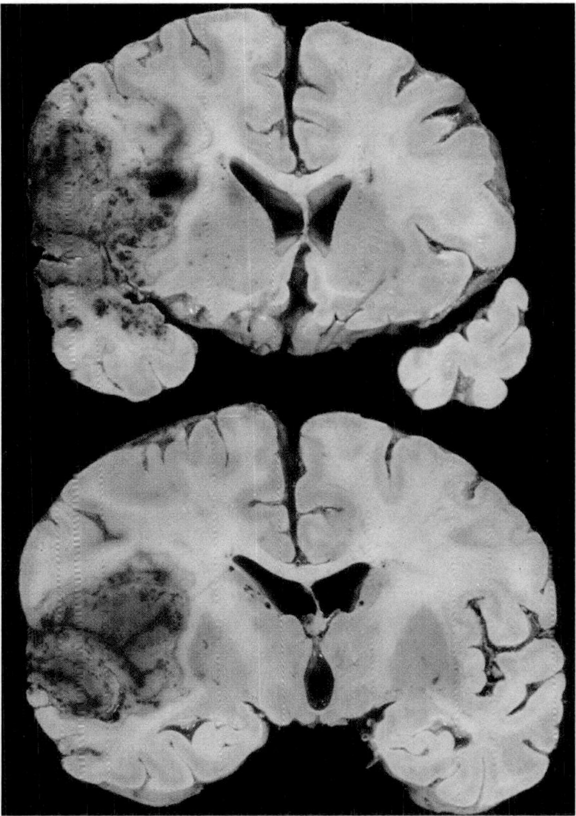

Figure 30–13 ■

Sections of the brain showing a large, discolored, focally hemorrhagic region in the left middle cerebral artery distribution.

anemic) infarcts are usually associated with thrombosis. The clinical management of patients with these two types of infarcts differs greatly: anticoagulation is contraindicated in hemorrhagic infarcts.

MORPHOLOGY. The macroscopic appearance of a **nonhemorrhagic infarct** changes in time. During the first 6 hours of irreversible injury, little can be observed. By 48 hours, the tissue becomes pale, soft, and swollen, and the corticomedullary junction becomes indistinct. From 2 to 10 days, the brain becomes gelatinous and friable, and the previously ill-defined boundary between normal and abnormal tissue becomes more distinct as edema resolves in the adjacent tissue that has survived. From 10 days to 3 weeks, the tissue liquefies, eventually leaving a fluid-filled cavity lined by dark gray tissue, which gradually expands as dead tissue is removed (Fig. 30–14).

On microscopic examination, the tissue reaction evolves along the following sequence: *After the first 12 hours,* ischemic neuronal change (red neurons; see earlier) and both cytotoxic and vasogenic edema predominate. There is loss of the usual tinctorial characteristics of white and gray matter structures. Endothelial and glial cells, mainly astrocytes, swell, and myelinated fibers begin to disintegrate. *Up to 48 hours,* neutrophilic emigration progressively increases and falls off. Phagocytic cells from circulating monocytes, adventitial histiocytes, and activated microglia are evident at 48 hours and become the predominant cell type in the ensuing *2 to 3 weeks.* The macrophages become stuffed with the products of myelin breakdown or blood and may persist in the lesion for months to years. As the process of liquefaction and phagocytosis proceeds, astrocytes at the edges of the lesion progressively enlarge, divide, and develop an extensive network of protoplasmic extensions. Reactive astrocytes can be seen as early as 1 week after the insult.

After several months, the striking astrocytic nuclear and cytoplasmic enlargement recedes. In the wall of the cavity, astrocyte processes form a dense feltwork of glial fibers admixed with new capillaries and a few perivascular connective tissue fibers. In the cerebral cortex, the cavity is delimited from the meninges and subarachnoid space by a gliotic layer of tissue, derived from the molecular layer of cortex. The pia and arachnoid are not affected and do not contribute to the healing process.

The microscopic picture and evolution of **hemorrhagic infarction** parallel ischemic infarction,

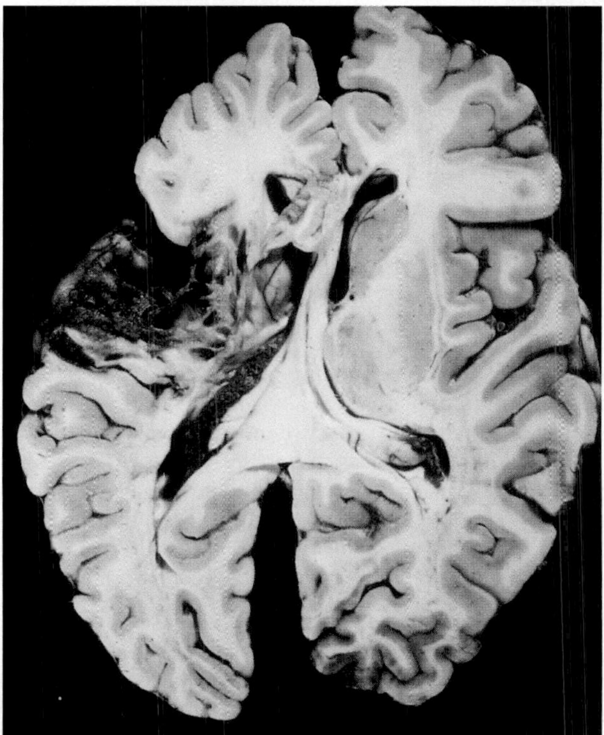

Figure 30–14 ■

Old cystic infarct. Destruction of cortex and surrounding gliosis.

but with the addition of blood extravasation and resorption. In patients receiving anticoagulant treatment, hemorrhagic infarcts may be associated with extensive intracerebral hematomas. Venous infarcts are often hemorrhagic and may occur after thrombotic occlusion of the superior sagittal sinus or other sinuses or occlusion of the deep cerebral veins. Carcinoma, localized infections, or other conditions leading to a hypercoagulable state place patients at risk for venous thrombosis.

Incomplete infarction occurs in focal cerebral ischemia when there is selective necrosis of neurons with relative preservation of glia and supporting tissues; it is reproduced in experimental animals by transient and incomplete focal ischemia and reperfusion.[38,39]

Spinal cord infarction may be seen in the setting of hypoperfusion or as a consequence of interruption of the feeding tributaries derived from the aorta. Occlusion of the anterior spinal artery is rarer and may occur as a result of thrombosis or embolism.

The biochemical changes that attend the cellular reactions in ischemia are discussed in Chapter 1. As regards nervous tissue, several special responses apply.[40] Recent work suggests that excitatory amino acid neurotransmitters such as glutamate, released during ischemia, cause cell damage by overstimulation and persistent opening of specific membrane channels, *N*-methyl-D-aspartate and kainate receptors. This may cause cell death through an uncontrolled influx of calcium ions, or through the neurotransmitter and potential toxin, nitric oxide. Inhibitors of these ion channels or of nitric oxide synthase protect against the effects of cerebral ischemia in some model systems and may have therapeutic potential in humans.[41]

Intracranial Hemorrhage

Hemorrhages may occur at any site within the CNS. In some instances, they may be a secondary phenomenon occurring, for example, within infarcts in arterial border zones or in infarcts caused by only partial or transient vascular obstruction. Primary hemorrhages within the epidural or subdural space are typically related to trauma and are discussed earlier with traumatic lesions. Hemorrhages within the brain parenchyma and subarachnoid space, in contrast, are often a manifestation of underlying cerebrovascular disease, although trauma may also cause hemorrhage in these sites.

INTRACEREBRAL (INTRAPARENCHYMAL) HEMORRHAGE

Spontaneous (nontraumatic) intraparenchymal hemorrhages occur most commonly in mid to late adult life, with a peak incidence at about age 60 years. Most are caused by rupture of a small intraparenchymal vessel. *Hypertension is the most common underlying cause of primary brain parenchymal hemorrhage,* accounting for more than 50% of cases of clinically significant hemorrhage. Conversely, brain hemorrhage accounts for roughly 15% of deaths among patients with chronic hypertension. Hypertension causes a number of abnormalities in vessel walls, including accelerated atherosclerosis in larger arteries; hyaline arteriolosclerosis in smaller vessels; and in severe cases, proliferative changes and frank necrosis of arterioles. Arteriolar walls affected by hyaline change are presumably weaker than are normal vessels and are therefore more vulnerable to rupture. In some instances, chronic hypertension is associated with the development of minute aneurysms, termed *Charcot-Bouchard microaneurysms,* which may be the site of rupture. Charcot-Bouchard aneurysms, not to be confused with saccular aneurysms of larger intracranial vessels, occur in vessels that are less than 300 μm in diameter, most commonly within the basal ganglia. In addition to hypertension, other local and systemic factors may cause or contribute to nontraumatic hemorrhage, including systemic coagulation disorders, open heart surgery, neoplasms, amyloid angiopathy, vasculitis, fusiform aneurysms, and vascular malformations.

MORPHOLOGY. Hypertensive intraparenchymal hemorrhage may originate in the putamen (50% to 60% of cases), thalamus, pons, cerebellar hemispheres (rarely), and other regions of the brain (Fig. 30–15). When the hemorrhages occur in the basal ganglia and thalamus, they are designated **ganglionic hemorrhages** to distinguish them from those that occur in the lobes of the cerebral hemispheres—**lobar hemorrhages.** Acute hemorrhages of either type are characterized by extravasation of blood with compression of the adjacent parenchyma. Old hemorrhages show an area of cavitary destruction of brain with a rim of brownish discoloration. On microscopic examination, the early lesion consists of a central core of clotted blood surrounded by a rim of brain tissue showing anoxic neuronal and glial changes as well as edema. Eventually, the edema resolves, pigment- and lipid-laden macrophages appear, and proliferation of reactive astrocytes is seen at the periphery of the lesion. The cellular events then follow the same time course observed after cerebral infarction.

Lobar hemorrhages[42] may arise in the setting of hemorrhagic diathesis, neoplasms, drug abuse, infectious and noninfectious vasculitis, and **amyloid (congophilic) angiopathy** (see discussion of Alzheimer disease).

SUBARACHNOID HEMORRHAGE AND RUPTURED BERRY ANEURYSMS

The most frequent cause of clinically significant subarachnoid hemorrhage is rupture of a *berry aneurysm.* Sub-

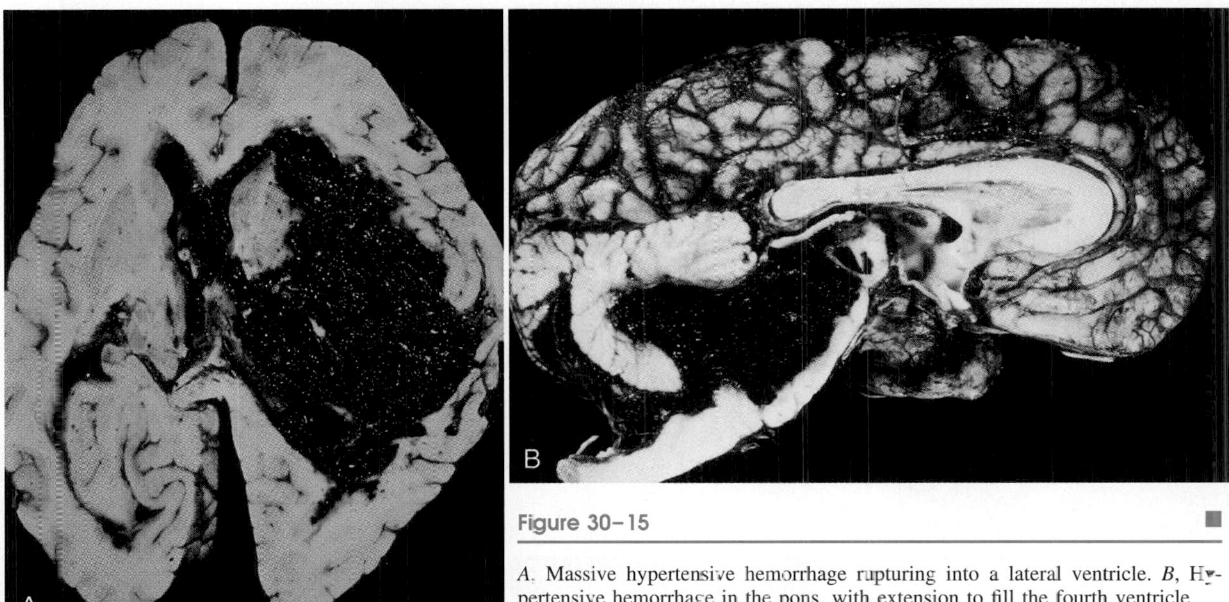

Figure 30–15

A, Massive hypertensive hemorrhage rupturing into a lateral ventricle. *B*, Hypertensive hemorrhage in the pons, with extension to fill the fourth ventricle.

arachnoid hemorrhage may also result from extension of a traumatic hematoma, rupture of a hypertensive intracerebral hemorrhage into the ventricular system, vascular malformation, hematologic disturbances, and tumors.

Berry aneurysm (saccular aneurysm, congenital aneurysm) is the most common type of intracranial aneurysm.[43] Ruptured berry aneurysm is the fourth most common cerebrovascular disorder, after atherosclerotic thrombosis, embolism, and hypertensive intraparenchymal hemorrhage. Other rarer types of aneurysm include atherosclerotic (fusiform; mostly of the basilar artery), mycotic, traumatic, and dissecting aneurysms; all of these chiefly involve the anterior circulation and ordinarily do not give rise primarily to subarachnoid hemorrhage.

Berry aneurysms, ruptured and unruptured, are found in about 2% of postmortem examinations[2]; a somewhat lower figure is reported from radiologic clinics. About 90% of berry aneurysms occur in the anterior circulation and are found near major arterial branch points (Fig. 30–16); multiple aneurysms exist in 20% to 30% of cases in autopsy series.

Pathogenesis of Berry Aneurysms. The etiologic basis of berry aneurysms is unknown. Although the majority of cases occur sporadically, genetic factors may be important in their pathogenesis. There is an increased risk of their occurrence among patients with heritable systemic disorders (such as autosomal dominant polycystic kidney disease, Ehlers-Danlos syndrome type IV, neurofibromatosis type 1, and Marfan syndrome) and with fibromuscular dysplasia of extracranial arteries and coarctation of the aorta. Cigarette smoking and hypertension (estimated to be present in 54% of patients) are accepted predisposing factors for the development of berry aneurysms. Although they are sometimes referred to as *congenital,* they are not identifiable at birth.

MORPHOLOGY. An unruptured berry aneurysm is a thin-walled outpouching at arterial branch points along the circle of Willis or major vessels just beyond. Berry aneurysms measure a few millimeters to 2 or 3 cm and have a bright red, shiny surface and a thin translucent wall (Fig. 30–17). Demonstration of the site of rupture requires careful dissection and removal of blood in the unfixed

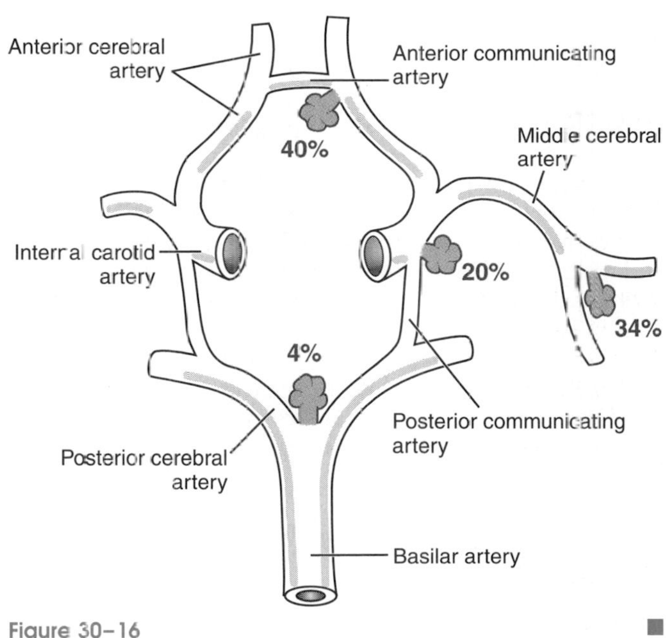

Figure 30–16

Common sites of berry aneurysms in the circle of Willis.

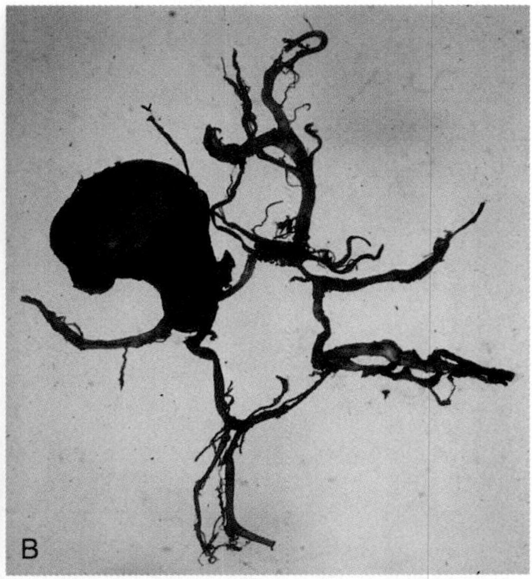

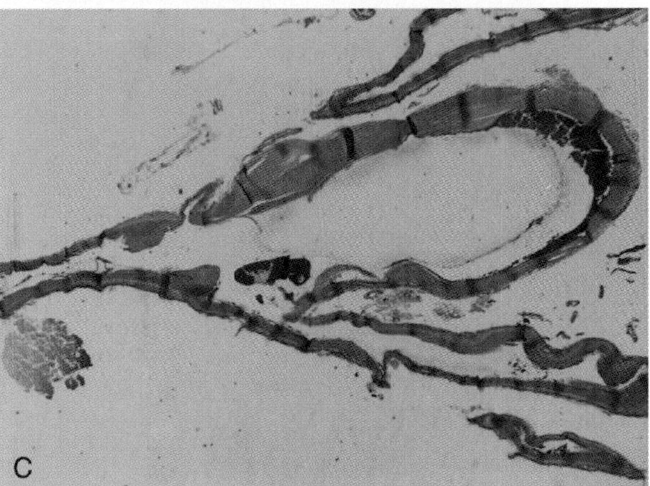

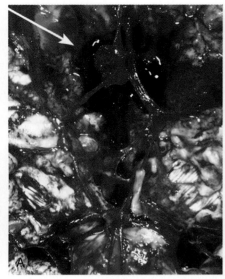

Figure 30–17

A, View of the base of the brain, dissected to show the circle of Willis with an aneurysm of the anterior cerebral artery (*arrow*). *B*, Dissected circle of Willis to show large aneurysm. *C*, Section through a berry aneurysm showing the hyalinized fibrous vessel wall (H&E).

brain. Atheromatous plaques, calcification, or thrombotic occlusion of the sac may be found in the wall or lumen of the aneurysm. Brownish discoloration of the adjacent brain and meninges is evidence of prior hemorrhage. The neck of the aneurysm may be either wide or narrow. Rupture usually occurs at the apex of the sac with extravasation of blood into the subarachnoid space, the substance of the brain, or both. The arterial wall adjacent to the neck of the aneurysm often shows some intimal thickening and gradual attenuation of the media as it approaches the neck. At the neck of the aneurysm, the muscular wall and intimal elastic lamina are usually absent or fragmented, and the wall of the sac is made up of thickened hyalinized intima. The adventitia covering the sac is continuous with that of the parent artery.

Clinical Features. Rupture of the aneurysm is the most frequent complication; 74% of patients with autopsy-proven aneurysms have evidence of aneurysmal rupture. Rupture with clinically significant subarachnoid hemorrhage is most frequent in the fifth decade and is slightly more frequent in females. The probability of rupture increases with the size of the lesion; aneurysms greater than 10 mm have a roughly 50% risk of bleeding per year. Rupture may occur at any time but is often after acute increases in intracranial pressure, such as with straining at stool or sexual orgasm. Blood under arterial pressure is forced into the subarachnoid space, and patients are stricken with sudden, excruciating headache, typically "the worse headache I've ever had," and rapidly lose consciousness. Between 25% and 50% of patients die with the first rupture, but most patients who survive improve and recover consciousness in minutes. Rebleeding is common in survivors, and it is currently not possible to predict in which patients rebleeding will occur. With each episode of bleeding, the prognosis is worse.

The clinical consequences of blood in the subarachnoid space can be separated into acute events, occurring in the hours to days after the hemorrhage, and late sequelae associated with the healing process. In the early post–subarachnoid hemorrhage period, regardless of the etiology of the hemorrhage, there is an increased risk of vasospastic injury involving vessels other than those originally injured. This vasospasm can lead to additional ischemic injury. This problem is of greatest significance in cases of basal subarachnoid hemorrhage, in which vasospasm can involve major vessels of the circle of Willis. Various mediators have been proposed to play a role in this reactive process; some data suggest a contribution from endothelin-1 acting from the adventitial side.[44] In the healing phase of subarachnoid hemorrhage, meningeal fibrosis and scarring occur, sometimes leading to obstruction of CSF flow as well as interruption of the normal pathways of CSF resorption.

VASCULAR MALFORMATIONS

Vascular malformations of the brain are classified into three groups: *arteriovenous malformations, cavernous angiomas,* and *capillary telangiectasias.*

Arteriovenous malformation is the most important type of vascular malformation. The lesion consists of a tangle of numerous, abnormally tortuous, misshapen vessels. Males are affected twice as frequently as females, and the lesion is most often recognized clinically between the ages of 10 and 30 years, presenting as a seizure disorder, an intracerebral hemorrhage, or a subarachnoid hemorrhage. The most common site is the territory of the middle cerebral artery, particularly its posterior branches, but they may occur anywhere along the midbrain, cerebellum, or spinal cord. Large arteriovenous malformations occurring in the newborn period can lead to congestive heart failure because of shunt effects, especially if the malformation involves the vein of Galen.

MORPHOLOGY. Arteriovenous malformations involve vessels in the subarachnoid space extending into brain parenchyma or may occur exclusively within the brain. In macroscopic appearance, they resemble a tangled network of wormlike vascular channels and have a prominent, pulsatile arteriovenous shunt with high blood flow through the malformation. On microscopic examination, they are composed of greatly enlarged blood vessels separated by gliotic tissue, often with evidence of prior hemorrhage. Some vessels can be recognized as arteries with duplication and fragmentation of the internal elastic lamina, while others show marked thickening or partial replacement of the media by hyalinized connective tissue.

Cavernous hemangiomas consist of greatly distended, loosely organized vascular channels with thin collagenized walls and are devoid of intervening nervous tissue (thus distinguishing them from capillary telangiectasias). They occur most often in the cerebellum, pons, and subcortical regions, in decreasing order of frequency, and have a low flow without arteriovenous shunting. Foci of old hemorrhage, infarction, and calcification frequently surround the abnormal vessels. **Capillary telangiectasias** are microscopic foci of dilated, thin-walled vascular channels separated by relatively normal brain parenchyma and occurring most frequently in the pons. **Venous angiomas** (varices) consist of aggregates of ectatic venous channels. **Foix-Alajouanine disease** (angiodysgenetic necrotizing myelopathy) is a venous angiomatous malformation of the spinal cord and overlying meninges associated with ischemic myelomalacia and slowly progressive neurologic symptoms most often referable to the lumbosacral cord.

Hypertensive Cerebrovascular Disease

The most important effects of hypertension on the brain include massive hypertensive intracerebral hemorrhage (discussed earlier), lacunar infarcts and slit hemorrhages, and hypertensive encephalopathy. Atherosclerosis and diabetes are frequently associated diseases.

LACUNAR INFARCTS

Hypertension affects the deep penetrating arteries and arterioles that supply the basal ganglia and hemispheric white matter as well as the brain stem. These cerebral vessels develop *arteriolar sclerosis,* and some go on to become occluded; the structural changes are similar to those described in vessels outside the CNS (Chapter 12). An important clinical and pathologic outcome of these arterial lesions is the development of single, or multiple, small cavitary infarcts—*lacunes*, lacunar state (*état lacunaire*) (Fig. 30–18). These are lakelike spaces, just a few millimeters wide (not more than 15 mm), which occur in the lenticular nucleus, thalamus, internal capsule, deep white matter, caudate nucleus, and pons, in descending order of frequency. On microscopic examination, they consist of cavities of tissue loss with scattered fat-laden macrophages

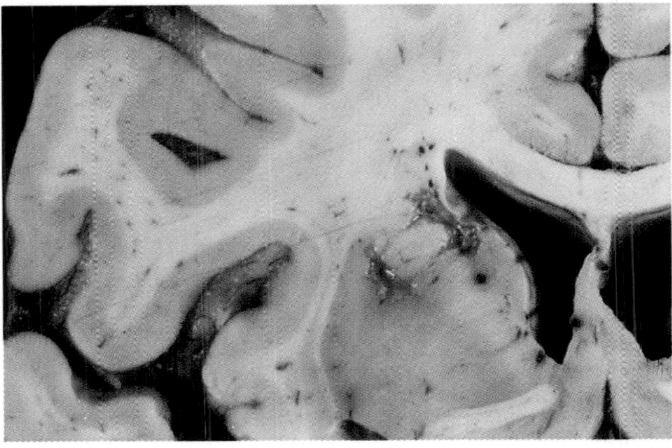

Figure 30–18

Lacunar infarcts in the caudate and putamen.

and surrounding gliosis. Depending on their location in the CNS, lacunes can either be clinically silent or cause severe neurologic impairment. Affected vessels may also be associated with widening of the perivascular spaces but without tissue infarction (*état criblé).*

SLIT HEMORRHAGES

Hypertension also gives rise to rupture of the small-caliber penetrating vessels and the development of small hemorrhages. In time, these hemorrhages resorb, leaving behind a slitlike cavity (*slit hemorrhage*) surrounded by brownish discoloration; on microscopic examination, slit hemorrhages show focal tissue destruction, pigment-laden macrophages, and gliosis.

HYPERTENSIVE ENCEPHALOPATHY

Acute hypertensive encephalopathy is a clinicopathologic syndrome arising in a hypertensive patient characterized by evidence of diffuse cerebral dysfunction, including headaches, confusion, vomiting, and convulsions, sometimes leading to coma. Rapid therapeutic intervention to reduce the accompanying increased intracranial pressure is required, as the syndrome often does not remit spontaneously. Patients coming to postmortem examination may show an edematous brain weighing more than normal, with or without transtentorial or tonsillar herniation. Petechiae and fibrinoid necrosis of arterioles in the gray and white matter may be seen microscopically.

Patients who during the course of many months and years suffer multiple, bilateral, gray matter (cortex, thalamus, basal ganglia), and white matter (centrum semiovale) infarcts in time develop a distinctive clinical syndrome characterized by dementia, gait abnormalities, and pseudobulbar signs, often with superimposed focal neurologic deficits. The syndrome, generally referred to as *vascular (multi-infarct) dementia,* is caused by multifocal vascular disease, consisting largely of (1) cerebral atherosclerosis, (2) vessel thrombosis or embolization from carotid vessels or from the heart, or (3) cerebral arteriolar sclerosis from chronic hypertension. When the pattern of injury preferentially involves expanses of the subcortical white matter with myelin and axon loss, the disorder is referred to as *Binswanger disease;* this distribution of vascular white matter injury needs to be distinguished clinically and radiologically from other diseases that affect the hemispheral white matter.

INFECTIONS

General aspects of the pathology of infectious agents, including pathogenetic mechanisms involving the CNS, are discussed in Chapter 9. To briefly recapitulate here, there are four principal routes of entry for infections of the nervous system.[45] *Hematogenous spread* is the most common means of entry; infectious agents ordinarily enter through the arterial circulation, but retrograde venous spread can occur through anastomotic connections between veins of the face and the cerebral circulation. *Direct implantation* of microorganisms is almost invariably traumatic; rarely it is iatrogenic, as when microbes are introduced with a lumbar puncture needle, or is associated with congenital malformations (such as meningomyelocele). *Local extension* occurs secondary to an established infection in an air sinus, most often the mastoid or frontal; an infected tooth; or a surgical site in the cranium or spine causing osteomyelitis, bone erosion, and propagation of the infection into the CNS. The fourth pathway is through the *peripheral nervous system* into the CNS, as occurs with certain viruses, such as rabies and herpes simplex. Damage to nervous tissue may be the consequence of direct injury of neurons or glia by the infectious agent or may occur indirectly through the elaboration of microbial toxins, destructive effects of the inflammatory response, or the influence of immune-mediated mechanisms.[45]

Acute Meningitis

Leptomeningitis or *meningitis,* as it is often called, refers to an inflammatory process of the leptomeninges and CSF within the subarachnoid space. *Meningoencephalitis* applies to inflammation of the meninges and brain parenchyma. Meningitis is usually caused by an infection, but *chemical meningitis* may also occur in response to a nonbacterial irritant introduced into the subarachnoid space. Infiltration of the subarachnoid space by carcinoma is referred to as *meningeal carcinomatosis* and by lymphoma as *lymphomatosis.* Infectious meningitis is broadly classified into *acute pyogenic* (usually bacterial), *aseptic* (usually viral), and *chronic* (most any infectious agent) on the basis of the characteristics of inflammatory exudate on CSF examination and the clinical evolution of the illness.

ACUTE PYOGENIC (BACTERIAL) MENINGITIS

The microorganisms that cause acute pyogenic meningitis vary with the age of the patient.[46,47] In neonates, the organisms include *Escherichia coli* and the group B streptococci; in infants and children, *Haemophilus influenzae*; in adolescents and in young adults, *Neisseria meningitidis*; and in the elderly, *Streptococcus pneumoniae* and *Listeria monocytogenes*. Patients typically show systemic signs of infection superimposed on clinical evidence of meningeal irritation and neurologic impairment, that is, headache, photophobia, irritability, clouding of consciousness, and neck stiffness. *A spinal tap yields cloudy or frankly purulent CSF, under increased pressure, with as many as 90,000 neutrophils/mm^3, a raised protein level, and a markedly reduced glucose content.* Bacteria may be seen on a smear or can be cultured, sometimes a few hours before the neutrophils appear. Untreated, pyogenic meningitis can be fatal; effective antimicrobial agents markedly reduce mortality.[48] In the immunosuppressed patient, purulent meningitis may be caused by other agents, such as *Klebsiella* or an anaerobic organism, and may have an atypical course and uncharacteristic CSF findings, all of which make the diagnosis more difficult.

MORPHOLOGY. The normally clear CSF is cloudy and sometimes frankly purulent; the exudate is evident within the leptomeninges over the surface of the brain (Fig. 30–19). The meningeal vessels are engorged and stand out prominently. The location of the exudate varies: in *H. influenzae* meningitis, for example, it is usually basal, whereas in pneumococcal meningitis, it is often densest over the cerebral convexities near the sagittal sinus. From the areas of greatest accumulation, tracts of pus can be followed along blood vessels on the surface of the brain. When the meningitis is fulminant, the inflammation may extend to the ventricles, producing ventriculitis.

On microscopic examination, neutrophils fill the entire subarachnoid space in severely affected areas and are found predominantly around the leptomeningeal blood vessels in less severe cases. In untreated meningitis, Gram stain reveals varying numbers of the causative organism, although they are frequently not demonstrable in treated cases. In fulminant meningitis, the inflammatory cells infiltrate the walls of the leptomeningeal veins with potential extension of the inflammatory infiltrate into the substance of the brain (focal cerebritis). Phlebitis may also lead to venous occlusion and hemorrhagic infarction of the underlying brain.

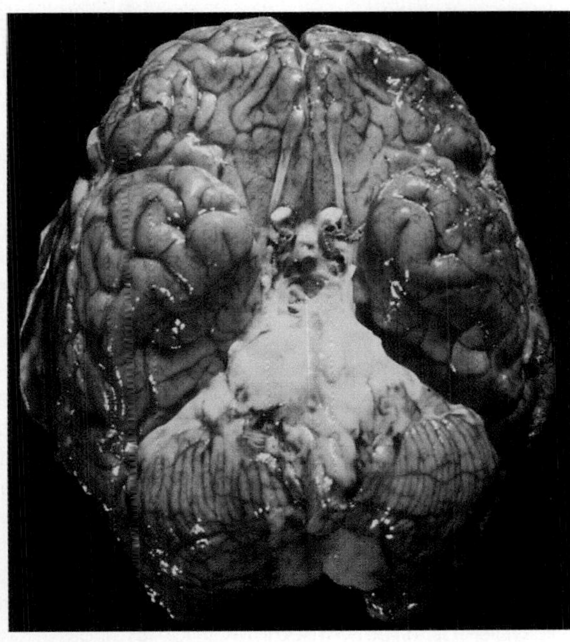

Figure 30–19

Pyogenic meningitis. A thick layer of suppurative exudate covers the brain stem and cerebellum and thickens the leptomeninges. (From Golden JA, Louis DN: Images in clinical medicine: Acute bacterial meningitis. N Engl J Med 333:364, 1994.)

Leptomeningeal fibrosis and consequent hydrocephalus may follow pyogenic meningitis, although if it is treated early, there may be little remaining evidence of the infection. In some infections, particularly in pneumococcal meningitis, large quantities of the capsular polysaccharide of the organism produce a particularly gelatinous exudate that encourages arachnoid fibrosis, **chronic adhesive arachnoiditis.**

ACUTE ASEPTIC (VIRAL) MENINGITIS

Aseptic meningitis is a misnomer, but it is a term used clinically to designate an illness comprising meningeal irritation, fever, and alterations of consciousness of relatively acute onset, generally of viral but rarely of bacterial or other etiology. The clinical course is less fulminant than that observed in pyogenic meningitis, and the CSF findings also differ between the two conditions. *There is a lymphocytic pleocytosis, the protein elevation is only moderate, and the sugar content is nearly always normal.* The viral aseptic meningitides are usually self-limiting and are treated symptomatically. In approximately 70% of cases, a pathogen can be identified, most commonly an enterovirus. Echovirus, coxsackievirus, and nonparalytic poliomyelitis are responsible for up to 80% of these cases.

MORPHOLOGY. There are no distinctive macroscopic characteristics except for brain swelling, seen in some instances. Pathologic material is limited, however, because recovery of patients is the rule. On microscopic examination, there is either no abnormality or a mild to moderate infiltration of the leptomeninges with lymphocytes.

An aseptic meningitis–like picture may develop subsequent to rupture of an epidermoid cyst into the subarachnoid space or the introduction of a chemical irritant therein—"chemical" meningitis. In these cases, the CSF is sterile, there is pleocytosis with neutrophils and a raised protein level, but usually the sugar content is normal.

Acute Focal Suppurative Infections

BRAIN ABSCESS

Brain abscesses may arise by direct implantation of organisms, local extension from adjacent foci (mastoiditis, paranasal sinusitis), or hematogenous spread (usually from a primary site in the heart, lungs, or distal bones or after tooth extraction). Predisposing conditions include *acute bacterial endocarditis,* which tends to produce multiple abscesses; *cyanotic congenital heart disease,* in which there is a right-to-left shunt and loss of pulmonary filtration of organisms; and *chronic pulmonary sepsis,* as can be seen with bronchiectasis. Streptococci and staphylococci are the most common offending organisms identified.[45,49]

MORPHOLOGY. On macroscopic examination, abscesses are discrete lesions with central liquefactive necrosis, a surrounding fibrous, collagenized response, and edema (Fig. 30–20). The most common brain regions affected, in descending order of frequency, are the frontal lobe, the parietal lobe, and the cerebellum. On microscopic examination, there is exuberant neovascularization around the necrosis that is responsible for the marked vasogenic edema and formation of granulation tissue. The collagen of the capsule is produced by fibroblasts derived from the walls of blood vessels. Outside the fibrous capsule is a zone of reactive gliosis with numerous gemistocytic astrocytes.

Cerebral abscesses are destructive, and patients almost invariably present clinically with progressive focal deficits in addition to the general signs of raised intracranial pressure. *The CSF is under increased pressure; the white cell count and protein level are raised, but the sugar content is normal.* A systemic or local source of infection may be apparent, or a small systemic focus may have ceased to be symptomatic. The increased intracranial pressure and progressive herniation can be fatal, and abscess rupture can lead to ventriculitis, meningitis, and sinus thrombosis. With surgery and antibiotics, the otherwise high mortality rate can be reduced to less than 10%.

SUBDURAL EMPYEMA

Bacterial or occasionally fungal infection of the skull bones or air sinuses can spread to the subdural space and produce a subdural empyema. The underlying arachnoid and subarachnoid spaces are usually unaffected, but a large subdural empyema may produce a mass effect. Further, a thrombophlebitis may develop in the bridging veins that cross the subdural space, resulting in venous occlusion and infarction of the brain. With treatment, including surgical drainage, resolution of the empyema occurs from the dural side, and if it is complete, a thickened dura may be the only residual finding. Symptoms include those referable to the source of the infection. In addition, most patients are febrile, with headache and neck stiffness, and if untreated may develop focal neurologic signs, lethargy, and coma. The CSF profile is similar to that seen in brain abscesses, because both are parameningeal infective processes. If diagnosis and treatment are prompt, complete recovery is usual.

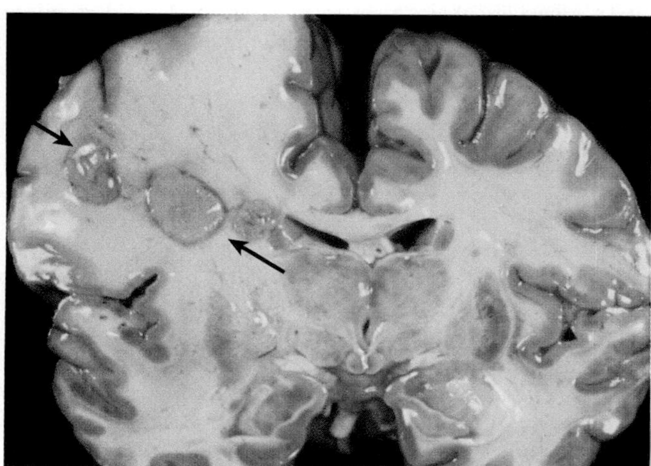

Figure 30–20

Frontal abscesses (*arrows*).

EXTRADURAL ABSCESS

Extradural abscess, commonly associated with osteomyelitis, often arises from an adjacent focus of infection, such as sinusitis or a surgical procedure. When the process occurs in the spinal epidural space, it may cause spinal cord compression and constitutes a neurosurgical emergency.

Chronic Bacterial Meningoencephalitis

TUBERCULOSIS AND MYCOBACTERIOSES

Patients with *tuberculous meningitis* usually have generalized complaints of a headache, malaise, mental confusion, and vomiting. *There is only a moderate CSF pleocytosis made up of mononuclear cells, or a mixture of polymorphonuclear and mononuclear cells; the protein level is elevated, often strikingly so; and the glucose content typically is moderately reduced or normal.*

The most serious complications of chronic meningitis are arachnoid fibrosis, which may produce hydrocephalus, and obliterative endarteritis with arterial occlusion and infarction of underlying brain. Because the process involves the spinal cord subarachnoid space, spinal roots may also be affected.

MORPHOLOGY. On macroscopic examination, the subarachnoid space contains a gelatinous or fibrinous exudate, most often at the base of the brain, obliterating the cisterns and encasing cranial nerves. There may be discrete, white granules scattered over the leptomeninges. The most common pattern of involvement is a diffuse **meningoencephalitis.**[47] On microscopic examination, there are mixtures of lymphocytes, plasma cells, and macrophages. Florid cases show well-formed granulomas, often with caseous necrosis and giant cells. Arteries running through the subarachnoid space may show **obliterative endarteritis** with inflammatory infiltrates in their walls and marked intimal thickening. Organisms can often be seen with acid-fast stains. The infectious process may spread to the choroid plexuses and ependymal surface, traveling through the CSF. In cases of long-standing duration, a dense, fibrous adhesive arachnoiditis may develop, most conspicuous around the base of the brain.

Another manifestation of the disease is the development of a single (or often multiple) well-circumscribed intraparenchymal mass **(tuberculoma)**, which may be associated with meningitis. A tuberculoma may be up to several centimeters in diameter, causing significant mass effect. On microscopic examination, there is usually a central core of caseous necrosis surrounded by a typically tuberculous granulomatous reaction, and calcification may occur in inactive lesions.

Infection by *Mycobacterium tuberculosis* in patients with acquired immunodeficiency syndrome (AIDS) is similar to that in non-AIDS patients. In addition, HIV-positive patients are also at risk for CNS infection by *Mycobacterium avium-intracellulare,* usually in the setting of disseminated infection.

NEUROSYPHILIS

Neurosyphilis is a tertiary stage of syphilis and occurs in only about 10% of patients with untreated infection.[47] Its major forms of expression are meningeal-meningovascular neurosyphilis, paretic neurosyphilis, and tabes dorsalis.

MORPHOLOGY. Meningovascular neurosyphilis is a chronic meningitis involving the base of the brain and, variably, also the cerebral convexities and the spinal leptomeninges; there may be an associated obliterative endarteritis (Heubner arteritis) accompanied by a distinctive perivascular inflammatory reaction rich in plasma cells and lymphocytes. Cerebral gummas may also occur in relation to meninges and extending into the cerebral hemispheres, diencephalon, or spinal cord.

Paretic neurosyphilis is caused by invasion of the brain by *Treponema pallidum* and is clinically manifested as an insidious but progressive loss of mental and physical functions with mood alterations (including delusions of grandeur), terminating in severe dementia **(general paresis of the insane)**. On microscopic examination, inflammatory meningeal lesions are associated with parenchymal damage in the cerebral cortex (particularly the frontal lobe but also affecting other areas of the isocortex) characterized by loss of neurons with proliferations of microglia (rod cells), gliosis, and iron deposits demonstrable with the Prussian blue stain (perivascularly and in the neuropil, presumably from damage to the microcirculation). The spirochetes can be demonstrated in tissue sections. There is often an associated hydrocephalus with damage to the ependymal lining and proliferation of subependymal glia—**granular ependymitis.**

Tabes dorsalis is the result of damage by the spirochete to the sensory nerves in the dorsal roots, which produces, among other features, impaired joint position sense and resultant ataxia (locomotor ataxia); loss of pain sensation, leading to skin and joint damage (Charcot joints); other sensory disturbances, particularly the characteristic "lightning pains"; and absence of deep tendon reflexes. On microscopic examination, there is loss of both axons and myelin in the dorsal roots, with pallor and atrophy in the dorsal columns of the spinal cord. It is not possible to demonstrate organisms in the cord lesions.

Although these three forms of expression of neurosyphilis have been described separately, patients often show incomplete or mixed pictures, notably the combination of tabes dorsalis and general paresis (taboparesis).

Patients with HIV infection are at increased risk for neurosyphilis, and the rate of progression and severity of the disease appear to be accelerated, presumably related to the impaired cell-mediated immunity. CNS involvement by *T. pallidum* in this setting may be manifested as asymptomatic infection, acute syphilitic meningitis, meningovascular syphilis, and rarely direct parenchymal invasion of the brain.[47]

NEUROBORRELIOSIS (LYME DISEASE)

Lyme disease is caused by the spirochete *Borrelia burgdorferi*, transmitted by various species of *Ixodes* tick (Chapter 9); involvement of the nervous system is referred to as neuroborreliosis. Neurologic symptoms are highly variable and include aseptic meningitis, facial nerve palsies, mild encephalopathy, and polyneuropathies.[45,50,51] The rare cases that have come to autopsy have shown a focal proliferation of microglial cells in the brain as well as scattered organisms (identified by Dieterle stain) in the extracellular spaces. Other findings include granulomas and vasculitis.

Viral Meningoencephalitis

Viral encephalitis (Chapter 9) is a parenchymal infection of the brain almost invariably associated with meningeal inflammation *(meningoencephalitis)* and sometimes with simultaneous involvement of the spinal cord *(encephalomyelitis)* and having a wide spectrum of clinical and pathologic expression.[45,52,53] *The most characteristic histologic features of viral encephalitides are perivascular and parenchymal mononuclear cell infiltrates (lymphocytes, plasma cells, and macrophages), glial cell reactions (including the formation of microglial nodules), and neuronophagia.* Direct indications of viral infection are the presence of viral inclusion bodies and, most importantly, the identification of viral pathogens by ultrastructural, immunocytochemical, and molecular methods.

The phenomenon of nervous system tropism that characterizes some viral encephalitides is particularly noteworthy; there are pathogenic viruses that infect specific cell types (such as oligodendrocytes), while others preferentially involve particular areas of the brain (such as medial temporal lobes, limbic system). The capacity of some viruses for *latency* is especially important in neurologic disease (see later, herpes zoster). Systemic viral infections in the absence of direct evidence of viral penetration into the CNS may be followed by an *immune-mediated disease*, such as perivenous demyelination (see later, acute disseminated encephalomyelitis). Intrauterine viral infection may cause *congenital malformations,* as occurs with rubella. A slowly progressive degenerative disease syndrome may follow many years after a viral illness; an example is *postencephalitic parkinsonism* after the viral influenza epidemic that occurred during and after the First World War.

ARTHROPOD-BORNE (ARBO) VIRAL ENCEPHALITIS

Arboviruses are an important cause of epidemic encephalitis, especially in tropical regions of the world, and are capable of causing serious morbidity and high mortality. In the Western hemisphere, the most important types are Eastern and Western equine, Venezuelan, St. Louis, and California; elsewhere in the world, pathogenic arboviruses include Japanese B (Far East), Murray Valley (Australia and New Guinea), and tick-borne (Russia and Eastern Europe).[52] All have animal hosts and mosquito vectors, except for the tick-borne type. Clinically, affected patients develop generalized neurologic deficits, such as seizures, confusion, delirium, and stupor or coma, and often focal signs, such as reflex asymmetry and ocular palsies. *The CSF is usually colorless but with a slightly elevated pressure and, initially, a neutrophilic pleocytosis that rapidly converts to lymphocytes; the protein level is elevated, but sugar content is normal.*

MORPHOLOGY. The arbovirus encephalitides differ in epidemiology and prognosis, but the histopathologic picture is similar among them, except for variations in the severity and extent of the lesions within the CNS. Characteristically, there is a lymphocytic (sometimes with neutrophils) meningoencephalitis with a tendency for inflammatory cells to occur perivascularly. Multiple foci of necrosis of gray and white matter are found; in particular, there is evidence of single-cell neuronal necrosis with phagocytosis of the debris **(neuronophagia).** Viral antigens can be detected in neurons by immunoperoxidase methods. In severe cases, there may be a necrotizing vasculitis with associated focal hemorrhages. Some cases have predominantly cortical involvement, whereas in others the basal ganglia bear the brunt of the disease as can be demonstrated with neuroradiographic studies.[54]

HERPES SIMPLEX VIRUS TYPE 1

HSV-1 produces an encephalitis that occurs in any age group but is most common in children and young adults. Only about 10% of the patients have a history of prior labial herpes ("fever blisters"). The most commonly observed clinical presenting symptoms in herpes (HSV-1) encephalitis are alterations in mood, memory, and behavior.

MORPHOLOGY. This encephalitis starts in, and most severely involves, the inferior and medial regions of the temporal lobes and the orbital gyri of the frontal lobes (Fig. 30–21). The infection is necrotizing and often hemorrhagic in the most severely affected regions. Perivascular inflammatory infiltrates are usually present, and Cowdry intranuclear viral inclusion bodies may be found in both neurons and glia. In patients with slowly evolving HSV-1 encephalitis, there is more diffuse involvement of the brain. Antiviral agents now provide effective treatment in many cases, with a significant reduction in the mortality rate. In some individuals, HSV-1 encephalitis follows a subacute course with clinical manifestations (weakness, lethargy, ataxia, seizures) that evolve during a more protracted period (4 to 6 weeks).

HERPES SIMPLEX VIRUS TYPE 2

HSV-2 also affects the nervous system and is responsible for most cases of *herpetic viral meningitis.* A generalized and usually severe encephalitis develops in as many as 50% of neonates born by vaginal delivery to women with active *primary* HSV genital infections. The dependence on route of delivery indicates that the infection is acquired during passage through the birth canal rather than transplacentally. HSV-1 causes a similar encephalitis in neonates. In AIDS patients, HSV-2 may rarely cause an acute, hemorrhagic necrotizing encephalitis.

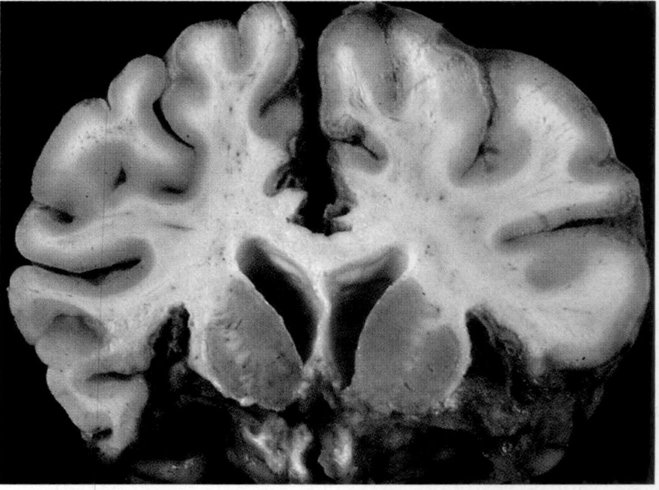

Figure 30–21 ■

Herpes encephalitis showing extensive destruction of inferior frontal and anterior temporal lobes. (Courtesy of Dr. T.W. Smith, University of Massachusetts Medical School, Worcester, MA.)

VARICELLA-ZOSTER VIRUS (HERPES ZOSTER)

The primary varicella infection presents as one of the childhood exanthems (chickenpox), ordinarily without any evidence of neurologic involvement. Reactivation in adults (commonly called shingles) usually manifests as a painful, vesicular skin eruption in the distribution of a dermatome (Chapter 9).

It is usually a self-limited process, but there may be a persistent postherpetic neuralgia syndrome in up to 10% of patients. Overt CNS involvement with herpes zoster is much rarer but can be more severe. Herpes zoster has been associated with a granulomatous arteritis; immunocytochemical and electron microscopic evidence of viral involvement has been obtained in a few of these cases. In immunosuppressed patients, herpes zoster may cause an acute *encephalitis* with numerous sharply circumscribed lesions characterized by early demyelination and subsequent necrosis. Inclusion bodies (Chapter 9) can be found in glia and neurons. Varicella-zoster virus infection accounts for about 12% of all systemic herpesvirus infections in patients with AIDS.

CYTOMEGALOVIRUS

This infection of the nervous system occurs in two groups of individuals: fetuses and the immunosuppressed. The outcome of in utero infection is periventricular necrosis that produces severe brain destruction followed later by microcephaly with periventricular calcification. CMV is the most common opportunistic viral pathogen in patients with AIDS, affecting the CNS in 15% to 20% of cases.[55]

MORPHOLOGY. In the immunosuppressed, the most common pattern of involvement is that of a subacute encephalitis, which may be associated with CMV inclusion-bearing cells (see Fig. 9–43). Although any type of cell within the CNS (neurons, glia, ependyma, endothelium) can be infected by CMV, there is a tendency for the virus to localize in the ependymal and subependymal regions of the brain. This results in a severe hemorrhagic necrotizing ventriculoencephalitis and a choroid plexitis. Prominent cytomegalic cells with intranuclear and intracytoplasmic inclusions can be readily identified by conventional light microscopy, immunocytochemistry, and in situ hybridization. These latter two techniques have also shown that normal-appearing, noncytomegalic cells at the edges of the lesions may contain virus.

POLIOMYELITIS

Poliovirus is a member of the picorna group of enteroviruses. While paralytic poliomyelitis has been effectively controlled by immunization in many parts of the world, there are still many regions where it remains a serious problem. In nonimmunized individuals, poliovirus infection causes a subclinical or mild gastroenteritis. In a small fraction of the vulnerable population, however, it secondarily invades the nervous system. Clinically, CNS infection manifests initially with meningeal irritation and a CSF picture of aseptic meningitis. The disease may progress no further or advance to involve the spinal cord. Attack of the anterior horns with *loss of motor neurons produces a flaccid paralysis with muscle wasting and hyporeflexia in the affected spinal segments that is the permanent neurologic residual of poliomyelitis.* In the acute disease, death can occur from paralysis of the respiratory muscles; a myocarditis sometimes complicates the clinical course. Permanent cranial nerve (bulbar) weakness is rare, as is any evidence of encephalitis, but severe respiratory compromise is an important cause of long-term morbidity.

MORPHOLOGY. Acute cases show mononuclear cell perivascular cuffs and neuronophagia of the anterior horn motor neurons of the spinal cord. In situ reverse transcriptase–polymerase chain reaction has shown poliovirus RNA in anterior horn cell motor neurons.[56] The inflammatory reaction is usually confined to the anterior horns but may extend into the posterior horns, and the damage is occasionally severe enough to produce cavitation. The motor cranial nuclei sometimes are involved. Postmortem examination in long-term survivors of symptomatic poliomyelitis shows loss of neurons and long-standing gliosis in the affected anterior horns of the spinal cord, some residual inflammation, atrophy of the anterior (motor) spinal roots, and neurogenic atrophy of denervated muscle.[57]

A late neurologic syndrome can develop in patients affected by poliomyelitis who had been stable during intervening years *(postpolio syndrome).* This syndrome, which typically develops 25 to 35 years after the resolution of the initial illness, is characterized by progressive weakness associated with decreased muscle bulk and pain.[58] There is no evidence, to date, of persistence of poliovirus genomes, and there is conflicting evidence regarding the re-emergence of an immune response.[59,60]

RABIES

Rabies is transmitted to humans by the bite of a rabid animal, usually a dog, although various wild animal populations form natural reservoirs. It causes a severe encephalitis. Exposure to bats, even without a bite, has now been identified as a risk factor for developing infection. The virus enters the CNS by ascent along the peripheral nerves from the wound site. The incubation period varies, depending on the distance between the wound and the brain (commonly between 1 and 3 months). Clinically, the disease manifests with nonspecific symptoms of malaise, headache, and fever, but the conjunction of these symptoms with local paresthesias around the wound is diagnostic. In advanced cases, the patient exhibits extraordinary CNS excitability; the slightest touch is painful, with violent motor responses progressing to convulsions. Contracture of the pharyngeal musculature on swallowing produces foaming at the mouth, which may create an aversion to swallowing even water. The former term for the disease, hydrophobia, describes this phenomenon. There is meningismus and, as the disease progresses, flaccid paralysis. Periods of alternating mania and stupor progress to coma and death from respiratory center failure.

MORPHOLOGY. On macroscopic examination, the brain shows intense edema and vascular congestion. On microscopic examination, there is widespread neuronal degeneration and an inflammatory reaction that is most severe in the basal ganglia, midbrain, and floor of the fourth ventricle, particularly in the medulla. The spinal cord and dorsal root ganglia may also be involved. Negri bodies, the pathognomonic microscopic finding, are cytoplasmic, round to oval, eosinophilic inclusions and can be found in pyramidal neurons of the hippocampus and Purkinje cells of the cerebellum, sites usually devoid of inflammation.[52,61] The presence of rabies virus can be detected within Negri bodies by ultrastructural and immunohistochemical examination.

HUMAN IMMUNODEFICIENCY VIRUS 1

As many as 60% of patients with AIDS develop neurologic dysfunction during the course of their illness, and in some, it dominates the clinical picture until death. (See Chapter 9 for a discussion of the epidemiology and pathogenesis of AIDS.) Neuropathologic changes have been demonstrated at postmortem examination in as many as 80% to 90% of cases.[62] These include direct or indirect effects of HIV-1, opportunistic infection, and primary CNS lymphoma (Chapter 15).

HIV-1 aseptic meningitis occurs within 1 to 2 weeks of seroconversion in about 10% of patients; antibodies to HIV-1 can be demonstrated, and the virus can be isolated from the CSF. The few neuropathologic studies of the early and acute phases of symptomatic or asymptomatic HIV-1 invasion of the nervous system have shown a mild lymphocytic meningitis, perivascular inflammation, and some myelin loss in the hemispheres.[63]

HIV-1 Meningoencephalitis (Subacute Encephalitis)

Patients affected with this remarkable neurologic disorder can manifest clinically with dementia referred to as AIDS-related cognitive-motor complex. The dementia begins insidiously with mental slowing, memory loss, and mood disturbances, such as apathy and depression. Motor abnormalities, ataxia, bladder and bowel incontinence, and seizures can also be present. Radiologic imaging of the brain may be normal or show some diffuse cortical atrophy, focal abnormalities of the cerebral white matter, and ventricular dilation.[64]

MORPHOLOGY. The brains of individuals with HIV-1 encephalitis with or without dementia show comparable findings. On macroscopic examination, the meninges are clear, and there is some ventricular dilation with sulcal widening but normal cortical thickness. The process is best characterized microscopically as a chronic inflammatory reaction with widely distributed infiltrates of **microglial nodules,** sometimes with associated foci of tissue necrosis and reactive gliosis (Fig. 30–22). The microglial nodules are also found in the vicinity of small blood vessels, which show abnormally prominent endothelial cells concurrent with perivascular foamy or pigment-laden macrophages. These changes occur especially in the subcortical white matter, diencephalon, and brain stem. An important component of the microglial nodule is the macrophage-derived **multinucleated giant cell.** In some cases, there is also a disorder of white matter characterized by multifocal or diffuse areas of myelin pallor with associated axonal swellings and gliosis.

HIV can be detected in CD4 mononucleate and multinucleate macrophages and microglia by ultrastructural immunoperoxidase and molecular methods. HIV infection has been reported in retinal and cerebral endothelial cells and astrocytes in some studies. There is considerable uncertainty as to whether neurons or oligodendrocytes are affected directly by HIV-1 or whether cellular damage occurs indirectly through the release of

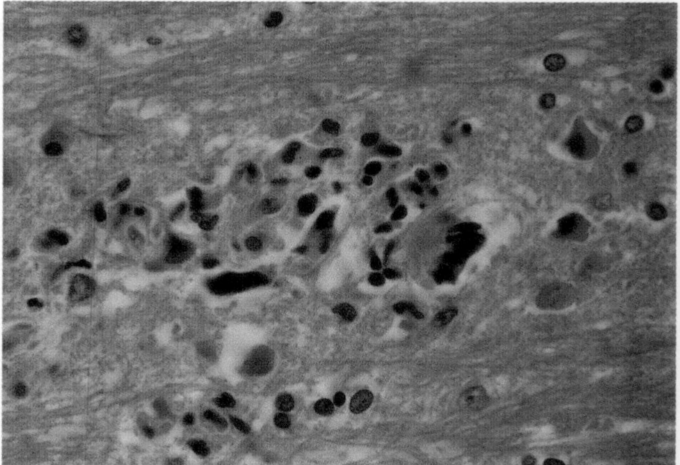

Figure 30–22

HIV-1 encephalitis. Note the microglial nodule and multinucleated giant cells.

toxic cytokines and alterations of the blood-brain barrier.[65] The pathogenesis of the dementing illness has not been fully elucidated[66] (see discussion in Chapter 9).

Vacuolar Myelopathy

This disorder of the spinal cord is found in 20% to 30% of unselected patients with AIDS in the United States, less often in Europe. The histopathologic findings resemble those of subacute combined degeneration, and abnormal utilization of vitamin B_{12} is suspected, though serum levels are normal. The pathogenesis of the lesion is unknown; it does not appear to be caused directly by HIV-1, and virus is not present within the lesions.[67]

Of related interest is the condition known as *tropical spastic paraparesis,* which occurs in several countries in the Caribbean, along the Indian Ocean, and in South America. Some cases show a severe lymphocytic meningomyelitis unlike that seen in vacuolar myelopathy. Virologic studies and polymerase chain reaction data have implicated human T-cell lymphotrophic virus I (HTLV-I).

AIDS-Associated Myopathy, Peripheral Neuropathy

Inflammatory myopathy has been the most often described skeletal muscle disorder in patients with HIV-1 infection. The disease is characterized by the subacute onset of proximal weakness, sometimes pain, and elevated levels of serum creatine kinase. The histologic findings include muscle fiber necrosis and phagocytosis, interstitial infiltration with HIV-positive macrophages, and in a few cases cytoplasmic bodies and nemaline rods. An acute, toxic, reversible myopathy with "ragged red" fibers and myoglobulinuria may also develop in patients treated with zidovudine (AZT).

The most commonly reported clinical syndromes of peripheral neuropathy include acute and chronic inflammatory demyelinating polyneuropathy, distal symmetric polyneuropathy, polyradiculopathy, mononeuritis multiplex, and rarely, sensory neuropathy due to ganglioneuronitis. The histopathologic findings observed in most of these cases include segmental demyelination, axonal degeneration, and epineurial and endoneurial mononuclear cell inflammation.

AIDS in Children

Neurologic disease is common in children with congenital AIDS. Clinical manifestations of neurologic dysfunction are evident by the first years of life and include microcephaly with mental retardation and motor developmental delay with spasticity of limbs. The most frequent morphologic abnormality is calcification of the large and small vessels and parenchyma within the basal ganglia and deep cerebral white matter. There is also loss of hemispheric myelin or delay in myelination; multinucleated giant cells and microglial nodules are also observed in many cases. HIV-1 virus is present in brain tissue.[68] Opportunistic infections of the CNS, including toxoplasmosis, CMV infection, progressive multifocal leukoencephalopathy, and cryptococcal meningitis, are relatively rare in infants and children with AIDS compared with adults.

PROGRESSIVE MULTIFOCAL LEUKOENCEPHALOPATHY

Progressive multifocal leukoencephalopathy is a viral encephalitis caused by a polyomavirus (JC virus, totally unrelated to Creutzfeldt-Jakob disease); because the virus preferentially infects oligodendrocytes, demyelination is its principal pathologic effect. The disease occurs almost invariably in immunosuppressed individuals in various clinical settings, including chronic lymphoproliferative or myeloproliferative illnesses, immunosuppressive chemotherapy, granulomatous diseases, and AIDS.[69,70] Although no systemic syndrome has been described, about 65% of normal people have serologic evidence of exposure to JC virus by the age of 14 years. It is not known with certainty whether progressive multifocal leukoencephalopathy results from a primary infection in a susceptible host or from the rekindling of an old infection, though the latter is suspected. Clinically, patients develop focal and relentlessly progressive neurologic symptoms and signs, and both computed tomography (CT) and magnetic resonance imaging (MRI) scans show extensive, often multifocal lesions in the hemispheric or cerebellar white matter.

MORPHOLOGY. The lesions consist of patches of irregular, ill-defined destruction of the white matter ranging in size from millimeters to extensive involvement of an entire lobe of the brain (Fig. 30–23). The cerebrum, brain stem, cerebellum, and occasionally the spinal cord can be involved. On microscopic examination, the typical lesion consists of a patch of demyelination in the center of which are scattered lipid-laden macrophages and a reduced number of axons. At the edge of the lesion are greatly enlarged oligodendrocyte nuclei whose chromatin is replaced by glassy amphophilic viral inclusion. These oligodendrocytes can be shown to contain viral antigens by immunohistochemistry (Fig. 30–23, *inset*), viral genome by in situ hybridization, and viral nucleocapsids by electron microscopy. Within the lesions, there are characteristic bizarre giant astrocytes with irregular, hyperchromatic, sometimes multiple nuclei. Reactive fibrillary astrocytes are scattered among the bizarre forms.

SUBACUTE SCLEROSING PANENCEPHALITIS

Subacute sclerosing panencephalitis (Dawson inclusion body encephalitis) is a rare progressive clinical syndrome characterized by cognitive decline, spasticity of limbs, and seizures. It occurs in children or young adults, months or years after an initial, early-age acute infection with measles. *Subacute sclerosing panencephalitis is thought to rep-*

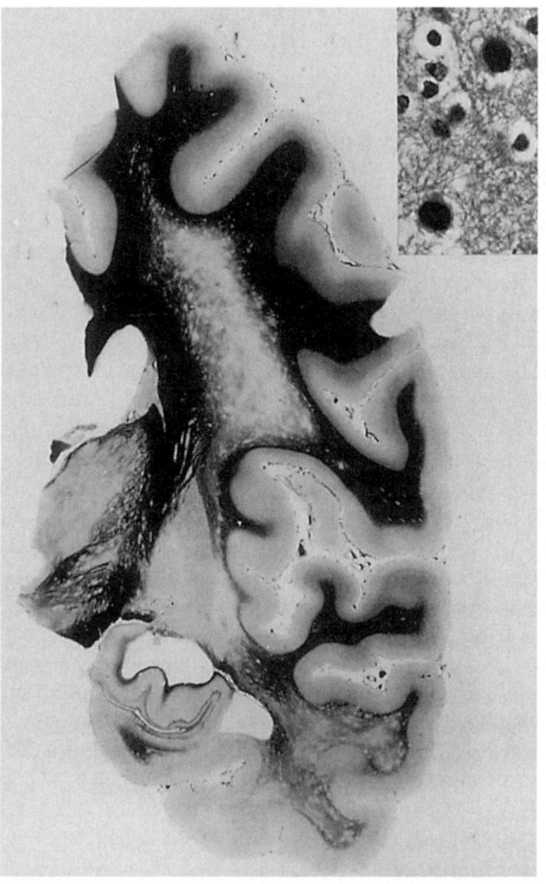

Figure 30–23 ■

Progressive multifocal leukoencephalopathy. Section stained for myelin showing irregular, poorly defined areas of demyelination, which become confluent in places. *Inset*, Enlarged oligodendrocyte nuclei stained for viral antigens.

resent persistent but nonproductive infection of the CNS by altered measles virus; changes in several viral genes have been associated with the disease. On microscopic examination, there is widespread gliosis and myelin degeneration; viral inclusions, largely within the nucleus, of oligodendrocytes and neurons; variable inflammation of white and gray matter; and neurofibrillary tangles.[71] Ultrastructural study shows that the inclusions contain nucleocapsids characteristic of measles, and measles virus antigen immunocytochemistry is positive. With widespread measles vaccination programs, the disease seems to have largely disappeared. However, there are still cases being reported around the world.

Fungal Meningoencephalitis

As with the systemic deep mycoses, fungal disease of the CNS is encountered primarily in immunocompromised patients in industrialized nations. The brain is usually involved only late in the disease, when there is widespread hematogenous dissemination of the fungus, most often *Candida albicans, Mucor, Aspergillus fumigatus*, and *Cryptococcus neoformans*. In endemic areas, pathogens such as *Histoplasma capsulatum*, *Coccidioides immitis*, and *Blastomyces dermatitidis* may involve the CNS after a primary pulmonary or cutaneous infection; again, this often follows immunosuppression.[72]

There are three basic patterns of fungal infection in the CNS: chronic meningitis, vasculitis, and parenchymal invasion. *Vasculitis* is most frequently seen with *Mucor* and *Aspergillus,* both of which have a marked predilection for invasion of blood vessel walls, but occasionally occurs with other organisms, such as *Candida*. The resultant vascular thrombosis produces infarction that is often strikingly hemorrhagic and that subsequently becomes septic from ingrowth of the causative fungus.

Parenchymal invasion, usually in the form of granulomas or abscesses, can occur with most of the fungi and often coexists with meningitis. The most commonly encountered are *Candida* and *Cryptococcus*. *Candida* usually produces multiple microabscesses, with or without giant cell granuloma formation. Although most fungi invade the brain by hematogenous dissemination, direct extension may also occur, particularly with *Mucor*, most commonly in diabetics with ketoacidosis.

Cryptococcal meningitis, observed now with increasing frequency in association with AIDS, may be fulminant and fatal in as little as 2 weeks or indolent, evolving over months or years. The CSF may have few cells but a high level of protein. The mucoid encapsulated yeasts can be visualized in the CSF by India ink preparations and in tissue sections by PAS and mucicarmine as well as silver stains.

MORPHOLOGY. With cryptococcal infection, the brain shows a chronic meningitis affecting the basal leptomeninges, which are opaque and thickened by reactive connective tissue and may obstruct the outflow of CSF from the foramina of Luschka and Magendie, giving rise to hydrocephalus. Sections of the brain disclose a gelatinous material within the subarachnoid space and small cysts within the parenchyma, which are especially prominent in the basal ganglia in the distribution of the lenticulostriate arteries. Parenchymal lesions consist of aggregates of organisms within expanded perivascular (Virchow-Robin) spaces associated with minimal or absent inflammation or gliosis. The meningeal infiltrates consist of chronic inflammatory cells and fibroblasts admixed with cryptococci. Well-formed granulomas are not seen ordinarily; in some cases, however, there is a marked chronic inflammatory and granulomatous reaction similar to that seen with *M. tuberculosis.*

Other Infectious Diseases of the Nervous System

Protozoal diseases (including malaria, toxoplasmosis, amebiasis, and trypanosomiasis), rickettsial infections (such as typhus and Rocky Mountain spotted fever), and metazoal diseases (especially cysticercosis and echinococcosis) may also involve the CNS and are discussed in Chapter 9.

Cerebral toxoplasmosis has assumed greater importance with the AIDS epidemic.[73] Infection of the brain by *Toxoplasma gondii* is one of the most common causes of neurologic symptoms and morbidity in patients with AIDS. The average incidence of CNS infection in most clinical and autopsy series ranges from 4% to 30%. The clinical symptoms are subacute, evolving during a 1- or 2-week period, and may be both focal and diffuse. CT and MRI studies may show multiple ring-enhancing lesions; however, this radiographic appearance is not pathognomonic, since similar findings may be associated with CNS lymphoma, tuberculosis, or fungal infections.

MORPHOLOGY. The brain shows abscesses, frequently multiple, most involving the cerebral cortex (near the gray-white junction) and deep gray nuclei, less often the cerebellum and brain stem, and rarely the spinal cord (Fig. 30–24). Acute lesions consist of central foci of necrosis with variable petechiae surrounded by acute and chronic inflammation, macrophage infiltration, and vascular proliferation. Both free tachyzoites and encysted bradyzoites may be found at the periphery of the necrotic foci. The organisms are usually seen on routine H&E or Giemsa stains, but they can be more easily recognized by immunocytochemical methods. The blood vessels in the vicinity of these lesions may show marked intimal proliferation or even frank vasculitis with fibrinoid necrosis and thrombosis. After treatment, the lesions consist of large, well-demarcated areas of coagulation necrosis surrounded by lipid-laden macrophages. Cysts and free tachyzoites can also be found adjacent to these lesions but may be considerably reduced in number if therapy has been effective. Chronic lesions consist of small cystic spaces containing small numbers of lipid- and hemosiderin-laden macrophages with surrounding gliosis. Organisms are difficult to detect in these older lesions.

Like CMV encephalitis, toxoplasmosis may also occur in the fetus. Primary maternal infection with toxoplasmosis, particularly if it occurs early in the pregnancy, may be followed by a cerebritis in the fetus, with the production of multifocal cerebral necrotizing lesions that may calcify, producing severe damage to the developing brain.

A rapidly fatal necrotizing encephalitis occurs with infection with *Naegleria* species, and a chronic granulomatous meningoencephalitis has been associated with infection with *Acanthamoeba.*[74] The amebae may sometimes be difficult to distinguish from histiocytes. Methenamine silver or PAS stains are helpful in visualizing the organisms, although definitive identification ultimately depends on combined immunofluorescence studies, morphology, and culture.

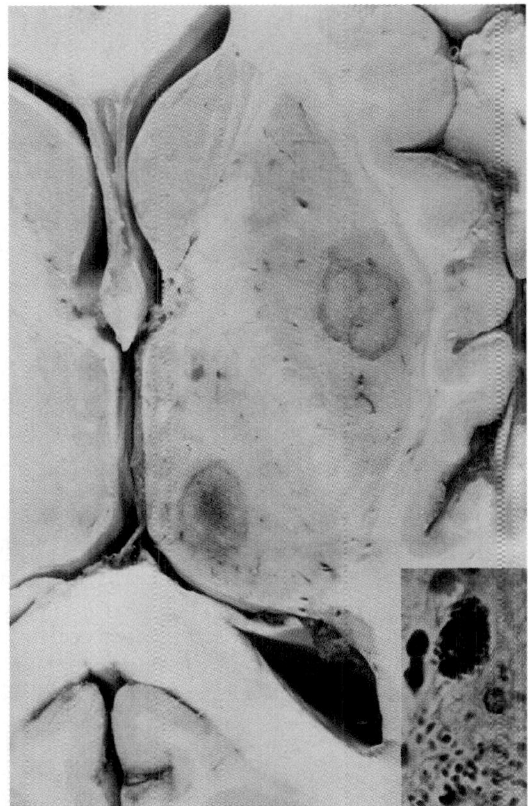

Figure 30–24 ■

Toxoplasma abscesses in the putamen and thalamus. *Inset, Toxoplasma* pseudocyst with bradyzoites and free tachyzoites.

TRANSMISSIBLE SPONGIFORM ENCEPHALOPATHIES (PRION DISEASES)

This group of diseases—which includes Creutzfeldt-Jakob disease (CJD), Gerstmann-Sträussler-Scheinker syndrome (GSS), fatal familial insomnia, and kuru in humans; scrapie in sheep and goats; mink transmissible encephalopathy; and bovine spongiform encephalopathy *(mad cow disease)*—share an etiologic basis that distinguishes them from other neurodegenerative and infectious diseases.[75] As the name implies, they are predominantly characterized by "spongiform change" caused by intracellular vacuoles in neural cells. Clinically, most of these patients develop progressive dementia. The most common type is CJD, which occurs in sporadic and familial forms. While differences exist among these disorders, *they are all associated with abnormal forms of a specific protein, termed prion protein* (PrP), *and are both infectious and transmissible.* For his discovery of prions, Prusiner won the 1997 Nobel Prize in Physiology and Medicine.

Pathogenesis and Molecular Genetics. PrP is a 30-kD normal cellular protein present in neurons. Disease occurs when the prion protein undergoes a conformational change from its normal α-helix isoform (PrP^c) to an abnormal β-pleated sheet isoform, usually termed either PrP^{sc} (for *scra-*

pie) or PrP^{res} (for protease *res*istant) (Table 30–1).[75a] Associated with the conformational change, the prion protein acquires relative resistance to digestion with proteases, such as proteinase K. The conformational change resulting in PrP^{sc} may occur *spontaneously at an extremely low rate* (resulting in sporadic cases) or at a *higher rate* if various mutations are present in PrP^{c}, such as occurs in familial forms of CJD and in GSS and fatal familial insomnia. PrP^{sc}, independent of the means by which it originates, then facilitates, in a cooperative fashion, comparable transformation of other PrP^{c} molecules (Fig. 30–25*A*). The infectious nature of PrP^{sc} molecules thus comes from their ability to corrupt the integrity of normal cellular components (Fig. 30–25*A*). Material prepared from sporadic cases of CJD or from the related familial disorders has been demonstrated to be infectious when it is inoculated into appropriate animal hosts.

The gene on chromosome 20, termed PRNP, which codes for PrP^{c} protein, has a single exon coding for the entire open reading frame and shows a high degree of conservation across species. Despite this conservation, infectious particles derived from one species are highly effective at transmitting disease in any host containing the gene for that species' normal protein. Engineered absence of a host *PRNP* gene renders an animal resistant to infection by PrP^{sc}.

Studies of the *PRNP* gene from cases of familial forms of these diseases have revealed interesting similarities and differences among them, which may shed some light on their variable clinical expression. In cases of familial CJD and GSS, a wide variety of disease-causing mutations have been identified. For example, in certain families with CJD and fatal familial insomnia, the disease is linked to a point mutation (D178N) in the *PRNP* gene (Fig. 30–25*B*). In addition, various polymorphisms have been found in the *PRNP* gene; of these, the Met/Val polymorphism at codon 129 has been found to influence disease pattern. The combination of Met at codon 129 in the same allele as the D178N mutation results in fatal familial insomnia, while a Val at codon 129 results in CJD.[76] Other influences of the codon 129 polymorphism have been observed in sporadic CJD: many patients with this disorder are homozygous at codon 129 for either Met or Val, while nearly half of control populations are heterozygous at this site, suggesting that heterozygosity at codon 129 is protective against development of the disease. Interestingly, this protection also applies against iatrogenic CJD.

Accumulation of PrP^{sc} in neural tissue appears to be the cause of the pathology in these diseases, but how this material causes the development of cytoplasmic vacuoles and eventual neuronal death is still unknown.

MORPHOLOGY. The progression of the dementia in CJD is usually so rapid that there is little, if any, macroscopic evidence of brain atrophy. On microscopic examination, the pathognomonic finding is a **spongiform** transformation of the cerebral cortex and, often, deep gray matter structures (caudate, putamen); this consists of a multifocal process that results in the uneven formation of small, apparently empty, microscopic vacuoles of varying sizes within the neuropil and sometimes in the perikaryon of neurons (Fig. 30–25*B*). In advanced cases, there is severe neuronal loss, reactive gliosis, and sometimes expansion of the vacuolated areas into cystlike spaces ("status spongiosus"). No inflammatory infiltrate is present. Electron microscopy shows the vacuoles to be intracytoplasmic and membrane bound in neuronal and glial processes. **Kuru plaques** are extracellular deposits of aggregated abnormal protein; they are Congo red–positive as well as PAS-positive and occur in the cerebellum in cases of GSS (Fig. 30–25*C*); they are present in abundance in the cerebral cortex in cases of variant CJD. Unlike other prion diseases, fatal familial insomnia does not show spongiform pathology. Instead, the most striking alteration is neuronal loss and reactive gliosis in the anterior ventral and dorsomedial nuclei of the thalamus; neuronal loss is also prominent in the inferior olivary nuclei.

Clinical Features

Creutzfeldt-Jakob Disease. CJD is a rare but well-characterized disease that manifests clinically as a rapidly progressive dementia. It is primarily sporadic (about 85% of cases) in its occurrence, with a worldwide annual incidence of about 1 per million; familial forms also exist. The disease has a peak incidence in the seventh decade. There are well-established cases of iatrogenic transmission, notably by corneal transplantation, deep implantation electrodes, and contaminated preparations of human growth hormone. The clinical picture is usually typical, with the initial subtle changes in memory and behavior followed by a rapidly progressive dementia, often with pronounced involuntary jerking muscle contractions on sudden stimulation (startle myoclonus). Signs of cerebellar dysfunction, usually manifested as ataxia, are present in a minority of patients. The disease is uniformly fatal, with an average duration of only 7 months, although a few patients have survived for several years.

Variant Creutzfeldt-Jakob Disease (vCJD). Starting in 1995, a series of cases with a CJD-like illness came to medical attention in the United Kingdom.[77] These new cases were clinically somewhat different from typical examples of CJD in several important respects: the disease affected young adults, behavioral disorders figured prominently in the early stages of the disease, and the neurologic syndrome progressed more slowly than what is usually observed in patients with CJD. When autopsy studies were performed, the neuropathologic findings and molecular features of these new cases were similar to CJD, suggesting a close relationship between the two illnesses. No alterations in the *PRNP* gene were found in any of these patients. The likely relationship between vCJD and human ingestion of beef from cows with bovine spongiform encephalopathy has raised serious public health issues.[78]

Gerstmann-Sträussler-Scheinker syndrome. GSS syn-

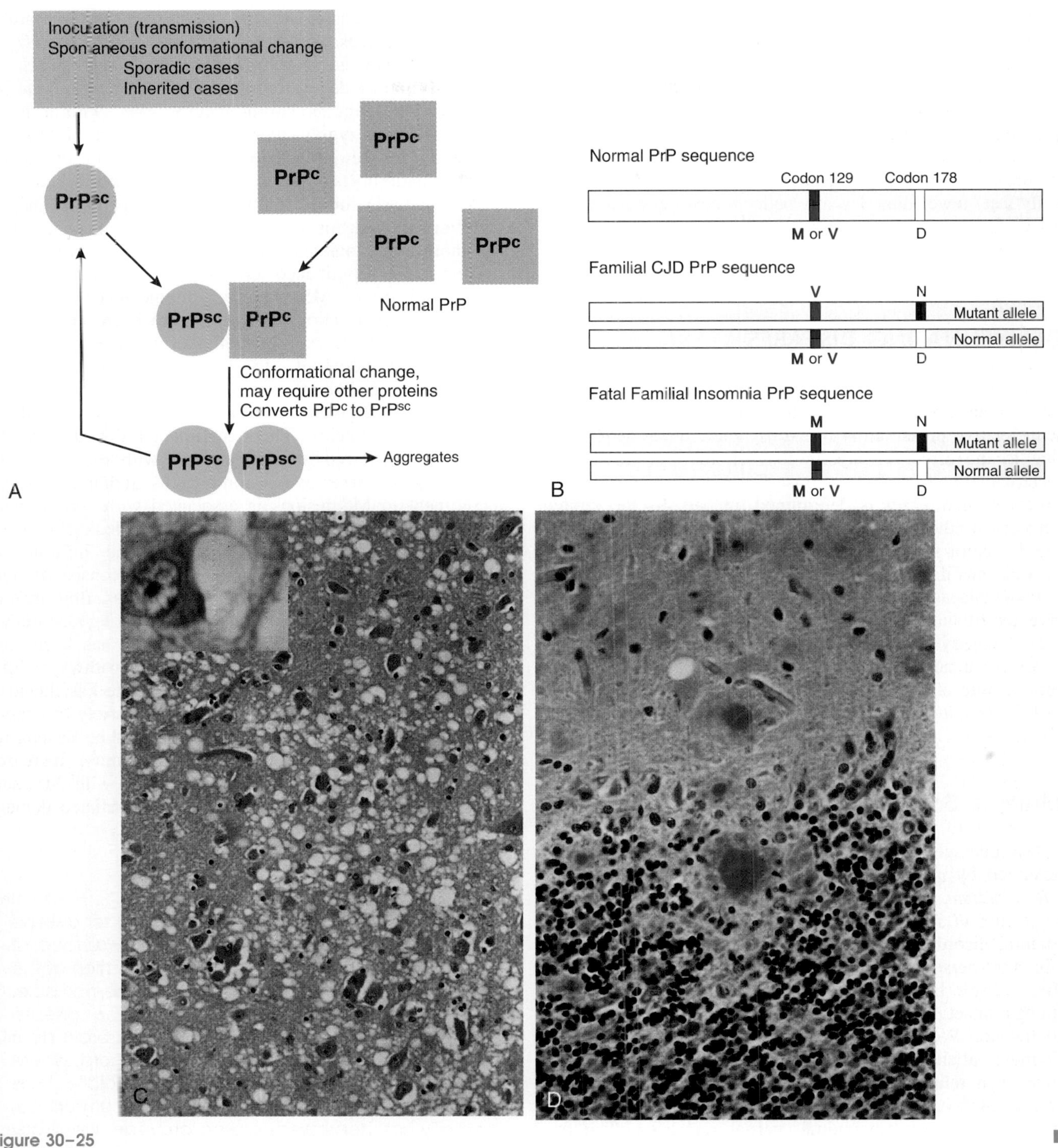

Figure 30–25

A, Proposed mechanism for the conversion of PrP^{c} through protein-protein interactions. The initiating molecules of PrP^{sc} may arise through inoculation (as in directly transmitted cases) or through an extremely low-rate spontaneous conformational change. The effect of the mutations in PrP (see *B*) is to increase the rate of the conformational change once PrP^{sc} is able to recruit and convert other molecules of PrP^{c} into the abnormal form of the protein. Although the model is drawn with no other proteins involved, it is possible that various other proteins play critical roles in the conversion of Prp^{c} to PrP^{sc}.

B, The basic structure of the PrP protein with important sites of mutation (codon 178) and disease-associated polymorphism (codon 129). In normal individuals, codon 178 encodes Asp (D) and codon 129 encodes either Met (M) or Val (V). In some familial forms of disease, the mutation changes codon 178 to Asn (D178N). When the allele containing the D178N mutation also has a Val at codon 129, the patient develops Creutzfeldt-Jakob disease (CJD). In contrast, when the D178N allele has Met at codon 129, the clinical disorder is fatal familial insomnia.

C, Histology of CJD showing spongiform change in the cerebral cortex. *Inset*, High magnification of neuron with vacuoles.

D, Cerebellar cortex showing *kuru plaques* (periodic acid–Schiff [PAS] stain) representing aggregated PrP^{sc}.

drome is an inherited disease with mutations of the *PRNP* gene that typically begins with a chronic cerebellar ataxia, followed by a progressive dementia. The clinical course is usually slower than that of CJD, with progression to death several years after the onset of symptoms.

Fatal Familial Insomnia. Fatal familial insomnia is named, in part, for the sleep disturbances that characterize its initial stages.[79] In the course of the illness, which typically lasts fewer than 3 years, patients develop other neurologic signs, such as ataxia, autonomic disturbances, stupor, and finally coma.

DEMYELINATING DISEASES

Demyelinating diseases of the CNS are acquired conditions characterized by a preferential damage to myelin, with relative preservation of axons. The clinical deficits are due to the effect of myelin loss on the transmission of electrical impulses along axons. The natural history of demyelinating diseases is determined, in part, by the limited capacity of the CNS to regenerate normal myelin and by the degree of secondary damage to axons that occurs as the disease runs its course.

Other disease processes can involve myelin. In progressive multifocal leukoencephalopathy, JC virus infection of oligodendrocytes results in loss of myelin (see infections section). In addition, there are inherited disorders that affect myelin synthesis and turnover. These disorders are termed *leukodystrophies* and are discussed with metabolic disorders.

Multiple Sclerosis

Multiple sclerosis (MS) is a demyelinating disorder characterized by *distinct episodes of neurologic deficits, separated in time, attributable to white matter lesions that are separated in space.* It is the most common of the demyelinating disorders, having a prevalence of approximately 1 per 1000 persons in most of the United States and Europe. The disease becomes clinically apparent at any age, although onset in childhood or after age 50 years is relatively rare. Women are affected twice as often as are men. In most patients with MS, the clinical course of the illness evolves as relapsing and remitting flare-up episodes of neurologic deficit during variable intervals of time (days to weeks), followed by gradual, partial remission. The frequency of relapses tends to decrease during the course of time, but there is a steady neurologic deterioration in a subset of patients.

Pathogenesis. The etiology and pathogenesis are not established, although environmental, genetic, and immune factors have been implicated. Different populations have distinct rates of MS, with some data showing an increase in incidence with distance away from the equator; however, groups living in relative proximity may have divergent rates. Individuals take on the relative risk of the environment in which they spent their first 15 years.[80,81] A transmissible agent has been proposed, but all attempts to identify a well-characterized virus have been unsuccessful.[82] Genetic influences are also clearly evident. The risk of developing MS is 15-fold higher when the disease is present in a first-degree relative. The concordance rate for monozygotic twins is approximately 25%, with a much lower rate for dizygotic twins. Genetic linkage of MS susceptibility to the DR2 extended haplotype of the major histocompatibility complex is also well established. The molecular basis for the influence of this particular haplotype on the risk of developing MS is unknown; other chromosome regions may be involved as well.

Given the prominence of chronic inflammatory cells within and around MS plaques, immune mechanisms that underlie the destruction of myelin have been the focus of much investigation. Experimental allergic encephalomyelitis is an animal model of MS in which demyelination and inflammation occur after immunization of animals with myelin, various myelin proteins, or certain peptides from these myelin proteins. The experimental disorder can be passively transferred to other animals with use of T cells that recognize these myelin components. Inflammatory cell recruitment to MS lesions is associated with certain cytokines and with the up-regulation of various leukocyte adhesion molecules on endothelial cells. The infiltrate in plaques and surrounding regions of brain consist of both T cells (CD8+ and CD4+) and macrophages. Both macrophages and T cells are thought to induce oligodendrocyte injury. Injury by cytotoxic CD4+ T cells has been suggested to occur through the Fas/Fas ligand pathway: oligodendrocytes in MS lesions express Fas while Fas ligand is present on the infiltrating T cells. From a variety of experiments, it is clear that development of MS-like lesions requires factors beyond cell-mediated immunity. Increased CSF immunoglobulin is found in patients with MS, and there is evidence for a role of antibody-mediated damage involving myelin oligodendroglial protein.

MORPHOLOGY. Since MS is a white matter disease and gray matter covers much of the surface of the hemispheres, macroscopic examination of the outer aspect of the cerebral gyri is unremarkable. On the other hand, evidence of the disease might be found on the surface of the brain stem (e.g., basis pontis) or along the spinal cord, where myelinated fiber tracts course superficially; here lesions appear as multiple, well-circumscribed, somewhat depressed, glassy, gray-tan, irregularly shaped **plaques,** both on external examination and on section (Fig. 30–26). In the fresh state, these have firmer consistency than the surrounding white matter **(sclerosis).** Plaques can be found throughout the white matter of the neuraxis; they may also extend into the gray matter structures as these often have myelinated fibers running through them, although their recognition within these regions is more difficult. The size of lesions varies considerably, from small foci recognizable only at microscopic examination to confluent plaques that involve large portions of the

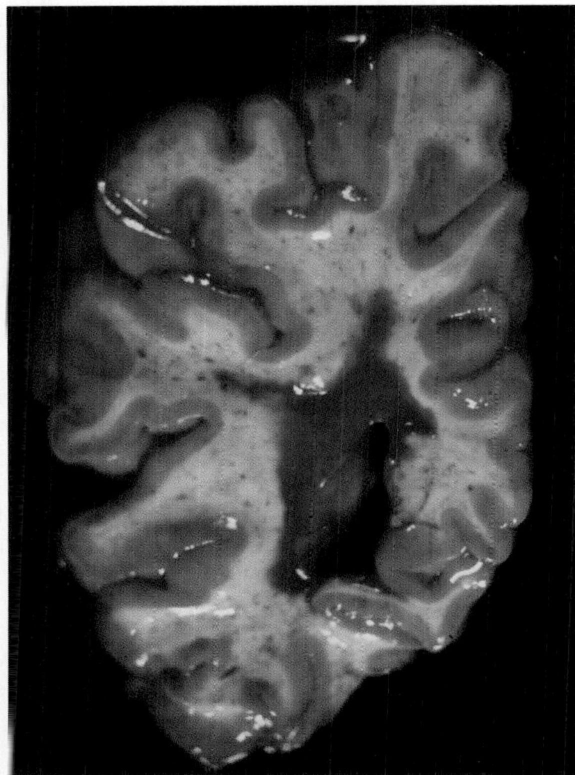

Figure 30–26

Multiple sclerosis. Section of fresh brain showing brown plaque around occipital horn of the lateral ventricle.

centrum semiovale. Plaques commonly occur beside the lateral ventricles and may be demonstrated to follow the course of paraventricular veins when the surface of the ventricle is inspected en face. They are also frequent in the optic nerves and chiasm, brain stem ascending and descending fiber tracts, cerebellum, and spinal cord.

The lesions have sharply defined borders at the microscopic level (Fig. 30–27*A*). In an **active plaque,** there is evidence of ongoing myelin breakdown with abundant macrophages containing lipid-rich, PAS-positive debris. Inflammatory cells, including both lymphocytes and monocytes, are present, mostly as perivascular cuffs, especially at the outer edge of the lesion (Fig. 30–27*B*). Small active lesions are often centered on small veins. Within a plaque, there is relative preservation of axons and depletion of oligodendrocytes. In time, astrocytes undergo reactive changes. As lesions become quiescent, there is a diminution of the inflammatory cell infiltrate and of macrophages. Within the center of an **inactive plaque,** little to no myelin is found and there is a reduction in the number of oligodendrocyte nuclei; instead, astrocytic proliferation and gliosis are prominent. Axons can be demonstrated in old gliotic plaques showing severe depletion of myelin, although they are also greatly diminished in number (Fig. 30–27*C*).

In some MS plaques—**shadow plaques**—the border between normal and affected white matter is not sharply circumscribed. In this type of lesion, some abnormally thinned-out myelin sheaths can be demonstrated, especially at the outer edges. This phenomenon has been interpreted either as evidence of partial and incomplete myelin loss or as remyelination by surviving oligodendrocytes. Abnormally myelinated fibers have also been observed at the edges of typical plaques. Although these histologic findings suggest a limited potential for remyelination in the CNS, the remaining axons within most MS plaques remain unmyelinated. The pathologic findings are remarkably similar regardless of the clinical tempo of disease progression. Autopsy studies and radiologic studies using MRI have demonstrated that subclinical forms of the disease exist and that some plaques may be clinically silent even in symptomatic patients.

Clinical Features. Although MS lesions can occur anywhere in the CNS and, as a consequence, may induce a wide range of clinical manifestations, certain patterns of neurologic symptoms and signs are commonly observed. Unilateral visual impairment during the course of a few days, due to involvement of the optic nerve *(optic neuritis, retrobulbar neuritis),* is a frequent initial manifestation of MS. However, only some patients (10% to 50%, depending on the population studied) with optic neuritis go on to develop MS. Involvement of the brain stem produces cranial nerve signs, ataxia, nystagmus, and internuclear ophthalmoplegia from interruption of the fibers of the medial longitudinal fasciculus. Spinal cord lesions give rise to motor and sensory impairment of trunk and limbs, spasticity, and difficulties with the voluntary control of bladder function.

Examination of the CSF in MS patients shows a mildly elevated protein level, and in one third of cases there is moderate pleocytosis. The proportion of gamma globulin is increased, and most MS patients show *oligoclonal bands.* This increase in CSF immunoglobulin is the result of proliferation of B cells within the nervous system; the target epitopes of these antibodies are widely variable.

Multiple Sclerosis Variants

Some individuals, especially Asians, develop a demyelinating disease similar to MS with presenting symptoms of bilateral optic neuritis and prominent spinal cord involvement. This disease is referred to as *neuromyelitis optica* or *Devic disease*. It may be rapidly and relentlessly progressive (in approximately 20% of cases), follow a relapsing-remitting course, or manifest as a single episode without subsequent relapses. The lesions in Devic disease are similar in histologic appearance to MS, although they are considerably more destructive and gray matter involvement of

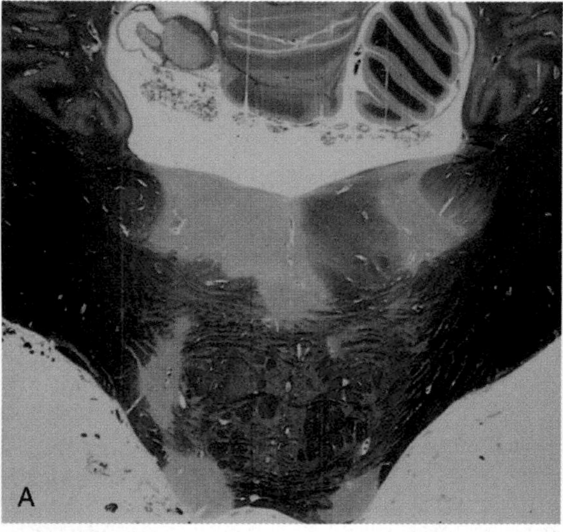

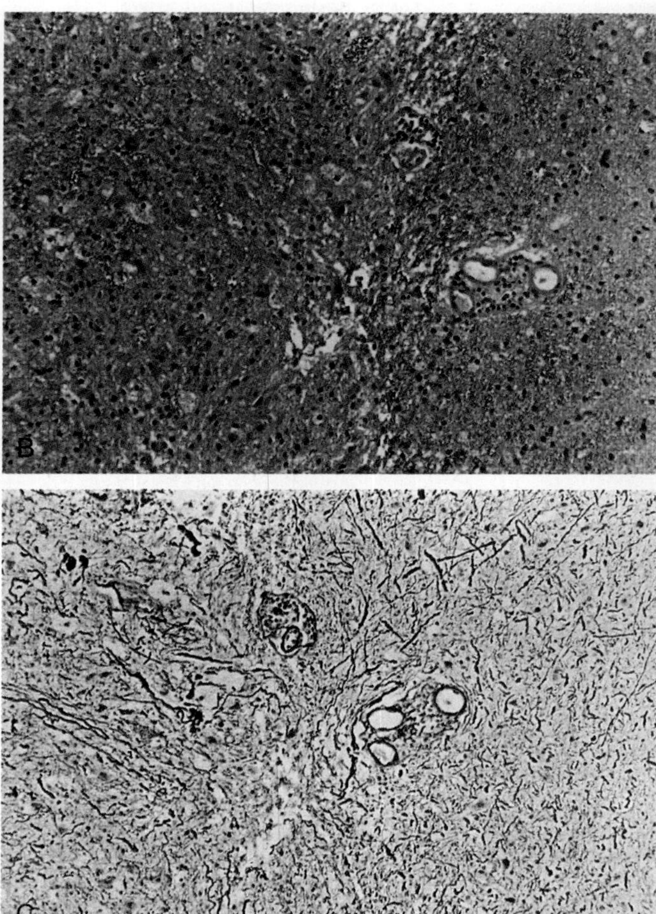

Figure 30–27

Multiple sclerosis. *A*, Unstained regions of demyelination (MS plaques) around the fourth ventricle. (Luxol fast blue PAS stain for myelin). *B*, Myelin-stained section shows the sharp edge of a demyelinated plaque and perivascular lymphocytic cuffs. *C*, The same lesion stained for axons shows relative preservation.

the spinal cord can be striking. Another variant, *acute MS (Marburg form),* tends to occur in young individuals and is characterized clinically by a fulminant course during a period of several months. On pathologic examination, the plaques are large and numerous, and there is widespread destruction of myelin with some axonal loss.

Acute Disseminated Encephalomyelitis and Acute Necrotizing Hemorrhagic Encephalomyelitis

Acute disseminated encephalomyelitis (ADEM, perivenous encephalomyelitis) is a monophasic demyelinating disease that follows either a viral infection or, rarely, a viral immunization. Symptoms typically develop a week or two after the antecedent infection and include evidence of diffuse brain involvement with headache, lethargy, and coma rather than focal findings, as seen in MS. Symptoms progress rapidly, with a fatal outcome in as many as 20% of cases; in the remaining patients, there is complete recovery.

Acute necrotizing hemorrhagic encephalomyelitis (ANHE, acute hemorrhagic leukoencephalitis of Weston Hurst) is a fulminant syndrome of CNS demyelination, typically affecting young adults and children. The illness is almost invariably preceded by a recent episode of upper respiratory infection; sometimes it is due to *Mycoplasma pneumoniae*, but often it is of indeterminate cause. The disease is fatal in many patients, but some have survived with minimal residual symptoms.

MORPHOLOGY. In ADEM, macroscopic examination of the brain shows only grayish discoloration around white matter vessels. On microscopic examination, myelin loss with relative preservation of axons can be found throughout the white matter. In the early stages of the disease, polymorphonuclear leukocytes can be found within the lesions; later, mononuclear infiltrates predominate. The breakdown of myelin is associated with the accumulation of lipid-laden macrophages.

ANHE shows histologic similarities with ADEM, including perivenular distribution of demyelination and widespread dissemination throughout the CNS (sometimes with extensive confluence of lesions). However, the lesions are much more devastating than those of ADEM and include destruction of small blood vessels, disseminated necrosis of white and gray matter with acute hemorrhage, fibrin deposition, abundant neutrophils, and scattered lymphocytes recognizable in less severely damaged areas and in foci of demyelination.

The lesions of ADEM are similar to those induced by immunization of animals with myelin components or with early rabies vaccines that had been prepared from brains of infected animals. This has suggested that ADEM may represent an acute autoimmune reaction to myelin and that ANHE may represent a hyperacute variant, although no inciting antigens have been identified.

Other Diseases with Demyelination

Central pontine myelinolysis is characterized by loss of myelin (with some preservation of axons and neuronal cell bodies) in a roughly symmetric pattern involving the basis pontis and portions of the pontine tegmentum but sparing the periventricular and subpial regions. Lesions may be found more rostrally; it is extremely rare for the process to extend below the pontomedullary junction. Extrapontine lesions in the supratentorial compartment occur in rare instances. The clinical presentation of central pontine myelinolysis is that of a rapidly evolving quadriplegia; radiologic imaging studies localize the lesion to the basis pontis. It occurs in a variety of clinical settings including alcoholism, severe electrolyte or osmolar imbalance, and orthotopic liver transplantation. The condition is believed to be caused by rapid correction of hyponatremia[83]; however, alternative pathogenetic hypotheses attribute the disorder to extreme serum hyperosmolarity or other metabolic imbalance.

Marchiafava-Bignami disease is a rare disorder of myelin characterized by relatively symmetric damage to the central fibers of the corpus callosum and anterior commissure.

DEGENERATIVE DISEASES

These are diseases of gray matter characterized principally by the *progressive loss of neurons* with associated secondary changes in white matter tracts. Two other general characteristics bring them together as a group. First, the pattern of neuronal loss is *selective, affecting one or more groups of neurons, while leaving others intact*. Second, *the diseases arise without any clear inciting event in patients without previous neurologic deficits*. The neuropathologic findings observed in the degenerative diseases differ greatly: in some there are intracellular abnormalities with some degree of specificity (e.g., Lewy bodies, neurofibrillary tangles), while in others there is only loss of the affected neurons. It is convenient to group the degenerative diseases according to the anatomic regions of the CNS that are *primarily* affected. Some degenerative diseases have prominent involvement of the cerebral cortex, such as Alzheimer disease; others are more restricted to subcortical areas and may present with movement disorders such as tremors and dyskinesias.

Degenerative Diseases Affecting the Cerebral Cortex

The major cortical degenerative disease is *Alzheimer disease*, and its principal clinical manifestation is *dementia*, that is, progressive loss of cognitive function independent of the state of attention. There are many other causes of dementia, including *Pick disease*, vascular disease (multi-infarct dementia), diffuse Lewy body disease, Creutzfeldt-Jakob disease, and neurosyphilis. *Dementia is not part of normal aging and always represents a pathologic process.*

ALZHEIMER DISEASE

Alzheimer disease is the most common cause of dementia in the elderly. The disease usually becomes clinically apparent as insidious impairment of higher intellectual function, with alterations in mood and behavior. Later, progressive disorientation, memory loss, and aphasia indicate severe cortical dysfunction, and eventually, in 5 to 10 years, the patient becomes profoundly disabled, mute, and immobile. Patients rarely become symptomatic before 50 years of age, but the progressive increase in the incidence of the disease in the succeeding decades has given rise to major medical, social, and economic problems in countries with a growing number of elderly individuals. When considered by age groups, the rates are 3% for 65 to 74 years, 19% for 75 to 84 years, and 47% for 85 years or more.[84] Most cases are sporadic, although at least 5% to 10% of cases are familial. Pathologic changes identical to those observed in Alzheimer disease occur in almost all patients with trisomy 21 who survive beyond 45 years, and a decline in cognition can be clinically demonstrated in many. Although pathologic examination of brain tissue remains necessary for the definitive diagnosis of Alzheimer disease, the combination of clinical assessment and modern radiologic methods allows accurate diagnosis in 80% to 90% of cases.

MORPHOLOGY. Macroscopic examination of the brain shows a variable degree of cortical atrophy with widening of the cerebral sulci that is most pronounced in the frontal, temporal, and parietal lobes. With significant atrophy, there is compensatory ventricular enlargement secondary to loss of parenchyma (Fig. 30–28). The major microscopic abnormalities of Alzheimer disease are **neurofibrillary tangles, senile (neuritic) plaques, and amyloid angiopathy.** All of these may be present to a lesser extent in the brains of elderly nondemented individuals. The diagnosis of Alzheimer disease is based on a combination of clinical and patho-

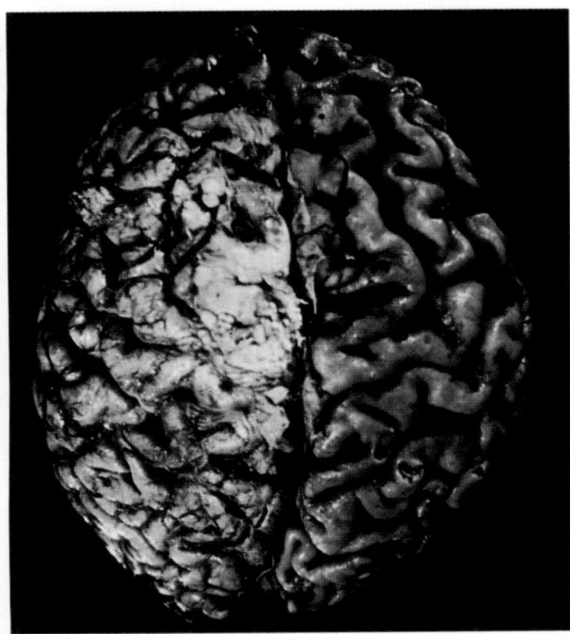

Figure 30–28

Alzheimer disease with cortical atrophy most evident on the right, where meninges have been removed. (Courtesy of Dr. E.P. Richardson, Jr, Massachusetts General Hospital, Boston, MA.)

logic features. Several different methods have been proposed, which include evaluation of different regions of the brain and various methods for estimating the frequency of plaques and tangles.[85–88]

Neurofibrillary tangles are bundles of filaments in the cytoplasm of the neurons that displace or encircle the nucleus. They often have an elongated "flame" shape; in some cells, the basket weave of fibers around the nucleus takes on a rounded contour (globose tangles). They are visible as basophilic fibrillary structures with H&E staining but are dramatically demonstrated by silver (Bielschowsky) staining (Fig. 30–29*A* and *B*). They are commonly found in cortical neurons, especially in the entorhinal cortex, as well as in other sites such as pyramidal cells of the hippocampus, the amygdala, the basal forebrain, and the raphe nuclei. Neurofibrillary tangles are insoluble and apparently difficult to proteolyze in vivo, thus remaining visible in tissue sections as "ghost" or "tombstone" tangles long after the death of the parent neuron.

Ultrastructurally, neurofibrillary tangles are composed predominantly of paired helical filaments along with some straight filaments that appear to have comparable composition. A major component of paired helical filaments is abnormally hyperphosphorylated forms of the protein **tau**, an axonal microtubule-associated protein that enhances microtubule assembly. Other antigens include MAP2 (another microtubule-associated protein), ubiquitin, and amyloid β-peptide (Aβ; see later). Paired helical filaments are also found in the dystrophic neurites that form the outer portions of neuritic plaques and in axons coursing through the affected gray matter—**neuropil threads.**

Although they are characteristic of Alzheimer disease, neurofibrillary tangles are not specific to this condition, being also found in progressive supranuclear palsy, postencephalitic Parkinson disease, and the amyotrophic lateral sclerosis–parkinsonism/dementia complex of Guam. They probably represent the endpoint of a number of different cellular pathophysiologic processes. The neurofibrillary tangle and its major components are a manifestation of abnormal organization of cytoskeletal elements in neurons of patients with Alzheimer disease.

Neuritic plaques are focal, spherical collections of dilated, tortuous, silver-staining neuritic processes (dystrophic neurites) surrounding a central amyloid core, often surrounded by clear halo (Fig. 30–29*C*). Neuritic plaques range in size from 20 to 200 μm in diameter; microglial cells and reactive astrocytes are present at their periphery. Plaques can be found in the hippocampus and amygdala as well as in the neocortex, although there is usually relative sparing of primary motor and sensory cortices (this also applies for neurofibrillary tangles). Comparable lesions can also be found in the corresponding regions of the brains of aged, nonhuman primates. The dystrophic neurites contain paired helical filaments as well as synaptic vesicles and abnormal mitochondria. The amyloid core, which can be stained by Congo red and by Bielschowsky silver methods, contains several abnormal proteins. **The dominant component of the plaque core is Aβ, a peptide of approximately 40- to 43-amino acid residues derived from a larger molecule, amyloid precursor protein (APP).** Other proteins—including components of the complement cascade, α1-antichymotrypsin, apolipoproteins, and a protein termed non-amyloid component of plaques (NACP)—are present in less abundance. Immunostaining for Aβ demonstrates the existence, in some patients, of amyloid peptide deposits of lesions lacking the surrounding neuritic reaction. These lesions, termed **diffuse plaques,** are found in superficial portions of cerebral cortex as well as in basal ganglia and cerebellar cortex. Commonly, when diffuse plaques are found in the cerebral cortex, they appear to be centered on small vessels or on clusters of neurons. Diffuse plaques may represent an early stage of neuritic plaque development: they may be present in the brains of individuals with clear-cut findings of Alzheimer disease or in isolation.

Amyloid angiopathy is an almost invariable accompaniment of Alzheimer disease; however, it can also be found in brains of individuals without

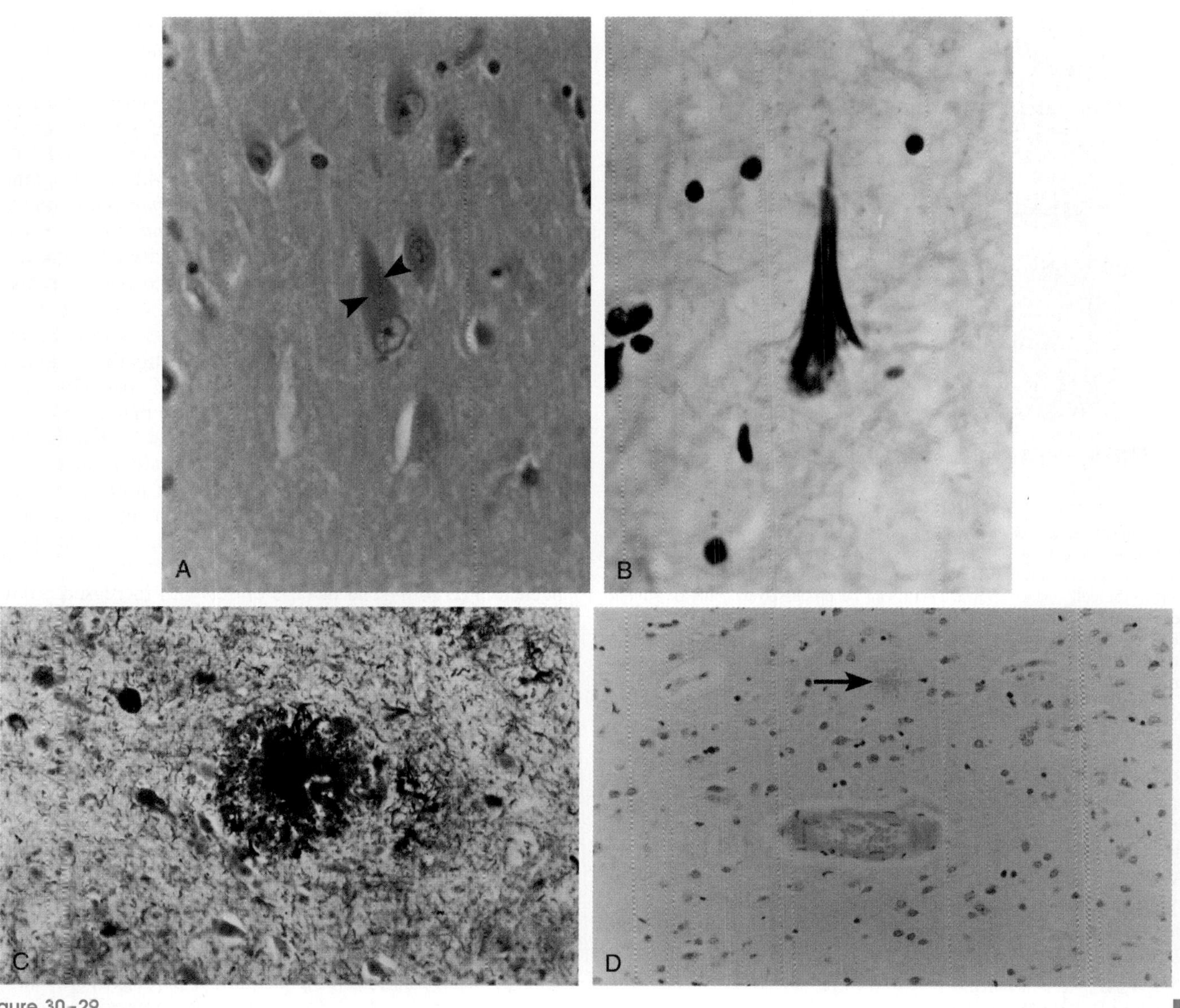

Figure 30-29

Alzheimer disease. *A*, Neurofibrillary tangles (*arrowheads*) are present within the neurons (H&E). *B*, Silver stain showing a neurofibrillary tangle within the neuronal cytoplasm. *C*, Neuritic plaque with a rim of dystrophic neurites surrounding an amyloid core. *D*, Congo red staining of the cerebral cortex showing amyloid deposition in the blood vessels and the amyloid core of the neuritic plaque (*arrow*).

Alzheimer disease (Fig. 30-29*D*). Vascular amyloid is derived from the same precursor as the amyloid cores of plaques (APP).

Granulovacuolar degeneration is the formation of small (5 μm in diameter), clear intraneuronal cytoplasmic vacuoles, each of which contains an argyrophilic granule. While it occurs with normal aging, it is most commonly found in great abundance in hippocampus and olfactory bulb in Alzheimer disease. **Hirano bodies**, found especially in Alzheimer disease, are elongated, glassy, eosinophilic bodies consisting of paracrystalline arrays of beaded filaments, with actin as their major component. They are found most commonly along hippocampal pyramidal cells.

Pathogenesis and Molecular Genetics. The pathogenesis of Alzheimer disease as well as the temporal and pathophysiologic relationships between the different morphologic changes described is being intensively investigated. While there is some disagreement regarding the best histologic correlate of dementia in patients with Alzheimer disease, the number of neurofibrillary tangles correlates better with clinical impairment than does the number of neuritic plaques. Biochemical markers that have been correlated with the degree of dementia include loss of choline acetyltransferase, synaptophysin immunoreactivity, and amyloid burden.

The Role of Amyloid (Aβ). Although amyloid-rich plaques correlate less well with dementia and clinical disease than do neurofibrillary tangles, most current work has

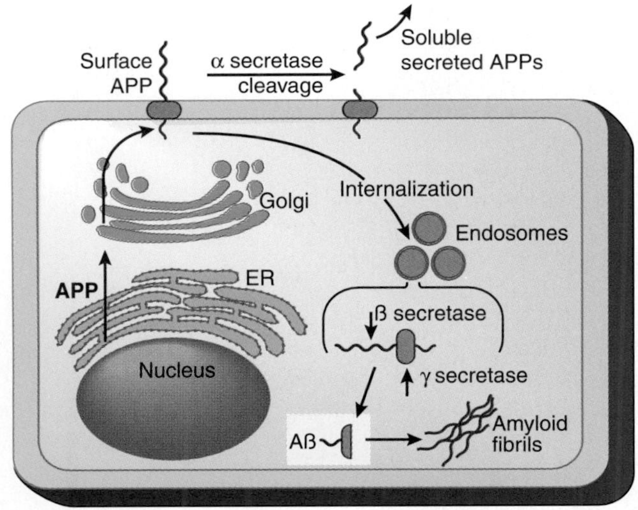

Figure 30–30

Amyloid precursor protein (APP) is a transmembrane protein: cellular trafficking of APP involves synthesis and maturation of APP through the endoplasmic reticulum (ER) and Golgi apparatus, with eventual expression in the cell surface. Surface APP can be processed to generate soluble secreted APP_s through α-secretase cleavage, or reinternalized into an endosomal compartment. Generation of Aβ by β- and γ-secretases may occur in the endosomal and other compartments. Aβ fragments form amyloid fibrils.

focused on the role of amyloid because of its relative specificity for Alzheimer disease and because of evidence from familial Alzheimer disease. The Aβ amyloid that is deposited in Alzheimer disease is derived from the larger APP. APP is a protein of uncertain cellular function that is synthesized with a single transmembrane domain and expressed on the cell surface (Fig. 30–30). A soluble form of APP can be released from the cell surface by proteolytic cleavage, by an enzyme termed α-secretase; these APP molecules cannot give rise to the Aβ fragment (Fig. 30–30). However, surface APP can also be endocytosed and then undergoes various forms of processing within distinct cellular compartments. One specific form results in the formation of the Aβ peptides; these are 40– to 43–amino acid fragments generated through cleavage at a site N-terminal to the start of the transmembrane domain by an enzyme called β-secretase and cleavage within the transmembrane domain by γ-secretase. There is mild variation in the endpoints of the proteolysis—the two predominant species generated have 40 (Aβ40) and 42 (Aβ42) amino acids. *The Aβ peptides aggregate and generate the amyloid that is found in the brain parenchyma and around vessels.* In vitro evidence suggests that Aβ and its aggregates are neurotoxic and thus may contribute to the pathogenesis of dementia.

A small minority of Alzheimer disease is familial (familial Alzheimer disease), and genetic investigations suggest a role for APP and its processing to Aβ peptides in the pathogenesis of these cases.[89,90] The gene that encodes APP is on chromosome 21, and several forms of familial Alzheimer disease have been linked to mutations in the *APP* gene (Table 30–2). These mutations are immediately outside of the Aβ region of the APP molecule and lead to increased production of Aβ. Furthermore, the development of Alzheimer disease in individuals with trisomy 21 has been related to a gene dosage effect with increased production of APP and subsequently Aβ. Another point mutation in *APP,* found in several Dutch pedigrees, gives rise to the accelerated deposition of amyloid in cerebral vessels with an increased risk of bleeding as well as dementia, a disease termed hereditary cerebral hemorrhage with amyloidosis (HCHWA-Dutch).

Presenilins. Two other genetic loci linked to early-onset familial Alzheimer disease have been identified on chromosomes 14 and 1 (Table 30–2); these probably account for the majority of early-onset familial Alzheimer disease pedigrees. The genes on these two chromosomes encode highly related intracellular proteins, *presenilin-1* and *presenilin-2.*[91] Two mechanisms are proposed for the role of presenilins. First, mutations in the presenilins increase production of Aβ, especially Aβ42, providing a pathogenetic link for the deposition of amyloid. Second, the presenilins are also targets for cleavage by caspase proteases activated during apoptosis, suggesting a role for these proteins in neuronal cell death.[92]

Table 30–2. GENETICS OF ALZHEIMER DISEASE

Chromosome	Gene	Mutations/Alleles	Consequences
21	Amyloid precursor protein (*APP*)	• Single missense mutations Double missense mutation Trisomy 21 (gene dosage effect)	• Early-onset FAD Increased Aβ production
14	Presenilin-1 (*PS1*)	• Missense mutations Splice site mutations	• Early-onset FAD Increased Aβ production
1	Presenilin-2 (*PS2*)	• Missense mutations	• Early-onset FAD Increased Aβ production
19	Apolipoprotein E (*APOE*)	• Allele ϵ4	• Increased *risk* of development of AD Decreased age at onset of AD

AD, Alzheimer disease; FAD, familial Alzheimer disease.

Apolipoprotein E. Distinct from these loci in which mutations cause Alzheimer disease, one allele ($\epsilon4$) of the apolipoprotein E (ApoE) gene on chromosome 19 increases the risk of Alzheimer disease and lowers the age at onset of the disease. Individuals with the $\epsilon4$ allele are overrepresented in populations of patients with Alzheimer disease compared with control populations. ApoE can bind $A\beta$ and is present in plaques, but how this allele increases the risk for Alzheimer disease is not established. A mutation in α_2-macroglobulin has also been found to increase the risk of Alzheimer disease.[129]

Clinical Features. The course of Alzheimer disease is slow but relentless, with a symptomatic course running more than 10 years. Initial symptoms are forgetfulness and other memory disturbances; with progression of the disease, other symptoms emerge including language deficits, loss of mathematical skills, and loss of learned motor skills. In the final stages of Alzheimer disease, patients may become incontinent, mute, and unable to walk. Intercurrent disease, often pneumonia, is usually the terminal event for these individuals.

PICK DISEASE

Pick disease (lobar atrophy) is a rare, distinct, progressive dementia characterized clinically by early onset of behavioral changes together with alterations in personality (frontal lobe signs) and language disturbances (temporal lobe signs).

MORPHOLOGY. The brain invariably shows a pronounced although frequently asymmetric atrophy of the frontal and temporal lobes with conspicuous sparing of the posterior two thirds of the superior temporal gyrus and only rare involvement of either the parietal or occipital lobe. The atrophy can be severe, reducing the gyri to a thin wafer ("knife-edge" appearance). This pattern of **lobar atrophy** is often prominent enough to distinguish Pick disease from Alzheimer disease on macroscopic examination. In addition to the localized cortical atrophy, there is also often bilateral atrophy of the caudate nucleus and putamen.

On microscopic examination, neuronal loss is most severe in the outer three layers of the cortex. Some of the surviving neurons show a characteristic swelling **(Pick cells)** or contain **Pick bodies,** which are cytoplasmic, round to oval, filamentous inclusions that are only weakly eosinophilic but stain strongly with silver methods. Ultrastructurally, these are composed of neurofilaments, vesiculated endoplasmic reticulum, and paired helical filaments that are immunocytochemically similar to those found in Alzheimer disease. Unlike the neurofibrillary tangles of Alzheimer disease, Pick bodies do not survive the death of their host neuron and do not remain as markers of the disease. In some cases with typical clinical history and macroscopic findings of lobar atrophy, it is not possible to find either Pick cells or Pick bodies; nonetheless, these cases are classified as Pick disease.

Degenerative Diseases of Basal Ganglia and Brain Stem

Diseases affecting these regions of the brain are frequently associated with movement disorders, including rigidity, abnormal posturing, and chorea. In general, they can be categorized as manifesting either a reduction of voluntary movement or an abundance of involuntary movement. The basal ganglia, and especially the nigrostriatal pathway, play an important role in the system of positive and negative regulatory synaptic pathways that serve to modulate feedback from the thalamus to the motor cortex. The most important disorders in this group are those associated with parkinsonism and Huntington chorea.

PARKINSONISM

Parkinsonism is a clinical syndrome characterized by diminished facial expression, stooped posture, slowness of voluntary movement, festinating gait (progressively shortened, accelerated steps), rigidity, and a "pill-rolling" tremor. *This type of motor disturbance is seen in a number of conditions that have in common damage to the nigrostriatal dopaminergic system.* Parkinsonism may also be induced by drugs that affect this system, particularly dopamine antagonists and toxins. The principal diseases that involve the nigrostriatal system are

- Idiopathic Parkinson disease
- Progressive supranuclear palsy
- Corticobasal degeneration
- Multiple system atrophy, a group of disorders that includes striatonigral degeneration, olivopontocerebellar atrophy, and the Shy-Drager syndrome
- Postencephalitic parkinsonism, which was observed in the wake of the influenza pandemic that occurred between 1914 and 1918 and is now vanishingly rare

IDIOPATHIC PARKINSON DISEASE (PARALYSIS AGITANS)

This diagnosis is made in patients with progressive parkinsonism in the absence of a toxic or other known underlying etiology. The disease appears in later life. Although there is no evidence for a genetic component in most cases, it can show autosomal dominant inheritance. In addition to the movement disorder, there are other less well-characterized changes in mental function, which may include dementia.

Pathogenesis. The dopaminergic neurons of the substantia nigra project to the striatum, and their degeneration in Parkinson disease is associated with a reduction in the striatal dopamine content. The severity of the motor syndrome is proportional to the dopamine deficiency, which can, at least in part, be corrected by replacement therapy with L-dopa (the immediate precursor of dopamine) since the striatum itself is not the primary target of the disease; unlike dopamine, L-dopa is able to cross the blood-brain barrier. Treatment does not, however, reverse the morphologic changes or arrest the progress of the disease, and with progression, drug therapy tends to become less effective and symptoms become more difficult to manage.

An acute parkinsonian syndrome and destruction of neurons in the substantia nigra follows exposure to MPTP (1-methyl-4-phenyl-1,2,3,6-tetrahydropyridine), a contaminant in the illicit synthesis of psychoactive meperidine analogs. Action by monoamine oxidase B is required for the toxicity of MPTP. Clinical trials with inhibitors of this enzyme show symptomatic improvement in patients with early-stage IPD.

In some pedigrees with autosomal dominant inheritance, mutations in the gene for α-synuclein have been linked to IPD.[93] This protein is present in presynaptic terminals and is the precursor protein for non-amyloid component of plaques, the non-amyloid protein found in plaques of Alzheimer disease (see earlier). In IPD it is found in the characteristic inclusion, the Lewy body.

MORPHOLOGY. On pathologic examination, the typical macroscopic findings are **pallor of the substantia nigra** (Fig. 30–31) and locus ceruleus. On microscopic examination, there is loss of the pigmented, catecholaminergic neurons in these regions associated with gliosis; Lewy bodies (Fig. 30–31*C*) may be found in some of the remaining neurons. These are single or multiple, intracytoplasmic, eosinophilic, round to elongated inclusions that often have a dense core surrounded by a pale halo. Ultrastructurally, Lewy bodies are composed of fine filaments, densely packed in the core but loose at the rim; immunocytochemical studies have shown the presence of neurofilament antigens within them as well as α-synuclein and ubiquitin. Lewy bodies may also be found in the cholinergic cells of the basal nucleus of Meynert, which is depleted of neurons (particularly in patients with abnormal mental function), as well as in other brain stem nuclei. Similar but less distinct inclusions are also found in cerebral cortical neurons, especially in the cingulate gyrus and the parahippocampal gyrus. These **cortical Lewy bodies** are demonstrable by immunohistochemistry for ubiquitin and α-synuclein.

Clinical Features. Given the well-characterized biochemical defect in IPD, therapy through neural transplantation has been attempted. Clinical improvement has been reported in patients with IPD or MPTP-induced Parkinson disease treated with stereotactic implants of fetal mesencephalic tissue into the striatum.[94,95] Other current neurosurgical approaches to this disease include the strategic placement of lesions elsewhere in the extrapyramidal system to compensate for the loss of nigrostriatal function.

About 10% to 15% of patients with IPD develop dementia, with increasing incidence with advancing age.[2] While many affected individuals also have pathologic evidence of Alzheimer disease (or, less frequently, other degenerative diseases), the dementia in others is attributed to widely disseminated Lewy bodies, particularly in the cerebral cortex but also involving the amygdala and brain stem neurons *(diffuse Lewy body disease).*

PROGRESSIVE SUPRANUCLEAR PALSY

This is an illness characterized clinically by truncal rigidity with dysequilibrium and nuchal dystonia; pseudobulbar palsy and abnormal speech; ocular disturbances, includ-

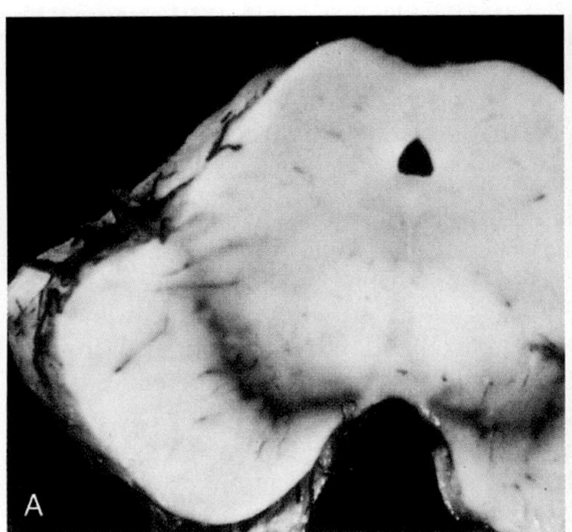

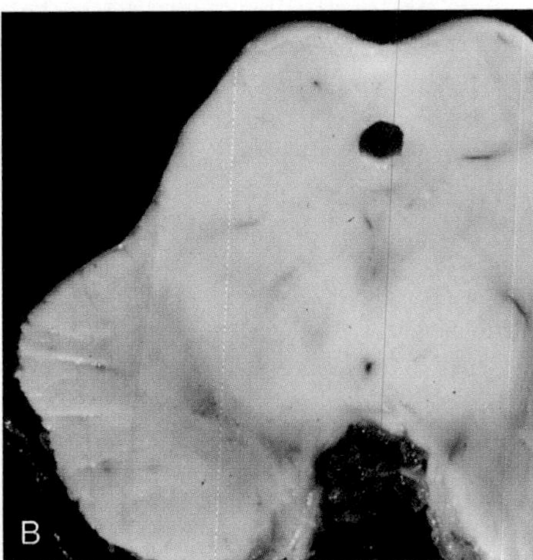

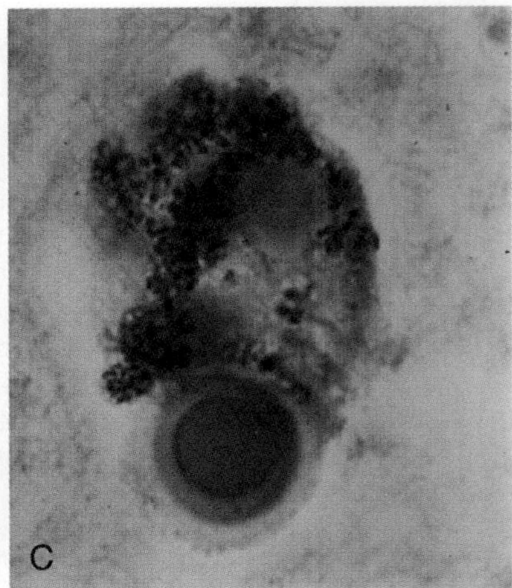

Figure 30–31

Parkinson disease (PD). *A*, Normal substantia nigra. *B*, Depigmented substantia nigra in idiopathic PD. *C*, Lewy bodies in a substantia nigra neuron stain bright pink. (*C*, Courtesy of Dr. R. Kim, V.A. Medical Center, Long Beach, CA)

ing vertical gaze palsy progressing to difficulty with all eye movements; and mild progressive dementia in most patients The onset of the disease is usually between the fifth and seventh decades, and males are affected approximately twice as frequently as are females; the disease is lethal within 5 to 7 years of onset.

MORPHOLOGY. There is widespread neuronal loss in the globus pallidus, subthalamic nucleus, substantia nigra, colliculi, periaqueductal gray matter, and dentate nucleus of the cerebellum. Neurofibrillary tangles are found in these affected regions, and cerebral cortical neurons have been found to contain tau protein. Although ultrastructural analysis reveals 15-nm straight filaments rather than the paired helical filaments found in Alzheimer disease, some epitopes (isoforms of tau protein) are shared with the tangles found in Alzheimer disease.

CORTICOBASAL DEGENERATION

This is a disease of the elderly, with considerable clinical and neuropathologic heterogeneity, characterized by extrapyramidal rigidity, asymmetric motor disturbances (jerking movements of limbs—"alien hand"), and sensory cortical dysfunction (apraxias, disorders of language); cognitive decline occurs late and only in some cases.[2,96,97] On macroscopic examination, there is cortical atrophy, mainly of the motor, premotor, and anterior parietal lobes. The regions of cortex show severe loss of neurons, gliosis, and *"ballooned" neurons* (neuronal achromasia) that can be highlighted with immunocytochemical methods for phosphorylated neurofilaments. Tau immunoreactivity has been found in astrocytes, basal ganglionic neurons, and, variably, in cortical neurons.[98, 99] The substantia nigra and locus ceruleus show loss of pigmented neurons and argyrophilic inclusions similar to those seen in progressive supranuclear palsy.

MULTIPLE SYSTEM ATROPHY

While this designation originally applied to a wide spectrum of neurodegenerative disorders affecting multiple neural "systems," it is now used to describe a group of disorders characterized by the presence of *glial cytoplasmic inclusions* typically within the cytoplasm of oligodendrocytes.[82] These inclusions can be demonstrated with silver impregnation methods and by immunostaining for various antigens (tau, ubiquitin, and αB-crystallin); they are ultrastructurally distinct from the inclusions found in other neurodegenerative diseases—they are composed primarily of 20- to 40-nm tubules. Similar inclusions may also be found in the cytoplasm of neurons, sometimes in neuronal and glial nuclei and in axons. It appears that glial cytoplasmic inclusions can occur in the absence of neuronal loss, suggesting that they may represent the primary pathologic event.[100,101]

The separate clinical entities striatonigral degeneration, Shy-Drager syndrome, and olivopontocerebellar atrophy, which can be classified within multiple system atrophy, are distinguished by clinical features and corresponding anatomic distribution of lesions, although clinical and pathologic overlap can be found in some cases.

Striatonigral Degeneration

Striatonigral degeneration is closely related to IPD clinically, but the movement disorder is relatively resistant to L-dopa treatment and the neuropathologic changes are different. On macroscopic examination, there is atrophy of the caudate nucleus and putamen; on microscopic examination, both nuclei show extensive neuronal loss, particularly of small neurons, and a marked gliosis. Loss of pigmented neurons also occurs, particularly in the zona compacta of the substantia nigra, but Lewy bodies are not seen. Because of this selective neuronal degeneration, both the dopaminergic projection (from the substantia nigra) and its target neurons (in the striatum) are lacking; L-dopa therapy cannot, therefore, bolster neurotransmission along this pathway, as is the case in the treatment of IPD. Some patients also evidence pontocerebellar degeneration or autonomic dysfunction.

Shy-Drager Syndrome

Shy-Drager syndrome is a clinical extrapyramidal syndrome that combines autonomic system dysfunction (orthostatic hypotension, impotence, disturbances of sweat and salivary gland secretion, pupillary abnormalities) and parkinsonism. Some cases are neuropathologically similar to IPD with Lewy bodies, while others resemble striatonigral degeneration with widespread neuronal loss. In all these syndromes, the sympathetic dysfunction is due to a degeneration of neurons in the intermediolateral column of the spinal cord.

Olivopontocerebellar Atrophy

Olivopontocerebellar atrophy is a cerebellar system degeneration that overlaps with the other cases of multiple system atrophy. Clinically, symptoms and signs include ataxia, eye and somatic movement abnormalities, dysarthria, and rigidity, although even within an affected pedigree, no two cases are exactly alike. The inheritance is no less varied; most cases are autosomal dominant, but others are autosomal recessive, and still others are nonfamilial. Macroscopic examination of the brain reveals shrinkage of the basis pontis due to loss of the pontine nuclei. The cerebellar cortex shows widespread depletion of Purkinje cells, especially in the lateral portions of the hemispheres. Secondary degenerative changes are found in the inferior olives (as in the cerebellar cortical atrophies).

HUNTINGTON DISEASE

Huntington disease (HD) is an inherited autosomal dominant disease characterized clinically by progressive movement disorders and dementia and histologically by neuronal degeneration of striatal neurons. The movement disorder chorea consists of jerky, hyperkinetic, sometimes dystonic movements affecting all parts of the body; patients may later develop parkinsonism with bradykinesia and rigidity. The disease is relentlessly progressive, with an average course of about 15 years to death.

Pathogenesis. The functional significance of the loss of striatal neurons is to dysregulate the basal ganglia circuitry that modulates motor output. The loss of the striatal inhibitory output, from the degeneration of GABA-containing neurons, to the external portion of the globus pallidus results in increased inhibitory input to the subthalamic nucleus. This inhibition of the subthalamic nucleus prevents it from exerting its regulatory effects on motor activity and thus leads to choreoathetosis. The structural basis of the cognitive changes associated with the disease remains unclear.

The *HD* gene, located on 4p16.3, encodes a predicted protein (huntingtin) of 348-kD molecular mass.[103] The coding region of the gene contains a polymorphic CAG trinucleotide repeat encoding a polyglutamine region of the protein. Normal *HD* genes contain 11 to 34 copies of the repeat; in disease-causing genes, the number of triplet repeats is increased. The disease is thus an example of the "triple repeat mutation" disorders discussed in Chapter 6. The larger the number of repeats, the earlier the onset of the disease. Repeat expansions occur during spermatogenesis, and paternal transmission is associated with early onset in the next generation *(anticipation;* Chapter 6). Newly occurring mutations are uncommon, and most apparently "sporadic" cases can be related to errors in paternal identification or the death of a parent before expression of the disease. Some unaffected fathers have expanded repeats that are further expanded during transmission to their children.

The biologic function of huntingtin and how mutations cause disease remain unknown but are the focus of much study.[104] The protein is clearly essential, as targeted gene disruption in the mouse has demonstrated an early embryonic lethal phenotype. In tissue from HD patients, both wild type and mutant protein are present. The expanded polyglutamine repeat appears to result in protein aggregation and formation of intranuclear inclusions (see Table 30-1 and Chapter 2). Furthermore, huntingtin has been suggested to be a potential target for caspase 3, a protease associated with neuronal apoptosis.

MORPHOLOGY. On macroscopic examination, the brain is small and shows striking atrophy of the caudate nucleus and, less dramatically, the putamen (Fig. 30-32). The globus pallidus may be atrophied secondarily, and the lateral and third ventricles are dilated. Atrophy is frequently also seen in the frontal lobe, less often in the parietal lobe, and occasionally in the entire cortex.

On microscopic examination, there is severe loss of striatal neurons; the most dramatic changes are found in the caudate nucleus, especially in the tail and portions nearer the ventricle. The putamen is less involved. Pathologic abnormalities develop in a medial to lateral direction in the caudate and from dorsal to ventral in the putamen. The nucleus accumbens is the best preserved structure. Both the large and the small neurons are affected, but loss of the small neurons generally precedes that of the larger. The medium-sized, spiny neurons that use γ-aminobutyric acid (GABA) and enkephalin or GABA and substance P as their neurotransmitters are especially affected. Two populations of neurons are relatively spared in the disease: the diaphorase-positive neurons that contain nitric oxide synthase and the large cholinesterase-positive neurons; both appear to serve as local interneurons. There is also fibrillary gliosis that is more extensive than in the usual reaction to neuronal loss. There is a direct relationship between the degree of degeneration in the striatum and the severity of clinical symptoms.[102]

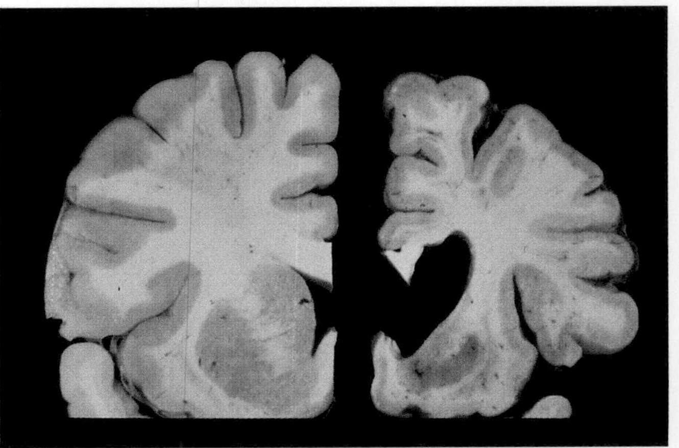

Figure 30-32

Huntington disease (HD). Normal hemisphere on the left compared with the hemisphere with HD on the right showing atrophy of the striatum and ventricular dilation. (Courtesy of Dr. J.-P. Vonsattel, Massachusetts General Hospital, Boston, MA.)

Clinical Features. The age at onset is most commonly in the fourth and fifth decades and is related to the length of the CAG repeat in the *HD* gene. Motor symptoms often precede the cognitive impairment. The movement disorder of HD is choreiform, with increased and involuntary jerky movements of all parts of the body; writhing movements of the extremities are typical. Early symptoms of higher cortical dysfunction include forgetfulness and thought and affective disorders, but there is progression to a severe dementia. HD patients have an increased risk of suicide, with intercurrent infection being the most common natural cause of death. Now that the genetic basis for the disease is known, it is possible to determine whether at-risk individuals carry the expanded repeat. This has made HD the focal point of discussion of ethical issues in genetic diagnosis.

Spinocerebellar Degenerations

This group of diseases affects, to a variable extent, the cerebellar cortex, spinal cord, peripheral nerves, and other regions of the neuraxis. The clinical spectrum includes cerebellar and sensory ataxia, spasticity, and sensorimotor peripheral neuropathy. This is a clinically heterogeneous group of illnesses that include several distinct diseases; these can be distinguished on the basis of their patterns of inheritance, age at onset, and pattern of signs and symptoms. Degeneration of neurons, without distinctive histopathologic changes, occurs in the affected areas and is associated with mild gliosis. Genetic analysis continues to redefine and subclassify these illnesses.

SPINOCEREBELLAR ATAXIAS

This is a group of genetically distinct diseases characterized by an autosomal dominant inheritance pattern; signs and symptoms referable to the cerebellum (progressive ataxia), brain stem, spinal cord, and peripheral nerves; and dystonia and parkinsonism, in some forms. Of the several genetically distinct types that have now been recognized, five (types 1–3, 6, and 7) are caused by unstable expansions of CAG repeats, which encode polyglutamine tracts in different proteins.[105] In addition, several other forms of spinocerebellar ataxia have been noted to demonstrate "anticipation," suggesting that they too may be caused by trinucleotide repeat expansions.

Friedreich Ataxia

This is an autosomal recessive progressive illness, generally beginning in the first decade of life with gait ataxia, followed by hand clumsiness and dysarthria. Deep tendon reflexes are depressed or absent, but an extensor plantar reflex is typically present. Joint position and vibratory sense are impaired, and there is sometimes loss of pain and temperature sensation and light touch. Most patients develop pes cavus and kyphoscoliosis. There is a high incidence of cardiac disease with cardiac arrhythmias and congestive heart failure. Concomitant diabetes is found in about 10% of patients. Most patients become wheelchair-bound within about 5 years of onset; the cause of death is intercurrent pulmonary infections and cardiac disease.

The gene for Friedreich ataxia has been mapped to chromosome 9q13, and in most cases there is a GAA trinucleotide repeat expansion in the first intron of a gene encoding a protein named frataxin.[106] Affected individuals inherit abnormal forms of the frataxin gene from both parents and have extremely low levels of the protein. In some cases of Friedreich ataxia, one of the mutant alleles harbors a missense or nonsense mutation.

MORPHOLOGY. The spinal cord shows loss of axons and gliosis in the posterior columns, the distal portions of corticospinal tracts, and the spinocerebellar tracts. There is degeneration of neurons in the spinal cord (Clarke column), brain stem (cranial nerve nuclei VIII, X, and XII), cerebellum (dentate nucleus, and the Purkinje cells of the superior vermis), and to some extent the Betz cells of the motor cortex. Large dorsal root ganglion neurons are also decreased in number; their large myelinated axons, traveling first in the dorsal roots and then in dorsal columns, therefore undergo secondary degeneration. The heart is enlarged and may have pericardial adhesions. Multifocal destruction of myocardial fibers with inflammation and fibrosis is detectable in about half the patients who come to autopsy examination.

Ataxia-Telangiectasia

Ataxia-telangiectasia (Chapter 8) is an autosomal recessive disorder characterized by an ataxic-dyskinetic syndrome beginning in early childhood, caused by neuronal degeneration predominantly in the cerebellum, and the subsequent development of telangiectasias in the conjunctiva and skin. Cells from patients with the disease show increased sensitivity to x-ray–induced chromosome abnormalities; these cells continue to replicate damaged DNA rather than stopping to allow repair or apoptosis. The ataxia-telangiectasia locus on chromosome 11q22–23 has been identified as a large gene, *ATM,* that encodes a protein with homology to phosphoinositol 3-kinases.[107] The carrier frequency of ataxia-telangiectasia has been estimated at 1%; in these individuals, the mutated ataxia-telangiectasia allele may underlie an increased risk of cancer, specifically breast cancer.

MORPHOLOGY. The abnormalities are predominantly in the cerebellum, with loss of Purkinje and granule cells; there is also degeneration of the dorsal columns, spinocerebellar tracts, and anterior horn cells and a peripheral neuropathy. Telangiectatic lesions have been reported in the CNS as well as in the conjunctiva and skin of the face, neck, and arms. The nuclei of cells in many organs (e.g., Schwann cells in dorsal root ganglia and peripheral nerves, endothelial cells, pituicytes) show a bizarre enlargement of the cell nucleus two to five times normal size and are referred to as **amphicytes.** The lymph nodes, thymus, and gonads are hypoplastic.

Clinical Features. The disease relentlessly progresses to death early in the second decade. Patients first come to medical attention because of recurrent sinopulmonary infections and unsteadiness in walking. Later on, speech is noted to become dysarthric and eye movement abnormalities develop. Many affected individuals develop lymphoid malignant disease (T-cell leukemia, T-cell lymphoma); gliomas and carcinomas have been reported in some.

Degenerative Diseases Affecting Motor Neurons

These are a group of inherited or sporadic diseases that in variable degrees of severity affect

- *Lower motor neurons* in the anterior horns of the spinal cord
- *Lower motor neurons* in certain cranial nerve nuclei (V, VII, IX, XII; but not those that control eye movements—III, IV, VI)
- *Upper motor neurons* (Betz cells) in the motor cortex

The disorders occur in all age groups, and the course of the illness is enormously variable—from slowly progressive or nonprogressive to rapidly progressive and fatal in a period of months or a few years. Denervation of muscles from loss of lower motor neurons and their axons results in muscular atrophy, weakness, and fasciculations; the corresponding histologic changes in nerve and muscle are discussed in Chapter 29. The clinical manifestations include paresis, hyperreflexia, spasticity, and extensor plantar responses (Babinski sign). Sensory systems and cognitive functions are unaffected, but types with dementia do occur.

AMYOTROPHIC LATERAL SCLEROSIS (MOTOR NEURON DISEASE)

This disease is characterized by neuronal muscle atrophy (amyotrophy) and hyperreflexia due to loss of lower motor and upper motor neurons in the anterior horns of the spinal cord and in corticospinal tracts, respectively.[108] The disease affects men slightly more frequently than women and becomes clinically manifest in the fifth decade or later. Five per cent to 10% of cases are familial, with autosomal dominant inheritance.

Pathogenesis. The etiology and pathogenesis of amyotrophic lateral sclerosis are unknown. For a subset of the familial cases, the genetic locus has been mapped to the copper-zinc superoxide dismutase gene *(SOD1)* on chromosome 21.[109] A wide variety of missense mutations have been identified that appear to generate an adverse gain-of-function phenotype. Growth factors can prevent developmentally regulated apoptosis of motor neurons as well as support the survival of motor neurons in vitro and may be involved in pathogenesis. Although no evidence has been found yet that alterations in growth factors cause amyotrophic lateral sclerosis, they continue to be investigated as potential therapeutic agents.

MORPHOLOGY. On macroscopic examination, the anterior roots of the spinal cord are thin; the precentral gyrus is somewhat atrophic in especially severe cases. Microscopic examination demonstrates a reduction in the number of anterior horn cell neurons throughout the length of the spinal cord with associated reactive gliosis and loss of anterior root myelinated fibers. Similar findings are found with involvement of the hypoglossal, ambiguus, and motor trigeminal cranial nerve nuclei. Skeletal muscles innervated by the degenerated lower motor neurons show neurogenic atrophy. Destruction of the upper motor neurons results in degeneration and pallor of myelin staining in the corticospinal tracts, particularly evident at the lower segmental levels but traceable throughout the corticospinal system with special studies (Fig. 30–33).

Clinical Features. Early symptoms include asymmetric weakness of the hands, manifest as dropping objects and difficulty performing fine motor tasks, and cramping and spasticity of the arms and legs. As the disease progresses, muscle strength and bulk diminish and involuntary contractions of individual motor units, termed *fasciculations,* occur. The disease eventually involves the respiratory muscles, leading to recurrent bouts of pulmonary infection. The severity of involvement of the upper and lower motor neurons is variable; the term *progressive muscular atrophy* applies to those relatively uncommon cases in which lower motor neuron involvement predominates. In some patients, degeneration of the lower brain stem cranial motor nuclei occurs early and progresses rapidly—referred to as *progressive bulbar palsy* or *bulbar amyotrophic lateral sclerosis).* In these individuals, abnormalities of deglutition and phonation dominate, and the clinical course is inexorable during a 1- or 2-year period. Familial cases develop symptoms earlier than most sporadic cases do, but the clinical course is comparable.

BULBOSPINAL ATROPHY (KENNEDY SYNDROME)

In most reported cases, this is an X-linked disease occurring in adult life characterized clinically by distal limb amyotrophy and bulbar signs such as atrophy and fasciculations of the tongue and dysphagia. Affected individuals manifest androgen insensitivity with gynecomastia, testicular atrophy, and oligospermia. On microscopic examination, there is degeneration of lower motor neurons in the spinal cord and brain stem. The fundamental defect appears to be CAG repeat expansion encoding a polyglutamine region within the androgen receptor; how this defect leads to neuronal degeneration is not known.

SPINAL MUSCULAR ATROPHY

This group of diseases affects mainly the lower motor neurons in children. It includes several entities with distinct patterns of inheritance and clinical course, discussed in Chapter 29.

INBORN ERRORS OF METABOLISM

A subset of genetic metabolic diseases affect the nervous system.[110] Some are covered earlier in this book (Chapter 6), but here their expression in the nervous system is briefly discussed. Many of these disorders express them-

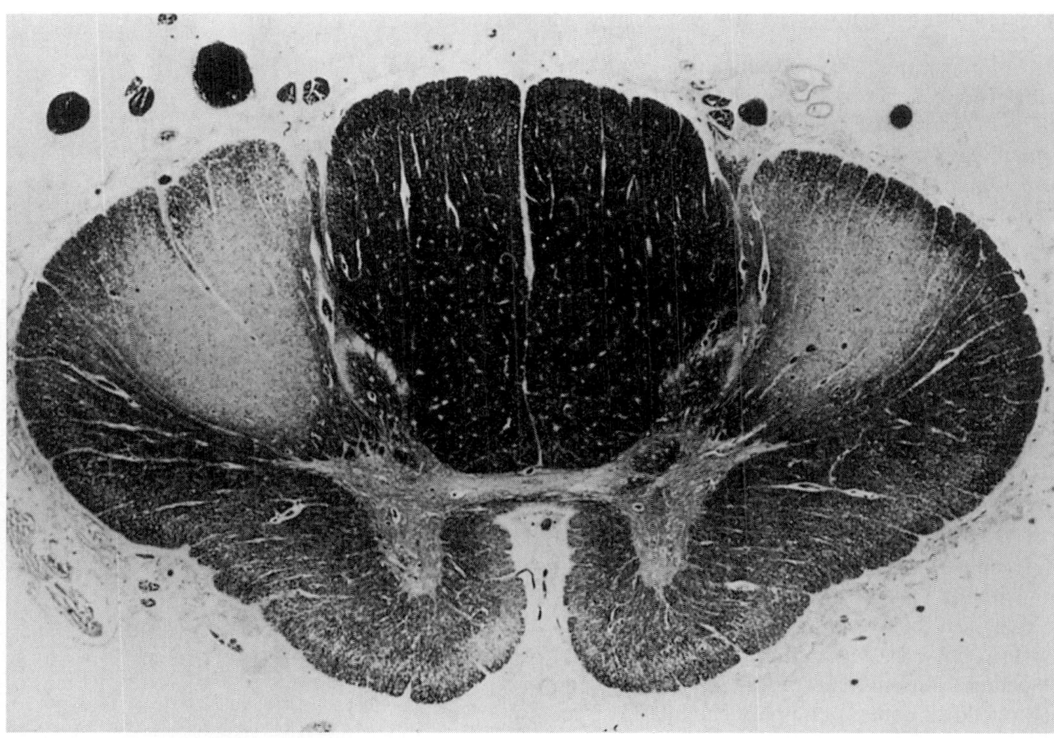

Figure 30–33 ■

Amyotrophic lateral sclerosis. Spinal cord showing loss of myelinated fibers (lack of stain) in corticospinal tracts. The anterior roots are smaller than the posterior; at higher magnification, loss of anterior horn neurons can also be seen (Woelcke stain for myelin).

selves in children who are normal at birth but who begin to miss developmental milestones during infancy and childhood.

- *Neuronal storage diseases* are mostly autosomal recessive diseases involving the deficiency of a specific enzyme of sphingolipid, mucopolysaccharide, or mucolipid catabolism. They are characterized by the accumulation of the substrate of the enzyme, often within neuronal lysosomes, leading to neuronal death. Cortical neuronal involvement leads to loss of cognitive function and may also cause seizures. The direct relationship between the accumulated material and cell injury and death is usually unclear.
- *Leukodystrophies* show a selective involvement of myelin (with either abnormal synthesis or turnover) and generally exhibit no neuronal storage defects. Some of these disorders involve lysosomal enzymes, while others involve peroxisomal enzymes. Diffuse involvement of white matter leads to deterioration in motor skills, spasticity, hypotonia, or ataxia. Although most are autosomal recessive disorders, adrenoleukodystrophy, an X-linked disease, is a notable exception. Subtypes, or variants, are recognized for many of these disorders. These variants may involve separate genetic loci and frequently follow the principle that *the earlier the age at onset, the more severe the deficiency and clinical course.*
- *Mitochondrial encephalomyopathies* are a group of disorders of oxidative phosphorylation, usually resulting from mutations in the mitochondrial genome. They typically involve gray matter as well as skeletal muscle (Chapter 29).

The mucopolysaccharidoses are discussed in Chapter 6.

Leukodystrophies

KRABBE DISEASE

This disease is an autosomal recessive leukodystrophy resulting from a deficiency of *galactocerebroside β-galactosidase*, the enzyme required for the catabolism of galactocerebroside to ceramide and galactose. The deficiency of galactocerebrosidase does *not* cause an identifiable accumulation of galactocerebroside, either in neurons or in white matter. Instead, it appears that an alternative catabolic pathway removes a fatty acid from this molecule, generating galactosylsphingosine, a cytotoxic compound that could cause oligodendrocyte injury.

The clinical course is rapidly progressive, with onset of symptoms often between the ages of 3 and 6 months. Survival beyond 2 years of age is uncommon. The clinical symptoms are dominated by motor signs, including stiffness and weakness, with gradually worsening difficulties in feeding. The brain shows loss of myelin and oligodendrocytes in the CNS and a similar process in peripheral nerves. Neurons and axons are relatively spared. A unique feature of Krabbe disease is the aggregation of macrophages around blood vessels as multinucleated cells—*globoid cells.*

METACHROMATIC LEUKODYSTROPHY

This disorder is transmitted in an autosomal recessive pattern and results from a deficiency of *arylsulfatase A.* This enzyme, present in a variety of tissues, cleaves the sulfate from sulfate-containing lipids (sulfatides), the first step in their degradation. Enzyme deficiency leads to an accumulation of the sulfatides, especially cerebroside sulfate; how this leads to myelin breakdown is not known. The gene for arylsulfatase A has been localized to chromosome 22q, and a wide range of mutations have been described.

Recognized clinical subtypes of the disorder include a late infantile form (the most common), a juvenile form, and an adult form. The two forms with childhood onset often present with motor symptoms and progress to greater deficits and death in 5 to 10 years. In the adult form, psychiatric or cognitive symptoms are the usual initial complaint, with motor symptoms coming later in the slower course of the disease. Although there is no known cure, promising results have recently been achieved with bone marrow transplantation.

The most striking histologic finding is demyelination with resulting gliosis (Fig. 30–34). Macrophages with vacuolated cytoplasm are scattered throughout the white matter. The membrane-bound vacuoles contain complex crystalloid structures composed of sulfatides; when bound to certain dyes such as toluidine blue, sulfatides shift the absorbance spectrum of the dye, a property called *metachromasia.* Similar changes in peripheral nerve are observed. The detection of metachromatic material in the urine is also a sensitive method of establishing the diagnosis.

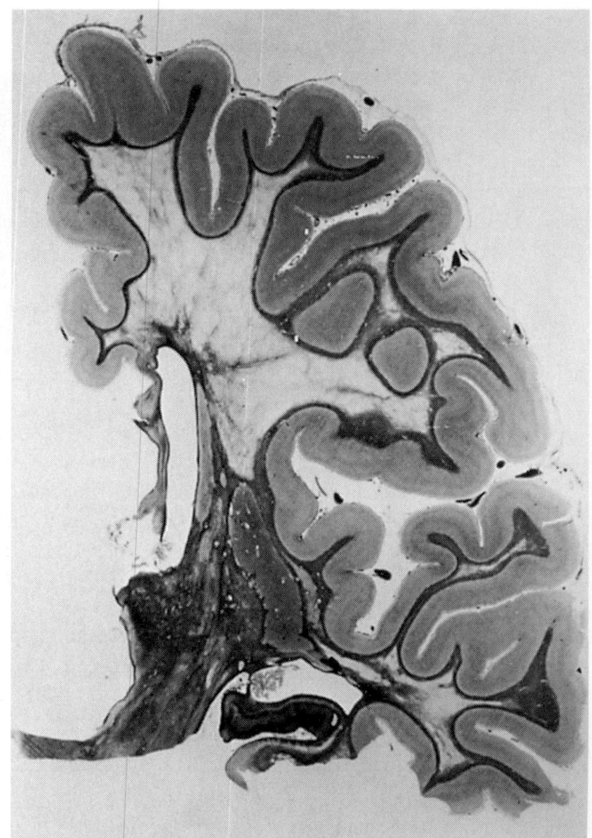

Figure 30–34 ■

Metachromatic leukodystrophy. Demyelination is extensive. The subcortical fibers in the cerebral hemisphere are spared (Luxol fast blue PAS stain for myelin).

ADRENOLEUKODYSTROPHY

This disorder, which has several clinically and genetically distinct forms, is a progressive disease with symptoms referable to myelin loss from the CNS and peripheral nerves as well as adrenal insufficiency. In general, forms with earlier onset have a more rapid course. The X-linked form usually presents in the early school years with neurologic symptoms and adrenal insufficiency. The disease is rapidly progressive and fatal. In individuals with later onset, the course is more protracted, and when it develops in adults, it is usually a slowly progressive disorder with predominantly peripheral nerve involvement developing for a period of decades. The *ALD* gene encodes a member of the ATP-binding cassette transporter family of proteins. However, there is little correlation between clinical course and the underlying mutations.

The disease is characterized by the inability to properly catabolize very long chain fatty acids (VLCFA) within peroxisomes, with elevation of levels of VLCFA in serum. There is loss of myelin, with relative preservation of the subcortical U fibers, accompanied by gliosis and lymphocytic inflammation. Atrophy of the adrenal cortex is present, and VLCFA accumulation can be seen in remaining cells.

PELIZAEUS-MERZBACHER DISEASE

This is an X-linked, invariably fatal leukodystrophy beginning either in early childhood or just after birth and characterized by signs and symptoms resulting from widespread white matter dysfunction. The disease has been shown to arise in most cases from defects in the gene encoding proteolipid protein *(PLP),* a major protein of CNS myelin.[110,111] Although myelin is nearly completely lost in the cerebral hemispheres, patches may remain, giving a "tigroid" appearance to tissue sections stained for myelin.

CANAVAN DISEASE

This disease results in a spongy degeneration of white matter with Alzheimer type II cells. Aspartoacylase activity has been recognized to be deficient in affected family members and is now thought to be the biochemical basis of this autosomal recessive disease.[110,112]

Mitochondrial Encephalomyopathies

LEIGH DISEASE

Usually an autosomal recessive disorder, this disease is characterized by lactic acidemia, arrest of psychomotor development, feeding problems, seizures, extraocular palsies, and weakness with hypotonia occurring between 1 and 2 years of age. Death usually occurs within 1 to 2 years. Various biochemical abnormalities have been found, all of which lie in the mitochondrial pathway for converting pyruvate to ATP. On histologic examination, there are multifocal asymmetric regions of destruction of brain tissue with a proliferation of blood vessels involving the periventricular gray matter of the midbrain, the tegmentum of the pons, and the periventricular regions of the thalamus and hypothalamus.

OTHER MITOCHONDRIAL ENCEPHALOMYOPATHIES

Myoclonic epilepsy and ragged red fibers is a maternally transmitted disease in which patients have myoclonus, a seizure disorder, and evidence of a myopathy. It has been associated with a mutation in the mtDNA gene for a mitochondrial-specific transfer RNA (tRNA), which appears to result in altered function of several of the oxidative complexes.

Mitochondrial encephalomyopathy, lactic acidosis, and stroke-like episodes is another syndrome, with a similar etiology, in which children have acute episodes of neurologic dysfunction, cognitive changes, and evidence of muscle involvement with weakness and lactic acidosis. Mitochondrial abnormalities can also be found in cerebral vessels.[123]

Leber hereditary optic neuropathy is an example of an mtDNA-based disease associated with a point mutation in the gene for a single enzyme, although nuclear genes influence the expression of the disease.

TOXIC AND ACQUIRED METABOLIC DISEASES

Toxic and acquired metabolic diseases are relatively common causes of neurologic illnesses. These diseases are discussed in Chapter 10, and only aspects that are of unique neurologic importance are discussed here.

Vitamin Deficiencies

THIAMINE (VITAMIN B_1) DEFICIENCY

As discussed earlier (Chapter 10), thiamine deficiency may result in the slowly evolving clinical disorder *beriberi.* In certain patients, thiamine deficiency may also lead to the development of psychotic symptoms that begin abruptly, a syndrome termed *Wernicke encephalopathy.* The acute stages, if unrecognized and untreated, may be followed by a prolonged and largely irreversible condition, *Korsakoff syndrome, characterized clinically by memory disturbances and confabulation.* Because the two syndromes are closely linked, the term Wernicke-Korsakoff syndrome is sometimes applied. The syndrome is particularly common in the setting of chronic alcoholism but may also be encountered in patients with thiamine deficiency resulting from gastric disorders, including carcinoma, chronic gastritis, or persistent vomiting. Treatment with vitamin B_1 may reverse manifestations of Wernicke syndrome, which is the basis for the treatment of abrupt-onset encephalopathy or coma with vitamin B_1.

MORPHOLOGY. Wernicke encephalopathy is characterized by foci of hemorrhage and necrosis, particularly in the mammillary bodies but also adjacent to the ventricle, especially the third and fourth ventricles. Early lesions show dilated capillaries with prominent endothelial cells. Subsequently, the capillaries leak red cells into the interstitium, producing hemorrhagic areas that are easily detectable macroscopically. With time, there is infiltration of macrophages and development of a cystic space with hemosiderin-laden macrophages as a permanent sign of the process. These chronic hemosiderin-laden lesions predominate in patients with Korsakoff syndrome. Lesions in the medial dorsal nucleus of the thalamus appear to be the best correlate of the memory disturbance.

VITAMIN B_{12} DEFICIENCY

The most severe and potentially irreversible effects of vitamin B_{12} deficiency are related to its nervous system lesions. The neurologic symptoms may present in the course of a few weeks, initially with slight ataxia and numbness and tingling in the lower extremities, but may progress rapidly to include spastic weakness of the lower extremities. Complete paraplegia may occur, usually only later in the course of the disease. With prompt vitamin replacement therapy, clinical improvement occurs; however, if complete paraplegia has developed, recovery is poor. On microscopic examination, vitamin B_{12} deficiency leads to a swelling of myelin layers producing vacuoles that begin segmentally at the midthoracic level of the spinal cord in the early stages. With time, axons in both the ascending tracts of the posterior columns and the descending pyramidal tracts degenerate. While isolated involvement of descending or ascending tracts may be observed in a variety of spinal cord diseases, the combined degeneration of both ascending and descending tracts of the spinal cord is characteristic of vitamin B_{12} deficiency and has led to the designation of the disorder as *subacute combined degeneration of the spinal cord.*

Neurologic Sequelae of Metabolic Disturbances

HYPOGLYCEMIA

Since the brain requires glucose and oxygen for its energy production, the cellular effects of diminished glucose resemble those of oxygen deprivation, as described earlier. Some regions of the brain are more sensitive to hypoglycemia than others are. There is a selective injury to large pyramidal neurons of the cerebral cortex, which, if it is severely involved, may result in pseudolaminar necrosis of the cortex, predominantly involving layers III to V. The hippocampus is also vulnerable to glucose depletion, as it is to hypoxia, and may show a dramatic loss of pyramidal neurons in Sommer sector (area CA1 of the hippocampus). Purkinje cells of the cerebellum are also vulnerable to hypoglycemia. If the level and duration of hypoglycemia are of sufficient severity, there may be widespread injury to many areas of the brain.

HYPERGLYCEMIA

Hyperglycemia is most commonly found in the setting of inadequately controlled diabetes mellitus and can be associated with either ketoacidosis or hyperosmolar coma. The patient becomes dehydrated and develops confusion, stupor, and eventually coma. The fluid depletion must be corrected gradually, otherwise severe cerebral edema may follow.

HEPATIC ENCEPHALOPATHY

The pathogenesis of hepatic encephalopathy or hepatic coma is discussed in Chapter 19. The cellular response in the CNS is predominantly glial. *Alzheimer type II changes* are evident in the cortex and basal ganglia and other subcortical gray matter regions, but there are no abnormalities in neurons.

Toxic Disorders

Cellular and tissue injury from toxic agents is discussed in Chapter 2. Aspects of several important toxic disorders that are of unique neurologic importance are discussed here.

CARBON MONOXIDE

Many of the pathologic findings that follow acute carbon monoxide exposure are those of hypoxia. Thus, selective injury of the neurons of layers III and V of the cerebral cortex, Sommer sector of the hippocampus, and Purkinje cells is the recognized consequence of carbon monoxide exposure. Bilateral necrosis of the globus pallidus may also occur and is more common in carbon monoxide–induced hypoxia than in hypoxia from other causes.

METHANOL

The pathologic findings of methanol toxicity are seen most often in the retina, where degeneration of retinal ganglion cells may cause blindness. Selective bilateral putamenal necrosis and focal white matter necrosis also occur when the exposure is severe. There is some evidence that formate, a major metabolite of methanol, may play a role in the retinal toxicity.

ETHANOL

The acute intoxication effects of ethanol are reversible, but chronic alcohol abuse is associated with a variety of neurologic sequelae. The "toxic" effects of chronic alcohol intake may be either direct effects of ethanol or secondary nutritional deficits. Cerebellar dysfunction occurs in about 1% of chronic alcoholics, associated with a clinical syndrome of truncal ataxia, unsteady gait, and nystagmus. The histologic changes are atrophy and loss of granule cells predominantly in the anterior vermis (Fig. 30–35). In advanced cases, there is loss of Purkinje cells and proliferation of the adjacent astrocytes *(Bergmann gliosis)* between the depleted granular cell layer and the molecular layer of the cerebellum. The fetal alcohol syndrome is discussed in Chapter 11.

RADIATION

Delayed effects of radiation present with rapidly evolving symptoms of an intracranial mass, including headaches, nausea, vomiting, and papilledema at an interval of months to years after irradiation.[114] The pathologic findings consist of large areas of coagulative necrosis with adjacent edema. The typical lesion is restricted to white matter, and all elements within the area undergo necrosis, including astrocytes, axons, oligodendrocytes, and blood vessels. Adjacent to the area of coagulative necrosis, proteinaceous spheroids may be identified, and blood vessels exhibit thickened walls with intramural fibrin-like material. In addition to necrosis, radiation can also induce tumors. Such tumors usually are not seen until years after radiation therapy and include poorly differentiated sarcomas, gliomas, and meningiomas.

Combined Methotrexate and Radiation-Induced Injury

Methotrexate toxicity most commonly develops when the drug has been administered in association with radiotherapy, whether synchronously or at separate times. The interval between the inciting events and the onset of symptoms varies considerably but may be as long as months. Symptoms often progress rapidly once they start, beginning with

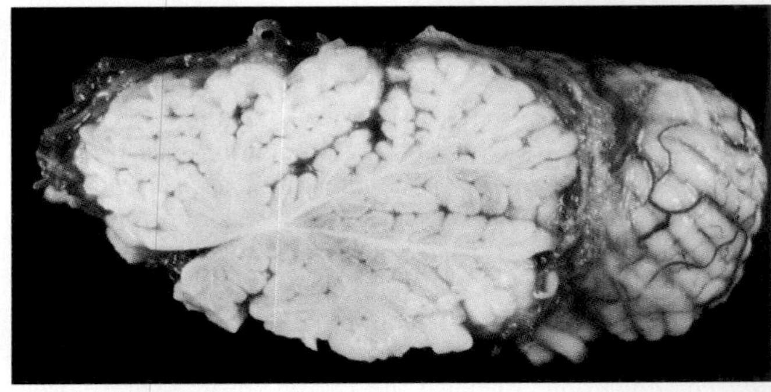

Figure 30–35

Alcoholic cerebellar degeneration. The anterior portion of the vermis (*upper portion of figure*) is atrophic with widened spaces between the folia.

drowsiness, ataxia, and confusion. While some patients recover function after the initial onset of symptoms, others may become comatose, and methotrexate neurotoxicity may rarely be responsible for the patient's death. The mechanisms of these delayed effects of methotrexate are unclear.

The basis of the symptoms are focal areas of coagulative necrosis within white matter, often adjacent to the lateral ventricles, but at times located in other areas of white matter. The necrosis may be distributed throughout the white matter or in the brain stem. Surrounding axons are often dilated to form axonal spheroids. Axons and cell bodies in the vicinity of the lesions undergo dystrophic mineralization, and there is adjacent gliosis.

TUMORS

The annual incidence of tumors of the CNS ranges from 10 to 17 per 100,000 persons for intracranial tumors and 1 to 2 per 100,000 persons for intraspinal tumors; about half are primary tumors, and the rest are metastatic. Tumors of the CNS account for 20% of all cancers of childhood. Seventy per cent of childhood CNS tumors arise in the posterior fossa, whereas a comparable number of tumors in adults arise within the cerebral hemispheres above the tentorium.[3,115–117]

Tumors of the nervous system have unique characteristics that set them apart from neoplastic processes elsewhere in the body. First, the distinction between benign and malignant lesions is less evident in the CNS than in other organs. Some glial tumors with histologic features of a benign neoplasm, including low mitotic rate, cellular uniformity, and slow growth, may infiltrate large regions of the brain, thereby leading to serious clinical deficits and poor prognosis. Second, the ability to surgically resect infiltrating glial neoplasms without compromising neurologic function is limited. Third, the anatomic site of the neoplasm can have lethal consequences irrespective of histologic classification; for example, a benign meningioma, by compressing the medulla, can cause cardiorespiratory arrest. Finally, the pattern of spread of primary CNS neoplasms differs from that of other tumors: even the most highly malignant gliomas rarely metastasize outside of the CNS. The subarachnoid space provides a pathway for spread, so that seeding along the brain and spinal cord can occur in highly anaplastic as well as in well-differentiated neoplasms that extend into the CSF pathways.

The four major classes of brain tumors are

- Gliomas
- Neuronal tumors
- Poorly differentiated neoplasms
- Meningiomas

Gliomas

Gliomas, derived from glial cells, include *astrocytomas, oligodendrogliomas,* and *ependymomas.*

ASTROCYTOMA

Several different categories of tumors derived from astrocytes are recognized, including fibrillary astrocytoma, glioblastoma multiforme, pilocytic astrocytoma, and pleomorphic xanthoastrocytoma as well as rarer types. These have characteristic histologic features, distribution within the brain, age groups typically affected, and clinical course.

Fibrillary (Diffuse) Astrocytomas and Glioblastoma Multiforme

These account for about 80% of adult primary brain tumors. Usually found in the cerebral hemispheres, they may also occur in the cerebellum, brain stem, or spinal cord, most often in the fourth through sixth decades. The most common presenting signs and symptoms are seizures, headaches, and focal neurologic deficits related to the anatomic site of involvement. Fibrillary astrocytomas show a spectrum of histologic differentiation that correlates well with clinical course and outcome.

MORPHOLOGY. **Diffuse fibrillary astrocytomas** are either well differentiated or evolve into less differentiated, higher-grade forms—**anaplastic astrocytoma and glioblastoma multiforme.** The macroscopic appearance of diffuse fibrillary astrocytoma is that of a poorly defined, gray, infiltrative tumor that expands and distorts the invaded brain (Fig. 30–36). These tumors range in size from a few centimeters to enormous lesions that replace an entire hemisphere. The cut surface of the tumor is either firm, or soft and gelatinous; cystic degeneration may be seen. In glioblastoma multiforme, variations in the gross appearance of the tumor from region to region is characteristic (Fig. 30–37). Some areas are firm and white, others are soft and yellow (the result of tissue necrosis), and yet others show regions of cystic degeneration and hemorrhage. The tumor may appear well demarcated from the surrounding brain tissue, but infiltration beyond the outer margins is always present.

Radiologic studies show mass effect as well as changes in the brain adjacent to the tumor, such as edema. High-grade astrocytomas have abnormal vessels that are "leaky" and are therefore demonstrable when contrast media are injected into the venous system.

On microscopic examination, well-differentiated fibrillary astrocytomas are characterized by a mild to moderate increase in the number of glial cell nuclei, somewhat variable nuclear pleomorphism, and an intervening feltwork of fine, GFAP-positive astrocytic cell processes that give the background a fibrillary appearance. The transition between neoplastic and normal tissue is indistinct, and tumor cells can be seen infiltrating normal tissue at some distance from the main lesion. Anaplastic astrocytomas show regions that are more densely cellular and have greater nuclear pleo-

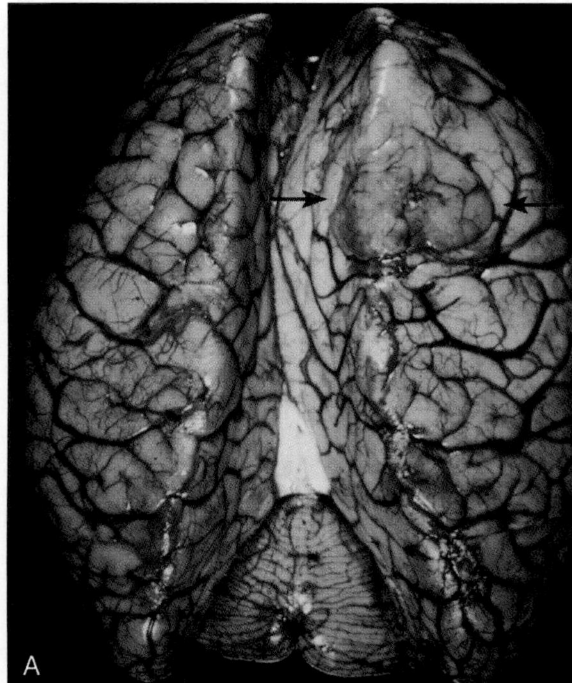

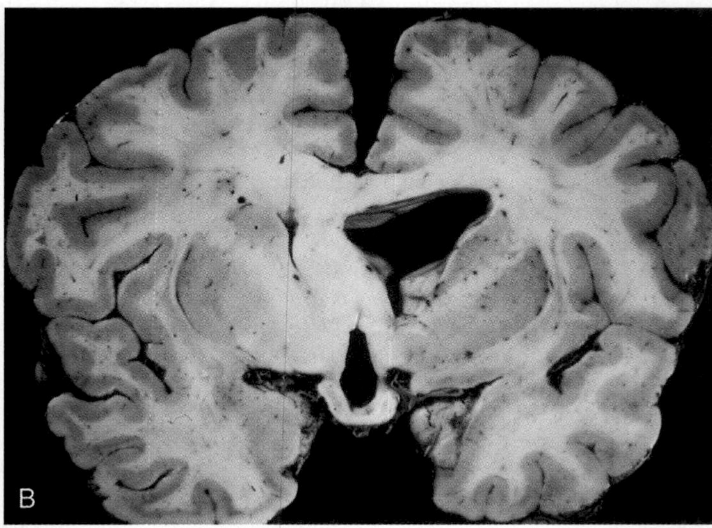

Figure 30–36

Well-differentiated astrocytoma. *A*, The right frontal tumor has expanded gyri, which led to flattening (*arrows*). *B*, Expanded white matter of the left cerebral hemisphere and thickened corpus callosum and fornices.

morphism from well-differentiated fibrillary astrocytoma; mitotically active cells or some vascular endothelial proliferation is also observed.

When the predominant neoplastic astrocyte shows a brightly eosinophilic cell body from which emanate abundant, stout processes, the term **gemistocytic astrocytoma** applies.

Glioblastoma multiforme has a histologic appearance similar to anaplastic astrocytoma with the additional features of *necrosis* and *vascular or*

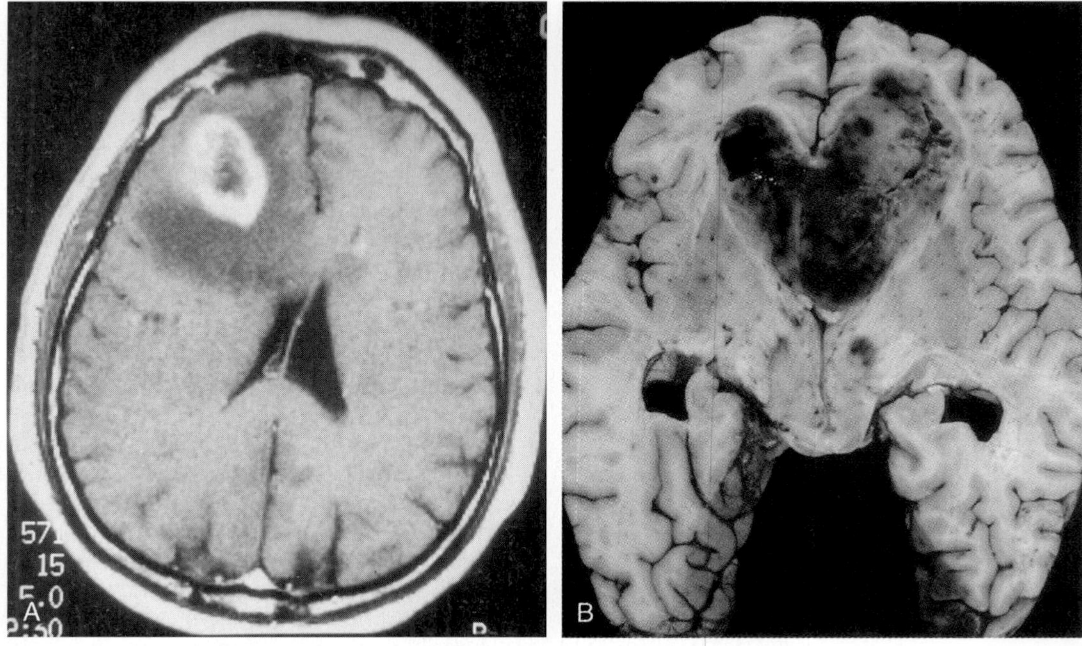

Figure 30–37

A, Computed tomographic (CT) scan of a large tumor in the cerebral hemisphere showing signal enhancement with contrast material and pronounced peritumoral edema. *B*, Glioblastoma multiforme appearing as a necrotic, hemorrhagic, infiltrating mass.

endothelial cell proliferation—tufts of piled-up vascular cells that bulge into the vascular lumen. When vascular cell proliferation is extreme, the tuft forms a ball-like structure, the **glomeruloid body** (Fig. 30–38). Vascular endothelial cell growth factor (VEGF), produced by malignant astrocytes, perhaps in response to hypoxia, contributes to this distinctive form of vascular change. Necrosis in glioblastoma multiforme, often in a serpentine pattern, occurs in areas of hypercellularity with highly malignant tumor cells crowded along the edges of the necrotic regions, producing a histologic pattern referred to as **pseudopalisading** (Fig. 30–38).

In the condition called **gliomatosis cerebri** multiple regions of the brain, in some cases, the entire brain, are infiltrated by neoplastic astrocytes.

Grading schemes for fibrillary astrocytomas have clinical utility in predicting prognosis and in fashioning treatment options. The three-tiered system of well-differentiated astrocytoma, anaplastic astrocytoma, and glioblastoma multiforme is commonly used; a four-tiered system (grades 1, 2, 3, and 4) based on the presence of specific histologic features (nuclear pleomorphism, mitoses, endothelial cell proliferation, and necrosis) is also prevalent.[3,117,118] The proliferation marker Ki-67 has also been used to discriminate between grades of anaplasia in astrocytomas as well as in other types of brain tumors.[119] Since the range of cellular anaplasia in fibrillary astrocytomas can be extremely variable from one region of the neoplasm to another, a single small biopsy specimen may not be representative of the tumor as a whole.

Molecular Genetics. Genetic alterations have been observed to be correlated with the progression of astrocytic tumors from low to high grade, which is part of the natural course of the disease in many patients.[120] Among the alterations most commonly found in the low-grade astrocytomas are inactivation of *p53* and overexpression of PDGF-A and its receptor. The transition to higher grade astrocytoma is associated with additional disruption of tumor-suppressor genes, the *RB* gene, the *p16/CDKNZA* gene, and a putative tumor suppressor on chromosome 19q.

About one third of glioblastomas show *p53* mutation; these glioblastomas, termed *secondary glioblastomas,* occur in younger patients whose tumors have progressed from a lower grade astrocytoma. Another third of glioblastomas do not show this change but rather have amplification of the epidermal growth factor receptor gene *(EGFR)*. This abnormality is typically found in older patients with a short clinical history and no evidence of progression from a lower grade astrocytoma, and the tumors are termed *primary,* or *de novo, glioblastoma.* The remaining third of glioblastomas show neither of these patterns of genetic alterations, and the changes associated with them remain to be discovered. These genetically distinct types of glioblastoma cannot be distinguished on histologic grounds, and it remains uncertain whether survival after diagnosis is different in these three groups.[121,122]

Clinical Features. The presenting symptoms of astrocytomas depend, in part, on the location of the lesion and its rate of growth. Astrocytomas have a tendency to become more anaplastic with time. With well-differentiated astrocytomas, the symptoms may remain static or progress only slowly during a number of years. Eventually, however, patients usually enter a period of more rapid clinical deterioration that is generally correlated with the appearance of

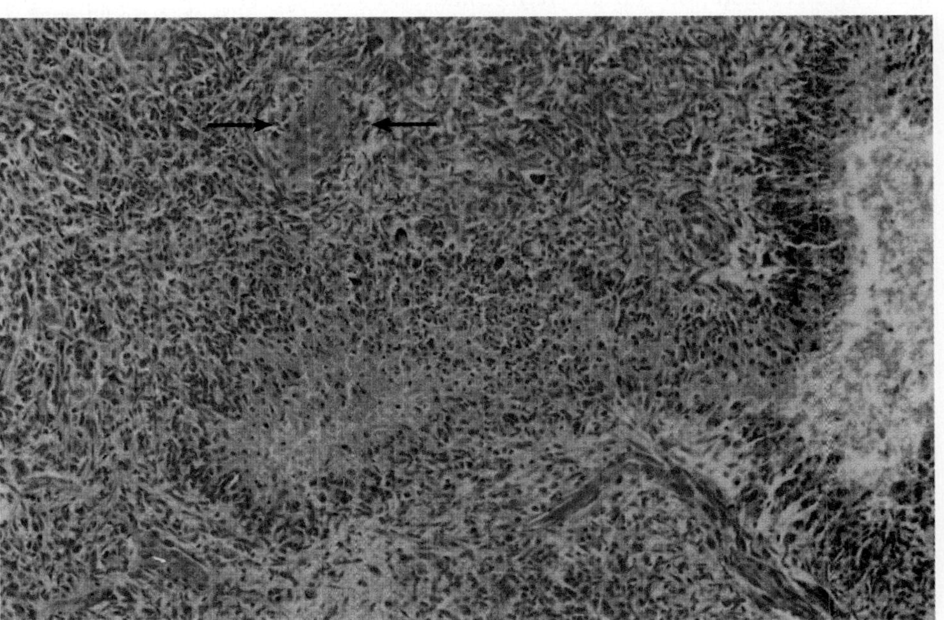

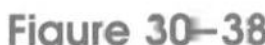

Figure 30–38 ■

Glioblastoma multiforme. Foci of necrosis with pseudopalisading of malignant nuclei and endothelial cell proliferation, leading to a "glomeruloid" structure (*arrows*).

anaplastic features and more rapid growth of the tumor. The prognosis for patients with glioblastoma is very poor. With current treatment, comprising resection when feasible together with radiotherapy and chemotherapy, the mean length of survival after diagnosis is only 8 to 10 months; less than 10% of patients are alive after 2 years. Survival is substantially shorter in older patients. Well-differentiated astrocytomas have a mean survival of more than 5 years.

Pilocytic Astrocytoma

These astrocytomas are distinguished from the others by their pathologic appearance and relatively benign behavior. They typically occur in children and young adults and are usually located in the cerebellum but may also appear in the floor and walls of the third ventricle, the optic nerves, and occasionally the cerebral hemispheres.

On macroscopic examination, a pilocytic astrocytoma is often cystic, with a mural nodule in the wall of the cyst (Fig. 30–39); if solid, it may be well circumscribed or, less frequently, infiltrative. On microscopic examination, the tumor is composed of bipolar cells with long, thin "hairlike" processes that are GFAP-positive; Rosenthal fibers and microcysts are often present. An increase in the number of blood vessels, often with thickened walls, is seen but does not imply an unfavorable prognosis; necrosis and mitoses are uncommon.

These tumors grow very slowly, and some patients have survived for more than 40 years after incomplete resection.

Pleomorphic Xanthoastrocytoma

This is a tumor that occurs most often relatively superficially in the temporal lobe of children and young adults usually with a history of seizures. On microscopic examination, the tumor consists of neoplastic astrocytes, sometimes lipidized and with bizarre forms, abundant reticulin deposits, and chronic inflammatory cell infiltrates. Anaplastic transformation occurs in some instances.

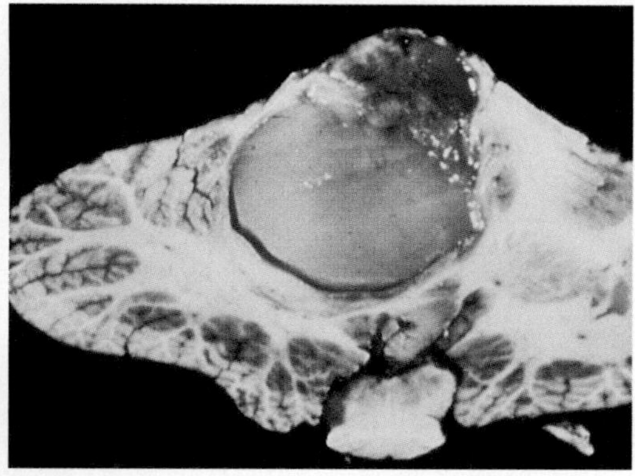

Figure 30–39 ■

Pilocytic astrocytoma in the cerebellum with a nodule of tumor in a cyst.

Brain Stem Glioma

A clinical subgroup of astrocytomas, these occur mostly in the first two decades of life and compose about 20% of primary brain tumors in this age group. At autopsy, about 50% of them have progressed to glioblastomas. With current radiotherapy, the 5-year survival rate for the composite group, which includes all grades of astrocytomas, is between 20% and 40%.

OLIGODENDROGLIOMA

These tumors constitute about 5% to 15% of gliomas and are most common in the fourth and fifth decades. Patients may have had several years of neurologic complaints, often including seizures. The lesions are found mostly in the cerebral hemispheres, with a predilection for white matter.

MORPHOLOGY. On macroscopic examination, oligodendrogliomas are well-circumscribed, gelatinous, gray masses, often with cysts, focal hemorrhage, and calcification. On microscopic examination, the tumor is composed of sheets of regular cells with spherical nuclei containing finely granular chromatin (similar to normal oligodendrocytes) surrounded by a clear halo of cytoplasm. The tumor typically contains a delicate network of anastomosing capillaries. The calcification, which is present in as many as 90% of these tumors, ranges from microscopic foci to massive depositions. At present, no diagnostically reliable immunohistochemical markers have been developed for oligodendroglioma.

Clinical Features. In general, patients with oligodendrogliomas have a better prognosis than that of patients with astrocytomas. Current treatment with surgery, chemotherapy, and radiotherapy has yielded an average survival of 5 to 10 years. Patients with anaplastic oligodendroglioma have a worse prognosis. The term *mixed glioma* has been employed to designate neoplasms consisting of oligodendroglioma and astrocytoma (or less often another gliomatous component).

EPENDYMOMA AND RELATED PARAVENTRICULAR MASS LESIONS

Ependymomas most often arise next to the ependyma-lined ventricular system, including the oft-obliterated central canal of the spinal cord. In the first two decades of life, they typically occur near the fourth ventricle and constitute 5% to 10% of the primary brain tumors in this age group. In adults, the spinal cord is their most common location.

MORPHOLOGY. In the fourth ventricle, ependymomas are typically solid or papillary masses extending from the floor of the ventricle (Fig. 30–40A). Although they are often better demarcated from adjacent brain than astrocytomas, their proximity to the vital pontine and medullary nuclei usually makes complete extirpation impossible. In the intraspinal tumors, this sharp demarcation sometimes makes total removal feasible. On microscopic examination, ependymomas are composed of cells with regular, round to oval nuclei with abundant granular chromatin. Between the nuclei, there is a variably dense fibrillary background. Tumor cells may form glandlike round or elongated structures ("rosettes," canals) that resemble the embryologic ependymal canal with long, delicate processes extending into a lumen (Fig. 30–40B); more frequently present are **perivascular pseudorosettes** (Fig. 30–40B) in which tumor cells are arranged around vessels with an intervening zone consisting of thin ependymal processes directed toward the wall of the vessel. About 50% of ependymomas can be shown immunocytochemically to contain GFAP. Most tumors are well differentiated, but anaplastic forms also occur.

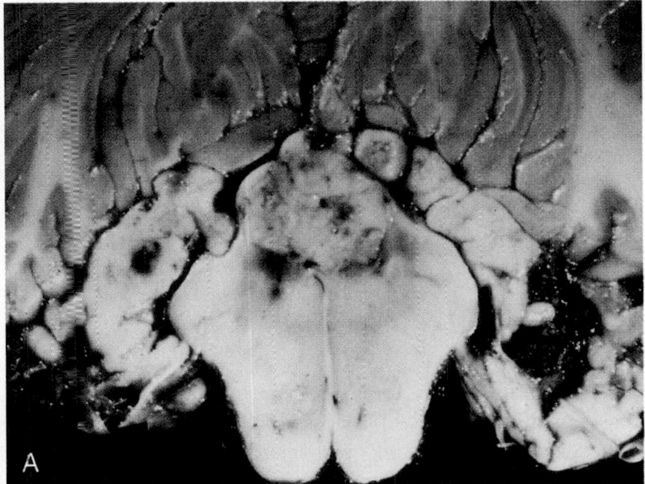

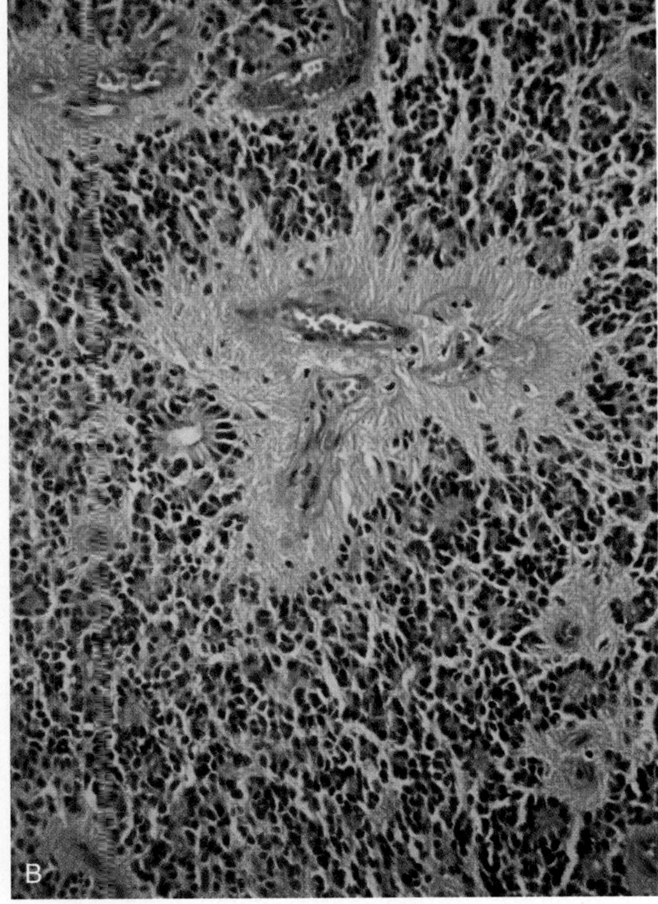

Figure 30–40

Ependymoma. *A*, Tumor growing into the fourth ventricle, distorting, compressing, and infiltrating surrounding structures. *B*, Microscopic appearance of ependymoma.

Clinical Features. Posterior fossa ependymomas often manifest with hydrocephalus secondary to progressive obstruction of the fourth ventricle rather than invasion of the pons or medulla. Prognosis is poor despite the slow growth of the tumor and the usual lack of histologic evidence of anaplasia. Because of their relationship to the ventricular system, CSF dissemination is a common finding. An average survival of about 4 years after surgery and radiotherapy has been reported.

- *Myxopapillary ependymomas* occur in the filum terminale of the spinal cord and contain papillary elements in a myxoid background, admixed with ependymoma-like cells. Cuboidal cells, sometimes with clear cytoplasm, are arranged around papillary cores containing connective tissue and blood vessels. The myxoid areas contain neutral and acidic mucopolysaccharides. Prognosis depends on completeness of surgical resection; if the tumor has extended into the subarachnoid space and surrounded the roots of the cauda equina, recurrence is likely.
- *Subependymomas* are solid, sometimes calcified, slow-growing nodules attached to the ventricular lining and protruding into the ventricle. They are usually asymptomatic and are incidental findings at autopsy, but if they are sufficiently large or strategically located, they may cause hydrocephalus. They are most often found in the lateral and fourth ventricles, and there, as is the case with other fourth ventricular tumors, are difficult for the neurosurgeon to remove. They have a characteristic microscopic appearance, with clumps of ependyma-appearing nuclei scattered in a dense, fine, glial fibrillar background.
- *Choroid plexus papillomas* can occur anywhere along the choroid plexus and are most common in children, in whom they are most often found in the lateral ventricles. In adults, they are more often found in the fourth ventricle. These tumors almost exactly recapitulate the structure of the normal choroid plexus and are markedly papillary growths. The papillae have connective tissue

stalks covered with a cuboidal or columnar epithelium. Clinically, choroid plexus papillomas usually present with hydrocephalus due either to obstruction of the ventricular system by tumor or to overproduction of CSF. An etiologic role for papovavirus has been shown in some studies.

There are rare cases of *choroid plexus carcinoma;* the histologic appearance of these lesions closely resembles adenocarcinoma. They are usually found in children; in adults, they need to be differentiated from the much more common metastatic carcinoma.

Colloid cyst of the third ventricle most often occurs in young adults. The cyst is attached to the roof of the third ventricle, thereby being capable of obstructing one or both of the foramina of Monro and, as a result, causing noncommunicating hydrocephalus, which may be rapidly fatal. Headache, sometimes positional, is an important clinical symptom. The cyst has a thin, fibrous capsule and a lining of low to flat cuboidal epithelium; it contains gelatinous, proteinaceous material.

Neuronal Tumors

Several types of CNS tumors contain mature-appearing neurons *(ganglion cells);* these may constitute the entire population of the lesion *(gangliocytomas).* More commonly, there is an admixture with a glial neoplasm, and the lesion is termed a *ganglioglioma.* Most of these tumors are slow growing, but the glial component occasionally becomes frankly anaplastic, and the disease then progresses rapidly.

MORPHOLOGY. Gangliocytomas are well-circumscribed masses with focal calcification and small cysts usually found in the floor of the third ventricle, the hypothalamus, or the temporal lobe. On microscopic examination, the neoplastic ganglion cells are present as clumps of cells separated by a relatively acellular stroma. The ganglioglioma has a macroscopic appearance similar to that of a glioma of comparable grade. It is most commonly found in the temporal lobe and may often have a cystic component. The neoplastic ganglion cells are irregularly clustered and have apparently random orientation of neurites. Binucleated forms are frequent. The neoplastic neurons can often be detected with the use of immunohistochemical reactions for neuronal proteins, neurofilaments, and synaptophysin.

Cerebral neuroblastomas are rare neoplasms that occur in the hemispheres of children and show highly aggressive clinical behavior. On microscopic examination, they resemble peripheral neuroblastomas (Chapter 11), being composed of small undifferentiated cells with characteristic Homer Wright rosettes. In contrast, **central neurocytoma,** typically, is a nonanaplastic neuronal neoplasm found within and adjacent to the ventricular system, characterized by evenly spaced, round, uniform nuclei resembling those of oligodendroglioma. Ultrastructural and immunohistochemical studies, however, reveal the neuronal lineage of the tumor cells.

Dysembryoplastic neuroepithelial tumor is a distinctive, nonanaplastic tumor of childhood often presenting as a seizure disorder, with a relatively good prognosis after surgical extirpation. This mixed glial-neuronal tumor is characterized by intracortical location, cystic changes, frequent association with dysplastic cortex, nodular growth, and the presence of well-differentiated "floating neurons" in a pool of mucopolysaccharide-rich fluid and surrounding neoplastic glia without anaplastic features.

Poorly Differentiated Neoplasms

Some tumors, although of neuroectodermal origin, express few if any of the phenotypic markers of mature cells of the nervous system and are described as poorly differentiated, or embryonal, meaning that they retain cellular features of primitive, undifferentiated cells. The most common is the *medulloblastoma,* which accounts for 20% of the brain tumors in children.

MEDULLOBLASTOMA

This tumor occurs predominantly in children and exclusively in the cerebellum. Neuronal and glial markers may be expressed, but the tumor is often largely undifferentiated.

MORPHOLOGY. In children, medulloblastomas are located in the midline of the cerebellum (Fig. 30–41*A*), but lateral locations are more often found in adults. Rapid growth may occlude the flow of CSF, leading to hydrocephalus. The tumor is often well circumscribed, gray, and friable and may be seen extending to the surface of the cerebellar folia and involving the leptomeninges (Fig. 30–41*B*). On microscopic examination, the tumor is usually extremely cellular, with sheets of anaplastic cells (Fig. 30–41*C*). Individual tumor cells are small, with little cytoplasm and hyperchromatic nuclei that are frequently elongated or crescent shaped. Mitoses are abundant, and markers of cellular proliferation, such as Ki-67, are detected in a high percentage of the cells. The tumor has the potential to express neuronal (neurosecretory granules or Homer Wright rosettes, as occur in neuroblastoma; Chapter 11) and glial (GFAP) phenotypes. At the edges of the main tumor mass, medulloblastoma cells have a propensity to form linear chains of cells infiltrating through cerebellar cortex to aggregate beneath the pia, pen-

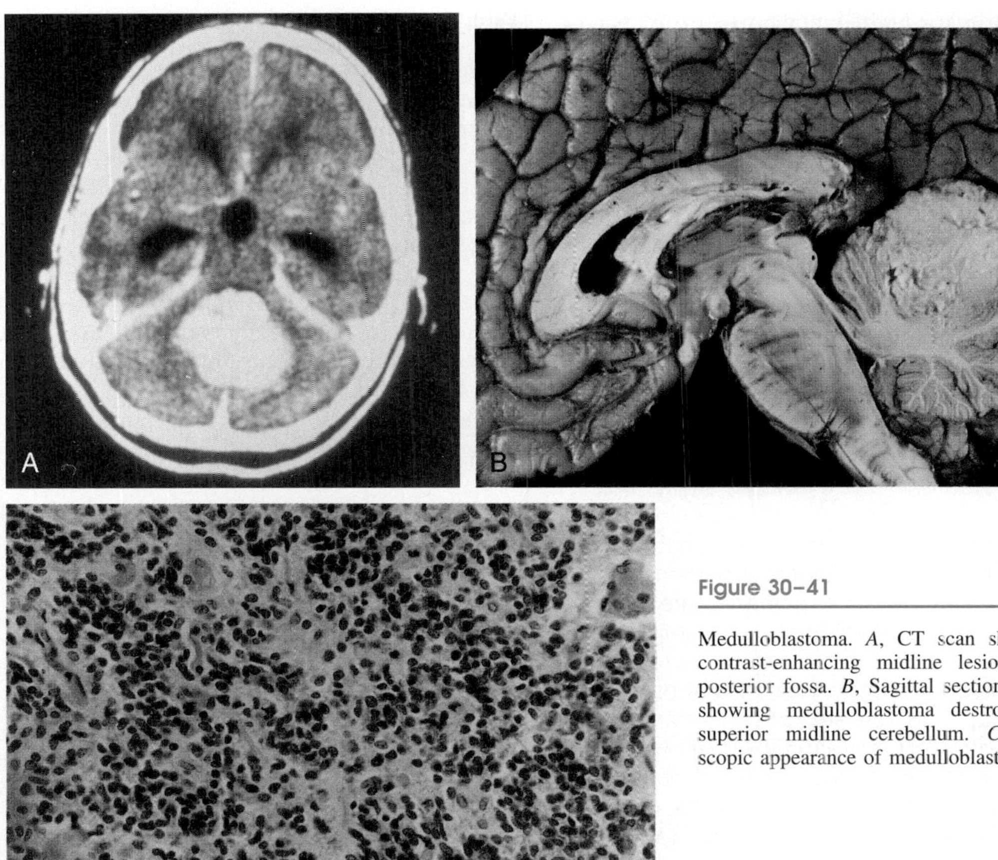

Figure 30–41

Medulloblastoma. *A*, CT scan showing a contrast-enhancing midline lesion in the posterior fossa. *B*, Sagittal section of brain showing medulloblastoma destroying the superior midline cerebellum. *C*, Microscopic appearance of medulloblastoma.

etrate the pia, and seed into the subarachnoid space. Extension into the subarachnoid space may elicit a prominent desmoplastic response. Dissemination through the CSF is a common complication, presenting as nodular masses elsewhere in the CNS, including metastases to the cauda equina that are sometimes termed "drop" metastases because of their direct route of dissemination through the CSF.

Clinical Features. The tumor is highly malignant, and the prognosis for untreated patients is dismal; however, it is an exquisitely radiosensitive tumor. Prognosis is also related to the amount of tumor resected, with better survival rates following complete resection. In addition, radiation of brain and spinal cord decreases the likelihood of recurrence. With total excision and radiation, the 5-year survival rate has been reported to be as high as 75%. The most common genetic alteration is loss of material from the short arm of chromosome 17. This often occurs in the setting of an abnormal chromosome derived from duplication of the long arm of chromosome 17 (isochromosome 17q or i(17q)).

Other Parenchymal Tumors

PRIMARY BRAIN LYMPHOMA

Primary brain lymphoma accounts for 2% of extranodal lymphomas and 1% of intracranial tumors. It is the most common CNS neoplasm in immunosuppressed patients, including those with AIDS. In nonimmunosuppressed populations, the age spectrum is relatively wide, and the frequency increases after 60 years of age.

The term *primary* reflects the distinction between these lesions and secondary involvement of the CNS by non-Hodgkin lymphoma arising elsewhere in the body (Chapter 15). Patients with primary brain lymphoma often have multiple tumor masses within the brain parenchyma; nodal, bone marrow, or extranodal involvement outside of the CNS is a rare and late complication. Conversely, non-Hodgkin lymphoma arising outside the CNS rarely involves the brain parenchyma; involvement of the nervous system, when it occurs in non-Hodgkin lymphoma, is manifested by the presence of malignant cells within the CSF and around intradural nerve roots and occasionally by the infiltration of superficial aspects of the cerebrum or spinal cord by malignant cells.

The majority of primary brain lymphomas are of B-cell origin. In immunosuppressed patients, all the neoplasms appear to contain Epstein-Barr virus genomes within the transformed B cells. Regardless of the clinical context in which it occurs, primary brain lymphoma is an aggressive disease with relatively poor response to chemotherapy compared with peripheral lymphomas.

MORPHOLOGY. Lesions are frequently multiple and often involve deep gray structures as well as white matter and cortex. Periventricular spread is common. The tumors are relatively well defined compared with glial neoplasms but are not as discrete as metastases and often show extensive areas of central necrosis. On cytologic study, the cells are nearly always those of a high-grade lymphoma (Chapter 15), most commonly large cell lymphoma, although immunoblastic sarcomas as well as small noncleaved cell patterns are also observed. Within lesions, malignant cells infiltrate the parenchyma of the brain and accumulate around blood vessels. Reticulin stains demonstrate that the infiltrating cells are separated from one another by silver-staining material; this pattern, referred to as hooping, is characteristic of primary brain lymphoma. A benign mixed T- and B-cell infiltrate, which often contains a plasmacytic component, can also be found adjacent to lesions.

GERM CELL TUMORS

Primary brain germ cell tumors occur along the midline, most commonly in the pineal and the suprasellar regions. They account for 0.2% to 1% of brain tumors in people of European descent but up to 10% in Japanese. Most occur in adolescents and young adults. Germ cell tumors in the pineal region show a strong male predominance, which is not seen in suprasellar lesions. It is not clear whether these tumors arise by the transformation of an otherwise normal resident population of germ cells, of a developmentally derived ectopic rest of germ cells, or of germ cells that migrated into the CNS late in development. Regardless of these uncertainties, germ cell tumors—like the lymphomas—share many of the features of their counterparts in the gonads. In contrast to lymphomas, however, CNS involvement by a gonadal germ cell tumor is not uncommon; thus, the presence of a non-CNS primary must be excluded before a diagnosis of primary germ cell tumor is made. The histologic classification of brain germ cell tumors is similar to that used in the testis (Chapter 23), but the tumor that is histologically similar to the seminoma in the testis is referred to as germinoma in the CNS. The responses to radiotherapy and chemotherapy roughly parallel those of similar histologic lesions at other sites. However, since the tumor frequently extends into the CSF, it can disseminate widely along the surface of the brain and within the ventricular system, complicating therapy.

PINEAL PARENCHYMAL TUMORS

These lesions arise from the specialized cells of the pineal gland (pineocytes) that have features of neuronal differentiation. The tumors range in histologic appearance from well-differentiated lesions *(pineocytomas)* with areas of neuropil, tumor cells with small round nuclei and no evidence of mitoses or necrosis, to high-grade tumors *(pineoblastomas)* of densely packed small cells with necrosis and frequent mitotic figures and little light microscopic evidence of neuronal differentiation. The highly aggressive pineoblastoma commonly spreads throughout the CSF space, is more commonly found in children, and may occur in patients with retinoblastoma.

Gliomas are also found in the pineal region, arising from the glial stroma of the gland. Low-grade gliomas at this site can be difficult to distinguish in a small biopsy from the glial reaction that can accompany non-neoplastic pineal region cysts.

Meningiomas

Meningiomas are predominantly benign tumors of adults, usually attached to the dura, that arise from the meningothelial cell of the arachnoid. Meningiomas may be found along any of the external surfaces of the brain as well as within the ventricular system, where they arise from the stromal arachnoid cells of the choroid plexus.

MORPHOLOGY. Meningiomas are usually rounded masses with a well-defined dural base that compress underlying brain but are easily separated from it (Fig. 30–42*A*). Extension into the overlying bone may be present. The surface of the mass is usually encapsulated with thin, fibrous tissue and may have a bosselated or polypoid appearance. Another characteristic growth pattern is the **en plaque** variant, in which the tumor spreads in a sheetlike fashion along the surface of the dura. This form is commonly associated with hyperostotic reactive changes in the overlying bone. The lesions range from firm and fibrous to finely gritty, or they may be extremely calcified with psammoma bodies. Gross evidence of necrosis or extensive hemorrhage is not present.

Several histologic growth patterns are described, but most carry little prognostic significance. These include **syncytial,** appropriately named for the whorled clusters of cells that sit in tight groups without visible cell membranes; **fibroblastic,** with elongated cells and abundant collagen deposition between them; **transitional,** which shares features of the syncytial and fibroblastic types; **psammomatous,** with numerous psammoma bodies, apparently forming from calcification of the syncytial nests of meningothelial cells (Fig. 30–42*B*); **secretory,** with PAS-positive intracytoplasmic droplets and intracellular lumens by electron microscopy; and **microcystic,** with a loose, spongy appearance. The **papillary** variant,

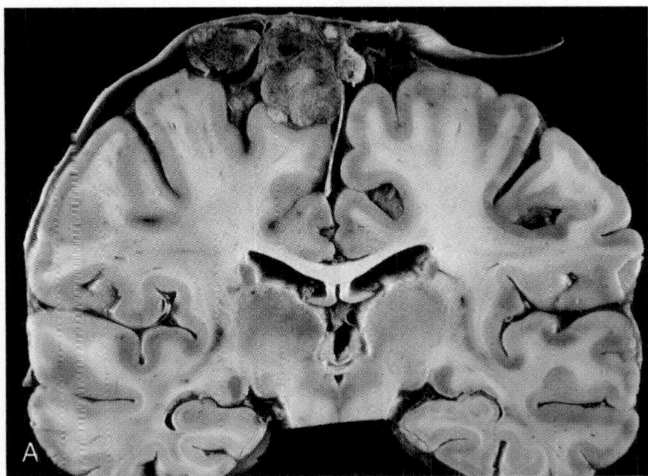

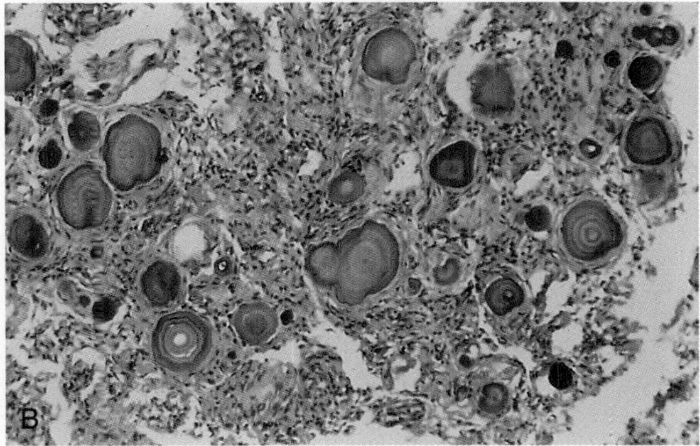

Figure 30-42

A, Parasagittal multilobular meningioma attached to the dura with compression of underlying brain. *B*, Meningioma with a whorled pattern of cell growth and psammoma bodies.

which has pleomorphic cells arranged around fibrovascular cores, has a higher propensity to recur. Xanthomatous degeneration, metaplasia, and moderate nuclear pleomorphism are common in meningiomas but have no prognostic significance.

By immunohistochemistry, meningiomas exhibit epithelial membrane antigen, in distinction to other tumors arising in this region. Keratin is restricted to lesions with the secretory pattern, and these tumors are also positive for carcinoembryonic antigen.

Malignant meningiomas are extremely rare tumors and may be difficult to recognize histologically. Features that support this diagnosis include infiltration of underlying brain, abundant mitoses with atypical forms, multifocal microscopic foci of necrosis, and loss of usual meningioma growth patterns.

The most common cytogenetic abnormality is loss of chromosome 22, especially the long arm (22q). The deletions include the region at 22q12 that harbors the *NF2* gene (see later). Indeed, 50% to 60% of meningiomas not associated with neurofibromatosis type 2 have mutations in the *NF2* gene. These genetic abnormalities are more common in meningiomas with fibroblastic or transitional histologic appearance.[123]

Clinical Features. Meningiomas are usually slow-growing lesions that present either with vague nonlocalizing symptoms or with focal findings referable to compression of underlying brain. Common sites of involvement include the parasagittal aspect of the brain convexity, dura over the lateral convexity, wing of the sphenoid, olfactory groove, sella turcica, and foramen magnum. They are uncommon in children and, in general, show a moderate (3:2) female predominance, although the ratio becomes 10:1 among patients with spinal meningiomas. Lesions are usually solitary, and their presence at multiple sites, especially in association with acoustic neuromas or glial tumors, suggests a diagnosis of neurofibromatosis type 2. The tumors often express progesterone receptors, and rapid growth during pregnancy has been reported.

Metastatic Tumors

Metastatic lesions, mostly carcinomas, account for approximately half of intracranial tumors in hospital patients. The five most common primary sites are lung, breast, skin (melanoma), kidney, and gastrointestinal tract, accounting for about 80% of all metastases. Some rare tumors (e.g., choriocarcinoma) have a high likelihood of metastasizing to the brain, whereas other more common tumors (e.g., prostatic carcinoma) almost never do even when they are metastatic to adjacent bone. The meninges are also a frequent site of involvement by metastatic disease. Metastatic tumors present clinically as mass lesions and may occasionally be the first manifestation of the cancer.

MORPHOLOGY. On macroscopic examination, intraparenchymal metastases form sharply demarcated masses, often at the gray matter–white matter junction, usually surrounded by a zone of edema. Meningeal carcinomatosis, with tumor nodules studding the surface of the brain, spinal cord, and intradural nerve roots, is associated particularly with small cell carcinoma and adenocarcinoma of the lung and carcinoma of the breast.

Paraneoplastic Syndromes

In addition to the direct and localized effects produced by metastases, *paraneoplastic syndromes* may involve the peripheral and central nervous systems, sometimes even preceding the clinical recognition of the malignant neoplasm.[124] These syndromes are discussed with diseases of peripheral nerves in Chapter 29; here we mention briefly only those affecting the CNS (Table 30–3).

Table 30–3. PARANEOPLASTIC SYNDROMES

Syndrome	Target	Tumor	Antigen	Potential Function
Subacute cerebellar degeneration	Purkinje cells	Breast, gynecologic cancer	Yo	Unknown
		Hodgkin disease	Tr	Unknown
		Small cell lung cancer	Hu	RNA-binding protein
Limbic encephalitis, brain stem encephalitis	Various neurons in limbic structures and brain stem	Small cell lung cancer	Hu	RNA-binding protein
Subacute sensory neuropathy	Dorsal root ganglion neurons	Small cell lung cancer	Hu	RNA-binding protein
Opsoclonus/myoclonus	Symptoms indicate brain stem, but exact target unknown	Breast, small cell lung cancer	Ri	Unknown
		Neuroblastoma	Unknown	—
Retinal degeneration	Photoreceptors	Small cell lung cancer, gynecologic cancer	Recoverin	cGMP-gated signal transduction during vision
Stiff-man syndrome	Spinal interneurons	Breast cancer	Amphiphysin	Role in synaptic vesicle function
Lambert-Eaton myasthenic syndrome	Neuromuscular junction (presynaptic terminals)	Small cell lung cancer	Presynaptic calcium channel	Allow influx of Ca^{2+} into terminals to allow neurotransmitter release

- *Paraneoplastic cerebellar degeneration:* the typical morphologic findings include destruction of Purkinje cells, gliosis, and a mild inflammatory infiltrate. The process appears to be an antibody-mediated injury of Purkinje cells and causes cerebellar signs and symptoms.
- *Limbic encephalitis* is characterized by subacute dementia. The pathologic findings are most striking in the anterior and medial portions of the temporal lobe and resemble an infectious process, with perivascular inflammatory cuffs, microglial nodules, some neuronal loss, and gliosis. A comparable process involving the brain stem can be seen in isolation or together with limbic system involvement.
- *Subacute sensory neuropathy* may be found in association with limbic encephalitis or in isolation. It is marked by loss of sensory neurons from dorsal root ganglia, again in association with inflammation.

The relationship among the underlying malignant process, the clinical features, and the antigens underlying the syndrome is complex. Some tumor types are associated with multiple types of autoantibodies, and the same antibodies can lead to different clinical syndromes. The most common tumor causing paraneoplastic syndromes is small cell carcinoma of the lung.

Peripheral Nerve Sheath Tumors

These tumors arise from cells of the peripheral nerve, including Schwann cells, perineurial cells, and fibroblasts. Many express Schwann cell characteristics, including the presence of S-100 antigen as well as the potential for melanocytic differentiation. As nerves exit the brain and spinal cord, there is a transition between myelination by oligodendrocytes and myelination by Schwann cells. This occurs within several millimeters of the substance of the brain; thus, peripheral nerve tumors can arise within the dura and may cause changes in adjacent brain or spinal cord. Tumors of comparable histogenesis and biologic behavior also arise along the peripheral course of nerves.

SCHWANNOMA

These benign tumors arise from the neural crest–derived Schwann cell and are associated with neurofibromatosis type 2 (see later). Symptoms are referable to local compression of the involved nerve.

MORPHOLOGY. Schwannomas are well-circumscribed, encapsulated masses that are attached to the nerve but can be separated from it (Fig. 30–43*A*). Tumors are firm, gray masses but may also have areas of cystic and xanthomatous change. On microscopic examination, tumors show a mixture of two growth patterns (Fig. 30–43*B*). In the **Antoni A** pattern of growth, elongated cells with cytoplasmic processes are arranged in fascicles in areas of moderate to high cellularity with little stromal matrix; the "nuclear-free zones" of processes that lie between the regions of nuclear palisading are termed Verocay bodies. In the **Antoni B** pattern of growth, the tumor is less densely cellular with a loose meshwork of cells along with microcysts and myxoid changes. In both areas, the cytology of the individual cells is similar, with elongated cell cytoplasm and regular oval nuclei. Electron microscopy shows basement membrane deposition encasing single cells and long-spacing collagen. Because the lesion displaces the nerve of origin as it grows, silver stains demonstrate that axons are largely excluded from the tumor, although they may become entrapped in the capsule. The Schwann cell origin of these tumors is borne out by their S-100 immunoreactivity. A variety of degenerative changes

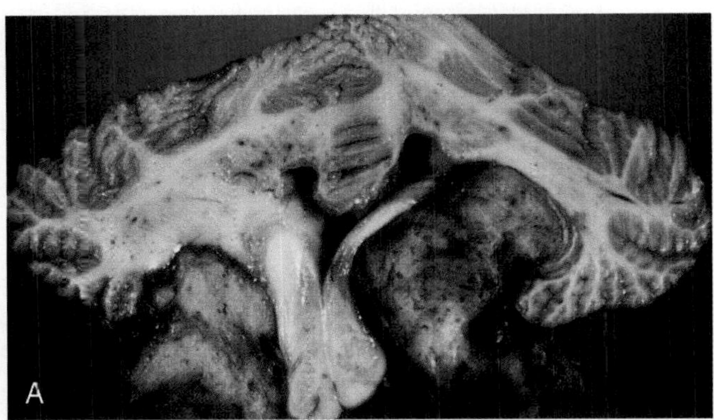

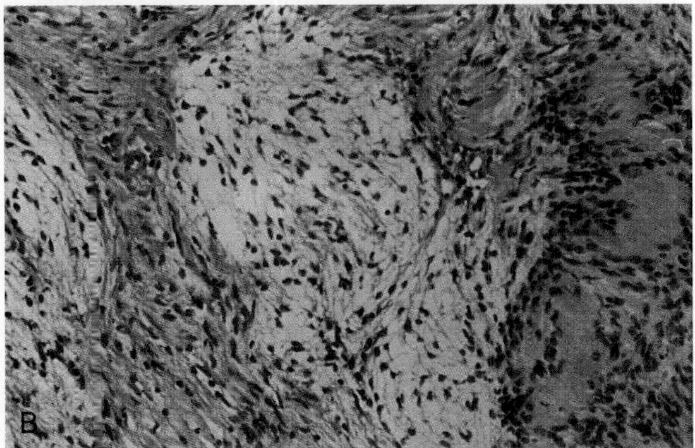

Figure 30-43

Schwannoma. *A*, Bilateral eighth nerve schwannomas. (Courtesy of Dr. K.M. Earle.) *B*, Tumor showing cellular areas (Antoni A), including Verocay bodies (*far right*), as well as looser, myxoid regions (Antoni B).

may be found in schwannomas, including nuclear pleomorphism, xanthomatous change, and vascular hyalinization. Malignant change is extremely rare in schwannomas, although local recurrence can follow incomplete resection.

Clinical Features. Within the cranial vault, the most common location is in the cerebellopontine angle, where they are attached to the vestibular branch of the eighth nerve (Fig. 30-43). Patients often present with tinnitus and hearing loss, and the tumor is often referred to as an acoustic neuroma. Elsewhere within the dura, sensory nerves are preferentially involved, including branches of the trigeminal nerve and dorsal roots. When extradural, schwannomas are most commonly found in association with large nerve trunks, where motor and sensory modalities are intermixed.

NEUROFIBROMA

Two histologically, and perhaps biologically, distinct lesions have been termed neurofibromas. The most common form occurs in the skin *(cutaneous neurofibroma)* or in peripheral nerve *(solitary neurofibroma).* These arise sporadically or in association with neurofibromatosis type 1 (see later). The skin lesions are evident as nodules, sometimes with overlying hyperpigmentation; they may grow to be large and become pedunculated. The risk of malignant transformation from these tumors is extremely small, and cosmetic concerns are their major morbidity. The second type is the *plexiform neurofibroma,* which is considered by some to occur only in patients with neurofibromatosis type 1. A major concern in the care of these patients is the difficulty in surgical removal of these plexiform tumors when they involve major nerve trunks, since they have a significant potential for malignant transformation.

MORPHOLOGY. ***Cutaneous Neurofibroma.*** Present in the dermis and subcutaneous fat, these well-delineated but unencapsulated masses are composed of spindle cells. Although they are not invasive, the adnexal structures are sometimes enwrapped by the edges of the lesion. The stroma of these tumors is highly collagenized and contains little myxoid material. Lesions within peripheral nerves are of identical histologic appearance.

Plexiform Neurofibroma. These tumors may arise anywhere along the extent of a nerve, although the large nerve trunk is the most common site. They are frequently multiple. At the site of each lesion, the host nerve is irregularly expanded, as each of its fascicles is infiltrated by the neoplasm. Unlike the case with schwannomas, it is not possible to separate the lesion from the nerve. The proximal and distal extremes of the tumor may have poorly defined margins, as fingers of tumor and individual cells insert themselves between the nerve fibers. On microscopic examination, the lesion has a loose, myxoid background with a low cellularity. A number of cell phenotypes are present, including Schwann cells with typical elongated nuclei and extensions of pink cytoplasm, larger multipolar fibroblastic cells, and a sprinkling of inflammatory cells, often including mast cells. Axons can be demonstrated within the tumor. Various ultrastructural and immunohistochemical studies have identified the neoplastic cells as showing markers of diverse lineages, including Schwann cells, perineurial cells, and fibroblasts.

MALIGNANT PERIPHERAL NERVE SHEATH TUMOR (MALIGNANT SCHWANNOMA)

These are highly malignant sarcomas that are locally invasive, frequently leading to multiple recurrences and eventual metastatic spread. Despite their name, these tumors do not arise from malignant degeneration of schwannomas. Instead, they arise de novo or from transformation of a plexiform neurofibroma. This fact provides the basis for their association with neurofibromatosis type 1. These tumors may also follow radiation therapy.

MORPHOLOGY. The lesions are poorly defined tumor masses with frequent infiltration along the axis of the parent nerve as well as invasion of adjacent soft tissues. Associated with the malignant nature of the neoplasm, necrosis is commonly present. On microscopic examination, a wide range of histologic findings can be encountered. Patterns reminiscent of fibrosarcoma or malignant fibrous histiocytoma may be found. In other areas, the tumor cells resemble Schwann cells, with elongated nuclei and prominent bipolar processes. Fascicle formation may be present. Mitoses, necrosis, and extreme nuclear anaplasia are common. Some but not all malignant peripheral nerve sheath tumors are immunoreactive for S-100 protein. In addition to the basic appearance of these tumors, a wide variety of "divergent" histologic patterns may be admixed, including epithelial structures, rhabdomyoblastic differentiation (termed **Triton tumors**), cartilage, and even bone. **Epithelioid malignant schwannomas** are aggressive variants derived from nerve sheaths and contain tumor cells having visible cell borders and epithelial type nests. They are immunoreactive for S-100 but not for keratin, the latter differentiating them from epithelial tumors.

Neurocutaneous Syndromes (Phakomatoses)

These are a group of inherited diseases characterized by the development of hamartomas and neoplasms throughout the body with particular involvement of the nervous system and skin. Many of the disorders are inherited in an autosomal dominant pattern and have been linked to tumor-suppressor genes. Symptoms are referable in part to the location of hamartomas or neoplasms; some patients are severely retarded, and seizure disorders are a serious problem in others. Most of these diseases (including *neurofibromatosis types 1 and 2, tuberous sclerosis complex,* and *von Hippel–Lindau disease*) are considered familial tumor syndromes, while others (such as *Sturge-Weber syndrome)* appear to be sporadic.

NEUROFIBROMATOSIS

(see also Chapter 6)

Type 1 Neurofibromatosis (NF1)

This autosomal dominant disorder is characterized by neurofibromas (plexiform and solitary), gliomas of the optic nerve, pigmented nodules of the iris *(Lisch nodules),* and cutaneous hyperpigmented macules *(café au lait spots).* It is one of the more common genetic disorders, having a frequency of 1 in 3000. Except for plexiform neurofibromas, the tumors that occur in NF1 are histologically comparable to those that occur sporadically. In patients with NF1, there is a propensity for the neurofibromas to undergo malignant degeneration at a higher rate than that observed for comparable tumors in the general population. This is especially true for plexiform neurofibromas.

The gene, located at 17q11.2, has been identified and encodes a protein termed *neurofibromin.* The protein contains a region homologous to one family of guanosine triphosphatase (GTPase)–activating proteins. This activity is presumed to allow neurofibromin to play a role in regulating signal transduction.[125] The protein is widely expressed, with the highest levels found in neural tissue. The *NF1* gene is a tumor-suppressor gene, based on evidence of loss of heterozygosity in tumors from NF1 patients. Mutations involving the *NF1* gene are of a wide variety of types, and there do not appear to be specific "hot spots" for changes. The clinical phenotype does not appear to correlate with the type or location of the mutation in the *NF1* gene, and the course of the disease is variable. Some individuals carry the gene and have no symptoms; others develop progressive disease with spinal deformities, disfiguring lesions, and compression of vital structures, including the spinal cord.

Type 2 Neurofibromatosis (NF2)

This is an autosomal dominant disorder in which patients develop a range of tumors, most commonly bilateral acoustic schwannomas and multiple meningiomas. Gliomas, typically ependymomas of the spinal cord, also occur in these patients. Many individuals with NF2 also have non-neoplastic lesions, which include nodular ingrowth of Schwann cells into the spinal cord (schwannosis), meningioangiomatosis (a proliferation of meningeal cells and blood vessels that grows into the brain), and glial hamartia (microscopic nodular collections of glial cells at abnormal locations, often in the superficial and deep layers of cerebral cortex). This disorder is much less common than NF1, having a frequency of 1 in 40,000 to 50,000.

The *NF2* gene is located on chromosome 22q12, and the gene product, merlin, shows structural similarity to a series of cytoskeletal proteins.[126] The protein is widely distributed throughout tissues, and its function remains uncertain. There is some correlation between the type of mutation and clinical symptoms, with nonsense mutations usually causing a more severe phenotype than missense mutations.

TUBEROUS SCLEROSIS

Tuberous sclerosis is an autosomal dominant syndrome characterized by the development of hamartomas and benign neoplasms involving the brain and other tissues. Hamartomas within the CNS occur as *cortical tubers* and subependymal hamartomas. Elsewhere in the body, lesions include renal angiomyolipomas, retinal glial hamartomas, and pulmonary and cardiac myomas. Cysts may be found at various sites, including the liver, kidneys, and pancreas. Cutaneous lesions include angiofibromas, leathery thickenings in localized patches (shagreen patches), hypopigmented areas (ash-leaf patches), and subungual fibromas. Genetic analysis is rendered complex because there are patients who are obligate carriers of the gene but have no evidence of the disease. Several distinct genetic loci have been identified at which mutations can cause tuberous sclerosis; however, the clinical and pathologic features caused by these different genes are indistinguishable. One tuberous sclerosis locus *(TSC1)* is found on chromosome 9q34, where it encodes a protein of unknown function (hamartin).[127] Another tuberous sclerosis locus *(TSC2)* is found on chromosome 16p13.3 and encodes a protein (tuberin) with homology to a GTPase-activating protein.[128]

MORPHOLOGY. Cortical hamartomas of tuberous sclerosis are firm areas of the cortex that, in contrast to the softer adjacent cortex, have been likened to potatoes, hence the appellation "tubers." These hamartomas are composed of haphazardly arranged neurons that lack the normal laminar organization of neocortex. In addition, some large cells express phenotypes intermediate between glia and neurons, with intermediate filaments of both neuronal (neurofilament) and glial (GFAP) types. These cells have large vesicular nuclei with nucleoli, resembling neurons, and abundant eosinophilic cytoplasm like gemistocytic astrocytes. Similar hamartomatous features are present in the subependymal nodules, where large astrocytic cells cluster beneath the ventricular surface. These multiple droplike masses that bulge into the ventricular system gave rise to the term "candle-guttering." In subependymal areas, a tumor unique to tuberous sclerosis (subependymal giant cell astrocytoma) occurs.

Treatment is symptomatic, including anticonvulsant therapy for control of seizures.

VON HIPPEL–LINDAU DISEASE

This is an autosomal dominantly inherited disease in which affected individuals develop tumors (capillary hemangioblastomas) within the cerebellar hemispheres, retina, and less commonly the brain stem and spinal cord. Patients may also have cysts involving the pancreas, liver, and kidneys and have a strong propensity to develop renal cell carcinoma of the kidney (Chapter 21). The disease frequency is 1 in 30,000 to 40,000.

The gene for von Hippel–Lindau disease, a tumor-suppressor gene, is located on chromosome 3p25–26 and encodes a protein (pVHL) that inhibits the "elongation" step during RNA synthesis. The gene product does this through interaction with two members (elongin B and elongin C) of a trimolecular complex through competition with the normal third member of the complex (elongin A). With mutations in pVHL, the ability to interact with the elongin B/C complex is lost, but how this defect causes the lesions is still unclear. Missense mutations, but not other types of mutations, are highly likely to result in a phenotype that includes, in addition to the vascular tumors, adrenal pheochromocytoma.

MORPHOLOGY. The cerebellar capillary hemangioblastoma, the principal neurologic manifestation of the disease, is a highly vascular neoplasm that occurs as a mural nodule associated with a large fluid-filled cyst. On microscopic examination, the lesion consists of a mixture of variable proportions of capillary-size or somewhat larger thin-walled vessels with intervening "stromal cells," cells of uncertain histogenesis characterized by vacuolated, lightly PAS-positive, lipid-rich cytoplasm and indefinite immunohistochemical phenotype.

Therapy is directed at the symptomatic neoplasms, including resection of the cerebellar hemangioblastomas and laser therapy for retinal hemangioblastomas. Partial nephrectomy is performed for renal carcinomas when these malignant neoplasms are bilateral. Polycythemia is associated with a hemangioblastoma in about 10% of cases; the tumor has been shown to be a source of erythropoietin in these cases, although the cell of origin of the growth factor is not known.

REFERENCES

1. Kandel E, et al: Principles of Neural Science. New York, Elsevier, 1991.
2. Adams RD, et al: Principles of Neurology, 6th ed. New York, McGraw-Hill, 1997.
3. Graham D, Lantos P (eds): Greenfield's Neuropathology, 6th ed. New York, Oxford University Press, 1997.
4. Parent A: Carpenter's Human Neuroanatomy, 9th ed. Baltimore, Williams & Wilkins, 1996.
5. Mountcastle V: The columnar organization of the neocortex. Brain 120:701–722, 1997.
6. Peters A, et al: The Fine Structure of the Nervous System: Neurons and Their Supporting Cells. Philadelphia, WB Saunders, 1991.
7. Cáccamo D, Rubinstein L: Tumors: application of immunohistochemical methods. In Garcia J (ed): Neuropathology: The Diagnostic Approach. St. Louis, Mosby, 1997, pp 193–218.
8. Garcia J, Mena H: Vascular diseases. In Garcia J (ed): Neuropathology: The Diagnostic Approach. St. Louis, Mosby, 1997, pp 263–320.
9. Koliatsos V, Price D: Axotomy as an experimental model of neuronal injury and cell death. Brain Pathol 6:447–465, 1996.
10. Chin SS-M, Goldman JE: Glial inclusions in CNS degenerative disease. J Neuropathol Exp Neurol 55:499–508, 1996.
11. Norenberg M: Astrocyte responses to CNS injury. J Neuropathol Exp Neurol 53:213–220, 1994.
12. Barron K: The microglial cell. A historical review. J Neurol Sci 134(Suppl):57–68, 1995.
13. Hickey WF, Kimura H: Perivascular microglial cells of the CNS are bone-marrow derived and present antigen in vivo. Science 239:290–292, 1988.
14. Keane R, Hickey WF (eds): Immunology of the Nervous System. New York, Oxford University Press, 1997.
15. Rowland LP, et al: Cerebrospinal fluid: blood-brain barrier, brain edema, and hydrocephalus. In Kandel ER, et al (eds): Principles of Neural Science. New York, Elsevier, 1991, pp 1050–1060.
16. Boyle C, et al: Prevalence and health impact of developmental disabilities in US children. Pediatrics 93:399–403, 1994.
17. Bayer S, et al: Embryology. In Duckett S (ed): Pediatric Neuropathology. Baltimore, Williams & Wilkins, 1995, pp 54–107.
18. O'Rahilly R, Müller F: The Embryonic Human Brain. New York, Wiley-Liss, 1994.
19. Friede RL: Developmental Neuropathology. Berlin, Springer-Verlag, 1989.

20. Harding B, Copp A: Malformations. In Graham D, Lantos P (eds): Greenfield's Neuropathology, 6th ed. New York, Oxford University Press, 1997, pp 397–533.
21. Perrimon N: Hedgehog and beyond. Cell 80:517–520, 1995.
22. Czeizel A, Dudás I: Prevention of the first occurrence of neural-tube defects by periconceptional vitamin supplementation. N Engl J Med 327:1832–1835, 1992.
23. Dobyns W: Lissencephaly and other malformations of cortical development. Neuropediatrics 26:132–147, 1995.
24. Mizuguchi M, et al: Lissencephaly gene product. Localization in the central nervous system and loss of immunoreactivity in Miller-Dieker syndrome. Am J Pathol 147:1142–1151, 1995.
25. Roessler E: Mutations in the human Sonic hedgehog gene cause holoprosencephaly. Nat Genet 14:357–360, 1996.
26. Volpe J: Neurology of the Newborn, 3rd ed. Philadelphia, WB Saunders, 1995.
27. Kinney H, Armstrong D: Perinatal neuropathology. In Graham D, Lantos P (eds): Greenfield's Neuropathology, 6th ed. New York, Oxford University Press, 1997, pp 536–599.
28. Graham D, et al: The nature, distribution and causes of traumatic brain injury. Brain Pathol 5:397–406, 1995.
29. Leestma J: Forensic neuropathology. In Garcia J (ed): Neuropathology: The Diagnostic Approach. St. Louis, Mosby, 1997, pp 475–527.
30. Knight B: Forensic Pathology, 2nd ed. New York, Oxford University Press, 1996.
31. Povlishock J, Jenkins L: Are the pathobiological changes evoked by traumatic brain injury immediate and irreversible? Brain Pathol 5: 415–426, 1995.
32. Tator C: Update on the pathophysiology and pathology of acute spinal cord injury. Brain Pathol 5:407–413, 1995.
33. Tator C, Koyanagi I: Vascular mechanisms in the pathophysiology of human spinal cord injury. J Neurosurg 86:483–492, 1997.
34. Caplan LR: Stroke. Boston, Butterworth-Heinemann, 1993.
35. Stehbens W, Lie J (eds): Vascular Pathology. London, Chapman & Hall, 1995.
36. Joutel A, et al: Notch3 mutations in CADASIL, a hereditary adult-onset condition causing stroke and dementia. Nature 383:707–710, 1996.
37. Tournier-Lasserve E, et al: Cerebral autosomal dominant arteriopathy with subcortical infarcts and leukoencephalopathy maps to chromosome 19q12. Nat Genet 3:256–259, 1993.
38. De Girolami U, et al: Selective necrosis and total necrosis in focal cerebral ischemia. Neuropathologic observations on experimental middle cerebral artery occlusion in the macaque monkey. J Neuropathol Exp Neurol 43:57–71, 1984.
39. Garcia JH, et al: Ischemic stroke and incomplete infarction. Stroke 27:761–765, 1996.
40. Auer R, Benveniste H: Hypoxia and related conditions. In Graham D, Lantos P (eds): Greenfield's Neuropathology, 6th ed. New York, Oxford University Press, 1997, pp 263–314.
41. Meldrum B: Cytoprotective therapies in stroke. Curr Opin Neurol 8: 15–23, 1995.
42. Molinari GF: Lobar hemorrhages. Where do they come from? How did they get there? Stroke 24:523–526, 1993.
43. Schievink W: Intracranial aneurysms. N Engl J Med 336:28–40, 1997.
44. Suzuki R, et al: The role of endothelin-1 in the origin of cerebral vasospasm in patients with aneurysmal subarachnoid hemorrhage. J Neurosurg 77:96–100, 1992.
45. Tyler K, Martin J: Infectious Diseases of the Central Nervous System. Philadelphia, FA Davis, 1993.
46. Durand ML, et al: Acute bacterial meningitis in adults. A review of 493 episodes. N Engl J Med 328:21–28, 1993.
47. Gray F: Bacterial infections. Brain Pathol 7:629–647, 1997.
48. Quagliarello V, Scheid W: Treatment of bacterial meningitis. N Engl J Med 336:708–716, 1997.
49. Chun CH, et al: Brain abscess: a study of 45 consecutive cases. Medicine (Baltimore) 65:415–431, 1986.
50. Garcia-Monco JC, Benach J: Lyme neuroborreliosis. Ann Neurol 37: 691–702, 1995.
51. Logigian EL, et al: Chronic neurologic manifestations of Lyme disease. N Engl J Med 323:1438–1444, 1990.
52. Esiri M: Viruses and rickettsiae. Brain Pathol 7:695–709, 1997.
53. Whitley RJ: Viral encephalitis. N Engl J Med 323:242–250, 1990.
54. Deresiewicz R, et al: Clinical and neuroradiographic manifestation of eastern equine encephalitis. N Engl J Med 336:1867–1874, 1997.
55. Morgello S, et al: Cytomegalovirus encephalitis in patients with acquired immunodeficiency syndrome. An autopsy study of 30 cases and a review of the literature. Hum Pathol 18:289–297, 1987.
56. Isaacson S, et al: Cellular localization of poliovirus RNA in the spinal cord during acute paralytic poliomyelitis. Ann N Y Acad Sci 753:194–200, 1995.
57. Kaminski H, et al: Spinal cord histopathology in long-term survivors of poliomyelitis. Muscle Nerve 18:1208–1209, 1995.
58. Dalakas M: The post-polio syndrome as an evolved clinical entity. Definition and clinical description. Ann N Y Acad Sci 753:68–80, 1995.
59. Melchers W, et al: The postpolio syndrome: no evidence for poliovirus persistence. Ann Neurol 32:728–732, 1992.
60. Munsat TL: Poliomyelitis—new problems with an old disease. N Engl J Med 324:1206–1207, 1991.
61. Mrak R, Young L: Rabies encephalitis in humans: pathology, pathogenesis and pathophysiology. J Neuropathol Exp Neurol 53:1–10, 1994.
62. Seilhean D, et al: The neuropathology of AIDS: the Salpêtrière experience and review of the literature, 1981–1993. Adv Pathol Lab Med 7:221–257, 1994.
63. Gray F, et al: Neuropathology of early HIV-1 infection. Brain Pathol 6:1–15, 1996.
64. Johnson R, et al: Quantitation of human immunodeficiency virus in brains of demented and nondemented patients with acquired immunodeficiency syndrome. Ann Neurol 39:392–395, 1996.
65. Shi B, et al: Apoptosis induced by HIV-1 infection of the central nervous system. J Clin Invest 98:1979–1990, 1996.
66. Lipton S: Neuropathogenesis of acquired immunodeficiency syndrome dementia. Curr Opin Neurol 10:247–253, 1997.
67. Tan S, et al: AIDS-associated vacuolar myelopathy. A morphometric study. Brain 118:1247–1261, 1995.
68. Sharer L, et al: In situ amplification and detection of HIV-1 DNA in fixed pediatric AIDS brain tissue. Hum Pathol 27:614–617, 1996.
69. Chaisson R, Griffin D: Progressive multifocal leukoencephalopathy in AIDS. JAMA 264:79–82, 1990.
70. Schmidbauer M, et al: Progressive multifocal leukoencephalopathy (PML) in AIDS and the pre-AIDS era. Acta Neuropathol 80:375–380, 1990.
71. Allen I, et al: The significance of measles virus antigen and genome distribution in the CNS in SSPE for mechanisms of viral spread and demyelination. J Neuropathol Exp Neurol 55:471–480, 1996.
72. Chimelli L, Mahler-Araújo B: Fungal infections. Brain Pathol 7: 613–627, 1997.
73. Porter SB, Sande MA: Toxoplasmosis of the central nervous system in the acquired immunodeficiency syndrome. N Engl J Med 327: 1643–1648, 1992.
74. Martinez A, Visvesvara G: Free-living, amphizoic and opportunistic amebas. Brain Pathol 7:583–598, 1997.
75. Prusiner SB: Human prion diseases and neurodegeneration. Curr Top Microbiol Immunol 207:1–17, 1996.
75a. Welch WJ, Gambetti P: Chaperoning brain diseases. Nature 392: 23–24, 1998.
76. Goldfarb L, et al: Fatal familial insomnia and familial Creutzfeldt-Jakob disease: disease phenotype determined by a DNA polymorphism. Science 258:806–808, 1992.
77. Will R, et al: A new variant of Creutzfeldt-Jakob disease in the UK. Lancet 347:921–925, 1996.
78. Prusiner SB: Prion diseases and the BSE crisis. Science 278:245–251, 1997.
79. Gambetti P, et al: Fatal familial insomnia and familial Creutzfeldt-Jakob disease: clinical, pathological and molecular features. Brain Pathol 5:43–51, 1995.
80. Compston A: Genetic epidemiology of multiple sclerosis. J Neurol Neurosurg Psychiatry 62:553–561, 1997.
81. Sadovnick AD, Ebers GC: Epidemiology of multiple sclerosis: a critical overview. Can J Neurol Sci 20:17–29 1993.
82. Allen I, Brankin B: Pathogenesis of multiple sclerosis—the immune diathesis and the role of viruses. J Neuropathol Exp Neurol 52:95–105, 1993.
83. Kleinschmidt-DeMasters BK, Norenberg MD: Rapid correction of

hyponatremia causes demyelination: relation to central pontine myelinolysis. Science 211:1068–1070, 1981.
84. Evans DA, et al: Prevalence of Alzheimer's disease in a community population of older persons: higher than previously reported. JAMA 262:2551–2556, 1989.
85. Braak H, Braak E: Neuropathological stageing of Alzheimer-related changes. Acta Neuropathol 82:239–259, 1991.
86. Khachaturian ZS: Diagnosis of Alzheimer's disease. Arch Neurol 42:1097–1105, 1985.
87. Mirra S, et al: The consortium to establish a registry for Alzheimer's disease (CERAD). Part II: Standardization of the neuropathologic assessment of Alzheimer's disease. Neurology 41:479–486, 1991.
88. Mirra SS, et al: Making the diagnosis of Alzheimer's disease. A primer for practicing pathologists. Arch Pathol Lab Med 117:132–144, 1993.
89. Lendon C, et al: Exploring the etiology of Alzheimer's disease using molecular genetics. JAMA 277:825–831, 1997.
90. Selkoe D: Cell biology of the β-amyloid precursor protein and the genetics of Alzheimer disease. Cold Spring Harb Symp Quant Biol 61:587–596, 1996.
91. Xia W, et al: Interaction between amyloid precursor protein and presenilins in mammalian cells: implications for the pathogenesis of Alzheimer disease. Proc Natl Acad Sci USA 94:8208–8213, 1997.
92. Kim TW, et al: Alternative cleavage of Alzheimer-associated presenilins during apoptosis by a caspase-3 family protease. Science 277: 373–376, 1997.
93. Polymeropoulos MH, et al: Mutation in the α-synuclein gene identified in families with Parkinson's disease. Science 276:204–2047, 1997.
94. López-Lozano J, et al: Long-term improvement in patients with severe Parkinson's disease after implantation of fetal ventral mesencephalic tissue in a cavity of the caudate nucleus: 5-year follow up in 10 patients. J Neurosurg 86:931–942, 1997.
95. Olanow C, et al: Fetal nigral transplantation as a therapy for Parkinson's disease. Trends Neurosci 19:102–109, 1996.
96. Rebeiz J, et al: Corticodentatonigral degeneration with neuronal achromasia. Arch Neurol 18:20–33, 1968.
97. Schneider J, et al: Corticobasal degeneration: neuropathologic and clinical heterogeneity. Neurology 48:959–969, 1997.
98. Feany M, Dickson D: Widespread cytoskeletal pathology characterizes corticobasal degeneration. Am J Pathol 146:1388–1396, 1995.
99. Feany M, et al: Neuropathologic overlap of progressive supranuclear palsy, Pick's disease and corticobasal degeneration. J Neuropathol Exp Neurol 55:53–67, 1996.
100. Papp M, et al: Glial cytoplasmic inclusions in the CNS of patients with multiple system atrophy (striatonigral degeneration, olivopontocerebellar atrophy, and Shy-Drager syndrome). J Neurol Sci 94:79–100, 1989.
101. Papp M, Lantos P: The distribution of oligodendroglial inclusions in multiple system atrophy and its relevance to clinical symptomatology. Brain 117:235–243, 1994.
102. Richardson E: Huntington's disease: some recent neuropathological studies. Neuropathol Appl Neurobiol 16:451–460, 1990.
103. The Huntington's Disease Collaborative Research Group: A novel gene containing a trinucleotide repeat that is expanded and unstable on Huntington's disease chromosomes. Cell 72:971–983, 1993.
104. Wellington C, et al: Toward understanding the molecular pathology of Huntington's disease. Brain Pathol 7:979–1002, 1997.
105. Koeppen AH: The hereditary ataxias. J Neuropathol Exp Neurol 57: 531–543, 1998.
106. Campuzano V, et al: Friedreich's ataxia: autosomal recessive disease caused by an intronic GAA triplet repeat expansion. Science 271: 1423–1427, 1996.
107. Blaese R: Genetic immunodeficiency syndromes with defects in both T- and B-lymphocyte function. In Scriver C, et al (eds): The Metabolic and Molecular Bases of Inherited Disease, 7th ed. New York, McGraw-Hill, 1995, pp 3895–3909.
108. Mitsumoto H, et al: Amyotrophic lateral sclerosis. Philadelphia, FA Davis, 1998.
109. Rosen DR, et al: Mutations in Cu/Zn superoxide dismutase gene are associated with familial amyotrophic lateral sclerosis. Nature 362: 59–62, 1993.
110. Scriver C, et al (eds): The Metabolic and Molecular Bases of Inherited Disease, 7th ed. New York, McGraw-Hill, 1995.
111. Sistermans EA, et al: Duplication of the proteolipid protein gene is the major cause of Pelizaeus-Merzbacher disease. Neurology 50: 1749, 1998.
112. Bartalini G, et al: Biochemical diagnosis of Canavan disease. Childs Nerv Syst 8:468–470, 1992.
113. Sparaco M, et al: Neuropathology of mitochondrial encephalomyopathies due to mitochondrial DNA defects. J Neuropathol Exp Neurol 52:1–10, 1993.
114. Gautin PH, et al: Radiation Injury to the Nervous System. New York, Raven Press, 1991.
115. Burger P, et al: Surgical Pathology of the Nervous System and Its Coverings, 3rd ed. New York, Churchill Livingstone, 1991.
116. Russell DS, Rubinstein LJ: Pathology of Tumors of the Nervous System, 5th ed. Baltimore, Williams & Wilkins, 1989.
117. World Health Organization: Histological Typing of Tumors of the Central Nervous System. Berlin, Springer-Verlag, 1993.
118. Daumas-Duport C, et al: Grading of astrocytomas. A simple and reproducible method. Cancer 62:2152–2165, 1988.
119. Hsu D, et al: Use of MIB-1 (Ki-67) immunoreactivity in differentiating grade II and grade III gliomas. J Neuropathol Exp Neurol 56: 857–865, 1997.
120. Louis D: A molecular genetic model of astrocytoma histopathology. Brain Pathol 7:755–764, 1997.
121. von Deimling A, et al: Subsets of glioblastoma multiforme defined by molecular genetic analysis. Brain Pathol 3:19–26, 1993.
122. Watanabe K, et al: Overexpression of the EGF receptor and p53 mutations are mutually exclusive in the evolution of primary and secondary glioblastomas. Brain Pathol 6:217–223, 1996.
123. Wellenreuther R, et al: Analysis of the neurofibromatosis 2 gene reveals molecular variants of meningioma. Am J Pathol 146:827–832, 1995.
124. Henson RA, Urich H: Cancer and the Nervous System. Oxford, Blackwell Scientific Publications, 1982.
125. Riccardi VM: The clinical and molecular genetics of neurofibromatosis-1 and neurofibromatosis-2. In Rosenberg RN, et al (eds): The Molecular and Genetic Basis of Neurological Disease. Boston, Butterworth-Heinemann, 1993, pp 837–853.
126. Trofatter JA, et al: A novel moesin-, ezrin-, radixin-like gene is a candidate for the neurofibromatosis 2 tumor suppressor. Cell 72: 791–800, 1993.
127. van Slegtenhorst M, et al: Identification of the tuberous sclerosis gene *TSC1* on chromosome 9q34. Science 277:805–808, 1997.
128. The European Chromosome 16 Tuberous Sclerosis Consortium: Identification and characterization of the tuberous sclerosis gene on chromosome 16. Cell 75:1305–1315, 1993.
129. Blacker D, et al: Alpha-2 macroglobulin is genetically associated with Alzheimer disease. Nat Genet 19:357–360, 1998.

31

The Eye

Daniel M. Albert and Thaddeus P. Dryja

CONGENITAL ANOMALIES
TRISOMY 13
TRISOMY 21
INFECTIOUS EMBRYOPATHIES
CONGENITAL RUBELLA SYNDROME
CONGENITAL SYPHILIS
CONJUNCTIVA
VITAMIN A DEFICIENCY
PINGUECULA AND PTERYGIUM
TRACHOMA
EPITHELIAL TUMORS
CORNEA
KERATITIS AND CORNEAL ULCERS
Herpetic Infections
HEREDITARY CORNEAL DYSTROPHIES
Stromal Dystrophies
Endothelial Dystrophy
UVEA
GRANULOMATOUS UVEITIS
Infectious Uveitis
Sarcoidosis
Sympathetic Ophthalmia
UVEAL MELANOMAS
LENS
CATARACTS
RETINA
RETINOPATHY OF PREMATURITY (RETROLENTAL FIBROPLASIA)
DIABETES MELLITUS
Background Retinopathy
Proliferative Retinopathy
HYPERTENSIVE AND ARTERIOSCLEROTIC RETINOPATHY
Hypertensive Retinopathy
Arteriosclerotic Retinopathy
RETINITIS PIGMENTOSA
MACULAR DEGENERATION
RETINAL DETACHMENT
RETINOBLASTOMA
VITREOUS
OPTIC NERVE
PAPILLEDEMA
OPTIC NEURITIS
OPTIC ATROPHY
TUMORS
GLAUCOMA
PHTHISIS BULBI AND THE END STAGE OF DIFFUSE OCULAR DISEASE

Ocular disorders are responsible for a great deal of morbidity. There are estimated to be between 27 and 35 million blind people in the world and probably another 13 million people with lesser degrees of visual impairment.[1] Mortality from primary ocular diseases is uncommon and is limited to malignancies developing in the eye, the orbit, or the lids.

The eye consists of a number of individual anatomic and functional elements (Fig. 31–1). In keeping with this, our discussion of the pathology of the eye covers the conjunctiva, cornea, uvea, lens, retina, vitreous, and optic nerve. All of these elements may respond to systemic disease. In some instances, as for example, the development of a cataract or glaucoma, the response may be unique for that part of the eye. Often the response is similar to that seen in other organs; for example, the blood vessels of the retina in hypertension are affected in a manner similar to that seen in the kidneys or the brain. Similarly, local infections as well as physical and chemical injuries of the eye may result in unique responses (as seen in the transparent and avascular cornea) or may parallel changes seen elsewhere. Pathologic processes in the lids are similar to those in other skin surfaces, and those in the conjunctiva may be closely related to changes in other mucous membranes.

A major proportion of blinding diseases is due to primary ocular disorders such as glaucoma, cataract, and macular degeneration, and these require specific discussion. Of the ocular tumors, melanomas deserve special mention because they differ significantly in their biologic behavior from cutaneous melanomas.[2] Retinoblastoma serves as a

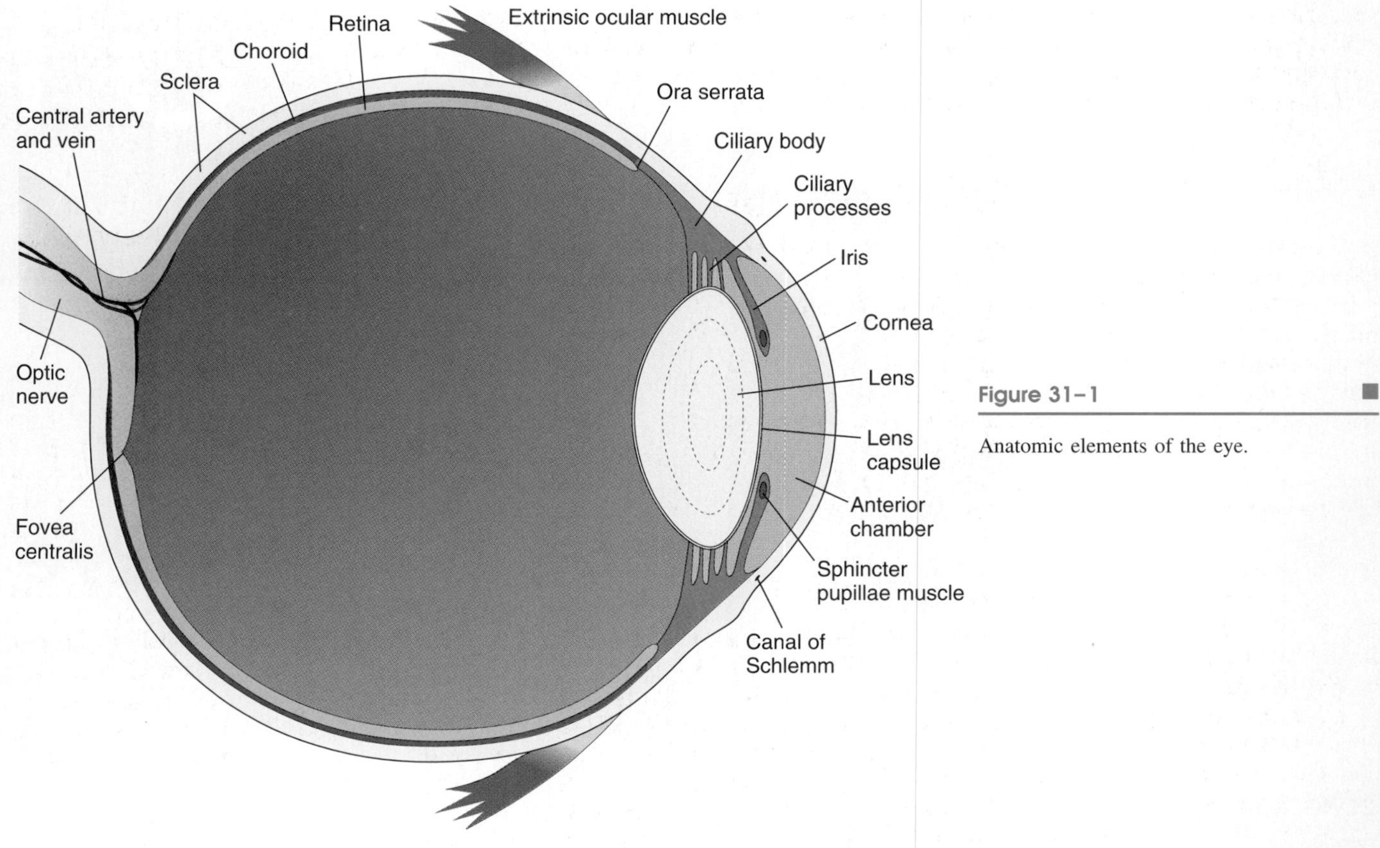

Figure 31–1

Anatomic elements of the eye.

prototype of a diverse group of human cancers caused by loss of function of suppressor cancer genes and is also reviewed.

CONGENITAL ANOMALIES

Chromosomal aneuploidies are often associated with ocular abnormalities. Among the most common are trisomy 13 and trisomy 21 (Chapter 6).

Trisomy 13

Severe ocular anomalies occur in almost all cases of trisomy 13. Abnormally small eyes (microphthalmos) are common. In rare instances, the eyes may be fused, resulting in a cyclopia-like condition known as *cyclopean synophthalmus*. The most characteristic findings are areas of defective formation of the iris and ciliary body (*colobomas*), *cataract*, and a persistence of the embryonic vasculature of the vitreous known as *persistent hyperplastic primary vitreous*. These features are present in 80% of eyes with trisomy 13. A striking finding seen in 65% of these eyes is cartilage present within the coloboma. In 75% of eyes, the retina contains tubular and rosette-like structures known as *retinal dysplasia*.[3] In 60% of cases, there is evidence of defective development of cornea, iris, and anterior chamber angle (termed *dysgenesis*), with associated congenital *glaucoma* in some instances.

Trisomy 21

The ocular findings in trisomy 21, while far less severe than in trisomy 13, are distinctive.[4] The eyes are usually set far apart (*hypertelorism*) and are associated with abnormalities of the lids, including oblique or arched palpebral fissures, epicanthus, and ectropion and eversion of the upper eyelids. A progressively cone-shaped cornea with ectasia of the central part (*keratoconus*), possibly secondary to knuckle-rubbing by the patients, and retinal dysplasia develop in many patients. The irides have a speckled appearance owing to the presence of ringlike foci of iris hypoplasia surrounding relatively normal iris stroma (*Brushfield spots*). In addition, the irides may show focal stromal hyperplasia. Flakelike lens opacities (a type of cataract) can develop in patients over 15 years of age.[5] Additional ocular abnormalities include esotropia, high myopia, hyperemic optic disc, retinal pigment epithelial atrophy, prominent whitened choroidal vessels, and chronic blepharoconjunctivitis.

INFECTIOUS EMBRYOPATHIES

A number of maternal infections during pregnancy may result in ocular abnormalities. Among the most severe are toxoplasmosis, cytomegalic inclusion disease, congenital rubella, and congenital syphilis. All are discussed except for rubella and syphilis in Chapter 9. Only the ocular findings in rubella and syphilis are reviewed here.

Congenital Rubella Syndrome

Ocular abnormalities found in the rubella syndrome[6] are cataract, congenital glaucoma, iris abnormalities, and a pigmentary disturbance of the retina known as *rubella retinopathy*. The rubella cataract is quite distinctive on histologic examination because of the retention of cell nuclei in the centrally located embryonic nucleus of the lens, an area in which the cell nuclei normally disappear well before birth. It has also been shown that the *rubella virus can survive within the lens for a number of years after birth.* Consequently, surgery on rubella cataracts may lead to the release of virus into the interior of the eye and cause uveitis or endophthalmitis.

The iris in congenital rubella syndrome has a poorly developed dilator muscle and a necrotic-appearing epithelium. In addition, chronic, nongranulomatous inflammation of the iris stroma is often present. These factors contribute to an inability of the iris to dilate normally and result in the clinical appearance of a *leathery* iris.

Rubella retinopathy is the most characteristic finding in this disorder. The principal defect is in the retinal pigment epithelium, which shows alternating areas of atrophy and hypertrophy; this gives rise to the clinically striking *salt-and-pepper* ophthalmoscopic appearance. In some cases, this retinal abnormality is progressive. Subretinal neovascularization may occur in some patients, usually between the ages of 10 and 18 years.

Congenital Syphilis

Although infrequently seen today, congenital syphilis results in marked ocular abnormalities.[7] The most common and characteristic finding is an inflammation of the stroma of the cornea (interstitial keratitis) occurring between 5 and 20 years of age. Initially the cornea becomes edematous and is infiltrated by lymphocytes and plasma cells. The involvement is often unilateral and may occupy only a sector of the cornea. Blood vessels grow into the deep cornea just anterior to the basement membrane of the endothelium (Descemet membrane). The inflammation typically lasts for 2 to 3 months. The edema and inflammatory cells disappear, but the blood vessels persist. They are usually not filled with blood (*ghost vessels*).

CONJUNCTIVA

Vitamin A Deficiency

Keratomalacia is a severe form of vitamin A deficiency characterized by diffuse, severe keratinization of all mucous membrane epithelia. In the eye, the corneal and conjunctival epithelia are involved (xerophthalmia). Hypovitaminosis A is also accompanied by *night blindness* first as a result of dysfunction of rod photoreceptors and later as a result of degenerative changes in the retina. The condition occurs principally in children. Secondary bacterial infection and corneal ulceration may occur with subsequent *corneal necrosis and perforation and panophthalmitis*. Keratomalacia is a leading cause of blindness in underdeveloped countries.[8]

Pinguecula and Pterygium

Pingueculae are raised yellowish lesions that characteristically occur in the conjunctiva near the nasal limbus of the cornea (Fig. 31–2). These are bilateral and are seen in middle-aged and elderly patients. On histologic examination, there are abnormal elastin and collagen fibers in the subepithelial tissue[9] (basophilic degeneration) resulting in gray-appearing material that stains positively for elastin but is insensitive to elastase.

A *pterygium* is histologically identical to pinguecula but grows as a winglike projection of vascularized tissue that extends onto the nasal cornea. Pterygia are usually bilateral but asymmetric. They cause dissolution of the anterior layer of the corneal stroma (Bowman membrane). The epithelium overlying pterygia or pingueculae may show a variety of secondary changes, including acanthosis, hyperkeratosis, and dyskeratosis.

Trachoma

Trachoma, one of the world's major causes of blindness, is caused by *Chlamydia trachomatis* (Chapter 9). It affects primarily the conjunctiva and corneal epithelium, ultimately causing cicatrization of this tissue. Its course can be divided into four stages (the McCallan classification).[10]

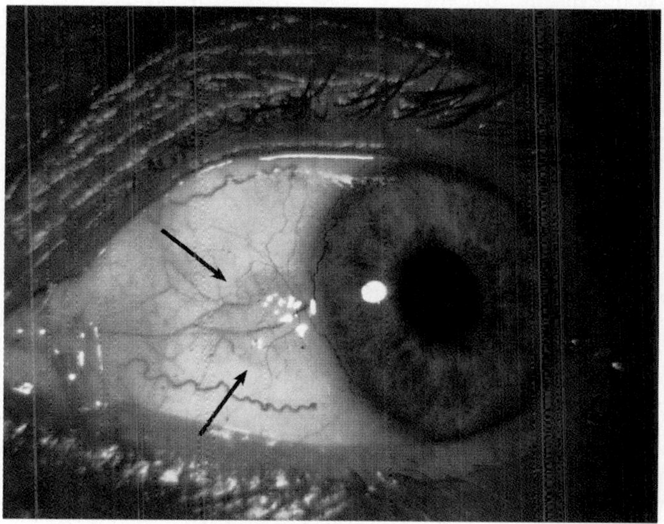

Figure 31–2 ■

Pinguecula (*arrows*) at the nasal limbus of the cornea.

Stage I is characterized clinically by the formation of conjunctival follicles (subepithelial conjunctival inflammatory infiltrates) and diffuse punctate inflammation of the cornea. Subsequently, there is growth of fibrovascular tissue in the substantia propria of the conjunctiva and onto the cornea (pannus). Microscopically, the corneal epithelium contains cytoplasmic inclusion bodies composed of microcolonies of elementary bodies and larger basophilic initial bodies (Fig. 31–3). Lymphocytes and plasma cells infiltrate the subepithelial tissue; polymorphonuclear leukocytes infiltrate the corneal and conjunctival epithelium.

In *stage II*, the inflammation becomes florid, with the further formation of follicles and epithelial thickening. The corneal pannus becomes more severe. Histologically, large macrophages with phagocytized debris (Leber cells) are seen in the conjunctiva, accompanying the epithelial hyperplasia with round cell infiltration and subepithelial edema.

In *stage III*, the follicles disappear, and cicatrization occurs, leaving in its wake inversion of the upper lid (cicatricial entropion) and misdirected lashes (trichiasis). On histologic examination, scattered lymphocytes and plasma cells can still be seen along with subepithelial scar tissue.

In *stage IV*, there is spontaneous arrest of the disease. The residual entropion and trichiasis lead to continuing corneal damage, however, denuding the epithelium and leaving the cornea vulnerable to infection and further opacification as a result of scarring.

Epithelial Tumors

Carcinoma in situ of the conjunctiva appears clinically either as an opaque, white, shiny lesion (leukoplakia) or as a fleshy mass.[11] Histologically the polarity of the epithelium is lost, and atypical pleomorphic cells are found throughout the entire thickness of the epithelium. Mitotic figures are commonly seen. The basement membrane of the epithelium is intact, and there is no invasion of the subepithelial tissue.

Squamous cell carcinoma shows the changes of carcinoma in situ, but there is also invasion by the tumor cells through the epithelial basement membrane into the superficial connective tissues.[12] Most commonly, squamous cell carcinoma of the conjunctiva shows only superficial invasion, deep invasion, and metastases are rarely seen.

Carcinoma composed of the mucus-secreting cells and squamous cells of the conjunctival epithelium (*mucoepidermoid carcinoma*) (Chapter 17) and *melanomas* of the conjunctiva also occur.

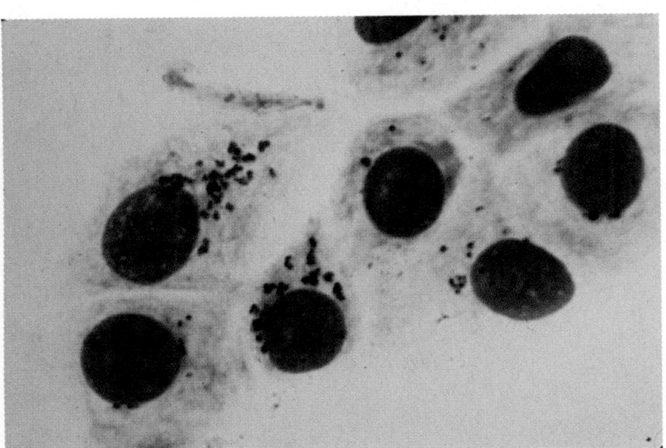

Figure 31–3

Trachoma. Corneal epithelial cells show cytoplasmic inclusion bodies (see text).

CORNEA

Keratitis and Corneal Ulcers

An inflammation of the corneal stroma that is under an intact corneal epithelium is called *stromal keratitis* or interstitial keratitis. Stromal inflammation with absent overlying epithelium is an *ulcer*. Corneal inflammations can be noninfectious (e.g., due to contact with abrasive chemicals or exposure to ultraviolet light) or infectious. Because of the cornea's hypocellularity and avascularity, numerous bacterial, viral, protozoal, and fungal agents, including types rarely considered pathogenic, can cause severe corneal infections. Risk factors predisposing to corneal ulcers include wearing contact lenses, exposure, and immune deficiency. Although corneal inflammations can respond to topical antibiotics and anti-inflammatory steroids, residual scarring of the cornea can decrease vision, necessitating corneal transplantation.

MORPHOLOGY. Histologically, numerous inflammatory cells are found in the corneal stroma. It is frequently difficult to identify precisely the types of inflammatory cells because their nuclei splay themselves out between the densely packed collagen lamellae of the stroma. The inflammatory cells and, if present, the infectious organisms can release proteases that digest the collagen lamellae of the stroma. If the stroma has melted away completely in one area, bare Descemet membrane is exposed to the tear film (a descemetocele). Perforation of this membrane leads to sudden hypotony of the eye, invasion of the infectious organisms into the globe, and often loss of the eye itself.

HERPETIC INFECTIONS

The most common cause of corneal ulcers is herpes simplex virus. They are usually unilateral and can often recur many times in the same eye. The classic clinical presentation is a *dendritic ulcer,* which is a thin epithelial defect in the shape of a branching set of connected, vermiform lines.

MORPHOLOGY. There is widespread epithelial edema, leading to bullae within the epithelium or between the epithelium and Bouman layer of

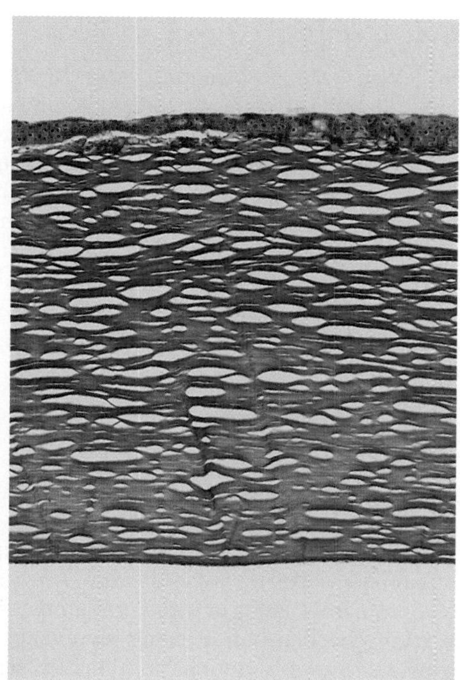

Figure 31–4

Granular dystrophy of the cornea (Masson trichrome stain).

stroma. In chronic cases, inflammation of the corneal stroma may take the form of a localized discoid opacity without ulceration **(disciform keratitis).** On histologic examination of a cornea with chronic recurrent herpetic keratitis, the stromal opacity is found to contain lymphocytes and plasma cells, sometimes with occasional multinucleated giant cells typically in the deep stroma near Descemet membrane. Intranuclear viral inclusion bodies are seen in corneal epithelial cells by light microscopy, and viral particles can be identified in the nucleus and cytoplasm of epithelial cells by electron microscopy. After resolution of the infection, and especially after many recurrences, the cornea may be left uninflamed but scarred and vascularized.

Hereditary Corneal Dystrophies

Hereditary corneal dystrophies are primary corneal disorders that are bilateral and usually symmetric. They are important clinically because they can cause severe visual loss that is reparable by corneal transplantation. Five clinically defined corneal dystrophies primarily involve the stroma; four of these are now known to be caused by different mutations in the same gene. Other dystrophies primarily affect the corneal epithelium or the endothelium.

STROMAL DYSTROPHIES

Granular dystrophy, lattice dystrophy, and *Avellino dystrophy* are autosomal dominant corneal stromal diseases caused by defects in the gene encoding *β-keratoepithelin.*[13] They all usually appear before age 20 and show a slow and continuous progression. *Granular dystrophy* is characterized by sharply defined, variably sized, white opacities in the anterior portion of the stroma. Histologically, these correspond to hyaline-like eosinophilic deposits best observed with the Masson trichrome stain (Fig. 31–4). By electron microscopy, these opacities consist of dense granules. *Lattice dystrophy* appears clinically as linear opacities forming a lattice configuration concentrated in the central portion of the anterior stroma. Histologically, these opacities (composed of amyloid) are eosinophilic, metachromatic, periodic acid–Schiff positive, and Congo red positive. The deposits in *Avellino dystrophy* have clinical and histologic features similar to both granular and lattice deposits. A fourth dystrophy, called *Reis-Bücklers dystrophy,* is due to a different mutation in the same gene.[13] The protein deposits in this dystrophy occur under the corneal epithelium and in Bowman layer of the anterior corneal stroma.

The most severe of the stromal dystrophies is *macular dystrophy,* which has an autosomal recessive mode of inheritance. The responsible genes have not yet been identified; however, a gene for one form is known to be on chromosome 16.[14] This disease presents clinically with diffuse cloudiness of the anterior stroma with aggregates of gray-white opacities in the axial region. Macular dystrophy usually results in severe impairment of vision by 30 years of age. This disorder is a localized corneal mucopolysaccharidosis (see Chapter 6), which appears to result from a defect in the catabolism of corneal keratan sulfate. Histologically, there are basophilic deposits that stain positive for acid mucopolysaccharides (Fig. 31–5).

ENDOTHELIAL DYSTROPHY

The most common dystrophy of the corneal *endothelium* is *Fuchs dystrophy.* It can be dominantly inherited. It presents clinically in middle age or in the elderly as edema of the corneal stroma consequent to the loss of endothelial cells, which normally function to pump water out of the

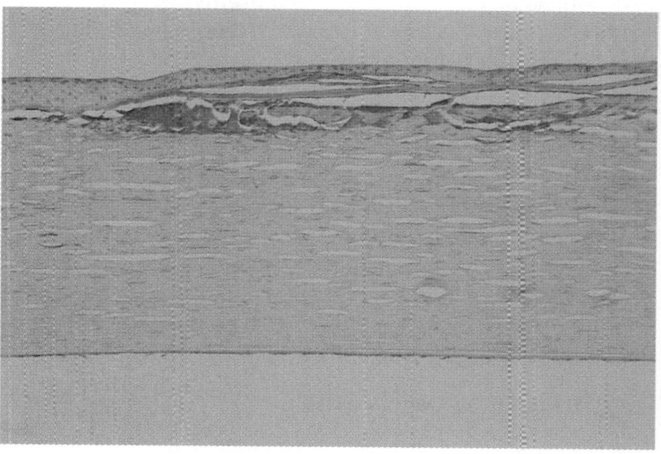

Figure 31–5

Macular dystrophy of the cornea. Alcian blue stains mucopolysaccharide deposits under the epithelium.

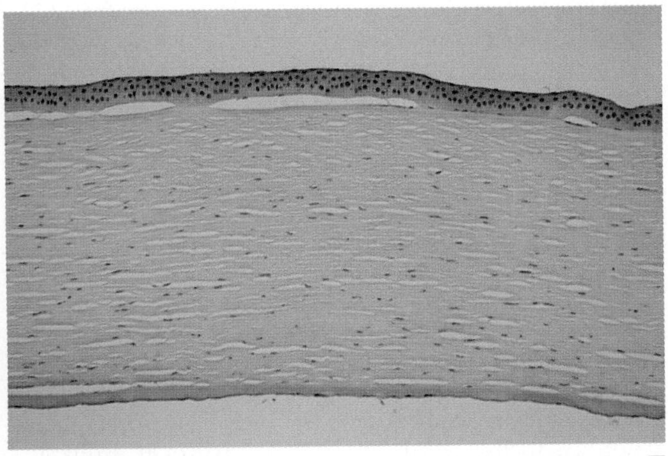

Figure 31–6

Fuchs dystrophy (H&E). Note the focal thickening of the basement membranes under the endothelium (*bottom*) and detachments of epithelium (*above*) from Bowman layer.

corneal stroma and keep it relatively dehydrated and clear. Histopathologically, bullous detachments of the epithelium from Bowman layer (bullous keratopathy) are seen. The attenuated endothelium rests on a diffusely, focally thickened Descemet membrane; the focal thickenings are called *guttata* and are seen best with the periodic acid–Schiff stain (Fig. 31–6).

UVEA

The uvea is a vascular coat that includes the choroid, ciliary body, and iris. Uveitis comprises a large and heterogeneous group of disorders that have in common inflammation of one or more portions of the uveal tract.[15] Uveitis is classified in several ways. Clinically, it is often convenient to separate cases of uveitis according to portions of the uveal tract involved (i.e., *iritis, cyclitis,* and *choroiditis*). Commonly, involvement of more than one part of the uvea and frequently the entire uvea (*panuveitis*) is seen. Another method of classification is based on etiology. Uveitis may result from trauma, systemic disease, or infection. In most cases, however, a definitive clinical cause cannot be found.

From a histologic standpoint, the two broad categories of uveitis are *granulomatous uveitis*, characterized by the presence of giant cells or epithelioid cells (or both), and *nongranulomatous uveitis*, in which only lymphocytes and plasma cells are the inflammatory components. Usually, histopathologic examination fails to reveal the cause of nongranulomatous uveitis. In cases of granulomatous uveitis, however, the etiologic agent can sometimes be identified.

Granulomatous Uveitis

Granulomatous uveitis is frequently caused by infectious agents. Alternatively, it may be idiopathic, have an autoimmune basis as in sympathetic ophthalmia, or be due to inflammatory diseases such as sarcoidosis.

INFECTIOUS UVEITIS

Infectious uveitis can be bacterial (tuberculosis, leprosy, syphilis, and tularemia); viral (cytomegalic inclusion disease and herpes zoster); fungal (blastomycosis, cryptococcosis, coccidioidomycosis, aspergillosis, phycomycosis, candidiasis, and histoplasmosis), or parasitic (onchocerciasis and toxoplasmosis). In all these disorders, the inflammation is not limited to the uvea but involves the retina and often the vitreous and sclera as well. In some cases, as in cytomegalic inclusion disease or toxoplasmosis, the infection primarily affects the retina and secondarily involves the choroid.

SARCOIDOSIS

Granulomatous uveitis is a common complication of sarcoidosis, occurring in about one third of patients with the disease. It is characterized by *mutton fat* deposits of chronic inflammatory cells on the cornea (*keratic precipitates*). Less commonly, granulomatous inflammation can be found involving the choroid. Retinal involvement in sarcoidosis is characterized by retinal periphlebitis with *candle wax drippings* on or near retinal vessels, retinal hemorrhages, and whitish masses in the adjacent vitreous. Retinal sarcoidosis is frequently associated with central nervous system sarcoidosis and carries a grave prognosis. Commonly, patients have granulomas in the conjunctiva, and thus conjunctival biopsy can be a relatively simple method for diagnosing sarcoidosis in a significant percentage of suspected cases. Histologically, discrete, noncaseating, granulomatous infiltrates are seen in the involved parts of the eye (Fig. 31–7), similar to lesions found elsewhere in the body in this disease (Chapter 16).

SYMPATHETIC OPHTHALMIA

Sympathetic uveitis is a rare but noteworthy disease that is an important consideration in the treatment of ocular trauma.[16] It is a bilateral diffuse granulomatous uveitis that is generally associated with penetrating injuries to one eye,

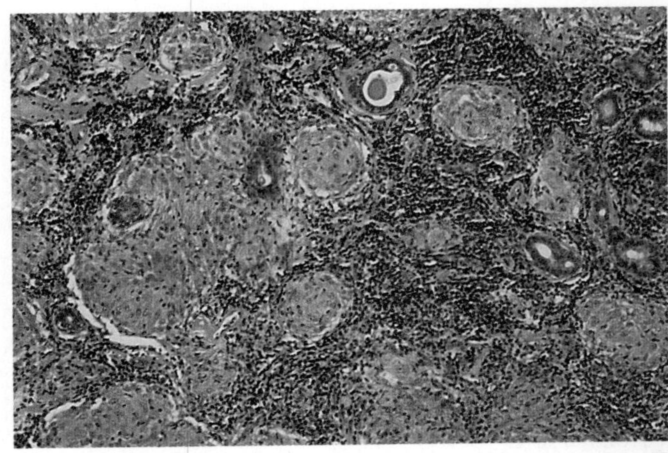

Figure 31–7

Sarcoidosis of the uvea (H&E). Note the granulomas with giant cells.

particularly those in which uveal prolapse or incarceration occurs. The cause is thought to be an autosensitivity against a putative antigen shared by the uveal melanocytes, retinal pigment epithelium, and neural retinal cells. Removal of the injured eye *before* the onset of sympathetic uveitis is the only method of preventing this disease.

Sympathetic uveitis rarely occurs earlier than 2 weeks after an ocular injury. Consequently a patient has only a few weeks after an ocular injury during which the ophthalmologist must weigh the likelihood of maintaining useful vision in the injured eye against the risk of developing this bilateral disease. After onset of inflammation, prompt removal of the injured eye (if blind) appears to result in milder inflammation in the noninjured or *sympathizing* eye.[17] Occasionally, however, the injured eye ends up as the eye with better vision, so judicious evaluation of the prognosis for vision in the injured eye is essential. The initial symptoms are loss of accommodation, blurred vision, and photophobia in the sympathizing eye. The earliest clinical signs are the appearance of keratic precipitates seen with the slit lamp and of choroidal infiltrates seen on fundus examination and fluorescein angiography.

MORPHOLOGY. The characteristic histopathologic signs are similar in both the injured (exciting) eye and the sympathizing eye: There is diffuse granulomatous uveal inflammation composed primarily of lymphocytes with clusters of epithelioid cells and sometimes giant cells. Plasma cells typically are scant. Early in the course, eosinophils may be seen. The inflammation primarily affects the choroid, which becomes markedly thickened (Fig. 31–8). There is sometimes mild involvement of the retina, usually appearing as a perivasculitis. Within the choroid, the choriocapillaris usually shows less severe inflammation. Although necrosis is not characteristic, pigment granules can be found in the macrophages, suggesting that disordered melanocytes play a role in the pathogenesis of the disease. In eyes in which the lens is injured, a form of granulomatous inflammation called *phakogenic endophthalmitis* may occur.

The course of the disease is generally protracted with flare-ups and remissions. Inflammation can usually be controlled with long-term immunosuppressive treatment.

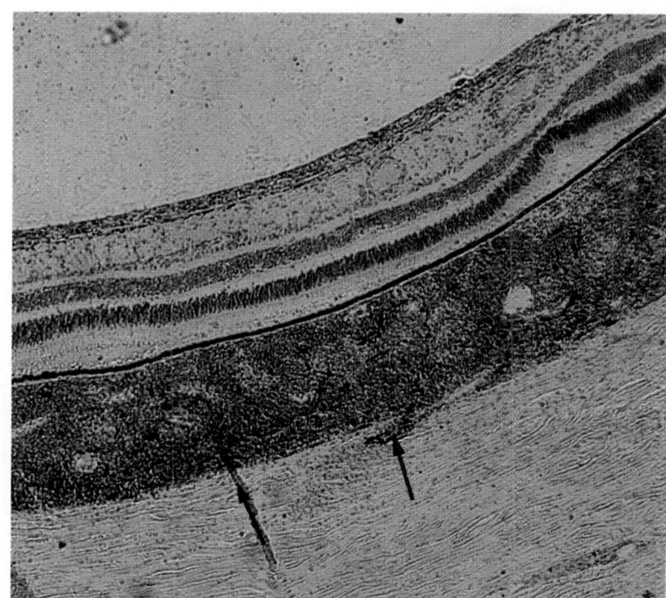

Figure 31–8 ■

Sympathetic ophthalmia showing thickening of the choroid with inflammatory cells (*arrows*).

Uveal Melanomas

Intraocular melanomas constitute the most common primary ocular malignancy in caucasians. Although we describe here melanomas of the uveal tract (i.e., the iris, ciliary body, and choroid), melanomas also occur on the skin of the lid, on the conjunctiva, and even within the orbit. Moreover, in addition to the *uveal melanocytes* (the cells giving rise to uveal melanomas), a second population of pigmented cells exists within the eye: the *pigment epithelium* of the iris, ciliary body, and retina. The pigment epithelium is embryologically part of the central nervous system derived from the neural tube. These cells can undergo non-neoplastic proliferation (reactive hyperplasia) in response to a variety of stimuli, but only rarely do they undergo malignant transformation. In contrast, the uveal melanocytes originate from the neural crest and possess long dendrite-like processes emanating from the center of the cell body, similar to dermal melanocytes. They do not undergo reactive hyperplasia, but are the origin of malignant melanomas of the eye.

The annual age-adjusted incidence of nonskin melanomas is 0.7 per 100,000 population in the United States, which is about one eighth that of melanoma of the skin. Ocular tumors constitute 80% of all the noncutaneous melanomas reported. The risk of ocular melanoma in whites is eightfold higher than in blacks.

Nevi are fairly common in the choroid, and most of these lesions are detected by chance during ophthalmic examinations. Most do not progress. Because histologic study is not feasible, some of the larger nevi are followed by periodic funduscopic examination for evidence of enlargement in circumference or thickness, which may indicate malignancy.

MORPHOLOGY. Most melanomas arise in the posterior choroid (see Fig. 31–9). They may spread laterally between the sclera and retina or may produce bulbous masses projecting into the vitreous cavity and pushing the retina ahead of them. The Callender classification, designed in 1931, relates histology to prognosis, and in somewhat modified form, remains in general use today as follows[19, 20]:

- **Spindle A melanomas** (Fig. 31–10*A*) have co-

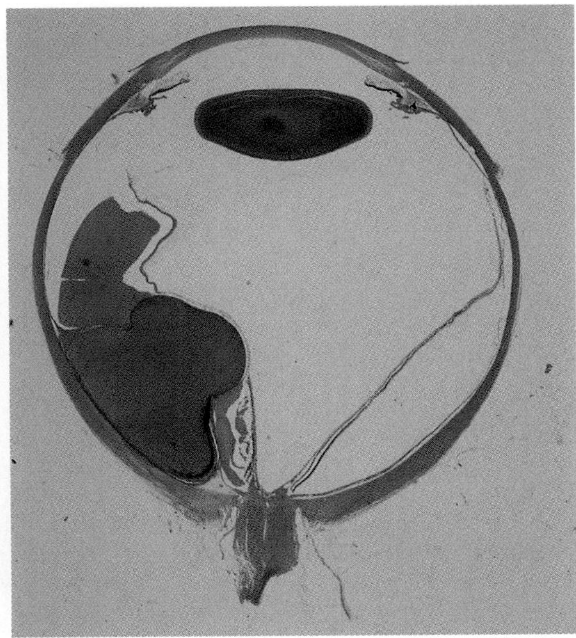

Figure 31–9

Malignant melanoma of the choroid. Note the collar button–shaped dark tumor on the left with adjacent pink proteinaceous exudate and detached retina. Optic nerve is at 6 o'clock, and the lens is at 12 o'clock.

hesive tumor cells with small, spindle-shaped nuclei containing a central dark strip that is seen by electron microscopy to be a nuclear fold. Nucleoli are not distinct, the cytoplasm is scant, and cell borders are difficult to identify. These constitute approximately 5% of ciliary body and choroidal melanomas. They have a good prognosis, with only 8% of patients dead from metastases 15 years after enucleation. (Because of the frequency of late metastases, 5-year cure rates are less useful prognostic parameters in ocular melanomas.)

- **Spindle B melanomas** are composed of cohesive cells having distinct spindle-shaped nuclei with prominent nucleoli. The cells contain more cytoplasm than those in the spindle A lesion, and cell borders are difficult to discern by light microscopy. This cell type constitutes approximately 40% of ciliary body and choroidal melanomas. The fascicular type of uveal melanoma is a subgroup of spindle B melanomas characterized by a palisading arrangement of the spindle-shaped cells, termed a **fascicular pattern**. These compose approximately 6% of choroidal melanomas. Spindle A and spindle B melanomas are the cell types seen in almost all iris melanomas. Approximately 15% of patients die from metastases 15 years after enucleation.
- **Epithelioid melanomas** are composed of poorly cohesive, large cells with round nuclei and prominent nucleoli. Abundant eosinophilic cytoplasm and well-demarcated cell borders are seen (Fig. 31–10*B*). This is the rarest type of the ciliary body and choroidal melanomas, occurring in only 3% of all cases. It has a poor prognosis, with 72% mortality after 15 years.
- **Mixed cell type melanomas** are neoplasms having spindle cells (usually spindle B) together

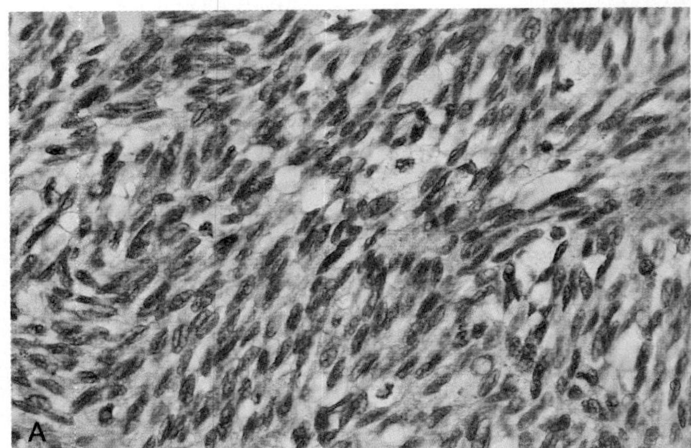

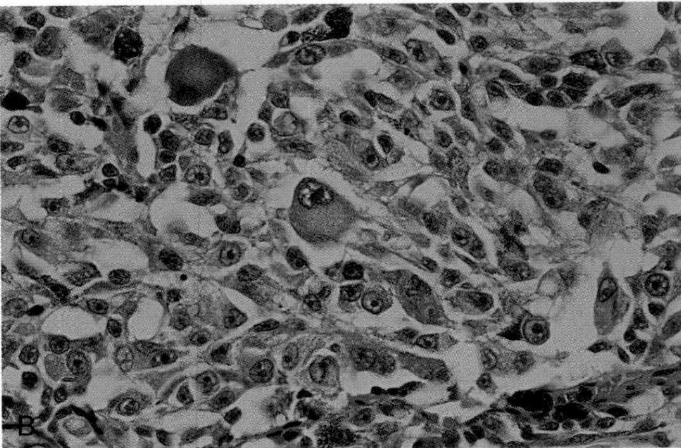

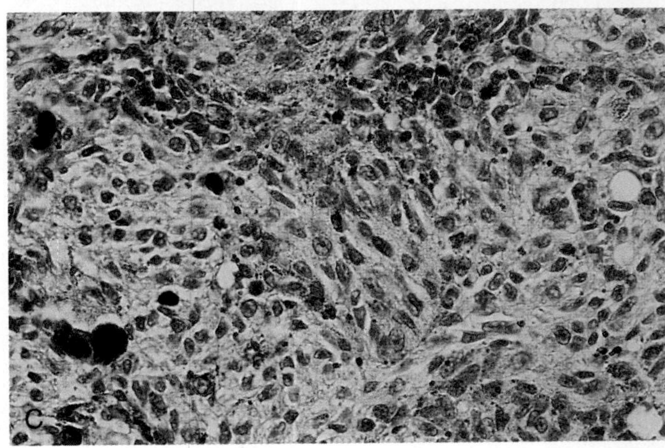

Figure 31–10

A, Spindle cell malignant melanoma. The cells have a spindle-shaped nucleus with nuclear fold, indistinct nuclei, and scant cytoplasm: the cell borders are difficult to discern. *B*, Epithelioid cell malignant melanoma. Large cells with round nuclei are seen. Tumors are poorly cohesive, with well-demarcated cell borders and eosinophilic cytoplasm. (H&E × 40.) *C*, Mixed cell malignant melanoma. Spindle cells and epithelioid cells are seen in the most common cell type of ocular melanoma.

with a significant epithelioid population (Fig. 31–10C). **This is the most common type of ciliary body and choroidal melanoma,** accounting for about 45% of these lesions. Approximately 60% of patients are dead after 15 years.

- **Necrotic melanoma** refers to a tumor so necrotic that the cell type cannot be identified. These compose only 7% of all ciliary body and choroidal tumors. The prognosis is similar to that for the mixed type.

In practice, uveal melanomas are often considered in two primary categories: the spindle cell variety (combining spindle A and spindle B types) and the non–spindle cell type (combining epithelioid, mixed, and necrotic types). Slightly less than 50% of ciliary body and choroidal malignant melanomas are of the spindle cell variety; these have a good prognosis, with about 73% survival at 15 years. A little more than 50% are of the non–spindle cell variety, with a prognosis of about 35% survival at 15 years. A number of other parameters have been correlated with survival. Features considered the most significant are cell type, largest dimension, scleral extension, and mitotic activity. Morphometry is also useful, with a high degree of pleomorphism of nucleoli indicating a poor prognosis. The configuration of blood vessels within the tumor has also been correlated with outcome.[21]

Clinical Features. An *iris melanoma* most commonly presents as a visible pigmented mass. It may be somewhat light in color. Distortion of the pupil is frequently seen. A *ciliary body melanoma* may elicit episcleral vascular injection over it, may interfere with accommodation, and may cause a localized cataract. Both iris and ciliary body melanomas can also cause glaucoma. *Choroidal melanoma* may appear as a pigmented lesion on routine ophthalmoscopic examination and may produce symptoms by causing retinal detachment, macular edema, or choroidal hemorrhage. A melanoma in any uveal region may extend through an emissary canal to the surface of the globe. There may be associated ocular inflammation.

For many years, enucleation was the primary treatment for all ocular melanomas. Because it became evident that iris melanomas are usually of the spindle cell type and of low malignancy, the current treatment is to observe melanomas arising from the iris and resect them only when intraocular spread threatens the eye. For ciliary body and choroidal melanomas, enucleation is still widely employed as treatment for large tumors (>15 mm in diameter) as well as for many medium-sized tumors (10 to 15 mm). Radiation delivered by proton beam or by a radioactive scleral plaque is being used increasingly in the treatment of small (<10 mm) and medium-sized choroidal and ciliary body melanomas.

The pattern of metastatic disease in ocular melanoma differs from that of cutaneous melanoma in that hepatic metastases predominate. Approximately 95% of patients with metastatic uveal melanoma have liver metastases, and in almost all of these, the liver is the first site affected with metastases.

LENS

Cataracts

Cataracts are opacities in the crystalline lens. They are a major cause of visual loss and blindness throughout the world. Among the many causes of cataracts are metabolic diseases such as diabetes mellitus, physical agents (ultraviolet light trauma, radiation therapy), ocular diseases (uveitis, glaucoma, intraocular tumors, retinitis pigmentosa), viruses (rubella), skin diseases (atopic dermatitis, scleroderma), drugs (corticosteroids), and aging. The most common type is idiopathic and develops in older individuals—so-called *senile cataracts.*[22]

Cataracts are examined by ophthalmologists using a slit-lamp biomicroscope. This permits observation of many of the same changes in vivo that the pathologist sees under the microscope after the lens is removed. Consequently, we first describe the changes that can be noted both on biomicroscopic examination of the patient and on light microscopic examination of the sectioned unstained lens. Following this, we discuss changes seen on histologic examination only.

- The most common change in the *aging* lens is *nuclear sclerosis* or compression of the lens fibers in the central (nuclear) portion of the lens. The borders of the individual nuclear fibers are indistinct, and the nucleus as a whole stands out from the cortex more distinctly than normal. As the process progresses, the nucleus may become brown (*brunescent cataract*). The earliest changes in the cortex are the appearance of wedgelike or spokelike opacities that occur first at the lens equator then progress into the anterior and posterior cortex (*cortical cataract*). Vacuoles often appear in the cortex of the lens, and clefts between lens fibers show an accumulation of opaque debris of degenerated lens material (Morgagni globules).
- Another common type of age-related cataract is marked by the development of granular opacities in the zone immediately anterior to the posterior capsule. These spread toward the periphery (*posterior subcapsular cataract*). A lens with an early or *immature cataract* frequently has an increased osmotic pressure as a result of the degenerated lens material and may imbibe water and swell (*intumescent cataract*). Eventually the entire lens may become involved in the degenerative process (*mature cataract*). The sclerotic nucleus may sink in the cortex when the latter becomes entirely liquefied (*morgagnian cataract*). Occasionally, cataractous lenses may shrink after the lens capsule and epithelium degenerate, and lenticular debris passes into the aqueous humor (*hypermature cataract*). As the lens capsule becomes more permeable, allowing lens material to escape, the lenticu-

lar debris is engulfed by macrophages that may obstruct the aqueous outflow, resulting in *phacolytic glaucoma.* Cataractous lenses may eventually calcify; less commonly, lens material is partially or completely reabsorbed, leaving the residual lens capsule. If cataract surgery is performed and some lens epithelium is left behind within the capsule, these cells may produce abnormal, opaque lens fibers that appear as large globules.

MORPHOLOGY. On histologic section, abnormalities of the epithelium may be seen. The most common finding is migration of lens epithelium under the posterior lens capsule. The epithelial cells may enlarge and appear vacuolated (bladder cells), they may undergo necrosis and be partially or totally absent, or they may undergo **fibrous metaplasia.** After routine extracapsular extraction of a cataract by a surgeon, the remaining anterior and posterior capsules of the lens may become apposed, while the epithelium at the periphery forms abortive lens fibers having a doughnut shape (**Soemmering ring cataract**).

RETINA

The retina has a complex structure but can be summarized as having a basic three-neuron organization (Fig. 31–11). An electrical impulse, generated by light impinging on the photoreceptor cell (rod or cone), is transmitted to cells of the inner nuclear layer (bipolar, horizontal, and amacrine cells). The neural impulses are transmitted, in turn, to the next retinal cell layer, which is composed of ganglion cells. The axons of the ganglion cells extend through the nerve fiber layer to the optic nerve and synapse in the brain in the lateral geniculate body or in the pretectal region.

Retinopathy of Prematurity (Retrolental Fibroplasia)

Retrolental fibroplasia was a leading cause of blindness in infants in the United States and other developed countries in the 1940s and the early 1950s, and it continues to occur with low but still disturbing frequency. It affects mostly premature infants who have been subjected to oxygen therapy. The major risk factors in this disease are the level and duration of oxygen exposure, the degree of prematurity at birth, and a carrier state for a defect in the Norrie disease gene.[23] The disease arises because the peripheral retinal vasculature, particularly on the temporal side, does not become fully formed until the end of fetal life. The least mature vessels are the most vulnerable to injury on exposure to oxygen. In infants of very low birth weight, the retinal vessels can apparently be injured by levels of arterial oxygen tension that are physiologic at term (i.e., approximately 90 mm Hg). The present ability to maintain infants weighing as little as 600 gm at birth has caused a rise in incidence of retrolental fibroplasia. The previously defined *safe* dose of oxygen (an ambient concentration of not more than 40%, which corresponds to a partial pressure in the arterial blood of 160 mm Hg) is now considered unsafe for extremely small infants. In addition, occasional examples of oxygen-induced retrolental fibroplasia at full term have been reported and are considered to be the result of a barely mature retinal vasculature in the extreme temporal periphery in some infants.

Pathogenesis and Pathology. The initial stage in the pathogenesis is a *vaso-obliterative phase* in which there is a functional constriction of the immature retinal vessels followed by structural obliteration.[24] The peripheral retina consequently fails to vascularize. On cessation of exposure to oxygen, the *vasoproliferative phase* ensues, in which there is an intense proliferation of vascular endothelium and fibroblasts and the formation of *new blood vessels.* This angiogenesis begins at the junction of the avascular and vascularized portions of the retina, and the new vessels break through the internal limiting membrane of the retina and grow into the vitreous. These changes become apparent about 5 to 10 weeks after cessation of exposure

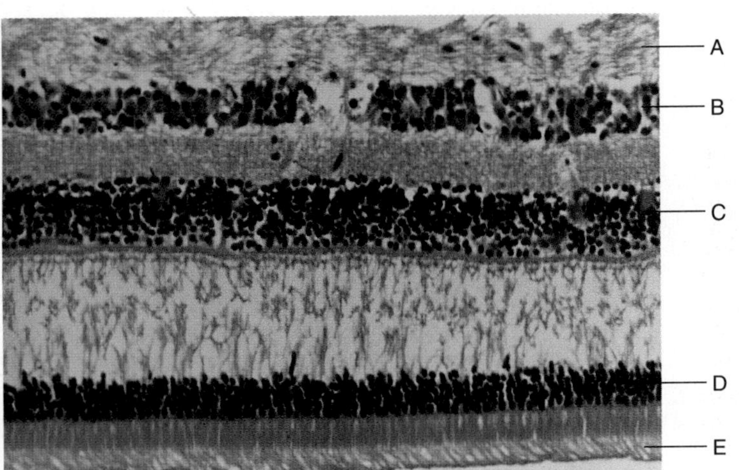

Figure 31–11

Normal retina. Layers from top down are *A*, nerve fiber layer, *B*, ganglion cell layer, *C*, inner nuclear layer, *D*, outer nuclear layer, and *E*, rods and cones. (Courtesy of Dr. Umberto De Girolami, Department of Pathology, Brigham and Women's Hospital, Boston, MA.)

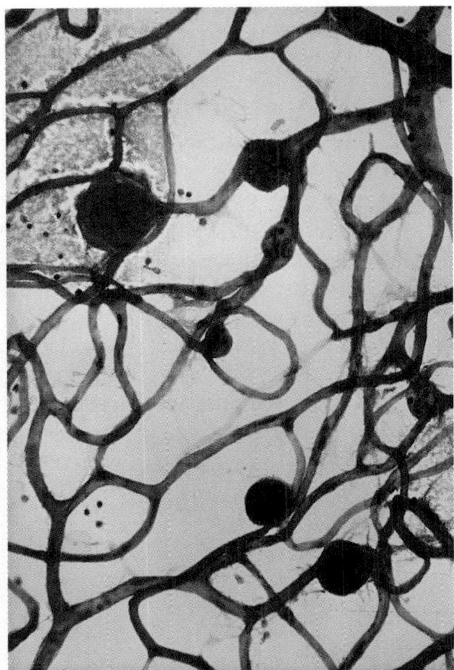

Figure 31–12

Diabetic retinopathy. Human retina from a case of advanced diabetic microangiopathy, after trypsin digestion. Note the several microaneurysms.

to oxygen. *There is an important role for vascular endothelial growth factor (VEGF) in these events.* High-oxygen therapy *inhibits* VEGF production and thus causes endothelial apoptosis, and the subsequent cessation of exposure to oxygen stimulates VEGF production and results in neovascularization (Chapter 11). In about 25% of cases, a cicatricial phase ensues, in which the fibrovascular component shrinks or contracts. The retrolental mass becomes increasingly pale, and retinal detachment occurs. The macula and posterior retinal vessels are displaced temporally, and areas of hemorrhage may be seen. Neovascularization of the iris may develop in later years, resulting in closed-angle glaucoma.

Diabetes Mellitus

The incidence of diabetic retinopathy rises with the duration of the metabolic defect. With advances in therapy, the life span of diabetic patients has improved, and the prevalence of secondary retinal disease has greatly increased. Approximately 60% of diabetic patients develop retinopathy 15 to 20 years after the original diagnosis. Diabetic retinopathy ranks with glaucoma, macular degeneration, and cataract as a major cause of blindness in the United States and Europe. Furthermore, about 2% of the diabetic population have a visual impairment (severe enough to be considered legally blind) that is attributable to retinopathy. There are two groups of changes in diabetic retinopathy known as *background* or *nonproliferative retinopathy* and *proliferative retinopathy*.[25]

BACKGROUND RETINOPATHY

Background retinopathy is the most common change and is characterized by a number of structural capillary alterations, as follows:

- *Capillary basement membrane changes* are identical to those described for diabetic microangiopathy in general (Chapter 20).[26]
- *Pericyte degeneration* is an almost invariable feature of diabetic retinopathy.[27] It has been postulated that the pericytes exercise a contractile function and that their loss plays a role in the formation of microaneurysms and arteriovenous shunts.
- *Capillary microaneurysms* are also a dramatic feature of diabetic retinopathy and are often its presenting clinical sign (Fig. 31–12). These are rare elsewhere in the body of the diabetic patient but do occur in several other retinal disorders. Microaneurysms are associated with excessive permeability and frequent rupture resulting in focal serous exudates and *hemorrhages*. Microaneurysms may develop thromboses and become occluded, and subsequent examination of the retina by fluorescein angiography may give a misleading impression of regression of the retinopathy.
- *Microvascular obstructions and nonperfusion of capillaries* occur in vessels in the posterior fundus that are lacking both pericytes and endothelium. Histologically, these vessels are seen as tubes of basement membrane. The nonperfusion provides a basis for the hypoxia that can later lead to proliferative retinopathy. *Cotton-wool* spots are often seen in these areas (Fig. 31–13), and scotomata occur owing to degeneration of nerve fibers and ganglion cells.
- *Arteriolar hyalinization* is thought to be due to increased endothelial permeability, insudation of plasma, and basement membrane thickening. Gradual narrowing of the

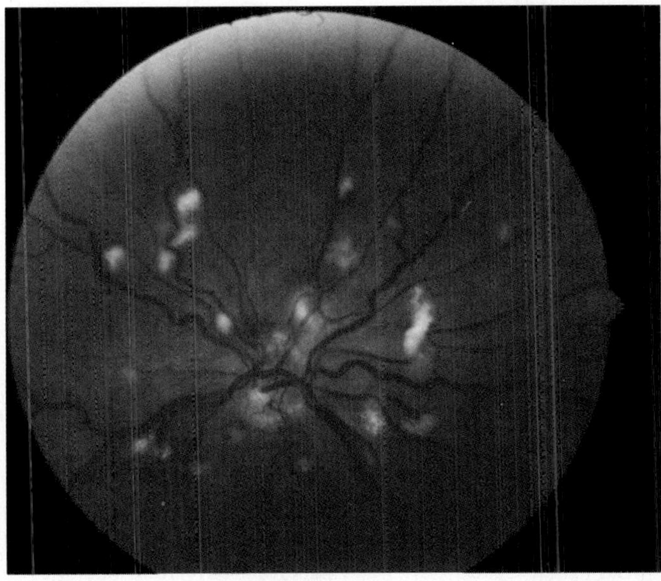

Figure 31–13

Funduscopic picture of fluffy, superficial, yellowish cotton-wool spots.

arteriolar lumen follows, particularly around the mouths of branch vessels. Occlusion of precapillary arterioles accounts for the cytoid bodies (see later) seen in approximately one third of diabetic retinas.

- *A gradual increase in retinal vein caliber* occurs. Additional venous abnormalities, occurring as a response to local ischemia, include the formation of venous loops as well as *beading* of the blood column within veins. Obstruction of the central retinal vein or of a retinal branch vein may occur in the preproliferative stage of diabetic retinopathy.

PROLIFERATIVE RETINOPATHY

Proliferative retinopathy is characterized by *neovascularization* and *fibroplasia*. The neovascularization occurs in response to severe ischemia and hypoxia of the retina. There is growing evidence, as we have seen, that ischemic retinal cells produce VEGF, which induces angiogenesis in diabetic and other retinal neovascular diseases.[28] The new vessels usually extend from the larger veins surrounded by areas of capillary closure, or they may arise from arterial vessels at the retinal periphery. The new capillaries contain both endothelial cells and pericytes but are incompletely formed and poorly supported. Initially, they proliferate within the potential space between the inner limiting membrane of the retina and the posterior face of the vitreous, where they have a flat appearance. Subsequently, they extend into the vitreous cavity. At this stage, bleeding is common as the vessels move with the normally shifting vitreous during eye movements. After a variable period, the neovascularization is followed by the development of fibrosis. At this stage, the neovascular membrane is referred to as *retinitis proliferans*. The fibrous component increases the traction on the underlying retina, often culminating in *retinal detachment*.

Hypertensive and Arteriosclerotic Retinopathy

Hypertensive and arteriosclerotic changes in the retinal vessels provide useful prognostic clues to the physician.[29,30]

HYPERTENSIVE RETINOPATHY

Hypertensive changes in the arterioles are characterized by narrowing and decrease in diameter of vessels. In acute severe hypertension, at the onset of malignant hypertension, these initially appear as focal *spasms*. In chronic hypertension, however, the narrowing is more diffuse. Histologically, they manifest a hyaline or *onion-skin* thickening of the arteriolar walls, as described in Chapter 12. Hypertensive retinopathy is categorized as follows:

- *Grade I*: Generalized narrowing of the arterioles
- *Grade II*: Grade I changes and focal arteriolar spasms
- *Grade III*: Grade II changes, flame-shaped hemorrhages, dot-and-blot hemorrhages, cotton-wool spots, and hard waxy exudates

Histologically, *flame-shaped hemorrhages* are extravasated erythrocytes within the retinal nerve fiber layer. Their typical shape results from the confinement of the red blood cells within spaces between the nerve fibers, which run in a parallel fashion. Dot-and-blot hemorrhages, in contrast, are seen in the inner nuclear layer with spreading to the outer plexiform layer. *Cotton-wool spots* are microinfarctions of the nerve fiber layer. Interruption of axonal flow produces clusters of ganglion cell axons that have undergone bulbous dilation at the site of ischemic damage or infarction. A swollen axon histologically assumes a shape resembling a cell—hence the term *cytoid (cell-like) body*. *Hard* or *waxy exudates* are composed of extravasated lipophilic material located in the outer plexiform layer.

- *Grade IV*: All grade III changes plus optic disc edema

ARTERIOSCLEROTIC RETINOPATHY

Arteriosclerotic retinopathy is also divided into four grades:

- *Grade I*: Increase in the arteriolar light reflex: Histologically, this corresponds to a subintimal hyaline deposition and a thickened arteriolar media and adventitia that causes the normally transparent arteriolar wall to become semiopaque.
- *Grade II*: Increase in the arteriolar light reflex plus arteriolar-venular crossing defects: At the site of crossing, the arteriole and venule share a common adventitia. The semiopaque wall of the arteriole obscures the venous blood column of the underlying venule. The various arteriovenous crossing changes are often collectively termed *arteriovenous nicking*.
- *Grade III*: Grade II lesions plus the presence of *copper-wire* arterioles: Here, as a result of subintimal hyaline deposition and thickening of the media and adventitia, the arteriolar wall is sufficiently opaque to reflect only a portion of the red color of the intravascular blood.
- *Grade IV*: Grade III changes plus the presence of *silver-wire* arterioles: The opacity resulting from the sclerotic changes in the arteriolar wall is now sufficient to obscure the intravascular blood entirely, giving a white or silver pattern of thickening of the media and adventitia.

Retinitis Pigmentosa

A variety of systemic and ocular diseases result in degeneration of the retina, characterized by a loss of visual receptors—rods and cones—usually accompanied by focal proliferations of the adjacent retinal pigment epithelium and migration of such cells into the sensory retina, where they appear as pigmented interstitial cells (*pigmentary retinopathy*).

Retinitis pigmentosa refers to one group of such pigmentary retinopathies that is hereditary, bilateral, and progressive. The disorder is inherited as an autosomal dominant recessive or sex-linked recessive trait or as a maternally inherited (mitochondrial) trait. Most patients have no other systemic or associated disease (*nonsyndromic retinitis pigmentosa*). In a minority of families, all affected individuals have other manifestations (*syndromic retinitis pigmentosa*), such as deafness (Usher syndrome) or obesity, short stature, hypogonadism, and polydactyly (*Bardet-Biedl syndrome*).

Within the nonsyndromic and within most syndromic forms of retinitis pigmentosa, there are mutations affecting different genes in different families.[31] For example, mutations in opsin and peripherin (photoreceptor proteins) occur in certain autosomal dominant families.[32]

Night blindness, as a result of the loss of rods, is usually an early symptom. Cone photoreceptors ultimately degenerate as well, leading to blindness in many cases. Because of the underlying genetic heterogeneity, there is a wide range of severity among patients with the disease. Some patients are severely visually handicapped before the age of 20; others experience little symptomatic visual deficit even after age 70; most have a severity in between these two extremes. The principal ophthalmoscopic findings in symptomatic patients are retinal pigmentation distributed in a branching reticulated pattern (bone-spicule pigmentation), a pale, waxy-appearing optic disc, and attenuation of the retinal blood vessels. A posterior subcapsular cataract is often present. Histologically the photoreceptors are few in number or absent. If some are present, their inner and outer segments are shortened or absent. The retinal pigment epithelium degenerates in some areas and proliferates and migrates into the neural retina in others.[33] The waxy pallor of the optic disc is due to a glial membrane that grows on the inner surface of the optic disc and spreads over the peripapillary retina.[34]

Macular Degeneration

The macula is the region of the posterior retina with a high density of photoreceptors and a high ganglion cell-to-photoreceptor ratio, which provides the fine visual acuity to which most humans are accustomed. It is the target for a variety of disorders. Factors that may predispose to degenerative lesions in this location include an absence of retinal vessels in the center of the macula (the *foveola*), the exclusive dependence of the foveola on the underlying choroidal circulation, the high density of both cone and rod photoreceptors and other retinal cell types, and a consequently high metabolic demand.

Age-related macular degeneration (formerly called *senile* macular degeneration) is the most common of the macular disorders. It is the most frequent cause of decreased vision in the elderly. There is evidence for both genetic and environmental (ultraviolet irradiation, drugs) components to its etiology,[35–37] but these are still not sufficiently well defined. Macular degeneration occurring in younger individuals is much less common and is more clearly of genetic origin.[38] For example, a photoreceptor cell-specific ATP-binding transport gene (*ABCR*) is mutated in one genetic form of macular degeneration of the young.[39]

MORPHOLOGY. Macular degeneration presents either as an atrophic form or as an exudative (*disciform*) degeneration.[40] In the atrophic form, Bruch membrane, the membrane between the retinal pigment epithelium and the choroid, is thickened generally and focally. The discrete thickenings are called *drusen*.[41] The choriocapillaris is often focally obliterated, and the pigment epithelium is atrophic and depigmented. The photoreceptors degenerate in the regions of atrophy of the retinal pigment epithelium. One complication of atrophic macular degeneration is the development of defects in Bruch membrane (Fig. 31–14). New vessels grow from the choroid through these defects into the subretinal space, creating the second form, *disciform macular degeneration*. Vascular membranes may form beneath the retina or overlying the retina. The new vessels leak and produce exudates and hemorrhage under the retina (*exudative macular degeneration*). Organization of the hemorrhage and exudate is accompanied by retinal pigment epithelial proliferation, fibrous metaplasia, and fibrous overgrowth. The end result is a fibrous scar in the macular region with degeneration of the neuroretina and permanent loss of central vision.

Retinal Detachment

A retinal *detachment* is a separation between the neurosensory retina and the retinal pigment epithelium. This is an opening of the potential space that is a vestige of the original cavity of the embryonic optic vesicle. Retinal detachments are common causes of blindness. Ophthalmologists recognize three major categories of retinal detachment:

- A *rhegmatogenous retinal detachment* arises when a break or tear in the retina allows vitreous fluid beneath the retina. The break or tear often results from contraction of vitreous collagen, which is attached to the inner surface of the retina (vitreous traction).

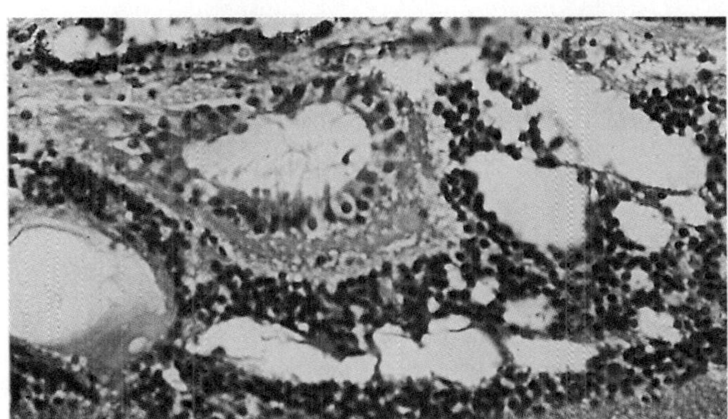

Figure 31–14 ■

Retina showing macular degeneration. Compare with normal retina in Figure 31–12.

- A *serous or exudative retinal detachment* occurs when fluid accumulates beneath an intact sensory retina. This arises secondarily from diseases such as choroidal malignant melanoma, malignant hypertension, and choroiditis (Fig. 31–15).
- *Traction detachments* develop after fibrous or glial membranes form in the vitreous. In some cases, the membranes contract and detach the retina without creating a retinal break. The membranes may form in diseases such as diabetic retinopathy or after penetrating or perforating ocular trauma or complicated intraocular surgery.

The earliest histopathologic change following retinal detachment is degeneration of the outer retinal layers because they are removed from their blood supply, the choriocapillaris.[42] Cystic degeneration follows in the outer plexiform layer. The cystic spaces may coalesce to form increasingly larger cysts. Glial proliferation frequently occurs in detached retinas. The subretinal space is filled with liquefied vitreous or serous fluid and may also contain inflammatory cells, blood, or tumor cells, depending on the nature of the detachment. In long-standing retinal detachment, the retinal pigment epithelium beneath the detached neural retina proliferates and may contribute to the membranes involving the retina.

Retinoblastoma

Retinoblastoma is the most common malignant eye tumor of childhood and is responsible for approximately 1% of all deaths from cancer in the age group of newborns to 15 years. Retinoblastoma is worldwide in distribution and affects all racial groups. Its frequency is approximately 1 in 17,000 live births. It is a tumor of infancy and childhood; cases with tumors present at birth are not exceptional. The risk for retinoblastoma decreases with age, with well over 90% of cases being diagnosed before the age of 7 years. It affects both sexes with equal frequency. The tumor is usually fatal once it spreads outside the eye and orbit. Most cases in developed countries are diagnosed before extraocular spread. Radiation therapy, laser photocoagulation, and cryotherapy are used to treat intraocular tumors in eyes with a potential for useful vision; in eyes with large tumors, enucleation is the preferred therapy.

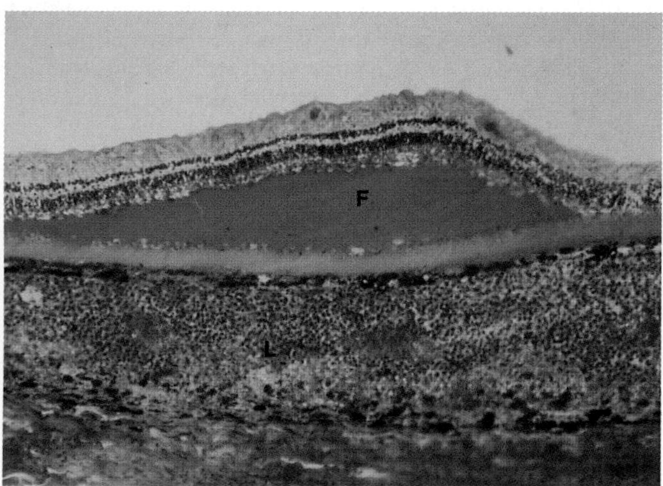

Figure 31–15

Retinal detachment caused by choroidal lymphoma. Note the infiltrate of lymphoma (L) in the choroid and the fluid collection (F) between the pigment epithelium and detached retina. (Courtesy of Dr. Umberto De Girolami, Department of Pathology, Brigham and Women's Hospital, Boston, MA.)

Molecular Genetics. Etiologically, retinoblastoma is unusual because it appears to be simply the result of defects in a single gene, the retinoblastoma gene (RB). If a mutant RB allele arises in the germ line, it can be transmitted as a dominant trait, and carriers are at high risk (>90% risk for most mutations) for retinoblastoma in childhood and for other cancers (e.g., osteosarcoma) later in life.[43] Most of such cases of *hereditary retinoblastoma* have tumors affecting both eyes (bilateral retinoblastoma); a small percent have, in addition, independently arising tumors, also occurring in childhood, either in the pineal gland or in the suprasellar or parasellar region (trilateral retinoblastoma).[44] A small number of carriers remain unaffected. Most patients with hereditary retinoblastoma have no previous family history of the disease because they have a new germ line mutation. In *nonhereditary retinoblastoma* (about 60 to 70% of all patients), the initial mutation affecting one copy of the RB gene arises in a somatic retinal cell or in a somatic cell that is a precursor of the developing retina. Almost all nonhereditary cases have only one tumor in one eye; they are *not* at increased risk for other cancers later in life.

In both hereditary and nonhereditary retinoblastoma, the retinoblastomas are clonal proliferations of sensitive retinal cells that have the initial germ line or somatic mutation affecting one RB allele and that also have lost the function of the remaining wild-type RB allele. The loss of the second RB allele can occur because of an independently arising somatic mutation, because of chromosomal nondisjunction or recombination occurring during mitosis, or because of epigenetic modification such as methylation of the promoter region.[45–49]

The RB gene is a prototype tumor-suppressor gene (Chapter 8). The loss of both allelic, wild-type copies of the respective *cancer-suppressor gene* appears to be a key step in malignant transformation. As we have seen, each tumor-suppressor gene underlies the origin of more than one tumor type, such as the RB gene causing retinoblastoma and osteosarcoma, or the neurofibromatosis type 2 gene causing acoustic neuroma or meningioma (Chapter 30).

MORPHOLOGY. Retinoblastoma is believed to arise from a cell of neuroepithelial origin in the retina. The tumors tend to be nodular masses, often with satellite seedings (Fig. 31–16). On light microscopic examination, undifferentiated areas of these tumors are composed of small, round cells with hyperchromatic nuclei and scanty cytoplasm. The resemblance of these cells to undifferentiated retinoblasts, which are precursors of the differentiated retinal cells, led to the use of the term **retinoblastoma**. Differentiated structures are found within many retinoblastomas, the most

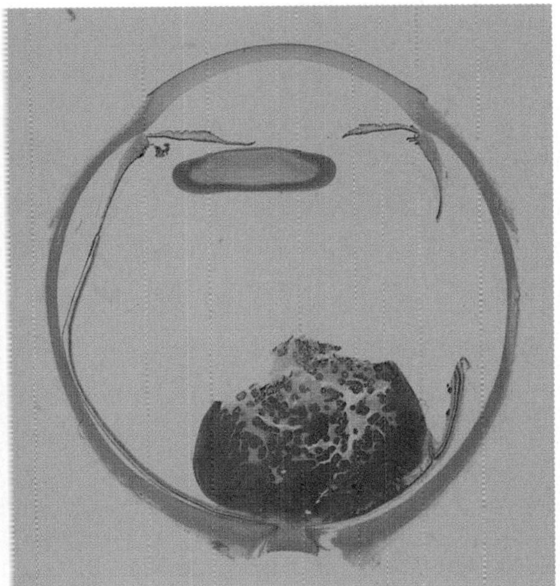

Figure 31–16

Retinoblastoma. Note poorly cohesive tumor in retina abutting optic nerve.

characteristic of these being the rosettes described by Flexner and Wintersteiner (Flexner-Wintersteiner rosettes) (Fig. 31–17). These structures consist of clusters of cuboidal or short columnar cells arranged around a central lumen. The nuclei are displaced away from the lumen, which by light microscopy appears to have a limiting membrane resembling the external limiting membrane of the retina. Photoreceptor-like elements protrude through the membrane, and some taper into fine filaments. Less common are the rosettes described by Wright; these are radial arrangements of cells around a central tangle of fibrils (Homer Wright rosettes). An additional differentiated structure in a few percent of tumors is the fleurette, which represents an attempt at photoreceptor differentiation by tumor cells.

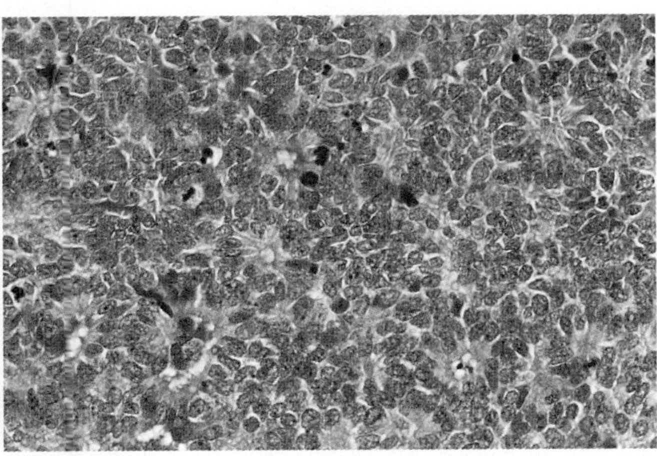

Figure 31–17

Higher-power view of retinoblastoma showing Flexner-Wintersteiner rosettes and numerous mitotic figures (H&E × 40).

Tumor cells may disseminate through the choroidal vasculature or may spread beyond the eye through the optic nerve or subarachnoid space. Bone marrow aspiration, peripheral blood smears, and cerebrospinal fluid examinations assess the extent of spread in patients with metastatic retinoblastoma. In advanced cases, the tumor may penetrate through the sclera and grow in the orbit. Metastases to the preauricular and cervical lymph nodes commonly follow overt extraocular extension. The most common sites of distant metastases are the central nervous system, skull, distal bones, and lymph nodes.

Spontaneous necrosis or regression of a retinoblastoma is marked by calcification and severe inflammation. The mechanism responsible for spontaneous necrosis, which is rare, is unknown. Rarely, tumors composed of uniformly benign-appearing cells exhibiting photoreceptor differentiation and the formation of fleurettes have been reported. These have been referred to as *retinocytomas* and are believed to be a benign variant of retinoblastoma.[50]

VITREOUS

The adult vitreous forms during the second month of embryonic development. It is composed of 99% water with the remainder being collagen and hyaluronic acid forming a hydrogel of high viscosity. Inflammatory cells in the vitreous can be a sign of infections of the eye (e.g., bacterial endophthalmitis), noninfectious inflammations (e.g., sarcoidosis), or tumors (e.g., ocular lymphoma). Amyloid deposits in the vitreous are almost always due to mutant forms of transthyretin[51] and are associated with familial amyloidotic polyneuropathy.[52]

OPTIC NERVE

Papilledema

Papilledema, or edema of the optic disc, classically is associated with increased intracranial pressure. There are several structural characteristics of the optic nerve that are believed to play a crucial role in the pathogenesis of papilledema.[53] The subarachnoid space surrounding the optic nerve is a direct extension of the subarachnoid space around the brain, with which it is normally in direct communication. Any increase in intracranial pressure is thus transmitted to the optic nerve. In addition, the central retinal vein draining the retina runs in the axial portion within the optic nerve for about 8 to 15 mm then exits from the nerve and crosses the meninges. At this point, it is vulnerable to occlusion from increased pressure in the subarachnoid space. The optic disc possesses a rich arterial blood supply from the central retinal artery and the choroidal arteries, supplied by the arterial circle of Zinn-Haller. The relevant differences between the arterial and venous pressure seem to be significant in the development of papilledema. Axonal swelling, however, appears to be the most important factor in the increase in tissue volume of the optic nerve head.

Acutely, there is edema and vascular congestion of the nerve head (Fig. 31–18). The physiologic cup is obliterated, and hemorrhages may be seen in the optic nerve or adjacent retinal nerve fiber layer. The sensory retina is displaced away from the edges of the optic disc by the edema, and folding of the retina and choroid are seen. With chronic papilledema, degeneration of nerve fibers, gliosis, and optic atrophy may occur.

Optic Neuritis

Grouped together under the term *optic neuritis* are many pathologic processes that are noninflammatory and are better described by the term *optic neuropathy.* Of major importance are the optic neuropathies of demyelinating diseases. These display similar histopathologic features to those found in the brain (Chapter 30).[54] Classically, these consist of loss of myelin and oligodendrocytes with relative preservation of axons. Other causes of optic neuritis include *systemic diseases*, such as sarcoidosis, collagen diseases, diabetes mellitus, and blood disorders; *ischemic diseases*, including temporal arteritis and atherosclerosis; *toxic conditions*, such as methyl alcohol or lead poisoning; spread of *inflammation* from the orbit or sinuses; and *infection.*

Optic Atrophy

The ultimate result of progressive optic nerve diseases is optic nerve atrophy. Variations in the findings depend on the pathogenic factors involved.[55] Common to all cases, however, are loss of both myelin and axis cylinders, glial proliferation (gliosis), thickening of the pial septa, and widening of the space separating the optic nerve and the meninges as a result of the loss of nerve parenchyma. In addition, the physiologic cup may appear wider or deeper than normal (Fig. 31–19).

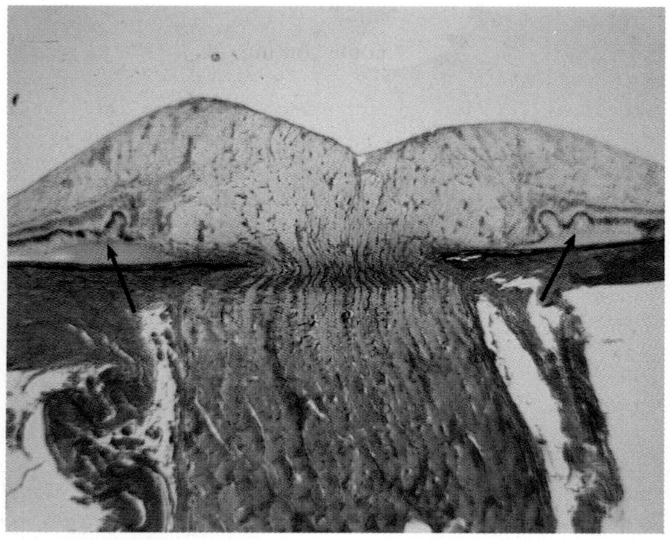

Figure 31–18

Papilledema showing displacement of the sensory retina (*arrows*).

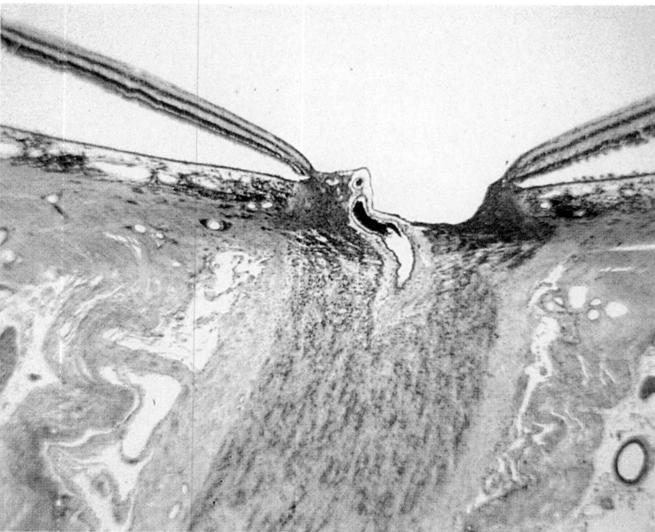

Figure 31–19

Optic atrophy: note the large optic cup (H&E × 10).

Tumors

The principal primary tumors of the optic nerve are gliomas and meningiomas. These are described in detail in Chapter 30. Less commonly, hemangiomas, hemangiopericytomas, and tumors arising from congenital rests may occur. Secondary tumors may extend into the optic nerve from adjacent or distant sites.

GLAUCOMA

Glaucoma is often mistakenly considered by nonophthalmologists to be a discrete disease entity. It is, in fact, several different diseases, many of which are characterized by an intraocular pressure sufficiently elevated to produce ocular tissue damage. Glaucoma is one of the leading causes of blindness in the United States. The three major categories of glaucoma are (1) angle-closure glaucoma, (2) open-angle glaucoma, and (3) congenital and juvenile glaucoma. The term *angle* refers to the angle of the anterior chamber formed by the junction of the uveal tract with the corneoscleral coat. This is the most important region of aqueous drainage.

Eyes that develop *primary angle-closure glaucoma* are anatomically predisposed to the condition. Most commonly, the eyes are smaller than normal and hyperopic. The surface of the peripheral iris is close to the inner surface of the trabecular meshwork, resulting in a narrow or shallow anterior chamber angle.

Primary open-angle glaucoma accounts for about two thirds of all glaucoma seen in whites and has an incidence of between 0.5 and 1%. The incidence of primary open-angle glaucoma in blacks is about 1.5%. The angle appears open but does not function properly in transporting aqueous humor out of the eye. The exact nature of the obstruction has not yet been elucidated.

Congenital glaucoma and *juvenile glaucoma* are thought to be hereditary in most cases, with both recessive and dominant forms documented,[56] although infectious causes are also possible (e.g., rubella). The incidence of congenital glaucoma is about 1:5000 to 1:10,000 live births. Genes responsible for dominant juvenile glaucoma,[57] recessive congenital glaucoma,[58] and Rieger syndrome (dysgenesis of the anterior segment of the eye with glaucoma)[59] have been identified. They belong to several classes of molecules, such as cytochromes and transcription factors. The mechanisms by which defects in these genes cause glaucoma are under investigation.

It is unknown how elevated intraocular pressure causes degeneration of the retinal ganglion cells and their axons (called *glaucomatous optic atrophy*) (Fig. 31–20) and consequent visual loss. Some experts speculate that in certain patients the elevated pressure may actually be an epiphenomenon, and the optic atrophy may be the result of a biochemical defect inherent to the ganglion cells. The occasional patient who develops glaucomatous optic atrophy in the absence of elevated intraocular pressure is evidence for this view. The more traditional explanation, however, is that the mechanical force of the intraocular pressure on the nerve fibers as they course around the margin of the cup of the optic nerve interferes with axoplasmic flow and produces axonal necrosis. In addition or alternatively, elevated intraocular pressure may impair the vascular supply of the optic nerve, thus leading to ischemic necrosis of nerve fibers.

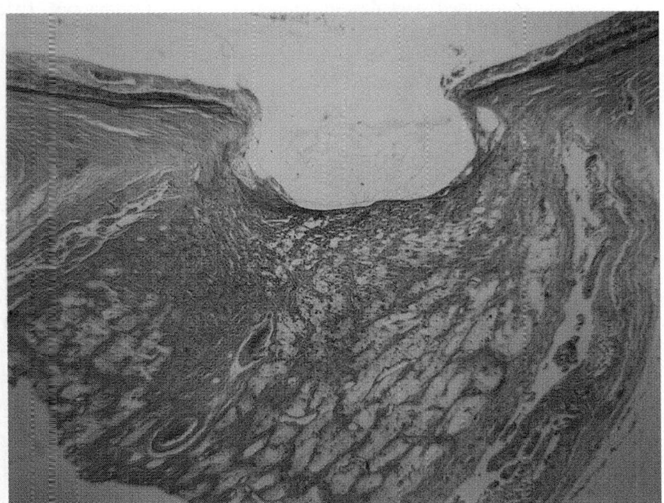

Figure 31–20

Glaucomatous cup. Note the characteristic excavation of the optic disc.

MORPHOLOGY. The loss of nerve fibers results in a characteristic cupped excavation of the optic disc (Fig. 31–20). As the nerve fibers disappear, the myelin in the retrobulbar portion of the nerve also vanishes, resulting in a decrease in the diameter of the nerve evident both on gross and on microscopic examination. The retina develops thinning of the nerve fiber layer, and the retinal ganglion cells degenerate. Additional changes in eyes with long-standing, greatly elevated pressure include intracellular and intercellular epithelial edema of the cornea, corneal stromal edema, degenerative pannus, and corneal scarring; cataracts; necrosis of the iris and the ciliary body stroma; atrophy, hyalinization, and shortening of the ciliary processes; and venous stasis in the retina, sometimes with occlusion of the central retinal vein. In infants with glaucoma, the corneoscleral coat may become stretched and thinned as a result of chronically elevated intraocular pressure, producing an enlargement of the entire eye (buphthalmos). In adult eyes, sustained elevation of pressure may lead to bulging of the cornea or sclera. These areas are often lined by atrophic uveal tissue and appear black when observed clinically (staphyloma).

PHTHISIS BULBI AND THE END STAGE OF DIFFUSE OCULAR DISEASE

With the exception of eyes enucleated because of intraocular tumors, most of the eyes sent to the pathology laboratory are removed because of blindness, pain, and disfigurement. The primary causes of the ocular changes are usually trauma, glaucoma, or intraocular inflammation. *End-stage* blind eyes are generally classified into one of three categories.[60] *Atrophy without shrinkage* refers to an eye of otherwise normal or enlarged size that has atrophy of the intraocular structures. An eye with long-standing glaucoma is an example of an eye in this category. If there is also atrophy of the globe, so that it is smaller than normal, the eye shows *atrophy with shrinkage. Phthisis bulbi* (Fig. 31–21) describes an eye with markedly thickened sclera and generalized disorganization of intraocular contents sufficiently severe to make them unrecognizable. The globe is small; the cornea is flattened, shrunken, and scarred. The lens, if not previously removed or extruded, may be displaced and shows cataractous changes, often with calcium deposition. Most phthisical eyes contain a dense fibrous membrane running across the ciliary body (cyclitic membrane). Intraocular bone formation is a characteristic finding in phthisis bulbi. This is a result of osseous metaplasia of the retinal pigment epithelium, and it forms without cartilage. A fatty marrow can be present

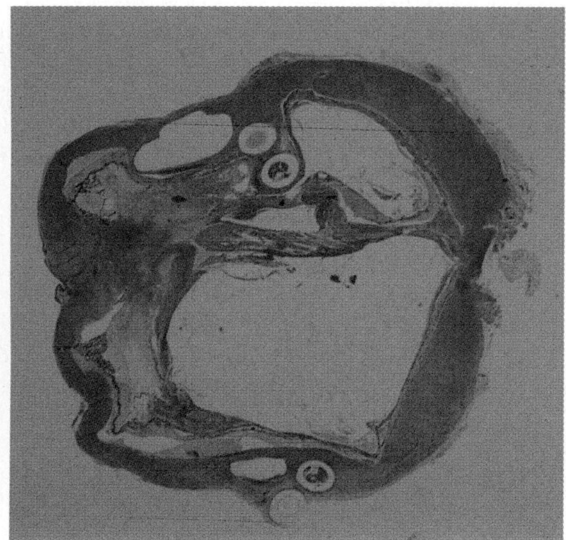

Figure 31–21

Phthisis bulbi. Note the markedly thickened sclera and disorganization of the intraocular contents.

within the bone, and particularly in younger individuals, the marrow may possess hematopoietic elements. The retina is usually detached and reduced to a gliotic scar, and the optic nerve is markedly atrophic.

REFERENCES

1. Kupfer C, et al: Leading causes of visual impairment worldwide. In Albert D, Jakobiec F (eds): Principles and Practice of Ophthalmology: Basic Sciences. Philadelphia, WB Saunders, 1994, p 1249.
2. Albert D: The ocular melanoma story. Am J Ophthalmol 123:729–741, 1997.
3. Lahav M, et al: Clinical and histopathological classification of retinal dysplasia. Am J Ophthalmol 75:648, 1973.
4. Jaeger EA: Ocular findings in Down's syndrome. Trans Am Ophthalmol Soc 78:808, 1980.
5. Robb RM, Marchevski A: A pathology of the lens in Down's syndrome. Arch Ophthalmol 96:1039, 1978.
6. Boniuk M, Zimmerman LE: Ocular pathology in the rubella syndrome. Arch Ophthalmol 77:455, 1967.
7. Contreras F, Pereda J: Congenital syphilis of the eye with lens involvement. Arch Ophthalmol 96:1052, 1978.
8. World Health Organization (ed): Global Situation: Vitamin A Deficiency. Expanded Program on Immunization Update. Geneva, World Health Organization, 1988.
9. Austin P, et al: Elastoplasia and elastodystrophy as the pathologic basis of ocular pterygia and pingueculae. Ophthalmology 90:96, 1983.
10. McCallan AF: The epidemiology of trachoma. Br J Ophthalmol 15: 369, 1931.
11. Spencer WH, Zimmerman LE: Conjunctiva. In Spencer WH (ed): Ophthalmic Pathology, 4th ed, Vol I. Philadelphia, WB Saunders, 1996, pp 38–125.
12. Blodi FC: Squamous cell carcinoma of the conjunctiva. Doc Ophthalmol 34:93, 1973.
13. Munier F, et al: Kerato-epithelin mutations in four 5q31-linked corneal dystrophies. Nat Genet 15:247–251, 1997.
14. Vance J, et al: Linkage of macular corneal dystrophy (MCD) to 16q: evidence that MCD types I and II are due to the same locus (abstract). Am J Hum Genet 57:A230, 1995.
15. Elliott J: Introduction to uveitis. In Albert D, Jakobiec F (eds): Principles and Practice of Ophthalmology: Clinical Practice, Vol I. Philadelphia, WB Saunders, 1994, pp 396–406.
16. Albert D, Diaz-Rohena R: Historical review of sympathetic ophthalmia and its epidemiology. Surv Ophthalmol 34:1–14, 1989.
17. Lubin JR, et al: Sixty-five years of sympathetic ophthalmia: a clinicopathologic review of 105 cases (1913–1978). Ophthalmology 87:109, 1980.
18. Scotto J, et al: Melanomas of the eye and other noncutaneous sites. J Natl Cancer Inst 56:489, 1976.
19. Yanoff M, Fine B: Ocular Pathology: A Text and Atlas, 3rd ed. New York, Harper & Row, 1989.
20. Callender GR: Malignant melanotic tumors of the eye: a study of histologic types in 111 cases. Trans Am Acad Ophthalmol 36:131, 1931.
21. Folberg R, et al: The prognostic value of tumor blood vessel morphology in primary uveal melanoma. Ophthalmology 100:1389–1398, 1993.
22. Eagle RJ, Spencer W: Lens. In Spencer W (ed) Ophthalmic Pathology: A Text and Atlas, 4th ed. Philadelphia, WB Saunders, 1996, pp 372–437.
23. Shastry B, et al: Identification of missense mutations in Norrie's disease gene associated with advanced retinopathy of prematurity. Arch Ophthalmol 115:651–655, 1997.
24. Garner A: Vascular disorders. In Garner AC, Klintworth GK (eds): Pathobiology of Ocular Disease. New York, Marcel Dekker, 1982, pp 1479–1575.
25. D'Amico DJ: Diseases of the retina. N Engl J Med 331:95–106, 1994.
26. Ashton N: Vascular basement membrane changes in diabetic retinopathy. Br J Ophthalmol 58:344, 1974.
27. Cogan DG, et al: Retinal vascular patterns: IV. diabetic retinopathy. Arch Ophthalmol 66:366, 1961.
28. Aiello L, et al: Vascular endothelial growth factor in ocular fluid of patients with diabetic retinopathy and other retinal disorders. N Engl J Med 331:1480–1487, 1994.
29. Scheie HG: Evaluation of ophthalmoscopic changes of hypertension and arteriorlar sclerosis. Arch Ophthalmol 49:117, 1953.
30. Wagener H, Keith N: Diffuse arteriolar disease with hypertension and associated retinal lesions. Medicine 18:317, 1939.
31. Berson E: Retinitis pigmentosa and related diseases. In Albert D, Jakobiec F (eds): Principles and Practice of Ophthalmology, Vol 2. Philadelpia, WB Saunders, 1994, pp 1214–1237.
32. Dryja T, Li T: Molecular genetics of retinitis pigmentosa. Hum Mol Genet 4:1739–1743, 1995.
33. Cogan D: Pathology [of retinitis pigmentosa]. Trans Am Acad Ophthalmol Otolaryngol 54:629–661, 1950.
34. Gartner S, Henkind P: Pathology of retinitis pigmentosa. Ophthalmology 89:1425, 1982.
35. Hyman L, et al: Senile macular degeneration: a case-control study. Am J Epidemiol 118:213–227, 1983.
36. Eye Disease Case Control Study Group: Antioxidant states and neovascular age-related macular degeneration. Arch Ophthalmol 111: 104–109, 1993.
37. Evans K, Bird A: The genetics of complex ophthalmic disorders. Br J Ophthalmol 80:763–768, 1996.
38. Felbor U, et al: Autosomal recessive Sorsby fundus dystrophy revisited: molecular evidence for dominant inheritance. Am J Hum Genet 60:57–62, 1997.
39. Allikemets R, et al: A photoreceptor cell-specific ATP binding transport gene (ABCR) is mutated in recessive Stargardt macular dystrophy. Nat Genet 15:236–245, 1997.
40. Green W, Enger C: Age-related macular degeneration: histopathologic studies. The 1992 Lorenz E. Zimmerman Lecture. Ophthalmology 100:1519–1535, 1993.
41. Klein R, et al: Prevalence of age-related maculopathy. Ophthalmology 99:933–943, 1992.
42. Machemer R, Kroll AJ: Experimental retinal detachment in the owl monkey: VII. photoreceptor protein renewal in normal and detached retina. Am J Ophthalmol 71:690, 1971.
43. Wong F, et al: Cancer incidence after retinoblastoma: radiation dose and sarcoma risk. JAMA 278:1272–1267, 1997.
44. Bader J, et al: Bilateral retinoblastoma with ectopic intracranial retinoblastoma: trilateral retinoblastoma. Cancer Genet Cytogenet 5:230–213, 1982.
45. Cavenee W, et al: Expression of recessive alleles by chromosomal mechanisms in retinoblastoma. Nature 305:779–784, 1983.

46. Dryja T, et al: Homozygosity of chromosome 13 in retinoblastoma. N Engl J Med 310:550–553, 1984.
47. Dryja T: Genetics of retinoblastoma. Curr Opin Pediatr 1:413–420, 1989.
48. Sakai T, et al: Allele-specific hypermethylation of the retinoblastoma tumor-suppressor gene. Am J Hum Genet 48:880–888, 1991.
49. Greger V, et al: Frequency and parental origin of hypermethylated RB1 alleles in retinoblastoma. Hum Genet 94:491–496, 1994.
50. McLean I: Retinoblastoma, retinocytoma, and pseudoretinoblastoma. In Spencer W (ed): Ophthalmic Pathology: A Text and Atlas. Philadelphia, WB Saunders, 1996, pp 1332–1380.
51. Burrell J, et al: Production and functional analysis of normal and variant recombinant human transthyretin proteins. B Biol Chem 267: 16595–16600, 1992.
52. Benson M, Wallace M: Amyloidosis. In Scriver C, et al (eds): The Metabolic Basis of Inherited Disease. New York, McGraw-Hill, 1989, pp 2439–2460.
53. Hayreh MS, Heyreh SS: Optic disc edema in raised intracranial pressure: I. evolution and resolution. Arch Ophthalmol 95:1237, 1977.
54. Arnold A, et al: Retinal periphlebitis and retinitis in multiple sclerosis: I. pathologic characteristics. Ophthalmology 91:255, 1984.
55. Sadun A: Optic atrophy and papilledema. In Albert D, Jakobiec F (eds): Principles and Practice of Ophthalmology: Clinical Practice, Vol 4. Philadelphia, WB Saunders, 1994, pp 2529–2538.
56. Raymond V: Molecular genetics of the glaucomas: mapping of the first five "GLC" loci. Am J Hum Genet 60:272–277, 1997.
57. Stone E, et al: Identification of a gene that causes primary open angle glaucoma. Science 275:668–670, 1997.
58. Stoilov I, et al: Identification of three different truncating mutations in cytochrome P4501B1 (CYP1B1) as the principal cause of primary congenital glaucoma (buphthalmos) in families linked to the GLC3 A locus on chromosome 2p21. Hum Mol Genet 6:641–647, 1997.
59. Semina E, et al: Cloning and characterization of a novel bicoid-related homeobox transcription factor gene, RIEG, involved in Rieger syndrome. Nat Genet 14:392–399, 1996.
60. Spencer W: Sclera. In Spencer W (ed): Ophthalmic Pathology: A Text and Atlas, Vol 1. Philadelphia, WB Saunders, 1996, pp 334–372.

Index

Note: Page numbers in *italics* refer to illustrations; page numbers followed by t refer to tables.

A

Abdominal pain, in acute pancreatitis, 907
Abetalipoproteinemia, 815
ABO (glycosyltransferase) gene, frameshift mutation in, 142, *142*
ABO isoimmunization, 473
Abortion, septic, 369–370
  spontaneous, 1079
Abrasion, 432, *432*
Abscess, 85, *85*
  amebic, 358–359, 867–868
  bone, 1232–1233, *1232*
  brain, 1315–1316, *1316,* 1323, *1323*
  Brodie, 1233
  cardiac, 574, *574*
  Chlamydia, 362
  extradural, 1316
  gonorrheal, 362
  hepatic, 358–359, 867–868
  Listeria, 378
  pancreatic, 907, 909
  perinephric, 974–975
  periodontal, 369–370
  pulmonary, 722, *723*
    in cystic fibrosis, 480
  ring, 574, *574*
  staphylococcal, 366–367, *367*
  streptococcal, 368
  subareolar, 1096–1097
  subdiaphragmatic, 841
  subhepatic, 841
  subperiosteal, 1232, *1232*
  Toxoplasma, 1323, *1323*
  tubo-ovarian, 1039
Absidia, 380–381
Acanthamoeba sp., 337t
Acantholysis, 1172
  in pemphigus, 1202, *1202, 1203*
Acanthosis, 1172
Acanthosis nigricans, 1180–1181
  paraneoplastic, 320, 321t
Accessory duct of Santorini, 903
Acetaminophen, adverse reactions to, 416
  hepatic necrosis with, 416
  in cell injury, 14–15
Acetylaminofluorene, in carcinogenesis, 309
Acetylcholine, in asthma, 713
Acetylcholine receptors, immune-mediated loss of, 1289
Acetylsalicylic acid. See *Aspirin (acetylsalicylic acid).*
Achalasia, 778–779, *778*
Achondrogenesis, 1220t
Achondroplasia, 1220–1221, 1220t
Acid aerosols, 417–418, 417t
Acid lipase, deficiency of (Wolman disease), 155t
Acid phosphate, deficiency of, 155t
Acid-fast stain, 345, 345t
Acidosis, metabolic, in renal osteodystrophy, 1229
Acinar cells, in acute pancreatitis, 906–907, *906*
Acinic cell tumor, 773
Acinus (acini), hepatic, 846, *846*
  pancreatic, 903, *903*
  pulmonary, 698, *708*
Acne vulgaris, 1206–1207, *1207*
Acoustic neuroma, 1352–1353, *1353*
Acquired immunodeficiency syndrome (AIDS), 236–251. See also *Human immunodeficiency virus (HIV) infection.*
  B-cell lymphoma in, 312
  candidiasis in, 247–248
  cervical carcinoma in, 250
  clinical features of, 247–251, 247t, *249*
  cryptococcal meningitis in, 1322
  cryptococcosis in, 248
  cytomegalovirus infection in, 248
  diarrhea in, 811
  diffuse large B-cell lymphoma in, 661–662
  epidemiology of, 236–238
  etiology of, 238–239, *238, 239*
  herpes simplex virus infection in, 248
  in children, 237, 1321
  infectious diarrhea in, 248
  Kaposi sarcoma in, 248–249, *249,* 535
  lymphoma in, 249–250
  Mycobacterium avium infection in, 352, *352*
  Mycobacterium tuberculosis infection in, 248, 351–352, 1317
  myocarditis in, 584
  natural history of, 245–247, *245,* 245t
  nephropathy in, 958
  neurosyphilis in, 1317
  opportunistic infections in, 247–248, 247t
  oral manifestations of, 759t
Acquired immunodeficiency syndrome (AIDS) *(Continued)*
  pathogenesis of, 239–245, *240–242, 244,* 245t
  peripheral neuropathy in, 1321
  Pneumocystis carinii pneumonia in, 247
  pneumonia in, 247, 726, 726t
  thrombocytopenia in, 636
  tuberculosis in, 248, 351–352, 1317
  vacuolar myelopathy in, 1321
Acrochordon, 1181
Acromegaly, somatotroph adenoma and, 1126
Actin, of sarcomere, 544
Actinic keratosis, 1184, *1185*
α-Actinin, 101, *101*
Actinomyces israelii, 334t, 369
Acute phase proteins, 86
Acute tubular necrosis (ATN), 969–971
  ischemic, 970, *970, 971*
  nonoliguric, 971
  pathogenesis of, 969–970, *969*
  toxic, 970–971, *970*
Acyl-coenzyme A dehydrogenase, deficiency of, in sudden infant death syndrome, 482
Adamantinomatous craniopharyngioma, 1129
Adaptation, 2, *3*
ADCC (antibody-dependent cell-mediated cytotoxicity), 191, *200,* 201
Addison disease, 1160–1161, *1161*
Additives, food, 436
Adenitis, vestibular, 1040
Adenocarcinoma, 262
  of bile ducts, 899–900
  of bladder, 1007
  of colon, *265,* 891, *891*
  of endometrium, 1061–1062, *1062*
  of esophagus, 786–787, *786*
  of fallopian tubes, 1065
  of gallbladder, 899, *900*
  of intestine, 827
  of ovary, 1072
  of vagina, 1046, *1046*
Adenofibroma, of ovary, 1072–1073, *1072*
Adenohypophysis. See *Pituitary gland, anterior.*
Adenoid cystic carcinoma, of salivary glands, 772–773, *773*
Adenolymphoma, 769, 771–772, *771*

Adenoma, 261
adrenocortical, 1153–1155, *1153,* 1155t, 1162
aldosterone-producing, 1155–1157, *1156, 1157*
adrenocorticotropic hormone–secreting, 1126–1127, 1153–1154, *1153*
aldosterone-producing, 1155–1157, *1156, 1157*
carcinoid, 747–748, *748*
follicle-stimulating hormone–secreting, 1127
gastric, 798, *798*
gonadotroph-secreting, 1127
growth hormone–secreting, 1126
hepatic, 887–888, *887*
oral contraceptives and, 416
intestinal, 827, *827,* 829–831, *829–831*
familial, 831, *831*
malignant change in, 830–831
tubular, 829–830, *829*
tubulovillous, 830
villous, 830, *830*
luteinizing hormone–secreting, 1127
null cell, 1127
of ampulla of Vater, 827, *827*
of nipple, 1104
of salivary glands, 770–771, *770*
pancreatic, 910
papillary, renal, 991
thyroid, 1142
parathyroid, 1148–1150, *1149*
pituitary, 1123–1127, *1124,* 1124t, *1125,* 1153–1154, *1153*
pleomorphic, 262, 770–771, *770*
prolactin-secreting, 1125–1126, *1125*
renal, 991
sebaceous, 1183t
thyroid, *265,* 1140–1142, *1141*
thyroid-stimulating hormone–secreting, 1127
Adenoma-carcinoma sequence, of intestine, 831–832
Adenomatoid tumor, of fallopian tubes, 1065
Adenomatous polyposis coli (APC) gene, 297, *297,* 832, *832*
Adenomyosis, of endometrium, 1057, *1057*
of gallbladder, 899
Adenosine, in type I hypersensitivity reaction, 197, *197*
Adenosine deaminase, deficiency of, gene mutation in, 147t
gene therapy in, 141
in severe combined immunodeficiency disease, 235
Adenosine triphosphate (ATP), depletion of, in cell injury, 5, *6*
Adenosis, of breast, 1099, 1101, *1101*
of vagina, 1046
Adenoviruses, 333t
gastrointestinal tract infection with, 354, 807t
Adhesins, bacterial, 341–343, *342*
Adhesions, intestinal, *825,* 826
Adhesive mediastinopericarditis, 588–589
Adnexal (appendage) tumors, 1182–1183, *1183,* 1183t, *1184*
Adrenal cortex, 1152–1163
adenoma of, 1153–1155, *1153,* 1155t, 1162
aldosterone-producing, 1155–1157, *1156, 1157*
carcinoma of, 1153–1155, 1155t, 1162–1163, *1162*
congenital hyperplasia of, 1157–1159, *1158*
cyst of, 1163
metastases to, adrenocortical insufficiency with, 1161
Adrenal cortex *(Continued)*
myelolipoma of, 1163
Adrenal gland. See also *Adrenal cortex; Adrenal medulla.*
amyloidosis of, 256
in shock, 137
Adrenal medulla, 1152–1153, 1163–1167
neuroblastoma of, 485–487, *486, 487,* 1166
pheochromocytoma of, 1164–1166, 1164t, *1165*
Adrenal virilism, 1157–1159, *1158*
Adrenalitis, 1160, *1161*
Adrenocortical insufficiency, 1159–1162, 1159t, *1160, 1161*
acute, 1159–1160
chronic (Addison disease), 1160–1161, *1161*
secondary, 1161–1162
Adrenocorticotropic hormone, hypersecretion of, 1153–1155, *1153,* 1155t
tumor production of, 1126–1127, 1153–1154, *1153*
Adrenogenital syndromes, 1157–1159, *1158*
Adrenoleukodystrophy, 1278t, 1340
Adriamycin, myocardial toxicity of, 580, 586
Adult polyglucosan body disease, 1297
Adult respiratory distress syndrome (ARDS), 700–703, 701t
clinical course of, 703
endotoxemia in, 701–702, *702*
hyaline membranes in, 701, *701*
pathogenesis of, 701–703, *702*
Adult T-cell leukemia/lymphoma, 656t, 670
Advanced glycosylation end products, in diabetes mellitus, 920, 920t
Adventitia, 494, *494*
Aflatoxins, 380
hepatocellular carcinoma and, 888–889
Aflatoxin B_1, 424, 424t
in carcinogenesis, 308, 309
African Kaposi sarcoma, 535
African sleeping sickness, *337*
African trypanosomiasis, 393
Agammaglobulinemia, X-linked, of Bruton, 232–233
Aganglionic megacolon, congenital, 805
Age. See also *Aging.*
cancer and, 273–275, 274t
maternal, trisomy 21 and, 170
Agenesis, definition of, 466
of corpus callosum, 1300, *1301*
of kidney, 936
of pancreas, 904
Age-related macular degeneration, 1371, *1371*
Aging, amyloidosis of, 253t, 254
atrophy with, 35
cellular, 45–48, *46, 47, 48*
timing of, 46–47, *46, 47*
Agranulocytosis, 200, 646–647. See also *Hypersensitivity reaction(s), type II (cytotoxic).*
Agricultural hazards, 422–424, 423t
Agyria, 1300
AIDS. See *Acquired immunodeficiency syndrome.*
Ail protein, of *Yersinia pseudotuberculosis,* 356
Air blast injury, 435
Air embolism, 131, 435
Air pollution, bronchogenic carcinoma and, 742
indoor, 418–419, 418t
outdoor, 416–418, 417t
Air-conditioner lung, 737
Airway. See *Respiratory tract.*
Alagille syndrome, 881
Albers-Schönberg disease, 1224–1225, *1224*
Albinism, 148
Albumin, in osmotic pressure, 115
Alcohol, breast cancer and, 1107
fetal effects of, 467
gastric cancer and, 799, 799t
myocardial toxicity of, 579–580
oral cancer and, 760
peptic ulcer disease and, 794
Alcohol abuse, 410–412, *410, 411,* 411t
cancer and, 273
cerebellar degeneration in, 1342, *1342*
dilated cardiomyopathy and, 579–580
thiamine deficiency in, 447
vitamin B_6 deficiency in, 449
Wernicke-Korsakoff syndrome in, 412, 447, 1341
Alcoholic cardiomyopathy, 579–580
Alcoholic liver disease, 869–873
cholestasis in, 872
cirrhosis in, 870–871, *870, 871,* 872
clinical course of, 872–873
collagen deposition in, 872
fatty liver in, 39, *39,* 869, *870,* 872
fibrosis in, 870
hepatitis in, 869–870, *870, 871,* 872
hyaline inclusions in, 27–28, *28*
iron distribution in, 874
Mallory bodies in, 869, *871*
mitochondria in, *27*
neutrophilic reaction in, 869
pathogenesis of, 871–872
prognosis for, 872
steatosis in, 869, *870*
Alcoholic myopathy, 1288
Aldosterone, biosynthesis of, *1152*
Alexander disease, 1297
Alginate, of *Pseudomonas,* 377
Aliphatic hydrocarbons, in occupational diseases, 419–420, 419t
Alkaline phosphatase, in cholestasis, 851
Alkaptonuria (ochronosis), 42, 162
Alkylating agents, in carcinogenesis, 309
Allele(s). See also *Gene(s).*
codominance of, 144
dominant negative, 145, 148
Allele-specific oligonucleotide hybridization, in genetic disorders, 183, *184*
Allergic gastroenteropathy, 793
Allergic rhinitis, 762
Allergy, 199. See also *Hypersensitivity reaction(s).*
in asthma, 713, *714*
in contact dermatitis, 1195t, 1196–1197, *1196*
Alpha (α) toxin, of *Clostridium perfringens,* 344, 368
of *Staphylococcus aureus,* 365
Alpha fetoprotein, in hepatocellular carcinoma, 891
in testicular germ cell tumors, 1024
in tumor diagnosis, 325, 325t
Alpha-cell tumors, 927
Alport syndrome, 962–963, *963*
Aluminum, in renal osteodystrophy, 1229
Alveolar macrophages, 698
in pneumonia, 718
Alveolar proteinosis, 739–740, *740*
Alveolar rhabdomyosarcoma, 1265–1266, *1265*
Alveolar septa, 698, *698*
Alveolitis, in diffuse interstitial disease, 727, 727t
Alveolus, 698, *708*

Alzheimer disease, 1296t, 1329–1333, *1330*
  amyloid deposition in, 252, 1331–1332, *1332,* 1332t
  apolipoprotein E in, 1333
  genetics of, 1332, 1332t
  granulovacuolar degeneration in, 1331
  Hirano bodies in, 1331
  neuritic plaques in, 1330, *1331*
  neurofibrillary tangles in, 28, 1330, *1331*
Alzheimer type II astrocyte, 1297
Amebiasis, 358–359, *358*
Ameboma, 358
Ameloblastoma, 761
Amenorrhea, in anorexia nervosa, 439
  in Turner syndrome, 175
Ames test, 307–308
Amides, in carcinogenesis, 309
Amines, aromatic, in carcinogenesis, 309
  vasoactive, in inflammation, 66–67, *66,* 77t
Amino acids, in cell injury, 11
Amiodarone, pulmonary effects of, 740, 740t
Amnion, infection of, 470
Amnion nodosum, 465
Amniotic band syndrome, 465, *465*
Amniotic fluid embolism, 131
Amphicytes, 1237
Ampulla of Vater, 892
  adenoma of, 827, *827*
Amputation neuroma, 1280, *1280*
Amylin, in type II diabetes mellitus, 918
Amyloid, composition of, 252
  Congo red–stained, 255, *255*
  hyaline appearance of, 45
  in Alzheimer disease, 252, 1331–1332, *1332,* 1332t
  in medullary thyroid carcinoma, 1146, *1146*
  in renal osteodystrophy, 1229
  structure of, 251–252, *251*
Amyloid angiopathy, in Alzheimer disease, 1310, 1330–1331, *1331*
Amyloid polyneuropathy, familial, 1277, 1278t
β_2-Amyloid protein, 252
Amyloid transthyretin, 252
Amyloidosis, 251–257, *251*
  cardiac, 256, *256,* 586
  clinical features of, 256–257
  endocrine, 253t, 254
  gastrointestinal, 256
  hemodialysis-associated, 253, 253t
  hemorrhage in, 634
  hepatic, 255–256
  heredofamilial, 253–254, 253t
  in multiple myeloma, 980
  localized, 253t, 254
  of aging, 253t, 254
  of nerves, 256
  pathogenesis of, 253t, 254–255, *254*
  primary, 252–253, 253t, 663
  protein misfolding in, 41
  reactive, 253 253t
  renal, 255, *255,* 968
  splenic, 255
Amyotrophic lateral sclerosis, 1338, *1339*
Analgesic nephropathy, 416, *977,* 978–979, *979,* 979t
Anaphase lag, 168
Anaphylaxis. See also *Hypersensitivity reaction(s), type I (anaphylactic).*
Anaplasia, 265–266, *265, 266,* 323, *323.* See also *Tumor(s).*
Anasarca, 113, 560
Ancylostoma duodenale, 394–395
Androblastoma, 1024, 1078, *1078*
Androgens, in nodular prostatic hyperplasia, 1027, *1027*
Androgen insensitivity syndrome (testicular feminization), 176
Androgenesis, in hydatidiform mole, 1085, *1086*
Anemia, 604–633, 605t
  aplastic, 630–632, *631, 632*
  blood loss, 605–606
  Fanconi, 169, 296
  hemolytic, 200, 605t, 606–621, *607*
    immune-mediated, 620–621, 620t
    in chronic lymphocytic leukemia, *659*
    in disseminated intravascular coagulation, 641
    in glucose-6-phosphate dehydrogenase deficiency, 610–611, *610, 611*
    in hereditary spherocytosis, 607–609, *609*
    in paroxysmal nocturnal hemoglobinuria, 619–620, *619*
    in sickle cell disease, 611–615, *612–614*
    in α-thalassemia, 618–619
    in β-thalassemia, 615–618, *615, 616,* 617t, *618*
    microangiopathic, 637
    trauma-induced, 621, *621*
  in liver disease, 632–633
  in renal failure, 633
  in Rh isoimmunization, 473–474
  iron deficiency, 118, 627–630, *627,* 627t, *628, 630*
  megaloblastic, 605t, 621–627, *622,* 623t
    in folate deficiency, 626–627, *626*
    in vitamin B_{12} deficiency, 623–626, 623t, *624*
  myelophthisic, 632
  of chronic disease, 630
  pernicious, 623–626, 623t, *624,* 791, 793
Anencephaly, 1300
Aneurysm, aortic, 524–528
    abdominal, 525–526, *525*
  berry, 525, 1310–1313, *1311, 1312*
    in polycystic kidney disease, 940
  blood flow effects of, 125
  Charcot-Bouchard, 1310
  dissecting, 524
  fusiform, 525
  mycotic, 128, 525
  rupture of, 526
  saccular, 525
  syphilitic, 526
  ventricular, after myocardial infarction, 563
Angelman syndrome, 180–181, *181*
Angiitis, leukocytoclastic, cutaneous, 517t, 521–522, *522*
Angina, agranulocytic, 647
Angina pectoris, 554
Angiodysplasia, intestinal, 823
Angiofibroma, nasopharyngeal, 763
Angiogenesis, 55
  angiopoietins in, 104–106, *105*
  growth factors in, 104–106, *105,* 105t
  in fibrosis, 103–106, *104, 105,* 105t
  in tissue repair, 103–106, *104*
  tumor, 301–302
  vascular endothelial growth factor in, 104–106, *105,* 105t
Angioma, spider, in hepatic failure, 852
  venous, 1313
Angiomatosis, bacillary, 534–535, *534*
Angiomyolipoma, 991
Angiopathy, amyloid, in Alzheimer disease, 1310, 1330–1331, *1331*
Angioplasty, balloon, 538–539, *538*
Angiopoietins, in angiogenesis, 104–106, *105*
Angiosarcoma, 537–538, *537*
  of breast, 1104
  of heart, 591
  of liver, 537, 888
Angiotensin, in hypertension, 512, *512*
Animal toxins, 424, 424t
Aniridia, PAX-6 gene in, 470
Anitschkow cells, in rheumatic fever, 570
  in rheumatic heart disease, 570
Ankylosing spondyloarthritis, 1252
Ankylosis, in rheumatoid arthritis, 1249
Ankyrin, gene for, 147t
Annuloaortic ectasia, 528
Anorexia, in cancer, 319–320
Anorexia nervosa, 439
Anovulatory cycle, 1056, *1056*
Anthracosis, 42, 730
Antibiotics, colitis with, 809–810, *810*
Antibody(ies), anticardiolipin, 126
  anticentromere, 227
  anti–DNA topoisomerase I, 227
  antigliadin, 813, 1205
  anti–glomerular basement membrane, 943–945, *944*
  anti–glutamic acid decarboxylase, 916
  anti–islet cell, *915,* 916
  antineutrophil, 516, 951
  antinuclear, 216, 217–218, 218t, 227
  antiphospholipid, 126
  antireticulin, 1205
  antirotavirus, 354
  antiviral, 344
  Donath-Landsteiner, 621
Antibody probes, 345, 345t
Antibody-dependent cell-mediated cytotoxicity, 191, *200,* 201
Anticardiolipin antibodies, 126
Anticentromere antibody, 227
Anticipation, in fragile X syndrome, 178
  in myotonia, 1283
Anticoagulants, endothelial, *119,* 120
Antidiuretic hormone, deficiency of, 1129
  inappropriate secretion of, 1129
Antigen(s), anatomic sequestration of, 215
  bacterial, 344
  B-cell recognition of, 190
  CALLA, 317
  hypersensitivity reaction to, 195–211. See also *Hypersensitivity reaction(s).*
  molecular sequestration of, 215
  nuclear, 216, 217–218, 218t
  ocular, 215
  oncofetal, 317, 325, 325t
  prostate-specific, 1032–1033
  self, 212–214, *213,* 215
  Smith (sm), 217, 218t
  T-cell recognition of, 189, *190,* 194, *194*
  tumor, 315–317, *316*
Antigen-antibody complex. See *Immune complexes.*
Antigenic drift, of influenza virus, 348
Antigenic shift, of influenza virus, 348
Antineutrophil cytoplasmic antibodies, in rapidly progressive glomerulonephritis, 951
  in vasculitis, 516
Antinuclear antibodies, 216, 217–218, 218t, 227
Antioxidants, 77
  in free radical inactivation, 13
  vitamin E as, 446
Antiphospholipid antibody syndrome, 126, 986
  in systemic lupus erythematosus, 218
Antiproteases, 76
Antithrombins, *119,* 120

α_1-Antitrypsin, 76
deficiency of, 148, 875–876, *876*
cell injury in, 38, *38,* 41
emphysema and, 709
gene mutation in, 147t
Antrum, of stomach, 787, *787*
Anus, imperforate, 804
Aorta, abdominal, aneurysm of, 525–526, *525*
aneurysm of, 524–528, *525*
syphilitic, 526
coarctation of, 596–597, *597*
cystic medial degeneration of, 527–528, *528*
dilation of, 149
dissection of, 526–528, *527–529*
in Marfan syndrome, 149
intimal tear of, 527, *527*
pediatric, fatty streaks in, 503
thoracic, aneurysm of, 526
Aortic arch, Takayasu arteritis of, 519–520, *519*
Aortic dissection, 526–528, *527–529*
Aortic incompetence, in Marfan syndrome, 149
Aortic valve, 545
atresia of, 597
bicuspid, calcification of, 568
dystrophic calcifications of, 43–44, *44*
Lambl excrescences of, 546, 591
sclerosis of, 568
stenosis of, calcific, 567–568, *567*
congenital, 597
subaortic, 597
supravalvular, 597
Aortitis, syphilitic, 364, 526
Aortocoronary bypass surgery, 539–540
APC gene, in cancer, 287t, 292–293
in colon cancer, 297, *297,* 832, *832*
Apgar score, 463–464, 463t
Aphthous ulcers, 757, *757*
in Crohn disease, 816
Aplasia, definition of, 466
Aplastic anemia, 630–632, *631, 632*
Aplastic crisis, in hereditary spherocytosis, 609
Apolipoprotein B, deficiency of, 815
Apolipoprotein E, in Alzheimer disease, 1333
Apoplexy, pituitary, 1124
Apoproteins, 505
Apoptosis, 2, 4, 18–25
after growth factor deprivation, 24–25
apoptotic bodies in, 19, *19*
bcl-2 gene in, 22–23, *23,* 294–295, *295*
biochemical features of, 20, *21*
caspases in, *22,* 23
chromatin condensation in, 19, *19*
cytoplasmic blebs in, 19
cytotoxic T-lymphocyte–stimulated, 24, 206
DNA damage–mediated, 25
DNA fragmentation in, 20, *21*
dysregulation of, 25
execution phase of, *22,* 23
Fas-Fas ligand–mediated, 23, *24,* 206, 212, *213*
failure of, 214
histology of, 19–20, *20*
in embryogenesis, 18
in Hashimoto thyroiditis, 1134
in hormone-dependent involution, 18
in immune reactions, 19, *20*
in myocardial ischemia, 556
in tumors, 19
in viral infection, 19
mechanisms of, 20–23, *22, 23*
mitochondrial function in, 21–23, *23*
morphology of, 19, *19*
myc gene in, 282
Apoptosis *(Continued)*
of cytotoxic T lymphocytes, 318–319
phagocytosis in, 19, 20, *22,* 23, 64
protein cross-linking in, 20
protein hydrolysis in, 20
Rb gene loss in, 290
regulation of, 21–22, *22, 23,* 277, 294–295, *295*
signaling pathways in, 21, *22*
tumor cell resistance to, 292
tumor necrosis factor receptors in, 23–24, *24*
tumor necrosis factor–induced, 23–24, *24*
vs. atrophy, 36
vs. necrosis, *18*
Appendage (adnexal) tumors, 1182–1183, *1183,* 1183t, *1184*
Appendicitis, 839–840, *839*
Appendix, 838–840
inflammation of, 839–840, *839*
mucinous cystadenocarcinoma of, 840, *840*
mucocele of, 840
normal, 838–839
pseudomyxoma peritonei of, 840
Arachidonic acid metabolites, in inflammation, 70–72, *71,* 71t, 77t
in leukocyte activation, 62
in type I hypersensitivity reaction, 198–199, *198,* 199t
Arachnoiditis, adhesive, chronic, 1315
Arboviruses, CNS infection with, 333t, 1318
ARDS. See *Adult respiratory distress syndrome (ARDS).*
Areola, 1094
Argentaffinoma. See *Carcinoid tumor.*
Ariboflavinosis, 447–448
Arnold-Chiari malformation, 1301, *1301*
Aromatic amines, in carcinogenesis, 309
Aromatic hydrocarbons, in carcinogenesis, 309
in occupational diseases, 419t, 420
Arrhythmias, after myocardial infarction, 562
in myocardial ischemia, 556
in sudden cardiac death, 564
Arrhythmogenic right ventricular cardiomyopathy, 581
Arsenic, in carcinogenesis, 274t, 309
in occupational diseases, 421t
Arterioles, 494
hyalinization of, 45
sclerosis of, 498
Arteriolitis, hypertension and, 983, *983*
Arteriolosclerosis, 498
diabetes mellitus and, 922, *922,* 924
hypertension and, 514–515, *515*
Arteriosclerosis, after heart transplantation, 598, *598*
malignant, 983
Mönckeberg (medial calcific sclerosis), 498
retinopathy with, 1370
Arteriovenous fistula, 498
Arteriovenous malformation, 1313
Arteritis, giant cell (temporal), 516–518, 517t, *518*
Heubner, 1317
in cerebrovascular disease, 1308
infectious, 524
Takayasu, 517t, 519–520, *519*
Artery(ies), 494–495, *494.* See also specific arteries.
abnormal venous communication with, 498
balloon angioplasty of, 538–539, *538*
collateral, 133
elastic, 494
fenestrations of, 494
graft replacement of, 539–540, *539*
Artery(ies) *(Continued)*
inflammation of, 515–524, 515t. See also *Arteritis; Vasculitis.*
intimal thickening of, 497, *497*
lamina of, 494
Mönckeberg medial calcific sclerosis of, 498
muscular, 494
sclerosis of, 498–509. See also *Atherosclerosis.*
tumors of, 531–538, 531t. See also specific tumors.
types of, 494
wall of, 494, *494*
endothelial cells of, 496–497, *496,* 496t
smooth muscle cells of, *495,* 497, *497*
Arthritis, 203, *203,* 1246–1257
enteropathic, 1252
gouty, 1253–1257, *1254–1256,* 1254t
in Reiter syndrome, 1252
in rheumatic heart disease, 572
infectious, 1253
Lyme, 389, 1253
psoriatic, 1252–1253
rheumatoid, 1248–1251. See also *Rheumatoid arthritis.*
suppurative, 1253
tuberculous, 1253
viral, 1253
Arthrogryposis, in congenital myopathy, 1285
Arthropods, bites by, 1210–1211
in viral encephalitis, 1318
Arthus reaction, 204
Arylamines, transitional cell carcinoma and, 1007
Arylsulfatases, deficiency of (multiple sulfatase deficiency), 155t
Arylsulfatase A, deficiency of (metachromatic leukodystrophy), 155t, 1340, *1340*
Asbestos, amphibole, 732
bronchogenic carcinoma and, 742
in buildings, 418, 418t
in carcinogenesis, 274t, 309
serpentine, 732
Asbestos bodies, 733, *733*
Asbestosis, 729t, 732–734, *733*
mesothelioma and, 751–752, *752, 753*
tumors in, 733
Ascaris, 336–337
Aschoff bodies, in rheumatic heart disease, 570, *570, 573*
Ascites, chylous, 531
in cirrhosis, 855, *855*
in right-sided heart failure, 550
in thecoma-fibroma, 1077–1078
Ascorbic acid. See *Vitamin C (ascorbic acid).*
Aspartoacylase, deficiency of, 1340
Aspartylglycosamine amide hydrolase, deficiency of, 155t
Aspartylglycosaminuria, 155t
Aspergilloma, 380
Aspergillosis, 380, *381*
Aspergillus, 380, *381*
Aspiration, pulmonary abscess and, 722
Aspirin (acetylsalicylic acid), adverse reactions to, 416
antiplatelet effect of, 637
asthmatic response to, 715
in inflammation, 71–72
nephropathy and, 416, *977,* 978–979, *979,* 979t
Reye syndrome with, 869
Asterixis, in hepatic encephalopathy, 853
Asteroid bodies, in sarcoidosis, 734

Asthma, 707t
  bronchial, 712–716, *715*
    allergy in, 199
    aspirin-related, 715
    atopic, 713–714, *714*
    clinical course of, 716
    drug-induced, 715
    extrinsic, 713
    intrinsic, 713
    nonatopic, 715
    occupational, 715
    pathogenesis of, 713–715, *714*
Astrocytes, 1296–1297, *1296*
  Alzheimer type II, 1297
  gemistocytic, 1297
Astrocytoma, 1343–1346, *1344–1346*
  platelet-derived growth factor production by, 279, 279t
Astroviruses, intestinal infection with, 807t
AT gene, 296
Ataxia, Friedreich, 1337
  spinocerebellar, 1296t, 1337
Ataxia-telangiectasia, 47, 1337
  DNA defects in, 296
Atelectasis, 699–700, *699*
Atheroemboli, 130, 502
Atheroma, 498–499
  in myocardial infarction, 553
Atheromatous plaque, 40, 499–503, 509
  blood flow effects of, 125, 129
  calcification of, 502
  components of, 500–501, *500, 501*
  distribution of, 499–500, 508
  fibrous cap of, 499, *500, 501,* 509
  hemorrhage into, 502
  histologic features of, 501–502, *501*
  in myocardial ischemia, 551–553, *552,* 553t
  necrotic core of, 499, *500, 501*
  renal, 986, *987*
  rupture of, 502
  size of, 499, *500*
  thrombosis with, 502–503
Atherosclerosis, 40, 79, 498–509, 551. See also *Coronary artery disease; Heart, ischemic disease of; Myocardial infarction.*
  age and, 504
  atheromatous plaque in, 499–503, *500, 501.* See also *Atheromatous plaque.*
  blood flow effects of, 125, 129
  Chlamydia pneumoniae and, 509
  cholesterol lowering in, 505
  cigarette smoking and, 506
  clinical features of, 498–499, *499,* 509
  diet and, 506
  dyslipoproteinemias and, 505, 505t
  endothelial injury in, 496–497, *496, 507,* *508*
  epidemiology of, 503–507, *504,* 504t, 505t
  fatty dots in, 503, *503*
  fatty streaks in, *502,* 503, 509
  genetic factors in, 504
  hemostatic factors and, 506
  homocystinuria and, 506
  hypercholesterolemia and, 508
  hyperlipidemia and, 504–506, 505t
  hypertension and, 506
  in cerebrovascular disease, 1308
  in diabetes mellitus, 506, 922, 924
  in sudden cardiac death, 564
  in transgenic mice, 506
  infection and, 509
  laminar shear stresses in, 508
  life-style factors in, 506
  lipids in, *495,* 508
Atherosclerosis *(Continued)*
  lipoprotein(a) and, 506
  macrophages in, 508–509
  monoclonal hypothesis of, 509
  mortality from, 498, 504
  natural history of, 498, *499*
  oligoclonality of, 509
  pathogenesis of, 507–509, *507, 510*
  patterns of, 498
  prevention of, 509
  response-to-injury hypothesis of, 507–509, *507*
  risk factors for, 503–507, *504,* 504t, 505t
    additive effects of, *504,* 506–507
  sex and, 504
  smooth muscle proliferation in, 509
  thrombosis with, 506. See also *Thrombosis.*
  vitamin E in, 446
Athlete's foot, 1210
Atmospheric pressure, injury and, 435–436
ATN, 2969–2971. See also *Acute tubular necrosis (ATN).*
Atomic bomb, cancer and, 310
Atopy, 199. See also *Hypersensitivity reaction(s), type I (anaphylactic).*
  in asthma, 713
ATPases, in cell injury, 6, *6*
Atresia, definition of, 466
  of aortic valve, 597
  of bile ducts, 898–899, *898*
  of duodenum, 804
  of esophagus, 777, *777*
  of pulmonary valve, 597
  of tricuspid valve, 596
  of vagina, 1045
Atrial natriuretic factor (peptide), 544
  in cardiac hypertrophy, 35
  in hypertension, 512
Atrial septal defect, 593–594, *593*
Atrial septum, lipomatous hypertrophy of, 590
Atrioventricular node, 544
Atrioventricular valves, 545. See also *Mitral valve; Tricuspid valve.*
Atrophy, 31, 35–36, *36*
  brown, 36, 546
  bulbospinal, 1338
  dentorubropallidolusian, 179t
  gastric, 792
  lobar, 1333
  multiple system, 1335
  muscle, 1274–1275, 1280–1281, *1281*
  olivopontocerebellar, 1335
  optic nerve, 1374, *1374,* 1375, *1375*
  pathologic, 35, *36*
  physiologic, 35
  spinal, 24, 1281, *1281,* 1338
  testicular, 874, 1015, *1015,* 1016
Auer rods, in acute myelogenous leukemia, 678, *678*
Auerbach plexus, absence of, 805
Auspitz sign, 1199
Autacoids, in inflammation, 70–72, *70*
Autoantibodies. See also *Antibody(ies); Autoimmune diseases.*
  in chronic lymphocytic leukemia, 659
  in rheumatoid arthritis, 1250
  in systemic lupus erythematosus, 219–220, *219*
  in type I diabetes mellitus, *915,* 916
Autocrine motility factors, in tumor invasion, 304, *304*
Autoimmune diseases, 79, 211–231, 211t. See also specific diseases.
  apoptosis failure in, 214
Autoimmune diseases *(Continued)*
  epitope unmasking in, 215
  genetic factors in, 215–216
  microbial agents in, 216
  molecular mimicry in, 215
  peripheral tolerance failure in, 214–215
  polyclonal lymphocyte activation in, 215
  sequestered antigens in, 215
  suppressor T cell failure in, 215
  T-cell anergy failure in, 214
Autoimmune gastritis, 791, 793
Autoimmune hepatitis, 868
Autolysis, 16
Autophagolysosome, 25
Autophagy, 25, *26*
Autosplenectomy, in sickle cell disease, 613, *614*
Avascular necrosis, 1231, *1231,* 1231t
Avellino dystrophy, 1363
Axons, 1269, *1270*
  degeneration of, *1270,* 1273, 1274–1275, *1274*
  diffuse injury of, 1304
  regeneration of, 1275, 1295
  segmental demyelination of, *1270,* 1273, 1274, *1274*
  sprouting of, *1270*
  unmyelinated, 1271
  wallerian degeneration of, 1274, *1274*
Axonal reaction, 1295
Azo dyes, in carcinogenesis, 309
Azotemia, 935
  in left-sided heart failure, 549

B

B lymphocytes. See *Lymphocyte(s), B.*
Babesia bovis, 337t
Babesia microti, 337t, 391, *391*
Babesiosis, 391, *391*
Bacillary angiomatosis, 534–535, *534*
Bacillus anthracis, 334t, 344
Bacteremia, 84
Bacteria, 332, 332t, 334t, 335, *335,* 341–344. See also *Infection* and specific organisms.
  adhesins of, 341–343, *342*
  antigens of, 344
  carbohydrate capsule of, 344
  cell injury by, 341–344, *342, 343*
  endotoxin of, 343
  exotoxins of, 343–344, *343*
  genome of, 330–331
  in endocarditis, 574, *575*
  in gastroenteritis, 807–809, 808t, *809*
  in myocarditis, 583–585, 584t
  Lancefield classification of, 330
  virulence of, 341–344, *342*
Bactericidal permeability increasing protein (BPIP), in phagocytosis, 64
Bacteriophages, 332
Bacteroides, 334t, 369–370
Bagassosis, 729t
BAGE genes, 316
Baker cyst, 1258
Balanoposthitis, 1012
Balantidium coli, 337t
Balloon angioplasty, 538–539, *538*
Balloon cells, in mucopolysaccharidoses, 160
Banti syndrome, 882
Bantu siderosis, 874
Barbiturates, 412
  hepatic adaptation to, 26, *27*
Bardet-Biedl syndrome, 1371

Baritosis, 729t
Barotrauma, 436
Barr body, 173
Barrett esophagus, 37, 781–782, *781, 782,* 786, *786*
Bartholin cyst, 1040
Bartonella, 334t, 534–535, *534*
Basal cell carcinoma, 1186–1187, *1187*
 ultraviolet radiation in, 310
Basal ganglia, degenerative disease of, 1333–1336, *1334, 1336*
Basement membrane, glomerular, 931–933, *932–934*
  antibodies to, 943–945, *944*
  ruptures in, 952, *952*
  thickening of, 943, 954, *954*
   in diabetes mellitus, 923, *923,* 966, *967*
 in diabetes mellitus, 922–923, *923,* 966, *967*
 in tissue repair, 90, 91
 tumor invasion of, 302–305, *303, 304*
Basophils, in type I hypersensitivity reaction, 196–197, *197*
Basophilia, 648t
Bat-wing deformity, 1300
B-cell receptor, 190
Bcg gene, in murine mycobacterial infection, 351
bcl-2 gene, in apoptosis, 22–23, *23,* 294–295, *295*
 in follicular lymphoma, 660, *661*
BCL6 gene, in diffuse large B-cell lymphoma, 661
BCR-ABL fusion gene, in chronic myelogenous leukemia, *680,* 681
bcr-c-*abl* gene, 282
Becker muscular dystrophy, 147t, 1281–1282, *1282, 1283*
Beckwith-Wiedemann syndrome, Wilms' tumor in, 488
Becquerel (Bq), 425
Bedbug bite, 1210–1212
Bee sting, 1210–1212
Bence Jones proteins, in amyloidosis, 252–253
 in multiple myeloma, 666, 980, 981, *981*
Bends, 131, 436
Benign prostatic hyperplasia, 1027–1029, *1027–1029*
Benzene, in cancer, 274t
Benzo[a]pyrene, in occupational diseases, 419t, 420
Berger disease, 961–962, *961,* 965t
Bergmann gliosis, 1297
 in alcohol abuse, 1342
Beriberi, 1341
 dry, *448*
 neuropathic, 1279
 wet, 447, *448*
Bernard-Soulier syndrome, 637
Berry aneurysm, 525, 1310–1313, *1311, 1312*
Berylliosis, 729t, 734
Beryllium, in cancer, 274t
 in occupational diseases, 421t
Beta (β) toxin, of *Clostridium perfringens,* 369
 of *Staphylococcus aureus,* 365
Beta-cell tumors, 926–927, *927*
Bezoar, 797, *797*
Bicarbonate, gastric secretion of, 788
Bile, composition of, 892, *892*
 hepatic formation of, 848–849, *849,* 892, *892*
 reabsorption of, 892
 secretion of, 891
 storage of, 891–892
Bile ducts, congenital dilations of, 899
 extrahepatic, 898–899
  atresia of, 898–899, *898*
  carcinoma of, 899–900
  cysts of, 899
  fibrosing cholangitis of, 879–880, *879*
  infection of, 898
  lithiasis of, 898
  obstruction of, 851–852
  paucity of, 881
 interlobular, 848
 intrahepatic, 877–881, 877t
  anomalies of, 880–881, *880*
  fibrosing cholangitis of, 879–880, *879*
  obstruction of, 851–852
  primary cirrhosis of, 878–879, *879*
  primary sclerosing cholangitis of, 879–880, *879*
  secondary cirrhosis of, 878, *878*
Biliary cirrhosis, 877t
 primary, 877t, 878–879, *879*
 secondary, 877t, 878, *878*
Biliary tract, 891–900. See also *Bile ducts; Gallbladder.*
 anatomy of, 892
 congenital anomalies of, 893, *893,* 899
 normal, 891–892, *892*
 obstruction of, 851–852, *852*
 tumors of, 899–900, *900*
Bilirubin, 43
 conjugated, 849–850
 hepatic processing of, 848–849, *849*
 serum, 850
 unconjugated, 849
Binge eating, 439
Binswanger disease, 1314
Bioaerosols, in indoor air, 418t, 419
Biologic effective dose, of chemicals, 405
Biomethylation, in toxicant metabolism, 406–407, *408*
Biopsy, bone marrow, 604
 endomyocardial, 579
Biotin, 440t
Birbeck granules, in histiocytosis X, *1190,* 1191
 in Langerhans histiocytosis, 685, *685*
Bird-breeder's lung, 729t
Birth. See also *Infant.*
 infection at, 470–471, *470*
 injury at, 464
 weight at, 460–462, *461*
Birthmark (nevus flammeus), 534
Bite, arthropod, 1210–1211
Bite cells, in G6PD deficiency, 610–611, *611*
Bitot's spots, in vitamin A deficiency, 441, *442*
BK moles, 1176–1177, *1177, 1178*
Black fever, 391–393, *392*
Bladder, 1000–1008
 adenocarcinoma of, 1007
 benign tumors of, 1008
 congenital anomalies of, 1000–1001, *1000, 1001*
 cystocele of, 998
 diverticula of, 1000, *1000*
 embryonal rhabdomyosarcoma of, 1008
 exstrophy of, 1000, *1001*
 infection of, 973
 inflammation of, 1001–1003, *1001, 1002*
 leiomyoma of, 1008
 malacoplakia of, 1002, *1002*
 metastatic tumors of, 1008
 normal, 997–998
 obstruction of, 1008, *1008*
 radiation injury to, 429
Bladder *(Continued)*
 rhabdomyosarcoma of, 1008
 sarcoma botryoides of, 1008
 sarcoma of, 1008
 Schistosoma haematobium infection of, 346, *347,* 397
 squamous cell carcinoma of, 1006–1007
 transitional cell carcinoma of, 1003–1008, 1003t, *1004–1006,* 1006t
Blast injury, 435
Blebs, cellular, 8, *9, 10,* 19
Bleeding. See also *Hemorrhage.*
 uterine, dysfunctional, 1055–1056, 1056t
  in gestational trophoblastic disease, 1086
Bleeding time, 633
Blindness, herpesvirus infection and, 360
 in Leber hereditary optic neuropathy, *180*
 in vitamin A deficiency, 441, *442*
Blister, 1172
Blood, loss of. See also *Hemorrhage.*
  anemia with, 605–606
 oxygen-carrying capacity of, 4
 tumor dissemination by, 270, *270*
Blood cells, 602–604, *603.* See also specific cell types.
Blood flow, in inflammation, *52,* 53
 in thrombus formation, 125
 laminar, 125
 wound healing and, 110
Blood group, infant-mother incompatibility in, 473–475, *474, 475*
Blood pressure, elevation of, 510–515, 511t. See also *Hypertension.*
 normal, 511t
 regulation of, 511–512, *511*
Blood-nerve barrier, 1271
Bloom syndrome, 296
Blue nevus, 1176t
Blue-dome cyst, 1099, *1099*
Body mass index, 452, *452*
Boil, 366–367
Bone(s), 1216–1246
 abscess of, 1232–1233, *1232*
 age-related change in, 1223, *1223*
 avascular necrosis of, 1231, *1231*
 basic multicellular unit of, 1218
 caisson disease of, 436
 calcification of, 44–45
 cells of, 1216–1217, *1216, 1217*
 congenital malformations of, 1220
 creeping substitution of, 1231
 developmental abnormalities of, 1220–1221
 diseases of. See also specific diseases.
  abnormal matrix in, 1221–1224, *1221,* 1222t, *1223,* 1223t, *1224*
  abnormal mineral homeostasis in, 1227–1229, *1228*
  infectious, 1232–1233, *1232*
  ischemic, 1231, *1231*
  osteoclast dysfunction in, 1224–1227, *1224–1227*
  trauma-induced, 1229–1231, *1230*
 eburnation of, in osteoarthritis, 1247, *1248*
 enchondral formation of, 1219, *1219*
 Ewing sarcoma of, 1244, *1244*
 fractures of, 1229–1231, *1230*
 giant cell tumor of, 1244–1245, *1245*
 growth of, 1218–1220, *1219*
  disorders of, 1220–1221
 growth plate of, 1219, *1219*
 heterotopic, 44
 in collagen disorders, 1221–1222, *1221,* 1222t

Bone(s) *(Continued)*
in hyperparathyroidism, 1150, 1228–1229, *1228*
in hyperthyroidism, 1132
in mucopolysaccharidoses, 1222
in multiple myeloma, 664, *664*
in myositis ossificans, 1262, *1262*
in renal osteodystrophy, 1229
in scurvy, 449–450, *450*
in vitamin deficiency, 1227–1228
infections of, 1232–1233, *1232*
intramembranous formation of, 1219
involucrum, 1232, *1232*
lamellar, 1217–1218, *1217, 1218*
in Paget disease, 1226–1227, *1226*
loss of, 1222–1224. See also *Osteoporosis.*
metaplastic, 1262, *1262*
mineralization of, 1216
normal, 1215–1220, *1216–1219,* 1218t
onion-skin appearance of, 1244
osteoblasts of, 1216–1217, *1216,* 1218
osteoclasts of, 1217, *1217*
osteocytes of, 1217
peak mass of, 1218, 1223, *1223*
proteins of, 1217–1218, 1218t
remodeling of, 1218, *1219*
repair of, 1229–1230, *1230*
sclerosis of, 1224–1225, *1224, 1225*
slow virus infection of, 1225–1227, *1226, 1227*
Treponema infection of, 1233
tuberculous infection of, 1233
tumors of, 1233–1244, 1234t
bone-forming, 1234–1237, *1235–1237*
cartilage-forming, 1237–1242, *1238–1241*
fibrous, 1242–1244, *1242, 1243*
in Paget disease, 1227
metastatic, 1245–1246
hypercalcemia and, 45, 1148
in prostate carcinoma, 1030, *1032*
vitamin D effects on, 441–444, *443*
von Recklinghausen disease of, 1228
woven, 1217, *1217*
Bone marrow, anatomy of, 604
biopsy of, 604
failure of, 632–633
in ariboflavinosis, 448
in Gaucher disease, 158, *159*
in idiopathic thrombocytopenic purpura, 635–636
in kwashiorkor, 439
in systemic lupus erythematosus, 224
transplantation of, 210–211
diarrhea after, 811
hepatic complications of, 884, *884,* 885–886
veno-occlusive disease after, 884, *884*
Bone morphogenetic proteins, in metaplasia, 37
Bony callus, 1230
Bordetella pertussis, 334t, 374–375, *374*
Borrelia burgdorferi, 334t, 338, 388–389, *388,* 1253, 1317
myocarditis and, 584
Borrelia recurrentis, 334t, 344
Borrelia spirochetes, 388
Borreliosis, 388
Botfly, 337–338
Botryomycosis, in agranulocytosis, 647
Botulinum toxin, 369
Botulism, 368, 369
Boutonneuse fever, 385t
Bowen disease, of penis, 1013, *1013*
of vulva, 1043, *1043*
Bowenoid papulosis, 1014, 1209
Brachial plexopathy, tumor-associated, 1279
Bradykinin, in inflammation, *68,* 69
Brain. See also *Central nervous system (CNS).*
abscess of, 1315–1316, *1316,* 1323, *1323*
atrophy of, 35, *36*
bridging veins of, 1305
contrecoup injury to, 1303–1304
contusion of, 1303–1304, *1303*
copper deposition in, 875
coup injury to, 1303–1304
cytotoxic edema of, 1298
diffuse axonal injury of, 1304
edema of, 116, 1298. See also *Hydrocephalus.*
embolism to, 1308
fungal infection of, 1316
giant cells in, 240, *240*
glucose supply to, 1341–1342
hemorrhage in, *117,* 118, 1302, 1305–1306, *1306,* 1310–1313, *1311, 1312*
herniation of, 1298, *1298, 1299*
in galactosemia, 477
in human immunodeficiency virus infection, 240, *240*
in left-sided heart failure, 549
in preeclampsia, 1083, *1084*
in preterm infant, 463
in protein-energy malnutrition, 439
in right-sided heart failure, 550
in shock, 136
in trisomy 21, 171
infarction in, 132
laceration of, 1303, *1303*
Niemann-Pick disease in, 158
perinatal injury to, 1302, *1302*
subfalcine herniation of, 1298, *1298*
tonsillar herniation of, 1298, *1298*
Toxoplasma abscess of, 1323, *1323*
transtentorial herniation of, 1298, *1298*
trauma to, 1302–1306, *1303, 1305, 1306*
sequelae of, 1305–1306
vascular malformations of, 1313
vasogenic edema of, 1298
Brain death, 1307
Brain stem, glioma of, 1346
Branchial cyst, 767
Branching enzyme, deficiency of, 160–161, *161*
BRCA genes, 292
in breast cancer, 1105, 1106, 1106t
in ovarian cancer, 1067
Breast, 1093–1117
adenosis of, 1099
angiosarcoma of, 1104
atypical ductal hyperplasia of, 1100, *1100*
atypical lobular hyperplasia of, 1100
carcinoma of, 1104–1117
angiogenesis in, 1115, *1117*
atomic bomb exposure and, 310
BRCA genes in, 292, 1105, 1106t
c-*erb B2* gene in, 286
classification of, 1107, 1107t
clinical course of, 1114–1115, *1116, 1117*
colloid, 1112, *1112*
diet and, 1107
distribution of, 1107
DNA index in, 1115, *1116*
ductal, *269*
in situ, 1107–1109, 1107t, *1108, 1109*
invasive, 1110, *1110*
environmental factors in, 1106–1107
epidemiology of, 1105–1106, 1106t
estrogen and, 1106
estrogen replacement therapy and, 414
Breast *(Continued)*
etiology of, 1106–1107
flow cytometry in, 1115, *1116*
genetic factors in, 1105, 1106, 1106t, 1107
grade of, 1115
hormonal factors in, 1106
hormone receptors in, 1115
in male, 1118
in situ, 1107–1110, 1107t, *1108, 1109*
ductal, 1107–1109, 1107t, *1108, 1109*
microinvasion with, 1109
lobular, 1109–1110, *1109*
incidence of, *272,* 1105
inflammatory, 1114, 1115
invasive, 1110–1112, *1110, 1111,* 1113–1114, *1114*
ductal, 1110, *1110*
lobular, 1110–1111, *1111*
lobular, in situ, 1109–1110, *1109*
invasive, 1110–1111, *1111*
lumpectomy for, 1116
lymph nodes in, 1114, 1115
mammographic appearance of, 1112–1113, *1113*
medullary, 1111, *1111*
metastatic, *269,* 1114, *1114,* 1115
models of, 1116
mortality with, *272,* 1105
oncogenes in, 280
oral contraceptives and, 415
papillary, 1112
peau d'orange skin change in, 1114
pesticides and, 422
prognosis for, 1115, *1116, 1117*
progression of, 1107
proliferative disease and, 1101–1102
risk factors for, 1105–1106
staging of, 1114
treatment of, lymphedema after, 115
tubular, 1112, *1112*
developmental abnormalities of, 1096
duct ectasia of, 1097, *1097*
epithelial hyperplasia of, 1100, *1100*
epithelial tumors of, 1104, *1105*
fat necrosis of, 1097–1098, *1098*
fibroadenoma of, 267, *268,* 1102–1103, *1103*
fibrocystic changes in, 1098–1100, *1099*
fibrosis of, 1098–1100
hypertrophy of, 34–35
inflammation of, 1096–1098, *1097, 1098*
lumps in, 1095, *1096*
lymphoma of, 1117
male, 1117–1118, *1118*
menstrual cycle–related changes in, 1094
normal, 1093–1095, *1094, 1095*
papilloma of, 1101–1102, *1102*
phyllodes tumor of, 1103–1104, *1105*
postmenopausal, 1095, *1095*
proliferative disease of, 1100–1102, *1100–1102*
radiation damage to, 429, *429*
sarcoma of, 1104
sclerosing adenosis of, 1101, *1101*
silicone implants for, 1098
size of, 1096
stromal tumors of, 1102–1104, *1103, 1104*
Brenner tumor, 1072–1073, *1072*
Brewer's lung, 380, *381*
Bridging veins, of brain, 1305
Brill-Zinsser disease, 385t
Brittle bone disease, 1221–1222, *1221,* 1222t
collagen in, 144–145

Brittle bone disease *(Continued)*
gene mutation in, 147t
gonadal mosaicism in, 181
Brodie abscess, 1233
Bronchial asthma, 712–716. See also *Asthma, bronchial.*
Bronchiectasis, 699, 707t, 716–717, *717*
Bronchioles, 698, *708*
in asthma, 715, *715*
infection of, 716–717, *717*
Bronchiolitis, 348, 707t, 711–712
Bronchiolitis obliterans, *736,* 738
in bronchitis, 712
in lung transplant rejection, 741
Bronchiolitis obliterans organizing pneumonia (BOOP), 738, *738*
Bronchioloalveolar carcinoma, 747, *747*
Bronchitis, chronic, 707t, 711–712, *712*
Bronchogenic carcinoma, 741–747. See also *Lungs, carcinoma of.*
Bronchopneumonia, 720–721. See *Pneumonia.*
Bronchopulmonary dysplasia, 472–473
Bronchopulmonary sequestration, 699
Brown atrophy, 36
of heart, 546
Brown tumor, in hyperparathyroidism, 1150, 1228, *1228*
Brucella abortus, 334t
Brucella melitensis, 334t
Brucella suis, 334t
Brugia malayi, 397–398, *398*
Brunn nests, 997
Brunner glands, 803
Brushfield spots, in trisomy 21, 1360
Bruton disease, 232–233
Bubonic plague, 387–388
Budd-Chiari syndrome, 883–884, *883*
Buerger disease, 523, *523*
Bulbospinal atrophy, 1338
Bulimia, 439
Bullae, 1172
pulmonary, 711, *711*
Bullous pemphigoid, 759t, 1203–1204, *1204*
Bundle of His, 544–545
Buphthalmos, 1375
Burkholderia cepacia, 376
Burkitt lymphoma, 485t, 655t, 662–663, *663*
Epstein-Barr virus in, 312, *313*
oncogenes in, 285, *285,* 286t
Burns, 433–434
blister from, 84, *85*
Curling ulcer in, 796
disseminated intravascular coagulation in, 641, *641*
electrical, 435
Pseudomonas aeruginosa in, 377
Burr cells, 815
Buschke-Löwenstein tumor, 1014
Byler syndrome, 851
Byssinosis, 729t, 737

C
C cells (parafollicular cells), 1131
C1 inhibitor, 69
deficiency of, 236
C2, deficiency of, 236
C3, activation of, 67–68, *67,* 77t
deficiency of, 236
C3b, in inflammation, 68
C3, in inflammation, 68, *68,* 70
C3 convertase, 69
C3a, in inflammation, 68
C3bi, in inflammation, 68
C3a, in inflammation, *68,* 70
C3b, in phagocytosis, 62
C4a, in inflammation, 68
C5, in inflammation, 68, 70
C5 convertase, 69
C5a, in inflammation, 68, 70
C5b–C9, in glomerulonephritis, 947, *947*
C3 nephritic factor, 959, *960*
c-*abl* gene, 282
c-*abl-bcr* gene, in chronic myelogenous leukemia, 285, *285,* 286t
Cachexia, in cancer, 319–320
tumor necrosis factor in, 74
E-Cadherin, in cancer, 293, 303
Cadmium, in cancer, 274t
in occupational diseases, 421, 421t
Caenorhabditis elegans, clock gene of, 47
insulin receptor gene of, 47
Café au lait spots, in McCune-Albright syndrome, 1243
in neurofibromatosis, 164
Cag pathogenicity islands, in *Helicobacter pylori* infection, 341
Caisson disease, 131, 436
Calcific sclerosis (Mönckeberg arteriosclerosis), 498
Calcification, 43–45, *44*
dystrophic, 18, 43–45, *44*
in analgesic nephropathy, *879,* 978
pathogenesis of, 44–45, *44*
in cell injury, 9
in mammary fibroadenoma, 1103
in pancreatitis, 908, *908*
in silicosis, 731, *732*
in systemic sclerosis, 228
membrane-facilitated, 44, *44*
metastatic, 45
of aortic valve, 567–568, *567*
of atheromatous plaque, 502
of cardiac valves, 567–568, *567*
of mitral annulus, *567,* 568
on mammography, 1113, *1113,* 1113t
Calciphylaxis, 1151
Calcitonin, 1131
in medullary thyroid carcinoma, 1145
Calcium, in cell injury, 6, *6*
in osteoporosis, 1223
metabolism of, 441–442
Calcium oxalate stone, 989, 989t, 990
Calcium pyrophosphate crystal deposition disease, 1257, *1257*
Calculi, gallbladder, 893–895, *894, 895,* 904
renal, 989–990, 989t, *990,* 999t
Caliciviruses, intestinal infection with, 807, 807t
CALLA antigen (CD10), 317
Call-Exner bodies, 1076, *1077*
Callus, bony, 1230
soft tissue, 1229
Calymmatobacterium donovani, 334t
Campomelic dysplasia, 1220t
Campylobacter, 334t, 355–356, 807–809, 808t
Canaliculi, bile, 848
Canals of Hering, 848
Canavan disease, 1340
Cancer. See *Carcinogens; Carcinogenesis; Tumor(s);* specific neoplasms, e.g., *Lymphoma.*
Cancer-suppressor genes, 286–294
in retinoblastoma, 275
protein products of, 287, 289–294, *289, 291*
Candidiasis, 332t, 378–379, *379*
CNS, 1322
Candidiasis *(Continued)*
esophageal, 782
genital, 1038t, 1039
in acquired immunodeficiency syndrome, 247–248
invasive, 379
oral, 757
Canker sores, 757, *757*
Cannabis sativa, abuse of, 413
Capillaries, 494–495
congestion of, 116
radiation damage to, 428
Capillary hemangioma, 532, *532*
Capillary microaneurysms, in diabetic retinopathy, 1369, *1369*
Caplan syndrome, 729t, 730, 733
Caput succedaneum, 464
Carbamates, 423, 423t
Carbon, cellular accumulation of, 42
Carbon monoxide, CNS effects of, 1342
in air pollution, 418, 418t
Carbon tetrachloride, toxic effects of, 14, *14, 15*
Carbonic anhydrase II, deficiency of, osteopetrosis with, 1225
Carcinoembryonic antigen (CEA), in tumor diagnosis, 325, 325t
Carcinogenesis, 305–315, 307t. See also *Tumor(s).*
chemical, 306–309, *306, 307*
initiation of, 306–308, *306, 307*
promotion of, *306, 307,* 308
diet and, 455–456
molecular basis of, 276–298, 296–298, *297, 298.* See also *Apoptosis; Cancer-suppressor genes; Oncogenes.*
radiation, 309–311, 426–427
viral, 311–315, *313, 314*
Carcinogens, chemical, 306–309, 307t
dietary, 455
immunosuppression with, 318
occupational, 273, 274t
Carcinoid tumor, 837, 837t
bronchial, 747–748, *748*
cardiac, 577–578, *577*
gastric, 802
intestinal, 835–837, *836,* 837t
pancreatic, 928
Carcinoma, 262. See also at specific sites, e.g., *Breast, carcinoma of.*
Carcinoma ex pleomorphic adenoma, 771
Carcinoma in situ, 266, *267*
Carcinomatosis, meningeal, 1314
Carcinosarcoma, of endometrium, 1063
Cardia, of stomach, 787, *787*
Cardiac cirrhosis, 117
Cardiac death, sudden, 564
Cardiac tamponade, 587
Cardiac valves, 545
disease of, 566–578, 567t. See also specific diseases.
prosthetic, 578, *578,* 578t
Cardiogenic shock, 134, 134t, 562
Cardiolipin, antibodies to, 126
Cardiomegaly, 544
Cardiomyopathy, 578–586, *578*
alcoholic, 579–580
dilated, 579–581
hypertrophic, 581–583, *582*
in pheochromocytoma, 1165–1166
ischemic, 564
peripartum, 580
restrictive, 583
thyrotoxic, 1131

Carditis, in rheumatic heart disease, 572
Caries, *Streptococcus* in, 367
Carney syndrome, 590
Carnitine, deficiency of, 1286–1287
Carnitine palmitoyltransferase, deficiency of, 1287
Caroli disease, 881
Carotid body tumor, 768–769, *768,* 1166
Carpal tunnel syndrome, 1280
Cartilage. See also *Bone(s).*
  articular, 1246
  ochronosis of, 42, 162
  tumor formation of, 1237–1242, *1238–1241*
Caruncle, 366–367
  urethral, 1009
Caspases, in apoptosis, 20, *22,* 23
Catalase, 13, 47
Cataracts, 1367–1368
  in diabetes, 1334
  in galactosemia, 476, 477
  in myotonic dystrophy, 1283
Catecholamines, cardiotoxicity of, 586
  in pheochromocytoma, 1165–1166
Catenin, E-cadherin linkage to, 303
β-Catenin, in tumorigenesis, 293
Caterpillar cells, in rheumatic heart disease, 570
Cathepsin D, in tumor invasion, 304
Cat-scratch disease, 83t
Cavernous hemangioma, *532,* 533, 1313
  of liver, 886
Cavernous lymphangioma (cystic hygroma), 533
  in Turner syndrome, 175
CD3, T-cell receptor linkage to, 189, *189*
CD8, 619
CD10 (CALLA antigen), in cancer, 317
CD34, in leukocyte adhesion, 57, 57t
CD44, in tumor dissemination, 305
CD55 (decay-accelerating factor), 619
CD59 (membrane inhibitor of reactive lysis), 69, 619–620
CDK4 gene, 1177
CDKN2 genes 1177
Celiac sprue, 813, *813,* 961
Cell(s), adaptations of, 2
  aging of, 4
  atrophy of, 2
  death of, 2–4, *3,* 4t, 18–25, 90, *90.* See also *Apoptosis; Necrosis.*
  differentiation of, 90, *90*
  genetic clock of, 46–47, *46, 47*
  hypertrophy of, 2, *3,* 34
  labile (continuously dividing), *90,* 91
  permanent (nondividing), *90,* 91–92
  regeneration of, 90
  stable (quiescent), *90,* 91
  stem, 91
  swelling of, vs. hypertrophy, 34
Cell cycle, *90,* 91–92
  checkpoints in, 96, *96*
  cyclin-dependent kinases in, 283, *283, 284*
  cyclins in, 283, *283, 284*
  ras gene in, 281
  Rb gene in, 289–290, *289*
  transforming growth factor-β in, 290, 293
Cell growth, 90–98, *90–93, 96,* 97t, *103*
  adaptation(s) in, 32–38
    atrophy as, 35–36, *36*
    hyperplasia as, 32–35, *32, 33*
    hypertrophy as, 33–35, *34*
    metaplasia as, 36–38, *37, 38*
  cell surface receptors in, 92–93, *93*
  collagen in, 98–99, *99,* 99t
Cell growth *(Continued)*
  contact inhibition of, 96
  cycle of, *90,* 91–92
  elastin in, 99–100
  extracellular matrix in, 98–102, *99–103,* 99t
  fibrillin in, 100
  fibronectin in, 100, *100*
  growth factors in, 97–98, 97t
  hyaluronan in, 102
  inhibition of, 96–97
  integrins in, 100–101, *101*
  intercellular signaling in, 92–95, *93–95.* See also *Intercellular signaling.*
  laminin in, 100
  matricellular proteins in, 101
  molecular events in, 92–95, *93–95*
  proliferative potential for, 91–92
  proteoglycans in, 101–102
  regulation of, 95–96, *96.* See also *Protooncogenes; Tumor-suppressor genes.*
    defects in, 162, 164
  signal transduction systems in, 92–95, *93–95*
  syndecan in, 102, *102*
  transcription factors in, 95
Cell injury, 2, *3,* 4–5. See also *Ischemia; Necrosis.*
  acetaminophen-induced, 14–15
  age-induced, 45–48, *46–48*
  amino acid loss in, 11
  ATP depletion in, 5, 9, *11*
  bacteria-induced, 341–344, *342, 343*
  calcification in, 9, 43–45, *44*
  calcium in, 6, *6*
  carbon accumulation in, 42
  carbon tetrachloride–induced, 14, *14, 15*
  chemicals in, 4, 14–15, *14, 15*
  cholesterol accumulation in, 40, *40*
  cytochrome *c* in, 6–7
  diphtheria toxin–induced, 343, *343*
  DNA damage in, 12
  drugs in, 14–15
  energy metabolism in, 7–8
  free radicals in, 5–6, *6,* 10, 12–15, *13–15,* 47, *48.* See also *Free radicals.*
  genetic defects in, 4
  glycogen accumulation in, 41–42
  hemosiderin accumulation in, 42–43, *43*
  hyaline change in, 45
  immunologic reactions in, 4
  in alpha$_1$-antitrypsin deficiency, 38, *38*
  in lysosomal storage disease, 38, *38*
  infectious agents in, 4
  intracellular accumulations in, 38–43, *38–43*
  irreversible, 8–11, *8–11*
    morphology of, 15–18, *16–18*
  lipid accumulation in, 38, *38,* 39–40, *39, 40*
  lipid peroxidation in, 12
  lipofuscin accumulation in, 42, *42*
  lysosomal catabolism in, 25–26
  lysosomal enzymes in, 8–9
  membrane permeability in, 6, 9–11, *11*
  mitochondrial damage in, 6–7, *7,* 9, *11*
  nitric oxide in, 12
  nutritional imbalances in, 4–5
  oxygen deprivation in, 4
  pH in, 9
  phospholipid loss in, 9–10, *11*
  physical agents in, 4
  pigment accumulation in, 38, *38,* 42–43, *42, 43*
  protein accumulation in, 40–41, *41*
  protein fragmentation in, 12
  protein synthesis in, 8
Cell injury *(Continued)*
  repair of, 47–48, *48*
  reperfusion, 11–12
  reversible, 7–8, *8–10*
    morphology of, *9, 10,* 15
  sodium in, 7
  subcellular response to, 25–28
  triglyceride accumulation in, 39–40, *39*
  ultrastructural features of, 8, *9,* 10, *10*
  virus-induced, 340–341, *341*
Cell membrane, lipid peroxidation of, 12
  permeability of, in cell injury, 6, 9–11, *11*
  phospholipid loss from, 9–10, *11*
Cellulitis, clostridial, 369, *369*
Centipede bite, 1210–1212
Central core disease, 1285t
Central nervous system (CNS). See also *Brain; Spinal cord.*
  amphetamine effects on, 413
  arbovirus infection of, 1318
  aspirin effects on, 416
  astrocytes of, 1296–1297, *1296*
  astrocytoma of, 1343–1346, *1344–1346*
  barbiturate effects on, 412
  Borrelia burgdorferi infection of, 1317
  carbon monoxide injury to, 1342
  cells of, 1294–1297, *1296*
  cytomegalovirus infection of, 1319
  degenerative diseases of, 1329–1338, *1330–1332,* 1332t, *1334, 1336, 1339*
  demyelinating diseases of, 1326–1329, *1327, 1328*
  ependymal cells of, 1297
  ependymoma of, 1346–1348, *1347*
  ethanol effects on, 412
  ethanol injury to, 1342, *1342*
  fungal infection of, 1322
  germ cell tumors of, 1350
  glial cells of, 1295–1297, *1296*
  gliomas of, 1343–1348, *1344–1347*
  hallucinogen effects on, 413
  herpes simplex virus infection of, 1318, *1318*
  human immunodeficiency virus infection of, 240, *240,* 244–245, 1320–1321, *1320*
  in diabetes mellitus, 924
  in Epstein-Barr virus infection, 373
  in hypoglycemia, 1341–1342
  in inborn errors of metabolism, 1338–1341, *1340*
  in systemic lupus erythematosus, 222–223
  in vitamin B_1 deficiency, 1341
  in vitamin B_{12} deficiency, 1341
  infection of, 1314–1323, *1315, 1316, 1323.* See also specific infections.
    fungal, 1322
    protozoal, 1323, *1323*
    viral, 1317–1322, *1318, 1320, 1322*
  lead effects on, 421
  lymphoma of, 1349–1350
  malformations of, 1299–1302, *1301*
  measles virus infection of, 1321–1322
  medulloblastoma of, 1348–1349, *1349*
  metastatic tumors of, 1351
  methanol injury to, 1342
  methotrexate injury to, 1342–1343
  microglia of, 1297
  Mycobacterium tuberculosis infection of, 1316–1317
  narcotic effects on, 413
  neuronal tumors of, 1348
  neurons of, 1294–1295
  oligodendrocytes of, 1297
  oligodendroglioma of, 1346

Central nervous system *(Continued)*
paraneoplastic syndromes of, 1351–1352, 1352t
pilocytic astrocytoma of, 1346, *1346*
pleomorphic xanthoastrocytoma of, 1346
poliovirus infection of, 1319
polyomavirus infection of, 1321, *1322*
poorly differentiated tumors of, 1348–1349, *1349*
prion infection of, 1323–1326, *1325*
rabies infection of, 1319–1320
radiation damage to, 430
radiation injury to, 1342–1343
stimulant effects on, 412–414, *413*
toxic injury to, 1342–1343, *1342*
Toxoplasma infection of, 1323, *1323*
trauma to, 1302–1306, *1303, 1305, 1306*
sequelae of, 1305–1306
Treponema pallidum infection of, 1317
tumors of, 1343–1355, *1344–1347, 1349, 1351,* 1352t, *1353.* See also specific tumors.
varicella-zoster virus infection of, 1319
vitamin E deficiency effects on, 446
Central pontine myelinolysis, 1329
Centrilobar necrosis, 117, *117*
Centroblasts, in follicular lymphoma, 660, *660*
Centrocytes, in follicular lymphoma, 660, *660*
Centronuclear myopathy, 1285t
Cephalhematoma, at birth, 464
Cephalosporins, in warm antibody hemolytic anemia, 620
Cerebral autosomal dominant arteriopathy with subcortical infarcts and leukoencephalopathy, 1308
Cerebral edema, 1298
Cerebral palsy, 1302
Cerebrospinal fluid (CSF), in acute aseptic meningitis, 1315
in acute pyogenic meningitis, 1314, 1315
in arthropod-borne viral encephalitis, 1318
in brain abscess, 1316
in poliomyelitis, 1319
ventricular accumulation of, 1298–1299, *1299*
Cerebrovascular disease, 1306–1314
arteritis in, 1308
atherosclerosis in, 1308
berry aneurysm in, 1310–1313, *1311, 1312*
collateral flow in, 1308
focal cerebral ischemia in, 1308–1310, *1309*
global cerebral ischemia in, 1307–1308
granulomatous angiitis in, 1308
hypertension in, 1313–1314, *1313*
hypertensive encephalopathy in, 1314
intracranial hemorrhage in, 1310–1313, *1311, 1312*
lacunar infarcts in, 1313–1314, *1313*
slit hemorrhage in, 1314
subarachnoid hemorrhage in, 1310–1313
vascular malformations in, 1313
Ceruloplasmin, in free radical inactivation, 13
in Wilson disease, 875
Cervicitis, 1038–1039, 1038t, 1047–1048, *1047, 1048*
Cervix, 1047–1053
adenocarcinoma of, 1053
adenosquamous carcinoma of, 1053
anatomy of, *1036,* 1037, *1037*
infection of, 1038–1039, 1038t, 1047–1048, *1047, 1048*
intraepithelial neoplasia of, 1049–1051, *1051, 1052*
polyps of, 1048, *1048*
Cervix *(Continued)*
squamous cell carcinoma of, 1051–1053, *1053*
clinical course of, 1053
human papillomavirus and, 311, 1049, *1050*
in acquired immunodeficiency syndrome, 250
oral contraceptives and, 415
Pap smear for, 322–323, *323*
pathogenesis of, 1049
Cestodes, 336–337
CFTR (cystic fibrosis transmembrane conductance regulator) gene, 478–479, *479*
Chagas disease, 393–394, 584, *585*
achalasia in, 778–779
megacolon in, 805
myocarditis in, 394
Chagoma, 393
Chancre, in syphilis, 363, *363*
in trypanosomiasis, 393
Channelopathy, 1285
Chaperones, in protein folding, 41, *41*
Charcot joints, 1317
Charcot-Bouchard aneurysms, 1310
Charcot-Leyden crystals, in asthma, 715
Charcot-Marie-Tooth disease, 1277–1278
Chédiak-Higashi syndrome, 64–65, 65t
Cheilosis, in ariboflavinosis, 448
Chemicals. See also *Carcinogenesis, chemical; Carcinogens, chemicals.*
at hazardous waste sites, 404, 404t
biologic effective dose of, 405
estrogenic, 422
in cell injury, 14–15, *14, 15*
in esophageal injury, 782
in type I diabetes mellitus, 917
metabolism of, 405–408, *406–408*
toxicity of, 404–408, *405–408*
Chemodectoma, 1166
Chemokines, 73, 192
C, 74
C-C, 74
C-X-C, 74
CX_3C, 74
in glomerulonephritis, 948
in inflammation, 74, 74t, 77t
Chemotaxis, leukocyte, *60,* 61, *61*
Chemotherapy, neutropenia with, 646–747
pulmonary effects of, 740, 740t
stem cell rescue with, 211
tumor cell resistance to, 292
tumor growth fraction and, 301, *301*
Chernobyl nuclear power plant, 427
Cherry-red spot, in Niemann-Pick disease, 158
in Tay-Sachs disease, 156
Chest deformity, in vitamin D deficiency, 444
Chickenpox, 373–374
Chief cells, in parathyroid adenoma, 1149–1150, *1149*
of parathyroid glands, 1147
of stomach, 788
Children. See also *Infant.*
acquired immunodeficiency syndrome in, 237
acute lymphoblastic leukemia/lymphoma in, 654–658, 655t, *657,* 657t, *658, 659*
Bordetella pertussis infection in, 374–375, *374*
congenital heart disease in, 591–597, 592t, *592–596.* See also specific diseases.
Corynebacterium diphtheriae infection in, 375, *375*
cystic fibrosis in, 477–481. See also *Cystic fibrosis.*
cytomegalovirus infection in, 376
Children *(Continued)*
Epstein-Barr virus infection in, 371–373, *372*
fatty streaks in, 503
fibrous tumors in, 484
ganglioneuroma in, 486
idiopathic thrombocytopenic purpura in, 636
infection in, 370–375, *370, 372, 374, 375*
measles virus infection in, 370, *370*
mortality rate for, 459–460, 460t
mumps virus infection in, 370–371
neuroblastoma in, 485–487, 485t, *486, 487*
poliovirus infection in, 373
tumors in, 482–489
benign, 483–484, *483, 484*
malignant, 484–491, 485t, *486, 487,* 488t, *489*
varicella-zoster infection in, 373–374, *374*
Waterhouse-Friderichsen syndrome in, 1160, *1160*
Wilms' tumor in, 485t, 487–489, *488,* 489t
Chlamydia pneumoniae, 361, 361t
atherosclerosis and, 509
Chlamydia psittaci, 361, 361t, 362
Chlamydia trachomatis, 332t, 360t
genital, 361–362, 361t, 1038t
in pelvic inflammatory disease, 357–358
ocular, 1361–1362, *1362*
Chlordane, 423, 423t
Chloride, epithelial transport of, in cystic fibrosis, 478, *478*
Chloroquine myopathy, 1288–1289
Chokes, 131, 436
Cholangiocarcinoma, 888, 889, 890–891, *890*
Cholangitis, 898
sclerosing, 877t, 879–880, *879*
Cholecystitis, 895–897, *896, 897*
Cholecystokinin, 903
Choledocholithiasis, 898
Cholelithiasis, 893–895, *894, 895*
cholesterol, 894, *895*
obesity and, 454
pigment, 894–895, *895*
Cholera, 357–358, *357*
Cholestasis, 848, 851–852, *852*
in alcoholic liver disease, 872
in pregnancy, 885
in secondary biliary cirrhosis, 878
neonatal, 876–877, 877t
Cholesteatoma, 767
Cholesterol, cellular accumulation of, 40, *40*
in atherosclerosis, 504–506, 505t
in gallstone formation, 893, 894, *895*
metabolism of, 151–152, *151, 152*
therapeutic lowering of, 505
Cholesterol emboli, 130, 502
Cholesterolosis, 40, *40,* 895
Chondroblastoma, 1239–1240, *1240*
Chondrocalcinosis, 1257, *1257*
Chondrocytes, in osteoarthritis, 1247
Chondroid syringoma, 1182, *1184*
Chondroitin sulfate, in mucopolysaccharidosis, 159–160
Chondroma, 261, 1238–1239, *1239*
Chondromyxoid fibroma, 1240, *1240*
Chondrosarcoma, 1240–1242, *1241,* 1260t
Chordae tendineae, 545
Chorioamnionitis, 470, 1082, *1083*
Choriocarcinoma, 1021, *1021,* 1023
gestational, 1087–1089, *1088*
ovarian, 1076
testicular, 1021, *1021,* 1023
Chorioretinitis, *Toxoplasma,* 383
Choristoma (heterotopia), 263
bone, 44

Choristoma (heterotopia) *(Continued)*
definition of, 483
duodenal, 789
neuronal, 1300
pancreatic, 789
Choroid, lymphoma of, *1372*
melanoma of, 1365–1367, *1366*
Choroid plexus, carcinoma of, 1348
papilloma of, 1347–1348
Christmas disease, 639–640
Chromaffin cells, 1163
Chromatin, in apoptosis, 19, *19*
Chromatolysis, central, 1295
Chromium, in carcinogenesis, 274t, 309
in occupational diseases, 421t, 422
Chromosome(s), analysis of, in acute lymphoblastic leukemia/lymphoma, 655, 655t
in acute myelogenous leukemia, 677
in adult T-cell leukemia/lymphoma, 656t
in angiocentric lymphoma, 656t
in Burkitt lymphoma, 655t, 662
in chronic lymphocytic leukemia, 655t, 659
in chronic myelogenous leukemia, 680–681, *680*
in diffuse large B-cell lymphoma, 655t, 661
in follicular lymphoma, 655t
in hairy cell leukemia, 656t
in large granular lymphocytic leukemia, 656t
in lymphoplasmacytic lymphoma, 656t
in mantle cell lymphoma, 656t, 668
in marginal zone lymphoma, 656t
in multiple myeloma, 655t, 664
in mycosis fungoides, 656t
in peripheral T-cell lymphoma unspecified, 656t
in plasmacytoma, 655t
in Sézary syndrome, 656t
in small lymphocytic lymphoma, 655t, 659
anaphase lag of, 168
deletion of, 169, *169,* 173
disorders of, 168–176, 466, 466t
fluorescence in situ hybridization analysis of, 166–168, *167*
fluorescent painting of, 166, 168, *168*
G banding of, 165–166, *166*
inversion of, 169, *169*
isochromosome formation of, 169–170, *169*
karyotype of, normal, 165–168, *166–168*
spectral, 168, *168*
terminology for, 166, *167*
mosaicism of, in intrauterine growth retardation, 461, *462*
nondisjunction of, 168
number of, aneuploid, 168
disorders of, 168–169, 170–173, *171, 172*
euploid, 168
paracentric inversion of, 169, *169*
pericentric inversion of, 169, *169*
Philadelphia, 285, *285*
postnatal evaluation of, 182
prenatal evaluation of, 182
reciprocal translocation of, *169,* 170
ring, 169, *169*
robertsonian translocation of, *169,* 170
sex. See also *X chromosome; Y chromosome.*
disorders of, 173–176, *175*
spectral karyotype of, 168, *168*
structure of, disorders of, 169–170, *169*
translocation of, *169,* 170
Chromosome(s) *(Continued)*
in oncogene activation, 284–286, *285,* 286t, 298
Chromosome 1, in neuroblastoma, 487
Chromosome 10, in thyroid carcinoma, 1143
Chromosome 15, maternal, in Angelman syndrome, 180–181, *181*
paternal, in Prader-Willi syndrome, 180–181, *181*
Chromosome breakage syndromes, 47, 169, 296, 1337
Chromosome 22q11 syndrome, 173
Chronic granulomatous disease, 65, 65t
Chronic obstructive pulmonary disease (COPD), 706–717, 707t. See also *Asthma; Bronchiectasis; Bronchitis; Emphysema.*
Churg-Strauss syndrome, 517t, 521–522
Chvostek sign, 1151
Chylocele, 1025
Chylopericardium, 531
Chylothorax, 531, 750t, 751
Cigarette smoking, 408–410, 409t, 712, *712*
atherosclerosis and, 506
bronchogenic carcinoma and, 741–742
cancer and, 273
emphysema and, 709
gastric carcinoma and, 799, 799t
oral cancer and, 760
passive exposure to, 410
peptic ulcer disease and, 794
periductal mastitis and, 1097
transitional cell carcinoma and, 1007
Cilia, defects of, in Kartagener syndrome, 716
Ciliary body, melanoma of, 1367
Circadian rhythms, in myocardial infarction, 551
Circle of Willis, berry aneurysm of, *1312*
Cirrhosis, 848, 853–855, *854*
alcoholic, 411–412, *411,* 411t, 869–871. See also *Alcoholic liver disease.*
ascites and, 855, *855*
biliary, 877t
primary, 877t, 878–879, *879*
secondary, 877t, 878, *878*
cardiac, 883
collagen deposition in, 854, *854,* 872
cryptogenic, 853
etiology of, 853
in chronic hepatitis, 866, *867*
Ito cells in, 254, *854*
portal hypertension and, 855–856, *855*
splenomegaly and, *855,* 856
Civatte bodies, 1200
Claudication, in thromboangiitis obliterans, 523
Clear cell adenocarcinoma, of ovary, 1072
clk-1 gene, 47
Clock genes, 47
Clonality, of tumors, 277, *277*
Cloning, 140, *140*
Clostridium botulinum, 334t, 368, 369
Clostridium difficile, 334t, 368, 369, 807–809, 808t
pseudomembranous colitis from, 809–810, *810*
Clostridium perfringens, 334t, 368–369, *369,* 807–809, 808t
necrosis with, 346
α toxin of, 344, 368
β toxin of, 369
δ toxin of, 368–369
Clostridium septicum, 334t
Clostridium tetani, 334t, 368, 369
Clotting. See *Coagulation.*
Cloverleaf cells, in adult T-cell leukemia/lymphoma, 670
Clubbing, of fingers, 320, 321t
CMM genes, in melanoma, 1177
CMV. See *Cytomegalovirus (CMV).*
CNS. See *Central nervous system (CNS).*
Coagulation, *121,* 122–124, *123, 124*
anticoagulation regulation of, 122–124, *124*
antithrombins in, 122, *124*
extrinsic pathway of, *121,* 122, 640
in inflammation, *68,* 69–70
intrinsic pathway of, *121,* 122, 640
protein C in, 122–123, *124*
protein S in, 122–123, *124*
vitamin K in, 446–447
Coagulation factors, deficiency of, 637–640, *638*
Coal workers' pneumoconiosis, 42, 729–730, 729t, *730*
Coarctation of aorta, *596,* 596–597
Coated pits, in lipoprotein clearance, 151, *152*
Cobalt, in occupational diseases, 421, 421t
Cocaine abuse, 412–414, *413*
Coccidioides immitis, 353, *353*
Cockayne syndrome, 47
Codeine abuse, 412
Codman triangle, 1237, *1238*
Cohnheim, Julius, 52
Coin lesion, 748
COL4A5 gene, 963
Colchicine, microtubule defects with, 27
Cold, common, 347–348, *347,* 762
Cold agglutinin immune hemolytic anemia, 620–621
Cold exposure, 435
Cold hemolysin hemolytic anemia, 621
Cold sore, 757
Colitis. See also *Enterocolitis.*
Clostridium difficile–induced, 809–810, *810*
collagenous, 810
ulcerative, 818–820, *819, 820,* 821t
Collagen, deficiency of, skeletal manifestations of, 1221–1222, *1221,* 1222t
genes for, 144–145, 147t, 150
in Ehlers-Danlos syndromes, 149–150
in hepatic cirrhosis, 854, *854,* 872
in osteogenesis imperfecta, 144–145
in silicosis, 731, *731, 732*
in systemic sclerosis, 226–228, *228*
of bone, 1217–1218, *1217*
of extracellular matrix, 98–99, *99,* 99t, *103*
of glomerular basement membrane, 931, 933, *933*
synthesis of, 98–99, *99,* 106, 106t
in fibrosis, 106, 106t
in wound healing, 108–109, *108*
types of, 98, 99t
Collagenase, in tissue remodeling, 107, *107*
type IV, in tumor invasion, 303–304, *304*
Collagenous colitis, 810
Collectins, in phagocytosis, 62
Colloid bodies, in lichen planus, 1200
Colloid carcinoma, of breast, 1112, *1112*
Colloid cyst, of cerebral ventricle, 1348
Coloboma, 1360
Colon. See *Intestine.*
Colony-forming units, 602–604, *603*
Colorado tick fever virus, 333t
Colorectal carcinoma. See *Intestine, carcinoma of.*
Columnar metaplasia, 37
Coma, in type I diabetes mellitus, 924–926, *925*
Comedocarcinoma, of breast, 1108, *1108*

Comedones, 1206–1207
Common cold, 347–348, *347,* 762
Common variable immunodeficiency, 233–234
Complement, deficiency of, 236
in systemic lupus erythematosus, 219
immune complex activation of, 203, *203*
in glomerulonephritis, 947
in inflammation, 67–69, *67,* 77t
in tuberculosis, 349
in type II hypersensitivity, 199–200
Complement receptors, in phagocytosis, 62
Concretio cordis, 589
Concussion, 1303
Condyloma, giant, 1014
Condyloma acuminatum, 1209
of penis, 1012, *1012, 1013*
of vulva, 1042, *1043*
Condylomata lata, 364
Congenital adrenal hyperplasia, 1157–1159, *1158*
Congenital heart disease, 591–597, 592t. See also specific types.
clinical features of, 592–593
etiology of, 592
incidence of, 592, 592t
left-to-right shunt in, 593–595, *593, 594*
obstructive, 596–597, *596, 597*
right-to-left shunt in, 595–596, *596*
Congenital malformation, 464–470, *465,* 466t, 467t, *468, 469.* See also *Malformation(s), congenital.*
Congestion, 116–117
hepatic, 116–117, *117*
pulmonary, 116
Congestive heart failure, 546–550, *547, 548.* See also *Heart, failure of.*
Conjunctiva, carcinoma in situ of, 1362
epithelial tumors of, 1362
in vitamin A deficiency, 1361
melanoma of, 1362
mucoepidermoid carcinoma of, 1362
pingueculae of, 1361, *1361*
pterygium of, 1361
squamous cell carcinoma of, 1362
trachoma of, 1361–1362, *1362*
Conjunctivitis, inclusion, 362
Conn syndrome, 1155–1157, *1156, 1157*
Connective tissue disease, mixed, 231
Consanguineous mating, in genetic disorders, 145
Consumer Products Safety Commission, 404
Contact dermatitis, 206, *206,* 1195t, 1196–1197, *1196*
Contaminants, food, 436
Contraceptives, oral, adverse reactions to, 414–416, 415t
Contraction bands, in myocardial infarction, 559, *561*
Contracture, 110
Contusion, 432–433, *432*
CNS, 1303–1304, *1303*
Coombs antiglobulin test, 620
Copper, deficiency of, 452t
hepatic accumulation of, 875
in Ehlers-Danlos syndromes, 150
in free radical generation, 12, *13*
Cor bovinum, 526
Cor pulmonale, 130, 549, 565–566, 565t, *566,* 703
Cord factor, of *Mycobacterium tuberculosis,* 349
Cornea, Avellino dystrophy of, 1363
copper deposition in, 875
endothelial dystrophy of, 1363–1364, *1364*
Cornea *(Continued)*
Fuchs dystrophy of, 1363–1364, *1364*
hereditary dystrophy of, 1363–1364, *1363, 1364*
herpesvirus infection of, 361
inflammation of, 1362–1363
lattice dystrophy of, 1363
macular dystrophy of, 1363, *1363*
Reis-Bücklers dystrophy of, 1363
stromal dystrophy of, 1363, *1363*
ulcer of, 1362–1363
Coronary artery(ies), 545
Coronary artery bypass graft surgery, 539–540
Coronary artery disease, 550–564. See also *Heart, ischemic disease of; Myocardial infarction.*
after heart transplantation, 598, *598*
epidemiology of, 551
in systemic lupus erythematosus, 223–224
pathogenesis of, 551–554, *552,* 553t
Coronaviruses, 333t, 354
Corpora amylacea, 1297
Corpora lutea, cystic, 1066
Corpus, of stomach, 787, *787*
Corpus callosum, agenesis of, 1300, *1301*
Corticobasal degeneration, 1335
Corticosteroids, peptic ulcer disease and, 794
Cortisol, biosynthesis of, *1152*
excess of, 1153–1155, *1153,* 1155t
Corynebacterium diphtheriae, 334t, 343, *343*
Costochondral junction, in vitamin D deficiency, 444, *445*
Cotton-wool spots, in retinopathy, 1369, *1369,* 1370
Councilman bodies, 19, 848
Cowden disease, breast cancer and, 1105
Cow's milk, type I diabetes mellitus and, 917
Coxiella burnetii, 384
Coxsackie B4 virus, in type I diabetes mellitus, 917
Coxsackievirus, 333t
CR3, in phagocytosis, 62
Craniopharyngioma, 1129
Craniorachischisis, 1220
Craniotabes, in vitamin D deficiency, 444
C-reactive protein, in febrile state, 86
in myocardial infarction, 506
Creatine kinase, in myocardial infarction, 561
Crescendo angina, 554
CREST syndrome (*c*alcinosis, *R*aynaud's phenomenon, *e*sophageal dysmotility, *s*clerodactyly, *t*elangiectasia), 226, 229
antibodies in, 218t, 227
Cretinism, 1133
Creutzfeldt-Jakob disease, 1297, 1323–1324, *1325*
Crigler-Najjar syndrome, 850–851, 850t
Crohn disease, 816–818, *817, 818,* 821t
complications of, 818
extraintestinal manifestations of, 818
fissures in, 816, *817*
granulomas in, 817, *818*
mucosal damage in, 817
pathogenesis of, 815–816
skip lesions in, 816
ulcers in, 816, 817, *817*
vs. ulcerative colitis, *819,* 821t
Crooke hyaline change, in Cushing syndrome, 1154
Cross-linkages, in collagen synthesis, 98–99, *99*
Crotalaria spectabilis, 705
Croup, 765
Crouzon syndrome, 1220t
Cryoglobulinemia, 968
Cryoglobulinemic vasculitis, 517t
Crypt cells, of intestine, 803
Cryptococcosis, 379–380, *380*
in acquired immunodeficiency syndrome, 248
Cryptococcus, 379–380, *380,* 1322
Cryptorchidism, 1015–1016, *1015*
Cryptosporidium, 337t, 382, *382*
Crystal arthropathy, 1253–1257. See also *Gout.*
CSF. See *Cerebrospinal fluid (CSF).*
Culture, 345, 345t
Cunninghamella, 380–381
Curie (Ci), 425
Curling ulcer, 796
Curschmann spirals, 715
Cushing disease, 1153, *1153*
Cushing syndrome, 1152–1155, *1153,* 1155t
diagnosis of, 1155
hemorrhage in, 634
paraneoplastic, 320, 321t
Cushing ulcer, 796
Cutaneous leukocytoclastic angiitis, 517t
Cutaneous lupus erythematosus, 1200–1201, *1200, 1201*
Cutaneous T-cell lymphoma, 1191, *1191*
Cyanosis, in left-to-right shunt, 593–595, *593, 594*
in right-to-left shunt, 595–596, *596*
of Raynaud disease, 524
Cyclic adenosine monophosphate pathway, for signal transduction, *93,* 94
Cyclins, in cancer, 282–284
in cell cycle, 95–96, *96,* 283, *283, 284*
Cyclin B/CDK1 complex, in cell cycle, 95–96, *96*
Cyclin D, in cancer, 283, 290
Cyclin-dependent kinases, 96, *96*
in cancer, 282–284
in cell cycle, 283, *283, 284*
inhibitors of, 283
Cyclin-dependent kinase inhibitors, in cell-cycle regulation, 96, *96*
Cyclooxygenases, in eicosanoid synthesis, 70, *71*
Cyclopean synophthalmus, 1360
Cyclophosphamide, cardiotoxicity of, 586
transitional cell carcinoma and, 1007
Cyclospora cayetanensis, 382
Cyclosporine, in transplantation, 210
Cylindroma, 1182, *1183*
CYP1A1 gene, 405
in lung cancer, 307
Cyst(s), adrenal, 1163
Baker, 1258
Bartholin, 1040
blue-dome, 1099, *1099*
branchial, 767
bronchogenic, 699
choledochal, 899
colloid, of cerebral ventricle, 1348
dermoid, 1181
Echinococcus granulosus, 395–396
epithelial, 1181
Gartner duct, 1045
hepatic, 880–881, *880*
in von Hippel-Lindau disease, 909
inclusion, epidermal, 1181
lymphoepithelial, 767
mammary, 1099, *1099*
mesenteric, 842
odontogenic, 761
ovarian, 1066–1067, *1066*
pancreatic, 909

Cyst(s) *(Continued)*
pilar, 1181
renal, 937–942, *938, 939, 941,* 941t
synovial, 1258
thymic, 691
thyroglossal tract, 767–768
thyroid, 1142, 1147
trichilemmal, 1181
tubal, 1065
urachal, 1001
ureteral, 998–999, *999*
vaginal, 1045
Cystadenocarcinoma, ovarian, 1069–1071, *1069–1071*
pancreatic, 910, *910*
Cystadenofibroma, ovarian, 1072
Cystadenoma, 261
ovarian, 1069, *1069*
pancreatic, 910
papillary, 261
Cystic fibrosis, 41, 477–481, *478–481*
genetic defects in, 143, *143,* 147t, 148, 478–479, *479*
hepatic abnormalities in, 480
pancreatic abnormalities in, 479–480, *481*
pathogenesis of, 478–479, *478, 480*
Pseudomonas infection in, 376, 377
pulmonary infection in, 479, 480, 481, *481*
Cystic fibrosis transmembrane conductance regulator (CFTR) gene, 143, *143,* 147t, 148, 478–479, *479*
Cystic hygroma, 533
Cystine stones, 989, 989t, 990
Cystitis, 1001–1003, *1001, 1002*
Cystitis cystica, 1002–1003
Cystitis glandularis, 1002–1003
Cytochrome C, cellular transit of, 294, *295*
Cytochrome *c,* in cell injury, 6–7
Cytochrome P-450–dependent monooxygenase system, in toxicant metabolism, 406, *407*
Cytogenetic disorders, 168–176, *169.* See also *Chromosome(s).*
Cytoid body, in hypertensive retinopathy, 1370
Cytokines, 98
autocrine effects of, 192
classes of, 73
endocrine effects of, 192
in asthma, 713, *714,* 715
in febrile state, 86
in glomerulonephritis, 948
in hepatocyte regeneration, 33, *33*
in Hodgkin disease, 674
in immune system, 191–192
in inflammation, 54, 73–74, *73,* 77t
in leukocyte adhesion, 57, 57t, *58*
in multiple myeloma, 664
in rheumatoid arthritis, 1250–1251
in type I diabetes mellitus, 916
in type I hypersensitivity reaction, 198
natural killer cell secretion of, 191
paracrine effects of, 192
pleiotropic effects of, 192
receptors for, 192
types of, 192
Cytology, in tumor diagnosis, 322–323, *323*
Cytomegalic inclusion disease, 376, *376*
Cytomegalovirus (CMV), 333t, 376, *376*
CNS, 376, 1319
congenital, 376
esophageal, 782
fetal, 467
in acquired immunodeficiency syndrome, 248
Cytoskeleton, abnormalities of, 27–28, *28*
Cytotrophoblastic cells, in choriocarcinoma, 1021, *1021*

D
Dacryocytes, in myelofibrosis with myeloid metaplasia, 684, *684*
Dandy-Walker malformation, 1301
Darier sign, 1192
Daunorubicin, cardiotoxicity of, 586
Dawson inclusion body encephalitis, 1321–1322
DCC gene, 293, *832,* 833
D-dimer, 123–124
DDT, 422–423, 423t
Deafness, in syphilis, 364
Decay-accelerating factor (CD55), 619
Decompression sickness, 131, 436
Deep vein thrombosis, 129. See also *Embolism; Thrombosis.*
Deer tick, 338, *338*
Defensins, in phagocytosis, 64
Deformation, congenital, 464–465. See also *Malformation(s), congenital.*
Degenerative joint disease, 1246–1257. See also *Arthritis.*
Dejerine-Sottas disease, 1278
Deleted in colon carcinoma gene, 293, *832,* 833
Delta agent, 861–862, *862, 863*
Delta toxin, of *Clostridium perfringens,* 368–369
Delta-cell tumor, 928
Dementia, 1329–1333. See also *Alzheimer disease.*
in Creutzfeldt-Jakob disease, 1324
in neurosyphilis, 1317
in progressive supranuclear palsy, 1334–1335
post-traumatic, 1305–1306
vascular (multi-infarct), 1314
Demyelinating polyradiculoneuropathy, inflammatory, 1275–1276
Demyelination, segmental, *1270,* 1273, 1274, *1274*
Dendritic cells, 191
follicular, 191, 243
human immunodeficiency virus infection of, 243, 250
in transplantation, 210
Dendrocytes, 1171
Dengue fever, 383
Dengue virus, 333t
Dense deposit disease, 959, *960*
Dentorubropallidoluysian atrophy, 179t
Denys-Drash syndrome, Wilms' tumor in, 488
Deoxyribonucleic acid (DNA), damage to, 310
chemical, 306, 308
repair of, 47–48, *48*
fragmentation of, in apoptosis, 20, *21*
mitochondrial, mutations in, 179–180
mutations in, 141–143. See also *Mutation(s).*
nucleotide excision repair of, 310
repair of, 47–48, *48,* 310
BRCA genes in, 292
defective, cancer and, 276
genes for, 277, 295–296
p53 gene in, 291, *291*
transfection of, 278, 297
ultraviolet ray effects on, 310
DeQuervain thyroiditis, 1135–1136, *1136*
Dermatan sulfate, in mucopolysaccharidosis, 159–160
Dermatitis. See also *Skin.*
atopic, 1195t
contact, 206, *206,* 1195t, 1196–1197, *1196*
drug-related, 1195t
eczematous, 1194–1197, *1195,* 1195t, *1196*
in ariboflavinosis, 448
in pellagra, 448, *449*
in zinc deficiency, 451, *452*
irritant, 1195t
Dermatitis herpetiformis, 1204–1205, *1205*
Dermatofibroma, 1187–1188, *1188,* 1264
Dermatofibrosarcoma protuberans, 1188
Dermatographism, 1192
Dermatomyositis, 229, 230, *230*
Dermatosis papulosa nigra, 1180
Dermis, *1171, 1172.* See also *Skin.*
dermatofibrosarcoma protuberans of, 1188
tumors of, 1187–1189, *1188*
vascular tumors of, 532–533, *532,* 534–535, *534,* 537–538, *537*
xanthoma of, 1189
Dermoid cyst, 1181
DES (diethylstilbestrol), in adenocarcinoma, 1046
Deshan disease, 452
Desmoid, 110, 1263
Desmoplasia, 261
Desmoplastic small round cell tumor, 1260t
Devic disease, 1327–1328
Dexamethasone suppression test, in Cushing syndrome diagnosis, 1155
Diabetes mellitus, 913–926
atherosclerosis and, 506
cellular glycogen in, 42
classification of, 913–914, 913t
complications of, 919–920, *919, 921*
advanced glycosylation end products and, 920, 920t
intracellular hyperglycemia and, *919,* 920
neuropathic, 924
nonenzymatic protein glycosylation and, 919–920, *919,* 920t
ocular, 924
renal, 922–923, *923, 924*
vascular, *921,* 922, *922*
glomerulosclerosis in, 966–968, *967*
glucose tolerance test in, 915
hyaline arteriolosclerosis in, 514
insulin-dependent (type I), 913, 913t
autoimmunity in, *915,* 916
β-cell loss in, 916
clinical features of, 924–926, *925*
environmental factors in, 916–917
genetic factors in, 915–916, *915*
HLA class II gene in, 915–916, *915*
immune system in, *915,* 916
insulitis in, 916, 920, *921*
ketoacidosis in, 924–926, *925*
mortality from, 926
pathogenesis of, 915–917, *915, 916*
T-cell anergy in, 214
transgenic mouse model of, 214
viruses in, 917
maturity-onset of young, 913, 918–919
microangiopathy in, 922–923, *923*
non–insulin-dependent (type II), 913, 913t
amylin in, 918
amyloidosis in, *921,* 922
β-cell degranulation in, 922
β-cell insulin secretion in, 917–918, *917*
clinical features of, 926
insulin resistance in, 918
mortality from, 926

Diabetes mellitus *(Continued)*
obesity in, 918
pathogenesis of, 917–918, *917*
pancreatic lesions in, 920, *921,* 922
peripheral nephropathy in, 966–968, *967*
peripheral neuropathy in, 1279, *1279*
retinopathy in, 1369–1370, *1369*
secondary, 913t
Dialysis, kidney, 941, 964
amyloidosis with, 253, 253t
Diaphragmatic hernia, 789
Diarrhea, 805–812, 806t. See also *Enterocolitis.*
after bone marrow transplantation, 811
bacterial infection in, 807–809, 808t, *809*
definition of, 805–806
drug-induced, 811
Entamoeba histolytica in, 811
Giardia lamblia in, 811, *811*
in abetalipoproteinemia, 815
in acquired immunodeficiency syndrome, 248, 811
in celiac sprue, 813
in cholera, 357–358
in disaccharidase deficiency, 815
in graft-verus-host disease, 811
in malabsorption syndromes, *214,* 806t, 812–815, 812t, *813*
in motility disorders, 806t
in pellagra, 448–449
in tropical sprue, 814
in Whipple disease, 814–815, *814*
infectious, 248, 806–810, 806t, 807t, 808t, *809*
osmotic, 806, 806t
radiation-induced, 811
rice-water, 357–358
secretory, 806, 806t
traveler's, 809
viral, 354–355, 806–807, 807t
Diatrophic dysplasia, 1220t
DIC, 640–642. See also *Disseminated intravascular coagulation (DIC).*
Diet, 436. See also specific minerals and vitamins.
disease and, 455
in atherosclerosis, 506
in breast carcinoma, 1107
in cancer prevention, 455–456
in carcinogenesis, 309
in colorectal carcinoma, 456, 833
in esophageal squamous cell carcinoma, 784–785, 785t
in gastric carcinoma, 799, 799t
in phenylketonuria, 476
life span and, 47
Diethylstilbestrol (DES), in adenocarcinoma, 1046
Diffuse alveolar damage, 700–703. See also *Adult respiratory distress syndrome (ARDS).*
Diffuse axonal injury, 1304
Diffuse Lewy body disease, 1334
DiGeorge syndrome (thymic hypoplasia), 173, 235, 691
Digestion, disorders of, 812–815, *813, 814*
Digits, glomus tumor of, 533–534
Dihydropteridine reductase, deficiency of, 476, *476*
Dihydrotestosterone, in benign prostatic hyperplasia, 1027, *1027*
Diphtheria, 343, *343*
oral manifestations of, 759t
peripheral nerve involvement in, 1276
Disaccharidase, deficiency of, 815
Discoid lupus erythematosus, 1200–1201, *1200, 1201*
Discs, intercalated, 544
Disomy, uniparental, 181
Disruption, congenital, 465, *465.* See also *Malformation(s), congenital.*
Disseminated intravascular coagulation (DIC), 129, 640–642, 640t, *641*
clinical course of, 642
hepatic sinusoid occlusion in, 882
in cancer, 321
in preeclampsia, 1083, *1084*
prognosis for, 642
Diverticulosis, 823–825, *824*
Diverticulum (diverticula), Meckel, 804–805, *805*
of bladder, 1000, *1000*
of esophagus, *778,* 779
of intestine, 823–825, *824*
of ureter, 998
Zenker, *778,* 779
DNA. See *Deoxyribonucleic acid (DNA).*
DNA helicase, in Werner's syndrome, 47
DNA probes, 345, 345t
DNA topoisomerase I, antibody to, 227
Dog tick, *338*
Döhle bodies, in neutrophilic leukocytosis, 648, *648*
Donath-Landsteiner antibody, 621
Dorsal root ganglion, varicella-zoster virus infection of, 373–374, *374*
Dose-response curve, for chemical toxicity, 405, *405*
Dot blot analysis, in genetic disorders, 183, *184*
Double minutes, in protooncogene amplification, 286, *286*
Down syndrome, 170–171, *171, 172*
G-banded karyotype of, *171*
ocular anomalies in, 1360
Doxorubicin, cardiotoxicity of, 580, 586
Drug(s), adverse reactions to, 148, 414–416, 415t, 634
fetal effects of, 467
hepatic toxicity of, 868–869, 869t
after bone marrow transplantation, 885
in cell injury, 4, 14–15
in iatrogenic lysosomal disease, 26
in warm antibody hemolytic anemia, 620
interstitial nephritis with, 977–979, *977, 979,* 979t
lupus erythematosus with, 218t, 224–225
neutropenia with, 646–647
pulmonary effects of, 740, 740t
smooth endoplasmic reticulum hypertrophy with, 26, *27*
thrombocytopenia with, 636
Drug abuse, 412–414, *413,* 413t
Dry eye, 769
Dubin-Johnson syndrome, 850t, 851, *851*
Duchenne muscular dystrophy, 147t, 1281–1282, *1282, 1284*
Duck fever, 737
Duct(s), accessory, of Santorini, 903
bile. See *Bile ducts.*
Gartner, cyst of, 1045
mammary, 1093, *1094*
ectasia of, 1097, *1097*
müllerian, 1036
of Luschka, 892
pancreatic, 903, *903*
obstruction of, 906, *906,* 908
thyroglossal, 1147
Ductus arteriosus, patent, *593,* 594, 596
Duncan's disease, 373
Duodenum, adenoma of, 827, *827*
atresia of, 804
Brunner glands of, 803
gastric heterotopia of, 789
stress ulcers of, 796–797
ulcers of, 793–796, *794, 795*
Dupuytren contracture, 1263
Duret hemorrhage, 1298, *1299*
Dusts, in lung disease, 727–734, *728,* 729t, *730–733*
Dutcher bodies, in lymphoplasmacytic lymphoma, 666
Dwarfism, thanatophoric, 1220t, 1221, 1300
Dysembryoplastic neuroepithelial tumor, 1348
Dysentery. See also *Diarrhea.*
amebic, 358
bacillary, 355, *355*
Dysgerminoma, 1075, *1075*
Dyskeratosis, 1172
Dyslipoproteinemias, atherosclerosis and, 505, 505t
Dysphagia, 776, 778
Dysplasia, definition of, 466
epithelial, 266, *267*
fibrous, 1242–1243, *1243*
Dyspnea, in left-sided heart failure, 549
Dystrophin, gene for, in dilated cardiomyopathy, 580
mutations in, 147t
in muscular dystrophy, 1282, *1282, 1284*

E

Ear, 766–767
bone deposition in, 767
inflammation of, 766–767
tumors of, 767
EBV. See *Epstein-Barr virus (EBV).*
Ecchymoses, 118
in idiopathic thrombocytopenic purpura, 636
Echinococcus, 336–337
Echinococcus granulosus, 395–396
Echovirus, 333t
Eclampsia, 1082–1084, *1084, 1085*
Ectasia, annuloaortic, 528
of mammary duct, 1097, *1097*
vascular, 534
Ecthyma gangrenosum, 377
Ectoparasites, 337–338, *338*
Ectopia lentis, in Marfan syndrome, 149
Ectopic pregnancy, 1079–1080, *1080*
Eczema, 1194–1197, *1195,* 1195t, *1196*
Edema, 113–116, *114,* 114t
cerebral, 116, 1298
clinical effects of, 116
congestion and, 116
generalized, 113, 560
hydrostatic pressure in, 114–115, *115*
in inflammation, 53–54
in nephrotic syndrome, 953
in right-sided heart failure, 550
in Turner syndrome, 175
lymphatic obstruction in, 115
of optic nerve, 1373–1374, *1374*
pitting, 116
plasma osmotic pressure in, 115
pulmonary, 116, 700
sodium retention in, 115–116
subcutaneous, 116
vs. hypertrophy, 34
water retention in, 115–116

Edwards syndrome, 171–173, *172*
E2F transcription factor family, in cell-cycle regulation, 96
Effusion, inflammatory, 84, *85*
pericardial, 550, 587
pleural, 550, 749–751, 750t
Ehlers-Danlos syndrome, 149–150
copper metabolism in, 150
gene mutation in, 147t
hemorrhage in, 634
Ehrlichia, 331, 384
Ehrlichiosis, 385t
Eicosanoids, in inflammation, 70–72, *71,* 71t, 77t
Eighth nerve deafness, 364
Eisenmenger syndrome, 592
Elastin, in aortic stenosis, 597
of extracellular matrix, 99–100
Electricity, injury from, 435
Electromagnetic field, 431
Electromagnetic radiation, 425
in carcinogenesis, 310–311
Elephantiasis, 115
Embolism, 127, *128,* 129–132
air, 131, 435
amniotic fluid, 131–132
cerebral, 1308
cholesterol, 130, 502
estrogen replacement therapy and, 414
fat, 130–131, *131*
from endocarditis, 574
gas, 435
in coronary artery occlusion, 555
oral contraceptives and, 415–416
paradoxical, 130, 555, 592
pulmonary, 130, *130,* 703–704, *703*
fibrous web from, 130
prevention of, 704
pulmonary abscess and, 722
renal, 986, *987*
saddle, 130, *130*
systemic, 130
with cardiac valve prostheses, 578
Embryo, 467–468, *468*
Embryonal carcinoma, 1020–1021, *1020*
Embryonal rhabdomyosarcoma, 1265, *1265*
of bladder, 1008
of vagina, 1046–1047, *1046*
Emery-Dreifuss muscular dystrophy, 1283t
Emphysema, 707–711, 707t
alveolar tears in, 711
α_1-antitrypsin deficiency and, 709
bullous, 711, *711*
centrilobular (centriacinar), 707–709, *708,* 710
cigarette smoking and, 709
clinical course of, 710
compensatory, 710
distal acinar (paraseptal), 709
incidence of, 709
irregular, 709, 710
panlobular (panacinar), *708,* 709, 710
pathogenesis of, 709–710, *709*
protease-antiprotease theory of, 709–710, *709*
senile, 710
Empty sella syndrome, 1128
Empyema, 721, 750
of gallbladder, 896
of sinus, 762–763
subdural, 1316
Encephalitis, arbovirus, 1318
cytomegalovirus, 376, 1319
hemorrhagic, necrotizing, 1328–1329
Encephalitis *(Continued)*
herpesvirus, 360, 1318, *1318*
JC virus, 1321, *1322*
limbic, 1352, 1352t
Naegleria, 1323
poliovirus, 1319
rabies, 1319–1320
varicella-zoster, 1319
Encephalocele, 1300
Encephalomyelitis. See also *Encephalitis.*
disseminated, acute, 1328–1329
Encephalomyopathy, mitochondrial, 1340–1341
Encephalopathy, hepatic, 853, 1342
hypertensive, 1314
hypoxic, 1307–1310
in left-sided heart failure, 549
multicystic, 1302
spongiform, 1296t, 1323–1326, *1325*
Wernicke, 1341
Encephalotrigeminal angiomatosis, 534
Enchondroma, 1238–1239, *1239*
Endocardial fibroelastosis, 584
Endocarditis, *Candida* in, 379
fungal, 574
in systemic lupus erythematosus, 127, *223,* 577, 765
infective, 572–576, *575*
artificial valves and, 578
renal manifestations in, 966
Libman-Sacks (noninfective, verrucous), *575,* 576–577, *576*
in systemic lupus erythematosus, 127, 223, *223*
thrombotic, in cancer, 321, 321t
Endocrine cells, of intestine, 803–804
of stomach, 788
Endocrine system. See specific glands and hormones.
Endocrinopathy, paraneoplastic, 320, 321t
Endocytosis, 25, *26*
Endodermal sinus tumor, 1075–1076, *1076*
Endometrioid tumors, of ovary, 1071–1072
Endometriosis, 1057–1058, *1058, 1059*
Endometritis, 1057, *1057*
Endometrium, adenocarcinoma of, 1061–1062, *1062*
adenomyosis of, 1057, *1057*
carcinoma of, 1061–1062, *1062*
estrogen replacement therapy and, 414
mortality rates with, *272*
oral contraceptives and, 415
carcinosarcoma of, 1063
complex hyperplasia of, 1060, *1060*
cyclic changes in, 1037–1038, *1054,* 1055, *1055*
oral contraceptives and, 1056
extrauterine, 1057–1058, *1058, 1059*
hyperplasia of, 33, 1059–1061, *1060*
inflammation of, 1057, *1057*
menopausal changes in, 1056
metaplasia of, 1060, *1060*
mixed müllerian tumors of, 1063
myosis of, 1065
papillary serous carcinoma of, 1062, *1062*
polyps of, 1058–1059, *1059*
sarcoma of, 1065
stromal tumors of, 1065
Endomyocardial fibrosis, 583–584
Endomyocarditis, Loeffler, 584
Endomyocardium, biopsy of, 579
Endomysium, 1273
Endoneurium, 1271
Endonucleases, in cell injury, 6, *6*
Endophthalmitis, phakogenic, 1365
Endoplasmic reticulum, smooth, hypertrophy of, 26, *27*
Endostreptosin, 949
Endothelial gaps, in inflammation, 54, *55*
Endothelin, *118,* 119
Endothelium, 496, 496t
activation of, 496–497, *496*
antibodies to, vasculitis and, 516
anticoagulant properties of, *119,* 120
antiplatelet properties of, 120
antithrombotic properties of, 120
dysfunction of, 496, 508
fibrinolytic properties of, *118,* 120
homocysteine effects on, 506
in atherosclerosis, 496–497, *496, 507,* 508
in disseminated intravascular coagulation, 640
in hemostasis, 119–120, *119*
in systemic sclerosis, 227, *227*
in thrombosis, 124–125, *124*
inflammation-related changes in, 53–55, *54, 55*
leukocyte adhesion to, 53, 57–61, 57t, *58, 59*
leukocyte pavementing of, 56–57, *56*
leukocyte-mediated injury to, 55
necrosis of, in inflammation, 55
nitric oxide of, 75–76, *75,* 77t. See also *Nitric oxide.*
permeability of, in inflammation, 53–55, *53–55*
procoagulant properties of, 119–120, *119*
prothrombotic properties of, 120
Endothelium-derived relaxing factor. See *Nitric oxide.*
Endotoxins, bacterial, 343
in adult respiratory distress syndrome, 701–702, *702*
in shock, 134–136, *134, 136*
Entamoeba histolytica, 337t, 346, 358–359, *358,* 811
Enteritis. See also *Gastroenteritis.*
bacterial, 355–356, *355*
Campylobacter, 355–356
eosinophilic, 793
Shigella, 355, *355*
viral, 354–355
Yersinia, 356
Enterobacter (Aerobacter) aerogenes, 334t
Enterobius vermicularis, 332t
Enterocolitis, 805–812, 806t
after bone marrow transplantation, 811
antibiotic-associated, 809–810, *810*
collagenous, 810
diversion, 812
drug-induced, 811
in acquired immunodeficiency syndrome, 811
infectious, 806–810, 807t, 808t, *809*
lymphocytic, 810
necrotizing, 809
neutropenic, 811–812
parasitic, 810–811
protozoal, 810–811, *811*
radiation-induced, 811
Enterocytozoon bieneusi, 337t
Enteropathic arthritis, 1252
Enteropathy, gluten-sensitive, 813, *813,* 961
Enterotoxins, bacterial, 807, 808t
Entrapment neuropathy, 1280
Environment, pollution of, 416–419, 417t, 418t
Environmental Protection Agency, 404
Enzymes, defects in, 146–148, *147,* 147t
in free radical inactivation, 13–14
lysosomal (acid hydrolases), 153–154, *153*

Enzymes *(Continued)*
of coagulation cascade, 122, *123*
pancreatic, 903–904
in acute pancreatitis, 905–907, *906*
Eosinophils, development of, *603*
in inflammation, 82, *82*
in type I hypersensitivity reaction, 198–199
reactive proliferations of, 648t
Eosinophilia, 648t
in inflammation, 86
in necrosis, 16, *16*
pulmonary, 738
Eosinophilic enteritis, 793
Eosinophilic gastritis, 793
Eosinophilic granuloma, 685
Eosinophilic pneumonia, 738
Eotaxin, in inflammation, 82
Ependymal cells, 1296, 1297
Ependymitis, granular, 1317
Ependymoma, 1346–1348, *1347*
Ephelis, 1174
Epidermal growth factor, 97
in hepatocyte regeneration, 33, *33*
Epidermal inclusion cyst, 1181
Epidermis, *1171, 1172.* See also *Skin.*
Epidermodysplasia verruciformis, 1209
Epidermolysis bullosa, 1205, *1206*
Epididymis, 1014–1015
inflammation of, 1016, *1016*
Epidural hematoma, 1304, *1305*
Epilepsy, myoclonus, triplet repeat mutations in, 179, *179,* 179t
Epimysium, 1273
Epineurium, 1271
Epispadias, 1012
Epithelial cyst, 1181
Epithelioid cells, in delayed-type hypersensitivity, 204, *205*
Epithelioma, sebaceous, 1183t
Epithelium, bacterial infection of, 343
dysplasia of, 266, *267*
renal, antibody-mediated injury to, 947, *947*
in minimal change disease, 954–956, *956*
vitamin A effects on, 441
Epstein-Barr virus (EBV), 333t
B lymphocyte infection by, 190
B-cell immortalization of, 312
in Burkitt lymphoma, 312, *313,* 662
in carcinogenesis, 312–313, *313*
in children, 371–373, *372*
in diffuse large B-cell lymphoma, 661
in Hodgkin disease, 674
in nasopharyngeal carcinoma, 313, 764
in rheumatoid arthritis, 1249
in X-linked lymphoproliferative syndrome, 318
Epulis, 758
c-*erb B1* gene, in cancer, 280
c-*erb B2* gene, 286, *316,* 317
in cancer, 280
c-*erb B3* gene, in cancer, 280
Ergotamine therapy, cardiac plaques in, 578
Erosion, cutaneous, 1173
Erysipelas, streptococcal, 368, *368*
Erythema, in systemic lupus erythematosus, 222, *223*
palmar, in liver failure, 852
Erythema chronicum migrans, 389
Erythema induratum, 1207–1208
Erythema multiforme, 759t, 1197–1198, *1197*
Erythema nodosum, 1207–1208
Erythroblastosis fetalis (hemolytic disease of newborn), 200, 473–475, *474, 475,* 849
Erythrocyte(s), 604–642
aplasia of, 632
deficiency of, 604–633, 605t. See also *Anemia.*
deformability of, 606, *607*
development of, *603*
in myelofibrosis with myeloid metaplasia, 685, *685*
Plasmodium falciparum infection of, 389–390, *390*
Erythrocytosis, 633, 633t
Erythroderma, 1198
Erythroplakia, 759–760
Erythroplasia of Queyrat, 1013–1014
Erythropoiesis, diminished, anemias of, 604–633, 605t. See also *Anemia.*
Escherichia coli, 334t, 343–344, 807–809, 808t
in hemolytic-uremic syndrome, 637
pili of, 342–343
Esophagogastric varices, in cirrhosis, 856
Esophagus, 776–787
achalasia of, 778–779, *778*
adenocarcinoma of, 786–787, *786*
atresia of, 777, *777*
Barrett, 37, 781–782, *781, 782,* 786, *786*
candidiasis of, 378, *379*
chemical-induced inflammation of, 782
congenital anomalies of, 777–778, *777*
diverticula of, *778,* 779
dysplasia of, 782
fistula of, 777, *777*
functions of, 776
hernia of, *778,* 779
herpes infection of, 361
in systemic sclerosis, 228
inflammation of, 780–783, *780–782*
lacerations of, *778,* 779–780
motor disorders of, 778–780, *778*
mucosa of, 776
normal, 776
polyps of, 783
reflux-associated inflammation of, 780–781, *780*
Schatzki rings of, 777–778
short-segment Barrett mucosa of, 781
sphincters of, 776
squamous cell carcinoma of, 783–786, *785,* 785t
squamous papilloma of, 783
stenosis of, 777–778
submucosa of, 776
tumors of, benign, 783
malignant, 783–787, *785,* 785t, *786*
varices of, 529–530, 783, *784*
in cirrhosis, 856
webs of, 777–778
Zenker diverticulum of, *778,* 779
Esthesioneuroblastoma, 764
Estrogen, adverse reactions to, 414–416, 415t
breast cancer and, 1106
in osteoporosis, 1223–1224
Estrogen replacement therapy, 414–416
Ethanol, 410–412, *410, 411,* 411t. See also *Alcoholic liver disease.*
CNS effects of, 1342, *1342*
Ethanol myopathy, 1288
Ethylene glycol, ingestion of, 412
Ethylene oxide, in cancer, 274t
Etiology, 1–2
Ewing sarcoma, 485t, 1244, *1244,* 1260t
EWS gene in, 285–286, 286t
Excoriation, 1172
Exocytosis, 64, 1173
Exoenzyme S, of *Pseudomonas,* 377
Exophthalmic ophthalmoplegia, 1287
Exotoxins, bacterial, 343–344, *343*
Exotoxin A, of *Pseudomonas,* 377
Extracellular matrix. See also *Basement membrane.*
collagen of, 98–99, *99,* 99t
elastin of, 99–100
fibrillin of, 100
fibronectin of, 100, *100*
hyaluronan of, 102
in angiogenesis, 106
in cell growth, 98–102, *99–103,* 99t
in fibrosis, 106, 106t
integrins of, 100–101, *101*
laminin of, 100, *100*
matricellular proteins of, 101
platelet adhesion to, 120–121, *120*
proteoglycans of, 101–102, *102*
tumor invasion of, 302–305, *303, 304*
Exudate, 53
fibrinous, 84, *85*
in inflammation, 53–54, *53*
purulent, 84–85, *85*
serous, 84, *85*
Eye(s), anatomy of, 1359, *1360*
congenital anomalies of, 1360
copper deposition in, 875
dryness of, 769
in ariboflavinosis, 448
in congenital syphilis, 1361
in diabetes mellitus, 924
in Graves disease, 1137, 1138
in hyperthyroidism, 1131, *1132*
in Marfan syndrome, 149
in rubella syndrome, 1361
in trisomy 13, 1360
in trisomy 21, 1360
in vitamin A deficiency, 441
infectious embryopathy of, 1360–1361
malignant melanoma of, 1365–1367, *1366*
Niemann-Pick disease in, 158
phthisical, 1375–1376, *1376*
radiation damage to, 430
retrolental fibroplasia of, 472
sarcoidosis of, 735
Eyelids, sebaceous carcinoma of, 1183

F

Fabry disease, 155t
Face, butterfly rash of, 368, *368*
Factitial panniculitis, 1208
Factor V, gene for, Leiden mutation in, 125
mutation in, 182–183, *183*
Factor VIII, deficiency of (hemophilia A), 147t, 639
Factor VIII–von Willebrand factor complex, deficiency of, 638, *638*
Factor IX, deficiency of (hemophilia B), 639–640
Factor X, 122, *123*
Factor Xa, 69
Factor XII (Hageman factor), *68,* 69, 70
Fallopian tubes, 1037, 1065
abscess of, 1039
cysts of, 1065
ectopic pregnancy of, 1079–1080, *1080*
inflammation of, 1065
tumors of, 1065
Familial adenomatous polyposis, 275, 831, *831*

Familial amyloid polyneuropathy, 252, 254, 1277
Familial cancer syndromes, 275–276, 275t
Familial hypercholesterolemia, atherosclerosis and, 505, 505t
  LDL receptor gene mutations in, 144, 147t, 148, 152–153, *153*
Familial Mediterranean fever, 253–254
Fanconi anemia, 169, 296
Farmer's lung, 729t, 737
Farnesyl transferase, *282*
  inhibitors of, 282
Fasciitis, nodular, 1261–1262, *1262*
Fascioscapulohumeral muscular dystrophy, 1283t
Fas-Fas ligand, in apoptosis, 23, *24,* 206, 212, *213,* 214
Fat, in carcinogenesis, 309
  stain for, 39–40
Fat embolism, 130–131, *131*
Fat necrosis, in breast, 1097–1098, *1098*
Fatal familial insomnia, 1326
Fatty acids, omega-3, 506
Fatty dots, in atherosclerosis, 503, *503*
Fatty liver, 38, *38,* 39, *39,* 847
  in alcoholic liver disease, 411, 869, *870,* 872
  in Wilson disease, 875
  of pregnancy, 884–885
Fatty streaks, in atherosclerosis, *502,* 503, *503,* 509
FBN1 gene, 148, 149
FBN2 gene, 148
FcγR, 62
Felon, 367
Fenfluramine therapy, cardiac lesions with, 578
Fenton reaction, 13, *13*
Ferritin, cellular accumulation of, 42–43, *43*
  in free radical inactivation, 13
Ferruginous bodies, 733
Fetal alcohol syndrome, 412, 467
α-Fetoprotein, in hepatocellular carcinoma, 891
  in testicular germ cell tumors, 1024
  in tumor diagnosis, 325, 325t
Fetor hepaticus, in hepatic failure, 852
Fetus. See also *Infant.*
  development of, 467–468, *468*
  drug effects on, 467
  ethanol effects on, 412
  infection in, 338–339, 467, 470–471
  maternal cigarette smoking and, 409
  radiation effects on, 467
  Toxoplasma gondii infection in, 383
Fever, 85–86, *86*
Fever blister, 757
Fiberglass, in indoor air, 418, 418t
Fibrillary glomerulonephritis, 968
Fibrillin, gene for, 147t
  in Marfan syndrome, 148–149
  of extracellular matrix, 100
Fibrin, *118,* 119
  in crescentic glomerulonephritis, 952
  in disseminated intravascular coagulation, 641–642
  in glomerulonephritis, 948
  in hemostasis, 122
  in pericarditis, 588
Fibrin split products, 123–124
  generation of, 123
  in inflammation, 69
Fibrinogen, in platelet aggregation, *120,* 122
Fibrinolysis, 123–124, *124*
Fibrinolytic system, in inflammation, *68,* 69
Fibrinopeptides, in inflammation, *68,* 69
Fibroadenoma, 267, *268,* 1102–1103, *1103*
Fibroblasts, proliferation of, 106, 106t, 1261–1262
Fibroblast growth factor, 97, 104, 106
  in tumorigenesis, 279t, 280
Fibroblastic meningioma, 1350
Fibrocystic changes, of breast, 1098–1100, *1099*
Fibroelastoma, papillary, cardiac, 590
Fibroelastosis, endocardial, 584
Fibroepithelial polyp, 1181
  of ureter, 999
Fibrohistiocytic tumors, 1264–1265, *1264*
Fibroids, uterine, *265, 271,* 1063–1064, *1063*
Fibroma, 261
  chondromyxoid, 1240, *1240*
  irritation, of buccal mucosa, 758
  nonossifying, 1242, *1242*
  pleural, 751
  renal, 991
Fibroma-thecoma, 1077–1078, *1077*
Fibromatoses, 110, 1262–1263
  in children, 484
Fibronectin, of extracellular matrix, 100, *100, 103*
  tumor cell attachment to, 303, *304*
Fibroplasia, 90
Fibrosa, of cardiac valves, 545
Fibrosarcoma, 1243–1244, 1263–1264, *1263*
Fibrosis, 102–107
  angiogenesis in, 103–106, *104, 105,* 105t
  endomyocardial, 583–584
  extracellular matrix in, 106, 106t
  fibroblast proliferation in, 106
  hepatic, 848
    congenital, 880, 881
  in chronic pancreatitis, 908
  in inflammation, 78, *78,* 84
  in systemic sclerosis, 227, *227*
  macrophage in, 106, 106t
  pipe-stem, in *Schistosoma* infection, 397, *397*
  pulmonary, 735–736, *736*
  radiation-induced, 426, 429, *429*
  retroperitoneal, 999–1000
  tissue remodeling in, 106–107, *107*
  transforming growth factor-β in, 98
Fibrous cap, of atheromatous plaque, 499, *500, 501,* 509
Fibrous capsule, of benign tumor, 267, *268*
Fibrous cortical defect, 1242
Fibrous dysplasia, of bone, 1242–1243, *1243*
Fibrous histiocytoma, 1243–1244
  benign, 1187–1188, *1188*
Fibrous tumors, in children, 484
Fibroxanthoma, atypical, 1264
Fibula, fracture of, 1230, *1230*
Fifth disease, 470, *470*
Filariasis, lymphatic, 397–398, *398*
Fimbriae, bacterial, 342
Fine-needle aspiration, in tumor diagnosis, 322
Fingers, clubbing of, 320, 321t
  glomus tumor of, 533–534
FISH, in tumor diagnosis, 324
Fish oil, in inflammation, 72
Fistula, arteriovenous, 498
  tracheoesophageal, 777, *777*
  vesicouterine, 1000
Flame cells, 665
  in trypanosomiasis, 393
Flatworms, 336–337
Flavin-containing monooxygenase system, in toxicant metabolism, 406, *407*
Flea bite, 1210–1212
Flexner-Wintersteiner rosette, in retinoblastoma, 1373, *1373*
Floppy baby syndrome, 1285
Floppy valve, in Marfan syndrome, 149
Flow cytometry, in tumor diagnosis, 324
Flower cells, in adult T-cell leukemia/lymphoma, 670
Flukes, 336–337
Fluorescence in situ hybridization, in cytogenetic analysis, 166–168, *167*
  in tumor diagnosis, 324
Fluoride, deficiency of, 452t
Fly bite, 1210–1212
FMR-1 gene, 143, 177
  mutations in, 177, 178
Foam cells, 40, *40*
  in Alport syndrome, 963
  in Niemann-Pick disease, 158
  of cholesterolosis, 40, *40*
  of fatty streaks, *40,* 41
Foamy histiocytes, in leprosy, 386
Focal proliferative glomerulonephritis, 962, *962*
Focal segmental glomerulosclerosis, 956–958, *957,* 965t
Foix-Alajouanine disease, 1313
Folate, 440t, 450–451
Folic acid, deficiency of, 626–627, *626*
Follicle-stimulating hormone, tumor secretion of, 1127
Follicular dendritic cells, 191
  human immunodeficiency virus infection of, 243
Follicular keratoses, inverted, 1180
Follicular lymphoma, 285, 286t, 655t, 659–661, *660, 661*
Food, safety of, 436
Food and Drug Administration, 404
Food poisoning, 356–357, 365
Forebrain, anomalies of, 1300, *1301*
Foreign body, wound healing and, 110
Foreign body granuloma, 83
Formaldehyde, in air pollution, 418, 418t
Foveolar cells, 787
Fractalkine, 74
Fracture(s), 1229–1231
  healing of, 1229–1230, *1230*
  in osteogenesis imperfecta, 1221, *1221,* 1222t
  in Paget disease, 1227
  infection of, 1231
  skull, 1302–1303
    at birth, 464
Fragile X syndrome, 177–179, *177, 179*
  trinucleotide repeat mutations in, 143
Francisella tularensis, 334t
Freckles, 1174
Free radicals, in cell injury, 5–6, *6,* 10, 12–15, *13–15,* 47, *48*
  in chronic pancreatitis, 908
  in toxicant metabolism, 406, *407*
  inactivation of, 12–14
  oxygen-derived, 76–77
  radiant energy–generated, 12
  reduction-oxidation reaction–generated, 12, *13*
Friedreich ataxia, 1337
  triplet repeat mutations in, 179, *179,* 179t
Frontal bossing, in vitamin D deficiency, 444
Fructose, in diabetes mellitus, *919,* 920
Fuchs dystrophy, 1363–1364, *1364*
α-Fucosidase, deficiency of, 155t
Fucosidosis, 155t
Fumigants, 423t
Fundus, of stomach, 787, *787*
Fungicides, 423t

Fungus (fungi), 335, *335, 336,* 354. See also *Infection.*
CNS infection with, 1322
cutaneous infection with, 1210
genital infection with, 1039
respiratory infection with, 352–353, *353*
Fungus ball, in aspergillosis, 380
Funisitis, 470
Furuncles, 366–367
Fusobacterium, 369

G
G banding, of chromosomes, 165–166, *166*
gag gene, of human immunodeficiency virus, 238, *239*
GAGE genes, 316
Gaisböck syndrome, 633
Galactocerebroside β-galactosidase, deficiency of, 1339
Galactokinase, deficiency of, 476–477, *477*
Galactosemia, 147, 476–477, *477*
Galactose-1-phosphate uridyl transferase, deficiency of, 147, 476–477, *477*
α-Galactosidase A, deficiency of (Fabry disease), 155t
Galactosylceramidase, deficiency of (Krabbe disease), 155t, 1339
Gallbladder, 893–897
adenomyosis of, 899
anatomy of, 892
carcinoma of, 899, *900*
cholelithiasis of, 893–895, *894, 895*
cholesterolosis of, 40, *40*
congenital anomalies of, 893, *893*
disease of, oral contraceptives and, 416
empyema of, 896
hydrops of, 895
inflammation of, 895–897, *896, 897*
mucocele of, 895
phrygian cap of, 893, *893*
porcelain, 897
stones of, 893–895, *894, 895*
pancreatitis with, 904
Gangliocytoma, 1348
Ganglion, of joint, 1258
Ganglioneuroma, 486
Ganglioside activator protein, deficiency of, 155t, 156, *156*
Gangliosidoses, 155t, *156.* See also *Tay-Sachs disease.*
Gangrene, 368–369, *369*
in diabetes mellitus, 922
pulmonary, 722
Gap junctions, in myocyte contraction, 544
Gardner syndrome, 831
osteoma in, 1235
Gardnerella, 1039
Garré, sclerosing osteomyelitis of, 1233
Gartner duct, cysts of, 1045
Gas embolism, 131, 435
Gastric glands, 787–788
atrophy of, 792
hyperplasia of, 797–798
Gastrinoma, 927
Gastritis, 789–793
acute, 789–790, *790*
autoimmune, 793
chronic, 790–793, 790t, *791, 792*
atrophy in, 792
dysplasia in, 792
Helicobacter pylori in, 790–791, 790t, *791,* 792, *792*
Gastritis *(Continued)*
hyperplasia in, 792
metaplasia in, 792, *792*
peptic ulcer disease and, 795
regenerative changes with, 791–792
eosinophilic, 793
ethanol-induced, 412
granulomatous, 793
lymphocytic, 793
Gastroenteritis. See also *Enteritis.*
bacterial, 807–809, 808t, *809*
uremic, 964
viral, 806–807, 807t
Gastroenteropathy, protein-losing, 798
Gastroesophageal reflux, 780–781, *780*
in systemic sclerosis, 228
Gastrointestinal tract. See also *Intestine; Stomach.*
amyloidosis of, 256
ethanol effects on, 412
in kwashiorkor, 439
infection of, 353–359
adenoviruses in, 354
bacterial, 354, 355–358, *355, 357*
barriers to, 353–354
Campylobacter in, 355–356
coronaviruses in, 354
Entamoeba histolytica in, 358–359, *358*
fungal, 354
Giardia lamblia in, 359, *359*
helminth, 354
Norwalk-like viruses in, 354
protozoan, 354, 358–359, *358*
rotavirus in, 354
Salmonella in, 356–357, *357*
Shigella in, 355, *355*
Vibrio cholerae in, 357–358, *357*
viral, 354–355
Yersinia in, 356
radiation damage to, 429
Gastroschisis, 804
Gaucher cells, 158, *159*
Gaucher disease, 155t, 158–159, *159*
Gene(s), clock, 47
linkage analysis of, 184–186, *185, 186*
mitochondrial, mutations in, 179–180
mutations in, 141–143, *141–143.* See also *Mutation(s).*
penetrance of, 144
pleiotropic, 144
variable expressivity of, 144
virulence, 341
Gene therapy, 141
Genetic disorders, 139–186. See also specific disorders.
consanguineous mating in, 145
cytogenetic, 168–176, *169.* See also *Chromosome(s).*
diagnosis of, 141, 182–186
direct, 182–184, *183, 184*
indirect, 184–186, *185, 186*
multifactorial, 164–165
mutations in, 141–143, *141–143.* See also *Mutation(s).*
single-gene (mendelian), 143–164
autosomal dominant, 144–145, 145t
autosomal recessive, 145, 145t
nonclassic, 176–182, *177–179,* 179t, *180*
X-linked, 146, 146t
Genital tract, female, 1036–1089. See also specific structures.
anatomy of, 1036–1038, *1037*
embryology of, 1036, *1036*
Genital tract *(Continued)*
infections of, 1038–1040, 1038t, *1039.* See also *Sexually transmitted diseases.*
male, 1011–1033. See also specific structures.
Genomic imprinting, 180–181, *181*
in Beckwith-Wiedemann syndrome, 488
Germ cell tumors, mixed, 1022–1024, *1023*
of brain, 1350
of ovary, 1073–1076, *1073–1076*
of testis, 1018–1024, 1018t, *1019–1023*
Germinoma, of pineal gland, 1168
Gerstmann-Sträussler-Scheinker syndrome, 1323–1326, *1325*
Gestational age, 460–461, *461*
Gestational choriocarcinoma, 1087–1089, *1088*
Gestational trophoblastic disease, 1084–1089, 1085t, *1086, 1087, 1088*
Ghon complex, 723, *723*
Ghost vessels, in congenital syphilis, 1361
Giant cell(s), in granulomatous inflammation, 83, *83*
in human immunodeficiency virus infection, 240, *240*
in measles virus infection, 370, *370*
in seminoma, 1020
in subacute thyroiditis, 1135–1136, *1136*
in tumors, 265–266
Giant cell (temporal) arteritis, 516–518, 517t, *518*
Giant cell granuloma, of gingiva, 758, *758*
Giant cell myocarditis, 585, *585*
Giant cell tumor, of bone, 1244–1245, *1245*
of tendon sheath, 1258–1259
Giant condyloma, of penis, 1014
Giant granules, in Chédiak-Higashi syndrome, 64
Giardia lamblia, 332t, 337t, 359, *359,* 811, *811*
Giardiasis, 359, *359*
Giardins, 359
Giemsa stain, 345, 345t
Gigantism, growth hormone–secreting adenoma and, 1126
Gilbert syndrome, 850t, 851
Gingiva, peripheral giant cell granuloma of, 758
pyogenic granuloma of, 758, *758*
Gingivostomatitis, 360, 757
Glands. See specific glands.
Glanzmann thrombasthenia, 122
Glaucoma, 1368, 1374–1375, *1375*
Gliadin, in celiac sprue, 813
in dermatitis herpetiformis, 1205
Glial cells, 1295–1297, *1296*
Glial cytoplasmic inclusions, 1335
Glial fibrillary acidic protein, 1296, *1296*
Glioblastoma multiforme, *1344,* 1345, *1345*
Glioma, 1343–1348, *1344–1347*
brain stem, 1346
Gliosis, 1297
in metachromatic leukodystrophy, 1340, *1340*
β-Globin gene, 142, *142*
Globoid cells, 1339
Glomerular filtration rate, in hypertension, 512
Glomeruloid body, *1344,* 1345
Glomerulonephritis, acute, 949–951, *950*
alternative complement pathway in, 947
anti–glomerular basement membrane, 943–945, 943t, *944*
basement membrane thickening in, 943
C5b-C9 in, 947, *947*
cell-mediated immune reactions in, 946
chemokines in, 948

Glomerulonephritis *(Continued)*
chronic, 963–964, *964,* 965t
circulating immune complexes in, *944,* 945–946, *946*
clinical manifestations of, 942, 942t
cytokines in, 948
endothelin in, 948
epithelial cell injury in, 947, *947*
fibrillary, 968
fibrin in, 948
Heymann, *944,* 945, 954
histology of, 942–943
hyalinization in 943
hypercellularity of, 942–943
immune complex deposition in, 943–946, 943t, *944, 946*
immunotactoid, 968
in amyloidosis, 968
in bacterial endocarditis, 966
in diabetic glomerulosclerosis, 966–968, *967*
in essential mixed cryoglobulinemia, 968
in Goodpasture syndrome, 968
in Henoch-Schönlein purpura, 965–966
in multiple myeloma, 968
in plasma cell dyscrasias, 968
in polyarteritis nodosa, 968
in systemic disease, 964–968, *967*
in systemic lupus erythematosus, 220, 221, *221,* 962, *962,* 965
in Wegener granulomatosis, 968
light-chain deposition in, 968
lymphocytes in, 947, *947*
macrophages in 947, *947*
membranoproliferative, 947, 958–960, *959–961,* 965t
membranous, 953–954, 965t
in systemic lupus erythematosus, 221, *221*
mesangial cells in, 947, *947*
monocytes in, 947, *947*
necrotizing, 962
nephrotic syndrome and, 952–953
neutrophils in, 947, *947*
nonglomerular antigens in, 945
pathogenesis of 943–948, 943t, *944, 946, 947*
platelets in, 947, *947*
poststreptococcal, 949–951, *950,* 965t
progression of, 948–949, *948, 949*
proliferative, acute (postinfectious), 949–951, *950*
diffuse, in systemic lupus erythematosus, 221, *221*
focal, 962, *962*
in systemic lupus erythematosus, 220–221, *220*
rapidly progressive (crescentic), 951–952, 951t, *952,* 965t
sclerosis in, 943
tubulointerstitial injury in, 948–949, *949*
Glomerulosclerosis, diffuse, 966–967, *967*
in diabetes mellitus, 923, *924*
intercapillary, 967
nodular, 967
segmental, focal, 956–958, *957,* 965t
collapsing, 958
malignant, 958
pyelonephritic scarring and, 977
renal ablation, 958
sequential, focal, 948, *948*
Glomerulus (glomeruli), 931–934, *932–934*
barrier function of, 934
basement membrane of, 931–933, *932–934*
antibodies to 943–945, *944*
diffuse thinning of, 963
Glomerulus (glomeruli) *(Continued)*
ruptures in, 952, *952*
thickening of, 943, 954, *955*
in diabetes mellitus, 966, *967*
compensatory hypertrophy of, 948, *948*
disease of, 942–968, 942t. See also *Glomerulonephritis; Glomerulosclerosis.*
epithelial cells of, 947, *947*
filtration function of, 934
hyalinization of, 943
hypercellularity of, 942–943
in poststreptococcal nephritis, 950, *950*
sclerosis of, 943
Glomus tumor, 533–534
Glossitis, 758
in ariboflavinosis, 448
in pernicious anemia, 625
Glucagonoma, 927
Glucocerebrosidase, deficiency of (Gaucher disease), 155t, 158–159, *159*
Glucocorticoids, in inflammation, 72
Glucoproteins, of extracellular matrix, 100, *100*
Glucose, homeostasis of, 914–915, *914*
metabolism of, life span and, 47
Glucose tolerance test, in diabetes mellitus, 915
Glucose transport (GLUT) proteins, 915
Glucose-6-phosphatase, deficiency of (von Gierke disease), 160, *161,* 163t
Glucose-6-phosphate dehydrogenase (G6PD), deficiency of, 610–611, *610, 611*
drug reactions in, 148
gene mutation in, 146
α-Glucosidase (acid maltase), deficiency of, 155t, 160–161, *161, 163,* 163t
Glucuronidation, in toxicant metabolism, 406, *408*
Glutamic acid decarboxylase, autoantibodies to, 916
Glutathione conjugation, in toxicant metabolism, 408, *408*
Glutathione peroxidase, in free radical inactivation, 13–14
Glutathione-s-transferase, in lung cancer, 307
Gluten, in dermatitis herpetiformis, 1205
Gluten-sensitive enteropathy, 813, *813,* 961
GlyCam-1, in leukocyte adhesion, 57, 57t
Glycogen, intracellular accumulation of, 41–42
metabolism of, 160, *161, 162*
Glycogen storage diseases (glycogenoses), 42, 155t, 160–162, *161–163*
Glycolysis, in cell injury, 7–8
Glycosaminoglycans, 101
Goblet cells, in bronchitis, 711, 712
of intestine, 803
Goiter, 1138–1140, *1140*
colloid, 1138
endemic, 1138–1139
intrathoracic, 1139
multinodular, 1139–1140, *1140*
nontoxic, diffuse (simple), 1138–1139
sporadic, 1139
Goitrogens, 1130–1131, 1138
Golgi apparatus, lysosomal enzyme processing in, 153–154, *153*
Gonadoblastoma, 1078
Gonorrhea, 362, 1017
Goodpasture syndrome, 739, 945, 951, 965t
Gout, 1253–1257, *1254–1256,* 1254t
nephropathy of, 980, *980*
Gp63, of *Leishmania,* 392
Graft-versus-host disease, diarrhea with, 811
esophagus in, 782
hepatic damage in, 885–886
with bone marrow transplantation, 210–211
Gram stain, 345, 345t
Granulation tissue, 102–103, *104,* 108, *108,* 109
exuberant, 110
Granules, alpha, 120, 121
atrial, specific, 544
azurophil, 76, *76*
Birbeck, 685, *685, 1190,* 1191
delta (dense bodies), 120, 121
giant, in Chédiak-Higashi syndrome, 64
hemosiderin, 43, *43*
lipofuscin, in atrophy, 36
lysosomal, 64, 76, *76*
specific, 76, *76*
toxic, 648
Granuloma, 83
eosinophilic, 685
foreign body, 83
immune, 83–84
in Crohn disease, 817, *818*
in *Histoplasma capsulatum* infection, 352, *353*
in pulmonary tuberculosis, 724, *724*
in sarcoidosis, 734–735, *734*
in *Schistosoma* infection, 396–397, *397*
in tuberculosis, 350–351, *351*
in type IV hypersensitivity, 204, *205*
of breast, 1098
of gingiva, 758, *758*
pyogenic, *532,* 533
Granuloma gravidarum, 533
Granulomatosis, Wegener, 517t, 522–523, *522*
renal manifestations of, 968
Granulomatous angiitis, in cerebrovascular disease, 1308
Granulomatous disease, chronic, 65, 65t
Granulomatous gastritis, 793
Granulomatous inflammation, 83–84, *83,* 83t, 346
Granulomatous thyroiditis, 1135–1136, *1135*
Granulosa luteal cysts, 1066
Granulosa-theca cell tumor, of ovary, 1076–1077, *1077*
Granzymes, of cytotoxic T lymphocytes, 206
Granzyme B, in apoptosis, 24
Graves disease, 1136–1138, *1138*
Gray (Gy), 425
Great arteries, transposition of, 595–596, *595–596*
Greig syndrome, 1220t
Grotton's lesions, in dermatomyositis, 229
Ground-glass nuclei, in papillary thyroid carcinoma, 1143, *1144*
Group A streptococci, in rheumatic fever, 570, 572
Growth factors, 73, 97–98, 97t
deprivation of, apoptosis after, 24–25
in fibroblast proliferation, 106, 106t
in signal transduction, 92–93, *93, 94*
in tumorigenesis, 279–280, 279t
receptors for, in tumorigenesis, 279t, 280
Growth hormone, tumor secretion of, 1126
Growth inhibitors, in hepatocyte regeneration, 33
Growth plate, of bone, 1219, *1219*
GTPase activating protein, 93
Guillain-Barré syndrome, 1275–1276
Gumma, syphilitic, 364, *364*
Gunshot wound, 433, *433*
Gynecomastia, 1117, *1118*

H
Haemophilus ducreyi, 334t
Haemophilus influenzae, 334t, 348–349

Hageman factor (factor XII), *68,* 69, 70
Hair follicles, 1171, *1171*
  lichen planus of, 1200
Hairball, 797, *797*
Hairy leukoplakia, 758–759
Hallucinogens, abuse of, 413
Halo nevus, 1176t
Halogenated hydrocarbons, in occupational diseases, 419t, 420
Hamartoma, 263
  definition of, 483
  in neurofibromatosis, 164
  in tuberous sclerosis, 1354–1355
  of iris, 164
  pulmonary, 748–749
  renal, 991
Handgun injury, 433, *433*
Hand-Schüller-Christian triad, 685
Hansen disease (leprosy), 385–386, *387*
Harrison groove, in vitamin D deficiency, 444
Hashimoto thyroiditis, 1133, 1133t, 1134–1135, *1135*
Hassall corpuscles, 691
Hay fever, 762
Hazardous waste sites, 404, 404t
HBx protein, in liver cancer, 314
Heart, 543–598. See also *Cardiac* entries; *Myocardium.*
  age-related changes in, 545–546, 546t
  amyloidosis of, 256, *256,* 586
  aortic valve of. See *Aortic valve.*
  basophilic degeneration of, 546
  blood supply to, 545
  brown atrophy of, 546
  carcinoid disease of, 577–578, *577*
  collateral circulation of, 545
    in nonlethal ischemia (preconditioning), 553, 561
  congenital disease of, 591–597, 592t. See also specific types.
    clinical features of, 592–593
    etiology of, 592
    incidence of, 592, 592t
    left-to-right shunt in, 593–595, *593, 594*
    obstructive, 596–597, *596, 597*
    right-to-left shunt in, 595–596, *596*
  dilation of, 544
  ethanol effects on, 412
  failure of, 546–550, *547, 548*
    after myocardial infarction, 563, *563,* 564
    cardiac hypertrophy in, 547–549, *547, 548*
    hepatic manifestations of, 117, 882–883, *883*
    hydrostatic pressure in, 114
    in dilated cardiomyopathy, 581
    left-sided, 549
    right-sided, 549–550
  fatty change in, 39–40
  great arteries of, transposition of, 595–596, *595*
  hemodynamic overload of, *34,* 35
  hypertensive disease of, 564–566, *565,* 565t, *566*
  hypertrophy of, *34,* 35, 544, 547–549, *547, 548.* See also *Cardiomyopathy, hypertrophic.*
    apoptosis in, 548
    compensatory mechanisms in, 548–549
    gene expression in, 548
    physiologic, 548
  in hyperthyroidism, 1131
  in malaria, 390
  in Marfan syndrome, 149
  in trisomy 21, 171
Heart *(Continued)*
  infection of, 572–576, *575.* See also *Endocarditis; Rheumatic fever.*
  ischemic disease of, 550–564. See also *Myocardial infarction.*
    angina pectoris in, 554
    chronic, 563, 564
    epidemiology of, 551
    pathogenesis of, 551–554
      fixed obstructions in, 551
      plaque change in, 551–553, *552*
      thrombus in, 553
      vasoconstriction in, 553–554, 553t
    sudden cardiac death in, 564
  left-to-right shunt of, 593–595, *593, 594*
  lipoma of, 590
  metastases to, 591, 591t
  mitral valve of. See *Mitral valve.*
  myocardium of, 544–545
  myxedema, 586
  myxoma of, 589–590, *590*
  normal, 544–546, 546t
  papillary fibroelastoma of, 590
  pressure hypertrophy of, 547, *547*
  radiation damage to, 429, *429*
  rhabdomyoma of, 591
  rheumatic disease of, 570–572, *571, 573, 575*
    blood flow alterations in, 125, 129
  rheumatoid disease of, 589
  right-to-left shunt of, 595–596, *596*
  sarcoma of, 591
  tigered effect in, 40
  transplantation of, 210, 598, *598*
    rejection of, 598, *598*
  tricuspid valve of. See *Tricuspid valve.*
  tumors of, 589–591, *590,* 591t
  valves of, 545
    disease of, 566–578, 567t. See also specific diseases.
    prosthetic, 578, *578,* 578t
  vegetations of. See also *Endocarditis.*
    infected, 572–576, *575*
    noninfected, 576–577, *576*
Heart attack. See *Myocardial infarction.*
Heartburn, 776
Heat cramps, 434
Heat exhaustion, 434
Heat stroke, 434–435
Heat-shock proteins, 41
  in tuberculosis, 349
Heavy-chain disease, 663
Heberden nodes, 1247–1248
Height, in Turner syndrome, 175
Heister, spiral valves of, 892
Helicobacter pylori, in chronic gastritis, 790–791, 790t, *791,* 792, *792*
  in gastric carcinoma, 315, 799
  in peptic ulcer disease, 793–794, *794*
  lymphoma and, 686
HELLP (*h*emolysis, *e*levated *l*iver enzymes, *l*ow *p*latelets) syndrome, 884
Helminths, 336–337
Hemangioendothelioma, 537
Hemangioma, 532–533, *532*
  capillary, 532, *532*
  cavernous, *532,* 533, 886, 1313
  differential diagnosis of, 1189
  in infant, 483, *483*
  sclerosing, 1264
Hemangiopericytoma, 538
Hemarthrosis, 118
Hematemesis, with esophageal varix rupture, 783
Hematocele, 1025
  of tunica vaginalis, 1025
Hematoma, 117–118
  dissecting, 526–528, *527–529*
  epidural, 1303, *1303,* 1304, *1305*
  in vitamin C deficiency, 449
  pulsating, 524
  subdural, 1305, *1306*
Hematopoiesis, 602–604, *603*
Hematuria, 935
  familial, 963
  in sickle cell disease, 987
Heme, degradation of, 848–849, *849*
Hemochromatosis, 586–587, 873–875, *874*
Hemoglobin, genetic defects in, *141,* 142, *142,* 147t
Hemoglobin H disease, 619
Hemoglobin S, 143–144
Hemoglobinuria, nocturnal, paroxysmal, 69, 619–620, *619*
Hemolysins, of *Trypanosoma cruzi,* 393
Hemolytic anemia. See *Anemia, hemolytic.*
Hemolytic disease of the newborn, 200, 473–475, *474, 475,* 849
Hemolytic-uremic syndrome, 636–637
  adult, 986
  childhood, 985–986
  idiopathic, 986
Hemopericardium, 118, 587
Hemoperitoneum, 118
Hemophilia A, 147t, 639
Hemophilia B, 639–640
Hemorrhage, 117–118, *117,* 633–642
  clotting factor abnormalities in, 637–640, *638*
  dot-and-blot, in hypertensive retinopathy, 1370
  Duret, 1298, *1299*
  flame-shaped, in hypertensive retinopathy, 1370
  ganglionic, 1310
  in amyloidosis, 634
  in Cushing syndrome, 634
  in disseminated intravascular coagulation, 641, *641*
  in drug reactions, 634, 636
  in drug-induced thrombocytopenia, 636
  in Ehlers-Danlos syndrome, 634
  in factor VIII deficiency, 639
  in factor IX deficiency, 639–640
  in Henoch-Schönlein purpura, 634
  in hereditary hemorrhagic telangiectasia, 634
  in HIV-associated thrombocytopenia, 636
  in idiopathic thrombocytopenic purpura, 635–636
  in infection, 634
  in platelet disorders, 634–637, 635t
  in polycythemia vera, 683
  in scurvy, 634
  in thrombotic microangiopathy, 636–637
  in vitamin C deficiency, 449
  in vitamin K deficiency, 447, 637–638
  in von Willebrand disease, 638–639
  into atheromatous plaque, 502
  intracerebral, *117,* 118
  intracranial, 118, *118,* 1305, 1310–1313, *1311, 1312*
    at birth, 464
    hypertensive, 1310, *1311,* 1314
    in infant, 1302
  lobar, 1310
  petechial, *117,* 118
  platelet abnormalities in, 634–637, 635t
  pulmonary, 738–739, *738*

Hemorrhage *(Continued)*
slit, 1314
subarachnoid, 1305, 1310–1313
vessel wall abnormalities in, 634
Hemorrhagic disease of newborn, 447
Hemorrhagic fever viruses, 333t
Hemorrhagic pericarditis, 589
Hemorrhagic shock, 118
Hemorrhoids, 530, 823
Hemosiderin, cellular accumulation of, 42–43, *43*
hepatic deposition of, 874, *874*
Hemosiderosis, 43
iron overload in, 586–587
pulmonary, idiopathic, 739
Hemostasis, 118–124, *118*
coagulation cascade in, *119, 121,* 122–124, *123, 124*
dysregulation of, 124–129, *124,* 125t, *127, 128*
endothelium in, 119–120, *119*
platelets in, *118,* 120–122, *120, 121*
tests of, 633–634
Hemostatic plug, *118,* 119, 121
Hemothorax, 118, 750, 750t
Henoch-Schönlein purpura, 517t, 961
hemorrhage in, 634
renal manifestations in, 965–966
Hepar lobatum, 364, *364*
Heparan sulfate, in mucopolysaccharidosis, 159–160
Heparin, thrombocytopenia with, 125–126
Hepatectomy, partial, experimental model of, 32–33, *32, 33*
Hepatic adenoma, 887–888, *887*
oral contraceptives and, 416
Hepatic artery, infarction of, 881–882, *882*
Hepatic encephalopathy, 853
Hepatic vein, obstruction of, 883–884, *883, 884*
veno-occlusive disease of, 884, *884*
Hepatitis, 848, 856–867, 856t
acute, 864, 865–866, *865, 866*
alcoholic, 411, *411,* 411t
apoptosis in, 866, *866*
asymptomatic, 864
autoimmune, 858
bridging necrosis in, 866
carrier state in, 864
chronic, 864–865, *865,* 866, *866, 867*
cirrhosis in, 866, *867*
fatty change in, 866
fulminant, 867
ground-glass hepatocytes in, 865, *865*
icteric phase of, 864
in alcoholic liver disease, 869–870, *870, 871,* 872
in Wilson disease, 875
interface, 866
neonatal, 876–877, 877t
in α_1-antitrypsin deficiency, 876
preicteric phase of, 864
sanded nuclei in, 865
Hepatitis A virus, 333t, 856–857, 856t, *857*
serologic diagnosis of, 857, *857*
Hepatitis B virus, 333t, 340, 856t, 857–859, *858, 859*
carrier of, 857, *858,* 859, 864
hepatitis D virus infection with, 862
hepatocellular carcinoma and, 888, 889
in carcinogenesis, 309, 313–314
integration of, 858
mutant strains of, 858
proliferation of, 857–858
Hepatitis B virus *(Continued)*
serologic diagnosis of, 858–859, *859*
structure of, 857, *858*
transmission of, 857
vaccine against, 889
vasculitis and, 516
Hepatitis C virus, 333t, 856t, 860–861, *860, 861, 866*
in hepatocellular carcinoma, 314, 888, 889
serologic diagnosis of, 861, *861*
structure of, 860, *860*
transmission of, 860
Hepatitis D virus, 333t, 856t, 861–862, *862, 863*
serologic diagnosis of, 852, *863*
Hepatitis delta virus, 861–862, *862, 863*
Hepatitis E virus, 333t, 856t, 862–863
Hepatitis G virus, 856t, 863–864
Hepatoblastoma, 888
Hepatocellular carcinoma, 888–891, *889*
clinical features of, 891
epidemiology of, 888
α-fetoprotein in, 891
fibrolamellar, 890, *890,* 891
fibrolamellar variant of, 891
hepatitis C virus in, 314
pathogenesis of, 888–889
spread of, 890–891
unifocal, 889, *889*
Hepatocytes, 846–847, *847.* See also *Liver.*
priming of, 33, *33*
regeneration of, 32–33, *32, 33*
Hepatocyte growth factor, in hepatocyte regeneration, 33, *33*
in tumor invasion, 304
Hepatorenal syndrome, 853
Herbicides, 423–424, 423t
Hereditary angioneurotic edema, 69
Hereditary chronic pancreatitis, 908
Hereditary corneal dystrophy, 1363–1364, *1363, 1364*
Hereditary exostosis, multiple, 1237–1238, *1238*
Hereditary hemorrhagic telangiectasia (Osler-Weber-Rendu disease), 531–532, 534, 634
Hereditary nephritis, 933, 962–963, *963*
Hereditary nonpolyposis colon cancer syndrome, 295–296, 831, 832–833
Hereditary optic neuropathy, 179–180, *180,* 1341
Hereditary peripheral neuropathy, 1277–1279, 1277t, 1278t
Hereditary spherocytosis, 147t, 607–609, *609*
Heredofamilial amyloidosis, 253–254, 253t
Heredofamilial congenital lymphedema, 531
Hermaphroditism, 176
Hernia, diaphragmatic, 789
hiatal, *778,* 779
intestinal, *825,* 826
Herniation, of brain, 1298, *1298, 1299*
Heroin abuse, 412
Herpesviruses, 333t
CNS, 1318, *1318*
corneal, 1362–1363
esophageal, 782
genital, 359–361, *360,* 360t, 1038–1039, 1038t
in acquired immunodeficiency syndrome, 248
mucosal, 346, *346*
oral, 757
Heterolysis, 16
Heterophagy, 25, *26*
Heterotopia (choristoma), bone, 44
definition of, 483
Heterotopia (choristoma) *(Continued)*
duodenal, 789
neuronal, 1300
pancreatic, 789
Heterotopic neurons, 1300
Hexosaminidase A, α subunit of, deficiency of (Tay-Sachs disease), 155–156, *156, 157*
β subunit of, deficiency of (Sandhoff disease), 155t, 156, *156*
gene for, mutations in, 142, *142,* 156, *156*
Heymann nephritis, *944,* 945, 954
Hidradenitis suppurativa, 367
Hidradenoma, papillary, vulvar, 1042
Hidradenoma papilliferum, 1182
chondroid, *1184*
High-altitude illness, 435
High-molecular-weight kininogen, in inflammation, *68,* 69
Hilus cell tumor, 1078
Hirano bodies, in Alzheimer disease, 1331
Hirschsprung disease, 805
Histamine, in asthma, 713
in inflammation, 66, *66,* 77t
in type I hypersensitivity reaction, 197, *197,* 198, 199t
Histiocytes, foamy, in leprosy, 386
sea-blue, in chronic myelogenous leukemia, 681
Histiocytoma, 1264
fibrous, 1243–1244
benign, 1187–1188, *1188,* 1264
malignant, 1264–1265, *1264*
Histiocytosis, Langerhans, 685–686
sinus, 650
Histiocytosis X, cutaneous, 1189–1191, *1190*
Histocompatibility antigens, 193–195, *193, 194*
Histoplasma capsulatum, 332t, 352, *353*
Histoplasmosis, 352, *353*
HIV. See *Human immunodeficiency virus (HIV).*
Hives (urticaria), 1194, *1194*
HLA DQw2, in celiac sprue, 813
HLA-DR1, in Crohn disease, 815
HLA-DR2, in ulcerative colitis, 815
hMSH genes, in colorectal carcinoma, 832–833
Hodgkin disease, 670–675
classification of, 672t
clinical course of, 674–675, 674t
Epstein-Barr virus in, 674
immunophenotype of, 672, 673
lymphocyte depletion type of, 672t
lymphocyte predominance type of, 672t, 673–674, *673*
mixed cellularity type of, 672t, 673, *673*
nodular sclerosis type of, 672, 672t, *673*
pathogenesis of, 674
staging of, 671–672, 672t
vs. Epstein-Barr virus infection, 372
vs. non-Hodgkin lymphoma, 674t
Holoprosencephaly, 1300, *1301*
Homeobox genes, 1218–1219
in congenital malformations, 469–470, *469*
Homeostasis, cellular, 2
Homer-Wright pseudorosettes, 486, *486*
Homer-Wright rosettes, 1373
Homicide, 431t, 433, *433*
Homocysteine, atherosclerosis and, 506
hereditary elevation of, 125
Homocystinuria, atherosclerosis in, 506
Homogeneous staining regions, in protooncogene amplification, 286, *286*
Homogentisic acid, cellular accumulation of, 42
Homogentisic oxidase, deficiency of (alkaptonuria), 162

Hookworm, 394–395
Hormones. See also specific hormones.
in systemic lupus erythematosus, 219
tumor expression of, 266–267, *267,* 319
wound healing and, 110
Horn cysts, 1180
Horner syndrome, with bronchogenic carcinoma, 747
Horseshoe kidney, 937
Howship lacunae, 1217
Hox genes, in congenital malformations, 469–470, *469*
hPMS genes, in colorectal carcinoma, 832–833
HPV. See *Human papillomavirus (HPV).*
HTLV-I, 314–315, *314,* 333t
HTLV-II, 333t
Human chorionic gonadotropin, in testicular germ cell tumors, 1024
Human Genome Project, 110
Human herpesvirus 8, in diffuse large B-cell lymphoma, 662
Human immunodeficiency virus (HIV), 333t
CD4+ T-lymphocyte infection by, 239–243, *240–242*
CNS infection with, 1320–1321, *1320*
dendritic cell infection with, 243
forms of, 238
genes of, 238–239, *239*
group M, 239
macrophage infection by, 240, 242–243
mother-to-infant transmission of, 237
occupational transmission of, 238
parenteral transmission of, 237
sexual transmission of, 237
structure of, 238, *238*
transmission of, 237–238
types of, 239
Human immunodeficiency virus (HIV) infection. See also *Acquired immunodeficiency syndrome (AIDS).*
acute phase of, 245–246, *245,* 245t
B lymphocytes in, 244
CD4+ cell count in, 247
CD4+ T-lymphocyte loss in, 240
chronic phase of, *245,* 245t, 246
crisis phase of, *245,* 245t, 246
giant cell formation in, 240, *240*
latent, 243
nephropathy with, 958
nonprogression of, 247
thrombocytopenia with, 636
viral load during, 246
Human leukocyte antigen (HLA) complex, 193–195, *193, 194*
class I, 193–194, *193*
class II, *193,* 194
autoimmune disease and, 216
disease associations of, 195, 195t
in rheumatoid arthritis, 216
in Sjögren syndrome, 193–195, *193, 194*
in systemic lupus erythematosus, 218–219
in transplantation, 210
in type I diabetes mellitus, 915–916, *915*
tumor expression of, 318
Human papillomavirus (HPV), 333t, 1208–1209, *1208*
genital infection with, 1012, *1012, 1013,* 1038t
hyperplasia with, 33
in carcinogenesis, 311–312
Human T-cell leukemia virus type 1 (HTLV-I), 314–315, *314,* 333t
Human T-cell leukemia virus type 2 (HTLV-II), 333t
Humerus, Paget disease of, 1227, *1227*
Humidifier lung, 737
Hunner ulcer, 1002
Hunter, John, 52
Hunter syndrome, 155t, 159–160
Huntingtin, 1336
Huntington disease, 145, 1296t, 1335–1336, *1336*
triplet repeat mutations in, 179, *179,* 179t
Hurler syndrome, 155t, 160
Hürthle cell, in Hashimoto thyroiditis, 1135, *1135*
Hürthle cell adenoma, 1142
Hutchinson teeth, 364
HX bodies, in Langerhans histiocytosis, 685, *685*
Hyaline arteriolosclerosis, in diabetes mellitus, 922, *922*
in hypertension, 514, *515*
Hyaline change, 45
Hyaline inclusions, in alcoholic liver disease, 27–28, *28*
Hyaline membrane disease (respiratory distress syndrome), 471–473, *472*
Hyalinization, of glomerulus, 943
Hyalinosis, in focal segmental glomerulosclerosis, 957, *957*
Hyaluronan, of extracellular matrix, 102
Hydatid disease, 395–396
Hydatidiform mole, 1084–1087, 1085t, *1086, 1087*
invasive, 1087, *1087*
Hydatids of Morgagni, 1065
Hydrocarbons, in carcinogenesis, 309
in occupational diseases, 419–420, 419t
Hydrocele, of tunica vaginalis, 1025
Hydrocephalus, 1298–1299, *1299,* 1305
Hydrocephalus ex vacuo, 1299
Hydrochloric acid, gastric secretion of, 788
Hydrogen peroxide, 12, *13.* See also *Free radicals.*
in inflammation, 76–77
Hydrogen peroxide–myeloperoxidase-halide system, in phagocytosis, 63, *63*
Hydromyelia, 1301–1302
Hydronephrosis, 988
Hydrops fetalis, 474, 474t, 475, 619
Hydrosalpinx, 1039
Hydrostatic pressure, in edema, 114–115, *114, 115*
Hydrothorax, 750, 750t
Hydroureter, 998
5-Hydroxyindoleacetic acid (5-HIAA), in carcinoid syndrome, 837, 837t
Hydroxyl radicals, 12, *13.* See also *Free radicals.*
in inflammation, 76–77
21-Hydroxylase, deficiency of, 1157–1159, *1158*
5-Hydroxytryptamine (serotonin), in carcinoid syndrome, 837, 837t
in inflammation, 67, 77t
Hygroma, cystic, 533
in Turner syndrome, 175
Hyper IgM syndrome, 234–235
Hyperaldosteronism, primary, 1155–1157, *1156, 1157*
secondary, 114
Hyperammonemia, 852
Hyperbilirubinemia, 850–851, 850t, *851*
Hypercalcemia, cancer-associated, 320, 321t, 1148
in multiple myeloma, 665
metastatic calcification in, 45
nephrocalcinosis with, 980
parathyroid hormone–related protein–induced, 1148
Hypercholesterolemia, atherosclerosis and, 504–506, 505t, 508
familial, atherosclerosis and, 505, 505t
LDL receptor gene mutations in, 144, 147t, 148, 152–153, *153*
Hypercoagulability, in thrombosis, 125–126, 125t
Hypercortisolism, 1152–1155, *1153,* 1155t
Hyperemia, 116–117
Hyperestrogenemia, 852
Hyperglycemia, CNS effects of, 1342
in diabetes mellitus, *919,* 920
Hyper-IgM syndrome, 190
Hyperinflation, compensatory, 710
Hyperinsulinemia, in obesity, 454
Hyperkeratosis, 1172, 1180
Hyperlipidemia, in atherosclerosis, 504–506, 505t
in nephrotic syndrome, 953
Hypermetabolism, with burns, 434
Hypernephroma, 991–993, *992–994.* See also *Renal cell carcinoma.*
Hyperoxaluria, 989, 989t, 990
Hyperparathyroidism, 1148–1151, *1149*
asymptomatic, 1150
brown tumor in, 1150, 1228, *1228*
metastatic calcification in, 45
primary, 1148–1150
secondary, 964, 1150–1151
skeletal manifestations of, 1228–1229, *1228*
Hyperphosphatemia, in renal osteodystrophy, 1229
Hyperpigmentation, in adrenocortical insufficiency, 1161
Hyperpituitarism, 1123–1127, *1124,* 1124t
Hyperplasia, 31, 32–35
compensatory, 32–33, *32, 33*
definition of, 466
hormonal, 32, 33
pathologic, 33
physiologic, 32–33, *32, 33*
Hyperpyrexia, malignant, 1285
Hypersensitivity, in asthma, 713
Hypersensitivity angiitis, 517t, 521–522, *522*
Hypersensitivity myocarditis, 584–585, *585*
Hypersensitivity pneumonitis, 737, *737*
Hypersensitivity reaction(s), 195–211
drug-induced, hemorrhage with, 634
in cell injury, 4
in transplant rejection, 206–211, *208, 209*
type I (anaphylactic), 195, 196–199, 196t
eosinophils in, 198–199
IgE antibodies in, 196–197, *197, 198*
in asthma, 713
local, 199
mast cells in, 196–198, *197, 198,* 199t
primary mediators of, 197–198, 199t
secondary mediators of, 198, 199t
systemic, 199
type II (cytotoxic), 195, 196t, 199–201
antibody-dependent, *200,* 201
antibody-mediated, *200,* 201, 201t
complement-dependent, 199–200, *200*
type III (immune complex–mediated), 195, 196t, 201–204, 201t
local, 204, *204*
systemic, 202–204, *202, 203*

Hypersensitivity reactions(s) *(Continued)*
  type IV (cell-mediated), 195, 196t, 204–206
    delayed-type, 204–206, *205, 206*
    T cell–mediated cytotoxicity in, 206
Hypersplenism, 689
Hypertelorism, in trisomy 21, 1360
Hypertension, 510–515, 511t
  benign, 511, 981–982, *982*
  encephalopathy with, 1314
  environmental factors in, 513
  genetic factors in, *512,* 513
  heart disease with, 564–565, *565*
  hyaline arteriolosclerosis and, 514, *515*
  hyperplastic arteriolosclerosis and, 514–515, *515*
  in atherosclerosis, 506
  in hyperaldosteronism, 1157
  in pheochromocytoma, 1165
  in preeclampsia 1083, *1084*
  malignant, 511, 982–984, *983,* 983t
  oral contraceptives and, 416
  pathogenesis of, 511–514, *512, 514*
  portal, 855–856, *855*
    esophageal varices with, 783
    idiopathic, 882
  pulmonary, 704–706, *706*
    in atrial septal defect, 594
  renovascular, 511, 512–513
  retinopathy with, 1370
  salt-sensitive, *512,* 513
  sodium retention in, 513
  vasoconstriction in, 513–514, *514*
Hyperthermia, 434–435, 1285
  malignant, 1285
Hyperthyroidism, 1131–1132, 1131t, *1132*
  clinical course of, 1131–1132
  heart in, 587
  in Graves disease, 1136, 1138
  in subacute thyroiditis, 1136
  with goiter, 1140
Hypertrophic cardiomyopathy, 581–583, *582*
Hypertrophic gastropathy, 797–798, *797*
Hypertrophic osteoarthropathy, 320, 321t
Hypertrophy, 31, 32–35, *34*
  definition of, 466
  vs. hyperplasia, 32
Hyperuricemia, nephrolithiasis with, 980
  nephropathy with, 979–980, *980*
Hyperviscosity syndrome, 125
  in lymphoplasmacytic lymphoma, 667
Hypoalbuminemia, in hepatic failure, 852
Hypocalcemia, in acute pancreatitis, 907
  in renal osteodystrophy, 1229
  in vitamin D deficiency, 444, 444t
Hypochondrogenesis, 1220t
Hypochondroplasia, 1220t
Hypogammaglobulinemia, of common variable immunodeficiency, 233–234
Hypoglycemia, CNS effects of, 1341–1342
Hypogonadism, female, 173, 174–176, *175*
  male, 174, 1016
Hypokalemia, in hyperaldosteronism, 1157
Hypoparathyroidism, 1151
Hypophysis. See *Pituitary gland.*
Hypopituitarism, 1127–1129, *1128*
Hypoplasia, definition of, 466
  renal, 936–937
  thymic (DiGeorge syndrome), 173, 235, 691
Hypoplastic left heart syndrome, 597
Hypoproteinemia, in edema, 115
Hypospadias, 1012
Hypothalamus, suprasellar tumors of, 1129
Hypothermia, 435
Hypothyroidism, 1132–1133, 1132t
  in Hashimoto thyroiditis, 1135
  in Turner syndrome, 175
  myocardial toxicity of, 587
  myopathy in, 1287
  with goiter, 1140
Hypotonia, congenital, 1285
Hypotrophy, definition of, 466
Hypoventilation syndrome, obesity and, 454
Hypovitaminosis A, 1361
Hypovolemic shock, 118, 134, 134t
Hypoxanthine guanine phosphoribosyl transferase, deficiency of, 1254–1255
Hypoxia, in cell injury, 4
  in cerebrovascular disease, 1307–1310
  p53 gene activation in, 292
  vs. ischemia, 4

I
I-cell disease, 155t
Ichthyosis, 1193, *1193*
Icterus, 848
α-L-Iduronidase, deficiency of (Hurler mucopolysaccharidosis), 155t, 160
L-Iduronosulfate sulfatase, deficiency of (Hunter mucopolysaccharidosis), 155t, 159–160
Ileostomy, colitis with, 812
Immersion blast injury, 435
Immotile cilia syndrome, 27
Immune complexes. See also *Hypersensitivity reaction(s), type III (immune complex–mediated).*
  in vasculitis, 516
  renal deposition of, 943–946, 943t, *944, 946.* See also *Glomerulonephritis.*
  tissue deposition of, 202–203, *202, 203*
Immune surveillance, 315
Immune system, 188–195. See also *Lymphocyte(s).*
  B lymphocytes of, 190, *190*
  cytokines of, 191–192
  deficiency syndromes of, 231–251. See also *Acquired immunodeficiency syndrome (AIDS).*
    primary, 231–236, *232,* 233t
  dendritic cells of, 191
  histocompatibility antigens and, 193–195, *193, 194,* 195t
  hypersensitivity reactions of, 195–211. See also *Hypersensitivity reaction(s).*
  in berylliosis, 734
  in Epstein-Barr virus infection, 371
  in filariasis, 397–398
  in giardiasis, 359
  in glomerulonephritis, 946
  in Graves disease, 1137
  in Hashimoto's thyroiditis, 1132, 1134–1135
  in hepatitis, 868
  in idiopathic pulmonary fibrosis, 735
  in *Leishmania* infection, 392
  in leprosy, 386
  in membranous glomerulonephritis, 959–960
  in minimal change disease, 955–956
  in multiple sclerosis, 1326
  in nephritis, 977–978, *977*
  in poststreptococcal (proliferative) glomerulonephritis, 949–950, *950*
  in rheumatic fever, 572
  in rheumatoid arthritis, 216, 1249–1250, *1250*
Immune system *(Continued)*
  in sarcoidosis, 734
  in systemic lupus erythematosus, 219–220, *219*
  in trisomy 21, 171
  in type I diabetes mellitus, *915,* 916
  in vasculitis, 203–204, *203, 204,* 516
  in vitamin A deficiency, 441
  infectious agent evasion of, 344, 344t
  intestinal, 804
  isotype switching in, 234
  macrophages of, 190–191
  microbe evasion of, 344, 344t
  natural, 191, *191, 192*
  natural killer cells of, 191, *191, 192*
  self-antigens in, 211–231. See also *Autoimmune diseases.*
  T lymphocytes of, 189, *189, 190*
  tolerance and, 212–214, *213*
  vitamin A effects on, 441
Immune tolerance, 212–214, *213*
  central, 212, *213*
  peripheral, 212, *213,* 214–215
Immune-mediated hemolytic anemia, 620–621, 620t. See also *Anemia, hemolytic, immune-mediated.*
Immunocytochemistry, in tumor diagnosis, 323–324, *323*
Immunodeficiency, 231–251. See also *Acquired immunodeficiency syndrome (AIDS).*
  B-cell lymphoma and, 661
  pneumonia and, 726, 726t
  primary, 231–236, *232,* 233t
Immunoglobulins, absence of, 232–233
  deficiency of, 233–234
  genes for, in lymphoma, 285
  in amyloidosis, 663
  in heavy-chain disease, 663
  in leukocyte adhesion, 57, 57t, *58*
  in multiple myeloma, 665–666, *665*
Immunoglobulin A (IgA), in dermatitis herpetiformis, 1205, *1205*
  in Henoch-Schönlein purpura, 965–966
  isolated deficiency of, 234
  mesangial deposition of, 961–962, *961*
Immunoglobulin A (IgA) nephropathy, 961–962, *961,* 965t
Immunoglobulin E (IgE), in asthma, 713, *714*
  in type I hypersensitivity reaction, 196–197, *197*
  in urticaria, 1194
Immunoglobulin G (IgG), deficiency of, 234–235
  Fc fragment of, in phagocytosis, 62
  in multiple myeloma, 665–666, *665*
  in pemphigus vulgaris, 1202, *1203*
  M component, 663
Immunoglobulin M (IgM), antigen binding to, 190
  elevated levels of, 234–235
  in Waldenström macroglobulinemia, 663
Immunophenotype, in acute lymphoblastic leukemia/lymphoma, 655, 655t, *657,* 657t
  in acute myeloblastic leukemia, *657*
  in adult T-cell leukemia/lymphoma, 656t
  in angiocentric lymphoma, 656t
  in Burkitt lymphoma, 655t, 662
  in chronic lymphocytic leukemia, 655t, 659
  in diffuse large B-cell lymphoma, 655t, 661
  in follicular lymphoma, 655t, 660, *660*
  in hairy cell leukemia, 656t, 668

Immunophentype *(Continued)*
in large granular lymphocytic leukemia, 656t
in lymphoplasmacytic lymphoma, 656t
in mantle cell lymphoma, 656t, 668
in marginal zone lymphoma, 656t
in multiple myeloma, 655t
in mycosis fungoides, 656t
in peripheral T-cell lymphoma unspecified, 656t, 669–670
in plasmacytoma, 655t
in Sézary syndrome, 656t
in small lymphocytic lymphoma, 655t, 659
Immunoproliferative small intestinal disease, 837
Immunosuppression. See also *Acquired immunodeficiency syndrome (AIDS).*
carcinogen-induced, 318
in transplantation, 210
Immunosurveillance, 318–319
Immunotactoid glomerulonephritis, 968
Imperforate anus, 804
Impetigo, 1210
Inappropriate secretion of antidiuretic hormone, 1129
Inclusions, cytomegalic, 376, *376*
in herpesvirus infection, 360, *360*
Inclusion conjunctivitis, 362
Inclusion cyst, 1181
Inclusion-body myositis, 229, *230,* 231
Infant. See also *Children.*
Apgar score in, 463–464, 463t
appropriate for gestational age, 460–461, *461*
birth injury in, 464
birth weight of, 460–461, *461*
congenital heart disease in, 591–597, 592t, *593–597.* See also specific diseases.
congenital malformation in, 464–470, *465,* 466t, 467t, *468, 469.* See also *Malformation(s), congenital.*
cystic fibrosis in, 477–481, *478–481*
cytomegalovirus infection in, 376
fibrous tumors in, 484
galactosemia in, 476–477, *477*
gestational age of, 460–461, *461*
hemangioma in, 483, *483*
hemolytic disease of, 200, 473–475, *474, 475,* 849
inborn errors of metabolism in, 475–481. See also specific disorders.
infection in, 470–471, *470*
intrauterine growth retardation of, 461–462, *462*
large for gestational age, 460–461, *461*
Listeria infection in, 378
lymphangiectasis in, 483–484
lymphangioma in, 483–484
mortality rate for, 459–460, 460t
phenylketonuria in, 475–476, *476*
postterm, 460
preterm, 460, 462–463, *463*
respiratory distress syndrome (hyaline membrane disease) in, 471–473, *472*
sepsis in, 471
small for gestational age, 460–462, *461, 462*
sudden death syndrome in, 481–482, 482t
teratoma in, 484, *484*
tumors in, 482–489
benign, 483–484, *483, 484*
malignant, 484–491, 485t, *486, 487,* 488t, *489*
Infarct of Zahn, 882
Infarction, 130, 132–137. See also *Ischemia.*
blood supply and, 133
cerebral, 1307–1310, *1309*
hepatic, 881–882, *882*
hypoxia and, 133
incomplete, 1310
intestinal, 820–823, *821–823*
mucosal, 822, *822,* 823
mural, 822, 823
transmural, 821–822, *822,* 823
myocardial, 554–564. See also *Myocardial infarction.*
oxygen tension and, 133
pulmonary, *133,* 703–704, *704*
red, 132, *133,* 1308, 1309–1310
renal, *133,* 987–988
septic, 132
spinal, 1310
splenic, *133,* 689–690, *689*
white, 132, *133,* 1308–1309, *1309*
Infection, 329–399. See also specific infection, e.g., *Pneumonia.*
agents of, bacterial, 332, 332t, 334t, 335, *335,* 341–344, *342, 343*
anaerobic, 369–370
gram-positive, 365–370, *366–369*
bacteriophage, 332
categories of, 331–338, 332t
chlamydial, 332t, 335
diagnosis of, 344–345, 345t
ectoparasite, 337–338, *338*
emerging, 331, *331,* 331t
fungal, 332t, 335, *335, 336*
helminth, 332t, 336–337
immune evasion by, 344, 344t
mycoplasmal, 332t, 335
prion, 332
protozoan, 332t, 335–336, *337,* 337t
rickettsial, 332t, 335
transmission of, 338–340, *339*
viral, 332, 332t, 333t, 340–341, *341*
atherosclerosis and, 509
bloodstream invasion by, 338
cardiac, 572–576, *575.* See also *Endocarditis.*
childhood, 370–375
Bordetella pertussis in, 374–375, *374*
Corynebacterium diphtheriae in, 375, *375*
Epstein-Barr virus in, 371–373, *372*
measles virus in, 370, *370*
mumps virus in, 370–371
poliovirus in, 373
varicella-zoster virus in, 373–374, *374*
clostridial, 368–369, *369*
contagious, 339
diagnosis of, 344–345, 345t
dissemination of, 338–339, *339*
fetal, 338–339
gastrointestinal, 344, 353–359
Ancylostoma duodenale in, 394–395
bacterial, 355–358, *355, 357*
barriers to, 353–354
Campylobacter in, 355–356
Entamoeba histolytica in, 358–359, *358*
Giardia lamblia in, 359, *359*
Necator americanus in, 394–395
parasitic, 358–359, *358, 359*
Salmonella in, 356–357, *357*
Shigella in, 355, *355*
Taenia solium in, 395–396, *395*
Vibrio cholerae in, 357–358, *357*
Infection *(Continued)*
viral, 354–355
Yersinia in, 356
hemorrhage with, 634
host barriers to, 338
in acquired immunodeficiency syndrome, 247–248, 247t
in adrenocortical insufficiency, 1160–1161, *1160*
in bronchiectasis, 716
in bronchitis, 712, *712*
in Bruton agammaglobulinemia, 233
in cell injury, 4
in common variable immunodeficiency, 234
in cystic fibrosis, 479, 480, 481, *481*
in hairy cell leukemia, 669
in hyper IgM syndrome, 234
in intrauterine growth retardation, 461
in isolated IgA deficiency, 234
in lung transplant patient, 741
in multiple myeloma, 665
in nephrotic syndrome, 953
in severe combined immunodeficiency disease, 235
inflammatory response to, 345–346, *345–347.* See also *Inflammation.*
nosocomial, 719
opportunistic, 334t, 375–383
Aspergillus in, 380, *381*
Candida spp. in, 378–379, *379*
Cryptococcus neoformans in, 379–380, *380*
Cryptosporidium parvum in, 382, *382*
cytomegalovirus in, 376, *376*
Legionella pneumophila in, 377–378
Listeria monocytogenes in, 378
Mucor in, 380–381, *381*
Pneumocystis carinii in, 381–382, *382*
Pseudomonas aeruginosa in, 376–377, *377*
Toxoplasma gondii in, 382–383
pathogenesis of, 340–344, *341–343*
historical studies of, 330–331, 330t
perinatal, 470–471, *470*
placental-fetal transmission of, 338, 470, *470*
respiratory, 347–353, 717–721. See also *Pneumonia.*
bacterial, 348–352, *350, 351*
Coccidioides immitis in, 353, *353*
fungal, 352–353, *353*
Haemophilus influenzae in, 348–349
Histoplasma capsulatum in, 352, *353*
influenza viruses in, 348
Mycobacterium tuberculosis in, 349–352, *350–352*
viral, 347–348, *347*
scar formation in, 347, *347*
secondary, 341
sexually transmitted, 359–365, 360t, 1038–1040, 1038t, *1039*
Calymmatobacterium donovani in, 360t
Chlamydia trachomatis in, 360t, 361–362, 361t
Haemophilus ducreyi in, 360t
herpesviruses in, 359–361, *360,* 360t
Neisseria gonorrhoeae in, 360t, 362
Phthirus pubis in, 360t
Treponema pallidum in, 360t, 362–364, *363*
Trichomonas vaginalis in, 360t, 364–365, *365*
sites of, 338, *339*

Infection *(Continued)*
  slow virus, 341
  staphylococcal, 365–367, *366, 367*
  streptococcal, 367–368, *368*
  TORCH, 470
  tropical, 383–399
    Chlamydia trachomatis in, 385
    dengue virus in, 383
    Leishmania in, 391–393, *392*
    Mycobacterium leprae in, 385–386, *387*
    Onchocerca volvulus in, 398–399, *399*
    Schistosoma in, 396–397, *396, 397*
    Trypanosoma in, 393–394
  vector-borne, 334t, 335, 339–340
    Babesia microti in, 391, *391*
    Borrelia in, 388–389, *388*
    Brugia malayi in, 397–398
    Onchocerca volvulus in, 398–399, *399*
    Plasmodium falciparum in, 389–391, *390, 391*
    Rickettsia spp. in, 383–385, *384, 385,* 385t
    Taenia solium in, 395–396, *395*
    Trichinella spiralis in, 394, *395*
    Wuchereria bancrofti in, 397–398, *398*
    Yersinia pestis in, 387–388
  viral. See also specific viruses.
    abortive, 340
    in subacute thyroiditis, 1135–1136, *1136*
    latent, 340
    persistent, 340
  with agranulocytosis, 647
  with burns, 434
  wound healing and, 110
  zoonotic, 340
Infectious arthritis, 1253
Infectious mononucleosis, 371–373, *372,* 759t. See also *Epstein-Barr virus (EBV).*
Inferior vena caval syndrome, 530
Inflammation, 50–87
  acute, 52–65, *52*
    abscess formation in, 78, *78*
    angiogenesis in, 55
    chemical mediators of, 65–78, *66,* 77t, 78t
      arachidonic acid metabolites as, 70–72, *71,* 71t, *72*
      chemokines as, 74, 74t
      cytokines as, 54, 73–74, *74*
      lysosomal granules as, 76, *76*
      neuropeptides as, 77
      nitric oxide as, 75–76, *75*
      oxygen-derived free radicals as, 76–77
      plasma proteases as, 67–70, *67, 68*
      platelet-activating factor as, 72, *72*
      vasoactive amines as, 66–67, *66*
    endothelial retraction in, 54
    fibrinous, 84, *85*
    fibrosis in, 78, *78,* 84
    immediate sustained response in, 55
    immediate transient response in, 54, *55*
    leukocyte extravasation in, 55–62, *56,* 57t, *58–61*
    leukocyte-induced tissue injury in, 64, 64t
    outcomes of, 78–79, *78, 79*
    phagocytosis in, 62–64, *63*
    resolution of, 78, *78, 79,* 84
    serous, 84, *85*
    transcytosis in, 54
    treatment of, 71–72
    ulceration in, 85, *85*
    vascular changes in, 53–55, *53–55*
    vesiculovacuolar organelle in, 54
Inflammation *(Continued)*
  chronic, 79–84, 346–347, *347*
    definition of, 79
    eosinophils in, 82, *82*
    etiology of, 79
    granulomatous, 83–84, *83*
    histologic features of, 79, *80*
    lymphatics in, 84
    lymphocytes in, 82, *82*
    mast cells in, 82
    mononuclear infiltration in, 79–82, *80, 81,* 81t
    suppurative, 84–85, *85*
    systemic effects of, 85–86, *86*
    ulcerations in, 85
  cytopathic-cytoproliferative, 346, *346*
  general features of, 50–52, *51*
  granulomatous, 346
  historical studies of, 52
  in infarction, 132
  mononuclear, 345–346, *346*
  necrotizing, 346
    in *Pseudomonas* infection, 377, *377*
  suppurative (polymorphonuclear), 345, *345*
Inflammatory bowel disease, 815–820. See also *Crohn disease; Ulcerative colitis.*
Inflammatory demyelinating polyradiculoneuropathy, 1275–1276
Influenza virus A, 333t, 348
Influenza virus B, 333t, 348
Influenza virus C, 348
Initiators, in chemical carcinogenesis, 306, *307*
Injury. See *Trauma.*
INK4 proteins, 283
Inositol-lipid pathway, for signal transduction, *93,* 95
Insect bites, 1210–1211
Insecticides, 422–423, 423t
Insertional mutagenesis, of protooncogenes, 278
Insulin. See also *Diabetes mellitus.*
  physiology of, 914–915, *914*
  receptors for, 915, 918
  resistance to, in obesity, 454
    in Turner syndrome, 175–176
    in type II diabetes mellitus, 918
Insulinoma, 926–927, *927*
Insulitis, 916
Integrins, in leukocyte adhesion, 57, 57t, *58*
  of extracellular matrix, 100–101, *101, 103*
  receptors for, 101
Intelligence quotient (IQ), in fragile X syndrome, 177
  in neurofibromatosis, 164
  in trisomy 21, 170
Intercalated discs, 544
Intercellular adhesion molecule 1 (ICAM-1), 57, 57t, 59
  rhinovirus binding to, 347, *347*
Intercellular signaling, 92–95, *93–95*
  autocrine, *91,* 92
  cell surface receptors in, 92–93, *93, 94*
  endocrine, *91,* 92
  paracrine, *91,* 92
Interferon-γ (IFN-γ), in delayed-type hypersensitivity, 205–206, *205*
  in inflammation, 82, *82*
Interleukins, 73
Interleukin-1 (IL-1), in febrile state, 86
  in inflammation, 73–74, *74,* 77t
  in rheumatoid arthritis, 1250–1251
Interleukin-2 (IL-2), in delayed-type hypersensitivity, *205,* 206
Interleukin-5 (IL-5), in Hodgkin disease, 674
Interleukin-6 (IL-6), in febrile state, 86
  in hepatocyte regeneration, 33, *33*
  in multiple myeloma, 664
Interleukin-12 (IL-12), in delayed-type hypersensitivity, 205, *205*
Interlobar artery, emboli of, 986, *987*
Intermediate filaments, abnormalities of, 27–28
Internalins, of *Listeria monocytogenes,* 378
Interstitial pneumonitis, 721–722
  desquamative, 736–737, *737*
Interstitium, pulmonary, 698
  renal, 934–935
Intestinalization, in pernicious anemia, 625
Intestine, 802–838
  adenoma of, 827, *827*
  adhesions of, 826
  anatomy of, 802
  angiodysplasia of, 823
  atresia of, 804
  blood supply of, 802
  carcinoid tumor of, 835–837, *836,* 837t
  carcinoma of, *265,* 827, *827,* 831–835, *832, 834, 835,* 835t
    adenoma development in, 830–831
    adenomatous precursors of, 831–833, *832*
    APC gene in, 287t, 292–293, 297, *297*
    clinical features of, 834–835
    DCC gene in, 293
    distribution of, 833–834, *834*
    epidemiology of, 833
    fat intake and, 456
    geographic factors in, 273, *273*
    hepatic metastases from, 891, *891*
    incidence of, *272*
    metastatic spread of, 835, *835,* 835t
    molecular genetics of, 832–833, *832*
    molecular model of, 297, *297*
    mortality rates with, *272*
    napkin ring constriction in, 834, *834*
    staging of, 835, 835t
    vitamin deficiencies and, 451
  celiac disease of, 813, *813*
  congenital anomalies of, 804–805
  diarrheal disease of, 805–812. See also *Diarrhea.*
  disaccharidase deficiency in, 815
  diverticular disease of, 823–825, *824*
  duplication of, 804
  endocrine cells of, 803–804
  enterocolitis of, 805–812, 806t
    after bone marrow transplantation, 811
    antibiotic-associated, 809–810, *810*
    collagenous, 810
    diversion, 812
    drug-induced, 811
    in acquired immunodeficiency syndrome, 811
    infectious, 806–810, 807t, 808t, *809*
    lymphocytic, 810
    necrotizing, 809
    neutropenic, 811–812
    parasitic, 810–811
    protozoal, 810–811, *811*
    radiation-induced, 811
  familial adenomatous polyposis of, *831,* 845, 1445
  gluten sensitivity of, 813, *813,* 961
  hemorrhoids of, 530, 823
  hernia of, 826
  Hirschsprung disease of, 805
  idiopathic inflammation of, 815–820. See also *Crohn disease; Ulcerative colitis.*
  infarction of, 820–823, *821–823*

Intestine *(Continued)*
mucosal, 822, *822*, 823
mural, 822, 823
transmural, 821–822, *822*, 823
intussusception of, 804, 826
ischemic disease of, 820–823, *821–823*
lymphoid tissue of, 804
lymphoma of, 837–838
malabsorption syndromes of, 812–815, 812t, *813*
malrotation of, 804
Meckel diverticulum of, 804–805, *805*
mesenchymal tumor of, 838
mucosa of, 802–803, *803*
necrotizing inflammation of, 809
obstruction of, 825–826, *825*, 825t
papilloma of, 261, *261*
peristalsis of, 804
polyp of, 261, *262*
polyps of, 827–831, *827–831*
regenerative capacity of, 803
stenosis of, 804
stricture of, 822, *823*
transplantation of, 811
tumors of, 826–838, 826t
vascular disorders of, 820–823, *821–823*
vasculature of, 802
villi of, 802–803, *803*
volvulus of, 826
Whipple disease of, 814–815, *814*
Intima, 494, *494*
thickening of, 497, *497*, 501. See also *Atherosclerosis.*
Intraepithelial neoplasia, of cervix, 1049–1051, *1051, 1052*
of prostate gland, 1031
of vulva, 1043, *1043*
Intrauterine growth retardation (IUGR), 461–462, *462*
Intrinsic factor, 788
autoantibodies to, 791
Intussusception, intestinal, 804, 826
Invasin, of *Yersinia pseudotuberculosis,* 356
Iodide, thyroid inhibition by, 1131
Iodine, deficiency of, 452t
in Graves disease, 1138
Iodine transporter, antibodies to, in Hashimoto thyroiditis, 1134
Ion channel myopathy, 1285
Ionizing radiation. See *Radiation.*
Iris, hamartoma of, 164
in neurofibromatosis, 164
melanoma of, 1367
Iritis, in sarcoidosis, 735
Iron, absorption of, 628–629, *628*
hepatic accumulation of, 873–875, *874*
in free radical generation, 12, *13*
metabolism of, 627–628, *627, 628*
myocardial toxicity of, 587
requirements for, 628, 629
systemic overload of, 43
Iron deficiency anemia, 118, 452t, 627–630, *627*, 627t, *628, 630*
Irritation fibroma, of buccal mucosa, 758
Ischemia, *3*, 7–12
ATP depletion in, 5
atrophy with, 35, 36
calcium imbalance in, 6, *6*
cardiac, 550–564. See also *Ischemic heart disease; Myocardial infarction.*
cerebral, 1307–1310, *1309*
focal, 1308–1310, *1309*
global, 1307–1308
free radicals in, 5–6, *6*
Ischemia *(Continued)*
intestinal, 820–823, *821–823*
irreversible, 8–11, *8–11*
membrane permeability defects in, 6
mitochondrial damage in, 6–7, *7*
renal, 969–971, *969–971*, 986
reversible, 7–8, *8–10*
vs. hypoxia, 4
Ischemia/reperfusion injury, 11–12
Ischemic heart disease, *3*, 550–564. See also *Myocardial infarction.*
angina pectoris in, 554
chronic, 563, 564
epidemiology of, 551
pathogenesis of, 551–554
fixed obstructions in, 551
plaque change in, 551–553, *552*
thrombus in, 553
vasoconstriction in, 553–554, 553t
sudden cardiac death in, 564
Islet cells, 911–913, *912*
amyloidosis of, *921*, 922
in type I diabetes mellitus, 916
Islet-cell tumor, 926–928, *927*
Isochromosome, 169–170, *169*
Isochromosome 12, in germ cell tumors, 1019
Isoimmunization, ABO, 473
Rh, 473–475, *474, 475*
Isolated IgA deficiency, 234
Isospora belli, 337t
Isotype switching, in immune response, 234
Ito cells, 847
in cirrhosis, 254, *854*

J
Jagziekte, 747
JAK (Janus kinases)/STAT (signal transducers and activators of transcription) pathway, *93*, 94–95
Jaundice, 848
in cholestasis, 851–852, *852*
in Rh isoimmunization, 473–474
neonatal, 850
pathophysiology of, 849–851, 850t
physiologic, 463, 850
JC virus, 333t
CNS infection with, 1321, *1322*
Joint(s), 1246–1259
crystal arthropathies of, 1253–1257. See also *Gout.*
cyst of, 1258
degenerative disease of, 1246–1257. See also *Arthritis.*
ganglion of, 1258
hemosiderin deposition in, 874
in alkaptonuria, 162
in Ehlers-Danlos syndromes, 150
in Marfan syndrome, 149
in systemic lupus erythematosus, 222
in systemic sclerosis, 228
normal, 1246
osteoarthritis of, 1246–1248, *1247, 1248*
rheumatoid arthritis of, 1248–1251. See also *Rheumatoid arthritis.*
sarcoma of, 1266–1267, *1267*
seronegative spondyloarthropathy of, 1252–1253
synovial, 1246
villonodular synovitis of, 1258–1259, *1258*
Joint mice, in osteoarthritis, 1247
Jones criteria, in rheumatic fever, 570
Juvenile intestinal polyps, 828, *828*
Juvenile rheumatoid arthritis, 1251–1252
Juxtaglomerular apparatus, 934

K
KAI-1 gene, 305
Kala-azar, 391–393, *392*
Kallikrein, 69
in inflammation, *68*, 69
Kaposi sarcoma, 535–537, *536*
in acquired immunodeficiency syndrome, 248–249, *249*
Kaposi sarcoma herpesvirus, 248–249, *249*
Kaposi varicelliform eruption, 361
Kartagener syndrome, 27, 716
sinusitis in, 763
Karyolysis, in necrosis, *9*, 16
Karyorrhexis, in necrosis, *9*, 16
Karyotype, 165–168, *166–168*, 182
Kawasaki syndrome (mucocutaneous lymph node syndrome), 517t, 521
Kayser-Fleischer rings, in Wilson disease, 875
Kearns-Sayre syndrome, 1287
Keloid, 110, *110*
Kennedy syndrome, 1338
Keratan sulfate, in mucopolysaccharidosis, 159–160
Keratin, staining for, 323, *323*
Keratinocytes, 1171, *1172*
Keratitis, 1362–1363
disciform, 1362–1363
epithelial, herpes, 361
stromal, herpes, 361
syphilitic, 364
Keratoacanthoma, 1181, *1182*
Keratoconjunctivitis sicca, 769. See also *Sjögren syndrome.*
Keratoconus, in trisomy 21, 1360
Keratomalacia, 1361
Keratoses, actinic, 1184, *1185*
follicular, inverted, 1180
seborrheic, 1179–1180, *1180*
Kernicterus, 474, 849
Ketoacidosis, diabetic, 924–926, *925*
Ketonemia, diabetic, 926
Ketonuria, diabetic, 926
Kidney. See also *Renal* entries.
agenesis of, 936
amyloidosis of, 255, *255*, 256, 968
dialysis-associated, 253, 253t
analgesic-induced injury to, 416, *977*, 978–979, *979*, 979t
angiomyolipoma of, 991
atheroembolic disease of, 986, *987*
autosomal dominant polycystic disease of, 937–940, *938, 939*, 941t
autosomal recessive polycystic disease of, 940, 941t
blood supply of, 931
blood vessels of, 931. See also *Renal artery(ies).*
calcium deposition in, 980
calyces of, 931
carcinoma of, 991–994, *992–994*. See also *Renal cell carcinoma.*
congenital anomalies of, 936–942, 941t
cortex of, 931
necrosis of, 987, *987*
cystic disease of, 937–942, 941t
autosomal dominant, 937–940, *938, 939*, 941t
autosomal recessive, 940, 941t
dialysis-associated, 941, 941t

Kidney (*Continued*)
dysplastic, 937, *938*
medullary, 940–941, *941*
simple, 941t, 942
dialysis of, 941, 941t, 964
amyloidosis with, 253, 253t
disease of, analgesic-induced, 416, *977,* 978–979, *979,* 979t
clinical manifestations of, 935–936, 936t
congenital, 936–942, *938, 939*
cystic, 937–942, 941t
glomerular, 942–968, 942t. See also *Glomerulonephritis; Glomerulus (glomeruli).*
neoplastic, 990–994, *992.* See also *Renal cell carcinoma.*
obstructive, 988–990, *988–990,* 989t
skeletal manifestations of, 1229
tubular, 968–981. See also *Acute tubular necrosis (ATN); Tubulointerstitial nephritis.*
vascular, 981–988. See also *Hypertension; Renal artery(ies).*
dysplasia of, cystic, 937, *938*
ectopic, 937
failure of, acute, 935
acute tubular necrosis in, 969–971, *969–971*
chronic, 935, 936, 936t
hyperparathyroidism in, 636–637, 964, 1151
in thrombotic microangiopathy in, 985–988, *985, 987*
metastatic calcification in, 45
postpartum, 986
fibroma of, 991
glomeruli of, 931–934, *932–934.* See also *Glomerulonephritis; Glomerulus (glomeruli).*
hamartoma of, 991
horseshoe, 937
hyaline arteriosclerosis of, 981–982, *982*
hypoplasia of, 936–937
in bacterial endocarditis, 966
in diabetes mellitus, 922–923, *923, 924,* 966–968, *967*
in essential mixed cryoglobulinemia, 968
in gout, 1256, 1257
in Henoch-Schönlein purpura, 965–966
in hypertension, 512, *512*
in left-sided heart failure, 549
in multiple myeloma, 665, 968, 980–981, *981,* 981t
in plasma cell dyscrasia, 968
in polyarteritis nodosa, 968
in preeclampsia, 1083, *1084*
in preterm infant, 463
in right-sided heart failure, 550
in shock, 136, 137
in sickle cell disease, 986–987
in systemic lupus erythematosus, 220–222, *220, 221, 961, 962,* 965
in systemic sclerosis, 228–229
in vitamin D metabolism, 441–442
in Wegener granulomatosis, 523, 968
infarction of, *133,* 987–988
interstitium of, 934–935. See also *Tubulointerstitial nephritis.*
ischemic injury to, 886, 969–971, *969–971*
medulla of, 931
cystic disease of, 940–941, *940,* 941t
normal, 931–935, *932–934*
oncocytoma of, 991
papillary adenoma of, 991
pyelonephritis of, 972–975, *972–975.* See also *Pyelonephritis.*

Kidney (*Continued*)
radiation injury to, 429
scars of, in pyelonephritis, 976, *975*
stones of, 936, 989–990, 989t, *990*
in hyperparathyroidism, 1150
in hyperuricemia, 979–980, 980, *980*
structure of, 931–935, *932–934*
transplantation of, rejection of, acute, 209–210, *209*
hyperacute, 207–208
tubules of, 934, 935–936
disease of. See *Acute tubular necrosis (ATN); Tubulointerstitial nephritis.*
tumors of, 990–994. See also *Renal cell carcinoma.*
Kimmelstiel-Wilson disease, 967
Kinases, cyclin-dependent, in cell cycle regulation, 95–96, *96*
Kinin system, in inflammation, *68,* 69
Kininase, 69
Kininogens, 69
KiSS-1 gene, 305
Klatskin tumor, 900
Klebsiella, 334t
Klinefelter syndrome (47,XXY), 174, 1016
Knockout mice, 140
FBN1, 148–149
Koch's postulates, 330
Koebner phenomenon, 1199
Koilocytosis, 1042
Koilocytotic atypia, 1042
Korsakoff syndrome, 447, 1341
Krabbe disease, 155t, 1339
K-*ras* gene, in colorectal carcinoma, *832,* 833
in pancreatic carcinoma, 910
Krukenberg tumor, 801
Kupffer cells, 847
Kuru plaques, 1324, *1325*
Kwashiorkor, 437–439, *438,* 438t

L
Labile cells, 91
Laceration, 432, *432*
Lacis cells, 934
Lacrimal gland, lymphocytic infiltration of. See *Sjögren syndrome.*
Lactase, deficiency of, 815
Lactate dehydrogenase, in testicular germ cell tumors, 1023–1024
Lactation, *1094,* 1095
Lactoferrin, in free radical inactivation, 13
in phagocytosis, 64
Lacunar cell, in Hodgkin disease, 671, *671*
Lacunar infarcts, 1313–1314, *1313*
Lafora bodies, 1297
Lambert-Eaton myasthenic syndrome, 1289
in bronchogenic carcinoma, 747
Lambl excrescences, 546, 591
Lamellar bone, 1217–1218, *1217, 1218*
in Paget disease, 1226–1227, *1226*
Laminin, of extracellular matrix, 100, *100, 103*
tumor cell attachment to, 303, *304*
Langerhans cells, 191, 1171, *1171*
ultraviolet light injury to, 1185
Langerhans histiocytosis, 685–686
Large for gestational age infant, 460–461, *461*
Laryngitis, 765
Laryngotracheobronchitis, 348
Bordetella, 374–375, *374*
Larynx, 765–766, *765*
carcinoma of, 765, *766*

Larynx (*Continued*)
inflammation of, 765
papillomatosis of, 766
reactive nodules of, 765
squamous papilloma of, 766, *766*
Late-phase reaction, in asthma, 713
Lattice dystrophy, 1363
LE cells, 219–220
Lead poisoning, 420–421, 421t, *422*
Leber hereditary optic neuropathy, 179–180, *180,* 1287, 1341
Left-to-right cardiac shunt, 593–595, *593, 594*
Legs, bowing of, in vitamin D deficiency, 445, *445*
thrombophlebitis of, 530
varicose veins of, 529–530, *529*
Legionella pneumophila, 334t, 377–378
Legionnaires disease, 377–378
Leigh disease, 1340–1341
Leiomyoma, 1266
of bladder, 1008
of esophagus, 783
of intestine, 838
of stomach, 802
of uterus, *264, 271,* 1063–1064, *1063*
Leiomyosarcoma, 1266
of intestine, 838
of stomach, 802
of uterus, *271,* 1064–1065, *1064*
Leishmania braziliensis, 337t
Leishmania donovani, 332t, 337t
Leishmania mexicana, 337t
Leishmania tropica, 337t
Leishmaniasis, 391–393, *392*
cutaneous, 392–393
mucocutaneous, 392
visceral, 392
Leishmanin test, 392
Length polymorphism analysis, in genetic disorders, 185–186, *186*
Lens, cataracts of, 1367–1368
in galactosemia, 476, 477
nuclear sclerosis of, 1367
Lentiginous, definition of, 1173
Lentigo, 1174
Leontiasis ossea, in Paget disease, 1227
Leprosy, 83t, 385–386, *387*
Leptin, in obesity, 454
Leptospira spp., 334t
Lesch-Nyhan syndrome, 148, 1254–1255
Letterer-Siwe disease, 685
Leukemia, c-*abl* gene in, 282
hairy cell, 656t, 668–669, *669*
in trisomy 21, 171
incidence of, *272*
lymphoblastic, acute, 485t, 654–658, 655t, *657,* 657
lymphocytic, chronic, 655t, 658–659, *658, 659*
definition of, 651
minimal residual disease monitoring of, 324
MLL gene in, 285, 286t
myelogenous, acute, *657,* 675–678, 676t, *676*
chronic, 680–682, *680*
c-*abl-bcr* gene in, 285, *285,* 286t
oncogenes in, 280
oral manifestations of, 759t
radiation-induced, 426–427
Leukemia/lymphoma, lymphoblastic, acute, 654–658, 655t, *657,* 657t
T-cell, adult, 656t, 670
Leukemoid reaction, 86, 648

Leukocyte(s), 645–688
activation of, *60,* 62
adhesion of, *56,* 57–61, 57t, *58*
apoptosis of, 64
chemotaxis of, *60,* 61, *61*
deficiency of, 646–647
development of, *603*
extravasation of, 55–62, *56*
hydrogen peroxide–deficient, 63–64
margination of, 53, 56–57, *56*
neoplastic proliferations of, 650–686. See also *Leukemia; Lymphoma.*
pavementing of, *56,* 57
phagocytosis by, 62–64, *63*
pseudopod of, 61, *61*
reactive proliferations of, 647–648, *648,* 648t, *649*
rolling of, *56,* 57
Leukocyte adhesion deficiency, 60, 64, 65t
Leukocyte adhesion molecules, 57–61, 57t, *58,* 62
Leukocytoclastic angiitis, 517t, 521–522, *522*
Leukocytosis, 647–648, *648,* 648t, *649*
in chronic myelogenous leukemia, 681, *681*
in inflammation, 86
Leukodystrophy, 1339–1340, *1340*
metachromatic, 155t, 1340, *1340*
Leukoerythroblastosis, in myelofibrosis with myeloid metaplasia, 684, *684*
Leukomalacia, periventricular, *1300,* 1302
Leukopenia, 86
Leukoplakia, hairy, 758–759
in squamous cell carcinoma, 1185
of oral soft tissues, 759–760, *760*
vulvar, 1040–1041
Leukotrienes, 70–71, *71, 72*
in asthma, 713
in type I hypersensitivity reaction, 198
Lewis, Sir Thomas, 52
Lewy bodies, 1295
in Parkinson disease, 1334, *1334*
Leydig cell tumor, 1024, 1078
Libman-Sacks (noninfective, verrucous) endocarditis, *575,* 576–577, *576*
in systemic lupus erythematosus, 127, 223, *223*
Lice, 1210–1212, *1211*
Lichen planopilaris, 1200
Lichen planus, 759t, 1199–1200, *1199*
Lichen sclerosis, vulvar, 1040–1041, *1041*
Lichenification, 1172
Liddle syndrome, *512,* 513
Li-Fraumeni syndrome, 290
Light-chain glomerulopathy, 968
Light-chain nephropathy, 980–981
Lightning injury, 435
Limb-girdle muscular dystrophy, 1282–1283, 1283t, 1284t
Limit dextrin, in glycogen metabolism, 160
Lindane, 423, 423t
Linear energy transfer, 425
Lines of Zahn, 126
Linitis plastica, 800–801, 802
Lip, pyogenic granuloma of, *532,* 533
Lipid(s), cellular accumulation of, 38, *38,* 39–40, *39, 40*
Lipid bodies, in eicosanoid synthesis, 70
Lipid myopathy, 1286–1287
Lipiduria, in nephrotic syndrome, 953
Lipoarabinomannan, of *Mycobacterium tuberculosis,* 349
Lipoblasts, 1261, *1261*
Lipodystrophy, partial, 959
Lipofuscin, 26
cellular accumulation of, 42, *42*
granules of, 36
neuronal, 1295
Lipoid nephrosis, 954–956, *956, 957,* 965t
Lipoma, 1260–1261
cardiac, 590
esophageal, 783
intestinal, 838
Lipophosphoglycans, of *Leishmania,* 391–392
Lipopolysaccharides, in septic shock, 134–136, *134, 136*
Lipoprotein(s), high-density, atherosclerosis and, 504–505
intermediate-density, metabolism of, 151, *151*
low-density, atherosclerosis and, 505, 505t
hepatic clearance of, 151, *152*
metabolism of, 151–152, *151, 152*
oxidized, 508
receptor for, defects in, atherosclerosis and, 505, 505t
gene for, mutations in, 144, 147t, 152–153, *153*
very low-density, metabolism of, 151, *151*
Lipoprotein(a), atherogenic effects of, 506
Liposarcoma, 1261, *1261*
Lipoteichoic acids, 341–342, *342*
Lipoxins, 71, *71*
Lipoxygenases, in eicosanoid synthesis, 70–71, *71*
Lisch nodules, in neurofibromatosis, 164
LISI gene, 1300
Lissencephaly, 1300
Listeria monocytogenes, 334t, 378
Listeriosis, 378
Lithostathine, in chronic pancreatitis, 908
Liver, 846–891
abscess of, 358–359, 867–868
acetaminophen-induced necrosis of, 416
acinus of, 846, *846*
adenoma of, 887–888, *887*
oral contraceptives and, 416
alcohol-induced disease of, 411–412, *411,* 411t, 869–873. See also *Alcoholic liver disease.*
amebic abscess of, 358–359
amyloidosis of, 255–256
angiosarcoma of, 888
bacterial infection of, 867
barbiturate effects on, 26, *27*
bile canaliculi of, 848
bile formation by, 848–849, *849*
bilirubin processing by, 848–849, *849*
carcinoma of, 888–891, *889, 890*
geographic factors in, 273, *273*
hepatitis B virus and, 313–314
metastatic, 270, *270,* 891, *891*
cardiac sclerosis of, 883
Caroli disease of, 881
cavernous hemangioma of, 886
cells of, 846–848
centrilobular necrosis of, 882–883, *883*
circulatory disorders of, 881–884, *882–884*
cirrhosis of, 853–855, *854.* See also *Cirrhosis.*
congestion of, 116–117, *117*
copper accumulation in, 875
Councilman bodies of, 848
degeneration of, 847
drug-induced disease of, 868–869, 869t
after bone marrow transplantation, 885
Liver *(Continued)*
failure of, 852–856, *854, 855*
fulminant, 867
fatty, 38, *38,* 39, *39,* 847
in alcoholic liver disease, 411, *411,* 869, *870,* 872
in Wilson disease, 875
of pregnancy, 884–885
fibrosis of, 848
congenital, 880, 881
in alcoholic hepatitis, 411–412, *411*
in heart failure, 117
focal nodular hyperplasia of, 886–887, *887*
helminthic infection of, 867–868
hemorrhagic necrosis of, 117, *117*
hemosiderin granules in, 43, *43*
hobnail appearance of, 870, *871*
hyaline inclusions of, 27–28, *28*
hyperplasia of, 886–887, *887*
immune-mediated injury to, 19–20, *20*
in α_1-antitrypsin deficiency, 875–876, *876*
in bone marrow transplantation, 884, *884,* 885–886
in cardiac failure, 882–883, *883*
in congenital syphilis, 364
in cystic fibrosis, 480
in Epstein-Barr virus infection, 373
in galactosemia, 476, *477*
in graft-versus-host disease, 885–886
in hairy cell leukemia, 668
in hemochromatosis, 873–874, *874*
in kwashiorkor, 439
in malaria, 390
in Niemann-Pick disease, 157–158, *157*
in pregnancy, 884–885, *885*
in preterm infant, 463
in Reye syndrome, 869
in right-sided heart failure, 550
in sarcoidosis, 735
in systemic lupus erythematosus, 224
in Wilson disease, 875
infection of, 856–868
bacterial, 867
helminthic, 867–868
parasitic, 867–868
viral. See *Hepatitis.*
inflammation of, 848. See also *Hepatitis.*
iron accumulation in, 873–875, 873t, *874*
microarchitecture of, 846–847, *846, 847*
necrosis of, 117, *117,* 847–848, 852
apoptosis-induced, 847–848
centrilobular, 882–883, *883*
ischemic, 847–848
lytic, 848
zonal distribution of, 848
nodular hyperplasia of, 886–887, *886, 887*
normal, 846–847, *846, 847*
nutmeg, 117, *117,* 883, *883*
parasitic infection of, 867–868
pipe-stem fibrosis of, in *Schistosoma* infection, 397, *397*
polycystic disease of, 880, *880,* 881, 940
pregnancy-associated disease of, 884–885, *885*
pyogenic abscess of, 867–868
regeneration of, 32–33, *32, 33,* 91, 848
sinusoids of, 846–847
occlusion of, 882
stellate cells of, 847
in cirrhosis, 854, *854*
stem cells of, 33
syphilitic gumma of, 364, *364*
toxin-induced disease of, 868–873, 869t

Liver *(Continued)*
- transplantation of, 210
  - complications of, 886
- vinyl chloride effects on, 420
- von Meyenburg complexes of, 880, 881

Lobar atrophy, 1333
Localized nodular tenosynovitis, 1258–1259
Lockjaw, 368
Loeffler endomyocarditis, 584
Loeffler syndrome, 738
Lower motor neuron, 1269–1270, *1270*
Lungs, 697–753. See also *Pulmonary; Respiratory* entries.
- abscess of, 722, *723*
- adenocarcinoma of, 743, 744, *744*
- age-related overdistention of, 710
- alveolar proteinosis of, 739–740, *740*
- alveolar walls of, 698, *698*
- atelectasis of, 699–700, *699*
- blood supply to, 698
- bronchiolitis obliterans organizing pneumonia of, 738, *738*
- brown induration of, 700
- bullae of, 711, *711*
- burns of, 434
- carcinoid tumor of, 747–748, *748*
- carcinoma of, 741–747
  - bronchioloalveolar, 747, *747*
  - cigarette smoking and, 409, 409t
  - classification of, 742–743, *743,* 743t, *744*
  - clinical course of, 745–746, *746,* 746t
  - etiology of, 741–742
  - glutathione-s-transferase in, 307
  - in asbestos workers, 733
  - incidence of, *272*
  - Lambert-Eaton myasthenic syndrome with, 1289
  - large cell, *744,* 745
  - metastatic, 749, *749*
  - molecular genetics of, 742
  - mortality rates with, *272,* 273, 745–746
  - non–small cell, 743
  - P-450 gene in, 307
  - paraneoplastic syndromes with, 320, 321t, 746–747
  - peripheral neuropathy with, 1280
  - small cell, 743, 744–745, *744*
  - spread of, 743–744, *743*
  - squamous cell, 743–744, *744*
  - staging of, 745, 745t
  - superior vena cava syndrome in, 745
- chronic obstructive disease of, 706–717, 707t. See also specific diseases, e.g., *Emphysema.*
- collapse of, 699–700, *699*
- congenital anomalies of, 699
- congenital overinflation of, 710
- congestion of, 116
- cysts of, 699
- desquamative interstitial pneumonitis of, 736–737, *737*
- diffuse alveolar damage to, 700–703. See also *Adult respiratory distress syndrome (ARDS).*
- diffuse interstitial diseases of, 726–740, 727t. See also specific diseases, e.g., *Pneumoconiosis.*
- drug-induced disease of, 740, 740t
- edema of, 116, 700, 700t
- embolism of, 703–704, *703*
- fibrosis of, 735–736, *736*
- gangrene of, 722
- hamartoma of, 748–749

Lungs *(Continued)*
- hemorrhage from, 738–739, *738*
- hemosiderosis of, 739
- honeycomb, 736
- hyaline membrane disease of, 471–473, *472*
- hypersensitivity pneumonitis of, 613, *737*
- in collagen vascular disorders, 739
- in congenital syphilis, 364
- in cystic fibrosis, 479, 480, 481, *481*
- in filariasis, 398
- in left-sided heart failure, 549
- in preterm infant, 462–463, *463*
- in shock, 136–137
- in systemic lupus erythematosus, 224
- in systemic sclerosis, 229
- in tuberculosis, 722–726. See also *Tuberculosis.*
- infarction of, *133,* 703–704, *704*
- infection of, 347–353, 717–721
  - bacterial, 348–352, *350–352,* 717–721. See also *Pneumonia, bacterial.*
  - *Coccidioides immitis* in, 353, *353*
  - fungal, 352–353, *353*
  - *Haemophilus influenzae* in, 348–349
  - *Histoplasma capsulatum* in, 352, *353*
  - in cystic fibrosis, 479, 480, 481, *481*
  - influenza viruses in, 348
  - *Mycobacterium avium* in, 352, *352*
  - *Mycobacterium tuberculosis* in, 349–352, *350, 351.* See also *Tuberculosis.*
  - rhinoviruses in, 347–348, *347*
  - viral, 347–348, *347*
- lobules of, 698
- maturation of, 462, *463*
- metastases to, 749, *749*
- neonatal respiratory distress syndrome of, 471–473, *472*
- neuroendocrine tumors of, 747–748, *748*
- normal, 697–698, *698*
- obstructive overinflation of, 710–711
- overinflation of, 710–711
- oxygen-induced dysplasia of, 472–473
- pneumonoconioses of, 727–734, *728,* 729t, *730*
- proteinosis of, 739–740, *740*
- radiation-induced disease of, 429, 740
- sarcoidosis of, 734–735, *734*
- scar cancer of, 742
- sequestrations of, 699
- staphylococcal abscess of, 367, *367*
- surfactant of, 471–473, *472*
- terminal respiratory unit of, 698, *708*
- transplantation of, 740–741, *741*
- tuberculosis of, 722–726. See also *Tuberculosis.*

Lupus anticoagulant, 218
Lupus band test, 1201, *1201*
Lupus erythematosus, cutaneous, 224, 1200–1201, *1200, 1201*
- discoid, 224
- drug-induced, 218t, 224–225
- pulmonary involvement in, 739
- systemic, 216–225. See also *Systemic lupus erythematosus (SLE).*

Lupus profundus, 1201
Luschka, ducts of, 892
Luteoma, pregnancy, 1078
Lyell disease (toxic epidermal necrolysis), 1198
Lyme disease, 388–389, *388,* 1253, 1317
- myocarditis in, 584

Lymph nodes, 645–646, *645*
- follicle of, *190*
- follicular hyperplasia of, 649–650, *650*

Lymph nodes *(Continued)*
- in acquired immunodeficiency syndrome, 250
- in Epstein-Barr virus infection, 372
- in inflammation, 84
- in sarcoidosis, 735
- in Sjögren syndrome, 226
- in systemic lupus erythematosus, 224
- marginal zone B-cell hyperplasia of, 649–650
- paracortical hyperplasia of, 650
- reticular hyperplasia of, 650

Lymphadenitis, 84
- in *Toxoplasma gondii* infection, 383
- nonspecific, 649–650, *650*

Lymphangiectasis, in infant, 483–484
Lymphangioma, 533
- in infant, 483–484

Lymphangiosarcoma, 537–538
Lymphangitis, 84, 530–531
Lymphangitis carcinomatosa, 749
Lymphatic filariasis, 397–398, *398*
Lymphatic system, 495
- in inflammation, 84
- obstruction of, 115, 531
- tumor metastases to, 269–270, *269*

Lymphedema, 115, 531
Lymphedema praecox, 531
Lymphocyte(s). See also *Immune system.*
- B, 190, *190*
  - antigen expression of, 654t
  - antigen recognition by, 190
  - antigen-independent activation of, 215
  - clonal anergy of, 213
  - clonal deletion of, 212, *213*
  - differentiation of, *653*
  - Epstein-Barr virus infection of, 190, 312
  - in human immunodeficiency virus infection, 244
  - monocytoid, 650
  - receptor of, 190
- deficiency of, 646
- development of, *603*
- granular, large. See *Natural killer cells.*
- in glomerulonephritis, 947, *947*
- in inflammation, 82, *82*
- of intestinal lymphoid tissue, 804
- T, 189–190, *190*
  - activated (immunoblasts), 650
  - antigen expression of, 654t
  - antigen recognition by, 189, *190,* 194, *194*
  - antigen sensitization of, in cancer, 318
  - antigen-independent activation of, 215
  - apoptosis of, 212–213, *213*
  - atypical, in Epstein-Barr virus infection, 371, *372*
  - CD4+, 189, *190*
    - activation of, 243
    - human immunodeficiency virus infection of, 239–243, *240–242*
    - in delayed-type hypersensitivity, 204–205, *205*
  - CD8+, 189, 194, *194*
  - CD3 protein expression by, 189, *189*
  - clonal anergy of, 212–213, *213*
    - failure of, 214
  - clonal deletion of, 212, *213*
  - cytotoxic, apoptosis of, 318–319
    - in apoptosis, 24, 206
    - in cancer, 317, *318*
    - in type IV hypersensitivity, 206
  - differentiation of, *653*
  - HTLV-I infection of, 314–315, *314*

Lymphocyte(s) *(Continued)*
in glomerulonephritis, 946
in Graves disease, 1137
in systemic lupus erythematosus, 219, *219*
in transplantation rejection, 207, *208*
receptor of, 189, *189*
suppressor, 214
loss of, 215
Lymphocytic colitis, 810
Lymphocytic gastritis, 793
Lymphocytic thyroiditis, 1136
Lymphogranuloma venereum, 361–362
Lymphoid neoplasms, 651–675, 685–686. See also *Leukemia; Lymphoma.*
antigen receptor genes in, 652–653
cellular origin of, 652, *653,* 654t
diagnosis of, 652
immune abnormalities with, 652
monoclonality of, 652–653
REAL classification of, 651–654, 652t, 655t, 656t
tissue patterns of, 653
Lymphokines, 73. See also *Cytokines.*
in inflammation, 82, *82*
Lymphoma, 485t, 651–654, 652t
angiocentric, 656t, 671
Burkitt, 485t, 655t, 662–663, *663*
Epstein-Barr virus in, 312, *313*
oncogenes in, 285, *285,* 286t
definition of, 651
follicular, 285, 286t, 655t, 659–661, *660, 661*
gastric, 802
gastrointestinal, 837–838
Hodgkin, 670–675. See also *Hodgkin disease.*
in acquired immunodeficiency syndrome, 249–250
in Sjögren syndrome, 226
incidence of, *272*
large B-cell, diffuse, 655t, 661–662, *661, 662*
lymphocytic, small, 655t, 658–659, *658, 659*
lymphoplasmacytic, 656t, 666–667, *667*
mantle cell, 285, 286t, 656t, 667–668, *668*
marginal zone, 315, 656t, 668
Mediterranean, 837
minimal residual disease monitoring of, 324
of brain, 1349–1350
of choroid, *1372*
of testes, 1024–1025
of upper airway, 763
oncogenes in, 285, 286t
sprue-associated, 837
T-cell, cutaneous, 1191, *1191*
peripheral, unspecified, 656t, 669–670, *669*
Lymphomatoid granulomatosis, 523
Lymphomatoid polyposis, 668
Lymphomatosis, meningeal, 1314
Lymphopenia, 646
Lymphotoxin, in delayed-type hypersensitivity, 206
Lynch syndrome, 831
Lysosomal acid phosphatase, deficiency of, 155t
Lysosomal enzymes, Golgi apparatus processing of, 153–154, *153*
Lysosomal granules, in inflammation, 76, *76*
release of, 64
Lysosomal storage diseases, 26, 147, 153–160, *153, 154*
Lysosomes, in atrophy, 36
in cell injury, 25–26
Lysozyme, in phagocytosis, 64
Lysyl hydroxylase, gene for, 150

M

M (membranous) cells, of intestinal lymphoid tissue, 804
M protein, of streptococci, 367
McArdle disease, 160, *161,* 163t
MacCallum plaques, in rheumatic heart disease, 572
McCune-Albright syndrome, 1243
α_2-Macroglobulin, 76
Macroglobulinemia, Waldenström, 663
Macromastia, 1096
Macro-orchidism, in fragile X syndrome, 177
Macrophage(s). See also *Leukocyte(s).*
activation of, 80, *81*
alveolar, 698
in diffuse interstitial disease, 727
in pneumonia, 718
antigen expression of, 654t
bacterial infection of, 343
cholesterol-laden, 40, *40*
foamy, 40, *40*
formation of, 80, *80, 603*
hemosiderin-laden, *738,* 739
human immunodeficiency virus infection of, 240, 242–243
immobilization of, 81, *81*
immune complex activation of, 203
immune functions of, 190–191
in adult respiratory distress syndrome, 702–703
in asbestosis, 732
in atherosclerosis, 508–509
in cancer, 318, *318*
in fibroblast proliferation, 106, 106t
in glomerulonephritis, 947, *947*
in inflammation, 79–82, *80, 81,* 81t
in pulmonary hemorrhage, *738,* 739
in silicosis, 731
in type IV hypersensitivity, 205, *205*
LDL receptors of, 152
Legionella pneumophila infection of, 377–378
proliferation of, 81, *81*
recruitment of, *81*
Macrophage infectivity potentiator, of *Legionella pneumophila,* 377
Macula, cherry-red spot of, in Tay-Sachs disease, 156
degeneration of, 1371, *1371*
Macular dystrophy, 1363, *1363*
Macule, 1172
Maffucci syndrome, 1239
MAGE genes, 315–316, *316*
Magnesium ammonium phosphate stones, 989, 989t, 990
Major basic protein, 64
Major histocompatibility complex. See *Human leukocyte antigen (HLA) complex.*
Malabsorption syndromes, 812–815, *813, 814*
Malacoplakia, 1002, *1002*
Malaria, 389–391, *390, 391*
Malassezia furfur, 1210
Malformation(s), congenital, 464–470
definition of, 464–466
environmental etiology of, 466–467, 466t
etiology of, 466–467, 466t
Malformation(s), congenital *(Continued)*
frequency of, 467, 467t
genetic etiology of, 466, 466t
homeobox genes in, 469–470, *469*
mechanisms of, 467–470, *468, 469*
PAX genes in, 470
Malignancy. See at *Tumor(s)* and specific malignancies.
Malignant hyperthermia (malignant hyperpyrexia), 1285
Malignant mixed müllerian tumors, of endometrium, 1063
Mallory body, 27–28, *28,* 869, *871*
Mallory-Weiss syndrome, *778,* 779–780
Malnutrition. See also specific minerals and vitamins.
in cell injury, 4–5
protein-energy, 437–439, *438,* 438t
in chronic pancreatitis, 908
MALToma, 315, 668
Mammography, 1112–1113, *1113,* 1113t
Manganese, deficiency of, 452t
α-Mannosidase, deficiency of, 155t
Mannosidosis, 155t
Mantle cell lymphoma, 285, 286t, 667–668, *667*
MAP kinases, 93, *94*
Maple bark disease, 737
Marasmus, 437, 438t, 439
Marble bone disease, 1224–1225, *1224*
Marchiafava-Bignami disease, 1329
Marek disease, 509
Marfan syndrome, 147t, 143–149, 528, 570
Marginal zone lymphoma, 315, 668
Marie-Strümpell disease, 1252
Marijuana, abuse of, 413
Mast cells, cytokine production by, 198
histamine release from, 66, *66,* 77t
in asthma, 713
in inflammation, 82, *82*
in type I hypersensitivity reaction, 195–198, *197, 198,* 199t
Mastitis, acute, 1096
granulomatous, 1098
periductal, 1096–1097
Mastocytosis, 1192–1193, *1192*
Matricellular proteins, 101
in angiogenesis, 106
Matrix γ-carboxyglutamic acid (GLA) protein, in dystrophic calcification, 45
Matrix metalloproteinases, in tissue remodeling, 106–107, *107*
Measles virus, 333t, 370, *370,* 759t
CNS infection with, 1321–1322
Meckel diverticulum, 804–805, *805*
Media, vascular, 494, *494*
Medial calcific sclerosis (Mönckeberg arteriosclerosis), 498
Mediastinopericarditis, 589
adhesive, 589
Mediastinum, tumors of, 749
Mediterranean lymphoma, 837
Medium-chain acyl-coenzyme A dehydrogenase, deficiency of, 482
Medullary carcinoma, of breast, 1111, *1111*
Medullary sponge kidney, 940, 941t
Medulloblastoma, 485t, 1348–1349, *1349*
Megacolon, aganglionic, congenital, 805
toxic, 818, *819*
Megakaryocytes, in essential thrombocytosis, 683, *683*
in myelodysplastic syndromes, 678, *679*
Megalencephaly, 1300
Megalin, 945

Megaloblastic anemia, 605t, 621–627, *622,* 623t
in folate deficiency, 626–627, *626*
in vitamin B_{12} deficiency, 623–626, 623t, *624*
Megaloureter, 998
Meig syndrome, 750, 1077–1078
Meissner plexus, absence of, 805
Melanin, cellular accumulation of, 42
Melanin pigment incontinence, 1174
Melanocytes, 1171, *1171*
hyperplasia of, 1174
loss of, 1173–1174, *1173*
Melanoma, malignant, 263, 1177–1179, *1178, 1179*
APC-β-catenin in, 293
dysplastic nevi and, 1177, *1178*
geographic factors in, 273
growth patterns of, 1178–1179, *1179*
incidence of, *272*
pigmentation of, 1178, *1179*
tyrosinase antigens of, 317
ultraviolet radiation in, 310
uveal, 1365–1367, *1366*
vulvar, 1045
Melasma, 1174
Membrane inhibitor of reactive lysis (CD59), 69, 619–620
Membrane-bound matrix metalloproteinases, in tissue remodeling, 107
Membranoproliferative glomerulonephritis, 947, 958–960, *959–961,* 965t
Membranous glomerulonephritis, 953–954, 965t
in systemic lupus erythematosus, 221, *221*
MEN1 gene, 149
Mendelian disorders, 143–164
autosomal dominant, 144–145, 145t
autosomal recessive, 145, 145t
nonclassic, 176–182, *177–179,* 179t, *180*
X-linked, 146, 146t
Mendelian Inheritance in Man, 143
Ménétrier disease, 797–798
Meningeal artery, rupture of, 1304, *1305*
Meningioma, 1350–1351, *1351*
Meningitis, 1314–1315, *1315*
aseptic, 1315
chemical, 1314
cryptococcal, 1322
herpes simplex, 1318
human immunodeficiency virus-1, 1320–1321, *1320*
pyogenic, 1314–1315, *1315*
tuberculous, 1316–1317
Meningocele, 1300
Meningoencephalitis, 1314
Acanthamoeba, 1323
bacterial, 1316–1317
fungal, 1322
human immunodeficiency virus-1 in, 1320–1321, *1320*
Mucor, 38
viral, 1317–1322, *1318, 1320, 1322*
Meningomyelocele, 1300
Menopause, atrophy with, 35
endometrial changes with, 1056
osteoporosis after, 1222–1224, *1223, 1224*
Menstrual cycle, 1037–1038, *1054,* 1055, *1055*
breast changes with, 1094
inadequate luteal phase of, 1056
Mental retardation, in fragile X syndrome, 177
in trisomy 21, 170
Mercury, in occupational diseases, 421t
Merkel cell carcinoma, 1187
Merlin, 164
Mesangial cells, 933–934
antibodies to, 946
in glomerulonephritis, 947
Mesenteric cysts, 842
Mesothelioma, in asbestos workers, 733
of fallopian tubes, 1065
of peritoneum, 842
of pleura, 751–752, *752, 753*
Metabolism, inborn errors of, 475–481. See also specific disorders.
wound healing and, 110
Metachromasia, 1340, *1340*
Metachromatic leukodystrophy, 155t, 1340, *1340*
Metal(s), in carcinogenesis, 309
in occupational diseases, 420–422, 421t
Metalloproteinases, in tissue remodeling, 106–107, *107*
tumor elaboration of, 303–304
Metaplasia, 31, 36–38, *37*
myeloid, myelofibrosis with, 683–685, *684*
Metastasis, tumor. See *Tumor(s), metastatic.*
Metastasis-suppressor genes, 305
Metchnikoff, Elie, 52
Methanol, CNS effects of, 1342
ingestion of, 412
Methotrexate, CNS effects of, 1342–1343
α-Methyldopa, in warm antibody hemolytic anemia, 620
Methysergide therapy, cardiac plaques in, 578
Mice, knockout, 140
FBN1, 148–149
transgenic, 140
Michaelis-Gutmann bodies, 1002, *1002*
Microabscess, in dermatitis herpetiformis, 1204, *1205*
in psoriasis, 1199, *1199*
Microalbuminuria, in diabetes mellitus, 967–968
Microaneurysm, in diabetes mellitus, 1369, *1369*
Microangiopathic hemolytic anemia, 637
Microangiopathy, diabetic, 922–923, *923*
thrombotic, 636–637, 985–988, *985, 987*
Microcystic adenoma, 910
Microcystic meningioma, 1350
Microencephaly, 1300
Microglia, 1296, 1297
Microglial nodules, 1297
in human immunodeficiency virus infection, 1320, *1320*
β_2-Microglobulin, 252
Microsatellite instability, in tumors, 295–296
Microsatellite repeats, in gene linkage analysis, 185–186, *186*
Microscopic polyangiitis, 517t, 521–522, *522*
Microtubules, abnormalities of, 27
Migrating thrombophlebitis, in cancer, 320–321, 321t
Mikulicz syndrome, 226, 735, 769
Milk leg, 530
Miller-Dieker syndrome, 1300
Milroy disease, 531
Minerals, deficiencies of, 451–452, *452*
Mineralocorticoids, of adrenal cortex, 1152, *1152*
Minimal change disease, 954–956, *956, 957,* 965t
Minisatellite repeats, in gene linkage analysis, 185–186
Mite bite, 1210–1212
Mitochondrial encephalomyopathy, 1340–1341
Mitochondrial encephalomyopathy, lactic acidosis, and stroke-like episodes, 1287, 1341
Mitochondrial myopathy, 26–27, *27,* 1287, *1288*
Mitochondrial permeability transition, in cell injury, 6–7, *7*
Mitochondrion (mitochondria), alterations in, 26–27, *27*
in alcoholic cirrhosis, *27*
injury to, 6–7, *7, 9, 11*
number of, 26
size of, 26, *27*
Mitogen-activated protein kinase pathway, for signal transduction, 93, *94*
Mitogillin, 380
Mitral annular calcification, *567,* 568
Mitral apparatus, 545
Mitral leaflets, intercordal ballooning of, 569, *569*
Mitral valve, annulus of, calcification of, *567,* 568
Lambl excrescences on, 546
myxomatous degeneration of, 568–570, *569*
prolapse of, 149, 568–570, *569,* 940
in Marfan syndrome, 149
in polycystic kidney disease, 940
stenosis of, blood flow alterations in, 125, 129
in rheumatic heart disease, 572
Mixed connective tissue disease, 231
Mixed müllerian tumors, 1063
MLL gene, in acute leukemia, 285, 286t
Mole, BK (dysplastic nevi), 1176–1177, *1177, 1178*
cutaneous, 1174–1176, *1175,* 1176t
Molluscum body, 1209, *1209*
Molluscum contagiosum, 1038t, 1209–1210, *1209*
Molluscum virus, 333t
Mönckeberg medial calcific sclerosis, 498
Monoblasts, in acute myelogenous leukemia, 676, *677*
Monoclonal gammopathy of uncertain significance, 666
Monocyte(s). See also *Macrophage(s).*
antigen expression of, 654t
development of, *603*
in glomerulonephritis, 947, *947*
LDL receptors of, 152
maturation of, 80, *80*
reactive proliferations of, 648t
recruitment of, 80–81
Monocytosis, 648t
Monokines, 73. See also *Cytokines.*
Mononucleosis, infectious, 371–373, *372,* 759t. See also *Epstein-Barr virus (EBV).*
Monostotic fibrous dysplasia, 1242–1243
Morton neuroma, 1280
Mosaicism, cellular, 168–169
in Klinefelter syndrome, 174
in trisomy 21, 170
in Turner syndrome, 174–175
gonadal, 181–182
placental, in intrauterine growth retardation, 461, *462*
Mosquito bite, 1210–1212
Motor and sensory hereditary peripheral neuropathy, 1277–1278
Motor neurons, degenerative diseases of, 1338, *1339*
lower, 1269–1270, *1270*
Motor unit, *1126,* 1269, *1270,* 1273–1275

Motor vehicle accidents, 431t
Mott cells, 393, 665
Mouse mammary tumor virus, 1107
Mouth. See *Oral cavity.*
Mucicarmine stain, 345, 345t
Mucin, as tumor antigen, 317
Mucinous carcinoma, of breast, 1112, *1112*
Mucinous cystadenocarcinoma, of appendix, 840, *840*
  of pancreas, 910, *910*
Mucinous cystadenoma, of appendix, 840
Mucocele, of appendix, 840
  of sinus, 763
Mucocutaneous lymph node syndrome (Kawasaki syndrome), 517t, 521
Mucoepidermoid carcinoma, 772, *772*
Mucolipidoses, 155t
Mucopolysaccharidoses, 155t, 159–160, 1222
Mucor, 380–381, *381,* 1322
Mucormycosis, 380–381, *381*
Mucosa-associated lymphoid tissue (MALT), 804
  tumors of, 315, 668
Mucous neck cells, 787
Mucous plugs, in asthma, 715
Mucoviscidosis, 477–481, *478–481.* See also *Cystic fibrosis.*
Mucus, in bronchitis, 711
Müllerian duct, 1036
Müllerian tumors, mixed, 1063
Multicystic encephalopathy, 1302
Multiple chemical sensitivity syndrome, 419
Multiple endocrine neoplasia (MEN) syndromes, 1166–1167, 1167t
  medullary thyroid carcinoma in, 1145, 1168
  parathyroid disorders in, 1149
  pheochromocytoma in, 1164, 1164t
Multiple hereditary exostosis, 1237–1238, *1238*
Multiple myeloma, 655t, 664–666, *665*
  renal involvement in, 968, 980–981, *981,* 981t
Multiple sclerosis, 1326–1327, *1327, 1328*
  Marburg form of, 1328
  myelin basic protein–reactive T cell clones in, 215
Multiple sulfatase, deficiency of, 155t
Multiple system atrophy, 1335
Mumps virus, 333t, 370–371, 1017
Munro microabscess, 1199, *1199*
Muscle(s), *1270.* See also *Muscle fibers.*
  chloroquine-induced disease of, 1288–1289
  congenital diseases of, 1285, 1286t, *1287*
  denervation atrophy of, 1274–1275, 1280–1281, *1281*
  disuse atrophy of, 1275
  drug-induced diseases of, 1288–1289
  ethanol-induced disease of, 412, 1288
  fibers of, 1272–1273, *1272, 1273,* 1273t
  in acquired immunodeficiency syndrome, 1321
  in Charcot-Marie-Tooth disease, 1277–1278
  in Dejerine-Sottas disease, 1278
  inflammatory diseases of, 229–231, *230,* 1287
    antinuclear antibodies in, 218t
  leiomyoma of, 1266
  leiomyosarcoma of, 1266
  lipid diseases of, 1285–1286
  mitochondrial diseases of, 1286–1287, *1288*
  pseudohypertrophy of, 1281
  regeneration of, 92
  reinnervation of, 1275
Muscle(s) *(Continued)*
  rhabdomyosarcoma of, *265,* 1265–1266, *1265*
  smooth, tumors of, 589–591, *589,* 591t
  steroid-induced diseases of, 1288
  thyrotoxic diseases of, 1287–1288
  toxic diseases of, 1287–1289
Muscle fibers, 1272–1273, *1272, 1273,* 1273t
  atrophy of, 1274–1275
  group atrophy of, *1273,* 1275
  hypertrophy of, 1275
  regeneration of, 1275
  reinnervation of, 1275
  segmental fibrosis of, 1275
  splitting of, 1275
  type grouping of, *1273,* 1275
Muscle spindles, 1273
Muscular dystrophy, 1281–1285
  autosomal, 1282–1284, 1283t, 1284t
  Becker, 1281–1282, *1282, 1283*
  Duchenne, 1281–1282, *1282, 1284*
  limb girdle, 1282–1283, 1283t, 1284t
  X-linked, 1281–1282, *1282, 1283*
Mushroom picker's lung, 737
Mutation(s), 141–143, 466. See also *Mendelian disorders.*
  chromosome, 141–142. See also *Chromosome(s).*
  frameshift, 142, *142,* 143
  gain of function, 145
  genome, 141
  in oncogene activation, 284
  loss of function, 144
  missense, 142, *142*
  point, *141,* 142, *142*
  trinucleotide repeat, 143
Mutton fat, in sarcoidosis, 1364
Myasthenia, paraneoplastic, 320, 321t
Myasthenia gravis, 1289
myc gene, in cancer, 282
c-*myc* gene, in bronchogenic carcinoma, 742
  in Burkitt lymphoma, 285, *285,* 286t, 312
N-*myc* gene, amplification of, 286, *286*
Mycobacterium avium-intracellulare, 334t
  in acquired immunodeficiency syndrome, 352, *352*
Mycobacterium bovis, 334t, 349
Mycobacterium intracellulare, 334t
Mycobacterium kansasii, 334t
Mycobacterium leprae, 334t, 385–386, *387,* 1276
Mycobacterium tuberculosis, 332t, 334t, 349–352, *350, 351.* See also *Tuberculosis.*
Mycobacterium ulcerans, 334t
Mycoplasma, 334t, 335
  genital infection with, 1039
Mycoplasma pneumoniae, 332t, 335, 721–722
Mycosis fungoides, 656t, 670, 1191, *1191*
Mycotoxins, 424, 424t
Myelin basic protein, 1270
Myelin basic protein–reactive T cell clones, in multiple sclerosis, 215
Myelin figures, in cell injury, 8, *9*
Myelin ovoids, in axonal degeneration, 1274
Myelin protein zero, 1270
  in Charcot-Marie-Tooth disease, 1277
  in Dejerine-Sottas disease, 1278
Myelodysplastic syndromes, 678–679
Myelofibrosis, myeloid metaplasia with, 683–685, *684*
Myeloid neoplasms, 675–686. See also *Leukemia, myelogenous; Myelodysplastic syndromes.*
Myelolipoma, adrenal, 1163
Myeloma, multiple, 655t, 664–666. See also *Multiple myeloma.*
Myelomeningocele, 1300
Myelopathy, vacuolar, in acquired immunodeficiency syndrome, 1321
Myeloperoxidase, in phagocytosis, 63, *63*
Myelophthisic anemia, 632
Myeloproliferative disorders, 679–685, *680–684.* See also specific disorders.
Myocardial fibers, in Pompe disease, *163*
Myocardial infarction, 129, 554–564
  after heart transplantation, 598
  apoptosis in, 556
  arrhythmias with, 562
  atheroma in, 553
  blood flow alterations in, 125
  cardiogenic shock after, 562
  circadian rhythms in, 551
  clinical features of, 561
  complications of, 562–563, *562, 563*
  contractile dysfunction with, 562
  contraction bands in, 559, *561*
  C-reactive protein in, 506
  creatine kinase in, 561
  estrogen replacement therapy and, 414–415
  expansion of, 563
  in diabetes mellitus, 922
  incidence of, 554–555
  inflammatory response in, 559, *560*
  myocardial rupture with, 562, *562*
  of right ventricle, 563
  oral contraceptives and, 416
  papillary muscle dysfunction with, 563
  pathogenesis of, 555–559
    coronary arterial occlusion in, 555
    myocardial response in, 555–559, *555,* 556t, *557,* 558t, *559, 560*
  pericarditis with, 562–563, *563*
  postreperfusion changes in, 559–561, *561*
  prevention of, 563
  prognosis for, 563
  reperfusion injury in, 559, 561
  risk factors for, 554–555
  septic, 574
  subendocardial, 554, 559
  thromboembolism with, 563
  thrombolytic therapy in, 559, 561
  thrombus in, 126–127, *127,* 552, 553, 553t
  transmural, 553, 554, 556–557, 558t
  triphenyltetrazolium chloride dye test in, 558, *559*
  ventricular aneurysm with, 563, *563*
  ventricular remodeling after, 563
  wavy fibers in, 558, *560*
Myocarditis, 584–586, 584t, *585*
  hypersensitivity, 584–585, *585*
  in Chagas disease, 394
  in rheumatic heart disease, 571
  in systemic lupus erythematosus, 223
  in trichinellosis, 394
Myocardium, 544–545. See also *Heart.*
  amyloid deposits of, 586
  catecholamine-induced injury to, 586
  disease of, 578–587, *578.* See also *Cardiomyopathy.*
  doxorubicin-induced injury to, 586
  drug-induced injury to, 586–587
  in thyroid disease, 587
  inflammation of, 584–586, 584t, *585*
  iron-induced disease of, 586–587
  ischemia of, 550–564. See also *Ischemic heart disease; Myocardial infarction.*

Myocardium *(Continued)*
  necrosis of, 16–17, *16, 17*
  rupture of, after myocardial infarction, 562, *562*
  stunned, 561
Myoclonic epilepsy and ragged red fibers, 1287, 1341
Myocytes, 544–545
  coagulation necrosis of, 16, *16*
  hypertrophy of, *34*, 35
  ischemic injury to, 2, *3*. See also *Ischemic heart disease; Myocardial infarction.*
  lipofuscin accumulation in, 42, *42*
Myocytolysis, in myocardial infarction, 559
Myofibers, in hypertrophic cardiomyopathy, 582, *582*
Myofibrils, 1272, *1272*
Myofibromatoses, in children, 484
Myofilaments, 1272, *1272*
Myometrium. See *Uterus.*
Myopathy. See at also *Muscle(s).*
  congenital, 1285–1286, 1285t
  ion channel, 1285
  lipid, 1286–1287
  mitochondrial, 1287
  toxic, 1287–1289
Myopericarditis, 588
Myosin, of sarcomere, 544
β-Myosin heavy chain, in cardiac hypertrophy, 35
Myositis, inclusion-body, 229, 231
Myositis ossificans, 37, 1262, *1262*
Myotonic dystrophy, 1283, 1285
  triplet repeat mutations in, 179, *179*, 179t
Myotonin protein kinase, 1283
Myxedema, 1133, 1138
Myxedema heart, 586
Myxoid chondrosarcoma, 1260t
Myxoma, 589–590, *589*

N

NADPH oxidase, genes for, in chronic granulomatous disease, 65, 65t
Naegleria, CNS infection with, 1323
Naegleria fowleri, 337t
NAIP gene, 1281
β-Naphthylamine, in carcinogenesis, 309
Narcotics, abuse of, 413
Nasopharynx, carcinoma of, 764, *764*
  Epstein-Barr virus in, 313
  inflammation of, 763
  tumors of, 763–764, *764*
Natural killer cells, 191, *191, 192*
  antigens of, 654t
  development of, *603*
  in cancer, 317–318, *318*
Necator americanus, 394–395
Neck, 767–768
  branchial cyst of, 767
  paraganglioma of, 768–769, *768*
  thyroglossal tract cyst of, 767–768
Necrosis, 2
  ATP depletion in, 5
  avascular, 1231, *1231*, 1231t
  calcium imbalance in, 6, *6*
  caseous, 17, *17*
  centrilobular, 117, *117*
  coagulative, 16–17, *16, 17*
  fat, 17–18, *18*
  free radicals in, 5–6, *6*
  gangrenous, 17
  hemorrhagic, 116–117, *117*
  hepatic, 117, *117*, 847–848, 852
Necrosis *(Continued)*
    apoptosis-induced, 847–848
    centrilobular, 882–883, *883*
    ischemic, 847–848
    lytic, 848
    zonal distribution of, 848
  liquefactive, 17, *17*
  mechanisms of, 5–7, *6, 7*
  membrane permeability defects in, 6
  mitochondrial damage in, 6–7, *7*
  morphology of, 15–18, *16–18*
  myocardial, 16–17, *16, 17*
  secondary, 19
  vs. apoptosis, *18*
Necrotizing arteriolitis, in hypertension, 983
Necrotizing glomerulitis, in hypertension, 983
nef gene, of human immunodeficiency virus, 238, *239*, 247
Neisseria gonorrhoeae, 334t, 362, 1038t
  in pelvic inflammatory disease, 1039–1040
  pili of, 342, *342*, 344
Neisseria meningitidis, 334t, 362
Nemaline myopathy, 1285t, *1286*
Nematodes, 336–337
Neointima, 497, *497*
Neonate. See *Infant.*
Neoplasm, 261. See also *Carcinogenesis; Tumor(s).*
Neovascularization. See *Angiogenesis.*
Nephritic syndrome, 935
Nephritis. See also *Glomerulonephritis.*
  anti–glomerular basement membrane antibodies in, 943–945, *944*
  hereditary, 933, 962–963, *963*
  Heymann, *944*, 945, 954
  immune complex, 945–946
  tubulointerstitial, 971–981, 972t
    drug-induced, 977–979, *977, 979*, 979t
    urinary tract infection and, 972–974, *972, 973*
Nephroblastomatosis, 488
Nephrocalcin, 990
Nephrocalcinosis, 930, 1150
Nephrolithiasis, 936, 989–990, 989t, *990*
  in hyperparathyroidism, 1150
  in hyperuricemia, 980
Nephronophthisis, 940–941, *941*, 941t
Nephropathy. See at *Kidney.*
Nephrosclerosis, benign, 981–982, *982*
  malignant, 982–984, *983*, 983t
Nephrosis, lipoid, 954–956, *956, 957*, 965t
Nephrotic syndrome, 115, 935, 952–953, 953t, 957, 959, 965t
Nerves. See *Central nervous system (CNS); Peripheral nerves.*
Nerve fiber, 1270, *1271*
Nerve sheath, tumors of, 1352–1354, *1353*
Nerve-cerebrospinal fluid barrier, 1271
Neural tube, defects of, 1299–1300
Neuraminidase, of *Trypanosoma cruzi*, 393
Neuroblastoma, 485–487, 485t, *486, 487*, 1166, 1348
  chromosome 1 in, 487
  N-*myc* gene amplification in, 286, *286*, 487, *487*
  olfactory, 764
  ploidy of, 487
  staging of, 486–487
Neuroborreliosis, 1317
Neurocytoma, 1348
Neurodegenerative diseases. See also *Alzheimer disease; Huntington disease; Parkinson disease.*
Neurodegenerative diseases *(Continued)*
  protein deposition in, 1295, 1296t
  protein misfolding in, 41
Neuroectodermal tumor, 1244, 1260t
Neuroendocrine tumors, 747–748, *748*
Neuroepithelial tumor, dysembryoplastic, 1348
Neurofibrillary tangles, 1295
  in Alzheimer disease, 28, 1330, *1331*
Neurofibroma, 164, 1353
Neurofibromatosis, 1354
  type 1 (von Recklinghausen disease), 147t, 162, 164, 293
  type 2 (acoustic neurofibromatosis), 162, 164
Neurofibromin, 147t, 164
Neurogenic shock, 134
Neurohypophysis. See *Pituitary gland, posterior.*
Neurokinin A, in inflammation, 77
Neuroma, acoustic, 1352–1353, *1353*
  in MEN-IIB, 1168
  Morton, 1280
  traumatic, 1280, *1280*
Neuromuscular junction, disease of, 1289
Neuromyelitis optica, 1327–1328
Neurons, 1294–1295
  degeneration of, 1295
  heterotopic, 1300
  in Tay-Sachs disease, 155–156, *157*
  inclusions of, 1295
  loss of, 91
  motor, degenerative diseases of, 1338, *1339*
    lower, 1269–1270, *1270*
  nitric oxide of, 75
  red, 1295
  tumors of, 1348
  ultrastructural features of, 1295
Neuronal apoptosis inhibitory protein, 24
Neuronal storage diseases, 1339
Neuronophagia, 1297
  in arthropod-borne viral encephalitis, 1318
Neuropathy. See *Peripheral neuropathy.*
Neuropeptides, in inflammation, 77
Neurosyphilis, 364, 1317
Neutropenia, 646–647
  colitis with, 811–812
  drug-induced, 646–647
Neutrophils. See also *Leukocyte(s).*
  azurophil granules of, 76, *76*
  deficiency of, 646–647
  immune complex activation of, 203, *203*
  in adult respiratory distress syndrome, 702, *702*
  in alcoholic liver disease, 869
  in glomerulonephritis, 947, *947*
  in inflammation, 86, 345, *345*
  in rheumatoid arthritis, 1249
  reactive proliferations of, 647–648, *648*, 648t, *649*
  specific granules of, 76, *76*
  toxic granules of, 648
Neutrophilia, in inflammation, 86
Nevus, dysplastic, 1176–1177, *1177, 1178*
  nevocellular, 1174–1176, *1175*, 1176t
Nevus flammeus, 534
NF-1 gene, 164, 293, 1355
NF-2 gene, 164, 293, 1351
Niacin, 440t, 448, *449*
Nickel, in carcinogenesis, 274t, 309
  in occupational diseases, 421t, 422
Niemann-Pick disease, 155t, 156–158, *157*
Night blindness, in retinitis pigmentosa, 1371
Nipples, 1094
  adenoma of, 1104
  congenital inversion of, 1096

Nipples *(Continued)*
Paget disease of, 1108–1109
papillomatosis of, 1104
supernumerary, 1096
Nitric oxide, antimicrobial activity of, 75–76
cytokine-inducible, 75
endothelial, 75
in cell injury, 12
in inflammation, 75–76, *75,* 77t
in platelet aggregation, *118,* 122
neuronal, 75
Nitrogen dioxide, in air, 417, 417t, 418, 418t
Nitrosamines, in carcinogenesis, 309
nm23 gene, 305
N-*myc* oncogene, in neuroblastoma, 487, *487*
Nocardia asteroides, 334t
Nocturnal dyspnea, paroxysmal, in left-sided heart failure, 549
Nocturnal hemoglobinuria, paroxysmal, 69, 619–620, *619*
Nodes of Ranvier, 1270
Nodular fasciitis, 1261–1262, *1262*
Nodule(s), 1172
in silicosis, 731, *732*
rheumatoid, 1249, *1249*
thyroid, 1140
typhoid, 357, *357*
Nodule of Arantius, 545
Nonbacterial thrombotic endocarditis, *575,* 576–577, *576*
Non-Hodgkin's lymphoma. See *Lymphoma.*
Nonossifying fibroma, 1242, *1242*
Nonsteroidal anti-inflammatory drugs (NSAIDs), diarrhea with, 811
in inflammation, 71–72
nephropathy with, 979
peptic ulcer disease and, 794
Norwalk agent, 333t
Norwalk-like viruses, 354, 807, 807t
Nose, 762–763
carcinoma of, 764, *764*
inflammation of, 762–763, *762*
necrotizing lesions of, 763
neuroblastoma of, 764
papilloma of, 763, *764*
plasmacytoma of, 763–764
polyps of, 762, *762*
tumors of, 763–764, *764*
NSAIDs. See *Nonsteroidal anti-inflammatory drugs (NSAIDs).*
Nuclear factor κB, in endothelial cell activation, 497
Null cell adenoma, 1127
Nutmeg liver, 117, *117,* 883, *883*
Nutrition, 436–452. See also specific minerals and vitamins.
in wound healing, 110
with burn injury, 434

O

O antigens, of bacteria, 344
O ring sign, in enchondroma, 1239
Obesity, 452–455, *452, 453*
cancer and, 273
in type II diabetes mellitus, 918
tumor necrosis factor in, 74
Obturator palsy, tumor-associated, 1279
Occupation, cancer and, 273, 274t
Occupational diseases, 404, 404t, 419–422, 419t, 421t, *422*
aromatic halogenated hydrocarbons and, 420
cigarette smoking and, 409
Occupational diseases *(Continued)*
herbicides and, 423–424
metals and, 420–422, 421t, *422*
pesticides and, 422–423, 423t
plastics and, 420
polymers and, 420
pulmonary, 727–734, *728,* 729t, *730*
rubber and, 420
volatile organic compounds in, 419–420, 419t
Occupational Safety and Health Administration, 404
Ochronosis (alkaptonuria), 42, 162
Oculopharyngeal muscular dystrophy, 1283t
Odontoma, 761
Okadoic acid, in tumor promotion, 308
Oligodendrocytes, 1296, 1297
Oligodendroglioma, 1346
Oligohydramnios (Potter) sequence, 465, *465*
Olivopontocerebellar atrophy, 1335
Ollier disease, 1239
Omega-3 fatty acids, in atherosclerosis, 506
Omphalocele, 804
Onchocerca volvulus, 398–399, *399*
Onchocerciasis, 398–399, *399*
Oncocytoma, mitochondria in, 27
of kidneys, 991
Oncofetal antigens, 317, 325, 325t
Oncogenes, 93, 277–286
activation of, 284–286, *285, 286,* 286t
nomenclature for, 278
protein products of, 279–284, 279t, *281, 283, 284*
recessive, 277
viral, 278
Oncoproteins, 279–284, 279t, *281, 283, 284*
Onion bulbs, in segmental demyelination, 1274, *1274*
Onycholysis, 1172
Onychomycosis, 1210
Ophthalmopathy, Graves, 1137, 1138
Ophthalmoplegia, exophthalmic, 1287
Opsonins, in phagocytosis, 62
Optic disc, in retinitis pigmentosa, 1371
Optic nerve, atrophy of, 1374, *1374*
glaucomatous, 1375, *1375*
edema of, 1373–1374, *1374*
tumors of, 1374
Optic neuritis, 1374
in multiple sclerosis, 1327
Optic neuropathy, 1374
Oral cavity, 756–761
aphthous ulcers of, 757, *757*
candidiasis of, 378, 757
cysts of, 761
dryness of, 758, 769
erythroplakia of, 760
hairy leukoplakia of, 758–759
herpes simplex virus infection of, 757
in systemic disease, 758–759, 759t
inflammation of, 756–758, *757*
leukoplakia of, 759–761, *760*
reactive lesions of, 758, *758*
squamous cell carcinoma of, 760–761, *761*
tumors of, 759–761, *760, 761*
Oral contraceptives, adverse reactions to, 414–416, 415t
Orchiopexy, 1016
Orchitis, granulomatous, 1017
mumps, 371, 1017
postvasectomy, 215
Organophosphates, 423, 423t
Organs of Zuckerkandl, 1164, *1164*
Ornithosis, 362
Orphan Annie nuclei, in papillary thyroid carcinoma, 1143, *1144*
Orthopnea, in left-sided heart failure, 549
Osler-Weber-Rendu disease (hereditary hemorrhagic telangiectasia), 531–532, 534, 634, 759t
Osmotic pressure, in edema, *114,* 115
Osteitis, dissecting, in hyperparathyroidism, 1228, *1228*
Osteitis deformans (Paget disease), 1225–1227, *1226, 1227*
Osteitis fibrosa, in hyperparathyroidism, 1228
Osteoarthritis, 1246–1248, *1247, 1248, 1254*
obesity and, 454
Osteoarthropathy, hypertrophic, 320, 321t
Osteoblasts, 1216–1217, *1216,* 1218
Osteoblastoma, 1235–1236
Osteocalcin, in dystrophic calcification, 45
Osteochondritis, syphilitic, 364
Osteochondroma, 1237–1238, *1238*
Osteoclasts, 1217, *1217*
Osteocytes, 1217
Osteodystrophy, renal, 1229
Osteogenesis imperfecta, 1220t, 1221–1222, *1221,* 1222t
collagen in, 144–145
gene mutation in, 147t
gonadal mosaicism in, 181
Osteoid, 1216
Osteoma, 261, 1235–1236, *1235*
Osteomalacia, 444–445, 444t, 1227–1228
Osteomyelitis, 1232–1233, *1232*
extradural abscess with, 1316
pyogenic, 1232, *1232*
sclerosing, of Garré, 1233
tuberculous, 1233
Osteonecrosis, 1231, *1231,* 1231t
Osteonectin, in dystrophic calcification, 45
Osteopenia, 445
Osteopetrosis, 1224–1225, *1224*
Osteopontin, 101
in dystrophic calcification, 45
Osteoporosis, 1222–1224, 1223t, *1224*
disuse, 1222
pathogenesis of, 1222–1224, *1223*
vs. osteomalacia, 445–446
Osteoprogenitor cells, 1216
Osteosarcoma, 1236–1237, *1236, 1237*
chondroblastic, 1237, 1241
platelet-derived growth factor production by, 279, 279t
Osteosclerosis, in myelofibrosis with myeloid metaplasia, 684
Otitis media, 766–767
Otosclerosis, 767
Oval fat bodies, in nephrotic syndrome, 953
Ovary(ies), 1066–1079
adenofibroma of, 1072–1073, *1072*
anatomy of, 1037
androblastoma of, 1078, *1078*
Brenner tumor of, 1072–1073, *1072*
carcinoma of, 1069–1072
clinical course of, 1073
endometrioid, 1071–1072
incidence of, *272*
mortality rates with, *272*
mucinous, 1070–1071, *1071*
oral contraceptives and, 415
risk factors for, 1067
serous, 1069–1070, *1069, 1070*
choriocarcinoma of, 1076
clear cell adenocarcinoma of, 1072
cystadenocarcinoma of, 1069–1070, *1069, 1070*

Ovary(ies) *(Continued)*
cystadenofibroma of, 1072
cystic follicles of, 1066
cystic teratoma (dermoid cyst) of, 262–263, *264*
cysts of, 1066–1067, *1066*
dysgerminoma of, 1075, *1075*
endodermal sinus tumor of, 1075–1076, *1076*
endometrioid tumors of, 1071–1072
germ cell tumors of, 1073–1076, *1073–1076*
gonadoblastoma of, 1078
granulosa luteal cysts of, 1066
granulosa-theca cell tumor of, 1076–1077, *1077*
hilus cell tumor of, 1078
in Turner syndrome, 176
Leydig cell tumor of, 1078
metastatic tumors of, 1079
mucinous tumors of, 1070–1071, *1071*
polycystic disease of, 1066–1067, *1066*
pregnancy luteoma of, 1078
radiation damage to, 430
serous cystadenoma of, 1069, *1069*
serous tumors of, 1069–1070, *1069, 1070*
Sertoli-Leydig cell tumor of, 1078, *1078*
sex cord–stromal tumor of, 1076–1079, *1077, 1078*
streak, 176
stromal hyperthecosis of, 1066–1067
teratoma of, 1073–1075, *1073, 1074*
thecoma-fibroma of, 1077–1078, *1077*
transitional cell carcinoma, 1073
tumors of, 1067–1079, 1067t, *1068,* 1068t
yolk sac tumor of, 1075–1076, *1076*
Ovotestes, 176
Ovulation, *1054,* 1055, *1055*
failure of, 1056, *1056*
Oxidative phosphorylation diseases, 1287, *1288*
Oxygen therapy, in respiratory distress syndrome, 472–473
Oxyphil cells, of parathyroid glands, 1147–1148
Ozone, 417, 417

P

P-450 gene, in lung cancer, 307
p53 gene, aflatoxin B1–related mutation of, 308
in angiogenesis, 302
in bronchogenic carcinoma, 742
in cancer, 290–292, *291*
in colorectal carcinoma, *832,* 833
in pancreatic carcinoma, 910
ultraviolet ray–induced mutation of, 310
p73 gene, 292
Paget disease, of bone (osteitis deformans), 1225–1227, *1226, 1227*
of nipple, 1107–1109, 1107t, *1108, 1109*
of vulva, 1044–1045, *1044*
Paget cell, 1109, *1109*
Pancarditis, in rheumatic heart disease, 571
Pancoast tumor, 747
Pancreas, 902–928
abscess of, 907, 909
acini of, 903, *903*
adenoma of, 910
agenesis of, 904
annular, 904
carcinoid tumors of, 928
carcinoma of, 910–911, *911*
hepatic metastasis from, *270*
Pancreas *(Continued)*
incidence of, *272*
mortality rates with, *272*
δ-cell tumor of, 928
α-cell tumors of, 927
β-cell tumors of, 926–927, *927*
congenital anomalies of, 904
cysts of, 909
cystadenoma of, 910
cystic tumors of, 909–910, *910*
ectopic, 904
endocrine, 911–928. See also *Diabetes mellitus.*
α cell of, 911–913, *912*
β cell of, 911, *912*
δ cell of, *912,* 913
D1 cell of, 913
enterochromaffin cell of, 913
enzymes of, 903–904
in acute pancreatitis, 905–907, *906*
exocrine, 902–904, *903*
gastrinoma of, 927
glucagonoma of, 927
hemosiderin deposition in, 874
heterotopic, 789
in cystic fibrosis, 479–480, *481*
inflammation of, 904–909, *905–908,* 905t
islet cell tumors of, 926–928, *927*
microcystic adenoma of, 910
mucinous cystadenocarcinoma of, 910, *910*
mumps virus infection of, 371
pseudocysts of, 907, 909, *909*
secretions of, 903–904
solid-cystic tumor of, 910
somatostatinoma of, 928
tumors of, 909–911, *910, 911*
VIPoma of, 928
Pancreas divisum, 904, 907
Pancreatic duct, 903, *903*
obstruction of, in acute pancreatitis, 906, *906*
in chronic pancreatitis, 908
Pancreatitis, 904–909
acute, 841, 904–907, *905,* 905t
clinical features of, 907, *907*
fat necrosis in, 17–18, *18,* 905, *905*
necrotizing, 905, *905*
pathogenesis of, 905–907, *906*
vs. chronic pancreatitis, *907*
chronic, 907–909
clinical features of, 908–909
hereditary, 908
pathogenesis of, 907–908
vs. acute pancreatitis, *907*
Pancytopenia, in hairy cell leukemia, 669
oral manifestations of, 759t
Panencephalitis, sclerosing, subacute, 1321–1322
Paneth cells, of intestine, 803
Panniculitis, 1207–1208
Pannus, in rheumatoid arthritis, 1249
Pantothenic acid, 440t
Pap smear, 322–323
Papillary adenoma, of kidney, 991
Papillary carcinoma, of breast, 1112, *1112*
Papillary craniopharyngioma, 1129
Papillary cystadenoma lymphomatosum, 769, 771–772, *771*
Papillary fibroelastoma, cardiac, 590
Papillary hidradenoma, of vulva, 1042
Papillary meningioma, 1350
Papillary muscle, dysfunction of, after myocardial infarction, 563
Papillary serous carcinoma, of endometrium, 1062, *1062*
Papillary thyroid carcinoma oncogene, 1143
Papilledema, 1373–1374, *1374*
Papillitis, necrotizing, in diabetes mellitus, 924
Papilloma, 261, *261*
large duct, of breast, 1104, *1105*
of choroid plexus, 1347–1348
of nose, 763, *764*
of urethra, 1009
sclerosing, of breast, 1101
small duct, of breast, 1101, *1102*
squamous, 1181
of esophagus, 783
Papillomatosis, 1172
of larynx, 766
of nipple, 1104
Papillomavirus. See *Human papillomavirus (HPV).*
Papule, 1172
Parafollicular cells (C cells), 1131
Paraganglioma, 768–769, *768,* 1166
Paraganglion system, 1163–1164, *1164*
Parainfluenza virus, 333t
Parakeratosis, 1172
Paralysis, periodic, thyrotoxic, 1287–1288
Paralysis agitans, 1333–1334, *1334*
Paramyotonia congenita, 1285
Paramyxovirus, in Paget disease, 1225–1226
Paraneoplastic syndromes, 320–321, 321t, 1351–1352, 1352t
with bronchogenic carcinoma, 746–747
Paraphimosis, 1012
Parasites, intestinal, 810–811
Parathyroid glands, 1147–1151
adenoma of, 1148–1150, *1149*
carcinoma of, 1149–1150
hyperfunction of, 1148–1151. See also *Hyperparathyroidism.*
hypofunction of, 1151
Parathyroid hormone, 1147
in renal osteodystrophy, 1229
Parathyroid hormone–related protein, 1218, 1219
in hypercalcemia, 320, 1148
Parietal cells, 787–788
autoantibodies to, 791, 793
Parking lot inclusions, in mitochondrial myopathy, 1287, *1288*
Parkinson disease, 1296t, 1333–1334, *1334*
Parkinsonism, 1333
Paronychia, 367
Parotid gland. See also *Salivary glands.*
inflammation of, 769
mixed tumor of, 262, *262*
pleomorphic adenoma of, 770–771, *770*
Parotitis, mumps, 371
Paroxysmal cold hemoglobinuria, 621
Paroxysmal nocturnal dyspnea, in left-sided heart failure, 549
Paroxysmal nocturnal hemoglobinuria, 69, 619–620, *619*
Partial thromboplastin time, 633
Particulates, in air, 417t, 418
Parvovirus, 333t
Parvovirus B19, transplacental infection with, 470, *470*
Patau syndrome, 171–173, *172*
Patent ductus arteriosus, *593,* 594
coarctation with, 596–597
Paterson-Kelly syndrome, 758, 778
Pathogenesis, 2
Pathogenicity islands, in bacterial virulence, 341
Pathology, 1–2
Pautrier microabscess, 1191, *1191*

PAX genes, 479
Paxillin, 101, *101*
PCP (phencyclidine), 413
Pediculosis, 1211–1212, *1211*
Peliosis hepatis, 883
Pelizaeus-Merzbacher disease, 1340
Pellagra, 448–449, *449*
Pelvic inflammatory disease, 1039–1040, *1039*
Pemphigoid, bullous, 1203–1204, *1204*
Pemphigus, 759t, 1201–1202, *1202, 1203*
Pemphigus erythematosus, 1202
Pemphigus foliaceus, 1202
Pemphigus vegetans, 1202
Pemphigus vulgaris, 200, 1202, *1202, 1203*
Penetrin, of *Trypanosoma cruzi,* 393
Penicillin, in warm antibody hemolytic anemia, 620
Penis, 1011–1014
  bowenoid papulosis of, 1012, 1209
  carcinoma in situ of, 1013–1014, *1013*
  carcinoma of, 1014, *1014*
  condyloma acuminatum of, 1012, *1012, 1013*
  congenital anomalies of, 1011–1012
  epispadias of, 1012
  erythroplasia of Queyrat of, 1013–1014
  fibromatosis of, 1263
  hypospadias of, 1012
  inflammation of, 1012
  phimosis of, 1012
  tumors of, 1012–1014, *1012, 1013*
Pentamidine, type I diabetes mellitus and, 917
Pepsinogen, 788
Peptic ulcer disease, 793–796, *794, 795,* 796t
Peptostreptococcus, 369
Percutaneous transluminal coronary angioplasty, 538
Perforin, in apoptosis, 24
  of cytotoxic T lymphocytes, 206
Pericardial effusion, 550, 587
Pericardial friction rub, 588
Pericarditis, 587–589, 587t, *588*
  after myocardial infarction, 562–563, *563*
  in systemic lupus erythematosus, 223
  in systemic sclerosis, 229
  uremic, 964
Pericardium, disease of, 587–589, 587t, *588*
  radiation damage to, 429, *429*
Pericytes, retinal, in diabetes mellitus, 1369
Perimysium, 1273
Perineurial barrier, 1271
Perineurium, 1271
Periodic acid–Schiff stain, 345, 345t
Periodic paralysis, thyrotoxic, 1288
Periostitis, syphilitic, 364
Peripheral myelin protein 22, 1270
  in Charcot-Marie-Tooth disease, 1277
  in Dejerine-Sottas disease, 1278
Peripheral nerves, 1269–1280, *1271.* See also *Peripheral neuropathy.*
  axonal degeneration of, 1274–1275, *1274*
  compression of, 1280
  demyelination of, 1274, *1274*
  laceration of, 1280
  regeneration of, 1275
  structure of, 1270–1271, *1271*
Peripheral neuroectodermal tumor, 485t
Peripheral neuropathy, diabetic, 924, 1279, *1279*
  hereditary, 1277–1279, 1277t, 1278t
    motor and sensory, 1277–1278
    sensory and autonomic, 1277, 1277t
  in acquired immunodeficiency syndrome, 1321
  in vitamin deficiencies, 1279
Peripheral neuropathy *(Continued)*
  infectious, 1276–1277
  inflammatory, 1275–1276
  metabolic, 1279
  nutritional, 1279
  optic, 1374
  paraneoplastic, 320, 321t, 1279–1280, 1352, 1352t
  toxic, 1280
  traumatic, 1280
  uremic, 1279
  viral, 1276–1277
Peripheral stem cell transplantation, 211
Peristalsis, intestinal, 804
Peritoneum, 841–842
  inflammation of, 841
  mesothelioma of, 752
Peritonitis, 841
  adhesions with, *825,* 826
Periventricular leukomalacia, *1300,* 1302
Pernicious anemia, 623–626, 623t, *624,* 791, 793
Peroxidase-dependent cooxidation, in toxicant metabolism, 406, *407*
Persistent hyperplastic primary vitreous, 1360
Pertussis toxin, 374
Pesticides, 422–423, 423t
Petechiae, *117,* 118
  in idiopathic thrombocytopenic purpura, 636
Petroleum products, in occupational diseases, 419t, 420
Peutz-Jeghers syndrome, 828, *828*
Peyer patches, 804
Peyronie disease, 1263
P-glycoprotein, in osteosarcoma, 1237
pH, in cell injury, 9
Phagocytosis, 25, *26,* 62–64, *63*
  frustrated, 64
  in apoptosis, 19, 20, *22,* 23
  in Chédiak-Higashi syndrome, 64–65
  nonopsonic, 62
  oxygen-dependent mechanisms of, 62–64, *63*
  oxygen-independent mechanisms of, 64
  surface, 64
Phagolysosomes, *26*
  in cell injury, 25–26
Phakogenic endophthalmitis, 1365
Phakomatoses, 1354–1355
Pharmacogenetics, 148
Pharyngitis, 763
  streptococcal, 368, 570, 572, *573*
Pharynx, carcinoma of, 764, *764*
  inflammation of, 763
  tumors of, 763–764, *764*
Phenacetin-induced nephropathy, 978–979, *979*
Phencyclidine (PCP), 413
Phenobarbital, barbiturate effects on, 26, *27*
Phentermine, cardiac valve lesions with, 578
Phenylalanine, tyrosine conversion of, 476, *476*
Phenylketonuria, 475–476, *476*
  gene mutation in, 147, 147t
Phenytoin, oral effects of, 759t
Pheochromocytoma, 1164–1166, 1164t, *1165*
Philadelphia chromosome, 285, *285*
Phimosis, 1012
Phlebothrombosis, 127, 129, 530
Phlegmasia alba dolens, 530
Phosphatidylserine, in apoptosis, 20
Phosphofructokinase, deficiency of, 160, *161*
Phosphoinositide-3-kinase pathway, for signal transduction, *93,* 94
Phospholipase, in cell injury, 6, *6*
Phospholipase C, of *Pseudomonas,* 377
Phosphorus, metabolism of, vitamin D in, 441–442
Phosphorylase, deficiency of (McArdle disease), 160, *161,* 163t
Phrygian cap, of gallbladder, 893, *893*
Phthisis bulbi, 1375–1376, *1376*
Phycomycetes, 380–381, *381*
Phyllodes tumors, 1103–1104, *1104*
Physical inactivity, in osteoporosis, 1223
Physis, 1219, *1219*
Phytobezoar, 797
Phytotoxins, 424, 424t
Pick disease, 1333
Pickwickian syndrome, 454
Pigeon breeder's lung, 737
Pigment, cellular accumulation of, 42–43, *42, 43*
Pigment cholelithiasis, 894–895, *895*
Pigment gallstones, 894–895, *895*
Pigmentation, disorders of, 1173–1179, *1173, 1175,* 1176t, *1177–1179*
  in adrenocortical insufficiency, 1162
Pigmented villonodular synovitis, 1258–1259, *1258*
Pilar cyst, 1181
Pili, bacterial, 342–343, *342*
Pineal gland, tumors of, 1168
Pinealoma, 1168
Pineoblastoma, 1168, 1350
Pineocytoma, 1168, 1350
Pingueculae, 1361, *1361*
Pinocytosis, 25
Pipe-stem fibrosis, in *Schistosoma* infection, 397, *397*
Pituitary gland, 1122–1129
  anterior, adenoma of, 1123–1127, *1124,* 1124t
      ACTH-secreting, 1126–1127, 1153–1154, *1153*
      FSH-secreting, 1127
      gonadotroph-secreting, 1127
      growth hormone–secreting, 1126
      LH-secreting, 1127
      null cell, 1127
      prolactin-secreting, 1125–1126, *1125*
      TSH-secreting, 1127
    carcinoma of, 1127
    normal, 1122–1123, *1123*
  Crooke hyaline change of, 1154
  empty sella syndrome of, 1128
  hyperfunction of, 1123–1127, *1124,* 1124t
  hypofunction of, 1127–1129, *1128*
  posterior, 1129
  Sheehan postpartum necrosis of, 642
PKD1 gene, 937–938, *938,* 939
PKD2 gene, 938, 939
PKD3 gene, 938
PKU (phenylketonuria), 475–476, *476*
Placenta, abnormalities of, 1080–1081, *1082, 1083*
  anatomy of, *1081*
  in intrauterine growth retardation, 461, *462*
  in preeclampsia, 1082, 1083, *1084*
  infection transmission by, 338, 470, *470*
  inflammation of, 1082, *1083*
  mosaicism of, in intrauterine growth retardation, 461, *462*
Placenta accreta, 1080–1081
Placental mosaicism, in intrauterine growth retardation, 461, *462*
Placental site trophoblastic tumor, 1089
Plague, 387–388

Plaques, 1172
  atheromatous, 499–503, *500, 501.* See also *Atheromatous plaque.*
  in Alzheimer disease, 1330, *1331*
  in multiple sclerosis, 1326–1327, *1327, 1328*
  kuru, 1324, *1325*
  pleural, 733, *733*
Plaque jaune, *1303,* 1304
Plasma cell, development of, *603*
  in inflammation, 82
Plasma cell dyscrasias, 651, 663–666, *665*
  renal manifestations of, 968
Plasma exchange, in diffuse pulmonary hemorrhage, 739
Plasma proteases, in inflammation, 67–70, *67, 68,* 77t
Plasmablasts, 664
Plasmacytoma, 555t, 666
  of nose, 763–764
Plasmids, 332
Plasmin, in coagulation, 123, *124*
  in inflammation, *68,* 69
Plasminogen, in coagulation, 124, *124*
Plasminogen activator(s), 124, *124*
  tissue-type (t-PA), 124, *124*
  urokinase-like (u-PA), 124, *124*
Plasminogen activator inhibitors, 124, *124*
  endothelial cell production of, 120
Plasmodium falciparum, 337t, 389–391, *390, 391*
  life cycle of, 389–390, *390*
Plasmodium malariae, 337t
Plasmodium ovale, 337t
Plasmodium vivax, 337t
Plastics, in occupational diseases, 419t, 420
Platelet(s), abnormalities of, bleeding with, 634–637, 635t
  activation of, in hemostasis, *118,* 119
  adhesion of, 120–121, *120*
    disorders of, 637
  aggregation of, 121–122, *121*
    disorders of, 637
    in hemolytic-uremic syndrome, 985
  alpha granules of, 120, 121
  aspirin effects on, 637
  contraction of, 121
  delta granules (dense bodies) of, 120, 121
  development of, *603*
  extracellular matrix adhesion of, 120–121, *120*
  giant, in essential thrombocytosis, 683, *683*
  immune-mediated destruction of, 635–636
  in glomerulonephritis, 947, *947*
  in hemostasis, *118,* 119, 120–122, *120, 121*
  inhibition of, 120
  secretions of, 121, 637
  serotonin release from, 67, 77t
Platelet count, 633
Platelet endothelial cell adhesion molecule 1 (PECAM-1), in leukocyte adhesion, 57, 57t, *58,* 61
Platelet-activating factor (PAF), in asthma, 713
  in inflammation, 72, *72,* 77t
  in type I hypersensitivity reaction, 198
Platelet-derived growth factor (PDGF), 97
  in angiogenesis, 105–106, *105*
  in myelofibrosis with myeloid metaplasia, 684
  in tumorigenesis, 279–280, 279t
Platybasia, in Paget disease, 1227
Pleura, 749–752
  effusion of, 749–751, 750t
    in right-sided heart failure, 550
    in systemic lupus erythematosus, 224
Pleura *(Continued)*
  fibroma of, 751
  gas in, 751
  inflammation of, 224, 749–751, 750t
  mesothelioma of, 751–752, *752, 753*
  metastatic carcinoma of, 751
  plaques of, in asbestosis, 733, *733*
  tumors of, 751–752, *752, 753*
Pleuritis, 749–751, 750t
  in systemic lupus erythematosus, 224
Plexogenic pulmonary arteriopathy, 705, *706*
Plummer syndrome, 1140
Plummer-Vinson syndrome, 758, 778
Plymphocytes, 666
Pneumoconiosis, 727–734
  coal workers', 729–730, 729t, *730*
  pathogenesis of, 727–729, *728,* 729t
Pneumocystis carinii pneumonia, 381–382, *382*
  in acquired immunodeficiency syndrome, 247
Pneumocytes, 698
Pneumolysin, of streptococci, 367
Pneumonia, atypical, primary, 721–722
  bacterial, 348–352, 717–721
    anatomic distribution of, 717, *717, 718*
    clinical course of, 721
    complications of, 721
    etiology of, 719–720
    host defense mechanisms in, 718–719
    in lung transplant patient, 741
    lobar, 717–718, *718*
    morphology of, 720–721, *720*
    patchy consolidation in, 717, *718*
    pathogenesis of, 718–719, *719*
    stages of, 720, *720*
  Chlamydia psittaci, 362
  eosinophilic, 738
  etiologic agents in, 719–720
  Haemophilus influenzae, 349
  herpes, 361
  in immunocompromised host, 247, 726
  Legionella, 377–378
  lipid, 721
  mycoplasmal, 721–722
  patchy consolidation in, 716, *717*
  pneumococcal, *345*
  Pneumocystis, 247, 381–382, *382*
  tuberculous, 726
  viral, 348, 721–722
  with burns, 434
Pneumonitis, cytomegalovirus, 376
  hypersensitivity, 737, *737*
  interstitial, 721–722
    desquamative, 736–737, *737*
  lupus, 739
  radiation, 740
  uremic, 964
Pneumothorax, 700, 751
Podocytes, 933, 947, *947*
Poison, in cell injury, 4
pol gene, 238, *239*
Poliomyelitis, 1319
Poliovirus, 333t, 373
  CNS infection with, 1319
Pollution, environmental, 416–418, 417t
Polyangiitis, microscopic, 517t, 521–522, *522*
Polyarteritis nodosa, 231, 517t, 520–521, *520,* 968
Polycyclic aromatic hydrocarbons, in carcinogenesis, 309
Polycystic kidney disease, autosomal dominant, 937–940, *938, 939,* 941t
  autosomal recessive, 940, 941t
Polycystin 1, 937–938, *938*
Polycythemia, 633, 633t
Polycythemia vera, 682–683, *682*
Polyglucosan body disease, 1297
Polymerase chain reaction (PCR), in genetic disorders, 182–184, *183, 185*
  in tumor diagnosis, 324
Polymers, in occupational diseases, 419t, 420
Polymicrogyria, 1300
Polymyositis, 229, 231
Polyneuropathy. See also *Neuropathy.*
  amyloid, familial, 1277, 1278t
  infectious, 1276–1277
Polyostotic fibrous dysplasia, 1243
Polyp(s), colonic, 261, *262*
  endocervical, 1048, *1048*
  endometrial, 1058–1059, *1059*
  esophageal, 783
  fibroepithelial, 1181
    of ureter, 999
  fibroid, inflammatory, 802
  gastric, 798
  intestinal, 827–831, *827–831*
    adenomatous, 827, *827,* 829–831, *829–831*
    hyperplastic, *827,* 828, *828*
    juvenile, 828, *828*
    non-neoplastic, *827,* 828, *828*
    Peutz-Jeghers, 828, *828*
  nasal, 762, *762*
  vocal cord, 765
Polyposis, lymphomatoid, 668
Polyradiculoneuropathy, demyelinating, inflammatory, 1275–1276
Pompe disease, 155t, 160–161, *161, 163,* 163t
Pores of Kohn, 698, *720*
Poroma, eccrine, 1182
Porphyria, 1206, *1206,* 1278t
Porta hepatis, 846
Portal hypertension, 783, 855–856, *855,* 882
Portal tracts, 846
Portal vein, obstruction of, 882
Portosystemic shunts, in cirrhosis, 855–856, *855*
Port-wine stain, 534
Posterior fossa, anomalies of, 1301, *1301*
Postpolio syndrome, 1319
Poststreptococcal (proliferative) glomerulonephritis, 949–951, *950,* 965t
Pott disease, 351, 1233
Potter (oligohydramnios) sequence, 465, *465*
Pouch of Douglas, 802
PRAD 1 protooncogene, 1149
Prader-Willi syndrome, 180–181, *181*
Precancerous conditions, 276
Preeclampsia, 884, *885,* 1082–1084
Pregnancy, ectopic, 1079–1080, *1080*
  fatty liver of, 884–885
  hepatic disease with, 884–885, *885*
  intrahepatic cholestasis of, 885
  luteoma in, 1078
  melasma in, 1174
  oral manifestations of, 758, *758,* 759t
  pituitary necrosis after, 642
  placental abnormalities in, 1080–1081, *1082, 1083*
  preeclampsia in, 884, *885,* 1082–1084
  pyogenic granuloma in, 533
  renal failure after, 986
  spontaneous termination of, 1079
  toxemia of, 642, 1082–1084, *1084, 1085*
  twin, 1081, *1082*
Preinfarction angina, 554
Prekallikrein, in inflammation, *68,* 69
Premature infant, intraparenchymal hemorrhage in, 1302

Premature infant *(Continued)*
periventricular leukomalacia in, *1300,* 1302
Prematurity, retinopathy of, 1368–1369
Preneoplastic disorders, 276
Presenilin, in Alzheimer disease, 1332, 1332t
Prevotella, 369–370
Primary sclerosing cholangitis, 877t, 879–880, *879*
Primitive neuroectodermal tumor, 1244, 1260t
Prinzmetal angina, 554
Prion diseases, 1296t, 1323–1326, *1325*
Prion protein, 332, 1323–1324, *1325*
PRNP gene, 1324
Pro-apoptotic protease activating factor, 22–23, *23*
Procallus, 1229
Progressive multifocal leukoencephalopathy, 1321, *1322,* 1326
Progressive supranuclear palsy, 1334–1335
Prolactin, tumor secretion of, 1125–1126, *1125*
Prolactinoma, 1125–1126, *1125*
Proliferation centers, in chronic lymphocytic leukemia, 658
Prolymphocytes, 659
in chronic lymphocytic leukemia, 658, *658*
Promoters, in carcinogenesis, 309
in chemical carcinogenesis, 306, *307,* 308
Propionibacterium acnes, 369, 1207
Propylthiouracil, in Graves disease, 1138
thyroid inhibition by, 1131
Prostaglandins, synthesis of, 70, *71*
Prostaglandin D_2, 70, *71*
in asthma, 713
in type I hypersensitivity reaction, 198
Prostaglandin E_2, 70, *71*
Prostaglandin $F_{2\alpha}$, 70, *71*
Prostaglandin G_2, 70, *71*
Prostaglandin H_2, 70, *71*
Prostaglandin I_2 (prostacyclin), 70, *71,* 122
Prostate, 1025–1033, *1025*
carcinoma of, 1029–1033, *1030, 1031*
clinical course of, 1031–1033, *1032*
etiology of, 1029–1030
geographic factors in, 273, *273*
grading of, 1031, *1032*
incidence of, *272,* 1029
metastases from, 1030, *1031, 1032*
morphology of, 1030–1031, *1030, 1031*
perineural invasion in, 1031, *1031*
prostate-specific antigen in, 1032–1033
treatment of, 1033
inflammation of, 1025–1027, *1026*
intraepithelial neoplasia of, 1031
nodular hyperplasia of, 1027–1029, *1027–1029*
bladder obstruction and, 1008, *1008*
clinical course of, 1028–1029
etiology of, 1027
incidence of, 1027
morphology of, 1027–1028, *1028, 1029*
pathogenesis of, 1027, *1027*
Prostate-specific antigen (PSA), in prostate carcinoma, 1032–1033
Prostatitis, 1025–1027, *1026*
Prosthetic heart valves, 578, *578,* 578t
Proteases, acid, 76
in angiogenesis, 106
in cell injury, 6, *6*
in inflammation, 67–70, *67, 68,* 77t
neutral, 76
tumor elaboration of, 303–304
Proteasome, in atrophy, 36
Protein(s), cellular accumulation of, 40–41, *41*
cross-linking of, in apoptosis, 20
degradation of, 36, 41
denaturation of, in necrosis, 16, *16*
folding of, defects in, 41, *41*
hydrolysis of, in apoptosis, 20
matricellular, 101
nonenzymatic glycosylation of, in diabetes mellitus, 919–920, *919,* 920t
of bone, 1217–1218, 1218t
Protein 4.1, gene for, 147t
Protein C, activation of, 120
in coagulation, 122–123, *124*
Protein S, in coagulation, 122–123, *124*
Protein-energy malnutrition, 437–439, *438,* 438t
atrophy with, 35
in chronic pancreatitis, 908
Protein-losing gastroenteropathy, 798
Protein-mobilizing factor, cancer cachexia and, 320
Proteinosis, alveolar, 739–740, *740*
Proteinuria, 935
in multiple myeloma, 981
in nephrotic syndrome, 952–953
in sickle cell disease, 987
renal tubular injury and, 948–949, *949*
renal tubule protein reabsorption droplets in, 40–41, *41*
Proteoglycans, of extracellular matrix, 101–102
Proteolipid protein, in Pelizaeus-Merzbacher disease, 1340
Proteus, 334t
in pyelonephritis, 977
Prothrombin, in coagulation, 122, *123*
Prothrombin time, 633
Protooncogenes, 92, 277–278
amplification of, 286, *286*
antigenicity of, 317
for growth factors, 279–280, 279t
for nuclear transcription proteins, 279t, 282
for signal-transducing proteins, 279t, 280–282
insertional mutagenesis of, 278
oncogene transformation of, 284–286, *285, 286,* 286t
Protozoa, 335–336, *337,* 337t
CNS infection with, 1322–1323, *1323*
gastrointestinal tract infection with, 358–359, *358, 359,* 810–811, *811*
Proud flesh, 110
Pruritus, in cholestasis, 851
Psammoma bodies, 43
in papillary thyroid carcinoma, 1143–1144
in renal cell carcinoma, 994
Psammomatous meningioma, 1350, *1351*
Pseudoaneurysm, 524
Pseudoarthrosis, 1231
Pseudocysts, pancreatic, 907, 909, *909*
Pseudogout, 874, 1257, *1257*
Pseudohermaphroditism, 176
Pseudo-Hurler polydystrophy, 155t
Pseudohypoparathyroidism, 1151
Pseudomembranous colitis, 809–810, *810*
Pseudomonas aeruginosa, 334t, 376–377, *377*
in cystic fibrosis, 479, 480
virulence factors of, 377
Pseudomonas cepacia, in cystic fibrosis, 480
Pseudomonas mallei, 334t
Pseudomonas pseudomallei, 334t
Pseudomyxoma peritonei, 1071, *1071*
Pseudo-Pelger-Huët cells, in myelodysplastic syndromes, 678, *679*
Pseudopod, of leukocyte, 61, *61*
Pseudorosettes, perivascular, 1347, *1347*
Pseudosarcomatous proliferations, reactive, 1262, *1262*
Psoriasis, 1198–1199, *1198, 1199*
Psoriatic arthritis, 1252–1253
PTC gene, 1186–1187
PTEN gene, 294
Pteroylmonoglutamic acid, deficiency of, 626–627, *626*
Pterygium, 1361
Pulmonary. See also *Lungs.*
Pulmonary embolism, 130, *130,* 703–704, *703*
fibrous web from, 130
prevention of, 704
pulmonary abscess and, 722
Pulmonary fibrosis, 735–736, *736*
Pulmonary hypertension, 704–706, *706*
Pulmonary stenosis, 597
Pulmonary surfactant, deficiency of, 471–473, *472*
Pulmonary valve, 545
atresia of, 597
Pulmonary vascular sclerosis, 704–706, *706*
Pulseless disease, 517t, 519–520, *519*
Punch-drunk syndrome, 1305–1306
Pure red cell aplasia, 632
Purine, metabolism of, 1254–1255, *1254*
Purpura, 118
Henoch-Schönlein, 517t, 961
hemorrhage in, 634
renal manifestations in, 965–966
nonthrombocytopenic, 634
thrombocytopenic, idiopathic, 635–636
thrombocytopenic, 636–637
thrombotic, 986
Pus, 53
Pustule, 1172
Pyelonephritis, 972–975, *972–975*
acute, 974–975, *974, 975*
chronic, 975–977, *976*
in diabetes mellitus, 924
obstructive, 975
papillary necrosis in, 974, *975*
vesicoureteral reflex in, 973–974, *973*
xanthogranulomatous, 977
Pyknosis, in necrosis, *9,* 16
Pyloric sphincter, 787, *787*
Pyloric stenosis, 789
Pyogenic granuloma, *532,* 533
Pyonephrosis, 974

Q

Q fever, 384, 385t, 721–722
Quiescent cells, 91
Quinsy sore throat, 368

R

Rabies virus, 333t, 1319–1320
Rad, 425
Radial scars, of breast, 1101
Radiation, biologic effects of, 425–426
carcinogenicity of, 309–311
CNS effects of, 1342–1343
fetal effects of, 467
injury from, 424t, 425–430
acute, 426, 426t, 427, *427,* 427t
cardiac, 429, *429*
cellular mechanisms of, 426–427, 426t
central nervous system, 430
cutaneous, 429, *429*
delayed, 426t, 428–430, *428, 429*

Radiation, injury from *(Continued)*
developmental abnormalities and, 428
esophageal, 782
fibrosis in, 426
gastrointestinal tract, 429
gonadal, 430
growth abnormalities and, 428
intestinal, 311
mammary, 429, *429*
mutations and, 428
ocular, 430
pulmonary, 429, 740
renal, 429
tumor development and, 426–427
urinary tract, 429
vascular, 428, *428*
sources of, 424–425, 424t
thyroid carcinoma and, 1142
ultraviolet, in carcinogenesis, 310
in systemic lupus erythematosus, 219, 222
injury from, 430–431, 430t, *431*
Radiation dermatitis, 429, *429*
Radiation sickness, 427
Radon, in air, 418, 418t
in cancer, 274t, 742
Raf protein, 93
RAGE genes, 216
Ragged red fibers, in mitochondrial myopathy, 1287, *1288*
Ramsay Hunt syndrome, 374
K-*ras* gene, in bronchogenic carcinoma, 742
ras genes, 280–282, *281,* 284
in chemical carcinogenesis, 308
in thyroid carcinoma, 1143
ultraviolet ray–induced mutation of, 310
Ras protein, activation of, 93
Rash, in measles virus infection, 370
in streptococcal infection, 368
in varicella-zoster virus infection, 374
Raynaud phenomenon, 524
Rb gene, 147t, 286–287, *288,* 1372
in cancer, 257t, 289–290, *289*
Rb protein, in cell-cycle regulation, 96
Reactive oxygen species. See *Free radicals.*
Reactive pseudosarcomatous proliferations, 1261–1262
Receptor(s), 92–93, *93, 94*
acetylcholine, immune-mediated loss of, 1289
angiopoietin, 105
autophosphorylation of, 92, *94*
cytokine, 92, *93*
dimerization of, 92, *94*
G protein–linked (seven-spanning), 92–93, *95*
LDL, gene for, 144, 147t, 152–153, *153*
serpentine, 74
Tie2, 105
tumor necrosis factor, in apoptosis, 23–24, *24*
tyrosine kinase, 92, *94*
vascular endothelial growth factor, 105
vitamin D, 147t
Rectum, blood supply of, 802
carcinoma of. See *Intestine, carcinoma of.*
Red blood cells. See *Erythrocyte(s).*
Reduction-oxidation reaction, in free radical generation, 12, *13*
Reed-Sternberg cell, in Hodgkin disease, 670–671, *671*
Reflux, vesicoureteral, congenital, 1000
Reflux esophagitis, 780–781, *780*
Reflux nephropathy, 975–976, *976*
Refsum disease, 1278t
Regional hemorrhagic fever viruses, 333t
Reid index, in bronchitis, 712
Reidel thyroiditis, 1136
Reis-Bücklers dystrophy, 1363
Reiter syndrome, 361, 1252
Relapsing febrile nodular panniculitis, 1208
Relapsing fever, 388
Relative biologic effectiveness, 425
Rem, 425
Renal. See also *Kidney.*
Renal ablation glomerulosclerosis, 948, *948*
Renal artery(ies), embolism from, 986, *987*
fibromuscular dysplasia of, 984, *984*
stenosis of, 984–985, *984,* 986
Renal cell carcinoma, 991–993, *992–994*
chromophobe, 992, 993
metastatic, 993
nonpapillary, 992, *992, 994*
papillary, 992, *992*
pulmonary metastases from, 749, *749*
venous spread of, 270
Renal osteodystrophy, 1229
Renal pelvis, 931
stone in, 990, *990*
urothelial carcinoma of, 994, *994*
Renal tubules, 934
acute necrosis of, 969–971. See also *Acute tubular necrosis (ATN).*
protein reabsorption droplets in, 40–41, *41*
thyroidization of, 976, *976*
Renal vein, renal cell carcinoma of, 270
thrombosis of, in nephrotic syndrome, 953
Renin-angiotensin system, in hypertension, *512,* 983
Renomedullary interstitial cell tumor, 991
Reperfusion injury, 11–12
Reserve cells, in metaplasia, 37
Residual bodies, 36
Respiratory distress syndrome (hyaline membrane disease), 471–473, *472*
Respiratory syncytial virus, 333t, 340–341
Respiratory tract. See also *Lungs.*
burns of, 434
infection of, 347–353
bacterial, 348–352, *350–352*
Coccidioides immitis in, 353, *353*
fungal, 352–353, *353*
Haemophilus influenzae in, 348–349
Histoplasma capsulatum in, 352, *353*
influenza viruses in, 348
Mycobacterium avium in, 352, *352*
Mycobacterium tuberculosis in, 349–352, *350, 351*
rhinoviruses in, 347–348, *347*
viral, 347–348, *347*
squamous metaplasia in, 37, *37*
Restriction fragment length polymorphism analysis, 184–185, *185*
Restrictocin, 330
ret gene, 280
RET protooncogene, 1143, 1145, 1167
Reticulin, antibodies to, in dermatitis herpetiformis, 1205
Retina, 1368–1373. See also *Retinopathy.*
congenital anomalies of, 1360
fibroplasia of, 1370
in Tay-Sachs disease, 156
layers of, 1368, *1368*
neovascularization of, 1370
rubella-related abnormalities of, 1361
sarcoidosis of, 1364
Retinal detachment, 1370, 1372, *1372*
Retinal vein, in diabetic retinopathy, 1370
Retinitis pigmentosa, 1370–1371
Retinitis proliferans, 1370
Retinoblastoma, 485t, 1372–1373, *1373*
genetic factors in, 147t, 275
pathogenesis of, 286–287, *288,* 290
two-hit hypothesis of, 286–287, *288*
Retinoic acid, 440, *440*
in cancer prevention, 455
teratogenicity of, 469–470, *469*
Retinoids, 439–440, *440.* See also *Vitamin A.*
Retinopathy, arteriosclerotic, 1370
hypertensive, 1370
in diabetes mellitus, 1369–1370, *1369*
of prematurity, 472, 1368–1369
pigmentary, 1370–1371
proliferative, 1370
Retrobulbar neuritis, in multiple sclerosis, 1327
Retrolental fibroplasia, 472, 1368–1369
Retroperitonitis, sclerosing, 841
rev gene, of human immunodeficiency virus, 238, *239*
Reye syndrome, 869
Rh isoimmunization, 473–475, *474*
Rhabdomyoma, cardiac, 591
Rhabdomyosarcoma, *265,* 485t, 1265–1266, *1265*
alveolar, 1265–1266, *1265*
embryonal, 1265, *1265*
of bladder, 1008
of vagina, 1046–1047, *1046*
of bladder, 1008
pleomorphic, 1266
Rheumatic fever, 570–572, *571, 573*
Rheumatoid arthritis, 1248–1251
clinical course of, 1251
diagnosis of, 1251
genetic factors in, 1249
heart in, 589
immune system in, 216, 1249–1250, *1250*
joint manifestations in, 1248–1249, *1248*
juvenile, 1251–1252
microbial agents in, 1249
pulmonary involvement in, 739
radiographic manifestations of, 1251, *1251*
skin manifestations in, 1249, *1249*
vascular manifestations in, 524, 1249
Rheumatoid spondylitis, 1252
Rhinitis, 762
Rhinoviruses, 333t, 347–348, *347*
Rhizopus, 380–381
Rhoptry, of *Plasmodium falciparum,* 389
Riboflavin, 447–448
Rice bodies, 1248–1249
Richter syndrome, 659
Rickets, 147t, 444–445, 444t, 1227–1228
Rickettsia spp., 334t, 335
Rickettsia prowazekii, 332t
Rickettsia spp., 383–385, *384, 385*
Rickettsialpox, 385t
Right-to-left cardiac shunt, 595–596, *596*
Ring fiber, in myotonic dystrophy, 1284
Ringed sideroblasts, in myelodysplastic syndromes, 678, *679*
Ristocetin aggregation test, 638
Robertsonian translocation, *169,* 170
Rocky Mountain spotted fever, 384, *385,* 385t
Rod cells, 1297
Rodenticides, 423t, 424
Roentgen, 425
Rokitansky-Aschoff sinuses, 892
Rosenthal fibers, 1297
Rotavirus, 333t, 354, 806, 807t
Rotor syndrome, 850t, 851
Roundworms, 336–337
Rubber, in occupational diseases, 419t, 420

Rubella retinopathy, 1361
Rubella virus, 333t, 467
Rubeola. See *Measles virus.*
Rugae, of stomach, 787, 797–798, *797*
Russell bodies, 41
in lymphoplasmacytic lymphoma, 666

S
SAA protein, in amyloidosis, 254–255, *254*
Saccular aneurysm, 525
Sacrococcygeal teratoma, 484, *484*
Salicylism, 416
Salivary glands, 769–773
acinic cell tumor of, 773
adenoid cystic carcinoma of, 772–773, *773*
inflammation of, 769
lymphocytic infiltration of, in Sjögren syndrome, 225, *226*
mixed tumor of, 262, *262*
mucoepidermoid carcinoma of, 772, *772*
pleomorphic adenoma of, 770–771, *770*
sarcoidosis of, 735
tumors of, 769–773, 769t, *770–773*
Warthin tumors of, 771–772, *771*
Salmonella, 334t, 807–809, 808t
Salmonella typhi, 334t, 356–357, *357*
Salmonellosis, 356–357
Salpingitis, 369–370, 1065
Salpino-oophoritis, 1039, *1039*
Salt-wasting syndrome, 1157
San Joaquin Valley fever complex, 353
Sandhoff disease, 155t
Sarcoglycan, in limb-girdle muscular dystrophy, 1284, 1284t
Sarcoidosis, 734–735, *734,* 1364, *1364*
Sarcolemma, 1272
Sarcoma, 261–262
cardiac, 591
clear cell, 1260t
Ewing, 1244, *1244*
Kaposi, 535–537, *536*
of bladder, 1008
of breast, 1104
of endometrium, 1065
osteogenic, 1236–1237, *1236, 1237*
synovial, 1260t, 1266–1267, *1267*
Sarcoma botryoides, of bladder, 1008
of vagina, 1046–1047, *1046*
Sarcomeres, 544, 1272, *1272*
Sarcoplasm, in myotonic dystrophy, 1284
Satellite cells, 1272
Scabies, *1211,* 1212
Scalded skin syndrome, staphylococcal, 365–366, 367
Scale, cutaneous, 1172
Scar, *104.* See also *Fibrosis.*
formation of, 106–107, *107,* 108–109, *108, 111*
in infection, 347, *347*
hypertrophic, 110, *110*
renal, in pyelonephritis, 976, *976*
Scarlet fever, 368, 759t
Scatter factor (hepatocyte growth factor), in hepatocyte regeneration, 33, *33*
Schatzki rings, 777–778
Schaumann bodies, 734
Schistosoma spp., infection of, 396–397, *397*
life cycle of, 396, *396*
Schistosoma haematobium, 346, *347,* 397
transitional cell carcinoma and, 1007
Schistosomiasis, 396–397, *396, 397*
Schwann cells, 1270, 1271, *1271*
in neurofibromatosis, 164
Mycobacterium leprae infection of, 1276
Schwannoma, 1352–1353, *1353*
malignant, 1353–1354
SCID (severe combined immunodeficiency disease), 235–236
gene mutation in, 147t
Scleroderma. See *Systemic sclerosis (scleroderma).*
Sclerosing adenosis, of breast, 1101, *1101*
Sclerosing cholangitis, 877t, 879–880, *879*
Sclerosing osteomyelitis of Garré, 1233
Sclerosing panencephalitis, subacute, 1321–1322
Sclerosing papilloma, of breast, 1101
Sclerosing retroperitoneal fibrosis, of ureters, 999–1000
Sclerosing retroperitonitis, 841
Sclerosis, calcific (Mönckeberg arteriosclerosis), 498
systemic, 226–229. See also *Systemic sclerosis (scleroderma).*
Scorpion bite, 1210–1212
Scrub typhus, 384–385, 385t
Scurvy, 449–450
hemorrhage in, 634
Sebaceous glands, *1171*
Seborrheic keratoses, 1179–1180, *1180*
Secretin, 903
Secretory meningioma, 1350
Selectins, in leukocyte adhesion, 57–58, 57t, *58*
Selenium, deficiency of, 451–452, 452t
Self-antigens, epitope crypticity of, 215
immune reactions against. See *Autoimmune diseases.*
molecular mimicry of, 215
tolerance to, 212–214, *213*
Semilunar valves, 545. See also *Aortic valve; Pulmonary valve.*
Seminoma, 263, 264, 1019–1020, *1019*
spermatocytic, 1020
vs. nonseminomatous germ cell tumor, 1023
Senescence, cellular, 46–47, *46, 47, 48*
Sensory neuropathy, 1277, 1277t
paraneoplastic, 1352, 1352t
Sepsis, in infant, 471
Listeria, 378
Septic shock, 134–136, *134,* 134t, *135*
Septum (septa), alveolar, 698, *698*
ventricular, sigmoid, 546
Sequence, congenital, definition of, 465, *465*
Sequestrins, of *Plasmodium falciparum,* 389–390
Serotonin (5-hydroxytryptamine), in carcinoid syndrome, 837, 837t
in inflammation, 67, 77t
Serratia marcescens, 334t
Sertoli cell tumor, 1024
Sertoli-Leydig cell tumor, 1078, *1078*
Serum amyloid A, in febrile state, 86
Serum amyloid P, in febrile state, 86
Serum sickness, 202–204, *202, 203*
Severe combined immunodeficiency disease (SCID), 235–236
autosomal recessive, 235
gene mutation in, 147t
X-linked, 235
Sex, genetic, 176. See also *X chromosome; Y chromosome.*
gonadal, 176
phenotypic (genital), 176
Sex cord–stromal tumor, 1076–1079, *1077, 1078*
Sex-determining region Y gene, 174
Sexually transmitted diseases, 359–365, 360t, 1038–1040, 1038t, *1039*
Chlamydia trachomatis in, 361–362, 361t
herpesvirus in, 359–361, *360*
Neisseria gonorrhoeae in, 362
Treponema pallidum in, 362–364, *363*
Trichomonas vaginalis in, 364–365, *365*
Sézary syndrome, 656t, 670
Sézary-Lutzner cells, 1191, *1191*
Sheep, jagziekte disease of, 747
Sherman's paradox, in fragile X syndrome, 177–178, *178*
Shiga toxin, 355
Shiga-like toxin, in hemolytic-uremic syndrome, 985, 986
Shigella, 334t, 355, *355,* 807–809, 808t, *809*
Shingles, 373–374, 1276–1277
Shock, 134–137, 134t
anaphylactic, 134
cardiogenic, 134, 134t, 562
clinical course of, 137
endotoxic, 134–136, *134*
hypovolemic, 118, 134, 134t
in acute pancreatitis, 907
irreversible phase of, 136
morphology of, 136–137
multiorgan system failure in, 136
neurogenic, 134
nonprogressive phase of, 136
progressive phase of, 136
septic, 134–136, *134,* 134t, *135*
stages of, 136
Shunt, cardiac, 591–596
left-to-right, 593–595, *593, 594*
right-to-left, 595–596, *595*
portosystemic, in cirrhosis, 855–856, *855*
Shy-Drager syndrome, 1335
Sialadenitis, 769
Sialolithiasis, 769
Sicca syndrome. See *Sjögren syndrome.*
Sick building syndrome, 419
Sickle cell disease, 611–615, *612–614*
blood flow alterations in, 125
gene mutation in, 143–144, 147t
hepatic sinusoid occlusion in, 882
nephropathy in, 979t, 986–987
Sickle cell trait, 143–144
Sideroblasts, ringed, in myelodysplastic syndromes, 678, *679*
Siderophages, in left-sided heart failure, 549
Siderosis, 729t
Sievert (Sv), 425
Sign of Leser-Trélat, 1180
Signal transduction systems, 93–95, *93–95*
cyclic adenosine monophosphate pathway, *93,* 94
in tumorigenesis, 279t, 280–282
inositol-lipid pathway, 94, *95*
JAK/STAT pathway, *93,* 94–95
mitogen-activated protein kinase pathway, 93, *94*
phosphoinositide-3-kinase pathway, *93,* 94
Silicone implants, for breast reconstruction, 1098
Silicosis, 729t, 730–732, *731, 732*
pathogenesis of, 728–729
Silver stains, 345, 345t
Singers' nodules, 765
Sinoatrial node, 544
Sinus histiocytosis, 650
Sinusitis, 762–763
Sinusoids, 495
Sipple syndrome (MEN-II), 1167, 1167t

Sjögren syndrome, 225–226, *226,* 758
antinuclear antibodies in, 218t
Skeletal muscle, 35, 1272–1273, *1272, 1273,* 1273t. See also *Muscle(s).*
Skin, 1170–1212
acanthosis nigricans of, 320, 321t, 1180–1181
acne vulgaris of, 1206–1207, *1207*
actinic keratosis of, 1184, *1185*
adnexal (appendage) tumors of, 1182–1183, *1183,* 1183t, *1184*
arthropod bites of, 1210–1211, 1212
atopic dermatitis of, 1195t
barrier function of, 338
basal cell carcinoma of, 1186–1187, *1187*
ultraviolet radiation in, 310
benign epithelial tumors of, 1179–1183, *1180, 1182–1184,* 1183t
benign fibrous histiocytoma of, 1187–1188, *1188*
blistering diseases of, 1201–1206, *1201–1206*
bullous pemphigoid of, 1203–1204, *1204*
burns of, 433–434
Pseudomonas infection in, 377
contact dermatitis of, 206, *206,* 1195t, 1196–1197, *1196*
dermatitis herpetiformis of, 1204–1205, *1205*
dermatofibroma of, 1187–1188, *1188*
dermatofibrosarcoma protuberans of, 1188
drug-related atopic dermatitis of, 1195t
eczema of, 1194–1197, *1195,* 1195t, *1196*
epidermolysis bullosa of, 1205, *1206*
epithelial cyst of, 1181
erythema chronicum migrans of, 389
erythema induratum of, 1207–1208
erythema multiforme of, 1197–1198, *1197*
erythema nodosum of, 1207–1208
fibroepithelial polyp of, 1181
fungal infection of, 1210
histiocytosis X of, 1189–1191, *1190*
hives of, 1194, *1194*
ichthyosis of, 1193, *1193*
impetigo of, 1210
in adrenocortical insufficiency, 1162
in ariboflavinosis, 448
in dermatomyositis, 229, *230*
in Ehlers-Danlos syndromes, 150
in filariasis, 398, *398*
in Graves disease, 1138
in hyperthyroidism, 1132
in McCune-Albright syndrome, 1243
in pellagra, 448, *449*
in situ carcinoma of, 1185
in systemic lupus erythematosus, 222, *223*
in systemic sclerosis, 228, *228*
in zinc deficiency, 451, *452*
inflammatory dermatoses of, 1193–1201
acute, 1193–1198, *1194, 1195,* 1195t, *1196*
chronic, 1198–1201, *1198, 1199*
irritant dermatitis of, 1195t
Kaposi varicelliform eruption of, 361
lice infestation of, 1211–1212, *1211*
lichen planus of, 1199–1200, *1199*
lupus erythematosus of, 1200–1201, *1200, 1201*
mastocytosis of, 1192–1193, *1192*
melanoma of, 310, 1177–1179, *1178, 1179*
Merkel cell carcinoma of, 1187
mite infestation of, *1211,* 1212
molluscum contagiosum of, 1209–1210, *1209*
Skin *(Continued)*
mycosis fungoides of, 1191, *1191*
papillomavirus infection of, 1208–1209, *1208*
peau d'orange change of, 1114
pemphigus of, 1201–1202, *1202, 1203*
pigmentation disorders of, 1173–1179, *1173, 1175,* 1176t, *1177–1179*
porphyria of, 1206, *1206*
protective function of, 1170–1173, *1171, 1172*
psoriasis of, 1198–1199, *1198, 1199*
radiation damage to, 429, *429*
sarcoidosis of, 735
seborrheic keratoses of, 1179–1180, *1180*
squamous cell carcinoma of, 266, *266,* 310, 1184–1186, *1186*
streptococcal erysipelas of, 368, *368*
T-cell lymphoma of, 670, 1191, *1191*
urticaria of, 1194, *1194*
vascular tumors of, 532–533, *532,* 534–535, *534,* 537–538, *537,* 1189
verrucae of, 1208–1209, *1208*
warts of, 1208–1209, *1208*
xanthoma of, 1189
Skin tag, 1181
Skull, fracture of, 1302–1303
at birth, 464
SLE. See *Systemic lupus erythematosus (SLE).*
Sleep, prion-associated disturbances of, 1326
Slit hemorrhages, 1314
Slow virus, 341
Small airway disease, 707t, 711–712
Small for gestational age infant, 460–462, *461, 462*
Small round blue cell tumor, 485, 485t. See also specific tumors.
Small round structured viruses, 807, 807t
Smith (sm) antigen, antibodies to, in systemic lupus erythematosus, 217, 218t
SMN gene, 1281
Smooth muscle, in atherosclerosis, 509
tumors of, 589–591, *589,* 591t
vascular, 497, *497*
Smudge cells, in chronic lymphocytic leukemia, 659, *659*
Soap-bubble lesions, in *Cryptococcus neoformans* infection, 380, *380*
SOD1 gene, 1338
Sodium, in cell injury, 7
renal retention of, in hypertension, 513
retention of, edema and, 115–116
Soemmering, cataract, 1368
Soft tissue tumors, 1259–1267, 1259t, 1260t. See also specific tumors.
Soldier's plaque, 589
Solid-cystic tumor, of pancreas, 910
Sorbitol, in diabetes mellitus, *919,* 920
Space of Disse, 846–847
SPARC (secreted protein acidic and rich in cystein) protein (osteonectin), 101
Spätapoplexie, 1305
Species, life span of, 47
Specific atrial granules, 544
Spectrin, gene for, 144, 147t
Spermatic cord, twisting of, 1017, *1017*
Spermatocele, 1025
Spermatozoa, postvasectomy release of, 215
Spherocytosis, hereditary, 147t, 607–609, *609*
Sphincter, esophageal, 776
pyloric, 787, *787*
Sphingolipidoses, 155t
Sphingomyelinase, deficiency of (Niemann-Pick disease), 155t, 156–158, *157*
Spider angioma, in hepatic failure, 852
Spider bite, 1210–1212
Spider cells, in rhabdomyoma, 591
Spider telangiectasia, 534
Spina bifida, 1300
Spinal cord, hydromyelia of, 1301–1302
in pernicious anemia, 625
malformation of, 1300
syringomyelia of, 1301–1302
trauma to, 1306
Spinal muscular atrophy, 24, 1281, *1281,* 1338
Spinobulbar muscular atrophy, 179t
Spinocerebellar ataxia, 179t, 1296t, 1337
Spiral valves of Heister, 892
Spirillum minus, 334t
Spitz nevus, 1176t
Spleen, 686–690
absence of, 690
accessory, 690
amyloidosis of, 255
enlargement of, 688, 688t
in cirrhosis, *855,* 856
in right-sided heart failure, 550
filtration function of, 687
hematopoiesis in, 688
immune function of, 687
in chronic myelogenous leukemia, 681, *681*
in diffuse large B-cell lymphoma, 662, *662*
in Epstein-Barr virus infection, 372–373
in follicular lymphoma, 660, *660*
in Gaucher disease, 158
in hairy cell leukemia, 668
in idiopathic thrombocytopenic purpura, 635
in myelofibrosis with myeloid metaplasia, 684, *689*
in polycythemia vera, 682, *682*
in systemic lupus erythematosus, 224
infarction of, *133,* 689, *689*
miliary tuberculosis of, 725–726, *725*
normal, 686–688, *687*
platelet sequestration in (hypersplenism), 635
red pulp of, 687, *687*
rupture of, 690
sarcoidosis of, 735
storage function of, 688
tumors of, 690
white pulp of, 687, *687*
Splenic artery, infarction of, 689, *689*
Spleniculi, 690
Splenitis, acute, nonspecific, 688–689
Splenomegaly, 688–689, 688t
congestive, 689
in cirrhosis, *855,* 856
in right-sided heart failure, 550
Spondylitis, rheumatoid, 1252
Spondyloarthritis, ankylosing, 1252
Spondyloarthropathy, seronegative, 1252–1253
Spongiform encephalopathy, 1296t, 1323–1326, *1325*
Spongiosa, of cardiac valves, 545
Spongiosis, 1173
in eczematous dermatitis, *1196,* 1197
Sprue, celiac, 813, *813,* 961
tropical, 814
Squamous cell carcinoma, 262
of bladder, 1006–1007
of cervix, 1051–1053, *1053*
of esophagus, 783–786, *785,* 785t
of penis, 1014, *1014*
of skin, 266, *266,* 310, 1184–1186, *1186*
of thymus, 692–693, *692*
of vagina, 1045–1046
of vulva, 1043–1044, *1044*

Squamous hyperplasia, of vulva, 1040–1042, *1041, 1042*
Squamous metaplasia, 36–37, *37*
Squamous papilloma, of esophagus, 783
Stable cells, 91
Staggers, 436
Stains, for infectious agents, 345, 345t
Stannosis, 729t
Staphylococcal scalded skin syndrome, 365–366, 367
Staphylococcus aureus, 334t, 365–367, *366, 367*
Staphylococcus epidermidis, 332t, 334t
Staphyloma, 1375
Starry sky pattern, in Burkitt lymphoma, 662, *663*
Starvation, self-induced, 439
Stasis, in inflammation, 53
Status marmoratus, 1302
Steatocystoma multiplex, 1181
Steatohepatitis, nonalcoholic, 873
Steatorrhea, in malabsorption syndromes, 812
Steatosis, 38, *38,* 39, *39,* 847
  in alcoholic liver disease, 869, *870,* 872
  in pregnancy, 884–885
  in Wilson disease, 875
Stein-Leventhal syndrome, 1066
Stem cells, 91, 602, *603*
  of liver, 33
Stenosis, aortic, 567–568, *567*
  esophageal, 777–778
  intestinal, 804
  mitral, 125, 129
    in rheumatic heart disease, 572
  pyloric, 789
  renal, 984–985, *984*
Steroid myopathy, 1288
Stevens-Johnson syndrome, 1197–1198
Stewart-Treves syndrome, 1104
Stickler syndrome, 1220t
Stomach, 787–802
  acid secretion of, 788
  adenoma of, 798, *798*
  anatomy of, 787–788, *787*
  benign tumors of, 798, *798*
  carcinoma of, 798–802, 799t, *800, 801*
    geographic factors in, 273, *273*
    in lymphoma, 315
    incidence of, *272*
    mortality rates with, *272*
  chief cells of, 788
  concretions of, 797, *797*
  congenital anomalies of, 788–789
  dilation of, 797
  endocrine cells of, 788
  foveolar cells of, 787
  glands of, 787–788
    atrophy of, 792
    hyperplasia of, 797–798
  heterotopic, 789
  hypertrophy of, 797–798, *797*
  inflammation of, 789–793. See also *Gastritis.*
  inflammatory fibroid polyp of, 802
  leiomyoma of, 802
  leiomyosarcoma of, 802
  lipoma of, 802
  lymphoma of, 802
  mucosa of, 787
    dysplasia of, 792, 799
    erosion of, 789–790, *790*
    hyperplasia of, 792
    metaplasia of, 792, *792*
Stomach *(Continued)*
  mucosal barrier of, 788
  mucous neck cells of, 787
  neuroendocrine cell tumors of, 802
  normal, 787–788, *787*
  pancreatic heterotopia of, 789
  parietal cells of, 787–788
  peptic ulcer disease of, 793–796, *794, 795,* 796t
  rugae of, 787, 797–798, *797*
  rupture of, 797
  stress ulcers of, 796–797, *796*
Stomatitis, herpetic, 757
Storage pool disease, 637
Strawberry mucosa, in trichomoniasis, 365
Streptobacillus moniliformis, 334t
Streptococcus, 367–368, *368*
  fibrillae of, 341–342, *342*
  glomerulonephritis and, 949–951, *950,* 965t
  in rheumatic fever, 570, 572, *573*
  virulence factors of, 367
Streptococcus pneumoniae, 332t, 334t
Streptococcus pyogenes, 334t
Stress ulcers, 796–797, *796*
Striatonigral degeneration, 1335
Stroke, 1306–1314. See also *Cerebrovascular disease.*
  obesity and, 454
Stromelysins, 107, *107*
Strongyloides, 336–337
Sturge-Weber syndrome, 534, 1164t
Subacute sclerosing panencephalitis, 1321–1322
Subarachnoid hemorrhage, 1305, 1310–1313
Subcutaneous tissues, edema of, 116
Subdural empyema, 1316
Subdural hematoma, 1305, *1306*
Subdural space, infection of, 1316
Subependymoma, 1347
Substance P, in inflammation, 77
Substantia nigra, in Parkinson disease, 1334, *1334*
Sudden cardiac death, 564
Sudden infant death syndrome, 481–482, 482t
Suicide, 431t
Sulfatidoses, 155t
Sulfur dioxide, in air, 417, 417t
Superantigens, 136, 215, 216
Superior vena cava syndrome, 530, 591, 745
Superoxide anion, 12, *13.* See also *Free radicals.*
  in inflammation, 76–77
Superoxide dismutases, in free radical inactivation, 13
  life span and, 47
Suprasellar region, tumors of, 1129
Surfactant, deficiency of, 471–473, *472*
Sweat glands, 1171, *1171*
Sympathetic ophthalmia, 1364–1365, *1365*
Synarthroses, 1246. See also *Joint(s).*
Syncytial meningioma, 1350
Syndecans, 102, *102*
Syndrome of inappropriate secretion of antidiuretic hormone, 1129
Synovitis, villonodular, 1258–1259, *1258*
Synovium, in rheumatoid arthritis, 1248–1249, *1248*
  in systemic sclerosis, 228
Synpolydactyly, 1220, 1220t
Syphilis, 83t, 362–364, *363*
  aortic aneurysms in, 526
  congenital, 338–339, 364, 1361
  false-positive serology for, 126
  infantile, 364
Syphilis *(Continued)*
  perinatal, 364
  secondary, *346,* 363–364
  skeletal, 1233
  testicular involvement in, 1017
Syphilitic aneurysm, 526
Syringobulbia, 1301–1302
Syringocystadenoma papilliferum, 1183t
Syringoma, 1182, 1183t, *1184*
Syringomyelia, 1301–1302
Systemic inflammatory response syndrome, 136
Systemic lupus erythematosus (SLE), 126, 216–225
  antinuclear antibodies in, 217, 218t
  antiphospholipid antibody syndrome in, 218
  cardiovascular system involvement in, 223–224, *223*
  clinical manifestations of, 220t, 224
  CNS involvement in, 222–223
  cutaneous abnormalities in, 222, *222*
  diagnosis of, 216, 217t
  drugs in, 219
  endocarditis in, 127, 223, *223*
  genetic factors in, 218–219
  glomerulonephritis in, 220–221, *220, 221,* 962, *962,* 965
  immunologic factors in, 219–220, *219,* 221, *222*
  joint involvement in, 222
  lymph nodes in, 224
  pathogenesis of, 216–220, 218t, *219*
  pericarditis in, 223
  pleural effusion in, 224
  pleuritis in, 224
  renal abnormalities in, 220–222, *220–222*
  sex hormones in, 219
  splenic enlargement in, 224
  tubulointerstitial lesions in, 222
  ultraviolet light in, 219, 222
  vasculitis in, 224, 524, *524*
  wire loop lesion in, 221, *222*
Systemic sclerosis (scleroderma), 226–229
  alimentary tract involvement in, 228
  antinuclear antibodies in, 218t
  clinical course of, 229
  cutaneous abnormalities in, 228, *228*
  musculoskeletal abnormalities in, 228
  pathogenesis of, 226–227, *227*
  pericarditis in, 229
  pulmonary involvement in, 229
  renal abnormalities in, 228–229

T

T lymphocytes. See *Lymphocyte(s), T.*
Tabes dorsalis, 1317
Taenia solium, 395–396, *395*
Takayasu arteritis, 517t, 519–520, *519*
Talin, 101, *101*
Tapeworms, 395–396, *395*
Target lesion, in *Aspergillus* infection, 380
tat gene, of human immunodeficiency virus, 238, *239*
Tattooing, 42
tax gene, 314–315
Tay-Sachs disease, 155–156, 155t, *156, 157*
  gene mutation in, 142, *142,* 147t
T-cell leukemia/lymphoma, 656t, 670
T-cell lymphoma, 669–670, *671,* 1191, *1191*
T-cell receptor, 189–190, *190*
Teeth, Hutchinson, 364
Telangiectases, 534
  capillary, 1313

Telomerase, in telomere stabilization, 46–47, *46*
Telomeres, cancer and, 296
  incomplete replication of, 46–47, *46*
  shortening of, 47, *47*
Telomere repeat binding proteins, in telomere stabilization, *46,* 47
Temperature, body, in inflammation, 86
Temporal (giant cell) arteritis, 516–518, 517t, *518*
Tenacins, 101
Tendon sheath, giant cell tumor of, 1258–1259
Tensegrity hypothesis, of cytokine signaling system, 101
Tensin, 101, *101*
Tension pneumothorax, 751
Teratoma, 262–263, 484, *484*
  benign, 1073–1074, *1074*
  malignant, 1074–1075, *1075*
  monodermal, 1074
  ovarian, 1073–1075, *1073, 1074*
  testicular, 1021–1022, *1022*
Testis (testes), 1014–1025
  atrophy of, 1015, *1015,* 1016
    in hemochromatosis, 874
  choriocarcinoma of, 1021, *1021,* 1023
  congenital anomalies of, 1015–1016, *1015*
  embryonal carcinoma of, 264, 1020–1021, *1020*
  germ cell tumors of, 1018–1024, 1018t, *1023*
  gonococcal infection of, 1017
  granulomatous (autoimmune) inflammation of, 1017
  hemorrhage infarction of, 1017, *1017*
  in fragile X syndrome, 177
  inflammation of, 1016–1017
  Leydig cell tumors of, 1024
  lymphoma of, 1024–1025
  mixed tumors of, 1022–1024, *1023*
  mumps infection of, 371, 1017
  nonseminomatous germ cell tumors of, 1022–1024, *1023*
  painless enlargement of, 1022
  seminoma of, 1019–1020, *1019*
  Sertoli cell tumors of, 1024
  sex cord–stromal tumors of, 1018t, 1024
  spermatocytic seminoma of, 1020
  syphilitic infection of, 1017
  teratoma of, 1021–1022, *1022*
  torsion of, 1017, *1017*
  tuberculosis of, 1017
  undescended, 1015–1016, *1015*
  yolk sac tumor of, 1021
Testosterone, biosynthesis of, *1152*
Tetanospasmin, 368
Tetanus toxin, 369
Tetany, in hypoparathyroidism, 1151
Tetralogy of Fallot, 595, *595*
α-Thalassemia, 147t, 148, 618–619
β-Thalassemia, 147t, 148, 615–618, *615, 616,* 617t, *618*
Thalidomide, fetal effects of, 467
Thanatophoric dwarfism, 1220t, 1221, 1300
Thecoma-fibroma, 1077–1078, *1077*
Thiamine, 440t, 447
  deficiency of, 447, *448,* 1279, 1341
Thin filaments, abnormalities of, 27
Thin membrane disease, 963
Three Mile Island nuclear power plant, 427
Thrombasthenia, 637
  Glanzmann, 122
Thrombin, *118,* 119
  in hemostasis, 121–122, *122*
  in inflammation, *68,* 69
  prothrombin conversion to, 122, *123*
  receptors for, 122
Thromboangiitis obliterans, 523, *523*
Thrombocytopenia, 200, 634–637, 635t
  dilutional, 635
  drug-induced, 636
  heparin-induced, 125–126
  HIV-associated, 636
  immunodeficiency with, 236
  petechiae with, 118
Thrombocytopenic purpura, thrombotic, 986
Thrombocytosis, essential, 683, *683*
Thromboembolism, 127, *128,* 129–132. See also *Embolism.*
Thrombolytic therapy, in myocardial infarction, 559, 561
Thrombomodulin, 120
Thrombophlebitis, 530
  migratory, 129, 530
    in cancer, 320–321, 321t
    in pancreatic carcinoma, 911
Thromboplastins, in disseminated intravascular coagulation, 641
Thrombosis, *118,* 119, 124–129
  arterial, 127, *127, 128,* 129
  blood flow abnormalities and, *124,* 125
  clinical correlation of, 129
  dissolution of, 127, *128*
  embolization of, 127, *128,* 129–132. See also *Embolism.*
  endothelial injury and, 124–125, *124*
  hepatic, 883–884, *883*
  hypercoagulability and, *124,* 125–126, 125t
  in myocardial infarction, 552, 553, 553t
  in polycythemia vera, 683
  morphology of, 126–127, *127*
  mural, 126–127, *127*
  organization of, 127, *128,* 129
  pathogenesis of, 124–127, *124,* 125t
  portal vein, 882
  propagation of, 127, *128*
  recanalization of, 127, 129
  renal, in nephrotic syndrome, 953
  venous, 127, 129
    outcome of, 127–129, *128.* See also *Embolism.*
  with atheromatous plaque, 502–503
  with atherosclerosis, 506
Thrombospondin, 101
  in apoptosis, 20
Thrombotic microangiopathy, 636–637, 985–988, *985, 987*
Thrombotic thrombocytopenic purpura, 986
  idiopathic, 986
Thromboxane A_2, synthesis of, 70, *71*
Thrombus, 124–129. See also *Thrombosis.*
  dissolution of, 127
  formation of, 124–127, *124,* 125t
  mural, 126–127, *127*
    after myocardial infarction, 563
  recanalization of, *128,* 129
Thrush, 378, 757
Thymomas, 691–693, *692*
Thymosin β15, in tumor invasion, 304
Thymus, 690–693
  aplasia of, 691
  cysts of, 691
  hyperplasia of, 691
  hypoplasia of (DiGeorge syndrome), 173, 235, 691
Thymus *(Continued)*
  in severe combined immunodeficiency disease, 235–236
  normal, 690–691
  radiation-induced injury to, 427, *427*
  tumors of, 691–693, *692*
Thyroglobulin, antibodies to, in Hashimoto thyroiditis, 1134
Thyroglossal duct, 1147
Thyroid gland, 1130–1131, *1130*
  adenoma of, *265,* 1140–1142, *1141*
  atypical adenoma of, 1142
  carcinoma of, 1142–1147
    anaplastic, 1147
    follicular, 1144–1145, *1144*
    ionizing radiation and, 310
    medullary, 1143, 1145–1147, *1146*
      familial, 1167
    papillary, 1143–1144, *1143*
    pathogenesis of, 1142–1143
  congenital anomalies of, 1147
  cysts of, 1142, 1147
  diseases of. See *Hyperthyroidism; Hypothyroidism.*
  enlargement of, 1138–1140, *1140*
  Hürthle cell adenoma of, 1142
  hyperfunction of, 1131–1132, 1131t, *1132.* See also *Hyperthyroidism.*
  hypofunction of, 1132–1134, 1133t. See also *Hypothyroidism.*
  inflammation of, 1134–1136, *1135, 1136*
  inhibition of, 1130–1131
  nodules of, 1140
  papillary adenoma of, 1142
  radioactive iodine uptake by, in hyperthyroidism, 1132
  thyroglossal duct of, 1147
Thyroid peroxidase, antibodies to, in Hashimoto thyroiditis, 1134
Thyroid storm, 1132
Thyroiditis, 1133–1136
  granulomatous (subacute), 1135–1136, *1135*
  Hashimoto, 1133, 1133t, 1134–1135, *1135*
  infectious, 1134
  lymphocytic, subacute, 1136
  Reidel, 1136
Thyroidization, of renal tubules, 976, *976*
Thyroid-stimulating hormone, in hyperthyroidism, 1132
  in hypothyroidism, 1133
  tumor secretion of, 1127
Thyroid-stimulating hormone receptor, antibodies to, in Graves disease, 1134, 1136–1137
    in Hashimoto thyroiditis, 1134
  in thyroid adenoma, 1140
Thyrotoxic myopathy, 1287–1288
Thyrotoxic periodic paralysis, 1288
Thyrotoxicosis, 1131–1132, 1131t, *1132.* See also *Hyperthyroidism.*
Thyroxine (T_4), 1130, *1130*
Tick, *338*
Tick bite, 1210–1212
Tie2 receptor, 105
Tinea barbae, 1210
Tinea capitis, 1210
Tinea corporis, 1210, *1211*
Tinea cruris, 1210
Tinea pedis, 1210
Tinea versicolor, 1210
Tissue factor, *118,* 119, 120
Tissue inhibitors of metalloproteinases, in experimental cancer treatment, 304
  in tissue remodeling, 107, *107*

Tissue repair, 89–111, *111*. See also *Cell growth; Wound, healing of.*
  angiogenesis in, 103–106, *104, 105,* 105t
  fibrosis in, 106, 106t
  remodeling in, 106–107, *107*
  wound healing in, 107–111, *108, 109*
Tissue-specific antigens, 317
Tobacco smoke, bronchogenic carcinoma and, 741–742
Tobacco use, 408–410, 409t. See also *Cigarette smoking.*
  oral cancer and, 760
  periductal mastitis and, 1097
Tolerance, immune, 212–214, *213*
    central, 212, *213*
    peripheral, 212, *213,* 214–215
Tongue, amyloidosis of, 256
  carcinoma of, 760–761, *761*
  hemangioma of, 532, *532*
  inflammation of, 758
Tonsillitis, 763
Tophi, in gout, 1254, 1256, *1256*
Total anomalous pulmonary venous connection, 596
Toxemia of pregnancy, 1082–1084, *1084, 1085*
Toxic epidermal necrolysis, 1198
Toxic megacolon, 805, 818, *819*
Toxic shock syndrome, 136
Toxic shock syndrome toxin-1 (TSST-1), 136, 366
Toxicity, chemical, 404–408, *405–408*
    dose-response curve for, 405, *405*
Toxins, hepatic toxicity of, 868–869, 869t
  natural, 424
Toxocara canis, 336–337
Toxoplasma gondii, 337t, 382–383
  CNS infection with, 1323, *1323*
Toxoplasmosis, 382–383, 1323, *1323*
  neonatal, 383
TPA, in tumor promotion, 308
Tracheoesophageal fistula, 777, *777*
Trachoma, 385, 385t, 1361–1362, *1362*
Transcription factors, in cancer, 279t, 282
  in metaplasia, 37
  structure of, 95
Transcytosis, in inflammation, 54
Transferrin, in free radical inactivation, 13
Transforming growth factor-α, 97
  in hepatocyte regeneration, 33, *33*
Transforming growth factor-β, 98
  in angiogenesis, 105–106, *105*
  in cell cycle, 290, 293
  in cell growth, 96–97
  in Hodgkin disease, 674
  in myelofibrosis with myeloid metaplasia, 684
Transforming growth factor-β receptor, in cancer, 293
Transfusion reaction, 200. See also *Hypersensitivity reaction(s), type II.*
Transgenic mice, 140
Transition metals, in free radical generation, 12, *13*
Transitional cell carcinoma, of bladder, 1003–1008, 1003t, *1004–1006,* 1006t
  of ovary, 1073
  of ureter, 999, *999*
Translocations, chromosome, *169,* 170
    in oncogene activation, 284–286, *285,* 286t
Transplantation, cardiac, *597,* 598, *598*
  HLA matching for, 210
  immunosuppressive therapy for, 210
  Kaposi sarcoma after, 535
Transplantation *(Continued)*
  lung, 740–741, *741*
  rejection of, 206–211
    acute, 209–210, *209*
    antibody-mediated, 207
    chronic, 210
    hyperacute, 207–208
    T cell-mediated, 207, *208*
Transposition of great arteries, 595–596, *595–596*
Transposons, 332
Trans-sialidase, of *Trypanosoma cruzi,* 393
Transthyretin, 252, 1277
Transudate, 53
Transverse myelitis, radiation-induced, 430
Trauma, 432–433, *432, 433*
  altitude-related, 435–436
  electrical, 435
  fat embolism after, 130–131, *131*
  hemolytic anemia with, 621, *621*
  peripheral neuropathy with, 1280
  thermal, 433–435
  to brain, 1302–1306, *1303, 1305, 1306*
  to spinal cord, 1306
  uveitis with, 215
Traveler's diarrhea, 809
Trematodes, 336–337
Trench foot, 435
Treponema carateum, 334t
Treponema pallidum, 334t, 362–364, *363.* See also *Syphilis.*
  CNS infection with, 1317
  skeletal infection with, 1233
Treponema pertenue, 334t, 1233
Trichilemmal cyst, 1181
Trichilemmoma, 1182
Trichinella spiralis, 332t, 394, *395*
Trichinellosis, 394, *395*
Trichobezoar, 797, *797*
Trichoepithelioma, 1182, 1183t
Trichofolliculoma, 1183t
Trichomonas vaginalis, 337t, 364–365, *365,* 1038t, 1039
Trichophyton sp., 332t
Tricuspid valve, atresia of, 596
Triglycerides, cellular accumulation of, 38, *38,* 39–40, *39, 40*
Triiodothyronine (T_3), 1130, *1130*
Trinucleotide repeat mutations, 143
Triphenyltetrazolium chloride dye test, in myocardial infarction, 558, *559*
Triplet repeat mutations, in fragile X syndrome, 177–178, *178*
  in Friedreich ataxia, 179, *179,* 179t
Trisomy 13 (Patau syndrome), 171–173, *172*
Trisomy 18 (Edwards syndrome), 171–173, *172*
Trisomy 21 (Down syndrome), 170–171, *171, 172*
  G-banded karyotype of, *171*
  ocular anomalies in, 1360
Triton tumor, 1354
Tropheryma whippelli, 814–815, *814*
Trophoblastic tumor, of placental site, 1089
Tropical pulmonary eosinophilia, 398
Tropical spastic paraparesis, 314, 1321
Tropical sprue, 814
Tropocollagen, 98
Troponin I, in myocardial infarction, 561
Troponin T, in myocardial infarction, 561
Trousseau sign, 530
  in hypoparathyroidism, 1151
  in pancreatic carcinoma, 911
Trousseau syndrome, 129
  in cancer, 320–321, 321t, 911
Truncus arteriosus, 596
Trypanosoma brucei, 337t
Trypanosoma cruzi, 332t, 337t, 393–394
  in myocarditis, 584, *585*
Trypanosoma gambiense, 332t, 337t
Trypanosoma rhodesiense, 337t
Trypanosomiasis, 393
Trypsin, in acute pancreatitis, 905–907, *906*
Tubercle, 83–84, *83*
Tuberculin reaction, 204–206, *205*
Tuberculoma, 1317
Tuberculosis, 83–84, *83,* 83t, 349–352, *350, 351*
  caseous necrosis in, 351
  disseminated, 351
  granuloma formation in, 350–351, *351*
  in acquired immunodeficiency syndrome, 248, 351–352
  in adrenocortical insufficiency, 1161
  in mice, 351
  inflammatory response in, 350, *350*
  intestinal, 807–809, 808t
  miliary, 351
  of CNS, 1316–1317
  pathogenesis of, 349–351, *350, 351*
  primary, 350–351, *351*
  pulmonary, 722–726
    clinical course of, 726
    fibrocaseous, 725
    miliary, 725–726, *726*
    primary, 723, *723, 724*
    progressive, *724,* 725–726, *726*
    secondary, 723–724, *724*
  secondary, 351
  skeletal, 1233
  testicular involvement in, 1017
Tuberculosis peritonitis, 841
Tuberculous salpingitis, 1065
Tuberous sclerosis, 1354–1355
  angiomyolipoma in, 991
Tubular carcinoma, of breast, 1112, *1112*
Tubulointerstitial nephritis, 971–981, 972t
  drug-induced, 977–979, *977, 979,* 979t
  urinary tract infection and, 972–974, *972, 973*
Tubuloreticular inclusion, in focal segmental glomerulosclerosis, 958
Tumor(s). See also *Carcinogenesis.*
  age and, 273, 274t, 275t
  alcohol and, 273, 412
  anaplastic, 265–266, *265, 266,* 323, *323*
  APC gene in, 287t, 292–293
  benign, 261, *261, 262,* 263t
    encapsulation of, 267, *268*
    malignant transformation of, 276
  cachexia with, 319–320
  caretaker genes in, 297, *298*
  chemoprevention of, 455–456
  chromosome translocation in, 284–286, *285,* 286t, 298
  cigarette smoking and, 273
  clinical features of, 319–325, 321t
  clonality of, 277, *277*
  cranial nerve palsy with, 1279
  cyclin D in, 283, 290
  desmoplasia of, 261
  diagnosis of, 322–325
    cytology in, 322–323, *323*
    flow cytometry in, 324
    histology in, 322
    immunocytochemistry in, 323–324, *323*

Tumor(s) *(Continued)*
molecular, 324
quick-frozen section for, 322
specimen for, 322
tumor markers in, 324–325, 325t
differentiation of, 264–267, *264–267,* 270t
DNA repair disorders and, 276
dysplasia and, 266, *267*
E-cadherin gene in, 293
environmental factors in, 273, 274t
epidemiology of, 271–276, *272, 273,* 274t, 275t
extracellular matrix invasion by, 302–305, *303, 304*
familial, 276
fibrous capsule of, 267, *268*
gatekeeper genes in, 297, *298*
genetic factors in, 275–276, 275t
geographic factors in, 273, *273*
germ cell, of testes, 1018–1024, 1018t, *1019–1023*
giant cells in, 265–266
grading of, 321–322
growth fraction of, 300–301, *301*
growth of, 267, 270t, 298–305. See also *Tumor growth.*
hematogenous dissemination of, 270, *270*
heredity and, 275–276, 275t
heterogeneity of, 302
homing of 305
hormonal effects of, 266–267, *267,* 319
host defense against, 315–319, *316, 318.* See also *Tumor immunity.*
hyperchromatic nuclei in, 265
incidence of, 271–273, *272, 273*
KAI-1 gene in, 305
KiSS-1 gene in, 305
latent period of, 301
local invasion of, 267–268, *268, 269,* 270t, 302–305, *303, 304*
lymphatic spread of, 269–270, *269*
metastatic 268–271, *269–271,* 270t, 305
calcification with, 45
minimal residual disease monitoring of, 324
mitotic figures in, 265, *266*
mixed, 262
molecular basis of, 276–298. See also *Apoptosis; Cancer-suppressor genes; Oncogenes.*
monoclonality of, 277, *277*
mortality rates with, 271–273, *272*
myc oncogene in, 282
NF-1 gene in, 293
NF-2 gene in, 293
nm23 gene in, 305
nomenclature for, 261–264, 263t
obesity and, 273, 455
occupation and, 244t, 273
of appendix, 840
of bladder, 1003–1008, 1003t, *1004–1006,* 1006t
of bone, 1233–1244, 1234t
of CNS, 1343–1355, *1344–1347, 1349, 1351,* 1352t, *1353*
of colorectum, 827–838, *827–832, 834–836*
of ear, 767
of esophagus, 783–787, *785,* 785t, *786*
of fallopian tubes, 1065
of intestine, 826–838, 826t
of kidney, 990–994
of larynx, 765, *766*
of liver, 887–891, *887, 889, 890*
of lung, 741–747, *743,* 743t, *744*

Tumor(s) *(Continued)*
of mediastinum, 749, *749*
of mouth, 759–761, *760, 761*
of muscle, 651–652, *1265*
of neck, 768–769, *768*
of nose, 763–764, *764*
of optic nerve, 1374
of ovary, 1067–1079, 1067t, *1068,* 1068t
of pancreas, 909–911, *910, 911*
of penis, 1012–1014, *1012, 1013*
of peritoneum, 842
of pineal gland, 1168
of pleura, 751–752, *752, 753*
of prostate, 1029–1033, *1030, 1031*
of salivary glands, 769–773, 769t, *770–773*
of small intestine, 826–827, 826t, *827*
of spleen, 690
of stomach, 798–802, *798,* 799t, *800, 801*
of testes, 1018–1024, 1018t, *1019, 1022, 1023*
of thymus gland, 691–693, *692*
of thyroid gland, 1142–1147, *1143, 1145–1147*
of ureters, 999, *999*
of urethra, 1009, *1009*
of urothelium, 994, *994*
of uterus, 1061–1065, *1062*
of vulva, 1042–1045, *1043, 1044*
organ tropism of, 305
p53 gene loss in, 290–292, *291*
p73 gene loss in, 292
paraneoplastic syndromes with, 320–321, 321t
parenchymal cells of, 261
pediatric, 482–489
benign, 483–484, *483, 484*
malignant, 484–491, 485t, *486, 487,* 488t, *489*
peripheral neuropathy with, 1279–1280
pleomorphic nuclei in, 265, *265*
predisposition to, 275–276, 275t
preneoplastic disorders in, 276
proteolytic enzyme secretion by, 303–304
PTEN gene in, 294
radiation and, 309–311
ras oncogene in, 280–282, *281,* 284
Rb gene in, 287t, 289–290, *289*
replication error phenotype of, 295
seeding of, 269
soft tissue 1259–1267, 1259t
staging of, 322
stromal cells of, 261
telomeres and, 296
transforming growth factor-β receptor in, 293
Trousseau syndrome in, 129, 320–321, 321t, 911
two-hit hypothesis of, 286–287
vascular, 532–533, *532,* 534–535, *534,* 537–538, *537,* 1189
VHL gene in, 293–294
viruses and, 311–315, *313, 314*
vitamin E and, 446
well-differentiated, 266, *266*
WT-1 gene in, 294
Tumor antigens, 315–317, *316*
Tumor growth, 267, 270t, 298–305
angiogenesis in, 301–302
extracellular matrix invasion and, 302–305, *303, 304*
kinetics of, 299–301, *300, 301*
metastases in, 305
rate of, 267

Tumor growth *(Continued)*
tumor heterogeneity and, 302
vascular dissemination and, 305
Tumor immunity, 315–319
effector mechanisms in, 317–319, *318*
immunosurveillance in, 318–319
tumor antigens in, 315–317, *316*
Tumor markers, in tumor diagnosis, 324–325, 325t
Tumor necrosis factor (TNF), cancer cachexia and, 320
in apoptosis, 23–24, *24*
in delayed-type hypersensitivity, *205,* 206
in disseminated intravascular coagulation, 640
in febrile state, 86
in hepatocyte regeneration, 33, *33*
in inflammation, 73–74, *74,* 77t
in rheumatoid arthritis, 1250–1251
Tumor necrosis factor receptors, in apoptosis, 23–24, *24*
Tumor-associated antigens, *316,* 317
Tumor-specific antigens, 315–316, *316*
Tumor-suppressor genes, 286–294
in retinoblastoma, 275
protein products of, 287, 289–294, *289, 291*
Tungsten carbide, in occupational diseases, 421, 421t
Tunica vaginalis, lesions of, 1025
Turban tumor, 1182, *1183*
Turner syndrome, 173, 174–176, *175*
mosaic variant of, 168
Twin pregnancy, 1081, *1082*
Twin-twin transfusion syndrome, 1081, *1082*
TXA_2, in platelet aggregation, 122
Typhlitis, 811–812
Typhoid fever, 356–357, *357,* 808
Typhoid nodule, 357, *357*
Typhus, 384, *384,* 385t
Tyrosinase, as tumor antigens, 317
deficiency of, 148
Tyrosine, phenylalanine conversion to, 476, *476*
Tyrosine kinase, Bruton, 232
nonreceptor-associated, in cancer, 282
Tyrosinemia, hereditary, hepatocellular carcinoma and, 889
Tzanck test, 757

U

Ubiquitin, in atrophy, 36
in protein degradation, 41
Ubiquitin-proteasome pathway, in cyclin degradation, 96, *96*
Ulcer(s), 85
aphthous, 757, *757*
corneal, 1362–1363
Curling, 796
Cushing, 796
cutaneous, 1173
gingival, with agranulocytosis, 647
in Crohn disease, 816, 817, *817*
in *Shigella* bacillary dysentery, 355, *355*
peptic, 793–796, *794, 795,* 796t. See also *Peptic ulcer disease.*
stress, 796–797, *796*
varicose, 129, 529
Ulcerative colitis, 818–820, *819, 820,* 821t
carcinoma and, 820
crypt abscess in, 819, *820*
mucosal damage in, 819–820, *819*

Ulcerative colitis *(Continued)*
pathogenesis of, 815–816
vs. Crohn disease, *819*, 821t
Ulegyria, 1302
Ultraviolet radiation, 430–431
cutaneous effects of, 430–431, 430t, *431*
in carcinogenesis, 310
in systemic lupus erythematosus, 219, 222
Umbilical cord, inflammation of, 470
Unstable angina, 555
Upper airway, 761–766. See also *Larynx; Nose; Pharynx.*
Urachus, patent, 1000
Uranium, bronchogenic carcinoma and, 742
Urate nephropathy, 979–980, *980*
Uremia, 637, 935
systemic complications of, 964
Uremic medullary cystic disease, 940–941, *941*, 941t
Ureter(s), 997–1000
bifid, 998
congenital anomalies of, 998
cysts of, 998–999, *999*
diverticula of, 998
double, 998
enlargement of, 998
inflammation of, 998–999, *999*
obstruction of, 999–1000, 999t
sclerosing retroperitoneal fibrosis of, 999–1000
tumors of, 999, *999*
Ureteritis, 998–999
Ureteritis cystica, 998–999, *999*
Ureteritis follicularis, 998
Ureteropelvic junction, obstruction of, 998
Urethra, carcinoma of, 1009, *1009*
caruncle of, 1009
infection of, 973
inflammation of, 1009
papilloma of, 1009
Urethritis, *Chlamydia trachomatis* in, 361–362, 361t
Uric acid stones, 989, 989t, 990
Urinary tract, 997–1009. See also *Bladder; Ureter(s); Urethra.*
infection of, 936
pyelonephritis and, 972–974, *972, 973*
tubulointerstitial nephritis and, 972–974, *972, 973*
normal, 997–998
obstruction of, 988–989, *988, 989*
Urokinase-type plasminogen activator, in tumor invasion, 304
Urolithiasis, 989–990, 989t, *990*
Uroplakins, 997
Urothelial carcinoma, 994, *994*
Urticaria (hives), 1194, *1194*
Urticaria pigmentosa, 1192
Uterus, 1054–1065. See also *Endometrium; Myometrium.*
anatomy of, 1037
dysfunctional bleeding from, 1055–1056, 1056t
hypertrophy of, 34, *34*
leiomyoma of, *264, 271,* 1063–1064, *1063,* 1266
leiomyosarcoma of, *271,* 1064–1065, *1064*
nodules of, 1065
prolapse of, 998
sarcoma of, 1065
Uvea, inflammation of, 1364–1365, *1364, 1365*
melanoma of, 1365–1367, *1366*
Uveitis, 1364–1365
granulomatous, 1364–1365, *1364, 1365*
Uveitis *(Continued)*
infectious, 1364
post-traumatic, 215
sympathetic, 1364–1365, *1365*

V

Vaccine, hepatitis B, 889
Vaccinia virus, 333t
Vacor, type I diabetes mellitus and, 917
Vacuolar myelopathy, in acquired immunodeficiency syndrome, 1321
Vacuoles, autophagic, in atrophy, 36
Vacuolization, 1173
Vagina, 1045–1047
adenocarcinoma of, 1046, *1046*
adenosis of, 1046
Candida infection of, 378
carcinoma of, 1045–1046
congenital anomalies of, 1045
embryonal rhabdomyosarcoma of, 1046–1047, *1046*
infection of, 1038–1039, 1038t
Valves, cardiac, 545
disease of, 566–578, 567t. See also specific diseases.
dystrophic calcifications of, 43–44, *44*
prosthetic, 578, *578,* 578t
thrombi of, 127
Variable surface glycoprotein, of *Trypanosoma,* 393
Varicella-zoster virus, 333t, 373–374, *374*
CNS infection with, 1319
peripheral nerve effects of, 1276–1277
Varicocele, 1025
Varicose veins, 529–530, *529*
Varix (varices), esophageal, 529–530, 783
in cirrhosis, 856
Vasa recta, 931
Vasa vasorum, 494
Vascular cell adhesion molecule 1 (VCAM-1), in leukocyte adhesion, 57, 57t
in rheumatoid arthritis, 1250
Vascular ectasias (telangiectases), 534, 1313
Vascular endothelial growth factor, 97–98
in angiogenesis, 104–106, *105,* 105t
in retinopathy of prematurity, 1369
Vascular (multi-infarct) dementia, 1314
Vascular permeability, in inflammation, 53–55, *53–55*
Vasculitis, 515–524, 515t
antineutrophil cytoplasmic antibodies in, 516
classification of, 515t, 516, 517t, *518*
cryoglobulinemic, 517t
drug-induced, 516
immune complex, 203–204, *203, 204,* 516
in connective tissue disorders, 524, *524*
in systemic lupus erythematosus, 224
pathogenesis of, 515t, 516
rejection, 209–210, *209*
rheumatoid, 524, 1249
viral infections in, 516
Vasculogenesis, 97, 103
Vasoactive amines, in inflammation, 66–67, *66,* 77t
Vasoconstriction, in hemostasis, *118,* 119
in hypertension, 513–514, *514*
in myocardial infarction, 553
Vasodilation, in inflammation, 53
Vater, ampulla of, 892
adenoma of, 827, *827*
Vegetations, cardiac, in Libman-Sacks endocarditis, *575,* 577
Vegetations, cardiac *(Continued)*
in rheumatic heart disease, 571–572, *571, 575*
infective, 572–576, *575*
noninfective, *575,* 576–577, *576*
Vein(s), 495. See also specific veins.
abnormal arterial communication with, 498
Velocardiofacial syndrome, 173
Ventricles, cerebral, cerebrospinal fluid accumulation in, 1298–1299, *1299*
colloid cyst of, 1348
ependymal cells of, 1297
Ventricular septal defect, *593,* 594, *594*
Venules, permeability of, in inflammation, 54, *55*
postcapillary, 495
Verocytotoxins, in hemolytic-uremic syndrome, 637, 985
Verrucae, 1208–1209, *1208*
Verrucous carcinoma, of penis, 1014
Vesicle, cutaneous, 1172
Vesicoureteral reflux, 973–974, *973*
congenital, 1000
Vesicouterine fistula, 1000
Vesiculovacuolar organelle, in inflammation, 54
Vestibular adenitis, 1040
VHL gene, 293–294
Vibrio cholerae, 332t, 334t, 357–358, *357,* 807–809, 808t
enterotoxin of, 343–344
vif gene, 238, *239*
Villonodular synovitis, 1258–1259, *1258*
Villus (villi), intestinal, 802–803, *803*
Vinculin, 101, *101*
Vinyl chloride, in carcinogenesis, 274t, 309
in occupational diseases, 419t, 420
VIPoma, 928
Viral arthritis, 1253
Virchow's triad, 124, *124*
Virilism, with congenital adrenal hyperplasia, 1157–1159, *1158*
Viruses, 332, 332t, 333t
antibody neutralization of, 344
antigenic variants of, 344, 344t
breast cancer and, 1107
cell injury by, 340–341, *341*
cell membrane penetration by, 340
cell receptor binding by, 340
hyperplasia with, 33
in autoimmune diseases, 216
in carcinogenesis, 311–315, *313, 314*
in congenital malformations, 467
in dilated cardiomyopathy, 579
in gastrointestinal tract infection, 354–355, 806–807, 807t
in myocarditis, 584–585, 584t
in rheumatoid arthritis, 1249
in type I diabetes mellitus, 917
nasal infection with, 762
replication of, 340
transplacental infection with, 470, *470*
Vision, loss of, herpesvirus infection and, 360
in Leber hereditary optic neuropathy, *180*
in vitamin A deficiency, 441, *442*
vitamin A in, 441
Vitamin A, 439–441, *440,* 440t
deficiency of, 441, *442,* 1361
in congenital malformations, 468–469, *468*
squamous metaplasia with, 37
functions of, 440–441
in cancer prevention, 455
toxicity of, 441

Vitamin B_1 (thiamine), 440t, 447
deficiency of, 447, *448,* 1279, 1341
Vitamin B_2 (riboflavin), 440t
Vitamin B_6 (pyridoxine), 440t, 449
Vitamin B_{12}, 440t
deficiency of, 1341
megaloblastic anemia with, 623–626, 623t, *624*
Vitamin C (ascorbic acid), 440t, 449–450
deficiency of, 449–450, *450, 451*
in collagen synthesis, 98
Vitamin D (calciferol), 440t, 441–446
deficiency of, *443,* 444, 444t, *445*
excess of, 45
functions of, 442, 444
metabolism of, 441–442, *443*
receptor for, 147t
Vitamin E (alpha-tocopherol), 440t, 446
Vitamin K, 440t, 446–447
deficiency of, 447, 637–638
Vitiligo, 1173–1174, *1173*
Vitreous, 1373
Vocal cords, polyps of, 765
squamous papilloma of, 766, *766*
Volatile organic compounds, in occupational diseases, 419–420, 419t
Volvulus, intestinal, 826
Von Gierke disease, 160, *161,* 163t
Von Hippel–Lindau disease, 1355
cysts in, 909
hemangiomas in, 533
Von Hippel-Lindau syndrome, pheochromocytoma in, 1164t
renal cell carcinoma in, 991–992
Von Recklinghausen disease, of bone, 1228
pheochromocytoma in, 1164t
Von Willebrand disease, 638–639
Von Willebrand factor, deficiency of, 638, *638*
endothelial cell production of, 120
vpr gene, 238, *239*
Vulva, 1040–1045
Bartholin cyst of, 1040
Bowen disease of, 1043, *1043*
carcinoma in situ of, 1043, *1043*
carcinoma of, 1042–1044, *1043, 1044*
condyloma acuminatum of, 1042, *1043*
infection of, 1038–1039, 1038t
inflammation of, 1040–1041, *1041*
intraepithelial neoplasia of, 1043, *1043*
lichen sclerosis of, 1040–1041, *1041*
melanoma of, 1045
Paget disease of, 1044–1045, *1044*
papillary hidradenoma of, 1042
squamous hyperplasia of, 1040–1042, *1041, 1042*
tumors of, 1042–1045, *1043, 1044*
verrucous carcinoma of, 1044
vestibular adenitis of, 1040

W
Waardenburg syndrome, 470, 1220t
PAX-3 gene in, 470
WAGR (*W*ilms' tumor, *a*niridia, *g*enital anomalies, and mental *r*etardation) syndrome, 488
Waldenström macroglobulinemia, 663
Wallerian degeneration, 1274, *1274*
Warm antibody hemolytic anemia, 620
Wart, 1208–1209, *1208*
Warthin tumor, 769, 771–772, *771*
Warthrin-Finkeldey cells, 370, *370*
Wasp sting, 1210–1212
Water retention, in edema, 115–116
Waterhouse-Friderichsen syndrome, 1160, *1160*
hemorrhage in, 642
Wavy fibers, in myocardial infarction, 558, *560*
Weber-Christian disease, 1208
Webs, esophageal, 777–778
Wegener granulomatosis, 517t, 522–523, *522*
renal manifestations of, 968
Weibel-Palade bodies, 57, *58,* 496
Weight, birth, 460–461, *461*
excess, 452–455, *452, 453*
loss of, in hyperthyroidism, 1132
Wen, 1181
Werdnig-Hoffmann disease, 1281
Wermer syndrome (MEN-I), 46, *46,* 1166–1167, 1167t
DNA helicase defect in, 47
Wernicke-Korsakoff syndrome, 412, 447, 1341
Wheal, 1172
Whipple disease, 814–815, *814*
White cells. See *Leukocyte(s).*
Whooping cough, 374–375, *374*
Wickham striae, 1199
Williams syndrome, 597
Wilms' tumor, 485t, 487–489, *488,* 489t
in Beckwith-Wiedemann syndrome, 488
in Denys-Drash syndrome, 488
Wilson disease, 875
Wire loop lesion, in systemic lupus erythematosus, 221, *222*
Wiskott-Aldrich syndrome, 236
Wolman disease, 155t
Wood smoke, in air, 418, 418t
Worms, 336–337
Wound, contraction of, 110
dehiscence of, 110
healing of, 107–111, *111*
by first intention, 107–109, *108*
by second intention, *108,* 109
pathologic aspects of, 110–111, *110*
strength recovery with, 109, *109*
systemic factors in, 109–110
ulceration of, 110
WT-1 gene, in cancer, 294
in Denys-Drash syndrome, 488
in urogenital development, 468
in WAGR syndrome, 488
WT-2 gene, in Beckwith-Wiedemann syndrome, 488
Wuchereria bancrofti, 332t, 397–398, *398*

X
X chromatin, 173
X chromosome, disorders of, 146, 146t, 173–176, *175*
fragile, 177–179, *177, 179*
inactivation of, 173
supernumerary, 176
Xanthelasma, 1189
Xanthogranulomatous pyelonephritis, 977
Xanthoma, 40, 1189
in cholestasis, 851
Xenoestrogens, 422
Xeroderma pigmentosum, 296, 310
Xerophthalmia, in vitamin A deficiency, 441
Xerosis, in vitamin A deficiency, 441
Xerostomia, 758, 769
X-linked agammaglobulinemia of Bruton, 232–233
X-linked lymphoproliferative syndrome, 373
Epstein-Barr virus infection in, 318
X-linked muscular dystrophy, 1281–1282, *1282, 1284*
X-rays, in carcinogenesis, 310–311
XYY syndrome, 174

Y
Y chromosome, sex-determining region Y gene of, 174
supernumerary, 174
Yeast, 378–380, *379, 380*
Yellow fever virus, 333t
Yersinia enterocolitica, 334t, 356, 807–809, 808t
Yersinia pestis, 334t, 387–388
Yersinia pseudotuberculosis, 356
Yolk sac tumor, 1021, 1075–1076, *1076*
Yop pathogenicity island, of *Yersinia,* 356

Z
Z bands, 1272, *1272*
Zahn, lines of, 126
Zebra bodies, in mucopolysaccharidoses, 160
Niemann-Pick disease in, 158
Zellballen, in carotid body tumor, 768, *768*
in pheochromocytoma, 1165
Zenker diverticulum, *778,* 779
Zinc, deficiency of, 451, *452,* 452t
Zollinger-Ellison syndrome, 927
in intestinal carcinoid tumor, 836
peptic ulcers in, 794
Zuckerkandl, organs of, 1164, *1164*